ANDERSON'S PATHOLOGY

ANDERSON'S PATHOLOGY

TENTH EDITION

Edited by:

Ivan Damjanov, M.D., Ph.D.
Professor and Chairman
Department of Pathology
University of Kansas School of Medicine
University of Kansas Medical Center
Kansas City, Kansas

■

James Linder, M.D.
Professor and Vice-Chairman
Department of Pathology and Microbiology
Associate Dean
College of Medicine
University of Nebraska Medical Center
Omaha, Nebraska

with 3366 illustrations, 1927 in color
Mary Jean McFadden
Illustrator

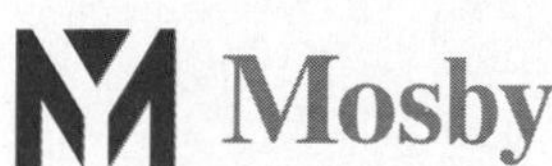

St. Louis Baltimore Boston Carlsbad Chicago Naples New York Philadelphia Portland
London Madrid Mexico City Singapore Sydney Tokyo Toronto Wiesbaden

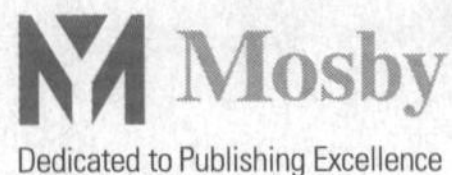

Dedicated to Publishing Excellence

A Times Mirror Company

Publisher: Anne S. Patterson
Senior Managing Editor: Lynne Gery
Project Manager: Dana Peick
Production Editor: Stavra Demetrulias
Manuscript Editor: Carl Masthay
Designer: Amy Buxton
Manufacturing Supervisor: Betty Richmond

TENTH EDITION

Printed in the United States of America
Composition by Clarinda Company
Color Separation by Color Dot Graphics, Inc.
Printing/binding by Von Hoffman Press, Inc.

Mosby-Year Book, Inc.
11830 Westline Industrial Drive
St. Louis, Missouri 63146

International Standard Book Number 0–8016–7236–8

95 96 97 98 99 / 9 8 7 6 5 4 3 2 1

Contributors

Nabil A. Abaza, D.M.D, Ph.D.
Professor of Pathology and Laboratory Medicine, and Professor of Oral and Maxillofacial Surgery, Medical College of Pennsylvania and Hahnemann University; Clinical Professor of Oral and Maxillofacial Surgery, School of Dental Medicine, University of Pennsylvania, Philadelphia, Pennsylvania
Chapter 50 Mouth, Teeth, and Pharynx

Jorge Albores-Saavedra, M.D.
Professor of Pathology, and Director, Division of Anatomic Pathology, University of Texas Southwestern Medical Center; Director, Division of Anatomic Pathology, Parkland Memorial Hospital, Dallas, Texas
Chapter 58 Gallbladder and Extrahepatic Biliary Ducts

D. Craig Allred, M.D.
Professor of Pathology, University of Texas Health Science Center at San Antonio, San Antonio, Texas
Chapter 70 Breast

Peter S. Amenta, M.D., Ph.D.
Associate Professor of Clinical Pathology and Chief of Pathology Service, Robert Wood Johnson Medical School and Robert Wood Johnson University Hospital, New Brunswick/Piscataway, New Jersey
Chapter 19 Repair and Regeneration

Mahul B. Amin, M.D.
Senior Staff, Department of Pathology and Bone and Joint Centre, Henry Ford Hospital, Detroit; Assistant Professor of Pathology, Case Western Reserve University School of Medicine, Cleveland, Ohio, and Clinical Assistant Professor of Pathology, Wayne State University School of Medicine, Detroit, Michigan
Chapter 67 Male Reproductive System

Robert E. Anderson, M.D.
Professor, Department of Laboratory Medicine and Pathology, University of Minnesota Medical School, Minneapolis, Minnesota
Chapter 23 Radiation Injury

Douglas C. Anthony, M.D., Ph.D.
Assistant Professor of Pathology, Harvard Medical School; Director of Neuropathology, Children's Hospital; Neuropathologist, Brigham and Women's Hospital, Boston, Massachusetts
Chapter 78 Peripheral Nervous System

Alberto G. Ayala, M.D.
Professor of Pathology, Deputy Chairman, and Director of Surgical Pathology, University of Texas, M.D. Anderson Cancer Center, Houston, Texas
Chapter 73 Bone Tumors

Shelina Babul, B.Sc.
Research and Education Coordinator, Cardiovascular Research Laboratory, Department of Pathology and Laboratory Medicine, St. Paul's Hospital, Vancouver, British Columbia, Canada
Chapter 2 Autopsy

Adam Bagg, M.D.
Assistant Professor of Pathology and Medicine, Director of Hematopathology, and Director, Hematology Laboratory, Georgetown University Medical Center, Washington, D.C.
Chapter 11 Diagnostic Molecular Pathology

Lewis A. Barness, M.D.
Professor of Pediatrics, University of South Florida College of Medicine and Emeritus Professor of Pediatrics, University of Wisconsin, Madison, Wisconsin
Chapter 14 Metabolic Diseases

Jay H. Beckstead, M.D.
Professor of Pathology, Oregon Health Sciences University, Portland, Oregon
Chapter 9 Histochemistry

Dwight A. Bellinger, D.V.M., Ph.D.
Associate Professor of Laboratory Animal Medicine and Pathology, University of North Carolina School of Medicine, Chapel Hill, North Carolina
Chapter 22 Hemostasis and Thrombosis

Morgan Berthrong, M.D.
Director Emeritus, Department of Pathology, Penrose/St. Francis Health Care System, Colorado Springs, Colorado; Professor Emeritus, Department of Pathology, University of Colorado School of Medicine, Denver, Colorado, and University of New Mexico School of Medicine, Albuquerque, New Mexico
Chapter 23 Radiation Injury

Nathan D. Bills, Ph.D.
Adjunct Assistant Professor of Pathology and Microbiology, University of Nebraska Medical Center, Omaha, Nebraska
Chapter 31 Nutritional Deprivation Diseases

David G. Bostwick, M.D.
Professor of Pathology and Consultant in Pathology, Department of Laboratory Medicine and Pathology, Mayo Medical School and Mayo Clinic, Rochester, Minnesota
Chapter 67 Male Reproductive System

Julia A. Bridge, M.D.
Associate Professor of Pathology and Microbiology, Pediatrics, and Orthopaedic Surgery; Director of Fragile X DNA Laboratory; Associate Director of Clinical Cytogenetics, University of Nebraska Medical Center, Omaha, Nebraska
Chapter 12 Cytogenetics

Richard D. Brunning, M.D.
Professor of Laboratory Medicine and Pathology, University of Minnesota Medical School; Head, Hematopathology Laboratory, University of Minnesota Hospital, Minneapolis, Minnesota
Chapter 41 Blood and Bone Marrow

David J. Bylund, M.D.
Adjunct Assistant Member, Department of Molecular and Experimental Medicine, The Scripps Research Institute, La Jolla; Director, Scripps Reference Laboratory, San Diego, California
Chapter 26 Autoimmunity and Autoimmune Diseases

Maria Luisa Carcangiu, M.D.
Associate Professor of Pathology and Obstetrics and Gynecology, Yale University School of Medicine and Yale New Haven Hospital, New Haven, Connecticut
Chapter 61 Thyroid Gland

John L. Carey III, M.D.
Division Head, Immunopathology, Henry Ford Health Care Corporation,

Farmington Hills, Michigan
Chapter 13 Flow and Imaging Cytometry

Wing (John) C. Chan, M.B., B.S., M.D.
Professor, Department of Pathology and Microbiology, University of Nebraska Medical Center, Omaha, Nebraska
Chapter 42 Lymph Nodes

Francis W. Chandler, D.V.M., Ph.D.
Professor, Department of Pathology, Medical College of Georgia, Augusta, Georgia
Chapter 37 Fungal Diseases

Gregorio Chejfec, M.D.
Professor of Pathology, Loyola University of Chicago, Stritch School of Medicine; Director, Anatomic Pathology, Loyola University Medical Center, Maywood; Chief, Pathology and Laboratory Medicine Service, Hines Veterans Administration Hospital, Hines, Illinois
Chapter 52 Esophagus

Stephen W. Chensue, M.D., Ph.D.
Associate Professor of Pathology, University of Michigan Medical School; Staff Pathologist, Veterans Affairs Medical Center, Ann Arbor, Michigan
Chapter 18 Inflammation

Arthur H. Cohen, M.D.
Professor of Pathology and Medicine, University of California, Los Angeles, School of Medicine; Attending Pathologist, Cedars-Sinai Medical Center, Los Angeles, California
Chapter 65 Kidney

Samuel M. Cohen, M.D., Ph.D.
Professor and Chairman, Department of Pathology and Microbiology, and Professor, Eppley Institute for Research in Cancer and Allied Diseases, University of Nebraska Medical Center, Omaha, Nebraska
Chapter 66 Lower Urinary Tract

Félix Contreras, M.D.
Professor of Pathology, Universidad Autónoma; Chairman, Department of Pathology, La Paz Hospital, Madrid, Spain
Chapter 71 Skin

Jeffrey Cossman, M.D.
Oscar Benwood Hunter Professor and Chairman, Department of Pathology, Georgetown University Medical Center; Pathologist-in-Chief, Georgetown University Hospital, Washington, D.C.
Chapter 11 Diagnostic Molecular Pathology

Richard J. Cote, M.D.
Associate Professor of Pathology, University of Southern California School of Medicine; Attending Pathologist, Kenneth Norris Jr. Comprehensive Cancer Center, Los Angeles, California
Chapter 8 Immunohistochemistry and Related Marking Techniques

John E. Craighead, M.D.
Professor of Pathology, University of Vermont College of Medicine; Attending Pathologist, Fletcher Allen Health Care, Burlington, Vermont
Chapter 49 Lung

Ivan Damjanov, M.D., Ph.D.
Professor and Chairman, Department of Pathology, University of Kansas Medical Center, Kansas City, Kansas
Chapter 32 Pathology of Obesity
Chapter 54 Small Intestine
Chapter 67 Male Reproductive System
Appendix-Table of Normal Values

Michael J. Davies, M.D.
Professor of Cardiovascular Pathology, University of London; Honorary Consultant, St. George's Hospital, London, United Kingdom
Chapter 45 Heart Disease in the Adult

Stephen J. DeArmond, M.D., Ph.D.
Professor of Pathology (Neuropathology) and Neurology, University of California, San Francisco, School of Medicine, San Francisco General Hospital, and San Francisco Veterans Administration Hospital, San Francisco, California
Chapter 40 Prions

Ronald A. DeLellis, M.D.
Professor of Pathology, Tufts University School of Medicine; Senior Pathologist, New England Medical Center, Boston, Massachusetts
Chapter 61 Thyroid Gland

J. Stephen Dumler, M.D.
Assistant Professor of Pathology, University of Maryland School of Medicine; Associate Director of Clinical Microbiology, University of Maryland Medical Center, Baltimore, Maryland
Chapter 35 Rickettsial and Chlamydial Diseases

Ralph C. Eagle, Jr., M.D.
Professor of Ophthalmology, Jefferson Medical College of Thomas Jefferson University; Director, Department of Pathology, Wills Eye Hospital, Philadelphia, Pennsylvania
Chapter 79 Eye and Ocular Adnexa

John N. Eble, M.D.
Professor of Pathology and of Experimental Oncology, Indiana University School of Medicine; Chief Pathologist, Richard L. Roudebush Veterans Affairs Medical Center, Indianapolis, Indiana
Chapter 65 Kidney

Jesse E. Edwards, M.D.
Clinical Professor of Pathology, University of Minnesota Medical School, Minneapolis; Senior Consultant, Registry of Cardiovascular Disease, United Hospital, St. Paul., Minnesota
Chapter 21 Circulatory Disturbances

William D. Edwards, M.D.
Professor of Pathology, Mayo Medical School and Mayo Graduate School of Medicine; Consultant, Division of Anatomic Pathology, and Clinical Appointment, Division of Cardiology, Mayo Clinic, Rochester, Minnesota
Chapter 46 Congenital Heart Disease

Samir K. El-Mofty, D.M.D., Ph.D.
Professor of Oral Pathology, Associate Professor of Pathology and Otolaryngology, Washington University School of Medicine; Attending Medical Staff, Barnes Hospital, Jewish Hospital, and St. Louis Children's Hospital; Consultant Pathologist, Veterans Administration Hospital, St. Louis, Missouri
Chapter 50 Mouth, Teeth, and Pharynx
Chapter 51 Salivary Glands

Luis F. Fajardo M.D.
Professor of Pathology, Stanford University School of Medicine, Stanford; Chief of Pathology and Laboratory Medicine, Veterans Affairs Medical Center, Palo Alto, California
Chapter 23 Radiation Injury

Lorraine A. Fitzpatrick, M.D.
Professor of Medicine, Consultant in Endocrinology and Metabolism, and Director, Bone Histomorphometry Laboratory, Mayo Clinic and Mayo Foundation, Rochester, Minnesota
Chapter 74 Metabolic and Nontumorous Bone Disorders

Howard S. Fox, M.D., Ph.D.
Assistant Member, Department of Neuropharmacology, The Scripps Research Institute, and Consultant, Department of Pathology, Scripps Clinic Medical Group, La Jolla; Assay Development, Scripps Reference Laboratory, San Diego, California
Chapter 26 Autoimmunity and Autoimmune Diseases

Stephen A. Geller, M.D.
Chairman, Department of Pathology and Laboratory Medicine, Cedars-Sinai Medical Center, and Professor, Department of Pathology and Laboratory Medicine, University of California, Los Angeles,

School of Medicine, Los Angeles, California
Chapter 28 Acquired Immunodeficiency Syndrome (AIDS)

Robert M. Genta, M.D.
Associate Professor of Pathology, Medicine, and Microbiology and Immunology, Baylor College of Medicine, Houston, Texas
Chapter 53 Stomach and Duodenum

Allen R. Gibbs, T.D., M.B., Ch.B., FRCPath
Consultant Pathologist, Llandough Hospital, Penarth; Honorary Clinical Teacher, University of Wales College of Medicine, Cardiff, United Kingdom
Chapter 49 Lung

Enid Gilbert-Barness, M.D.
Professor of Pathology and Pediatrics, University of South Florida College of Medicine, Tampa, Florida; Professor Emeritus of Pathology and Pediatrics; Distinguished Medical Alumni Professor Emeritus, University of Wisconsin Medical School, Madison, Wisconsin
Chapter 14 Metabolic Diseases

Douglas R. Gnepp, M.D.
Professor of Pathology, Rhode Island Hospital, and Brown University School of Medicine, Providence, Rhode Island
Chapter 51 Salivary Glands

John R. Goldblum, M.D.
Staff Pathologist, Cleveland Clinic Foundation, Cleveland, Ohio
Chapter 55 Appendix

Neal S. Goldstein, M.D.
Anatomic Pathologist, William Beaumont Hospital, Royal Oak, Michigan
Chapter 44 Thymus and Mediastinum

John G. Gruhn, M.D.
Associate Professor of Pathology, Rush Medical College, Chicago, Illinois
Chapter 63 Adrenal Glands

Yezid Gutierrez, M.D.
Associate Professor of Pathology, Institute of Pathology, Case Western Reserve University School of Medicine; Adjunct Staff, Department of Microbiology, Cleveland Clinic Foundation, Cleveland, Ohio
Chapter 38 Protozoal Diseases
Chapter 39 Metazoan Diseases

Sheryl Haggerty, Ph.D.
Assistant Professor, Department of Pathology and Microbiology, University of Nebraska Medical Center, Omaha, Nebraska; American Foundation for AIDS Research Scholar
Chapter 36 Viral Diseases

Christopher J. Harrison, M.D.
Associate Professor of Pediatrics and Medical Microbiology, Creighton University School of Medicine; Associate Professor of Pediatrics, and Clinical Staff, University of Nebraska Medical Center; Hospital Epidemiologist and Active Staff, Children's Hospital; Active Staff, St. Joseph Hospital, Omaha, Nebraska
Chapter 36 Viral Diseases

Reid R. Heffner, Jr., M.D.
Professor and Associate Chairman, Department of Pathology, State University of New York at Buffalo School of Medicine and Biomedical Sciences, Buffalo, New York
Chapter 76 Skeletal Muscle

Philipp U. Heitz, M.D.
Professor and Chairman, Department of Pathology, University of Zürich, Zürich, Switzerland
Chapter 64 Diabetes and Endocrine Pancreas

Steven H. Hinrichs, M.D.
Associate Professor, Department of Pathology and Microbiology, Department of Orthopaedic Surgery, and Eppley Research Institute; Director of Virology and Director of Molecular Diagnostics, University of Nebraska Medical Center; Associate Faculty, Pediatric Infectious Disease, Creighton University School of Medicine, Omaha, Nebraska
Chapter 15 Molecular Basis of Human Disease
Chapter 36 Viral Diseases

Charles S. Hirsch, M.D.
Professor and Chairman, Department of Forensic Medicine, and Professor, Department of Pathology, New York University School of Medicine; Chief Medical Examiner, City of New York, New York
Chapter 5 Forensic Pathology

Dikran S. Horoupian, M.D.
Professor, Department of Pathology; and Director, Neuropathology Division, Stanford University School of Medicine, Stanford, California
Chapter 77 Central Nervous System

Eva Horvath, Ph.D.
Associate Professor of Pathology, St. Michaels Hospital, University of Toronto Faculty of Medicine, Toronto, Ontario, Canada
Chapter 60 Pituitary Gland

Aubrey J. Hough, Jr., M.D.
Professor and Chairman, Department of Pathology, University of Arkansas College of Medicine, Little Rock, Arkansas
Chapter 75 Joints

Kamal G. Ishak, M.D., Ph.D.
Chairman, Department of Hepatic and Gastrointestinal Pathology, Armed Forces Institute of Pathology, Washington, D.C.; Clinical Professor of Pathology, Uniformed Services University for the Health Sciences and Medical Care, Bethesda, Maryland; Professorial Lecturer, Mount Sinai School of Medicine, New York, New York
Chapter 57 Liver

J. Charles Jennette, M.D.
Professor of Pathology and Medicine, and Director, Nephropathology Laboratory, University of North Carolina School of Medicine, Chapel Hill, North Carolina
Chapter 47 Vascular System

Jose Jessurun, M.D.
Associate Professor of Pathology, University of Minnesota Medical School, Minneapolis, Minnesota
Chapter 58 Gallbladder and Extrahepatic Biliary Ducts

Sonny L. Johansson, M.D., Ph.D
Professor and Director of Anatomic Pathology, Department of Pathology and Microbiology, and Professor, Eppley Institute for Research in Cancer and Allied Diseases, University of Nebraska Medical Center, Omaha, Nebraska
Chapter 66 Lower Urinary Tract

William W. Johnston, M.D.
Professor of Pathology, Chief, Division of Anatomic Pathology, and Head, Section of Cytopathology, Duke University School of Medicine, Durham, North Carolina
Chapter 4 Cytopathology

Vijay V. Joshi, M.D., FRCPath
Professor of Pathology and Clinical Professor of Pediatrics, East Carolina University School of Medicine, Greenville, North Carolina; Consultant in Pediatric Pathology, Beth Israel Medical Center, New York, New York
Chapter 28 Acquired Immunodeficiency Syndrome (AIDS)

Dagmar K. Kalousek, M.D., FRCPC, FCCMG
Professor of Pathology, The University of British Columbia Faculty of Medicine; Director of Cellular Pathology Program, Department of Pathology, B.C. Children's Hospital, Vancouver, British Columbia, Canada
Chapter 16 Developmental Pathology

David G. Kaufman, M.D., Ph.D.
Professor of Pathology, University of North Carolina School of Medicine,

Chapel Hill, North Carolina
Chapter 17 Cell Injury and Cellular Adaptations

James K. Kelly, M.B.
Chief, Anatomical Pathology, Greater Victoria Hospital Society, Victoria, British Columbia, Canada
Chapter 56 Large Intestine and Anus

Thomas Kirchner, M.D.
Professor and Chairman, Institute of Pathology, University of Erlangen, Erlangen, Germany
Chapter 44 Thymus and Mediastinum

Robert Kisilevsky, M.D., Ph.D., FRCPC
Professor, Departments of Pathology and Biochemistry, Queen's University Faculty of Medicine; Attending Staff, Departments of Pathology, Kingston General and Hotel Dieu Hospitals, Kingston, Ontario, Canada
Chapter 20 Amyloidosis

John M. Kissane, M.D.
Professor of Pathology and of Pediatrics, Washington University School of Medicine; Pathologist, Barnes and Affiliated Hospitals, Children's Hospital, and Jewish Hospital, St. Louis, Missouri
Chapter 33 Bacterial Diseases

Gordon K. Klintworth, M.D., Ph.D.
Professor of Pathology, Joseph A.C. Wadsworth Research Professor of Ophthalmology, and Director of Research, Duke University Eye Center, Durham, North Carolina
Chapter 79 Eye and Ocular Adnexa

Günter Klöppel, M.D., Ph.D.
Professor and Director, Department of Pathology, University of Kiel, Kiel, Germany
Chapter 64 Diabetes and Endocrine Pancreas

Paul Komminoth, M.D.
Department of Pathology, University of Zürich, Zürich, Switzerland
Chapter 64 Diabetes and Endocrine Pancreas

Kalman Kovacs, M.D., Ph.D., D.Sc., FRCPC, FCAF, FRC(Path)
Professor, Department of Pathology, St. Michaels Hospital, University of Toronto Faculty of Medicine, Toronto, Ontario, Canada
Chapter 60 Pituitary Gland

Charles Kuhn III, M.D.
Professor of Pathology, Brown University Program in Medicine, Providence, Rhode Island; Pathologist-in-Chief, Memorial Hospital of Rhode Island, Pawtucket, Rhode Island
Chapter 49 Lung

Ernest E. Lack, M.D.
Professor of Pathology and Director of Anatomic Pathology, Georgetown University School of Medicine, Washington, D.C.
Chapter 63 Adrenal Glands

Benjamin Landing, M.D.
Professor Emeritus, Pathology and Pediatrics, University of Southern California School of Medicine; Research Pathologist, Children's Hospital of Los Angeles, Los Angeles, California
Chapter 14 Metabolic Diseases

Russell M. Lebovitz, M.D., Ph.D.
Assistant Professor, Departments of Pathology and Cell Biology, Baylor College of Medicine, Houston, Texas
Chapter 24 Neoplasia

Juan Lechago, M.D., Ph.D.
Professor of Pathology, Baylor College of Medicine; Director, Surgical Pathology, The Methodist Hospital, Houston, Texas
Chapter 53 Stomach and Duodenum

Michael W. Lieberman, M.D., Ph.D.
The W. L. Moody Jr. Professor and Chairman, Department of Pathology, Baylor College of Medicine, Houston, Texas
Chapter 24 Neoplasia

James Linder, M.D.
Professor and Vice-Chairman, Department of Pathology and Microbiology, University of Nebraska Medical Center, Omaha, Nebraska
Chapter 4 Cytopathology
Chapter 6 Informatics

Craig E. Litz, M.D.
Associate Professor, Department of Laboratory Medicine and Pathology, University of Minnesota Medical School, Minneapolis, Minnesota
Chapter 41 Blood and Bone Marrow

Ricardo V. Lloyd, M.D., Ph.D.
Professor of Pathology and Senior Associate Consultant, Mayo Clinic and Mayo Foundation, Rochester, Minnesota
Chapter 60 Pituitary Gland

Daniel S. Longnecker, M.D.
Professor, Department of Pathology, Dartmouth Medical School, Hanover, and Dartmouth-Hitchcock Medical Center, Lebanon, New Hampshire
Chapter 59 Pancreas

Bruce Mackay, M.D., Ph.D.
Professor of Pathology, University of Texas, M.D. Anderson Cancer Center, Houston, Texas
Chapter 7 Electron Microscopy

Alberto Marchevsky, M.D.
Clinical Professor of Pathology, University of California, Los Angeles, School of Medicine; Director, Division of Anatomic Pathology, Cedars-Sinai Medical Center, Los Angeles, California
Chapter 44 Thymus and Mediastinum

Rodney S. Markin, M.D., Ph.D.
Professor of Pathology and Microbiology and of Surgery, Department of Pathology and Microbiology, University of Nebraska Medical Center, Omaha, Nebraska
Chapter 6 Informatics
Chapter 57 Liver

Antonio Martinez-Hernandez, M.D.
Professor, Department of Pathology, University of Tennessee College of Medicine; Chief, Pathology and Laboratory Medicine Service, Veterans Affairs Medical Center, Memphis, Tennessee
Chapter 19 Repair and Regeneration

Alexander Marx, M.D.
Lecturer in Pathology, University of Würzburg, Würzburg, Germany
Chapter 44 Thymus and Mediastinum

John S. McClure, M.D.
Pathologist, Unity Hospital, Allina Laboratories, Fridley, Minnesota
Chapter 41 Blood and Bone Marrow

Miles M. McFarland, M.D.
Clinical Assistant Professor of Pathology, Medical College of Pennsylvania and Hahnemann University, Philadelphia, Pennsylvania
Chapter 50 Mouth, Teeth, and Pharnyx

Bruce M. McManus, M.D., Ph.D.
Professor and Head, Department of Pathology and Laboratory Medicine, University of British Columbia Faculty of Medicine; Chairman, Department of Pathology and Laboratory Medicine, St. Paul's Hospital, Vancouver, British Columbia, Canada
Chapter 2 Autopsy
Chapter 30 Pathology of Prosthetic Materials and Devices
Chapter 45 Heart Disease in the Adult

Neil Scott McNutt, M.D.
Professor of Pathology, Cornell University Medical Center; Director,

Dermatopathology Division, Department of Pathology, Cornell University Medical Center and The New York Hospital; Consultant in Pathology, Memorial Sloan-Kettering Cancer Center, New York, New York
Chapter 71 Skin

Wayne M. Meyers, M.D., Ph.D.
Chief, Mycobacteriology Branch, Armed Forces Institute of Pathology, Washington D.C.; Research Affiliate, Tulane University, New Orleans, Louisiana
Chapter 34 Mycobacterial Diseases

Leslie Michaels, M.D., FRCPath, FRCPC
Professor Emeritus, University of London; Department of Histopathology, UCL Medical School, London, United Kingdom
Chapter 80 Ear

Markku Miettinen, M.D.
Associate Professor of Pathology, Jefferson Medical College of Thomas Jefferson University; Attending Pathologist, Thomas Jefferson University Hospital, Philadelphia, Pennsylvania
Chapter 72 Soft Tissue Tumors

Stacey E. Mills, M.D.
Professor of Pathology and Associate Director of Surgical Pathology, University of Virginia Health Sciences Center, Charlottesville, Virginia
Chapter 3 Surgical Pathology

Sean Moore M.B., B.Ch., FRCPC
Professor of Pathology, McGill University Faculty of Medicine; Consultant Pathologist, Royal Victoria Hospital, Montreal, Quebec, Canada
Chapter 47 Vascular System

Hans Konrad Mueller-Hermelink, M.D.
Professor and Chairman, Institute of Pathology, University of Würzburg, Würzburg, Germany
Chapter 44 Thymus and Mediastinum

Robert M. Nakamura, M.D.
Chairman Emeritus, Department of Pathology, Scripps Clinic and Research Foundation, La Jolla, California
Chapter 26 Autoimmunity and Autoimmune Diseases

Cynthia C. Nast, M.D.
Associate Professor of Pathology, University of California, Los Angeles, School of Medicine; Associate Pathologist, Cedars-Sinai Medical Center, Los Angeles, California
Chapter 65 Kidney

Richard S. Neiman, M.D.
Professor of Pathology and Laboratory Medicine and of Medicine; Director of Hematopathology, Department of Pathology and Laboratory Medicine, Indiana University Medical Center, Indianapolis, Indiana
Chapter 43 Spleen

Christian Nezelof, M.D.
Professor Emeritus d'Anatomie Pathologique, Faculté de Médecine de Paris, Consultant Pathologist, Hôpital Saint-Vincent de Paul, Paris, France
Chapter 1 The History of Pathology: An Overview
Chapter 27 Primary Immunodeficiencies

Gerard J. Nuovo, M.D.
Associate Professor of Pathology and Obstetrics and Gynecology, State University of New York at Stony Brook, Stony Brook, New York
Chapter 10 In Situ Hybridization

Attilio Orazi, M.D.
Associate Professor of Pathology and Laboratory Medicine, Indiana University School of Medicine; Director of Immunohistochemistry, Indiana University Medical Center, Indianapolis, Indiana
Chapter 43 Spleen

Nelson G. Ordóñez, M.D.
Professor of Pathology, Director of Immunocytochemistry Section, University of Texas, M.D. Anderson Cancer Center, Houston, Texas
Chapter 7 Electron Microscopy

David A. Owen, M.B., B.Ch., FRCPath, FRCPC
Professor of Pathology, University of British Columbia Faculty of Medicine; Head, Division of Anatomical Pathology, Vancouver Hospital and Health Sciences Centre, Vancouver, B.C., Canada
Chapter 56 Large Intestine and Anus

Robert E. Petras, M.D.
Chairman, Department of Anatomic Pathology, The Cleveland Clinic Foundation, Cleveland, Ohio
Chapter 55 Appendix

Edwina J. Popek, D.O.
Assistant Professor of Pathology, Baylor College of Medicine; Perinatal and Placental Pathologist, Texas Children's Hospital, Houston, Texas
Chapter 69 Placenta

James M. Powers, M.D.
Professor of Pathology and Neurology, Associate Chair for Education, and Director, Neuropathology Unit, University of Rochester, Rochester, New York
Chapter 77 Central Nervous System

Jaime Prat, M.D., FRCPath
Professor of Pathology, Autonomous University of Barcelona; Director, Department of Pathology, Hospital de la Santa Creu i Sant Pau, Barcelona, Spain
Chapter 68 Female Reproductive System

Stanley B. Prusiner, M.D.
Professor of Neurology and of Biochemistry and Biophysics, University of California, San Francisco, School of Medicine, San Francisco, California
Chapter 40 Prions

Stanley J. Radio, M.D.
Associate Professor of Pathology and Director, Cytology and Cardiovascular Registry, Department of Pathology and Microbiology, University of Nebraska Medical Center, Omaha, Nebraska
Chapter 29 Transplantation Pathology
Chapter 30 Pathology of Prosthetic Materials and Devices

Juhani Rapola, M.D.
Chief of Pathology Unit, Children's Hospital, University of Helsinki, Helsinki, Finland
Chapter 14 Metabolic Diseases

A. Kevin Raymond, M.D.
Associate Professor of Pathology, University of Texas, M.D. Anderson Cancer Center, Houston, Texas
Chapter 73 Bone Tumors

Robert L. Reddick, M.D.
Brinkhous Professor of Pathology, University of North Carolina School of Medicine, Chapel Hill, North Carolina
Chapter 22 Hemostasis and Thrombosis

Janardan K. Reddy, M.D.
Magerstadt Professor and Chairman, Department of Pathology, Northwestern University Medical School; Attending Pathologist, Northwestern Memorial Hospital, Chicago Illinois
Chapter 17 Cell Injury

Jae Y. Ro, M.D., Ph.D.
Professor of Pathology, University of Texas, M.D. Anderson Cancer Center, Houston, Texas
Chapter 73 Bone Tumors

Seymour Rosen, M.D.
Director of Surgical Pathology and Senior Pathologist, Department of Pathology, Beth Israel Hospital; Professor of Pathology, Harvard Medical School, Boston, Massachusetts
Chapter 47 Vascular System

Sanford I. Roth, M.D.
Professor of Pathology, Northwestern University Medical School; Attending Pathologist, Northwestern Memorial Hospital, Chicago, Illinois
Chapter 62 Parathyroid Glands

Jürgen Roth, M.D., Ph.D.
Professor of Cell and Molecular Pathology, Division of Cell and Molecular Pathology, Department of Pathology, University of Zürich, Zürich, Switzerland
Chapter 64 Diabetes and Endocrine Pancreas

Jonathan W. Said, M.D.
Professor of Pathology, University of California, Los Angeles, School of Medicine; Associate Pathologist, Cedars-Sinai Medical Center, Los Angeles, California
Chapter 28 Acquired Immunodeficiency Syndrome (AIDS)

Carolyn M. Salafia, M.D.
Associate Professor of Pathology and of Obstetrics and Gynecology, Georgetown University Medical Center, Washington, D.C.; Section Head, Perinatal Pathology, Perinatology Research Faculty, National Institute of Child Health and Human Development, Bethesda, Maryland
Chapter 69 Placenta

George E. Sale, M.D.
Professor of Pathology, University of Washington School of Medicine; Member and Pathology Program Head, Fred Hutchinson Cancer Research Center, Seattle, Washington
Chapter 29 Transplantation Pathology

Avery A. Sandberg, M.D., D.Sc.
Senior Medical Director, Genetrix, Inc., and Vice-President and Director of Cancer Center, Southwest Biomedical Research Institute, Scottsdale; Senior Clinical Lecturer, University of Arizona College of Medicine, Tucson, Arizona
Chapter 12 Cytogenetics

Gail M. Schauer, M.D.
Clinical Assistant Professor, Departments of Pathology and Obstetrics and Gynecology, The Ohio State University College of Medicine; Director, Autopsy Service, Columbus Children's Hospital, Columbus, Ohio
Chapter 16 Developmental Pathology

Bertram Schnitzer, M.D.
Professor of Pathology and Director of Hematopathology, University of Michigan Medical Center, Ann Arbor, Michigan
Chapter 42 Lymph Nodes

Sydney S. Schochet, Jr., M.D.
Professor of Pathology, Neurology and Neurosurgery, West Virginia University School of Medicine, Morgantown, West Virginia
Chapter 76 Skeletal Muscle

Thomas A. Seemayer, M.D.
Professor of Pathology and Microbiology and of Pediatrics, University of Nebraska Medical Center, Omaha, Nebraska; Adjunct Professor of Pathology, McGill University Faculty of Medicine, Montreal, Quebec, Canada
Chapter 1 The History of Pathology: An Overview
Chapter 27 Primary Immunodeficiencies

Stewart Sell, M.D.
Professor, Department of Pathology and Laboratory Medicine, University of Texas Medical School, Houston, Texas
Chapter 25 Immunopathologic Mechanisms

Francis E. Sharkey, M.D.
Associate Professor of Pathology, University of Texas Health Science Center; Consulting Pathologist, Audie Murphy Memorial Veterans Administration Hospital, San Antonio, Texas
Chapter 70 Breast

Herschel Sidransky, M.D.
Professor and Chairman, Department of Pathology, George Washington University Medical Center, Washington, D.C.
Chapter 31 Nutritional Deprivation Diseases

Jerome H. Smith, M.S., M.Sc. Hyg., M.D.
Professor and Director of Pathology Education, Department of Pathology, University of Texas Medical Branch, Galveston, Texas
Chapter 39 Metazoan Diseases

Bruce R. Smoller, M.D.
Associate Professor of Pathology and Dermatology, Stanford University Medical Center; Director, Dermatopathology, Stanford University Hospital, Stanford, California
Chapter 71 Skin

Dale C. Snover, M.D.
Professor and Director of Anatomic Pathology, Department of Laboratory Medicine and Pathology, University of Minnesota Medical School, Minneapolis, Minnesota
Chapter 29 Transplantation Pathology

Lucia Stefaneanu, Ph.D.
Assistant Professor of Pathology, St. Michaels Hospital, University of Toronto Faculty of Medicine, Toronto, Ontario, Canada
Chapter 60 Pituitary Gland

Jerome B. Taxy, M.D.
Associate Pathologist, Lutheran General Hospital, Park Ridge, Illinois; Clinical Associate Professor of Pathology, Northwestern University Medical School, Chicago, Illinois
Chapter 48 Upper Respiratory Tract

Clive R. Taylor, M.A., M.D., D. Phil, FRCPath
Professor and Chair, Department of Pathology and Laboratory Medicine University of Southern California School of Medicine; Director of Laboratories, Los Angeles County-University of Southern California Medical Center, University Hospital, and Norris Cancer Hospital and Research Institute, Los Angeles, California
Chapter 8 Immunohistochemistry and Related Marking Techniques

Jack L. Titus, M.D., Ph.D.
Clinical Professor of Laboratory Medicine and Pathology, University of Minnesota Medical School, Minneapolis; Director, Registry of Cardiovascular Diseases, United Hospital, St. Paul, Minnesota
Chapter 21 Circulatory Disturbances

Monica D. Traystman, Ph.D.
Assistant Professor of Pathology and Microbiology and Pediatrics; Eppley Research Institute, University of Nebraska Medical Center, Omaha, Nebraska
Chapter 15 Molecular Basis of Human Disease

Robert L. Trelstad, M.D.
Professor and Chairman, Department of Pathology, Robert Wood Johnson Medical School, New Brunswick/Piscataway, New Jersey
Chapter 19 Repair and Regeneration

Philip T. Valente, M.D.
Associate Professor of Pathology and of Obstetrics and Gynecology, University of Texas Health Science Center at San Antonio; Director of Cytology, University Hospital and Audie Murphy Veterans Administration Hospital, San Antonio, Texas
Chapter 70 Breast

F. Stephen Vogel, M.D.
Professor of Pathology, Emeritus, Duke University School of Medicine, Durham, North Carolina; Clinical Professor of Pathology, Medical College of Georgia, Augusta, Georgia
Chapter 78 Peripheral Nervous System

Franz von Lichtenberg, M.D.
Professor of Pathology, Emeritus, Harvard Medical School; Senior Pathologist, Brigham and Women's Hospital, Boston, Massachusetts
Chapter 38 Protozoal Diseases

David H. Walker, M.D.
Professor and Chairman, Department of Pathology, University of Texas

Medical Branch; Director, Center for Tropical Diseases, Galveston, Texas
Chapter 35 Rickettsial and Chlamydial Diseases

Peter A. Ward, M.D.
Godfrey D. Stobbe Professor and Chairman, Department of Pathology, University of Michigan Medical School and Hospitals, Ann Arbor, Michigan
Chapter 18 Inflammation

John C. Watts, M.D.
Chief, Surgical Pathology, Department of Anatomic Pathology, William Beaumont Hospital, Royal Oak, Michigan, Clinical Associate Professor of Pathology, Wayne State University School of Medicine, Detroit, Michigan
Chapter 37 Fungal Diseases

David S. Weinberg, M.D., Ph.D.
Associate Professor of Pathology, Harvard Medical School; Pathologist, and Medical Director, Hematology Laboratory, Brigham and Women's Hospital, Boston, Massachusetts
Chapter 13 Flow and Imaging Cytometry

Lawrence M. Weiss, M.D.
Director of Surgical Pathology, Department of Pathology, City of Hope National Medical Center, Duarte, California
Chapter 42 Lymph Nodes

Sharon W. Weiss, M.D.
James French Professor of Pathology and Director of Anatomic Pathology, University of Michigan Hospitals, Ann Arbor, Michigan
Chapter 72 Soft Tissue Tumors

William W. West, M.D.
Associate Professor of Pathology, University of Nebraska School of Medicine; Pathologist in Chief, Veterans Administration Hospital, Omaha, Nebraska
Chapter 49 Lung

Mark R. Wick, M.D.
Professor of Pathology and Director of Surgical Pathology, Washington University School of Medicine; Associate Director of Anatomic Pathology, Washington University Medical Center, St. Louis, Missouri
Chapter 3 Surgical Pathology

Washington C. Winn, Jr., M.D., M.B.A.
Professor of Pathology, University of Vermont College of Medicine; Director, Clinical Microbiology, Department of Pathology and Laboratory Medicine, Fletcher Allen Health Care, Burlington, Vermont
Chapter 33 Bacterial Diseases

James L. Wisecarver, M.D., Ph.D.
Associate Professor, Department of Pathology and Microbiology, and Medical Director, Transplant Immunology Laboratory, University of Nebraska Medical Center, Omaha, Nebraska
Chapter 25 Immunopathologic Mechanisms

Gail L. Woods, M.D.
Professor of Pathology with joint appointmnents in Internal Medicine and Microbiology and Immunology, University of Texas Medical Branch, Galveston, Texas
Chapter 34 Mycobacterial Diseases

Anjana V. Yeldandi, M.D.
Assistant Professor of Pathology, Northwestern University Medical School; Staff Pathologist, Veterans Administration Lakeside Hospital, and Attending Pathologist, Northwestern Memorial Hospital, Chicago, Illinois
Chapter 17 Cell Injury and Cellular Adaptations

Iain D. Young, M.D., C.M., FRCPC
Associate Professor of Pathology, Queen's University Faculty of Medicine; Attending Staff, Departments of Pathology, Kingston General and Hotel Dieu Hospitals, Kingston, Ontario, Canada
Chapter 20 Amyloidosis

Ross E. Zumwalt, M.D.
Professor of Pathology, University of New Mexico School of Medicine; Chief Medical Investigator, State of New Mexico, Albuquerque, New Mexico
Chapter 5 Forensic Pathology

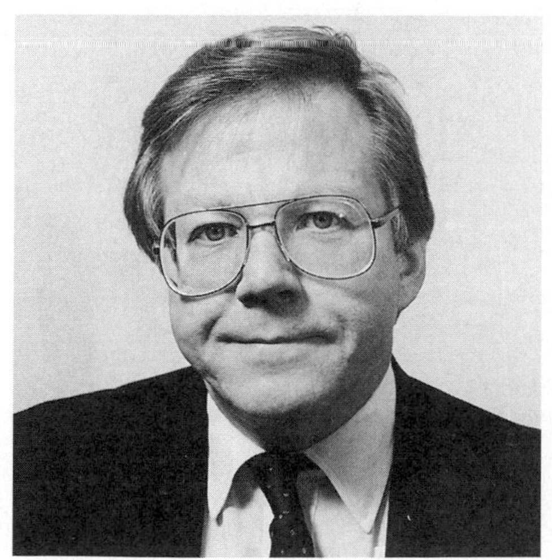

David T. Purtilo, M.D.
1939-1992

"The only solid piece of scientific truth about which I feel totally confident is that we are profoundly ignorant about nature. . . It is this sudden confrontation with the depth and scope of ignorance that represents the most significant contribution of twentieth-century science to the human intellect"

—Lewis Thomas (1913-1993), *The Medusa and the Snail,* The Viking Press, 1979, New York

This book is dedicated to David T. Purtilo, M.D., friend and mentor of pathologists throughout the world, in the spirit of bridging the ignorance that we face in our struggle to understand, diagnose, and treat disease.

Preface

The first edition of *Anderson's Pathology* appeared in 1948. As the first modern multiauthored textbook of pathology, it was enthusiastically greeted and almost immediately adopted as the standard textbook for graduate and postgraduate medical education. Generations of physicians grew up on *Anderson's Pathology,* and many of them still practice medicine remembering fondly the book that has introduced them to clinical medicine. During the next 40-plus years, the book saw eight editions published, the first six of which were edited by Dr. W.A.D. Anderson. For the seventh edition Dr. John M. Kissane became the co-editor and after Dr. Anderson's death on January 20, 1986, Dr. Kissane prepared the ninth edition. The baton has been passed now to us.

Few textbooks have names as resonant as *Anderson's Pathology.* It was thus with considerable trepidation that we accepted the publisher's invitation to devise a major revision of this venerable textbook and redesign it for the new generations of physicians who will be practicing in the 21st century. At the end of the project we are, nevertheless, pleased that we undertook it. On behalf of all our contributors we are proud to present the 10th edition, confident that it will herald a new era in the history of this textbook.

In order to restore the luster and popularity of the original edition, we had to make some drastic changes, both in the content and in the design. First of all, we expanded the text. This was achieved by increasing the number of pages and by a more judicious use of space. The number of chapters was increased from 42 in the ninth edition to 80 in the tenth edition. The group of outstanding contributors was increased proportionally, from 58 to 170. With this redesign we were in a position to give every contributor a smaller and presumably more manageable task. The contributors were asked, in turn, to provide more details and cover the assigned topics in greater depth. For example, alimentary tract pathology, which previously was presented in a single chapter, is now subdivided into five smaller chapters, and hematopathology has been subdivided into three chapters.

The first chapter deals with the history of pathology: we are standing on the shoulders of our predecessors and we thought that new generations of physicians should know that they are not working in a vacuum but are continuing in the tradition of true giants. The subsequent chapters deal with techniques that are essential for the practice of pathology. It would be inconceivable to study modern pathology without a solid understanding of these techniques. We also believe that the study of pathology requires solid understanding of basic pathologic processes, which are discussed in considerable detail.

The diseases that affect the entire body and those that have a common cause or pathogenesis have been grouped together. Although these chapters were conceived as overviews in which not all the diseases could be discussed at extreme length, they still provide a solid foundation—a starting point from which the interested physician can proceed further. Nevertheless, we feel that there are few books like this one, in which one will find a general overview of the pathology of Mendelian disorders and a description of a rare disease such as hyperpipecolicacidemia in the same subdivision.

The last part of Volume One and all of Volume Two are devoted to diseases of organ systems. In addition to lesions seen by the surgical pathologist, these chapters deal also with "medical" diseases. Whenever it was appropriate the specific diseases were discussed in terms of their etiology, pathogenesis, and clinical significance. Numerous tables, diagrams, and black and white or color photographs were included as a supplement to enhance the message of the written text.

In contrast to previous editions, which were illustrated almost exclusively with black and white photographs, this edition contains many color illustrations. To make the material more readable and esthetically pleasing, the text has been enhanced by a four-color design. We anticipate that the colors will break the monotony, highlight the salient features, and enable the reader to grasp the visually enhanced message more efficiently. Two-color computer-generated graphic illustrations have been designed with the same aim in mind.

By design the tenth edition of *Anderson's Pathology* is a detailed book. Obviously it is too big for sophomore medical students, although we assume that some students looking for a good reference text might buy it as a source book and a "companion for life." We anticipate that the primary users of the book will be residents in pathology and related disciplines, and practicing pathologists. Specifically, we had in mind residents looking for a comprehensive textbook of pathology that is "one notch higher" than their sophomore pathology textbook. We hope that they will use this book as their primary text while preparing for the specialty boards, but also annotate it and keep it handy as they enter pathology practice. Practicing pathologists will find in it authoritative reviews of new information. They could use it also as a quick reference or a guide for more detailed reading. Educators who want to be one step ahead of their students should find in it enough material to enliven their lectures or seminars. Finally, although we do not expect our clinical colleagues to read it cover to cover, we hope that they will find it useful for consultation and reference.

The electronic media revolution has had a major impact on our thinking and has changed both our way of life and how we practice pathology. To meet the requirements of new generations of pathologists more comfortable with computers than books, we will produce a CD-ROM version of *Anderson's Pathology.* Like the Habsburg king, Charles V of Austria, who was known in Spain as Carlos I, the first CD-ROM version will also be known under two names, depending on the constituents who are using it. Since history does not teach us how to prognosticate, we do not know which dynastic branch will survive longer. We hope that both the printed and the electronic version will have their own followers. We are very eager to learn which format will be more popular.

We hope that the readers will react favorably to our team effort. To produce an even better book in the next edition we are soliciting comments and criticism from the readers. We can be reached via the internet at **idamjano@kumc.wpo.ukans.edu** and **jlinder@unmc.edu.** We are asking not only for creative suggestions for revisions but also entries and references that could help us in updating the text. We are inviting all pathologists to keep us informed of their important new publications and encourage them to deposit the references of their papers, along with a brief descriptor, into our e-mail bags. Furthermore, we are inviting junior (and not so junior) pathologists who would like to be considered as contributors for future editions of the textbook to send us their credentials.

We are pleased that so many outstanding pathologists agreed to share their time and expertise in completing this tenth edition. Without their dedication, this book would not exist. Our thanks are directed also to the publisher and especially Susan Gay, Lynne Gery, Stavra Demetrulias, and Dana Peick.

The support we received at our respective insitutions and from our families was invaluable. Judith Russell and Sandra Dixon-Ross deserve all the credit for the work done at Thomas Jefferson University, Philadelphia, where the entire project was conceived and begun. Cynthia Van Derbur has our thanks for the work done at the University of Kansas Medical Center. I (ID) thank also my wife, Andrea Damjanov, for her encouragement, dedication, and understanding, even when I did not deserve it.

At the University of Nebraska Medical Center our sincere thanks go to Valerie Gunderson, who provided the major organizational support for the textbook in addition to typing many of the chapters, proofreading, and extensive correspondence with contributors. I (JL) thank Samuel M. Cohen, M.D., Ph.D., Chairman of the Department of Pathology and Microbiology, and Harold M. Maurer, M.D., Dean of the College of Medicine, for providing an atmosphere that allowed us to complete a project of this scope. The project would not have been possible without the support of faculty and resident colleagues at the University of Nebraska Medical Center, particularly Dr. Thomas Seemayer, who provided invaluable guidance on many chapters. Finally, I thank my wife, Wendy Linder, M.D., and our children, Emily, Kari, and Eric Linder, for their patience and support.

Ivan Damjanov
James Linder

Contents

VOLUME ONE

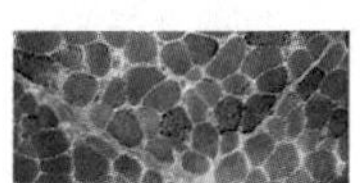

PART ONE METHODS IN PATHOLOGY

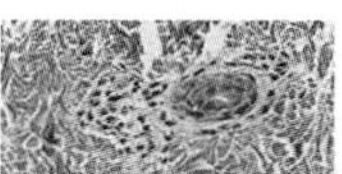

PART TWO SYSTEMIC PATHOLOGY

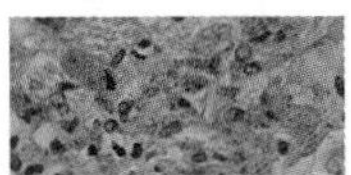

PART THREE INFECTIOUS DISEASES

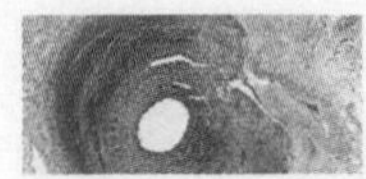

PART FOUR DISEASES OF THE BLOOD, HEART, AND LUNGS

VOLUME TWO

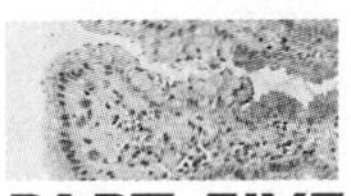

PART FIVE DISEASES OF THE DIGESTIVE SYSTEM

ANDERSON'S PATHOLOGY

1 The History of Pathology: An Overview

Christian Nezelof
Thomas A. Seemayer

Since the beginning of time, people have wished to know more about the causes of the evils and afflictions that befell them. The answers to these basic queries have evolved with time and reflect the main philosophical, religious, and scientific concepts, as well as the technical possibilities, of the day.

THE BASIS OF PATHOLOGY

Pathology, (from the Greek *pathos,* meaning 'suffering' and *logos,* meaning 'word', the discipline that deals with the causes and mechanisms of human diseases, originated from the above mentioned fundamental physical and metaphysical concerns and hence can be considered to be as old as medicine itself. For this reason, pathology is one of the basic medical sciences and is vital to the understanding of disease and hence its appropriate treatment.

To relate the history of pathology is not simply to express our debt to our predecessors, but also to acknowledge the different stages and the unpredictable ways through which progress has been made in the understanding of human diseases. The gradual shift over centuries from a divine or astrologic interpretation to a molecular approach not only fulfills the most ambitious expectations of the early philosophers but also offers a unique opportunity to analyze dynamically both the major breakthroughs and the deductive errors that have occurred along this journey. This historical approach can also be of value to facilitate a more critical evaluation of recently forwarded concepts in medicine.[1-14]

It is important to realize that, like medicine, *pathology is not a clearly delineated science.* It owes its development to successive intellectual and technical borrowings from nearby disciplines such as anatomy, physiology, physics, chemistry, microbiology, immunology, genetics, and cell and molecular biology. For this reason, pathology reflects closely the body of knowledge gradually acquired in each of these disciplines.

THE CONCEPT OF DISEASE

Disease, which can be defined as "any condition of the organism which limits life in either its power, enjoyment or duration" (R. Reynolds 1866), is as old as life itself. Ancient Egyptian, Assyrian, Chinese, Indian, and Hebrew writings make clear reference to the existence of afflictions such as tumors, cysts, fractures, and dislocations in humans and animals. However, these reports remained purely descriptive. The first attempts to establish a causal relationship for human disease are found in the medieval writings of Ibn-Sina, also known as Avícenna (980-1037). These expressed the metaphysical desire to put forward a complete system able to encompass all facets of the visible world, mainly as it affects living things leading to disease. In this approach, physical events such as temperature, storms, wind, and air (from the Italian *malaria,* 'bad air') were frequently mentioned as etiologic agents of human disease.

DISEASES AND RELIGIOUS BELIEFS

In this early period, diseases were linked with contemporary metaphysical and religious beliefs. This supernatural concept regarded illness as the work of malefic spirits, the "evil eye," or as the punishment delivered by touchy gods. These beliefs established primitive and tenacious links between medicine and religion and opened the way for the mediatory activity of priests, believed to possess the exclusive power to obtain, through their prayers and sacrifices, the kindness of the gods and the relief of pain. This close connection between medicine and religion has been found throughout the world and is embodied in the Old Testament. It persisted for a long time in almost all religions and was marked by the "specialization" of certain gods such as Aesculapius, Greek Asklēpios who became tutelary god of medicine, or christian saints reputed for the cure of specific diseases.

THE HELLENIC PERIOD: A RATIONAL APPROACH TO DISEASE

The Hellenic civilization, through its philosophers Socrates, Plato, and Aristotle, introduced a more coherent and rationalistic approach to the interpretation and understanding of natural phenomena. Although not entirely liberated from supernatural, astrologic, and magical beliefs, medicine benefited from this trend, which advocated the pursuit of knowledge for its own sake. Thus the healing arts became dissociated from theology and philosophy. Hippocrates (460-377 B.C.) personified Hellenic medicine and, even today, represents the paradigm of a physician combining adherence to observation, clinical accuracy, ethics, and creativity. According to Hippocrates, health was the expression of a state of harmony based on an equilibrium achieved through the balancing of extremes. Any disturbance of this equilibrium resulted in an illness. Later, Galen (131-201 A.D.) substantiated the concept of disequilibrium and postulated that illness originated from an imbalance between four constituent humors (fluids): sanguine (blood), phlegmatic or lymphatic (believed to be the product of the brain), biliary (liver), and melancholic (black bile from the spleen).

This humoral theory had the advantage of being remarkably flexible, offering a plausible answer to any medical problem. For this reason, it was well accepted and propagated by the Romans, notably Cornelius Celsius, throughout the Roman Empire, which extended from Asia Minor to Gaul and beyond. So successful was the humoral, or galenic, theory, that it exerted an almost exclusive influence for nearly 14 centuries.

THE MEDIEVAL PERIOD: THE TIME OF WIDESPREAD EPIDEMICS

The medieval period was characterized by a step backward, the recurrence of supernatural beliefs, the return of astrologic and alchemic practices, and the emergence of supernatural beings such as elves, devils, and witches. The latter were mostly invoked by Teutonic tribes and believed to be responsible for any affliction from a severe pain to "St. Vitus's dance," the latter thought to stem from demonic possession. The frequent occurrence of widespread and devastating epidemics reinforced the popular belief of divine punishment and hence the inquisitorial and often oppressive influence of the Christian churches over the lives of their adherents. Indeed, belief in the supremacy of the soul, regarded as an infinite divine property, resulted in a disdainful attitude toward the body and the frequent prescription of exercises of mortification. For this very reason, the anatomical (Greek *ana*, 'up' and *temnein*, 'to cut') dissection of a human body was regarded as "a violation of the temple of the soul" and, indeed, strictly forbidden. From the fourteenth to the seventeenth centuries, the practice and teaching of the healing arts remained entrenched on the learning by rote of the imperfectly translated and transcribed writings of Galen's texts and the blurred concept of *vitalism*. According to this theory, life was the manifestation of some "vital substance" *(élan vital)* that was under the control of the soul. The soul, or *anima* could give life to inanimate matter and maintain the body in a state of equilibrium, or *tonus*. Any modification in this tonus could result in disease. Vitalism, essentially advocated by certain German philosophers, spread throughout Europe and, until the nineteenth century, remained as a dominant concept, impeding the development of other ideas.

In this apparently homogeneous chorus, some dissident voices were heard. They came from a few philosophers, as well as physicians. René Descartes in France and Francis Bacon in England advocated, respectively, the value of doubt and the necessity for an experimental approach as the means of advancing learning (1605). The Swiss Paracelsus (1493-1541) extolled the relevance of clinical examination and the superiority of facts over theories. He was regarded as a rebel and had to travel through various European countries to escape medical and religious persecution. In this context, Girolamo Fracastoro (Latinized Fracastorius; 1483-1553), a classmate of Copernicus, appeared; he was one of the most ingenious and intuitive of modern medical theorists. Physician, poet, astronomer, and mathematician, he turned his attention to epidemics and postulated prophetically in his work *De Contagione et Contagiosis Morbi* that epidemics could result from the transfer from host to host of diminutive living agents, "a *contagium vivum*." Incidentally, he introduced in an epic poem the name of syphilis to designate the great pox (*grosse vérole*, *morbus gallicus*) believed to have been imported by members of the Columbus crew. Syphilus, a mythologic, handsome, but irreverent shepherd, was punished with the disease by Apollo.

THE RENAISSANCE: THE EMERGENCE OF ANATOMY

The Renaissance was characterized by a reaction against this theologic hegemony and a desire to rediscover the spiritual values and rationalistic approach of the Hellenic civilization.

The Renaissance originated in Italy and radiated throughout Europe in the fifteenth and early sixteenth centuries. This period was characterized by a ferment of intellectual activity and by a series of technical and economic advances such as the invention of the printing press, the compass, and the rudder; through them, there followed the discovery of new worlds. Overall, this period was characterized by the search for new forms of beauty and truth. As such, science was often overshadowed by the arts.

The dominant influence of this time was Leonardo da Vinci (1452-1519), a universal mind who first applied himself to human anatomy making drawings of muscles and embryos and molds of cardiac chambers. His work combined art and precision and established the value of accurate description as a cornerstone of the scientific approach. Five years before da Vinci

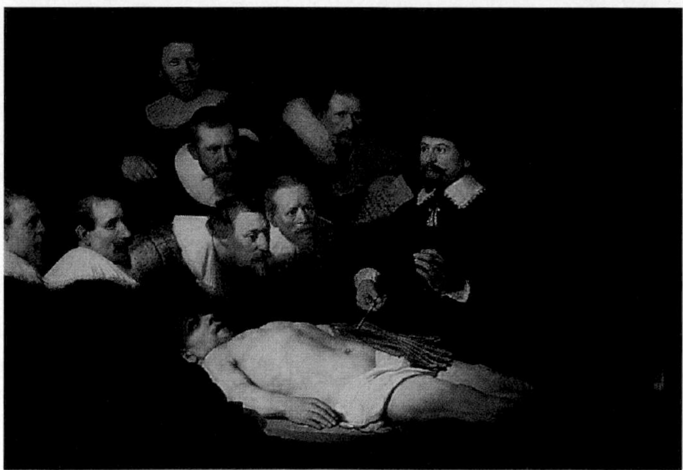

Fig. 1-1 The famous *Leçon d'Anatomie du Docteur Tulp* by Rembrandt (1632) reveals the authority and influence of the teacher as well as the respectfully attentive attitude of the spectators. (From Mauritshuis Museum, The Hague, The Netherlands.)

died, Vesalius (1514-1564) was born in Brussels. He moved early to Padua, a satellite city of Venice, at the time the most renowned medical center in Europe. Among other activities, Vesalius performed anatomical dissections of the bodies of executed criminals and extensively examined the skeleton, vessels, and nerves. With the assistance of von Calcar, he produced beautiful graphic plates reproducing his findings. Published as *De Humanis Corporis Fabrica* (1543), these plates represent the first scientific contribution to the study of normal human anatomy.

In the wake of Vesalius and his pupils Fallopius and Fabricius, the practice of anatomic dissection became, curiously enough, a fashionable activity attracting not only physicians but also notables and nosy spectators. For this activity, special postmortem amphitheaters were built and soon became the centers of medical teaching, staffed by dignified professors (Fig. 1-1). The curiosity about the composition of the human body, the events accompanying the end of life, and the possible site of the soul were some of the motivations behind this craze for anatomic dissection. Moreover, the acquisition of knowledge of the normal components of the human body constituted the necessary foundation for the birth and development of morbid anatomy.

THE EMERGENCE OF MORBID ANATOMY: G.B. MORGAGNI

Although Vesalius reported cases of aneurysms and Benivieni, a Florentine surgeon, recorded various visceral abnormalities, the credit for launching morbid anatomy (pathologic anatomy) as a science could be ascribed to Giovanni Battista Morgagni (1682-1777). Morgagni, known in Padua as his "Anatomical Majesty," divided his time between patients, clinical examination, and anatomic dissection. His monumental book *De Sedibus et Causis Morborum per Anatomen Indagatis*,[15] published in 1761 and based on 700 postmortem reports, condensed his threefold experience and represented the first scientific and comprehensive approach to human diseases. In addition to Morgagni, and often independently, many contemporary European physicians and surgeons contributed to the emergence of the clinicopathologic methodology and the propagation of medical knowledge. Most of them are today forgotten. History has retained only the names of a few who either influenced the understanding and definition of some human diseases or introduced a new technical approach to the investigation of patients or diseased organs. Among them are Hermann Boerhaave (1668-1738), who taught in Leyden, and Leopold Auenbrugger (1722-1809), who studied chest diseases; the latter, a descendant of a family of Austrian coopers, suggested percussion as a valuable means of clinical investigation.

All these contributions inaugurated the clinicopathologic methodology based on the correlation between bedside observations and the changes discovered in the postmortem room. This approach was of decisive importance for the following reasons:

1. It contributed to the definition of the term *lesion*, a word designating some characteristic anatomic change present in a diseased organ.
2. It introduced an anatomic concept and method to current practice aimed at expressing symptoms in terms of lesions, such as ulcer, effusion, sclerosis, and enteritis.
3. It offered the possibility of constructing for an illness a coherent schema including cause, lesions, symptoms, and outcome, namely, a clinicopathologic entity or, better named, a "disease."

THE DEVELOPMENT OF THE CLINICOPATHOLOGIC METHODOLOGY

The intense yet disorderly intellectual activity that accompanied and followed the French Revolution offered the opportunity to distance oneself from Latin, pioneer medical research, and introduce revolutionary concepts in the understanding of human diseases. Without the benefit of microscopic examination, Marie François Xavier Bichat (1771-1802), using only water, acids, alkalis, and maceration, put forward the idea that organs were composed of a limited number of building materials or tissues and postulated prophetically that morbid anatomy could be divided into two parts: systemic alterations restricted to one or two tissues (general pathology) and changes localized to one organ (special pathology).

However, this period was dominated clearly by the personality of René Laënnec (1781-1826). Laënnec was essentially a general practitioner eager to know the nature of the diseases that afflicted his patients. Long before the advent of the microscope and the notion of the existence of microorganisms, he ingeniously hypothesized that puzzling varieties of lung lesions, as diverse as tubercles, miliary lesions, caseous nodules, and pleural effusions could represent different expressions of the same disease, which he called *tuberculosis* on the basis of the similarity with potato tubercles. Among other achievements, he described as separate entities bronchial dilatation, bronchiectasis, as well as a chronic sclerotic liver disease that he called *cirrhosis*. His invention of the stethoscope stemmed from his need to establish a convenient bridge between the anatomic pulmonary changes and their auscultatory manifestations. In the wake of Laënnec came Pierre Bretonneau (1778-1862), who described diphtheria and typhoid fever; Gaspard Bayle (1774-1816), who first reported on cardiac auscultation; Pierre Louis (1782-1872), who worked on tuberculosis; Guillaume Dupuytren (1777-1835), a skilled surgeon who described the characteristics of some fractures; and Jean Cruveilhier (1791-1874), a pupil of Dupuytren who published one of the first complete works on the pathologic anatomy of the human body.

The first comprehensive English textbook of pathologic anatomy was published in the United Kingdom by Matthew Baillie (1761-1823), a pupil of the great English anatomist and naturalist John Hunter (1718-1793). In this treatise,[16] Baillie insisted on the fact that the most accurate morphologic description is not an end in itself but only a step in the search for the cause of a disease and the establishment of a reliable classification of human diseases. Later, in the middle and second half of the nineteenth century, the British School of Pathology with men such as Thomas Hodgkin, Richard Bright, Thomas Addison, James Paget, and Joseph Lister flourished and spread its influence to the distant parts of the British Empire.

However, it was in German-speaking countries that morbid anatomy reached its apogee. The leader was Carl von Rokitansky (1804-1878). Von Rokitansky, a self-taught pathologist, contrary to his predecessors, dealt solely with postmortem examinations performed in the central morgue of Vienna. It is said that he performed personally more than 30,000 autopsies during his scientific life. More significantly, he was the leader of a prolific Austrian school of pathology that included Hans Kundrat for his contribution to lymphogranulomatosis, Carl Sternberg, known for the description of the particular cells encountered in Hodgkin's disease, Hans Chiari and Richard Paltauf for their contributions to liver pathology, Anton Weichselbaum for his interest in microorganisms, and Karl Landsteiner (see below) in immunohematology.

THE ADVENT OF THE MICROSCOPE AND THE EMERGENCE OF CELL PATHOLOGY

Although the magnifying capacities of lenses had been demonstrated early on by Antonie van Leeuwenhoeck (1632-1723) and had made possible detailed descriptions of the spleen, epithelial surfaces, renal glomeruli, and capillary network by the great anatomic pathologist[17] Marcello Malpighi (1624-1694), the extensive utilization of the microscope took place only in the second half of the nineteenth century. Indeed, the combination of two lenses with a light condenser, invented by the German physicist Ernst Abbe (1868), allowed for immersion examination and higher magnification. In addition, the manufacture of high-quality knives and the emergence of the chemical dye industry permitted the development of enhanced methods of processing and staining and the possibility of obtaining, through microtomy, countless new thinly cut surfaces to study. This technical progress was a prerequisite for the development of histology, cytology, and cell biology. In fact, the notion of the cell (from Latin *cella,* 'small room, storehouse') demonstrated earlier by the English physicist Robert Hooke on the examination of fine sections of cork (1667), had been forgotten and was resurrected two centuries later through the works of the French botanist R.J.H. Dutrochet (1824) and the German zoologist Theodor Schwann (1839). Very soon, the cell came to be regarded as the "unit of living matter" (Herbert Spencer) or the primary representative of life (Claude Bernard) and became the focus of a new science, cell biology.

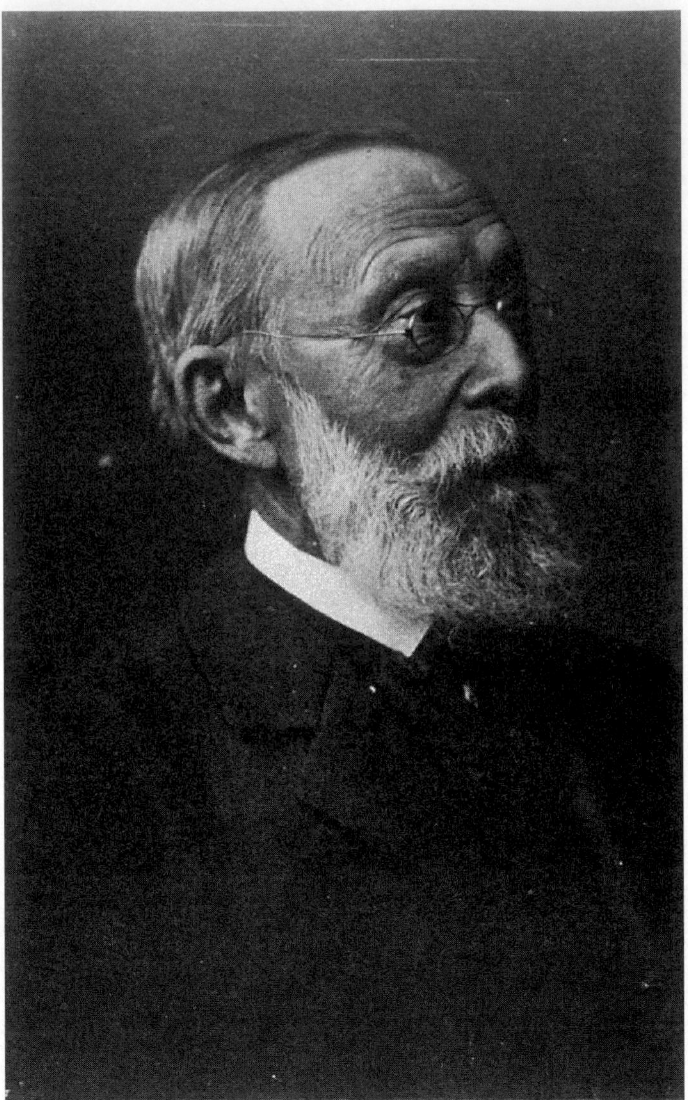

Fig. 1-2 Rudolph Virchow (1821-1905) pioneered histopathology as a method of investigation of diseased tissues. Portrait of the scientist when he was director of the Institute of Pathology at La Charité Hospital in Berlin (1900).

The credit for initiating the study of pathologic changes of the cell and regarding histopathology and cytopathology as fundamental methods of investigation rightly belongs to the German pathologist Rudolph Virchow (1821-1905) (Fig. 1-2). Working with the hypothesis *"omnis cellula e cellula"* (every cell derives from a cell), Virchow demonstrated that a variety of gross pathologic modifications could be reduced to basic cellular changes. With his mentor, Johannes Müller (1801-1858), he postulated that neoplastic proliferations took their origin and characteristics from the cellular and tissular counterparts in normal or embryonal organisms, thereby inaugurating the histogenetic approach to the classification of tumors. He drew a clear distinction between the homogeneous character of neoplastic proliferations and the heterogeneity of the reactive and inflammatory processes. Virchow published his master work *Die Cellularpathologie in ihrer Begründung auf physiologische und pathologische Gewebelehre* in 1858 in Berlin.[18]

Through his work, Virchow anchored pathology firmly in the morphologic disciplines. Today, he is considered as the pioneer of histopathology and the father of modern pathology. Virchow's creative work was pursued by his numerous and brilliant disciples who promoted morbid histology as a fundamental medical science. The names of some are well known as they left traces in the history of medicine: Edward von Rindfleisch, Friedrich von Recklinghausen, and Robert Rössle.

THE CONTRIBUTION OF NONMORPHOLOGIC SCIENTIFIC DISCIPLINES TO PATHOLOGY

Very soon, physicians and morbid anatomists realized that even the most accurate anatomic dissections could not explain the causes of common symptoms such as fever, dropsy, or coma, to name but a few. They felt the necessity to delve beyond static morphologic examination, to explore the dynamic aspect of lesions, to enlarge their methods of investigation, and to employ the conceptual and technical advances being made in physiology, chemistry, and physics. This trend resulted in the emergence and development of two different branches of pathology: experimental pathology and the detection of physiologic and chemical pathologic abnormalities in the living body, that is, pathophysiology.

The advent of experimental pathology originated from the desire to study dynamically, in living animals, the different steps in the development of a lesion and their accompanying functional changes and, in this way, to establish the mechanisms central to the progression of an induced disease. By demonstrating the crucial role of the liver in the regulation of blood sugar, Claude Bernard (1813-1878) was one of the pioneers of pathophysiology. Experimental pathology and pathophysiology played an important role in the identification of metabolic and nutritional diseases and led to the demonstration of the critical role of some essential substances, called *vitamins.* At the same time, the theoretical progress made by Lavoisier, Priestley, Berzelius, Dalton, and others in the chemical analysis of organic components made possible the development of microanalytical methods to measure certain blood constituents, such as glucose, and urea. This methodology allowed for the detection of chemical modifications underlying conditions such as diabetes mellitus and Bright's (chronic renal) disease, thereby providing the biochemical basis for a clear definition of metabolic diseases.

Along the same line, the tremendous advances made in the last part of the nineteenth century in physiology, physics, and chemistry were extended to provide a better knowledge of the living cell. This shift in thinking led to the development of new morphologic methods of cell investigation and was rapidly applied to all of pathology:

- Tissue and cell culture (R.G. Harrison 1907), which permitted the utilization of vital staining to study cell differentiation.
- The development of the electron microscope (Ruska and von Lorries 1933), which provided an ultrastructural view of cell constituents.
- Ultracentrifugation and differential centrifugation (Bensley and Hoerr 1934), which allowed for cell fractionation and the isolation of large quantities of nuclei, mitochondria, and enzymatic substrates such as lysosomes (de Duve 1963).
- Cytochemistry and histochemistry initiated by Robert Feulgen (1924) and developed by Lucien Lison (1936), George Gomori (1941), and A. Pearse (1960), which permitted the localization in fresh or fixed material of chemical compounds or enzymes at the cellular or tissular level. The combination of these different techniques, complemented by immunologically derived methods, made cell biology a mature and fully integrated discipline (Novikoff 1960) and provided a solid basis on which to study and interpret pathologic changes.

THE EMERGENCE OF SURGICAL PATHOLOGY: THE CONTRIBUTION OF NORTH AMERICA

For historical reasons, the activity of most pathologists had been long centered around the postmortem amphitheater and the pathologic museums housing specimens of teaching value. Moreover, in German-speaking countries, separate buildings, each an institute of pathology *(pathologisches institut)*, distinct from the hospital wards, were created and soon become the centers of intense research and teaching activities, the reputation of which spread over the world. In contrast, in Latin countries, there was not such a sharp physical separation of pathology from clinical medicine.

For a long time, this activity had been the work of practicing physicians and surgeons, eager, as Morgagni or Laënnec, to know more about the causes and the mechanisms of the diseases that affected their patients. For instance, Jean-Martin Charcot (1825-1893), Pierre-Paul Broca (1824-1880), Charles Brown-Séquard (1817-1894), and Constantin von Economo (1886-1931) were brilliant neurologists, yet creative pathologists. The diseases and anatomic regions they described are contained in several chapters that follow.

When it was recognized that pathologists were able to anticipate postmortem findings and put forward reliable diagnoses solely on the examination of the histologic changes present in samples of living tissues, this led to the surgical biopsy and the emergence of the discipline of surgical pathology.[19] Long a descriptive, retrospective, and academic science, pathology was becoming a prospective and practical discipline. With the clinical awareness of this capacity, pathology entered a new era, enlarging dynamically its range of activities and becoming an essential element in the daily management of human diseases. Although the surgeons Carl Ruge and Johann Veit in the 1870s in Berlin and Friedrich August von Esmarck in Kiel introduced surgical biopsy as an essential tool of diagnosis, the emergence and the development of surgical pathology as a discipline were mostly the work of American pathologists: Francis Delafield (1841-1915), William Henry Welch (1850-1934), James Ewing (1866-1943), Arthur Purdy Stout (1885-1967), and Lauren Ackerman (1905-1993).

The development of frozen-section procedures, popularized in 1895 by the Canadian pathologist Thomas Stephen Cullen,[20] made available a rapid, almost instant diagnosis during surgery and anchored firmly and perhaps definitively the pathology department close to the operating room. As a result, the routine workings of the pathology department progressively evolved into a diagnostic activity.

In this medium, the morphologic examination of cells (more easily available than samples of tissues) assumed a gradual importance. Blood cells were the first to be investigated. The application of aniline dyes, especially the methylene blue eosinate stain of Ehrlich, led to the staining procedures of Artur Pappenheim (1902), May-Grünwald (1902), and Gustav Giemsa (1914) and a reliable classification of blood and bone marrow cells. It was only later that the exfoliative, brush, touch, and aspiration cytology techniques were developed, with the aim of detecting malignant cells. Inaugurated in 1927 by the Rumanian, Victor Babès, the practice of exfoliative cytology was developed and popularized by an American anatomist of Greek descent, George Papanicolaou. Since then, the study of "Pap smears" has become an important field of activity in all pathology departments for the detection of early cervical neoplasia. Indeed, cytopathology is now recognized as a distinct subspecialty of pathology; textbooks, such as those of Leopold Koss, a distinguished student of Papanicolaou, are now essential components of a departmental library.

DISCOVERY OF THE EXISTENCE OF MICROORGANISMS: THE EMERGENCE OF BACTERIOLOGY

The recognition that some diseases could be related to the presence and proliferation of minute parasitic "animalcules," or microorganisms, also occurred in the second half of the nineteenth century. Unexpectedly, this discovery was made, not by a biologist or a physician, but by a French chemist, Louis Pasteur (1822-1895), who investigated the events accompanying lactic and acetic acid fermentation and the transmission of contagious diseases affecting silkworms and sheep. The identification, thanks to the heightened resolution of the microscope, of minute disease agents and the demonstration of their transmission from one animal to another dismissed the long-held notion of spontaneous generation and opened the door to experiments that showed that these organisms were pathogenic. Moreover, this discovery led to a profound revolution in the understanding of certain human diseases and offered, at last, a solid and verifiable basis for the old and frightening notion of contagion. Under the influence of Pasteur and his numerous disciples and colleagues, Émile Roux, Pierre Bretonneau, Albert Calmette, A.J.E. Yersin in France, Joseph Lister in Scotland, Robert Koch in Germany, Gerhard Hansen in Norway, Anton Weichselbaum in Austria, Simon Flexner in the USA, and many others, bacteriology was developing as an autonomous science and having repercussions of its own. Apart from the fact that bacteriology provided a reliable basis for the etiologic identification and classification of human infectious diseases, it opened the door to aseptic procedures and, spearheaded by Lister, the development of safer surgery. Equally important, it challenged the supremacy and exclusivity of morphologic investigations in establishing disease etiology, introduced new means to study disease, and led to the discovery of penicillin in 1928 by the Scottish microbiologist Alexander Fleming.

The recognition that certain microbes could be responsible for specific diseases offered a new dimension to pathology and suggested also that agents unseen with the light microscope might exist. The discovery of the "filterable infectious principle" called *virus* (in Latin, 'slimy liquid, poison') likewise came from a quite distant field, botany. Indeed, the first identification of a virus was made by a Russian bacteriologist, Dmitri Iosifovich Ivanovsky, in 1892 and subsequently confirmed a few years later by Dutch botanist M.V. Beijerinck (1851-1931) in his study of mosaic, a disease affecting tobacco leaves. The isolation of the tobacco mosaic virus was the first step in the identification of countless human and animal viruses. Not only did this offer a satisfactory explanation to some worldwide epidemics such as influenza, but also it made it possible to investigate, through the study of bacteriophages (Frederick W. Twort 1915), the most elementary forms of life and the transmission of genetic characteristics.

IMMUNOLOGY: A SPIN-OFF FROM THE STUDY OF INFECTIOUS DISEASES

One of the unexpected spin-offs from the study of infectious diseases was the emergence of the discipline of immunology. The fact that, in the spread of epidemics, some individuals managed to escape infection and appeared protected, in other words, "immunized" (from the Latin *immunius,* meaning 'exempt'), had been mentioned by Fracastorius several centuries ago, yet the nature of the defenses against these agents could not be analyzed until they were identified.

The step-by-step advances in the analysis of the mechanisms underlying host defenses resulted in a better understanding of the immune response, but it also led to the discovery of utterly different states such as immune tolerance and its opposite, allergic and anaphylactic reactions. In addition, it provided the scientific basis for immunization, a concept that had been accepted since Edward Jenner (1749-1823), solely on empirical observations. Finally, advances in this domain contributed greatly to the classification of immunodeficiency disorders and autoimmune diseases and allowed for the development of new immunologic tools of investigation.

Here again, these advances were closely dependent on progress in other domains, which facilitated the serologic and cytologic techniques of investigation. The results obtained from these different methods fueled, at the end of the nineteenth and the early part of the twentieth centuries, great controversy opposing the advocates of the predominant role of humoral factors and those favoring cellular mechanisms in the struggle against microbes.

By discovering the antimicrobial property of some fractions of blood serum, Paul Ehrlich (1854-1916) and Emil von Behring (1854-1917) in Germany and Jules Bordet (1870-1961) in Belgium gave credence to the concepts of antibodies and complement. Several years later, these elements were demonstrated by physical methods: electrophoresis (Tiselius 1939), ultracentrifugation (Cohn 1947), immunoprecipitation (Ouchterlony 1948), and immunoelectrophoresis (Williams and Grabar 1955). Refinements in the knowledge of antibodies resulted rapidly in decisive progress. Taking advantage of their specific affinity for antigens, the evaluation of antibodies made possible the detection of foreign or endogenous antigenic substances in the blood and tissues. The best illustration of this property was the discovery of blood agglutinins and the subsequent identification of the three main blood groups in 1900 by a Viennese pathologist, Karl Landsteiner (1863-1943)[21] (Fig. 1-3). Later, when he was in New York, he and others demonstrated the immunologic basis of Rh incompatibility. The characterization of the blood groups was indeed the first proof of the philosophical concept regarding the uniqueness of the indi-

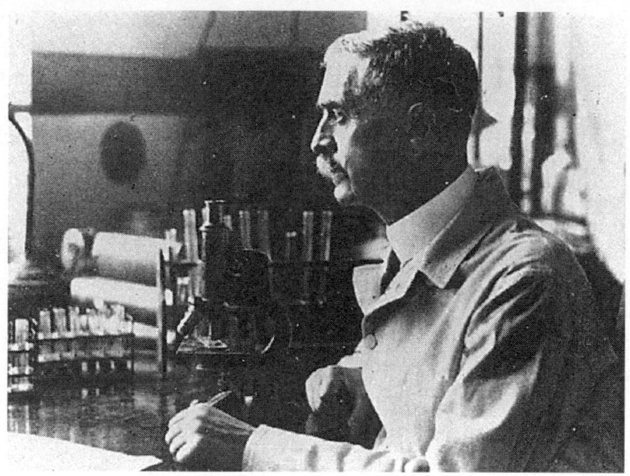

Fig. 1-3 Karl Landsteiner (1863-1943) in his laboratory at the Institute of Pathology in Vienna, where he put forward the concept of the existence of various human blood groups, a discovery for which he received the Nobel prize.

vidual, one that was further developed between 1950 and 1953 by Burnet[22] and Billingham.[23] This concept was based mainly on the similarity between the phenomena associated with the rejection of a graft and those connected with the immunologic defense mechanisms against invading microbes. The body's ability to distinguish between self and nonself provided the basis for the identification of the major histocompatibility complex (MHC) present in all vertebrates (Benacerraf,[24] McDevitt[25]) and termed "HLA (human leukocyte antigens)" in humans (Dausset[26]). The recognition of the MHC not only led to a better understanding of the immune response, but also opened the way for tissue and organ transplantation.

In contrast, progress in cell-mediated immunity had been slower. Ilya Metchnikoff (1845-1916), a Russian zoologist working closely with Pasteur in Paris, recognized the existence and importance of a phenomenon that he called "phagocytosis" in the struggle against microbes. However, the crucial immunologic role of the small lymphocyte was not identified until 1961, when the English physiologist J. Gowans,[27] among others, demonstrated that hypersensitivity manifestations could be transmitted by lymphocytes drained from the thoracic duct and showed that lymphocyte-deprived animals could become tolerant to allografts. These findings ushered in a new era in the understanding of the immune response. The experimental demonstration of the thymus[28,29] and the bursa of Fabricius[30] as the primary ontogenic lymphoid organs subsequently introduced a fundamental distinction between T cell–derived cellular immunity and B cell–derived humoral immunity. It soon become clear that cooperation between these two populations of cells, mediated by the MHC and the participation of antigen presenting cells, was necessary for mounting a satisfactory immune response.[31]

DEVELOPMENT OF IMMUNOLOGY-BASED METHODS OF INVESTIGATION

Not only did the immunologic approach allow tremendous advances to be made in the identification and understanding of some hitherto obscure illnesses, but it also provided new tools for the investigation of diseased tissues. Based on the ability to generate a great assortment of antibodies in animals and the close affinity between these antibodies and their respective antigens, immunohistochemical techniques were developed for the detection of antigens in tissues or cells in suspension. Fluorescent compounds coupled with animal antisera were elaborated, and such a combination established immunofluorescence as the first immunohistochemical procedure,[32] which was rapidly applied in the routine diagnosis of immunologically mediated diseases of the kidney and the skin. The replacement of fluorescein by enzymes, such as horseradish peroxidase, secondarily revealed by a chromogen, opened the way for immunoenzymatic methodology.

Numerous refinements were proposed to address the issues of sensitivity and specificity and the most convenient methods for diagnostic use. The generation of monoclonal antibodies through cell hybridization by Köhler and Milstein[33] greatly improved the specificity of these techniques but concomitantly decreased their sensitivity. Numerous methods to increase sensitivity have been developed. These exploit new enzyme markers, such as alkaline phosphatase, preformed peroxidase antiperoxidase (PAP) complexes, or the high affinity of avidin for biotin in the avidin-biotin-peroxidase complex (ABC) method.

Techniques derived from immunology made possible not only the "in situ" detection of certain molecules but also allowed for the quantitative evaluation of circulating cells and antigenic substances. Flow-cytometry methodology was developed in 1953[34] for counting cells in suspension. Coupled with laser and computer-based technologies in the fluorescence-activated cell sorter (FACS), it is now possible to separate different cell populations and isolate a small subpopulation from a complex mixture. This methodology has been found most useful in characterizing blood and tissue lymphoid cells.

In a different way, the quantitative methods known as RIA (radioimmunoassay) and ELISA (enzyme-linked immunoabsorbent assay) are also based on an antigen-antibody reaction coupled with the use of a scintillation liquid or a chromogenic solid substrate. These methods allow for the detection and quantification of minute amounts of a given molecule and have formed the basis for progress in various fields of medicine. By contrast, methods for investigating cell-mediated immunity such as the mixed lymphocyte culture (MLC) and tests for evaluating lymphoid proliferation and cell cytotoxicity have had a more restricted influence.

ADVANCES IN THE UNDERSTANDING OF GENETIC DISEASES

It had long been recognized that certain diseases recur in some families, certain geographic areas, or at specific periods of the year. These observations offered the basis for early epidemiologic investigations and provided the subsoil for the classical distinction between nature-linked and nurture-linked diseases, conditions known today respectively as hereditary (or genetic) and environmental diseases.

The recognition that certain external malformations and diseases were restricted to some families and recurred from generation to generation indicated that "something" was transmitted from parents to their offspring, and this was designated by the legal term *heredity*. For a long time, the principles of such transmission remained mysterious. Unexpectedly, the first insight came from the observations made by a Moravian botanist and monk, Gregor Mendel, drawn from his work on breeding and crossbreeding a common edible pea.[35] These observations, which formed the basis of what is today accepted as the Mendelian laws, were at first neglected and forgotten, then rediscovered and popularized 60 years later by the Dutch botanist Hugo de Vries. The American biologist Thomas Morgan (1866-1945), working on the hereditary transmission of the phenotypical characteristics of the rapidly multiplying fruit fly *Drosophila melanogaster,* first threw light on the nature of inheritance. He demonstrated the crucial role of chromosomes and postulated the existence of genetic units: genes.[36] For a long time, investigations on the transmission of external characteristics had been restricted to plants, insects, protozoons, or fungi such as yeast, simply because of their low numbers of chromosomes. Nevertheless, these studies resulted in the notions of dominant and recessive genes, sex-linked transmission, and notably the occasional occurrence of sudden changes, known as *mutations*, in the genetic program.

In humans, although the hereditary transmission of external malformations had been recognized for centuries, the crucial role of genetic factors in the genesis of internal illnesses has only recently been recognized. This was first exposed in 1923 by Garrod in his book *Inborn Errors of Disease*.[37] Not only did this approach give some support for the old concept of a constitutional predisposition for certain diseases, but it also contributed to establishing the importance of biochemical mechanisms in numerous metabolic diseases and led to the concept, with the soon-to-appear field of molecular biology, of "one gene, one enzyme"[38] and a scientific approach to metabolic disorders.

CHROMOSOME IDENTIFICATION

The name *chromosome* was coined in 1888 by the zoologist Heinrich Waldeyer to designate isolated fragments of nuclear chromatin observed during mitosis and meiosis. Based on the work of numerous botanists and zoologists, it was assumed that chromosomes represented permanent elements ensuring the genetic continuity of the somatic and germ cells and were characteristic of each species. Using cultured cells of fetal lung, Tjio and Levan reported in 1956[39] that the diploid number (2n) of chromosomes in humans was 46 and not 48, as had been believed for more than 30 years. Countless studies using squash preparations, short-term lymphocyte or tissue cultures, coupled with hypotonic shock and colchicine, fixed the size, number, and morphology of each of these 23 chromosomes. Down syndrome, the trisomy of chromosome 21, discovered in 1959 by Lejeune,[40] was the first chromosomal abnormality identified, one of a long series of changes observed, involving either the number, shape, or banding pattern of each chromosome. Initially, most of these abnormalities were associated with severe congenital malformations, sexual abnormalities, and spontaneous abortions. Subsequently, after the discovery by Nowell and Hungerford in 1960 of an abnormality involving chromosome 21, known as the *Philadelphia chromosome* (later recognized as a translocation 9;22) in chronic myelogenous leukemia,[41] chromosomal changes such as translocations, breakpoints, deletions, and inversions have been found to be specific for many malignancies, a matter of no small diagnostic and prognostic importance. In addition, by defining the presence of a constant breakpoint in a defined chromosomal region, the karyotypic investigations of neoplastic cells consolidated the linkage between malignancies and genomic abnormalities and facilitated the mapping of normal and abnormal genes.

Investigators worldwide were soon localizing abnormal genes along the chromosomes. This endeavor was facilitated by parallel developments in molecular biology along with genetic linkage studies. In 1971, by staining of chromosomes with quinacrine, a chemical with an affinity for the nucleotide guanine, it was possible to distinguish all 23 pairs of human chromosomes by their banding patterns. With refinements of stainings and "stretching out" chromosomes, the technology is now able to identify at least 2000 bands, attaining a resolution of 10 million base pairs. The detection of a given karyotypic abnormality has frequently been the first step in the cloning of an abnormal gene, as in Duchenne's myopathy and cystic fibrosis. In a different approach, the possibility of obtaining, through the action of a virus or a chemical agent, hybrid somatic cells with different chromosomal complements (human and mouse) allows for the selection of certain human chromosomes to study their abnormality and possible metabolic effects. The more recent use of yeasts, primitive prokaryotes almost devoid of noncoding introns, has led to the development of Yeast Artificial Chromosomes (YACs) and their libraries central to the human genome project.

THE DISCOVERY OF THE STRUCTURE OF DNA

For years, cytologists were convinced that the basophilic material, chromatin, present in the chromosomes and interphase nucleus, was the substance responsible for genetic continuity. It was known early on that chromatin was composed of a complex combination of proteins and nucleotides arranged in a long linear array. As early as 1924, Feulgen and Rossenbeck developed an efficient cytochemical method that allowed for not only the detection, but also to some extent the quantitation of nucleic acids. However, the role of nucleic acids and their associated proteins in genetic transmission remained unclear until 1944, when Avery at the Rockefeller Institute established in experiments with the pneumococcus that DNA was the true genetic material.[42] In 1953, James Watson, an American biologist, and Francis Crick, an English chemist, working in the laboratory of Maurice Wilkins in Cambridge, England, proposed "a radically different structure for the salt of deoxyribonucleic acid" (DNA). This discovery stemmed from both intuition and critical analysis of the x-ray crystallographic images of wet and dry DNA obtained from Rosalind Franklin.[43] The structure proposed (in one of the most concise scientific papers ever written) was that of two paired complementary strands of nucleic acids coiled in a double-helix arrangement and organized in an antiparallel fashion.[44] The duplicate organization of the DNA molecules gives rise to important properties: their self-replication, each strand serving as a template to generate a complementary strand through the association of base pairs,[45] and their capacity to deliver a coded message through the intermediary of a complementary single-stranded messenger RNA.[46] This seminal discovery, unquestionably the most important in all of science up to now, provided at last the evidence to support the hitherto theoretical concept of the gene.

DNA ENGINEERING AS A TOOL OF INVESTIGATION

DNA appeared to be a very flexible and dynamic molecule. Indeed, in her study of maize, Barbara McClintock had shown that genes can move along chromosomes, "jumping genes," creating a certain fluidity to genetics.[47] This set the stage for subsequent discoveries, among others, of the shuffling of immunoglobulin and T-cell receptor genes in lymphoid ontogeny. The Nobel committee in awarding the prize in 1983 regarded her work over decades as "one of the two greatest discoveries in genetics." The other was the elucidation of the structure of DNA. DNA could be "replicated, sliced, stitched, spliced, and repaired" through the action of physical agents (temperature) and enzymes such as nucleases, ligases, transcriptases, and topoisomerases. This malleability offered vast possibilities for the field of DNA engineering. In particular, restriction endonucleases, able to cut DNA at specific sequences,[48-50] made it possible to generate fragments of various lengths that could be separated by size and transferred to a membrane for analysis following the method of Southern.[51] The isolation and use of reverse transcriptase,[52,53] a retroviral enzyme, allowed DNA to be synthesized from an RNA template. This advanced the understanding of the biology of retroviruses and facilitated progress in DNA cloning. The splicing of small DNA fragments (from 10^3 to 10^6 base pairs) into self-replicating vectors such as plasmids,[54] bacteriophages, and more recently yeasts also allowed multiple DNA copies to be obtained, and in such a way facilitated the dissection of the human genome. With this technology, a rational methodology for exploring DNA polymorphisms was proposed to establish genetic maps of the human genome.[55]

In a different way, the utilization of a thermoresistant DNA polymerase, as proposed by Mullis,[56] coupled with automated thermocyclers made possible the generation of countless copies of a selected DNA sequence. This polymerase chain reaction (PCR) currently represents a rapid, highly sensitive, commonly employed, and inexpensive method of DNA investigation, thereby contributing to the "democratization of molecular biology" as Joshua Lederberg said.

DNA PROBES FOR IN SITU HYBRIDIZATION

DNA recombinant technology offered the possibility of constructing certain oligonucleotides, which in turn can be labeled and used as DNA probes, able to target homologous complementary sequences in a complex system. This property formed the basis of the widely used molecular hybridization techniques. The use and increasing availability of labeled DNA probes opened the way for the development of in situ hybridization methodology. Radioactive DNA probes were first used in 1978[57] for the prenatal diagnosis of hemoglobinopathies. More recently, fluorescent DNA probes have been elaborated. The fluorescence in situ hybridization (FISH) technique has rapidly become an invaluable tool for the visualization of chromosomal subregions and is useful in detecting chromosomal abnormalities, not only in karyotypes but also in interphase nuclei.

DNA METHODOLOGY IN GENETIC DISEASE

DNA recombinant technology not only furnished qualitative and quantitative clues to the genetic relationships between diverse species and showed the extreme diversity of individuals of the same species, but also provided invaluable tools for the identification of microorganisms, the dissection of the human genome, and the understanding of many genetic and neoplastic conditions. Numerous investigators have estimated that between 50,000 and 100,000 genes are buried in the 3 billion base pairs of the human genome. In 1993, some 5000 genetic loci have been identified for the over 4000 known human genetic diseases.[58]

DNA METHODOLOGY IN NEOPLASIA: ONCOGENES AND TUMOR SUPPRESSOR GENES

In addition to genetic diseases, molecular investigations have provided valuable insights into the nature of the mechanisms underlying neoplastic changes. As early as 1914, the German zoologist Theodor Boveri hypothesized the existence of genetic and chromosomal changes in carcinogenesis.[59] Later, the identification of mutational changes, either spontaneous or induced by x-rays or chemical agents, substantiated this hypothesis and provided the basis for the development of experimental oncology.

One of the biggest breakthroughs came unexpectedly from studies of retroviruses. Peyton Rous reported in 1911 that an unusual sarcoma in chickens could be induced by cell-free filtrates.[60] The significance of this finding was appreciated only decades later, when retroviruses were recognized to be latent RNA viruses that had to be activated to become oncogenic. These data led to the hypothesis of the existence of proviruses and viral oncogenes (v-*onc*), believed to be responsible for the development of anarchic cellular growth. The discovery of reverse transcriptase made it possible to demonstrate that retroviruses integrated into the cellular genome by recombination with cellular DNA sequences. Surprisingly, homologous DNA sequences were later found in normal and uninfected cells.[61] These homologous sequences were found to have a pivotal role in the cellular growth and differentiation of eukaryotes and, by analogy, were called *protooncogenes*, or *cellular oncogenes* (c-*onc*). More than 50 c-oncogenes have been identified, yet only 20 v-*onc* have so far been recognized. Their precise chromosomal localization was soon identified, often at "fragile sites" where breakpoints and translocations occurred preferentially in neoplasia.[62]

Within the past decade, a new family of cancer genes has been defined. In contrast to oncogenes, which exert a biologic effect through a gain of function, tumor suppressor genes make their presence known through loss of function. First described in retinoblastoma,[63] the loss of both functional alleles of these genes is central to uncontrolled cell proliferation because their mutated nuclear protein products are no longer able to exert appropriate controls on the cell cycle. An ever-expanding list of these genes along with their mutations continues to unfold in diverse pediatric and adult cancers. Their existence was predicted some time ago by Knudson,[64] based on an epidemiologic study of familial and sporadic retinoblastoma.

CONCLUDING REMARKS

This chapter is a prelude to the several thousand pages that follow. In the sections to come, you will discover that pathology embraces all disciplines of medicine and draws heavily on the physical sciences. The modern pathologist is called upon to integrate these multiple disciplines on a daily, indeed case-by-case, basis. The cornerstone of pathology resides in morbid anatomy, the foundation upon which the discipline was founded. Yet this is but a foundation, and for that reason this introduction was constructed to reflect that, to be relevant, pathologists must be conversant with and employ techniques stemming from diverse fields of scientific endeavor. In this overview, the works of 34 Nobel laureates have been cited. While only two (Sir Howard Florey and Karl Landsteiner) were pathologists, all of their contributions have a great influence on modern-day pathology. The necessity to grow beyond morbid anatomy, perhaps, is one reason we continue to be enamored with our specialty. In short, we remain lifelong students of the mechanisms of disease, as were our predecessors.

REFERENCES

1. Majno G: *The healing hand: man and wound in the ancient world,* Cambridge, Mass, 1975, Harvard University Press.
2. Kiple KF, editor: *The Cambridge world history of human disease,* Cambridge, England, 1993, Cambridge University Press.
3. Sournia JC: *Histoire de la médecine et des médecins,* Paris, 1991, Ed. Larousse.
4. Florey H: *General pathology based on lectures delivered at the Sir William Dunn School of Pathology,* Oxford University, London, 1962, Lloyd-Luke.
5. Klemperer P: Pathologic anatomy at the end of the eighteenth century, *J Mount Sinai Hosp* 24:589, 1957.
6. Klemperer P: The pathology of Morgagni and Virchow, *Bull Hist Med* 32:24, 1958.
7. Pérez-Tamayo R: *Mechanisms of disease: an introduction to pathology,* Philadelphia, 1961, Saunders.
8. Rössle R: Das Virchowsche Archiv 100 Jahre alt, *Virchows Arch* 315:1, 1948.
9. Long ER: *A history of American pathology,* Springfield, Ill, 1962, Charles C Thomas.
10. Nezelof C: The European roots of pathology, *Pathol Res Pract* 190:103, 1994.
11. Bendiner E: Andreas Vesalius: man of mystery in life and death, *Hosp Pract* 21:199, 1986.
12. Laënnec RTH: *Traité de l'auscultation médiate et des maladies du poumon et du cœur,* Paris, 1879, Ed. Asselin.
13. Lesky E: *Carl von Rokitansky: selbstbiographie und antrittsrede,* Vienna, 1960, Hermann Böhlans.
14. Bendiner E: Renaissance medicine: alchemy and astrology, art and anatomy, *Hosp Pract* 24:247, 1989.
15. Morgagni JB: *De sedibus et causis morborum per anatomen indagatis,* Venice, 1762.
16. Baillie M: *The morbid anatomy of some of the most important parts of the human body,* London, 1793, J. Johnson.
17. Scarani P, Salvioli GP, Eusebi V: Marcello Malpighi (1628-1694): a founding father of modern anatomic pathology, *Am J Surg Pathol* 18:741, 1994.
18. Virchow R: *Die Cellularpathologie in ihrer Begrundung auf physiologische und pathologische Gewebe,* Berlin, 1858, A Hirschwald.
19. Rosen G: Beginnings of surgical biopsy, *Am J Surg Pathol* 1:361, 1977.
20. Cullen TS: A rapid method of making permanent sections from frozen specimens by the use of formalin, *Johns Hopkins Hosp Bull,* p 67, 1895.
21. Landsteiner K: Zur Kenntnis der antifermentativen, lytischen und agglutinierenden Wirkungen des Blutserums und der Lymphe, *Zentralbl Bakteriol* 27:357, 1900.
22. Burnet FM, Fenner F: *The production of antibodies,* ed 2, London, 1950, Macmillan.
23. Billingham RE, Brent L, Medawar PB: Actively acquired tolerance of foreign cells, *Nature* 172:603, 1953.
24. Benacerraf B, Paul WE, Green I: The immune response of guinea pigs to hapten-poly-L-lysine conjugates as an example of the genetic control of the recognition of antigenicity, *Cold Spring Harb Symp Quant Biol* 32:569, 1967.
25. McDevitt HO, Chinitz A: Genetic control of the antibody response: relationship between immune response and histocompatibility (H-2) type, *Science* 175:273, 1972.
26. Dausset J, Svejgaard A: *HLA and disease,* Baltimore, 1977, Williams and Wilkins.
27. Gowans JL: The immunological activity of lymphocytes. In Wolstenholme GEW, O'Connor M, editors: *Biological activity of the leucocyte,* London, 1961, Churchill.
28. Miller JFAP: Immunological function of the thymus, *Lancet* 2:748, 1961.
29. Good RA, Dalmasso AP, Martínez C et al: The role of the thymus in development of immunologic capacity in rabbits and mice, *J Exp Med* 116:773, 1962.
30. Glick B, Chang TS, Jaap RG: The bursa of Fabricius and antibody production, *Poultry Sci* 35:224, 1956.
31. Mosier DE: A requirement for two cell types for antibody formation, *Science* 158:1573, 1967.
32. Coons AH, Creech HJ, Jones RN et al: The demonstration of pneumococcal antigens in tissues by the use of fluorescent antibody, *J Immunol* 45:159, 1942.
33. Köhler G, Milstein C: Continuous cultures of fused cells secreting antibody of predefined specificity, *Nature* 256:495, 1975.
34. Coulter WH: High speed automated blood cell counter and cell analyzer, *Proc Natl Elec Conf* 12:1034, 1956.
35. Mendel GJ: Versuche über Pflanzenhybriden, *Verhandlungen des Naturforschenden Vereins,* Brünn, 1865.
36. Morgan TH: Sex-limited inheritance in *Drosophila, Science* 32:120, 1910.
37. Garrod AC: *Inborn errors of metabolism,* London, 1923, Henry Frowde.
38. Beadle GW, Tatum EL: Genetic control of biochemical reactions in *Neurospora, Proc Natl Acad Sci USA* 27:499, 1941.
39. Tjio HJ, Levan A: The chromosome numbers of man, *Hereditas* 42:1, 1956.
40. Lejeune J, Gautier M, Turpin MR: Étude des chromosomes somatiques de neuf infants mongoliens. *CR Acad Sci* (Paris) 248:1721, 1959.
41. Nowell PC, Hungerford DA: A minute chromosome in human chronic granulocytic leukemia, *Science* 132:1497, 1960.
42. Avery OT, Macleod CM, MacCarty M: Studies on the chemical nature of the substances inducing transformation of pneumococcal types, *J Exp Med* 79:137, 1944.
43. Franklin RE, Gosling RG: Molecular configuration in sodium thymonucleate, *Nature* 171, 740, 1953.
44. Watson JD, Crick FHC: Molecular structure of nucleic acids: a structure for deoxyribose nucleic acid, *Nature* 171:737, 1953.
45. Chargaff E: Structure and function of nucleic acids as cell constituents, *Fed Proc* 10:654, 1951.
46. Watson JD, Crick FHC: Genetic implications of the structure of deoxyribonucleic acid, *Nature* 171:964, 1953.
47. McClintock B: Chromosome organization and genic expression, *Cold Spring Harb Symp Quant Biol* 16:13, 1951.
48. Linn S, Arber W: Host specificity of DNA produced by *Escherichia coli,* X: in vitro restriction of phage fd replicative form, *Proc Natl Acad Sci USA* 59:1300, 1968.
49. Smith HO, Wilcox KW: A restriction enzyme from *Hemophilus influenzae, J Mol Biol* 51:379, 1970.

50. Danna K, Nathans D: Specific cleavage of simian virus 40 DNA by restriction endonuclease of *Hemophilus influenzae, Proc Natl Acad Sci USA* 68:2913, 1971.
51. Southern EM: Detection of specific sequences among DNA fragments separated by gel electrophoresis, *J Mol Biol* 98:503, 1975.
52. Baltimore D: Viral RNA-dependent DNA polymerase, *Nature* 226:1209, 1970.
53. Temin HM, Mizutani S: RNA-dependent DNA polymerase in virions of Rous sarcoma virus, *Nature* 226:1211, 1970.
54. Cohen SA, Chang A, Boyer H et al: Construction of biologically functional bacterial plasmids in-vitro, *Proc Natl Acad Sci USA* 70:3240, 1973.
55. Botstein D, White RL, Skolnick M et al: Construction of a genetic linkage map in man using restriction fragment length polymorphisms, *Am J Hum Genet* 32:314, 1980.
56. Mullis KB, Faloona FA: Specific synthesis of DNA in vitro via a polymerase-catalyzed chain reaction, *Methods Enzymol* 155:335, 1987.
57. Kan YM, Dozy AM: Antenatal diagnosis of sickle-cell anemia by DNA analysis of amniotic-fluid cells, *Lancet* 2:910, 1978.
58. McKusick VA: *Mendelian inheritance in man: catalogs of autosomal dominant, autosomal recessive, and X-linked phenotypes*, ed 10, Baltimore, 1992, Johns Hopkins University Press.
59. Boveri T: *Zur Frage der Entstehung maligner Tumoren*, Jena, 1914, Fisher.
60. Rous P: A sarcoma of the fowl transmissible by an agent separable from the tumor cells, *J Exp Med* 13:397, 1911.
61. Spector D, Varmus HE, Bishop JM: Nucleotide sequences related to the transforming gene of ASV are present in DNA of uninfected vertebrates, *Proc Natl Acad Sci USA* 75:4102, 1978.
62. Nowell PC, Croce EM: Chromosomes, genes and cancer, *Am J Pathol* 125:8, 1986.
63. Cavenee WK, Dryja TP, Phillips RA et al: Expression of recessive alleles by chromosomal mechanisms in retinoblastomas, *Nature* 305:779, 1983.
64. Knudson AG Jr: Mutation and cancer: statistical study of retinoblastoma, *Proc Natl Acad Sci USA* 68:820, 1971.

Part One

METHODS IN PATHOLOGY

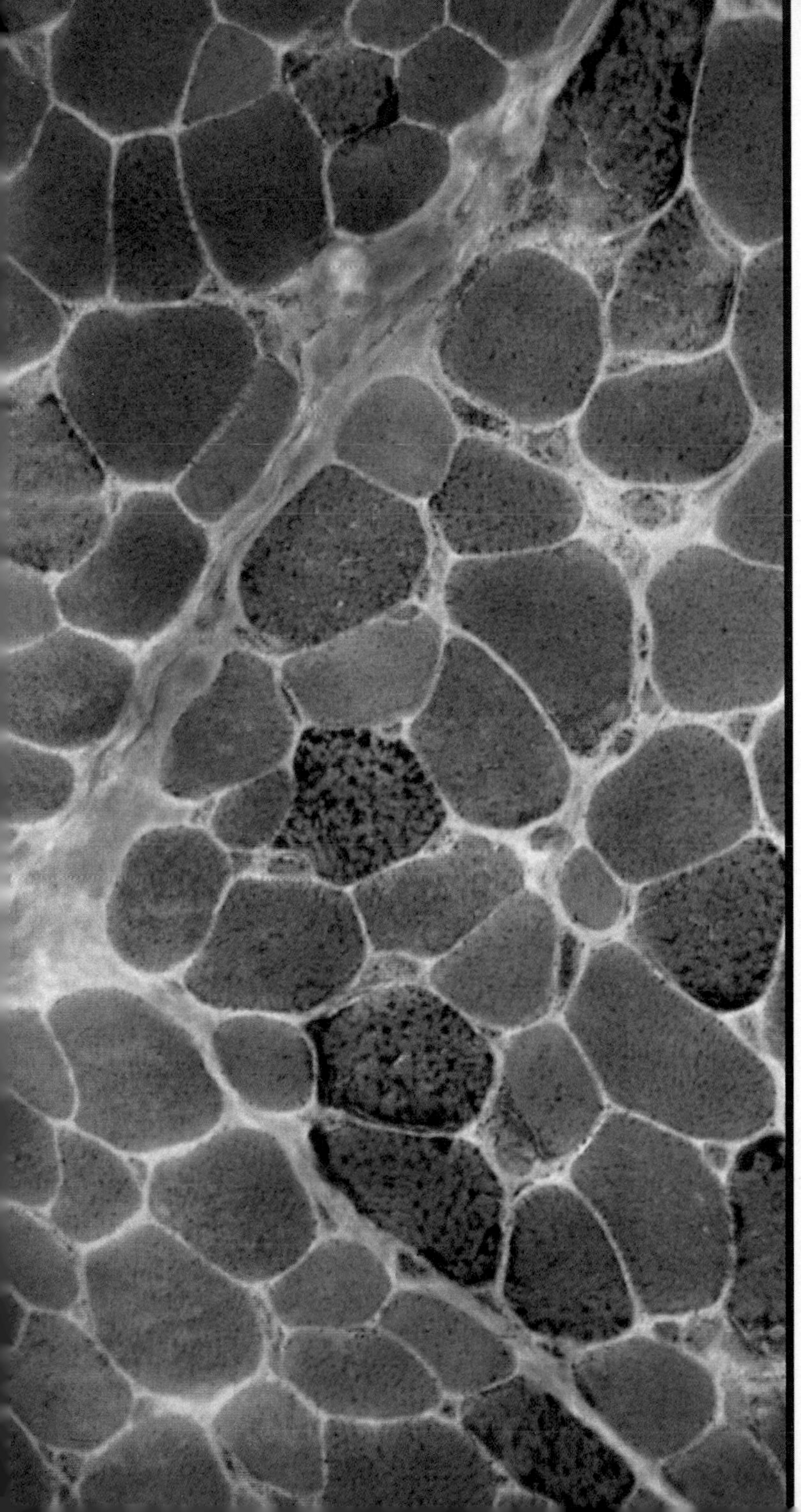

2 The Autopsy

Bruce M. McManus
Shelina Babul

STOP THE AUTOPSY! LIFE'S TOO SHORT

Don't spend the time, money, energy, expertise. . . . Life's too short.
Whether an old lady, transplant recipient, or something we abort.
To cut 'em open, pull 'em apart, and find out what's inside
Would bring new discomfort to the ignorance we hide.
Just how coarse and callous can an eager pathologist be
To exhort, "Tumor!" or whate'er different than "it" clinically be.
Leave well enough alone, good sir, quietly under wraps,
Let high technology pave the way to countless errors and traps!
We can't afford the cost of "morgues," 'cept for deaths by gun or knife
Care and counseling, discovery and truth, small reward for examined life.
Lord, keep us strong with vitamin E and foods chock-full of claims.
We may die, but when we do, we'll hide the facts in flames.

The parable of the autopsy is perhaps more poignant and recounted than any in the field of pathology and laboratory medicine. Since the inception of formal autopsies, recognition of their worth has been widely voiced, while at the same time they have been progressively more ill supported. The autopsy has served medicine in numerous ways and continues to play evolving roles in a time when technologies have dramatically improved and when new diseases, naturally occurring or iatrogenic, continue to arise on the medical horizon. Thus, despite broad-based appreciation of autopsies as a means of diagnosis and discovery, and of quality control, support for the autopsy, fiscally, professionally, and administratively, has remained inappropriately and dismally low, in the face of increasing complexity in medical care (Fig. 2-1). False confidence in clinical diagnosis has been heightened by highly advanced imaging techniques available in certain centers. The ultimate fate of the autopsy as a diagnostic tool will depend heavily on the organized efforts of pathology. Vigorous committee work, public outreach, and cross-disciplinary conferences will stand to thwart the adversities that mitigate against sensible use of the autopsy in medicine.

The bounty of understanding derived from autopsies was demonstrated most vividly through the early decades of this century. Despite recent loss of focus on the autopsy's virtues, most would agree that the examination of one's palmar lifeline is not sufficient as a "guesstimation" of the timing or cause of death, or establishment of contributory factors. The autopsy remains the singular opportunity for a comprehensive and indeed final history and physical and laboratory examination.

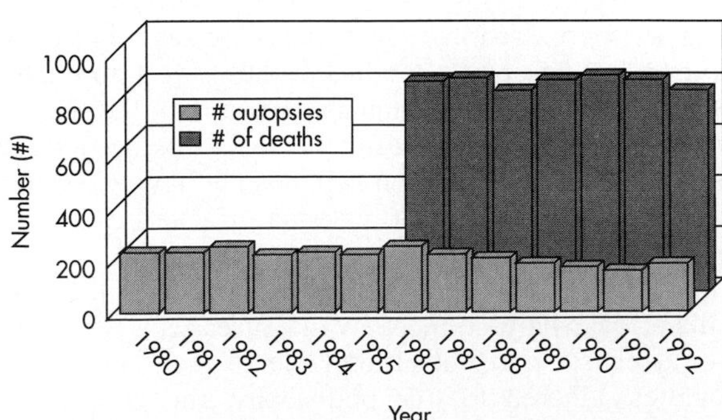

Fig. 2-1 Histographic representation of very low and declining autopsy rates in a typical large, busy tertiary care center. The autopsy rate has slipped below 20%.

If the autopsy process is promoted and undertaken with renewed commitment and finesse, it could lead medicine into the next millennium with fortified appreciation for the pathobiologic nature of disease and with enhanced opportunities for prevention and therapy.

Public perception of the autopsy and that of anatomic pathologists and their assistants responsible for the autopsy is fettered by images from late-night movies of Dr. Frankenstein and his friends. Such images have been reinforced by several factors, not the least of which is the turning away of pathologists themselves from the vital activity of autopsy pathology. The reasons for deflection of attention away from the autopsy is to be addressed in detail. It suffices to say here that the lack of remuneration for autopsy examinations performed outside of forensic settings has reinforced the sense of worthlessness that the postmortem examination has garnered recently. Placement of autopsy rooms in basements and subbasements, the lack of provision for adequate "viewing" rooms for family members of the deceased, and less than an esthetic presentation of autopsies have spurred devaluation of the autopsy. The use of the term *morgue* to refer to the autopsy room or suite promotes the view of autopsies as unattractive and distasteful. Finally, the concept that modern medicine has obviated the need for detailed pathologic examinations has permeated medical training programs and has contributed to a sense of extraneous virtue that autopsies now carry in many healthcare institutions.

This chapter is devoted to several issues pertinent to the survival of the autopsy. Discussion will highlight certain historical vignettes and provide a critical examination of the fundamental purposes of the autopsy, an inquiry as to why autopsy rates have declined, an assessment of other challenges facing the autopsy, a résumé of suggestions and ideas as to how and why autopsy rates might be improved, and finally a prospect for the future of autopsies in medical care.

HISTORICAL CONTEXT

Ancient times

Several treatises of the autopsy are available for perusal and greater depth of study.[1–12] A historical synopsis in the context of medical history may also be helpful.[13] In its most remote sense, the autopsy has been related rather vaguely to the doctrine of animism.[1] The ancient gods and other spiritual forces were believed to be in control of what happened on Earth, and as such the "supernatural" empowered the "natural." Animistic thinking was expressed in many forms. One school of thought, haruspicy (hepatoscopy), predicted the future through the investigation of entrails of animals, particularly the liver. This process of divination allowed the ancients gradually to accumulate a wealth of information that, despite having a religious or spiritual context, was of potential relevance to human anatomy and the autopsy.

A distinct and apparently opposite conceptual framework, naturalism,[1] was built on the view that diseases were the result of natural causes and not attributable to the "supernatural." Hippocrates adhered to this philosophy, the conception of which fostered the formative phase of medical science. At the time of their early cultural prominence, the Greeks conceived that "physiology" encompassed physics, physiology, and anatomy, as we know them currently. These sciences were taken together to compose the natural, or "pure," sciences of the Greek scholars. Anatomy was studied only in this "pure" sense and not in the pathologic sense.

Human dissections were known to have been advocated as early as 1000 B.C.[1,14] Several hundred years later, Mediterranean people conjured up the solidist theory of disease or illness to replace the theory of humors.[1] The solidists believed that diseases and illnesses were attributable to abnormalities of solid organs. It is perhaps of note that the humors and the solid organs together constitute a primitive version of fluids and organ systems, which indeed would be the frame of reference for understanding diseases today. However, in early Greek life, the two bodily components, solid organs and fluids (humors), were considered separately as a basis of health or disease. Hippocrates recognized the hollow, spongy, and solid organs and that the organs contained or took up fluids. It is perhaps not surprising that the solidists' theory of disease eventually dominated, considering the relative ease with which one could observe a pathologic change in an organ as opposed to a fluid and the lack of understanding of a circulation or meaningful relationship between the humors.

Medieval period

The medieval period was vacuous in many regards, a characteristic not excluding medical science. Autopsies, though conspicuous by their infrequence, were performed regularly in circumstances when criminal behavior was questioned.[1] This practice represents the remote basis for forensic pathology as we currently know it. The pathologic investigation of potential murders, suicides, accidents, and possible iatrogenic deaths remains today as having greater financial, political, and ethical priority than investigation of "natural" disease-related deaths. Religious objections to autopsies were pervasive in Europe during the Middle Ages. The Church is said to have abhorred blood, thus prohibiting surgery on the living or the dead. This abhorrence seems antithetical considering the bloodshed that occurred over centuries of religious wars. As an exception to religious aversion to blood and the autopsy, an autopsy was ordered when Pope Alexander died unexpectedly in 1410,[14] and later the papistry decreed the dissection of people dying with the plague. Another factor underlying the limited number of autopsies during this period was the medieval public's general repugnance of anatomy. Appreciation for the human form and the details of anatomy would await the great anatomists like Andreas Vesalius. The brilliance of Rembrandt's *Lesson in Anatomy by Doctor Tulp*, in 1632, is perhaps the strongest reflection of emergence from the darkness of medieval times, a collision of artistry and anatomic detail that invigorated art, science, and medicine.

Renaissance

Other works in the Renaissance period brought new life to the autopsy. Benivieni's publication in 1507[15] *Some Remarkable Hidden Causes of Disease and of Cures* presented information on 110 patients, 15 of whom had autopsy examination to confirm or deny clinical impressions. It is fascinating that in 1533 in the territory that would become known as the Dominican Republic female conjoined twins were born as a thoracopagus joined in the lower thorax and upper abdomen. At baptism, the priest was uncertain as to whether there was one soul or two. The father had noted that one infant would cry while the other was quiet and one might sleep while the other was awake. Thus two baptisms were performed. The priest, being still uneasy, advocated an autopsy when the infants died at 8 days of age in hopes of settling the issue of one soul versus two. Two sets of internal organs were identified, an indication that there were probably two souls.[1] This anecdote perhaps represents one of the few occasions in which religion was a basis of an autopsy and definitely represented a way of thinking distinct from that of the "dark" ages. Theophilus Bonetus's monumental work *Sepulchretum sive Anatomica Practica* followed in 1679 and included descriptions of 3000 autopsies. Thereafter, Hermann Boerhaave (1668-1738) wrote two monographs dealing with autopsy methodology,[16,17] and Giovanni Battista Morgagni (1682-1771) popularized the fledgling activity of clinicopathologic correlation.[18] It is of no small consequence that such correlations ultimately became a mainstay of clinical teaching conferences in university hospitals around the world.

Premodern period

Marie François Xavier Bichat (1771-1802), known by some as the father of histology, provided fresh intellectual and compassionate ingredients common to the eighteenth century, when medicine was reaching a major turning point. Bichat studied anatomy, physiology, and pathology as well as providing bedside care to patients. Through his comprehensive involvement in these arenas, he was able to gain insight into disease processes at greater depths.[19,20] During this period, medical science was advanced by a host of other great physicians (Fig. 2-2). Jean Nicolas Corvisart des Marets (1755–1821) made extensive contributions to our understanding of the pathology of cardiovascular diseases. René Théophile Hyacinthe Laënnec, whose work included description of the clinical and pathologic features of tuberculosis, further illustrated commitment to an anatomic basis of medical care. This basis was fortified by the renowned contemporaries in pathology Carl von Rokitansky[21] and Rudolf Virchow.[22]

In a somewhat sardonic fashion, the question may be posed, Who was more important in laying the groundwork for medical and pathologic breakthroughs of the twentieth century, von Rokitansky or Virchow? Rokitansky (1804-1878), as important as he was to the establishment of anatomic pathology as a discipline and as skillful as he was in gross pathologic studies, attempted to make pathophysiologic correlations based on gross findings alone. The resultant derivations were insufficient to explain disease processes. In his defense, one might consider that the lack of coherent and broad-based knowledge in medical science mitigated against a proper or complete interpretation of gross pathologic findings. Virchow, in his brilliance, drew relationships between gross and microscopic findings and their relationship to the clinical picture. Inadvertently, however, in the face of his eminent and charismatic influence, he led generations of "high-powered" pathologists into the pitfall of utilizing histologic still life as a singu-

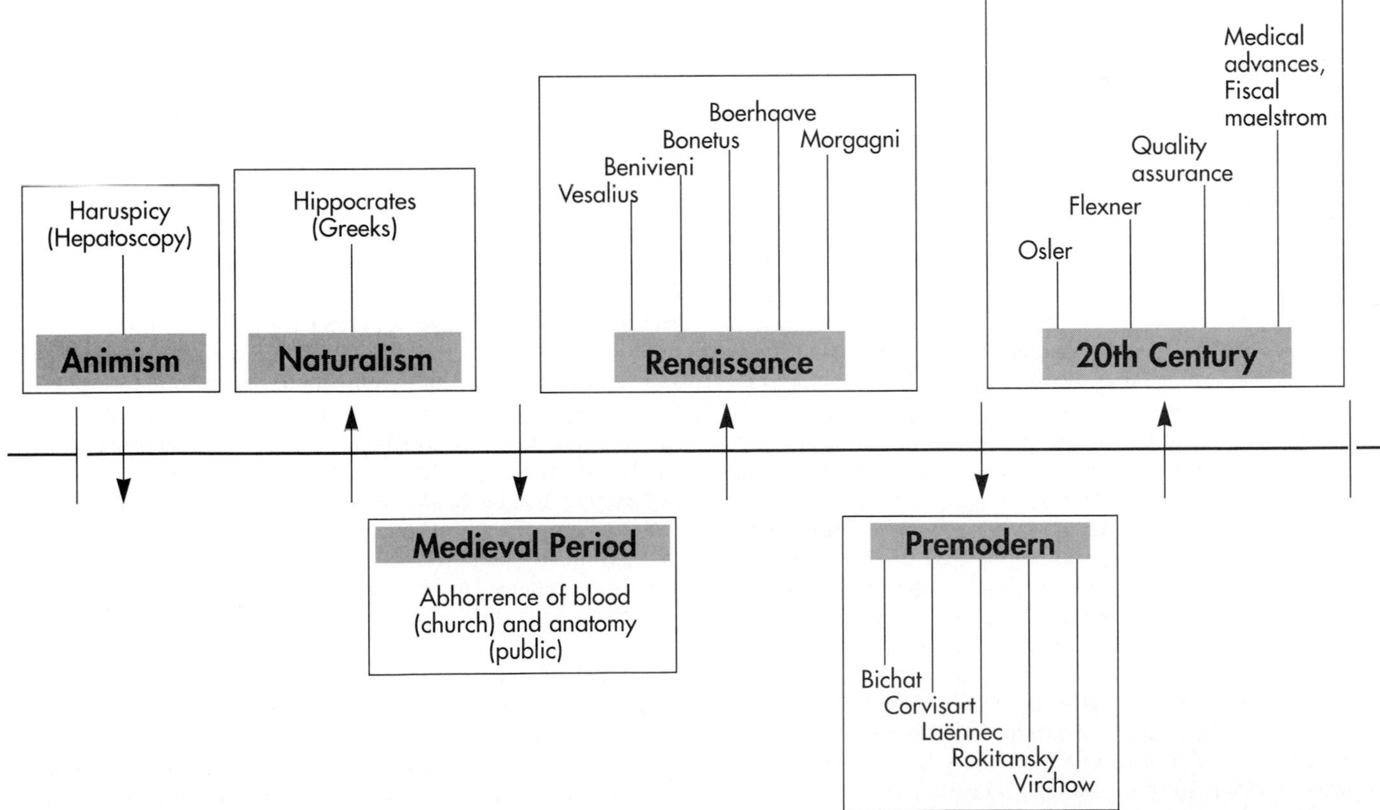

Fig. 2-2 Historical footprints from early civilization until the present depicting several notable periods and people who have contributed to the history of the autopsy.

lar tool to understand disease causation and pathobiologic processes. Morphologic pursuit by way of the light microscope remains as a centerpiece in pathologic diagnosis, but this approach is not sufficient for contemporary diagnostics. Microscopy is evolving and will take on new roles as applications change.

Rokitansky, Virchow, and their colleagues made profound contributions to current thinking, approaches, and methodology in pathology and medicine. Of particular note, Rokitansky's encrustation theory of atherogenesis, the covering over of microthrombi by vessel-wall endothelium as a contributor to plaque development (refined by Duguid), is of great relevance to current concepts of atherothrombosis. On the other hand, Virchow, supporting the lipid imbibition theory of atherogenesis, has also been validated by evidence in the present century. His drawings of smooth muscle foam cells are classic and seemingly timeless.

On a separate issue, the historical basis of autopsy technique is a legacy of practicality and tradition. Of interest, the "Rokitansky method" of abdominal and thoracic block extraction is in fact the technique employed by LeTulle.[6] The method of Rokitansky was actually organ-by-organ dissection. Either approach or some variation may be entirely adequate, depending on the disease, its expression, and the intention of the autopsy.

Twentieth century

An anatomic basis of human disease was a dominant theme in medicine toward the end of the last century. Influence of physicians in the mold of Bichat and Sir William Osler was represented in textbooks of medicine, in clinicopathologic conferences, and through the cross-disciplinary foundation of physicians' medical practices. Physicians frequently performed autopsies on their own patients. Many of Osler's great treatises included thorough correlations between clinical course of disease and his personal observations made at autopsy examination. His textbook editions in the early part of this century reflected the autopsy as a key process in medical education. Discovery of cause of death and acquisition of insight into pathogenesis were foremost on the list of objectives at the autopsy table. The concept of quality assurance through the autopsy was emerging. The landmark survey of medical education programs across the United States and Canada by Abraham Flexner in 1910 would lead to many recommendations and reform.[23] The report is still heralded as a major factor in the improvement and standardization of medical education in both countries. Among those recommendations, a minimum percentage of autopsies on patients dying in a given hospital stood a long test of time. Hospital-based medicine saw the autopsy as an important measure of its general quality. In the first decades of the twentieth century, the autopsy rate in hospitals across the United States was quite stable and generally at a high level. However, coincident to the escalating development of chemistry and hematology as specialties and with the emergence of fields such as immunology, the laboratory physician's attention was diverted more and more from studies of anatomic pathology. In particular, attention was diverted from the autopsy. The attraction of new laboratory specialties and the evolution of clinical pathology as a laboratory focus initiated a decline in autopsy rates that would continue virtually to the present day (Fig. 2-3). The broad development of laboratory technologies in recent years and the

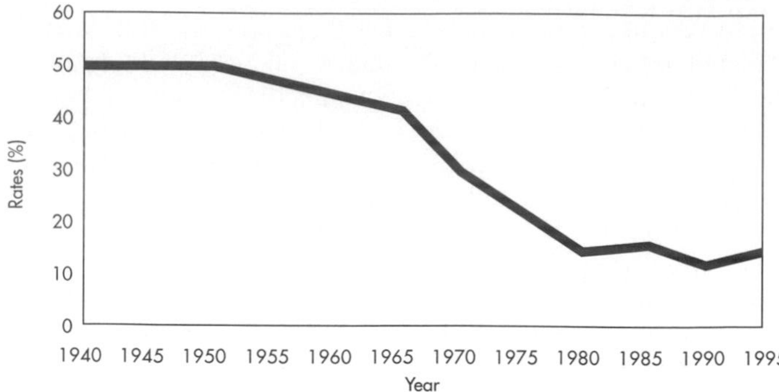

Fig. 2-3 Composite data from investigations covering a 43-year period. A progressive decline in autopsy rates beginning in the 1950s and accelerating through the subsequent two decades is quite evident.

promise of new vistas in biotechnology and molecular genetics will make returning the focus to the autopsy even more difficult than before.

Immense thought, reflection, and published fact and fiction have emerged in concern regarding steadily declining rates for autopsies in the United States and elsewhere.[24–30] Recent history has included extensive analyses demonstrating the continued high rates of discrepancy between major clinical diagnoses and those obtained at autopsy. These reminders are of great significance considering the pervasive use of new technologies and therapies and the breadth of biologic principles now applied to medicine. The message is clear: we simply need the autopsy to continue checking on our clinical acumen. We will never be perfect despite excellent historical data collection and the application of the most revealing technologies. More is to be said of this issue shortly. The natural and unnatural presentation of disease processes is such that the human mind, even with tremendous informational support, cannot reach such ideals in diagnosis. Thus, for quality assurance alone, the autopsy is desperately needed. Quality assurance, however, does not in any way represent the entirety of need for autopsies.

PURPOSES OF THE AUTOPSY

Further to the foregoing commentary, the definition of purpose underlying autopsies in the nonforensic setting includes a focus on the needs of medicine itself, society at large, and the family of the deceased (Fig. 2-4). Insofar as medicine is concerned and as alluded to above, the quality assurance and educational mandates are the strongest (Table 2-1). The role of autopsy in investigation should not be understated, however, and is considered in Chapter 5. The need to check clinical diagnoses and the approximate value of historical data, to check the precision of various diagnostic instruments, and to check the efficacy of operative and nonoperative therapies[24] may be foremost reasons for autopsies. A most discerning series of studies on the practical need for continued and enhanced autopsy programs was conducted by Goldman and associates.[31] Their work clearly indicates the lack of improvements in clinical abilities to make the correct diagnoses of common diseases over three different eras of medical care and corresponding advancement of technologic support.[31] Thus the capacity of a "good" physician working in a strong environ-

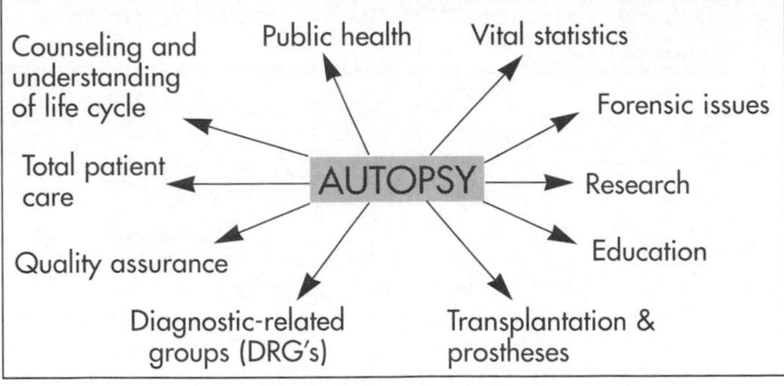

Fig. 2-4 The autopsy has a pervasive influence on medical care, medical science, society in general, and the family of the deceased. The influence ranges from intangible understandings of the life cycle and the relationship between life and death to the facilitation of organ retrieval and transplantation. One may group the points of influence into those pertinent to medical care (diagnostic-related groups, quality assurance, and total patient care), the body of medical science (research, education, transplantation, and prostheses), society (public health, vital statistics, forensic issues), and the family (counseling and understanding the life cycle).

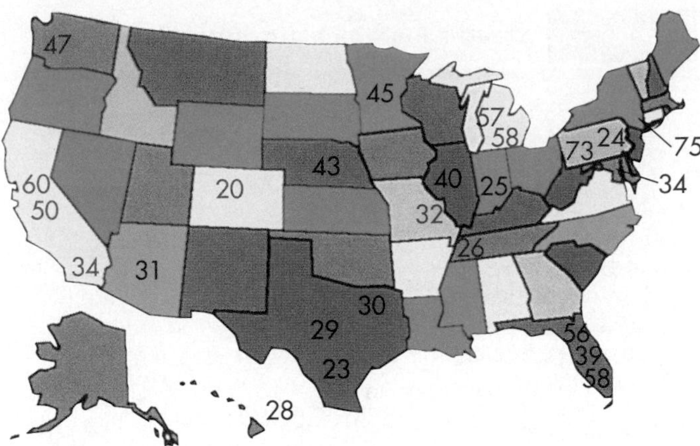

Fig. 2-5 Representative portrayal of the percentage of natural deaths leading to forensic autopsies. The data represent multiple jurisdictions in 19 states. There is an impressive frequency of natural deaths on these forensic services. The opportunities for education of pathology residents and for discovery are immense.

Table 2-1 The value of the autopsy

Assure quality control of medical care
Establish or confirm cause of death
Confirm, modify, or refute clinical diagnoses
Monitor therapeutic responses
Evaluate new operative, pharmacologic, and diagnostic approaches
Enhance education
Foster research
Discover new or previously unrecognized diseases
Provide essential information on disease manifestations
Provide essential organs and tissues for research and transplantation
Heighten total patient care
Offer general psychoemotional benefits to the family
Establish basis of genetic counseling
Improve public health
Investigate and identify environmental, occupational, and life style–related diseases
Evaluate new prostheses, (e.g., cardiac, vascular, orthopedic)
Allow forensic diagnoses
Improve hospital reimbursements and efficiency through more accurate diagnostic-related groups (DRGs)
Improve accuracy of vital statistics
Provide information and assistance to legal and judicial systems

ment with modern diagnostic amenities (clinical laboratory, imaging, and so on) is not sufficient to exclude the possibility of errant diagnoses.

In addition to ascertaining clinicopathologic differences, the development of new understanding of old diseases and provision of the opportunity to discover new diseases should be emphasized. Data are obtained at autopsy regarding the effect of different drugs, procedures, and operations, the nature of which exceed the simple evaluation of clinical efficacy. Of great importance, the autopsy provides a critical interface between pathologists and organ-retrieval groups and a similar role with respect to tissues for transplantation and, until recently, provided extracts for therapeutic purposes (pituitary growth hormone[32]). A carefully administered and organized autopsy database can provide crucial information about the demography and epidemiology of disease processes. An effort to establish a national autopsy data bank[33,34] in the United States never quite came to fruition. A variety of logistical, fiscal, and other issues have prevented this goal from being realized. However, registries of autopsy material targeting different disease processes have become an invaluable resource in clinical research and in the linkage of traditional pathologic approaches to studies of gene expression or genetic abnormalities. It is of conceptual importance that the autopsy does not represent a search for "zebras" or five-legged horses but rather a detailed evaluation of commonly occurring, proteanly presenting illnesses and diseases as well as evaluation of therapies and interventions. Thus the fundamental purpose of the autopsy is quality assurance for medicine through direct case relevance and through indirect educational relevance. The autopsy provides an opportunity to review collated clinical information including that derived from the historical, physical, and laboratory studies. All this information can be considered in terms of gross and microscopic examination of key organs. In an optimal setting, an autopsy by itself is a clinicopathologic conference for the autopsist and for those who participate actively in the autopsy process. The autopsy is of general as well as specific value, depending on the nature of the autopsy service and the patients to be evaluated. Of note, forensic services, often regarded as places where people who were found in harm's way are examined, in actuality offer tremendous opportunities for education and discovery of natural causes of disease and death[35] (Fig. 2-5). Thus, these values of autopsies, including the characterization of a range of known diseases and those that yet defy particular classification, may be met on both nonforensic and forensic services. Only the discerning and ingenious will be the discoverers of "new" diseases. The remainder of us will do well to distinguish properly already known causes of death or disability from other more elusive abnormalities. Finding the unifying thread of thought in a given autopsy rests on proper preparatory work in human anatomy and physiology as well as

Table 2-2 Deaths for which autopsy is indicated

Unknown and unanticipated medical complications
Cause of death not known with certainty on clinical grounds
Help to relieve concerns and provide reassurance to the family or public
Unexpected or unexplained deaths
Occurring during or after any dental, medical, or surgical diagnostic procedure
Apparently natural and not subject to a forensic medical jurisdiction
Natural deaths subject to but waived by forensic medical jurisdiction
High-risk infectious and contagious disease
Obstetric deaths
Neonatal and pediatric deaths
Disclose a known or suspected illness that may bear on survivors or recipients of transplant organs
Known or suspected environmental or occupational hazards
Patients who have participated in clinical trials

an understanding of immunology, infectious diseases, biochemistry, and genetics.

In the absence of certainty, decisions to obtain autopsy permission still must be made. Multiple purposes may be served by general guidelines for requesting an autopsy, and the College of American Pathologists (1988) has proposed circumstances when such should occur (Table 2-2).

WHY AUTOPSY RATES HAVE DECLINED

Autopsy, defined as 'seeing for oneself', implies being able to go directly into the human body and visualize the amazing variability of human responses to disease and injury. Unfortunately, as alluded to earlier, the autopsy is a learning experience on the decline. Over the years, a sharp downturn in the number of autopsies has been evident, fluctuating from year to year and from institution to institution (Fig. 2-3). Even in hospitals with vigorous autopsy programs and rates much higher than the average at any given time in recent history, the percentage of deaths coming to autopsy continues to decline.[36-38] Reasons most often cited include attitudes of pathologists, clinicians, and families, laboratory time constraints, clinicians' fear of legal liability and of "being wrong," costs, newer diagnostic tests, as well as the decision by the Joint Commission on Accreditation of Healthcare Organizations (JCAHO) to eliminate the recommended minimum 20% autopsy rate for community and 25% for teaching hospitals.[32,39-41] All these factors here contributed to the diminishing rate (Table 2-3). As a consequence, patient care, several facets of education, clinical and basic research, and the quality control of medical care have been compromised.

From the perspective of clinicians, autopsies are no longer needed as frequently because diagnostic confidence is higher and because little or no information will be obtained that is not readily available by sophisticated clinical tests. In addition, clinicians at times believe that the lack of knowledge of pathologists leads to inaccurate interpretation as well as an inadequate communication and clinical feedback. Fear of malpractice suits from errors uncovered at autopsy and the attitude

Table 2-3 Probable reasons for declining autopsy rates

Attitudes (clinicians, pathologists, families, administrators, politicians)
Time constraints and competing responsibilities of pathologists
Physicians' fears of legal liability and of being wrong
Costs (professional, overhead)
Modern medical technology building false confidence
Lack of Joint Commission on Accreditation of Healthcare Organizations (JCAHO, USA) autopsy requirements (since 1971)
Lack of inclusion of autopsy findings in death certificate documentation, as well as in published clinical case reports
Unnecessary "complete" autopsies as opposed to partial autopsies
Inability to request permission from bereaved families appropriately

that a patient's death represents a physician's failure play a big part in this declining interest. *Ergo*, "we don't like to be confronted with our mistakes—no one does."[42] Asking permission from the bereaved next of kin is also difficult for the clinical physician, who fears negative reactions from an upset family. Last, the lack of appreciation of the value in knowledge of etiology, pathogenesis, and treatment of human diseases as derived from the autopsy is also a reason for depreciated values and lower rates of autopsy request by physicians.

From the pathologist's standpoint, greater interest in other activities has placed autopsies as a low priority. Lack of appreciation of the pathologist by clinical physicians further hinders autopsy rates. Families of deceased members perceive the autopsy as a time-consuming procedure, impeding the burial process. Information obtained at autopsy is inadequately relayed to these families, and sometimes it takes months before conclusive critical details can be clarified. The attitude and feeling of discomfort related to the cutting and potential mutilation of a loved one during an autopsy also blocks consent. Religious attitudes should not play a significant role in the reasoning for refusal of an autopsy, though such considerations are often cited.[43] Almost all cultures can accept an autopsy when explained properly.

Currently, hospital administrators and accreditors view autopsies as unfavorable, expensive, non-reimbursable trade, the costs of which include body transportation, facility maintenance, professional fees (forensic), routine histology, special testing, radiographic and photographic documentation, and consultation fees. Since most administrators believe that their foremost aim is to achieve cost-effective health care and efficient allocation of resources, they look at the autopsy as one more short-term loss leader. The long-term benefits are typically beyond their vision.

So what are the consequences of a low point in autopsy rates? Assessment of the quality of medical care remains impaired, since the autopsy functions as a key quality control tool and a verification mechanism in seeking quality in diagnostics. Ultimate salutary effects on clinical practice may be achieved by steady use of the autopsy. Clinicians will continue to err, undiagnosed contagious disease will be missed, accidental deaths and homicides will go undetected, environmental hazards and iatrogenic diseases will remain unrecognized, and death certificates will continue to be imprecise. All this will occur, even with the autopsy being done, and done well. The major consequence of medicine without sufficient autopsies is that both patient care and progress in medical science will be impeded. Biomedical and epidemiologic research is hindered, since data on new diseases and responses to drugs and surgical interventions will be limited. Organs, tissues, and extracts will also be unavailable. Medical student education will be hampered. Both the public and the health professions must be reeducated, not only as to the value of the autopsy, but also as to the practical mechanisms for reinstatement of the autopsy in the core of medical practice.

ADDITIONAL CHALLENGES FOR THE AUTOPSY

All "stakeholders" in regard to the autopsy have major challenges. These challenges lie at the heart of the diminished autopsy rates observed almost universally across North America. The dimensions of the issues involved are myriad. There are issues in common between administrators, clinical physicians, pathologists, and families, and each stakeholder also has particular hurdles to face in mustering support for and actively promoting autopsy performance.

Economic factors

Administratively, the economic factors are most pressing and represent the key factors in the impairment of autopsy programs and their role in medicine. Numerous analyses regarding the economics of the autopsy have been performed. The general categories of fiscal concern include the actual costs associated with the autopsy, the indeterminant cost savings in medical care as a result of application of autopsy-generated knowledge, the lack of professional reimbursement (apart from forensic settings), and the current atmosphere of general constraint in the economics of health care delivery.

The costs of autopsies include those that relate to the maintenance of a facility, those related to the performance of each individual examination, and those potentially associated with professional remuneration. Maintenance of facilities includes the physical space, the key pieces of equipment, and those environmental requirements related to lighting and regulation of temperature and air quality. The costs of supplies relative to an autopsy service include both those that are consumed for each individual autopsy and those that are necessary to keep the autopsy service running regardless of how many cases are performed. The fact that autopsy suites in many institutions have long periods of inactivity brings out the paradox that the unit cost per autopsy, given all costs related to the service, may actually decrease as a result of increased utilization. This is particularly so considering that there is no professional fee associated with the autopsy in the nonforensic setting. Thus, to a certain limit, an increased autopsy rate provides a greater sense of efficiency in use of capital expenditures that are necessary simply to keep the facility open. On the other hand, the costs associated with documentation through laboratory testing, postmortem X-ray films, and special diagnostic approaches will be increased with each case done, and this increase will be proportionate to the level of sophistication applied by the autopsist and the general programmatic philosophy. Those institutions dedicated to discovery, which serve as a basis for educational programs (residencies and postgraduate pathology education) and for clinical research, will find that obtaining in-depth autopsy diagnoses is a mentally, physically, and temporally demanding process. The burden of such discovery is unfortunately accompanied by a substantial monetary price tag.

Financial expenditures, as we have noted, cannot be immediately translated into economic benefits. Measures of wellbeing in a given family, or the likelihood of better care of future similar patients, and healthier, longer lives with decreased hospitalization and treatment, diminished loss of work productivity, and diminished spread of disease in the community at large are difficult to establish as benefits of the autopsy. Also the intimation that autopsy performance will result in improved resource allocation to better diagnose or better treat certain diseases is in theory plausible, but in fact difficult to prove. These indistinct results or outcomes represent significant challenges for all parties interested in a viable future for the autopsy.

Lack of professional reimbursement for nonforensic autopsies has driven many pathologists from the autopsy room.[44] Anywhere from 2 to 20 hours may be expended on a given autopsy case depending on its level of complexity and other extenuating medical or medicolegal factors. The time commitment is huge and requires a level of expertise held only by anatomic pathologists. Unfortunately, the historical paradigm of autopsies for "free" has been a factor in the disallowance of the autopsy from reimbursement through the usual channels of third-party payer or government programs.[45,46] The cost of autopsy has been analyzed in many jurisdictions and estimates range from as low as $1000 per autopsy to as high as $2500 per autopsy for those carried out in university-teaching hospitals.[47] This cost includes little if any reimbursement for staff pathologists. Resident pathologists are paid salaries or stipends that are not pertinent to this calculation. Failure of the system to reward the autopsy means that little motivation can be generated for the busy anatomic pathologist who, like other professionals, does not live by wit alone. This serious overriding financial issue has been addressed in innumerable publications.[2,24,45,46,48-50] Certain studies have suggested that autopsy performance in a given hospital and reclassification of diagnoses on the basis of autopsy as opposed to clinical impressions alone would or could lead to increased reimbursement to the hospital for patients of certain levels of acuity.[51] This objective evidence and line of argument has fallen on deaf ears.

Other major challenges for administrators relate to the generally shrinking budgets from government sources at all levels of organization and the necessitated focusing of efforts on areas of excellence. Because of the philosophical overtone related to the autopsy, it is perhaps never going to be considered a program where achievement of excellence is a mandate strong enough to drive a solid financial plan. The autopsy is one of several procedures that may be performed after death along with transplant organ retrieval and assessment of new operative techniques. Willingness of government and administrators to provide support for "after-death" procedures will be based on their appreciation of the continuum between life and death and the informed enthusiasm of laboratorians and clinical physicians.

Other challenges in the realm of autopsy technique, communications regarding the autopsy, and mutual understanding of relevant terminologies are matters that face clinical physicians, pathologists, and families. The results of poor technique, poor communication, or poor mutual understanding of terminologies related to autopsy and death also become administrative problems when public image or medicolegal boundaries are affected.

Methodologic and technical factors

Careful conduct of the autopsy examination is not a new matter for discussion. Particular issues must be faced in special groups;[11,52-54], however, the general approaches are broadly applicable (Fig. 2-6). Robertson in 1925[55] emphasized the necessity of careful autopsy conduct, organ preservation, and microscopic examination. The actual strategy of autopsy examination has undergone increasing scrutiny as renewed emphasis on its role in clinical audit has been brought to bear. Whether the autopsy is performed in situ with organ-by-organ dissection and return of organs to the body immediately after sampling for histology or there is near-complete exenteration with more detailed sectioning and review by other laboratory physicians at departmental conferences is not the essential issue in technique or methodology. Certainly, when pathogenesis of organ-specific disease is in question, a "miniautopsy"[56,57] or "limited autopsy"[58] may suffice. However, most illnesses involve multiple organs and are systemically involved. A "complete" autopsy is indicated under these circumstances.

Focus on autopsy rates is not sufficient,[1] and the need for the highest quality preparatory work, dissection, interpretation, and clinical correlation in turn demands a certain amount of speciality and attention by the autopsist. If pathologists are going to gain favor with other medical professionals and those stakeholders beyond the limits of the healthcare establishment, they must convince others of the highly sophisticated nature of the autopsy approach. This is accomplished through appropriate triage of tissue, cells, and fluids, as well as superlative photographic documentation. There is no excuse in the 1990s for marginal documentation of pathologic features utilizing poor photographic or esthetic approaches. The video display and recording systems now available, provide the pathologist and other physicians with an opportunity to document and review anatomic specimens in a way heretofore impossible. The careful observations of our predecessors in a previous century, often recorded in drawings by their own hand, emphasize, however, that elaborate modern technology will not save the day either. Attention to detail will.

Technique issues with regard to the autopsy are of equal importance to financial matters but of a different dimension. As noted earlier, it has been reiterated many times[1,55] that sufficiency of the autopsy cannot be measured by rates alone. Although rates may be driven down by other factors, poor execution of the autopsy is the ultimate Achilles' heel. Thus, services whereupon autopsies are performed without high standards and rigor may lead to little new insight regarding

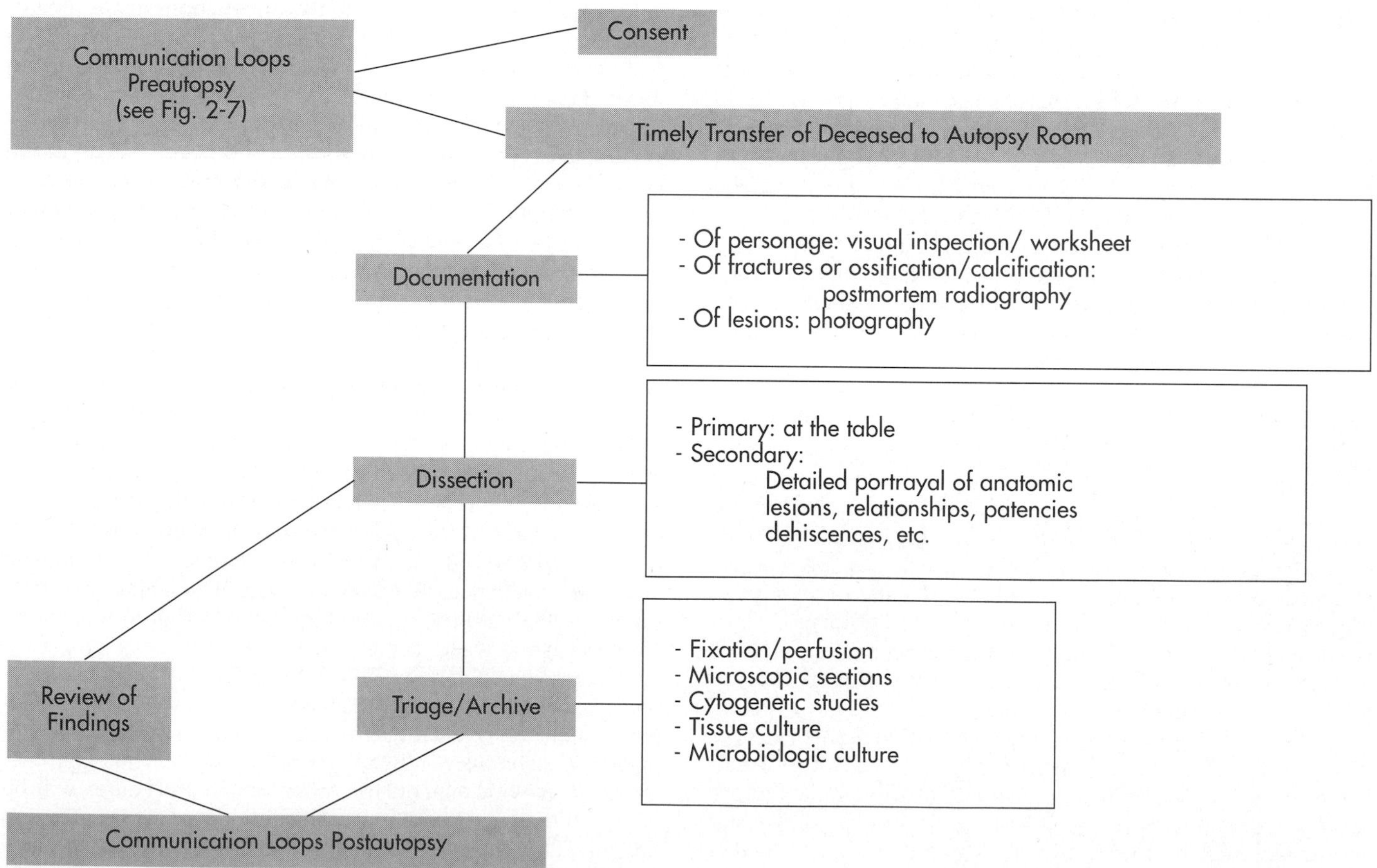

Fig. 2-6 Fundamental concept of the autopsy procedure and techniques as might be followed in a non-forensic hospital setting. The steps in the process include communication loops before and after autopsy (see Fig. 2-7).

pathogenesis, cause of death, or other issues and may be strong arguments against the promotion of the autopsy in general. The procedural fastidiousness of pathologists' assistants and the residents and staff pathologists is part of the answer. In addition, it is critical that pathologists approach dissection and triage of tissues with relevance to a patient's clinical disease process. Thus the manner of sectioning (in relation to imaging), the manner of preservation (in relationship to molecular, biologic, and genetic studies), the assessment of tissue and organ relationships (in the context of a complicated operative procedures), the composite use of tissues and fluids (in the consideration of occult infectious, toxic, inflammatory, or metabolic diseases), or the careful review of clinical tests and patient course (to target the overall procedure) may be less than first rate. General quality assurance indicators should be charted and responded to in the conduct of autopsy programs (Table 2-4). Regular review of final reports and slides by peers in a given department will greatly strengthen the quality assurance process if corrective action is a functional component. When any of these matters are not addressed with maximum compulsion, the chances for a less-than-revealing autopsy examination are heightened. Thus, although pathologists often relate the fact that the autopsy may reveal diagnoses not suspected clinically or may in some other way discredit clinical impressions, the possibility that an autopsy is performed less well than any number of clinical examinations certainly exists. When this occurs, the reputation of the autopsy as a diagnostic tool suffers. The autopsy examination is already considered less valuable than other in vivo diagnostic procedures. Thus, whether laboratory physicians like it or not, they must achieve quality of techniques of performance of autopsy that are superior in comparison to any in vivo technique to garner the support autopsies deserve. The paradox is that lack of support for and interest in the autopsy at the current time mitigates against the kind of superior performance that is necessary for self-sustenance.

Technique-related issues do not begin and end in the autopsy room or with the performance of the gross dissection. Technique includes preparatory review of clinical data and materials, the enlightened archive or triage of suspect tissues, cells, and fluids, the post-hoc re-review of various materials, and the seeking of other expert clinical and scientific opinions when necessary. This kind of comprehensive analysis is best carried out in a teaching hospital environment. There will be times when simple documentation of a more or less immediate cause of death will suffice. However, the manifestations of disease are unnervingly diverse and establishment of "simple" cause of death often exceeds our capabilities.

The greatest potential risk to pathologists and their colleagues in relationship to the autopsy are the microorganisms that may have infected a patient before death and that are carried to the autopsy room. Although the particular value of postmortem cultures in the detection of a variety of bacterial, fungal, parasitic, and viral organisms remains somewhat uncertain,[59–62] there is the possibility that virulent organisms including Creuzfeldt-Jakob disease, hepatitis viruses, tubercle bacilli and other mycobacteria, human immunodeficiency viruses (HIV), and others may be transmitted at the time of autopsy or examination of autopsy tissues.[63–66] The possibility of transmitting hepatitis B virus and tuberculosis appears relatively high as compared with the possibility of other infectious agents that pathologists may be exposed to in the context of a postmortem examination. As well, recent observations indicate that HIV type I may persist in human tissues and fluids for several days.[63,64,67] At times, patients with unsuspected infectious diseases will come to death and autopsy. Such patients represent a greater potential threat than those in whom the clinical infective process was defined and followed to the end.

The concern about Creuzfeldt-Jakob disease was highlighted by evident transmission of the organism to two neurohistology technicians.[68] Fixation of brain tissue in phenolized formalin was recommended. The safety procedures only minimally affected histologic stains. The approach of using 15% phenol in formalin with fixation for several weeks apparently can render a brain infected with Creuzfeldt-Jakob organism noninfective.[65] Disinfection of Creuzfeldt-Jakob organism is best accomplished with steam heating, sodium hypochlorite, and sodium hydroxide.[69] Recently, several others have suggested devices to prevent aerosolization of potentially infectious particulate matter released upon opening of the cranial vault.[70-72] Other policies and procedures to be implemented in the pathology laboratory to reduce the risk of infection of personnel by contact with infected specimens or aerosols include rigorous attention to gloving, face (eye, nose, and mouth) protection, the effectiveness of certain disinfectant solutions, the process of disinfection of surgical instruments, hand washing, laboratory clothing, ban on eating, drinking, smoking, cosmetic use, and contact lenses in the autopsy suite, proper handling of sharp instruments including needles, proper pipette technique, care with centrifugation, care with disposable items and specimens as well as reusable items, and proper handling of laboratory records.[73]

For certain, a cavalier approach to autopsy-related infection of professional staff cannot be tolerated and would be fiduciarily compromising. Every effort to contain high-risk autopsies and autopsy tissues to the utmost and to draw attention to personal and general safety must be expected.

Table 2-4 Useful indicators for an autopsy quality assurance program

Indicator
Discrepancies between pathologic and final diagnosis
Lack of documentation by x-ray, photography and other tests
Evidence of pathologic misdiagnosis in final autopsy reports
Specimens with no clinical information sent to Pathology
Number of:
Autopsies
Cases sent to reference autopsy laboratory or registry
Incident reports
Patient complaints
Physician complaints
Staff complaints
Outstanding survey deficiencies (JCAHO, CAP, AABB, state)
Mislabled specimens
Results of family satisfaction questionnaires
Infection rates

Adapted from Dunham WG, Quilan A, Krolikowski FJ, Reuter K: *CAP Today*, 24, June 1986.

Communication issues

Embedded in issues of technique is the matter of communication. Communication loops (Fig. 2-7) are numerous in the life cycle of the autopsy. The manner in which clinical physicians

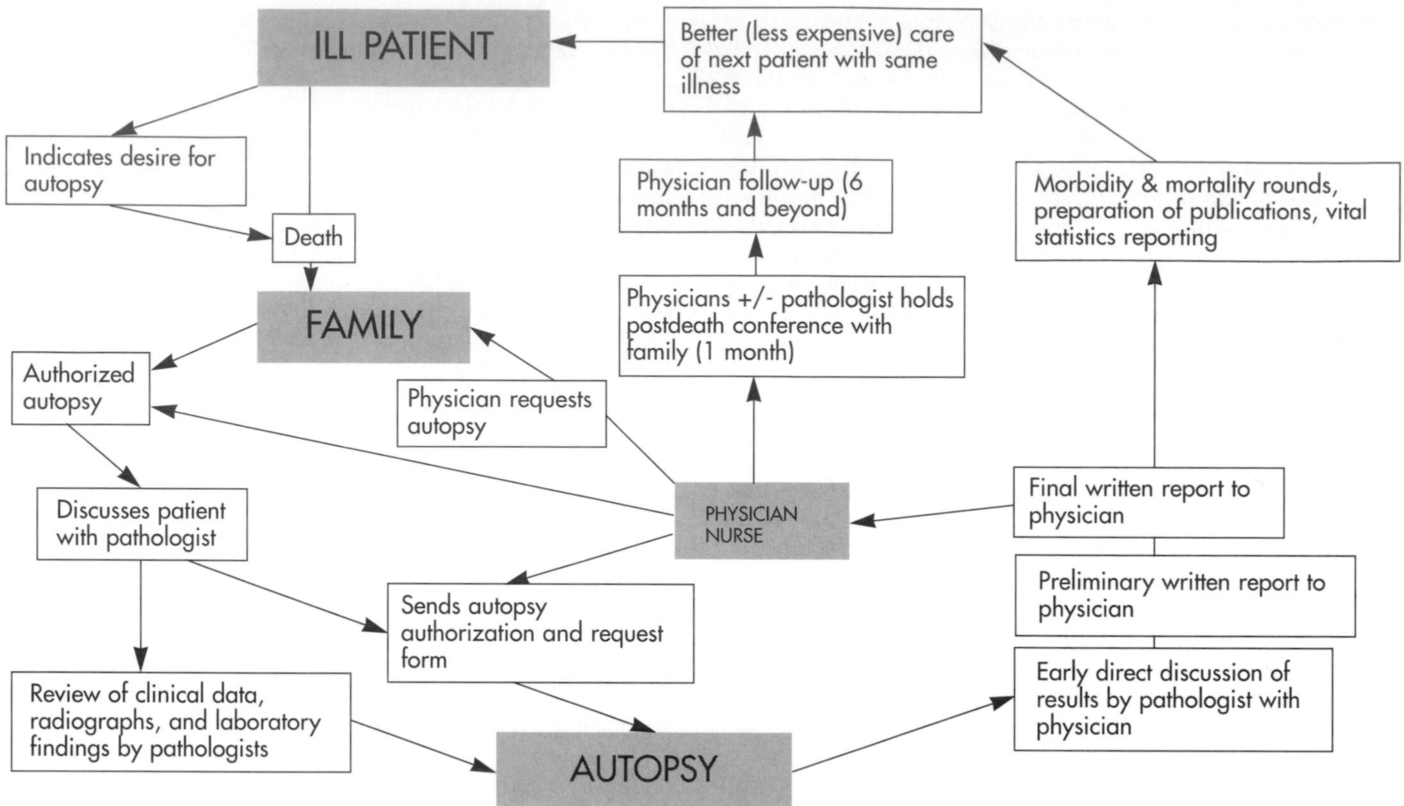

Fig. 2-7 Success with respect to the autopsy depends on multiple interpersonal interactions, which may be termed *communication loops*. These interactions are complex and begin with the personal physician and nursing staff interacting with a patient and his or her family. Once a death has occurred this initial communication loop will be a major factor in subsequent interactions, the authorization process, the effectiveness of the autopsy, the transmission of accurate and timely information to various stakeholders, and the ultimate effect on the family and on medical care.

Table 2-5 Critical elements for success in obtaining an autopsy

Attitude	Autopsy is routine. Permission will be requested in every death. Autopsy can be viewed as a positive option, offered to every family.
Availability	Attending staff availability is an important resource to house staff or nursing staff when concerns arise regarding appropriateness of the request or if reluctance is voiced. It is helpful to offer expectations of what might be learned in the autopsy.
Timing	Avoid requesting an autopsy in proximity to the pronouncement of death. Coordinate the closure and grieving process with other involved staff. Be patient with families.
Absolve guilt	Autopsy may remove concern about possible genetic defects. Especially in sudden or unexpected death, the autopsy may answer questions that, if left unanswered, generate guilt. Eliminate suspicion and provide reassurance.
Benefit to others	Families may take solace in the possibility that other persons might benefit (from new knowledge or organ donation).
Nursing and ancillary support	Families benefit from a primary caregiver in a stressful time. They are generally most open to those persons with whom they have developed a relationship, however brief.
Bereavement programs	Continued long-term support helps families deal with grief. A sensitive and timely sharing of autopsy results can be an important part of this process.

have related personally to families in the course of an illness, the nature of the illness, the nature of the patient, and other factors may determine the success of requests for autopsy (Table 2-5). Authorization of the autopsy depends on a miniloop between the ill patient and the family. Clear understanding of the desire or need for the autopsy among family members, including the patient, will be a catalyst for the autopsy-request process. Physicians and nurses will greatly influence the type of request that is ultimately approved by the family. The discussion loop between physicians and pathologists before and during the autopsy ensure attack of the most troubling clinicopathologic issues. The issuance of an autopsy request form that supplements the authorization and includes key pieces of clinical data may enhance the effectiveness of the autopsy. As noted earlier, the review of relevant clinical data by the pathologist is also expected. These interactions and events feed into the autopsy procedure itself and determine the nature of early verbal communications and later written communications regarding the autopsy results. The quality of the autopsy will also dictate the manner in which the physician may subsequently do a follow-up study with the family.

The utilization of a family-oriented conference by the caring physician, related nursing staff, and pathologist in the early postmortem period (at approximately 1 month), and later on, will have a significant positive effect on the family's psychoemotional status. The potential for benefit to a family includes a better understanding of certain environmental or genetic risk factors. The role of the postmortem conference has been championed by several pathologists.[3,74,75] The nature of this professional and at times personal interaction will assist in the grieving process, potentially allay guilt of family members, assuage anger and bring realistic light to the process of health, illness, and disease, and clarify the relationship between life and death. The particular role of the family practitioner in this setting should be emphasized. Because of the typically longstanding relationship between the family doctor and family, early and ongoing clarification regarding a loved one's death and general counseling with respect to familial risks may best be carried out in primary care offices. Additional counseling can occur through specialists when genetic determinants are overriding or other critical environmental influences are at play. The communication loop between physicians and families after a death (and autopsy) has a major influence on the public perception of care-giving institutions and their professionals. The concept of a "decedent affairs office"[74] has not received the attention that it deserves and would greatly influence communities served by hospitals. If one reflects for a moment on a hypothetical hospital with 500 active beds in which 500 deaths occur yearly and in which 200 autopsies are performed, the postmortem follow-up process would, over a period of 10 years, have an effect on 5000 immediate families. Of these families, 2000 would have had the benefit of a well-interpreted autopsy. The benefits of a well-conducted postmortem interaction could include a positive influence on the viability of healthcare institutions themselves. This kind of image-related dialog has potentially important fiscal implications. Humanistic efforts in the context of postmortem conferences have never been attended to in these broad public relations and fiscal terms.

The linkage of other postmortem procedures, including organ retrieval, to the autopsy is one way to enhance the appreciation of the value of such postmortem interventions. Sanner[76-78] has recently studied in depth, in a Swedish population, the willingness of people to have organs retrieved from themselves or their family members or to have an autopsy on themselves or family members. The results indicate a relatively high acceptance of the possibility of an autopsy by the public in the Swedish population. The research emphasizes the distinction between the willingness to have an autopsy and the discomfort the public may feel in authorizing an autopsy. The discomforts identified (Table 2-6) are numerous, but they represent fantastic opportunities for the health professions to ameliorate these concerns and to further the cause of organ donation for transplantation, as well as the autopsy examination. Before Sanner's work, information regarding personal perceptions about the autopsy has been based mainly on studies of medical students, physicians, other caring professionals, and persons who had recently experienced the death of a loved one.[79-84] Lay public perceptions of autopsy were scant.[85,86] The need for professional attention to public uneasiness with respect to all medical interventions is highlighted by the work of Sanner and her efforts focusing on the autopsy and on organ retrieval.

Table 2-6 Emotional discomforts in authorization of an autopsy by family

Discomfort with cutting the dead body
Fear of being desrespectful to the dead
Anxiety about offending Nature
Fear of objections from next of kin
Concern about biomedical development
Resistance to revealing one's diseases
Anxiety about offending God
Distrust of doctors and healthcare system
Apprehension about the funeral being influenced
Fear of not being dead
Other discomforts

Terminology

Challenges regarding the utilization of terminology relate primarily to the transmission of diagnoses into autopsy reports, final discharge summaries, and vital statistics ledgers. Well-known heterogeneity of vital-statistics reporting in most developed countries leads to considerable question about the validity of causes of death and other contributory factors. Efforts of the College of American Pathologists and other organizations to bring clarity to cause of death[87] and to standardize approaches to death certificate completion will improve this situation. The need to understand the distinction between immediate, proximate, and remote causes of death, mechanisms of death, and manner of death should be stressed to medical students at key points in their educational programs. The confusion of cause of death with mechanism of death is frequent. Fundamental definitions related to terminologies implicit in death and autopsy are summarized in Fig. 2-8.

General considerations

Solutions to the challenges that face the autopsy are particular to the challenge. The financial challenges may be approached through several initiatives. The designation of reimbursable diagnostic-related groups for autopsy-related findings,[51] possibly somewhat different for pediatric versus adult autopsies and possibly different for the apparent complexity of the illness, would seem mandatory to maintain the autopsy. The possibility of inclusion of autopsies in reimbursement plans will depend heavily on a change in insight of many observers. There is a clear need for professional remuneration for those performing nonforensic autopsies. The concept of core or centralized autopsy facilities servicing several hospitals in a community should be pursued. The possibility of centralized

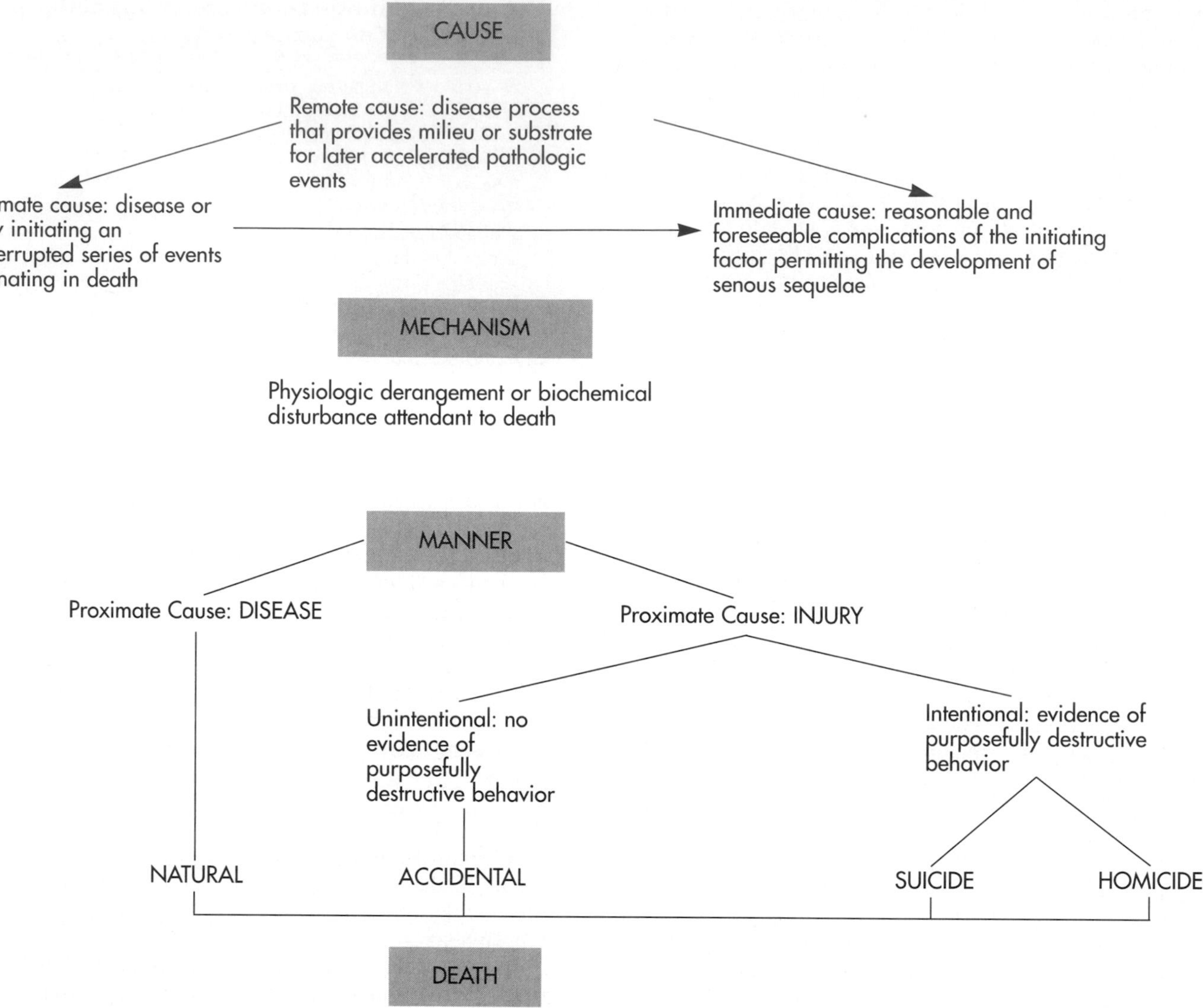

Fig. 2-8 Challenges in communication lie with understanding basic terminology about the causes, mechanisms, and manner of death. Remote cause may or may not be known depending on the patient, whereas the immediate cause is also less likely to be determined than the proximate cause. The most frequent distinction between cause and mechanism that needs to be made is the concept of an event leading to death versus an event attendant to death (ventricular rupture versus ventricular fibrillation after rupture). Nonforensic deaths are natural deaths when the proximate cause is disease.

autopsies in resident teaching programs could include a well-defined interdisciplinary autopsy conference at a single facility, with video-transmission to other relevant sites. There are logistical impediments to implementation of such programs; however, the fact that autopsy suites are not fully occupied in a normal day indicates that facilities should be consolidated when possible. This maneuver would lead to a greater possibility of standardization as well as better-trained, overall less expensive staff coverage, and a heightened quality assurance program for medicine in a given community.

Guidelines for autopsy performance have been developed by the College of American Pathologists.[88] These guidelines are aimed at practical matters in obtaining autopsy permission, dealing with funerals, unusual (protective) precautions, gross and histologic examination, special studies, quality control, and quality assurance. If adopted and adapted to local circumstance, these thoughtful recommendations will serve to address many challenges facing the autopsy.

HOW AND WHY TO IMPROVE AUTOPSY RATES

To renew adequate levels of use of the autopsy in medicine, major changes must be undertaken to reestablish its importance and value to society. The potentially major values of the autopsy have been introduced earlier (see Table 2-1). Information in this realm must be conveyed to administrators, clinical physicians, anatomic pathologists, and families in a concise, understandable, simple, and diplomatic manner. The philosophical and informational gap between the groups must be narrowed through institution of effective and efficient communication pathways. A host of strategies may improve autopsy

Table 2-7 Methods to improve autopsy rates

Identify champion of quality assurance
Utilize autopsy reports for potential revision of patient care practices (value-added care)
Campaign to educate the medical professional and society as a whole, to make them aware of autopsy discoveries that have contributed to medical knowledge
Stress excellence of educational tools for clinicians, pathologists, and researchers
Emphasize evaluation of new techniques, procedures, or medication for patient care
Improve the process of obtaining consent
- Ask for permission at every death
- Institute a nonphysician autopsy advocate

Improve communication of autopsy results
- Shorter reports with more expert information
- More timely completion
- Improve communication loops (see Fig. 2-7)
- Oral communication of results

Establish a national autopsy database, or at least major registries
Obtain reimbursement for the autopsy
- Link reimbursement to autopsy performance standards

Institute regulatory requirements

rates (Table 2-7). Health sciences programs might structure more educational activities around the autopsy, and more of these need to be cross disciplinary and patient focused. The establishment of "subspecialty" training in medical pathology[24] may ensure more accurate diagnostic examinations and allow for more expert analysis. Methods for obtaining consent for an autopsy also need to be modified. In Scandinavia, permission has been obtained upon hospital admittance, unless the family specifies differently by signing a form refusing postmortem examination within 12 hours of admittance.[24] Physicians must also be better educated with respect to approaching the family on this matter. Monetary support for the autopsy must be instituted to illuminate the way for hospital administrators and accreditors, on the one hand, and for pathologists, on the other. The autopsy procedure itself does allow for "limited" versus "complete" autopsies. The "limited" autopsy may reduce the problems of time and cost while assuaging family discomforts about the autopsy. However, the organismic approach to medicine and the autopsy[89] has solid rationale and speaks in favor of more "complete" than "partial" autopsies.

Although the subject of the quality assurance role of the autopsy in medicine makes some physicians and pathologists uncomfortable, it is crucially important.[90-93] The manner in which the quality assurance procedures are conducted and purveyed is equally crucial. The general unwillingness of physicians, including pathologists, to accept that they have made an error in diagnosis or interpretation is a stumbling block in the proper use of quality assurance data emanating from such diagnostic services as surgical pathology, autopsy pathology, radiology, and the like. The risk of finger pointing and unnecessary implication of guilt with respect to missed diagnoses impairs the process of applying new insights derived from clinical and autopsy discrepancies in a positive fashion. Thus it is fundamental that clinical physicians and pathologists engage in a continuous dialog regarding diagnostic discrepancies with a view to improving the education of their protégés[94-96] and for the betterment of future care. If one does not adhere to this tenet, the improvement of medical care through the autopsy tool will not be plausible. Cabot recognized the need for autopsies to detect clinical diagnostic oversights well over 90 years ago.[97]

The extent of discrepancies between clinical diagnosis and autopsy diagnosis varies widely from study to study (Table 2-8).[98-100] In compilations by Nemetz and associates[101] and Wheeler[25] the possibility of a missed clinical diagnosis ranged from as little as 4% to as much as 66%. Obviously, the patient mix, the observing clinician, the observing pathologist, the manner of definition of discrepancy, and other factors contribute to the wide range of discrepancies reported in any

Table 2-8 Malignant neoplasms missed clinically: discovered at autopsy

Author(s) (year)	Total deaths in series	Diagnoses of neoplasms	Percent (%) missed clinically
Bethrong (1984)	1846	182 carcinomas of the prostate, 101 clinically occult	55.5
Stemmermann (1982)	1376	813 tumors in elderly Hawaiian Japanese, 327 clinically occult	40
Gobbato et al (1982)	1405	Malignant neoplasm undiagnosed	27
Mandard et al (1981)	111	Discovery at autopsy of second primary tumor in patients with esophageal cancer	21
Asnaes and Paaske (1980)	807	Malignant neoplasm undiagnosed	4
Cechner et al (1980)	415	Bronchogenic carcinoma, clinically occult	28

Adapted from Nemetz PN, Ludwig J, Kurland LT: *Am J Pathol* 128:362, 1987.

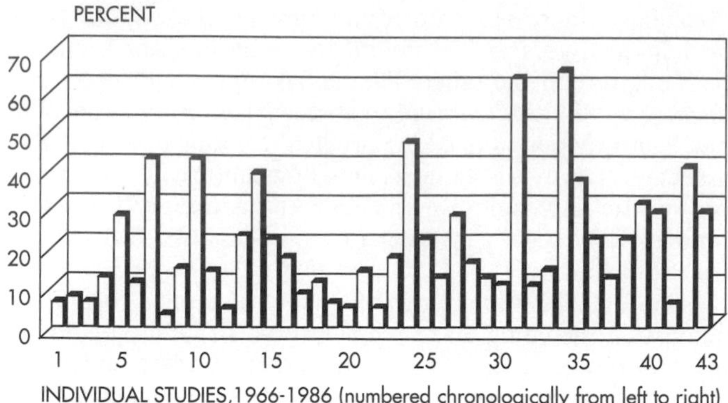

Fig. 2-9 Composite summary of studies of discrepancies between clinical and autopsy diagnoses over a 20-year period. As evidenced, the percentage of discrepancies ranges from as low as a few percent to as high as 66%. In general, 10% to 20% of cases have a significant discrepancy (one in which if the diagnosis had been made in life a difference in the course of the patient would have been expected).

Table 2-9 Autopsy diagnoses commonly missed clinically

Pneumonia
Pulmonary embolus
Acute pancreatitis
Mesenteric thrombosis
Vascular aneurysm
Infective endocarditis
Myocardial infarction
Hepatic cirrhosis
Neoplasm

Table 2-10 Importance of death certificates

Information provides basis for state and national mortality statistics used to:
- assess general health of population
- evaluate medical treatment success
- examine medical problems with higher prevalence in certain demographies and to identify where medical research can have the greatest effect
- identify public health problems and evaluate established programs to help these problems
- allocate healthcare services and follow-up studies of infant and maternal deaths and infectious diseases
- identify disease cause
- evaluate diagnostic and therapeutic technique
- identify leading causes of death
- identify potential life-years lost to diseases or injury
- provide information for epidemiologic studies
- identify geographical areas with increased death rates from certain causes of death
- serve as the primary means for evaluating health at the local level

Adapted from Kircher T, Anderson RE: *JAMA* 258:349, 1987.

given series. However, it is important to emphasize that there is usually a 10% to 20% discrepancy rate (modal discrepancy of 43 studies reviewed by Nemetz[36] and Wheeler[25] (Fig. 2-9). Numerous studies have a greater discrepancy rate. Although the definition of discrepancy does vary, most studies utilize a definition wherein the observation made at autopsy and not made clinically would have altered significantly the therapy and possible longevity of the patient. Although the precise number of discrepancies will not be known and the ultimate effect must be considered at the individual patient level, the important fact remains that an expectation of discrepancy should be potent motivation for the use of the autopsy as a positive tool in the quality assurance of medicine. This is not a novel concept but rather reflects the reiterations of many wise people. The fact that the discrepancy rate applies to common illnesses (Table 2-9), including myocardial infarcts, is suggestive of the need for vigilant comparison of what occurred or was observed clinically and what was established at autopsy. The potential effect of autopsy discrepancies on vital statistics encompassed in death certificates also cannot be overestimated (Table 2-10).[102] If one considers that in the United States in 1980 less than 9% of deaths from cardiovascular disease (classified by death certificate) or cancer were accompanied by autopsy, the possibility of significant misclassification of immediate, proximate, or even remote causes of death is considerable. Although perfection will remain elusive, a larger experience of autopsy observations in representative diseases and in particularly troubling or frequent disorders will enhance the likelihood that what is recorded on death certificates has some relationship to reality.

As noted in Table 2-9, along with myocardial infarcts, various pneumonias are frequently missed at autopsy or mistaken for pulmonary embolism. The reverse is also true. Abdominal catastrophes including acute pancreatitis, mesenteric thrombosis, and vascular aneurysm rupture are easily missed in a patient who has had a short period of observation or in whom complications or multiple disorders pertain. As well, infective endocarditis, in the patient with structural heart disease, intravenous drug abuse, or without apparent risk factors remains a significant challenge despite greatly enhanced imaging modalities. On first face, the clinical differential diagnosis must indicate endocarditis; otherwise it will easily be missed. Other occult processes with protean presentations, including solid organ injury and aberrant repair processes, like cirrhosis of the liver, and the broad range of neoplasms, may also fool even the most careful clinical observer and astute radiologist.

Factors that may contribute to differences in antemortem and postmortem diagnoses have been discussed.[103] The autopsy rate at a particular institution will influence the likelihood of detecting certain kinds of lesions in certain types of patients. Also, the age of the patient in a given institution will influence the likelihood of finding discrepancies with regard to certain types of lesions. In addition, it is well known that pediatric patients are most likely to be autopsied, young adult patients somewhat less likely to be autopsied, older adult patients even less likely, and the elderly the least likely.[104] Thus the particular illnesses or lesions most common in each of these age groups will be affected by the autopsy rate within each category. The same effect can be seen on the basis of patient sex. Across all age groups, males are considerably more likely to be autopsied than women.[47] The person classifying the discrepancies will obviously influence the identification of such clinical-autopsy differences. However, it is important to emphasize that among studies now published, whether by clinicians, pathologists, or multidisciplinary groups, all investigators come up with significant discrepancies between the diagnoses in life and those after death. Thus the overriding fact is that discrepancies will be found, should be expected, and must be utilized to decrease the frequency of repeat discrepancy within a given institution and within a given practice group. Finally, the likelihood that discrepancies will occur relates to the divergent manifestation of common diseases, as noted earlier.

Penner[49] emphasized other factors at play in determination of clinical-to-autopsy discrepancies. He highlighted the insufficient clinical data that may be derived from history, physical examination, or special examinations conducted in laboratories. In this regard, he emphasized the obvious fact that there may be insufficient time to carry out the optimum clinical evaluation (as when someone arrives moribund in the emergency room or has a short admission after an ill-defined illness). He also points out the potential for "deficient value judgments in relation to the state of the art," a potentially perjorative outlook. Certainly, different physicians will interpret the same findings differently; some will recognize a Chevrolet when they see it, and others will not.

Discovery is underemphasized as a benefit of the autopsy. It is utterly amazing how many conditions or diseases have been identified or recognized during the last half of this century. Thus, "new" diseases will be discovered, partly because the spark of insight will be emitted from a wary observer about a case that just doesn't fit any known category, partly because the expression of diseases may change with altered virulence of an organism or susceptibility of a subset of people or patients and partly because of changing environments, therapies, and genetic milieus. Striking examples of new discoveries include Reye's syndrome,[105] hypertrophic cardiomyopathy,[106] Legionnaires' disease and related pneumonias,[107] Hantavirus-related respiratory failure,[108] and many others. A partial legacy of knowledge generated by the autopsy is synopsized in Table 2-11.[2,5,109-111]

POSTSCRIPT

The autopsy must be advocated by nonpathologists as a key element in the rapidly evolving medical landscape. Numerous "pressure points" for autopsy advocacy can be easily identified (Fig. 2-10). The champions of autopsy in clinical care should be clinical leaders who understand the key reasons for and methods necessary to obtain and communicate the results of an autopsy. The education of the public through brochures, videos, properly framed articles, and other venues will bring the autopsy back to usefulness. It is worth noting in the simplest of terms that no animal model experimentation could be conducted successfully, with full force and with competitive funding, unless it was based on a strong plan for the gross, microscopic, cellular, and molecular examination of tissues taken at autopsy. Of interest, the models used have typically well-characterized susceptibilities, well-characterized interventions, and well-defined temporal courses, and yet the autopsy is still essential to garner key steps in the experimental process. On the other hand, expensive human clinical trials are conducted utilizing taxpayers' money in support of peer-review organizations and from industries without any attention to the essential value of autopsy observations to be made on patients who do not survive the trial, whether in the control or in the experimental group. Thus, most clinical trials are limited in their pathobiologic capabilities by the lack of availability of human tissues, cells, and fluid at different time points of disease and therapy. Even more unbelievable and in contrast to well-controlled animal experiments and quite well-defined clinical trials from only somewhat characterized clinical populations, the average patient comes to a hospital with a modestly understood disease process of uncertain time of onset and with complex and often changeable therapies and dies with a high likelihood of never having an autopsy. This whole contradictory situation should be emphasized in the process of trying to bring solutions to the general autopsy malaise. The use of postautopsy follow-up study as a humane and medically and institutionally self-serving process should be pursued with a vengeance.

Table 2-11 Clinical lessons from the autopsy

Infectious	Viral hepatitis, myocarditis, micrococcal enterocolitis, Hantavirus lung disease, Whipple's disease, disseminated candidiasis, Legionnaires' disease
Toxicologic and physical agents	Radiation injury, radiation nephritis, diethylene glycol nephropathy, occupational lung diseases, anthracycline cardiomyopathy, hypervitaminoses, industrial hazards, urethane poisoning (liver, bone marrow)
Genetic, inherited, and congenital	Fibrocystic disease of pancreas, taxonomy of congenital and acquired heart disease, collagen diseases, cirrhosis and alpha-1-antitrypsin deficiency, adrenoleukodystrophy
Perinatal disorders	Erythroblastosis fetalis, storage (metabolic) diseases, perinatal deaths, amniotic pulmonary embolism, postpartum pituitary necrosis (Sheehan's disease)
Endocrine and metabolic	Hyperparathyroidism, diabetic glomerulosclerosis, secondary hemochromatosis, glycogen storage diseases, cardiac amyloidosis, carcinoid heart disease
Inflammatory diseases	Lipoid pneumonia, Reye's syndrome, rheumatic heart disease, diffuse interstitial fibrosis of lung
Preneoplastic and neoplastic diseases	Myeloid metaplasia, posttransplantation lymphoproliferative disorder, bone tumors (radium water and chloride)
Iatrogenic	Consequences of hormone therapy, chemotherapy for cancer

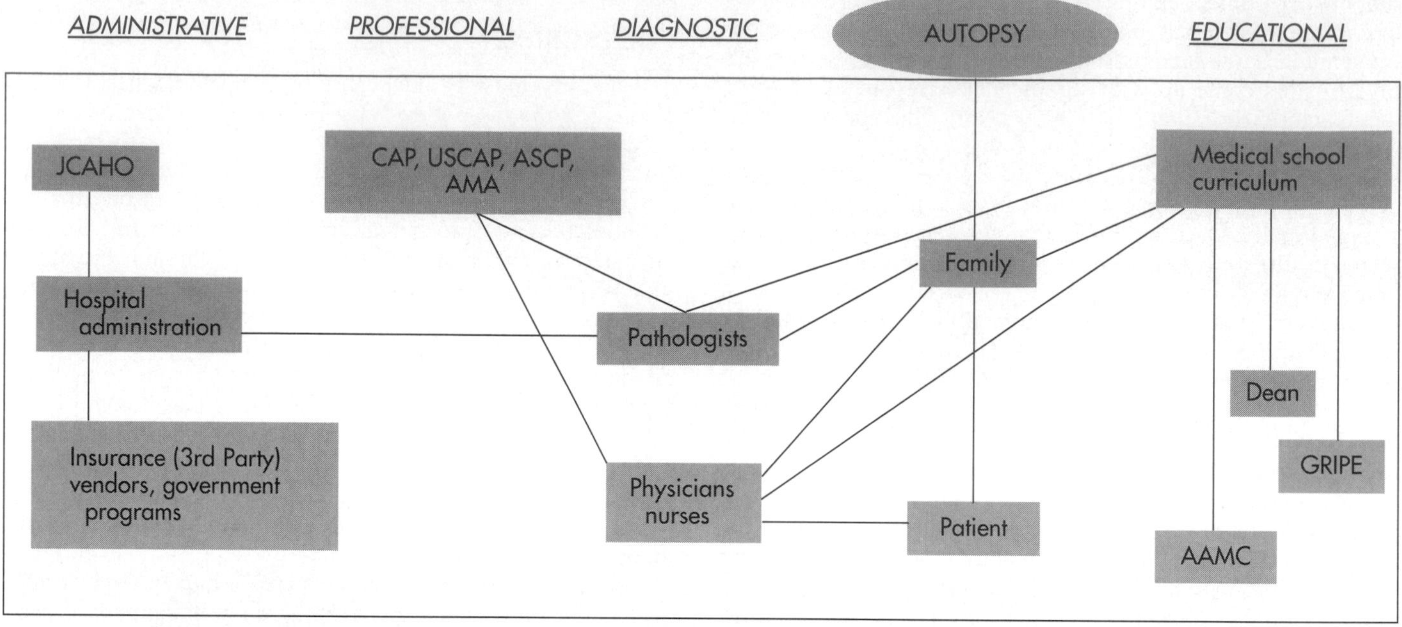

Fig. 2-10 In the effort to improve the use of the autopsy in medicine, there are numerous opportunities to bring pressure to bear. The administrative, professional, diagnostic, educational, and community focuses of pressure, if orchestrated effectively, may enhance the status of the autopsy. *AAMC,* American Association of Medical Colleges; *AMA,* American Medical Association; *ASCP,* American Society of Clinical Pathologists; *CAP,* College of American Pathologists; *GRIPE,* Group for Research in Pathology Education; *JCAHO,* Joint Commission on Accreditation of Healthcare Organizations; *USCAP,* United States and Canadian Academy of Pathology.

REFERENCES

1. King LS, Meehan CM: A history of the autopsy, *Am J Pathol* 73:514, 1973.
2. McManus BA, Beneke JA: The autopsy in medical science and clinical practice: where have we been and where are we going? *Nebr Med J* 71:184, 1986.
3. College of American Pathologists: *Autopsy: performance and reporting,* Northfield, Ill, 1990, College of American Pathologists.
4. Symposium on the autopsy: a professional obligation dissected, *Hum Pathol* 21:127, 1990.
5. The autopsy, *Arch Pathol Lab Med* 108:429, 1984.
6. Ludwig J: *Current methods of autopsy practice,* Philadelphia, 1979, Saunders.
7. Hill RB, Anderson RE: *The autopsy—medical practice and public policy,* Boston, 1988, Butterworth.
8. Anderson RE, Hill RB: The autopsy in academic medical centers in the United States, *Hum Pathol* 19:1369, 1988.
9. Goldman L: Diagnostic advances and the value of the autopsy: 1912-1980, *Arch Pathol Lab Med* 108:501, 1984.
10. King DW: Potential of the autopsy, *Arch Pathol Lab Med* 108:439, 1984.
11. Valdes-Dapena M, Huff D: *Perinatal autopsy manual,* Washington, DC, 1983, Armed Forces Institute of Pathology.
12. Sundstroem C: *The autopsy in clinical practice and research: problems and possibilities,* Stockholm, 1993, Swedish Medical Research Council.
13. Clendening L: *Source book of medical history,* New York, 1942, Dover Publications.
14. Gordon PL: The autopsy revisited, *Arch Pathol Lab Med* 109:305, 1985.
15. Benivieni A: *De abditis ac mirandis morborum et sanationum causis.* Translated by D Singer, with a bibliographical appreciation by ER Long, Springfield, Ill, 1954, Charles C Thomas.
16. Boerhaave H: Atrocis, nec descripti prius, morbi historia, Hermann Boerhaave opera omnia medica. Translated in Derbes VJ, Mitchell RE: Hermann Boerhaave's Atrocis, nec descripti prius, morbi historia, *Bull Med Lib Assoc* 43:217, 1955.
17. Boerhaave H: Atrocis, rarissimique morbi historia altera. Translated in Smith MW: Description of another dreadful and unusual disease drawn up by Hermann Boerhaave, *J Hist Med Allied Sci* 23:331, 1968.
18. Morgagni JB (1769): *The seats and causes of diseases, investigated by anatomy.* Translated by Alexander B, Miller et al, London, 1769.
19. Bichat X: *Anatomie générale, appliquée à la physiologie at à la médicene,* Vols. 1-4, Paris, 1801, Brosson, Gabon & Co.
20. Bichat X: *Discours préliminaire. Traité d'anatomie descriptive,* Paris, Brosson, 1801-1803, Gabon & Co.
21. Rokitansky C: Tuberculosis. In *A manual of pathological anatomy,* London, 1884, Syndenham Society.
22. Virchow R: Post-mortem examination with especial reference to medico-legal practice. Translated from the second German edition by TP Smith, Philadelphia, 1880, Presley Blakiston.
23. Flexner A: Medical education in the United States and Canada: a report to the Carnegie Foundation for the Advancement of Teaching, *Bulletin* 4, 1910, 1960.
24. Roberts WC: The autopsy: its decline and a suggestion for its revival, *N Engl J Med* 299:332, 1978.
25. Wheeler MS: One resident's view of the autopsy, *Arch Pathol Lab Med,* 106:311, 1982.
26. Cohen M, Schiff G: Declining rate of autopsies, *N Engl J Med* 310(19):1266, 1984.
27. Brooks JP, Dempsey J: How can hospital autopsy rates be increased? *Arch Pathol Lab Med* 115:1107, 1991.
28. Smith RD, Zumwalt RE: One department's experience with increasing the autopsy rate, *Arch Pathol Lab Med* 108:455, 1984.
29. Collins JA: The importance of autopsies in geriatric medicine, *Geriatrics* 36:35, 1981.
30. Price RA, McCormick WF: The declining rate and its significance for neuropathology: two viewspoints, *J Neuropathol Exp Neurol* 40:489, 1981.
31. Goldman L, Sayson R, Robbins S et al: The value of the autopsy in three medical eras, *N Engl J Med* 308:1000, 1983.
32. Robinson MJ: Autopsy: unending controversy, *NY State J Med* 76:761, 1976.

33. Carter JR, Nash NP, Cechner RL, Platt RD: Proposal for a national autopsy data bank, *Am J Clin Pathol* 76(suppl):597, 1981.
34. Carter JR: National autopsy data bank: potentially useful to so many, for so little, *Pathologist* 548, Oct. 1981.
35. Hirsch CS: Forensic pathology and the autopsy, *Arch Pathol Lab Med* 108:484, 1984.
36. McPhee SJ, Bottles K: Autopsy: moribund art or vital science? *Am J Med* 78:107, 1985.
37. McManus BM, Suvalsky SD, Wilson JE: A decade of acceptable autopsy rates: Does concordance of clinician and pathologist views explain relative success? *Arch Pathol Lab Med* 116:1128, 1992.
38. Pollock DA, O'Neil JM, Parrish RG et al: Temporal and geographic trends in the autopsy frequency of blunt and penetrating trauma deaths in the United States, *JAMA* 269:1525, 1993.
39. Editorial: The JCAH and the autopsy, *Hum Pathol* 16:1, 1985.
40. Joint Commission on Accreditation of Hospitals JCAHO, Board of Commissioners Revision: *Accreditation manual for hospitals,* Oak Brook Terrace, Ill, 1971.
41. Prutting J: Abolition of percentage requirement for accreditation of hospitals, *NY State J Med* 72:2507, 1972.
42. Spice B: Technological advances linked to autopsy drop, *Albuquerque New Mexico Tribune* a-1, a-3, Nov. 27, 1984.
43. Geller SA: Religious attitudes and the autopsy, *Arch Pathol Lab Med* 108:494, 1984.
44. Shapiro MJ: Reimbursement for autopsies: a personal view, *Arch Pathol Lab Med* 108:473, 1984.
45. Dunham WG, Quilan A, Krolikowski FJ, Reuter K: Quality assurance programs cope with today's demands, *Pathologist*, 24, June 1986.
46. Pontius EE: Financing mechanisms for autopsy, *Am J Clin Pathol* 69:245, 1978.
47. Beneke JA, Suvalsky SD, McManus BM: The autopsy in medical science and clinical practice: what are we doing in Nebraska? *Nebr Med J* 71:222, 1986.
48. Clark M: AMA asked to take action on autopsy, *CAP Today* 4:5, 1990, (College of American Pathologists).
49. Penner DW: Cost effectiveness of the autopsy in maintaining and improving the standard of patient care, *Am Soc Clin Pathol* 69:250, 1978.
50. Schned AR, Mogielnicki P, Stauffer ME: A comprehensive quality assessment program on the autopsy service, *Am J Clin Pathol* 86:133, 1986.
51. Guariglia P, Abrahams C: The impact of autopsy data on DRG reimbursement, *Hum Pathol* 16:1184, 1985.
52. Beckwith JB: The value of the pediatric postmortem examination, *Pediatr Clin North Am* 36:29, 1989.
53. Curran R, Hunt AC, Keeling JW: Problems with perinatal pathology, *Br Med J* 284:1469, 1982.
54. Darby JM, Stein K, Grenvik A, Stuart SA: Approach to management of the heartbeating brain dead organ donor, *JAMA* 261:2222, 1989.
55. Robertsson HE: Better postmortem service, *J Lab Clin Med* 10:486, 1925.
56. Mini-necropsy, *Lancet* 2:1026, 1981.
57. Mini-necropsy, *Lancet* 2:1235, 1981.
58. Dorsey DB: Limited autopsies: defined benefits, limited costs, *Arch Pathol Lab Med* 108:469, 1984.
59. Dolan CT, Brown AL, Ritts RE: Microbiological examination of postmortem tissues, *Arch Pathol Lab Med* 92:206, 1971.
60. Wilson WR, Dolan CT, Washington JA: Clinical significance, *Arch Pathol Lab Med* 94:244, 1972.
61. Dolan CT, Trump BF, McDowell EM et al: Special autopsy methods: microbiology, electron microscopy, chromosome study, chemistry, and roentgenology. In Ludwig J, editor:, *Current methods of autopsy practice*, ed 2, Philadelphia, 1979, Saunders.
62. Baley JE, Kliegman RM, Fanaroff AA: Disseminated fungal infections in very low-birth-weight infants: clinical manifestations and epidemiology, *Pediatrics* 73:144, 1984.
63. Reichert CM: New safety considerations for the acquired immunodeficiency syndrome autopsy, *Arch Pathol Lab Med* 116:1109, 1992.
64. Douceron H, Deforges L, Gherardi R et al: Long-lasting postmortem viability of human immunodeficiency virus: a potential risk in forensic medicine practice, *Forensic Sci Int* 60:61, 1993.
65. Brumback RA: Case records of the Massuchusetts General Hospital weekly clinicopathological excercises, *N Engl J Med* 303:1162, 1980.
66. Brown JW: Laboratorians: on the front lines of exposure, *Med Lab Observer* 54, August 1991.
67. Bankowski MJ, Landay AL, Staes B et al: Postmortem recovery of human immunodeficiency virus type I form plasma and mononuclear cells: implications for occupational exposure, *Arch Pathol Lab Med* 116:1124, 1992.
68. Creutzfeldt-Jakob disease: autopsy safety protocol urged, *CAP Today*, 2:4, 50, 1988 (College of American Pathologists).
69. Brown P: Guidelines for high risk autopsy cases: special precautions for Creutzfeldt-Jakob disease. In Hutchins G, editor: *Autopsy: performance and reporting*, Northfield, Ill, 1990, College of American Pathologists.
70. MacArthur S, Schneiderman H: Infection control and the autopsy of persons with human immunodeficiency virus, *Am J Infect Control* 15:172, 1987.
71. Trexler PC, Gilmour AM: Use of flexible plastic film isolators in performing potentially hazardous necropsies, *J Clin Pathol* 36:527, 1983.
72. Towfighi J, Roberts AF, Foster NE, Abt AB: A protective device for performing cranial autopsies, *Hum Pathol* 20:288, 1989.
73. Grizzle WE, Polt SS: Guidelines to avoid personnel contamination by infective agents in research laboratories that use human tissues, *J Tiss Cult Meth* 11:191, 1988.
74. Smith JH, Haque AK, Gilmer PR, Jekielek S: A solution to declining autopsy rates: the decedent affairs office, *Pathologist* 40(7):22, 1986.
75. Valdes-Dapena M: The post-autopsy conference with families, *Arch Pathol Lab Med* 108:497, 1984.
76. Sanner MA: In perspective of declining autopsy rate: attitudes of the public, *Arch Pathol Lab Med* 118:878, 1994.
77. Sanner MA: Attitudes toward autopsy, organ donation, and transplantation: a model for understanding reactions to medical procedures after death, *JAMA* 271:284, 1994.
78. Sanner MA: Attitudes toward organ donation and transplantation, *Soc Sci Med* 38:1141, 1994.
79. Heckerling PS, Williams MJ: Attitudes of funeral directors and embalmers toward autopsy, *Arch Pathol Lab Med* 116:1147, 1992.
80. Wilkes MS, Link RN, Jacobs TA et al: Attitudes of house officers toward the autopsy, *J Gen Intern Med* 5:122, 1990.
81. Webster JR, Derman D, Kopin J et al: Obtaining permission for an autopsy: its importance for patients and physicians, *Am J Med* 186:325, 1989.
82. McGoogan E, Cameron HM: Clinical attitudes to the autopsy, *Scot Med J* 23:19, 1978.
83. Gardner R, Peskin L, Katz JL: The physician, the autopsy request, and the consent rate, *J Med Educ* 48:636, 1973.
84. McPhee SJ, Bottles K, Lo B et al: To redeem them from death: reactions of family members to autopsy, *Am J Med* 80:665, 1986.
85. Brown HG: Lay perceptions of autopsy, *Arch Pathol Lab Med;*108:446, 1984.
86. Brown HG: Perceptions of the autopsy: views from the lay public and program proposals, *Hum Pathol* 21:154, 1990.
87. Autopsy Committee: *Protocol for writing cause-of-death statements for natural causes,* Northfield, Ill, 1994, College of American Pathologists.
88. Hutchins GM, Glenn GC: Practice guidelines for autopsy pathology, *Arch Pathol Lab Med* 118:18, 1994.
89. Corrigan GE: Autopsy goals and the concept of the organism, *Arch Pathol Lab Med* 99:453, 1975.
90. Anderson RE: The autopsy as an instrument of quality assessment, *Arch Pathol Lab Med* 108:490, 1984.
91. Anderson RE, Hill RB, Gorstein F: A model for the autopsy-based quality assessment of medical diagnostics, *Hum Pathol* 21:174, 1990.
92. Gambino SR: The autopsy: the ultimate audit, *Arch Pathol Lab Med* 108:444, 1984.

93. Report of the Joint Working Party of the Royal College of Pathologists, Royal College of Physicians of London and Royal College of Surgeons of England, Edinburgh: *The autopsy and audit,* London, 1991, Royal College of Pathologists.
94. Lundberg GD: Medicine without the autopsy, *Arch Pathol Lab Med* 108:449, 1984.
95. Anderson RE, Fox RC, Hill RB: Medical uncertainty and the autopsy: occult benefits for students, *Hum Pathol* 21:128, 1990.
96. Berthrong M: The autopsy as a vehicle for the lifetime education of pathologists, *Arch Pathol Lab Med* 108:506, 1984.
97. Cabot RC: Diagnostic pitfalls identified during a study of three thousand autopsies, *JAMA* 59:2295, 1912.
98. Landefeld CS, Chren MM, Myers A et al: Diagnostic yield of the autopsy in a university hospital and a community hospital, *N Engl J Med* 318:1249, 1988.
99. Landefeld CS, Goldman L: The value of autopsy in modern oncology, *Eur J Cancer Clin Oncol* 25:607, 1988.
100. McFarlane MJ: The necessity of studying mortality and necropsy data of adults, *Arch Pathol Lab Med* 111:783, 1987.
101. Nemetz PN, Ludwig J, Kurland LT: Assessing the autopsy, *Am J Pathol* 128:362, 1987.
102. Kircher T, Anderson RE: Cause of death: proper completion of the death certificate, *JAMA* 258:349, 1987.
103. Battle RM, Anderson RE, Key BR, Hill RB: Factors influencing discrepancies between pre- and post-mortem diagnoses, *JAMA* 258:339, 1987.
104. Ahronheim JC, Bernhole AS, Clark WD: Age trends in autopsy rates, *JAMA* 250:1182, 1983.
105. Reye RDK, Morgan G, Baral J: Encephalopathy and fatty degeneration of the viscera, *Lancet* 2:749, 1963.
106. Teare RD: Asymmetrical hypertrophy of the heart in young adults, *Br Heart J* 20:1, 1958.
107. Schurrmann D, Ruf B, Fehrenbach FJ et al: Fatal legionnaires' pneumonia: frequency of legionellosis in autopsied patients with pneumonia from 1969 to 1985, *J Pathol* 155:35, 1988.
108. Duchin JS, Koster FT, Peters CJ et al: Hantavirus pulmonary syndrome: a clinical description of 17 patients with a newly recognized disease. The Hantavirus Study Group, *N Engl J Med* 330:949, 1994.
109. Wissler RW: The value of the autopsy for understanding cardiovascular disease: past, present and future, *Arch Pathol Lab Med* 108:479, 1984.
110. Cannon PR: Clinical lessons learned in the morgue, *JAMA* 161:730, 1956.
111. Garcia JH, Wilmes FJ: Autopsy: the path to progress, *Pathologist* :793, 1983, *Ala J Med Sci* 21:290, 1984.

3 SURGICAL PATHOLOGY

Mark R. Wick
Stacey E. Mills

Any chapter written on the topic of surgical pathology must, by definition, be only a superficial and predominantly philosophical consideration of this increasingly broad subject. Today, there are no fewer than five major American textbooks that are entirely devoted to "general" surgical pathology[1-5] and countless books dealing with individual organs. Similar monographs have also been assembled by editors and authors from outside the United States. Although the field of surgical pathology as we know it today is relatively new in the practice of medicine, the knowledge base from which it grew continues to expand at a dizzying pace. The latter phenomenon has, perforce, mandated that practitioners in pathology today must develop special expertise in selected topics. This is true even if the setting in which they work is a general hospital laboratory. Hence "surgical pathology" is currently not a mere facet of the practice of pathology but is rather a distinct, largely independent, and ever-more-demanding discipline, requiring high and ever-increasing levels of expert knowledge. The philosophical and practical frameworks for this subspecialty have been discussed previously by several authors.[1,3,6] This chapter summarizes and expands on such information, and it presents the authors' admittedly personalized views of its current application.

HISTORY AND SCOPE OF SURGICAL PATHOLOGY

Surgical pathology was a largely unknown enterprise a century ago. Laboratory physicians were then regarded as stuffy, nonclinical academicians who were concerned only with the "morbid anatomy" of the autopsy room and the nuances of histology. In fact, the now obvious concept that pathologic findings postmortem bear a strong relationship to antemortem clinical observations was a "revolutionary" idea. This concept was actually introduced in the seventeenth and eighteenth centuries by Severino and Morgagni.[6-8] Nonetheless, it took Sir William Osler, one of the greatest internists in history, to promulgate and champion the latter idea[9] before physicians granted it growing (but grudging) acknowledgment. Had it not been for the fact that Osler himself had begun his career as a pathologist, it would likely have required even more time to establish the premise that cataloguing the morphologic aspects of disease had vicarious benefits for *living* patients.

Emotional and technical factors also delayed the entry of pathologists into proactive medical decision making. Many surgeons who were held in high regard at universities and in the community at large had gone on record with the statement that the microscope was unnecessary to distinguish diseased from normal tissues, particularly if a malignancy was suspected.[10,11] After the development of effective anesthesia literally opened the body to the surgeon's scalpel, many mutilating procedures were undoubtedly performed needlessly as a byproduct of this dogma. Often, pathologists were not afforded any opportunity to study excised tissues at all because they were discarded after cursory examination by the surgeon. In this context, "pathologic" diagnoses were assigned more by mandate than by method. One had to rely solely on the operator's impressions of the surgical findings and his or her estimation of their meaning for the patient.

The somewhat tenuous early interface between surgery and pathology has been traced eloquently by Underwood.[6] He attributes publication of the first microscopic illustrations of human tumors (drawings) to a text by Sir Everard Home in 1830, followed shortly by another by Johannes Müller in 1838. These books did not really present any pragmatic aspects of the emerging new field of medical microscopy but instead were again concerned with its theoretical aspects. It remained for two physicians, J.H. Bennett and F. Donaldson, working more or less simultaneously, on opposite sides of the Atlantic, to invigorate cytohistopathology by giving it a definite clinical application.[12,13] Interestingly, both of these men employed what would now be called "touch-imprint" preparations rather than actual tissue sections, yielding slides more akin to those currently seen in fine-needle aspiration cytology than those used in classic surgical pathology. Cytologic examination was also preferred by Lionel Beale, an eminent professor of medicine in London who authored *The Microscope in Medicine* in 1854.[14]

As also related by Underwood, the major obstacle that retarded general acceptance of the "biopsy" (from the Greek *bios,* meaning 'life' and *opsis,* meaning 'appearance') as a valuable procedure was the disaster surrounding the diagnosis of the "Kaiser's cancer." German Kaiser Frederick III had developed a laryngeal tumor in 1887, which was sampled surgically by Sir Morell Mackenzie. In an ensuing comedy of errors that unfortunately has been repeated at other intervals throughout history, the tissue was sent to a pathologist who had little familiarity with biopsy interpretation but was a professional icon, Professor Rudolph Virchow of Berlin, rather than individuals (such as Bennett or Beale) who were "children of a lesser god" but nonetheless experienced ones! Predictably, the case was botched. The biopsy specimens were interpreted as benign, but within a year it became obvious that the Kaiser did indeed have an advanced laryngeal malignancy that was to take his life.[15] Accusatory fingers were pointed in all directions, and the ultimate conclusion held throughout England and Europe (and supported by Virchow's negativistic statements[16]) was that biopsy procedure and "surgical pathology" were inherently unreliable. Moreover, existing technology for the handling and sectioning of human tissues was not highly developed. Embedding specimens in wax did not come into general use until the latter 1800s, and histotechnology was still rudimentary. Frozen sections and cytologic smears were preferred as much more procedurally amicable preparations.[17]

Fortunately, surgeons in the United States were more optimistic about such matters. At the turn of the twentieth century, there had already been reports from American medical centers on the use of frozen sections in examining biopsy specimens,[18] and it was even suggested that this activity could be carried on while the patient was still in the operating theater.[19] As pathology flourished globally as a respected area of medicine that integrated clinical practice and basic science, technical developments in biologic staining methods were rapidly forthcoming between the years of 1900 and 1930.[17]

In fact, during this period it quickly became evident that a sufficient body of knowledge was growing outside of traditional autopsy-based "morbid anatomy," such that special expertise regarding pathologic processes in living patients was needed.[6] Surprisingly, however, only a few physicians whose training and background theretofore had been devoted to laboratory science, that is, "pathologists," seemed willing to develop the new area of "surgical" pathology.

This paradox fostered the growing involvement of clinical practitioners, usually surgeons, in the morphologic evaluation of specimens sent to the laboratory from the operating room. It was therefore a common scenario to find the division of surgical pathology and its faculty members within the department of *surgery.* At many large medical centers, this approach was in effect as recently as the 1950s.[20] There have been several titanic intellects and dynamic personalities in the field, some of whom originally came from backgrounds in primary clinical training. They included but were not limited to such familiar names as James Ewing and later Fred Stewart at the Memorial Sloan-Kettering Cancer Center (New York), Pierre Masson of the University of Montreal (Montreal, Quebec, Canada), Arthur Purdy Stout and Raffaele Lattes of Columbia University (New York), and Lauren Ackerman at Washington University (St. Louis, Missouri).[1,20,21-23]

Professor William Boyd, another important pioneering figure, had been educated as a psychiatrist in Scotland but he acquired somewhat involuntary training in pathology because of the needs of British physicians and the Royal Army Medical Corps during World War I.[24] This experience changed Boyd's career plans after the armistice, and he accepted a teaching position as chief of pathology at the Manitoba Medical College in Canada. The upshot of these events was the publication of *Boyd's Surgical Pathology* in 1925, representing the first textbook that addressed the specific needs of the surgeon and his or her interaction with the laboratory.[25] This monograph went through several subsequent editions and was widely referenced; it was supplanted only in the 1950s through the appearance of *Ackerman's Surgical Pathology,* now in its eighth edition.[1]

Today, the scope of surgical pathology is broad. It encompasses traditional morphologic analysis of all organ systems and has relevance to immediate patient care, as well as many related adjunct enterprises including cytopathology, electron microscopy, immunopathology, cytometry, telepathology and other modes of electronic information transfer, and "molecular" pathology.[26] Information derived from such disciplines is used in the close communication that surgical pathologists must have with attending physicians concerning the tissue changes seen in their patients. Furthermore, the "surgeon" of record is currently as likely to be an internist or a pediatrician as a surgical specialist because technology now affords virtually all clinicians the means to obtain biopsy samples with relative ease and safety. The proactive, problem-solving nature of most surgical pathologists has revitalized the autopsy room as well because they conduct a substantial portion of modern postmortem examinations done throughout the United States.[27]

THE SURGICAL PATHOLOGY LABORATORY

The day has long passed when clinicians could personally take each specimen to the laboratory after having procured it and speak at length to the pathologist about the circumstances of the case and the suspected disease processes. The essentials of this communication are still vital, but they now must be obtained in a much more terse and stylized fashion. Request forms that accompany surgical pathology specimens should be designed to survey the major historical, physical, and operative findings that are associated with each specimen (Fig. 3-1). Furthermore, it must be assured by both the pathologist and the clinician that such forms are thoroughly and accurately completed before submission of the tissue to surgical pathology. The paperwork is unacceptable if it is merely labeled "lesion," or if it simply restates the operative procedure that was performed. The latter statements reflect our strong belief that there is absolutely no place for "gamesmanship" in surgical pathology, where a diagnosis is expected from the pathologist, in the total absence of contributory information from the clinician. It is deplorably true that some surgeons currently will agree to perform a procedure without garnering even the most rudimentary knowledge of the general condition of the patient. Under those circumstances, the name of another clinician who does possess this information must be sought for necessary telephone contact by the pathologist.

BARNES

E9

TISSUE EXAM REQUEST

Unit: ______________________

Date: ______________________

Age: ______________________

Birthdate: ______________________

Sex: ______________________

(If handwritten, name, address, & registration number)

CLINICAL HX:

OB/GYN: Last Menses: Date Ovulation: G: P: AB: Hormone RX:

OPERATIVE PROCEDURE AND FINDINGS:

DIAGNOSIS:

SPECIMEN:

SURGEON: ______________________ 1st ASSISTANT: ______________________

Filled out by: ______________________

Form 114-9 Rev. 3/90

Fig. 3-1 Representative specimen request form used for submission of tissues removed in the clinic or the operating room and sent to surgical pathology department.

Accessioning procedures

Accessioning is the entry point of specimens into the surgical pathology laboratory. As with submitting clinicians, accessioning personnel similarly must be impressed with the need for scrupulous attention to the proper, unambiguous identification of the specimen and accurate transfer of this information to the pathology data base. Under no circumstances should a tissue sample ever be accepted for examination when it has no identification attached to it or if the identifying data are contradictory or otherwise questionable. Furthermore, incomplete specimens also must be declined, as exemplified by one that is said on accompanying paperwork to consist of three parts but is represented by only one on receipt.

Paramedical technicians working in pathology must understand the many pitfalls that attend their duties and the ways in which these problems can be avoided. For example, a patient in English-speaking countries who is named "John Smith" may have 20, 30, or more cohorts in the pathology data base with the same first and last names. It is furthermore conceivable that one or more of these people might have an identical type of tissue specimen under concurrent evaluation. The need scrupulously to check middle initials, birth dates, social security numbers, hospital registration numbers, and any other available demographic information is obvious in such cases. Failure to do so invites diagnostic disaster for physician and patient alike. Likewise, batches of biopsy specimens of the same type and general description (for example, prostatic needle biopsy specimens received en masse from a urology clinic) must be handled with maximum caution throughout the accessioning process. If two samples of the same type are transposed through carelessness at this stage, there may be no way (short of rebiopsy or application of costly special technology[28,29]) to determine later which one came from which patient. When possible, modern provisions for specimen identification, including bar codes and other computer-driven information,[30] should be given strong consideration as compared with handwritten or typewritten labels. Indeed, both types of identifier may be affixed to each tissue container, and this redundancy seems to be the best of all approaches.

The "gross room"

Delivery of surgical specimens from the operating rooms to the pathology laboratory accessioning area and from there to the "gross" (prosection) room should ideally be done several times throughout the day. At each step in the transfer from one area of the hospital to another, identifying paperwork and specimen labels must be meticulously checked to verify that there are no errors. The pathologist who is charged with direction of the gross room must assume ultimate responsibility for this function, though it is often delegated today to physicians' assistants who are employed in the prosection area.

All personnel working in the gross room should be familiar with the proper prosection of all types of surgical specimens, or, at the very least, they must be supervised closely by professional superiors who have such knowledge. The details of macroscopic pathology and dissection, packaging of gross specimens as archival teaching tools, use of special tissue fixatives and decalcification solutions, labeling and submission of tissue blocks for microscopic examination and adjunctive special studies, specimen photography and radiology, and other functions of persons working in the gross room have been covered well elsewhere[1,3] and are far beyond the scope of this discussion. Suffice it to say that competent surgical pathologists must be fully versed in all these duties and must perform them appropriately. As an aside, there is nothing more maddening than having no macroscopic specimen photograph to show clinical staff members at teaching conferences. Similarly, specimen radiographs of breast biopsy specimens and paraffin blocks of them are not only of interest to surgeons and radiologists seeking to localize pathologic mammary calcifications, but also they play a definite role in assuring these physicians that the proper area of tissue has, in fact, been excised and sampled microscopically.[31]

In recent times, at least one commercial speech-recognition system has appeared for the handling of gross room dictations. This device can "learn" the voice patterns of those who are dictating, matching them with a relatively extensive electronic vocabulary of pathologic and clinical terms, measurements, and other data.[32] Contextual templates in such systems accommodate most "common" specimens, such as gallbladders, prostatic needle biopsy samples, and endoscopic biopsy samples of the gut. The end product is a transcribed (typed) gross pathology report that has the advantages of reproducibility, rapidity, and relative freedom from the influence of human foibles. Nonetheless, there may be problems with the ability of systems such as this to recognize the pronunciation of certain individuals, and although their vocabularies are substantial, they are not exhaustive. Despite these drawbacks, it is likely that nonhuman transcription devices will be used increasingly in the future.[33,34]

Besides the technical aspects of gross room functions, pathologists today must be fully versed in the occupational hazards that are encountered in this section of the laboratory and in attendant governmental and professional regulations. For example, it is now recognized that formaldehyde has undeniably adverse effects on the health of persons who inhale it on a regular basis.[35,36] Hence, regulations have established ventilation requirements and limit the ambient concentration of formaldehyde fumes in hospital laboratories.[37] These statutes mandate that regular monitoring programs must be established and documented in each institution. Similarly, specimens that prove to be infected with mycobacteria, hepatitis viruses, human immunodeficiency virus (HIV), and other transmissible agents are numerous. For this reason, it is absolutely necessary that all gross-room personnel adhere to strict protective measures in the handling of *all* tissues. This is particularly important when specimens must be cut with the aid of band saws and other relatively crude electrical instruments. Universal precautions always must be followed, and protective gowns or aprons, rubber gloves, and goggles always must be worn in the gross room and discarded or cleaned regularly. Microbicidal solutions with activity against hepatitis virus and HIV should be applied liberally to bench tops and prosecting instruments after each use,[38] and, in general, the laboratory must be kept clean and orderly. Washable covers may be necessary for telephone receivers and computer terminals to accomplish this goal. Formal infection-control procedures also should be developed by all hospitals to deal with inadvertent mucosal exposure of gross-room workers to body fluids, as well as knife cuts and puncture wounds incurred while prosecting.[39] Similarly, potentially hazardous chemical exposures must be dealt with in a prescribed fashion using facilities (for example, emergency showers and chemical neutralizers) and written protocols that are readily accessible in the laboratory.

Histology and other laboratories

As with the passage of specimens from the accessioning area to the gross room, submission of tissue cassettes from the gross room to the histology laboratory must be done in a careful and programmatic fashion. Each gross-room prosector should "sign off" electronic or handwritten lists of cassettes, each of which must be labeled with a unique case number and an alphanumeric block designation, with the histology technologist or technologists who will be responsible for processing them. The use of special fixatives should be clearly communicated, along with any singular requests for wax-embedding procedures, microtomy, or special stains. Instruction for the orientation of tissue for embedding must be provided if at all unclear; otherwise, valuable tissue will be lost through sectioning. All these provisos can be acknowledged by the technologist by their simply initialing and dating the request forms. In those surgical pathology laboratories not yet using computer-driven histology requests, tissue cassette forms should have one or two carbon copies so that the submitter and laboratory personnel each have one for easy reference and tracking of cases in progress.

The modern histology laboratory must be proficient at handling all types of surgical pathology specimens and the production of high-quality hematoxylin and eosin–stained sections. Given the many biochemical processing steps that all tissue samples must go through, quality control in histotechnology is a complicated and demanding area.[40] However, it is still unfortunately true that poor slide preparation is a leading cause of misdiagnosis, indicating that many institutions continue to fall short of expected performance levels in histology.[41] Rigorous "in-service" presentations (continuing technical education) must be established in each laboratory, and these should be accompanied by a meaningful, daily quality assurance program. In these regards, it behooves the pathologist to play a consistent role in such activities, rather than providing only occasional (and usually negative) comments on slide quality. The reader is referred to the excellent textbook *Histotechnology: a self-instructional text* by Carson for further details.[40]

The importance of histochemistry, immunohistochemistry, molecular diagnostics, and electron microscopy to surgical pathology is substantial and discussed elsewhere in this book. Whether every histology laboratory elects to offer a full range of "special" (histochemical and immunohistochemical) stains is a decision that must be made in concert by technical supervisors and surgical pathologists. However, it is our opinion that transmittal of tissue sections or blocks to reference laboratories for particularly difficult or seldom-performed technical procedures is the most logical and cost-effective approach to this topic. Similarly, electron microscopic studies and "molecular" analyses (for example, in situ hybridization; Southern, western, or northern blotting techniques; polymerase chain reaction–based assays) of selected cases are best done by laboratories and technical personnel with substantial experience and day-to-day involvement with such procedures. Those institutions that choose to maintain such facilities on site must, of course, adhere to the same standards of quality practice that are applied in the general histology laboratory.

THE SURGICAL PATHOLOGY REPORT

The principal aim of surgical pathology is obviously that of the accurate and clinically meaningful diagnoses of specimens taken from living patients. Nevertheless, if a diagnostic interpretation made by the pathologist is not expeditiously and clearly transmitted to the physician caring for the patient in question, it may be almost useless. In the past, this issue was a much less pressing one because patients enjoyed longer hospital stays after surgical or biopsy procedures and interactions among clinical consultants could take place at a more relaxed pace. Currently, however, there is a significant urgency in obtaining a tissue diagnosis so that all physician inputs considered necessary to optimal patient care can be marshaled during hospitalizations that are being greatly foreshortened by fiscal considerations.

This problem has begun to alter prior practice patterns in surgical pathology in a potentially serious fashion. For example, frozen-section consultation (discussed below) has recently experienced a sizable increase in utilization, as surgeons push to obtain diagnoses earlier and earlier. Whereas this approach is certainly understandable, given the economic pressures mentioned above, it is not altogether supportable or commendable because of the inherent error rate attached to the use of the cryostat or freezing microtome.[42]

Rosai has described one method (established by Lauren Ackerman) for communication of pathologic diagnoses, which is used in some institutions with residency programs in laboratory medicine.[1] This relies on a hierarchy of housestaff members, with a "hot-seat fellow," or chief resident, occupying a central and crucial position. In the latter paradigm, all microscopic sections are delivered to that one house officer, who examines them and records his or her diagnoses for each case. These may then be communicated orally to clinicians calling the laboratory for information. Afterwards, the slides are distributed to other residents and fellows for final interpretation by staff members, and ultimate diagnoses are again returned to the "hot seat" for case closure, formal dictation, transcription, and generation of written reports.

The "hot-seat" system has proved of value in residency and fellowship teaching, but it undeniably adds time to the case sign-out process. Another proved but also time-consuming approach used in some academic centers is to return the microscopic slides to the prosecting resident. This individual then has time (usually an afternoon and early evening) to review the cases, review appropriate prior specimens from the patient, study the pathology literature concerning possible diagnoses, and make tentative interpretations. The cases are then signed out with an on-call faculty member the next morning, with the prosecting resident responsible for report dictation and proofreading.

The time-consuming nature of these training approaches, in concert with increasing pressure for rapid diagnosis has unfortunately prompted some academic centers to employ sign-out procedures more like those used in community hospital laboratories. In those settings, microscopic slides often are delivered directly to the faculty pathologists who are responsible for dictating final diagnoses, which are promptly transcribed. Residents and fellows either see the cases for the first time with the faculty member during the sign-out time and not being allowed more generous time for independent study or, even worse, are given the cases after faculty review, with appropriate diagnoses indicated. Such completed cases usually carry all the allure of yesterday's newspaper, and, in our opinion, this approach is detrimental to resident training.

The transcription of surgical pathology reports, likewise, has become a time-pressured activity, insofar as some practitioners have resorted to the use of "stock" dictations for common specimens and common diagnoses; these are simply identified for the transcriptionist by a code number. Others have opted to delete traditional microscopic descriptions from most reports, reserving them only for those cases (such as liver and renal biopsies done for medical diseases) in which diagnoses cannot be properly conveyed or in which unique aspects of the clinical or pathologic findings mandate a special comment.[3] We wish to emphasize that decisions on reporting formats are solely those of the pathologist, *if* it has been assured that all data necessary for timely clinical decision-making have been provided. The fatuous equation made by some clinicians between the worth of the institutional laboratory and the mere length or complexity of its surgical pathology reports has no validity.

The latter topics have admittedly undergone considerable evolution in the past decade. Whereas it was previously perfectly acceptable for surgical pathologists simply to make correct diagnoses, they must now provide detailed information relating to possible pathogenesis, response to specific therapies, and prognosis.[43-45] It appears that the best approach to this demand, at least for neoplastic diseases, is the use of programmatic templates for pathology reports. Some of these yield a terse, synoptic, final product[46] (Fig. 3-2), whereas others are more elaborate checklists designed to generate a prose-style report[47] (Fig. 3-3). Either provision can be applied to traditional typewriter-mediated transcription or computer-facilitated systems, though the latter are infinitely more efficient. An important advantage to programmatic templates and synoptic reporting is uniformity in the staging and grading of tumors. For large tissue resections, the pathologic stage is often specified according to the TNM system, which assigns stage according to the size and extent of the tumor (*T*) and the presence or absence of metastasis (*M*) and lymph node spread (*N*) (Table 3-1). Given existing electronic imaging capabilities, digitalized gross and microscopic pictures of any given specimen can even be incorporated into the permanent report and stored in computer memory[48] (Fig. 3-4).

As discussed in Chapter 6, the end point in measuring the turnaround time (TAT) of a test is when the physician receives the report. Many laboratories will measure the TAT of surgical pathology as the difference from time of signout and specimen accessioning, not taking into account unreliable surface-mail delivery. Well-designed information systems will allow the clinical staff to view the surgical pathology diagnosis immediately after sign-out. Another electronic advance, the telephone-mediated facsimile device (fax), also has proved to be useful in the distribution of surgical pathology reports. Some pathology computer systems now make provision for direct fax transmittals in batches from electronic memory, circumventing the need to print "hard" copies of the reports. Obviously, there are some problems relating to the confidentiality of reports sent in this fashion, but these appear to be remediable with appropriate system "passwords" entered by fax recipients.[49]

ROLES OF SURGICAL PATHOLOGISTS

As alluded to earlier, the surgical pathologist must be more than a mere provider of diagnostic labels. His or her fulfillment of a more expansive role in hospital practice has *always* distinguished the laboratorian of value from more mundane cohorts. This area is considered in the following sections of this chapter.

General clinical consultation

Because of his or her de facto role as a non–primary care physician, the surgical pathologist is, by definition, a consultant in all respects. The act of consultation in this context is the procurement of a tissue sample to be analyzed and is therefore a more implicit one than that experienced by other "secondary" providers such as radiologists or anesthesiologists.

It is because of the indirect, or "user-transparent," nature of such consultative activities that many clinicians have become misinformed or misdirected in their interactions with the surgical pathology laboratory. For example, it is currently rather common for specimens to be submitted with unsolicited demands for certain special studies or processing requirements. This practice ignores and, in fact, insults the expertise of the physician (pathologist) recipient and should be discouraged. It is tantamount to a pathologist telling a surgeon which knots to tie or which instrument to use. As outlined by Silverberg,[3] pathologists have the right to demand that decisions on tissue processing and interpretation of biopsy specimens be theirs alone. But, they also must assume the obligation to provide all clinically relevant pathologic information on each case and to perform all studies that are relevant and can legitimately be expected.

Intraoperative consultations (IOC) represent very special circumstances in which the pathologist is asked to provide special expertise. A surgeon's general tendency is to equate IOC with the performance of frozen-section examinations, but, here again, the laboratory physician has the prerogative to decide whether cryostat sections are the best means of specimen examination or, indeed, whether any microscopic examination is necessary. In fact, this point has been addressed specifically by several authors in the past with the conclusion that cytologic preparations (fine-needle aspirates; "scrape," "crush," or "imprint" smears) are actually safer for laboratory personnel (in dealing with potentially infectious tissues), faster to make, as accurate, and of considerably higher morphologic quality than frozen sections.[50-53] These two generic categories of tissue preparation were found to be complementary by Mair and associates, with an overall accuracy of 99.5% when they were used together.[53] The major area of superiority of frozen section over cytologic examinations is that of determining the adequacy of surgical margins.[3,52,53]

Traditionally, the major justification for an IOC has been that the surgeon has reached a point in the procedure where morphologic information is necessary for immediate operative planning. Thus, it is important for the surgical pathologist to educate himself or herself regarding the consequences of assorted frozen-section diagnoses. Even more essentially, the skilled pathologist must engage in active interposition to help the surgeon make any number of dichotomous decisions in the surgical suite. As mentioned earlier, there are now chronologic and "cost-effectiveness" factors to consider in deciding on the

Large Bowel (Colon and Rectum) - Colectomy and AP Resections for Carcinoma

1. ____ A neoplasm is present (C1)
   ____ There is no residual carcinoma (prior therapy was extirpative) (**T0**) (C0)

2. The tumor is located in the:
   ____ appendix (C1)
   ____ cecum (C2)
   ____ ascending colon (C3)
   ____ hepatic flexure (C4)
   ____ transverse colon (C5)
   ____ splenic flexure (C6)
   ____ descending colon (C7)
   ____ sigmoid colon (C8)
   ____ rectum (C9)
   ____ dentate (pectinate) line (C10)

3. The principal histologic pattern is:
   ____ adenocarcinoma, enteric type (C11)
   ____ adenocarcinoma, enteric type with mucinous component comprising ≤50% of the tumor (C12)
   ____ adenocarcinoma, with mucinous component comprising >50% of the tumor (C13)
   ____ adenocarcinoma, signet-ring cell type (C14)
   ____ adenocarcinoma, small cell type (C15)
   ____ adenosquamous carcinoma (C16)
   ____ squamous cell (epidermoid) carcinoma (C17)
   ____ neuroendocrine carcinoma, small cell type (C18)
   ____ neuroendocrine carcinoma, large cell type (C19)
   ____ carcinoid tumor (C20)
   ____ carcinoma, mixed type (specify types and relative proportions):
   ____
   ____ (C21)
   ____ other (specify): ________________________________ (C1A)
   ____

4. The lesion is:
   ____ well differentiated (C22)
   ____ moderately differentiated (C23)
   ____ poorly differentiated (C24)
   ____ undifferentiated (C25)

5. Tumor Size
   The maximum tumor diameter (luminal aspect) is: ____ cm (C26)
   The maximum tumor thickness is: ____ cm (C27)

Fig. 3-2A Sample synoptic checklist for resections done for colorectal carcinomas. The responsible housestaff and staff members in surgical pathology select and check the appropriate entries on the working draft.

6. Specimen Margins

The length of the specimen is: ____ cm (C28)
The distance from the tumor to the proximal margin is: ____ cm (C29)
The distance from the tumor to the distal margin is: ____ cm (C30)
The distance from the tumor to the closest margin is: ____ cm (C31)
(unoriented specimens only)
The distance from the tumor to the radial soft-tissue margin is: ____ cm (C32)
(rectal carcinomas and AP resections only)

7. Tumor Staging

Depth of Invasion:
____ the depth of invasion cannot be assessed **(TX)** (C33)
____ tumor is confined to the lamina propria **(Tis)** (C34)
____ tumor invades into submucosa **(T1)** (C35)
____ tumor invades into the muscularis propria **(T2)** (C36)
____ tumor invades through muscularis propria into subserosa or into nonperitonealized soft tissues **(T3)** (C37)
____ tumor penetrates serosal surfaces **(T3)** (C38)
____ tumor invades regional organs or adjacent structures **(T4)**: (C39)
  ____ a tumor fistula is not present (C40)
  ____ a tumor fistula is present (C41)
____ tumor involves retroperitoneal soft tissue or abdominal wall **(T4)** (C42)

Nodal Involvement:
The total number of lymph nodes examined is: ____ (if zero:**NX**) (C43)
____ no lymph node metastases are present **(N0)** (C44)
____ metastases are present in less than four (4) nodes **(N1)** (C45)
____ metastases are present in four (4) or more nodes: (C46)
  ____ involved nodes are not along a named vascular trunk **(N2)** (C47)
  ____ involved nodes are along a named vascular trunk **(N3)** (C48)
The total number of involved lymph nodes is: ____ (C49)
____ extranodal soft-tissue metastases are present **(N3)** (C50)
(does not include extracapsular spread of nodal metastasis)

Distant Metastases:
____ no distant metastases are reportedly present **(M0)** (C51)
____ liver metastases are identified **(M1)** (C52)
____ metastases to distant sites other than liver are identified **(M1)** (C53)

8. TNM Stage (AJCC/UICC) Based on this information, the tumor is:

____ Stage 0 **(Tis;N0;M0)** (C54)
____ Stage I **(T1 or T2;N0;M0)** (C55)
____ Stage II **(T3 or T4;N0;M0)** (C56)
____ Stage III (any **T;N1,2 or 3;M0)** (C57)
____ Stage IV (any **T;**any **N;M1)** (C58)

9. Presence of Other Neoplastic Lesions

Adenomatous Changes in Primary Carcinoma Site:
____ a preexisting neoplastic polyp is not present at the primary lesion site (C59)
____ a preexisting polyp is present at the primary lesion site (specify type):
________________________________ (C60)

Adenomatous Changes Distant to Primary Site:
____ no separate neoplastic polyps are present (C61)
____ separate neoplastic polyps are present (C62)
the number of polyps is: ____
the histologic type of the polyp(s) is (are): ____________________

Fig. 3-2A *(Continued)*

defensibility of IOC, but laboratory physicians should never compromise their abilities to deliver a definitive final diagnosis by the expediencies of an injudicious frozen section. Hence they do have the right to decline to perform an IOC if, in their best judgment, it is contraindicated. As an example, it would be patently foolish to undertake detailed histologic diagnosis of a small-cell pulmonary neoplasm by frozen section of a tiny transbronchial biopsy sample (Fig. 3-5). Experience has likewise shown that frozen-section examinations of breast biopsy samples and thyroid nodules are fraught with difficulty and carry a relatively high risk of error. This problem relates to tissue distortion induced by the procedure itself and also to sampling artifact. Some surgeons also may request an IOC merely because they are curious about the results (but will not depend on them for any short-term decisions), or they wish to "take a break" from operating room tedium. As emphasized by Ackerman and Ramirez,[54] both indications are inappropriate and may be rightly challenged, inasmuch as agreement to do the IOC may well delay providing results to other surgeons operating at the same time.

Another area of practice in which surgical pathologists are directly engaged as consultants is that of fine-needle aspiration (FNA).[55] This procedure is typically both performed and interpreted by pathologists, at the request of clinical physicians.[56,57] It has proved to be an extremely useful technique for relatively noninvasive sampling of virtually all tissue sites, particularly if it is done with radiologic support. As mentioned above, FNA also can be utilized in the frozen-section laboratory to replace or supplement cryostat sections.[53] From the vantage point of the pathologist, its advantages in each of these settings are those of superior morphologic detail, rapidity, and enhanced volumetric sampling.[58] In some centers, clinicians also perform FNA biopsies; however, if the resulting slide preparations are suboptimal, the pathologist should attempt to educate the operator on proper technique, or, preferably, substitute for him or her.[57]

Surgical pathologists often serve as consultants for one another as well by specific request or when reviewing materials on patients who have had a surgical procedure at one institution and are referred to another. In these instances, common courtesy obligates the originator of the specimens to send a complete representation of the case (hematoxylin and eosin–stained slides, special stains, written reports, etc.), and in turn the recipient provides a similarly comprehensive consultative report and returns a copy of it to the first pathologist. Clinicians often want sections of controversial cases reviewed beyond the confines of their own hospitals. Pathologists may acquiesce to this request, but they should retain the prerogative of choosing the outside consultant. The latter proviso reflects the reality that clinicians may be poorly informed or uninformed regarding the expertise of particular pathologists at other medical centers and tend to make their choices based on overall, *institutional* reputations or the stature of their analogous clinical department at another center. Under no circumstances should specimens ever be given to researchers or others to do with as they wish, because of the huge potential for diagnostic confusion that this action generates. Diagnostic material is the property and *responsibility* of surgical pathology.

Quality control

There are very few physicians in any medical center who are positioned more favorably than surgical pathologists regarding quality assurance issues. Because of the certainty that a tissue diagnosis provides, the appropriateness and accuracy of other procedures and the efficacy of treatment may be judged by comparison. Thus pathologists often serve in key roles on hospital "tissue committees," "tumor boards," and general quality control review organizations. There, in concert with clinical colleagues, decisions on prospective patient management and retrospective assessments of care are made.

In a more immediate sense, the surgical pathologist must also keep abreast of new developments in clinical diagnosis and treatment so that "continual quality improvement" (CQI) of general hospital services may take place. The need for often expensive, new procedures must be carefully monitored by pathologists, not only in their own departments, but in others as well. Clinical physicians requesting the services of a surgical pathologist should expect to present evidence that the results of such a consultation will be used in a cogent fashion, rather than contributing to factual "fishing expeditions," which may attend difficult cases. Similarly, demands to perform largely experimental tests on tissue specimens, under the guise of clinical applicability, can and should be questioned seriously by laboratory physicians. The pertinent literature should be reviewed and analyzed, and the assay in question should be performed only if it appears to provide unique and independently valuable information. These decisions are often unpopular with clinical colleagues, but they are an integral part of the pathologists' function as "gatekeepers" of healthcare resources.

A stringent protocol of internal quality assurance also is expected of surgical pathologists. When they practice as a group, difficult or potentially controversial cases should be shown to several people intramurally and a record of this activity should be included in the report. When a dissenting opinion arises as a result, the case may be referred to an extramural consultant, as mentioned above, with similar documentation. Other intradepartmental areas for ongoing quality control include histologic preparations and special techniques; mislabeling, mishandling, and loss of specimens in the accessioning area and the gross room; adequacy of specimen labeling; congruence of frozen section and permanent section diagnoses; and turnaround times for final diagnostic reports. Guidelines relative to many of these parameters have been published by the Association of Directors of Anatomic and Surgical Pathology.[59,60]

As a final entry in this section, it should be noted that several opportunities exist currently for surgical pathologists to participate in organized, continuing education programs and assessments of professional performance that are sponsored by national societies in pathology.[61,62] These represent excellent avenues for additional documentation of individual diagnostic competence and quality assurance, and they are highly recommended.

Tissue archivist

Because of the intensity with which applied biomedical research is being conducted today on a worldwide scale, surgical pathologists, particularly at academic medical centers, are commonly deluged with requests (and demands) to relinquish portions of excised specimens for investigative uses. The drawbacks to unquestioning participation in such ventures again relate to compromises that may result in the ability to evaluate optimally the tissue in question. As examples, tumors for which precise mea-

BARNES HOSPITAL
WASHINGTON UNIVERSITY MEDICAL CENTER
LAUREN V. ACKERMAN LABORATORY
OF SURGICAL PATHOLOGY

Surg. Path. No.:

Name:

GROSS

The specimens are received in two containers of formalin, both labeled with the patient's name. The first container is labeled "right colon" and contains a partial ileocolectomy specimen that measures 28 cm in total length (fixed state) with the ileum measuring 9 cm and the right bowel measuring 18.5 cm. Adjacent to the ileocecal valve is a cupped, solid pink-tan tumor mass, with rolled edges. The luminal aspect of the tumor is pink-tan and shiny and measures 4.7 x 2.6 cm. The maximal depth of invasion is 0.6 cm. The tumor appears to invade through muscularis propria into the surrounding subserosal tissue. Further lesions are not appreciated with the uninvolved bowel mucosa being shiny, tan and plicated. A large piece of omental fat, measuring 15 x 7 x 1 cm, is attached to the distal resection margin. Multiple lymph nodes are found. Labeled: A1 through A3, tumor; B1, proximal margin; B2, distal margin; C, random colon; D, random ileum; and peri-ileal lymph node; E, possible omental lymph nodes; F1 through F3, pericolonic lymph nodes. Jar 2.

The second container is labeled "ileal pouch" and contains two segments of bowel, oriented perpendicularly to each other, with one of the segments inserting into the mid portion of the other. These segments each measure 3 cm in length by 2 cm in cross sectional diameter. A small amount of peri-ileal fat is attached to the specimen. The serosal surfaces are pink-tan, shiny, and smooth. At the anastomosis site, the mucosa is mildly hyperemic but the mucosa away from the anastomotic site is unremarkable, tan and plicated. One of the segments of bowel is consistent with ileum while the other is consistent with colon. Multiple sutures are noted at the anastomotic site. No lesions are seen. Labeled G, tissue from anastomotic site. Jar 2. (cs/sam)

COMMENT

SYNOPTIC REPORTING FORM FOR CARCINOMAS OF LARGE BOWEL

1. A neoplasm is PRESENT (C1)

2. The LOCATION of the tumor is the:
   Cecum (C2)

3. The HISTOLOGIC TYPE of the tumor is:
   Adenocarcinoma, enteric type (C11)

Fig. 3-2B The synoptic checklist (p. 39) is transformed by the transcriptionist's key strokes into a final format, which is incorporated into the formal surgical pathology report for that case.

surements have apparent staging or diagnostic value (such as carcinomas of the breast, carcinomas of the lung, parathyroid adenomas) can obviously not be analyzed properly if large portions of them have been cut away in the operating room and sent to a research laboratory before review by a pathologist. Similarly, confinement of certain lesions (such as follicular thyroid neoplasms, thymomas) within capsular boundaries has a direct bearing on diagnosis or prognosis but may be impossible to evaluate if the specimen has been violated.

Thus pathologists have traditionally and rightly insisted on having departmental representatives serve as members of institutional human studies committees, cooperative oncology groups, and other organizations that make research requests for human tissues. Decisions on such matters must be made that do not place the clinical evaluation process at risk. They also should maintain the integrity of institutional tissue archives that are required by most hospital bylaws and state statutes of limitation.

BARNES HOSPITAL
WASHINGTON UNIVERSITY MEDICAL CENTER
LAUREN V. ACKERMAN LABORATORY
OF SURGICAL PATHOLOGY

Surg. Path. No.

Name:

COMMENT (continued)

4. The GRADE of the tumor is
   Moderately-differentiated (C23)

5. The MAXIMUM TUMOR DIAMETER (luminal aspect) is 4.7 cm. (C26)
   The MAXIMUM TUMOR THICKNESS is 0.6 cm. (C27)

6. SPECIMEN MARGINS
   The length of the specimen is 27 cm. (C28)
   The distance from the tumor to the proximal margin is 9 cm. (C29)
   The distance from the tumor to the distal margin is 13 cm.

7. TUMOR STAGING
   DEPTH OF INVASION
   Tumor penetrates serosal surfaces (T3) (C38)
   NODAL INVOLVEMENT:
   The total number of lymph nodes examined is: 13.
   Metastases are present in less than four nodes (N1) (C45)
   The total number of involved lymph nodes is 2. (C49)
   DISTANT METASTASES:
   No distant metastases are identified (M0) (C51)

8. TNM STAGE (AJCC/UICC) Based on this information, the tumor is:
   Stage III (T3/N1/M0) (C57)

9. PRESENCE OF OTHER NEOPLASTIC LESIONS - None.

{End of Report}

11/19/93 sam

Mitchell Ryan
Gross Pathologist

Mark Wick, M.D.

Fig. 3-2B ***(Continued)***

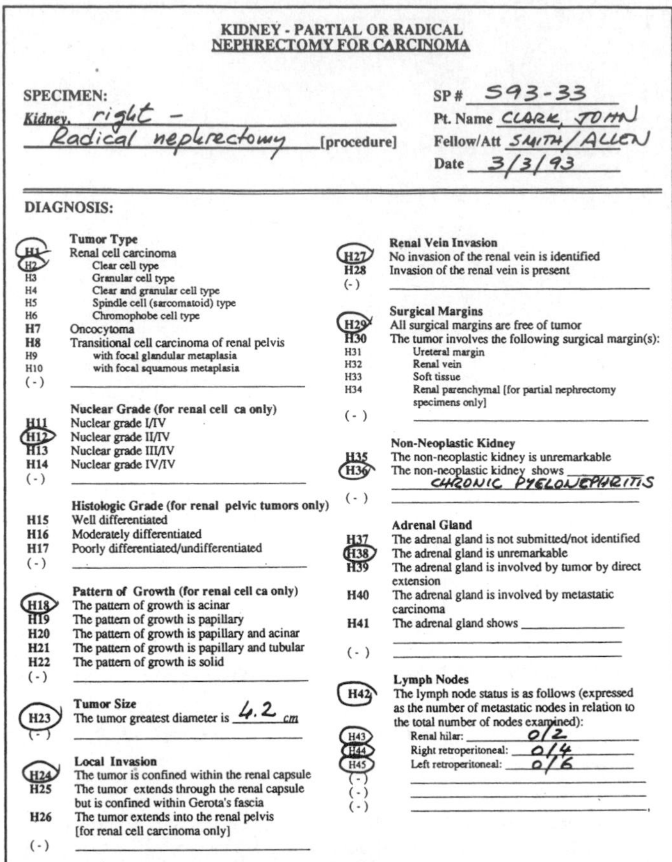

KIDNEY - PARTIAL OR RADICAL
NEPHRECTOMY FOR CARCINOMA

SPECIMEN:
Kidney, right -
Radical nephrectomy [procedure]

SP # S93-33
Pt. Name CLARK, JOHN
Fellow/Att SMITH/ALLEN
Date 3/3/93

DIAGNOSIS:

Tumor Type
H1 Renal cell carcinoma
H2 Clear cell type
H3 Granular cell type
H4 Clear and granular cell type
H5 Spindle cell (sarcomatoid) type
H6 Chromophobe cell type
H7 Oncocytoma
H8 Transitional cell carcinoma of renal pelvis
H9 with focal glandular metaplasia
H10 with focal squamous metaplasia
(-) ________

Nuclear Grade (for renal cell ca only)
H11 Nuclear grade I/IV
H12 Nuclear grade II/IV
H13 Nuclear grade III/IV
H14 Nuclear grade IV/IV
(-) ________

Histologic Grade (for renal pelvic tumors only)
H15 Well differentiated
H16 Moderately differentiated
H17 Poorly differentiated/undifferentiated
(-) ________

Pattern of Growth (for renal cell ca only)
H18 The pattern of growth is acinar
H19 The pattern of growth is papillary
H20 The pattern of growth is papillary and acinar
H21 The pattern of growth is papillary and tubular
H22 The pattern of growth is solid
(-) ________

Tumor Size
H23 The tumor greatest diameter is 4.2 cm
(-) ________

Local Invasion
H24 The tumor is confined within the renal capsule
H25 The tumor extends through the renal capsule but is confined within Gerota's fascia
H26 The tumor extends into the renal pelvis [for renal cell carcinoma only]
(-) ________

Renal Vein Invasion
H27 No invasion of the renal vein is identified
H28 Invasion of the renal vein is present
(-) ________

Surgical Margins
H29 All surgical margins are free of tumor
H30 The tumor involves the following surgical margin(s):
H31 Ureteral margin
H32 Renal vein
H33 Soft tissue
H34 Renal parenchymal [for partial nephrectomy specimens only]
(-) ________

Non-Neoplastic Kidney
H35 The non-neoplastic kidney is unremarkable
H36 The non-neoplastic kidney shows CHRONIC PYELONEPHRITIS
(-) ________

Adrenal Gland
H37 The adrenal gland is not submitted/not identified
H38 The adrenal gland is unremarkable
H39 The adrenal gland is involved by tumor by direct extension
H40 The adrenal gland is involved by metastatic carcinoma
H41 The adrenal gland shows ________
(-) ________

Lymph Nodes
H42 The lymph node status is as follows (expressed as the number of metastatic nodes in relation to the total number of nodes examined):
H43 Renal hilar: 0/2
H44 Right retroperitoneal: 0/4
H45 Left retroperitoneal: 0/6
(-) ________
(-) ________
(-) ________

Fig. 3-3 Alternative reporting form, intended to yield a prose-style final report for malignant tumors of the kidney. This sample form yields the following diagnosis: Kidney, right, radical nephrectomy: renal cell carcinoma, clear cell type, nuclear grade 2/4. The pattern of growth is acinar. The greatest tumor diameter is 4.2 cm. The tumor is confined within the renal capsule. No invasion of the renal vein is identified. All surgical margins are free of tumor. The nonneoplastic kidney shows chronic pyelonephritis. The adrenal gland is unremarkable. The lymph node status is as follows (expressed as the number of metastatic nodes in relation to the total number of nodes examined): renal hilar: 0/2; right retroperitoneal: 0/4; left retroperitoneal: 0/6. (From Rosai J: *Am J Clin Pathol* 100:240, 1993.)).

The long-term "banking" of tissue specimens, particularly neoplasms, in liquid nitrogen or ultracold refrigerators is to be encouraged. Such specimens may assume great importance over time, particularly with the increasing development of molecular biologic techniques of potential clinical relevance. Under appropriate conditions, such material may also be used for more purely research or investigative purposes. However, such tissue *must always* remain under the ultimate control of surgical pathologists because they assume the responsibility and long-term liability for diagnoses based on this material. *Under no circumstances* should researchers, clinicians, or others not trained in surgical pathology be allowed to remove tissue from a surgical specimen before its examination by a surgical pathologist. As discussed above, to do so is to court disaster for both the patient and the pathologist.

Medicolegal consultation

The foregoing comments serve to introduce another important function of surgical pathologists—that of serving as maintenance personnel for the legal integrity of pathologic materials and records at any given medical center. It is required that a permanent record of all specimen evaluations be kept in the pathology laboratory, at least for as long as is dictated by existing statutes. This has become progressively more difficult in recent years, as patients increasingly seek consultants' opinions at other hospitals and are enrolled in regional or national treatment protocols that require outside review of pathologic specimens.

The risks of tissue blocks being exhausted by requests for slide recuts and the certainty that many slides sent away for review will be lost are perplexing outgrowths of augmented specimen entropy. In this context, it is likely that there will be increasing institutional dependence on electronic data archives in pathology in the future. Properly labeled photographic images of gross and microscopic specimens can be stored on "compact disc–read only memory" (CD-ROM) devices that are space efficient and resistant to damage.[63] Similarly, microfiche or computer text-entry documents can replace paper case records.

Table 3-1 TNM staging of breast cancer

T = Primary tumor		
TX	Primary tumor not assessable	
T0	No evidence of primary tumor	
Tis	Carcinoma in situ	
T1	Primary tumor < 2 cm	
	T1a	< 0.5 cm
	T1b	0.5 to < 1.0 cm
	T1c	> 1.0 to 2.0 ≤ cm
T2	Primary tumor > 2 to 5 ≤ cm	
T3	Primary tumor > 5 cm	
T4	Direct extension to skin or chest wall	
	T4a	Extension to chest wall
	T4b	Cutaneous edema
	T4c	Both T4a and T4b
	T4d	Inflammatory carcinoma
N = Regional lymph nodes		
NX	Regional nodes not assessable	
N0	No regional nodal metastasis	
N1	Metastasis to mobile ipsilateral axillary nodes	
N2	Metastasis to fixed ipsilateral axillary nodes	
N3	Metastasis to ipsilateral internal mammary nodes	
M = Distant metastasis		
MX	Distant metastasis not assessable	
M0	No distant metastasis	
M1	Distant metastasis present	

Stage grouping			
Stage 0	Tis	N0	M0
Stage I	T1	N0	M0
Stage II	T0	N1	M0
	T1	N1	M0
	T2	N0	M0
	T2	N1	M0
	T3	N0	M0
Stage III	T0	N2	M0
	T1	N2	M0
	T2	N2	M0
	T3	N1-2	M0
	T4	any N	M0
	any T	N3	M0
Stage IV	any T	any N	M1

Name: DOE, Sara
*Hosp. No.:*123456
Loc.: 5W *Age:* 34
Ser.: URO *Sex:* F

Accession No: S89-10000

Accession Date: 05/13/89
Physician(s): Harrison, John
Referral Physician(s)

Surgical Pathology
University of Nebraska Hospital and Clinic
Department of Pathology and Microbiology
42nd & Dewey Avenue, Omaha, NE 68105
(402) 559-4186 Fax: (402) 559-6018

Diagnosis:
Left Nephrectomy with renal artery stenosis

History:
The patient is a 34 year old female with hypertension.

Source/Gross:
The specimen consists of a kidney measuring 7x5x3cm and weighing 150gms. The surface of the kidney is smooth. On bisection the renal parenchyma , calyceal system and renal pelvis is unremarkable. Attached to the kidney is 3cm of unremarkable ureter. The renal vein measures 2cm in length and is likewise unremarkable. The renal artery measures 3.5cm in length and ranges from 0.4cm to 0.2cm in diameter. An area of apparent renal artery stenosis is present 1.5 cm from the distal surgical margin.

Microscopic:
Sections reveal normal renal parenchyma with tubules in a back to back configuration. Glomeruli are present in normal number and configuration. Parenchymal blood vessels show mild focal thickening of the intima. Sections of the grossly observed stenotic area reveals fibromuscular hyperplasia with near total occulusion of the lumen.

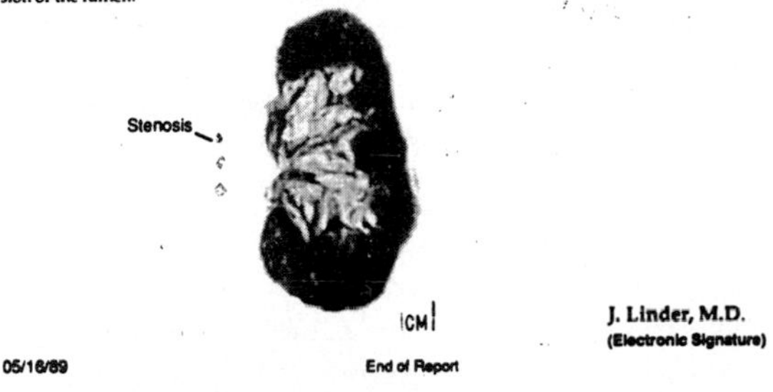

J. Linder, M.D.
(Electronic Signature)

05/16/89 End of Report

Fig. 3-4 Example of surgical pathology report containing a digital gross photographic image of the specimen. (From Linder J: *Am J Clin Pathol* 94(suppl 1):530, 1990.)

In keeping with their generally consultative activities in the medical community at large and their broadly based knowledge, surgical pathologists are commonly engaged to provide objective opinions for attorneys in matters of litigation. Topics for possible medicolegal consultations are broad and include personal injury, particularly concerning various environment-related diseases having characteristic tissue manifestations, putative malpractice in laboratory medicine, and questions of malpractice in selected clinical areas, regarding the necessity for and procurement of diagnostic tissue specimens. In addition, the pathologist's general expertise regarding the natural history of disease processes may be of considerable value in assessing claims regarding the potential effects of treatment modalities and treatment "delays" on the course of disease. Details of the law in these areas clearly exceed our ability to discuss them here, and they can be found in other references specifically addressing such issues.[3,64]

Education

When asked, most surgical pathologists relate having chosen this area of practice because of its intellectual challenges, broad scope of operations, and breadth of contact with other specialty groups. There are really no restrictions on the anatomic sources from which modern-day specimens may be obtained, and, in that sense, the pathologist is one of the last true "generalists" in medicine.

For these reasons, surgical pathologists find themselves engaged, on a daily basis, in reviewing pathologic observations with many physicians, presenting their findings at interdepartmental hospital conferences, and interacting closely with clinical services in choosing optimal patient management. There is probably no area of the hospital where students, residents, and colleagues can obtain as much information or correlate it as well with other patient-related studies as they can in the laboratory.[65] Astute clinicians are acutely aware of this fact, and often seek such consultations. It is for all these individuals—teachers and students alike[66]—that this chapter has been written.

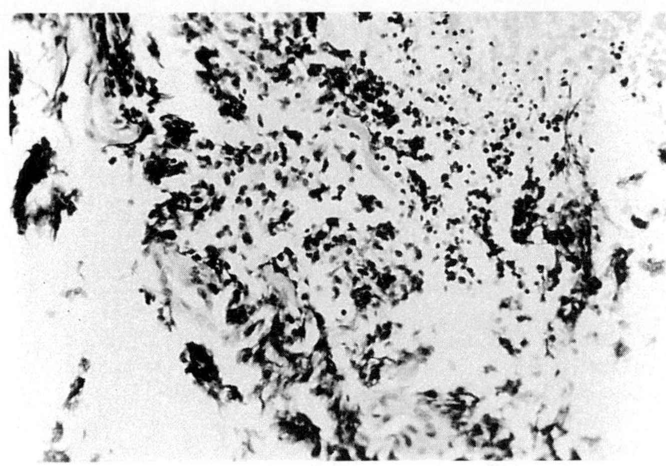

Fig. 3-5 Example of unacceptable distortion introduced by cryostat sectioning of a small cell tumor of the bronchus. This procedure also consumed the entire specimen, leaving none for permanent section examination.

REFERENCES

1. Rosai J, editor: *Ackerman's surgical pathology,* ed 7, St. Louis, 1989, Mosby.
2. Sternberg SS, editor: *Diagnostic surgical pathology,* ed 2, New York, 1994, Raven Press.
3. Silverberg SG, editor: *Principles and practice of surgical pathology,* ed 2, New York, 1990, Churchill-Livingstone.
4. Coulson WF, editor: *Surgical pathology,* ed 2, Philadelphia, 1983, Lippincott.
5. Karcioglu ZA, Someren A, editors: *Practical surgical pathology,* Lexington, Mass, 1985, Collamore Press.
6. Underwood JCE, editor: *Introduction to biopsy interpretation and surgical pathology,* ed 2, London, 1987, Springer-Verlag.
7. Sheldon H: *Boyd's introduction to the study of disease,* ed 9, Philadelphia, 1984, Lea & Febiger.
8. Castiglioni A: *A history of medicine,* New York, 1947, Knopf.
9. Osler W: *The evolution of modern medicine,* New Haven, Conn, 1921, Yale University Press.
10. Fechner RE: One century of mammary carcinoma *in-situ:* what have we learned? *Am J Clin Pathol* 100:654, 1993.
11. Bloodgood JC: The clinical and pathological differential diagnosis of diseases of the female breast, *Am J Med Sci* 135:157, 1908.
12. Bennett JH: Introductory address to a course of lectures on histology and the use of the microscope, *Lancet* 1:517, 1845.
13. Donaldson F: The practical application of the microscope to the diagnosis of cancer, *Am J Med Sci* 25:43, 1853.
14. Beale LS: *The microscope in medicine,* London, 1854, Churchill.
15. Ober WB: The case of the Kaiser's cancer, *Pathol Annu* 5:207, 1970.
16. Virchow R: Professor Virchow's report on the portion of growth removed from the larynx of H.I.H. the Crown Prince of Germany by Dr. M. MacKenzie on June 28th, *Br Med J* 2:199, 1887.
17. Wright JR: The development of the frozen section technique, the evolution of surgical biopsy, and the origins of surgical pathology, *Bull Med Histol* 59:295, 1985.

18. Cullen TS: A rapid method of making permanent specimens from frozen sections by the use of formalin. *Johns Hopkins Hosp Bull,* p. 67, Baltimore, 1895.
19. Wilson LB: A method for the rapid preparation of fresh tissues for the microscope, *JAMA* 45:1737, 1905.
20. Azar HA: Arthur Purdy Stout (1885-1967): the man and the surgical pathologist, *Am J Surg Pathol* 8:301, 1984.
21. Fenoglio CM: Raffaele Lattes, M.D, *Am J Surg Pathol* 4:107, 1980.
22. Seemayer TA: The life and legacy of Professor Pierre Masson, *Am J Surg Pathol* 7:179, 1983.
23. Dehner LP: Lauren Vedder Ackerman, M.D. (1905-1993), *Am J Clin Pathol* 100:709, 1993.
24. McManus JFA: William Boyd: a biographical sketch, *Am J Surg Pathol* 3: 377, 1979.
25. Boyd W: *Surgical pathology,* Philadelphia, 1925, Saunders.
26. Fechner RE: Anatomic pathology in the 1980's: a decade of new information and new challenges, *Am J Clin Pathol* 96(suppl 1):S10, 1991.
27. Anderson RE, Hill RB: The current status of the autopsy in academic medical centers in the United States, *Am J Clin Pathol* 92(suppl 1):S31, 1989.
28. Ritter JH, Sutton TD, Wick MR: The use of immunostains to ABH blood group antigens to resolve problems in the identity of tissue specimens, *Arch Pathol Lab Med* 118:293, 1994.
29. Shibata D: Identification of mismatched fixed specimens with a commercially-available kit based on the polymerase chain reaction, *Am J Clin Pathol* 100:666, 1993.
30. McNeely MDD: Advances in medical informatics during the 1980's, *Am J Clin Pathol* 96(suppl 1):S33, 1991.
31. Frappart L, Remy I, Lin HC et al: Different types of microcalcifications observed in breast pathology: correlations with histopathological diagnosis and radiological examinations of operative specimens, *Virchows Arch (A)* 410:179, 1986.
32. Tischler AS, Martin MR: Generation of surgical pathology reports using a 5000-word speech recognizer, *Am J Clin Pathol* 92(suppl 1):S44, 1989.
33. Chambers AL: Speech technology in the emergency room, *Speech Technol* 4:50, 1987.
34. Robbins AH, Horowitz DM, Srinivasan MK et al: Speech-controlled generation of radiology reports, *Radiology* 164:569, 1987.
35. Weaver VM, McDiarmid MA, Guidera JA et al: Occupational chemical exposures in an academic medical center, *J Occup Med* 35:701, 1993.
36. Partanen T: Formaldehyde exposure and respiratory cancer—a meta-analysis of the epidemiologic evidence, Scand J Work Environ Health 19:8, 1993.
37. Occupational Safety and Health Administration: Occupational exposure to formaldehyde, *Fed Reg* 52:46168, 1987.
38. Bankowski MJ, Landey AL, Kessler S: Postmortem recovery of human immunodeficiency virus type I from plasma and mononuclear cells: implications for occupational exposure, *Arch Pathol Lab Med* 116:1124, 1992.
39. Orient JM: Assessing the risk of occupational acquisition of the human immunodeficiency virus: implications for hospital policy, *South Med J* 83:1121, 1990.
40. Carson FL: *Histotechnology: a self-instructional text,* Chicago, 1990, ASCP Press.
41. Thompson SW, Luna LG: *An atlas of artifacts,* Springfield, Ill, 1978, Charles C Thomas, Publisher.
42. Oneson RH, Minke JA, Silverberg SG: Intraoperative pathologic consultation: an audit of 1,000 recent consecutive cases, *Am J Surg Pathol* 13:237, 1989.
43. Wick MR: Oncogene analysis in diagnostic pathology: a current perspective, *Am J Clin Pathol* 97(suppl 1):S1, 1992.
44. Linden MD, Torres FX, Kubus J, Zarbo RJ: Clinical application of morphologic and immunocytochemical assessments of cell proliferation, *Am J Clin Pathol* 97(suppl 1):S4, 1992.
45. Quinn CM, Wright NA: The clinical assessment of proliferation and growth in human tumors: evaluation of methods and applications as prognostic variables, *J Pathol* 160:93, 1990.
46. Markel SF, Hirsch SD: Synoptic surgical pathology reporting, *Hum Pathol* 22:807, 1991.
47. Rosai J: Standardized reporting of surgical pathology diagnoses for the major tumor types: a proposal, *Am J Clin Pathol* 100:240, 1993.
48. Linder J: Overview of digital imaging in pathology: the fifth wave, *Am J Clin Pathol* 94(suppl 1):S30, 1990.
49. Wick MR, Mills SE: Unpublished observations on the CoMed/CoPath[R] Commercial Pathology Computer System, 1993.
50. Bloustein PA, Silverberg SG: Rapid cytologic examination of surgical specimens, *Pathol Annu* 12(2):251, 1977.
51. Costa M, Sidawy MK: Diagnosis of benign follicular lesions of the thyroid: intraoperative cytology, *Mod Pathol* 2:521, 1989.
52. Sakai Y, Lauslahti K: Comparison and analysis of the results of cytodiagnosis and frozen section during operation, *Acta Cytol* 13:359, 1969.
53. Mair S, Lash RH, Suskin D, Mendelsohn G: Intraoperative surgical specimen evaluation: frozen section analysis, cytologic examination, or both? A comparative study of 206 cases, *Am J Clin Pathol* 96:8, 1991.
54. Ackerman LV, Ramirez GA: The indications for and limitations of frozen section diagnosis: a review of 1269 consecutive frozen section diagnoses, *Br J Surg* 46:336, 1959.
55. Koss LG, Woyke S, Olszewski W, editors: *Aspiration biopsy: cytologic interpretation and histologic bases,* ed 2, New York, 1992, Igaku-Shoin.
56. Japko L: Aspiration biopsy: the pathologist as hands-on consultant, *Diagn Cytopathol* 2:233, 1986.
57. Grohs HK: The interventional cytopathologist: a new clinician-pathologist hybrid, *Am J Clin Pathol* 90:351, 1988.
58. Layfield LJ, Tan P, Glasgow BJ: Fine needle aspiration of salivary gland lesions: comparisons with frozen sections and histologic findings, *Arch Pathol Lab Med* 111:346, 1987.
59. Association of Directors of Anatomic & Surgical Pathology: Standardization of the surgical pathology report, *Am J Surg Pathol* 16:84, 1992.
60. Association of Directors of Anatomic & Surgical Pathology: Recommendations on quality control and quality assurance in anatomic pathology, *Hum Pathol* 22:1099, 1991.
61. Zarbo RJ: Interinstitutional assessment of colorectal carcinoma surgical pathology report adequacy: a College of American Pathologists' Q-probes study of practice patterns from 532 laboratories and 15,940 reports, *Arch Pathol Lab Med* 116:1113, 1992.
62. Kraemer BB: Quality assurance activities of the College of American Pathologists, *Acta Cytol* 33:434, 1989.
63. Nathwani BN, Heckerman DE, Horvitz EJ, Lincoln TL: Integrated expert systems and videodisc in surgical pathology: an overview, *Hum Pathol* 21:11, 1990.
64. Mason JK: Special medicolegal considerations in pediatric pathology, *Leg Med* 1:1, 1992.
65. McBroom HM, Ramsay AD: The clinicopathologic meeting: a means of auditing diagnostic performance, *Am J Surg Pathol* 17:75, 1993.
66. Gorstein F, Trelstad R: The pathologist as student and educator, *Hum Pathol* 21:1, 1990.

4 Cytopathology

James Linder
William W. Johnston

The origins of cytopathology date back more than a century. As early as the second quarter of the nineteenth century, European microscopists observed morphologic differences between human cells in health and disease. Subsequently, case studies in the late 1800s and early 1900s demonstrated that cancer could be diagnosed by the study of cells shed in body fluids and obtained by aspiration.[1] Particularly notable were studies in the late 1920s and early 1930s by Martin Ellis, Stewart, and Ewing on the aspiration biopsy of human tumors[2] and the landmark report by Papanicolaou and Traut in 1943 on the detection of carcinoma of the uterine cervix in vaginal smears.[3] The latter, of course, came to be known as the "Pap smear."

Pioneers of cytologic methods made a key observation that holds true today: *The power of cytopathology lies in its simplicity.* Diagnoses can be made by the study of spontaneously exfoliated cells, as obtained from the uterine cervix, lung, or urinary tract; cells that are mechanically dislodged by scraping, washing, or brushing; and cells and tissue fragments that are easily collected by needle aspiration of superficial or deep masses, such as those that occur in the thyroid and breast or lung and liver. Surprisingly, though, many years passed between the early descriptions of the cytologic method and its broad acceptance as either a screening test or a diagnostic tool. There were multiple reasons for this delay, but the major ones rested in the reluctance of pathologists in general to accept the basic principle on which cytopathology rested: morphologic changes in individual cells reflect the disease processes present in the tissues from which they are derived. Many pathologists simply refused to recognize the existence of a "cancer cell" that could be distinguished from a benign cell. In the Western world, microscopic examination of tissues had become established as the standard for cancer diagnosis.

Cytopathology has moved to center stage in contemporary anatomic pathology. Here it occupies two distinctly different roles, serving either as a screening test or as a diagnostic procedure. The Papanicolaou smear, or cervicovaginal smear, is the classic example of a screening test, and it has had unparalleled success in the detection of cellular abnormalities of the cervix before they progressed to invasive carcinoma. Since the late 1940s, the incidence and mortality for invasive carcinoma of the cervix have declined 70% to 75% in the United States. The widespread use of the Papanicolaou smear is generally cited as the major factor influencing these trends.[4]

The success of the Papanicolaou smear ultimately fostered interest in other cytologic procedures, including examination of cellular material from the respiratory tract, body cavity fluids, cerebrospinal fluid, brushing of various body sites, and "rediscovery" of fine-needle aspiration biopsy (FNAB) first in Europe then in the United States. As these procedures were being performed in symptomatic patients, the role of cytopathology as a diagnostic procedure began to emerge.

As a diagnostic procedure, cytologic examination is usually undertaken when there is a clinical suspicion of disease. For example, a lung mass may be sampled to determine if the mass is attributable to infection, cancer, or other causes. Nowhere is the diagnostic power of cytopathology more evident than in the case of FNAB. In most organs, the concordance between cytopathologic diagnosis by FNAB and open tissue biopsy reaches or exceeds 95%. This concordance should not be unexpected because each method relies on a relatively defined set of rules and concepts to discriminate between different diseases. However, cytopathology has not been uniformly accepted as a diagnostic tool. Many physicians retain the view that cytopathology can only guide the further evaluation of the patient, for example, suggesting when an open biopsy is needed. Unfortunately, this view is furthered by some pathologists who routinely refuse to render a definitive cytologic diagnosis. A pathologist does little to enlighten his or her clinical colleague by labeling a 10 cm lung mass as "suspicious." This approach only adds to the cost of medical care, without tangible benefit to the patient. With the increased use of diagnostic cytopathology in the 1990s, a practical question has emerged: What degree of confidence should be assigned to a cytologic diagnosis? The proposition raised by this question is whether definitive therapy should be based solely on the cytologic diagnosis. There is no simple yes or no answer because the physician offering therapy to a patient must consider the clinical history, results of the physical examination, other laboratory studies, and body site of the lesion. For instance, in the presence of a positive "Pap" smear, biopsy confirmation and staging before therapy are traditional. In contrast, a definitive cancer diagnosis by FNAB of lung cancer in a patient with supporting clinical signs and x-ray findings is a justifiable basis for therapy. A philosophy held by most cytopathologists is that a cytopathologic diagnosis should carry the same level of accuracy as a histopathologic diagnosis. With this view, because surgery or chemotherapy may result from the cytopathologic diagnosis, it is paramount that the pathologist understand the morphologic criteria that distinguish benign from malignant conditions.

The remainder of the chapter is a discussion of three major topics: the morphologic basis for cytopathologic diagnosis, specimen collection and staining, and selected body sites where cytologic diagnosis is useful. A discussion of all aspects of cytopathology is beyond the scope of this chapter, but many excellent general or specialized textbooks of cytopathology are available.[5-13]

PRINCIPLES OF CYTOMORPHOLOGY

For the purposes of diagnostic cytopathology, cells can be categorized morphologically into five groups: normal, reactive, degenerate, dysplastic, and neoplastic. To assign cells into these categories, the cytopathologist evaluates various morphologic features. Although the essence of cytopathology lies in the evaluation of the fine structural detail of cells, evaluation should begin with an appraisal of the cellular specimen under the microscope at low or medium magnification. Here, depending on the type of specimen, the cytopathologist will make initial assessments related to the adequacy of the material for diagnostic interpretation. The degree of cellularity of the specimen is an important criterion, particularly in FNAB when the differential diagnosis lies between a benign versus a malignant tumor. The assessment of the individual cells is based on several parameters, such as cell size, cell shape, the ratio of nuclear area to cytoplasmic area, cytoplasmic qualities such as staining or the presence or absence of mucin, nuclear qualities including the size, shape, and distribution of chromatin and the number, size, and shape of nucleoli. The statements that follow refer to cells stained by the Papanicolaou method, which is preferred by most American pathologists because it provides an excellent rendition of nuclear morphology and differential staining of the cytoplasm.

In the general evaluation of the cell, there are three broad principles: (1) morphologic features of the nucleus are most critical to discriminate benign cells from malignant cells, (2) cytoplasmic features generally provide clues that are suggestive of the manner of cell differentiation (such as squamous versus glandular), and (3) a cytologic diagnosis almost always requires the consideration of multiple morphologic features for proper classification of cells. A corollary to this last statement is that the diagnosis of malignancy always requires the consideration of multiple features. No single cytologic feature is diagnostic of malignancy.

A discussion of the practical use of these morphologic features to classify cells accurately follows.

The normal cell

Illustrated in Figs. 4-1 to 4-4 are normal cells from three different body sites: mature squamous cells and endocervical cells from the uterine cervix, ciliated columnar cells from the

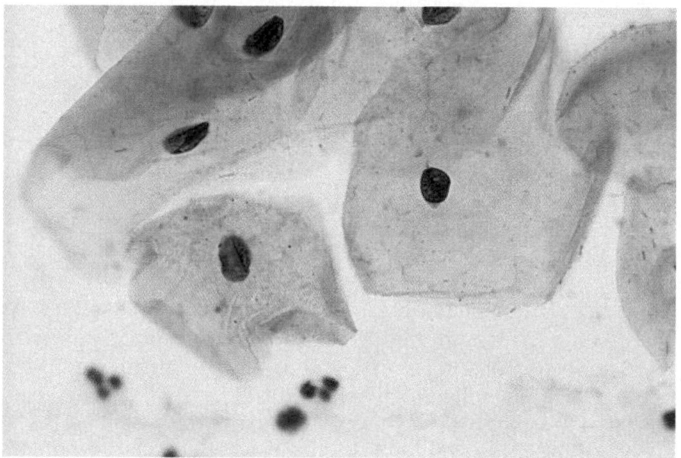

Fig. 4-1 Normal intermediate squamous cells from the uterine cervix. (Papanicolaou stain.)

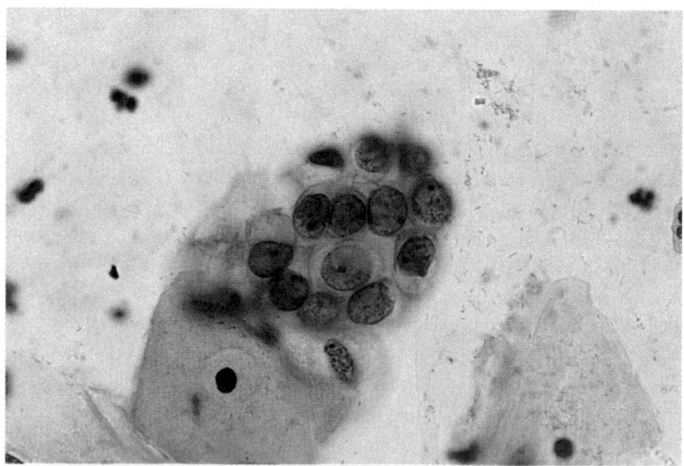

Fig. 4-2 Normal columnar cells from the endocervix. (Papanicolaou stain.)

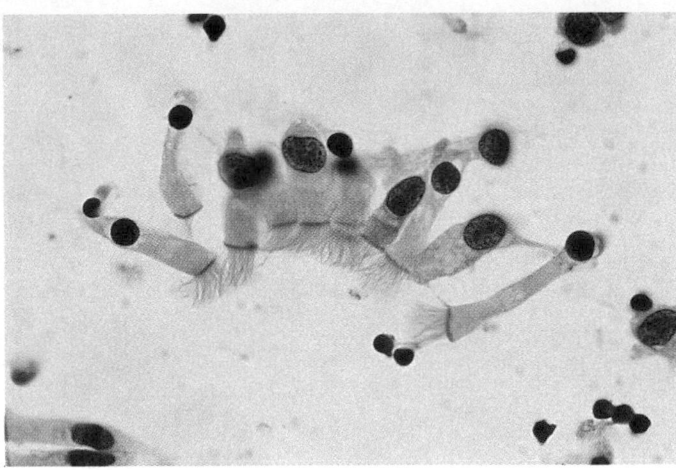

Fig. 4-3 Normal ciliated columnar cells from the bronchus. (Papanicolaou stain.)

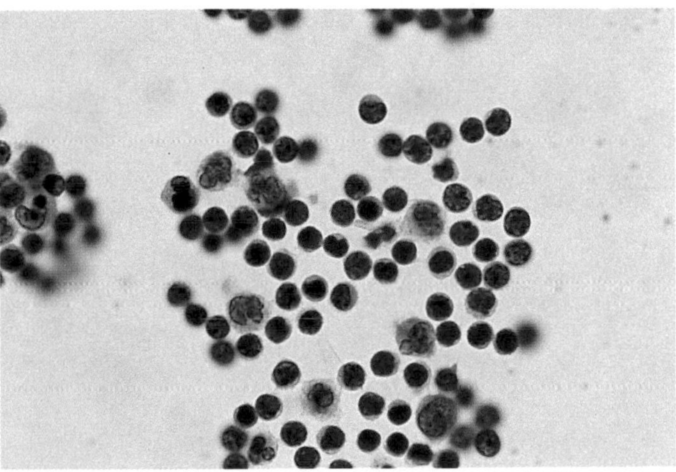

Fig. 4-4 Mature lymphocytes and macrophages in pleural effusion. (Papanicolaou stain.)

bronchus, and mature lymphocytes and macrophages from a pleural effusion. It is evident that the appearances of normal cells differ enormously according to their origin. They may be large, small, rectangular, round, polygonal, or spindle shaped. The amount of cytoplasm may be scanty, or it may be abundant. Yet there are features that are characteristic of normal cells. Frost, when describing the normal cells, stresses the principles of roundness, uniformity, and predictability.[11] The location of nuclei in cells is of some diagnostic importance; for example, in columnar cells they are basally located, whereas in squamous cells they are centrally placed. Normal nuclei tend to be round or oval. Nuclear chromatin is typically evenly dispersed, a feature that one best assesses by mentally dividing the nucleus into quadrants and comparing the chromatin mass within each quadrant. In normal cells, the amount of chromatin within each quadrant is relatively equal, though in some normal cells, notably lymphocytes, substantial clumping of chromatin is present. Some of the chromatin is deposited along the nuclear envelope. This defines the boundary between the nucleus and cytoplasm, which is referred to by the light microscopist as the "nuclear membrane." In normal cells this membrane is uniform in thickness.

Nucleoli may be present, or absent, in normal cells. Their presence indicates that the cells are metabolically active, producing protein or ribosomal RNA. The number, size, and shape of nucleoli have diagnostic utility. The number of nucleoli within cells of a benign proliferating population should be approximately equal. Nucleoli are generally small, as opposed to the macronucleoli of some malignant cells. Nucleoli of nonneoplastic cells are rounded or slightly polygonal, instead of the sharp, angulated nucleoli that may characterize malignant neoplasms. Study of the cytoplasm of the cell may provide valuable information about its differentiation. The cytoplasm of mature squamous cells is abundant and wafer thin around a centrally placed nucleus. Orangeophilia or eosinophilia indicates keratin production. The cytoplasm of columnar cells may be finely or coarsely vacuolated, an indication of the production of serous or mucous secretory products. Identification of various cytoplasmic pigments may give information about differentiation and cell function. The presence of true cilia in a cell is a powerful marker for benignancy.

The reactive cell

Benign cells may reflect responses to many different external stimuli by profound changes in their morphology. The resultant cell forms have been called by various names including reactive cells, irritated cells, hyperplastic cells, hypertrophic cells, and proplastic cells.[5,6,10,11] These reactive cells are exceedingly common and are to be found in all body sites accessible to sampling by cytologic methods. The provocative stimuli are of multiple and various causes and include mechanical trauma, various toxic and noxious external environmental agents, infectious organisms, drugs, ionizing radiation, and chemotherapeutic agents. The cellular response to these insults is characterized by cellular enlargement, nuclear enlargement, and increase in nuclear activity. The last is characterized by increasing granularity and hyperchromasia of the chromatin, thickening of the nuclear membrane, and increase in size and number of nucleoli. Pleomorphism in cell size may occur, but the relative shapes remain uniform. In extreme examples of this reactive process the cells may begin to mimic the changes of dysplastic and even malignant cells. In particular, reactive changes in cells in response to ionizing irradiation and anticancer chemotherapeutic agents can be so severe as to make their distinction from cancer cells impossible morphologically. Examples of various types of reactive cells are depicted in Figs. 4-5 to 4-8.

In the event that the stimuli are violent enough to provoke cell death, a proliferation of reparative cells may result. Because reparative cells are actively dividing and synthesizing protein, morphologic evidence of extreme nuclear activity may be present. Again, distinction between these changes and malignancy may be very difficult. Examples of reparative changes in cells are illustrated in Fig. 4-9.

The degenerate cell

Although cell degeneration and death are normal at the end of a cell's life-span, they may also be an indicator of injury. Cell degeneration is significant to the cytopathologist because of its potential to be misinterpreted as malignancy. During degeneration the nucleus may become swollen and portions of the cytoplasm lost. This imparts the impression of an elevated nuclear to cytoplasmic ratio. Also, during degeneration the chromatin may begin to clump and become hyperchromatic

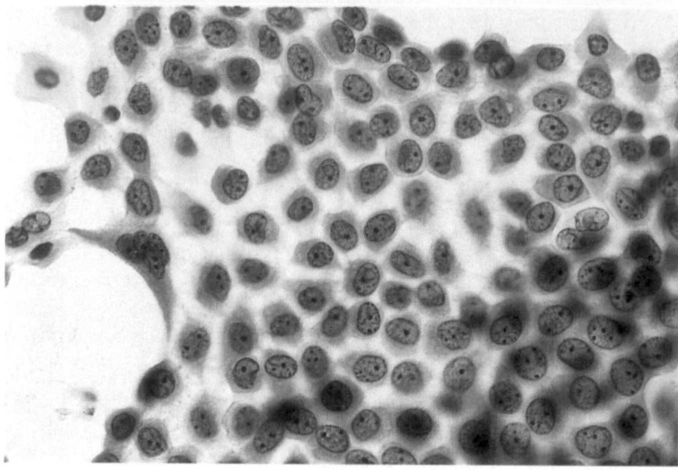

Fig. 4-5 Reactive mesothelium in pleural effusion. (Papanicolaou stain.)

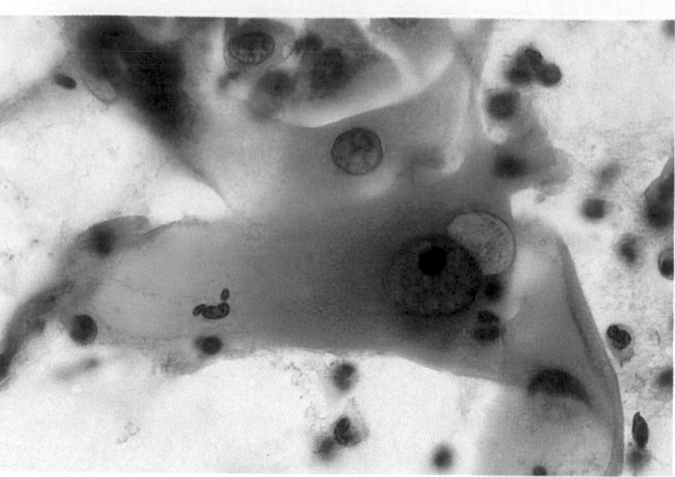

Fig. 4-8 Cellular changes in squamous cells from the vagina in response to ionizing irradiation. (Papanicolaou stain.)

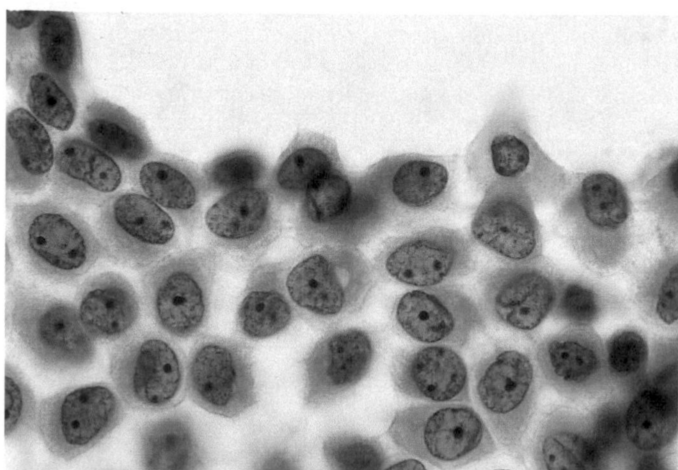

Fig. 4-6 Reactive mesothelium in pleural effusion. (Papanicolaou stain.)

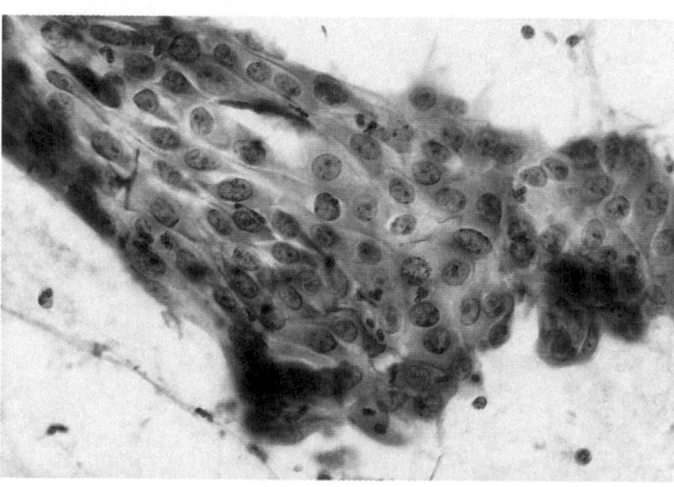

Fig. 4-9 Reparative changes in squamous cells from the uterine cervix. (Papanicolaou stain.)

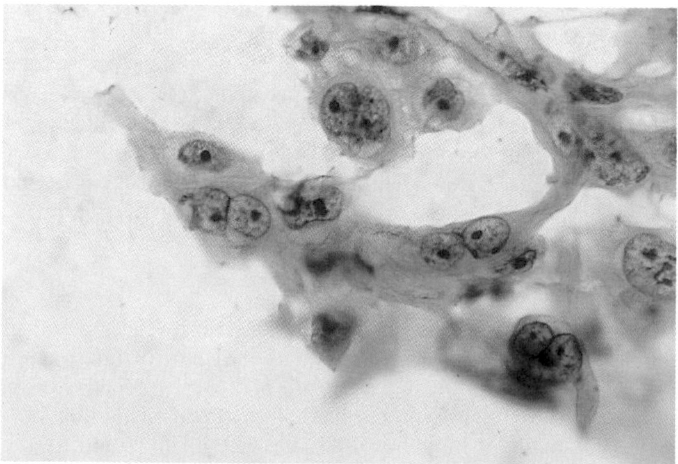

Fig. 4-7 Cellular changes in cells from the bronchus in response to ionizing irradiation. (Bronchial brushing; Papanicolaou stain.)

(karyorrhexis) and the nuclear membrane may become wrinkled. Condensation of the chromatin (karyopyknosis) can be misinterpreted as "ink-dot" nuclei present in some cells from squamous cell carcinoma.

An example of the cell degeneration that may be present in the parabasal cells in vaginal atrophy is shown in Fig. 4-10. Examples of cellular degenerative changes provoked by viral infections are illustrated in Figs. 4-11 to 4-15. These virally induced changes are highly characteristic and virtually diagnostic for the viral agent.

The dysplastic cell

In one standard medical dictionary, dysplasia is defined as "abnormal tissue development." The term is applied to 30 separate diseases, with dysplasia of the uterine cervix being the only one among these referring to a biologic state related to cancer. In the practice of contemporary pathology, the term *dysplasia* most often refers to squamous dysplasia of the uterine cervix, though it is also being used with increasing frequency when one is referring to lesions of the respiratory, gas-

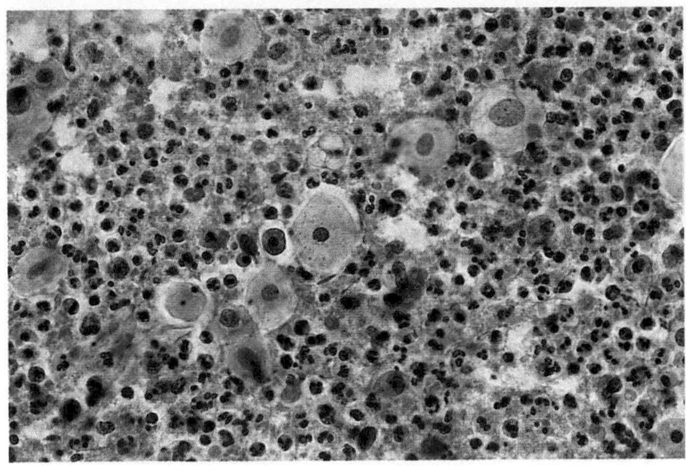

Fig. 4-10 Vaginal atrophy with inflammation, degeneration, and necrosis. (Papanicolaou stain.)

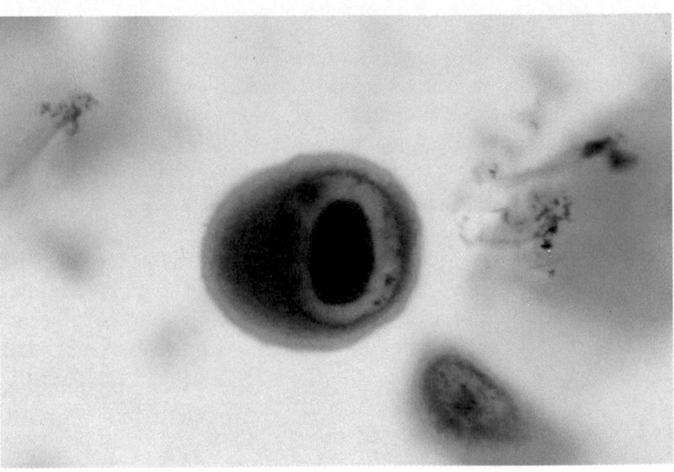

Fig. 4-13 Cytomegalovirus infection. (Bronchial brushing; Papanicolaou stain.)

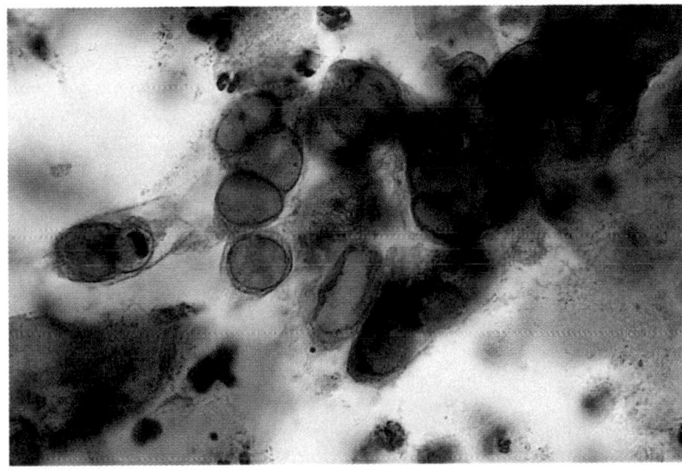

Fig. 4-11 Herpes simplex virus infection. (Papanicolaou smear; Papanicolaou stain.)

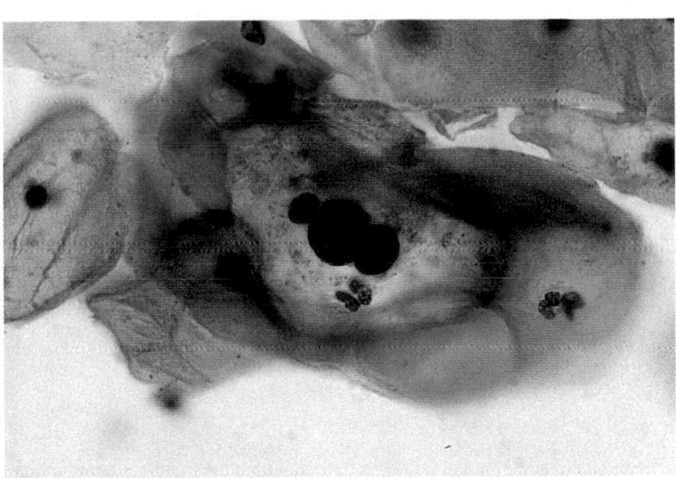

Fig. 4-14 Human *Papillomavirus* infection. (Papanicolaou smear; Papanicolaou stain.)

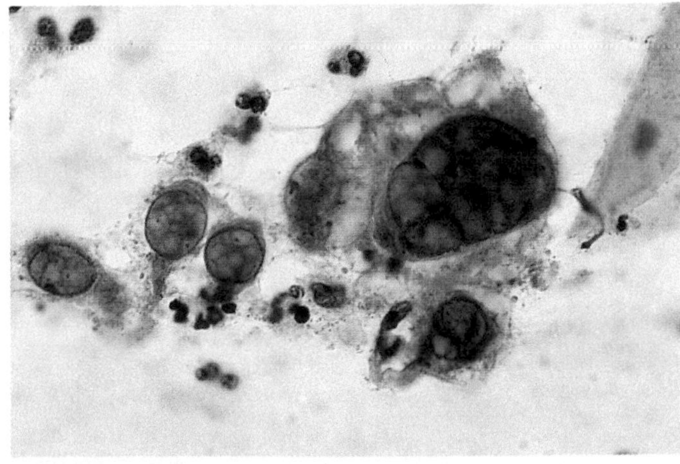

Fig. 4-12 Herpes simplex virus infection. (Papanicolaou smear; Papanicolaou stain.)

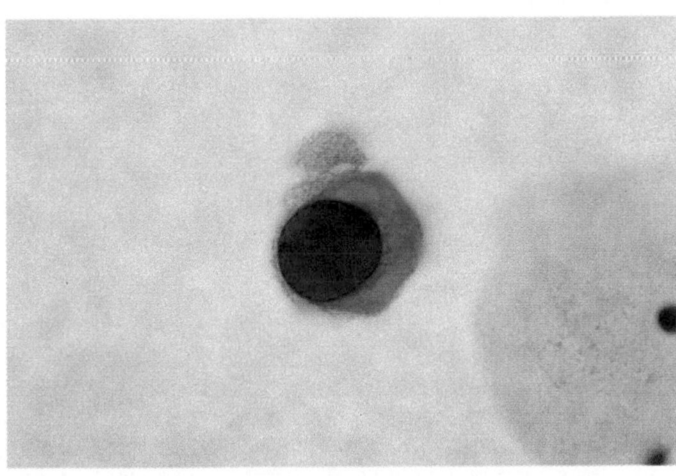

Fig. 4-15 *Polyomavirus* infection. (Urine; Papanicolaou stain.)

trointestinal, and urinary tracts. The cytopathologic concept of dysplasia can be traced back to Papanicolaou's original descriptions of what he termed "dyskaryosis."[12] Cells in a state of gradual transition from normalcy to frank malignancy were described as "dyskaryotic." Their nuclei were characterized by increasing nuclear enlargement, uniform coarsening and hyperchromasia of the chromatin, and thickening of the nuclear membrane. Their cytoplasm exhibited an increasing failure to mature and differentiate. The end stage of this process was considered to be the cell of in situ carcinoma. None of these cellular changes, however, was of a severity equal to that observed in malignant cells from invasive cancer. The term *dysplasia* as applied to these dyskaryotic cells exfoliating from lesions of the uterine cervix was introduced by Reagan in 1953[14] and defined further by an international committee on nomenclature whose recommendations were published in 1962.[15] Out of their deliberations resulted the following definitions:

Carcinoma in situ: Only those cases should be classified as carcinoma in situ which, in the absence of invasion, show a surface lining and epithelium in which, throughout its whole thickness, no differentiation takes place. The process may involve the lining of the cervical glands without thereby creating a new group. It is recognized that the cells of the uppermost layers may show some slight flattening. The very rare case of an otherwise characteristic carcinoma in situ which shows a greater degree of differentiation belongs to the exception for which no classification can provide.

Dysplasia: All other disturbances of differentiation of the squamous epithelial lining of the surface and of glands are to be classified as dysplasia. They may be characterized as of high or low degree, terms which are preferable to suspicious and non-suspicious, as the proposed terms describe the histologic appearance and do not express an opinion.

Patten has defined dysplasia of the uterine cervix as "a spectrum of heteroplastic reactions involving stratified squamous or squamous-like (metaplastic) epithelium."[16] He elaborates further: "Fundamentally, the dysplastic reaction is characterized by a combination of hyperplasia and a block in normal differentiation of the component cells as they reach the uppermost cell layers. The resultant effect is a greater number of cells per unit area and abnormally large nuclei in the upper layers of the involved epithelium."

The degree of dysplasia may be qualified as mild, moderate, or severe. This subjective assessment is subject to interobserver and intraobserver variation, prompting recommendations that dysplasia be quantified as either "low grade" or "high grade." The classification and grading of dysplasia are discussed later in this chapter with reference to the female reproductive tract. Some examples of dysplasias of the uterine cervix of varying degrees of severity are illustrated in Figs. 4-16 to 4-18.

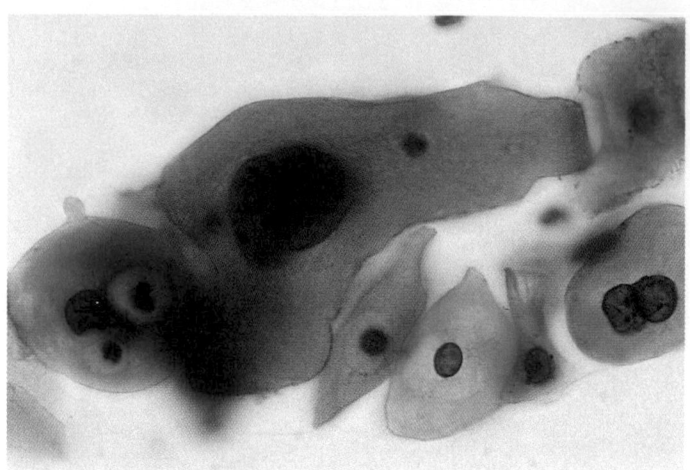

Fig. 4-16 Mild dysplasia of uterine cervix (LSIL, CIN-1; see p. 61 for codes). (Papanicolaou stain.)

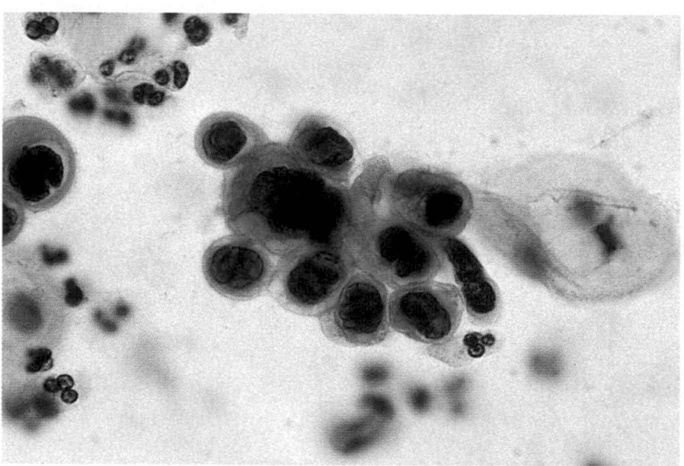

Fig. 4-17 Severe dysplasia of uterine cervix (HSIL, CIN-3). (Papanicolaou stain.)

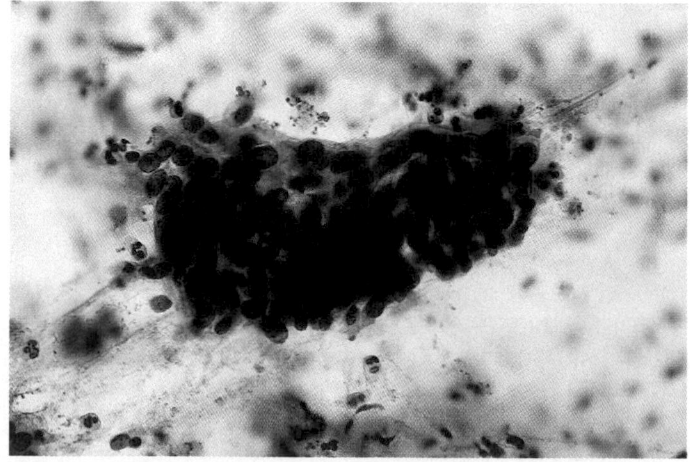

Fig. 4-18 Carcinoma in situ of uterine cervix (HSIL, CIN-3). (Papanicolaou stain.)

The neoplastic cell

The interpretation of a cell as malignant is a statement by the cytopathologist that the cell has the biologic ability to invade tissues and metastasize. It was stated earlier in this chapter that no single morphologic feature allows prediction of malignancy. This concept cannot be overemphasized because grievous diagnostic errors occur when this simple concept is ignored. Major criteria for malignancy are summarized in

Table 4-1. The cytologic features that define a cell as malignant are found principally within the nucleus. Malignant nuclei are abnormally enlarged and often highly variable among a population of cells. They may show extreme abnormalities of nuclear shape, with sharp angulations and deep divot holes or folding of the nuclear membrane. This membrane, which is uniform in thickness in a benign cell, can be variably thick and thin in the malignant nucleus. Likewise, the chromatin may be unevenly distributed as sharply angulated shapes in malignant nuclei, and so certain quadrants contain overly abundant chromatin whereas in others it is relatively scant. Associated with the chromatin abnormalities there may be extreme clearing of the parachromatin areas and variation in the size and shape of these cleared areas within the nucleus. Nucleoli, when present, can assist in the identification of a cell as malignant. When there is pronounced nucleolar enlargement or sharp angulation to the nucleolus, or when there are extreme variations in the numbers of nucleoli between cells, these features favor an interpretation of malignancy.

Aside from the evaluation of single cells, a diagnosis of malignancy is aided by comparisons between individual cells in the overall cell population. Pleomorphism of nuclear and cytoplasmic morphology is the rule, rather than the exception, for a diagnosis of malignancy. Intercellular molding and the presence of inappropriate organelles formed by tissue fragments are two additional criteria of great significance. The malignant cells depicted in Figs. 4-19 and 4-20 illustrate many of the features of malignancy described in this text.

Determining whether a cell is malignant is but one part of the clinical question. Classifying the type of malignancy (such as carcinoma, lymphoma) determines the therapy that the patient will receive. This decision is based on morphologic features within the cell cytoplasm and upon relationships between cells. Figs. 4-21 and 4-22 contrast the appearance of cytoplasm in squamous cell carcinoma of the lung, and adenocarcinoma of the lung. Characteristically, cells with squamous differentiation have dense cytoplasmic orangeophilia with the Papanicolaou stain. This staining quality is found in malignant squamous cells from many body sites. In contrast, the cells of adenocarcinoma have cyanophilic staining and may demonstrate mucin-containing vacuoles in the cytoplasm.

The size of malignant cells and their relationship to one another also help to determine differentiation. Cells from so-called small-cell undifferentiated carcinomas of the lung and

Table 4-1 **Criteria for malignancy in cells**

I. **Nuclear features**
  A. Chromatin
    1. Hyperchromatic
    2. Abnormally hypochromatic (some adenocarcinomas)
    3. Irregularly dispersed as sharply angulated masses
    4. Parachromatin abnormally cleared
  B. Nuclear membrane
    1. Pronounced thickening abruptly merging with pronounced thinning
    2. Pronounced angularity in outline
  C. Nucleolus
    1. Increase in size and number
    2. Pronounced irregularity in shape
    3. Variation in size, shape, and number from cell to cell
    4. Perinucleolar clearing
  D. Mitotic activity
    1. Significant only if abnormal mitotic figures present
II. **Cytoplasmic features**
  A. Decreased with respect to total cell volume (usually expressed as increase in nuclear-to-cytoplasmic ratio)
  B. Abnormal maturation and differentiation
III. **Nuclear and cytoplasmic relationships**
  A. Increase in relative volume of the cell occupied by the nucleus
  B. Tendency of nuclear and cytoplasmic membranes to parallel one another at a uniform distance apart for long components of the cell perimeter
IV. **Intercellular relationships**
  A. Pleomorphism in size and shape
  B. Intercellular nuclear-cytoplasmic molding
  C. Inappropriate formation of organelles and acini, papillary fronds, or morulas
V. **Background changes**
  A. Clean
    1. Intraepithelial neoplasia
    2. Metastatic cancer
  B. Dirty (necrosis, inflammation, and old blood)
    1. Invasive cancer

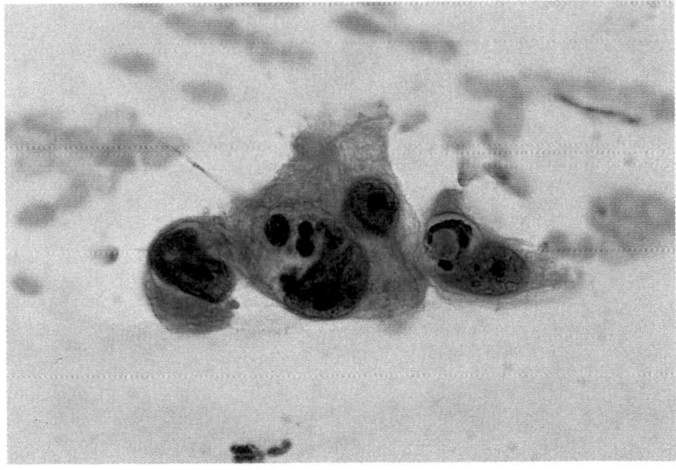

Fig. 4-19 Adenocarcinoma in endocervix. (Papanicolaou stain.)

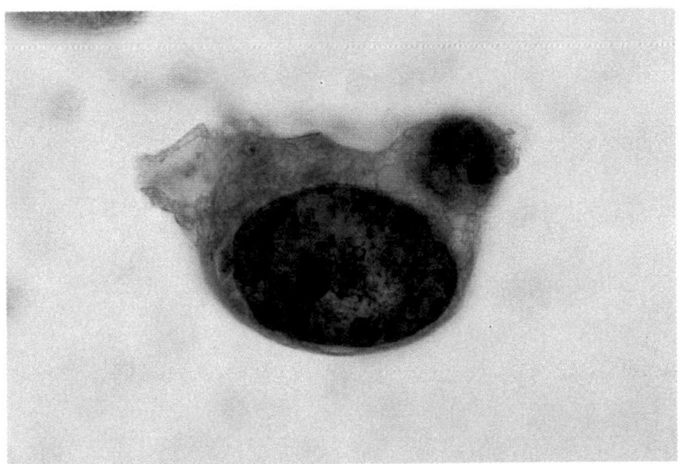

Fig. 4-20 Poorly differentiated squamous cell carcinoma in lung. (Bronchial washing; Papanicolaou stain.)

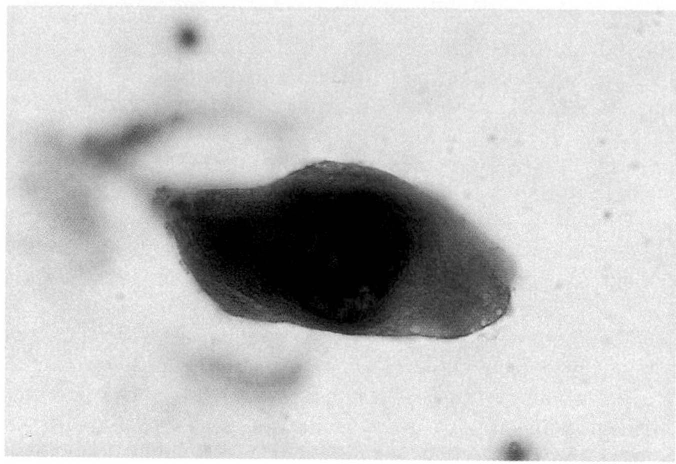

Fig. 4-21 Keratinizing squamous cell carcinoma in lung. (Bronchial brushing; Papanicolaou stain.)

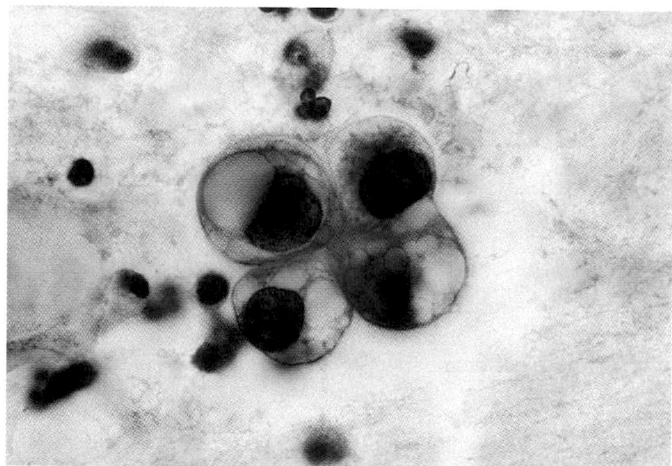

Fig. 4-22 Adenocarcinoma in lung. (Sputum; Papanicolaou stain.)

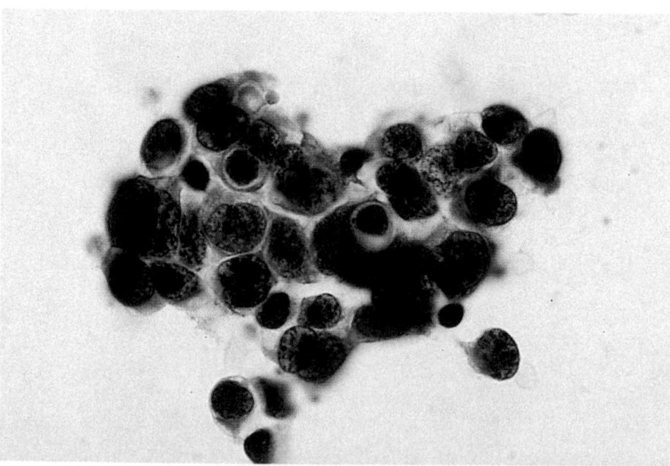

Fig. 4-23 Small-cell undifferentiated carcinoma in lung. (Bronchial brushing; Papanicolaou stain.)

other body sites have a diameter smaller than the diameter of those from squamous cell carcinoma and adenocarcinoma arising in those organs. Cell size and shape, the relative lack of cytoplasm, and a tendency of the cells to mold around one another are important diagnostic features for this type of malignancy (Fig. 4-23).

PREPARATION OF THE CELLULAR SPECIMEN

As is the case for all the biomedical sciences that depend on microscopic anatomy, diagnostic accuracy in cytology rests upon a foundation of excellence in cytopreparatory techniques. A cellular specimen that has been prepared for cytologic diagnosis exhibits an abundance of well-preserved and meticulously stained diagnostic cellular material, has been prepared rapidly and with relative ease, and will remain preserved for permanent slide storage.[17]

The staff in the cytopathology laboratory must play an active role in ensuring proper collection of specimens. This may include formal in-service lectures, a constant dialog with the clinical staff to comment on the adequacy of collected materials, and a manual of written instructions for specimen procurement available in all clinics and wards. The method of specimen collection differs according to body site. Major collection methods depend on spontaneous cell exfoliation, mechanical scraping, brushing, or lavage of an epithelial surface, body cavity or organ, and fine-needle aspiration of suspicious masses.

Exfoliation

Spontaneously exfoliated cells are the mainstay of cytologic diagnosis, principally because of their ease of collection. Among the earliest demonstrations of the cytologic method were the diagnosis of lung cancer in cells exfoliated into sputum.[1] Similarly, the cervical Papanicolaou smear depends on cell exfoliation, albeit with the gentle coaxing by brush or spatula. Exfoliated cells are usually prepared for cytologic examination by the careful spreading of cellular material onto a glass slide. If Papanicolaou staining is anticipated, this slide should be fixed in 95% alcohol, or with a suitable spray fixative within 10 seconds after smearing. Delays in fixation cause air-drying, which compromises the nuclear detail that can be revealed by the Papanicolaou stain. Alternatively, the slides may be allowed to air-dry, for staining with Wright-Giemsa or Diff-Quik stains.

Brushing techniques

Brushing is the favored method for collecting many specimens. In the uterine cervix, the transformation zone, or squamocolumnar junction, is best sampled by a brush. Brushing of the esophagus, stomach, lung, or colon is commonly performed during endoscopic examination. Endoscopic brushing can specifically sample a visible lesion. A major pitfall in the evaluation of brush specimens is the risk of misinterpretation of a sample as abnormal, simply because many cells are present. Although brushing techniques characteristically recover large numbers of cells, that in itself does not indicate that the sample is malignant. Cells with morphologic features of malignancy must be present. The high yield of cells by brush techniques is an important consideration for cytopathologists who are accustomed to endocervical samples collected with a swab. In brushing, the better preservation of endocervical cells and their large number can cause an erroneous diagnosis of endocervical dysplasia or adenocarcinoma.

Body fluids

Cells within fluids are commonly collected from tapping of the subarachnoid space for cerebrospinal fluid, from tapping of pleural, pericardial, and peritoneal effusions, from spontaneously voided urine, or from lavage of the lung, stomach, or other body cavity. Common methods for processing this fluid include membrane filtration and cytocentrifugation. Either technique may render specimens suitable for morphologic analysis. Advantages of membrane filtration are superior cell preservation, minimization of cell loss, and the accurate display of the three-dimensional relationships in cells. A disadvantage to membrane filtration is the trapping of extraneous debris and the potential for poor visualization of cells if excessive amounts of protein are trapped in the filter. Cytocentrifugation techniques are popular because of the ease with which specimens are prepared. Excessively bloody specimens may require lysis before being processed. The potential for cell loss is present, and unless careful technique is followed, cells are often distorted by air-drying.

Another option for processing fluid-based specimens relies on recently described monolayer methods. These techniques, originally developed to support the processing of fluid-based gynecologic specimens, are also suitable for nongynecologic materials. These methods, which rely on either density-gradient centrifugation or filtration, yield a relative monolayer of cells well suited for staining and cytologic evaluation. An example of a monolayer prepared from cellular material from the uterine cervix is illustrated in Fig. 4-24.

Fine-needle aspiration biopsy

Needles ranging from 20 to 27 gauge fall under the umbrella of "fine-needle" aspiration. There are several options for preparing cells procured by FNAB. Typically the aspirated material is expressed directly onto a glass slide for preparation of smears that are then either fixed in 95% ethanol for Papanicolaou staining or air-dried for a Romanovsky stain. It is also a common practice to rinse the needle used in the aspiration procedure. This fluid is suitable for processing by membrane filtration or cytocentrifugation. Finally, needle aspiration may yield small tissue fragments that can be used to prepare a cell block for tissue sectioning and hematoxylin and eosin staining.

Staining procedures

The most widely used procedures for the fixation and staining of cytologic specimens are fixation in ethanol or other chemically related alcohols and staining by the Papanicolaou method.[18] This stain embodies the following features: There is a good nuclear stain that demonstrates the detailed structure of the nucleus. The nuclear stain is hematoxylin, which renders chromatin and nuclear membranes blue to purple and nucleoli red, pink, or orange. Differential counterstains bring out certain qualities inherent in the cytoplasm and at the same time provide sharp contrast for the nuclei. The conterstains are orange G, which colors the cytoplasm either yellow or orange if keratin is present, and a polychrome mixture consisting of eosin, light green, and Bismarck brown. The latter stain is no longer used in many laboratories. Cells that have an acidophilic cytoplasm show an affinity for the eosin and take on various shades of pink to yellow. Those with a basophilic cytoplasm are stained pale blue (cyanophilically) or greenish-blue by the light green, a basic stain. Most cornified superficial squamous cells are acidophilic or orangeophilic, whereas other types of cells are most likely to be basophilic. Brown staining from Bismarck brown may be seen in such materials as glycogen, keratohyaline granules, and some microorganisms, particularly fungi. And finally the combination of alcohol fixation with the alcohol-soluble counterstains provides for the preservation of the transparency of the cytoplasm to permit good visualization of underlying cells, since there are often clusters of overlapping cells in cytologic preparations.

Air-dried preparations may be stained by the Wright-Giemsa or Diff-Quik stains. This staining procedure is particularly popular as an adjunct in the evaluation of fine-needle aspiration materials that have been air-dried. A particular advantage of this staining procedure is the ease and rapidity with which it can be performed. It also stains mucins and other mucopolysaccharides metachromatically and as such enhances the diagnosis of adenocarcinoma and tumors that contain

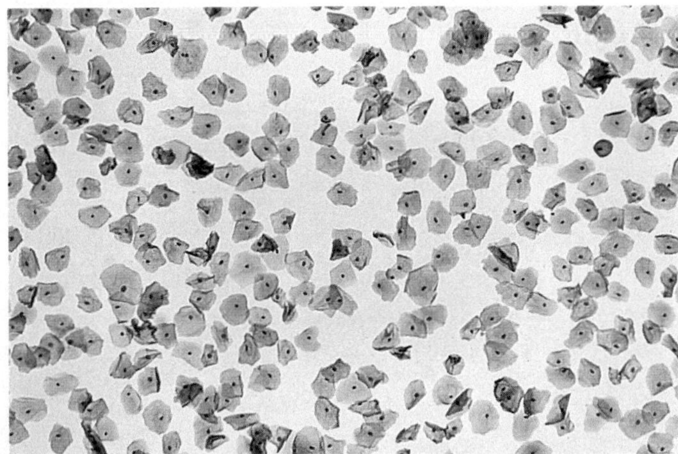

Fig. 4-24 A monolayer of cellular material from the uterine cervix prepared from an automated device. (Papanicolaou stain.)

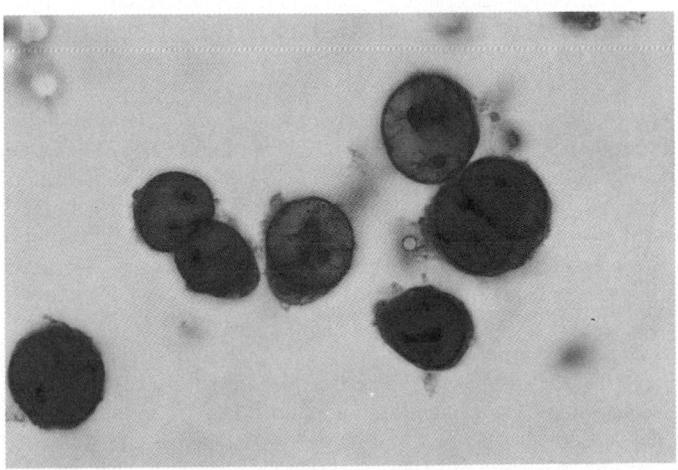

Fig. 4-25 Malignant melanoma cells obtained by fine-needle aspiration biopsy of lymph node. (Toluidine blue.)

stroma and ground substances, such as pleomorphic adenoma of salivary gland (see Fig. 4-65), fibroadenoma of the breast, and adenoid cystic carcinoma.

In supravital staining a drop of a specimen is mixed with toluidine blue or similar stain and mounted under a coverslip. This procedure is particularly well-suited toward evaluation of the adequacy of cytologic specimens. An example of malignant melanoma cells obtained by FNAB and stained by this material is shown in Fig. 4-25.

INFECTIOUS DISEASES

The cytologic identification of infectious organisms may be made in specimens from all the body sites that provide material for cytologic evaluation. Viruses, fungi, and other organisms occur with varying levels of frequency in these body sites, and their morphology is largely independent of the specimen source. The cytologic appearance of the more common organisms is described below. A complete discussion of infectious diseases is found in Chapters 33 to 40.

Cellular manifestations of infectious diseases

In some infectious diseases cellular manifestations of host response to the insult may appear in cytologic specimens. The inflammatory component may be relatively nonspecific, consisting of a mixed inflammatory exudate of neutrophils, lymphocytes, plasma cells, and macrophages. Eosinophils may be suggestive of an allergic response; large numbers of neutrophils may support the suspicion of acute suppurative inflammation or abscess. Perhaps one of the more specific inflammatory responses that can be appreciated in cytologic specimens is granulomatous inflammation. Such changes may be recognized by the presence of epithelioid cells and Langerhans giant cells. A necrotic background corresponding to caseous necrosis may also be present. FNAB offers the added advantage of tissue fragments in which intact tuberculoid granulomas may be seen, particularly if these fragments are examined through paraffin sections of cell blocks. In all these inflammatory reactions, careful search for infectious organisms should be made. Special stains for general bacteria, acid-fast bacteria, fungi, and parasites should be obtained when appropriate. Viral infections may produce changes of diagnostic significance in epithelial cells and are discussed in more detail in the section on viral infections, p. 59.

Fungal infections

Many of the mycotic infections are readily detectable by cytologic methods. In these diseases the etiologic agent is visible and in some cases has a morphology on which a specific diagnosis may be based. The detection of these fungi in a stained cytologic specimen may be the first clue to the nature of the patient's problems. The more common ones are discussed here.

Blastomyces dermatitidis

Infection with *Blastomyces dermatitidis* may closely resemble the appearance and progression of lung cancer. In well-developed cases, the x-ray films show unilateral, dense, irregular shadows that frequently are indistinguishable from those produced by an infiltrating neoplasm. In cytologic materials that have been fixed in 95% alcohol and stained by the Papanicolaou technique, the organism appears as single or budding spherical cells 8 to 15 μm in diameter with thick, refractile walls. The thickness of these walls may impart to these forms a "double-contoured" appearance. No hyphae are seen. Single budding is characteristic, and the bud has a tendency to remain in close apposition to the mother cell such that a flattening of the two surfaces occurs. The wall is highly refractile and may stain a pale blue-green. The presence in itself of these organisms is diagnostic for infection.[19]

Cryptococcus neoformans

The budding yeast of *Cryptococcus neoformans* has been reported in cytologic preparations from many body sites. Although capable of producing primary infection, the organism more frequently is a secondary invader in the debilitated. Single budding is characteristic of this yeast, with the single bud pinching itself off, leaving a greatly attenuated isthmus of attachment to the mother cell and thus assuming a tear-drop shape. The cell is ovoid to spherical, thick-walled, and 5 to 20 μm in diameter. It is usually surrounded by a gelatinous capsule, which may require special stains for visualization (periodic acid–Schiff, mucicarmine, or alcian blue). However, frequently, even with Papanicolaou staining alone, the capsule can be visualized. It may stain faintly cyanophilically or be seen as a nonstaining space between cell body and displaced mucus. The latter effect is similar in principle to an India ink preparation.[20] An example of cryptococcus in sputum is shown in Fig. 4-26.

Coccidioides immitis

Spherules and endospores of *Coccidioides immitis* have been reported in cytologic preparations of sputum, bronchial washings, and fine-needle aspiration biopsy specimens. In Papanicolaou-stained material the spherule appears as a nonbudding, spherical, thick-walled structure, measuring 20 to 60 μm in diameter. Staining characteristics are variable and of little aid in identification. The spherules may be empty or contain endospores. The latter are round, nonbudding structures measuring 1 to 5 μm in diameter. It is easy to confuse the empty spherules with nonbudding forms of *Blastomyces dermatitidis*. Occasionally, arthrospores may be present in sputum; they must be differentiated from those of *Geotrichum*.[21,22]

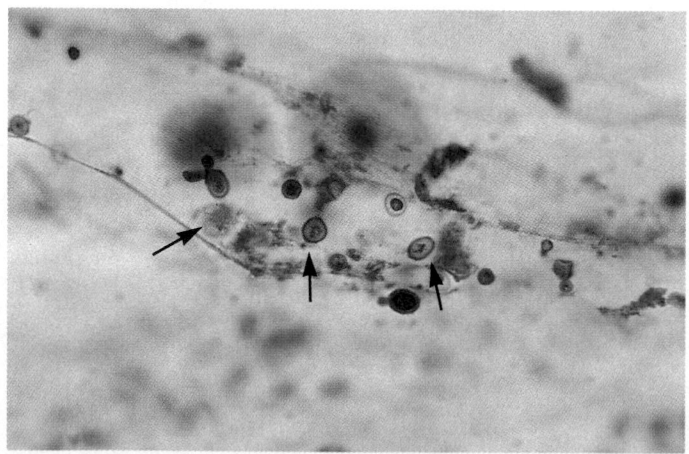

Fig. 4-26 Cryptococcus neoformans. The arrows indicate the yeastlike organisms. (Sputum; Papanicolaou stain.)

Histoplasma capsulatum

Histoplasma capsulatum is seen in sputum, bronchial washings, fine-needle aspiration biopsy specimens, and gastric washings from patients with symptoms. The organism is so small as to make recognition on Papanicolaou-stained specimens difficult. With special staining (particularly methenamine silver) it may be visualized as a 1 to 5 μm round to oval budding yeast. For diagnostic purposes it must be intracellular in macrophages or neutrophils. Some small budding yeasts present as contaminants are remarkable in their resemblance to *Histoplasma,* but they are usually found extracellularly only.[22]

Candida species

Species of *Candida* (most frequently *Candida albicans*) are the most frequently encountered fungi in cytologic specimens. Because of this frequency, their clinical significance must be very carefully assessed. All *Candida* species may appear as small, oval, 2 to 4 μm budding yeasts. Occasionally they may elongate into pseudohyphal forms with additional budding at the points of constriction. Although their presence in pulmonary material is not usually significant, it may reflect an overwhelming candidiasis in the compromised host.

Aspergillus species

Aspergillus (most frequently *Aspergillus fumigatus*) is seen most often in sputum. Its most characteristic presentation is that of thick, septate hyphae with 45 degree angle brushlike branching. The mycelial growth in pulmonary aspergillosis only rarely is associated with the presence of conidiophores, or fruiting heads, so that confusion with phycomycosis may occur; however, fungi producing the latter disease are not septate. The presence of septate, branching hyphae in cytologic material is strong morphologic evidence of infection. An example of this phenomenon is depicted in Fig. 4-27. Cultures alone may indicate *Aspergillus* in the absence of true infection. Occasionally conidiophores may be seen. Mycetomas of the lung produced by *Aspergillus* as well as other fungi may produce pronounced cellular atypias easily mistaken for squamous cell carcinoma. Occasionally their presence may be associated with the production of crystals of calcium oxalate.[23] Identification of oxalate crystals in the cytologic specimen may be the first clue to the presence of *Aspergillus*.

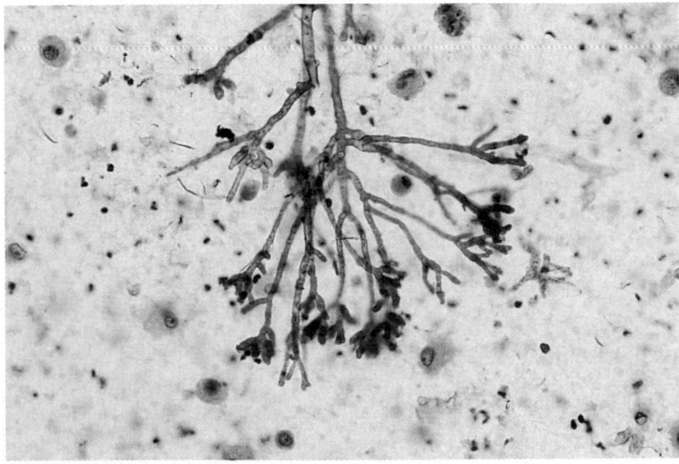

Fig. 4-27 *Aspergillus* species. (Bronchial brushing; Papanicolaou stain.)

Phycomycetes

Phycomycosis is an acute fungus infection occurring in the debilitated patient with diabetes mellitus, leukemia, or lymphoma, and in those patients receiving steroids, chemotherapy, and antibiotics. The disease is characterized by inflammation and vascular thrombosis secondary to invasion of blood vessels by the organism. The disease was originally called mucormycosis because of the belief that the phycomycete *Mucor* was the sole infectious agent. However, in more recent years additional multiple phycomycetes, including *Absidia, Rhizopus, Mortierella,* and *Basidiobolus,* have been isolated from disease. Thus the name "phycomycosis" is now used to describe more correctly the disease. The fungus is characterized by ribbonlike, nonseptate, branching hyphae. They may vary widely in width from 6 to 50 μm. Culture is necessary to identify which fungus is causing the infection.

Parasitic infections

A growing number of parasites are being diagnosed in cytologic material. The two most important ones, *Pneumocystis carinii* (although taxinomically a possible fungus) and *Strongyloides stercoralis,* are discussed here.

Pneumocystis carinii

In recent years, the incidence of *Pneumocystis carinii* pneumonia has been increasing and is now recognized as occurring potentially in any situation of impaired immune response. More particularly, it is seen in infants who are premature or debilitated, in immunologic disorders, in immunoglobulin defects, and in the presence of therapy with corticosteroids and chemotherapy. Currently it is being seen as an infectious complication in patients with acquired immunodeficiency syndrome. The introduction of effective therapeutic drugs has greatly increased the clinical importance of an antemortem diagnosis. On methenamine-silver stains the organism is seen mainly as a spherical cyst measuring 6 to 8 μm in diameter or approximately the diameter of an erythrocyte. Certain variations of this form can be seen. The organism can be cup shaped, crescent shaped, or crinkled. Depending on the surface of the organism that is exposed to view, one can see small interior structures that take the forms of rings, dots, or commas.[24-28] Some laboratories prefer a Giemsa stain for identification of this organism. In this situation one is able to identify up to eight trophozoites occurring within the cyst. These structures are about 0.5 to 1.0 μm in diameter, are easily overlooked, and may be confused with granules or cell fragments.

Recently there has been a renewed interest in the initial recognition of *Pneumocystis carinii* in smears stained by the Papanicolaou method. Greaves and Strigle have described these organisms in such smears as presenting in the form of casts of alveoli.[29] These casts are composed of masses of organisms packed together with a smooth border around the periphery of the mass representing the molding induced by the alveolar walls. Tinctorial characteristics of these masses vary from eosinophilic to cyanophilic. In the experience of the authors, these casts may be seen in sputum, bronchial material, bronchoalveolar lavage, and fine-needle aspiration biopsy specimens. They may be extremely numerous in the presence of massive infection such as that seen in patients with acquired immunodeficiency syndrome and are conclusively diagnostic for *Pneumocystis carinii*. Ghali and associates have reported apple-green fluorescence of these masses in Papanicolaou-stained smears when exposed to ultraviolet radiation.[30] Examples of *Pneumocystis* organisms stained with methenamine silver and by the Papanicolaou method are shown in Figs. 4-28 and 4-29. An example of simultaneous infections with *Pneumocystis* and cytomegalovirus is shown in Fig. 4-30.

Strongyloides stercoralis

Respiratory infection with *Strongyloides stercoralis* has been seen mostly in patients who are receiving very heavy steroid therapy for such conditions as rheumatoid arthritis, renal transplantation, and severe asthmatic bronchitis. Pulmonary infection is produced when the filariform larvae migrate through the intestinal wall into the bloodstream and finally penetrate into the alveolar spaces. There a hemorrhagic pneumonia is produced. The organisms are readily identified in the bloody sputum expectorated by these patients. The filariform larvae observed measure 400 to 500 μm in length and exhibit a closed gullet and a slightly notched tail. In extreme cases, filariform larvae, rhabditiform larvae, and ova may all be seen in the alveoli.[31]

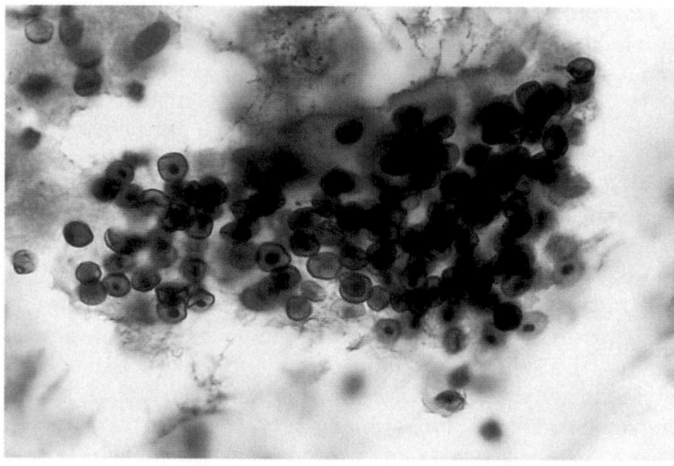

Fig. 4-28 *Pneumocystis carinii.* (Bronchial brushing; methenamine silver stain.)

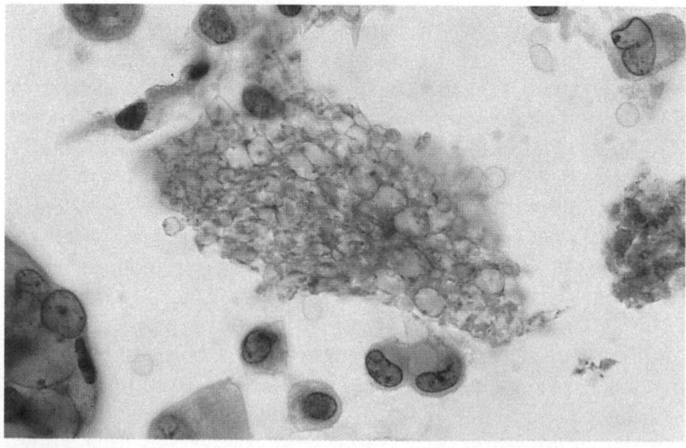

Fig. 4-29 *Pneumocystis carinii.* (Bronchial brushing; Papanicolaou stain.)

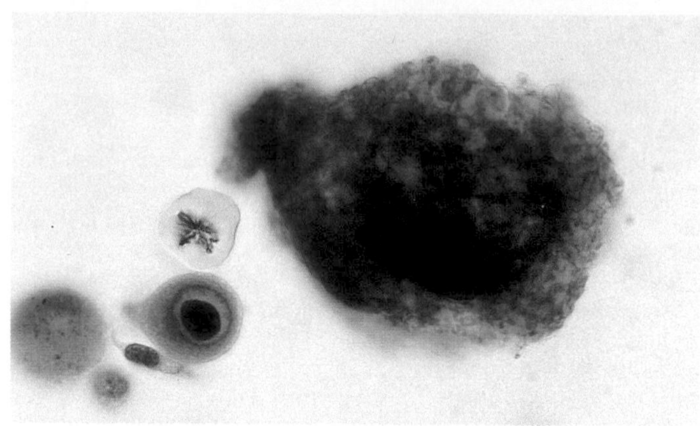

Fig. 4-30 Simultaneous infections with *Pneumocystis carinii* and cytomegalovirus. (Bronchial brush; Papanicolaou stain.)

Other parasites

Also described in the cytologic literature are diagnoses of echinococcosis,[32] *Paragonimus kellicotti*,[33] *Entamoeba gingivalis*,[34] *Paragonimus westermani*[35] and *Dirofilaria immitis*.[36]

Bacterial infections

Although most infections produced by bacteria do not lend themselves to primary diagnosis by conventional cytologic methods, there are a few instances in which cytologic diagnosis may be extremely helpful.

Gram-positive and Gram-negative bacteria

It is not at all uncommon for specimens from the female reproductive system and lung to show bacillary and coccal forms of bacteria. The presence of bacteria in a cytologic specimen from a fine-needle aspiration biopsy may be of extreme importance.

Opportunistic infections with *Legionella pneumophila* and *Legionella micdadei*[37] are worthy of note because they appear to be increasing in frequency. *Legionella* is an extremely small gram-negative rod. Specimens of sputum, bronchial material, and particularly fine-needle aspiration biopsy specimens stained by the Dieterle method of silver impregnation may reveal the organisms; however, much greater sensitivity in detection of this organism is being achieved by immunofluorescence microscopy utilizing anti-*Legionella* antibodies, which are now commercially available.

Acid-fast bacteria

The search for acid-fast organisms in a cytologic specimen is likely to be the most rewarding among those patients in whom there is either suggestive morphologic evidence of granulomatous inflammation with necrosis or in whom there is an extremely suggestive clinical history. Patients infected with *Mycobacterium avium-intracellulare* may show large alveolar macrophages that on acid-fast stain will reveal large numbers of branching acid-fast bacilli. Cell blocks prepared from fine-needle aspirates are useful for acid-fast staining when it is suspected that a tuberculous lesion has been aspirated. Fluorescence microscopy with auramine O may also reveal the organisms. Nocardiosis should be suspected when a fine-needle aspiration biopsy specimen reveals the presence of delicate branching filamentous rods with an inflammatory reaction manifesting mainly as neutrophils. Positive acid-fast stains will further enforce this diagnosis.

Viral infections

There are many reports describing cellular changes in association with several different viral infections, including adenovirus, herpes simplex, herpes zoster, measles, cytomegalovirus, *Polyomavirus,* parainfluenza respiratory syncytial virus, and human *Papillomavirus.*[38-49] Most frequently observed are the changes seen in association with infection with herpes simplex virus. The hallmark of cellular alteration produced by herpes is that of cells with multiple molded nuclei that may either contain eosinophilic irregular inclusion bodies or exhibit a peculiar type of nuclear degeneration that appears as slate-gray, homogenized nuclear contents (Figs. 4-11 and 4-12). Cells infected by the cytomegalovirus are larger and may show some multinucleation, but they have fewer nuclei and none of the molding as seen in herpes simplex. Large amphophilic, smooth, intranuclear inclusions surrounded by very prominent halos and clear-cut margination of chromatin on the inner surface of the nuclear membrane are present. Within the nucleus cytomegalovirus particles take on a protein envelope and migrate out into the cytoplasm where they present as cytoplasmic inclusions, which are manifested by a textured appearance to the cytoplasm (Figs. 4-13 and 4-30).

The cytomorphology of cells from the female reproductive tract infected with human *Papillomavirus* (HPV) is now widely recognized.[38] The biologic relationship between genital HPV infections and the subsequent development of cancer is discussed in Chapter 24. The hallmark of infection of cells from the female reproductive tract with HPV is the koilocyte. The koilocyte is an abnormal intermediate or superficial squamous cell so named originally by Koss and Durfee because of its peculiar perinuclear cavity.[50] The edges of this cavity are irregular but clear and are bounded by a dense cytoplasm. The nuclear changes may vary from those of degeneration to those associated with dysplasia. The lesion from which these cells are shed is a condyloma. In the Bethesda Classification, cellular changes associated with HPV infection are grouped with the squamous intraepithelial neoplastic lesions. Examples of cellular changes induced by infection with HPV are illustrated in Figs. 4-14 and 4-31 to 4-35.

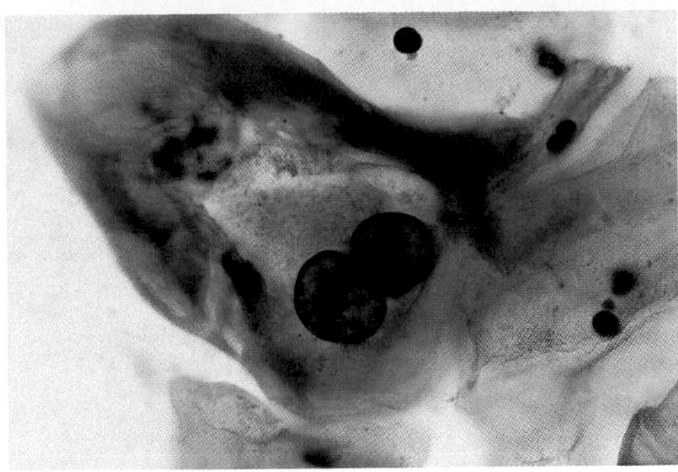

Fig. 4-32 HPV infection (LSIL with HPV). (Papanicolaou smear; Papanicolaou stain.)

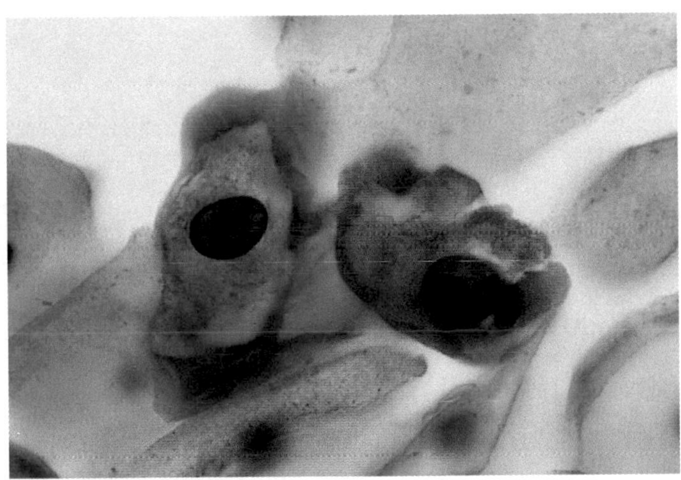

Fig. 4-33 HPV infection (LSIL with HPV). (Papanicolaou smear; Papanicolaou stain.)

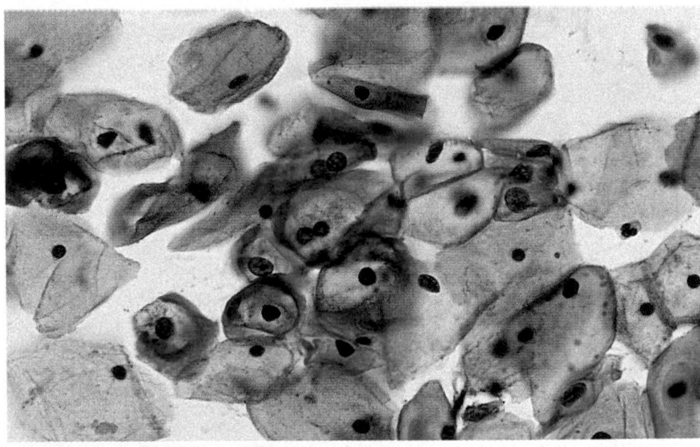

Fig. 4-31 Human *Papillomavirus* (HPV) infection (LSIL with HPV; see p. 61 for codes). (Papanicolaou smear; Papanicolaou stain.)

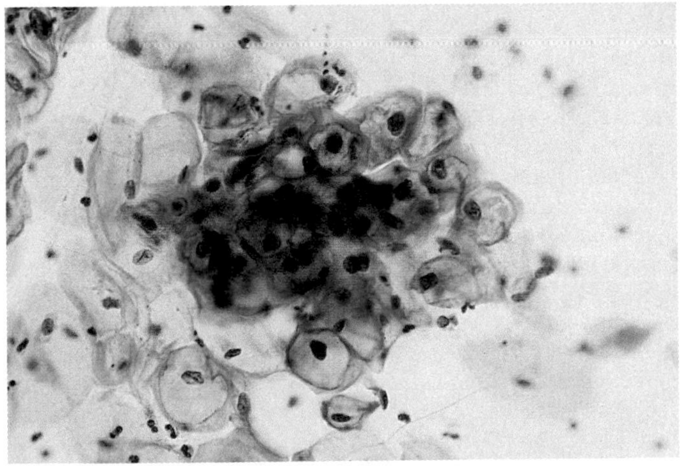

Fig. 4-34 HPV infection (LSIL with HPV). (Papanicolaou smear; Papanicolaou stain.)

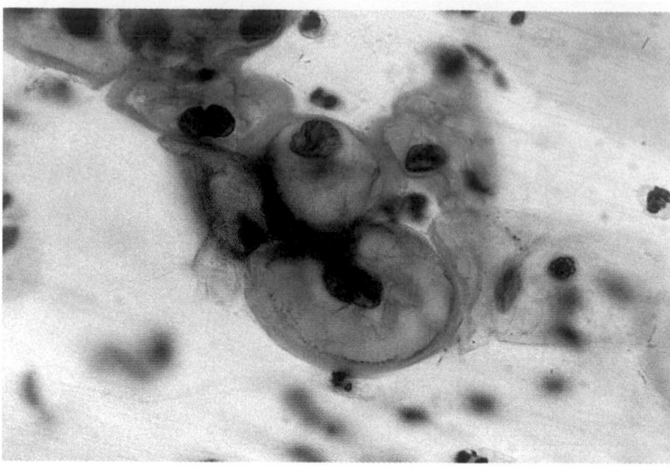

Fig. 4-35 HPV infection (LSIL with HPV). (Papanicolaou smear; Papanicolaou stain.)

FEMALE REPRODUCTIVE TRACT

Papanicolaou and Traut first successfully introduced clinical cytopathology of the female reproductive tract to the medical and scientific world in 1943.[3] Since that time the use of the Papanicolaou smear as a screening test for early cervical cancer has had remarkable success and has spread throughout the world. Despite this, however, the United States Department of Health and Human Services in 1991 reported the development of invasive cervical cancer in approximately 13,000 women and death from it in 4500.[51] It is clear from these data that there will continue to exist a great need for this screening test.

Although clinical cytopathology as applied to the female reproductive tract is a powerful tool for the detection of a wide variety of benign atypias, inflammatory changes, and infectious organisms, for cytohormonal evaluation of the endocrine status of the patient, and for detection of adenocarcinoma of the endometrium and a wide variety of other neoplasms, its major role is as a screening test for invasive and preinvasive cervical cancer. This discussion emphasizes that role.

Adequacy of the Papanicolaou smear

Because the major focus of the Papanicolaou smear is upon the earliest possible diagnosis of cervical cancer and its precursors, the most common site of origin of these lesions, the squamocolumnar junction, or transformation zone, must be adequately sampled. Although there continues to be controversy regarding what cellular components must be present to constitute an adequate or satisfactory Papanicolaou smear, the report from the Criteria Committee of the 1991 Bethesda System Workshop provides a statement of consensus from a group of experts in the field of cytopathology and is quoted in part here: "Well-preserved and well-visualized squamous epithelial cells should be spread over >10% of the slide surface. An adequate endocervical/transformation zone component should consist, at a minimum, of two clusters of well-preserved endocervical and/or squamous metaplastic cells, with each cluster composed of a minimum of at least five appropriate cells. This definition applies to specimens from both premenopausal and postmenopausal women with a cervix except in the situation of pronounced atrophy in which metaplastic and endocervical cells often cannot be distinguished from parabasal cells. In cases of pronounced atrophic changes, the absence of an identifiable endocervical/transformation zone component does not effect the specimen-adequacy categorization of a specimen otherwise determined to be "satisfactory for evaluation."[52]

To obtain an adequate specimen, one must sample both the cervix and the endocervix. Several reports in the literature have analyzed the relative efficacy of various sampling devices now available on the market. One report that is fairly typical of the conclusions reached is summarized here. Boon and associates analyzed the performance of five sample takers in a screening program, each of whom had made approximately 5000 smears, and of the five sampling methods each had used: spatula alone (method A), Cytobrush and spatula (method B), Cytopick (method C), cotton swab and spatula (method D), and Cervex brush (method E). The differences between the sample takers and the sampling methods were significant both in the detection of grade III cervical intraepithelial neoplasia (CIN III) and in the production of smears containing endocervical cells (EC+). The data obtained were believed to establish firmly the importance of the presence of endocervical cells for smear adequacy. The results of this study indicated that method B (Cytobrush and spatula) and method C (Cytopick) gave superior results in the preparation of EC+ smears and in the detection of CIN III and thus should be used in population-screening programs and that methods A and D should not be used for cervical cytologic sampling in such programs.[53]

The two samples obtained from the cervix and endocervix can be applied either to two halves of one glass microscopic slide or to two separate slides. Experience and expertise on the part of the sample taker are necessary to ensure that the cellular samples are evenly spread over the slides and that rapid fixation without any air-drying occurs. Fixation by immediate immersion of the smears into 95% ethanol is most desirable, but satisfactory results can also be obtained by correct use of any one of the several commercial spray fixatives now available.

Cytologic nomenclature

From the period of the first introduction of the Papanicolaou smear as a screening test for cervical cancer during the late 1940s and early 1950s up to the present, the diagnostic terminology used to describe the cellular changes present on the smear has undergone a gradual but unremitting series of evolutionary changes. The earliest, introduced by Papanicolaou himself, was described by him as follows:

> Smears cannot always be judged as positive or negative. There are cases in which cytologic findings are inconclusive. A classification taking into consideration the relatively large group of questionable smear findings is therefore necessary.
>
> One may often experience great difficulty in classifying cells that deviate from the normal type but show no malignant characteristics. An intermediate class between the entirely normal and the suspicious groups appears thus to be necessary.
>
> A similar need for subdivision exists in the positive group. There are instances in which the results are of an overwhelmingly positive character, leaving no doubt as to their final interpretation. On the

other hand, there are cases in which there is strong but not fully convincing evidence of malignancy.

These considerations led us to the acceptance of the following system of classification for cytologic findings, consisting of five groups: *Class I*—Absence of atypical or abnormal cells. *Class II*—Atypical cytology but no evidence of malignancy. *Class III*—Cytology suggestive of, but not conclusive for, malignancy. *Class IV*—Cytology strongly suggestive of malignancy. *Class V*—Cytology conclusive for malignancy.[12]

Criticisms that this classification was being used differently by various laboratories and was failing to correspond to the histologic features of the lesions represented on the smears led to the introduction of terminology that attempted to be predictive of the histology. Thus the terms *dysplasia (mild, moderate, severe)* as introduced by Reagan and *carcinoma* in situ *(CIS)* began to be substituted for the old Papanicolaou classification system in many laboratories.[14] This dysplasia-CIS classification system was not without its own critics. The very definitions in themselves were challenged, and it was impossible to achieve a consensus among experts with respect to morphologic criteria necessary for diagnosis and correlation between the cytology and the histology.

In 1968 Richart introduced the term *cervical intraepithelial neoplasia (CIN)*. This term was reflective of his concept that preinvasive neoplastic lesions of the uterine cervix represented a continuum of disease that progressed toward invasive cancer. Furthermore, dysplasia and carcinoma in situ, rather than representing separate diseases as originally proposed by Reagan and associates, was a part of the range of disease progression. Richart's CIN-1 corresponded to mild dysplasia and class III; CIN-2 corresponded to moderate dysplasia and class III; and CIN-3 corresponded both to severe dysplasia and class III and to carcinoma in situ and class IV.[54]

By 1988 all these classifications, plus many modifications, were in use throughout the world, resulting in confusion in communications among clinicians, pathologists, and researchers. In December 1988, the National Cancer Institute convened a workshop of experts to study the current status of terminology and to consider possible solutions. The result of this workshop was the Bethesda System (TBS) of classification of cervical and vaginal cytology. An updated and revised classification has been published more recently.[52] The Bethesda System classification is reproduced in Table 4-2.[55] A comparison between this system and earlier ones described here is summarized in Table 4-3. The most significant development in nomenclature in TBS is the creation of the broad categories of atypical squamous and glandular cells of undetermined significance (ASCUS and AGUS) and of low-grade squamous intraepithelial lesion (LSIL) and high-grade squamous intraepithelial lesion (HSIL). LSIL encompasses class III, mild dysplasia, CIN-1, and infections with human *Papillomavirus*. HSIL encompasses classes III and IV, moderate dysplasia, severe dysplasia, and carcinoma in situ, and CIN-2 and CIN-3. An essential feature of the Bethesda System is that each gynecologic specimen should have three elements: (1) a comment on the adequacy of the material, (2) a comment on whether the specimen is broadly classifiable as normal or abnormal, and then, if it is abnormal, (3) a descriptive diagnosis of the abnormality. A significant variation from popular reporting methods was the development of two classifications for intraepithelial neoplasia—so-called low-grade squamous epithelial lesions (LSIL) and high-grade lesions (HSIL). These categories were offered in response to observations that there was substantial variability between pathologists in discriminating between certain abnormalities such as moderate and severe dysplasia. The Bethesda

Table 4-2 The Bethesda System

Adequacy of the specimen
Satisfactory for evaluation
Satisfactory for evaluation but limited by __________ (Specify reason)
Unsatisfactory for evaluation __________ (Specify reason)
General categorization (optional)
Within normal limits
Benign cellular changes: See descriptive diagnosis
Epithelial cell abnormality: See descriptive diagnosis
Descriptive diagnoses
Benign cellular changes
Infection
Trichomonas vaginalis
- Fungal organisms morphologically consistent with *Candida* spp.
- Predominance of coccobacilli consistent with shift in vaginal flora
- Bacteria morphologically consistent with *Actinomyces* spp.
- Cellular changes associated with herpes simplex virus
- Other*

Reactive changes
Reactive cellular changes associated with:
- Inflammation (includes typical repair)
- Atrophy with inflammation ("atrophic vaginitis")
- Radiation
- Intrauterine contraceptive device (IUD)
- Other

Epithelial cell abnormalities
Squamous cell
- Atypical squamous cells of undetermined significance: Qualify†
- Low-grade squamous intraepithelial lesion (LSIL) encompassing: HPV* mild dysplasia/CIN 1
- High-grade squamous intraepithelial lesion (HSIL) encompassing: moderate and severe dysplasia/CIS, CIN-2 and CIN-3
- Squamous cell carcinoma

Glandular cell
- Endometrial cells, cytologically benign in a postmenopausal woman
- Atypical glandular cells of undetermined significance: Qualify†
- Endocervical adenocarcinoma
- Endometrial adenocarcinoma
- Extrauterine adenocarcinoma
- Adenocarcinoma, NOS

Other malignant neoplasms: specify
Hormonal evaluation (applies to vaginal smears only)
- Hormonal pattern compatible with age and history
- Hormonal pattern incompatible with age and history: Specify
- Hormonal evaluation not possible due to: Specify

*Cellular changes of human *Papillomavirus* (HPV)—previously termed *koilocytotic atypia* and *condylomatous atypia*—are included in the category of LSIL.
†Atypical squamous or glandular cells of undetermined significance should be further qualified, if possible, as to whether a reactive or premalignant-malignant process is favored.
NOS, Not otherwise specified.

Table 4-3 Comparison of cytologic nomenclature classifications

Papanicolaou	Reagan	Richart	Bethesda
Class I—Absence of atypical or abnormal cells	Normal cellular pattern	Normal cellular pattern	Within normal limits
Class II—Atypical cytology but no evidence of malignancy	Benign cellular changes	Benign cellular changes	Benign cellular changes
Class III—Cytologic features suggestive of, but not conclusive for, malignancy	Mild dysplasia	Cervical intraepithelial neoplasia, CIN-1	Atypical squamous cells of undetermined significance (ASCUS). Atypical glandular cells of undetermined significance (AGUS) Low-grade squamous intraepithelial lesion (including infections with human *Papilloma virus*) (LSIL)
Class IV—Cytologic features strongly suggestive of malignancy	Moderate dysplasia	CIN-2	High-grade squamous intraepithelial lesion (HSIL)
	Severe dysplasia	CIN-3	
	Carcinoma in situ		
Class V—Cytologic features conclusive for malignancy	Invasive cancer	Invasive cancer	Invasive cancer

System has not been without its critics. Morever, most troublesome has been the category *atypical squamous cells of undetermined significance (ASCUS),* which some writers believe has been overused by some pathologists.

The Bethesda concept of ASCUS and AGUS is an area of clinical cytopathology that merits particular attention because herein lies the problem of the diagnosis and clinical management of patients in whose Papanicolaou smears atypical epithelial cells of uncertain significance are encountered. As previously discussed, it is well established that many reactive, reparative, and atypical but benign epithelial cellular changes can be induced by various inflammatory processes and other irritants. For example *Trichomonas vaginalis* infections have been recognized since the earliest years of clinical cytology as being capable of inducing violent reactive changes in both squamous and glandular epithelial cells. In addition to these well-recognized areas of reactive cellular patterns, however, there are other changes that are much more difficult to interpret. In TBS the term *ASCUS* is used to define a group of squamous cell abnormalities that cannot be explained on the basis of inflammatory or reactive processes but yet lack the criteria for a diagnosis of a LSIL, or mild dysplasia. This category of cellular changes does have both diagnostic and prognostic significance because studies have shown that patients on whom the diagnosis of ASCUS is rendered may indeed have a squamous intraepithelial lesion or go on to develop one.

The term *AGUS* in a fashion comparable to *ASCUS* defines atypical glandular changes that exceed those expected in benign reparative reactions but that are not diagnostic for adenocarcinoma. The most common sites of origin of AGUS are endocervix and endometrium. Unfortunately because of the lack of scientific information about the pathobiology of lesions exfoliating ASCUS and AGUS, many patients are probably being needlessly subjected to further diagnostic studies with colposcopy, directed biopsy, and endocervical and endometrial curettage.

Normal histology and cytology

The normal histology and cytology of the female reproductive tract has been described extensively.[3,5-6,11-12,56] The vagina and ectocervix are covered by a nonkeratinizing stratified squamous epithelium. Under normal biologic conditions, superficial cells, intermediate cells, and parabasal cells may exfoliate from this epithelium and may be found on the Papanicolaou smear. The relative proportions of these three cell types to one another will vary according to the hormonal status of the patient when the vagina and cervix are sampled. In the normal adult female, the cells present will consist almost entirely of superficial and intermediate cells. Parabasal cells may also be shed in the prepubescent or postmenopausal periods and in response to inflammatory insults. The superficial cell is the most mature cell of the squamous epithelium and is usually abundant in cellular specimens from the uterine cervix or vagina. It is relatively large and polygonal with a small, dense, centrally placed nucleus without discernible structure. The cytoplasm is wafer thin and transparent. The Papanicolaou stain will show an intense orangeophilia or eosinophilia as a reflection of keratin production in the cytoplasm. Intermediate cells are also abundant in specimens obtained from the uterine cervix or vagina. The intermediate cell is polygonal in form with a thin waferlike cytoplasm. The cytoplasm usually stains cyanophilically but may also be eosinophilic. The nucleus is larger than that of the superficial

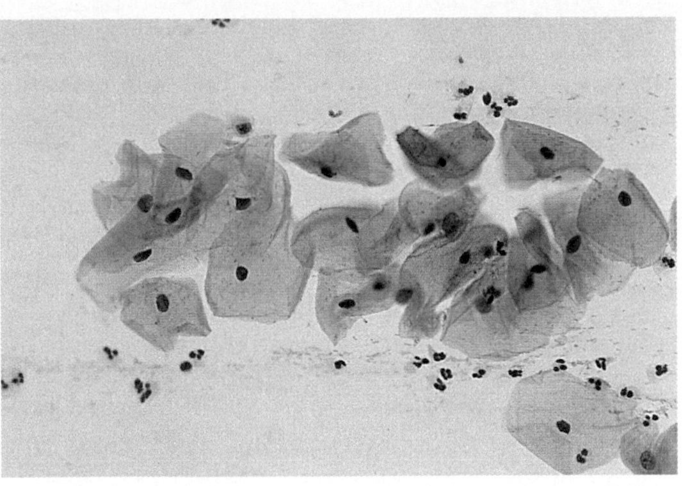

Fig. 4-36 Normal Papanicolaou smear showing intermediate and superficial squamous cells. (Papanicolaou stain.)

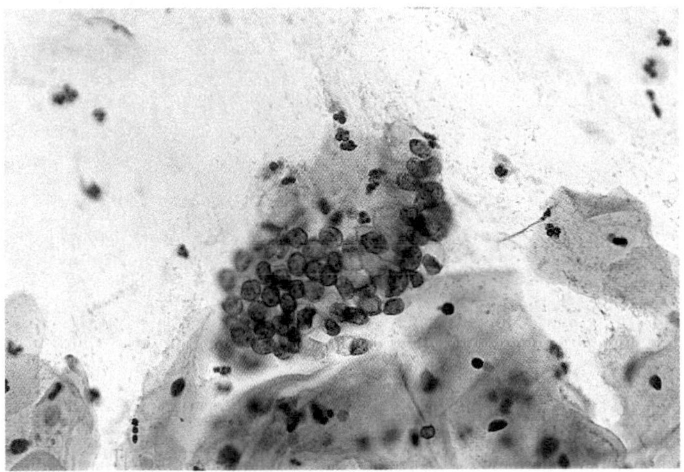

Fig. 4-37 Normal columnar cells from the endocervix. (Papanicolaou stain.)

cell and has a delicate reticulated structure to the chromatinic material (Figs. 4-1 and 4-36). The parabasal cell is characterized by a round vesicular nucleus similar to that seen in the intermediate cell. The cytoplasm is thick and cyanophilic.

The endocervical canal and the glands opening into it are lined by tall, columnar epithelium. At least two varieties of columnar cells are represented. One is a secreting columnar cell and the other is a ciliated columnar cell. When viewed on cross section, the columnar cells have a rectangular or prismatic form, and when viewed *en face,* they are polygonal in shape. The nucleus is round or oval and varies in its location depending on the phase of hormonal activity. With abundant mucin production, the nucleus may lie at the base of the cell and be indented. The columnar cells originating in the endocervix occur in smears as isolated cells or in small sheets. Isolated cells may have the form of typical columnar epithelium with an asymmetrically placed nucleus or they may have a prismatic form. The cytoplasm may be either eosinophilic or cyanophilic. The nuclear chromatin is very finely granular and uniformly dispersed. A small nucleolus may be present. When viewed *en face,* the columnar cells have a polygonal form and

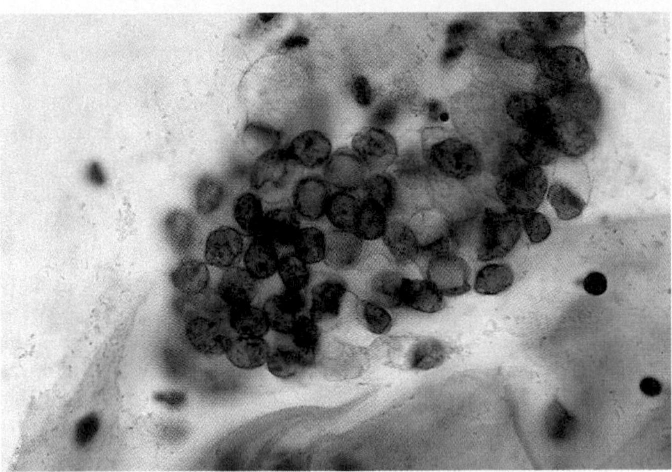

Fig. 4-38 Normal columnar cells from the endocervix. (Papanicolaou stain.)

the sheet of cells has a honeycomb arrangement (Figs. 4-2, 4-37, and 4-38).

The endometrial canal and the glands that open into it are lined by columnar epithelium. It merges almost imperceptibly with the epithelium lining the endocervical canal in the vicinity of the internal uterine opening. This epithelium is made up of columnar secreting and ciliated forms. It undergoes definite cyclic changes in response to ovarian hormones and is in large part exfoliated at the time of menstruation. The cells shed from the endometrium include both epithelial cells and stromal cells. When present in Papanicolaou smears, they may appear in small ball-like groups. Because normally they are exfoliating from a menstruating endometrium, they may appear quite degenerate with indistinct cytoplasmic membranes. The nuclei appear round to oval, with reticulated chromatin, and a small nucleolus may be present. The cell cytoplasm is more commonly cyanophilic than eosinophilic. Stromal cells resembling macrophages may also be present.

Squamous metaplasia of the endocervix is defined as focal or extensive replacement of the glandular epithelium of the endocervix by stratified squamous epithelium. This alteration occurs most frequently at the squamocolumnar junction, which is also the most frequent site for cervical intraepithelial neoplasia and invasive cancer. The metaplastic cells observed in Papanicolaou smears will reflect the maturity of the metaplastic epithelium from which they are being shed. Cells from immature squamous metaplasia will be seen as single cells or as small sheets. The cells may be round, oval, or spindle shaped and formed with numerous cytoplasmic processes, giving them a "spidery" appearance. The cells are similar to but generally smaller than true parabasal squamous cells.

Dysplasia of the uterine cervix

As has been stated in prior portions of this chapter, dysplasia of the uterine cervix defines an abnormality of the squamous or metaplastic epithelium that is characterized by progressive abnormalities of the nucleus and loss of the ability of the cytoplasm to mature. Dysplasias traditionally are graded as mild, moderate, and severe. Mild dysplasia (CIN-1, LSIL) characterizes an abnormal epithelium that is composed of immature dyskaryotic squamous cells composing approximately one third of the thickness of the abnormal epithelium extending up from the basal layer to the surface. The upper one third is composed of mature dyskaryotic squamous cells that may show varying degrees of dyskeratosis of the cytoplasm. With moderate dysplasia (CIN-2, HSIL), the immature cells extend upward through two thirds of the thickness of the epithelial layer. The cells composing the upper third of the layer reveal nuclear abnormalities and maturation defects more advanced than those seen with the mild dysplasia. In severe dysplasia (CIN-3, HSIL), the immature cells extend up through greater than two thirds of the epithelium thickness. As the lesion of carcinoma in situ (CIN-3, HSIL) is approached, all evidence of cell maturation and differentiation disappears.

The dysplastic cells that are present on the Papanicolaou smear will reflect the cellular alterations on the surface of the dysplastic epithelium from which they are exfoliated. In mild dysplasia, the dysplastic cells resemble either superficial or intermediate squamous cells but with enlarged nuclei displaying features of dyskaryosis previously described (Fig. 4-16). In moderate dysplasia, the abnormal cells are predominantly polygonal in configuration, the cytoplasm stains cyanophilically, and nuclear dyskaryosis is more advanced. Cytoplasm is less waferlike than in the cells with mild dysplasia and has begun to thicken up. With severe dysplasia, the exfoliated cells are relatively small and oval or round with some polygonal forms. The cytoplasm usually stains intensively cyanophilically, and the nuclei show extremely advanced changes of dyskaryosis (Fig. 4-17). As the severity of the lesion increases, the quantity of abnormal cells per slide increases from an average of 50 cells with mild dysplasia to an excess of 300 cells in severe dysplasia. With all levels of severity, the cells are most frequently observed to occur singly but may also be seen in small sheets. In carcinoma in situ, syncytial groupings in addition to single cells are identified (Fig. 4-18).[57,58]

Invasive carcinoma

Wentz and Reagan have classified invasive squamous cell carcinoma of the uterine cervix as keratinizing squamous cell carcinoma, large cell nonkeratinizing squamous cell carcinoma, and small cell carcinoma.[59] The overall histologic features of keratinizing squamous cell carcinoma are those of a well-differentiated squamous cell carcinoma. A single well-formed epithelial pearl includes a neoplasm in the category of the keratinizing carcinoma. Large cell nonkeratinizing squamous cell carcinoma is composed of relatively large neoplastic cells forming sheets. Epithelial pearl formation is absent, though isolated cell keratinization may be present in some cases. Small-cell carcinoma is characterized by a predominance of uniformly small cells forming sheets with poorly defined cytoplasmic outlines and extremely high nuclear to cytoplasmic ratios.

The cytopathology of keratinizing squamous cell carcinoma is characterized by the presence of few to many tumor cells lying in a clean slide background. The abnormal cells are mainly occurring as single cells. Relatively large malignant squamous cells with prominent cellular pleomorphism and pronounced variation in size including the formation of caudate and spindle cell forms are common. Prominent nucleoli are rare. In nonkeratinizing carcinoma, large numbers of tumor cells will be shed, and the slide background will show a tumor diathesis. The cells are present either as single forms or as syncytial groups. The cells are relatively large and uniform with many macronucleoli. Isolated cell dyskaryosis may be occasionally present. Small-cell carcinomas exfoliate many abnormal cells with a slide background exhibiting a tumor diathesis. The abnormal cells are present both singly and as syncytia. The cells are relatively uniform and small, with extremely high nuclear to cytoplasmic ratios and prominent nucleoli present in many of the cells.[16] Examples of squamous cell carcinoma are depicted in Figs. 4-39 and 4-40.

Adenocarcinomas of the endocervix compose approximately 5% of primary malignant neoplasms of the cervix. Their exfoliated cells are found most frequently in the endocervical sample obtained by endocervical brushing. The exfoliation from this tumor is characterized by the presence of large numbers of elongated columnar malignant cells occurring both singly and in sheets in a highly characteristic side-by-side arrangement of the malignant cells. The nuclear chromatin is hyperchromatic and coarsely granular with one or more macronucleoli present. It may be extremely difficult from the smear alone to differentiate between adenocarcinoma in situ and invasive adenocarcinoma. In the latter, larger numbers of tumor cells are present in a background of tumor diathesis on the slide.[16,57,60,61] Examples of endocervical adenocarcinoma are shown in Figs. 4-19, 4-41, and 4-42.

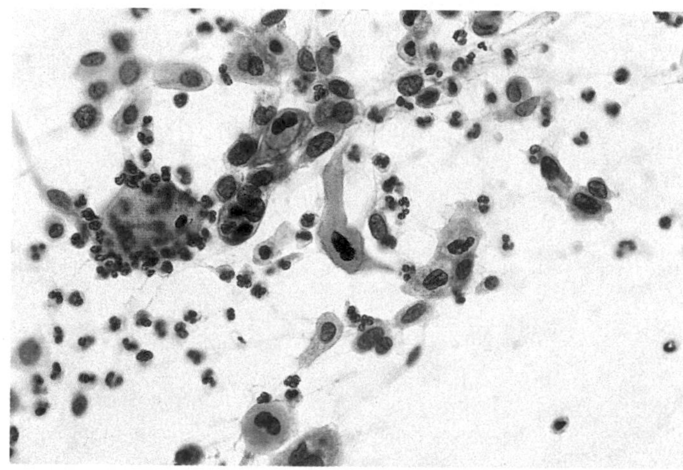

Fig. 4-39 Squamous cell carcinoma of the uterine cervix. (Papanicolaou stain.)

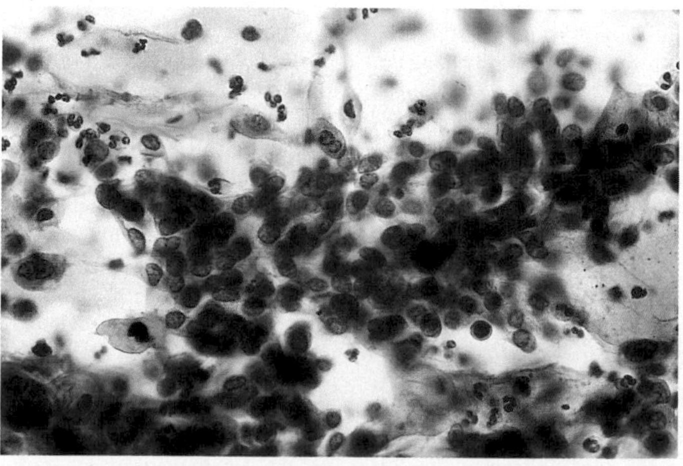

Fig. 4-40 Squamous cell carcinoma of the uterine cervix. (Papanicolaou stain.)

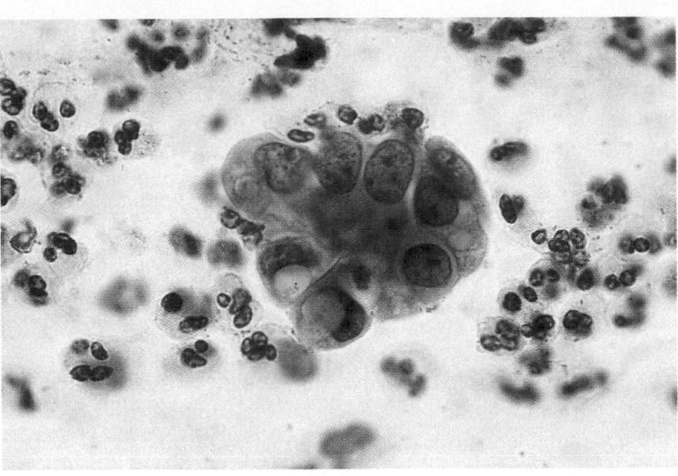

Fig. 4-41 Adenocarcinoma of endocervix. (Papanicolaou stain.)

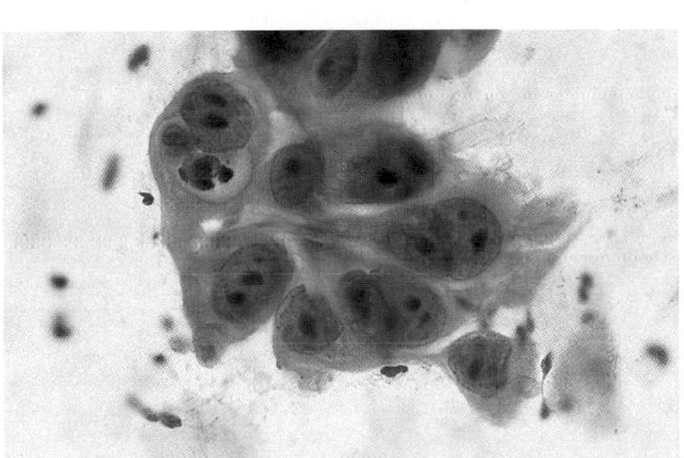

Fig. 4-42 Adenocarcinoma of endocervix. (Papanicolaou stain.)

Adenocarcinomas of the endometrium may exfoliate diagnostic cells into the Papanicolaou smear. If present, they will most likely be observed in either the endocervical sample or the vaginal pool sample. Because of its low specificity for the detection of endometrial adenocarcinoma, the Papanicolaou smear is not an effective screening tool for this lesion. When present in smears, tumor cells exfoliating from endometrial adenocarcinomas may vary in number from a few scattered cells to many malignant cells. The size of these cells, the size of their nuclei, and the degree of nuclear abnormalities correlate with the degree of differentiation present in the primary tumor. The presence of even benign-appearing endometrial cells in the Papanicolaou smear of a postmenopausal woman is cause for concern and merits further evaluation of the patient for possible endometrial cancer.[62,63]

Occasionally malignant tumor metastatic to the female reproductive tract may be manifested by the exfoliation of malignant cells into the Papanicolaou smear. The most common of these are adenocarcinomas of the ovary and breast (Fig. 4-43).

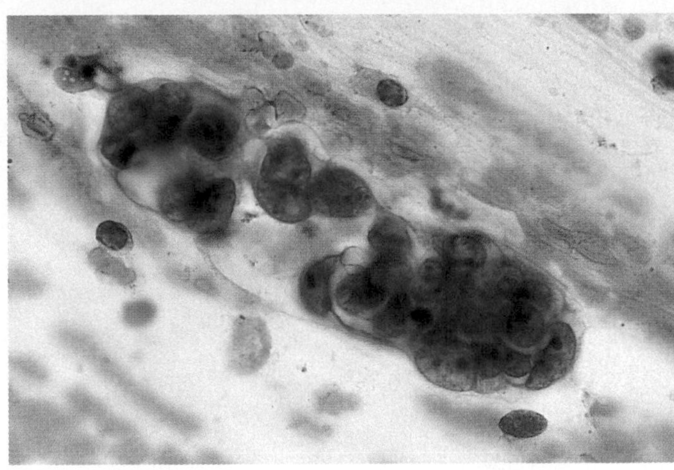

Fig. 4-43 Adenocarcinoma of the ovary in a Papanicolaou smear. (Papanicolaou stain.)

Accuracy of the Papanicolaou smear

In 1989, Koss characterized the Papanicolaou test for cervical cancer detection as "a triumph and a tragedy."[64] The "triumph" was the remarkable contribution of this screening test to the prevention of cervical cancer. The "tragedy" was the not infrequent failure of the Papanicolaou smear to detect neoplastic disease states extant in the patient being tested. Stated more simply, the Papanicolaou smear is an imperfect screening test and has a significant error rate. Thus repetition of the procedure at regular intervals (usually 1 year) in the same patient is a major key to its success. The scientific literature is replete with studies that report these error rates expressed in terms of false-negative rate (sensitivity) and false-positive rate (specificity).[58] Depending on which study is being cited, the reported false-negative rates vary from 6% to 55%. Several informative studies are summarized here.

In 1985, Gay and associates, on review of the Papanicolaou smears from 339 patients with histologically confirmed carcinoma in situ, or invasive cancer, found 66 that had been reported as negative. On rescreen, sampling errors accounted for 62%, screening errors for 16%, and interpretive errors (by the pathologist) for 22%. When the 39 cases attributable to sampling error were subtracted, the false-negative rate fell to 8.1% (sensitivity 91.9%).[65]

In 1987 van der Graaf and associates reported on a review of 555 cervical smears, originally classified as Papanicolaou classes I and II, from women in whom 3 years later cytologic findings consistent with moderate dysplasia, severe dysplasia, carcinoma in situ, and invasive cancer were diagnosed. The initial diagnosis proved to be underestimated in 17.5% of the smears. The two diagnoses correlated in 70.2% of the smears, whereas 12.3% of the smears that contained no abnormality were judged to be inadequate for making a diagnosis, probably representing sampling errors.[66]

Using a large computerized data base of 748,871 cytologic screenings of 277,842 women over a 10-year period, Soost and associates in 1991 examined the value of screening. Only subsequent histologic examinations within 1 year were accepted to validate positive initial cytologic diagnoses; only two subsequent cytologic screenings within the next 3 years were accepted to validate negative initial cytologic diagnoses that had not been followed by a histologic examination. From these data, the predictive value of a negative cytologic examination was determined to be 99.8%; the predictive value of a positive cytologic examination was 73.4% for an initial diagnosis of mild-to-moderate dysplasia, 90.6% for a diagnosis of severe dysplasia/carcinoma in situ, 94.5% for a diagnosis of carcinoma in situ or microinvasive carcinoma, and 95.5% for an initial diagnosis of invasive carcinoma. Extrapolation from the validated cases to the entire screened population showed an overall sensitivity of 80% and a specificity of 99.4% for cytologic screening for cervical cancer.[67]

A current ongoing study at Duke University Medical Center, Durham, North Carolina, has been evaluating in a prospective fashion the correlation between the Papanicolaou smear and a concomitant cervical biopsy. Up to now 2498 cases have been reviewed, with a false-negative cytology rate attributable to sampling of 7.2% and a false-negative cytology rate attributable to screening or interpretive error of 0.64%.[68]

RESPIRATORY TRACT

The diagnosis of cellular specimens from the respiratory tract is established throughout the world as a vital diagnostic procedure in the evaluation of any patient with a suspected lung lesion in which morphologic confirmation is indicated. At present, most of the major medical institutions throughout the world utilize some combination of various cytologic specimens in the diagnostic work-up of a patient with suspected lung cancer. Sputum continues to be the most frequently examined specimen, but bronchial washings and brushings, bronchoalveolar lavages (BAL), and FNAB are gaining irreplaceable positions in the use of cytology. These procedures used appropriately in concert have the capability of both diagnosing and classifying correctly most of the common lung neoplasms. Sputum examined as multiple specimens will show the more central tumors, whereas bronchial brushings and FNABs will show the remaining ones, usually presenting as the more peripheral or even subpleural lesions. Recalling the histogenesis of primary lung cancers is a very persuasive aid for comprehending exactly why it is that cytologic diagnosis of the respiratory tract has been so successful. The reason is mainly that most primary lung cancers arise from the epithelium lining the respiratory passages and have the potential of shedding cancer cells into specimens of sputum or of having their cells harvested for cytologic diagnosis by methods of fiberoptic bronchoscopy, BAL, or FNAB. But it is also this same epithelial lining that is the origin of the fact that several atypical but benign cellular changes could be confused with cancer by the unwary observer. Knowledge of these atypias is absolutely mandatory if the cytopathologist is to avoid the pitfalls of false-positive cancer diagnoses, which ultimately result in the compromise of the credibility and reliability of the cytopathology laboratory.

Neoplastic conditions

Among the nonneoplastic lesions that occur in the lung, major considerations are reactive and reparative reactions, infections, and interstitial lung diseases. The lung contains an enormous diversity of cells, which when stimulated or irritated assume abnormal morphology, which can be mistaken for neoplasia. These cellular changes have been described in the section on the reative cell.

Abnormal but benign squamous cells may be exfoliated in the presence of many diseases of the mouth. Infection, inflammation, and ulceration may release parabasal cells. These may be confused with metaplasia. Chronic mucosal irritation with leukoplakia may produce masses of anucleate squames. The rare disease pemphigus may result in the exfoliation of extremely abnormal-appearing immature squamous cells with enlarged nuclei and centrally placed macronucleoli. These cells are easily mistaken for cancer cells.[69]

Squamous metaplasia of the lung describes the replacement of the ciliated pseudostratified bronchial epithelium normally lining the trachea and bronchi by a truly stratified and flattened epithelium. Cells from squamous metaplasia may occur as single cells or as small tissue fragments. As fragments, they are grouped in a uniform, monolayered cobblestone-like arrangement with striking uniformity between the cells. Some fragments may exhibit flattening of one surface, presumably that which was adjacent to the lumen of the bronchus. Although they resemble maturing squamous cells, they are smaller and possess a higher nuclear to cytoplasmic ratio. Because squamous metaplasia mimics maturing squamous epithelium, metaplastic cells of varying degrees of maturity may be present. The nuclei may be intensely karyopyknotic. Squamous metaplasias are capable of undergoing changes characterized by increasing degrees of nuclear abnormality. These metaplasias exhibit an increase in the nuclear to cytoplasmic ratio, thickening of the nuclear membrane, increasing granularity and hyperchromasia of the chromatin, and the appearance of nucleoli. These abnormalities have been called by various names, including "atypical squamous metaplasia" and "squamous metaplasia with dysplasia." They have been observed in the presence of longstanding chronic irritation of the tracheobronchial tree, particularly in cigarette smokers, and they are believed by many investigators to antedate the appearance of carcinoma of the lung. In about 60% of patients, however, these atypical metaplastic cells are associated with nonneoplastic conditions of the lung, most notably pneumonia.[70] Intracavitary fungus balls of the lung produced by *Aspergillus* as well as other fungi and viral infections may produce surprising metaplastic atypias easily mistaken for squamous cell carcinoma.[71]

Squamous metaplasia is antedated by a beginning proliferation of reserve or basal cells. As this proliferation continues, it begins to form a multilayered epithelium that intervenes between the columnar epithelial cells and the basement membrane. As these reserve cells gradually mature, there is produced an epithelium that more and more resembles a stratified squamous epithelium. In cytologic materials, reserve cell hyperplasia is recognized by the presence of tissue fragments composed of small, uniform, tightly cohesive cells possessing darkly stained nuclei and a thin rim of cyanophilic cytoplasm. There is nuclear molding, but uniformity exists throughout the fragment. There is no tendency toward fragmentation of the cluster. There is no necrosis. At times reserve cell hyperplasia may be very alarming in appearance and must be distinguished from small-cell undifferentiated carcinoma. Other small cell neoplasms, such as leukemias and lymphomas, should not be confused with reserve cell hyperplasia because they characteristically exfoliate into the respiratory material as single cells.

Reserve cell hyperplasia may be present in all types of respiratory specimens but is most frequent in bronchial brushings.

So-called reactive cells of bronchial epithelium may occur in response to a wide variety of insults, varying from microorganisms to environmental toxins. These altered cells are characterized by pronounced nuclear enlargement, coarsening of the chromatin pattern, and one or more enlarged nucleoli. Nuclear enlargement may be at a magnitude of 10 to 20 times the diameter of a normal bronchial cell nucleus.

Another extremely common response to irritation is the presence of multinucleation; however, the nuclei are small and mirror images of one of another. Although such cells may appear after a wide variety of insults, they are most commonly seen after instrumentation.

Koss and Richardson were among the first investigators to note the diagnostic pitfall posed by hyperplasia of bronchial epithelium.[72] These changes may occur in association with many of chronic diseases of the lung, including tuberculosis, bronchiectasis, chronic bronchitis, and asthma. Naylor and Railey described a patient with chronic asthmatic bronchitis in whom papillary tissue fragments exfoliating from hyperplastic bronchial epithelium were noted and incorrectly diagnosed as adenocarcinoma. These tissue fragments have come to bear the name "Creola bodies" in honor of the patient in whom they were seen.[73] They may be seen in the sputum and bronchial brushings from 42% of cases of asthmatic bronchitis. The cytologic presentation is that of papillary clusters of cells partially covered on the surface by well-differentiated, ciliated respiratory epithelium. There is some nuclear molding between individual cells, though chromatin and nucleolar structures remain relatively unremarkable. At times nuclear detail may be obscured because of the thickness of the tissue fragment. A varying number of vacuolated mucus cells may also be present in these fragments. The key to their benignancy is to be found in the finely granular chromatin pattern, regular uniform nucleoli, and the presence of cilia. Examples of bronchial hyperplasia are illustrated in Figs. 4-44 and 4-45.

Although the utilization of several modern laboratory techniques has enabled one to differentiate a variety of subtypes of terminal bronchiolar and alveolar cells, conventional light microscopic examination of cytologic specimens in the absence of disease does not often permit the observer to appreciate these various cell types. These cells are relatively small and, when present in cytologic material, appear as rounded single cells with finely vacuolated cytoplasm and centrally placed nuclei with one or two small nucleoli. Some may bear cilia. With such morphology they are usually interpreted as alveolar macrophages. Among various specimen types, they are likely to be most commonly encountered in BALs and FNAs, and if they are reactive or hyperplastic, they may be a diagnostic pitfall for false-positive cancer diagnoses in these specimens.

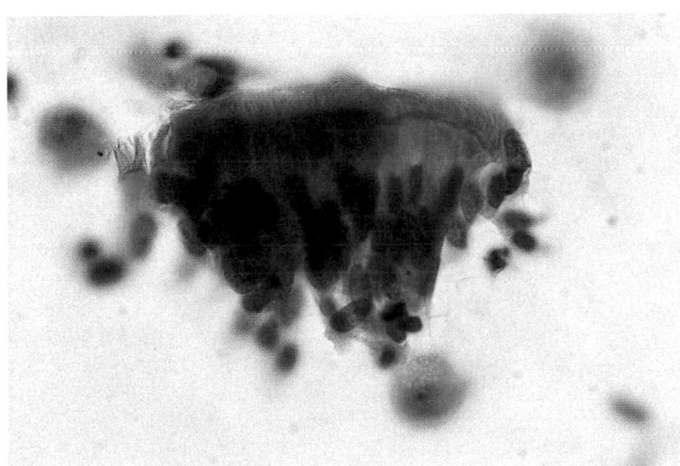

Fig. 4-44 Hyperplasia of bronchial epithelium. (Bronchial brush; Papanicolaou stain.)

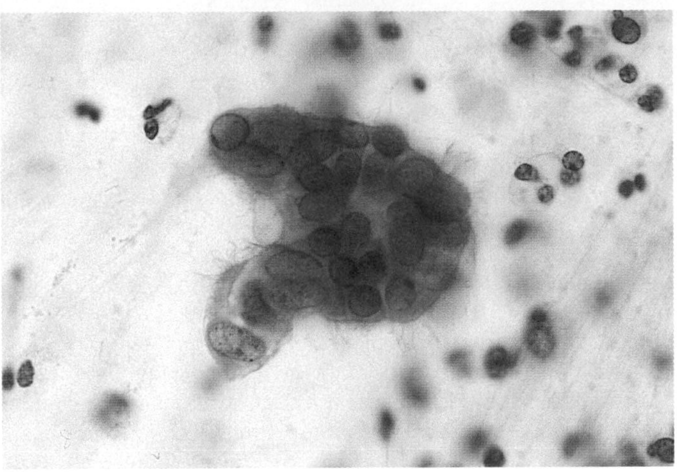

Fig. 4-45 Hyperplasia of bronchial epithelium. (Bronchial brush; Papanicolaou stain.)

In the presence of insult, type II pneumocytes may enlarge, proliferate, and produce differential diagnostic problems. In such circumstances they may be present either as single cells or as small papillary tissue fragments composed of enlarged cells with prominent nucleoli. Hyperdistended vacuoles may be present in the cytoplasm. Differential diagnosis of such cells then becomes a rather formidable problem of determining whether these cells are coming from one of the benign disease processes, or whether they are actually derived from an adenocarcinoma.[74-76] Pulmonary infarcts are cited in the literature as being particularly prone to give rise to such cells in sputum[76]; however, in the experience of the authors, they are most frequently encountered in association with pneumonias of various forms and causes. Frable has stressed the diagnostic distinction between the poorly preserved cell clusters associated with infarcts and the well-preserved cells forming ball-like clusters without molding but with deep depth of focus that are originating in bronchioloalveolar carcinoma.[77-79] Stanley and associates have studied hyperplasia of type II pneumocytes in acute lung injury, utilizing the technique of sequential bronchoalveolar lavage.[80] Some nuclear abnormalities were noted, including increased ratio to cytoplasm, multiplicity, angulation of nuclear membranes, chromatin clumping and clearing, and macronucleoli. Individual cells were believed to resemble those of malignant lymphoma, adenocarcinoma, or malignant melanoma. They concluded that an attempt at distinction between benign and malignant on the basis of morphologic observations alone may be insufficient to diagnose the disease process correctly.

Severe morphologic changes in benign cells of the lung and upper respiratory tract may occur at varying intervals after treatment with ionizing radiation or with a variety of drugs. These cells may be so severely altered that they may be mistaken for cancer cells. Knowledge of a history of prior therapy with such agents is the best safeguard against an erroneous cancer diagnosis. Cellular alterations in response to radiation therapy may involve both squamous cells and columnar cells and are characterized by cytomegaly with both cytoplasmic and nuclear enlargement, multinucleation, macronucleoli, and cytoplasmic vacuolization (Fig. 4-7). An acute radiation response can stimulate such cellular changes both within the area that had been irradiated or at a remote site. Epithelial abnormalities may persist and run a gamut from focal areas of squamous metaplasia of the lining bronchial cells to severe squamous atypia. A false-positive diagnosis of squamous cell carcinoma on specimens of sputum and bronchial material is a potential dangerous pitfall in such patients.

Some drugs used for anticancer chemotherapy may be associated with the production of severe changes in the lung parenchyma. These drugs include busulfan, cyclophosphamide, chlorambucil, melphalan, bleomycin, carmustine, (1,3-bis[2-chlorethyl]-1-nitrosourea, BCNU), methotrexate, and azathioprine. The toxic injury to the lung is that of diffuse alveolar damage. The initial phase of this damage manifests as pulmonary edema and hemorrhage. The striking feature of this phase, which permits this type of alveolar damage to be differentiated from that resulting from causes other then from these drugs, is the presence of atypical epithelial cells in great abundance. It has been shown by Bedrossian and associates that these atypical cells are in fact abnormal type II pneumocytes that have undergone degranulation and loss of lamellar bodies.[81] These atypical pneumocytes may shed into sputum or be harvested in brushings, BALs,[82] or FNAB.

The morphology of infectious agents that occur in cytologic specimens from the lung is described earlier in this chapter and in Chapters 36 and 37.

Cytology techniques are also used to identify the so-called interstitial lung diseases, which cytologically have as their major components different types of inflammatory cells, such as eosinophils, lymphocytes, or neutrophils, depending on the type of disorder. Idiopathic pulmonary fibrosis, eosinophilic granuloma, and sarcoidosis may sometimes be identified through the cytologic examination of bronchoalveolar lavage fluid.[82]

Malignant neoplasms

Squamous cell carcinoma

Invasive squamous cell carcinomas usually exfoliate large numbers of diagnostic neoplastic cells into the cytologic specimen. In sputum the neoplastic cells occur singly and in loose clusters. Tissue fragments are rare. Intact keratin pearls and intercellular bridges, though important in the histologic diagnosis of squamous cell carcinoma, are uncommonly observed. Pronounced cellular pleomorphism is characteristic of these tumors, and bizarre cytoplasmic shapes of almost infinite variety may occur. Classic forms such as the caudate, or "tadpole," cell, the fiber or spindle cell, and the "third type" of cell similar in morphology to those seen in squamous cell carcinoma of the cervix are present. The nuclei exhibit enlargement and noticeable hyperchromasia with a tendency toward pyknosis. When the chromatin pattern is preserved, it is arranged into irregular, sharp-bordered clumps with abnormal clearing of the parachromatin. As a result of the densely staining chromatin, nucleoli are observed less frequently than in other types of malignant neoplasms. They may, however, be conspicuously large in some cells. Their presence is more frequently associated with squamous cell carcinomas of a lesser degree of differentiation. Nuclear to cytoplasmic ratios may vary from extremely high to very low because of the great variability in the amount of cytoplasm produced by these cells. Keratinization of the cytoplasm is indicated by an intense hyaline appearance with either a bright orangeophilic staining or a deep cyanophilia. Ectoendoplasmic ringing as described by Frost is another striking feature of abnormal keratinization in the cytoplasm.[11] In bronchial specimens and FNAB, keratinizing squamous cell carcinomas exhibit findings similar to those in sputum, though tissue fragments are more common.

As the differentiation of the squamous cell carcinoma decreases, nuclear and cytoplasmic features of squamous differentiation are also less apparent. In sputum, poorly differentiated squamous cell carcinomas present as single cells and cell clusters, whereas in bronchial brushing specimens and FNAs, there is a noticeable tendency toward formation of large irregular sheets of cells. The only cytologic evidence of squamous differentiation may lie in the sharp appearance of the cytoplasmic borders and in the tendency of the cells to form a monolayer. The cytoplasm of these cells is generally cyanophilic. Care must be taken to ensure that these neoplasms are not confused with tissue reparative reactions. In the latter, nucleoli are prominent and multiple, but chromatin pattern and ratio of nucleus to cytoplasm are normal. Cells remain tightly cohesive, and the necrosis is absent. Examples of squamous cell carcinoma are illustrated in Figs. 4-20, 4-21, and 4-46 to 4-51.

Adenocarcinoma

Depending on their location and size, adenocarcinomas may exfoliate large numbers of diagnostic cells, few cells, or no cells at all. Small peripheral tumors are least likely to provide diagnostic material in sputum or bronchial specimens. Although the cellular pattern reflective of the adenocarcinoma group is readily identified in specimens of respiratory material,

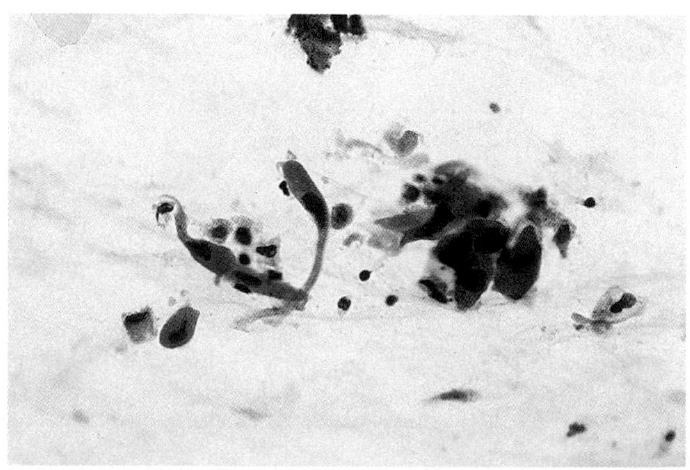

Fig. 4-46 Keratinizing squamous cell carcinoma in lung. (Sputum; Papanicolaou stain.)

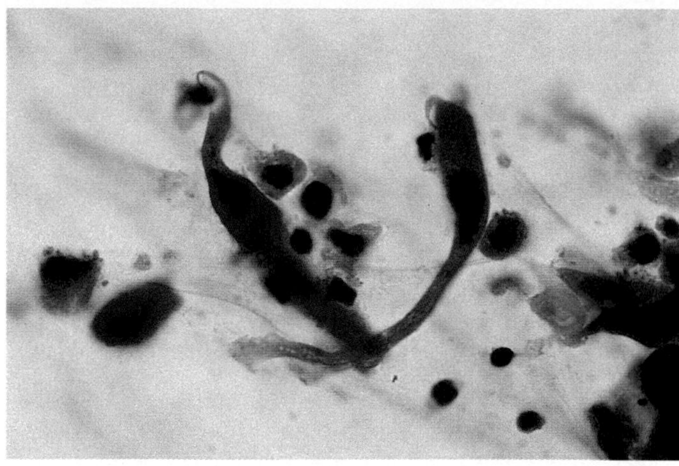

Fig. 4-47 Keratinizing squamous cell carcinoma in lung. (Sputum; Papanicolaou stain.)

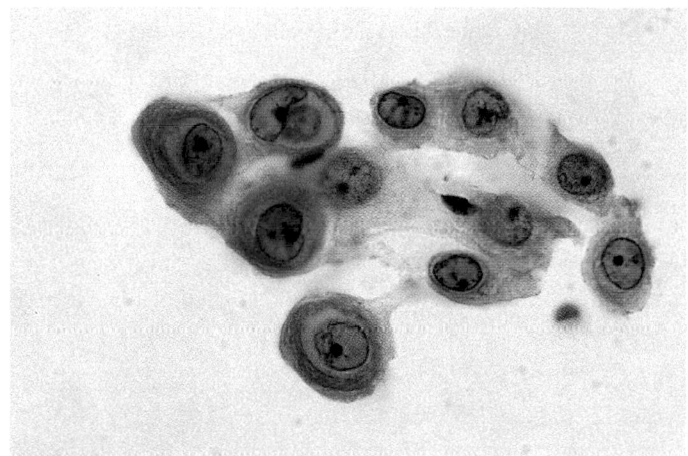

Fig. 4-48 Keratinizing squamous cell carcinoma in lung. (Bronchial brush; Papanicolaou stain.)

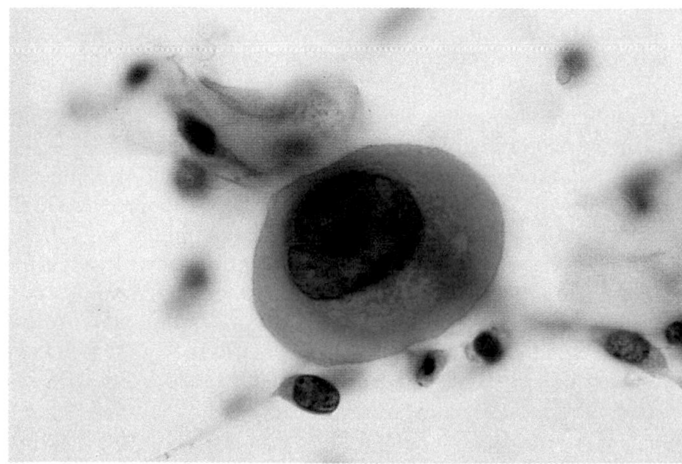

Fig. 4-49 Keratinizing squamous cell carcinoma in lung. (Bronchial brush; Papanicolaou stain.)

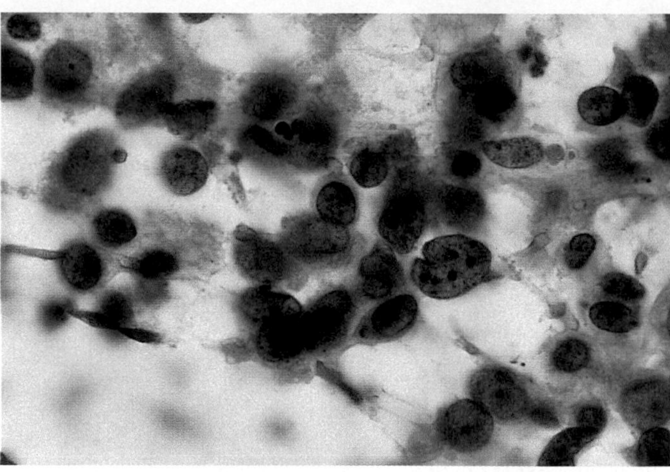

Fig. 4-50 Poorly differentiated squamous cell carcinoma in lung. (Bronchial brush; Papanicolaou stain.)

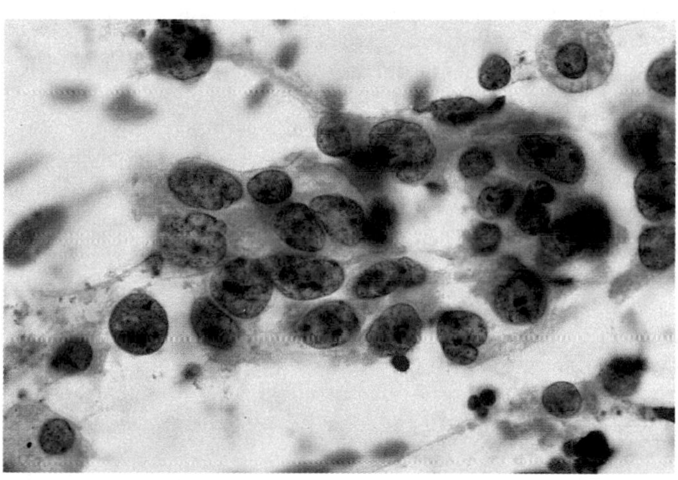

Fig. 4-51 Poorly differentiated squamous cell carcinoma in lung. (Bronchial brush; Papanicolaou stain.)

attempts to further classify the adenocarcinoma into acinar, papillary, or bronchioloalveolar cell types are less successful. Adenocarcinomas present in cytologic material with both single cells and cell clusters. The chromatin in well-differentiated tumors is typically finely granular to powdery in appearance. The nuclei are enlarged and round to oval with varying degrees of nuclear membrane abnormalities. They may, however, be so bland in appearance that one must rely on other features, such as variation of cell size and shape, cell crowding and disorganization within groups, and lack of cohesion to establish a diagnosis of malignancy. In many adenocarcinomas of the acinar type, the presence of centrally placed macronucleoli is a prominent feature. The cytoplasm may vary in appearance from homogeneous to extremely vacuolated. The vacuoles may be multiple and small, imparting a delicate foamy appearance to the cytoplasm, or may be large, causing indentation and margination of the nucleus. In well-differentiated neoplasms, the cells may assume a columnar shape, whereas in other cases, many cells will exhibit extremely high nuclear to cytoplasmic ratios and will be recognized only as undifferentiated malignant tumor cells. Cell groups in specimens of adenocarcinoma may consist of ball-like clusters, papillary fragments, loose clusters, or true acini with central lumens. With decreasing differentiation of the neoplasm, one sees increasing nuclear hyperchromasia, coarsening of chromatin, more irregular nuclear contours, and greater cellular pleomorphism, such that the cytomorphology begins to merge with that of large cell undifferentiated carcinoma.

The histologic diagnosis of bronchioloalveolar carcinoma is based upon a predominant pattern of growth of cuboidal or columnar cells along alveolar or fibrovascular septa.[83] Although this pattern may sometimes be appreciated in FNAB,[84] one obviously does not have benefit of this architectural feature in sputum or bronchial specimens. There are, however, some cytologic features that are typical of bronchioloalveolar carcinomas and that may allow one to suggest this diagnosis in cytologic material.[85] Like other adenocarcinomas, bronchioloalveolar carcinoma tends to exfoliate both as single cells and cell groups. The nuclei are characteristically round to oval and uniform in size, with finely granular or powdery chromatin and small inconspicuous nucleoli. A minority of cases, however, will show prominent nucleoli. Nuclear folds are commonly present, and in some cases intranuclear cytoplasmic invaginations will be observed. The cytoplasm varies in amount from modest to abundant and, like that of other adenocarcinomas, may be homogeneous, granular, finely vacuolated, or distended by single or multiple large vacuoles. Smith and Frable[86] and others[84,85] have emphasized the extreme depth of focus in the three-dimensional cell clusters of bronchioloalveolar carcinoma. Papilla-shaped fragments lacking fibrovascular cores are also common. In some cytologic preparations numerous nonpigmented macrophage-like cells will be present. It may be extremely difficult or impossible to determine in individual cases whether these cells represent tumor cells or macrophages. Illustrations of adenocarcinoma are shown in Figs. 4-22 and 4-52 to 4-54.

Large cell undifferentiated carcinoma

Large cell undifferentiated carcinomas exfoliate large numbers of diagnostic cells and present in respiratory specimens both as single cells and as tissue fragments. The single cells are large and possess multiple criteria for malignancy, including high nuclear to cytoplasmic ratios, great aberrations in the chromatin patterns, abnormal nuclear contours, and multiple, enlarged, irregular nucleoli. Cytoplasm may be wispy or homogeneous with a tendency toward cyanophilia, but there is no evidence of keratinization, and there is insufficient cytoplasmic differentiation to warrant a diagnosis of adenocarcinoma (Fig. 4-55). The large tissue fragments, which may be present, lack any recognizable architectural pattern such as squamous pearls, acini, or papillary structures. Occasionally seen is the giant cell carcinoma variant of large cell undifferentiated carcinoma, so named because of the presence of many multinucleated tumor giant cells. Additional differential diagnostic considerations for large cell undifferentiated carcinoma would include metastatic undifferentiated carcinomas, amelanotic malignant melanomas, sarcomas, chemotherapy changes, and radiation changes. Benign irradiated epithelial cells may possess very large nuclei, but their equally abundant cytoplasm should help to differentiate them from tumor cells. Previously irradiated neoplasm may

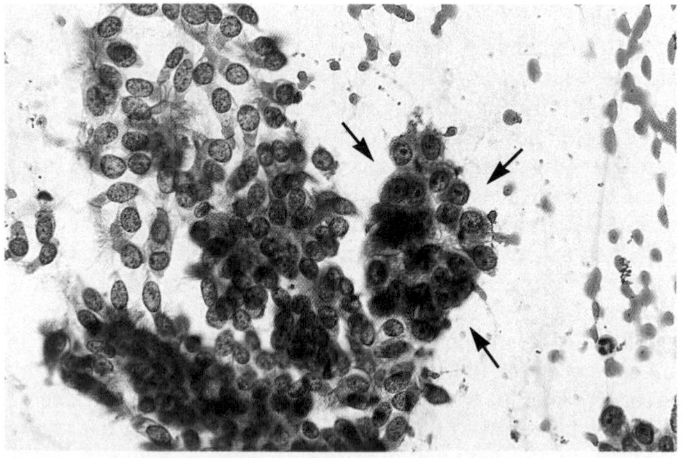

Fig. 4-52 Adenocarcinoma in lung *(arrows)*, contrasted with ciliated columnar epithelial cells. (Bronchial brush; Papanicolaou stain.)

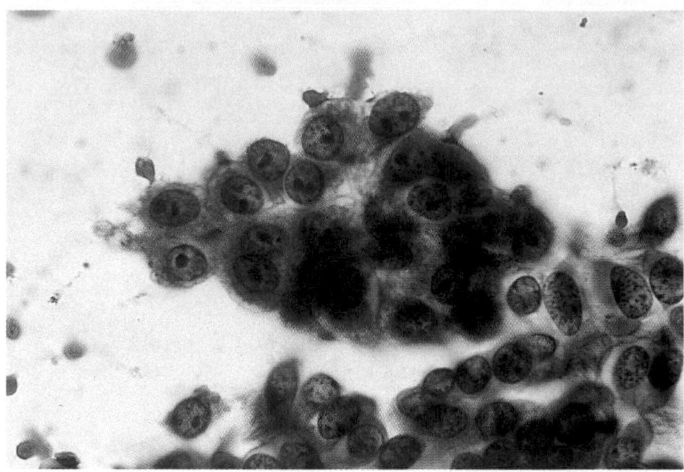

Fig. 4-53 Adenocarcinoma in lung. (Bronchial brush; Papanicolaou stain.)

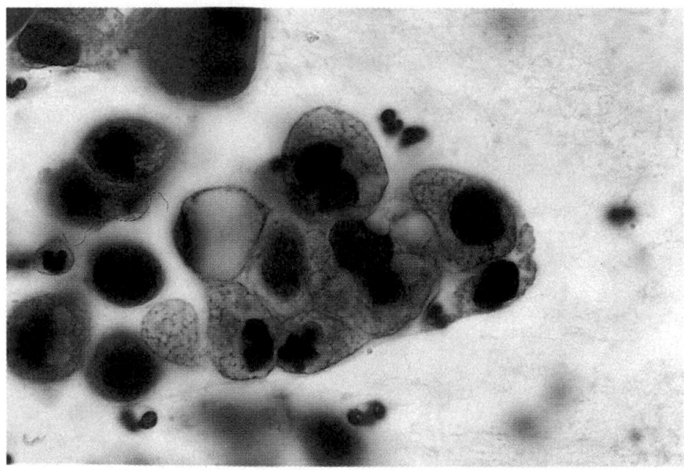

Fig. 4-54 Adenocarcinoma in lung. (Bronchial brush; Papanicolaou stain.)

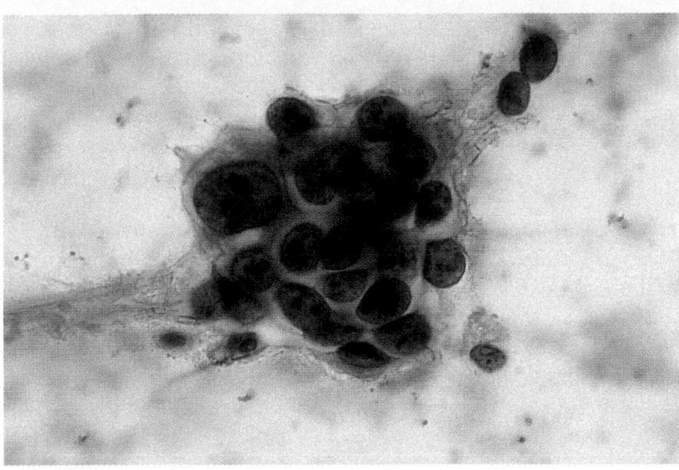

Fig. 4-55 Large cell undifferentiated carcinoma in lung. (Bronchial brush; Papanicolaou stain.)

exhibit bizarre giant cells indistinguishable from those observed in giant cell carcinoma. All the non–small cell carcinomas of the lung may exfoliate only large anaplastic malignant tumor cells into the cytologic specimens, and so the cytologic diagnosis of large cell undifferentiated carcinoma is made.

Small cell undifferentiated carcinoma

The individual cell from small cell undifferentiated carcinoma varies from approximately one and one half times to two times the size of a lymphocyte. It is round to oval, possessing a centrally placed nucleus with a uniform but deeply staining chromatin pattern and a very high nuclear to cytoplasmic ratio. Nucleoli are occasionally visible but are generally inconspicuous. In specimens of freshly prepared sputum, large numbers of tumor cells may be found entrapped in strands of mucus. A most characteristic presentation results with clusters of these small tumor cells exhibiting extreme molding superimposed upon irregular nuclear outlines. Because this tumor is highly prone to necrosis, the cellular specimen will frequently reflect this, with cells exhibiting karyopyknosis, disintegration of the cytoplasm, and the formation of cyanophilic masses of necrotic debris (Fig. 4-23). Cells of the intermediate cell subtype of small cell undifferentiated carcinoma possess slightly larger nuclei with a larger rim of cytoplasm and, on occasion, conspicuous nucleoli.

Diagnostic accuracy

The diagnostic accuracy of cytologic methods in the detection of lung cancer will vary according to the site and size of the tumor and the cytologic method chosen for the diagnostic procedure. Sensitivity reports for the detection of primary malignancies from one satisfactory specimen of sputum have varied from 27% to 42%. With multiple specimens the sensitivity rises to a reported range of 57% to 89%. Reported sensitivity for single bronchial specimens obtained by washing or brushing varies from 61% to 77%. For sputum and bronchial material, specificity has been reported consistently as 98%, or greater. Sensitivity for FNAB has been reported in the range of 75% to 95%, and specificity as 99% or greater.[69]

BODY CAVITY FLUIDS

The body cavities are those spaces lined by parietal and visceral serous membranes covered by a single layer of mesothelium and comprise the pleural, pericardial, and peritoneal cavities. In the absence of underlying disease, these spaces contain less than 5 ml of a fluid consisting of small amounts of protein, electrolytes, hyaluronic acid, and other substances. The cellular components are extremely low, consisting of a few mesothelial cells, lymphocytes, macrophages, and other rare cells derived from the circulating blood or lymphatics. One of the major functions of this fluid appears to be that of lubricating the parietal and visceral serosal surfaces and thus supporting normal anatomic movements. Normally this fluid is turned over rapidly, a process in which fluid production is equalled by fluid absorption. A variety of nonneoplastic diseases or conditions may produce effusions through either altered fluid dynamics, protein content, or capillary permeability. The formation of a truly malignant effusion, that is, one that contains malignant tumor cells, is dependent on the invasion through the serosal membrane by cancer so that the mesothelial lining is penetrated. This can occur by direct extension from a primary or metastatic cancer lying in the periphery of a visceral organ, or by lymphatic or vascular metastases. Effusions associated with cancer but devoid of tumor cells may be produced when malignant tumors alter hydrostatic pressures, capillary permeability, and protein content but do not penetrate the mesothelial lining.

Effusions are extremely common and constitute a significant proportion of all cytologic specimens being examined in any laboratory of a large general hospital. The major purpose of cytologic examination of specimens of effusion fluid is to determine whether malignant tumor cells are present. If it is determined that neoplastic cells are present, two additional objectives are to define cell type and tissue or organ of origin. The diagnostic accuracy of such examinations is dependent on several factors, but most noteworthy are the level of training and experience in pathology and cytopathology of the examiner, the quality of preservation and cellular display of the specimen of fluid, and the nature of the disease involving the pleural membranes.[87]

Nonneoplastic diseases

In the absence of cancer, effusions may be produced by a wide variety of abnormalities and insults. In most of these cases, the cellular response is quite nonspecific and will show varying proportions of mesothelial cells, macrophages, erythrocytes, lymphocytes (Fig. 4-4), neutrophils, and other leukocytes. Studies in the literature have shown that certain diseases may occasionally show cellular changes in the effusion that will reflect their presence. Examples of these include infections such as tuberculosis,[88] blastomycosis,[89] aspergillosis,[89] viral infections,[46-49] echinococcosis,[90] cryptococcosis, and strongyloidiasis.[91] Noninfectious nonneoplastic diseases include rheumatoid arthritis,[92] lupus erythematosus,[93] eosinophilic pleural effusion,[94] pleural endometriosis,[95] and sickle cell disease.[96]

From the standpoint of diagnostic interpretation, the major practical problem that the cytopathologist encounters is the distinction between reactive mesothelial cells and cancer cells. When the mesothelial lining is injured or destroyed, the mesothelial cell reacts by both hyperplasia and hypertrophy of irritated mesothelium and regeneration of destroyed mesothelium. In a typical fluid specimen one will observe large numbers of mesothelial cells growing both singly and as cell clusters. Individual cells will exhibit enlargement, occasional binucleation, or even multinucleation, and prominent nucleoli (Figs. 4-5 and 4-6). Fluid imbibition may produce cytoplasmic vacuolization mimicking adenocarcinoma. Pulmonary infarction, uremia, polyserositis, irradiation,[97] and chemotherapy are but a few examples of situations that may result in the presence of extremely bizarre mesothelial cells. For the experienced examiner the absence of true nuclear evidence of malignancy and the rarity of cellular organoid formations should preclude an erroneous diagnosis of cancer.

Neoplastic diseases

In prior sections of this chapter emphasis has been placed upon the presence of excellent malignant criteria in well-displayed and well-preserved cells in support of a conclusive cytologic diagnosis of cancer. Indeed the diagnosis of cancer made from a cellular specimen should be at the same level of confidence as one made from the examination of a paraffin section of tissue. Such conservatism and assuredness are particularly crucial when one is evaluating specimens of body cavity fluid. A cytologic diagnosis of cancer on such a specimen presents extremely grave evidence that the cancer has become widely disseminated and may trigger major therapeutic decisions without further attempts to verify the diagnosis.

Of importance, in addition to the search for excellent criteria of malignancy in individual cells, is the finding of true tissue fragments composed of these putative tumor cells. Individual reactive mesothelial cells, though mimicking cancer, are much less likely to be found in large cell-based tissue aggregates. The following types of tissue fragments are of particular help in establishing a diagnosis of cancer: true acinar formations, papillary fronds, small cells forming tightly molded cellular chains, and ball-like clusters of cells forming a true external community border. Epithelial cell cancers are those most likely to shed tissue fragments into the body cavity fluids. The lymphomas and leukemias usually present as single small cells. The sarcomas also usually show single tumor cells with poorly defined cytoplasm. Occasionally either intracellular or intercellular changes may aid in the determination of differentiation or organ of origin. Examples are intracellular evidence of the presence of mucin, keratin, melanin, hyaluronic acid, acid phosphatase, glycogen, and fat and cross-striations and intercellular formations such as psammoma bodies, rosettes, Call-Exner bodies, osteoid, and cartilage.

Many studies in the literature report on the frequency and accuracy of cytologic detection of cancer cells in effusions drawn from patients with known cancers,[98-104] and in such patients cancer cells will be found in 50% to 60% of such cases and in 90% of such cases, the cancer diagnosis will be definitely established after examination of one specimen. The most common tumors will be adenocarcinomas and lymphoid malignancies. Squamous cell carcinomas, though very common primary neoplasms, will be recognized with much less frequency.

In the experience of one of the authors in the cell typing of 766 consecutive specimens of pleural malignant effusions, a cytologic diagnosis of adenocarcinoma was by far the most common one rendered.[103] It constituted more than 50% of the diagnoses made and was more than four times more frequent than the next two most common diagnoses: the lymphoma-leukemia group and large cell undifferentiated carcinoma. The lung was the most common organ of tumor origin. The next four neoplastic groups or organ sites encountered in order of descending frequency were lymphomas and leukemias, breast, female genital tract, and gastrointestinal tract. In more than 16% of patients cited in this series, the primary site of the neoplasm was never determined. It is not at all uncommon for a malignant effusion to be the first clinical manifestation of unknown cancer that has already spread. For this reason alone, cytologic examination of all effusions is mandatory, regardless of the clinical diagnosis. Frequently the cytologic diagnosis will help disclose cell type and probable organ primary. But even when this is not possible and further clinical studies fail to find the primary cancer, the cytopathologic diagnosis has correctly uncovered the true nature of the patient's disease. Appropriate palliative radiation therapy and chemotherapy can then be begun without further delay.

In peritoneal effusions in adult women the most common organ sites in order of decreasing frequency are reported as ovary, breast, gastrointestinal tract, and lymphoma. In peritoneal malignant effusions in adult men it is gastrointestinal tract and lymphoma. In children the most common sites for all effusions are leukemia-lymphoma, Wilms' tumor, neuroblastoma, embryonol, rhabdomyosarcoma, and Ewing's sarcoma.[5]

In some patients cellular changes are so specific as to permit not only an unequivocal diagnosis of cancer, but also a definitive identification of the tumor differentiation and organ of primary origin. Several examples follow. Small cell undifferentiated carcinomas are characterized by a highly specific morphology, which almost always permits a definitive cytologic diagnosis.[105] In one series reported, all effusion specimens from the patients with small cell undifferentiated carcinoma were correctly diagnosed as showing malignant cells from small cell undifferentiated carcinoma of the lung.[103] An example of small cell undifferentiated carcinoma in a pericardial effusion is illustrated in Fig. 4-56. Conclusive studies in the literature and the personal experience of the authors justify the conclusion that cytologic studies on effusions are able to differentiate between lymphoma or leukemia and inflammatory exudates in over 75% of cases. Furthermore, with an even

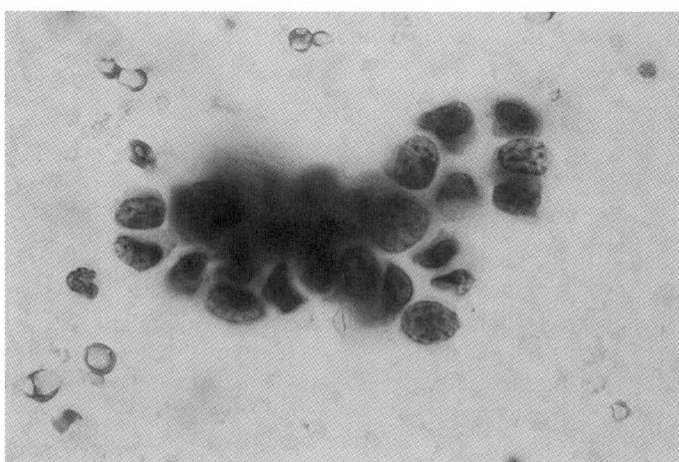

Fig. 4-56 Small cell undifferentiated carcinoma of lung in pericardial effusion. (Papanicolaou stain.)

higher level of accuracy such studies can differentiate between the lymphoma and leukemia group and other types of malignancies.[106,107] Adjunct studies with cell markers make possible the further classification of the various neoplastic types.[108] Neoplastic cells in effusions shed from metastatic breast cancer may exhibit cellular features that permit a correct identification of the primary organ site.[109,110] Distinctive diagnostic features for ductal carcinoma include large polygonal cells with vesicular nuclei and centrally placed macronucleoli; cellular aggregates forming organoid structures—solid ball-like clusters and hollow spheres, cellular chains described variously as "Indian filing" and "Chinese lettering," and tissue fragments with cells molded into "owl-eyed" configurations (Fig. 4-57). Particular interest has focused on the unique presentation in body cavity fluids of metastatic lobular carcinoma. The cells are present as single small cells with occasional small tissue fragments. The cytologic picture of lymphoma may be suggested. The ovarian carcinomas in their metastases may have a highly distinctive morphology. Malignant tissue fragments composed of cells with greatly hyperdistended secretory vacuoles, macronucleoli, and psammoma bodies should always be suggestive of certain organ primaries—adenocarcinomas of the ovary or endometrium, bronchioloalveolar carcinoma of the lung, and papillary adenocarcinoma of the thyroid (Fig. 4-58). Additional examples of other malignant neoplasms are illustrated in Figs. 4-59 to 4-61. The malignant cells containing mucin and presenting as "signet-ring" forms are diagnostic for this tumor type (Fig. 4-59).

The epithelial type of diffuse mesothelioma is the sole neoplasm arising as a primary neoplasm of the serous membranes that is of concern to the cytopathologist. Malignant effusions from this neoplasm, through generally uncommon in most hospitals, may present a more frequent problem in differential diagnosis in those institutions receiving patients who have worked in shipyards or other industries with heavy exposure to asbestos. There is considerable controversy in the literature regarding the ease and accuracy of the cytologic diagnosis of mesothelioma.[111-115] The typical cytologic specimen of fluid from such a tumor will exhibit many large atypical cells with prominent nucleoli occurring both singly and as papillary clusters. Multinucleation is common. The clusters may show a

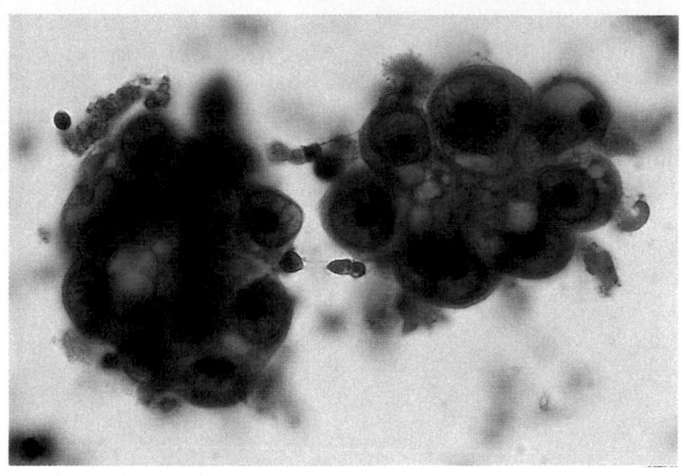

Fig. 4-58 Adenocarcinoma of the ovary in peritoneal effusion. (Papanicolaou stain.)

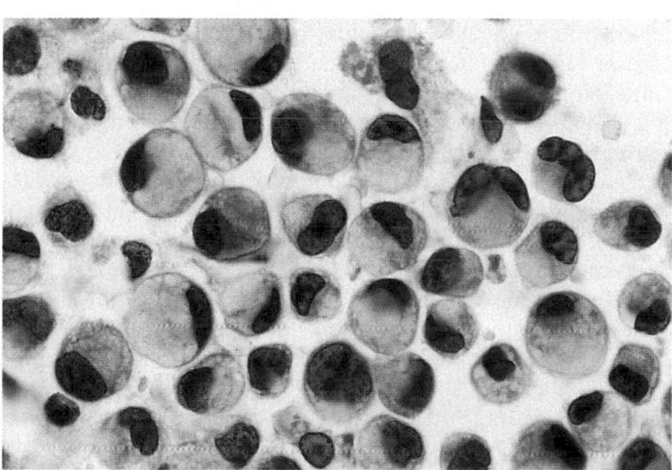

Fig. 4-59 Mucus-producing adenocarcinoma of "signet-ring" type in pleural effusion. (Papanicolaou stain.)

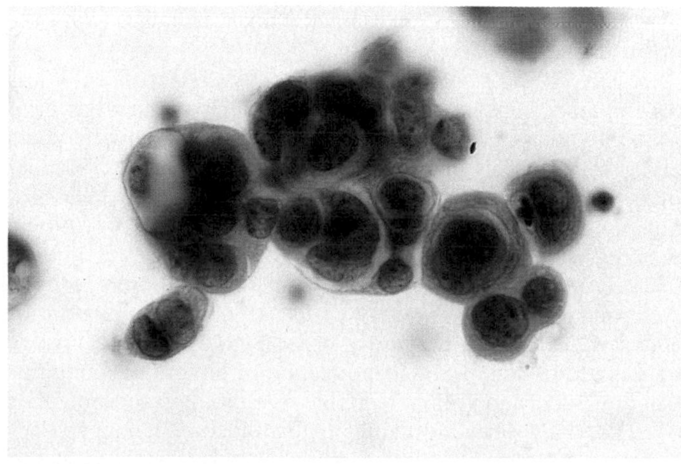

Fig. 4-57 Ductal carcinoma of the breast in pleural effusion. (Papanicolaou stain.)

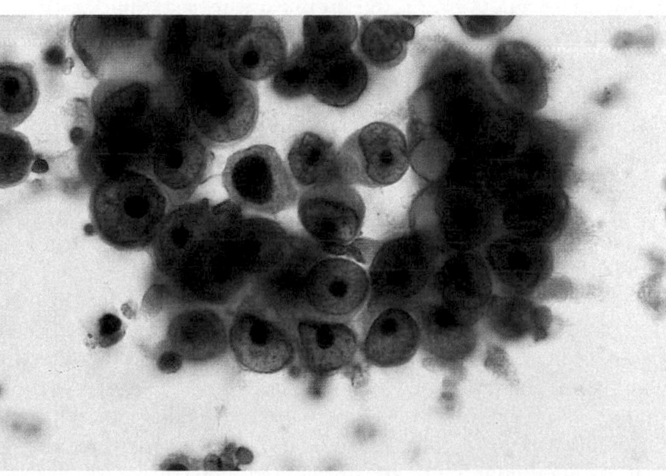

Fig. 4-60 Adenocarcinoma of endometrium in peritoneal effusion. (Papanicolaou stain.)

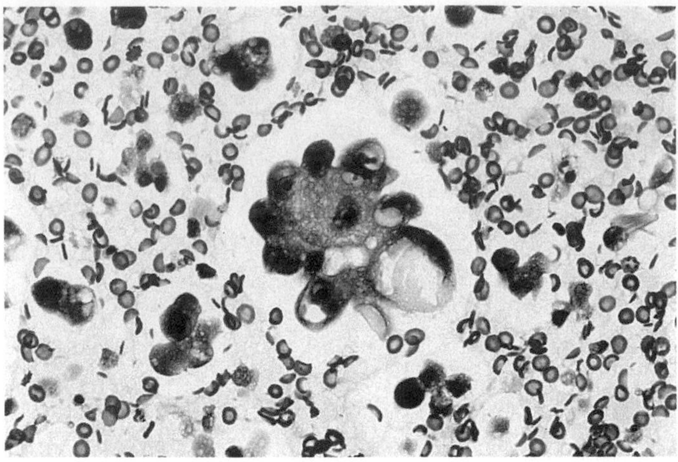

Fig. 4-61 Adenocarcinoma of the endometrium in peritoneal effusion. Same case as in Fig. 4-60 but showing the malignant cells displayed in a cell block preparation. (Hematoxylin and eosin stain.)

knobby border and finely vacuolated cytoplasm. The diagnostic dilemmas are those of differentiating between mesothelioma, reactive mesothelium, and adenocarcinoma. Special stains and some immunoperoxidase markers may be of some help. Alcian blue, before and after treatment with hyaluronidase, periodic acid–Schiff stain, before and after treatment with diastase, and mucicarmine may aid the differential diagnosis by demonstrating the presence of hyaluronic acid or mucin. Positive staining of the cells with antibodies to carcinoembryonic antigen, epithelial membrane antigen (EMA), tumor-associated glycoprotein (TAG-72), and Leu-M1 antigen strongly favor a diagnosis of adenocarcinoma over mesothelioma or reactive mesothelium.[116-120]

OTHER BODY SITES

In addition to the body sites previously discussed where clinical cytopathology plays a significant diagnostic role, several others lend themselves to the techniques of conventional exfoliative cytology. They include the gastrointestinal tract,[121,122] urinary tract,[123-127] and the central nervous system.[128-131] The applications of cytopathology in these sites are briefly summarized here.

Gastrointestinal tract

Cytopathology plays a useful but relatively limited role in the evaluation of lesions of the esophagus, stomach, colon, and rectum. Major indications are for viral or fungal infections of the esophagus and carcinomas of this organ or stomach.

Fungal infections, mainly caused by *Candida* species, and viral infection, usually caused by herpes simplex, are the most common causes for infectious esophagitis. When present, organisms or diagnostic cellular changes are readily identified by characteristic features previously discussed. Barrett's esophagus, the presence of glandular cells in the lower portion of the esophagus above the gastroesophageal sphincter, may be diagnosed by cytologic methods. The cytologic picture is that of glandular cells in sheets and clusters with varying degrees of cellular atypia and inflammation. Squamous cell carcinoma is the most common malignant neoplasm of the esophagus. Histologically the tumor may range from well to poorly differentiated. Morphologic features are similar to squamous cell carcinoma of the lung and other body sites. Adenocarcinoma may also arise in the esophagus, either from Barrett's esophagus or from extension from the gastric cardia.

By far the most important use of cytopathology in the evaluation of lesions of the stomach is that of endoscopically directed brushing for detection of cancer of the stomach. Adenocarcinoma is the most common malignant neoplasm arising in the mucosa and is most frequently characterized by the formation of tubules or papillae. The malignant cells shed may vary from small to large and may exhibit mucin production. The cytopathology of these tumors reflects the histology. Individual nuclei display irregular chromatin distribution and a single enlarged and rounded nucleolus. Cytoplasm may be abundant in well-differentiated tumors and stain positively for mucin. These cells must be differentiated from the atypical but benign ones that may arise in acute gastritis, gastric atrophy, and peptic ulceration. The signet-ring form of adenocarcinoma is quite distinctive but uncommon.

Cytopathologic techniques (usually brushing) have been sucessfully employed in the evaluation of benign inflammatory and malignant diseases of the colon and rectum. They are particularly useful in the presence of severe inflammatory disease such as ulcerative colitis in which the development of colon cancer is a major concern. The brushing technique permits sampling of multiple sites in a rapid and noninvasive manner. Thus a cytologic mapping of suspicious areas can be easily achieved.

Urinary tract

Although the cytologic evaluation of urine has been reported to be of use in many benign diseases and malignant neoplasms of the urinary tract, the most important indication for its use is in the detection of malignant tumors arising in the urothelium. In this respect it may serve as a screening tool for the evaluation of patients who are asymptomatic but who are at high risk for the development of bladder cancer, as a diagnostic procedure in symptomatic patients, and as a follow-up procedure for detecting possible recurrence of urothelial malignancies in patients previously treated. For screening purposes the voided urine is the most frequently utilized specimen. In symptomatic patients and in patients being followed, additional useful specimens include catheterized urine, bladder washings, and washings and brushings from the ureter and renal calyces.

A very accurate and realistic assessment of the place of urinary cytology in the evaluation of urothelial tumors has been stated by Koss: "Papillary urothelial tumors may be lined either by morphologically normal urothelium or by a urothelium with only slight cellular or nuclear abnormalties. For obvious reasons, such tumors cannot be identified in cytologic material with any degree of certainty. Thus the general concept that all malignant or potentially malignant tumors can be identified in cytologic material because they are made up of abnormal cells does not apply here. Cytology of the urinary tract is useful only in the identification of tumors or conditions that are associated with perceptible morphologic abnormalities of cells. This pertains mainly to papillary and nonpapillary carcinoma in-situ and related atypical hyperplasia."[5] An example of a urothelial carcinoma of high grade present in urine is illustrated in Fig. 4-62.

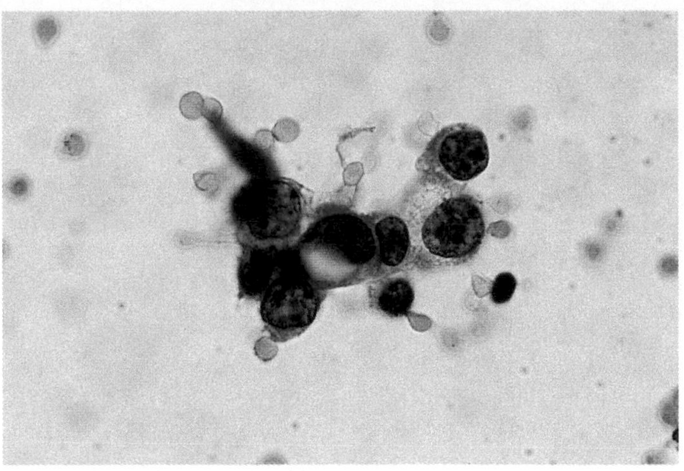

Fig. 4-62 Urothelial carcinoma in urine. (Papanicolaou stain.)

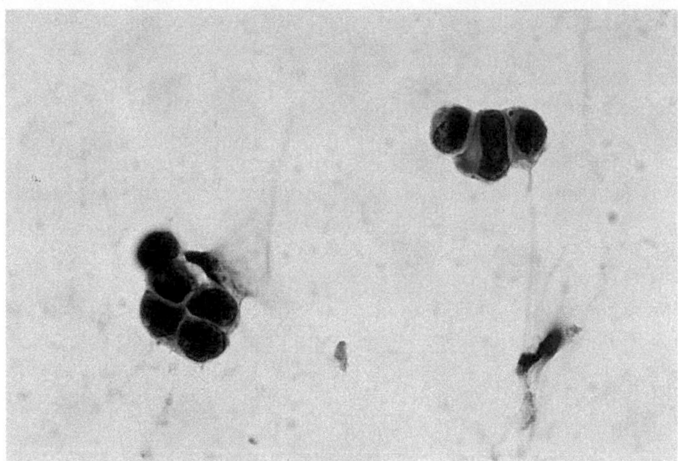

Fig. 4-63 Medulloblastoma in cerebrospinal fluid. (Papanicolaou stain.)

Adenocarcinomas of the renal parenchyma and prostate may occasionally shed diagnostic cells into the urine. Unfortunately this event signals evidence of far-advanced disease that usually has already manifested itself with earlier signs and symptoms.

Cerebrospinal fluid

The major indications for cytologic examination of cerebrospinal fluid are suspicion of malignancy (primary or metastatic) and infection. Samples of the cerebrospinal fluid may be obtained by sampling of the ventricular space or, more commonly, through spinal tap in the lumbosacral region. These specimens are best suited to allow detection of disseminated malignancy (carcinomatosis) of the subarachnoid space, or infection.

All the common fungal infections may be identified by examination of the cerebrospinal fluid. Of these, *Cryptococcus neoformans* is the most common and usually appears as a variably sized, budding yeast with a thick mucopolysaccharide capsule. It is uncommon to identify the direct cytopathic effects of central nervous system viral infection. More commonly, indirect evidence of viral infection is seen as represented by a pleocytosis of inflammatory cells. Bacterial infection should be suspected if large numbers of polymorphonuclear leukocytes are present, but organisms will rarely be seen in the Papanicolaou stain. If such infections are suspected, appropriate samples should be taken for microbiology and Gram-stain procedures.

An important consideration in the examination of cerebrospinal fluid is the potential contamination by cells from the bone marrow or neoplastic cells from peripheral blood or from other patients. Megakaryocytes and myeloid blast cells, in particular, if introduced into the specimen from the vertebral marrow, can appear sufficiently atypical to raise concern regarding metastatic tumor. In patients with leukemia, contamination of the fluid with peripheral blood containing blast forms may be a major pitfall. Although both primary and metastatic malignant neoplasms may be found in the cerebrospinal fluid, malignant cells in the cerebrospinal fluid are most frequently representative of metastatic malignancy, with the histologic types paralleling the most common tumors affecting men and women: lung and breast. The morphology of these tumors in the cerebrospinal fluid generally parallels that of the primary neoplasms. Except for medulloblastomas, it is uncommon for primary brain tumors to shed into the cerebrospinal fluid. The cytomorphology of medulloblastoma is highly characteristic and virtually diagnostic. An example is depicted in Fig. 4-63.

FINE-NEEDLE ASPIRATION BIOPSY

As has been summarized previously in this chapter, the discipline of cytopathology is founded on the basis of the diagnostic interpretation of changes occurring within individual cells that exfoliate spontaneously or are harvested by some mechanical device (usually a brush) from epithelial linings. In contrast, the discipline of surgical pathology is based mainly on the studies of alterations in architecture of intact tissues. Changes in individual cells are of secondary importance. Fine-needle aspiration biopsy (FNAB) is the bridge between these two morphologic disciplines. A fine needle inserted into a mass under investigation samples both individual cells and tiny tissue biopsy specimens. Thus, when the pathologist views a specimen obtained by FNAB, the observations of histoarchitecture and alterations in individual cells combine to produce a powerful diagnostic tool. Where one further considers that, in addition to its high accuracy, FNAB is rapid, simple, and relatively inexpensive and has a very low morbidity, one can understand why FNAB has achieved such widespread use since its reintroduction.

FNAB may be divided into that performed on superficial organs and tissues and that performed on the internal and deep-seated organs and tissues.

FNAB of superficial organs

FNAB of superficial organs is most frequently directed at breast, thyroid, salivary glands, lymph nodes, eyes, or any other palpable mass.[132-142] The greatest advantage from this procedure is achieved when the cytopathologist personally performs the aspiration of the mass, prepares specimens for immediate microscopic study, and renders an immediate opinion about the satisfactoriness of the specimen for diagnosis. By this procedure, the cytopathologist is able to talk directly to the patient, palpate the mass, and directly guide the passage of the needle into it. The major advantages include a significant drop in the number of unsatisfactory specimens and a striking increase in the sensitivity and specificity of the diagnoses rendered. Sensitivities and specificities for FNAB of superficial organs are summarized in Table 4-4. Illustrations of cellular specimens obtained by FNAB of the parotid gland are shown in Figs. 4-64 and 4-65, by FNAB of the thyroid in Fig. 4-66, and by FNAB of the breast in Figs. 4-67 and 4-68.

FNAB of deep-seated organs

Giant strides in radiologic technology such as modern fluoroscopy and computerized axial tomography have made it possible to pass a needle into virtually any mass present in any of the deep-seated organs. The resultant diagnostic procedure now in many situtations obviates the need for major surgery with exploratory laparotomy. The advantages gained through lowered patient morbidity and mortality and monetary savings are both obvious and enormous.

The scientific literature is now replete with numerous publications that document the sucesses of FNAB in such

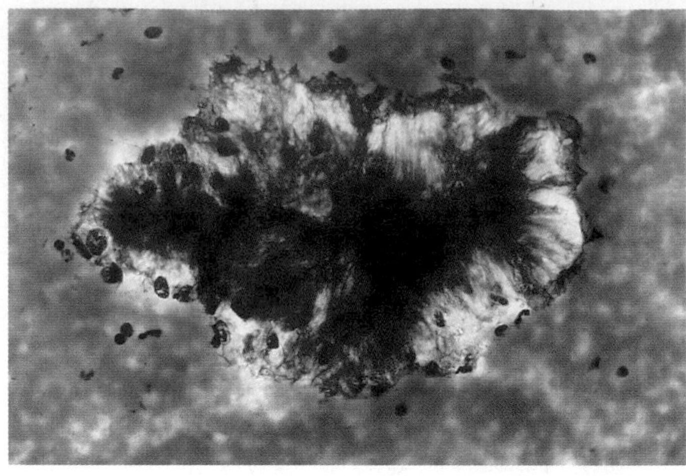

Fig. 4-65 Pleomorphic adenoma of parotid gland from FNAB of parotid gland mass. Notice the metachromasia of the stroma. (Diff-Quik stain.)

Table 4-4 Accuracy of fine needle aspiration biopsy

Organ or tissue	Sensitivity (%)	Specificity (%)
Superficial Organs		
Breast	73-95	87-100
Thyroid	88-99	80-100
Salivary glands	66-100	96-99
Lymph nodes	87-100	88-99
Deep Organs		
Lung	75-95	98-100
Liver	92-96	98-100
Pancreas	61-100	97-100
Kidney	68-93	96-100
Prostate	94-98	96-98
Central nervous system	87-90	99-100
Bone and soft tissues	67-100	98-100

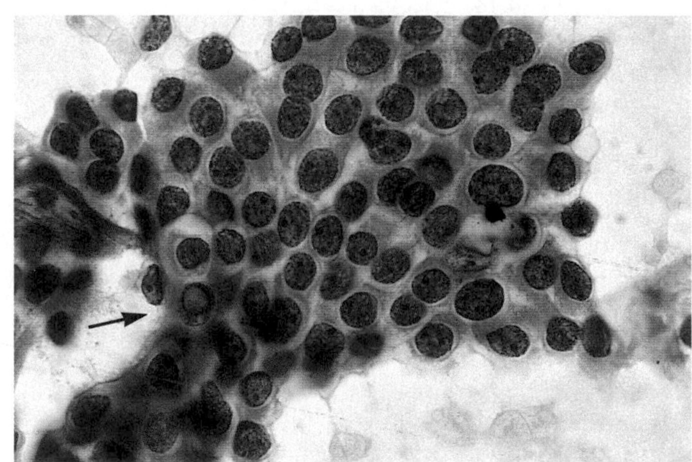

Fig. 4-66 Papillary carcinoma of thyroid gland from FNAB of thyroid gland mass. *Arrow,* Intranuclear cytoplasmic protrusion ("Little Orphan Annie eye") diagnostically important. (Papanicolaou stain.)

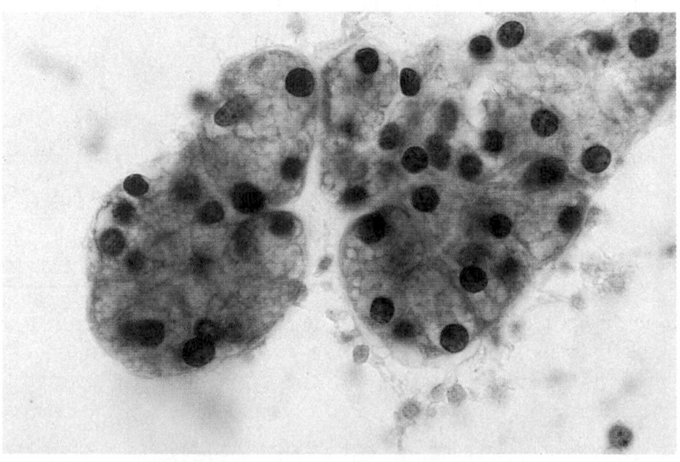

Fig. 4-64 Normal parotid acinar tissue from fine-needle aspiration biopsy of parotid gland. (Papanicolaou stain.)

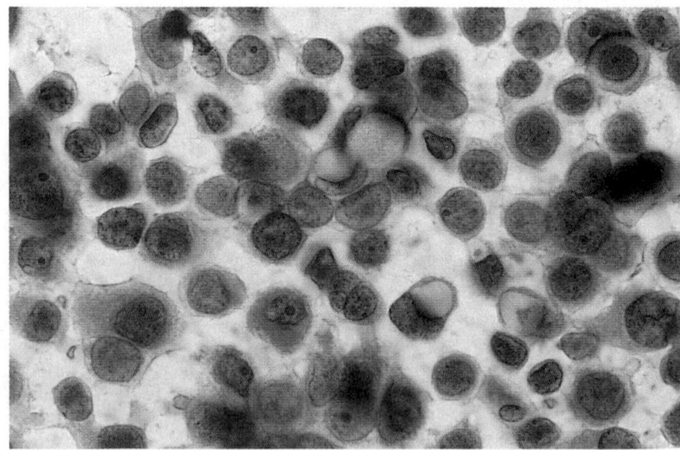

Fig. 4-67 Adenocarcinoma of the breast in FNAB from breast mass. (Papanicolaou stain.)

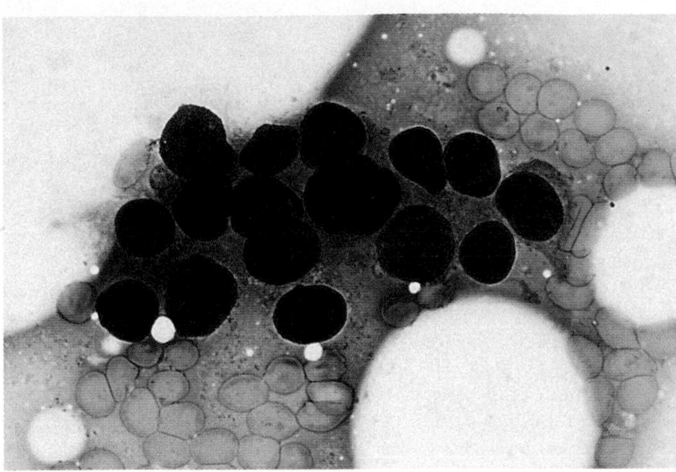

Fig. 4-68 Adenocarcinoma of the breast in FNAB from breast mass. (Diff-Quik stain.)

deep-seated organs as the lung, mediastinum, liver, pancreas, kidney, adrenal, spleen, ovary, bone, soft tissues, and central nervous system.[143-148] Selected sensitivities and specificities for these are summarized in Table 4-4.

REFERENCES

General

1. Grunze H, Spriggs AI: *History of clinical cytology,* Darmstadt, West Germany, 1980, G-I-T Verlag, Ernst Giebeler
2. Martin HE, Ellis EB: Biopsy by needle puncture and aspiration, *Ann Surg* 92:169, 1930.
3. Papanicolaou GN, Traut HF: *The diagnosis of uterine cancer by the vaginal smear,* New York, 1943, Commonwealth Fund.
4. U.S. Department of Health and Human Services: *Implementation of the Breast and Cervical Cancer Mortality Prevention Act: a progress report,* Washington, DC, 1991.
5. Koss LG: *Diagnostic cytology and its histopathologic bases,* ed 4, Philadelphia, 1992, Lippincott.
6. Bibbo M: *Comprehensive cytopathology,* Philadelphia, 1991, Saunders.
7. Frable WJ: *Thin-needle aspiration biopsy,* Philadelphia, 1983, Saunders.
8. Koss LG, Woyke S, Olszewski W: *Aspiration biopsy: cytologic interpretation and histologic bases,* ed 2, New York, 1992, Igaku-Shoin.
9. Keebler CM, Somrak TM, editors: *The manual of cytotechnology,* ed 7, Chicago, 1993, ASCP Press.
10. Wied GL, Keebler CM, Koss LG et al, editors: *Compendium on diagnostic cytology: tutorials of cytology,* ed 7, Chicago, 1992, ASCP Press.
11. Frost JK: The cell in health and disease. In Wied GL, editor: *Monographs in clinical cytology,* ed 2, Basel, 1986, Karger.
12. Papanicolaou GN: *Atlas of exfoliative cytology,* Cambridge, Mass, 1954, Harvard University Press.
13. Naib ZM: *Exfoliative cytopathology,* ed 2, Boston, 1976, Little, Brown.

Principles of cytomorphology

14. Reagan JW, Siedermann IL, Saracusa Y: The cellular morphology of carcinoma in-situ and dysplasia or atypical hyperplasia of the uterine cervix, *Cancer* 6:224, 1953.
15. Wied GL: An international agreement on histological terminology for lesions of the uterine cervix, *Acta Cytol* 6:236, 1962.
16. Patten S: Diagnostic cytopathology of the uterine cervix. In Wied GL, editor: *Monographs in clinical cytology,* Basel, 1978, Karger.

Preparation of the cellular specimen

17. Keebler, CM: Cytopreparatory techniques. In Bibb M, editor: *Comprehensive cytopathology,* Philadelphia, 1991, Saunders.
18. Papanicolaou GN: A new procedure for staining vaginal smears, *Science* 95:438, 1942.

Infectious diseases

19. Johnston WW, Amatulli J: The role of cytology in the primary diagnosis of North American blastomycosis, *Acta Cytol* 14:200, 1970.
20. Gupta RK: Diagnosis of unsuspected pulmonary cryptococcosis with sputum cytology, *Acta Cytol* 29:154, 1985.
21. Guglietti LC, Reingold IM: The detection of *Coccidioides immitis* in pulmonary cytology, *Acta Cytol* 12:332, 1968.
22. Johnston WW: Pulmonary cytopathology in the compromised host. In Greenberg SD, editor: *Lung pathology for the clinician,* New York, 1982, Thieme-Stratton.
23. Reyes CV, Kathuria S, MacGlashan A: Diagnostic value of calcium oxalate crystals in respiratory and pleural fluid cytology: a case report, *Acta Cytol* 23:65, 1979.
24. Kim H, Hughs WT: Comparison of methods for identification of *Pneumocystis carinii* in pulmonary aspirates, *Am J Clin Pathol* 60:462, 1973.
25. Pintozzi RL, Blecka LJ, Nanos S: The morphologic identification of *Pneumocystis carinii, Acta Cytol* 23:35, 1979.
26. Lobenthal SW, Hajdu SI, Urmacher C: Cytologic findings in homosexual males with acquired immunodeficiency, *Acta Cytol* 27:597, 1983.
27. Orenstein M, Weber CA, Heurich AE: Cytologic diagnosis of *Pneumocystis carinii* infection by bronchoalveolar lavage in acquired immune deficiency syndrome, *Acta Cytol* 29:727, 1985.
28. Fleury J, Escudier E, Pocholle M-J et al: Cell population obtained by bronchoalveolar lavage in *Pneumocystis carinii* pneumonitis, *Acta Cytol* 29:721, 1985.
29. Greaves TS, Strigle SM: The recognition of *Pneumocystis carinii* in routine Papanicolaou-stained smears, *Acta Cytol* 29:714, 1985.
30. Ghali VS, Garcia RL, Skolom J: Fluorescence of *Pneumocystis carinii* in Papanicolaou smears, *Hum Pathol* 15:907, 1984.
31. Humphreys K, Hieger LR: *Strongyloides stercoralis* in routine Papanicolaou-stained sputum smears, *Acta Cytol* 23:471, 1979.
32. Garrett M, Herbsman H, Fierst S: Cytologic diagnosis of echinococcosis, *Acta Cytol* 21:553, 1977.
33. McCallum SM: Ova of the lung fluke *Paragonimus kellicotti* in fluid from a cyst, *Acta Cytol* 19:279, 1975.
34. Dao AH: *Entamoeba gingivalis* in sputum smears, *Acta Cytol* 29:632, 1985.
35. Willie SM, Snyder RN: The identification of *Paragonimus westermani* in bronchial washings: case report, *Acta Cytol* 21:101, 1977.
36. Hawkins AG, Hsiu J-G, Smith RM III et al: Pulmonary dirofilariasis diagnosed by fine needle aspiration biopsy: a case report, *Acta Cytol* 29:19, 1985.
37. Walker AN, Walker GK, Feldman PS: Diagnosis of *Legionella micdadei* pneumonia from cytologic specimens, *Acta Cytol* 27:252, 1983.
38. Gupta PK: Microbiology, inflammation and viral infections. In Bibbo M, editor: *Comprehensive cytopathology,* Philadelphia, 1971, Saunders.
39. Nash G, Foley FD: Herpetic infection of the middle and lower respiratory tract, *Am J Clin Pathol* 54:857, 1970.
40. Frable WJ, Kay S: Herpesvirus infection of the respiratory tract: electron-microscopic observation of the virus in cells obtained from a sputum cytology, *Acta Cytol,* 21:391, 1977.
41. Beale AJ, Campbell WA: A rapid cytological method for the diagnosis of measles, *J Clin Pathol* 12:335, 1959.
42. Koprowska I: Intranuclear inclusion bodies in smears of respiratory secretions, *Acta Cytol* 5:219, 1961.
43. Warner NE, McGrew EA, Nonos S: Cytologic study of the sputum in cytomegalic inclusion disease, *Acta Cytol* 8:311, 1964.
44. Jain U, Mani K, Frable WJ: Cytomegalic inclusion disease: cytologic diagnosis from bronchial brushing material, *Acta Cytol* 17:467, 1973.
45. Naib ZM, Stewart JA, Dowdle WR et al: Cytological features of viral respiratory tract infections, *Acta Cytol* 12:162, 1968.
46. Elson CE, Vick WW, Shelburne JD, Johnston WW: Viral peritonitis caused by herpes simplex virus type II, *Acta Cytol* 33:726, 1989.
47. Perry MD, Elmore PD, Johnston WW: Unusual benign pericarditis, *Acta Cytol* 29:947, 1985.
48. Goodman ZD, Gupta PK, Frost KJ, Erozan Y: Cytodiagnosis of viral infections in body cavity fluids, *Acta Cytol* 23:204, 1979.

49. Charles RE, Katz RL, Ordóñez NG, Mackay B: Varicella-zoster infection with pleural involvement, *Am J C Pathol* 85:522, 1986.
50. Koss LG, Durfee GR: Unusual patterns of squamous epithelium of the uterine cervix: cytologic and pathologic study of koilocytotic atypia, *Ann NY Acad Sci* 63:1245, 1956.

Female reproductive tract

51. U.S. Department of Health and Human Services: *The National Strategic Plan for the Early Detection and Control of Breast and Cervical Cancer,* Washington, DC, 1991.
52. The 1988 Bethesda System for reporting cervical/vaginal cytologic diagnoses. *Hum Pathol* 21:704, 1992,
53. Boon ME et al: Analysis of five sampling methods for the preparation of cervical smears, *Acta Cytol* 33:843, 1989.
54. Richart RM: Cervical intraepithelial neoplasia, *Path Annu* 8:301, 1973.
55. The Bethesda System for Reporting Cervical/Vaginal Cytologic Diagnoses, *Acta Cytol* 37:115, 1993.
56. Frost JK: Gynecologic and obstetric clinical cytopathology. In Novak ER, Woodruff JD, editors: *Novak's Gynecologic and obstetric pathology,* ed 8, Philadelphia, 1979, Saunders.
57. Meisels A, Morin C: Cytopathology of the uterine cervix, In Johnston WW, editor: *ASCP theory and practice of cytopathology I,* Chicago, 1991, ASCP Press.
58. Vooijs GP: Benign proliferative reactions, intraepithelial neoplasia and invasive cacner of the uterine cervix. In Bibbo M, editor: *Comprehensive cytopathology,* Philadelphia, 1991, Saunders.
59. Wentz WB, Reagan JW: Survival in cervical cancer with respect to cell type, *Cancer* 12:384, 1959.
60. Reagan JW, Ng AP: *The cells of the uterine adenocarcinoma.* In Wied GL, editor: *Monographs in clinical cytology,* vol 1, 2nd rev ed, Basel, 1973, Karger.
61. Pacey NF: Glandular neoplasms of the uterine cervix. In Bibbo M, editor: *Comprehensive cytopathology,* Philadelphia, 1991, Saunders.
62. Ng AP: Endometrial hyperplasia and carcinoma and extrauterine cancer. In Bibbo M, editor: *Comprehensive cytopathology,* 1991, Philadelphia, Saunders.
63. Tao L-C: Cytopathology of the endometrium: direct uterine sampling. In Johnson WW, editor: *ASCP theory and practice of cytopathology,* ed 2, Chicago 1993, ASCP Press.
64. Koss LG: The Papanicolaou test for cervical cancer detection: a triumph and a tragedy, *JAMA* 261:737, 1989.
65. Gay JD et al: False-negative results in cervical cytologic studies, *Acta Cytol* 29:1043, 1985.
66. vad der Graaf Y et al: Screening errors in cervical cancer cytologic screening, *Acta Cytol* 31:434, 1987.
67. Soost H-J et al: The validation of cervical cytology, *Acta Cytol* 35:8, 1991.
68. Ibrahim S et al: The clinical effects of prospective correlation of Pap smears and concomitant biopsies, *Mod Pathol* 7:38A, 1994 (Abstract).

Respiratory tract

69. Johnston WW, Elson CE: Respiratory tract. In Bibbo M, editor: *Comprehensive cytopathology,* Philadelphia, 1991, Saunders.
70. Johnston WW: Ten years of respiratory cytopathology at Duke University Medical Center. III. The significance of inconclusive cytopathologic diagnoses during the years 1970-1974, *Acta Cytol* 26:759, 1982.
71. Louria DB, Lieberman PH, Collins HS, Blevins A: Pulmonary mycetoma due to *Allescheria boydii, Arch Intern Med* 121:748, 1966.
72. Koss LG, Richardson HL: Some pitfalls of cytological diagnosis of lung cancer, *Cancer* 8:937, 1955.
73. Naylor B, Railey C: A pitfall in the cytodiagnosis of sputum of asthmatics, *J Clin Pathol* 7:84, 1964.
74. Berkheiser JW: Bronchiolar proliferation and metaplasia associated with bronchiectasis, pulmonary infarcts and anthracosis, *Cancer* 12:499, 1959.
75. Berkheiser JW: Bronchiolar proliferation and metaplasia associated with thromboembolism: a pathological and experimental study, *Cancer* 16:205, 1963.
76. Bewtra C, Dewan N, O'Donahue WJ, Jr: Exfoliative sputum cytology in pulmonary embolism, *Acta Cytol* 27:489, 1983.
77. Frable WJ, Johnston WW: *Respiratory cytology: transparencies, explanatory text and self-evaluative test,* International Slide Sets, XIX, Chicago, 1974, Tutorials of Cytology.
78. Johnston WW, Frable WJ: Cytopathology of the respiratory tract: a review, *Am J Pathol* 84:371, 1976.
79. Johnston WW Frable WJ: *Diagnostic respiratory cytopathology,* Paris and New York, 1979, Masson.
80. Stanley MW, Henry-Stanley MJ, Galj-Peczalska KJ, Bitterman PB: Hyperplasia of type II pneumocytes in acute lung injury: cytologic findings of sequential bronchoalveolar lavage, *Am J Clin Pathol* 97:669, 1992.
81. Bedrossian CWM: Iatrogenic and toxic injury. In Dail DH, Hammar SP, editors: *Pulmonary pathology,* New York, 1988, Springer-Verlag.
82. Linder J, Rennard SI: *Bronchoalveolar lavage,* Chicago, 1988, ASCP Press.
83. Manning JT, Spjut HJ, Tschen JA: Bronchioalveolar carcinoma: the significance of two histopathologic types, *Cancer* 54:525, 1984.
84. Silverman JF, Finley JL, Park HK et al: Fine needle aspiration cytology of bronchioalveolar-cell carcinoma of the lung, *Acta Cytol* 29:887, 1985.
85. Elson CE, Moore SP, Johnston WW: Morphologic and immunocytochemical studies of bronchioloalveolar carcinoma at Duke University Medical Center, 1968-1986, *Anal Quant Cytol and Histol* 11:261, 1989.
86. Smith JH, Frable WJ: Adenocarcinoma of the lung: cytologic correlation with histologic types, *Acta Cytol* 18:316, 1974.

Body cavity fluids

87. Naylor B: Pleural, peritoneal and pericardial fluids. In Bibbo M, editor: *Comprehensive cytopathology,* Philadelphia, 1991, Saunders.
88. Spieler P: The cytologic diagnosis of tuberculosis in pleural effusions, *Acta Cytol* 23:374, 1979.
89. Covell JL, Lowry EH Jr, Feldman PS: Cytologic diagnosis of blastomycosis in pleural fluid, *Acta Cytol* 26:833, 1982.
90. Jacobson ES: A case of secondary echinococcosis diagnosed by cytologic examination of pleural fluid and needle biopsy of pleura, *Acta Cytol* 17:76, 1973.
91. Avagnina MA, Elsner B, Iotti RM, Re R: *Strongyloides stercoralis* in Papanicolaou-stained smears of ascitic fluid, *Acta Cytol* 24:36, 1980.
92. Nosanchuk JA, Naylor B: A unique cytologic picture in pleural fluid from patients with rheumatoid arthritis, *Am J Clin Pathol* 50:330, 1968.
93. Seaman AJ, Christerson JW: Demonstration of LE cells in pericardial fluid: report of a case, *JAMA* 149:145, 1952.
94. Veress JF, Koss LG, Schreiber K: Eosinophilic pleural effusions, *Acta Cytol* 23:40, 1979.
95. Zaatari GS, Gupta PK, Bhagavan BS, Jarboe BR: Cytopathology of pleural endometriosis, *Acta Cytol* 26: 227, 1982.
96. Dekker A, Graham T, Bupp P: The occurrence of sickle cells in pleural fluid: report of a patient with sickle cell disease, *Acta Cytol* 19:251, 1975.
97. Fentanes de Torres E, Guevara CE: Pleuritis by radiation: report of two cases, *Acta Cytol* 25:427, 1981.
98. Saphir O: Cytologic diagnosis of cancer from pleural and peritoneal fluids, *Am J Clin Pathol* 19:309, 1949.
99. Foot NC: The identification of types and primary sites of metastatic tumors from exfoliated cells in serous fluids, *Am J Pathol* 30:661, 1954.
100. Grunze H: The comparative diagnostic accuracy, efficiency and specificity of cytologic technics used in the diagnosis of malignant neoplasm in serous effusions of the pleural and pericardial cavities, *Acta Cytol* 8:150, 1964.
101. Murphy WM, Ng AB: Determination of primary site by examination of cancer cells in body fluid, *Am J Clin Pathol* 58:479, 1972.
102. Spieler P, Gloor F: Identification of types and primary sites of malignant tumors by examination of exfoliated tumor cells in serous fluids: comparison with the diagnostic accuracy on small histologic biopsies, *Acta Cytol* 29:753, 1985.
103. Johnston WW: The malignant pleural effusion, *Cancer* 56:905, 1985.
104. Spriggs AI, Boddington MM: Atlas of serous fluid cytopathology, In Gresham GA editor: *Current histopathology,* vol 14, Oordrecht, 1989, Kluwer.
105. Spriggs AI, Boddington MM: Oat-cell bronchial carcinoma identification of cells in pleural fluid, *Acta Cytol* 20:525, 1976.

106. Melamed MR: The cytological presentation of malignant lymphomas and related diseases in effusions, *Cancer* 16:413, 1963.
107. Billingham ME, Rawlinson DG, Berry PF, Kempson RL: The cytodiagnosis of malignant lymphomas and Hodgkin's disease in cerebrospinal, pleural and ascitic fluids, *Acta Cytol* 19:547, 1975.
108. Yam LT, Lin DG, Janckila AJ, Li C-Y: Immunocytochemical diagnosis of lymphoma in serous effusions, *Acta Cytol* 29:833, 1985.
109. Ashton PR, Hollingsworth AS Jr, Johnston WW: The cytopathology of metastatic breast cancer, *Acta Cytol* 19:1, 1975.
110. Danner DE, Gmelich JT: A comparative study of tumor cells from metastatic carcinoma of the breast effusions, *Acta Cytol* 19:509, 1975.
111. Naylor B: The exfoliative cytology of diffuse malignant mesothelioma, *J Pathol Bacteriol* 86:293, 1963.
112. Berge T, Grontoft O: Cytologic diagnosis of malignant pleural mesothelioma, *Acta Cytol* 9:207, 1965.
113. Roberts GH, Campbell GM: Exfoliative cytology of diffuse mesothelioma, *J Clin Pathol* 25:577, 1972.
114. Tao L-C: The cytopathology of mesothelioma, *Acta Cytol* 23:209, 1979.
115. Triol JH, Conston AS, Chandler SV: Malignant mesothelioma: cytopathology of 75 cases seen in a New Jersey community hospital, *Acta Cytol* 28:37, 1984.
116. Sehested M, Ralfkjer E, Rasmussen J: Immunoperoxidase demonstration of carcinoembryonic antigen in pleural and peritoneal effusions, *Acta Cytol* 27:124, 1983.
117. To A, Dearnaley DP, Ormerod G et al: Epithelial membrane antigen: its use in the cytodiagnosis of malignancy in serous effusions, *Am J Clin Pathol* 77:214, 1982.
118. Johnston WW, Szpak CA, Lottich SC et al: Use of a monoclonal antibody (B72.3) as an immunocytochemical adjunct to diagnosis of adenocarcinoma in human effusions, *Cancer Res* 45:1894, 1985.
119. Szpak CA, Johnston WW, Roggli V et al: The significance of monoclonal antibody (B72.3) in the diagnostic distinction between malignant mesothelioma of the pleura and adenocarcinoma of the lung, *Am J Pathol* 122:252, 1986.
120. Warnock ML, Stoloff A, Thor A: Differentiation of adenocarcinoma of the lung from mesothelioma, *Am J Clin Pathol* 133:30, 1988.

Other body sites

121. Shu Y-J: The cytopathology of esophageal carcinoma, In Johnston WW, editor: *Masson monographs in diagnostic cytopathology,* Paris, 1985, Masson.
122. Husain OAN: Alimentary tract (esophagus, stomach, colon, rectum). In Bibbo M, editor: *Comprehensive cytopathology*, Philadelphia, 1991, Saunders.
123. Holmquist N: *Diagnostic cytology of the urinary tract.* In Wied GL, editor: *Monographs in clinical cytology,* Basel, 1977, Karger.
124. Schumann GB, Weiss MA: *Atlas of renal and urinary tract cytology and its histopathologic bases,* Philadelphia, 1981, Lippincott.
125. Tweeddale DN: *Urinary Cytology,* Boston, 1977, Little, Brown.
126. Murphy WM: *Atlas of bladder carcinoma,* Chicago, 1986, ASCP Press.
127. Kern WH: Urinary tract. In Bibbo M, editor *Comprehensive cytopathology,* Philadelphia, 1991, Saunders.
128. Kölmel HW: *Atlas of cerebrospinal fluid cells,* New York, 1976, Springer-Verlag.
129. Jager WA den: *Color atlas of C.S.F. cytopathology,* Philadelphia, 1980, Lippincott.
130. Rosenthal DL: *Cytology of the central nervous system.* In Wied GL, editor: *Monographs in clinical cytology,* Basel, 1994, Karger.
131. Bigner SH, Johnston WW: *Cytopathology of the central nervous system.* In Johnston WW, editor: *ASCP theory and practice of cytopathology,* vol 3, Chicago, 1994, ASCP Press.

Fine-needle aspiration biopsy

132. Kaminsky DB: Applications of thin-needle aspiration biopsy in a community hospital. In Johnston WW editor: *Masson series in diagnostic cytopathology,* New York, vol 2, 1981, Masson.
133. Zajicek J: Aspiration Biopsy Cytology. Part 1. Cytology of supradiaphragmatic organs. In Wied GL, editor: *Monographs in clinical cytology,* Karger, vol 4, Basel, 1974, Karger.
134. Schmidt WA, editor: *Cytopathology annual 1993,* Baltimore, 1993, Williams & Wilkins.
135. Kline TS: *Handbook of fine needle aspiration biopsy cytology,* St Louis, 1981, Mosby.
136. Oertel Y: *Fine-needle aspiration of the breast,* Boston, 1987, Butterworth.
137. Feldman PS, Covell JL: *Fine needle aspiration cytology and its clinical applications: breast and lung,* Chicago, 1985, ASCP Press.
138. Silverman JF: Breast. In Bibbo M, editor: *Comprehensive cytopathology,* Philadelphia, 1991, Saunders.
139. Davidson HG, Campora RG: Thyroid. In Bibbo M, editor: *Comprehensive cytopathology,* Philadelphia, 1991, Saunders.
140. Löwhagen T, Tani EM, Skoog L: Salivary glands and rare head and neck lesions. In Bibbo M, editor: *Comprehensive cytopathology,* Philadelphia, 1991, Saunders.
141. Das DK: Lymph nodes. In Bibbo M, editor: *Comprehensive cytopathology,* Philadelphia, 1991, Saunders.
142. Rosenthal DL, Mandell DB, Glasgow BJ: Eye. Philadelphia, In Bibbo M, editor: *Comprehensive cytopathology,* Philadelphia, 1991, Saunders.
143. Dahlgren S, Nordenstrom B: *Transthoracic needle biopsy,* St Louis, 1966, Mosby.
144. Bonfiglio T: Transthoracic thin needle aspiration biopsy. In Johnston WW, editor: *Masson series in diagnostic cytopathology,* Paris and New York, 1983, Masson.
145. Zajicek J: Aspiration biopsy cytology. Part 2. Cytology of infradiaphragmatic organs. In Wied GL, editor: *Monographs in clinical cytology,* Basel, 1979, Karger.
146. Katz RL: Kidney, adrenal and retroperitoneum. In Bibbo M, editor: *Comprehensive cytopathology,* Philadelphia, 1991, Saunders.
147. Skoog L, Tani EM, Löwhagen T: Prostate. In Bibbo M, editor: *Comprehensive cytopathology,* Philadelphia, 1991, Saunders.
148. Hajdu SI: Soft tissue and bone. In Bibbo M, editor: *Comprehensive cytopathology,* Philadelphia, 1991, Saunders.

5 Forensic Pathology

Charles S. Hirsch
Ross E. Zumwalt

With the exception of forensic pathology, all special competence or subspecialty areas of pathology practice (such as neuropathology, pediatric pathology, cytopathology, and hematopathology) have arisen and evolved to meet scientific or medical needs. Forensic pathology, on the other hand, exists to meet the needs of government.

Any government with an interest in the lives of its citizens must have a compelling interest in their deaths. Forensic pathology fulfills part of that governmental interest by investigating and evaluating sudden, unexpected, suspicious, and violent deaths as well as fatalities occurring in special, legally defined circumstances, such as those in public institutions, from occupational diseases, from communicable diseases that threaten public health, or from complications of diagnostic and therapeutic procedures. The specifics of the foregoing generalities are not uniform in the United States and are contained in state, county, and municipal laws and codes. Hence all pathologists involved full or part time in forensic practice should be familiar with the statutes that define their responsibility and authority.

BASIC CONCEPTS

Three fundamental terms and the concepts embodied in their understanding underlie many discussions in this chapter. To ensure clarity we begin with definitions and explanations of those terms.[1,2]

Manner of death. The manner of death[1] is an explanation of how the cause arose, either naturally or violently. Natural deaths are defined as those caused exclusively by disease. We emphasize that exclusive means 100%. If an injury of any sort causes or contributes to death, the fatality cannot be classified as natural and is, instead, classified as violent. In this context, violence is not synonymous with foul play because violent deaths include accidents and suicides as well as homicides. Our definition of injury is not restricted to mechanical trauma such as beating, shooting, or stabbing. Injury includes all modalities of physical trauma (mechanical, electrical, heat, cold, and changes of atmospheric pressure) and almost all modalities of chemical trauma. We qualify chemical injury with an "almost" because by convention we classify the natural complications of chronic substance abuse (ethanol, opiates) as natural diseases. Further, a death attributable to acute and chronic alcoholism is still classified as natural because the ethanol intoxication of the fatal episode is conceptually an acute exacerbation of a chronic disease. Paradoxically, fatal opiate intoxication of a person who is a chronic intravenous drug abuser is classified as a violent (usually accidental) death.

When insufficient information is available to make a determination with reasonable certainty, the medicolegal official has the option to classify the manner of death as undetermined.

Cause of death. The cause of death[1] is the disease, injury, or combination of disease and injury responsible for the fatality. Whenever possible, causes of death should be *etiologically specific* diseases or injuries. The *underlying,* or *proximate, cause of death* is that which in a natural and continuous sequence, unbroken by an efficient intervening cause, brings about the result and without which the result would not have occurred. *Immediate causes of death* are complications of the underlying cause, temporally interposed between underlying causation and its subsequent result. There may be many immediate causes and they may occur over a prolonged interval, but none absolves the proximate cause of its ultimate responsibility. For example, if a person dies from infected decubitus ulcers and chronic urinary tract infections 20 years after sustaining a spinal cord injury that caused paraplegia or quadriplegia, the foregoing complications are the immediate causes and the spinal cord injury is the proximate cause of death. The manner of such a death is violent, to be classified according to the circumstances of the injury.

Mechanism of death. Mechanisms of death[1] are the *etiologically nonspecific* alterations of physiology and biochemistry whereby the causes exert their lethal effects. Common mechanisms of death include congestive heart failure, cardiac arrhythmias, septicemia, disseminated intravascular coagulation (DIC), exsanguination, asphyxiation, hepatic failure, renal failure, the adult respiratory distress syndrome (ARDS), and emaciation. "Multiple organ failure" is a pathologically nonspecific, end-stage, clinical conglomerate that occurs in patients who receive prolonged intensive care.

Mechanisms require the etiologic clarification of an underlying disease or injury because many diseases and injuries can cause death by the same mechanism. For example, fatal cardiac arrhythmias can occur as a consequence of any type of heart disease, electrocution, mechanical trauma, drug reactions, poisoning, and a wide variety of metabolic abnormalities.

Since medical treatment frequently is directed at management of mechanisms, treating physicians often are not focused on underlying causes of death. As a result, after complex illnesses, treating physicians usually report that death was caused by sepsis with DIC, ARDS, or that all-encompassing, uninformative designation "multiorgan failure." Appropriate analysis of such fatalities requires identification of an etiologically specific response to the question, "Caused by what?"

OBJECTIVES OF THE MEDICOLEGAL AUTOPSY

An old adage holds that "dead men tell no tales." The day-to-day experience of the forensic pathologist proves the adage incorrect. Dead men "speak" eloquently when interrogated appropriately. So do dead women and dead babies. The six questions that compose the forensic pathologist's "dialog with the dead" summarize the objectives of the medicolegal autopsy.

Who are you? Identification of the dead is a logical starting point in the criminal investigation of most homicides and is required for civil and humanitarian reasons. Families need to know that the identification of their dead relatives is reliable or the grieving process is interrupted and aggravated.

From a practical standpoint, identification is required to issue a death certificate, and in many respects a death certificate is a far more useful instrument than a birth certificate is. Most of us can get through life very nicely without a birth certificate, but if our survivors do not have a valid death certificate, they face complex, lengthy, legal tangles in attempting to collect life insurance, settle an estate, and get on with their lives.

Personal recognition is the most commonly used form of postmortem identification. The person making the identification is required to sign an affidavit or its equivalent and to provide proof of their own identity. Personal recognition as a means of identification runs well-known risks of mistaken positive identification, denial of identity, or fraudulent misrepresentation of identity. However, mistakes or misrepresentations are rare in the reality of routine experience.

When decomposition or mutilation preclude personal recognition, the preferred methods of objective identification are fingerprinting, dental comparison, or x-ray filming of the body. Fingerprints have the advantage of existing in large data bases, which can be searched by automated processes in many jurisdictions, and do not require a suspected identity of the decedent. Antemortem dental records or an x-ray film of any part of the body frequently are compared with their postmortem counterparts and serve to establish or to exclude suspected identification. DNA profiling and comparison with DNA from relatives also can establish identity and is particularly useful in instances of extreme mutilation that render fingerprinting and dental or x-ray comparison impossible. Other means of conclusive identification include individual scars, tattoos, or any other personal characteristic, such as the detailed anatomy of the external ear as demonstrated on antemortem photographs of a suspected decedent. Personal items such as clothing and jewelry can be worn by anyone, and they are unreliable identifiers without supporting evidence.

When did you die? All the biologic postmortem changes that form the basis for our estimates of the postmortem interval are governed by the characteristics of the decedent and the environment in which the body rests. Temperature is the most important variable to be considered because heat accelerates and cold retards the onset and development of all postmortem changes, except cooling of the body.

Salient individual characteristics that influence postmortem temperature include body temperature at the time of death, decedent's phenotype, and clothing or other body covering. All persons do not have normal body temperature at the time of death. Those who are febrile when they die develop postmortem changes more rapidly than usual, and conversely those who have a subnormal temperature develop postmortem changes more slowly than usual. Fat persons retain body heat longer than the lean. Persons who are clothed or covered with bedding retain heat longer than those who are nude and exposed.

Severe bacterial infections, particularly if associated with septicemia, can provide an antemortem head start on putrefaction. Likewise, diseases or injuries that disrupt or perforate the gastrointestinal tract provide early postmortem egress for the bacterial flora that cause putrefaction. Miscellaneous factors that retard postmortem decomposition include exsanguination and burning of the body.

The most important environmental factor influencing postmortem changes is temperature. Freezing preserves the body, and a hot environment accelerates decomposition. A hot, humid environment leads to putrefaction, which can be fully manifest as bloating, discoloration, and purging in as little as 18 hours under appropriate circumstances (such as death in a closed car parked in full sun on a hot, humid day). Death in a hot, dry environment leads to mummification. Death in a cool, moist environment results in a peculiar form of decomposition characterized by the formation of adipocere. Other environmental factors that influence the development of postmortem changes include the heat-conducting efficiency of the surroundings (air, water, or soil) and of the surface on which the body rests (metal, fabric, or synthetic); humidity; and the presence or absence of wind or air currents passing over the body.

In the reality of forensic practice, we use all the available data to derive a range for the postmortem interval. The shorter the interval, the smaller is the range. If a person has been dead only a few hours, we should come pretty close. If a person has been dead a few days, we do well to come within a day. When death occurs weeks, months, or years before our examination, we have a progressively expanded range.

In arriving at our estimate of the postmortem interval, we also consider a nearly infinite, common-sense set of associated environmental factors. When was the person last seen alive or spoken to? For how long has the telephone been unanswered? Are dirty dishes on the kitchen table soiled with the remnants of last night's dinner or this morning's breakfast? Is the stomach still filled with food known to have been eaten at a specific time? How many days of newspapers have accumulated on the front porch?

As difficult as it may be to determine the time of death, the pathologist's task in this regard can be greatly complicated when injury and death are not contemporaneous. Mortally wounded persons can lay incapacitated or comatose for many hours before death. In such instances the autopsy must estimate the postinjury survival interval as well as the postmortem interval in order to provide police investigators a range of time during which the victim sustained the ultimately fatal injuries. Failure to recognize the postinjury survival interval can cause the pathologist to provide an erroneous and seriously misleading estimate of when the injury was sustained. In fact, the assailant may have an "ironclad alibi" for the time of death.

Where did you die? Recognizing that the scene of discovery of a body is not the scene of death can provide valuable investigative information. Environmental observations, such as drag marks across dirty surfaces, are the commonest clues that lead to the deduction that a body has been moved after death. In unusual instances, the body provides unmistakable evidence that it has been moved. These instances usually rest upon the observation of rigor mortis or livor mortis in defiance of gravity.

Firmly developed rigor mortis in opposing groups of muscles that act diametrically on a joint cause fixation of the motion of that joint, with resultant resistance to movement of the joint by postmortem manipulation or the force of gravity. Consequently, if a person dies in a sitting position with hips and knees flexed and remains in that position for the several hours required for rigor mortis to envelop the lower body, the lower extremities will remain flexed as long as rigor mortis persists and the joints are not forcefully extended. If the previous subject is moved from the seated position to a supine position on the floor, the hips and knees will remain flexed, holding the lower extremities in defiance of gravity.

Livor mortis, a purple discoloration of dependent surfaces of the body except for the weight-bearing contact surfaces, is caused by gravitational settling of blood in capillaries after cessation of circulation. If a body is moved shortly after the onset of livor mortis, previously dependent, livid body surfaces will blanch spontaneously as blood drains away under the force of gravity. However, if livor mortis has persisted for several hours in its original distribution and blood has congealed in cutaneous and subcutaneous capillaries, it becomes partially and then completely fixed in its original distribution. Consequently, blood cannot drain from capillaries if a previously dependent surface is moved to a nondependent position.

Why did you die? Determining the cause of death is an obvious objective of the medicolegal autopsy. Since the autopsy is a structurally based procedure, dependent primarily on techniques that demonstrate abnormal morphology, those causes and mechanisms of death that are structurally demonstrable are simple to identify at autopsy. Consequently, in most deaths attributable to mechanical trauma the cause of death is unmistakable. At the other extreme, causes and mechanisms of death that are entirely functional derangements are impossible to demonstrate at autopsy. Between the foregoing two extremes lie a gamut of diseases, injuries, and intoxications that can be demonstrated either morphologically or chemically but have functional lethal mechanisms that must be inferred rather than seen or measured. Such inferences must rest upon the foundation of an entire case study, including the decedent's history, the circumstances and environment of death, and all the postmortem studies. The autopsy and other postmortem studies, no matter how meticulous or detailed, cannot be competent substitutes for a complete case study. In fact, forensic pathologists solve more of their difficult medicolegal problems with their telephones than they do with their microscopes. The history and circumstances can dominate over the pathology and toxicology in an appropriate evaluation of some deaths, and the autopsy should be regarded as a laboratory test. (See the discussion of sudden unexpected deaths from natural causes, p. 83).

The importance of history and circumstances to medicolegal problem solving cannot be overemphasized. In this regard, we urge that whenever possible the pathologist seek *primary sources* of historical and circumstantial information. Forget the erroneous notion that medically trained persons are the only legitimate and reliable sources of information. Medical professionals usually relate second-hand or third-hand information that they get from ambulance personnel or police officers, who originally got it from a bystander. Furthermore, medical professionals add an additional layer of obfuscation because they process the information and pass on their conclusions rather than the original observations. In a sense, our professional colleagues give us the editorials. What we need to solve our problems is not the medical editorials but the news that comes from persons who have first-hand knowledge derived from what they saw and heard. The certainty with which autopsies determine causes of deaths attributable to disease is discussed in the following section on sudden unexpected deaths from natural causes.

What happened? The medicolegal autopsy can provide an abundant variety of information that helps to reconstruct the fatal episode. What were the relative positions of victim and assailant? Was the decedent shot at close or distant range? Was the wounded victim capable of voluntary movement after sustaining the ultimately fatal injury? Does the victim have injuries consistent with a struggle before infliction of the lethal wound? Had the victim been using ethanol, cocaine, or opiates, and what was the influence of those substances on the person's behavior? Was the fatal head injury caused by a blow or a fall with cranial impact?

Answering questions typified by the foregoing examples, the forensic pathologist contributes importantly to the adjudication of contested issues in criminal trials. Such answers often are straightforward and noncontroversial, and their legal significance may be completely unknown to the pathologist. In essence, the importance of the answers resides in the objective yardsticks that they provide to measure the reliability and credibility of intensely controversial statements made by criminal defendants or by witnesses to the killing. The statements of each such witness may be correct, confused, honestly mistaken, intentionally misleading, or some combination of the foregoing. The answers provided by the autopsy can help to sort out the range of credible and reliable to incredible and unreliable.

Who did it? Contrary to the depictions of written and video fiction, the pathologist rarely answers the "Who did it?" question. Determinations of time and place of death can help to evaluate whether a suspect had the opportunity to kill the victim. More often, evidence obtained by the pathologist at autopsy provides other scientific participants in the investigation the opportunity to incriminate or exclude a suspect. For example, samples obtained by the pathologist during the autopsy on the victim of a fatal sexual assault are used by the forensic biologist to exclude or match the DNA recovered from a blood sample taken from a suspect. Bullets recovered at autopsy are used by the firearms examiner to link a suspect gun to the slaying or to link multiple gunshot victims to the same weapon.

SUDDEN, UNEXPECTED DEATHS FROM NATURAL CAUSES

Translation of pathologic, chemical, and historical data into an opinion titled "cause of death" is accomplished with a variable degree of certainty in natural fatalities. The following classification is a useful framework to demonstrate the certainty with which an autopsy discloses the causes of deaths from disease.

Class 1. The autopsy discloses the cause of death with 100% certainty because the pathologic findings are inconsistent with continued life. We obtain such a high degree of certainty when the cause and mechanism of death are structurally demonstrable. Common examples of this class include ruptured myocardial infarct with hemopericardium and cardiac tamponade, ruptured aortic aneurysm with exsanguination into a body cavity, and spontaneous intracerebral hemorrhage with primary or secondary involvement of the brainstem. Despite the overt lethality of each of the foregoing examples, frequently we must exclude the participation of cocaine intoxication in the pathogenesis of the disorder before concluding that death resulted entirely from natural causes. Class 1 cases account for only approximately 5% of natural deaths in medicolegal autopsy populations. Therefore, in the remaining 95%, the autopsy fails to reveal structural changes that are inconsistent with continued life.

Class 2. The autopsy discloses a disease with lethal potential, sufficiently advanced to provide a competent explanation for the death, but without the development of a complication that produces a structurally demonstrable mechanism of death. Common examples of class 2 findings include almost any type of advanced, chronic heart disease, chronic lung diseases, and natural sequelae of chronic alcoholism. In medicolegal autopsies, approximately 90% of natural fatalities are class 2 cases.

The certainty with which we can conclude that the observed class 2 findings are the cause of death is determined by the history and circumstances surrounding death and by toxicologic findings. Virtually identical instances of potentially lethal disease can range from incontrovertible explanations for the death to incidental findings completely unrelated to the cause of death. For example, when a person with multifocal, occlusive coronary atherosclerosis is witnessed by reliable observers to "drop dead," autopsy discloses no other disease that can cause sudden death, and subsequent toxicologic studies are negative, the pathologist can conclude confidently that death resulted from a cardiac arrhythmia attributable to arteriosclerotic heart disease. The cardiac arrhythmia is a functional derangement that cannot be measured at autopsy, but its occurrence is inferred by the history and circumstances surrounding death, the presence of a disease known to cause sudden death by that mechanism, and the exclusion of other causes. On the other hand, if the same person with the same heart was found dead in bed after the ingestion of an obviously lethal overdose of secobarbital, the heart disease would be an incidental autopsy finding, noncontributory to death.

Class 3. The autopsy discloses a disease with lethal potential, not sufficiently advanced to be regarded as a competent explanation for death under ordinary circumstances. However, a compelling history and the exclusion of other causes lead to the conclusion that the observed marginal pathologic findings are responsible for the fatality. For example, a sedentary, overweight man is witnessed to collapse and die immediately after shoveling his driveway after the first major snowfall of winter. Autopsy is completely unremarkable except for multifocal, moderate coronary atherosclerosis with no focus of more than 60% stenosis at any level in his epicardial coronary arteries. Microscopic examination and toxicology show negative results. Despite the marginal lethality of his coronary atherosclerosis, one must conclude that the sudden death resulted from arteriosclerotic heart disease after unaccustomed, strenuous physical exertion.

Fatalities in class 3 are infrequent, but conceptually the example is very important. Class 3 deaths teach us that occasionally the history and circumstances dominate over the autopsy in medicolegal decisions. Most pathologists reflexly rebel against such a notion, but to reject the concept is to deny reality in the name of objectivity.

Class 4. The decedent has a lethal disease that is not structurally demonstrable. The death is evaluated on the basis of history and the exclusion of other causes. The disease most frequently implicated in this class is epilepsy. In most medicolegal autopsy populations, the majority of persons with a well-documented clinical diagnosis of epilepsy have a structurally normal brain. We can conclude that such a person died from epilepsy if the history and circumstances are consistent with that conclusion and the autopsy and toxicologic studies fail to disclose a reasonable alternative explanation.

Class 5. The cause of death is undetermined after autopsy and toxicologic studies. Despite competent investigations, complete autopsies, and state-of-the-art toxicology support, a small proportion of deaths cannot be attributed to any identifiable cause. The proportion of deaths in class 5 in a medicolegal jurisdiction is governed by the selection of cases for autopsy, by the competence of personnel at every level of the process, and by the inclusion or exclusion of sudden infant death syndrome fatalities in the tabulation of undetermined causes. The importance of this class of deaths lies not in its frequency but in its existence. Even in excellent medicolegal offices, staffed by superb professionals, there always will be occasional reminders of the limitations of our science and art. We are, after all, relying on a structurally based autopsy to study functional disorders that define the difference between life and death.

SUDDEN INFANT DEATH SYNDROME

Sudden infant death syndrome (SIDS) is defined as the sudden death of an infant under 1 year of age that remains unexplained after a thorough case investigation, including performance of a complete autopsy, examination of the death scene, and review of the clinical history.[3] The SIDS victim usually is found dead some time after being put to bed. More than 90% die before 6 months of age; the median age is 11 weeks. The incidence is approximately 1.5 per 1000 live births and has declined slowly in the past several decades. Still, SIDS is the most common cause of death in infants under 6 months of age beyond the neonatal period.[4] Deaths occur more often in the winter months. Infant risk factors include male sex (50% higher than females), prematurity, low birth weight, low

APGAR scores, and minority race. High-risk maternal factors are smoking and age less than 20 years. Other maternal risk factors include unmarried status, late or little prenatal care, high parity, not breast feeding, substance abuse, and little education. These maternal risk factors correlate with low socioeconomic status and are compellingly suggestive of a less than optimum in utero environment.[4,5]

The cause of SIDS remains unknown, though there is no paucity of hypotheses. Proving a cause will be difficult, since the mechanism of death probably is asphyxia or a fatal physiologic biochemical abnormality during sleep that does not cause any anatomic abnormality.

Historically, SIDS was believed to be the result of suffocation or accidental overlying. Another early and now discredited theory was airway blockage by an enlarged thymus (status thymicolymphaticus). More current theories have included fulminant infections, hypersensitivity reactions (especially to cow's milk), toxins, trace element deficiency, hormonal imbalances, developmental abnormalities, and mechanical obstruction of the airway.[6] Recent interest has focused on developmental apnea and sleep position.

Proponents of the developmental apnea theory postulate that infants die because they "forget to breathe." These infants also are believed to have had repeated episodes of nonfatal apnea.[7] Support for this theory comes from investigators who have found subtle anatomic differences between SIDS and control infants suggestive of repetitive hypoxia.[8,9]

Comparison of SIDS rates between countries with different cultural practices for infant sleep positions has led to a great deal of interest in the possible role of the prone sleep position as a causative factor in SIDS.[10,11] In particular, sleeping face down on soft bedding and being swaddled seem to increase the risk for SIDS. The mechanism of death is postulated to be carbon dioxide narcosis from rebreathing exhaled air in a pocket formed by the soft bedding and the prone position.[12]

The pathologic findings in SIDS are nonspecific. Frequently, there is pulmonary edema, and when found dead, infants often have white froth or pink, blood-tinged froth around their mouth and nose and staining their bed clothes. Agonal aspiration of gastric contents is another common finding and is not a cause of death. Petechiae of the thymus, epicardium, and pleura are usually present (Fig. 5-1). However, their presence is not diagnostic of SIDS, and their absence does not exclude the diagnosis.[5]

The diagnosis of SIDS is made after a careful review of the circumstances of death and the exclusion of a competent cause of death by a complete autopsy. Occasionally, it is difficult to decide if a mild inflammation represents a competent cause of death or an incidental finding.[5] For example, most forensic pathologists do not regard the finding of chronic otitis media as a competent cause of death that would exclude the diagnosis of SIDS.

The most common conditions to consider in the differential diagnosis include pneumonia, meningitis, congenital heart disease, metabolic disorders such as medium-chain acyl-CoA dehydrogenase deficiency,[13] homicidal smothering, accidental asphyxia, and poisoning. Infections and congenital abnormalities usually can be excluded by an autopsy and by postmortem cultures and chemical analyses. Suspicion of homicidal or accidental asphyxia must be addressed by an investigation of the circumstances of the death. An autopsy on an asphyxiated infant may be identical to that of a SIDS victim. Poisoning can be identified if a toxin is suspected and the appropriate toxicologic tests are performed.

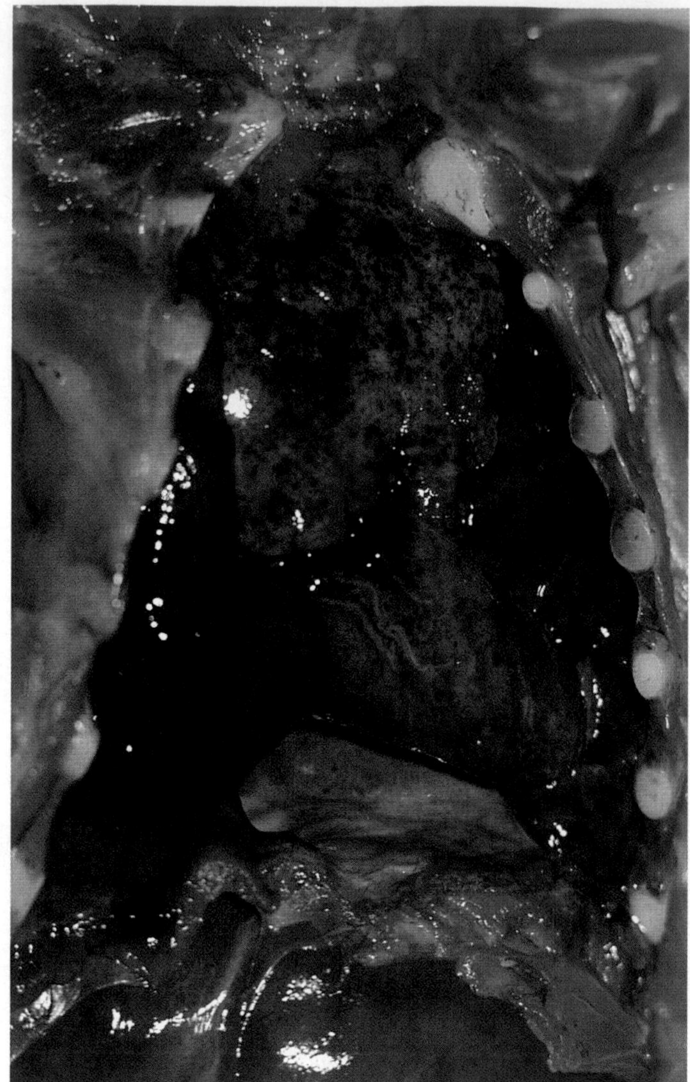

Fig. 5-1 Sudden infant death syndrome (SIDS) fatality. Thoracic viscera in situ with petechiae of thymus, epicardium, and pleura.

PHYSICAL INJURIES

Physical injuries include those caused by mechanical trauma, increases or decreases of atmospheric pressure, sound waves, heat (local and systemic), cold (local and systemic), and electricity. In terms of morbidity and mortality, mechanical trauma is more important by an order of magnitude than all other modalities of physical injury combined. Therefore more than half of this chapter is devoted to mechanical trauma.

Mechanical trauma

Force or mechanical energy is that which changes the state of rest or uniform motion of matter. When force applied to any part of the body results in a harmful disturbance in function or structure, a mechanical injury is said to have been sustained.

The most common manifestation of such an injury is a disruption in the continuity of tissue, or a wound. The force responsible for wound production is usually liberated incident to a collision between the body and some external mass and may be derived from the motion of the body itself, from the motion of the other participant in the collision, or from both.

Wounding by mechanical trauma is governed by (1) the amount of force transmitted to the tissues, (2) the rate of application of force to the tissues, (3) the surface area involved in energy transfer, and (4) the characteristics of the target area.

Physical principles

Amount of force. The kinetic energy or wound-producing capacity that an object has in consequence of its motion is determined by its weight and velocity. In the case of simple forward motion, this force may be computed by the formula $MV^2/2g$, in which M = weight, V = velocity, and g = the acceleration of gravity. It is important to note that the kinetic energy of a moving object increases arithmetically in relation to its weight and geometrically in relation to its velocity. If two objects, one weighing twice as much as the other, are traveling at the same velocity, the kinetic energy of the former will be twice that of the latter; however, if they weigh the same but one is traveling twice as fast as the other, the energy will be four times as great. Wounding by bullets provides an important application of this principle to an understanding of the resulting injuries. Bullets fired from military and hunting rifles commonly have muzzle velocities three to four times as great as those fired from handguns. Consequently, such high-velocity bullets have kinetic energies 9 to 16 times greater than their low-velocity counterparts.

One should not infer that the kinetic energy and the wound-producing factor of a mass in motion are necessarily identical. Only that part of the total energy of motion actually utilized in changing the state of rest or uniform motion of the tissues is capable of contributing to injury production. Unexpended force, possessed by the source of energy after the impulse of collision, is still capable of doing work and has not contributed to injury production. Force of impact utilized to induce uniform motion of the tissues or to displace or deform the object that has struck the tissue is likewise noninjurious, since it has been expended for work other than disturbing the uniform state of rest or motion of the tissues.

In addition to the kinetic energy of forward motion, an object may possess energy by reason of the fact that it is rotating on its own axis. Such energy frequently is possessed by a flying missile and adds to the wound-producing capacity of bullets. The extra energy possessed by a spinning object may be calculated from the formula $IW^2/2g$, in which I = the rotary inertia or $Mr^2/2g$ (r = radius of cross section and M = weight), W = the angular velocity in radians per second, or $2\pi \times$ number of rotations/second, and g = the acceleration of gravity.

Rate of energy transfer. The duration of impulse or period of energy transfer is an important factor in determining how much of the force of an impact will be expended in the causation of uniform or noninjurious motion and how much in the causation of nonuniform or potentially injurious movement of the tissues. Athletes are aware of the desirability of prolonging the duration of impulse. To diminish the amount of force likely to be expended in the production of nonuniform or disruptive movement of tissues, the tumbler rolls with his fall, the ballplayer moves his gloved hand with the caught ball, and the fighter endeavors to move with his opponent's blow. Protracted deceleration probably accounts in large measure for the occasional and seemingly miraculous survival of people who have fallen from great heights.

Surface area. Another important factor in determining the wound-producing capacity of an impact is the size of the surface area to which the force is applied. The larger the area through which a given amount of impact force is transmitted, the less will be its intensity. Thus an impulse of a certain number of foot-pounds might cause uniform tissue displacement without injury when acting over a large area and yet be capable of causing severe disruption of tissue when acting through an area comparable to the edge or point of a knife.

Target area. Many other factors may modify the disruptive effects of impacts even when they are similar in respect to the amount of energy expended, the duration of impulse, and the area of collision contact. Among these is the extent to which the force may be intensified by lever action or by hydrostatic effect. A small force applied near the end of a liver will be greatly intensified as the fulcrum is approached. This phenomenon is particularly important in relation to the production of fractures of long bones. Similarly, a relatively small compression of a large hollow viscus may displace a sufficient volume of fluid to rupture the wall of a less voluminous communicating structure. Differences in the elasticity, plasticity, or inertia of tissues are of great importance with respect to whether a given force will produce disruptive change. Liver is ordinarily more friable and more readily disrupted by distortion than lung or muscle is. A hyperplastic and friable spleen may be torn to pieces by an impact that would be harmless to a normal spleen. The capillary fragility of persons with certain vitamin deficiencies is often greater than that of the normal person.

The foregoing discussion of the mechanics of injury production by the energy of motion has concerned disruption of tissue or wound production. Although a wound is the most common manifestation of injury caused by the energy of motion, it is by no means the only one. Force has been defined as that which changes the state of rest or uniform motion of matter. The application of force to the surface of the body may alter subsurface relationships sufficiently to cause severe functional disturbance even though no cutaneous wound is produced. In fact, many victims of fatal blunt trauma have no externally visible wound. This pertains especially to persons with head injuries whose scalp is shielded by thick hair or a hat and to persons who sustain chest and abdominal impacts over a broad area.

Also, the application of pressure in many situations may cause harmful interference with the function of the compressed or displaced tissue even though the force is insufficient to produce a wound. Mechanical obstruction of the air passages for more than a few minutes is likely to cause death from systemic anoxia. A tight tourniquet applied for 30 minutes may result in ischemic necrosis of a limb. Furthermore, as in many other areas of pathology, traumatically induced functional disturbances can be profound, or even lethal, yet not structurally demonstrable. For example, the term "instantaneous physiologic death" can be used to describe the rapidly fatal outcome of a blunt impact to the chest that fails to mark the skin, causes no fractures of the sternum or ribs, and does not produce a cardiac contusion.[1] Such deaths probably result from ventricular fibrillation, a structurally traceless lethal mechanism.

Local effects of mechanical violence

Wounds. As previously indicated, a wound is a mechanically produced interruption in the continuity of tissue. There are several anatomic types of such disruptive lesions, for which distinctive terms are used.

Abrasion. An abrasion (scratch or scrape) represents the tearing away of epidermal cells by friction or crushing. Such a defect may or may not penetrate to the corium. Although an abrasion may provide a portal of entry for infection, such a wound is ordinarily of little pathologic significance beyond the fact that it provides objective evidence that force has been applied to the surface of the body. The direction of motion responsible for an abrasion can frequently be recognized by the manner in which the partially detached sheets of epidermis have been rolled on themselves at the distal end of the defect (Fig. 5-2). In some instances the nature of the abrading object can be recognized by the distribution and configuration of the epidermal defects.

Laceration. The word *laceration* is commonly misused as a synonym for a cut (or incised wound). A laceration is a split or tear and represents the effect of excessive stretching of tissue. Although any tissue may be disrupted in this manner, such injuries most commonly involve the integument, particularly where it is stretched over bone, as in the hands or over the skull. Lacerations of skin caused by the unidirectional displacement and stretching that occur incident to the impact of an obliquely directed force are likely to be linear or curved, whereas those produced by the multidirectional radial displacement of a crushing impact oriented at a right angle to the skin may be linear or stellate. The latter commonly have crushed, abraded margins; such an injury is an "abraded laceration" (Fig. 5-3). Linear lacerations may be so cleanly disrupted as to resemble an incised wound. In such a circumstance it may be necessary to identify the attenuated strands of tissue that bridge the margins of the defect in order to recognize it as a laceration (Fig. 5-4). In the case of curved or angular lacerations of the skin, the apex of the angle or the convexity of the curve will face the direction from which the force was applied.

The force of an external impact may lacerate internal structures without damage to the skin or subcutaneous tissue (Fig. 5-5). Thus ligaments, muscles, or blood vessels are frequently lacerated by excessive stretching with or without superficial injury. Compression of fluid or gas in hollow viscera may cause laceration and perforation of their walls (Fig. 5-6). Soft tissues adjacent to the site of a fracture are usually lacerated by the broken ends of the bone.

Contusion. A contusion or bruise is an injury in which the force of an impact is transmitted through the skin to the underlying tissues with sufficient intensity to disrupt the walls of small blood vessels and to cause interstitial bleeding without disruption of the epidermis (Fig. 5-7).

Usually the interstitial bleeding is so superficial as to be almost immediately visible through the skin. However, a bruise may be so deep that either hours elapse before the extravasated blood becomes superficial enough to be visible or it is never seen from the surface. An external impact may cause extensive bruising of internal viscera without damage to the skin or subcutaneous tissue.

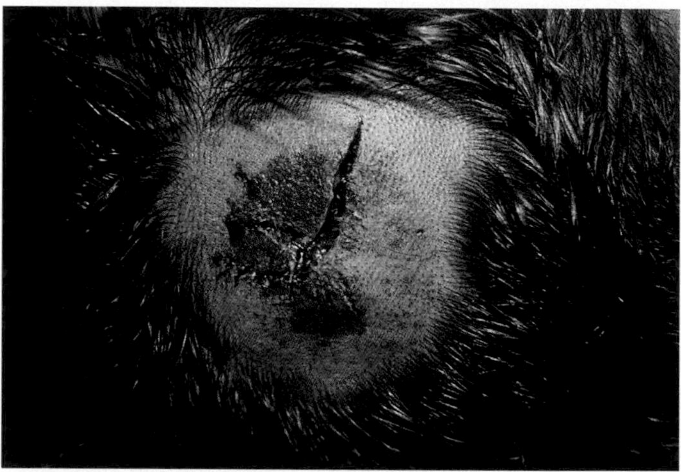

Fig. 5-3 Abraded laceration of scalp caused by impact of circumscribed object with force directed perpendicularly to skin. Abrasion resulted from crushing of epidermis, and stellate laceration was caused by stretching of skin over subjacent bone.

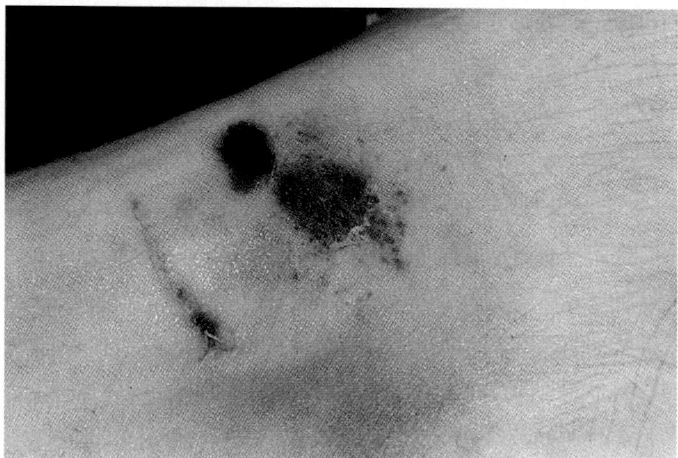

Fig. 5-2 Abrasion of left medial malleolus of a pedestrian who was "knocked out of his shoes" when struck by auto. Force acting on ankle as it left the shoe was directed distally and nearly parallel to the surface. Heaping of epidermis on lower margin of injury reflects direction and orientation of abrading force.

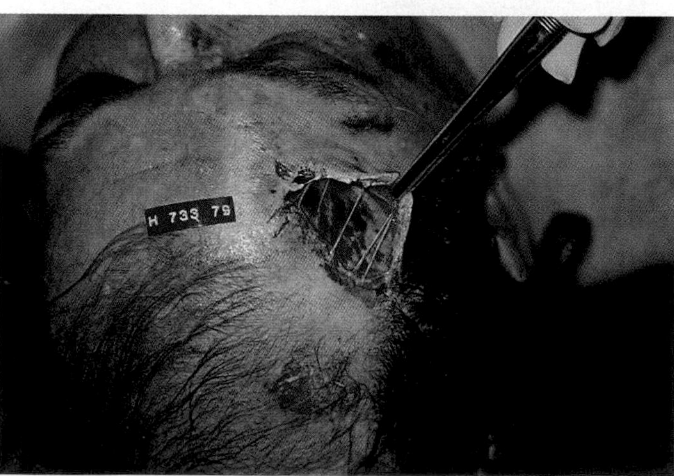

Fig. 5-4 Linear laceration of forehead with undermining of distal margin. Strands of tissue bridging defect indicate that injury is a laceration rather than an incised wound because a cutting instrument cannot leave intact tissue above its deepest penetration.

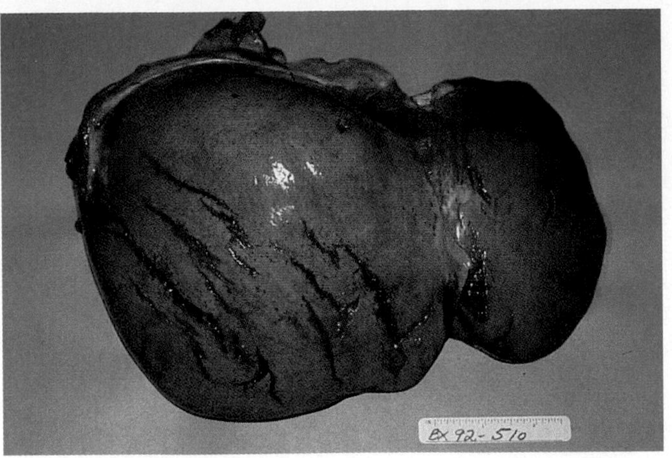

Fig. 5-5 Multiple lacerations of liver caused by compression of upper abdomen or chest. Similar injuries are common without external wounds or fractures.

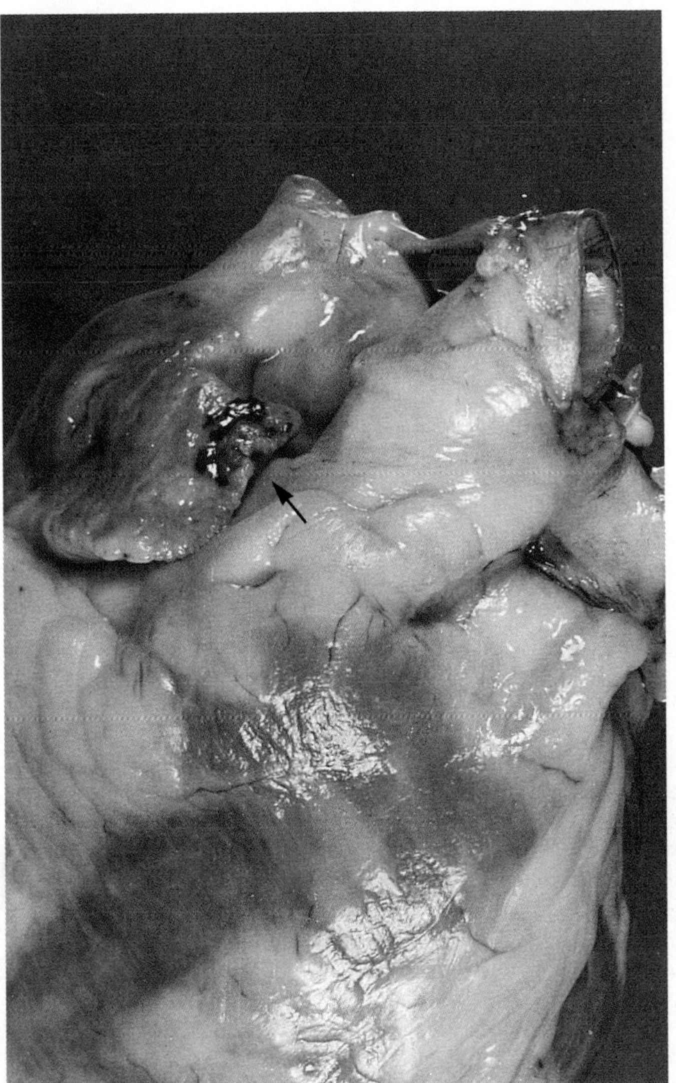

Fig. 5-6 "Blowout" laceration of right atrial appendage *(arrow)*, the sole cardiac injury in young woman who fell from a height and landed on her chest. Compression of right atrium during diastole caused hydrostatic transmission of pressure into atrial appendage with laceration of its tip. Death resulted from hemopericardium with tamponade.

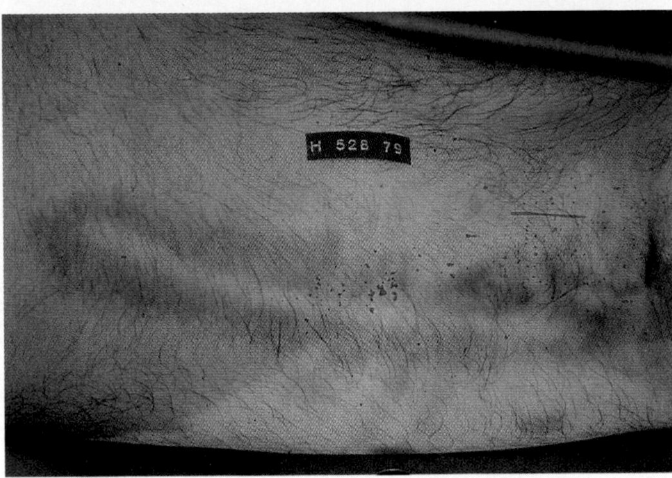

Fig. 5-7 Contusions caused by one impact with cylindrical object on posterior area of thigh. Linear pale mark indicates point of impact, which was subjected to uniform compressive stress. Adjacent, parallel, linear contusions correspond to areas of maximal shearing stress along edges of striking object.

Individuals vary enormously in their susceptibility to mechanical disruption of small blood vessels. Persons with certain dietary deficiencies or blood dyscrasias are likely to sustain remarkably extensive contusions as a result of relatively mild impacts.

Incision. An "incised wound" (or cut) is one produced by the pressure and friction against skin or other tissues by an instrument having a sharp edge. By definition an incised wound is longer than it is deep. "Stab wounds" are deeper than they are long. In these types of injury the tissues are uniformly displaced to either side of the cutting edge with the result that the primary damage is limited largely to the immediate vicinity of the defect.

Penetrating injury. The impact of an appropriately shaped resistant object against the skin may produce a defect so deep and of such relatively small diameter that its outstanding characteristic is penetration. Slender sharp objects and flying missiles are the most common causes of such injuries. Although the majority of penetrating wounds involve the skin and subcutaneous tissue, the broken end of a bone often causes penetrating injury without involving the integument.

Fracture. Any force that tends to change the state of uniform motion or rest of the body is likely to disrupt its least plastic tissue, the bony skeleton. A fracture is a mechanically produced disruption in the continuity of bone. Such osseous defects vary from a simple linear break, caused by excessive bending, to an explosive comminution caused by the impact of a high-velocity projectile. Of particular importance in the mechanics of fracture production is the transmission of force from the site of external application and its intensification at a distant point through lever action. One should not assume that the stress responsible for a fracture is necessarily of unusual magnitude or of external origin. A relatively minor stress may cause "pathologic fractures" of diseased bones.

Traffic injuries. Because traffic injuries are so common and exemplify the physical principles involved in blunt wound production, they deserve separate consideration.[15]

Injuries to vehicle occupants. The most straightforward situation with respect to the fate of vehicle occupants is a head-on crash without ejection. Such a collision with another vehicle or fixed object (such as a bridge abutment) causes the car to decelerate rapidly or come to a dead stop. The occupants are, of course, moving at the same speed and in the same direction as the vehicle at the instant of its crash. However, because they are not riveted to the vehicular frame, they do not decelerate and stop with it. Instead, they continue on their forward course as masses in motion until they meet an opposing force. The latter force is exerted by their impact against the vehicle interior. To recapitulate, the first collision involves the vehicle and some other object; the second collision involves the occupant and the interior of the vehicle, and this is the injury-producing energy transfer. Other types of vehicular crash (such as side impacts) add a complicating factor in that the initial collision changes the vehicle's direction as well as its speed. In these more complex situations, the occupants move toward the point of vehicular crash en route to their decelerating impact with the car's interior.

The extent and severity of resulting injuries are determined by the initial velocity of the occupant, the rate of the occupant's deceleration, the nature and distribution of the opposing force that causes occupant deceleration, and the part of the body involved in energy transfer. As with other modalities of mechanical violence, rapid energy transfer and concentration of force over a small area produce more injurious, nonuniform displacement of tissues than does slowly applied, widely distributed force. All types of occupant safety systems, whether some form of restraining belt or an air bag, a collapsible steering column, padded interior panels, or recessed knobs and buttons, are designed to prolong the energy transfer of deceleration, to distribute the decelerating force over the broadest or sturdiest possible area of the occupant's body, and to prevent unrestrained movement (and ejection) of the occupant after the vehicular crash.

Injuries to the head and neck commonly result from impacts against the windshield, side windows, or upper part of the vehicular frame. Trunk injuries are caused by decelerating impacts against the steering wheel (Fig. 5-8) or column, dashboard, or back of the front seat in the case of rear-seat passengers. Injuries of the lower limbs are frequently produced by impacts against the dashboard, foot compression against the floor, or entanglement of the feet in pedals or beneath the seats. Arm fractures can be produced when an occupant braces for a front-end collision by gripping the steering wheel or the dashboard.

Improperly worn safety belts can cause or contribute to patterns of injury.[16,17] Lap belts should be worn over the pelvic area so that the sturdy iliac crests absorb the stress of deceleration. If they are worn loosely or high, the force thereby transmitted to the abdomen can injure virtually any structure between the diaphragm and pelvis (Fig. 5-9). Likewise, an improperly worn shoulder strap, resting against the side of the neck rather than the upper chest, can cause severe cervical injury.

Occupant ejection from the vehicle allows for second or additional impacts with the road and other objects, greatly increasing the likelihood of serious injury or death. A crash that causes such severe deformity of the vehicle interior that the occupants are crushed is a nonsurvivable accident.

Injuries to pedestrians. Pedestrian fatalities are of three general types, with an approximately equal incidence. One third are children who carelessly dart into the path of a moving vehicle; one third are elderly persons who may have defective vision or hearing, which usually is coupled with diminished agility; and one third are healthy adults who commonly are under the influence of ethanol or drugs. Pedestrians sustain injuries when they are run over, "run under," or violently slammed aside.

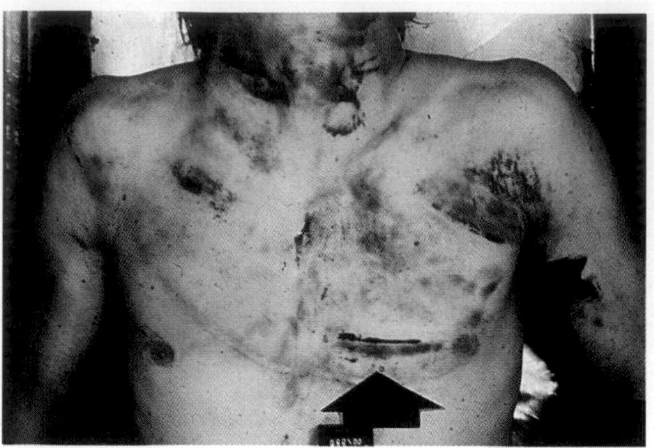

Fig. 5-8 Multiple contusions and abrasions on chest of driver killed in head-on collision. Curved abrasion *(arrow)* resulted from impact against steering wheel. (Courtesy Office of the Chief Medical Examiner, Baltimore, Md.)

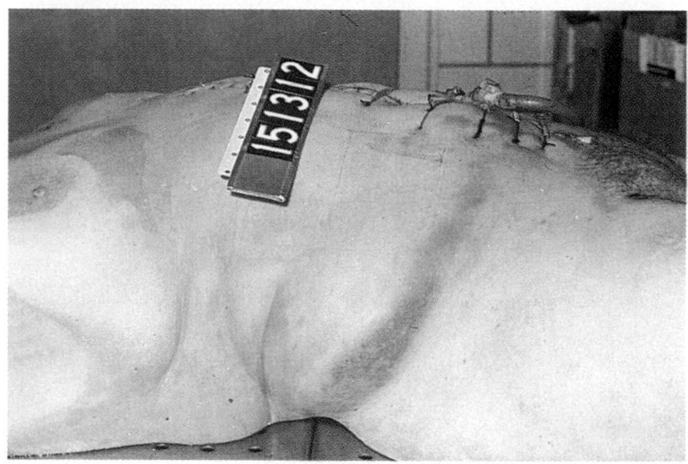

Fig. 5-9 Bandlike contusion extending across right flank and lower abdomen of driver who sustained mesenteric and small intestinal lacerations in a head-on collision. Patterned bruise and visceral injuries probably resulted from force applied to trunk by way of improperly worn lap belt.

A person is run over in one of two circumstances; either he is lying in the path of a moving vehicle or his center of gravity lies below the point of impact with the vehicle. The latter situation arises with children and crouching adults or when the involved vehicle is a bus or truck whose front end is high and broad. Tire tread marks on the victim's skin or clothing can be conspicuous or subtle, but the injured area almost invariably shows underlying avulsions of subcutaneous fat and severe crushing. An exception to the foregoing sometimes occurs when the victim is lying on a surface that yields, such as soft dirt or grass.

It is far more common for pedestrians to be run under than run over.[15] This occurs when an upright adult is struck by a moving vehicle below his center of gravity. Compound ("bumper") fractures of the lower legs are the classic stigmas of such impacts, but the thighs, hips, and low back are other common areas of initial impact.[18] As a result of the primary impact, the pedestrian's legs are thrown forward and elevated. His next impact usually occurs when he strikes the automobile hood or roof, after which he bounces to the pavement. The point or points of secondary impact with the vehicle are determined by the victim's height and weight and the speed and configuration of the moving vehicle. If the auto is moving rapidly, it may pass completely beneath the victim, who is tossed high into the air and comes down on the road. The majority of pedestrian fatalities result from head injuries.

Victims who walk or run into the side of a moving vehicle usually are hurled aside. They may impact against a wide variety of nearby objects before hitting the ground and generally sustain head injuries.

Injuries to cyclists. Cyclists sustain injuries when they are struck by motor vehicles, when they drive into a vehicle or some other object, or when they lose their balance and fall. The cyclist who is hit by a moving vehicle is the mechanical equivalent of a "sitting pedestrian," and the principles governing injury in this circumstance are similar to those mentioned previously. The cyclist who hits another object is the mechanical equivalent of an unrestrained, open-vehicle occupant who is "launched" when he continues in forward motion after his cycle is stopped by its decelerating impact. As with pedestrians, the vulnerability of cyclists allows for multiple severe injuries of more than one body area, though craniocerebral trauma is the leading cause of cyclist fatalities.

Common medicolegal problems associated with traffic injuries. TOXICOLOGY. Blood ethanol and drug determinations should be done on all teenage and adult victims of traffic accidents who survive their injuries for less than 24 hours. Tests for carboxyhemoglobin are indicated when vehicles catch fire or when there is a possibility that the car had a defective exhaust system or extensive rusting of its undersurface. On the latter basis, we have seen fatal asphyxia by carbon monoxide in occupants of a car parked in an open area with its engine running.

In any victim of a fatal traffic incident, the pathologist should save at least 50 ml of blood and urine, all available bile, stomach content, and generous samples of liver, kidney, and brain. Toxicologists have adequate means to dispose of samples they do not need, but none can retrieve a specimen that went down the drain or into an incinerator. Nothing frustrates the toxicologist more than a 5 to 10 ml sample of blood accompanied by an all-encompassing request that it be analyzed for "drugs."

IDENTITY OF DRIVER. When all vehicle occupants are ejected, important medicolegal questions may arise concerning the identity of the driver. Patterns of injury may provide the answer, and comparison of the victims' blood groups with the location of blood stains in the car may be helpful. Hair samples should be plucked from any hair-bearing area that is injured. The victims' clothing should be preserved carefully for evidentiary evaluation by trained personnel. In this regard, smooth-soled shoes should be examined, since they may show patterned imprints imparted by forces transmitted through the brake or accelerator pedals or the floor mats.

HIT-SKIP (HIT AND RUN) PEDESTRIANS. Samples of blood and hair should be saved as mentioned previously. In addition, fragments of metal, glass, or paint are usually present on the victim's clothing and may be on or in the victim's body. Reconstruction of the accident situation may hinge on correlation of the victim's impact areas with damage to the suspected vehicle. It should be standard practice to measure the height or impact areas on the lower limbs above the level of the heels. The presence of cataracts or optic atrophy occasionally helps to explain why an elderly pedestrian walked into the path of an oncoming vehicle, thereby exonerating an innocent driver.

Firearm injuries. *Guns and bullets.* Pulling the trigger on a loaded gun causes the firing pin to strike the cartridge base, detonating the primer. The latter event causes ignition of gunpowder in the cartridge. Gunpowder combustion produces rapidly expanding gas, the pressure of which propels the bullet.

A bullet's diameter, or caliber, can be expressed in hundredths of an inch or in millimeters. Fig. 5-10 shows representative handgun bullets of commonly available calibers. The .25- and .45-caliber bullets have full copper jackets, and the .38-caliber bullet on the right has a partial copper jacket. The .22-caliber bullet has been coated with a thin film of copper ("copper wash"), which is not a discrete jacket. The specimens arranged on the bottom row of Fig. 5-10 are bullets that have been deformed and fragmented as a result of their passage through a hard object such as bone. A misshapen partial jacket, which has been separated from the bullet core after contact with a hard object, is shown at the far right of the bottom row. Deformed bullets and fragments such as these present irregular surfaces to the tissues in their path. Consequently, they are likely to expend all of their energy in wound production. From the standpoint of "wounding efficiency," the residual kinetic energy possessed by a bullet as it exits from the victim is wasted because it has not been utilized in injury production.

During the manufacture of handgun and rifle barrels, a rifling tool cuts a series of spiral grooves in their interiors. The elevated surfaces between the grooves are called "lands." Because the interior diameter of the barrel is slightly smaller than the bullets intended for use in the gun, the fired bullet entering the breech end of the barrel is gripped by the lands, which impart a spin to it as it passes through the barrel. This

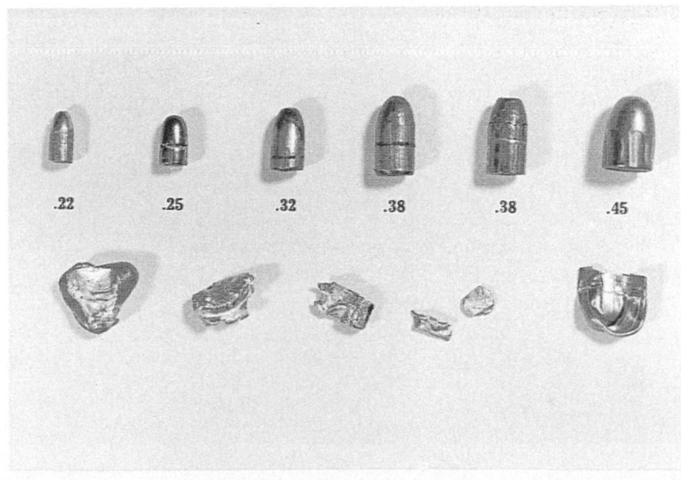

Fig. 5-10 *Top row,* Bullets of commonly available calibers for handguns. *Bottom row,* Deformed bullets, misshapen bullet fragments, and a deformed partial jacket (see text).

spin about its long axis produces the bullet's gyroscopic stability while it is in flight.

In addition to the bullet, a variety of particulate matter emerges from the muzzle of a fired gun. The smallest particles are the residue of completely burned gunpowder and take the form of a black, dustlike material. These particles are so light that they generally travel only 6 to 8 inches from the gun muzzle. As a result, targets shot at ranges closer than 6 to 8 inches usually show a zone of black fouling, or smudging, surrounding the bullet perforation (Fig. 5-11). Larger particles emerging with or behind the bullet consist of partially burned or unburned gunpowder, metal shavings, and other debris or lubricant from the barrel interior or bullet surface. Since these particles are larger and heavier than the dustlike residue of completely burned powder, they travel farther. In flight they take the form of tiny individual missiles, each creating a punctate impression on or in the target. Collectively, these individual marks are referred to as "stippling," or "tattooing" (Fig. 5-12). Most handguns produce stippling up to ranges of 1½ to 3 feet.

Cutaneous entrance wounds. In reference to muzzle-target distance, we use the following classification for handgun and rifle wounds.[19] "Contact" shots are those in which the muzzle of the gun touches the target. When the muzzle is pressed firmly against the skin so that all of the powder residue is blasted *into* the tissue, the wound is classified as "tight contact" (Fig. 5-13). If the seal between muzzle and skin is imperfect, a "loose contact" wound results in which powder residue is deposited *on* the cutaneous surface as well as being blasted *into* the wound track (Fig. 5-14). In either instance the expanding gas that follows the bullet augments the severity of the injury. When the muzzle does not touch the target but is sufficiently close to produce fouling, the wound is "close range." Wounds having stippling but no fouling are "intermediate range," and those beyond the range of stippling are "distant." In reference to cutaneous wounds, the foregoing criteria are inappropriate when the skin is not the primary target. Passage of a bullet through thick hair, clothing, or some other object before it strikes the skin may filter some or all of the powder residue, shielding the skin from fouling and stippling (Fig. 5-11).

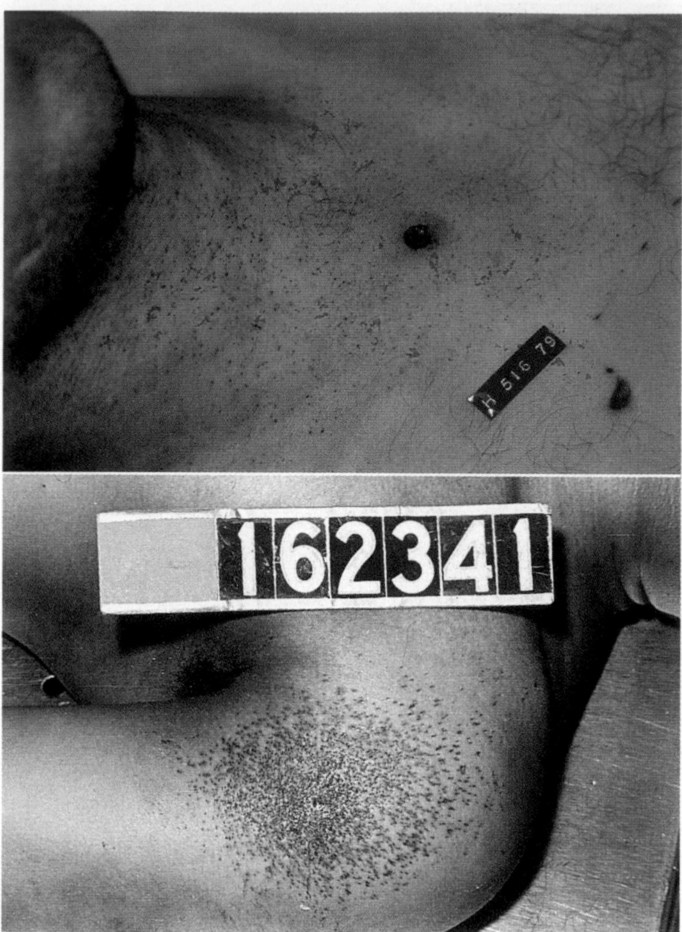

Fig. 5-12 A, Entrance gunshot wound of neck with sparse, fine stippling, typical of flake gunpowder. Skin of chest was shielded by shirt. (Skin defect at lower right corner is an artifact of medical treatment.) **B,** Entrance gunshot wound with conspicuous, dense stippling, typical of ball gunpowder.

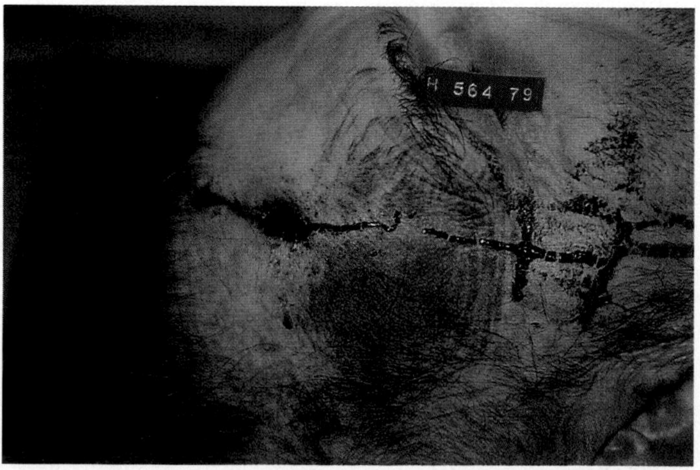

Fig. 5-11 Entrance gunshot wound, right side of forehead, with fouling of lateral right area of forehead. Skin above and medial to fouling shielded by hat.

The appearance of a contact-range gunshot wound is determined by the amount of gunpowder in the cartridge (load), the characteristics of the firearm, the firmness of the seal between muzzle and skin, and the part of the body that is shot. If sufficient expanding gas is blasted into an area with underlying firm bony support (such as the head), the skin is torn loose from its attachment and lacerated (Fig. 5-13, *A*). Such wounds are commonplace with contact-range wounds produced by handguns of .32 caliber or greater. Smaller-caliber handgun ammunition often does not produce sufficient gas to lacerate the skin. Instead it may elevate the skin from its support and press it back against the face of the gun, imparting a "muzzle stamp" to the skin surrounding the gunshot perforation (Fig. 5-13, *B*). If the arrangement of the tissues is such that the explosive force can be decompressed *internally*, as is likely with contact wounds of the chest or abdomen, the external characteristics of the cutaneous wound may resemble those of a distant wound.

Typical distant cutaneous entrance wounds are abraded perforations whose central defect is slightly smaller than the bul-

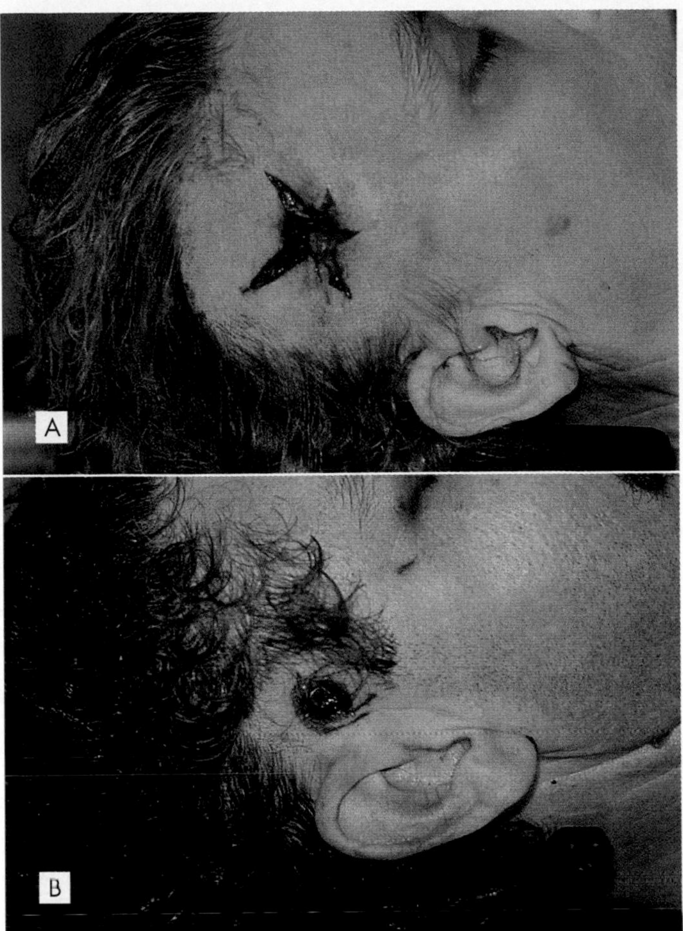

Fig. 5-13 Typical tight contact-range gunshot wounds with no escape of powder residue onto cutaneous surfaces adjacent to perforations. Expanding gas blasted into wound, **A**, caused extensive lacerations. In **B**, gas elevated scalp and pressed it against gun, producing a "muzzle stamp," but quantity of gas was insufficient to lacerate skin. Internally both wounds contain gunpowder residue, visible in **A** because of lacerated margins but not visible in external view of **B**.

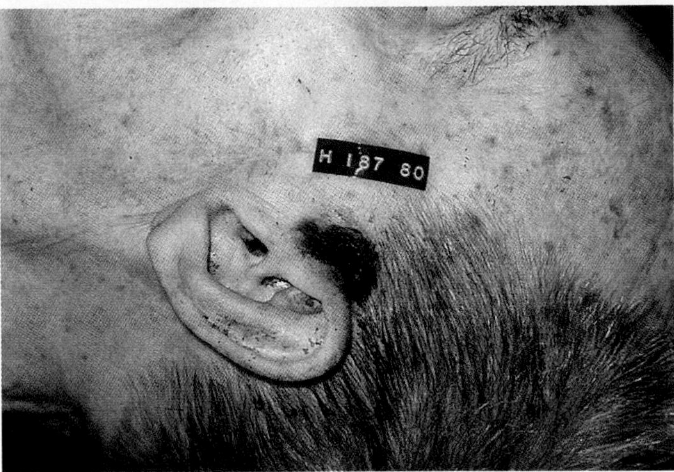

Fig. 5-14 Loose contact-range gunshot wound with imperfect seal between muzzle and skin, allowing escape of gas and powder residue onto cutaneous surface adjacent to perforation. *Arrow* indicates centrally located perforation. Internally, tracks of such wounds contain powder residue.

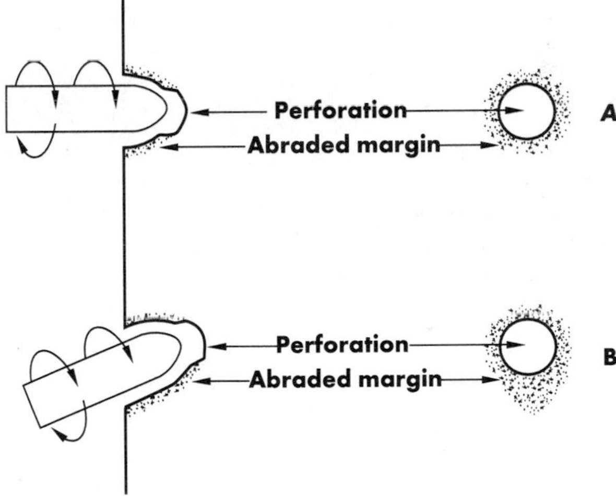

Fig. 5-15 Schema of mechanism whereby spinning bullets cause abraded defects when they perforate an elastic structure such as skin. Bullet striking at a right angle, **A**, creates a uniform margin of abrasion, whereas bullet approaching at an acute angle, **B**, leaves asymmetric abrasion that is widest on the side from which the bullet approached.

let diameter. This characteristic appearance is the combined result of the bullet's forward motion and the skin's elasticity. In the process of perforating the skin, the bullet initially indents and stretches it. The epidermis in contact with the margin of the moving bullet is scraped away, creating a rim of abrasion about the perforation. The outer circumference of the abrasion collar may be soiled by lubricant or dirt ("gray ring"), which must not be misinterpreted as fouling. Bullets striking the skin at right angles usually produce a uniform margin of abrasion (Figs. 5-15 and 5-16), whereas those that strike at an angle of less than 90 degrees leave asymmetric abrasions whose widest margin indicates the direction from which the bullet approached the skin (Fig. 5-17).

Atypical entrance gunshot wounds are those having unusual configurations, which commonly include lacerated margins and alteration of the typical abrasion collar described previously. Such anomalies occur in a variety of circumstances. Alterations of a bullet's normal gyroscopic spin and exaggerations of its yaw may be produced by defective guns or faulty ammunition, ricochet off a solid object, or passage of a bullet through some other target before it strikes the skin. In the last instance, if the primary target is close to the victim or is a personal item, such as spectacles or jewelry, fragments of the article may act as secondary missiles, which complicate the bullet perforation. In like fashion, primary perforation of a victim's hand or arm may render a wound of reentrance on his trunk or face decidedly atypical (Fig. 5-18). Finally, when the skin of the target area has a texture or contour different from that of ordinary skin, its wound (of entrance or exit) may have a totally different appearance. Examples of such areas include the eyelids, nose, lips, external ears, penis, scrotum, and fingertips.

"Rifle wounds" usually differ from those inflicted by handguns because the former typically are caused by bullets with

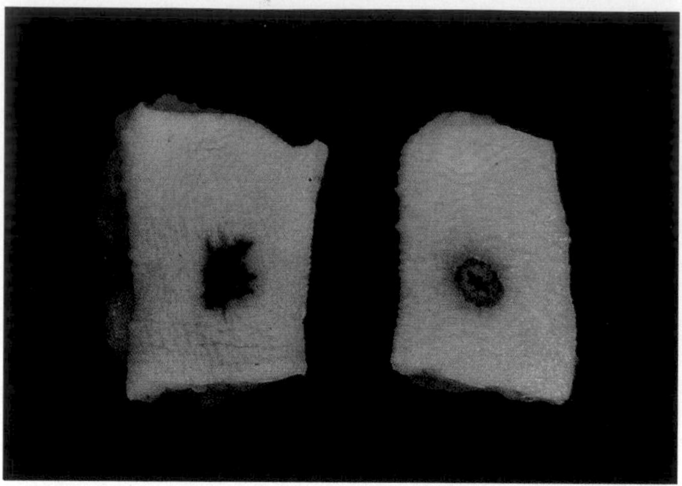

Fig. 5-16 Cutaneous entrance *(right)* and exit wounds made by same bullet. Symmetric, uniform margin of abrasion surrounding entrance perforation indicates that bullet approached at a nearly right angle. Exit wound is a lacerated, nonabraded perforation.

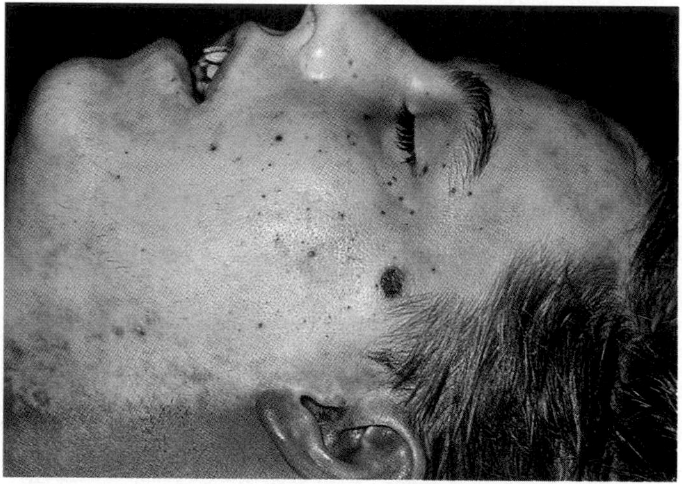

Fig. 5-17 Left preauricular entrance gunshot wound with sparse stippling of anterior check and eyelids; path of bullet front to back. Wide anterior margin of abrasion and minimal abrasion of remaining margins.

much greater kinetic energy. Commonly available handguns loaded with standard ammunition generally fire bullets with an initial muzzle velocity of 600 to 1000 feet per second, whereas rifle bullets frequently are in the range of 2000 to 3000 feet per second. Since a bullet's kinetic energy varies with the square of its velocity, a tripling of velocity increases its energy by a factor of 9.

Contact-range wounding with military and powerful civilian rifles causes massively destructive or explosive injuries. Distant wounding with these weapons will, in many instances, produce cutaneous wounds of entrance and exit that are atypical and larger than those inflicted by handguns (Fig. 5-19). Although distant rifle wounds may resemble handgun injuries externally, they generally inflict far more visceral trauma than handgun bullets do (Fig. 5-20). Small-caliber, low-velocity civilian rifle wounds may be similar to those produced by handguns.

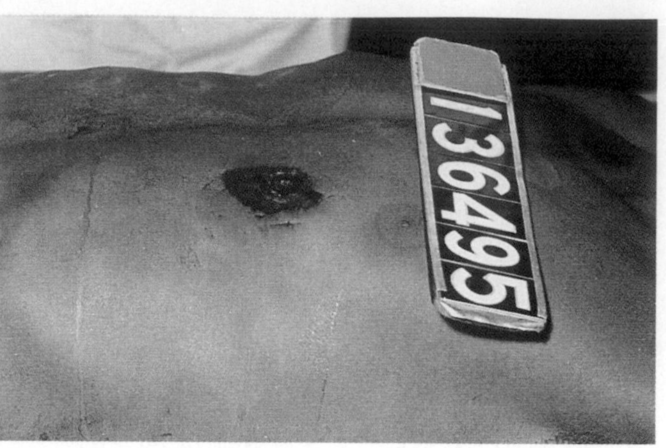

Fig. 5-18 Gunshot wound of reentrance in left inframammary area. Before striking decedent's chest, bullet perforated his right hand, passing from dorsum to palm, with exit defect on thenar eminence. At instant of wounding, palmar surface of his hand was resting against the chest. Oval abrasion, asymmetrically surrounding perforation, relflects configuration of his thenar eminence.

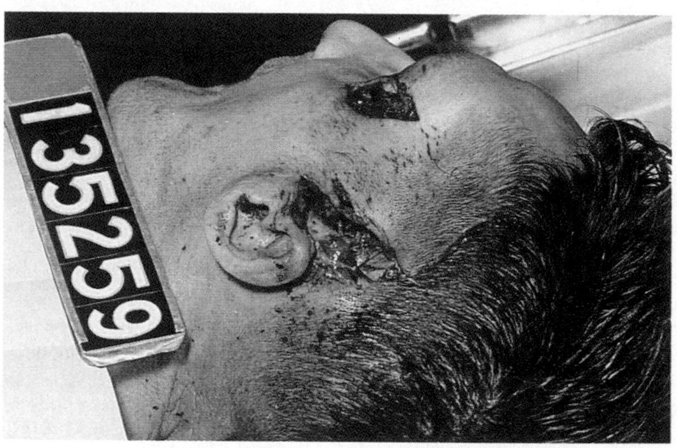

Fig. 5-19 Instantly fatal, distant-range, high-velocity (.30-caliber rifle) bullet wound of head. Entrance defect is adjacent to lateral aspect of left eyebrow, and exit defect is located above superior attachment of auricle. Skin between entrance and exit wounds has been torn loose from its attachments and shows tiny, stretch type of lacerations. (Dark spots on and behind ear are dry blood rather than stippling.) Subjacent skull was shattered, and multiple bone fragments ("secondary missiles") penetrated brain.

Cutaneous exit wounds. When a bullet leaves the body, it is traveling at a slower speed and is frequently deformed. It normally produces an irregularly lacerated wound with everted edges (Fig. 5-16). A slowly moving bullet may leave only a small, easily overlooked slit in the skin. The surface of an exit wound lacks the marginal epidermal abrasion that characterizes an entrance wound unless the skin was somehow supported at the moment it was perforated by the exiting missile. Support of this type can be provided by elastic bands of undergarments, belts, articles in pockets, or a firm external surface, such as a wall or the floor, against which the cutaneous surface was resting when perforated. With high-velocity bullets, the exit wound is usually larger than the entrance wound.

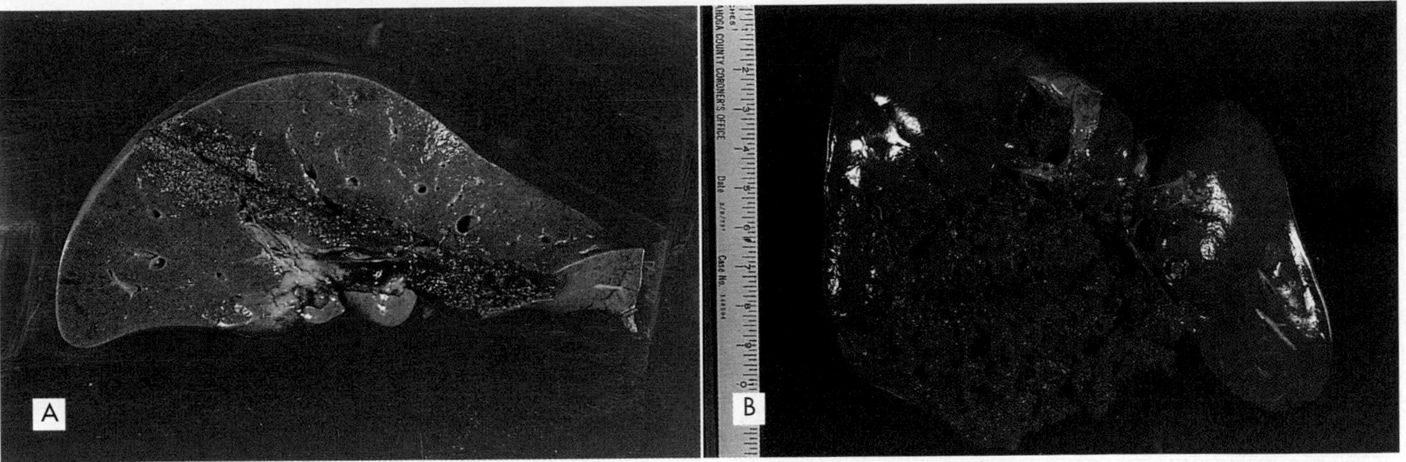

Fig. 5-20 Wound tracks through liver caused by low-velocity .38-caliber revolver bullet, **A,** and high-velocity .30-caliber rifle bullet, **B.** In **A,** zone of tissue damage is much larger than diameter of bullet but is far less destructive than hepatic fragmentation in **B.** Striking contrast between the two specimens exemplifies the dominance of velocity over weight in determining wounding potential because the .38-caliber revolver bullet was slightly heavier than the .30-caliber rifle bullet.

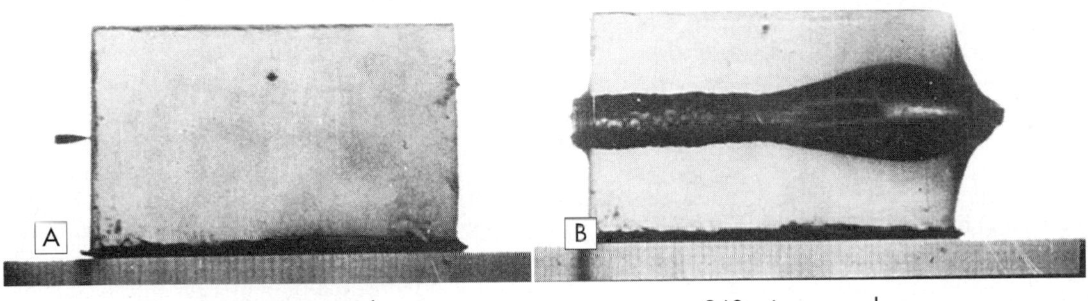

Fig. 5-21 Temporary cavity formation in gelatin block. **A,** A 7.62 mm rifle bullet approaching from left at velocity of 2800 feet/second. **B,** At 360 microseconds, bullet is approximately two thirds through the block and temporary cavitation has started. **C,** At 2160 microseconds, maximum formation of temporary cavity after bullet has left the block. Depending on the tolerance of the tissue to stretching stress, the entire area of temporary cavitation may be devitalized. (Courtesy Armed Forces Institute of Pathology.)

Internal injuries produced by gunfire have peculiar and important characteristics caused principally by the velocity of the wounding missile and the nature of the target area. Tissues in direct contact with the bullet are crushed and devitalized as they are perforated. Such crushing results in a permanent cavity or wound track. Radial or centrifugal displacement of force from the path of the bullet causes temporary cavitation of tissue and generates potentially damaging, stretching stress at a considerable distance from the bullet track (Figs. 5-20 and 5-21).[20] Any fragmentation of the projectile can augment wound production by providing points of weakness where the stretching effect is focused rather than being uniformly absorbed by the tissue.[21] Rigid tissues and structures are more susceptible to injury by stretching than soft, elastic tissues such as muscle. One of the more commonly encountered manifestations of radially transmitted forces from bullets is comminution of the orbital plates, which occurs frequently in association with transcerebral passage of projectiles (Fig. 5-17). Bullet perforations in bones are characteristically conical, with the entrance defect being smaller than the corresponding exit (Fig. 5-22).

Medicolegal evidence in death by gunfire. Frequently, the only opportunity to acquire reliable evidence as to the circumstances in which the injury occurred or to establish the identifying characteristics of the responsible weapon is provided by the autopsy. Such evidence may be readily lost or destroyed unless it is looked for and preserved. Loss or destruction of such medical and paramedical evidence can be disastrous. Thus failure to recognize powder residue in the interior of a wound may lead to

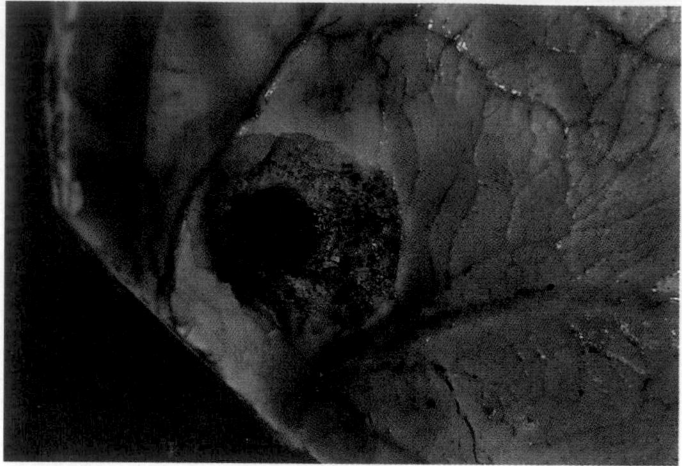

Fig. 5-22 Entrance perforation of skull made by .38-caliber bullet, viewed from the inner table, showing bone beveling in direction of flight and exemplifying principle that fractures dissipate forces acting on bone. In entrance wound of skull, bullet first strikes and fractures outer table. Force is dissipated as it is transmitted through bony trabeculas and therefore is exerted over larger area on inner table, causing larger perforation of the latter. Beveling is reversed in exit wounds, with the larger defect on outer table of skull. Most bones develop morphologically similar defects when perforated by bullets.

the exclusion of suicide and give support to the erroneous suspicion that murder has been committed. Failure to distinguish an entrance wound from an exit wound may seriously distort the official investigation of a homicidal incident.

GENERAL CONSIDERATIONS. A detailed examination and description of all skin wounds, all associated holes in the clothing, and such changes in either as might have resulted from powder residue should be routine practice in all cases of death by gunfire. It is common for a bullet that has passed through the body to be found in the clothing. The dimensions and precise location of each wound, each hole in clothing, and each area of fouling or stippling should be recorded with their locations related to standard anatomic landmarks as well as to the standing height of the victim. Color photographs are an indispensable supplement to the descriptive text.

BULLETS OR FRAGMENTS OF BULLETS. Any bullet or fragment of a bullet (sufficiently large to be recovered) in the body should be retrieved, even though no reason for preserving the bullet is anticipated at the time of operation or autopsy. Each bullet should be placed in its own properly labeled container and saved. In cases where more than one bullet or fragment of bullet are recovered, each should be identified in relation to the entrance wound with which it is associated.

Although the need for exercising care in the handling of projectiles and projectile fragments recovered from a victim should be common knowledge, many surgeons and some pathologists still make the mistake of extracting and handling such objects in the unprotected jaws of metal instruments or of scratching identifying initials across rifling marks on the sides of the bullet. Fig. 5-23 shows two bullets, each of which has been inscribed with the victim's initials, J.D.H. The specimen on the left is improperly marked because the initials obliterate some of the rifling striations. The correctly initialed specimen on the right has been marked on its base.

Because bullets often migrate or travel considerable distances from their entrance sites, autopsies of persons who have died from gunfire should be performed in locales where x-ray facilities are available. In the case of a perforating wound, where the bullet has emerged from the victim and has been lost, it may be extremely important to collect bullet fragments that have been sheared off in passing through a bone or deposited along the track of the wound. X-ray examination is often essential to locate such metallic debris. Subsequent identification of the chemical composition of the fragment or fragments may establish that it could or could not represent a certain type or branch of ammunition.

DIRECTION OF FIRE. In a case of death by gunfire, it is necessary to verify the direction from which the bullet came. If there is only one surface wound (that is, entrance defect) and the bullet is still in the victim, the problem is simplified. With low-power handguns, the bullet frequently is palpable beneath the skin of the side of the body opposite to the site of entrance. Skin offers greater resistance to perforation than any tissue other than bone or tooth.

If more than one hole is present in the skin, entrance must be distinguished from exit. The gross appearances of typical and atypical entrance and exit wounds have been described already; Adelson[14] has reported the histopathologic characteristics of cutaneous gunshot wounds. Also, one should be aware that bullet defects in clothing frequently are easier to orient as entrance or exit wounds than the corresponding perforations of the victim's skin are.

If bullet wounds in the skin (entrance or exit) have been altered or destroyed as a result of putrefaction or other postmortem change or surgery, it may still be possible to recognize the direction in which the bullet was traveling by the manner

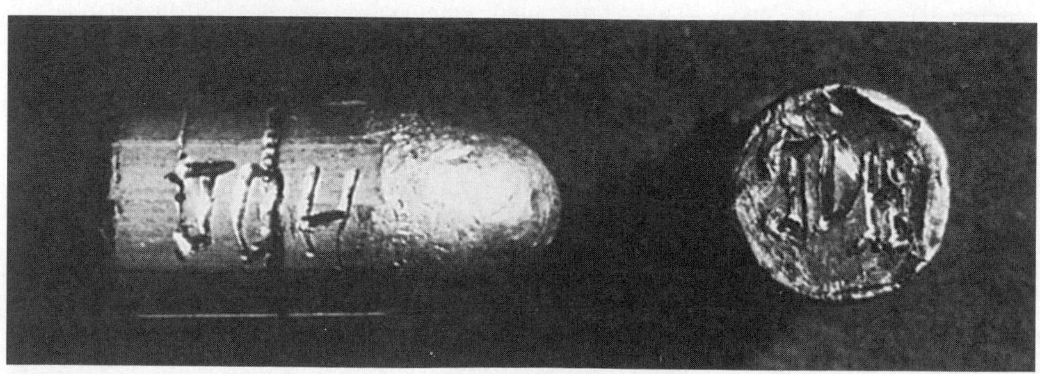

Fig. 5-23 Two nonjacketed .38-caliber bullets, each bearing initials J.D.H. Specimen on left is marked improperly because initials obscure rifling striations ("autograph" of gun from which it was fired). Specimen on right has been properly marked on its base.

in which bones have been fractured. In passing through a bone, a bullet characteristically produces a larger defect at the site of exit than at the site of entrance (Fig. 5-22). It also displaces fragments of bone in the direction of its flight.

RANGE OF FIRE. The evidence needed to establish the distance between the gun and the target when the shot was fired has been mentioned in connection with entrance wounds. Gray-black powder residue beneath the periosteum of the outer table of the skull or on the underlying dural margins is seen often with contact gunshot wounds of the head. Blotting of the wound with paper towels may help demonstrate powder soiling by removing excess blood. Removal of blood by this means must be done with care because contact or near-contact wounds produced by some ammunition may result in minimal surface fouling that is easily overlooked. The potential importance of such evidence for reconstructing the fatal incident is so great that the decedent should be examined by the pathologist before clothing has been removed and before the skin has been washed. If the clothing is dark, it may need to be photographed with infrared technique or tested chemically to disclose the presence or absence of combustion residues. When gunshot wounds are sustained through clothing, range of fire determinations rest on an evaluation of the garments rather than the person's skin. The effectiveness with which clothing shields the skin from powder residue is determined by the range of fire, characteristics of the gunpowder, number of layers of cloth perforated, and tightness of weave of the fabric.

Contact wounds in areas with underlying skeletal muscle (such as the chest) commonly show a zone of pink discoloration in muscle surrounding the wound-track. This is attributable to an uptake of carbon monoxide by myoglobin and probably also to a staining of muscle by nitrites in powder residue. The pink discoloration fades when the muscle is exposed to air.

NUMBER AND SEQUENCE OF SHOTS FIRED. The number of entrance wounds may not coincide with the number of bullets that have been fired into the body. Since the *number* of shots fired is often a matter of critical medicolegal importance, the causes of such "discrepancies" deserve investigation. The most common circumstance in which there may be a disparity between the number of bullets fired and the number of entrance wounds occurs when a bullet passes through an arm or hand before entering the trunk or head (Fig. 5-18). In such circumstances it is obvious that a single bullet can produce two or more entrances. Another type of discrepancy arises when a bullet strikes a compact bone and splits into two or more pieces. In such circumstances there may be more than one exit wound for a single hole of entrance. In rare instances, two bullets enter the same cutaneous perforation. This can occur with tandem or "piggyback" bullets or in contact-range wounding when the muzzle of the gun is pressed against a previous site of entrance. Bullets can be coughed up, expectorated, vomited, or defected when their tracks terminate in an air passage or the gastrointestinal tract, explaining the occasional situation in which there is an entrance wound without a corresponding exit defect and no bullet in the body.

TIME AND DEGREE OF DISABILITY AFTER GUNSHOT INJURY. Great caution should be exercised in estimating the immediate disabling effects of a bullet wound. Through-and-through wounds of the heart commonly fail to cause immediate disability. Only when there is massive destruction of the motor area of the central nervous system or of the brainstem or cervical cord, or when the heart or aorta has been extensively damaged can it be said "with reasonable medical certainty" that the injury was immediately and totally disabling.

Shotgun wounds. Shotguns are smooth-bore weapons that fire a charge composed of one or more projectiles plus wadding. The single-projectile shotgun ammunition, called a "rifled slug," is encountered rarely in human wounding and will not be considered further. Pellets in shotgun shells vary in size from 0.36 inch (000 buckshot) to 0.05 inch (number 12 shot). In our jurisdiction, the most frequently encountered sizes of shot in civilian wounding are from 0.10 to 0.15 inch in diameter, and average loads contain 100 to 250 such pellets. Police "riot guns" usually are loaded with large-sized buckshot.

Shotgun "gauge" formerly was defined as the number of spherical lead balls, each of the same diameter as the bore, required to weigh 1 pound. In actual measure a 12-gauge shotgun has a bore diameter of 0.729 inch and a 16-gauge bore is 0.662 inch in diameter. Bore diameter also can be expressed in thousandths of an inch—for example, .410 ("four-ten").

Choke refers to constriction of the muzzle end of the barrel and is designed to reduce pellet dispersion. The amount of choke varies from "full" to none. It is measured functionally by the percentage of shot falling in a 30-inch circle when the weapon is fired at a distance of 40 yards and ranges from 65% to 75% for full choke to 25% to 35% in the case of an unchoked cylinder bore. Choke either is added to the barrel during the manufacturing process or can be controlled with a variable choke adapter.

Contact-range shotgun wounds of the trunk are round or oval, smoothly marginated defects that may or may not contain an abundance of powder residue. Contact wounds in the interior of the mouth or against the scalp frequently produce explosive semidecapitation. The appearance of shotgun wounds beyond contact range is determined by the muzzle-target distance, barrel choke and length, shot size, and presence or absence of clothing or other intermediate objects in the path of the charge. Consequently, an estimate of range of fire in a given case is made with considerable latitude unless appropriate experimental test firings have been done. Generally speaking, at ranges beyond 3 to 6 feet the charge begins to separate, producing a skin defect with ragged margins, often referred to as a "rat hole." Next, a few pellets create individual satellite perforations adjacent to the major defect. As the distance lengthens, the main defect becomes smaller, more satellite perforations appear, and the spread of satellite perforations increases. Beyond approximately 5 yards, the wound pattern consists mainly of individual perforations with or without wad injuries in the form of circular, nonpenetrating abrasions.

Passage of the shotgun charge through clothing or any intermediate object, no matter how flimsy, accelerates the pellet spread and renders the skin pattern inappropriate for estimating range of fire. An x-ray film of the victim showing the spread of pellets cannot be utilized to estimate range of fire because the final distribution of pellets may be identical in contact and distant wounds.

Shotgun pellets usually do not exit from the body except for the following situations: contact wounds of the head that cause virtual explosions; tangentially oriented wounds, either close or distant, where part or all of the charge follows a short track through the body; wounding of a thin part of the body, such as the neck or a limb; and wounding by large-sized buckshot.

Local sequelae of mechanical injury. The mechanical disruption of living tissue is attended and followed by various local disturbances, the nature of which depends in part on the site and severity of the disruptive lesion and in part on the organism's capacity to react.

Hemorrhage. Hemorrhage is an immediate and inevitable sequel to mechanical disruption of living vascularized tissue. Blood continues to flow from the damaged vessels until prevented from doing so by thrombosis, vasoconstriction, or equalization of intravascular and extravascular pressures (through a drop in the former or a rise in the latter).

In the case of damage to the small vessels (capillaries, arterioles, venules), vasoconstriction is a more important mechanism than thrombosis in the induction of hemostasis. This is also true when vessels, whether large or small, are lacerated or crushed. When a vessel is incised or injured in such a manner that the disturbance is limited to the site of the defect, hemostasis is more dependent on the occurrence of thrombosis.

In noncommunicating injuries such as may occur with fracture or other forms of internal laceration, the opposition offered by the surrounding intact tissue to the accumulating mass of extravascular blood is an important mechanism of hemostasis. When injury has caused a state of shock, the fall in systemic blood pressure contributes to other factors in preventing further loss of blood.

Mechanical disturbances resulting from an extravascular accumulation of blood may be caused by distention, compression, or obstruction. Pain is an outstanding manifestation of distention of tissue by hemorrhage. It may be the first evidence of the accumulation of a relatively small amount of blood beneath the periosteum or immediately below the peritoneum. The most important compressive effects of extravasated blood are those seen in relation to intracranial and intrapericardial hemorrhage. The rapid accumulation of as little as 50 ml in the former situation or 150 ml in the latter may be fatal by its compressive effect. The importance of the rate of hemorrhage in determining such a mechanical effect is revealed by the fact that a considerably larger amount of blood can be tolerated in either situation if it has accumulated slowly. In the case of a slowly developing subdural hemorrhage, more than 100 ml may accumulate before signs of increased intracranial pressure become apparent. If the pericardium is distended slowly, a liter or more of fluid may be tolerated without the occurrence of fatal cardiac tamponade.

One of the best examples of obstructive disturbance caused by extravasated blood may occur when blood is aspirated into the lower air passages. The foam created by mixing blood and air in such a situation may be sufficiently obstructive to cause asphyxiation, though the lungs need not be heavier than normal.

The preceding paragraphs have been concerned with early mechanical disturbances caused by the extravascular accumulation of blood. The possibility of late mechanical disturbances attributable to secondary edema incident to the presence of blood in tissue spaces should not be ignored. One of the best examples of this phenomenon is the progressive expansion of a subdural hematoma. Although the space originally consumed by such a hemorrhage may fail to cause a significant amount of cerebral compression, the subsequent imbibition of fluid by the hematoma or secondary spontaneous bleeding from capillaries contained in newly formed granulation tissue sometimes gives rise to a progressively incapacitating or even fatal rise in intracranial pressure.

Pigmentary changes are a striking feature of the deterioration of blood at the site of hemorrhage. As the oxyhemoglobin is reduced, the color of the injured tissue changes from red through purple to blue. In the case of small extravasations, either the erythrocytes are ingested by phagocytes and transported from the site of injury or the products of their disintegration in situ are carried away by the lymph so rapidly that secondary pigmentary changes are inconspicuous. If the mass of extravasated blood is large or its disposal is delayed by inadequate lymph flow, the iron is separated from the globin after hemolysis in situ and the pigment is subsequently converted to bilirubin and biliverdin, with chromatic changes ranging through brown, green, and yellow. In addition to these color changes, two types of crystalline derivatives of hemoglobin may be identified on microscopic examination: hematoidin and hemosiderin. (For further discussion of hemoglobin pigments, see Chapter 9.)

Chronologic changes in the gross and microscopic appearances of contusions can provide the basis for important medicolegal interpretations. However, caution is in order when making such interpretations because of variability in temporal evolution of the gross appearances of bruises and of the histopathologic inflammatory responses. Such variability is governed by the vascularity of the injured locus, the quantity of blood accumulating in the tissues, the integrity of the overlying skin, and the factors that combine to define the host response to injury.

Aseptic inflammation. Unless immediately fatal, a mechanical injury of living tissue is almost invariably followed by a series of local reactive changes producing the phenomenon of aseptic inflammation. The extent to which the inflammatory reaction progresses or eventually disturbs the tissue usually depends on the severity and location of the injury that elicited it. The inflammatory cycle in such instances probably is set in motion and maintained by a variety of chemical and physical alterations. (Inflammation and wound healing are discussed in detail in Chapters 18 and 19.)

Other local circulatory disturbances. Attention already has been directed to the circulatory disturbances that may be induced by an expanding hematoma and to those that occur incident to vascular participation in the phenomenon of inflammation. Various other factors may contribute to local disturbances in circulation after a mechanical injury.

One of these is the occurrence of regional vascular spasm of sufficient extent and severity that the original injury is enlarged by the occurrence of secondary ischemic necrosis. Generalized ischemic of a limb may result from reactive spasm of large and apparently unwounded arteries after the occurrence of an injury whose disruptive effects were local. Nonthrombotic ischemia apparently from vasospasm is sometimes responsible for the progressive enlargement, by infarction, of relatively small primary injuries of the brain or kidney.

Similar enlargement of the original scope of injury may result from the propagation of a thrombus from the site of a disruptive vascular injury or from stasis and thrombosis caused by posttraumatic vascular compression by edema or interstitial hemorrhage. In the case of disabling injuries, the inactivity imposed by disability is an additional cause of stasis and may be responsible for thrombosis in the region of injury or in the lower extremities.

Intravascular stasis may be sufficient to cause thrombosis independent of preceding injury to the affected vessel. Although it is unlikely that thrombosis will occur in a normal vessel, the lining of a vessel does not remain normal for long after the blood within it has ceased to flow. Degeneration of the lining endothelium and edema of the intima occur concomitantly with stasis. Platelets adhere to the damaged lining. In larger vessels, clot formation begins at the periphery of the stream and progresses toward the center until the obstruction is complete. In small vessels, much or most of the fluid elements of the blood diffuse through the vascular wall, leaving the distended lumen occluded by a solid, sausagelike mass of closely packed erythrocytes.

Local infection. Any injury that disturbs the continuity of the protective and especially adapted layer of cells that stands between the organism and its external environment, whether it be the integument or the mucous membrane lining an internal passage, may create a portal of entry for infection. The infective agent may be carried into the tissues on the surface of the instrument that was responsible for the wound, or it may subsequently gain access to the tissues because of the existence of a wound.

Under nonsurgical conditions, any instrument responsible for the production of a mechanical injury is likely to be contaminated with pathogenic organisms. Soil is an important source of such contamination, and *Clostridium tetani* and *Clostridium welchii* are among the more important pathogenic inhabitants of soil. Streptococci, staphylococci, *Proteus vulgaris, Pseudomonas aeruginosa,* and *Escherichia coli* are commonly present on the skin. Pathogenic organisms that may be present on mucous membranes of the body include streptococci, pneumococci, meningococci, *Haemophilus influenzae, Klebsiella pneumoniae, E. coli, Corynebacterium diphtheriae,* and *C. welchii.*

The creation of an external portal of entry is by no means the only mechanism by which mechanical violence may render the site of an injury vulnerable to infection. Even though primary wound infection does not take place, a locus of diminished resistance may be established. Delayed infection of the injured tissue by way of the bloodstream may occur because of the creation of conditions favorable to bacterial growth at the wound site.

Systemic effects of mechanical injury

Almost immediately incapacitating systemic anoxia may be the direct consequence of an injury if its primary effect is such as to interfere with respiration or systemic circulation. Certain types of disruptive injury of the brain or heart may thus be the direct and immediate cause of fatal systemic disturbance. One should not conclude, however, that wounds of these structures are invariably fatal. As long as the brainstem escapes damage, extensive and disruptive cerebral injury may be survived. Through-and-through stab or bullet wounds of the heart are sometimes survived, and even those that eventually cause death may not be immediately incapacitating.

It is a fact, however, that even though the function of the damaged tissue is not normally concerned with such basic physiologic processes as respiration, circulation, nutrition, or elimination, such an injury may be responsible for systemic disturbances by any of several mechanisms.

Although the cause and nature of such disturbances are described in detail in various other places in this book, it is not unduly repetitive to bring them to the reader's attention at this time.

Primary shock. A mechanical injury to any part of the body may elicit a reflex vasodilatation and a fall in blood pressure of sufficient severity to cause collapse, loss of consciousness, and in some instances death. This type of posttraumatic circulatory disturbance constitutes the syndrome of primary or neurogenic shock. Pressure on the carotid sinuses, a blow to the epigastrium or a testicle, puncture of the pleura, a dilatation of the rectum may lead to sufficient fall in blood pressure to result in unconsciousness and occasionally in death. The reduction in blood pressure in such circumstances is caused by vasodilatation rather than by heart failure or a reduction in blood volume.

Secondary shock. Secondary shock is the state of circulatory failure that results from an excessive reduction in blood volume. It occurs whenever the amount of blood or plasma that has escaped from damaged vessels exceeds the limits of physiologic compensation. The vascular damage responsible for the escape of blood or plasma may be local and attributable to the direct effects of trauma or may be generalized and attributable to infection or some other systemic complication of what was originally a local injury.

Vasoconstriction is the initial homeostatic reaction to reduced blood volume. This may or may not be sufficient to maintain blood pressure, depending on the amount of blood lost. The secondary compensation is a movement of extravascular fluid into the vascular system, with hemodilution that may or may not be compensated by the mobilization of the erythrocyte reserves from the bone marrow and spleen. In its initial stages, shock is reversible. Severe and uncompensated shock may become irreversible as a result of widespread hypoxic parenchymatous injury. If bleeding or plasma loss continues, compensation fails and the volume of circulating blood decreases. When the pressure falls below a certain critical level, the vasomotor centers become anoxic and the resulting vasodilatation leads to rapid circulatory collapse and death.

The amount of hemorrhage necessary to produce circulatory collapse is governed by the rate of blood loss, the person's general cardiovascular condition, and the presence or absence of other factors, such as alcohol or drug intoxication, that may predispose to hypotension. In otherwise healthy persons, rapid loss of one third of the blood volume causes hemorrhagic shock, and death ensues when half of the blood volume is lost rapidly. Slow bleeding permits the occurrence of previously mentioned physiologic compensations and allows larger volumes of blood to be lost without causing shock or death.

In cases of death from acute massive hemorrhage, the most significant postmortem changes are gross rather than microscopic and consist in generalized pallor of tissue, collapse of the great veins, and a flabby, shrunken, gray spleen.

Shock kidney. Irreversible renal injury leading to anuria and death as a complication of secondary shock first attracted general attention during World War II. It did so because of the frequency with which persons who had sustained severe crushing injuries as a result of being caught in buildings demolished by air raids subsequently became anuric and died of renal insufficiency. Examination disclosed segmental obstruction of the renal tubules by pigmented casts, which were particularly conspicuous in the lower portions of the nephrons. It was first believed that the extensive crushing of skeletal muscle was responsible for the renal lesion. Subsequent studies, however, indicated that the essential damage to the kidney in such circumstances was probably attributable primarily to the renal ischemia that occurs during and may be prolonged beyond the posttraumatic episode of systemic hypotension. Any injury that is followed by secondary shock is capable of causing renal damage if the state of shock is sufficiently severe or protracted. If the original injury is associated with extensive muscle injury or intravascular hemolysis, the renal casts tend to be conspicuous by reason of their brown pigment. The injury is not confined to the lower reaches of the nephrons, and the casts represent the result rather than the cause of renal injury (see Chapter 65).

Shock lung. The term *shock lung* probably is a misnomer because shock alone fails to explain the pathogenesis of a variety of nonspecific pulmonary abnormalities that occur in injured persons. Lung injury from shock can be regarded as one of the local and systemic causes of the adult respiratory distress syndrome. In addition to chest wall and lung injuries, such patients may have aspiration of gastric content with pneumonia or lung abscess, bronchopneumonia, septicemia, fat embolism, large or small thromboemboli, embolism of cellular aggregates in massive blood transfusions, cardiac failure, fluid overloads, retained secretions, abdominal distention, atelectasis, and all the complications of prolonged mechanical ventilation.

Pulmonary pathologic changes understandably are variable and include alveolar and interstitial edema, thickening and fibrosis of alveolar septa, interstitial lymphocytic infiltrates, and alveolar hyaline membranes in various stages of organization. Obliterative changes in the pulmonary microvasculature, attributable to fibrin and platelet thromboemboli, commonly complicate disseminated intravascular coagulation and multiple transfusions. Bacterial, fungal, and viral pulmonary infections are common complications of trauma associated with coma, burns, debility, or inactivity.

General adaptation syndrome. The frequent occurrence of a posttraumatic neuroendocrine disturbance in the form of an evanescent hyperglycemia has long been recognized. That the neuroendocrine reaction to an injury may be such as to modify significantly the injury's total effect on the organism was not fully appreciated before the investigations of Selye.[22]

It is postulated that a wide variety of damaging stimuli may cause the pituitary gland to discharge an excessive amount of corticotropic hormone, which in turn leads to an outpouring of cortical hormones from the adrenal glands. Pathologic evidence of this effect on the adrenal glands is partial or complete depletion of lipid from the cortical cells within the first few days after an injury. That the reaction is part of a defense mechanism can be inferred from the fact that cortical hormone may cause a rapid release of antibodies from lymphoid tissue. The pathologic evidence of this effect is the rapid involution of thymus and lymphoid tissue.

Embolism. Fat droplets of sufficient size to obstruct capillaries may be found in the blood after almost any kind of disruptive injury involving adipose tissue and particularly after fractures of long bones. Unless the number and size of the emboli are such that fat-distended arterioles and capillaries are seen in every low-power field of lung, their lethality is doubtful. Usually when droplets and cylinders of fat are numerous in the pulmonary capillaries, emboli will also be found in the brain and kidneys (Fig. 5-24). Scully[23] found that only when the cerebral vessels are obstructed are fat emboli capable of causing death. In massive fat embolism, clinical features of the fat embolism syndrome, respiratory distress, and petechiae are present within 3 days of the injury.[24]

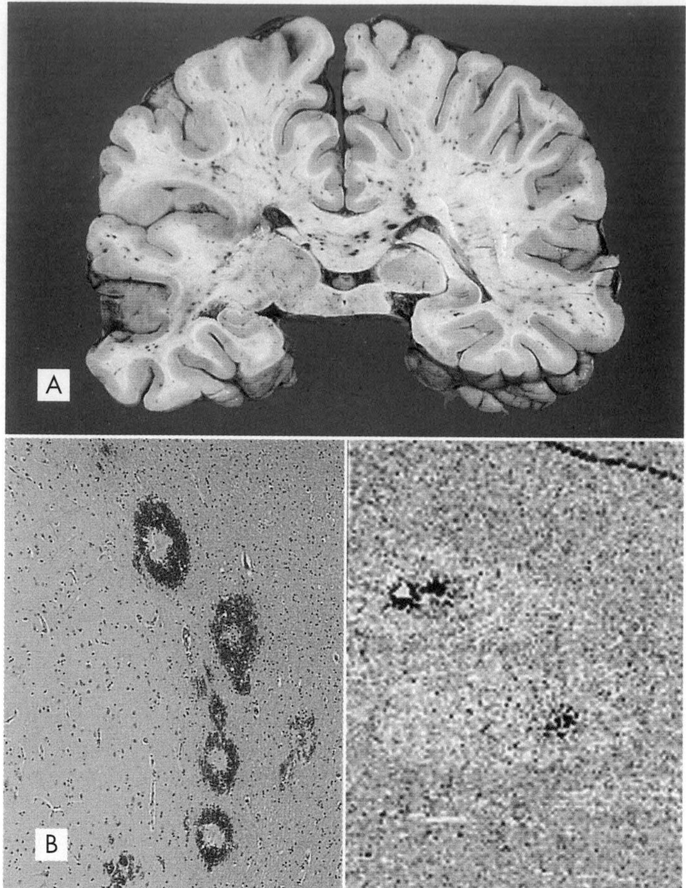

Fig. 5-24 A, Cerebral fat embolism. Coronal section of cerebral hemispheres with multiple small hemorrhagic infarcts producing gross appearance of white matter petechiae. Fat emboli are more numerous in gray matter, but richer vascularity of gray matter provides sufficient collateral circulation to prevent infarction from such microscopic-caliber emboli. **B,** Cerebral fat embolism. *Left,* Hemorrhagic mircroinfarcts in white matter near junction of cortex with subcortical white matter. *Right,* Microinfarcts in cerebral white matter, with arterioles obstructed by fat emboli. (Oil Red O).

Controversy exists regarding the origin of the fat. Originally it was believed that fat released from the damaged adipose tissue (or bone marrow) at the site of injury was forced or aspirated into the central ends of the lacerated value. That this does happen is indicated by the occasional finding of organized masses of myeloid tissue in the pulmonary vessels of persons who have died after fractures. However, the amount of fat found in the pulmonary vascular bed in some instances is far in excess of what might plausibly be derived from the site of injury.

Lehman and Moore[25] were among the first researchers to suggest that the phenomenon of posttraumatic fat embolism was the result of a change in the droplet size of the endogenous plasma lipids. Support for this point of view has been provided by the work of LeQuire and associates,[26] who found that the cholesterol content of the embolic fat was much higher than that of adipose tissue. More recent investigations have demonstrated posttraumatic alterations in lipid metabolism and mobilization. Elevated plasma levels of free fatty acids (FFA) and macroglobules and prolonged shifts in lipoprotein composition distinguish those patients at risk for developing fat embolism.[27,28] Pulmonary fat embolism occurring independent of mechanical violence may be encountered in association with such diverse conditions as diabetes mellitus, extensive cutaneous burns, and decompression sickness.[29]

A detached blood clot is another type of embolism frequently caused by mechanical injury. Venous thrombosis may occur as a direct result of trauma to a vein or as a result of stasis caused by edema or inactivity. Thus the thrombus may form at the site of injury or at some remote place in the body. The spontaneous detachment of such a thrombus frequently results in fatal pulmonary embolism.

A third type of embolism that may be caused by mechanical injury results from the entrance of air into the circulating blood. The most common portals of entry for fatal air embolism are the dilated veins of the gravid uterus. Large amounts of air may be sucked into the uterine veins during orogenital sex[30] or an attempt to empty the uterus by instrumentation or by irrigation. Air embolism may result from tubal insufflation, from the insufflation of a nongravid uterus, from the injection of air into the peritoneal cavity, or from incision or laceration of veins anywhere in the body. Iatrogenic air embolism may occur with disconnection of intravenous catheters or intraoperatively, particularly in procedures of the posterior cranial fossa. Small amounts of air may enter the veins and be carried to the lung without causing significant disturbance. If the amount of air is large, however, the right side of the heart and the pulmonary arteries become occluded by foam, and death results from acute circulatory failure. As a result of penetrating injuries of the lungs, air may be carried to the left side of the heart and thence to the systemic circulation, where it causes death as the result of cerebral or coronary air embolism.[31] The autopsy diagnosis of fatal cardiac air embolism can be substantiated by a postmortem x-ray film or opening the heart under water.

Injuries caused by changes in atmospheric pressure

The biologic consequences of changes in atmospheric pressure are dependent on two physical properties of gases:

1. The volume of gas contained in an elastic membrane increases in size as the surrounding barometric pressure is reduced.
2. The solubility of a gas in a liquid solvent (such as blood) is proportional to the partial pressure of that gas in the ambient atmosphere.

These two characteristics of gases in general are responsible for the signs and symptoms created by "trapped" and "evolved" gases that are observed with sudden changes in barometric pressure.

Gases may be trapped in body cavities that are usually in free communication with the ambient atmosphere if ready passage of air into and out of the cavity is blocked. Thus, in the presence of acute upper respiratory tract inflammation with resultant edema and swelling of the mucous membrane, the sinus orifices and eustachian tubes may be blocked or narrowed so that equalization of pressures within the paranasal air sinuses or middle ear cavities and the outside atmosphere is delayed or prevented. The clinical consequences may be severe.

Sufficient decrease in atmospheric pressure leads to expansion of gastric and intestinal gases with resultant abdominal distension. Expansion progresses until deflation occurs as a result of gaseous eructations or the passage of flatus or both.

Injuries associated with changes in atmospheric pressure may be seen in underwater use of a caisson, in high-altitude climbing or flight, or most commonly in diving with *s*elf-*c*ontained *u*nderwater *b*reathing *a*pparatus (scuba). The three characteristics of an episode of abnormal atmospheric pressure that determine its injurious effects on humans are as follows:

1. Direction and magnitude of change
2. Rate of change
3. Duration of change

Decreased atmospheric pressure

The human organism tolerates an increase in atmospheric pressure better than a decrease of equal magnitude. Thus the atmospheric pressure of the human environment can be tripled without harm, and yet a lowering of the pressure by as little as 50% incident to elevation to an altitude of 20,000 feet results in severe systemic hypoxia and may cause death.

Rapid accentuation of hypoxia as a result of diminished barometric pressure is followed by strong peripheral vasoconstriction with consequent shifting of a large portion of the blood volume to the pulmonary circuit. This hemodynamic disturbance leads to pulmonary arterial hypertension associated with anoxic damage to pulmonary capillary endothelium and alveolar pneumocytes. The result of the combined action of these two responses to the abnormal physical environment is the so-called high-altitude pulmonary edema and high-altitude cerebral edema.[32,33] The pulmonary edema fluid is characterized by high molecular weight proteins, erythrocytes, and alveolar macrophages without significant neutrophil accumulation and is a result of loss of integrity of the endothelial-epithelial barrier with a transient leak in the pulmonary circulation.[34]

Acute high-altitude pulmonary edema usually occurs between 3 and 48 hours after exposure to altitudes above 3000 meters, especially if severe physical exertion has taken place in the unaccustomed environment. This illness poses a particular hazard to those who climb or ski at high altitudes. Therefore most instances occur in athletic young adults who are otherwise healthy. The condition is also a threat to those who live and work permanently at high altitudes, especially if they are faced with repeated reentry into the hypoxic environment after trips to lower altitudes. Fatalities can be indistinguishable clinically from fulminant pneumonia. At autopsy the lungs are congested and have interstitial and alveolar edema. Hyaline membranes may be present.[35]

In addition to decreased barometric pressure and decreased partial oxygen pressure encountered at high altitudes, there is often a simultaneous exposure to decreased environmental temperature and increased ultraviolet irradiation. A further source of physiologic stress is the decreasing humidity of air at high altitudes. This factor in concert with the hyperventilation that accompanies even moderate physical exertion can lead to rapid dehydration with resultant extreme thirst. The combination of hyperventilation and profuse diaphoresis can bring about a moderate degree of hypokalemic alkalosis. These multiple physical and biochemical assaults may give rise to acute mountain sickness, a syndrome characterized by headache, palpitations, nausea, anorexia, weakness, and insomnia.

Exposure to increasing altitudes activates various adaptive mechanisms that permit the body to tolerate the changes. The types and degrees of adaptation depend on many factors, including duration of exposure, level of physical activity, age, and general physical condition. Persons with limited cardiorespiratory reserve may experience dyspnea, nausea, and insomnia at altitudes as low as 1500 meters above sea level.

Increased atmospheric pressure

Injuries associated with increased atmospheric pressure usually occur during the return from elevated to normal barometric pressure. The rate at which the atmospheric pressure changes—more particularly, the rate at which it is decreased—is an exceedingly important factor in injury production. Unless barometric pressure is lowered slowly to normal, decompression sickness (also known as dysbarism, caisson disease, the bends, the staggers, or the chokes) may occur. A very rapid change from normal to subnormal pressure, as may occur during rapid ascent in supersonic aircraft, may also cause decompression sickness.

An increase in atmospheric pressure results in a net flow of nitrogen, which makes up four fifths of the inspired air, from the alveoli through the blood in which the gas dissolves, to tissue. When the return to normal pressure is slow, the loss of gas from tissue is analogous to gas uptake. However, if the return to normal pressure is rapid, gas bubbles form in tissue and blood because nitrogen evolves faster than it can be transported to the lungs and expired.[36]

Some degree of microscopic bubble formation probably occurs whenever the tissue partial pressure of nitrogen even moderately exceeds that in the surrounding atmosphere. However, symptom-producing bubbles (decompression sickness) will not occur until the partial pressure of nitrogen is more than twice that of the surrounding atmosphere.[37] (At the ocean's surface a diver and his viscera are under a pressure of 1 atmosphere [760 mm Hg], and 1 additional atmosphere of pressure is added for each 33 feet he descends.[38]

The nature and severity of decompression sickness are determined by the rate and location of nitrogen release. Disability and death may supervene within minutes or hours after decompression. Pulmonary and central nervous system involvement dominate in the causation of sudden fatalities. Subacute or chronic effects of decompression are characterized by lower limb, bladder, and rectal paralysis from demyelination of the dorsal and lateral columns of the inferior thoracic spinal cord rather than the upper cord or brain.[39] In divers and tunnelers with a history of the bends and persistent joint symptoms, foci of aseptic necrosis have usually developed in bones. Venous gas embolism with resultant vascular obstruction is the most likely basis for the localized areas of osseous destruction. Because of the solubility of nitrogen in fat, obesity predisposes to the development of decompression sickness.[40]

With the acute decompression seen in rapid ascent of a scuba diver who fails to exhale, mediastinal interstitial emphysema, subcutaneous emphysema, pneumothorax, and *arterial* air embolism may follow rupture of distended pulmonary alveoli from expanding intrapulmonary air. The air embolism is the most serious consequence because of the possibility of cerebrovascular involvement with the production of such phenomena as hemiplegia, confusion, blindness, unconsciousness, and death.[41] Inasmuch as the incident occurs in an aquatic environment, the victim may drown. It is of interest that this series of catastrophic events can occur during rapid ascent in water from a depth of only 10 feet.

Rapid descent in an aircraft or rapid ascent during a scuba dive can lead to sinus barotrauma, so-called aerosinusitis and aero–otitis media with rupture of the tympanum. As the air in the intracranial spaces expands during ascent (1 volume of air at sea level becomes 2 volumes at 18,000 feet and 4 volumes at 33,000 feet), it passes easily through the natural ostia of the sinuses to equilibrate with the ambient barometic pressure. During *descent,* air must enter the sinuses through the ostia to equalize the intrasinus pressure with the *increasing* atmospheric tension. When sinus ostia and nasal mucosa are normal, the air exchange occurs efficiently and promptly. (Similar dynamic changes occur in all the hollow body structures that communicate with the exterior.)

However, if a sinus ostium is obstructed by tenacious mucus (a "mucus plug"), edematous mucosa, or a bony structural deformity, the defect may act as a cork during descent, effectively occluding the orifice, which is now under negative pressure. The negative pressure in the sealed-off sinus cavity is resolved by the sinus's filling with fluid transudate or blood. Indeed, if the pressure changes are especially rapid or severe, the mucous membrane may be stripped from the sinus wall with formation of a hematoma. The frontal sinus is most vulnerable to barotrauma because of the long, narrow bony nasofrontal defect with its dependent position on the floor of the sinus and the lack of accessory ostia.[42]

Although most cases of sinus barotrauma occur with compression (rapid descent in an aircraft or in diving), a considerable pressure disequilibrium can occur during *ascent* if the same type of interference exists with the passage of air *out* of the sinus.[43]

Explosions

The term *blast injury* designates the disruptive effects of the sudden changes in pressure that result from an explosion. If the force of the explosion is transmitted through the air, the term *air blast* is employed; if through water, *immersion blast,* and if through more or less rigid structures, *solid blast.*[44]

The shock wave of an air blast is a sound wave of very high pressure that emanates radially from an explosive source at the speed of sound. The air pressure is highest in the region of the explosion and falls rapidly, almost exponentially, as the distance from the blast increases. The amount of injury inflicted depends on the peak pressure and to a lesser degree on the duration of the shock wave.[45] In the case of an air blast the compression tends to be unilateral, and its principal effect is on the side of the body that faces the explosion. Here, much of the energy is reflected, but at least part is transmitted through the tissues and strikes the subjacent organs during the succeeding millisecond or less. Solid organs are virtually incompressible and consequently undergo little or no internal displacement. They vibrate as a whole and so escape serious injury. However, organs that contain air or gas respond differently because they *are* compressible and contain gas-liquid interfaces. Compression generates displacement, and whenever tissues of different density exist side by side, the amount of displacement varies from point to point, causing distention and tearing. An air blast also gives rise to surface phenomena such as epithelial shredding. Lesions tend to be most severe at tissue junctions. When loose, poorly supported tissues attached to dense unyielding tissues are displaced beyond their elastic limits, they are lacerated or otherwise damaged. Differences in fixation, cohesion, compressibility, and inertia on the part of the various components of the body result in nonuniform response to the displacing force and in widespread disruptive change. Thus the walls or compartments of hollow viscera are particularly susceptible to blast injury.

The lungs are especially vulnerable to blast injury. Alveolar septa are torn, permitting neighboring alveoli to coalesce, with ensuing emphysema. Alveolar parenchyma shears away from vascular structures, and alveolar epithelium is shredded. At the same time, bronchiolar epithelium is stripped from its basement membrane. These lesions lead to destruction of the fluid-air barrier. Blood and edema fluid escape into the alveoli, and air is forced into pulmonary vessels as a result of the formation of alveolar-venous fistulas. Cerebral air embolism attributable to the aspiration of air by disrupted pulmonary veins may be an important component of such an injury. Visible damage ranges from petechiae to massive hemorrhages and extensive areas of hemorrhagic edema. The hemorrhages tend to be more severe in the pulmonary parenchyma underlying the intercostal spaces, with the lung tissue beneath the protecting ribs being comparatively only slightly damaged. At autopsy, the pleural surfaces show alternating light and dark bands, the former corresponding to the ribs ("rib markings") and the latter to the intercostal spaces. Diffuse injuries of both the thoracic and the abdominal viscera may occur and may be sustained with little or no external evidence of trauma. Hemorrhage may occur in the gastric wall and elsewhere. The greater the degree of distention of the viscus when the shock waves strike, the more severe the injury.[46]

Since a blast wave is a sound wave of high intensity, it is obvious that the ear, built specifically for the reception of sound, is likely to be damaged by explosions. The pressure pulse approaching the human ear is concentrated as it passes down the external auditory canal so that the pressure on the tympanic membrane is approximately 20% higher than that just outside the ear. Injuries to the ears range from hyperemia and punctate bruising of the intact tympanic membrane to laceration of the membrane and damage to the cochlea. Membrane laceration usually occurs when the pressure rises to 15 psi and typically is associated with bleeding into the middle ear.[47]

In the case of an immersion blast, a shock wave is propagated at approximately the speed of sound in water (1450 m/second). Since water is much less compressible than air, corresponding pressures are much higher in a water shock wave than in those produced in air. Injury can occur from the shock wave or from the subsidiary pulse when the shock wave is reflected, for example, from the surface or from the bottom. The sequel of the pressure pulse injury is hemorrhage and laceration of air-containing organs. Lung damage of the type already described under air blast is a constant feature in deaths. Small perforations of the gut, especially of the cecum, may occur, and there may be subperitoneal contusions.[45]

In the case of solid blast, the disruptive force of the explosion is transmitted to the body through those parts that are in contact with an agitated rigid structure, such as the deck of a ship or the wall of an air raid shelter. Most solid blast injuries involve fractures of the lower extremities with considerable soft-tissue damage.[48]

One should bear in mind that proximity to either air or immersion blast may result in virtual destruction of the body by the extreme air or water turbulence induced by the blast. Flying missiles may add an infinite variety of wounds to those induced by turbulence and compression. These lesions are called *secondary blast* injuries; they result from missiles energized by blast pressure and winds and are distinguished from the "primary blast" injuries caused by the blast per se. In civilian explosions, including terrorist bombings, most deaths are caused by injuries from high-velocity fragments and falling debris (secondary blast injuries).[49]

Blast injuries sustained incident to atomic bomb explosion may be complicated by exposure to excessive heat and ionizing radiation. The cutaneous burns incurred in this manner are often unique by reason of the extremely high intensity and short duration of the hyperthermic episode. The injurious effects of ionizing radiation frequently require weeks to years for the development of signs and symptoms.

Injuries caused by sound waves

Noise

Permanent hearing loss resulting from excessive exposure to noise has long been recognized as an occupational hazard in industry. Such hearing defects develop with chronic exposure when the "work noise" exceeds the critical level of 80 to 90 decibels (dB).[50] It is less well known that many noise levels encountered in the community exceed standards found injurious in industry. For example, animals exposed to live rock music for 2½ hours in a discotheque had loss of sensory cells in the organ of Corti. The average sound pressure level measured in the discotheque was 107 dB.[51]

Chemical and structural changes in the spiral ganglion and hair cells have been demonstrated during exposure to sound, and exposure to sound levels of the degree produced by home food blenders causes noticeable changes in the hair cells, which characteristically show cytoplasmic vacuolization and swelling with compression of their nuclei and changes in their shape.[52]

In human autopsy studies no clear histologic picture has been identified in which morbid anatomic changes can be correlated with clinical hearing loss. Postmortem changes in the organ of Corti are the rule and complicate attempts to find such relationships.

Studies of persons subjected to high noise levels have revealed that long-term exposure to acoustic insult first affects hearing in the range between 3000 and 6000 hertz (Hz, cycles per second), whereas hearing for frequencies below 3000 Hz and above 8000 Hz remains essentially normal for long periods of time. High-frequency receptors deteriorate with age, and the burden of extra noise increases the wear.[53]

Ultrasound

Ultrasonic vibrations are those above limits of hearing of the human ear. Although ultrasound can be generated at frequencies exceeding 1000 megahertz (MHz), in current medical practice the useful range is generally from 900 kilohertz (kHz) to 6 MHz. The medical literature has been almost unanimous in suggesting that there is little or no danger associated with diagnostic or therapeutic exposure of current levels.[54] Reports that diagnostic levels of ultrasound produced chromosomal damage in vitro and retarded rapidly growing tissue have not been confirmed in human cells.[55]

High-frequency ultrasound producing intensities many times that used in diagnostic or therapeutic procedures may cause biologic changes by increasing tissue temperature or producing tissue microcavitation. Wittenzellner[56] carried out self-experiments by irradiating both thighs in the frequency range of 20 to 800 kHz. Postirradiation changes in the skin receiving 800 kHz for 25 minutes included an acute inflammatory infiltrate and intraepidermal vesicles. Twenty-five years later the irradiated skin showed no significant signs.

Recently, shock waves have been employed as a treatment for renal calculus disease. These generated shock waves differ from ultrasound in having a positive-pressure front of multiple frequencies with a steep onset rather than a sinusoid waveform.[57] Although theoretically designed to be propagated through the body without energy loss or damage to body tissue, morphologic and functional renal changes attributed to kidney contusion resulting in edema and extravasion of urine and blood into the interstitial, subcapsular, and perirenal spaces have been described.[58]

Injuries from heat and cold

Despite humans' ability to survive wide variations in environmental temperature, internal temperature must be maintained within a narrow range to avoid thermal injury. Cellular injury or death occurs if tissue temperature is maintained at a level more than 5° C above or more than 15° C below that which is normal for the blood. The severity of injury caused at any given temperature tends to be proportional to the duration of the hypothermal or hyperthermal episode. The somatic function of circulation is more susceptible to irreversible disturbance by dysthermia than are the individual cells of the body, and hence somatic death may result from a systemic alteration in temperature that would not cause cellular death if it were localized.

The skin is the principal site of heat loss during exposure to a cold environment or of heat gain during exposure to a hot environment. The respiratory membranes are rarely injured by heat or cold—and then only when the alteration of air temperature is so extreme that the skin is burned or frozen.[59,60]

Local hypothermia

Chilling of tissue retards the metabolic activity of the cells and may cause irreversible cellular change attributable to intracellular ice formation. This is not to imply, however, that hypothermal injury is dependent on the occurrence of congelation. The most important injurious effects of chilling are alterations in the walls and contents of the small blood vessels. A brief period of severe tissue hypothermia or a protracted period of mild tissue hypothermia may injure capillary endothelium sufficiently to cause transudation of fluid and edema. Superficially, such edema may lead to extensive vesication. The threshold for edema formation incident to chilling varies greatly among individuals.

If chilling is rapid and severe, the tissue may be rendered ischemic so quickly that evidence of vascular injury does not become apparent until the temperature rises and circulation is reestablished. Intense hyperemia is usually the immediate response to restitution of circulation after hypothermia. The hyperemia is followed by edema as soon as sufficient time has elapsed for plasma to diffuse through the cells of the injured vessels.

During a protracted episode of nonfreezing hypothermia such as that causing immersion or trench foot or after a brief episode of freezing hypothermia such as that causing frostbite, the local vascular injury may be so severe that the capillaries and even the larger vessels become plugged by tightly packed masses of erythrocytes. The nature and severity of the subsequent changes are determined by the extent and permanence of the ensuing ischemia. If the vascular occlusion is extensive, complete infarction in the form of moist or dry gangrene takes place. If the necrotic tissue becomes moist and dark colored, one can infer that infarction was preceded or accompanied by some degree of vascular patency. If the necrotis tissue becomes dry and mummified, one can infer that vascular occlusion was complete from the beginning.

Most if not all of the residual injury from protracted nonfreezing hypothermia can be attributed to the ischemia that results from the vascular occlusion. Atrophic and degenerative changes are seen in the epidermis, sweat glands, nerves, subcutaneous fat, and skeletal muscle, with proliferation of fibrous connective tissue in all situations.

Systemic hypothermia

If the area exposed to cold is relatively small, a severe local injury may be sustained without significant lowering of the blood temperature. If the area of exposure is large, the body temperature may be lowered sufficiently to cause death from circulatory failure even though no local injury has been sustained. Circulation fails when the temperature of the blood is reduced to approximately 20° C. Immersion in cold water or exposure to a rapidly moving current of cold air may lower the body temperature to a fatal level in a remarkably short time. However, prolonged exposure to cool temperatures may also result in hypothermia, particularly in susceptible elderly persons with impaired homeostatic reactions or with chronic disease. The full extent of the problem of hypothermia in the elderly is not recognized because of the limited awareness of the hazard of mildly cold temperatures to the elderly and the focus on the medical complications of the hospitalized victim of the exposure.[61] There are no histologic or anatomic changes that can be regarded as pathognomonic of death from systemic hypothermia. However, autopsy examinations of some persons who have died after accidental hypothermia have demonstrated widespread thromboses and visceral infarction along with acute, necrotizing pancreatitis (Fig. 5-25).

Circulatory stasis and ischemia are probably responsible for the vascular phenomena and for the acute pancreatitis that has been observed in experimental and clinical situations. In accidental hypothermia the pancreatitis usually occurs when exposure to cold is prolonged, with coma preceding death.[62,63]

Local hyperthermia

Humans are far more susceptible to injury from an increase in tissue temperature than from a corresponding decrease.

Cutaneous burns. An elevation of tissue temperature by even a few degrees above that which is normal for the blood may be injurious. At any given temperature the nature and extent of the resulting injury are determined by the duration of the hyperthermal episode. During episodes of low intensity (40° to 45° C), injury is the result of accelerated metabolism of the hyperthermal tissue, and ordinarily many hours are required before irreversible changes have occurred. The higher the temperature, the shorter is the time required to cause cell death.[64,65] Transepidermal necrosis occurs if the epidermal temperature is brought to and maintained at 70° C or higher for a second or less, whereas transepidermal temperature elevation to 50° C for periods as long as 10 minutes may or may not destroy the epidermis.

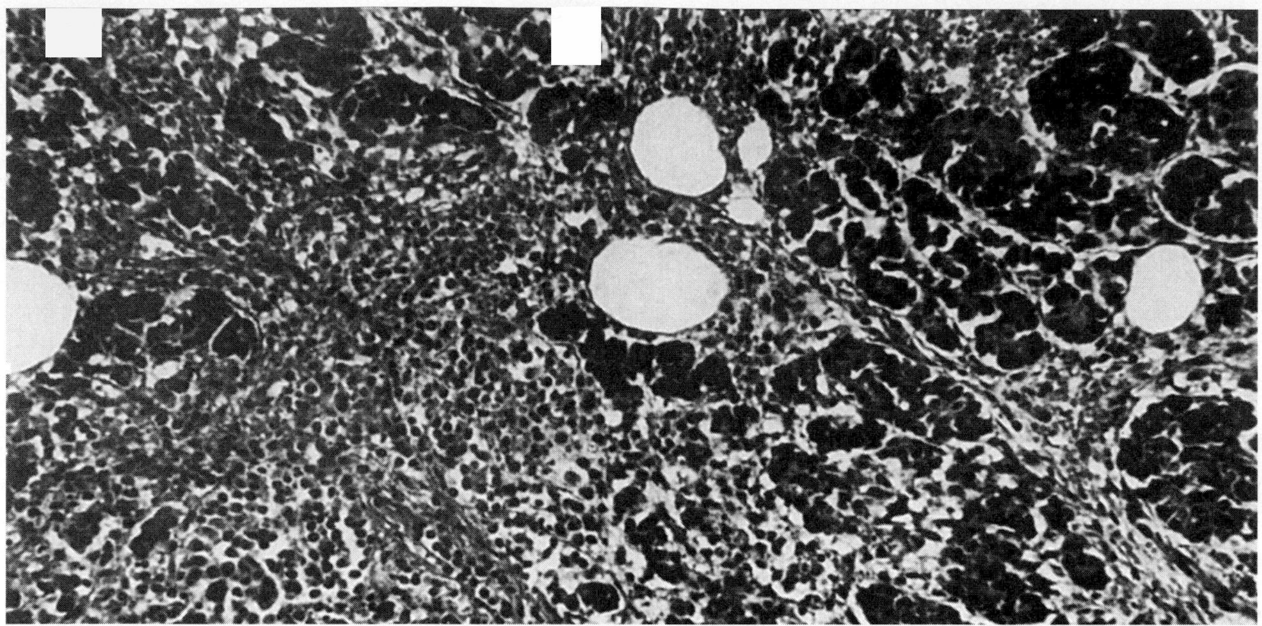

Fig. 5-25 Pancreas from 85-year-old man who died approximately 24 hours after being found in a snowbank and who suffered from exposure. Parenchyma is abundantly infiltrated with acute inflammatory cells.

The earliest evidence of hyperthermal injury is functional rather than structural. Capillaries and small blood vessels become dilated as the tissue temperature is raised, the permeability of the capillary walls is increased, and the fluid components of the blood leave the vessel and enter the interstitial spaces, with resulting edema. When thermal edema occurs in the superficial portion of the skin, the fluid may collect beneath the epidermis, with resulting vesiculation.

The earliest cytologic evidence of hyperthermal injury is a redistribution of the fluid and solid components of the nuclei, followed by nuclear swelling attributable to the imbibition of fluid, rupture of the nuclear membranes, and finally pyknosis. Since the rise in tissue temperature incident to exposure of the surface of the skin to excessive heat is greatest at the surface and becomes progressively less as the distance from the surface is increased, it is apparent that any given burn will include a wide range of thermal effects. The cytoplasm of thermally injured cells becomes at first granular and later homogeneously coagulated. The collagen tends to lose its fibrillar character and to take on the appearance of a more or less homogeneous gel. The pH of the thermally denatured cells falls, as indicated by their increased affinity for basic stains.

Cutaneous burns may be designated as either first, second, or third degree or now more commonly as partial thickness or full thickness. Partial-thickness burns result in no permanent damage to the dermis and include both first- and second-degree burns from the older classification (Figs. 5-26 and 5-27). If vesication occurs with partial-thickness burns, regeneration of epithelium is generally rapid and is derived in part from the margin of the burned area and in part from the underlying hair follicles. Full-thickness burns are those in which there has been sufficient damage to the dermis to interfere with epithelial regeneration.

The irreversibly injured dermis must be disposed of before a new layer of epithelium can be regenerated. The organization and repair of the damaged dermis are accomplished by growth of new fibrous connective tissue and often result in extensive scar formation.

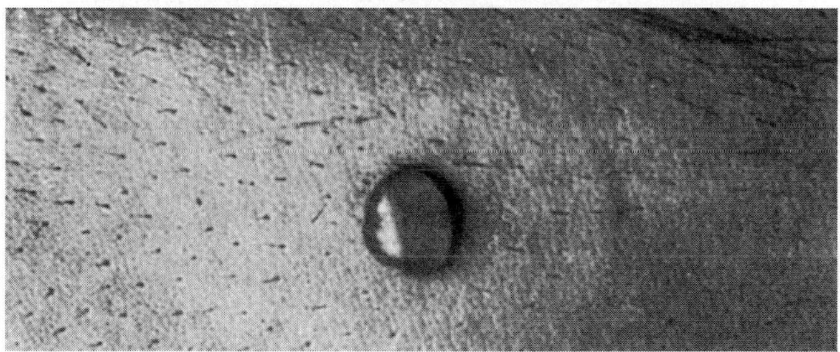

Fig. 5-26 Experimentally produced partial-thickness (second-degree) burn of human skin caused by maintaining surface temperature at 45°C for 3 hours. There is transepidermal necrosis with vesication. Irreversible dermal injury was minimal, and epidermal regeneration was complete in 10 days.

The flash burn resulting from exposure to the tremendous caloric flux of the first 0.6 second of the fireball of the atomic bomb explosion differs from the ordinary relatively low temperature burn in several respects.[66,67] Despite carbonization of the epidermis and subjacent dermis, the zone of injury may be shallow and sharply demarcated.

Vascular reaction with hyperemia and edema is inevitable if the tissue hyperthermia has been sufficient to be injurious, and this reaction frequently occurs before the duration or the intensity of the exposure has been great enough to cause other perceptible evidence of injury.

In the case of exposure to intense heat, the superficial vessels may become so rapidly fixed in a state of contraction that neither edema nor hyperemia is visible from the surface. In such an event, the reactive vascular changes will occur at a lower level but with no less severity. One of the most important systemic effects of extensive cutaneous burning is sec-

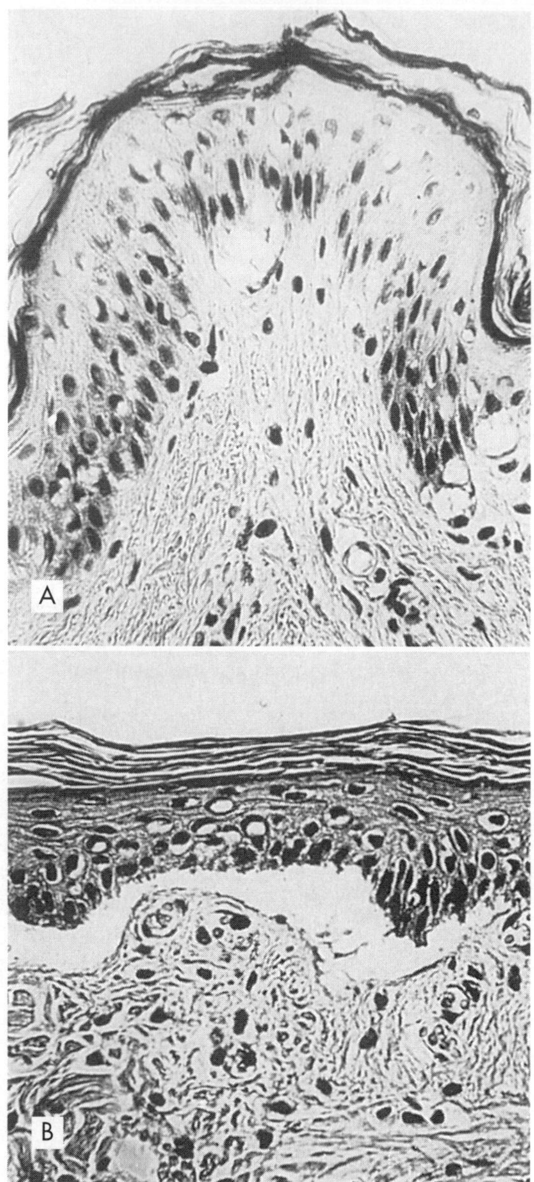

Fig. 5-27 Partial-thickness cutaneous burns. **A,** Mild burn (first degree). Although epidermis is damaged, it is not completely destroyed. Many nuclei are swollen and show eccentric displacement of chromatin. Minute vesicles have formed at junction of dermis and epidermis. **B,** More severe burn (second degree). Vesication is complete. Entire thickness of epidermis is necrotic and detached from relatively uninjured dermis.

ondary shock brought on by hemoconcentration from loss of plasma at the site of injury.

Thermally denatured tissue elicits an aseptic inflammatory reaction, represents a foreign body, and must undergo lysis and organization or be sloughed off as a sequestrum. Before organization or sequestration, it provides a favorable medium for bacterial growth and predisposes the adjacent tissue to infection.

The use of topical antibacterial agents in current burn therapy show bacterial growth and usually prevent infection by the common bacteria that colonize burn wounds. However, the later appearance of resistant microorganisms, bacterial, fungal, and viral, often causes invasive infection and systemic sepsis, which combined remain the leading immediate cause of death among hospitalized burn patients.[68]

Systemic disturbances caused by cutaneous burns. Burning of the surface of the body may result in a wide variety of secondary disturbances. Such an injury may precipitate the development of primary or neurogenic shock with rapid peripheral circulatory collapse leading to syncope or death. The progressive loss of plasma from the burned surface or into the damaged tissue beneath it may result in hemoconcentration and secondary shock.

Patients with third-degree burns experience an average water loss of 0.35 ml/cm^2 of burned area per day during the first week.[69] It is a reasonable inference that the hemoconcentration, low blood pressure, and systemic anoxia of secondary shock predispose not only to phlebothrombosis, particularly in immobilized limbs, but also to the occurrence of the degenerative changes so commonly observed in the kidneys, liver, and adrenal glands of burned persons.

Although the precise cause of the ulcers that sometimes develop in the proximal portion of the small intestine of severely burned persons is not known, local mesenteric thrombosis and mucosal infarction would appear to constitute a plausible explanation.

Erythrocytes break down rapidly in vitro at temperatures over 50° C and in vivo at temperatures over 42.5° C, and intravascular hemolysis usually takes place if the hyperthermal episode has been of sufficient intensity or duration to destroy the epidermis. Free plasma hemoglobin is excreted rapidly by the kidneys, where it may be precipitated in the lower segments of the nephrons to form obstructive casts similar to those formed as a result of a mismatched transfusion.

The combined effects of these pigmented casts and the irreversible tubular damage caused by prolonged shock result in the renal failure so often associated with severe burns.

Since most cutaneous burns are associated with fire, the possibility of inhalation injury must be considered in most burn victims. Many homes and other buildings are built and furnished with synthetic materials that give off copious smoke and toxic gases when burned. In addition to carbon monoxide, victims of cutaneous burns may be exposed to such toxic gases as cyanide, hydrogen chloride, and acrolein. Upper airway occlusion may result from thermal damage or edema secondary to burns from soluble toxic gases. Lower airway obstruction may occur as the result of sloughing of mucosa, bronchospasm, or peribronchial edema. At the alveolar level, inactivation of surfactant with subsequent atelectasis and an increase in pulmonary capillary permeability further impair ventilation-perfusion abilities.[70,71]

Systemic hyperthermia

The temperature of the body may be raised to an injurious level either by the inflow of heat from without or by the body's failure to eliminate the heat developed by metabolic processes. A general rise in the temperature of the circulating blood to a level higher than 42.5° C leads to profound functional disturbances, including the following:

1. Generalized vasodilatation with resulting reduction in effective blood volume as a consequence of the disparity between the newly expanded capacity of the circulatory apparatus and the unchanged quantity of the fluid (blood) available to fill it
2. Rapid pulse and dilatation of the heart with impairment of cardiac efficiency
3. Stimulation of the respiratory centers, manifested first by tachypnea, later by irregularity, and finally by suspension of respiratory activity

It is difficult to determine which of these several physiologic effects of systemic hyperthermia may contribute most to somatic deterioration and death. It is of interest in this connection that a heart-lung preparation fails when the temperature of the perfusate reaches approximately 42.5° C.

Heatstroke is the result of uncontrolled overproduction of body heat or impairment of the body's ability to lose heat; it occurs most frequently in susceptible persons exposed to unusually hot conditions. Heat is dissipated principally by evaporative cooling through sweating and by cutaneous vasodilatation with increased cardiac output. The more labile thermoregulatory mechanism of small children and, particularly, the elderly renders them vulnerable to heatstroke; heatstroke rates are 10 to 12 times higher in persons older than 65 years than in younger adults. Other factors that predispose persons to heatstroke include alcoholism, any skin disease or injury that impairs or prevents sweating, cardiovascular disease, general debility, coexistence of a febrile disorder, dehydration, obesity, anticholinergic drugs, and some medications that are used to treat psychiatric disorders (such as chlorpromazine, fluphenazine, promazine, and haloperidol). Environmental risk factors include hot temperature, high humidity, and the entire complex of living conditions in poorly insulated urban housing, especially the multistory buildings of slums.[72]

Heatstroke also can occur in healthy persons who exert themselves with such intensity that the heat produced by skeletal muscles cannot be dissipated quickly enough to cool the body. This exertional heatstroke occurs in unacclimated athletes, such as football players during spring training, or in military recruits who undergo basic training in summer. Athletes wearing heavy equipment or impervious plastic sweatsuits increase their risk. Autopsy findings in heatstroke deaths are nonspecific and are governed by the survival interval, treatment, and previous condition of the victim.

Delayed systemic disturbances from systemic hyperthermia include widely distributed degenerative changes in the parenchymatous viscera and particularly in the brain.[73]

Electrical injury

Electrical injury does not occur unless some part of the body completes the circuit between two conductors. An electrician supported by an insulated boom may safely handle a high-tension conductor because he is isolated from the ground.

The path of a current through the body tends to follow the most direct route between the contact points. The current may cause injury or death by altering the function of a vital organ (for example, throwing the heart into ventricular fibrillation or paralyzing the respiratory center), by stimulating strong (and occasionally tetanic) muscular contractions, or by creating large quantities of heat (electrothermal effect).

When conditions (contacts) are appropriate for the flow of current through the body (or tissues), the occurrence and nature of the harmful effects created by its passage depend on the following:

1. The kind of current (direct or alternating)
2. The amount of current (amperage)
3. The electromotive force (voltage)
4. The amount of resistance offered by the tissues in the path of the current
5. The actual path of the current between the sites of contact
6. The duration of current flow
7. The surface area of contact

An alternating current is more effective in the production of physiologic disturbances than a direct current is, and some alternating frequencies are more disturbing than others. The 60-cycle alternating current commonly available for domestic and industrial use lies in the frequency range that is particularly disturbing to the respiratory centers of the brain and to the heart, where it can induce fibrillation by interacting with the vulnerable phase of the cardiac cycle. Increasing the duration of current flow increases the risk of disrupting the vulnerable phase. One of the major dangers of alternating current is its tetanizing effect, so that a person becomes "locked" to the contact until the circuit is broken. Since the amount of current necessary to cause tetany may be less than that necessary to cause fibrillation, he may succumb to a current that would otherwise not be lethal.

The amount of current that will flow through the body when it becomes part of a circuit is determined by the formula $C = V/R$, in which C is the current in amperes, V is potential in volts, and R is the resistance in ohms with which the body opposes the flow of the current. Thus the higher the voltage or the lower the resistance, the greater the flow of current. The usual currents available for domestic use have a fixed potential of either 110 volts or 220 volts. Therefore the resistance R is the major variable in determining the flow of current in an electrical accident in the home. The resistance of the human body may be reduced to less than 40 ohms under particularly favorable conditions (large areas of electrode contact against a moist skin surface). Since a 60-cycle alternating current as small as 100 milliamperes, applied at the body surface and passing through the trunk, can be sufficient to cause ventricular fibrillation, household currents with a potential of 110 volts greatly exceed the threshold for fatal electrocution.

Currents applied to the body surface tend to disperse over multiple pathways as they pass through the trunk. Therefore the amount of current passing through the heart will be considerably less than the amount of current on the surface of the body. The result is that currents far lower than 100 milliamperes, currents in the microampere range, can cause fibrillation if directly applied at the heart. Persons susceptible to such "microshocks" are those with indwelling catheters, particularly cardiac catheters hooked to monitors where there is a potential of leakage of current along the catheter.[74,75]

That the path taken by the current is of critical importance in determining whether a fatal shock will occur is indicated by the fact that, in electroshock therapy, transcranial current flow as great as 1 ampere may be survived without injury.

In general, the severity of the disturbance caused by the flow of a given amount of current between similar external contacts is proportional to the duration of flow. Certainly the generation of heat bears a linear relationship to time. Physiologic disturbances that are evanescent after a momentary shock may be rendered irreversible by a longer period of electrical exposure.

Electrical burns

The amount and place of heat formation incident to the flow of a given amount of electricity through the body are determined by the resistance that the tissue offers to the current. Most of the resistance offered by the human body to an electrical current is that of the skin and the interface between skin and external conductor. Thus electrothermal burns are ordinarily limited to the skin and the immediately subjacent tissue.

Thin skin is less resistant to the flow of electricity than thick skin is, and moist skin offers less resistance than dry skin does. Heavily callused dry skin may provide a resistance-protection of several hundred thousand ohms. Because of this fact, persons with callused hands often handle with impunity live wires that would be exceedingly dangerous if brought into contact with a less-resistant portion of the body surface.

If the contact between the skin and an external conductor is large, the generation of heat in terms of calories per square centimeter of surface per second may be too low to produce a burn, and yet the amperage may be more than enough to paralyze respiration or circulation. On the other hand, if the skin contact is a small one such as may occur by touching the end of a live wire, the amount of heat generated in a few cubic millimeters of epidermis may be sufficient to produce a burn even though the total amperage has been insufficient to cause a significant degree of physiologic disturbance. The significance of the surface area of contact is best exemplified by what is observed in low-voltage incidents. A child sucking on a live cord may sustain deep labial burns without suffering systemic effects because contact is limited to the mouth, whereas a person lying in a bathtub who touches an ungrounded electrical element of identical voltage may well be killed immediately without the production of any localized injuries.

In a study of 108 electrocutions by low voltage (less than 1000 volts), electrical burns were absent in over 40% of the cases.[76] In the absence of electrical burns the determination of a fatal electrical shock may depend on the circumstances of the death and an "autopsy" of the electrical source.

Typical low-voltage cutaneous electrical burns are small, circumscribed, indurated lesions that have a central, depressed, gray or black focus of charring surrounded by a zone of grayish white discoloration (Fig. 5-28). The latter change represents coagulation necrosis of the skin and often is surrounded by a narrow areola of erythema. Microscopically there is an abrupt transition from normal to burned skin. The burn commonly shows microvesicles in the epidermis, separation of the lower epidermis, and transcutaneous coagulation extending into the dermis. Epidermal nuclei are pyknotic, elongated, and aligned in a parallel or palisading fashion, often referred to as "nuclear streaming" (Fig. 5-29). High-voltage burns usually have large areas of contact and generate sufficient heat to produce extensive, deep charring that may amputate extremities (Fig. 5-30). Ignition of clothing is a frequent concomitant of contact with high-voltage electrical current and results in the superimposition of ordinary burning on electrical injury.

Arcing of the current may produce pitlike defects on the surface of hair or epidermis that are rarely, if ever, produced by other forms of heat. Metallic constituents of the external conductor may be deposited in or on the surface of an electrical burn, and their presence may help to establish the kind of electrode with which the skin was in contact. In the case of alternating current, such metallic deposits may be present at both sites of contact. With direct current the deposits will occur only at the site of contact with the negative electrode.

In persons who survive high-voltage electrical injury, the size of the primary burn does not change, but a surrounding zone of secondary ischemic necrosis may enlarge progressively in the days or weeks after the incident. Such ischemic progression results primarily from thrombosis of arterioles and arteries whose intima was damaged when they served as con-

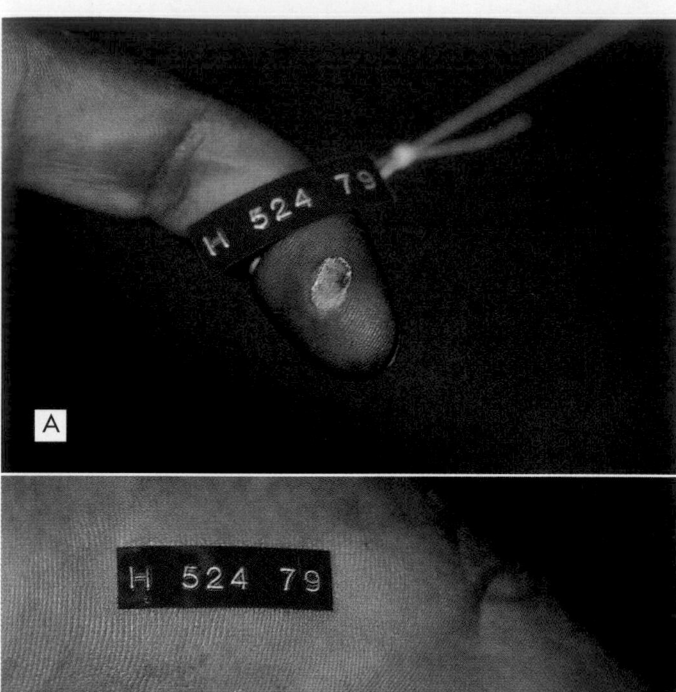

Fig. 5-28 Typical low voltage electrical burns. **A,** Entrance at left index finger. **B,** Exit at sole of right foot.

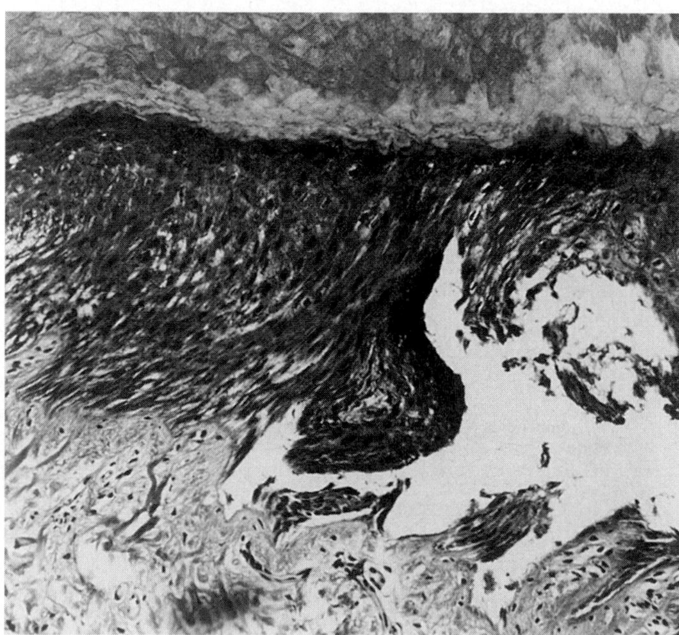

Fig. 5-29 Low-voltage electrical burn of hand. Epidermal separation *(right)* and nuclear streaming *(left)*.

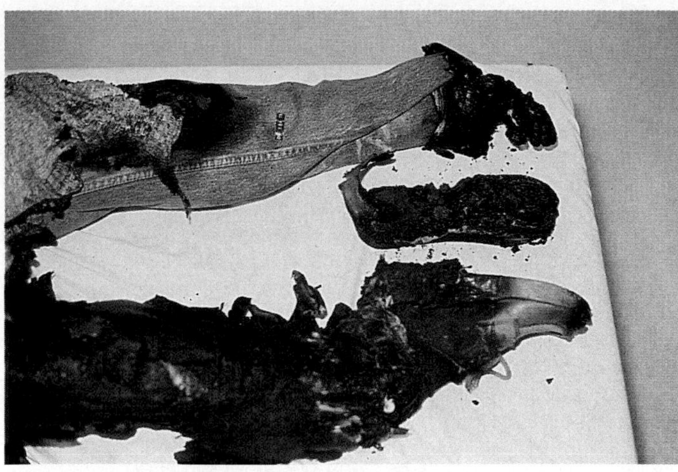

Fig. 5-30 High-voltage electrical burns of lower extremities in young woman who came into contact with downed 13,000-volt power line. There is extensive charring, with partial amputation of left foot and heat fractures of right tibia and fibula. Shoes and clothing were ignited, with superimposed thermal trauma.

duits for the transmission of electricity. These arterial sequelae may necessitate repeated débridement or amputations before the circulatory state is stabilized.

Electrothermal injuries should not be confused with the burns caused by contact with an object that has been rendered hot by a short circuit. If a short circuit occurs through a metallic conductor, the flow of current through it may be so great that even with a potential of 110 volts its temperature is raised almost immediately to the melting point. Contact with such a superheated conductor will cause severe and instantaneous burning even though no electricity flows through the skin. When a current of 110 volts flows through the skin, the resistance is ordinarily so great that there is insufficient amperage for rapid elaboration of heat. Rarely does a current of 110 volts produce a large electrothermal injury of the skin unless the contact is maintained for a considerable period of time.

Apart from injuries caused by heat production and the explosive effects of currents of extremely high voltage, there are no tissue changes that can be regarded as consistently pathognomonic of electricity. Attention has already been directed to the facts that an electrical current flowing through the brainstem may cause death by inhibition of the respiratory centers and that electricity flowing through the heart may cause death by central circulatory failure. Victims of fatal accidental electrocution resulting from a transthoracic current pathway have spoken rationally and continued breathing up to 15 seconds after contact with the electrical circuit was broken. This is typical of ventricular fibrillation or asystole from any cause such as coronary arteriosclerosis. During this interval, they complained of such symptoms as "tightness" in the chest, difficulty in breathing, a sensation of "strangulation," and a feeling of the heart pounding fiercely against the chest wall.[77]

Whether death results from ventricular fibrillation or from respiratory paralysis is immaterial from the standpoint of the production of characteristic gross or microscopic alterations in the viscera. In neither instance are there internal organic lesions that indicate the cause or mechanism of death. In both circumstances, somatic death is likely to be preceded by a brief period of intense systemic anoxemia, which may lead to the occurrence of petechiae in the serous membranes and central nervous system.

Myoglobinuria of the type that occurs after muscle injury from crushing force or excessive exercise is occasionally encountered in survivors of electric shock. It is a consequence of tissue damage caused by heat generation and coagulation necrosis, both of which are functions of current intensity (amperage), duration and pathway of current flow, tissue resistance, and grounding of the victim.

The myoglobinuria is usually associated with renal tubular necrosis with resulting oliguria or even anuria. The extremely high voltage and amperage characteristics of lightning (see the following) render the survivor of a lightning stroke a likely candidate for this life-threatening, posttraumatic sequel.[78]

Lightning

When a bolt of lightning approaches the earth or a grounded conductor, it tends to break up into many paths of varying intensity. In such circumstances a person struck by lightning may become the conductor of a current so small that his injury is superficial and inconsequential or so large as to be fatal with or without extensive burning (Fig. 5-31). In some instances the current produces an arborescent cutaneous hyperemia that resembles a fern (Fig. 5-32). That some of the electrical energy of a bolt of lightning has produced a superficial injury does not preclude the simultaneous passage of a fatal current through the body with severe burning at the sites of entrance, exit, or both.

In addition to skin burns of varying degrees of severity, victims of lightning may suffer fractures and ruptures of blood vessels and abdominal viscera. The enormous energy (as much as 10^9 volts) of a lightning bolt may cause injury by direct effect of the current or by the expanded (and returning) air resulting in blastlike injuries.[79] Current passing through the body may cause either ventricular fibrillation or respiratory paralysis. Instances of fetal electrocution with maternal survival have been reported in which the path of electrical current passed through the gravid uterus after a lightning strike.[80,81]

In addition to thermal injuries, persons surviving lightning strikes may develop diverse serious complications such as myoglobinuria, cardiac arrhythmias and infarction, peripheral nerve lesions, and tympanic membrane rupture.[82]

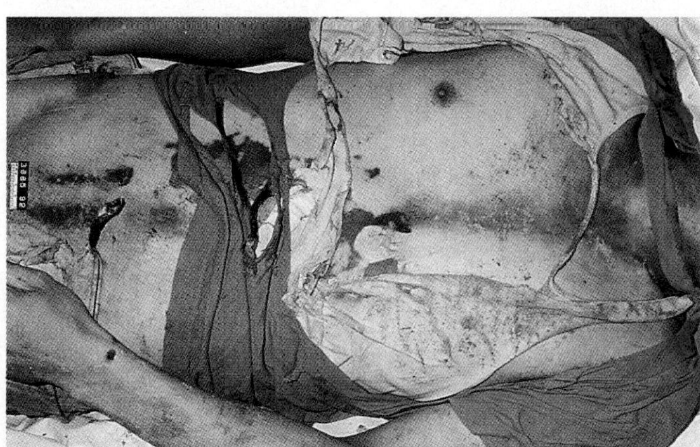

Fig. 5-31 Lightning death with torn and partially burned clothing and cutaneous burn of anterior trunk.

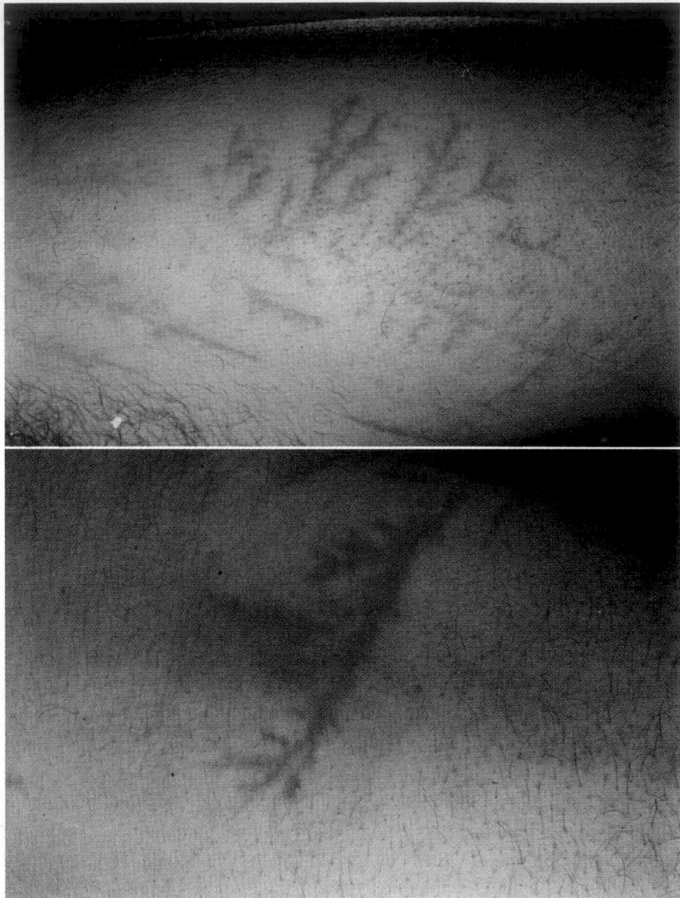

Fig. 5-32 Arborescent, "fern" pattern on skin from lightning strike.

A broad variety of ocular injuries can develop in survivors of lightning strikes. These include cataracts, corneal ulcers (occasionally going on to perforation), iridocyclitis, hyphema, and vitreous hemorrhage. In rare instances, choroidal ruptures, chorioretinitis, macular tears, retinal detachments, and even optic nerve injury have been recorded.[83]

REFERENCES

1. Adams VI, Hirsch CS: Trauma and disease. In Spitz WU: *Spitz and Fisher's medicolegal investigation of death,* ed 3, Springfield, Ill, 1993, Charles C Thomas.
2. Hirsch CS, Adams VI: Sudden and unexpected death from natural causes in adults. In Spitz WU: *Spitz and Fisher's medicolegal investigation of death,* ed 3, Springfield, Ill, 1993, Charles C Thomas.
3. Willinger M, James LS, Catz C: Defining the sudden infant death syndrome SIDS: deliberations of an expert panel convened by the National Institute of Child Health and Human Development, *Pediatr Pathol* 11:677, 1991.
4. Hoffman HJ, Damus K, Hillman L, Krongard E: Risk factors for SIDS: results of the National Institute of Child Health and Human Development SIDS cooperative epidemiological study, *Ann N Y Acad Sci* 533: 13, 1988.
5. Valdes-Dapena M et al: *Histopathology atlas for the sudden infant death syndrome,* Washington, DC, 1993, Armed Forces Institute of Pathology.
6. Valdes-Dapena M: The pathologist and the sudden infant death syndrome, *Am J Pathol* 106:118, 1982.
7. Steinschneider AS: Prolonged apnea and the sudden infant death syndrome: clinical and laboratory observations, *Pediatrics* 50:646, 1972.
8. Naeye RL: Hypoxemia and the suddent infant death syndrome, *Science* 186: 837, 1974.
9. Naeye RL: The sudden infant death syndrome: a review of recent advances, *Arch Pathol Lab Med* 101:165, 1977.
10. Kattwinkle J, Brooks J, Myerberg D: Positioning and SIDS: AAP task force on infant positioning and SIDS, *Pediatrics,* 89: 1120, 1992.
11. Guntheroth KG, Spires PS: Sleeping prone and the risk of sudden infant death syndrome, *JAMA* 267:2359, 1992.
12. Gilbert-Barness EF, Barness LA: Sudden infant death syndrome: is it a cause of death? *Arch Pathol Lab Med*: 117:124, 1993.
13. Rinaldo P et al: Medium-chain Acyl-CoA dehydrogenase deficiency, *N Engl J Med* 319:1308, 1988.
14. Adelson L: A microscopic study of dermal gunshot wounds, *Am J Clin Pathol* 35:393, 1961.
15. Ryan GA: Injuries in traffic accidents, *N Engl J Med* 276:1066, 1967.
16. Fletcher BD, Brogdon BG: Seat-belt fractures of the spine and sternum, *JAMA* 200:167, 1967.
17. Sube J, Ziperman HH, McIver WJ: Seat belt trauma to the abdomen, *Am J Surg* 133:346, 1967.
18. Spitz WU: Essential postmortem findings in the traffic accident victim, *Arch Pathol* 90:451, 1970.
19. Zumwalt RE, Hirsch CS: Medicolegal interpretation of gunshot wounds, *Am J Emerg Med* 5:133, 1987.
20. Department of the Army: *Wound ballistics,* Washington, DC, 1962, Superintendent of Documents.
21. Fackler ML: Wound ballistics: a review of common misconceptions, *JAMA* 259:2730, 1988.
22. Selye H: Stress and disease, *Science* 122: 625, 1955.
23. Scully RE: Fat embolism in Korean battle casualties: its incidence, clinical significance and pathologic aspects, *Am J Pathol* 32:379, 1956.
24. Williams AG, Mettler FA, Jr, Christie JH, Gordon RE: Fat embolism syndrome, *Clin Nucl Med* 7:497, 1986.
25. Lehman EP, Moore RM: Fat embolism including experimental production without trauma, *Arch Surg* 14:621, 1927.
26. LeQuire VS, Shapiro JL, LeQuire CB et al: A study of the pathogenesis of fat embolism based on human necropsy material and animal experiments, *Am J Pathol* 35, 1959.
27. Schnaid E, Lamprey JM, Viljoen MJ et al: The early biochemical and hormonal profile of patients with long bone fractures at risk of fat embolism syndrome, *J Trauma* 27:309, 1987.
28. Treiman N, Waisbrod V, Waisbrod H: Lipoprotein electrophoresis in fat embolism, *Injury* 13:108, 1981.
29. Sevitt S: *Fat embolism,* London, 1962, Butterworth.
30. Bray P, Myers RAM, Cowley RA: Orogenital sex as a cause of nonfatal air embolism in pregnancy, *Obstet Gynecol* 61:653, 1983
31. King MW, Aitchison JM, Nel JP: Fatal air embolism following penetrating lung trauma: an autopsy study, *J Trauma* 24:753, 1984.
32. Heath, D, Williams DR: The lung at high altitude, *Invest Cell Pathol* 2:147, 1979.
33. Roy SB, Guleria JS, Khanna PK et al: Haemodynamic studies in high altitude pulmonary oedema, *Br Heart J* 31:52, 1969.
34. Schoene RB, Hackett PH, Henderson WR et al: High altitude pulmonary edema: characteristics of lung lavage fluid, *JAMA* 256:63, 1986.
35. Heath D, Williams DR: *Man at high altitude,* Edinburgh, 1977, Churchill Livingstone.
36. Strauss RH, Yount DE: Decompression sickness, *Am Sci* 65:598, 1977.
37. Neuman TS, Spragg RG, Wagner PD, Moser KM: Cardiopulmonary consequences of decompression stress, *Respir Physiol* 41:143, 1980.
38. Strauss RH, Prockop LD: Decompression sickness among scuba divers, *JAMA* 223:637, 1973.
39. Fryer DI: Pathological findings in fatal sub-atmospheric decompression sickness, *Med Sci Law* 2:110, 1962.
40. Whitcraft DD, III, Karas S: Air embolism and decompression sickness in scuba divers, *JACEP (J Am Coll Emerg Physicians)* 5:355, 1976.
41. Leitch DR, Green RD: Pulmonary barotrauma in divers and the treatment of cerebral arterial gas embolism, *Aviat Space Environ Med* 57:931, 1986.

42. Weissman B, Green RS, Roberts PT: Frontal sinus barotrauma, *Laryngoscope* 82:2160, 1972.
43. Idicula J: Perplexing case of maxillary sinus barotrauma, *Aerospace Med* 43:891, 1972.
44. Cohen J, Biskind GR: Pathologic aspects of atmospheric blast injuries in man, *Arch Pathol* 42:12, 1946.
45. Rawlins JSP: Physical and pathophysiological effects of blast, *Injury* 9:313, 1978.
46. Decandole CA, Blast injury, *Can Med Assoc J* 96:207, 1967.
47. Hill JF: Blast injury with particular reference to recent terrorist bombing incidents, *Ann R Coll Surg Engl* 61:4, 1979.
48. Barr JS, Draeger RH, Sager W: Solid blast personnel injury: a clinical study, *Milit Surg* 98:1, 1946.
49. Marshall TK: Explosion injuries in forensic medicine. In Tedeschi CG, Eckert WG, Tedeschi LG, editors: *Forensic medicine,* Philadelphia, 1977, Saunders.
50. Schwetz F: The critical intensity for occupation noise, *Acta Otolaryngol* 89:358, 1980.
51. Bohne BA, Ward PH, Fernandez C: Rock music and inner ear damage, *Am Fam Physician* 15:117, 1979.
52. Doughterty JD, Welsh OL: Community noise and hearing loss, *N Engl J Med* 275:759, 1966.
53. Sataloff J, Vassalo J, Menduke H: Occupational healing loss and high frequency thresholds, *Arch Environ Health* 14:832, 1967.
54. Baker ML, Dalrymple GV: Biological effects of diagnostic ultrasound: a review, *Radiology* 126:479, 1978.
55. Liebeskind D, Bases R, Elequin F et al: Diagnostic ultrasound: effects on the DNA and growth patterns of animal cells, *Radiology* 131: 177, 1979.
56. Wittenzellner R: Tissue damaging effects of ultrasound, *Ultrasonics* 14:281, 1976.
57. Chaussey C, Schuller J, Schmiedt E et al: Extracorporeal shock-wave lithotripsy (ESWL) for treatment of urolithiasis, *Urology* 23 (special issue):59, 1984.
58. Kaude JV, Williams CM, Millner MR et al: Renal morphology and function immediately after extracorporeal shock-wave lithotripsy, *AJR* 1450:305, 1985.
59. Moritz AR, Henriques FC, Jr, McLean R: Effects of inhaled heat on air passages and lungs, *Am J Pathol* 21:311, 1945.
60. Moritz AR, Weisiger JR: Effects of cold air on air passages and lungs: experimental investigation, *Arch Intern Med* 75:233, 1945.
61. Moss J: Accidental severe hypothermia, *Surg Gynecol Obstet* 162:501, 1986.
62. Read AE, Emslie-Smith D, Gough KR, Holmes R: Pancreatitis and accidental hypothermia, *Lancet* 2:1219, 1961.
63. Savides EP, Huffband BI: Hypothermia, thrombosis and acute pancreatitis, *Br Med J* 1:614, 1974.
64. Moritz AR: Studies of thermal injury: pathology and pathogenesis of cutaneous burns, experimental study, *Am J Pathol* 23:915, 1947.
65. Moritz AR, Henriques FC, Jr: Studies of thermal injury: relative importance of time and surface temperature in causation of cutaneous burns, *Am J Pathol* 23:695, 1947.
66. Leibow AA, Warren S, DeCoursey E: Pathology of atomic bomb casualties, *Am J Pathol* 25:853, 1949.
67. Pearse HE, Kingsley HD: Thermal burns from atomic bombs, *Surg Gynecol Obstet* 98:385, 1954.
68. Luterman A, Dacso CC, Curreri PW: Infections in burn patients, *Am J Med* 81(suppl. 1A):45, 1986.
69. Davies JWL, Lamke LO, Liljedahl SO: A guide to the rate of nonrenal water loss from patients with burns, *Br J Plast Surg* 27:325, 1974.
70. Cohen MA, Guzzardi LJ: Inhalation of products of combustion, *Ann Intern Med* 12:628, 1983.
71. Witten MG, Quan SF, Sobonya RE, Lemen RJ: New developments in the pathogenesis in smoke inhalation induced pulmonary edema, *West H Med* 148:33, 1988.
72. Jones TS, Liang AP, Kilbourne EM et al: Morbidity and mortality associated with the July 1980 heat wave in St. Louis and Kansas City, Mo., *JAMA* 247:3327, 1982.
73. Anderson RJ, Reed G, Knochel J: Heatstroke, *Adv Int Med* 28:115, 1983.
74. Leeming MN: Protection of the electrically susceptible patient, *Anesthesiology* 38:370, 1973.
75. Leonard PF: Characteristics of electrical hazards, anesthesia and analgesia, *Curr Res* 51:798, 1972.
76. Wright RK, Davis JH: The investigation of electrical deaths: a report of 220 fatalities, *J Forensic Sci* 25:514, 1980.
77. Walter CW: Is death from accidental electric shock instantaneous? *JAMA* 221:922, 1972.
78. Yost JW, Olmes FF: Myoglobinuria following lightning stroke, *JAMA* 228:1147, 1974.
79. Brown KL: Electrical injuries, *J Trauma* 4:608, 1964.
80. Guha-Ray DK: Fetal death at term due to lightning, *Am J Obstet Gynecol* 134:103, 1979.
81. Weinstein L: Lightning: a rare cause of intrauterine death with maternal survival, *South Med J* 72:103, 1979.
82. Amy BW, McManus WF, Goodwin CW, Jr, Pruitt BA: Lightning injury with survival in five patients, *JAMA* 253:243, 1985.
83. Taussig HB: "Death" from lightning—and the possibility of living again, *Ann Intern Med* 68:1345, 1968.

6 Informatics

Rodney S. Markin
James Linder

FEATURES OF LABORATORY INFORMATION SYSTEMS
- Advantages
- Hardware
- Software

SELECTION OF AN INFORMATION SYSTEM
- Evaluation of current needs and operations
- Evaluation and selection of available systems
- Contract negotiations
- Implementation of an information system

EMERGING TECHNOLOGIES
- Speech recognition
- Image management
- Pathologist's workstation

Informatics describes the combination of basic and applied sciences to the processing of data and information.[1] When applied to medically related information, the term "medical informatics" is used. The scope of medical informatics includes clinical science, computer science, decision science, aspects of engineering, library science, and information science.

During the past 10 years medical informatics has grown, fueled by a new generation of physicians and stunning advances in computer hardware and software. Informatics has been recognized as an essential element of healthcare. Nursing, pharmacy, and other allied health professions have embraced the technology as well. As interest grows and the boundaries between healthcare and other disciplines fade, the term "healthcare informatics" will encompass the expanse of healthcare computing interests.

The practice of pathology produces vast amounts of *data,* which are communicated to physicians and others. As these individuals process the data, it becomes *information* that guides clinical decisions. The data and their availability influence greatly the decisions made in the care of the patient. Arising from these thoughts is the concept of the pathologist as information manager, first articulated by Bruce Friedman in 1987[2] and further refined by Weinstein[3] and Korpman.[4] These authors have expressed that there is a logical progression from the pathologist as laboratory department information manager to a hospital or campus level information officer.

In the role as an *information officer,* the pathologist would evaluate information and technology and develop and install software that would add value to the current data stream passed to the laboratory customer. The skills developed in planning for the growth of the clinical laboratory can be applied to information systems. In the changing financial environment, formulating a plan to implement new information-handling tools and technologies in the clinical laboratory is paramount. The pathologist with interest in and knowledge of these systems can provide that function.

One of the emerging disciplines that has reached into all aspects of business and medicine is decision support. Decision support in the clinical laboratory has been slow to develop, focusing mainly on expert systems research.[5] The future development of decision support in the clinical laboratory will focus on two areas—test performance and medical utility.

Test performance has been an area of interest in the clinical laboratory for the past 20 years.[6] Previous evaluations were limited to sensitivity and specificity; however, over the last 10 years, receiver-operator characteristic (ROC) curve analysis has been used.[7] The use of ROC curves and other industrial applications is a classic example of where informatics can bridge the gap between clinical medicine and decision analysis.

The *medical utility* of testing and test results is also a component of medical informatics. The application of cost-effectiveness analysis to clinical laboratory testing and other medical procedures has also entered clinical medicine through this emerging discipline. These analyses have been performed on a variety of tests[8-10] in an effort to determine methods to reduce costs. The application of rigorous numerical analysis to clinical testing and medical procedures should be performed by the informatician—the pathologist.

The introduction of expert systems during the past several years has followed the development of computer hardware. The application of a knowledge base to clinical problems is the next logical step in "informating" the medical record and clinical medical practice. The use of expert systems in medical decision making will be highly dependent on the clinical laboratory and anatomic pathology results. This situation puts the pathologist in a unique position to act as information manager.

Neural networks are also being applied to medical problem solving.[11-17] Conceptually, neural nets are artificial neurons arranged in logical layers "connected" to each other by elicitation of either positive (excitatory) or negative (inhibitory) inputs. The sum of the inputs is passed to the next layer until they reach the output layer. The proposed flexibility of neural nets is based on the "education" of the network—the potential to learn from multiple passes of data through the network. One of the successful applications of neural nets to clinical practice has been the laboratory diagnosis of myocardial infarction.[17] Furlong and colleagues[17] have applied neural networks to the diagnosis of myocardial infarction using serial cardiac enzyme determinations. The results were comparable when evaluated against the human "expert."

Models for training in medical informatics have been proposed by several authors[6,18-20] including informatics rotations in pathology residency programs. A universal theme is the development of computer proficiency (computer literacy) during the training period. These skills include the general understanding of hardware and network connections, the ability to use electronic mail (E-mail) and Internet access. In addition, competence in the use of word processing, software, spreadsheets, and database software, as well as statistics and graphic tools, has been suggested.

In the future, informatics will be recognized as a distinct discipline in medical practice. The pathologist is in a unique position to capitalize on the current opportunities because of the long experience of laboratory computerization. The advantages of laboratory information systems (LIS) as a tool for the pathologist are summarized below.

FEATURES OF LABORATORY INFORMATION SYSTEMS

Advantages

Access to information

Repetitive access to diagnostic information is required in most departments, laboratories, and areas of the hospital or clinic. The ability to access rapidly a tissue diagnosis or test result improves patient care. The access to the diagnosis or test result through a computer network and distribution mechanisms is a significant advantage of an LIS.

Turnaround time

The turnaround time of any laboratory test is the elapsed time from specimen collection to the reporting of the result. For example, the turnaround time in surgical pathology includes transfer of the specimen to the pathology department, specimen acquisition and its electronic accessioning, gross examination, histologic processing, microscopic examination, report dictation, report transcription, report printing, proofreading, and distribution of report (Fig. 6-1). An LIS can shorten turnaround time by improving processing of the specimen, transcription, distribution of results, and billing. Although these individual processes may represent only a small fraction of the turnaround time, they also indirectly affect other components of the examination. For example, if the patient's historical information is available, the pathologist may be able to render a diagnosis with less delay.

Productivity and financial management

As healthcare resources become constrained, it is increasingly important to monitor the work load and optimize productivity of all laboratory staff, such as technologists, transcriptionists, and pathologists. Information systems can improve productivity by use as a management tool to collect data regarding the work load, turnaround time, and, potentially, cost accounting (usually coupled with an inventory system).

The ability to access large volumes of data using the information system is a critical component of the LIS functionality. The ability of the LIS to provide data at several different organizational levels for analysis by the user is also very important. Most information systems deliver the utilities necessary to provide a limited analysis in the form of standard reports. The ability to extract data into formats that are easily imported into more sophisticated analysis programs (databases and spreadsheets) is also useful.

Regulatory compliance

Accreditation agencies are creating and enforcing more rules and regulations that apply to the practice of pathology and the operation of the laboratory. Compliance with these regulations and the accreditation agencies' requests for data will require us either to manually account for specific types of cases, that is, correlation of biopsy and cytologic diagnosis of squamous carcinoma of the cervix, or to utilize an information system to extract that information. In the future, correlations with clinical findings, anatomic pathology diagnoses, and utilization levels and patterns may be requested or even required. Including this information in an LIS will allow rapid collection of such data. This is increasingly essential to enable the laboratory to perform quality assurance in both anatomic and clinical pathology.

Research support

The value of information systems in conducting medical research cannot be understated. The ability to analyze large quantities of data, collected over a prolonged period of time, is of great value. Databases can be used to perform statistical analysis comparing various parameters. Particularly powerful are systems in which the laboratory system is linked with clinical information, so that outcome analysis can be performed for assessment of the value of different laboratory tests, or therapeutic interventions.

Hardware

The hardware components of an LIS are described as follows.

The *central processing unit* (CPU) of a computer executes the logical commands within software. CPUs differ in design, functionality, and speed of executing these commands. The speed of the processor may be designated by two different measures: million cycles per second (megahertz, or MHz) or million instructions per second (MIPS), the latter being the most common measure of the processor power. MIPS are a function of both the inherent processor speed and the type of software instructing the processor.

Processor power is the key to an LIS. The relationship between the number of users and the size of the CPU should be understood. Generally, there are two types of processes that will be occurring: foreground and background processes. The foreground processes are those interactive events instituted by users. Background processes are those that are either spawned by the main program or by a user during an interactive session and run in the "background" without the user's knowledge. The total number of processes that may be handled at any one time by the CPU include both foreground and background

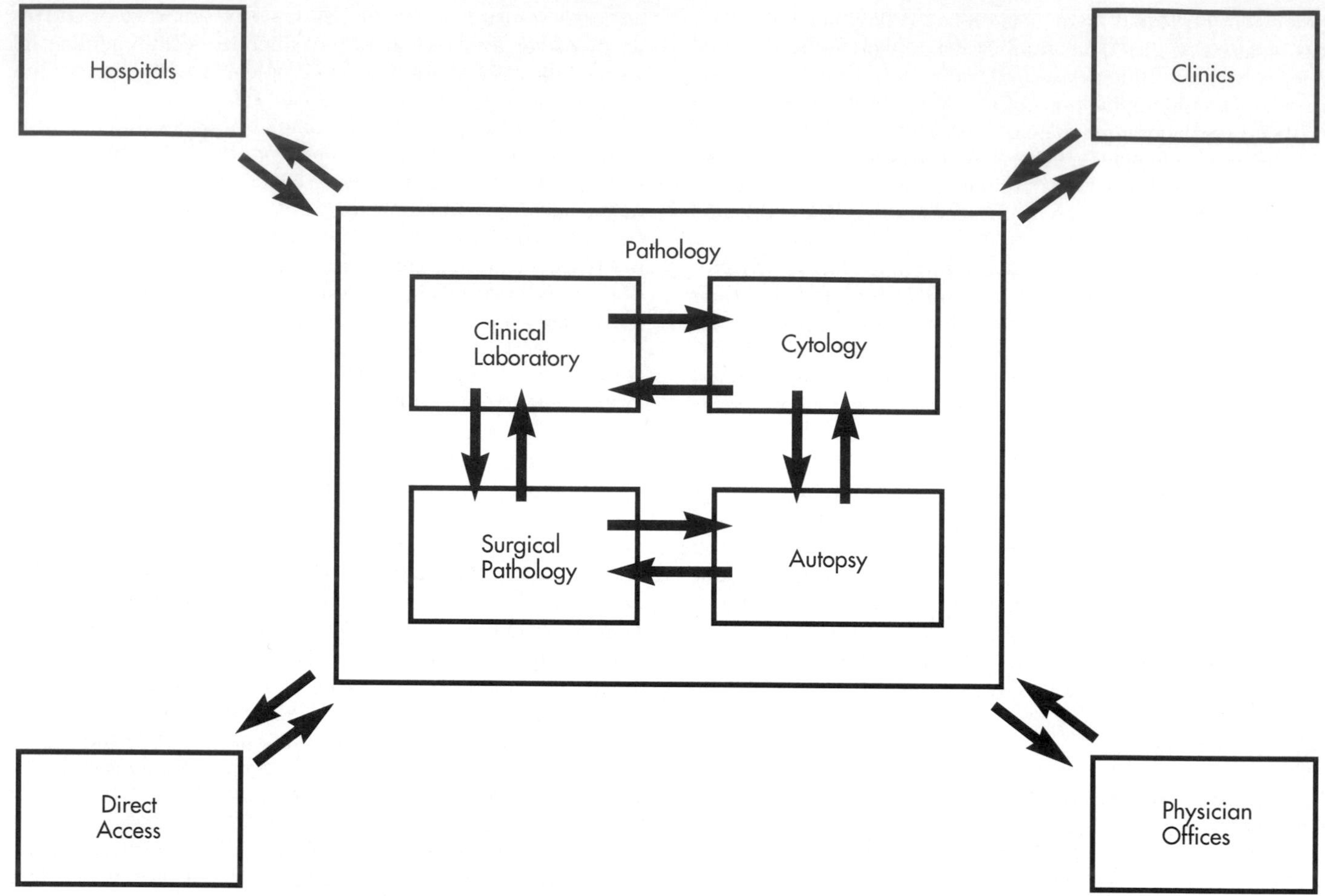

Fig. 6-1 Process steps and their relationship to turnaround time at points where information systems can make improvements.

processes. Correct determination of the number of both processes is important to avoid undersizing the system.

Poor system performance is reflected by delayed response time when using the system. The response time is influenced by several factors including traffic across the CPU bus and processor speed. Upgrading to a faster, more powerful CPU will improve poor system performance as concurrently foreground and background processes increase. Desirable hardware configurations allow for an upgradable CPU.

Electronic *storage* of information is a key feature of the LIS because it provides a permanent, easily accessible record. At the time of this writing most laboratory systems that are in use have finite storage capacity. A superior design allows for storage of complete anatomic pathology reports and relevant clinical laboratory data. The amount of storage space required to support a new installation is difficult to predict. An effective design may be to use several types of storage media, including a fixed-disk medium for recently acquired data (to allow for short access time) and optical media for archival data.

Terminals on the system may be of two types: "dumb" terminals (cathode ray tubes, CRTs) or "smart" terminals (PCs/workstations). The "dumb" terminals (CRTs) are generally used with a network or multiplexed system. The terminals initiate (by the user) a process on the CPU. The major advantage of dumb terminals is that they are inexpensive.

Personal computers are superior because in addition to functioning as a terminal for the mainframe, they can function as an independent workstation for data analysis. Some workstations extract information from a central CPU/data repository (server) and use those data in a process that originates in the workstation CPU (client). The data are then sent back to the server and stored on the disk drive. This transfer of data sent to and from a central server and a remote process is called "client-server technology". This technology is increasingly used. Workstations may also be used to support other functions, such as word processing, spreadsheets, and database, independent of the main CPU.

Network communications

During the last decade computer networks proliferated, providing a conduit for the increasing amount of information available in digital form. Networks of various types connect computers with terminals, printers, modems, and other devices. The definition of a network by the Institute of Electrical and Electronics Engineers (IEEE) is *"a data communications system allowing a number of independent devices to communicate directly with each other, within a moderately sized geographic area over a physical communication channel of moderate data rates."*

Networks require some type of dedicated or nondedicated public telecommunication facilities (phone lines) or dedicated high-speed communication lines such as T1 (1.5 megabytes/second), T3 (45 megabytes/second) lines, frame-relay, and asynchronous transfer mode (ATM). The latter provides for very high speed network communications (100 megabytes/second).

Networks can be termed "wide-area networks (WANs)" or "local-area networks (LANs)" according to the geographic separation of their users. As technologies improve and constraints on space decline, these two types of networks will appear to converge. To a user operating a PC serving as a workstation in the client-server paradigm, there is no difference to the user between local-area networks and wide-area networks.

Network hardware includes the physical medium over which the communication signals are transmitted and the connectors or adaptors required to connect to that physical medium. Physical medium may consist of twisted pair copper wire, coaxial cable of varying sizes, or fiber-optic cables. The type of physical medium coupled with the software technology will limit the speed at which communications may occur.

Several standards serve as the basis for network technologies. Ethernet, first developed by Xerox at the Palo Alto Research Center, serves as the basis for the standard IEEE 802.3. Ethernet and Ethernet-like networking schemes, many of which are compatible with the IEEE 802.3 definition, are offered by a variety of vendors. Ethernet typically uses a bus technology as shown in Fig. 6-2. Ethernet applications operate at speeds up to 10 megabytes/second and are dependent on the transmission media (such as wire, cable, fiber optic) used.

Token Ring technology is based upon the IEEE 802.5 standard developed by International Business Machines (IBM). Token Ring technology is used in both wide-area and local-area networks. A Token Ring network may be used to cross very high speed media including fiber-optic cables with transmission speeds up to 100 megabytes/second. As suggested by the name, a Token Ring network uses a ring topology for its physical media (Fig. 6-2).

Novelle Incorporated offers a network operating system product called NetWare. NetWare may be used with Ethernet, token ring, and other architectures that follow the IEEE standards. The Novelle product provides a number of functions including file sharing, printer sharing, electronic mail remote access, and interconnection between different types of local area networks. The Novelle products may be used in information applications either to provide or to enhance functionality of other vendors' products.

Networks provide a bridge to integrate the laboratory system into an existing information system environment. In other words, network-to-system communication or terminal-to-system communication allows for communication where devices have a similar status in the system. The primary reason for employing a local area network is to improve productivity through the automation of routine job functions and improve the manageability of information through reduced duplication and improved accessibility. Using an anatomic pathology information system achieves both of these goals. Fig. 6-2 demonstrates some of the common topologies of LANs.

Refer to the monograph titled *Local Area Networks, Architectures and Implementations*, by James Martin,[21] for a more detailed discussion of networks and how they function.

Software

The basic functionality of the software used to automate data and information handling in pathology includes registration, demographics (admissions-discharge-transfer [ADT]), and order entry. Basic functionality also includes the entry of results and the printing of reports. Functionality of registration should be defined based upon the needs of the hospital for billing and results reporting and for billing of individual pathology fees. Data for registration demographics and order entry should be accomplished either through direct entry into the system or through an interface with another information system.

Specialized functions

Specialized functions of the information system serve anatomic pathology and clinical laboratory functions.

The anatomic pathology functions usually contain modules or subsections for surgical pathology, cytology, and autopsy pathology. The anatomic pathology systems usually function in a significantly different manner from that of those designed for the general clinical laboratory. Anatomic pathology reports are usually composed of text as narrative descriptions of clinical, gross, microscopic pathologic diagnoses and, in some cases, diagnostic clinical information. Coding mechanisms such as SNOMED (College of American Pathologists, Skokie, Illinois) are used to subclassify or organize cases based upon key words in their narrative descriptions. Databases in which diagnoses have been recorded may be searched by standardized code, such as the standardized nomenclature of medicine (SNOMED) or by a natural language search to identify key words within the diagnosis. Depending on the accuracy of SNOMED coding, most objective comparisons will find that natural language searching techniques are more complete but more time consuming.

Clinical laboratory functions usually produce a high volume of discrete results that fit into numerical reference ranges or are positive or negative results. Certain applications, including the Blood Bank, are now regulated by the Food and Drug Administration (FDA) and have highly complex rules and regulations. A standard bar-code identification system has been implemented for banks of the Blood Bank and the disbursing of blood products. Blood banking is a particular liability for the clinical laboratory operation, since blood products are disbursed as a product from the laboratory.

The microbiology component of the clinical laboratory is also a specialized function because of the nature of the tests being performed. The turnaround times for microbiology results are variable, depending on the growth attributes of the organism, as compared with other results in the laboratory, which may be derived by simple sampling and analysis. Microbiology subsystems require the ability to retain orders and report results as late as 6 to 8 weeks.

Interfaces

An interface is an electronic or mechanical mechanism for data transfer between information systems. The most common interfaces are billing interface and an admissions-discharge-

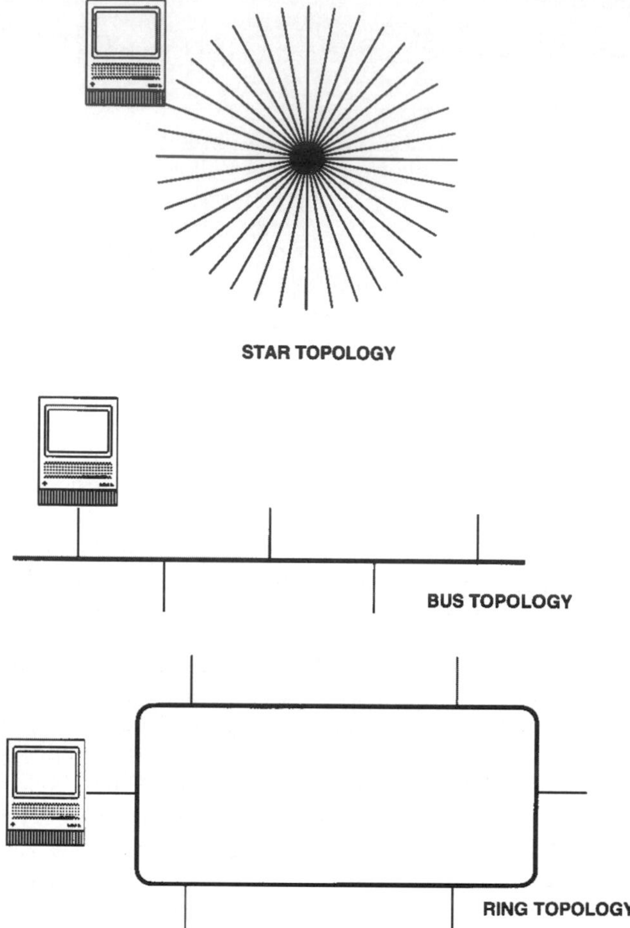

Fig. 6-2 Examples of basic network configurations: bus topology, ring topology, star topology.

Table 6-1 ADT/OE interface

ADT—admission-discharge transfer date
Patient number
Patient name
Age
Sex
Patient location
Attending physician
Insurance information *
OE—order entry
Patient number
Ordering physician
Ordering location
Order date
Order time
Test ordered (codified)

*The insurance information passed and the format that it is presented in will be dependent on the elements collected and the entity that does the billing.

Table 6-2 Billing interface components

Patient number—unique identifier for patient
Encounter number—unique identifier for visit
Patient name—for tracking purposes
Date of service—date specimen received in laboratory
Patient Social Security number (SSN)—for some systems
Physician rendering service—for physician of record
ICD-9 code, if available*
Patient location: inpatient, outpatient, outside patient
CPT code (or unique charge identifier–procedure code)
CPT Code
CPT Code
. . .†

CPT, current procedural terminology
*Some insurers require ICD - 9 code for clinical diagnoses
†Multiple charge codes may be appended to record up through the physical length of the record. Additional charges will be appended to another record.

transfer (ADT) between the hospital admitting system or hospital information system (HIS) and the LIS.

The ADT interface is the key to decreasing turnaround time. ADT data usually comes from the hospital admitting system or hospital information system. Transfer of ADT data to the LIS by means of a network saves the time of personnel working in either the gross room or transcription area because these data need not be reentered for each specimen. The usual information that comes across an ADT interface is listed in Table 6-1.

When all components are purchased from the same vendor (both CP, clinical pathology, and AP, anatomic pathology), interfaces between the two systems are nonexistent. Systems or models from the same vendor usually share the same data files, reporting, and billing mechanisms. This eliminates a substantial amount of work and maintenance when this sharing is done. When it does not occur, an interface between the LIS and HIS may be necessary. The typical billing interface data elements are listed in Table 6-2.

Result reporting

Reporting of results is accomplished by either printed reports or by electronic transmission of results to another LIS or HIS. Table 6-3 outlines the components of a results-reporting interface. The results are transmitted with a heading that contains information regarding the specimen and order so that the results may be linked to the patient. The results are sent as either a single component or a linked list of components that represent test codes as part of a battery or profile.

An anatomic pathology report is shown in Chapter 3. Styles and formats of reports vary depending on the type of tests performed and the frequency of the results reported. Most inpatient reports with results from the clinical laboratory are presented in row and column formats much like a spreadsheet. Outpatient clinical results are presented as single-entry items with defined reference range values. Anatomic pathology report forms are highly variable, but they usually contain the same basic components. Fig. 6-3 shows a prototype format of laboratory results displayed by frequency and nature.

Printing of reports may occur based upon the type of patient, either inpatient or outpatient, and the requirements of the individual customers of the laboratory operation. Remote printing of reports may be accomplished using either printers in remote locations that are directly connected to the IS network, or remote printers that are connected to the LIS network through a modem connection or through the use of facsimile transmission (fax). The most commonly used remote printing option is currently a remote printer that contains a built-in modem.[22] The modem is connected to a telephone line, usually provided by the laboratory, and results based on a mutually agreed upon time frame between the laboratory and the customer are sent. The advantages to a system such as this are that the laboratory has control over the type of paper used and the type of printing equipment utilized. The disadvantages are the cost of the paper, the cost of remote repair, and the cost of the telephone line.

An alternative means for result reporting is the use of the facsimile machine. Many LIS allow transmission directly to the customer's facsimile machine. The lack of security and access to the results need to be investigated before one uses a fax machine to send results. There are several advantages for both the customer and the laboratory in using the facsimile machine: reduced space, decreased number of phone lines to maintain, decreased maintenance for the laboratory of client instrumentation, and space.

Table 6-3 Results reporting interface data elements

Report number
Order number
Battery code
Test code*
Test result*
Reference range*
Test code*
Test result*
Reference range*

*Repeating elements that are dependent on the presence of a battery code and the number of test codes in that battery.

SELECTION OF AN INFORMATION SYSTEM

Evaluation of current needs and operations

Accurate understanding of the current needs and operations of the laboratory is essential for proper selection of an LIS.

The financial considerations with respect to procuring a laboratory information system are significant. The purchase of an LIS is by far the most expensive single capital acquisition of a clinical laboratory. Several cost-analysis and cost-justification studies of the implementation of an LIS into the clinical laboratory have been published.[23-38] These articles discuss the tangible (financial) and intangible benefits of the LIS and the problems encountered in the evaluation of those benefits.[22,25,27,33,38]

The tangible benefits include a savings in the time required to perform specific tasks,[39] including specimen processing, results reporting (including calculation of results), and administration and management. The total number of hours that are expended each year for these individual tasks is significant. The return on investment (ROI) for such a system may be around 5 to 7 years.[40]

The intangible benefits of an IS purchase and implementation have been described and are summarized in Table 6-4.[23,41-43] The most important is improved service through decreased turnaround time for test-result reporting, increased legibility of reports, reduced transcription errors, flexibility of result reporting, and elimination of duplicate test orders or requests, all leading to better patient care.

Evaluation and selection of available systems

Evaluation and selection of available systems is an arduous task. New IS vendors are constantly entering the marketplace.

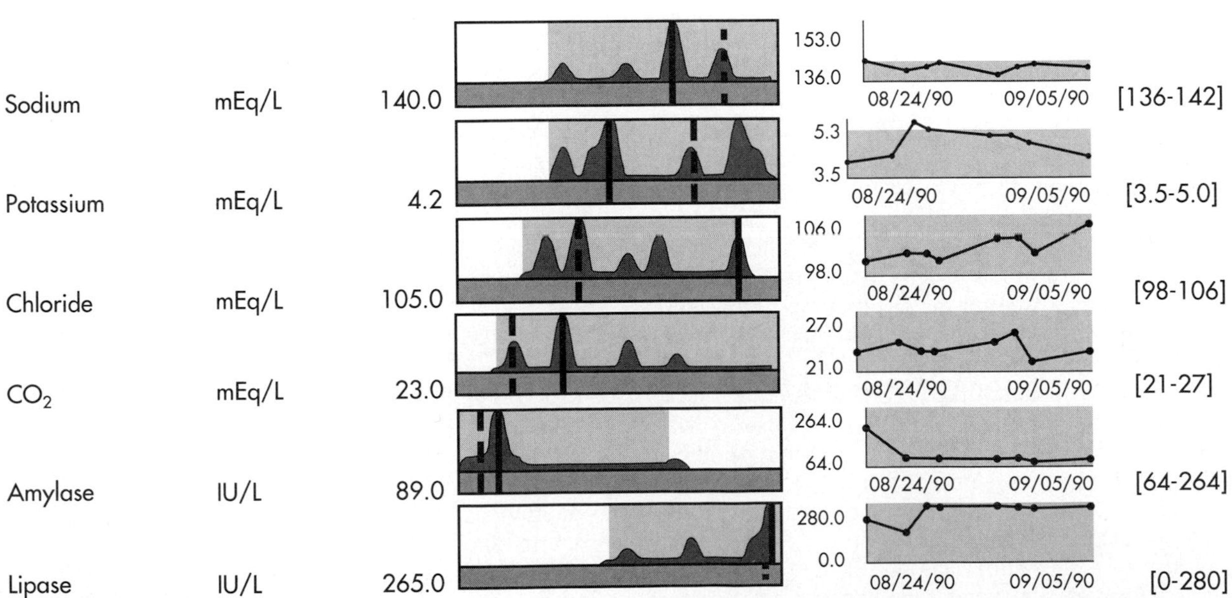

Fig. 6-3 Prototypical clinical laboratory reports with numeric and graphic representation of clinical laboratory data. In the plots on the left the shadowed area represents the normal range. The current value is shown numerically, and by the *solid black line*. The most recent is shown by the *dashed line*. On the right the values over a 2 week period are displayed.

Table 6-4 Intangible benefits

Decreased turnaround time
Improved report formats
Increased access to results
Improved access to results on clinical results
Reduced transcription errors
Reduction in duplicate testing
Printing of pending lists
Printing of overdue lists
Access of data for research
Reporting of work load of laboratory section
Improved charge capture
Specialized reports for transplant services
Research data for research efforts outside pathology department
Reference laboratory support
Graphic reports
User group
Computer proficiency for employees
Home and outside access to data and results

At the same time, a variety of established vendors have mature markets and have the potential of going out of business. Various publications provide annual lists and updates on LIS vendors, including *CAP Today, Healthcare Informatics,* and *Medical Laboratory Observer (MLO).*

Contract negotiations

The process of contract negotiations may be simple and swift, or complex and lengthy. The vendor should provide a contract defining the services previously decided upon, except for the price. Before the selection process the pathologist should have defined a budget, which will become a tool for negotiation.

The actual negotiation of the contract may be performed by members of the purchasing department, the director or associate director of information services, the chief financial officer (CFO) or chief information officer (CIO) of the hospital or institution, or the director of laboratories. Ideally, input and assistance will be provided by all those mentioned above, since they all have different experiences and perspectives.

A strategy should be developed before negotiations. Every institution has acquisition rules it must follow in the process. The rules should be understood by all involved in the process. An itemized list that includes the rules and the functional and financial limits of the institution and the functional limits of the laboratory should be prepared for the negotiation. At this point, the negotiating firm must agree that a compromise is one of the goals of the negotiations. A fair contract should be negotiated. The buyer must be cognizant of the need for the vendor to pay its expenses and make a profit. The vendor should also be aware of the financial constraints of doing business with a healthcare entity in the current financing environment. The development of an adversarial relationship at the outset may not lead to a mutually beneficial relationship in the future.

The payment of a substantial amount of the contract price at signing will provide the vendor with necessary funds to implement the installation. To ensure the proper performance of the vendor, a performance bond and last-payment holdback may be incorporated into the contract to ensure completion of the project. Before and during the negotiations, the use of legal counsel with experience in LIS contracts is essential.

Implementation of an information system

The responsibility to implement an LIS may be the pathology department's, or delegated to a computer or engineering support service. The pathologist assuming a leadership role in implementing the system is the most effective way to achieve desired results. Some of the important considerations with regard to implementing the system include the physical plant, training, and system support.

Physical plant

Considerations of the physical plant and the layout of the network is primarily determined by the physical location of both terminals and printers with respect to a CPU/server. The CPU/server for the LIS may be located within the pathology department or in a remote location such as a campus or hospital computer room. In the first case, the network or mechanism of communications between terminals or workstations in the CPU and the server may be limited to a small area. The most efficient way to set up a physical network layout is to determine the location for all devices (printers and terminals) throughout the department. The configuration and location of the network can then be laid out to bridge the devices. Certain physical restrictions may apply to both the physical plant and the media (wires and cables) used to operate the network.

The installation of the network is usually the responsibility of the client. A reliable contractor should be sought to install the local area network. In addition, they usually provide a warranty.

Training

Training is a very important issue; if you can't use the system, it is useless. Training and training schedules vary by vendor. Usually, training is a one-time proposition, at the vendor's office, designed to provide a large amount of information in a short period of time. It is therefore important to identify key people at the level of the pathologist, transcriptionist, histologist, and the pathologist assistants who may act as resource personnel in the local area. Usually system managers are available for both global and specific user and system support.

System support

The support of your system will be highly dependent on the level of departmental involvement and the availability of resources. Internal support for LIS operations is desirable to maximize features and functionality.

EMERGING TECHNOLOGIES

Speech recognition

Computerized speech recognition allows computers to transform the spoken word into text or to recognize spoken words to execute commands within a computer program. This is not synonymous with voice recognition, which refers to frequency patterns, such as voice prints, which are relatively unique to an individual. Speech-recognition systems are classified as either speaker dependent or speaker independent. The former requires a training period so that the system becomes accustomed to the accents and speech inflections of the speaker. Speaker-independent systems require less or no training periods. Systems have different abilities to recognize types of dictation. In order of increasing sophistication, dictation can be viewed as discrete speech, trigger phrases, or continuous speech. Discrete-speech systems require momentary pauses between individual words. Trigger-phrase systems come close to emulating continuous speech; these systems recognize words or phrases that trigger the incorporation of complete sentences or paragraphs into the final text. Continuous-speech systems, as the name implies, permit dictation at rates equivalent to that obtained by a tape recorder and human transcriptionist.

Aside from the type of speech that is recognized, the vocabulary of the system is a measure of its power and potential functionality. Currently, systems in the emergency room, radiology room, and pathology settings have lexicon capacities exceeding 5000 words. Between 70% and 90% of surgical pathology material can be handled by vocabulary of this size. Systems with vocabularies exceeding 30,000 words—far larger than that of the most erudite pathologist—are under development.

Speech-recognition systems have been demonstrated to function in the anatomic pathology work environment.[44] Shorter turnaround times and savings of secretarial staffing have been observed.

The cost of speech-recognition systems is rapidly decreasing, and the cost is influenced by the size of the vocabulary, the degree of speaker dependence, and whether the system supports discontinuous or continuous speech. When considering cost, one must remember that it may be necessary to have several workstations with speech recognition if multiple individuals are dictating gross or microscopic material simultaneously.

Image management

Both pathology and radiology departments depend on imaging technology to diagnose disease. The radiologist uses a variety of imaging instruments dependent on x-ray radiation, sound waves, magnetic resonance, or emitted particles to reconstruct images that will be interpreted by the radiologist. The pathologist depends on the images formed by the microscope because its optics magnify tissue sections that have been appropriately processed and stained to highlight differences in the biochemical composition of the tissue. Aside from a diagnosis, the written consultation report often goes to great lengths to recreate a mental picture of the gross or microscopic images in support of the written diagnosis.

Digital images can be captured by techniques described in Chapter 13. Insight into what this technology may mean to the pathology department can be drawn from the experience in the radiology department. Concerted efforts are underway in the radiology departments to move toward "filmless" environments where archives of radiographs are stored in the digital format. The advantage of digitally stored material is that it consumes far less space, is more readily accessible and permanent (since it can't be lost when "checked out" of the department), and can be transmitted either within the hospital or to remote viewing sites. Similar arguments can be made for the archiving of digital images in pathology.

A further aspect of digital images is the ability to transmit these images for remote consultation or educational purposes. "Telepathology" has been added to the lexicon of pathologists in recent years to describe the transmission of images for diagnostic or educational uses.

The fundamental challenge in either telepathology or teleradiology is rapidly moving a vast amount of information from one point to another. Several approaches have been taken, including direct line-of-sight microwave transmission, satellite systems, standard telephone lines, coaxial cables, and broad-bandwidth telephone systems.

At the time of this writing, the "information superhighway" is a major topic in the popular literature. The essential concept is a broad-band communication network capable of transmitting large volumes of text, sound, and image information at a nearly instantaneous rate. The *Internet* is cited as the prototype. The Internet is best described as a network of networks, of which the NSFNET is the major backbone. This is a high-speed data transmission network capable of transmitting approximately 45 million bits per second, roughly equivalent of 1000 typewritten pages each second. Internet access is widely available at universities and medical centers. Many commercial providers are also available.

Although accessing the Internet is easy, navigating and finding specific files may be difficult. Various event services, such as the Internet Gopher and Archie provide software tools to World Wide Web (WWW) and Veronica.

The full potential of the Internet as an adjunct in medicine and the transmission of medical information has not been realized. The Internet has been used to transmit images and perform real-time clinical consultation. The use of this technology will rapidly expand in the 1990s.

Pathologist's workstation

In order for the pathologist to manage the inflow and outflow of information from the department it is mandatory that the information be readily accessible and under his or her control. Again, drawing on the experience of radiologists in recent years, Image Management and Communication Systems (IMACS) have been used to integrate hospital information, radiology information, and digital archives of radiographic images. This integration allows the radiologist rapidly to review multiple current or previous images on patients.

The salient features of this workstation are that it integrates diverse clinical information from clinic, hospital, pharmacy, and radiology information systems (Table 6-5). Thus, when a slide was presented for review, a complete clinical profile could be obtained. A workstation would have hypertext mod-

Table 6-5 Characteristics of a physician's workstation

Access to patient data from the following departments:
- Clinical laboratory
- Anatomic pathology
- Radiology
- Pharmacy
- Operating room
- Respiratory therapy
- Hospital system

Access to information database, such as MedLine and Micromedix (Pharmacy)

Access to experts systems and diagnostic aids

User-information wing-speech recognition or touch-screen or pen-based operation

Ability to capture archive, retrieve, and manipulate digital images

Connected to a network, ideally with a unique Internet address

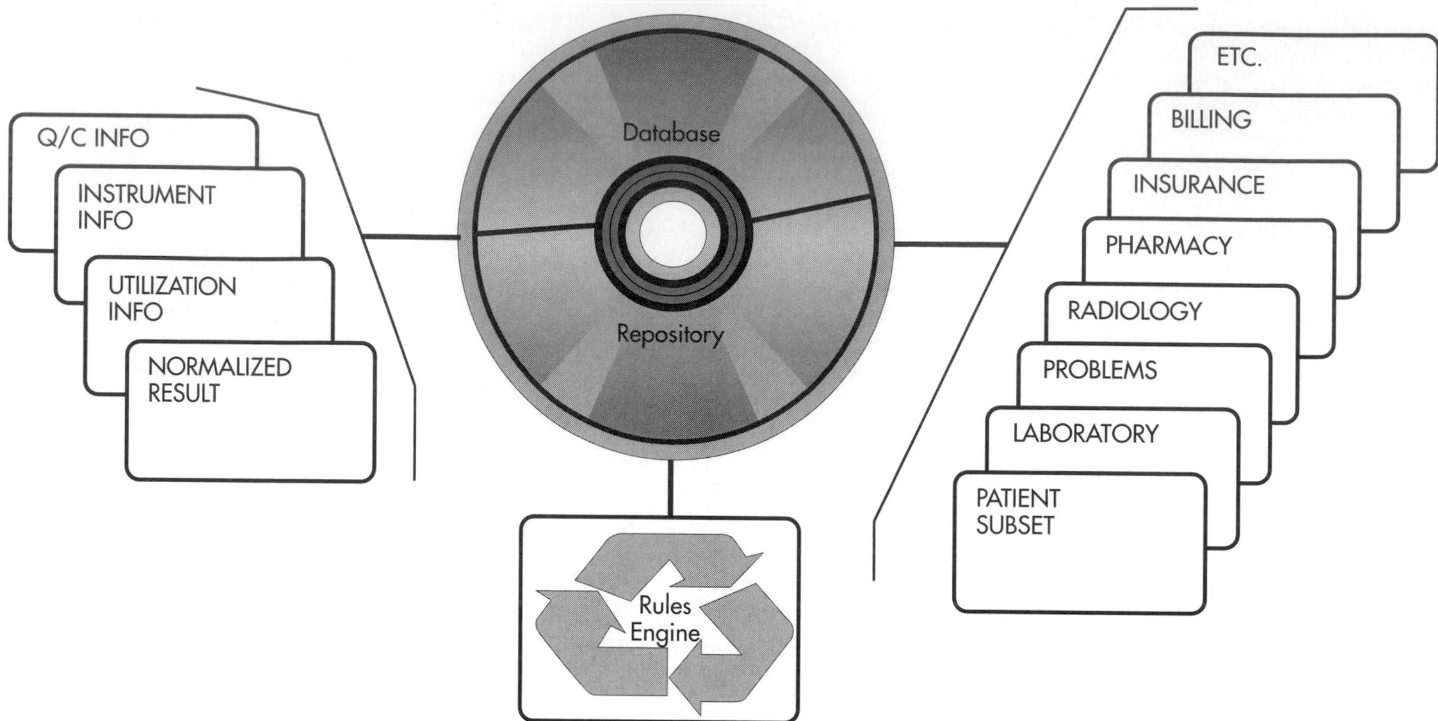

Fig. 6-4 Flow of information within a patient care operation including data from the clinical laboratory, anatomic pathology, and other departments and clinics in the hospital.

ules, making available to the pathologist general and specialty textbooks in surgical pathology, image archives of images, and online access to literature databases (Fig. 6-4). Although not specifically linked to the anatomic system, expert systems or image analysis could be incorporated.[45]

REFERENCES

1. Greenes RA, Shortliffe ED: Medical informatics: an emerging academic discipline and institutional priority, *JAMA* 263:1114, 1990.
2. Friedman BA: Laboratory information systems and the competency trap. In Greenes RA, editor: *Proceedings of the 12th Annual Symposium on Computer Applications in Medical Care,* New York, 1988, IEEE Computer Society Press.
3. Weinstein RL, Bloom, KJ: The pathologist as an information specialist, *Hum Pathol* 21:4, 1990.
4. Korpman RA: Using the computer to optimize human performance in healthcare delivery: the pathologist as medical information specialist, *Arch Pathol Lab Med* 111:637, 1987.
5. Buffone GJ, Beck JR: Informatics: a subspecialty in pathology, *Am J Clin Pathol* 100:75, 1993.
6. Galen RS, Gambino SR: Beyond normality: the predictive value and efficiency of medical diagnoses, New York, 1975, John Wiley & Sons.
7. Beck JR, Shultz EK: The role of relative operating characteristic (ROC) curves in test performance evaluation, *Arch Pathol Lab Med* 110:13, 1986.
8. Beck JR, Appleton PE, Shultz EK: Cost-effectiveness of thyroid testing strategies. In Kerkhof PLM, van Dieijen-Visser MP, editors: *Laboratory data and patient care,* New York, 1988, Plenum Press.
9. Kocjan G: Evaluation of the cost effectiveness of establishing a fine needle aspiration cytology clinic in a hospital out-patient department, *Cytopathology* 2:13, 1991.
10. Ransohoff DF, Lang CA, Kuo HS: Colonoscopic surveillance after polypectomy: considerations of cost effectiveness, *Ann Intern Med* 114:177, 1991.
11. Kratzer MA, Ivandic B, Fateh-Moghadam A: Neuronal network analysis of serum electrophoresis, *J Clin Pathol* 96:134, 1992.
12. O'Leary TJ, Mikel UV, Becker RL: Computer-assisted image interpretation: use of a neural network to differentiate tubular carcinoma from sclerosing adenosis, *Mod Pathol* 5:402, 1992.
13. Astion M, Wilding P: Application of neural networks to the interpretation of laboratory data in cancer diagnosis, *Clin Chem* 38:34, 1992.
14. Dawson AE, Austin RE Jr, Weinberg DS: Nuclear grading of breast carcinoma by image analysis, *Am J Clin Pathol* 95:S92, 1991.
15. Wied GL, Dytch H, Bibbo M et al: Artificial intelligence-guided analysis of cytologic data, *Anal Quant Cytol Histol* 12:417, 1990.
16. Dytch HE, Wied GL: Artificial neural networks and their use in quantitative pathology, *Anal Quant Cytol Histol* 12:379, 1990.
17. Furlong JW, Dupuy ME, Heinsimer JA: Neural network analysis of serial cardiac enzymes data: a clinical application of artificial machine intelligence, *Am J Clin Pathol* 96:134, 1991.
18. Friedman CP, Oxford GS, Juliano EL: A collaborative institutional model for integrating computer applications in the medical curriculum, *Proc Annu Symp Comput Appl Med Care,* p. 752, 1991.
19. Haber MH, Clifford SS, Britton CT: A management informatics rotation for pathology residents, *Am J Clin Pathol* 95(suppl 1):S38, 1991.
20. Friedman BA: Informatics as a separate section within a department of pathology, *Am J Clin Pathol* 94(suppl 1):S2, 1990.
21. Martin J: *Local area networks, architectures and implementations* (a monograph), Englewood Cliffs, NJ, 1989, Prentice Hall.
22. Markin RS: Remote reporting of laboratory results: a marketing tool, *Informatics in Pathol* 2:23, 1987.
23. Westlake GE: Cost analysis and cost justification of automated data processing in the clinical laboratory, *Clin Lab Med* 3:63, 1983.
24. Abson J, Prall A, Wootton JD: Data processing in pathology laboratories, *Clin Biochem* 14:323, 1977.
25. Brecher G, Loken HF: The laboratory computer—Is it worth its price? *Am J Clin Pathol* 57:527, 1971.
26. Cole GW: Biochemical test profiles and laboratory system design, *Hum Pathol* 11:424, 1980.
27. Grams RR: Cost analysis of a laboratory information system (LIS), *J Med Syst* 10:27, 1977.
28. Grann RP: Failure to learn from failure: evaluating computer systems in medicine. In *Proceedings of the Fourth Annual Symposium on Computer Appli-*

cations in Medical Care, Washington, DC, 1980, Institute of Electrical and Electronics Engineers.

29. Hendricks EJ, Langhofer BS: A community hospital laboratory computer system, *Am J Clin Pathol* 77:297, 1982.
30. Johnson HL: Does it pay to interface instruments with a computer? *Med Lab Observer,* p. 85, 1978.
31. Jorgensen JH, Holmes P, Williams WL et al: Computerization of a hospital clinical microbiology laboratory, *Am J Clin Pathol* 69:605, 1978.
32. Kobernick SD, Mandell GH: Implementing a laboratory computer system: a case history, *Am J Clin Pathol* 61:122, 1974.
33. Lame K: Cost justification of laboratory computer systems. In Westlake G, editor: *Automation and management in the clinical laboratory,* Baltimore, Md, 1972, University Park Press.
34. Lincoln TL, Korpman RA: Computers, health care, and medical information science, *Science* 17:257, 1980.
35. Makey DG, Corle DK, Byar DP et al: A computerized reference laboratory, *Med Instrum* 13:46, 1979.
36. Nussbaum B, Minckler T, Roby R et al: Economic impact of a computer based centralized organization in a clinical laboratory, *Am J Clin Pathol* 67:149, 1977.
37. Scalfani JJ, Ramkissoon RA: The acquisition of a laboratory information system, *J Med Syst* 5:281, 1981.
38. Workload recording method and personnel management manual, Northfield, Ill, 1991, College of American Pathologists.
39. Winsten D: Why spend the money? Justification of laboratory information systems, *Clin Lab Med* 11:105, 1991.
40. Markin RS, Hald DL: Cost justification of a laboratory information system: an analysis of projected tangible and intangible benefits, *J Med Syst* 16:281, 1992.
41. Lincoln TL, Aller RD: Acquiring a laboratory computer system: vendor selection and contracting, *Clin Lab Med* 11:21, 1991.
42. Wolfe HB: Cost-benefit of laboratory computer systems, *J Med Syst* 10:1, 1986.
43. Erler BS, Chein K, Marchevsky AM: An image analysis workstation for the pathology laboratory, *Mod Pathol* 6:612, 1993.
44. Tischler AS, Martin MR: Generation of surgical pathology report using a 5,000-word speech recognizer, *Am J Clin Pathol* 92(4 suppl 1):S44, 1989.
45. Weilert M: Implementing information systems, *Clin Lab Med* 11:41, 1991.

7 Electron Microscopy

Bruce Mackay
Nelson G. Ordóñez

The electron microscope has made enormous contributions, and it continues to provide new information to our understanding of the structure and function of normal and diseased tissues. Its role in routine diagnostic pathology is, however, quite selective.

During its development in Germany in the 1930s, the role of electron microscopy (EM) in medicine, biology, and the material sciences was questioned.[1] It required years of refinement of techniques related to tissue fixation, staining, and sectioning before EM became available for routine specimen analysis in the early 1960s. Once pathologists began to study diseased tissues using EM, a plethora of information accumulated in the medical literature. From this time until the mid 1980s, EM was the mainstay technique to aid in the diagnosis of surgical biopsies that were unresolved by light microscopy.

Immunohistochemistry has greatly diminished the use of ultrastructural studies in surgical pathology. Immunohistochemistry has several advantages over EM as a routine diagnostic tool. It is more accessible, through the use of commercially available kits; a special microscope is not required; immunohistochemical stains are easily compared with hematoxylin-eosin sections; and one may examine many more cells than are usually studied in electron microscopic preparations.[2]

The role of EM is now restricted to selected areas of diagnostic pathology. A common application is the study of renal biopsy specimens in conjunction with immunofluorescent procedures and conventional light microscopy. Some tumors of uncertain histogenesis, after inconclusive light microscopic and immunohistochemical study, may be characterized at the ultrastructural level. Other tissues and cells are studied by EM on occasion: liver, heart, nerve, macrophages (storage disorders), and respiratory epithelium (ciliary dysfunction) are among them. Immunocytochemistry[3] and in situ hybridization[4] can be performed with EM to reveal the subcellular location of antigens. Thus EM constitutes a valuable tool in pathology research.

Aside from cost and technical factors that limit the use of EM in many small hospitals, there is a growing shortage of pathologists who are sufficiently experienced in ultrastructural pathology. A specialist in renal pathology may be knowledgeable in the ultrastructure of the kidney yet be unable to evaluate problematic tumors. The range of ultrastructural changes that can be encountered among human tumors is particularly broad. Therefore the pathologist who interprets diagnostic EM must be familiar with the differential diagnosis by light microscopy. The electron microscopic study of clinical specimens should be performed by a pathologist. Allowing a technician to take random photographs of specimens, which are then perused by the pathologist, can lead to erroneous and missed diagnoses. As emphasized, the information from ultrastructural studies must always be correlated with routine light microscopy, clinical and radiologic data, and immunohistochemistry. The surgical pathologist is the sole physician with sufficient breadth of expertise to integrate this diverse information.

TECHNICAL ISSUES

Electron microscopes

The types of electron microscopes used in diagnostic and experimental pathology are the transmission electron microscope (TEM), the scanning electron microscope (SEM), and the analytical electron microscope.

TEM, the technique best known to pathologists, relies on the passage of a beam of electrons through ultrathin sections of tissues. During staining, the sections have been impregnated with heavy-metal atoms (such as osmium and uranium) that bind to different subcellular organelles. The resolution of TEMs can be as fine as 0.2 nm, but most diagnostic EM is conducted at a relatively low magnification, which ranges from 2000× to 10,000×.

The SEM provides a three-dimensional view of tissues, though the technique is largely confined to providing views of surface architecture[5]; its resolution is inferior to that of the TEM.[6] The SEM provides impressive images of cell surfaces[7-12] and the topographic relationships of components of tissues. Fig. 7-1 shows podocytes with their foot processes ensheathing capillaries in a renal glomerulus. However, in most instances the experienced pathologist can deduce the same information about the surface of a tissue from the two-dimensional images obtained with the TEM and at the same time is able to derive unique and often critical information on the organelle composition of the cells or tissues. The educational contribution of the SEM is nonetheless considerable.

Analytical electron microscopy provides information on the elemental composition of material within tissues.[13-18] Many exogenous materials will incite inflammation (such as granulomas) or be etiologically linked to human disease (such as asbestosis, silicosis). Such materials have characteristic emission spectra, as determined by their constituent elements.

Immunoelectron microscopy allows the precise localization of cellular and subcellular products in tissues. A marker, conjugated to an antibody, serves to identify an antigen within tissues. The markers include peroxidase, ferritin, and gold particles. The latter are now widely used[19] because they are available in different diameters, which permit visualization of more than one antigen.[20] Immunoelectron microscopy is not used for routine diagnosis because most clinical issues can be answered by immunohistochemical studies of paraffin tissue. Immunoelectron microscopy is, however, a valuable research tool because of the precision with which substances can be localized on or within cells.[21-26]

Electron microscopy, to be properly employed as a diagnostic tool, requires attention to details so that a clinically relevant report is provided. A representative sample of tissue must be selected, correctly fixed and processed, and then examined by a pathologist who is familiar with the corresponding light microscopy, the clinical situation, and differential diagnostic issues.

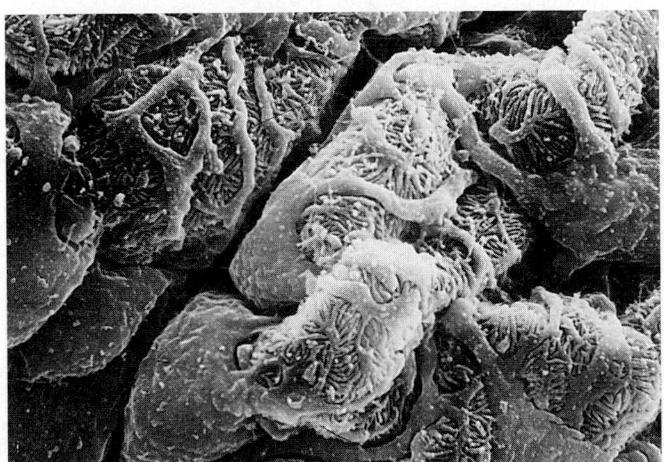

Fig. 7-1 With the scanning electron microscope podocytes are seen ensheathing capillaries of a renal glomerulus. The cytoplasmic arms of the podocytes have many slender secondary processes.

Specimen procurement

Tissue should be obtained for diagnostic electron microscopy whenever it is suspected that the diagnosis will be a problem by light microscopy. The suspicion may arise from difficulty interpreting previous biopsy specimens, the clinical history, or examination of a frozen section or rapid smear. Tissue can be routinely set aside in glutaraldehyde in small labeled bottles, available near the grossing or frozen section area. The tissue can be retained in glutaraldehyde, for weeks if necessary, and then processed if needed for diagnosis.

In larger diagnostic departments where electron microscopy is performed regularly and there is a constant flow of specimens, one may choose to process the electron microscopy tissue daily. If the tissue is already embedded in plastic and examination of the paraffin sections reveals that ultrastructural study is indicated, it is possible to section and examine the electron microscopy specimen and give a verbal opinion within an hour of the request being made.

The importance of specimen collection to diagnostic EM cannot be overemphasized. Minimization of sampling and fixation artifacts is critical. Artifacts that are tolerable by light microscopy interfere with electron microscopy. Tissue preservation must be impeccable for visualization of ultrastructural details. The material that is provided for ultrastructural examination must be representative of the disease. If it is poorly preserved or if it shows degenerative or artifactual changes, the effectiveness of the study may be severely impaired. The area or areas for study must be carefully chosen. There is limited opportunity to be selective when the material is from a fine-needle aspiration biopsy, though immediate screening of a rapid smear can confirm that the aspirated material is suitable. There is again little choice for selection with a core biopsy, but examination of a touch preparation of the surface at specimen collection can provide an indication that the tissue is representative and viable. For renal biopsies, both ends of the core are submitted to ensure that glomeruli are obtained. When material for EM is being selected from a surgical specimen, areas of the surface that show signs of degeneration, necrosis, hemorrhage, or artifactual change must be avoided. The suitability of material can be confirmed by a frozen section or touch preparation of an adjacent slice, but care must be taken to avoid drying of the surface from which tissue is taken for ultrastructural study.

Fixation

Fixatives employed in EM penetrate tissues slowly. Autolytic damage to the cells proceeds until halted by fixation. If an EM fixative penetrates tissue at a rate of 0.5 mm per hour, the specimen should be no more than 1 mm thick if it is to be fixed completely within half an hour. Thus only small thin pieces of solid tissues should be placed into a fixative. Ideally, from solid tissue, a tapering wedge not more than 1 mm in greatest thickness should be sliced off with a fresh scalpel blade and immediately immersed in the fixative solution; once fixation is complete, the slice can be cut up into small cubes about 1 mm in size. The practice of mincing fresh tissue should be avoided, since it is liable to introduce crushing artifact.

Buffered glutaraldehyde is widely used to fix tissues for EM, but tissues fixed in it are brittle and difficult to cut in paraffin blocks. Therefore, some pathologists prefer a mixture of formalin and glutaraldehyde if there is a possibility that paraffin sections may be required. Since the tissue specimen must be small to allow rapid penetration of the fixative, it is preferable to place a small piece of tissue in glutaraldehyde for the electron microscopy and treat the tissue for light microscopy in the usual way. A buffered solution of glutaraldehyde in a strength of 2% to 4% is suitable. After the tissue has been fixed, it is rinsed in buffer and then postfixed in a buffered solution of osmium tetroxide, which enhances the contrast in the sections. It is then dehydrated in graded alcohols and embedded, commonly in an epoxy resin. The customary procedure is to process tissue in one day so that it will be available for sectioning on the following morning. It is possible to shorten the processing time, so that the entire sequence from acquiring the specimen to examining it with the electron microscope can be achieved within 5 hours.[27] This calls for constant attention by a technician and is too labor intensive for routine work in a busy laboratory.

If glutaraldehyde-fixed material was not procured, wet formalin-fixed tissue or even paraffin-embedded tissue may suffice. Wet tissue, provided it has been fixed promptly in buffered formalin, is often quite suitable for ultrastructural study, though the quality of preservation is inferior to that obtained in glutaraldehyde. In selecting formalin fixed tissue for electron microscopy, an area that is likely to be fixed well from the outer surface of a slice should be chosen. Tissue that has been embedded in paraffin is never satisfying to the electron microscopist because of considerable distortion. Sometimes, however, paraffin tissue can provide important data,[28] such as the presence of cell-to-cell junctions or cytoplasmic granules in an unknown neoplasm. Before taking tissue from a paraffin block, the corresponding light microscopic section should be examined so that the best portion of the block can be mapped. A few square millimeters are removed from the block with a scalpel blade, deparaffinized in several changes of xylene, and processed and embedded as for other EM specimens.

Certain types of specimens require special processing for EM. For the more common specimens, these methods are described briefly.

Percutaneous renal biopsy

The complete evaluation of a *percutaneous renal biopsy* requires division of the tissue for light microscopy, immunofluorescent studies, and EM. To ensure that cortical glomeruli are represented in tissue processed for each study, 1 to 2 mm pieces from both ends of the core are placed in glutaraldehyde. The remainder of the core may be sliced longitudinally to provide material for immunofluorescence and paraffin embedding.

Fine-needle aspiration biopsy

There is increasing use of percutaneous *fine-needle aspiration* for tumor diagnosis. Immunohistochemical stains and EM can readily be performed on aspirated material.[29,30] For EM, the preferred method is to express the aspirate directly into buffered glutaraldehyde, with gentle agitation of the specimen bottle to maintain dispersion of the cells and prevent clot formation. The fixed specimen can then be filtered through a fine, 20 μm mesh screen, which allows passage of most of the peripheral blood cells while retaining many of the larger tumor cells and tissue fragments.[31,32] Cells are washed from the filter with buffer and then pelleted by centrifugation. The pellet is processed as for solid tissue.

Bone marrow aspirate

If a heparinized *bone marrow aspirate* is expressed into glutaraldehyde and then centrifuged, peripheral blood cells will greatly outnumber the other cells, so that it is virtually impossible to locate the cells of interest for EM study. The preferred method is to centrifuge the heparinized aspirate in a hematocrit tube and then to remove the buffy coat. If the procedure is performed carefully, the cells will remain together in a wormlike coil, which can be cut into small pieces after fixation.[33] A more elegant method is to centrifuge the aspirate in a tube of larger bore and then to gently layer fixative on the buffy coat; once fixation is complete, the disk can be gently dislodged and transferred to buffer. A gradient separation of different cells can often be detected in sections of these disks.[34]

Core biopsies of bone

Core biopsies of bone are a challenge because decalcifying agents cause severe damage to the structure of the cells. Often, decalcified tissue is unsuitable for ultrastructural evaluation. It is possible but inconvenient to section undecalcified bone for electron microscopy. It is therefore preferable to first fix the core biopsy specimen in glutaraldehyde. The softer marrow tissue can be dislodged with a fine needle under a dissecting microscope and then processed in routine fashion.

Body fluids

If a *fluid specimen,* such as urine, cerebrospinal fluid, or effusion is not frankly bloody, it can be centrifuged to provide a pellet of cells, which are then fixed in glutaraldehyde for electron microscopy. When the effusion is hemorrhagic, many of the erythrocytes can be removed with a brief hemolysis, followed by rinsing in buffer. Correlation of the ultrastructural findings with the routine light microscopic preparations is particularly important with specimens from effusions, since mesothelial cells and macrophages are invariably present and they can readily be confused with tumor cells.

Tissue sectioning

After the tissue has been embedded in plastic, the blocks are sectioned at a thickness of approximately 1 μm. These so-called *thick* or *semithin sections* are usually stained with either methylene blue or toluidine blue. Examination of the semithin sections of the plastic-embedded tissue is important, since it verifies that the blocks selected are representative of the disease process. For example, with a renal biopsy, blocks containing glomeruli that are involved by the disease process but not globally sclerosed are chosen. The quality of tissue preservation can also be assessed, since with severe artifactual distortion a diagnosis may not be possible. If artifacts are patchy, it is often possible to select unaffected areas. Semithin sections from more than one block of a case should be examined to ensure that the best available area is selected. Plastic sections offer more detail than paraffin-embedded sections. Scrutiny of the semithin sections will sometimes help to narrow the differential diagnosis. The actual number of blocks that are cut varies with the specimen and the preferences of the pathologist. For most tumor specimens, two blocks are initially sufficient, and generally only one will be thin sectioned.

Once blocks for ultrastructural examination are selected, thin sections are cut by use of a diamond knife. The technician who cuts the thin sections should have viewed the semithin sections together with the pathologist who is to perform the ultrastructural study. If the selected blocks are only partially representative, the technician must note the areas of the block that can be sacrificed when the block face is trimmed to a size suitable for thin sectioning. The architecture of the tissue in the semithin sections provides a useful guide when viewing the thin sections. At the ultrastructural level, it is not always easy to be certain that cells being examined are part of the pathologic process. In a tumor specimen, for example, a reactive fibroblast can closely resemble a sarcoma cell; a plump endothelial cell may simulate a carcinoma cell; or a macrophage might be mistaken for a lymphoma cell.

The electron microscopist must be aware of the different types of artifacts that can be produced in thin sections during the preparation of the tissues or the sectioning and staining. Delay in fixation results in alterations in the mitochondria and other parts of the cells. Drying of the tissues during dehydration produces uneven densities and blurs the structural detail. Imperfect permeation of the tissue by the plastic embedding medium causes holes in the section. Chatter and knife marks on the sections make them difficult to evaluate. Contamination from the staining procedure can also interfere with the interpretation. The thin sections will have been stained to increase the electron density of the tissues and give the image more contrast. The staining process involves immersing the grid bearing the sections in solutions of the stains, commonly lead citrate and uranyl acetate, and small particles from the stain are sometimes deposited on the sections.

The pathologist performing the EM will, as a rule, have developed impressions from the clinical history and examination of routine light microscopy. In every renal biopsy, particular attention to the filtration barrier is needed. For tumor specimens, a differential diagnosis has probably already been formulated, based on the age of the patient, location of the tumor, any other clinical or radiologic information, the light microscopic appearance, and immunohistochemistry if it has been performed. The differential diagnosis may focus the attention of the pathologist on particular aspects of the structure of the tumor cells, though all the features of the tissue should be examined. It is vital that the observations from the electron microscope be evaluated together with the routine light microscopy and interpreted in the context of the clinical situation. It may be possible to suggest a firm diagnosis from EM alone, but misinterpretation of the ultrastructural findings is all too easy.

ULTRASTRUCTURAL DIAGNOSIS OF NONTUMOR BIOPSIES

Renal biopsies

EM has aided the classification of kidney disease, in particular, and has also contributed to a better understanding of the pathogenesis of glomerular disease.[35-46] EM reveals all the structural details of the glomerulus. Epithelial and endothelial cells, basement membrane, and mesangium can be clearly seen and objectively evaluated. Alterations in these normal components or any extraneous material (such as amyloid) can be accurately assessed. Many lesions that cannot be discerned by light microscopy can be readily evaluated with the electron microscope. An example is minimal change disease, in which the glomeruli appear normal by light microscopy, but ultrastructurally there is extensive epithelial foot process loss and microvillus formation, which are the characteristic features seen in this condition (Fig. 7-2).

EM is the best method available with which to evaluate the thickness and structure of the glomerular basement membrane. The diffuse decrease in its thickness that occurs in patients with benign familial hematuria is easily recognized,[36] as is the increase in the thickness that takes place in diabetic glomerulopathy.[37] The characteristic splitting and reticulation of the lamina densa in patients with hereditary nephritis (Alport's syndrome),[38] and the accumulation of collagen-like fibrils in the basement membrane in patients with hereditary onycho-osteodysplasia (nail-patella syndrome)[39] are structural changes that can be identified only with the electron microscope.

Although the presence of immune complex deposits can be detected by immunofluorescence, it is only with the use of the electron microscope that their exact location within the glomeruli can be determined (Fig. 7-3). The ultrastructural morphologic feature of the immune complex deposits can also provide some clues regarding the cause and pathogenesis of glomerular lesions. Subepithelial dome-shaped deposits ("humps") are often associated with postinfectious glomerulonephritis. Deposits with a fingerprint-like interior are usually seen in lupus nephritis, whereas fibrillar or tubular deposits may indicate cryoglobulinemia[41] or immunotactoid glomerulopathy.[42] Intranuclear tubular inclusions characteristic of lead nephropathy may be detected with EM (Fig. 7-4). Other aspects of renal disease are discussed in Chapter 65.

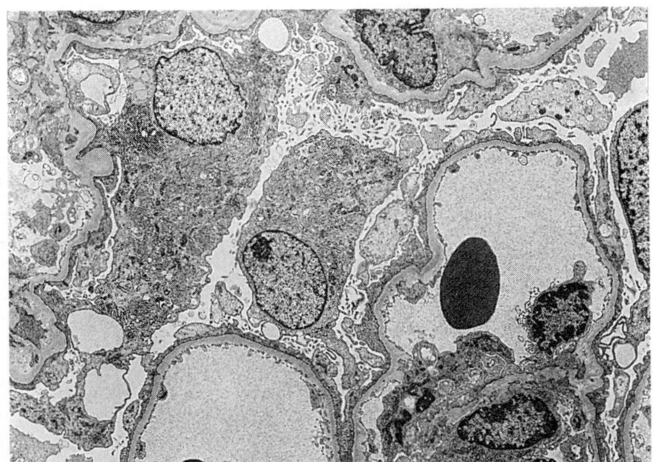

Fig. 7-2 With the transmission electron microscope, the detailed structure of the diseased glomerulus can be examined. The figure shows extensive loss of foot processes of the podocytes in a case of minimal change glomerulopathy.

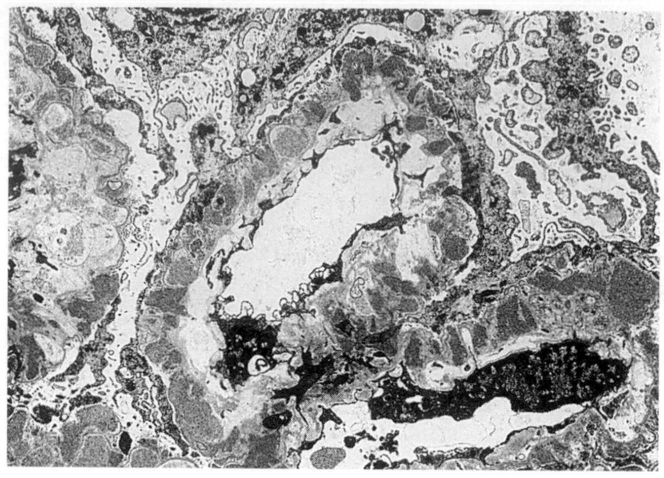

Fig. 7-3 Glomerular deposits are partially encircled by basement membrane material in a case of type III membranous nephropathy.

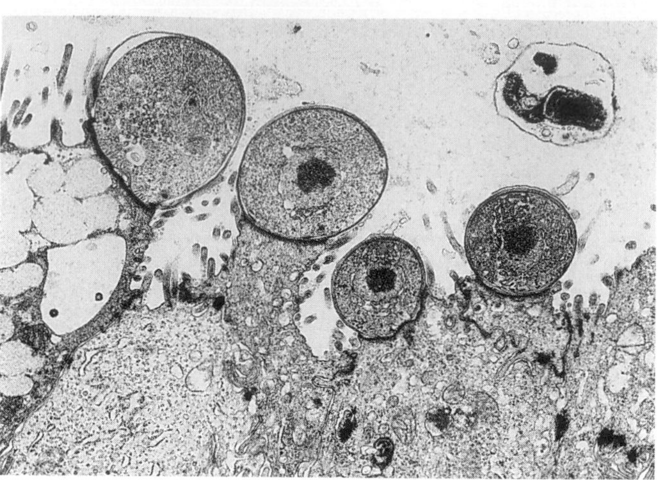

Fig. 7-5 Cryptosporidia attached to the apices of epithelial cells of the large intestine.

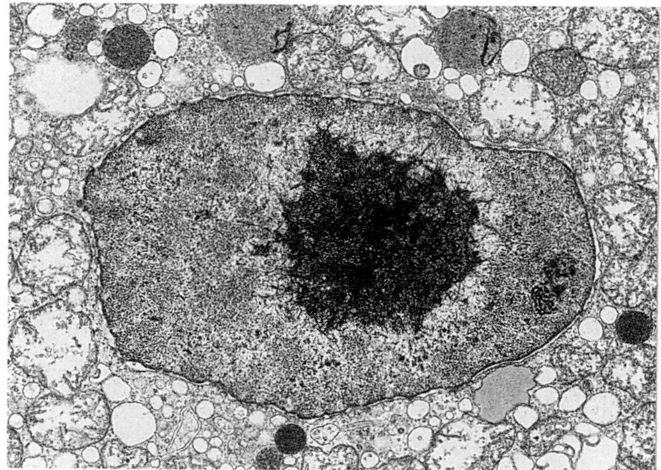

Fig. 7-4 An intranuclear inclusion (renal tubular) from a rat with lead nephropathy.

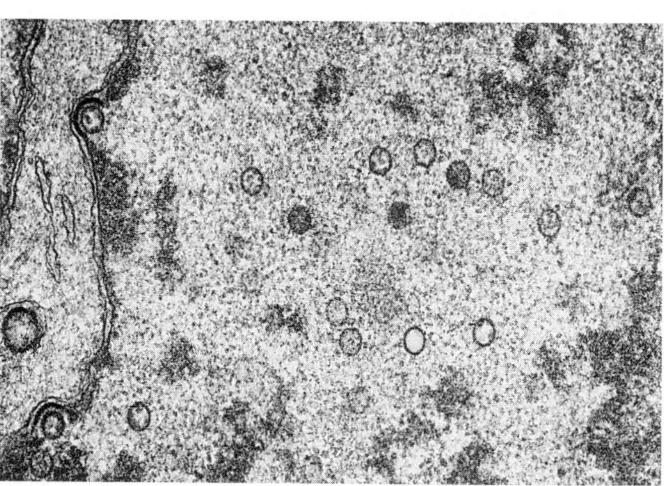

Fig. 7-6 Viral capsids in the nucleus of a varicella–zoster–infected cell from pleural fluid. Two nuclear projections contain viruses with their envelopes continuous with the inner nuclear membrane.

Liver biopsies

Ultrastructural studies improved our understanding of the cellular pathology of liver disease.[47] Specific deposits characterize Wilson's disease and hemochromatosis.[48] Alpha-1-antitrypsin inclusions can be identified in hepatocytes in partial alpha-1-antitrypsin deficiency and chronic liver disease.[49] Glycogen storage disorders and drug-induced liver disease may be characterized by EM.

Microorganisms

TEM has furthered our understanding of viruses and other microorganisms. However, from a practical standpoint, it is exceedingly rare to examine surgical pathology material by EM for microorganisms. One exception is the EM detection of intestinal cryptosporidia[50,51] (Fig. 7-5). A strong indication of their presence is necessary before the study is undertaken.[52] Particularly, now that viruses can be identified in paraffin sections with immunohistochemical or molecular diagnostic methods, this role for EM has diminished greatly. In microbiology laboratories, negative staining of fluid specimens is a rapid method with which to reveal the presence and structure of viruses in secretions, fluids, and feces (Fig. 7-6).[53-55] The electron microscope was instrumental in the initial classification of the human immunodeficiency virus and the Hanta virus outbreak.[56,57]

EM will likely prove valuable for other "new" diseases.

Storage diseases

The accumulation of material within cells characterizes the lipidoses and glycogen storage disorders. EM can visualize such material in biopsy specimens of the skin, brain, rectum, muscle, or nerve.[58-62] In Gaucher's disease, an autosomal recessive disorder of lipid metabolism, abnormal glucocerebrosides accumulate in reticuloendothelial cells in the liver, spleen, lymph nodes, and bone marrow.[63] Sphingomyelin is present in the cells in Niemann-Pick disease.[64] In Fabry's disease, glycolipid produces distinctive lamellar inclusions in many tissues including heart, kidney (Fig. 7-7), and skin.[65]

Amyloidosis, though technically not a storage disease, has distinctive ultrastructural features,[66,67] illustrated in Chapter 20. Lysosomal inclusions appear in cells within the lungs and other tissues in patients with amiodarone pulmonary toxicity.[68]

Respiratory tract biopsies

Documentation of abnormal fine structure of cilia has been used to assess ciliary dysfunction, such as the immotile cilia syndrome.[69,70] The procedure is of questionable value because abnormal ciliary ultrastructure can follow inflammation and occur in normal individuals. Technically, the procedure is difficult and time consuming, since only perfect cross sections through the shaft of the cilium are suitable for evaluation. Many cilia have to be examined before enough are obtained for an adequate assessment. The total needed is arbitrary, but at least 100 true cross sections should be scrutinized in high-magnification micrographs. The material for this study may be obtained from the nasal cavity, but the anterior portion of the cavity should be avoided because here the epithelium is often not ciliated. Rubbing the mucosa with a small brush is an effective method with which to obtain surface cells for EM.

Several abnormalities in ciliary structure have been described. The most obvious structural deviation and the easiest to assess is alterations in the number and pattern of the microtubules that compose the axoneme of the cilium. Normally, nine pairs of peripheral microtubules are evenly distributed around a central doublet, and radial spokes hold them in position. Fused cilia show duplication of the complement of microtubules. Defects in the radial spokes are presumably responsible for the microtubules moving out of position. Study of the dynein arms is difficult, since they are not clearly seen in many micrographs. Respiratory cilia can also be evaluated by various in vivo and in vitro methods.[71]

Skeletal muscle biopsies

Although many alterations in skeletal muscle can be seen at the ultrastructural level, the changes are relatively nonspecific. Nemaline rods are distinctive in nemaline rod myopathy, but they are also seen in some normal skeletal muscle fibers and in a small proportion of cardiac muscle fibers. Disarray of the myofibrils occurs within fibers in congenital multicore disease (Fig. 7-8). Inclusions within myofibrils accompany lysosomal and nonlysosomal storage disorders including Fabry's disease, Pompe's disease, and neuronal ceroid lipofuscinosis. Paracrystalline inclusions occur in various myopathies, including Luft's disease and thyrotoxic periodic paralysis, and in some metabolic disorders. Inclusions with a filamentous appearance have been found within the cytoplasm and nucleus in inclusion body myositis, and at high magnification a tubular substructure has been identified.[72]

Cardiac biopsies

The major indications for examining a biopsy of myocardium with the electron microscope are to search for indications of rejection in a transplant patient[73,74] and to detect and quantitate cardiotoxicity in patients who are receiving anthracycline. Other alterations that may be detected in these biopsy specimens are the presence of amyloid[75] and occasionally of tumor.

Several blocks are selected for thin-sectioning because myocardial abnormalities in cardiotoxicity may be focal and blocks may contain extensive blood clot or fat. Dense core granules within the cytoplasm of the muscle fibers (Fig. 7-9) are an indication that the biopsy has probably been taken from the atrium, the site of atrial natriuretic factor. The features of anthracycline cardiotoxicity are vacuole formation, attributable to dilatation of the sarcoplasmic reticulum, disarray leading to loss of myofibrils (Fig. 7-10), and frank degeneration with accumulation of lysosomes within the cytoplasm of the muscle fibers (Fig. 7-11). Of these, the most reliable indicator of drug induced cardiotoxicity appears to be dropout of the myofibrils. Nemaline rods are sometimes found within the myocardial fibers, yet their presence is not known to be an indicator of cardiotoxicity (Fig. 7-12). The numbers of fibers involved by the different types of change are noted, and the totals are used to provide a numerical grade that indicates the severity of the cardiotoxicity.[76]

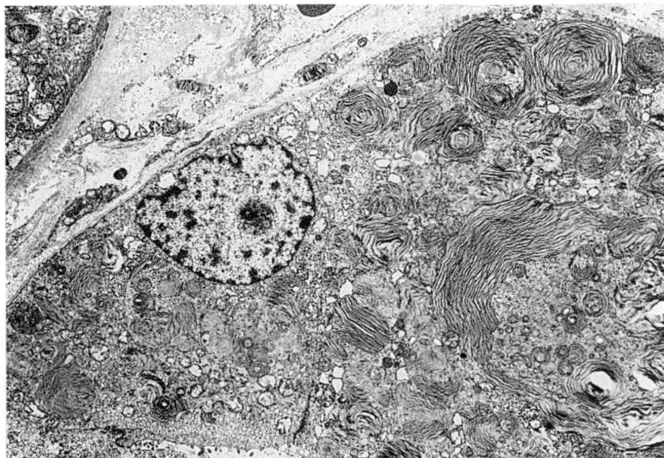

Fig. 7-7 Many inclusions composed of concentric membranes are present within the cytoplasm of renal tubule cells from a patient with Fabry's disease.

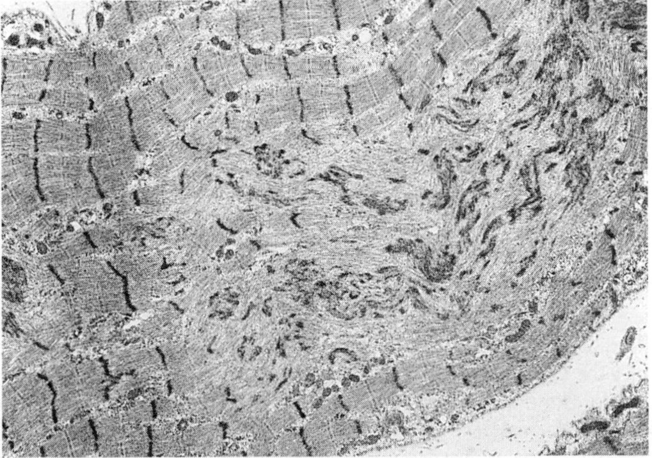

Fig. 7-8 Disarray and streaming of the myofilaments and Z-band material within a skeletal muscle fiber in congenital multicore disease.

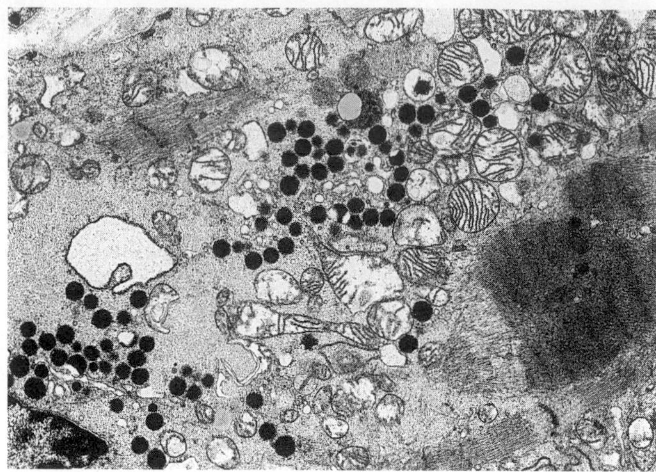

Fig. 7-9 Peptide-containing dense core granules in the cytoplasm of an atrial muscle fiber obtained by endomyocardial biopsy.

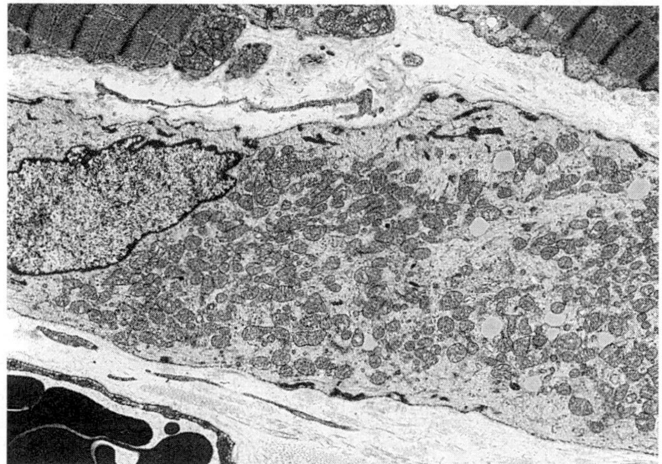

Fig. 7-10 Severe loss of myofibrils in a myocardial muscle fiber from a patient with doxorubicin (Adriamycin) cardiomyopathy.

Brain biopsies

EM is sometimes useful to identify herpes or other viral infections of the brain. Viral particles may be identified in the affected brain cells in subacute sclerosing panencephalitis and progressive multifocal leukoencephalopathy. The electron microscope is a useful adjunct to routine light microscopy and immunocytochemistry in the study and diagnostic evaluation of various central nervous system neoplasms.[77-79]

Peripheral nerve biopsies

Structural damage to peripheral nerves is readily assessed by EM but the changes that are seen are relatively nonspecific. Damage to mitochondria and accumulation of myelin figures may be produced by some metabolic disorders, toxins, and dietary deficiencies. In the rare entity, giant axonal neuropathy, there are extensive aggregates of neurofilaments. A concentric replication of Schwann cell cytoplasm admixed with collagen and basal lamina material is found around axons in the peripheral neuropathy of the Dejerine-Sottas type and in Refsum's disease.[80]

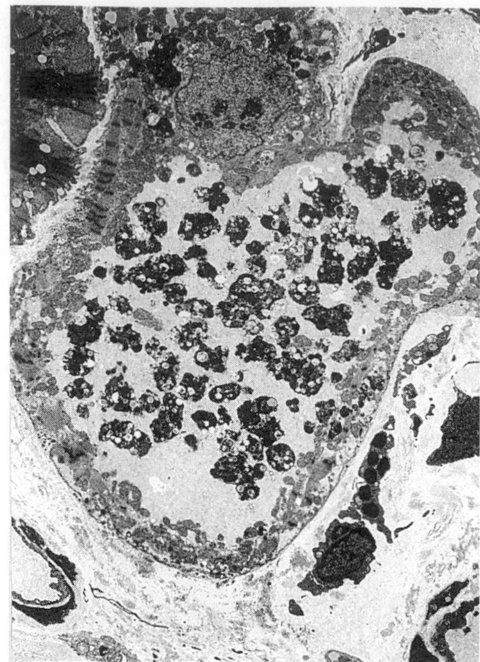

Fig. 7-11 Many lysosomes are present in the cytoplasm of this muscle fiber from the heart of a patient with doxorubicin (Adriamycin) cardiomyopathy.

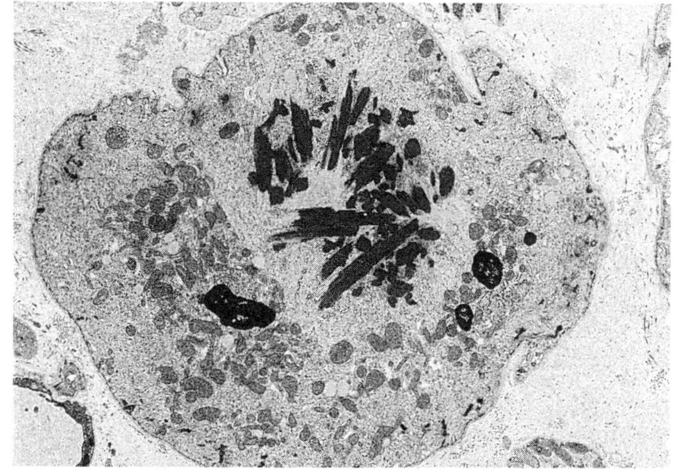

Fig. 7-12 Nemaline rods in a myocardial muscle fiber.

ULTRASTRUCTURE OF TUMORS

TEM plays an important but selective role in the diagnostic study of tumors. The electron microscope will always provide some relevant information on a problematic tumor, and it sometimes is the only method whereby a firm diagnosis can be reached. Often, ultrastructural study will serve to condense a differential diagnosis that has been reached by light microscopy and immunohistochemistry. The following summary of tumor ultrastructure provides some examples wherein diagnostic EM can be useful and describes features that are characteristic of different tumors.

A systematic approach first requires examination of the stroma, with the size, shape, and relationships of the tumor cells being noted. If they are in contact with one another, the presence and type of any *cell junctions* is important. The cell surfaces are viewed for *surface specializations* such as microvilli. It can be difficult to gauge the *shape* of cells in thin two-dimensional sections, but if sufficient cells are present for study, it is usually possible to determine whether they are uniformly round or irregular. It is important to detect the presence of cytoplasmic extensions, since these are often well developed on cells of neural tumors. The shape of the nucleus and size and density of the nucleoli can be assessed effectively in semithin sections by light microscopy, but they are seen more clearly with the electron microscope. Moreover, the occurrence of specializations in the nuclear surface such as pockets, or the presence of intranuclear inclusions, can be determined.

Substantial morphologic information regarding the tumor cells is found in the cytoplasm. Put otherwise, the lineage of a given cell is often reflected in its cytoplasm, even in neoplastic cells. It may take the form of the number or paucity of the organelles, or their relative proportions, or deviations from their normal structure. Dense bodies within the cytoplasm are often informative, but the pathologist must distinguish lysosomes from protein secretory products. Any other secretory material that is present and any abnormal components of the cytoplasm are documented. It is not feasible in this short summary to attempt to enumerate all the features that the pathologist might find, but some of the more important are described below. The enormous range and variety of the fine structure of cells, normal and abnormal, is impressively conveyed in the text *Ultrastructural Pathology of the Cell and Matrix* by Ghadially.[81]

Epithelial tumors

In addition to establishing that a particular tumor is a carcinoma, ultrastructural features may provide a clue to the origin of metastatic tumors.

The cells of epithelial tumors are usually connected to one another by sites of *junctional specialization*. The desmosome is the most recognized junction seen in epithelial tumors; in its mature form it is readily identified. Desmosomes are found in carcinomas of all types though they are best seen in squamous tumors (Fig. 7-13, *A*), where they can be numerous. As tumors dedifferentiate, however, the cell junctions become fewer in number and more primitive in their structure (Fig. 7-13, *B*). In a poorly differentiated carcinoma, the only junctions may be mere thickenings or densities of the apposed cell membranes.

Other cell junctions in epithelial tumors include junctional complexes of adenocarcinoma, which include tight junctions at the luminal surface and zonula adherens. With dedifferentiation, the tight junctions may persist. Cytokeratin filaments are found in squamous carcinoma cells (Fig. 7-13) though, like the junctions, they tend to become sparse with loss of differentiation. They are not usually prominent in glandular neoplasms or in small cell carcinomas.

The ultrastructural appearance of squamous carcinoma is the same, regardless of its site of origin. Differences in the amount of keratin are of no aid in determining the primary site if the tumor is metastatic. The electron microscopist can identify the origin of some metastatic glandular neoplasms, since the cells may be forming a secretory product that betrays the cell type.[82] Other features of the cells are of more limited value. Uniform microvilli are found in neoplastic gastrointestinal epithelial cells (Fig. 7-14), but they can appear in neoplasms of other foregut derivatives, including the biliary passages, and they are occasionally encountered in a tumor of the respiratory tract or ovary. Thus, although a picket fence-like array of microvilli on metastatic adenocarcinoma cells will indicate gastrointestinal origin, other possibilities must also be considered. Clusters of microvilli can be found by EM in some adenocarcinomas that appear solid in paraffin sections (Fig. 7-15). A basal lamina is sometimes present on malignant epithelial cells though it may be incomplete. Replication of the basal lamina is a feature of some salivary

Fig. 7-13 A, Connections between neighboring cells can be seen in this well-differentiated squamous cell carcinoma of the lip. *Inset,* One of the connecting strands is shown in greater detail and a desmosome is visible.

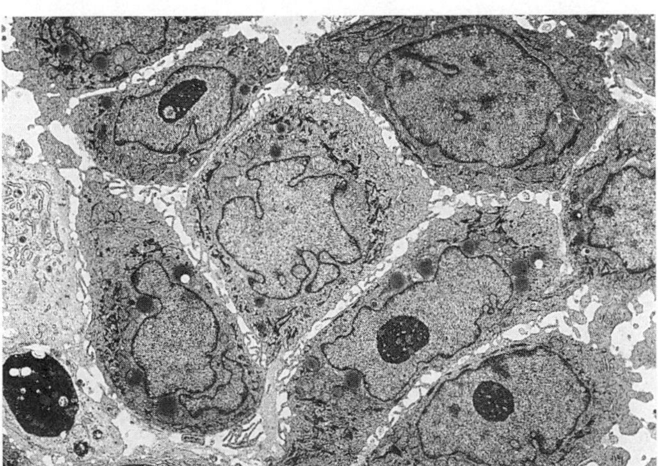

Fig. 7-13 B, Squamous cell carcinoma. The tumor is only moderately differentiated and desmosomes are inconspicuous, but cytokeratin is plentiful within the cytoplasm of the tumor cells.

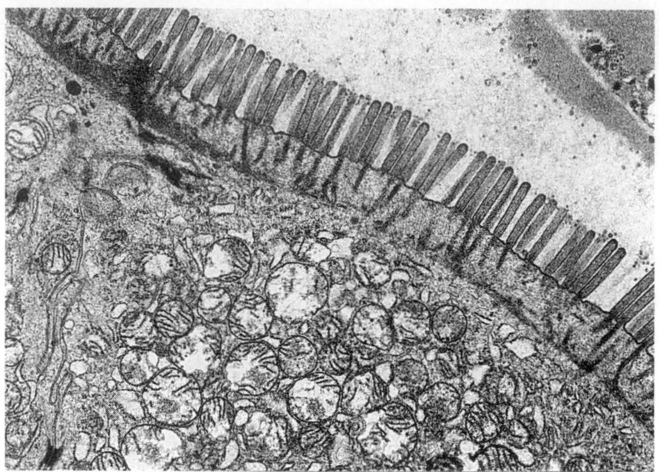

Fig. 7-14 The microvilli on cells of adenocarcinomas of the gastrointestinal tract often present this picket fence-like array. Actin filaments from the interior of the microvilli form a terminal web in the apical cytoplasm.

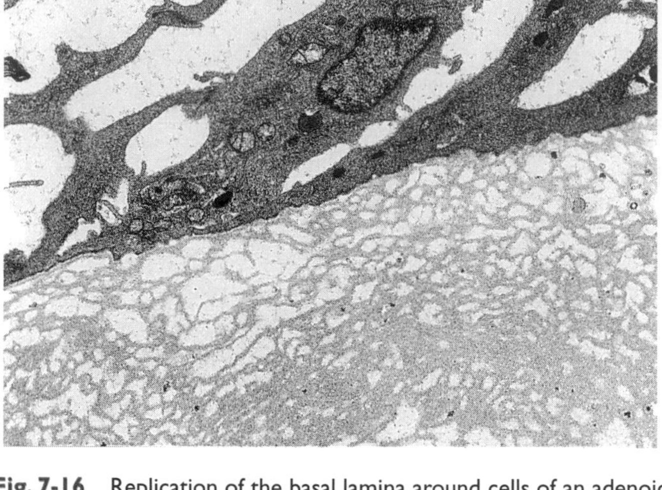

Fig. 7-16 Replication of the basal lamina around cells of an adenoid cystic carcinoma of the parotid gland.

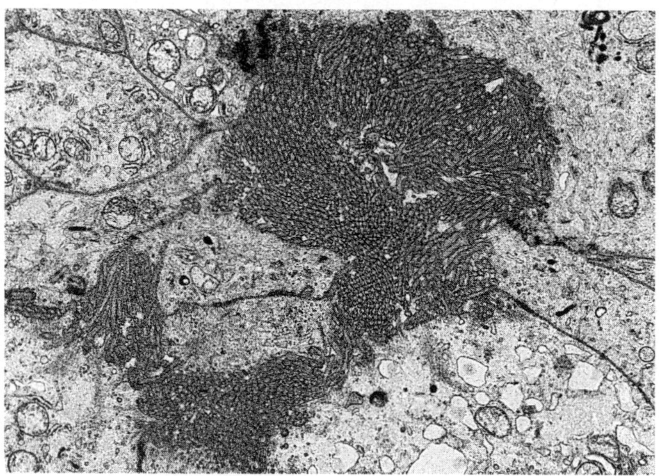

Fig. 7-15 This adenocarcinoma appeared solid in paraffin sections, but microvilli were clearly visible with the electron microscope.

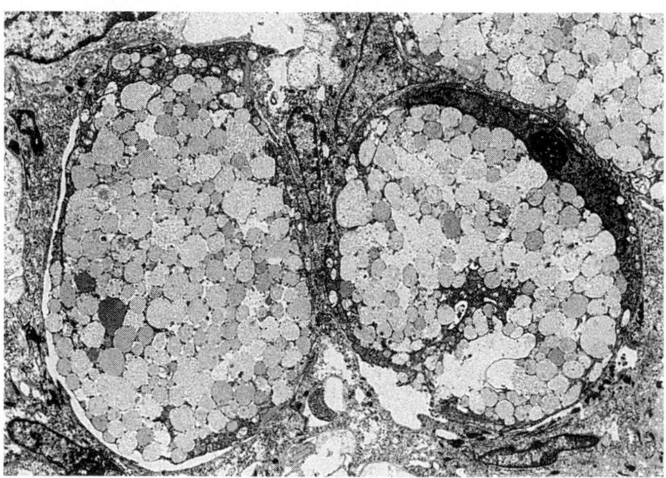

Fig. 7-17 Mucin droplets occupy the cytoplasm of cells of Paget's disease involving the vulva.

tumors, as shown in the adenoid cystic carcinoma in Fig. 7-16.

Useful information is often obtained from the quantity and appearance of the endoplasmic reticulum, ribosomes, and mitochondria in tumor cells. Extensive ribosome-bearing reticulum is typical of cells of protein-secreting tumors. The cells usually contain dense-core granules, which represent the stored secretion. The cisternae of the reticulum may align in parallel, and this feature is seen particularly well in plasma cells and some exocrine cells such as those of the pancreas. In endocrine cells, short cisternae will frequently be arranged in stacks. In contrast, the reticulum is typically sparse, and many of the ribosomes lie free within the cytoplasm in cells of lymphoid and hematopoietic neoplasms. Mitochondria vary in their size, shape, number, and appearance in different tumors. Among the more distinctive variations are the large dense intramatrical mitochondrial inclusions, probably consisting of lipid, that are seen in some adrenocortical and renal tumors[83] and the large number of mitochondria in oncocytic cells.[84]

Mucin in carcinoma cells may take the form of discrete droplets (Fig. 7-17) or form diffuse, electron-lucent zones within the cytoplasm. Glycogen can also be recognized readily by EM, though it is relatively ubiquitous among tumors and of limited value in differential diagnosis. Protein secretions take the form of dense granules that accumulate within the cytoplasm. Before concluding that dense bodies in the cytoplasm of a metastatic carcinoma are secretory granules, it is necessary to consider the possibility that they may be lysosomes. The distinction is not always possible, but true secretory granules tend to be numerous in many cells of a tumor and to be fairly uniform in shape, size, and internal composition. Lysosomes, in contrast, will often be irregular in size and shape and have a heterogeneous interior.

Secretory granules tend to fall within a limited range of diameters for a particular cell type. The size of the granules is therefore useful. The appearance of the granules is of less value, though some distinctive appearances are seen among endocrine tumors. Pheochromocytoma cells, for example, often contain granules with ovoid, loose-fitting limiting membranes and eccentrically placed cores (Fig. 7-18), and a beta cell islet cell tumor may have granules with crystalline cores.

The approximate size of secretory granules can be gauged when one compares them with the mitochondria. Extremely accurate measurement is obtained when a morphometric analysis is performed on the electron micrographs. Such studies show that although the granules in tumor cells are slightly smaller than those in the corresponding normal cells, most of the granules within the cells of endocrine neoplasms fall within a range of 100 to 400 nm in diameter (Fig. 7-19). In contrast, the granules in an exocrine cell carcinoma are distinctly larger. Those in the acinic cell carcinoma of the parotid shown in Fig. 7-20 averaged close to 600 nm. Salivary tumors and pulmonary bronchioloalveolar adenocarcinomas are other examples of tumors whose cells contain granules of this size.

Cells that produce steroid secretion have certain unique ultrastructural characteristics that are often recapitulated in their tumors. Two features are of particular note. The endoplasmic reticulum is often smooth surfaced, forming slender anastomosing tubules or flattened cisternae (Fig. 7-21), and mitochondria may possess tubular (Fig. 7-22) rather than the usual shelflike cristae. Both features may be present in tumor cells, but they are not always found and occasionally they are seen in other tumors, and so correlation with the light microscopy and clinical information is always necessary.

Mesothelioma

As well as satisfying the inquiries of clinicians, a diagnosis of mesothelioma may be of considerable interest to members of the legal profession. The clinical and radiographic findings coupled with routine light microscopy or cytologic features of a pleural effusion may suffice to establish that a particular tumor is a mesothelioma, yet this tumor displays a broad range of morphology. In part, this stems from the ability of the multipotential submesothelial mesenchymal cell to differentiate into cells with an epithelial morphology and phenotype.[85] A neoplasm arising from the pleura may therefore be composed

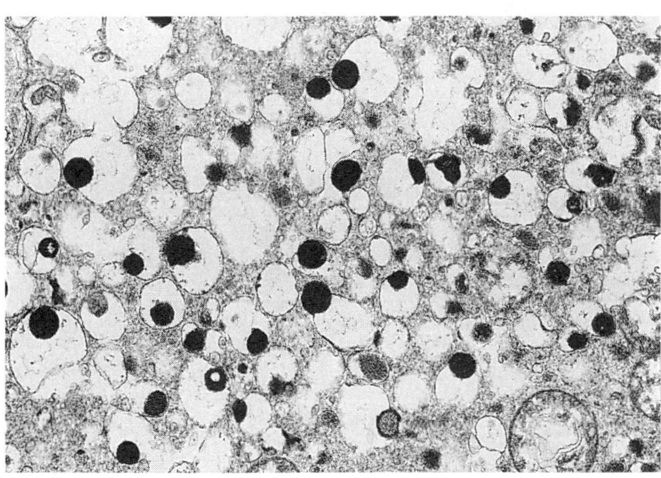

Fig. 7-18 Many of the granules in pheochromocytoma cells have ovoid limiting membranes and eccentrically positioned dense cores.

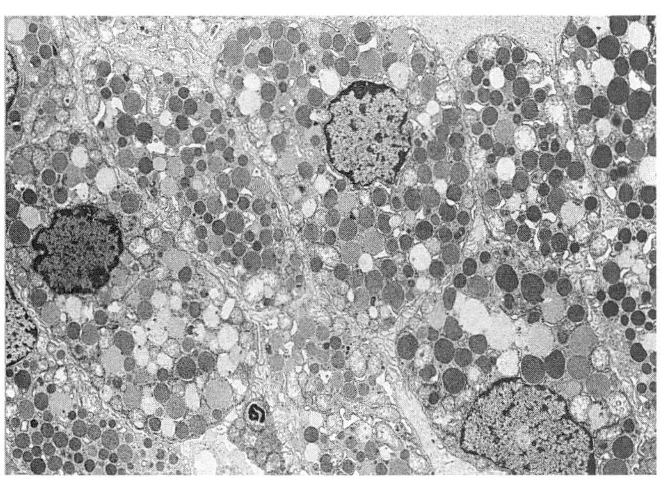

Fig. 7-20 The granules in the cells of an acinic cell carcinoma of the parotid gland appear similar in size to those of the carcinoid in the preceding figure, but the magnification of this photograph is lower and the granules in this tumor are almost twice as large.

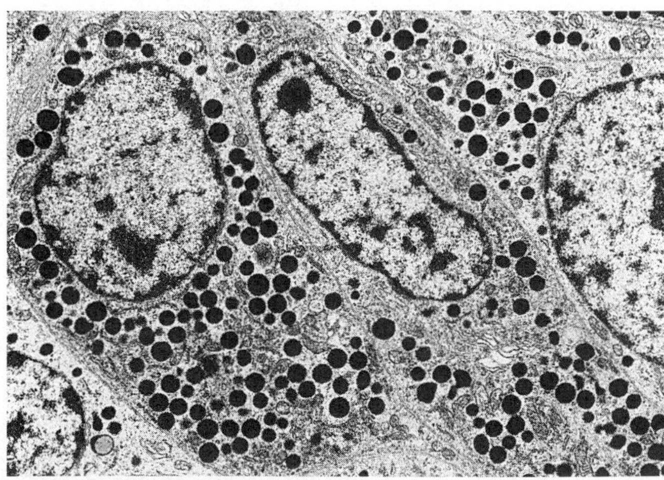

Fig. 7-19 Numerous round, relatively uniform granules are present within the cytoplasm of the cells of this bronchial carcinoid tumor.

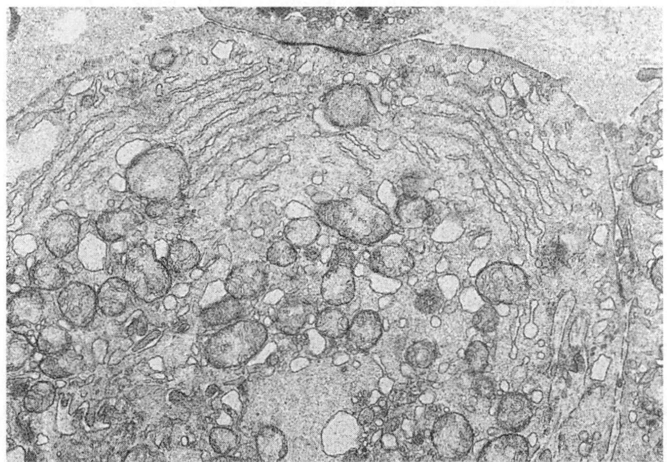

Fig. 7-21 The endoplasmic reticulum in this cell from an interstitial cell tumor of the testis is forming parallel cisternae whose membranes are devoid of ribosomes.

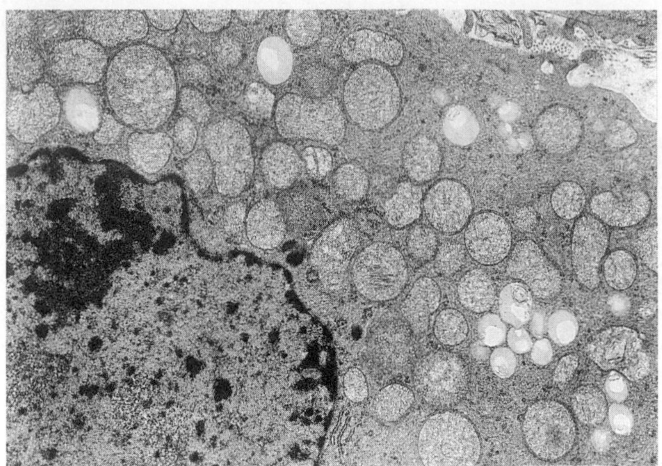

Fig. 7-22 Mitochondria with tubular cristae from an adrenocortical adenoma.

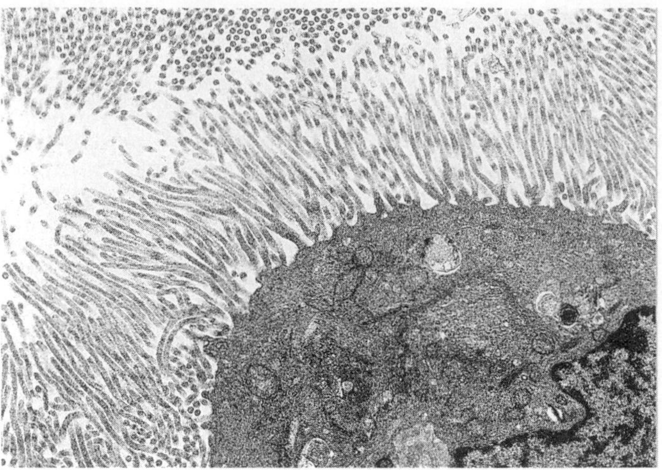

Fig. 7-23 The characteristic long, slender, often branching and curving microvilli of mesothelioma.

of spindle cells with the features of fibroblasts or myofibroblasts or be purely epithelial; transitional forms and mixed variants occur. The transformation of the submesothelial mesenchymal cell is accompanied by alterations in its immunostaining properties from being vimentin-positive through a phase in which the cells show evidence for low molecular weight cytokeratin but no longer for vimentin. Later on, they may revert to the mature epithelial phenotype characterized by staining for high molecular weight keratin.

Spindle cell tumors of the pleura may be composed of cells that ultrastructurally are fibroblasts or myofibroblasts. The spindle cells of some solitary fibrous tumors of the pleura appear mesenchymal by EM, but they may not possess the extensive endoplasmic reticulum of the classic fibroblast or show myofibroblastic differentiation. In transitional forms of mesothelioma, spindle cells may even disclose hints of an epithelial structure in the presence of small lumens bordered by microvilli.

Most malignant tumors of the pleura are epithelial mesotheliomas that form glandlike or papillary structures, nests, or solid sheets of cells. Immunohistochemical studies will aid in separating the glandular and papillary mesothelioma from adenocarcinomas, since the latter will usually mark with anticarcinoembryonic antigen, B72.3, or Leu-M1. Mesotheliomas are negative for these markers (see Chapter 8). The ultrastructural appearance of mesothelioma is also characteristic,[86] since the cells frequently show microvilli that are similar to those seen on the normal mesothelial surface. They are profuse and closely packed, forming a luxuriant array that tends to clothe many of the free surfaces of the cells rather than lining circumscribed acini, and it is common to find a layer of microvilli filling narrow clefts between neighboring cells. The microvilli are slender, and they curve and often branch (Fig. 7-23). In their fully developed form, the microvilli can be ascribed to mesothelial cells with considerable confidence, but with dedifferentiation, they become shorter and lose their distinctive features, and separation of an epithelial mesothelioma from an adenocarcinoma becomes difficult and ultimately impossible. Some dedifferentiated mesotheliomas cannot be distinguished from poorly differentiated carcinomas.

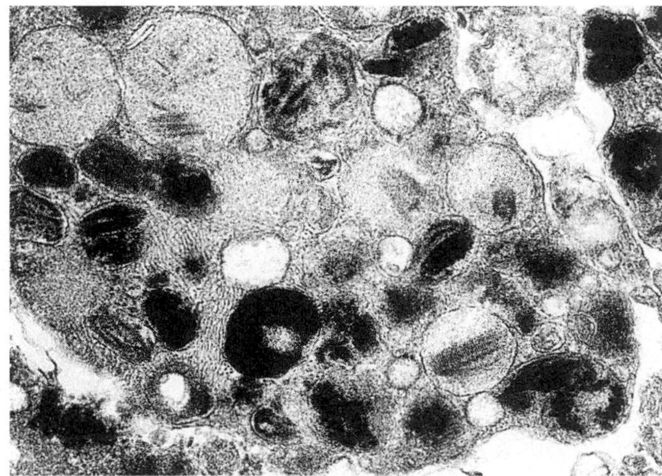

Fig. 7-24 A cutaneous melanoma cell containing many melanosomes in varying stages of maturation. The fine periodicity of the type II premelanosome can be seen.

Melanoma

The wide variety of forms that melanoma cells can present in light microscopy is recapitulated ultrastructurally. Most melanomas mark with anti-S-100 protein or the HMB-45 monoclonal antibody. However, some do not, and diagnosis may then require EM to demonstrate melanosomes, the hallmark of melanoma. Melanosomes are cytoplasmic organelles within which melanin is formed through the action of tyrosinase. Melanosomes have a well-defined sequence of maturation. The earliest form is a vacuole, roughly the size of a primary lysosome. Electron-dense material condenses in its interior to produce a rodlike core with a fine periodicity, and as the melanin is progressively deposited on this framework, the periodic structure is gradually obscured until in the mature melanosome it can no longer be seen (Fig. 7-24). The mature melanosome cannot be reliably distinguished from a lysosome, and so it is the identification of the premelanosome with its barred structure that establishes that dense bodies are melanosomes. The recognition of numerous dense bodies within the cytoplasm of cells of a suspected melanoma at low magnification will lead the electron microscopist to screen at higher magnifications searching for premelanosomes. Melanosomes and premelanosomes are not pathognomonic of melanoma because they occasionally occur in other tumors. Many nevus cells contain them, and nevi can occur in extracutaneous locations including mucosal surfaces, lymph nodes, and meninges. Carcinomas arising in or spreading to the skin may contain melanosomes, sometimes in considerable numbers. They are also found, albeit rarely, in cells of Schwann cell tumors, where their presence can be attributed to the common embryologic heritage of the melanocyte and Schwann cell.

A problem arises with the melanoma in which the cells are devoid of premelanosomes. If only mature melanosomes are found by ultrastructural examination, the diagnosis may be strongly suspected, but it cannot be confidently given. The index of suspicion may be heightened when one observes certain fine structural features, such as the presence of parallel arrays of microtubules within cisternae of the endoplasmic reticulum, but this is an uncommon finding, seen in fewer than 5% of melanomas; moreover, it is not unique to melanoma. EM may nonetheless be useful in the differential diagnosis by exclusion of other tumors that could not be ruled out by other means.

Melanoma cells may manifest their common ancestry with Schwann cells by undergoing a type of neural transformation in which they develop greatly elongated cytoplasmic extensions and become organized into bundles. This type of alteration is seen in some desmoplastic melanomas, and it has been referred to as neurotropic, or neurosarcomatous, transformation.[87] The cells tend to lose their melanosomes but may retain immunostaining properties. The range of morphology of melanoma extends to balloon cell, myxoid, and signet-ring types. Soft-tissue melanomas presumably arise from melanocytes that have become sequestered within soft tissues in the course of their embryologic migration to the skin. In these tumors, it is usually not difficult to find some melanosomes and premelanosomes, and the nucleoli are often particularly large and dense.[88]

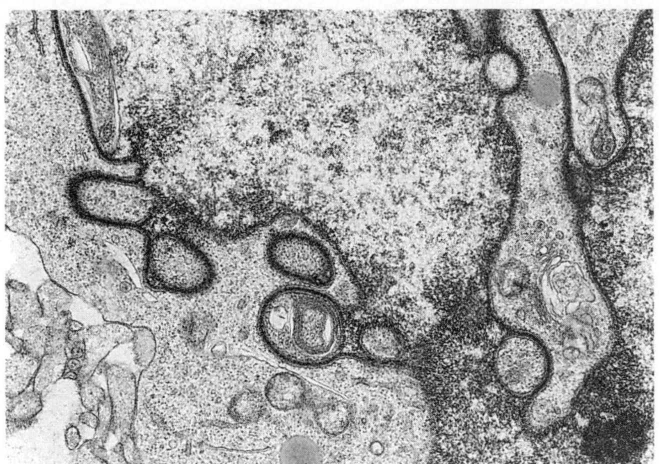

Fig. 7-25 Nuclear pockets in a large cell lymphoma cell.

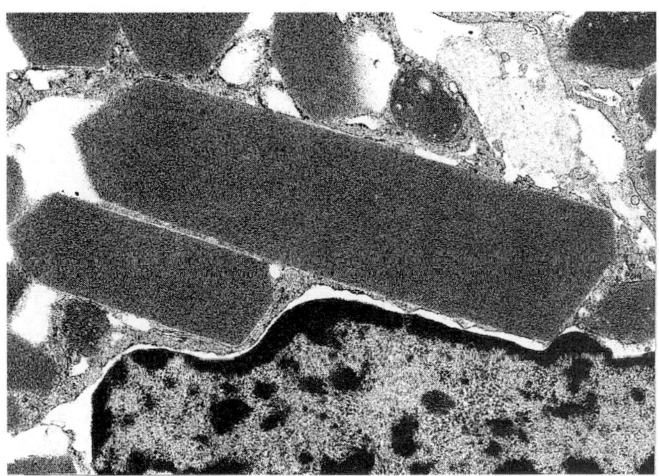

Fig. 7-26 Many crystals were present in the cells of this lymphoplasmacytic lymphoma, which had formed diffuse lung infiltrates.

Hematopoietic and lymphopoietic tumors

Immunohistochemical and molecular procedures are the usual approach to the diagnosis and subclassification of tumors in this category. In an assessment of the light microscopic appearance of the cells, high magnification examination of the semithin plastic-embedded sections can often be informative, since the nuclear morphology and profiles can be assessed with considerable precision.

The proliferating cells of leukemias and lymphomas will often have distinctive features at the ultrastructural level, such as nuclear pockets (Fig. 7-25), and a few are sufficiently singular to be of value in diagnosis. Even when the cells are closely packed, there is no good evidence of attachment sites between them: at most, a rare tiny density of the apposed cell membranes is identified. Larger specializations are seen in some histiocytes, however. In many lymphomas, there is a notable lack of endoplasmic reticulum, and the cytoplasm is filled with free ribosomes. Mitochondria are also sparse, but lipid droplets can be present in some undifferentiated and large cell lymphomas. With immunoblastic transformation, the cisternae of the endoplasmic reticulum become abundant and organized, leading ultimately to the orderly parallel organization that is seen in the plasma cell.

Dense bodies within cells of leukemias and lymphomas range from the small lysosomes of a granulocytic sarcoma to large crystalline bodies in some plasma cells[89] (Fig. 7-26). One of the best known structures in this category is the Birbeck granule, which occurs in Langerhans cells.[90] This is a cytoplasmic rod-shaped body with an internal periodicity. These bodies are evidently endocytotic organelles that transport antigens from receptors on the cell surface to the interior of the cell where they fuse with saccules of the Golgi complex producing a racket-like configuration (Fig. 7-27). Their presence, in the correct clinical setting, establishes the diagnosis of Langerhans cell histiocytosis.

Soft-tissue tumors

The range of fine structure that can be encountered within sarcomas is particularly extensive, and there are many unique features that can be used to classify the tumors when such is difficult by light microscopy.[91]

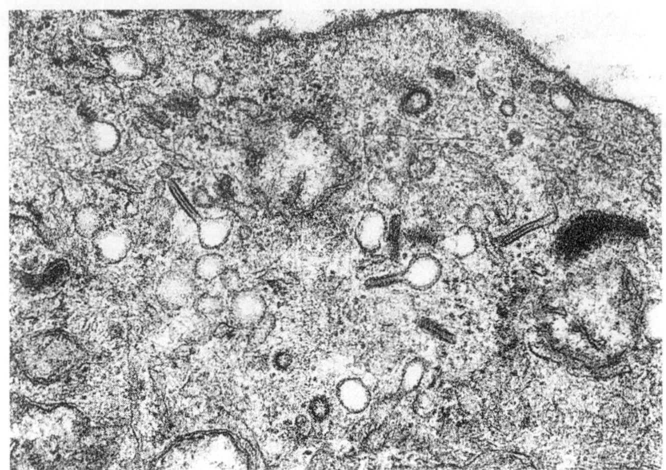

Fig. 7-27 Birbeck granules from a case of Langerhans cell histiocytosis. Two of the granules show the distinctive racketlike configuration.

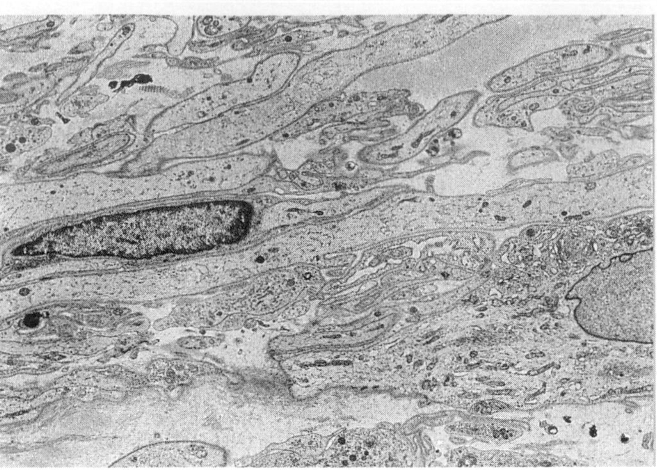

Fig. 7-28 Long cytoplasmic extensions of schwannoma cells are sectioned in different planes.

It is beyond the scope of this chapter to detail the fine structure of the different tumors of the soft tissues. The following paragraphs offer only a brief summary of some of the major features.

In part, the variation from one tumor to another results from production of different amounts or types of ground substance by the neoplastic cells. There also can be overlap in the structural properties of the cells, as exemplified by the occurrence of smooth muscle myofilaments in some neoplastic fibroblasts, or skeletal muscle myofilaments in a dedifferentiated chondrosarcoma. The histogenesis of many soft-tissue tumors is uncertain, causing difficulty in classification. The tendency to subdivide sarcomas into categories and append descriptive names based on differences in the light microscopic appearance may not be easily reconciled with the fine structure.

A significant structural feature of sarcomas is cytoplasmic intermediate filaments. They are not unique to this category of neoplasm but are found more often and in greater quantities than in most other neoplasms. The intermediate filaments can be grouped into different types based on their molecular composition; immunohistochemical methods are extremely useful to identify the different filament types in tumor cells. Keratin is principally found in epithelial cells. But it may also occur in certain sarcomas, notably the epithelial cells of synovial sarcomas, and in epithelioid sarcomas; rare instances are recorded of keratin immunoreactivity in other sarcomas including leiomyosarcoma and rhabdomyosarcoma. To the electron microscopist, the filaments may be nonspecific as in epithelioid sarcoma, or specific as in myogenic tumors, and the latter can be separated into smooth and skeletal muscle types.

Some soft-tissue neoplasms have more or less unique ultrastructural features that can aid in their identification. The long cytoplasmic extensions of schwannian tumors are distinctive (Fig. 7-28). Among the more striking cytoplasmic findings are the lysosomes of a granular cell tumor, found also in the uncommon malignant examples, the arrays of microtubules within cisternae in some extraskeletal myxoid chondrosarcomas, and the crystals of an alveolar soft part sarcoma. In contrast, a minority of soft-tissue sarcomas are composed of cells that lack any specific features that would serve to place them within a defined subcategory. Although this may be suspected by light microscopy, it is only by ultrastructural examination of the cells that such a tumor can be confidently placed in the category of primitive sarcoma. Clinicopathologic studies have not yet been conducted to determine if there is prognostic significance in this designation.

Central nervous system tumors

EM can complement routine light microscopy in the diagnostic evaluation of a tumor of the central nervous system. Among the gliomas, there are overlapping features, such that a clear separation of astrocytes and oligodendroglial cells is not always possible. A hallmark of a typical ependymoma in paraffin sections is an acellular zone around small vessels. With the electron microscope, this is seen to be formed by many concentrically oriented processes of the tumor cells, which are rich in intermediate filaments. An undulating basal lamina will often be present at the periphery of the band of processes, where it abuts on the perivascular collagen. Most ependymomas also contain lumens; microvilli and cilia may be found within them (Fig. 7-29). Small lumens filled with microvilli will not be identified by the light microscopist. Similar features occur in extra-axial ependymomas, and EM is useful in their identification, since mature cilia are uncommon in tumors.

The tendency of neurogenic cells to develop cytoplasmic processes is exemplified in meningiomas. The cell surface often undulates, and processes may curve elaborately, creating a filigree pattern when the cells are loosely distributed, or multicurving surfaces if they are apposed. A basal lamina is sometimes found. Many meningioma cells contain nonspecific intermediate filaments, and some cells are large with plentiful cytoplasm that is replete with filaments. Cell junctions are common between the tumor cells, and there are often well-formed desmosomes.

Small round cell tumors

The convenient umbrella term *small round cell tumors* encompasses several defined entities, as well as some tumors

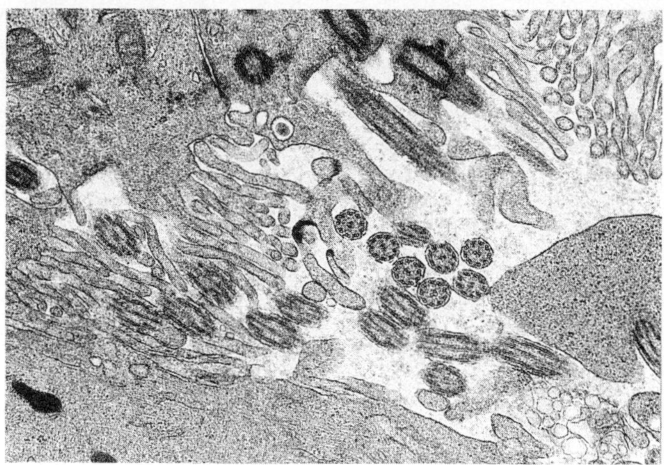

Fig. 7-29 Cilia and microvilli from an ependymoma.

that morphologically fit within the group but cannot be further characterized. By light microscopy, the tumors have in common a population of uniform small cells, typically spherical but sometimes ovoid or even elongated, with a central nucleus that is similar in shape to the cell. A pattern may be discerned by light microscopy, as in the rosettes of a neuroblastoma, but often the cells form contiguous sheets, rendering classification difficult. With immunohistochemistry, some tumors can be confidently classified (see Chapter 8).

In the assessment of a small round cell tumor that cannot be classified by other means, EM is particularly valuable. It may reveal no evidence of differentiation other than lakes of cytoplasmic glycogen, findings that are in keeping with a diagnosis of Ewing's tumor; yet various other features can be informative. For example, the dendritic processes of neuroblastoma cells containing microtubules and small dense-core granules that vary in frequency but can readily be recognized by the electron microscopist. Although myofilaments of skeletal muscle type are not always present in an embryonal or alveolar rhabdomyosarcoma, finding them will confirm the diagnosis that usually will have been made or suspected from the results of immunostaining or molecular analyses.

REFERENCES

1. Ruska E: *The early development of electron lenses and electron microscopy* (translated by T. Mulvey), Stuttgart, 1980, S. Hirzel Verlag.
2. Mackay B, Ordóñez NG: Pathological evaluation of neoplasms with unknown primary tumor site, *Semin Oncol* 20:206, 1993.
3. Tomita T, Watanabe I, Rengachary SS: Immunoelectron microscopy for growth hormone and prolactin in pituitary adenomas, *Hum Pathol* 18:367, 1987.
4. Binder M, Tourmente S, Roth J et al: In situ hybridization at the electron microscopy level: localization of transcripts on ultrathin sections of Lowicryl K4M–embedded tissue using biotinylated probes and protein A–gold complexes, *J Cell Biol* 102:1646, 1986.

Types of electron microscopes

5. Boyde A, Reid SA: A new method of scanning electron microscopy for imaging biological tissues, *Nature* 302:522, 1983.
6. Joy DC, Pawley JB: High-resolution scanning electron microscopy, *Ultramicroscopy* 47:80, 1992.
7. Beals TF: Scanning electron microscopy of body fluids, *Diagn Cytopathol* 8:266, 1992.
8. Akhtar M, Ali MA, Sackey K et al: Aspiration cytology of neuroblastoma: light microscopy with transmission and scanning electron microscopic correlations, *Diagn Cytopathol* 4:323, 1988.
9. Ng WL, Chan KW, Ma L: A scanning electron microscope study of isolated glomeruli in glomerulonephritis, *Pathology* 15:139, 1983.
10. Burton GJ: Scanning electron microscopy of intervillous connections in the mature human placenta, *J Anat* 147:245, 1986.
11. Horn T, Henriksen JH, Christoffersen P: The sinusoidal lining cells in "normal" human liver: a scanning electron microscopic investigation, *Liver* 6:98, 1986.
12. Baskerville A, Dowsett AB, Cook RW et al: *Pneumocystis carinii* pneumonia in simian immunodeficiency virus infection: immunohistological and scanning and transmission electron microscopical studies, *J Pathol* 164: 175, 1991.
13. Roggli VL, Pratt PC, Brody AR: Asbestos fiber type in malignant mesothelioma: an analytical scanning electron microscopic study of 94 cases, *Am J Ind Med,* 23:605, 1993.
14. Tvedt KE: Analytical electron microscopy—a diagnostic tool? [editorial], *Ultrastruct Pathol* 15:iii, 1991.
15. Irie H, Mori W: Long term effects of thorium dioxide (Thorotrast) administration on human liver: ultrastructural localization of thorium dioxide in human liver by analytical electron microscopy, *Acta Pathol* 34:221, 1984.
16. Pooley RD, Ranson DL: Comparison of the results of asbestos fibre dust counts in lung tissue obtained by analytical electron microscopy and light microscopy, *J Clin Pathol* 39:313, 1986.
17. McMahon JT: Analytical electron microscopy in pneumoconiosis, *Cleveland Clin Q* 52:530, 1985.
18. Izutsu K, Wilkinson L, Oda D et al: Comparison of elemental concentrations in the acinar cells of the human labial salivary gland, *Arch Oral Biol* 36:727, 1991.
19. Silver MM, Hearn SA: Postembedding immunoelectron microscopy using protein A-gold, *Ultrastruct Pathol* 11:693, 1987.
20. Holm R, Newland J: Double-staining methods at the ultrastructural level applying colloidal gold conjugates, *Ultrastruct Pathol* 12:279, 1988.
21. Kawana S, Segawa A: Confocal laser scanning microscopic and immunoelectron microscopic studies of the anatomical distribution of fibrillar IgA deposits in dermatitis herpetiformis, *Arch Dermatol* 129:456, 1993.
22. Isola J, Helen H, Kallioniemi OP: Immunoelectron-microscopic localization of a proliferation-associated antigen Ki-67 in MCF-7 cells, *Histochem J* 22:498, 1990.
23. Linke RP, Hugh D, Casanova S et al: Immunoelectron microscopic identification of human AA-type amyloid: exploration of various monoclonal AA-antibodies, methods of fixation, embedding and of other parameters for the protein-A gold method, *Lab Invest* 61:692, 1989.
24. Thiry M: Immunoelectron microscope localization of bromodeoxyuridine incorporated into DNA of Ehrlich tumor cell nucleoli, *Exp Cell Res* 179:204, 1988.
25. Mimura R, Hansmann ML, Lennert K: Immunoelectron microscopic localization of immunoglobulin in B-cell lymphomas, *Virchows Arch B Cell Pathol* 52:207, 1986.
26. Berg KK, Scheithauer BW, Felix I et al: Pituitary adenomas that produce adrenocorticotropic hormone and alpha-subunit: clinicopathological, immunohistochemical, ultrastructural, and immunoelectron microscopic studies in nine cases, *Neurosurgery* 26:397, 1990.

Technical Procedures

27. Baic D, Baic B: A fast method for processing biopsy material for electron microscopy, *Ultrastruct Pathol* 6:347, 1984.
28. Wang N, Minassian H: The formaldehyde-fixed and paraffin-embedded tissues for diagnostic transmission electron microscopy, *Hum Pathol* 18:715, 1987.
29. Dardick I, Hazdi HM, Brosko C et al: A quantitative comparison of light and electron microscopic diagnoses in specimens obtained by fine-needle aspiration biopsy, *Ultrastruct Pathol* 15:105, 1991.
30. Strausbauch P, Neill J, Dabbs DJ et al: The impact of fine-needle aspiration biopsy on a diagnostic electron microscopy laboratory, *Arch Pathol Lab Med* 113:1354, 1989.
31. Akhtar M, Bakry M, Nash EJ: An improved technic for processing aspiration biopsy for electron microscopy, *Am J Clin Pathol* 85:57, 1986.

32. Mackay B, Fanning T, Bruner J et al: Diagnostic electron microscopy using fine needle aspiration biopsies, *Ultrastruct Pathol* 11:659, 1987.
33. Mackay B, Katz R: Tissue procurement for diagnostic electron microscopy, *Texas Soc Electron Microsc J* 4:5, 1982.
34. Mills AE, Emms M, Licata SG: A simple technique for preparation of bone marrow or peripheral blood buffy coat cells for electron microscopy, *Ultrastruct Pathol* 14:173, 1990.

Renal biopsies

35. Habib R: A story of glomerulopathies: a pathologist's experience, *Pediatr Nephrol* 7:336, 1993.
36. Dische FE: Measurement of glomerular basement membrane thickness and its application to the diagnosis of thin-membrane nephropathy, *Arch Pathol Lab Med* 116:43, 1992.
37. Gundersen JH, Gotzsche O, Hirose K et al: Early structural changes in glomerular capillaries and their relationship to long-term diabetic nephropathy, *Acta Endocrinol* 97(suppl):19, 1981.
38. Bernstein J: The glomerular basement membrane abnormality in Alport's syndrome, *Am J Kidney Dis* 10:222-229, 1987.
39. Morita T, Laughlin LO, Kawano K et al: Nail-patella syndrome: light and electron microscopic studies in the kidney, *Arch Intern Med* 131:271, 1973.
40. Ehrenreich T, Churg J: Pathology of membranous nephropathy, *Pathol Annu* 3:145, 1968.
41. Feiner H, Gallo G: Ultrastructure in glomerulonephritis associated with cryoglobulinemia: a report of six cases and review of the literature, *Am J Pathol* 88:145, 1977.
42. Korbet SM, Schwartz MM, Lewis EJ: Immunotactoid glomerulopathy, *Am J Kidney Dis* 17:247, 1991.
43. West CD: Idiopathic membranoproliferative glomerulonephritis in childhood, *Pediatr Nephrol* 6:96, 1992.
44. Anders D, Agricola B, Sippel M et al: Basement membrane changes in membranoproliferative glomerulonephritis: II. Characterization of a third type by silver impregnation of ultrathin sections, *Virchows Arch* 376:1, 1977.
45. Noel LH, Droz D, Ganeval D et al: Renal granular monoclonal light chain deposits: morphological aspects of 11 cases, *Clin Nephrol* 21:263, 1984.

Other types of specimens

46. Sheehan HL: Renal morphology in preeclampsia, *Kidney Int* 18:241, 1980.
47. Phillips MJ, Latham PS, Poucell-Hatton S: Electron microscopy of human liver diseases. In Saluff L, Saluff ER:, *Diseases of the liver*, ed 7, Philadelphia, 1993, Lippincott.
48. Goldblatt PJ, Gunning WT III: Ultrastructure of the liver and biliary tract in health and disease, *Ann Clin Lab Sci* 14:159, 1984.
49. Lindmark B, Millward-Sadler H, Callea F et al: Hepatocyte inclusions of alpha-1-antichymotrypsin in a patient with partial deficiency of alpha-1-antichymotrypsin and chronic liver disease, *Histopathology* 16:221, 1990.
50. Perrone TL, Dickersin GR: The intracellular location of cryptosporidia [letter], *Hum Pathol* 14:1092, 1983.
51. Lefkowitch JH, Krumholz S, Feng-Chen KC et al: Cryptosporidiosis of the human small intestine: a light and electron microscopic study, *Hum Pathol* 15:746, 1984.
52. Osborne BM, Butler JJ, Mackay B: Ultrastructural observations in cat scratch disease, *Am J Clin Pathol* 87:739, 1987.
53. Doane FW: Immunoelectron microscopy in diagnostic virology, *Ultrastruct Pathol* 11:681, 1987.
54. Reed KD, Fowler CB, Brannon RB: Ultrastructural detection of herpes-type virions by negative staining in oral hairy leukoplakia, *Am J Clin Pathol* 90:305, 1988.
55. Charles RE, Katz RL, Ordóñez, NG et al: Varicella-zoster infection with pleural involvement, *Am J Clin Pathol* 85:522, 1986.
56. Orenstein JM: Ultrastructural pathology of human immunodeficiency virus infection, *Ultrastruct Pathol* 16:179, 1992.
57. O'Hara CJ, Groopman JE, Federman M: The ultrastructural and immunohistochemical demonstration of viral particles in lymph nodes from human immunodeficiency virus-related and non-human immunodeficiency virus-related lymphadenopathy syndromes, *Hum Pathol* 19:545, 1988.
58. Sancho S, Navarro C, Fernandez JM et al: Skin biopsy findings in glycogenosis III: clinical, biochemical, and electrophysiological correlations, *Ann Neurol* 27:480, 1990.
59. Hug G, Soukup S, Ryan M et al: Rapid prenatal diagnosis of glycogen-storage disease type II by electron microscopy of uncultured amniotic-fluid cells, *N Engl J Med* 310:1018, 1984.
60. Takahashi K, Naito M, Suzuki Y: Genetic mucopolysaccharidoses, mannosidosis, sialidoses, galactosialidosis, and I-cell disease: ultrastructural analysis of cultured fibroblasts, *Acta Pathol Jpn* 37:385, 1987.
61. Vogler C, Rosenberg HS, Williams JC et al: Electron microscopy in the diagnosis of lysosomal storage diseases, *Am J Med Genet*, Suppl 3:243, 1987.
62. Ceuterick C, Martin JJ: Electron microscopic features of skin in neurometabolic disorders, *J Neurol Sci* 112:15, 1992.
63. Cervos-Navarro J, Zimmer C: Light microscopic and ultrastructural study on CNS lesions in infantile Gaucher's disease, *Clin Neuropathol* 9:310, 1990.
64. Sane SY: Urinary sediment in storage diseases: differential diagnosis of Nieman-Pick disease by cytologic means, *Diagn Cytopathol* 6:122, 1990.
65. Simon M, Frey H, Gruler H et al: Glycolipid storage material in Fabry's disease: a study of electron microscopy, freeze-fracture, and digital image analysis, *J Struct Biol* 103:40, 1990.
66. Cohen AS, Connors LH: The pathogenesis and biochemistry of amyloidosis, *J Pathol* 151:1, 1987.
67. Bourgeois N, Buyssens N, Goovaerts G: Ultrastructural appearance of amyloid, *Ultrastruct Pathol* 11:67, 1987.
68. Dake MD, Madison JM, Montgomery CK et al: Electron microscopic demonstration of lysosomal inclusion bodies in lung, liver, lymph nodes, and blood leukocytes of patients with amiodarone pulmonary toxicity, *Am J Med* 78:506, 1985.
69. Mierau GW, Agostini R, Beals TF et al: The role of electron microscopy in evaluating ciliary dysfunction: report of a workshop, *Ultrastruct Pathol* 16:245, 1992.
70. Lurie M, Rennert G, Goldenberg S et al: Ciliary ultrastructure in primary ciliary dyskinesia and other chronic respiratory conditions: the relevance of microtubular abnormalities, *Ultrastruct Pathol* 16:547, 1992.
71. Pysher TJ, Neustein HB: Ciliary dysmorphology, *Perspect Pediatr Pathol* 8:101, 1984.
72. Tome FMS, Fardeau M, Lebon P, Chevallay M: Inclusion body myositis, *Acta Neuropathol* (Berlin) 7:(Suppl)287, 1981.
73. Pardo-Mindán FJ, Lozano MD, Contreras-Mejota F et al: Pathology of heart transplant through endomyocardial biopsy, *Semin Diagn Pathol* 9:238, 1992.
74. Rowan RA, Billingham ME: Pathologic changes in the long-term transplanted heart: a morphometric study of myocardial hypertrophy, vascularity, and fibrosis, *Hum Pathol* 21:767, 1990.
75. Frenzel H, Schwartzkopff B, Kuhn H et al: Cardiac amyloid deposits in endomyocardial biopsies, light microscopic, ultrastructural, and immunohistochemical studies, *Am J Clin Pathol* 85:674, 1986.
76. Mackay B, Ewer MS, Carrasco CH, Benjamin RS: Assessment of anthracycline cardiomyopathy by endomyocardial biopsy. *Ultrastruct Pathol* 18:203, 1994.
77. Scheithauer BW, Bruner JM: The ultrastructural spectrum of astrocytic neoplasms, *Ultrastruct Pathol* 11:535, 1988.
78. Sarkar C, Roy S, Tandon PN: Oligodendroglial tumors: an immunohistochemical and electron microscopic study, *Cancer* 61:1862, 1988.
79. Dehner LP, Abenoza P, Sibley RK: Primary cerebral neuroectodermal tumors: neuroblastoma, differentiated neuroblastoma, and composite neuroectodermal tumor, *Ultrastruct Pathol* 12:479, 1988.
80. Dick AD, Jagger J, McCartney AC: Refsum's disease: electron microscopy of an iris biopsy, *Br J Ophthalmol* 74:370, 1990.
81. Ghadially FN: *Ultrastructural pathology of the cell and matrix*, ed 3, Stoneham, Mass, 1988, Butterworth.

Tumors

82. Herrera GA, Reimann BEF: Electron microscopy in determining origin of metastatic adenocarcinomas, *South Med J* 77:1557, 1984.

83. El-Naggar AK, Evans DB, Mackay B: Oncocytic adrenal cortical carcinoma, *Ultrastruct Pathol* 15:557, 1991.
84. Kataoka R, Hyo Y, Hoshiya T et al: Ultrastructural study of mitochondria in oncocytes, *Ultrastruct Pathol* 15:231, 1991.
85. Bolen JW, Hammar SP, McNutt MA: Serosal tissue: reactive tissue as a model for understanding mesotheliomas, *Ultrastruct Pathol* 11:251, 1987.
86. Dardick I, Jabi M, McCaughey WTE et al: Diffuse epithelial mesothelioma: a review of the ultrastructural spectrum, *Ultrastruct Pathol* 11:503, 1988.
87. DiMaio S, Mackay B, Smith JL et al: Neurosarcomatous transformation in malignant melanoma, *Cancer* 50:2345, 1982.
88. Benson JD, Kraemer BB, Mackay B: Malignant melanoma of soft parts: an ultrastructural study of four cases, *Ultrastruct Pathol* 8:57, 1985.
89. Yamamoto T, Hishida A, Honda N et al: Crystal-storing histiocytosis and crystalline tissue deposition in multiple myeloma, *Arch Pathol Lab Med* 115:351, 1991.
90. Osborne BM, Mackay B: Inguinal lymphadenopathy in a 52 year old male, *Ultrastruct Pathol* 3:187, 1982.
91. Mackay B: Electron microscopy of soft tissue tumours. In Fletcher CDM, McKee PH, editors: *Pathobiology of soft tissue tumours,* New York, 1990, Churchill Livingstone.

8 Immunohistochemistry and Related Marking Techniques

Richard J. Cote
Clive R. Taylor

Immunohistochemistry is, as the name implies, a marriage of two disciplines—immunology and histology. The immunohistochemical technique is used not only to determine if a tissue expresses (or does not express) a particular antigen, but also to determine the antigenic status of particular cells within that tissue and the microanatomic (cellular) location of the antigen. Immunohistochemistry uses antibodies to distinguish the antigenic differences between cells. These differences can specifically identify the lineage of cell populations, define biologically distinct populations of cells within the same lineage, and identify functional differences between cells and can even be used to identify infections. The key to immunohistochemistry is the exquisite specificity of antibodies for particular antigens. Although immunohistochemistry is used by a variety of disciplines to study a wide range of questions, in this chapter we discuss the application of this technology in surgical pathology, where immunohistochemistry has had a profound and fundamental impact on the practice of pathology.[1]

Surgical pathology is an inherently subjective discipline. Although "standard" histologic criteria can be described for virtually all diagnoses, in fact overlap among different entities and dissimilarities among the same entity can be enormous. This is compounded by the subjective evaluation by the individual pathologist, each of whom varies in skill, training, experience, patience, and local habits. Not only is there substantial variation among pathologists at different institutions, but there are also variations among pathologists at the same institution. Indeed, the opinion of a single pathologist can vary depending on a variety of external factors and pressures. In the clinical laboratory, intralaboratory variation can be minimized through a variety of quality assurance programs. However, these programs are less easily applied to surgical pathology.[2]

Unlike many precise assays and numerical results (with normal reference ranges) that emanate from the clinical laboratory, the surgical pathology report itself also invites clinical misinterpretation,[3] not only because of its inherent subjectivity (alluded to above), but also because it is a narrative report in a nonstandard format. Recommendations have been made as to the standard content of surgical pathology reports in certain conditions.[4] However, in most cases the organization of a surgical pathology report is as much a reflection of the institution at which the pathologist trained as anything else.

The implication then is that the subjectivity that is inherent to the surgical pathology diagnostic process may result in a lack of reproducibility among pathologists.[5] Rigorous studies of the accuracy and reliability of histopathologic diagnosis, comparing surgical pathologists across a broad range of diseases, are rare. However, where such studies have been performed the results clearly indicate that there is cause for concern. In the diagnosis of malignant lymphoma, the agreement for certain diagnostic criteria was less than 30% for practicing pathologists and did not exceed 50% even among "experts."[6,7] Diagnostic discordance has also been observed in the assessment of dysplasias in the colon[8,9] and "borderline" lesions in the breast.[10-12] Attempts to utilize histologic criteria for the grading of tumors in order to predict prognosis are fraught with an even greater degree of difficulty, and the reproducibility of findings is poor among different pathologists or even for the same pathologist over time.[13]

Surgical pathologists have long recognized the subjectivity of their discipline. One response has been to seek additional

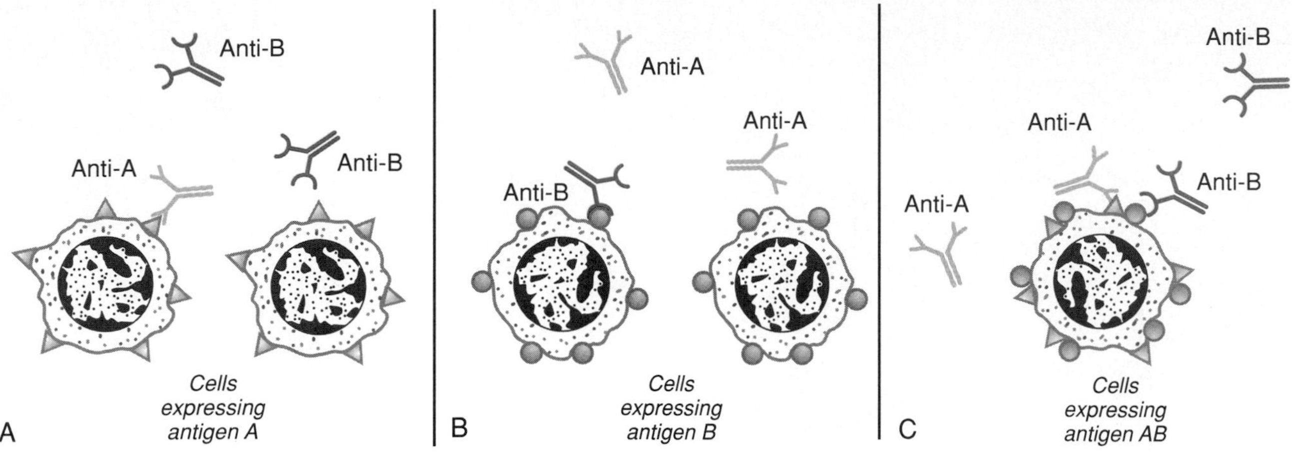

Fig. 8-1 Antigen-antibody binding in tissue sections. Antigen-antibody binding is governed by matching up reciprocal "charge-shape" structures. **A,** Antibody binds with the determinants in antigen A. Anti-B antibody does not bind. The reverse occurs in **B. C,** A molecule bears both determinants A and B, and both anti-A and anti-B antibodies bind.

staining techniques, using so-called special stains, that enhance cell recognition by development of tinctorial differences between the various types of normal and abnormal cells. Charles Culling[14] attributed the beginning of histochemistry to a mid–nineteenth century essay by Raspail entitled "Essai de chimie microscopique appliqué à la physiologie." The goal of histochemistry, as summarized by Culling, has not changed: "The object of staining tissue sections is to impart colour and therefore contrast to specific tissue constituents." In a similar vein, Lillie[15] stated that, "the purpose of staining is to make more evident various tissue and cell constituents and extrinsic materials." In essence, therefore, histochemistry, as discussed in Chapter 9, provides an additional discriminatory function, serving as a supplement to the morphologic criteria upon which the surgical pathology diagnosis is based.

The object of immunohistochemistry is to use antibodies to identify antigens, which "therefore contrast specific tissue constituents." The advantage of immunohistochemistry over histochemistry is of course the degree of specificity imparted by antibodies (Fig. 8-1). Coons, Fagraeus, and others[16,17] demonstrated that antibodies labeled with fluorescent compounds could localize their corresponding antigens in tissue sections. Avrameas[18] replaced the fluorescent label with an enzymatic label (horseradish peroxidase), which, in the presence of a suitable colorogenic substrate system, allowed visualization of the enzymatically labeled antibody by routine light microscopy (Fig. 8-2). Initially, frozen sections were employed because tissue processing was believed to destroy antigens. In a quest for improved morphologic detail, cold alcohol fixation and special processing methods (the Sainte-Marie technique)[19] were utilized to preserve antigens that were believed to be destroyed in formalin-fixed, paraffin-embedded tissues. An inability to identify murine and human lymphoma cells in either paraffin or frozen sections using immunofluorescence techniques led to the application of labeled antibody methods (immunoperoxidase) to formalin-fixed paraffin sections[20,21] (Fig. 8-3). A measure of success was achieved utilizing anti-immunoglobulin antibodies of high quality, thereby revealing a potential for the development of stains based upon the antigenic composition of cells, independent of existing morphologic criteria. Demonstration of viral antigens in paraffin sections[22] further reinforced the notion that certain antigens did, in fact, survive the fixation process. Over the subsequent two decades the number of antigens demonstrable in routinely processed paraffin sections has risen exponentially. Of the several hundred antigens described, many are of value to the surgical pathologist (Table 8-1); the most generally useful antibodies at present are those that can be used in paraffin-embedded tissue.

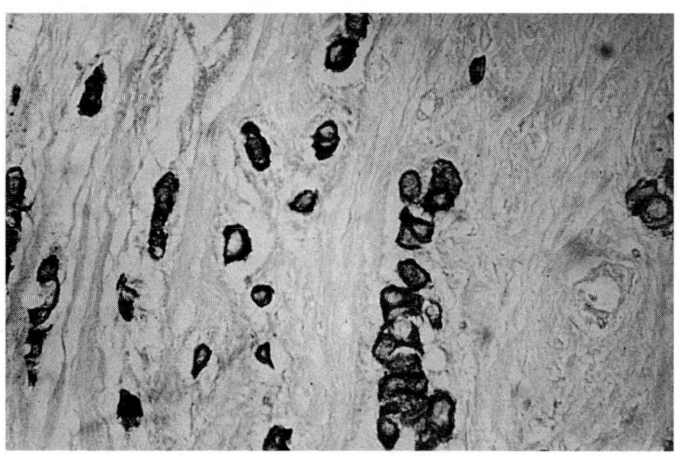

Fig. 8-2 The chromogens normally used in immunohistochemical reaction are diaminobenzidine tetrahydrochloride (DAB) and aminoethyl carbazole (AEC). Other chromogens include alpha-naphthol pyronine, alkaline phosphatase, glucose oxidase, and immunogold. This figure demonstrates the use of immunogold as the chromogen.

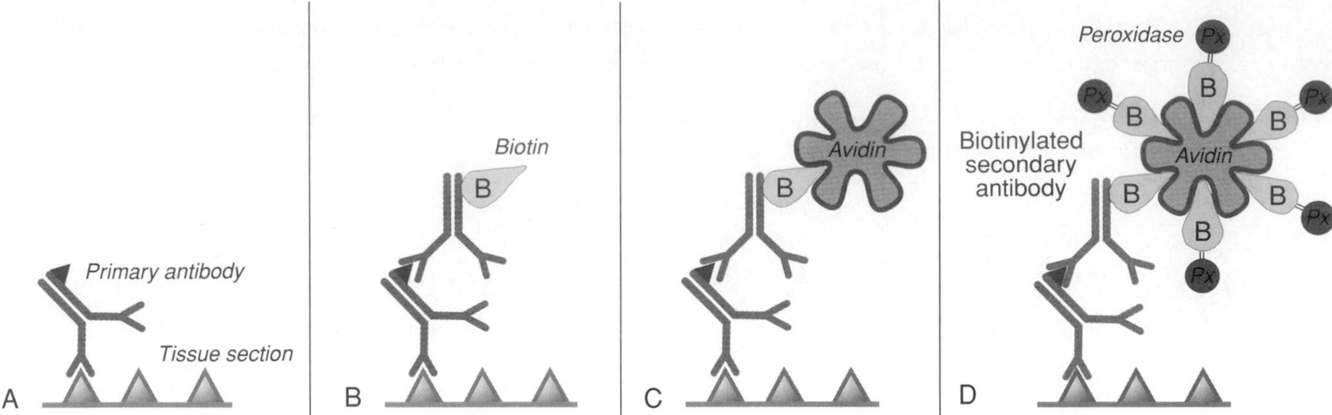

Fig. 8-3 **A,** Avidin-biotin conjugate (ABC) immunohistochemical detection method. The biotinylated secondary antibody (**Panel B**) serves to link the primary antibody (**Panel A**) to a large preformed complex of avidin, biotin, and peroxidase (**Panels C,D**). *B,* biotin; *Px,* peroxidase.

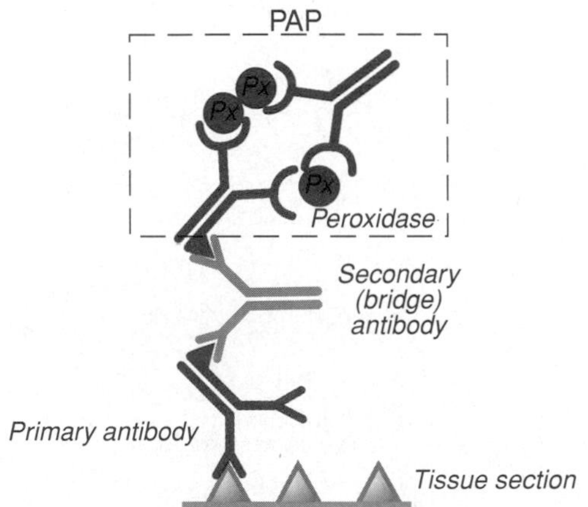

Fig. 8-3 **B,** Peroxidase-antiperoxidase (PAP) method. PAP reagent is a preformed stable immune complex; it is linked to the primary antibody by a "bridging" antibody.

From these modest beginnings immunohistochemistry has expanded beyond expectation. In 1974 and 1975 there were approximately 6 published papers pertaining to immunoperoxidase staining of paraffin sections. In 1992 a computer literature search identified more than 15,000 such articles. Immunohistochemistry has become an essential part of surgical pathology, both in the facilitation of cell recognition in circumstances where the diagnosis is uncertain based upon the hematoxylin and eosin (H&E) stain alone and in helping to determine the biologic potential of tumors.

IMMUNOHISTOCHEMISTRY AS A LABORATORY TEST

Immunohistochemistry has the potential of transforming surgical pathology from a subjective "art" to an objective science, based on the way cells can be recognized by microscopic methods. Although this potential has been almost universally recognized, it has not been universally fulfilled. In large part, this failure derives from the same tendency toward imprecision that was described for "surgical pathology." Immunohistochemical reproducibility is compromised, not only by a lack of standardization of reagents, protocols, and technical performance, but also by variance in interpretation.[23] Nevertheless, laboratories may yet achieve technical excellence in the performance of the assay through consideration of each of the components of the idealized total test (Table 8-2).

Test selection

Given the choice of a vast array of antibodies that can be used in immunohistochemistry, the problem is in choosing wisely. Such guidance to the practicing pathologist is found in the accumulated literature and in a limited number of textbooks[1,24-28] that address the use of immunohistochemistry.

Immunohistochemical tests should be employed with a defined objective in mind. It is sound practice first to develop a differential diagnosis based on clinical data and the morphologic findings in H&E preparations. The question should then be asked, "Are there any antibodies that will refine the differential diagnosis?" For each antibody that is considered, the pathologist should question the importance of a positive or negative result. To accomplish this step the pathologist must have extensive knowledge of the staining patterns of the primary antibodies under consideration and an awareness of any technical limitation imposed by tissue fixation or the immunohistochemical procedure. The principles of test selection are discussed later in this chapter.

Specimen preparation

Although the indications for requesting histopathologic examination (test selection) are well understood ("to get a tissue diagnosis"), protocols for specimen acquisition and preparation are often imprecise, both in design and execution. In some institutions specimens are taken fresh from the operating room to the histopathology laboratory; this approach potentially provides the most rigorous control over the processing of tissues. More often, however, specimens taken in the operating room are dropped whole (regardless of size) into formalin of unknown freshness and unknown pH, for an unknown period of time, before the specimen reaches the laboratory.

Table 8-1 Selected antigens that are successfully demonstrated in paraffin sections

Hormones
ACTH
GH
LH
LTH
FSH
TSH
Parathormone
Calcitonin
Thyroxine
Thyroglobulin
hCG
beta-hCG
Testosterone
Estradiol
Progesterone
Insulin
Glucagon
Somatostatin
VIP
Gastrin
Secretin
Motilin
Neurotensin
Cholecystokinin
Renin
Vasopressin
Oxytocin
Neurophysin
Bombesin

Receptors
Transferrin receptor
Estrogen receptor
Progesterone receptor
Androgen receptor

Other tissue components
Laminin
Fibronectin
Collagens
Amyloid A protein
Cell adhesion molecules

Other cellular components
Lysozyme (muramidase)
Lactoferrin
Transferrin
Ferritin
Hemoglobin A

Other cellular components—*Cont'd*
Hemoglobin F
Myoglobin
Actin
Myosin
Keratins
Alpha$_1$-antitrypsin
Alpha$_1$-antichymotrypsin
Alpha-fetoprotein
Carcinoembryonic Ag
Mammary epithelial membrane Ag
Hepatorenal Ag
Pancreatic Ag
Melanoma Ag (HMB 45)
Prostatic acid phosphatase
Prostate specific Ag
Glial fibrillary acidic protein
Tyrosine hydroxylase
Myelin basic protein
Enolases
Adenosine deaminase
Terminal deoxynucleotideal transferase
Carbonic anhydrase
Cathepsin D
Factor VIII–related Ag
Creatine kinase
Intestinal mucin Ags
HLA Ags
Blood group Ags
Surfactant apoprotein
S-100 Ag
Neurofilament
Vimentin
Desmin
Mucin Ags
Celomic Ags
Endocrine granule Ags
Gross cystic disease protein
Cu-18 breast related Ag
OC125 (ovarian) celomic Ag
Synaptophysin
Placental alkaline phosphatase
Colon ovarian tumor Ag (CoTA)

Infectious agents
Herpes virus I and II
Hepatitis B surface Ag/core Ag
Mouse mammary tumor virus Ag

Infectious agents—*Cont'd*
Rubella virus
Measles virus
Respiratory syncytial virus
Buffalo pox virus
Legionella sp
Klebsiella sp
Group B streptococcus
Influenza virus
Poliovirus
Varicella-zoster virus
Cytomegalovirus (CMV)
SV 40
Human *Papillomavirus*
Polyomavirus
Chlamydia sp
Mycoplasma sp
Trichomonas sp
Toxoplasma sp
Trichophyton sp
Amebas
Mycobacteria sp
Leishmania sp
Fasciola sp
HTLVI
Hepatitis delta virus
HIV

Immunoglobulin components
Kappa, lambda light chains
Gamma, alpha, mu, delta, epsilon heavy chains
J chain
Secretory component
C1, C2, C3, C4

Leukocyte antigens
CD markers 1 to 78
Nonassigned markers: e.g., BLA 36, MB 2

Oncogenes/products
bcl-2
Her-2/*neu*/C-*erb* 2
p53 suppressor gene

Nuclear proliferation antigens
Ki-67
PCNA
p105

Modified from Taylor CR, Cote RJ: *Immunomicroscopy: a diagnostic tool for the surgical pathologist,* ed 2, Philadelphia, 1994, Saunders.

Once in the pathology laboratory, all is not necessarily well either. Specimens usually are not processed immediately but are accumulated into batches. During the "cutting-in" process, blocks are not prepared to uniform size, and they are not placed in standard amounts of fresh formalin (or other fixative). Tissue blocks may then remain in fixative for 12 hours to 36 hours or more, until placed on the autoprocessor, where again there is considerable variation in exposure to formalin and other reagents according to the processing cycle (for example, weekend cycles are routinely prolonged). Great variation therefore exists within individual institutions and certainly across institutions. All of this may matter little for diagnosis by routine H&E staining, but these variations may be disastrous for immunohistochemistry.

It has become increasingly clear that much of the variation in immunohistochemical test results observed between different laboratories and even within the same laboratory from day-to-day stems from irregularities in specimen handling, particularly fixation. The type of fixative is of great importance[1,29]; however, whatever the optimal fixative may be, formalin remains by far the most widely used fixative and is likely to remain so into the near future. Although the physicochemical

Table 8-2 The Total Test—Immunohistochemistry

Elements of testing process	Quality assurance issues	Responsibility
Clinical question and test selection	Indications for immunohistochemistry; selection of stain(s)	Surgical pathologist: sometimes clinician
Specimen acquisition and management	Specimen collection, fixation processing, sectioning	Clinician pathologist and technologist
Technology and methodology	Reagents, protocols, sensitivity, specificity	Pathologist and technologist
Analytical issue	Qualifications of staff Intralaboratory and interlaboratory proficiency testing of procedures	Pathologist and technologist
Results: validation and reporting	Criteria for positivity and negativity in relation to controls Content and organization of report Turnaround time	Pathologist and technologist
Interpretation, significance	Experience and qualification of pathologist Proficiency testing of interpretational aspects Diagnostic, prognostic significance Appropriateness and correlation with other data	Surgical pathologist or clinician, or both

effects of different fixatives on different antigens are not well understood, it is generally apparent that *many antigens are adversely affected by prolonged fixation.* The first and perhaps the most important step to standardize the fixation process is to restrict fixation of any tissue to a maximum of 24 hours, including that time spent within the automated processor. Uniform fixation is a common starting point upon which to build a standardized, reproducible immunohistochemical procedure. Other influential factors such as differences in pH of the formalin, different fixatives, and different temperatures can then be evaluated as isolated variables. Indeed, their separate evaluation is an essential part of establishing any new immunohistochemistry laboratory.

Technology issues

Standards for the "quality control" of individual reagents are well established in the clinical laboratory and require similar attention in immunohistology laboratories. Recent changes in the College of American Pathologists (CAP) certification criteria (Table 8-3) emphasize the need to validate every reagent and each new lot of reagents. Such validation is desirable because commercial reagents used in immunohistochemistry may be of uncertain origin, composition, concentration, and specificity.[1,2,23,24,30] Often no information is provided as to performance characteristics in formalin-fixed, paraffin embedded tissues. Even when such data are provided, it is still incumbent on the pathologist to perform in-house validation studies, remembering that fixation and processing methods employed by the manufacturer are unlikely to be identical to those methods in use in the hospital laboratory. The recent collaborative effort of the Biologic Stain Commission and the Food and Drug Administration in providing a set of guidelines for standard package inserts for manufacturers[2,30] represents a great step forward (Table 8-4).

It must be emphasized that *immunohistochemical tests performed in the absence of the appropriate controls are valueless and even dangerous.* Minimal controls should include a tissue known to express the particular antigen of interest, processed in a manner analogous to the unknown tissue (the positive control), and a second section of the test specimen in which the primary antibody is replaced either by diluent or, better, by an irrelevant antibody of the same isotype, from the same species, and at the same concentration (the negative control). In the positive control, only those cells expected to express the antigen should show positivity; all other cells and structural elements should be negative. In the negative control, there should be no specific staining. The "sausage" technique, where samples of multiple tissues are gathered into a single tissue block, is a useful control method.[31]

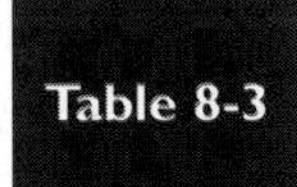

Table 8-3 Areas covered by the revised and extended College of American Pathologists' inspection program for immunohistochemistry

Procedure manual for immunohistochemistry (NCCLS format)
Manual addresses all methods and antibodies currently in use
Manual addresses fixative or fixatives and types of specimens
Tissue-processing temperature defined and monitored as appropriate*
Storage conditions of immunoreagents
pH of the buffers routinely monitored
Positive and negative controls for each antibody
Control slides or tissue stored properly to assure antigen retention
Records of results of controls
All reagents properly labeled are dated
Records for evaluation of new antibody lots and new antibodies
Maintenance records of any automated stainer
Daily records of the quality of immunohistochemical stains
Representative stains should be reviewed and found to be acceptable by the inspector
Immunohistochemistry slides should be on file†

Modified from Taylor CR: *Biotechnic Histochem* 67:323, 1992.
NCCLS, National Committee for Clinical Laboratory Standards.
*The laboratory should also be in compliance with relevant sections from other anatomic pathology criteria, including Histology Laboratory, Collection and Accessioning, and Laboratory Safety.
†Stains performed on referred cases may be returned to the referring source.

Table 8-4 **Quality controls for use in immunohistochemistry as recommended by the Biologic Stain Commission and Food and Drug Administration**

Type of control	Antigen (analyte)	Antibody (reagent)	Purpose
Positive	Nonpatient tissue or cells containing antigen to be detected and quantified and with known expected result Fixed processed in same way as patient sample Fixed processed in manner shown to preserve antigen under analysis	Antibody reagent (of the kit) constituted in same way as intended for patient sample	Control of all steps of the analysis Training user for appearance of positive reaction Comparison for semiquantitation of reaction Validates all steps of analysis including fixation and processing Validates all steps of analysis, except fixation or processing used by individual laboratory
Negative (specific)	Tissues or cells expected to be negative by antibody (of kit)	Antibody reagent (of kit) constituted in same way as intended for patient sample	Detection of unintended antibody cross-reactivity to cells or cellular components
Negative (nonspecific)	Patient tissue with components that are the same as tissue to be studied Processed in same way as patient sample	Diluent (as used with antibody) without antibody Antibody not specific for antigen of interest in same diluent as used with kit antibody	Detection of unintended background staining

Positive and negative controls, performed as above, test the integrity of the total immunohistochemical system and the function in the day-to-day validation of an assay. However, in developing an immunohistochemical protocol, one always needs to evaluate the separate reagents in a multistep procedure. This process can be complex and time consuming, involving the determination of the specificity, and the optimal working dilution of primary antibodies, secondary or bridge antibodies, labeling reagents, and substrates, together with appropriate incubation times, temperatures, buffers, and any predigestion or antigen-enhancement procedures that may be utilized.[1]

Those unwilling to perform such extensive procedures may purchase all-inclusive kits, which provide the immunohistochemistry components at working dilutions deemed appropriate by the manufacturer, together with recommended working protocols. These kits are formulated for effectiveness on tissues available to the manufacturer; they may perform well on tissues processed by the purchasing laboratory, but inferior results can result from different fixation and processing protocols. Adjustment of certain steps of the kit protocol may be (and often are) necessary. However, it may be difficult to achieve satisfactory results because the working dilutions of the kit components are sometimes near the critical limit of sensitivity. Any departure from the protocol recommended by the manufacturer mandates a total revalidation of the whole procedure by the performing laboratory.

Automated immunostaining systems are also becoming widely available and offer certain potential advantages over existing manual techniques.[1] By providing uniform reaction conditions at equilibrium and by standardizing reagents, automated immunohistochemistry should impart standardization, improve reproducibility, facilitate interlaboratory comparisons, reduce reagent expenses, and increase technician productivity. Efforts toward the automation of immunohistochemistry date back to the 1980s.[32] Published data and anecdotal experience indicates that automated immunostaining systems can produce high-quality results.[32-38] However, it is important to recognize that if automated systems are to be employed they may represent a departure from the recommended antibody protocols and thus require complete revalidation of all tests by the performing laboratory.

Analytical issues

The quality of the immunohistochemical tests performed within each laboratory should be evaluated on a regular basis against internal controls (the "reference standards").[1,39,40] Also, external proficiency testing has now been extended to the immunohistochemistry laboratory.[39] It should be noted that this testing program, which principally uses unstained paraffin sections that are sent to each laboratory, tests the reagents, the performance of the staining protocol, and the basic interpretation of the results, but it does *not* test the degree to which "in-house" tissues may be adversely affected by fixation and processing.

Results and reporting

Although immunohistochemistry may help to determine whether a specific antigen is expressed, certain limitations exist. As described previously, many factors influence the results, including tissue fixation (type and duration), processing, the antibody employed (concentration, specificity, and sensitivity), and the detection system used. All these factors must be considered by the pathologist in interpreting the findings. Negative, weak, or uninterpretable results should lead to consideration of repeating the test after the use of antigen retrieval.[40a,b] One measure of antigen preservation is to test for expression of the intermediate filament vimentin, a fixation-sensitive protein, which is typically expressed by vascular or connective components; this technique can often serve as an internal indicator of conservation or loss of antigenicity.[40] Test results may also be affected by technical artifacts and by the nature of the tissue under study. For example, if tumor cells are crushed, false-positive, nonspecific staining may be encountered. Nonviable areas of tissue from a necrotic tumor may also be a source of false-positive results, attributable in part to leakage of serum proteins (such as immunoglobulins). Moreover, the subcellular distribution of immunoreactivity is critical to the interpretation of immunohistochemical results. For example, leukocyte common antigen, cluster of differentiation 45 (LCA/CD45) shows membranous staining, whereas antibodies to estrogen and progesterone receptors produce nuclear staining; when unexpected staining patterns are observed with an antibody, the results should be discounted.[1]

Because many variables can compromise the immunohistochemical procedure, the results of a single immunohistochemical stain can be misleading; the use a panel of several antibodies is preferable to a single test. Interpretation should be undertaken in conjunction with the morphologic findings and any other clinical or pathologic information available.

There are no uniform, published criteria defining "positivity" in the interpretation of immunohistochemical tests. Evaluation of positivity is subjective, requiring experience and an understanding of the anticipated *patterns of staining* for each antibody. With more than 100 antibodies routinely available in large laboratories, this represents a considerable commitment for any pathologist so engaged. Also, positivity should be described only in the presence of appropriate controls; just as in the clinical laboratory, if the controls have not performed as anticipated, the assay should be repeated.

The immunohistochemical report, like the surgical pathology report, is generally in narrative form, though some laboratories simply report immunohistochemical results in tabular form without qualitative description. This practice is to be discouraged, unless the pattern and distribution of the stain are also clearly described. In addressing this problem, the Biologic Stain Commission Steering Committee concluded that significant advantages would accrue from a standardized report format, one including a listing of all the tests performed, details of the reagents employed, a description of the patterns of staining, the results of the appropriate controls, and comments on the interpretation and significance[41] (Table 8-5). The diagnostic and prognostic significance of particular markers is in constant evolution as experience in their use accrues; the implications of certain immunoreactivity patterns should be incorporated into the final report as well.

Table 8-5 The immunohistochemistry report

1. Patient demographics and specimen identification data
2. Reference to the diagnostic problem (that is, differential diagnosis)
3. Nature of specimen analyzed (frozen, fine-needle aspiration, paraffin section, and fixative*)
4. Statement of all stains used with details of all primary antibodies (designate specificity and clone where appropriate†)
5. Findings, both positive and negative, for all stains; sufficient details of patterns and controls to justify the interpretation‡
6. The immunohistochemistry report should not stand alone but should be integrated into the final surgical pathology report

*Details of fixation and detection systems should be kept on record in the performing laboratory and should be incorporated in the report where they are an essential part of the interpretative process (such as whether enzyme digestion or antigen retrieval was employed, or B5 versus formalin fixation for certain leukocyte antigens).

†For example "anti-T-cell" is not acceptable; it should read "T-cell antibody UCHL-1 (CD45 RO)" or "antipankeratin" should read "antikeratin cocktail (AE-1 + Cam 5.2 + 34βE12 + 35βH11)."

‡Detailed control records should be retained in the performing laboratory. Findings may also be stated in the report where they are contributory. For example, in a breast tumor that is negative for estrogen receptor the presence of residual normal breast epithelium that shows positivity is significant. Similarly, in an anaplastic large cell tumor showing absence of staining for leukocyte common antigen (CD45), the presence of intermingled LCA-positive small lymphocytes should be described.

Interpretation

Many studies have now shown that immunohistochemistry has an essential role in diagnostic pathology; the need for immunohistochemical studies to help resolve diagnostic problems (such as tumor of unknown origin) or to help to determine therapy (such as estrogen and progesterone receptor status) are increasingly well recognized. Furthermore, the failure to perform the appropriate immunohistochemical tests in cases where there is diagnostic doubt might well be interpreted as professional negligence.

As long ago as 1985, one study revealed an alarmingly high rate of misdiagnosis of anaplastic tumors when conventional morphologic criteria alone were utilized in their classification.[42] After reevaluation using immunohistologic methods, the diagnosis was changed in almost 50% of 120 such tumors. In a separate study of 200 cases,[43] it was concluded that immunohistochemistry contributed to the diagnosis in a similar percentage of cases. In a subsequent study of more than 500 poorly differentiated round-cell or spindle-cell tumors,[44] immunohistochemistry "provided a definitive diagnosis in 70% of the former and 92% of the latter." Banks,[45] in reviewing case material collected over a 1-year period, concluded that immunohistochemistry was essential to the diagnosis in 55% of cases where such special stains were performed. Given this experience within tertiary referral centers, it might be anticipated that a community surgical pathologist would confront a requirement for immunohistochemical studies less frequently, in perhaps 10% to 25% of tumors. Even the decision not to use immunohistochemistry must be predicated upon a firm understanding of the power and, in addition, the limitations of the technique as experienced within each individual laboratory.[38]

In the future, greater efficacy in the use of immunohistochemistry may derive from the application of more formal "appropriateness criteria," which are presently being developed. These shall be coupled with analyses of outcome, relevance to therapy, and cost effectiveness to fashion criteria similar to those proposed by the Rand Corporation[46] for such procedures as coronary angiography. Evaluation of the effectiveness of automation, including automated image analysis of stained slides,[47] will also be included in these analyses.

LIMITATIONS OF IMMUNOHISTOCHEMISTRY

Experience

The practical details of performing immunohistochemical tests have been set forth by many investigators. There is no uniformly superior method, and different modifications may be required under different circumstances.

Whichever method is adopted, however, there is little doubt that experience is critical in standardizing the procedure, including the selection and proper dilution of all the necessary reagents and the regular performance of all the appropriate controls (Table 8-4).

Interpretation, too, has its foundation in experience. Nevertheless, the immunohistochemical analysis is far more objective than routine morphologic examination. Indeed, immunohistochemistry is elevating surgical pathology to an entirely new level of specificity and is allowing the pathologist to provide information that is not available by morphologic evaluation alone.

Availability of antibodies

The paucity of antibodies with a high degree of specificity for cellular and tissue antigens was a serious limitation until recently. In part, this has been remedied by the increased use of techniques to manufacture pure antigen preparations, permitting the production of high-affinity polyclonal antisera, which are then purified by means of multiple absorption procedures to attain the specificity necessary for immunohistologic techniques. More significant, however, has been the refinement of the hybridoma technique for monoclonal antibody production, which has provided specific high-affinity reagents for the detection of numerous antigens. The sensitivity of monoclonal antibodies, which are directed against a single epitope on an antigen, tends to be more adversely affected by fixation-induced antigen alterations than that of polyclonal antisera, which recognize many epitopes. This compromises the function of monoclonal antibodies in routinely processed tissues and thereby limits their widespread utilization in surgical pathology. Nonetheless the vast majority of antibodies used on routinely processed tissues are monoclonal antibodies.[1]

Antigen loss

The specificity of an antibody for a particular antigen and its ability to react with that antigen require the preservation of the antigen's configuration. Clearly, fixation and paraffin-embedding, with their induction of alterations in three-dimensional "charge-shape" patterns and with the protein cross-links they incur, may have deleterious effects on antigenicity. There is a growing realization today, however, that these processes are not so catastrophic to antigens as once believed. Although much has yet to be learned about the precise effects of different fixatives on different antigens, a large number of antigens are now demonstrable in paraffin sections (Table 8-1). Table 8-6 summarizes the degree of preservation of immunoglobulin reactivity witnessed under different conditions of fixation. These observations, however, may not necessarily apply equally to other antigens.

Table 8-6 Preservation of immunoreactivity of immunoglobulin in plasma cells after different fixation procedures

Quality of preservation	Fixation procedures
Good	Mordants including Zenker's, Bouin's, and B-5 fixatives
Intermediate	10% formalin*
Poor	Oxidizing dichromates, permanganates

Modified from Banks PM: *J Histochem Cytochem* 27:1192, 1979.

*In our experience 10% *fresh* buffered formalin also gives excellent results provided that fixation is not prolonged unnecessarily. As a general rule, *fixation should be for the minimum time consistent with good morphology.*

CURRENT APPLICATIONS OF IMMUNOHISTOCHEMISTRY

Analysis of tumors of uncertain origin

A tumor cannot be staged and appropriate therapy cannot be determined without a specific classification. Generally, tumors are classified histogenetically (such as epithelial, mesenchymal, or neural) or by their tissue of origin (such as breast, colon, lung). Most tumors can be readily characterized in such a fashion. At times, however, a tumor may defy classification, as when (1) the tumor is first found as a metastatic deposit and the primary site cannot be determined; (2) the tumor is so poorly differentiated that it exhibits no specific morphologic features; and (3) the tumor has a morphologic appearance that is compatible with more than one distinct tissue (for example, it could be either of epithelial or lymphoid origin).

The magnitude of this problem is significant. The diagnosis of "metastatic cancer of unknown primary site" is the eighth most common cancer diagnosis and may represent up to 15% of cancers at large hospitals.[48] These cases can clearly benefit from the type of information that can be provided by the application of immunohistochemistry. However, even when an "expert" has rendered a specific diagnosis, on the basis of an H&E stain alone, morphologic ambiguity may lead to misdiagnosis in a significant percentage of "difficult" cases.[38,42-44,49]

Immunohistochemical methods have revolutionized the approach to tumors of uncertain origin. Many antibodies recognize antigens that are expressed by cells of specific histogenesis (Table 8-1). The antibodies with widest use are those that indicate the embryologic origin of cells (such as epithelial, mesenchymal, neural). The great effect of this technology is difficult to overstate: the majority of undifferentiated (anaplastic) tumors can now be classified using immunohistochemistry.[42-44,49]

There has been less success in the development of "tissue-specific" markers that can allow identification of the origin of metastatic tumors. Most of these antigens are not tissue specific. For example, although GCFDF-15 is expressed primarily by breast epithelium, it also is expressed by a small number of other tissues.[51]

Furthermore, immunohistochemical studies usually do *not* discriminate between neoplastic and nonneoplastic lesions, or between benign and malignant cells. These distinctions continue to be made by conventional cytomorphologic criteria. There are few exceptions to this general rule. For example, atypical B-cell proliferations may have immunohistochemical features of clonality (such as only kappa or lambda light-chain immunoglobulins on the cell surface); when this occurs, they are usually assumed to be malignant.

Finally, caveats related to fixation, performance, and interpretation must be considered in the assessment of tumors of uncertain origin. The absence of staining in a poorly preserved tissue does not provide conclusive information.

Selection of antibodies

Although many different antibodies are available, it is neither sensible nor practical to test all unknown tumors with a large number of antibodies, only some of which may provide useful information in a particular case. On the other hand, the use of only one or two antibodies will rarely provide information adequate to support a specific diagnosis and can produce misleading results that delay the final diagnosis. Antibodies should be chosen to affirm or exclude considerations in the differential diagnosis. This *problem-oriented approach* is based on the selection of appropriate *panels* of antibodies to resolve the diagnostic problem. The factors that must be weighed in the selection of an appropriate panel of antibodies including the clinical history, morphologic features of the tumor, results of other tests (such as serologic or radiologic), and the relative frequency of different tumor types. The primary panel of antibodies should include those that characterize major categories of epithelial, mesenchymal, neural, or hematopoietic neoplasms. Based on the results of the initial immunohistochemical study, additional antibodies are chosen to identify more definitively the specific tumor type.

The algorithms that follow are designed to include well-characterized antibodies and to address frequent problems of differential diagnosis (Table 8-7).

Intermediate-filament expression

Intermediate filaments form the cytoskeleton of normal and neoplastic cells. The pattern of expression of intermediate filaments is characteristic of different cells and thus useful in the classification of undifferentiated neoplasms.[1] There are five major subclasses of intermediate filaments: *keratins, vimentin,*

Table 8-7 Antigens of value for analysis of anaplastic tumors

	General categorization	
	First tier	Second tier
Epithelial tumors (carcinomas)	Pankeratin	High molecular weight keratins Low molecular weight keratins EMA B72.3 CEA NSE
Mesenchymal tumors (sarcomas)	Vimentin	Desmin Factor VIII
Special groups		
Melanomas	Vimentin S-100	HMB45 NSE
Germ cell tumors	Pankeratin Vimentin	PLAP AFP hCG Ferritin
Neural/neuroendocrine tumors	NSE (pankeratin) NF	Chromogranin Leu-7 Synaptophysin GFAP
Lymphomas	LCA	Pan-B Pan-T Kappa and lambda light chains R-S cell markers Histiocytic markers

Modified from Taylor CR, Cote RJ: *Immunomicroscopy: a diagnostic tool for the surgical pathologist,* ed 2, Philadelphia, 1994, Saunders.
AFP, Alpha-fetoprotein; *CEA,* carcinoembryonic antigen; *EMA,* epithelial membrane antigen; *GFAP,* glial fibrillary acidic protein filaments; *hCG,* human chorionic gonadotropin; *LCA,* leukocyte common antigen (CD45); *NF,* neurofilament; *NSE,* neuron-specific enolase; *PLAP,* placental alkaline phosphatase; *R-S,* Reed-Sternberg cell.

desmin, neurofilament (NF), and glial fibrillary acidic protein (GFAP). Most neoplasms show predominant expression of one intermediate filament, though coexpression of filament proteins occurs, and is an important consideration in the differential diagnosis. Carcinomas usually express keratin; sarcomas, melanomas, and lymphomas typically contain vimentin; myogenic tumors show the presence of desmin and vimentin; glial tumors are predominantly positive for GFAP; neural tumors express neurofilament. Some tumors characteristically coexpress more than one intermediate filament, and others may rarely exhibit no, or very low, intermediate-filament expression. The detection of intermediate filaments is one of the most important and productive ways of characterizing the histogenesis of cells and thus in classifying "tumors of uncertain origin." Anaplastic neoplasms can be broadly characterized into tumors that are keratin positive (carcinomas, mesotheliomas, and some germ cell tumors) and those that are vimentin positive (sarcomas, lymphomas, or melanomas) or NF and GFAP positive (certain neuroendocrine, neural, and astrocytic tumors).

Keratin-positive tumors

Because keratins are present in almost all epithelial cells, they are highly sensitive markers for malignant cells of epithelial origin (that is, carcinomas). Antikeratin antibodies may also aid detection of micrometastases in bone marrow or lymph nodes (discussed later in the chapter).[52-56] There are more than 20 different subtypes of human keratin proteins that differ by their molecular weight and isoelectric point.[57] Specific monoclonal antibodies have been developed against many of these, and immunohistochemical studies have shown that some carcinomas have characteristic keratin profiles. In general, there is a correlation between the complexity of the epithelium from which the tumor is derived and the complexity of the keratin subunits expressed. During embryogenesis, the low molecular weight (or nonsquamous) keratins appear earlier in development; the higher molecular weight (or squamous) keratins appear later with the formation of more complex stratified epithelia. In human neoplasias, the low molecular weight keratins predominate in tumors derived from more simple nonstratified epithelia (such as breast carcinomas and gastrointestinal adenocarcinomas), whereas the high molecular weight keratins predominate in tumors derived from stratified epithelia (such as squamous cell carcinomas). Tumors such as pulmonary adenocarcinomas, derived from pseudostratified columnar respiratory epithelium, contain cytokeratins of both high and low molecular weight, with a predominance of the latter.

Monoclonal antibodies that predominantly recognize low molecular weight and acidic cytokeratins include AE1, AE3, Cam 5.2, and 35βH11. Because low molecular weight keratins are present in most epithelial cells, these antibodies can be used (either individually or in "cocktails") as broad-range markers of epithelial derivation. By contrast, 34βE12 (K903)[58] allows detection of primarily high molecular weight keratins (Fig. 8-4).

Monoclonal antibodies against the keratin subtypes may help determine the histogenesis of certain poorly differentiated neoplasms (Fig. 8-5). For example, hepatocellular carcinomas (positive for AE3 and Cam 5.2 but negative for AE1) can be separated from adenocarcinoma metastatic to the liver (positive for AE1).[59] As monoclonal antibodies to other keratin sub-

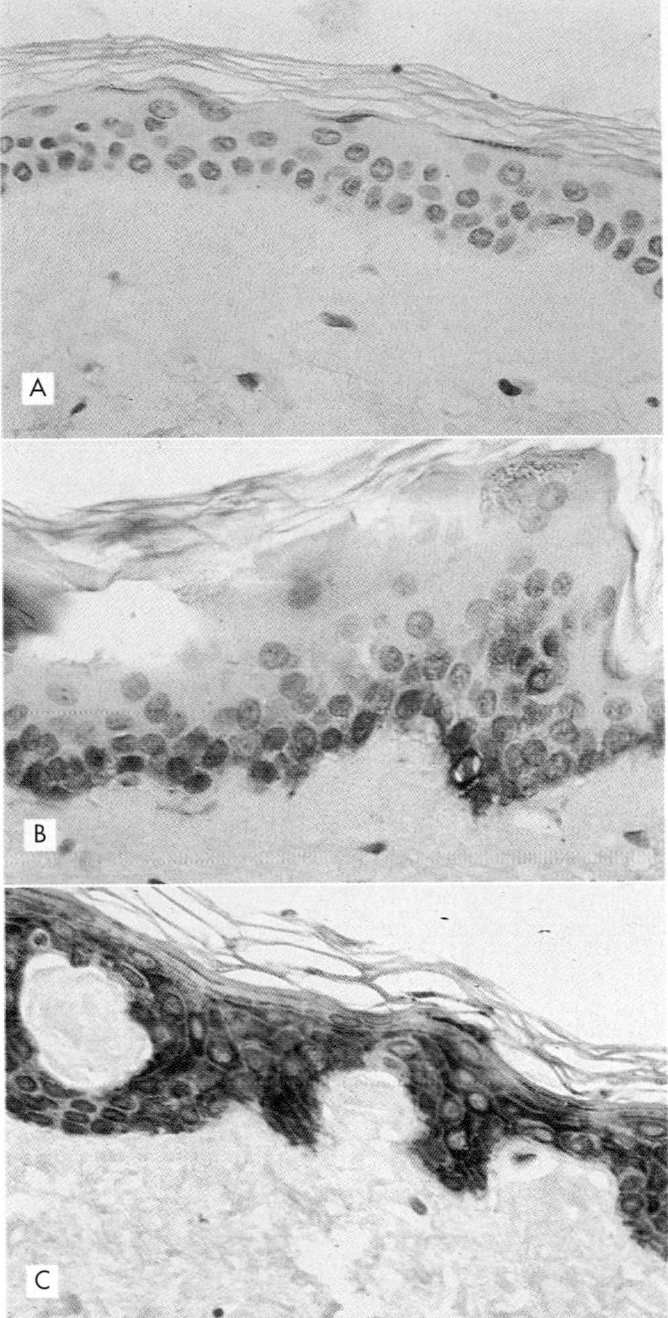

Fig. 8-4 Range of cytokeratin expression demonstrated in squamous and glandular epithelium of skin. **A,** Squamous epithelium stained with antibody Cam 5.2, which recognizes the low molecular weight cytokeratins 8 (52 KD) and 18 (45 kD). Squamous epithelium shows little or no expression of these cytokeratins. **B,** The basal cells of squamous epithelium show reactivity with antibody AE-1, which recognizes the low molecular weight cytokeratins 19 (40 kD), 16 (48 kD), 14 (50 kD), and 11 (56.5 kD). **C,** All layers of squamous epithelium express the cytokeratins recognized by antibody 34βE12, which reacts with high molecular weight cytokeratins 1 (68 kD), 5 (58 kD), 10 (56 kD), and 11 (56.5 kD). Higher molecular weight and more basic keratins are expressed in the upper layers of squamous epithelium.

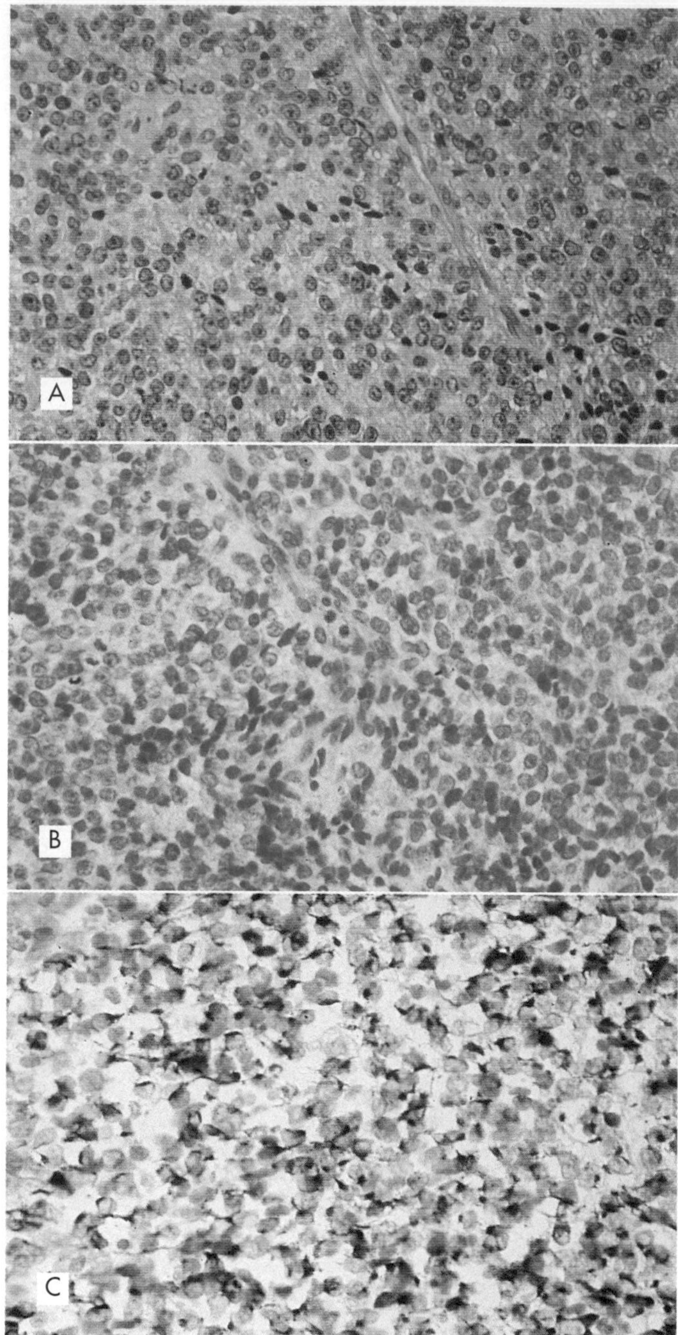

Fig. 8-5 Biopsy from a mass in the mediastinum. Histologic examination of this lesion revealed a malignancy of uncertain histogenesis, **A.** Immunohistochemical examination of this tumor revealed that it did not express lymphoid markers, including CD45, **B.** However, the tumor cells demonstrated strong reactivity with anticytokeratin antibodies, **C.** These results demonstrated the epithelial nature of this tumor; further work-up revealed a primary lung carcinoma. In **B,** notice the presence of normal lymphocytes showing immunoreactivity for CD45 *(center of field).* Internal controls such as these can be critical in the evaluation of the results of an immunohistochemical test.

types become better characterized, it may be possible to distinguish the different types of carcinoma more effectively.

Although keratin expression is characteristic of epithelial cells, nonepithelial neoplasms may in rare instances show aberrant expression of keratin. Such tumors include lymphomas[60] (especially anaplastic large cell lymphoma), various sarcomas,[61,62] gliomas,[63] epithelioid vascular tumors,[64] and melanomas.[65] Although these anomalies are encountered infrequently, their presence emphasizes the importance of using panels of several antibodies in the evaluation of an anaplastic or undifferentiated tumor. Finally, mesotheliomas are keratin-positive tumors. They may be reliably distinguished from other anaplastic epithelial tumors but only by application of a panel of antibodies (Table 8-8).

Keratin-negative, vimentin-positive tumors

The keratin-negative, vimentin-positive undifferentiated tumors are mesenchyme-derived neoplasms, including lymphomas, melanomas, some sarcomas, and certain neural tumors (Fig. 8-6). Several antibodies, discussed later in the chapter, are useful in further characterizing the keratin-negative, vimentin-positive tumor.

Lymphomas. Lymphomas are often diagnosed as undifferentiated malignant neoplasms. A large-cell lymphoma may be difficult to differentiate from carcinoma or melanoma by morphologic criteria alone. Anaplastic large-cell lymphomas (Ki-1 or CD30 positive) may sometimes also show keratin or epithelial membrane antigen (EMA) positivity. Similarly, small-cell lymphomas often resemble other tumors, such as small-cell undifferentiated carcinoma (Tables 8-9 and 8-10). Thus immunohistochemistry can be invaluable for determining the proper therapy for patients with lymphoma. Also, immunohistochemistry may aid the subclassification of non-Hodgkin's lymphoma into groups of different prognostic significance (such as B-cell versus T-cell) (Figs. 8-7 and 8-8). Another important application of the technique is phenotyping to determine the immunoglobulin light-chain expression on lymphocytes. Using these techniques (discussed more fully in Chapter 42) one can distinguish between a malignant and a benign lymphoid proliferation by demonstration of light-chain or heavy-chain restriction, so-called monoclonal patterns (Fig. 8-9).

Leukocyte common antigen (LCA/CD45) is an excellent screening marker for lymphoid cells, including the non-Hodgkin's lymphomas. Staining is characteristically membranous (Fig. 8-10). However, some lymphoid neoplasms may be LCA negative, and a few nonlymphoid neoplasms show non-specific cytoplasmic staining for LCA. The phenotype of LCA-positive cells can be further delineated by more specific lymphoid markers, including those for T-lymphocytes (UCHL-1, CD3, L60, and MT1), B-lymphocytes (L26, LN1, LN2, MB1, and MB2), and immunoglobulin heavy or light chains.[1] Although these markers are best used on fresh or frozen tissue, many work on paraffin-embedded material (Table 8-9).

Immunohistochemistry is also helpful in the identification of Hodgkin's disease. Markers for Reed-Sternberg cells include Leu-M1 (CD15), Ber H2 (Ki-1, CD30), and BLA36 (Fig. 8-11).[1] Note that in lymphocyte-predominant Hodgkin's disease the Reed-Sternberg cells differ in phenotype and are CD15, CD30 negative but CD45, CD20 (B-cells) and BLA36 positive. B-cell markers may also be positive when sensitive techniques are used. "True histiocytic lymphomas," neoplastic proliferation of macrophages, can be identified by positive

Table 8-8 **Antibodies of value in the differential diagnosis of malignant mesothelioma**

Antibody	Mesothelioma	Adenocarcinoma	Sarcoma (including lymphoma, melanoma)
High MW keratins	++	+/–	–
Low MW keratins	++	++/+++	–
Vimentin	+/++	– (+)*	+
CEA	– (<30%+)	– to +++†	–
EMA	+/++	++/+++	– (rare +)
B72.3	– (10%+)	+/++	–
Leu-M1	–	–/++(50%)	– (rare +)
Ber EP4	–	+	–
Others‡	–	(+)	(+)

Modified from Taylor CR, Cote RJ: *Immunomicroscopy: a diagnostic tool for the surgical pathologist,* ed 2, Philadelphia, 1994, Saunders.
CEA, Carcinoembryonic antigen; *EMA,* epithelial membrane antigen; *MW,* molecular weight.
*Vimentin-positive adenocarcinomas include some but not all carcinomas of kidney, thyroid, endometrium, and salivary glands; others rarely.
†Dependent on type of adenocarcinoma: rarely strongly positive in prostate; almost always positive and intense in gastrointestinal tract–derived adenocarcinomas.
‡Other antibodies may be employed if specific types of nonmesothelial tumors are suspected, that is, prostatic acid phosphatase, if prostate; thyroglobulin, if thyroid; and so forth.

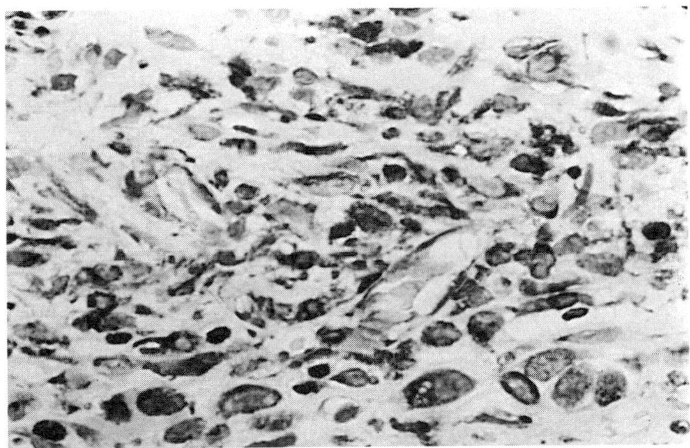

Fig. 8-6 Spindle cell tumor showing intense reactivity with antibody to vimentin intermediate-filament protein.

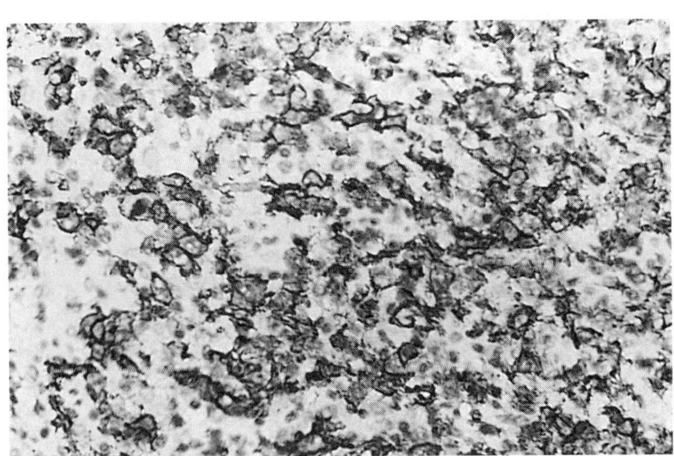

Fig. 8-7 Poorly differentiated neoplasm showing membrane reactivity with monoclonal antibody UCHL-1. These results demonstrate the T-lymphocyte origin of this neoplasm; final diagnosis was T-cell immunoblastic lymphoma.

staining with macrophage markers, such as HAM56, KP1 (CD68), or lysozyme.

Melanomas. Melanomas, termed the "great simulators" of diagnostic pathology,[66] always enter into the differential diagnosis of a poorly differentiated malignant neoplasm. Traditionally, Fontana-Masson or other silver-based stains for melanin and for the ultrastructural detection of melanosomes have assisted in the diagnosis. These approaches have been supplanted by immunohistochemistry, which is more specific than silver stains and more rapid than electron microscopy.

Melanomas typically have no cytoplasmic keratin but do mark with antivimentin. Other useful melanoma markers include antibodies to S-100 protein and to melanosomes (HMB45). S-100 is a sensitive melanoma marker, in that it reacts with the majority of cells in most tumors. Nuclear reactivity is always observed when one is testing melanomas for S-100 expression (Fig. 8-12). However, S-100 lacks specificity for melanoma and it also labels benign nevus cells, Langerhans histiocytes, many sarcomas (liposarcomas and chondrosarcomas), neural tumors (schwannomas, neurofibromas, and granular cell tumors), and certain carcinomas, such as those derived from the salivary gland, breast, and lung.[67,68]

The identity of an S-100-positive neoplasm as a melanoma can be confirmed by its reaction with HMB45,[69] a more specific marker for melanoma. HMB45 decorates melanoma cells with a finely granular cytoplasmic pattern (Fig. 8-12); however, it is less sensitive than S-100, reacting with 70% to 90% of cases, and the reactivity observed with this antibody may be only focal.[70,71] Moreover, its specificity is not absolute; positivity has been reported, albeit very rarely, in some nonmelanocytic tumors, including breast carcinomas and plasmacytomas.[70,72] Anti-HMB45 should therefore be used with antibodies for S-100 protein and vimentin. In anaplastic tumors marking with all three antibodies but not keratin, the probability of melanocytic origin is high.

Sarcomas and soft-tissue tumors. The differential diagnosis of poorly differentiated spindle cell neoplasms includes spindle-cell carcinoma, melanoma, sarcomatoid mesothelioma, lymphoma, and sarcoma. Although electron microscopy has some value in resolving these considerations, the long

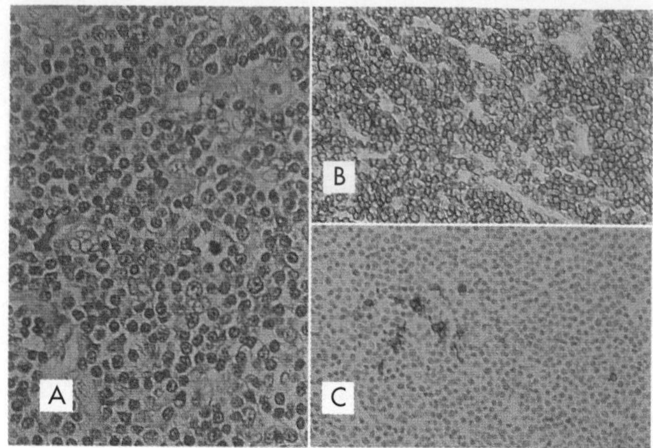

Fig. 8-8 Immunohistochemical staining for T- and B-lymphocytes in paraffin sections. H and E section **(A)** show diffuse lymphoma. UCHL-1 (CD45RO-anti-T-cell) gives staining of lymphoma cells **(B)**, while L26 (CD20-anti-B-cell) identifies scattered residual B-cells. This is a T-cell lymphoma (chromogen diamino benzidine stained using BioTek Techmate automated immunostainer).

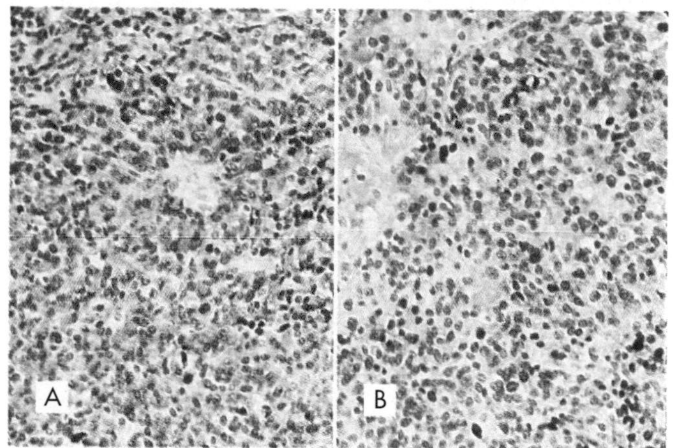

Fig. 8-9 Plasmacytoma showing a monoclonal staining pattern for IgA-κ, **A,** with negative immunoreactivity for IgG, IgM, and λ light chain, **B.** (From Taylor CR, Cote RJ: *Immunomicroscopy: a diagnostic tool for the surgical pathologist,* ed 2, Philadelphia, 1994, Saunders.)

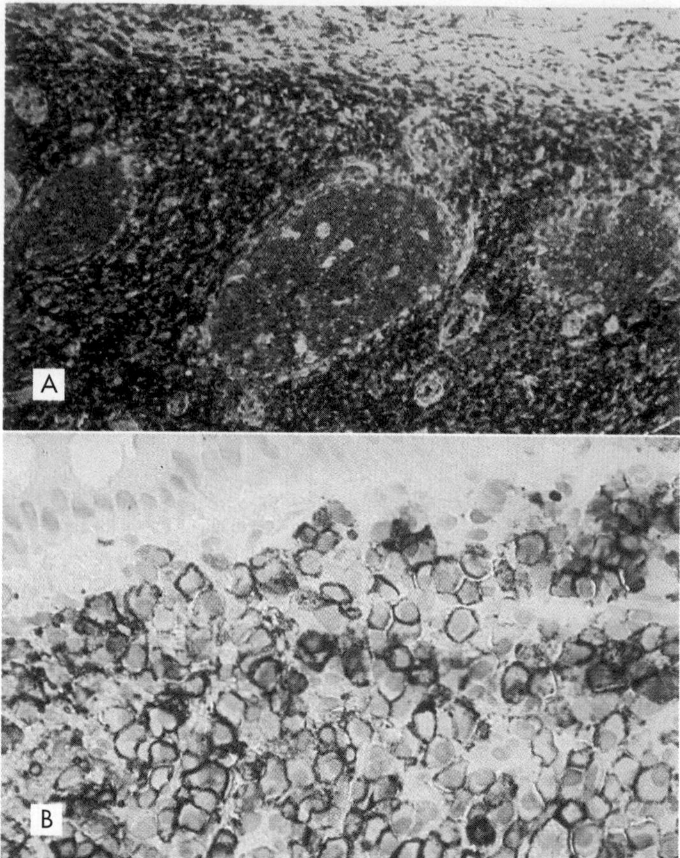

Fig. 8-10 Leukocyte common antigen showing characteristic cell surface membrane staining in normal lymph node, **A,** and in an intestinal B-cell lymphoma, **B.** Counterstain hematoxylin, immunoperoxidase with 3,3′-diaminobenzidine as chromogen. (From Taylor CR, Cote RJ: *Immunomicroscopy: a diagnostic tool for the surgical pathologist,* ed 2, Philadelphia, 1994, Saunders.)

turnaround time is limiting. Immunohistochemical analysis provides information more rapidly and may delineate the type of sarcoma, such as myogenic tumors, fibrohistiocytic tumors, tumors with neural differentiation, vascular sarcomas, or others. A diagnosis of sarcoma is worth considering when a neoplasm expresses vimentin but not keratin, LCA, and HMB45.

Myogenic sarcomas react with antibodies to muscle-specific actin (such as HHF35)[73] and desmin. Both muscle-specific actin and desmin are expressed in normal smooth and striated muscle and in tumors derived from these tissues, such as leiomyosarcomas and rhabdomyosarcomas[74,75] (Fig. 8-13). Myogenic sarcomas can be further characterized immunohistochemically. For example, antibodies against smooth muscle actin[76] show preferential reactivity with leiomyosarcomas (note that myoepithelial cells also stain). Alveolar soft-part sarcomas typically coexpress vimentin and desmin.[77] Tumors derived from skeletal muscle often also contain myoglobin; positive immunoreactivity for muscle-specific actin, desmin, and myoglobin indicates that the tumor in question may be a rhabdomyosarcoma.

Fibrohistiocytic tumors, including malignant fibrous histiocytoma (MFH), are the most common form of soft-tissue sarcomas in adults. The histology of MFH is that of a large-cell pleomorphic neoplasm, occasionally resembling anaplastic carcinoma or other sarcomas. MFH reacts with vimentin and lacks significant reactivity for keratin. Other defining features are expression of alpha-1-antitrypsin, alpha-1-antichymotrypsin, HAM56, and KP1 (CD68). These are useful in distinguishing MFH from other sarcomas[78] (Table 8-10). In fact, alpha-1-antichymotrypsin is such a sensitive marker for MFH that one should reconsider this diagnosis should the tumor fail to react with this antibody. However, alpha-antichymotrypsin is not specific for MFH, occurring in other sarcomas, some carcinomas, and melanomas.[78-80]

Neurogenic tumors, including malignant peripheral nerve sheath tumors and schwannomas, are composed mostly of elongated spindle cells with wavy cytoplasm. Because malignant peripheral nerve sheath tumors often contain epithelioid areas, they may be confused with carcinomas. Immunohistochemical tests that define a neural origin include S-100,

Table 8-9 Principal antibodies against lymphoid cells effective in paraffin section*

Antibody	Cluster of differentiation (CD)	T-cells	B-cells	Monocytes (Histiocytes)	Others
LCA	CD45	+	+	+	G
UCHL-1	CD45RO	+	– (+)	–	Plasma cells, G
MT2	CD45RA	– (+)	+ (–)	–	G
MT1, Leu-22	CD43	+	– (+)	– (+)	Plasma cells, G
MB1, KiB3	CD45RA	– (+)	+	+ (–)	G
L26	CD20	–	+	–	Dendritic RC
LN1	CD75	–	+	–	R-S cells
LN2	CD74	–	+	+	R-S cells
Ber H2 (Ki-1)	CD30	– (+)†	–(+)†	–	R-S cells
Leu-M1	CD15	–	–	– (+)	G, R-S cells
BLA36	–	–	(+)[2]	–	R-S cells
KP1	CD68	(+)	–	+	–
Ig	–	–	–	–	Plasma cells
PCNA‡	–	–	(+)†	(+)†	(+)†

*Note that fixatives also influence results: brief fixation is best, and B5 is better than formalin for some antibodies (such as LN1 and LN2).
†Expressed in dividing cells.
‡PCNA (proliferating cells nuclear antigen) is being superseded by antibody MIB1, which detects Ki-67 proliferation antigen in paraffin sections. (Data from Taylor CR, Cote RJ: *Immunomicroscopy: a diagnostic tool for the surgical pathologist,* ed 2, Philadelphia, 1994, Saunders.)
G, Granulocytes; *Ig,* immunoglobulin; *LCA,* leukocyte common antigen; *RC,* reticulum cells; *R-S,* Reed-Sternberg cells.
Polyclonal CD3 and beta-F1 (anti–T-cell receptor beta chain): both detect T-cells in paraffin sections but in our experience miss many cases (especially large cell), leading to a preference for CD43 and CD45RO reagents. An excellent CD3 antibody has recently become available.
Leu-7 (HNK-1, CD57) has limited application for natural killer (NK) cells.

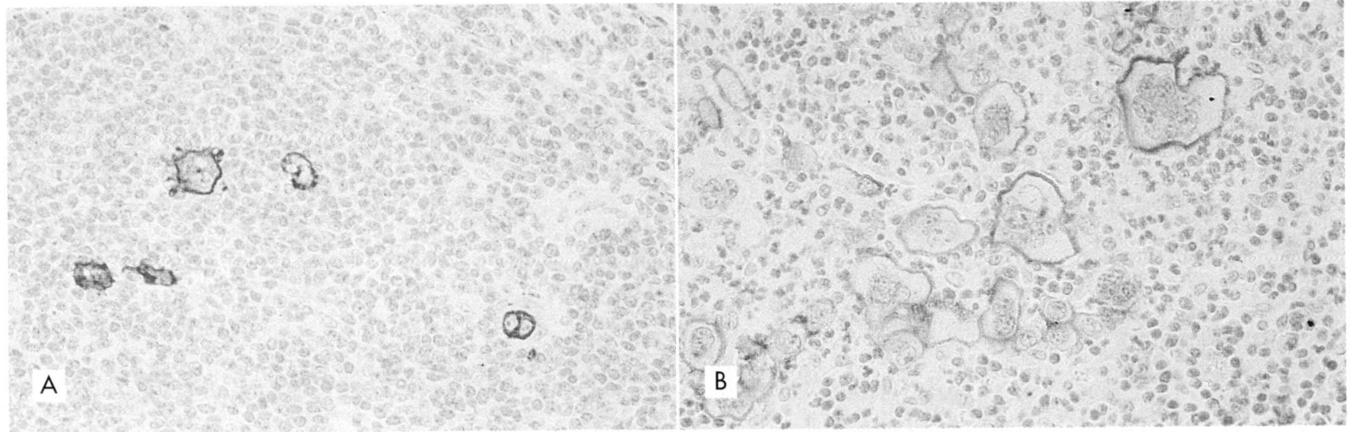

Fig. 8-11 CD30 antigen (Ki-1) is expressed by Reed-Sternberg cells in Hodgkin's disease, **A.** Although this antibody can be helpful in confirming the diagnosis of Hodgkin's disease, Ki-1 is also expressed in anaplastic large cell lymphomas, **B.**

myelin basic protein (MPB), and Leu-7.[81,82] Although most benign neurogenic tumors (schwannomas and neurofibromas) contain S-100, less than half of malignant peripheral nerve sheath tumors contain detectable S-100 protein.[83] It is important to note that S-100 is not a specific marker for schwannomas, and positivity has been described in a variety of neoplasms.

Vascular tumors, including angiosarcoma, also occur among the poorly differentiated malignant neoplasms. Normal and neoplastic vessels can be identified with endothelial markers, such as factor VIII–related antigen (von Willebrand's factor) (Fig. 8-14) and *Ulex europaeus* 1 (UEA) lectin. Antibodies to factor VIII–related antigen react only with endothelial cells and megakaryocytes and are therefore more specific than UEA. The latter is, however, more sensitive.[84,85] Antibodies to the human progenitor cell antigen (CD34) have the curious property of marking endothelial cells, and they can aid in the identification of vascular tumors.

Other tumors to be considered in the differential diagnosis of an anaplastic spindle cell tumor include liposarcomas, chondrosarcomas, osteogenic sarcomas, fibrosarcomas, synovial sarcomas, and epithelioid sarcomas (Table 8-10). Liposarcomas are the second most common type of soft-tissue tumor in adults. Although certain variants (such as myxoid liposarcomas) may be diagnosed by histologic criteria alone, the diagnosis of pleomorphic liposarcomas is aided by immunohistochemistry. The majority of liposarcomas react with both vimentin and S-100 but are nonreactive for HMB45,

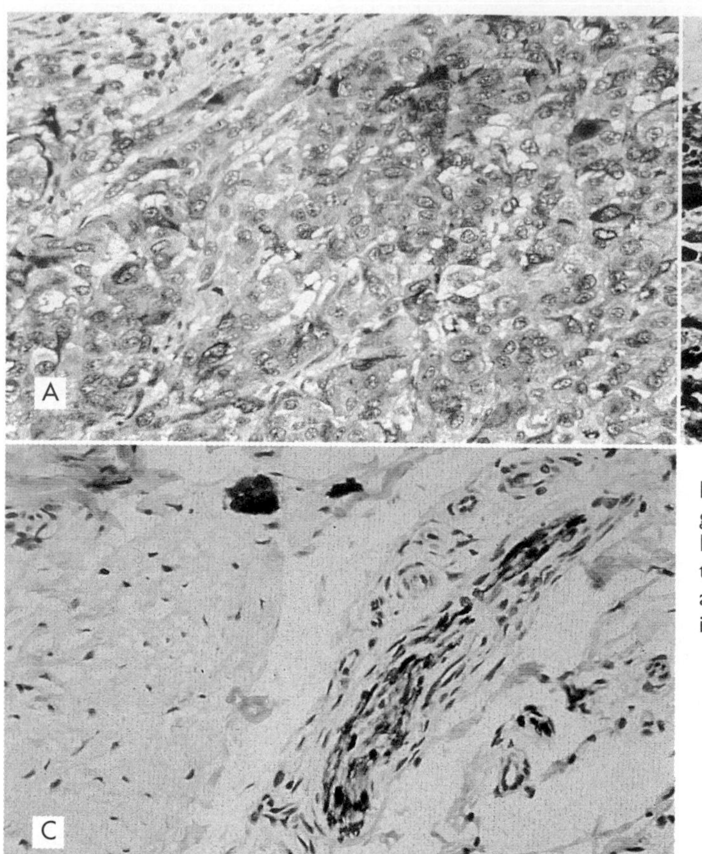

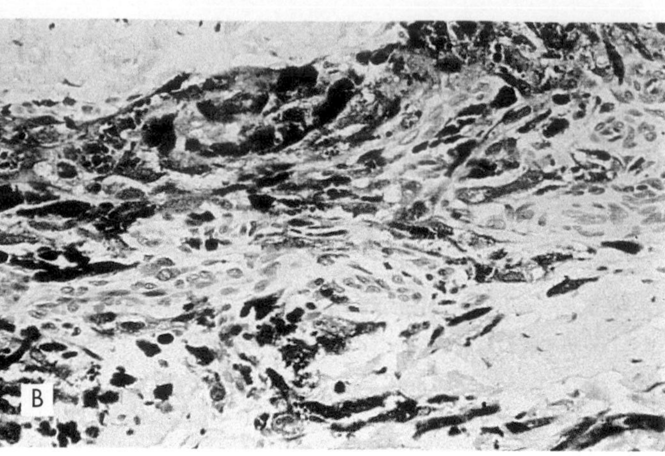

Fig. 8-12 Cells of melanocytic origin express characteristic antigens. This melanoma expresses the melanosome-associated antigen HMB45, **A,** and protein S-100, **B.** In the same section, the antibody to protein S-100 also reacts with nerves, which express the S-100 antigen, **C.** This demonstrates the use of internal controls in immunohistochemical staining.

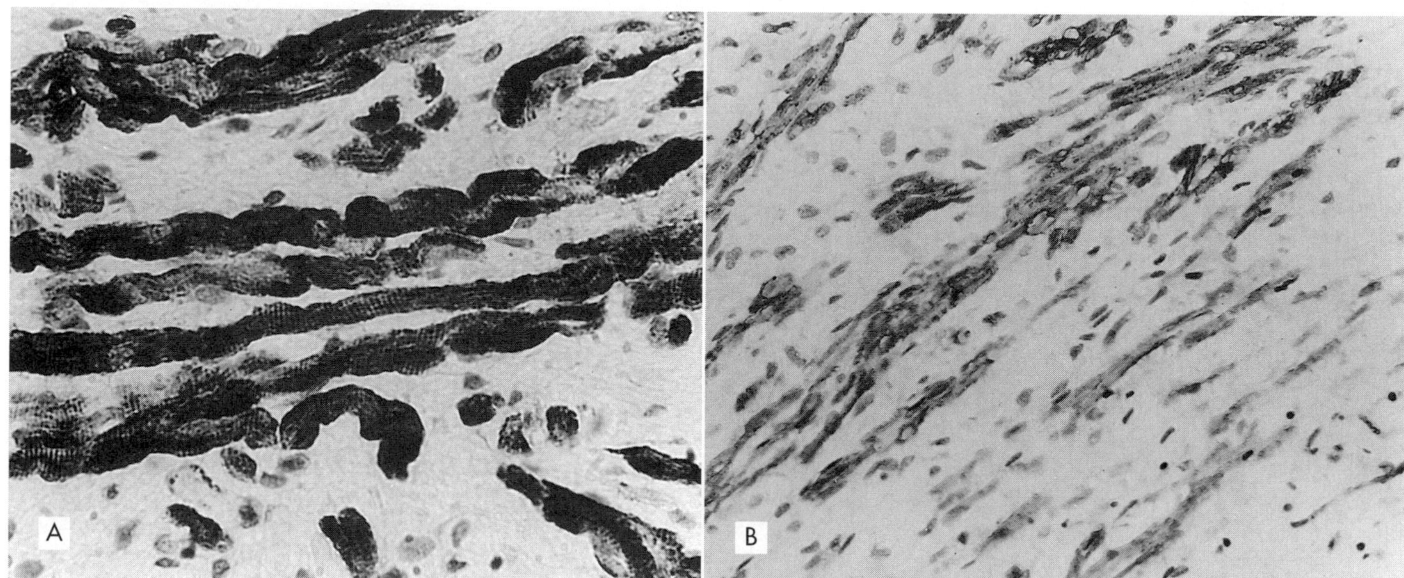

Fig. 8-13 Spindle-cell tumor of the liver showing reactivity with antibodies specific for desmin intermediate filaments, **A,** and muscle-specific actin (HHF35), **B.** Notice the localization of desmin reactivity to cross striations, **A.** These results demonstrate the myogenic nature of this tumor. Final diagnosis was rhabdomyosarcoma. (From Cote RJ, Urmacher C: *Am J Surg Pathol* 14:784, 1990.)

Table 8-10 Patterns of immunohistochemical staining for vimentin-positive tumors—sarcomas

Tumor	Pan-K	Vim	FVIII	S-100	NSE	Myog	Actin	SMA	Des	Other
Lymphomas	–	+	–	–	–	–	–	–	–	LCA
Melanoma	–	+	–	+	–	–	–	–	–	HMB-45
Muscle cell										
Leiomyosarcoma	– (+)	+	–	–	–	–	+	+	(+)	
Rhabdomyosarcoma	–	+	–	–	–	–	+	–	+	
Alveolar soft-part sarcoma	–	+	–	–	–	–	(+)	–	+	
Vascular										CD34 *Ulex*
Angiosarcoma	–	+	+	–	–	–	(+)	–	–	Lectin
Kaposi's sarcoma	–	+	+	–	–	–	(+)	–	–	CD3
Ewing's sarcoma*	–	+	–	–	(+)	–	–	–	–	
Liposarcoma	–	+	–	+	–	–	–	–	–	
Fibrosarcoma	–	+	–	–	–	–	–	–	–	
Malignant fibrous histiocytoma	–	+	–	+	–	–	–	–	–	HAM56
"Neural tumor related"										
Schwannoma†	–	+	–	+	+	–	–	–	–	
Granular cell tumor	–	+	–	+	+	–	–	–	–	
Osteosarcoma	–	+	–	–	–	–	–	–	–	Osteonectin, UJ13A
Chondrosarcoma	–	+	–	+	–	–	–	–	–	
Spindle cell sarcoma										
Synovial	+	+	–	–	–	–	–	–	–	
Epithelioid	+	+	–	–	–	–	–	–	–	
Chordoma	+	+	–	+	–	–	–	–	–	

Modified from Taylor CR, Cote RJ: *Immunomicroscopy: a diagnostic tool for the surgical pathologist,* ed 2, Philadelphia, 1994, Saunders.
*Ewing's tumor is a member of the peripheral neuroectodermal tumor group (PNET) with neural features; other antibodies are helpful (such as HBA71).
†Malignant nerve sheath tumors often lose expression of S-100 and neuron-specific enolase (NSE).
(+) indicates focal reactivity in a subset of cases.
CD, Cluster of differentiation; *Des,* desmin; *FVIII,* factor VIII; *LCA,* leukocyte common antigen; *Myog,* myoglobin; *NSE,* neuron-specific enolase; *Pan-K,* pancytokeratin; *SMA,* smooth muscle–associated actin; *Vim,* vimentin.

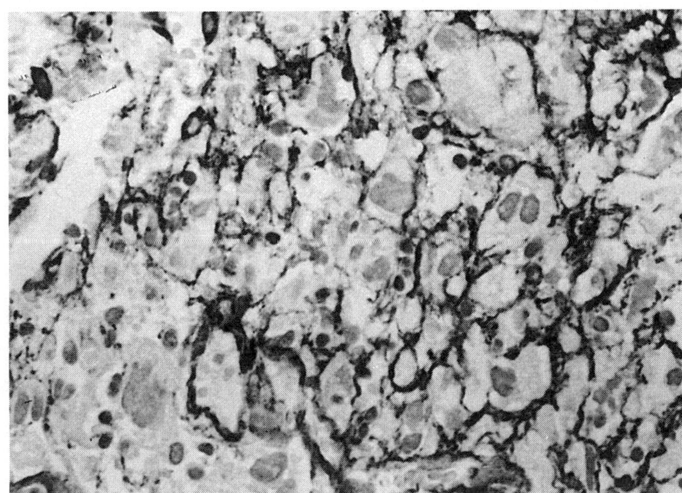

Fig. 8-14 Poorly differentiated tumor showing reactivity with antibody to factor VIII related antigen. This result demonstrated the endothelial origin of this tumor; final diagnosis was angiosarcoma.

in contrast to most melanomas. The same holds true for chondrosarcomas.[86] Osteosarcomas react with vimentin. Antibodies to the so-called osteonectin, or osteosarcoma antigens,[87] may also assist in the diagnosis. An antibody (UJ13A) that stains neuroblastoma cells and osteogenic sarcoma has been described.[88] Fibrosarcomas are rare neoplasms that express only vimentin.

Neural and neuroendocrine tumors

Neural and neuroendocrine tumors may be categorized into three main types, depending on the predominant intermediate filament within the cytoplasm: *Neural tumors* include neuroblastomas, paragangliomas, and pheochromocytomas.[89] These tumors express neurofilament, neuron-specific enolase (NSE), chromogranin (approximately 40%), and synaptophysin.[90-92] *Neuroepithelial tumors* coexpress keratin and neuroendocrine markers; they include carcinoids, Merkel cell carcinomas, and small-cell undifferentiated carcinoma. *Neural neoplasms of mesenchymal origin,* including primitive neuroectodermal tumors (PNET), Ewing's sarcomas, and medulloblastomas typically contain vimentin and variably express NSE and Leu-7.[93]

Although NSE is a sensitive marker for neuroendocrine tumors, it is not specific, being present in many other tumors.[94] For example, carcinoma of the prostate may mark with both NSE and Leu-7.[95] Chromogranin and synaptophysin are more specific markers of neuroendocrine neoplasms, but these antibodies are less sensitive than NSE (Fig. 8-15). Chromogranin content correlates with the degree of tumor differentiation; therefore it is a less useful marker for poorly differentiated neuroendocrine tumors, such as small-cell undifferentiated carcinoma.[96-99] Leu-7 and bombesin are also employed as broad-range neuroendocrine markers but are also not specific.[98,99]

GFAP-positive tumors

Glial fibrillary acid protein (GFAP) is a 51-kilodalton intermediate filament expressed by glial cells. It is present in anaplastic tumors, including astrocytomas, ependymomas, medulloblastomas, some oligodendrogliomas, and choroid plexus tumors.[100,101] Intracerebral tumors that are generally nonreactive with antibodies to GFAP include meningiomas, lymphomas, and metastatic carcinomas. GFAP expression has also been described in a few extracerebral neoplasms, including pleomorphic adenomas of the salivary gland,[102] neurofibromas, and schwannomas.[103]

The unknown primary

As discussed previously, immunohistochemistry often delineates the embryologic histogenesis of a poorly differentiated malignant neoplasm and may occasionally assist the determination of the primary site of a metastatic tumor.

Insight as to cellular origin is often provided by antigens that are related to the functional characteristics of anaplastic tumors (Table 8-11 and Fig. 8-16). For example, cells of melanocytic origin can be identified by the expression of the melanosome-associated antigen HMB45.[69] Cells of myogenic origin can be identified by the expression of contractile actin proteins, desmin, and myoglobin.[73-76] Breast epithelium can be identified by expression of proteins associated with milk production (such as lactalbumin).[104,105] Antigens of relative tissue specificity have also been characterized for thyroid follicular

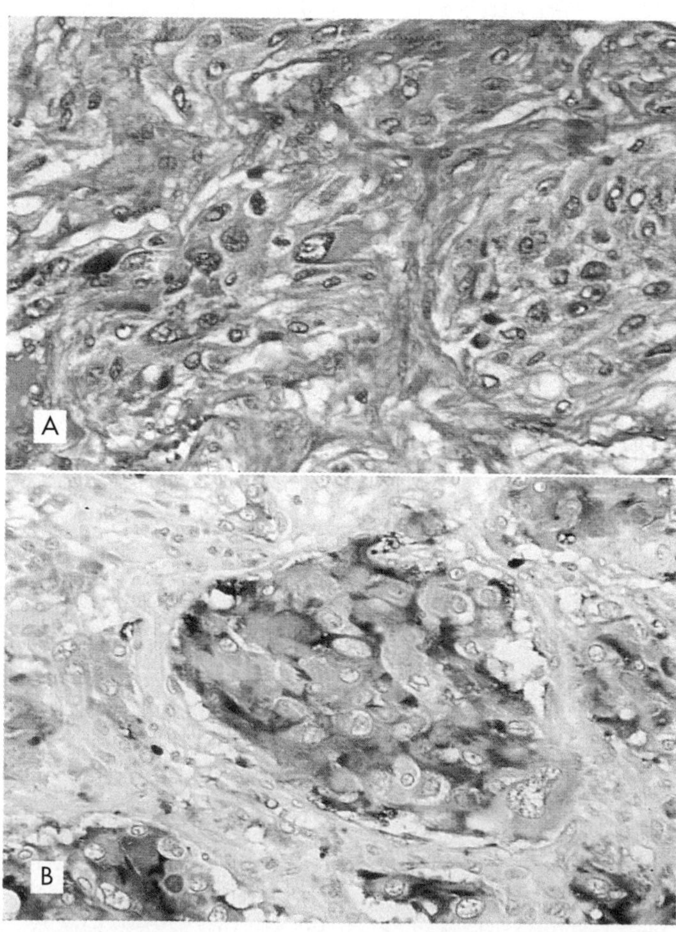

Fig. 8-15 Pheochromocytomas are neuroendocrine neoplasms arising in the adrenal medulla. **A,** Histologic section of a typical pheochromocytoma. **B,** These tumors can be marked with neurospecific enolase (NSE).

Table 8-11 Antigen and antibodies of value in determination of specific tumor types cell origin

Epithelial tumors	Mesenchymal tumors
Breast	***Myogenous tumors***
Alpha-Lactalbumin	Actin
GCDP-15	Smooth muscle–specific actin
Estrogen/progesterone (ER/PR)	Desmin
	Myoglobin
	Fibrohistiocytic tumors
Liver	Lysozyme
Alpha-fetoprotein (AFP)	HAM56
HepBSAg	
Keratin (Cam 5.2)	***Endothelial tumors***
Thyroid	Factor VIII
Thyroglobulin	*Ulex* lectin
Calcitonin	CD34
Prostate	***Melanomas***
Prostatic acid phosphatase (PAP)	S-100
Prostate specific antigen (PSA)	HMB45
Ovary	***B-cell lymphomas***
OC125	LCA, L-26, LN1, LN2, MB1, MB2
Mesothelioma	Immunoglobulins, kappa, lambda
Keratins	
Leu-M1, CEA, Ber EP4, B72.3 } negative expression	***T-cell lymphomas***
	LCA, UCHL-1, L60, MT1
	Reed-Sternberg cells
	Ki-1, L-26, Leu-M1, BLA36
	Histiocytic lymphoma
	KP1, HAM56, lysozyme
Germ cell tumors	**Neuroendocrine tumors**
Human chorionic gonadotropin (HCG)	Neuron-specific enolase (NSE)
Alpha-fetoprotein (AFP)	Chromogranin
	Synaptophysin
	Pituitary
	ACTH, PRL, GH, LH, FSH, TSH
	Pancreas
	Insulin, gastrin, vasoactive intestinal polypeptide, somatostatin, glucagon

Modified from Taylor CR, Cote RJ: *Immunomicroscopy: a diagnostic tool for the surgical pathologist,* ed 2, Philadelphia, 1994, Saunders.

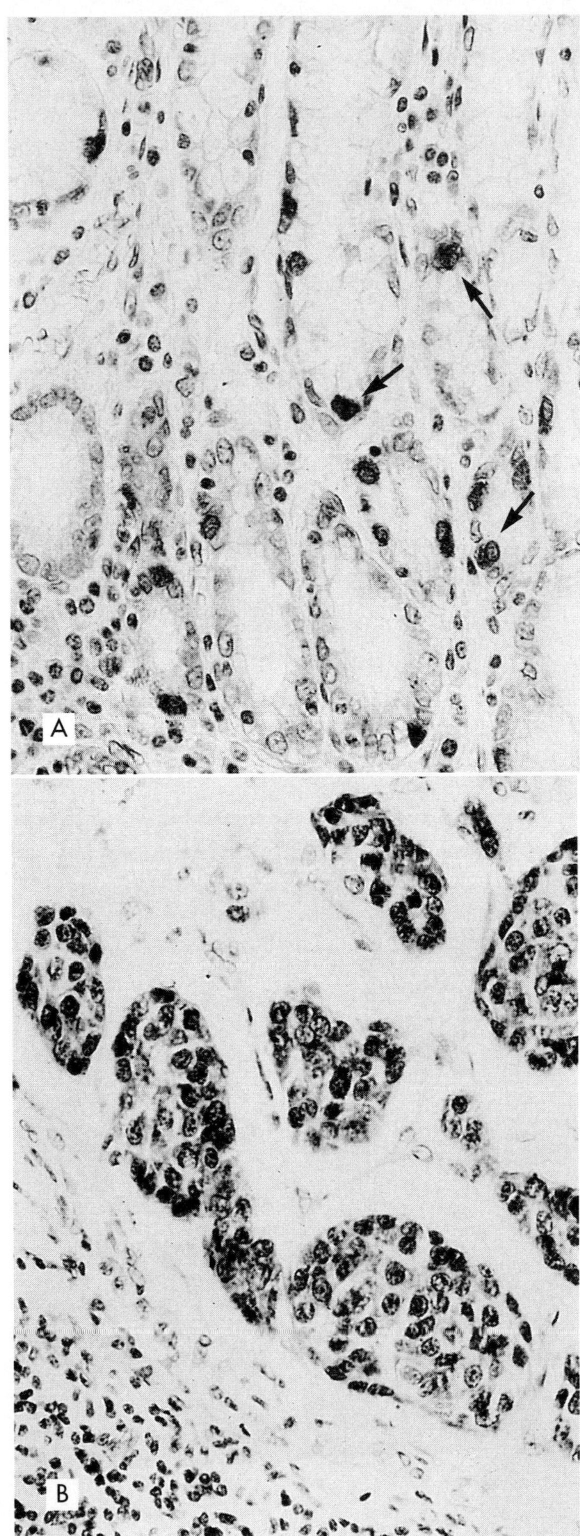

Fig. 8-16 Immunohistochemical detection of gastrin expression in the normal stomach, **A.** Notice the scattered G (gastrin-containing) cells within these glands (*arrows*). **B,** Neuroendocrine neoplasm in duodenal wall showing immunoreactivity with antibodies to gastrin, confirming the diagnosis of gastrinoma. (From Taylor CR, Cote RJ: *Immunomicroscopy: a diagnostic tool for the surgical pathologist,* ed 2, Philadelphia, 1994, Saunders.)

epithelium and C cells (thyroglobulin and calcitonin),[106-108] neuroendocrine cells (NSE, chromogranin, and synaptophysin) (Fig. 8-15),[109-113] and pancreatic islet cells (such as insulin and glucagon).[114-117]

A few antigens of unknown function, such as prostate-specific antigen (PSA), are specific for particular cell types (Fig. 8-17).[118,119] Finally, a small number of tumors are specifically associated with viral infection, such as hepatocellular carcinoma (hepatitis B) and squamous cell carcinoma (human *Papillomavirus*).

Antigens characteristic of particular tissues are provided in Table 8-11. Although tumors derived from those tissues can be identified by specific antigen expression, many tissues have no unique marker (such as lung, colon, and fat). The goal of immunohistochemistry in these instances is to define the embryologic histogenesis of the lesion (such as epithelial versus mesenchymal). Furthermore, the expression of tissue-specific antigens tends to diminish with tumor dedifferentiation.

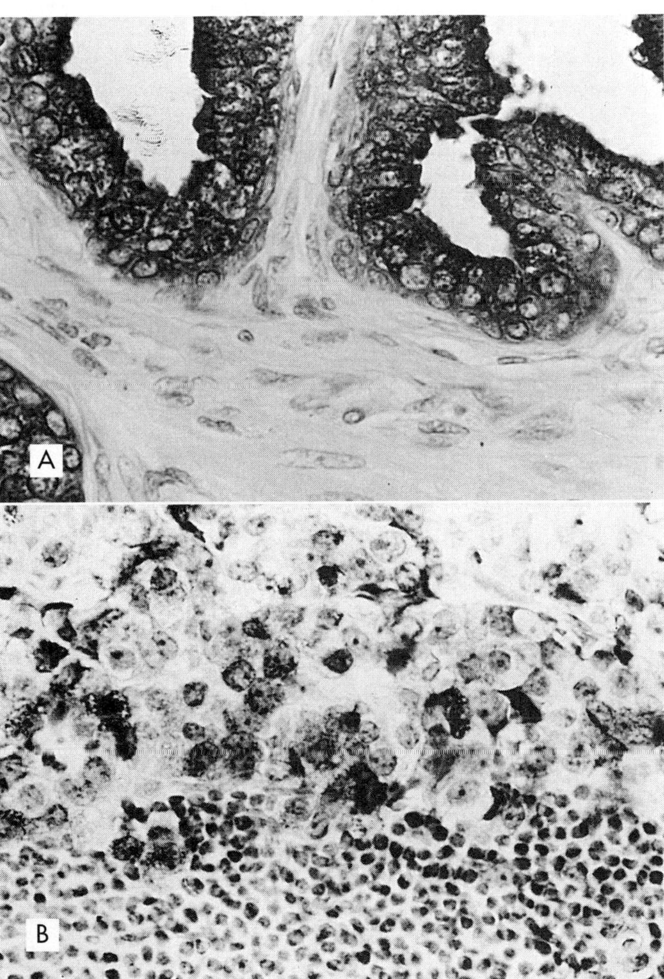

Fig. 8-17 The prostate expresses several characteristic antigens. **A,** Normal prostate epithelium showing positive cytoplasmic with antibody to prostate-specific antigen (PSA). **B,** This anaplastic tumor reacts with antibodies to PSA, confirming the diagnosis of prostate origin for this tumor. (From Taylor CR, Cote RJ: *Immunomicroscopy: a diagnostic tool for the surgical pathologist,* ed 2, Philadelphia, 1994, Saunders.)

Unfortunately the anaplastic tumors that are the most difficult to morphologically recognize are the least likely to express the antigens useful in their identification. For example, although 60% to 70% of breast tumors express GCDFP-15,[120,121] (Fig. 8-18) the more poorly differentiated breast cancers generally do not express this antigen. The same holds true for expression of alpha-lactalbumin and estrogen receptor. Therefore the absence of a tissue-specific antigen within a tumor does not rule out its derivation from that tissue. Here again, panels of antibodies can be extremely helpful.

Finally, many of the antigens listed in Table 8-11 are not completely tissue specific. For example, although GCDFP-15 is preferentially expressed by cells of the breast, other cells (such as salivary epithelium) also express this antigen.[120] Again, the use of antibody panels can minimize the chance of misinterpreting such staining patterns.

Prognostic markers in cancer

The goal of the surgical pathologist is to provide information that defines the clinical outcome, based on specific clinical and pathologic parameters. Staging criteria, for example, are used to evaluate virtually every type of solid tumor and are important not only in predicting prognosis, but also in selecting therapy. Indeed, one of the outstanding achievements of modern medicine is the ability to predict the behavior of tumors based on specific clinical and pathologic criteria. However, tumor stage and grade provide only general estimates of outcome for a particular patient. For example, in the case of breast cancer, the single most important prognostic parameter is the presence or absence of metastases to the axillary lymph nodes. However, patients without nodal metastases have a low but definite risk for recurrence. Other patients, who should seemly have high risk of recurrence by virtue of lymph node metastases, do not develop systemic metastases. The current clinical and pathologic staging parameters do not identify precisely those individuals destined to relapse.

These considerations are motivating efforts to identify enzymes, oncogenes, or tumor-suppressor genes, the presence or absence of which may more accurately predict the biologic behavior of tumors. Such studies represent a fundamental shift in the means by which tumor behavior is defined, a change from outcome-based analysis to one founded upon tumor biology.

The immunohistochemical analysis of tumors is undergoing a profound shift in emphasis. Although initial studies focused on the use of immunohistochemistry to define tumor histogenesis (as discussed earlier), the aim of much of the current research in immunohistochemistry is to reveal the biologic potential of tumors, thus providing a more scientific basis for tumor management (Table 8-12).

Microinvasion and pseudoinfiltration

Microinvasion of a carcinoma is generally defined as infiltration through the underlying basement membrane. Antibodies to basement membrane components assist in the evaluation of basement membrane integrity; the two most commonly used antibodies target either collagen type IV or laminin.[122,123] With an intact basement membrane, invasion is unlikely. In benign tissues, however, the basement membrane may appear slightly discontinuous when studied by immunohistochemical procedures. Microinvasion should be diagnosed only when the basement membrane is lost or grossly disrupted.

Benign pseudoinfiltrative lesions, which can be extremely difficult to distinguish from infiltrating carcinoma, are particu-

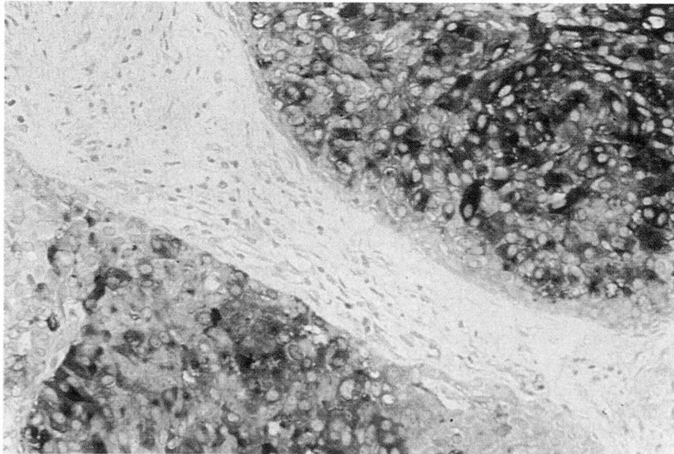

Fig. 8-18 Breast epithelium and the majority of breast carcinomas express the antigen GCDFP-15. This infiltrating duct carcinoma demonstrates strong immunoreactivity with antibody to GCDFP-15.

Table 8-12 Immunohistochemical analysis of cancer: prognosis and approaches to therapy

Tumor staging	**Tumor-suppressor gene products**
Microinvasion	Rb (retinoblastomer gene)
Detection of bone marrow micrometastases	p53
Detection of lymph node micrometastases	DCC (gene deleted in colon cancer)
	NF-1 (neurofibromatosis type 1)
	Wilms' tumor gene
	NM23
	Metastatic potential
Tumor-associated antigens	Laminin receptor
Tn	Type IV collagenase
Carcinoembryonic antigen (CEA)	Cathepsin D
Glycosylation antigens	OA519
Blood-group antigens	
Tumor cell proliferation	**Predictors of response to therapy**
Ki-67	Estrogen receptor (ER)
Proliferating cell nuclear antigen (PCNA)	Progesterone receptor (PR)
	Androgen receptor (AR)
	pS2
	MDR (multidrug resistance)
Oncogenes/growth factors and receptors	
Her-2/*neu*	
ras	
N, c-*myc*	
c-*kit*	
INT-2/HST-1	
EGFR (epidermal growth factor receptor)	
TGF-α, β (transforming growth factor)	

larly common in the breast and prostate. A basement membrane that circumscribes the suspicious cell groups is suggestive of a benign or in situ process. Also, many types of normal glandular epithelial cells are circumscribed by a basal cell layer. In the case of breast tissue, the basal cell layer is composed of myoepithelial cells. Myoepithelial cells are readily identified with antibodies to muscle-specific actin.[73] The presence of myoepithelial cells around "infiltrating" tubular elements is suggestive of a benign process (such as sclerosing adenosis or radical scar). Their absence is not diagnostic of malignancy, however, because breast myoepithelial cells may often be discontinuous in their distribution and thereby not captured in solitary planes of section.[124]

In the case of the prostate, the basal cells can be distinguished from the luminal cells by virtue of their expression of a different set of cytokeratin intermediate filaments. Several antibodies that have been described react with the unique, high molecular weight cytokeratins expressed by basal cells to the exclusion of the low molecular weight cytokeratins expressed by luminal cells.[125-127] These immunoreactivity patterns may be used to distinguish benign from malignant prostatic epithelial lesions because basal cells can be identified in nearly all benign glandular proliferations of the prostate but are never present at the periphery of malignant glands[126-131] (Fig. 8-19).

Occult micrometastasis

After pioneering studies at the Ludwig Institute and Royal Marsden Hospital in London, England,[132] several groups have described the use of immunohistochemistry to identify otherwise occult micrometastases of carcinoma within the bone marrow and lymph nodes.[133-138] Although most of these studies have focused on breast carcinoma, many other tumors are now under investigation.[139-145] These studies take advantage of the ability of antibodies to distinguish cells of different histogenesis; in this case, epithelial (carcinoma) cells from the normal constituents of the bone marrow and lymph nodes.

Bone marrow

Many antibodies with specificity for epithelia have been used to detect metastatic carcinoma cells in the bone marrow,[132-138] in exploitation of the fact that the normal bone marrow compartment contains no epithelial elements.[135] By such means, occult micrometastases have been detected in the bone marrow of patients with a variety of tumors, including carcinomas of the colon, prostate, ovary, and lung, as well as neuroblastoma.[132-145]

With breast carcinoma, immunohistochemistry can demonstrate occult micrometastases in the bone marrow in approximately 25% to 30% of low-stage (operable) patients (Fig. 8-20). Several studies have addressed the clinical significance of bone marrow micrometastases in breast cancer. The presence of occult micrometastases has been correlated with other known predictors of prognosis, including lymph node status and stage of disease.[132,134,135,137,138] In addition, the presence of bone marrow micrometastases has independent significance in identifying a population of patients at increased risk for disease progression.[133,136,138,146] Of particular note is the work of Dearnaley and associates,[146] who followed a cohort of breast cancer patients for a median of 9.5 years and found that the majority (85%) of patients who had occult bone marrow micrometastases detected at the time of surgery developed overt metastases, whereas dissemination occurred in only one third of those with no evidence of bone marrow micrometastases. Bone marrow micrometastases are also associated with increased risk for disease progression in patients with colon and lung carcinoma.[139,140,144,145]

Occult lymph node metastases

Regional lymph node metastases are the single most important prognostic factor for most tumors. Routine histopathologic examination of lymph nodes may understate the prevalence of such metastases, however, and Gusterson and Ott have calculated that a pathologist has only a 1% chance of identifying a metastatic focus of breast cancer of a diameter of three cells in cross section within a histologic section of a lymph node.[147] Others have identified a false-negative rate in the detection of metastatic carcinoma within lymph nodes evaluated by conventional histologic means alone.[148] Fully 8% to 30% of node-

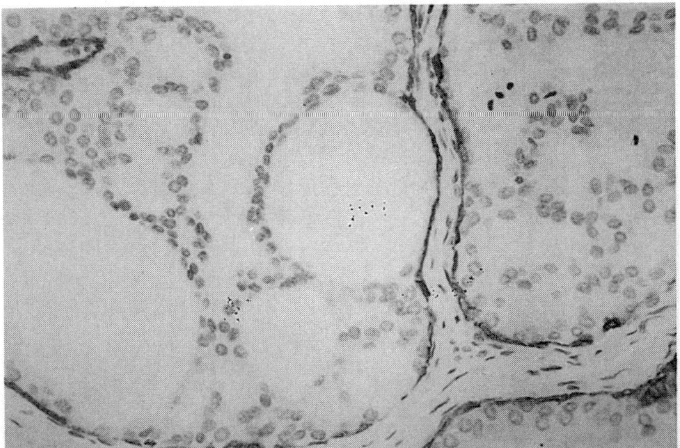

Fig. 8-19 Cribriform hyperplasia of the prostate. The basal cells lining the glands demonstrate reactivity with antibody 34βE12 (K903). Notice that the luminal epithelial cells show no detectable expression of the cytokeratins identified by 34βE12. The presence of a basal cell layer indicates that this is a benign lesion.

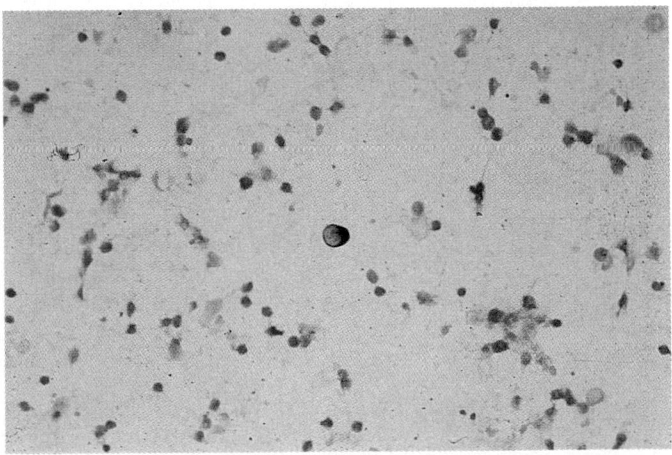

Fig. 8-20 Bone marrow from a patient with stage I carcinoma of the breast. This patient had no clinical or pathologic evidence of metastatic spread of tumor. With use of a cocktail of anticytokeratin monoclonal antibodies, rare positive cells were seen in the bone marrow, consistent with carcinoma. Notice that the surrounding normal bone marrow elements show no immunoreactivity.

negative breast cancer patients will be found to harbor occult micrometastases using more rigorous histomorphologic or immunohistochemical means (Fig. 8-21).[142-161] Similar data exist for carcinomas of colon, lung, and prostate and for melanoma.[162-165,165a]

Although numerous studies have approached the problem of the detection of occult lymph node metastases,[148-165] there is surprising disagreement regarding the prognostic importance of these occult tumor deposits, particularly with reference to breast cancer. Most of the studies have involved too few patients to address the issue with statistical power.

More recently, however, investigators from the Ludwig Institute and International Breast Cancer Study Group performed a more definitive study on the importance of occult lymph node metastases in patients with node-negative breast cancer.[152] Serial sections from paraffin blocks containing lymph nodes from 921 patients were examined by routine histologic methods. Nine percent of these patients had occult lymph node metastases not detected by routine histopathologic examination. These patients had a poorer disease-free state ($p = 0.003$) and overall survival ($p = 0.002$) after a 5-year median follow-up study, relative to those patients whose nodes remained negative after serial sectioning. Recent 6-year median follow-up data show even more conclusive evidence regarding this prognostic significance.[166] Studies using immunohistochemical methods to detect occult lymph node metastases have shown that this information is prognostically significant.[156,158,161]

Definitive comparative analyses of methods to detect micrometastases are now ongoing;[159] data emerging from these studies indicate that immunohistochemical methods may be superior to histologic examination of lymph node serial sections. Its significance has already been found to be clinically important in patients with stage I melanoma,[162] Dukes B colon carcinoma,[164] and early stage non–small cell lung carcinoma.[165]

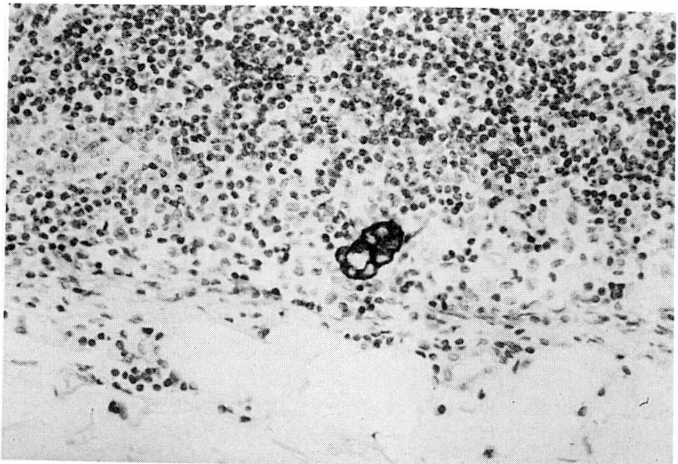

Fig. 8-21 Section of an axillary lymph node from a patient with breast carcinoma. No tumor was identified in any axillary lymph nodes from this patient after routine histologic analysis. However, using a cocktail of antiepithelial monoclonal antibodies, a small cluster of carcinoma cells was seen in this lymph node in the subcapsular sinus.

"Tumor" antigens

One of the most fascinating, complex, and controversial areas of immunohistochemistry has been the study of antigenic changes that are associated with malignant transformation and tumor progression. From the perspective of the immunohistopathologist, these changes can be classified into four general categories: (1) new expression of tumor-specific antigens; (2) microanatomic changes in the cellular distribution of antigens; (3) changes (increase or decrease) in the level of antigen expression, including changes associated with differentiated cellular functions; and (4) alterations in the biochemical nature of antigens, particularly changes in glycosylation patterns of glycoprotein and glycolipid antigens.

The expression of *tumor-specific* antigens has been a focus of intense research.[167] These include mutated oncogene and tumor-suppressor gene products, such as p53 protein. For virtually all antigens, however, tumor specificity is not absolute; for example, mutations in the p53 gene have been described in premalignant lesions from the prostate and breast. Furthermore, the detection of mutated p53 protein is not based on the mutation itself but rather on the increased accumulation of the protein that results from the mutation.

The *microanatomic distribution* of antigens in normal cells is often different from that of their malignant counterparts' cells. Epithelial differentiation antigens, particularly cell surface antigens, such as CEA, B72.3, and EMA, have an apical or luminal distribution in benign cells. However, in malignant epithelial cells these antigens show a less discrete cellular distribution surrounding the entire cell membrane and with increased expression in the cytoplasm. These changes result from increased expression (and therefore accumulation) of the antigens and failure of active transport and membrane insertion of the antigens in neoplastic cells. Although these changes are characteristic of malignant cells, this feature is not specific enough to be diagnostic of malignancy.[168-171]

Increased *antigen expression* is a feature of some tumor cells. Well-characterized examples exist for epithelial tumors, where glycoprotein antigens that are expressed in excess include Tn, CEA, OC125, and others.[168,172-175] Unfortunately, these changes are relative and not tumor specific. The differences in the level of antigen expression between normal and malignant cells can be profound. Many of these antigens that were originally believed to be tumor specific are not, but early assay methods were too insensitive to detect low-level antigen expression on normal cells. Most serum tumor markers belong to this class of antigens (that is, low-level expression by normal cells, increased expression by tumor cells).

Just as some antigens have increased expression on neoplastic cells, so too other antigens have decreased expression by malignant cells. The most important examples are those antigens that are associated with the differentiated function of the cell of origin, such as GCDFP-15 (breast), thyroglobulin, and calcitonin. Although many tumors continue to produce the same products as their benign counterparts, these characteristics can be lost as the tumor becomes more undifferentiated. For example, well-differentiated breast carcinomas will often express GCDFP-15, but poorly differentiated breast carcinomas will do so less often.[120] A similar situation exists with regard to the expression of thyroglobulin by thyroid carcinomas. In fact, decreased expression of thyroglobulin by thyroid tumors is associated with a poorer prognosis.[108,176]

An interesting example of a change in antigen expression that accompanies malignant transformation and progression is that of intermediate-filament expression seen in epithelial tumorigenesis. Dedifferentiation of epithelial tumors is characteristically accompanied by decreased expression of cytokeratins (which are intermediate filaments specific for epithelial differentiation), with a concomitant increase in the expression of the intermediate filament vimentin. This coordinated change is well illustrated by cells of adrenocortical origin: normal adrenocortical cells express cytokeratins but not vimentin (at detectable levels), whereas adrenocortical carcinomas consistently show vimentin expression but generally do not express cytokeratin.[177,178] Interestingly, adrenocortical adenomas usually demonstrate expression of both cytokeratins and vimentin.[177]

Changes in the pattern of *glycosylation* of glycoproteins and glycolipids occur in many neoplasms.[179-181] Tumor cells can show aberrant, often truncated glycosylation compared to normal cells, as in the case of blood group–related antigens.[181] The blood group antigens are carbohydrates that are expressed on epithelial cells, endothelial cells, and red blood cells. Changes in blood group antigen expression can take several forms. For example, the major blood group antigens (A, B, H) are not expressed by normal colonic epithelium but are expressed (according to the blood type of the individual) by the majority of colonic adenocarcinomas.[182] In contrast, normal urothelium (generally) expresses ABH antigens, whereas malignant urothelial cells show loss of ABH expression. However, Lewis type of blood group antigens (Le^x and Le^y), which are not found on normal urothelium, are expressed by the majority of urothelial tumors.[183,184] These changes are consistent and have been used to aid in the diagnosis and screening of urothelial carcinomas. The identification of Le^x by exfoliated urothelial cells significantly improves the detection of urothelial tumors and can be used as an early marker of bladder cancer recurrence.[184] Finally, alteration in blood group antigen expression has been described in other epithelial tumors and has even been found to predict outcome for some tumor types.[185,186]

A detailed discussion of the antigenic changes that have been associated with malignant transformation and tumor progression is beyond the scope of this chapter. Indeed, a detailed knowledge of the particular tumor in question is required because the same antigenic change can have entirely different meaning in different cell types (for example, loss of ABH expression is associated with malignant urothelium, and normal colonic epithelium). Nevertheless, the study of antigenic changes is important to tumor analysis and provides fundamental insights for understanding the biologic differences between benign and malignant cells.

Tumor cell proliferation

Cell proliferation correlates with clinical outcome in many tumors. However, quantitating proliferation by counting of mitotic figures is not easily learned or reproducible between different pathologists. There have been attempts, therefore, to find more objective methods for measuring tumor cell proliferation. Methods have included measurement of tritiated thymidine or bromodeoxyuridine (BrdU) incorporation into tumor cell DNA[187-191] and measurement of the proportion of cells in the synthetic (S) phase of the cell cycle (S-phase fraction) by flow cytometry[192-203] (see Chapter 13).

A promising approach is immunohistochemical assessment of proliferative potential by the detection of nuclear proteins related to DNA replication.[204] The principle advantage of this method over flow cytometric techniques is that it permits concurrent morphologic examination of the tissue.

Two extensively studied proliferation-related markers are Ki-67 and PCNA (proliferating cell nuclear antigen, or cyclin)[205-207] (Fig. 8-22). Ki-67 is a nuclear antigen that is present in cells in the active phases of the cell cycle (that is, G_1, S, G_2, and mitosis) but is absent in G_0 (resting, or quiescent; "gap") cells. PCNA shows a distribution in the cell cycle that is similar to Ki-67 (that is, absent in G_0 cells), though its degree of expression differs. Interestingly, human autoantibodies reacting to PCNA have been described.

There is a strong correlation between thymidine labeling and the proportion of cells exhibiting Ki-67 or PCNA expression.[192-194,205,206] As expected, the proportion of cells showing Ki-67 or PCNA reactivity is greater than that identified by thymidine labeling; the reason is that these antigens are present in a broader range of cells (G_1, S, G_2, and mitosis) than that detected by labeling with thymidine (S-phase only). In addition, there appears to be less intraspecimen variability in

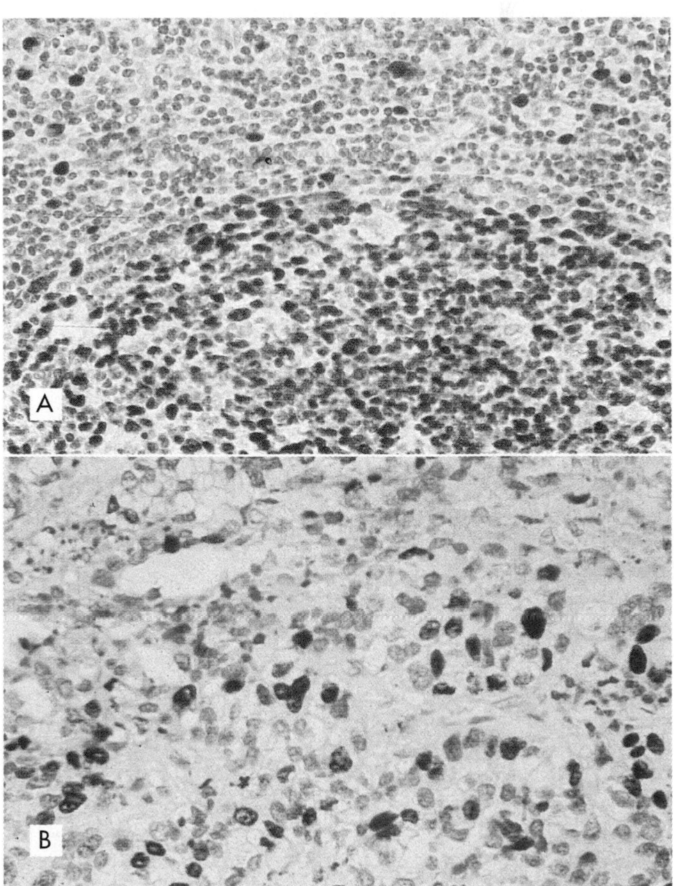

Fig. 8-22 Immunohistochemical detection of proliferation associated antigens. **A,** Proliferating cell nuclear antigen (PCNA) in normal lymph node. Notice the density of PCNA-positive cells in the hyperplastic germinal center, where the majority of cells are proliferating. **B,** Detection of the Ki-67 antigen in paraffin-embedded tissue using antibody MIB-1.

growth fraction estimates when assessed by Ki-67 or PCNA versus thymidine labeling.[192-194] Immunohistochemical assessment of proliferation is highly correlated with S-phase fraction analysis obtained by flow cytometry, particularly in aneuploid tumors.[192-194] Some discrepancies have been observed, particularly in diploid cell populations, a finding attributed to the relatively slow decrease in Ki-67 and PCNA expression in cells as they enter into G_0. Staining in these cells is faint, relative to the replicating cell population.

Ki-67 and PCNA immunoreactivity correlates well with morphologic features of cell proliferation as well, particularly mitotic index and tumor grade, and in breast tumors their expression is related to other markers of differentiation and prognosis. For example, there is a strong inverse association between proliferation rate as assessed by Ki-67/PCNA immunoreactivity and estrogen-progesterone expression.[207] On the other hand, there is a positive association between increased proliferation rate and p53 gene abnormalities.[208] Finally, in patients with breast, prostate, colon, lung, liver, and gastric carcinomas, as well as some lymphomas and sarcomas, there is now substantial evidence that increased proliferation, as assessed by immunohistochemical analysis using Ki-67 or PCNA, allows identification of patients whose tumors are more likely to progress; a high Ki-67/PCNA labeling index identifies patients who have a significantly shorter disease-free and overall survival.[209-219]

There are technical advantages of using proliferation-related markers like Ki-67 and PCNA. They can be used in tissue sections, an important consideration when one is dealing with small tumors. Analysis of proliferation by thymidine labeling or flow cytometry is not able to distinguish benign from malignant cells in tumors with irregular admixtures of these elements. In cases in which the proportion of benign to malignant cells is high (as is often the case), an aberrant proliferation index (in this case, too low) may be obtained. Because the immunohistochemical analysis occurs in a morphologic context, the tumor cell population of interest can be identified and distinguished from the surrounding benign tissue, allowing for a more precise assessment of proliferation in the tumor cells themselves. Finally, tumors may show geographic variations in the proliferation rate; nonmorphologic methods cannot produce an assessment of this heterogeneity, whereas this can be reliably done with immunohistochemical methods.

Recently, antibodies to other cell cycle-related proteins have been developed, such as cyclin A, cyclin D1, and p21.[219a,b] These may allow a finer dissection of the cell cycle and a better understanding of proliferation and tumor progression.

Oncogenes, growth factors, and receptors

There is now considerable evidence that autocrine and paracrine factors, at least some of which may be mediated by the action of oncogenes, play a significant role in oncogenesis, as well as in normal tissue growth and differentiation (see ch. 24). For several of these factors, immunohistochemical analysis is a primary method of evaluation.

***Her-2/*neu.** Her-2/*neu* (or c-*erb* B-2) is a protooncogene first isolated from chemically induced rat ganglioneuroblastomas. The gene codes for a protein (185 KD) that shows homology with the epidermal growth factor receptor (EGFR) and displays tyrosine kinase activity. A putative ligand for the Her-2/*neu* receptor protein, termed *heregulin,* has recently been described; it binds to and activates the receptor and is similar to proteins in the epidermal growth factor (EGF) family.[220]

Amplification of the gene coding for Her-2/*neu* has been described in breast, ovarian, prostate, gastric, salivary gland, lung, colon, and squamous cell carcinomas.[221-231] Overall, 25% to 30% of primary breast cancers and about one third of primary ovarian cancers demonstrate amplification of the gene. These patients appear to have an increased rate of recurrence and decreased survival.[221,228] The amplification of the Her-2/*neu* gene is accompanied by increased expression of the protein gene product, which can be detected in frozen or paraffin sections by immunohistochemical techniques.[221,228]

There is near uniform correlation between gene amplification and immunohistochemical reactivity for Her-2/*neu* on frozen sections, such that immunohistochemistry has become the standard method for analysis of Her-2/*neu* gene amplification (Fig. 8-23).[221,228,232] However, there are several important caveats. About 10% of breast cancers show immunohistochemical reactivity for Her-2/*neu* but show no gene amplification, a finding attributed to increased gene expression (increased mRNA). Also, there appears to be some loss of antigen after routine (formalin/paraffin) fixation and processing. As a result, some tumors with low levels of amplification may not be detected immunohistochemically. Newer techniques of antigen retrieval, however, have substantially improved this situation. Finally, the intracellular localization of the immunohistochemical reactivity is critical to its assessment. When overexpressed, the protein accumulates at the cell membrane and is seen as a crisp membrane stain; a cytoplasmic staining pattern is not associated with protein or gene overexpression.[221,228] The meaning of the cytoplasmic stain is unclear and does not appear to be attributable simply to "background," or nonspecific, reactivity.

Although Her-2/*neu* overexpression and amplification has been described in several tumor systems, it has been most extensively studied in the breast. Her-2/*neu* overexpression occurs in 25% to 30% of primary breast carcinomas and is

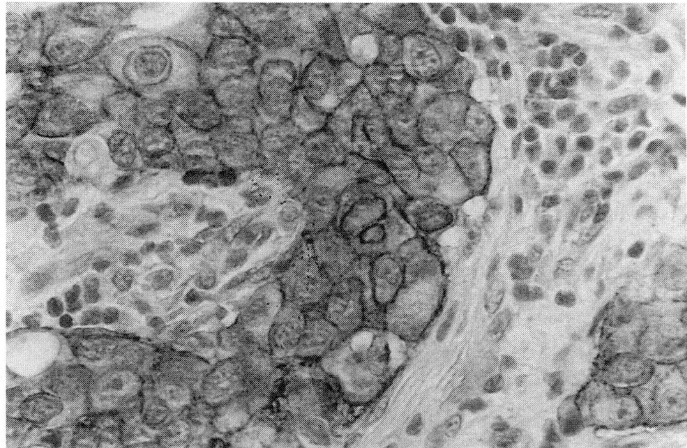

Fig. 8-23 Infiltrating ductal carcinoma of the breast demonstrating overexpression of Her-2/*neu* oncoprotein. Overexpression of the protein is associated with amplification of the Her-2/*neu* gene. The presence of membrane reactivity (as seen here) indicates protein (and thus gene) overexpression; cytoplasmic reactivity is not related to Her-2/*neu* expression.

restricted to cancer cells; overexpression is not seen in normal breast epithelium.[233] There is an inverse association of Her-2/*neu* amplification and the expression of estrogen and progesterone receptors. Her-2/*neu* overexpression is also associated with high-grade tumors.[234,235]

The relationship of Her-2/*neu* overexpression and prognosis is more controversial. The weight of evidence strongly indicates, however, that overexpression may be an important adverse prognostic factor in node-positive breast cancer.[221,228,236] The relationship of Her-2/*neu* overexpression to prognosis in node-negative breast cancer is less clear, though several studies have recently reported that Her-2/*neu* overexpression is associated with poorer disease-free and overall survival in such patients.[228,237,238] Another potentially important association has recently been described; Her-2/*neu* overexpression may identify patients who will not respond to conventional adjuvant chemotherapy but who may gain advantage from alternative forms of chemotherapy.[238,238a]

Her-2/*neu* overexpression has been studied in several other tumor types. It appears to be associated with a poorer prognosis in patients with ovarian carcinoma.[221,226] Overexpression of undetermined significance has been observed in salivary gland tumors, squamous cell carcinomas of the head and neck, gastric carcinomas, and prostate carcinomas,[222-225,227] whereas gene amplification has not been identified in cases of non–small cell lung carcinoma or colon cancer.[229-231]

Other oncogenes. Although antibodies to virtually all oncogene products have been developed, their applications in immunohistochemical analyses of tumor behavior remain at an early stage, save for the study of Her-2/*neu* and of several oncogenes important in hematopoietic malignancies. Although alterations of virtually every oncogene described have been associated with one human tumor or another, a relationship to differentiation, prognosis, and progression has been demonstrated for very few.

The *ras* oncogene is a good case in point. Once believed to be perhaps the single most important genetic event in cancer, mutations in the ras gene and increased expression of the ras product have been associated with a wide variety of tumor types.[239-249] For some types of tumors (such as pancreatic carcinoma) mutations in the ras gene are detected in the majority of examples studied. The primary event is generally a point mutation, which takes place at a few characteristic sites. Immunohistochemical analysis of *ras* has been compromised by the failure to develop antibodies that reliably distinguish mutated forms from the wild type of *ras* gene product, which manifests as a 21 kD protein with GTPase activity. Attention has consequently been focused on the immunohistochemical analysis of the amplification of the ras gene product. Despite early reports to the contrary, this has not proved to be of prognostic value in most cases.[250,251]

Alterations of the *myc* family of protooncogenes (c-*myc* and N-*myc*) have been associated with increased cellular proliferation. In the case of small cell lung carcinoma, both c-*myc* and N-*myc* amplification have been associated with poor prognosis.[252] N-*myc* amplification may also allow identification of small cell lung carcinomas that will show a poor response to chemotherapy;[252] thus assessment of N-*myc* amplification may be important in developing an effective treatment plan.

Epidermal growth factor receptor (EGFR) belongs to a family of growth factor receptors involved in normal cell growth. It shares structural and functional characteristics with the Her-2/*neu* gene product, including a transmembrane localization and kinase activity. Binding of EGFR by its ligand produces proliferative activity in cells. That ligand (EGF) is one of a family of polypeptide growth factors and has significant homology with transforming growth factor-alpha (TGF-α). Both EGF and TGF-α cause activation of EGFR, with subsequent internalization, and both may bind to EGFR in endocrine, paracrine, or autocrine manners.[253-256]

EGFR is present in a wide variety of tissues, with predominant (but not exclusive) expression in epithelial cells.[254,257] When expressed, EGFR may localize to the cell membrane or cytoplasm, and it has been postulated that the localization has physiologic significance in determining the availability of the receptor for the ligand.[257] Expression of EGFR on the cell surface allows for signal transduction in response to binding of available ligand, whereas loss of such expression indicates loss of responsiveness to the ligand. Cytoplasmic localization, on the other hand, identifies cells that maintain the capacity to bind ligand (for example, by autocrine mechanisms or by the induction of membrane localization by physiologic stimuli) but do not respond to external (circulating) ligand.[257]

The expression of EGFR has been examined by immunohistochemistry in a wide variety of tissues. In many cases, increased expression of EGFR may be related to tumor progression (such as breast, esophageal, adrenocortical, lung, bladder, thyroid, and gastric carcinomas).[258-265] In the case of gastric carcinomas, those tumors that express both EGFR and EGF have a worse prognosis than those with neither EGFR nor EGF expression or those with EGFR expression only, an indication of an autocrine mechanism of proliferation activation.[265]

Oncogenes in lymphoma. The *bcl*-2 protooncogene is located distally to a cluster of breakpoints on chromosome 18, such that the t(14;18) translocation frequently results in juxtaposition of *bcl*-2 with an immunoglobulin heavy-chain gene on chromosome 14. In such circumstances the *bcl*-2 gene appears to be deregulated, synthesizing excess amounts of a 25 kD protein that localizes to the inner mitochondrial membrane. In some instances, the t(14;18) translocation also appears to be associated with abnormalities of heavy-chain gene function and of immunoglobulin production in neoplastic cells. Functionally, *bcl*-2 protein prolongs the survival of cells by interfering with the process of normal programmed cell death (apoptosis), whereby redundant lymphoid cells in the immune response are deleted.[266-268] Immunohistochemical studies of normal lymph nodes using antibody to *bcl*-2 protein (clone 124) reveal expression in memory cells, resting cells, and other long-lived lymphoid cells.[269,270] This is illustrated particularly well in reactive follicles within these nodes, where long-lived follicular mantle B-cells typically express *bcl*-2, reflecting the presumptive inhibition of apoptosis by high levels of *bcl*-2, whereas rapidly proliferating germinal center cells show little *bcl*-2 expression, reflecting their high rate of apoptotic cell death in the absence of *bcl*-2.[270,271] Although this is the typical appearance in normal reactive centers, neoplastic follicules characteristically differ by virtue of the intense staining for *bcl*-2 within cells of both the mantle zone and neoplastic follicle center. The presence of the characteristic t(14:18) translocation in many follicular center cell lymphomas exhibiting abnormal *bcl*-2 expression has led to the hypothesis that this translocation and consequent abnormal activation of *bcl*-2 may be the seminal event leading to neoplastic transformation in this subset of B-cell tumors. Indeed, there is experimental evidence in support of a role of elevated *bcl*-2 activity in lymphoma genesis, in that increased *bcl*-2 expression, accompanied by c-*myc* activation, induces aggressive B-cell lymphomas in transgenic mice.[272]

Although some investigators are convinced of the role of *bcl*-2 in lymphoma and its close association with the t(14;18) translocation,[273,274] others have claimed that increased expression of *bcl*-2 is not specific for the t(14;18) translocation, arising by other means in certain instances, and that it may not be diagnostic of follicular center cell malignancy, particularly in light of the findings that the t(14;18) translocation occurs early in normal B-cell development and that it may be found infrequently (1 in 10^5 cells) in normal lymph nodes.[275-277] Finally, *bcl*-2 expression in non-Hodgkin's lymphoma may be without prognostic significance.[275,276]

Although *bcl*-2 expression is observed in 80% to 90% of cases of follicular center cell lymphomas,[278] it may also be observed in 20% or more of diffuse lymphomas, including some T-cell lymphomas and a small number of Ki-1–positive anaplastic large cell lymphomas, and within the Reed-Sternberg cells in some cases of Hodgkin's disease.[279-281] As noted above, although many lymphomas show elevated *bcl*-2 levels, not all of these show a demonstrable translocation of t(14;18). In these cases, it has been postulated that other disregulatory mechanisms may be in effect. For example, recent studies have shown that the latent membrane protein (LMP-1) of Epstein-Barr virus (EBV) can induce expression of *bcl*-2 in EBV-infected cells.[282] Abnormalities of a number of other oncogenes and tumor-suppressor genes (that is, c-*myc*, *bcl*-1, p53, and Rb) have been observed in malignant lymphomas, but the immunohistochemical data in reference to them are limited.[283,284]

Tumor-suppressor genes and gene products

The existence of tumor-suppressor genes (also known as "antioncogenes") was first suggested by Knudson in 1971,[285] who explained the epidemiology of retinoblastoma by postulating a recessive retinoblastoma (Rb) gene that normally acts to inhibit the formation of the tumors. Mutations in both alleles coding for this gene lead to the development of retinoblastoma. The primary characteristics of tumor-suppressor genes are that (1) they encode normal cellular products believed to be involved in growth control or differentiation and (2), since the abnormality is recessive, both the alleles must be inactivated for loss of function (that is, loss of tumor suppression) to occur. This is in contrast to the abnormalities described for oncogenes, which are dominant, and thus require mutation in only one allele.

The loss of function of both alleles of a tumor-suppressor gene can occur in a variety of ways, including (1) loss of the entire gene, as in deletion of a large region of the chromosome; (2) loss of a portion of the gene because of minor deletions or translocations; (3) a mutation in the gene, including a point mutation, which may result in a change of only a single amino acid in the gene product; and (4) loss of gene expression.[286]

Several putative tumor-suppressor genes have been identified, including the Rb gene, p53, DCC (deleted in colon cancer), the Wilms' tumor gene, and the neurofibromatosis type 1 gene (NF1).[285-290] NM23 may also be an example of a tumor-suppressor gene.[291] The two best characterized are the Rb and the p53 genes; the gene products for these have also been identified and studied by immunohistochemical methods. Both p53 and Rb gene products are believed to be involved in growth control through regulation of transcription; wild type of p53 protein has been shown specifically to activate transcription (which may then lead to production of products that control cell growth).[292] Both are nuclear phosphoproteins, and there is evidence that phosphorylation may inactivate the Rb protein. In addition, a variety of viral oncoproteins, including SV40 T antigen, E1A from adenovirus, and E6 from human *Papillomavirus,* bind to and neutralize Rb and p53 proteins. More recently, there has been described a cellular oncoprotein (MDM2) that binds to and may neutralize the p53 protein.[293]

Although tumor-suppressor gene alterations may be critical events in malignant transformation and tumor progression, most human cancers are multifactorial in causation. Loss of tumor-suppressor gene function represents only one event in a multistep process, which may include activation of oncogenes, loss of tumor-suppressor genes, and antigenic changes that allow the cell to escape immune recognition.

Rb. The Rb gene is located on chromosome 13q14 and spans a region of more than 200,000 bases, including 27 exons. The Rb protein has a molecular weight of 105,000 daltons, and several antibodies have been developed to recognize specific parts of this protein.[294,295] The Rb gene is the only tumor suppressor that has been shown to suppress tumor formation directly. Alterations in this gene have been described in many human tumors, including retinoblastoma, osteosarcoma, other sarcomas, leukemias, lymphomas, and certain carcinomas, including those derived from breast, lung, prostate, bladder, kidney, and testis.[294,296-307] Rb gene alterations have been associated with increasing tumor grade and stage in a variety of tumors.[299,300,303] In the case of breast carcinoma, alterations in the Rb gene have been associated with other signs of progression, such as loss of hormone receptor expression.[308] Furthermore, there is growing evidence that Rb alterations may identify primary tumors that are at higher risk of developing metastases.[308]

It is now clear that genetic alterations in the Rb gene correlate with loss of expression of Rb protein as determined by immunohistochemical methods.[294-296,307] In fact, it has been suggested that immunohistochemical analysis of Rb protein may detect Rb gene inactivation more rapidly, specifically, and reliably than direct screening of DNA for gene abnormalities.[309] Assessment of Rb gene loss by immunohistochemistry is based upon the absence of detectable nuclear staining for Rb protein. This is in contrast to the immunohistochemical staining pattern seen in tumors with altered p53, in which staining is increased (see below).

p53. The p53 protein was originally described as a nuclear protein (53,000 daltons) expressed in methylcholanthrene-induced mouse sarcomas but not in normal mouse cells.[310] Originally believed to be a cellular oncoprotein specifically expressed by tumor cells, it is now included in the tumor-suppressor family.[311] p53 protein is expressed by all normal cells, but the half-life of the wild ("normal") type of protein is so short (6 to 30 minutes) that it does not accumulate to levels high enough to be detected by standard immunohistochemical techniques;[312] mutant p53 protein, by contrast, has an extended half-life, accumulates, and is readily detectable in the cell nucleus (Fig. 8-24).

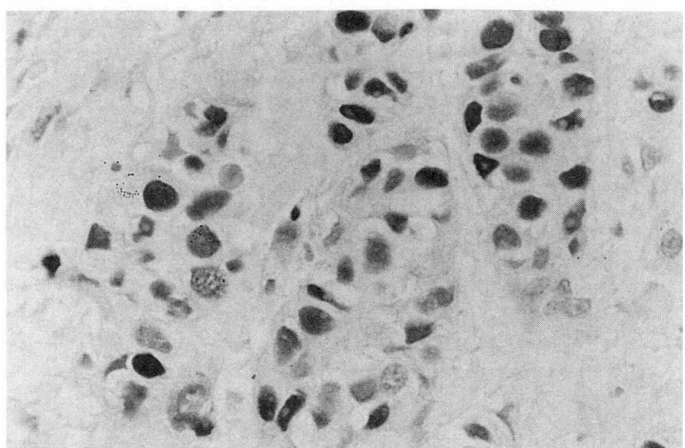

Fig. 8-24 Infiltrating ductal carcinoma of the breast showing nuclear immunoreactivity with the anti-p53 antibody Ab 1801. Notice that the tumor cells show heterogeneous expression of the antigen and the surrounding normal stroma cells show no detectable immunoreactivity. Point mutations in the p53 gene result in a protein product that has a significantly longer half-life than the wild type of p53 protein. The mutated p53 protein accumulates in the nucleus at high enough levels to be detected by standard immunohistochemical techniques; this is the basis for the immunohistochemical detection of p53 mutations.

The p53 gene is located on chromosome 17p13.1. Alterations of the p53 gene, identified by cytogenetic, molecular, and immunohistochemical methods, are the most common genetic abnormalities seen in human cancer and have been described in a wide variety of human tumor types, including colon, bladder, lung, breast, and other carcinomas, as well as astrocytomas, leukemias, sarcomas, and mesotheliomas.[286,313-318] Loss of p53 suppressor function usually results from complete loss of one allele associated with a point mutation in the second allele.[316] This generally occurs in such a way that the mutant p53 gene continues to be expressed but lacks the regulatory activity of the wild type of p53. However, mutant p53 protein has several important properties: it can bind to and neutralize residual wild type of p53 proteins (that is, it has antisuppressor or oncogenic effects), and it is a metabolically stable protein, with a long half-life.

There is increasing evidence that the immunohistochemical detection of p53 protein in the nucleus identifies cells that have mutations in the p53 gene.[319-321] However, a small percentage of tumors having p53 gene mutations do not show detectable p53 nuclear accumulation by immunohistochemistry.[321] Explanations for this include: (1) the mutations in these tumors may have resulted in loss of protein expression; therefore p53 protein did not accumulate; (2) the mutations may have disrupted the binding sites or sites of the anti-p53 antibody; and (3) p53 antigen–binding sites may have been lost or disrupted as a result of tissue processing and fixation.[321]

The greatest source of discrepant results are tumors that demonstrated detectable p53 nuclear accumulation by immunohistochemistry but in which p53 gene alterations or mutations were not found by molecular methods.[321] This has several possible explanations, which are not necessarily mutually exclusive: (1) when the entire gene is not examined by molecular methods, immunohistochemical analysis of p53 accumulation may more accurately reflect the true incidence of p53 mutations; (2) tumors are composed of both neoplastic and benign cells intermingled in various proportions. If the proportion of tumor cells (containing the p53 mutation) is relatively low, compared to normal cells (containing wild type of p53), molecular analysis may not detect the mutation in the tumor because of a dilutional effect;[314] (3) the antibodies used to detect p53 protein react with both the wild type and the mutant forms. It is possible that the immunohistochemical assay detects the accumulation of the wild type of p53 in some cases. For example, binding of wild type of p53 to viral oncoproteins or oncogene products not only inactivates p53, but stabilizes it as well. Thus the immunohistochemical analysis of p53 may not only be more sensitive than molecular methods in detecting p53 gene alterations, but also may detect important alterations in p53 function that do not involve mutations at the gene level.[321]

When p53 nuclear reactivity is detected by immunohistochemistry, significant heterogeneity in the staining pattern (percentage of reactive tumor cell nuclei) is observed, even within the same tumor type. Although some of the variation may be attributable to differences in fixation, there is now evidence that this may be attributable to a property of the mutant p53 protein.[321] As discussed, mutant p53 protein has a significantly longer half-life than the wild type of protein has. However, the half-lives of the mutated forms are not uniform and vary with different sites of mutation. The heterogeneity in the staining pattern is apparently attributable (at least in part) to different sites of mutation; although some mutations result in a protein with an extremely long half-life (resulting in intense immunoreactivity in most of the tumor cells), other mutations result in a protein with a shorter half-life (resulting in weaker immunoreactivity, demonstrable in fewer tumor cells).[321]

Another possible source of heterogeneous staining is that some cells in a tumor may have a mutant p53 gene whereas others do not. Although this mechanism has been suggested for some tumors (particularly astrocytomas)[314], it is not common because p53 mutation is apparently an early event in most of the common tumors, such as breast, prostate, and bladder carcinoma.[321,322]

Because of the importance of p53 alterations in human cancer and the ease of detecting p53 mutations by molecular or immunohistochemical techniques, p53 alterations have been the focus of intense examination. As with Rb alterations, p53 alterations are associated with tumors of high histologic grade and tumors with a high proliferative index (again, an association suggestive of a relationship between tumor-suppressor genes and control of cell growth).[323-326] In the case of breast tumors, p53 alterations are associated with loss of hormone receptor expression and hormone-independent tumor growth (as are Rb alterations), again an indication that tumors that lose normal growth controls may do so because they become independent of normal growth regulators.[308,327-329] There is growing evidence that, at least for some types of tumors, p53 alterations identify patients with shorter disease-free interval and poorer overall survival.[321,330,330a] In the case of breast and bladder carcinoma, the association between p53 alterations and prognosis appears strongest in the earliest stage tumors, thus emphasizing the potential value of p53 examination in the assessment of the future behavior of the tumor. It appears that in many tumors, p53 alterations are an early event in tumorigenesis and can be detected in in situ carcinomas (in the case of breast and bladder carcinoma)[321-331] or even in dysplastic lesions (in prostate and colon carcinoma).[320] Thus tumors that are at highest risk for progression may be identified even before becoming invasive.

Invasion and metastases

Metastasis is a multistep process involving tumor cell interactions with the extracellular matrix and disruption of basement membranes. As described earlier, benign lesions have continuous basement membranes that separate an epithelium from its surrounding interstitial stroma, whereas carcinomas are associated with disrupted or absent basement membranes. Once in the stroma, tumor cells undergo further systemic dissemination via the lymphatic and blood vessels. The initial step in this process, that is, the attachment of tumor cells to the extracellular matrix, is mediated by interactions of specific glycoproteins in the matrix with receptors, such as laminin receptor, present on the plasma membrane of tumor cells. Invasive cells then secrete or induce the secretion of proteolytic enzymes that degrade the components of the extracellular matrix (such as laminin, heparin) and the underlying basement membrane (such as type IV collagen, laminin, and heparin sulfate proteoglycan), thereby facilitating migration of tumor cells away from the primary site.[332]

The importance of tumor cell interactions with the extracellular matrix is illustrated by the distribution of laminin receptor in invasive carcinoma. Increased expression of a 67 kD laminin receptor, at both the mRNA and protein levels, is associated with the metastatic phenotype in several human cancers, including colon and breast carcinoma.[333] Hormones that regulate growth of breast cancer cells increase the expression of laminin receptor in hormone receptor–positive breast cancer cells. Using immunohistochemical methods with an affinity-purified antibody against a cDNA-derived laminin receptor peptide, cells from benign breast tissue were found to express low levels of laminin receptor;[333] immunoreactivity was primarily cell membrane associated but was also present in the cytoplasm. Further, the progression from in situ ductal and in situ lobular carcinomas to their infiltrating counterparts was associated with an increase in the percentage of tumor cells that expressed laminin receptor.[334] Thus, as cells progress from benign to malignant phenotypes, or from in situ to invasive phenotypes (that is, as cells become more aggressive and more likely to metastasize), the expression of laminin receptor is increased. Increased expression of the laminin receptor is not only associated with the mechanism of metastasis, but may also be a measurable marker of the metastatic phenotype in cells still at their primary site.

Recent work on the mechanisms of metastasis has shown that invasive tumor cells have increased levels of proteolytic activity, when compared with normal tissue or noninvasive tumors. Particular interest has focused on type IV collagenase. At least two forms (72 kD and 92 kD isozymes) of type IV collagenase have been described. Evidence indicates that levels of the 72 kD form correlate with invasiveness in a variety of human tumors, including hepatomas, melanomas, and sarcomas and in various carcinomas, such as gastric, colorectal, and breast.[334,335]

Immunohistochemical approaches for predicting response to therapy

Certain receptors cell surface may provide an understanding of how tumors may respond to certain types of therapy. The responsiveness of breast and prostate carcinoma to hormonal manipulation is the classic example. More recently, a transmembrane protein, encoded by the so-called multidrug resistance (MDR) gene, has been found to identify cells that are resistant to specific types of chemotherapy. This protein acts as a "pump" to remove toxins (including certain chemotherapeutic agents) before they can act to kill the cell. Finally, the expression of certain proteins (principally oncogene products) has been associated with resistance to some types of chemotherapy, either by direct or indirect mechanisms. All of these can be assessed by immunohistochemical methods.

Estrogen and progesterone receptors

The observation that certain tumors, principally those derived from reproductive organs (breast, prostate, endometrium, and ovary), are under the growth regulation of steroid sex hormones (estrogens and androgens) has had a fundamental effect upon the therapeutic approach to these tumors. Seminal work by Beatson,[336] Huggins and Hodges,[337] and Jensen and colleagues[338] demonstrated that the growth of certain tumors (breast and prostate carcinoma, in particular) is dependent on the presence of circulating factors (estrogens, androgens) and that removal of the source of these hormones (by oophorectomy or orchiectomy) could result in dramatic tumor remissions. The growth regulation of the tumors was found to be mediated through the expression of specific receptors for the circulating hormones; tumors expressing high levels of the receptor tended to respond to hormone ablation therapy, whereas tumors that expressed low levels of the receptor tended to be unresponsive to such therapy (that is, these tumors demonstrate hormone-independent growth).[338] These observations paved the way for rational, patient-specific cancer treatment, based on specific biologic characteristics of the tumor cells.

Until recently, the primary method for determination of hormone-receptor expression was based on the binding of labeled hormones (such as estradiol, progestins, or androgen) to receptors present in tissue homogenates (the so-called cytosol-based assays).[338] These assays provide a "quantitative" measurement of hormone-receptor content in tissues. Prediction of response to hormone-ablation therapy by this method is imperfect, however, because a sampling error frequently results in the contamination of the cytosol extract by nonneoplastic stromal and epithelial elements, which may obscure the true receptor content of the tumor cells. Also, the cytosol-based assays are technically exacting, require biologically active hormone receptor (which is present only in fresh or frozen tissue), and may be affected by the presence of endogenous hormones (which compete with the radiolabeled ligands for the receptor). Early on, it was hoped that the development of the means to directly determine receptor content in histologic preparations of tissues might be expected to resolve some of these difficulties (Table 8-13).

Immunohistologic detection of receptor expression in tissue sections can theoretically be achieved either indirectly, by utilizing the biologic binding activity of the receptor for the steroid with subsequent detection of the bound steroid molecule by an antisteroid antibody,[339,340] or directly, by immunologic reactivity of the receptor protein with an antireceptor antibody.[341-343] Both methods discriminate between receptor sites confined to tumor cells and those localizing to nonneoplastic components. Furthermore, the exact proportion of

Table 8-13 Problems with standard (biochemical) steroid hormone binding assays

False-negative results
Improper specimen collection and handling.* Specimen must be collected fresh and snap frozen because of lability of receptor.
Poor sampling of tissue*—cannot directly determine if tumor cells are in the sample.
Low concentration* of tumor cells because of sclerosis or necrosis.
Receptor sites* occupied by endogenous hormone.
False-positive results
Hormone/ligand* can bind to nonreceptor cellular proteins (such as albumin).
Tumor heterogeneity.* Although some tumor cells may be receptor positive, the majority may be negative.
Change in hormone receptor content when primary lesions are compared with metastases.
Positive result* attributable to receptor expression by surrounding normal tissue.

*Can be addressed by immunohistochemical detection of steroid hormone receptors.

tumor cells showing reactivity is made evident. The ability to assess receptor expression morphologically at the cellular level is important. A tumor in which only 10% of the tumor cells are positive, but strongly so, would be expected to respond differently to hormonal manipulation from another tumor in which all the tumor cells are weakly positive, yet both tumors could give identical results on a cytosol-based assay (Table 8-13). With the availability of monoclonal antibodies that recognize epitopes on estrogen, progesterone, and androgen-receptor proteins (antireceptor antibodies), this direct approach has supplanted the aforementioned methods utilizing antibodies to the steroid hormones (Figs. 8-25 and 8-26) and has proved superior to the standard cytosol (biochemical) assays.

Immunohistochemical assays can be used on extremely small tissue specimens, including cytologic preparations of cells, (such as fine-needle aspirates, FNA), and on core needle biopsy specimens. This is particularly important in the evaluation of receptor content of metastatic disease, in which one might hesitate to perform a formal biopsy.

Immunohistochemical detection of estrogen receptors initially was restricted to frozen tissue, but techniques now allow use of routinely processed, formalin-fixed, paraffin-embedded tissue. Comparative studies of these cytosol assays with the immunohistochemical antireceptor assays[344-354] reveal high concordance, ranging from 77% to more than 90%. Discordance, when present, is usually limited to borderline cases and often results from heterogeneity of receptor expression, tissue-sampling errors (scant tumor cells available for the assay), or the presence of endogenous hormone that binds to the receptor, thus making it unavailable for assay (this binding may occur in premenopausal patients, who can have substantial levels of circulating hormone, or in patients being treated by endocrine therapy)[355,356] and, therefore, can lead to "false"-negative biochemical test results. "False"-positive biochemical results have been attributed to the binding of the labeled hormone ligand to nonreceptor proteins, or to the presence of receptor-positive normal tissues admixed with receptor-negative carcinoma. Immunohistochemical assays then may better reflect the receptor status of the tumor than assays that utilize tissue homogenates do (see Table 8-14).

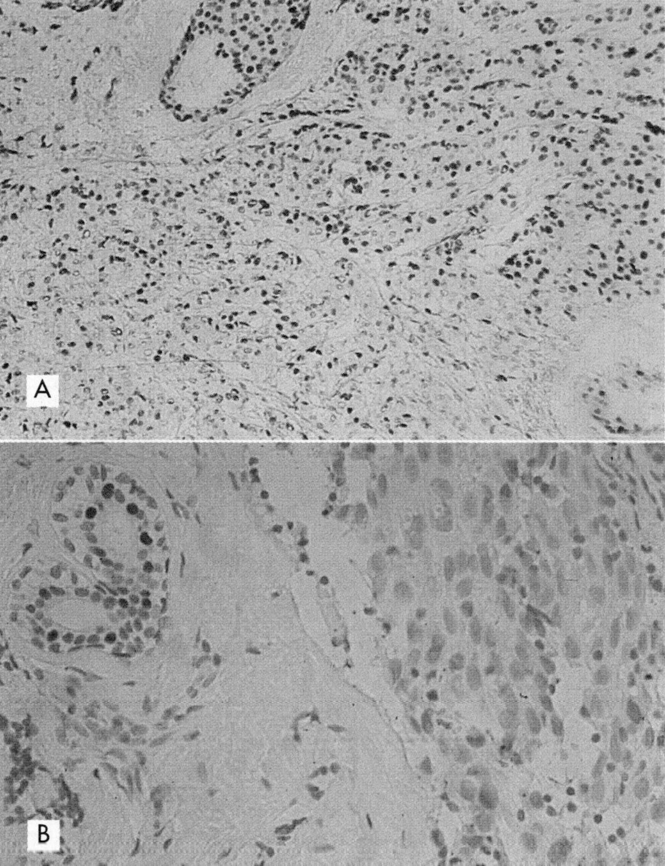

Fig. 8-25 Breast carcinoma assessed for estrogen receptor expression using the antireceptor monoclonal antibody. **A,** This tumor shows intense homogeneous nuclear reactivity with the anti–estrogen receptor monoclonal antibody. The immunoreactivity demonstrates specific nuclear localization; any cytoplasmic reactivity would be discounted. In this case, use of the immunohistochemical assay allows for assessment of estrogen receptor expression in both the infiltrating and in situ component of this tumor. **B,** In this section from a different tumor, the infiltrating ductal carcinoma *(on right)* does not show significant immunoreactivity with the antireceptor antibody. However, adjacent normal ducts show positive nuclear reactivity. The presence of significant amounts of nontumor tissue, which expresses hormone receptor, could lead to a false-positive result when one is using biochemical assays, which do not allow for the morphologic evaluation of the tissue being tested.

The results of immunohistochemical assays for both estrogen-receptor and progesterone-receptor expression have been shown to be well correlated with prognosis (disease-free survival and overall survival) in patients with breast cancer,[357-359] and they also correlate with other putative prognostic factors, such as tumor grade, ploidy, and stage.[356,360-363] Well-differentiated tumors and tumors of low stage are more likely to be estrogen and progesterone receptor positive. The correlation of immunohistochemically determined estrogen/progesterone receptor content with histologic characteristics is better than that with biochemically determined receptor content. The immuno-

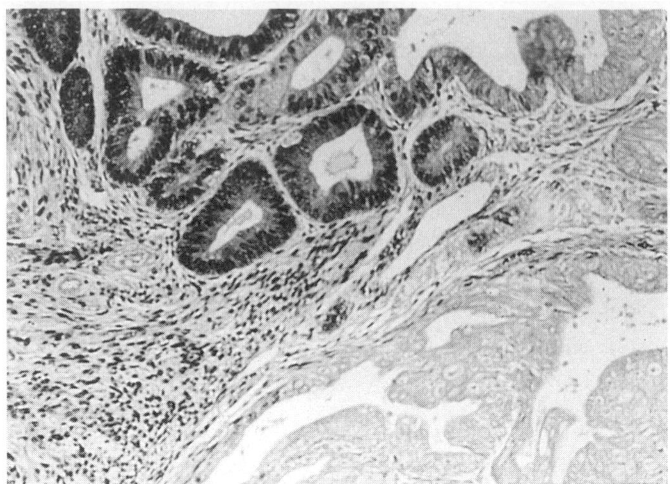

Fig. 8-26 Endometrial carcinoma showing positive nuclear immunoreactivity with anti–progesterone receptor monoclonal antibody. Notice that both glandular epithelium and myometrium show hormone receptor expression. This tumor shows variable immunoreactivity in morphologically distinct areas, with the more poorly differentiated areas showing less intense staining, thus indicating decreased receptor expression.

Table 8-14 Advantages of immunohistochemical assays for detection of steroid hormone receptors

Can be used on small samples, even those too small for routine biochemical methods
Can be used on fine-needle aspiration and cytology preparations
Can be used on both frozen and routinely processed formalin-fixed, paraffin-embedded tissue
Can allow assessment of different populations of cells (such as in situ versus invasive components)
Can directly assess heterogeneity of receptor expression
Since the assay is histologic, it can distinguish tumor cells from other cell populations and determine if the specimen was appropriately collected
Produces a permanent histologic record or result that can be reviewed in the future
Can take advantage of internal positive and negative controls in most tissue samples to assess quality of each test
Speed; results can be obtained more quickly than with standard assays
More predictive of prognosis than standard biochemical assays
More predictive of response to hormonal therapy than standard biochemical assays

histochemical determination of estrogen and progesterone receptor expression may better reflect the biologic features of tumor cells than biochemical determinations of receptor content.[360-363] The identification by immunohistochemistry of a significant decrease in receptor-positive tumor cells is associated with increasing proliferative cell fractions, increased Her-2/*neu* oncogene amplification, and EGFR expression.[360-363]

Immunohistochemical antireceptor assays allow prediction of the response of breast cancer to hormonal treatment.[364-366] Tumors that express no estrogen or progesterone receptors have a low probability of responding to hormonal manipulation, whereas estrogen receptor– and progesterone receptor–positive tumors have a high probability of responding to such treatment. Furthermore, when compared with standard biochemical tests, the antireceptor assays are significantly better at allowing a prediction of the likelihood of tumor response to hormonal manipulation.[367-371] Although immunohistochemical assays do not provide the quantitative end point of the biochemical assays, the use of semiquantitative measures, which take into account receptor heterogeneity and intensity of immunoreactivity, show an excellent correlation with prognosis and response to therapy.[368]

Derivation of clinically meaningful data from these immunohistochemical assays, however, demands interpretive rigor based on familiarity with the specific reaction patterns to be anticipated. In particular, the specific cellular localization of immunoreactivity is important. Unlike the biochemical assays, in which the receptor was localized to cell cytoplasm, or the earlier "indirect" immunohistochemical receptor ligand assays (see above), which showed nuclear and cytoplasmic localization of reactivity, immunohistochemical assays using antireceptor (estrogen, progesterone, and androgen receptor) antibodies have demonstrated nuclear localization of staining. Cytoplasmic reactivity is considered nonspecific. These results are in concordance with the demonstrated nuclear localization for the steroid sex hormone receptors, along with a wide variety of other hormone receptors, such as those for vitamin D and thyroid hormone.

Androgen receptor

Prostate carcinomas can express androgen receptor, a finding grounded in the empiric observation by Huggins and Hodges that antiandrogen therapy could control the growth of prostate carcinomas, often in a dramatic fashion.[337] Today, androgen ablation therapy through orchiectomy, endocrine therapy, or both, is a fundamental treatment step in patients with advanced prostate carcinoma. However, approximately 25% of patients are unresponsive to such therapy. Nevertheless, measurement of androgen receptor levels has not routinely been performed in cases of prostatic carcinoma, primarily because prostate carcinomas are notoriously difficult to recognize and sample grossly.

One of the primary problems with some of the early studies of androgen receptor measurements in prostate cancer was that many used cytosolic tissue extracts. Later studies confirmed a nuclear localization for androgen receptor, and it has now been shown that the measurement of nuclear androgen receptor, unlike cytosolic receptor, is predictive of response to endocrine therapy and prognosis.[372-374] In fact, nuclear receptor levels have been shown to be independent of both tumor grade and stage in the prediction of progression of disease.[374-376]

Monoclonal and polyclonal antibodies specific for the androgen receptor have been developed and used to study receptor distribution in normal and malignant tissues.[377-383] Both benign and malignant prostatic epithelia express nuclear androgen receptor. In the case of prostatic carcinoma, the heterogeneity in receptor expression observed within tumors, as assessed biochemically, has been confirmed by immunohistochemical techniques using antiandrogen receptor antibodies.[379,381,382] However, only limited studies have been conducted examining the relationship of the immunohistochemical detection of androgen receptors with response to endocrine therapy and prognosis.[383]

Drug resistance

P-glycoprotein. P-glycoprotein (P-170) is a transmembrane protein of 170 KD that has been associated with both intrinsic and acquired resistance to certain chemotherapeutic agents, particularly anthracyclines and vinca alkaloids. P-170 is an energy-dependent "pump" that functions in drug efflux, reducing intracellular accumulation of chemotherapeutic drugs and thus conferring the so-called multidrug resistance (MDR) phenotype on cells expressing increased levels of this protein. P-glycoprotein is encoded by a family of so-called MDR genes; however, only the protein encoded by the MDR 1 gene appears to induce the MDR phenotype.[384,385]

As studied by molecular or immunochemical means, the expression of P-glycoprotein has been observed in tumors that show a high degree of intrinsic drug resistance, such as renal, colon, and adrenocortical carcinomas.[384-387] In these cases, high levels of expression of P-glycoprotein have also been observed in the normal tissues from which these tumors are derived. In fact, renal proximal tubular cells have become a standard positive control in the immunohistochemical analysis of P-glycoprotein expression.[386,387] The physiologic function of P-glycoprotein may be inferred from its normal tissue distribution; for example, P-glycoprotein shows high levels of expression on endothelial cells of the blood-brain barrier and in renal proximal tubular cells.[386,387] Both of these cell types have, as a primary function, the movement of toxic substances across membranes.

Tumors responsive to chemotherapy generally show a low incidence of P-glycoprotein expression.[386] In fact, those solid tumors that are most responsive to systemic chemotherapy (such as seminomas and embryonal carcinomas) rarely show detectable expression of P-glycoprotein.[386] Tumors from patients previously treated with chemotherapy show frequent elevation of P-glycoprotein, an indication that the MDR phenotype may be induced by exposure to chemotherapy.[388-390] Detection of elevated P-glycoprotein expression may identify tumors likely to be resistant to conventional chemotherapy and thus provide a rationale for the provision of alternative treatments for these patients. Immunohistochemical evaluation of P-glycoprotein expression appears to be the analytical method of choice, primarily because it allows the discrimination of P-glycoprotein expression in tumor cells from that in normal cells.

It has also been suggested that P-glycoprotein may have other effects on cell behavior. P-glycoprotein expression is increased in colon carcinoma cells that compose the "leading" or invasive edge of the tumor.[391] Furthermore, P-glycoprotein expression is associated with blood vessel invasion and lymph node metastases in patients with colon cancer. P-glycoprotein, then, may play a role in tumor progression.

Only two MDR genes are known to be present in humans (MDR 1 and MDR 3), but only the MDR 1 gene product confers the MDR phenotype. One of the most widely used antibodies to P-glycoprotein, C219, reacts with both the MDR 1 and MDR 3 gene product. Several antibodies specific for the MDR 1 gene product have now been described, however, including HYB-241, HYB-612 (Hybridtech), and C494. Although most studies have used frozen tissue sections because of the observed loss of P-glycoprotein reactivity after routine processing, several studies have more recently described successful applications within routinely processed, paraffin-embedded material.

Other predictors of drug resistance. As described above, the expression of certain oncogene products identifies tumors that are resistant to particular types of chemotherapy. Overexpression of Her-2/*neu* by breast cancers is associated with resistance to conventional chemotherapy regimens containing cyclophosphamide, methotrexate, and fluorouracil (CMF).[237] Similarly, increased expression of N-*myc* by small cell lung carcinomas and by neuroblastomas has been associated with lack of response to chemotherapy and rapid progression of disease.[252] Whether or not overexpression of Her-2/*neu* or-N*myc* itself contributes to the provocation of drug resistance or is simply a manifestation of an increasingly aggressive phenotype remains unclear. In either case, these markers may have utility in the determination of the most effective course of treatment for these cancers.

The determination of drug resistance by the identification of specific cellular products (such as P-glycoprotein) in preserved (frozen or routinely processed) tissue specimens by immunohistochemistry represents a considerable simplification compared with the alternative "clonogenic" techniques for the assessment of drug resistance, in which the response of cultured tumor cells to myriad chemotherapeutic agents is gauged by several means.[392,393] Most importantly, the immunohistochemical assays do not require viable tumor. Immunohistochemical analysis offers the added advantage that the entire population of cells within a representative portion of the tumor can be assessed, unlike the clonogenic assay, in which specific clones of cells may be selected. Finally, the expression of the product on tumor cells can be distinguished from that on normal cells by immunohistochemical means; such is not the case in the culture assay.

The ability to predict specifically the response of individual tumors to chemotherapeutic agents could have a profound effect on the way treatment decisions for patients with cancer are made. It is not difficult to envision the day when the specificity of tumor therapy approaches that presently exercised in the treatment of microbial diseases, with drug selection based upon the resistance patterns of individual tumors to specific agents. Thus treatment decisions will become less organ based and will better reflect the biology of individual tumors.

Infections

Until recently, the armamentarium of special stains available to the surgical pathologist for identification of infectious agents in tissue sections was essentially limited to Gram stains, various acid-fast stains, and periodic acid–Schiff or silver stains for fungi. The availability of antibodies against microbial antigens and, more recently, of nucleic acid probes targeting microbial DNA or RNA has bred the development of a wide range of immunohistochemical or in situ hybridization techniques for the detection of specific types of organisms within fixed paraffin sections. By these means, a large number of organisms may now be reliably demonstrated in a manner directly useful to the surgical pathologist (Table 8-15). Although culture techniques remain the most important method for the diagnosis of many specific infections, many studies have demonstrated the superiority of immunohistochemical methods to both culture and the morphologic identification of cytopathic changes for the detection of certain infectious agents, such as cytomegalovirus (CMV).[394,395]

Early antigens of CMV can frequently be identified by immunohistochemistry before the virus appears in culture and

Table 8-15 Infectious agents for which antibodies are available for use in paraffin section

Adenovirus	Influenza
Aspergillus spp.	*Klebsiella spp.*
Baboon endogenous virus	*Legionella spp.*
Blastomyces	*Leishmania spp.*
Borrelia burgdorferi	Lymphocytic choriomeningitis virus
Buffalo pox virus	Measles antigen
Campylobacter jejuni	Moloney's virus
Campylobacter coli	Mouse mammary tumor virus antigen
Campylobacter spp.	Mycobacteria
Candida spp.	*Mycoplasma*
Chlamydia spp.	*Parainfluenza*
Coccidioides immitis	*Pneumocystis carinii*
Coronavirus	Poliovirus
Cryptococcus neoformans	Polyomavirus
Cryptosporidium spp.	*Pseudomonas aeruginosa*
Cytomegalovirus	Rabies virus
Distemper virus	Respiratory syncytial virus
Entamoeba histolytica	Rotavirus
Epstein-Barr virus	Rubella virus
Escherichia coli	*Salmonella*
Fasciola hepatica	*Shigella spp.*
Friend's virus	Shope's fibroma virus
Giardia lamblia	*Staphylococcus*
Hepatitis A virus	*Streptococcus*
Helicobacter pylori	SV40 virus
Hepatitis B core antigen	*Toxoplasma gondii*
Hepatitis B surface antigen	*Treponema pallidum*
Hepatitis C virus	Trichomonas spp.
Herpes simplex virus 1 and 2	*Trichophyton spp.*
Histoplasma capsulatum	Varicella-zoster virus
Human immunodeficiency virus (HIV-1)	*Yersinia*
Human *Papillomavirus*	

From Taylor CR, Cote RJ: *Immunomicroscopy: a diagnostic tool for the surgical pathologist,* ed 2, Philadelphia, 1994, Saunders.

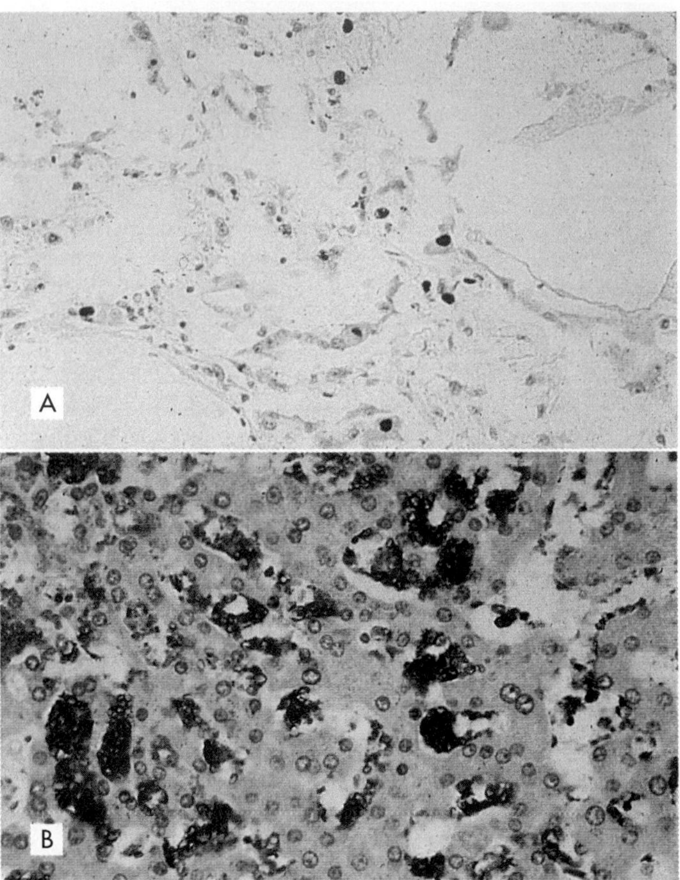

Fig. 8-27 Immunohistochemical detection of infectious disease. **A,** Identification of early and late antigens of cytomegalovirus (CMV) in the lung. Notice that the typical inclusions of CMV are not seen in this section. **B,** Immunohistochemical detection of *Pneumocystis carinii* in the liver of a patient with AIDS. This antibody (2G2) identifies both the cyst and the trophozoite forms. The GMS (silver) stain, typically used to detect *Pneumocystis* organisms, identifies only the cyst form, which will represent as few as 10% of the total volume of organisms.

before its characteristic inclusions become apparent to the surgical pathologist (Fig. 8-27, *A*). In addition, immunohistochemical methods can be used to identify specifically and rapidly several organisms that are difficult to grow in culture, such as *Helicobacter pylori, Histoplasma capsulatum,* certain mycobacteria, and *Pneumocystis carinii*[396-404] (Fig. 8-27, *B*). In situ hybridization methods offer similar advantages but tend to be technically more demanding than immunohistochemical procedures. There are some data to indicate that immunohistochemistry may be more sensitive than in situ hybridization in some instances, though this is probably a reflection of the varying quality of the technique and reagents available for use in the application of either method in the identification of specific organisms. With regard to human *Papillomavirus* (HPV), immunohistologic studies provide a sensitive method of screening, whereas in situ hybridization offers a higher degree of specificity for the distinction of different subtypes of HPV, which may be of prognostic significance.[405-408]

Both immunohistochemistry and in situ hybridization are applicable not only to formalin-fixed, paraffin-embedded sections, but also to materials derived from fine-needle aspiration biopsies and various cytologic preparations. Such broad applicability is of particular value in searching for evidence of infection by CMV or *Pneumocystis* in biopsy or sputum samples from transplant patients or in immunodeficient individuals, in whom the need for therapeutic intervention is urgent. At present, immunohistochemical methods for the detection of HPV, CMV, and *Pneumocystis* are the most widely employed in routine practice. Other applications, however, are rapidly entering general use. Current diagnostic applications are summarized in Table 8-15; the list is likely to grow as research applications are translated into diagnostic practice. A more extensive treatment of the subject is to be found in the review by Cartun.[1]

REFERENCES

General

1. Taylor CR, Cote RJ: *Immunomicroscopy: a diagnostic tool for the surgical pathologist,* ed 2, Philadelphia, 1994, Saunders.
2. Taylor CR: Quality assurance and standardization in immunohistochemistry: a proposal for the annual meeting of the Biological Stain Commission, June, 1991, *Biotechnic Histochem* 67:110, 1992.

3. Taylor CR, Kledzik G: Immunohistologic techniques in surgical pathology: a spectrum of "new" special stains, *Hum Pathol* 12:590, 1981.
4. American Society of Clinical Pathologists: Q probes program, Chicago, 1994, the society.
5. Hensen DE: Studies in observer variation, *Arch Pathol Lab Med* 115:991, 1991.
6. Kim H, Zelman RJ, Fox MA et al: Pathology panel for lymphoma clinical studies: a comprehensive analysis of cases accumulated since its inception, *J Natl Cancer Inst* 68:43, 1982.
7. Stehl HV, Vroom TM, Blok P et al: Therapy-relevant discrepancies between diagnoses of institutional pathologists and experienced hematopathologists in the diagnosis of malignant lymphoma, *Pathol Res Pract* (Stuttgart) 184:242, 1989.
8. Dixon MF, Brown LJ, Gilmour HM et al: Observer variation in the assessment of dysplasia in ulcerative colitis, *Histopathology* 13:385, 1988.
9. Melville DM, Jass JR, Morson BC et al: Observer study of the grading of dysplasia in ulcerative colitis: comparison with clinical outcome, *Hum Pathol* 20:1008, 1989.
10. Palli D, Bianchi S, Linell F et al: Histologic classification of breast cancer in Sweden and Italy: a comparison between two pathologists, *Tumori* 78:247, 1992.
11. Schnitt SJ, Connolly JL, Tavassoli FA et al: Interobserver reproducibility in the diagnosis of ductal proliferative breast lesions using standardized criteria, *Am J Surg Pathol* 16:1133, 1992.
12. Rosai J: Borderline epithelial lesions of the breast, *Am J Surg Pathol* 15:209, 1991.
13. Ooms EC, Anderson WA, Alons CL et al: Analysis of the performance of pathologists in the grading of bladder tumors, *Hum Pathol* 14:140, 1983.
14. Culling CFA: *Handbook of histopathological and histochemical techniques*, ed 3, London, 1974, Butterworth.
15. Lillie RD, Fullmer HM: *Histopathologic technic and practical histochemistry*, New York, 1975, McGraw-Hill.
16. Coons AH, Creech HJ, Jones RN: Immunological properties of an antibody containing a fluorescent group, *Proc Soc Exp Biol* 47:200, 1941.
17. Fagraeus A: Plasma cellular reaction and its relation to formation of antibodies in vitro, *J Immunol* 58:1, 1948.
18. Avrameas S: Coupling of enzymes to proteins with glutaraldehyde: use of the conjugates for the detection of antigens and antibodies, *Immunochemistry* 6:43, 1969.
19. Sainte-Marie G: A paraffin embedding technique for studies employing immunofluorescence, *J Histochem Cytochem* 10:250, 1962.
20. Taylor CR: The nature of Reed-Sternberg cells and other malignant cells, *Lancet* 2:802, 1974.
21. Burns J, Hambridge M, Taylor CR: Intracellular immunoglobulins: a comparative study of three standard tissue processing methods using horseradish peroxidase and fluorochrome conjugates, *J Clin Pathol* 27:584, 1974.
22. Nayak NC, Sachdeva R: Localization of hepatitis B antigen in conventional paraffin sections of the liver, *Am J Surg Pathol* 81:479, 1975.

Immunohistochemistry as a laboratory test

23. Wick MR: Quality assurance in diagnostic immunohistochemistry (Editorial), *Am J Clin Pathol* 92:844, 1989.
24. DeLellis RA: *Advances in immunohistochemistry*, New York, 1984, Masson.
25. Jasani B, Schmid KW: *Immunocytochemistry in diagnostic histopathology*, Edinburgh, 1993, Churchill Livingstone.
26. True LD: *Atlas of diagnostic immunohistopathology*, Philadelphia, 1990, Lippincott.
27. Elias JM: *Immunohistopathology: a practical approach to diagnosis*, Chicago, 1990, ASCP Press (American Society of Clinical Pathologists).
28. Filipe MI, Lake BD: *Histochemistry in pathology*, New York, 1990, Churchill Livingstone.
29. Banks PM: Diagnostic applications of an immunoperoxidase method in hematopathology, *J Histochem Cytochem* 27:1192, 1979.
30. Taylor CR: Report of the Immunohistochemistry Steering Committee of the Biological Stain Commission: "proposed format: package insert for immunohistochemistry products," *Biotechnic Histochem* 67:323, 1992.
31. Battifora H, Mehta P: The checkerboard tissue block: an improved multitissue control block, *Lab Invest* 63:722, 1990.
32. Lindeman J, Von Gise H, Smid L et al: Evaluation of the automation of immunoenzymatic procedures in a routine histo/cytopathological laboratory, *Histopathology* 6:739, 1982.
33. Stark E, Faltinat D, Von der Fecht R: An automated device for immunocytochemistry, *J Immunol Methods* 107:89, 1988.
34. Brigati D, Budgeon LR, Unger ER et al: Immunocytochemistry is automated: development of a robotic workstation based upon the capillary action principle, *J Histotechnol* 11:165, 1988.
35. Tubbs RR, Bauer TW: Automation of immunohistology, *Arch Pathol Lab Med* 113:653-657, 1989.
36. Grogan TM: Automated immunohistochemical analysis, *Am J Clin Pathol* 98:S35, 1992.
37. Grogan TM, Casey TT, Miller PC et al: Automation of immunohistochemistry. In Weinstein RS, Graham AR, Anderson RE et al, editors: *Advances in pathology and laboratory medicine*, St Louis, 1993, Mosby.
38. Taylor CR: Exaltation of experts: concerted efforts in the standardization of immunohistochemistry, *Hum Pathol* 25:2, 1994.
39. Corwin D: Personal communication, June 1993, *College of American Pathologists*.
40. Battifora H: Assessment of antigen damage in immunohistochemistry: the vimentin internal control, *Am J Clin Pathol* 96:669, 1991.

40a. Shi S-R, Key ME, Kalra KL: Antigen retrieval in formalin-fixed, paraffin embedded tissues: an enhancement method for immunohistochemical staining based on microwave oven heating of tissues sections, *J Histochem Cytochem* 39:741,1991.

40b. Shi S-R, Imam SA, Young L et al: Antigen retrieval immunohistochemistry under the influence of pH using monclonal antibodies, *J Histochem Cytochem* 43:193,1995.

41. Banks PM: Incorporation of immunostaining data in anatomic pathology reports, *Am J Surg Pathol* 16:808, 1992.
42. Gatter KC, Alcock C, Heryet A et al: Clinical importance of analyzing malignant tumours of uncertain origin with immunohistochemical techniques, *Lancet* 1:1302, 1985.
43. Leong AS-Y, Wright J: The contribution of immunohistochemical staining in tumor diagnosis, *Histopathology* 11:1295, 1987.
44. Leong AS, Wannakrirot P: A retrospective analysis of immunohistochemical staining in identification of poorly differentiated round cell and spindle cell tumors—results, reagents and costs, *Pathology* (Sidney) 24:254, 1992.
45. Banks PM: Presentation to the trustees, *Biologic Stain Commission Annual Meeting* 1993 (abstract).
46. Hilborne LH, Nathan LE: Quality of assurance in an era of cost containment, *Am J Clin Pathol* 96(suppl 1):S6, 1991.
47. Fritz P, Hones J, Lutz D et al: Quantitative immunohistochemistry: standardization and possible application in research and surgical pathology, *Acta Histochem Suppl* 37:213, 1989.

Analysis of tumors of uncertain origin

48. Altman E, Cadman E: An analysis of 1539 patients with cancer of unknown primary site, *Cancer* 57:120, 1986.
49. Lauder I, Holland D, Mason DY et al: Identification of large cell undifferentiated tumors in lymph nodes using leukocyte common and keratin antibodies, *Histopathology* 8:259, 1984.
50. Mazoujian G, Bodian C, Haagensen DE Jr, Haagensen CD: Expression of GCDFP-15 in breast carcinomas: relationship to pathologic and clinical factors, *Cancer* 63: 2156, 1989.
51. Wick MR, Lillemoe TJ, Copland GT et al: Gross cystic disease fluid protein-15 as a marker for breast cancer: immunohistochemical analysis of 690 human neoplasms and comparison with alpha-lactalbumin, *Hum Pathol* 20:281, 1989.
52. Redding WH, Coombes RC, Monaghan P et al: Detection of micrometastases in patients with primary breast cancer, *Lancet* 2:1271, 1983.
53. Cote RJ, Rosen PP, Hakes TB et al: Monoclonal antibodies detect occult breast carcinoma metastases in bone marrow of patients with early stage disease, *Am J Surg Pathol* 12:333, 1988.

54. Cote RJ, Rosen PP, Lesser ML et al: Prediction of early relapse in patients with operable breast cancer by detection of occult bone marrow micrometastases, *J Clin Oncol* 9:1749, 1991.
55. Schlimok G, Funke I, Bock B et al: Epithelial tumor cells in bone marrow of patients with colorectal cancer: immunocytochemical detection, phenotypic characterization, and prognostic significance, *J Clin Oncol* 8:831, 1990.
56. Sedmak DD, Meineke TA, Knechtges DS et al: Prognostic significance of cytokeratin-positive breast cancer metastases, *Mod Pathol* 2:516, 1989.
57. Moll R, Franke WW, Schiller DL, Geiger BA-K: The catalog of human cytokeratins: patterns of expression in normal epithelia, tumors and cultured cells, *Cell* 31:11, 1982.
58. Gown AM, Vogel AM: Monoclonal antibodies to human intermediate filament proteins: III. Analysis of tumors, *Am J Clin Pathol* 84:413, 1985.
59. Johnson DE, Herndier BG, Medeiros LJ et al: The diagnostic utility of keratin profiles of hepatocellular carcinoma and cholangiocarcinoma, *Am J Surg Pathol* 12:187, 1988.
60. de Mascarel A, Merlio JP, Coindre JM et al: Gastric large cell lymphoma expressing cytokeratin but no leukocyte common antigen: a diagnostic dilemma, *Am J Clin Pathol* 91:478, 1989.
61. Brown DC, Theaker JM, Banks PM et al: Cytokeratin expression in smooth muscle and smooth muscle tumours, *Histopathology* 11:477, 1987.
62. Miettinen M: Immunoreactivity for cytokeratin and epithelial membrane antigen in leiomyosarcoma, *Arch Pathol Lab Med* 112:637, 1988.
63. Ng CS, Chan JK, Hui PK, Lau WH: Large B-cell lymphomas with a high content of reactive T cells, *Hum Pathol* 20:1145, 1989.
64. Gray MH, Smoller BR, McNutt NS, Hsu A: Immunohistochemical demonstration of factor XIIIa expression in neurofibromas: a practical means of differentiating these tumors from neurotized melanocytic nevi and schwannomas, *Arch Dermatol* 126:472, 1990.
65. Zarbo RJ, Gown AM, Nagle RB et al: Anomalous cytokeratin expression in malignant melanoma: one- and two-dimensional western blot analysis and immunohistochemical survey of 100 melanomas, *Mod Pathol* 3:494, 1990.

65a. Haluska FG, Brufsky AM, Canellos GP: The cellular biology of the Reed-Sternberg cell, *Blood* 84:1005, 1994.

66. Nakhleh RE, Wick MR, Rocamora A et al: Morphologic diversity in malignant melanomas, *Am J Clin Pathol* 93:731, 1990.
67. Dwarakanath S, Lee AKC, DeLillis RA et al: S100 protein positivity in breast carcinomas: a potential pitfall in diagnostic immunohistochemistry, *Hum Pathol* 18:1144, 1987.
68. Drier JK, Swanson DL, Cherwitz DL, Wick MR: S100 protein immunoreactivity in poorly differentiated carcinomas: immunohistochemical comparison with malignant melanoma, *Arch Pathol Lab Med* 111:447, 1987.
69. Duray PH, Palazzo J, Gown AM, Ohuchi N: Melanoma cell heterogeneity: a study of two monoclonal antibodies compared with S-100 protein in paraffin sections, *Cancer* 61:2460, 1988.
70. Leong A-Y, Milios J: An assessment of a melanoma-specific antibody (HMB-45) and other immunohistochemical markers of malignant melanoma in paraffin-embedded tissues, *Surg Pathol* 2:137, 1989.
71. Pelosi G, Bonetti F, Colombari R et al: Use of monoclonal antibody HMB-45 for detecting malignant melanoma cells in fine needle aspiration biopsy samples, *Acta Cytol* 34:460, 1990.
72. Bonetti F, Colombari R, Manfrin E et al: Breast carcinoma with positive results for melanoma marker (HMB-45): HMB-45 immunoreactivity in normal and neoplastic breast, *Am J Clin Pathol* 92:491, 1989.
73. Gown AM, Vogel AM, Gordon D, Lu PL: A smooth muscle–specific monoclonal antibody recognizes smooth muscle actin isozymes, *J Cell Biol* 100:807, 1985.
74. Azumi N, Ben Ezra J, Battifora H: Immunophenotypic diagnosis of leiomyosarcoma and rhabdomyosarcoma with monoclonal antibodies to muscle-specific actin and desmin in formalin-fixed tissue, *Mod Pathol* 1:469, 1988.
75. Tsukada T, McNutt MA, Ross R, Gown AM: HHF35, a muscle actin–specific monoclonal antibody II. Reactivity in normal, reactive, and neoplastic human tissues, *Am J Pathol* 127:389, 1987.
76. Skalli O, Ropraz P, Trzeciak A et al: A monoclonal antibody against a smooth muscle actin: a new probe for smooth muscle differentiation, *J Cell Biol* 103:2787, 1986.
77. Mukai K, Torikata C, Iri H et al: Histogenesis of alveolar soft part sarcoma: an immunohistochemical and biochemical study, *Am J Surg Pathol* 10:212, 1986.
78. DuBoulary CEH: Demonstration of alpha-1-antitrypsin and alpha-1-antichymotrypsin in fibrous histiocytomas using the immunoperoxidase technique, *Am J Surg Pathol* 6:559, 1982.
79. Fisher C: The value of electron microscopy and immunohistochemistry in the diagnosis of soft tissue sarcoma: a study of 200 cases, *Histopathology* 16:441, 1990.
80. Leader M, Collins PM, Henry KA: Anti-1-antichymotrypsin staining of 194 sarcomas, 38 carcinomas, and 17 malignant melanomas: its lack of specificity as a tumor marker, *Am J Surg Pathol* 11:133, 1987.
81. Gould VE, Lee I, Wiedenmann B et al: Synaptophysin: a novel marker for neurons, certain neuroendocrine cells and their neoplasms, *Hum Pathol* 17:979, 1986.
82. Wick MR, Swanson PE, Scheithauer BW, Manivel JC: Malignant peripheral nerve sheath tumor, an immunohistochemical study of 62 cases, *Am J Clin Pathol* 87:425, 1987.
83. Weiss SW, Langloss JM, Enzinger FM: Value S100 protein in the diagnosis of soft tissue tumors with particular reference to benign and malignant schwann cell tumors, *Lab Invest* 49:299, 1983.
84. Alles JU, Bosslet K: Immunocytochemistry of angiosarcomas: a study of 19 cases with special emphasis on the applicability of endothelial cell specific markers to routinely prepared tissues, *Am J Clin Pathol* 89:463, 1988.
85. Ordóñez NG: Comparison of *Ulex europaeus* I lectin and factor VIII–related antigen in vascular lesions, *Arch Pathol Lab Med* 129:132, 1984.
86. Tetu B, Ordóñez NG, Ayala AG, Mackay B: Chondrosarcoma with additional mesenchymal component (dedifferentiated chondrosarcoma) II: an immunohistochemical and electron microscopic study, *Cancer* 58:287, 1986.
87. Schulz A, Jundt G, Berghaeuser KH et al: Immunohistochemical study of osteonectin in various types of osteosarcoma, *Am J Pathol* 132:233, 1988.
88. Oppedal BR, Brandtzaeg P, Kemshead JT: Immunohistochemical performance testing of monoclonal antibodies to neuroblastoma cells on normal adrenals, spin and sympathetic ganglia, and neural crest tumours, *Histopathology* 11:351, 1987.
89. Triche TJ: Neuroblastoma and other childhood neural tumors: a review, *Pediatr Pathol* 10:175, 1990.
90. Ishiguro Y, Kato K, Ito T et al: Enolase isozymes as markers for differential diagnosis of neuroblastoma, rhabdomyosarcoma, and Wilms' tumor, *Gann* 75:53, 1984.
91. Wilson BS, Lloyd RV: Detection of chromogranin in neuroendocrine cells with a monoclonal antibody, *Am J Pathol* 115:458, 1984.
92. Caillaud JM, Benjelloun S, Bosq J et al: HNK-1–defined antigen detected in paraffin-embedded neuroectoderm tumors and those derived from cells of the amine precursor uptake and decarboxylation system, *Cancer Res* 44:4432, 1984.
93. Gould VE, Jansson DS, Molenaar WM et al: Primitive neuroectodermal tumors of the central nervous system: patterns of expression of neuroendocrine markers, and all classes of intermediate filament proteins, *Lab Invest* 62:498, 1990.
94. Vinores SA, Bonnin JM, Rubinstein LJ, Marangos PJ: Immunohistochemical demonstration of neuron-specific enolase in neoplasms on the CNS and other tissues, *Arch Pathol Lab Med* 108:536, 1984.
95. Wahab ZA, Wright GL: Monoclonal antibody (anti-Leu 7) directed against natural killer cells reacts with normal, benign, and malignant prostate tissues, *Int J Cancer* 36:677, 1985.
96. Wilson BS, Lloyd RV: Detection of chromogranin in neuroendocrine cells with a monoclonal antibody, *Am J Pathol* 115:458, 1984.
97. Miettinen M: Immunohistochemical spectrum of rhabdomyosarcoma and rhabdomyosarcoma-like tumors: expression of cytokeratin and the 68 kD neurofilament protein, *Am J Surg Pathol* 12:120, 1989.
98. Bunn PA, Jr, Linnoila I, Minna JD et al: Small cell lung cancer, endocrine cells of the fetal bronchus, and other neuroendocrine cells express the

Leu-7 antigenic determinant present on natural killer cells, *Blood* 65:764, 1985.

99. Said JW, Vimadalal S, Nash G et al: Immunoreactive neuron-specific enolase, bombesin, and chromogranin as markers for neuroendocrine lung tumors, *Hum Pathol* 16:236, 1985.
100. Chen Y, Zhang Y: Use of monoclonal antibodies to glial fibrillary acidic protein in the cytologic diagnosis of brain tumors, *Acta Cytol* 33:922, 1989.
101. Perentes E, Rubinstein LJ: Recent applications of immunoperoxidase histochemistry in human neuro-oncology: an update, *Arch Pathol Lab Med* 111:796, 1987.
102. Achtstaetter T, Moll R, Anderson A et al: Expression of glial filament protein (GFP) in nerve sheaths and non-neural cells re-examined using monoclonal antibodies, with special emphasis on the co-expression of GFP and cytokeratins in epithelial cells of human salivary gland and pleomorphic adenomas, *Differentiation* 31:206, 1986.
103. Kawahara E, Oda Y, Ooi A et al: Expression of glial fibrillary acidic protein (GFAP) in peripheral nerve sheath tumors: a comparative study of immunoreactivity of GFAP, vimentin, S100 protein and neurofilament in 38 schwannomas and 18 neurofibromas, *Am J Surg Pathol* 12:115, 1988.
104. Clayton F, Ordóñez NG, Hanssen GM et al: Immunoperoxidase localization of lactalbumin in malignant breast neoplasms, *Arch Pathol Lab Med* 106:268, 1982.
105. Lee AK, DeLellis RA, Rosen PP et al: Alpha-lactalbumin as an immunohistochemical marker for metastatic breast carcinomas, *Am J Surg Pathol* 8:93, 1984.
106. Deftos LJ, Bone HG, Parthemore JG: Immunohistological studies of medullary thyroid carcinoma and C cell hyperplasia, *J Clin Endocrinol Metab* 51:857, 1980.
107. Wilson NW, Pambakian H, Richardson TC et al: Epithelial markers in thyroid carcinoma: an immunoperoxidase study, *Histopathology* 10:815, 1986.
108. Ordóñez NG, El-Naggar AK, Hickey RC et al: Anaplastic thyroid carcinoma, Immunocytochemical study of 32 cases, *Am J Clin Pathol* 96:15, 1991.
109. Lewin KJ, Riddell RH, Weinstein WM: Endocrine cells. In Lewin KJ, editor: *Gastrointestinal pathology and its clinical implications,* New York, 1992, Igaku Shoin.
110. Bordi C, Pilato FP, D-Adda T: Comparative study of seven neuroendocrine markers in pancreatic endocrine tumours, *Virchows Arch [A]* 413:387, 1988.
111. Gould VE, Lee I, Wiedenmann B et al: Synaptophysin: a novel marker for neurons, certain neuroendocrine cells and their neoplasms, *Hum Pathol* 17:979, 1986.
112. Said JW, Vimadalal S, Nash G et al: Immunoreactive neuron-specific enolase, bombesin, and chromogranin as markers for neuroendocrine lung tumors, *Hum Pathol* 16:236, 1985.
113. Wilson BS, Lloyd RV: Detection of chromogranin in neuroendocrine cells with a monoclonal antibody, *Am J Pathol* 115:458, 1984.
114. Mikhaĭlov I, Aleksiev B, Zhablenska R et al: Combined ultrastructural and immunocytochemical studies of pancreatic endocrine tumors, *Arkh Patol* 53:14, 1991.
115. Mukai K, Grotting JC, Greider MH et al: Retrospective study of 77 pancreatic endocrine tumors using the immunoperoxidase method, *Am J Surg Pathol* 6:387, 1982.
116. Cohen C, Budgeon LR: Commercial immunoperoxidase kits in the study of 13 pancreatic islet-cell tumors, *Am J Clin Pathol* 78:364, 1982.
117. Klempa I, Helmstadter V, Feurle G et al: [Endocrine tumors of the gastrointestinal and pancreatic systems: multiple endocrine adenoma from another viewpoint], *Chirurg* 51:321, 1980.
118. Frankel AE, Rouse RV, Wang MC et al: Monoclonal antibodies to a human prostate antigen, *Cancer Res* 42:3714, 1982.
119. Kuriyama M, Loor R, Wang MC et al: Prostatic acid phosphatase and prostate-specific antigen in prostate cancer, *Int Surg Oncol* 5:347, 1982.
120. Wick MR, Lillemoe TJ, Copland GT et al: Gross cystic disease fluid protein-15 as a marker for breast cancer: immunohistochemical analysis of 690 human neoplasms and comparison with alpha-lactalbumin, *Hum Pathol* 20:281, 1989.
121. Mazoujian G, Bodian C, Haagensen DE Jr, Haagensen CD: Expression of GCDFP-15 in breast carcinomas: relationship to pathologic and clinical factors, *Cancer* 63:2156, 1989.

Prognostic markers in cancer

122. Birembaut P, Caron Y, Adnet JJ, Froidart JM: Usefulness of basement membrane markers in tumoural pathology, *J Pathol* 145:283, 1985.
123. Charpin C, Lisitzky JC, Jacquemier J et al: Immunohistochemical detection of laminin in 98 human breast carcinomas: a light and electron microscopic study, *Hum Pathol* 17:355, 1986.
124. Gusterson BA, Warburton MJ, Mitchell D et al: Distribution of myoepithelial cells and basement membrane proteins in the normal breast and in benign and malignant breast diseases, *Cancer Res* 42:4763, 1982.
125. Gown AM, Vogel AM: Monoclonal antibodies to human intermediate filament proteins. II. Distribution of filament proteins in normal tissues, *Am J Pathol* 114:309, 1984.
126. Guinan P, Shaw M, Targonski P et al: Evaluation of cytokeratin markers to differentiate between benign and malignant prostatic tissue, *J Surg Oncol* 42:175, 1989.
127. Sherwood ER, Theyer G, Steiner G et al: Differential expression of specific cytokeratin polypeptides in the basal and luminal epithelia of the human prostate, *Prostate* 18:303, 1991.
128. Hedrick L, Epstein JI: Use of keratin 903 as an adjunct in the diagnosis of prostate carcinoma, *Am J Surg Pathol* 13:389, 1989.
129. Ronnett BM, Epstein JI: A case showing sclerosing adenosis and an unusual form of basal cell hyperplasia of the prostate, *Am J Surg Pathol* 13:866, 1989.
130. Sakamoto N, Tsuneyoshi M, Enjoli M: Sclerosing adenosis of the prostate: histopathologic and immunohistochemical analysis, *Am J Surg Pathol* 15:660, 1991.
131. Shah IA, Schlageter MO, Stinnett P, Lechago J: Cytokeratin immunohistochemistry as a diagnostic tool for distinguishing malignant from benign epithelial lesions of the prostate, *Mod Pathol* 7:98, 1991.
132. Redding WH, Coombes RC, Monaghan P et al: Detection of micrometastases in patients with primary breast cancer, *Lancet* 2:1271, 1983.
133. Mansi JL, Berger U, Easton D et al: Micrometastases in bone marrow in patients with primary breast cancer: evaluation as an early predictor of bone metastases, *Br Med J* 295:1093, 1987.
134. Schlimok G, Funke I, Holzmann B et al: Micrometastastic cancer cells in bone marrow: in vitro detection with anti-cytokeratin and in vivo with anti-17-1A monoclonal antibodies, *Proc Natl Acad Sci USA* 84:8672, 1987.
135. Cote RJ, Rosen PP, Hakes TB et al: Monoclonal antibodies detect occult breast carcinoma metastases in bone marrow of patients with early stage disease, *Am J Surg Pathol* 12:333, 1988.
136. Cote RJ, Rosen PP, Lesser ML, et al: Prediction of early relapse in patients with operable breast cancer by detection of occult bone marrow micrometastases, *J Clin Oncol* 9:1749, 1991.
137. Porro G, Menard S, Tagliabue E et al: Monoclonal antibody detection of carcinoma cells in bone marrow biopsy specimens from breast cancer patients, *Cancer* 61:2407, 1988.
138. Diel IJ, Kaufmann M, Goerner R et al: Detection of tumor cells in bone marrow of patients with primary breast cancer: a prognostic factor for distant metastases, *J Clin Oncol* 10:1534, 1992.
139. Schlimok G, Funke I, Bock B et al: Epithelial tumor cells in bone marrow of patients with colorectal cancer: immunocytochemical detection, phenotypic characterization, and prognostic significance, *J Clin Oncol* 8:831, 1990.
140. Lindemann F, Schlimok G, Dirschedl P et al: Prognostic significance of micrometastatic tumour cells in bone marrow of colorectal cancer patients, *Lancet* 340:685, 1992.
141. Mansi JL, Berger U, Wilson R et al: Detection of tumor cells in bone marrow of patients with prostatic carcinoma by immunocytochemical techniques, *J Urol* 139:545, 1988.
142. Bretton PR, Melamed MR, Fair WR, Cote RJ: Detection of occult micrometastases in the bone marrow of patients with prostate carcinoma, *The prostate* 25:108, 1994.

143. Cain JM, Ellis GK, Collins C et al: Bone marrow involvement in epithelial ovarian cancer by immunocytochemical assessment, *Gynecol Oncol* 38:442, 1990.
144. Frew AJ, Ralfkiaer N et al: Immunocytochemistry in the detection of bone marrow metastases in patients with primary lung cancer, *Br J Cancer* 53:555, 1986.
145. Leonard RCF, Duncan LW, Hay FG: Immunocytological detection of residual marrow disease at clinical remission predicts metastatic relapse in small cell lung cancer, *Cancer Res* 50:6545, 1990.
146. Dearnaley DP, Ormerod MG, Sloane JP: Micrometastases in breast cancer: long-term follow-up of the first patient cohort, *Eur J Cancer* 27:236, 1991.
147. Gusterson BA, Ott R: Occult axillary lymph-node micrometastases in breast cancer, *Lancet* (336):434, 1990.
148. Neville AM: Breast cancer micrometastases in lymph nodes and bone marrow are prognostically important, *Ann Oncol* 2:13, 1991.
149. Saphir O, Amromin GD: Obscure axillary lymph-node metastasis in carcinoma of the breast, *Cancer* 1:238, 1948.
150. Pickren JW: Significance of occult metastases, *Cancer* 14:1266, 1961.
151. Fisher ER, Saminoss S, Lee CH et al: Detection and significance of occult axillary node metastases in patients with invasive breast cancer, *Cancer* 42:2025, 1978.
152. International (Ludwig Institute) Breast Cancer Study Group: Prognostic importance of occult axillary lymph node micrometastases from breast cancers, *Lancet* (335):1565, 1990.
153. Wells CA, Heryet A, Brochier J et al: The immunocytochemical detection of axillary micrometastases in breast cancer, *Br J Cancer* 50:193, 1984.
154. Bussolati G, Gugliotta P, Morra I et al: The immunohistochemical detection of lymph node metastases from infiltrating lobular carcinoma of the breast, *Br J Cancer* 54:631, 1986.
155. Byrne J, Waldron R, McAvinchey D et al: The use of monoclonal antibodies for the histopathological detection of mammary axillary micrometastases, *Eur J Surg Oncol* 13:409, 1987.
156. Trojani M, Mascarel I, Bonichon F et al: Micrometastases to axillary lymph nodes from carcinoma of breast: detection by immunohistochemistry and prognostic significance, *Br J Cancer* 55:303, 1987.
157. Apostolikas N, Petraki C, Agnantis ND: The reliability of histologically negative axillary lymph nodes in breast cancer, *Pathol Res Pract* 184:35, 1989.
158. Sedmak DD, Meineke TA, Knechtges DS et al: Prognostic significance of cytokeratin-positive breast cancer metastases, *Mod Pathol* 2:516, 1989.
159. Cote RJ, Chaiwun B, Qu J et al: Prognostic importance of occult lymph node metastases in patients with breast cancer, *Proc Am Assoc Cancer Res* 33:202, 1992.
160. Nasser IA, Lee KC, Bosari S et al: Occult axillary lymph node metastases in "node-negative" breast carcinoma, *Hum Pathol* 24:950, 1993.
161. Hainsworth PJ, Tjandra JJ, Stillwell RG, et al: Detection and significance of occult metastases in node-negative breast cancer, *Br J Surg* 80:459, 1993.
162. Cochran AJ, Wen DR, Morton DL: Occult tumor cells in the lymph nodes of patients with pathological stage I malignant melanoma, *Am J Surg Pathol* 12:612, 1988.
163. Hering F, Rist M, Roth J et al: Does microinvasion of the capsule and/or micrometastases in regional lymph nodes influence disease-free survival after radical prostatectomy? *Br J Urol* 66:177, 1990.
164. Greenson JK, Isenhart CE, Rice R et al: Identification of occult micrometastases in pericolic lymph nodes of Dukes' B colorectal cancer patients using monoclonal antibodies against cytokeratin and CC49, *Cancer* 73:563, 1994.
165. Chen Z-L, Perez S, Holmes EC et al: Frequency and distribution of occult micrometastases in lymph nodes of patients with non–small-cell lung carcinoma, *J Natl Cancer Inst* 85:493, 1993.
165a. Freeman JA, Esrig D, Grossfeld GD et al: Incidence of occult lymph node metastases in pathologic stage C (pT3N0) prostate cancer, *J Urol*, 1995 (In press).
166. Neville AM, Price KN, Gelber RD et al: Axillary node micrometastases and breast cancer, *Lancet* 337:110, 1991.
167. Old LJ: Cancer immunology: the search for specificity—G.H.A. Clowes Memorial Lecture, *Can Res* 41:361, 1980.
168. Kuhajda FP, Offutt LE, Mendelsohn G: The distribution of carcinoembryonic antigen in breast carcinoma: diagnostic and prognostic implications, *Cancer* 52:1257, 1983.
169. Barry JD, Koch TJ, Cohen C et al: Correlation of immunohistochemical markers with patient prognosis in breast carcinoma: a quantitative study, *Am J Clin Pathol* 82:582, 1984.
170. Dearnaley DB, Sloan JP, Imrie S et al: Detection of isolated mammary carcinoma cells in marrow of patients with primary breast cancer, *J R Soc Med* 76:359, 1983.
171. Cardiff RD, Taylor CR, Wellings SR, et al: Monoclonal antibodies in immunoenzyme studies of breast cancer, *Ann N Y Acad Sci* 420:140, 1983.
172. Springer GF, Taylor CR, Howard DR et al: Tn, a carcinoma-associated antigen, reacts with anti-Tn of normal human sera, *Cancer* 55:561, 1985.
173. Springer GF: Tn epitope (*N*-acetyl-D-galactosamine alpha-*O*-serine/threonine) density in primary breast carcinoma: a functional predictor of aggressiveness, *Mol Immunol* 26:1, 1989.
174. Howard DR, Taylor CR: A method for distinguishing benign from malignant breast lesions utilizing antibody present in normal human sera, *Cancer* 43:2279, 1979.
175. Papsidero LD, Croghan GA, O'Connell MJ et al: Monoclonal antibodies (F36/22 and M7/105) to human breast carcinoma, *Cancer Res* 43:1741, 1983.
176. Venkatesh YS, Ordóñez NG, Schultz PN et al: Anaplastic carcinoma of the thyroid: a clinicopathologic study of 121 cases, *Cancer* 66:321, 1990.
177. Cote RJ, Cordon-Cardo C, Reuter VE et al: Immunopathology of adrenal and renal cortical tumors: coordinated change in antigen expression is associated with neoplastic conversion in the adrenal cortex, *Am J Pathol* 136:1077, 1990.
178. Henzen-Logmans SC, Stel HV, Van-Muijen GN et al: Expression of intermedial filament proteins in adrenal cortex and related tumors, *Histopathology* 12:359, 1988.
179. Hakamori S, Kannagi R: Glycosphingolipids as tumor-associated differentiation markers, *J Natl Cancer Inst* 71:231, 1982.
180. Hakamori, S: Aberrant glycosylation in cancer cell membranes as focused on glycolipids: overview and perspectives, *Cancer Res* 45:2405, 1985.
181. Lloyd KO: Blood group antigens as markers for normal and abnormal differentiation and malignant change in human tissues, *Am J Clin Pathol* 87:129, 1987.
182. Cordon-Cardo C, Lloyd KO, Sakamoto J et al: Immunohistologic expression of blood-group antigens in normal human gastrointestinal tract and colonic carcinoma, *Int J Cancer* 37:667, 1986.
183. Cardon-Cardo C, Victor RE, Lloyd KO et al: Blood group–related antigens in human urothelium: enhanced expression precursor, Le^x, and Le^y determinants in urothelial carcinoma, *Cancer Res* 48:4113, 1988.
184. Sheinfeld J, Reuter VE, Fair WR, Cordon-Cardo C: Expression of blood group antigens in bladder cancer: current concepts, *Semin Surg Oncol* 8:308, 1992.
185. Wolf GT, Carey TE, Schmaltz SP et al: Altered antigen expression predicts outcome in squamous cell carcinoma of the head and neck, *J Natl Cancer Inst* 82:1566, 1990.
186. Byrne M, Thrane PS, Dabelsteen E: Loss of expression of blood group antigen H is associated with cellular invasion and spread of oral squamous cell carcinomas, *Cancer* 66:2118, 1990.
187. Meyer JS, Friedman E, McCrate MM, Bauer WC: Prediction of early course of breast carcinoma by thymidine labeling, *Cancer* 51:1879, 1983.
188. Hoshino T, Nagashima T, Murovic J et al: Proliferative potential of human meningiomas of the brain: a cell kinetics study with bromodeoxyuridine, *Cancer* 58:1466, 1986.
189. Meyer JS, McDivitt RW, Stone KR et al: Practical breast carcinoma cell kinetics: review and update, *Breast Cancer Res Treat* 4:79, 1984.
190. Tubiana M, Pejovic MH, Chavaudra N et al: The long-term prognostic significance of the thymidine labelling index in breast cancer, *Int J Cancer* 33:441, 1984.
191. Silverstini R, Daidone MG, Di Fronzo G et al: Prognostic implications of labelling index versus estrogen receptors and tumor size in node-negative breast cancer, *Breast Cancer Res Treat* 7:161, 1986.

192. Kamel OW, Franklin WA, Ringus JC, Meyer JS: Thymidine labeling index and Ki-67 growth fraction in lesions of the breast, *Am J Pathol* 134:107, 1989.
193. Deshmukh P, Ramsey L, Garewal HS: Ki-67 labeling index is a more reliable measure of solid tumor proliferative activity than tritiated thymidine labeling, *Am J Clin Pathol* 94:192, 1990.
194. Isola JJ, Helin HJ, Helle MJ, Kallioniemi O-P: Evaluation of cell proliferation in breast carcinoma: comparison of Ki-67 immunohistochemical study, DNA flow cytometric analysis, and mitotic count, *Cancer* 65:1180, 1990.
195. Koss LG, Bogdon C, Herz F et al: Flow cytometric measurements of DNA and other cell components in human tumors: a critical appraisal, *Hum Pathol* 20:528, 1989.
196. Clark GM, Dressler LG, Owens MA et al: Prediction of relapse or survival in patients with node-negative breast cancer by DNA flow cytometry, *N Engl J Med* 320:627, 1989.
197. Hedley DW: Developments in the use of flow cytometry as a guide to the prognosis of cancer, *Diagn Oncol* 1:2, 1991.
198. Chang K-J, Enker WE, Melamed M: Influence of tumor cell DNA ploidy on the natural history of rectal cancer, *Am J Surg* 153:184, 1987.
199. Kokal W, Sheibani K, Terz J, Harada JR: Tumor DNA content in the prognosis of colorectal carcinoma, *JAMA* 255:3123, 1986.
200. Witzig TE, Loprinzi CL, Gonchoroff NJ et al: DNA ploidy and cell kinetic measurements as predictors of recurrence and survival in stages B2 and C colorectal adenocarcinoma, *Cancer* 68:879, 1991.
201. Wolley RC, Schreiber K, Koss LG et al: DNA distribution in human colon carcinomas and its relationship to clinical behavior, *J Natl Cancer Inst* 69:12, 1982.
202. Lehman J, Krug H: Flow-through fluorocytophotometry of different brain tumors, *Acta Neuropathol* 49:123, 1980.
203. Spaar FW, Ahyai A, Spaar U et al: Flow-cytometry of nuclear DNA in biopsies of 45 human gliomas and after primary culture in vitro, *Clin Neuropathol* 5:157, 1986.
204. Lloyd RV, Wilson BS, Varani J et al: Immunocytochemical characterization of a monoclonal antibody that recognizes mitosing cells, *Am J Pathol* 121:275, 1985.
205. Dawson AE, Norton JA, Weinberg DS: Comparative assessment of proliferation and DNA content in breast carcinoma by image analysis and flow cytometry, *Am J Pathol* 136:1115, 1990.
206. van Dierendonck JH, Wijsman JH, Keijzer R et al: Cell-cycle–related staining patterns of anti-proliferating cell nuclear antigen monoclonal antibodies: comparison with BrdUrd labeling and Ki-67 staining, *Am J Pathol* 138:1165, 1991.
207. Di Stefano D, Minganzzini PL, Schucchi L et al: A comparative study of histopathology, hormone receptors, peanut lectin binding, Ki-67 immunostaining, and nucleolar organizer region–associated proteins in human breast cancer, *Cancer* 67:463, 1991.
208. Cattoretti G, Rilke F, Andreola S et al: P53 expression in breast cancer, *Int J Cancer* 41:178, 1988.
209. Wintzer HO, Zipfel I, Schulte-Moenting J et al: Ki-67 immunostaining in human breast tumors and its relationship to prognosis, *Cancer* 67:421, 1991.
210. Sahin AA, Ro J, Ro JY et al: Ki-67 immunostaining in node-negative stage I/II breast carcinoma: significant correlation with prognosis, *Cancer* 68:549, 1991.
211. Harper MD, Glynne-Jones E, Goddard L et al: Relationship of proliferating cell nuclear antigen (PCNA) in prostatic carcinomas to various clinical parameters, *Prostate* 20:243, 1992.
212. Mayer A, Takimoto M, Fritz E et al: The prognostic significance of proliferating cell nuclear antigen, epidermal growth factor receptor, and *mdr* gene expression in colorectal cancer, *Cancer* 71:2454, 1993.
213. Fujii M, Motoi M, Saeki H et al: Prognostic significance of proliferating cell nuclear antigen (PCNA) expression in non–small cell lung cancer, *Acta Med Okayama* 47:103, 1973.
214. Kitamoto M, Nakanishi T, Kira S et al: The assessment of proliferating cell nuclear antigen immunohistochemical staining in small hepatocellular carcinoma, *Cancer* 72:1859, 1993.
215. Mori M, Kakeji Y, Adachi Y et al: The prognostic significance of proliferating cell nuclear antigen in clinical gastric cancer, *Surgery* 113:683, 1993.
216. Jain S, Filipe MI, Hall PA et al: Prognostic value of proliferating cell nuclear antigen in gastric cancer, *J Clin Pathol* 44:655, 1991.
217. Woods AL, Hall PA, Shepherd NA et al: The assessment of proliferating cell nuclear antigen (PCNA) immunostaining in primary gastrointestinal lymphomas and its relationship to histological grade S+G_2+M phase fraction (flow cytometric analysis) and prognosis, *Histopathology* 18:21, 1991.
218. Yu CCW, Hall PA, Fletcher CDM et al: Haemangiopericytomas: the prognostic value of immunohistochemical staining with a monoclonal antibody to proliferating cell nuclear antigen (PCNA), *Histopathology* 19:29, 1991.
219. Oda Y, Hashimoto H, Takeshita S, Tsuneyoshi M: The prognostic value of immunohistochemical staining for proliferating cell nuclear antigen in synovial sarcoma, *Cancer* 478:485, 1993.
219a. Bodey B, Williams RT, Carbonaro-Hall DA et al: Immunocytochemical detection of cyclin A and cyclin D in formalin-fixed, paraffin-embedded tissues: novel, pertinent markers of cell proliferation, *Mod Path* 7:846, 1994.
219b. Carbonarro-Hall D, Williams R, Wu L et al: G1 expression and multistage dynamics of cyclin-A in human osteosarcoma cells, *Oncogene* 8:1649, 1995.
220. Holmes WE, Sliwkowski MX, Akita RW et al: Identification of Heregulin, a specific activator p185*erb*B2, *Science* 256:1205, 1992.
221. Slamon DJ, Godolphin W, Jones LA et al: Studies of the Her-2/*neu* proto-oncogene in human breast and ovarian cancer, *Science* 244:707, 1989.
222. Riviere A, Becker J, Loening T: Comparative investigation of c-*erb*B2/*neu* expression in head and neck tumors and mammary cancer, *Cancer* 67:2142, 1991.
223. Stenman G, Sandros J, Nordvist A et al: Expression of the *erb*B2 protein in benign and malignant salivary gland tumors, *Genes Chromosom Cancer* 3:128, 1991.
224. Ware JL, Maygarden SJ, Koontz WW et al: Immunohistochemical detection of c-*erb*B-2 protein in human benign and neoplastic prostate, *Hum Pathol* 22:254, 1991.
225. McCann A, Dervan PA, Johnston PA et al: c-*erb* B-2 oncoprotein expression in primary human tumors, *Cancer* 65:88, 1990.
226. Yu D, Wolf JK, Scanlon M et al: Enhanced c-*erb*B-2/*neu* expression in human ovarian cancer cells correlates with more severe malignancy that can be suppressed by E1A, *Cancer Res* 53:891, 1993.
227. Sasano H, Date F, Imatani A et al: Double immunostaining for c-*erb*B-2 and p53 in human stomach cancer cells, *Hum Pathol* 24:584, 1993.
228. Press MF, Pike MC, Chazin VR, et al: Her-2/*neu* expression in node-negative breast cancer: direct tissue quantitation by computerized image analysis and association of overexpression with increased risk of recurrent disease, *Cancer Res* 53:4960, 1993.
229. Schneider PM, Hung MC, Chiocca SM et al: Differential expression of the c-*erb*B-2 gene in human small cell lung cancer, *Cancer Res* 49:4968, 1989.
230. Weiner DB, Nordberg J, Robinson R et al: Expression of the *neu* gene–encoded protein (p185*neu*) in human non–small cell carcinomas of the lung, *Cancer Res* 50:421, 1990.
231. D'Emilia J, Bulovas K, D'Ercole K et al: Expression of the c-*erb*B-2 gene product (p185) at different stages of neoplastic progression in the colon, *Oncogene* 4:1233, 1989.
232. Berger U, Wilson ST, McClelland RA et al: Comparison of an immunocytochemical assay for progesterone receptor with a biochemical method of measurement and immunocytochemical examination of the relationship between progesterone and estrogen receptors, *Cancer Res* 49:5176, 1989.
233. De Potter CR, Van Daele S, van de Vijver MJ et al: The expression of the *neu* oncogene product in breast lesions and in normal fetal and adult human tissues, *Histopathology* 15:351, 1989.
234. Slamon DJ, Clark GM, Wong SG et al: Human breast cancer: correlation of relapse and survival with amplification of the HER-2/*neu* oncogene, *Science* 235:177, 1987.
235. Wright C, Angus B, Nicholson S et al: Expression of c-*erb*B-2 oncoprotein: a prognostic indicator in human breast cancer, *Cancer Res* 49:2087, 1989.

236. Tandon AK, Clark GM, Chamnes GC et al: HER-2/*neu* oncogene protein and prognosis in breast cancer, *J Clin Oncol* 7:1120, 1989.
237. Allred DC, Clark GM, Tandon AK et al: HER-2/*neu* in node-negative breast cancer: prognostic significance of overexpression influenced by the presence of in situ carcinoma, *J Clin Oncol* 10:599, 1992.
238. Gusterson BA, Gelber RD, Goldhirsch A et al: Prognostic importance of c-*erb*B-2 expression in breast cancer, *J Clin Oncol* 10:1049, 1992.
238a. Muss HB, Thor, AD, Berry DA et all: c-*erb*-2 expression and response to adjuvant therapy in women with node positive early breast cancer, *N Eng J Med* 330:1260, 1994.
239. Williams ARW, Piris J, Spandidos DA et al: Immunohistochemical detection of the *ras* oncogene p21 product in an experimental tumour and in human colorectal neoplasms, *Br J Cancer* 52:687, 1985.
240. Kerr IB, Lee FD, Quintalla M et al: Immunocytochemical demonstration of p21 *ras* family oncogene product in normal mucosa and in premalignant and malignant tumours of the colorectum, *Br J Cancer* 52:695, 1985.
241. Viola MV, Fromowitz F, Oravez S et al: *ras* oncogene p21 expression is increased in premalignant lesions and high grade bladder carcinoma, *J Exp Med* 161:1218, 1985.
242. Viola MV, Fromowitz F, Oravez S et al: Expression of *ras* oncogene p21 in prostate cancer, *N Engl J Med* 314:133, 1986.
243. Varma VA, Austin GE, O'Connell AC: Antibodies to *ras* oncogene p21 proteins lack immunohistochemical specificity for neoplastic epithelium to human prostate tissue, *Arch Pathol Lab Med* 113:16, 1989.
244. Ghosh AK, Moore M, Harris M: Immunohistochemical detections of *ras* oncogene p21 product in benign and malignant mammary tissue in man, *J Clin Pathol* 39:428, 1986.
245. Noguchi M, Hirohashi S, Shimasato Y et al: Histological demonstration of antigens reactive with anti-p21 *ras* monoclonal antibody (RAP-5) in human stomach cancers, *J Natl Cancer Inst* 77:379, 1986.
246. Johnson TL, Lloyd RV, Thor A: Expression of *ras* oncogene p21 antigen in normal and proliferative thyroid tissues, *Am J Pathol* 127:60, 1987.
247. Mizukami Y, Nonomura A, Hashimoto T et al: Immunohistochemical demonstration of *ras* p21 oncogene product in normal, benign, and malignant human thyroid tissues, *Cancer* 61:873, 1988.
248. Nonomura A, Ohta G, Hayashi M et al: Immunohistochemical localization of *ras* p21 and carcinoembryonic antigens (CEA) in cholangiocarcinoma, *Liver* 7:142, 1987.
249. Rodenburg CJ, Koelma IA, Nap M et al: Immunohistochemical detection of the *ras* oncogene product p21 in advanced ovarian cancer: lack of correlation with clinical outcome, *Arch Pathol Lab Med* 112:151, 1988.
250. Wick MR: Immunohistologic detection of *ras* oncogene products: specific or spurious? *Arch Pathol Lab Med* 113:13, 1989.
251. Samonitz WS, Paull G, Hamilton SR: Reported binding of monoclonal antibody RAP-5 to formalin-fixed tissue sections is not indicative of *ras* p21 expression, *Hum Pathol* 193:1115, 1988.
252. Funa K, Steinholtz L, Nou E, Bergh J: Increased expression of N-*myc* in human small cell lung cancer biopsies predicts lack of response to chemotherapy and poor prognosis, *Am J Clin Pathol* 88:216, 1987.
253. Carpenter G, Cohen S: Epidermal growth factor, *Annu Rev Biochem* 48:193, 1979.
254. Cohen S: The epidermal growth factor (EGF), *Cancer* 51:1787, 1983.
255. Todaro GJ, Fryling C, De Larco JE: Transforming growth factors produced by certain human tumor cells: polypeptides that interact with epidermal growth factor receptors, *Proc Natl Acad Sci USA* 77:5258, 1980.
256. Massague J: Epidermal growth factor–like transforming growth factor. II. Interaction with epidermal growth factor receptors in human placenta membranes and A431 cells, *J Biol Chem* 258:1614, 1983.
257. Damjanov I, Mildner B, Knowles BB: Immunohistochemical localization of the epidermal growth factor receptor in normal human tissues, *Lab Invest* 55:588, 1986.
258. Sainsbury JRC, Farndon JR, Needham GK et al: Epidermal-growth-factor receptor status as predicator of early recurrence of and death from breast cancer, *Lancet* 1:1398, 1987.
259. Nicholson S, Richard J, Sainsbury C et al: Epidermal growth factor receptor (EGFr); results of a 6 year follow-up study in operable breast cancer with emphasis on the node negative subgroup, *Br J Cancer* 63:146, 1991.
260. Yano H, Shiozaki H, Kobayashi K et al: Immunohistologic detection of the epidermal growth factor receptor in human esophageal squamous cell carcinoma, *Cancer* 67:91, 1991.
261. Kamio T, Shigematsu K, Sou H et al: Immunohistochemical expression of epidermal growth factor receptors in human adrenocortical carcinoma, *Hum Pathol* 21:277, 1990.
262. Neal DE, Marsh C, Bennett MK et al: Epidermal growth factor receptors in human bladder cancer: comparison of invasive and superficial tumours, *Lancet* 1:366, 1985.
263. Duh Q-Y, Gum ET, Gerend PL et al: Epidermal growth factor receptors in normal and neoplastic thyroid tissue, *Surgery* 98:1000, 1985.
264. Kanamori A, Abe Y, Yajima Y et al: Epidermal growth factor receptors in plasma membranes of normal and diseased human thyroid glands, *J Clin Endocrinol Metab* 68:899, 1989.
265. Sugiyama K, Yonemura Y, Miyazaki I: Immunohistochemical study of epidermal growth factor and epidermal growth factor receptor in gastric carcinoma, *Cancer* 63:1557, 1989.
266. Swerdlow SH, Utz GL, Williams ME et al: Bcl-2 protein in centrocytic lymphoma; a paraffin section study, *Leukemia* 7:1456, 1993.
267. Ambinder RF, Griffin CA: Biology of the lymphomas: cytogenetics, molecular biology, and virology, *Curr Opin Oncol* 3:806, 1991.
268. Korsmeyer SJ: Bcl-2: an antidote to programmed cell death, *Cancer Surv* 15:105, 1992.
269. Korsmeyer SJ: Chromosomal translocation in lymphoid malignancies reveal novel proto-oncogenes, *Annu Rev Immunol* 10:785, 1992.
270. Limpens J, de Jong D, van Krieken JH et al: Bcl-2/JH rearrangements in benign lymphoid tissues with follicular hyperplasia, *Oncogene* 6:2271, 1991.
271. Chleq-Deschamps CM, LeBrun DP, Huie P et al: Topographical dissociation of BCL-2 messenger RNA and protein expression in human lymphoid tissues, *Blood* 81:293, 1993.
272. McDonnel T, Deane N, Platt FM et al: bcl-2-immunoglobulin transogenic mice demonstrate extended B cell survival and follicular lymphoproliferation, *Cell* 57:79, 1989.
273. Hockenbery D, Nunex G, Milliman C et al: Bcl-2 is an intermitochondrial membrane protein that blocks programmed cell death, *Nature* 348:334, 1990.
274. Korsmeyer SJ, McDonnell TJ, Nuñez G et al: Bcl-2: B cell life, death and neoplasia, *Curr Top Microbiol Immunol* 166:203, 1990.
275. Pezzella F, Tse AG, Cordell JL et al: Expression of the bcl-2 oncogene protein is not specific for the 14;18 chromosomal translocation, *Am J Pathol* 137:225, 1990.
276. Pezzella F, Jones M, Ralfkiaer E et al: Evaluation of bcl-2 protein expression and 14;18 translocation as prognostic markers in follicular lymphoma, *Br J Cancer* 65:87, 1992.
277. de Jong D, Limpens J, van Krieden J et al: t(14;18) translocation in benign lymphoid tissues with follicular hyperplasia, *Br J Cancer* 65(suppl. 16):S14, 1992.
278. Zutter M, Hockenbery D, Silverman GA et al: Immunolocalization of the Bcl-2 protein within hematopoietic neoplasms, *Blood* 78:1062, 1991.
279. LeBrun DP, Kamel OW, Cleary ML et al: Follicular lymphomas of the gastrointestinal tract: pathologic features in 31 cases and bcl-2 oncogenic protein expression, *Am J Pathol* 140:1327, 1992.
280. Aisenberg AC: Utility of gene rearrangements in lymphoid malignancies, *Annu Rev Med* 44:75, 1993.
281. Doussis IA, Pezella F, Lane DP et al: An immunocytochemical study of p53 and bcl-2 protein expression in Hodgkin's disease, *Am J Clin Pathol* 99:663, 1993.
282. Larsen CJ, Seite P, Hillion J et al: Some recent aspects of the molecular biology of human lymphoma, *Nouv Rev Fr Hematol* 35:37, 1993.
283. Koch K, Tesch H, Eidt S et al: Analysis of c-*myc*, *bcl*-1 and *bcl*-2 translocations in human lymphoma by pulsed-field gel electrophoresis, *Leuk Lymphoma* 7:463, 1992.
284. Ginsberg A, Raffeld M, Cossman J: Mutations of the retinoblastoma gene in human lymphoid neoplasms, *Leuk Lymphoma* 7:359, 1992.
285. Knudson AG Jr: Mutation and cancer: statistical study of retinoblastoma, *Proc Natl Acad Sci USA* 68:820, 1971.
286. Cote RJ, Jhanwar SC, Novick S, Pellicer A: Genetic alterations of the p53 gene are a feature of malignant mesotheliomas, *Cancer Res* 51:5410, 1991.

287. Nowell PC, Croce CM: Chromosomes, genes and cancer, *Am J Pathol* 125:7, 1986.
288. Knudson AG: Hereditary cancer, oncogenes and anti-oncogenes, *Cancer Res* 1437:1443, 1985.
289. Hansen MF, Cavenee WK: Genetics of cancer predisposition, *Cancer Res* 47:5518, 1987.
290. Francke U: A gene for Wilms' tumor? *Nature* 343:692, 1990.
291. Leone A, McBride OW, Weston A et al: Somatic allelic deletion of nm23 in human cancer *Cancer Res* 51:2490, 1991.
292. Farmer G, Bargonetti J, Zhu H et al: Wild-type p53 activates transcription in vitro, *Nature* 358:83, 1992.
293. Oliner JD, Kinzler KW, Meltzer PS et al: Amplification of a gene encoding a p53-associated protein in human sarcomas, *Nature* 358:80, 1992.
294. T'Ang A, Varley JM, Chakraborty S et al: Structural rearrangement of the retinoblastoma gene in human breast carcinoma, *Science* 242:263, 1988.
295. Xu H-J, Hu S-X, Cagle P-T et al: Absence of retinoblastoma protein expression in primary non–small cell lung carcinomas, *Cancer Res* 51:2735, 1991.
296. Bookstein R, Shew J-Y, Chen PL et al: Suppression of tumorigenicity of human prostate carcinoma cells by replacing a mutated RB gene, *Science* 247:712, 1990.
297. Strohmeyer T, Reissmann P, Cordon-Cardo C et al: Correlation between retinoblastoma gene expression and differentiation in human testicular tumors, *Proc Natl Acad Sci USA* 88:6662, 1991.
298. Cheng J, Scully P, Shew JY et al: Homozygous deletion of the retinoblastoma gene in an acute lymphoblastic leukemia (T) cell line, *Blood* 75:730, 1990.
299. Cordon-Cardo C, Wartinger D, Petrylak D et al: Altered expression of the retinoblastoma gene product: prognostic indicator in bladder cancer, *J Natl Cancer Inst* 84:1251, 1992.
300. Logothetis CJ, Xu HJ, Ro JY et al: Altered retinoblastoma protein expression and known prognostic variables in locally advanced bladder cancer, *J Natl Cancer Inst* 84:1256, 1992.
301. Friend SH, Bernards R, Rogelj, D et al: A human DNA segment with properties of the gene that predisposes to retinoblastoma and osteosarcoma, *Nature* 323:643, 1986.
302. Reissmann PT, Simon MA, Lee W-H et al: Studies of the retinoblastoma gene in human sarcomas, *Oncogene* 4:839, 1989.
303. Cance WG, Brennan MF, Dudas ME et al: Altered expression of the retinoblastoma gene product in human sarcomas, *N Engl J Med* 323:1457, 1990.
304. Horowitz JM, Park SH, Bogenmann E et al: Frequent inactivation of the retinoblastoma anti-oncogene is restricted to a subset of human tumor cells, *Proc Natl Acad Sci USA* 87:2775, 1990.
305. Wunder JS, Czitrom AA, Kandel R et al: Analysis of alterations in the retinoblastoma gene and tumor grade in bone and soft-tissue sarcomas, *J Natl Cancer Inst* 83:194, 1991.
306. Anglard P, Tory K, Brauch H et al: Molecular analysis of genetic changes in the origin and development of renal cell carcinoma, *Cancer Res* 51:1071, 1991.
307. Lee EY, To H, Shew JY et al: Inactivation of the retinoblastoma susceptibility gene in human breast cancers, *Science* 241:218, 1988.
308. Drobnjak M, Cote RJ, Saad AD et al: p53 and Rb alterations in primary breast carcinoma: correlation with hormone receptor expression and lymph node metastases, *Int J Oncol* 2:173, 1993.
309. Borg A, Zhang Q-X, Alm P et al: The retinoblastoma gene in breast cancer: allele loss is not correlated with loss of gene protein expression, *Cancer Res* 52:2991, 1992.
310. DeLeo AB, Jay G, Apella E et al: Detection of a transformation-related antigen in chemically induced sarcomas and other transformed cells of the mouse, *Proc Natl Acad* 76:2420, 1979.
311. Finlay CA, Hinds PW, Levine AJ: The p53 proto-oncogene can act as a suppressor of transformation, *Cell* 57:1083, 1989.
312. Reich NC, Oren M, Levine AJ: Two distinct mechanisms regulate the levels of a cellular tumor antigen p53, *Mol Cell Biol* 3:2143, 1983.
313. Nigro JM, Baker SJ, Preisinger AC et al: Mutations in the p53 gene occur in diverse human tumour types, *Nature* 342:705, 1989.
314. Sidransky D, Mikkelsen T, Schwechheimer K et al: Clonal expansion of p53 mutant cells in associated with brain tumor progression. *Nature* 355:846, 1992.
315. Fujimoto K, Yamada Y, Okajima E et al: Frequent association of p53 gene mutation in invasive bladder cancer, *Cancer Res* 52:1393, 1992.
316. Baker SJ, Fearson ER, Nigro JM et al: 17 detections and p53 gene mutations in colorectal carcinomas, *Science* 244:217, 1989.
317. Takahashi T, Nau MM, Chiga I et al: p53: a frequent target for genetic abnormalities in lung cancer, *Science* 246:491, 1989.
318. Iggo R, Gatter K, Bartek J et al: Increased expression of mutant forms of p53 oncogene in primary lung cancer, *Lancet* 335:675, 1990.
319. Bartek J, Iggo R, Gannon J, Lane DP: Genetic and immunochemical analysis of mutant p53 in human breast cancer cell lines, *Oncogene* 5:893, 1990.
320. Kikuchi-Yanoshita R, Konishi M, Ito S et al: Genetic chances of both p53 alleles associated with conversion from colorectal adenoma to early carcinoma in familial adenomatous polyposis and non-familial adenomatous polyposis patients, *Cancer Res* 52:3965, 1992.
321. Esrig D, Spruk CH III, Nichols PW et al: p53 nuclear protein accumulation correlates with mutations in the p53 gene, tumor grade and stage in bladder cancer, *Am J Pathol* 1389, 1993.
322. Davidoff AM, Kerns B-J, Inglehart JD et al: Maintenance of p53 alterations throughout breast cancer progression, *Cancer Res* 51:2605, 1991.
323. Davidoff AM, Humphrey PA, Iglehart JD et al: Genetic basis for p53 overexpression in human breast cancer, *Proc Natl Acad Sci USA* 88:5006, 1991.
324. Ostrowski JL, Sawan L, Wright HC et al: p53 expression in human breast cancer related to survival and prognostic factors: an immunohistochemical study, *J Pathol* 164:75, 1991.
325. Iwaya K, Tsuda H, Hiraide H et al: Nuclear p53 immunoreaction associated with poor prognosis of breast cancer, *Jpn J Cancer Res* 82:835, 1991.
326. Thor AD, Moore DH, Edgerton SM et al: Accumulation of p53 tumor suppressor gene protein: an independent marker of prognosis in breast cancers, *J Natl Cancer Inst* 84:845, 1992.
327. Cattoretti G, Rilke F, Andreola S et al: p53 expression in breast cancer, *Int J Cancer* 57:353, 1988.
328. Cattoretti G, Andreola S, Clemente C et al: Vimentin and p53 expression on epidermal growth factor receptor-positive, oestrogen receptor-negative breast carcinomas, *Br J Cancer* 57:353, 1988.
329. Varley JM, Brammar WJ, Lane DP et al: Loss of chromosome 17p13 sequences and mutation of p53 in human breast carcinomas, *Oncogene* 6:413, 1991.
330. Sarkis AS, Dalbagni G, Cordon-Cardo C et al: Nuclear overexpression of p53 protein in transitional cell bladder carcinoma: a marker for disease progression, *J Natl Cancer Inst* 85:53, 1993.
330a. Esrig D, Elmajian D, Groshen S et al: Accumulation of nuclear p53 and tumor progression in bladder cancer, *N Eng J Med* 331:1259, 1994.
331. Walker RA, Dearing SJ, Lane DP, Varley JM: Expression of p53 protein in infiltrating and in situ breast carcinomas, *J Pathol* 165:203, 1991.
332. Liotta LA, Stetler-Stevenson WG, Steeg PS: Cancer invasion and metastasis: positive and negative regulatory elements, *Cancer Invest* 9:543, 1991.
333. Castronovo V, Colin C, Claysmith AP et al: Immunodetection of the metastasis-associated laminin receptor in human breast cancer cells obtained by fine-needle aspiration biopsy, *Am J Pathol* 137:1373, 1990.
334. D'Errico A, Garbisa S, Liotta LA et al: Augmentation of type IV collagenase, laminin receptor, and Ki67 proliferation antigen associated with human colon, gastric, and breast carcinoma progression, *Mod Pathol* 4:239, 1991.
335. Monteagudo C, Merino MJ, San-Juan J et al: Immunohistochemical distribution of type IV collagenase in normal, benign, and malignant breast tissue, *Am J Pathol* 136:585, 1990.

Immunohistochemical approaches for predicting response to therapy

336. Beatson GT: On the treatment of inoperable cases of carcinoma of the mamma: suggestions for a new method of treatment, with illustrative cases, *Lancet* 2:104; 162, 1896.

337. Huggins C, Hodges CV: Studies on prostatic cancer. I. The effect of castration, of estrogen and of androgen injection on serum phosphatases in metastatic carcinoma of the prostate, *Cancer Res* 293:297, 1941.
338. Jensen EV, Green GL, Closs LE et al: Receptors reconsidered: a 20 year perspective, *Rec Progr Horm Res* 38:1, 1982.
339. Pertschuk LP, Tobin EH, Tanapat P et al: Histochemical analysis of steroid hormone receptors in breast and prostatic carcinoma, *J Histochem Cytochem* 28:799, 1980.
340. Taylor CR, Cooper CL, Kurman RJ et al: Detection of estrogen receptor in breast and endometrial carcinoma by the immunoperoxidase technique, *Cancer* 47:2634, 1981.
341. Greene GL, Nolan C, Engler JP et al: Monoclonal antibodies to human estrogen receptor, *Proc Natl Acad Sci USA* 77:5115, 1980.
342. Press M, Greene GL: Localization of progesterone receptor with monoclonal antibodies in the human progesterone receptor, *Endocrinology* 122:1165, 1988.
343. Press MF, Greene GL: Immunocytochemical localization of estrogen and progesterone receptors. In RA De Lellis, editor; *Advances immunohistochemistry*, New York, 1988, Raven Press.
344. King WJ, Desombre ER, Jensen EV et al: Comparison of immunocytochemical and steroid-binding assays for estrogen receptor in human breast tumors, *Cancer Res* 45:293, 1985.
345. McCarty K Jr, Szabo E, Flowers JL et al: Use of a monoclonal anti–estrogen receptor antibody in the immunohistochemical evaluation of human tumors, *Cancer Res* 46:4244s, 1986.
346. Hanna W, Mobbs BG: Comparative evaluation of ER-ICA and enzyme immunoassay for the quantitation of estrogen receptors in breast cancer, *Am J Clin Pathol* 91:182, 1989.
347. Bevilacqua P, Pea M, Gasparini G: Immunocytochemical detection of progesterone receptor by monoclonal KD-68 antibody in operable breast cancer: correlations with biochemical assay, pathological features and cell proliferative rate, *Eur J Cancer Clin Oncol* 25:1595, 1989.
348. Berger U, Wilson ST, McClelland RA et al: Comparison of an immunocytochemical assay for progesterone receptor with a biochemical method of measurement and immunocytochemical examination of the relationship between progesterone and estrogen receptors, *Cancer Res* 49:5176, 1989.
349. Masood S, Dee S, Goldstein JD: Immunocytochemical analysis of progesterone receptors in breast cancer, *Am J Clin Pathol* 96:59, 1991.
350. Shintaku IP, Said JW: Detection of estrogen receptors with monoclonal antibodies in routinely processed formalin-fixed paraffin sections of breast carcinoma: use of DNase pretreatment to enhance sensitivity of the reaction, *Am J Clin Pathol* 87:161, 1987.
351. Shimada A, Kimura S, Abe K et al: Immunocytochemical staining of estrogen receptor in paraffin sections of human breast cancer by use of monoclonal antibody: comparison with that in frozen sections, *Proc Natl Acad Sci USA* 82:4803, 1985.
352. Hiort O, Kwan PW, DeLellis RA: Immunohistochemistry of estrogen receptor protein in paraffin sections, *Am J Clin Pathol* 90:559, 1988.
353. Paterson, DA, Reid CP, Anderson TJ et al: Assessment of oestrogen receptor content of breast carcinoma by immunohistochemical techniques on fixed and frozen tissue and by biochemical ligand binding assay, *J Clin Pathol* 43:46, 1990.
354. Andersen J, Orntoft TF, Poulsen HS: Immunohistochemical demonstration of estrogen receptors (ER) in formalin-fixed, paraffin-embedded human breast cancer tissue by use of a monoclonal antibody to ER, *J Histochem Cytochem* 36:1553, 1988.
355. Parl FF, Posey Y: Discrepancies of the biochemical and immunohistochemical estrogen receptor assays in breast cancer, *Hum Pathol* 19:960, 1988.
356. Toi M, Nakamura T, Wada T et al: The discrepancy between immunocytochemical and biochemical assay of estrogen receptor in breast cancer patients treated by endocrine therapy, *Jpn J Surg* 19:768, 1989.
357. Desombre ER, Thorpe SM, Rose C et al: Prognostic usefulness of estrogen receptor immunocytochemical assays for human breast cancer, *Cancer Res* 46(suppl):4256s, 1986.
358. Kinsel LB, Szabo E, Greene GL, Konrath JA-L Jr: Immunocytochemical analysis of estrogen receptors as a predictor of prognosis in breast cancer patients: comparison with quantitative biochemical methods, *Cancer* 49:1052, 1989.
359. Reiner A, Neumeister B, Spona J et al: Immunocytochemical localization of estrogen and progesterone receptor and prognosis in human primary breast cancer, *Cancer Res* 50:7057, 1990.
360. Helle M, Helin M, Isola J, Helin H: Immunohistochemical versus biochemical estrogen-receptor and progesterone-receptor analysis: correlation with histological parameters, *J Cancer Res Clin Oncol* 115:361, 1989.
361. Di Stefano D, Minganzzini PL, Schucchi L et al: A comparative study of histopathology, hormone receptors, peanut lectin binding, Ki-67 immunostaining, and nucleolar organizer region–associated proteins in human breast cancer, *Cancer* 67:463, 1991.
362. Helin ML, Helle MJ, Helin HJ, Isola JJ: Proliferative activity and steroid receptors determined by immunohistochemistry in adjacent frozen sections of 102 breast carcinomas, *Arch Pathol Lab Med* 113:854, 1989.
363. Fernandes BJ, Yao XY, Hao Y et al: DNA content and estrogen receptors in primary carcinoma of the breast, *Can J Surg* 34:349, 1991.
364. Coombes RC, Berger U, McCleland RA et al: Prediction of endocrine response in breast cancer by immunocytochemical detection of oestrogen receptor in fine-needle aspirates, *Lancet* 2:701, 1987.
365. Andersen J, Thorpe SM, King WJ et al: The prognostic value of immunohistochemical estrogen receptor analysis in paraffin-embedded and frozen sections versus that of steroid binding assays, *Eur J Cancer* 26:442, 1990.
366. McClelland RA, Berger LS, Powles TJ et al: Immunocytochemical assay for estrogen receptor: relationship to outcome of therapy in patients with advanced breast cancer, *Cancer Res* 46(suppl):4241s, 1986.
367. Pertschuk LP, Eisenberg KB, Carter AC, Feldman JG: Immunohistologic localization of estrogen receptors in breast cancer with monoclonal antibodies, *Cancer* 55:1513, 1985.
368. McCarty KS Jr, Miller LS, Cox EB et al: Estrogen receptor analyses, *Arch Pathol Lab Med* 109:716, 1985.
369. Allred DC, Bustamante MA, Daniel CO et al: Immunocytochemical analysis of estrogen receptors in human breast carcinomas: evaluation of 130 cases and review of the literature regarding concordance with biochemical assay and clinical relevance, *Arch Surg* 125:107, 1990.
370. Pertschuk LP, Feldman JG, Eisenberg KB et al: Immunocytochemical detection of progesterone receptor in breast cancer with monoclonal antibody: relation to biochemical assay, disease-free survival, and clinical endocrine response, *Cancer* 62:342, 1988.
371. Pertschuk LP, Kim DS, Nayer K et al: Immunocytochemical estrogen and progestin receptor assays in breast cancer with monoclonal antibodies: histopathologic, demographic, and biochemical correlations and relationship of endocrine response and survival, *Cancer* 66:1663, 1990.
372. Trachtenberg J, Walsh PC: Correlation of prostatic nuclear androgen receptor content with duration of response and survival following hormonal therapy in advanced prostatic cancer, *J Urol* 127:466, 1982.
373. Ghanadian R, Auf G, Williams G et al: Predicting the response of prostatic carcinoma to endocrine therapy, *Lancet* 2:1418, 1981.
374. Benson RC, Gorman PA, O'Brien PC et al: Relationship between androgen receptor binding activity in human prostate cancer and clinical response to endocrine therapy, *Cancer* 59:1599, 1987.
375. Gonor SE, Lakey WH, McBlain WA: Relationship between concentrations of extractable and matrix-bound nuclear androgen receptor and clinical response to endocrine therapy for prostatic adenocarcinoma, *J Urol* 131:1196, 1984.
376. Fentie DD, Lakey WH, McBlain W: Applicability of nuclear androgen receptor quantification to human prostatic adenocarcinoma, *J Urol* 135:167, 1986.
377. Demura T, Kuzumaki N, Oda A et al: Establishment and characterization of monoclonal antibody against androgen receptor, *J Steroid Biochem* 33:845, 1989.
378. Chang C, Whelani CT, Popovich TC, Kokontis J: Fusion proteins containing androgen receptor sequences and their use in the production of poly- and monoclonal anti-androgen receptors antibodies, *Endocrinology* 123:1097, 1989.
379. Takeda H, Chodak G, Mutchnik S et al: Immunohistochemical localization of androgen receptors with mono- and polyclonal antibodies to androgen receptor, *J Endocrinol* 126:17, 1990.

380. Ruizeveld de Winger JA, Trapman J, Vermey M et al: Androgen receptor expression in human tissues: an immunohistochemical study, *J Histochem Cytochem* 39:927, 1991.
381. Masai M, Sumiya H, Akimoto S et al: Immunohistochemical study of androgen receptor in benign hyperplastic and cancerous human prostates, *The Prostate* 17:293, 1990.
382. Ruizeveld de Winter JA, Trapman J, Brinkmann AO et al: Androgen receptor heterogeneity in human prostatic carcinomas visualized by immunohistochemistry, *J Pathol* 161:329, 1990.
383. Sadi MV, Barrack ER: Determination of growth fraction in advanced prostate cancer by Ki-67 immunostaining and its relationship to the time to tumor progression after hormonal therapy, *Cancer* 67:3065, 1991.
384. Kartner N, Ling V: Multidrug resistance in cancer, *Sci Am* 260:44, 1989.
385. Dalton WS, Grogan TM: Does p-glycoprotein predict response to chemotherapy, and if so, is there a reliable way to detect it? *J Natl Cancer Inst* 83:80, 1991.
386. Cordon-Cardo C, O'Brien JP, Boccia J et al: Expression of the multidrug resistance gene product (p-glycoprotein) in human normal and tumor tissues, *J Histochem Cytochem* 38:1277, 1990.
387. Cordon-Cardo C, O'Brien JP, Casals D et al: Multidrug-resistance gene (p-glycoprotein) is expressed by endothelial cells at blood-brain barrier sites, *Proc Natl Acad Sci USA* 86:695, 1989.
388. Schneider J, Bak M, Efferth T et al: P-glycoprotein expression in treated and untreated human breast cancer, *Br J Cancer* 60:815, 1989.
389. Ro J, Sahin A et al: Immunohistochemical analysis of p-glycoprotein expression correlated with chemotherapy resistance in locally advanced breast cancer, *Hum Pathol* 21:787, 1990.
390. Verrelle P, Meissonnier F, Fonck Y et al: Clinical relevance of immunohistochemical detection of multidrug resistance p-glycoprotein in breast carcinoma, *J Natl Cancer Inst* 83:111, 1991.
391. Weinstein RS, Jakate SM, Dominguez JM et al: Relationship of the expression of the multidrug resistance gene product (p-glycoprotein) in human colon carcinoma to local tumor aggressiveness and lymph node metastasis, *Cancer Res* 51:2720, 1991.
392. Hamburger AW, Salmon SE: Primary bioassay of human tumor stem cells, *Science* 197:461, 1977.
393. Weisenthal LM, Marsden JA, Dill PL, Maculuso CK: A novel dye exclusion method for testing in vitro chemosensitivity of human tumors, *Cancer Res* 43:749, 1983.

Infections

394. Cartun RW, Pedersen CA, Cole SR et al: Identification of CMV in formalin-fixed, paraffin-embedded tissues: comparison of immunocytochemistry and in situ DNA hybridization, *Mod Pathol* 2:15A, 1989.
395. Jiwa M, Steenbergen RDM, Zwaan FE et al: Three sensitive methods for the detection of cytomegalovirus in lung tissue of patients with interstitial pneumonitis, *Am J Clin Pathol* 93:491, 1990.
396. Engstrand L, Pahlson C, Gustavsson S, Schwan A: Monoclonal antibodies for rapid identification of *Campylobacter* pyloritis, *Lancet* 2:1402, 1986.
397. Cartun RW, Kryzmowski GA, Pedersen CA et al: Immunocytochemical identification of *Helicobacter pylori* in formalin-fixed gastric biopsies, *Mod Pathol* 4:498, 1991.
398. Klatt EC, Cosgrove M, Meyer PR: Rapid diagnosis of disseminated histoplasmosis in tissues, *Arch Pathol Lab Med* 110:1173, 1986.
399. Mshana RN, Humber DP, Harboe M et al: Demonstration of mycobacterial antigens in nerve biopsies from leprosy patients using peroxidase-antiperoxidase immunoenzyme technique, *Clin Immunol Immunopathol* 29:359, 1983.
400. Barbolini G, Bisetti A, Colizzi V et al: Immunohistologic analysis of mycobacterial antigens by monoclonal antibodies in tuberculosis and mycobacteriosis, *Hum Pathol* 20:1078, 1989.
401. Cote RJ, Rosenblum M, Telzak EE et al: Disseminated *Pneumocystis carinii* infection causing extrapulmonary organ failure: clinical, pathologic and immunohistochemical analysis, *Mod Pathol* 3:25, 1990.
402. Kovacs JA, Gill V, Swan JC et al: Prospective evaluation of a monoclonal antibody in diagnosis of *Pneumocystis carinii*, *Lancet* 2:1, 1986.
403. Kovacs JA, Halpern JL, Lundgren B et al: Monoclonal antibodies to *Pneumocystis carinii*: identification of specific antigens and characterization of specific antigens and characterization of antigenic differences between rat and human isolates, *J Infect Dis* 159:60, 1989.
404. Kovacs JA, Ng VL, Masur H et al: Diagnosis of *Pneumocystis carinii* pneumonia: improved detection in sputum with use of monoclonal antibodies, *N Engl J Med* 318:589, 1988.
405. Lorincz AT, Temple GF, Kurman RJ et al: Oncogenic association of specific human papillomavirus types with cervical neoplasia, *J Natl Cancer Inst* 79:671, 1987.
406. Burmer GC, Parker JD, Bates J et al: Comparative analysis of human papillomavirus detection by polymerase chain reaction and Virapap/Viratype kits, *Am J Clin Pathol* 94:554, 1990.
407. Tase T, Okagi T, Clarke BA et al: Human papillomavirus DNA in adenocarcinoma in situ, microinvasive adenocarcinoma of the uterine cervix, and coexisting cervical squamous intraepithelial neoplasia, *Int J Gynecol Pathol* 8:8, 1989.
408. Felix JC, Wright TC: Analysis of lower genital tract and lesions suspicious for condyloma by in situ hybridization and consensus sequence PCR for the detection of HPV, *Arch Pathol Lab Med* 118:39, 1994.

9 Histochemistry

Jay H. Beckstead

Histochemistry has been defined by Pearse as "the identification, localization and quantification, in cells and tissues and by chemical or physical tests, of specific substances, reactive groups, and enzyme-catalyzed substances."[1] Thus, any chemical procedure that localizes a substance within cells or tissues for subsequent microscopy is a histochemical technique. In this broad sense histochemistry encompasses immunologic and molecular biologic techniques when they are combined with histology.

The origins of histochemistry can be traced back directly to the French botanist François-Vincent Raspail, who according to Pearse[1] in 1825 was the first to fully appreciate the power of combining a chemical reaction with the microscopic observation of tissues and cells. Despite this auspicious beginning in 1825, progress was slow and soon became even slower as aniline dyes came into use in histology (1862-1929). These dyes revolutionized histology but were used largely without any effort to understand the chemistry involved. There was a resurgence of interest in the 1930s because of the publication of Lison's *Histochimie Animale*. Interest remained high from the 1940s through the 1970s, but more recently classical histochemistry has been overshadowed by the development of immunohistochemical procedures, in situ hybridization, and molecular biologic techniques.

Most pathologic diagnoses are made on histologic tissue sections stained with hematoxylin and eosin. Supplementation with a variety of special histochemical stains is often required. The past 20 years have witnessed an explosion of new techniques, immunohistochemistry first and foremost, that have somewhat overshadowed traditional approaches to tumor diagnosis. This naturally raises the question of what histochemical techniques remain useful. An associated question is, Are there new nonimmunologic, non–nucleic acid based procedures that have value today? The answer to both questions is yes. Many histochemical procedures remain useful and new techniques with diagnostic utility have been developed.

PRINCIPLES OF HISTOCHEMISTRY

Histochemical procedures are based on the simple premise that tissues or cells, when placed in a solution (or series of solutions) chemically react with the solution to produce a colored insoluble end product. The amount and location of the end product can then be evaluated in the context of the cell or tissue.

Classical histochemical reactions are generally based on one of four principles: (1) simple ionic interactions, (2) reactions of aldehydes with Schiff's reagent or silver compounds, (3) coupling of aromatic diazonium salts with aromatic residues on proteins or hormones, and (4) conversion of the primary reaction product of an enzyme acting on a substrate to form a colored precipitate. Some substances cannot be identified directly by these reactions. Often, one can localize them indirectly by changing them chemically (as by oxidation). Specificity of histochemical reactions can be partially controlled by modifying the reaction conditions (such as changing pH by using highly specific substrates or inhibitors).

Ideally, the following conditions should be met to ensure accurate assessment of a histochemical reaction: (1) Tissue preparation should not influence the location or preservation of the component tested; (2) all the reagents should penetrate into the cells or tissues at the same rate; (3) the reaction should be relatively specific; (4) the final colored reaction product should be precipitated immediately and be stable.

A variety of biochemical substances are present in any cell, but some specialized cells may contain relatively unique substances or unusual amounts of a particular substance. These generally fall into five groups: (1) nucleic acids, (2) proteins and peptides (enzymes, hormones), (3) mucosubstances, (4) lipids, and (5) inorganic salts. Many of these substances can be relatively localized using traditional histochemical procedures. Immunologic reactions or in situ hybridization can be utilized to specifically identify specific protein or nucleic acid sequences. Another technique that can be exploited is the selective binding of lectins to various carbohydrate groups.

APPLICATIONS IN SPECIFIC ORGANS

Nervous system

Histochemistry plays an important role in the evaluation of disorders of the nervous system, both peripheral and central.

This is particularly true in some demyelinating, degenerative or storage disorders.

In *demyelinating diseases* there is a degenerative process that may be secondary to axonal damage (Wallerian) or primary as the result of a variety of demyelinating diseases where the myelin sheath is selectively injured. Representative demyelinating diseases that deserve to be studied by histochemistry are listed in Table 9-1 but are also discussed in Chapters 77 and 78.

Although the etiology and pathogenesis are highly varied, the effects on myelin are similar and may be demonstrated by a variety of techniques. Normal myelin is hydrophilic, but injury converts the polar phospholipid into hydrophobic lipid droplets (cholesterol esters). This conversion requires the activity of phagocytic cells and is thus delayed approximately 10 days after the injury. The changes are readily demonstrable in frozen sections by using enzyme histochemical reactions for lysosomal enzymes and neutral lipid stains. These reactions can be performed in combination, e.g., β-galactosidase–oil red O.[2]

In fixed tissues, staining for myelin with Luxol fast blue is the most generally useful procedure.[3] The dye binds strongly to normal myelin, which contrasts with the unstained areas of demyelination (Fig. 9-1). This technique is, however, not as successful at localizing actively demyelinating sites.

Histochemical reactions are moderately useful in the diagnosis of diseases of *neuronal degeneration*. Chromatolysis, the characteristic feature of neuronal degeneration, is identifiable in routine sections. In selected instances histochemical reactions can add diagnostic information. In Parkinson's disease the "Lewy bodies" can be identified with the NaOH–dichromate acid–hematin reaction.[4] The plaques of Alzheimer's disease stain with Congo red and the neurons in Pick's presenile dementia contain a ganglioside that reacts with a modified periodic acid–Schiff (PAS) procedure.[5]

Metabolic disorders of the nervous system encompasses a variety of hereditary diseases caused by deficiencies in enzymes involving lipid or mucopolysaccharide metabolism. Although histochemical methods cannot precisely identify the storage products involved, the combination of clinical history, histologic changes, and histochemical reactions usually is sufficient for diagnostic purposes. More precise definition requires biochemical assay procedures that are available in specialized laboratories. An overview of important metabolic disorders involving the nervous system is given below and detailed in Ch. 14.

The *gangliosidoses* (Tay-Sachs and others) have similar histochemical changes even though a variety of different enzyme defects are involved. The neurons of both the central and the peripheral nervous system become ballooned by the presence of excess gangliosides. The material is frequently extracted during tissue processing, but staining of frozen tissue sections reveals a strong diastase-resistant PAS reaction. A metachromatic reaction can be demonstrated with Feyrter's thionin method. In G_{MI}-gangliosidosis a pronounced reduction in β-galactosidase can be demonstrated histochemically.

Batten's disease (ceroid lipofuscinosis) is a group of disorders with neuronal deposits of lipofuscin-like substances. The neurons containing these materials stain strongly with PAS and Sudan black (Fig. 9-2). They can be differentiated from the gangliosidoses by the resistance of the material to extrac-

Table 9-1 Demyelinating diseases

Central nervous system
Multiple sclerosis
Subacute sclerosing panencephalitis
Postvaccinial encephalomyelitis
Progressive multifocal leukoencephalopathy
Creutzfeldt-Jakob disease
Subacute combined degeneration
Marchiafava-Bignami disease
Grinker's myelopathy
Peripheral nervous system
Diabetic neuropathy
Diphtheritic neuropathy
Guillain-Barré syndrome
Wallerian degeneration (secondary)
Dejerine-Sottas disease

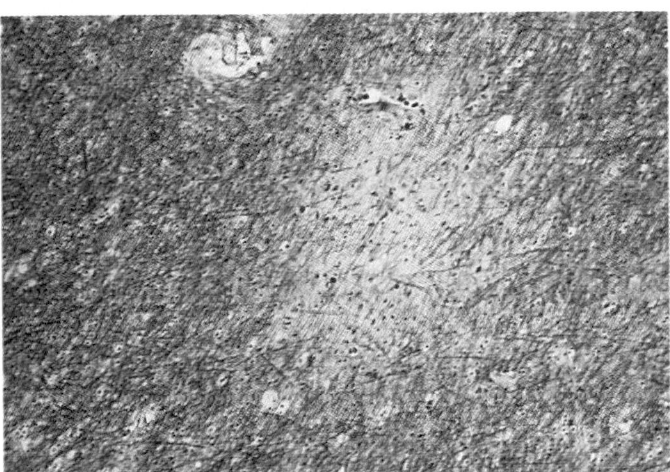

Fig. 9-1 Luxol fast blue strongly stains the normal myelin within the white matter of the CNS. The unstained plaque of demyelination in this case of progressive multifocal leukoencephalopathy contrasts sharply against this background.

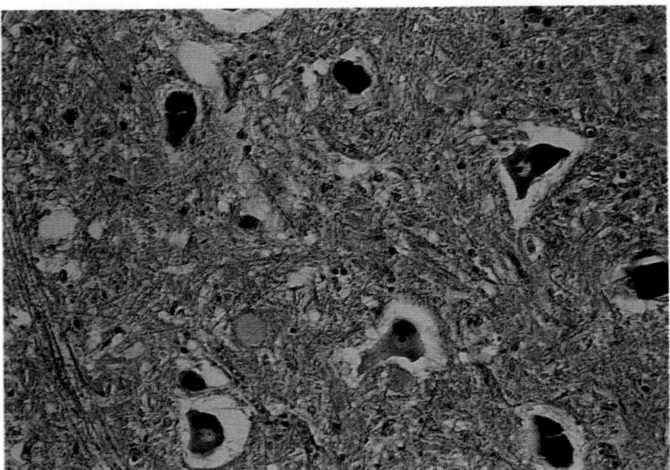

Fig. 9-2 The neurons in this case of Batten's disease are strongly labeled with Sudan black because of their content of abnormal lipofuscin-like substances.

tion by a chloroform/methanol solution.[6] These disorders can be diagnosed most conveniently by histochemical examination of ganglion cells in a rectal biopsy.

In *Krabbe's leukodystrophy* (galactocerebrosidase deficiency) perivascular collections of globoid cells are seen in the white matter in association with demyelination. These cells are strongly PAS positive, are weakly positive with Sudan black, and show a strong acid phosphatase reaction. The globoid cells are not seen in the peripheral nervous system, but strong staining of Schwann cells with acid phosphatase in association with demyelination is highly supportive of this diagnosis.

A defect in aryl sulfatase A results in the accumulation of galactocerebroside sulfate in macrophages and other cells in a variety of tissues. These substances are metachromatic with a variety of dyes (acid cresyl violet, toluidine blue) in frozen sections, resulting in the name "metachromatic leukodystrophy." Deposits can be demonstrated in Schwann cells of peripheral nerves (by skin biopsy) and kidney tubules more conveniently than in the central nervous system (Fig. 9-3).

The group of diseases shows neuronal ballooning only in types A and C. The sphingomyelin, cholesterol, ganglioside mixture stored in type A are metachromatic with Feyrter's thionin, are positive with PAS, stain blue with ferric hematoxylin, and are strongly PAS positive. The same reactions are present in macrophages, which can be more conveniently observed in bone marrow or other sites. The unrelated type C disorder shows variable neuronal storage of a water-soluble oligosaccharide. The material is strongly positive with PAS in celloidin-protected frozen sections. The cells are also strongly positive with acid phosphatase and metachromatic with Feyrter's thionin. Sudan black staining gives negative results. The neurons of the gastrointestinal tract show the same changes and since they are more accessible they are more easily evaluated histochemically.

Pompe's disease (acid α-glucosidase deficiency) results in the accumulation of glycogen in many different cell types, including some neurons and astrocytes. Affected neurons are accessible by biopsy in the gastrointestinal tract. The nervous system is generally not affected in the adult form of the disease.

In some types of *mucopolysaccharidosis* the neurons show ballooning changes, but the storage material appears to be a mixture of gangliosides and not a mucopolysaccharide. Neurons in frozen sections are positive with PAS, Sudan black, and Luxol fast blue. Mucopolysaccharides can be demonstrated in perivascular regions by toluidine blue in frozen sections.

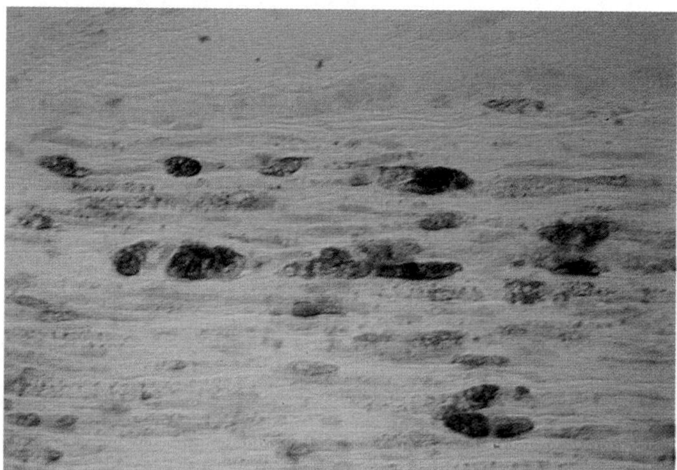

Fig. 9-3 In this nerve from a patient with metachromatic leukodystrophy, the Schwann cells stain brownish black (that is, metachromatically) with the dye acid cresyl violet.

Skeletal muscle

Histochemical techniques remain absolutely essential for the diagnostic evaluation of muscle biopsy specimens. Despite the apparent morphologic similarity between various muscle fibers, they are remarkably heterogeneous. These differences are readily demonstrable using histochemical techniques and can be used to investigate muscle disorders.[7] Almost all the currently utilized procedures are carried out on cryostat sections of fresh frozen tissue. Muscle biopsy specimens must be carefully oriented to obtain cross sections of the fibers, and they should be trimmed to assure rapid and complete freezing. Freezing is generally optimal using isopentane cooled to −150° C in liquid nitrogen to prevent ice-crystal formation, which disrupts muscle fibers and causes artifacts. Ten-micrometer sections cut at approximately −20° C are considered ideal.

Basic muscle fiber typing is the first goal of the evaluation, and myofibrillar ATPase with acidic and basic preincubations is the most useful technique for this purpose. Muscle fibers are generally divided into groups based on their contractile properties, slow-twitch (type 1) and fast-twitch (type 2). Type 1 fibers have low levels of ATPase and high levels of mitochondrial oxidative enzymes. These features make them more fatigue resistant. Type 2 fibers have low levels of mitochondria oxidative enzymes and high myophosphorylase activity so that they can utilize anaerobic glycolysis. Using these enzymes, we can divide histochemically stained fibers into two basic types and three subtypes (Table 9-2). The proportions of fiber types vary from muscle to muscle, but they are randomly distributed within a single muscle (Fig. 9-4).

A secondary aim of muscle histochemical procedures is to monitor the health of the fibers by examining marker enzymes. For the examination of mitochondria, succinate dehydrogenase (SDH) is the most suitable enzyme, but NADH dehydrogenase can also be utilized. Myofibrillar ATPase serves as a marker for abnormalities of the myofibrils. Acid phosphatase or α-naphthyl acetate esterase can be useful stains to enumerate phagocytic cells in inflamed muscle.

The more common metabolic disorders can be screened using the PAS reaction or Sudan black for glycogen or lipids respectively. A variety of specific enzyme defects can be investigated by demonstration of the catalytic activity of the

Table 9-2 Muscle fiber typing discovered at autopsy

	Type of muscle fibers			
	Type I	Type 2A	Type 2B	Type 2C
ATPase				
pH 10.2 preincubation	−	++	+++	+
pH 4-3 preincubation	+++	−	−	+
Succinate dehydrogenase	+++	++	+	++
Myophosphorylase	+	++	+++	+

enzyme, such as myophosphorylase, phosphofructokinase, cytochrome oxidase and myoadenylate deaminase.

Serial sections of muscle biopsy specimens allow accurate comparisons and should include, as a minimum, treatment with ATPase with acidic and basic preincubations, SDH, and myophosphorylase.[7] In addition, sections stained with hematoxylin and eosin and Masson's trichrome should be examined to correlate histochemical and histologic features.

For a more detailed discussion of muscle pathology, consult Chapter 76.

The muscle biopsy examination can provide diagnostic information about a variety of *denervating disorders*. In normal muscle, fiber types are randomly arranged. If relatively few motor nerves are affected, the atrophic fibers will be scattered, but as more units become affected groups of atrophic fibers are found. If these become reinnervated by branches of a single nerve, a group of uniform fiber type results; this is a valuable diagnostic feature in biopsy specimens where reinnervation masks the atrophy morphologically[8] (Fig. 9-5). Reinnervation may also result in an increase in type 2C fibers and a change in the mitochondrial enzyme activity to produce "target" fibers.[9]

The *muscular dystrophies* are also evaluated by histochemical techniques. In Duchenne muscular dystrophy there is an increase in the proportion of type 1 fibers, loss of the clear separation of type 1 and 2 fibers in ATPase preparations, and a decrease in type 2B fibers. The early manifestations of disease are myocyte necrosis, which is well demonstrated by lysosomal enzyme techniques. Becker's muscular dystrophy is characterized by a predominance of similar type 1 fibers but lacks the 2B deficit and the blurring of distinctions between type 1 and type 2 fibers. Additional common features are the presence of "moth-eaten fibers" in mitochondrial enzyme preparations, which are caused by irregularities in the distribution of mitochondria,[8] and "ring fibers," seen in ATPase and PAS preparations, which are caused by the displacement of peripheral myofibrils. These changes may also be seen in other chronic dystrophies.

Myotonic dystrophy causes atrophy of type 1 fibers and hypertrophy of type 2A and 2B fibers, numerous "ring fibers," and sarcoplasmic masses outside the rings. Fiber typing in myotonia congenita reveals a great decrease in type 2B fibers. Muscle histochemistry is also diagnostically critical in several congenital myopathies, including central core disease where NADH dehydrogenase preparations reveal the characteristic absence of central staining.[10] In the centronuclear myopathies, the abnormal type 1 fibers are well demonstrated by enzyme histochemistry.

The work-up of metabolic myopathies requires special histochemical techniques. In the glycogenoses, muscle fibers, show vacuolization caused by glycogen accumulation, which can be demonstrated with the PAS reaction. These changes are particularly prominent in glycogenosis type 2 and type 3. In type 5 glycogenosis (McArdle's disease), the absence of myophosphorylase is readily demonstrated histochemically[11] (Fig. 9-6). In lipid storage disorders, intracellular deposition of lipid in skeletal muscle is a common but relatively nonspecific feature. Enzyme defects in the respiratory chain underlie a variety of disorders commonly grouped as mitochondrial myopathies. A morphologic hallmark, the "ragged red fiber" (Fig. 9-7) seen on the Gomori trichrome stain, is caused by the peripheral clustering of mitochondria.[12] These changes can be more specifically demonstrated with SDH or NADH dehydrogenase reactions. Although many of the specific underlying enzyme defects in these disorders are difficult to demonstrate histochemically, cytochrome oxidase deficiencies can be reliably detected using the technique of Seligman.[13]

Enzyme histochemical techniques may occasionally be useful in the evaluation of *endocrine myopathies*. In Cushing's syndrome and exogenous glucocorticoid excess, selective type 2 atrophy is usually demonstrable. These same fibers are also deficient in myophosphorylase. Similar changes may also be seen in diabetes. Thyroid abnormalities can change the proportions of type 1 and 2 fibers through an effect on ATPase.

Histochemical techniques in lysosomal enzyme are useful for the work-up of biopsy specimens from inflammatory myopathies. In juvenile dermatomyositis, the damage is perifascicular but may be difficult to recognize in the absence of active inflammation. The damage to the muscle fibers is reflected in a central loss of ATPase and mitochondrial enzyme activity. Later in the disease, regeneration may obscure diagnostic features, but the distribution of regenerating fibers can

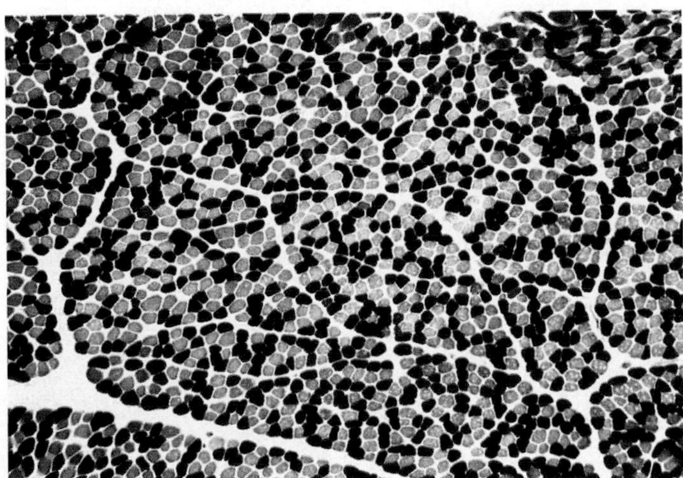

Fig. 9-4 Normal skeletal muscle stained with ATPase with a preincubation at pH 9.4. The random distribution of the light type I fibers and dark type 2 fibers is easily seen in this frozen section.

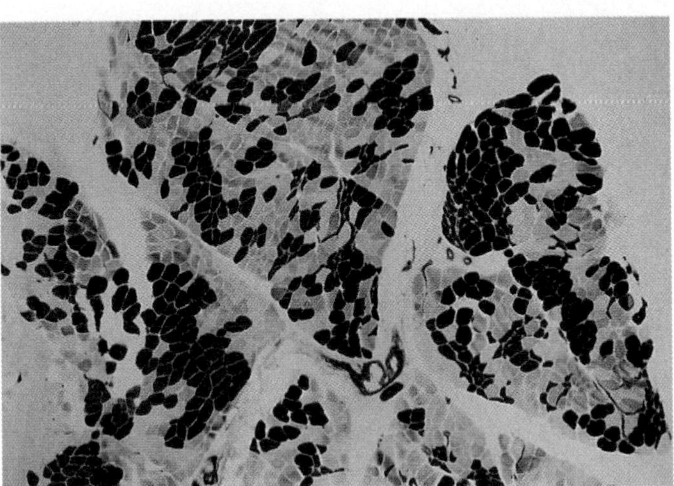

Fig. 9-5 Denervation and reinnervation may mask muscle atrophy morphologically, but the distinct grouping of dark fibers and light fibers in this ATPase preparation contrasts strongly with the normal distribution (Fig. 9-4).

be highlighted by use of methyl green–pyronin staining. These same features may also be seen in adult dermatomyositis. The demonstration of muscle fiber damage may also be important in separating these disorders from polymyopathies where inflammation is not associated with muscle damage. In the relatively recently described entity inclusion body myositis, the characteristic inclusions are highlighted by a modified trichrome stain on frozen sections.[14]

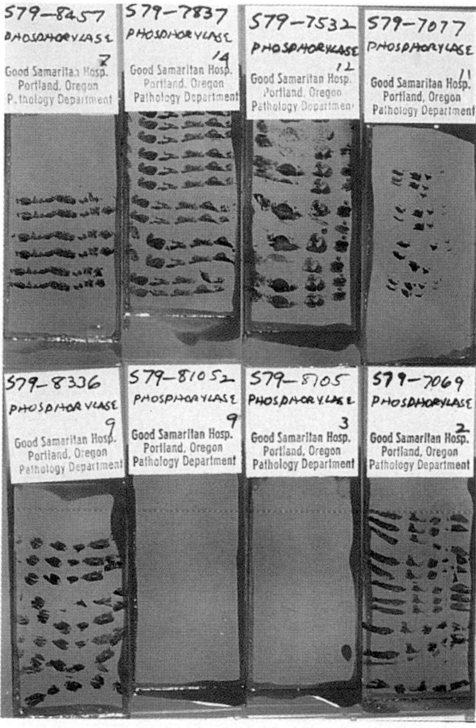

Fig. 9-6 A myophosphorylase reaction on frozen sections of skeletal muscle shows strong dark staining in the sections of normal muscle, whereas the two slides from a patient with McArdle's disease show no staining.

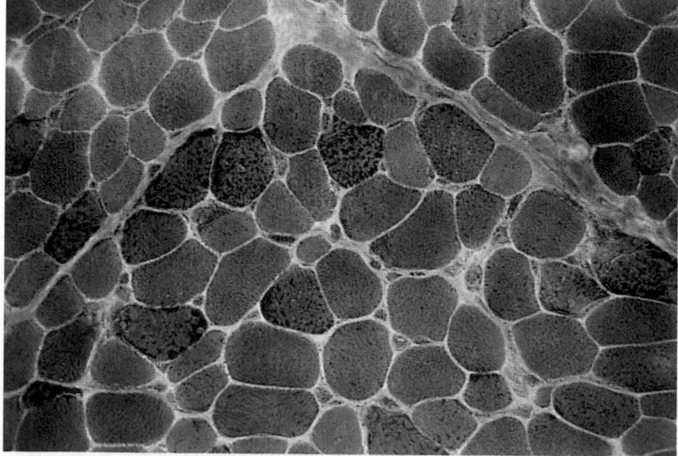

Fig. 9-7 A ragged red fiber seen in a Gomori trichrome stain. The peripheral clustering of mitochondria results in the ragged red staining on the periphery of the muscle fiber in the mitochondrial myopathies.

Hematopoietic system

The use of histochemical techniques in the evaluation of hematopoietic disorders has decreased with the advent of immunohistochemistry. However, histochemistry remains critically important in the diagnosis of leukemia and can be useful in other disorders as well. Histochemical techniques can provide an alternative to and can be used in combination with immunohistochemical procedures in studies of hematopoietic tissues. This often provides better definition of normal architecture and pathologic processes. Enzyme histochemistry can be readily applied to frozen sections and even fixed, embedded sections in paraffin or plastic if the tissues are properly processed.[15-18]

The human bone marrow is a loose mixture of hematopoietic precursors and fat cells. The subtle organization of bone marrow can be clarified with histochemical techniques.[17] Under normal conditions, the marrow contains relatively few reticulin fibers. The marrow is not structureless, however. Staining for alkaline phosphatase reveals a population of slender branched stromal cells whose processes form a framework for the marrow (Fig. 9-8). The normal population of macrophages, including those that form the erythroid islands, is readily revealed by a variety of lysosomal enzyme reactions, such as acid phosphatase and α-naphthyl-butyrate esterase. Myeloid cells are easily stained with chloracetate esterase even in routine paraffin sections, providing an excellent method for identifying the distribution of these cells and to reveal disturbances in this distribution (Fig. 9-9).

Like the marrow, lymph nodes have an unobtrusive structural framework that can be revealed by histochemical techniques.[17] Reticulin fibers are somewhat more prominent in the lymph node than in the bone marrow. A reticulin stain can be used to demonstrate the delicate framework of the lymph node. Alterations in the architecture of the node may be important diagnostic clues. Enzyme histochemistry can provide a more precise look at the supporting cells. Alkaline phosphatase-positive branched reticular cells, similar to those in the marrow, are present in the paracortex. The follicular stromal cell (dendritic reticulum cell) stains strongly with 5′-nucleotidase, and the macrophages in both compartments and the sinuses are identifiable with lysosomal

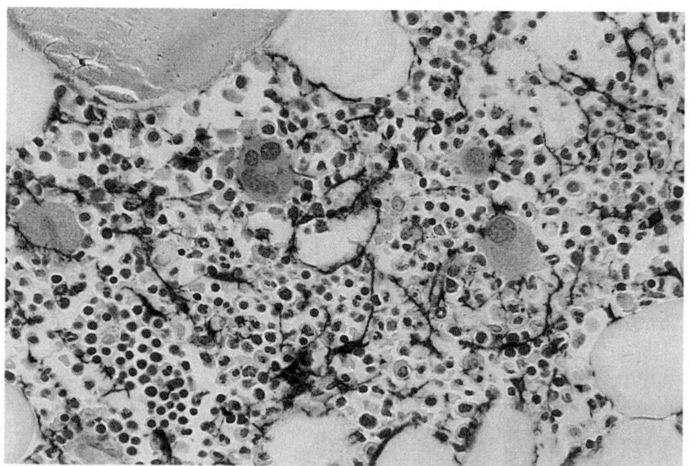

Fig. 9-8 A normal bone marrow reacted for alkaline phosphatase reveals a branching network of stromal cells stained blue.

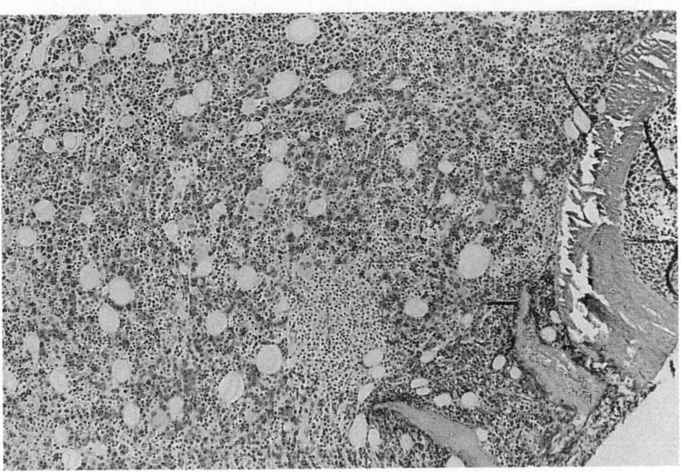

Fig. 9-9 A bone marrow after reaction for chloroacetate esterase demonstrates strong red reaction product in the cytoplasm of neutrophils and their precursors. A small focus of metastatic lymphoma contrasts sharply with this background because of the absence of staining.

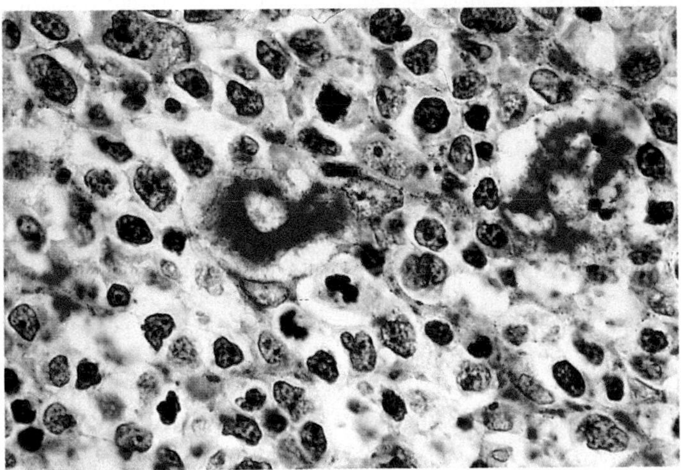

Fig. 9-10 Acid phosphatase reaction in the paracortex of a reactive lymph node. The red reaction product strongly labels the macrophages.

enzymes (Fig. 9-10). Vascular structures also show relatively specific enzyme profiles.[19]

In *metabolic disorders,* abnormal storage of cell products often occurs in macrophages within the spleen, lymph nodes, bone marrow, or liver. Lymphoid cells and granulocytes may also be affected by metabolic disorders. Histochemical evaluation of these tissues, including peripheral blood, may be useful in the diagnosis and evaluation of these disorders.[20] A classic example is *Gaucher's disease.* The abnormal glucocerebroside in macrophages results in modest PAS positivity, a weak reaction with Sudan black, and strong reactivity with acid phosphatase. They are most easily accessible in the bone marrow but may be massively present in the spleen and lymph nodes as well.

The morphology of macrophages in *Niemann-Pick* disease is relatively characteristic. These cells contain large amounts of sphingomyelin, cholesterol, and ganglioside, causing them to stain pale blue with Sudan black and exhibit red birefringence in polarized light. The cells stain dark blue with the ferric hematoxylin method. The PAS reaction is quite variable, but acid phosphatase reactions dramatically accentuate the foamy nature of the cells in the bone marrow, spleen and lymph nodes. In the adult form of the disease, the sea-blue histiocyte seen in routine Romanovsky-stained preparations of air-dried material may be much more numerous. These cells stain dark gray with Sudan black and are acid phosphatase positive.

In *G_{M1}-gangliosidosis type 1,* numerous large foamy storage cells are present in hematopoietic tissues and lymphocytes with cytoplasmic vacuoles occur in peripheral blood. Specific storage material is not demonstrable, but the cells can be accentuated with acid phosphatase. Storage cells are much less frequent in type 2 and the vacuolated lymphocytes are not seen. The storage cells are like those in Gaucher's disease in appearance with similar histochemistry. In both disorders, however, histochemical deficiency of β-galactosidase can be demonstrated.[21]

Wolman's disease (cholesteryl ester storage disease) is characterized by a deficiency of acid esterase. In this disorder, foamy macrophages in the bone marrow contain abundant neutral fat that imparts strong staining with oil red O or Sudan black. Small fatty vacuoles with similar staining properties can be demonstrated in peripheral blood lymphocytes. The enzyme defect can be demonstrated histochemically in tissue sections if nonspecific esterases are inhibited.[22]

Cystine crystals can be demonstrated in the macrophages of patients with *cystinosis* in alcohol-fixed smears stained in alcoholic basic fuchsin. Polarization shows characteristic rectangular birefringent crystals.

Mucopolysaccharidoses are not readily identifiable in tissues or blood, though vacuolated lymphocytes with metachromatic staining reactions are seen in most forms. In type 7, however, the specific β-glucuronidase deficit can be identified histochemically in both lymphocytes and neutrophils from the peripheral blood.[23]

Storage cells may be seen in a variety of other uncommon disorders. More importantly, it should be remembered that foamy macrophages can also be seen in many acquired conditions, including hyperlipidemias, hematologic disorders, and some infectious diseases and as a result of drug treatment.

Gastrointestinal tract

Histochemical procedures play a relatively limited role in the evaluation of inflammatory disorders in the gastrointestinal tract, except for bacteriologic and parasitologic stains for the demonstrations of pathogens.

Mucins in the gastrointestinal tract are either neutral or acidic (sialomucins or sulfomucins). PAS–Alcian blue stain neutral mucins magenta and acid mucins blue or purplish blue.[24] In the stomach, the mucins are almost exclusively neutral with only trace amounts of acid mucins. The small intestine contains predominantly acidic sialomucins, whereas the large intestine shows sulfomucins in the lower two thirds of the crypts and sialomucins in the upper third and on the surface.

The sialomucins stain purplish blue because they react with both the PAS and Alcian blue, whereas the sulfomucins stain predominantly blue because the PAS reaction is quite weak. If necessary, sialomucins may be further separated from the sul-

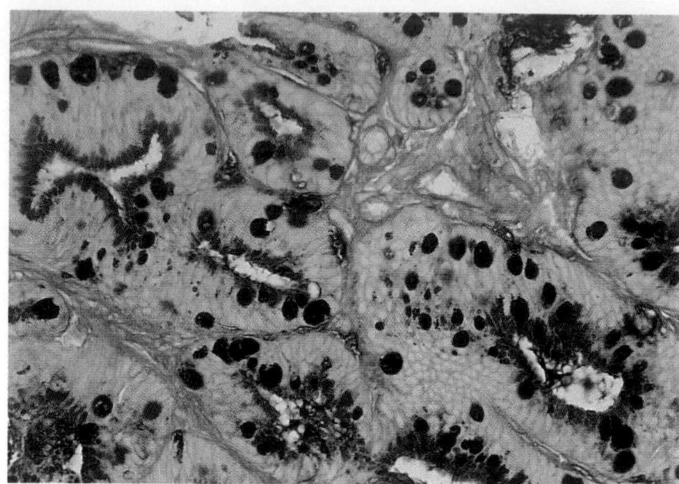

Fig. 9-11 The metaplastic epithelium in a patient with Barrett's esophagus shows mixture of neutral mucins (magenta) and acid mucins (blue) with the PAS-Alcian blue stain.

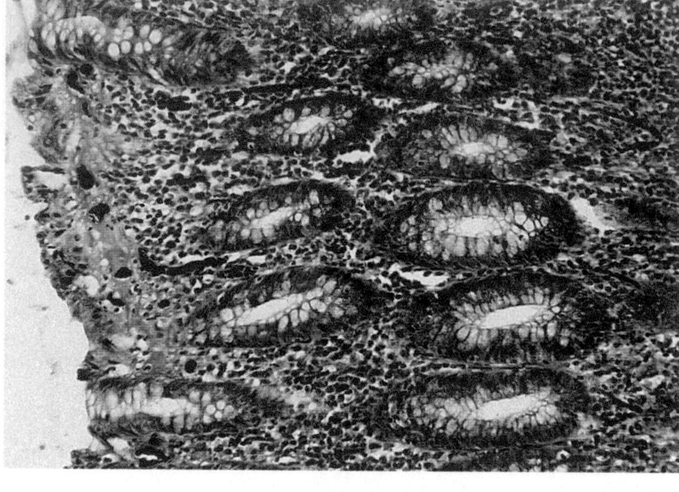

Fig. 9-12 The subepithelial collagen layer is emphasized by the trichrome stain in this case of collagenous colitis.

fomucins by use of the Alcian blue stain at pH 0.5 or the high iron diamine stain.[25] Both reactions stain sulfomucins but are negative in sialomucins.

The mucin staining pattern may assist the differential diagnosis of inflammatory bowel disease.[26] In Crohn's disease, mucin secretion with a normal staining pattern is usually seen even in the presence of pronounced chronic inflammation. In ulcerative colitis, mucin secretion is frequently absent, though it may be present in the resolving stage. In the solitary rectal ulcer syndrome, mucins are altered and sialomucins predominate.[27] Although several of studies have shown some association of altered mucin patterns with dysplasia in the intestine,[28] the clinical value remains unproved.

Metaplastic and reactive changes may also be accentuated by histochemical techniques. In the esophagus, reflux is usually accompanied by basal zone hyperplasia.[29] The PAS reaction can improve evaluation by staining the glycogen in the mature squamous cells while leaving the basal zone unstained. Glandular epithelium of *Barrett's esophagus* is a form of incomplete intestinal metaplasia which is best demonstrated with PAS–Alcian blue (pH 2.5) staining. With this approach, one can show a mixture of neutral mucins (PAS positive) and acid mucins (Alcian blue positive)[30] (Fig. 9-11). Accurate identification of Barrett's esophagus type of mucosa is important because of the increased incidence of adenocarcinoma associated with this change. Intestinal metaplasia of small bowel, or large bowel, or mixed type may be seen in the stomach with atrophic gastritis and gastric atrophy. The mucin staining pattern corresponds to the morphologic pattern and may be useful in confirming the histologic diagnosis.[31] Gastrin cell hyperplasias (primary or secondary) can be identified by an argyrophilic/argentaffin (e.g., Grimelius) stain when specific immunologic stains are not available.

Recognition of collagenous colitis is facilitated by the use of the trichrome stain for collagen. This stain improves the definition of the thickened subepithelial collagen layer characteristic of this disorder[32] (Fig. 9-12).

The diagnosis of *Hirschsprung's disease* requires the documented absence of ganglion cells in the distal portions of the colon. Many pathologists approach this diagnosis by using 50 serial hematoxylin and eosin–stained sections, a labor-intensive method. However, it is well established[33] that enzyme histochemical techniques for acetylcholinesterase in frozen sections can definitively establish the diagnosis with a single tissue section. Staining with this enzyme clearly demonstrates an increase in acetylcholinesterase-positive nerve fibers in the muscularis mucosa and submucosa. In normal biopsy specimens, ganglion cells, including "immature" ganglion cells, are strongly stained and easily identified. These changes are present regardless of the patient's age, though they become more prominent with time.

Pseudo-obstructions are uncommon motility disorders caused by diseases affecting either nerves or smooth muscle. Neural abnormalities most commonly can be grouped as hyperganglionosis or hypoganglionosis. The increase and decrease, respectively, of nerve fibers and ganglion cells is best demonstrated with the acetylcholinesterase stain. Abnormalities may also be identified by silver stains on en face sections (Smith technique).[34] Changes in the smooth muscle are usually accompanied by an increase in connective tissue, which can be demonstrated with any of the common connective tissue stains.

Histochemistry is an alternative to the traditional morphologic approach[35] to the diagnosis of intestinal malabsorption.[36,37] Cryostat sections of small bowel mucosa distal to the duodenum are the best materials for diagnosis. PAS stains can be used to identify Whipple's disease and to delineate the increase in goblet cells associated with celiac disease, protein intolerance, and cystic fibrosis. The most important part of the evaluation is the examination of brush-border enzymes. A semiquantitative evaluation using histochemical techniques for disaccharidase (lactase, sucrose and trehalase) is usually sufficient for clinical purposes. These techniques can be utilized to identify disaccharidase deficiencies and to follow the response of patients with celiac disease to treatment.

Liver

Histochemical stains are standard in the histologic examination of the liver biopsy. Reticulin preparations and collagen stains more accurately demonstrate the liver's structural framework and fibrotic reactions to pathologic processes. The PAS stain,

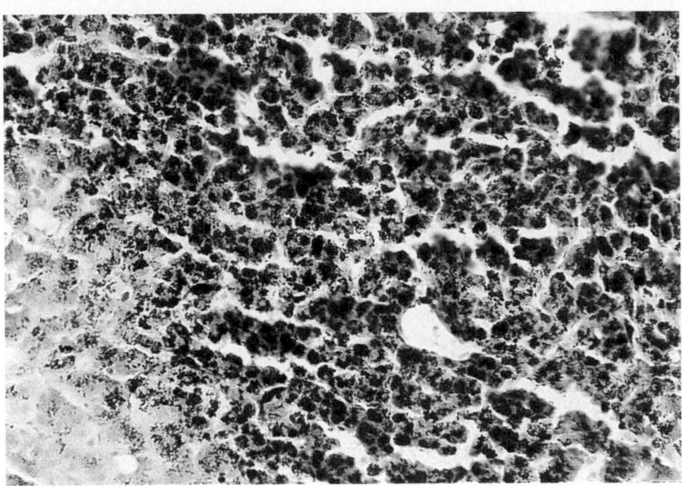

Fig. 9-13 The blue Perls reaction nearly obscures the parenchyma of the liver in this case of hemochromatosis.

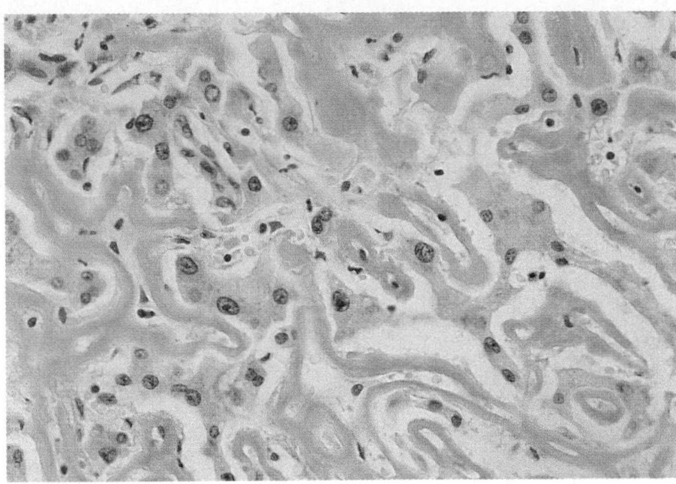

Fig. 9-14 The pink amyloid sinusoidal deposit in this Congo red stain after pretreatment with potassium permanganate strongly indicates that this is primary (AL type).

with and without prior diastase digestion allows assessment of glycogen stores and may highlight cytoplasmic inclusions and ceroid pigment within hepatocytes. The Perls reaction for iron serves as an inexpensive practical tool for evaluating the extent and distribution of iron stores in the liver[38] (Fig. 9-13).

The presence of *copper*, stained directly by *p*-dimethylaminobenzylidine rhodamine,[39] or copper-associated proteins, stained according to the orcein method,[40] may be useful in the diagnosis of adults with biliary disorders. Copper is excreted in bile and it will accumulate in the liver in biliary obstruction. Both copper-associated protein and copper should normally be absent from the adult liver, but deposits are commonly seen in the periportal region in patients with primary biliary cirrhosis or primary sclerosing cholangitis.[41] The density of the deposits increases with the stage of the disease. Most other disorders that may lead to cirrhosis show little or no deposition before the onset of cirrhosis, and when cirrhosis develops, the deposits are smaller and show a patchy distribution. The rare disorder Indian childhood cirrhosis shows striking, diffuse copper deposition.[42] Patchy deposits are observed in the cirrhotic stage of Wilson's disease but are typically absent in the earlier stages.[43]

In *α-l-antitrypsin deficiency*, the abnormal protein cannot be exported from the hepatocytes. In routine paraffin sections, eosinophilic globules of various sizes that are strongly PAS positive after diastase digestion are observed. This can then be confirmed immunohistochemically with antibodies to α-l-antitrypsin.

Amyloid deposits in the liver are best demonstrated by Congo red or crystal violet stains. Primary (AL type) amyloidosis is resistant to pretreatment with potassium permanganate and generally shows a sinusoidal distribution (Fig. 9-14), whereas with secondary amyloidosis (AA type), pretreatment abolishes the congo red reaction and the distribution is usually vascular.[44]

The diagnosis of *Reye's syndrome* can be confirmed histochemically. The liver shows a panlobular microvesicular fatty infiltration, which can be demonstrated with oil red O staining, and a severe depletion of glycogen, confirmed with the PAS reaction. More specifically, there is an almost complete loss of succinate dehydrogenase activity in frozen sections of the liver[45] as a result of the accompanying damage to the mitochondria. This combination of changes may also be seen in Jamaican vomiting sickness and valproic acid toxicity. Microvesicular fatty change may also be seen in acute fatty liver of pregnancy, alcoholic foamy degeneration, and lipid storage disorders but without the loss of succinated dehydrogenase activity. Succinate dehydrogenase activity may be lost also in toxic conditions (such as mushroom poisoning) because of mitochondria damaged.

Victoria blue B and similar stains[40] for hepatitis B surface antigen (HB_sAg) have largely been replaced by immunohistochemical methods.

The liver is a mirror of several metabolic diseases,[46] either because hepatocytes contain an abnormal storage product or because macrophages lining hepatic sinusoids contain storage products. Histochemical techniques can often provide a presumptive diagnosis, though biochemical assay is frequently required for a definitive diagnosis.

In the *glycogen storage diseases*, the liver usually shows changes in the distribution and type of glycogen. Routine histologic processing will extract variable amounts of glycogen; thus it is not suited as the primary procedure in suspected glycogen storage disorders. Frozen sections protected with a coat of celloidin before PAS staining allow accurate estimation of the glycogen stores present. In type 0 (glycogen synthetase deficiency) and type I (glucose-6-phosphatase deficiency), the liver is enlarged and fatty, but type 0 shows a severe reduction or absence of glycogen and type I shows an increased amount of normal glycogen. The infantile form of type II (Pompe's disease) shows an excess of monoparticulate (more soluble) glycogen in the hepatocytes and Kupffer cells. Type III (amylo-1,6-glucosidase deficiency) has an excessive amount of a highly soluble form of glycogen stored in the hepatocytes. A highly insoluble form of glycogen (amylopectin) is stored in the hepatocyte with type IV (branching enzyme deficiency) resulting in a pale cytoplasmic inclusion body that stains with PAS, Lugol's iodine or colloidal iron stains. Type VI (liver phosphorylase kinase deficiency) characteristically shows a pronounced excess of normal glycogen in hepatocytes. Types V and VII show no abnormalities in the liver.

Glucose-6-phosphatase (glycogen storage disease type I) can be histochemically demonstrated to be absent in type IA[47] but not in types IB and IC. Lysosomal acid phosphatase activity demonstrated histochemically is normal or only slightly decreased in the glycogen storage disorders, except in type II where it is greatly and characteristically increased in both the hepatocytes and the Kupffer cells.

Lipid storage disorders can also involve the liver. Gaucher's disease results in enlarged Gaucher-like changes in the Kupffer cells and Gaucher cells in the portal areas (Fig. 9-15). The staining reactions are the same as in other sites (see above). The hepatocytes are not affected. In *Niemann-Pick disease,* the hepatocytes, as well as the Kupffer cells, are large and foamy. Stains for fat, cholesterol, and sphingomyelin are positive, whereas the acid phosphatase reaction dramatizes the foamy character of the cells. In the cholesteryl ester storage diseases, the liver is enlarged and distinctly orange, and the hepatocytes are filled with lipid. The cells are positive with stains for lipids and cholesterol and in frozen sections the absence of acid esterase can be demonstrated.[48]

In *G_{M1}-gangliosidosis,* the absence of the β-galactosidase enzyme can be readily demonstrated with the indoxyl method in frozen sections.[49] Changes in the liver are generally not obvious in the juvenile form of the disease despite the absence of the enzyme. The infantile form, however, shows pronounced vacuolation of the hepatocytes and Kupffer cells, but fat cannot be demonstrated.

Acid mucopolysaccharides are present in the hepatocytes and Kupffer cells of patients with all types of mucopolysaccharidosis. These substances are extremely water soluble but may be demonstrated with the method of Haust and Landing[50] in frozen sections. In fucosidosis a variety of saccharide-containing substances are found in hepatocytes, Kupffer cells, and bile duct epithelium. These are very soluble and difficult to demonstrate histochemically. Mannosidosis shows a similar distribution of soluble foamy material in lesser amounts. Acid phosphatase reaction accentuates the deposits.

Skin

Histochemical procedures are routinely used in dermatopathology. The PAS reaction has multiple applications including the detection of fungal elements, demonstration of basement membrane thickening in lupus erythematosus, identification of deposits in porphyria and diabetes, and diagnosis of some cutaneous neoplasms (granular cell tumor, Paget's disease). A variety of conditions (follicular mucinosis, myxedema) result in mucin accumulation within the skin; these are usually glycosaminoglycans, well demonstrated by the Alcian blue reaction. Amyloid stains and reactions for pigments and minerals (see above) may also be useful. The demonstration of mast cells in urticaria pigmentosa is best shown by the chloracetate esterase method, though toluidine blue and Alcian blue (pH 1.0) can also be used.

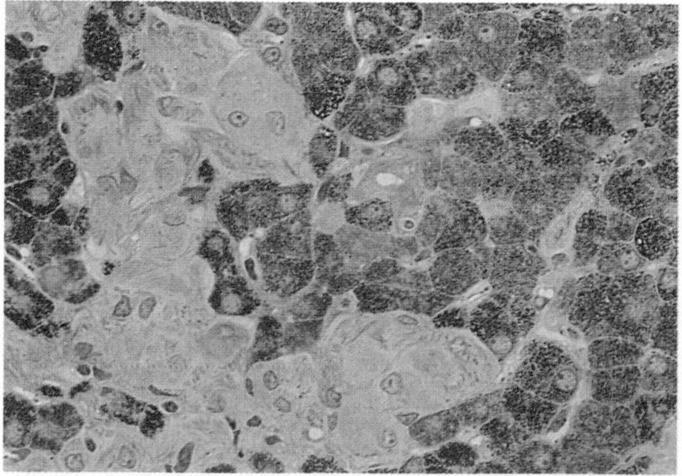

Fig. 9-15 The pale, weakly PAS-positive Gaucher cells contrast well with the hepatocytes.

Cardiovascular system

Histochemical methods for fat and enzymes have historically contributed to our understanding of atherosclerosis, but are rarely utilized today for diagnostic purposes. Some histochemical techniques can be useful at the gross level in autopsy pathology. The oil red O reaction can be performed on washed arteries to demonstrate the extent of early atheromatous changes. This may be particularly useful in young patients and to demonstrate the effects of pulmonary hypertension. The nitro blue tetrazolium (NBT) reaction is a reliable, easily performed method for the gross identification of early myocardial infarction. The endogenous dehydrogenase of the myocardium rapidly reduce the substrate and produce dark blue staining of the myocardium. Areas of ischemia fail to stain, making the area of infarction easily visible. The reaction appears as early as 1 hour after occlusion and remains demonstrable for as long as 3 days after death. Amyloid deposits within the heart may be demonstrated by the Congo red reaction or other amyloid stains. PAS stains can be used to demonstrate the myocardial deposits of glycogen seen in some glycogen storage diseases (types II, III, IV). Some metabolic cardiomyopathies (drug and alcohol) result in the accumulation of triglycerides in the myocardium which can be demonstrated by oil red O or the Sudan black B reaction.

Genitourinary system

Histochemical techniques are routinely used for the evaluation of glomerular diseases. Most renal pathologists require the examination of silver (Jones), PAS, and Masson's trichrome stains in addition to the standard hematoxylin and eosin, on all renal biopsy specimens. The silver stain reliably labels the basement membrane, which facilitates its examination. Many glomerular deposits stain with the PAS reaction, whereas the trichrome identifies areas of fibrosis. Amyloid is best demonstrated with Congo red stain.

In addition to its utility in tumor diagnosis (see p. 185), histochemical procedures can aid in the diagnosis of malakoplakia anywhere in the urinary tract. The characteristic Michaelis-Gutmann bodies are PAS positive and Alcian blue positive and may contain stainable iron.

Respiratory system

Histochemical techniques are often used in the differential diagnosis of pulmonary neoplasms and infections (see p. 185), but there are other, less common specific applications. Histochemical methods can be useful in the diagnosis of some pneumoconioses. These include the naphthochrome B method for beryllium, the Perls and alizarin reactions that stain iron and calcium respectively, which are deposited on asbestos fibers, the Morin method for zirconium, chromoxane pure black B for aluminum, dimethylglycoxine method for nickel, Perl's reaction for iron, and the alizarin method for calcium. The rare disorder pulmonary alveolar proteinosis is characterized by a homogeneous PAS-positive protein within the alveolar spaces.

TUMOR DIAGNOSIS

Histochemical techniques are still used in the diagnosis of tumors (Table 9-3), though immunohistochemical procedures have become more popular.

The use of a basement membrane/collagen stain to emphasize the basic architecture of a tissue or a neoplasm is a time-honored approach that remains of value.[51] Such stains may serve as a useful first approximation before one embarks on a large immunohistochemical work-up. Several choices of stains, including PAS, silver (reticulin) stains, van Gieson's, or even trichrome, can be used. Epithelial tumors contain little or no basement membrane material, but reticulin stains frequently emphasize the groups of cells so often seen in epithelial tumors. Hematopoietic tumors generally contain little reticulin but may infiltrate as individual cells through preexisting structures. Many mesenchymal tissues, including Schwann cells, muscle cells, fat cells, and blood vessels, show basement membranes surrounding individual cells. The same appearance is frequent in the tumors derived from these cells, though malignant cells may lose the ability to produce these materials.

In some tissues, focal loss of basement membrane may help confirm stromal invasion; for example, tubular carcinoma of the breast lacks basement membranes, but radial scars and sclerosing adenosis (which may be confused with tubular carcinoma) have well-defined basement membranes. Unfortunately, staining of these structures may not be completely reliable, and such uncertainty decreases its diagnostic utility. Identification of vascular invasion can also be aided by stains, like the elastic van Gieson, that emphasize vascular structures.

The identification of cellular differentiation by histochemistry remains useful but less specific than immunohistochemical procedures. Procedures to demonstrate mucins and glycogen are the most commonly used reactions. The PAS reaction stains glycogen, neutral mucins and the carbohydrate portions of glycoproteins and glycolipids. The PAS stain may be performed with or without prior digestion of the tissue by diastase (salivary α-amylase). Glycogen is digested by diastase, which causes a loss of PAS staining. Glycoproteins, glycolipids, and glycomucins, however, retain PAS reactivity even after diastase treatment. Diastase pretreatment is essential to confirm that PAS-positive material in a cell is not glycogen.

Alcian blue (pH 2.5) is the best stain for the acid mucins that are produced by mesenchymal cells. These stains can assist differential diagnosis (Tables 9-3 and 9-4). Mucicarmine is a commonly used but relatively insensitive stain for epithelial mucin. The combined Alcian blue–PAS is the best general mucin stain. Highly sulfated mucins, positive with high iron diamine, are present in adenocarcinoma of the prostate, but not in benign epithelium. The PAS reaction also stains the secretory granules of acinic cell carcinoma of the salivary glands.

Staining for bile (van Gieson's) can be helpful in confirming a hepatocellular carcinoma.

Neuroendocrine tumors (such as pheochromocytoma, paraganglioma, Merkel cell tumor, medullary thyroid carcinoma, carcinoids, and small cell carcinomas) have dense core granules, which are *argyrophilic* and usually can be stained indirectly by silver stains (Grimelius). Carcinoids of midgut origin and melanocytic tumors are *argentaffin* and can reduce silver salts directly (Masson-Fontana). These cells can also be identified by diazonium salt procedures. Melanin can be differentiated by its response to bleaching. Tumors of the adrenal medulla (pheochromocytoma) typically change color with chromate-containing fixatives and green cytoplasmic granules are seen with a Giemsa stain.

Traditional stains are of limited value in the identification of mesenchymal tumors. Collagen and fat can be demonstrated, but this is usually not diagnostically important. Large amounts of glycogen are typical of Ewing's sarcoma but is not diagnostic. Cross-striations can be satisfactorily demonstrated using a PTAH stain in muscle tumors, but only a minority show sufficient differentiation.

Table 9-3 Histochemical differential diagnosis

	PAS with diastase	Alcian blue pH 2.5	Alcian blue pH 2.5 with hyaluronidase
Adenocarcinoma	+	–/+	–/+
Mesothelioma	–	+	–
Myxoid mesenchymal tumors without cartilagenous differentiation	–	+	–
Myxoid mesenchymal tumor with cartilagenous differentiation	–	+	+/–

Table 9-4 Mucins and glycogen in tumors

	Neutral mucins	Acid mucins	Glycogen
Prostate carcinoma	–	–	–
Small cell carcinoma	–	–	–
Transitional cell carcinoma	–	–	+/–
Melanoma	–	–	+/–
Squamous carcinoma	–	–	+/–
Breast carcinoma	–	–	+/–
Hepatocellular carcinoma	–	–	+
Embryonal carcinoma	–	–	+
Seminoma	–	–	++
Osteogenic sarcoma	–	+	–
Rhabdomyosarcoma	–	+	+
Liposarcoma	–	+	–
Neurogenic tumors	–	+	–
Smooth muscle tumors	–	+	–/+
Renal carcinoma	–/+	–	–
Ovarian carcinoma	+/–	+/–	+/–
Endometrial carcinoma	+	+	–/+
Mucoepidermoid carcinoma	+	+	–
Colloid carcinoma	+	+	–
GI tract carcinoma	+	+	–

Enzyme histochemical procedures are used most extensively in diagnostic *hematopathology.* The FAB classification of acute leukemias[52] relies extensively on well-performed enzyme cytochemical reactions for classification. The presence or absence of myeloperoxidase may be the single most important ancillary test in the diagnosis of acute leukemias (Fig 9-16). Other enzymes useful in the subclassification of acute leukemia include naphthol AS-D chloracetate esterase (CAE) as a marker of neutrophilic differentiation. The presence of tartrate-resistant acid phosphatase (TRAP) in hairy cell leukemia (Fig. 9-17) and not in most proliferations likely to be confused with it is another enzyme histochemical procedure that is widely utilized.[53] Chloracetate esterase is also a useful marker in the identification of mast cell proliferations. Alkaline phosphatase staining on mantle-cell lymphomas[54] led in part to their recognition as distinct entities, though utilization diagnostically is infrequent. Enzyme stains can also provide some differential diagnostic aid in histiocytic disorders and Hodgkin's disease.[55-57] Many of these procedures have not been widely applied clinically because of the difficulties in obtaining reliable enzyme histochemical reactions in fixed paraffin-embedded tissues (except for CAE). Although it has been demonstrated that these enzymes can be well preserved in fixed plastic-embedded tissues,[17] these techniques have not become widely adopted either.

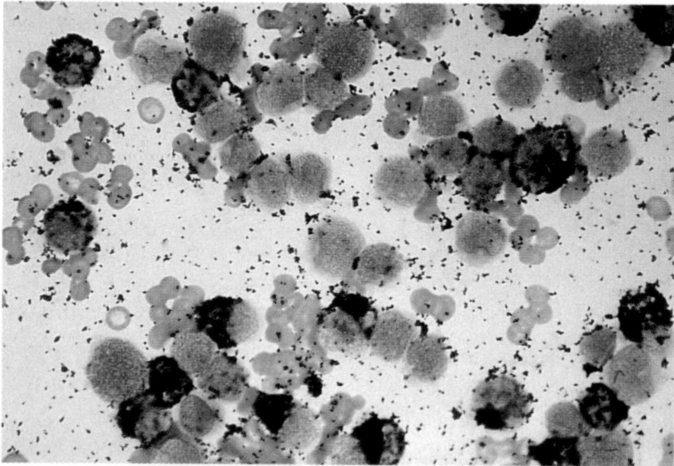

Fig. 9-16 This acute myelogenous leukemia shows a strong black reaction with the diaminobenzidine procedure, which demonstrates myeloperoxidase.

Although there was considerable interest in the use of enzyme histochemistry in the diagnosis of solid tumors in the 1950s and 1960s,[58] these techniques are rarely utilized because of the problems cited above and specificity of the enzymes. Alkaline phosphatase can be quite useful in confirming the diagnosis of a germ cell malignancy (and can even be useful in the recognition of in situ lesions)[59] (Fig. 9-18). Alkaline phosphatase is also present in almost all osteogenic sarcomas and may serve as a useful adjunct in diagnosis. Enzyme histochemistry has diagnostic utility in chordomas,[60] thyroid neoplasms,[61] and hepatic tumors[62] as well.

Lectin procedures

Carbohydrate moieties form important and frequently unique portions of many proteins. Many of these carbohydrates can be specifically and readily identified by their ability to bind to lectins. Lectins are carbohydrate binding proteins of nonimmune origin; although widespread in nature most of those used in pathology are of plant origin. By labeling the lectins with an enzyme or biotin, they can be used as probes for the localization of a specific carbohydrate group. Because carbohydrates are quite resistant to fixation, interest in exploiting them as tools in biology has been high.[63]

Their use in diagnostic pathology has not become widespread, though some useful applications are well recognized. The lectin *Ulex europaeus* (UEA I) is an extremely useful marker of endothelial cells (Fig. 9-19) and tumors derived from them.[64] Its use in determining vascular invasion has also been reported.[65] Peanut agglutinin (PNA) has been shown to be a useful marker in Langerhans cell granulomatosis[66,67] and Hodgkin's disease.[68-70] More recently, another lectin, *Bauhinia purpurea,* has also been shown to have utility in the diagnosis of Hodgkin's disease.[71] A variety of reports have suggested some value prognostically or diagnostically in carcinomas,[72-76] germ cell tumors,[77,78] sarcomas,[79-81] melanomas,[82] and tumors of childhood.[83-85]

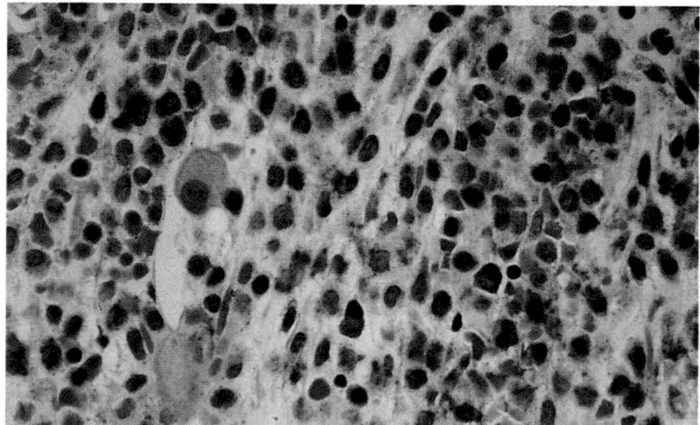

Figure 9-17 A bone marrow biopsy specimen reacted for tartrate resistant acid phosphatase. The red reaction product (tartrate-resistant acid phosphatase, TRAP) demonstrates presence of hairy cell leukemia.

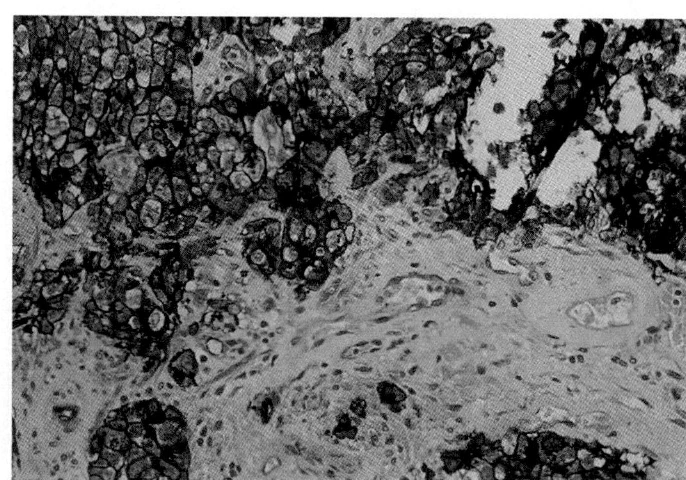

Fig. 9-18 Strong blue reaction product labels the membranes of this seminoma when tested for alkaline phosphatase.

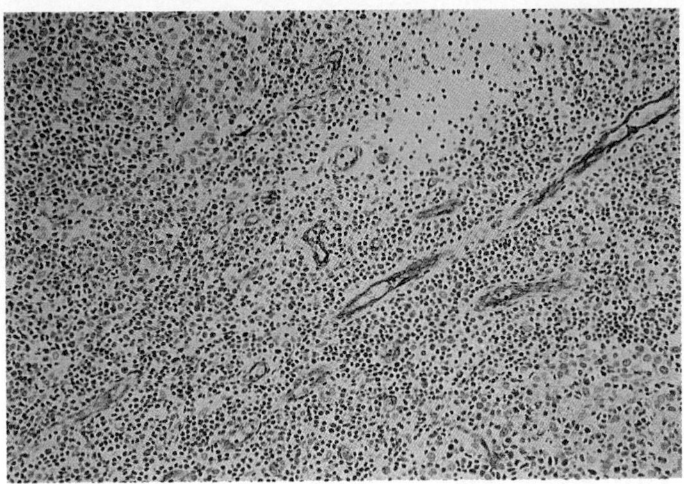

Fig. 9-19 The lectin *Ulex europaeus* (UEA I) labels the endothelial cells of this lymph node when the peroxidase tag is developed by the diaminobenzidine reaction.

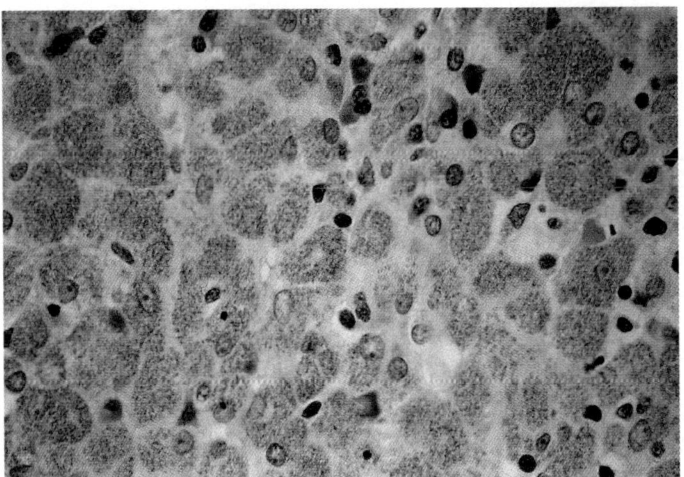

Fig. 9-20 A lymph node from a patient with the acquired immunodeficiency syndrome shows a massive number of acid-fast bacilli.

Nucleolar organizer

There has been considerable recent interest in the diagnostic and prognostic utility of stains for the chromosomal regions associated with ribosomal RNA genes. These have become known as "nucleolar organizer regions" (NORs). The proteins associated with these regions stain with colloidal silver procedure in routine paraffin sections and become readily visible.[86] Differences in the size and number of these stained NORs have been investigated in a wide variety of neoplasms.[87-90] The number of NORS correlates with the S-phase proliferation fraction in many neoplasms. They appear to have some value in separating hyperplastic and dysplastic lesions from malignancies and high-grade from low-grade tumors, but additional work is necessary to confirm these interesting observations.[91]

Table 9-5 Organisms and histochemical methods

Organism	Recommended methods
Bacteria	Tissue Gram stain
Mycobacterium tuberculosis and nontuberculosis mycobacteria	Fite stain
Legionella species	Dieterle's
Fungi	PAS, digested Silver methenamine
Spirochetes and *Rochalimaea* species	Warthin-Starry Dieterle's Steiner and Steiner
Protozoons	May-Grunwald-Giemsa
Pneumocystis carinii	Silver methenamine

OTHER APPLICATIONS

Infectious disease

Histochemical techniques remain the most commonly utilized method of identifying organisms in tissue sections. Although precise identification of organisms is rarely possible with these methods, their diagnostic utility is unquestionable. A presumptive diagnosis of bacterial, fungal, or parasitic infection can be made quickly and treatment instituted pending more precise microbiologic methods (Fig. 9-20). Most pathology laboratories maintain a standard repertoire of stains. The precise staining methods are summarized in several texts.[92,93] Table 9-5 lists general groups of organisms and appropriate histochemical methods. Stains for viral inclusions, though historically useful, have been largely replaced by more specific immunohistochemical techniques.

For most organisms a variety of staining methods is appropriate. Laboratories would do best to concentrate on doing a few stains well rather than developing multiple techniques. The most important element in these stains is good control tissues containing adequate numbers of organisms. Also, the identification of organisms in tissue usually requires the study of multiple sections at high magnification.

Minerals and pigments

Although not commonly required in diagnostic practice, the identification of pigments and minerals may occasionally be important. A variety of histochemical methods that can aid in the identification of these materials in tissue sections are available.[92-94] Methods commonly utilized are listed in Table 9-6.

Table 9-6 Methods for minerals and pigments

Substance	Recommended method
Calcium	GBHA* method Alizarin method
Copper	Rubeanic acid
Lead	Acid-fast inclusion bodies
Iron	Perls' reaction
Starch	PAS
Bilirubin	van den Bergh reaction
Melanin	Masson-Fontana

*Glynoxal-bis(2-hydroxyanil).

REFERENCES

General Histochemistry

1. Pearse AGE: Historical introduction. In *Histochemistry, theoretical and applied,* vol 1, Edinburgh, 1980, Churchill Livingstone.

Specific organs

Nervous system

2. High OBB: Degenerative diseases of the central and peripheral nervous system. In Filipe MI, Lake BD, editors: *Histochemistry in pathology,* Edinburgh, 1983, Churchill Livingstone.
3. Kulver H, Barrera A: A method for the combined staining of cells and fibers of the nervous system, *J Neuropathol Exp Neurol* 12:400, 1953.
4. den Hartog Jager WA: Sphingomyelin in Lewey inclusion bodies in Parkinson's disease, *Arch Neurol* 21:615, 1969.
5. Adams CWM, Bayliss OB: Histochemical observations on the localization and origin of sphingomyelin, cerebroside and cholesterol in normal and atherosclerotic artery, *J Pathol Bacterial* 85:113, 1963.
6. Lake BD, Hall NA, Patrick AD: Dolichyl pyrophosphate oligosaccharides are increased in Batten's disease, *Proc R Microscop Soc* 23:45, 1988.

Skeletal muscle

7. Dubowitz V, Brooke MH: *Muscle biopsy: a modern approach,* London, 1973, Saunders.
8. Brooke MH, Engel WK: The histologic diagnosis of neuromuscular disease: a review of 79 biopsies, *Arch Phys Med Rehabil* 47:99, 1966.
9. Engle WK: Muscle target fibers, a newly recognized sign of denervation, *Nature* 191:389, 1961.
10. Dubowitz V, Pearse AGE: Oxidative enzymes and phosphorylases in central core disease of muscle, *Lancet* 2:23, 1960.
11. Pearson CM, Rimber DG, Mommaerts WF: Defect in muscle phosphorylase: a newly defined human disease, *Clin Res* 7:298, 1959.
12. Engle WK: 'Ragged-red fibers' in ophthalmoplegia syndromes and their differential diagnosis, Proc 11th Int Congr Muscle Diseases, Nov, 1971, Perth, Australia, ICS No 237, Amsterdam, *Excerpta Medica* (Abstract).
13. Seligman AM, Karnovsky MJ, Wasserkrug HL, Hanker JS: Nondroplet ultrastructural demonstration of cytochrome oxidase activity with a polymerizing osmiophilic reagent, diaminobenzidine (DAB), *J Cell Biol* 38:1, 1968.
14. Yunis EJ, Samaha FJ: Inclusion body myositis, *Lab Invest* 25:240, 1971.

Hematopoietic system

15. Fujimori T, Mochino T, Miura M, Katayama I: Enzyme histochemistry on paraffin embedded tissue sections, *Stain Technol* 56:355, 1981.
16. Chilosi M, Pizzolo G, Menestrina F et al: Enzyme histochemstry on normal and pathologic paraffin-embedded lymphoid tissue, *Am J Clin Pathol* 76:729, 1981.
17. Beckstead JH, Halverson PS, Ries CA, Bainton DF: Enzyme histochemistry and immunohistochemistry on biopsy specimens of pathologic human bone marrow, *Blood* 57:1088, 1981.
18. Beckstead JH: The evaluation of human lymph nodes, using plastic sections and enzyme histochemistry, *Am J Clin Pathol* 80:131, 1983.
19. Turner RR, Beckstead JH, Warnke RA, Wood GS: Endothelial cell phenotypic diversity: in situ demonstration of immunologic and enzymatic heterogenity that correlates with specific morphologic subtypes, *Am J Clin Pathol* 87:569, 1987.
20. Lake BD: Blood, bone marrow, spleen and lymph nodes in metabolic disorders. In Filipe MI, Lake BD, editors: *Histochemistry in pathology,* Edinburgh, 1990, Churchill Livingstone.
21. Lojda Z: Indigogenic methods for glycosidases. II. An improved method for β-D-galactosidase and its application to localization studies of the enzymes in the intestine and in other tissues, *Histochemie* 23:266, 1970.
22. Lojda Z: Studies on glycyl-proline naphthylamidase. I. Lymphocytes, *Histochemistry* 54:299, 1977.
23. Peterson L, Nelson A, Parkin J: Mucopolysaccharidosis type VII: a morphologic, cytochemical and ultrastructure study of the blood and bone marrow, *Lab Invest* 44:5 (abstract), 1981.

Gastrointestinal system

24. Mowry RW: Alcian blue techniques for the histochemical study of acidic carbohydrates, *J Histochem Cytochem* 6:82, 1958.
25. Spicer SS: Diamine methods for differentiating mucosubstances histochemically, *J Histochem Cytochem* 13:211, 1980.
26. Filipe MI: Value of histochemical reactions for mucosubstances in the diagnosis of certain pathological conditions in the colon and rectum, *Gut* 10:577, 1969.
27. Ehsanullah M, Filipe MI, Gazzard B: Morphological and mucous secretion criteria for differential diagnosis of solitary ulcer syndrome and non-specific proctitis, *J Clin Pathol* 35:26, 1982.
28. Ehsanullah M, Filipe MI, Gazzard B: Mucin secretion in inflammatory bowel disease: correlation with disease activity and dysplasia, *Gut* 23:485, 1982.
29. Collins BJ, Elliott H, Sloan JM et al: Oesophageal histology in reflux oesophagitis, *J Clin Pathol* 38:1265, 1985.
30. Lee RG: Mucins in Barrett's esophagus: a histochemical study, *Am J Clin Pathol* 81:500, 1984.
31. Segura DI, Montero C: Histochemical characterization of different types of intestinal metaplasia in gastric mucosa, *Cancer* 52:498, 1983.
32. Jessurun J, Yardley JH, Giardiello FM et al: Chronic colitis with thickening of the subepithelial collagen layer (collagenous colitis): histopathologic findings in 15 patients, *Hum Pathol* 18:839, 1987.
33. Lake BD, Puri P, Nixon HH, Claireaux AE: Hirschsprung's disease: an appraisal of histochemically demonstrable acetylcholinesterase activity in suction rectal biopsy specimens as an aid to diagnosis, *Arch Pathol Lab Med* 102:244, 1978.
34. Smith B: The neuropathology of pseudo-obstruction of the intestine, *Scand J Gastroenterol* 71(suppl):103, 1982.
35. Piris J: Malabsorption and protein intolerance. In Whitehead R, editor: *Gastrointestinal and oesophageal pathology,* Edinburgh, 1989, Churchill Livingstone.
36. Lojda Z: Proteinases in pathology: usefulness of histochemical methods, *J Histochem Cytochem* 29:481, 1981.
37. Lojda Z: The importance of protease histochemistry in pathology, *Histochem J* 17:1063, 1985.

Liver

38. Lee R: *Diagnostic liver pathology,* St. Louis, 1993, Mosby.
39. Lindquist RR: Studies on the pathogenesis of hepatolenticular degeneration, *Arch Pathol* 87:370, 1969.
40. Shikata T, Uzawa T, Yoshiwara N et al: Staining method of Australia antigen in paraffin sections: detection of cytoplasmic inclusion bodies, *Jpn J Exp Med* 44:25, 1974.
41. Salaspuro M, Sipponen P: Demonstration of an intracellular copper-binding protein by orcein staining in long-standing cholestatic liver disease, *Gut* 17:787, 1976.
42. Nayak NC, Ramalingaswami V: Indian childhood cirrhosis, *Clin Gastroenterol* 4:333, 1975.
43. Scheinburg JH, Sternlieb I: *Wilson's disease,* Philadelphia, 1984, Saunders.
44. Looi L-M, Sumithran E: Morphologic differences in the pattern of liver infiltration between systemic AL and AA amyloidosis, *Hum Pathol* 19:732, 1988.
45. Bove KE, McAdams AJ, Partin JC et al: The hepatic lesion in Reye's syndrome, *Gastroenterology* 69:685, 1975.
46. Scriver CR, Beandet AL, Sly WS, Valle D, editors: *The metabolic basis of inherited disease,* New York, 1989, McGraw-Hill.
47. Chiquoine AD: The distribution of glucose-6-phosphatase ion liver and kidney, *J Histochem Cytochem* 1:429, 1953.
48. Lake BD, Patrick AD: Wolman's disease: deficiency of E-600 resistant acid esterase activity with storage of lipids in lysosomes, *J Pediatr* 76:262, 1970.
49. Lake BD: An improved method for the detection of β-galactosidase activity and its application to G_{M1}-gangliosidosis and mucopolysaccharidosis, *Histochem J* 6:211, 1974.
50. Haust MD, Landing BH: Histochemical studies in Hurler's disease. A new method for localization of acid mucopolysaccharide and an analysis of "lead acetate" fixation, *J Histochem Cytochem* 9:79, 1961.

Tumor diagnosis

51. D'Ardenne AJ: Use of basement membrane markers in tumor diagnosis, *J Clin Pathol* 42:449, 1989.

52. Bennett JM, Catovsky D, Daniel MT et al: Proposals for the classification of the acute leukemias, *Br J Haematol* 33:451, 1976.
53. Yam LT, Janckila AJ, Li C-Y, Lam WKW: Chemistry of tartrate-resistant acid phosphatase: fifteen years' experience, *Leukemia* 1:285, 1987.
54. Nanba K, Jaffe ES, Braylan RC et al: Alkaline phosphatase–positive malignant lymphoma: a subtype of B-cell lymphomas, *Am J Clin Pathol* 68:535, 1977.
55. Turner RR, Wood GS, Beckstead JH et al: Histiocytic malignancies: morphologic, immunologic and enzymatic heterogeneity, *Am J Surg Pathol* 8:485, 1984.
56. Beckstead JH, Warnke R, Bainton DR: Histochemistry of Hodgkin's disease, *Cancer Treat Rep* 66:609, 1982.
57. Beckstead JH, Wood GS, Turner RR: Histiocytosis X cells and Langerhans cells: enzyme histochemical and immunologic similarities, *Hum Pathol* 15:826, 1984.
58. Burstone MS: *Enzyme histochemistry and its application in the study of neoplasms,* New York, 1962, Academic Press.
59. Beckstead JH: Alkaline phosphatase histochemistry in human germ cell neoplasms, *Am J Surg Pathol* 7:341, 1983.
60. Bottles K, Beckstead JH: Enzyme histochemical characterization of chordomas, *Am J Surg Pathol* 8:443, 1984.
61. Cohen MB, Miller TR, Beckstead JH: Enzyme histochemistry and thyroid neoplasia, *Am J Clin Pathol* 85:668, 1986.
62. Cohen MB, Beckstead JH, Ferrell LD, Yen TSB: Enzyme histochemistry of hepatocellular neoplasms, *Am J Surg Pathol* 10:789, 1986.

Lectin histochemistry

63. Damjanov I: Lectin cytochemistry and histochemistry, *Lab Invest* 57:5, 1987.
64. Ordóñez NG, Batsakis JG: Comparison of *Ulex europaeus* I lectin and factor VIII–related antigen in vascular lesions, *Arch Pathol Lab Med* 108:129, 1984.
65. Stephenson TJ, Griffiths DWR, Mills PM: Comparison of *Ulex europaeus* I lectin binding and factor VIII–related antigens as markers of vascular endothelium in follicular carcinoma of the thyroid, *Histopathology* 10:251, 1986.
66. Ree JH, Kadin ME: Peanut agglutinin: a useful marker for histiocytosis X and interdigitating reticulum cells, *Cancer* 57:282, 1986.
67. Hadjin I, Zhang W, Gordon GB: Peanut agglutinin binding as a histochemical tool for the diagnosis of eosinophilic ganuloma, *Arch Pathol Lab Med* 110:719, 1986.
68. Moller P: Peanut lectin: a useful tool for detecting Hodgkin cells in paraffin sections, *Virchows Arch* (A) 396:313, 1982.
69. Hsu SM, Jaffe ES: Leu M1 and peanut agglutinin stain the neoplastic cells of Hodgkin's disease, *Am J Clin Pathol* 82:29, 1984.
70. Ree JH, Neiman RS, Martin AW et al: Paraffin section markers for Reed-Sternberg cells: a comparative study of peanut agglutinin, Leu-M1, LN-2, and Ber-H2, *Cancer* 63:2030, 1989.
71. Sarker AB, Akagi T, Jeon JH et al: *Bauhinia purpurea*—a new paraffin section marker for Reed-Sternberg cells of Hodgkin's disease. A comparison with Leu-M1 (CD15), LN2 (CD74), peanut agglutinin, and Ber-H2 (CD30), *Am J Pathol* 141:19, 1992.
72. Leathem AJ, Brooks SA: Predictive value of lectin binding in breast cancer recurrence and survival, *Lancet* 1:1054, 1987.
73. Walker RA, Hawkins RA, Miller WR: Lectin binding and steroid receptors in human breast carcinomas, *J Pathol* 147:103, 1985.
74. Limas C, Lange P: T-antigen in normal and neoplastic urothelium, *Cancer* 58:1236, 1986.
75. Söderström KO: Lectin binding to prostate adenocarcinoma, *Cancer* 60:1823, 1987.
76. Yen Y, Schmiemann C, Damjanov I: Lectin histochemistry of adenocarcinomas, *Arch Pathol Lab Med* 112:791, 1988.
77. Teshima S, Hirohashi S, Shimosato Y et al: Histochemically demonstrable changes in cell surface carbohydrates of human germ cell tumors, *Lab Invest* 50:271, 1984.
78. Malmi R, Söderström KO: Lectin bindng to carcinoma in situ cells of the testis: a comparative study of CIS germ cells and seminoma cells, *Virchows Archiv A, Pathol Anat Histopathol* 413:69, 1988.
79. Uedo T, Aozasa K, Yamamura T et al: Lectin histochemistry of malignant fibrohistiocytic tumors, *Am J Surg Pathol* 11:257, 1987.
80. Leader M, Collins M, Patel J, Henry K: Staining for factor VIII related antigen and *Ulex europaeus* agglutinin I (UEA I) in 230 tumors: an assessment of their specificity for angiosarcoma and Kaposi's sarcoma, *Histopathology* 10:1153, 1986.
81. Beckstead JH, Wood GS, Fletcher V: Evidence for the origin of Kaposi's sarcoma from lymphatic endothelium, *Am J Pathol* 119:294, 1985.
82. Kohchiyama A, Oka D, Ueki H: Differing lectin-binding patterns of malignant melanoma and nervocellular and Spitz nevi, *Arch Dermatol Res* 279:226, 1987.
83. Hennigar RA, Sens DA, Spicer SS et al: Lectin histochemistry of nephroblastoma (Wilm's tumour), *Histochem J* 17:1091, 1985.
84. Yeger H, Baumal R, Harason P, Phillips MJ: Lectin histochemistry of Wilm's tumor: comparison with normal adult and fetal kidneys, *Am J Clin Pathol* 88:278, 1987.
85. Kahn HJ, Baumal R, Thorner PS, Chan H: Binding of peanut agglutinin to neuroblastomas and ganglioneuromas: a marker for differentiation of neuroblasts into ganglion cells, *Pediatr Pathol* 8:83, 1988.

Nucleolar organizer

86. Ploton D, Menager M, Jeannesson P et al: Improvements in the staining and in the visualization of the argyrophilic proteins of the nucleolar organizer regions at optical level, *Histochem J* 18:5, 1986.
87. Egan MJ, Crocker J: Nucleolar organizer regions in cutaneous tumors, *J Pathol* 154:247, 1988.
88. Egan MJ, Raafat F, Crocker J, Smith K: Nucleolar organizer regions in small cell tumours of childhood, *J Pathol* 153:275, 1988.
89. Crocker J: Histochemistry of malignant lymphomas: review of conventional histochemical, enzyme histochemical, and argyrophil nucleolar organizer region stains, *J Histotech* 15:185, 1992.
90. Delahunt B, Mostofi FK, Sesterhenn IA et al: Nucleolar organizer regions in seminoma and intratubular malignant germ cells, *Mod Pathol* 3:141, 1990.
91. Walker RA: The histopathological evaluation of nucleolar organizing regions, *Histopathology* 12:221, 1988.

Infectious disease, minerals, and pigments

92. Sheehan DC, Hrapchak BB: *Theory and practice of histotechnology,* St. Louis, 1980, Mosby.
93. Bancroft JD, Stevens A: *Theory and practice of histological techniques,* Edinburgh, 1990, Churchill Livingstone.
94. Filipe MI, Lake BD: *Histochemistry in pathology,* Edinburgh, 1990, Churchill Livingstone.

10 In Situ Hybridization

Gerard J. Nuovo

INTRODUCTION

In situ hybridization is a molecular hybridization technique well suited for the surgical pathologist. The technique allows localization of nucleic acid sequence, viral RNA or DNA, or cellular RNA or chromosomal DNA. It involves the specific hybridization of a labeled nucleic acid probe to complementary target sequences in tissue, followed by visualization of the location of the probe. In situ hybridization is applicable in many areas of biology and medicine. It is valuable in genetic studies, allowing analysis of temporal and spatial regulation of gene expression. As well, in situ hybridization is used diagnostically in medicine to identify viral sequences in tissue and provide insight into the pathogenetic mechanisms of viral infections. The technique can also be applied to the physical mapping of the genome and identification and interpretation of chromosomal rearrangements. The feature that distinguishes it from the other hybridization-based methodologies—filter hybridization and thermal cycling techniques (polymerase chain reaction [PCR], DNA ligase, etc.)—is that sample DNA is not extracted but rather detected directly in the intact cell. Indeed, it can be argued that surgical pathology training is mandatory to interpret the localization of the target DNA or RNA evident in in situ hybridization. This statement also applies to the new technique of PCR in situ hybridization, which is also discussed.

A major drawback of in situ hybridization, relative to filter hybridization and PCR, is its relatively low sensitivity (Table 10-1). Fig. 10-1 compares the in situ hybridization of three different cervical cancer cell lines that contain 1, 20, and 600 copies of human *papillomavirus* (HPV) DNA per cell, respectively. Notice that the one copy of HPV DNA in SiHa cells is detectable by in situ hybridization only after PCR amplification, as is discussed below. There are many conditions where there is only a single copy of the target DNA or RNA in every 100 cells but not more than one or a few copies in a given cell and thus detectable by filter hybridization or PCR but not detectable by in situ hybridization analysis. Several classical examples are evident in viral infections. For example, in low-grade squamous intraepithelial lesions of the cervix, more than 1000 copies of HPV DNA or RNA can occur in a cell (Fig. 10-2). However, in occult HPV infection (without evidence of cervical disease) or in cervical cancer, the number of HPV genomes in squamous cells may be one or very few copies and thus detectable only by filter hybridization or PCR (Fig. 10-2).

Table 10-1 Relative sensitivities of the different hybridization-based techniques

Test	Detection threshold	Type of specimen
Filter hybridization (Southern blot or slot blot)	1 copy/100 cells	Fresh
In situ hybridization	10 copies/cell	Fresh or fixed
Polymerase chain reaction (PCR)	10 copies/tissue	Fresh or fixed
PCR in situ hybridization	1 copy/cell	Fixed

Human immunodeficiency virus type 1 (HIV-1) provides another example. After viral entry into a cell, the RNA genome serves as a template for synthesis of a complementary copy of DNA (cDNA) by reverse transcriptase. The viral RNA is destroyed, and the DNA is integrated into the human genome, where it can remain latent for years. The latent virus may not be detected by in situ hybridization but could be detected by PCR. However, when the virus is "activated," it may synthesize many (>50) copies of its RNA, which can then be detected by in situ hybridization.

RNAs, either as mRNAs or RNA viruses, are also often difficult to detect by in situ hybridization. This reflects, in part, the fact that a given RNA molecule can direct the synthesis of multiple copies of its protein, and thus large numbers are not needed for its effect.

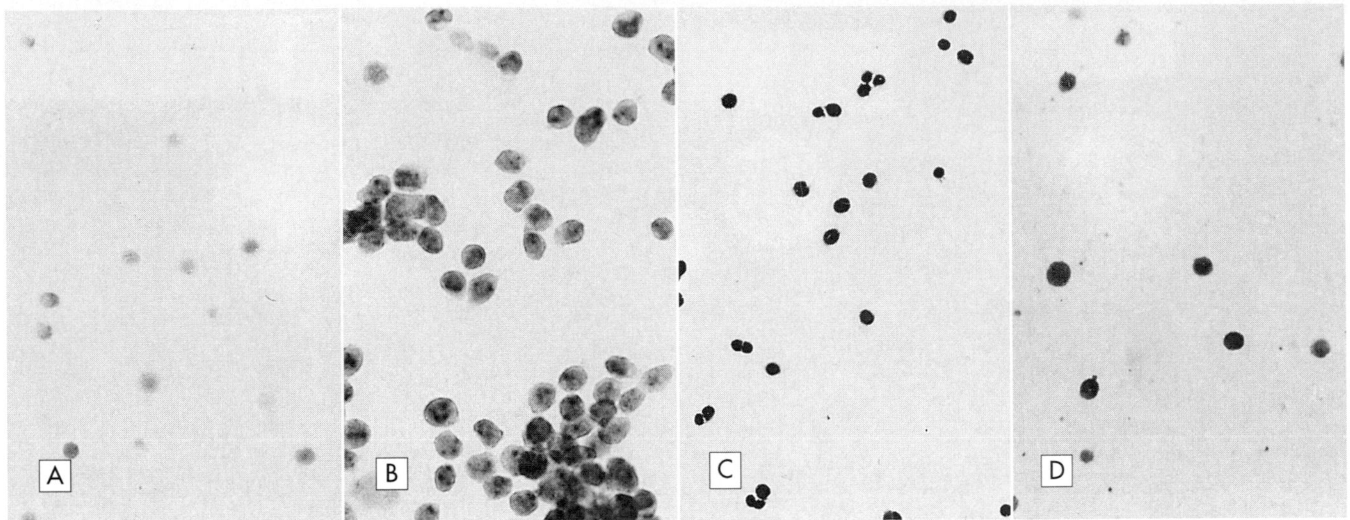

Fig. 10-1 Detection of HPV DNA in cell lines by in situ hybridization. HPV DNA is not detected by in situ hybridization in SiHa cells that contain 1 copy of HPV 16, **A.** The virus is detectable by the in situ assay in HeLa cells (20 copies of HPV 18), **B,** and a much stronger signal is seen in Caski cells (600 copies of HPV 16), **C.** HPV DNA is detectable in the SiHa cells if the PCR in situ hybridization test is used, **D.**

A misconception regarding in situ hybridization is that radiolabeled probes (usually ^{35}S or ^{3}H) are required to maximize sensitivity. Although this statement may have been true in 1988, advances in nonisotopic labeling and, more importantly, detection systems have greatly enhanced the sensitivity of in situ hybridization using probes labeled with biotin or digoxigenin.

The first section of this chapter deals with the essentials for performing in situ hybridization. This is followed by a discussion of the utility of in situ hybridization in the diagnosis of viral infection and in the characterization of other diseases. Recent books offer more thorough discussion of in situ hybridization techniques.[1,2]

METHODS

The laboratory

If the laboratory is to be used for RNA studies, it is essential to have a clean, dust-free work space that is also ribonuclease (RNase) free. All glassware must be washed, treated with 0.1% diethylpyrocarbonate (DEPC), autoclaved, and then wrapped in aluminum foil, before being baked in an oven at 180° C (4 hours to overnight) to eliminate residual RNases. All solutions must be treated with 0.1% DEPC before autoclaving. (DEPC, which deactivates proteins by alkylation, is a potential carcinogen and should be handled in a fume hood. DEPC is broken down to CO_2 and ethanol when autoclaved.) All plasticware should be sterile, disposable, and RNase free. Clean, disposable, and preferably talc-free gloves should be worn at all times when one is handling glassware, reagent containers, and appliance handles. With formalin-fixed tissues, precautions against RNases are less critical until after protease digestion; formalin cross-linking protects RNA from degradation. If the investigator plans to use radioactive probes, strict adherence to institutional guidelines for proper storage, handling, and disposal of radioisotopes and waste is mandatory. The considerations on equipping a laboratory for in situ hybridization and the handling of radioactive materials have been reviewed.[3]

Glass slides

Considering the number of steps required before one may directly visualize small segments of nucleic acids within a cell with in situ hybridization, it is interesting to note that a major technical advancement in the field had nothing to do with the dynamics of probe entry and hybridization but simply with the preparation of the glass slide. Coating the slide with an organosilane solution improves tissue adherence from about 10% to over 99%. Silane-coated slides are available commercially from many sources. Other methods of enhancing the adherence of tissues to glass slides include the use of gelatin, polylysine, Denhardt's solution, or glue.[2] However, these are less effective methods when compared to silane coating.

Tissue fixation

In situ hybridization can be conducted on frozen or fixed tissue, or on cell smears. A limitation with frozen tissue is poor morphology, such that it is not nearly as crisp as with fixed, paraffin-embedded tissues. Also, pretreatment with protease (commonly, proteinase K), which increases accessibility of the target nucleic acid sequence and substantially improves that signal obtained, may lead to further morphologic degradation of frozen tissue. Further, in most cases only fixed tissues are available.

The choice of fixative is critical for successful in situ hybridization. Buffered formalin (pH 7.0) is an excellent fixative for in situ hybridization. Fixation times of several hours to several days reproducibly yield strong hybridization signals. The hybridization signal is reduced by half if unbuffered formalin is used. More dramatic reductions in the intensity of the hybridization signal may be seen with fixatives that contain heavy metals, such as mercury (Zenker's solution) or picric

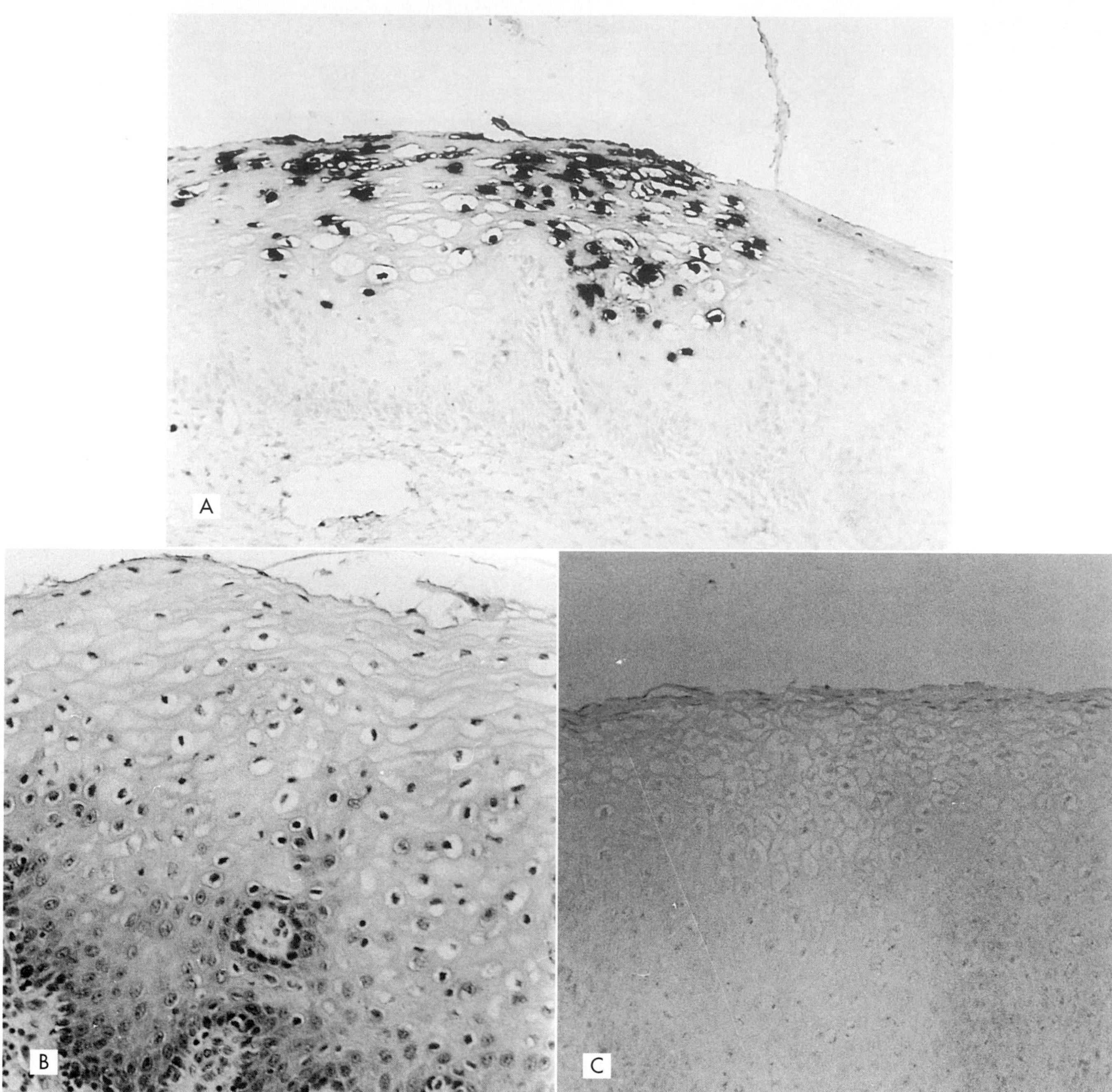

Fig. 10-2 Correlation of HPV copy number with the histologic findings. Low-grade cervical SILs are often associated with large numbers of HPV in a given cell, and that association results in an intense in situ hybridization signal, **A.** However, the viral numbers are much less in occult HPV infection such that, although the virus was detected in this tissue that appeared normal (negative for SIL) histologically, **B,** by PCR, it was not detected by in situ hybridization, **C.**

acid (Bouin's solution), though the extent of the inhibitory effect depends on the length of fixation time. Two hours of fixation in Bouin's solution has a minimal effect on the intensity of the hybridization signal, which may be completely eradicated after overnight (15-hour) fixation; intermediate results are seen after 8 hours of Bouin's fixation. The pronounced reduction in the intensity of the hybridization signal is associated with another interesting effect. The signal is lost at high stringency, even when one is certain that the probe and target are completely homologous. This indicates that picric acid and heavy metals may cause conformational changes that interfere with the binding of probe to the target.[1]

Protease digestion

Fixatives that cross-link proteins and nucleic acids may hinder penetration of the probe to the target nucleic acid molecule. Different methods have been used to facilitate probe entry, including treatment with chemicals, such as HCl, photofluor, and sodium sulfite. However, most of the interest has focused on pretreatment with proteases.

The different types of commercial proteases (such as pepsin, trypsin, proteinase K, Pronase) are equivalent for in situ hybridization. Determining the proper concentration of the protease and digestion time requires some trial and error. Insufficient protease treatment does not suitably enhance the hybridization signal. Too much protease treatment is easy to recognize because the tissue morphology will be destroyed; this is more likely to occur with proteinase K digestion. As a general rule, pepsin pretreatment (2 mg/ml) for 12 to 25 minutes works well for tissues fixed for 8 to 24 hours in 10% buffered formalin. It is recommended that the investigator choose one protease and use it exclusively so as to be familiar with its nuances. Another caveat is that the effectiveness of protease treatment is tissue specific. The optimal concentration of protease and incubation time for the tissue of interest should be determined by titration using a positive control probe for hybridization. Proteinase K has been used successfully at concentrations ranging from 0.25 to 1.0 mg/mL depending on the type of tissue.[2]

A reliable measure of the adequacy of protease pretreatment, as well as the other conditions in in situ hybridization, is with the use of "positive control probes." These probes detect targets in each cell of the tissue and therefore should produce a hybridization signal in every cell if the in situ hybridization was correctly done. A useful control probe is specific for the repetitive *alu* sequence that comprises about 5% of the total human genome. If this probe does not yield a hybridization signal in most cells, some condition or conditions, possibly protease digestion, are not adequate. When this occurs, it is recommended that one follow the flow chart presented in Fig. 10-3.

Probe labels

Probes may be labeled with radioisotope (^{3}H, ^{35}S, ^{32}P, or ^{125}I) and detected by autoradiography, or they may be labeled nonradioactively with a hapten and detected immunocytochemically.[4] Of the radioisotopes, ^{35}S is used most frequently, since it yields the best compromise between speed, sensitivity, resolution, and low background labeling. Different labeled probes can be used in combinations to allow simultaneous detection of two or more targets.[5] Nonradioisotope labeling (digoxigenin or biotin) offers a safer work environment, faster signal detection, and are easier to use than radiolabeled probes. Digoxigenin-labeled probes are detected with alkaline phosphatase–conjugated, antidigoxygenin antibody. Biotin-labeled probes may be detected by use of a streptavidin–alkaline phosphatase conjugate system.

Probe synthesis and probe cocktail mixture

Probes for in situ hybridization fall into two categories, genomic probes and oligonucleotide probes (oligoprobes). Genomic probes are made from DNA segments that are often greater than 1000 base pairs in length. Genomic probe synthesis and labeling is usually done by random priming, nick translation, or PCR. Longer probes may lead to weaker signals, possibly because they penetrate cross-linked tissue less efficiently. Probes of 50 to 250 base pairs in length have been used successfully. The length of the probe is determined by the concentration, of the primer or by the amount of DNAse in the reaction for probes labeled by random priming or nick translation, respectively. Primer selection dictates the length of probes produced by PCR. Oligoprobes are much shorter, usually 20 to 40 base pairs in length. They are produced synthetically, in house, or commercially, without the requirement of cloning techniques. A disadvantage of oligoprobes is their relative insensitivity, relative to longer probes. Oligonucleotides can be labeled to high specific activity by 3′-end tailing with terminal deoxynucleotidyl transferase (TdT). Many excellent kits for probe labeling are commercially available.

The function of the formamide and relatively low salt concentration is to facilitate denaturing of the probe and target DNA.

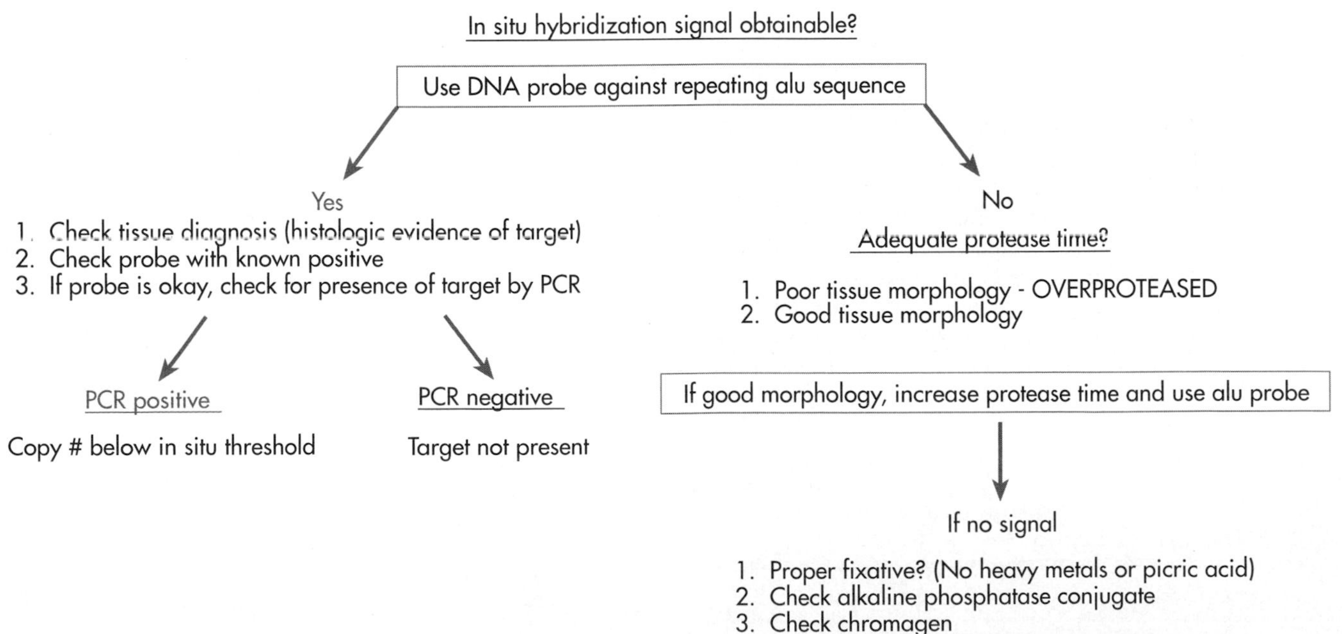

Fig. 10-3 Flow chart for negative result with in situ hybridization, detailing a step-by-step approach to follow if a hybridization signal is not evident with in situ analysis.

Dextran sulfate is commonly used to increase the effective concentration of the probe and thus the rate of hybrid formation.

The most important difference between the oligoprobe and genomic probe cocktail mix is the formamide concentration. The single-strand oligoprobe does not need to be denatured, hence the lower formamide concentration. Also, during the 2-hour hybridization step (see below), 50% formamide would block hybridization of the 20 to 40 base pair oligoprobe and its target, precluding any hybridization signal. Blocking is much less likely if the formamide concentration is 10%. Under these conditions, the temperature at which the adhered oligoprobe and target DNA would separate (the *Tm*) would likely be above the temperature of the hybridization step (37° C), as evident from the following formula for Tm for DNA probes:

$$\text{Tm} = 81.5° \text{ C} + 16.6 \log [\text{Na}] \text{ (as molarity)} + 0.41 \text{ (\% G + C content)} - 0.61 \text{ (\% formamide)} - \text{(500/number of base pairs in the DNA/DNA hybrid)}.$$

Specifically, if the formamide concentration is 10% (with the [Na^+] at 0.1 M, the G + C content at 50%, and the probe size at 25 base pairs), the Tm is 59° C, as compared to 34° C if the formamide concentration is 50%. A more detailed description of Tm and its importance in hybridization and the posthybridization wash is discussed in recent monographs.[1,2]

Posthybridization wash

With radioactive probes, the posthybridization wash is a key step, because of the background problems inherent with ^{35}S-labeled probes. Probe that is nonspecifically bound to the membranes and nontarget nucleic acids produces enough background to render the slide uninterpretable. This is less of a concern with the biotin and digoxigenin nonisotopic systems. Hence, the washing step, which removes the probe that is bound to molecules other than the target DNA or RNA, is much simplified.

Oligoprobes and genomic probes require different posthybridization wash conditions. Because the number of base pairs in the probe-target complex is less for oligoprobes, the temperature where background is removed is closer to the temperature where the signal is lost. This is reflected in the recommended posthybridization wash conditions listed in Table 10-2. The melting point of the genomic probe–target complex is higher, and so one could increase the temperature of the wash to 70° C and still retain the hybridization signal. However, for an oligoprobe, the signal would be lost at a temperature of 55° C if the salt concentration is 15 mM. Thus a salt concentration much higher (150 mM) for the posthybridization wash is recommended when one is using an oligoprobe. Still, a high salt concentration risks seeing background with the oligoprobe because of the relatively low temperature.

Table 10-2 Posthybridization washes for in situ hybridization

Genomic probe	Oligoprobe
15 mM NaCl	150 mM NaCl
0.1% bovine serum albumin	0.1% bovine serum albumin
55° to 65° C for 10 minutes	45°to 55° C for 10 minutes

Detection system

After the posthybridization wash, one is left with a target/probe complex. Labeled nucleotides are incorporated into the probe. This section deals only with digoxigenin-labeled nucleotides and reflects my experience that ^{35}S-, ^{3}H-, or ^{32}P-labeled probes offer no advantages over the nonradioactive systems.

There are many ways to localize the alkaline phosphatase target–probe complex. A wide variety of chromagens are available, allowing one to select a blue, red, or yellow precipitate (with other colors becoming available), which is either water soluble or insoluble. Chromagens that fluoresce, because of the activity of alkaline phosphatase, are also available. A commonly used chromagen is 5-bromo-4-chloro-3-indolylphosphate in the presence of nitroblue tetrazolium (NBT-BCIP), which yields a blue precipitate. The choice of counterstain depends largely on the chromagen used. For NBT-BCIP, we prefer a pale pink nuclear counterstain called "nuclear fast red" (Fig. 10-4). A summary of an in situ hybridization protocol using digoxigenin-labeled probes is provided in Table 10-3.

Table 10-3 Protocol for in situ hybridization

Tissue preparation
1. Place several 4 μm of paraffin-embedded sections on a glass slide.
2. Wash slides in xylene for 5 minutes, then 100% ethanol for 5 minutes, and then air dry.

Probe cocktail
See text.

Denaturing of probe and target DNA
1. Add 10 μl of the probe to a given tissue section.
2. Overlay with plastic coverslip cut slightly larger than tissue section.
3. Place slide on hot plate at 95° to 100° C for 5 minutes.
4. Remove bubbles over tissue gently with a toothpick.

Hybridization and washing
1. Place slides in humidity chamber at 37° C for 2 hours.
2. Remove coverslips and place slides in "wash solution" (see Table 10-2 for oligoprobe versus genomic probe).
3. Wipe off excess wash solution and put slides in a humidity chamber. Do not let slides dry out.

Detection
1. Add digoxigenin–alkaline phosphatase conjugate (1:200 dilution) to tissue sections in humidity chamber.
2. Incubate for 30 minutes at 37° C.
3. Wash slides at room temperature for 3 minutes in a solution of 0.1 M Tris HCl (pH 9 to 9.5) and 0.1 M NaCl (detection reagent solution).
4. Place slides in detection reagent solution to which NBT-BCIP has been added.
5. Incubate slides for 30 minutes to 2 hours, checking results periodically under microscope.

Counterstain and coverslip
1. Wash slides for 1 minute in distilled water.
2. Counterstain for 5 minutes in nuclear fast red solution.
3. Wash slides for 1 minute in distilled water × 2.
4. Place slides for 1 minute in 95% ethanol.
5. Place slides for 1 minute in 100% ethanol.
6. Place slides in xylene for at least 1 minute.
7. Coverslip using Permount and glass coverslip.
8. View under microscope.

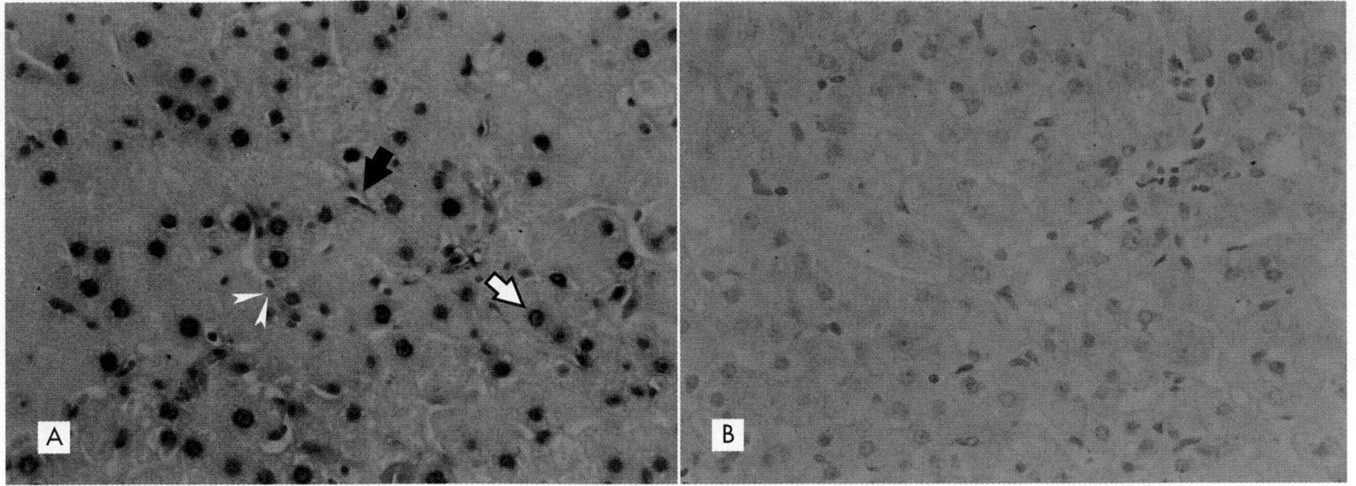

Fig. 10-4 Molecular analysis for hepatitis cDNA in liver tissue. Diffuse lymphoid infiltrates, steatosis, and "activated" sinusoidal Kupffer cells were evident on histologic examination. **A,** Most of the hepatocytes *(open arrow)* in this lobule demonstrated a signal after RT in situ PCR with use of the hepatitis C–specific primers (the blue signal is positive, and the red is the negative nuclear fast red counterstain). Notice the positive Kupffer cell *(closed arrow)* and negative endothelial cells *(double arrow,* with pink being negative). **B,** The staining was lost if "nonsense" (measles-specific) primers were used, if RT in situ PCR was preceded by RNase digestion, or if the RT step was omitted.

Troubleshooting

Background is the most common problem encountered with in situ hybridization. Background is the result of nonspecific binding of the probe to nontarget molecules. One example is the presence of a hybridization signal with a specific probe in a tissue that does not contain the target. The absence of the target could be confirmed by PCR. Another example of background would be a hybridization signal when the labeled plasmid vector is employed (the plasmid is the vehicle used to clone the probe of interest). Two simple and logical ways to deal with background are to decrease the concentration of the probe or to increase the stringency of the posthybridization wash, or to do both. If the background is a problem, first try decreasing the concentration of the salt in the posthybridization wash by half and increase the wash time by 10-minute intervals. If it still persists, try decreasing the probe concentration tenfold.

Poor tissue morphology is another common problem. The major cause of this problem is overtreatment with protease. Decreasing the time of protease digestion (by intervals of 3 minutes) or decreasing the protease concentration tenfold will solve this problem. Some investigators include an RNase digestion step in the wash sequence to eliminate unbound, single-stranded probe to reduce the background.

Tissue sections should not fall off silane-coated slides. A loss greater than 5% indicates incorrect silanization of the slides. The most obvious potential problem with in situ hybridization is the absence of a hybridization signal. In this author's experience, which has focused on HPV, a common finding when asked to review HPV-negative in situ results that "should be HPV-positive" is that the tissue was incorrectly diagnosed as condyloma/squamous intraepithelial lesion, and thus should be HPV-negative by in situ hybridization (see below). A flow chart-type of protocol for dealing with a negative hybridization signal is provided in Fig. 10-3. In any case, positive controls should be included in each run (i.e., tissue known to be infected with the target organism, and positive control probe specific for the alu sequence will confirm the relative success of the in situ hybridization run).

APPLICATIONS OF IN SITU HYBRIDIZATION

Viral infection

Human papillomavirus

In situ hybridization has furthered the understanding of the role of HPV in lower genital tract squamous intraepithelial lesions (SILs).[6-8] The following issues were clarified with in situ hybridization: (1) HPV DNA is more abundant in the cells toward the surface that show perinuclear halos and nuclear atypia; (2) HPV DNA is present in much higher copy numbers in low-grade SILs than in high-grade SILs and invasive cancers; (3) the diversity of HPV types is much greater in cervical SILs than in vulvar and penile SILs. This point is of particular interest but is poorly understood. HPVs 6 and 11 are relatively rare in low-grade cervical SILs, whereas they are detected in over 95% of the histologically equivalent lesion of the vulva. HPV 16, the most common HPV type in genital tract cancers, is, as expected, the most common type in high-grade lesions. However, it is also the most common HPV type in low-grade cervical SILs but is rarely found in low-grade vulvar (and penile) lesions. A practical consideration of these data is that one would need probes of only HPVs 6, 11, and 16 for study of vulvar and penile lesions. However, without additional probes, one may miss as much as 50% of the HPV types in cervical SILs.

Occult HPV infection is defined as the presence of the virus in the absence of clinical or pathologic evidence of the infection. Most studies have focused on the cervix and have demonstrated that, with use of slot blot or Southern blot analysis, the rate of occult infection is about 10%. When PCR is employed, a higher rate of about 30% has been found. As noted above, studies of occult infection analyzing HPV by in situ hybridization have shown that the virus is rarely detected with this technique. There are two possible explanations. First,

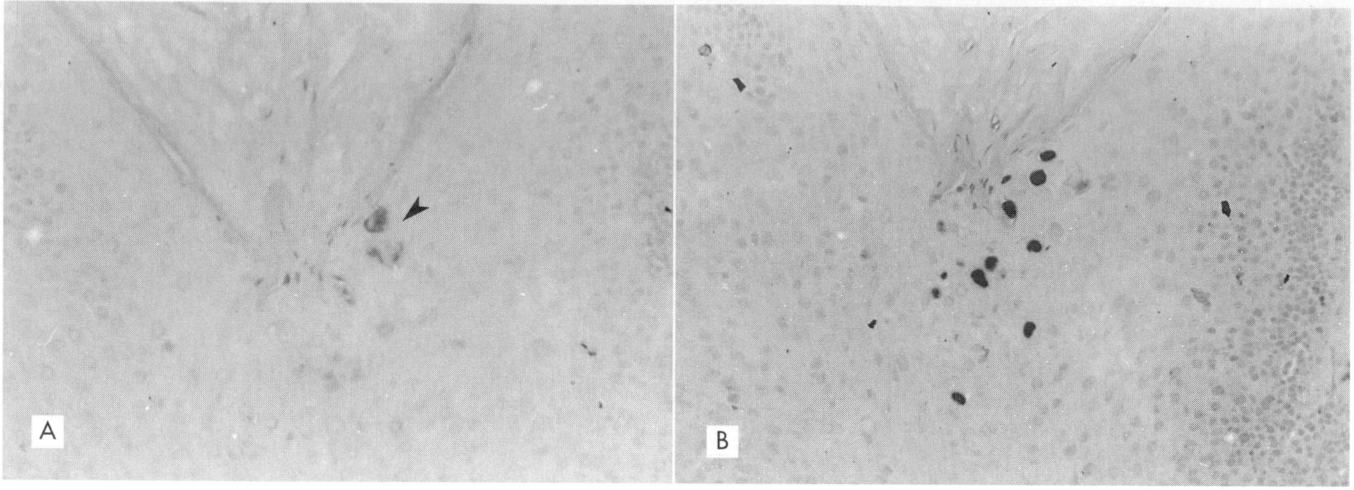

Fig. 10-5 Detection of HPV DNA by PCR in situ hybridization in an equivocal penile biopsy specimen. The biopsy sample was from a penile lesion clinically suggestive of a low-grade SIL (condyloma). **A,** HPV DNA was detected in a few cells by standard in situ hybridization. **B,** Many more cells had detectable HPV DNA when PCR in situ hybridization was done on the serial section.

occult infection may be associated with rare HPV types, which have poor homology, to the more common types recognized by the probe, and thus they escape detection. However, though rare, uncharacterized types have been shown to be associated with occult infection, in many instances more common types, such as HPVs 6, 11, or 16, are found. The second and more tenable explanation is that occult infection is associated with low numbers of the virus per cell, that is, below the detection threshold of the in situ hybridization assay (Fig. 10-2). It follows that in situ hybridization analysis is a poor technique to use in the study of invasive cancers or occult infection but is as good as Southern blot or PCR for the detection of HPV DNA in low-grade SILs.

In situ hybridization analysis of equivocal tissue biopsy specimens can provide useful information. A major diagnostic problem for the pathologist is differentiating "nonspecific" changes from low-grade SIL. The detection rate of HPV DNA by in situ hybridization in low-grade SILs is 90% to 95%, compared to 1% for tissues grossly and microscopically unremarkable. Hence the test offers high sensitivity and specificity. For equivocal vulvar or penile lesions, the rate of HPV detection by in situ hybridization is about 8%; the rate for equivocal cervical lesions is 1% to 2%. This disparity likely reflects the observation that cervical low-grade SILs show more conspicuous cytologic changes than comparable lesions of the vulva and penis do. Whatever the explanation, two diagnostically relevant points may be made from this information. First, for equivocal tissues, in situ hybridization analysis for HPV DNA is a reliable way to distinguish mimics from "true" SILs because the detection rate is basically 0% in normal tissues and over 90% in SILs. Second, for vulvar and penile tissues, one needs probes for only HPVs 6, 11, and 16. For cervical tissues, probes for at least 14 distinct HPV types are needed to achieve a detection rate for SILs of >90%.

In situ hybridization may aid the analysis of equivocal vulvar and penile tissues that are equivocal for HPV infection. In about 10% of cases HPV DNA will be detected when the classical histologic changes of a low-grade SIL are not seen (Fig. 10-5). Because in situ hybridization requires at least 20 viral genomes per cell for detection, one may assume that the virus is actively proliferating in the HPV-positive equivocal tissues. This should be contrasted with HPV detection by slot or Southern blot hybridization or PCR, where the virus may be present in low numbers and in a quiescent state but still be detected. In such situations it is unclear whether the virus is pathogenetic. However, if active viral synthesis is occurring, it is possible that changes noted on pathologic examination, even if nonspecific, such as parakeratosis or papillomatosis, may be directly induced by the virus.

A technique whereby the extreme sensitivity of PCR is combined with the cell-localizing ability of in situ hybridization has been described. Using PCR in situ hybridization, one HPV viral genome in a given cell can be detected.[1,9] This allows one to locate cells containing virus in occult infection. If the virus cannot be detected by PCR in situ hybridization, it is highly unlikely that it is present in the tissue section.

Progressive multifocal leukoencephalopathy: the JC virus

The emergence of AIDS has dramatically increased the incidence of progressive multifocal leukoencephalopathy (PML), a rare demyelinating disease caused by the JC virus (so named after the patient from whom it was first isolated). This papovavirus is related to HPV. The JC virus actively proliferates in PML, probably reflecting the immunosuppressed state of the patient. The classical histologic changes of PML are enlarged oligodendroglial nuclei, but inflammation is usually minimal (Fig. 10-6). The diagnostic, enlarged oligodendroglial nuclei are often difficult to find, whereas demonstration of JC virus by in situ hybridization is diagnostic.[10-12] JC virus may also be detected in the cerebrospinal fluid by PCR, a finding that correlates well with in situ hybridization.[13]

Cytomegalovirus (CMV)

CMV is the most common opportunistic viral infection in patients with AIDS, affecting many organs, including the brain, eye, kidney, lung, esophagus, and colon. The cytologic changes of CMV are distinctive, eosinophilic intranuclear inclusions, defined by a clear zone from peripheral chromatin clumping, and basophilic cytoplasmic inclusions (Chapter 36).

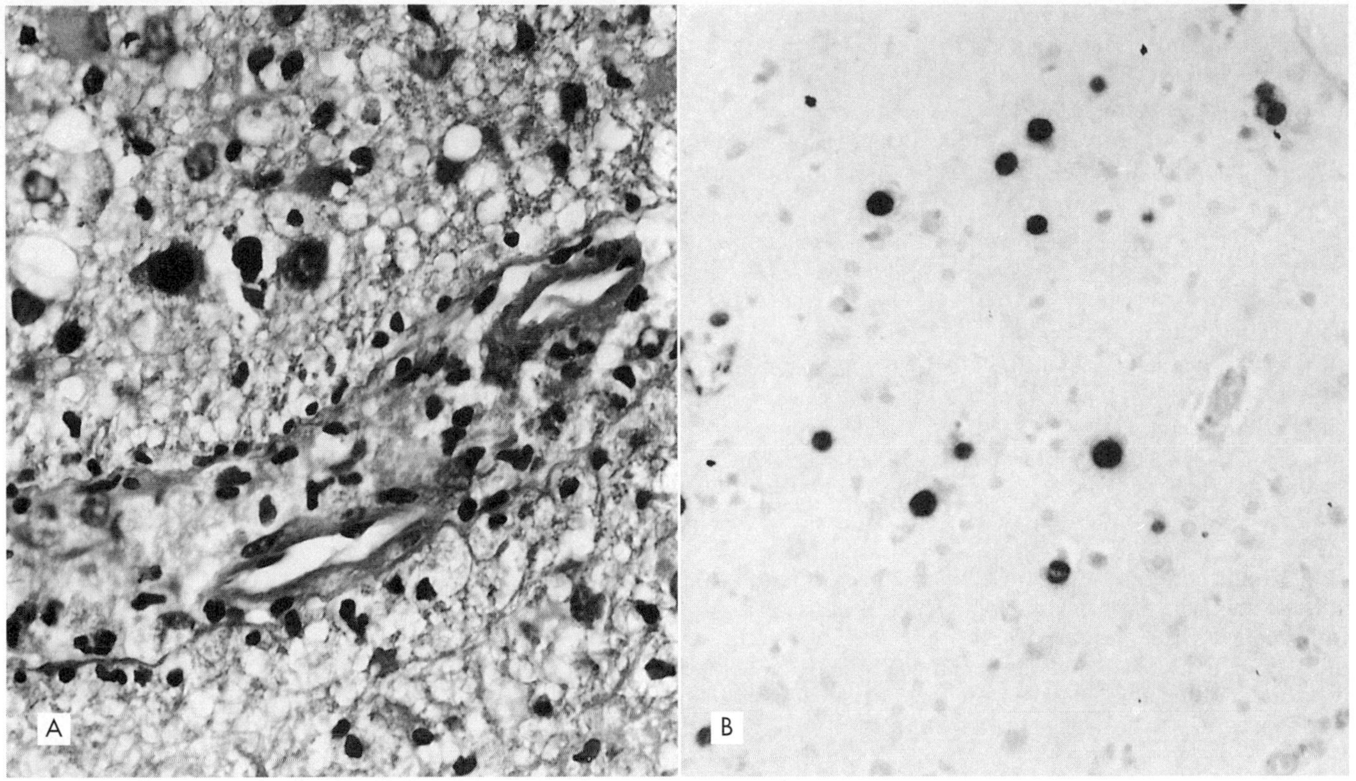

Fig. 10-6 Detection of JC virus by in situ hybridization. **A**, The tissue is from the central nervous system of an AIDS patient in which enlarged atypical oligodendroglial cells were suggestive of progressing multifocal leukoencephaly. **B**, Detection of the JC virus by in situ hybridization confirmed the diagnosis.

In situ hybridization of such cells yields an invariably intense hybridization signal, indicative of hundreds or thousands of copies of viral genomes in the nucleus. However, many more cells are infected by CMV than is evident by morphology. In situ hybridization can increase the sensitivity of CMV detection in lung, liver, and gastrointestinal specimens[14-17] and in diseases of uncertain cause, such as nonspecific villitis.[17]

Epstein-Barr virus (EBV)

Infection with EBV, a DNA virus and a member of the Herpetoviridae family usually causes asymptomatic seroconversion, or infectious mononucleosis. EBV is also etiologically linked to Burkitt's lymphoma and nasopharyngeal carcinoma, to lymphoproliferative disorders in congenital immunodeficiency, and in immunosuppressed transplant recipients. In situ hybridization has proved useful in establishing that such lymphoid infiltrates are attributable to EBV.[19-21]

Hepatitis C infection

The histologic changes of hepatitis C infection, the etiologic agent of many cases of posttransfusion hepatitis, are not specific, occurring in other viral hepatides and conditions, such as autoimmune hepatitis.

Studies of hepatitis C RNA with cDNA-RNA in situ hybridization have suggested that the viral RNA can be found in scattered periportal hepatocytes and not in inflammatory cells or damaged bile duct epithelium.[22,23] Viral RNA was detectable with in situ hybridization soon after infection but was not detectable with this methodology in the livers of infected chimpanzees 3 weeks after the onset of infection. This finding indicates that the viral copy number may decrease as the disease progresses. However, the virus is readily detectable by RT in situ PCR. PCR-amplified viral cDNA occurs in hepatocytes in a perilobular distribution and in scattered Kupffer cells (Fig. 10-4). Positive signal is usually located in a perinuclear pattern within cells with occasional cytoplasmic positivity. Occasional bile duct epithelium cells located in portal tracts with an inflammatory infiltrate also display a positive signal. The absence of a signal in lymphocytes and endothelium-lining cells provides for a negative internal control (specific cell types in a tissue that lack the target of interest), and is very important in interpreting the results of PCR in situ hybridization because it serves to demonstrate the specificity of the results.

Human immunodeficiency virus (HIV-1)

The diagnosis of HIV infection is usually made by serologic tests, by western blotting, or by molecular diagnostic methods. PCR in situ hybridization may allow documentation of viral infection in tissues obtained from the kidney, skeletal muscle, cervix, lymph nodes, or the central nervous system, where the AIDS patient has related symptoms.[24,25]

HIV-1 can integrate into the host genome and remain in a latent state. A critical event in HIV-1–related pathogenesis is the shift from latent to active infection, manifested by viral transcription. In situ hybridization would not be expected to detect the latent infection. However, even the activated infection may not be detected by in situ hybridization because the virus often does not make many copies of its RNA. By combining PCR in situ hybridization with RT in situ PCR, one can detect HIV-1 infection in situ and differentiate between latent and activated infection. These analyses have shown that:

1. Activated HIV-1 infection is invariably found in the endocervical aspect of the transformation zone of the cervix.[24]

The virus is mostly in macrophages at the mucosal border and around the deep lymphatics, which may reflect spread of the virus from the cervix to the regional lymph nodes and then to the rest of the body.

2. HIV-1 myopathy is associated with activated HIV-1 infection of macrophages and myocytes in areas of muscle necrosis.[1]
3. AIDS dementia is associated with activated viral infection of neurons, astrocytes, and microglial cells, whereas HIV-1 is present as a latent infection in microglial cells in AIDS patients without CNS symptoms.[23]
4. In the asymptomatic patient, HIV-1 infects up to 50% of the CD4 cells in lymph nodes and 1% to 10% of the CD4 cells in the peripheral blood. As the disease progresses, 80% to 90% of these cells at these sites contain activated HIV-1 infection.[1]

Other viral infections

In situ hybridization has proved useful in documenting other viral infections where cytomorphologic features in tissue may be inapparent. These include adenovirus,[17] herpes simplex virus,[27,28] and measles virus.[30] The technique may be particularly useful when multiple viral infections occur simultaneously.[28]

Other applications

Aside from aiding the diagnosis of infection, in situ hybridization has shown extreme promise in the identification of chromosomal disorders. Fluorescent in situ hybridization (FISH), discussed in Chapter 12, utilizes fluorescently labeled probes to detect numerical abnormalities of chromosome copies, rearrangements, and translocations. This method may supplement or replace several types of cytogenetic analysis.

In situ hybridization has also been proposed in the analysis of certain human tumors[30,31] as a rapid and sensitive assay for the study of oncogenes.[32]

REFERENCES

1. Nuovo GJ: *PCR in situ hybridization: protocols and applications,* ed 2, New York, 1993, Raven Press.
2. Wilkinson DG: *In situ hybridization: a practical approach,* New York, 1992, Oxford University Press.
3. Blumberg DD: *Methods Enzymol* 152:3, 1987.
4. Nuovo GJ: A comparison of different in situ hybridization methodologies (biotin and ^{35}S based) for the detection of HPV DNA, *Lab Invest* 61:471,1989.
5. Gentilomi G, Musiani M, Zerbini M et al: Double in situ hybridization for detection of herpes simplex virus and cytomegalovirus DNA using non-radioactive probes, *J Histochem Cytochem* 40:421, 1992.
6. Nuovo GJ: *Cytopathology of the female genital tract: an integrated approach,* Baltimore, 1993, Williams & Wilkins.
7. Crum CP, Nuovo GJ: *Genital papillomaviruses and related neoplasms,* New York, 1991, Raven Press.
8. Nuovo GJ, Friedman D, Richard RM: In situ hybridization analysis of HPV DNA: segregation patterns of lesions of the female genital tract, *Gynecol Oncol* 36:256, 1990.
9. Nuovo GJ, Becker J, MacConnell P et al: Histological distribution of PCR-amplified HPV 6 and 11 DNA in penile lesions, *Am J Surg Pathol* 16:269, 1992.
10. von Einsiedel RW, Fife TD, Aksamit AJ et al: Progressive multifocal leukoencephalopathy in AIDS: a clinicopathologic study and review of the literature, *J Neurol* 240:391, 1993.
11. Mori M, Kurata H, Tajima M et al: JC virus detection by in situ hybridization in brain tissue from elderly patients, *Ann Neurol* 29:428, 1991.
12. Hair LS, Nuovo GJ, Powers JM: Progressive multifocal leukoencephalopathy in patients with human immunodeficiency virus infection, *Hum Pathol* 23:663,1992
13. Moret H, Guichard M, Matheron S et al: Virological diagnosis of progressive multifocal leukoencephalopathy: detection of JC virus DNA in cerebrospinal fluid and brain tissue of AIDS patients, *J Clin Microbiol* 31:3310, 1993.
14. Iwa N, Sasaki M, Yutani C et al: Detection of cytomegalovirus DNA in pulmonary specimens: confirmation by in situ hybridization in two cases, *Diagn Cytopathol* 8:357, 1992.
15. Weiss RL, Snow GW, Schumann GB et al: Diagnosis of cytomegalovirus pneumonitis on bronchoalveolar lavage fluid: comparison of cytology, immunofluorescence, and in situ hybridization with viral isolation, *Diagn Cytopathol* 7:243, 1991.
16. Delvenne P, Margiotta M, Nuovo GJ: Comparison of in situ hybridization and immunochemistry for the detection of cytomegalovirus infection, *J Histotech* 16:27, 1993.
17. Nuovo MA, Nuovo GJ, Becker J: Correlation of concomitent viral infection and mortality in patients with pneumocystis pneumonia: an analysis by in situ hybridization and PCR, *Diag Mol Pathol* 2:200, 1993.
18. Greco MA, Wieczorek R, Sachdev R et al: Phenotype of villous stromal cells in placentas with cytomegalovirus, syphilis, and nonspecific villitis, *Am J Pathol* 141:835, 1992.
19. Berg LC, Copenhaver CM, Morrison VA et al: B-cell lymphoproliferative disorders in solid-organ transplant patients: detection of Epstein-Barr virus by in situ hybridization, *Hum Pathol* 23:159, 1992.
20. Randhawa PS, Jaffe R, Demetris AJ et al: The systemic distribution of Epstein-Barr virus genomes in fatal post-transplantation lymphoproliferative disorders: an in situ hybridization study, *Am J Pathol* 138:1027, 1991.
21. Strickler JG, Rooney MT, d'Amore ES et al: Detection of Epstein-Barr virus by in situ hybridization with a commercially available biotinylated oligonucleiotide probe, *Mod Pathol* 6:208, 1993.
22. Embretson J, Zupancic M, Beneke J et al: Analysis of human immunodeficiency virus infected tissues by amplification and in situ hybridization reveals latent and permissive infections at single cell resolution, *Proc Natl Acad Sci USA* 90:357, 1993.
23. Nuovo GJ, Gallery F, Bravin A: In situ detection of PCR-ampliphied HIV-1 nucleic acids and tumor necrosis factor RNA in the central nervous system, *Am J Pathol* 144:659, 1994.
24. Nuovo GJ, Forde A, MacConnell P, Fahrenwald R: In situ detection of PCR-amplified HIV-1 nucleic acids and tumor necrosis factor cDNA in cervical tissues, *Am J Pathol,* 143: 40, 1993.
25. Nuovo GJ, Lidonocci K, MacConnell P, Lane B: Intracellular localization of PCR-amplified hepatitis C cDNA, *Am J Pathol,* 17: 683, 1993.
26. Haruna Y, Hayashi N, Hiramatsu N et al: Detection of hepatitis C virus RNA in liver tissues by an in situ hybridization technique, *J Hepatol* 18:96, 1993.
27. Tomita T, Chiga M, Lenahan M et al: Identification of herpes simplex virus infection by immunoperoxidase and in situ hybridization methods, *Virchows Arch A, Pathol-Anat Histopathol* 419:99, 1991.
28. Strickler JG, Manivel JC, Copenhaver CM et al: Comparison of in situ hybridization and immunohistochemistry for detection of cytomegalovirus and herpes simplex virus, *Hum Pathol* 21:443, 1990.
29. Nuovo MA, Nuovo GJ, MacConnell P, Steiner G: Analysis of Paget's disease of bone for the measles virus using the reverse transcriptase in situ polymerase chain reaction technique, *Diagn Mol Pathol* 1: 256, 1993.
30. Varagona G, Brown D, Haase A et al: Increased steady-state levels of alpha-fetoprotein mRNA in hepatocellular carcinoma: an analysis by in situ hybridization, *Liver* 12:62, 1992.
31. Shorrock K, Roberts P, Pringle JH et al: Demonstration of insulin and glucagon mRNA in routinely fixed and processed pancreatic tissue by in situ hybridization, *J Pathol* 165:105, 1991.
32. Nuovo GJ, MacConnell P, French D: Correlation of the in situ detection of PCR-ampliphied metalloprotease cDNA and their inhibitors with prognosis in cervical carcinoma, *Cancer Res* 55:267, 1995.
33. Loda M: Polymerase chain reaction-based methods for detection of mutations in oncogenes and tumor supressor genes, *Hum Pathol* 25:564, 1994.

11 Diagnostic Molecular Pathology

Adam Bagg
Jeffrey Cossman

The rapid transition and application of molecular biologic techniques, once the exclusive realm of research laboratories, to diagnostic pathology, has resulted in the availability of indispensable tools for a multitude of uses in the diagnostic laboratory. One of the major advantages of these techniques is that they allow for tissue analysis and diagnosis without requiring an evaluation of the disease phenotype or the associated protein defect. Their power lies in the ability to sensitively and specifically detect abnormalities at the level of DNA (or RNA), rather than by studying the protein products or morphologic expression of the abnormal gene. Indeed, diagnosis can be established in the absence of morphologic changes or discernible protein expression.

It is now accepted that most diseases, whether congenital or acquired, have a genetic basis. Although conventional teaching considered genetics only in the context of congenital or inherited diseases, the term *genetic* is now understood to be applicable to acquired diseases as well. Acquired diseases occur as a consequence of the expression of "abnormal" genes, such as the creation of an aberrant gene (as in neoplasia) or related to their pathologic presence (such as infectious diseases). Accordingly, DNA/RNA-based molecular techniques have utility in virtually every area of diagnostic pathology, including neoplastic disorders, infectious diseases, inherited conditions, and the determination of identity (including forensic pathology, paternity testing, and transplantation).

The purpose of this chapter is to detail the molecular diagnostic and molecular genetic methodologies of relevance in a molecular diagnostic laboratory as well as to discuss the interpretation of molecular method–based assays. The first section is a description of methods of broad application to molecular diagnostics, and the second deals with specific methodologies.

FUNDAMENTALS OF TECHNIQUES

Structure of a molecular diagnostic laboratory

A diagnostic molecular laboratory, as with any other diagnostic laboratory, must have established procedures for accessioning samples, techniques, procedures to monitor work flow, issuing of reports, and quality assurance. There are, however, many components that are unique to a molecular diagnostics laboratory.[1,2] These include the following: (1) *Personnel.* Given the ongoing transition of molecular technology from research to diagnostic laboratories, an essential member of the staff is a research-trained scientist whose experience in molecular biology is crucial for the troubleshooting peculiar to molecular biology. (2) *Specimen bank.* In many clinical situations, particularly in oncology, there is a need for retrospective studies, such as comparing current (posttreatment) samples with previous (presentation) samples. To facilitate such analyses, it is important that a user-friendly banking system be established for easy access to previously collected material. (3) *Specialized equipment.* Specific equipment, not normally present in a clinical laboratory but usually found in a research laboratory, is essential for a diagnostic molecular laboratory. A partial list of some of the equipment required is presented in Table 11-1. Depending on the work flow, some duplication of equipment is necessary. This is particularly crucial in laboratories where polymerase chain reaction (PCR) assays are performed, as a consequence of the need to physically separate preamplification and postamplification work areas (see p. 206). A variety of

Table 11-1 Equipment required for a molecular diagnostics laboratory

Freezers (−20° and −70° C)
Vortex mixers
Horizontal and angle-head microcentrifuges
Spectrophotometer (ultraviolet)
Electrophoresis (agarose and polyacrylamide) apparatus and power supply
Ultraviolet transilluminator
Autoradiography cassettes
Dark room with automated x-ray film processor
Laminar flow hoods
Thermocycler
Oligonucleotide synthesizer
DNA-sequencing equipment
Light boxes
Computer hardware and software

Table 11-2 Reagents and supplies used in molecular diagnostics

Phenol and chloroform for nucleotide extraction
Guanidium isothiocyanate for RNA extraction
dNTPs (unlabeled and ^{32}P labeled or biotin labeled)
Ethidium bromide for gel staining
Kits for labeling reactions (nick translation, random hexamer, end labeling)
Polymerases, including *Taq* polymerase
Microcentrifuge tubes
Positive displacement pipettes
Supplies for radiation safety

relatively unique reagents and supplies are required for molecular biology assays, and some of those more commonly used are listed in Table 11-2.

DNA and RNA extraction

Originally, DNA and RNA extraction was only optimally achieved from fresh or frozen, unfixed tissue, limiting the sources from which molecular analyses could be performed. Currently, however, virtually all pathologic material is suitable for nucleotide extraction, and methods now in practice yield DNA from formalin-fixed, paraffin-embedded tissues,[3] and RNA from small volumes of whole blood[4] or glass slides.[5] Indeed, DNA and RNA can be isolated from a single cell, amplified, and analyzed[6] (see below).

Generally, DNA extraction is simpler to perform than RNA extraction.[7] The initial step involves the lysis of the cells, usually performed with a detergent such as sodium dodecyl sulfate (SDS). Proteinase K is used both to release the DNA from the chromatin and to destroy DNAases. DNAases can also be inhibited through their heat sensitivity (65° C for 5 minutes) or with high concentrations of the chelating agent EDTA. Cellular macromolecules, including proteins, are removed by extraction of the sample in phenol or chloroform, or both, which also function to inactivate and remove any excess proteinase (which would otherwise interfere with the subsequent action of the restriction endonucleases required for DNA digestion). After this extraction step, the DNA is concentrated by ethanol precipitation in the presence of acetate salts. The DNA is then brought into solution with a buffer or distilled water, and its concentration is assessed by measurement of the optical density of the solution at a wavelength of 260 nm (ultraviolet light). The sample is then ready for further processing, or it can be stored for long periods of time. If stored for a period up to 1 year, a 4° C refrigerator is sufficient, but for longer periods, −20° C freezing is required.

Table 11-3 Strategies for dealing with RNAases

Dry heating of glass supplies, >200° C for 2 hours (autoclaving alone insufficient)
1M NaOH for plastic ware
Triple distilled water
Diethylpyrocarbonate addition (used less frequently)
Designated laboratory area for RNA work
Disposable gloves, with frequent changing
Guanidium isothiocyanate

By contrast to DNA extraction, RNA extraction[8] is complicated by the need to remove ubiquitously present RNAases, which may be endogenous or exogenous, or both. Endogenous ribonucleases are those normally found in the tissues from which the RNA is extracted, and certain specimens such as placenta, tumors, and liver contain abundant amounts of RNAase. The serum component of tissue culture media is also richly endowed with RNAases, and so thorough cell washing is required before lysis. The skin (and hence all laboratory equipment that is touched by bare hands) contains nucleases and is the usual source of exogenous RNAases. Numerous strategies exist for the removal and inhibition of this major nemesis of the molecular biologist (Table 11-3).

The chaotropic agent guanidium isothiocyanate (GITC) is one of the most effective reagents for RNA extraction. In addition to temporarily inhibiting RNAases, it also facilitates the removal of proteins from RNA. GITC, in conjunction with acid phenol, is popularly used for routine RNA extraction.[9] As for DNA, RNA is also quantitated by measurement of optical density at 260 nm. Although DNA may be suitably stored at 4° C, RNA is not so robust and needs to be kept at much lower temperatures (−70° C).

More recently developed extraction techniques, which lend themselves to automation, have simplified matters considerably, allowing for the rapid yield of DNA and RNA.

Preparation of DNA for analysis

Digestion

The DNA obtained from the extraction step is somewhat unwieldy, mainly because of its high molecular weight, and usually needs to be further processed to allow for optimal analysis. An invaluable tool in molecular diagnostics is the restriction endonuclease (RE), which facilitates the production of small fragments of DNA that are amenable to easier manipulation and analysis.[10] These REs are obtained from bacteria (from which they derive their names, such as *Hind III* is derived from *H*emophilus *in*fluenza strain *d* and was the third *[III]* RE isolated from this bacterium), and they specifically recognize stretches of DNA between 4 and 10 base pairs long, catalyzing the cleavage of the DNA molecule wherever the specific sequence occurs in the genome. Most REs in routine use recognize a 6 base-pair sequence, which is almost always palindromic. The cleavage of the DNA by REs results in the generation of a heterogeneous mixture of different-sized pieces of DNA, called "restriction fragments." Although the digestion step is performed in a tube, usually a small microcentrifuge tube, the separation of these fragments is achieved by agarose gel electrophoresis. With the appropriate buffer, pH, and electric field, the DNA fragments will separate according to their size. Conventional gel electrophoresis, with a linear electric field, can segregate DNA fragments up to approximately 25 kilobases in size. Alternative strategies, such as pulsed-field gel electrophoresis (PFGE), are required for separating larger DNA fragments, up to a few hundred kilobases long.[11] This form of electrophoresis utilizes a current that alternates directions. These larger DNA fragments are generated through the use of infrequently cutting REs, such as *NotI*. The infrequent cutters have to recognize 8 base-pair sequences, which statistically occur less frequently (every 4^8 base pairs) than the 6 base-pair (every 4^6 base pairs) sequences recognized by the conventionally used REs, and hence yield larger DNA fragments.

Electrophoresis of RNA is also based upon size separation in an electric field, but the different and complex secondary structure of RNA molecules, in particular related to intramolecular hybridization, requires formaldehyde denaturing gels.

Denaturation

Most molecular diagnostic techniques exploit the Watson-Crick base-pairing and complementary nature of DNA. This refers to the double stranding (ds) of DNA, with one strand always and predictably complementary to the opposite strand. Adenine (A) is always bound to thymidine (T), and guanine (G) is always bound to cytosine (C). Many molecular biologic assays involve the separation of these strands, exposing the bases, which allows the specific binding of an added stretch of nucleotides, either in the form of a probe (for the actual detection of a sequence of interest) or a primer (a critical component of the polymerase chain reaction, see below). Separation of the DNA strands (by denaturation or melting) is usually achieved by heating. The temperature required to dissociate this double-stranded molecule is predictable and depends on the relative GC content of the DNA molecule (G-C bonds are stronger, because of 3 hydrogen bonds between the two molecules, as compared with A-T, which is held together by 2 hydrogen bonds). Electrophoretic gels are clearly not suitable for denaturation by heating, and so alkaline solutions are employed to separate the dsDNA strands required for probe hybridization.

Preparation of RNA for analysis

Many but not all of the techniques analyzing RNA require the enrichment of mRNA, that component of RNA that is transcribed from DNA and translated into protein. Enrichment is necessary since mRNA accounts for only 1% of the total cellular RNA and is performed by exploiting the presence of the poly(A) tail present on the mRNA. This is achieved with a column or beads of oligo(dT)-cellulose and subsequent elution of the mRNA.[12]

Transfer

The electrophoretic gel used to separate the fragments of DNA (or various-sized species of mRNA) is not amenable to probe hybridization, and hence these nucleotide fragments need to be transferred to a solid support where specific probing can be performed. The transfer of DNA through capillary action onto this solid support (membrane or filter) is called Southern blotting,[13] named after its original developer. This eponymous description has subsequently been expanded upon to describe the terms for RNA blotting (northern blot), protein blotting (western blot), and protein-DNA blotting (southwestern blot). Transfer by capillary action is usually performed overnight, but it may be facilitated by vacuum and electrotransfer. The time taken for standard capillary transfer can also be significantly reduced under alkaline conditions.[14] It is not always necessary to digest and electrophorese DNA before transfer to the membrane: the unmanipulated DNA may be simply spotted, or dotted, onto the membrane (dot-blot). Dot-blotting is performed to determine whether a genetic sequence (normal or abnormal) is present or absent, without any requirement for knowing the size of the fragment to which the probe is hybridizing. Manifolds may be used to enhance this transfer through wells (slot-blot). Once the DNA sample has been transferred, it needs to be immobilized onto the membrane to ensure that it remains present during the washing step of probing and also to allow for repeat analyses using different probes. Traditionally used membranes are made from nitrocellulose, in which the DNA is immobilized by baking. However, nylon membranes, to which the DNA is cross-linked by ultraviolet light, are currently more popular because they are hardier and easier to work with, particularly for stripping and reprobing. Charge-based membranes need no further treatment to facilitate DNA binding.

Probes and probing

A probe refers to a stretch of nucleotides (from a few base pairs to a few thousand base pairs) that is used to detect a specific region of DNA or RNA, as a function of its complementarity to the target sequence.[15] A prerequisite is some fundamental knowledge of the base sequence of the target. Probes vary in both size and source (Tables 11-4 and 11-5).

Those derived from native DNA are referred to as genomic probes and essentially mirror a region of DNA and may include both exonic (that part of the gene that is transcribed into mRNA and contains the coding regions that will be translated into protein) and intronic (nontranscribed part of the gene, or intervening sequence) regions. A probe derived from RNA is a cDNA probe (in that the DNA is synthesized from the RNA by the enzyme reverse transcriptase in a *complementary* fashion) and will, by definition, recognize only exons. Whereas genomic DNA and cDNA probes are derived from cellular material, a third form of probe is synthesized in the laboratory. These oligonucleotide probes are typically much shorter than the other two types of probes (usually 15 to 30 bases). Synthetic oligonucleotide probes can be designed to

Table 11-4 Types of probes

Type	Source
Genomic DNA	Cloned cellular DNA
cDNA	Reverse transcribed cellular mRNA
Oligonucleotide	DNA synthesizer
Riboprobe	In vitro transcription system

distinguish between normal and abnormal genomic sequences, referred to as allele-specific oligonucleotide (ASO) probes (see the discussion of mutational analysis, p. 209). Riboprobes, or labeled RNA probes, are made using in vitro transcription systems (that is, they are transcribed from DNA), using RNA polymerase and labeled ribonucleotides. These riboprobes are used primarily for in situ hybridization (ISH).

A variety of vectors are available for the propagation of probes (Table 11-5), so that sufficient amounts can be generated for the actual probing, with the form of vector dependent on the size of the probe.

The concept of probe binding to target exploits the complementary nature of DNA, alluded to above, with this binding (hybridization)[16] essentially being the corollary of denaturation. Indeed, before one adds a dsDNA probe to a membrane, it needs to be denatured (usually by boiling) to allow for the exposure of the nucleotides required for hybridization. Single-stranded probes (oligonucleotides) do not require a denaturing step. The binding of probe or primer DNA to the target DNA is temperature dependent. Generally, for genomic probes, optimal binding occurs at temperatures in the range of 25° C below the Tm (temperature at which 50% of the dsDNA is separated/bound) of the target DNA-probe hybrid. By contrast, temperatures of only 5° C below the Tm are suitable for oligonucleotide probes. Two considerations need to be balanced in this context: lower temperatures will increase binding, enhancing the sensitivity, whereas an increase in temperature will decrease the binding (referred to as *increased stringency*) and hence enhance specificity. The opposite of stringent hybridization conditions is referred to as relaxed. Other factors also affect DNA denaturation and binding (Table 11-6), such as ionic strength of the solution and the concentration of formamide, and these are varied depending on the specific application. The ionic strength of a hybridization solution is usually provided by the buffer SSC (a mixture of sodium chloride and sodium citrate). Genomic probes often require the addition of dextran sulfate to optimize the rate of hybridization, but this reagent can be omitted in reactions using oligonucleotide probes. Modifications of conventional hybridization include sandwich assays using solid supports, affinity-based hybrid collection performed in solution, and reversed hybridization in which the sample is labeled rather than the probe or probes, which can be immobilized and used as a panel.

Stringency factors are manipulated, not only at the hybridization stage of the procedure, but also at the time of washing. These factors are usually altered in the washing stage, to increase the stringency. For example, although the salt concentration used for hybridization is of the order of 5 × SSC, a much lower concentration, such as 0.1 × SSC, may be used for washing.

Detection systems. Probes need to be further manipulated by the artificial incorporation of a label, allowing for the detection of the specific binding of the probe to the target sequence (Table 11-7). The initial labeling step is performed before hybridization.

Nick translation is one method of labeling DNA probes,[17] in which the enzyme DNAase is added to the probe, to create breaks or "nicks" in the dsDNA, at the site of the phosphodiester bond. A second enzyme, DNA polymerase I, is then employed to remove nucleotides at the site of the nicks and replace them with free nucleotides (some of which have been modified to allow for their detection; see below) which have been added to the reaction mixture. A second, and perhaps more popular method for probe labeling, is random hexamer priming, in which the double-stranding (ds) probe is first denatured. Subsequently, random hexamers (arbitrary stretches of six nucleotides) are added to serve as templates for DNA synthesis. The polymerase used for random hexamer labeling is not the same as that used in nick translation (this latter poly-

Table 11-5 Probe propagation

Vector or source	Approximate maximum probe size (bp)
DNA synthesizer	50
Thermocycler	1000
Plasmid	6000
Bacteriophage	20,000
Cosmid	45,000
YAC	1,000,000

bp, base pair; *cosmid,* combination of *cos* site of bacteriophage and a plas*mid; YAC,* yeast artificial chromosome, of particular utility in fluorescent in situ hybridization.

Table 11-6 Factors affecting hybridization and stringency

	When variable is increased or present	
Variable	Hybridization	Stringency
Temperature	↓	↑
Salt concentration (SSC)	↑	↓
Denaturing agent (formamide)	↓	↑
HMW polymer (dextran SO_4)	↑	–*

*Dextran sulfate affects the rate of reaching binding equilibrium, rather than stringency per se.

Table 11-7 Detection systems

- Methods of labeling
  - Nick translation
  - Random hexamer priming
  - End labeling (kinase, terminal deoxynucleotidyl transferase [Tdt], or polymerase)
  - Polymerase chain reaction
- Visualization
  - Isotopic
    - ^{32}P, ^{3}H, ^{35}S
  - Nonisotopic
    - Biotin-avidin
    - Digoxigenin
    - Enzymes (phosphatase, peroxidase)
    - Chemiluminescence

Table 11-8 Comparison of different probe-labeling systems

Parameter	^{32}P	Digoxigenin	Chemiluminescence
Shelf life of labeled probe	<6 weeks	>1 year	>6 months
Hybridization time	>16 hours	>6 hours	1 hour
Detection time	usually days	12-16 hours	1 hour
Sensitivity (detection limit for single-copy genes)	10^{-14} grams	10^{-13} grams	10^{-8} grams

merase has exonuclease activity, which removes nucleotides). Rather, a fragment of DNA polymerase I (the Klenow fragment), which does not have exonuclease activity, is used to incorporate the free nucleotides to fill the gaps between the random hexamers. The added nucleotides, in any labeling system, first have to be modified, to facilitate detection. This modification may be isotopic or nonisotopic. ^{32}P-triphosphates are used for isotopic labeling, whereas biotin (incorporated into a nucleotide) can be used for nonisotopic detection.[17]

After appropriately stringent washing (to remove nonspecifically bound probe), the specific binding of the probe needs to be visualized, and the method depends on how the probe was initially labeled. For radioactively labeled probes, autoradiography is used, in which the membrane is exposed to an x-ray film at −70° C, often for periods as long as 10 to 14 days. The hybridization of the probe to specific target sequences is detected by subsequent development of the x-ray film. For in situ hybridization (see Chapter 10), isotopes different from ^{32}P are used, such as ^{3}H and ^{35}S. These isotopes have lower energy emissions than ^{32}P does, and their relatively retarded travel through the photographic emulsion optimizes intracellular localization. Biotin is visualized with avidin- or streptavidin-labeled enzyme (and substrate), which exploits the binding of these compounds to the biotin.[18] Binding of biotin-labeled probes can also be measured spectrophotometrically, by evaluation of the change in color generated by the addition of a chromogenic substrate for the enzyme. The biotin may be substituted with another compound, digoxigenin. This steroid hapten is then detected by use of antidigoxigenin conjugated to an enzyme. A third strategy for visualizing probe binding to target is through chemiluminescence, which can be detected either luminometrically or on photographic film as for autoradiography. Although nonradioactive probe systems are somewhat less sensitive than those using radioisotopes, their advantages include the avoidance of radioactive hazard, stability of reagents over longer periods, shorter assay time, and relative inexpense of reagents (Table 11-8).

SPECIFIC TECHNIQUES

DNA analysis

There are several ways in which DNA can be analyzed, and a few of the more commonly used methods are detailed here.[19] The analysis of amplified DNA is discussed on page 206, concerning the polymerase chain reaction.

Slot- and dot-blots

For slot-blot and dot-blot hybridizations, the DNA sample is directly bound to the membrane, without prior digestion and electrophoresis, but the sample still needs to be denatured so that hybridization can occur. This application is ideally suited to assaying multiple samples and also for semiquantitation, using serial dilutions of template DNA.

Southern blot

Southern blotting is similar in principle to slot and dot blotting, but there are prior steps of DNA digestion and separation of the fragments by size, allowing for the identification of specifically sized DNA fragments (Fig. 11-1).

In addition to the requirement for denaturation, usually performed by alkaline (NaOH) treatment of the gel, it is often necessary to partially hydrolyze the DNA to facilitate the transfer of the larger DNA fragments. This latter step, called *depurination,* is achieved by incubation of the gel in a mild acid (HCl) solution. The depurinated and denatured DNA fragments are carried by capillary action from the gel to the membrane. After this, the DNA is fixed onto the membrane by baking (nitrocellulose) or with ultraviolet light (nylon). The membrane is now ready to be probed.

Two broad types of probes can be used. The differences here are defined not in terms of their origin alluded to in Table 11-4, but rather in terms of their hybridization target. These probes can be considered *specific,* if they are homologous to a known gene, or *linked,* if they are likely to be associated with or near a gene, which may be *unknown,* but is believed to be associated with a particular disease or locus. These two types of analyses are also referred to as *direct* and *indirect* analysis, respectively. With direct analysis, the gene that is responsible for the disease or condition being studied has been relatively well characterized, whereas in indirect analysis the incriminating gene has not been identified, and its presence, or abnormalities thereof, can be inferred by the use of linked probes.

Linkage analysis

The use of linked probes is termed *linkage analysis.*[20] An allele is defined as being linked to the disease-causing gene if it is found in affected individuals at a frequency greater than that expected by chance alone. Linkage-analysis studies have been most applicable to the study of inherited diseases. It is important to remember that the marker allele is not, in itself, the cause of the disease but provides a useful tool to indirectly track genes. Linkage analyses are limited in that they can be employed only when polymorphisms exist at a particular locus. Another prerequisite is that there must be a family with several affected individuals, all of whom are available for study. In addition, another limitation is that not all affected families will be informative for a particular linked polymorphic marker.

RFLP and VNTR

Two broad categories of polymorphisms can be detected at the DNA level (Fig. 11-2). These restriction fragment length poly-

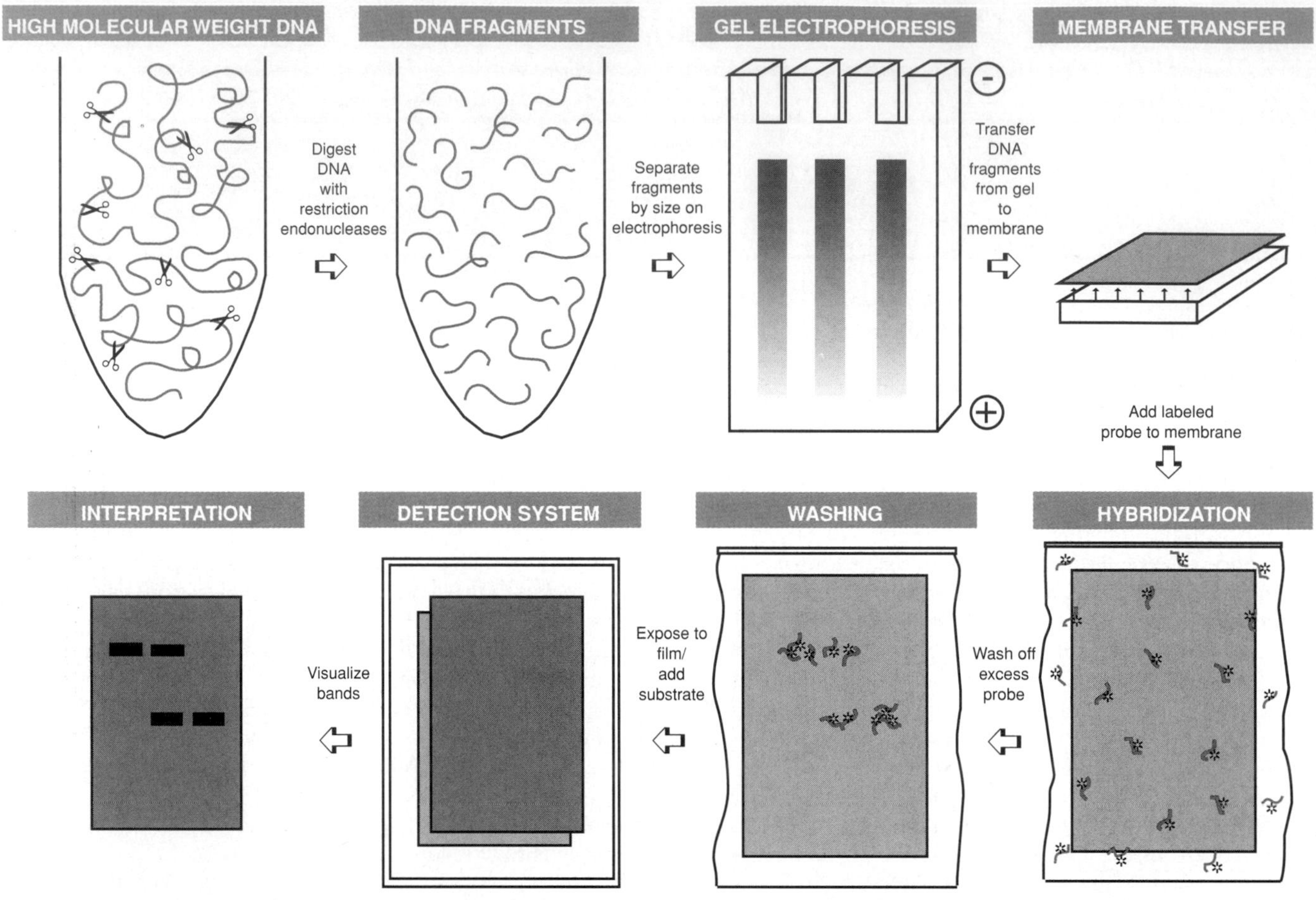

Fig. 11-1 Southern blotting. Diagram of the steps involved in conventional Southern blot analysis. Although the actual Southern blot component refers specifically to the membrane transfer step *(upper right),* the whole procedure, from DNA digestion to detection, is generically referred to as *Southern analysis.*

morphisms (RFLPs) may be attributable to, among others, single base mutations or to variable number of tandem repeats (VNTRs).[21] An RFLP refers to a specific fragment of DNA, created by restriction endonuclease (RE) digestion of the genomic DNA, which differs in length from one individual to another or at the two alleles of the gene in a single individual. RFLPs occurring as a consequence of nucleotide differences, which are found at approximately 1 base per 200 and which result in the creation or loss of a RE digestion site, have proved to be useful in linkage analysis. The nucleotide substitutions most often are neutral in that they have no functional significance (usually occurring in noncoding regions or introns) and are inherited in a mendelian fashion. VNTRs, on the other hand, are composed of short sequences of DNA that are repeated multiple times, and they are also referred to as *minisatellite DNA sequences.*[22] This phenomenon can be used to generate an individual specific Southern blot pattern and is exploited for DNA fingerprinting for identity determination (see below). These tandemly repeated sequences of DNA range in length (approximately 35 base pairs long) and occur approximately once every 30 to 60 kilobases. It is believed that they play a functional role in recombination or gene regulation. Even smaller than minisatellites of the VNTR are the recently described microsatellites, which are probably even more polymorphic, with each locus capable of producing numerous alleles varying in length by as few as 2 base pairs.

So, linked probes recognize regions in and around genes, without our necessarily understanding that gene's function or having any knowledge of what it is that the probe recognizes. The distance between the two loci (that recognized by the linked probe and the actual disease-associated gene) is measured in units called *centimorgans* (cM). One cM is defined as a stretch of DNA that has a 1% chance of recombination at the time of meiosis and is roughly equivalent to 10^6 base pairs. For example, if the linked region is separated from the gene by 5 cM, there is a 5% chance of recombination (and hence potential for loss of linkage) at meiosis. These highly variable genetic markers initially serve to evaluate families with a particular hereditary disease and provide an indirect method of not only tracking the segregation of the gene through generations, but also for the localization of the gene to a particular chromosome and ultimately to identify the gene responsible for the disease. This strategy of *positional cloning* has led to the identification of the genes responsible for, among others, chronic granulomatous disease, cystic fibrosis, neurofibromatosis, fragile X syndrome, myotonic dystrophy, Charcot-Marie-Tooth syndrome, and Kallman's syndrome (see the discussion of inherited genetic diseases, p. 215). In other situations (such as adult polycystic kidney disease), genetic linkage markers have a diagnostic sensitivity of greater than 95%, despite the fact that the causative gene has not yet been isolated.

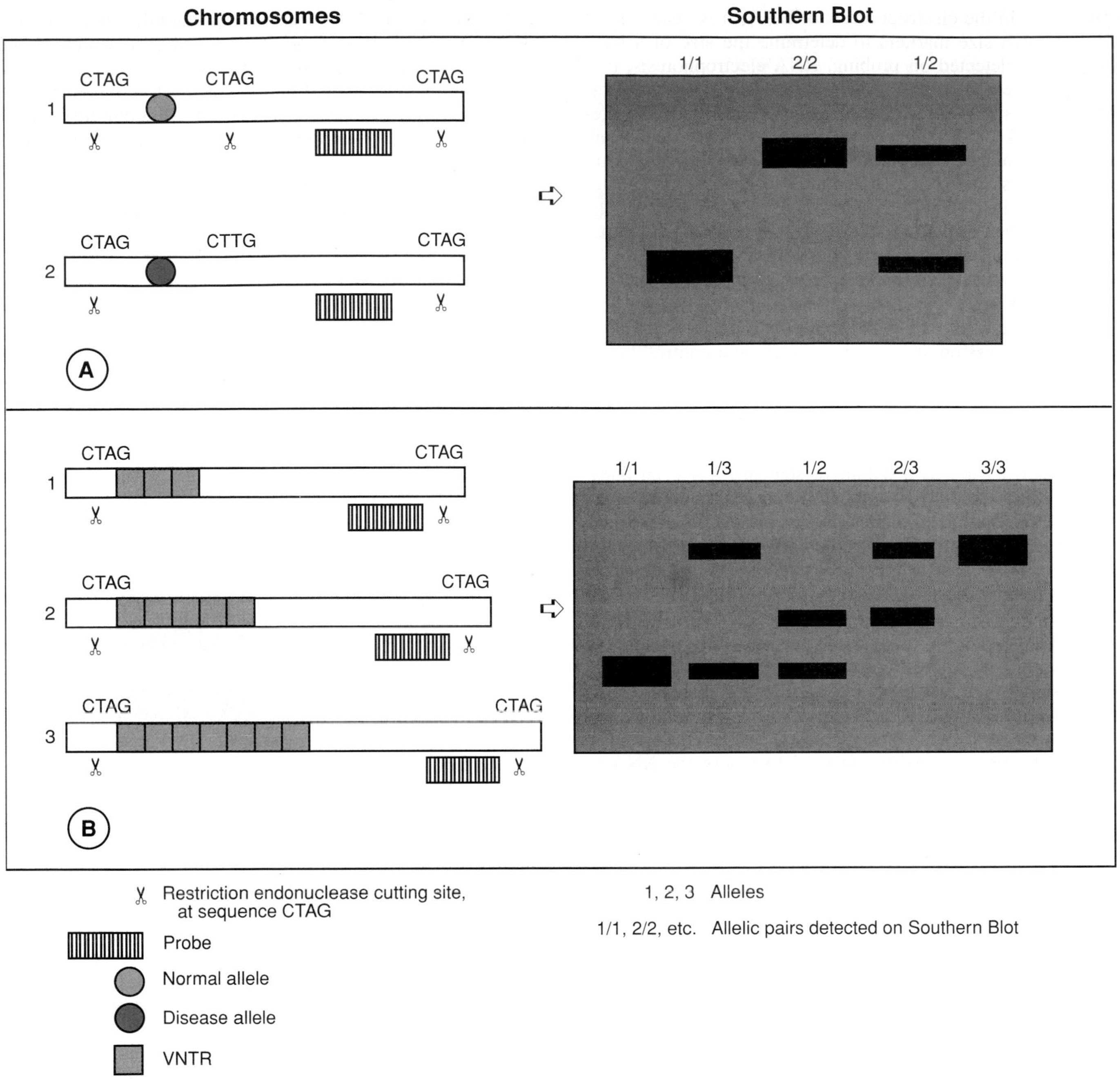

Fig. 11-2 **A**, Restriction fragment length polymorphisms attributable to a single base substitution (A→T). This results in the loss of the sequence (CTAG) recognized and cut by the restriction endonuclease, so that a different sized fragment will hybridize with the probe. There are three possible Southern blot profiles, depending on whether the substitution is present (one or both alleles) or absent. In this example, allele 2 is associated with a particular disease, and hence can be used for linkage analysis. **B**, Restriction fragment length polymorphisms are attributable to a variable number of tandem repeats. In this situation, different-sized fragments are generated because of the presence of repeat sequences (*stippled boxes*). No change occurs at the actual site of restriction endonuclease digestion (as in **A**), with the different fragment sizes being generated because of the digestion sites being closer together or farther apart. Five of the possible combinations are shown in Southern blot.

RNA analysis

Northern blotting[23] is the RNA equivalent of Southern blotting, but there are several critical procedural differences related to the inherent differences between RNA and DNA. For example, no restriction enzyme digestion is needed. Since RNA is single stranded, one would assume that denaturation is not required. However, the complex secondary structure of RNA molecules necessitates a denaturing step. Instead of heating or alkaline treatment used for DNA denaturation, RNA is most commonly denatured with formaldehyde or formamide (formaldehyde is often included in the gel, whereas formamide is usually added to the RNA sample before loading for elec-

phenotype or function of the protein. Mutations may be transmitted in the germ line or they may be somatically acquired. The presence of a mutation may be inferred indirectly, using linkage analysis and RFLPs, referred to earlier. There are, however, numerous approaches available for the direct detection of mutations[44] (Table 11-11).

Many of these procedures, whether screening or diagnostic, have been greatly facilitated by PCR, which has significantly influenced both the speed and sensitivity of these assays. Indeed, preamplification of the target sequence is an integral part of most assays. LCR and ARMS are discussed in the previous section on PCR. ARMS is a particularly sensitive method for mutational detection, being able to discern rarely occurring mutants in the background of a huge excess of the normal allele.

Direct sequencing. This is the standard for the detection of single base substitutions. The two most commonly employed methods are the chemical technique of Maxam and Gilbert[45] and the dideoxy chain termination method of Sanger.[46] The latter method is currently more popular. These techniques are somewhat cumbersome, though they can now be automated[47] by commercially available instruments.

SSCP. The single stranded conformation polymorphism assay is a relatively simple technique, useful in the initial screening for mutations.[48] DNA segments are obtained either by RE digestion of genomic DNA or by PCR amplification of a defined sequence. This DNA sample is then denatured (by alkaline treatment or heating) and electrophoresed in a neutral/nondenaturing polyacrylamide gel. Nucleotide substitution, presumably by alteration of the conformation of the ssDNA, causes a mobility shift of that fragment. It is always important to run wild type DNA at the same time, to look for differences between the band patterns of the normal and test DNA. The presence of an abnormal band in the latter indicates that there is a mutation, and this band can be cut out of the gel and subsequently directly sequenced.

DGGE. Denaturing gradient gel electrophoresis is able to separate DNA strands of less than 1 kilobase in length that contain single mutations.[49] These DNA strands are first generated by PCR and then separated by polyacrylamide gel electrophoresis. However, as compared with SSCP, the gel contains a linear gradient of DNA denaturants (urea, formamide). DNA migration is retarded when it is melted (denatured) by the denaturant, with the melting property being a function of the nucleotide sequence. A modification of conventional DGGE is thermal gradient gel electrophoresis, in which both a temperature and chemical denaturing gradient exists within the gel.

ASO probing. The DNA product obtained from PCR is dot blotted onto a solid support filter. Two different probes are used for the hybridization: one that recognizes the normal allele and another that will only hybridize to the gene containing the mutation.[50] The specific binding of the allele specific oligonucleotide (ASO) is ensured by appropriately stringent hybridization and washing, such that only a completely complementary oligonucleotide probe will bind stably to the different target sequences. If the number of possible alleles is very large, reverse dot blotting can be used. In this format, a panel of oligonucleotide probes is immobilized onto the filter and allowed to hybridize to a labeled PCR product. Applications of this reverse technique include HLA and forensic testing, and diagnosis of beta-thalassemia and cystic fibrosis, where numerous different mutations occur.[51]

Mismatch cleavage. In one of these methods for screening for mutations, the ribonuclease protection assay,[52] PCR-generated fragments are hybridized with a radioactively labeled RNA probe. This is then treated with RNAase A, which will digest the DNA-RNA duplex at regions where mutations occur, in turn resulting in the accessibility of the unbound nucleotide to the action of the ribonuclease. An alternative mismatch cleavage strategy is chemically based.[53] In this method, chemicals are used to modify mispaired bases, which are then susceptible to cleavage by another chemical agent. Whatever method is used (enzymatic or chemical), the position of the mismatch (cleavage) site is discerned when the DNA fragments are sized on a denaturing gel.

Table 11-11 Methods for detecting point mutations

Methods for detecting point mutations
Direct sequencing
Single-stranded conformation polymorphism (SSCP)
Denaturing gradient gel electrophoresis (DGGE)
Allele specific oligonucleotide (ASO)
Mismatch cleavage
Ligase chain reaction (LCR)
Amplification refactory mutation system (ARMS)

Fluorescent in situ hybridization

Fluorescent in situ hybridization allows for the detection of, among others, chromosomal translocations, deletions, monosomies and trisomies, in interphase nuclei.[54] It can be conceived of as a methodologic bridge between conventional cytogenetics and molecular genetics and is further discussed in Chapters 10 and 12.

Quality control in molecular diagnostics

The rapid and recent emergence of molecular diagnostic assays as well as the availability of automated and nonisotopic techniques have resulted in a dramatic increase in the number of laboratories performing the tests alluded to in the previous sections. Concomitant with this new technology, it is absolutely essential that rigorous quality assurance practices be adopted to ensure the reliability of these new assays.[55] Such a quality assurance (QA) program, as with any other QA program, needs to be all pervasive, beginning with appropriately qualified personnel. As noted before, given the ongoing transition of these technologies from basic science to clinical diagnostics, a key member of staff is the research-trained molecular scientist, who has both the training and practical experience to troubleshoot these emerging techniques. Training and certification for such individuals are currently being implemented by the American Board of Medical Genetics and also by the recent recognition of medical genetics as a specialty area by the American Medical Association. In addition, the American Board of Pathology is actively considering adding molecular diagnostics as a certified specialty. This will ensure that the performance and interpretation of molecular diagnostic assays will be achieved by appropriately educated and trained medical personnel.

A key to assuring optimal quality is clear documentation and retention of gel photographs and autoradiograms for each patient, with aberrant band sizes, restriction enzymes, and probes used being recorded in easily retrieved reports. This is particularly relevant in molecular oncologic assays, in which a comparison with the original diagnostic material is often required to gauge the efficacy of the therapy.

There are several laboratory safety issues that are unique to a molecular diagnostic laboratory because some of the reagents commonly used are particularly hazardous. These include phenol (which is caustic, with the potential for causing painful burns), as well as ethidium bromide, ultraviolet radiation, and ^{32}P (which are all mutagens). Appropriate safety equipment needs to be used by all staff exposed to these, and there should also exist frequent monitoring and surveys of both personnel and work areas, particularly when ^{32}P is being used.

In Southern blot–based assays, which form a significant component of molecular diagnostic assays performed in pathology laboratories, there are four constituents that need to be optimally controlled[56]: (1) the target material, (2) the probe, (3) the hybridization reaction, and (4) signal detection. For Southern blot assays, at least 10^6 nucleated cells are required for an adequate DNA yield, though for PCR-based assays, far fewer cells would suffice. It is important for a pathologist to review the submitted specimen both for its adequacy and representative nature, though the latter is less of an issue given the enhanced sensitivity of these techniques over conventional morphologic assessment. There are several ways to determine the adequacy of the DNA yielded. These include ethidium bromide–stained gels and optical density readings, with both able to provide quantitative and qualitative (presence of intact high-molecular-weight DNA and a 260:280 nm ratio respectively) information. As with any other diagnostic assay, the inclusion of both positive and negative controls is essential to ensure the sensitivity and specificity respectively. Negative controls for Southern blot assays usually consist of normal human DNA (from placenta), whereas for PCR-based assays, given the exquisite sensitivity and risk of contamination, a negative control usually entails running a mock reaction without any template but with all the other required reagents. Another quality control measure for PCR-based tests is to determine whether a nontest sequence (DNA or RNA) can be amplified to demonstrate that there are amplifiable nucleotides present.

Strict quality control also needs to be maintained with the variety of probes now available for diagnostic use. It is crucial to have good documentation of various factors related to the probe, in particular an RE map of the gene it detects. This provides information on the expected germ-line fragments generated with the different enzymes. Furthermore, it is recommended that more than one RE be used (usually three are used) to avoid the misdiagnosis of positivity because of an RFLP.

As discussed in the section on hybridization, numerous variables affect the binding of the probe to the target sequence. These factors, which include the temperature and ionic strength of the hybridization mixture, need to be monitored to assure consistency and appropriate stringency, both at the time of hybridization and at washing. Scintillation counting is performed to determine that probes incorporating ^{32}P have been adequately labeled. This is expressed in counts per minute per microgram (cpm/µg) of probe, referred to as the specific activity of that particular labeled probe (3×10^8 cpm/µg is considered to be a reasonable minimum activity). Ideally, a final report should also include the lowest level of sensitivity attained using that probe, based upon serial dilutions of positive control target sequence.

PCR-based diagnosis has its own peculiar quality assurance components, related to its remarkable sensitivity. Many different practices need to be adopted in laboratories performing such assays, all related to minimizing the risk of contaminating reagents with the target sequence. Integral components include the geographic separation and use of separate designated equipment in the preamplification and postamplification parts of the procedure, as well as the inclusion of negative controls at numerous points during the assay.

One can achieve intralaboratory proficiency to some degree by realizing that molecular diagnostic assays need to be interpreted in the appropriate context. This entails an evaluation of the results together with other diagnostic tests, whether they are conventional morphology and histology, immunophenotypic, or karyotypic studies. Furthermore, it is crucial to be aware of the many caveats of molecular diagnostics (one example is the phenomenon of cross-lineage antigen receptor gene rearrangements; see the discussion below on neoplasia), an awareness gleaned from a thorough and continuing familiarity with the emerging literature in the area. External auditing programs, to measure interlaboratory proficiency, are currently being implemented by the College of American Pathologists.

APPLICATIONS

The specificity, rapidity, and sensitivity of the techniques described here has led to a diagnostic revolution, and many laboratories now perform these molecular diagnostic techniques on a routine basis. Given the safety and cost concerns associated with the use of radioactive label–based assays, many formats are evolving toward the use of techniques that avoid these compounds. This includes the use of nonisotopic labeling systems or PCR without the need for blotting and hybridization. The introduction of these alternative strategies should further accelerate the technologic adaptation of these assays to routine diagnosis.

Virtually every area of diagnostic pathology has been enhanced by the availability and application of these assays, which is briefly detailed here. The four areas on which their effect has been most evident are neoplasia, infectious diseases, hereditary diseases, and identity determination. This is the format that is used for subsequent discussion. A complementary way to approach molecular diagnostic applications is one based on the molecular assays available for answering specific molecular questions (such as what techniques are appropriate to look for, among others, the presence of a gene or a point mutation in a gene), and this is briefly summarized in Table 11-12. As the research effort to map the human genome progresses, and more and more "disease" genes are characterized, we can anticipate a similar progression in the application of molecular diagnostics to pathology.

Neoplasia

Since most malignancies occur because of acquired genetic events and are clonal, they are particularly suitable for molecular-based diagnostic studies.[57] These acquired somatic mutations generally affect genes physiologically involved in cell growth, proliferation, and differentiation (the protooncogenes and tumor suppressor genes), and they are recapitulated in the clonal progeny of single cells. Indeed, the molecular dissection of genetic events in tumors has led to the discovery of a variety of "novel" genes, which has enhanced our understand-

Table 11-12 Molecular diagnostic strategies

Strategy	Techniques*	Examples
Presence or absence of a gene	SB, NB, ISH, PCR	**Infectious diseases** (diagnosis, epidemiology) **Identity determination** (forensics, organ transplantation)
Point mutation in a gene	RED, SB, PCR, ASO, SSCP, SEQ	**Inherited disease** (sickle cell disease, cystic fibrosis, Lesch-Nyhan syndrome) **Neoplasia** (oncogene [*ras*], tumor suppressor gene [p53, retinoblastoma]) **Pharmacology** (AIDS treatment resistance-polymerase mutations)
Abnormality of a region of a gene (other than a point mutation, such as insertions and deletions)	SB, PCR, FISH	**Inherited disease** Type II von Willebrand's Disease, Trinucleotide repeat syndromes [fragile X syndrome, Myotonic dystrophy, Huntington's chorea, Kennedy's syndrome], Duchenne's muscular dystrophy, Prader-Willi and DiGeorge syndromes
Monosomy or trisomy	FISH	**Congenital** (Down syndrome) **Acquired** (malignancies)
Rearrangement of a gene	SB, PCR	**Lymphoid malignancies** (diagnosis, minimal residual disease detection)
Translocation of a gene	SB, PCR, FISH	**Malignancies**
Creation of a novel gene	NB, PCR	**Malignancies** (chronic myelocytic leukemia, acute promyelocytic leukemia, pre–B-cell acute lymphocytic leukemia)

**ASO,* Allele specific oligonucleotide hybridization; *DGGE,* denaturing gradient gel electrophoresis; *FISH,* fluorescence in situ hybridization; *ISH,* in situ hybridization; *NB,* northern blot; *PCR,* polymerase chain reaction (DNA or cDNA); *RED,* restriction endonuclease digestion; *SB,* Southern blot; *SEQ,* sequencing; *SSCP,* single-stranded conformational polymorphism.

ing of normal cell biology. Although molecular diagnostic studies have historically been more applicable to hematologic malignancies,[58] their application to the evaluation of nonhematologic/solid tumors is rapidly evolving. These two groups of cancers are discussed separately.

Table 11-13 Molecular genetic assays in hematologic malignancies

Documentation of clonality
Assignment of lineage
Oncogene involvement
Molecular cytogenetics
Mutational analysis
Minimal disease detection

Hematologic malignancies

A variety of questions can be answered by the molecular analysis of hematologic malignancies (Table 11-13).

Antigen receptor gene rearrangements. The unraveling of the mechanisms of antigen receptor gene rearrangements (immunoglobulin genes in B-cells, and T-cell receptor genes in T-cells) and the cloning of probes of these regions has been pivotal to both the documentation of clonality and the assignment of lineage.[59] In T-cell proliferations and in B-cell proliferations that lack immunoglobulin expression (which would have allowed an analysis of the ratio of kappa:lambda-bearing cells), an analysis of the configuration of these genes is essential for the documentation of clonality and hence neoplasia. A variety of hematologic malignancies, the lineage of which was unclear based on morphology and immunophenotypic studies, have had lineages assigned to them based on finding clonal antigen receptor gene rearrangements. For example, the finding of immunoglobulin heavy-chain gene rearrangements in 100% of "common" acute lymphoblastic leukemia and hairy cell leukemia was used to firmly establish these leukemias as being of B-cell lineage.

However, antigen receptor gene rearrangements, in isolation, can be misleading if used for lineage assignment. It is now well recognized that "cross-lineage" rearrangements are not uncommon: immunoglobulin gene rearrangements are found in immature T-cell malignancies, and T-cell receptor gene rearrangements are seen in precursor B-cell malignancies. Both "crossover" types of rearrangement occur in a small but significant proportion of cases of acute nonlymphoblastic leukemia. Hence, antigen receptor gene rearrangements should always be evaluated in the context of conventional morphology, cytochemistry, and immunophenotyping. Although immunoglobulin heavy-chain gene rearrangements not uncommonly occur in non–B-cell malignancies, with very few exceptions, immunoglobulin light-chain gene rearrangements are essentially specific for documenting B-cell lineage. Antigen receptor gene rearrangements have been traditionally evaluated with standard Southern blot methodology with its attendant disadvantages of a requirement for high-molecular-weight DNA, use of radioactive materials, and lengthy turnaround time. These disadvantages have been overcome, to some degree, by the advent of PCR-based assays for documentation of the rearrangement of these genes.[60] In addition to providing answers in much shorter periods of time, formalin-fixed, paraffin-embedded tissue is amenable to PCR analysis, since there is no longer a requirement for high-molecular-weight DNA. Furthermore, although Southern blot analysis has the ability to detect a single neoplastic cell in the background of 25 to 50 normal cells, PCR's level of sensitivity is such that it is able to detect one neoplastic cell admixed with 100,000 normal cells.

Molecular cytogenetics. Many hematologic malignancies carry specific, nonrandom cytogenetic abnormalities. The determination of the genes affected by these karyotypic abnormalities has allowed for the development of molecular methods to detect their involvement.[61] Broadly, this may be achieved in one of three ways: on standard Southern analysis (such as c-*myc* and *bcl-2* rearrangements in Burkitt's and follicular non-Hodgkin's lymphoma respectively); northern analysis (aberrant *abl* and *pml* transcripts in chronic myeloid leukemia and acute promyelocytic leukemia respectively); and by PCR (Table 11-14). In addition to their diagnostic utility, a number of cytogenetic abnormalities provide prognostic information. In the context of pediatric acute lymphoblastic leukemia, the presence of t(1;19), t(9;22), or t(4;11) is associated with a poor prognosis, while in de novo adult acute nonlymphoblastic leukemia, the t(8;21), t(15;17), and inv(16) abnormalities are associated with a relatively favorable outcome. In patients with diffuse large cell non-Hodgkin's lymphoma, *bcl-6* rearrangements are associated with a good prognosis, while *bcl-2* rearrangements portend a relatively poor outcome.[61a]

The translocations noted in Table 11-14 are all detectable by PCR amplification of cDNA (RT-PCR), since the breaks occur in introns, except for the t(14;18) translocation, in which the breaks are exonic. The submicroscopic deletion of a region of chromosome 1p in acute T-lymphoblastic leukemia (involving the *scl* and *sil* loci), can also be discerned by DNA-PCR. All these translocations can also be documented by molecular methods other than PCR, including standard Southern analysis. There are, in addition, numerous other translocations currently amenable only to Southern analysis. These include *myc* in the t(8;14) of Burkitt's lymphoma, *bcl-1* in the t(11;14) of mantle cell lymphoma and *bcl-3* in the t(14;19) found in a minority of patients with chronic lymphocytic leukemia.

The ability to perform PCR on DNA (or cDNA) is dependent on the clustering and a knowledge of the sequences of the genes that flank the break points of a chromosomal translocation, so that primers can be designed to amplify only the translocation, if present, but they will not amplify any non-translocated gene or genes. Thus, in addition to the enhanced sensitivity afforded by PCR amplification, these assays are specific for specific translocations. The specificity can be exploited for diagnostic purposes, and the sensitivity can be used in several different scenarios. The ability to detect low numbers of tumor cells (not discerned by morphology, immunophenotyping, or Southern analysis) may be used to (1) discover occult disease for staging purposes,[62] (2) determine the efficacy of ex vivo purging of involved bone marrow in patients treated with autologous bone marrow transplantation,[63] and (3) monitor for minimal residual disease and detect early relapse after therapy[64] (including chemotherapy and bone marrow transplantation). The finding of a positive signal by PCR does not provide any information regarding the viability or proliferative capacity of the cell (indeed, a positive signal may be obtained from extracellular DNA) and hence needs to be interpreted with some caution. In many malignancies a positive result after therapy is, in itself, not indicative of minimal disease or relapse. Rather, the presence of sustained (greater than 6 months) or quantitatively increasing positivity is predictive of recurrence.

Detection of clonality. In addition to the use of antigen receptor gene rearrangements and molecular cytogenetics, there are other molecular methods to document clonality. These techniques exploit the presence of polymorphisms of regions of the X chromosome and are analogous to the original G6PD isoenzyme studies, which were previously used to document clonality. As with these original isoenzyme studies, their limitation is that they are informative only if the patient is both female and polymorphic. However, some are particularly useful, such as those wherein numerous alleles are present (using the M27β or human androgen receptor probe) resulting in a very high heterozygosity rate.[65] Curiously, some diseases considered nonmalignant, such as aplastic anemia, have been shown to be clonal with these techniques and perhaps fall into the realm of neoplastic diseases.[66]

Mutational analysis. The molecular analysis of mutations has also provided diagnostic and prognostic insights in hematologic malignancies. Among others, mutations of *ras* genes[67] have been suggested to be an indication of evolution of myelodysplastic syndromes into acute leukemia and, when found in acute lymphoblastic leukemia, are predictive of an increased risk of relapse. Mutations of the c-*fms* protooncogene (macrophage colony–stimulating factor receptor) are more commonly seen in acute nonlymphoblastic leukemia of monoblastic lineage.

Table 11-14 Translocations in hematologic malignancies amenable to polymerase chain reaction (PCR) detection

Disease	Translocation	Genes involved
Chronic myelocytic leukemia	t(9;22)	abl-bcr
Acute lymphoblastic leukemia	t(9;22)	abl-bcr
Follicular non-Hodgkin's lymphoma	t(14;18)	IgH-bcl-2
Anaplastic large cell lymphoma	t(2;5)	ALK-NPM
Acute nonlymphoblastic leukemia (FAB M2)	t(8;21)	eto-aml-1
Acute promyelocytic leukemia (FAB M3)	t(15;17)	pml-rarα
Acute myelomonoblastic leukemia with abnormal eosinophils (FAB M4E)	inv(16)	CBFβ-MYH11
Acute mixed lineage leukemia	t(4;11)	af4-mll
Acute nonlymphoblastic leukemia (basophilia)	t(6;9)	can-dek
Pre–B-cell acute lymphoblastic leukemia	t(1;19)	PBX1-E2A

Oncogenic viruses. Oncogenic viruses can also be studied at a molecular level in hematologic malignancies, including EBV in endemic Burkitt's and AIDS-associated non-Hodgkin's lymphoma and Hodgkin's disease, and HTLV-I in adult T-cell leukemia/lymphoma.

Nonhematologic malignancies

Cytogenetic studies are less feasible in solid tumors as compared with hematologic malignancies. However, the advent of molecular probes has helped circumvent these technical problems.[68] Nevertheless, there are currently fewer well-defined molecular defects amenable to diagnostic and prognostic use, though the emerging technology should dictate some evolution in this field. Indeed, one group of tumors in which numerous nonrandom and specific chromosomal translocation have recently been identified are soft tissue sarcomas.[68a,b] RT-PCR assays of these translocations (Table 11-15) are particularly useful in reaching accurate diagnoses that are otherwise difficult to make using histologic and immunophenotypic criteria.

The stepwise nature of carcinogenesis has been well documented in colon carcinoma, in which several sequential genetic events appear crucial to the development of full-blown malignancy.[69] In some families predisposed to colon cancer, the following sequence of events occurs: (1) loss of the FAP gene from chromosome 5q, (2) mutation of K-*ras* on chromosome 12p, (3) loss of the DCC gene from chromosome 18q, and (4) loss of p53 on chromosome 17p, which is associated with the evolution of adenoma to carcinoma. The identification and tracking of these events has obvious diagnostic and therapeutic relevance.

Regarding familial cancers, in the rare Li-Fraumeni syndrome, germ-line inheritance of p53 mutations has been documented as the probable predisposing event.[70] Indeed, in tumors generally, acquired mutations of p53, a tumor suppressor gene, have been shown to be the single commonest genetic defect.[71] Germline abnormalities of other tumor suppressor genes have also been identified in other rare familial cancers, including the Rb and WT genes in retinoblastoma and Wilm's tumor respectively. Mutations affecting a number of other recently identified genes have been shown to be involved in the predisposition to a variety of cancers. These include BRCA1[71a] (breast and ovary), BRCA2[71b] (breast), and RET[71c] (some forms of multiple endocrine neoplasia and familial medullary, thyroid carcinoma). Most of the mutations affecting the BRCA1 gene result in the formation of a truncated protein,[71d] and may lead to the development of a simple diagnostic test for screening of first-degree relatives of affected individuals. Overall, however, the majority of the mutations observed in protooncogenes and tumor suppressor genes are acquired events in tumors rather than being inherited in the germline, and they provide both diagnostic and prognostic information. For example, acquired mutations of the *ras* gene in adenocarcinoma of the lung are associated with a poor outcome.[72]

The frequent occurence of p53 mutations in cancers in general can be elegantly exploited in a number of clinical scenarios. In patients with cancer of the lung, tumor cells can be detected in the sputum in situations where cytologic evaluation failed to detect tumor cells.[72a] Histopathologic assessment of surgical margins in patients with squamous cell carcinoma of the head and neck is an important prognostic factor. However, local recurrence occurs in many patients with microscopically negative surgical margins, leading to treatment failure and death of the patient. The advent of an assessment of "molecular margins" through a molecular evaluation of p53 mutations may dramatically refine the prediction of local recurrence of the tumor.[72b] In addition to p53, another recently identified tumor suppressor gene, CDKN2 (also referred to as p[16] or MTS1), has been found to be mutated or deleted in a broad spectrum of malignancies,[72c] and similarly may prove to be useful in the detection of minimal numbers of tumor cells. Furthermore, many patients with apparently localized prostatic cancer who are candidates for surgery may be upstaged using RT-PCR of prostate specific antigen (PSA) in the peripheral blood.[72d]

In addition to mutational analysis, the finding of gene amplification in some solid tumors has been shown to have prognostic relevance. Increased copies of N-*myc* is associated with a poor prognosis in neuroblastoma,[73] whereas amplification of *erb*B-2/HER-2/*neu* portends a poor outcome in breast cancer.[74] In some solid tumors, overexpression of the MDR1 gene (multiple drug resistance 1), which can occur in the absence of gene amplification, is associated with resistance to conventional chemotherapy.[75] Deletions of genetic material have been used to distinguish various glial tumors, and such genotypic analyses can be used to supplement their histologic characterization.[76] Generally, deletions and insertions of genetic material in solid tumors can be documented with FISH, and the "reverse" technique of comparative genomic hybridization (CGH),[76a] with the latter method not requiring specific probes. In small round cell tumors of childhood, often an area of some diagnostic dilemma, molecular analysis may be helpful. Here, detection of the expression of the muscle specific gene, MYOD1, appears to be specific for rhabdomyosarcoma.[77] Furthermore, embryonal and alveolar subtypes of rhabdomyosarcoma can be distinguished by DNA analysis.[78] Increased expression of WT1 mRNA and protein can be used as a specific molecular marker of malignant mesothelioma, and can aid in distinguishing this from other pleural tumors.[78a] Molecular studies in solid tumors can identify the presence of oncogenic viruses, including HPV 16 and 18 in invasive cervical and other genital carcinomas, HBV in hepatoma, and EBV in nasopharyngeal carcinoma. Finally, a quantitative and qualitative assessment of the actual DNA content[79] in tumor cells (using DNA intercalating dyes such as propidium iodide) can provide useful prognostic information,

Table 11-15 Translocations in soft tissue tumors amenable to reverse transcription polymerase chain reaction (RT-PCR) detection

Disease	Translocation	Genes involved
Ewing's sarcoma	t(11;22)	EWS-FLI1
Peripheral neuroectodermal tumor	t(21;22)	EWS-ERG
Desmoplastic small round cell tumor	t(11;22)	EWS-WT1
Alveolar rhabdomyosarcoma	t(2;13)	PAX3-FKHR
	t(1;13)	PAX7-FKHR
Clear cell carcinoma	t(12;22)	EWS-ATF-1
Myxoid liposarcoma	t(12;16)	CHOP-TLS

regarding DNA ploidy and S-phase value, in a variety of solid tumors.

Infectious diseases

There are three areas in which molecular diagnostic tests have application to infectious disease, namely, (1) actual diagnosis, (2) epidemiologic studies, and (3) identification of previously unknown infectious agents.

Diagnosis

Numerous commercial gene probes and PCR assays are now available for the diagnosis of infectious diseases.[80,80a] Several of these exploit the existence of 16S ribosomal RNA, which serves as a convenient and universal hybridization target for at least two reasons. First, this rRNA contains sequences that are specific for individual microbial taxa, and, second, in each organism the rRNA exists in thousands of identical copies, which serve as a natural form of amplification of the target sequences. Table 11-16 contains a partial list of microorganisms that can be detected using molecular diagnostic assays.

Many of the techniques now use PCR,[81] or adaptations thereof. This has proved to be particularly useful in situations where there is a need to document early infection (such as CMV in immunocompromised patients,[82] including those after bone marrow transplantation and infection with HIV; transmissible viruses [HIV and hepatitis B and C] in the context of seronegative blood donors), and HIV infection in neonates. In addition, PCR-based assays are useful discriminants in the context of "indeterminate" results obtained from HIV immunoblots.[83] Low-risk HPV types 6 and 11 can be distinguished from high-risk HPV genotypes, such as 16 or 18, by in situ hybridization applied to cellular material.[84]

The choice between conventional culture techniques and probe-based assays will be dictated to some degree by the diagnostic and clinical scenario, with each having pros and cons.[85,85a] The rapidity and sensitivity of tests using probes is somewhat offset by their ability to detect only one organism at a time (though this could be overcome by the use of multiple primers or probes[86]) and by their lack of amenability to antimicrobial sensitivity testing.

Table 11-16 Partial list of microorganisms detected by molecular techniques

Viral	Other
Herpes simplex virus	*Mycobacterium* (*M. tuberculosis* and atypical)
Human herpes virus 6	*Neisseria sp.*
Epstein-Barr virus	*Helicobacter sp.*
Cytomegalovirus	*Escherichia coli*
Hepatitis B virus	*Legionella sp.*
Hepatitis C virus	*Treponema sp.*
Human immunodeficiency virus 1 and 2	*Mycoplasma sp.*
Human T-cell leukemia virus (HTLV) I and II	*Rickettsia sp.*
Papillomavirus	*Chlamydia sp.*
Parvovirus	*Borrelia* (Lyme disease) *sp.*
Picornavirus	*Toxoplasma sp.*
Coxsackievirus	*Trypanosoma sp.*
Rotavirus	*Plasmodium*
	Leishmania sp.
	Candida sp.

Epidemiology

Molecular methods have proved to be invaluable in answering many epidemiologic questions that arise in the context of outbreaks of infectious diseases.[87] They provide information in determining whether a single strain or multiple strains are involved, as well as helping to identify the possible reservoir and routes of transmission. Other epidemiologic applications include the ability to identify hypervirulent strains and to track an infectious agent that may be difficult to culture. Several different techniques may be employed for these purposes. Plasmid profile analysis or plasmid fingerprinting entails the extraction of plasmids from bacteria, followed by gel electrophoresis, and this has been considered to be the standard for defining bacterial strains.[88] Genomic fingerprinting is performed on microorganisms that lack plasmids. This technique uses conventional restriction endonuclease (RE) digestion and visualization of band patterns either in agarose gels or after specific hybridization.[89] Useful probes for hybridization include random chromosomal fragments or rRNA or DNA probes. Ribotyping has been shown to be particularly useful in the study of epidemics. Pulsed field gel electrophoresis (PFGE), using infrequent cutters, has also been shown to be a useful epidemiologic tool. PCR, followed by sequencing, has epidemiologic applications as well. The detection of mutations in an infectious agent in a group of patients may provide information regarding the transmission of a specific strain from an index patient as well as in identifying those with increased virulence. This was used to prove the transmission of HIV from a Florida dentist to his patients, in the now notorious and well-publicized case.[90]

Identification of "new" organisms

Some syndromes exist in which an infectious cause has been strongly suspected. The identification of possible causative agents eluded investigators until the advent of molecular assays. The usual strategy employed for the identification of previously unknown agents has been to use generic 16S rRNA primers to amplify and subsequently characterize the incriminating microorganism. These techniques have documented *Rochalimaea henselae* as the cause of bacillary angiomatosis[91] and *Ehrlichia chaffeensis* as the agent of human ehrlichiosis[92] and also have been used in determining the cause of Whipple's disease.[93]

Inherited genetic diseases

As a consequence of the rapid pace with which the human genome is being mapped, molecular diagnosis has become increasingly applicable to the detection of more and more hereditary diseases.[94] Molecular assay–based diagnosis is now available for many diseases for which few if any methods were previously available. Well over 300 inherited diseases have now been mapped to specific regions in the genome and are actually or potentially amenable to DNA-based detection.[95] A partial list of these disorders is presented in Table 11-17.

There are three areas in which molecular diagnosis can be exploited in inherited diseases: (1) carrier testing, (2) prenatal diagnosis, and (3) direct diagnosis of the disease. The major applications are in the first two areas because molecular diagnosis is usually less relevant for diagnosis when the phenotype is already manifest. Prenatal diagnosis is currently most often performed on chorionic villus sampling, which is obtained in a

Table 11-17 Partial list of inherited diseases amenable to DNA-based diagnosis

Albinism
α-1-antitrypsin deficiency
Ataxia telangiectasia
Congential adrenal hyperplasia
Chronic granulomatous disease
Cystic fibrosis
Familial hypercholesterolemia
Fragile X syndrome
Gaucher's disease
Hemophilia A and B
Huntington's disease
Mucopolysaccharidoses
Muscular dystrophies
Myotonic dystrophy
Neurofibromatosis
Osteogenesis imperfecta
Phenylketonuria
Porphyria
Sickle cell disease
Tay-Sachs disease
Thalassemia (α and β)
von Willebrand's disease

relatively safe manner in the first trimester of pregnancy, allowing for early abortion if indicated. With the advent of in vitro fertilization, it is now feasible to perform preimplantation testing.[96] This allows for embryos to be biopsied when all cells are still totipotent. One cell may be sufficient for a number of different PCR-based diagnoses,[96a] and the remaining cells can be successfully reimplanted.

Two broad strategies exist for molecular diagnosis. These are linkage analysis or direct analysis, referred to in the previous section on probes (p. 203). Linkage analysis allows for disease genes to be indirectly tracked through families by exploiting the existence of polymorphisms occurring in their vicinity. The association of a disease with a related genetic haplotype is known as *linkage dysequilibrium*. However, molecular diagnosis is rapidly evolving from linked analyses to direct detection as the specific genes are cloned and characterized and mutations are identified. The actual technology used for the molecular based detection of a disease is also dictated by a knowledge of the pattern of mutations that occur, based upon information derived from population genetics. So, for example, many recessively inherited diseases that have a strong ethnic association (such as sickle cell anemia) are usually caused by small mutations that are often identical in all carriers. By contrast, those diseases that have a dominant or X-linked pattern of inheritance usually occur as a consequence of different and usually unpredictable mutations in different families.

The hemoglobinopathies were the first diseases diagnosable by molecular analysis,[97] though these initial studies were linked in that RFLP analysis was required. One of the more common hemoglobinopathies, sickle cell anemia (which has a heterozygosity rate of 8% among African-Americans), provides a paradigm for the evolution of molecular diagnostic analyses. Contemporary studies for sickle cell anemia diagnosis use direct analysis, almost always requiring PCR amplification of that part of the β-globin gene involved as a first step. The substitution of A for T at codon 6 may be recognized in one of two easy ways.[98] Since this mutation results in the loss of a RE digestion site *(DdeI)*, it is simple to distinguish the mutant from the normal allele depending on whether the RE is able to digest the PCR product into two pieces, which can then be determined by conventional gel electrophoresis. The other strategy is to use dot blotting and ASO probing,[99] using different oligonucleotides, that will specifically recognize only the normal or mutant allele. Another common hemoglobinopathy, beta-thalassemia, in contrast to sickle cell disease, can be caused by greater than 50 different mutations.[100] However, certain mutations tend to occur more frequently in specific ethnic groups, such that one can target which mutations to look for in a given family, based upon their ethnicity.

Cystic fibrosis occurs in about 1 in 2500 whites, with a carrier frequency (heterozygosity) of 4%. Whereas more than 20 different mutations in the associated gene, the cystic fibrosis transmembrane conductance regulator (CFTR), have been documented, one specific defect is much more common than others.[101] This abnormality is a 3 base-pair deletion resulting in the loss of a single amino acid at position 508 (denoted ΔF508, as the amino acid lost is phenylalanine, which is abbreviated *F*). This defect is found in about 75% of United States carriers but is more frequent in people of northern European descent (>80%) and less common in Ashkenazi Jews (30%). It is easy to detect this common mutation using preamplification of the flanking sequence by PCR. The 3 base-pair difference in size between the normal and mutant allele can be resolved by use of polyacrylamide gel electrophoresis. Detection of the other mutations is usually more difficult, but if the specific mutation in a given family is already known, the defect is obviously easier to detect in that particular family. Automated analysis of commonly occurring mutations has facilitated large scale evaluation, with an attendant lowering of costs and enhanced sensitivity.[101a] For some families, where the exact defect remains unknown, linkage analysis may be required, with its attendant limitations.

In Duchenne's muscular dystrophy and the related disease, Becker's muscular dystrophy, 65% of patients have a deletion in the dystrophin gene, which can be rapidly screened for by using PCR.[102] Since only about two thirds of patients have this detectable deletion, linkage analysis is currently required to detect the other one third of carriers. However, the dystrophin gene is enormous (>2 million base pairs) and the use of indirect analysis, with intragenic, as well as proximal and distal markers, is associated with significant problems of recombination. This then necessitates the use of multiple markers to statistically improve the diagnostic accuracy. Multiplex PCR amplification,[103] using multiple primer sets to amplify as many as nine exons of the dystrophin gene in a single reaction, overcomes many of the problems related to mutational heterogeneity and is thus useful for screening purposes. Analysis for these muscular dystrophies is further complicated by the estimation that up to one third of isolated cases are attributable to new mutations.

Hemophilia A and B are similarly heterogeneous in the number of mutations causing these coagulopathies.[104] Also, the large sizes of the factor VIII and IX genes precludes a rapid analysis of all their exons. Consequently, carrier detection and prenatal diagnosis of the conditions is often reliant upon indirect linkage analysis with RFLPs (p. 203) and requires that numerous members of the family be available for analysis. Molecular defects in the von Willebrand factor gene, resulting in the various forms of von Willebrand's disease, are also heterogeneous and include both large deletions and missense mutations.[105]

The aforementioned examples are single gene disorders, which, depending on the heterogeneity of mutations, may be simply, or with some labor, diagnosed using molecular methods. Other hereditary diseases, however, are probably attributable to multiple gene defects and are hence more difficult to document. For example, in coronary vascular disease, mutations in the LDL receptor and ApoB genes, as well as polymorphisms of the ApoE and Apo(a) loci, can all contribute to the risk.[106] PCR-based HLA typing has also been very informative in detecting the specific alleles of HLA class II loci associated with several autoimmune diseases. As our knowledge of these multigenic syndromes evolves, DNA-based diagnosis is likely to play a greater role.

Identity determination

Molecular techniques can be used to assign identity in several areas of relevance to pathology. The three areas in which they are best established are in the context of (1) transplantation, (2) forensic pathology, and (3) parentage testing, which is discussed below (Table 11-18).

Other areas of potential application, which will not be detailed here, include twin zygosity testing, determination of maternal contamination of fetal samples obtained for prenatal diagnosis, military usage where "DNA dog tags" may play an invaluable role in the identification of casualties of war, and detection of potential mix-up of clinical specimens in pathology laboratories.

Transplantation

There are at least five areas in which molecular assays have application to the realm of transplantation: (1) tissue antigen matching, (2) the rapid detection of life-threatening infections that develop in these immunocompromised patients, (3) ensuring the effective purging of neoplastic disease before autologous transplantation, (4) tracking the engraftment process, and (5) monitoring for recurrent disease. The first two mentioned roles have almost universal application to most forms of transplantation, and the latter three are of particular application to bone marrow transplantation. The role of molecular technologies in ensuring the adequacy of purging bone marrow of malignancy before autologous transplantation, in the monitoring of residual disease, and in the detection of infectious diseases are discussed in prior sections.

Table 11-18 Molecular applications of identity determination

Transplantation
Tissue antigen matching
Tracking engraftment
Forensic pathology
Parentage testing
Twin zygosity
Maternal contamination in prenatal diagnosis
Military usage of DNA dog tags
Specimen mix-ups

Tissue antigen matching is critical to ensure sustained engraftment and prevention of graft-versus-host-disease and to optimize reconstitution of the immune system, particularly after bone marrow transplantation. This matching of HLA gene products is traditionally performed using complement-mediated immunologic assays (especially for HLA class I characterization) and the mixed lymphocyte reaction (MLR) for a functional assessment of HLA class II discrepancies. However, the advent and application of molecular genetic assays to characterize HLA genes has yielded a much finer resolution.[107,107a] Indeed, molecular typing, particularly at the HLA-D loci, has been shown to supersede the conventional methods at several levels: (1) Molecular assays can detect discrepancies not otherwise discerned, and it is clear that conventional assays greatly underestimate the degree of polymorphism. In one study, over one half of potential donor-recipient pairs called identical by serotyping were not matched by molecular typing.[108] (2) The restricted expression of HLA class II antigens on only some cell types (in particular B-cells and monocyte-macrophages) has limited the conventional methods. (3) In some patients with leukemia, expression of these antigens may be lost. Molecular assays are not compromised by these limitations, and, in fact, the predictive value of molecular matching may well exceed that of the conventional assays, and their application should lead to the ultimate goal of reaching transplantation success paralleling that achieved in identical twins. However, a corollary of these advantages is that the criteria for donor selection based upon molecular genetic matching have led to a level of complexity, the relevance of which still needs to be determined.

Technologically, molecular antigen matching uses three primary but related methods. All three have an initial PCR step to amplify the HLA locus to be studied. The three methods employed are the use of ASO probes,[109] sequence-specific priming,[110] and restriction fragment length polymorphisms (RFLP) analysis.[111] ASO and sequence-specific priming are performed for the initial screening of prospective donors and are considered relatively low-resolution methods. High-resolution typing is performed by PCR-RFLP and is used to identify and select the most appropriate donor. The ASO-based detection employs one of two methods, conventional dot-blotting or reverse dot-blotting, with the latter probably more appropriate in this setting.[112] These techniques have been performed to identify potential donors on hairs sent in the mail from family members of a patient!

In the context of bone marrow transplantation, even in patients in whom HLA genotypically identical marrows have been transplanted, other genes can be evaluated to document donor cell engraftment. For sex-mismatched transplants, the task is relatively simple and can be performed using Barr-body detection, conventional cytogenetics, FISH analysis, and either X or Y chromosome–specific molecular probes.[113] In non–sex mismatched transplants, other genetic differences can be determined.[112] Specific oligonucleotides to other polymorphic regions can be used to detect these differences. Also, minisatellite probes, which are locus specific for hypervariable regions, can determine whether circulating cells are of donor or recipient origin.[114] Furthermore, molecular probes can be used to determine the clonality of the reconstituting bone marrow cells and the recapitulation of the immune response.[115]

Forensic testing

The highly polymorphic nature of DNA can be exploited for the determination of an individual's (almost) unique genotype and has been used to link suspects with crimes. These genotypic studies are based upon an analysis of the variable number of tandem repeats (VNTR) regions, alluded to earlier. Many of these analyses require only minute specimens (microliters of blood or semen, and single hair follicles), after prior PCR amplification using primers that flank the regions that contain these VNTRs. VNTR analysis can be performed using single-locus or multilocus probes and are used to generate complex band patterns for each individual, analogous to a uniquely identifying bar code, the so-called DNA fingerprint.[116] The areas containing VNTRs may be minisatellite or microsatellite regions containing tandem repeats of either 33 to 37 base pairs, or 2 to 4 base pairs, respectively. In the MVR (minisatellite variable repeat) approach, identity can be determined based upon both length and sequence variation at some loci.[117] Biologic evidence found at crime scenes can be analyzed by testing for polymorphisms at the HLA-DQα locus, and a reverse dot blot kit is available for this.[118] In addition to being useful for specimen identification, DNA analysis can determine the identity of abducted or lost children.

Although the above are nuclear DNA-based analyses, characterized by mendelian inheritance, mitochondrial DNA (which is maternally inherited) can also be analyzed for forensic purposes.[119] Mitochondrial DNA is "naturally amplified" in cells, with many mitochondria per cell and several copies of DNA per mitochondrion. These multiple copies enhance the probability of recovering mitochondrial DNA, as opposed to nuclear DNA, from forensic samples.

The lack of identity between the specimen and the suspect is used for exclusion, whereas the presence of a match indicates probability of identity. Clearly, the more polymorphic the genetic region and the more markers analyzed, the greater is the probability of determining identity. However, it is important to appreciate that the credibility of these assays is still evolving. The controversy of these tools is not related to laboratory procedures but rather to the debate over the related genetic and statistical population issues.[120] Nevertheless, there are ongoing efforts directed at technical refinement, standardization, and quality assurance. Another crucial component of such tests is that the collection, transfer, and storage of specimens, the so-called chain of evidence, be well documented.

Parentage testing

Conventional serologic and protein polymorphism testing has been used to *exclude* relationships with certainty but has been much less reliable in the *establishment* of a relationship. DNA typing now provides some clarification in this area.[121] DNA typing for parentage testing is based on the fundamental principle that each individual inherits one allele, for any given locus, from each parent, and this simple concept has proved to be invaluable in the resolution of parentage disputes. Many of the methodologies used for parental determination are identical to those alluded to in the previous section on forensic testing. With the advent of PCR-based techniques and study of mitochondrial DNA it is even possible to perform retrospective analysis on postmortem tissue in order to assign parentage. In an extension of the traditional parentage dispute, these techniques can be used to clarify the identity of neonates inadvertently switched at birth, and can resolve immigration disputes based upon putative parentage.

THE FUTURE

The swift and widespread effect of molecular diagnostics on medical practice testifies to the high likelihood that it will remain a major tool well into the future. Rather than passing as a fashionable substitute for conventional diagnostics, molecular diagnostics has begun to reveal its true power as an adjunct technology with high specificity and extraordinary sensitivity. Furthermore, the capacity to detect presymptomatic disease changes strategies for patient care. However, any vision of improved diagnosis and early intervention must include serious thought regarding the effect on society. As we enter an era of conflicting demands of improved health care but with lower cost, what is the prognosis for molecular diagnostics? Will it aid in the selection of therapy? What are the ethical choices to be made regarding the detection of disease susceptibility in an otherwise healthy individual? We will discuss these issues and the implications of this emerging new technology on clinical diagnostic medicine.

New technologies

On the horizon are emerging technologies and improvements that involve developments in laboratory instrumentation, computerization, automation, as well as new laboratory techniques, probes, and other disease markers.[122] These technologic advances are being supported by the U.S. Human Genome Project.[123] To meet its goal of mapping and substantially sequencing the human genome, the development of new gene technology is recognized as essential to the success of the project.

Sample preparation is being simplified to decrease the time and cost of nucleic acid analysis. A variety of DNA/RNA extraction kits have become available to reduce what was once a several-day extraction procedure involving organic solvents and ultracentrifugation to a matter of minutes. This improvement, coupled with the ability of DNA amplification techniques, such as PCR, enables the rapid preparation of virtually any tissue sample type ranging from fixed, paraffin-embedded tissue to a drop of blood obtained with a needle stick. Automation of much of the Southern blot procedure and PCR has meant improvements in reliability of results and a decrease in hands-on time. Under consideration are further robotic applications[124] such as solution hybridization (rather than immobilized blot hybridization), DNA "chips" for rapid detection of DNA sequences,[125] and for DNA amplification technology, a combined amplification and readout utilizing emitted light as a signal. Indeed, handheld diagnostic units may become available for use at the bedside and in doctors' offices.[125a] Ultimately, sample preparation, technical processing, and data analysis and recording will likely be performed mechanically. Data recording and storage has been accomplished by digitized image analysis with mass data storage on magnetic or optical media. One can envision rapid data retrieval by computer, which would significantly aid in research and teaching. Moreover, patient data could be electronically incorporated into diagnostic pathology reports with image transfer to the referring physician or to the consultant for further analysis. Such image analysis in data storage has broad applications to hybridization studies, DNA amplification, and in situ techniques, such as fluorescent in situ hybridization.

With the many rapid advances in molecular biology, it seems likely that novel approaches to develop diagnostic molecular markers will continue to find their way into diagnostic medicine. Several alternative examples of DNA amplification technology have been described earlier in this chapter. In addition to these new methods, we are witness to an almost logarithmic rate of progress in the discovery of new molecular disease markers, particularly at the nucleic acid level. Inasmuch as virtually any disease is amenable to diagnosis at the molecular level, we are far from reaching the full range of diagnostic applications of molecular assays. We can expect a continued proliferation of new genetic probes for genetic disease, cancer, and infectious disease and, in parallel, an increasing dependence on the use of these probes for precise and accurate diagnosis. Furthermore, the selection of therapy[126] for many disease processes will be made on the basis of the specific molecular lesion or disease subtype demonstrated by molecular diagnostics. For example, the choice of antibiotic could be based on the DNA typing of drug-resistant microorganisms. Targeted gene therapy for cancer is being intensively developed, and its success will most certainly depend on precise identification of the target molecule. Identity testing at the molecular level will continue to have a significant influence in the legal system but may also find its way as an advantage to ensuring the identity of patient laboratory specimens, thereby minimizing the problem of switched specimens.

Regulation

As with any sophisticated technology in clinical medicine, molecular diagnostics must be used properly and with great care for quality assurance of methodology and interpretation. Diagnostic pathology and pathologists trained in the use and interpretation of molecular diagnostics will be needed to safely apply this new technology to clinical decision making. In recognition of this, national cooperative pathology groups have begun to meet the challenge by initiating the organization of leaders in molecular diagnostics to establish guidelines for certification and quality assurance. Organizations such as the College of American Pathologists (CAP) and the National College of Clinical Laboratory Scientists (NCCLS) have begun to establish quality standards in proficiency testing for parentage testing, forensic identity, in situ hybridization, and molecular oncology.[127] The Interlaboratory Comparison Program of the CAP has implemented the first Molecular Oncology Survey, which should serve as a model for future molecular diagnostic laboratory proficiency testing. In addition to quality assurance and proficiency testing, credentialing of qualified specialists to perform molecular diagnostics is essential. Molecular diagnostics represents a major advance in diagnostic pathology. It is truly more than just another special stain but, rather, a new window on the diagnosis of disease that spans virtually all areas of diagnostic pathology. Accordingly, the American Board of Pathology and equivalent boards in other countries must seriously consider the creation of a credentialed specialty in molecular diagnostic pathology. This would at once ensure quality of a field that requires special characteristics and would demonstrate that it is a field inherent to pathology.

Economics

As we approach a time of major change in healthcare delivery and financing, a new technology like molecular diagnostics must have demonstrable economic value. Specifically, it should improve patient outcome without unduly increasing overall costs. Indeed, PCR-based assays may be, somewhat surprisingly, relatively economically performed.[128] Recognizing that it is very difficult to measure the cost-benefit ratio for this technology, one can still envision that precise diagnosis before the initiation of interventional therapy, will save time and avoid additional diagnostic tests or ineffective treatments. The ability to perform diagnostic molecular pathology examination on small tissue samples may have a measurable effect by lessening the extent of a surgical procedure required to obtain diagnostic material, such as fine needle aspiration versus open biopsy of an internally located mass.

Although the future for financing laboratory-based diagnostics remains uncertain at this point, there is room for optimism that certain molecular diagnostic tests will be considered essential for patient care. The costs of these tests may be reduced through labor-saving devices, by reducing the excessive charges made by suppliers, and by eliminating royalty fees, such as the tax on collections for PCR levied by a company that holds the patent for the technique.

Ethical implications

Molecular diagnostics, in particular DNA-based technology, has changed the way we think about diagnosing disease. Our ability to detect disease susceptibility in clinically disease-free individuals raises challenging new questions for the healthcare community.[129] What will a "preexisting condition" mean to an individual's ability to obtain health insurance? Or, will this be circumvented through a new national health plan? What choices will an individual make when informed that a devastating disease will almost certainly strike in the future? Questions such as these can have a severe effect on the major life decisions for patients and parents of children carrying disease susceptibility markers and for decisions to make about the yet unborn. Issues such as these are already on the table and affect healthy individuals as well as those being monitored for treated disease. Indeed, the Human Genome Project is addressing these issues through its Ethical, Legal and Social Implications (ELSI) component.[130] Now is the time we must proceed thoughtfully and responsibly as we use this powerful new technology.

REFERENCES

Structure of a molecular diagnostic laboratory

1. Garrett CT, Rodriguez ER, Comerford J, Sarago C: Establishing a molecular diagnostic laboratory, *Adv Pathol Lab Med* 5:35, 1992.
2. Lai-Goldman M, Ross DW: Establishing a molecular diagnostics laboratory, *Clin Immunol News* 8:111, 1990.

DNA and RNA extraction

3. Reed TJ, Reid A, Wallberg K et al: Determination of B-cell clonality in paraffin-embedded lymph nodes using the polymerase chain reaction, *Diagn Mol Pathol* 2:42, 1993.
4. Macfarlane DE, Dahle CE: Isolating RNA from whole blood: the dawn of RNA-based diagnosis, *Nature* 362:186, 1993.
5. Akoury DA, Seo JJ, James CD, Zaki SR: RT-PCR detection of mRNA recovered from archival glass slide smears, *Mod Pathol* 6:195, 1993.
6. Brady G, Barbara M, Iscove N: Representative in vitro cDNA amplification from individual hematopoietic cells and colonies, *Methods Mol Cell Biol* 2:17, 1990.

7. Berger SL, Kimmel AR: Guide to molecular cloning techniques. Section II: General methods for isolating and characterizing nucleic acids, *Methods Enzymol* 152:33, 1987.
8. Berger SL: Preparation and characterization of RNA: Overview, *Methods Enzymol* 152:215, 1987.
9. Chomczynski P, Sacchi N: Single-step method of RNA isolation by acid guanidium thiocyanate-phenol-chloroform extraction, *Anal Biochem* 161: 156, 1987.

Preparation of DNA for analysis

10. Brooks JE: Properties and uses of restriction endonucleases, *Methods Enzymol* 152:113, 1987.
11. Smith CL, Cantor CR: Pulsed-field gel electrophoresis of large DNA molecules, *Nature* 319:701, 1986.

Preparation of RNA for analysis

12. Sambrook J, Fritsch EF, Maniatis T: *Molecular cloning: a laboratory manual.* Section 7: Extraction, purification and analysis of messenger RNA from eukaryotic cells, Plainview, NY, 1989, Cold Spring Harbor Laboratory Press.

Transfer

13. Southern EM: Detection of specific sequences among DNA separated by gel electrophoresis, *J Mol Biol* 98:503, 1975.
14. Chomczynski P: One-hour downward alkaline capillary transfer for blotting DNA and RNA, *Anal Biochem* 201:134, 1992.

Probes and probing

15. Narayanan S: Overview of principles and current uses of DNA probes in clinical and laboratory medicine, *Ann Clin Lab Sci* 22:353, 1992.
16. Keller GH, Manak MM: Hybridization formats and detection procedures. In *DNA probes,* New York, 1989, Stockton Press.

Detection systems

17. Sambrook J, Fritsch EF, Maniatis T: *Molecular cloning: a laboratory manual.* Section 10: Preparation of radiolabeled DNA and RNA probes, Plainview, NY, 1989, Cold Spring Harbor Laboratory Press.
18. Diamindis EP, Christopoulos TK: The biotin-(strept) avidin system: principles and application in biotechnology, *Clin Chem* 37:625, 1991.

DNA analysis

19. Sambrook J, Fritsch EF, Maniatis T: *Molecular cloning: a laboratory manual.* Section 9: Analysis and cloning of eukaryotic genomic DNA, Plainview, NY, 1989, Cold Spring Harbor Laboratory Press.
20. Botstein D, White RL, Skolnick M, Davis RW: Construction of a genetic linkage map in man using restriction fragment length polymorphisms, *Am J Hum Genet* 32:314, 1980.
21. Langlois S: Genetic diagnosis based on molecular analysis, *Pediatr Clin North Am* 39:91, 1992.
22. Armour JA, Jeffreys AJ: Recent advances in minisatellite biology, *FEBS Lett* 310:113, 1992.

RNA analysis

23. Alwine JC, Kemp DJ, Stark GR: Methods for detection of specific RNAs in agarose gels by transfer to diazobenzyloxymethyl paper and hybridization with DNA probes, *Proc Natl Acad Sci USA* 74:5350, 1977.
24. Moorman AF, De Boer PA, Vermeulen JL, Lamers WH: Practical aspects of radioisotopic in situ hybridization on RNA, *Histochem J* 25:251, 1993.

Protein analysis

25. Sambrook J, Fritsch EF, Maniatis T: *Molecular cloning: a laboratory manual.* Section 18: Detection and analysis of proteins expressed from cloned genes, Plainview, NY, 1989, Cold Spring Harbor Laboratory Press.

Polymerase chain reaction and other amplification systems

26. Eisenstein B: The polymerase chain reaction: a new method of using molecular genetics for medical diagnosis, *N Engl J Med* 322:178, 1990.
27. Templeton NS: The polymerase chain reaction: history, methods and applications, *Diagn Mol Pathol* 1:58, 1992.
28. Erlich HA: *PCR technology: principles and applications for DNA amplification,* New York, 1989, Stockton.
29. Kwok S, Higuchi R: Avoiding false positives with PCR, *Nature* 339:237, 1989.
30. Kawasaki ES, Clark SS, Coyne MY et al: Diagnosis of chronic myeloid and acute lymphocytic leukemias by detection of leukemia-specific mRNA sequences amplified in vitro, *Proc Natl Acad Sci USA* 85:5698, 1988.
31. Maurer J, Thiel E: Rapid detection of chimeric *bcr/abl* mRNAs in acute lymphoblastic and chronic myeloid leukemia by the polymerase chain reaction, *Blut* 61:350, 1990.
32. Bagasra O, Seshamma T, Pomerantz RJ: Polymerase chain reaction in situ: intracellular amplification and detection of HIV-1 proviral DNA and other specific genes, *J Immunol Methods* 158:131, 1993.
33. Meijerink JPP, Smetsers TFCM, Raemaekers JMM et al: Quantitation of follicular non-Hodgkin's lymphoma cells carrying t(14;18) by competitive polymerase chain reaction, *Br J Haematol* 84:250, 1993.
34. Handyside AH, Lesko JG, Tarin JJ et al: Birth of a normal girl after in vitro fertilization and preimplantation diagnostic testing for cystic fibrosis, *N Engl J Med* 327:905, 1992.
35. Trumper LH, Brady G, Bagg A et al: Single-cell analysis of Hodgkin and Reed-Sternberg cells: molecular heterogeneity of gene expression and p53 mutations, *Blood* 81:3097, 1993.
36. Sano T, Smith CL, Cantor CR: Immuno-PCR: very sensitive antigen detection by means of specific antibody-DNA conjugates, *Science* 258:120, 1992.
37. Huang SH, Hu YY, Wu CH, Holcenberg J: A simple method for direct cloning cDNA sequence that flanks a region of known sequence from total RNA by applying the inverse polymerase chain reaction, *Nucleic Acids Res* 18:1922, 1990.
38. Ohara O, Dorit RL, Gilbert W: One sided polymerase chain reaction: the amplification of cDNA, *Proc Natl Acad Sci USA* 86:5673, 1989.
39. Mazars GR, Moyret C, Jeanteur P, Theillet CG: Direct sequencing by thermal asymmetric PCR, *Nucleic Acids Res* 19:4783, 1991.
40. Barany F: Genetic disease detection and DNA amplification using cloned thermostable ligase, *Proc Natl Acad Sci USA* 88:189, 1991.
41. Newton CR, Graham A, Heptinstall LE et al: Analysis of any point mutation in DNA: the amplification refractory mutation system (ARMS), *Nucleic Acids Res* 17:2503, 1989.
42. Cahill P, Foster K, Mahan DE: Polymerase chain reaction and Q beta replicase amplification, *Clin Chem* 37:1482, 1991.
43. Kwoh DY, Davis GR, Whitfield KM et al: Transcription-based amplification system and detection of amplified human immunodeficiency virus type 1 with a bead-based sandwich hybridization format, *Proc Natl Acad Sci USA* 86:1173, 1989.

Mutational analysis

44. Forrest S, Cotton RGH: Methods of detection of single base substitutions in clinical genetic practice, *Mol Biol Med* 7:451, 1990.
45. Maxam AM, Gilbert W: A new method for sequencing DNA, *Proc Natl Acad Sci USA* 74:560, 1977.
46. Sanger F, Nicklen S, Coulson AR: DNA sequencing with chain-terminating inhibitors, *Proc Natl Acad Sci USA* 74:5463, 1977.
47. Landegren U, Kaiser R, Caskey CT, Hood L: DNA diagnostics: molecular techniques and automation, *Science* 242:229, 1988.
48. Orita M, Iwahana H Kanazawa H et al: Detection of polymorphisms of human DNA by gel electrophoresis as single-strand conformation polymorphism, *Proc Natl Acad Sci USA* 86:2766, 1989.
49. Fischer SG, Lerman LS: DNA fragments differing by single base-pair substitutions are separated in denaturing gradient gels: correspondence with melting theory, *Proc Natl Acad Sci USA* 80:1579, 1983.
50. Saiki RK, Chang CA, Levenson CH et al: Diagnosis of sickle cell anemia and β-thalassemia with enzymatically amplified DNA and nonradioactive allele-specific oligonucleotide probes, *N Engl J Med* 319:537, 1988.

51. Saiki RK, Walsh PS, Levenson CH, Erlich HA: Genetic analysis of amplified DNA with immobilized sequence-specific oligonucleotide probes, *Proc Natl Acad Sci USA* 86:6230, 1989.
52. Myers RM, Larin Z, Maniatis T: Detection of single base substitutions by ribonuclease cleavage at mismatches in RNA:DNA duplexes, *Science* 230:1242, 1985.
53. Cotton RGH, Rodrigues NR, Campbell RD: Reactivity of cytosine and thymine in single-base-pair mismatches with hydroxylamine and osmium tetroxide and it application to the study of mutations, *Proc Natl Acad Sci USA* 85:4397, 1988.

FISH

54. Leversha MA: FISH and the technicolour revolution: molecular cytogenetics and its application in chromosome analysis today, *Med J Aust* 158: 545, 1993.

Quality control

55. Farkas DH: *Molecular biology and pathology: a guidebook for quality control,* San Diego, 1993, Academic Press.
56. Lovell MA: Quality control in diagnostic molecular immunology, *Clin Immunol News* 10:150, 1990.

Applications to neoplastic disease

57. Bishop JM: Molecular themes in oncogenesis, *Cell* 64:235, 1991.
58. Medeiros LJ, Bagg A, Cossman J: Application of molecular genetics to the diagnosis of hematopoietic neoplasms. In Knowles DM, editor: *Neoplastic hematopathology,* Baltimore, 1992, Williams & Wilkins.
59. Cossman J, Uppenkamp M, Sundeen J et al: Molecular genetics and the diagnosis of lymphoma, *Arch Pathol Lab Med* 112:117, 1988.
60. Inghirami G, Szabolcs, Yee HT et al: Detection of immunoglobulin gene rearrangement of B cell non-Hodgkin's lymphomas and leukemias in fresh, unfixed and formalin-fixed, paraffin-embedded tissue by polymerase chain reaction, *Lab Invest* 68:746, 1993.
61. Gray JW: Molecular cytogenetic analysis of human tumors, *Ann NY Acad Sci* 677:194, 1993.

61a. Offit K, LeCoco F, Louie DC et al: Rearrangement of the *bcl-6* gene as a prognostic marker in diffuse large-cell lymphoma, *N Engl J Med* 331:74, 1994.

62. Gribben JG, Freedman AS, Woo SD et al: All advanced stage non-Hodgkin's lymphomas with a polymerase chain reaction amplifiable breakpoint of *bcl-2* have residual cells containing the *bcl-2* rearrangement at evaluation and after treatment, *Blood* 78:3275, 1991.
63. Negrin RS, Kiem HP, Schmidt-Wolf IGH et al: Use of the polymerase chain reaction to monitor effectiveness of ex vivo tumor cell purging, *Blood* 77:654, 1991.
64. Gehly, GB: Diagnosis of minimal residual disease in bone marrow transplant patients, *Clin Lab Med* 12:129, 1992.
65. Hodges E, Howell WM, Boyd Y, Smith JL: Variable X-chromosome DNA methylation patterns detected with probe M27 beta in a series of lymphoid and myeloid malignancies, *Br J Haematol* 77:315, 1991.
66. Janssen J, Buschle M, Layton M et al: Clonal analysis of myelodysplastic syndromes: evidence of multipotent stem cell origin, *Blood* 73:248, 1989.
67. Carter G, Hughes CD, Clark RE et al: RAS mutations in patients following cytotoxic therapy for lymphoma, *Oncogene* 5:411, 1990.
68. Cossman J: *Molecular genetics in cancer diagnosis,* New York, 1990, Elsevier.

68a. Sreekantaiah C, Ladanyi M, Rodriguez E, Chaganti RSK: Chromosomal abberations in soft tissue tumors. Relevance to diagnosis, classification, and molecular mechanisms, *Am J Pathol* 144:1121, 1994.

68b. Barr FG, Chatten J, D'Cruz CM et al: Molecular assays for chromosomal translocations in the diagnosis of pediatric soft tissue sarcomas, *JAMA* 273:553, 1995.

69. Cho KR, Vogelstein B: Genetic alterations in the adenoma-carcinoma sequence, *Cancer* 70:1727, 1992.
70. Malkin D, Jolly KW, Barbier N et al: Germline mutations of the p53 tumor-suppressor gene in children and young adults with second malignant neoplasms, *N Engl J Med* 326:1309, 1992.
71. Vogelstein B, Kinzler KW: p53 function and dysfunction, *Cell* 70:532, 1992.

71a. Miki Y, Swensen J, Shattuck-Eidens D et al: A strong candidate for the 17q-linked breast and ovary cancer susceptibility gene *BRCA1, Science* 266:66, 1994.

71b. Wooster R, Neuhausen S, Mangion J et al: Localization of a breast cancer susceptibility gene, *BRCA2,* to chromosome 13q 12-13, Science 265:2088, 1994.

71c. Goodfellow PJ: Inherited cancers associated with the RET protooncogene, *Curr Opin Genet Devel* 4:446, 1994.

71d. Shattuck-Eidens D, McClure M, Simard J et al: A collaborative survey of 80 mutations in the *BRCA1* breast and ovarian cancer susceptibility gene. Implications for presymptomatic testing and screening, *JAMA* 273:535, 1995.

72. Slebos RJC, Kibbelaar RE, Dalesio O et al: K-*ras* oncogene activation as a prognostic marker in adenocarcinoma of the lung, *N Engl J Med* 323:561, 1990.

72a. Mao L, Hruban RH, Boyle JD et al: Detection of oncogene mutations in sputum precedes diagnosis of lung cancer, *Cancer Res* 54:1634, 1994.

72b. Brennan JA, Mao L, Hruban RH et al: Molecular assessment of histopathological staging in squamous-cell carcinoma of the head and neck, *N Engl J Med* 332:429, 1995.

72c. Nobori T, Miura K, Wu DJ et al: Deletions of the cyclin-dependent kinase-4 inhibitor gene in multiple human cancers, *Nature* 368:753, 1994.

72d. Katz AE, Olsson CA, Raffo AJ et al: Molecular staging of prostatic cancer with the use of an enhanced reverse transcriplase-PCR assay, *Urology,* 43:765, 1994.

73. Joshi VV, Cantor AB, Brodeur GM et al: Correlation between morphologic and other prognostic markers of neuroblastoma: a study of histologic grade, DNA index, N-*myc* gene copy number, and lactic dehydrogenase in patients in the Pediatric Oncology Group, *Cancer* 71:3173, 1993.
74. Farkas DH, Long JC, Schulz R et al: Laboratory analysis for HER-2/*neu* gene amplification and protein overexpression, *Lab Med* 24:557, 1993.
75. Faqua SAW, Moretti-Rojas IM, Schneider SL et al: P-glycoprotein expression in human breast cancer cells, *Cancer Res* 47:2103, 1987.
76. James CD, Carlbom E, Dumanski JP et al: Clonal genomic alterations in glioma malignancy stages, *Cancer Res* 48:5546, 1988.

76a. Houldsworth J, Chaganti RSK: Comparative genomic hybridization: an overview, *Am J Pathol* 145:1253, 1994.

77. Scrable H, Witte D, Shimada H et al: Molecular differential pathology of rhabdomyosarcoma, *Genes Chromosom Cancer* 1:23, 1989.
78. Crist WM, Kun LE: Common solid tumors of childhood, *N Engl J Med* 324:461, 1991.

78a. Amin KM, Litzky LA, Smythe WR et al: Wilms' tumour 1 susceptibility (WT1) gene products are selectively expressed in malignant mesothelioma, *Am J Pathol* 146:344, 1995.

79. Seckinger D, Sugarbaker E, Frankfurt O: DNA content in human cancer, *Arch Pathol Lab Med* 113:619, 1989.

Applications to infectious disease

80. Engleberg NC, Eisenstein BI: Detection of microbial nucleic acids for diagnostic purposes, *Annu Rev Med* 43:147, 1992.

80a. Makimura K, Murayama SY, Yamaguchi H: Detection of a wide range of medically important fungi by the polymerase chain reaction, *J Med Microbiol* 40: 358, 1994.

81. Woods CR, Versalovic J, Koeuth T, Lupski JR: Whole-cell repetitive element sequence-based polymerase chain reaction allows rapid assessment of clonal relationships of bacterial isolates, *J Clin Microbiol* 31:1927, 1993.
82. Smith KL, Dunstan RA: PCR detection of cytomegalovirus: a review, *Br J Haematol* 84:187, 1993.
83. Jackson JB, MacDonald KL, Cadwell J et al: Absence of HIV infection in blood donors with indeterminate western blot tests for antibody to HIV-1, *N Engl J Med* 322:217, 1990.
84. Amortegui AJ, Meyer MP: In-situ hybridization for the diagnosis and typing of human papillomavirus, *Clin Biochem* 23:301, 1990.

85. Relman DA: The identification of uncultured microbial pathogens, *J Infect Dis* 168:1, 1993.

85a. Noordhoek GT, Kolk AH, Bjune G et al: Sensitivity and specificity of PCR for detection of mycobacterium tuberculosis: a blind comparison study among seven laboratories, *J Clin Microbiol* 32:277, 1994.

86. Dattagupta N, Rae PMM, Huguenel ED et al: Rapid identification of microorganisms by nucleic acid hybridization after labeling the test sample, *Anal Biochem* 177:85, 1989.

87. Lupski JR: Molecular epidemiology and its clinical application, *JAMA* 270:1363, 1993.

88. Mayer LW: Use of plasmid profiles in epidemiologic surveillance of disease outbreaks and in tracing the transmission of antibiotic resistance, *Clin Microbiol Rev* 1:228, 1988.

89. Tompkins LS: The use of molecular methods in infectious diseases, *N Engl J Med* 327:1290, 1992.

90. Update: transmission of HIV infection during an invasive dental procedure—Florida, *MMWR* 40:21, 1991.

91. Regnery RL, Anderson BE, Clarridge JE III et al: Characterization of a novel *Rochalimaea* species, *R. henselae* sp. nov., isolated from blood of a febrile, human immunodeficiency virus-positive patient, *J Clin Microbiol* 30:265, 1992.

92. Anderson BE, Sumner JW, Dawson JE et al: Detection of the etiologic agent of human ehrlichiosis by polymerase chain reaction, *J Clin Microbiol* 30:775, 1992.

93. Relman DA, Schmidt TM, MacDermott RP, Falkow S: Identification of the uncultured bacillus of Whipple's disease, *N Engl J Med* 327:293, 1992.

Applications to inherited disease

94. McKusick VA, Amberger JS: The morbid anatomy of the human genome: chromosomal localization of mutations causing disease, *J Med Genet* 30:1, 1993.

95. Wagener C, Epplen JT, Erlich H et al: Molecular biology techniques in the diagnosis of monogenic diseases, *Clin Chem Acta* 225:535, 1994.

96. Critser ES: Preimplantation genetics: an overview, *Arch Pathol Lab Med* 116:383, 1992.

96a. Snabes MC, Chong SS, Subramanian SB et al: Preimplantation single-cell analysis of multiple genetic loci by whole-genome amplification, *Proc Natl Acad Sci USA* 91:6181, 1994.

97. Kan YW, Globus MS, Dozy AM: Prenatal diagnosis of alpha-thalassemia: clinical application of molecular hybridization, *N Engl J Med* 295:1165, 1976.

98. Saiki RK, Scharf S, Faloona F et al: Enzymatic amplification of β-globin genomic sequences and restriction fragment analysis for diagnosis of sickle cell anemia, *Science* 230:1350, 1985.

99. Saiki RK, Bugawan TL, Horn GT et al: Analysis of enzymatically amplified β-globin and HLA-DQα DNA with allele specific oligonucleotide probes, *Nature* 324:163, 1986.

100. Kazazian HH: The thalassemia syndromes: molecular basis and prenatal diagnosis in 1990, *Semin Hematol* 27:209, 1990.

101. Beaudet AL: Genetic testing for cystic fibrosis, *Pediatr Clin North Am* 39:213, 1992.

101a. DeMarchi JM, Beaudet AL, Caske CT, Richards CS: Experience of an academic reference laboratory using automation for analysis of cystic fibrosis mutations, *Arch Pathol Lab Med* 118:26, 1994.

102. Caskey CT, Pizzuti A, Fu YH et al: Triplet repeat mutations in human disease, *Science* 256:784, 1992.

103. Beggs AH, Koenig M, Boyce FM, Kunkel LM: Detection of 98% of DMD/BMD gene defects by polymerase chain reaction, *Hum Genet* 86:45, 1990.

104. Tuddenham EGD, Cooper DN, Gitschier J et al: Haemophilia A: database of nucleotide substitutions, deletions, insertions and rearrangements of the factor VIII gene, *Nucleic Acids Res* 19:4821, 1991.

105. Ginsburg D: The von Willebrand factor gene and genetics of von Willebrand's disease, *Mayo Clin Proc* 66:506, 1991.

106. Talmud P, Tybjaerg-Hansen A, Bhatnagar D et al: Rapid screening for specific mutations in patients with a clinical diagnosis of familial hypercholesterolemia, *Atherosclerosis* 89:137, 1991.

Applications to identity determination

107. Kukuruga D, Eisenbrey AB: Role of molecular tools in tissue transplantation, *Lab Med* 24:589, 1993.

107a. Begovich AB, Erlich H: HLA typing for bone marrow transplantation. New polymerase chain reaction-based methods, *JAMA* 273:586, 1995.

108. Baxter-Lowe LA, Eckels DD, Ash R et al: The predictive value of HLA-DR oligotyping for MLC responses, *Transplantation* 53:1352, 1992.

109. Scharf S, Griffith R, Erlich H: Rapid typing of DNA sequence polymorphism at the HLA-DRB1 locus using the polymerase chain reaction and nonradioactive oligonucleotide probes, *Hum Immunol* 30:190, 1991.

110. Olerup O, Zetterquist H: HLA-DR typing by PCR amplification with sequence-specific primers (PCR-SSP) in 2 hours: an alternative to serological DR typing in clinical practice including donor-recipient matching in cadaveric transplantation, *Tissue Antigens* 39:225, 1992.

111. Ota M, Seki T, Fukushima H et al: HLA-DRB1 genotyping by modified PCR-RFLP method combined with group-specific primers, *Tissue Antigens* 39:187, 1992.

112. Bugawan TL, Begovich AB, Erlich HA: Rapid HLA-DPB typing using enzymatically amplified DNA and nonradioactive sequence specific oligonucleotide probes, *Immunogenetics* 32:231, 1990.

113. Lawler M, McCann SR, Conneally E et al: Chimaerism following allogeneic bone marrow transplantation: detection of residual host cells using the polymerase chain reaction, *Br J Haematol* 73:210, 1989.

114. Roth MS, Antin JH, Bingham J et al: Use of polymerase chain reaction–detected sequence polymorphisms to document engraftment following allogeneic transplantation, *Transplantation* 49:714, 1990.

115. Nash R, Storb R, Neiman P: Polyclonal reconstitution of human marrow after allogeneic bone marrow transplantation, *Blood* 72:2031, 1988.

116. Debenham PG: DNA fingerprinting, *J Pathol* 164:101, 1991.

117. Jeffreys AJ, MacLeod A, Tamaki K et al: Minisatellite repeat coding: a digital approach to DNA typing, *Nature* 354:204, 1991.

118. Blake E, Mihalovich J, Higuchi R et al: Polymerase chain reaction (PCR) amplification and human leukocyte antigen (HLA)-DQα oligonucleotide typing on biological evidence samples: casework experience, *J Forensic Sci* 37:700, 1992

119. Skolnick AA: Mitochondrial DNA studies help identify lost victims of human rights abuses, *JAMA* 269:1911, 1993.

120. Weir BS: Population genetics in the forensic DNA debate, *Proc Natl Acad Sci USA* 89:11654, 1992.

121. Walker RH, Crisan D: DNA technology: the fourth generation in parentage testing, *Transfusion* 31:383, 1991.

The future

122. Felder RA, Boyd JC, Margrey K et al: Robotics in the medical laboratory, *Clin Chem* 36:1534, 1990.

123. Collins F, Galas D: A new five year plan for the U.S. Human Genome Project, *Science* 262:43, 1993.

124. Felder RA: Prospective role of automation and robotics in routine diagnostic applications of PCR, *Ann Biol Clin* 51:332, 1993.

125. Fodor SPA, Rava RP, Huang XC et al: Multiplexed biochemical assays with biological chips, *Nature* 364:555, 1993.

125a. Gershon D: DNA diagnostic tools for the 21st century, *Nature Med* 1:102, 1995.

126. Samara G, Sawicki MP, Hurwitz M, Passaro E: Molecular biology and therapy of disease, *Am J Surg* 165:720, 1993.

127. *Current surveys in molecular pathology,* Northfield, Ill, 1993, College of American Pathologists.

128. Gunther KE, Cohn RJ, Mendelow BV: Polymerase chain reaction in cancer diagnosis, *S Afr Med J* 83:514, 1993.

129. Billings PR, Kohn MA, de Cuevas M et al: Discrimination as a consequence of genetic testing, *Am J Hum Genet* 50:476, 1992.

130. Caskey CT: Presymptomatic diagnosis: a first step toward genetic health care, *Science* 262:49, 1993.

12 Cytogenetics

Julia A. Bridge
Avery A. Sandberg

HUMAN CHROMOSOMES

Chromosomes, as they appear in a metaphase spread, consist of tightly coiled DNA and protein. Although different numbers, sizes, and shapes of chromosomes characterize different species, considerable gene homology also exists. Study of the evolution of human chromosomes has revealed 99% homology between chromosomes of humans and those of our closest relatives—the chimpanzee, gorilla, and orangutan. It is believed that the gene content of certain individual chromosomes has remained the same throughout mammalian development.[1] In other words, there is evidence of gene conservation of a duration of approximately 125 million years.[2]

Human somatic cells were for many years believed to contain 48 chromosomes. In 1956, Tjio and Levan described the correct number of chromosomes as 46.[3] The human *diploid* cell (46 chromosomes) contains 22 pairs of *autosomes,* identical in males and females, and two *sex chromosomes,* XX in the female and XY in the male. Each member of a pair of chromosomes consists of the same linear sequence of genes (homologous chromosomes, or *homologs*). The individual gene loci on each chromosome, referred to as *alleles,* may be the same or may differ in DNA sequence, yielding a variety of functioning gene product possibilities.

Meiosis

There are two types of cell division, meiosis and mitosis. *Meiosis* is the reduction division that gives rise to male and female *gametes* (sperm and oocytes respectively). Male and female gametes differ from other human cells in that they contain only 23 chromosomes, *haploid* cells. This process is necessary for normal fertilization for if the sperm and oocyte united with a complement of 46 chromosomes each, the result would be a zygote containing 92 chromosomes.

Meiosis consists of two stages; meiosis I and meiosis II (Fig. 12-1). In the first stage of meiosis each chromosome replicates into two *sister chromatids* (identical strands of DNA joined by a centromere) followed by the alignment of homologous chromosomes in pairs. This latter process is called *synapsis* and is unique for the meiotic form of division. *Crossing-over,* exchange of homologous segments between two of the four chromatids, takes place during synapsis. Crossing-over allows for the wide range of genetic combinations in the gamete. Genes located close to one another are more likely to be passed together than genes located farther apart. This is an important phenomenon when one is considering gene mapping and linkage studies. Approximately one or two exchanges occur per chromosome (30 to 40 exchanges total) during meiosis.

When synapsis is complete, the homologous chromosomes separate to opposite poles. This is followed by meiosis II, in which the centromeres of the sister chromatids divides resulting in the gametes, each with 23 chromosomes. The sex of the offspring is determined by the paternal chromosomal contribution. In sperm, each haploid set includes either an X or a Y chromosome whereas all ova contain a single X. If an ovum is fertilized by an X-bearing sperm, a female zygote will result; if by a Y-bearing sperm, a male zygote.

Mitosis

Mitosis is the process of cell division in which the genetic material of a cell is divided equally between two daughter cells and is identical to the parental cell. Five primary phases

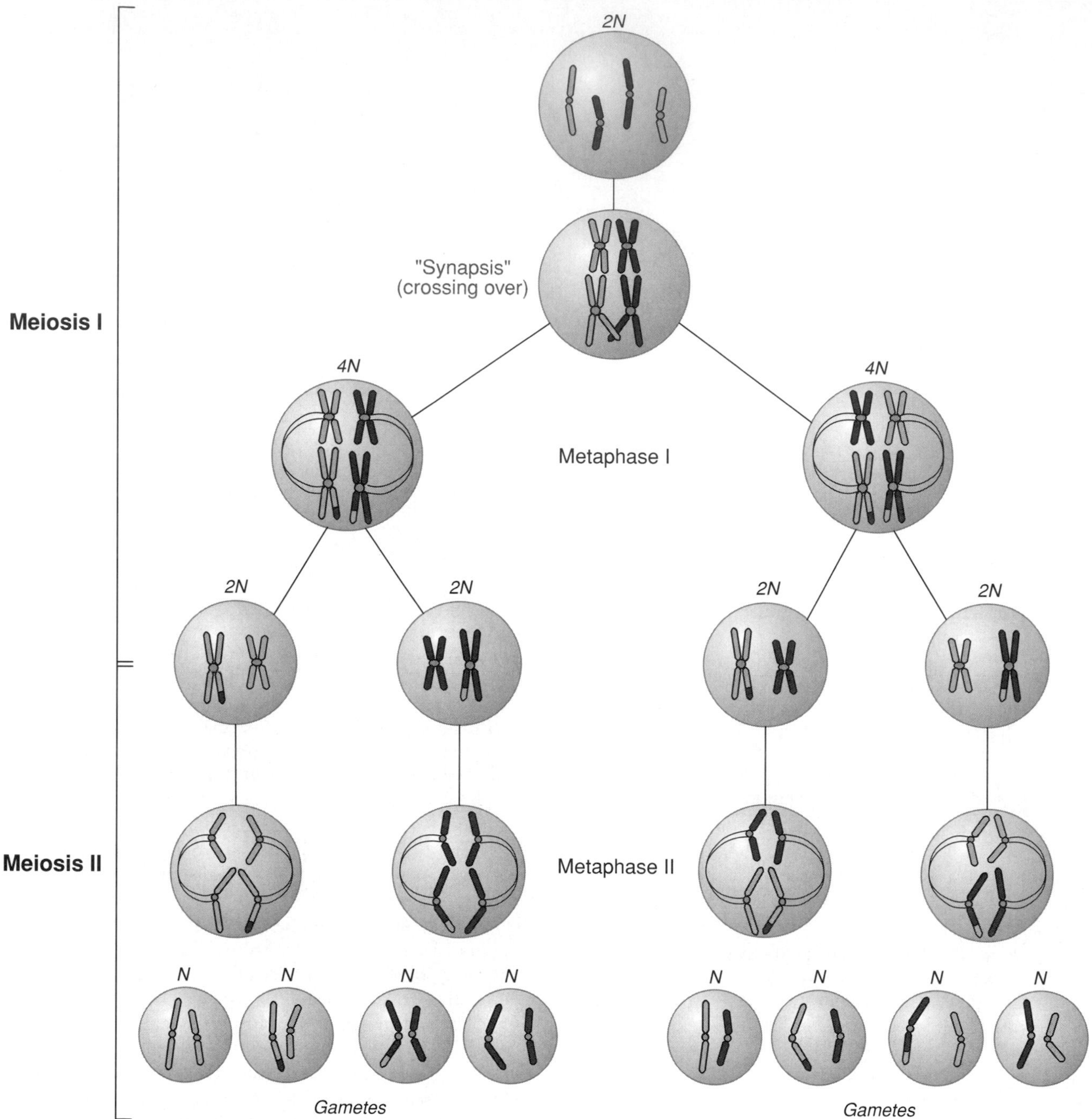

Fig. 12-1 The two stages of meiosis shown diagrammatically with two pairs of chromosomes. A single crossing-over in one pair is illustrated (meiosis I). Eight gamete arrangements are possible after sister chromatid separation in meiosis II.

are recognized in mitosis: *prophase, prometaphase, metaphase, anaphase,* and *telophase.* Each chromosome replicates in *interphase,* or more specifically during the *S phase* (DNA synthesis) of the cell cycle (Fig. 12-2). G1 (gap 1) and G2 (gap 2) stages are essentially resting phases (no DNA synthesis or cellular division is occurring). G1 and G2 together with the S phase constitute *interphase.*

A replicated chromosome consists of two sister chromatids connected by a primary constriction called the *centromere.* Mitotic spindle fibers (microtubules) attach to the centromeres of replicated chromosomes and pull each sister chromatid to the opposite pole during anaphase (Fig. 12-3). Two daughter nuclei are formed at the completion of each cell cycle.

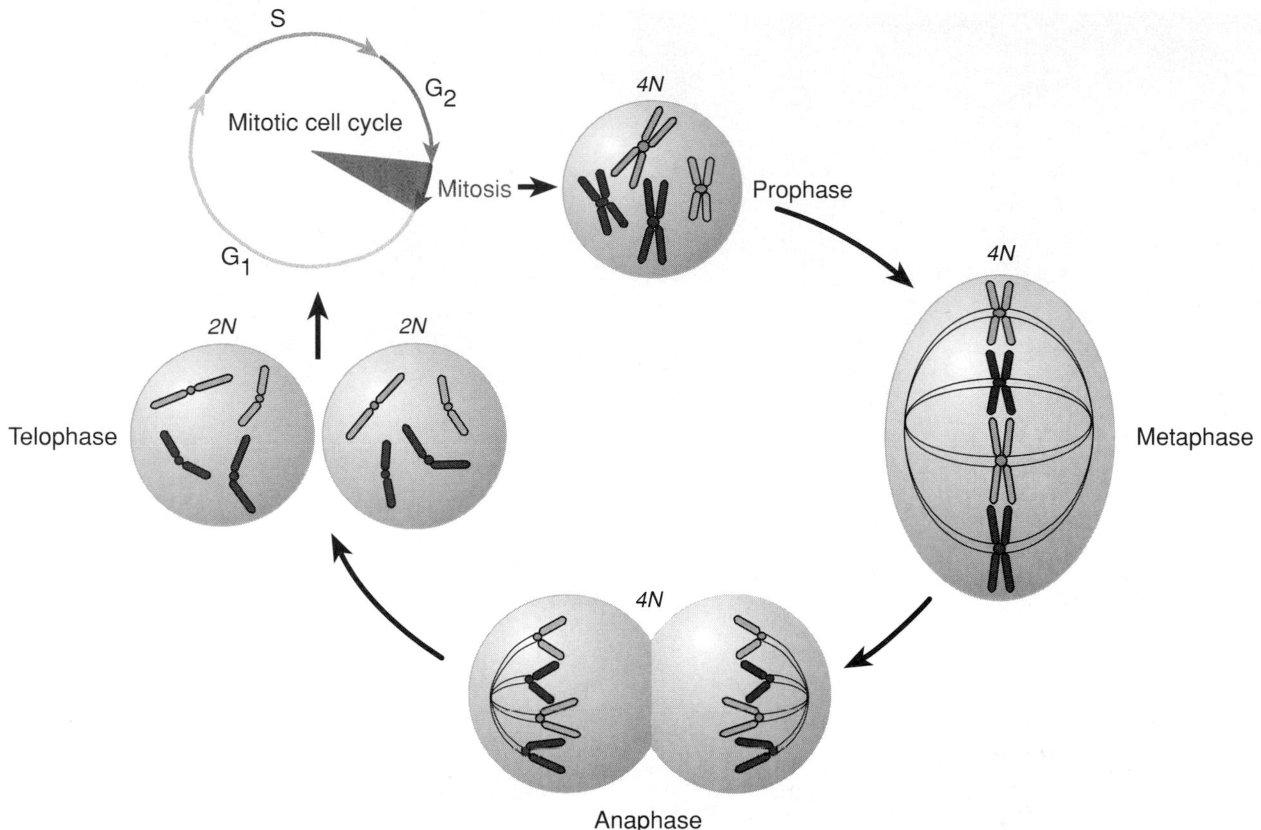

Fig. 12-2 Mitosis, the cellular division phase of the cell cycle. Contraction of the chromosomes and disappearance of the nucleolus in prophase with lining up of the chromosomes on the equatorial plane and microtubule attachment during metaphase. Sister chromatid separation and the formation of two independent daughter cells takes place in anaphase and telophase.

THE NORMAL KARYOTYPE

A *karyotype* is the somatic chromosomal complement of an individual or species. For the human, a normal karyotype consists of 46 chromosomes aligned in a standard sequence on the basis of size, centromere location, and banding pattern (Fig. 12-4). One can produce karyotypes by photographing a metaphase spread under a microscope, manually cutting out the chromosomes from the photograph, and arranging and pasting them in order. Automated or computerized systems have been developed in recent years to facilitate analysis by eliminating the need for photography and other darkroom activities as well as the manual preparation of the karyotype. The karyotype is one of the basic tools of the cytogeneticist.

Certain properties of the chromosomes are identified to assist in distinguishing each pair (Fig. 12-5). For example, chromosomes can be segregated into three groups on the basis of centromere location, an important identifying chromosomal feature. The *centromere* divides the chromosome into a short (upper) arm and a long (lower) arm. The short arm is referred to as the *p (petit) arm,* and the long arm as the *q arm.* The distal ends of each chromosome are termed *telomeres.*

A *metacentric* chromosome is one in which the centromere is located in the middle of the chromosome and includes chromosomes 1, 3, 16, 19, and 20. In contrast, an *acrocentric* chromosome (chromosomes 13, 14, 15, 21, and 22) is one in which the centromere is located near the end of the chromosome. The remainder of the chromosomes are known as *submetacentric* with centromeres located in between the middle and the end. The short arm of the acrocentric chromosome differs from other chromosomes in that it has a small knob of chromatin called a *satellite* connected to it by a thin stalk. The *stalks,* also known as secondary constrictions, are composed of genes for 18S and 28S ribosomal RNA (rRNA) and form the nucleolus of the resting cell.[4]

Cell culture

To produce a karyotype, one must obtain cells capable of growth and division. Different types of samples commonly analyzed in a clinical cytogenetic laboratory and basic principles of analysis are summarized in Table 12-1.

Amniotic fluid

One can analyze fetal cells by obtaining amniotic fluid (cell types cultured include those derived from amnion, skin, and urogenitory, respiratory, and alimentary systems), chorionic villi (cell types cultured include those derived from the mesenchymal core of the villus and trophoblastic cells), or blood (percutaneous umbilical blood sampling, PUBS). All will produce cells acceptable for cytogenetic analysis; however, each

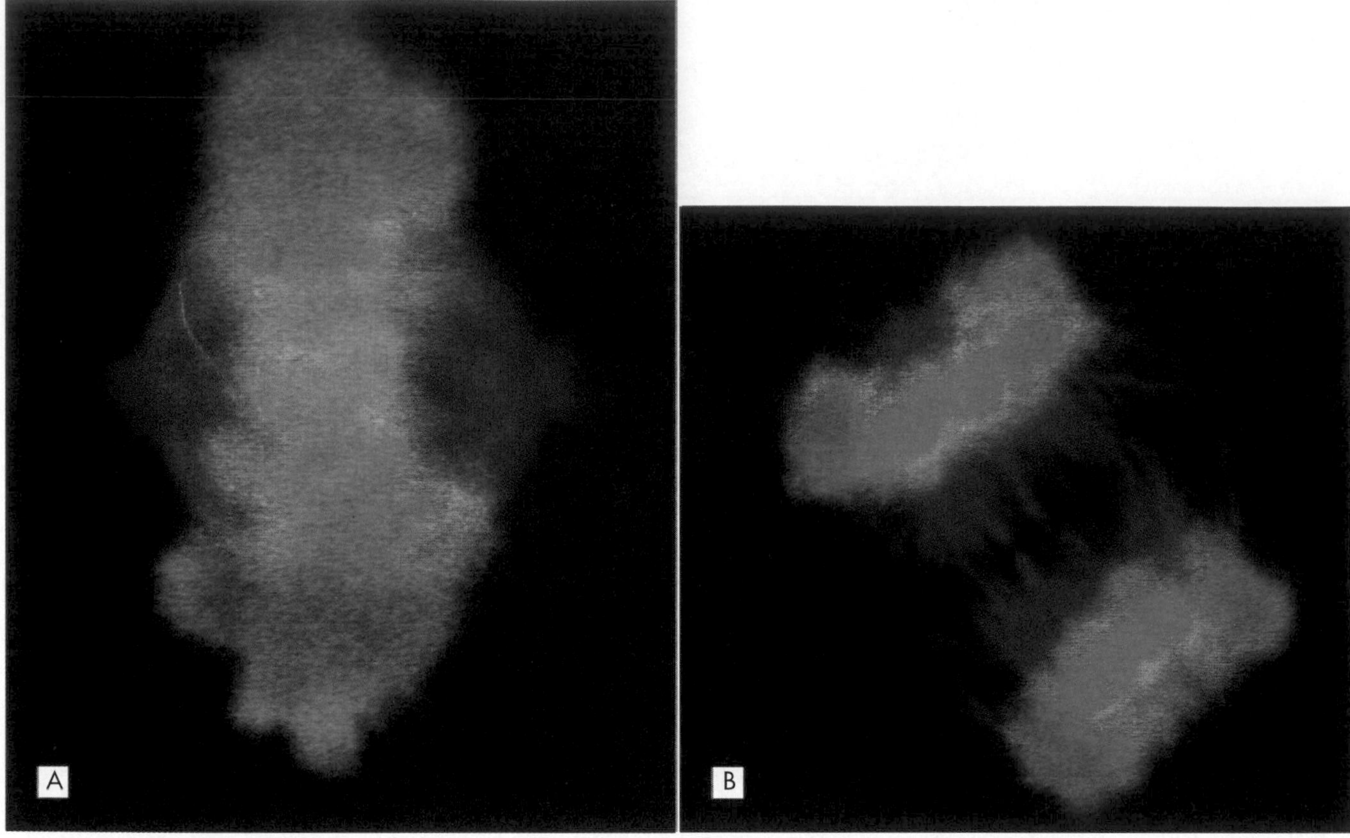

Fig. 12-3 **A,** CHO (Chinese hamster ovary) cell in metaphase of mitosis showing the chromosomes in green and microtubules in red or yellow-orange. **B,** CHO cell in anaphase of mitosis showing the chromosomes in green and microtubules in red or yellow-orange. (Courtesy Dr. David L. Spector, Cold Spring Harbor Laboratory, Cold Spring Harbor, NY.)

tissue and the associated laboratory procedures have intrinsic qualities that make them more or less appropriate to different clinical situations. For amniotic fluid an optimum quantity of 20 milliliters (ml) is obtained by amniocentesis performed at or after 14 weeks of gestation. On the average, obstetric complications are encountered in less than 0.5% of cases.[5] The specimen is divided equally, and parallel cultures are established. Two cultures per patient sample are customary in case a problem, such as contamination, occurs with one sample; the other can serve as a "backup."

A variety of culture mediums are commercially available for culturing amniotic fluid as well as other specimen types. Individual laboratories may differ based on personal preferences. Typically, amniotic fluid specimens require 8 to 14 days of culture before harvest. Dividing cells are arrested in metaphase by the addition of *colchicine* or *colcemid (deacetylmethylcolchicine)*. These are agents that inhibit microtubule formation, thus obstructing the completion of the mitotic cycle. Subsequently, cells are exposed to a *hypotonic solution* to induce swelling of the cell for enhanced spreading of the chromosomes. The metaphase cells are then fixed, most commonly with a 3:1 methanol/glacial acetic acid mixture, and stained by one of several banding techniques. The chromosomes are analyzed under a microscope and photographed. A karyotype is constructed by manual or automated means.

Table 12-1 Successive steps in cytogenetic analysis

Sample procurement
Amniotic fluid
Chorionic villi
Skin, fibroblasts
Peripheral blood lymphocytes
Products of conception
Bone marrow
Lymph nodes
Solid tumors
Sample preparation and culture
Arrest of cellular division (colchicine)
Hypotonic swelling and lysis of cells
Cell fixation
Slide preparation
Staining (banding)
Microscopic analysis and photography
Karyotype production
Interpretation

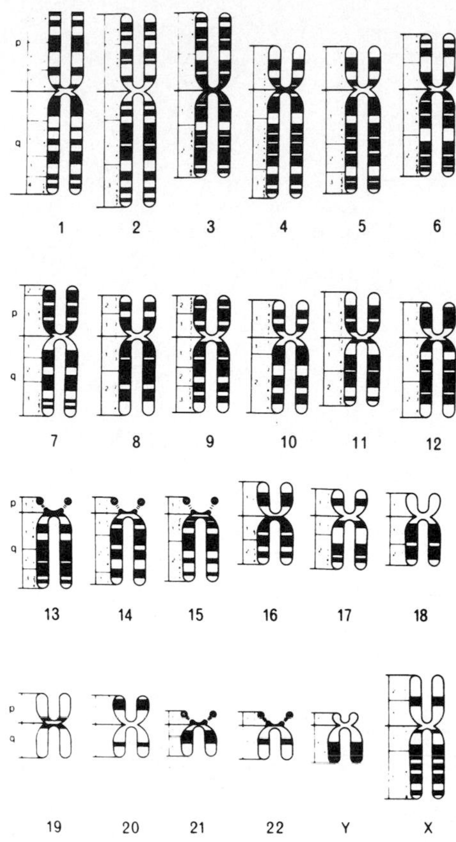

Fig. 12-4 Schema of chromosomes (G banded) according to the Paris Conference (ISCN 1985; see references 19 and 20).

Chorionic villus sampling

A distinct advantage of chorionic villus sampling (CVS) is the earlier gestational age at which the specimen may be collected (8 to 12 weeks of gestation). A sample may be obtained transcervically or transabdominally with ultrasound guidance. Collection of vascularized and budding villi of the chorion frondosum is essential for a successful fetal cell culture representation. Moreover, separation of maternally derived tissue such as maternal blood, decidua, and cervical mucus is a critical step in the preparation of the culture to prevent maternal cell contamination and the serious consequence of erroneous interpretation. Villous material can be separated from other tissues under a dissecting microscope. Two separate approaches based on the analysis of two different cell populations can be performed. These include a rapid technique to visualize spontaneous metaphases in the cytotrophoblast layer (results in 1 to 3 days) and a long-term culture of the mesenchymal cells (requiring 6 to 14 days in culture). The basic steps of cellular division arrest, harvest, fixation, staining, and karyotype production are similar to those outlined for amniotic fluid samples.

Fetal blood sampling

Fetal blood may be obtained by PUBS as early as the seventeenth gestational week. Although analysis of fetal blood yields the most reliable results (sample obtained is totally fetal in origin), the risks of obstetric complications are relatively high. The two most common indications for this form of analysis include determination of isoimmune hemolytic disease and rapid fetal karyotyping.[6] With respect to the latter, fetal blood sampling is invaluable in ascertaining whether chromosomal mosaicism as determined by analysis of amniotic fluid or chorionic villi is representative of the fetus or is an extraembryonic abnormality confined to the placenta.

Peripheral blood

Peripheral blood is one of the easiest and most accessible specimens for cytogenetic analysis and normally is productive of a large quantity of quality mitoses. Peripheral blood is commonly obtained for the determination of constitutional chromosomal disorders such as Down syndrome (trisomy 21) or the somatic chromosomal abnormalities of neoplastic cells of patients with hematologic malignancies. A sample is usually collected by venipuncture and mixed with sodium or lithium heparin to prevent clotting. The specimen is centrifuged, allowing the white cells to form a separate layer (buffy coat). Peripheral blood lymphocytes are separated and stimulated to grow in culture with the addition of *mitogens* (mitogens are not necessary for the chromosomal analysis of spontaneously dividing neoplastic cells). Examples of these growth stimulating or in vitro mitotic agents include tuberculin purified protein, tetanus toxoid, diphtheria toxoid, smallpox vaccine, leukocyte antiserum, pollen extract, yeast extract, living or dead donor cells (histocompatibility mismatched), various tissue antigens, Epstein-Barr virus (EBV), and plant antigens such as concanavalin A, pokeweed mitogen (PWM), phorbol ester (TPA), and phytohemagglutinin (PHA).[7] Peripheral blood lymphocytes are usually cultured for 72 hours before the addition of colchicine and the remaining steps of analysis. Note that the success or failure of the culture is dependent on adequate numbers of lymphocytes in the peripheral blood. Clinical factors such as the presence of myeloproliferative or myelodysplastic disorders, infections, or drugs may affect analysis untowardly.

Prophase or *prometaphase* analysis of synchronized cells provides a high degree of chromosomal resolution not achieved with standard metaphase analysis (*high-resolution analysis*). With this technique, cells are arrested at an earlier stage of mitosis (prophase or prometaphase) when the chromosomes are not so contracted and display more bands.[8] This permits the detection of subtle abnormalities and rearrangements such as the small chromosomal segments lost in each of the *microdeletion syndromes* (Fig. 12-6). For high-resolution analysis, dividing cells are blocked in synthesis with the addition of *amethopterin (methotrexate),* a folic acid antagonist. The block is subsequently released with a thymidine-rich medium, and the cells are allowed to proceed in synchrony to complete division. Knowledge of the timing of the cell cycle allows initiation of harvest when a large proportion of the cells are in prophase or prometaphase.

Skin fibroblasts

A skin-punch biopsy, which typically yields a specimen 4 mm in diameter, is commonly performed for the cytogenetic analysis of skin. Skin obtained from deceased patients frequently includes spontaneously aborted or induced pregnancy termination fetuses. *Products of conception* are the evacuated contents of the uterus after termination of an early pregnancy or the spontaneously aborted material collected after early fetal death. The latter specimen consists of variably recognizable fetal parts and remnants of the sac and placenta. Although some fetal specimens may be severely autolyzed (depending

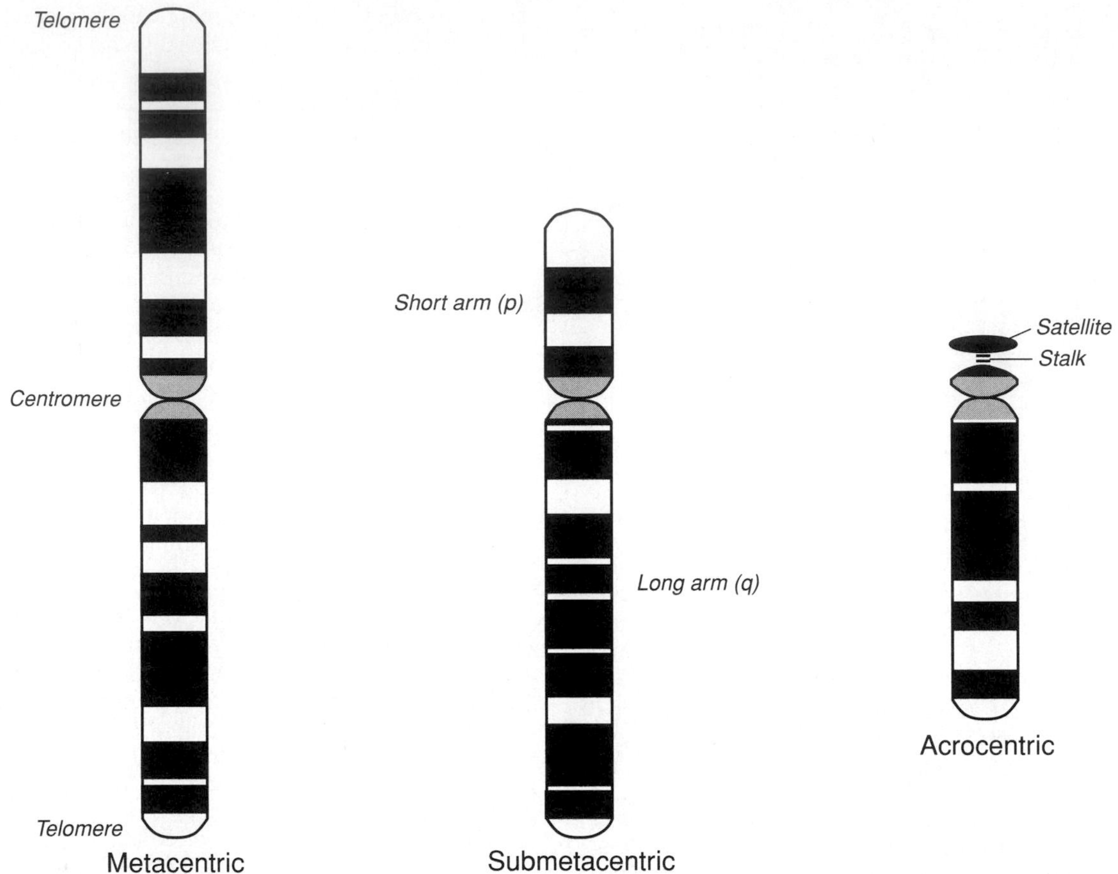

Fig. 12-5 Chromosomal properties and types as defined by size and centromere location.

on the time elapsed between death and specimen collection), it is important not to be dissuaded from attempting culture because the placenta will have recently been attached to the maternal circulation and may still contain viable cells. Additionally in some instances, molecular cytogenetic techniques may be used (fluorescence in situ hybridization), which do not require cell culture.

The predominant cell type cultured in these specimens is the *fibroblast,* a spindle-shaped mesenchymal cell. Because the sample received is often a solid or whole piece of tissue, a cell suspension of the specimen must be prepared first. This is achieved by mechanical mincing of the specimen into small pieces or exposure of it to an enzymatic treatment such as collagenase for disaggregation. The cells are subsequently placed in culture medium and cultured for 1 to 3 weeks.

Bone marrow

Bone marrow is the optimal source of dividing cells in hematologic malignancies and related conditions.[9] Approximately 1 ml of heparinized bone marrow is adequate for analysis. It is preferable to process a sample without delay; however, specimens originating from the marrow can be successfully processed when sent over long distances (usually received in the cytogenetic laboratory within 24 hours after withdrawal of the marrow). No sample (bone marrow, amniotic fluid, peripheral blood) should be frozen or sent in dry ice. Freezing of the cells precludes their division in vitro.

Bone marrow cellularity varies from patient to patient. Thus the volume of specimen established for culture may differ individually (in part related to the underlying clinical disorder). After 24 to 48 hours of culture, marrow specimens can be harvested for analysis. Although several agents have been used to increase the yield of metaphases in marrow specimens, up to now none of these, except for mitogenic agents in chronic lymphocytic leukemia (CLL), has been shown to be truly useful.

Bone marrow specimens can also be processed without resorting to culture conditions. These so-called *direct cytogenetic preparations* may be used if there is a need to determine the results as quickly as possible. In some instances, results obtained from immediately processed samples such as an acute lymphoblastic leukemia (ALL) specimen are often superior. (Specimens are processed within 15 minutes of sample retrieval.) In addition, direct processing of bone marrow specimens can be used to establish congenital chromosomal anomalies when expeditiousness is necessary. Blood obtained from the umbilical cord may also serve this same purpose.

Lymph nodes

Cytogenetic analysis of the various clinicohistopathologic types of lymphoma generally requires the culturing of involved lymph node tissue. (Bone marrow is a relatively poor source of material for analysis of lymphoma.[9]) Cultures are short term (24 to 48 hours) and dependent on growth pattern, which can be monitored under an inverted phase microscope. The optimal length follows the appearance of small, regular, and spherical clumps of cells. Stimulation of lymph node cells by various mitogenic agents for B- and T-cells may be useful under some circumstances, though lymphoma cells are not often responsive to such stimulation.

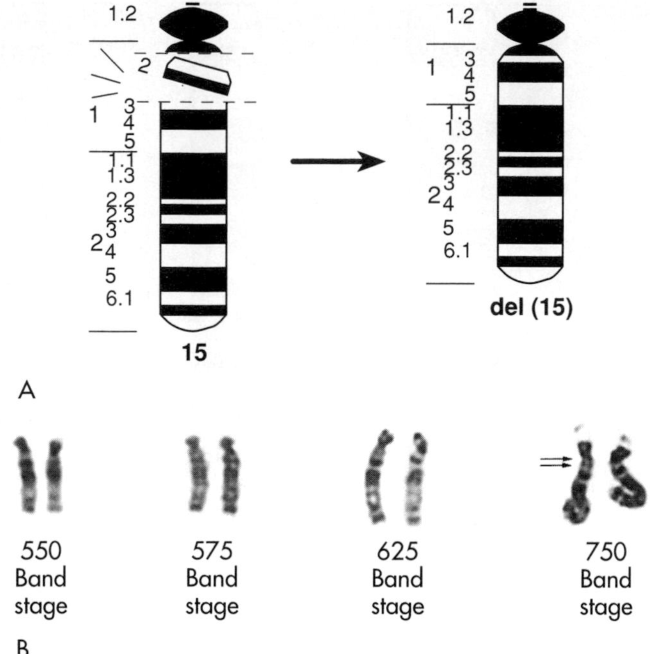

Fig. 12-6 Prader-Willi syndrome is an example of a microdeletion disorder, characterized by a deletion of 15q11-q13 most readily recognizable with high-resolution analysis. **A,** Schema illustrating the normal 15 homolog on the left and the deleted 15 on the right. **B,** Four sets of chromosome 15 in increasing band stage (550, 575, 625, and 750). The normal 15 homolog is on the left of each set, and the deleted 15 is on the right. Notice that with higher resolution the deleted segment is easier to distinguish.

Solid tumors

A solid tumor sample submitted for cytogenetic analysis should be representative of the neoplastic process and preferably be part of the specimen submitted for pathology.[9,10] If several specimens from the same tumor are available, each should be processed separately because some neoplasms have been shown to be heterogeneic.[11] Ideally, a 1 to 2 cm^3 sample (approximately 0.5 to 1.0 g) is provided for analysis. Small biopsy specimens (less than 500 mg) can also be successfully analyzed but may require prolonged culture to produce enough cells for examination. If only a tiny piece of tissue is available, it may be best to use an explant method of culturing. Analogous to a skin sample, a cell suspension must be prepared. Culture times will vary dependent on the tumor type and rate of growth. Success in the cytogenetic analysis of solid tumor specimens is enhanced by the frequent (at least daily) examination of the cultured cells under an inverted phase microscope to establish the peak of mitotic activity.

CHROMOSOMAL BANDING PATTERNS

Before the banding era, chromosomes appeared as solid, dark linear structures. Chromosomes were divided into seven groups (A to G) on the basis of individual size and centromere location (Fig. 12-7). In the 1970s, new techniques were developed that produced unique alternating light and dark staining patterns for each chromosome, called *bands*.[12-14] The most commonly used banding technique today is Giemsa banding (Giemsa stain) or *G-banding*. With traditional G-banding (cells arrested in metaphase) approximately 350 to 550 bands are detected per haploid set. One band represents approximately 5 to 10×10^6 base pairs (bp) of DNA. A further advancement in the evaluation of chromosomes was the development of *high resolution* or *prophase/ prometaphase analysis*. With this approach, dividing cells are arrested in an earlier mitotic phase, prophase, or prometaphase. In these stages additional bands are observed because the chromosomes are not so contracted as in metaphase and there is less coalescence of bands. More than 850 bands per haploid set are seen in this form of analysis.

A uniform system of designating bands produced with different staining techniques in human chromosomes was introduced at a conference in Paris in 1971.[15,16] Such a system is necessary for various purposes: designating breakpoints in structurally aberrant, rearranged, or deleted chromosomes and defining the location of genes on chromosomes, for example. The system for numbering chromosome bands proposed by the Paris conference and adopted universally by cytogeneticists starts by dividing the short and long arms into a number of *regions,* each defined as an area of a chromosome lying between two adjacent landmarks. Landmarks are defined as consistent and distinct morphologic features important for identifying chromosomes. (Actually landmarks, like bands, are features of staining rather than morphologic features in the strict sense of the word.) Regions are numbered consecutively from the centromere to the telomere on each arm; within each region the individual bands are numbered in the same direction. Thus the complete designation of a band would consist of the chromosome number, a letter to indicate the short or long arm, a number for the region, and a number for the band; for example, Xq21 refers to the long arm of chromosome X, region 2, band 1.

It was realized at the time of the Paris Conference report that bands might require subdividing, and provision was made for this simply by adding, after a full stop (= a period), further figures from 1 upwards to indicate subbands and if necessary sub-subbands. Thus Xq21 could be divided into Xq21.1, Xq21.2, and Xq21.3, and the last further divided into Xq21.31, Xq21.32, and Xq21.33 (Fig. 12-8). The wisdom of this provision for almost unlimited expansion became apparent with the development of high-resolution banding. The 1981 report of the standing committee on Human Cytogenetic Nomenclature was concerned entirely with the numbering of bands in prophase chromosomes.[17]

The principal techniques that demonstrate the different classes of bands are *G-*, *Q-*, and *R-banding* (Table 12-2). All use the same principle of chromatin denaturation or enzymatic digestion followed by the incorporation of a DNA-specific dye.[18] All produce a pattern of dark and light bands of various sizes throughout the length of the chromosomes; G- and Q-banding produce essentially the same pattern (a brightly fluorescent Q-band is darkly stained with G-banding), whereas that produced by R-banding is complementary, that is, it produces dark (positive) bands where there would be negative G- or Q-bands. Thus, it is not possible to refer to positive or negative bands without stating the method used to demonstrate these bands. The *International System for Cytogenetic Nomenclature* summarizes these banding patterns,[19-21] supersedes all previous guides to nomenclature, and is a fundamental reference in all cytogenetic laboratories.

G-banding

G-banding is undoubtedly the most widely used banding technique. This is attributable to the relative ease and reliability of

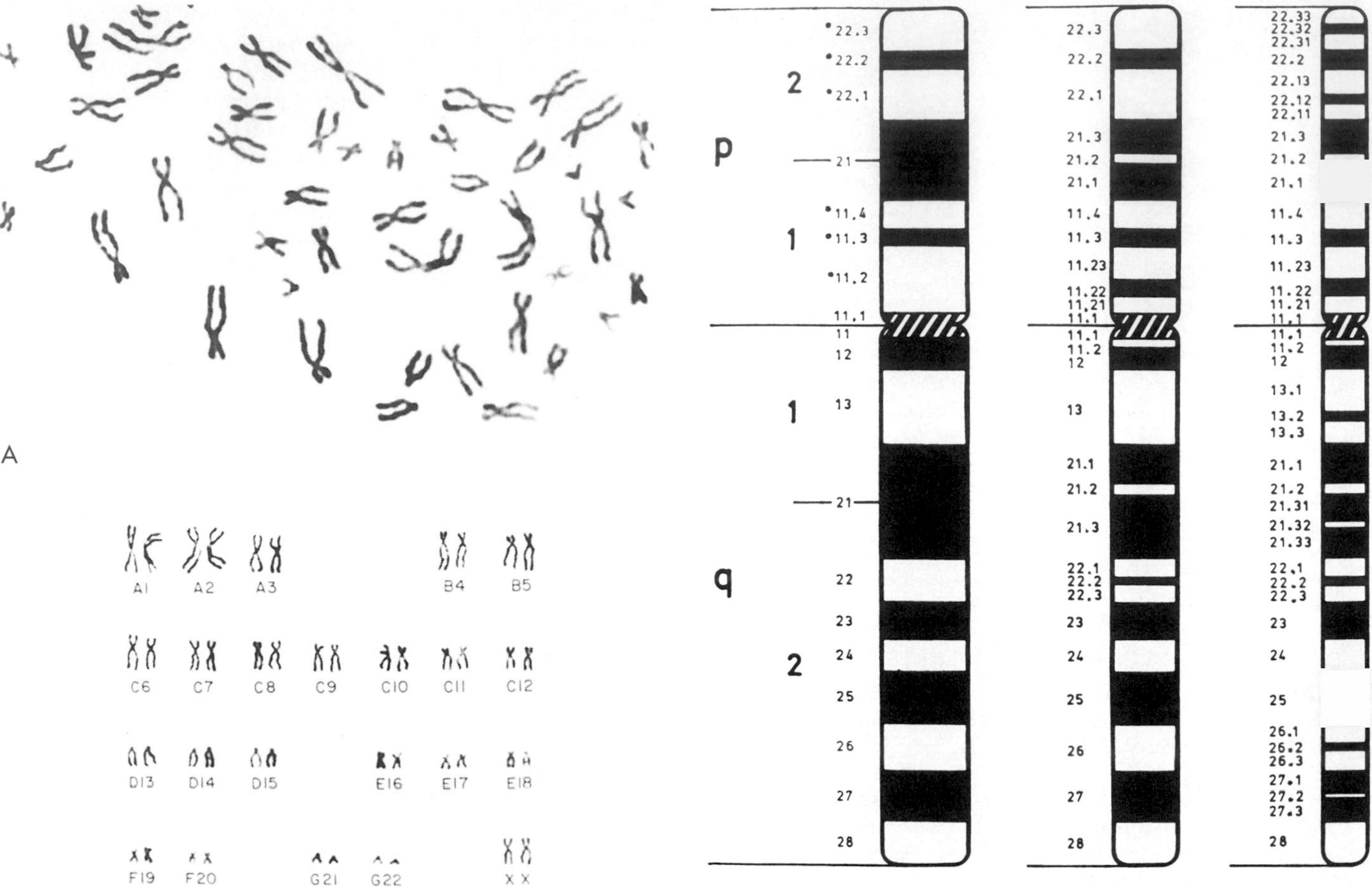

Fig. 12-7 **A,** Normal nonbanded ("solid-stained") metaphase spread from a lymphocyte culture. **B,** Representative karyotype demonstrating grouping of chromosomes (A to G) based on centromere location and chromosome size.

Fig. 12-8 Three different levels of chromosomal band resolution of the X chromosome. The chromosome *on the left* represents a 400-band level stage (400 bands per haploid set); *center,* a 550-band level stage, and *right,* an 850-band level stage.[19,20]

Table 12-2 **Definition of banding methods, according to Paris Conference (ISCN 1985)**

Banding method	Definition
C	Methods that demonstrate "constitutive heterochromatin." A C-band is a unit of chromatin stained by these methods.
Q	Methods using quinacrine mustard or quinacrine to demonstrate bands along chromosomes.
G	Techniques that demonstrate bands along the chromosomes using a Giemsa dye mixture.
R	The "reverse-staining Giemsa method," which gives patterns opposite in staining intensity to those obtained by G-staining methods.

From *ISCN: An international system for human cytogenetic nomenclature: birth defects,* Original Article Series 21(1), New York, 1985, March of Dimes Defects Foundation, and from Hardner DG, Klinger HP, editors: *ISCN 1985: An international system for human genetic nomenclature,* Basel, 1985, Karger.

performing the technique, observation of the results, and the permanence of the preparations. It is a form of identifying chromosomes (Figs. 12-9 and 12-10), in contrast to certain other methods that may draw attention to specific features of chromosomes such as heterochromatin but are of limited value for identification. The fields of application of G-banding are defining karyotypes and locating breakpoints in clinical conditions, in cancer cells, in evolutionary studies, and in gene mapping. In all these fields the use of G-banding, as well as other techniques for demonstrating euchromatic bands, has been indispensable.

The term *G-banding* arose because of the use of Giemsa dye mixture to stain such bands after appropriate treatment of the chromosomes. The treatment consists in exposure of the chromosomes to a salt solution at 60° C or to trypsin to denature the chromosomal proteins. The bands produced are believed to reflect both the structural composition and function of the chromosomes.[22] Adenine and thymidine

(A+T)–rich segments of DNA, which appear to contain few transcribed genes and are late-replicating in the S-phase, correspond to dark G-bands or brightly fluorescing Q-bands.[23,24] In contrast, light-staining G-bands or dark Q-bands parallel early-replicating DNA, have a lower AT content (guanosine and cytosine, G+C, predominant), and are rich in active genes. The band distribution of genes has been studied by "universal" gene markers such as mRNA and the gene-rich, G+C-rich H3 fraction of DNA (localized by in situ hybridization), DNAase hypersensitivity, and digestion by restriction enzymes known to show selectivity for the CpG islands associated with active genes (detected by in situ nick translation).[25] These notions of gene-rich negative G bands is also supported by the clinical and cytogenetic association of viable trisomy disorders (that is, trisomies 21, 18, and 13) that display bright Q-bands (dark G-bands) and are late replicating. Dark and light G-bands may also be different in protein composition. Differential extraction of protein during fixation and banding pretreatments from different regions of the chromosome may be important in the mechanism by which G-bands are obtained.[26]

Marker chromosomes (chromosomes whose exact origin cannot be identified) may have segments that do not band with the G-banding technique but instead show a uniform and intermediate level of staining with Giemsa after treatment that produced a typical G-banding pattern elsewhere on the chromosomes. These distinctive segments are called *homogeneously staining regions,* or HSR. It has been shown that HSR together with *double minute chromosomes* (dmin) (Fig. 12-11), minute chromosome-like bodies lacking centromeres, are a manifestation of DNA amplification, particularly of genes associated with resistance to drugs. In tumor cells,

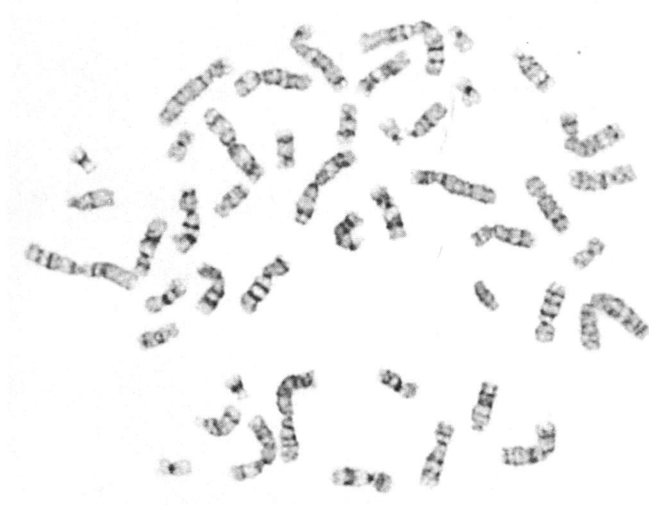

Fig. 12-9 G-banded metaphase of a normal cell showing the bands of all normal chromosomes.

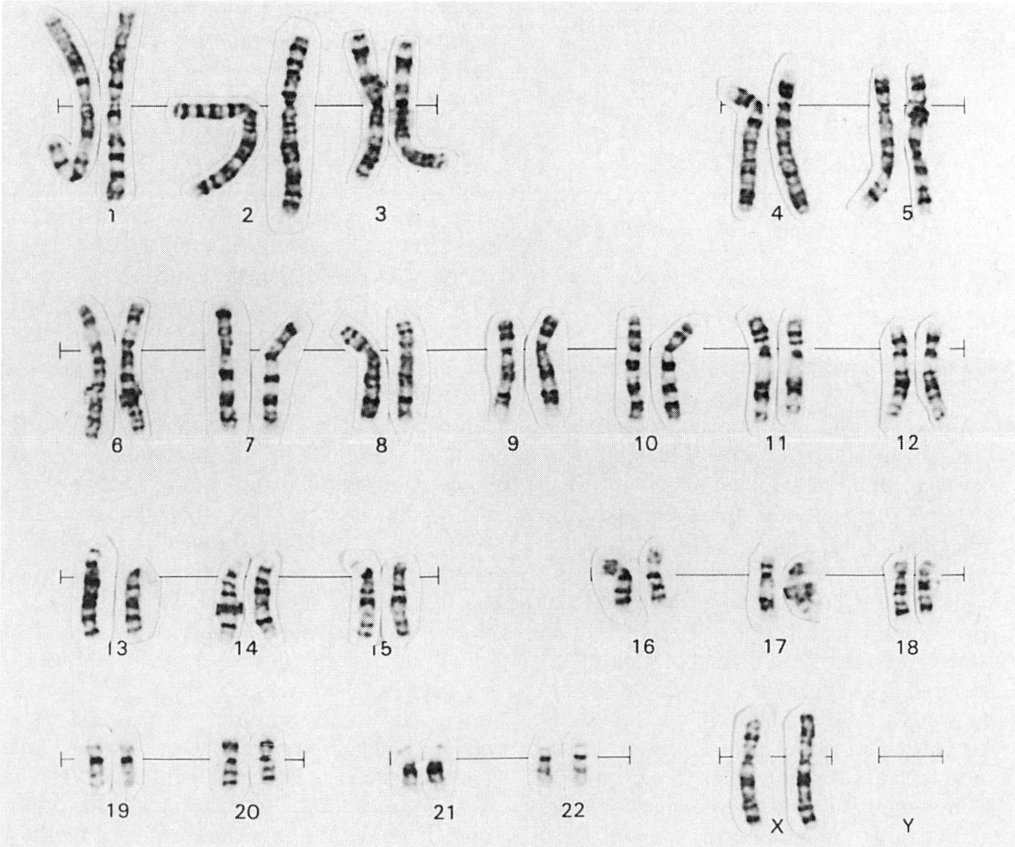

Fig. 12-10 G-banded karyotype of a normal female cell showing the banding patterns of the various chromosomes. Identical patterns characterize homologous chromosomes.

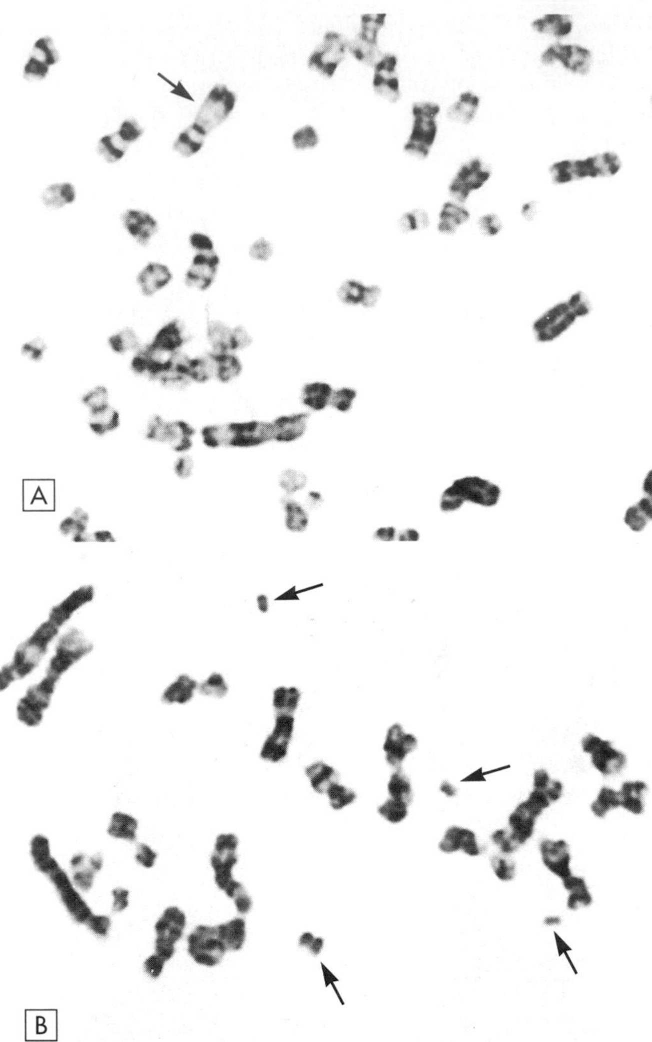

Fig. 12-11 **A,** Homogeneously staining region (HSR) on the short arm of chromosome 11 (*arrow*). **B,** Multiple double minutes (dmin) (*arrows*) in a neoplastic metaphase cell.

HSR and dmin are often associated with oncogene amplification.

It seems paradoxical that, despite its immense value, relatively little is known about certain aspects of G-banding. For example, although it is apparent that a relationship exists between the different types of bands and gene density, base composition, and replication timing, the functional basis for the interdependence of these features of chromosome structure and behavior is not known.[18] Therefore it is fortunate that although at present G-banding is applicable only to a limited group of organisms, that group happens to include the mammals and particularly humans, the species in which we are most interested. If this were not so, G-banding would be little more than a curiosity instead of the essential tool it has become. Thus the deficiencies in knowledge regarding G-banding mechanisms are more than counterbalanced by the immense practical value of this form of analysis.

Q-banding

Q-bands are fluorescent patterns produced on chromosomes after staining with quinacrine mustard or quinacrine (Fig. 12-12). The acridine dye quinacrine dihydrochloride binds to DNA by intercalation or by external ionic binding.[26] This method was first introduced by Caspersson and coworkers in 1968[27] and is thus the oldest of the modern banding techniques, as well as one of the simplest and most versatile. Q-banding patterns can be demonstrated throughout the length of the human chromosomes and were the basis of the standard description of the banded human karyotype. Although Q-banding is now only one of a large number of banding methods, it remains important, not only for the many pioneering discoveries made with this technique, but also because it is still a practical technique in many fields. Like all fluorescence methods, Q-banding suffers from the impermanence and faintness of the image and also from the requirement for special microscopes. These disadvantages are greatly outweighed by the advantages: in particular, its simplicity. Chromosome preparations are stained in a solution of the dye, mounted in an appropriate aqueous fluid, and viewed with a fluorescence microscope. None of the parameters of Q-banding appears to be critical, and a reasonable result can generally be obtained without difficulty. However, as with any other banding method, good chromosome preparations are required for the best results. Despite Caspersson's original remarks of the relative merits of quinacrine versus quinacrine mustard for Q-banding, it is generally believed that there is little practical difference between the two, and most workers now use quinacrine, which is more readily available, cheaper, and safer to handle than the mustard. The most serious disadvantage of quinacrine as compared to its mustard is its greater tendency to fade when illuminated.

There are two types of Q-bands in human chromosomes: *heterochromatic* and *euchromatic*. The former are highly fluorescent bands as compared to the dull euchromatic bands, though the former bands show a good deal of polymorphism. Most of this variation is in band size, but in certain chromosomes there is also variation in brightness, as in the short arms and satellites of the acrocentric chromosomes. The distal long arm of the Y chromosome is visible not only in metaphases, but also in interphase nuclei. The brightness of the fluorescence of Q-bands appears to be related to the presence of A+T-rich DNA and corresponds to the other properties described for G-bands.

R-banding

Shortly after the introduction of Q-banding, other techniques were developed. One of these, *R-banding,* relied on chromosome preparations that were heated in phosphate buffer at 87° C and then stained with Giemsa.[14] The stained chromosomes in R-banding showed a pattern of bands that were complementary to that obtained with G- and Q-banding; that is, bands strongly stained with Giemsa were equivalent to those showing pale G-bands or weak quinacrine fluorescence in Q-banding. One serious disadvantage of the original R-banding method was the very pale staining, and so phase microscopy was required to examine the preparations adequately. The introduction of acridine orange (instead of Giemsa stain) solved this problem (Fig. 12-13). Apart from giving much better contrast than the original Giemsa staining method, the acridine orange methods have revealed color heteromorphisms in certain segments of the human chromosomes.

R-bands contain most of the genes, are G+C rich, and replicate early in the S phase. One of the advantages of R-banding

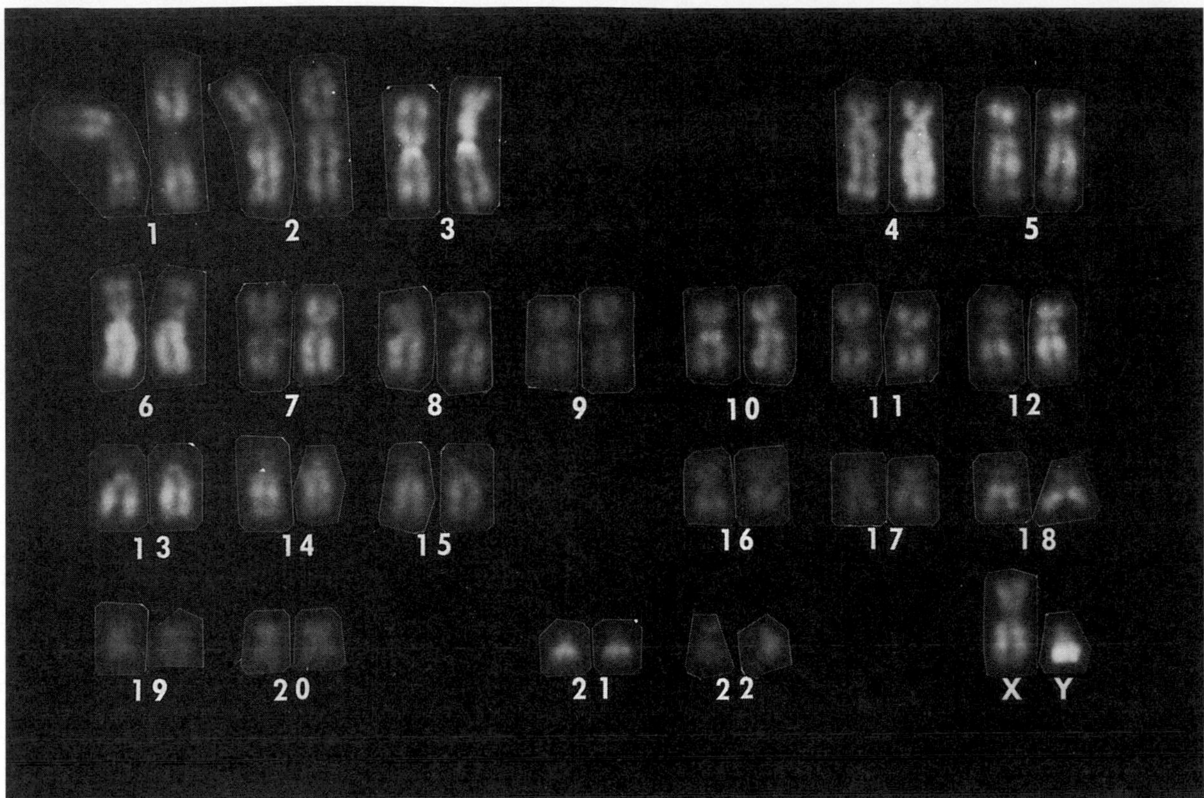

Fig. 12-12 Q-banded karyotype of a normal male cell demonstrating the various bands with the long arm of the Y chromosome showing its unique staining.

is that the ends of chromosomes (termini) are strongly stained. This is of great benefit in studying translocations or other structural anomalies involving the distal ends of chromosomes. Techniques have been introduced in which the intensity of the R-bands is reduced but the terminal bands are still strongly stained (*T-bands*). T-bands are the highest in gene density; 58% of the R-band genes map to T-bands.[28] T-bands account for only 37% of R-band DNA.

C-banding

Constitutive heterochromatin comprises approximately 20% of the human genome and is composed of satellite and nonsatellite repetitive DNA sequences.[14] Constitutive heterochromatin appears to be genetically inert (does not contain mendelian genes and is not transcribed). This form of chromatin stains dark in nondividing (interphase cells) and remains condensed. In the interphase cell, these dark-staining masses of chromatin are called *chromocenters*.

C-banding selectively stains constitutive heterochromatin. In humans, C-bands are located at all centromeres and the distal long arm of the Y chromosome (Fig. 12-14). These regions, particularly on chromosomes 1, 9, 16, and Y, may vary in size (are heteromorphic). These variations, or *heteromorphisms*, are classified into five size categories, levels 1 to 5 (very small, small, intermediate, large, and very large).[16] C-bands also vary in their position with respect to the centromere. On this basis they are classified into five levels, 1 to 5 (NI, no inversion; MIN, partial inversion—minor; HI, half inversion; MAJ, partial inversion—major; and CI, complete inversion).[29] Heteromorphisms of C-bands have no proved clinical significance, but because they are inherited from parent to child they can be used as familial markers. These heteromorphisms as well as satellite polymorphisms may also be used to distinguish donor and recipient cells of the same sex in patients after bone marrow transplant.

Arrighi and Hsu[30] originally described a method of producing C-banding utilizing an alkali, sodium hydroxide (NaOH). Sumner[14] modified the technique by substituting barium hydroxide, $Ba(OH)_2$, a milder alkali, for NaOH, which resulted in less chromosomal distortion and was less time consuming. It has been shown that approximately 60% of DNA is extracted during the C-banding procedure and that certain DNA-associated proteins closely involved in constitutive heterochromatin condensation provide resistance to extraction.[31] The basic procedure includes an initial acid treatment to depurinate the DNA, followed by exposure to the alkali—NaOH or $Ba(OH)_2$—resulting in DNA denaturation, and a final treatment to break down the denatured DNA chain at the depurinated sites by exposure to hot salt.

Chromosomal aberrations involving the heterochromatic regions on the long arms of chromosomes 1, 9, and 16 and the short arms of the acrocentric chromosomes and Yq are often regarded as normal variants because carriers have no associated deleterious effects. One example is the commonly observed inversion involving the centromere of chromosome 9, inv(9)(p11q12) (Fig. 12-15). This inversion is seen in approximately 1% of all individuals tested by cytogenetic laboratories.

Nuclear organizer region (NOR) banding

The *nucleolus* is a highly basophilic body in the cell nucleus that is involved with the production and assembly of ribosomal

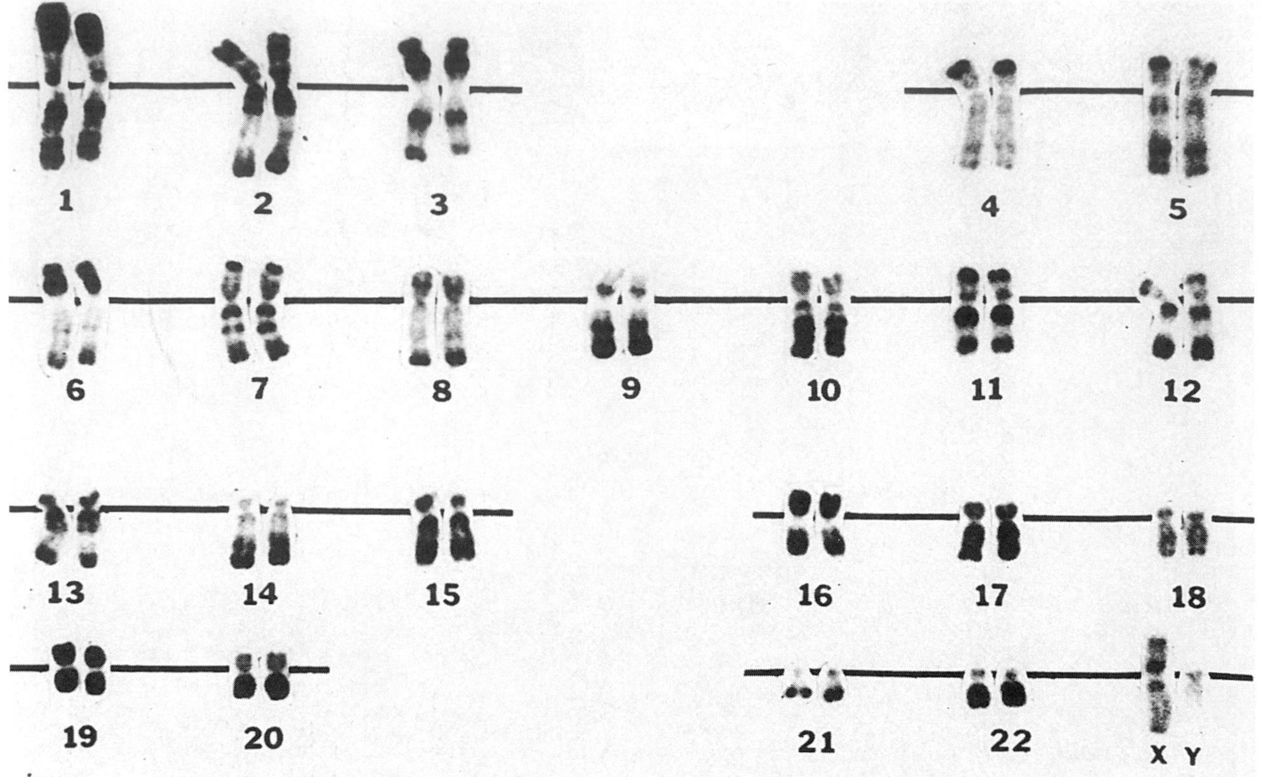

Fig. 12-13 R-banded karyotype of a normal male cell showing the prominent banding of the telomeric regions at the end of chromosomes.

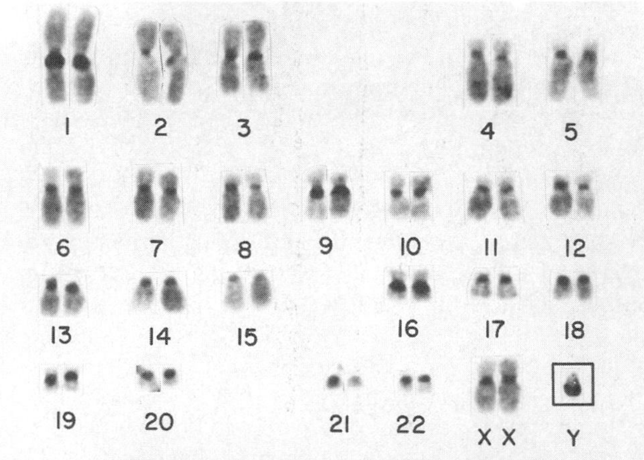

Fig. 12-14 C-banded karyotype of a normal female cell. Notice the prominent C-bands of chromosomes 1, 9, and 16 and the variation in the size of these bands between homologs. *Inset,* The staining of a male Y chromosome, particularly prominent in the long arm.

subunits. Specific chromosomal regions that form and maintain the nucieoli are called *nucleolar organizer regions* (NORs). These regions are located on the stalks of the acrocentric chromosomes (chromosomes 13, 14, 15, 21, and 22) and contain the genes for 18S and 28S rRNA. They can be stained by use of a Giemsa stain (N-banding) or silver impregnation (Ag-NOR banding).[32,33] Specifically linked, structural, nonhistone NOR proteins theoretically remain after DNA, RNA, and histones are extracted by the N-banding method. The Ag-NOR banding method stains a protein associated with rDNA-containing structures.[34] The exact function of this protein is unknown.

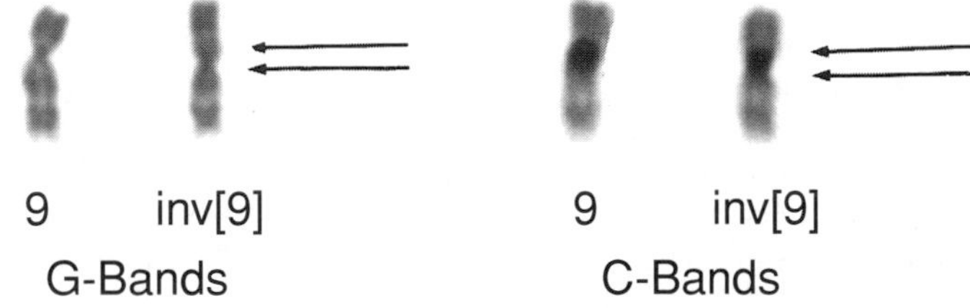

Fig. 12-15 Partial G- and C-banded karyotypes of the commonly encountered inversion 9, that is, inv(9)(p11q12). Normal homolog is on the left and inv(9) on the right.

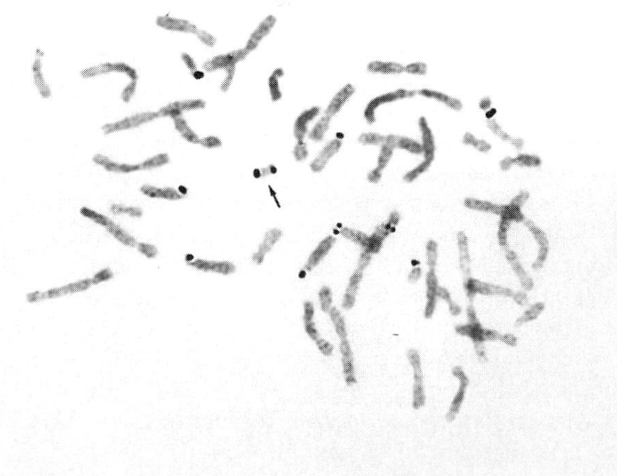

Fig. 12-16 Nuclear organizing region-(NOR) banded metaphase cell from an individual with a small bisatellited marker chromosome *(arrow).*

NOR-banding, similar to C-banding is useful for the identification of heritable polymorphisms. It is also important in defining precise breakpoints involving acrocentric chromosomes in structural rearrangements. NOR-banding is particularly valuable in distinguishing small bisatellited marker chromosomes of acrocentric origin from others of similar size and morphology[35] (Fig. 12-16). Furthermore, NOR activity in human male meiosis and in malignant cells can be evaluated with these techniques.

MOLECULAR CYTOGENETIC ANALYSIS

In situ hybridization

A revolutionary tool in the analysis and characterization of chromosomes and chromosomal abnormalities has been the development of *in situ hybridization* (ISH) techniques. *Hybridization* refers to the binding or annealing of complementary DNA or RNA sequences. This approach permits the detection of specific nucleic acid sequences in morphologically preserved chromosomes, cells, or tissue sections. Gene activity at the DNA, mRNA, and protein level can be examined in combination with immunocytochemistry.

In situ hybridization techniques originated in studies such as those described by Gall and Purdue,[36] who used labeled 18 and 28S ribosomal RNA probes to detect genes in nucleoli of *Xenopus laevis* (an African frog). In early studies, radioisotopes were utilized as labels for nucleic acids, and detection of hybridized sequences was attained with autoradiography. Localization of genes in these studies was found with multiple gene copies, making detection easier because a large signal was generated by the many labeled probe molecules within a small chromosome region.

As technology advanced, detection by enzymatic and fluorescent means became available for quick and safe analysis. Haptenated probes (labeled with biotin, digoxigenin, or dinitrophenol) are frequently detected with one of three sets of distinguishable fluorophores emitting green (fluorescein), red (rhodamine, or Texas Red), or blue (7-amino-4-methylcoumarin-3-acetic acid [AMCA], or Cascade Blue). Concurrent hybridization with two or more of these different haptens and fluorophores allows for simultaneous assessment of two or more sequences (or whole chromosomes) of interest (Fig. 12-17). Combinatorial labeling of probes with two or more different reporters (such as fluorescein with rhodamine) further increases the number of distinguishable targets. In addition, improvements in the sensitivity of the procedure have been dramatic, thereby permitting the detection of small unique or low copy-number gene sequences (as small as 500 base pairs).[37,38]

The applications of ISH are numerous. With this approach an investigator can (1) map the DNA sequences on specific chromosomes; (2) directly detect repositioning of sequences between chromosomes or within a particular chromosome as a result of a chromosomal rearrangement (one example would be the *bcr-abl* rearrangement commonly seen in chronic myelogenous leukemia, Fig. 12-18); (3) uncover small rearrangements that are not detectable with standard karyotype analysis (the presence of a microdeletion can be detected by the absence of signal on one of a homologous chromosome pair, Fig. 12-19); (4) detect and characterize breakpoints using probes for defined DNA sequences; and (5) detect numerical chromosomal abnormalities in interphase or metaphase cells.[10,11] For example, with omission of cell culture, an expedited prenatal diagnosis for Down syndrome can be performed on interphase cells of amniotic fluid or chorionic villi, using a probe specific for the sequence on chromosome 21 (21q22) necessary to be present in three copies for the Down syndrome phenotype (Fig. 12-20).

ISH compensates for several limitations of conventional cytogenetic analysis. For example, cytogenetic analysis is dependent on the production of high-quality metaphase preparations. The use of chromosome-specific probes with ISH can

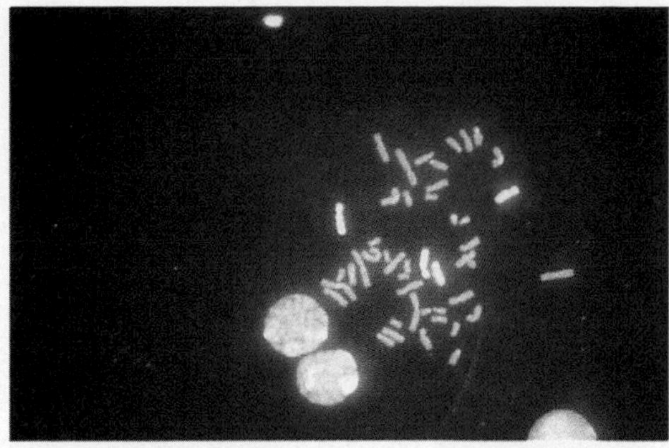

Fig. 12-17 Multicolor fluorescence in situ hybridization (FISH) utilizing chromosome-specific paint probes. Chromosome 4 is labeled with Spectrum Orange (Life Technologies, Gaithersburg, Md.) and chromosome 10 with Spectrum Green. The remainder of the chromosomes or nucleus is counterstained with DAPI.

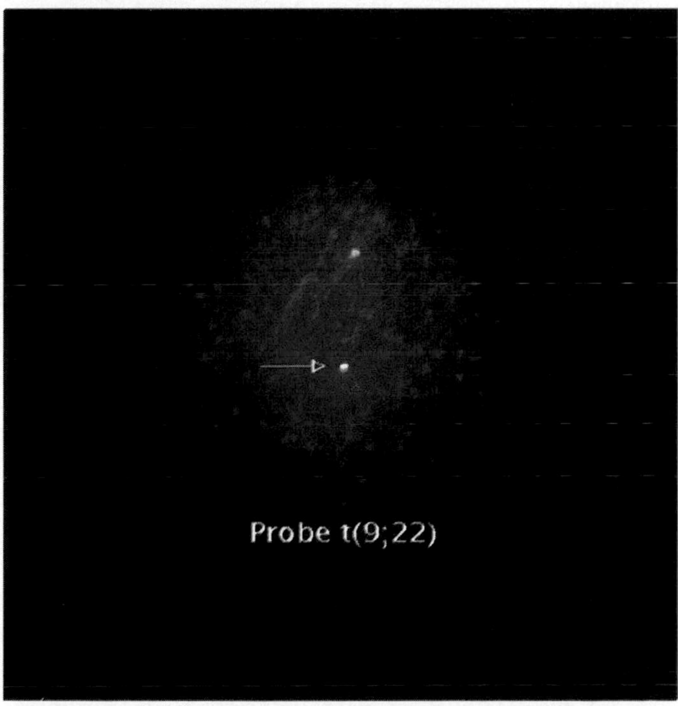

Fig. 12-18 Chronic myelogenous leukemia (CML) is characterized by a reciprocal exchange of chromosomal material (translocation) between chromosomes 9 and 22. Probes specific for the involved regions, that is, *abl* gene (chromosome 9) and *bcr* (breakpoint cluster region chromosome 22), are labeled with a green and red–emitting signal respectively (ONCOR, Gaithersburg, Md.). If a translocation is present (bringing *abl* and *bcr* into proximity), a yellow-white signal is seen, as in this cell from a patient with CML.

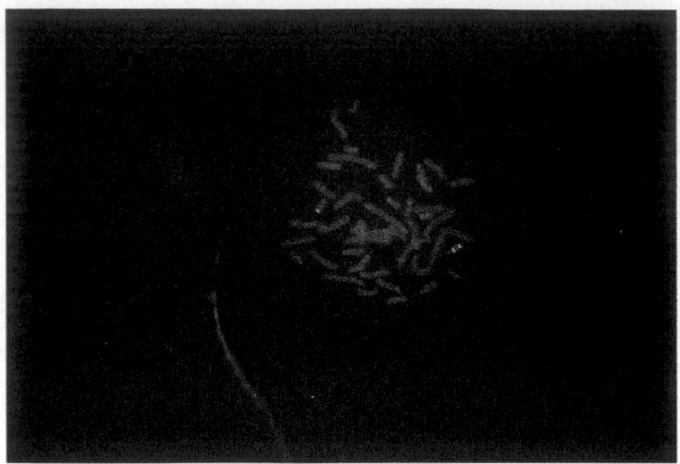

Fig 12-19 A deletion of q11.22 (DiGeorge syndrome, a microdeletion syndrome characterized by absent thymus and parathyroids) is seen on one of the chromosome 22 homologs and is appreciated by the absence of a yellow-green signal (labeled probe specific for that gene sequence) on the long arm. A centromeric probe for chromosome 22 is used simultaneously to assist in identifying these chromosomal homologs of interest.

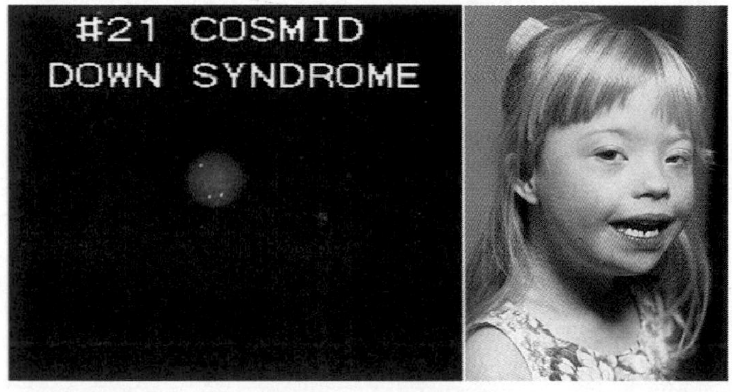

Fig. 12-20 A probe specific for the chromosome 21 sequence responsible for the Down syndrome phenotype is seen in three copies, **A,** in cells of patients shown cytogenetically to be trisomic for chromosome 21, **B.** (Photograph of patient courtesy Drs. A. Olney and M. MacDonald, University of Nebraska Medical Center, Omaha, Nebr.)

Fig. 12-21 An alpha satellite probe specific for chromosome 15 was used to assist in identifying a marker chromosome (chromosome of unidentifiable origin), *lower left.* The two normal chromosome 15 homologs are also identified.

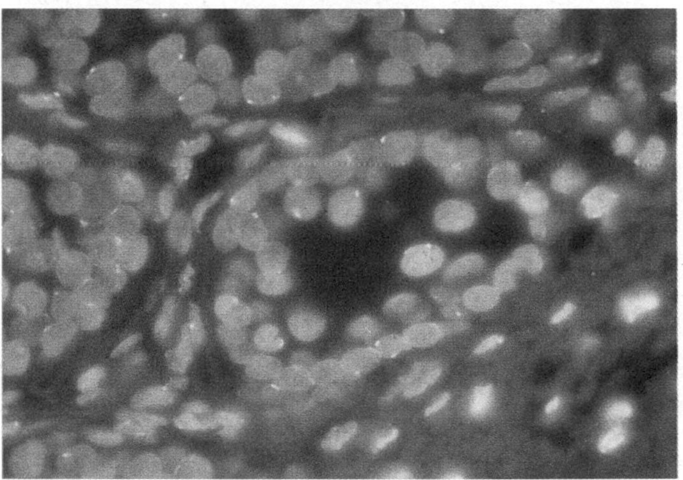

Fig. 12-22 Fluorescence in situ hybridization (FISH) utilizing X (green signal) and Y (red signal) chromosome-specific probes on paraffin-embedded tissue section of normal testis. Notice tubule in center.

identify chromosomes and chromosomal abnormalities that are not definable with standard techniques (Fig. 12-21). Dividing cells are also essential for traditional cytogenetic analysis, as well as the necessity of establishing a tissue culture in most instances. With ISH it is possible to analyze interphase cells or terminally differentiated cells and specimens with a low mitotic rate.

Probes that are frequently utilized for ISH, particularly in the determination of aneuploidy, are specific for a type of DNA called *alpha satellite DNA*. This type of DNA is unique in three respects: it is present at the (peri)centromeric region of each chromosome, it is specific for each chromosome, and it is present in high copy number.[39] Alpha-satellite DNA is organized as tandem repeats of unique 171 base-pair sequences that are present in as many as 5000 copies. Other types of probes include *whole chromosome probes (paint probes)* and *region-specific probes*.

Paint probes in combination with *competition in situ suppression hybridization* (CISS hybridization), utilized to visualize an entire chromosome in either metaphase or interphase cells, are generated by bulk isolation of inserts into plasmid vectors, interspersed repetitive-sequence polymerase chain reaction (PCR) using hybrid cell lines containing only the human chromosome of interest, linker-primer PCR on small numbers of flow-sorted chromosomes, vector PCR on libraries prepared in plasmid vectors, and PCR amplification of bacteriophage library inserts.[11] Region or band-specific probes may be constructed by use of microdissection and microcloning techniques and PCR to amplify the minute amount of dissected chromosomal material. Fluorescent ISH (FISH) can be performed on cytologic specimens such as cytospin or cytologic touch preparations and on surgically obtained pathologic specimens such as paraffin-embedded tissue sections (Figs. 12-22 and 12-23).

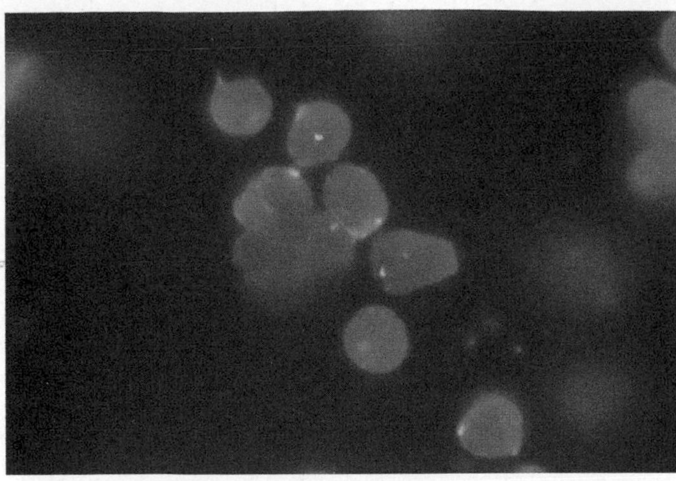

Fig. 12-23 Higher magnification of FISH testicular tissue section shown in Fig. 12-22.

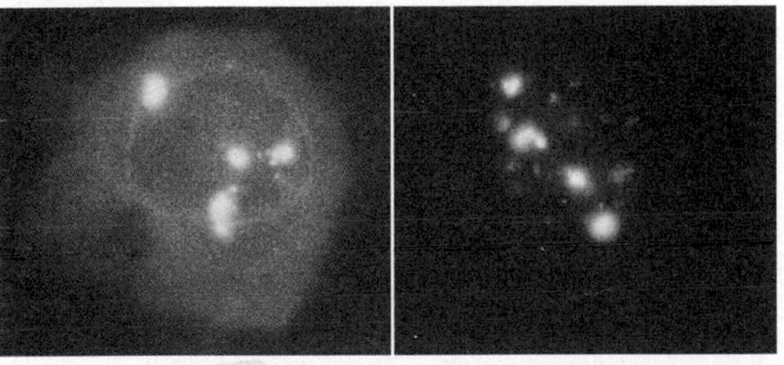

Fig. 12-24 Combined immunocytochemical and molecular cytogenetic approach. In this example of a dedifferentiated chondrosarcoma with a rhabdomyosarcomatous component, a desmin-positive aneuploid cell is present on the left. The cytoplasmic portion of the cell is immunoreactive for desmin *(red)* and four signals *(green)* are seen representative of the α-satellite region of chromosome 7. (Bridge JA, et al: *Am J Pathol* 144:215, 1994). On the right is a desmin-negative aneuploid cell. Only the four signals *(green)* representative of chromosome 7 copy number are detected in this field.

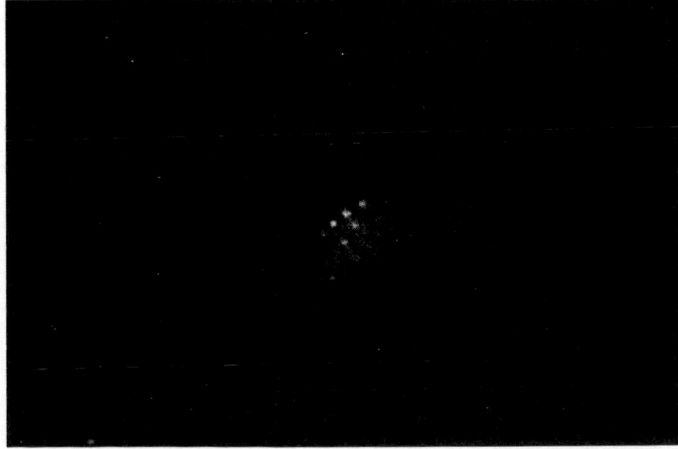

Fig. 12-25 The combined immunocytochemical and molecular cytogenetic approach can also be performed on cytologic touch preparations as in this case of malignant melanoma. The cytoplasmic portion of the cell is immunoreactive for S-100 protein (red) and seven signals *(green)* are seen representative of the α-satellite region of chromosome 7.

Many modifications or variations of ISH exist. One unique method combines ISH with cellular immunophenotyping. When these two forms of analysis are executed simultaneously, determination of the cellular lineage of a specific abnormal cell is possible[40,41] (Figs. 12-24 and 12-25). Knowledge of the histologic derivation of an aneuploid cell is important in developing novel therapeutic modalities that could selectively target the neoplastic population within a specific malignancy.

CHROMOSOMAL ABNORMALITIES

Nomenclature

The field of human cytogenetics has over the years developed its own symbols, glossary, and nomenclature. Aspects of the nomenclature and symbols likely to be encountered in the bulk of articles dealing with cytogenetic changes in human conditions are presented in Table 12-3. For more information regarding these areas the reader may consult the *International System for Human Cytogenetic Nomenclature*.[19-21]

Numerical abnormalities

The number of chromosomes in a normal *haploid* gamete is 23, or N. A *diploid* complement is the equivalent of 46 chromosomes, or 2N. *Euploid* refers to an exact multiple of N; for example, a *triploid* complement, or 3N, would consist of 69 chromosomes, and a *tetraploid* complement, or 4N, would consist of 92 chromosomes. Changes in the number of individual chromosomes as opposed to sets of chromosomes may also be encountered. The term *aneuploidy* indicates a noneuploid state such as the loss of a single chromosome, *monosomy,* or the gain of a single chromosome, *trisomy.* A chromosome complement with two extra identical chromosomes is *tetrasomic.*

The most common mechanism responsible for aneuploidy is *nondisjunction* or the failure of chromosomes to separate normally during cell division. Nondisjunction may occur in the first or second stage of meiosis (Fig. 12-26) or in mitosis. When nondisjunction occurs during the first stage of meiosis, two of four gametes have both the parental chromosomes that failed to separate and two gametes lack any chromosome copies, *nullisomic.* Nondisjunction in the second meiotic stage results in a gamete with two identical copies of the same chromosome, one nullisomic gamete, and two gametes with normal chromosome copy number. If fertilization occurs between a nullisomic gamete and a normal gamete, the result is a monosomic conceptus. The outcome of a fertilization between a gamete retaining both paternal and maternal members of a pair of chromosomes, or both copies of either the paternal or maternal chromosome and a normal gamete, is an offspring trisomic for that chromosome. Nondisjunction occurs frequently though the exact cause is not known. One percent to 3% of human sperm are aneuploid,[42] and it is well recognized that the risk of meiotic nondisjunction increases with increasing maternal age. Most aneuploid conceptuses spontaneously abort early in a pregnancy, usually before recognition of the pregnancy.

The occurrence of nondisjunction in mitosis results in *mosaicism,* a condition in which an individual has two or more cell lines of different chromosomal constitution derived from the same zygote. Mitotic nondisjunction can be striking in malignant cells, resulting in greatly abnormal chromosomal complements.

Table 12-3 Nomenclature

del	Deletion, or loss, of a chromosome segment. EXAMPLE: del(13)(q14) = deletion of band 14 located on the long arm of chromosome 13.
der	Structurally abnormal chromosome created by the rearrangement of two or more chromosomes or more than one rearrangement in the same chromosome.
dup	Duplication, a replicated or duplicated chromosome segment next to itself; if in the same orientation = *direct* duplication (*dir dup*); if inverted = *inverted* duplication (*inv dup*).
i	Isochromosome, a symmetric chromosome composed of duplicated long or short arms formed after misdivision of the centromere in a transverse plane. EXAMPLE: i(5)(p10), duplication of the short arm of chromosome 5 with loss of the long arm.
ins	Insertion, a chromosomal segment from one chromosome is inserted into a nonhomologous chromosome; similar to a duplication, an insertion can be direct or inverted. EXAMPLE: dir ins(10;3)(q22;p14p24) = a direct insertion of the chromosomal segment of a short arm of chromosome 3 (p14-p24) into chromosome 10 at q22.
inv	Inversion, a segment of a chromosome is reversed 180 degrees; a *paracentric* inversion does not involve the centromere in the inversion, a *pericentric* inversion does (a break in each chromosomal arm is necessary). EXAMPLE: inv(2)((p14q22) is a pericentric inversion involving the centromere of chromosome 2.
p	Short arm of a chromosome (from French *petit*).
q	Long arm of a chromosome (letter following *p*).
t	Translocation, a *reciprocal* translocation is an exchange of chromosomal material between two or more nonhomologous chromosomes (may be balanced or unbalanced); a *Robertsonian* translocation involves acrocentric chromosomes with fusion at the centromere and loss of the short arms and satellites. EXAMPLE: t(9;11)(q31;q21.1) denotes a reciprocal translocation involving breaks at band 31 on the long arm of chromosome 9 and at band 21.1 on the long arm chromosome 11 with exchange of the segments distal to those breakpoints.
+ (plus sign)	Added chromosome (+8) or chromosomal segment (8q+).
− (minus sign)	Lost (deleted) chromosome (−7) or chromosomal segment (5q−).

Structural abnormalities

Structural abnormalities of chromosomes result from chromosomal breakage and rejoining of the broken ends to form new combinations. The number of structural variations possible are endless. Structural abnormalities may originate in meiosis or mitosis.

Structural abnormalities may be classified as *balanced* or *unbalanced*. If there is no change in the total number of genes or genetic material present after a structural alteration, the abnormality is designated as balanced. An unbalanced abnormality, however, arises when the rearrangement results in loss or gain of genetic material or information. If the abnormality is stable (capable of passing through cell division) and balanced, the individual carrying such an abnormality will be *phenotypically* (clinically or morphologically) normal. These individuals, however, have an increased risk of producing chromosomally unbalanced offspring.

Translocations

One frequently observed form of a balanced rearrangement is the *balanced translocation*. There are two major types of translocations, *reciprocal* and *Robertsonian* (Fig. 12-27). In a reciprocal translocation, chromosomal material is exchanged between two or more nonhomologous chromosomes. A break occurs in one arm of each chromosome, and the chromosomal segments distal to the breakpoints trade positions. Fusion of two acrocentric chromosomes at the centromere with loss of the short arms and satellites characterizes a Robertsonian translocation.

Reciprocal translocations are relatively common and are seen in approximately 1 in 500 individuals. Reciprocal translocations are often recognized in either the female or male partner of a couple after the birth of a chromosomally unbalanced child or for evaluation of fertility problems or repeated miscarriages. Specifically, if a woman has had two or more spontaneous abortions, the likelihood that one of the partners is a translocation or inversion carrier is 2% to 5%.[43] The translocation is reciprocal in approximately two thirds of these individuals and Robertsonian in the other third.

The meiotic segregation of reciprocal translocation chromosomes is illustrated in Fig. 12-28. In the first stage of meiosis, the four chromosomes with segments in common pair in a cross-shaped, *quadriradial* figure. With the first meiotic cell division, the four chromosomes can separate from this configuration in several different ways. In *alternate segregation*, alternate centromeres travel to opposite poles. This is the only pattern of segregation that can yield a genetically complete gamete (with either a karyotypically normal chromosomal complement or one containing the reciprocal translocation). All other modes of segregation are referred to as "malsegregation."

Adjacent 1 and *adjacent 2* forms of segregation result in chromosomally unbalanced gametes. In adjacent 1 segregation, chromosomes with alike (homologous) centromeres separate into different daughter cells. This is the most common mode of malsegregation in the children of reciprocal translocation carriers. In this form of malsegregation, offspring are partially trisomic for one of the translocation chromosomes and partially monosomic for the other. In adjacent 2 segregation, chromosomes with unalike (nonhomologous) centromeres separate into different daughter cells.

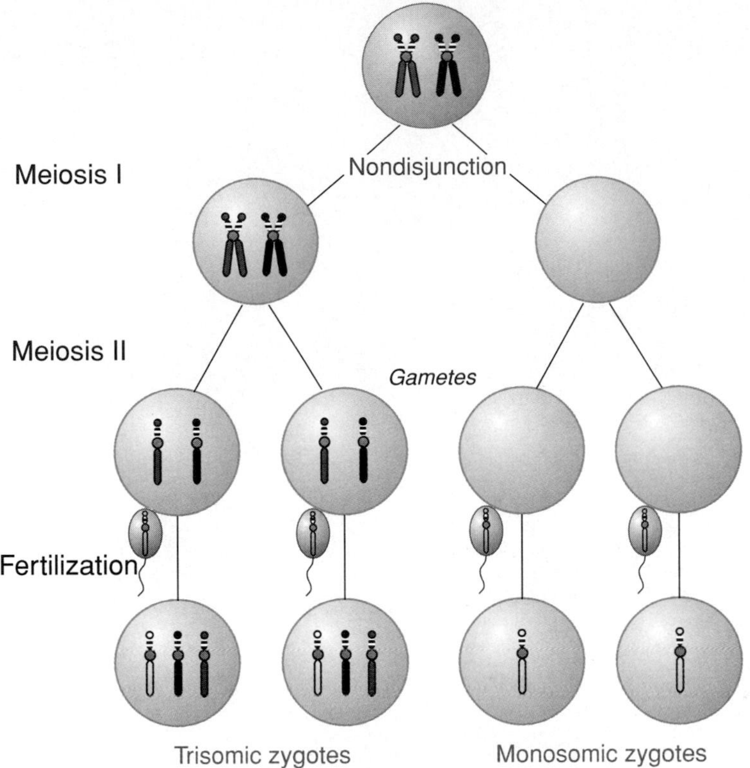

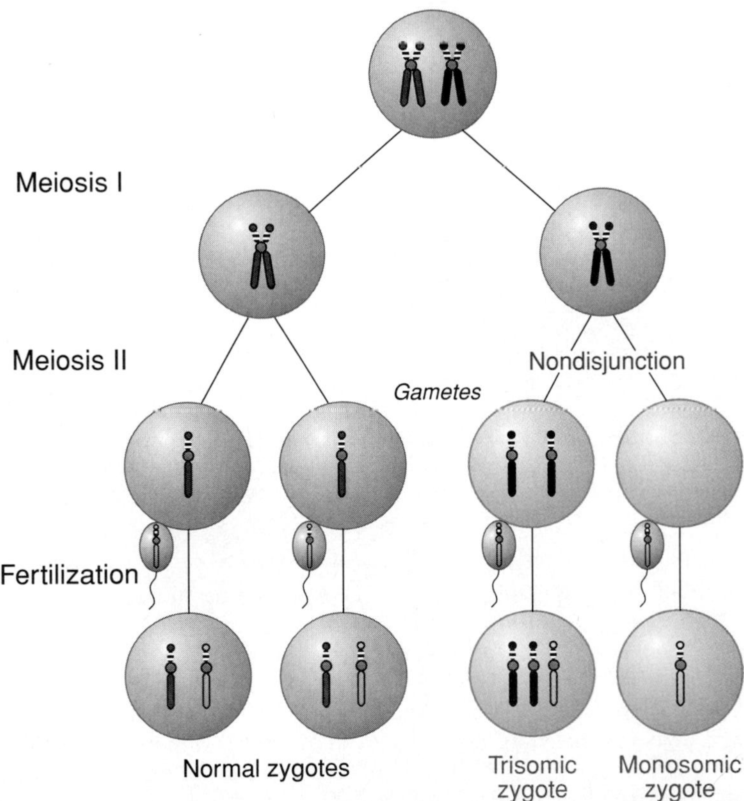

Fig. 12-26 Meiosis I and meiosis II nondisjunction. If nondisjunction occurs in meiosis I, gametes receive either both the parental copies or no copies of a particular chromosome. If fertilization follows, the resulting zygote will either be trisomic or monosomic for a particular chromosome. If nondisjunction occurs in meiosis II, abnormal gametes will either contain two copies of one parental chromosome or undergo total loss.

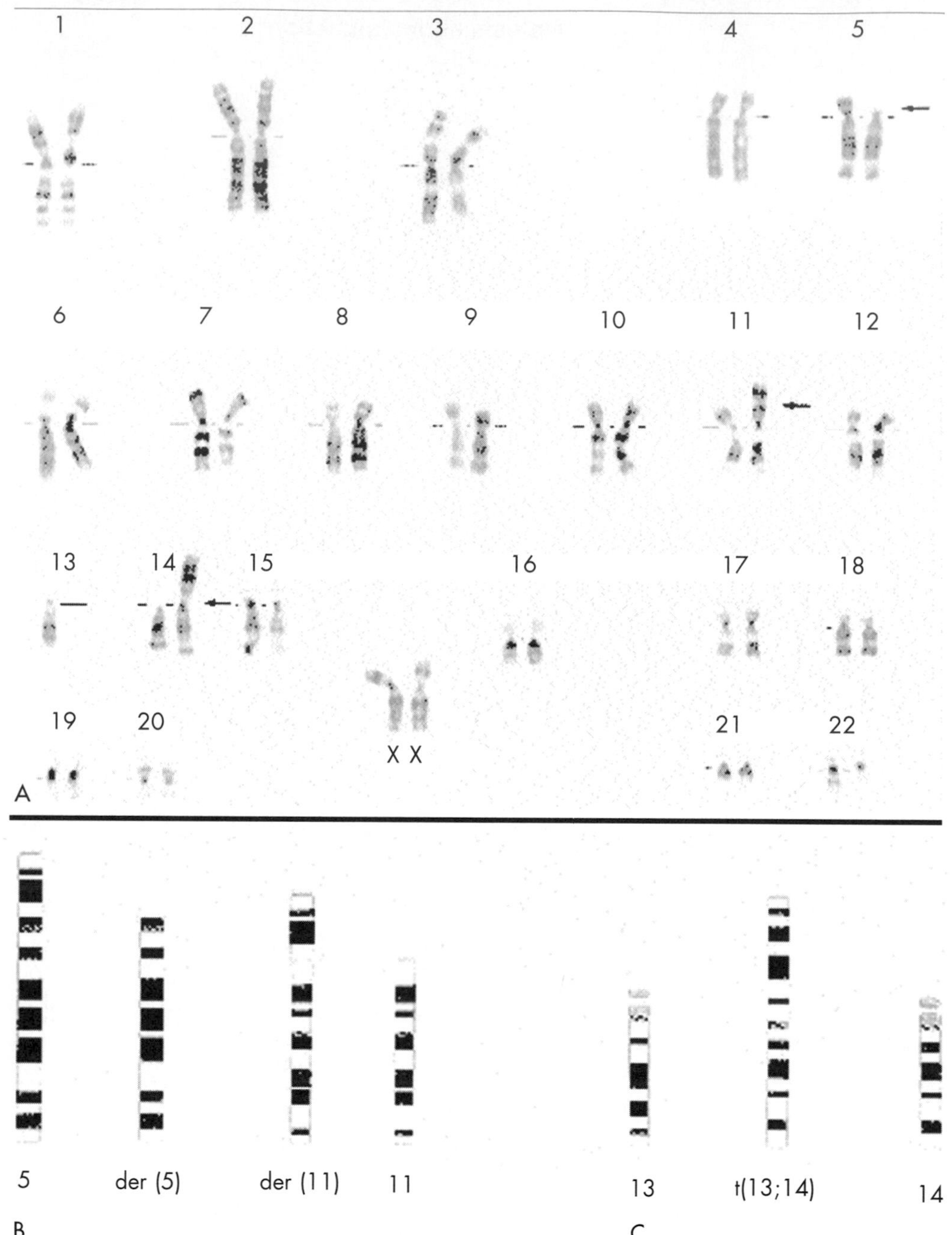

Fig. 12-27 **A,** G-banded karyotype of a phenotypically normal individual with a reciprocal translocation between chromosomes 5 and 11 and a 13;14 Robertsonian translocation. **B,** Schema of t(5;11) with normal 5 and 11 homologs on the outside and derivatives 5 and 11 in between. **C,** Schema of t(13;14) with normal homologs on each side of the translocation.

Fertilization of gametes produced in adjacent 2 segregation results in an offspring nearly monosomic for one of the two aberrant chromosomes and partially trisomic for the other. The clinical outcome associated with this form of segregation is generally so severe as to be incompatible with life. Thus, liveborn offspring are rarely seen succeeding adjacent 2 segregation.

Other possible meiotic segregation patterns include 3-to-1 and 4-to-1 nondisjunction events. With *3-to-1 segregation,* gametes with either 22 or 24 chromosomes are formed. Offspring may receive two normal chromosomes of the quadrivalent and one of the translocation chromosomes (*tertiary trisomy*), the two translocation chromosomes and one of the normal chromosomes (*interchange trisomy*), or only one of the translocation chromosomes (*tertiary monosomy*). *Interchange monosomy* is almost never viable. Three to 1 segregation (three chromosomes to one pole and one to the other) is seen in 5% to 6% of the offspring of carriers with the 11;22 translocation—t(11;22)(q23;q11)—but is otherwise rare (Fig. 12-29).[44] Four to 1 segregation is a nonviable state.

A Robertsonian translocation may occur between nonhomologous or homologous chromosomes. The chromosomes in a *nonhomologous Robertsonian translocation* will configurate in a trivalent form at meiosis. Three different avenues of seg-

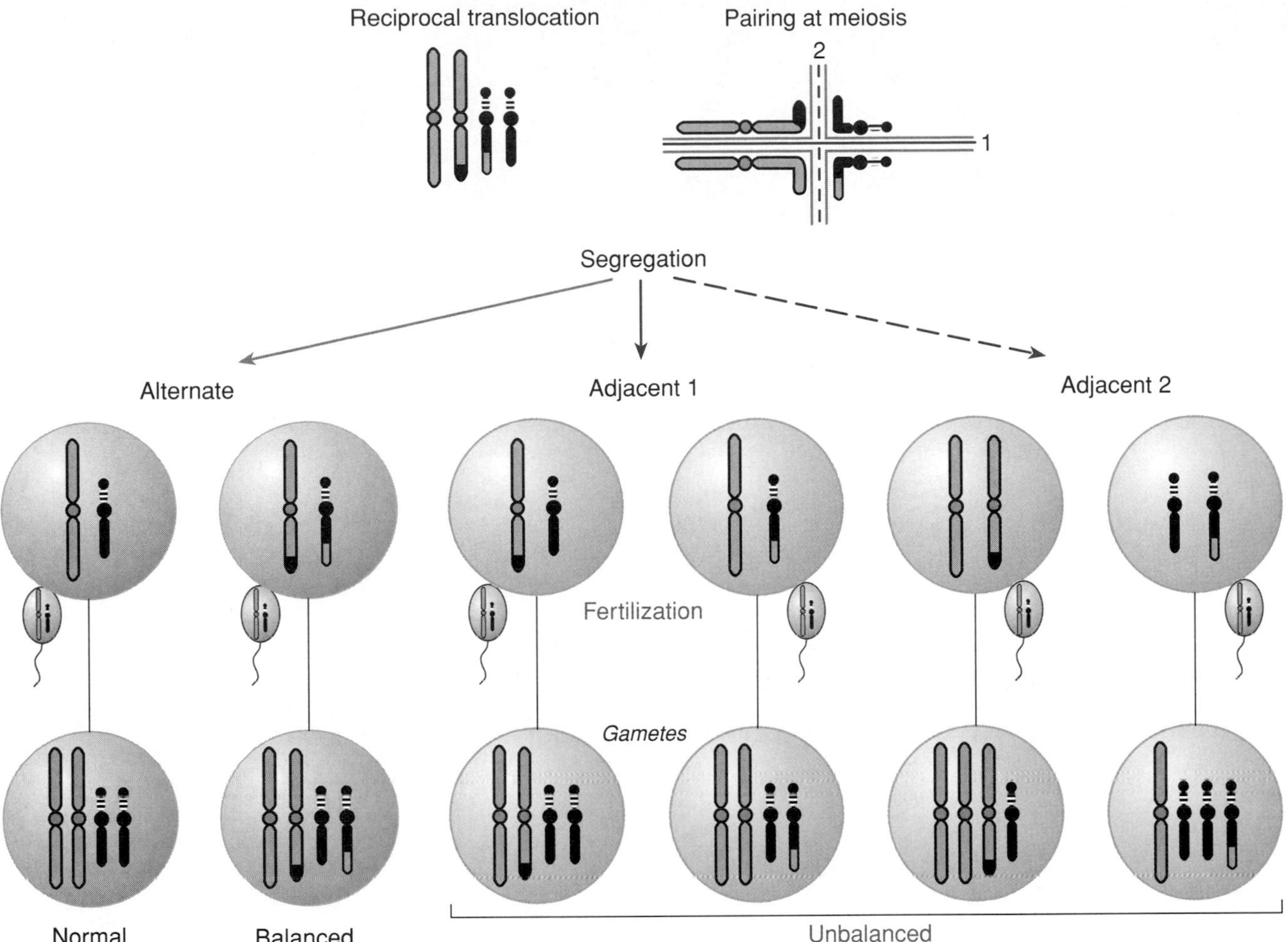

Fig. 12-28 Meiotic segregation of a reciprocal translocation. Alternate segregation results in genetically complete gametes (either with a karyotypically normal chromosomal complement or one containing the reciprocal translocation). Adjacent forms of segregation result in chromosomally unbalanced gametes.

regation are possible, as illustrated in Fig. 12-30. *Alternate segregation* in a Robertsonian translocation results in one normal gamete and one gamete with the translocation chromosome (balanced translocation karyotype). Clinically normal offspring are produced with fertilization of either of these gametes. The outcome of *adjacent segregation* is two gametes with a normal chromosome and the translocation chromosome (consequently, an extra copy of one acrocentric chromosome) and two gametes with one normal chromosome (therefore, loss of one acrocentric chromosome).

Interestingly, the six different gamete possibilities in nonhomologous Robertsonian translocation segregation do not appear to occur with equal frequency. Indeed, translocation trisomy 13 is hardly ever seen.[45] Moreover, nearly 99% of offspring of males with a chromosome D;21 translocation are karyotypically normal or are balanced translocation carriers, whereas a female D;21 translocation carrier has a 10% to 15% risk of having a child with Down syndrome (trisomy 21) (Fig. 12-31)[46] The segregation patterns of a *homologous Robertsonian translocation* (involving both chromosomes of a single chromosome pair) are limited to two. Neither one can produce a balanced chromosomal gamete. Either the gamete will receive the translocation chromosome and with fertilization yield an offspring trisomic for that chromosome or will not receive the translocation chromosome leading to a monosomic conceptus. Progeny trisomic for chromosomes 13 and 21 may be viable but never any of the other unbalanced homologous Robertsonian translocation possibilities.

Inversion

There are two types of inversions, *paracentric* and *pericentric* (Fig. 12-32). A *paracentric inversion* occurs when there are two breaks on one arm of a single chromosome and the chromosomal segment between those two breaks is reconstituted at 180°. This form of inversion does not involve the centromere. A *pericentric inversion* differs from a paracentric inversion in that it does involve the centromere. In this type of inversion, one break occurs on one chromosomal arm and the other break on the other chromosomal arm of a single chromosome. Carriers of either type of inversion are usually phenotypically normal because typically all of the genetic material is retained (balanced); such material is simply rearranged differently. Analogous to carriers of balanced translocations, however, individuals with inversions are at an increased risk of producing chromosomally unbalanced

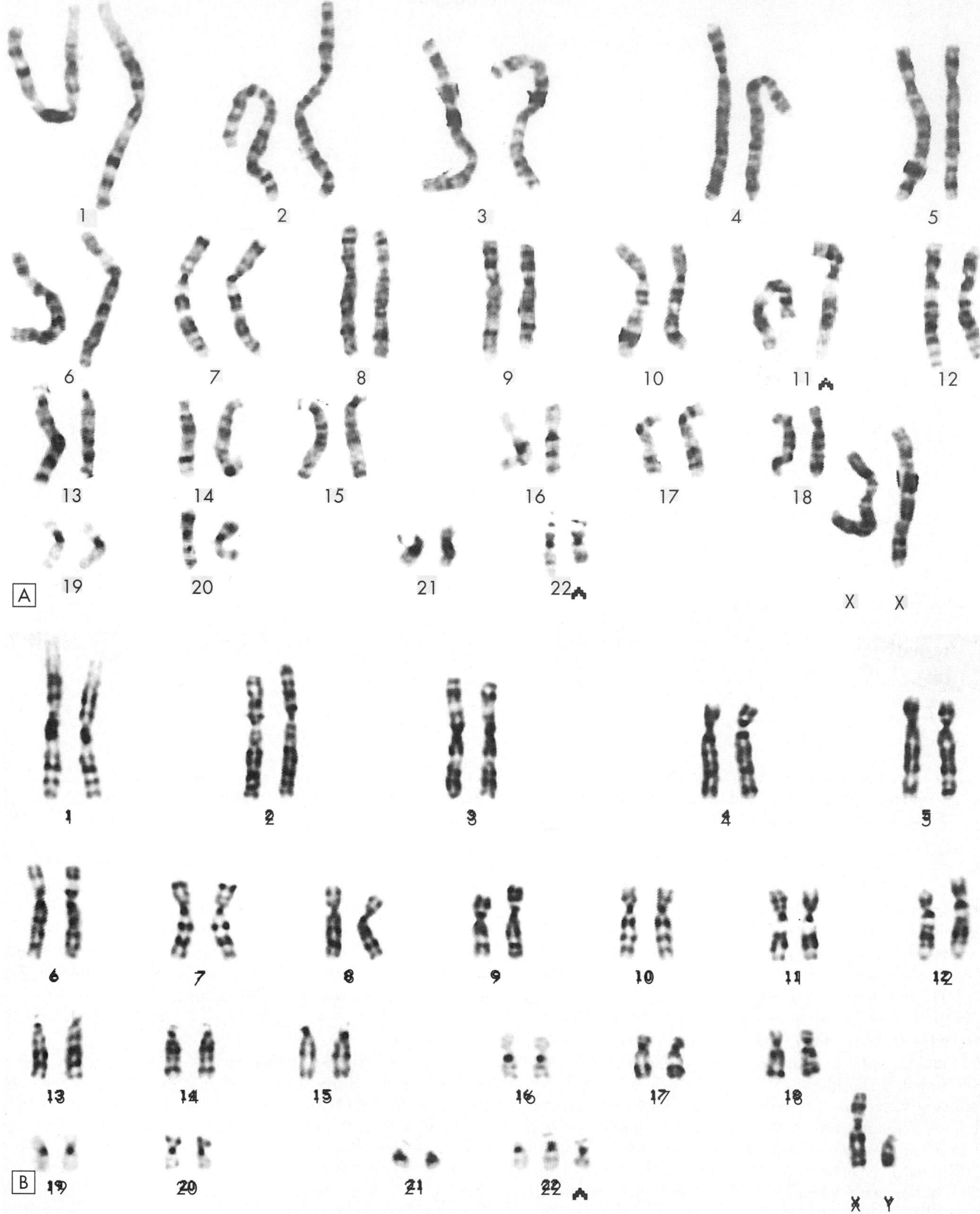

Fig. 12-29 **A,** Karyotype of a female with an 11;22 translocation, that is, t(11;22) (q23;q11). **B,** Karyotype of an unbalanced offspring of the above female resulting from 3:1 segregation.

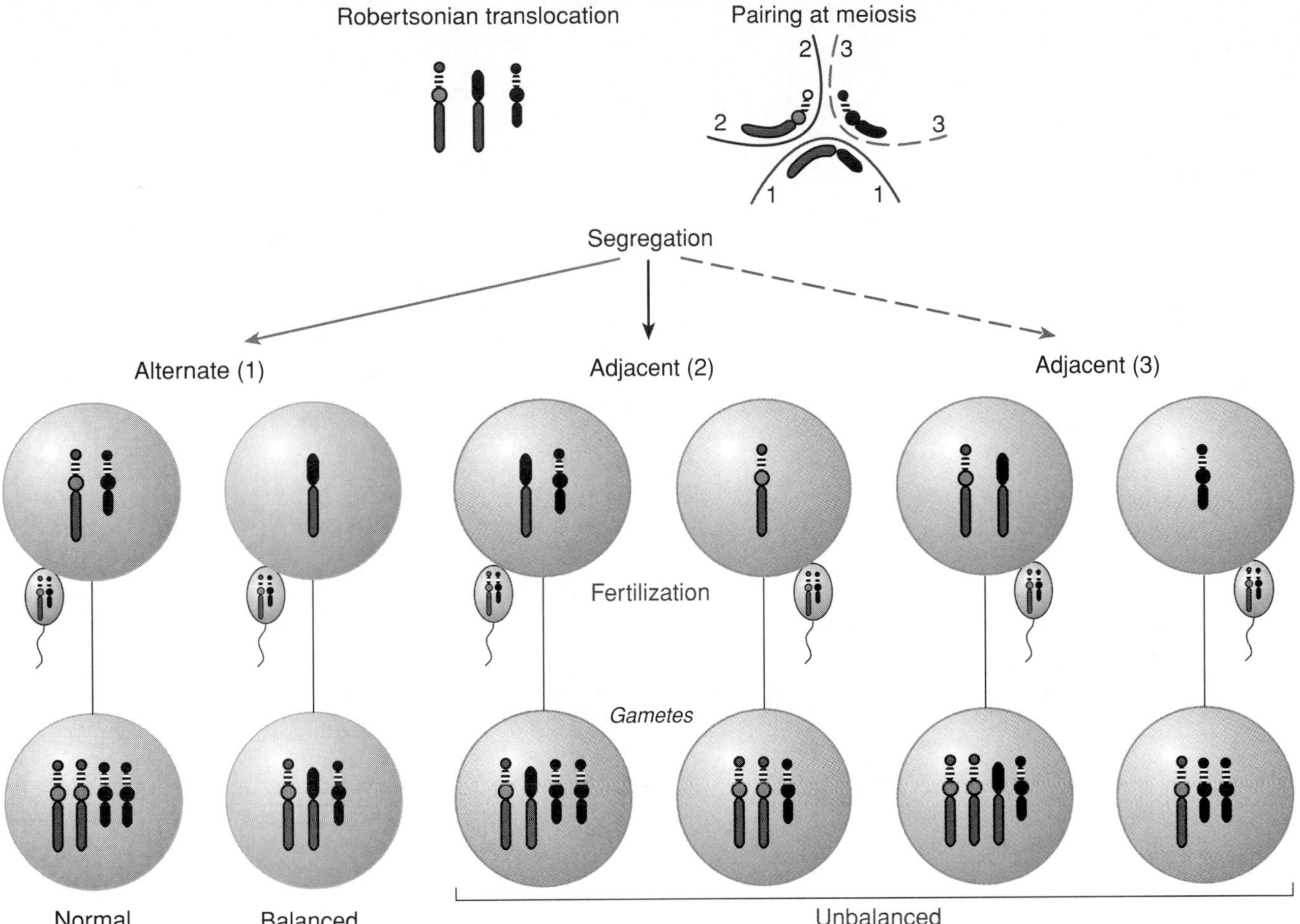

Fig. 12-30 Meiotic segregation of a Robertsonian translocation. Alternate segregation results in genetically complete gametes (either with a karyotypically normal chromosomal complement or one containing the robertsonian translocation). Adjacent forms of segregation result in chromosomally unbalanced gametes (either monosomic or trisomic for one acrocentric chromosome).

progeny. Excluding inversions involving constitutive heterochromatin such as the common variant inv(9)(p11q12), inversions are seen in about 1 in 1000 individuals.[47]

Chromosomes with large inverted segments characteristically form a loop *(inversion loop)* to pair in meiosis I. Crossing-over or recombination may occur within the loop, resulting in both normal or balanced gametes and unbalanced gametes. The unbalanced gametes produced after recombination of a paracentric inversion are either dicentric or acentric and are rarely capable of yielding viable offspring. Thus the risk of a paracentric inversion carrier having a chromosomally unbalanced child is small. A pericentric inversion may recombine to form gametes with both duplication and loss of chromosomal segments. These chromosomal segments are distal to the inversion, and depending on the size of the inversion, the risk of having a chromosomally unbalanced child may be quite high. Overall, however, the risk of a pericentric inversion carrier producing an abnormal offspring is 1% to 10%.[46]

Deletions and duplications

A *deletion* is the loss of a chromosomal segment (Fig. 12-33). If the deletion results in loss of the distal end of a chromosome, it is called a *terminal deletion,* requiring only one chromosomal break. If the loss is within the chromosome (not to include one of the distal ends), it is called an *interstitial deletion,* requiring two chromosomal breaks. Deletions may arise as the result of (1) chromosomal breakage with loss of the acentric fragment, (2) abnormal translocation segregation or inversion recombination, or (3) unequal crossing-over between sister chromatids or misaligned homologous chromosomes.

A *duplication* results in partial trisomy for the involved chromosomal segment. Similar to deletions, duplications may arise as a consequence of unequal crossing-over between sister chromatids or misaligned homologous chromosomes. A duplication may also be generated during the meiotic segregation of a pericentric inversion; however, a deleted chromosome will also be seen in most of these cases.

High-resolution chromosomal analysis and in situ hybridization techniques have enabled the detection of very small deletions and duplications not previously recognized with standard cytogenetic analysis (see Figs. 12-6 and 12-19). A group of different disorders showing either a microdeletion or a small duplication have been identified with these

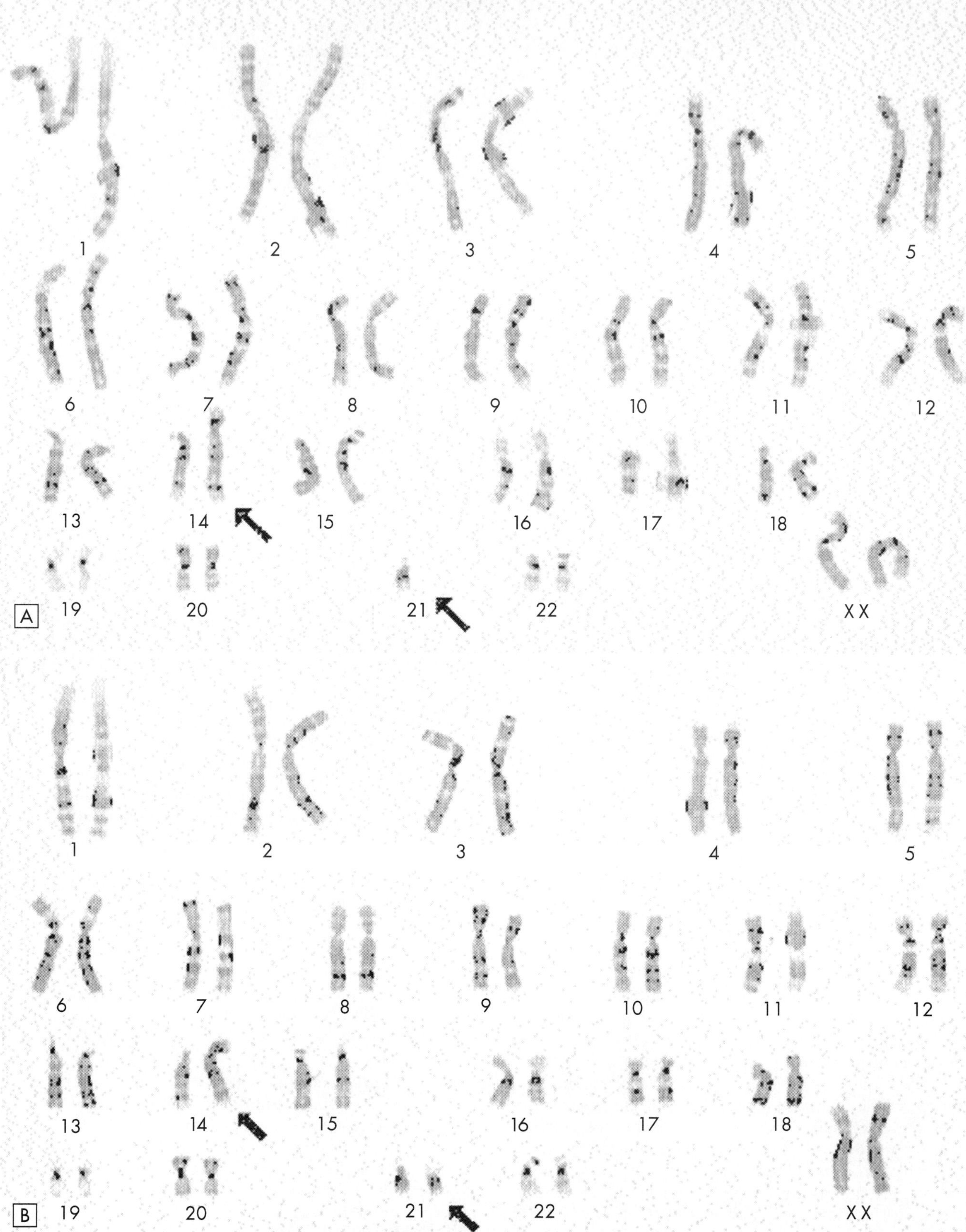

Fig. 12-31 Karyotype of a mother with a 14;21 translocation. **B,** Karyotype of offspring trisomic for chromosome 21 (Down syndrome) as a result of adjacent segregation.

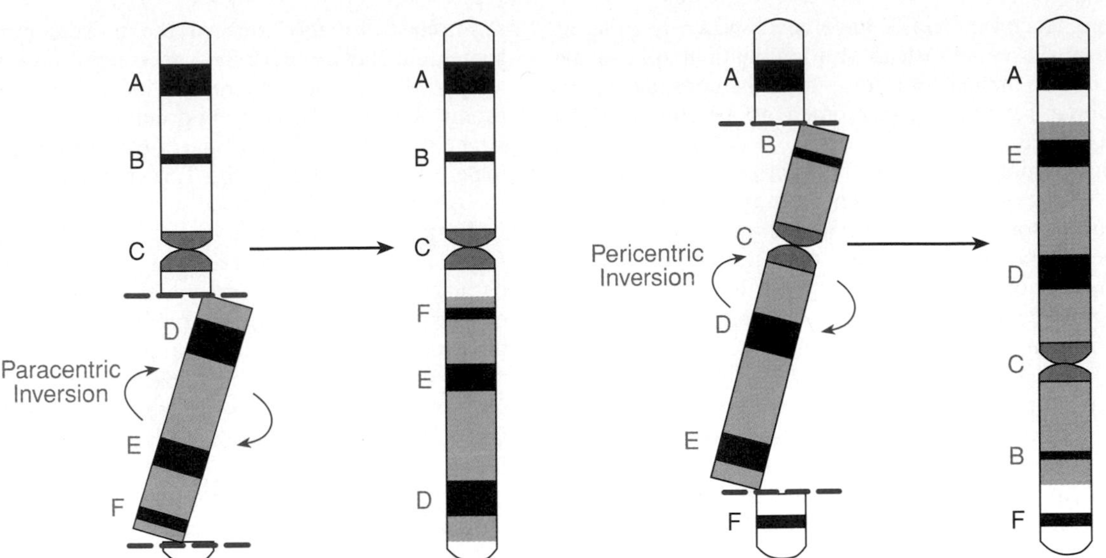

Fig. 12-32 A paracentric inversion *(left)* does not involve the centromere, in contrast to a pericentric inversion *(right)*, which does.

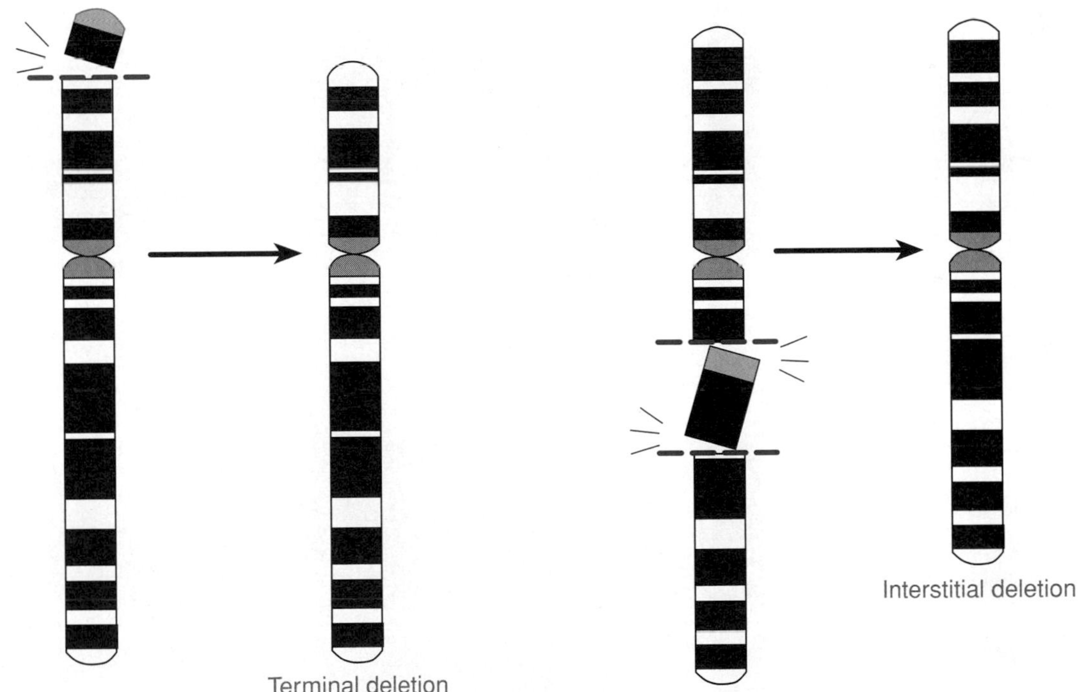

Fig. 12-33 Terminal deletion resulting in loss of the distal end of a chromosome *(left)*. Interstitial deletion *(right)*, requiring two chromosomal breaks and resulting in loss within a chromosome.

approaches. These disorders are entitled *contiguous gene syndromes* because the multisystem abnormalities seen in these syndromes are attributable to the involvement of positionally adjacent (not functionally related) genes.

Insertions

Insertions are manifested by either a segment of one chromosome introduced into a different chromosome *(interchromosomal insertion)* or into another part of itself *(intrachromosomal insertion)*. A segment can be inserted upright *(direct insertion)* or inverted *(inverted insertion)*. Because insertions require three chromosomal breaks instead of just one or two, they are rare. Similar to other carriers of structural abnormalities, insertion carriers are at risk of producing different types of recombinant conceptuses (partial monosomy or trisomy) in addition to normal and carrier products.

Isochromosomes

An *isochromosome* is composed of either two identical short arms or two identical long arms arranged in a mirror-image configuration. Isochromosomes have been shown to arise as the result of a transverse instead of a longitudinal split of the centromere during meiosis or mitosis or as the consequence of a translocation adjacent to the centromere of one chromosomal arm to its homolog.

One copy (partial monosomy) of a chromosomal arm and three copies of the other chromosomal arm (partial trisomy) of the same chromosome would be seen in an individual with 46 chromosomes carrying an isochromosome. If, in addition to an isochromosome, both normal homologs of the same chromosome were present, an individual would be partially tetrasomic for that particular chromosomal arm participating in the isochromosome.

Isochromosomes are frequently seen as a feature of a malignant chromosomal complement. Isochromosomes can also be seen constitutionally, however, and have reportedly been detected involving a variety of different autosomes. For example, mosaic tetrasomy for the short arm of chromosome 12 is compatible with life and is referred to as Pallister-Killian syndrome. Probably, one of the most common isochromosomes clinically reported is an isochromosome for the long arm of the X chromosome in individuals with Turner syndrome (Fig. 12-34). This abnormality is one of a few different structural abnormalities of the X chromosome seen in approximately 15% of patients with Turner syndrome.

Ring chromosomes

Ring chromosomes are rare but have been found for every chromosome. Ring chromosomes are formed when a break occurs on each arm of a chromosome followed by fusion of the exposed ends to create a circular structure. The distal fragments are lost because they lack a centromere. Ring chromosomes may also arise as the result of telomere-to-telomere fusion.[48] A ring chromosome originating by this mode loses little if any chromatin.

In mitosis ring chromosomes are often unstable, undergoing sister chromatid exchange and generating smaller or larger rings (sometimes containing more than one cen-

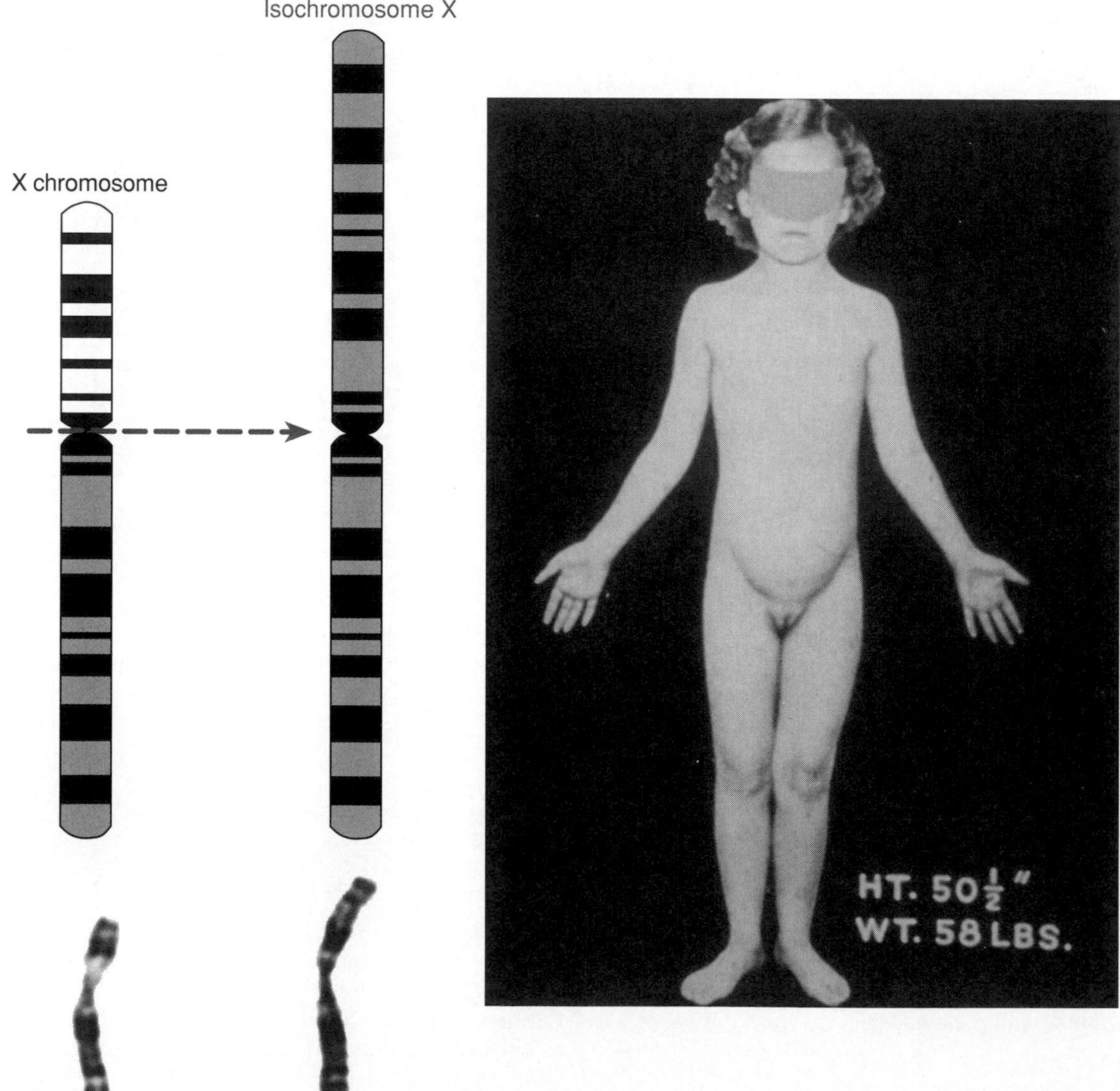

Fig. 12-34 Schema of the formation of an isochromosome Xq *(upper left)*. Partial karyotype of normal X homolog and i(X)(q10) *(lower left)*. An individual with the lower left complement has phenotypical Turner syndrome *(right)*. (Photograph of patient with Turner syndrome is from original series described by Dr. Henry Turner; courtesy Dr. G.B. Schaefer, University of Nebraska Medical Center, Omaha, Nebr.)

tromere). In some cells, the ring chromosomes may be lost altogether. Individuals with ring chromosomes may be severely mentally retarded with multiple congenital anomalies or only mildly delayed or clinically normal. The phenotypic variability is dependent on how much (if any) chromosomal material is lost in the formation of the ring chromosome and the stability of the ring chromosome after conception, during mitosis.

CLINICAL ABNORMALITIES

Spontaneous abortions

About one in every 200 live-born children is chromosomally abnormal, most with significant physical and mental impairment. By the time of birth, however, over 95% of chromosomally abnormal conceptuses have been aborted spontaneously. Fully 50% of aborted fetuses are chromosomally abnormal. Most of these are a result of aneuploidy.

More is known about the occurrence and effects of aneuploidy in the human population than any other group of animals.[49-63] This is not necessarily because it occurs more frequently in humans but because of its readily recognized clinical effects, which are always severe except when it occurs in some mosaics. Trisomy has been identified for all the human autosomes except chromosome 1. Generally, trisomies result in spontaneous abortions. Table 12-4 summarizes some of the available data. Appreciable numbers of live births occur only for the autosomal trisomies 13, 18, and 21, and these children are always abnormal.[64-66] Mosaic trisomies of these chromosomes are more likely to survive to term than those that are not. Postzygotic loss of a trisomy 13 and 18 that result in placental mosaics increase the survival rate of these trisomic fetuses to term.

Trisomies are to be expected to result from nondisjunction during meiosis, and this is borne out by the observations that the incidence of disomies and other chromosomal abnormalities in sperm from healthy males is 8% to 9% and even higher in human oocytes. Nondisjunction should result in an equal number of monosomic and trisomic zygotes after fertilization, but monosomics are rare, an indication either that the monosomic lethality may be expressed earlier than the trisomic one before conception is recognized or that gametes lacking a chromosome may be nonfunctional to begin with. As mentioned, trisomy of chromosome 1 has not been seen, an indication that abortions may be occurring before the conception is recognized, since disomy of this chromosome has been noted in gametes.

Sex chromosomal aneuploidy also accounts for a significant number of spontaneous abortions. Abnormalities encountered include XXX, XXY, XYY, and in particular 45,X (Turner syndrome), which is the single most common abnormality detected in spontaneous abortions (Table 12-5). Overall, in order of frequency, 45,X, triploidy (Fig. 12-35), and trisomy 16 are responsible for the majority of chromosomally aberrant spontaneous abortions. Note that trisomy 16 is the most common trisomy in abortuses but is never seen in live births.

Autosomal disorders

In general, the severity of an abnormal phenotype secondary to a chromosomal imbalance parallels the aberrant gene dosage (excess gene copy or loss of gene copy). Most chromosomal disorders, however, have three primary features in common: mental retardation, growth retardation, and somatic abnormalities. Although anomalies of nearly every chromosome have been reported, some are distinctly more common than others and are associated with well-recognized phenotypes. Many abnormalities are encountered with greater frequency in women over 35 years of age (Table 12-6).

Down syndrome (trisomy 21)

Down syndrome is the most common chromosomal disorder. It affects approximately 1 in 700 to 800 newborns and is a major cause of mental retardation. As previously mentioned, the incidence is higher in children born to mothers 35 years of age and older. For example, the incidence is 1 in 25 liveborn children of mothers older than 45 years of age.[67]

The specific location on chromosome 21 believed to be responsible for the characteristic Down syndrome phenotype

Table 12-4 Frequency of chromosome abnormalities in various samples

Condition of polyploidy	Age of pregnancy (weeks)	Approximate percentage of abnormal karyotypes in sample				
		Total	Trisomy	Disomy	Monosomy	Structural
Spontaneous abortions	<12	61.5	33.0	9.4	2.5	16.2
	6-25	30.5	16.5	7.4	1.3	5.3
	<20	51.9	27.0	9.3	<3.6	12.0
	<6-28	53.9	33.0	10.1	2.5	8.3
	0-18	46.3	22.7	11.3	2.0	10.3
	<6-25	38.5	21.1	6.9	1.5	8.0
Induced abortions	5-15	3.2	1.8	—	0.4	1.0
	<10	6.4	4.4	0.7	0.2	1.1
Stillbirths and neonatal deaths	>28	5.1	4.0	0.1	0.8	0.2
	>28	5.6	3.8	0.2	1.4	0.2
	>20	7.2	5.9	—	0.7	0.7
Live births		0.6	0.3	0.01	0.3	—
		0.65	0.3	0.01	0.3	—

Modified from Mange MP, Mange EJ: *Genetics: human aspects*, Sunderland, Mass., 1990, Sinauer Associates, Inc.

Table 12-5 Chromosomal abnormalities occurring in recognized human abortuses

Type of abnormality	Percentage of chromosomally abnormal abortuses	Percentage survival to term
Trisomies of autosomes		
16	15	0
13, 18, and 21	9	15
All others	27	~0
Sex chromosomal abnormalities XXY, XYY, XXX	1	75
45,X	18	1
Triploidy	17	~0
Tetraploidy	6	0
Structural abnormalities (such as translocations, balanced and unbalanced)	7	~55

Modified from: Hassold TJ: *Trends Genet* 2:105, 1986.

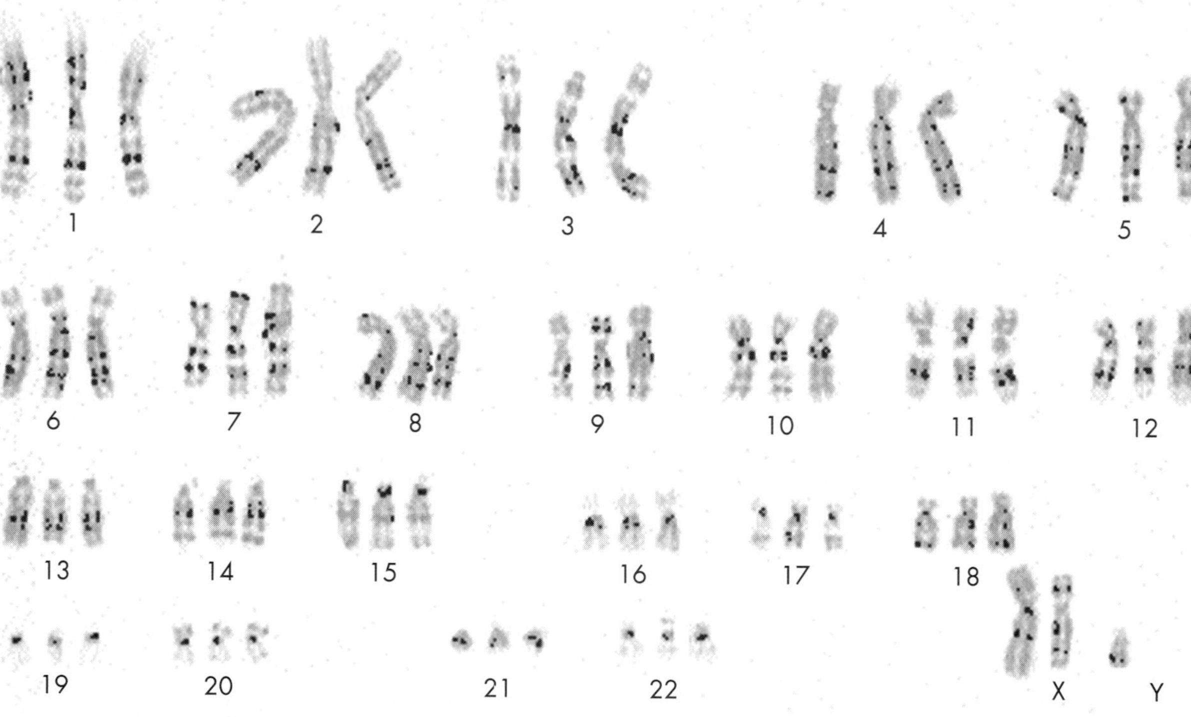

Fig. 12-35 Triploid (69,XXY) karyotype from a spontaneously aborted fetus.

(mental retardation, flat facies and occiput, upward slanting palpebral fissures, epicanthic folds, and variable cardiac defects) when present in three copies is 21q22.[68] This is important because not all individuals with Down syndrome have three copies of the entire chromosome 21.

The chromosomal basis for approximately 95% of individuals with Down syndrome is trisomy 21. Approximately 4% of cases of Down syndrome are the result of unbalanced translocations. These translocations are usually inherited from one of the parents who is a balanced translocation carrier by means of abnormal segregation. Translocations between chromosome 21 and a D group chromosome (chromosomes 13, 14, and 15) are the most commonly responsible parental translocations (roughly 60%). The remainder (40%) involve only the G group chromosomes (chromosomes 21 and 22). A 21;21 translocation is seen in approximately 80% of these cases and most commonly arises as a de novo event. One percent of Down syndrome cases are mosaic.

Trisomy 18 and trisomy 13

Two other relatively common disorders seen at birth as the result of an extra autosomal chromosome are *trisomy 18* and *trisomy 13*. The prospect for survival for an infant with either disorder beyond 1 year is grim. Trisomy 18 is characterized by multiple abnormalities including severe mental and growth retardation, prominent occiput, low-set ears, micrognathia, rockerbottom feet, and serious cardiac anomalies. Severe mental and growth retardation are also features of trisomy 13 as well as serious central nervous system malformations (arrhinencephaly and holoprosencephaly, Fig. 12-36), microph-

Table 12-6 Detection of chromosome anomalies at amniocentesis in pregnancies of women over 35 years of age compared with rates determined from surveys of the newborns

Type of chromosome abnormality	Prenatal diagnoses (%)	Newborn surveys including all maternal ages	
		%	Fraction
Autosomal abnormalities			
Trisomy 21	1.16	0.12	1 in 700
Trisomy 18	0.23	0.01	1 in 3000
Trisomy 13	0.07	0.01	1 in 5000
t(13q14q)	0.05	0.07	
Other balanced structural rearrangements	0.18	0.12	
Extra marker chromosome	0.06	0.02	
Other unbalanced structural rearrangements	0.08	0.06	
Sex chromosome abnormalities			
47,XXX	0.25f	0.10f	1 in 800f
47,XXY	0.33m	0.09m	1 in 700m
47,XYY	0.07m	0.09m	1 in 800m
45,X	0.09f	0.01f	1 in 2500f
Other unbalanced	0.05	0.06	

Modified from Jonasson and based on data from Hook EB, Hamerton JL: In Hook EB, Porter IH, editors: *Population cytogenetics: studies in humans,* New York, 1977, Academic Press, and from Ferguson-Smith MA, Yates JRW: *Prenat Diagn* 4 (special issue): 5, 1984.
Rates for females, *f*; rates for males, *m*.

thalmia, iris coloboma, or absence of the eyes, cleft lip and palate, rockerbottom feet, and polydactyly. Internally, cardiac and renal anomalies are also common.

Similar to trisomy 21, trisomy 18 and trisomy 13 are more commonly seen in offspring of older mothers and are most frequently the result of a nondisjunctional event. For trisomy 18, approximately 10% are mosaics. These individuals are not so severely affected (having a longer life-span) and are born to mothers of normal maternal age. Approximately 20% of cases of trisomy 13 are secondary to unbalanced Robertsonian translocations and mosaicism.[69] This figure is significantly higher than that observed in Down syndrome.

Cri-du-Chat (5p) syndrome

Other serious autosomal abnormalities may be of a structural nature. The cri-du-chat syndrome, so called because an affected infant's cry is reminiscent of a mewing cat, is caused by a partial deletion of 5p. The size of the deletion may vary in different patients; however, the critical segment (the absence of which is responsible for the phenotype) is 5p15 (Fig. 12-37).

The majority of cases of cri-du-chat syndrome are sporadic, but, in approximately 10% of patients one parent is a balanced translocation carrier.[70] In another 10%, the patients show other abnormalities such as rings, translocations, and mosaicism.

Sex chromosome disorders

The sex chromatin body

In 1949 Barr and Bertram described the occurrence of a tiny dark granule adjacent to the nuclear membrane in the neuronal nuclei of female but not male cats.[71] It was soon established that this difference extended to other tissues and to other mammals, including humans. These granules, known as *sex chromatin* or *Barr bodies,* represent one X chromosome that is condensed and inactive in the female. A simple technique allowing visualization of Barr bodies in cells obtained from buccal smears was quickly developed. Investigators studying patients with abnormal sexual development or infertility, or both, noted that the number of sex chromatin bodies differed in these patients from individuals of the same sex with normal sexual development and fertility. For example, short infertile females (Turner syndrome) had no Barr bodies.

Cytogenetic analysis shed definitive light on the origin of the sex chromatin body. Individuals with three X chromosomes had at most two sex chromatin bodies (Fig. 12-38); individuals with four X chromosomes had at most three, and with five Xs there were at most four sex chromatin bodies per cell. Thus the maximum number of sex chromatin bodies per cell is always one less than the number of X chromosomes.

Inactivation of the X chromosome

In 1961 Lyon proposed the X-inactivation hypothesis (*Lyon hypothesis*), such that in somatic cells of normal females (but not males) one X chromosome is randomly inactivated (inert, not participating in the manufacturing of RNA).[72] This theory was based on genetic studies showing that the coats of female mice heterozygous for X-linked fur color genes (two nonallelic, mutant coat color genes) were patchy mosaics of the two colors. It also advanced the concept of equal expression of genes located on the X chromosome in males and females. In patients with extra X chromosomes, all but one X chromosome are inactivated.[73] As stated, the inactivated X chromosome or chromosomes can be seen in interphase cells as Barr or sex chromatin bodies.

The chromatin that makes up the sex chromatin body or the inactive X chromosome is referred to as *facultative heterochromatin* (in contrast to constitutive heterochromatin described earlier). Facultative heterochromatin appears in one or the other X chromosome, at random, in females at about the blastula stage.

Importantly, inactivation of the X chromosome is not always random. A structurally aberrant X chromosome, such

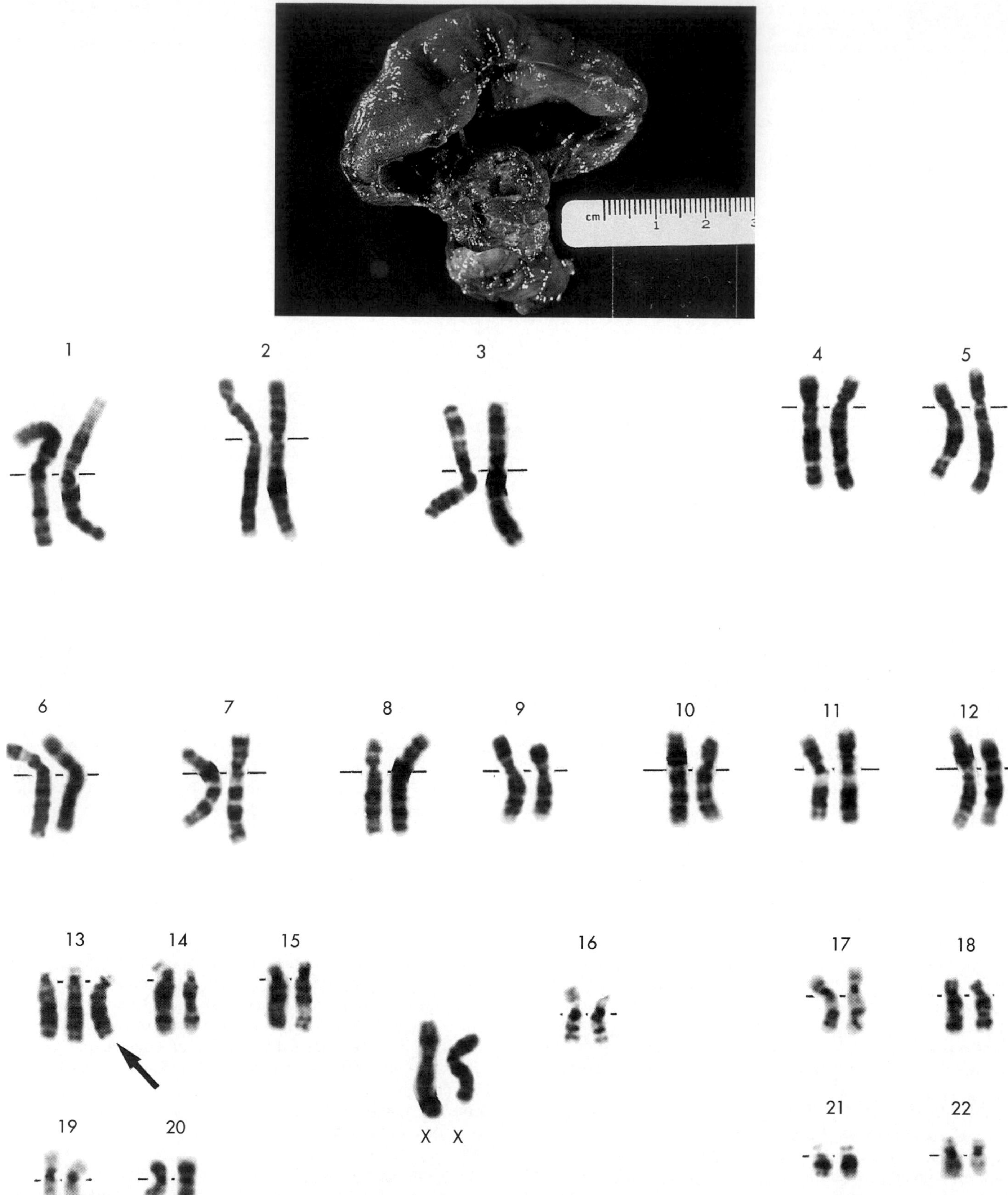

Fig. 12-36 Holoprosencephaly is a feature of trisomy 13 (karyotype below).

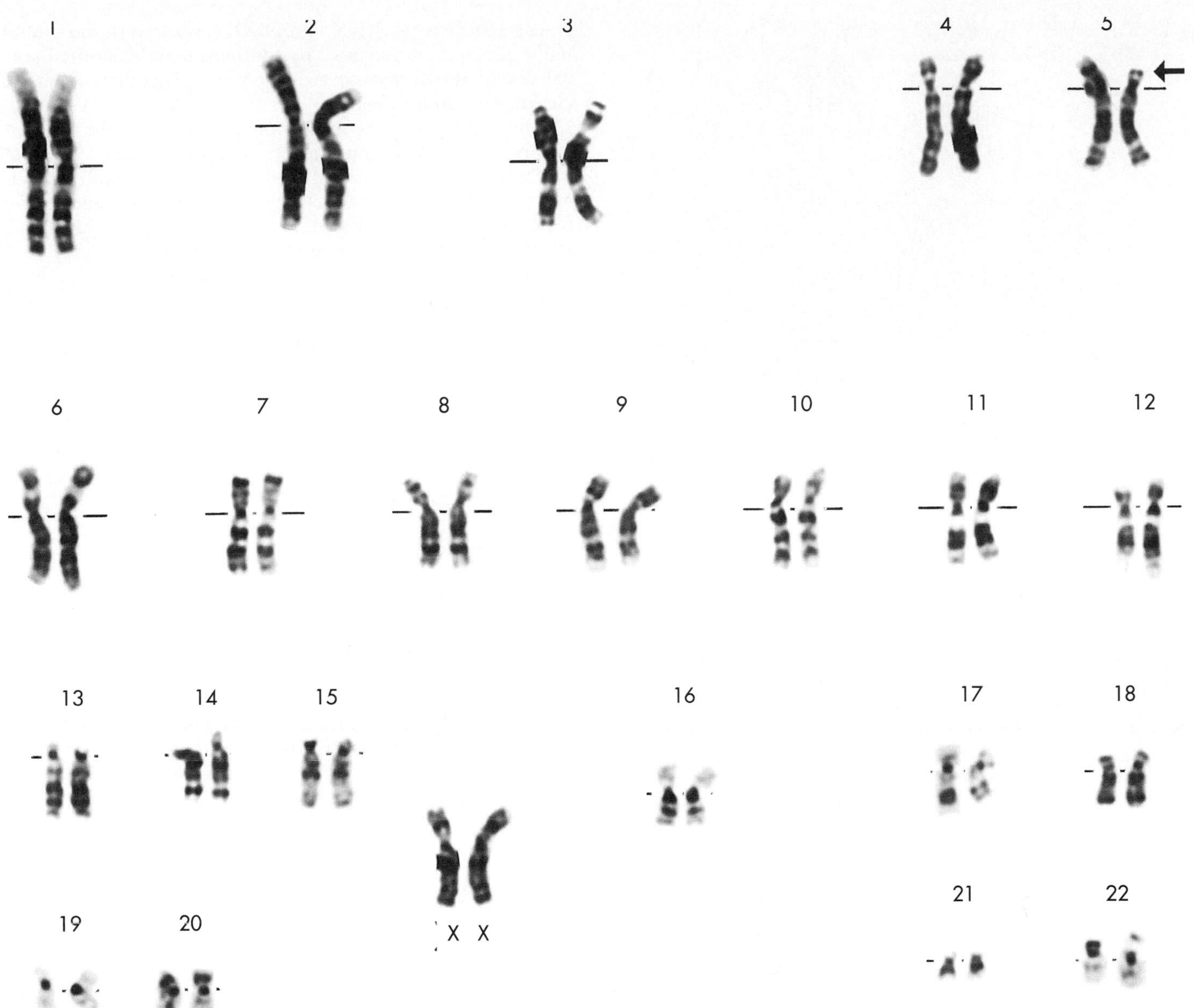

Fig. 12-37 Deletion of the distal portion of the short arm of chromosome 5 (to include 5p15) resulting in cri-du-chat (5p–) syndrome.

as an isochromosome X, is almost always preferentially inactivated. One exception is if the aberrant X chromosome is the result of an X-autosome translocation, and then it is usually the normal X chromosome that is inactivated.

Turner syndrome (45,X)

Analogous to autosomal disorders, sex chromosome disorders can be numerical or structural and may exhibit mosaicism. In *Turner syndrome,* a 45,X chromosomal complement is most commonly responsible. Other variants, however, are also frequently seen, accounting for approximately 47% of Turner syndrome cases. (Table 12-7).[74] Interestingly though, these variants may present differently phenotypically. For example, individuals with a deletion of the short arm of the X chromosome have short stature and other somatic abnormalities accompanying the syndrome. On the other hand, females with a deletion of the long arm of chromosome X have only gonadal dysfunction, an indication that genes necessary for ovarian development and preservation are located on this arm. Some Turner syndrome variants are fertile.

As mentioned, 45,X is the single most common chromosomal complement detected in spontaneous abortions. Paternal nondisjunction appears to be most frequently responsible because the X chromosome present is usually of maternal origin. It is not known why the majority of 45,X fetuses do not make it to term when this syndrome is seemingly compatible with life.

An XY cell line may be found in up to 5% of Turner syndrome patients. These individuals may have undergone virilization or are phenotypically male and have testicular tissue or a dysgenic gonad. They are often at a high risk of developing a malignancy (dysgerminoma). A 45,X/46,XY mosaic individual arose as a male who underwent mitotic nondisjunction with loss of the Y chromosome.

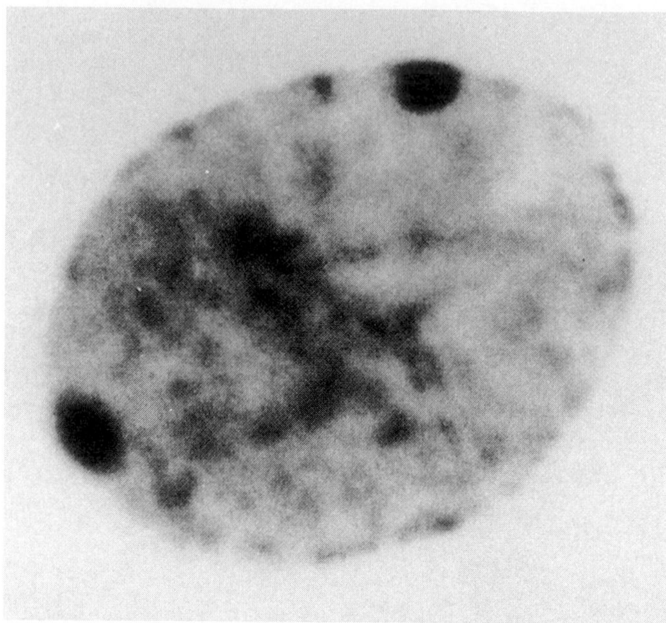

Fig. 12-38 A cell with two Barr (sex chromatin bodies) representative of a female with XXX or a male with XXXY.

Table 12-7 Types and relative percentages of chromosomal abnormalities in Turner syndrome

45,X	53%
45,X/46,XX mosaics	15%
46,X,i(Xq)	10%
45,X/46,X,i(Xq) mosaics	8%
46,XXq– or 46,XXp– deletions	6%
Other 45,X/? mosaics	8%

Data from Hook EB, Warburton D: *Hum Genet* 64:24 1983.

Trisomy, tetrasomy, and pentasomy X

As the number of X chromosomes increases beyond two in the female in the respective syndromes *trisomy X* (47,XXX), *tetrasomy X* (48,XXXX), and *pentasomy X* (49,XXXXX) so does the likelihood for retardation in both mental and physical development. The majority of trisomy X females have severe learning disabilities but are phenotypically normal (and may be above normal in height). Almost all cases arise as the result of maternal meiosis I nondisjunction (associated with advanced maternal age). Although theoretically one might expect trisomy X females to be at increased risk of producing a chromosomally abnormal offspring, no such risk has been demonstrated. Apparently, only normal ova, with a single X, are produced.[75]

Klinefelter syndrome

Individuals with *Klinefelter syndrome* typically have a 47,XXY chromosomal constitution. This syndrome, occurring in approximately 1 in 1000 live male births, is characterized by infertility (postpubertal testicular atrophy with hyalinization of tubules and azoospermia), learning difficulties and a slightly decreased IQ, and increased stature with relatively long legs. Similar to females with extra copies of the X chromosome (that is, 47,XXX, 48,XXXX, and so on), the probability of mental retardation, dysmorphism, and abnormal sexual development increases with increasing numbers of the X chromosome in the male.

Klinefelter syndrome most commonly arises as the result of paternal meiosis I nondisjunction (approximately 50% of cases), followed by maternal meiosis I nondisjunction (associated with advanced maternal age), and the remainder being meiosis II or postzygotic mitotic errors. A nondisjunctional event occurring in mitosis results in mosaicism. Roughly 15% of Klinefelter patients have a mosaic karyotype. These individuals are variable in phenotype, and some may be fertile.

Klinefelter syndrome was the first human sex chromosome abnormality to be reported. This syndrome seen in individuals with a male phenotype and a 47,XXY chromosome constitution provided an explanation for the mechanism of sex determination. It was realized that the presence or absence of the Y chromosome, not the X chromosome, was responsible for determining sex. In particular, a gene assigned to the short arm of the Y chromosome, the *testis-determining factor (TDF),* plays the critical role in sexual differentiation of the gonad in early embryonic life.[76-78]

47,XYY Syndrome

The chromosomal constitution *47,XYY* occurs in approximately 1 in 1000 male live births. This abnormality arises as the result of nondisjunction in paternal meiosis II, producing YY sperm. XYY males are phenotypically tall and are prone to severe acne. These individuals have a normal IQ but have an increased risk for mild learning disabilities.[79] Fertility is normal. As with XXX females, there appears to be no increased risk of producing chromosomally abnormal offspring.[79]

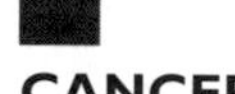

CANCER

Cancer is a genetic disease resulting from deviations of the normal genetic mechanisms that regulate cell growth. These deviations manifest themselves in many different ways,

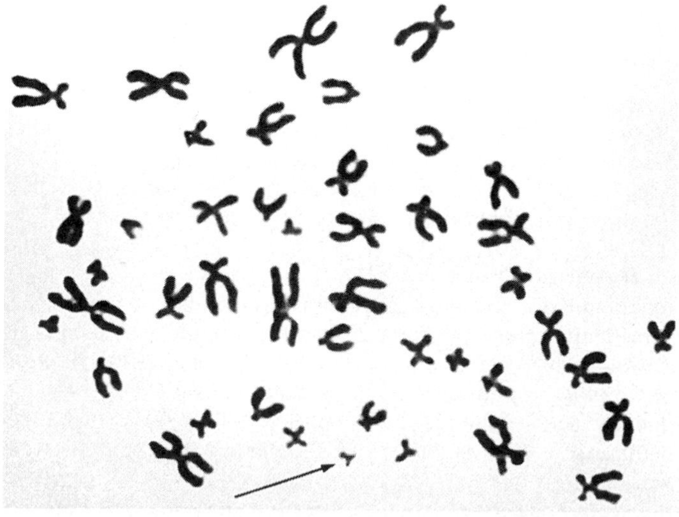

Fig. 12-39 Unbanded metaphase of bone marrow showing the Ph chromosome *(arrow),* characteristically seen as a small (minute) chromosome in chronic myelogenous leukemia.

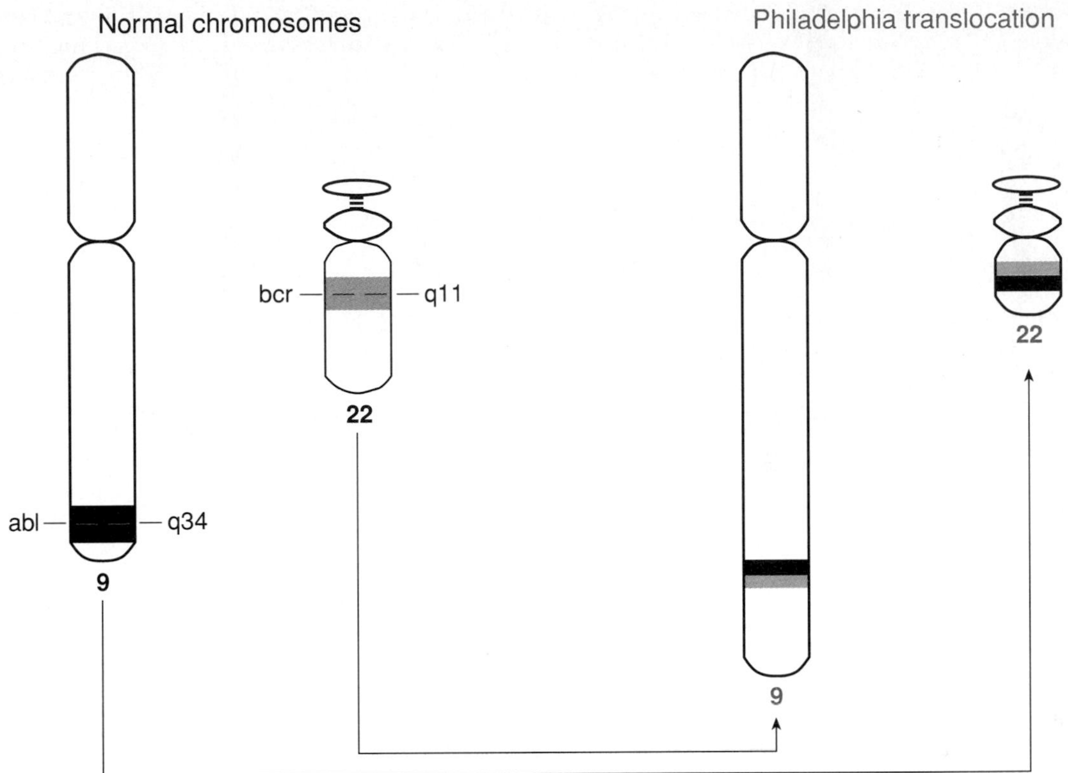

Fig. 12-40 Schema of the Philadelphia (Ph) translocation seen in chronic myelocytic leukemia. The Ph chromosome results from an exchange of materials between chromosomes 9 and 22, that is, t(9;22)(q34;q11). Since chromosome 22 gives up much more of its long arm than that translocated to it from chromosome 9, chromosome 22 becomes much abbreviated and known as *Ph*.

including alteration of the normal chromosomal complement. These changes may be numerical (that is, whole chromosomes are lost or gained) or structural (chromosomal material is rearranged, deleted, or duplicated).

Chronic myelogenous leukemia was the first neoplastic disease to be associated with a specific chromosomal abnormality (Fig. 12-39). This was a shorter-than-normal chromosome 22 (the *Philadelphia,* or *[Ph], chromosome*), which was identified in 1960.[80] With the evolution of banding techniques, the Ph chromosome was later redefined as a reciprocal translocation occurring between chromosomes 9 and 22, called t(9;22)(q34;q11).[81] The Ph chromosome is a paradigm of a cancer-associated translocation.[82] Normally, the abl gene located at 9q34 encodes for a protein of 145 kilodaltons (kD). The *BCR (breakpoint cluster region) gene* located at 22q11 encodes for a protein of 160 kD. As a result of the 9;22 translocation, there is created a chimeric gene that encodes for an abnormal protein of 210 kD (Fig. 12-40). The Ph translocation and subsequent abnormal protein production is considered responsible for the development of chronic myelogenous leukemia.

The Ph translocation has also been observed in acute nonlymphocytic leukemia (ANLL) and acute lymphocytic leukemia (ALL). Molecular studies of the translocation, however, have revealed that the Ph breakpoint in ALL is usually located proximally to that of CML and is associated with an abnormal mRNA and protein different from those in chronic myelogenous leukemia. A Ph translocation similar to that in ALL can be seen in some cases of ANLL. Thus these molecular studies indicate that Ph chromosomes, which cytogenetically appear identical, show differences when examined molecularly.[83]

Translocations are common not only in the leukemias, but also in mesenchymal neoplasms (sarcomas), where they are often the sole karyotypic change. Anomalous juxtaposition of genetic material can occur as the result of a translocation generating a chimeric gene,[9,11,84-87] such as that described above for the Ph chromosome. These altered genes and abnormal protein production are believed to be responsible for the induction of abnormal cellular proliferation. These genes are referred to as *oncogenes.*

Deletions represent another structural chromosomal anomaly frequently encountered in neoplasia. Deletions or loss of chromosomal material are common in epithelial adenocarcinomas (such as those of the large bowel, lung, breast, and prostate) and bladder carcinoma. More than one deletion is often detected in these different malignancies and may represent the stepwise process of genetic changes leading to malignant transformation (Fig. 12-41).[88] Deletion of chromosome 13 is observed cytogenetically or by molecular means in retinoblastoma (a malignancy of the cells of the retina). Deletion of a critical segment on the long arm of this chromosome (to include the retinoblastoma gene, Rb) results in loss of cellular mitotic regulation (Fig. 12-42). The Rb gene is an example of a *tumor suppressor gene.*[89]

The chromosomal abnormalities observed in cancer are often multiple and complex (include many numerical and structural abnormalities). In general, as additional chromosomal aberrations develop in any condition, the disease tends to progress, requiring a reevaluation of therapeutic approaches. Readers should be aware, however, that exceptions are seen with regular frequency. An example would be the lipoma, a

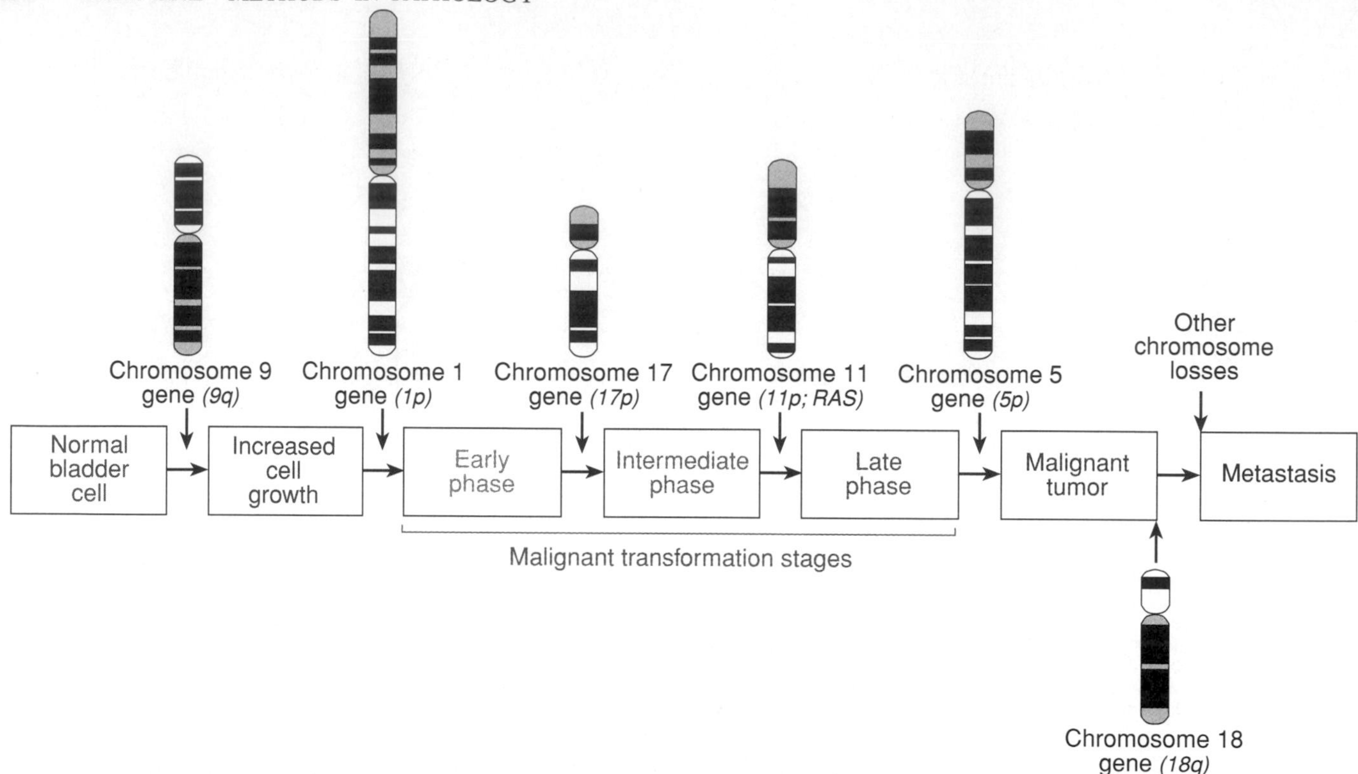

Fig. 12-41 Suggested pathway for the development of bladder cancer through a series of genetic events involving primarily tumor suppressor genes (particularly on chromosomes 9, 1, 17, and 5) and some oncogenes (such as ras on chromosome 11). The ordered accumulation of these changes gives rise to tumors that eventually become malignant. With each progressive involvement of a gene or genetic change, the affected cell becomes less and less responsive to normal control mechanisms, ultimately resulting in a tumor capable of invasion or metastasis. The chromosomes shown to be involved are based on our present knowledge, and this scheme or parts of it may have to be modified or abandoned as more cogent information is obtained on events in bladder cancer. Furthermore, the scheme shown may apply to only a subtype of bladder cancer. In addition to the deletions shown in this figure, loss of heterozygosity in bladder cancer has been described for 2q, 3p, 4q, 13q, 18q, and 21q. Numerical changes may affect chromosomes 1, 7, 9, 10, 11, and 20.

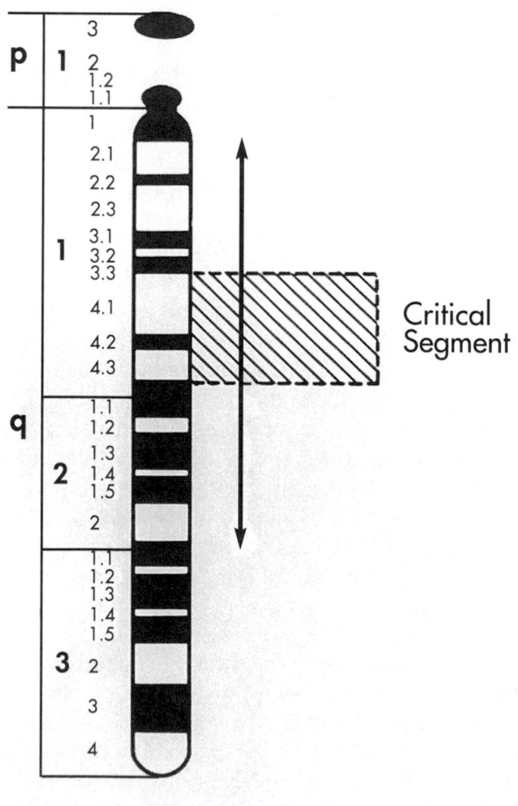

Fig. 12-42 Schema of the 13q– (deletion in the long arm of chromosome 13) seen in hereditary retinoblastoma. The range of deletions described in the literature is shown by the *arrows* and the critical segment, necessary for retinoblastoma development, as a *hatched area*.

benign tumor of adipose tissue, in which complex abnormalities have been described in a number of cases.[9]

Cytogenetic analysis has provided insight into the histopathogenesis of certain types of neoplasms for which the derivation was previously unknown. For example, Ewing sarcoma (a tumor of uncertain histopathogenesis) has been shown to share a functionally identical chromosomal rearrangement involving chromosomes 11 and 22 with peripheral neuroepithelioma, esthesioneuroblastoma, and Askin tumor (tumors with evidence of a neural origin), indicating a common mechanism of oncogenesis and a similar tissue of origin for these distinct clinicopathologic entities.[40]

A direct, potentially decisive role in the examination of benign and malignant tumors is provided through chromosomal analysis (Table 12-8). For example, the histologic classification of mesenchymal neoplasms, especially the so-called high-grade lesions, often presents a challenge to the surgical pathologist. Many cases defy histologic classification even with the aid of electron microscopy and immunohistochemistry, which can be plagued by problems such as sampling errors or overlapping mesenchymal features. An accurate diag-

Table 12-8 Chromosomal changes diagnostic of the tumor involved

Tumor	Chromosomal abnormality
	Translocations
Myxoid liposarcoma	t(12;16)(q13;p11)
Rhabdomyosarcoma (alveolar)	t(2;13)(q37;q14) or t(1;13)(p13;q14)
Leiomyoma	t(12;14)(q14-15;q23-24)
Lipoma	t(12)(q14)
Ewing's sarcoma	t(11;22)(q24;q12)
Synovial sarcoma	t(X;18)(p11;q11)
Pleomorphic adenoma	t(3;8)(p21;q12) or t(9;12)(p13;q13)
Clear cell sarcoma (malignant melanoma of soft parts)	t(12;22)(q13;q12 or 13)
Desmoplastic small round-cell tumor	t(11;22)(p13;q11.2 or 12)
	Deletions and other changes
Germ-cell tumors	i(12)(p10)
Meningioma	−22/22q−
Retinoblastoma	13q−
Wilms' tumor	11p−
Kidney tumors	3p−

From Sandberg AA: *CA* 44:136, 1994.

nosis is essential for optimal therapy. Cytogenetic analysis not only may be used to supplement conventional pathologic examination in the differentiation of mesenchymal neoplasms (Fig. 12-43), but may be vital when other investigations fail.

Fluorescence in situ hybridization (FISH) is a valuable complement to traditional cytogenetic analysis in the examination of tumors.[10] For instance, FISH techniques are useful in following patients when material for cytogenetic analysis is sparse or inadequate, such as during chemotherapy or after bone marrow transplantation. FISH analysis can also be used to establish the source of cells after bone marrow transplantation when the donor and the host cells are of different sex (Fig. 12-44). FISH can be performed on fresh tumor tissue, exfoliative cells of such tumors, and embedded and archival specimens.

In summary, the multistep process of malignant transformation is complex. Cytogenetic and molecular genetic analyses have led to a greater understanding of carcinogenesis. Techniques for the identification of characteristic chromosomal changes that are specific for certain histologic types of cancer have served as important diagnostic tools. Cytogenetic analysis is not a panacea for histopathology, but it is a powerful adjunct that can complement conventional microscopy in the formulation of an accurate diagnosis. Examination of these chromosomal changes at the molecular level has led to the identification of specific genes and the development of new tests for the diagnosis of these disease processes.

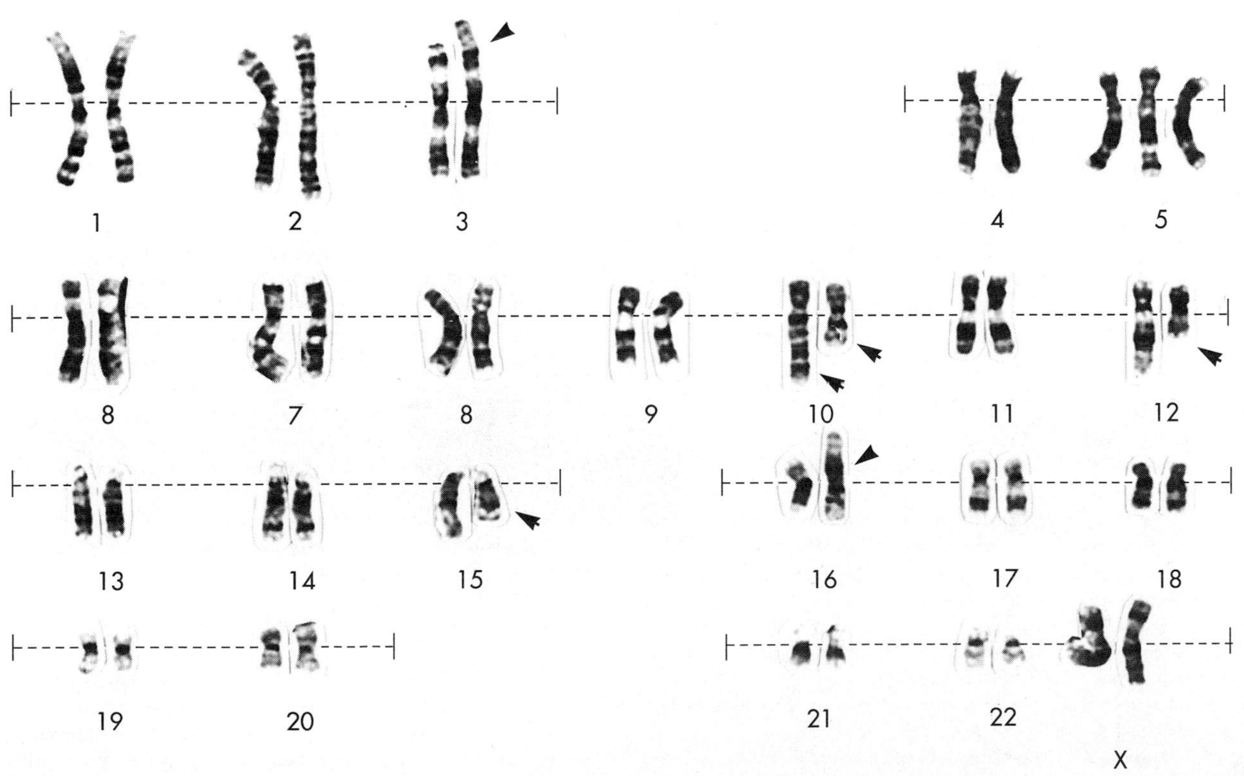

Fig. 12-43 Karyotype of a cell from a myxoid liposarcoma showing the characteristic translocation, t(12;16)(q13;11), of this type of tumor. Additional abnormalities involving chromosomes 3, 5, 10, and 15 are also present as secondary changes. Other solid tumors for which specific changes have been described are shown in Table 12-8.

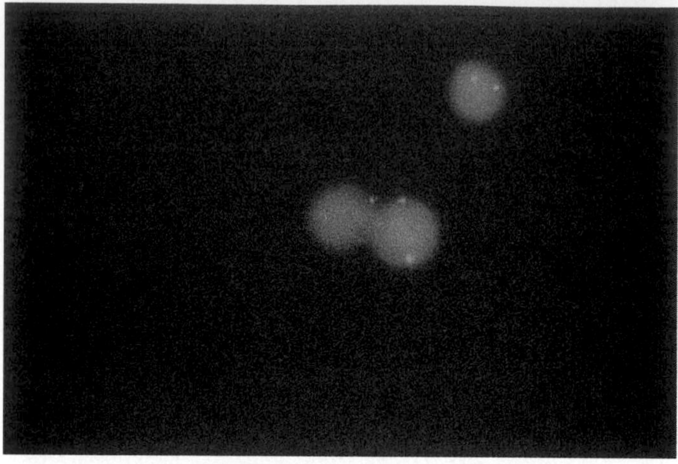

Fig. 12-44 Fluorescent in situ hybridization (FISH) after sex-mismatched bone marrow transplantation. The X-chromosome probe is represented by a green signal and the Y-chromosome probe by a red signal. In this case, a male recipient had received a bone marrow transplant from a female donor but as evidenced by this FISH (XY cells are seen) has undergone disease relapse.

REFERENCES

1. Yunis JJ, Prakash O: The origin of man: a chromosomal pictorial legacy, *Science* 215:1525, 1982.
2. Seuánez HN: *The phylogeny of human chromosomes,* Berlin, 1979, Springer.
3. Tjio JH, Levan A: The chromosome number of man, *Hereditas* 42:16, 1956.
4. Miller OJ: Nucleolar organizers in mammalian cells. In Bennett MD, Bobrow M, Hewitt G, editors: *Chromosomes Today,* London, 1981, Allen & Unwin.
5. National Institute of Child Health and Human Development Amniocentesis Registry: The safety and accuracy of midtrimester amniocentesis, DHEW publication no. (NIH) 78-190. Washington, DC, 1978, United States Department of Health, Education and Welfare.
6. Craparo FJ, Weiner S, Ludomirski A: Fetal blood sampling, *Curr Opin Obstet Gynecol* 2:265, 1990.
7. Gosden CM, Davidson C, Robertson M: Lymphocyte culture. In Rooney DE, Czepulkowski BH, editors: *Human cytogenetics: a practical approach,* Oxford, 1992, Oxford University Press.
8. Yunis JJ: High resolution of human chromosomes, *Science* 191:1268, 1976.
9. Sandberg AA: *The chromosomes in human cancer and leukemia,* ed 2, New York, 1990, Elsevier.
10. Sandberg AA, Bridge JA: Techniques in cancer cytogenetics: an overview and update, *Cancer Invest* 10:163, 1992.
11. Sandberg AA, Bridge JA: *The cytogenetics of bone and soft tissue tumors,* Austin, 1994, RG Landes Co.
12. Caspersson T, Lomakka G, Zech L: The 24 fluorescence patterns of the human metaphase chromosomes—distinguishing characters and variability, *Hereditas* 67:89, 1971.
13. Sumner AT, Evans HJ, Buckland RA: New technique for distinguishing between human chromosomes, *Nature, New Biology* 232:31, 1971.
14. Sumner AT: *Chromosome Banding,* London, 1990, Unwin Hyman.
15. Paris Conference (1971): Standardization in human cytogenetics, *Cytogenetics* 11:313, 1972.
16. Paris Conference (1971), supplement (1975): Standardization in human cytogenetics, *Cytogenet Cell Genet* 15:201, 1975.
17. ISCN: An international system for human cytogenetic nomenclature: high resolution banding, *Cytogenet Cell Genet* 31:1, 1981.
18. Craig JM, Bickmore WA: Chromosome bands: flavours to savour, *BioEssays* 15:349, 1993.
19. *ISCN: An international system for human cytogenetic nomenclature,* Birth Defects: Original Article Series 21(1), New York, 1985, March of Dimes Defects Foundation.
20. Hainden DG, Klinger HP, editors: ISCN 1985: An international system for human cytogenetic nomenclature. Basel, 1985, Karger.
21. Mitelman F, editor: *ISCN (1991): Guidelines for cancer cytogenetics. supplement to an international system for human cytogenetic nomenclature,* Basel, 1991, Karger.
22. Holmquist G, Gray M, Porter T, Jordan J: Characterization of Giemsa dark- and light-band DNA, *Cell* 31:121, 1982.
23. Yunis JJ: Interphase deoxyribonucleic acid condensation, late deoxyribonucleic acid replication, and gene inactivation, *Nature* 205:311, 1965.
24. Bickmore WA, Sumner AT: Mammalian chromosome banding: an expression of genome organization, *Trends Genet* 5:144, 1989.
25. Sumner AT, de la Torre J, Stuppia L: The distribution of genes on chromosomes: a cytological approach, *J Mol Evol* 37:117, 1993.
26. Benn PA, Perle MA: Chromosome staining and banding techniques. In Rooney DE, Czepulkowski BH, editors: *Human cytogenetics: a practical approach,* Oxford, 1992, Oxford University Press.
27. Carpersson T, Farber S, Foley GE et al: Chemical differentiation along metaphase chromosomes, *Exp Cell Res* 49:219, 1968.
28. Holmquist GP: Evolution of chromosome bands: molecular ecology of noncoding DNA, *J Mol Evol* 28:469, 1989.
29. Verma RS, Dosik H, Lubs HA: Size and pericentric inversion heteromorphisms of secondary constriction regions (h) of chromosomes 1, 9, and 16 as detected by CBG technique in Caucasians, *Am J Med Genet* 2:331, 1979.
30. Arrighi FE, Hsu TE: Localization of heterochromatin in human chromosomes, *Cytogenetics* 10:81, 1971.
31. Burkholder GD, Duczek LL: The effect of chromosome banding techniques on the proteins of isolated chromosomes, *Chromosoma* 87:425, 1982.
32. Matsui S-I, Sasaki M: Differential staining of nucleolus organizers in mammalian chromosomes, *Nature* 246:148, 1973.
33. Goodpasture C, Bloom SE: Visualization of nucleolar organizer regions III. Mammalian chromosomes using silver staining, *Chromosoma* 53:37, 1975.
34. Spector DL, Ochs RL, Busch H: Silver staining, immunofluorescence, and immunoelectron microscopic localization of nucleolar phosphoproteins B23 and C23, *Chromosoma* 90:139, 1984.
35. Verma RS, Babu A: Banding techniques. In *Human chromosomes: manual of basic techniques,* New York, 1989. Pergamon Press.
36. Gall J, Pardue ML: Formation and detection for RNA-DNA hybrid molecules in cytological preparations, *Proc Natl Acad Sci USA* 63:378, 1969.
37. Mathew S, Murty VVVS, Hunziker W, Chaganti RSK: Subregional mapping of 13 single-copy genes on the long arm of chromosome 12 by fluorescence in situ hybridization, *Genomics* 14:775, 1992.
38. Bhatt B, McGee J O'D: Chromosomal assignment of genes. In Polak JM, McGee J O'D, editors: *In situ hybridization: principles and practice,* New York, 1990, Oxford Science.
39. Anastasi J: Interphase cytogenetic analysis in the diagnosis and study of neoplastic disorders, *Am J Clin Pathol* 95:22, 1991.
40. Bridge JA: Cytogenetic and molecular cytogenetic techniques in orthopaedic surgery, *J Bone Joint Surg* 75A:606, 1993.
41. Bridge JA, DeBoer J, Travis J et al: Simultaneous interphase cytogenetic analysis and fluorescence immunophenotyping of dedifferentiated chondrosarcoma: implications for histopathogenesis, *Am J Pathol* 144:215, 1994.
42. Martin RH, Rademaker AW, Hildebrand K et al: Variation in the frequency and type of sperm chromosomal abnormalities among normal men, *Hum Genet* 77:108, 1987.
43. Castle D, Bernstein R: Cytogenetic analysis of 688 couples experiencing multiple spontaneous abortions, *Am J Med Genet* 29:549, 1988.
44. Islelius L, Lindsten J, Aurias A et al: The 11q;22q translocation: a collaborative study of 20 new cases and analysis of 110 families, *Hum Genet* 64:343, 1983.
45. Mori MA, Huertas H, Pinel I et al: Trisomy 13 in the child of two carriers of a 13/15 translocation, *Am J Med Genet* 20:17, 1985.
46. Gardner RJM, Sutherland GR: *Chromosome abnormalities and genetic counseling,* New York, 1989, Oxford University Press.
47. VanDyke DL, Weiss L, Robertson JR, Babu VR: The frequency and mutation rate of balanced autosomal rearrangements in man estimated from prenatal genetic studies for advanced maternal age, *Am J Hum Genet* 35:301, 1983.
48. Kosztolanyi G: Does "ring chromosome" exist? An analysis of 207 case reports on patients with a ring autosome, *Hum Genet* 75:174, 1987.

49. Wagner RP, Maguire MP, Stallings RL: In *Chromosomes: a synthesis,* New York, 1993, Wiley-Liss.
50. Mange AP, Mange EJ: *Genetics: Human Aspects,* Sunderland, Mass, 1990, Sinauer Associates.
51. Boué A, Boué J, Gropp A: Cytogenetics of pregnancy wastage, *Adv Hum Genet* 14:1, 1985.
52. Creasy MR, Crolla JA, Alberman ED: A cytogenetic study of human spontaneous abortions using banding techniques, *Hum Genet* 31:177, 1976.
53. Carr DH, Gedeon M: Population cytogenetics of human abortuses. In Hook EB, Porter IH, editors: *Population cytogenetics: studies in humans,* New York, 1977, Academic Press.
54. Kajii T, Ferrier A et al: Anatomic and chromosomal anomalies in 639 spontaneous abortuses, *Hum Genet* 55:87, 1980.
55. Hassold T, Chen N, Funkhouser J et al: A cytogenetic study of 1000 spontaneous abortions, *Ann Hum Genet* 55:151, 1980.
56. Warburton D, Kline J, Stein Z, Strobino B: Cytogenetic abnormalities in spontaneous abortions of recognized conceptions. In Porter IH et al, editors: *Perinatal genetics: diagnosis and treatment,* Orlando, Fla, 1986, Academic Press.
57. Kajii T, Ohama K, Mikamo K: Anatomic and chromosomal anomalies in 944 induced abortuses, *Hum Genet* 43:247, 1978.
58. Yamamoto M, Watanabe M: Epidemiology of chromosomal anomalies at the early stage of pregnancy. In *Contribution to epidemiology and biostatistics?*1:101, 1979.
59. Hassold TJ: Chromosome abnormalities in human reproductive wastage, *Trends Genet* 2:105, 1986.
60. Machin GA: Chromosome abnormality and perinatal death, *Lancet* 1:549, 1974.
61. Bauld RG, Sutherland R, Bain AD: Chromosome studies in investigation of stillbirths and neonatal deaths, *Arch Dis Child* 49:782, 1974.
62. Hook EB, Hamerton JL: The frequency of chromosome abnormalities detected in consecutive newborn studies, differences between studies, results by sex and by severity of phenotypic involvement. In Hook EB, Porter IH editors: *Population cytogenetics: studies in humans,* New York, 1977, Academic Press.
63. Hsu LYF: Prenatal diagnosis of chromosome abnormalities. In Milunsky A, editor: *Genetic disorders and the fetus: diagnosis, prevention, and treatment,* New York, 1986, Plenum Press.
64. Hook EB, Cross PK: Rates of mutant and inherited structural cytogenetic abnormalities detected at amniocentesis: results on about 63,000 fetuses, *Ann Hum Genet* 51:27, 1987.
65. Hook EB, Cross PK, Regal RR: The frequency of 47,+21, 47,+18, and 47,+13 at the uppermost extremes of maternal ages: results on 56,094 fetuses studied prenatally and comparisons with data on livebirths, *Hum Genet* 68:211, 1984.
66. Schreinemachers DM, Cross PK, Hook EB: Rates of trisomies 21, 18, 13 and other chromosome abnormalities in about 20,000 prenatal studies compared with estimated rate in live births, *Hum Genet* 61:318, 1982.
67. Ferguson-Smith MA, Yates JRW: Maternal age specific rates for chromosome aberrations and factors influencing them: report of a collaborative European study on 52,965 amniocenteses, *Prenat Diagn* 4(Special Issue):5, 1984.
68. Watkins PC, Tanzi RT, Cheng SV, Gusella JF: Molecular genetics of human chromosome 21, *J Med Genet* 24:257, 1987.
69. Grouchy J de: Clinical cytogenetics: autosomal disorders. In Busch H, editor: *The cell nucleus,* New York, 1974, Springer.
70. Niebuhr E: The cri-du-chat syndrome, *Hum Genet* 44:227, 1978.
71. Barr ML, Bertram EG: A morphological distinction between neurons of the male and female, and the behavior of the nucleolar satellite during accelerated nucleoprotein synthesis, *Nature* 163:676, 1949.
72. Lyon MF: Gene inactivation in the X chromosome of the mouse (*Mus musculus L*), *Nature* 190:372, 1961.
73. Lyon MF: The William Allan Memorial Award Address: X-chromosome inactivation and the location and expression of X-linked genes, *Am J Hum Genet* 42:8, 1988.
74. Hook EB, Warburton D: The distribution of chromosomal genotypes associated with Turner syndrome: live birth prevalence rates and evidence for diminished fetal mortality and severity in genotypes associated with structural X abnormalities or mosaicism, *Hum Genet* 64:24, 1983.
75. Neri G: A possible explanation for the low incidence of gonosomal aneuploidy among the offspring of triplo-X individuals, *Am J Med Genet* 18:357, 1984.
76. Berta P, Hawkins JR, Sinclair AH et al: Genetic evidence equating SRY and the testis determining factor, *Nature* 348:448, 1990.
77. Fechner PY, Marcantonio SM, Jaswaney V et al: The role of the sex determining region Y gene in the etiology of 46,XX maleness, *J Clin Endocrinol Metab* 76:690, 1993.
78. Lukusa T, Fryns JP, Van den Berghe: The role of the Y chromosome in sex determination, *Genet Couns* 3:1, 1992.
79. Netley CT: Summary overview of behavioral development in individuals with neonatally identified X and Y aneuploidy. In Ratcliffe SG, Paul N, editors: *Prospective studies on children with sex chromosome aneuploidy,* Birth Defects: Original Article Series 22(3):293, 1986.
80. Nowell PC, Hungerford DA: A minute chromosome in human granulocytic leukemia, *Science* 132:1497, 1960.
81. Rowley JD: A new consistent chromosomal abnormality in CML identified by quinacrine fluorescence and Giemsa staining, *Nature* 243:290, 1973.
82. Rowley JD: The Philadelphia chromosome translocation: a paradigm for understanding leukemia, *Cancer* 65:2178, 1990.
83. Sandberg AA: Cancer cytogenetics for clinicians, *CA* 44:136, 1994.
84. LeBeau MM: Cytogenetic analysis of hematological diseases. In Barch MJ, editor: *The ACT cytogenetic laboratory manual,* New York, 1991, Raven Press.
85. Heim S, Mitelman F: *Cancer Cytogenetics,* New York, 1987, Alan R Liss, Inc.
86. Rowley JD, Aster JC, Sklar J: The clinical applications of new DNA diagnostic technology on the management of cancer patients, *JAMA* 270:2331, 1993.
87. Rowley JD, Aster JC, Sklar J: The impact of new DNA diagnostic technology on the management of cancer patients, *Arch Pathol Lab Med* 117:1104, 1993.
88. Vogelstein B, Fearson ER, Hamilton SR et al: Genetic alterations during colo-rectal tumor development, *N Engl J Med* 319:525, 1988.
89. Knudson AG: Antioncogenes and human cancer, *Proc Natl Acad Sci USA* 90:10, 1993.

13 Flow and Imaging Cytometry

David S. Weinberg
John L. Carey

Microscopic examination of cells and tissues is the central function of surgical pathology and cytology. The resulting diagnoses are based on subjective interpretation of observed features. There are many instances, however, in which objective measurements of cell and tissue features provide important diagnostic or prognostic information, as is described below. Although the human visual system and brain excel in tasks requiring recognition of previously learned patterns (such as human faces), we are not well adapted for quantitation, finding the tasks either too tedious (that is, counting mitoses) or too difficult (that is, judging the size of cells). Also, there are physical limits to our visual systems that can make it difficult or impossible to perceive image features accurately. In all these instances, computer analysis of images can be of considerable aid to the pathologist. In addition, computerization of images may find important applications in the archiving and sharing of diagnostic findings through storage and transmission of images rather than glass slides. This technology, developed in response to the needs of the aerospace industry, has found many other important applications in industry and medicine, especially in diagnostic radiology. In this chapter, the basic technology of flow and imaging cytometry is explained, and examples of current and future applications in diagnostic pathology are presented.

FLOW CYTOMETRY AND DIAGNOSTIC PATHOLOGY

Flow cytometric (FCM) analysis has allowed detailed insights into the cellular biology of normal, reactive, and neoplastic tissues. In addition, clinical correlation has led to the establishment of FCM for diagnosis and prognosis in a limited range of disorders, summarized in Table 13-1.

As one will see, most clinically relevant flow assays deal with leukocytes, erythroid cells, and their precursors. This is not surprising, given the need for single-cell suspensions for FCM and a tradition of the use of more dedicated cytometry in blood and related tissues (such as a complete blood cell count). FCM-based assays have been described for other tissues. However, except for DNA content analysis, these are not currently clinical standards of practice. This reflects the rarity of these diseases or the questionable clinical significance of the flow studies.

The purpose of this section on flow cytometry is to review concisely the clinically relevant technology and applications to the diagnosis and prognostication of human disease. Some nonstandard assays will be described, given their potential to become truly clinically useful with future validation. For those interested in more complete and descriptive reviews of the technology and applications, references are included on several authoritative texts.[1-5]

Table 13-1 Uses of flow cytometric analysis

Assistance in the diagnosis and prognostication of leukemias and lymphomas
Definition of prognosis, and the stage of and the need for therapeutic intervention in HIV-infected patients
Determination of DNA ploidy and proliferation fraction in certain neoplasms
Enumeration of reticulocytes
Detection of autoantibodies to platelets and neutrophils

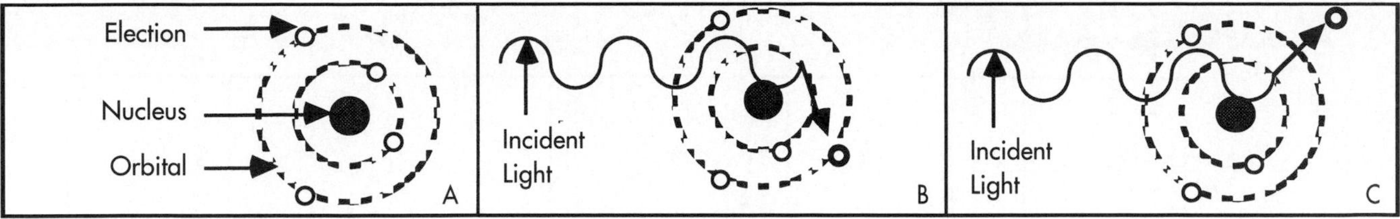

Fig. 13-1 Bohr theory. Basic Bohr model of the atom, **A.** Stable stimulation of atom, **B.** Ionization (photobleaching), **C.**

METHODOLOGY IN FLOW CYTOMETRY

Fluorescence

Fluorescence is defined as the immediate emission of light from a molecule (fluorochrome) that has absorbed light energy (excitation light). Because only part of the absorbed energy is reemitted, the wavelength of the fluorescence light is greater than the excitation light. This process can be visualized with a simplified Bohr model. The nucleus of the atom is surrounded by an electron cloud, which has distinct orbitals, shown here for simplicity as concentric rings (Fig. 13-1, *A*). The higher the orbital, the greater the energy of the electron. If the electron is excited by absorbing a photon of light, it will move to a higher orbital (Fig. 13-1, *B*). If the excitation is sufficiently great (the photon is energetic enough), the electron will escape from the atom entirely, leaving a charged atom (such as, an ion; Fig. 13-1, *C*).

In fluorescence, the excitation light is absorbed by the electron, which increases the energy of the electron and raises it to a higher orbital. This electron is not stable at this higher energy level, however, and quickly reverts to the lower orbital (Fig. 13-2). During this reversion, the electron will give off some of its energy as light, which is the fluorescence. The difference between the peak intensity of the incident and the fluorescent light is called the *Stokes shift*. The more clinically useful fluorochromes have relatively large Stokes shifts.

Fluorescent light is *not* of one wavelength. Rather, it is a spectrum with "shoulders" that are usually surprisingly far away from the most common ("peak") wavelength (Fig. 13-3). As a result, the spectral ranges of different fluorochromes often overlap to a significant extent. This is not a problem when only one fluorochrome is used. However, the simultaneous analysis of two or more "markers" bound to different fluorochromes may be complicated by spectral overlap and resultant false-positive results (see the subsequent discussion of fluorescence compensation).

Cytometry

Light sources

Lasers are the light source of choice for clinical cytometry. This is particularly true with the newer air-cooled lasers, which are much more reliable and cheaper. Although alternative sources of excitation light are available (such as a mercury arc, halogen lamps), the less focused light and broader spectrum of excitation lead to relatively decreased resolution and increased autofluorescence as compared to lasers. The laser used on most clinical cytometers is the argon type, with a 488 nm wavelength. This allows excitation of a variety of fluorochromes (such as fluorescein isothiocyanate [FITC], phycoerythrin [PE], tandem conjugates) as well as certain DNA-binding dyes (propidium iodide).

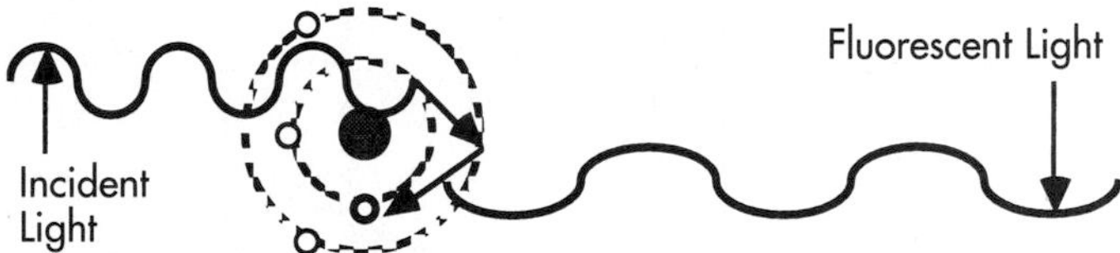

Fig. 13-2 Fluorescence. Unstable photostimulation of atom, with reemission of light (fluorescence) when electron returns to base orbital.

Filters

The practical use of fluorescence involves the selective separation/elimination of incident and fluorescence light. The light detectors in most cytometers are not specific for any one type of light. Optical barriers (filters) and mirrors are used for this purpose in both manual microscopic and automated-flow cytometric fluorescence analysis. Most of these barriers are called *secondary filters* because they are positioned between the cell stream and the photon detectors.[6]

There are three principle types of secondary filters: barrier, band pass, and dichroic mirrors.[7] Band-pass filters will allow light between the stated values to pass through. The longer and shorter wavelengths will be absorbed. Barrier filters will block light above or below a certain unique value and will allow the other wavelengths to pass through. "Long-pass" barrier filters allow wavelengths longer than the stated value to pass through, blocking those with shorter wavelengths. "Short-pass" barrier filters do just the opposite. Dichroic mirrors are used to split a spectrum of light, directing them in two different directions. Light is not absorbed or blocked to any significant extent with these filters. In flow cytometers, these are used to initially separate different wavelengths of fluorescence light, as well as to separate the side-scatter incident (laser) photons from any fluorescence photons (see below).

Cytometer

Flow cytometric analysis in its most general form would include any instrument that analyzes a stream of individual cells from a cell suspension. However, in current usage, the term *flow cytometer* means an instrument that interrogates individual cells by light so as to determine intrinsic (light scatter/cell size and granularity) and extrinsic characteristics (fluorescence/antibody, and nuclei acid dye binding) of the cells. The latter usually involves antibodies, which are bound to a fluorochrome (direct conjugation). Other extrinsic fluorescence markers involve the metabolism of compounds. In this

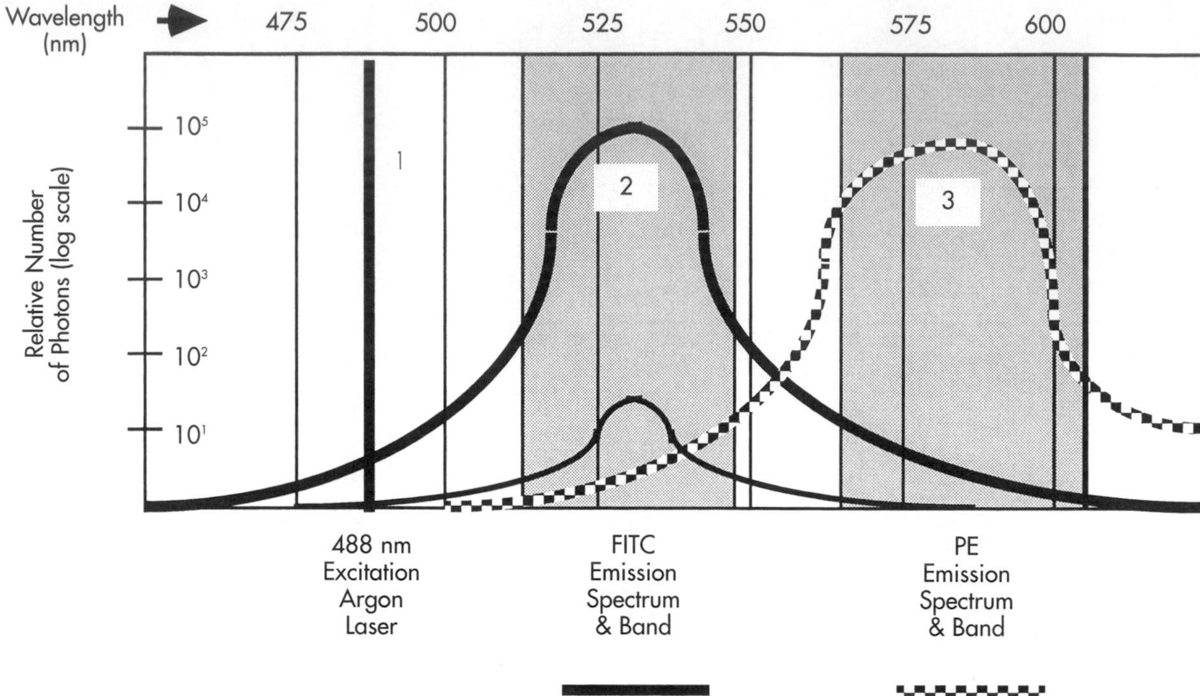

Fig. 13-3 Basic fluorochrome excitation and emission spectra. *X*-axis is photon wavelength; *y*-axis is log scale of number of photons; *line 1* is laser wavelength; *curve 2* and *curve 3* are the relative numbers of the different photons given off by fluorescein isothiocyanate and phycoerythrin fluorochromes when excited by an argon laser.

process, these markers may (1) become fluorescent, (2) become nonfluorescent, or (3) be eliminated from the cell. Changes in the fluorescence over time or after stimulation can then be used to infer the presence or absence of certain functions (such as an oxidative burst in neutrophils or an elimination of cytotoxic drugs in neoplastic cells).

The flow cytometer is a sophisticated mixture of fluidics, optics, light detectors, and computers[6] (Fig. 13-4). The cell suspension is funneled by the instrument into a single cell stream, which passes through the laser light. There is a characteristic scattering of the laser light by the cells that gives information as to intrinsic cellular parameters. These include cell size or volume and granularity. The former is proportional to the amount of laser light slightly deflected from parallel to the incident beam (low-angle or forward light scatter). A photomultiplier tube (PMT) is set up in line with the incident laser beam, which is usually blocked by a light barrier (obscuration bar). Thus only laser photons at a low angle to the incident beam can be detected.

Some incident laser photons pass into the cytoplasm and are deflected by cytoplasmic granules or the nucleus. Light scatter proportional to this is best observed at approximately 90 degrees to the incident beam and is known as 90-degree, side, or orthogonal, light scatter. This is usually separated from any fluorescent light by a combination of dichroic mirrors and barrier filters. Highly irregular cellular membrane (nuclear and cytoplasmic) can also result in increased 90-degree light scatter.

Forward and side light scatter are examples of intrinsic parameters measured by flow cytometry. They do not require specific probes to be measured. Immunofluorescence data are examples of extrinsic parameters because they require fluorochrome-bound antibody probes to define antigenic characteristics. The current generation of bench-top flow cytometers usually will measure two or three different fluorescence bands (hence fluorochrome-labeled markers) simultaneously. The fluorescence light is usually observed along the same axis as the 90-degree light scatter, so as to minimize any incident laser light. As before, the 90-degree laser and various fluorescence photons are separated by a combination of dichroic mirrors, barrier, and band-pass filters.

Fluorescence compensation

The increased application of simultaneous multiantigen analysis in clinical laboratories, primarily for cell-surface phenotyping, has necessitated implementation of procedures to minimize interference of fluorescent signals with one another (that is, compensate for overlapping emission spectra). This prevents a strong fluorescent signal from one parameter from falsely resulting in a positive signal for the second parameter.[6] This lack of overlap is important not only for antigen immunophenotyping, but also for two-color DNA content analysis.[8]

As either the FITC ("green") or PE ("red") fluorescence gets stronger, the false dual emission of the FITC or PE fluorochrome becomes apparent (Fig. 13-4). This is attributable to the "tail end" of the emission spectrum having a sufficient number of photons to be detected. This may give the false impression of dual antigen expression with immunofluorescence analysis.

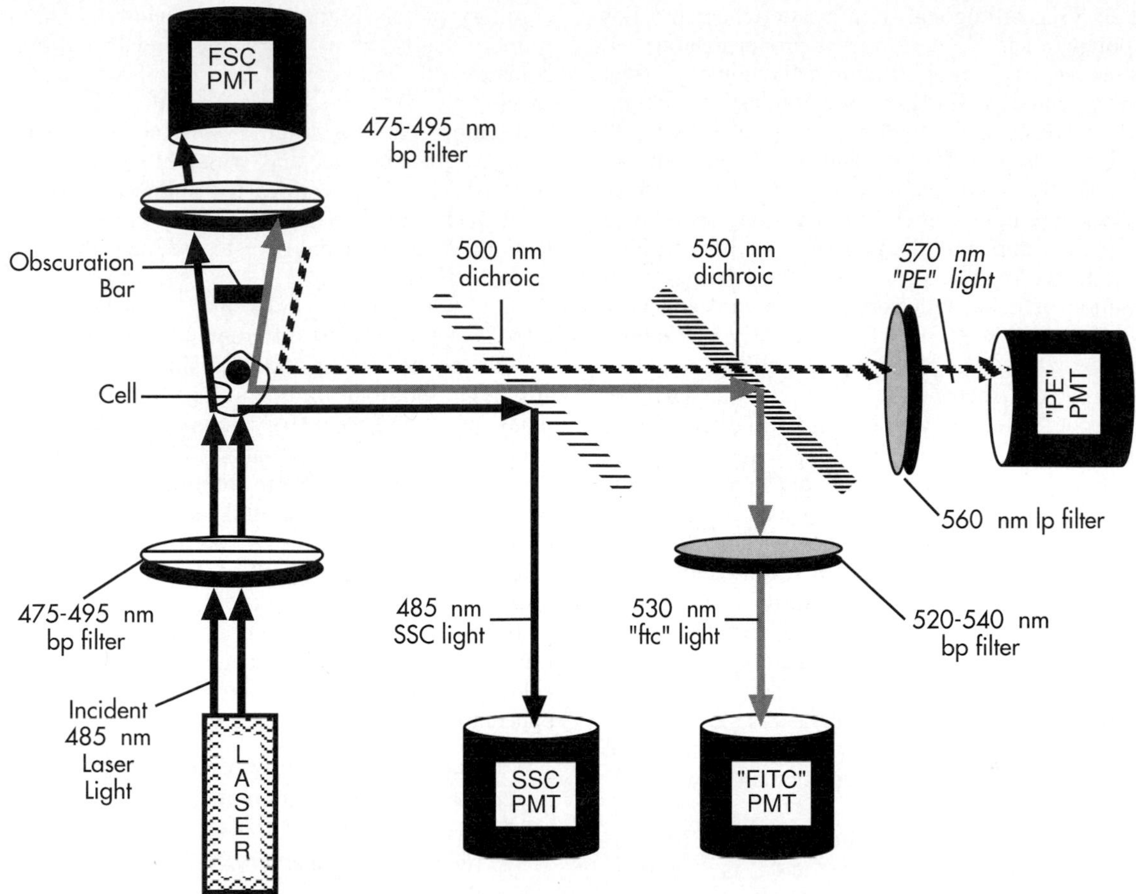

Fig. 13-4 Basic "two-color" flow cytometer configuration.

After the instrument is properly aligned and calibrated, the multifluorochrome-stained cell suspensions are run. To set fluorescence compensation, there should be a single strongly positive population for each fluorochrome, plus one lacking any of the test fluorochromes. Usually the instrument initially appears undercompensated, with both positive populations having apparent partial or complete dual immunofluorescence. Using electronic addition or subtraction, one aligns the peaks of the positive populations with the negative populations, as shown above. Should one have excess compensation, the positive populations appear squashed against their respective axes. The latter may give rise to a false-negative result (such as $CD5^-$ CLL; $CD10^-$ CLL; that is, 'negative common acute lymphoblastic leukemias').

Sample preparation

The type of sample will determine what mode of purification is utilized. Peripheral blood and bone marrow may be directly stained with antibodies ("whole blood" technique), followed by erythrocyte lysis. However, cell suspensions of marrow and disaggregated solid tissue often have a significant amount of debris or nonviable cells. Such samples often benefit from density-gradient (such as ficol hypaque) purification. This technique will retain most of the mature lymphocytes, monocytes, and immature hematolymphoid precursors at the interface between the plasma and the ficol layers. The mature myeloid cells, erythrocytes, and erythroid precursors sink to the bottom along with dead or aggregated cells.

A small number of diagnostic cells that may be lost from the ficol-purified tissues are usually not clinically significant, given current diagnostic classifications and treatment. Nevertheless, a Giemsa- or Leishman-stained cytospin preparation of the purified cell suspensions should be examined to assess for the representativeness of the suspension and for possible loss of diagnostically significant mononuclear cell populations.

The decision to perform flow cytometric analysis, and the type and extent of markers to be run (such as antibodies) will be based upon the morphologic and clinical differential diagnosis. For evaluations that require multiple markers, the use of simultaneous two- or three-color analysis has become widely accepted. The data derived from such an approach are often more precise and informative and are probably more cost effective than single-color methods.

Acquisition and analysis of data

The proper selection of the cell population to be analyzed and interpretation of the resultant flow cytometric data are obtained by careful correlation with the cellular morphology of the original tissue specimen or the stained cytospin of the purified cell suspension. This is particularly true and important with lymph node and marrow specimens. Such samples may have heterogeneous populations or have lost the diagnostic (malignant) population during isolation, staining, and washing.

The selection of cells to be analyzed on the cytometer is usually based upon the low-angle (forward; FALS; FSC) and side (90-degree; SSC; orthogonal) light scatter characteristics of the major populations.[9,10] The former is proportional to cell size, whereas the latter is in proportion to cell complexity (that is, cytoplasmic granularity, nuclear convolutions). In peripheral blood leukocytes, one usually sees three major cell groups: lymphoid cells (low forward and 90-degree scatter—mostly T, B, and NK cells), monocytoid cells (intermediate forward and 90-degree light scatter—mostly monocytes, some T, B, and NK cells), and granulocytes (intermediate to high forward and 90-degree light scatter). In addition, there is often a small population of cells with very low forward and very low to intermediate side scatter ("RBC"). This is a heterogeneous mixture of erythrocytes, platelets, and debris.

The standard two-parameter light-scatter analysis will usually allow the proper selection of the cells of interest. This is primarily true for lymphocyte analysis or when the malignant population predominates. However, there are times when the light-scatter populations are not clear because of either technical problems or samples with a wide variety of cell types (such as bone marrow). The populations of interest can be identified at the time of data acquisition by "backgating" a fluorescent parameter (as with CD45, CD19, CD3) compared to the forward or the side light scatter.[11,12] Data acquisition on only the population of interest can then proceed. Alternatively, one can collect the data from 20,000 unselected cells and save the data electronically (LIST mode). This allows the laboratorian to later gate electronically upon the various populations to determine their immunophenotypes.

The interpretation of the immunofluorescence histograms and dot plots should be attempted only if there is the appropriate reactivity with negative and positive controls.[6,13] The computation of the number of cells staining for a given marker is relatively straightforward if the positive staining is bright and the fluorescence peak of the positive cells is distinct from those of the antigen-negative population or the cells stained with the negative control, or both types. A variety of analytical methods may be used for these calculations. These include subtraction of histograms, curve-match subtraction, and simple integration of the areas under the histogram beyond a cutoff marker, which is determined using the negative control. All these techniques have their limitations.

As a rule, all single-parameter histograms and multiparameter contour and dot plots should be visually inspected. It is well known that nonspecific staining among polyclonal and even isotype-matched monoclonal antibodies can have significant small shifts in the nonspecifically stained fluorescence peaks.[13] The situation of "dim-positive" staining with the positive peak being ≤0.5 log more fluorescent than the negative control peak *and* with both extensive overlapping may very well represent variations in nonspecific staining among reagent antibodies. Lastly, when analyzing the immunophenotypic results, one should also pay attention to the intensity of the positive peak in addition to the percentage of antigen-positive cells.

APPLICATIONS OF FLOW CYTOMETRY

Immunophenotyping

Flow cytometric analysis can rapidly provide detailed antigen profiles of various hematolymphoid neoplasias. However, some clinically relevant applications are much more limited. A corollary of this is that immunophenotypic analysis is not a primary diagnostic or prognostic modality. Rather, traditional hematoxylin and eosin and Giemsa-stained morphology remains the definitive standard for the diagnoses of leukemia and lymphoma. In addition, nonmorphologic parameters, such as stage, patient age, and white blood cell count, are well established as key features for defining prognosis and treatment plans. Last but not least, these more traditional parameters are often less expensive to ascertain than immunophenotypic profiles.

The widespread availability of monoclonal antibodies directly conjugated to different fluorochromes has allowed a significant increase in the precision of immunophenotyping. Although multiple fluorochromes have been available for many years, the recent development of chromogens that are excitable by the standard argon laser has allowed bench-top flow cytometers to perform these analyses routinely. In addition to allowing a more definitive typing of all leukocyte populations, multicolor analysis can decrease the number of tube cells needed to run a panel of antibodies. The latter may be useful in cases where there is a paucity of cells.

From the above observations, it is clear that the laboratorian must have a question that routine morphologic and clinical data do not answer. These usually arise from the histologic appearance of the tumor and are most often the following:

- Is a neoplasm of leukocyte origin (lineage)?
- Is a leukocyte proliferation neoplastic (clonality)?
- What is the differentiation (type) of leukemia or lymphoma (myeloid versus lymphoid; Hodgkin's versus non-Hodgkin's)?

If such an approach is taken, immunophenotypic analysis is able to aid significantly in diagnosis in approximately 40% to 50% of cases where it is applied.[14,15]

As a general rule, immunophenotypic analysis is most useful when one is defining tumors arising from tissues that are developmentally quite distinct (epithelial to carcinoma versus leukocyte to lymphoma). On the other hand, neoplasms of the same or very closely related lineages often have a significant overlap of antigen phenotypes. In the latter instance, even multicolor immunoanalysis may not be sufficiently specific on a case-by-case basis.

A practical result of the above considerations is that lineage is best defined by a multi–antibody panel. Traditionally, this includes antibody to at least two different lineage-associated or lineage-restricted antigens for each of the major cell lines in the clinical differential. Such an approach will help overcome the lack of absolute sensitivity and specificity of any one antigen for a particular cell line.

The interpreter should expect to see the appropriate pattern of both positive and negative immunoreactivities. Attention should also be directed at the intensity of the positive peak in addition to the percentage of cells expressing the antigen. As always, careful consideration of the patient's clinical history and morphologic appearance of the tumor, along with the composite antigen profile, is required to render a diagnosis.

Chronic lymphoid leukemias

There are two major rationales for phenotyping the lymphocytic leukemias and related lymphomas.[16] The most common is to differentiate between an early stage of lymphoid leukemia and a persistent reactive lymphocytosis. The other is to help differentiate between clinically significant subtypes of an otherwise diagnostic mature lymphoid leukemia.[17]

The definition of B-cell clonality is primarily determined by the *population* expression of surface or cytoplasmic immunoglobulin light chains (kappa and lambda). The light-chain ratio will help define clonality and define B-cell lineage. This is most reliably seen using two- or three-color immunofluorescence assays. These allow one to define transmembrane-bound immunoglobulin clearly from nonspecifically bound immunoglobulin (Fc receptor bound).

Some malignant B-cell proliferations (such as large cell lymphomas) may lack detectable immunoglobulin.[18] Although this is significantly correlated with a malignant B-cell proliferation, further evidence should be sought to confirm malignancy (such as morphology and immunoglobulin gene rearrangement). Other indirect immunophenotypic evidence of B-cell clonality would include coexpression of differentiation and activation antigens on an atypically large proportion of the cells in a particular tissue compartment.[19] The assumption in these cases is that only monoclonal proliferations would result in such an atypical immunophenotype.

The definition of T-cell clonality by immunoanalysis is more difficult. Currently, there is no reliable analog of kappa and lambda light-chain expression for the TCR (T-cell receptor) protein on T-cell populations. Only indirect immunophenotypic evidence of T-cell clonality is currently well defined. The best defined would be the lack of expression of one or more "pan"–T-cell antigens ('cluster of differentiation': CD2, 3, 4[+8], 5, 7, TCR).[18] To a lessor degree, one may also use atypical coexpression of differentiation antigens, similar to the approach with B-lineage leukemias.[16]

To type lymphoid leukemias efficiently, one must keep in mind the relevant differential diagnosis, as well as the relative frequency of the various types. A lymphocytosis usually falls into four major diagnostic possibilities: reactive or the B-lineage chronic lymphocytic, prolymphocytic, and small cleaved cell leukemias.[20,21] Given the infrequent occurrence of T-cell neoplasia in the United States, the antigen profile should be directed at the relevant differential for B-cell leukemias, with one reliable "pan"–T-cell marker. If there is significant clinical or morphologic evidence suggestive of T lineage, inclusion of more pan–T-cell and T-subset markers (CD2, 3, 4, 5, 7, 8, 16, or 56) would be appropriate.

Acute leukemias

The delineation between acute lymphoblastic (ALL) and myeloblastic leukemias (AML) is important, given the differences in therapy and overall prognosis. Although this usually can be performed with routine morphologic and cytochemical analysis, a small minority of cases still have an undifferentiated phenotype by these techniques. In addition, approximately 1% to 5% of cases of "cytomorphologic" ALL are really undifferentiated (M0) or megakaryocytic (M7) AMLs.[22-24] These entities require immunophenotyping for correct diagnosis[25,26] The advent of immunophenotypic analysis has also significantly enhanced the reliability of ALL diagnosis, which are largely diagnoses of exclusion in the French-American-British (FAB) classification. A good general rule is to perform immunophenotypic analysis if the acute leukemia is undifferentiated or is probably ALL.

Immunophenotyping has undoubtedly narrowed the diagnostic gray areas of the traditional FAB classification, but it has also created new gray areas (such as acute mixed lineage leukemia).[25,27-31] The good news is that some of these have *partially* independent prognostic significance, thus allowing a more refined definition of patient prognosis (reviewed by Carey and Hanson[16]).

A reasonable "base" acute leukemia immunophenotyping panel includes:

- B lineage: CD19, kappa, lambda
- T lineage: CD5, CD7
- T and B lineage: CD10, TdT (terminal deoxynucleotidyl transferase)
- Myelomonocytic lineage: CD13, CD14, CD33
- "Blasts": CD34

Such a panel will reliably identify better than 95% of all AMLs and ALLs, as well as define additional prognostically important subsets. Should the initial results not be diagnostic, the addition of antibodies to megakaryocytic (CD41, CD61), erythroid (glycophorin A), leukocyte common antigen (CD45), or additional T (CD1, CD2), B (CD20, cytoplasmic CD22), and myelomonocytic antigens (CD14, CD24, cytoplasmic myeloperoxidase) may be helpful. However, no one antigen or combination of antigens are 100% specific or sensitive for any lineage. Thus careful correlation with morphologic, cytochemical, and clinical information is essential.

Non-Hodgkin's lymphomas and plasmacytic neoplasias

Plasma cell leukemia, multiple myeloma, plasmacytoma, and Waldenström's macroglobulinemia are the major entities in secretory B-cell malignancies.[32-34] These malignancies do not often cause a diagnostic dilemma because of their obvious plasmacytic differentiation and monoclonal proteins in the serum or urine. However, anaplastic variants of plasma cell leukemia and myeloma and small cell variants of Waldenström's macroglobulinemia may not be easily recognizable. Because these B-cell tumors have differing prognoses, immunophenotypic analysis may allow a more definitive diagnosis.[19,35]

Immunophenotyping is primarily used for defining benign tissue lymphoid infiltrates from non-Hodgkin's lymphoma (NHL) and defining the lineages of hematolymphoid neoplasms that are histogenetically quite far apart. However, many NHLs have overlapping immunophenotypic profiles, even when 10 or 20 antigens are evaluated. Thus, for a particular patient's NHL, this usually precludes a definitive grading based only upon antigen phenotype. Immunophenotyping is only able to allow reliable prediction of NHL grades when they have distinct lineages (such as true histiocytic lymphoma) or stages of maturation (lymphoblastic lymphomas; "Ki-1" anaplastic large cell lymphomas).

Hodgkin's disease

The immunoanalysis of Hodgkin's disease is almost entirely done by in situ techniques (immunohistochemistry or cytochemistry). This reflects the widespread experience that it is nearly impossible to get any significant number of Reed-Sternberg (RS) cells into a mononuclear suspension. The utility of immunoanalysis in the differential diagnosis of Hodgkin's disease has been significantly enhanced by the advent of antibodies to formalin-resistant antigens. It may be difficult to identify RS cells cytologically in some frozen sections. However, they can usually be quite easily visualized in formalin-fixed tissue (reviewed by Carey and Hanson[16]). Usually, the combination of anti-CD15, anti-CD30, and anti-CD45, along with a morphologic examination, can reliably confirm or refute the diagnosis of Hodgkin's disease.

Proliferation antigens

Although most flow cytometric measurements of cell proliferation are made by mathematical determination of the S-phase fraction, proliferation antigen expression may be quantitated by flow cytometry.

The best example is the Ki67 protein. This nuclear antigen, which is essentially absent in G_0, is first expressed in the G_1 phase and then is variably present throughout S, G_2, and M. The Ki-67 proliferation index (% cells Ki-67$^+$) has been evaluated most widely on NHLs and breast carcinomas. Schwartz[36,37] and Hall[38] have both demonstrated good correlation between the grade of the NHL and Ki-67 proliferative fraction and with nuclear DNA content.

However, the prognostic utility of Ki-67 proliferative fraction in NHL is controversial. Some studies have shown that high fractions have a favorable prognosis,[38,39] whereas others found the opposite.[40] In addition, the methods of analysis (immunohistochemistry, flow cytometry), grade of NHLs, and cutoff criteria for proliferative fraction have varied in all cases. Standardization of the technique, along with large prospective studies, will be needed to assess definitively whether the Ki-67 proliferative fraction has a truly independent and clinically significant role in NHLs.[41]

Proliferating cell nuclear antigen (PCNA)

Proliferating cell nuclear antigen (PCNA) is otherwise known as cyclin. It is the 36 kD delta-subunit of DNA polymerase and is found here during the G_1 through M phases of the proliferation cycle, peaking in the S phase.[42,43] The antigen can be detected by both in situ[44] and flow cytometric methods.[42,43] PCNA-proliferative fractions in fixed tissue directly correlate with mitotic activity of breast and colon carcinomas[44] and with NHL grade.[45] However, as with Ki-67 and other proliferation-associated antigens, further work is required to elucidate more clearly any prognostic values for leukemia, lymphomas, and other neoplasms.

Other proliferation-associated antigens

The p105 antigen, a nuclear matrix–associated protein, is present at low levels in G_0 and progressively increases in quantity during G_1 to M.[46,47] One study of sarcomas did not find any correlation between histologic grade, DNA, or Ki67 proliferative fraction.[48] Any value in the prognostication of NHLs must await further large prospective studies.

Other proliferation-related antigens (4F2, CD25, CD71) are expressed on the cell membrane at the beginning of the G_1 to S phases of cell proliferation.[49] Holte and associates[50] reported a significant correlation between the percentage of 4F2$^+$ cells in low-grade NHLs and poor patient survival. There have been no reports of a significant association between treatment responses or survival and CD25 or CD71 expression.

Immunodeficiency

HIV/AIDS

The acquired immunodeficiency syndrome (AIDS) is the result of infection of leukocytes and other cells by the human immunodeficiency viruses (HIV) 1 and 2 as discussed in Chapter 28.

The HIV virus infects cells expressing the CD4 antigen.[51,52] The latter, a binding protein for an HLA-Dr, serves as the binding site for the HIV. The most prominent cell affected is the CD4$^+$ T-lymphocyte, which is essential for controlling the upregulation and downregulation of the cellular and humoral immune systems. The CD4 lymphocytes are destroyed over time, with the degree of destruction being directly related to HIV viral proliferative and burden.[53]

The CD4$^+$ T-cell concentration in HIV+ patients is the *single* most reliable laboratory parameter for assessment of the effects of HIV infection. It is able to predict *disease progression* in HIV-infected patients.[54,55] Although somewhat controversial, it is now recommended that HIV+ individuals with CD4$^+$ T-cell concentrations of less than 500/μL be given antiretroviral therapy to slow the progression of the infection. The use of interferon to augment T-cell numbers has also been attempted. The CD4$^+$ lymphocyte concentration is also predictive of the risk of particular infectious and neoplastic sequels and the patient's prognosis when these occur.[56-59] Based on these observations, the CD4$^+$ lymph concentration is used to initiate prophylactic therapy.[60-62]

Primary immunodeficiency

The laboratory approach to the evaluation of suspected immunodeficiency is most effective when approached from a consideration of basic clinical and blood parameters.[63] The age of onset, sex, and any abnormal anatomic features and family history are the crucial pieces of historical data. The type of infectious agent (viral versus pyogenic bacterial versus fungal) and site are also vital clues. Finally, consideration of these and the basic blood cell and serum immunoglobulin and complement values will allow a concise differential diagnosis and, if indicated, direct any follow-up testing.

Flow cytometry is strictly an adjuvant testing modality, primarily to enumerate lymphocytes (Table 13-2). The panel should be directed at the relevant differential diagnosis. Rarely, phagocytic deficiencies of surface adhesion molecules or oxidative burst functions arise.[64] These can be screened for by standard immunophenotypic or specialized fluorescence metabolic flow assays.[65]

Transplantation

End-stage renal disease (ESRD), a complex medical problem, is increasing in the United States.[66] It is most often treated with dialysis. However, ESRD patients with successful kidney transplants have a more favorable prognosis than those receiving dialysis. Successful transplantation results in an enhanced quality of life compared to the dialyzed ESRD patients and is less expensive in the long term. The principle side effects of solid organ transplantation are allograft failure and the increased incidence of infection and malignancy.[67-69] These problems revolve around the delicate balancing of immunosuppression to allow host tolerance of the allograft without significant impairment of the immune surveillance or drug toxicity. The correct diagnosis of the cause of allograft failure

Table 13-2 Use of leukocyte antigens in immunodeficiency disorders

White blood cell subset	Antibodies	Rationale
Pan-T	CD2, 3, 5, 7	*T-cell quantity:* SCID, DiGeorge's, Nezelof's, ADA, PNP, WAS, AT, CMC
T Subset	CD4, 8	*T-cell subset:* HIV infection, SCID, DiGeorge's
	MHC I (HLA-A,B,C)	*Absence:* bare lymphocyte syndrome
	gp39	*Mutant protein ligand for CD40:* Hyper-IgM syndrome
B	CD19, 20	*B-cell quantity:* Bruton's, SCID, CVID, DiGeorge's, WAS, AT
	kappa, lambda	*Absence:* Kappa and lambda light-chain deficiency
	IgG, IgA, IgM	*Isotype switch/secretion defect:* Hyper-IgM syndrome; CVID
	MHC II (HLA-D)	*Absence:* some bare lymphocyte syndrome
Polymorphonuclear neutrophil and monocyte	CD11; sialyl-CD15,18	*Absence:* adhesion molecule deficiency
	MHC II (HLA-D)	*Absence:* some bare lymphocyte syndrome
Platelet	CD42	*Absence:* Wiskott-Aldrich syndrome

ADA, Adenosine deaminase deficiency; *AT,* ataxia-telangiectasia; *CD,* cluster of differentiation; *CMC,* chronic mucocutaneous candidiasis; *CVID,* common variable immunodeficiency; *HIM,* hepatitis-infectious mononucleosis; *HLA,* human leukocyte antigen; *MHC,* major histocompatibility complex; *PNP,* purine nucleoside phosphorylase deficiency; *SCID,* severe combined immunodeficiency syndrome; *WAS,* Wiskott-Aldrich syndrome.

is important because inappropriate changes in immunosuppression can lead to loss of graft or death from infection.[70-72] Core or fine-needle aspiration biopsy of the graft may aid in defining the cause of allograft failure and may contain features predictive of ultimate graft survival.[73-75] However, the diagnostic and prognostic value of standard histology during acute graft dysfunction has limitations, as discussed in Chapter 29.

Allograft dysfunction

The absolute blood T-cell count (CD3$^+$) may be important because transplanted patients with T-cell counts below 100 to 200/μL have been reported to have a lower risk of acute cellular rejection (ACR).[76] However, others have failed to observe such a correlation with similar[77] or different[78] immunosuppressive therapy. Further, when the absolute T-cell count is above 150/μL, the concentration of CD2$^-$ or CD3$^-$ positive cells often fails to be predictive of the following[76,79-81]:

- Risk of onset of ACR in stable allograft patients
- That the cause of a renal failure episode is attributable to ACR, or
- Reversibility of an ACR

Single antigen analysis of the major T-cell subsets has not proved to be useful in the evaluation of allograft failure. Multiple studies have indicated that the absolute CD4$^+$ or CD8$^+$ cell concentrations are not:

- Diagnostic of ACR[77,82]
- Predictive of ACR onset[77,87,82]
- Predictive of ACR reversibility[78]

Most studies, regardless of mode of immunosuppressive therapy, indicate that the pretransplant CD4/CD8 ratio cannot be predictive of the risk of ACR,[80,83-86] graft failure,[87,88] or resistance to ACR therapy.[87] During the first months after transplantation, some studies found that alterations in the CD4/CD8 ratio were predictive of the diagnosis of ACR as the cause of a clinically apparent allograft failure[77,82,85,89,90] or the risk of ACR before the clinical onset of a allograft failure.[85,87,91-93] However, others found no such correlation, regardless of type of immunosuppressive therapy.[77-79,87,94]

The enumeration of small yet functionally significant T subsets can be more accurately done by simultaneous two-antigen (two-color) analysis. This may be significant because the number of activated T-cells (CD2$^+$/DR$^+$ or CD3$^+$/DR$^+$) may be a better predictor of ACR. In a small series, Hayes and associates[95] reported a significant decrease in blood activated T-cells (CD2$^+$/DR$^+$) 3 to 4 days before the clinical onset of ACR, followed by an increase in this population at onset. In this series, these findings were not dependent on the mode of immunosuppressive therapy. Hayashi and associates[96] reported a similar increase in T activation at the onset of ACR. In addition, Gross and associates[97] found that the percentage of CD8$^+$/DR$^+$ cell increased before clinical onset of ACR. However, this finding was also seen with acute viral infections, as with cytomegalovirus.

Analysis of the subsets of CD8$^+$ T-cells, which contain the Ts and Tc precursors and effectors, might be expected to aid in predicting ACR. Using the definition of Ts as either CD8$^+$/CD11b$^+$ or CD8$^+$/CD57$^+$ lymphoid cells, increased Ts cells are seen in stable renal allografts, both early and long term (>5 years). Gross and associates[97] found that a decrease in Ts cells (CD8$^+$/CD11b$^+$) was seen during the week preceding the onset of clinical ACR. This increased risk of ACR was best predicted by the ratio of activated CD8$^+$ cells to Ts (CD8$^+$/DR$^+$: CD8$^+$/CD11b$^+$). However, similar changes were seen with acute viral infections.

Most studies up to now indicate that virtually all lymphoid cells in rejecting allografts are T-cells[98-105] and that increased numbers of intragraft T-cells are a sensitive marker of ACR.[100] The B- and plasma cells total less than 5% to 10% of interstitial leukocytes seen in ACR and have no significant association with the diagnosis of ACR, viral infection, acute vascular rejection (AVR), or chronic rejection.[102-104,106] Most[104,105,107,108] but not all[102] reports indicate that monocytes and macrophages predominate during severe or longstanding ACR.

The ability of the relative composition of the major T-cell subsets to define the *risk* or *cause* of allograft failure is unclear. The changes in CD4$^+$ cells during ACR[98,99,103,106] and the ability of the CD4/CD8 ratio or localization of the CD4$^+$ and CD8$^+$ cells to allow prediction of the histologic severity or reversibility of ACR is controversial.[98,101-104,106]

Analysis for markers of T, B, or monocyte activation may aid in defining pathologically significant mononuclear cell infiltrates from those not associated with graft dysfunction. Increased numbers of DR^+, $CD38^+$, $CD15^+$, $CD25^+$, or transferrin receptor$^+$ cells are seen during ACR and are consistent with increased activated T-cells or macrophages.[98,99,105,106] In addition, Cunningham and Ascher[86] noted increased activated Ts and Tc cells ($CD8^+/DR^+$) and activated macrophages ($CD14^+$/DR bright$^+$) in the graft during ACR.

Anti-CD3 therapy

The monoclonal antibody recognizing one of the epitopes of the CD3 molecule has become a potent drug for treating de novo and steroid-resistant solid organ allograft rejection[69,109-113] In addition, some centers have used OKT3 as one of their primary prophylactic immunosuppressives. Although other anti–T-cell monoclonals have been used in such a setting (CD25, CD2, CD4, CD8), none has yet gained the wide acceptance of OKT3.

OKT3 functions by causing either the destruction of some T-cells (ADCC) or inducing immune paralysis.[111,114-118] The latter occurs by either the elimination or steric blockage of the CD3 and associated T-cell antigen receptor (TCR) molecules on the T-cell surface. This results in T immune paralysis by incapacitating the antigen *TCR*CD3 pathway of T-cell activation.

The flow cytometric evaluation of OKT3 therapy primarily deals with verifying the loss of detectable CD3 antigen on T-cells. The usual pattern is an abrupt decrease in $CD2^+3^+(4^+$ or $8^+)$ T-lymphocytes within the first few hours after initiation of OKT3 therapy. However, by the second day, there are circulating $CD2^+3^-(4^+$ or $8^+)$ T-cells detectable. These may be present in normal or decreased concentrations.[117]

Detailed studies have indicated that, usually, the CD3 molecule is still present on the T-cells.[114-116,118] The OKT3 antibody block binding of any other anti-CD3 or anti-TCR antibody. In a small number of cases, dim CD3 immunostaining can be seen. These cells lack detectable TCR, and the patients almost always are in the process of reversing the rejection.

These observations indicate that the OKT3 has resulted in effective T-cell immune paralysis and that the dim CD3 T-cells are functionally inactive. Landay and others[115] have suggested that both $CD3^+$ and TCR^+ T-cell counts be done to identify the immune paralyzed dim $CD3^+/TCR^-$ from presumably dim $CD3^+/TCR^+$ immunocompetent T-cells. However, I have noted that (1) virtually all the time, when dim $CD3^+$ T-cells are seen in the setting of OKT3 therapy, there is clinically effective immune paralysis and (2), in this light, determination of serum BUN and creatinine would be more timely and cost effective.

The other flow cytometric assay involved in OKT3 immunosuppressive therapy is the monitoring of the production of anti-OKT3 antibodies.[120-123] Because OKT3 is a murine protein, there is usually an immune response mounted to it. However, this is seen only rarely during the first 14-day round of treatment if low-dose azathioprine and corticosteroids are given in association with the OKT3. More commonly, during retreatment for rejection, an alloimmune response is seen.

The anti-OKT3 humoral immune response can be divided into two basic groups: (1) an anti-idiotypic antibody and (2) an anti-isotypic antibody.[120,123] The former binds to the antigen-recognition site of OKT3 and effectively blocks its therapeutic activity. The anti-isotypic anti-OKT3 binds to non–antigen recognition sites and does not neutralize the OKT3 immunosuppressive activity.

Assays for both such types of anti-OKT3 antibodies can be performed by ELISA or flow cytometric procedures.[119,120,123] Such tests do not need to be performed on a patient prior to his or her first course of OKT3. However, before reexposure to the drug, assays for serum anti-OKT3 should be performed. If no activity or only IgM or low-titer anti-isotypic OKT3 are present, the patient will probably respond appropriately to therapy. The only difference from a de novo treatment is with low-titer anti-isotypic/anti-OKT3, where the reduction of $CD3^+$ T-cells and rise in serum OKT3 levels may be more gradual.[122]

In a patient previously treated with OKT3, a high-titer anti-isotypic or anti-idiotypic anti-OKT3 is associated with a low rate of reversal of rejection.[122] In such instances, alternative methods of antirejection therapy should be considered. Last, these patients undergoing a second round of anti-OKT3 treatment should be monitored more closely as to the level of the circulating $CD3^+$ lymphocytes.

Autoantibodies

Autoimmune thrombocytopenia

The differential diagnosis of thrombocytopenia is a relatively common clinical dilemma. An autoimmune etiology (ITP) is part of this. Traditionally, ITP has been largely a diagnosis of exclusion, combined with morphologic evidence of adequate marrow megakaryopoiesis. The rapid detection of either circulating or platelet-bound antibody is a significant piece of direct evidence supporting an autoimmune cause. Correlation with the overall clinical and laboratory picture is essential because such autoantibodies may be seen with thrombotic thrombocytopenia purpura, transfusion- and pregnancy-induced alloimmunization, and certain drug therapy.[124]

A variety of methods for detection of antiplatelet antibodies have been described. The flow method is usually a one- or two-color assay, utilizing an FITC-labeled anti–human IgG antibody. The primary advantage of the flow cytometric immunofluorescence method is the ability to analyze rapidly and objectively a large number of platelets, despite a low in vivo concentration. Although the method is not a simple assay to quality control, the predictive value of a positive result in the correct clinical setting is quite high.[124]

Autoimmune and alloimmune neutropenia

Autoimmune neutropenia (AIN) is a relatively rare disorder.[125] Usually the clinical history and blood and marrow morphology are sufficient to determine the cause of neutropenia. Antineutrophil antibodies have been found in most cases of AIN. Alloimmune neutropenia may be a response either to in utero (neonatal alloimmune neutropenia) or transfusion-related exposure.

The flow cytometric method for detection of either circulating antineutrophil or neutrophil-bound immunoglobulin is very similar to that used for platelets.[2,125] The primary difference is that the neutrophils are more labile, necessitating more rapid and fastidious processing. The advantage of the flow cytometric method over others is essentially the same as with platelets: objectivity, speed, and the ability to assay low concentrations of neutrophils. However, the data currently do not support the utility of any one method over the other.[125]

Nucleic acids

Reticulocytes

Reticulocytes are nearly mature red blood cells that contain residual amounts of ribonucleic acid (RNA). These are relative measures of the level of erythropoiesis. Along with the degree and quality of anemia, the reticulocyte concentration can allow the clinician to ascertain whether the marrow is responding appropriately to peripheral loss (bleeding, hemolysis) or is being directly suppressed (iron deficiency, primary or secondary neoplasias).

The utilization of flow cytometry for reticulocyte quantitation is a classic "win-win" situation. It applies an essential, relatively high volume assay to the flow cytometer, thus diversifying and enhancing this technology's medical worth. In return, the cytometer offers a rapid, objective assay, with a decrease in overall "hands-on" labor.

Most flow cytometric assays utilize either thiazole orange or auramine O.[126] These flow cytometric reticulocyte counts exhibit excellent precision and accuracy, both from a clinical and a laboratory standpoint. The primary difficulty is the method's inability to distinguish Howell-Jolly bodies from reticulocytes. In such instances, a manual assay is required.

DNA ploidy and proliferation fraction

Standard nonsurgical therapy of tumors focuses on the relative vulnerability of rapidly dividing neoplastic cells to various chemical and radiation modalities. Thus assessment of tumor proliferation may allow insights into the possible effectiveness of cytoreductive therapy. Further, the proliferation fraction or DNA ploidy measurements may correlate with the intrinsic biologic aggressiveness of the neoplasm. Last, the demonstration of identical (clonal) genetic lesions would be direct evidence of a neoplastic process, though it would neither be absolutely diagnostic nor necessarily imply that a tumor was malignant.

The percentage of the neoplastic cells in the proliferative phases of the cell cycle (G1, S, G2, M) can be approximated by many techniques. Counting mitoses is subjective and labor intensive. Measurement of DNA synthesis using radiolabled nucleotides is objective. However it cannot delineate the different phases of the cell cycle and requires use of radioactive substances. Fluorescent molecules, such as propidium iodide (PI) and 4,6-diamidino-2-plenylindole (DAPI), stoichiometrically bind to available DNA sites and allow an objective determination of the percentage of cells with S (>2N, <4N) or G_2+M (4N) DNA content.

These latter procedures cannot determine the fraction of cells in G_1, a critical phase when the cell commits itself to proliferate. Several nuclear and membrane antigens have recently been defined and are directly or indirectly associated with cell proliferation (see below). They define not only the actual DNA synthetic and postsynthetic phases of the cell cycle, but also include the G_1 time period. In addition to being able to be quantitated by either in situ or flow cytometric methods, these are measured by an antigen-antibody reaction. The latter is a technique more familiar to most clinical laboratories and hence is more likely to be performed competently.

DNA quantitation methodology

The quantitation of DNA appears relatively straightforward. Suspensions of cells or purified nuclei are permeabilized. After pretreatment with RNAase, an intercalating dye (such as propidium iodide) infiltrates and binds stoichiometrically to the DNA. When analyzed on a flow cytometer, the amount of PI fluorescence is proportional to the DNA content of the cells. From this, the DNA ploidy and proliferation fraction can be directly determined. However, it is not all so straightforward.

Several aspects of flow DNA analysis conspire to limit its clinical effectiveness (reviewed by Zarbo[8]). First, it is often true that not all the cells in the suspension are neoplastic. Unfortunately, light scatter (because of size, granularity, or membrane irregularity) cannot reliably differentiate benign cells from malignant cells. Two-color techniques, using PI and a FITC-conjugated antibody against either cytokeratin, leukocyte common antigen (CD45), or T/B lineage–associated antigens, can allow one to significantly separate benign from neoplastic cells. Unfortunately, this cannot be applied to isolated nuclear suspensions from either archival or fresh tissue.

The use of archival tissue (such as formalin-fixed paraffin-embedded tissue blocks) for DNA analysis has been quite popular because of the ability quickly to correlate DNA ploidy and proliferation fraction with clinical outcome. However, there is a significant increase in the number of cases with increased background debris or decreased resolution of nuclear DNA content. In these instances, the ability to ascertain proliferation fraction or a mildly DNA aneuploid population is greatly decreased. As mentioned above, nuclear preparations of archival tissue also stripped the cytoplasm away, thus precluding the use of two-color techniques to limit the analysis to neoplastic cells.

Variation of the accessibility of the DNA of the cells can make different populations with diploid DNA content appear to be aneuploid. This may reflect in vivo differences (proliferative or activation states; different lineages) or in vitro differences (differing degrees of fixation; storage conditions; enzyme or detergent preparations for DNA staining). This has led to the recommendations for using well-established techniques on optimally prepared tissue and two-color techniques.

Other methodologic problems compromise the efficacy of flow DNA literature. In particular, differing methods of data analysis and definitions of aneuploidy and proliferation fraction complicate the comparison of differing studies. Also, the variable documentation of grade or stage of tumor, along with other pertinent clinical features (such as age), limit not only the conclusions of the authors but also the comparison to other papers.

The best recommendation is that individual flow laboratories contact and discuss the application of tumor DNA content analysis with the relevant clinical staff. The key question is whether significant changes in clinical prognostication or therapy will be dictated by the data. If so, the lab should coordinate with the surgical pathology and surgical staff to assure the availability of fresh tissue. Only if the latter is accomplished can one employ the most precise and accurate methods for tumor DNA ploidy and proliferation fraction determinations.

Leukemia and lymphoma

There currently is no widely accepted utility for DNA quantitation in Hodgkin's disease, or the chronic lymphoid, myeloid, or acute myelogenous leukemias (reviewed by Carey and Hanson[16]). The primary application has been toward the mature non-Hodgkin's lymphomas,[127-133] myeloma,[134-136] and childhood acute lymphoblastic leukemias.[137] The conclusions of the individual studies have been somewhat contradictory, a result not surprising given the variety of methods used. A fair conclusion at this time is that, though promising, DNA ploidy or proliferation fraction is not included in any national or international clinical grading scheme for prognosis, hence treatment, of leukemia and lymphoma.

Gastrointestinal tumors

DNA ploidy and proliferative fraction have been extensively studied in gastrointestinal tumors for their ability to be predictive of recurrence and overall survival (reviewed by Zarbo and Linden[138]). Currently, only in colonic carcinomas does DNA analysis appear to have well-documented value. In this instance, a lower proliferative fraction in early-stage disease is significantly associated with decreased recurrence and increased survival. The prognostic role of aneuploidy in colon carcinoma is more controversial.

There has been an extensive amount of work done on other carcinomas and smooth muscle tumors of the gastrointestinal tract. Many studies have shown a univariant relationship between proliferative fraction and DNA ploidy in these tumor systems. Aneuploidy, but not proliferation fraction, has been the parameter most often associated with more adverse prognosis (increased recurrence; decreased survival). However, a consensus has not been apparent, nor have many studies continued to show significance with multivariant analysis. Further prospective studies are needed, using optimal techniques to confirm or refute definitively whether DNA content analysis is clinically relevant in these tumors.

Genitourinary tumors

Tumors of the urinary bladder and prostate gland are among the most common in humans. Given their frequency and the morbidity and mortality associated with surgical and chemotherapy, additional nonmorphologic parameters would be quite valuable. Many investigators have found that DNA aneuploidy and increased proliferation fraction are associated with increased recurrence or decreased survival in early-stage transitional cell carcinoma of the bladder (reviewed by Zarbo and Linden[138]). A similar conclusion has been reached with DNA aneuploidy and survival in renal cell carcinomas.

It currently is unclear whether DNA ploidy is independently predictive of survival in prostate carcinoma. However, increased proliferative fraction and DNA aneuploidy are predictive of decreased survival with metastatic testicular neoplasia and ovarian carcinoma, respectively.[138] DNA aneuploidy appears also to be predictive of increased recurrence and decreased survival with uterine adenocarcinoma. However, a clear consensus of methodology and definitions of DNA aneuploidy are necessary to validate these observations fully and allow them to be used optimally to direct clinical treatment.

Breast carcinoma

Breast carcinoma is a particularly difficult neoplasm to treat optimally, given its propensity for early occult metastasis, which may not become clinically evident for several years to decades. Besides morphologic grade, other markers have been sought to define the risk for such metastases (such as estrogen and progesterone receptors). Multiple studies have now shown that the proliferation fraction in stage I and II breast carcinomas is inversely associated with recurrence of disease (reviewed by Furlong[139]). A similar trend is seen with DNA aneuploidy, though this may partially reflect its association with higher grades, which usually have larger proliferation fractions.

Cytogenetics and other molecular techniques

The membrane antigens, changes in proliferation status, and presence of gross DNA lesions (DNA aneuploidy) are external manifestations of multiple lesions at the level of the genome. As such, standard flow cytometric analysis is somewhat limited in its ability to define the fundamental pathologic changes leading to neoplasia and to allow prediction of its biologic aggressiveness.

Standard manual molecular techniques, such as polymerase chain reaction and molecular blotting, provide for more sensitive assessment of genetic abnormalities. These are rather expensive and, with few exceptions, very time consuming. However, as pointed out by McCoy,[140] the combination of flow cytometry and molecular assays can give rise to sensitive, semiautomated methods for the detection of such genetic lesions in thousands of cells.

Approaches include nucleic acid probes for particular chromosomes or genes. These may use the neoplastic cells for targets (fluorescence in situ hybridization, FISH). A novel variant is to bind biotinylated DNA of known sequences to avidin-labeled beads and then measure for the binding or presence of fluorescence-labeled PCR products from neoplastic cells.[141] Like many cutting-edge tests, the major problem remains with defining clinically relevant applications within the overall framework of diagnostic medicine.

Functional assays

Oxidative burst

Neutrophils kill phagocytosed cells by a complex method called the *oxidative burst*. This generates oxidizing products, such as free radicals and hydrogen peroxide. If any of this complex mechanism is defective, the individual's neutrophils may be unable to destroy ingested organisms. A classic example of such is chronic granulomatous disease.[64] The ability of a given individual's neutrophils to generate an oxidative burst can be measured by the oxidation of dichlorofluorescein diacetate (DCFH-DA) to dichlorofluorescein (DCF).[2] The DCFH-DA is a nonfluorescent molecule and is taken up into the cell membrane. Here, the acetate is cleaved off, resulting in DCFH. The latter is oxidized by H_2O_2 into DCF, which is fluorescent. The degree of fluorescence, compared to a normal control, can be used in the diagnostic evaluation for chronic granulomatous disease.[64]

Phagocytosis

Rare congenital immune deficiencies are attributable to defects in neutrophil and monocyte phagocytosis.[64] In addition, acquired phagocytic defects may be seen. Such disorders can be estimated by ingestion of FITC-labeled bacteria as measured by flow cytometry.[2] By comparing these results to normal controls, one can gauge the degree of enhancement or impairment of a patient's neutrophil and monocyte phagocytic functions.

Tumor drug resistance

Similar to bacteria, tumors often develop resistance to various anticytotoxic agents during the course of therapeutic induction (reviewed by Furlong[139] and by McCoy and Carey[142]). These may be attributable to mutations in metabolic proteins, rendering these proteins less likely to be bound antimetabolites. Others, like the p170 multiple drug resistance protein, act like pumps to allow the cells to excrete a broad variety of cytotoxic drugs. Flow cytometric assays, by immunoassay or fluorescent metabolites, can measure the presence of such proteins, retention of cytotoxin-related molecules, or their catabolism. Although such assays are fascinating, convincing demonstration of true clinical relevance is still lacking.

PRINCIPLES AND TECHNIQUES OF IMAGE ANALYSIS

Instrumentation

The central technique in computerized image analysis is the conversion of continuous (analog) image information to discontinuous (digital) information, a form of data that can be stored and manipulated by digital computers.[143,144] Basically, most image analysis systems consist of the following components (Fig. 13-5): (1) a video camera, mounted on a light microscope, that sends out a continuous (analog) video signal; (2) an image capture board, which converts the analog video signal to discrete digital values and stores these values in specific memory locations in a frame buffer; (3) a computer, which houses the image capture board, provides an interface for the user, and performs a variety of mathematical operations on the stored image data; (4) a video monitor, which displays the live or captured video image; (5) storage media (magnetic disc, optical disc); (6) user-interface devices (keyboard, mouse, pad, light pen, and so forth), and (7) system software.[145] Each of these components is briefly discussed.

Most applications for image analysis make use of video cameras mounted on standard light microscopes, though fluorescence images or scanning electron microscopic images may be used as well.[146-148] The video cameras are usually solid-state devices in which the light from the image is focused on an array of light sensors that convert light intensity at all points of the image to proportional voltage signals. Monochrome cameras contain a single sensor chip to record light intensity, whereas some color cameras employ three chips to record separately the red, green, and blue components of the image (RGB color). The output from the camera consists of an analog video signal, which usually conforms to a set of standards developed for the video industry (NTSC or RS170 in the United States). This video signal, through voltage variation, represents the light intensity along each scan line of a television image, with approximately 500 such lines representing a full frame of the video image. The illusion of a continuous image is produced by displaying two interlaced fields (composed of every other scan line) each 1/60 second, to produce a full frame of video each 1/30 second.

This video signal can be directly displayed on a video monitor, as is done for live video display for group viewing. For image analysis, the video signal is sent to the *image capture board* containing an analog-to-digital (A/D) converter, which rapidly samples the continuous-voltage signal and assigns a numerical value to the voltage at discrete points along each video line (Fig. 13-6). Commonly, such A/D converters sample 512 points along each line and assign values from 0 (pure black) to 255 (highest intensity) to the light levels. These light values are referred to as *gray levels*. For RGB (color) cameras, the light intensity for each primary color is similarly converted to digital form. More frequent image sampling or greater numbers of gray levels can be obtained, depending on the image system hardware and the requirements for analysis. The numerical gray scale values for each point of the image are stored in specific memory locations (that is, frame buffer) in the image capture board, which can be accessed by the host computer. Each picture element, or "pixel," comprises a square fragment of the image and is represented as a discrete digital value representing the light intensity at that point (Fig. 13-6). A "captured" image represented by 512 horizontal and vertical samples, for example, would contain 262,144 pixels. These digital values form the substrate for all subsequent computer evaluations and manipulations of the image.

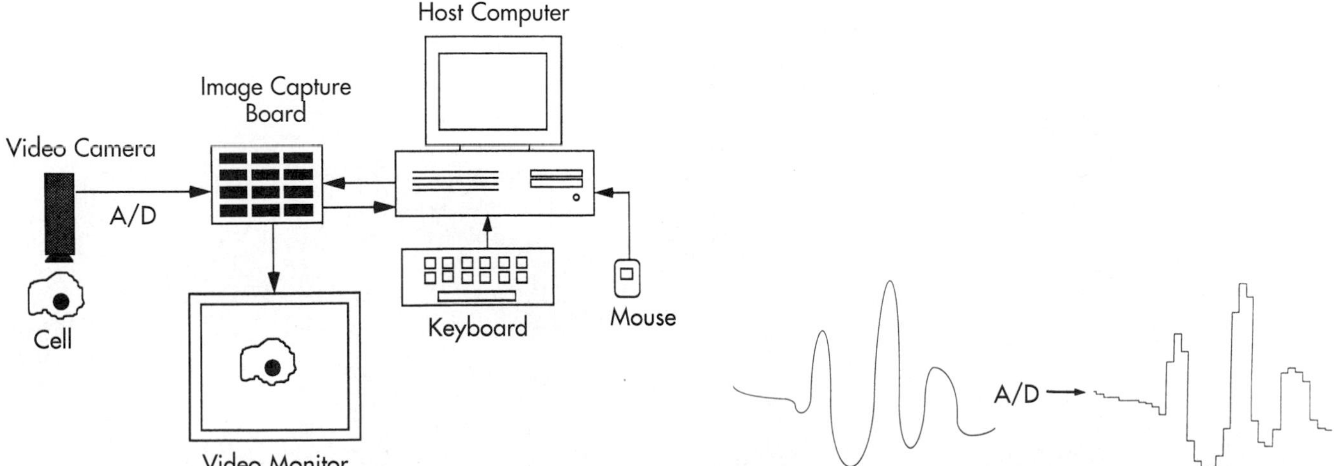

Fig. 13-5 *Left,* Components and configuration of a typical image analysis system. For analysis of cells and tissues, the video camera is coupled to a microscope (not shown). (Redrawn from Bauer KD, Duque RE, Shankey TV: *Clinical flow cytometry: principles and application,* Baltimore, 1993, Williams & Wilkins.). *Right,* Digitized analog video signal. The continuous voltage signal from a single scan line of a standard video output, which varies according to light intensity, is sampled at discrete intervals, with the voltage at each point assigned a numerical value (gray level).

The pixel values can be altered by the host computer either before or after they are stored in the frame buffer. One of the most useful such manipulations for image quantitation is the conversion of light-intensity values to optical density (OD), based on previous instrument calibration.[149] The imaging system can then be used as a microspectrophotometer to measure the concentrations of dyes staining cells or tissues because concentration is directly proportional to OD, according to the Beer-Lambert law. This method is used to measure nuclear DNA content, as will be discussed. Also, the pixel values can be altered to affect the video display of the image, for example, by assigning different colors to gray-scale values ("pseudocolor"). Because the human eye can discern far greater numbers of colors than gray levels, pseudocolor can be used to reveal subtle variations in light intensity that cannot be otherwise perceived. Information can be derived from the color content of the image either by using selective optical filters in the light pathway or by converting the red, green, and blue signals from a color camera into hue, saturation, and intensity components. Using this method, specific ranges of color within the image can be selected for further analysis.

Image processing and analysis

The captured image, now in digital form, can be subjected to manipulation by the host computer, using software applications designed for this purpose. The stored pixel values may be altered individually ("point processing") or in groups ("neighborhood processing") using computer algorithms in a manner designed to alter the displayed image and to reveal or suppress certain image features.[143] *Image processing* may be used to remove noise or artifacts from the image, subtract uneven background illumination, improve image contrast (by transforming

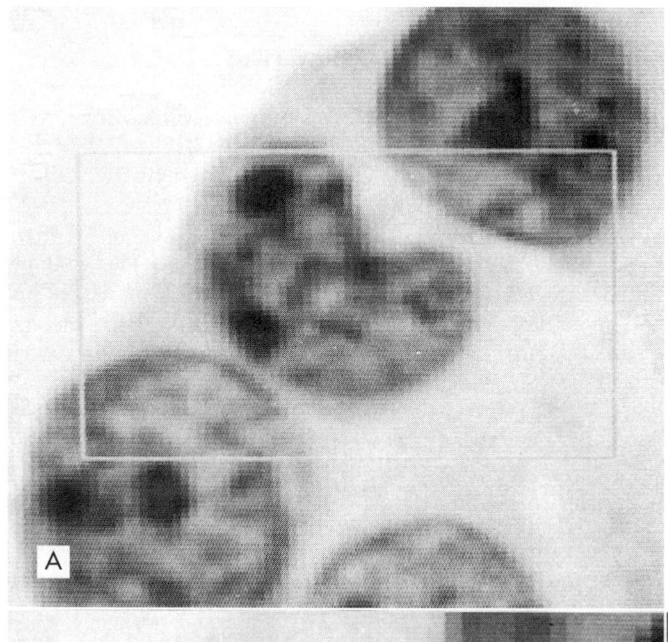

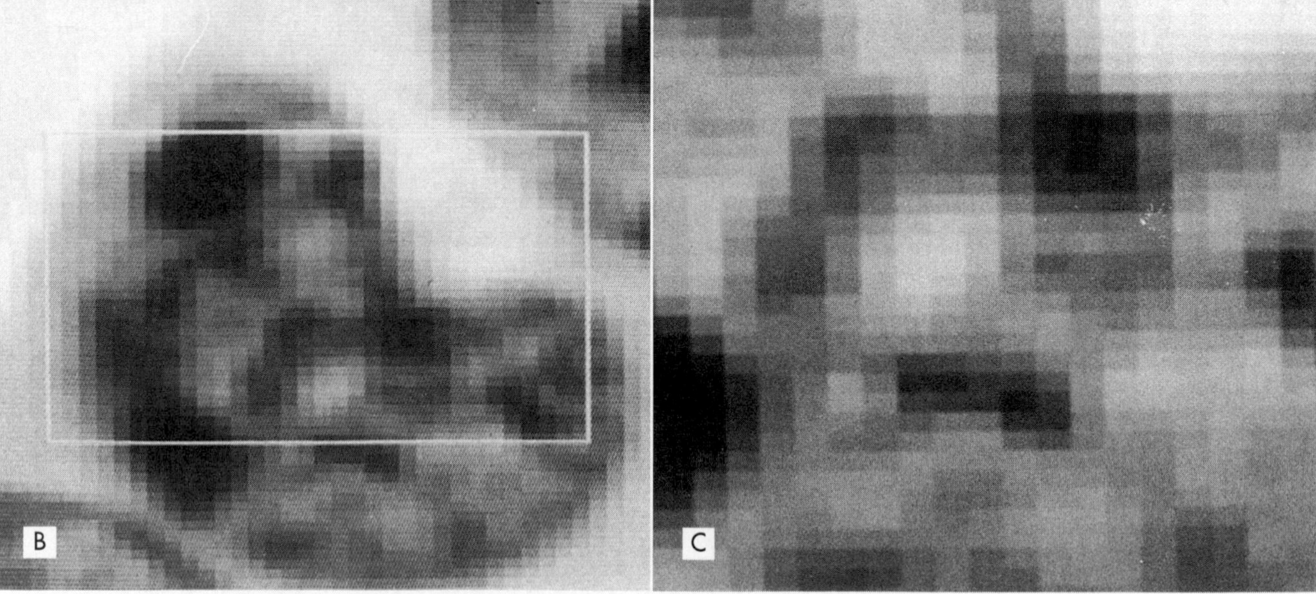

Fig. 13-6 Digitized image of breast cancer cells. Progressive enlargement of the digitized image reveals individual pixels, seen best in **C,** each displaying a single level of light intensity (gray level). The location and digital value of the gray level (typically 0 to 256) for each pixel is stored in computer memory.

gray values to a wider range), or to average ("smooth") regions of the image. Image processing using a variety of computer algorithms is usually required before meaningful measurements can be made because the desired objects (such as tissues, cells, or nuclei) must be distinguished from background, or the edges of the objects must be outlined. It may also be important to separate objects that overlap or touch so that they will be separately evaluated. *Quantitative digital image analysis* is the process of computerized measurement of these digitally captured and processed images. There are a vast number of such measurements that can be experimentally performed on cells and tissues, some of which are direct (such as distance, area) and others of which are mathematically derived (such as ratio of cell area to perimeter).[150] Many of these measurements, such as counting grains in autoradiograms or measuring the depth of invasion of cutaneous melanoma, could be performed by tedious manual methods but are performed more rapidly and reliably by image analysis. Other measurements that required analysis of optical density, such as DNA analysis, cannot be performed by manual methods and require image analysis. Image texture, which results from local variations in pixel values, can also be measured by image analysis and may provide important descriptive information about the nuclear chromatin pattern.[151,152] Immunohistochemical staining reactions may also be quantitated by use of image analysis, as will be described. Some of the more clinically useful parameters that can be measured by image analysis are listed in Table 13-3. Depending on the system software, the measurements of the image features for each object are stored in computer files and can be used for graphic display or statistical analysis. Different classes of objects can be designated by the operator (such as lymphocytes and tumor cells) so that comparisons can be made between different types of cells. Alternatively, the computer may be used to discern different classes of objects based on similarities and differences in image features, as will be discussed later. The measurements typically are performed rapidly on each object within the microscopic field, though the speed of analysis depends greatly on the computer hardware and software configurations.

Table 13-3 Clinically useful cellular parameters measured by image analysis*

Parameter
Morphometry
Nuclear diameter, circumference, area
Cytoplasmic diameter, circumference, area
Nuclear shape (roundness, contour index)
Ratio nucleus to cytoplasm area
Distance (such as thickness, vessel caliber)
Fractal dimension (architectural complexity)
Texture (chromatin)
Percentage positivity (immunohistochemistry)
Counting
Numbers of cells or nuclei
Grains (autoradiography)
Optical density
Sum optical density (for DNA by Feulgen stain)
Average optical density
Standard deviation (texture)

*This list is far from complete. Many additional direct and mathematically derived measurements can be performed, depending on the needs and imagination of the investigator.

Sample preparation for image analysis

A great variety of cell and tissue preparations may be used for image analysis. Cytologic samples suitable for imaging can be obtained from smears, touch preparations, or cytocentrifuge preparations. Nuclei isolated by enzyme digestion of paraffin-embedded tissues ("Hedley preparations") can be evaluated for DNA ploidy in this manner.[153,154] Attempts to minimize cell debris and cellular overlap are important for successful image analysis. Tissue sections may also be employed, though the problems of cell overlap and artifacts induced by tissue sectioning present greater analytic difficulties. However, viewing cells in the context of the tissue architecture can provide important information and can help to distinguish more easily benign from malignant tissue components, for example. Also, measurement of architectural features on tissue sections may provide important diagnostic information.[155] The quality and uniformity of the staining reactions used to reveal the cell or tissue features of interest are important, and adequate controls and standards are required for accurate clinical measurements.

Technical comparison of flow cytometry and image analysis

In some regards, image analysis and flow cytometry represent complementary technologies for measuring cellular features, though certain relative advantages and disadvantages are inherent in each method.[156,157] A comparison of the technical features of image analysis and flow cytometry is shown in Table 13-4.

One of the principle limitations in flow cytometry is the requirement for single cell or nuclear suspensions, which can be difficult to achieve for solid tissues.[158] In this regard, although blood and body fluids may provide ideal preparations for flow cytometry, such as those for lymphocyte phenotyping, solid tumors and tissue may prove more problematic. In addition to the technical problems of making single cell suspensions from tissues, the final suspension may not be representative of the tissue, and intact tumor cells may be few in number or difficult to distinguish from benign tissue components. Also, some specimens may be too small to provide adequate cells for flow cytometry. Image analysis can circumvent these problems because several options that require minimal sacrifice of diagnostic tissue are available for specimen preparation. The morphologic features of cells or tissue architecture can be directly observed by use of image analysis and can be used selectively to analyze cells or foci of interest; flow cytometry provides minimal morphologic information, limited mainly to light-scatter signals. Also, compared to flow cytometry, far greater numbers of cellular features can be measured by image analysis, providing powerful tools for multiparameter classification of cells. Therefore, image analysis may have distinct advantages over flow cytometry for the analysis of solid tumors, sparse or small specimens, or in situations where preservation of tissue architecture is essential. In addition, although studies on archival tissues by flow cytometry are mostly limited to quantitative DNA analysis, paraffin blocks may be used for many types of retrospective studies using image analysis.

One of the principle advantages of flow cytometry is the rapid rate of analysis, typically 300 to 1000 cells per second. This speed allows the rapid accumulation of information on large numbers of cells, typically 10,000 or more, which

Table 13-4 Comparison of technical features of flow cytometry and image analysis

Feature	Flow cytometry	Image analysis
Speed	Rapid, large numbers of cells (10,000 to 20,000)	Relatively slow, fewer cells (100 to 200)
Measurements	Fluorescence, light scatter	Fluorescence, visible light
Specimens	Single cell suspensions	Cytospins, cytology, touch imprints, tissue sections
Morphometry	Light scatter	Large numbers of measurements
Gating	Based on light scatter, fluorescence	Direct morphologic identification
Morphologic correlations	None	Direct correlation with cell morphology and tissue histology
Archival studies	Limited to DNA for paraffin, or cryo-preserved cells	Paraffin blocks, frozen tissue or cells, glass slide material
Subset analysis	Based on cell markers or light scatter, or both types	Based on morphology or cell markers
Rare events	Difficult to detect	May select for rare events

Modified from Bauer KD, Duque RE, Shankey TV: *Clinical flow cytometry,* Baltimore, 1993, Williams & Wilkins.

greatly adds to the precision and statistical significance of the measurements. In contrast, image analysis is relatively slow, and far fewer events are recorded (100 to 200 individual cells). However, some types of image measurements may be performed on microscopic fields containing hundreds of cells, and so the sample size in some applications may include thousands of cells. Further advances in the speed and automation of image analysis may help to overcome these limitations.[159] It is clear, though, that flow cytometry is better suited for such clinical applications as phenotyping of peripheral blood and bone marrow cells, reticulocyte counting, and evaluation of platelets. Also, controls and standards for clinical measurements are better established for flow cytometry than for image analysis.[155,160]

For laboratories having access to both technologies, the decision to use either flow cytometry or image analysis (or both) will depend greatly on the type and quantity of specimen, the type of measurement desired, and the experience of the laboratory.

Table 13-5 Routine clinical applications of flow cytometry and image analysis

Test*	Flow cytometry	Image analysis
DNA content	+	+
Tumor cell proliferation		
S-phase fraction	+	–
Nuclear antigens	–	+
Phenotyping		
Lymphocyte subsets	+	–
Leukemia	+	–
Lymphoma	+	–
Reticulocyte counts	+	–
Antiplatelet antibodies	+	–
Estrogen/progesterone receptor	–	+
Oncoproteins	–	+
Karyotyping	–	+
Cell classification	–	+

Modified from Bauer KD, Duque RE, Shankey TV: *Clinical flow cytometry,* Baltimore, 1993, Williams & Wilkins.

*For every example listed, methods for both flow cytometry and image analysis have been demonstrated. However, the list is intended to reflect the most commonly used technology.

CLINICAL APPLICATIONS OF IMAGE ANALYSIS

Some of the more common clinical applications for both flow cytometry and image analysis are listed in Table 13-5. It is clear that although either technology can be used for some applications some assays are uniquely suited for image analysis. Some of these applications are described below.

Morphometry

Morphometry is the process of measuring cellular and tissue architectural features with regard to size (area, volume), shape, numbers of objects, and distances. Although there is great interest in using morphometry as an aid to diagnosis in surgical pathology,[161] there are surprisingly few current applications in routine practice.[145] Mitotic count is used to distinguish benign from malignant soft-tissue tumors and as a component of some grading systems for breast cancer.[162 164] The measured depth of invasion in malignant melanoma is a well-established prognostic factor. In neuropathology, measurement of axonal and myelin cross-sectional areas and distribution of muscle-fiber diameter are useful in the diagnosis of neuromuscular disease[165,166] (Fig. 13-7). The nuclear contour index, used to measure the complexity of nuclear infolding, helps to confirm the extreme "cerebriform" appearance of lymphocytes in mycosis fungoides with the Sézary syndrome.[167,168] For many of these applications, digital image analysis can replace tedious manual methods.

A large number of morphologic parameters can be measured directly, including cell or nuclear diameter, circumference, area, and texture. To these obvious features can be added a great number of mathematically derived features, most of which cannot be readily discerned by eye.[155] Many investigations have been performed to discover the combinations of features that can be used to distinguish normal and abnormal cells in various organs, with the ultimate hope of using these objective measurements as diagnostic aids.[155,169] This

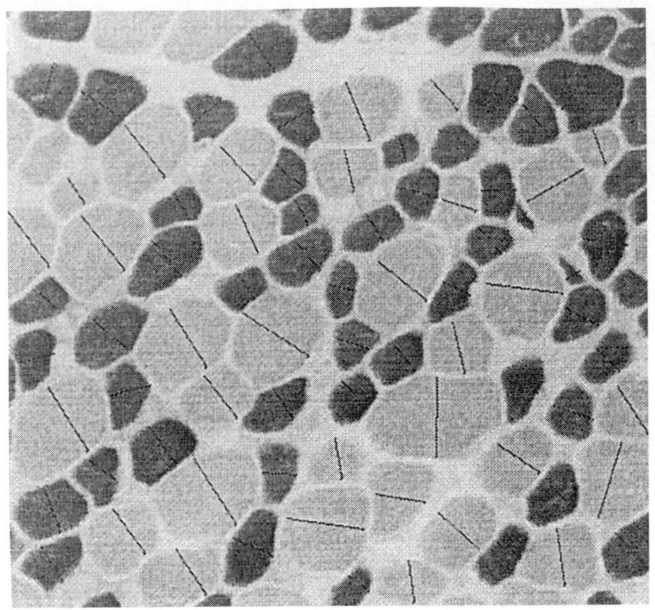

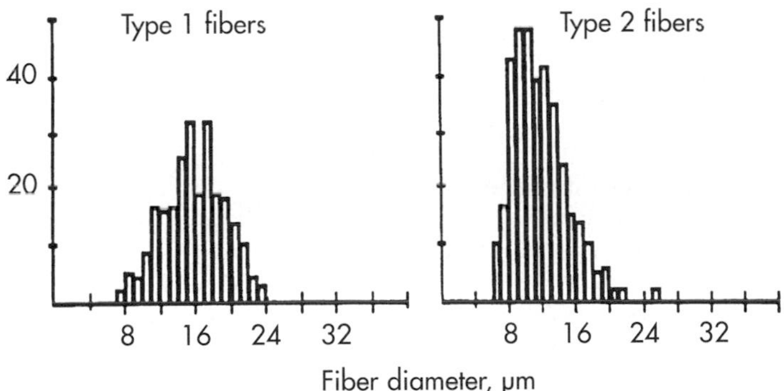

Fig. 13-7 *Top,* Digitized image of a muscle biopsy specimen from a 2-year-old male with encephalopathy and muscle atrophy, stained histochemically for ATPase activity (pH 9.4). The type 2 fibers (darkly stained) appear smaller than type I fibers, though some of the type I fibers also appear atrophic. *Bottom,* Histogram showing the fiber-size distribution for both fiber types. Since the normal fiber diameter distribution expected at 2 years of age is a bell-shaped curve with average diameter 18 μm, this histogram shows that type I fibers are mildly atrophic and are variable in size, with some being as small as 8 μm. By comparison, the type 2 fibers are atrophic with a more uniform distribution, the majority being 8 to 12 μm in diameter. Atrophy of type 2 fibers is attributable to cerebral dysfunction in this case but may also be seen in steroid myopathy and with disuse (Courtesy Douglas C. Anthony, M.D., Ph.D., Brigham and Women's Hospital, Boston).

approach relies heavily on statistical evaluation of multiparameter data.[155,166] Advances in this area have been slowed by several problems: (1) the lack of standardization and availability of the necessary computer hardware and software, (2) the time-consuming aspect of interactive image analysis, and (3) the significant overlap that is commonly observed among feature measurements, making definite classification uncertain in too many cases.[145] However, technologic advances will overcome many of these obstacles, as has been demonstrated in the area of automated cervical cytology.

DNA ploidy analysis

Quantitative nuclear DNA measurement is the most frequent clinical application of image analysis. The Feulgen stain, which binds to DNA in a stoichiometric fashion by a Schiff base reaction, is most often used for DNA measurement.[170,171] The optical density of the stained nucleus at the appropriate wavelength of light is directly proportional to DNA content.[149] As mentioned in the technical section, it is possible to use image analysis to measure optical density, and the sum of the optical densities of all the pixels composing the image of the cell nucleus is used to calculate the DNA content, based on prior instrument calibration.[172] An external standard, such as a tumor cell line or normal human cells with known DNA content, are used as controls for staining, and nonmalignant cells within the specimen can be used as internal diploid controls. DNA measurement is best performed on cytologic specimens or nuclear preparations from fresh or paraffin-embedded tissues, but even tissue sections may be studied for DNA ploidy in this manner. As for flow cytometry, accurate DNA measurements required great attention to technical details, including specimen preparation, staining, instrumentation, and the proper use of controls and standards.

Even though far fewer nuclei are measured by use of image analysis than by flow cytometry, the DNA histograms obtained by both methods on individual specimens are usually very similar (Fig. 13-8). Most studies have shown approximately a 90% concordance between DNA ploidy obtained by flow cytometry and image analysis.[156,173-175] Differences in DNA ploidy detected by flow cytometry and image analysis are probably attributable to one or more technical factors. The histograms obtained by flow cytometry usually exhibit somewhat better peak resolution, and near-diploid aneuploid peaks observed by flow cytometry may be difficult to detect by image analysis.[176,177] On the other hand, rare aneuploid cells may be more readily detected by image analysis because of the advantage of visual identification of atypical cells in cytologic preparations.[178] Again, limitations of sample size, such as sparsely cellular body fluids, may dictate that image analysis, which requires fewer cells, be used to measure DNA ploidy in some cases.

The DNA histogram obtained by image analysis usually contains too few events in the S-phase region to provide a reliable measure of cell proliferation. Instead, immunocytochemical stains for proliferation-associated nuclear antigens may be used for this purpose.

Quantitative immunohistochemistry: general principles

Although immunohistochemical stains are usually evaluated qualitatively (and subjectively), there are occasions in which the measurement of staining might prove useful. This is especially true for tumor markers, which have prognostic or therapeutic importance, because precise levels of staining or the proportion of positive tumor cells may be useful for stratifying patients. Although staining can be measured using tedious manual counting or semiquantitative methods, image analysis affords a rapid and objective means of accomplishing this task. For solid tumors, image analysis of tissue sections provides a means for distinguishing benign and malignant tissue components, ensuring that the measurements are tumor specific. Optical density measurements may be used in an attempt to

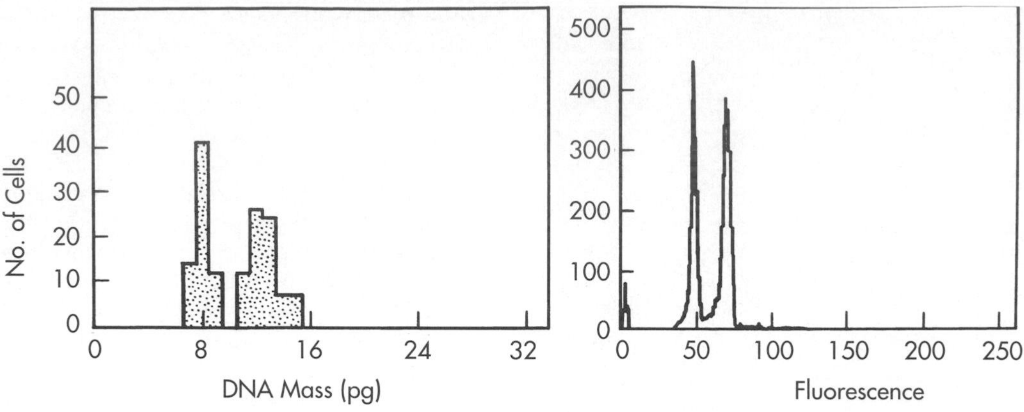

Fig. 13-8 DNA histograms obtained in a case of breast cancer from image analysis of Feulgen-stained cells, *left*, and flow cytometry, *right*. Both histograms reveal the presence of a hyperdiploid population of DNA aneuploid cells *(arrow)* in addition to diploid cells, with similar DNA index (*A* = 1.45, *B* = 1.55) (From Dawson AE, Norton JA, Weinberg DS: *Am J Pathol* 136:1115, 1990).

measure the concentration of antigen, but the variability and nonlinearity of the enzymatic reactions used in the stain-detection systems can prove difficult to overcome. Measurements of percentage positivity of cells, nuclei, or area are more commonly used, because staining above a defined threshold can be established using appropriate control antibodies. Standards regarding methods of staining and measurement have not yet been developed for clinical practice. However, several clinical applications for quantitative immunocytochemistry have emerged and are briefly discussed.

Cell proliferation

The fraction of tumor cells synthesizing DNA, or proliferative fraction, has prognostic significance for many common malignancies, including lymphoma and breast cancer.[179-183] Although a variety of methods may be used to measure tumor cell proliferation, the measurement of the S-phase fraction of the flow cytometric DNA histogram is most common. However, there are some technical problems associated with this method that can limit its accuracy. The problems of obtaining a representative cell sample in suspension has already been discussed. In addition, the tumor cells can be variably diluted by normal stromal and inflammatory cells, which can greatly influence the result, especially for diploid tumors.[184] The presence of cell debris and multiple populations of cells having overlapping DNA histograms can greatly complicate the computer measurement of the S-phase portion of the histogram.[154] For these reasons, it may be an advantage to observe tumor cell proliferation in tissue sections. Mitosis counting has found some limited applications in surgical pathology but is tedious and has poor reproducibility.[162,163] The use of previously discussed proliferation-associated nuclear markers, measured by image analysis, may circumvent some of these problems.[185]

The antibody Ki-67 stains a nuclear antigen that is absent in resting (G_0 phase) cells. It appears during mid- to late G_1 phase, and is expressed throughout the cell cycle[186,187] Another marker commonly used is PCNA (proliferating cell nuclear antigen), a 36 kD protein present in the nuclei of proliferating cells, and one that is an accessory protein to DNA polymerase-delta.[188-191] Other studies have used antibodies to DNA polymerase-alpha.[192] Staining using antibodies to these markers can be used to detect the proliferating cell fraction of malignant tumors in tissue sections so that morphologic correlations can be made. Image analysis can then be used to make tumor-specific measurements of proliferation either by counting the percentage of positive nuclei or by the more rapid method of calculating the percentage of staining of the total tumor nuclear area. One performs this latter method by analyzing the image first at one wavelength of light, which reveals all cell nuclei (usually stained with methyl green), and then viewing the same scene at another wavelength, which makes visible only the immunostaining reaction product. Superimposed maps of all cell nuclei and positive staining are used to determine the percentage of nuclear area staining positive for the nuclear antigen[193] (Fig. 13-9). In this manner, the tumor can be widely sampled to derive a measurement of the proliferative fraction. The prognostic significance of these proliferation-associated markers has been demonstrated for several tumor types, including breast cancer.[194-198] Image analysis affords a rapid and objective means for providing the necessary quantitation.

Hormone receptor analysis

Antibodies to estrogen and progesterone receptor may be used to detect hormone receptors in breast cancer and to provide an alternative to standard biochemical methods.[199] Immunohistochemical staining requires far less tissue and allows histologic correlation, which are important considerations in the evaluation of breast cancer, as discussed in detail in Chapter 70. These receptors are expressed in the nuclei of tumor cells, and quantitation may be performed using image analysis in a manner similar to that described for other nuclear antigens previously.[200,201] Good correlation with the biochemical method has been demonstrated,[202,203] and quantitation by image analysis can provide objective measurements, especially in tumors showing borderline levels of staining.

Other tumor markers

The overexpression of oncogenes can be detected by immunohistochemical staining for oncoproteins, such as Her-2/*neu* and p53, and image analysis has been used to quantitate this staining.[204-206] The intensity of the staining reaction is relevant to this application, and attempts have been made to calibrate the staining using cell lines having known levels of oncoprotein

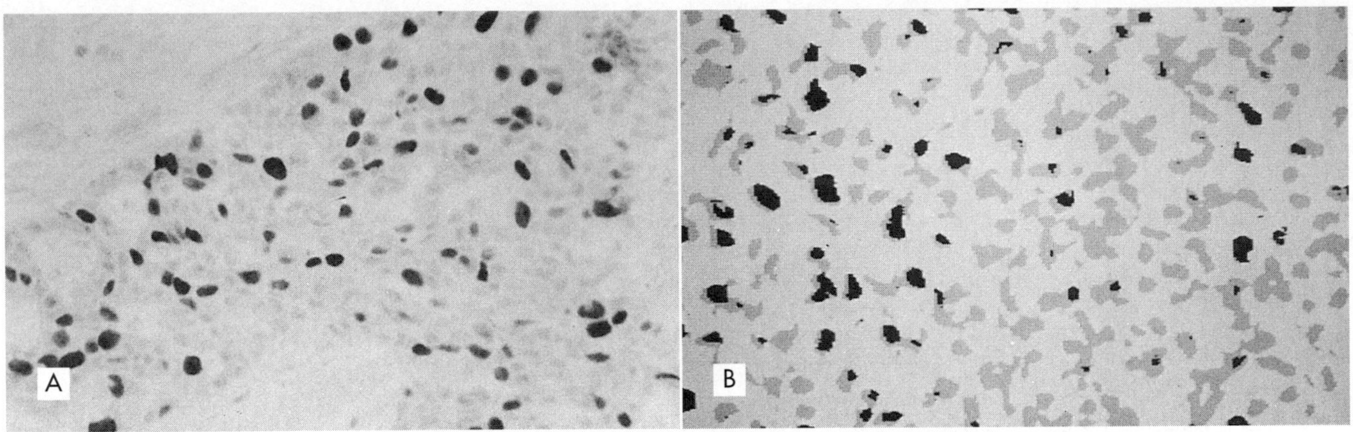

Fig. 13-9 **A,** Tissue section from a case of breast cancer stained with Ki-67 antibody to detect proliferating (cycling) cells. Darker appearing nuclei are stained positive. **B,** "Nuclear map" method for measuring nuclear Ki-67 staining. The image shows the field from a case of non-Hodgkin's lymphoma, with the location of all nuclei (counter-stained with methyl green) mapped from an image captured using a 650 nm filter (pale areas) and the location of sites of Ki-67 staining (immunoperoxidase reaction, brown) detected using a 500 nm filter (dark areas). The percentage of nuclear area occupied by the staining reaction is calculated. A similar approach can be used to measure any nuclear antigen, such as estrogen receptor.

expression. A similar approach has been used to measure the expression of multiple drug resistance, using antibodies to p-glycoprotein.[207] The level of expression of these tumor markers has prognostic and therapeutic significance, and image analysis can provide the necessary objective means of measurement.

AUTOMATED CYTOLOGY

Automation of cervical cytology has long been one of the major goals of microscopic image analysis, and attempts to develop a commercial instrument for this purpose have been under development since the 1950s.[208] More recently, the need for increased quality control in cytology as well as the problem of decreasing numbers of cytology technologists have made the need for some automation in cytology even more apparent. The technology of image analysis has progressed very rapidly in recent years, and advances in computer technologies and artificial intelligence software have helped to speed developments in this area. The decrease in size and cost of the necessary computer systems have made this field commercially viable, and several companies at the time of this writing are pursuing approval by the Food and Drug Administration (FDA) to market such instruments. The main goal of most systems is to provide automated prescreening, with final diagnosis of nonnormal slides still to be based on human observation.

The systems currently under development rely either on the conventional cervical Pap smear[209] or on new sample preparation methods that create a uniformly distributed monolayer of cells within a defined area on a glass slide.[210] This improved method of sample preparation helps to avoid cell overlap and clumps and makes the task of image analysis easier. The image analyzer scans the slide (unaided) and measures several cytologic features, such as the ratio of the nuclear and cytoplasmic areas, nuclear size and shape, and chromatin texture. These multiple cell parameters are then analyzed by the computer to classify each cell as either normal or abnormal, based on limits established for cervical epithelial cells. The cell-classification schemes are based either on statistical analysis of the multiparameter data,[149,155] or on artificial intelligence programs referred to as "neural networks."[211-214] Neural networks represent a nonalgorithmic form of computer analysis in which individual image features are entered into a multilayered networks of data processors ("nodes," or "neurons") that are highly interconnected (Fig. 13-10), with an "output" resulting from the interaction of inputs and outputs among the preceding layers of neurons. There are many possible architectures for neural networks, which are generally designed to excel at pattern-recognition tasks. These systems learn to produce correct outputs based on learning from a teaching set of examples and are then capable of accurately classifying new objects. Neural network systems have already found many important applications, such as automated speech recognition and automated inspection, and will undoubtedly find important medical applications.

The specific designs of automated cytology systems will differ with regard to the sample preparation method, types of image feature measurements, and computer methods for image classification. However, preliminary data indicate that any of several approaches to cytology automation may perform satisfactorily.

IMAGES AS INFORMATION: TELEPATHOLOGY

Images and descriptions of images are the raw data from which surgical pathologists and cytologists make their diagnoses. Documenting and sharing these images for the purposes of teaching and consultation with clinical colleagues are also important functions in the practice of pathology. Most of these images for documentation and teaching are obtained by standard photography of gross and microscopic findings. However, many technologies are converging in the area of telecommunications, and they can vastly expand the ways in which pathologists use and share images.

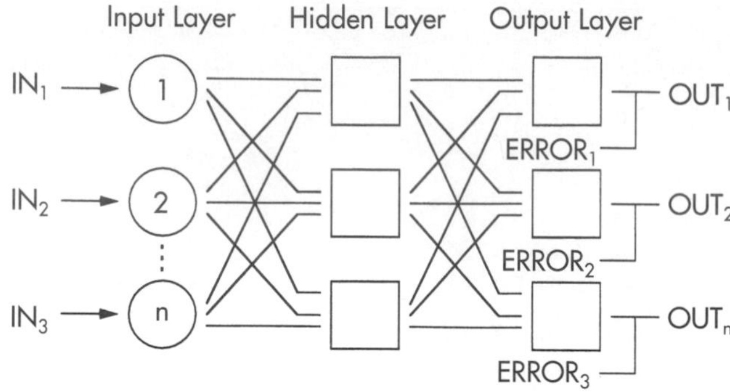

Fig. 13-10 Neural network architecture. The various computational elements of the network ("neurons") are arranged in multiple layers, with each neuron connected to all others in subsequent layers (feedforward network). The inputs to each neuron are additive and can be altered by assignation of a weight to each signal. The output of each neuron is determined by a nonlinear transfer function applied to the final input value. The input layer receives data elements, such as cell measurement parameters, and the output layer provides an answer, such as membership in a particular cell class. Training of the network takes place by use of known examples, with the output corrected by altering the weights to each neuron based on the magnitude of the incorrect response (backpropagation method). Training proceeds until the strengths of the interconnections are optimized to provide correct answers. Subsequent unknown inputs are then classified based on the output of the network. Many different types of neural network architectures have been developed for specific types of classification and analysis problems.

In the most simple application, the analog output from a video camera can be used to share "live" microscopic images for teaching conferences or for transmitting diagnostic findings to clinicians, such as those from the frozen section room to the surgical suite. However, computer digitization of images allows for many additional functions. Archives of digitized images can be saved in a variety of computer memory storage devices (magnetic or optical) and retrieved for use at a later time. Such digitized images, combined with appropriate computer software, can form the basis of computer educational programs and may prove useful for teaching pathology in a more efficient and effective manner, and such programs are already available using images stored in analog form on laser discs.[215,216] Digital imaging can greatly expedite the process of karyotyping, since digital cutting and pasting can replace the tedious task of manual cutting and arranging of photographic images of chromosomes (as discussed in chapter 12) and, in some instances, perform automated classification.[217] Digitized images of serial sections of tissue can be used to perform three-dimensional reconstructions of pathologic processes,[166] and images from confocal microscopy can similarly be manipulated to visualize tissue and cellular morphology in three dimensions.[218]

Importantly, digitized images of gross and microscopic pathology can be sent over telecommunications networks to workstations at distant sites, vastly expanding the communication and consultation capability of pathologists.[219,220] Such "telepathology" systems will speed the transmission of diagnostic information and will greatly decrease our dependence on transporting fragile glass slides. The chief barriers to the routine use of digitized images in pathology are related to the immense amounts of data in full-color high-resolution images, which affect computer data storage capacity and speed of transmission. However, rapid advances in data compression and high-speed telecommunications should make it possible in the near future for most centers to send and receive stored or live images of quality sufficient for diagnosis. Many telepathology systems in the United States and other countries are being developed,[221] and it is expected that this technology will become widely available in the near future.

REFERENCES

1. Keren DF, Hanson CA, Hurtubise PE, editors: *Flow cytometry and clinical diagnosis,* ed 2, Chicago, 1994, ASCP Press.
2. Robinson JP, editor: *Handbook of flow cytometry methods,* ed 2, New York, 1993, Wiley-Liss.
3. Melamed MR, Lindmo T, Mendelsohn ML, editors: *Flow cytometry and sorting,* ed 2, New York, 1990, Wiley.
4. Darzynkiewicz Z, Crissman H, editors: *Flow cytometry,* San Diego, 1990, Academic Press (Wilson L, ed, *Methods in Cell Biology,* vol 33).
5. *Fluorescent microbead standards,* Research Triangle Park, NC, 1988, Flow Cytometry Standards Corp.
6. McCoy JP Jr: Basic principles in clinical flow cytometry. In Keren DF, Hanson CA, Hurtubise PE, editors: *Flow cytometry and clinical diagnosis,* ed 2, Chicago, 1994, ASCP Press.
7. *Fluorescent microbead standards,* Research Triangle Park, NC, 1988, Flow Cytometry Standards Corp.
8. Zarbo RJ: Quality control issues and technical considerations in flow cytometric DNA and cell cycle analysis of solid tumors. In Keren DF, Hanson CA, Hurtubise PE, editor: *Flow cytometry and clinical diagnosis,* ed 2, Chicago, 1994, ASCP Press.
9. Hansen W, Hoffman R, Healey K: Light scatter as an adjunct to cellular immunofluorescence in flow cytometric systems, *J Clin Immunol* 2:32S, 1982.
10. Salzman G, Crowell J, Martin J et al: Cell classification by laser light scattering: identification and separation of unstained leukocytes, *Acta Cytol* 19:374, 1973.
11. Borowitz MJ, Guenther KL, Shults KE, Stelzer GT: Immunophenotyping of acute leukemia by flow cytometric analysis: use of CD45 and right-angle light scatter to gate on leukemic blasts in three-color analysis, *Am J Clin Pathol* 100:534, 1993.
12. Nicholson JKA, Jones BM, Hubbard M: CD4 T-lymphocyte determinations on whole blood specimens using a single-tube three color assay, *Cytometry* 14:685, 1993.
13. McCoy JP Jr, Carey JL, Krause JR: Quality control in flow cytometry for diagnostic pathology: I. Cell surface phenotyping and general laboratory procedures, *Pathol Patterns* 93(suppl. 1):S27, 1990.
14. Carey JL, Linden MD, Maeda K, Hawley R: Evaluation and reproducibility of criteria for leukemia and lymphoma immunophenotyping triage and interpretation by a quality assurance program, *Am J Surg Pathol* 100(3):338, 1993.
15. Kamat D, Laszewski M, Kemp J, Goeken J: The diagnostic utility of immunophenotyping and immunogenotyping in the pathologic evaluation of lymphoid proliferations, *Mod Pathol* 3(2):105, 1990.
16. Carey JL, Hanson CA: Flow cytometric analysis of leukemia and lymphoma. In Keren DF, Hanson CA, Hurtubise PE, editor: *Flow cytometry and clinical diagnosis,* ed 2, Chicago, 1994, ASCP Press.
17. Bennett J, Catovsky D, Danial M-T et al: Proposals for the classification of chronic (mature) B and T lymphoid leukemias, *J Clin Pathol* 42:567, 1989.
18. Picker L et al: Immunophenotypic criteria for the diagnosis of non-Hodgkin's lymphoma, *Am J Pathol* 128:181, 1987.
19. Anderson K et al: Expression of human B cell–associated antigens on leukemias and lymphomas: a model of human B cell differentiation, *Blood* 63:1424, 1984.
20. Tefferi A, Li C-Y, Phyliky R: Immunotyping in chronic lymphocytosis: review of the natural history of the condition in 145 adult patients, *Mayo Clin Proc* 63:801, 1988.
21. Batata A, Shen B: Immunophenotyping of subtypes of B-chronic (mature) lymphoid leukemia: a study of 242 cases, *Cancer* 70(10):2436, 1992.

22. Sobol R et al: Adult acute lymphoblastic leukemia phenotypes defined by monoclonal antibodies, *Blood* 65:730, 1985.
23. Lee E, Pollak A, Leavitt R et al: Minimally differentiated acute nonlymphocytic leukemia: a distinct entity, *Blood* 70(5):1400, 1987.
24. Miro J, Zipf T, Pui C-H et al: Acute mixed lineage leukemia: clinicopathologic correlations and prognostic significance, *Blood* 66(5):1115, 1985.
25. Cheson B, Cassileth P, Head D et al: Report of the National Cancer Institute–sponsored workshop on definitions of diagnosis and response in acute myeloid leukemia, *J Clin Oncol* 8(5):813, 1990.
26. Bennett J et al: Proposed revised criteria for the classification of acute myeloid leukemia, *Ann Intern Med* 103:626, 1985.
27. Borowitz MJ, Gockerman JP, Moore JO et al: Clinicopathologic and cytogenic features of CD34 (My 10)-positive acute nonlymphocytic leukemia, *Am J Clin Pathol* 91:265, 1989.
28. Cantú-Rajnoldi A, Putti C, Saitta M et al: Co-expression of myeloid antigens in childhood acute lymphoblastic leukaemia: relationship with the stage of differentiation and clinical significance, *Br J Haematol* 79:40, 1991.
29. Urbano-Ispizua A, Matutes E, Villamor N et al: The value of detecting surface and cytoplasmic antigens in acute myeloid leukaemia, *Br J Haematol* 81:178, 1992.
30. Thomas X, Campos L, Archimbaud E et al: Surface marker expression of acute myeloid leukaemia at first relapse, *Br J Haematol* 81:40, 1992.
31. Sobol RE, Mick R, Royston I et al: Clinical importance of myeloid antigen expression in adult acute lymphoblastic leukemia, *N Engl J Med* 316:1111, 1987.
32. Barlogie B, Epstein J, Selvanayagam P, Alexanian R: Plasma cell myeloma—new biological insights and advances in therapy, *Blood* 73(4):865, 1989.
33. Kosmo M, Gale R: Plasma cell leukemia (Review), *Semin Hematol* 24:202, 1987.
34. Dimopoulos MA, Alexanian R: Waldenström's macroglobulinemia, *Blood* 83(6):1452, 1994.
35. Strickler JG, Audeh MW, Copenhaver CM, Warnke RA: Immunophenotypic differences between plasmacytoma/multiple myeloma and immunoblastic lymphoma, *Cancer* 61:1782, 1988.
36. Schwartz B, Pinkus G, Bacus S et al: Cell proliferation in non-Hodgkin's lymphomas: digital image analysis of Ki-67 antibody staining, *Am J Pathol* 134(2):327, 1989.
37. Schwartz B, Weinberg D, Pinkus G: Image analysis quantitation of proliferation in non-Hodgkin's lymphomas, *Mod Pathol* 1:82A, 1988.
38. Hall P et al: The prognostic value of Ki67 immunostaining in non-Hodgkin's lymphoma, *J Pathol* 154:223, 1988.
39. Slymen D, Miller T, Lippman S et al: Immunobiologic factors predictive of clinical outcome in diffuse large-cell lymphoma, *J Clin Oncol* 8(6):986, 1990.
40. Chott A, Augustin I, Wrba F et al: Peripheral T-cell lymphomas: a clinicopathologic study of 75 cases, *Hum Pathol* 21:1117, 1990.
41. Brooks DJ, Garewal HS: Measures of tumor proliferative activity, *Int J Clin Lab Res* 22:196, 1992.
42. Kurki P, Ogata K, Tan E: Monoclonal antibodies to proliferating cell nuclear antigen (PCNA) / cyclin as probes for proliferating cells by immunofluorescence microscopy and flow cytometry, *J Immunol Methods* 109:49, 1988.
43. Kurki P, Lotz M, Ogata K, Tan E: Proliferating cell nuclear antigen (PCNA) / cyclin in activated human T lymphocytes, *J Immunol* 138:4114, 1987.
44. Robbins B, de la Vega D, Ogata K et al: Immunohistochemical detection of proliferating cell nuclear antigen in solid human malignancies, *Arch Pathol Lab Med* 111:841, 1987.
45. Kamel OW, LeBrun DP, Davis RE et al: Growth fraction estimation of malignant lymphomas in formalin-fixed paraffin-embedded tissue using anti-PCNA/cyclin 19A2, *Am J Pathol* 138(6):1471, 1991.
46. Bauer K, Clevenger C, Williams T, Epstein A: Assessment of cell cycle–associated antigen expression using multiparameter flow cytometry and antibody-acridine orange sequential staining, *J Histochem Cytochem* 34:245, 1986.
47. Clevenger C, Epstein A, Bauer K: Modulation of nuclear antigen p105 as a function of cell-cycle progression, *J Cell Physiol* 130:336, 1987.
48. Swanson SA., Brooks JJ: Proliferation markers Ki-67 and p105 in soft-tissue lesions, *Am J Pathol* 137(6):1491, 1990.
49. Cotner Y, Williams J, Christenson L et al: Simultaneous flow cytometric analysis of human T cell activation antigen expression and DNA content, *J Exp Med* 157:461, 1983.
50. Holte H, Davies C, Kvaløy S et al: The activation-associated antigen 4F2 predicts patient survival in low-grade B-cell lymphomas, *Int J Cancer* 3(5):590, 1987.
51. Ho D, Pomerantz R, Kaplan J: Pathogenesis of infection with human immunodeficiency virus, *N Engl J Med* 317:278, 1987.
52. Mock D, Roberts N: Proposed immunopathogenic factors associated with progression from human immunodeficiency virus seropositivity to clinical disease (review), *J Clin Microbiol* 25:1817, 1987.
53. Schnittman S, Greenhouse J, Psallidopoulos M et al: Increasing viral burden in CD4+ T cells from patients with human immunodeficiency virus (HIV) infection reflects rapidly progressive immunosuppression and clinical disease, *Ann Intern Med* 113(6):438, 1990.
54. de Wolf F, Lange J, Houweling J et al: Appearance of predictors of disease progression in relation to the development of AIDS, *AIDS* 3:563, 1989.
55. Nicholson J, Jones B, Echenberg D et al: Phenotypic distribution of T cells of patients who have subsequently developed AIDS, *Clin Immunol Immunopathol* 43:82, 1987.
56. Buckley R, Braffman M, Stern J: Opportunistic infections in the acquired immunodeficiency syndrome, *Semin Oncol* 17:335, 1990.
57. Pluda J, Yarchoan R, Jaffe E et al: Development of non-Hodgkin lymphoma in a cohort of patients with severe human immunodeficiency virus (HIV) infection on long-term antiretroviral therapy, *Ann Intern Med* 113(4):276, 1990.
58. Stein DS, Korvick JA, Vermund S: $CD4^+$ lymphocyte cell enumeration for the prediction of clinical course of human immunodeficiency virus disease: a review, *J Infect Dis* 165:353, 1992.
59. Mitsuyasu R: Clinical variants and staging of Kaposi's sarcoma, *Semin Oncol* 14:13, 1987.
60. Centers for Disease Control: Guidelines for prophylaxis against *Pneumocystis carinii* pneumonia for children infected with human immunodeficiency virus, *MMWR* 40(RR-2), 1991.
61. Centers for Disease Control: Recommendations for prophylaxis against *Pneumocystis carinii* pneumonia for adults and adolescents infected with human immunodeficiency virus, *MMWR* 41(RR-4), 1992.
62. Centers for Disease Control: Recommendations on prophylaxis and therapy for disseminated *Mycobacterium avium* complex for adults and adolescents infected with human immunodeficiency virus, *MMWR* 42(RR-9):17, 1993.
63. Stiehm ER: Immunodeficiency disorders: general considerations. In Stiehm ER, editor: *Immunologic disorders in infants and children,* ed 3, Philadelphia, 1989, Saunders.
64. Quie PG, Abramson JS: Disorders of the polymorphonuclear phagocytic system. In Stiehm ER, editor: *Immunologic disorders in infants and children,* ed 3, Philadelphia, 1989, Saunders.
65. Robinson JP, editor: *Handbook of flow cytometry methods,* Lafayette, Ind, 1990, Purdue Research Foundation.
66. Monaco A: Clinical kidney transplantation in 1984, *Transplant Proc* 17:5, 1985.
67. Penn I: Cancers after cyclosporine therapy, *Transplant Proc* 20:276, 1988.
68. Penn I: Tumors arising in organ transplant recipients, *Adv Cancer Res* 28:31, 1978.
69. Monaco A, Goldstein G, Barnes L: Use of Orthoclone OKT3 monoclonal antibody to reverse acute renal allograft rejection unresponsive to treatment with conventional immunosuppressive regimens, *Transplant Proc* 19(suppl. 1):28, 1987.
70. Dummer J, Hardy A, Poorsattar A et al: Early infections in kidney, heart and liver transplant recipients on cyclosporine, *Transplantation* 36(259), 1983.
71. Fiche M, Soulilou J, Bignon J et al: T lymphocyte monitoring in kidney transplant recipients undergoing cytomegalovirus infection or rejection episodes, *Transplantation* 37:421, 1984.
72. Richardson W, Colvin R, Cheesemen S et al: Glomerulopathy associated with cytomegalovirus viremia in renal allografts, *N Engl J Med* 305:57, 1981.

73. Matas A, Sibley R, Mauer M et al: The value of needle renal allograft biopsy. I. A retrospective study of biopsies performed during putative rejection episodes, *Ann Surg* 197:226, 1983.
74. Parfrey P, Kuo Y, Hanley J et al: The diagnostic and prognostic value of renal allograft biopsy, *Transplantation* 38:586, 1984.
75. von Willebrand E, Hayry P: Fine needle aspiration cytology of the transplanted kidney. In Morris J, editor: *Kidney transplantation,* ed 3, Philadelphia, 1988, Saunders.
76. Cosimi A, Colvin R, Burton R et al: Use of monoclonal antibodies to T-cell subsets for immunologic monitoring and treatment in recipients of renal allografts, *N Engl J Med* 305:308, 1981.
77. Ellis T, Lee HM, Mohanakumar T: Alterations in human regulatory T lymphocytes subpopulations after renal allografting, *J Immunol* 127:2199, 1981.
78. van Es A, Tanke H, Baldwin W et al: Ratios of T lymphocyte subpopulations predict survival of cadaveric renal allografts in adult patients on low dose corticosteroid therapy, *Clin Exp Immunol* 52:13, 1983.
79. Birkeland S: Immunological monitoring of renal transplant patients treated with prednisolone/azathioprine or cyclosporine A, *Transplant Proc* 17:2543, 1985.
80. Carter N, Cullen P, Thompson J et al: Monitoring lymphocyte subpopulations in renal allograft recipients, *Transplant Proc* 15:1157, 1983.
81. Pullis C, Waltzer W, Arnold A et al: Differential effects of cyclosporine and azathioprine on host cell populations in renal allograft recipients, *Transplant Proc* 19:1596, 1987.
82. Burton R: Lymphocyte monitoring in renal transplantation, *Transplant Proc* 16:983, 1987.
83. Toledo-Pereya L, Atalia S: Pretransplant T cell subsets do not predict rejection, *Transplant Proc* 17:2569, 1985.
84. Mazaheri R, Laupacis A, Keown P et al: Lymphocyte subsets in the allograft recipient: correlation of helper to suppressor ratio with clinical events, *Transplant Proc* 14:676, 1982.
85. Daniel V, Opelz B, Dreikorn K: Lymphocyte subpopulations in kidney transplant patients with different types of immunosuppression, *Transplant Proc* 17:2554, 1985.
86. Cunningham T, Ascher N: Effect of prerenal transplant OKT4-OKT8 ratio and immunosuppression protocol on posttransplant viral infections, *Transplant Proc* 17:633, 1985.
87. Lewis R, Kirchner K, Preuss T et al: Serial monitoring of T-cell subset ratios with monoclonal antibodies in steroid- and antithymocyte globulin-treated patients with renal alltransplants, *Clin Immunol Immunopathol* 31:241, 1984.
88. Helling T, Cross D, Shield C: Low pretransplant OKT4/OKT8 ratios do not adversely affect patients and allograft survival following renal transplantation, *Transplant Proc* 17:2550, 1985.
89. Mazaheri R, Laupacis A, Keown P et al: Lymphocyte subsets in the allograft recipient: correlation of helper to suppressor ratio with clinical events, *Transplant Proc* 14:676, 1982.
90. Kerman R, Flechner S, Van Buren C et al: Role of suppressor cells in cyclosporine-treated allograft recipients, *Transplant Proc* 19:1580, 1987.
91. Colvin R, Cosimi A, Burton R et al: Circulating T-cell subsets in 72 human renal allograft recipients: the OKT4+/OKT8+ cell ratio correlates with reversibility of graft injury and glomerulopathy, *Transplant Proc* 15:1166, 1983.
92. Binkley W, Valenzuela R, Braun W et al: Flow cytometry quantification of peripheral blood (PB) T-cell subsets in human renal allograft recipients, *Transplant Proc* 15:1163, 1983.
93. Senitzer D, Sawyer T, Clifford S et al: Daily lymphocyte subset monitoring of kidney transplant recipients treated with prednisone in combination with azathioprine or cyclosporine, *Transplant Proc* 17:2558, 1985.
94. Kerman R, Van Buren C, Payne W et al: Monitoring of T-cell subsets and immune events in renal allograft recipients, *Transplant Proc* 15:1170, 1983.
95. Hayes J, Valenzuela R, Novick A et al: Correlation between two-color flow cytometry quantitation of activated T cells and acute allgraft rejection, *Transplant Proc* 19:1605, 1987.
96. Hiyashi R, Sakakibara I, Suzuki S et al: Two-color flow cytometric techniques as a diagnostic tool for rejection of renal transplantation, *Transplant Proc* 19:1603, 1987.
97. Gross U, Thomas F, Matthews C et al: In vivo–in vitro correlates of human rejection using flow cytometry with two-color fluorescence on peripheral blood mononuclear cells, *Transplant Proc* 19:1609, 1987.
98. Hall B, Bishop G, Farnsworth A et al: Identification of the cellular subpopulations infiltrating rejecting cadaver renal allografts, *Transplantation* 37:564, 1987.
99. Walzer W, Miller F, Arnold A et al: Identification of mononuclear cell populations infiltrating human renal allografts, *Transplant Proc* 19:1629, 1987.
100. McWhinnie D, Azevedo L, Carter N et al: Diagnosis of renal allograft rejection by analysis of infiltrating cell profiles: an assessment of cyclosporine, azathioprine/prednisolone and triple therapy, *Transplant Proc* 19:1633, 1987.
101. McWhinnie D, Carter N, Taylor H et al: Is the T4/T8 ratio an irrelevance in renal transplantation monitoring? *Transplant Proc* 17:2548, 1985.
102. Platt J, LeBien T, Michael A: Interstitial mononuclear cell populations in renal graft rejection, *J Exp Med* 155:17, 1982.
103. Hammer C, Land W, Stadler J et al: Lymphocyte subclasses in rejection kidney grafts detected by monoclonal antibodies, *Transplant Proc* 15:356, 1985.
104. Hancock W, Thomson N, Atkins R: Composition of interstitial cellular infiltrate identified by monoclonal antibodies in renal biopsies of rejection human renal allografts, *Transplantation* 35:458, 1983.
105. Hancock W: Analysis of intragraft effector mechanisms associated with human renal allograft rejection: immunohistological studies with monoclonal antibodies, *Immunol Rev* 77:61, 1984.
106. van Es A, Meyer C, Oljans P et al: Mononuclear cells in renal allografts, *Transplantation* 37:134, 1984.
107. Hayry P, von Willebrand E: Monitoring of human renal allograft rejection with fine-needle aspiration cytology, *Scand J Immunol* 13:87, 1981.
108. von Willebrand E: Fine-needle aspiration cytology of human renal transplants, *Clin Immunol Immunopathol* 17:309, 1980.
109. Cosimi A: Clinical development of Orthoclone OKT3, *Transplant Proc* 19(suppl. 1):7, 1987.
110. Birkeland S, Svendsen V, Rohr N et al: Use of monoclonal antibodies to T cells (OKT3) for treatment of acute cellular rejection after renal transplantation, *Transplant Proc* 20(3):451, 1988.
111. Goldstein G: Overview of the development of orthoclone OKT3: monoclonal antibody for therapeutic use in transplantation, *Transplant Proc* 19(suppl. 1):1, 1987.
112. Klein J, McLeish K, Bunke C et al: Use of OKT3 monoclonal antibody in the treatment of acute cardiac allograft rejection, *Transplantation* 45:727, 1988.
113. Norman D, Shield C, Barry J et al: A U.S. Clinical Study of Orthoclone OKT3 in renal transplantation, *Transplant Proc* 19(suppl 1):21, 1987.
114. Carreno M, Miller J, Esquenazi V et al: Are OKT3 binding sites on T cells modulated or merely converted (blindfolded) by OKT3 during therapy? *Transplant Proc* 21(1):987, 1989.
115. Gebel H, Lebeck L, Jensik S et al: Discordant expression of CD3 and T-cell receptor antigens on lymphocytes from patients treated with OKT3, *Transplant Proc* 21(1):1745, 1989.
116. Gebel H, Lebeck L, Jensik S et al: T cells from patients successfully treated with OKT3 do not react with the T-cell receptor antibody, *Hum Immunol* 26:123, 1989.
117. Delmonico F, Colvin R, Fuller T et al: T cell subset alterations in OKT3-treated patients, *Transplant Proc* 17(1):628, 1985.
118. Kerr P, Atkins R: The effects of OKT3 therapy on infiltrating lymphocytes in rejecting renal allografts, *Transplantation* 48:33, 1989.
119. Bach J-F, Chatenoud L: Immunologic monitoring of orthoclone OKT3-treated patients: the problem of anti-monoclonal immune response, *Transplant Proc* 19(suppl 1):17, 1987.
120. Chatenoud L, Baudrihaye M, Chkoff N et al: Restriction of the human in vivo immune response against the mouse monoclonal antibody OKT3, *J Immunol* 137:830, 1986.
121. Caillat-Zucman S, Blumenfeld N, Legendre C et al: The OKT3 immunosuppressive effect: in situ antigenic modulation of human graft–infiltrating T cells, *Transplantation* 49:156, 1990.
122. First M, Schroeder T, Hurtubise P et al: Immune monitoring during retreatment with OKT3, *Transplant Proc* 21(1):753, 1989.

123. Jaffers G, Fuller T, Cosimi A et al: Monoclonal antibody therapy: anti-idiotypic and non–anti-idiotypic antibodies to OKT3 arising despite intense immunosuppression, *Transplantation* 41:572, 1986.
124. Huard TK: Clinically useful nontraditional applications of flow cytometry. In Keren DF, Hanson CA, Hurtubise PE, editors: *Flow cytometry and clinical diagnosis,* ed 2, Chicago, 1994, ASCP Press.
125. McCullough J, Press C, Clay M, Kline W: *Granulocyte serology: a clinical and laboratory guide,* Chicago, 1988, ASCP Press.
126. Hanson CA: Reticulocyte analysis by flow cytometry. In Keren DF, Hanson CA, Hurtubise PE, editors: *Flow cytometry and clinical diagnosis,* ed 2, Chicago, 1994, ASCP Press.
127. Christensson B, Tribukait B, Linder I-L et al: Cell proliferation and DNA content in non-Hodgkin's lymphoma, *Cancer* 58:1295, 1986.
128. Lenner P, Roos G, Johansson H et al: Non-Hodgkin's lymphoma: multivariate analysis of prognostic factors including fraction of S-phase cells, *Acta Oncol* 26:179, 1987.
129. Bauer K, Merkel D, Winter J et al: Prognostic implications of ploidy and proliferative activity in diffuse large cell lymphomas, *Cancer Res* 46:3173, 1986.
130. Williamson J, Grigor I, Smith M et al: Ploidy, proliferative activity, cluster differentiation antigen expression and clinical remission in high grade non-Hodgkin's lymphoma, *Histopathogy* 11:1043, 1987.
131. Shackney S, Levine A, Fisher R et al: The biology of tumor growth in the non-Hodgkin's lymphomas, *J Clin Invest* 73:1201, 1984.
132. Kerrigan D, Grogan T, Spier K et al: Analysis of diffuse large cell lymphoma with immunophenotypic and clinical correlation, *Lab Invest* 47, 1988.
133. Wooldridge T, Grierson H, Weisenburger D et al: Association of DNA content and proliferative activity with clinical outcome in patients with diffuse mixed cell and large cell non-Hodgkin's lymphoma, *Cancer Res* 48:6608, 1988.
134. Bunn P, Krasnow S, Makuch R et al: Flow cytometric analysis of DNA content of bone marrow cells in patients with plasma cell myeloma: clinical implications, *Blood* 59:528, 1982.
135. Witzig T, Gonchoroff N, Katzman J et al: Peripheral blood B cell labeling indices are a measure of disease activity in patients with monoclonal gammopathies, *J Clin Oncol* 6(6):1041, 1988.
136. Greipp P, Katzmann J, O'Fallon W, Kyle R: Value of β_2-microglobulin level and plasma cell labeling indices as prognostic factors in patients with newly diagnosed myeloma, *Blood* 72(1):219, 1988.
137. Look T, Roberson P, Williams D et al: Prognostic importance of blast cell DNA content in childhood acute lymphoblastic leukemia, *Blood* 65:1079, 1985.
138. Zarbo RJ, Linden MD: DNA analysis of gastrointestinal and genitourinary tract neoplasms. In Keren DF, Hanson CA, Hurtubise PE, editors: *Flow cytometry and clinical diagnosis,* ed 2, Chicago, 1994, ASCP Press.
139. Furlong JW: DNA analysis of breast, lung, central nervous system, endocrine, and head and neck tumors. In Keren DF, Hanson CA, Hurtubise PE, editors: *Flow cytometry and clinical diagnosis,* ed 2, Chicago, 1994, ASCP Press.
140. McCoy JP Jr: Clinical molecular cytometry: merging flow cytometry with molecular biology in laboratory medicine. In Keren DF, Hanson CA, Hurtubise PE, editors: *Flow cytometry and clinical diagnosis* ed 2, Chicago, 1994, ASCP Press.
141. Barker RL, Worth CA, Peiper SC: Cytometric detection of DNA amplified with fluorescent primers: applications to analysis of clonal bcl-2 and IgH gene rearrangements in malignant lymphomas, *Blood* 83(4):1079, 1994.
142. McCoy JP Jr, Carey JL: Recent advances in flow cytometric techniques for cancer diagnosis and prognosis. In Herberman RB, Mercer DW, editors: *Immunodiagnosis of cancer,* ed 2, New York, 1990, Marcel Dekker.
143. Gonzalez RC, Wintz P: *Digital image processing,* Reading, Mass, 1977, Addison-Wesley.
144. Wells WA, Rainer RO, Memoli VA: Basic principles of image processing, *Am J Clin Pathol* 98:493, 1992.
145. Marchevsky AM, Gil J, Jeanty H: Computerized interactive morphometry in pathology: current instrumentation and methods, *Hum Pathol* 18:320, 1987.
146. Inoue S: *Video microscopy,* New York, 1986, Plenum Press.
147. Arndt-Jovin DJ, Robert-Nicoud M, Kaufman SJ et al: Fluorescence digital imaging microscopy in cell biology, *Science* 230:247, 1985.
148. Taylor DL, Nederlof M, Lanni F et al: The new vision of light microscopy, *Am Scientist* 80:322, 1992.
149. Bacus JW, Grace LJ: Optical microscope system for standardized cell measurements and analyses, *Appl Optics* 26:3280, 1987.
150. Wied GL, Bartels PH, Bahr GF et al: Taxonomic intracellular system (TICAS) for cell indentification, *Acta Cytol* 12:180, 1968.
151. Young IT, Verbeek PW, Mayall BH: Characterization of chromatin distribution in cell nuclei, *Cytometry* 7:467, 1986.
152. Dawson AE, Cibas ES, Bacus JW et al: Chromatin texture measurement by Markovian analysis: the use of nuclear models to define and select texture features, *Analyt Quant Cytol Histol* (In press).
153. Hedley DW, Friedlander ML, Taylor IW et al: Method for analysis of cellular DNA content of paraffin-embedded pathological material using flow cytometry, *J Histochem Cytochem* 31:1333, 1983.
154. Hedley DW: Flow cytometry using paraffin-embedded tissue: five years on, *Cytometry* 10:229, 1989.
155. Wied GL, Bartels PH, Bibbo M et al: Image analysis in quantitative cytopathology and histopathology, *Hum Pathol* 20:549, 1989.
156. Weinberg DS: Relative applicability of image analysis and flow cytometry in clinical medicine. In Bauer KD, Duque RE, editors: *Flow cytometry: principles and applications,* Baltimore, 1992, Williams & Wilkins.
157. Auer G, Askensten U, Ahrens O: Cytophotometry, *Hum Pathol* 20:518, 1989.
158. Pallavicini MG, Taylor IW, Vindelov LL: Preparation of cell/nuclei suspensions from solid tumors for flow cytometry. In Melamed MR, Lindmo T, Mendelsohn ML, editors: *Flow cytometry and sorting,* New York, 1990, Wiley-Liss.
159. Bartels PH: Computer-generated diagnosis and image analysis, *Cancer* 69:1636, 1992.
160. Landay A, Auer R, Duque R et al: *Clinical applications of flow cytometry: quality assurance and immunophenotyping of peripheral blood lymphocytes (NCCLS doc H42-P, vol 9, no 13),* Villanova, Penn, 1989, National Committee for Clinical Laboratory Standards.
161. Gil J: Image analysis in pathology: what are the issues? *Hum Pathol* 20:203, 1989.
162. Baak JPA: Mitosis counting in tumors (editorial), *Hum Pathol* 21:683, 1990.
163. Ellis PSJ, Whitehead R: Mitosis counting: a need for reappraisal, *Hum Pathol* 12:3, 1981.
164. Russell WO, Cohen J, Enzinger FM et al: A clinical and pathologic staging system for soft tissue sarcomas, *Cancer* 40:1562, 1977.
165. Castleman KR, Chui LA, Martin TP et al: Quantitative muscle biopsy analysis, *Monogr Clin Cytol* 9:101, 1984.
166. Pesce CM: Defining and interpreting diseases through morphometry, *Lab Invest* 56:568, 1987.
167. Shum DT, Roberts JT, Smout MS et al: The value of nuclear contour index in the diagnosis of mycosis fungoides: an assessement of current ultrastructural morphometric diagnosis criteria, *Cancer* 57:298, 1986.
168. McNutt NS, Crain WR: Quantitative electron microscope comparison of lymphocyte nuclear contours in mycosis fungoides and in benign infiltrates in the skin, *Cancer* 47:698, 1981.
169. Hall TL, Fu YS: Applications of quantitative microscopy in tumor pathology, *Lab Invest* 53:5, 1985.
170. Wied GL: *Introduction to quantitative chemistry,* vol 1, New York, 1966, Academic Press.
171. Gill JE, Jotz MM: Further observations on the chemistry of pararosanaline-Feulgen staining, *Histochemistry* 46:147, 1976.
172. Taylor SR, Titus-Ernstoff L, Stitely S: Central values and variation of measured nuclear DNA content in imprints of normal tissues determined by image analysis, *Cytometry* 10:382, 1989.
173. Bauer TW, Tubbs RR, Edinger MG et al: A prospective comparison of DNA quantitation by image and flow cytometry, *Am J Clin Pathol* 93:322, 1990.
174. Claud RD, Weinstein RS, Howeedy A et al: Comparison of image analysis of imprints with flow cytometry for DNA analysis of solid tumors, *Mod Pathol* 2:463, 1989.

175. Dawson AE, Norton JA, Weinberg DS: Comparative assessment of proliferation and DNA content in breast carcinoma by image analysis and flow cytometry, *Am J Pathol* 136:1115, 1990.
176. Wilbur DC, Zakowski MF, Kosciol CM et al: DNA ploidy in breast lesions: a comparative study using two commercial image analysis systems and flow cytometry, *Anal Quant Cytol Histol* 12:28, 1990.
177. Fallenius AG, Askensten UG, Skoog LK et al: The reliability of microspectrophotometric and flow cytometric nuclear DNA measurements in adenocarcinomas of the breast, *Cytometry* 8:260, 1987.
178. Schneller J, Eppich E, Greenebaum E et al: Flow cytometry and Feulgen cytophotometry in evaluation of effusions, *Cancer* 59:1307, 1987.
179. Braylan RC, Diamond LW, Powell ML et al: Percentage of cells in the S phase of the cell cycle in human lymphoma determined by flow cytometry: correlation with labeling index and patient survival, *Cytometry* 1:171, 1980.
180. Bauer KD, Merkel DE, Winter JN et al: Prognostic implications of ploidy and proliferative activity in diffuse large cell lymphomas, *Cancer Res* 46:3173, 1986.
181. Clark GM, Dressler LG, Owens MA et al: Prediction of relapse or survival in patients with node-negative breast cancer by DNA flow cytometry, *N Engl J Med* 320:627, 1989.
182. Silvestrini R, Daidone MG, Gasparini G: Cell kinetics as a prognostic marker in in node-negative breast cancer, *Cancer* 56:1982, 1985.
183. Sigurdsson H, Baldetorp B, Borg A et al: Indicators of prognosis in node-negative breast cancer, *N Engl J Med* 322:1045, 1990.
184. Frankfurt OS, Greco WR, Slocum HK et al: Proliferative characteristics of primary and metastatic human solid tumors by DNA flow cytometry, *Cytometry* 5:629, 1984.
185. Weinberg DS: Proliferation indices in solid tumors, *Adv Pathol Lab Med* 5:163, 1992.
186. Gerdes J, Lemke H, Baisch H et al: Cell cycle analysis of a cell proliferation-associated human nuclear antigen defined by the monoclonal antibody Ki-67, *J Immunol* 133:1710, 1984.
187. Gerdes J, Schwab U, Lemke H et al: Production of a mouse monoclonal antibody reactive with a human nuclear antigen associated with cell proliferation, *Int J Cancer* 31:13, 1983.
188. Miyachi K, Fritzler MJ, Tan EM: Autoantibody to a nuclear antigen in proliferating cells, *J Immunol* 121:2228, 1978.
189. Bravo R: Synthesis of the nuclear protein cyclin (PCNA) and its relationship with DNA replication, *Exp Cell Res* 163:287, 1986.
190. Bravo R, Frank R, Blundell PA, et al: Cyclin/PCNA is the auxiliary protein of DNA polymerase-delta, *Nature* 326:515, 1987.
191. Ogata K, Kurki P, Celis JE et al: Monoclonal antibodies to a nuclear protein (PCNA/cyclin) associated with DNA replication, *Exp Cell Res* 168:475, 1987.
192. Nakamura H, Morita T, Masaki S et al: Intracellular localization and metabolism of DNA polymerase alpha in human cells, Exp Cell Res 151:123, 1984.
193. Schwartz BR, Pinkus G, Bacus S et al: Cell proliferation in non-Hodgkin's lymphomas: digital image analysis of Ki-67 staining, *Am J Pathol* 134:327, 1989.
194. Bouzubar N, Walker KJ, Griffiths K et al: Ki67 immunostaining in primary breast cancer: pathological and clinical association, *Br J Cancer* 59:943, 1989.
195. Wintzer H-O, Zipfel I, Schulte-Monting J et al: Ki-67 immunostaining in human breast tumors and its relationship to prognosis, *Cancer* 67:421, 1991.
196. Shahin AA, Ro J, Ro JY et al: Ki-67 immunostaining in node-negative stage I/II breast carcinoma: significant correlation with prognosis, *Cancer* 68:549, 1991.
197. Brown RW, Allred DC, Clark GM et al: The prognostic significance of cell-cycle kinetics measured by Ki-67 immunohistochemistry in node-negative breast cancer, *Lab Invest* 64:10A, 1991 (Abstract).
198. Veronese SM, Gambacorta M, Gottardi O et al: Proliferation index as a prognostic marker in breast cancer, *Cancer* 71:3926, 1993.
199. Greene GL, Jensen EV: Monoclonal antibodies as probes for estrogen receptor detection and characterization, *J Steroid Biochem* 16:353, 1982.
200. Bacus S, Flowers JL, Press MF et al: The evaluation of estrogen receptor in primary breast carcinoma by computer-assisted image analysis, *Am J Clin Pathol* 90:233, 1988.
201. Bacus SS, Goldschmidt R, Chin D et al: Biologic grading of breast cancer using antibodies to proliferating cells and other markers, *Am J Pathol* 135:783, 1989.
202. Allred DC: Should immunohistochemical examination replace biochemical hormone receptor assays in breast cancer? *Am J Clin Pathol* 99:1, 1993.
203. Allred DC, Bustamante M, Daniel CO et al: Immunocytochemical analysis of estrogen receptors in human breast carcinomas: evaluation of 130 cases and a review of the literature regarding concordance with the biochemical assay and clinical relevance, *Arch Surg* 125:107, 1990.
204. Czerniak B, Herz F, Wersto RP et al: Quantitation of oncogene products by computer-assisted image analysis and flow cytometry, *J Histochem Cytochem* 38:463, 1990.
205. Bacus SS, Chin D, Stern RK et al: HER-2/*neu* oncogene expression, DNA ploidy and proliferation index in breast cancers, *Anal Quant Cytol Histol* 14:433, 1992.
206. Bacus SS, Ruby SG, Weinberg DS et al: HER-2/*neu* oncogene expression and proliferation in breast cancers, *Am J Pathol* 137:103, 1990.
207. Grogan T, Dalton W, Rybski J et al: Optimization of immunocytochemical P-glycoprotein assessment in multidrug-resistant plasma cell myeloma using three antibodies, *Lab Invest* 63:815, 1991.
208. Herman CJ, Bunnag B: Goals of the cytology automation program of the National Cancer Institute, *J Histochem Cytochem* 24:2, 1976.
209. Bartoo GT, Lee JSJ, Bartels PH et al: Automated prescreening of conventionally prepared cervical smears: a feasibility study, *Lab Invest* 66:116, 1992.
210. Hutchinson ML, Cassin CM, Ball HG: The efficacy of an automated preparation for cervical cytology, *Am J Clin Pathol* 96:300, 1991.
211. Wasserman PD: *Neural computing: theory and practice*, New York, 1989, Van Nostrand Reinhold.
212. Roberts L: Are neural networks like the human brain? *Science* 243:481, 1989.
213. Anderson JA, Rosenfeld E: *Neurocomputing: foundations of research*, Cambridge, Mass, 1988, MIT Press.
214. Dawson AE, Austin R, Weinberg DS: Nuclear grading in breast carcinoma by image analysis: classification by multivariate and neural network analysis, *Am J Clin Pathol* 95(suppl 1):S29, 1991.
215. Henry JB: Computers in medical education: information and knowledge management, understanding, and learning, *Hum Pathol* 21:998, 1990.
216. Nathwani BN, Heckerman DE, Horvitz EJ et al: Integrated expert systems and videodisc in surgical pathology: an overview, *Hum Pathol* 21:11, 1990.
217. Castleman K, Wall R: Automatic systems for chromosome identification. In Caspersson T, Zech L, editors: *Chromosome identification*, New York, 1973, Academic Press.
218. Shotton DM: Confocal scanning optical microscopy and its applications for biological specimens, *J Cell Science* 94:175, 1989.
219. Weinstein RS, Bloom KJ, Rozek LS: Telepathology: long-distance diagnosis, *Am J Clin Pathol* 91(suppl 1):S39, 1989.
220. Weinstein RS: Prospects for telepathology, *Hum Pathol* 17:433, 1986.
221. Parsons DF: Progress and problems of interhospital consulting by computer networking, *Ann N Y Acad Sci* 670:1, 1992.

Part Two

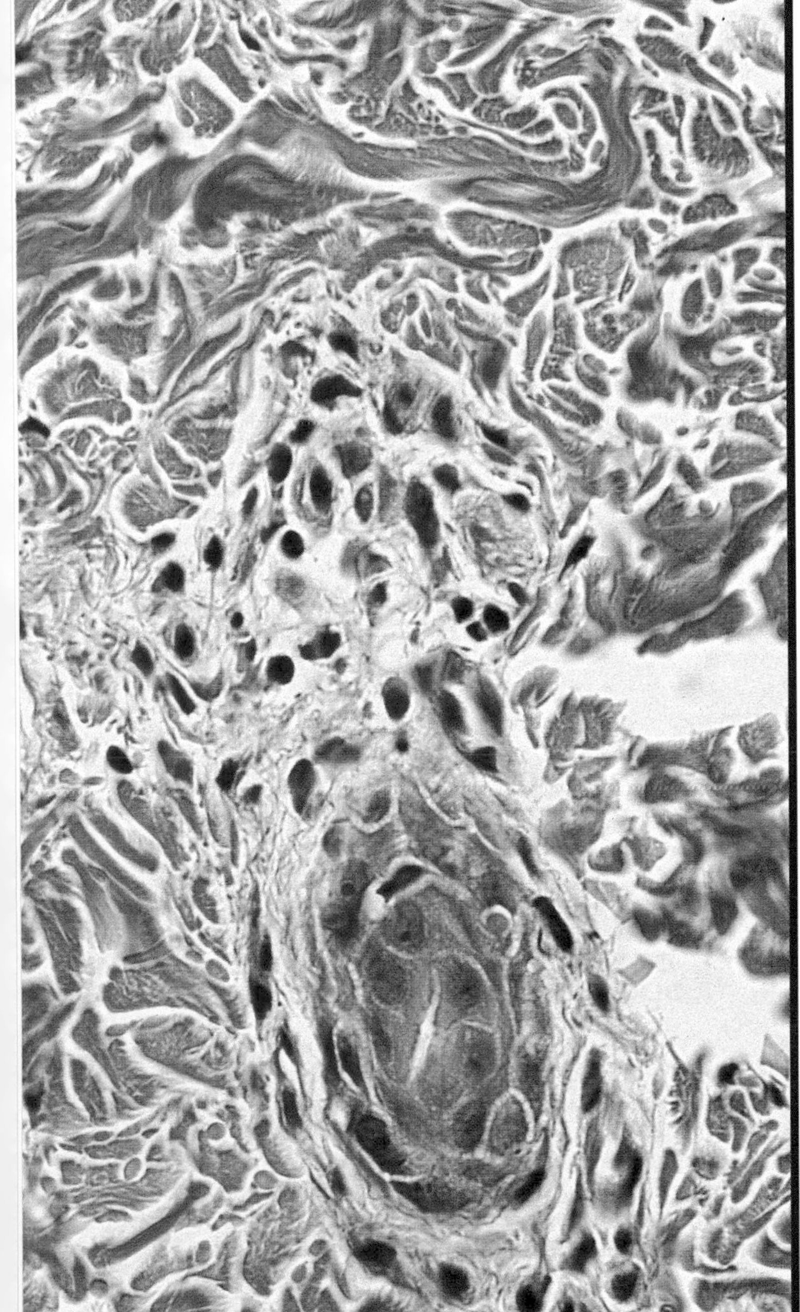

SYSTEMIC PATHOLOGY

Glycogenosis type II (Pompe's disease)

The original description of this glycogenosis included early onset cardiomegaly, heart failure, hypotonia, and death by 1 to 2 years of age.[26] Since then, other forms of type II glycogenoses have been described.

This group of glycogenoses is unique by featuring a *lysosomal accumulation* of glycogen, as opposed to the diffuse cytoplasmic deposition as seen in all other forms of glycogenoses. Indeed, this was the first inborn lysosomal disease to be clearly defined.[27] The condition stems from mutations in the gene encoding alpha-1,4-glucosidase (acid maltase)[28] leading to the profound reduction of this lysosomal enzyme.[29] Glycogen accumulates in the heart (Fig. 14-1), skeletal muscle, and many other cells, including lymphocytes. The condition is uniformly fatal, because of intractable heart failure.

In addition to the infantile form, both childhood and adult variants exist. In these, skeletal muscle is preferentially involved; biopsy reveals excessive muscle lysosomal glycogen and acid maltase deficiency. Since the heart is unaffected, these patients solely feature variable degrees of skeletal muscle weakness.

Lastly, one rare variant IIb, in which a lysosomal glycogen storage disease exists without deficiency of acid maltase, has been described.[30] The enzyme involved has not yet been characterized. In many instances, the condition, which appeared to be restricted to the myocardium,[31] allows for survival to the second decade.

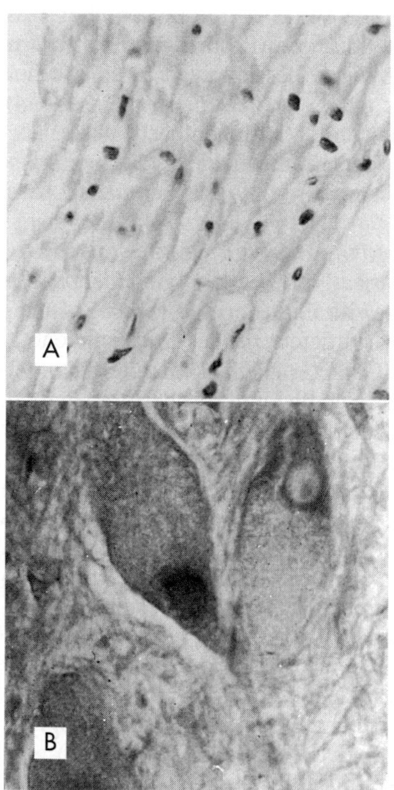

Fig. 14-1 **A,** Heart in Pompe's glycogenosis 2. The accumulations of glycogen-filled lysosomes in the heart in infantile "acid maltase" deficiency are perinuclear and central in the cardiac muscle fibers but are more peripheral and subsarcolemmal in skeletal muscle fibers. **B,** Brainstem neurons in Pompe's glycogenosis 2 showing cytoplasmic swelling and a finely vacuologranular appearance of cytoplasm imparted by the accumulation of glycogen-filled lysosomes.

Glycogenosis III (Forbes' disease, Cori's disease)

Glycogenosis III, originally described in 1956,[32] stems from a deficiency of amylo-1,6-glucosidase, the glycogen debrancher enzyme.[33] For most patients, both liver and skeletal muscle are involved; some feature hepatomegaly and hypoglycemia only; others manifest muscle weakness and wasting; rarely, only the heart may be involved. Up to now, six subtypes have been described. At affected sites, the glycogen molecules contain an excessive number of branching points. In general, the clinical features are mild, and most patients survive into adulthood; in a few, hepatic fibrosis and even cirrhosis may develop.

Glycogenosis IV (Andersen's disease, brancher deficiency)

The rare glycogenosis IV, described in 1952,[34] stems from mutations of the gene encoding amylo-(1,4 to 1,6) transglucosidase (brancher enzyme). As a result, there is a deficiency of this branching enzyme.[35] The main involvement is hepatic; children develop portal hypertension and cirrhosis in early life after the massive hepatic accumulation of this abnormal glycogen. Some have been successfully treated with liver transplantation.[36]

The material that accumulates is a starchlike linear glucose polymer with distinctive histologic and histochemical features (strong periodic acid–Schiff stain, resistant to diastase, positive iodine stain imparting a bluish color to the deposits, and positive colloidal iron stain) (Fig. 14-2). This condition is said to be the most common hepatic glycogenosis in Mexico, whereas Hers glycogenosis (see below) is the most common in Europe.

Glycogenosis V (McArdle's disease)

Glycogenosis V, a pure myopathy,[37] stems from deficiency of skeletal muscle glycogen phosphorylase.[38] Molecular studies of chromosome 11 have shown considerable molecular hetero-

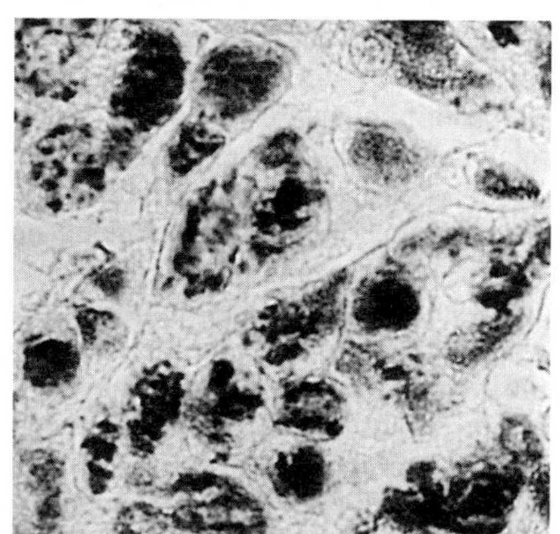

Fig. 14-2 Colloidal iron stain of hepatocytes in glycogenosis 4 (brancher enzyme deficiency). The mechanism of the colloidal iron staining of the linear starchlike glucose polymer that accumulates in hepatocytes, macrophages, and other cell types in this disease is not established.

geneity of the phosphorylase gene.[39] Compared with many other glycogenoses, the clinical features are rather mild manifesting as muscle pain, myoglobinuria, and muscle weakness. Strenuous exercise has been associated with rhabdomyolysis and acute tubular necrosis leading to acute renal failure.

Glycogenosis VI (Hers' disease)

The liver is the sole site of glycogen accumulation resulting from the hepatic deficiency of glycogen phosphorylase.[40] The clinical syndrome is that of mild hypoglycemia, hepatomegaly, and growth retardation. The prognosis is excellent.

Glycogenosis VII (Tarui disease)

The rare myopathy glycogenosis VII stems from deficiency of phosphofructokinase.[41] Clinical features mimic McArdle's disease. Some patients experience hemolysis, a fact explained by the presence of a closely related mutated enzyme in the erythrocyte.

Glycogenosis VIII

The variant glycogenosis VIII represents the only X-linked glycogenosis. The defect, a deficiency of hepatic phosphorylase kinase, results in one of the mildest of the glycogenoses.[42] In addition to hepatomegaly and growth retardation, there is mild elevation of serum cholesterol and triglycerides. By adulthood, these biochemical abnormalities disappear. A rare variant is also described with a cerebral palsy–like phenotype.

Glycogenosis O

The rare condition glycogenosis O features fasting hypoglycemia and hyperketonemia because of a deficiency of hepatic glycogen synthase.[43] The liver features a sharp reduction of glycogen stores. As these stores are reduced, it is regarded as glycogenosis O.

Other polysaccharide storage diseases

The three entities presented in this category all produce cytoplasmic bodies called "Lafora bodies," considered to be composed of polyglycosans. All are neurologic diseases, one causing myoclonic epilepsy,[44,45] one a motor neuron defect progressing to tetraparesis as well as peripheral neuropathy, and one producing bulbar signs. That the biochemical defects involve a "branching enzyme," possibly similar to that involved in glycogenosis IV, has been proposed, but the pathogenesis of these disorders is unclear.

Lysosomopathies

In 1955, DeDuve and coworkers, in a landmark series of experiments, discovered the lysosome as a cellular organelle. These single membrane-bound organelles, rich in acid hydrolases, are responsible for the degradation of an assortment of compounds including mucopolysaccharides, sphingolipids, and glycoproteins. Substances targeted for degradation include both exogenous as well as endogenous materials. Defective degradation may stem not only from a mutation of a gene encoding a particular enzyme, but also from genes encoding proteins central to the transport of substances to or from the lysosome, the activator protein for an enzyme or the formation of a recognition marker on an enzyme that directs it to the lysosome.

The first lysosomal storage disease to be defined was glycogenosis, type II,[29] in 1963. Since then, the list of lysosomopathies has expanded to include the mucopolysaccharidoses, glycoproteinoses, sialidoses, certain lipid storage diseases, sphingolipidoses, sulfatide lipidoses, gangliosidoses, mucolipidoses, and a short list of "other neurolipidoses."

Mucopolysaccharidosis

Mucopolysaccharides (MPS) are large molecules with a protein core to which are attached repetitive units of sulfated hexuronate or hexosamine disaccharides. Gene defects negating specific enzyme activities result in diverse phenotypes stemming from the accumulation of partially degraded fragments. The nature of material that accumulates may be correlated with specific tissue sites. Hence, bone involvement is associated with keratan sulfate storage; visceral and bone involvement are seen with dermatan sulfate; central nervous system involvement reflects heparan sulfate accumulation. The diagnosis of these conditions is based upon the age of onset, severity of symptoms, clinical phenotype, radiologic findings, characterization of the urinary mucopolysaccharide, and, if need be, characterization of the specific enzyme defect in blood leukocytes or fibroblast cultures. All are transmitted as autosomal recessive disorders except for MPS type II which is X linked. Bone marrow transplantation has been performed for many of these conditions with variable results.

Hurler's syndrome

The prototype and most severe condition, Hurler syndrome (MPS-1H), results in the faulty degradation of mucopolysaccharides,[46] stemming from the deficiency of alpha-L-iduronidase.[47] The clinical phenotype is complex and makes its appearance late in the first year of life with the development of coarse facial features. With time, corneal clouding, gingival hyperplasia, hepatosplenomegaly, upper airway obstruction as the result of thickening of the nasal mucous membranes, cor pulmonale, heart valve thickening, myocardiopathy, central nervous system deterioration, mental retardation, and diffuse radiographic bony changes (dysostosis multiplex) ensue. The clustering of bone lesions may include an elongated, enlarged skull (dolichocephaly), a thick calvarium, an abnormally shaped sella, hypoplasia of the anterior superior lower thoracic and lumbar vertebral bodies, dorsal kyphosis, thick ribs, metacarpal thinning and thickening, abnormal angulation of the distal humerus and ulna, flaring of the iliac bones, coxa valga, and hypoplasia of the odontoid process. On electron microscopy, the stored material appears finely granular, contained within vacuoles. Later on, the joints become stiff and contractures develop, rendering the child severely handicapped. Death usually occurs from cardiopulmonary involvement. This pleiotropic syndrome stems from the excessive accumulation of heparan and dermatan sulfate. If performed early, bone marrow transplantation may be beneficial.[48]

Scheie's syndrome

An allelic form of mutation (same gene locus, different mutation),[49] known as *Scheie syndrome* (MPS-1S), results in the accumulation of dermatan sulfate alone. As a result, the manifestations are considerably more mild with a later onset, corneal clouding, and joint involvement, yet with normal mentation and stature. Some children have aortic valvular problems; however, most live a near-normal life-span.

Compound syndrome

Rarely, a compound Hurler-Scheie phenotype may occur with a possibly different allelic mutation in the alpha-L-iduronidase locus. The phenotype produced is intermediate between the Hurler and Scheie syndromes.[50]

Hunter's syndrome

The sole X-linked entity (all others are autosomal recessive) in this category is Hunter's syndrome (MPS-II). Stemming from a mutation in the gene encoding iduronosulfate sulfatase,[51] levels of the enzyme are reduced,[52] and both heparan and dermatan sulfate accumulate in a multitude of tissues. The clinical phenotype may be severe or mild; the former resembles Hurler's syndrome yet appears later (1 to 2 years), progresses more slowly, and is devoid of corneal clouding. On electron microscopy, the stored material, particularly within neurons, is striated, giving rise to the term *zebra bodies*. Although fatal, survival is extended one decade beyond that for Hurler's syndrome. The milder form resembles Scheie's syndrome. The diagnosis can be established by enzyme analysis of fibroblasts, leukocytes, amniotic cells, and even chorionic villi.

Sanfilippo's syndrome

The group of four disorders known as Sanfilippo's syndrome (MPS-III) are ascribed to mutations involving four different genes[53-56] that lead to the accumulation of heparan sulfate. In each, the clinical features are similar. Children present around 3 years of age with coarse facial features, developmental delay, and behavioral problems. Mental retardation and progressive central nervous system involvement ensue. Although joint stiffness, hepatosplenomegaly and osseous lesions occur, they are less severe than that witnessed in Hurler's syndrome. Most survive about two decades.

Morquio syndrome

In Morquio syndrome (MPS-IV), the skeletal system is the target of disease attributable to the accumulation of keratan sulfate and chrondroitin-6-sulfate. Two forms, types A and B, stem from the deficiency of *N*-acetylgalactosamine-6-sulfate sulfatase[57] and beta-galactosidase[58] respectively. The latter gene is allelic with those causing the three G_{M1}-gangliosidases so that compound genetic disorders in this category will presumably be demonstrated. Children present with short stature and joint laxity in the first year of age. Osseous lesions give rise to hearing impairment and restrictive cardiorespiratory problems. Hypoplasia of the odontoid process and atlantoaxial subluxation lead to cervical cord compression, often requiring posterior spinal fusion. Most patients die in their twenties from cardiorespiratory failure.

Scheie's syndrome

Scheie syndrome, originally classified as MPS-V, is now reclassified as MPS-1S.

Maroteaux-Lamy syndrome

Deficiency of arylsulfatase B[59,60] leads to the accumulation of dermatan sulfate and the Maroteaux-Lamy syndrome (MPS-VI). Severe, intermediate, and mild forms exist. The severe form is similar to Hurler syndrome, whereas the mild form resembles Scheie syndrome. This form of MPS features the most striking inclusions in circulating white blood cells.

Sly syndrome

Deficiency of beta-glucuronidase[61] results in the accumulation of heparan, keratan, chondroitin-4 sulfate, and chondroitin-6 sulfate. Sly syndrome (MPS-VII), has a variable phenotype and best resembles a mild form of Hurler syndrome.

MPS VIII syndrome

Lastly, keratan and heparan sulfaturia (MPS-VIII) stems from a deficiency of glucosamine-6-sulfate sulfatase.[62] Complex bony lesions (dysostosis multiplex) and psychomotor retardation are its manifestations.

Glycoproteinoses

By definition, glycoproteins feature a peptide core to which oligosaccharide chains are attached. Deficiency of specific lysosomal acid hydrolases results in the failure to remove carbohydrate residues from the oligosaccharide chains. Since similar chains are present in sphingolipids and mucopolysaccharides, several types of material may be accumulated in these conditions. Indeed, the clinical features for the group of glycoproteinoses are not unlike those described for the sphingolipidoses, mucolipidoses, and mucopolysaccharidoses. As with the mucopolysaccharidoses, the urine contains excessive amounts of the oligosaccharide characteristic for the disease.

Fucosidosis

Deficiency of alpha-fucosidase[63,64] leads to the multisystem accumulation of fucose-containing sphingolipids, glycoproteins, and oligosaccharides. The condition fucosidosis presents in infancy with short stature, dysostosis multiplex, epilepsy, coarse facial features, diffuse angiokeratomas, hepatosplenomegaly, and cardiac problems.[65] The children, generally of Italian or Spanish descent, usually die in the first decade. A milder form has been described with less severe manifestations.

Mannosidoses

Deficiency of alpha-mannosidase[66] leads to mannosidosis,[67] characterized by the accumulation of mannose-containing glycoproteins. In the severe form, multiple systems are affected, resulting in hypotonia, hepatosplenomegaly, cataracts, dysostosis multiplex, deafness, and coarse facial features. The condition is lethal during the first decade of life. A mild form, allowing for survival into young adulthood, has been described.

Beta-mannosidosis

More rarely, beta-mannosidase may be deficient,[68] with or without an associated reduction of heparan sulfamidase. The former condition features psychomotor retardation with angiokeratomas. The latter has a phenotype akin to the Sanfilippo A syndrome.

Geleophysic dysplasia

An uncommon form of dwarfism has been ascribed to the accumulation of an as yet undefined glycoprotein. The children who inherit this defect were described as having "laughable faces"; hence, the name "Geleophysic (*geloios* 'laughable; humorous'; *physis* 'nature') dwarfism."[69] Phenotypes vary, yet most feature dysostosis multiplex and storage material in the liver, skin, and heart valves. The material accumulates within lysosomes and has staining properties of a glycoprotein.

Alpha-1-antitrypsin deficiency

By far, the most common example of a glycoprotein storage condition is alpha-1-antitrypsin deficiency. Alpha-1-antitrypsin is a glycoprotein of 50 kD molecular weight that is synthesized in the liver. Accounting for 80% of the serum α_1-globulin, it functions as a protease inhibitor. The hepatic and pulmonary complications stemming from its deficiency are covered in Chapters 57 and 49, respectively.

Lysosomal transport disorders

Sialic acid disorders (sialidoses)

The cherry-red spot—myoclonus syndrome, formerly considered in this group of conditions, is now coded as mucolipidosis 1.

Infantile sialic acid storage disease with sialuria is considered not to result from lysosomal acid hydrolase deficiency but from a defect in transport of sialic acid out of lysosomes;[70,71] the abnormal gene is presumably in allelic relation with that for the Finnish Salla disease. In each, patients store excessive amounts of unbound *N*-acetylneuraminic acid in lysosomes and excrete large amounts in their urine. The infantile form features hepatosplenomegaly, dysostosis multiplex, coarse facial features, and severe mental and motor retardation.[72,73] Death occurs in early life. Patients with Salla disease[74,75] present with ataxia and psychomotor delay in the first year of life. Although the life-span is only slightly affected, intelligence is severely impaired.

The disorder called *French type of sialuria,* the mechanism of which has not been established, appears not to be a lysosomal storage disease.

Nephrosialidosis produces cytoplasmic storage with vacuolation in a very wide range of cell types; the pattern of glomerular crescent formation seen in the disease is distinctive.

Lysosomal lipid storage diseases

Cholesterol esters/triglyceride storage

Cholesterol esters and triglycerides are hydrolyzed by lysosomal acid lipase. Deficiency of two allelic forms of the enzyme[76-78] results in Wolman disease and cholesterol ester storage disease. The most severe form is Wolman disease, which presents in early life and is lethal by 6 months of age. Children feature failure to thrive, hepatosplenomegaly, adrenal calcifications and necrosis, and widespread deposition of cholesterol esters and triglycerides.[79-82] The material, on electron microscopy, features homogeneous lipid with cholesterol clefts. The allelic form, cholesterol ester storage disease, presents much later with atheromas, hepatomegaly, and portal hypertension. The foam cells, characteristic of Wolman disease, are not a feature of the mild allelic version of this gene defect.

Farber's disease

The condition known as Farber's disease[83] was originally regarded as a lipogranulomatosis process, based upon the histologic features. It is now known to reflect the deficiency of ceramidase[84] leading to the accumulation of ceramide and other gangliosides in the skin, lymph nodes, brain, and viscera. The histologic response to these extraneous substances is the production of a lipogranuloma. The defect may present at any age. As with all such conditions, early onset implies a more widespread and even lethal condition. Biopsy specimens of periarticular tissues are particularly diagnostic.

Gaucher's disease

In Europe, it is customary for graduating physicians to present a doctoral thesis. Such was the case for Phillipe L.E. Gaucher, who, in 1882, described a peculiar splenic epithelioma.[85] The work was continued by others: the description of a storage material in reticuloendothelial cells,[86] its solubility in alcohol, and its identification as a cerebroside.[87]

It is now known that deficiency of beta-glucocerebrosidase[88,89] results in the accumulation of glucocerebroside in the reticuloendothelial system. The condition that results, Gaucher's disease, exists in several forms that relate to the age at presentation and whether neurons are involved.

The most common, indeed the most frequent of the sphingolipid disorders, is type 1, adult, chronic, nonneuropathic Gaucher's disease. The mutated gene is prevalent in Jewish people of Eastern European ancestry. A typical presentation is that of hypersplenism with pancytopenia and splenomegaly. As well, a characteristic radiologic expansion of the distal femoral cortex (Erlenmeyer-flask deformity) occurs in two thirds of the cases. Both the liver and the bone marrow (Fig. 14-3) are involved; the latter may lead to a leukoerythroblastic peripheral blood picture stemming from the ingress of Gaucher's cells, large histiocytes with abundant "wrinkled" cytoplasm. On electron microscopy, the lysosomal inclusions have an elongated, tubular shape. Similar cells are seen in the spleen and liver. This is one condition (apart from those affecting the prostate), in which serum acid phosphatase is elevated. The hypersplenism may necessitate splenectomy; if so, immunization and antibiotics may be necessary as prophylaxis against infection. In general, patients live a normal life-span with this variant.

In contrast, type 2 disease (acute, infantile neuronopathic form) presents in early life with the systemic reticuloendothelial involvement of type 1 disease and rapid central nervous system dysfunction. Although neuronal cerebroside storage is not a feature, the brain is the site of extensive neuronal cell death, reactive gliosis, and the perivascular accumulation of Gaucher's cells. The central nervous system deterioration is manifest by strabismus, trismus, and retroflexion of the head. Death occurs by 2 years of age. The condition is believed to stem from an unstable enzyme precursor.[90]

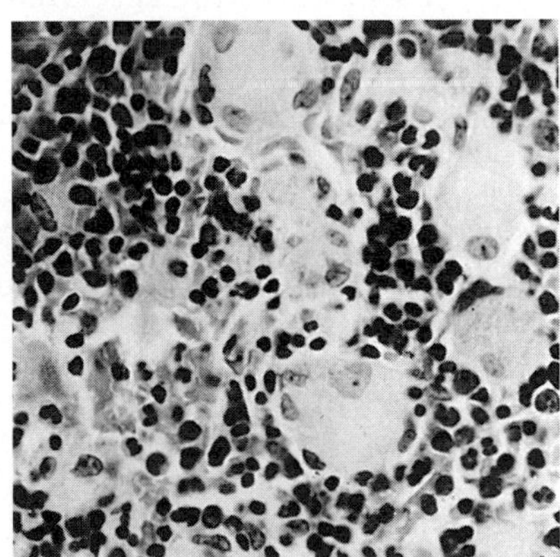

Fig. 14-3 Bone marrow of young child with "adult" Gaucher's I (glucocerebroside storage) disease showing macrophages with greatly enlarged cytoplasm, some (such as the lower cell on the midright) with the streaky, "wrinkled-paper" appearance produced by the greatly elongated storage lysosomes of this disease.

The hybrid form, type III (a feature common to most of the conditions covered in this section), blends features of types 1 and 2. This subacute neuronopathic or juvenile form has been described in ancestry from Norrbotten, a county in northern Sweden. Patients present in childhood with hepatosplenomegaly, followed later by central nervous system deterioration. Death occurs in early adulthood. Patients with types II and III disease share the same mutation (leu 444 to pro 444) in the gene. The phenotypic differences are ascribed to a nonfunctional allele in type II patients.[91]

Krabbe's disease

In the form of "globoid cell" leukodystrophy called *Krabbe's disease,* the deficiency of beta-galactosidase[92-94] leads to the accumulation of galactosylceramide in the peripheral and central nervous system. The "globoid cells," microglial macrophages, are large, multinucleated, and distended with PAS-positive material. On electron microscopy, the inclusions consist of hollow, twisted tubular structures.

The infantile form[95] is rapidly progressive with spasticity and irritability progressing to hypotonia, blindness, deafness, epilepsy, and peripheral neuropathy. The brain is the site of severe atrophy, gliosis, demyelination, and the accumulation of the diagnostic cell.[96] Death occurs by 2 years of age.

The later-onset variants[97,98] present in childhood, yet subsequently undergo diverse, progressive neurologic complications.

Fabry's disease

In contrast to other conditions described in this section, Fabry's disease is X-linked. The condition is attributable to deficiency of alpha-galactosidase A.[99-103] The defect is reflected by the accumulation of glycosphingolipids in tissues throughout the body: eyes, heart, skeletal muscle, central and autonomic nervous system,[104] endothelium, smooth muscle, and kidneys. On electron microscopy, the lysosomes are packed with a granular material, often in lamellar arrays. A common presentation is that of painful paresthesia of the hands and feet and episodic abdominal pain. Both corneal and lens lesions ensue. Angiokeratomas may be numerous,[105] though they are not pathognomonic because they are present in a wide variety of storage diseases. Renal involvement, presenting with the nephrotic syndrome, attributable to the accumulation of the lipids in the glomerular epithelial cells, may progress to renal failure by the mid-thirties. The latter has led to renal transplantation.[106]

Sphingomyelin storage diseases

Niemann-Pick disease

The index report[107] in the early part of this century is ascribed to a Berlin pediatrician, Albert Niemann, followed by the description of additional cases by Ludwig Pick.[108] The salient finding was a foam cell accumulation in tissues, yet one different from that described by their Parisian predecessor, Gaucher.

Within this group exist an assortment of disorders characterized by hepatosplenomegaly and the accumulation of sphingomyelin, gangliosides, and cholesterol in the brain, ganglion cells, macrophages, and diverse viscera (Figs. 14-4). The lysosomal stored material features a loose "opening-rose" lamellar pattern (Fig. 14-5). The phenotype is related to the organ and tissue distribution. In each, lipid-filled foam cells predominate; "sea-blue" histiocytes may also be demonstrated. The latter are not pathognomonic for this condition, since they are seen in other storage diseases. Of the five types (A, B, C, D, E), two (types A and B)[109] are the consequence of a deficiency of sphingomyelinase. In type C, defects in the esterification of cholesterol have been identified.[110] In contrast, the deficient enzyme has not been characterized for types D and E.

The most common and severe variant is type A, the acute neuronopathic form. These patients, often of Eastern European Jewish ancestry, present early in life with hepatosplenomegaly and a rapidly progressive deterioration of the central nervous system. Often the skin is pigmented yellow-brown, lymph nodes are enlarged, and ocular manifestations (cherry-red macula and corneal opacifications) are evident. Few survive beyond 4 years of age.

The type B (an allelic variant of type A)[111,112] features a similar pattern of visceral involvement as type A yet spares the central nervous system. These children present at a later age with isolated splenomegaly. In time, a more generalized vis-

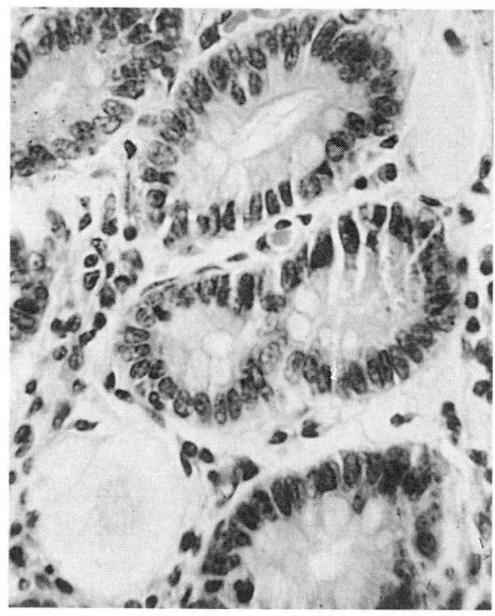

Fig. 14-4 Axonal "torpedos" and macrophages with pale, swollen "foam cell" cytoplasm in mucosa of small intestine of patient with Niemann-Pick disease.

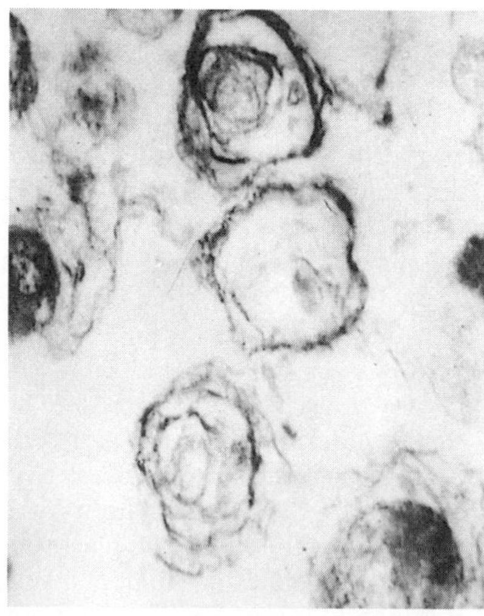

Fig. 14-5 Electron micrograph of cell in interstitial tissue of testis in Niemann-Pick disease, showing loose lamellar pattern of storage lysosomes in this disease. (Courtesy Dr. S. Kamoshita, Tokyo.)

ceral pattern of involvement is manifest, yet many patients survive several decades.

The chronic neuronopathic or juvenile form (type C) presents with diverse neurologic symptoms (ataxia, seizures, loss of previously learned speech) at about 5 years of age. Although hepatosplenomegaly is present, it is less pronounced than that in types A and B. Studies of cell lines from these patients have revealed a block in cholesterol esterification. The diagnosis may also be established by cytochemical staining with filipin, which demonstrates an intravesicular cholesterol storage material. Although it is not rapidly fatal, few patients survive beyond 15 years.

Types D and E have been shown to have normal levels of sphingomyelinase. The D variant was described in a large kindred of French Acadians in Nova Scotia.[113] Patients with type E disease feature moderate degrees of hepatosplenomegaly and marrow involvement. The two differ since neurologic involvement is present in type D disease but not in type E.

Last, a new variant[114] has been described in children with neonatal jaundice, hepatosplenomegaly, vertical supranuclear ophthalmoplegia, and sea-blue histiocytes. The children, from a Spanish-American family of the southwest United States, featured low (30% of normal) levels of sphingomyelinase in cultured fibroblasts.

Sulfatide lipidoses

Metachromatic leukodystrophy

Deficiency of arylsulfatase A (cerebroside sulfatase)[115-118] results in the accumulation of cerebroside sulfatide in the white matter of the central and peripheral nervous system and, to a lesser extent, in the kidney, gallbladder, and other organs (Fig. 14-6). The deposition in the white matter leads to spongy degeneration, reactive gliosis, demyelination, and atrophy. Thus this represents largely a disease of myelin metabolism. The name is derived from the brown metachromasia obtained when the acidic sulfatides are stained with acetic acid–cresyl violet. The diagnosis can be established by the demonstration of metachromatic cells derived from renal tubular epithelium in the urinary sediment.

Three phenotypes are defined; all stem from allelic mutations in the gene encoding arylsulfatase A. As demonstrated with other diseases, the most severe form features an infantile presentation. Less virulent but equally fatal expressions manifest in a juvenile or even adult form. All exhibit diffuse neurologic disturbances stemming from involvement of the brain, brainstem, cerebellum, and spinal cord.[119] Genetic heterogeneity is manifest in some patients with later onset disease who feature normal activity of arylsulfatase A but decreased levels of the corresponding activator protein, saposin B.[120]

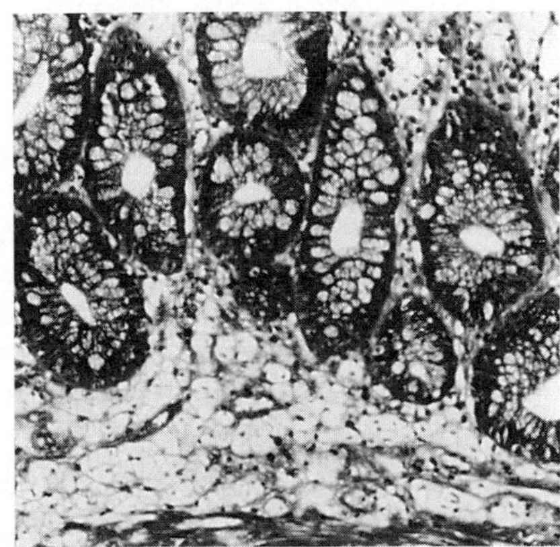

Fig. 14-6 Vacuolar histiocytosis of lamina propria of the colon in juvenile metachromatic leukodystrophy. The nature of the material stored in these cells, which does not stain for sulfatide, is not established. (Cresyl violet stain)

Multiple sulfatase deficiency (Austin disease)

The widespread deficiency of multiple lysosomal and nonlysosomal sulfatases (arylsulfatase A, B, and C) produces a composite clinical phenotype with features of metachromatic leukodystrophy, the mucopolysaccharidoses, and steroid sulfatase deficiency. Children present early in life with dysostosis multiplex, coarse facial features, ichthyosis, weakness, psychomotor delay, and deafness. Most die in the first decade of life.[121]

The gangliosidoses

The group of autosomal recessive diseases called *gangliosidoses* stems from the incomplete degradation of ganglioside molecules because of deficient (mutant) lysosomal acid hydrolases or because of the lack of an activator protein central to enzyme-lipid interaction. Three major groups have been defined; within each, subgroups exist. The designations G_{M1} and G_{M2} and so forth stem from the Svennerholm classification and are based on the number of sialic acid residues coupled to the oligosaccharide chain and by the number (5-*n*) of neutral sugars within the chain.

G_{M1}-gangliosidosis

Structural mutations in the gene, acid beta-glucosidase,[122-125] are central to diverse phenotypes within this group. The most severe form, type 1, generalized gangliosidoses, was defined by Landing in 1964.[126] Previously, such children were believed to have Hurler disease or a variant thereof, given their coarse facial features, joint stiffness, angiokeratomas, hepatosplenomegaly, and dysostosis multiplex.

More ominous, however, was the extensive central nervous system involvement that featured the accumulation of gangliosides in neurons, as well as in cultured fibroblasts and histiocytes in lymph nodes, bone marrow, spleen, and liver, and renal tubular epithelium. The stored material is less lamellar (in electron microscopic images) than that seen in G_{M2}-gangliosidosis. The precocious onset and severity of symptoms correlate with early demise, usually before 2 years of age.

Type 2 (juvenile G_{M1}-gangliosidosis), presumably an allelic mutation to type 1, presents somewhat later and features predominantly central nervous system involvement.[127] The diverse manifestations, simulating a mucopolysaccharidosis as seen in type 1 disease, are not manifest. Death occurs before the end of the first decade.

Type 3 (adult-onset G_{M1}-gangliosidosis), also presumably an allelic mutation to Type 1,[128] is uncommon and features a diverse phenotype. Common threads include angiokeratomas, blindness, mental deterioration, myoclonic seizures, and ataxia.

G_{M2}-gangliosidosis, type 1 (Tay-Sachs disease)

The phenotype type 1, affects many tissues, including the eye and central nervous system. Not surprisingly, the name it bears stems from its recognition as being unique because of the British ophthalmologist Warren Tay[129] and the American neurologist Bernard Sachs,[130] at the end of the 19th century. The matter rested until 1939, when Klenk identified in such patients a high concentration of neuronal sialic acid glycolipids, which he called "gangliosides."[131] The central theme to these conditions (there was no longer a single entity but a family known) was ascribed to Svennerholm,[132] Makita and Yamakawa,[133] Ledeen and Salsman,[134] Okada and O'Brien,[135] Sandhoff,[136] and Hultberg.[137] The last three sources identified the enzyme deficiency.

This group comprises eight entities (and is still increasing in number!). The diverse clinical phenotypes stem from mutations in the genes coding for beta-hexosaminidases or a sphingomyelin activator protein. As a consequence, the accumulation of lysosomal G_{M2}-ganglioside and glycosphingolipids leads to progressive cerebral degeneration. The number of phenotypes relates to the structure of beta-hexosaminidase, which has an alpha-subunit and a beta-subunit, each encoded by separate genes. Combinations of these subunits leads to isoenzyme diversity. To stabilize the enzyme-substrate complex, a G_{M2} activator protein is essential.

Formerly, Tay-Sachs disease was regarded as a clear-cut expression of a gangliosidosis. Now, at least three forms are known; two feature mutations of the alpha-subunit of beta-hexosaminidase (types B[135-137] and B1[138]), and another stems from mutation of the gene for *saposin,* the hexosaminidase activator protein (AB form).[139] The prototype, form B, manifests a striking incidence in children of Eastern European Jewish origin. Since the alpha but not beta subunit is mutated, the total amount of beta-hexosaminidase is normal. Although normal at birth, affected children develop (in the first year of life) hypotonia and psychomotor retardation. The central nervous system degeneration proceeds rapidly, and spasticity and blindness soon follow. The classical "cherry-red macula," now known to be present in many storage diseases, was first described with Tay-Sachs disease. It is noteworthy, that the red macula represents a normal segment of the retina rendered vivid by contiguous white areas, which contain the stored material. Given the magnitude of generalized neuronal dysfunction, respiratory problems are common and pneumonia by 3 years of age is the usual cause of death.

G_{M2}-gangliosidosis, type 2 (Sandhoff disease)

Five phenotypes are listed within this group, which features a total deficiency of beta-hexosaminidase leading to the extensive neuronal and visceral storage of G_{M2}-gangliosides, glycolipids, glycoproteins, and oligosaccharides.[140] Both alpha- and beta-subunit mutations are described for the beta-hexosaminidase gene.[141,142] Some may be diagnosed after rectal biopsy, which discloses large, lipid-rich ganglion cells in the autonomic plexes. On balance, the clinical phenotypes mimic Tay-Sachs disease. The storage material in all forms of G_{M1}- and G_{M2}-gangliosidoses features, on electron microscopy, a characteristic tightly circumferential onionskin pattern, the membranous cytoplasmic bodies (Fig. 14-7). Infantile, juvenile, and adult forms have been described; each follows the progression described for the previously described storage diseases.

Galactosialidosis

Galactosialidosis is associated with the deficiency of both alpha-neuramidase and beta-galactosidase.[143] To be functional, each enzyme requires coupling by a protective protein. Deficiency of the latter gives rise to a phenotype that includes coarse facial features and dysostosis multiplex. Congenital, juvenile and adult forms exist.

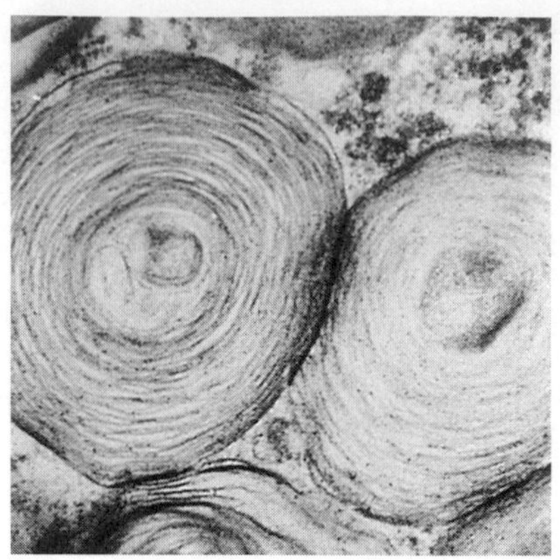

Fig. 14-7 Electron micrograph of tightly lamellar "membranous cytoplasmic body" storage lysosomes typical of G_{M2}-ganglioside storage from teenaged patient with juvenile G_{M2}-ganglioside storage disease.

Other neural lipidoses

Cerebrotendinous xanthomatosis

The rare, autosomal recessive lipid-storage disease called *cerebrotendinous xanthomatosis* is characterized by the deposition of cholesterol and cholestanol (the 5-alpha-dihydroxy derivative of cholesterol), most prominently in the brain, lungs, Achilles tendon, and blood vessels. Children present in their teens with cerebellar ataxia, spinal cord symptoms, cataracts, and premature atherosclerosis.[144] The demonstration of elevated levels of cholesterol in the serum and tendons establishes the diagnosis. The defect resides in the deficiency of a mitochondrial cytochrome P-450, the C27-steroid 26-hydroxylase.[145] Treatment is with the cholesterol-chelating drug chenodroxycholic acid. Death is related to progressive neurologic involvement ascribed to the deposition of the storage material in the brainstem.

Mucolipidoses

The mucolipidoses (ML) are a group of recessively inherited lysosomal storage diseases characterized by the intracellular, lysosomal accumulation of both mucopolysaccharides and lipids.

Mucolipidoses have been divided into four main groups, I, II, III, IV (Table 14-2) by McKusick[9] and Gilbert-Barness.[146]

Diagnosis of ML is suspected clinically because of the phenotypic appearance of the child including coarse facial features, mental retardation, dysostosis multiplex, and the lack of mucopolysacchariduria. It is confirmed histopathologically and biochemically by identification of the substrates.[147] Deficiency of *N*-acetylneuraminidase has been identified in ML I, also called *sialidosis III.*[148-150] Hepatocytes, macrophages, hepatic and splenic sinusoidal lining cells, neurons, and renal glomerular and collecting tubular epithelial cells are most severely affected in ML I.[148] ML II more severely affects mesenchymal tissues (such as cartilage), whereas neurons show the most striking changes at the ultrastructural level. Both placental trophoblast and stromal cells are involved in ML I,

Table 14-2 Mucolipidoses

Disease	Enzyme defect or deficiency
Mucolipidosis I (sialidosis III)	Glycoprotein-specific *N*-acetylneuraminidase
Mucolipidosis II (I-cell)	(GcNaC-phosphotransferase) *N*-acetylglucosamine-phosphotransferase
Mucolipidosis III (pseudo-Hurler disease)	(GcNaC-phosphotransferase) *N*-acetylglucosamine-phosphotransferase
Mucolipidosis IV (sialolipidosis)	Unknown?; ganglioside sialidase?

GcNac, Glycoprotein-specific *N*-acetylneuraminic acid.

II,[151,152] and IV.[153] Multiple cellular lysosomal enzyme deficiencies in conjunction with elevated serum levels of specific enzymes are features of ML II and III. Few tissues have been studies from cases of ML III and IV.

The accumulated cytoplasmic acid mucopolysaccharide exhibits histochemical characteristics of a weakly sulfated compound, producing a positive reaction with Hale's colloidal iron, alcian blue at pH 2.5, and toluidine blue at pH 2.0, but a negative reaction with Alcian Blue at pH 1.0.[147]

By electron microscopy, lysosomes contain finely granular to flocculent, moderately electron-dense material as the preponderant component of stored mucopolysaccharides. Osmiophilic multilamellar bodies and fragments of membrane-like profiles are characteristic of lipid compounds. The membranous structures are typically found within lysosomes of visceral tissues in the classic mucopolysaccharidoses but are more common in the mucolipidoses that contain both mucopolysaccharide and lipid. The storage vacuoles in brain cells in the mucolipidoses, as in the lipidoses and mucopolysaccharidoses, are filled predominantly with osmiophilic membranous bodies and lamellar arrays.[147]

Mucolipidosis II (I-cell disease)

I-cell disease was first differentiated from the Hurler syndrome by the absence of mucopolysacchariduria.[154] It was designated I ('inclusion')-cell disease because of numerous phase-dense inclusions in the cytoplasm of cultured fibroblasts from affected individuals (Fig. 14-8). Similar inclusions have since been seen in cells from patients with ML I and pseudo-Hurler polydystrophy (ML III).[155]

Multiple lysosomal enzymes in ML II are deficient in cultured fibroblasts[156,157] with an increased concentration in culture medium,[157,158] serum, and other body fluids. The recognition marker for the intracellular transport of lysosomal acid hydrolase that is absent in ML II has been identified as mannose-6-phosphate.[159,160]

The diagnosis of both ML II and ML III can be confirmed[161] by measurement of the activities of lysosomal enzymes in serum or in cultured fibroblasts. Ten- to twentyfold increases in beta-hexosaminidase, iduronate sulfatase, and arylsulfatase A are characteristic of both ML II and ML III.[162,163]

ML II, like Hurler syndrome, is characterized by severe psychomotor retardation with coarse facial features. Gingival hyperplasia is a more striking feature than the gingivae in the

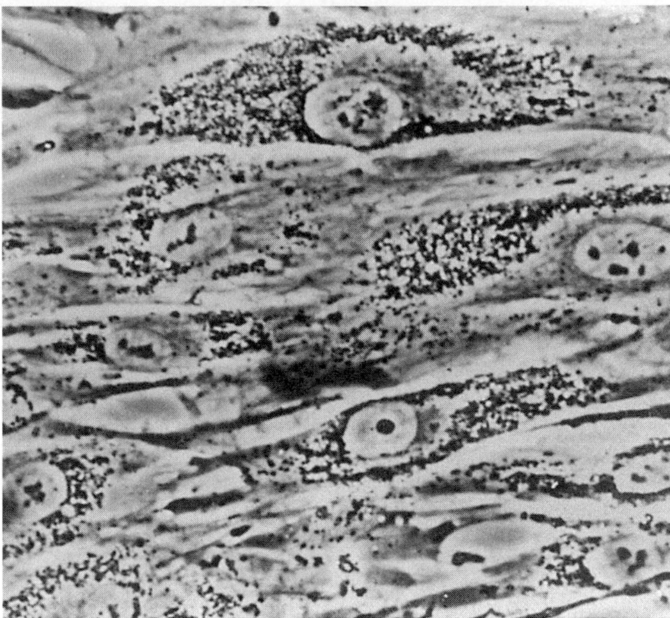

Fig. 14-8 Cultured fibroblasts showing coarse granules in I-cell disease. (Phase contrast microscopy.)

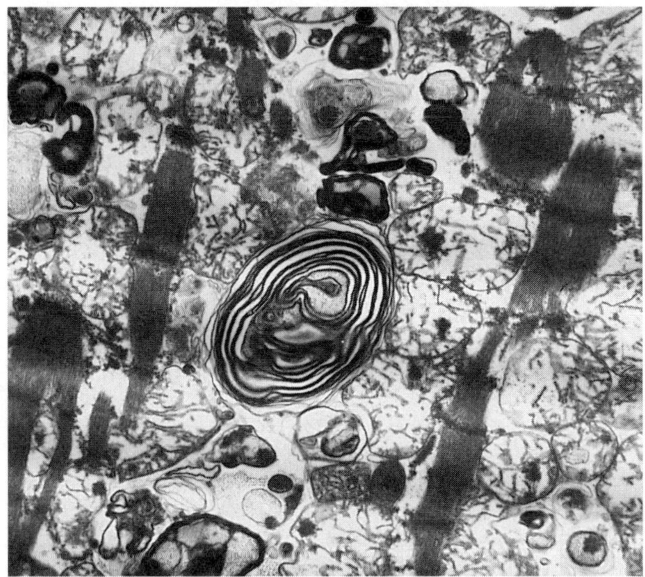

Fig. 14-9 Electron micrograph of myocardium showing membranous lamellar profile. (Uranyl acetate and lead citrate.)

Hurler syndrome.[164-166] Hepatomegaly is prominent, but splenomegaly is minimal. Cardiomegaly, cardiac murmurs, and aortic insufficiency are common.[167]

The heart is uniformly hypertrophied. The mitral and aortic valve leaflets are extremely thick, rigid, retracted, and distorted. The aorta, the major aortic branches, and the coronary vessels are thickened by yellow subintimal plaques.[168] The individual myocardial cells appear vacuolated because of the accumulation of lipid and mucosubstances. The ultrastructure of the myocardial cells reveals cellular distortion, sarcolemmal inclusions of osmiophilic dense bodies and membranous lamellar bodies, ringlike structures, and reticulogranular deposits (Fig. 14-9). The pulmonary arteries may show similar changes.

Hepatocytes, Kupffer cells, glomerular and tubular epithelial cells, and bone marrow lymphocytes contain inclusions.[168] By electron microscopy, there is lysosomal accumulation of reticulogranular material and laminated membranous bodies arranged in parallel or concentric lamellae, some in myelin-like configurations with a periodicity of 5 to 6 nm.

If death occurs after 5 years of age, the brain is small. The leptomeninges over the cerebral convexity are usually thickened, opaque, and gelatinous. There may be atrophy of the cerebral cortex with widening of sulci and slight atrophy of the vermis of the cerebellum. Cortical neurons are diminished in number. Most anterior horn motor neurons of the spinal cord contain PAS-positive granules.[168] By electron microscopy, nerve cells and Purkinje cells contain scattered pleomorphic inclusions from 0.6 to 2 nm in greatest dimension. Some inclusions contain stacked linear membranes, circular and hemicircular profiles, globules and granules, all of considerable electron opacity.

Prenatal diagnosis has been accomplished in the mucolipidoses I, II, and IV and is possible in mucolipidosis III. Amniocentesis or chorionic villous sampling can be used for diagnosis.

AMINO ACID DISORDERS

Phenylketonuria

Inherited as an autosomal recessive trait, phenylketonuria has an incidence of 1 in 15,000 live births. The classical form is attributable to deficiency of the enzyme phenylalanine hydroxylase, encoded by chromosome region 12q22q24.1.[169] A variant includes a deficiency of the phenylalanine hydroxylase cofactor tetrahydrobiopterin. In the classical form, untreated infants become mentally retarded, develop seizures, and have a mousy odor to the urine and eczema. The Guthrie test is to screen for phenylketonuria.

Pathologically, demyelination and gliosis occur in the white matter of the brain with the presence of lipid-laden macrophages. Extensive neuronal loss occurs with a reduction in the number of dendritic processes on the Purkinje cells.[170]

Patients treated for phenylketonuria who reach reproductive age may give birth to an infant with severe abnormalities including microcephaly, growth retardation, and congenital cardiac defects.

Hereditary tyrosinemia

Type I hereditary tyrosinemia has an incidence of 1 per 100,000 to 200,00 except in Quebec, where for unknown reasons the incidence is 8 per 100,000 live births. This autosomal recessive disorder attributable to deficiency of fumarylacetoacetate hydrolase.[171] Acute tyrosinemia is evident within the first weeks of life, with failure to thrive, vomiting, fever, diarrhea, hepatomegaly, and decreasing liver function. The patient with chronic tyrosinemia carries the risk of developing hepatocellular carcinoma.[169] Infants with this disorder have increased levels of plasma methionine, prolonged prothrombin time, increased alpha-fetoprotein, and urinary excretion of succinyl acetone and succinyl acetoacetate. Prenatal detection is possible by definitive enzyme analysis of cultured amniotic fluid cells or from chorionic villous sampling. The presence of succinyl acetone in amniotic fluid and high concentrations of alpha-fetoprotein in cord blood of affected newborn infants is suggestive that liver changes may occur in utero.[170]

Tyrosinemia type II, attributable to a deficiency of hepatic tyrosine aminotransferase, is also inherited as an autosomal recessive trait. Because the major manifestations are in the skin and eyes, it is described as *oculocutaneous tyrosinemia*. Children demonstrate mental retardation, corneal ulcers, and palmar and plantar hyperkeratosis. Tyrosinemia and tyrosinuria are present. Treatment with a low phenylalanine–low tyrosine diet may affect a cure.

Pathology

Tyrosinemia principally affects the liver and kidney. The liver is large, with pseudoacinar arrangements of hepatocytes. Regenerative nodules, which are frequently dysplastic, may give rise to hepatocellular carcinoma.[171] A lobular fibrosis, diffuse fibrosis, or cirrhosis may develop.[172] The kidneys may be enlarged with cortical tubular ectasia and focal tubular calcification. Islet-cell hyperplasia of the pancreas, hypophosphatemic rickets, and mineralization of blood vessels may occur.

The skin biopsy of patients with tyrosinemia type II may show acanthosis or hyperkeratosis and parakeratosis. Ultrastructurally, 2 to 3 μm lipidlike granules with 10 nm filaments intermixed with myelin-like figures may be seen. Mitochondria may appear edematous.

Hepatic encephalopathy, meningitis, or liver failure is the usual fatal outcome. Liver transplantation has been the treatment of choice.

Alcaptonuria

Alcaptonuria, inherited as an autosomal recessive trait, is attributable to the accumulation of homogentisic acid, a byproduct of phenylalanine and tyrosine metabolism. It is attributable to a defect or absence of the enzyme homogentisic acid oxidase. The connective tissues are pigmented, usually gray to bluish-black grossly but ochre microscopically. Usually, pigment deposition does not occur until the end of the first decade of life. Pigmentation is visible in the sclera, ears, cartilage, and joints. Deposition of homogentisic acid in the connective tissue underlies arthritis, and in the heart, cardiac failure. Homogentisic acid itself is not colored, but oxidation by homogentisic acid polyphenol oxidase forms the ochronotic pigment.

Cystinosis

There are three forms of cystinosis, which, as a unifying feature, share a defect in carrier-mediated transport of cystine. Children with the *nephropathic* form of cystinosis are usually normal at birth but develop renal tubular damage similar to Fanconi's syndrome by 1 year of age. They develop polyuria, growth failure, rickets, photophobia, and decreased pigmentation. Renal failure is a common cause of death. The *juvenile* form has similar signs and symptoms, only later in life. Benign cystinosis is characterized by minimal cystine accumulation and a normal life expectancy.

Cystine crystals form within the lysosomes of most organs but particularly in cells of the reticuloendothelial system. Cystinosis is diagnosed by elevated cystine content of leukocytes or cultured fibroblasts. Cystine crystals can be seen in the cornea and in the bone marrow. The retina may demonstrate retinopathy with depigmentation. Hypothyroidism occurs in some children with cystinosis. Renal transplantation is effective in treating the renal disease. Prenatal diagnosis is possible by amniocentesis or chorionic villous sampling.

Cystinuria

Cystinuria is a relatively common inborn error of transport of the amino acids cystine, ornithine, lysine, and arginine. Excess urinary excretion of these amino acids causes the formation of cystine calculi. No other tissue disorder has been detected. Untreated patients may develop renal failure.

Homocystinuria

Three distinct pathophysiologic mechanisms may underly homocystinuria, an autosomal recessive disorder. The classic, type I form is attributable to a deficiency of cystathionine β-synthetase. The type II form is attributable to defects in methylcobalamin reactions, whereas type III reflects a deficiency of methylene tetrahydrofolate reductase. In each, homocysteine and other metabolites of methionine accumulate in the body. Patients are usually tall and marfanoid and develop dislocated optic lenses, osteoporosis, mental retardation, and thromboemboli in small and large vessels.

Infarcts are found in the brain and elsewhere. Arterial walls show pronounced fibrous thickening of the intima, splitting of the muscle fibers of the media, and elastic fragmentation resulting in a basket-weave pattern. The vascular change may progress to advanced arteriosclerosis. Treatment includes dietary restriction of sulfur-containing amino acids, supplemental vitamin B_6, folate, and betaine.

Maple sugar urine disease

Maple sugar urine disease, so named because of the odor of maple syrup in urine, sweat, and saliva, is an autosomal recessive disorder of defective metabolism of the branched-chain amino acids leucine, isoleucine, and valine. The estimated incidence is 1 per 120,000 to 1 per 400,000 live births. The disease is manifested during the first week of life, with vomiting, convulsions, and coma. Intermittent or late forms of the disease may be precipitated by a high-protein diet or by infection. A thiamine-responsive type has been described. The diagnosis is made by plasma amino acid analysis and urinary organic acid determinations. Analysis of the branched-chain decarboxylase may be performed on leukocytes, fibroblasts, or amniotic fluid cells.

The liver, kidney, and brain may be enlarged, and the liver contains increased amounts of glycogen. Renal cortical cysts may be present, and the brain shows hypomyelinization particularly in the pons and medulla. On frozen sections crystals within vacuoles may be seen in the liver and other organs.[173]

Nonketotic hyperglycinemia

Nonketotic hyperglycinemia is an autosomal recessive disorder with an incidence of 1 in 55,000 births. Defective glycine cleavage activity in the brain and diminished enzyme activity in the liver cause the accumulation of glycine in blood, cerebrospinal fluid, and the brain.[174,175] Diagnosis is made by the determination of plasma glycine, which may be only slightly elevated, and elevated cerebrospinal fluid glycine. Infants with this disorder develop severe mental retardation, seizures, and death usually in the first 6 months of life. Some forms of the disease have a later onset, with varying degrees of retardation. In the brain, changes include hypomyelinization and spongiosis. The liver may appear normal or show nonspecific steatosis.

ORGANIC ACIDEMIAS

Organic acidemias are usually manifested during childhood. If symptoms begin in the neonatal period, the course may be fulminant with severe central nervous system dysfunction, coma, seizures, and death. In older infants and children, the disease may be episodic, with exacerbations after infections that may be reminiscent of Reye's syndrome. Acidosis with hyperammonemia and hypoglycemia may be present.

Major organic acidemias are attributable to the accumulation of isovaleric, propionic, methylmalonic, or glutaric acid. These disorders are suspected if serum acid concentrations are elevated. The diagnosis is verified by enzyme analysis of fibroblasts, leukocytes, or amniocytes. Pathologic changes are nonspecific though hemorrhages may occur in the viscera and steatosis in the liver.[176] Congenital anomalies may accompany glutaricacidemia.[177,178]

Sulfite oxidase deficiency

Sulfite oxidase deficiency is attributable to deficiency of molybdenum cofactor and is inherited as an autosomal recessive trait. Patients have severe neurologic abnormalities including mental retardation and develop dislocated ocular lenses. Sulfite, thiosulfate, sulfocystine, taurine, xanthine, and hypoxanthine are excreted in the urine. Extensive neuronal loss, demyelination of the white matter, gliosis, and diffuse spongiosis are manifested as a severe encephalopathy. Prenatal diagnosis is made by a sulfite oxidase assay in a culture of amniotic cells or from chorionic villus sampling. No effective treatment is known.

Pyruvate dehydrogenase deficiency

Pyruvate dehydrogenase participates in the oxidation of glucose and fatty acids and provides acetylcoenzyme A (acetyl-CoA) for the citric acid cycle. Pyruvate dehydrogenase is a protein complex with three main catalytic domains, E_1, E_2, and E_3. Defects of the E_1 alpha-subunit are inherited in an X-linked fashion; males with E_1 alpha-deficiency have a partial deficiency. Females may carry a more severe mutation. A defect of pyruvate dehydrogenase results in a variable phenotype including lacticacidosis in the early neonatal period, ataxia, and developmental delay in infancy. Subtle dysmorphic features are similar to the fetal alcohol syndrome[178] including a narrow head with frontal bossing, wide nasal bridge, upturned nose, long philtrum, and flared nostrils. Agenesis of the corpus callosum and cardiac defects have occurred.[179] Pyruvate dehydrogenase deficiency has been found in Leigh encephalopathy.[180]

FATTY ACID BETA-OXIDATION DEFECTS

The major metabolic flux of long-chain fatty acids is through the beta-oxidation system of the mitochondria, present in all cells except the mature erythrocyte. Access of the fatty acid to the beta-oxidation enzymes requires a carnitine-dependent transport system to cross the mitochondrial membrane.

Fatty acids are activated to acyl-CoAs at the outer mitochondrial membrane, converted to acylcarnitines by carnitine palmitoyl transferase (CPT) I, transported across the inner mitochondrial membrane by a translocase, and the fatty acid acyl-CoA regenerated by CPT II. The fatty acid acyl-CoA then undergoes beta-oxidation to generate acetyl-CoA. Beta-oxidation proceeds through a series of steps resulting in the release of acetyl-CoA and a fatty acid acyl-CoA derivative, which is shorter by two carbon groups than the original fatty acid. The enzymes of beta-oxidation are categorized as long-chain acyl-CoA dehydrogenase (LCAD)(C12), medium-chain acyl-CoA dehydrogenase (MCAD)(C6-C10), and short-chain acyl-CoA dehydrogenase (SCAD)(C4-6).

Inherited defects in the beta-oxidation pathway include LCAD, MCAD, and SCAD deficiency, inherited as autosomal recessive traits. Patients may present with episodes of hypoglycemia especially after fasting, but ketosis does not occur. In MCAD-deficiency medium-chain length metabolites are excreted, whereas in SCAD deficiency short-chain length fatty acid metabolites are excreted. Carnitine esters are increased, and free carnitine levels are low in the plasma, skeletal muscle, and liver. Coma may be a presenting sign. Pathologically there is fatty infiltration of the liver cells, muscle cells, and cardiac myocytes. The enzyme defects can be demonstrated in fibroblasts and leukocytes.

Carnitine deficiency

Carnitine deficiency impairs fatty acid transport across the mitochondrial membrane. Primary carnitine deficiency is classified into myopathic and systemic forms. In the myopathic form, progressive skeletal muscle weakness with myocyte lipid accumulation is found. Serum carnitine concentration is normal, but muscle carnitine is low. Systemic carnitine deficiency is characterized by low serum and tissue carnitine concentration and is responsive to supplemental carnitine.

Symptoms of cardiomyopathy, muscle weakness, hypotonia, hypoglycemia, hypoketonemia, and coma implicate a carnitine deficiency in many tissues including heart, skeletal muscle, and liver. Lipid accumulates in skeletal muscle in type I myocytes, liver, and frequently the cardiac muscle cells. Electron microscopy demonstrates abnormal mitochondria. Secondary carnitine deficiency may be associated with varied defects of intermediary metabolism.

UREA CYCLE DEFECTS

Ornithine transcarbamylase deficiency

Ornithine transcarbamylase (OTC) deficiency is an X-linked dominant disorder. Hemizygous males die in neonatal life, and the heterozygous females have a variably severe expression. In infants, hyperammonemia and oroticaciduria are noted, with reduction in plasma citrulline. The diagnosis may be made by enzyme assay of liver tissue. Prenatal diagnosis may be achieved by analysis of amniocytes.[181] In males, the liver is enlarged with focal cellular necrosis and steatosis. In older heterozygous females, the liver exhibits focal piecemeal necrosis, inflammation, steatosis, and fibrosis. Peroxisomal swelling and matrix rarefaction are the usual ultrastructural changes; mitochondria are usually normal. The central nervous system changes include Alzheimer type II astrocytes and spongiosis with hypomyelination and cerebellar heterotopias.

Carbamyl phosphate synthetase deficiency

Carbamyl phosphate synthetase (CPS) deficiency is an autosomal recessive disorder, usually characterized by a fulminant course in the newborn with hyperammonemia. Plasma citrulline and arginine levels are reduced. Prenatal diagnosis is possible by DNA analysis of amniocytes and enzyme assay of liver tissue. Pathologically the liver may show mild steatosis and focal cellular necrosis and progress to mild portal fibrosis.[182] Ultrastructurally, mitochondria may be normal, swollen, or pleomorphic with dense deposits in the matrix and abnormal cristae. Concentric endoplasmic reticulum with loss of microvilli may be present.[182] Alzheimer type II astrocytic changes and spongiosis are the usual findings in the central nervous system.

Citrullinemia

The autosomal recessive disorder citrullinemia causes pronounced hyperammonemia, with low plasma arginine and high plasma citrulline levels because of a deficiency of argininosuccinate synthetase. Enzyme assays may be performed on fibroblast or amniotic cell cultures. Neuropathologic changes are similar to those of the other urea cycle disorders. Steatosis and cellular necrosis may be found in the liver though cholestasis is more common.

Hyperornithinemia, hyperammonemia, homocitrullinuria syndrome (Haust)

The hyperornithinemia, hyperammonemia, homocitrullinuria (HHH) syndrome is an autosomal recessive disorder characterized by postprandial or intermittent hyperammonemia with increased plasma ornithine concentration and homocitrullinuria. Symptoms may begin in the newborn period or any time through adulthood. Hypotonia, seizures, or mental delay may occur.

Liver biopsy or light microscopy shows no abnormalities, but with electronmicroscopy, liver mitochondria are elongated with bizarre shapes and contain crystalloid structures. Abnormal mitochondria may also be found in muscle and leukocytes.

Argininosuccinicaciduria

Argininosuccinicaciduria (ASA) is an autosomal recessive disorder attributable to deficiency of argininosuccinic lyase. In the newborn, hyperammonemia develops with increased argininosuccinic acid in plasma and urine and elevation of plasma citrulline levels. Hepatomegaly and increased levels of transaminases are present. Microvesicular steatosis may be confused with Reye's syndrome. However, the mitochondrial changes seen in Reye's syndrome are not present. In the brain, hypomyelination and Alzheimer type II cells are present.

Argininemia

Argininemia is an inherited autosomal recessive disorder caused by deficiency of arginase and is characterized by progressive spastic diplegia, mental retardation, hyperammonemia that is usually mild, hepatomegaly, and elevation of transaminases. The hepatocytes may be swollen. Mitochondria are normal. Symptoms usually do not occur until after infancy in this disorder.

PEROXISOMAL DISORDERS

The peroxisomal diseases are genetically determined disorders, caused either by the failure to form or to maintain the peroxisome or by a defect in the function of a single peroxisomal enzyme (Table 14-3).

Peroxisomes play an important role in fatty acid oxidation.[183] Peroxisomal fatty acid oxidation is not dependent on carnitine[184] and is of particular importance for the oxidation of saturated very-long-chain fatty acids (VLCFA).[185] Abnormally high levels of VLCFAs in tissues and body fluids occur in many patients with peroxisomal disorders.

Peroxisomes contain a group of enzymes that oxidize a variety of substrates and thereby form hydrogen peroxide. The H_2O_2 thus formed is efficiently decomposed within the organelle by catalase, which is present in high concentration.

Peroxisomal disorders can be subdivided into two major groups. In the first, the organelle fails to be formed or to be maintained, resulting in the defective function of multiple peroxisomal enzymes. This defect is observed in Zellweger's syndrome, neonatal adrenoleukodystrophy, infantile Refsum's disease, and hyperpipecolicacidemia. In the second group there is a genetically determined deficiency of a single peroxisomal enzyme, and the peroxisome structure is intact; examples include X-linked adrenoleukodystrophy, acatalasemia, and others.

Rhizomelic chondrodysplasia punctata (RCDP) is placed in neither group because, at present, there is no general agreement concerning the peroxisomal defect in this disorder. It is characterized by mental retardation, rhizomelic shortening of the long bones, cataracts, and microcephaly.

As a result of complementation studies, these disorders are determined to be genetically heterogeneous and indicate that the relationships between phenotype and genotype are complex. For instance, Zellweger syndrome with its characteristic and consistent phenotype can be associated with at least four distinct genotypes.

Several diagnostic procedures aid the diagnosis of peroxisomal disorders.

1. Increased levels of very-long-chain saturated fatty acids in plasma,[186] red blood cells,[187] or cultured skin fibroblasts.[188] Elevated levels of saturated VLCFAs are the main abnormality in X-linked adrenoleukodystrophy, and this assay is indispensable for the diagnosis of this disorder.[189] VCLFA levels are also elevated in peroxisomal disorders,[190] except RCDP.[191]

Table 14-3 Abnormalities present in disorders of peroxisomes

Peroxisomes absent or reduced in number
Deficiency of catalase
Deficient synthesis and reduced tissue levels of plasmalogens
Defective oxidation and abnormal accumulation of very-long-chain fatty acids
Deficient oxidation and age-dependent accumulation of phytanic acid
Defects in certain steps of bile acid formation and accumulation of bile acid intermediates
Defects in oxidation and accumulation of L-pipecolic acid
Increased urinary excretion of dicarboxylic acids

2. Diminished levels of plasmalogen in red blood cells and defective plasmalogen synthesis is a feature in all the disorders of peroxisome biogenesis[192-195] and represents the most striking single abnormality in RCDP.[196]

3. Elevated pipecolic acid levels in plasma are present in nearly all patients with disorders of peroxisomes.

4. Elevated levels of plasma phytanic acid are the prime and characteristic abnormality in Refsum disease.[196]

5. For the demonstration of absent or abnormal peroxisomes in liver biopsy specimens by electron microscopy,[197] an elegant procedure has recently been described in which peroxisomal enzyme activities and immunoblot studies of peroxisomal fatty acid oxidation enzymes were performed in a rectal mucosal biopsy specimen.[198]

Prenatal diagnosis

Except for hyperoxaluria type 1, all peroxisomal disorders can be identified prenatally in the first or second trimester of pregnancy by chorion villus samples or in amniocytes by measurement of VLCFA[199] in cultured amniocytes or cultured chorion villus cells and assays of plasmalogen synthesis.[200] Direct utilization of chorion villus samples makes it possible to obviate the delay imposed by the requirement for tissue culture.

X-linked adrenoleukodystrophy

X-linked adrenoleukodystrophy was the first peroxisomal disorder to be described and is the most common. The basic defect in X-linked adrenoleukodystrophy is a specific impairment in the capacity to degrade VLCFAs,[201] a function that has been localized to the peroxisome.[185] Evidence indicates that the defect may involve the impaired capacity to activate VLCFAs, that is, defective function of the enzyme lignoceroyl-CoA synthetase.[202-206]

Development is usually normal until 4 to 8 years of age. Males exhibit a behavioral deficit that is progressive with emotional outbursts. Later, there is progressive deterioration until death, usually by 10 years.[189,207,208]

Adrenal insufficiency is the presenting manifestation in 15% to 30% of boys.[189,207,208] The adrenal glands are small, and cells in the zona fasciculata contain cytoplasmic lipid inclusions with a characteristic lamellar structure.[209] These inclusions consist of cholesterol esterified with saturated VLCFAs, such as hexacosanoic (C26:0) and tetracosanoic (C24:0) acids.[210] The same type of lipids accumulate in the central nervous system, causing severe demyelination that initially affects the posterior parietal or occipital regions.[189,207,208] Perivascular infiltration by lymphocytes is similar to that observed in multiple sclerosis. White matter involvement causes characteristic abnormalities in computed tomographic (CT) or magnetic resonance imaging (MRI) studies[209] caused by demyelination in the posterior portion of the brain, with a garland of accumulated contrast material.

The X-linked ALD gene has been mapped to the terminal segment of the long arm of the X chromosome (Xq28).[211] It is linked to an anonymous DNA probe (DXS52), and this is of diagnostic value particularly for the identification of heterozygotes.[212]

Zellweger syndrome

Zellweger syndrome is inherited as an autosomal recessive trait characterized by the absence of peroxisomes. Newborn infants with the Zellweger syndrome have a typical facies, neonatal seizures, and eye abnormalities. Infants with the Zellweger syndrome rarely live more than a few months.

Some atypical cases of the Zellweger syndrome (Versmold variant) have hypertonia and may live longer.[185,213] Increased serum iron content and evidence of tissue siderosis are diagnostically helpful.[214,215]

Major abnormalities are present in the liver, kidney, and brain. The hallmark finding is the absence of peroxisomes in the liver and kidney.[216] The defect is also present in cultured skin fibroblasts[217] and amniocytes.[218] The brain shows a striking and characteristic disorder of neuronal migration involving the cerebral hemispheres, the cerebellum, and the inferior olivary nucleus.[219,220] Other brain abnormalities include focal lissencephaly and other cerebral gyral abnormalities, heterotopic cerebral cortex, olivary nuclear dysplasia, defects of the corpus callosum, numerous lipid-laden macrophages and histiocytes in cortical and periventricular areas, and dysmyelination.[219]

The liver is usually enlarged and fibrotic with micronodular cirrhosis in one third of cases.[221,222] The kidneys show persistent fetal lobulations, and cortical renal cysts are frequent.[221,222] Numerous other abnormalities have been described.[223-227]

Neonatal adrenoleukodystrophy

Neonatal adrenoleukodystrophy (NALD) is a slightly less severe illness than the Zellweger syndrome, with fewer dysmorphic features. Peroxisomes in hepatocytes[228] or cultured skin fibroblasts[217] are not so severely diminished in number; thus VLCFA accumulation is less severe than in Zellweger syndrome. Patients may have micropolygyria[229] or only mild neuronal migrational defects and heterotopias.[230] Renal cysts are not observed in NALD.

Most NALD patients have an impaired adrenal cortisol response to ACTH stimulation, but overt adrenal insufficiency is infrequent. Their biochemical abnormalities are similar to those in patients with Zellweger syndrome.

Hyperpipecolicacidemia

The clinical features of hyperpipecolicacidemia closely resemble those of Zellweger syndrome in which there is also excretion of pipecolic acid; electron microscopy, however, shows the presence of peroxisomes in the liver, suggestive of a functional disorder of the peroxisome. Complementation studies have suggested that hyperpipecolicacidemia is allelic, with one form of Zellweger syndrome and with the infantile form of Refsum syndrome.[231,232]

Hyperoxaluria type I

There are two types of genetically determined hyperoxaluria. The type 1 form is somewhat more common and exhibits hyperoxaluria with increased excretion of glycolic and glyoxylic acid, whereas the type 2 form is accompanied by increased excretion of L-glyceric acid.[233] The mode of inheritance is autosomal recessive.

Patients have a deficiency of the enzyme alanine: glyoxylate aminotransferase, which catalyzes the conversion of glyoxylate to glycine. This reaction results in the accumulation of glyoxylate, which is also converted to oxalic acid. The enzyme is localized in the peroxisome.[234,235]

In hyperoxaluria type 1 renal calculi are common, with deposition of oxalate crystals in the kidneys, bones, conduction system of the heart, and testes. Patients experience progressive renal failure, multiple fractures, and death before 20 years of age. Diagnosis depends on demonstration of excessive quantities of glyoxylate, oxalate, and glycolic acid in the urine. The specific enzyme defect can be demonstrated by percutaneous liver biopsy. Kidney transplantation is of limited benefit because of the reaccumulation of oxalate crystals in the transplanted kidney.[233]

Acatalasemia

The majority of persons with acatalasemia are free of symptoms.[236] The disorder appears to be heterogeneous. The human catalase gene has been cloned[237] and mapped to chromosome 11p13.[238] Deletions in this region may be associated with Wilms tumor, aniridia, and hypocatalasemia.[238]

Classic Refsum disease

In classic Refsum disease, inherited as autosomal recessive, there is an isolated defect of phytanic acid oxidation. This leads to accumulation of phytanic acid in tissues and body fluids.[196] Peroxisome structure and function are intact.[239] Manifestations include retinitis pigmentosa, hearing loss, peripheral neuropathy, and cerebellar ataxia. Cardiac arrhythmias or conduction defects may occur when phytanic acid levels are very high. A rare, autosomal recessive form, termed *infantile Refsum disease,* has been described.[230]

Rhizomelic chondrodysplasia punctata (RCDP)

Rhizomelic chondrodysplasia punctata (RCDP) is autosomal recessive and differs from the single-enzyme disorders, since at least two and possibly three separate peroxisomal functions are deficient. In RCDP there is a profound defect in plasmalogen synthesis, more severe than that in Zellweger syndrome, defective phytanic acid oxidation, and failure to process the thiolase enzyme.[191,240,241] Levels of VLCFA, bile acids, and pipecolic acid are normal. Peroxisome structure is abnormal. Peroxisomes may be absent in many hepatocytes or be huge and irregularly shaped.

MITOCHONDRIAL DISORDERS

Mitochondria are present in all eukaryotic cells that depend on the aerobic metabolism. A disease caused by abnormal mitochondrial energy production was first described in 1962 by Luft and colleagues.[242] Mitochondrial cristae divide the mitochondria into separated compartments, each harboring specific biochemical structures. The largest compartment inside the mitochondrion is called a *matrix.* Its many functions include the citric acid (Krebs) cycle and fatty acid oxidation pathways. The mitochondrial genome and its protein synthetic machinery for mitochondrially coded polypeptides is also confined to the matrix.

Mitochondria are unique cytoplasmic organelles by virtue of having their own genome, the mitochondrial DNA (mtDNA). The mtDNA of all cells has its origin in the unfertilized ovum. Although spermatozoa contain mitochondria, no paternal mtDNA has been demonstrated in the human zygote. Consequently, mtDNA is inherited exclusively from the mother.[243] Maternal or cytoplasmic inheritance has several unique features differing from the mendelian traits.[244] When mutant mtDNA is present in the ovum, it is transmitted to all offspring, resulting in larger numbers of affected individuals than in autosomal dominant traits. The clinical traits will differ, reflecting unequal distribution of normal and abnormal mitochondria.

Mitochondrial function involves hundreds of enzymes performing active transportation and oxidation of substrates while generating ATP. Inherited defects of each of the main biochemical sets of reactions are known. The majority of them are inherited as Mendelian traits, with autosomal recessive transmission being the most common. Mitochondrial inheritance provides for ranges of mitochondrial diseases.[245-249]

The contemporary classification,[245] based on the biochemical defects, is linked with the molecular genetic findings of the patients. All disorders caused by mitochondrial DNA defects and intergenomic signaling defects impair respiratory chain or oxidative phosphorylation.

Pathology

Clinical and laboratory findings in mitochondrial disorders are diverse. Lacticacidemia is a common laboratory finding in mitochondrial dysfunction. Diagnosis of mitochondrial disorders is multidisciplinary. The key diagnostic procedures include detailed enzyme determinations and molecular analysis of mtDNA. The enzyme defects are usually assayed in fresh muscle samples, but cultured fibroblasts have proved very rewarding in problematic cases, and they provide fresh cells for repeated enzyme measurements. Analysis of mtDNA is a relatively easy procedure in modern laboratories. With the aid of the polymerase chain reaction it is possible to show the changes in the mtDNA from very small samples. Old paraffin embedded tissue specimens have shown to be an excellent source of mtDNA.

The morphologic changes associated with mitochondrial dysfunction are divided into two groups. In the first, abnormalities are associated directly with altered number and structure of the mitochondria. Secondary degenerative and destructive changes are attributable to impaired function of the mitochondria.

Electron microscopy reveals an increased number and size of mitochondria. Especially characteristic are giant mitochondria, with concentric tubular, reticular, lamellar, or otherwise dissociated cristae.[250] The mitochondrial matrix may be swollen and contain large spherical dense bodies, vacuoles, or crystals. The rectangular crystals are often arranged in blocks of parallel crystals, "parking-lot" configuration. They contain proteins, and at least two different types of crystals are known.[250]

Information gained from light and electron microscopic investigation of suspected mitochondrial disorders is usually limited. The changes are confined to the defects of the respiratory chain or of oxidation-phosphorylation coupling, but they are not present in disorders of substrate utilization.[246] In many disorders of the oxidative phosphorylation mitochondria are morphologically normal. On the other hand, ragged red fibers (RRF) and accompanying electron microscopic findings are occasionally seen in a small proportion of muscle fibers in neuromuscular disorders other than mitochondriopathies. Zidovudine, a drug used to treat AIDS, causes myopathy with RRF.[251] Absent or weak histochemical cytochrome oxidase (COX) activity is seen in some but not in all mitochondrial disorders because of complex IV defects. Moderately increased fat droplets and glycogen are often seen in association of RRF, but extensive fatty infiltration of the muscle and liver is more characteristic for carnitine-transport defects and impaired fatty acid oxidation.[252]

Subacute *necrotizing encephalomyelopathy* (SNE), or Leigh syndrome, is relatively common in association with defects of oxidative phosphorylation. It is characterized by symmetric basal lesions extending from the thalamus to the pons, inferior olives of the medulla, and posterior columns of the spinal cord.[253] Histologically, SNE shows necrosis astrocytosis and vascular proliferation. A few cases of SNE have been described in association of defects of the pyruvate dehydrogenase complex, but most are caused by dysfunction of the respiratory chain, often a COX defect.[254]

A distinctive pattern of destructive brain lesions is seen in mitochondriopathies caused by deletions and *point mutations* of the mtDNA, Kearns-Sayre, myopathy-encephalopathy-lacticacidosis-stroke (MELAS), and myoclonic epilepsy–ragged red fibers (MERRF) syndromes.[255] Status spongiosus, neuronal degeneration, gliosis, demyelinization, necrosis, and mineral deposits are seen in various grades and localizations of brain in these disorders.

Secondary changes in tissues other than brain and muscle are poorly known and related to the clinical picture of the diseases.[256-258]

DISORDERS OF METAL METABOLISM

Neonatal iron storage disease

Neonatal iron storage disease, or perinatal hemochromatosis, is an uncommon disorder. It is clinically and pathologically defined by severe liver disease of intrauterine onset associated with extrahepatic siderosis that spares the reticuloendothelial system.[259-263] Attempts to identify a primary disorder of iron handling in neonatal hemochromatosis have not been successful, and evidence now indicates that hemochromatotic siderosis in the perinate may be a sequel of intrauterine liver disease. Several laboratory abnormalities are present.[264]

The presence of hyperferritinemia supports the diagnosis of neonatal hemochromatosis. An autosomal recessive or codominant inheritance has been postulated; alternatively, this disorder may be related to a latent maternal viral infection affecting the fetal liver.[259] Grossly, the liver weighs less than normal, is fibrotic and cirrhotic, and may be bile stained. Cholestasis and giant cell transformation are found in all cases, and there is massive accumulation of iron in liver cells[265] with lesser quantities in biliary epithelium and Kupffer cells. Diffuse interacinar fibrosis, cholangiolar proliferation and cirrhosis may be present at birth.[263,267,268] Hyperplasia and hypertrophy of the islets of Langerhans are constant findings. Iron may accumulate in extrahepatic sites.[268,269]

Wilson's disease

Wilson disease is an inborn error of copper metabolism with autosomal recessive inheritance. The basic defect has not been defined, but there is abnormal copper metabolism. Elevated levels of serum and hepatic copper and decreased liver serum ceruloplasmin are characteristic, though in some cases the serum ceruloplasmin values may be normal. Although a normal serum copper concentration excludes Wilson's disease, an elevated concentration is not diagnostic because serum copper may be increased in other forms of liver disease, especially cholestatic disorders and chronic active hepatitis. Incorporation of radioactive copper into ceruloplasmin is considered the most reliable test for Wilson's disease.

Most symptoms reflect hepatic involvement, such as acute hepatitis and hepatic failure in the very young patient. Hemolytic anemia, central nervous system signs, and Kayser-Fleischer rings develop during the course of the disease.

Pathology

The pathologic effects on the liver, kidneys, and brain are considered to be directly related to the accumulation of copper ions.

In the precirrhotic stage of Wilson's disease, the changes resemble a chronic, active hepatitis with focal necrosis, scattered acidophilic bodies, and moderate to severe steatosis.[270] Glycogenated nuclei in periportal hepatocytes are a typical finding in Wilson's disease. Kupffer's cells are hypertrophied and may contain hemosiderin. In later stages, periportal fibrosis, portal inflammation, and finally cirrhosis occur.

Submassive or massive hepatocellular necrosis may occur; the clinical and biochemical findings in such cases may resemble those of chronic active hepatitis.[270-273]

The cirrhosis of Wilson's disease is macronodular, or macronodular and micronodular, with periportal fibrosis, cholangiolar proliferation, and lymphocytic infiltration.[274]

The presence of copper may not be cytochemically demonstrable in the precirrhotic stage. In young, asymptomatic patients, the copper is diffusely distributed in the cytoplasm but later accumulates in lysosomes.[275] Rhodamine and rubeanic acid stains specifically detect the presence of copper.[276,277] Copper-associated protein can be stained with orcein or aldehyde fuchsin.[278,279]

The ultrastructural changes in Wilson's disease are pathognomonic.[270,280,281] The mitochondria show pronounced pleomorphism, intracristal spaces widen, and microcysts form at the tips of the cristae.[280] Copper deposits are extremely electron dense.

A major copper-binding protein in Wilson's disease is metallothionein. It has been suggested that the liver damage in Wilson's disease may be attributable to the toxic ionic form of copper, which saturates the binding sites of metallothionein.[282]

Treatment has been the use of penicillamine as a chelating agent; however, more recently the use of succimer has been more effective. If advanced liver disease occurs, transplantation will be effective and curative.

Menkes syndrome

Inherited as an X-linked recessive trait of copper metabolism, Menkes' kinky hair syndrome is characterized by a defect in intestinal copper absorption resulting in a low serum level of copper and ceruloplasmin in male infants.[283,284] The phenotype is characterized by sparse, coarse, and brittle hair (pili torti),[285] pudgy cheeks, and skeletal changes including wormian bones, metaphyseal widening, particularly of the ribs and femora and lateral spurs, progressive cerebral deterioration with seizures, and widespread arterial elongation and tortuosity attributable to deficiency of copper-dependent cross-linking in the internal elastic membrane of the arterial wall. By histofluorescence, for the identification of catecholamines, peculiar torpedo-like swellings of catecholamine-containing axons are seen in the peripheral nerve tracts and there are reduced numbers of adrenogenic fibers in the midforebrain.[286] Progressive neurologic deterioration leads to death in infancy.

OTHER METABOLIC DISORDERS

Neuronal ceroid-lipofuscinosis (Batten disease)

Neuronal ceroid-lipofuscinoses (NCL) encompass disorders sharing features of progressive psychomotor retardation and accumulation of large amounts of lipopigments in neural and extraneural cells. Historically, NCL was included in amaurotic family idiocy (AFI), a familial progressive neurologic disease characterized by impaired psychomotor development, blindness, and early death.[287] The group was later divided into Tay-Sachs disease (G_{M2}-gangliosidosis discussed previously) and NCL. The term *neuronal ceroid-lipofuscinosis* was coined by Zeman and Dyken,[288] who demonstrated that the autofluorescent lipopigment showed tinctorial characteristics of ceroid and lipofuscin in histologic specimens.

Because of the long history of AFI, different types and variants of the disease have carried a surfeit of eponymic designations. Neuronal ceroid-lipofuscinosis and Batten disease are common names. The different syndromes are separated by descriptive adjectives, such as infantile and juvenile. Current names of the different syndromes with some favored eponym are presented in Table 14-4. Uncommon and very rare variants of NCL are described in special reviews.[289,290]

NCL occurs worldwide. It is the most common hereditary neurodegenerative disorder in children, with an estimated incidence of 1:12,500 in the USA.[291] The lipopigments in NCL accumulate in the lysosomes, but the metabolic derangement causing the storage phenomenon is unknown. Whether the discovery of accumulation of the normal subunit c of ATP-synthase in the stored material of NCL helps to unravel the biochemical pathogenesis of these disorders remains to be seen.[292] DNA-linkage studies have shown that the gene responsible for juvenile NCL is located in chromosome 16 (16p12)[293] and that of infantile NCL in chromosome 1 (1p32),[294] whereas the gene for the late infantile NCL is excluded from both of these chromosomes.

Pathology

The accumulating lipopigment is autofluorescent (Fig. 14-10), stains positively with PAS, Sudan black B, oil red O, and acid fuchsin. Only slight differences in the staining characteristic of the lipopigment in different syndromes have been noted.[295] The lipopigment granules show intense acid phosphatase activity, and they are encased by a trilaminar unit membrane in electron microscopy indicating lysosomal resid-

Table 14-4 Neuronal ceroid-lipofuscinosis (NCL), or Batten disease

Type of NCL	Abbreviations and synonyms
Infantile	INCL; Santavuori-Haltia
Late infantile	LINCL; Jansky-Bielschowsky
Juvenile	JNCL; Spielmeyer-Sjögren
Adult	Kufs' disease

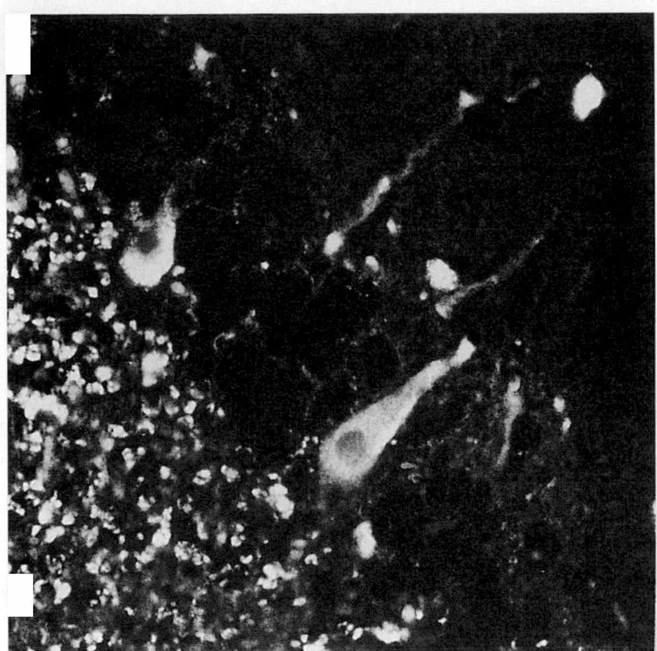

Fig. 14-10 A section of the cerebellum of juvenile neuronal ceroid-lipofuscinosis (NCL). Autofluorescent material is present in the cell bodies and dendrites of the Purkinje cells as well as in the cells of the granular layer.

ual body structure. Lipopigments are very resistant to polar and nonpolar solvents, rendering them visible in ordinary paraffin sections.

Ultrastructurally the lipopigment contains residual bodies, or cytosomes, of variable morphology. According to the fine structure, the cytosomes can be divided into three principal types (Table 14-5). The first type is homogeneous, electron dense, and finely granular without any, or only occasional, membranous structures. Some of the cytosomes seem to be formed as spherical globules about 0.2 to 0.5 μm in diameter. They are called *granular osmiophilic deposits* (GROD). The deposits of the second type are more elaborate and show crescentic or horseshoe-shaped dark profiles. The curved profiles consist of stacks of lamellae with alternating dark and light lines of about 4 μm in thickness. Each stack contains from two to six pale and dark lines. These bodies are called *cytosomes with curvilinear profiles* (CCP). The third type forms structures superficially resembling fingerprints and are therefore named "cytosomes with fingerprint profiles" (CFP). They are composed of groups of curved parallel paired dark lines separated by a thin clear space. The fine structure of the NCL cytosomes may occasionally be modified or distorted, and in some cases different so-called membranous bodies may be seen,[296] but one or the other of the basic patterns usually prevails.

The diagnosis of a clinical syndrome based solely on the ultrastructural findings is not warranted.[290]

Infantile NCL (Santavuori-Haltia)

The clinical onset of the disorder infantile NCL (Santavuori-Haltia) is between 8 and 14 months of age. It runs a relentless, rapid course of psychomotor deterioration, and the patients become unresponsive at about 3 years of age and bedridden until death ensues between 6 and 15 years of age.[297]

The neuropathology[298,299] shows extremely atrophic brains at autopsy and weighing from 250 to 400 g. Extreme degrees of gyral atrophy are present, and the atrophic cortex can hardly be distinguished from the shrunken and tough white matter encircling the dilated ventricles. The cerebellum is likewise very atrophic.

The neurons accumulate lipopigments early, and there are signs of neuronal destruction together with astrocytosis and macrophagocytosis. Both astrocytes and macrophages harbor lipopigments. After this stage up to 4 years of age, subtotal loss of cortical neurons is evident, and the cortex is occupied by astrocytes and large amounts of macrophages. The white matter undergoes demyelinization. After 4 years of age the cerebral cortex is totally devoid of neurons, axons, and myelin sheaths. The retina degenerates to the same extent as the cerebral cortex. In the spinal cord and autonomic ganglion cells the cytoplasm is filled with the storage material, but neuronal destruction is not seen.

The storage cytosomes can be detected by electron microscopic investigation of skin,[300,301] ocular conjunctiva,[302] skeletal muscle,[303] rectal mucosa,[304] and lymphocytes.[305] Electron microscopic investigation of the skin biopsy specimen is probably the most used diagnostic method. Diagnostic cytosomes of INCL are most easily found in the cytoplasm of the endothelial cells in different organs. Investigation of the autonomic ganglion cells of the rectal mucosal biopsy specimens is also rewarding.[304]

Late infantile NCL (Jansky-Bielschowsky)

The classical late infantile NCL (LINCL) has its clinical onset between 2 and 4 years of age. Symptoms include epilepsy, followed by rapid deterioration of vision and psychomotor functions. The patient enters a vegetative stage 2 to 4 years after the onset and dies soon thereafter.[306]

The macroscopic neuropathologic findings are similar to those of INCL but are considerably milder. The neuroepithelium and ganglionic nerve cells of the retina are destroyed and are accompanied by optic atrophy.[307]

Table 14-5 **Electron microscopic types of cytosomes in neuronal ceroid-lipofuscinosis (NCL)**

Cytosome	Abbreviation	Predominant disease
Granular osmiophilic deposits	GROD	INCL
Cytosomes with curvilinear profiles	CCP	LINCL
Cytosomes with fingerprint profiles	CFP	JNCL
Combination of CCP and CFP		Adult NCL
Unspecific electron-dense inclusions		All types

Diagnosis is made by electron microscopic investigation of skin, conjunctiva, rectal mucosa, or lymphocytes. The prevailing electron microscopic inclusion is that of CCP. In skin, inclusions are common in the epithelium of the secretory coils of sweat glands, but they are also easily found in the variety of cells of skin specimens.

Juvenile NCL (Spielmeyer-Sjögren)

Juvenile NCL is a slowly progressing neurologic disease. Impaired vision usually becomes evident between 4 and 7 years. Mental retardation develops slowly. Parkinsonian motor dysfunction and seizures appear late in the disease. There is a wide clinical variation of JNCL. Some patients die in the first years of the second decade, and some live to 40 years of age.[308]

The brains of JNCL patients are less atrophic than those of INCL and LINCL. Yellow brown discoloration of the moderately narrowed gray matter of the cerebral cortex is present. The white matter is slightly atrophic but not so severely demyelinized as in LINCL and INCL.

In the cortical neurons, the proximal axons are distended by the lipopigment, whereas in the Purkinje cells, the dendritic processes are distended.

As in the other types of NCL, lipopigment accumulation is easily found in many extraneural cells, best appreciated by the electron microscopic investigation of the biopsy specimens.[309] One manifestation of the extraneural storage, not requiring electron microscopy, is the presence of vacuolated blood lymphocytes. Vacuolated lymphocytes are not seen in NCL other than in JNCL.

In electron microscopy the cytosomes show predominantly fingerprint profiles (FP), but mixtures of curvilinear (Fig. 14-11) and fingerprint profiles (Fig. 14-12) in the same cytosome are common, and cytosomes containing curvilinear profiles (CP) are also found. This applies particularly to many extraneural tissues.[304] In skin biopsy specimens the diagnostic cytosomes are sometimes exclusively in the secretory coils of sweat glands, and a biopsy specimen without the sweat glands may render false-negative results.[309] Although the CCP and GROD are usually tightly packed within the lysosomal membrane, part of the FP inclusions are within cytoplasmic vacuoles with an abundant clear space around them. This is the case in the lymphocytes and in the autonomic ganglion cells of the gut wall.[310,311]

Adult NCL (Kufs disease)

Adult NCL is the least common type of the classical NCL. Clinically and genetically heterogeneous, there are at least two clinical types, one with progressive myoclonus epilepsy and another with abnormal behavior and dementia.[312] Both autosomal recessive and dominant patterns of inheritance are known.[313] The usual age of clinical onset is about 30 years, but occurs occasionally in adolescence. A distinct feature is that Kufs' disease patients do not become blind. The patients live long with their disease.

Brains show slight atrophy. The cortex shows dark yellow discoloration. The cerebellum is macroscopically atrophic in autopsied cases. Histologic investigation reveals mild and patchy loss of neurons and almost total disappearance of the Purkinje cells in the cerebellum.[314,315]

Presence of cytosomes with FP and CP in skeletal muscle, perivascular smooth muscle cells of several visceral organs, and eccrine sweat glands have been reported.[312,313,315]

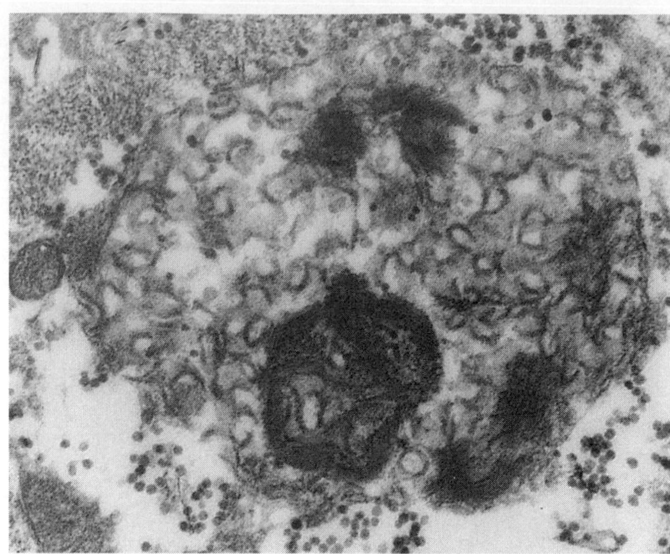

Fig. 14-11 A storage inclusion of late infantile NCL showing curvilinear profiles together with some poorly defined electron-dense material.

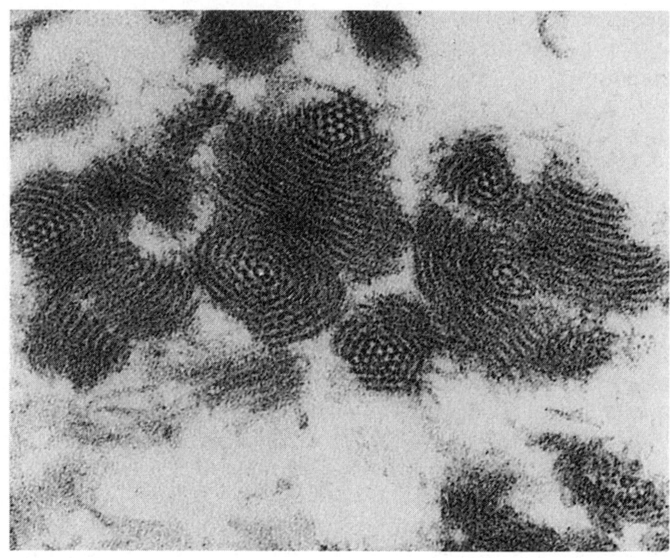

Fig. 14-12 Contents of a storage inclusion of juvenile NCL showing the fingerprint pattern.

Prenatal diagnosis of NCL

Prenatal diagnosis of each of the childhood types of NCL has been made. Electron microscopic demonstration of typical cytosomes has been demonstrated in free-floating amniotic cells of a pregnancy at risk for LINCL[316] and another pregnancy at risk of JNCL showed fingerprint inclusions in the trophoblastic cells of a chorion villus specimen.[317] A large number of pregnancies at risk for INCL have been subjected to chorionic villus biopsy in the first trimester of pregnancy and the specimens studied by electron microscopy. The affected fetuses show typical GROD in the endothelial cell cytoplasm of the chorionic villi. GRODs are found in the central nervous system and visceral organs of the fetuses after termination of the pregnancy.[318]

Another approach to the prenatal diagnosis is DNA-linkage analysis of the chorionic villus specimens. Prenatal diagnosis of INCL has been made simultaneously with electron microscopy and DNA linkage in increasing numbers of risky pregnancies with fully concordant results.[319] Prenatal diagnosis of JNCL is also possible by employing the DNA linkage studies.

Differential diagnosis of NCL

Differential diagnosis in variant types having the clinical onset in the age range of JNCL but with the clinical picture more like LINCL is problematic.[320]

The electron microscopy must be interpreted with caution. The presence of one or the other of the typical cytosomes in several cells confirms the diagnosis of NCL, but this does not fully separate the different types. Normal cells contain occasional inclusions reminiscent of those in NCL, and the electron microscopist must be aware of them.[321,322]

An overview of the main clinical and neurophysiologic findings of different types of NCL are presented in Table 14-6.

All types of NCL are found worldwide; some, however, are clustered in certain populations. JNCL has an unusually high prevalence in Sweden.[323] Another cluster of LINCL and a variant of JNCL are found in the small population of Newfoundland.[324] INCL is unusually common in the population of Finland with an incidence of 1:20,000.[308] Worldwide the JNCL and LINCL are the most common types.

The clinical and neurophysiologic features of NCL are shown in Table 14-5.

Cystic fibrosis of pancreas

Cystic fibrosis is a common metabolic disorder inherited as autosomal recessive trait and characterized by steatorrhea and malnutrition, resulting from pancreatic exocrine insufficiency, combined with severe pulmonary disease and disturbances in the secretion of sweat glands and mucus-secreting glands. In whites it is estimated to occur in 1 in 2000 to 1 in 3000 liveborn infants with equal sex occurrence.

The defect has now been clearly identified as a mutation of a specific gene, the cystic fibrosis transmembrane regulator (CFTR) gene, on chromosome 7. The most common mutation results in a protein defective in phenylalanine at position 508, referred to as ΔF508; in addition, more than 120 other mutations have been identified.

The pathology has been extensively reviewed. The most severe form of the disease is meconium ileus in which meconium is so viscid it results in intestinal obstruction and even rupture leading to meconium peritonitis. The *pancreas* in a severe case contains dilated and cystic ducts filled with inspissated secretion. The acini may be completely destroyed by fibrosis; the islets are usually intact. Nasal polyps, salivary glands, duodenum, small bowel, and appendix are the sites of accumulation of eosinophilic secretions. The *lung* changes also present a wide range. Grossly, there are always alternating zones of emphysema and atelectasis, depending on whether the obstruction by viscid secretions has been partial or complete. Secondary infection is usually attributable to *Staphylococcus aureus* or *Pseudomonas aeruginosa* and leads to severe bronchitis and bronchiectasis. In longstanding cases, especially where vitamin A lack and infection coexist, there is often squamous metaplasia of the tracheobronchial mucosa. At the time of death, the entire tracheobronchial tree is usually filled with dense purulent material. In 90% of cases, this yields a pure culture. In the *liver* a focal biliary cirrhosis occurs in 10% of infants up to 3 months and 25% over 1 year of age.

The standard methods of diagnosis rely on either detection of abnormal chloride secretion in sweat or, in newborns, on elevated immunoreactive trypsinogen and, for prenatal diagnosis, measurement of microvillar enzymes in amniotic fluid.

Table 14-6 Clinical and neurophysiologic features of neuronal ceroid-lipofuscinosis (NCL)

Feature	INCL	LINCL	JNCL	Adult NCL
Age of onset	8-18 months	2-4 years	4-8 years	30 years
Mental retardation	Early	Late	Late	Late
Visual failure	Relatively early	Late	Early, leading symptom	Not present
Ataxia	Moderate to severe	Pronounced	Pronounced	Variable
Myoclonius	Constant	Constant	Mild to moderate	Severe, leading symptom in part of the patients
Nonambulant	8-30 months	3-5 years	13-28 years	Over 35 years
Retinal pigment aggregations	Not present	Rare	Constant	Not present
EEG	Isoelectric by 3 years	Spikes inducible	Unspecific by low photic stimulation	Sensitivity to low photic stimulation
VEP Flash-evoked visual potential	Abolished 2 to 4 years	Early high	Early abnormal	High
SEP Somatosensory evoked potential	Low	High	Variable	Variable, high
Vacuolated lymphocytes*	Negative	Negative	Positive	Negative
Age at death	8-14 years	6-15 years	13-40 years	Over 40 years

*Cases from the past have been diagnosed with this material.
INCL, infantile form; *LINCL*, late infantile form; *JNCL*, juvenile form.

However, DNA probes are the most valuable diagnostic procedures. DNA can be isolated and used in a polymerase chain reaction to detect the ΔF508 (the most common mutation in the white population), Δ1507, G551D, R553X, and S549N mutations. With these DNA analyses up to 95% of all cystic fibrosis mutations can be detected.

Alpha-1-antitrypsin (Alpha-1-antiprotease) deficiency

Alpha-1-antitrypsin (α_1-AT), a glycoprotein of molecular weight 52 kD, is a major plasma protease inhibitor and accounts for 80% of serum X_1 globulin. The physiologic substrate is elastase, particularly important for the integrity of the lower respiratory tract. The Pi locus (protease inhibitor) for α_1-AT is on chromosome 14 at 14 q32.1, close to the locus for the Pi alpha-1-chymotrypsin. α_1-AT shows considerable genetic variability; there are more than 60 genetic variants. For the most common variants, letters are used according to their electrophoretic mobility F (fast), S (slow), Z (very slow). The normal phenotype is PiMM and has 100% activity. The phenotype of the most severe form of α_1-AT deficiency is PiZZ with 10% to 20% activity. α_1-AT is retained in the cytoplasm of the cell. In children, liver involvement is most frequent where the hepatocytes contain eosinophilic hyalin-like globules usually in periportal hepatocytes. With periodic acid–Schiff staining followed by diastase, the inclusions are easily visualized as brilliant pink globules in the cytoplasm. In newborn infants, the intracytoplasmic inclusions may be fine, granular, and indistinguishable from other granules such as bile. Immunohistochemical stains are useful to confirm the identity of the material using an antibody to α_1-AT. By electron microscopy the storage material is present within the cisternae of the endoplasmic reticulum. The most common type of liver involvement is characterized by conjugated hyperbilirubinemia, raised serum aminotransferases, and frequently hepatosplenomegaly. In addition to giant cell transformation, hepatocellular injury, and fibrosis, cholestasis and bile duct proliferation can be seen in liver biopsy specimens. Liver cell carcinoma has been reported in this disease.

In adults α_1-AT is most frequently associated with panlobular emphysema in the lower lobes of the lung. In PiZZ patients, the incidence of cirrhosis or emphysema is approximately 40%.

REFERENCES

1. Garrod AE: *Inborn errors of metabolism,* London, 1909, Oxford Press.
2. Beaudet AL, Scriver CR, Sly WS et al: Genetics and biochemistry of variant human phenotypes. In Scriver CR, Beaudet AL, Sly WS, et al, editors: *The metabolic basis of inherited disease,* ed 6, New York, 1989, McGraw-Hill.
3. Fernandes J, Saudubray J-M, Tada K, editors: *Inborn metabolic diseases: diagnosis and treatment,* Berlin, 1990, Springer-Verlag.
4. Applegarth DA, Dimmick JE, Toone JR: Laboratory detection of metabolic disease, *Pediatr Clin North Am* 36:49, 1989.
5. Ishak KG, Sharp HL: Metabolic errors and liver disease. In MacSween RNM, Anthony PP, Scheuer PJ, editors: *Pathology of the liver,* Edinburgh, 1987, Churchill Livingstone.
6. Vogler C, Rosenberg HS, Williams JC et al: Electron microscopy in the diagnosis of lysosomal storage diseases, *Am J Med Genet Suppl* 3:243, 1987.
7. O'Brien JS, Bernett J, Veath ML et al: Lysosomal storage disorders: diagnosis by ultrastructural examination of skin biopsy specimens, *Arch Neurol* 32:592, 1975.
8. Kronick JB, Scriver CR, Goodyer PR et al: A perimortem protocol for suspected genetic disease, *Pediatrics* 71:960, 1983.

Storage diseases

9. McKusick VA: *Mendelian inheritance in man: catalogue of autosomal dominant recessive and X-linked phenotypes,* ed 10, Baltimore, 1994, John Hopkins University Press.
10. Scriver CR, Beaudet AL, Sly WS, Valle D, editors: *The metabolic and molecular bases of inherited disease,* ed 7, New York, 1995, McGraw-Hill.
11. Muller C: Xanthomata, hypercholesterolemia, angina pectoris, *Acta Med Scand Suppl* 89:75, 1938.
12. Brown MS, Goldstein JL: A receptor-mediated pathway for cholesterol homeostasis, *Science* 232:34, 1986.
13. Breckenridge WC, Little JA, Steiner G et al: Hypertriglyceridemia associated with deficiency of apolipoprotein C-II, *N Engl J Med* 298:1265, 1978.
14. Mahley RW, Innerarity TL, Rall SC Jr et al: Lipoproteins of special significance in atherosclerosis: insights provided by studies of type III hyperlipoproteinemia, *Ann NY Acad Sci* 454:209, 1985.
15. Fredrickson DS: The inheritance of high density lipoprotein deficiency (Tangier disease), *J Clin Invest* 43:228, 1964.
16. Bassen FA, Kornzweig AL: Malformation of the erythrocytes in a case of retinitis pigmentosa, *Blood* 5:381, 1950.
17. Salt HB, Wolff OH, Lloyd JK et al: On having no beta-lipoprotein: a syndrome comprising abetalipoproteinemia, acanthocytosis, and steatorrhea, *Lancet* 2:325, 1960.
18. Norum KR, Gjone E: Familial serum-cholesterol esterification failure: a new inborn error of metabolism, *Biochem Biophys Acta* 144:698, 1967.
19. Carlson LA: Fish eye disease: a new familial condition with massive corneal opacities and dyslipoproteinemias: clinical and laboratory studies in two afflicted families, *Eur J Clin Invest* 12:41, 1982.
20. von Gierke E: Hepato-nephro-megalia Glykogenia (Glycogenspeicherkrankheit der Leber und Nieren), *Beitr Pathol Anat* 82:487, 1929.
21. Cori GT, Cori CF: Glucose-6-phosphatase of the liver in glycogen storage disease, *J Biol Chem* 199:661, 1952.
22. Howell RR, Stevenson RE, Ben-Menachem Y et al: Hepatic adenomata with type I glycogen storage disease, *J Nucl Med* 19:354, 1978.
23. Malatack JJ, Finegold DN, Iwatsuki S et al: Liver transplantation for type I glycogen storage disease, *Lancet* 1:1073, 1983.
24. Narisawa K, Igarashi Y, Otomo H et al: A new variant of glycogen storage disease type I probably due to a defect in the glucose-6-phosphate transport system, *Biochem Biophys Res Commun* 83:1360, 1978.
25. Arion WJ, Lange AJ, Walls HE et al: Evidence for the participation of independent translocases for phosphate and glucose-6-phosphate in the microsomal glucose-6-phosphate system, *J Biol Chem* 255:10396, 1980.
26. Pompe JC: Over idiopatische hypertrophie van het hart, *Ned T Geneesk* 76:304, 1932.
27. Hers HG: Inborn lysosomal diseases, *Gastroenterology* 48:625, 1965.
28. Martiniuk F, Mehler M, Tzall S et al: Extensive genetic heterogeneity in patients with acid alpha glucosidase deficiency as detected by abnormalities of DNA and mRNA, *Am J Hum Genet* 47:73, 1990.
29. Hers HG: α-glucosidase deficiency in generalized glycogen storage disease (Pompe's disease), *Biochem J* 86:11, 1963.
30. Danon MJ, Oh SJ, DiMauro S et al: Lysosomal glycogen storage disease with normal acid maltase, *Neurology* 31:51, 1981.
31. Antopol W, Boas EP, Levison W et al: Cardiac hypertrophy caused by glycogen storage disease in a 15-year-old boy, *Am Heart J* 20:546, 1940.
32. Forbes GB: Glycogen storage disease: report of a case with abnormal glycogen structure in liver and skeletal muscle, *J Pediat* 42:645, 1953.
33. Illingworth B, Cori GT, Cori CF: Amylo-1,6-glucosidase in muscle tissue in generalized glycogen storage disease, *J Biol Chem* 218:123, 1956.
34. Andersen DH: Familial cirrhosis of the liver with storage of abnormal glycogen, *Lab Invest* 5:11, 1956.
35. Brown BI, Brown DH: Lack of an α-1,4-glucan 6-glycosyl transferase in a case of type IV glycogenosis, *Proc Natl Acad Sci US* 56:725, 1966.
36. Selby R, Starzl TE, Yunis E et al: Liver transplantation for type IV glycogen storage disease, *N Engl J Med* 324:39, 1991.
37. McArdle B: Myopathy due to a defect in muscle glycogen breakdown, *Clin Sci* 10:13, 1951.

38. Schmid R, Mahler R: Chronic progressive myopathy with myoglobinuria: demonstration of a glycogenolytic defect in the muscle, *J Clin Invest* 38:2044, 1959.
39. Servidei S, Schanske S, Zeviani M et al: McArdle's disease: biochemical and molecular genetic studies, *Ann Neurol* 24:774, 1988.
40. Hers HG, Van Hoof F: Glycogen storage diseases: type II and type VI glycogenosis. In Dickens F, Randle PJ, Whelan WJ, editors: *Carbohydrate metabolism and its disorders,* New York, 1968, Academic Press.
41. Tarui S, Okuno G, Ikura Y et al: Phosphofructokinase deficiency in skeletal muscle: a new type of glycogenosis, *Biochem Biophys Res Commun* 19:517, 1965.
42. Huijing F: Phosphorylase kinase deficiency, *Biochem Genet* 4:187, 1970.
43. Lewis GM, Spencer-Peet J, Stewart KM: Infantile hyperglycemia due to inherited deficiency of glycogen synthase in the liver, *Arch Dis Child* 38:40, 1963.
44. Harriman DGF, Millar JHD: Progressive familial myoclonic epilepsy in 3 families: its clinical features and pathological basis, *Brain* 78:325, 1955.
45. Busard BLSM, Gabreels-Festen AAWM, Renier WO et al: Axilla skin biopsy: a reliable test for the diagnosis of Lafora's disease, *Ann Neurol* 21:599, 1987.
46. Fratantoni JC, Hall CW, Neufeld EF: The defect in Hurler's and Hunter's syndromes: faulty degradation of mucopolysaccharide, *Proc Natl Acad Sci USA* 60:699, 1968.
47. Matalon R, Dorfman A: Hurler's syndrome, an alpha-L-iduronidase deficiency, *Biochem Biophys Res Commun* 47:959, 1972.
48. Hobbs JR, Hugh-Jones K, Barrett AJ et al: Reversal of clinical features of Hurler's disease and biochemical improvement after treatment by bone marrow transplantation, *Lancet* 2:709, 1981.
49. Scheie HG, Hambrick GW Jr, Barness LA: A newly recognized forme fruste of Hurler's disease (gargoylism), *Am J Ophthalmol* 53:753, 1962.
50. Jensen OA, Pedersen C, Schwartz M et al: Hurler-Scheie phenotype: report of an inbred sibship with tapeto-retinal degeneration and electron-microscopic examination of the conjunctiva, *Ophthalmologica* 176:194, 1978.
51. Wilson PJ, Morris CP, Anson DS et al: Hunter syndrome: isolation of an iduronate-2-sulfatase cDNA clone and analysis of patient DNA, *Proc Natl Acad Sci USA* 87:8531, 1990.
52. Bach G, Eisenberg F Jr, Cantz M et al: The defect in the Hunter syndrome: deficiency of sulfoiduronate sulfatase, *Proc Natl Acad Sci USA* 70:2134, 1973.
53. Matalon R, Dorfman A: Sanfilippo A syndrome: sulfamidase deficiency in cultured skin fibroblasts and liver, *J Clin Invest* 54:907, 1974.
54. O'Brien JS: Sanfilippo syndrome: profound deficiency of alpha-acetylglucosaminidase activity in organs and skin fibroblasts from type-B patients, *Proc Natl Acad Sci USA* 69:1720, 1972.
55. Klein U, Kresse H, von Figura K: Sanfilippo syndrome type C: deficiency of acetyl-CoA: alpha-glucosaminide *N*-acetyltransferase in skin fibroblasts, *Proc Natl Acad Sci USA* 75:5185, 1978.
56. Kresse H, Paschke E, von Figura K et al: Sanfilippo disease type D: deficiency of *N*-acetylglucosamine 6 sulfate sulfatase required for heparan sulfate degradation, *Proc Natl Acad Sci USA* 77:6822, 1980.
57. Singh J, DiFerrante NM, Niebes P et al: *N*-acetylgalactosamine-6-sulfate sulfatase in man: absence of the enzyme in Morquio disease, *J Clin Invest* 57:1036, 1976.
58. O'Brien JS, Gugler E, Giedion A et al: Spondyloepiphyseal dysplasia, corneal clouding, normal intelligence and acid beta-galactosidase deficiency, *Clin Genet* 9:495, 1976.
59. Barton RW, Neufeld EF: A distinct biochemical deficit in the Maroteaux-Lamy syndrome (mucopolysaccharidosis VI), *J Pediat* 80:114, 1972.
60. Stumpf DA, Austin JH, Crocker AC et al: Mucopolysaccharidosis type VI (Maroteaux-Lamy syndrome). I. Sulfatase B deficiency in tissues, *Am J Dis Child* 126:747, 1973.
61. Sly WS, Quinton BA, McAlister WH et al: Beta-glucuronidase deficiency: report of clinical, radiologic and biochemical features of a new mucopolysaccharidosis, *J Pediatr* 82:249, 1973.
62. DiFerrante NM, Ginsburg LC, Donnelly PV et al: Deficiencies of glucosamine-6-sulfate or galactosamine-6-sulfate sulfatases are responsible for different mucopolysaccharidoses, *Science* 199:79, 1978.
63. Patel V, Watanabe I, Zeman W: Deficiency of alpha-L-fucosidase, *Science* 176:426, 1972.
64. Zielke K, Veath ML, O'Brien JS: Fucosidosis: deficiency of alpha-L-fucosidase in cultured skin fibroblasts, *J Exp Med* 136:197, 1972.
65. Willems PJ, Gatti R, Darby JK et al: Fucosidosis revisited: a review of 77 patients, *Am J Med Genet* 38:111, 1991.
66. Carroll M, Dance N, Masson PK et al: Human mannosidosis—the enzymic defect, *Biochem Biophys Res Commun* 49:579, 1972.
67. Ockerman PA: A generalized storage disorder resembling Hurler's syndrome, *Lancet* 2:239, 1967.
68. Jones MZ, Dawson G: Caprine beta-mannosidosis: inherited deficiency of beta-D-mannosidase, *J Biol Chem* 256:5185, 1981.
69. Spranger JW, Gilbert EF, Tuffli GA et al: Geleophysic dwarfism—a "focal" mucopolysaccharidosis? (Letter) *Lancet* 1:97, 1971.
70. Mancini GMS, Verheijen FW, Galjaard H: Free *N*-acetylneuraminic acid (NANA) storage disorders: evidence for defective NANA transport across the lysosomal membrane, *Hum Genet* 73:214, 1986.
71. Blom HJ, Andersson HC, Seppala R et al: Defective glucuronic acid transport from lysosomes of infantile free sialic acid storage disease fibroblasts, *Biochem J* 268:621, 1990.
72. Montreuil J, Biserte G, Strecker G et al: Description d'un nouveau type du méliturie: la sialurie, *C R Acad Sci* [D] (Paris) 265:97, 1967.
73. Stevenson RE, Lubinsky M, Taylor HA et al: Sialic acid storage disease with sialuria: clinical and biochemical features in the severe infantile type, *Pediatrics* 72:441, 1983.
74. Renlund M, Aula P, Raivio KO et al: Salla disease: a new lysosomal storage disorder with disturbed sialic acid metabolism, *Neurology* 33:57, 1983.
75. Renlund M, Kovanen PT, Raivio KO et al: Studies on the defect underlying the lysosomal storage of sialic acid in Salla disease: lysosomal accumulation of sialic acid formed from *N*-acetyl-mannosamine or derived from low density lipoprotein in cultured mutant fibroblasts, *J Clin Invest* 77:568, 1986.
76. Patrick AD, Lake BD: Deficiency of an acid lipase in Wolman's disease, *Nature* 222:1067, 1969.
77. Sloan HR, Fredrickson DS: Enzyme deficiency in cholesteryl ester storage disease, *J Clin Invest* 51:1923, 1972.
78. Hoeg JM, Demosky SJ Jr, Pescovitz OH et al: Cholesteryl ester storage disease and Wolman disease: phenotypic variants of lysosomal acid cholesteryl ester hydrolase deficiency, *Am J Hum Genet* 36:1190, 1984.
79. Wolman M, Sterk VV, Gatt S et al: Primary family xanthomatosis with involvement and calcification of the adrenals: report of two more cases in siblings of a previously described infant, *Pediatrics* 28:742, 1961.
80. Crocker AC, Vawter GF, Neuhauser EBD et al: Wolman's disease: three new patients with a recently described lipidosis, *Pediatrics* 35:627, 1965.
81. Schiff L, Schubert WK, McAdams AJ et al: Hepatic cholesterol ester storage disease, a familial disorder. I. Clinical aspects, *Am J Med* 44:538, 1968.
82. Beaudet AL, Ferry GD, Nichols BL Jr et al: Cholesterol ester storage disease: clinical, biochemical, and pathological studies, *J Pediatr* 90:910, 1977.
83. Farber S, Cohen J, Uzman LL: Lipogranulomatosis: a new lipo-glycoprotein "storage" disease, *J Mt Sinai Hosp* 24:816, 1957.
84. Sugita M, Dulaney JT, Moser HW: Ceramidase deficiency in Farber's disease (lipogranulomatosis), *Science* 178:1100, 1972.
85. Gaucher P: De l'epithelioma primitif de la rate, thèse Paris, 1882.
86. Marchand F: Über sog idiopathische Splenomegalie - Typus Gaucher. *Muench Med Wochenschr* 54:1102, 1907.
87. Lieb H: Der Zucker im Cerebrosid der Milz bei der Gaucher Krankheit, *Hoppe - Seyler's Z Physiol Chem* 171:211, 1924.
88. Patrick AD: A deficiency of glucocerebrosidase in Gaucher's disease, *Biochem J* 97:17C, 1965.
89. Brady RO, Kaufer JN, Shapiro D: Metabolism in glucocerebrosides. II. Evidence of enzymatic deficiency in Gaucher's disease, *Biochem Biophys Res Commun* 18:221, 1965.
90. Beutler E, Kuhl W: Glucocerebrosidase processing in normal fibroblasts and in fibroblasts from patients with type I, type II, and type III Gaucher disease, *Proc Natl Acad Sci USA* 83:7472, 1986.

91. Grace ME, Smith F, Lathan T et al: Gaucher disease: a molecular basis for the type 2 and type 3 phenotypes (Abstract), *Am J Hum Genet* 47(suppl):A156, 1990.
92. Bachhawat BK, Austin J, Armstrong D: A cerebroside sulphotransferase deficiency in a human disorder of myelin, *Biochem J* 104:15C, 1967.
93. Suzuki K, Suzuki Y: Globoid cell leucodystrophy (Krabbe's disease): deficiency of galactocerebroside beta-galactosidase, *Proc Natl Acad Sci USA* 66:302, 1970.
94. Ben-Yoseph Y, Hungerford M, Nadler HL: The nature of mutation in Krabbe disease, *Am J Hum Genet* 30:644, 1978.
95. Krabbe K: A new familial infantile form of diffuse brain-sclerosis, *Brain* 39:74, 1916.
96. Andrews JM, Cancilla PA, Grippo J et al: Globoid cell leukodystrophy (Krabbe's disease): morphological and biochemical studies, *Neurology* 21:337, 1971.
97. Kolodny EH, Raghavan S, Krivit W: Late-onset Krabbe disease (globoid cell leukodystrophy): clinical and biochemical features of 15 cases, *Dev Neurosci* 13:232, 1991.
98. Young E, Wilson J, Patrick AD et al: Galactocerebrosidase deficiency in globoid cell leucodystrophy of late onset, *Arch Dis Child* 47:449, 1972.
99. Sweeley CC, Klionsky B: Fabry's disease: classification as a sphingolipidosis and partial characterization of a novel glycolipid, *J Biol Chem* 238:3148, 1963.
100. Brady RO, Gal AE, Bradley RM et al: Enzymatic defect in Fabry's disease: ceramidetrihexosidase deficiency, *N Engl J Med* 276:1163, 1967.
101. Romeo G, Migeon BR: Genetic inactivation of the alpha-galactosidase locus in carriers of Fabry's disease, *Science* 170:180, 1970.
102. Bernstein HS, Bishop DF, Astrin KH et al: Fabry disease: six gene rearrangements and an exonic point mutation in the alpha-galactosidase gene, *J Clin Invest* 83:1390, 1989.
103. Klint JA: Fabry's disease: alpha-galactosidase deficiency, *Science* 167:1268, 1970.
104. Cable WJL, Kolodny EH, Adams RD: Fabry disease: impaired autonomic function, *Neurology* 32:498, 1982.
105. Fabry J: Ein Beitrag zur Kenntnis der Purpura haemorrhagica nodularis (Purpura papulosa hemorrhagica Hebrae), *Arch Dermatol Syph* 43:187, 1898.
106. Clement M, McGonigle RJS, Monkhouse PM et al: Renal transplantation in Anderson-Fabry disease, *J R Soc Med* 75:557, 1982.
107. Niemann A: Ein unbekanntes Krankheitsbild, *Jahrb Kinderheilkd* 79:1, 1914.
108. Pick L: Über die lipoidzellige Splenohepatomegalie Typus Niemann-Pick als Stoffwechselerkrankung, *Med Klin* 23:1483, 1927.
109. Brady RO, Kanfer JN, Mock MB et al: The metabolism of sphingomyelin. II. Evidence of an enzymatic deficiency in Niemann-Pick disease, *Proc Natl Acad Sci USA* 55:366, 1966.
110. Pentchev PG, Comly ME, Kruth HS et al: A defect in cholesterol esterification in Niemann-Pick disease (type C) patients, *Proc Natl Acad Sci USA* 82:8247, 1985.
111. Levran O, Desnick RJ, Schuchman EH: Niemann-Pick disease: a frequent missense mutation in the acid sphingomyelinase gene of Ashkenazi Jewish type A and B patients, *Proc Natl Acad Sci USA* 88:3748, 1991.
112. Levran O, Desnick RJ, Schuchman EH: Niemann-Pick type B disease: identification of a single codon deletion in the acid sphingomyelinase gene and genotype/phenotype correlations in type A and B patients, *J Clin Invest* 88:806, 1991.
113. Winsor EJT, Welch JP: Genetic and demographic aspects of Nova Scotia Niemann-Pick disease (type D), *Am J Hum Genet* 30:530, 1978.
114. Wenger DA, Barth G, Githens JH: Nine cases of sphingomyelin lipidosis, a new variant in Spanish-American children, *Am J Dis Child* 131:955, 1977.
115. Austin J, McAfee D, Armstrong D et al: Abnormal sulphatase activities in two human diseases (metachromatic leukodystrophy and gargoylism), *Biochem J* 93:15C, 1964.
116. Cravioto H, O'Brien J, Lockwood R et al: Metachromatic leukodystrophy (sulfatide lipidoses) cultured in vitro, *Science* 156:243, 1967.
117. Greene H, Hug G, Schubert WK: Arylsulfatase A in the urine and metachromatic leukodystrophy, *J Pediatr* 71:709, 1967.
118. Polten A, Fluharty AL, Fluharty CB et al: Molecular basis of different forms of metachromatic leukodystrophy, *N Engl J Med* 324:18, 1991.
119. Greenfield JG: Form of progressive cerebral sclerosis in infants associated with primary degeneration of interfascicular glia, *Proc R Soc Med* 26:690, 1933.
120. Inui K, Emmett M, Wenger DA: Immunological evidence for deficiency in an activator protein for sulfatide sulfatase in a variant form of metachromatic leukodystrophy, *Proc Natl Acad Sci USA* 80:3074, 1983.
121. Austin J: Studies in metachromatic leukodystrophy. XII. Multiple sulfatase deficiencies, *Arch Neurol* 28:258, 1973.
122. MacBrinn MC, Okada S, Ho MW et al: Generalized gangliosidosis: impaired cleavage of galactose from a mucopolysaccharide and a glycoprotein, *Science* 163:946, 1969.
123. Kaback MM, Sloan HR, Sonneborn M et al: Gm(1) gangliosidosis type I: in utero detection and fetal manifestations, *J Pediatr* 82:1037, 1973.
124. O'Brien JS: Molecular genetics of G_{M1} beta-galactosidase, *Clin Genet* 8:303, 1975.
125. O'Brien JS, Norden AGW: Nature of the mutation in adult beta-galactosidase deficient patients, *Am J Hum Genet* 29:184, 1977.
126. Landing BH, Silverman FN, Craig JM et al: Familial neurovisceral lipidosis: an analysis of eight cases of a syndrome previously reported as "Hurler-variant", "pseudo-Hurler disease" and "Tay-Sachs disease with visceral involvement," *Am J Dis Child* 108:503, 1964.
127. Derry DM, Fawcett JS, Andermann F et al: Late infantile systemic lipidosis (major monosialogangliosidosis; delineation of two types), *Neurology* 18:340, 1968.
128. Wenger DA, Goodman SI, Myers GB: Beta-galactosidase deficiency in young adults (Letter), *Lancet* 2:1319, 1974.
129. Tay W: Symmetrical changes in the region of the yellow spot in each eye of an infant, *Trans Ophthalmol Soc UK* 1:155, 1881.
130. Sachs B: A family form of idiocy, generally fatal associated with early blindness, *J Nerv Ment Dis* 21:475, 1896.
131. Klenk E: Beiträge zur Chemie der Lipidosen. I. Niemann-Pick'sche Krankheit und amaurotische Idiotie, *Hoppe-Seyler's Z Physiol Chem* 262:128, 1939/40.
132. Svennerholm L: The chemical structure of normal human brain and Tay-Sachs gangliosides, *Biochem Biophys Res Commun* 9:436, 1962.
133. Makita A, Yamakawa T: The glycolipids of the brain of Tay-Sachs disease: the chemical structure of globoside and main ganglioside, *Jpn J Exp Med* 33:361, 1963.
134. Ledeen R, Salsman K: Structure of the Tay-Sachs ganglioside, *Biochemistry* 4:2225, 1965.
135. Okada S, O'Brien JS: Tay-Sachs disease: Generalized absence of a beta-D-*N*-acetylhexosaminidase component, *Science* 165:698, 1969.
136. Sandhoff K: Variation of β-*N*-acetylhexosaminidase-pattern in Tay-Sachs disease, *FEBS Lett* 4:351, 1969.
137. Hultberg B: *N*-acetylhexosaminidase activities in Tay-Sachs disease, *Lancet* 2:1195, 1969.
138. Ohno K, Suzuki K: Mutation in G_{M2}-gangliosidoses B1 variant, *J Neurochem* 50:316, 1988.
139. Li S-C, Kihara H, Serizawa S et al: Activator protein required for the enzymatic hydrolysis of cerebroside sulfate, *J Biol Chem* 254:10592, 1979.
140. Krivit W, Desnick RW, Lee J et al: Generalized accumulation of neutral glycosphingolipids with Gm_2 ganglioside accumulation in the brain: Sandhoff's disease (variant of Tay-Sachs disease), *Am J Med* 52:763, 1972.
141. Srivasta SK, Beutler E: Hexosamine-A and hexosamine-B: studies in Tay-Sachs and Sandhoff's disease, *Nature* 241:463, 1973.
142. Chern CJ, Beutler E, Kuhl W et al: Characterization of heteropolymeric hexosamidase A in human X mouse hybrid cells, *Proc Natl Acad Sci USA* 73:3637, 1976.
143. Adria G, Stricinglio P, Pontcrelli G et al: Infantile neuraminidase and β-galactosidase deficiencies (galactosidase) with mild clinical course. In *Perspectives in inherited metabolic diseases,* vol 4, Milan, 1981, Ermes.
144. Harlan WR Jr, Still WJ: Hereditary tendinous and tuberous xanthomatosis without hyperlipidemia: a new lipid-storage disorder, *N Engl J Med* 278:416, 1968.

145. Cali JJ, Russell DW: Characterization of human sterol 27-hydroxylase: a mitochondrial cytochrome P-450 that catalyzes multiple oxidation reactions in bile acid biosynthesis, *J Biol Chem* 266:7774, 1991.
146. Gilbert-Barness E, Barness LA: The mucolipidoses. In Landing B, Haust M, Bernstein J, Rosenberg H, editors: *Perspectives in pediatric pathology,* vol 17, *Genetic metabolic diseases,* Basel, 1993, Karger.
147. Aylsworth A, Thomas G, Hood J et al: A severe infantile sialidosis: clinical, biochemical, and microscopic features, *J Pediatr* 96:662, 1980.
148. Spranger J, Gehler J, Cantz M: Mucolipidosis I—a sialidosis, *Am J Med Genet* 1:21, 1977.
149. Spranger J: Mini review: inborn errors of complex carbohydrate metabolism, *Am J Med Genet* 28:489, 1987.
150. Martin J, Leroy J, Farriaux J et al: I-cell disease (mucolipidosis II), *Acta Neuropathol* 33:385, 1975.
151. Powell H, Benirschke K, Favara B et al: Foamy changes of placental cells in fetal storage disorders, *Virchows Arch [A]* 396:191, 1976.
152. Rapola J, Aula P: Morphology of the placenta in fetal I-cell disease, *Clin Genet* 11:107, 1977.
153. Sekels E, Ornoy A, Cohen R et al: Mucolipidosis IV: fetal and placental pathology, *Monogr Hum Genet* 10:47, 1978.
154. DeMars RI, Leroy JG: The remarkable cells cultured from a human with Hurler's syndrome: an approach to visual selection for in vitro genetic studies, *In Vitro* 2:107, 1967.
155. Taylor HA, Thomas GH, Miller CS et al: Mucolipidosis III (pseudo-Hurler polydystrophy): cytological and ultrastructural observations of cultured fibroblast cells, *Clin Genet* 4:388, 1973.
156. Leroy JG, Jo M, McBrinn MC et al: I-cell disease: biochemical studies, *Pediatr Res* 6:752, 1972.
157. Hickman S, Neufeld EF: A hypothesis for I-cell disease: defective hydrolases that do not enter lysosomes, *Biochem Biophys Res Commun* 49:922, 1972.
158. Wiesmann UN, Lightbody J, Vasella F et al: Multiple enzyme deficiency due to enzyme leakage, *N Engl J Med* 284:109, 1971.
159. Kaplan A, Achord DT, Sly WS: Phosphohexosyl components of a lysosomal enzyme are recognized by pinocytosis receptors on human fibroblasts, *Proc Natl Acad Sci USA* 74:2026, 1977.
160. Distler J, Hieber V, Sahagian G et al: Identification of mannose 6-phosphate in glycoproteins that inhibit the assimilation of beta-galactosidase by fibroblasts, *Proc Natl Acad Sci USA* 76:4325, 1979.
161. Gabel CA, Costello CE, Reinhold VN et al: Identification of methylphosphomannosyl residues as components of the high mannose oligosaccharides of *Dictyostelium discoideum* glycoproteins, *J Biol Chem* 259:13762, 1984.
162. Herd JK, Dvorak AD, Wiltse HE et al: mucolipidosis type III: multiple elevated serum and urine enzyme activities, *Am J Dis Child* 132:1181, 1978.
163. Liebaers I, Neufeld EF: Iduronate sulfatase activity in serum, lymphocytes and fibroblasts: simplified diagnosis of the Hunter syndrome, *Pediatr Res* 10:733, 1976.
164. Patriquin HB, Kaplan P, Kind HP et al: Neonatal mucolipidosis II (I-cell disease): clinical and radiologic features in three cases, *Am J Roentgenol* 129:37, 1977.
165. Cipolloni C, Boldrini A, Donti E et al: Neonatal mucolipidosis II (I-cell disease): clinical, radiological and biochemical studies in a case, *Helv Paediatr Acta* 35:85, 1980.
166. Whelan DT, Chang PL, Cockshott PW: Mucolipidosis II: the clinical, radiological and biochemical features in three cases, *Clin Genet* 24:90, 1983.
167. Satoh Y, Sakamoto K, Fujibayashi Y et al: Cardiac involvement in mucolipidosis: importance of non-invasive studies for detection of cardiac abnormalities, *Jpn Heart J* 24:149, 1983.
168. Gilbert EF, Dawson G, ZuRhein GM et al: I-cell disease, mucolipidosis II, pathological, histochemical, ultrastructural and biochemical observations in four cases, *Z Kinderheilkd* 114:259, 1973.

Amino acid disorders

169. Weinberg AG, Mize CE, Worthen HG: The occurrence of hepatoma in the chronic form of hereditary tyrosinemia, *J Pediatr* 88:434, 1976.
170. Hostetter MK, Levy HL et al: Evidence for liver disease preceding amino acid abnormalities in hereditary tyrosinemia, *N Engl J Med* 36:1190, 1983.
171. Kvittingen EA: Hereditary tyrosinemia type I: an overview, *Scand J Clin Lab Invest* 46(suppl)184:27, 1986.
172. Hardwick DF, Dimmick JE: Metabolic cirrhoses of infancy and early childhood, *Perspect Pediatr Pathol* 3:103, 1976.
173. Roels H: Pathology of aminoacidurias, *Monogr Hum Genet* 6:79, 1972.
174. Perry TL, Urquhart N et al: Nonketotic hyperglycinemia: glycine accumulation due to absence of glycine cleavage in brain, *N Engl J Med* 292:1269, 1975.
175. Tada K, Hayasaka K: Non-ketotic hyperglycinaemia: clinical and biochemical aspects, *Eur J Pediatr* 146:221, 1987.
176. Bohm N, Kiessling M, Lehner JW: Multiple acyl-CoA dehydrogenation deficiency (glutaric aciduria type II), congenital polycystic kidneys, symmetric warty dysplasia of the cerebral cortex in two newborn brothers, *Eur J Pediatr* 139:60, 1982.
177. Hokanson JT, O'Brien WE, Ademoto J et al: Carrier detection in ornithine transcarbamylase deficiency, *J Pediatr* 93:75, 1978.
178. Wilson GN, de Chadarevian J-P, Kaplan P et al: Glutaric aciduria type II: review of the phenotype and report of an unusual glomerulopathy, *Am J Med Genet* 32:395, 1989.
179. Robinson BH, MacMillan H, Petrova-Benedict R et al: Variable clinical presentation in patients with defective E_1 component of pyruvate dehydrogenase complex, *J Pediatr* 111:525, 1987.
180. Zimmerman A, Bachmann C, Colombo JP: Ultrastructural pathology in congenital defects in the urea cycle: ornithine transcarbamylase and carbamyl phosphate synthetase deficiency, *Virchows Arch* [A] 93:321, 1981.
181. Old JM, Briand PL et al: Prenatal exclusions of ornithine transcarbamylase deficiency by direct gene analysis, *Lancet* 1:73, 1985.
182. Zimmerman A, Moll C, Bachmann C: Liver fibrosis in carbamoyl-phosphate synthetase deficiency, *Pediatr Pathol* 7:191, 1987.

Peroxisomal diseases

183. Moser HW: Peroxisomal diseases, *Adv Pediatr* 36:1, 1989.
184. Lazarow PB: Rat liver peroxisomes catalyze the beta oxidation of fatty acids, *J Biol Chem* 253:1522, 1978.
185. Singh I, Moser AE, Goldfischer S et al: Lignoceric acid is oxidized in the peroxisome: implications for the Zellweger cerebro-hepato-renal syndrome and adrenoleukodystrophy, *Proc Natl Acad Sci USA* 81:4203, 1984.
186. Moser HW, Moser AB, Frayer KK et al: Adrenoleukodystrophy: increased plasma content of saturated very long chain fatty acids, *Neurology* 31:1241, 1981.
187. Tsuji S, Suzuki M, Ariga T: Abnormality of long chain fatty acids in erythrocyte membrane sphingomyelin from patients with adrenoleukodystrophy, *J Neurochem* 36:1046, 1981.
188. Moser HW, Moser AB, Kawamura N et al: Adrenoleukodystrophy: elevated C26 fatty acid in cultured skin fibroblasts, *Ann Neurol* 7:542, 1980.
189. Moser HW, Moiser AB, Singh I et al: Adrenoleukodystrophy: survey of 303 cases: biochemistry, diagnosis and therapy, *Ann Neurol* 16:628, 1984.
190. Moser AE, Singh I, Brown FR III et al: The cerebro-hepato-renal (Zellweger) syndrome: increased levels and impaired degradation of very long fatty acid and prenatal diagnosis, *N Engl J Med* 310:1114, 1984.
191. Hoefler G, Hoefler S, Watkins PA et al: Biochemical abnormalities in rhizomelic chondrodysplasia punctata, *J Pediatr* 112:726, 1988.
192. Datta NS, Wilson GN, Hajra AK: Deficiency of enzymes catalyzing the biosynthesis of glycerol-ether lipids in Zellweger syndrome: a new category of metabolic disease involving the absence of peroxisomes, *N Engl J Med* 311:1080, 1984.
193. Schrakamp G, Roosenboom CFP, Schutgens RBH: Alkyl dihydroxyacetone phosphate synthase in human fibroblasts and its deficiency in Zellweger syndrome, *J Lipid Res* 26:867, 1985.
194. Wanders RJA, van Weringth G, Schrakamp G et al: Deficiency of acyl-CoA; dihydroxyacetone phosphate acyltransferase in thrombocytes of Zellweger patients: a simple postnatal test, *Clin Chim Acta* 151:217, 1985.
195. Roscher A, Molzer B, Bernheimer H et al: The cerebro-hepato-renal (Zellweger) syndrome: an improved method for the biochemical diagnosis and its potential for prenatal diagnosis, *Pediatr Res* 19:930, 1985.
196. Steinberg D: Phytanic acid storage disease (Refsum's disease): In Scriver CR, Beaudet Al, Aly WS et al, editors. *The metabolic basis of inherited disease,* ed 6, New York, McGraw Hill, 1995.

197. Roels F, Goldfischer S: Cytochemistry of human catalase: the demonstration of hepatic and renal peroxisomes by a high temperature procedure, *J Histochem Cytochem* 27:1471, 1979.
198. Shimozawa N, Suzuki Y, Orii T et al: Diagnosis of Zellweger syndrome by rectal biopsy: immunoblot of peroxisomal beta oxidation enzyme and activity of dihydroxyacetone phosphate acyltransferase in rectal mucosa, *Clin Chim Acta* 175:345, 1988.
199. Bjorkhem I, Folk O: Assay of the major bile acids in serum by isotope dilution-mass spectrometry, *Scand J Clin Invest* 43:163, 1983.
200. Hajra AK, Datta NS, Jackson LG et al: Prenatal diagnosis of Zellweger cerebro-hepato-renal syndrome, *N Engl J Med* 312:445, 1985.
201. Singh I, Moser AB, Moser HW et al: Adrenoleukodystrophy: impaired oxidation of very long chain fatty acids in white blood cells, cultured skin fibroblasts and amniocytes, *Pediatr Res* 18:286, 1984.
202. Hashmi M, Stanley W, Singh I: Lignoceroyl-CoASH ligase: enzyme defect in fatty acid beta oxidation system in X-linked childhood adrenoleukodystrophy, *FEBS Lett* 196:247, 1986.
203. Wanders RJA, van Roermund CWT, van Wijland MJA et al: X-linked adrenoleukodystrophy: defective peroxisomal oxidation of very long chain fatty acids but not of very long chain fatty acyl-CoA esters, *Clin Chim Acta* 165:321, 1987.
204. Wanders RJA, van Roermund CWT, van Wijland MJA et al: Direct demonstration that the deficient oxidation of very long chain fatty acids in X-linked adrenoleukodystrophy is due to an impaired ability of peroxisomes to activate very long chain fatty acids, *Biochem Biophys Res Commun* 153:618, 1988.
205. Lazo O, Contreras M, Hashmi M et al: Peroxisomal lignoceroyl-CoA ligase deficiency in childhood adrenoleukodystrophy and adrenomyeloneuropathy, *Proc Natl Acad Sci USA* 85:7647, 1988.
206. Brushan A, Singh RP, Singh I: Characterization of rat brain microsomal acylcoenzyme A ligases: different enzymes for the synthesis of palmitoyl-coenzyme A and lignoceroyl-coenzyme A, *Arch Biochem Biophys* 246:374, 1986.
207. Schaumburg HH, Powers JH, Raine CS et al: Adrenoleuko-dystrophy: a clinical and pathological study of 17 cases, *Arch Neurol* 32:577, 1975.
208. Moser HW, Naidu S, Kumar AJ et al: Adrenoleukodystrophy: toward a biochemical definition of a disease with varied presentations, *CRC Crit Rev Neurobiol* 3:29, 1987.
209. Kumar AJ, Rosenbaum AE, Naidu S et al: Adrenoleukodystrophy: correlating MR imaging with CT, *Radiology* 165:497, 1987.
210. Igarashi M, Schaumburg HH, Powers J et al: Fatty acid abnormality in adrenoleukodystrophy, *J Neurochem* 26:851, 1976.
211. Migeon BA, Moser HW, Moser AB et al: Adrenoleukodystrophy: evidence for X-linkage, inactivation, and selection favoring the mutant allele in heterozygous cells, *Proc Natl Acad Sci USA* 78:5066, 1981.
212. Aubourg PR, Sack GH, Meyers DA et al: Linkage of adrenoleuko-dystrophy to a polymorphic DNA probe, *Ann Neurol* 21:349, 1987.
213. Friedman A, Betzhold J, Hong R et al: Clinico-Pathologic Conference: a three-month-old infant with failure to thrive, hepatomegaly and neurological impairment, *Am J Med Genet* 7:171, 1980.
214. Versmold HT, Bremer HJ et al: A metabolic disorder similar to Zellweger syndrome with hepatic acatalasia and absence of peroxisomes, altered content and redox state of cytochromes, and infantile cirrhosis with hemosiderosis, *Eur J Pediatr* 124:261, 1977.
215. Vitale L, Opitz JM, Shahidi NT: Congenital and familial iron overload, *N Engl J Med* 280:642, 1969.
216. Goldfischer S, Moore CL, Johnson AB et al: Peroxisomal and mitochondrial defects in the cerebro-hepato-renal syndrome, *Science* 182:62, 1973.
217. Arias JA, Moser AB, Goldfischer SL: Ultrastructural and cyto-chemical demonstration of peroxisomes in cultured fibroblasts from patients with peroxisomal deficiency disorders, *J Cell Biol* 100:1789, 1985.
218. Lazarow PB, Small GM, Santos M et al: Zellweger syndrome amniocytes: morphological appearance and a simple sedimentation for prenatal diagnosis, *Pediatr Res* 24:63, 1988.
219. Volpe JJ, Adams RD: Cerebro-hepato-renal syndrome of Zellweger: an inherited disorder of neuronal migration, *Acta Neuropathol* 20:175, 1972.
220. Evrard P, Caviness VS Jr, Prats-Vinas J et al: The mechanism of arrest of neuronal migration in the Zellweger malformation, an hypothesis based upon cytoarchitectonic analysis, *Acta Neuropathol* (Berl) 41:109, 1978.
221. Heymans HS: Cerebro-hepato-renal (Zellweger) syndrome: clinical and biochemical consequences of peroxisomal dysfunction (thesis), University of Amsterdam, 1984.
222. Bernstein J, Brough AJ, McAdams AJ: The renal lesions of syndromes of multiple congenital malformations: cerebro-hepato-renal syndrome, Jeune asphyxiating thoracic dystrophy, tuberous sclerosis, Meckel syndrome, *Birth Defects* 10:35, 1974.
223. Goldfischer S, Powers JM, Johnson AB et al: Striated adrenocortical cells in cerebro-hepato-renal (Zellweger) syndrome, *Virchows Arch [A]* 401:355, 1983.
224. Cohen SMZ, Brown FR III, Martyn L et al: Ocular histopathological and biochemical studies of the cerebro-hepato-renal (Zellweger) syndrome and its relation to neonatal adrenoleukodystrophy, *Am J Ophthalmol* 96:488, 1984.
225. Poznanski AK, Nosanchuk JS, Baublis J et al: The cerebro-hepato-renal syndrome (CHRS) Zellweger's syndrome, *AJR Am J Roentgenol* 109:313, 1970.
226. Williams JP, Secrest L, Fowler GW et al: Roentgenographic features of the cerebro-hepato-renal syndrome of Zellweger, *AJR Am J Roentgenol* 115:607, 1972.
227. Hong R, Horowitz SD, Borzy MF et al. The cerebro-hepato-renal syndrome of Zellweger: similarity to and differentiation from the DiGeorge syndrome, *Thymus* 3:97, 1981.
228. Vamecq J, Draye JP, van Hoof F et al: Multiple peroxisomal enzymatic deficiency disorders: a comparative biochemical and morphological study of Zellweger cerebro-hepato-renal syndrome and neonatal adrenoleukodystrophy, *Am J Pathol* 125:524, 1986.
229. Ulrich J, Herschkowitz N, Heitz P et al: Adrenoleukodys-trophy: preliminary report of a connatal case, *Acta Neuropathol* 43:77, 1978.
230. Aubourg P, Scotto J, Rocchiccioli F et al: Neonatal adrenoleukodystrophy, *J Neurol Neurosurg Psychiatry* 49:77, 1986.
231. Torvik A, Torp S, Kase BF et al: Infantile Refsum's disease: a generalized peroxisomal disorder: report of a case with postmortem examination, *J Neurol Sci* 85:39, 1988.
232. Brul S, Westerweld A, Strigland et al: Genetic heterogeneity in the cerebrohepatorenal (Zellweger) syndrome and other inherited disorders with a generalized impairment and peroxisomal functions: a study using complementation analysis, *J Clin Invest* 81:1710, 1988.
233. Williams HE, Smith LH Jr: Primary hyperoxaluria. In Stanbury JB, Wyngaarden JB, Fredrickson DS, et al, editors. *The metabolic basis of inherited disease,* ed 5, New York, 1983, McGraw-Hill.
234. Danpure CJ, Jennings PR: Peroxisomal alanine: glyoxylate aminotransferase deficiency in primary hyperoxaluria type I, *FEBS Lett* 201:20, 1986.
235. Nakatani T, Kawasaki Y, Minatogawa Y et al: Peroxisome localized human hepatic alanine-glyoxylate aminotransferase and its application to clinical diagnosis, *Clin Biochem* 18:311, 1985.
236. Eaton JM: Acatalasemia. In Scriver CR, Beaudet AL, Sly WS et al, editors: *Metabolic basis of inherited disease,* ed 6, New York, McGraw-Hill, 1995.
237. Quan F, Komeluk RG, Tropak MB et al: Isolation and characterization of the human catalase gene, *Nucleic Acids Res* 14:5321, 1986.
238. Junien C, Turleau C, de Grouchy J et al: Regional assignment of catalase (CAT) gene to band 11p13: association with the aniridia–Wilms' tumor–gonadoblastoma (WAGR) complex, *Ann Genet* 23:165, 1980.
239. Wanders RJA, Heymans HSA, Schutgens RBH et al: Peroxisomal functions in classical Refsum's disease: comparison with infantile form of Refsum's disease, *J Neurol Sci* 84:147, 1988.
240. Heymans HSA, Oorthuys JWE, Nelck G et al: Rhizomelic chondro-dysplasia punctata: another peroxisomal disorder, *N Engl J Med* 313:187, 1985.
241. Heymans HSA, Oorthuys JWE, Nelck G et al: Peroxisomal abnormalities in rhizomelic chondrodysplasia punctata, *J Inherited Metab Dis* 9(suppl 2):329, 1986.

Mitochondrial disorders

242. Luft R, Ikkos D, Palmieri G et al: A case of severe hypermetabolism of nonthyroid origin with a defect in the maintenance of mitochondrial

respiratory control: a correlated clinical, biochemical, and morphological study, *J Clin Invest* 41:1776, 1962.
243. Giles RE, Blanc H, Cann HM et al: Maternal inheritance of human mitochondrial DNA, *Proc Nat Acad Sci USA,* 77:6715, 1980.
244. Wallace DC: Diseases of the mitochondrial DNA, *Annu Rev Biochem* 61:1175, 1992.
245. De Vivo DC: The expanding clinical spectrum of mitochondrial diseases, *Brain Dev* 15:1, 1993.
246. DiMauro S, Bonilla E, Lombes A et al: Mitochondrial encephalomyopathies, *Neurol Clin* 8:483, 1990.
247. De Vivo DC, DiMauro S: Mitochondrial defects of brain and muscle, *Biol Neonate* 1:54, 1990.
248. Salo MK, Rapola J, Somer H et al: Reversible mitochondrial myopathy with cytochrome c oxidase deficiency, *Arch Dis Child* 67:1033, 1992.
249. Tritschler HJ, Bonilla E, Lombes A et al: Differential diagnosis of fatal and benign cytochrome c oxidase–deficient myopathies of infancy: an immunohistochemical approach, *Neurology* 41:300, 1991.
250. Stadhouders AM, Sengers RC: Morphological observations in skeletal muscle from patients with a mitochondrial myopathy, *J Inherit Metab Dis* 1:62, 1987.
251. Arnaudo E, Dalakas M, Shanske S et al: Depletion of muscle mitochondrial DNA in AIDS patients with zidovudine-induced myopathy, *Lancet* 337:508, 1991.
252. Hale DE, Bennett MJ: Fatty acid oxidation disorders: a new of metabolic diseases, *J Pediatr* 121:1, 1992.
253. van Erven PMM, Cillessen JP, Eekhoff EM et al: Leigh syndrome, a mitochondrial encephalo(myo)pathy: a review of the literature, *Clin Neurol Neurosurg* 89:217, 1987.
254. Lombes A, Nakase H, Tritschler HJ et al: Biochemical and molecular analysis of cytochrome c oxidase deficiency in Leigh's syndrome, *Neurology* 41:491, 1991.
255. Sparaco M, Bonilla E, DiMauro S et al: Neuropathology of mitochondrial encephalomyopathies due to mitochondrial DNA defects, *J Neuropathol Exp Neurol* 52:1, 1993.
256. Trijbels JM, Sengers RC, Ruitenbeek W et al: Disorders of the mitochondrial respiratory chain: clinical manifestations and diagnostic approach, *Eur J Pediatr* 148:92, 1988.
257. Robinson BH, Lactic acidemia. In Scriver CR, Beaudet AL, Sly WS, et al, editors: *The metabolic basis of inherited disease,* ed 6, New York, 1989, McGraw-Hill.
258. Munnich A, Rustin P, Rotig A et al: Clinical aspects of mito-chondrial disorders, *J Inherit Metab Dis* 15:448, 1992.

Disorders of metal metabolism

259. Knisely AS, Magid MS, Dische MR et al: Neonatal hemochromatosis. In Gilbert EF, Opitz JM, editors. *Genetic aspects of development pathology,* New York, 1987, Alan R Liss.
260. Silver MM, Beverley DW, Valberg LS et al: Perinatal hemochromatosis: clinical, morphologic, and quantitative iron studies, *Am J Pathol* 128:538, 1987.
261. Witzleben CL, Uri A: Perinatal hemochromatosis: entity or end result? *Hum Pathol* 20:335, 1989.
262. Knisely AS: Neonatal hemosiderosis. In Barness LA, editor: *Advances in pediatrics,* St Louis, 1990, Mosby.
263. Moerman P, Pauwels P, Vandenberghe K et al: Neonatal hemo-chromatosis, *Histopathology* 17:345, 1990.
264. Hamill RL, Woods JC, Cook BA: Congenital atransferrinemia: a case report and review of the literature, *Am J Clin Pathol* 96:213, 1991.
265. Bassett ML, Halliday JW, Powell LW: Value of hepatic iron measurements in early hemochromatosis and determination of the critical iron level associated with fibrosis, *Hepatology* 8:24, 1986.
266. Silver E, Cutz LS, Valberg M et al: Hepatic morphology in perinatal hemochromatosis compared with liver disease in the newborn caused by proven and presumptive inborn metabolic errors, *Pediatr Pathol Abstr* 12:248, 1992.
267. Silver MM, Cutz E, Valberg LS et al: Hepatic morphology in perinatal hemochromatosis compared with healing massive necrosis in the perinatal liver, *Pediatr Pathol Abstr* 12:249, 1992.
268. Hoogstraten J, DeSa DG, Knisely AS: Fetal liver disease may precede extrahepatic siderosis in neonatal hemochromatosis, *Gastroenterology* 98:1699, 1990.
269. Phillips MJ, Poucell S, Patterson J et al: *The liver: an atlas and text of ultrastructural pathology,* New York, 1987, Raven Press.
270. Scheinberg IH, Sternlieb I: *Wilson's disease,* Philadelphia, 1984, Saunders.
271. Archer GJ, Monie RDH: Wilson's disease and chronic active hepatitis, *Lancet* 1:486, 1977.
272. Scott J, Gollan JL, Samourian S, Sherlock S: Wilson's disease presenting as chronic active hepatitis, *Gastroenterology* 74:645, 1978.
273. Stromeyer FW, Ishak KG: Histology of the liver in Wilson's disease: a study of 34 cases, *Am J Clin Pathol* 73:12, 1980.
274. Ishak KG: Pathology of inherited metabolic disorders. In Balistreri WF, Stocker JT, editors: *Pediatric hepatology,* Washington, DC, 1990, Hemisphere Publishing.
275. Goldfischer S, Sternlieb I: Changes in the distribution of hepatic copper in relation to the progression of Wilson's disease (hepatolenticular degeneration), *Am J Pathol* 53:883, 1968.
276. Irons RD, Schenk EA, Lee JCK: Cytochemical methods for copper, *Arch Pathol Lab Med* 101:298, 1977.
277. Lindquist RR: Studies on the pathogenesis of hepatolenticular degeneration, II: cytochemical methods for localization of copper, *Arch Pathol* 87:370, 1969.
278. Jain S, Scheuer PJ, Archer BB et al: Histological demonstration of copper and copper-associated protein in chronic liver diseases, *J Clin Pathol* 31:784, 1978.
279. Salaspuro M, Sipponen P: Demonstration of an intracellular copper-binding protein by orcein staining in long-standing cholestatic liver disease, *Gut* 17:787, 1976.
280. Phillips MJ, Poucell S, Patterson J, Valencia P: *The liver: an atlas and text of ultrastructural pathology,* New York, Raven Press, 1987.
281. Sternlieb I: Evolution of hepatic lesion in Wilson's disease (hepatolenticular degeneration), *Prog Liver Dis* 4:511, 1972.
282. Nartey NO, Frei JV, Cherian MG: Hepatic copper and metalothionein distribution in Wilson's disease (hepatolenticular degeneration), *Lab Invest* 57:397, 1987.
283. Danks DM, Campbell PE et al: Menkes' kinky hair syndrome: an inherited defect in copper absorption with widespread effects, *Pediatrics* 50:188, 1972.
284. Danks DM, Stevens BJ et al: Menkes' kinky hair syndrome, *Lancet* 1:1100, 1972.
285. Menkes JH, Alter M, Steigleder GK et al: A sex-linked recessive disorder with retardation of growth, peculiar hair, and focal cerebral and cerebellar degeneration, *Pediatrics* 29:764, 1962.
286. Uno H, Arya S, Laxova R et al: Menkes' syndrome with vascular and adrenergic nerve abnormalities, *Arch Pathol Lab Med* 107:286, 1983.

Other metabolic disorders

287. Zeman W: Historical development of the nosological concept of amaurotic familial idiocy. In Vinken PJ, Bruyn GW, editors: *Handbook of neurology,* Amsterdam, 1970, North Holland.
288. Zeman W, Dyken P: Neuronal ceroid-lipofuscinosis (Batten's disease): relationship to amaurotic family idiocy? *Pediatrics* 44:570, 1969.
289. Dyken PR: The neuronal ceroid lipofuscinoses, *J Child Neurol* 4:165, 1989.
290. Rapola J: Neuronal ceroid-lipofuscinoses in childhood. In Landing BH, Haust MD, Bernstein J et al, editors: *Perspectives in pediatric pathology,* Basel, 1993, Karger.
291. Rider JA, Rider DL: Batten disease: past, present and future, *Am J Med Genet, Suppl* 5:21, 1988.
292. Hall NA, Lake BD, Patrick AD: Recent biochemical and genetic advances in our understanding of Batten's disease (ceroid-lipofuscinosis), *Dev Neurosci* 13:339, 1991.
293. Callen DF, Baker E, Lane S et al: Regional mapping of the Batten disease locus (CLN3) to human chromosome 16p12, *Am J Hum Genet* 49:1372, 1991.
294. Järvelä I, Schleutker J, Haataja L et al: Infantile neuronal ceroid lipofuscinosis (CLN1) maps to the short arm of chromosome 1, *Genomics* 9:170, 1991.

295. Lake BD: Lysosomal enzyme deficiencies. In Adams JH, Corsellis JAN, Duchen LW, editors: *Greenfield's neuropathology,* London, 1984, Edward Arnold.
296. Goebel HH, Zeman W, Patel VK et al: On the ultrastructural diversity and essence of residual bodies in neuronal ceroid-lipofuscinosis, *Mech Ageing Devel,* 10:53, 1979.
297. Santavuori P: Clinical findings in 69 patients with infantile type of neuronal ceroid lipofuscinosis. In Armstrong D, Koppang N, Rider JA, editors: *Ceroid-lipofuscinosis (Batten's disease),* Amsterdam, 1982, Elsevier Biomedical Press.
298. Haltia M, Rapola J, Santavuori P: Infantile type of so-called neuronal ceroid-lipofuscinosis: histological and electron microscopical studies, *Acta Neuropathol* (Berl) 26:157, 1973.
299. Haltia M: Infantile neuronal ceroid-lipofuscinosis: neuropathlogical aspects. In Armstrong D, Koppang N, Rider JA, editors: *Ceroid-lipofuscinosis (Batten's disease),* Amsterdam, 1982, Elsevier Biomedical.
300. Martin JJ, Jacobs K: Skin biopsy as a contribution to diagnosis in late infantile amaurotic idiocy with curvilinear bodies, *Eur Neurol* 10:281, 1973.
301. Ceuterick Ch, Martin JJ, Casaer P et al: The diagnosis of infantile generalized ceroid-lipofuscinosis (type Hagberg-Santavuori) using skin biopsy, *Neuropädiatrie* 7:250, 1976.
302. Libert J: Diagnosis of lysosomal storage disorders by the ultrastructural study of conjunctival biopsies, *Pathol Annu* 15(Pt1):37, 1980.
303. Carpenter S, Karpati G, Andermann F: Specific involvement of muscle, nerve, and skin in late infantile and juvenile amaurotic idiocy, *Neurology* 22:170, 1972.
304. Rapola J, Santavuori P, Savilahti E: Suction biopsy of rectal mucosa in the diagnosis of infantile and juvenile types of neuronal ceroid lipofuscinoses, *Hum Pathol* 15:352, 1984.
305. Haynes ME, Manson JI, Carter RF et al: Electron microscopy of skin and peripheral blood lymphocytes in infantile (Santavuori) neuronal ceroid lipofuscinosis, *Neuropädiatrie* 10:245, 1979.
306. Boustany R-MN, Alroy J, Kolodny EH: Clinical classification of neuronal ceroid-lipofuscinosis subtypes, *Am J Med Genet, Suppl* 5:47, 1988.
307. Goebel H, Zeman W, Damaske E: An ultrastructural study of the retina in the Jansky-Bielschowsky type of neuronal ceroid lipofuscinosis, *Am J Ophthalmol* 83:70, 1977.
308. Santavuori P: Neuronal ceroid-lipofuscinoses in childhood, *Brain Dev* 10:80, 1988.
309. Carpenter S, Karpati G, Andermann F et al: The ultrastructural characteristics of the abnormal cytosomes in Batten-Kufs' disease, *Brain* 100:137, 1977.
310. Aula P, Rapola J, Andersson LC: Distribution of cytoplasmic vacuoles in blood T and B lymphocytes in two lysosomal disorders, *Virchows Arch [B]* 18:263, 1975.
311. Schwendemann G, Colmant HJ, Elze K-L et al: Juvenile type of generalized ceroid-lipofuscinosis (Spielmeyer-Sjögren syndrome), *Neuropädiatrie* 9:28, 1978.
312. Berkovic SF, Andermann F, Andermann E et al: Kufs disease: clinical features and forms, *Am J Med Genet, Suppl* 5:105, 1988.
313. Martin JJ: Adult type of neuronal ceroid lipofuscinosis, *Dev Neurosci* 13:331, 1991.
314. Boehme DH, Cottrell JC, Leonberg SC et al: A dominant form of neuronal ceroid-lipofuscinosis, *Brain* 94:745, 1971.
315. Goebel HH, Braak H: Adult neuronal ceroid-lipofuscinosis, *Clin Neuropathol* 8:109, 1989.
316. MacLeod P, Dolman C, Nickel R et al: Prenatal diagnosis of neuronal ceroid lipofuscinosis, *N Eng J Med* 310:595, 1984.
317. Conradi NG, Uvebrant P, Hökegård K-H et al: First-trimester diagnosis of juvenile neuronal ceroid lipofuscinosis by demonstration of fingerprint inclusions in chorionic villi, *Prenat Diagn* 9:283, 1989.
318. Rapola J, Salonen R, Ämmälä P et al: Prenatal diagnosis of the infantile type of neuronal ceroid lipofuscinosis by electron microscopic investigation of human chorionic villi, *Prenat Diagn* 10:553, 1990.
319. Järvelä I, Rapola J, Peltonen L et al: DNA-based prenatal diagnosis of the infantile form of neuronal ceroid lipofuscinosis (INCL, CLN1), *Prenat Diagn* 11:323, 1991.
320. Santavuori P, Rapola J, Nuutila A et al: The spectrum of Jansky-Bielschowsky disease, *Neuropediatrics* 22:135, 1991.
321. Goebel HH, Schulz F: The ultrastructural variability of non-specific lipopigments, *Acta Neuropathol* (Berl) 48:227, 1979.
322. Carpenter S: Morphological diagnosis and misdiagnosis in Batten-Kufs disease, *Am J Med Genet, Suppl* 5:85, 1988.
323. Sjögren T: Die juvenile amaurotische Idiotie: klinische und erblichkeitsmedizinische Untersuchungen, *Hereditas* (Lund) 14:197, 1931.
324. Andermann E, Jacob JC, Andermann F et al: The Newfoundland aggregate of neuronal ceroid-lipofuscinosis, *Am J Med Genet, Suppl* 5:111, 1988.

15 Molecular Basis of Human Disease

Monica D. Traystman
Steven H. Hinrichs

Nomenclature

allele One of the alternative forms of a gene at a particular locus. Allelic heterogeneity is the presence of several different mutant alleles at the same gene locus that result in the same or similar clinical phenotypes.

genotype The entire genome or genetic constitution of an individual. At the gene locus, the genotype refers to the types of alleles present in an individual.

haplotype A defined combination of alleles within a specific region of a chromosome. A haplotype is usually determined by restriction fragment length polymorphism analysis in which the results define the orientation of the markers on each chromosome. The marker pattern can then be used to determine the inheritance of each chromosome in a family in association with a disease gene (linkage analysis) or used to determine the frequency in a population of a particular marker pattern (linkage disequilibrium) with known mutations.

heterozygous A variation in the DNA sequence of a gene between the two chromosomes of an individual (that is, one chromosome has the normal or "wild type" of sequence, whereas the other chromosome has a different sequence, which can be as small as a single base change); an individual is considered to be a heterozygous carrier of a mutation if one chromosome has a disease causing DNA sequence change and the other chromosome has the normal sequence. An individual who has two different DNA mutant alleles at a particular locus is a compound heterozygote. In contrast, an individual who has a different mutant allele at two different individual loci is a double heterozygote.

homozygous The same DNA sequence of a gene appearing on both chromosomes; for a mutation to be homozygous the same sequence changes appear on both chromosomes in an individual.

housekeeping genes Genes that are constitutively expressed in most or all cells, since their products are necessary for essential cell functions.

kindred An extended family pedigree, which may include several families within a generation or multigenerational families.

nondisjunction The failure of two homologous chromosomes to separate during meiosis I or two chromatids of a chromosome to separate during meiosis II or mitosis resulting in the transmission of both to one daughter cell while the other daughter cell receives neither.

phenotype The clinical expression of the interaction of the gene or genes of an individual with the environment.

polymorphism Any change in the genomic DNA sequence that results in two or more alternative genotypes that are each maintained at a frequency greater than that caused by mutation alone. A genetic locus is polymorphic if the rarer allele has a frequency of at least 0.01, and so heterozygotes carrying this allele occur at a frequency greater than 0.02.

sibship All the brothers and sisters within a single family.

THE ROLE OF MOLECULAR GENETICS IN PATHOLOGY

Molecular diagnostic techniques, as described in Chapter 11, have greatly influenced every aspect of clinical diagnosis. It is now apparent that several mechanisms may underlie disease, such as a mutation in the genome, an RNA processing defect, an alteration in the level of expression, or a structural defect in a particular protein. Different types of defects determine the type of specimen required for diagnosis, as well as the way in which the specimen is processed. The comment "Fix the specimen in formalin for processing in the morning" is not an acceptable approach.

When molecular analyses are requested as part of a clinical evaluation that includes a tissue biopsy, retention of a portion of the specimen in a frozen condition may be critical. DNA is relatively stable, and degradation occurs over minutes to hours rather than seconds to minutes as in the case for mRNA. Even the normal delay in transport of a specimen from the operating room to the surgical pathology suite may result in considerable loss in RNA integrity, whereas DNA degradation is usually not affected. Thus, if the genetic question is at the level of RNA, the specimen is best collected in the operating room and immediately frozen in a dry ice bath and then transferred to a −80°C freezer. DNA and RNA can be recovered from formalin-fixed material; however, the cross-linking that occurs in fixation invariably results in shorter fragments or a reduction in size of the RNA. Fig. 15-1 demonstrates the reduction in size occurring with DNA over time. If the target for study is relatively short, less than 500 base pairs in length, and abundant in quantity, then diagnostic information can still be obtained after fixation; however, processing is more tedious than that with longer forms. DNA and RNA are recovered through the disruption of cellular membranes in an ionic or nonionic detergent followed by degradation of the proteins composing cellular components as well as the protein matrix containing histones and protamine that protect DNA. Subsequently the genetic material is extracted from the contaminating proteins on the basis of the solubility of DNA in water. DNA can be separated from RNA on the basis of its differential solubility salt solution. It should be recognized that studies examining extracted DNA, RNA, or protein need a means to standardize the results relative to single cells.

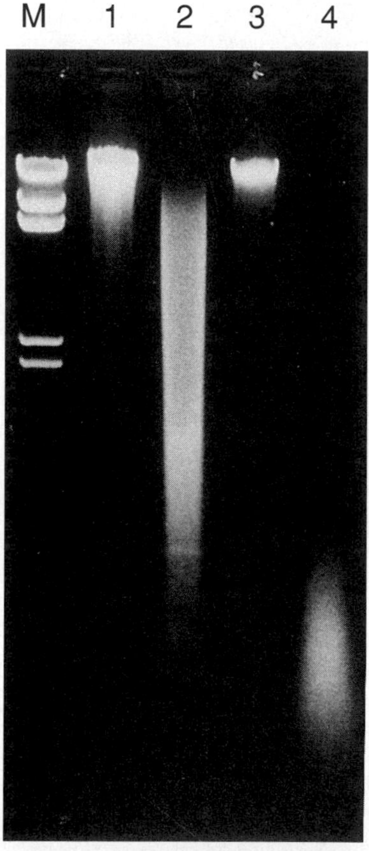

Fig. 15-1 Evaluation of DNA integrity following various methods of processing. Lane M; lambda DNA digested by HIND III, which generates fragment sizes of 564, 2027, 2322, 4361, 6557, 9416, and 23,130 base pairs. Lane 1, human lymphocyte DNA prepared from freshly collected cells using standard protocols. Lane 2, DNA from lymphocyte preparation from lane 1, following digestion with restriction enzymes EcoRI. Note repetitive bands above and below the 564-based pair marker. Lane 3, DNA preparation of kidney tissue fixed in ethanol immediately following resection. DNA extraction occurred two months after fixation. Note that DNA migrates as high molecular mass or size, essentially identical to freshly prepared lymphocyte DNA in lane 1. Lane 4, DNA preparation of kidney tissue fixed in formalin for 4 hours and embedded in paraffin, followed by storage for 2 months. Note the DNA fragments are of much smaller size with the majority being less than 500 base pairs.

The inappropriate application of any new technique can provide results that not only are irrelevant to the clinical problem, but may also mislead and confuse. The potential for misuse therefore exists with molecular biology as it has with any other new technology. As the role for oncogenes was first being elucidated, great claims were made for their diagnostic and even therapeutic potential. When H-*ras* and K-*ras* oncogenes were detected in bladder and colon cancers, it was believed that they would have diagnostic significance for these types of tumors. Although subsequent studies have shown the essential role of these genes in cell regulation, there has not been good correlation with any specific tissue type, tumor morphology, or prognostic significance. It is important and reasonable to ask whether genetic diagnostic techniques have any relevance to clinical problems that require tissue diagnosis. The most widely accepted applications of molecular techniques are in the field of hematology, which has greatly benefited from the pioneering work of many researchers (see Chapters 41 and 42). Basic research has led to the development of tests with clinical application. Commercial assays are under FDA evaluation; the widespread use of molecular biology–based tests will occur when more commercial assays have been approved. Although many applications exist for both cancer diagnostics and genetic disorders, the list of commercial tests available is largely composed of assays for infectious diseases. In situ hybridization, immunohistochemistry, in situ polymerase chain reaction (PCR), and reverse dot blot (a modification of a blot procedure) have been used, for example, to detect components of human papillomavirus (HPV) that identify the specific type. Familiarity and understanding of these assays are essential to aid the laboratorian in test utilization and cost-effective diagnostic procedures.

There are also situations where it is not necessary to extract the genetic material but rather to study the DNA or RNA in situ. In situ hybridization or in situ PCR may be employed (Chapter 10). In general, 10% formaldehyde is a sufficient fixative for in situ hybridization and detection of DNA or RNA. However, the length of exposure to the fixative should be minimized and the specimen processed and embedded in paraffin as soon as possible. Transfer of a specimen to 80% alcohol has been suggested and is optimal if done after 2 to 3 hours of fixation in formalin. Detection of viral genome in a specific morphologic lesion is the most common application of in situ hybridization techniques. In situ hybridization or in situ PCR has been used to detect components of HPV that are capable of allowing one to assign or determine a specific subtype of HPV associated with a particular clinical entity. The retention of tissue samples for subsequent molecular biology techniques should be considered no different from saving a small fragment for electron microscopy.

A significant advantage of molecular analysis is increased discrimination between similar diseases. There are numerous examples where subclassification of malignant neoplasms by specific morphologic criteria has aided in the prediction of prognosis and outcome. Combination therapies based on subcategories of tumors have been developed. It is anticipated that as the molecular basis of disease is understood, specific therapeutic modalities will be further refined. Other examples are found in the evaluation of a patient with muscular dystrophy or in patients with cystic fibrosis (see Chapter 14). Molecular studies on muscular dystrophy have demonstrated the basis for clinical variations in disease phenotype. The identification of functional domains within the dystrophin molecule showed how different clinical phenotypes correlate with alterations on the DNA level that result in translation of a truncated protein product that either provides some function or is degraded and results in no function. As the complexities of cystic fibrosis are becoming understood, it is apparent that it is a heterogeneous disease that affects many organ systems. The primary systems involved include the pulmonary and gastrointestinal, show a wide range of severity in clinical phenotype. Currently, more than 500 unique mutations have been documented, and they consist of alterations within the DNA-coding and RNA-splicing regions. Therapy is being affected in unpredictable ways. For example, the buildup of viscous mucins admixed with DNA from lysed epithelial and inflammatory cells leads to plugged bronchioles and an expanding spiral of disease. The presence of inflammatory cells adds to the disorder since DNA from lysed cells is extremely viscous. Treatment with an enzyme routinely used in the laboratory to digest DNA has had therapeutic benefit for accomplishing the same purpose in vivo. The enzyme DNAase is administered in an aerosol form to digest the DNA from lysed cells. Thus molecular techniques not only document the presence of a specific disease entity, but also are used to analyze the full range of disease and also lay the groundwork for potential treatment.

The essential concept for understanding how molecular genetic analysis provides an evaluation of the full range of disease is based on the relationship between events at the DNA versus RNA level and how they are reflected at the protein level. The detailed description of the anatomy of a gene and the processes involved are presented. Not only is the gene sequence important but the regulatory components of a gene are also critical to correct function. Dysfunction can occur when alterations are present within the DNA coding for the gene as well as when there are alterations in the regulation of RNA production.

In all these examples, the potential for a problem exists long before an individual may become symptomatic. It is anticipated that the greatest influence of molecular diagnostics will come from screening for genes that are correlated with an increased risk of cancer, heart disease, or other disorders, such as the human nonpolyposis cancer gene and colon carcinoma.

The ability to characterize genetic defects and the development of therapeutic strategies results in the need for testing strategies during the various points of the natural history of a disease. One test strategy may be important during a presymptomatic period, whereas other test strategies are used during the asymptomatic and therapeutic periods. Presymptomatic testing is influenced by a history of familial genetic disease. Some genetic tests have great specificity and are capable of detailing specific mutations; however, because of their complexity and labor-intensive procedures, they are not appropriate for mass population screening. However, given sufficient clinical information, a testing panel, such as that required for evaluation of cystic fibrosis, can be used appropriately and provides clinically relevant information. Pretreatment as well as posttreatment molecular characterizations assist in the management of patients undergoing solid organ or bone marrow transplantation. HLA typing can be determined at a molecular level, for both the patient's and the transplant donor's DQ and DR status. After bone marrow reconstitution with an allogeneic donor, it may be useful to determine whether cells are of donor or of recipient origin.

Molecular techniques are also useful in the monitoring of special populations, including patients at high risk of developing a specific disorder but who are asymptomatic or presymptomatic as well as those individuals who are at risk for disease relapse after therapy. The ethnic background of populations influences genetic testing. Northern Europeans have a higher incidence of the ΔF508 mutation found in cystic fibrosis. Individuals of African descent are well known to have a high incidence of sickle cell disease. Other correlations are listed in Table 15-1.

The identification of genes responsible for maintenance of DNA and prevention of the introduction of mutations has accelerated the importance of monitoring patients at high risk for disease. Thus, patients with the Li-Fraumeni syndrome or the Lynch syndrome, which involves breast cancer as well as many other disease conditions, may benefit from an exact determination of their genetic status. Since molecular markers exist for identification of a specific population of neoplastic cells, it is possible to search on a predetermined schedule for the reappearance of tumor cells after therapy. Several examples exist in the lymphoma field, and the potential exists in other fields such as breast cancer and colon cancer. The association of specific viruses, particularly the human papillomaviruses, with different risk categories for development of neoplastic lesions is another example of the screening of high-risk presymptomatic patients. Although therapy is based on the morphologic appearance of a lesion such as those occurring in the uterine cervix, the detection of a high-risk *Papillomavirus* type, such as type 16 and type 18, has been proposed as meriting more frequent follow-up study. In comparison, the detection of an HPV subtype with a lower risk for development of carcinoma may indicate that frequent clinical evaluations are not warranted.

GENETIC DISEASE INHERITANCE

Chromosomal disorders

Chromosomal disorders are attributable to an abnormal number or structure of any of the 44 autosomes (22 homologous pairs) or two sex chromosomes (female, XX; male, XY) or

Table 15-1 Selected examples of significant genetic disorders

Disorders	Incidence
Autosomal dominant	
Familial hypercholesterolemia	~1/500 heterozygotes
Huntington's disease	Variable, 4 to 8/100,000; much higher in some small, isolated populations
Myotonic dystrophy	Most common autosomal dominant muscular dystrophy; ~1/10,000 up to 1/1000 in some populations
Neurofibromatosis type I	~1/3000 to 1/5000
Autosomal recessive	
Adenosine deaminase deficiency	Rare
α_1-antitrypsin deficiency	~1/3000 to 1/20,000
Cystic fibrosis	~1/2000 in some white populations; very rare in Asians
Osteogenesis imperfecta	~1/15,000 for most common type
Phenylketonuria	Variable; 1/5000 to 1/200,000; most common in western Europeans
Sickle cell anemia	Common mutation in equatorial Africa; ~1/400 American blacks affected
Tay-Sachs disease	~1/3000 in Ashkenazi Jews; much lower in other populations
Thalassemia	Most common single-gene disease; found in regions where malaria is endemic
X-Linked	
Duchenne muscular dystrophy	~1/3000 to 1/3500 males
Fragile X syndrome	~1/1500 males; ~1/2000 to 1/3000 females
Glucose-6-phosphate dehydrogenase deficiency	Ethnic variation; very common (1/4 to 1/20 males) in some populations
Hemophilia A	~1/10,000 males
Carcinoma	
Retinoblastoma	~1/14,000
Wilms' tumor	~1/10,000
Multifactorial	
Congenital malformations	
Cleft lip with or without cleft palate	1/250 to 1/600; ethnic variation
Congenital heart disease	1/125 to 1/250
Neural tube defects	1/100 to 1/500; ethnic variation
Adult diseases	
Cancer, some forms	>1/3 (exclusive of skin cancer)
Coronary artery disease	Heterogeneous; variable frequency; up to 1/15 in Western populations; currently declining
Diabetes mellitus	Heterogeneous; 1/10 to 1/20 adults; less common in children
Mitochondrial	
Leber's hereditary optic neuropathy	Rare

Modified from Thompson MW, McInnes RR, Willard HF: *Genetics in medicine,* ed 5, Philadelphia, 1991, Saunders.

both. Survey data have established the following statistics to show the significance of the contribution of chromosomal disorders to the genetic basis of disease. Fifty percent of all spontaneous abortions are the result of a chromosomal abnormality. Chromosomal abnormalities have been observed in 0.5% to 0.7% of all liveborn infants. A more thorough discussion of the genetic abnormalities associated with the inheritance of these types of disorders can be found in Chapter 12.

Single-gene disorders

Single-gene disorders are attributable to one or more types of mutations that occur at a single gene locus. Different gene changes found at the same gene locus produce alternative forms (alleles) of the mutant gene. These alternative forms result in allelic heterogeneity, and so each different allele results in an abnormal phenotype. A single gene alteration may be found on only one of two chromosomes (such as autosomal dominant or X-linked disorders), or on both chromosomes (such as autosomal recessive disorders). Single-gene disorders range in frequency from 1/500 (seen in familial hypercholesterolemia) to rare diseases such as adenosine deaminase deficiency. Cumulative data from many investigations of single-gene disorders have provided insights into the diversity of genetic mechanisms that produce disease. These mechanisms include single base substitutions, deletions, insertions, duplications, and amplifications. These mechanisms are discussed below, with pertinent examples of the phenotypes. Examples of some of the more significant single gene disorders are shown in Table 15-1. Currently, from a total of more than 6000 documented genes, 3000 single-gene disorders have been cataloged by Dr. Victor A. McKusick in *Mendelian Inheritance in Man* (1994) (Fig. 15-2). This data base is the largest cataloged reference of genetic disorders available.[1] Several other key reference books dealing with these disorders have been published.[2-9]

Multigenic disorders

Multigenic disorders result from a genetic defect in more than one gene and tend to be inherited without a distinctive inheritance pattern within a single family (Table 15-1). The clinical phenotype is a result of the cumulative effects of these multiple defects. In addition to genetic factors, nongenetic factors may play a significant role in the development of disease. Smoking, diet, stress, and the physical environment may influ-

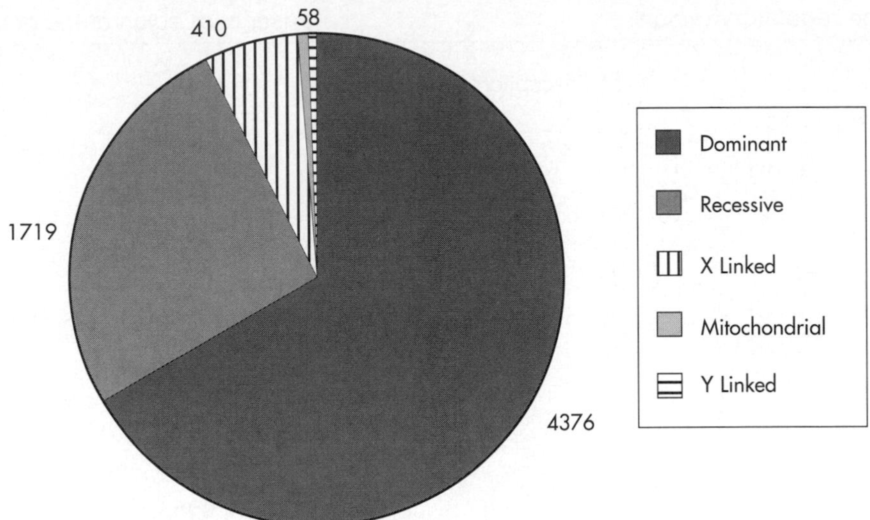

Fig. 15-2 The number of documented patterns and types of inheritance (as of February 1994). (Adapted from McKusick VA: *Mendelian inheritance in man,* ed 11, Baltimore, 1994, Johns Hopkins University Press.)

ence the severity of the phenotypic expression. Well-studied multigenic disorders include some cancers, coronary artery disease, and diabetes mellitus. In some disorders within this group, a series of mutational events must occur before the development of clinical disease. This has been observed in some colon and breast cancers.

Somatic cell disorders and cancer

Most common cancers contain mutations in somatic cells, (not found in germ cells—ovum or sperm). DNA mutations are more frequently acquired, rather than inherited, as a result of one or more mutational mechanisms. The primary mutational event or events appear to be random, affecting a single cell that divides to produce a clonal cell mass. A series of mutational events may be required before the development of cancer (see Chapter 24). Predisposition to these events may be determined by the individual's genetic background and environment. Therefore the single-gene disorder model of Mendelian inheritance cannot be used as a model in many cases. There are approximately 100 examples of single-gene disorders in which cancer is a prominent component of the disorder. The majority of these types of cancers are inherited in an autosomal dominant pattern. Most cancers must be studied using a multifactorial model that includes genetic and environmental components to perform risk analyses. Not until all the genes that are involved in the development of a particular cancer are identified can the mechanisms for the genetic predisposition and their relationship to environmental factors be understood.

FREQUENCY OF GENETIC DISORDERS

Genetic disease, once believed to be a rare occurrence, is a major cause of morbidity and mortality.

Baird and associates in one of the largest surveys done in British Columbia, which included over 1 million births,[10] showed that 5% (1 in 20 individuals) of the population under 25 years of age developed a significant disease associated with a genetic disorder of chromosomal, single-gene, or multigene abnormality. Others have published reports on the causes of mortality in over 12,000 children in the United Kingdom.[11,12] Genetic disease was found to contribute to 38% and 42%, respectively, of the deaths among these children. Studies of the frequency of genetic disease in pediatric populations have shown that in Montreal (36%) and in Seattle (>53%), many of the diseases that were diagnosed on admission were believed to have a genetic component.[13,14] These studies illustrate the significant financial and medical burden that genetic disease places on society. With the continued documentation of new genes and their associated diseases and the identification of all the genes involved in a multigenic disorder the importance of genetic disorders will become even more apparent.

GENE ANATOMY

The cloning and sequencing of a large number of genes has provided insights into general gene anatomy. Most genes, with some variation, have a structure similar to the one seen in Fig. 15-3. Gene structures provide insight into gene function and into differences among genes. The structure of a gene establishes its anatomical compartments, which can then be studied to determine the location, frequency, and diversity of mutations that result in an altered protein product or altered expression. The anatomy of a gene can also be used to study the relationships between newly discovered genes and well characterized gene families; potential function may be suggested when compared to other known genes.

The standard depiction of a gene includes regulatory sequences on the left (enhancer/silencer and promoter) and transcribed sequences on the right. Typically the upper strand is shown with the gene oriented in a 5′ to 3′ direction. This terminology refers to the free phosphate group of the 2-deoxyribose sugars of the upper strand being placed to the left and the unattached 3′ hydroxyl group being placed to the right. This established notation denotes the order of the gene in relationship to the direction of transcription. The 5′-phosphate and 3′-hydroxyl radicals on the sugar molecules are the internu-

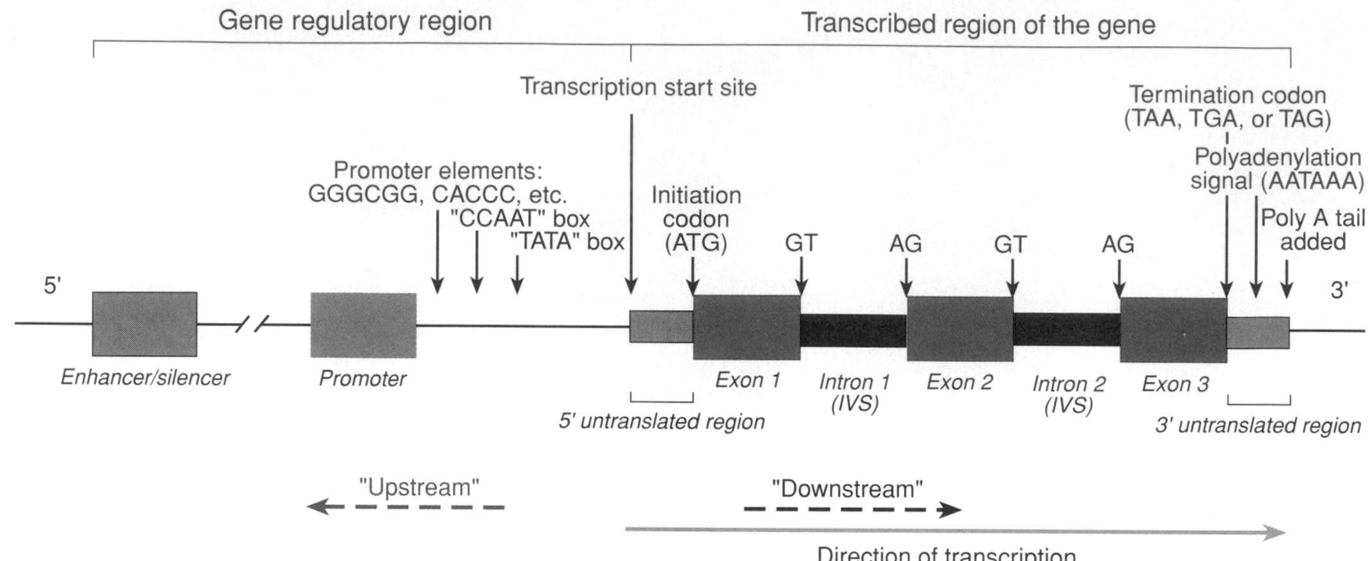

Fig. 15-3 Anatomy of a gene and its associated regulatory region.

cleotide attachment regions for the phosphodiester bonds. This sugar-phosphate polymer provides the backbone to which the nucleotides are attached. If both strands are presented, the top strand of a DNA sequence is read from left to right, 5′ to 3′, and by convention contains the sequence of the messenger RNA or coding strand. The lower strand is read from right to left in a 3′ to 5′ direction and is the template strand from which the DNA sequence will be transcribed into RNA. The bidirectional polarity of the DNA sequence is denoted as being antiparallel. By convention, the sense strand is used for the published sequence so that it can easily represent the sequence of the RNA transcribed.

The sequence of a gene includes four types of nucleotide bases that consist of the purines adenine (A) and guanine (G) and the pyrimidines cytosine (C) and thymidine (T). These bases form Watson-Crick pairing between the two DNA strands in a known pattern (that is, A=T and C=G). This double-stranded molecule contains the inherited genetic information in a double helix. Accumulated data from known gene sequences have shown that some nucleotide sequences occur more frequently together, representing landmarks and sequence signals for initiation, termination, and processing involved in transcription. The proportion of A=T- and C=G-rich areas in a sequence varies among genes. DNA regions that are C=G rich are 50% stronger because they are paired by three bonds versus the two bonds of A=T pairs. C=G-rich DNA requires a higher melting temperature to unstack and denature than A=T-rich regions do. These interactions can be important for determining hybridization conditions for different types of probes, for designing PCR primers, and for sequencing DNA (Chapter 11).

The promoter

The promoter region is defined as the sequences that are involved in the initiation of transcription. This region can generally be found within 300 base pairs (bp) of the transcription start site. This region may contain several DNA elements that include the TATA box, the CCAAT box, and other relatively generic sequences that determine where the RNA polymerase binds and transcription starts. The start point for transcription contains the "cap site," since a modified 7-methylguanosine is added to the 5′ end of the nascent mRNA to maintain its integrity after completion of transcription.

Many human genes contain a TATA box whose sequences are conserved. This region is located about 30 bp 5′ of the start site of transcription. Based on data from both studies of *Escherichia coli* and human promoters the consensus sequence for this AT-rich region is TATAAT, and it serves to position and stabilize the RNA polymerase at the start site. The CCAAT box is located about 80 bp upstream from the start site and may not be present in all genes. Another regulatory sequence that is frequently found in housekeeping genes in place of both the TATA and CCAAT boxes is a GC-rich sequence, the consensus sequence of which is GGGCGG.

Enhancers/silencers

DNA sequence elements that increase or decrease the level of transcription of a gene are called *enhancers* or *silencers*, respectively. These sequences act in *cis*, upon an adjacent promoter to regulate transcription. Each of these elements can influence transcription whether they are 5′ or 3′ to a gene or located within a gene. They can act even when they are great distances from the promoter and oriented in a forward or reverse position. An example is the locus control region (LCR) associated with the β-globin gene and positioned about 13 kb 5′ of the start site. This region consists of a cluster of four regulatory regions (HS1-4) each made up of 200 to 400 bp that contain sequences that interact with common transcription factors and erythroid-specific transcription factors.

Exons

The regions of the gene that are transcribed into messenger RNA, and subsequently translated into a functional protein product, are termed the *exons*. The DNA sequences in exons are conserved from generation to generation within a species and may be conserved between closely related species. This conservation in sequence is critical for the maintenance of the structure and function of the protein being coded. An alteration in even a single nucleotide may result in a disease-producing mutation if it results in an altered protein product. The number and size of exons within a gene and among genes varies greatly. The largest known human gene at present, the dystrophin gene on the X chromosome, is composed of 2 million bases and has 75 exons. The exons vary in size from 100 to 300 bp, with an average size of 150 bp. The retinoblastoma gene, which is 200 kbp in length and has 27 exons, is an example of the variation of exon size. The size of the smallest exon is 31 bp and the largest is 1000 bp. The Factor VIII gene, also considered to be a large gene at 186 kbp, has 26 exons, which range from 69 to 313 bp for the smaller exons and 1958 to 3106 bp for the two largest ones.

Introns

The DNA sequence intervening between two exons is called the *intron*. This sequence may not be conserved among species as that found in exons, since variations in an intron do not alter the protein product. Introns are spliced out during the processing of the messenger RNA into a mature message. The exception to this statement is discussed below under splicing. Because of normal sequence variation among individuals, the sequence differences in introns can be used to advantage for restriction fragment length polymorphism (RFLP) analysis (Chapter 11). As with exons, introns can vary considerably in length. The genes encoding the histones do not have any introns. Examples of genes that have exceptionally long introns include a 35,000 bp intron in the dystrophin gene and a 220,000 bp intron in the *bcl-2* gene. Introns are the regions that are spliced out during the processing of the messenger RNA into a mature message.

Splicing

Splicing is the process through which introns are removed and exons are joined. Signal sequences that direct the mRNA-processing enzymes to the correct region of RNA sequence found at the 5′ and 3′ regions of each intron. The signal at the 5′ end of an intron is usually GT (the *splice donor*) and the signal at the 3′ end of the intron is AG (the *splice acceptor*). Adjacent to these signal sequences are several nucleotides that together with the signal sequences occur in a consistent pattern. At these two defined points the introns are clipped out, and the exons are brought together to result in a mature messenger RNA (mRNA). If the nucleotides at either one of these signal sites are altered, one of three events will occur. First, the entire intron could remain as part of the sequence in the partially processed mRNA. This would result in a longer then predicted mRNA. Second, an alternative splice site called a *cryptic splice site* that has the common signal sequence noted above but is found elsewhere in the intron or in the preceding exon could be chosen during the splicing process. Third, the splicing at that site may have a reduced efficiency, resulting in the first or second events occurring for some of the mRNAs. This would result in a longer or shorter processed mRNA. Each of these situations would result in an altered protein product that would be truncated and either partially functional or degraded depending on the location of the mutation. A normal process called *alternative splicing* occurs in some genes. This process involves the alternative selection of exon combinations in a gene that results in different mature mRNAs. Different protein products may result that have highly homologous regions. Splicing sequences are found in transcribed genes that may not be used. The consistent correct choice for splicing indicates that other factors in addition to the splice-site sequences may be important for this process.

Polyadenylation

Mature mRNAs contain a series of adenosine residues that signal the end of the message and provide stability for transport of the mature mRNA out of the nucleus to the endoplasmic reticulum. After one of the translation termination signal sequences, UAA, UAG, or UGA, in mRNA, the consensus *polyadenylation sequence* is found in the 3′ untranslated region and consists of AAUAAA or a similar sequence. A string of adenosine residues are added after this sequence to the end of the mRNA.

PATTERNS OF INHERITANCE

Autosomal dominant disorders

Genetic disorders with autosomal dominant inheritance represent more than one half of the 6000 known mendelian phenotypes. This group of disorders is characterized by several distinguishing characteristics. First, the family pedigree shows a vertical inheritance pattern (Fig. 15-4) in which the disorder is passed from generation to generation, usually by an individual who is genotypically a heterozygote. Homozygotes are rarely seen in autosomal dominant disorders, but this situation could be suspected in a family pedigree if all the children were affected and none were normal. Such a pedigree demonstrates that no matter which affected chromosome from the homozygous parent or parents was inherited, a child would have the disease. The exception to this would be the occurrence of a new mutation in the gamete of an unaffected parent, or a situation in which the phenotypic expression of a disorder was inapparent or was mild in some individuals. A child of an affected parent has a 50% risk of inheriting the disorder. Although each pregnancy is considered as an independent event, the expected 1:1 ratio among a sibship may vary in families. In a family of four children only 1 of 4 may be affected in one family, whereas 3 of 4 may be affected in another family with the same disorder. Phenotypically normal individuals do not transmit the disorder to their children. Mild phenotypic expression or lack of penetrance of the disease are limitations of this characteristic. Within each generation, both males and females can be affected, and both males and females are equally likely to transmit the disorder to their children. Examples of autosomal dominant disorders include neurofibromatosis 1, Huntington's disease, colonic polyposis, polycystic kidney disease, and Marfan's syndrome.

Autosomal recessive disorders

Autosomal recessive disorders are less common than autosomal dominant disorders, accounting for about one third of the Mendelian disorders. Autosomal recessive disorders have several distinctive characteristics. First, the mode of transmission is characterized by a horizontal inheritance pattern (Fig. 15-5) in which the disorder is observed in the offspring of an individual family in a pedigree but not in the parents. An affected

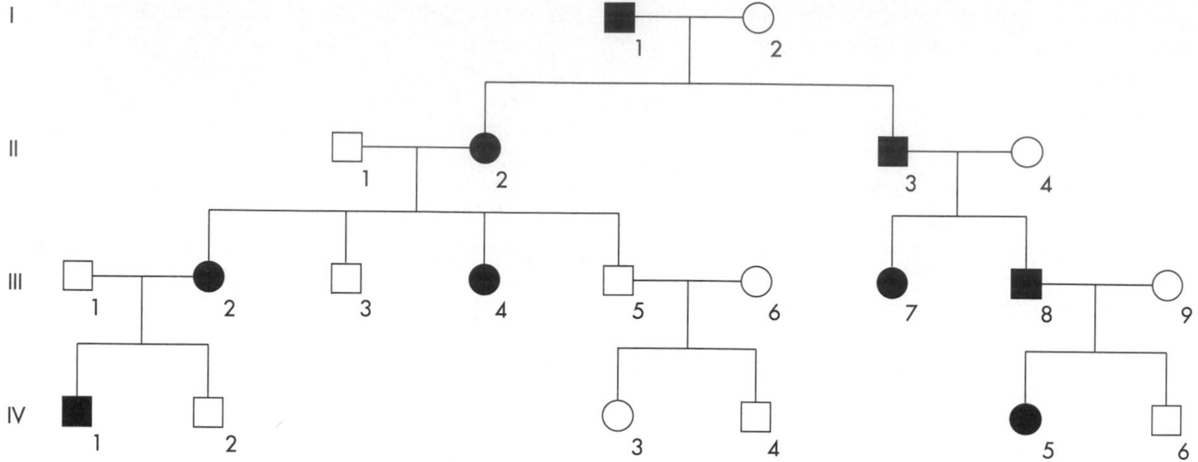

Fig. 15-4 Autosomal dominant inheritance (*box,* male; *circle,* female; *shaded,* affected).

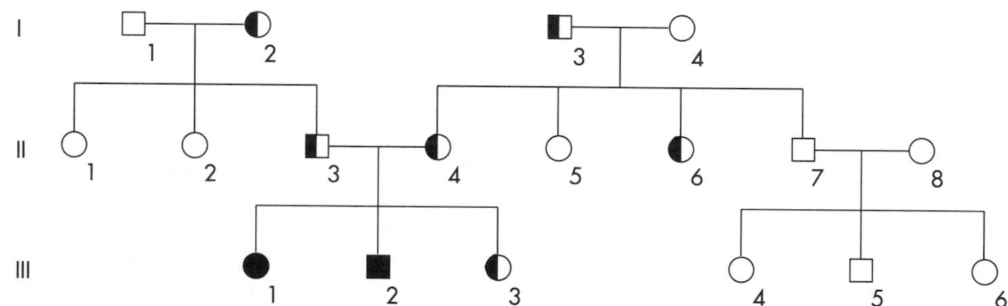

Fig. 15-5 Autosomal recessive inheritance (*box,* male; *circle,* female; *shaded,* affected).

individual, who is homozygous for a disorder, has inherited a disease allele from each heterozygous parent. In autosomal recessive disorders heterozygotes are usually not phenotypically recognizable; only the homozygotes express a clinical phenotype. Second, the horizontal mode of transmission means that affected individuals are usually observed within the sibship of a single family in the same generation among families of a kindred. Third, with each pregnancy there is a 1 in 4 (25%) chance of having an affected individual. Males and females have an equal chance of being affected. The frequency of a carrier having an affected child is determined by the frequency of heterozygotes and the frequency of mutant alleles in a population. An increased frequency of an autosomal recessive disorder within a kindred can be observed in two situations. The first is intermarriage between close relatives (that is, consanguinity). The second occurs when the mutant allele frequency is high within a given population, such as cystic fibrosis in individuals of northern European extraction or sickle cell anemia among individuals of African origin.

X-linked disorders

X-linked diseases are associated with mutations in the X chromosome and have a distinctive inheritance pattern (Fig. 15-6). Both X-linked dominant and X-linked recessive traits can be observed with this inheritance pattern. The family pedigree is distinctive in that there is a lack of male-to-male-transmission. In families where the father is affected, all his daughters will be heterozygous, and they are therefore called *obligate carriers*. In general, heterozygotes do not express the disease clinically, but in rare cases, if a female does manifest the disease, it is termed *X-linked recessive.* These manifesting females have been observed in cases of hemophilia A and B, Duchenne muscular dystrophy, and several X-linked eye diseases, which include color blindness. The mechanism for this clinical phenotype is attributable to the lack of inactivation of the X chromosome that carries the mutation. Normal X inactivation, called *lyonization,* occurs in somatic cells in females randomly, approximately 3 days after fertilization. This results in the inactivation of one or the other X chromosome, which produces a mosaic pattern of hemizygous function of the alternate chromosome among the cells within each female. Rarely, an X-linked disease can be seen in a homozygous female whose father was affected and whose mother was a heterozygote for

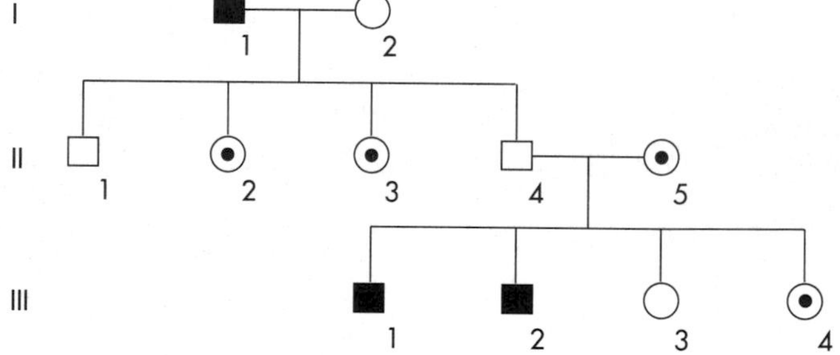

Fig. 15-6 X-linked inheritance (*box,* male; *circle,* female).

the disease. Many immunodeficiency disorders arise from abnormalities on the X chromosome (see Chapter 27).

NonMendelian inheritance

NonMendelian inheritance patterns include mitochondrial inheritance, mosaicism, uniparental disomy, and genomic imprinting. *Mitochondrial inheritance* is attributable primarily to maternal transmission, which results in disease transmission to both males and females, and a lack of disease transmission from males (Fig. 15-7). Diseases arising from mutations in mitochondrial DNA (mtDNA) frequently show a variable phenotypic pattern. This is attributable to the random inheritance of variable proportions of normal and mutant mitochondria. Although the majority of mitochondrial proteins are encoded by genes in the nucleus, subunits of mitochondrial enzymes are encoded in mtDNA found in cytoplasm. The enzymes are used in the oxidative phosphorylation (respiratory) pathway. Several diseases have been associated with mutations in these genes, as discussed in Chapter 14, including Leber's hereditary optic neuropathy (LHON), myoclonic epilepsy with ragged-red fiber disease (MERRF), mitochondrial encephalomyopathy with lacticacidosis and strokelike symptoms (MELAS), and Kearns-Sayre syndrome (KSS). More recently, mutations in mitochondrial DNA have also been demonstrated in patients with late-onset diabetes mellitus, Parkinson's, Alzheimer's, and Huntington's diseases.[15]

Mosaicism occurs in an individual in which two or more genetically different cell lines are generated from a single zygote. This condition has been documented in several different genetic diseases in both males and females, including hemophilia A, Duchenne muscular dystrophy, neurofibromatosis I, and ornithine transcarbamylase deficiency. A typical example is found in the normal female, as a result of X inactivation (Lyonization), discussed previously. However, in the disease one observes two types of mosaicism, which includes somatic and germline mosaicism. The most prominent disease associated with somatic mosaicism is cancer. Data from many studies indicate that a tumor is the result of unregulated proliferation of a single malignant cell that produces a clone of cells. The original evidence of the clonal nature of tumors was obtained from tumors in women who were heterozygous for the X-linked enzyme glucose-6-phosphate dehydrogenase (G6PD). Because of lyonization, one or the other of the G6PD alleles was inactivated. The origin of either active X allele (that is, maternal or paternal) could then be determined and associated with the cell lines derived from each tumor. Results showed that one or the other but not both G6PD alleles were found to be expressed in each tumor, demonstrating the clonal nature of the tumor.

The second type of mosaicism involves mutations that occur in germline during gametogenesis. During the early development of one parent, a somatic mutation occurs in a germline cell during a series of mitotic divisions, for females about 30 divisions and for males several hundred, before meiosis. This mutation is then expanded through clonal proliferation and represents a portion of the final gametes in that parent. As a result of this process one or more germline cells carrying a mutation may by chance be selected to contribute to an individual who manifests a particular disease. Examples of diseases that in some cases have arisen from germline mosaicism include osteogenesis imperfecta, hemophilia A, and Duchenne muscular dystrophy.

Two newer concepts of nonMendelian inheritance are uniparental disomy and genomic imprinting. Uniparental disomy involves the presence of a disomic cell line in which there are two parental chromosomes of the same type, derived from the same parent. When the two chromosomes represent a duplication of the same chromosome, the condition is called "isodisomy." If the two chromosomes represent the homologs from one parent, the condition is called "heterodisomy." This condition has been observed in both males and females and in both somatic and sex chromosomes. The first case of uniparental disomy was reported by Spence and associates, and involved a female cystic fibrosis patient with short stature.[16] This case represented an example of isodisomy involving chromosome 7. Additional examples of uniparental disomy have been documented in Prader-Willi syndrome and hemophilia A.

Genomic imprinting involves the differential expression of either the maternal or the paternal chromosome that influences the expression of a particular genetic disorder. Until recently, the parental origin of a chromosome was not believed to be significant in determining the phenotypic expression of a genetic disorder. Up to now, classical Mendelian inheritance was based on independent assortment and random recombination of parental alleles that allow an equal opportunity for each parent to transmit an autosomal gene or a female to transmit either of her X chromosomes. The significance of the origination of the parental chromosome was recognized in studies of patients with Prader-Willi syndrome and Angelman syndrome. Both genetic disorders involve deletions on the long arm of chromosome 15 (15q11q13). In many patients with Prader-Willi, the deletions occur on the paternal chromosome, allowing similar regions from the maternal chromosome to influence phenotypic expression. In contrast, patients with Angelman syndrome have a strikingly different clinical phenotype. In this syndrome, the deletions occur in the same region on 15q of the maternal chromosome, allowing similar regions on the paternal chromosome to influence phenotypic expres-

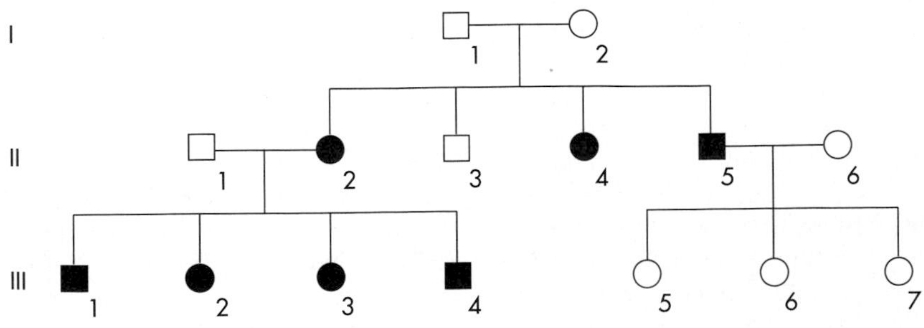

Fig. 15-7 Mitochondrial inheritance (*box,* male; *circle,* female; *shaded,* affected).

sion. An additional unique finding documented by Nicholls and colleagues in two Prader-Willi patients was the inheritance of both homologs of the maternal chromosome and neither of the paternal chromosomes.[17] This represented an example of uniparental disomy and further showed the significance of the intricate influence that each parental chromosome contributes in normal gene expression.

CONCEPTS OF GENE REGULATION

Transcription

Proteins are the functional molecules that carry out the encoded messages of DNA. The production of protein is a highly controlled process within an organism, and these processes are regulated at the level of RNA production (transcription) or at the level of protein production (translation). Diseases may arise through disruption of transcriptional regulation of gene expression at multiple levels, resulting in abnormal human embryogenesis and development, selected physiologic abnormalities, or neoplasia. The most significant mechanisms for controlling RNA production from DNA are at the level of transcription, though RNA processing and RNA stability can also affect the overall level of protein present within a cell. The production of mRNA from DNA templates is accomplished through the activity of RNA polymerase II. RNA polymerases I and III account for production of ribosomal and transfer RNA respectively. In order for the full activity of RNA polymerase II to occur, a transcriptionally active complex must form at specific sites along the DNA. One of the most important features of a gene that is capable of transcription is for it to be within an open chromatin domain or euchromatin. This is in contrast to heterochromatin, which is highly condensed and probably exists in a confirmation that is not accessible to polymerase II and the associated transcription factors. However only a small number of the sequences within euchromatin are transcribed.[18-20]

In addition to the structural features that provide for the correct conformation of DNA, the process of transcription involves multiple events. The assembly of a transcriptionally active complex includes the binding of polymerase II with DNA and has been shown to be influenced by the DNA sequences downstream of the site of initiation as well as the presence of numerous basal factors and associated proteins termed "transcription factors." The basal factors include TFIIA, TFIIB, TFIID, TFIIE, TFIIF, TFIIH, and TFIIJ.[21,22] These factors must appropriately assemble and thereby provide for association of polymerase II to DNA before transcription. These factors are collectively referred to as the *transcription initiation complex* (TIC), the assembly of which is the rate-limiting step in transcription of many genes. Before assembly of the TIC, the regulatory element is conditioned by the presence of numerous other transcription factors. These transcription factors may either bind directly to the DNA at sequence-specific binding sites or may interact with other transcription factors and accelerate or impede their attachment or complex formation to binding sites. Transcription factors are capable of acting in *trans,* or at a distance, upon the expression of genes separate from the one producing the factor. The DNA sequences to which some of these transcription factors bind are usually *cis* acting, since they influence transcription within the gene they are located. Even so, an enhancer may be located considerably upstream or downstream from the site at which RNA transcription begins.[23]

Transcription factors may have a positive or a negative influence on the rate of transcription and are thus termed *activators* or *repressors.* The viral proteins E6 and E7 associated with human *Papillomavirus* have been shown to have a disruptive effect through binding to and subsequent removal of a normally abundant repressor protein. The activity of transcription factors can also be altered through other mechanisms, including common chromosomal translocations. Translocations result in the production of a "Frankenstein protein" that otherwise does not normally exist, and yet it is able to overcome the multiple layers of regulation involved in transcription. Abnormalities may occur through translocation that affect either the DNA sequence-specific binding site, the regulatory domain of a transcription factor, or the deregulation of its normal level of expression (Fig. 15-3).[24]

Transcription factors play important roles in tissue-specific gene expression. They may either collectively or individually contribute to tissue-specific gene expression. Since any one cell contains a wide array of transcription factors in which gene transcription is orchestrated, the overrepresentation of one group of factors (instruments) may greatly affect the overall production. Simply stated, the group of transcription factors found in a tissue may determine production of liver proteins as opposed to pancreas protein production. Alternatively, certain tissues have been found to contain a unique transcription factor not found in other cell types.

Transcription factors have both distinct components and common features. Four large superfamilies of transcription factors have been identified: the *helix loop helix,* the *leucine zipper,* the *zinc finger,* and the *homeodomain factors.* Common among these transcription factors is a component that conveys the DNA-binding activity, a second element that facilitates the dimerization or formation of combination units, and a possible third domain that accounts for features conveying activation such as phosphorylation sites. Transcription factors often dimerize, such that two individual units combine to form the active molecule. This dimerization may occur within a region in which the amino acid leucine is present at every seventh residue and is a key feature of factors in the leucine zipper family. Alternatively, dimerization may occur within the α-helices found in the helix loop helix motif.

DNA binding can be accomplished either through formation of a tetrahedron complex with zinc that conveys DNA-binding properties, such as that found in the zinc finger superfamily, or alternatively the DNA-binding domain consists of a region with numerous basic amino acid residues. An additional property of transcription factors is that they may form heterodimers composed of two different factors within the same subfamily, rather than homodimers. Such an example is the *fos-jun* dimer, which recognizes the AP-1 binding site. Alternatively, *jun* may homodimerize, but *fos* does not have this capability. It should be noted that both of these transcription factors were first recognized as viral oncogenes with transforming capability long before their actual cellular functions were found. Through the process of alternative splicing or alternative initiation various forms of these transcription factors are also generated. Such isoforms may contain the dimerization domains but lack the DNA-binding capability of the larger transcription factors and therefore may act as inhibitors of transcription. For example, IP-1, which contains a leucine zipper, can dimerize with either *fos* or *jun,* but because a DNA-binding domain is absent in IP-1, its association with other factors results in a nonfunctional heterodimer.

Several important concepts related to transcription factors and the DNA sites to which they bind must be considered. First, the DNA protein binding sites are modular units that work in tandem with multiple other units in the same vicinity. Second, transcription factors that bind to these DNA elements may either have a positive or a negative influence on the overall level of transcription and in some cases may have no effect. Third, the activity of the transcription factor can be influenced by extracellular factors such as cyclic AMP, calcium levels, or serum factors. Thus the process of transcription regulation forms a bridge between external factors and demands of the environment with the inherent capability of a cell to respond as encoded by its DNA.

A classic example of abnormal transcription resulting in a pathologic condition is that of hemoglobinopathies. In hereditary persistence of fetal hemoglobin, the production of gamma globin persists into adult life. The mechanism for this persistence has been shown to be attributable to a single base mutation within the gamma globin gene-transcription initiation site. A mutation in the promoter from GATA to GATG affects in some way the overall activation state of the promoter even though the transcription factor GATA1 is capable of binding to either sequence. One form of hemophilia B has been shown to be caused by an alteration within the transcription initiation site.[25,26] A mutation within the binding site for C/EBP results in production of Factor IX at levels less than 1% of normal until puberty, when the levels rise to 60% of normal activity. This situation illustrates another feature of transcriptional regulation: the effect that certain hormones or mediators have on cell signaling. Hormones or chemicals such as cyclic AMP may exert their influence through affecting transcriptional pathways. In the case of Leyden hemophilia B the production of steroid hormones during maturation results in activation of the androgen receptor, a known transcription factor that either influences the binding of C/EBP or directly activates transcription of factor IX.

Steroid hormones may influence transcription in other ways resulting in altered expression of certain genes. Estrogen, dihydrotestosterone, glucocorticoids, mineralocorticoids, vitamin D, thyroid hormone, and retinoic acid are hormones, the action of which is mediated through their effects on transcription factors. Each of these hormones is capable of binding to their receptor within the cytoplasm, which is subsequently transported to the nucleus where the effects on transcription occur. Thus it is reasonable that the production of these hormones may result in a wide variety of other genes being expressed, recognized phenotypically by feminization or masculinization. Abnormalities in the androgen receptor have been shown to be responsible for the testicular feminization syndrome. Testicular feminization or androgen insensitivity occurs in genotypic 46 XY males in which the androgen-receptor component of the transcription factor is mutated and rendered incapable of binding testosterone.[27]

Abnormalities have also been documented in the vitamin D receptor, the thyroid hormone receptor, and the glucocorticoid receptor. These mutations result in a hereditary vitamin D–resistant rickets in which secondary hyperparathyroidism may also appear. In this case the vitamin D_3 receptor, also a member of the zinc finger transcription family, contains a mutation rendering it unable to bind vitamin D_3 or alternatively incapable of activating transcription.

The Wilms' tumor locus on the short arm of chromosome 11 contains a gene that illustrates how transcription factors play a role in embryogenesis as well as in neoplasia. The Wilms' tumor gene (WT1) is expressed at high levels in embryonic kidney. It has been proposed that WT1 may inhibit cellular proliferation through its competition with the activity of a second transcription factor that binds to the same DNA-recognition sequence. In the case of Wilms' tumor when the WT1 transcription factor is absent or altered, the activity of the early growth response-1 (EGR1) gene product results in cellular proliferation, eventually recognized as neoplasia.[28,29] Similarly, the retinoblastoma (Rb) gene product has several important roles related to cell proliferation. However, the Rb protein does not bind to DNA but rather has its effect on other transcription factors present within the cell, one of which is E2F. Rather than directly competing for binding to the DNA-recognition site, as in the case of WT1 and Wilms' tumor, the Rb protein prevents E2F from binding to its sequence. E2F is a transcription factor that influences the expression of a wide variety of genes involved in cell replication. The importance of phosphorylation can also be demonstrated in this system, in that phosphorylation of Rb results in the release of E2F whereas nonphosphorylated Rb retains its ability to bind E2F. As discussed in Chapter 13 certain viral proteins such as E1A and T antigen exert their influence through binding of Rb with the subsequent increase in activity of E2F.

Whereas some transcription factors are global in their effect and are found in multiple cell types, other transcription factors are limited in their expression. One of the most elegant examples of this occurs within the superfamily of transcription factors that includes the PIT, OCT, and UNC families. Whereas OCT1 is expressed in a wide variety of cell types, the expression of OCT2 appears to be cell-type specific and limited to expression in B-cells. As discussed earlier, transcription factors can work in concert only with other factors, and OCT2 is not solely responsible for expression of immunoglobulins from B-cells but rather contributes in some currently undetermined way. With each experimental discovery an additional level of complexity is discovered. In the case of immunoglobulin gene expression other factors, termed "coactivators," are proving to be important, such as the OCA-B factor from B-cells. Thus tissue-specific transcription factors may not be the on/off switch of gene expression, but rather influence the timing of events leading to the expression of immunoglobulins.[30]

Translation

Translation is the process whereby the nucleic acid sequence of RNA is decoded and converted into proteins through the assembly of amino acids. In this system, the template is mRNA from which the information stored in three consecutive nucleotides or codons is used to select the corresponding amino acid. By convention, DNA is written with an upper strand proceeding from the 5′ end to the 3′ end and a lower strand proceeding from 3′ to 5′. RNA is generated from the lower strand and is therefore identical to the upper strand of DNA, except that uracil is substituted in RNA for thymidine in DNA. Since the machinery for translation of protein from RNA is present in the cytoplasm and the genetic material is present within the nucleus, the RNA serves as a messenger bringing the information from one compartment into the next.

Thus, RNA is analogous to a floppy disk on which information on the computer can be taken to a distant site for printing. The translation process occurs along the endoplasmic reticulum by ribosomes, which are also composed of RNA. Ribosomes have subunits identified by their sedimentation properties as 60S and 40S. A third RNA molecule termed *transfer RNA* brings the appropriate amino acid to the mRNA ribosome complex termed the *polysome*. Since the ribosome can accommodate two tRNA molecules with the corresponding amino acids at any one time, the stage is set for linking of the two amino acids through a peptide bond. Since the polysome moves from the 5′ end to the 3′ end of the mRNA, proteins are assembled in the direction from the amino terminus to the carboxy terminus. Since the codons are composed of three separate nucleotides, the positioning of the beginning of translation is very important. Codons that represent the initiation site for translation, such as AUG, have been identified. The conversion of codons to protein proceeds directly from the AUG start sequence with every subsequent three nucleotides representing the next amino acid. In the absence of such an initiation site the DNA could have three possible reading frames. However, the other reading frames are commonly blocked by the presence of termination codons, such as UAA, UAG, and UGA, which do not allow for continuation of the translation process. Thus, it can be understood how single changes in the nucleotide sequence can lead to the addition or deletion of an appropriate initiation site, can add a termination signal, or shift the entire reading frame. The introduction of such mutations accounts for a large number of the genetic defects described below.

SMALL STRUCTURAL CHANGES IN DNA

A variety of different mutation types are found among the genes that have been characterized to date. Mutations range in size from the smallest structural change in DNA, which involves the substitution of a single nucleotide, to the deletion or insertion of thousands of nucleotides. Mutations, which include missense, nonsense, frameshift, insertion, deletion, duplication, amplification, and translocation, can be found singly or in combination in a particular gene. The use of mutation analysis to characterize the location, diversity, and frequency of mutations in a gene provides insight into the normal structure and function of a gene, the mechanisms of its regulatory response and control regions, the regions of critical interactive sites of the protein product, and possible strategies for therapeutic modalities. In the following paragraphs, different types of mutations are defined and examples of each are given.

The smallest structural change in DNA involves the substitution, addition, or deletion of a single nucleotide. If a single nucleotide within a codon is changed, such as CGT to CAT (Arg to His), the result is an exchange of one amino acid for another. This is a *missense mutation*. A full-length protein product is produced, which may have an altered structure that prevents proper function. Common diseases that result from missense mutations include sickle cell anemia, alpha- and beta- thalassemia, cystic fibrosis, and alpha-1-antitrypsin deficiency. If a single nucleotide that changes the reading code of the DNA sequence from an amino acid to a stop codon, such as AGA to TGA (Arg to STOP) is substituted, the result is the termination of transcription, resulting in an incomplete protein product. These *nonsense mutations* are seen in cystic fibrosis, hemophilia A, and neurofibromatosis 1. *Frameshift mutations* arise from the insertion or deletion of one or two nucleotides in a codon of the DNA sequence. These mutations alter the reading frame, resulting in the substitution of different amino acids in the protein product. As a result of the changed reading frame in the messenger RNA, a premature STOP codon or codons are frequently introduced generating a truncated protein that has altered function or is degraded if it occurs early in protein synthesis. Examples of this type of mutation occur in Duchenne muscular dystrophy, alpha-thalassemia (hemoglobin Cranston) and beta-thalassemia (hemoglobin Constant Spring). If a deletion or insertion of three nucleotides in the DNA sequence that code for an amino acid occurs, the result is an in-frame mutation. The final protein product will be shorter or longer and may not function properly because of its altered folding properties. This type of mutation is found in the ΔF508 mutation of cystic fibrosis, a common change in 67% to 75% of cystic fibrosis (CF) chromosomes. It results from a three base-pair deletion that codes for phenylalanine. The protein product that is produced remains in the endoplasmic reticulum and does not go to the Golgi for further processing.

Deletions and insertions of DNA also occur in a wide range of sizes in several diseases. In Duchenne and Becker muscular dystrophy, the most common type of mutation, seen in approximately 65% of patients, is a deletion. Out-of-frame deletions are characteristic of Duchenne muscular dystrophy and result in little or no dystrophin being synthesized. In contrast, in-frame deletions are characteristic in a majority of Becker muscular dystrophy patients. This type of mutation results in a shortened protein product that is semifunctional. In hemophilia A, a variety of sizes of deletions ranging from 2 to greater than 210 kilobase pairs have been documented throughout the factor VIII gene. Examples of insertions in DNA that result in disease are found in Tay-Sachs disease and hemophilia A. The most common mutation found in Tay-Sachs patients consists of a four base-pair insertion in the hexosaminidase A gene that causes a premature stop codon that results in a lack of protein production. In hemophilia A, two cases involving the insertion of an L1 sequence of 3.8 and 2.3 kilobase pairs, respectively, in the factor VIII gene have been documented.

LARGE STRUCTURAL CHANGES IN DNA

Large structural changes in DNA consist of translocations, deletion/duplications, and amplifications. These changes occur in well-recognized disorders, including Down syndrome, t(14;21); Burkitt lymphoma, t(8;14)(q24;32); and chronic myelogenous leukemia, t(9;22)(q34;11). Approximately 4% of Down syndrome cases are attributable to an unbalanced translocation of two acrocentric chromosomes. In greater than 50% of these cases, the translocation results from a de novo event in the parent during gametogenesis, and the balance of cases are attributable to inheritance. This translocation involves the fusion of the long arms of chromosomes 14 and 21. For Burkitt lymphoma, the reciprocal exchange is between the long arms of chromosomes 8 and 14. The break on chromosome 8 is in the q24 region, where the *myc* oncogene is located, and on chromosome 14, at q32, where the immunoglobulin heavy-chain gene is located. In chronic myelogenous leukemia, the breakpoints occur on chromosome 9, the Philadelphia chromosome, at q34, where the *abl* oncogene maps, and chromosome 22q11, where the breakpoint cluster region *(bcr)* gene maps.

Another mutation causing large DNA rearrangements involves a combination of deletion and duplication. This type of mutation is the result of unequal crossing over during meiosis I or mitosis. Misalignment and exchange of chromosomal material between homologous chromosomes produces a duplication on one chromosome and a deletion on the other. This type of DNA rearrangement is believed to be responsible for the deletions found in alpha-thalassemia, beta-thalassemia (hemoglobin Gun Hill), X-linked color-vision defects, variation in the number of normal copies of the green visual-pigment gene within the red and green visual-pigment gene cluster, and growth hormone deficiency.

A final type of mutation, only recently documented in human DNA, involves the amplification and expansion of an unstable trinucleotide repeat. These triplet repeat regions may be found within the gene or at the 5′ or 3′ flanking regions. In affected individuals the size of the expansions vary among disease types but range from several hundred to several thousand repeats. Diseases such as fragile X, myotonic dystrophy, spinal and bulbar muscular dystrophy, and Huntington's disease are examples of this type of mutation.

REFERENCES

1. McKusick VA: *Mendelian inheritance in man: catalogs of autosomal dominant, autosomal recessive, and X-linked phenotypes,* ed 12, Baltimore, 1995, Johns Hopkins University Press.
2. Vogel F, Motulsky AG: *Human genetics: problems and approaches,* ed 2, Berlin, 1986, Springer-Verlag.
3. Alberts B, Bray D, Lewis J et al: *Molecular biology of the cell,* ed 3, New York, 1994, Garland Publishing,.
4. Scriver CR, Beaudet AL, Sly WS, Valle D: *The metabolic basis of inherited disease,* ed 7, New York, 1995, McGraw-Hill Information Services Co.
5. Gelehrter TD, Collins FS: *Principles of medical genetics,* Baltimore, 1990, Williams & Wilkins.
6. Lewin B: *Genes V,* Oxford, 1994, Oxford University Press.
7. Murray RK, Granner DK, Mayes PA, Rodwell VW: *Harper's biochemistry,* ed 22, Norwalk, Conn, 1994, Appleton & Lange.
8. Thompson MW, McInnes RR, Willard HF: *Genetics in medicine,* ed 5, Philadelphia, 1991, Saunders.
9. Watson JD, Gilman M, Witkowski J, Zoller M: *Recombinant DNA,* ed 2, New York, 1992, Scientific American Books, WH Freeman.
10. Baird PA, Anderson TW, Newcombe HB, Lowry RB: Genetic disorders in children and young adults: a population study, *Am J Hum Genet* 42:677, 1988.
11. Carter CO: Changing patterns in the causes of death at the Hospital for Sick Children, *Great Ormond Street J* 11:65, 1956.
12. Roberts DF, Chavez J, Court SDM : The genetic component in child mortality, *Arch Dis Child* 45:33, 1970.
13. Scriver CR, Neal JL, Saginur R, Clow A: The frequency of genetic disease and congenital malformation among patients in a pediatric hospital, *Can Med Assoc J* 108:1111, 1973.
14. Hall JG, Powers EK, McIlvaine RT, Ean VH: The frequency and financial burden of genetic disease in a pediatric hospital, *Am J Med Genet* 1:417, 1978
15. Wallace DC: Mitochondrial genetics: a paradigm for aging and degenerative diseases? *Science* 256:628, 1992.
16. Spence JE, Perciaccante RG, Greig GM et al: Uniparental disomy as a mechanism for human genetic disease, *Am J Hum Genet* 42:217, 1988.
17. Nicholls RD, Knoll JH, Butler MG, et al: Genetic imprinting suggested by maternal heterodisomy in nondeletion Prader-Willi syndrome, *Nature* 342:281, 1989.
18. Forrester WC, Epner E, Driscoll MC et al: A deletion of the human β-globin locus activator region (LAR) causes a major alteration in chromatin structure and replication across the entire β-globin locus, *Genes Dev* 4:1637, 1990.
19. Emerson, BM : Gene expression in hematopoietic cells: the β-globin gene. In Karin M, editor: *Gene expression: general and cell-type-specific,* Boston, 1993, Birkhauser.
20. Roberts SGE, Green MR: The basic transcriptional machinery. In Karin M, editor: *Gene expression: general and cell-type-specific,* Boston, 1993, Birkhauser.
21. Briggs MR, Kadonaga JT, Bell SP et al: Purification and biochemical characterization of the promotor-specific transcription factor Sp1, *Science* 234:47, 1986.
22. Busch SJ, Sassone-Corsi P: Dimers, leucine zippers and DNA binding domains, *Trends Genet* 6:36, 1990.
23. Thompson CC, McKnight SL: Anatomy of an enhancer, *Trends Genet* 8:232, 1992.
24. Foulkes NS, Sassone-Corsi P: More is better: activators and repressors from the same gene, *Cell* 68:411, 1992:
25. Crossley M, Brownlee GG: Disruption of a C/EBP binding site in the factor IX promoter is associated with hemophilia B, *Nature* 345:444, 1990.
26. Crossley M, Ludwig M, Stowell KM et al: Recovery from hemophilia B Leyden: an androgen-responsive element in the factor IX promotor, *Science* 257:377, 1992.
27. Evans RM : The steroid and thyroid hormone receptor superfamily, *Science* 240:889, 1988.
28. Schleif R: DNA binding by proteins, *Science* 241:1182, 1988.
29. Rauscher FJ, Morris JF, Tournay OE et al: Binding of the Wilms' tumor locus zinc finger protein to the EGR-1 consensus sequence, *Science* 250:1259, 1990.
30. Verrijzer CP, Van der Vliet PC: POU domain transcription factors, *Biochim Biophys Acta* 1173:1, 1993.

16 Developmental Pathology

Dagmar K. Kalousek
Gail M. Schauer

SCOPE OF DEVELOPMENTAL PATHOLOGY

Developmental pathology may be broadly defined as the study of processes and problems related to growth, differentiation, and maturation from the time of fertilization through adulthood. In more practical terms, the discipline is concerned with developmental problems presenting in the embryo, fetus, and infant. The emphasis on embryonic development is an essential feature that sets developmental pathology apart from other areas of pathology. Our understanding of normal and abnormal human development is dependent on the general advances in developmental biology. Each species has unique variations, but the basic developmental patterns recur and interspecies comparisons are helpful. The fruit fly, frog, and chick were mostly used for early comparative studies. More recently, the nematode and mouse have served as models for specific aspects of development.[1]

Early embryonic pattern formation is essential to developing complex organisms, and the genes that produce the patterns appear to have been conserved through evolution. In *Drosophila,* the genetic program that guides the orientation of embryonic cells to produce patterns of anteroposterior, ventrodorsal, and segmentation have been elucidated. The process involves sequential transcription of a variety of homeotic genes in the cells defining a particular area. The coding regions of homeotic genes include almost identical DNA sequences that are 180 base pairs long—homeoboxes—that encode closely related polypeptide regions. These polypeptide regions impart to their proteins the ability to bind to certain DNA sequences that regulate transcription of many genes that are important in embryonic development. In fact, sequential production of these proteins is believed to underlie the cascade that guides the orderly events necessary for creation of a new organism. mRNA molecules containing transcribed homeobox sequences are found in embryonic mouse cells soon after fertilization. Various cell surface markers and receptors, along with the characteristics of the neighboring cells, play important roles in the progressive determination of cell identity. As embryonic cells differentiate into progenitors of specific tissues they become programmed to give rise to only a limited number of adult cell types. When such "limited" cells divide, their daughter cells inherit their restricted fate.[2] The ultimate goal of developmental pathology is to understand how genetic as well as environmental influences subvert the normal processes of embryonic and fetal development, thereby resulting in developmental defects.

One unique aspect of developmental pathology that has increased dramatically in importance in the past decade is its central role in genetic counseling regarding recurrence risk for specific developmental problems in future pregnancies. The heightened utilization of amniocentesis, chorionic villi, and fetal blood and urine sampling have facilitated the recognition of developmental abnormalities prenatally, particularly during the fetal period when morphologic findings are subtle.

Normal standards for embryonic development and many fetal physiologic measurements based on combined noninvasive and invasive laboratory studies are being established. Equally important information for genetic counseling is being derived from the study of spontaneous abortion, stillbirth, and neonatal death. Pregnancy loss during the embryonic period, up to 10 weeks of gestation, is termed "early spontaneous abortion" and that between 10 and 20 weeks gestation, "late spontaneous abortion." Stillbirth is broadly defined as delivery of a fetus that has died before birth after 20 weeks of gestation. Among stillbirths a distinction is frequently made between fetal deaths occurring before onset of labor, intrauterine death, and those that occur during labor or parturition, intrapartum death. The absence of changes of maceration usually implies intrapartum death.

The field of developmental pathology is quite broad, and therefore not all of the entities that rightly belong to its province are discussed. Liberal reference is of necessity made to chapters that are discussions of related issues, in particular cytogenetics, hereditary metabolic disease, developmental defects of individual organs systems, and the placenta.

The specialist in developmental pathology spends much time gaining knowledge of normal requirements for fertility, embryonic, fetal, and placental development and growth, human genetics, and the normal physiology of adaptation to extrauterine life. Against this background, the developmental pathologist learns to identify aberrations from normal and to carefully describe, catalogue, and make efforts to assign the abnormalities to a causal mechanism or mechanisms. The most important attributes in an individual performing postmortem examination of a malformed fetus or infant are attention to detail, facility of description, and thoroughness in collecting tissues for histology and ancillary studies. If these are employed in the initial examination, the literature and consultation can point to the correct diagnostic and prognostic category, even in the absence of specialized training. The establishment of a differential diagnosis can be aided by reference to encyclopedias of birth defects,[3-5] syndromology texts,[6,7] and, where available, computerized syndrome identification systems.[8]

Concepts and definitions

In developmental pathology, "congenital" is perhaps the most often used term and engenders much confusion in the uninitiated. "Congenital" means simply 'present at birth.' The term suggests nothing about cause. The terms "hereditary" and "inborn" are used interchangeably and refer to traits that can be transmitted genetically from parents to their offspring. Some such heritable traits arise for the first time in an individual because of a new mutation; thus one can have a heritable disorder that was not derived from one's parents but that would be transmissible to one's offspring. The *phenotype* of an individual is the collection of traits that can be seen or measured and that can be described without reference to the genetic composition of the individual. For a given abnormal phenotype, one or a few abnormalities represent the pertinent traits for a diagnosis, and these may be used to name the phenotype, as in the "multiple lethal pterygium phenotype." In contrast, the *genotype* of an individual is the sum of genetic material that determines the phenotype. A genotype can be studied either by microscopic examination of chromosomes using routine or molecular cytogenetic studies and by molecular techniques that directly identify defects in individual genes (Chapter 15).

Many terms used by developmental pathologists to describe grossly identifiable developmental abnormalities reflect their presumed pathogenesis and relationship to other observed abnormalities.[9] By definition, a *malformation* arises during the initial formation of a structure and may affect an organ or a large body region. An example of a common malformation is autosomal recessive polydactyly. Malformations are caused by genetic or environmental influences or by a combination of the two. Some malformations represent components of a *developmental field defect,* that is, an intrinsic abnormality affecting several parts of the embryo that develop in a coordinated and perhaps interdependent fashion. Utilization of the developmental field concept helps to explain why certain malformations occur together and requires understanding of the complex interactions between cells and tissues in the process of morphogenesis.[7] Two pathogenetically different mechanisms that also result in abnormal morphogenesis are *deformation* and *disruption.* Forces extrinsic to the embryo or fetus that impinge upon or disrupt a normal process of development result in these two types of abnormalities. *Deformations* occur when mechanical forces act to alter the form, shape, or position of a body part, as in clubfoot in a fetus developing within an abnormally small uterine cavity. *Disruptions* are usually more severe, resulting from the breakdown of normal developmental processes, usually with tissue destruction. Examples of this are digital amputations and facial clefting resulting from amniotic bands entangling the embryo or fetus. When an intrinsic or extrinsic process interrupts normal organization of cells into tissues, a *dysplasia* or *dyshistiogenesis* is said to result.

Individual congenital lesions may be found as isolated single defects in otherwise normal individuals, but frequently they are present in combination. Multiple anomalies, when found in a recognizable pattern with a known pathogenesis, are called a *syndrome.* For example, the abnormalities resulting from fetal infection with rubella virus are grouped under the entity "congenital rubella syndrome." The presence of an extra chromosome 21 results in a diagnostic phenotype with characteristic morphologic features called "trisomy 21 syndrome," or "Down syndrome." A recognized pattern of deformations or disruptions that result from a single preexisting abnormality, either known or inferred, is called a "sequence." For example, the positional, deformational, and dysmorphic features that result from persistent lack of normal amniotic fluid volume form the "oligohydramnios sequence." Although the oligohydramnios itself may have resulted from one of several causes, such as persistent rupture of the placental membranes, or fetal bilateral renal agenesis, the phenotypic features that define the sequence are the same in both instances. An *association* is also a pattern of anomalies that is nonrandom, for which a common pathogenetic mechanism cannot be presently discerned. The assumption is that the inciting cause of an association will eventually, through study, be understood. The VATER association is a frequently cited example, named as an acronym for the most common features, namely, vertebral anomalies, anal atresia, tracheoesophageal fistula, and radial or renal anomalies.

Etiology of developmental defects

Developmental defects in humans are caused by genetic and environmental factors.

Genetic disorders may be transmitted from parents to offspring by various mechanisms. Classical Mendelian genetics recognizes several dose-related forms of inheritance, including *autosomal dominant, autosomal recessive,* and *X-linked.* An *autosomal dominant* mutant gene is expressed phenotypically when a single copy of the gene is present, even if a complementary normal copy is present. Affected individuals are *heterozygous* for the abnormal gene. In these diseases, an affected parent has a 50% chance of passing the defective gene and therefore the disease to each child. Huntington's disease is one example. By contrast, *autosomal recessive* disorders are expressed fully only when both copies of a particular gene are abnormal, and the affected individual is then *homozygous* for the defective gene. Cystic fibrosis is an example of an autosomal recessive disease. Usually, both unaffected parents (called "carriers") of an affected homozygote are heterozygotes for the gene, and their risk of having another affected offspring is 25%. *X-linked* genes are located on the X chromosome and therefore are present only in single copies in males. Random inactivation of one X chromosome in females accounts for the similar quantities of X-linked gene products in normal XX females and XY males. Males are therefore obligate homozygotes for X-linked genes and express diseases because of gene mutations on their lone X chromosome, inherited from the mother. Females generally express X-linked diseases only when two copies of the mutant gene are received.

Apart from classical Mendelian genetic mechanisms there are now recognized several types of nonMendelian genetic information transmission, which include cytoplasmic inheritance, genomic imprinting, uniparental disomy, and mosaicism. These new genetic concepts have far-reaching implications for our understanding of developmental defects and intrauterine survival.

Cytoplasmic inheritance refers to derivation of cytoplasmic components, such as mitochondria, solely from the mother because they are present in the ovum but not in the portion of sperm that contributes to the zygote. Serious brain and muscle disorders are known to be inherited from unaffected carrier mothers, who have both normal and abnormal mitochondria. The affected fetus inherits by chance a preponderance of abnormal mitochondria, which may function poorly in oxidative metabolism. *Genomic imprinting* refers to the concept that certain genes are imprinted, or expressed differently, based on the sex of their parent of origin. Genomic imprinting appears to be accomplished in the process of egg and sperm production, and so certain genes when received by the offspring from sperm are expressed differently from those received from the egg. In the normal individual who receives one complete copy of each chromosome from each parent, imprinting produces gene expression that is assumed to be complementary. Only certain chromosomal regions and genes seem to be affected by genomic imprinting. The most often cited examples of human disease resulting from abnormal genomic imprinting are the Prader-Willi and Angelman syndromes.[10] These two distinct clinical syndromes are caused by separate but closely placed genes in a region of the proximal long arm of chromosome 15. The loss of this region on the paternal chromosome 15 yields Prader-Willi syndrome, whereas the same loss on the maternal chromosome gives the Angelman syndrome.

The existence of genomic imprinting makes the parental origin of chromosomes very important. The condition in which both chromosomes in a pair are inherited from one parent is called "uniparental disomy." Uniparental disomy will produce an abnormal phenotype only if the involved pair carries an imprinted region or gene. To extend the above example, uniparental disomy for the paternal chromosome 15 pair will result in the Angelman syndrome, whereas maternal uniparental disomy for the same chromosome will give the Prader-Willi syndrome.

The last category of nonmendelian inheritance is *mosaicism,* which is the presence of both normal cells and abnormal cells, carrying either a chromosomal aberration or gene mutation, within a single conceptus. Mosaicism always arises *after* fertilization as the result of a mutation in an embryonic progenitor cell. Depending on the timing of the mutation, it may be confined to certain tissues, that is, present only in placental tissue, present only in embryonic-fetal somatic cells, present only in germ cells, or generalized. *Confined placental mosaicism* for a chromosome mutation has been recognized in 2% of viable pregnancies after 11 weeks of gestation. Its identification in placenta often signals the presence of uniparental disomy in the fetus, since a proportion of such pregnancies will have confined placental mosaicism as a result of "trisomic zygote rescue." This is a process through which a pregnancy that begins as a trisomic zygote undergoes a later postzygotic mitotic error with loss of one of the trisomic chromosomes in embryonic progenitors, with enhanced viability for the embryo or fetus.[11]

Somatic mosaicism results from a gene mutation or chromosome abnormality arising in embryonic cells. Somatic mosaicism may produce "patchy" disorders such as Albright's polyostotic fibrous dysplasia in which dysplastic cells have an abnormal genotype, or asymmetric growth in which the hypoplastic side may show a chromosomal defect.

Germ-line mosaicism, on the other hand, occurs when an individual develops both normal and mutation-carrying germ-line cells and does not express detectable somatic mosaicism. The importance of this concept is that such parents may have more than one child who expresses the same assumed "new" mutation but may be perfectly normal themselves.[12]

Some defects appear to have a familial predisposition but do not follow the rules of either Mendelian or nonMendelian inheritance. These defects are often single isolated disorders such as cleft lip or neural tube defects. They represent the interactions of many additive genetic and environmental factors and therefore are called "multifactorial." The recurrence risk for this type of defect is empirically determined and is usually increased among first-, second-, and third-degree relatives.

Conditions that show multiple anomalies are the most difficult to evaluate. When identified in a fetus or infant, multiple anomalies should be fully catalogued and correlated by body region, developmental field, timing of their embryonic origin, and presumed mechanism so that a differential diagnosis for the underlying cause or syndrome may be delineated. Multiple anomalies are often caused by chromosome defects or environmental factors but may be attributable to poorly understood single-gene defects.

Environmental influences on embryonic and fetal development, representing the second major source of developmental defects in humans, are innumerable. The gravid uterus and in fact the entire maternal body itself can be thought of as an environment for the developing conceptus, acting in part as an imperfect filter to eliminate harmful external influences on the fetus. Substances such as ethanol, thalidomide, and insulin, some infections such as cytomegalovirus or rubella, maternal metabolic diseases such as phenylketonuria, as well as physical forces such as heat and ionizing radiation, when demonstrated to cause fetal damage, are called "teratogens." The joint foundations of modern teratology, which is the study of environmental influences on embryonic and fetal development, focus epidemiologic research in human populations and animal models to screen environmental influences and elucidate the mechanisms of a teratogen's actions. There are intrinsic problems with studies of teratogenicity in humans, stemming from the uncontrollability of "natural experiments"

Table 16-1 Known teratogenic agents in humans

Environmental agents	Maternal illness or anomalies (cont)	Drugs (cont)
Ionizing radiation	Phenylketonuria	Anticonvulsants
Infections	Lupus or other autoimmune disorders	Phenobarbitol
AIDS	Myotonic dystrophy	Phenytoin
Cytomegalovirus	Myasthenia gravis	Trimethadione
Herpesvirus	Thyroid disease	Valproic acid
Rubella virus	Virilizing tumors	Antithyroid drugs
Syphilis	Fever	Cocaine
Toxoplasmosis	Uterine compression	Diethystilbestrol (DES)
Varicella-zoster virus	Multiple gestation	Folic acid antagonists
Hyperthermia	Uterine anomaly	Methotrexate
Mercury	Oligohydramnios	Aminopterin
Polychlorinated biphenyls (PCBs)	**Drugs**	Streptomycin
Maternal illness or anomalies	Alcohol	Tetracycline
Metabolic imbalance	Alkylating agents	Thalidomide
Diabetes mellitus	Aminoglycosides	Vitamin A derivatives
Endemic cretinism	Androgens	Warfarin
Galactosemia		

Modified from Hall JG: Developmental defects in stillborn and newborn infants. In Dimmick JE, Kalousek DK, editors: *Developmental pathology of the embryo and fetus*, Philadelphia, 1992, Lippincott.

involving accidental or inadvertent *exposure* to purported teratogens. Relatively few human teratogens have been unequivocally identified; rarely are the mechanisms of their action understood (Table 16-1). Many chemicals, in particular, are suspected of causing fetal damage, but convincing evidence is sparse. Numerous therapeutic drugs have known patterns of fetal effects but dose-effect relationships are frequently unpredictable, probably because of maternal metabolic factors that are undelineated.

PATHOLOGY OF EMBRYONIC DEVELOPMENT

It is not possible to assess accurately the total embryonic loss rate in humans, since many embryos fail to implant or are lost before the mother recognizes that she is pregnant. Some 15% to 20% of clinically recognized pregnancies result in spontaneous abortion (SA). SA can be subdivided into early, corresponding to the embryonic period of development (8 weeks), and late, covering the previable fetal period (9 to 18 weeks). Most SA occur during the embryonic period, and most are attributable to chromosomal errors. The significance of pathologic examination of early SA lies in providing an answer to two basic questions the parents ask when the pregnancy fails. These are "Why did it happen?" and "Will it happen again?" The same questions are asked whether the loss occurs early or late in pregnancy. The increasing concern about early pregnancy losses reflects the fact that pregnancies are often well planned and delayed to the fourth decade of the mother's life when fertility is declining. Understanding the underlying cause of early pregnancy loss helps the obstetrician in the management of future pregnancy and allows for accurate genetic counseling for the couple if necessary. It is the pathologist who receives the complete specimen of SA and must make decisions regarding the extent of the investigation.

Detailed clinical history including number of successful pregnancies, abortions, stillbirths, general health history, and exposure to drugs and teratogens must be sought if not included with the specimen. When the history indicates previous pregnancy losses, stillbirths, or infertility, or when the couple has a specific history of known metabolic or molecular hereditary disease, the pathologist must initiate additional investigations. These include, depending on history, sampling for chromosomal analysis, microbiologic investigation, electron microscopy, and direct tissue analysis or cell culture for molecular or biochemical investigations. The gross and microscopic examination documenting the development of gestational sac, presence or absence of the embryo, cord, and yolk sac, and the evaluation of normal or abnormal embryonic development represent a standard approach to any early SA. The use of an inverted dissecting microscope in the examination of chorionic villi and embryonic morphology is essential, as is histologic evaluation of chorionic villi, fetal membranes, and umbilical cord.

Chromosomal abnormalities

Chromosomal abnormalities are present in over 60% of conceptuses aborted in the earlier weeks of development.[13] The most common defects are trisomies, monosomy X, and polyploidy. Structural rearrangements and chromosomal mosaicism are less prevalent (Table 16-2).

Trisomies are mainly attributable to a meiotic error occurring predominantly in the maturing oocyte. Cytogenetic analysis of human ova has shown that close to 20% are aneuploid. The frequency of chromosomal errors in sperm is also high, about 14%, but the types of abnormalities are different, mainly structural defects.[14] With increasing maternal age, the frequency of aneuploid eggs also increases,[15] and subsequently SA with chromosomal trisomies are more common in mothers over 35 years of age. Trisomies involving each chromosome have been described in early SA. Their frequency varies greatly (Table 16-3). It has been shown that having an early SA with trisomy does not predispose a couple to a liveborn trisomic infant and that those couples with trisomic abortion are more likely to have a successful next pregnancy than couples with chromosomally normal loss. This is most likely attribut-

Table 16-2 Types of chromosomal abnormalities in 2743 spontaneous abortions

Type	Number	Frequency (%)
Chromosomal trisomy	1411	52.0
Sex chromosome monosomy	538	20.0
Polyploidy	588	21.0
Structural abnormality	104	3.5
Mixoploidy (mosaicism)	89	3.5
Other	13	0.5

Modified from Creasy MR: The cytogenetics of spontaneous abortion in humans. In Beard RW, Sharp F, editors: *Early pregnancy loss,* New York, 1988, Springer-Verlag.

Table 16-3 Relative frequency of different trisomies in spontaneous abortions

Trisomic chromosome	Observed frequency (%)
3, 5, 6, 11, 12, 17, 19	<1
2, 4, 7, 8, 9, 10, 14, 20, X	1-5
13, 15, 18, 21, 22	5-10
16	30

Modified from Warburton D, Stein Z, Kline J, Susser M: Chromosome abnormalities in spontaneous abortions: data from the New York City Study. In Porter IH, Hook EB: editors: *Human embryonic and fetal death,* New York, 1980, Academic Press.

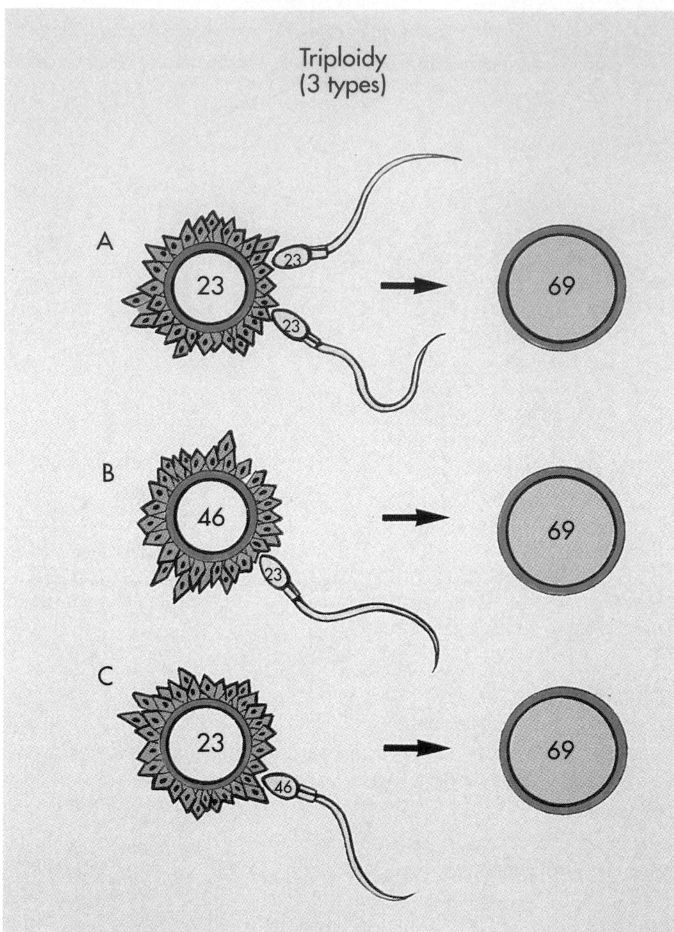

Fig. 16-1 Diagram showing the origin of chromosomal triploidy. The commonest is type *A*. Notice that in types *A* and *C* there is dominance of paternal genome whereas in B 46 chromosomes originate from the ovum (mother).

able to the randomness of aneuploidy in human gametes versus the habitual nature of genetic or maternal factors involved in nonchromosomal loss.

Chromosomal monosomy is the result of fertilization with a nullisomic gamete, deficient for a particular chromosome. Such gametes have been documented for various chromosomes in both males and females. However, only monosomy for X chromosome and chromosome 21 have been recorded in large cytogenetic studies of SA.[15] This finding is explained by the presumed inability of embryos that are monosomic for chromosomes other than X or 21 to develop beyond early implantation. Monosomy X is the second most common chromosome defect in early SA (Table 16-2), whereas monosomy 21 is a rare finding.

Chromosomal *triploidy* results from abnormal fertilization (Fig. 16-1). The commonest cause of triploidy is double fertilization of a haploid ovum. The fertilization of diploid ovum or diploid sperm is less common. It has been estimated that 1% of all human conceptions are triploid. When a haploid egg is fertilized by two sperms or by a diploid sperm, the resulting chromosomal complement (69 chromosomes) is dominated by paternal genetic information (46 chromosomes originating from the father). The opposite is true for fertilization of a diploid ovum by a haploid sperm. Because of genomic imprinting the phenotype of paternally dominated triploidy differs from the maternally dominated one. Paternally dominated triploidy is often called partial hydatidiform mole.[16] It is characterized by abundant cystically dilated chorionic villi and an embryo with a characteristic phenotype, consisting of retarded limb development, facial dysplasia, subectodermal symmetric hemorrhages, and frequently an open neural tube defect.[17] On histologic examination of the gestational sac, the presence of hydropic chorionic villi with blood vessels containing nucleated red blood cells and focal hyperplasia of trophoblast, villous swelling with cistern formation, scalloping of villous outline, and trophoblastic inclusions represents a diagnostic phenotype of paternally dominated triploidy. In contrast, maternally derived triploid SA cannot be distinguished histologically from any other chromosomally abnormal early spontaneous abortion.

There are two mechanisms by which chromosomal *tetraploidy* may arise (Fig. 16-2). The more common is abnormal cleavage: during the first postzygotic cell cycle the DNA is replicated, but the actual nuclear division does not take place. This results in 92 chromosomes. Less commonly, fertilization of a haploid egg by three haploid sperms occurs, and such products of conception share a similar phenotype with paternally dominated triploidy.

The phenotype of any chromosomally abnormal early SA specimen is not diagnostic except for paternally dominated triploidy[18] and tetraploidy. The correlation of gross embryonic morphology and karyotype in complete specimens (intact chorionic sac) of early SA is shown in Table 16-4. There is an excellent correlation between an abnormal karyotype and

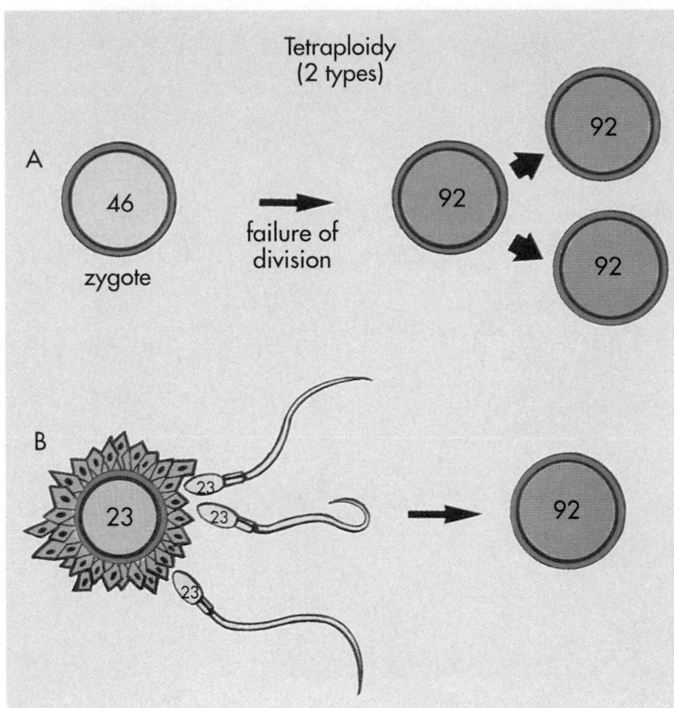

Fig. 16-2 Diagram showing the origin of chromosome tetraploidy. The failure of the first division is believed to be the most common type.

Table 16-4 Frequency of abnormal cytogenetics in early spontaneous abortion specimens

Morphology of specimen	Abnormality (%)
Embryos with growth disorganization	56
Embryos with localized defect or defects	93
Normal embryos	20

Modified from Kalousek DK: Anatomic and chromosome anomalies in specimens of each spontaneous abortion: seven year experience. In Gilbert EF, Opitz JM, editors: *Genetic aspects of developmental pathology,* New York, Alan R. Liss for the National Foundation–March of Dimes, BD:OAS XXIII(1): 153-168, 1987.

localized embryonic defects, yet no correlation between embryonic growth disorganization and the karyotypic abnormalities. Similarly, in the evaluation of ruptured chorionic sacs from which the embryos have been lost, except for the above-described phenotype for paternally dominated triploidy (partial hydatidiform mole), there is no histologic correlation with either a normal or an abnormal karyotype.

Developmental embryonic defects

Embryos are not easy to evaluate without an intimate knowledge of normal embryonic development. There are several excellent textbooks and atlases the pathologist can use to guide the evaluation of embryonic development.[19,20] It is most important to remember that only the structures that are developed at a given embryonic stage can be evaluated. For example, the diagnosis of syndactyly cannot be made until stage 22, when embryonic fingers are normally individually separated. External examination of embryos therefore provides data for determining their developmental stage. The examination consists of detailed evaluation of characteristic facial, limb, and body features under the dissecting microscope (Fig. 16-3). The embryonic age is established by correlation of crown-rump (CR) length and developmental stage. An observed difference greater than 14 days between the developmental age, thus derived, and the gestational age, calculated from the last menstrual period, most often reflects the length of retention in utero after embryonic death. *The CR length of the embryo is the single most important embryonic measurement.* Any discrepancy between embryonic length and specific developmental milestones points to the existence of a developmental defect. For example, if a fresh, well-preserved embryo has a CR length of 25 mm and shows unfused frontonasal or maxillary prominences, the diagnosis of facial clefts is appropriate. However the same finding in an embryo with a 15 mm CR length would be consistent with normal development for that stage.[17]

Damaged and severely macerated embryos cannot be fully evaluated. Their developmental age can be estimated based on the development of specific structures (eye, hand), but a defect should not be diagnosed, since maceration of embryonic tissue can be indistinguishable from or may mimic frequent defects such as neural tube defect, facial clefting, or absence of limbs.

Among complete specimens the commonest finding is disorganized embryonic development (GD, 'growth disorganization') represented either by an empty chorionic sac (GD_1) or a nodular, cylindric, or stunted embryo ($GD_{2\text{-}4}$). These embryos are illustrated in Figs. 16-4 to 16-7. GD_1 is characterized by a complete lack of any embryo. Occasionally, an amniotic sac may be identified (Fig. 16-4). GD_2 embryos are represented by a 2 to 3 mm nodule of disorganized embryonic tissue attached to the amniotic membrane without any body stalk or umbilical cord formation (Fig. 16-5). GD_3 embryos show recognizable retinal pigment, which allows the identification of the cranial end. They have a rudimentary body stalk and measure 5 to 7 mm in length. Usually no other differentiation is seen (Fig. 16-6). GD_4 embryos have not only retinal pigment, but also a dysplastic face and a small cranium. Limb buds are less developed than what would be expected for normal embryos of a 10 to 15 mm CR length. The body stalk is usually short but identifiable. Other external features expected in a normal embryo of this length are missing (Fig. 16-7).

Many embryologists and obstetricians have described various developmental defects in human embryos.[21] Although it is critical to observe and record these abnormalities, their simple description does not provide any guide to the obstetrician and geneticist in future pregnancies unless their cause is established. From the point of view of genetic counseling and future reproductive success, the most important group of early SA specimens (though the least frequent) are the specimens with embryos that appear to follow the normal overall developmental design but show localized developmental defects (Figs. 16-8 to 16-10). These are often embryos with facial clefts, polydactyly, neural tube defects, or microcephaly. The role of the pathologist in these cases is to establish the cause of the defect. For example, if the embryo shows an open neural tube defect (NTD), the defect may be of multifactorial, chromosomal, or recessive mutant gene origin. The risk of NTD recurrence in any future pregnancy of the couple depends on the cause of the defect. Multifactorial NTD has recurrence risk of 2%, chromosomal because of simple trisomy 1%, triploidy 0%, and chro-

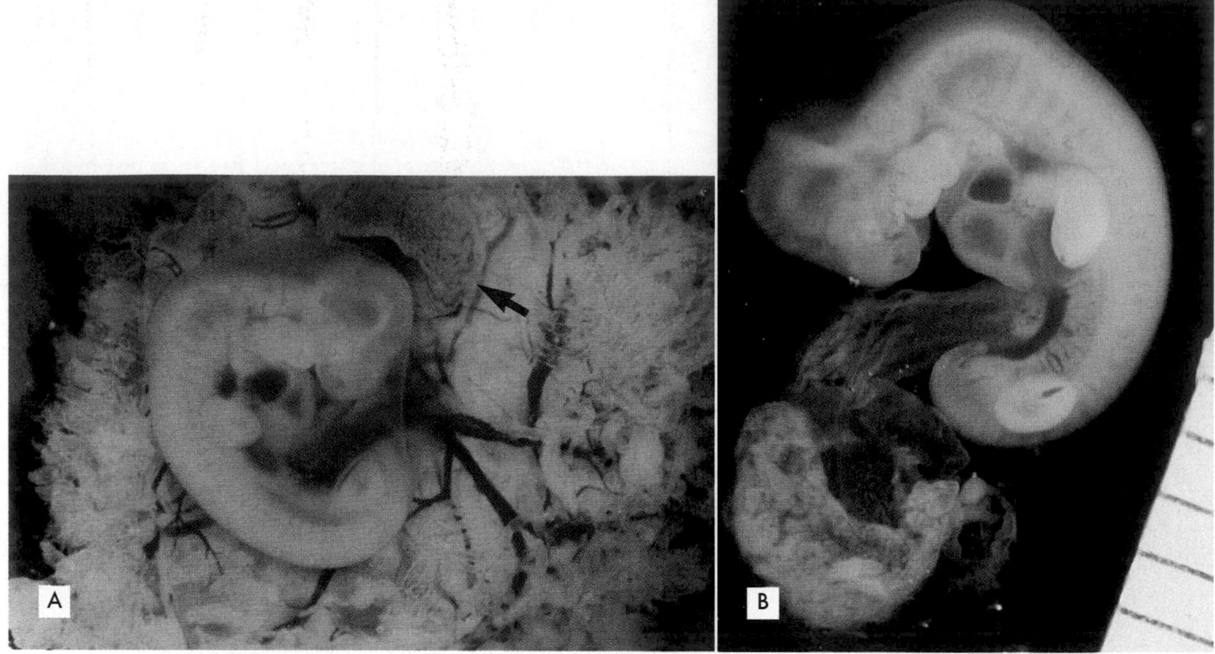

Fig. 16-3 **A**, A normal human embryo stage 13 inside the intact amniotic sac and in an opened chorionic sac. Arrow indicates the yolk sac. **B**, The same embryo removed from the gestational sac. Attached to body stalk is a part of the amniotic sac and a yolk sac. Notice well developed embryonic body curvature and advanced development of the upper limb compared to the lower limb. These two features are usually absent in abnormal embryos.

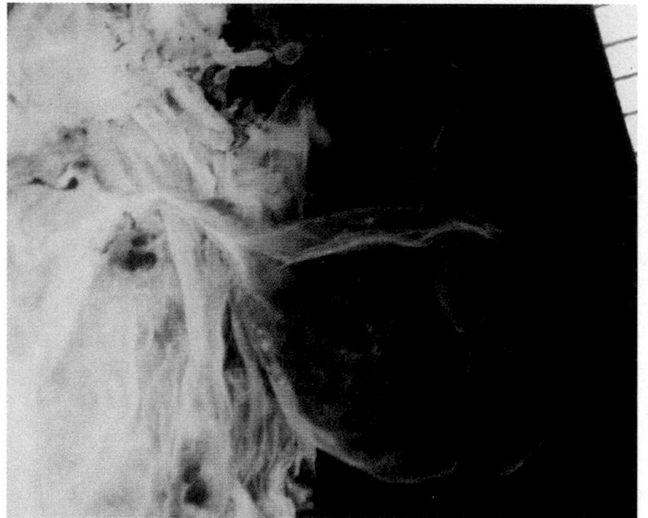

Fig. 16-4 Abnormal monozygotic twin pregnancy with two empty amniotic sacs and one chorionic sac with sparse villi (GD_1). (*GD* is 'growth disorganization'.)

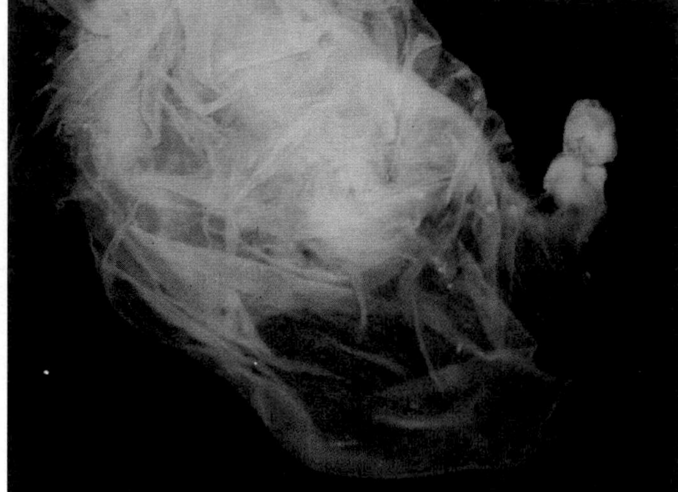

Fig. 16-5 Amniotic membrane with attached disorganized nubbin of embryonic tissue (GD_2) cytogenetically diagnosed as trisomy 14.

mosomal translocation (when one parent carries a Robertsonian translocation) 10%. A recessive mutant gene causing NTD, such as that in Meckel syndrome, has a 25% recurrence risk (Table 16-5). Therefore, both detailed morphologic examination and cytogenetic analyses are indicated when a NTD is detected in an early SA specimen.[17]

Placental and embryonic interaction

Placental and embryonic interaction as an aspect of developmental pathology has not received a great deal of attention. The question is not whether any interaction exists, but rather how intensive this interaction is and what form it assumes. We know that intrauterine death causes a collapse of embryonic vessels in placental villi, fibrosis of villous stroma, and clumping of trophoblast. However, we do not know when and to what degree abnormal function of the placental tissue actually contributes to embryonic death. Studies of confined placental mosaicism in which only the placenta and not the embryo proper contains aneuploid cells show us that the interaction must be bidirectional.

Confined placental mosaicism is defined as a dichotomy between the chromosomal constitution of the placental tissues

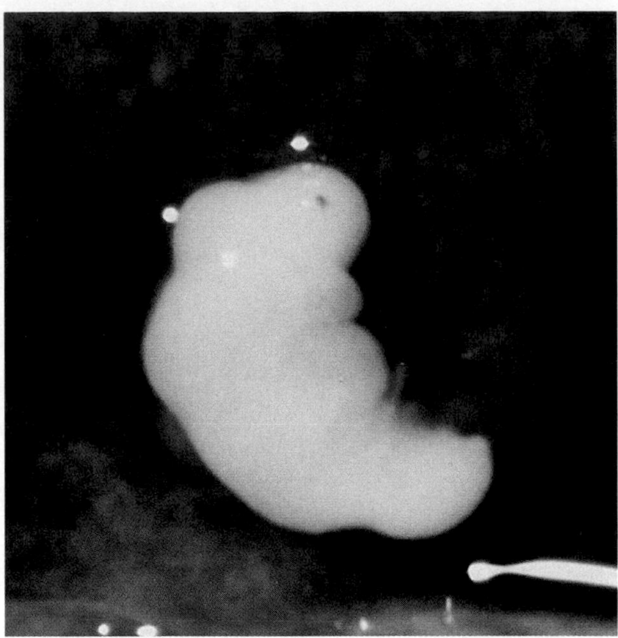

Fig. 16-6 Typical embryonic disorganization in which a cranial end of the embryo can be distinguished (GD_3).

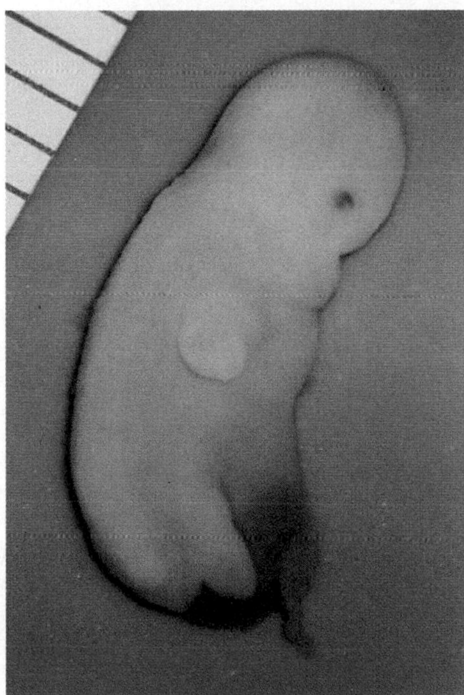

Fig. 16-7 Human embryo measuring 14 mm in length and showing abnormal delayed development of head and limbs (GD_4). Cytogenetically diagnosed as 69,XXX.

versus the embryonic-fetal tissues. It can assume three different forms as shown in Fig. 16-11. Each type of confined placental mosaicism affects a different cell lineage or several lineages and shows distinct clinical consequences, dependent on the specific chromosome involved and gestation. For example, type I can be found in both diploid and aneuploid gestations (Fig. 16-12). In diploid pregnancies with this type of mosaicism, a higher pregnancy loss rate has been observed. On the

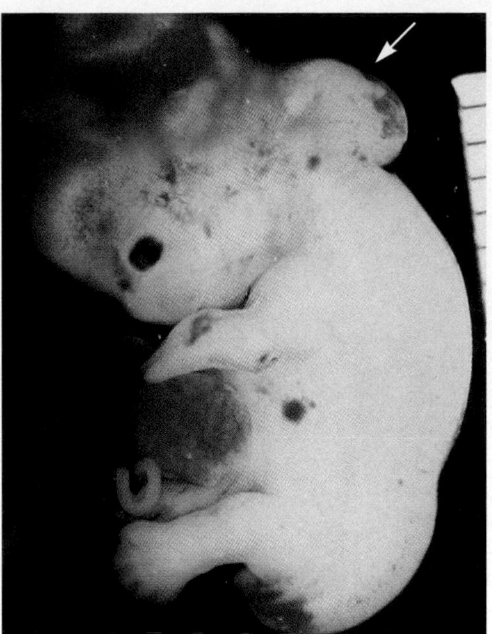

Fig. 16-8 Human embryo stage 19 with occipital encephalocele (*arrow*).

other hand, nonmosaic trisomy 13 and 18 fetuses show enhanced intrauterine survival when diploid-trisomic mosaicism is found in the trophoblast.[22]

There are data to support the proposal that numerous trisomic zygotes are "rescued" by a postzygotic mitotic mutation, giving rise to a dichotomy between the placenta and the fetus (type III confined placental mosaicism). In these pregnancies, both trophoblast and chorionic stroma show chromosomal aneuploidy, whereas the fetus is diploid.[23] The frequency with which various chromosomes are involved in placental aneuploidy corresponds to the frequency with which specific chromosomal aneuploidies are observed in spontaneous abortions.[24] The most common confined placental trisomy is trisomy 16. The clustering of chromosomally abnormal cell lines in the placental progenitors has been experimentally shown in chimeric mouse embryos (Fig. 16-13).

It is important to note that in one third of "rescued" trisomic pregnancies a loss of the extra chromosome will result in uniparental disomy (Fig. 16-14). Uniparental disomy may or may not affect the embryonic-fetal development, depending on whether the involved chromosome pair carries imprinted DNA segment (or segments) (Fig. 16-15). In "rescued" trisomic pregnancies, there is an increased rate of pregnancy complications, including fetal intrauterine growth restriction, pregnancy-associated hypertension, and intrauterine fetal death. However, it is not clear how many of these complications result from fetal uniparental disomy and how many from abnormal functioning of the aneuploid placenta.[11]

PATHOLOGY OF PREVIABLE FETAL DEVELOPMENT

Late spontaneous abortion, occurring between 9 and 18 weeks of development, is much less common than early SA; however, the parents and clinicians are generally more distressed

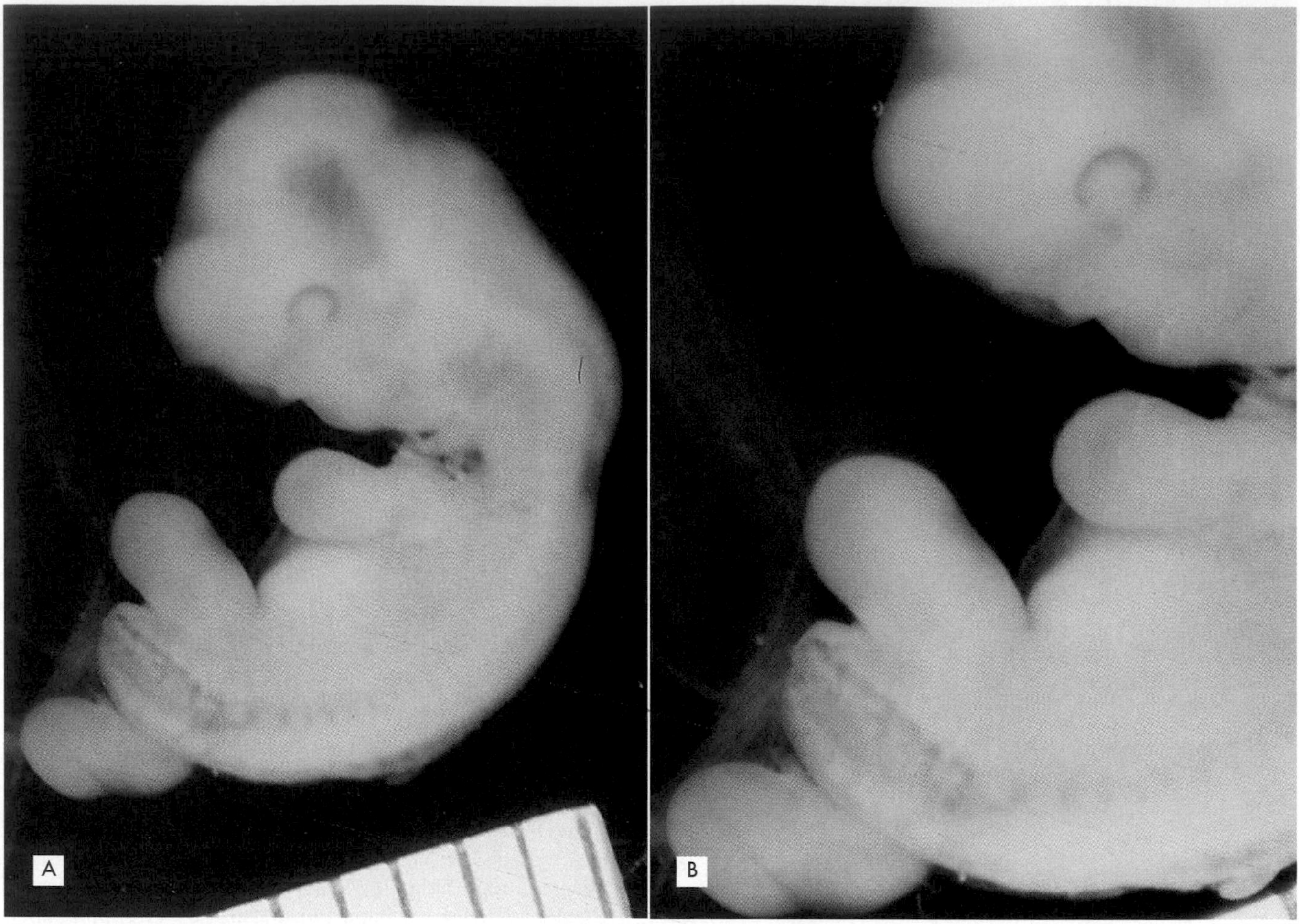

Fig. 16-9 **A**, Damaged and partially degenerated triploid embryo stage 16, showing a large open neural tube defect in the lumbosacral area. **B**, A close up view of the defect. Notice increased vascularization around the edges of the defect.

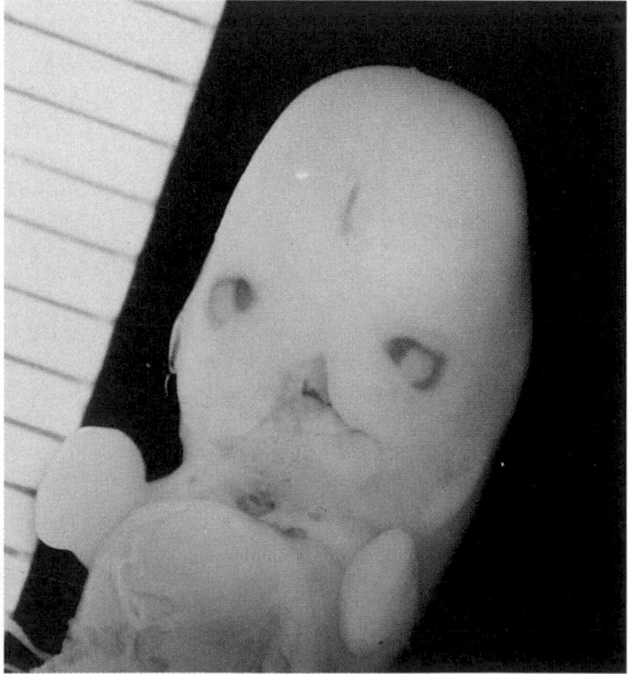

Fig. 16-10 Damaged incomplete triploid embryo approximately stage 19 with a large midline upper lip cleft.

Table 16-5 **Etiology of common neural tube defects and their recurrence risk in subsequent pregnancies**

Etiology	Defect	Risk of recurrence
Amnion rupture syndrome	Encephalocele-like	0
Triploidy	Myelocele	0
Trisomy 13	Myelocele	1-10
Multifactorial inheritance	Anencephaly	2-4
	Myelocele	
	Encephalocele	
Meckel-Gruber syndrome	Encephalocele	25

Modified from Kalousek DK et al: *Pathology of the human embryo and previable fetus: an atlas,* New York, 1990, Springer-Verlag.

by late than by early SA. The fetus, unlike the embryo, is fully formed and its examination need not differ from a neonatal autopsy. When younger fetuses are examined, a magnifying glass or a good quality dissecting microscope is useful. The causes of late SA are quite different from the causes of embryonic loss. The frequency of chromosomal defects among spontaneously aborted fetuses is much lower compared to that during the embryonic period.[25] A large number of late SA are

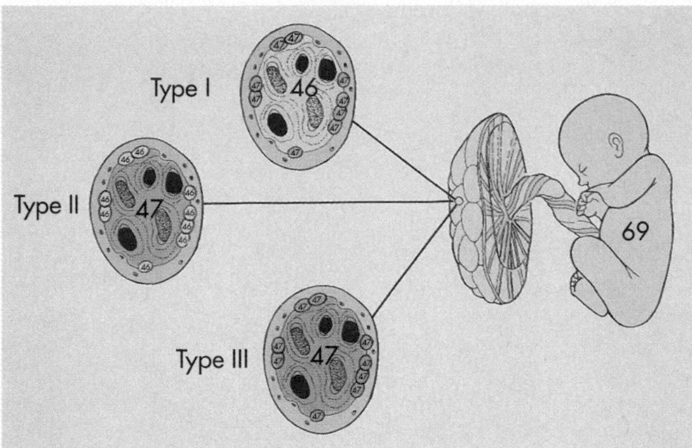

Fig. 16-11 Diagram of 3 types of confined placental mosaicism. In type I, the chromosomally abnormal cell line is confined to trophoblast, in type II to villous stroma, and in type III both trophoblast and extraembryonic stroma are different from the fetus.

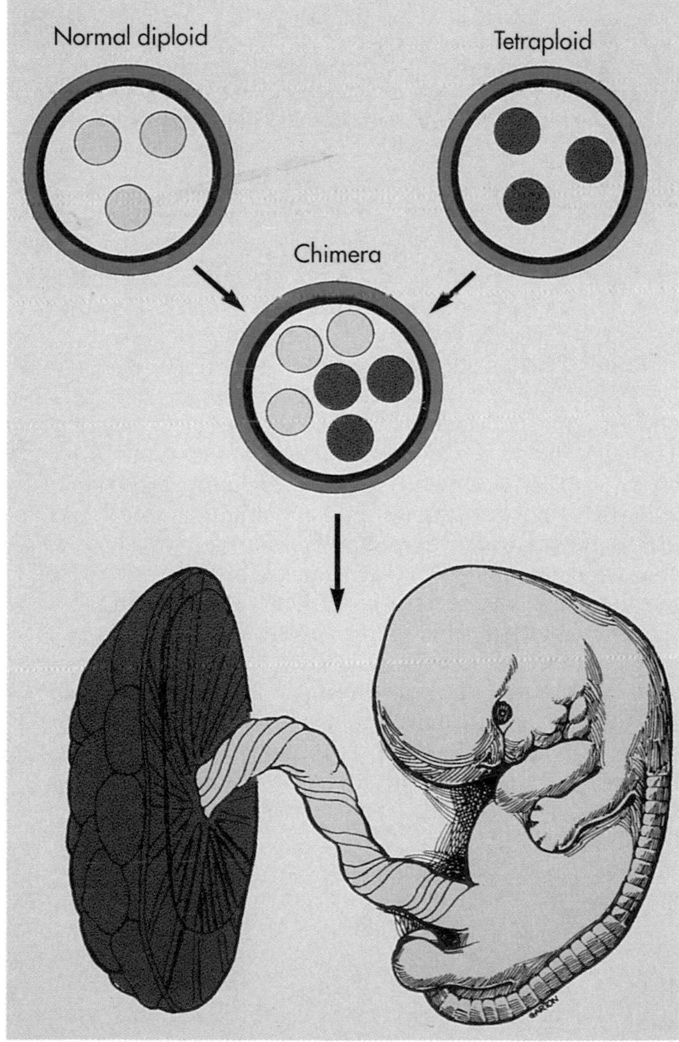

Fig. 16-12 Summary of experiments with chimeric mice embryos showing that the abnormal cell line in chimeric preimplantation embryos is usually expressed in the placental tissues whereas normal diploid progenitors cluster to form the embryo proper.

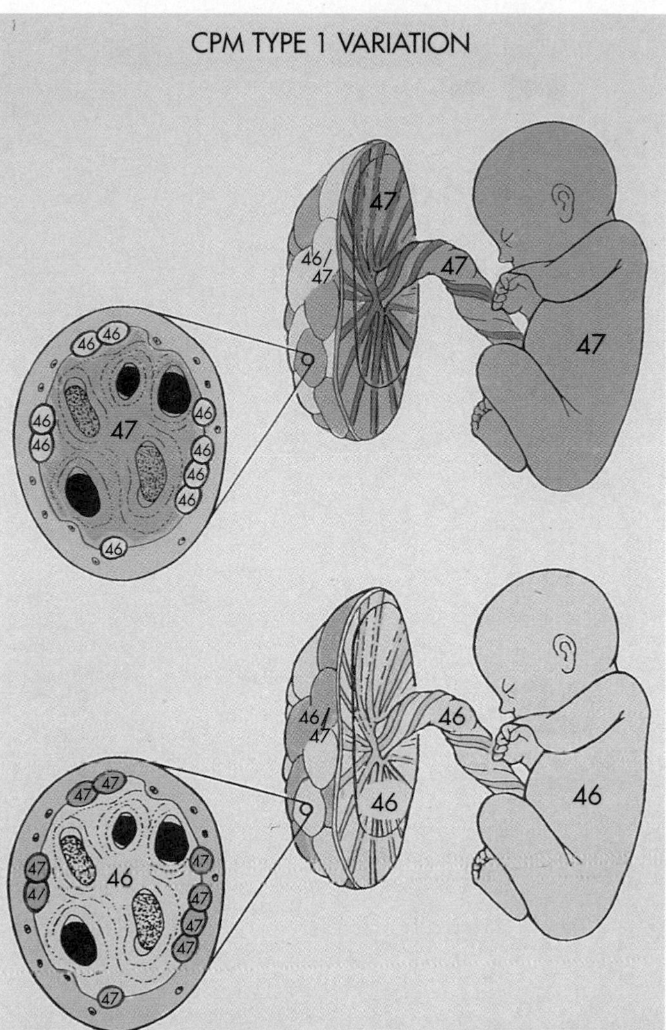

Fig. 16-13 Confined placental mosaicism type I can be found in both diploid and aneuploid pregnancies. In diploid pregnancies its presence seems to be associated with a higher pregnancy loss, whereas in aneuploid gestation the presence of a diploid cell line in the trophoblast appears to be necessary for intrauterine survival of the trisomic fetus into the third trimester. This has been documented for trisomy 13 and 18 stillbirth or live birth.

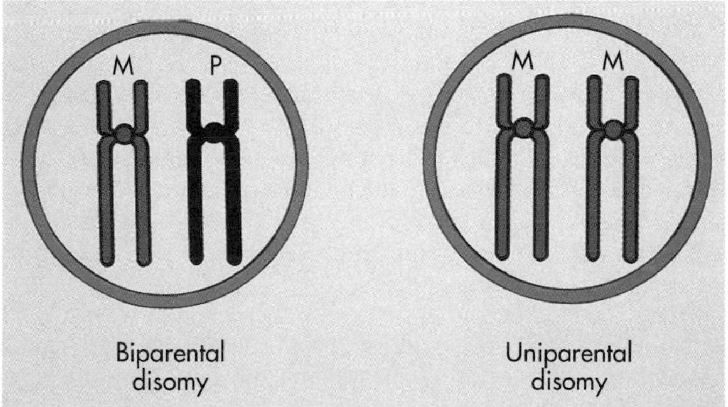

Fig. 16-14 Normally each chromosome pair in a diploid chromosomal complement has one member derived from the mother and one from the father. This is known as "biparental disomy." When both chromosomes are derived from the same parent, uniparental disomy results.

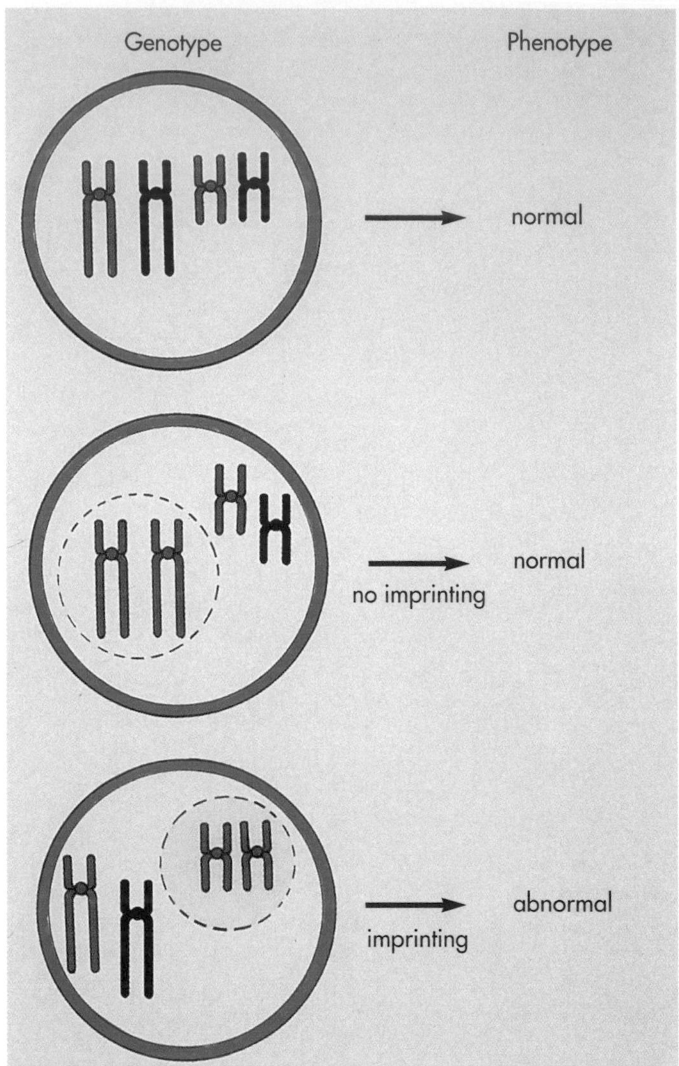

Fig. 16-15 This diagram shows the significance of genomic imprinting in uniparental disomy. When a chromosomal pair does not carry an imprinted segment of DNA, there is no phenotypic effect of uniparental disomy *(middle genotype)*. However, when genomic imprinting affects DNA carried by the chromosomal pair that is present in a uniparental state, the phenotype is abnormal because the expression on each chromosome should be different and "black chromosome" expression is missing *(bottom genotype)*.

caused by placental defects and many remain unexplained at the present. Immunologic causes of fetal intrauterine death are widely discussed, but the hard evidence for their existence is lacking, as are routine tests the pathologist can use to evaluate them. One exception is maternal lupus[26] and the immunologically related anticardiolipin antibody syndrome,[27] in which recurrent SAs are seen.

Late abortion specimens, 9 to 18 development weeks or 11 to 20 gestational weeks, consist of an identifiable fetus and a placenta, and each can be examined separately. Both the fetus and placenta should be submitted fresh, without fixation, as quickly as possible to the pathology department so that cytogenetic, microbiologic, or biochemical studies can be initiated when required. Fixation should be used only if refrigeration is not available and if a delay of several days in delivery is anticipated. In such cases, a small piece of aseptically collected fetal skin and a segment of the placenta, including the chorionic villi and the amnion, should be separately submitted in tissue culture media for the cytogenetic laboratory.[17]

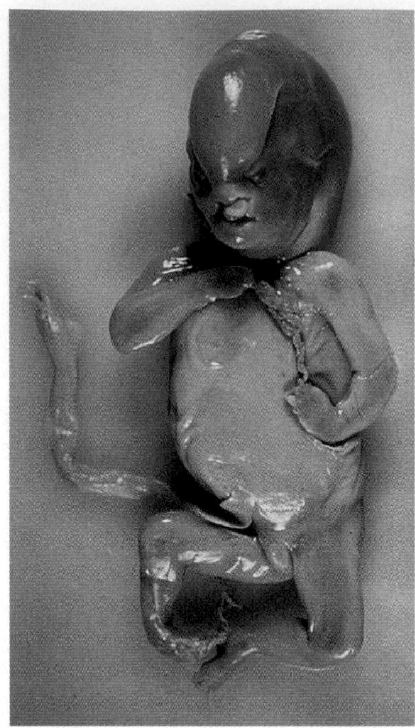

Fig. 16-16 Macerated male fetus, 14½ developmental weeks, with characteristic features of amnion rupture sequence. Notice deep bilateral cleft lip and palate extending into the nostrils and amputation of fingers and toes of all four limbs with tethering by amniotic bands.

Routine examination of the fetus consists of both an external and an internal examination, a radiologic examination, a photographic documentation, and a histologic examination. The fetus should be weighed and measurements of CR length, crown-heel (CH) length, and head circumference should be recorded. The CR length is the main criterion used for establishing the fetal developmental age. Various tables are available for determining developmental age from foot and hand lengths. These can be used instead of the CR length when the specimen is incomplete or fragmented and in dwarfing conditions, or they can be used in addition to the CR length to verify its accuracy.[17] Macerated and damaged fetuses should not be ignored, even though they may appear to be grossly distorted. Despite molding and distortion, such external malformations as neural tube defect, cleft lip and palate, syndactyly, polydactyly, amputations, and constrictions can be easily diagnosed (Fig. 16-16).

The internal examination should not be directed only toward the diagnosis of such obvious abnormalities as organ agenesis, a diaphragmatic hernia, malrotation of intestine, or a cleft palate. Meticulous dissection, identical to that for the perinatal autopsy, should identify all internal malformations, including congenital heart defects. In cases in which abnormal morphogenesis has been identified on external examination (Fig. 16-17), the incidence of internal developmental defects is high; the likelihood of finding a major internal malformation, however, is only 2% if no external malformation is present. All internal

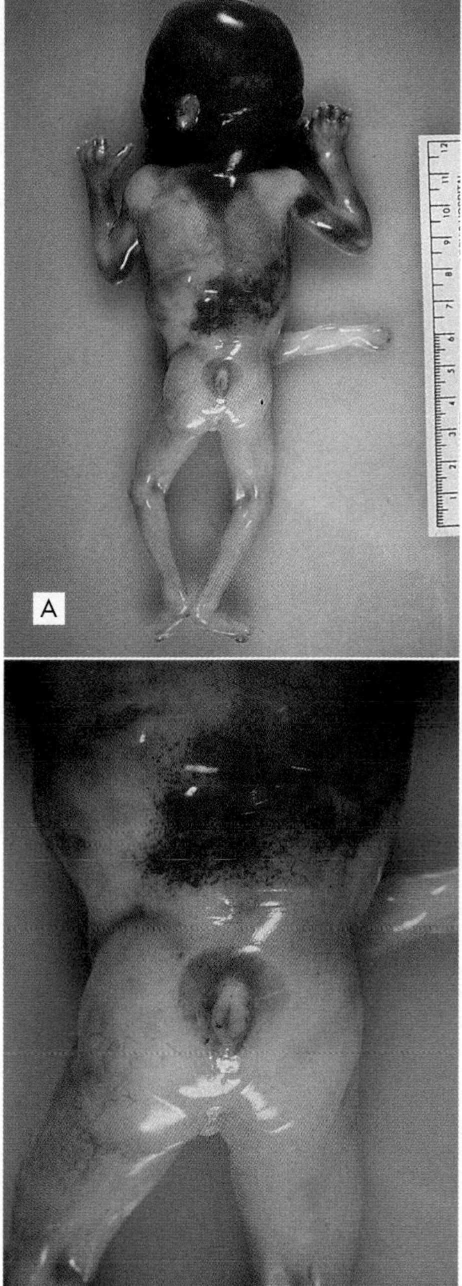

Fig. 16-17 **A**, Well-preserved female fetus at 15 developmental weeks, with sacral meningocele. **B**, A close-up of the spinal defect.

organs should be weighed, and the weight should be compared with normal values to estimate developmental age and possible hypoplasia or hyperplasia.[28] Full examination of the brain is feasible only in nonmacerated fetuses because it is often completely liquefied in macerated fetuses. If softened, brain tissue should be removed after fixation in situ, with a widely open skull and dura in 10% formaldehyde or Bouin fixative for at least a week.[17]

Artifactual abnormalities are frequently found in fetuses that are either spontaneously aborted or terminated in the second trimester of pregnancy. A common artifact, the tearing of skin and muscle, is caused by delivery trauma. It can occur anywhere in the fetal body, but it is most frequent in the abdominal, thoracic, and neck areas. Disruption of developmental abnormalities such as an omphalocele sac or an encephalocele sac require that the pathologist be familiar with this type of artifact and direct a search for vestiges of the sac around the circumference of the defect. Autolysis and degeneration interfere with the evaluation of normal development. In early fetuses, it is difficult to distinguish between opened eyes as a result of eyelid degeneration and a primary defect in eyelid closure. A similar difficulty arises in the evaluation of the lower lumbar and sacral areas in macerated fetuses (9 to 11 weeks) when the widening of the spinal canal attributable to autolysis may mimic an open neural tube defect. Another artifactual defect seen in macerated retained fetuses is the "pseudo–primitive neuroectodermal tumor." This artifact resembles an invasive tumor yet is the result of a squeezing of the brain tissue into the spinal canal and along the spinal nerves into the retroperitoneal and retropleural spaces or the neck area.[17]

Photographic documentation of all detected developmental defects is mandatory. The importance of recording fetal abnormalities photographically cannot be overstressed. It identifies the range of abnormalities within a particular syndrome, allows comparisons to be made, and makes reevaluation of the case or evaluation by consultant syndromologists possible.

Morphologic assessment of the abnormal fetus should also routinely include a radiographic examination to determine the developmental age of bone and to document skeletal anomalies (Fig. 16-18). Fetal radiography is most useful in the examination of fetal skeletal dysplasia. However, even when a skeletal defect is not suspected, a routine radiographic examination permits detection of anomalies that are difficult to demonstrate by dissection; these include abnormal vertebrae or hypoplasia/aplasia of individual bones.[29]

The placenta of conceptuses of 9 to 18 developmental weeks consists of an umbilical cord, extraembryonic membranes, a chorionic plate, and villi; each component should be carefully examined. Essential points in placental examination are placental weight, evaluation of both fetal and maternal placental surface, placental shape, site of insertion and length of the umbilical cord, the number of cord vessels, and the appearance of the placental membranes. A histologic evaluation of membranes, the cord, chorionic villi, and the fetal and the maternal surfaces and any detected focal abnormalities should also be routinely made. It should be remembered that, in all cases of fetal intrauterine death and prolonged retention, the placenta still contains viable cells that can be used to initiate cell cultures for both metabolic disease diagnosis and cytogenetic studies, as well as for DNA studies.

Chromosomal abnormalities

Trisomy 21

Even though the majority of spontaneous abortions with trisomy 21 occur during the embryonic stage of development, some also take place during the early part of fetal development. Spontaneously aborted trisomy 21 fetuses tend to be younger (8 to 14 weeks of development) and have either nuchal or generalized edema, whereas electively aborted trisomy 21 fetuses rarely show any nuchal or generalized edema. Most of the trisomy 21 fetuses seen by a pathologist come from pregnancy terminations after prenatal diagnosis.

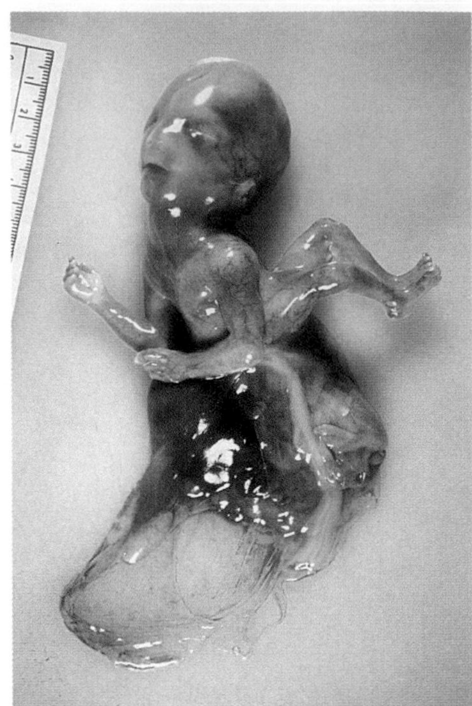

Fig. 16-18 Male fetus, 14½ developmental weeks with limb–body wall complex. X-ray examination allows better evaluation of severe scoliosis and detection of lumbar dysraphism.

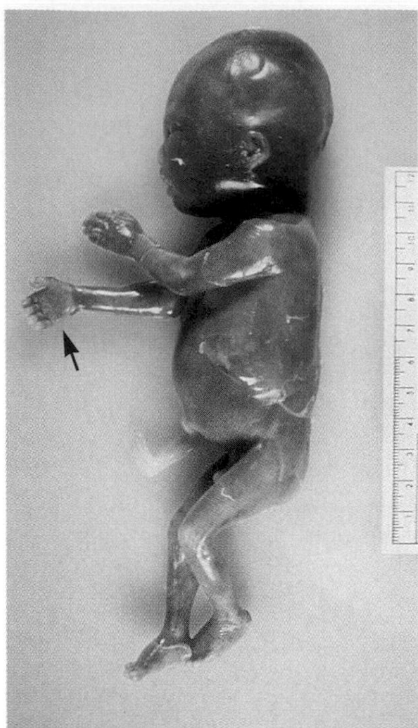

Fig. 16-19 Trisomy 21 male fetus at 16 developmental weeks showing simian crease *(arrow)*, clinodactyly of fifth fingers, and mild posterior nuchal edema.

The most frequent external abnormalities in previable fetuses with trisomy 21 are found in the hands and manifest as clinodactyly of the fifth fingers, because of hypoplasia or aplasia of the midphalanx verified radiographically, and a single palmar crease (Fig. 16-19). An increased space between the first and second toes is sometimes seen before 20 weeks of gestational age. Femur length is often shortened. This varies from a mild to a pronounced decrease in length; this decrease in femur length is sometimes used as part of the sonographic screening for trisomy 21. It is not unusual for the fetus with trisomy 21 to have either no external abnormalities or to have only single palmar creases or clinodactyly of the fifth fingers.[17] A flat occiput and upslanting palpebral fissures are seen in about one third to one fourth of the specimens, yet a protruding tongue is an uncommon finding.

Internal developmental defects are infrequent in fetal trisomy 21, except for cardiovascular malformations and abnormal lobation of the lungs. The most common heart abnormalities are atrioventricular septal defects, atrial septal defect (ASD), and ventricular septal defect (VSD). Although large cystic and calcified Hassall corpuscles in the thymus in trisomy 21 appear to be a constant anomaly in older fetuses and newborns, they are not found in previable fetuses.[30] Multiple anomalies of the brain described in trisomy 21 newborns include brachycephaly and hypoplasia of the superior temporal gyrus, brainstem, medulla, and cerebellum. Usually, none of these defects is recognizable in the previable trisomy 21 fetuses. Table 16-6 lists the incidence and type of abnormalities present in fetuses with trisomy 21.

Table 16-6 Frequent abnormalities in trisomy 21 fetuses

Head and face	
Upslanting palpebral fissures	22%
Lowset ears	10%
Flat occiput	33%
Protruding tongue	13%
Neck	
Edema, cystic hygroma, ascites	30%
Hands and feet	
Clinodactyly of the fifth finger	83%
Absent or small midphalanx in the fifth finger after 16 weeks	78%
Simian crease	38%
Increased space between the first and second toes	20%
Cardiovascular system	
Heart abnormalities	68%
Respiratory system	
Abnormal lobation of lungs	47%

Modified from Kalousek DK et al: *Pathology of the human embryo and previable fetus: an atlas,* New York, 1990, Springer-Verlag.

Trisomy 18

Prenatal growth retardation is the most common finding in trisomy 18 fetuses. Typical craniofacial features include a triangular face with a small chin. The occiput is not yet prominent, but the ears may be low set. In a majority of previable fetuses the appearance of hands and feet is characteristic (Fig. 16-20). The second and fifth fingers usually overlap the third and fourth. This is believed to be caused by a displacement of the finger extensor tendons over the metacarpophalangeal joints and is not seen in macerated fetuses or before 14 weeks of gestation. In the lateral view, the feet have prominent heels with a rocker-bottom appearance, because of vertical taluses in one third of fetuses.

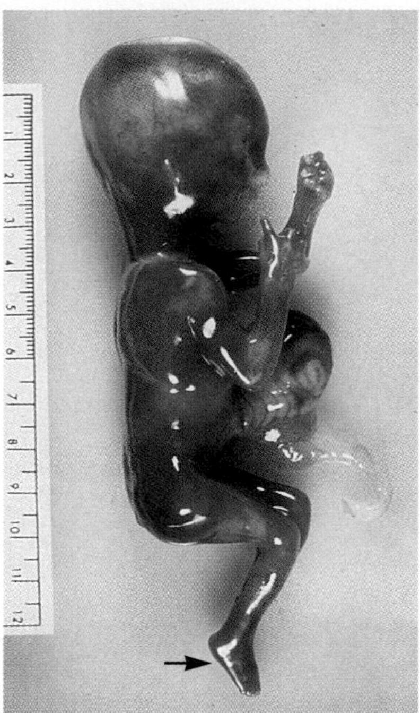

Fig. 16-20 Female fetus with trisomy 18 at 14 developmental weeks. Notice typical positioning of hand and rocker-bottom feet *(arrow)*. Omphalocele is found in a third of fetuses with trisomy 18.

Table 16-7 Frequent abnormalities in trisomy 18 fetuses

Head and face	
Micrognathia	29%
Low-set ears	25%
Triangular face	21%
Cleft lip or palate, or both	12%
Neck	
Cystic hygroma, edema	25%
Extremities	
Fingers two and five overlap fingers three and four	50%
Rocker-bottom feet	33%
Clinodactyly of the fifth finger	21%
Clubfeet	17%
Joint contractures, with webbing	12%
Duplicated or absent thumb	12%
Cardiovascular system	
Any heart defect	96%
Polyvalvar dysplasia	62%
Aortic coarctation and tubular hypoplasia	21%
Ventricular septal defect	19%
Atrial septal defect	17%
Respiratory system	
Abnormal lobation of lungs	37%
Hypoplasia of lungs	12%
Gastrointestinal system	
Omphalocele	33%
Eventration of diaphragm	20%
Meckel's diverticulum	12%
Gut malrotation	12%
Tracheoesophageal fistula	12%
Urogenital system	
Horseshoe kidney	33%
Kidney hypoplasia with dilated or double ureter	8%

Modified from Kalousek DK et al: *Pathology of the human embryo and previable fetus: an atlas*, New York, 1990, Springer-Verlag.

Diagnostic cardiac defects are nearly always present, with polyvalvular dysplasia being the most frequent finding. Omphalocele and renal abnormalities are common. Neural tube defects may be found but are not common. No difference in the type or frequency of abnormalities found in the spontaneously and the therapeutically aborted group has been found. Table 16-7 lists the incidence and most frequent types of abnormalities present in fetuses with trisomy 18.

Trisomy 13

Most of the abnormalities typical of trisomy 13 newborns are present in the previable fetus as well. Craniofacial abnormalities include holoprosencephalic defects, microcephaly, microphthalmia, cleft lip or palate, and scalp defects. Postaxial polydactyly in one or more limbs and cardiac abnormalities are usually present. Neural tube defects, malrotation of the intestine with or without omphalocele, and variable renal anomalies such as microcysts involving nephrons and collecting tubules, nodular renal blastema, and renal dysplasia are commonly seen. Compared to other autosomal trisomies, fetuses with trisomy 13 show more severe craniofacial, skeletal, and brain abnormalities. No difference in the type or incidence of abnormalities has been observed in trisomy 13 fetuses spontaneously or therapeutically aborted. Table 16-8 reports the incidence of common types of abnormalities found in fetuses with trisomy 13.

Monosomy X

Monosomy X fetuses usually have a large posterior nuchal cystic hygroma with generalized edema and hypoplasia of the preductal aortic arch (Fig. 16-21). It has been postulated that generalized edema and cystic hygroma are the result of hypoplasia or aplasia of the lymphatic vessels and a failure of the jugular lymph sacs and the jugular vein to communicate. It has been suggested that preductal aortic hypoplasia may also be secondary to altered blood flow caused by lymphatic underdevelopment.

Posterior cervical hygroma has been described in many genetic and nongenetic syndromes. These include trisomies 13, 18, and 21, lethal multiple pterygium syndrome, Noonan's syndrome, Roberts' syndrome, and Cowchock syndrome. However, in 45,X fetuses, cervical hygroma is always accompanied by generalized edema and preductal aortic hypoplasia, which is not true for other conditions with cystic hygroma.[17]

Although a constant feature of adult 45,X women is infertility and 45,X newborns show small fibrotic streak gonads, some ova can be identified in all the fetal ovaries from affected previable fetuses. It has been postulated that ova in 45,X fetuses initially develop normally but that impaired follicular development caused by the absence of the second X chromosome leads to gradual loss of ova during the gestation. Table 16-9 lists common abnormalities in 45,X fetuses.

Triploidy

During the fetal period, if the supernumerary chromosomal set is paternal in origin, placental changes characteristic of partial

Table 16-8 Frequent abnormalities in trisomy 13 fetuses

Head and face	
Microcephaly	55%
Hypoplastic or absent nose	55%
Cleft lip and palate	55%
Small eyes	44%
Low-set ears	33%
Hypotelorism	33%
Holoprosencephaly	22%
Parietal scalp defect	11%
Cyclopia	11%
Encephalocoele	11%
Absent uvula	11%
Extremities	
Postaxial polydactyly (hands)	77%
Postaxial polydactyly (feet)	11%
Cardiovascular system	
Any heart defect	77%
Tetralogy of Fallot	33%
Ventricular septal defect and atrial septal defect	22%
Isolated ventricular septal defect	22%
Double-outlet right ventricle	11%
Mitral valve atresia	11%
Bicuspid aortic valve	11%
Respiratory system	
Abnormal lobation of lungs	55%
Hypoplasia of lungs	33%
Gastrointestinal system	
Malrotation of the small bowel	33%
Umbilical hernia or omphalocele	11%
Urogenital system	
Small penis	50%
Horseshoe kidney	22%
Enlarged kidneys (unexplained)	11%
Hydronephrosis	11%
Extra splenic tissue	22%
Meningomyelocele or myelocele	20%

Modified from Kalousek DK et al: *Pathology of the human embryo and previable fetus: an atlas,* New York, 1990, Springer-Verlag.

hydatidiform moles are usually found; if the extra set is maternal in origin, the placenta is usually small and fibrotic.[31] The majority of triploid abortions in the previable fetal period show a placental phenotype that is consistent with a maternal origin of the extra set. The typical phenotype of fetal triploidy, with severe intrauterine growth retardation and a large fetal head, includes a small fibrotic placenta (Fig. 16-22). Therefore, the frequency of maternal dominance in the fetal period contrasts with the embryonic triploidy loss, which shows mainly the placental phenotype consistent with a paternal origin of the extra set. The conclusion drawn from this observation is that maternally dominated triploidy is more likely to survive beyond the embryonic period. Most triploid fetuses, in addition to severe intrauterine growth retardation and large head, show a cleft palate, syndactyly between the third and the fourth fingers, and heart defects. Ambiguous genitalia are common among fetuses with a 69,XXY karyotype. It is interesting to note that the more rare, large cystic placentas are usually seen with the microcephalic, well-nourished triploid fetus. These fetuses originate from a double paternal and a single maternal complement. There seems to be no difference in type

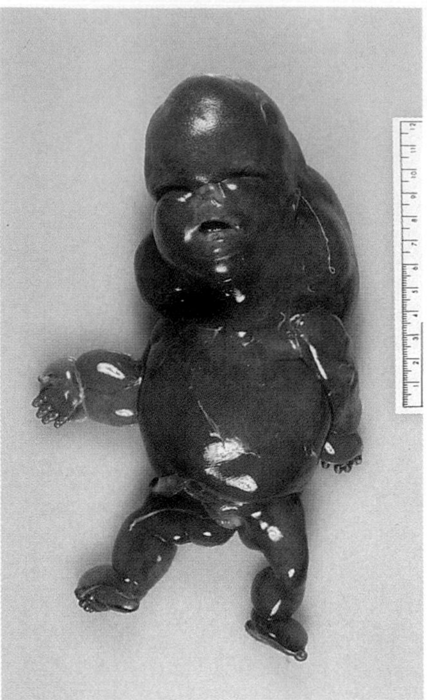

Fig. 16-21 Typical appearance of female fetus with monosomy X, 19½ developmental weeks. Notice bilateral posterior cervical hygroma and generalized edema.

Table 16-9 Common abnormalities in 45,X fetuses

External findings	
Nuchal cystic hygroma or nuchal edema	100%
Generalized edema	100%
Cardiovascular system	
Hypoplasia of preductal aortic arch	100%
Bicuspid aortic valve	38%
Persistent left superior vena cava	19%
Respiratory system	
Incomplete lung lobation	62%
Urogenital system	
Horseshoe kidney	52%
Gastrointestinal system	
Malrotation of the bowel	19%

Modified from Kalousek DK et al: *Pathology of the human embryo and previable fetus: an atlas,* New York, 1990, Springer-Verlag.

and frequency of internal developmental defects between maternally and paternally derived triploid fetuses.

The frequently observed abnormalities in the triploid fetuses are listed in Table 16-10.

Developmental fetal defects

The morphologic evaluation of developmental defects in previable fetuses is easier than the evaluation of embryonic defects. *The morphogenesis of all structures, except for brain, teeth, and external genitalia, is finished by the end of the eighth week.*

When chromosomally defective fetuses abort, they usually show classic phenotypic abnormalities as described above. Most spontaneously aborted diploid fetuses are morphologically normal. When developmental defects are present in chro-

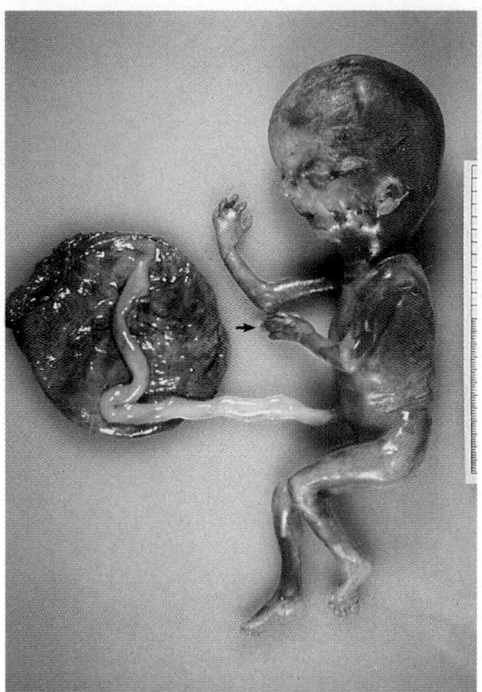

Fig. 16-22 Typical appearance of a second-trimester fetus with chromosomal triploidy. This male fetus is 18½ developmental weeks. Notice relative macrocephaly, obvious intrauterine growth retardation, third and fourth finger syndactyly on left hand *(arrow)*, and a small noncystic placenta. This phenotype is characteristic for maternally dominated triploidy.

Table 16-10 Abnormalities in triploid fetuses

Head and face	
Large head	75%
Cleft palate	50%
Low-set ears	25%
Small mandible	25%
Cleft lip	16%
Neck	
Edema	16%
Extremities	
Syndactyly between the third and fourth fingers	58%
Clinodactyly of the fifth finger	16%
Syndactyly between the toes	50%
Cardiovascular system	
Any heart defect	66%
Atrial septal defect and ventricular septal defect	25%
Ventricular septal defect isolated	25%
Valve dysplasia	25%
Atrioventricular septal defect	16%
Aortic stenosis	16%
Respiratory system	
Hypoplastic lungs	66%
Abnormal lobation and fissurization of lungs	66%
Gastrointestinal system	
Malrotation of small bowel	33%
Imperforate anus	8%
Urogenital system	
Ambiguous genitalia	58%
Horseshoe or hypoplastic kidney	8%
Adrenal gland	
Severe hypoplasia	75%
Lumbrosacral neural tube defect	16%
Placenta	
Cystic dilatation of placental villi	8%
Small placenta	92%
Oligohydramnios	16%

Modified from Kalousek DK et al: *Pathology of the human embryo and previable fetus: an atlas,* New York, 1990, Springer-Verlag.

mosomally normal spontaneously aborted fetuses, they are frequently attributable to abnormal development of the amniotic membranes, seen in disorders such as limb body wall defects or the early amnion rupture sequence.[17] The twinning process is also associated with a higher frequency of fetal problems because of structural placental abnormalities, as when fetal hydrops is caused by placental vascular anastomoses, which provide a route for shunting between twins.

A different group of structural defects is seen in fetuses that have been electively aborted because of prenatally detected abnormalities. Sonography is frequently the modality used to detect such problems; however, there is increasing use of fetal blood sampling and other clinical laboratory tests on fetal urine, amniotic fluid, and maternal blood to detect biochemical defects that may accompany nonspecific ultrasound abnormalities. Findings in this group of fetuses vary from small choroid plexus cysts to massive dilatation of the urinary bladder because of urethral obstruction. As the resolution of sonographic examination is continuously improving, the range of detected abnormalities in previable fetuses is increasing. Fetal echocardiography allows early prenatal diagnosis of many congenital cardiac defects.

After pregnancy termination for a prenatally diagnosed abnormality, the developmental defects are often easy to confirm, unless the abortion procedure is unduly destructive. The confirmation of prenatally demonstrated defects is important in providing quality control for the prenatal diagnostician but is not the pathologist's most critical task. The determination of the cause of developmental defects, for the purpose of providing accurate reproductive counseling for the family, is the ultimate goal of the postmortem investigation. For example, in a pregnancy terminated for prenatally diagnosed holoprosencephaly, the abnormality should be confirmed morphologically and any additional findings should be fully characterized; however, cytogenetic analysis is the most important test to perform successfully. There is a variety of chromosomal abnormalities associated with holoprosencephaly, but both autosomal dominant and recessive forms also exist, and referral for genetic counseling should be made with the karyotype results so that accurate recurrence risks can be provided to the family and prenatal testing for future pregnancies planned. Similarly, when a sonographic diagnosis of facial cleft and encephalocele is made, and the pathologic examination shows extensive amniotic bands causing the fetal disruption (clefting) and deformation (encephalocele), the pathologist must be clear and explicit in the report, indicating the cause of the lesions and their low risk of recurrence.

Although the majority of prenatally diagnosed defects are confirmed easily, some sonographic abnormalities, such as mild ventriculomegaly or hydrocephalus, may be difficult to confirm. Appropriate diagnostic criteria are still being developed in sonographic diagnosis of fetal brain lesions; therefore postdelivery reexamination of the brain by ultrasound is recommended before brain fixation and removal in suspected cases. In both electively and spontaneously aborted pregnancies, the recording of negative findings is important for genetic counseling and future follow-up study of the family.

Increased utilization of biochemical screening of maternal serum for abnormal levels of various proteins and hormones will not only lead to expansion of the range of prenatally detectable fetal defects, but will also improve the sensitivity of prenatal diagnosis for known fetal defects. Abnormal levels of alpha-fetoprotein indicate several specific fetal defects, such as neural tube defect, skin disorder, renal dysfunction, and body-wall defect, and also raise the possibility of a chromosomal abnormality in either the placenta or the fetus, or both.

FETAL INFECTIONS

Infectious causes of spontaneous abortion, fetal malformations, and stillbirth are numerous and varied. Our understanding of the pathophysiology of intrauterine infection in causing fetal abnormality and pregnancy loss has been seriously hampered by the large number of microorganisms associated with placental and fetal pathology.[32] The fact that many maternal infections are asymptomatic or have nonspecific symptoms has also interfered with our ability to draw causal inferences. Microbiologic diagnoses are further complicated because many putative fetal pathogens may reside normally in the maternal genital tract as commensal flora (such as group B streptococci and *Mycoplasma*). Also, obtaining appropriate, noncontaminated embryonic, fetal, and placental samples for culture in both early and late pregnancy loss is difficult. Special culture or detection techniques are required for some organisms (such as *Chlamydia* and *Mycoplasma*) and interpretations of microbial growth in cultures are often complicated by the presence of multiple microorganisms.

Bacterial infections

Bacterial infections in the fetus are more frequently recognized than viral, parasitic, or fungal infections.[33] In most cases, acquisition of the organism is believed to be from the maternal genital tract by an ascending route. Premature rupture of membranes or a sudden spontaneous abortion may be the first indication of intrauterine infection. Although the maternal genital tract is probably the most common route for an ascending infection, there are several other possibilities, including (1) hematogenous spread of maternal infection, (2) iatrogenic infection introduced during prenatal procedures such as amniocentesis, and (3) direct infection from the maternal peritoneal cavity. In addition, bacteria can be carried asymptomatically in the male urogenital tract and can infect the conceptus by the ascending route after sexual intercourse in pregnancy. It has been reported that intact membranes do not prevent bacteria from gaining access to the amniotic fluid, contrary to former assumptions.

Bacterial infection of the uterine contents during a previable second-trimester pregnancy usually leads to pregnancy loss. The most frequent organisms found associated with ascending intrauterine infection are listed in Table 16-11. The typical manifestation of bacterial infection is acute inflammation of the placental membranes and the chorionic plate, decidua, and umbilical cord. The predominant inflammatory process is termed *chorioamnionitis* because the first signs of inflammation are usually found beneath the amnion and along the surface of the chorion (Fig. 16-23).

Table 16-11 Bacterial pathogens associated with chorioamnionitis

Gram positive	Gram negative	Other bacteria
Group B streptococci	*Bacteroides* sp.	*Ureaplasma urealyticum*
Listeria monocytogenes	Coliform bacteria	*Chlamydia* sp.
Coagulase-negative staphylococci	*Haemophilus* sp.	*Mycoplasma hominis*
Viridans streptococci	*Brucella* sp.	*Treponema pallidum*
Group D streptococci	*Neisseria gonorrhoeae*	*Borrelia* sp.
Anaerobic gram-positive cocci	*Campylobacter* sp.	*Mobiluncus* sp.
Lactobacilli	*Fusobacterium* sp. Miscellaneous non-fermentative bacteria (*Pseudomonas, Aeromonas*)	*Gardnerella vaginalis*

Modified from Kalousek DK et al: *Pathology of the human embryo and previable fetus: an atlas,* New York, 1990, Springer-Verlag.

Whether the infection occurs before rupture of the membranes by invasion of the amniotic sac through devitalized membranes over the cervical os or gains access secondary to membranes rupture in most cases is not clear.[34] Once bacteria are in the amniotic sac, they incite maternal leukocyte migration from the intervillous space toward the amniotic cavity. The accumulation of neutrophils leads to a loss of translucency of the membranes, which become creamy yellow. Most bacteria infect the membranes diffusely. Inhalation and ingestion of infected amniotic fluid by the fetus (amniotic infection syndrome) can be diagnosed microscopically by sectioning of the fetal lungs and stomach, which will contain neutrophils in amniotic fluid. When infection spreads to the fetus in this manner, it can cause intrauterine aspiration pneumonia with interstitial neutrophils, or develop into septicemia. Intrauterine death may occur before spontaneous abortion[35] when the infecting agent is strongly virulent, as is frequently the case with group B streptococci.

Acute chorioamnionitis frequently induces labor, presumably because the neutrophils and bacteria that are present release phospholipases, which in turn enzymatically release arachidonic acid from the fetal membranes. The arachidonic acid rapidly converts to prostaglandin E_2 and to $F_{2\alpha}$. Prostaglandin E_2 causes the cervix to dilate and $F_{2\alpha}$ initiates uterine contractions.

The genital *Mycoplasma hominis* and *Ureaplasma urealyticum* were implicated in the cause of repeated spontaneous abortion after it was shown that the organisms were isolated more often from the cervix and endometrium of habitual aborters than from those of controls. The isolation of genital mycoplasmas in conceptuses spontaneously lost before 20 weeks of gestation has been described, and colonization of endometrium, placental membranes, and amniotic fluid by

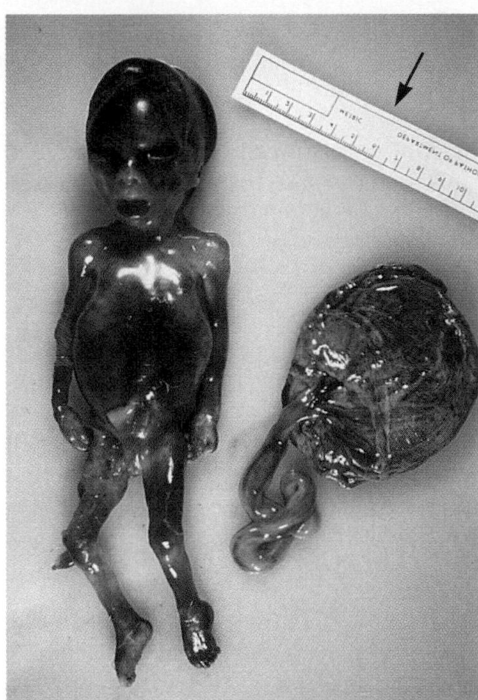

Fig. 16-23 Products of conception at 19 developmental weeks showing severe amniotic infection syndrome caused by culture-proved *Escherichia coli* and *Streptococcus faecalis*. Chorioamnionitis and focal villitis were found microscopically.

genital mycoplasmas has been demonstrated in patients with clinical intraamniotic infection and stillbirth.[36] Colonization of the female genital tract by *Chlamydia trachomatis* is commonly described, but no significant evidence of *Chlamydia* involvement in early pregnancy loss has been reported.[37]

In many cases of intrauterine bacterial infection, the infection extends into the decidua basalis, from which bacteria may reach the fetus hematogenously by being shed into the intervillous blood. Hematogenously acquired infections are less commonly associated with pregnancy loss or intrauterine fetal death than ascending infections are. The villi appear to form an effective barrier to the transfer of most bacteria but do not seem to hinder passage of *Listeria monocytogenes* and *Treponema pallidum*. *Listeria monocytogenes* can be a devastating prenatal infection[38] with a characteristic gross and histologic pattern of granulomatous lesions in fetus and placenta. Severely infected fetuses may be hydropic, showing the typical granulomatous lesions and microabcesses affecting skin and multiple viscera. Longstanding infections can show calcification of lesions as well, and placental lesions should be present.

Infection with *Treponema pallidum* is likely to be queried by the obstetrician on the basis of maternal serology and symptoms. Congenital syphilis can present at autopsy in a fetus with profound changes or may be quite subtle, and even unconfirmable, depending on the timing of infection and subsequent fetal death. Syphilis infects the fetus by hematogeneous spread from the mother with primary or secondary disease, and although organisms have been recovered from first trimester abortuses, the endothelial inflammatory lesions in the fetus that result in the classic findings appear to develop only with active infection after about 16 weeks gestation.

Mycobacterium tuberculosis as a congenital infection is rare. Spread from the mother is by the hematogeneous route, and characteristic caseating lesions in liver are therefore most common. Acid-fast stains should demonstrate characteristic organisms.

Viral infections

Several modes of transmission are involved in the pathogenesis of intrauterine viral infection.[32] The most commonly recognized mechanism is transplacental transmission during maternal viremia. Viruses may also be transmitted by means of latently infected endometrial or cervical cells, or an endogenous retrovirus may be carried by maternal or paternal germ cells.

Since spontaneous abortion is a rare complication of maternal viral disease, chronic fetal disease is the usual result of viral intrauterine infection. A fetus exposed to a chronic viral intrauterine infection usually has several characteristic features. Growth retardation and destructive brain lesions are frequent findings. Hepatomegaly and splenomegaly with focal necrosis constitute typical features of most chronic viral intrauterine infections.

Rubella virus

Fetal infection can result from maternal rubella viremia. Spontaneous abortion was found in only 8% of 477 women whose pregnancies were complicated by rubella and not terminated. The type of fetal malformation caused by intrauterine rubella infection is related to the time of the infection.[39,40] Fetuses infected before 11 weeks of gestation are always malformed, with heart defects and deafness being present in about 85% of fetuses and infants. Isolated deafness has been reported in 35% of those survivors infected between 13 and 16 weeks of gestation, yet no defects attributable to rubella have been found in fetuses infected after this period. Since definitive prenatal diagnosis of fetal infection is not widely available, the pathologist should carefully examine the fetus for any signs of fetal infection after pregnancy termination for suspected rubella infection. Fresh tissue from the heart, brain, liver, and placenta should be submitted for rubella culture, antigen detection, and nucleic acid hybridization.

Herpes group viruses

The herpes group of viruses includes cytomegalovirus (CMV), herpes simplex virus (HSV), varicella-zoster virus (VZV), and Epstein-Barr virus (EBV). The complexity of the diseases in this group makes it difficult to evaluate fetal infection, since it may be attributable to primary maternal infection or (less commonly) to the reactivation of an old infection during pregnancy. As a general rule, primary maternal herpes virus infection during pregnancy is more likely to cause fetal morbidity or mortality. Maternal antibody status (IgG and IgM) can be helpful in diagnosing and distinguishing primary and reactivated infections.

Of this group, *cytomegalovirus* is most commonly associated with intrauterine infection[41] (Fig. 16-24). The manifestations of fetal CMV infection include intrauterine growth retardation, hepatosplenomegaly, hepatitis with hyperbilirubinemia, pneumonitis, encephalitis, cerebral calcification, and microcephaly. Placental changes include villitis, with prominent plasma cell infiltrate, focal villus necrosis, and hemorrhage.

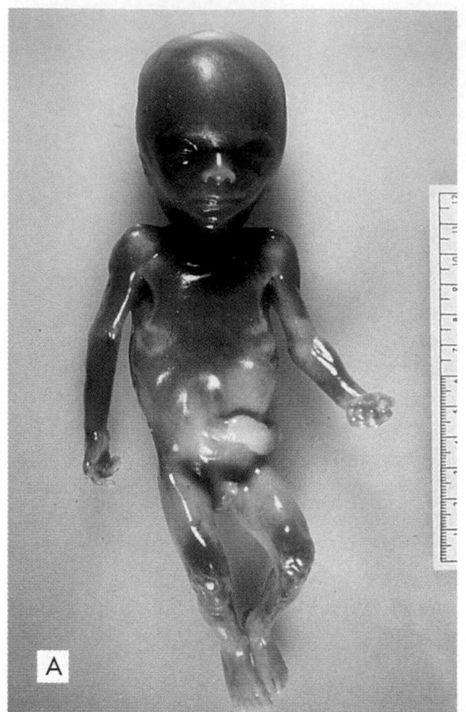

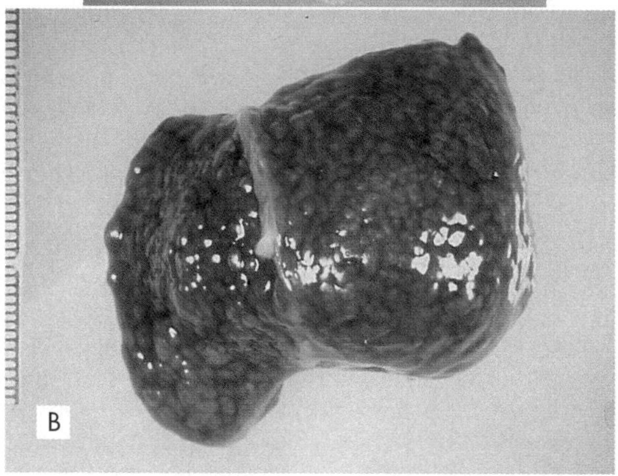

Fig. 16-24 **A**, Male fetus at 16 developmental weeks with prenatally diagnosed hydrocephalus. Autopsy showed diffuse cytomegalovirus infection involving placental and fetal tissues, including brain. **B**, Disseminated intrauterine cytomegalovirus infection with involvement of liver. Notice that the liver is enlarged and shows a nodular surface as a result of parenchymal necrosis and regeneration. Microscopically typical inclusions were found in both hepatocytes and biliary duct epithelium.

The majority of HSV fetal infections are caused by herpes simplex virus type 2 after rupture of membranes or during passage of the fetus through an infected birth canal.[42] Rarely, the fetus may become infected after a primary maternal infection during pregnancy. Developmental defects include microcephaly, intracranial calcifications, chorioretinitis, and microphthalmia.

Approximately 95% of women of child-bearing age have serologic evidence of past *varicella-zoster virus* infection.[42] Although congenital varicella and the pattern of anomalies associated with it are recognized, primary varicella infection in pregnancy and fetal loss are rare.

There are no convincing reports in the literature of Epstein-Barr virus infection associated with fetal loss.

Influenza virus

A causal relationship between influenza virus and developmental defects remains unclear. High rates of fetal loss, however, were reported in the influenza pandemic of 1918 to 1920, especially when the disease was complicated by maternal pneumonia.[32]

Enteroviruses

Enteroviruses include Coxsackieviruses A and B, ECHO virus, poliovirus, and all of the picornavirus group. None of these viruses has been positively associated with an increase in developmental defects.[32] Spontaneous abortion has been observed after documented Coxsackievirus A16 infection and poliovirus infection in the first trimester, but causal association has not been established.

Hepatitis viruses

No increase in fetal loss or in the frequency of developmental defects has been reported with maternal hepatitis caused by the known viruses A, B, C, or D, though neonatal disease acquired in utero or intrapartum can occur.[32]

Parvovirus

Spontaneous abortion with fetal hydrops is reported to result from some maternal infections with parvovirus B19,[43] the cause of "fifth disease," also called erythema infectiosum. The hydrops fetalis seen in this infection is the result of anemia caused by red blood cell destruction by virus. Histologic features consist of excessive iron pigment in the liver, hepatitis, a leukoerythroblastic reaction, and eosinophilic nuclear inclusions in hematopoietic cell nuclei. In situ hybridization with labeled viral DNA is best for confirmation of the diagnosis.

Human immunodeficiency virus

Congenital human immunodeficiency virus (HIV) infections (AIDS) have been reported, and an estimate of in utero transmission is in the range of 50% to 65%. Transplacental transmission has been demonstrated by positive virus cultures from aborted 14- to 20-week fetuses and from cord blood. The exact pathway of transmission remains unknown, but transplacental passage by a cell-associated virus is likely. There are no well-documented cases of HIV infection causing specific dysmorphic features or malformations. The rate of pregnancy loss in otherwise healthy HIV-infected mothers appears to be increased.[44]

Fungal infections

Despite the frequency and ease with which fungi, specifically *Candida* species, are isolated from the genital tracts of pregnant patients, antenatal fetal fungal infections are rare. Discrete rounded yellow plaques varying in size from 0.5 to 2 mm seen on the umbilical cord surface and membranes represent pathognomonic gross changes. As the organisms penetrate the surface epithelium of the cord and amnion, they evoke an intense cellular response by polymorphonuclear and mononuclear cells. Evidence of inflammatory changes affecting the chorionic villi or decidual plate is not generally found. This is usually an incidental finding in an otherwise normal pregnancy that has resulted in a normal newborn.

CONTROL OF FETAL GROWTH AND INTRAUTERINE GROWTH RESTRICTION

Fetal growth is a complex, dynamic process that is only partially understood. The intrinsic growth potential of the conceptus is expressed separately in an interdependent fashion by the fetus and its placenta, and both can be modified by environmental and maternal factors. Fetal growth velocity changes throughout gestation, with gains for weight and length following slightly different curves. At the end of embryogenesis (the eighth week of pregnancy) the fetus is 3.0 cm long and weighs 2.8 g; by term the fetus is expected to measure on average 50 cm and weigh 3500 g. The greatest increases in length are found in the twentieth week of pregnancy, at 2.5 cm per week. The greatest increases in weight occur from the thirty-fifth week of pregnancy onward. The fetal weight is approximately doubled in the final 8 weeks of pregnancy.

Growth factors are of much greater significance for intrauterine differentiation and body growth than growth hormone. Several different "families" of growth factors, usually polypeptides, have been described.[45] It has been estimated that intrauterine fetal growth is determined 30% to 60% by fetal genes.[46,47] This estimate is in keeping with recurrent findings of chromosomal abnormalities in a proportion of fetuses with intrauterine growth restriction.[48] It is important to keep in mind that finding a diploid karyotype in a fetus with intrauterine growth restriction does not mean that a genetic cause of growth failure does not exist. A diploid fetus may have an identifiable genetic disorder such as uniparental disomy, or a monogenic disorder. As stated above, in cases of fetal uniparental disomy, it is not clear how much of the intrauterine growth failure is attributable to accompanying placental mosaicism and how much is attributable to uniparental disomy and genomic imprinting (Figs. 16-14 and 16-15).

There are two main groups of monogenic disorders associated with abnormal intrauterine growth. These are constitutional skeletal dysplasias[49] and disorders of connective tissue.[50] In addition, there are numerous syndromes of unknown cause such as Russell-Silver syndrome, Rubinstein-Taybi syndrome, and Cornelia de Lange syndrome, which are characterized by intrauterine growth failure.

Although intrauterine growth disturbance caused by environmental factors may be present in up to 40% to 70% of cases, little is known about the mechanisms by which factors such as maternal alcohol consumption, infections, or drug exposure influence fetal growth. The effect of maternal smoking has been studied extensively, and placental and uterine vascular constriction resulting in reduced placental blood flow is believed to cause reduced fetal growth. A similar mechanism is presumed to cause intrauterine growth restriction with maternal eclampsia. At the other extreme, maternal hyperglycemia induces fetal pancreatic islet cell hyperplasia, and the resulting increased fetal glucose uptake in part causes the macrosomia that accompanies poorly controlled maternal diabetes.

Different patterns of restricted fetal growth have been observed, which primarily distinguish between symmetrically small head and body proportions and small body measurements with normal brain and head size. These two patterns have also been called *proportionate (symmetrical)* versus *disproportionate (asymmetrical) fetal growth restriction*. It has been generally accepted that these patterns differentiate between intrinsic fetal versus placental causes of reduced fetal growth, respectively.[51] However, the situation now appears to be considerably more complex, and this generalization may be useful statistically but fails in the evaluation of the individual case.[52] Our understanding of the factors involved in fetal growth restriction is improving with increased application of prenatal sonography and karyotyping. When either pattern of prenatal fetal growth restriction is diagnosed, a careful sonographic evaluation by the obstetrician for associated malformations in the fetus and placenta, and estimations of amniotic fluid volume are generally made. Placental function may be evaluated by Doppler ultrasound of umbilical vessels, and fetal karyotype should be determined by amniocentesis, chorionic villi, or fetal blood sampling. The likelihood of a fetal chromosomal or genetic abnormality to account for the growth restriction is increased when there are localized fetal defects, normal or increased amniotic fluid volume (which may be caused by defective fetal swallowing or gastrointestinal atresias), and normal uteroplacentofetal blood flow by sonographic measurements.[52] The specific chromosome abnormality present influences the pattern of growth restriction. Triploidy causes severe early disproportionate growth retardation, whereas other chromosome disorders cause proportionately reduced fetal growth before 30 weeks, with disproportion apparently developing in later gestation. As discussed above, some forms of confined placental mosaicism may cause fetal growth restriction; this makes *placental* cytogenetic analysis invaluable in studies of fetal growth restriction.

When growth retardation is caused by placental insufficiency, there are abnormalities in sonographically determined uteroplacental function and reduced amniotic fluid volume on the basis of decreased renal perfusion and low fetal urine production. All body measurements tend to be below the expected ranges, with some sparing of head circumference relative to body measurements. The likelihood of fetal chromosomal abnormality in this group is much lower, and major malformations are unusual. When a growth-retarded fetus and its placenta are examined at autopsy, the pattern of growth restriction should be noted and correlated with abnormalities in fetus and placenta and with placental weight and development. A karyotype obtained from placental tissue is critical in determining if placental mosaicism plays a role in a case of otherwise unexplained fetal growth restriction, even when a normal fetal karyotype has been obtained by fetal blood sampling.

STILLBIRTH

The main goal in the evaluation of a case of late fetal death is identification of the underlying cause of death, so that meaningful information for future pregnancy management can be obtained. A complete examination of both the stillborn fetus and its placenta will provide the pathologist with the greatest chance to make meaningful diagnoses. It is important to keep in mind the distinction between cause and associations, mechanisms, and final common pathways that lead to fetal death. Many cases of stillbirth will show gross and histologic features that indicate an acute asphyxial mechanism of death, but the cause for the asphyxia may be less apparent. In other cases, a finding known to be associated with stillbirth, such as fetal trisomy 21, may be present, but the mechanism of death will remain unidentified. *The later the gestational age at the time of stillbirth, the more likely the cause is related to the placenta or umbilical cord, and the more likely the examination of the fetus will show only changes of asphyxia.* Asphyxia is a common mechanism of fetal death as a result of a great number of underlying causes. One of the most easily recognizable gross features that indicates asphyxia is meconium discharge by the fetus after 28 to 30 weeks of gestation in utero. The evidence for this can be found in the form of yellow-green pasty material on the skin and placental surfaces and a granular yellow pigmented or eosinophilic material in the lungs. Hypoxia is a stimulant to deep inspiratory efforts in the fetus, which then draws amniotic fluid with all its cellular and noncellular particulate matter, including meconium, deep into the lungs. This finding has less significance in a term or postterm stillbirth, when discharge of meconium may reflect the physiologic maturation of the bowel more than severity of asphyxic stress.

Petechial hemorrhages of skin and viscera, particularly in areas subject to increased capillary pressure, can be seen in the asphyxiated fetus. Intracranial hemorrhages are frequently also seen in the setting of asphyxia and may be in the germinal eminence, with or without rupture into the lateral ventricle, or may be subarachnoid or within the falx.

The "complete" stillbirth autopsy is identical to the previable fetal examination described above. Maceration, defined as the degenerative changes that occur after fetal death and before delivery, is a common finding in stillborn fetuses and their placentas. Because of the implications the maceration changes may have for timing fetal death and correlating with clinical history, useful patterns of morphologic changes for estimating the duration of intrauterine retention of a dead fetus before delivery have been established[53-55] (Table 16-12). Fig. 16-25 shows features of moderate maceration in a malformed fetus.

To avoid unnecessary costs, ancillary studies should be chosen to reflect those most likely to be useful in providing information to aid future pregnancy counseling. Any fetus with malformations should have full-body anteroposterior and lateral x-ray films taken (Fig. 16-26). If fetal metabolic disease is suspected, or in cases of unexplained hydrops, tissue samples of placenta, fetal liver, spleen, and skeletal muscle should be snap frozen and stored at –70°C for biochemical or DNA studies. A fibroblast culture from fetal or placental tissue should also be initiated, since many enzyme defects can be measured in fibroblasts. Ultrastructural study of the placental villi or of fetal tissues can be helpful in confirming biochemical disorders, including those with abnormal storage products, or organelle pathology. Catalogs of prenatally diagnosed diseases and tables of metabolic diseases that manifest during fetal life are available.[56,57] Referral laboratories with special research and service interests in many heritable metabolic diseases can be found.

The most controversial (because of the high cost) of the ancillary studies to be considered in evaluation of the stillbirth

Table 16-12 Timetable of changes of maceration following intrauterine fetal death

Duration of retention equal to or greater than:	Gross fetal examination	Histology of fetal organs: loss of nuclear basophilia in:	Histology of placenta
4 hours		Individual renocortical tubular cells	
6 hours	Desquamation of 1 cm patches; brown or red discoloration of umbilical stump		Villus intravascular karyorrhexis
12 hours	Desquamation on face, back, or abdomen		
18 hours	Desquamation of 25% of body, or two or more body regions		
24 hours	Brown or tan skin discoloration on abdomen	Individual liver cells Inner one half of myocardium	
36 hours	Any cranial compression		
48 hours	Desquamation of >50% of body	Outer one half of myocardium	Multifocal vascular luminal fibroblast septation or obliteration
72 hours	Desquamation of >75% of body		
96 hours		Some bronchial epithelial cells All cells in liver	
1 week	Widely open mouth	Tracheal cartilage All gastrointestinal tract cells All adrenal cells	
2 weeks	Mummification, that is, dehydration, compression, tan color		Extensive vascular luminal changes (see 48-hour findings) Extensive fibrosis of terminal villi

Data from Genest DR, Williams MA, Greene MF: Estimating the time of death in stillborn fetuses: I. Histologic evaluation of fetal organs: an autopsy study of 150 stillborns, *Obstet Gynecol* 80(4):575, 1992; II. Histologic evaluation of the placenta: a study of 71 stillborns, *Obstet Gynecol* 80(4):585, 1992; III. External fetal examination: a study of 86 stillborns, *Obstet Gynecol* 80(4):593, 1992.

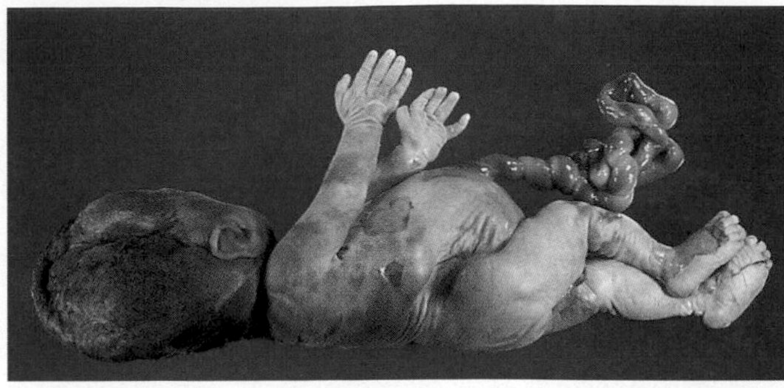

Fig. 16-25 This 29-week-gestation stillborn fetus with vertebral defects, imperforate anus, tracheoesophageal fistula, and radial and renal dysplasia (VATER association) shows evidence of moderate maceration in the form of patchy skin slippage, collapse of the head, and dark discoloration of the umbilical cord.

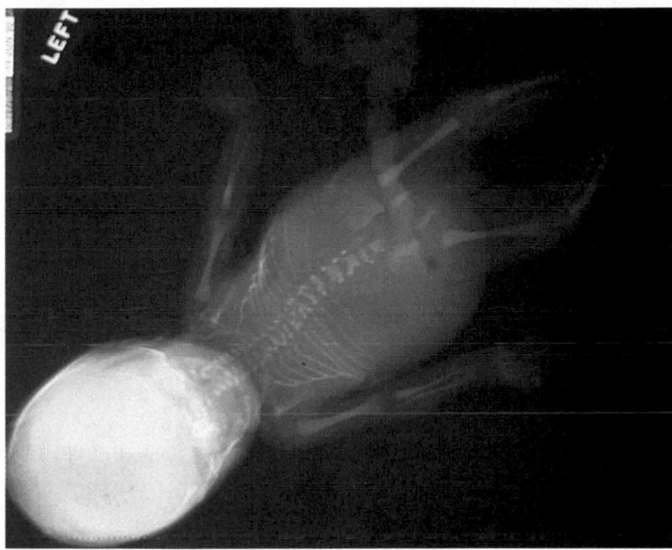

Fig. 16-26 Radiograph of same fetus as in Fig. 16-25 shows the obvious multiple vertebral anomalies, illustrating the importance of radiographs in the evaluation of any fetus with anomalies.

autopsy is routine cytogenetics. The benefits are well established and will therefore be stressed. Firstly, both a normal and an abnormal karyotype provide important data in any case of stillbirth. Studies have revealed an abnormal karyotype in 5% to 10% of stillbirths. A stillborn with minor dysmorphic features may have an abnormal karyotype with implications for genetic counseling, such as an unbalanced translocation inherited from a balanced carrier parent. Some severe anomalies, such as holoprosencephaly, occur on a sporadic basis when associated with a simple trisomy 13 but are autosomal recessive or even autosomal dominant in familial syndromes in which the chromosomal complement is normal. Only a fetal chromosome study can distinguish between the chromosomal, sporadic form and one that may carry a significant recurrence risk. An important point to keep in mind when one is choosing tissue for chromosomal analysis in stillbirth is that the placenta, being in direct contact with the maternal circulation, remains more viable after fetal demise and for that reason is the best tissue to sample for any cytogenetic study after stillbirth. Amnion and chorion will often yield fibroblast cultures even when advanced maceration of the fetus is present. In cases of otherwise unexplained intrauterine growth restriction, cytogenetic analysis of the chorionic villi and amnion may provide evidence of confined placental mosaicism to explain the restricted growth and the stillbirth. If placental cultures show an abnormal karyotype in mosaic form, formalin-fixed fetal tissue can be subsequently analyzed by DNA-specific probes using in situ hybridization to ascertain the fetal chromosome complement without the need for viable fibroblast cultures.[58] Such interphase techniques are suited to answering specific questions about particular chromosomes and the growing number of genes with available probes.

The question often arises whether a particular fetal demise was preventable. The pathologist is then asked to determine whether an acute or a chronic condition caused the death. An increase of fetal adrenal cortex lipid accumulation appears to correlate with an increased likelihood of chronicity, though the amount of time required to produce significant fatty change has not been well established. An absence of fat within the fetal adrenal cortex, however, is accepted as indicating a precipitous event leading to fetal death. Other features that indicate chronic fetal compromise appear to be stress involution of the thymus, with lymphoid depletion, prominence and perhaps karyorrhexis of Hassall's corpuscles, and increased cortical histiocytosis. A modest increase in circulating fetal nucleated red blood cells in the absence of findings suggestive of a specific hemoglobinopathy or hemolysis also is suggestive of ongoing fetal stress of unknown duration. These changes are not specific to any underlying cause for the fetal stress but indicate a period of fetal morbidity before death.

The rates of stillbirth as determined in many countries over the past 3 decades have been remarkably similar and constant over time, on the order of 6 to 12 per 1000 live births per year. The risk of stillbirth is dramatically greater in multiple gestations, up to seven times that of singleton pregnancies.[59] Modest increases have been seen in mothers past 34 years of age or below 20 years, mothers of high parity, and those who received inadequate prenatal care, used illicit drugs, or had severe pregnancy-related hypertension. Low maternal weight, previous history of pregnancy loss, and smoking in older mothers have been significantly associated with stillbirth,[60] as have a variety of pregnancy complications, including maternal insulin-dependent diabetes[61] and urinary tract infection.[62] Obstetric factors contributing to stillbirth include breech presentation, particularly in preterm deliveries, and obvious causes such as placental abruption, umbilical cord prolapse, and birth trauma. Fetal factors that are found at increased frequency in stillbirth include intrauterine growth restriction, as well as congenital malformations as a group.[60] Numerous classification systems have been devised for categorizing stillbirth. Some systems have been based solely on clinical history, others on necropsy data only, and yet others have attempted to correlate clinical findings with pathologic evidence. Table 16-13 is a compilation and homogenization of several studies[61-67] that tabulated and classified stillbirths by presumed "cause." The most frequently assigned "cause" was "unknown" ranging from 9% to 50% in individual studies. Antepartum hemorrhage was the single largest known cause of stillbirth, frequently attributable to premature separation of the placenta, accounting for 12% to 17%.

Table 16-13 Pathology findings and background data in seven studies of stillbirth

Reference	Fretts et al, 1992	Lofgren et al, 1982	Hovatta et al, 1983	Machin, 1975	Magani et al, 1990	Morrison and Olsen, 1985	Whitfield et al, 1986
Locale	Montreal	Malmö	Helsinki	South London	Galway	Manitoba	Glasgow
Study period	1961-1988	1974-1980	1974-1979	1970-1973	1972-1982	1977-1982	1979-1982
Stillbirths	709	84	243	346	325	765	161
Total deliveries	88,651	17,983	39,318	35,000	27,072	98,927	13,446
Stillbirth rate/1000	8.3	4.7	6.2	10.0	12.0	7.7	12.0
Minimum gestational age/ weight for inclusion	500 g	28 wk	26 wk	28 wk	20 wk	20 wk	
Causes of death(%)							
Anomalies	11.0	7.0	16.9	21.1	20.3	10.2	13.1
Infection	6.1	3.6	2.1	<1.0	2.5		3.1
Isoimmunization	2.3	0	3.3	<1.0	7.7		5.6
Fetal growth retardation	14.6	11.9			6.8	11.2	8.1
Abruptio placentae	12.4		14.4		15.7	15.4	17.4
Intrapartum asphyxia	7.0	8.3	3.3	28.0			
Maternal diabetes	2.5	1.2			<1.0	4.8	
Maternal hypertension	1.9	6.0	7.4		15.7	7.5	9.9
Other causes	13.0	7.0	18.0	<1.0	19.1	18.7	3.1
Unexplained antepartum causes	29.2	50.0	9.1	6.1	11.4	19.3	13.1
Cord complication		4.8	11.9				
Large placental infarction			10.7				
Fetal bleeding			2.9				
Antepartum hypoxia with birth trauma				3.2			
Placental insufficiency						7.5	
Trauma						1.7	
Postmaturity						3.7	
"Spontaneous preterm" delivery (20 to 28 weeks)							26.7

Fetal causes

The intrauterine environment allows the fetus to tolerate many fetal abnormalities that are lethal after birth, and this fact accounts for the low frequency of stillbirths attributable directly to an exclusive, fetal cause. Some chromosomal and genetic syndromes are associated with an increased incidence of stillbirth, but for many of these the mechanism of death is unclear.[58] The finding of anomalies that are diagnostic for such a syndrome aids in directing genetic and pregnancy counseling. Known mechanisms of fetal death related to fetal genetic abnormalities include metabolic diseases that presumably interfere with transport across the placental barrier, such as those causing hydrops[57] (Table 16-14). Fetal malformations, in contrast to functional abnormalities affecting metabolism, infrequently result in fetal death. Those that do usually have obvious structure-function relationships, such as large fetal vascular malformations or hypoplastic left heart syndrome causing hydrops attributable to fetal heart failure. Fetal cardiovascular defects with functional effects, such as fetal arrhythmia, are the most common heart malformations to which fetal death can be attributed.[68] When attributing fetal death directly to a fetal malformation, one would be prudent to ascertain the frequency of liveborns with similar malformations, since liveborn infants can be delivered without kidneys, lungs, or cerebral cortex, or with severe malformations of the skeletal, hepatobiliary, gastrointestinal, and endocrine systems.

As the frequency, accuracy, and sophistication of prenatal diagnostic techniques increases, our understanding of the functional events that can lead to fetal death will vastly improve. Persistent fetal arrhythmias that have led to high-output fetal heart failure, hydrops, and death have been reported. Postcordocentesis fetal death attributable to unremitting bradycardia is explained by a vasoreactive reflex brought on by umbilical cord trauma. Placental vascular Doppler studies can allow prediction of abnormal placental blood flow and correlation of it with abnormal fetal growth and ultimately with fetal death.

Placental causes

Placental and umbilical causes of fetal demise are the most common as a group. *Therefore any stillbirth evaluation is grossly inadequate if a complete examination of placenta and cord is not undertaken.* Frequently, with these causes, the autopsy findings in the fetus will be only those of asphyxia. The obvious lesions are tight umbilical cord knots, placental abruptions, and large placental infarctions. As the majority of these lesions are also discovered incidentally in lesser forms at delivery of live born normal infants, the putative culpability of an umbilical knot or placental infarction in causing fetal death needs to be carefully established, and no significant abnormalities other than those of acute asphyxia should be present in the fetus. Chapter 69, discussing the placenta, addresses these issues in greater detail.

The placenta is also the site of an underrecognized cause of fetal death: fetomaternal bleeding. Although not always apparent, significant fetal pallor and relative bloodlessness at autopsy should raise the question of this entity. The Kleihauer-Betke test should be a part of the obstetric protocol for every stillbirth. This test, which assesses the volume of fetal blood in the maternal circulation, is the only reliable test to prove this mechanism of intrauterine death. Even maternal blood drawn after the delivery of an unexpected stillborn can yield a meaningful result.[69]

Infections play a major role in stillbirth, and most infections cause fetal death because of their placental effects, by inciting premature delivery and compromising placental function. Chorioamnionitis with common pathogenic bacteria has been discussed in the foregoing section on pathology of the previable period and in Chapter 69. Fetal death is frequently intrapartum because severely premature fetuses are ill equipped to withstand the stress of labor. In utero death before the onset of labor of a fetus with amniotic infection syndrome is usually ascribed to fetal sepsis, which manifests histologically as intrauterine interstitial pneumonia. When fetal sepsis is absent, a reactive vasoconstrictive phenomenon in the umbilical or fetal surface vessels in response to inflammation has been postulated to account for intrauterine asphyxia. Viral infections infrequently cause fetal death but may lead to pregnancy termination because of prenatally diagnosed abnormalities, including hydrops.

Table 16-14 Metabolic causes of hydrops fetalis

Gaucher's disease
G_{M1}-gangliosidosis
Sialidosis
Salla disease
Wolman disease
β-Glucuronidase deficiency
Morquio syndrome
Neuraminidase deficiency
Myotonic dystrophy
Perinatal iron storage syndrome
Carnitine deficiency

From Clark LA et al: Pathology of inherited metabolic diseases. In Dimmick JE, Kalousek DK: editors: *Developmental pathology of the embryo and fetus,* Philadelphia, 1992, Lippincott.

Maternal causes

Maternal disorders that adversely affect pregnancy outcome are varied, ranging from uterine anomalies to autoimmune phenomena. These disorders can be roughly divided into those that are specifically related to pregnancy, such as preeclampsia, and those that may preexist, such as maternal lupus erythematosus. A category termed *maternal exposures* is also warranted to account for the effects of smoking, drug and alcohol use, and undesired effects of prescribed medications. Several diseases, such as diabetes, may straddle these categories, as when preexistent glucose intolerance requires insulin during pregnancy. The mechanisms leading to fetal death attributable to maternal diabetes are poorly understood as is the case with respect to many other diseases. Some basic facts are known. For example, pregnancy-related hypertension induces placental-bed vascular changes that compromise placental flow and thus fetal growth and health. Whether there is a primary "vasculopathy" accompanying the hypertension is open to debate.

The most common cause of fetal death in trauma is maternal death.[70] Evidence of direct fetal trauma is frequently absent in such cases, since the gravid uterus offers relatively effective mechanical protection to the fetus and placenta; however, maternal shock or cardiac arrest can quickly cause fetal asphyxia. Blunt trauma to the abdomen can also cause fetal death by direct fetal trauma with massive hemorrhage, or, more often, through placental separation with subsequent fetal exsanguination and asphyxia. Abruptio placentae and fetal death may not occur immediately in such cases, with reports of up to a 5-day interval between maternal trauma and the diagnosis of abruption. Obviously, the ongoing clinical condition of the mother in nonfatal maternal trauma is pertinent to the pathophysiology of late placental abruption after trauma. Microscopic examination of any retroplacental clot and a search for hemosiderin in such a case may aid in establishing the timing of placental separation. Uterine rupture is a less common cause of fetal death in direct maternal abdominal trauma. Penetrating injury to the maternal abdomen can injure the fetus, placenta, or cord, with obvious results.

Fetal hydrops

Significant subcutaneous edema accompanied by serous effusion in the fetus is termed *fetal hydrops*. The differential diagnosis of prenatally identified fetal hydrops is extremely broad[71] and is beyond the scope of this chapter. Table 16-15 is a summary of major nonimmunological disease categories associated with fetal hydrops and gives an idea of the range of individual disorders that can present at autopsy with a picture of hydrops.[72] Table 16-16 lists cardiac malformations associated with fetal hydrops. Fig. 16-27 shows a hydropic newborn with a prenatally diagnosed cystic adenomatoid malformation of the lung. Prenatally diagnosed fetal hydrops that progresses to fetal death frequently is accompanied by volumes of clinical, hematologic, serologic, and other data derived from maternal and prenatal fetal tests, many of which will exclude the more common causes such as TORCH infections (toxoplasmosis, rubella, cytomegalovirus, and herpes simplex) (Fig. 16-28), hemoglobinopathies, isoimmunization, and major malformations and chromosomal abnormalities in the fetus itself. If such studies have not been undertaken prenatally, the pathologist should consult with the referring obstetrician to ensure obtaining maternal serology specimens, Kleihauer-Betke testing, maternal hemoglobin electrophoresis, and other tests as indicated by the clinical history or postmortem examination. The postmortem examination should include the studies listed in Table 16-17.[72]

Birth trauma

Birth trauma is a diminishing cause of stillbirth that draws the pathologist into potential legal conflicts out of proportion to its incidence. Some fetal anomalies, such as the lethal form of osteogenesis imperfecta, and certain cases of congenital contractural deformities, such as severe pterygia, predispose to fetal trauma during uncomplicated delivery. The unsuspected delivery of a macrosomic macerated stillborn fetus can lead to severe disruption of fetal soft tissues and even bones and joints, which must be distinguished by the pathologist from fatal fetal injury.

Fetal death caused by mechanical trauma has an incidence of 0.2 to 0.7 per 1000 births.[73] Cranial and intracranial injuries associated with significant hemorrhage are the most commonly lethal forms of birth trauma. Preterm as well as term fetuses are affected in proportion to their numbers. It is important to distinguish at autopsy between deforming but nonlethal injuries, such as *caput succedaneum* (an edematous swelling of the skin and superficial fascia of the presenting

Table 16-15 Associations with nonimmunological fetal hydrops: analysis of 594 cases

Cases	Number	Percentage
Cardiovascular abnormalities	**111**	**18.7**
Cardiac malformations	57	
Arrhythmias	29	
Fetal angioma	6	
Placental angioma	5	
Arterial pathology	5	
Rhabdomyoma of heart	6	
Cardiomyopathy	3	
Noncardiovascular anomalies	**83**	**14.0**
Adenomatoid malformation of lung	12	
Pulmonary sequestration	6	
Pulmonary lymphangiectasis	1	
Diaphragmatic hernia	9	
Renal anomaly	17	
Skeletal	19	
Not otherwise specified	18	
Jejunal atresia	1	
Chromosome anomaly	**82**	**13.8**
45,X	25	
Trisomy 21	19	
Trisomy 18	8	
Trisomy 13	2	
Triploidy	1	
Not otherwise specified	3	
"Cystic hygroma"	24	
Monochorionic twin pregnancy	**61**	**10.3**
Twin-twin transfusion	54	
Acardia or acephaly	7	
Infection	**32**	**5.3**
Cytomegalovirus	8	
Parvovirus	4	
Myocarditis	2	
Not otherwise specified	16	
Toxoplasmosis	1	
Rubella	1	
Fetal anemia	**25**	**4.2**
Alpha-thalassemia	16	
Fetomaternal hemorrhage	4	
Not otherwise specified	5	
Tumors	**17**	**2.9**
Teratoma	11	
Neuroblastoma	3	
Other	3	
Hepatic pathology	**8**	**1.4**
Giant cell hepatitis	5	
Other	3	
Genetic metabolic disease	**6**	**1.0**
Meconium peritonitis	**6**	**1.0**
Obstructed venous return from placenta	**2**	
Unexplained	**161**	**27.1**
TOTAL	594	100%

Data from Keeling JW: Hydrops fetalis and other forms of excess fluid collection in the fetus. In Wigglesworth JS, Singer DB, editors: *Textbook of fetal and perinatal pathology*, Boston, 1990, Blackwell Scientific Publications.

Table 16-16 Cardiac malformations associated with fetal hydrops

Hypoplastic left heart
Atrioventricular septal defect
Hypoplastic right heart
Antenatal closure of foramen ovale
Ebstein malformation
Antenatal closure of ductus arteriosus

From Taylor GP: Cardiovascular system. In Dimmick JE, Kalousek DK, editors: *Developmental pathology of the embryo and fetus,* Philadelphia, 1992, Lippincott.

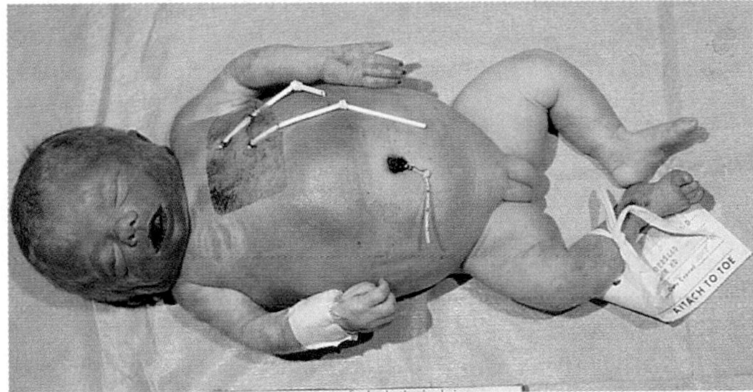

Fig. 16-27 This hydropic newborn had prenatal diagnosis of a cystic adenomatoid malformation of the left lung with consequent severe hypoplasia of the right lung because of the space-occupying malformation. The chest tubes were placed to try to drain both the pleural space and the cystic lesion in the left side of the chest.

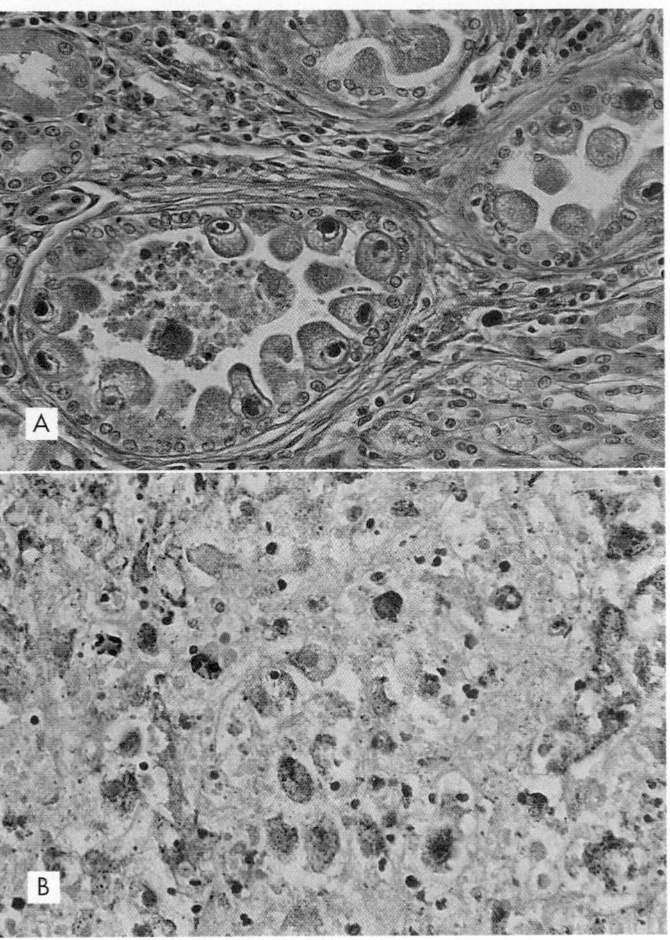

Fig. 16-28 **A**, Both nuclear and cytoplasmic viral inclusions can be seen in renal tubular cells from this late-gestation fetus with congenital cytomegalovirus infection. **B**, Herpes simplex was cultured from postmortem material from this premature hydropic infant who survived 3 days. This micrograph shows immunohistochemical staining for herpes simplex virus in a section of liver necrosis.

Table 16-17 Antemortem and postmortem evaluation of fetal hydrops

Investigation of the mother	Ultrasonography	Postmortem examination
Hemoglobin, Kleihauer	Severity of hydrops	Photographic record
Alpha-fetoprotein	Multiple pregnancy	Weights and measurements
ABO and rhesus group	Fetal heart rate and rhythm	Radiologic examination
Hemolysins, hemagglutinins	Fetal anomaly	Malformation
Minor blood group antigens	Heart	Cardiac
Serologic tests for syphilis	Other	Other
Glucose tolerance test	Placenta	Karyotype
Autoantibodies	Thickness/abnormality	Effusions
	?Virus culture	Culture
		Biochemical analysis
		Virus culture/TORCH screen
		Blood group and antibodies
		Lung weight
		Histologic examination
		Examination of placenta
		Tissue for DNA extraction
		Fetal/placental

Modified from Keeling JW: Hydrops fetalis and other forms of excess fluid collection in the fetus. In Wigglesworth JS, Singer DB, editors: *Textbook of fetal and perinatal pathology,* Boston, 1990, Blackwell Scientific Publications. *TORCH,* Toxoplasmosis, rubella, cytomegalovirus, and herpes simplex infection.

part of the fetal scalp), and lethal hemorrhage, which leads to fetal death by exsanguination, disruption of central nervous system function, or both.[74]

The most common of the lethal cranial hemorrhages is that occurring in the *subgaleal* tissues deep to the occipitofrontalis muscle, *subaponeurotic hemorrhage*. This lesion can coexist with subperiosteal hemorrhage of the outer table of the skull, called *cephalohematoma* (Fig. 16-29). Both these lesions are seen in fatal cranial hemorrhages because of vacuum extraction in cases of dystocia. Skull fracture during delivery is uncommon, because of the intrinsic deformability of the fetal skull both by molding at fibrous sutures and actual bending of the relatively soft skull bones during labor and delivery. Associated hemorrhage and injury to the brain are usually the clinically significant lesions when a skull fracture is discovered in a stillborn. *Subdural hemorrhage* is identified at autopsy as a sheet of blood clot over the convexities or the structures of the posterior fossa. Subdural hemorrhages can arise by several mechanisms, with bleeding stemming from injury to dural venous sinuses or, more often, the bridging veins that traverse the space between the subarachnoid space and these sinuses. *Subarachnoid hemorrhage* alone is not evidence of cranial trauma, because it most frequently results from asphyxia and is often seen in association with multiple sites of parenchymal bleeding in other organs in this context.

Large *visceral hemorrhages* originating in organs such as liver, spleen, kidney, and adrenals, and from spinal injuries, are the most common lethal results of birth trauma found in the rest of the body. Significant but less easily quantified hemorrhage can develop in muscles. It is often difficult to establish the precise significance of visceral or muscle hemorrhage in causing fetal death because large but unmeasurable quantities of blood can collect in interstitial tissues.

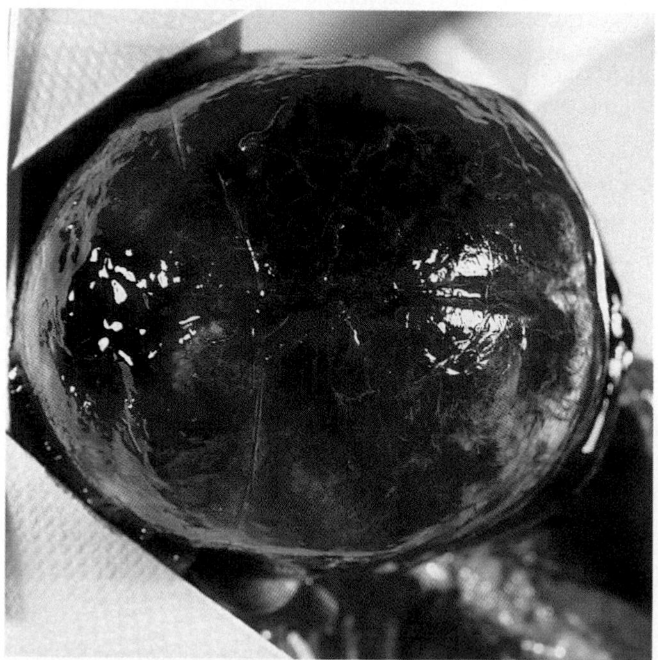

Fig. 16-29 The scalp has been reflected, revealing large cephalohematomas on the upper occipital and mostly left parietal regions in this 4-day-old term newborn. The difficult vaginal delivery was assisted by a vacuum extractor, which also abraded the scalp. Severe birth asphyxia with anoxic brain damage was the cause of death.

Spinal trauma is associated with excessive manipulation and torsion of the fetal head during breech delivery. Spinal cord damage can coexist with tentorial tears and other causes of posterior fossa hemorrhage. Whenever mechanically induced injuries are discovered in an intrapartum stillborn, careful attention to hemorrhage and microscopic damage to the brachial plexus is recommended. Likewise, *fractures* of long bones, the clavicle in particular, can easily be overlooked in the autopsy suite unless routine radiographs are examined before dissection is completed. The degree of surrounding soft-tissue bleeding is a clue to determine whether fractures occurred before or after fetal death in cases of intrapartum stillbirth.

PREMATURITY

Preterm birth is the most common factor that interferes with the successful establishment of extrauterine life. Therefore, the postmortem evaluation of any fetus or neonate should include an explicit assessment of fetal maturity using standard physical criteria,[75] weights and measurements, brain gyral development, histologic development of organs,[76] and radiographs. The most accurate estimate of gestational age will take into account many of these factors,[76] with emphasis being put on those that appear unaffected by malformations or by acquired diseases or lesions. A preterm infant is generally defined as one born before 37 completed weeks of gestation.

Preterm delivery is most frequently caused by preterm onset of labor, often accompanied by rupture of membranes and amniotic infection. Maternal hypertension, intrauterine growth restriction, and multiple gestations are other specific clinical conditions commonly leading to preterm delivery.

Adaptation to extrauterine life

At the time of birth, the fetus becomes an infant who is legally an individual and who must be physiologically independent of the function of its mother and placenta to survive. Some of the adaptations required must take place rapidly, such as air breathing for gas exchange. Although adaptation in many other systems, such as full development of the immune system, proceeds at a more leisurely pace, the requirements for commencement of successful enteral nutrition and hydration also begin at birth. The infant must rely on its own systems and enzymes for absorbing and metabolizing nutrients and for producing excretory products. After birth, any persistent deficiency in these functions can no longer be compensated for by the placenta and will become apparent as metabolic disease.

The development of functional lung maturity has been the focus of intense investigation. In utero, the lung must develop sufficient internal surface area, appropriate relationships between the vasculature and airspaces to permit adequate gas exchange, and surfactant secretion needed to allow full inflation as well as to reduce the pressures required to maintain residual volumes. At the initiation of air breathing, physiologic changes begin in the lung and the cardiovascular system. When relatively oxygen-rich air enters newborn lungs to replace the liquid that has filled them in utero, there is increasing relaxation of pulmonary arterial tone, as well as uncoiling of lung capillaries with full inflation. These changes translate into a dramatic reduction of right-sided cardiac pressures, away from the relatively balanced pressures present during fetal life. This results in functional closure of the normal foramen ovale, which together with the ductus arteriosus functioned as an in utero right-to-left shunt; the ductus arteriosus thus begins to constrict in response to the increased arterial oxygen tension. The relative thickness of the left ventricular myocardium increases for months after birth to follow the functional requirements of the high-pressure systemic circulation. Anything that perturbs the orderly progression of these adaptive changes will have potential consequences for the healthy growth and subsequent development of the heart and lungs.

Respiratory system pathology

The successful transition to air breathing in the premature neonate is complicated by functional immaturity of all components of the lung. Attention has been focused on surfactant deficiency as a major cause of neonatal *respiratory distress syndrome* (RDS),[77] also called "hyaline membrane disease" (HMD) for the hallmark histologic feature (Fig. 16-30). Yet, anatomical and functional immaturity of alveolar walls and airways also contribute to the additional findings seen at autopsy in premature infants, such as pulmonary interstitial emphysema and pneumothorax.

HMD appears to be directly related to a deficiency of pulmonary surfactant, which is most often but not always seen in the setting of prematurity. The clinical picture of HMD includes immediate or early respiratory distress requiring mechanical ventilation. X-ray findings show increased density of lung parenchyma with air bronchograms. At autopsy, the lungs are heavy, dense, and relatively airless. Evidence of pneumothorax should be sought before the chest cavity is opened, particularly when mechanical ventilation has been used. Severe interstitial emphysema may be obvious as subpleural blebs, or as a prominent pattern of air-filled lines along interlobular septa. The histologic hallmark, the hyaline membrane, is an eosinophilic crust composed of proteinaceous fluid, necrotic epithelial debris, and sometimes fibrin, which lines the terminal and respiratory bronchioles and alveolar ducts. The most important and clinically relevant feature, however, is widespread airspace collapse, which correlates with the pathophysiology and with the gross impression of an airless lung. Other features that can usually be seen include scattered hemorrhages, both interstitial and intra-alveolar, and dilated lymphatics in interlobular septa. When significant neonatal jaundice has been present, hyaline membranes may be pigmented, appearing even in unstained sections as bright yellow.

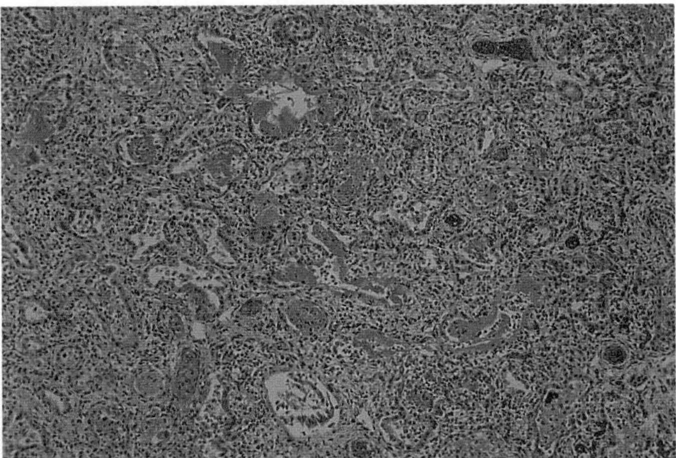

Fig. 16-30 Thick eosinophilic hyaline membranes line the terminal bronchioles of this 25-week-gestation infant who survived for 8 days on mechanical ventilation. Other areas of the lung were hemorrhagic. Premature rupture of membranes and chorioamnionitis necessitated delivery.

Pulmonary interstitial emphysema (PIE)[77] is a serious complication of neonatal RDS, occurring especially with the use of high-pressure mechanical ventilation. Up to 30% of extremely premature (under 1500 g) neonates with RDS will develop this complication. Barotrauma is the mechanism leading to PIE in ventilated infants, and prematurity of the airways increases the risk of development of PIE versus pneumothorax, which is more likely to be seen in term infants. In PIE, smaller airways rupture and leak air into interstitial tissues, particularly into the interlobular septa and the peribronchiolar, perivascular, and pleural connective tissues. Intrapleural air may form blebs seen on the lung surface; these may reach several centimeters in size, and pneumothorax, pneumomediastinum, or pneumopericardium may develop consequent to rupture. Histologically, PIE manifests as large, empty, or mildly hemorrhagic cavities in connective tissue of the lung or pleura, sometimes demonstrating an endothelial lining when air has dissected into lymphatics. There may be destruction of adjacent lung parenchyma, and in longstanding cases coming to late autopsy, a giant cell (macrophage) reaction to air may be seen.

Massive pulmonary hemorrhage occurs in a similar group of immature neonates, especially in growth-restricted premature infants. At autopsy, the lungs are heavy and may appear diffusely or focally hemorrhagic, with blood present in larger airways. Histologically, intra-alveolar and often interstitial blood in large quantities is seen. The pathophysiology of this lesion is not well established, though hypoxic capillary damage seems a likely contributor.

Bronchopulmonary dysplasia (BPD)[77,78] is defined *clinically* as the continuing requirement for mechanical ventilation and oxygen therapy subsequent to RDS for a period longer than 1 month from birth. In nonsurvivors of RDS, characteristic changes of early stages of BPD are seen at autopsy before 1 month of age. The pathophysiology of BPD is not well understood: both mechanical ventilation and oxygen toxicity, probably mediated through free-radical damage, have been implicated separately and in combination. Affected infants have usually been born prematurely, and there is a strong correlation with low birthweight, with the incidence of BPD approaching 40% in very low birthweight neonates near 1000 g.

Bronchopulmonary dysplasia is a progressive disease. Large, cobblestoned, focally overinflated and atelectatic lungs are the expected gross findings in longstanding BPD. Secondary changes include cardiac hypertrophy, frequently biventricular but not uncommonly univentricular, with equal involvement of right or left. The histologic picture varies with the stage of the lesion,[79] and changes are summarized in Table 16-18 Infants with BPD are at risk for additional late complications including structural problems such as honcycomb lung and tracheal stenosis, as well as functional abnormalities including apnea and reactive airways disease. Fig. 16-31 shows the histology of longstanding BPD in an infant who succumbed to cor pulmonale.

Cardiovascular system pathology

The changes required in the transition from the fetal to the adult type of circulation have been described above. One cir-

Table 16-18 Pathologic changes in bronchopulmonary dysplasia

Stage	Pulmonary findings	Cardiac findings
Exudative, and early reparative (1 to 2 weeks)	Hyaline membranes Bronchial necrosis Bronchiolitis obliterans Bronchiolectasis Early septal fibrosis Mucosal dysplasia and necrosis of trachea and bronchi Interstitial edema, with or without emphysema	Patent ductus arteriosus
Subacute, fibroproliferative	Bronchiolitis obliterans Bronchiolectasis	
Chronic fibroproliferative (months)	Gross appearance like cobblestones Interstitial fibrosis Smooth muscle proliferation Honeycomb lung Vascular wall thickening No bronchiolitis obliterans or bronchiolectasis Mucosal metaplasia, trachea, bronchi, bronchioles Muscular hyperplasia, trachea, bronchi	With or without left ventricular hypertrophy With or without cor pulmonale
Longstanding "healed" (months to years)	Alveolar septal fibrosis Pulmonary vascular hypertensive changes, low grade Pleural fibrosis	Biventricular hypertrophy with or without myocardial or endocardial fibrosis

Based on Stocker JT, Dehner LP: Acquired pulmonary disease in the pediatric age group. In Dail DH, Hammer SP, editors: *Pulmonary pathology,* New York, 1987, Springer-Verlag.

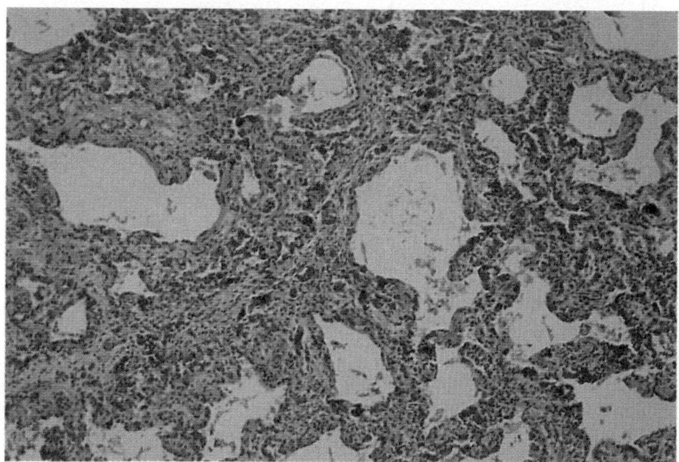

Fig. 16-31 The diffuse thickening and fibrosis of the interstitium is evident in this section of lung from a 5-month-old infant who had been delivered at 25 weeks of gestation. The infant remained hospitalized throughout life. The cause of death was acute cor pulmonale with ischemic myocardial damage.

culatory consequence of prematurity and especially of severe HMD is persistence of a *patent ductus arteriosus,* which allows continued left-to-right shunting, providing abnormally high pulmonary pressures and flow while compromising systemic arterial perfusion. Normal neonates appear to complete *functional* closure of the ductus within 4 days of birth, which can be seen at autopsy as plication or wrinkling of the luminal surface, with or without thrombosis; anatomical closure with complete obliteration demonstrable histologically takes weeks to months. The incidence of functional ductal patency is inversely related to gestational age. The progression of histologic changes that lead to ductal obliteration have been described.[80] Prolonged functional patency of the ductus has been implicated as a risk factor for the development of bronchopulmonary dysplasia and necrotizing enterocolitis.

A related clinical entity is *persistent pulmonary hypertension of the newborn* (PPHN), which because of its similar presentation to the above entity, has been called *persistence of the fetal circulation* (PFC). It is characterized by an abnormal continuation of the high pulmonary vascular resistance present during fetal life, with the resultant compromise of pulmonary perfusion and gas exchange. The ductus arteriosus and often the foramen ovale continue to function as right-to-left shunts because of the high pulmonary vascular resistance. There is a primary, idiopathic form of PPHN, for which the underlying cause is obscure. There are multiple causes for this condition as a secondary process, which can be divided into three categories:

1. Normal pulmonary vascular anatomy, with secondary failure of the expected postnatal decrease in resistance, as with hyperviscosity
2. Excessive prenatal muscularization of distal pulmonary vasculature, as seen with certain congenital cardiac lesions and with meconium aspiration

3. Developmental abnormalities of the lung that result in decreased capillary area for gas exchange, as in pulmonary hypoplasia, and a specific anomaly termed "malalignment of lung vessels." Careful examination (including detailed histologic evaluation of lung microanatomy) of the cardiorespiratory system is called for in cases of PPHN.

Premature closure of the ductus arteriosus or foramen ovale in utero occurs rarely and predisposes to fetal congestive heart failure, secondary underdevelopment of left-sided cardiac structures (atrium, valves, ventricle, and aorta), and possible hydrops, stillbirth, or early neonatal death. Careful cross-sectional histologic examination of the unprobed ductus is necessary to establish the diagnosis of premature ductal closure if there is any lumen visible at the aortic or pulmonary ends in a suspected case.

Central nervous system (CNS) pathology

The brain is probably the organ that is most vulnerable to the stresses imposed by extremely premature birth. The infant brain is large relative to body size, and the high water content together with lack of significant connective tissue or myelin at early gestational ages render it fragile and exceptionally susceptible to damage by mechanical forces. The blood-brain barrier is incompletely developed in early life, allowing exposure of the premature brain to substances that would be retained within a more mature circulation. The immaturity of the fetal brain and its vasculature also predisposes to vessel rupture.

Three groups of CNS lesions are associated with prematurity or its treatment:

1. Metabolic lesions, such as kernicterus
2. Germinal matrix and intraventricular hemorrhage
3. Periventricular leukomalacia

Kernicterus is defined as the grossly visible yellow-staining and microscopically apparent damage of specific brain nuclei as a result of hyperbilirubinemia. It is now relatively uncommon but must be recognized when present. The possible causes of neonatal hyperbilirubinemia are many, but the typical normal but premature infant will have prolonged "physiologic jaundice" on the basis of immaturity of liver function, combined with excessive hemolysis attributable to the decreased life-span of preterm red blood cells. The susceptibility of the brain to hyperbilirubinemia seems to be related to the degree of prematurity. Survivors may develop persistent brain dysfunction, with "minimal" to significant mental retardation, seizures, debilitating motor symptoms, choreoathetosis, and variable pyramidal tract signs.

Germinal matrix hemorrhage, with or without rupture into the lateral or third ventricle, or *intraventricular hemorrhage* (IVH), occurs in up to 30% of newborns below 35 weeks of gestational age and in up to 70% of very low birth weight infants (1000 g).[81] The germinal matrix is a transient mass of immature neurons, glia, and blood vessels in the subependymal region over the head of the caudate, between the caudate and the thalamus, and in the roof of the temporal horn and lateral wall of the occipital horn. This vulnerable structure persists until 33 to 34 weeks of gestation, by which time most neurons have migrated outward toward the cortical surface. Factors predisposing to hemorrhage in this area include the immaturity of the abundant capillary vessels.

The role of various mediators of capillary permeability, including prostacyclin and the fibrinolytic system, and transient abnormalities of capillary and platelet function in the first hours of life have been questioned. Conditions resulting from prematurity of other systems and leading to alterations of cerebral blood flow are significantly associated with the development of IVH (Table 16-19). IVH usually occurs within the first few hours of life but has also been observed in stillborn infants. Therapeutic interventions are aimed at prevention, so that one can avoid the physiologic variations known to be risk factors.

Gross CNS disorders in premature infants with germinal matrix hemorrhage range from small, contained hemorrhages within the germinal matrix (Fig. 16-32) to massive hemorrhage that fills the ventricular system, spilling out first into the subarachnoid space of the posterior fossa and eventually into the basal cisterns and the spinal subarachnoid space. Microscopically, in fresh lesions there will be variable destruction of the germinal matrix with dilatation of capillaries or additional focal hemorrhages in intact germinal matrix tissue that

Table 16-19 Risk factors for the development of intraventricular hemorrhage

Obstetric factors
Breech delivery
Birth asphyxia and hypotension
Infant factors
Prematurity with:
Immature cerebrovascular autoregulation
Poorly supported germinal matrix vascular rete
Impaired platelet and capillary interaction
Respiratory distress syndrome and hypoxia
Hypothermia
Hypercapnia and acidosis
Blood pressure lability
Pneumothorax

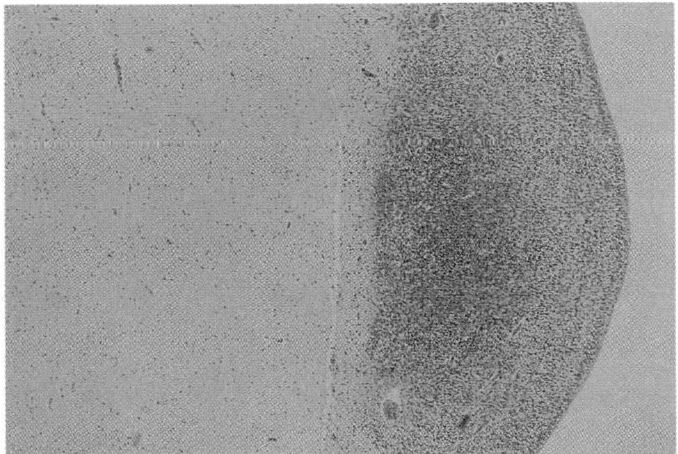

Fig. 16-32 A small germinal matrix hemorrhage is present in this 28-week-gestation infant who survived 3 days on mechanical ventilation. The small dark cells are neuroblasts that have not yet migrated toward the cortical surface. The ependyma is to the right and the periventricular white matter is to the left of the germinal eminence in this section.

remains. Older unruptured germinal matrix hemorrhages may still contain liquid blood, and their subacute nature can be determined by the numbers of hemosiderin-laden macrophages they contain. Surrounding such a lesion will be a mass of reactive glia, forming a persistent subependymal pseudocyst.

Periventricular leukomalacia (PVL)[81,82] frequently coexists with intraventricular hemorrhages in premature infants. It is the sequel to hypoxic and ischemic deep white matter damage. The high incidence of periventricular leukomalacia (30% to 80%) is most likely attributable to the prolonged survival of extremely premature infants to an age that has permitted the development and recognition of these subacute lesions. Grossly, PVL manifests as sharply demarcated chalky white areas in the subependymal white matter, particularly at the angles of the ventricles. Histologically, the appearance of these lesions is time dependent, with the earliest consisting of coagulation necrosis, showing nuclear pyknosis and some rarefaction of the tissue (Fig. 16-33). Proliferation of astrocytes can be seen in lesions with a few days duration and conspicuous neuraxonal swellings. There is accumulation of lipid-laden macrophages, with cavitation and glial proliferation around the periphery leading to cyst formation over a period of weeks. Calcification in axons around the periphery is common. Secondary hemorrhage into these lesions can occur and may be massive.

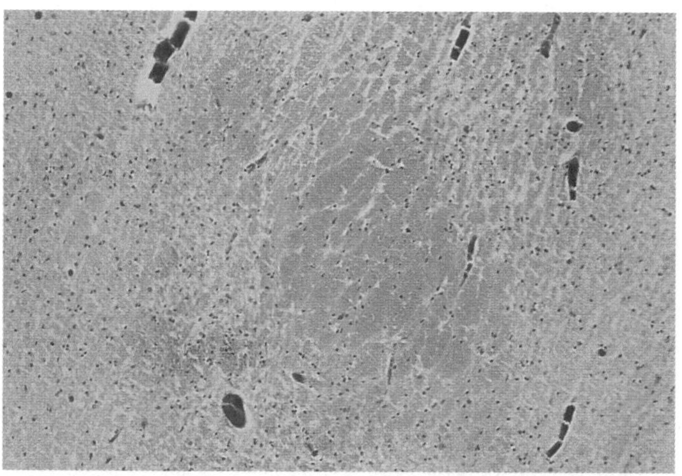

Fig. 16-33 Hypoxic and ischemic encephalopathy was evident from birth in this 9-day-old premature infant with periventricular leukomalacia. The section shows a new lesion, which consists of coagulation necrosis of the axons with disappearance of nuclei in the white matter. These lesions are easier to appreciate and appear darker than the surrounding white matter in sections stained with Luxol fast blue/PAS such as this.

Hypoxic damage to the *cerebral cortex* is more commonly seen in asphyxiated term newborns, whereas hypoxic neuronal damage in the thalamus, basal ganglia, brainstem, and cerebellar and midbrain nuclei are seen at all gestational ages.

Gastrointestinal tract pathology

Although the anatomical development of the gut and liver are seemingly complete by midgestation, functional immaturity, which can compromise the success of enteral feeding, persists until 30 weeks of gestational age. The motility of the small bowel, in particular, is known to remain disorganized until around 30 weeks of gestation. Neurologic factors preclude successful sucking and swallowing in small premature infants. Absorptive mechanisms are also not fully operational until the early-to-mid third trimester and may require the presence of appropriate intraluminal contents (such as colostrum) to stimulate necessary enzymes such as lactase. The liver in premature infants is functionally immature, lacking glucuronyl transferase and the ability to conjugate bilirubin effectively. This contributes to the increased frequency and duration of "physiologic" jaundice seen in premature infants.

The most common gastrointestinal problem that the pathologist sees as a result of prematurity is *necrotizing enterocolitis* (NEC),[83,84] characterized by ischemic necrosis and nonspecific inflammation of bowel wall. Regional bowel ischemia, invasion of microorganisms from the bowel lumen, and osmotic effects of food on the intestinal epithelium appear to be involved in the development of NEC. Immaturity of mesenteric vascular control may be a predisposing factor. No single specific bacterial pathogen has been overwhelmingly associated with NEC, though many have been found to be present

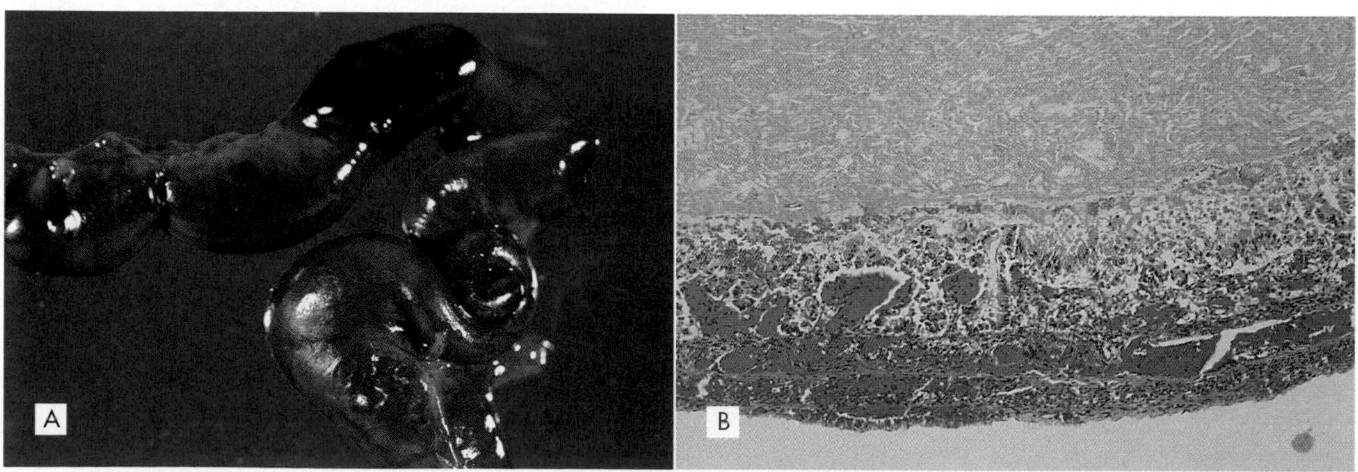

Fig. 16-34 **A**, This segment of necrotic terminal ileum, cecum, and ascending colon is from a 2-day-old premature infant. **B** shows hemorrhagic ischemic necrosis of all layers of bowel wall at low magnification. The lumen contains meconium.

and proposed as causal agents. Any serious neonatal illness that predisposes to hypoxia in a premature infant can lead to NEC, including birth asphyxia, respiratory distress syndrome, sepsis, congenital heart disease, or polycythemia. Clinical intervention is primarily directed toward prevention by the use of delayed enteral feedings and prophylactic antibiotics in at-risk infants. Segmental resection of necrotic bowel is often a last resort (Fig. 16-34), with survivors of extensive NEC being left with short bowel syndrome.

REFERENCES

Scope of developmental pathology

1. Gilbert SF: *Developmental biology*, ed 2, Sunderland, Mass, 1988, Sinauer Associates.
2. Berg P, Singer M: *Dealing with genes: the language of heredity*, Oxford, 1992, Blackwell Scientific Publications.
3. Buyse ML, editor: *Birth defects encyclopedia*, ed 2, Dover, Mass, 1993, Center for Birth Defects Information Services, Inc.
4. Bergsma D, editor: *Birth defects compendium*, ed 2, New York, 1979, The National Foundation — March of Dimes, Alan R. Liss, Inc.
5. McKusick VA: *Mendelian inheritance in man: catalogs of autosomal dominant, autosomal recessive, and X-linked phenotypes*, ed 10, Baltimore, 1992, Johns Hopkins University Press.
6. Jones KL: *Smith's recognizable patterns of human malformations*, ed 4, Philadelphia, 1988, Saunders.
7. Stevenson RE, Hall JG, Gordman RM, editors: *Human malformations and related anomalies*, Oxford Monographs on Medical Genetics No. 27, New York, 1993, Oxford University Press.
8. London Dysmorphology Database, Oxford, UK, 1993, Oxford Electronic Publications, Oxford University Press.
9. Spranger J, Benirschke K, Hall JG et al: Errors of morphogenesis: concepts and terms, *J Pediatr* 100:160, 1982.
10. Hall JG: Genomic imprinting: review and relevance to human diseases, *Am J Hum Genet* 46:857, 1990.
11. Kalousek DK, Langlois S, Barrett I et al: Uniparental disomy for chromosome 16 in humans, *Am J Hum Genet* 52:8, 1993.
12. Austin KD, Hall JG: Nontraditional inheritance, *Pediatr Clin North Am* 39:335, 1992.

Pathology of embryonic development

13. Warburton D, Byrne J, Canki N: *Chromosome anomalies and prenatal development: an atlas.* Oxford Monographs on Medical Genetics no. 21, New York, 1991, Oxford University Press.
14. Martin RH, Ko E, Redemaker A: Distribution of aneuploidy in human gametes: comparison between human sperm and oocytes, *Am J Med Genet* 39:321.
15. Jacobs P, Hassold T: Chromosome abnormalities: origin and etiology in abortions and livebirths. In Vogel F, Sperling K, editors: *Human Genetics*, Berlin, 1987, Springer-Verlag.
16. Jacobs PA, Szulman AE, Funkhouser J et al: Human triploidy: relationship between parental origin of the additional haploid complement and development of partial hydatidiform mole, *Ann Hum Genet* 46:223, 1982.
17. Kalousek DK, Fitch N, Paradice B: *Pathology of the human embryo and previable fetus: an atlas*, New York, Heidelberg, Tokyo, 1990, Springer-Verlag.
18. Rehder H, Coerdt W, Egger R et al: Is there a correlation between morphological and cytogenetic findings in placental tissue from early missed abortions? *Hum Genet* 82:377, 1989.
19. O'Rahilly R, Muller F: *Developmental stages of human embryos*, Publication 637, Washington, DC, 1987, Carnegie Institution.
20. Moore KL, Persaud TVN: *The developing human: clinically oriented embryology*, ed 5, Philadelphia, 1993, Saunders.
21. Poland BJ, Miller JR, Harris M et al: Spontaneous abortion: a study of 1961 women and their conceptuses, *Acta Obstet Gynecol Scand* (suppl 102):5, 1981.
22. Kalousek DK, McGillivray BC, Barrett I: Placental mosaicism and intrauterine survival of trisomies 13 and 18, *Am J Hum Genet* 44:338, 1989.
23. Kalousek DK: Confined placental mosaicism and intrauterine growth restriction, *Placenta* 1995. (In press.)
24. Jacobs PA: The chromosome complement of human gametes, *Oxf Rev Reprod Biol* 14:47, 1992.

Pathology of previable fetal development

25. Craver RD, Kalousek DK: Cytogenetic abnormalities among spontaneously aborted previable fetuses, *Am J Med Genet* (suppl 3):113, 1987.
26. Petri M, Allbritton J: Fetal outcome of lupus pregnancy: a retrospective case-control study of the Hopkins Lupus Cohort, *J Rheumatol* 20(4):650, 1993.
27. Birdsall M, Pattison N, Chamley L: Antiphospholipid antibodies in pregnancy, *Aust NZ J Obstet Gynaecol* 32(4):328, 1992.
28. Tanimura T, Nelson T, Hollingsworth RR et al: Weight standards for organs from early human fetuses, *Anat Rec* 171:226, 1971.
29. Ornoy A, Borochowitz Z, Lachman R et al: *Atlas of fetal skeletal radiology*, St. Louis, 1988, Mosby.
30. Gilbert EF, Arya S, Laxova R et al: Pathology of chromosome abnormalities in the fetus: pathologic markers, *Birth Defects OAS* 23:293, 1987.
31. McFadden DE, Kalousek DK: Fetal triploid phenotypes: correlation with parental origin of extra haploid set, *Am J Med Genet* 38:535, 1991.
32. Anderson JD, Thomas EE, Cimolai N: Infections and the conceptus. In Dimmick JE, Kalousek DK, editors: *Developmental pathology of the embryo and fetus*, Philadelphia, 1992, Lippincott.
33. Benirschke K, Robb JA: Infectious causes of fetal death, *Clin Obstet Gynecol* 30(2):284, 1987.
34. Rudbeck Røge H, Henriques U: Fetal and perinatal infections, *Pathol Res Pract* 188:135, 1992.
35. Madan E, Meyer M, Amortequi A: Chorioamnionitis: a study of organisms isolated in perinatal autopsies, *Ann Clin Lab Sci* 18(1):39, 1988.
36. Quinn PA, Butany J, Chipman M et al: A prospective study of microbial infection in stillbirths and early neonatal death, *Am J Obstet Gynecol* 151:238, 1985.
37. McGregor JA, French JI: *Chlamydia trachomatis* infection during pregnancy, *Am J Obstet Gynecol* 164(6 pt 2):1782, 1991.
38. McLauchlin J: Human listeriosis in Britain, 1967–85, a summary of 722 cases. 1. Listeriosis during pregnancy and in the newborn, *Epidemiol Infect* 104:181, 1990.
39. Miller E, Craddock-Watson JE, Pollock TM: Consequences of confirmed maternal rubella at successive stages of pregnancy, *Lancet* 2(8302):781, 1982.
40. Freij BJ, South MA, Sever JL: Maternal rubella and the congenital rubella syndrome, *Clin Perinatol* 15:247, 1988.
41. Stagno S, Whitley RJ: Herpesvirus infections of pregnancy. I. Cytomegalovirus and Epstein-Barr virus infections, *N Engl J Med* 313:1270, 1985.
42. Stagno S, Whitley RJ: Herpesvirus infections of pregnancy. II. Herpes simplex virus and varicella-zoster virus infections, *N Engl J Med* 313:1327, 1985.
43. Hall SM (study coordinator), Public Health Laboratory Service Working Party of Fifth Disease: Prospective study of human parvovirus (B19) infection in pregnancy, *BMJ* 300:1166, 1990.
44. Temmerman M, Plummer F, Mirza NB et al: Infection with HIV as a risk factor for adverse obstetrical outcome, *AIDS* 4:1087, 1990.
45. Hollenberg MD: Growth factors, their receptors and development, *Am J Med Genet* 34:35, 1989.
46. Magnus P, Berg K, Bjerkedal T et al: Parental determinants of birth weight, *Clin Genet* 26:397, 1984.
47. Milner RDG: Mechanisms of overgrowth. In Shep F, Fraser RB, Milner RDG, editors: *Fetal growth,* London, 1989, Springer-Verlag.
48. Schinzel A: *Catalogue of unbalanced chromosome aberrations in man*, Berlin, 1983, Walter de Gruyter.
49. Maroteaux P: International nomenclature of constitutional disorders of bones with bibliography, *Birth Defects OAS XXII* 4:1, 1986.
50. Beighton P, de Paepe A, Danks D et al: International nosology of heritable disorders of connective tissue, *Am J Med Genet* 29:581, 1988.
51. Brar HS, Rutherford SE: Classification of intrauterine growth retardation, *Semin Perinatol* 12:2, 1988.

52. Snijders RJM, Sherrod C, Gosden CM et al: Fetal growth retardation: associated malformations and chromosomal abnormalities, *Am J Obstet Gynecol* 168(2):547, 1993.

Stillbirth

53. Genest DR, Williams MA, Greene MF: Estimating the time of death in stillborn fetuses: I. Histologic evaluation of fetal organs: an autopsy study of 150 stillborns, *Obstet Gynecol* 80:575, 1992.
54. Genest DR: Estimating the time of death in stillborn fetuses. II. Histologic evaluation of the placenta: a study of 71 stillborns, *Obstet Gynecol* 80:585, 1992.
55. Genest DR, Singer DB: Estimating the time of death in stillborn fetuses. III. External fetal examination: a study of 86 stillborns, *Obstet Gynecol* 80:593, 1992.
56. Weaver DD: *Catalog of prenatally diagnosed conditions*, ed 2, Baltimore, 1992, Johns Hopkins University Press.
57. Clark LA, Dimmick JE, Applegarth DA: Pathology of inherited metabolic diseases. In Dimmick JE, Kalousek, DK, editors: *Developmental pathology of the embryo and fetus*, Philadelphia, 1992, Lippincott.
58. Schauer GM, Kalousek DK, Magee JF: Genetic causes of stillbirth, *Semin Perinatol* 16:341, 1992.
59. Lammer EJ, Brown LE, Anderka MT et al: Classification and analysis of fetal deaths in Massachusetts, *JAMA* 261:1757, 1989.
60. Ferraz EM, Gray RH: A case-control study of stillbirths in northeast Brazil, *Int J Gynaecol Obstet* 34:13, 1990.
61. Fretts RC, Boyd, ME, Usher RH et al: The changing pattern of fetal death, 1961-1988, *Obstet Gynecol* 76:35, 1992.
62. Hovatta O, Lipasti A, Rapola J et al: Causes of stillbirth: a clinicopathological study of 243 patients, *Br J Obstet Gynaecol* 90:691, 1983.
63. Lofgren O, Pohlberger S: Perinatal mortality: changes in the diagnostic panorama, 1974-1980, *Acta Paediatr Scand* 72:327, 1982.
64. Machin GA: A perinatal mortality survey in south-east London, 1970-73: the pathological findings in 726 necropsies, *J Clin Pathol* 28:428, 1975.
65. Magani IM, Rafla NM, Mortimer G et al: Stillbirths: a clinicopathological survey (1972-1982), *Pediatr Pathol* 10:363, 1990.
66. Morrison I, Olsen J: Weight-specific stillbirths and associated causes of death: an analysis of 765 stillbirths, *Am J Obstet Gynecol* 152:975, 1985.
67. Whitfield CR, Smith NC, Cockburn F et al: Perinatally related wastage: a proposed classification of primary obstetric factors, *Br J Obstet Gynaecol* 93:694, 1986.
68. Taylor GP: Cardiovascular system. In Dimmick JE, Kalousek DK, editors: *Developmental pathology of the embryo and fetus*, Philadelphia, 1992, Lippincott.
69. Owen J, Stedman CM, Tucker TL: Comparison of predelivery versus post-delivery Kleihauer-Betke stains in cases of fetal death, *Am J Obstet Gynecol* 161:663, 1989.
70. Lifschultz BD, Donoghue ER: Fetal death following maternal trauma: two case reports and a survey of the literature, *J Forensic Sci* 36:1740, 1991.
71. Machin GA: Hydrops revisited: literature review of 1,414 cases published in the 1980s, *Am J Med Genet* 34:366, 1989.
72. Keeling JW: Hydrops fetalis and other forms of excess fluid collection in the fetus. In Wigglesworth JS, Singer DB, editors: *Textbook of fetal and perinatal pathology*, Boston, 1990, Blackwell Scientific Publications.
73. Mangurten HH: Birth injuries. In Fanaroff AA, Martin RJ, editors: *Neonatal-perinatal medicine*, St. Louis, 1992, Mosby.
74. Keeling JW: Intrapartum asphyxia and birth trauma. In Keeling JW, editor: *Fetal and neonatal pathology*, New York, 1987, Springer-Verlag.
75. Ballard JL, Novak KZ, Driver M: A simplified score for assessment of fetal maturation of newly born infants, *J Pediatr* 95:769, 1979.
76. Naeye RL, Kelly JA: Judgement of fetal age. III. The pathologist's evaluation, *Pediatr Clin North Am* 13:849, 1966.
77. Stocker JT, Dehner LP: Acquired neonatal and pediatric diseases. In Dail DH, Hammar SP, editors: *Pulmonary pathology*, New York, 1988, Springer-Verlag.
78. Bonikos DS, Bensch KG, Northway WH Jr et al: Bronchopulmonary dysplasia: the pulmonary pathologic sequel of necrotizing bronchiolitis and pulmonary fibrosis, *Hum Pathol* 7:643, 1976.
79. Stocker JT: Pathologic features of longstanding "healed" bronchopulmonary dysplasia: a study of 28 3-to 40-month-old infants, *Hum Pathol* 17:943, 1986.
80. Silver MM, Freedom RM, Silver MD et al: The morphology of the human newborn ductus arteriosus: a reappraisal of its structure and closure with special reference to prostaglandin E_1 therapy, *Hum Pathol* 12:1123, 1981.
81. Volpe JJ: Intraventricular hemorrhage and brain injury in the premature infant: neuropathology and pathogenesis, *Clin Perinatol* 16:361, 1989.
82. Friede RL: Periventricular infarcts. In *Developmental Neuropathology*, New York, 1975, Springer-Verlag.
83. Tait RA, Kealy WF: Neonatal necrotising enterocolitis, *J Clin Pathol* 23:1090, 1979.
84. Kliegman RM, Walsh MC: Neonatal necrotizing enterocolitis: pathogenesis, classification, and spectrum of illness, *Curr Probl Pediatr* 17:219, 1987.

17 Cell Injury and Cellular Adaptations

Anjana V. Yeldandi
David G. Kaufman
Janardan K. Reddy

Most pathologic processes begin with cell injury, and all forms of loss of function emanate from cell injury and cell death. The extent and types of cell injury can determine whether the cell and the tissue in which it resides are restored to normal, whether the cell dies and disappears, or whether residual effects persist as evidence of injury. In regard to cell injury, the most important consideration is survival of the whole organism, not necessarily the survival of an individual cell or even groups of cells. Injured cells may recover (reversible injury) or die (irreversible cell injury). The dead cells may be shed from the organism, or they are disintegrated and dissolved by proteolytic mechanisms for salvage and reutilization of the essential molecules such as amino acids. In some tissues, like the intestine, skin, trachea, and bronchi, cells are normally shed from the epithelium on a continuing basis through programmed cell division, differentiation, and death. Cell injury and cell death are often responses of the living organism to toxic chemicals, to bacterial, viral, and parasitic infections, and to hypoxia or anoxia. These responses are not always undesirable; for example, many drugs exert their overall beneficial action by damaging selected cell populations.

Cells can manifest injury in a variety of ways, but the number of morphologic manifestations of injury are finite and are encountered repetitively in numerous disease entities. The reversible or irreversible injury to cells and tissues can be caused by several factors or etiologic agents. Cellular reactions to stress or injury vary depending on the type, duration, and severity of injury induced. The consequences of cell injury also depend, to a large extent, on a variety of factors, including the intrinsic nature of cells and tissues involved, in particular, their differentiated state, and their ability to divide and replicate. An understanding of the causes and mechanisms of reversible and irreversible cell injury is a prerequisite for an appreciation of the biologic basis of disease processes. It is valuable for determining the therapeutic regimen, in anticipating the short-term and long-term sequelae of a given pathologic process, and in implementing effective preventive measures.

Cell death is the state in which cells are incapable of sustaining essential cellular functions, including transmembrane potential, energy generation, homeostatic control, motility, uptake of materials, synthesis, export, cell communication, excitability, and reproduction. Either cell death is an irreversible event that can occur under normal physiologic conditions as part of a process by which cells and tissues maintain their cell numbers and vitality (homeostatic mechanism), or it can be the ultimate result of cell injury. In the latter case cell death frequently has a fundamental role in the development (pathogenesis) of various diseases. We distinguish these two modes of cell death as apoptosis and necrosis respectively.

Apoptosis (programmed cell death) is an active process of cellular self-destruction, and the importance of this process is increasingly recognized both in physiologic regulation and in pathologic conditions. Apoptosis is usually manifested as the death of an individual cell or cells in a given cell population. The process exhibits certain distinct morphologic and molecular features such as cell shrinkage, chromatin condensation, internucleosomal DNA fragmentation, and activation or inactivation of specific gene functions. *Necrosis* is the more common form of cell death occurring in a tissue or organ in a living organism and usually encompasses large groups of cells. Necrosis is the common result of an irreversible cell injury caused by ischemia, toxic chemicals, or other harmful agents. Necrosis also occurs as a result of various parasitic, bacterial, fungal, and viral infections and the body's response to these agents. In contrast to apoptosis, where the morphologic features of injury are predominantly nuclear at the time of onset, necrotic cells exhibit concomitant nuclear and cytoplasmic disintegration. These cytoplasmic changes are characterized by severe swelling and degeneration of plasma membrane and cytoplasmic organelles. The term *oncosis* (Greek *onkos* meaning 'swelling') has been proposed recently to describe cell swelling preceding necrosis with the suggestion that it be used as a counterpart to apoptosis.[1]

Alterations of nuclear abnormalities include *pyknosis* (condensation), *karyorrhexis* (fragmentation), and *karyolysis* (dissolution). *Autolysis* (self-digestion) is the result of liberation of hydrolytic enzymes from lysosomes in dead and dying cells. Such enzymes rapidly degrade intracellular materials, including organelles, other cellular membrane systems, and macromolecules. As autolysis proceeds, the cell cytoplasm becomes homogeneous in appearance and intensely eosinophilic on routine hematoxylin and eosin staining. Progression of autolysis culminates in the loss of cellular details and tissue architecture. Autolysis proceeds rapidly in cells with a high content of hydrolytic enzymes or zymogens, such as those of pancreas and gastric mucosa. The onset of autolysis in heart, liver, and kidney is somewhat slower because of intermediate levels of lysosomal or proteolytic enzymes. Fibroblasts with relatively few lysosomes degenerate slowly after their death. Cell death can also occur after immersion of living tissue into denaturing agents such as formalin, glutaraldehyde, or absolute alcohol; because the hydrolytic enzymes are also denatured by these fixatives, such tissues are well preserved with cellular and organizational integrity and are not subject to autolytic degradation.

ETIOLOGIC FACTORS AND MECHANISMS

Cells are complex units the survival and function of which depend on the delicate balance between intracellular and extracellular events. Fundamental knowledge of the morphologic and functional reactions of cells and tissues to various injurious agents and genetic defects is critical for the understanding of disease processes and for instituting preventive and therapeutic measures.

There are many ways that a cell can be injured. Loss of availability of necessary substrates in critical cell metabolism pathways can injure cells; an example is the loss of oxygen that results in hypoxia and causes ischemic injury. Cells can be injured by microbial agents and by the body's responses to these invaders. Examples include the toxins and enzymes secreted by certain bacteria or fungi that inhibit metabolic pathways and dissolve cellular structures. Viruses may co-opt cell metabolic enzymes and processes for their own replication, and this may impair the production of necessary proteins, lipids, and nucleic acids for the maintenance of the cells. Efforts to contain or destroy microbial agents may lead to cell injury through the release of lytic enzymes, free radicals, and other reactive oxygen species used to kill microbes by the neutrophils and macrophages drawn into the infected area. This process may be facilitated by the cells and antibodies of the immune system. Immune mechanisms are also designed to exclude other exogenous biologic materials, dissolve cell debris, and eliminate abnormal cells such as those that arise in cancers. Unfortunately, they may also injure cells when these mechanisms inappropriately affect the normal cells of the host organism. Antibodies and cells of the immune system act primarily by damaging cell membranes, and this affects water and ion fluxes, ion concentration, and cell polarization. The oxygen radicals that are released by these cells can consume cell antioxidants and lead to damage of other cell macromolecules including lipids in the cell membranes and the DNA in the chromosomes and mitochondria.

Ionizing radiation also acts primarily by the generation of oxygen radicals within cells and tissues (see Chapter 23). The quantity and intensity of radical generation is related to the energy level of the ionizing radiation. In this case, damage to nucleic acids may be prominent and includes chromosomal alterations, but peroxidation of membrane lipids with alterations of the integrity of the lipid membrane may result. Other forms of radiation such as ultraviolet radiation have a very narrow macromolecular target because of their preferential transfer of energy to nucleic acid bases.

The mechanisms of cell injury by chemicals are varied. Nature and humans have evolved a vast number of chemicals that can nonselectively affect the structures and metabolic processes of all cells or can have very narrow effects on the unique processes of single specific cell types. Selective effects on particular cells have been used in the development of some of these chemicals as drugs. Other exposures to injurious chemicals can come through the food, water, and air that we need for life, as well as through other natural products and synthetic chemicals produced by humans. Different chemicals can have specific effects on cell membranes, interfere with ion pumps, poison steps in energy metabolism, block the production of metabolic products, or inhibit macromolecular synthesis. Chemicals that have their greatest effects on protein synthesis may manifest their most significant injuries in cells and tissues in which proteins are synthesized in great quantity, like the liver or pancreas. Other agents may have profound effects on cells in the brain or breast because of their greater lipophilicity. Some of the chemicals are damaging in their native form as they enter the body, but others are converted into injurious agents by the metabolic processes of the body.

How can diverse elements such as hypoxia, chemicals, infectious agents, genetic disturbances, and other etiologic factors elicit seemingly complex disturbances in cells, some of which lead to irreversible damage and cell death, whereas others are transient and reversible? Critical analysis of the complex cellular, biochemical, and molecular perturbations induced by a variety of injurious agents provides insight as to the role of certain common mechanistic principles of cell injury and cell death. The final common pathway of irreversible cell injury concerns the ability of the cell to maintain an intact membrane that allows the partition of ions and maintenance of a sufficient transmembrane potential. Chemicals and other agents capable of causing injury to cells can violate the membrane integrity through direct effects on cell membranes or pumps by the generation of energy, or through the nucleic acids that are involved in the synthesis of the structural proteins or enzymes that are involved in these processes.

Hypoxia

Cells use oxygen to generate energy and carry out metabolic processes. *Anoxic* and *hypoxic* injury are caused by absolute and relative deficiency of oxygen respectively. If oxygen is not available for use by cells in sufficient quantity, that is, if the cells are hypoxic, these processes fail to generate sufficient amounts of energy, or fail to metabolize substrates adequately. The result of these failures is cell injury. The cell injury that results can be reversible if the failure of these processes is brief in duration or mild in extent, or it can be lethal if of sufficient duration or severity. Hypoxia typically results from ischemia, which occurs when the oxygenated arterial blood supply to cells or tissues is interrupted either by occlusion of the artery from within by thrombus or embolism, or by physical disruption by external compression of the vessel, or when it is cut as in cases of trauma. If cells are deprived of oxygen, they are unable to generate sufficient energy to maintain the ion pumps of the cell membranes. As a result, the cell cannot maintain the partition of monovalent and divalent anions and cations that characterize the inside and outside of normal living cells. With this loss of ion partition comes the loss of the electrostatic potential across the membrane, and an accumulation of water within the cell. The latter change gives rise to one of the most characteristic changes of an injured cell, cloudy swelling, as described below.

Ischemia and the hypoxia of cells and tissues is the basic mechanism of some of the most important forms of human pathologic conditions.[2–4] Ischemia in the heart, usually caused by the obstruction of coronary artery blood flow, may cause ischemic injury and infarction of the myocardium. Myocardial infarction, colloquially, a "heart attack," is currently the leading cause of death in the United States and many other countries. Similarly, in the brain, ischemic injury resulting from obstruction of blood flow may lead to infarctions. These lesions, colloquially, "strokes," are another major cause of death in economically advantaged countries. Ischemia can develop at any site where blood flow to a tissue is completely or severely compromised and may result from venous as well as arterial obstruction. Some sites in the body are more prone to develop ischemia and infarction (so-called watershed areas) because the blood supply to these areas is completely or largely through a single artery or vein, with little collateral circulation (see Chapter 77). Ischemic injury can result when the blood supply is blocked acutely by external compression or internal obstruction. It can also result from the gradual reduction of blood flow through a vessel by intrinsic vascular diseases. In this case, there is a slowly evolving decrease in the caliber of the vessels until the carrying capacity of the vessel fails to meet the blood flow needs of the tissue under conditions of increased demand.

It is instructive to consider information that has been acquired about hypoxia and ischemic injury through experimental studies. The most studied and simplest experimental model is experimental hypoxia in the heart, induced by ligation of coronary arteries, to investigate the physiologic and morphologic consequences of the obstructed blood flow. Soon after ligation, pallor develops in the area of the heart with obstructed blood flow. This area of the myocardium no longer contracts during systole, but rather is distended by the contraction elsewhere in the chamber. This results in reduction of the effective pumping capacity of the chamber, with less blood passing through the valve and more blood being recirculated within the chamber.

The cellular consequences of ischemia and hypoxia that have been determined in this model offer insights about the gross manifestations observed. The loss of oxygen flow to the myocardial cells causes cessation of mitochondrial oxidative phosphorylation. The lack of oxygen as a terminal electron carrier for the mitochondrial respiratory chain precipitously interrupts electron flow, causing the respiratory chain to become reduced as opposed to its normal aerobic oxidized state. This leads to reduction of pyridine nucleotides, resulting in an increase in the intracellular NADH/NAD ratio. The cessation of oxidative phosphorylation rapidly leads to depletion of cell stores of adenosine triphosphate (ATP) and creatine phosphate. Myocardial muscle cells use ATP to provide the energy for movement of Ca^{2+} between sarcoplasmic reticulum cisternae and the sarcoplasm. In the sarcoplasm the Ca^{2+} binds to actin and myosin and leads to contraction of the muscle and converting ATP to ADP in the process. Thereafter the actin and myosin return to their uncontracted state. Restoration of the capacity to contract again requires the active pumping of Ca^{2+} back into the sarcoplasmic reticulum and the rephosphorylation of ADP to ATP, and these processes require energy that is usually generated by oxidative metabolism in the mitochondria. Myocardial cells have small cellular stores of ATP and can regenerate some ATP from creatine phosphate or from anerobic glycolysis. But these cell reserves are soon depleted in the absence of oxygen. This deficit of ATP interferes with the capacity of the affected area of the heart to participate in contraction and leads to hemodynamic consequence on heart function. It should be noted that these effects may occur in a relatively few minutes, long before sustained hypoxia is manifested by morphologic changes demonstrable by conventional microscopy. In fact, it usually takes a much longer time with sustained severe hypoxia for the deficit in ATP to be manifest as morphologically detectable injured cells. The sustained deprivation of ATP leads to the failure of cell ion pumps that transport Na^+, K^+, Ca^{2+}, and H^+ (Fig. 17-1). With the loss of membrane potential and loss of regulation channels, water enters the cells, leading to edema and the swelling of their mitochondria. If the ischemic injury is reversed within even as much as 20 to 30 minutes, these cells may recover from the injury.

Reoxygenation injury. Reoxygenation injury is defined as cellular injury caused by reintroduction or restoration, or reperfusion of physiologic concentrations of oxygen to viable cells that have been exposed to injurious but nonlethal or reversible anoxic or hypoxic conditions. Reoxygenation injury is a complex process in which anoxia and oxidative stress cause paradoxical effects. Reoxygenation injury results from the generation of highly reactive oxygen intermediates such as hydroxyl radical and superoxide. Hypoxic episode leads to accumulation of xanthine from ATP metabolism; hypoxia also results in proteolytic cleavage of xanthine dehydrogenase to xanthine oxidase. When the oxygen supply is restored by reperfusion, the accumulated xanthine is rapidly oxidized by xanthine oxidase, leading to the generation of toxic reactive oxygen intermediates. Reoxygenation also leads to the generation of superoxide by mitochondrial electron carriers. In addition, the entry of polymorphonuclear leukocytes (PMLs) into the injured tissue after reperfusion accentuates the injury because these cells also generate free radicals.

Protection against reoxygenation injury is possible to a certain extent by antioxidants such as superoxide dismutase and vitamin E. In the myocardial injury, if ischemia persists for a longer time and then perfusion is restored, the actin and myosin contract severely, forming the "contraction bands" or "rigor bands" that are a sign of irreversible cell injury (see

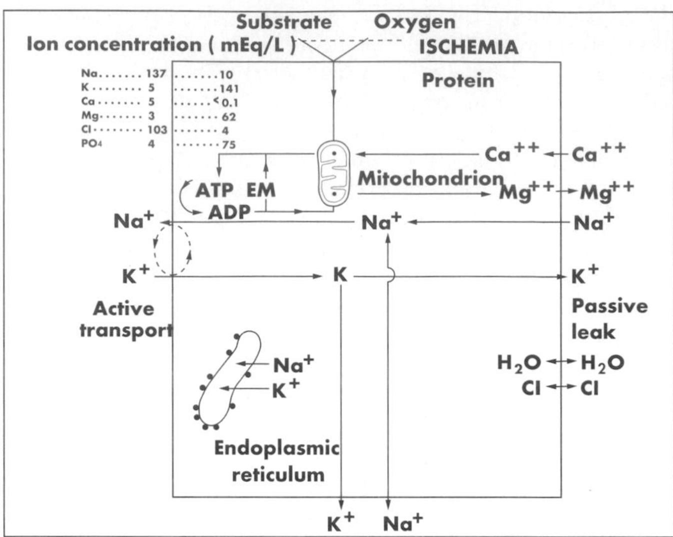

Fig. 17-1 Factors responsible for control of cell volume. High intracellular concentration of protein requires continuous active pumping of ions (largely sodium and potassium ions) and passive outward diffusion of water to counteract the tendency for water to enter cells because intracellular osmolality is higher than that in the extracellular space. Control is mediated by vectorial transport enzyme associated with cell membranes, particularly the plasma membrane, that are driven by dephosphorylation of high-energy compounds such as adenosine triphosphate (ATP). *Upper left,* Extracellular and intracellular concentrations of various ions in "normal" cells are shown; maintenance of the intracellular concentration of various ions requires expenditure of considerable work against a chemical gradient. Energy in the form of ATP is supplied by aerobic glycolysis and mitochondrial phosphorylation (oxidative phosphorylation). The latter reaction or reactions are highly sensitive to alterations of substrate and oxygen concentration and are interrupted by ischemia. When the pump is effective, it pumps sodium ions at a rate to balance their entry into the cell by passive leak, which in turn, regulates inward passive diffusion of water and thus the cell volume. Notice that active transport of sodium and potassium ions also occurs in intracellular membrane systems such as endoplasmic reticulum. *EM,* Embden–Meyerhof pathway. (From Scarpelli D, Trump BF: *Cell injury,* Bethesda, Md, 1974, Universities Associated for Research and Education in Pathology, Inc.)

Chapter 30). If hypoxia is sustained for a longer time, whether perfusion is restored or not, the cell membranes become permeable to cell macromolecules, and cells lose enzymes and other components. The membrane leakiness predisposes to the release of enzymes into the extracellular space with absorption into the circulation. In cardiac ischemia the injured myocytes are leaky, releasing lactate dehydrogenase (LD) and creatine kinase (CK), which then appear in serum. CK is a dimer that consists of skeletal muscle (M) subunit and or brain (B) subunit. LD is a tetramer consisting of heart (H) and skeletal muscle (M) subunits; LD in myocardium is a homodimer of H subunits (LD_1) that is released into the circulation. In normal serum the LD_1 is less than LD_2 (skeletal muscle type of LD). Elevation of MB isozymes of CK accompanied by elevation of LD_1 isozyme occurs in 48 hours after chest pain with diaphoresis, tachycardia, and hypotension in patients suffering from myocardial ischemia. In myocardial infarct LD_1 is released into the circulation from damaged myocardium, resulting in the elevation of serum levels of LD_1 and causing

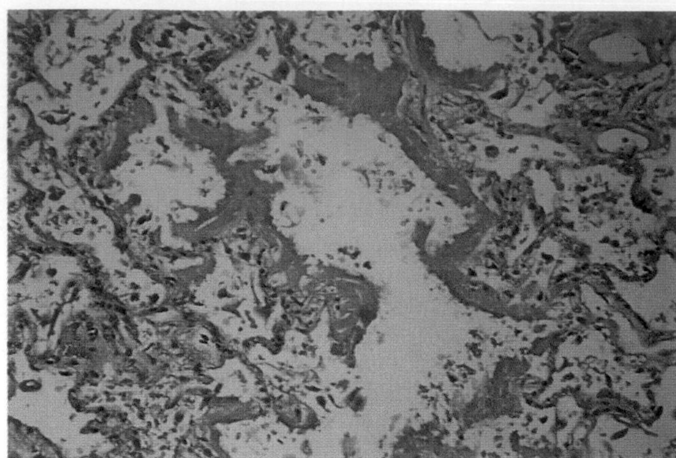

Fig. 17-2 Diffuse alveolar damage. Lung from an adult who died with adult respiratory distress syndrome complicating gram-negative septicemia and endotoxic shock. Notice the pink staining exudate outlining the alveolar spaces; these hyaline membranes represent proteins including fibrin that have leaked out of the necrotic vessel walls.

an "LD flip" ($LD_1 > LD_2$). It is important to note that LD flip does not usually occur in reversible myocardial injury. With irreversible damage, the synthetic processes of the cells would cease, and lysosomes would become activated for the autodigestive degradation of the cell.

Oxygen-radical injury and hyperoxia

Oxygen is essential for the survival of cells, and tissues and cells are injured when it is not present in sufficient quantities. Therapy with oxygen is beneficial in certain clinical situations, but oxygen carries a definite risk of injury. Thus, cells can be injured when they are exposed to excess oxygen, as in treatments with oxygen at high partial pressures, particularly when such treatments are prolonged. Similar effects may occur when the natural protectants of cells against the deleterious effects of activated oxygen species (that is, antioxidants) are deficient in quantity.[5-8]

An important mode of exposure to excess oxygen is clinical treatment with oxygen, typically for internal problems in the lung that block diffusion of oxygen into the capillaries of the alveolar septa. Humans can tolerate 100% oxygen for 24 to 48 hours with little pulmonary damage, but prolonged hyperoxia leads to lung injury. Under hyperoxic conditions intracellular oxygen concentrations rise, leading to accelerated generation of superoxide anion ($O_2^{\dot{-}}$). In bacterial sepsis (endotoxic shock), tissue trauma, acute pancreatitis, and necrotizing pulmonary infections, severe intravascular stasis of PMLs can occur within the lung. These neutrophils liberate oxygen radicals and damage capillary endothelium, causing diffuse alveolar damage (Fig. 17-2). Some of these radicals will escape the protective effects of the cellular antioxidants and will damage the cells. With high levels of reactive oxygen species the cellular antioxidant capacity may be overwhelmed, and above a threshold level, excessively high amounts of cell damage may occur. There are also forms of ionizing radiation (see below) that generate oxygen radicals in a dose-dependent manner that can overwhelm cellular defense mechanisms. Furthermore, it should be recognized that PMLs, T-lymphocytes, and macrophages generate reactive oxygen species as their means of killing exogenous biologic or physical materials or abnormal cells.

Mechanistically the genesis of oxygen radicals may begin when an electron is added to molecular oxygen to yield the superoxide ion (O_2^-) within mitochondria, by membrane oxidase of phagocytic cells, and by other enzymes in microsomes and peroxisomes. In addition to O_2^-, the other oxidizing species include hydrogen peroxide (H_2O_2), the hydroxyl radical (OH^-), hypochlorous acid (HOCl), singlet oxygen, chloramines, peroxyradicals, and peroxynitrite ion ($ONOO^-$). Superoxide dismutase enzymes (SOD) converts O_2^- to H_2O_2. When H_2O_2 interacts with ferrous iron, it abstracts an electron from the iron and forms a highly reactive $OH^\cdot$, while the ferrous form is oxidized to ferric form; this classical chemical process is known as the *Fenton reaction*.

$$Fe^{2+} + H_2O_2 \rightarrow Fe^{3+} + OH^\cdot + OH^-$$

The H_2O_2 generated by enzymatic dismutation of $O_2^{\bar{}}$ can interact with O_2 to generate OH through the *Haber–Weiss reaction:*

$$H_2O_2 + O_2^{\bar{}} \rightarrow OH^\cdot + OH^- + O_2$$

Macrophages, Kupffer's cells and vascular endothelium can generate nitric oxide (NO), a biologically potent chemical mediator and an active free radical. NO is formed by the conversion of L-arginine to L-citrulline by NO synthase. NO reacts with O_2 to form the peroxynitrite ion ($ONOO^-$). Radicals formed from NO are known to inhibit mitochondrial respiration.

The potency and biologic toxicity of different reactive oxygen species varies considerably. O_2 is relatively weak and diffuses poorly across cell membranes. H_2O_2 is also a weak oxidant, but it can readily diffuse into the cytoplasm from organelles where it is produced and also across plasma membranes. On the other hand, $OH^\cdot$ that is generated is an extremely reactive chemical that phagocytes use to attack microbes or necrotic cell debris, but it can also attack vital molecules within living cells and lead to cell injury or cell death. It is worthy of note that ionizing radiation produces $OH^\cdot$ along with a variety of other ionic and free radical forms of water and, to a lesser extent, other cellular molecules.

Although the reactive products like $OH^\cdot$ quickly interact with other cellular molecules to exert their damaging effects in the cell, it is the fact that they are stable enough to have mobility within the cell, rather than just rejoining with the remainder of H_2O or H_2O_2 immediately, that makes them so damaging to the cell. The $OH^\cdot$ radicals persist sufficiently long to travel to cell structures like membranes, proteins, or nucleic acids and attack them.[5,6] As noted below for carbon tetrachloride, the addition of a free radical to unsaturated cell membrane lipids can lead to the propagation of the radical through the membrane lipids, damaging many molecules until the reaction is damped by antioxidants. Where this changes the integrity of the membrane sufficiently to permit influx of water and Na^+ and Ca^{2+} ions, the effect on the cell can be produced. These cells can be recognized by their enlarged size and their pale, cloudy, and granular cytoplasm. If the extent of their loss of membrane integrity is sufficient, the cells are irreversibly injured, and they die soon thereafter.

Although most oxyradicals do not add to DNA, the $OH^\cdot$ is unique in that it does so very readily in vivo. The unique reactivity of the $OH^\cdot$ is attributable to its very high electrophilicity and high reactivity to penetrate the shield of the easily abstracted H atom in the sugar moieties and to reach the DNA bases. These energetic $OH^\cdot$ radicals attack DNA, yielding altered bases or single- or double-strand breaks. Interaction of $OH^\cdot$ with DNA also results in the formation of 8-hydroxydeoxyguanine residues, which are considered to be markers of radical damage.

Cells have a variety of mechanisms for repairing DNA damage, and much of this damage may be removed or reversed to preserve the viability of the cells. To the extent that the damage is not repaired, however, the results may be as gross as loss of portions of chromosomes after the next mitosis. The radicals also may cause more subtle base modifications that may be converted to base substitutions in DNA during the next round of DNA replication; such sequence changes can be silent or can have profound effects on cell function. If the effects of these changes are lethal, it typically takes more time and often one or more additional rounds of cell proliferation before the cell succumbs to the lethal effects of the genetic changes.

Reactive oxygen species cause cell injury by oxidation of critical cellular macromolecules such as proteins, DNA, and lipids. Reactive oxygen species can also oxidize thiols, leading to the formation of protein disulfides and protein mixed disulfides.[5-8] Reactive oxygen species are also known to interact with cytoskeletal elements and interfere with mitochondrial oxidative phosphorylation and cause ATP depletion. Of considerable interest, however, is that $OH^\cdot$ and other reactive oxygen species interact with polyunsaturated fatty acids (PUFA) in a rapid-fire fashion to yield highly destructive PUFA radicals, lipid hydroperoxy radicals, and lipid hydroperoxides. This process is known as *lipid peroxidation.* The lipid peroxides are decomposed by transition metals, such as iron to yield conjugated dienes, pentane, and ethane, which can be measured and serve as indicators of lipid peroxidation. Furthermore, toxic reactants such as 4-hydroxynonenal and malondialdehyde are also generated during lipid peroxidation. Lipid peroxidation propagates to sites distant from the original injury, resulting in widespread membrane damage.

Chemical agents

There are a vast number of naturally occurring and synthetic chemicals that can injure or kill cells. In most cases whether a cell is unaffected or is injured or killed is influenced by the dose of the chemical to which the cell is exposed. For some chemicals, particularly for some natural toxins, these amounts may be very small. When one considers the toxic or injurious effects of chemicals as a group, it is necessary to recognize the diversity of the chemical agents and thus their mechanisms of action and the types of cells they affect. Some chemicals affect a particular cell type with enough selectivity that their effects appear to be limited to that one cell type. Other chemicals are universal in their effects and can act on any cell type that they encounter. An example of a selectively toxic agent is curare toxin, which poisons the transmission of signals between motor neurons and muscle cells by acting at the synaptic junction between them. At the other extreme is cyanide, which acts by poisoning the oxygen transfer reactions in the mitochondria and reducing the generation of energy within any cell. In the first case, the chemical may lead to the death of the person because the muscle cells may become nonfunctional because of failure of neuronal stimulation. This has dramatic effects physiologically, but morphologic evidence of the primary lesion may be absent. In the latter case, the loss of energy generation may result in the failure of cell membrane ion pumps with the loss of intracellular and extracellular ion partition, reduction in cell membrane potential, and influx of water into the cell. The hydropic appearance of the most severely affected cells indicates that the membrane integrity of the cells may have been compromised, but it gives little indication about which agent with similar mechanism of action produced the effect. The following deals with sequential biochemical and other functional and structural changes that occur in injury caused by certain representative types of chemical agents.

Carbon tetrachloride. Toxic injury of the liver is a common outcome of ethanol abuse, exposure to certain industrial chemicals, or, to a lesser extent, exposure to therapeutic drugs or naturally occurring toxicants such as aflatoxins. Carbon tetrachloride (CCl_4) is a classic example of an industrial toxin that produces liver cell injury and exemplifies general principles of chemically induced cell injury.[9-11] Cell injury by CCl_4 is not caused by the chemical itself but rather by products produced from the chemical by the body's drug-metabolizing cytochrome P-450 enzyme system. The P-450 enzymes typically oxidize diverse endogenous and exogenous chemicals in an effort to facilitate their inactivation and excretion as more water-soluble molecules. This is typically accomplished by reduction of the iron in the cytochrome from ferric (+++) ion to ferrous (++) ion with transfer of an electron and addition of molecular oxygen to the substrate chemical while the chemical is associated with the enzyme, followed by release of a stable product from the enzyme.

In the case of CCl_4 the product of the reaction with the P-450 is a trichloromethyl free radical (CCl_3) that is stable enough to dissociate from the cytochrome P-450 but rapidly reacts with other molecules in the immediate vicinity of its formation. This leads to the reductive cleavage of carbon-chlorine bond as follows:

$$CCl_4 + e \rightarrow CCl_3^{\cdot} + Cl^{\cdot}$$

Since the P-450 enzymes are associated with intracellular membranes, the free-radical product of CCl_4 typically attacks the unsaturated lipids of the membranes, abstracting a hydrogen atom, and creating a lipid free radical within the membrane:

$$-CH_2-\overset{H}{C}=\overset{H}{C}- + CCl_3^{\cdot} \rightarrow -CH_2-C^{\cdot}=\overset{H}{C}- + CCl_3H$$

$$-CH_2-C^{\cdot}=\overset{H}{C}- + CCl_3^{\cdot} \rightarrow -CH_2-CH=\overset{H}{C}^{\cdot} + CCl_3H$$

Molecular oxygen reacts with the lipid free radical, leading to the formation of lipid peroxides, which in turn break down to form aldehydes, ketones, malonaldehyde, and other products that alter the membrane. In the process, the free radical is transferred to an adjacent lipid molecule. Once begun, this process rapidly spreads through the lipid in an autocatalytic manner and progresses to produce widespread local damage to the membranes.

Although these initial effects of CCl_4-induced cell injury are not detectable by conventional histologic methods, within a few hours of exposure, neutral lipids (triglycerides) begin to accumulate as osmiophilic droplets in liver parenchymal cells. Eventually, these small microvesicular lipid droplets coalesce to form larger aggregates that fill the cytoplasm. Grossly, the liver is observed to enlarge and become pale to yellowish in color. It is believed that the lipid accumulates in the liver cells because the radical-induced damage in the liver impairs the synthesis of proteins including the lipid acceptor protein that couples triglyceride to phospholipids to form lipoproteins. In the absence of formation of lipoproteins, the neutral lipids accumulate in the liver, yielding the histologic and gross pathologic alterations.

Metabolic products of CCl_4 also injure mitochondria, resulting in partial to total decoupling of oxygen consumption and the generation of ATP from ADP. With a progressive deficit in the supply of ATP, the cells cease to pump ions adequately to preserve the transmembrane differential in sodium and calcium ions. Water diffuses into the cells, and they swell to yield the large, pale, finely granular cells that have been called "balloon cells." As the cell injury progresses, the influx of calcium leads to the precipitation of calcium salts in the matrix of the swollen mitochondria. This is observed histologically as basophilic granules in the cytoplasm. The extent of basophilia increases with time and severity of damage and typically reflects the dead and dying liver cells.

Carbon tetrachloride also results in injury to the nucleus and nucleolus, presumably as a result of free-radical metabolic products. Histologically, this is initially observed as marginated and clumped nuclear chromatin. Later the nucleus undergoes progressive changes in which it becomes shrunken and densely basophilic (pyknosis), then the chromatin becomes fragmented (karyorrhexis), and finally the chromatin is dissolved (karyolysis). The clumping of chromatin is believed to reflect the altered intracellular ion concentrations and lowered pH that follows the failure of membrane ion pumps because of the deficit of ATP. The deficit of ATP and the altered ion concentrations inhibit nuclear macromolecular synthesis. This deprives the cells of synthesis of new enzymes and proteins to replace those that are being lost through the failing membrane. The influx of calcium and the lowered pH because of lacticacidosis causes the activation of nuclear nucleases that participate in the fragmentation and lysis of the DNA.

Acetaminophen (paracetamol, Tylenol). Acetaminophen (*N*-acetyl-*p*-aminophenol), is a commonly used analgesic and antipyretic. Although most of the therapeutically administered dose of this compound is detoxified in the liver by sulfation and glucuronidation and excreted, a minute amount of acetaminophen is oxidized by the cytochrome P-450–dependent monooxygenase system to *N*-acetyl-*p*-benzoquinoneimine (NABQI). NABQI is a highly reactive electrophile and an oxidant that is effectively detoxified by conjugation with GSH. Thus the adverse effects of acetaminophen are extremely rare. Nonetheless, as the dose of acetaminophen increases, the rate of formation of NABQI increases with concomitant depletion of GSH. This results in the failure of detoxification of NABQI; an increase in the level of this toxic electrophile causes destruction of nucleophilic macromolecules in the cell. Acetaminophen intoxication also results in lipid peroxidative damage, which correlates with its hepatotoxicity. The acetaminophen-induced hepatotoxicity is accentuated by alcohol.

Alcohol. Alcohol (ethanol), consumed in moderation, is a mood-modifying or pleasant sensation–enhancing substance that has its cultural origins in antiquity.[12] If chronically abused, it damages a variety of organs and is responsible for a significant degree of morbidity and mortality in the world. Alcohol is a less potent toxicant than CCl_4, but even a single episode of excessive ingestion of alcohol can significantly alter hepatic function; this effect is typically rapidly reversible with abstinence. Chronic ethanol consumption causes injury and death of hepatocytes.

Ethanol is rapidly absorbed from the stomach and small intestine and is detected in the blood within a few minutes. It is metabolized to acetaldehyde in the liver by three different pathways.[12-14] The major pathway involves the conversion of ethanol to acetaldehyde by alcohol dehydrogenase. The second pathway involves the microsomal ethanol-oxidizing system, which utilizes cytochrome P-450–IIE1; this pathway is highly active in the chronic alcoholic. The third pathway involves the peroxisomal catalase. All these reactions yield acetaldehyde, which is then rapidly metabolized by aldehyde dehydrogenase, resulting in the formation of acetate. The metabolism of alcohol generates NADH from NAD^+. The depletion of NAD^+ results in a net increase in the NADH/NAD^+ ratio in the hepatocyte, which leads to oxidative stress and lipid peroxidation. The high level of NADH favors the reduction of pyruvate to lactate, decreased gluconeogenesis, and high intracellular concentrations of α-glycerophosphate in the hepatocyte. These metabolic disturbances lead to decreases in fatty acid oxidation and promotes increased synthesis of fatty acids and their esterification to triglycerides. These changes lead to lipid accumulation in hepatocytes and fatty liver.

Chronic alcoholism affects a variety of organs, but the most frequently observed disorder is in the liver. Fatty metamorphosis of hepatocytes in the centrilobular zone is seen within a few days of consumption of alcohol. Chronic ethanol abuse causes extensive fatty accumulation in the liver. In addition, the hepatocytes with and without fatty metamorphosis may reveal accumulations of intermediate filaments, known as *"Mallory body,"* or *alcoholic hyalin.* These are brightly eosinophilic intracytoplasmic inclusions consisting of prekeratin intermediate filaments. Neutrophil infiltration into the liver lobule can occur in the chronic alcoholic *(alcoholic hepatitis)* as a consequence of chemoattractants generated by ethanol metabolism and also is attributable to the presence of Mallory bodies. These activated neutrophils further contribute to tissue oxidative injury by releasing oxygen radicals.

Alcoholic intake also predisposes to reductions in the antioxidant mechanisms. Depletion of GSH and vitamin E are commonly associated with alcohol abuse; the depletion of these protective molecules can account for the adverse drug reactions such as the accentuated hepatic necrosis caused by acetaminophen in the alcoholic.

Radiation

All flora and fauna are exposed to ionizing radiation emanating from natural sources such as cosmic radiation and naturally occurring radionuclides. In addition to natural environmental sources of ionizing radiation over which we have no control, we are exposed to radiation from a variety of manmade sources, including diagnostic radiology and therapeutic, industrial, and fallout radiation. Radiation is widely used in the treatment of malignant neoplastic conditions. Whole-body irradiation is also extensively used in the preparation for bone marrow transplantation in patients with leukemia or lymphoma and in some cases before organ transplantation to minimize immune rejection of the grafted organ.

Ionizing radiation exists in many different forms (see Chapter 23). The effects of ionizing radiation on cells begins with the absorption of energy by cellular macromolecules and water.[15,16] There is excitation of atoms to form ions, resulting in a series of localized physicochemical perturbations in the cell. Water, the major component of cells, absorbs energy from ionizing radiation to a greater extent than other macromolecules do. The interaction of ionizing radiation with water results in the formation of ionizing water molecules, H_2O^+ and H_2^-, which dissociate to form $H^\cdot$ and $OH^\cdot$ free radicals. These free radicals then react with other elements in the cell, causing cell injury.

Ionizing radiation rarely causes instant cell death. Rapidly proliferating cells and tissues are more prone to quickly reveal radiation-induced damage, as compared to conditionally dividing cells. Although the reactive free radicals such as $OH^\cdot$ interact with various nucleophiles, the critical target for killing is the DNA of the cells. High doses of ionizing radiation damage many cell organelles and rapidly induce cell injury characterized by swelling and vacuolization of the cytoplasm, rupture of the nucleus and nucleolus, pyknosis, karyorrhexis, karyolysis, and cytolysis. These alterations are essentially similar to those seen in any acutely injured cell and must be considered nonspecific reactions to injury.

DNA damage with ionizing radiation varies considerably; the changes include single-strand breaks, damage to individual bases, intrastrand cross-links, interstrand cross-links, and very rarely double-strand breaks. 8-Hydroxydeoxyguanine adducts in DNA are also encountered in tissues exposed to ionizing radiation. Several DNA repair mechanisms exist in cells to remove deleterious DNA lesions and repair correctly. Nonetheless, misrepair may lead to mutations, and neoplastic transformation is a long-term complication of ionizing radiation.

Immunologic mediators and processes

The immune system has as its major role to destroy or contain biologic or physical materials that are perceived as being "foreign" to the body. The cells of the immune system accomplish this either by generating antibodies that interact with materials or cells at a distance from cells that generated them *(humoral mechanisms)* or by the effects of cells acting locally through the production of reactive oxygen species and growth regulatory factors *(cellular mechanisms).* Although the antibodies may injure or kill cells directly, they also may act by targeting cells for killing by cellular immune mechanisms. When these normal protective mechanisms inappropriately attack cells of the body, they produce immune-mediated cell injury. The immune-mediated cell injury is either a primary event (such as autoimmune) or a secondary response to another process (such as viral hepatitis). The cellular components of immune system vary considerably and play different roles in cell injury. A broad perspective of the mechanism by which inflammatory cells contribute to cell injury is therefore essential.

Immunologically mediated cell killing results in either necrosis or apoptosis. These immunologic mechanisms were presumably developed to enable the body to resist the effects of microbes and other materials that it recognizes as foreign. Nonetheless, these same cells and mechanisms may act inappropriately against normal cells and structures and result in injury or death of these cells. Such *autoimmune* processes are believed to be major features of several diseases as diverse as systemic lupus erythematosus, juvenile diabetes, rheumatic heart disease, and multiple sclerosis (see Chapter 26). Because of the selectivity of the immune system, these diseases are characterized by attack on specific cell types and the later consequences of such earlier specific attacks. Cytotoxic lymphocytes contribute to a wide variety of immune-mediated cell injury patterns. The likely mechanism involves T-cell recognition of the target cell, leading to T-cell activation and release of *perforin* (pore-forming protein). Perforin acts in concert with other hydrolytic enzymes to damage the target cell plasma membrane. The injury to plasma membrane causes influx of Ca^{2+} into the cell, leading to necrosis. An alternative mechanism, proposed recently, involves *calcium influx–independent* lymphocyte-mediated cell killing. This mechanism postulates perforin-independent permeabilization of plasma membrane. The damage to plasma membrane is considered secondary to endonuclease activation and DNA hydrolysis. Additional information is necessary to unravel this unorthodox apoptotic process of immune-mediated cell injury. The cytotoxic T-cell–mediated apoptosis is unorthodox in that it does not require RNA and protein synthesis. The contribution of the target cell receptor, possibly APO/Fas system, to the receptor-mediated lymphocyte cytotoxic killing remains to be explored.

Neutrophils are a common inflammatory cell in many conditions and can participate in cell injury (such as alcoholic hepatitis; anoxic/hypoxic cell injury). Neutrophils are recruited to sites of injury by cytokines, leukotrienes, and other products such as adhesion molecules P and E selectins. These selectins initiate rolling of neutrophils on endothelial cells, which then promotes adherence of neutrophils to endothelial cells by means of the neutrophil CD11/CD18 protein and the intercellular cell adhesion molecules (ICAM 1 and 2) on endothelium. After this adhesion, the activated neutrophils release H_2O_2 and hypochlorous acid. Resident and wandering macrophages also contribute to the generation of reactive oxygen intermediates, including the production of NO radicals. To the extent that the cell injury and killing is mediated by reactive oxygen species generated by the immune system cells, the same mechanisms apply as for injuries attributable to reactive oxygen species. One point to note, however, is that these cells can produce relatively high levels of reactive oxygen in a localized area, and this can cause severe localized damage to the cells that they attack. The cells that the body dispatches to engage in this oxygen radical attack are terminally differentiated and destined to die immediately or soon after their attack; for this reason they are not adversely affected by the genetic damage to themselves that may result from the oxygen radicals they unleash. These cells typically produce other secreted products, cytokines, that signal other immune cells to migrate to the region of their attack and in this manner sustain the process (see Chapter 18).

As noted above, the reactive oxygen species have high affinity for electron-dense regions, such as the double bonds in unsaturated fatty acids in cell membranes. These sites can be peroxidated by the reactive oxygen species, thus changing the intrinsic properties, including flexibility of the fatty acid and the membrane in this area. Peroxidation of the membrane can also be propagated by chain reaction until terminated by antioxidants. Thus considerable alteration of the membrane can occur locally, particularly if the cellular reserves of antioxidants are low or have been consumed. Local damage to the cell membrane, if sufficiently severe, can result in a segment of membrane where ion partition between the inside and outside of the cell cannot be maintained, with the loss of membrane polarization and the entry of water into the cell. If these changes are limited, the cell may be injured but may recover from the injury. If the changes are sufficiently extensive, the cell dies.

Infectious agents

Humans come into contact with a variety of microorganisms at every stage of existence. Indeed many microorganisms exist as "commensals" or "normal flora" of skin, oropharynx, respiratory tract, gastrointestinal tract, and genital tract. In these locations the host-parasite relationships are complex, and these normal flora rarely give rise to infectious problems. Disease ensues when this delicate relationship is perturbed in favor of the microorganism; opportunistic infections then arise, especially in conditions where there is immunosuppression. For example, a tear in the epidermis of skin or the mucosa of the lower intestinal tract can permit the entry of the normal flora into the wound, enabling such flora to become infectious. In acquired immunodeficiency syndrome (AIDS) or with widespread malignancy, the compromised immune system makes the patient susceptible to a wide range of infections. When exposed to pathogenic organisms such as some viruses, bacteria, fungi, and protozoan parasites that are not found in normal healthy individuals, the chances of developing disease are certainly greater. This susceptibility depends to some extent upon the virulence of the microorganism, the dose of the infectious agent, genetic susceptibility of the individual, and the immune status, among others.

Mechanisms of cell injury by bacterial toxins, extracellular bacteria, facultative intracellular bacteria, mycobacteria, fungi, viruses, and protozoan parasites are described in Chapters 33 to 39. Cell injury produced by infectious agents, in particular bacteria, is attributable to toxins (both *endotoxins* and *exotoxins*) elaborated by these biologic agents. Host factors may also contribute to cell injury in infections. *Exotoxins* are diffusible bacterial polypeptides secreted by the infectious organism into the surrounding tissues. Bacterial exotoxins are designated "cytolytic" type when they interfere with permeability properties of cell membranes, or called "bipartite" toxins, when they bind to a specific receptor on the target cell by the binding region (B region) of the toxin molecule, and then enter the cell to release the toxic A region, which causes cell injury. Cytolytic toxins are generated by many pathogenic bacteria such as *Clostridium difficile, Clostridium perfringens, Escherichia coli, Staphylococcus aureus,* and *Streptococcus pyogenes.* Mechanisms by which cytolytic exotoxins cause membrane damage may vary but the general theme appears to be that they degrade membrane phospholipids (phospholipase activity), or enhance the formation of discrete transmembrane pores (pore-forming toxins). These membrane changes culminate in cell lysis. Pseudomembranous colitis is a classical example of cytotoxicity caused by cytotoxins produced by *C. difficile*. The bipartite exotoxins, such as the one produced by *Corynebactrium diphtheriae* (diphtheria toxin), have been well characterized. Diphtheria toxin causes cellular damage in heart, lungs, liver, and kidneys by inhibiting protein synthesis. This is accomplished by binding of the B region of the toxin to membrane receptor to facilitate entry of the toxin into the cell, proteolytic nicking, and thiol reduction to yield A and B fragments. The A fragment of the toxin causes ADP-ribosylation of elongation factor 2 (EF2), leading to inhibition of protein synthesis.

Endotoxins of bacteria are lipopolysaccharides (LPS) in nature and are constituents of the outer membrane of gram-negative bacteria. LPS may induce an array of biologic changes including activation of complement, induction of cytokines, and activation of clotting mechanisms. Gram-negative septicemia may lead to endotoxic shock because of the release of LPS.

Many viruses injure cells. Some of the viruses exhibit tropism. After entry into the host, viruses reach the target organ and replicate to produce disease. Hepatitis viruses (A, B, C, D, and E viruses) are hepatotrophic; rabies virus and polio virus target brain, and coxsackievirus B4 exhibits tropism for the pancreatic β cells.[17] Cytomegalovirus, on the other hand, can affect many different cell types. As discussed in detail (in Chapter 36), viruses can injure and kill cells *directly by cytopathic effect,* or *indirectly by eliciting a host immune response.* The direct viral cytopathic effect may be the result of the virus co-opting the host cell macromolecular synthetic machinery for its own use and impairing the host transcriptional and translational processes. Viruses suppress the host mRNA synthesis and interfere with other vital cellular functions, which lead to plasma membrane damage and cell death. Poliovirus is an example of a virus causing a direct cytopathic effect. The indirectly cytopathic viruses trigger a series of immune responses. The viruses replicate, and viral capsular proteins are synthesized in the susceptible cell. The progeny viruses are then released from such a cell without affecting the cell's survival. Nonetheless, some of the viral proteins not utilized in the assembly of virus particles become exposed on the external surface of the cellular plasma membrane. These foreign proteins on the host cell plasma membrane are recognized by the immune system, and the cytotoxic T-cells then participate in killing the infected cell by the cytotoxic or apoptotic mechanisms.

Genetic factors

Cell injury resulting from defects in single genes is now well recognized. These genetic alterations may lead to disturbances in the maintenance of cell homeostatic regulation, synthesis, transport and secretion of macromolecules, and the catabolism and turnover of specific proteins. The mutant proteins may lead to a loss or a gain in function. In the current context of cell injury, two examples of genetic disease are worth citing. First, mutations in the gene encoding Cu/Zn superoxide dismutase may result in a gain in function; this altered superoxide dismutase appears to play a role in motor neuron disease of familial amyotrophic lateral sclerosis (ALS).[18,19] Transgenic mice expressing mutant Cu/Zn SOD ($Gly^{93} \rightarrow Ala^{93}$) develop disease prevalently affecting motor neurons. The cascade of events leading to motor neuron death in familial ALS is not fully elucidated. The mutant SOD appears to make motor neurons selectively vulnerable to motor neuron disease. The second example is the single mutation in the alpha-1-antitrypsin gene, which leads to the synthesis in liver of an abnormal protein that cannot be secreted.[20] This leads to alpha-1-antitrypsin deficiency in serum and liver cell injury as a result of massive intracellular accumulation of the mutant protein.

REVERSIBLE CELL INJURY AND INTRACELLULAR ACCUMULATIONS

Reversible injury

Cells exist in a dynamic milieu that requires virtually continuous control mechanisms with expenditure of energy to maintain homeostasis. The metabolic control depends on the functional integrity of various membranes, organelles, and compartments of the cell, such as the plasma membrane, endoplasmic reticulum, Golgi complex, mitochondria, lysosomes, peroxisomes, nuclear membrane, chromatin, nucleoplasm, and nucleolus. At the molecular level, the integrity and functions of these membranes are precisely controlled by a variety of gene products, ions, and intracellular and extracellular signals. A cell's capacity to rapidly and effectively regulate its internal environment and function to adapt to perturbations in extracellular milieu is crucial for its survival. Cells die when they can no longer maintain the integrity of their cell membranes and when the partitioning of water and ions and with them the potential energy or change across the membranes is sufficiently disrupted so as not to be restorable.[21-24]

The fine regulation of cell volume depends on the continuous function of active-transport systems for a variety of ions. The ionic composition and protein concentrations of the cell interior differ greatly from those of the extracellular fluid. These fundamental differences between the interior and exterior of the cell would lead to a passive diffusion of water into the cell, which would be considerable and detrimental, if unopposed by active transport of sodium ions into the extracellular fluid and the intracellular uptake of potassium ions by the sodium-potassium ATPase pumps. It is essential to remember that maintenance of these critical plasma membrane ion-channel functions prevent the cell from reaching the Gibbs-Donnan equilibrium in which ingress of water into the cell would lead to massive swelling and its eventual death. Thus a lack of energy-producing substrates, poisoning of mitochondrial energy-generating pathways, disruption of cell-membrane ion pumps, and even the interruption of transcriptional and translational mechanisms involved in the generation of the proteins that function in these roles can impair membrane function and integrity. The net effect of any of these mechanisms is the accumulation of water within the cell and a change in intracellular ions to more closely resemble the concentrations in extracellular fluids.

As pointed out earlier, the cellular reactions to stress vary depending on the type, duration, and severity of injury induced. Also important is the type and metabolic state of the cell, since cells such as hepatocytes and pancreatic acinar cells that are metabolically highly active are more susceptible to injury. If injury is severe and surpasses the capacity of the cellular protective mechanisms to counter, cell death commonly occurs. If the injury is not severe to cause cell death, temporary impairment of cell function or structural damage to the cellular organelles or to the DNA could result. Such cells may recover completely or may die if they sustain further damage. The response to acute cell injury can range from a minimal and reversible disturbance of cell volume to massive irreversible swelling with a concomitant loss of cell function, disintegration of plasma membrane, and cell death. The factor or factors that ultimately determine whether a cell will survive *(reversible injury)* or succumb *(irreversible injury)* remain unknown, and even the morphologic features that allow one to predict reversibility or irreversibility of cell injury are not clearly definable. The factors responsible for the point beyond which survival of the cell is no longer possible—the point of no return—also remain to be delineated (Fig. 17-3).

The morphologic alterations resulting from nonlethal injury to the cell were referred to in the past as "degeneration" to denote progressive deterioration of cells and "infiltration" to describe intracellular or extracellular accumulations of normal or abnormal substances. These designations provide little information on the nature of such alterations. The nonlethal alterations are now known as reversible injury. The first such alteration is *cellular swelling* or *hydropic change,* caused by the influx of water into the cell. Morphologically these changes are typically reflected in an enlargement of the cells and their organelles with a reduction in the clarity of contrast of cellular organelles. Cells with hydropic change are characterized by a large, pale cytoplasm and sometime slightly enlarged but normally located nucleus. This initial event, occurring almost immediately after exposure of a cell to a noxious environment, is a loss of cell volume control, which is rapidly followed by a decrease in the optical density of the cytoplasm because of intracellular swelling (hydropic change) and eventual accumulation of lipid droplets (fatty change). Cells with hydropic swelling reveal dilated endoplasmic reticulum cisternae, disaggregation of polysomes from the rough endoplasmic reticulum signifying decreased protein synthesis, blebbing of the plasma membrane to generate focal extensions of the cytoplasm, which may be pinched off and released into the extracellular matrix, and swelling of mitochondria because of dysfunction of energy gradient and inability to maintain mitochondrial volume. These changes are essentially reversible, and the cells can fully recover provided that there is cessation of the injurious stimulus. Nonetheless, further injury results in continued damage to mitochondria such as high-amplitude swelling and the appearance of mitochondrial matrix densities rich in phospholipid content and in enormous blebbing of membranes, which are generally considered signs of onset of the so-called point of no return, or impending irreversibility. If the noxious agent is particularly toxic and the exposure is sufficiently prolonged to be lethal, additional alterations are seen: violent movements of the plasma membrane followed by the development of bizarre pseudopods and blebs of the plasma membrane, nuclear swelling, condensation of nuclear chromatin *(pyknosis),* dissolution of the nucleus *(karyolysis),* and finally lysis of the cell *(cytolysis).*

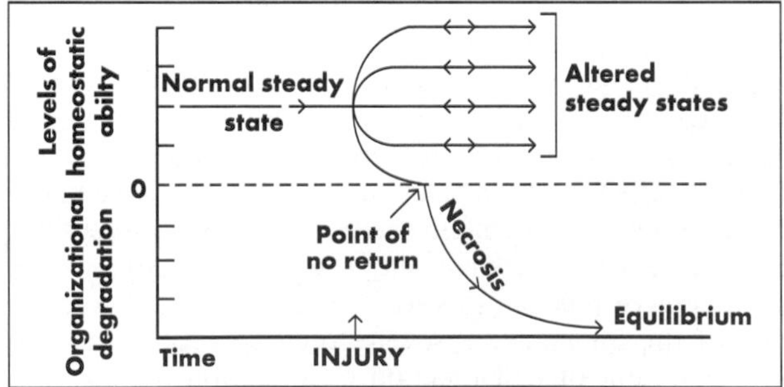

Fig. 17-3 In the "normal" steady state a cell is able to maintain a homeostasis (internal milieu) that allows optimum function. When injury occurs, the cell alters its steady state and function; if injury is sufficiently intense and protracted, it is unable to maintain its homeostasis at a level sufficient for function compatible with life, and cell death results. (From Scarpelli D, Trump BF: *Cell injury,* Bethesda, Md, 1974, Universities Associated for Research and Education in Pathology, Inc.)

Intracellular accumulations

A fundamental property of cells is their capacity to adapt to an adverse environment, especially when the environmental alterations develop slowly and are not of sufficient intensity to be lethal, at least at their onset. Many biologic processes culminating in cellular or organismal adaptations are mediated through feedback control mechanisms that initiate and modulate structural and functional alterations to allow cell survival under adverse conditions. Cellular adaptations are a common and integral part of many disease states. In some instances, it is difficult to ascertain what a pathologic response is and what an extreme adaptation to an excessive functional demand represents. It should be recalled that in the early stages of a successful adaptive response cells may be capable of enhanced function. When injury is sublethal and sustained, cells and tissues tend to accumulate substances in abnormal quantities, a phenomenon referred to as "infiltration" and "inclusions." Most commonly such accumulations consist of molecules that are normally present, such as triglycerides, glycogen, calcium, uric acid, melanin, and bilirubin. Alternatively, the abnormal substances accumulated may be either endogenous or exogenous in origin. The abnormal endogenous accumulations include materials such as amyloid. More rarely in diseases attributable to defective genes, cell products such as proteins, lipids, or sugars accumulate protein, an example of which is the abnormal accumulation of alpha-1-antitrypsin deficiency. In addition, exogenous materials such as mineral dusts, pigments, and certain heavy metals may accumulate in the cytoplasm of cells after their introduction into the body by inhalation, ingestion, or injection.

The basic processes of ingestion, digestion, and storage of materials by cells involves their complex interactions of cell membranes and their fusion with lysosomes. Ingestion involves the inward flow of plasma membrane, which eventually encloses either fluid *(pinocytosis)* or particulate material *(heterophagocytosis)* that is internalized in the cytoplasm though still enclosed in a membrane-limited vacuole. As the vacuole *(phagosome)* moves inward, its membrane fuses with that of a preexisting lysosome, whereupon hydrolytic enzymes are released into the phagosome, interacting with and digesting the enclosed material. Because of the rapidity of pinocytosis, phagocytosis, phagosome movement, and fusion with lysosomes, certain types of cells may ingest and digest prodigious amounts of material. When the material is ingested in amounts so large that they exceed the capacity of lysosomes to digest them, or if the material is degraded slowly or not at all, it tends to accumulate in the cytoplasm, a condition known as "lysosomal overloading."

Lysosomal overloading may occur rapidly if not all the ingested material is subject to attack by digestive enzymes or more slowly, sometimes a matter of years, if only a small proportion of ingested material is undigested. Digestion of biologic material leads to the formation of soluble substances such as small peptides, amino acids, and sugars, which are reutilized by the cell. Accumulation of material may cause the organs involved to become enlarged and firm; in the case of pigments the tissues may be strikingly colored. When the storage of material is excessive, cells may be mechanically compromised and their functions may be impaired to the point that cell death occurs. Lysosomal overloading can also result from material originating within the cell, for example, the indigestible material resulting from focal cytoplasmic degradation, a process referred to as *autophagy* ("self-eating"). Autophagy is probably a normal cellular event responsible for the turnover of cell organelles and membranes. The following deals with various intracellular accumulations encountered with certain forms of cell injury.

Lipids (fatty metamorphosis, steatosis)

Many cells normally contain varying amounts of fat in the form of minute fat droplets, which may or may not be recognizable at the light microscopic resolution. Abnormal amounts of fat, mostly in the form of triglycerides, accumulating in the cytoplasm of parenchymal cells, is referred to as *steatosis, fatty metamorphosis,* or *simply fatty change*. Such triglyceride accumulations in cells are prominent at the light microscopic level and can become obvious or appreciable at the gross level, in an organ such as liver, if the cellular fatty change is considerable. Fatty change can occur in any parenchymatous organ. It is commonly seen in the liver in view of its major role in lipid metabolism. Fatty metamorphosis of liver is a common occurrence after excess alcohol consumption, which is most likely the commonest cause of fatty liver (Fig. 17-4). Other causes of fatty liver include protein-calorie malnutrition, injury by hepatotoxins and hepatotoxic chemicals (such as aflatoxins, carbon tetrachloride), hypoxia or anoxia, diabetes mellitus, obesity, total parenteral nutrition, Reye's syndrome, and tetracycline sensitivity, particularly in pregnant women, among others. The pathogenesis of fatty liver varies according to the causative factor. Triglyceride excess in liver cells can be the sum of any of the following disturbances: (1) increased fatty acid entry into liver cells, (2) excess production of fatty acids from acetate, (3) reduced oxidation of fatty acids, (4) increased retention of triglycerides caused by inadequate complexing of triglycerides with apoprotein molecules to form lipoproteins, and (5) decreased release of lipoproteins from hepatocytes.

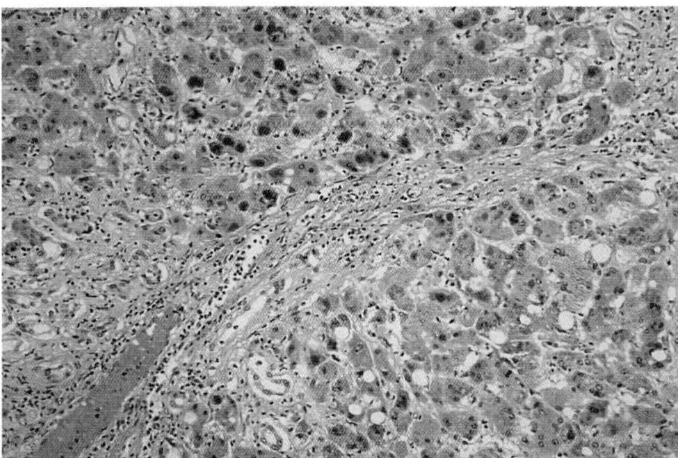

Fig. 17-4 Mallory bodies (alcoholic hyaline) in liver parenchymal cells. Hepatocyte cytoplasm contains eosinophilic inclusions. Mallory body consists of a perinuclear aggregate of filamentous material (mostly intermediate cytokeratin filaments) in the cytoplasm of hepatocyte.

Two morphologically distinct patterns of fatty change as discussed in Chapter 57 can be recognized in liver parenchymal cells—microvesicular and large droplet (macrovesicular) fatty change—though such clear-cut demarcations may not always be evident.[13] *Microvesicular fatty change* is seen as numerous small fat droplets or vesicles in the hepatocyte cytoplasm without any overt alterations in the nuclear morphology or location. The nucleus remains essentially in the center of the cell, unlike in large droplet fatty change where the nucleus is eccentrically located or peripherally displaced. The *large droplet fatty change* typically presents as a large single fatty vacuole occupying the entire hepatocyte cytoplasm, displacing the cytoplasm and the nucleus. The cytoplasm frequently appears as a ring at the periphery of the large fatty vacuole, and the nucleus is pushed to one corner, giving the cell a "signet-ring" appearance. The cells with large droplet fatty change are usually larger than normal. The microvesicular fatty change signifies acute toxic hepatocellular injury, whereas the large droplet fatty change is chronic, seen in malnutrition and chronic alcohol abuse. Fatty change in liver is reversible; nonetheless continued fatty metamorphosis caused by chronic alcohol intake can cause liver cell death.

Fatty change can also occur in other organs such as heart and kidney in severe anemia and chronic protein-calorie malnutrition. Multiorgan fatty metamorphosis (liver, heart, and kidney) is seen in children with Reye's syndrome.

Fatty change, or steatosis, at the cellular level should be distinguished from fatty infiltration occurring in some tissues and organs. Infiltration by fat cells, or adipocytes, in the interlobular space in pancreas and between muscle fibers in skeletal and cardiac muscle produces some commonly encountered examples of fatty infiltration.

Glycogen and carbohydrates

Pathologic accumulations of glycogen occur in the tissues of patients with diabetes mellitus in whom the normal cellular uptake of glucose is impaired. Excessive storage of glycogen is also found in genetic diseases in which there is absence of one or another of the enzymes that constitute the Embden-Meyerhof glycolytic pathway, or when an abnormally structured glycogen is synthesized that cannot be degraded by glycolytic enzymes. Intracellular accumulations of glycogen impart a vacuolated appearance to the cytoplasm. Since accumulations of glycogen morphologically resemble those of water *(hydropic swelling)* and fat (triglyceride under the light microscope), one of the following tests is necessary to establish that the deposit is glycogen: (1) application of the periodic acid–Schiff test in which glycogen is stained a reddish purple (tissues previously digested with diastase to digest glycogen serve as negative controls) or (2) quantitative analysis of the glycogen content of affected tissues. Massive intracellular deposits of glycogen occurring in glycogen storage disease cause affected organs such as the liver, kidney, or heart to be greatly enlarged and their function to be compromised.

In diabetes mellitus, glycogen deposits are encountered in the epithelium of the distal segment of the proximal convoluted renal tubules and the descending loop of Henle, hepatocytes, beta cells of the pancreatic islets, and cardiac muscle. Accumulation in the kidney occurs when the degree of glycosuria leads to levels of glucose in the glomerular filtrate that exceed the rate at which glucose is reabsorbed by epithelial cells of the renal tubules.

Excessive intracellular deposits of glycogen develop in patients with genetic disorders, designated as glycogen storage diseases, characterized by lysosomes with specific enzyme deficiencies that render them incapable of metabolizing glycogen. Abnormal metabolites accumulate in neurons of the central nervous system, as well as parenchymal cells of the liver, kidney, and heart. As in the other storage diseases attributable to gene defects, involvement may become so severe that it is incompatible with life.

Protein and proteinaceous products

Accumulation of globular and filamentous proteins within the cells is not a common occurrence. When proteins are abnormal, they tend to accumulate within the cell in appreciable amounts; the rate of accumulation exceeds the proteolytic degradation or capacity to excrete. A typical example of protein droplet accumulation is observed in the proximal convoluted tubular epithelium of the kidney in severe proteinuria. In nephrotic syndrome and other conditions where there is excess leakage of protein from the glomerular capillaries, some of it is reabsorbed by the lining epithelium of the proximal tubules by pinocytosis. The reabsorbed protein accumulates within the lysosomes and appears as eosinophilic hyaline granules by light microscopy.

Mallory's alcoholic hyaline (Mallory body) in hepatocytes is an example of intracellular protein accumulation in which cytokeratin filaments (intermediate filaments) accumulate as dense intermingled, serpentine aggregates in the cytoplasm (Fig. 17-4). These appear as amorphous eosinophilic masses at the light microscopic level. Mallory bodies are characteristic of alcoholic liver disease. Nonetheless, they are seen also in many other conditions, such as hepatocellular carcinomas, Wilson's hepatolenticular degeneration, Indian childhood cirrhosis of the liver, and others. Mallory bodies are also seen in hepatocytes in response to cytoskeletal damaging chemicals such as colchicine, phalloidin, and griseofulvin. The classical *neurofibrillary tangle* found in the brain in Alzheimer's disease is also an example of filamentous inclusion, consisting of a complex of neurofilaments and microtubule-associated proteins.

One classic example of intracellular protein accumulation is alpha-1-antitrypsin deficiency, an autosomal recessive disorder in which an abnormal alpha-1-antitrypsin is synthesized by the hepatocytes. In this condition, a mutation is responsible for a single amino acid substitution of Glu342 to Lys342. This mutant protein in misfolded and cannot be excreted from the rough endoplasmic reticulum, resulting in massive globular accumulations within the cytoplasm of liver cells. Hepatocellular death, cellular regeneration, and fibrosis ensue, eventually resulting in the development of cirrhosis of the liver and in some children hepatocellular carcinomas (see Chapters 14 and 57).

Amyloid

Amyloid deposition is associated with advanced aging and with a variety of chronic diseases, especially those accompanied by chronic infection and inflammation, disturbances of immune and autoimmune reactions, excessive tissue breakdown, wasting, and certain neoplasms.[25] These varied disorders can lead to cell damage and death (see Chapter 20).

Urate

In mammals the purine moieties of nucleic acids and nucleotides are catabolized and appear in urine as uric acid or allantoin.[26,27] In humans and hominoid primates, uric acid is the major end product of purine catabolism because of the absence of urate oxidase (uricase) attributable to deleterious mutations in the gene.[28] As a result uric acid is the end product of purine metabolism in the human and in hominoid primates. Other mammals have urate oxidase in the liver and excrete allantoin as the end product. Dalmatian dogs, though possessing urate oxidase, excrete uric acid because of a defect in the renal tubular reabsorption of uric acid.

In humans, uric acid is present as the monosodium salt in plasma at pH 7.4, and its levels approach the saturation point. The solubility of monosodium urate in body fluid is approximately 6.4 mg/dl. In general the serum urate concentration is quite stable, with the average being approximately 5 mg/dl in postpubertal males and 4.1 mg/dl in postpubertal females. Although the intake of foods rich in nucleoprotein, such as liver, thymus, pancreas, and certain fish, tends to increase the serum urate concentration whereas the restriction of such foods tends to reduce it, the influence of exogenous purine on the serum urate concentration is considered minor. There is a complex interrelated balance among the production of purine nucleotides, catabolism of purine-containing compounds to produce free purine, oxidation of purine to uric acid by xanthine oxidase, tubular reabsorption of urate, and finally tubular secretion of urate. Disturbances of this balance can result in hyperuricemia and deposition of sodium urate crystals in the tissues, leading to painful acute arthritis, chronic gouty arthritis, tophus formation, and nephritis. Hyperuricemia is the cardinal biochemical feature of the group of clinical disorders collectively referred to as "gout." Ninety-five percent of the cases occur in males.

Persistent hyperuricemia results in the deposition of urate in tissues, cell injury, and an inflammatory reaction.[27] Microcrystals of monosodium urate are phagocytized by leukocytes and eventually enter lysosomes. This is followed by increased permeability of the lysosomal membrane, which leads to leakage of hydrolytic enzymes. Since urate crystals are not degradable by lysosomal enzymes, they remain after the digestion of dead cells and cellular debris. Labilization of lysosomes may play an important pathogenetic role in chronic gout, particularly in the severe damage that occurs in the joint space and articular surfaces of joints. The crystals of monosodium urate initiate an inflammatory reaction by virtue of their physical presence in the interstitial fluid and tissues. Urate crystals cause the emigration of inflammatory cells to crystalline deposits in tissues and tissue spaces by activating the complement system. The combination of these events precipitates the clinically well-known severe inflammatory reaction seen in acute bouts of gout. These are characterized by the development of hot, swollen, and very painful joints, especially those of the great toe. The most effective drug for treatment of an acute attack of gout is the plant alkaloid colchicine, which is a potent stabilizer of the lysosomal membrane and, furthermore, inhibits leukocyte motility and function by interfering with microtubules in the cytoplasm.

Continued deposition of urate results in the formation of characteristic tophi; these are firm, nodular, subcutaneous deposits of urate crystals surrounded by foreign-body giant cells and fibrosis. When such deposits are preserved by fixation of tissue in absolute alcohol, urate crystals can be demonstrated as brilliantly doubly refractile crystals by polarized light (birefringence). They can also be demonstrated by a silver-containing stain as brown-black crystals. Urate deposition tends to occur in relatively avascular tissues, such as cartilage, epiphyseal bone, and periarticular structures. In chronic gouty arthritis, both cartilage and subchondral bone are destroyed. Proliferation of fibrous tissue and marginal bone tissue leads finally to crippling immobilization of the joint. Urate deposits also occur in the kidney, leading to severe renal damage. Crystals of monosodium urate monohydrate are needle shaped and are arranged radially in small, sheaflike clusters (Fig. 17-5). Calcific material may be deposited in the matrix, rendering such deposits radiopaque. The tissues in which urate deposits commonly occur are those rich in mucopolysaccharides. Some authorities have suggested that the release of lysosomal enzymes from leukocytes may alter protein-mucopolysaccharide conjugates in connective tissues and so urates are preferentially deposited in this matrix.

A mouse model for hyperuricemia and gout has been developed by disruption of the urate oxidase gene in the mouse by homologous recombination in embryonic stem cells. Unlike the human situation, urate oxidase deficiency in mice causes pronounced hyperuricemia and urate nephropathy.

Pigments

Pigments are colored substances present in most living forms, including humans, and are widely distributed in our environment both as pollutants and as artifacts of cultural practices such as the smoking of tobacco and the tattooing of skin. Pigments are generally classified into two broad categories: (1) *endogenous pigments,* which are normal constituents of cells and tissues, such as tyrosine and tryptophan-derived pigments, such as melanin, argentaffin substances, and adrenochromes; hemoproteins, which include porphyrins, hemoglobin, and hemosiderin (ferritin); and lipid-rich pigments such as lipofuscin and ceroid; and (2) *exogenous pigments* introduced into the body from without, such as anthracotic pigments, mineral dusts containing silica and oxides of iron, ingested iron, lead, and silver salts, and the various pigments that are used in tattooing the skin.

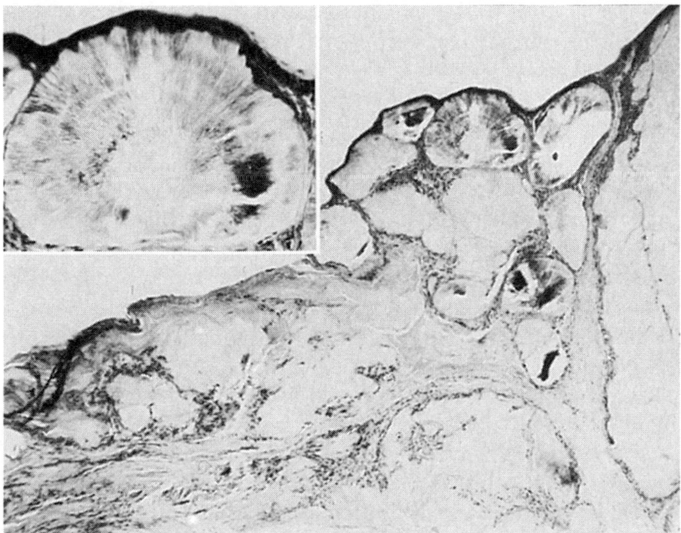

Fig. 17-5 Deposits of urate crystals in connective tissue of skin in patient with gout. Large nodular deposits are surrounded by thin strands of connective tissue with inflammatory foci. *Inset,* Higher magnification of a deposit shows radial arrays of urate crystals.

Melanin. Melanin (derived from the Greek word *melas,* meaning 'black') is a brown-black pigment synthesized by melanocytes from tyrosine. In humans, as in lower animals (the ink of cuttlefish and the cutaneous pigment cells of some animals), melanin serves a protective function. The radioprotective function of melanin in humans is well recognized. The skin of individuals adapted to long exposure to sunlight contains much more melanin than does the skin of those living in northern latitudes where such exposure is much less. This is believed to be an important factor in the widely differing incidences of skin cancer in these two population groups; skin cancer, which is virtually unknown among blacks, is a common neoplasm in fair-skinned whites. Measurements of sheets of stratum corneum for their effectiveness in screening out ultraviolet radiation have shown that such material derived from blacks is much more effective than that from less-pigmented people. Ultraviolet radiation, which stimulates the synthesis of melanin, is also highly absorbed by the pigment as part of the protective mechanism. In addition, since melanin's properties indicate that it is a stable free-radical scavenger and that its free-radical content increases after exposure to ultraviolet radiation, it may protect by capturing injurious free radicals formed by the action of ultraviolet rays on skin.

Melanin is formed by the oxidation of tyrosine to dihydroxyphenylalanine (dopa), a reaction catalyzed by tyrosinase, a copper-containing enzyme. Dopa is further oxidized to indole-5,6-quinone (dopachrome), which in turn is converted by oxidation-reduction to 5,6-dihydroxyindole, which is polymerized to a highly insoluble substance.

A generalized increase in skin melanin commonly occurs with continued exposure to sunlight; more rarely it is seen in persons with Addison's disease, an adrenocortical insufficiency resulting from destruction of the adrenal cortex. The mechanism by which melanogenesis is stimulated in such cases is an interesting facet of comparative endocrinology. In the lower animals, melanin formation is under control of a polypeptide hormone called melanin-stimulating hormone (MSH), which is localized in the pars intermedia of the pituitary. Its existence has not been unequivocally established in humans, in whom melanogenesis appears to be stimulated by adrenocorticotropic hormone (ACTH). The loss of adrenocortical hormones in Addison's disease leads to a loss of feedback control of ACTH secretion, and so it continues to be secreted at high levels. The melanin-stimulating properties of ACTH are no doubt related to the fact that a segment of the molecule bears a strong chemical homology to MSH through an identical amino acid sequence.

Increased melanogenesis is also seen in patients with proliferative lesions of melanocytes, including benign nevi and malignant melanoma.

Albinism is an inherited disorder of melanin metabolism in which there is a decrease or absence of the pigment in the skin and choroid of the eye. It occurs in both lower animals and mammals, including humans. Careful histologic and ultrastructural studies of the skin of albinos have definitely established that although melanocytes are present and show an essentially normal structure and complement of cell organelles, including premelanosomes, the latter are devoid of melanin. The condition may be diffuse, involving all the skin, the eyes, and the hair, or it may be localized to a certain site or sites (piebalding). Such curious distributions are attributable to the fact that the genetic defect is limited to only a specific group or groups of precursor melanocytes that migrate during embryonic development from the neural crest to peripheral sites where albinism is localized. Patients with oculocutaneous albinism have poor vision and severe photophobia. The hair is blond, often with a slight reddish cast, and the skin is exquisitely sensitive to sunlight, becoming rapidly erythematous on exposure. Chronic exposure invariably leads to the development of precancerous lesions of the skin that ultimately evolve into squamous and basal cell cancers. Leukoderma is another condition in which amelanotic patches of skin develop. These progressively expanding lesions do not contain melanocytes. The cause of this condition is not known, but an autoimmune-based melanocyte death is postulated.

Hemosiderin. Iron enters the plasma from tissue stores, from the intestinal mucosa, and from reticuloendothelial cells, which remove and destroy aged and damaged red cells. Plasma iron then enters the bone marrow where it is used for synthesis of hemoglobin. Iron is stored in tissues in essentially two forms: *ferritin,* which is not apparent with light microscopy but is visualized with electron microscopy as a tetrad aggregation of intensely electron-dense particles, and *hemosiderin,* which is composed of large, irregular aggregates of ferritin that are insoluble and appear as coarse, brown cytoplasmic granules. The granules can be demonstrated to contain ferric iron because they form a deep blue product, ferric ferrocyanide, on reaction of tissue with an acid solution of potassium ferrocyanide (Prussian blue reaction). The equilibrium between storage and plasma iron depends on the degree of transferrin saturation by iron. Low plasma-iron levels and reduced saturation shift the equilibrium so that iron is mobilized from stores to the plasma; when the converse is true, iron moves from plasma to tissue stores.

Local accumulations of hemosiderin *(hemosiderosis)* occur regularly around areas of bruising and hemorrhage and in lungs and spleen subjected to the protracted congestion that accompanies recurrent heart failure. In each instance the pigment is localized in cells of the reticuloendothelial system. In the lungs hemosiderin-laden macrophages are appropriately referred to as "heart failure cells." The pigment imparts a deep brown color to tissues and organs when it is present in high concentrations. The generalized form of iron accumulation attributable to systemic overload of iron, manifesting as excessive hemosiderin deposits in parenchymal cells and leading in the long run to cell injury and cell death, is called *hemochromatosis* (Fig. 17-6). Iron overload can be either *primary (hereditary) hemochromatosis* because of a genetic abnormality in iron absorption, or *secondary hemochromatosis* because of an acquired iron overload. In primary hemochromatosis, as much as 80 g of iron can accumulate in the body by 40 or 50 years of age because of abnormal iron absorption from the intestine. This condition is characterized by the micronodular (pigmentary) cirrhosis of liver, bronze discoloration of the skin, and diabetes mellitus. Secondary hemochromatosis is most commonly encountered in individuals who have received repeated blood transfusions or more rarely after prolonged parenteral administration of iron; it can also occur in patients with chronic ineffective erythropoiesis (such as thalassemia major), presumably from increased absorption of dietary iron across the duodenal mucosa. Alcohol ingestion when carried to extremes can lead to hemosiderosis because of the augmentation of iron uptake by alcohol; wines, which are rich in iron, place the alcoholic in double jeopardy. In the South African Bantu there is an added interesting facet in that the alcoholic beverages *(kaffir beer)* are conventionally prepared in iron pots, which probably serve as an abundant source of additional dietary iron (estimated to be as high as 100 mg per day). Although iron deposition in hemosiderosis is initially limited to the reticuloendothelial system, with time the parenchymal cells of the liver, kidney, and heart are also affected, and the condition becomes clinically and pathologically indistinguishable from primary hemochromatosis.

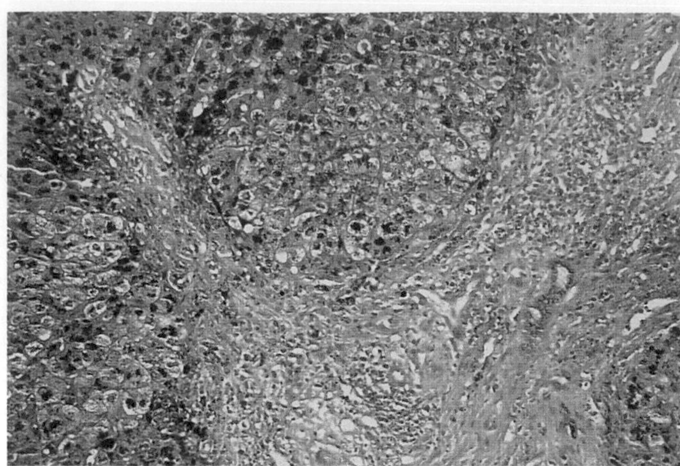

Fig. 17-6 Hemochromatosis. A Prussian blue stain for iron demonstrates considerable hemosiderin in cells in a cirrhotic liver.

Iron accumulation in tissues is common in chronic alcoholics, but alcohol consumption may occasionally help to unmask a genetic predisposition to primary hemochromatosis. In general, iron accumulation in alcoholism remains confined to the reticuloendothelial system, and hepatic scarring is more prominent than tissue accumulation of iron, whereas in primary hemochromatosis the reverse is true. Occasionally, however, a precise diagnosis is difficult.

Hematin. Hematin is a brown-black pigment derived from hemoglobin. Although its precise composition has not yet been determined, it is known to contain heme iron in the ferric form. The pigment is associated most commonly with a severe hemolytic crisis after transfusion of incompatible blood or chronic parasitization of red blood cells by malarial protozoa. It is usually found in the cytoplasm of reticuloendothelial cells. This pigment is not stained by the Prussian blue reaction despite the presence of ferric iron; this anomaly is believed to be attributable to the presence of an as yet unknown material, perhaps a protein that has formed a complex with the iron so that it is unable to react.

Bilirubin. Bilirubin is a non–iron-containing yellow pigment derived from the porphyrin ring of the heme moiety of hemoglobin; it is a product of red blood cell destruction by cells of the reticuloendothelial system. Bilirubin is essentially water insoluble and is kept in solution in blood plasma by binding to albumin. Since it is formed normally as a result of the turnover of red cells, there is an efficient pathway in the body for its metabolic conversion and ultimate excretion. Circulating

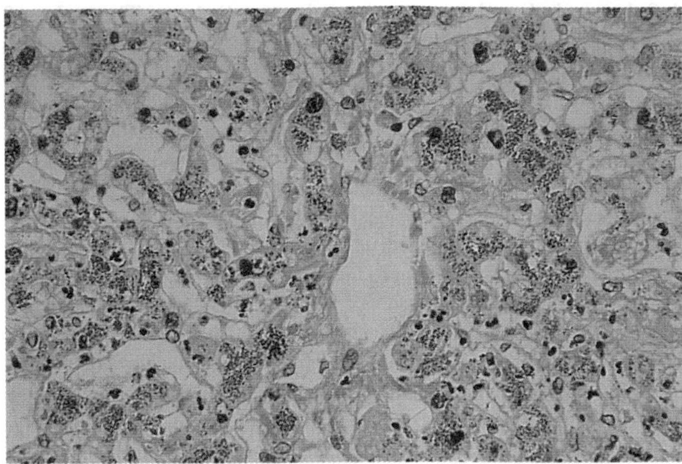

Fig. 17-7 Lipofuscin granules in liver in a 90-year-old male. Notice the fine golden cytoplasmic granules in hepatocytes.

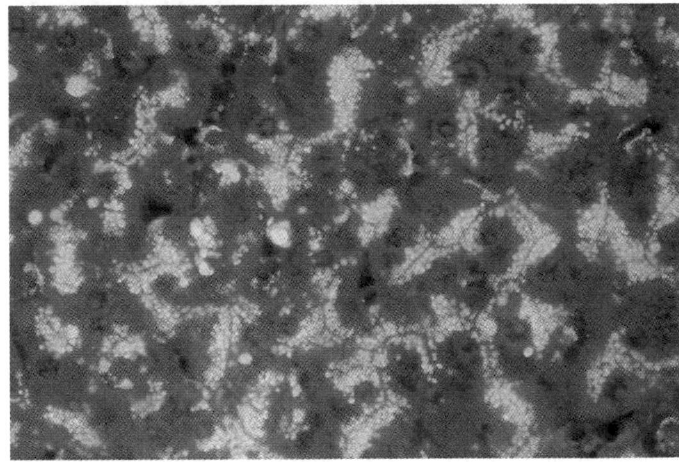

Fig. 17-8 Autofluorescence of lipofuscin in liver parenchymal cells.

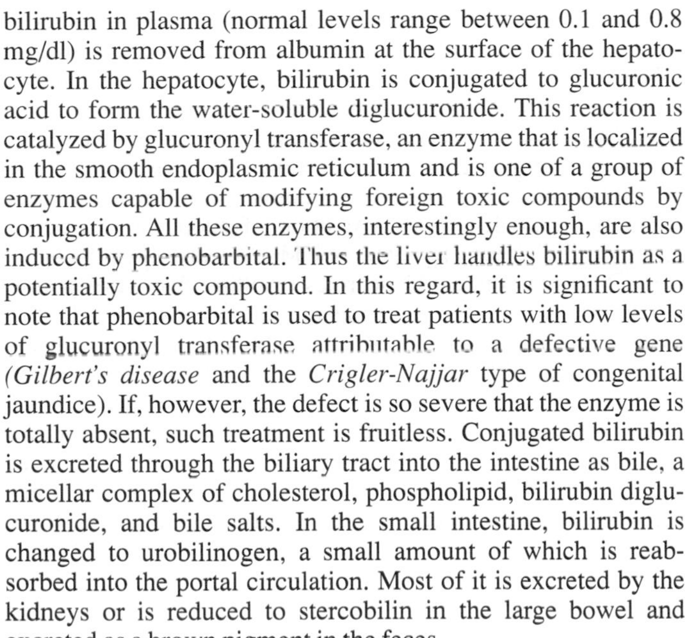

bilirubin in plasma (normal levels range between 0.1 and 0.8 mg/dl) is removed from albumin at the surface of the hepatocyte. In the hepatocyte, bilirubin is conjugated to glucuronic acid to form the water-soluble diglucuronide. This reaction is catalyzed by glucuronyl transferase, an enzyme that is localized in the smooth endoplasmic reticulum and is one of a group of enzymes capable of modifying foreign toxic compounds by conjugation. All these enzymes, interestingly enough, are also induced by phenobarbital. Thus the liver handles bilirubin as a potentially toxic compound. In this regard, it is significant to note that phenobarbital is used to treat patients with low levels of glucuronyl transferase attributable to a defective gene (*Gilbert's disease* and the *Crigler-Najjar* type of congenital jaundice). If, however, the defect is so severe that the enzyme is totally absent, such treatment is fruitless. Conjugated bilirubin is excreted through the biliary tract into the intestine as bile, a micellar complex of cholesterol, phospholipid, bilirubin diglucuronide, and bile salts. In the small intestine, bilirubin is changed to urobilinogen, a small amount of which is reabsorbed into the portal circulation. Most of it is excreted by the kidneys or is reduced to stercobilin in the large bowel and excreted as a brown pigment in the feces.

Jaundice is a condition in which the level of bilirubin in plasma is greater than 2 mg/dl and the skin and scleras are yellow. The organs of patients with jaundice are deeply stained, being yellow early and becoming dark green in more protracted cases. Bilirubin is present in cells as dark mahogany brown to green droplets; in liver, bile fills the sinusoids, canaliculi, and ductules. Because of its lipid solubility and structure, bilirubin has the potential for inducing cell injury, a fact that has been documented clinically, especially in the case of kernicterus. *Kernicterus* occurs in premature infants with severe Rh incompatibility or infection; in this condition, very high levels of bilirubin exert toxic effects on neurons in the basal ganglia. This occurs because the blood-brain barrier in newborn infants, unlike that in adults, is permeable to bilirubin. In obstructive jaundice the kidneys are intensely bile stained with bile casts in the renal tubules and renal tubular damage. This condition is called *cholemic nephrosis*. However, the precise mechanism or mechanisms by which cytotoxicity occurs are not clear. In the body, albumin has a significant protective effect by binding free bilirubin, a fact amply supported by experimental studies in which it was shown that albumin-bound bilirubin is nontoxic to tissue-culture cells and that albumin is capable of extracting significant amounts of cell-bound bilirubin from such cells. Free bilirubin exerts two effects—uncoupling of oxidative phosphorylation and a loss of cell proteins—suggestive of a primary effect on the inner membrane of mitochondria and other cell membranes, including the plasma membrane. Clearly, that one does not encounter overt evidence of significant cell injury in most cases of jaundice is probably the result of the protective effects of serum albumin and conjugation.

Lipofuscin. Lipofuscin is an insoluble lipid pigment present in cells of elderly persons and those with malnutrition or a chronic wasting disease. It is also known as "wear-and-tear," or "aging," pigment. It is a golden-brown intracellular granular pigment found in hepatocytes, cardiocytes, and neurons (Figs. 17-7) It represents the accumulation of indigestible membrane material in lysosomes after autophagy. Ingested material may accumulate when the rate of autophagy exceeds the capacity for digestion or when it has been chemically altered, as by lipid peroxidation, which would render it resistant to enzymatic degradation. Organs containing large amounts of lipofuscin are deep brown; in the heart, this is referred to as "brown atrophy." This condition appears to correlate directly with age; however, since such pigment can also accumulate rapidly with extensive tissue wasting, it seems prudent not to attribute its presence strictly to aging. Lipofuscin exhibits yellowish autofluorescence (Fig. 17-8).

Exogenous pigments (mineral dusts). The presence of considerable amounts of inhaled pigmented particulate materials in the lungs of most persons, especially those in urban centers, attests to the contaminated state of the environment.

Acute or chronic occupational or environmental exposure to harmful dust particles can lead to cell injury (see Chapter 49). *Pneumoconiosis* results from an accumulation of dust in the lungs, and such dusts usually produce fibrogenic reaction in the lung. Pneumoconiosis of coal workers is a serious condition encountered in anthracite coal miners. It develops over a period of years and leads to excessive deposition of black pigment in the lung, the impairment of respiratory function, and the development of emphysema. This indicates that the

Necrosis

Necrosis (Gr. *nekrōsis,* 'deadness') is the cumulative morphologic range of changes indicative of cell death in a living tissue or an organism and is caused by the progressive degradative action of hydrolytic enzymes on a cell or cells and on tissues. If the injury is sufficiently prolonged or severe, it exceeds the threshold of irreversibility and results in death of the injured cell. Necrosis can affect a single cell or groups of cells or part of an organ. In the extreme case, especially as the result of a severe toxic or ischemic episode, an entire organ may become necrotic. The process of necrosis reflects the near simultaneous enzymatic degradation of the cellular organelles, resulting in a loss of structural integrity, and the denaturation of proteins and other macromolecules. Necrotic cells display features of cytoplasmic disintegration with disruption of plasma membrane and organellar membranes. The early or immediate nuclear changes in necrosis range from *pyknosis,* where the nuclei show shrinkage, and *karyorrhexis,* which manifests as nuclear fragmentation, to *karyolysis* characterized by diminished or disappearing basophilia leading to ghost nuclei. During later stages of necrosis, the nuclei become completely indistinct and unrecognizable. The degradative enzymes are frequently those released from the lysosomes of the irreversibly damaged or dead cells resulting in autolysis or self-digestion. In contrast to apoptosis in which cell dissolution does not elicit an inflammatory reaction, the necrotic tissue provokes an inflammatory response and the recruited leukocytes and macrophages further contribute to the enzymatic degradation of the necrotic tissue. Such a process with tissue destruction and dissolution facilitated by exogenous cells is referred to as "heterolysis" (in contrast to autolysis). Morphologic variants of necrosis include coagulative necrosis, liquefactive necrosis, caseous necrosis, and enzymatic fat necrosis. This morphologic distinction is of some value in ascertaining whether the necrotic process is predominantly attributable to protein denaturation *(coagulative necrosis)* or enzymatic digestion *(liquefactive necrosis).* The type of necrosis that follows cell death is in part determined by the richness of the lysosomal enzymes in a given cell type or organ; that is, coagulative necrosis is typically encountered in the myocardium of the heart after an ischemic injury, whereas in the central nervous system the necrosis is frequently liquefactive. Finally, the type of necrosis occasionally provides a clue about the underlying cause of necrosis, such as caseous necrosis being observed usually in fungal and mycobacterial infections.

Coagulative necrosis

In humans, this type of necrosis is most frequently caused by irreversible focal injury after sudden cessation of blood flow (ischemia) in organs such as the heart, kidney, and spleen. Less common causes of coagulative necrosis are cell death by potent bacterial toxins, phenol, mercurials, and other corrosive chemicals. The process of coagulation necrosis has been well documented in ischemic injury to the myocardium. Irreversibly injured myocytes explosively swell and contract with reoxygenation. This event is typically described as contraction band necrosis (Fig. 17-12). Foci of coagulation necrosis vary in their gross appearance depending on their age. The tissue has an opaque appearance likened to that of boiled meat and is dry. Fresh coagulation necrosis is pale, firm, and slightly swollen; as it progresses, it becomes more yellowish in color from increasing numbers of inflammatory cells and softer in consistency from autolysis (Fig. 17-13). Histologically, foci of early coagulation necrosis contain cells that are slightly more eosinophilic than normal with little or no alteration of cellular detail. As necrosis progresses, dead cells are swollen; their cytoplasm appears densely eosinophilic as a result of granular debris of insoluble denatured proteins. The nuclei become indistinct in cells undergoing coagulative necrosis, and the cells resemble faint "ghost" outlines (Fig. 17-14). Eventually the necrotic focus becomes infiltrated with inflammatory cells, which participate in the digestion of dead cells (Fig. 17-15). This salvage process leaves behind residual cellular debris and sets the stage for repair of the tissue.

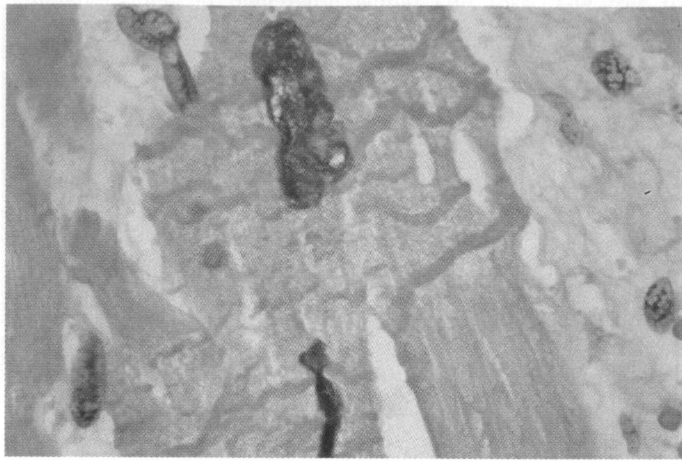

Fig. 17-12 Irreversible injury to myocardium. Contraction band necrosis in heart in patient who died of a "heart attack." Contraction bands form as a result of reperfusion of ischemic myocardium.

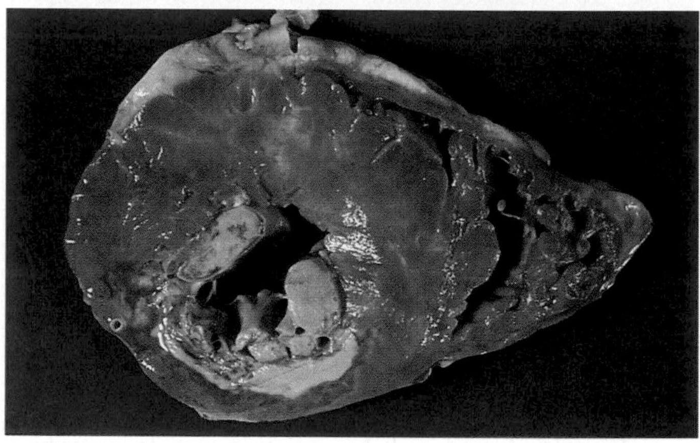

Fig. 17-13 Coagulative necrosis of myocardium of posterior wall of left ventricle of heart. A large anemic *(white)* infarct is readily apparent; notice also the necrosis of papillary muscle.

Liquefactive necrosis

The term *liquefactive necrosis* is applied to necrotic degradation of tissue that rapidly undergoes softening and liquefaction because of the action of hydrolytic enzymes. Proteolytic digestion of dead parenchymal, stromal, and extracellular matrix material by enzymes released from dead cells, invading leukocytes, and the plasma results in the liquefaction of necrotic tissue. Liquefactive necrosis is most characteristic in the central

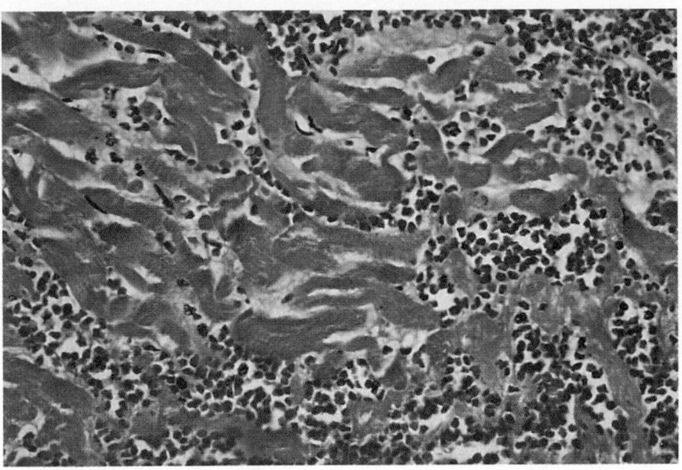

Fig. 17-14 Acute myocardial infarct (24 to 36 hours after ischemia). Coagulative necrosis of cardiac myocytes and extravasation of erythrocytes. The striations and nuclei of myocytes have disappeared.

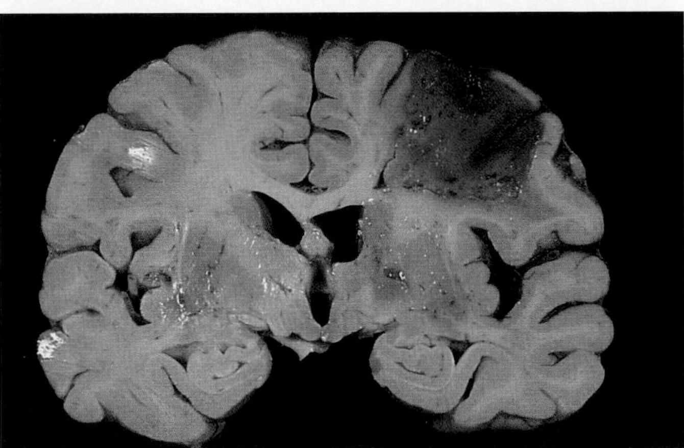

Fig. 17-16 Liquefacte necrosis of the brain developed at a large cerebral infarct caused by ischemia.

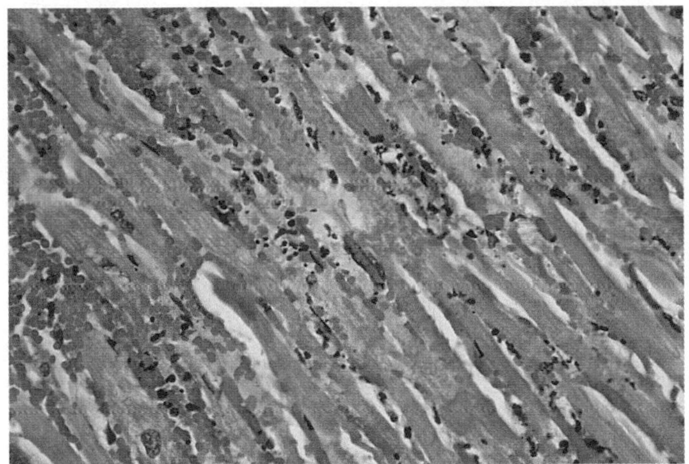

Fig. 17-15 Coagulate necrosis of myocardium (72 hours after myocardial infarction). Myocardial fibers are anucleate and lack normal cross striations. Notice the presence of an early neutrophilic inflammatory cell infiltrate. Presence of acute polymorphonuclear leukocytes indicate that myocardial cell death occurred during life.

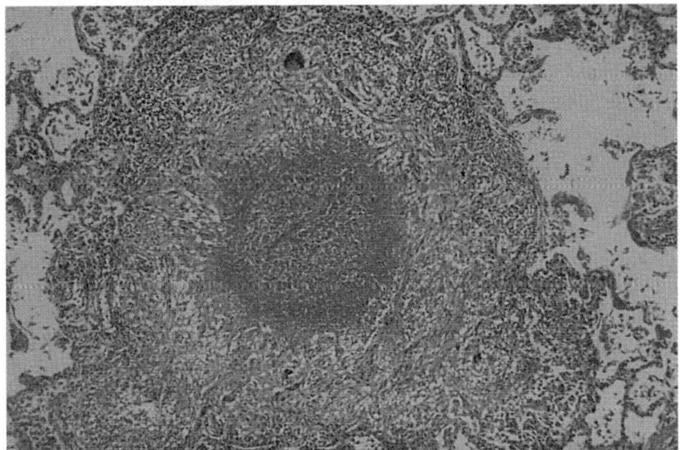

Fig. 17-17 Granuloma with central caseous necrosis typical of pulmonary tuberculosis.

nervous system after ischemic or hypoxic injury to the brain after arterial occlusion or after massive cerebral trauma, in which dead brain tissue is softened (encephalomalacia) and converted into a cystic fluid–filled space or spaces. Grossly the necrotic area of the brain is soft, and the center is liquefied. As time passes, there develops a cystic space, the walls of which are defined by nonnecrotic tissue. Histologically the content of the cystic space consists of necrotic cell debris among which can be seen glial cells containing phagocytized material. The cyst wall is lined by a network of proliferating capillaries and numerous glial cells (Fig. 17-16). Liquefactive necrosis is also commonly seen secondary to a bacterial infection of a devitalized tissue and in bacterial abscesses filled with collections of fluid pus consisting of necrotic bacteria, leukocytes, and degenerating tissue cells. Wet gangrene is also an example of liquefactive necrosis, where ischemic tissue (frequently in the lower extremity) is invaded by anaerobic bacteria such as *Clostridium* species with liquefaction of dead tissue by bacterial proteases.

Caseous necrosis

Caseous necrosis is a variant of coagulative necrosis most commonly encountered when cell death is attributable to certain mycobacteria (such as *Mycobacterium tuberculosis*) or fungal organisms (such as *Histoplasma capsulatum,* and coccidioidomycosis). Some degree of liquefactive necrosis is also encountered in the center of a large caseous necrotic lesion. Grossly, such foci are yellowish white and sharply circumscribed from the surrounding normal tissues. The necrotic tissue is soft, granular, and friable, reminiscent of dry cheese, hence the term *caseous*. Microscopically, the caseous necrosis appears as an amorphous, eosinophilic, granular focus that is surrounded by inflammatory cells, epithelioid macrophages, and the Langerhans' type of multinucleate giant cells (Figs. 17-17 and 17-18).

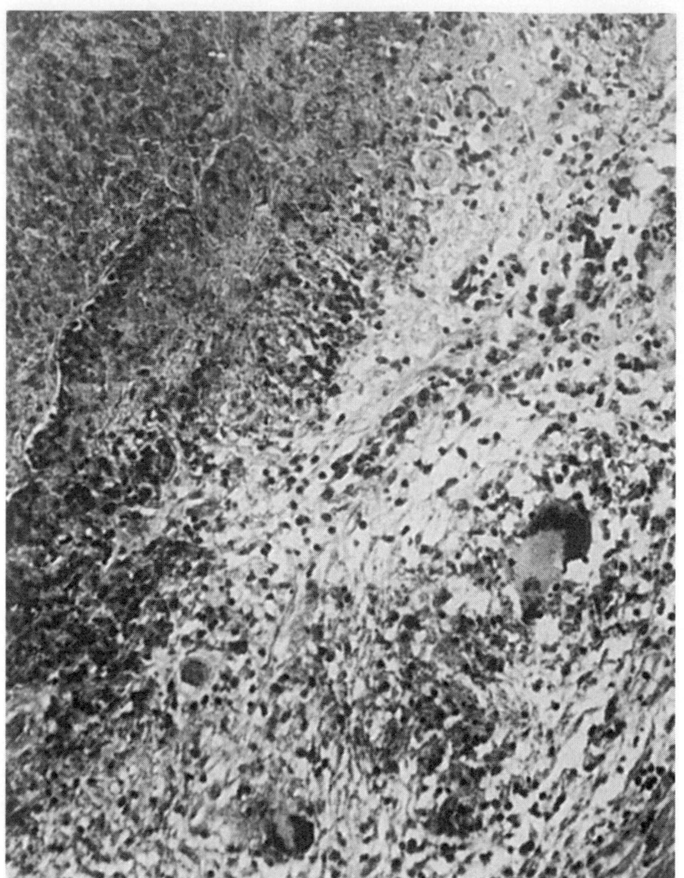

Fig. 17-18 Caseous necrosis in a patient with widespread pulmonary tuberculosis; area of necrosis appears at the right with an adjacent zone of inflammation including multinucleated Langerhans' type of giant cells.

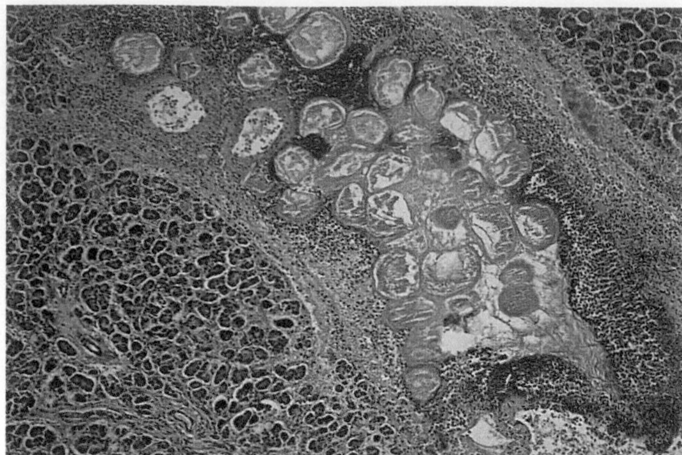

Fig. 17-19 Fat necrosis of pancreas. Interlobular adipocytes are necrotic; these are surrounded by acute inflammatory cells.

The necrosis is, in part, attributable to the severe histotoxic macrophage–mediated hypersensitivity reaction directed toward high molecular weight lipoid substances, such as wax D and tuberculoprotein, present in the cell walls of tubercle bacilli (see Chapter 25). Because of limited growth of capillary-sized blood vessels from the surrounding normal tissues into the area of necrosis, intense scarring around such foci, and the inhibition of intracellular hydrolytic enzymes by certain chemical components of mycobacteria, the caseous material remains in situ in tissues for long periods. The protracted process of caseous necrosis usually leads to pathologic calcification.

Enzymic fat necrosis

Enzymatic fat necrosis is peculiar to adipose tissue, usually in adipose tissue contiguous to the pancreas. Acute pancreatitis results in leakage of lipase and other proteases secondary to acute injury of pancreatic acinar tissue, as occurs after obstruction of pancreatic ducts. When the extent of pancreatic injury is severe, fat necrosis may be widespread, affecting extra-abdominal adipose tissue such as that in the anterior mediastinum and bone marrow. The necrotic foci consist of necrotic fat cells in which the triglycerides have been hydrolyzed by pancreatic lipase into fatty acids and glycerol. The fatty acids are subsequently converted into soaps (saponification) by reaction with calcium, magnesium, and sodium ions. As the concentration of calcium and magnesium in soaps increases in the necrotic cells and tissue, the deposits become firmer and chalky white. In severe cases of acute pancreatitis the peripancreatic, omental, and abdominal fat may show extensive areas of fat necrosis because of the release of activated pancreatic enzymes into the peritoneal cavity. In such instances, these necrotic areas of fat serve as calcium sinks leading to the development of serum hypocalcemia and in the extreme can result in tetany. Grossly, fat necrosis appears as firm minute yellow-white deposits in peripancreatic and mesenteric adipose tissue. Histologically, necrotic fat cells are distinguishable as pale outlines, and their cytoplasm is filled with an amorphous-appearing, faintly basophilic material (soap) (Fig. 17-19). Traumatic fat necrosis is seen in the adipose tissue of breast, thigh, and other locations, where the physical blunt injury can cause damage to the adipocytes with release of triglycerides and subsequent hydrolysis by the tissue or serum lipases. The sequence of events leading to enzymatic fat necrosis in a case of acute pancreatitis are as follows: Necrosis of acinar cells → Release and activation of lipase and other zymogens → Cell injury and death of fat cells → Hydrolysis of triglycerides → Formation of glycerol and fatty acids → Mineralization of fatty acids → Saponification (formation of soaplike chalky material).

Gangrenous necrosis

Gangrenous necrosis is not a different category of necrosis but a clinically distinct variant of coagulation necrosis. It is characteristically localized to the soft tissues of the lower extremities (leg, foot, toes) that have been compromised by protracted hypoxia and ischemia, which leads indeed to coagulation necrosis. However, since the extent of vascular occlusion is frequently global in the lower limbs, which impedes or prevents the migration of leukocytes in to the areas of coagulation necrosis, it is called *gangrenous necrosis* because the dead tissue is not digested and removed but remains mummified. We recognize two types of gangrenous necrosis: *dry gangrene,* when the necrotic mummified tissue remains desiccated as a result of the lack of proteolytic enzymes, and *wet gangrene,* if the overlying skin is devitalized permitting the entry of bacteria, fluid, and leukocytes to cause extensive liquefaction.

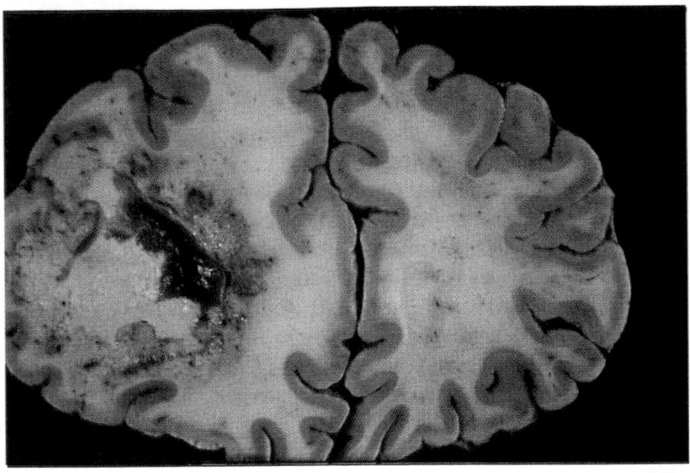

Fig. 17-20 Tumor necrosis. This tumor in the brain shows extensive necrosis in the center.

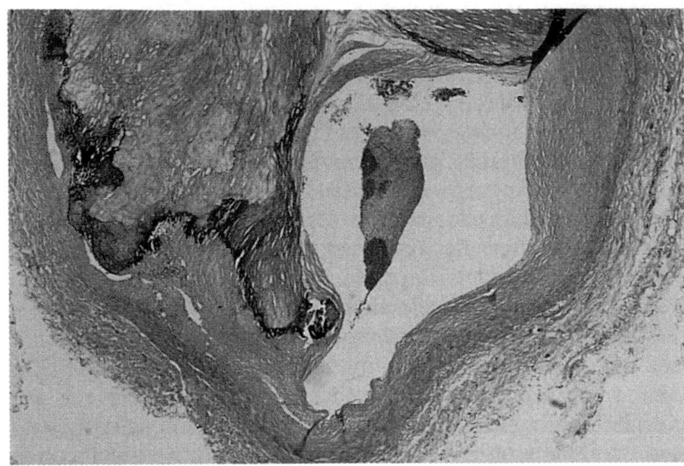

Fig. 17-21 Dystrophic calcification in atherosclerotic coronary artery.

Tumor necrosis

Cell death in tumors is frequently in the form of necrosis and is easily recognizable grossly in large tumors (Fig. 17-20). Apoptosis is also a recognizable feature in both small and large tumors and is amenable to quantitation using the immunolabeling methods aimed at recognizing the damaged DNA. Factors responsible for tumor cell death include hypoxia (in that "tumors outgrow their blood supply"); irregularities in the production of a tumor angiogenic factor or factors (TAF) resulting in the inability of neovascularization (angiogenesis) to keep "pace" with the growth rate of tumors; the action of cytotoxic T-cells and natural killer cells; elaboration of tumor necrosis factors (TNF) by activated monocytes/macrophages; the elaboration of apoptotic factors by dying tumor cells; and therapeutic interventions. Thus the extent of necrosis encountered in any given tumor is based on the interplay of many factors.

Pathologic calcifications

Abnormal deposition of calcium salts, together with trace quantities of iron, magnesium, and other mineral salts in cells and tissues that are normally not mineralized, is designated *pathologic (ectopic) calcification*. Calcification of dead and dying cells and tissues is a common finding in human pathologic conditions.[39] Pathologic calcification, when it occurs in a normal tissue and is not preceded by cell injury or cell death, is a relatively infrequent occurrence seen most commonly in hypercalcemic states. Pathologic calcification is subdivided into two categories: *dystrophic calcification* and *metastatic calcification*. In addition, cell injury and cell death in some specialized tissues, such as skeletal muscle, can initiate a process of cell proliferation and differentiation resulting in new bone formation.[40] This is referred to as *pathologic (ectopic) ossification*.

Dystrophic calcification

Dystrophic calcification occurs in dead, dying, or degenerating tissues and is generally associated with normal serum calcium levels. Tissue necrosis invariably precedes the process of dystrophic calcification. Calcium is deposited in necrotic tissues such as atheromatous plaques (Fig. 17-21), healing or healed tuberculous and fungal granulomas, old scars, degenerating and damaged heart valves and cusps, parasitic lesions (toxoplasmosis of brain and hydatid cysts), and degenerating tumors (leiomyoma, teratomas, ovarian cysts, squamous cell carcinomas) among others. Occasionally, a dead fetus in ectopic abdominal pregnancy may be completely calcified or ossified, appearing as a fossil (lithopedion, or 'stone child'). Dystrophic calcification appearing in a certain characteristic form (psammoma bodies) in some lesions may have diagnostic implications, as in papillary carcinomas of thyroid. Areas of dystrophic calcification appear grossly as fine or large gray granules with gritty or eggshell consistency. Large calcified lesions, especially calcified tuberculous or histoplasmotic lymph nodes, impart a feeling of a stone or calculus. Histologically, dystrophic calcification presents essentially a nondescript, amorphous, granular, or lamellated basophilic pattern in routine hematoxylin and eosin–stained tissue sections. Since calcium deposition is initiated in a dying or necrotic cell, the distinction of intracellular and extracellular calcium deposits in a dystrophic lesion becomes difficult. The mechanism of calcification in this entity is most likely a process of slow diffusion of calcium into the necrotic lesion leading to progressive accumulation. This mechanism is, in part, based on the fact that serum calcium levels are usually within normal limits in these individuals and that denatured proteins in dead or irreversibly damaged cells and tissues preferentially bind phosphate ions, which in turn react with calcium ions to form a precipitate of calcium phosphate. Thus, necrotic tissue serves as a calcium sink. Initiation of a calcium phosphate nidus usually occurs in mitochondria or microsomal vesicle and then progresses through crystal propagation.

Metastatic calcification

Metastatic calcification is a distinct entity of considerable clinicopathologic significance. Unlike in dystrophic calcification, in this form of pathologic calcification cell or tissue death is not prerequisite. Metastatic calcification occurs in normal tissues in pathophysiologic conditions associated with increased serum levels of inorganic phosphate ions (hyperphosphatemia) in extracellular milieus in disease states where there is hyperphosphatemia either alone or with hypercal-

extensive period of differentiation to carry on the numerous synthetic, catabolic, and transport functions characteristic of the liver in adults. The extent to which liver cells respond to the perturbation of hepatectomy can be emphasized if one recalls that in the normal liver in an adult less than 1% of the cells in the liver are synthesizing DNA at any one time, whereas at the peak of regeneration about 80% of the cells are in the cell-proliferation cycle and undergo DNA synthesis. The liver cell proliferation occurring after partial hepatectomy is coordinately regulated by changes in the expression of several growth factor genes (TGF–α, TGF–β, and HGF), early growth responsive genes (c–*fos*, c–*jun*, and c–*myc*), and cytokines such as TNF.[56]

This process can be arbitrarily divided into three phases: *initiation phase,* which prepares the cells to commit to DNA synthesis; *proliferative phase,* during which cells begin to synthesize the DNA and actively divide; and the *growth inhibitory phase,* which essentially senses that the restoration of liver cell mass has occurred and sets in motion the events to stop further cell proliferation. Evidence supports the view that priming for compensatory hyperplasia after partial hepatectomy is initiated by cytokines, metabolic disturbances, and immediate early growth–responsive genes. This is followed by the readily recognizable cell proliferation mediated mostly by growth factors such as TGF–α, HGF, and EGF (epidermal growth factor). The mitoinhibitory function during the third, or growth inhibition, phase in liver is mostly attributable to the elaboration of TGF–β by nonparenchymal cells of liver. Thus, compensatory hyperplasia occurring after partial hepatectomy is a well-orchestrated and precisely controlled process.

Hyperplasia also occurs as a response to injury when the injury has been sufficiently severe and prolonged to have caused cell death. The loss of cells in epithelial surfaces and in liver and kidney triggers DNA synthesis, which is followed by mitosis. The process by which cell loss is converted into a signal for augmented cell growth is a complex multistep process. In the case of the liver, liver cell regeneration resulting from injury and cell death caused, for example, by ccl_4, involves the production of specific growth factors that stimulate the remaining hepatocytes through a receptor-mediated series of intracellular events, to synthesize new cell components and ultimately divide to produce more liver cells. Regeneration of the renal tubules after injury with mercuric chloride has shown that the proliferative response leads to an increase in the rate of DNA synthesis. Increased mitoses become apparent about 20 hours after the administration of mercuric chloride and reach a peak on the third day. Proliferating epithelial cells rapidly reline the renal tubules and largely complete this stage by the fifth day. By the ninth day the mitotic index has returned to its normal preinjury level. The glomerular filtration rate drops to a low level by the fifth day and returns to normal by the ninth day. Tubular reabsorption does not return to normal levels until the twentieth day after the initial injury, an indication that considerable differentiation of the epithelial cells must occur before they are capable of effective transport.

In tissues exhibiting steady-state cell renewal, hyperplasia is also a very common occurrence and is invariably attributable to persistent mitogenic signals conveyed by decreased function or by some other pathologic process. In epidermis of skin and in gastrointestinal and respiratory mucosa chronic inflammatory conditions and other injurious insults cause persistent hyperplasia. Psoriasis, chronic eczematous dermatitis, calluses or corns, warts (verruca vulgaris), and ulcerative colitis are some of the examples of pathologic hyperplasia encountered in tissues where there is steady-state cell renewal. In these tissues not only is hyperplasia attributable to increased cell proliferation, but there also may be a concomitant decrease in cell differentiation and cell loss.

Of considerable relevance is the distinction between *mitogen-induced cell proliferation* and *compensatory cell proliferation.* The former is not preceded by death of some cells, whereas the latter is frequently triggered by the loss of some cells or part of a tissue. These two types of regenerative response are well characterized in liver in which compensatory hyperplasia is induced by partial hepatectomy or carbon tetrachloride administration, and primary mitogenic response is caused by certain hepatomitogens, namely, lead nitrate, ethylene dibromide, and certain potent peroxisome proliferators such as Wy-14643 and ciprofibrate. Although mitogen-induced primary cell proliferation is not known to increase the risk of cancer, the compensatory hyperplastic cell proliferation triggered by cell death is strongly implicated in the carcinogenic process. It is important to keep in mind that mitogenesis can predispose to increased mutagenic events in the replicating DNA of dividing cells. Rapidly proliferating cells are also more prone to mutagenic damage caused by chemical and other carcinogens.

Thus far we have limited our discussion of hyperplasia to instances of repair and regeneration. Neoplasia is a major condition in which hyperplastic growth plays a central role. Hyperplasia associated with neoplasia differs from that just described in that growth-regulatory mechanisms become dysregulated because of genetic changes in the cells. The growth advantage of neoplastic cells operates to the disadvantage of the host because it is often accompanied by either loss or abnormality of cell function and in the case of malignant tumors leads ultimately to death. The process of neoplasia is discussed in Chapter 24.

Hypoplasia

Hypoplasia in the strictest sense connotes a reduction in the size of an organ or tissue because of a reduction in the number of cells as a result of developmental perturbations. This definition implies that hypoplasia is congenital and can affect all organs or tissues during fetal development, whether they are composed primarily of nonreplaceable cells (heart, skeletal muscle, brain), conditionally dividing cells (liver, kidney, lung, pancreas), or steady-state renewing cell types (epidermis, gastrointestinal and respiratory mucosa, bone marrow). One such example is pulmonary hypoplasia in which there is incomplete or defective development of the lung, which results in reduced size attributable in part to diminished numbers of alveolar units. Pulmonary hypoplasia is attributable frequently to an associated malformation that compromises the thoracic space. This thwarts the lung development and manifests clinically as respiratory distress in full-term infants within minutes after birth.

Hypoplasia does not usually occur in adult tissues or organs. Any diminution in the size in adult life of a normally developed organ that is composed of either nonreplaceable or conditionally dividing cells, because of reductions in size or number of cells, indeed reflects atrophy and not hypoplasia. Nevertheless, in tissues with steady-state renewal such as epidermis or gastrointestinal mucosa, if reductions in cell number occur sometime during the adult life because of protracted physiologic or pathologic stimuli, such a change is sometimes referred to as *hypoplasia* instead of *atrophy*. Since these tissues consist of constantly renewing cell types, reductions in stem cell divisions as a result of attrition of these progenitor cells reduce the overall population density. Hypoplasia in the adult intestine may occur as a result of prolonged parenteral feeding leading to disuse hypoplasia or disuse atrophy of intestinal mucosa. A variety of chronic skin disease such as lupus erythematosus or lichen atrophicus also manifest hypoplasia because of reduced cell proliferation.

Metaplasia

Metaplasia (Gr. *metaplasis,* 'reconstruction, transformation') is a reversible process of transformation or transdifferentiation in which one type of differentiated cell type is replaced by another differentiated cell type usually in response to abnormal stimuli. Metaplasia presents as patches of ectopic tissue caused by disturbances in the cellular lineage in which precursor cells differentiate along a different pathway and not between two terminally differentiated cells themselves. For example, in the tracheobronchial mucosa, normally the basal stem cells divide and their progeny go through predicted patterns of differentiation to yield ciliated columnar cells and goblet cells. In chronic cigarette smokers, the irritation by the noxious ingredients present in the smoke causes a change in the normal differentiation process of the progenitor cells of the respiratory epithelium through a different pathway of differentiation to generate more resistant squamous epithelium. In essence metaplasia is a change in commitment of differentiation of precursor cells in a given tissue to form a different tissue. Such patches of metaplasia are reversible in due course after elimination of the causative factor. Nonetheless, in the context of cells that have attained definitive phenotypes of a particular kind, such as the squamous phenotype in respiratory epithelium in squamous metaplasia, the options for reversibility of a terminally differentiated squamous cell are limited. Consequently, squamous metaplastic patches are eliminated by loss of these differentiated squamous cells and by restoration of normal differentiation process or lineage in the respiratory epithelium.

Metaplastic changes occur in epithelium (epithelial metaplasia) as well as in connective tissue (connective tissue metaplasia) and are generally patchy in distribution. Epithelial metaplasia represents change of one type of epithelium to another type of epithelium, whereas connective tissue metaplasia refers to change of one type of connective tissue to another type of connective tissue. Metaplastic transformation of epithelium to connective tissue or vice versa, though possible, is rare. If it occurs at all, it has to be attributed to the presence in such tissues of multipotential stem cells that are capable of differentiating into both epithelial and mesenchymal derivatives.

Epithelial metaplasia is a common adaptive response and is usually associated with chronic irritation, cigarette smoking, infections, chronic inflammation, and vitamin A deficiency. Most or all surface epithelia are renewable tissues in which there is perpetual cell proliferation or turnover. In these tissues, it is believed that the stem cells and other progenitor cells divide, and their progeny go through a series of less differentiated to more differentiated phenotypes, ultimately developing into terminally differentiated cells, which are destined to die. Metaplastic epithelium is the culmination of a change in the differentiation pathway to which the stem cell progeny commit. *Squamous metaplasia* is the most common adaptive response that occurs in the respiratory tract as a result of chronic irritation by cigarette smoke; the mucous and ciliated epithelial cells are replaced by patches of stratified squamous epithelial cells. The squamous epithelium is more resistant than the normal ciliated respiratory epithelium of the tracheobronchial tree but is functionally inferior because it cannot perform the normal mucus-transport functions because of lack of cilia. Thus squamous metaplasia represents an attempt by the host to repair or prepare an epithelial tissue that has been damaged by environmental toxicants with a more resistant tissue. The evolution of the metaplastic process in the tracheobronchial tree in the chronic smoker commences with a proliferation of basal reserve cells into a multilayered epithelium that intervenes between the columnar epithelium and the basement membrane. These reserve cells do not mature into respiratory epithelium but differentiate into stratified squamous cell phenotype. Squamous metaplasia is also encountered in other locations such as pancreatic ducts (vitamin A deficiency, stones in the pancreatic ducts), gallbladder (mechanical irritation caused by gallstones), urinary bladder (urinary bladder calculi, chronic cystitis, parasitic infections such as schistosomiasis), intrahepatic bile ducts (chronic infections, liver flukes), and in the endocervix.

Squamous metaplasias may be capable of undergoing progressive evolutionary changes toward squamous cell carcinoma if the offending insult or insults persist. These changes include increasing degrees of nuclear abnormality, increase in the nuclear-cytoplasmic ratio, thickening of the nuclear membrane, increasing granularity, increasing hyperchromasia of the chromatin, enlarged and prominent nucleoli, atypical or disorganized orientation, and increased mitotic activity and dysplasia. Such an atypical and dysplastic metaplastic epithelium is generally believed to antedate the appearance of carcinoma in situ and the carcinoma of the lung. Thus, this metaplastic change appears to have an essential role in the histogenesis of squamous cell carcinomas in a tissue or organ that does not normally possess squamous epithelium.

Glandular metaplasia generally refers to a change of the squamous epithelium to glandular epithelium as in Barrett's esophagus, in which the stratified squamous epithelium of the esophagus is replaced by gastric columnar epithelium (Fig. 17-25). The development of Barrett's esophagus is attributed to chronic heartburn resulting in a reflux of acid contents of the stomach into the esophagus, causing injury to the squamous epithelium of esophagus. This necessitates the replacement of susceptible squamous epithelium of the lower third of esophagus with gastric acid–resistant glandular epithelium. Barrett's esophagus develops in 1 in 10 individuals with severe chronic heartburn, and in 10 years 1 in 10 of these with Barrett's esophagus develop adenocarcinoma of the esophagus. Glandular metaplasia of urothelium can occur in chronic cystitis or pyelitis. Nests of glandular epithelium, consisting of goblet cells and Paneth cells, give rise to cystitis glandularis. Another form of glandular metaplasia is the intestinal metaplasia in the stomach, associated with chronic gastric ulcers. In this condition there is essentially a complete transformation of gastric mucosa to small intestinal crypts, which may be eventually responsible for the development of carcinomas of the intestinal type in the stomach.

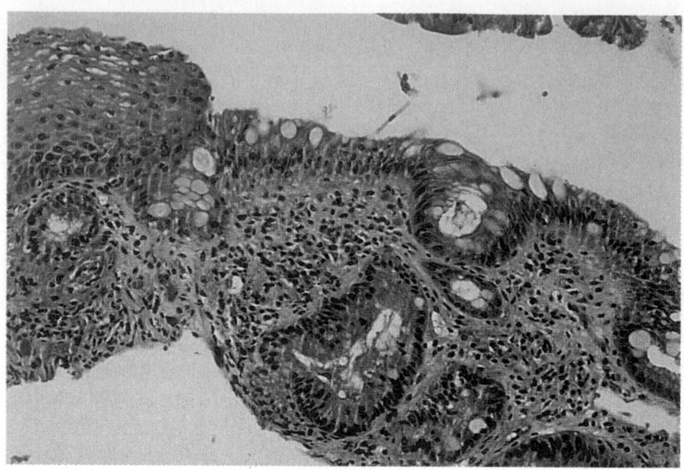

Fig. 17-25 Glandular metaplasia in Barrett's esophagus. In this condition the stratified squamous epithelium of esophagus is replaced by gastric mucosa.

Another type of unique metaplasia or transdifferentiation is the differentiation of hepatocytes in the pancreas. In rats subjected to chronic copper deficiency there is almost global loss of pancreatic acinar cells caused by apoptosis by about 8 to 10 weeks. Return to normal diet after depletion of pancreatic acinar cell population results in the proliferation of ductal and periductal cells, which then differentiate into phenotypically characteristic hepatocytes.[59,60] These pancreatic hepatocytes resemble parenchymal cells of liver and express hepatocyte-specific gene products. This metaplastic change is attributed to the presence of bipotential stem cells in pancreas, which are normally dormant but when stimulated to divide can make a commitment to differentiate into hepatocytes in the pancreas.

Epithelial metaplasia, in particular the glandular metaplasias such as the differentiation of hepatocytes in pancreas, indicates that during embryonic development gastric, intestinal, hepatic, and urothelial epithelia arise from the same or contiguous endoderm, there is a possibility that precursor cells, capable of differentiating into any of these populations, could persist into the adult life. Such cells may commit themselves to differentiate toward a desired metaplastic version when there is chronic tissue damage.

Connective tissue metaplasias depict many different transformations or transdifferentiations between mesodermally derived tissues. These are characterized by conversion of fibroblast-derived soft tissue into muscle, cartilage, chondrocytes or osteoblasts including bone formation with and without bone marrow elements (Fig. 17-26). A fibroblast, or a cell looking like a fibroblast, or a primitive/stem cell–like mesodermal cell, is most likely the precursor cell capable of undergoing metaplastic conversion to other types of mesenchymal tissues. Fibroblasts are believed to give rise to bone tissue in many parts of the body subsequent to physically induced injury and in surgical or burn scars. The plasticity of fibroblast descendants in culture to convert into a variety of mesenchymal derivates such as cartilage, smooth muscle, and adipocytes has been demonstrated by a 24-hour exposure of mouse fibroblasts to 5-azacytidine, a DNA-hypomethylating agent. In particular the smooth muscle lineage has been shown to be attributable to activation of the specific transcription factors such as MyoD, which can activate the entire panoply of smooth muscle gene expression. Bone formation in muscle, referred to as myositis ossificans, is also frequently observed after injury. Osseous metaplasia with bone marrow elements is also seen in calcified arterial walls, in the lung parenchyma, and in certain benign mesenchymally derived tumors such as uterine leiomyomas. This type of osseous metaplasia is attributed to the elaboration of two proteins, namely, osteogenin and bone marrow morphogenetic protein.

The clinical relevance of metaplasias depends on the type and location of metaplastic change, the reversibility of such an alteration, and the persistence of chronic injury. Metaplastic epithelium is prone to undergo malignant transformation and is the histogenetic basis for the development of squamous cell carcinomas in the lung and adenocarcinomas in the esophagus because these organs do not normally contain squamous epithelium and glandular epithelium respectively. Tissues with metaplastic epithelium are susceptible to infections. In some cases, secretions such as hydrochloric acid by metaplastic gastric tissue in an inappropriate location such as the Meckel's diverticulum of small intestine can cause ulceration and bleeding. Although most metaplastic alterations are usually reversible after cessation of chronic insult (as when one abstains from smoking), connective tissue metaplasia, in particular osseous metaplasia, persists even after the cause has been eliminated. Likewise, pancreatic hepatocytes persist in the pancreas and remain as a stable phenotype.

Dysplasia

Dysplasia implies bad development or abnormal formation (from the Greek *dys,* 'bad' or 'difficult'; *plasis,* 'forming, molding'). As an adaptive response dysplasia signifies abnormal or atypical hyperplasia and sometimes atypical metaplasia; thus dysplastic change refers to an alteration in the size, shape, and organization of the cellular components of hyperplastic or metaplastic tissue. Dysplastic changes can occur in both epithelial and mesenchymal tissues. The cells in a dysplastic focus exhibit increased mitotic activity in addition to pronounced pleomorphism and hyperchromasia. The compo-

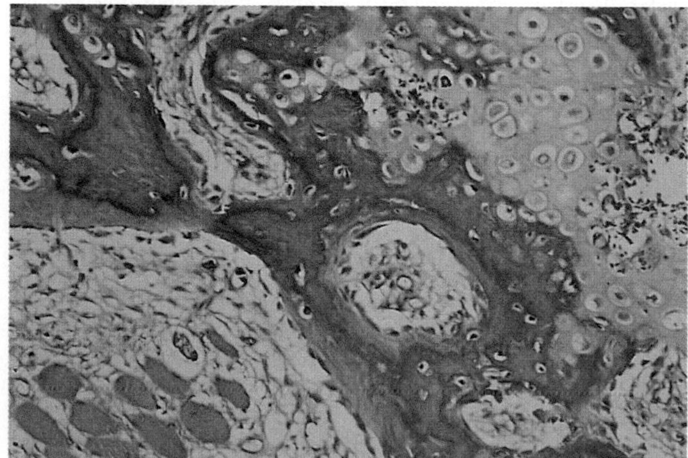

Fig. 17-26 Osseous metaplasia in myositis ossificans.

nent cells show disorganization of the spatial architecture. Dysplastic alterations commonly occur in the de novo or metaplastic squamous epithelium. Dysplasia also occurs in the glandular epithelium in ulcerative colitis and in regenerative nodules in cirrhotic livers. Some dysplastic alterations may be reversible with removal of the causative stimuli. Dysplasia is of considerable concern when present in the epithelium of the uterine cervix and in the squamous metaplastic foci of the bronchial epithelium and is often a precursor lesion to the development of malignancy. In essence dysplasia is an extreme example of adaptive response that triggers the excessive growth of abnormal cells and is more aggressive and biologically ominous. Indeed, dysplasia sometimes refers to an unequivocal neoplastic transformation in the epithelium without penetration into the lamina propria. In gastric mucosal dysplasia cytologic features of neoplasia without invasion are generally observed. The dysplastic alterations in Barrett's esophagus and ulcerative colitis are graded as indefinite, low grade, and high grade; the high-grade dysplasia essentially replaces the designation carcinoma in situ (see Chapter 24).

REFERENCES:

1. Majno G, Joris I: Oncosis and necrosis: an overview of cell death, *Am J Pathol* 146:3, 1995.
2. Reimer KA, Ideker RE: Myocardial ischemia and infarction, *Hum Pathol* 18:462, 1987.
3. Jennings RB, Reimer KA: Lethal myocardial ischemic injury, *Am J Pathol* 102:241, 1981.
4. Venkatachalam MA et al: Salvage of ischemia cells by impermeant solute and ATP, *Lab Invest* 49:1, 1983.
5. Stadtman ER: Protein oxidation and aging, *Science* 257:1220, 1992.
6. Martin GR et al: Aging—causes and defenses, *Annu Rev Med* 44:419, 1993.
7. Yu BP: Oxidative damage by free radicals and lipid peroxidation in aging. In Yu BP, editor: *Free radicals in aging,* Boca Raton, Fla, 1993, CRC Press.
8. Brog DC: Oxygen free radicals and tissue injury. In Tarr M, Samson F, editors: *Oxygen free radicals in tissue damage,* Boston, 1993, Birkhauser.
9. Smuckler EA, Benditt EP: Studies on CCl_4 intoxication III: a subcellular defect in protein synthesis, *Biochemistry* 4:671, 1965.
10. Rosser BG, Gores GJ: Liver cell necrosis: cellular mechanisms and clinical implications, *Gastroenterology* 108:252, 1995.
11. Moslen MT: Protection against free radical–mediated tissue injury. In Moslen MT, Smith CV, editors: *Free radical mechanisms of tissue injury,* Boca Raton, Fla, 1992, CRC Press.
12. Rubin E, editor: *Alcohol and the cell,* New York, 1987, New York Academy of Sciences.
13. Lee RJ: Fatty change and steatohepatitis. In Lee RJ, editor: *Diagnostic liver pathology,* St. Louis, 1994, Mosby.
14. Takahashi T, Lasker JM, Rosman AS, Lieber CS: Induction of cytochrome P-4502E1 in the human liver by ethanol is caused by a corresponding increase in encoding messenger RNA, *Hepatology* 17:236, 1993.
15. Cormack DV, Johns HE: Electron energies and ion densities in water irradiated with 200 keV, 1 MeV and 25 MeV radiation, *Br J Radiol* 25:369, 1952.
16. Cleaver JE: DNA repair and radiation sensitivity in human (xeroderma pigmentosum) cells, *Int J Radiat Biol* 18:557, 1970.
17. Purcell RH: Hepatitis viruses: changing patterns of human disease, *Proc Natl Acad Sci USA* 91:2401, 1994.
18. Rosen DR, Siddique T, Patterson D et al: Mutations in Cu/Zn superoxide dismutase gene are associated with familial amyotrophic lateral sclerosis, *Nature* 362:59, 1993.
19. Gurney ME, Pu H, Chiu AY et al: Motor neuron degeneration in mice expressing a human CuZn superoxide dismutase mutation, *Science* 264:1772, 1994.
20. Sifers RN, Carlson JA, Clift SM et al: Tissue specific expression of the human alpha–1–antitrypsin gene in transgenic mice, *Nucleic Acids Res* 15:1459, 1987.
21. Farber JL: The role of calcium in cell injury, *Chem Res Toxicol* 3:503, 1990.
22. Schanne FAX, Kane AB, Young EE, Farber JL: Calcium dependence of toxic cell death: a final common pathway, *Science* 206:700, 1979.
23. Farber J: Membrane injury and calcium homeostasis in the pathogenesis of coagulative necrosis, *Lab Invest* 47:114, 1982.
24. Bonventre J: Mechanisms of ischemic renal failure, *Kidney Int* 43:1160, 1993.
25. Glenner GG: Amyloid deposits and amyloidosis: the beta–fibrilloses, *N Engl J Med* 302:1283; 1333, 1980.
26. Kelley WN, Wyngaarden JB: Enzymology of gout, *Adv Enzymol* 41:1, 1974.
27. Weissman G: Crystals, lysosomes and gout, *Adv Intern Med* 19:239, 1974.
28. Yeldandi AV, Yeldandi V, Kumar S et al: Molecular evolution of the urate oxidase–encoding gene in hominoid primates: nonsense mutations, *Gene* 109:281, 1991.
29. Kerr JFR, Wyllie AH, Currie AR: Apoptosis: a basic biologic phenomenon with wide-ranging implications in tissue kinetics, *Br J Cancer* 26:239, 1972.
30. Wyllie AH, Kerr JFR, Currie AR: Cell death: the significance of apoptosis, *Int Rev Cytol* 68:25, 1980.
31. Hockenbery DM, Oltvai Z, Yin X-M et al: *Bcl–2* functions in an antioxidant pathway to prevent apoptosis, *Cell* 75:241, 1993.
32. Hockenbery D: Defining apoptosis, *Am J Pathol* 146:16, 1995.
33. McCarthy NJ, Smith CA, Williams GT: Apoptosis in the development of the immune system: growth factors, clonal selection, and *bcl–2*, *Cancer Metastasis Rev* 11:157, 1992.
34. Oltvai ZN, Korsmeyer SJ: Checkpoints of dueling dimers foil death wishes, *Cell* 79:189, 1994.
35. Williams GT, Smith CA: Molecular regulation of apoptosis: genetic controls on cell death, *Cell* 74:777, 1993.
36. Reed JC: *bcl–2* and the regulation of programmed cell death, *J Cell Biol* 124:1, 1994.
37. Carson DA, Ribeiro JM: Apoptosis and disease, *Lancet* 341:1251, 1993.
38. Vaux D: Towards an understanding of the molecular mechanisms of physiological cell death, *Proc Natl Acad Sci USA* 90:786, 1993.
39. Schoen FJ et al: Calcification: pathology, mechanisms and strategies of prevention, *J Biomed Mater Res* 22:A1, 1988.
40. Sawyer JR, Myers MA, Rosier RN, Puzas JE: Heterotopic ossification: clinical and cellular aspects, *Calcif Tissue Int* 49:208, 1991.
41. Tsutsui T et al: Cytoskeletal role in the contractile dysfunction of hypertrophied myocardium, *Science* 260:682, 1993.
42. Boheler KR, Schwartz K: Gene expression in cardiac hypertrophy, *Trends Cardiovasc Med* 2:176, 1992.
43. Simpson PC: Proto-oncogenes and cardiac hypertrophy, *Annu Rev Physiol* 51:189, 1988.
44. Hammerman MR, O'Shea M, Miller SB: Role of growth factors in regulation of renal growth, *Annu Rev Physiol* 55:305, 1993.
45. Fine LG, Norman J: Cellular events in renal hypertrophy, *Annu Rev Physiol* 51:19, 1989.
46. Jones AL, Fawcett DW: Hypertrophy of the agranular endoplasmic reticulum in hamster liver induced by phenobarbital, *J Histochem Cytochem* 14:215, 1966.
47. Reddy JK, Rao MS: Peroxisome proliferation and hepatocarcinogenesis. In Vainio H, Magee PN, McGregor DB, McMichael AJ, editors: Mechanism of carcinogenesis in risk identification, Lyon, 1992, International Agency for Research on Cancer.
48. Reddy JK, Mannaerts GP: Peroxisomal lipid metabolism, *Annu Rev Nutr* 14:343, 1994.
49. Baserga R: *The biology of cell reproduction,* Cambridge, 1985, Harvard University Press.
50. Cheng H, LeBlond CP: Origin, differentiation and renewal of the four main epithelial cell types in the mouse small intestine, *Am J Anat* 141:461, 1974.
51. Fausto N: Liver stem cells. In Arias IM et al, editors: *The liver: biology and pathobiology,* New York, 1993, Raven Press.
52. Sell S: Liver stem cells, *Mod Pathol* 7:105, 1994.

53. Rhim JA, Sandgren EP, Degen JL et al: Replacement of diseased mouse liver by hepatic cell transplantation, *Science* 263:1149, 1994.
54. Coni P, Simbula G, De Prati AC et al: Differences in the steady-state levels of c-*fos*, c-*jun* and c-*myc* messenger RNA during mitogen-induced liver growth and compensatory regeneration, *Hepatology* 17:1109, 1993.
55. Furlong RA: The biology of hepatocyte growth factor/scatter factor, *BioEssays* 14:613, 1992.
56. Fausto N, Webber EM: Liver regeneration. In Arias IM et al, editors: *The liver: biology and pathobiology,* New York, 1993, Raven Press.
57. Matsumoto K, Nakamura T: Hepatocyte growth factor: molecular structure, roles in liver regeneration, and other biological functions, *Crit Rev Oncog* 3:27, 1992.
58. Michalopoulos GK, Zarnegar R: Hepatocyte growth factor, *Hepatology* 15:149, 1992.
59. Rao MS, Dwivedi RS, Yeldandi AV et al: Role of periductal and ductular epithelial cells of the adult rat pancreas in pancreatic hepatocyte lineage: a change in the differentiation commitment, *Am J Pathol* 134:1069, 1989.
60. Reddy JK, Rao MS, Yeldandi AV et al: Pancreatic hepatocytes: an in vivo model for cell lineage in pancreas of adult rat, *Dig Dis Sci* 36:502, 1991.

18 Inflammation

Stephen W. Chensue
Peter A. Ward

For centuries humans have intuitively identified inflammation with fire, undoubtedly, as a result of the experience of redness, heat, and pain associated with its occurrence. Interestingly, scientific investigation of inflammation has extended this analogy. At the microscopic level, inflammation is described as an accumulation of leukocytes that "spread" within tissues and then ultimately "burn out" and heal or lead to "smoldering" conditions. Similarly, at the molecular level, leukocytes use an oxidative mechanism, in essence a form of biologic fire, that destroys microorganisms and damages tissues. Despite the essential truth of our intuitive sense of inflammation, the objective understanding has come slowly.

At least since the eighteenth century, inflammation has been considered a manifestation of immunity, but the mechanisms governing inflammatory events have remained enigmatic until recent decades. During the late nineteenth and much of the twentieth centuries, important advances were made with regard to manipulating humoral immunity as evidenced by the development of vaccines and the use of antiserum.[1] These great advances tended to overshadow the role of phagocytic cells in resistance to infection as promoted by the famed zoologist Élie Metchnikoff.[2] Likewise, histopathologists such as Rudolf Virchow and Julius Cohnheim speculated that cellular and vascular components of inflammation were critical elements, but they could not ascertain their full significance or relationship to humoral immunity. It is now understood that inflammation is a dynamic interaction of humoral and cellular reponses. Recently, studies of inflammation have focused on revealing the "molecular language" that dictates the observed events. Clearly there is a complex array of both humoral and cellular signals that determine the quality, intensity, and duration of inflammation.

Inflammation is best defined in teleologic terms. Specifically, it is a series of molecular and cellular responses acquired during evolution designed to eliminate foreign agents and promote repair of damaged tissues. Unfortunately, these responses are not infallible. Pathogens have concurrently evolved mechanisms to avoid elimination; new pathogens occasionally emerge from the environment, and under some circumstances aberrant immunoinflammatory responses damage the host (see Chapters 25 and 27). The complexity of the immunoinflammatory system is a reflection of millions of years of environmental challenges. It is becoming apparent that the system is not simple but rather a complex composite of responses that were assembled opportunistically and when elicited may synergize or antagonize each other.

For the histopathologist, the inflammation observed in tissue specimens represents only a single frame of an unfolding process that is dynamic and complex. Although it is beyond the scope of this chapter to provide an exhaustive review of the many aspects of inflammation, it does describe the basic elements and patterns of inflammation and provide current understanding of underlying mechanisms. The aim is to supply one with a theoretical and practical understanding of inflammation in dynamic terms. This knowledge should enrich the understanding of inflammation in clinical and research settings.

PATTERNS OF INFLAMMATION

It is appropriate to begin with a presentation of the various histologic patterns of inflammation, keeping in mind that the microscopic picture is a function of at least three factors. The first is the *nature of the inciting agent,* which might include bacteria, fungi, multicellular parasites, viruses, foreign bodies, chemical irritants, particulate allergens, transplanted tissues, and self-tissue components. Some of these elicit characteristic tissue responses. The second is the *time of observation.* Because inflammation is a dynamic process, its morphology varies according to the time of observation, and asynchronous lesions, even in the same individual, will likely have different appearances. For example, an early acute lesion will be highly cellular, differing from older, largely acellular lesions in the stages of fibrosis. The third factor is the *immune status of the host.* A host previously immunized to a specific pathogen can

production. Lymphoid cells are major components of delayed-type hypersensitivity reactions and in tissue responses to viral infections (Fig. 18-7, *A*). At times, lymphoid-rich responses become diagnostic dilemmas, when there is a question of lymphoma. Special studies may be indicated to differentiate the reactive from the neoplastic infiltrate. Under some conditions plasma cells dominate a response, as in syphilitic lesions and infections involving ducts and surface epithelia (Fig. 18-7, *B*). Interestingly in some neoplasms, especially carcinomas and melanomas, an associated stromal lymphoplasmacytic response may indicate a better prognosis. The basis of the infiltrate is speculative and may be in response to antigens, growth factors, or homing signals released by the tumor.

Mixed-cell responses

As mentioned above, chronic inflammatory responses most commonly involve a variety of leukocyte types as well as proliferation of local tissue elements. The mixed type of inflammation accompanies many conditions at many sites. Chronic ulcerative colitis is a notable example of this heterogeneous pattern of inflammation in which there is ongoing acute cryptitis with neutrophil infiltration and an interstitial lymphoplasmacytic infiltrate admixed with varying numbers of mononuclear phagocytes and eosinophils (Fig. 18-8). Ulcer sites often show repair and regenerative changes with proliferation of fibroblasts, vessel components, and epithelium. It is not difficult to imagine the complexity of events that must occur to coordinate the recruitment and function of so many cell types.

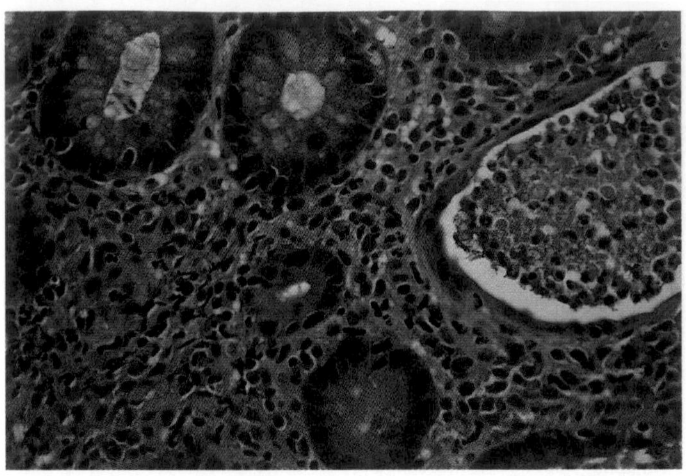

Fig. 18-8 Mixed type of inflammatory reaction. Neutrophilic crypt abscesses and stromal lymphoplasmacytic infiltrates with scattered eosinophils are present in this case of ulcerative colitis.

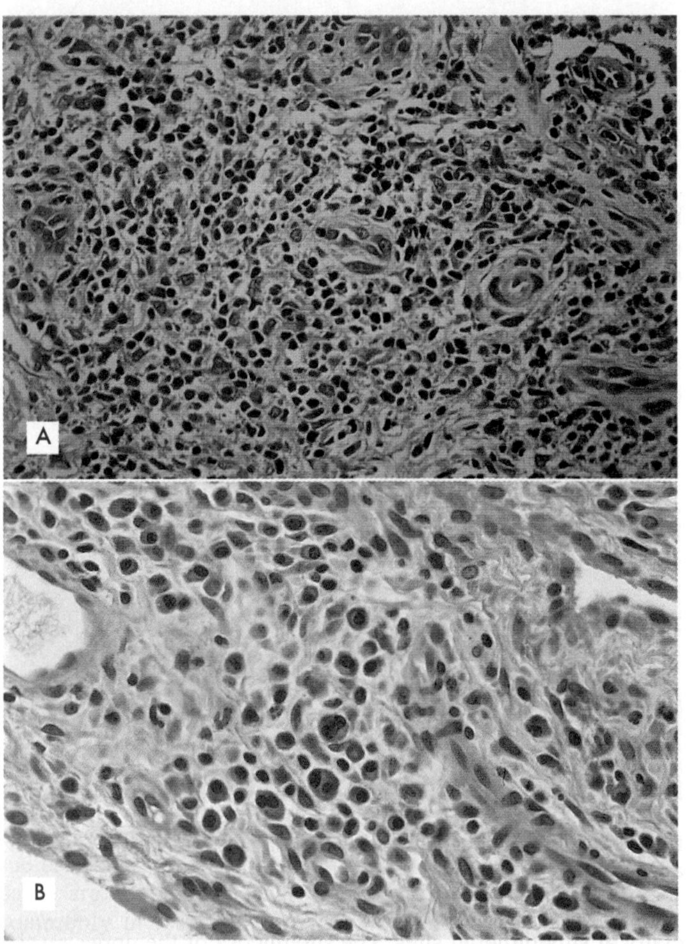

Fig. 18-7 Lymphoplasmacytic inflammation. **A,** Numerous perivascular lymphocytes are present in the dermal delayed hypersensitivity response. **B,** Plasma cells dominate the inflammation of chronic rheumatoid synovitis.

Granulomatous responses

The *granuloma* is a specialized form of chronic inflammation, defined as a focal accumulation of leukocytes in which macrophages and their derivatives, epithelioid and multinucleate giant cells, are fundamental elements.[3] One may assume that the primary function of the granuloma is to sequester and if possible destroy an offending agent. Granulomas occur in many conditions (Table 18-1) and have been classified into hypersensitive and nonimmune types.[4] The former involve a lymphocyte-mediated response to specific antigens, whereas the latter do not require antigen-specific lymphocytes. Characteristically, the hypersensitive type of granulomas form in response to infectious agents (such as *Mycobacterium* species and fungi). Nonimmune granulomas usually form in response to poorly digestible substances, either extrinsic (such as silica and sutures) or intrinsic (such as keratin). Finally, there are many granulomatous diseases that appear to be of the hypersensitive type but are of unknown cause. Sarcoidosis is the outstanding example of this response. Granulomas are also observed in some connective tissue disorders (such as rheumatoid arthritis) and can spontaneously occur in some individuals with malignancies such as Hodgkin's lymphoma and carcinomas, but the role of lymphocytes is not known.

Despite the constant feature of macrophages, granulomas display significant variety of histologic appearances, depending on the disease or etiologic agent. For example, it is well known that granulomas of *Mycobacterium tuberculosis* often show pronounced central caseous necrosis (Fig. 18-9, *A*). This contrasts with sarcoidal granulomas, which consist primarily of epithelioid macrophages and lymphocytes with little to no necrosis (Fig. 18-9, *B*). Granulomas induced by foreign bodies may consist almost entirely of epithelioid cells and multinucleate giant cells (Fig. 18-9, *C*), whereas those induced by parasites or their ova may contain a large component of eosinophils. The *Chlamydia* and bacteria that cause lymphogranuloma venereum and cat-scratch disease, respectively,

Table 18-1 Granulomatous diseases

Bacterial	**Helminthic**
Tuberculosis	Schistosomiasis
Leprosy	Trichiniasis
Brucellosis	Filariasis
Salmonellosis	Capillariasis
Listeriosis	**Foreign body-types**
Syphyllis	Foreign body pneumonitis
Q fever	Silica granulomatosis
Metal induced	**Unknown cause**
Berylliosis	Sarcoidosis
Zirconium granulomatosis	Crohn's disease
Fungal	Wegener's granulomatosis
Histoplasmosis	Giant cell arteritis
Blastomycosis	Primary biliary cirrhosis
Coccidiomycosis	Granuloma annulare
Hypersensitivity pneumonitis	Rheumatoid arthritis
Viral, Chlamydial	
Cat-scratch fever	
Lymphogranuloma venerum	

induce granulomas with a characteristic central neutrophilic abscess surrounded by macrophages and other mononuclear cells.

The nature of the granulomatous response is also a function of the immune status of the host. This is illustrated by the miliary form of *M. tuberculosis* and the lepromatous form of *M. leprae* infections in which granulomas become small and disseminated with impaired sequestration capacity. A similar phenomenon is observed in HIV-infected individuals in whom the granulomatous response is defective, resulting in smaller less compact lesions (Fig. 18-9, *D*). It is generally accepted that these histologic changes reflect impaired or altered T-cell function required for effective hypersensitive-type granuloma formation.

HUMORAL AND CELLULAR PARTICIPANTS OF INFLAMMATION

Understanding inflammation requires a knowledge of the varied components of the process. Although the recruited cellular components are the most readily observed, it is well established that fluid-phase molecular systems or humoral factors have an essential role in initiating and promoting subsequent cellular

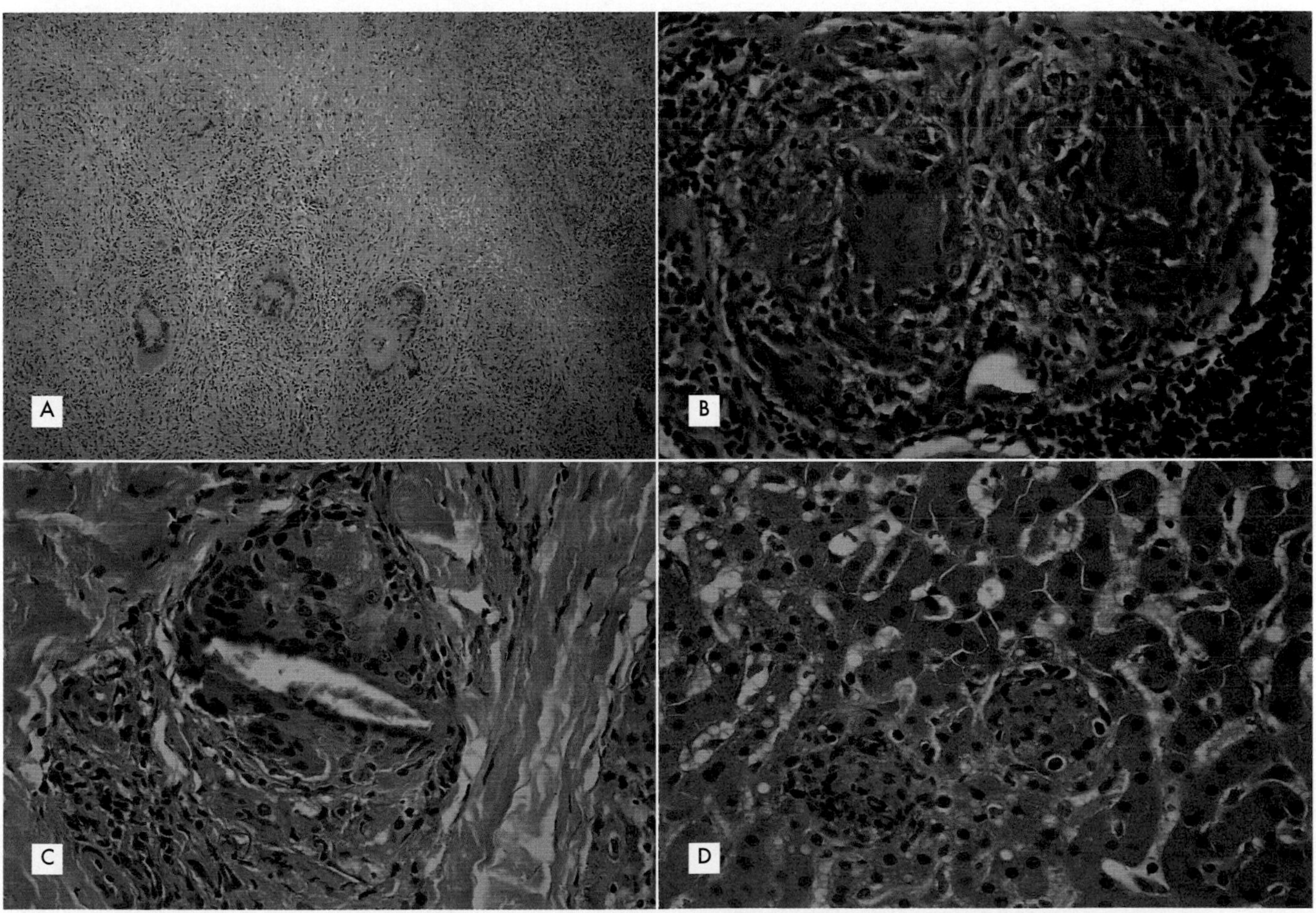

Fig. 18-9 Granulomatous inflammation. **A,** Caseating granulomas of *Mycobacterium tuberculosis* infection. Notice multinucleate giant cells *(middle)* and caseation *(upper right.)* **B,** Sarcoid granulomas, closely packed with many epithelioid and giant cells. **C,** Foreign-body granuloma with central crystalloid foreign body. **D,** Small hepatic *Mycobacterium avium-intracellulare* granulomas in patient with HIV infection.

events. In addition, it is becoming apparent that cellular participants of inflammation include not only blood-borne leukocytes but also stromal components of organs. The following discussion overviews the functions of these various components.

Humoral elements

Coagulation and fibrinolytic factors

Although the primary function of clotting mechanisms is to maintain vascular integrity, this system also plays important roles in microbial resistance and inflammation. The formation of a clot or *coagulum* at a site of infection acts to contain microbes and to provide a framework for host cell infiltration and growth. The importance of this function in host resistance is illustrated by the fact that phagocytic leukocytes produce procoagulant products that can participate in the formation of localized coagula. In addition, pathogenic bacteria such as *Staphylococcus aureus* have specifically evolved coagulases to counter this function.

By-products of the activated clotting system also act as molecular signals to induce vasopermeabilty and attract host leukocytes. Since the detailed aspects of the clotting and fibrinolytic systems are described in Chapter 19, only those features relating to inflammation are noted here. It is well known that the clotting system consists in a series of blood-borne proenzymes, or *zymogens,* that can be activated in a cascade fashion ultimately to generate thrombin from prothrombin (factor II). The active enzyme thrombin cleaves fibrinogen (factor I) to fibrin, which polymerizes to form a coagulum (Fig. 18-10). The fibrinopeptides A and B generated by that cleavage are chemotactic and induce vasopermeabilty, promoting fluid and cellular accumulation.[5,6]

The events leading to the formation of a clot likewise trigger the generation of regulatory molecules that limit its extension and ultimately degrade the clot. Fibrinolytic derivatives also contribute to inflammatory events. The enzyme primarily responsible is plasmin, which is derived from its precursor, plasminogen. Plasmin cleaves polymerized fibrin at specific sites producing the D-D dimer and E fragments that promote vasopermeability.[7,8]

Kinins

Kinins are polypeptides with potent vasoactive properties that induce vasopermeability, smooth muscle contraction, and enhancement of leukocyte margination.[9] The kinins are released after proteolytic cleavage of plasma precursor proteins, called *kininogens,* existing in high- and low-molecular-weight forms. The cleavage is mediated by serine proteases, termed *kallikreins,* which are derived from tissues or from the

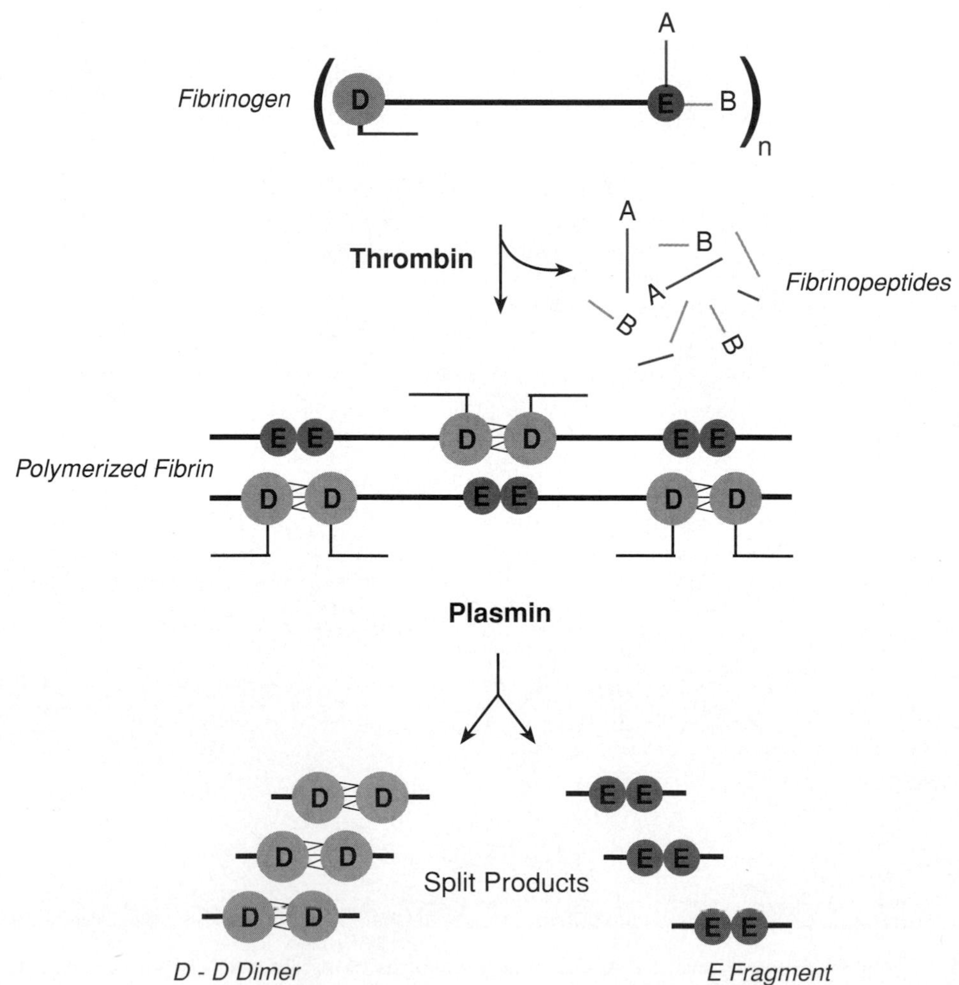

Fig. 18-10 Coagulation-related proinflammatory products. Cleavage products of clot formation, (fibrinopeptides) and dissolution, (fibrin split products) have vasoactive and chemotactic properties.

plasma by the *contact activation system*. This system is a collection of four plasma proteins, Hageman factor (HF, or coagulation factor XII), prekallikrein (PK), high-molecular-weight kininogen (HMWK), and coagulation factor XI. The contact activation system is initiated when there is exposure to negatively charged organic or inorganic surfaces. Moreover, through HF and coagulation factor XI there is a close relationship with the activation of the intrinsic clotting pathway. It is well known that genetic deficiencies of components of the contact activation system result in clotting abnormalities. HF in noncovalent association with PK and HMWK bind to the charged surface and are reciprocally activated, resulting in the generation of kallikrein, an active serine protease that releases the major kinin, bradykinin, from HMWK by site-specific proteolysis (Fig. 18-11). The system is self-amplifying and is under regulation by plasma protease inhibitors such as C1 inhibitor, antithrombin III, α_1-antitrypsin, α_2-antiplasmin, and α_2-macroglobulin. Tissue kallikreins were originally identified in glandular and vascular tissues. In addition, neutrophil-derived lysosomal enzymes can cleave HMWK, and thus inflammatory cells potentially contribute to kinin generation.[10]

Complement factors

The complement system is a major complex of plasma proteins comprising a group of proteases that circulate in zymogen form that are activated in a self-amplifying cascade fashion.[11] Unlike the coagulation, fibrinolytic, and kinin systems, the complement system is not directly related to blood-clotting functions. Instead, it appears specifically to promote microbial killing and elimination as well as produce vasoactive and chemotactic peptides. There are two activation pathways described for the complement system (Fig. 18-12). The *classical pathway* is initiated by immune complexes of complement-fixing immunoglobulin isotypes, IgM, IgG1, IgG2, or IgG3. The *alternative pathway* is initiated by negatively charged surfaces, particulate polysaccharides, fungi, bacteria, viruses, and aggregated immunoglobulins, especially of the IgA isotype. Both pathways require activation of the C3 component (with C3b representing the major product involved in the activation process) and lead to the eventual activation of C5 and assemblage of the membrane attack complex (MAC). The last is composed of factors C5 through C9, which, when deposited on the target cell membrane, cause lysis by disrupting membrane integrity. It should be noted that several factors that regulate complement are integral membrane proteins. These factors, such as decay-accelerating factor, vary among species and determine target cell sensitivity to lysis by the MAC. Nevertheless, lysis is not the only outcome of complement activation. The C3b and iC3b cleavage products act as an *opsonin,* binding to microbial surfaces and promoting attachment and phagocytosis by leukocytes, to be discussed later under Phagocytosis. The precise chemistry of complement activation has been described in detail[11] and is not reviewed here. Instead, this discussion focuses on the properties of the inflammation-related by-products of the complement pathways.

As shown in Fig. 18-12, complement activation involves the generation of peptide cleavage products. Three of these, C3a, C4a, and C5a, are highly cationic molecules with molecular weights of 9, 9, and 11.2 kD respectively. These *anaphylatoxins* induce vascular permeability (causing edema), smooth muscle contraction, and histamine release, events associated with anaphylaxis. Of these peptides, C5a has the greatest potency and has the additional properties of inducing directed migration of leukocytes and fibroblasts (chemotaxis) as well as increasing leukocyte adherence and functional activation.[12] The anaphylatoxins appear to be regulated by plasma carboxypeptidase N, which cleaves arginyl residues from C5a and C3a, resulting in the much less potent *des-arg* forms of the molecules.

Immunoglobulins

The immunoglobulins have been subject to intense investigation since their discovery over a century ago. It is widely known that they are antibodies, specialized serum proteins with the capacity to specifically bind target molecules (antigens) by noncovalent interactions.[13] Immunoglobulins are produced after appropriate antigenic stimulation of B lympho-

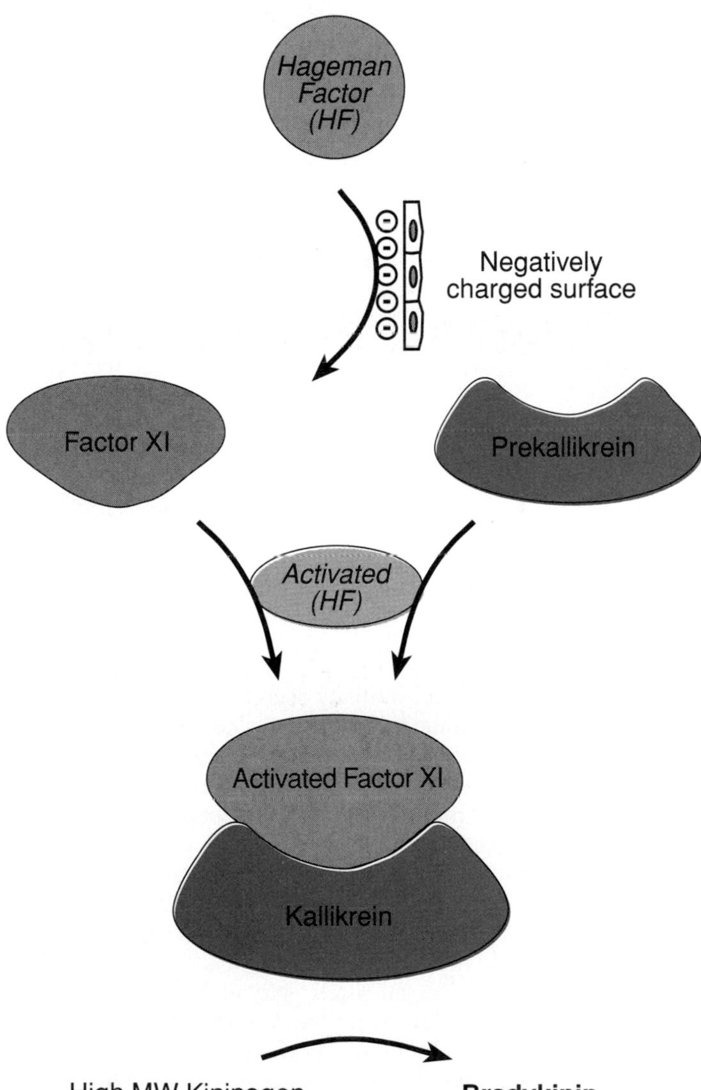

Fig. 18-11 Pathway of plasma-derived kinin generation. Interaction of Hageman factor with negatively charged surfaces results in activation of coagulation factor XI and conversion of prekallikrein to kallikrein. The resulting activated complex enzymatically cleaves HMWK releasing bradykinin, a peptide with potent vasoactive properties.

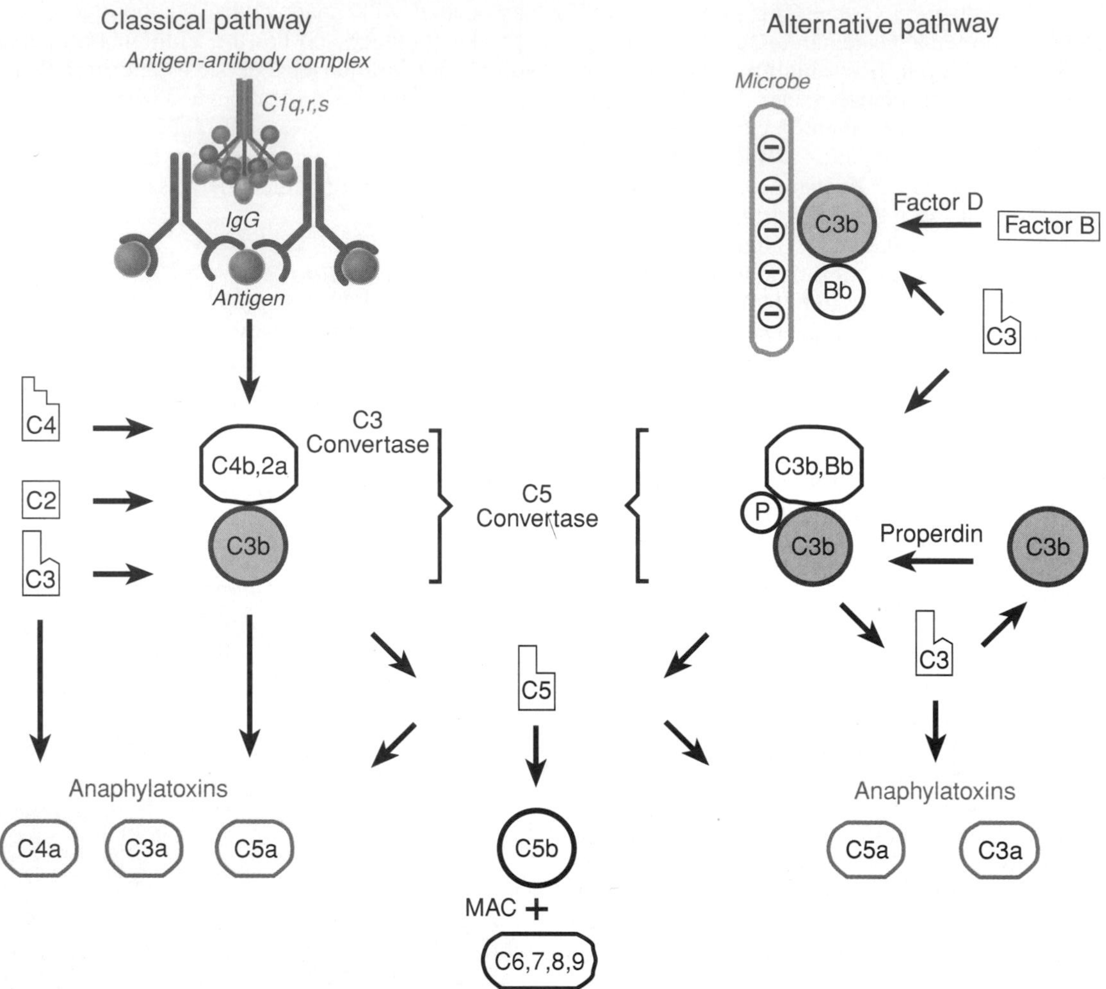

Fig. 18-12 Pathways of plasma-derived anaphylatoxin generation. Circulating complement components can be activated by two pathways. The classical pathway is initiated by antibody-antigen complex, whereas the alternative pathway is initiated by interaction with negatively charged surfaces. Both pathways result in the assembly of C5 convertases that generate C5a fragment, the most potent chemotactic and vasoactive anaphylatoxin. Other cleavage products such as C4a and C3a have a lesser degree of activity.

cytes, which mature to antibody-secreting plasma cells. The main function of immunoglobulins is to neutralize viruses and toxins as well as to promote killing and phagocytosis of bacteria and other microorganisms. However, certain immunoglobulin isotypes have more specialized functions, and most can contribute to inflammation. The five major classes of human immunoglobulins, their isotypes, major properties, and relative concentrations in serum are shown in Table 18-2.

The dominant serum immunoglobulin class is IgG followed by IgA and IgM. IgD is a minor serum component, and its more important role is in B-cell activation, as a membrane receptor for antigen. As mentioned, when complexed with antigen, IgG1, IgG2 , IgG3, and IgM have the capacity to trigger complement activation by the classical pathway and thereby generate proinflammatory anaphylatoxins. IgA is in mucus secretions and bile and is believed to provide mucosal immunity. However, IgA can also trigger complement activation by the alternative pathway. As is discussed later, and in Chapter 25, IgG1 and IgG3 are the primary immunoglobulins that interact with leukocyte Fc receptors, allowing for antigen-specific "arming" of inflammatory cells. Fc receptors have been described for most of the immunoglobulin isotypes, Fcμ, Fcγ, Fcα, Fcε. There are subclasses of these receptors that have distinct cellular distributions and effector functions.

IgE is a minor serum component but has potent proinflammatory function because it binds to specific membrane receptors of inflammatory cells. The high-affinity IgE receptor FcεRI is expressed by mast cells[14] and basophils, whereas the low-affinity receptor FcεRII is expressed by eosinophils, monocytes, platelets, and some B-lymphocytes.[15,16] Cross-linking of mast cell bound IgE by antigen triggers the release of histamine and other proinflammatory compounds having vasoactive and chemoattractant properties. These mediators are discussed in greater detail below.

Blood-borne cells

Neutrophils

Polymorphonuclear leukocytes (PMNs), or polymorphonuclear neutrophils, are the primary phagocytic cells involved in host resistance to bacterial infection. Individuals with acquired or congenital abnormalities of PMNs are subject to recurrent bacterial infections. These cells, characterized by their lobulated

Table 18-2 Immunoglobulins and their properties

Isotype	IgG1	IgG2	IgG3	IgG4	IgA1	IgA2	IgM	IgD
Concentration (mg/ml)	3-10	1-7	0.2-2.0	0.1-1.3	0.7-2.3	0.1-0.5	0.5-2.0	0.005-0.2
Classic C′ + activation	+	++	–	–	–	+++	–	
Alternative C′ activation	±	+	±	±	?	+++	±	–
Defined Fc receptor	+	+	+	+	+	+	+	–

nucleus and granular cytoplasm, represent the largest population (40% to 60%) of blood leukocytes and circulate for about 10 hours after release from the bone marrow. Under steady-state conditions, there is a large marrow-storage pool of PMNs, and about 55% of the released population is marginated by loose attachment to endothelium. PMNs are derived from myeloid precursors in the bone marrow, and during maturation, they develop cytoplasmic granules that contain a variety of molecules with antimicrobial activities.[17] Table 18-3 summarizes the constituents of the major PMN-associated granules. The primary (azurophilic granules) develop early during the promyelocytic stage, whereas secondary (specific granules) accumulate during the late myelocytic and metamyelocytic stage of PMN maturation. The major constituents of these granules are enzymes that can digest bacterial structural components as well as degrade host tissues. Both types of granules can empty into phagocytic vacuoles that form around engulfed material. In addition, the contents of specific granules can also be deposited extracellularly, an important consideration in damage to host tissues. Also, myeloperoxidase of primary granules is among a group of enzymes that generate toxic oxygen metabolites, with microbicidal properties, that are important in the molecular events of inflammation. Tertiary granules or C particles appear to be released during the initial stage of PMN chemotaxis and contain enzymes that promote migration of PMNs through the connective tissue framework.[18] Because of the activity of degradative enzymes and oxygen metabolites, PMN-rich responses are usually associated with significant bystander damage of host tissues.

Through a wide variety of membrane receptors, PMN functions can be regulated. For example, receptors for complement fragment C3b and the immunoglobulin Fc region allows for more efficient phagocytosis of particles coated with these molecules. Receptors (integrins) for endothelial cell membrane proteins (addressins) and interstitial matrix proteins allow for local adherence of PMNs to sites of inflammation. Other receptors for chemotactic molecules (such as C5a) and cytokines lead to PMN activation and directed migration. Products of PMNs can also amplify inflammatory responses and regulate the activity of other cells. For example, granule plaminogen activator and membrane phospholipases promote vascular permeability and chemotaxis by respectively generating fibrin split products and metabolites of arachidonic acid. There is also some evidence that PMNs have partial capacity for active protein synthesis, releasing biologically active cytokines with local and systemic effects.[19]

Table 18-3 Polymorphonuclear leukocyte granules

Granule	Synonym	Constituent
Primary	Azurophil	Myeloperoxidase Lysozyme Bacterial permeabilizing protein Defensins Seprocidins (serine protease–like) Elastase Cathepsin G Proteinase 3 Azurocidin Acid hydrolases
Secondary	Specific	Lysozyme Collagenase Gelatinase Lactoferrin Plasminogen activator Histaminase Vitamin B_{12}–binding proteins Cytochrome *b* β_2-Microglobulin
Tertiary	C particles	Gelatinase Acid hydrolases

Monocytes and mononuclear phagocytes

Mononuclear phagocytes (MP), also known as "macrophages" or "histiocytes," are distributed throughout virtually all tissues.[20] The MP arise from monoblasts in the marrow, and they are released into the circulation as monocytes, where they remain for about 25 hours. As with PMNs there is a large (about 75%) marginated pool. The monocytes then migrate to tissues and become part of the tissue (fixed) macrophage population. These are found in high concentrations within the vasculature of the liver, spleen, and lungs, where they remove effete cells and foreign particles from the blood. Tissue macrophages are also associated with lymphoid tissue and bone marrow where they assist the regulation of immune responses and hematopoiesis. Animal studies indicate that tissue macrophages turnover every 4 to 15 days depending on their location. Mononuclear phagocytes may be quite heterogeneous, with specialized functions, but it is not known if this heterogeneity simply reflects cells at different stages of maturation. Unlike PMNs, MP are longer lived and secrete a vast repertoire of bioactive products,[21] partially listed in Table 18-4. These cells also display a unique capacity to adapt to varied environmental challenges, a characteristic that is often enhanced and directed by signals provided by reactive lymphocytes as well as by humoral and bacterial products.

Mononuclear phagocytes occur in varying numbers in nearly all forms of inflammation and likely participate in every stage of the inflammatory process. Local tissue macrophages can potentially initiate inflammation by producing cytokines in response to bacterial products such as endotoxin.[21,22] Cytokines such as interleukin-1 and tumor necrosis factor can induce expression of endothelial adhesion molecules, which begin local recruitment of circulating leukocytes. Other chemotactic molecules such as IL-8 and leukotriene B4 can further attract inflammatory cells. In addition, MP can amplifiy their contribution by proliferating at sites of inflammation.

Phagocytosis of microbes is a major function of MP, requiring the stages of attachment, engulfment, and destruction of the offending agent. Although MP bear receptors for carbohydrates that allow for nonspecific attachment to target particles, the attachment and engulfment process is greatly enhanced when the object is coated with activated complement fragments or immunoglobulins, a condition called "opsonization." MP bear membrane receptors for immunoglobulin Fc component and C3b, allowing for both recognition and tight attachment.[23] The destruction stage consists in fusion of the phagosome and lysosome, with release of attacking enzymes and reactive oxygen metabolites. This process is enhanced when the MP is activated.[24] Activation is defined in terms of enhanced functions, as compared to an initial baseline value, and occurs when the MP is exposed to molecular signals (such as interferon-γ, endotoxin, and monocyte chemotactic protein-1). The activated state can vary, depending on the signal, but involves increased synthesis of enzymes, membrane receptors, and cytokines.

An important function of the activated MP is antigen processing and antigen presentation.[25] After phagocytosis or endocytosis, exogenous proteins are degraded into peptides and transported to the membrane in association with class II major histocompatibility (MHC) antigens. Activation signals induce MP to synthesize class II MHC proteins encoded in the D region of the MHC gene complex located on chromosome 6. The membrane-exposed complex of foreign and MHC antigens then serves to activate antigen-specific helper ($CD4^+$) T-lymphocytes.

As mentioned, MP are constituents of granulomas and can differentiate into epithelioid macrophages and multinucleate giant cells.[26] The former is a specialized MP with abundant cytoplasm that sometimes acquires spindled and palisaded appearances within granulomas. They likely sequester and degrade irritating agents with secreted enzymes but have poor phagocytic capacity. Multinucleate giant cells result from MP fusion, a process that can be induced in vitro with cytokines such as interferon-γ.[27] Such cells can contain multiple nuclei, which sometimes distribute themselves peripherally, forming so-called *Langhans* giant cells (Fig. 18-13). These are more commonly seen in highly active immune type of granulomas. Like epithelioid cells, giant cells are weakly phagocytic but produce secretory products and likely help to sequester agents.

Table 18-4 Secretory products of mononuclear phagocytes

Plasma-related proteins	Leukotrienes
Coagulation factors	Hydroxyeicosaenoic acids
Factors II, III, V, VII, IX, X	Platelet activating factor and lysophospholipids
Thrombospondin	**Matrix proteins**
Prothrombinase	Fibronectin
Complement components	Thrombospondin
C1-C5	Proteoglycans
Factors B and D	**Enzymes**
Properdin	Proteases
C3b inactivator	Collagenases
Serum amyloids A and P	Elastase
Apolipoprotein E	Plasminogen activator
Haptoglobin and transcobalamin II	Cathepsins B, L, H, N
Cytokines and growth factors	Angiotensin convertase
Interleukins (IL-1a, IL-1b, IL-6)	Phospholipase A2
IL-1 receptor antagonist	Hyaluronidase
Tumor necrosis factor-alpha	β-Galactosidase
Chemokines (IL-8, MCP-1, *gro*, IP-10)	β-Glucuronidase
Growth- and colony stimulating factors	Nucleases
Transforming growth factor-β	Ribonucleases
Platelet-derived growth factor	Sulfatases
Fibroblast growth factor	Lysozyme
Angiogenesis factor	Acid phosphatases
G-CSF and GM-CSF	Amylase
Erythropoietin	**Enzyme inhibitors**
Lactoferrin	α_2-Macroglobulin
Oxygen and nitrogen metabolites	α_1-Antiprotease
O_2^-, H_2O_2, OH^-	α1-Antichymotrypsin
Hypohalous acids	Lipomodulin
NO, NO_2, NO_3	Fibrinolysis inhibitors
Active lipid products	**Other active molecules**
Arachidonate metabolites	Vitamin D_3
Prostaglandins	Glutathione
Prostacyclin	Nucleic acid derivatives

Lymphocytes

Lymphocytes are critical cells of the immune system, conferring the ability for antigen-specific recognition and regulating the functional capacity of other leukocytes.[28] Morphologically, resting lymphocytes are simple mononuclear cells with a small amount of cytoplasm containing few organelles. Activated or transformed lymphocytes have increased cytoplasm and synthetic capacity. Based upon function and membrane antigen markers, lymphocytes are classified into B-cells and T-cells. B-cells are responsible for immunoglobulin production and humoral immunity. T-cells are responsible for cell-mediated immunity and can regulate humoral responses. During gestation, prelymphocytes derived from the yolk sac become B-cells or T-cells upon receiving maturation signals in the bone marrow or thymus, respectively. Each lymphocyte undergoes gene rearrangements to acquire membrane antigen receptors with unique specificity. The B-cell antigen receptor is a transmembrane immunoglobulin molecule of IgD or IgM isotype. The T-cell receptor is a immunoglobulin-related protein, consisting of a heterodimer of α and β or γ and δ transmembrane proteins.[29,30] The α/β T-cells are dominant in numbers but, depending on the organ, γ/δ T-cells can compose up to 30% of

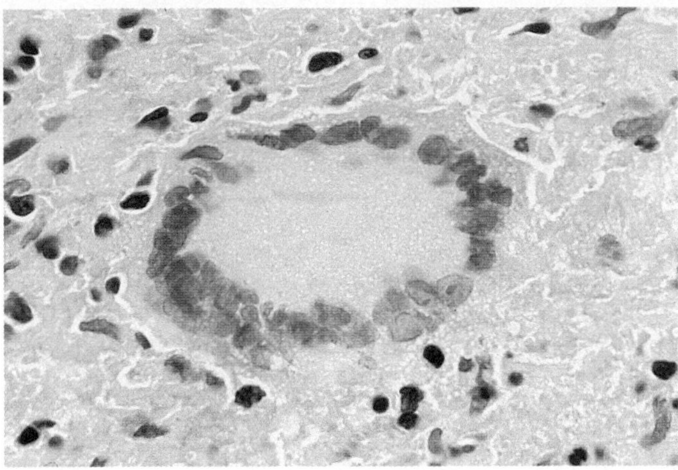

Fig. 18-13 Langhans giant cell commonly seen in granulomas of tuberculosis.

lymphocytes. The γ/δ T-cells have a more restricted antigen recognition repertoire and appear to respond largely to bacterial antigens.[30] Compared to α/β T-cells, they have less capacity to recognize histocompatibility antigens during graft rejection. The α/β T-cells are further classified into helper cells bearing the CD4 membrane marker and suppressor/cytotoxic cells bearing the CD8 marker.[31] CD4-bearing cells amplify proliferation, promote Ig synthesis, and mediate delayed type of hypersensitivity inflammation. CD8-bearing cells suppress proliferation and Ig production and mediate cell-mediated cytotoxic responses. The γ/δ T-cells also express CD4 or CD8, but many express neither marker.[30]

Mature lymphocytes constantly circulate between the blood and lymphatics.[32] Lymph nodes, spleen, and skin/mucosal lymphoid tissues provide sites for potential contact of lymphocytes with foreign antigen. Lymphocyte populations display homing characteristics, tending to return more often to certain lymphoid tissues. For example, isolated intestinal lymphocytes recirculate preferentially to the gut upon parenteral adoptive transfer. This strategy places lymphocytes with appropriate antigen receptors at sites most exposed to the target antigen. The homing process requires lymphocyte-endothelial interactions involving membrane adherence molecules such as *L-selectin* discussed below.

Activation of B- and T-cells requires antigen-receptor cross-linking.[33] Some polymeric antigens, such as lipopolysaccharide, will directly stimulate B-cells to proliferate. Smaller antigens require antigen-presenting cells (usually macrophages) with added receptor counterreceptor interactions for optimal B-cell stimulation. Differentiation factors derived from T-cells promote B-cells to become Ig-secreting plasma cells. Unlike B-cells, T-cells recognize antigen only in the context of MHC membrane antigens. Specifically, $CD4^+$ helper T-cells are activated by antigen plus class II MHC proteins and $CD8^+$ T-cells by antigen plus class I MHC proteins. Both populations secrete a variety of bioactive molecules, called "cytokines," or "lymphokines," which modulate functions of target cells. The anamnestic response is attributable to the expansion of antigen-specific T and B memory cell populations, which consequently mount a more rapid and augmented response to secondary challenge.

Natural killer (NK) cells are lymphoid cells that mark with CD2 but are nonreactive with CD4 or CD8 antibodies. A characteristic of NK cells are large cytoplasmic granules; thus the term *large granular lymphocytes* is used synonymously.[34] They have the capacity to kill certain virally infected and tumor cells in vitro. NK cells also produce cytokines and may be important in providing a form of limited antigen-nonspecific immunity.

Eosinophils

Eosinophils (EOS) are peripheral blood leukocytes with bilobed or trilobed nuclei and distinctive cytoplasmic granules that bind eosin dye and appear as crystalloid structures by transmission electron microscopy. These bone marrow–derived cells develop from stem cells in response to colony-stimulation factors such as interleukin-5.[17] Under normal physiologic conditions they compose less than 5% of circulating leukocytes. Their absolute number or relative percentage can be significantly increased with allergic responses and during helminthic infections.[35] EOS are major participants in the inflammation associated with these conditions. Like PMNs, EOS have a variety of receptors for complement components and IgG that allow for activation and antigen-directed effector function. In addition, EOS bear IgE receptors and can be induced to express MHC class II antigens, allowing for antigen-presenting capacity.[16,36]

Compared to PMNs, EOS are weakly phagocytic, and their effector functions result mainly from degranulation. The EOS granules are well studied and contain a variety of biologically active proteins[36] (Table 18-5). Major basic protein (MBP), the dominant granule protein, is bactericidal and toxic to helminthic parasites. MBP also causes degranulation of mast cells and thereby potentially exacerbates inflammation. EOS also produce lipid-derived proinflammatory mediators such as leukotrienes and platelet activating factor.

Basophils and mast cells

Basophils and mast cells are widely recognized as important inflammatory cells.[37] Both are are derived from the bone marrow and contain granules that stain strongly with basic dyes.[38,39] However, basophils circulate in the blood (though less than 0.5% of the leukocyte population) and are recruited during allergic responses, whereas mast cells reside and

Table 18-5 Eosinophil granule proteins

Protein	Molecular weight (kilodaltons)	Action
Major basic protein	14	Helminthotoxin, histamine-releasing factor, bactericidal
Eosinophil cationic protein	20	Helminthotoxin, histamine-releasing factor, bactericidal, neurotoxin
Eosinophil-derived neurotoxin	18	Neurotoxin, inhibits lymphocyte proliferation
Eosinophil peroxidase	66	Generates microbicidal hypohalous acids Histamine-releasing factor

mature in tissues. Like eosinophils, the function of basophils and mast cells depends on the release of preformed granule-derived mediators as well as de novo synthesis of mediators. Basophilic granules contain histamine, proteoglycans, carboxypeptidase A, serine proteases, glycosidases, and sulfatases. Histamine is derived from the the amino acid histidine and causes vascular dilatation and leakage by stimulating the H_1 receptor on vascular smooth muscle and endothelium.[40] The enzyme components of the granules likely loosen the intercellular matrix for the arrival of leukocytes. In addition to these preformed products, basophils and mast cells produce a variety of lipid and protein mediators with proinflammatory activities, including chemotactins, cell-activating, and cell-growth factors.[37] Tissue mast cells are not homogeneous. For example, the enzymes within granules of mucosal and connective tissue mast cells are different from each other. Thus, the range of mast cell activities is specialized for their anatomic location.

It is well known that mast cells and basophils bear receptors for IgE and degranulate when this cytophilic antibody is cross-linked by antigen. But, other factors such as mechanical trauma, complement C5a, eosinophil-derived cationic protein, and certain bacterial products can cause mast cell degranulation. Also, a novel group of low-molecular-weight proteins with chemotactic properties (such as platelet factor 4, monocyte chemotactic protein, and Regulated upon Activation, Normal T-cell Expressed and Secreted [RANTES]) have potent histamine-releasing activity.[41] Thus mast cells can promote inflammation in the absence of IgE-mediated activation and likely initiate inflammatory events under many circumstances.

Platelets

In addition to their important role in hemostasis, platelets can participate in all stages of inflammation.[42] These flat, anuclear cellular fragments are shed from bone marrow megakaryocytes and contain a large array of enzymes and granule components with potential inflammation-related activities (Table 18-6). Moreover, inflammatory conditions are often associated with thrombocytosis and an enhanced coagulation state.

Platelets become activated upon contact with exposed matrix elements after tissue injury and undergo a release reaction involving stages of adherence, shape change, and aggregation. The released products include chemotactic agents such as platelet-derived growth factor (PDGF), platelet factor 4 (PF4) and 12-hydroxyeicosatetraenoic acid (12-HETE). Activated platelets also promote adherence of leukocytes and generation of the highly chemotactic C5a fragment. Other platelets products such as PDGF are chemotactic and support growth of fibroblasts and smooth muscle cells, presumably promoting tissue repair.[43] Membrane Fc receptors for IgG and IgE allow them to recognize antigens by way of surface-bound immunoglobulin with subsequent aggregation and activation. The presence of bound IgE is suggestive of participation of platelets in allergic responses. Platelets also have antimicrobial and antiparasitic activities in vitro (such as beta-lysin and nitric oxide release), thus potentially playing a direct role in host resistance to infection. They also have the capacity to assimilate and store serotonin (5-hydroxytryptamine), a largely gut-derived neurotransmitter with the capacity to regulate vascular tone, vasopermeability, and promote platelet aggregation.[44]

Table 18-6 Platelet-derived inflammatory products

Alpha granule components
Adherence promoting
Fibronectin
Fibrinogen
von Willebrand factor
Thrombospondin
Lysosome associated membrane protein
Granular membrane protein 140
Chemotactic
Platelet-derived growth factor
Platelet factor 4
Growth factors
Transforming growth factors α and β
Basic fibroblast growth factor
Platelet-derived growth factor
Coagulation and complement modulators
Factors D and H
Plasminogen
$Alpha_2$ plasmin inhibitor
Dense granule components
Aggregation promoting
Adenosine diphosphate (ADP)
Serotonin and calcium
Arachidonate metabolites
Aggregation promoting
Thromboxane A_2
Chemotactic
12-HETE

Stromal elements

Endothelial cells, fibroblasts, and smooth muscle cells

Until recently, vessels and connective tissues were believed to be passive participants of inflammation, being largely involved in repair functions. There is mounting evidence that these cells actually play an active role in inflammation. Not only do these cells respond to the molecular signals of leukocytes, but they also modulate leukocyte functions.

Endothelial cells cover the luminal surfaces of all vessels and form the first barrier between blood-borne elements and the interstitium; they are crucial cells in inflammation.[45] These cells display both morphologic and functional heterogeneity depending on their anatomic location. This is exemplified by the specialized cuboidal postcapillary endothelium of lymph nodes that bears receptors for circulating lymphocytes and is responsible for lymphocyte-homing capacity.[46] Under normal conditions, endothelial cells produce factors that regulate vascular tone and coagulation. Three major factors include prostacyclin (PGI_2),[47] a vasodilator and antithrombotic agent; nitric oxide radical (NO·),[48] also a vasodilator and antithrombotic agent; and endothelin,[49] a peptide vasoconstricting agent. As is discussed later, after injury or infection endothelial cells undergo functional and phenotypic changes, such as the expression of receptors (addressins), that allow adherence and recruitment of leukocytes. In addition, the "activated" endothelium can synthesize leukocyte-activating and chemotactic mediators such as platelet-activating factor and interleukin-8, consequently linking leukocyte adhesion to activation.[50]

Fibroblasts, myofibroblasts, and smooth muscle cells will produce proinflammatory mediators in response to bacterial endotoxin or endogenous molecular signals such as interleukin-1 (IL-1) and tumor necrosis factor (TNF). For example, IL-1 and TNF induce fibroblasts to synthesize monocyte chemotactic protein, colony-stimulating factors, complement components, and interleukin-6.[51-53] Hence, connective tissue cells have the capacity to sustain and modulate inflammation.

Matrix Proteins

The cellular components of tissues are embedded in intercellular matrix. The matrix is composed of various collagens, elastins, hyaluronic acid, proteoglycans, and other glycoproteins. The latter include fibronectins,[54] tenascin,[55] and vitronectin.[56] The primary function of these compounds is structural, but they also can play an active role in inflammation. Polymorphonuclear leukocytes bear receptors for matrix proteins, and when bound to matrix, they display enhanced granule secretion, LTB_4 synthesis, and respiratory burst.[57] Likewise, γ/δ T-cells bear receptors for vitronectin, allowing it to act as an accessory activation signal.[58] Many proinflammatory proteins can bind to matrix elements, and recent evidence indicates that chemotactic proteins may be at least temporarily immobilized in matrix, forming a trail of chemotactic "scent" for migrating leukocytes.

MOLECULAR BASIS OF INFLAMMATORY EVENTS

Cytokines

It is not surprising that inflammatory responses involving the participation of numerous cell types would require a means of communication. This communication occurs through a complex network of molecular mediators or cytokines that direct all stages of the response from initiation to repair. Many of these molecules are biochemically characterized, but there is still much to be learned regarding their relative participation in vivo. Moreover, cytokines are often pleiotropic and functionally redundant, confounding their classification. Defining the specific biologic activity of cytokines is likewise difficult because many act by triggering a cascade of other mediators that exert the ultimate biologic effect. Some of the cytokines were previously alluded to, but this discussion will provide a systematic introduction of the major cytokines involved in inflammatory events and conclude with an overview of their role in inflammation.

In the broadest definition, cytokines are cellular products with the capacity to alter target cell functions in an autocrine, paracrine, or endocrine manner. This definition includes polypeptides, neuropeptides, lipids, vasoactive amines, nucleotides, and even metabolites of oxygen and nitrogen. Some authors consider only the polypeptide mediators to be cytokines (listed in Tables 18-7 and 18-8). However, this section includes a discussion of both polypeptide mediators and the important lipid mediators of inflammation. The major vasoactive amines, histamine, and serotonin are described on p. 403 and the oxygen and nitrogen metabolites are discussed on p. 408.

Lipid-derived mediators

The arachidonic acid (AA) metabolites are the best-studied lipid mediators, and virtually all cells involved in the inflammatory response have the capacity to generate at least some form of AA derivative. Arachidonic acid is normally part of the lipid membrane and is released by the action of phospholipase A_2.[59] The free AA can be metabolized by two major enzymatic pathways, cyclooxygenase or lipoxygenase (Fig. 18-14). Whereas cyclooxygenases can be found in a wide variety of tissues, lipoxygenases are largely restricted to leukocytes and their derivatives.[60] The major cyclooxygenase products include prostaglandins (PGE_2, $PGF_{2\alpha}$, and PGD_2), prostacycline (PGI_2), and thromboxane (TXA_2). The last two are important in regulating coagulation. Endothelium-derived PGI_2 and platelet-derived TXA_2 respectively inhibit and promote platelet aggregation. With regard to inflammation, PGE_2 increases blood flow and synergizes with other factors to induce vascular permeability and hyperalgesia.[61,62] PGE_2 potentially also has antiinflammatory effects, since it elevates cAMP levels and inhibits effector functions of inflammatory cells.[63]

The major lipoxygenase products include leukotrienes (LTB_4, LTC_4, LTD_4, and LTE_4) and hydroxyeicosatetraenoic acids (HETEs). LTB_4, is a potent proinflammatory mediator with activity at nanomolar concentrations. It induces PMN leukocyte chemotaxis, chemokinesis, degranulation, and adherence to endothelial cells.[64] LTC_4, LTD_4, and LTE_4 induce histamine-independent bronchial smooth muscle contraction, vasopermeability, and mucus production.[65] Not surprisingly, they are detectable in respiratory secretions during allergic and asthmatic states.[66] The HETEs such as 5-HETE and 12-HETE are monohydroxylated AA derivatives that are chemotactic for PMNs and eosinophils.[67,68] Concentrations of these com-

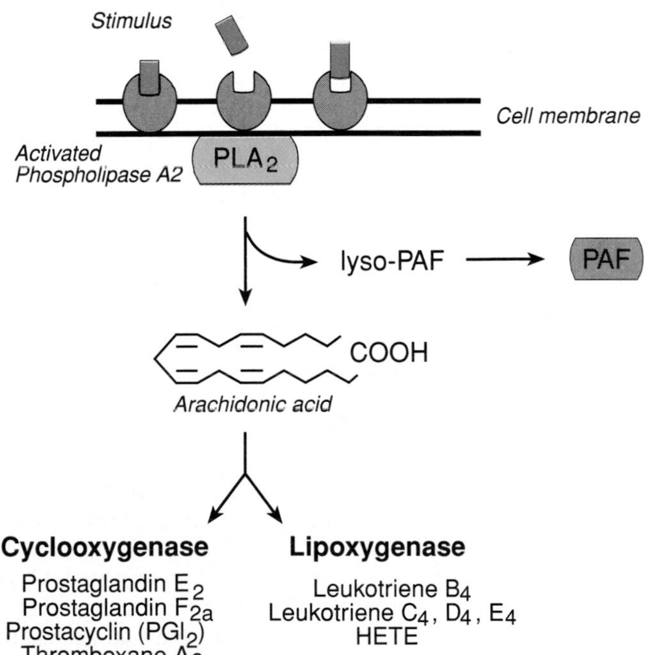

Fig. 18-14 Pathways of arachidonic acid (AA) metabolism. Activated phospholipase A_2 cleaves AA from the membrane, which can be metabolized by way of cyclooxygenation or lipoxygenation, depending upon cell type and stimulus. Platelet-activating factor (PAF) is generated concurrently upon phospholipase activation. Cyclooxygenase derivatives tend to influence coagulation and vascular tone. Lipoxygenase products tend to have chemotactic and secretagogue activity and contract airway smooth muscle.

Table 18-7 Polypeptide cytokines

Cytokine	Molecular weight (kilodaltons)	Major sources	Major activities
Interferons			
IFN-α and IFN-β	16-20	Myeloid and stromal cells	Antiviral, activates phagocytes
IFN γ	20-24	Lymphoid cells	Antiviral, activates phagocytes, induces class I and class II MHC antigens and IgG2α
Interleukins			
IL-1	17-18	Mostly MP but also many other cells	Promotes lymphocyte growth, cytokines, adhesion molecules, fever, acute-phase protein synthesis
IL-2	15-18	Lymphocytes	Promotes lymphocyte growth, NK-cell activity, and phagocyte activation
IL-4	15-19	Lymphocytes	Promotes lymphocyte growth, IgE and IgG1 synthesis, Fcε, adhesion molecules
IL-5	20	Lymphocytes	Promotes B-cell differentiation, eosinophil growth, IgE synthesis
IL-6	21-28	Leukocytes, stromal and epithelial cells	Promotes lymphocyte growth, Ig synthesis, acute-phase protein synthesis, thrombopoiesis
IL-7	25	Stromal and epithelial cells	Promotes B-cell precursor growth, T-cell growth and hematopoiesis
IL-9	32-39	Lymphocytes	Promotes T-cell growth
IL-10	35-40	Lymphocytes and MP	Promotes B-cell and mast-cell growth; inhibits IFN-γ, TNF, and IL-1 synthesis
IL-11	23	Stromal cells	Promotes lymphocyte growth and hematopoiesis
IL-12	65-75 dimer	Lymphocytes and MP	Promotes NK cell and cytotoxic T-cells; opposes IL-10 actions
IL-13	16-19	Lymphocytes	Promotes lymphocyte growth, IgE synthesis
Colony-stimulation factors			
IL-3	14-15	Lymphocytes	Stimulates myeloid and erythroid differentiation
GM-CSF	13-14	MP, stromal cells, and endothelium	Stimulates PMN, monocyte and eosinophil growth, phagocyte activation
G-CSF	19-20	Leukocytes, stromal, endothelial and epithelial cells	Stimulates PMN differentiation
M-CSF	70-90 dimer	Leukocytes, stromal, endothelial and epithelial cells	Stimulates monocyte growth
Cytotoxins			
TNF-α	17	Mostly macrophages	Cytotoxic for some tumor cells; promotes adhesion molecules, fibroblast growth, fever, cachexia, and acute-phase proteins
TNF-β	17	Lymphocytes	Activities similar to those of alpha form

Fcε, Fc receptor for IgE; *G*, granulocyte; *GM*, granulocyte-macrophage (or monocyte); *Ig*, immunoglobulin; *M*, monocyte or macrophage; *MP*, macrophage; *NK*, natural killer, *PMN*, polymorphonuclear leukocyte; *TNF*, tumor necrosis factor.

pounds are elevated in inflamed joints of patients with rheumatoid arthritis and in psoriatic skin lesions, and such elevation is suggestive of a role for HETEs in these chronic diseases.[68]

Platelet-activating factor (PAF) is a membrane phospholipid derivative (1-*O*-alkyl-2-acetyl-*sn*-glycerol-3-phosphocholine) generated after activation of phospholipase A_2 and often released concomitantly with AA metabolites. In addition to its platelet-aggregating effects, PAF is detectable in a wide variety of inflammatory lesions and is known to activate or promote selected functions of PMNs, mononuclear phagocytes, eosinophils, and basophils.[69] Interestingly, PAF can be expressed on the membranes of endothelial cells and exerts activation effects without entering the fluid phase. PAF also has demonstrated endocrine acitivities and may play a role in the physiologic regulation of vascular tone, uterine contractility, and hepatic glycogenolysis.[70]

Polypeptide mediators

There are many polypeptide cytokines, but because of their pleiotropic effects, they are difficult to classify and have acquired a confusing nomenclature. This section is a discussion of some of the properties of the major groups of polypeptide cytokines (Table 18-7).

Interferons (IFN) were originally defined by their capacity to inhibit viral replication but are now known to alter the function of many target cells. The type I (IFN-α/β) and type II (IFN-γ) interferons have independent, species-specific receptors. Type I α/β-IFNs are a heterogeneous but homologous group of 16 to 20 kD proteins.[71] The IFN-αs are derived mainly from myeloid cells, whereas IFN-βs are derived from stromal cells. IFN-γ, also known as immune IFN, is a 20 to 24 kD protein that is largely lymphocyte derived.[72] On the whole, IFNs have the capacity to activate PMNs and mononuclear phagocytes as well as support B-lymphocyte growth. Comparatively, IFN-γ is a much more potent inducer of class I and II major histocompatibility antigens than the IFN-α/βs are and consequently is likely more important in promoting antigen-presentation to T-cells.

Interleukins are a variety of polypeptide mediators that modulate leukocyte activity. The term "interleukin" was intended to bring a standard usage to a confusion of nomenclature that was based upon specific biologic activities. For example, interleukin-1 was previously known as lymphocyte-activating factor, endogenous pyrogen, and osteoclast-activating factor.

As reflected by its various names, IL-1 is a highly pleiotropic cytokine.[73] This 17.5 kD molecule exists in α and β forms. It was originally described as a product of mononuclear phagocytes, but other cells including PMNs, lymphocytes, keratinocytes, glial cells, endothelial cells, and other stromal cells are potential sources. Microbial products (endotoxin, viruses, yeast) and other cytokines can induce IL-1 synthesis. Its known in vitro proinflammatory biologic activities include stimulation of T-lymphocyte proliferation, prostaglandin synthesis, chemokine synthesis, and expression of endothelial adhesion molecules. In vivo, IL-1 appears to contribute to neutophilic leukocytosis, fever, and acute-phase protein production. IL-1 also induces glucocorticoid release, which potentially provides an immunoregulatory feedback circuit. Mononuclear phagocytes also produce IL-1 receptor antagonist protein, a natural inhibitor IL-1 that tempers the biologic effects of IL-1.[74]

Interleukin-2 is a 15 to 17.5 kD product of stimulated T-cells.[75] Its first described biologic effect was its capacity to support the growth of antigen-stimulated T-cells, and it appears to be required for an effective immune response. Many other biologic activities are now known, including stimulation of B-cells, natural killer cells, and mononuclear phagocytes. IL-2 also induces the lymphokine-activated killer cell phenomenon in which lymphocytes are activated to kill tumor cells in an antigen-independent manner. IL-2 responsiveness requires expression of IL-2 receptors, which include low-, intermediate-, and high-affinity types. After antigen stimulation, resting lymphocytes rapidly express IL-2 receptors, permitting subsequent IL-2 supported proliferation.

Interleukin-4 is a 15 to 19 kD product of stimulated T-cells and was first described as a B-cell growth factor.[76] Subsequent studies indicated that it was also a T-cell growth factor and, like IL-2, could induce its own receptor. Rodent studies indicate that IL-4 is produced by a subset of T helper cells called "Th2 cells" that appear to play a crucial role in allergic responses and resistance to parasites. IL-4 messenger RNA transcripts have been detected at sites of allergic cutaneous reactions and its known biologic activities support a role in allergy. It causes immunoglobulin isotype switching to IgE, induces Fcε receptors, contributes to mast cell growth, and stimulates expression of adhesion molecules, which promote binding of lymphocytes and eosinophils. IL-4 also downregulates many effector functions of mononuclear phagocytes, such a IL-1 and TNF production, but upregulates IL-1 receptor antagonist synthesis and MHC expression, such that a role in modifying the specific nature of the inflammatory response is indicated.

Interleukin-5 is a 20 kD product of stimulated T-cells and was first described as a B-cell differentiation factor.[77] IL-5, like IL-4, is produced by Th2 cells and plays a role in allergic responses by inducing selective differentiation of eosinophils from marrow stem cells and promoting IgE synthesis. In addition to stimulating eosinophil growth and maturation, IL-5 assists eosinophil chemotaxis.

Interleukin-6 is a 21 to 28 kD cytokine produced by a host of cell types including lymphocytes, mononuclear phagocytes, PMNs, fibroblasts, keratinocytes, and endothelial cells.[78] IL-6 is highly pleiotropic and induces a wide array of biologic effects. It induces immunoglobulin synthesis, promotes IL-2 production, triggers thymocyte proliferation, and supports hematopoiesis, particularly thrombopoiesis. Beyond these activities, IL-6 is among several cytokines that contribute to acute-phase protein synthesis by hepatocytes, including fibrinogen, C-reactive protein, haptoglobin, and serum amyloid A.

Interleukin-7 is a 25 kD protein originally described to promote growth of immature B-cell precursors.[79] Its role in inflammation is unknown, but it also can act as a T-cell growth factor and induce endothelial adhesion molecule expresssion. Interleukin-9 is a 32 to 39 kD cytokine and T-cell growth factor; its role in inflammation is likewise not yet known.[80] Similarly, interleukin-11, a 23 kD cytokine, is a stromal-derived growth factor for lymphocytes and hematopoietic cells, but its relative contribution to inflammation is not known.[81]

Interleukin-10 is a 35 to 40 kD protein produced by Th2 cells, mononuclear phagocytes, and B-cells.[82] It has potent capacity to suppress cytokine production by Th1 cells and thereby is likely an important regulatory molecule. Similar to IL-4, IL-10 suppresses IL-1 and TNF production by monocytes and impairs their capacity to present antigen to Th1 cells effectively. IL-10 is also a B-cell stimulant, promoting proliferation, differentiation, and antibody production. It also synergizes with IL-3 and IL-4 to stimulate mast cell growth.

Interleukin 12 is a heterodimeric lymphocyte and macrophage-derived cytokine with 35 and 40 kD subunits.[83] It was originally found to synergize with IL-2 in the generation of cytotoxic lymphocytes. IL-12 also stimulates natural killer lymphocytes, enhances IFN-γ production, and induces Th1 immune responses. Overall, its functions oppose those of IL-10 and is part of a cytokine immunoregulatory network (see the discussion of cross-regulatory cytokines on p. 412).

Interleukin-13 is a 16 to 19 kD product of Th2 cells with partial homology to IL-4 that shares many of the functional properties of IL-4.[84] Like IL-4, it would be expected to take part in allergic reponses, but its relative contribution is unknown.

The colony-stimulation factors (CSFs) are a group of cytokines that primarily stimulate hematopoiesis.[85] The myeloid growth factors are most relevant to inflammation and include interleukin-3, granulocyte-monocyte CSF, granulocyte CSF, and monocyte CSF. IL-3 is a 14.6 kD protein derived from activated T-cells that stimulates growth of all myeloid and erythroid lineages. GM-CSF is a 14.3 kD protein that stimulates neutrophil, eosinophil, and some erythroid differentiation; it is produced by mononuclear phagocytes, fibroblasts, and

Table 18-8 Supergene family of human chemokines (cytokines)

C-X-C group	C-C group
Interleukin-8	Monocyte chemotatic protein
gro/MGSA	RANTES
Macrophage inflammatory protein-2	LD78
Platelet factor 4	ACT-2
IP-10	I-309

endothelial cells. G-CSF and M-CSF are more restricted in their effects, stimulating mainly neutrophil and monocyte growth, respectively. Both G-CSF and M-CSF are produced by several cell types such as mononuclear phagocytes, stromal cells, endothelial cells, and some epithelial cells. The CSFs regulate the supply of leukocytes that can participate in inflammatory responses. Some have been reported to induce the expression of other cytokines and enhance leukocyte functional activities, thereby potentially participating directly in inflammation. Synthetic versions of colony-stimulating factors, produced by recombinant DNA technology, are useful in reducing the duration of neutropenia associated with cancer chemotherapy.

Two important cytotoxic cytokines are tumor necrosis factor (TNF-α) and lymphotoxin (TNF-β).[86,87] TNF-α was first discovered in the plasma of animals challenged with bacterial endotoxin and was found to cause necrosis of tumor cells in vivo and in vitro. TNF-α is a 17 kD protein that normally exists as a trimer and is produced primarily by activated mononuclear phagocytes. Like IL-1 it is a highly pleiotropic cytokine and most of its functions overlap with those of IL-1. Parenteral adminstration of TNF causes fever, leukopenia, and hypotension. Animal studies indicate that it may be a critical mediator of septic shock and the cachexia of chronic disease. TNF has many inflammation-related actions including the induction of multiple cytokines, adhesion molecule expression, bone and cartilage resorption, fibroblast proliferation, collagen synthesis, angiogenesis, and acute-phase protein synthesis. Lymphotoxin, or TNF-β is also a 17 kD protein but produced by activated T-lymphocytes. Despite a 32% homology to TNF-α, it shares the same receptors and consequently has similar activities.

In addition to the potent chemotactic signals previously discussed (LTB4 and C5a), there is another group of recently described chemotactic polypeptides. These chemokines belong to a supergene family of homologous molecules that are derived from a variety of cells types and can be induced by endotoxin or cytokine stimulation (such as IL-1 and TNF).[88] These small molecules are often basic and generally less than 15 kilodaltons. Based upon the relative position of two cysteine residues, they are classified in C-X-C or C-C subgroups (Table 18-8). Members of the C-X-C family tend to be chemotactic for neutrophils, of which interleukin-8 is the best studied example. The C-C family tends to be chemotactic for mononuclear cells, and monocyte chemotactic protein is representative of this group. In addition to being chemotactic, many of the chemokines induce histamine release from mast cells, thus evoking other features of inflammation such as edema. Presently, the full range of biologic activities of these molecules is unknown.

Another class of compounds with the capacity to modulate inflammatory events are the neuropeptides.[89] These peptides, produced by neural and neuroendocrine tissues, were originally believed to act purely as neurotransmitters and endocrine-growth signals. Examples include substance P, somatostatin, and vasoactive intestinal peptide (VIP). Recent evidence indicates that not only do leukocytes bear receptors for these compounds, but some can also produce them. In general, substance P has proinflammatory actions such as enhancing mast cell degranulation, cytokine production by T-cells, and leukocyte functional activities. In contrast, somatostatin and VIP tend to inhibit lymphocyte responses.

An important component of the inflammatory reaction is the proliferation of fibroblasts and deposition of collagen. Many cytokines have fibrogenic activity that govern this process, including platelet-derived growth factor (PDGF), transforming growth factor β (TGF-β), and fibroblast growth factors (acidic FGF and basic FGF).[90] These compounds are produced by a variety of cells, but all can be produced by stimulated mononuclear phagocytes. It should be noted that TGF-β has immunoregulatory properties and downregulates several proinflammatory functions (such as oxygen metabolite synthesis). It also induces immunoglobulin heavy-chain switching to the IgA isotype.

Cytokine receptors and signal transduction

Cytokines interact with target cells through specific transmembrane protein receptors. The structure and amino acid sequence of many of the known cytokine receptors are characterized. Based upon shared structural features, they are classified into three major families, the Ig (immunoglobulin-like) superfamily, the hematopoietic receptor family, and the nerve growth factor–like (NGF) receptor family.[91] Table 18-9 summarizes the family distribution of some of the cytokine receptors and their physical characteristics. The precise mechanisms by which cytokine signals are transduced into cellular responses are unknown. However, the stimulation of many of the receptors is associated with phosphorylation events

Table 18-9 Human cytokine receptor families

Family and receptor	Molecular weight (kilodaltons)	Kinase acceptor
Immunoglobulin-like family		
IL-1	80	yes
IL-6	80	?
Hematopoietin receptor family		
IL-2b	80	yes
GM-CSF	85	?
IL-4	140	no
IL-7	75	?
Nerve growth factor receptor family		
TNF(p55)	55	?
TNF(p75)	75	?

GM-CSF, Granulocyte and monocyte–colony stimulating factor; *IL,* interleukin; *TNF,* tumor necrosis factor.

believed to involve protein kinase C or other protein kinases.[92] Phosphorylation modulates the proteins and triggers subsequent intracellular enzymatic and binding events. These events lead to induction and activation of nuclear transcription regulation factors such as NF-κB. Some receptors, like the IL-1 receptor, appear to be internalized after cytokine binding and are transported to the nucleus, where presumably gene-transcription events are initiated. Some receptors such as those for chemotactic molecules are associated with guanine nucleotide binding proteins, or G-proteins;[93] these stimulate phospholipases that generate second messengers for calcium mobilization and secretory events.

Cytokine overview

At our present level of understanding, it is difficult to place the cytokines into an easily comprehensible scheme. One approach is to consider them in terms of their relationship to the stages of immunoinflammatory events. As shown in Fig. 18-15, four stages can be defined—initiation, recruitment, removal, and repair. These stages are not necessarily sequential but more likely represent concurrent events. Likewise, although certain cytokines dominate in some stages, there is clearly overlap between stages because of cytokine pleiotropism. For example, as Fig. 18-15 indicates, IL-1 and TNF may participate in all stages. With this caveat in mind, certain generalizations can be surmised. The arachidonic acid metabolites, histamine, neuropeptides, and plasma-derived activation products likely play an important role in the initiation of responses. Sustained recruitment is believed to be mediated by chemokines and colony-stimulation factors that direct the local accumulation and supply of leukocytes. Many interleukins and interferons mediate leukocyte activation and antibody synthesis, promoting removal of foreign agents. Finally, growth factors participate in the resolution phase by directing the repair of damaged tissues. Some of the repair-related factors such as TGF-β may actively inhibit the effector functions of inflammatory cells, thereby preventing further bystander tissue damage and promoting the transformation to the repair stage.

Cellular and molecular events of inflammation

The vascular response

Vessels and tissue perfusion are critical to inflammation. Increased perfusion (vasodilatation) and edema (vascular leakage) are among the earliest events after acute tissue injury or insult. Under homeostatic conditions, fluid is steadily transported across vessels and removed by the lymphatics. The rate of flow is determined by hydrostatic and oncotic pressures. When this system is imbalanced, *noninflammatory edema* can result as in the pulmonary edema associated with congestive heart failure or lymphedema caused by lymphatic obstruction. In contrast, *inflammatory edema* is an active response to injury or allergen exposure. There are three described patterns of inflammation-related vascular leakage as derived from experimental models.[94] Although under most circumstances these patterns cannot be distinguished histologically, it is useful to understand them, since they likely reflect differing molecular mechanisms of vascular leakage. The first is the immediate transient response and occurs within 10 minutes after mild injury and resolves thereafter. Traditionally, it was described in terms of the "triple response." There is initially a transient vasoconstriction of precapillary arterioles succeeded by their dilatation resulting in increased perfusion. Next, there is a third phase of increased permeability of small to medium-sized postcapillary venules. At the molecular level these events are dictated by a host of plasma and cell-derived vasoactive mediators including histamine, serotonin, neuropeptides, prostaglandins, leukotrienes, kinins, complement fragments, and coagulation cleavage products (Fig. 18-16) These mediators bind to specific receptors on vascular smooth muscle and endothelium. The relaxation of prearteriole smooth muscle results in vasodilatation, whereas contraction of endothelial cells causes formation of intercellular gaps and fluid loss. The second pattern is the immediate sustained response and results from injury that damages vascular structural integrity. Under these circumstances, any type of vessel may be affected, with leakage occurring immediately and lasting for hours to days depending on the severity of injury. Finally, the third pattern is the delayed-prolonged response

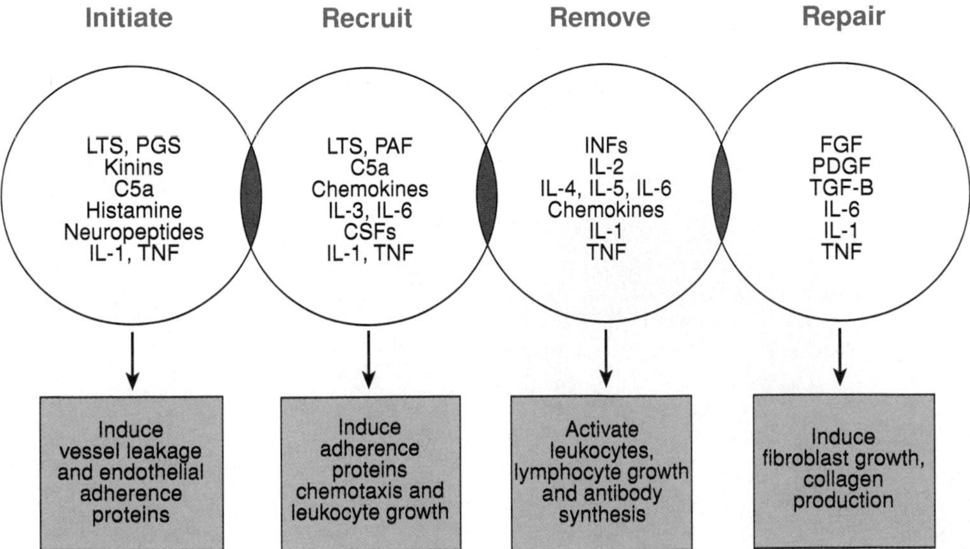

Fig. 18-15 Stages of immune and inflammatory responses. Cytokines can be associated with the stage of the response they most influence. Some cytokines can affect all stages; others are more restricted in their activity.

and is induced by irradiation, bacterial toxins, and delayed-type hypersensitivity reactions. It is characterized by vascular leakage in capillaries and venules and occurs hours after the initial stimulus. Presumably, the cells or cytokines that mediate this response must be recruited or synthesized de novo.

Margination and adherence

The accumulation of blood-borne leukocytes at a site of inflammation requires a complex series of interactions between endothelium and leukocytes. Under homeostatic conditions a variable portion of circulating leukocytes is normally transiently attached to endothelium of postcapillary venules and constitutes the marginated pool. In areas of developing inflammation, the initial vascular dilatation and leakage slows blood flow and promotes the local margination of leukocytes.

The next stage of inflammation requires the committed adherence of leukocytes to endothelium and involves a series of receptor-counterreceptor interactions. Two major classes of membrane adherence proteins have been described. The proteins of the first, termed "selectins," bind carbohydrate ligands expressed by leukocytes and endothelium.[95,96] Those of the second, termed "integrins," bind specific target proteins.[97-99] The known inflammation-related selectins, integrins, and their target molecules are summarized in Table 18-10. There are three known types of selectins—L-selectin, E-selectin, and P-selectin. L-selectin is constitutively expressed by all leukocytes and appears to play a role in lymphocyte homing and PMN recruitment. E-selectin, also known as ELAM-1, is synthesized by endothelial cells after stimulation with cytokines or endotoxin and promotes leukocyte adhesion during acute inflammation. P-selectin is stored in the alpha granules of platelets and Weibel-Palade bodies of endothelial cells and is mobilized from granules after activation with histamine or thrombin. It likewise promotes adhesion events involving platelets, leukocytes, and endothelium during acute inflammation. The selectin target ligands are carbohydrate moieties, commonly sialylated and fucosylated glycoproteins expressed by leukocytes and endothelium. One example, sialyl Lewis X (sLex), is expressed by PMNs and monocytes and is a ligand for E-selectin.

The integrins are a more sophisticated family of adhesion-related leukocyte membrane glycoproteins consisting of noncovalently associated heterodimers of alpha- and beta-polypeptide chains. Eleven alpha and seven beta (β1 to β7) subunits are known and occur in various combinations. Subfamilies are defined by the beta unit and desigated as β_1 integrins, β_2 integrins, β_3 integrins, and so forth. The β_1 integrins include a group of six heterodimers, also known as VLA-1 to VLA-6, that are expressed by lymphocytes, monocytes, and some myeloid cells. This subfamily primarily binds to matrix proteins such as laminin, fibronectin, and collagen types I and IV. One would assume that these integrins allow for interactions with matrix that likely aid migration and modulate cell functions. One of these integrins, VLA-4, also interacts with endothelial vascular cell adhesion molecule-1 (VCAM-1); the expression of this molecule is induced by cytokines and allows adhesion of lymphocytes, monocytes, and eosinophils in areas of inflammation. VCAM-1 is among a family of membrane proteins structurally related to immunoglobulins (the immu-

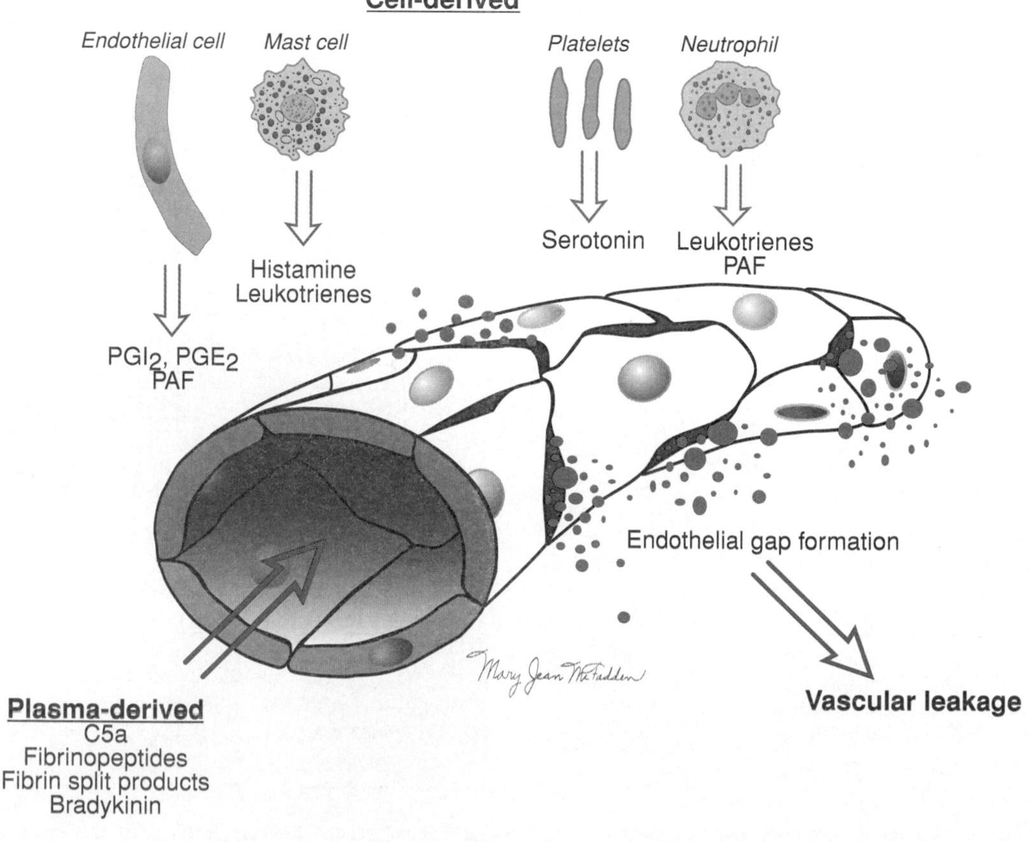

Fig. 18-16 Plasma- and cell-derived products inducing vascular permeability.

Table 18-10 Selectins and integrins

Molecule	Cells expressing	Counterreceptor and target cells
Selectins		
L-selectin (LAM-1 or LECAM-1)	PMNs, eosinophils, monocytes, lymphocytes	Sialyl-fucosyl-sulfated glycoproteins (endothelium)
E-selectin (ELAM-1)	Activated endothelial cells	Sialyl Lewis X (PMNs, monocytes)
P-selectin (GMP-140)	Activated platelets and endothelial cells	Sialyl Lewis X–like (PMNs, monocytes)
Integrins		
VLA-4 (α4β1)	Lymphocytes, monocytes, eosinophils	VCAM-1 (activated endothelium)
LFA (CD11a/CD18)	PMNs, monocytes, lymphocytes	ICAM-1, 2, and 3 (activated and unstimulated endothelium and other cells)
Mac-1 (CD11b/CD18)	PMNs, eosinophils, monocytes	ICAM-1 (activated and unstimulated endothelium and other cells)
P150,95 (CD11c/CD18)	PMNs, monocytes	Unknown

CD, Cluster designation; *ELAM*, endothelial leukocyte adhesion molecule; *GMP*, granule membrane protein; *ICAM*, intercellular adhesion molecule; *LAM*, leukocyte adhesion molecule; *LECAM*, lectin-cellular adhesion molecule; *LFA*, lymphocyte function–associated antigen; *Mac*, macrophage associated antigen-1; *PMN*, polymorphonuclear leukocytes; *VCAM*, vascular cell adhesion molecule; *VLA*, very late activation antigen.

Table 18-11 Immunoglobulin superfamily of addressins

Molecule	Cells expressing	Counterreceptor and target cells
ICAM-1	Endothelium and some epithelial cells	Mac-1 and LFA-1 (leukocytes)
ICAM-2	Endothelium	LFA-1 (leukocytes)
ICAM-3	Leukocytes	LFA-1 (leukocytes)
VCAM-1	Activated endothelium	VLA-4 (lymphocytes, monocytes, eosinophils)
PECAM-1	Endothelial junctional areas	Undefined ligand on endothelium, leukocytes, platelets

ICAM, Intercellular adhesion molecule; *LFA*, lymphocyte function-associated antigen or CD11a/CD18; *Mac-1*, macrophage associated antigen-1 or CD11b/CD18; *PECAM*, platelet-endothelial cell adhesion molecule; *VCAM*, vascular cell adhesion molecule; *VLA*, very late activation antigen.

noglobulin superfamily), which take part in cell-cell adhesion events (Table 18-11)

The β_2 integrins, also known as the leukocyte, integrins are among the best studied because of their apparent role in inflammation. The β_2 chain is common to this group and bears a specific antigenic moiety recognized by CD18-specific monoclonal antibodies. Monoclonal antibody reagents specific for three different alpha-chains define the three members of this subfamily—CD11a/CD18, CD11b/CD18, and CD11c/CD18 also known as lymphocyte function antigen-1, (LFA-1), Mac-1, and p150,95, respectively. The importance of these molecules is demonstrated clinically in patients who have absent or functionally impaired CD18 (leukocyte adhesion defect) and suffer from life-threatening microbial infections. It should be noted that there is a second type of adhesion defect in which sialyl Lewis X, the ligand for E and P selectins, is defective and likewise results in recurrent infections.

LFA-1 (CD11a/CD18) is expressed by lymphocytes, granulocytes, monocytes, and macrophages. Ligand binding to LFA-1 allows for both adhesion and augmented functional activities of leukocytes such as cell-mediated cytotoxicity and cytokine production. The LFA-1 counterreceptors are members of the immunoglobulin superfamily of glycoproteins, intercellular adhesion molecules (ICAM-1, ICAM-2, and ICAM-3) (Table 18-11). ICAM-1 is expressed by many tissues including endothelial, epithelial, and stromal cells. Normally, basal expression is low, but during inflammatory and immune responses, microbial products and cytokines such as IL-1 and TNF upregulate expression of ICAM-1 and promote local binding and activation of leukocytes. In contrast, ICAM-2, another LFA-1 counterreceptor, is constituitively expressed and not upregulated by cytokines, but it also appears to contribute to leukocyte-endothelial cell adhesion. ICAM-3 is expressed by lymphocytes and may play a role in lymphocyte adhesion and activation. PECAM-1 is also expressed constitutively at endothelial intercellular junctions and appears to participate in leukocyte transmigration through endothelial gaps.

Mac-1 (CD11b/CD18) is expressed by granulocytes, monocytes, macrophages, and natural killer cells but not by T- or B-lymphocytes. Counterreceptors for Mac-1 include ICAM-1, complement fragment iC3b, fibronectin, coagulation factor X, and certain bacterial glycoproteins. Because of its complement binding capacity, Mac-1 is also known as the type 3 complement receptor (CR3), and it confers the capacity of leukocytes to adhere to cells and particles coated with iC3b. Binding of Mac-1 also results in enhanced PMN leukocyte functions such as oxygen metabolite synthesis and phagocytosis. Monocytes constitutively express high levels of Mac-1, whereas PMNs rapidly mobilize this protein from intracellular stores upon stimulation with chemotactic agents.

The p150,95 (CD11c/CD18) integrin is located primarily on monocytes, macrophages, and NK cells. Like Mac-1, it binds to iC3b and appears to contribute to adhesion functions, but its full range of activities is unknown. Interestingly, p150,95 expression is greater on macrophages than on monocytes, an indication that its function may be maturation-associated.

Endothelial-leukocyte adhesion can also be mediated by a juxtacrine mechanism.[69] As mentioned above, one of the important products of activated endothelial cells is platelet-activating factor (PAF), which can be expressed in the membrane. PAF receptors of circulating leukocytes recognize and bind to the membrane PAF, allowing for both adhesion and leukocyte activation. The latter event promotes further interaction with β_2 integrins resulting in yet stronger adherence.

As shown in Fig. 18-17 *A,* the process of leukocyte adherence is believed to occur in sequential stages. Initial activation of endothelium by locally released microbial products (such as lipopolysaccharide) or cytokines (such as TNF and IL-1) results in the expression of E-selectin, and leukocytes begin loosely attaching to endothelial cells. Meanwhile, there is also upregulation of PAF, ICAM-1, and VCAM-1 expression along with the release of other products such as chemokines that promote leukocyte activation. The activated leukocytes display increased integrin expression as well as enhanced affinity for endothelial adherence molecules, resulting in strengthened binding and local aggregation. The cells then can respond to local chemotactic stimuli and begin transendothelial migration. Fig. 18-17, *B,* is a photomicrograph showing leukocyte adherence and local transmigration.

Chemotaxis

Leukocyte migration into the interstitium requires the crossing of several barriers, including endothelium, basement membrane, perivascular myofibroblasts, and matrix components. This directed migration, called "chemotaxis," occurs in response to chemotactic molecules generated in the vicinity of tissue insult and should be differentiated from simple increased random motion or chemokinesis. Both phenomena can be studied in vitro by observing the passage of cells through a porous membrane or gel matrix. Using this approach, several potent chemotactic agents are now known such as LTB4, PAF, C5a, chemokines (such as IL-8.), and bacterium-derived formylated peptides (such as fMLP, *N*-formyl-methionylleucyl phenylalanine). All stimulate chemotaxis at subnanomolar concentrations. At higher concentrations (>10 nM), IL-8, C5a, and fMLP also act as secretagogues causing granule release and respiratory burst. Specific receptors for each of the major chemotactic agents have been described in detail.[100-102] All are transmembrane proteins with a series of intracellular and extracellular loops. The third intracellular loop and final carboxy terminus are associated with a cytoplasmic G-protein that couples the chemoattractant binding to the cellular response (Fig. 18-18). The G-protein is a heterotrimeric molecule that binds guanine triphosphate (GTP) and then activates a phospholipase C, which cleaves membrane phosphatidylinositol.[103] The resulting cleavage products are inositol 1,4,5-trisphosphate (IP-3) and 1,2-diacylgycerol (DAG). The IP-3 mediates calcium mobilization, which appears to be involved in leukocyte motility and subsequent activation of other phospholipases. The accumulation of DAG is linked to the activation of protein kinase C and secretory events, as well as the activation of phospholipase A_2 and consequent arachidonic acid metabolism. As mentioned above, the nonlipid chemoattractants stimulate secretory responses at higher concentrations, an action that seems related to their capacity to induce sustained DAG accumulation. It should be noted that there are several other GTP-binding proteins that are linked to leukocyte functions. For example, *rac*1 and *rac*2 are low molecular weight G-proteins that are tied to the respiratory burst response through activation of NADPH-oxidase.[104]

In vitro studies indicate that leukocytes may move by forward projection of cytoplasm (lamellipodia) that are anchored and used to pull the rearward portions of the cell. This motion involves dynamic assembly and disassembly of actin subunits, which is dependent on gradients of intracellular calcium.[105] Actin filaments are concentrated in cytoplasmic projections and in zones of phagocytic engulfment. Polymerization is regulated by several proteins that inhibit assembly such as gelsolin, profilin, acumentin, and macrophage capping protein. These proteins are believed to contain the polymerization process allowing for localized changes in the cytoskeleton. The importance of actin is revealed by the effect of cytochalasin B, a fungus-derived agent that disrupts actin polymerization and blocks both directed leukocyte motility and phagocytosis. Interestingly, the secretagogue activity of the nonlipid chemotactic compounds is promoted by cytochalasin, indicating that secretion occurs by an actin-independent mechanism. Leukocyte motion also involves contractile events that are believed to require actin-myosin interactions, but the role of myosin is presently unknown.

Movement of leukocytes through the tissue framework appears to involve integrin-mediated attachments to matrix elements, allowing anchoring of cytoplasmic projections (Fig. 18-19). In addition, enzymes released by leukocytes potentially digest and remodel matrix elements to assist their movement. Thus there is a teleologic basis for the association of chemotaxis with secretory events.

Effector functions

Leukocytes arriving to a site of tissue injury or infection are equipped with an array of mechanisms that eliminate offending microbes and remove damaged or aberrant tissue components. Depending on the nature of the insult, differing mechanisms are invoked. For example, bacterial infections are eliminated by both extracellular release of microbicidal factors and phagocytosis with intraphagosome release of toxic agents. Virally infected cells can be killed directly by cytotoxic lymphocytes, by antibody-dependent cell-mediated killing, or by complement-dependent lysis. Large multicellular parasites must be killed by extracellular release of digestive and toxic agents. This section is a discussion of the major classes of leukocyte effector functions, phagocytosis, secretory responses, and cell-mediated cytotoxicity.

Phagocytosis

Attachment. The first stage of phagocytosis requires energy-independent attachment to the target particle.[106] As mentioned previously, this step is greatly enhanced when the particle is coated with opsonins. The classic opsonins are immunoglobulin and complement-activation fragments (C3b, iC3b, and C4b). In addition to these classical opsonins, there are several serum acute-phase proteins that have opsonin activity, such as mannose binding protein and lipopolysaccharide binding protein, that directly bind yeast and bacterial cell wall components. In the absence of opsonins, macrophages

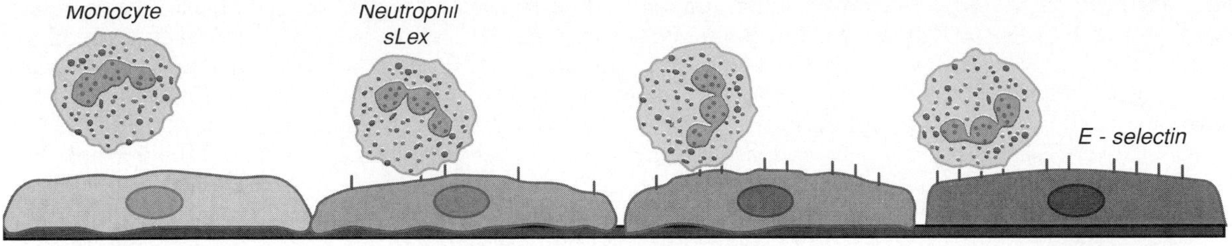

1. "Rolling" with sLex - E - selectin interactions with activated endothelium.

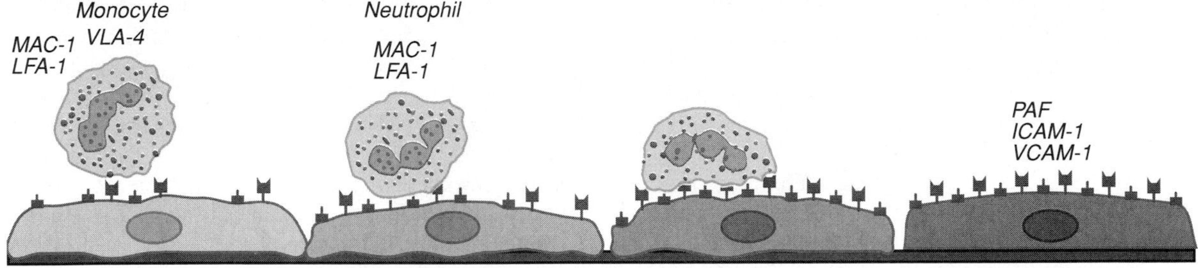

2. Juxtacrine interactions with activation, increased expression of ICAM and VCAM with intergrin binding.

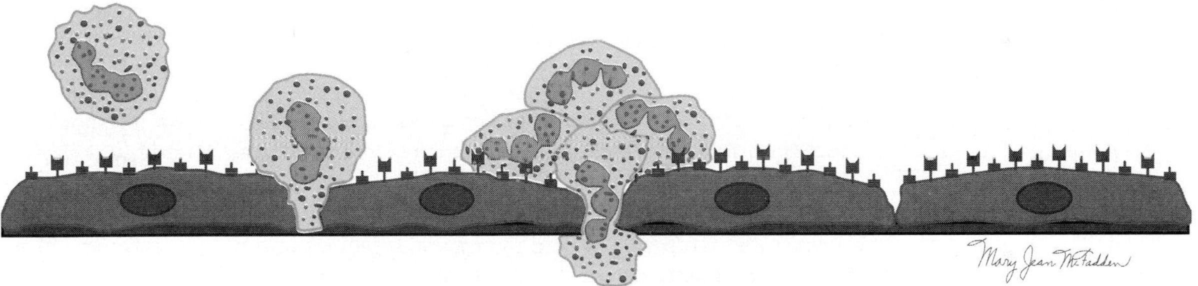

3. Strengthened adhesion with aggregation and transmigration.

A

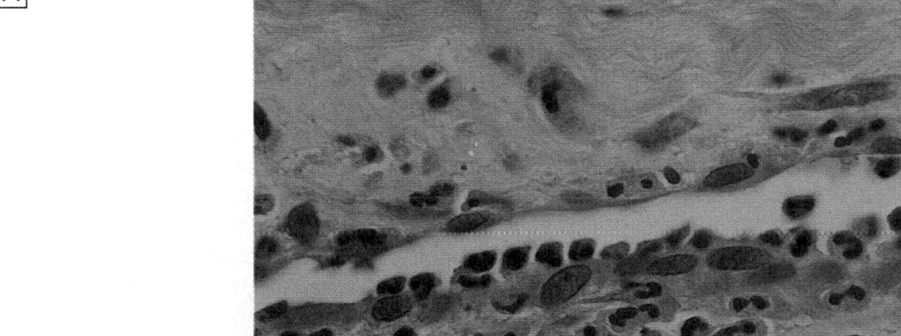

Fig. 18-17 Leukocyte-endothelial adherence during inflammatory responses. **A,** Stages of leukocyte adherence and aggregation. **B,** Photomicrograph showing leukocyte adherence and transmigration in an area of inflammation.

bear receptors for mannose-fucosyl carbohydrate residues that allow attachment to certain yeasts and bacteria. Attachment by way of the classic opsonins is mediated by Fc and complement receptors expressed by leukocytes. Leukocytes bear a variety of Fc receptors with differing Ig isotype specificities; the IgM (Fcμ), IgG (Fcγ), and IgA (Fcα) receptors all can play a role in attachment, but IgG1 and IgG3 are the dominant Ig opsonins. There is heterogeneity among Fc receptors for IgG as well as cell-specific expression. For example, the Fcγ RI is expressed primarily by monocytes and macrophages; it binds IgG1 and IgG3 with high affinity. The low-affinity IgG1/IgG3 binding Fcγ RII is expressed by all leukocytes. An intermediate-affin-

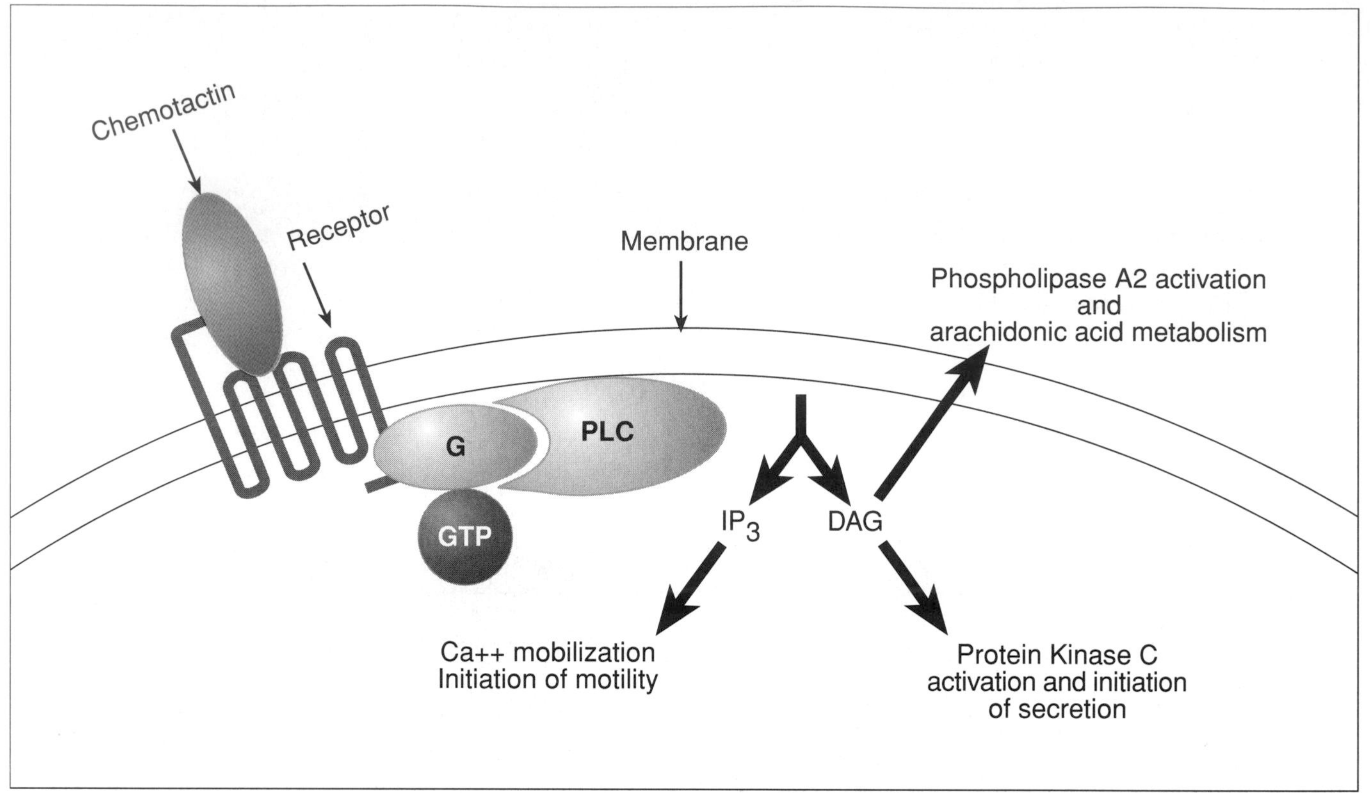

Fig. 18-18 Stimulus-response coupling after binding of chemotactin to its receptor. Activation of membrane-associated G-proteins leads to phospholipase C activation and the generation of inositol trisphosphate (IP-3) and diacylglycerol (DAG), compounds influencing motility and secretion, respectively.

ity IgG1/IgG3 binding Fcγ RIII has two forms; the A form is expressed mainly by PMNs and the B form is found on macrophages and NK cells. Likewise, a variety of complement receptors (CR) are known. CR1 and CR3 are expressed by most phagocytic cells and are important in opsonin-mediated phagocytosis. CR1 binds C3b with high affinity, whereas CR3 avidly binds the C3bi degradation product of C3b. CR3 is identical to the Mac-1 integrin that binds ICAM-1 and consequently plays a role in both phagocytosis and endothelial adhesion. FcR and CR expression or activity are regulated by cytokines. Interferon-γ profoundly upregulates the expression of Fcγ RI but simultaneously deactivates binding capacity of CR. In contrast, other cytokines such as chemotactins and TNF transiently enhance CR3 binding activity.

Engulfment. The engulfment stage of phagocytosis is an energy-dependent active cellular process. The phagocyte extends flat actin-rich pseudopods around the particle, and they ultimately meet and pinch off to form an intracellular phagosome containing the particle. The particle must be fully opsonized, since the membrane moves over the surface by recognizing the opsonin molecules. The process of engulfment is activated in the presence of matrix proteins, that is, fibronectin and laminin, that bind a leukocyte β_3 integrin, called the "leukocyte response integrin." Additionally, low molecular weight products of T cells can also activate phagocytosis. The major features of phagocytosis are summarized in Fig. 18-20.

Secretion. Upon engulfment, the phagocyte enters a secretory phase in which preformed granules begin to fuse with the phagosome and the plasma membrane, discharging enzymes and microbicidal factors into the phagosome and extracellular environment. Again, the importance of these mechanisms is illustrated by congenital abnormalities of leukocyte granules, such as Chédiak-Higashi syndrome and neutrophil-specific granule deficiency, diseases associated with severe recurrent infections.[107,108] The mechanisms of secretion are largely unknown, but similar to motility induction, there is involvement of G-proteins, protein kinases, and calcium ion fluxes. Evidence indicates that the various types of intracellular granules (lysosomes, specific granules, azurophilic granules, and so forth) are mobilized independently.[109] Particularly, the specific or secondary granules of PMNs are more accessible for extracellular release, whereas the azurophilic granules may preferentially fuse with phagosomes.

In addition to the preformed, granule-stored products, phagocytic leukocytes and in particular mononuclear phagocytes begin de novo synthesis and secretion of a variety of active compounds. These include enzymes (such as hydrolases, elastase, collagenase, and plasminogen activator), cytokines (such as IL-1, IL-6 TNF, IFN-α/β, CSFs, PDGF, and TGF-β), active lipid mediators (such as prostaglandins, leukotrienes, and PAF) and oxygen metabolites (such as O_2^-, H_2O_2, and HOCl).[21] The range of activity and nature of these products indicate that leukocyte secretory efforts are directed at both the immediate destruction of invading microbes and the regulation of other cellular participants.

Although leukocytes produce a variety of oxygen-independent antimicrobial factors such as lysosomal hydrolases, bactericidal/permeability increasing factor, defensins, and cationic proteins, the production of reactive oxygen metabolites is

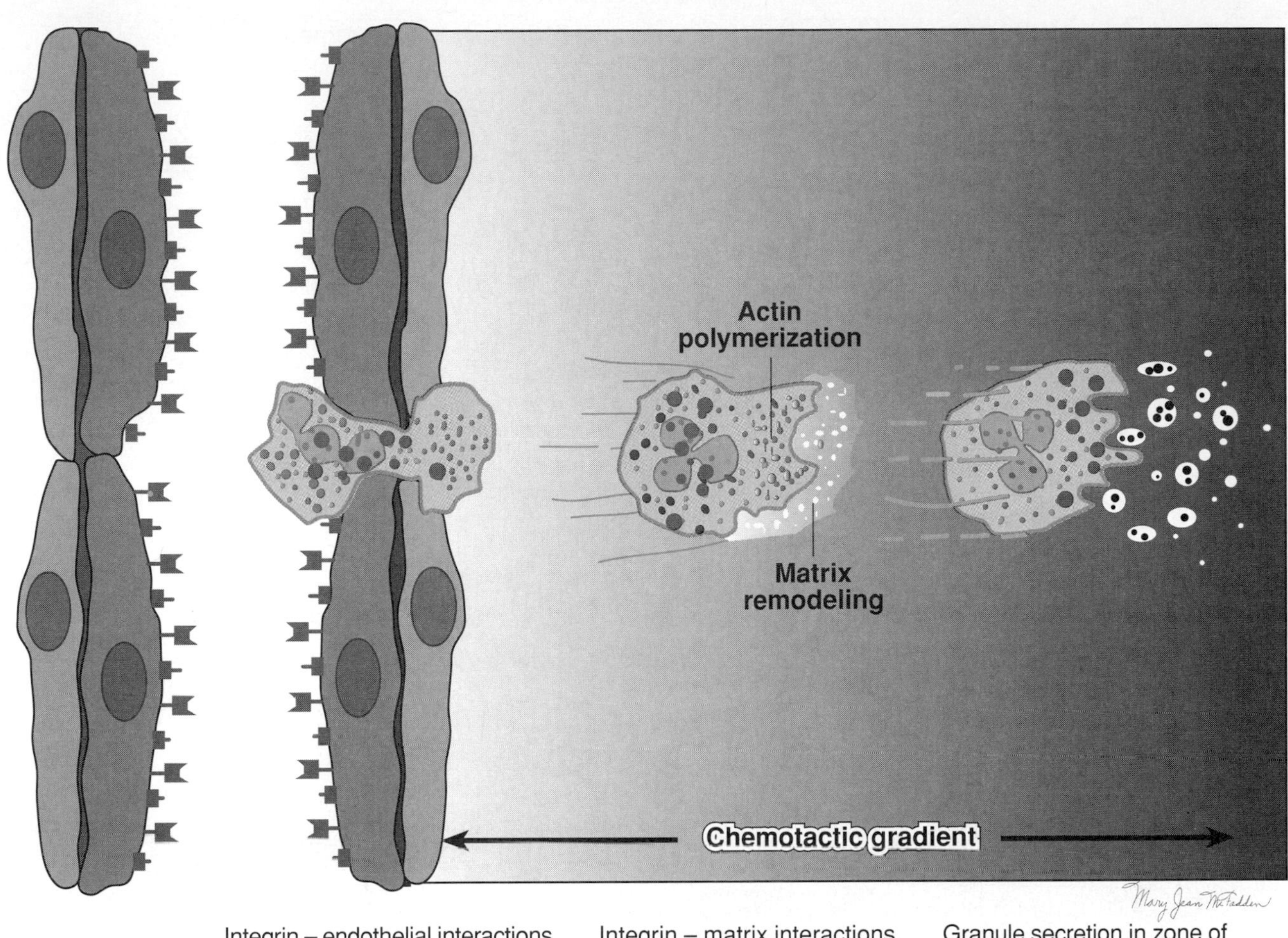

Fig. 18-19 Stages of leukocyte chemotaxis and secretion.

clearly a critical mechanism of microbial killing.[110, 111] Stimulation of phagocytic leukocytes is associated with a phase of increased oxygen consumption known as the "respiratory burst." Hypoxia blocks this response and causes impaired microbicidal activity.[112] Central to this response is NADPH oxidase, an enzyme complex that is assembled by adduction of cytoplasmic cofactors to the cell membrane and catalyzes transfer of electrons from NADPH to molecular oxygen.[113,114] Congenital defects of this enzyme result in the disease syndrome called "chronic granulomatous disease of childhood" (CGD), characterized by repeated and often fatal bacterial, especially catalase-producing *Staphlyococcus* spp. and sometimes fungal infections.[115] As illustrated in Fig. 18-21, NADPH-oxidase generates superoxide anion (O_2^-) which undergoes dismutation to form hydrogen peroxide (H_2O_2). The latter is then utilized by myeloperoxidase or eosinophil peroxidase in the presence of halide ion (Cl^-, I^-, or Br^-) to generate toxic hypohalous acids (HOCl, HOI, or HOBr). Some phagocytosed microbes (such as streptococci and pneumococci) aid in their own destruction by producing H_2O_2 themselves. Individuals with CGD are usually resistant to these organisms. Hydroxyl radical ($OH^{\cdot}$) is another highly reactive oxygen metabolite that can be derived from H_2O_2 by O_2^--mediated reduction (the Haber-Weiss reaction) or in the presence of ferrous ion (Fe^{2+}) (the Fenton reaction). The oxygen metabolites cause cell death by halogenation and oxidation of critical proteins, lipids, hemes, and nucleotides.

The production of reactive oxygen metabolites is especially required for the elimination of microbes that can grow within phagosomes of mononuclear phagocytes. Major examples of these organisms include *Mycobacterium tuberculosis, Histoplasma capsulatum,* and *Listeria* monocytogenes. Elimination of these organisms is promoted by cytokines such as interferon-γ that enhance the capacity of phagocytes to produce oxygen metabolites.

Recently, there has been growing interest in the role of nitric oxide ($NO^{\cdot}$) in inflammatory responses. It was previously mentioned that endothelial cells produce NO as a vascular relaxation factor.[48] Experimental models using mouse macrophages have demonstrated that activated macrophages also produce NO as a byproduct of the oxidation of arginine with formation of citrulline (Fig. 18-22). The NO or its derivatives oxidizes iron-sulfur centers in target cells, resulting in impaired DNA synthesis and cell respiration; NO has been shown to have tumoricidal, fungicidal, and antiparasitic action.[116] The role of NO in human resistance to microbes is not fully known.

Unfortunately, many of the secreted enzymes and oxygen metabolites are not discriminating, and when released into the extracellular environment they also cause damage to host tis-

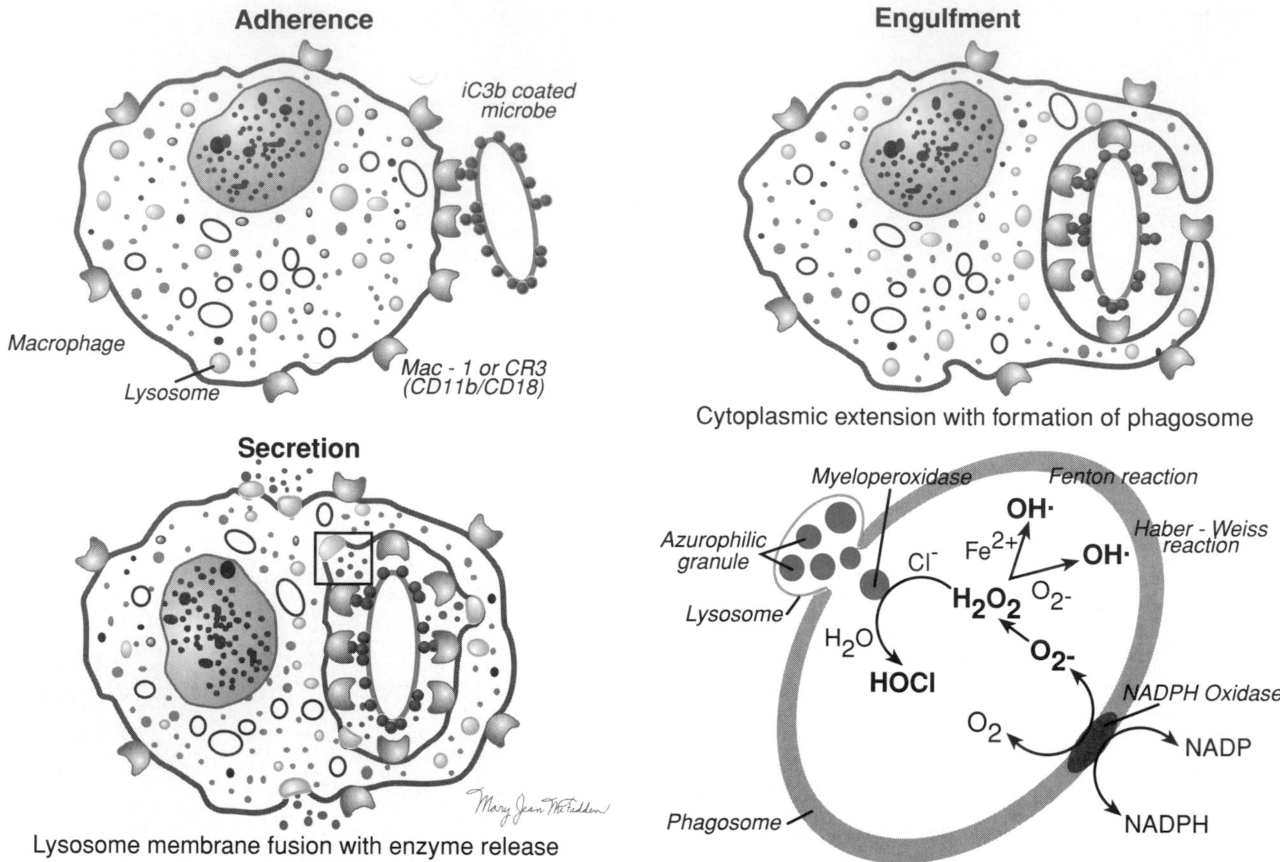

Fig. 18-20 Stages of phagocytosis of opsonized particle. Adherence is followed by engulfment and secretion. The biochemical reactions in the boxed area of the secretory cell are illustrated at lower right.

sues. The host is equipped with several mechanisms to limit this damage, as discussed later regarding regulation of inflammation.

Cell-mediated cytotoxicity

The effector functions discussed so far usually involve PMNs, eosinophils, or MP and are mainly designed to kill and eliminate bacteria, fungi, and parasites. Virally infected and neoplastic cells represent difficult challenges for the immune system. Elimination of these cells requires recognition of aberrant or altered membrane antigens followed by killing of the target cell. This function can be executed by MP if they are directed by their Fc receptors loaded with antibodies specific for the target antigen, a mechanism known as antibody-dependent cell-mediated cytotoxicity (ADCC).[117] Killing by this mechanism involves the production of toxic oxygen metabolites that are presumably spilled directly onto the target cell.

Antibody-independent cell-mediated cytotoxicity is a relegated function of cytotoxic lymphocytes.[118] Two classes of lymphocytes with cytotoxic function are known—natural killer (NK) and cytotoxic T-lymphocytes (CTL). As mentioned above, the latter are CD8+ T-cells that are generated from small agranular lymphocytes after exposure to antigens in the context of class I histocompatibility molecules. These cells enter a memory pool, since there is an anamnestic response upon reexposure to antigen. In contrast, NK cells represent a non-T, non-B-cell population of large lymphocytes with cytoplasmic granules. In the peripheral blood they compose about 5% of the lymphoid population. They do not have MHC-restricted antigen-specific receptors or display memory responses like T-cells, but they do express Fc receptors and thereby can execute ADCC. Most notably, NK cells have the capacity to directly interact with and kill a wide variety of cells including tumor cells, virus-infected cells, and subpopulations of normal immature cells. NK cells respond to cytokine activation and are largely responsible for what is known as lymphokine-activated killer cell (LAK) activity, an enhanced cytotoxic activity after exposure of blood lymphoid cells to IL-2.[119] NK cells also produce IFN and through its action may enhance other immune responses. Killing by both NK and CTL requires initial binding to the target cell but the precise nature of the target structure recognized by NK cells is unknown (Fig. 18-23). Likewise, the killing mechanism or mechanisms of these cells are unclear, but it is known that NK cell granules contain a cytolytic protein called "cytolysin" and CTL contain an identical protein called "perforin." These proteins are related to the C9 complement component and similarly disrupt ion transport by creating characteristic circular pores in target cells.[120] One can assume that the specificity of killing is completely at the recognition stage.

Regulation of inflammation

It is evident from the above discussions that invocation of inflammatory responses unleashes a multitude of plasma and cell-derived molecules with potentially damaging effects on host tissues. These effects are observed most dramatically in the hypersensitivity disease states (see Chapter 25, Immunopathology) and chronic inflammatory conditions. To minimize

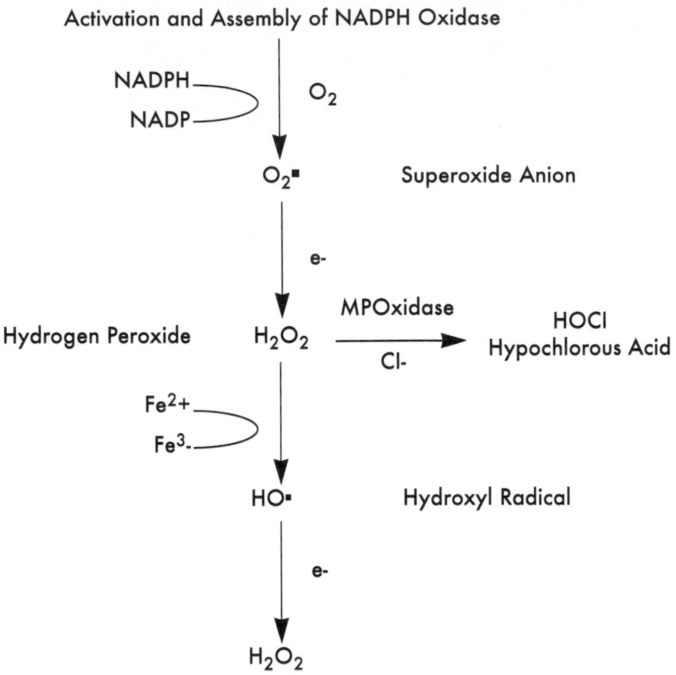

Fig. 18-21 Phagocyte-derived toxic oxygen products generated after NADPH oxidase assembly.

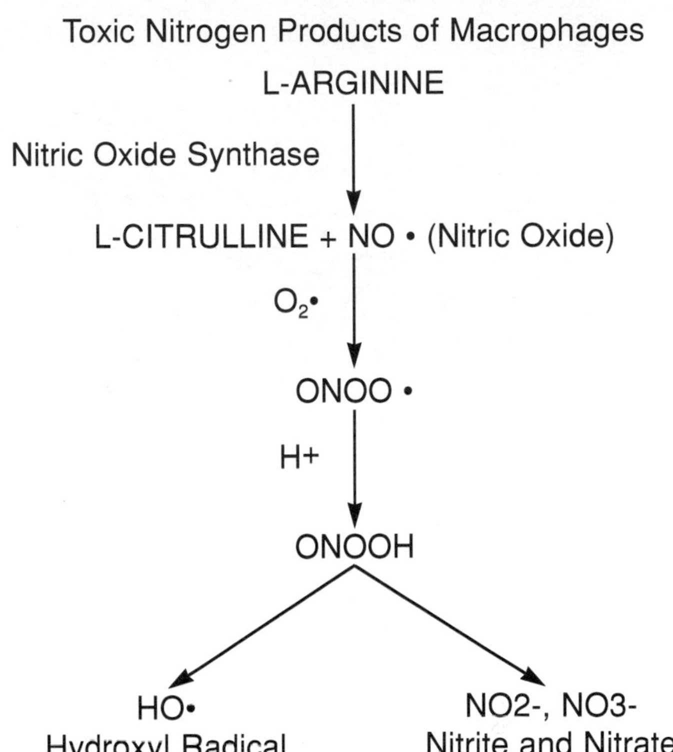

Fig. 18-22 Macrophage-derived toxic nitrogen products generated after nitric oxide synthase induction and activation.

the self-damaging effects of inflammation, the host applies a variety of mechanisms to contain and when possible eventually resolve inflammation.

The acute phase proteins

Infection and tissue trauma are associated with characteristic changes in the levels and composition of plasma proteins.[121,122] When combined with fever and leukocytosis this reaction is known as the "acute-phase response." The bulk of plasma proteins are derived from the liver, which synthesizes acute-phase proteins (APP) in response to circulating cytokines produced during inflammation. IL-6 and to a lesser extent IL-1 appear to be important cytokines responsible for APP synthesis.[123] Table 18-12 lists some of the major APP and their functions. Although some of these proteins, such as C-reactive protein and C3, have opsonic activity and directly participate in microbial resistance, others play a regulatory role. For example, α_1-antitrypsin and ceruloplasmin respectively help to inactivate proteases and reactive oxygen metabolites secreted by leukocytes. Activated humoral factors such as bradykinin are also regulated by α_1-antitrypsin and α_2-macroglobulin. Congenital deficiency of α_1-antitrypsin results in severe lung and liver disease because of the chronic injury from repeated inflammatory events.

Table 18-12 **Acute-phase proteins**

Protein	Function
α_1-Antitrypsin	Antiproteinase
α_1-acid glycoprotein	Transport protein
Cysteine protease inhibitor	Antiproteinase
Haptoglobin	Binds hemoglobin
Fibrinogen	Coagulation factor
C-reactive protein	Activates complement
Complement factor 3	Opsonin
Mannose binding protein	Opsonin
LPS binding protein	Opsonin
Ceruloplasmin	O_2 metabolite scavenger
Hemopexin	Heme binding protein
Serum amyloid A	Apolipoprotein
Serum amyloid P	Unknown

Glucocorticoids

The antiinflammatory effect of corticosteroids is well known and indeed levels of endogenous glucocorticoids (GC) increase in response to infection or trauma. Cytokines such as IL-1 and TNF have the capacity to induce GC synthesis and thereby may act in a feedback manner to regulate inflammation.[124] GCs inhibit a broad range of inflammatory functions including the production of cytokines, histamine release, phagocytosis, oxygen-metabolite release and immunoglobulin production.[125] GCs also enhance the production of APP and increase IL-6 and IL-1 receptor expression. The precise mechanism or mechanisms of GC antiinflammatory actions are unknown, but like many other tissues, leukocytes bear glucocorticoid receptors, which can be translocated to the nucleus where they signal the transcription of target genes.

Analysis of the regulatory effects of GCs is complicated by the fact that in vitro and in vivo effects do not always correlate. For example, GCs reduce immunoglobulin production in vivo but enhance it in vitro. Similarly, there is clear evidence that GCs inhibit leukocyte production of arachidonic acid

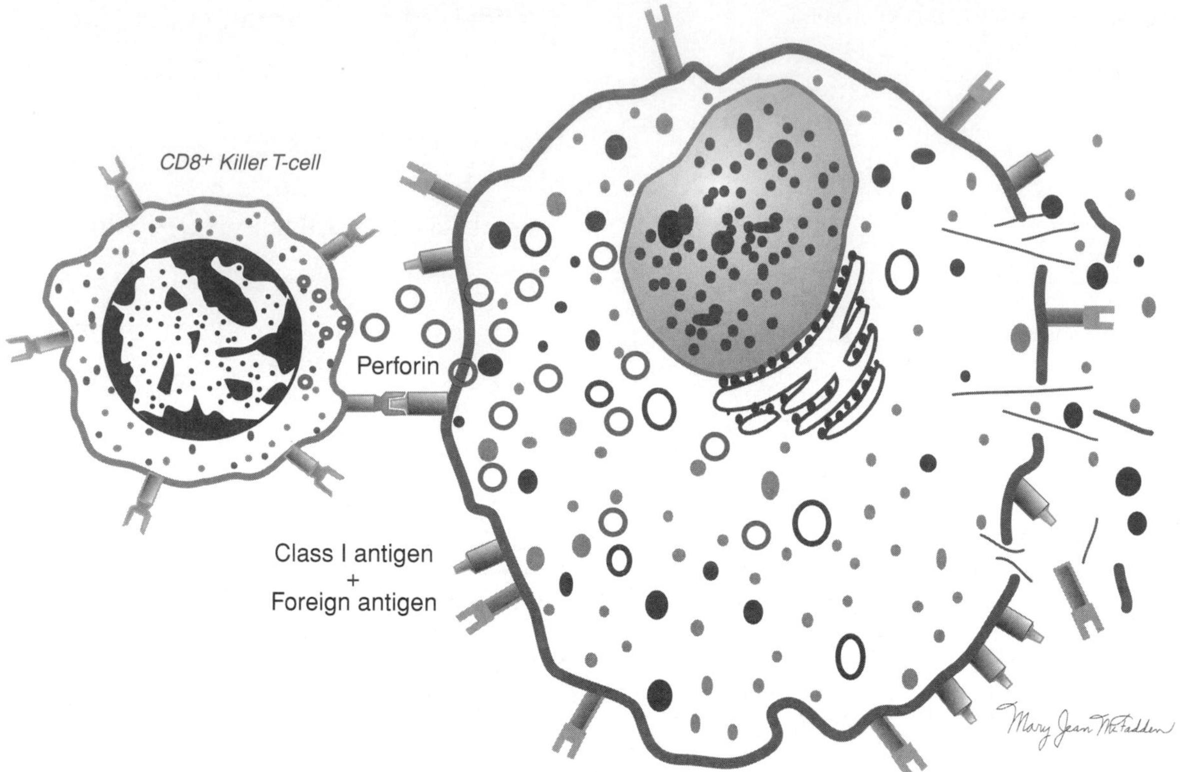

Fig. 18-23 CD8$^+$ T-cell–mediated cytotoxicity. Killer T-cell binds to target cell by means of antigen and class I MHC membrane proteins and then releases perforin, which permeabilizes the membrane and kills the target cell.

metabolites in vitro; this effect is attributed to the induction of a regulatory 40 kD cytoplasmic protein called "lipocortin," a phospholipid binding protein that regulates the activity of phospholipase A_2.[126] Despite this finding, glucocorticoids do not appear to inhibit arachidonate metabolism when adminstered to human volunteers. Clearly, the mechanisms by which GCs regulate inflammation are complex and will require further elucidation.

Shed receptors and receptor antagonists

There is mounting evidence indicating that cytokine activity is modulated by shed cytokine receptors and endogenous receptor antagonists. Free cytokine receptors are detectable in the serum of individuals with a variety of inflammatory diseases. Interleukin-2 receptors are detectable in the serum of patients with chronic inflammatory conditions[127] such as sarcoidosis, tuberculosis, rheumatoid arthritis, and Crohn's disease. Similarly, TNF receptors are detectable in the serum of patients with systemic lupus erythematosus.[128] In general, the presence of the soluble receptors directly correlates with disease activity, but experimental evidence indicates that they may help to neutralize cytokine effects. For example, in a mouse model of experimental pneumonitis, administration of exogenous soluble TNF receptor inhibited acute inflammation induced by locally instilled bacterial endotoxin.[129]

Cytokine action can also be modulated by naturally occurring cytokine receptor antagonists. Mononuclear phagocytes are a major source of the broad-range cytokine, IL-1; these cells also produce a partially homologous protein known as IL-1 receptor antagonist (IL-1 ra).[74,130] This protein binds to the two known types of IL-1 receptors and effectively blocks the action of IL-1. Under experimental conditions IL-1 ra can temper symptoms of endotoxic shock[131] and appears to act as an endogenous inhibitor of inflammation.[132]

Suppressor cells

Cellular immunologists have long recognized a population of suppressor T-cells with the capacity to inhibit the functions of other T-cells as well as those of B-cells. Despite numerous studies the precise mechanisms of regulation have remained obscure. However, there appears to be a complex network of CD4$^+$ and CD8$^+$ T-cells that acquire the capacity to recognize specific lymphocyte antigen receptor sites, or idiotypes, of the target lymphocytes to be suppressed.[133] These anti-idiotypic cells in turn neutralize the action of effector lymphocytes either by direct elimination or by production of soluble factors that block antigen recognition. Suppressor T-cells inhibit immunoglobulin production and the hypersensitivity type of inflammation; they are generally considered to be of the CD8 phenotype, but CD4 cells may be required for their generation.

Cross-regulatory cytokines

The particular manifestation of an immunoinflammatory response is also influenced by cytokine cross-regulation.[134] As alluded to previously, CD4$^+$ and likely CD8$^+$ T-cells can be divided into subpopulations based upon the profiles of cytokines that they produce.[135] Type 1, or Th1, cells produce IFN-γ and IL-2 and are believed to be required for effective responses to intracellular pathogens such as *Mycobacteria* spp.

and *Listeria* spp. Type 2, or Th2, cells produce IL-4, IL-5, and IL-10 and are involved in antibody responses and the allergic type of inflammatory responses. A dominant Th2 response to an intracellular pathogen results in ineffective parasite removal and potential death of the host.[136] Depending on the cytokine environment a Th1 or Th2 response can predominate. IFN-γ and IL-12 promote the development of Th1 cells and inhibit Th2 cells. Conversely, Th2 cytokines, IL-4 and IL-10, promote Th2 cell maturation and inhibit Th1 cells. The dominant response is determined by the nature of the antigen and host genetic factors. There are likely other lymphocyte populations with characteristic cytokine profiles, and their potential roles in the induction and modulation of inflammation are presently under investigation.

Finally, a note should be made regarding mediators with both inflammatory and regulatory functons. Prostaglandin E_2 and prostacyclin are vasoactive but also cause elevation of cAMP levels in leukocytes, which inhibits many of their effector functions such as phagocytosis, synthetic events, and secretion.[62] Histamine likewise is a potent proinflammatory mediator, but it can also stimulate H_2 receptor–bearing suppressor cells.[137] Transforming growth factor-β is angiogenic as well as chemotactic for fibroblasts and macrophages, but it also inhibits the growth and function of many leukocytes and stromal cells.[138] Hence, inflammation likely depends upon a balance of proinflammatory and antiinflammatory signals that constantly changes as the response evolves and resolves.

REFERENCES

1. Burnet, FM, Fenner R: *The production of antibodies,* Melbourne, 1949, Macmillan.
2. Metchnikoff E: *Immunity to infective diseases,* London, 1905, Cambridge University Press.

Patterns of inflammation

3. Boros DL: Granulomatous inflammation, *Prog Allergy* 24:183, 1978.
4. Warren KS: A functional classification of granulomatous inflammation, *Ann NY Acad Sci* 278:7, 1976.

Humoral and cellular participants of inflammation

Humoral elements

5. Kay AB, Pepper DS, McKenzie R: The identification of fibrinopeptide B as a chemotactic agent derived from human fibrinogen, *Br J Haematol* 27:669, 1974.
6. Senior RM, Skogen WF, Griffin GL, Wilner GD: Effects of fibrinogen derivatives upon the inflammatory response: studies with human fibrinopeptide B, *J Clin Invest* 77:1014, 1986.
7. Movat HZ: Chemical mediators of the vascular phenomena of the acute inflammatory response, *Med Clin North Am* 56:541, 1976.
8. Saldeen T, Ryan JW, Ragnarsson U: A peptide formed by fibrinolysis increases microvascular permeability and inhibits angiotensin converting enzyme, *Adv Exp Med Biol* 156:829, 1983.
9. Cochrane CG, Griffin JH: The biochemistry and pathophysiology of the contact system of plasma, *Adv Immunol* 33:241, 1982.
10. Movat HZ, Habal FM, MacMorine DRL: Neutral proteases of human PMN leukocytes with kininogenase activity, *Int Arch Allergy Appl Immunol* 50:257, 1976.
11. Müller-Eberhard HJ: Molecular organization and function of the complement system, *Annu Rev Biochem* 57:321, 1988.
12. Hugli TE, Müller-Eberhard HJ: Anaphylatoxins: C3a and C5a, *Adv Immunol* 26:1, 1978
13. Burton DR: Structure and function of antibodies: In Calabi R, Neuberger MS, editors: *Molecular genetics of immunoglobulin,* Amsterdam, 1987, Elsevier Science Publishers.
14. Metzger H, Alcaraz G, Hohman R et al: The receptor with high affinity for immunoglobulin E, *Annu Rev Immunol* 4:419, 1986.
15. Capron A, Ameisen JC, Joseph M et al: New functions for platelets and their pathologic implications, *Int Arch Allergy Appl Immunol* 77:107, 1985.
16. Capron M, Spiegelberg HL, Prin L et al: Role of IgE receptors in effector functions of human eosinophils, *J Immunol* 40:416, 1984.

Blood-borne cells

17. Bainton DF: Developmental biology of neutrophils and eosinophils. In Gallin JI, Goldstein IM, Snyderman R, editors: *Inflammation: basic principles and clinical correlates,* New York, 1992, Raven Press.
18. Dewald B, Bretz U, Baggiolini M: Release of gelatinase from a novel secretory compartment of human neutrophils, *J Clin Invest* 70:518, 1982.
19. Cicco N, Lindemann A, Content J et al: Inducible production of interleukin-6 by human polymorphonuclear neutrophils: role of granulocyte-macrophage colony-stimulating factor and tumor necrosis factor alpha, *Blood* 75:2049, 1990.
20. van Furth R, van Zwet TL: Production and migration or monocytes and kinetics of macrophages. In van Furth R, editor: *Mononuclear phagocytes: biology of monocytes and macrophages,* Dordrecht, 1992, Kluwer Academic Publishers.
21. Nathan CF: Secretory products of macrophages, *J Clin Invest* 79:319, 1987.
22. Adams DO, Hamilton TA: Molecular bases of macrophage activation: diversity and its origins. In *The natural immune system,* vol 2, Oxford, 1992, Oxford University Press.
23. Gordon S, Perry VH, Rabinowitz S et al: Plasma membrane receptors of the mononuclear phagocyte system, *J Cell Science* 9(suppl):1, 1988.
24. Cohn ZA: The activation of mononuclear phagocytes: fact, fancy and future, *J Immunol* 121:813, 1978.
25. Germain RN, Margulies DH: The biochemistry and cell biology of antigen processing and presentation, *Annu Rev Immunol* 11:403, 1993.
26. Adams DO, Hamilton TA: The activated macrophage and granulomas, *Curr Top Pathol* 79:151, 1989.
27. Möst JH, Neumayer HP, Dierich MP: Cytokine-induced generation of multinucleate giant cells in vitro requires interferon-gamma and expression of LFA-1, *Eur J Immunol* 20:1661, 1990.
28. Paul WE: Development and function of lymphocytes. In Gallin JI, Goldstein IM, Snyderman R, editors: *Inflammation: basic principles and clinical correlates,* New York, 1992, Raven Press.
29. Marrack P, Kappler J: The T-cell receptor, *Science* 238:1073, 1987.
30. Haas W, Pereira P, Tonegawa S: Gamma/delta T-cells, *Annu Rev Immunol* 11:637, 1993.
31. Littman DR: The structure of the T-4 and T-8 genes, *Annu Rev Immunol* 5:561, 1987.
32. Duijvestijn A, Hamann A: Mechanisms and regulation of lymphocyte migration, *Immunol Today* 10:23, 1989.
33. Clark EA, Lane PJL: Regulation of human B-cell activation and adhesion, *Annu Rev Immunol* 9:97, 1991.
34. Herberman RB, Reynolds CW, Ortaldo JR: Mechanism of cytotoxicity by natural killer (NK) cells, *Annu Rev Immunol* 4:651, 1986.
35. Weller PF: The immunobiology of eosinophils, *N Engl J Med* 324:1010, 1991.
36. Gleich, GJ, Adolphson CR, Leiferman KM: Eosinophils. In Gallin JI, Goldstein IM, Snyderman R, editors: *Inflammation: basic principles and clinical correlates,* New York, 1992, Raven Press.
37. Metcalfe DD, Costa JJ, Burd PR: Mast cell and basophils. In Gallin JI, Goldstein IM, Snyderman R, editors: *Inflammation: basic principles and clinical correlates,* New York, 1992, Raven Press.
38. Metcalfe D: The molecular control of cell division, differentiation, commitment and maturation in haematopoietic cells, *Nature* 339:27, 1989.
39. Kirshenbaum AS, Kessler SW, Goff JP, Metcalfe DD: Demonstration of the origin of human mast cells from CD34+ bone marrow progenitor cells, *J Immunol* 146:1410, 1991.
40. Holgate ST, Robinson C, Church MK: Mediators of immediate hypersensitivity. In Middleton E Jr, Reed CE, Ellis EF et al, editors: *Allergy: principles and practice,* ed 4, St Louis, 1993, Mosby.
41. Kuna P, Reddigari SR, Schall TJ et al: RANTES, a monocyte and T-lymphocyte chemotactic cytokine releases histamine from human basophils, *J Immunol* 149:636, 1992.

42. Weksler BB: Platelets, In Gallin JI, Goldstein IM, Snyderman R, editors: *Inflammation: basic principles and clinical correlates,* New York, 1992, Raven Press.
43. Sporn MB, Roberts AB: Peptide growth factors and inflammation, tissue repair and cancer, *J Clin Invest* 78:329, 1986.
44. Verbeuren TJ: Synthesis, storage, release and metabolism of 5-hydroxytryptamine in peripheral tissues. In Fozard JR, editor: *The peripheral actions of 5-hydroxytryptamine,* New York, 1989, Oxford University Press.

Stromal elements

45. Pober JS, Cotran RS: The role of endothelial cells in inflammation, *Transplantation* 50:537, 1990.
46. Shimizu Y, Newman W, Tanaka Y, Shaw S: Lymphocyte interactions with endothelial cells, *Immunol Today* 13:106, 1992.
47. Marcus AJ: The eicosanoids in biology and medicine, *Lipid Res* 25:1511, 1984.
48. Moncada S, Palmer RJM, Higgs EA: The discovery of nitric oxides as the endogenous nitrovasodilator, *Hypertension* 12:365, 1988.
49. Luscher TF: Endothelin: systemic arterial and pulmonary effects of a new peptide with potent biologic properties, *Am Rev Respir Dis* 146:S56, 1992.
50. Strieter RM, Kunkel SL, Showel HJ et al: Endothelial cell gene expression of a neutrophil chemotactic factor by TNFα, LPS and IL-1b, *Science* 243:1467, 1989.
51. Strieter RM, Wiggin R, Phan SH et al: Monocyte chemotactic peptide gene expression by cytokine treated human fibroblasts and endothelial cells, *Biochem Biophys Res Commun* 162:694, 1989.
52. Fibbe WE, Van Damme JV, Billiau A et al: Human fibroblasts produce granulocyte CSF, macrophage CSF, and granulocyte-macrophage CSF following stimulation by interleukin 1 and poly(rI)-poly(rC), *Blood* 72:860, 1988.
53. Walther Z, May LT, Sehgal PB: Transcriptional regulation of the interferon β_2/B-cell differentiation factor BSF-21 hepatocyte-stimulating factor gene in human fibroblasts by other cytokines, *J Immunol* 140:974, 1988.
54. Ruoslahti E: Fibronectin and its receptors, *Annu Rev Biochem* 57:375, 1988.
55. Erickson HP, Bourdon MA: Tenascin: an extracellular matrix protein prominent in specialized embryonic tissues and tumors, *Annu Rev Cell Biol* 5:71, 1989.
56. Ruoslahti E, Suzuki S, Hayman EG et al: Purification and characterization of vitronectin, *Methods Enzymol* 144:430, 1987.
57. Nathan C, Scrimal S, Farber C et al: Cytokine-induced respiratory burst of human neutrophils: dependence on extracellular matrix proteins and CD11/CD18 integrins, *J Cell Biol* 109:1341, 1989.
58. Roberts K, Yokoyama WM, Kehn PJ et al: The vitronectin receptor serves as an accessory molecule for the activation of a subset of γ/δ T cells, *J Exp Med* 173:231, 1991.

Molecular basis of inflammatory events

Cytokines

59. Marcus AJ: Eicosanoids: transcellular metabolism. In Gallin JI, Goldstein IM, Snyderman R, editors: *Inflammation: basic principles and clinical correlates,* New York, 1988, Raven Press.
60. Williams TJ: Prostaglandin E_2, prostaglandin I_2 and the vascular changes of inflammation, *Br J Pharmacol* 65:517, 1979.
61. Wedmore CV, Williams TJ: Control of vascular permeability by polymorphonuclear leukocytes in inflammation, *Nature* 289:646, 1981.
62. Zurier RB: Role of prostaglandin E in inflammation and immune responses, *Adv Prostaglandin Thromboxane Leukotriene Res* 21:947, 1990.
63. Lewis RA, Austen KF: The biologically active leukotrienes: biosynthesis, metabolism, receptors, functions, and phamacology, *J Clin Invest* 73:889, 1984.
64. Smith MJH, Ford-Hutchinson AW, Bray MA: Leukotriene B: a potential mediator of inflammation, *J Pharm Pharmacol* 32:517, 1980.
65. Samuelson B: Leukotrienes: mediators of immediate hypersensitivity reactions and inflammation, *Science* 220:568, 1983.
66. Warlaw AJ, Hay H, Cromwell O et al: Leukotrienes, LTC4 and LTB4, in bronchioalveolar lavage in bronchial asthma and other respiratory diseases, *J Allergy Clin Immunol* 84:19, 1989.
67. Goetzl EJ, Pickett WC: The human PMN leukocyte chemotactic activity of complex hydroxyeicosatetraenoic acids (HETEs), *J Immunol* 125: 1789, 1980.
68. Goetzl EJ: Mediators of immediate hypersensitivity derived from arachidonic acid, *N Engl J Med* 303:822, 1980.
69. Zimmerman GA, Prescott SM, McIntyre TM: Platelet activating factor: a fluid phase and cell-associated mediator of inflammation. In Gallin JI, Goldstein IM, Snyderman R, editors: *Inflammation: basic principles and clinical correlates,* New York, 1992, Raven Press.
70. Barnes PJ, Page CP, Henson PM: *Platelet activating factor in health and disease,* Oxford, 1989, Blackwell Publishers.
71. Stewart WE: *The interferons,* New York, 1979, Springer-Verlag.
72. Farrar MA, Schreiber RD: The molecular cell biology of interferon-γ and its receptor, *Annu Rev Immunol* 11:571, 1993.
73. Durum SK, Schmidt JA, Oppenheim JJ: Interleukin 1: an immunological perspective, *Annu Rev Immunol* 3:263, 1985
74. Carter DB, Deibel MR, Dunn CJ et al: Purification, cloning, expression and biologic characterization of an interleukin-1 receptor antagonist protein, *Nature* 344:633, 1990.
75. Smith K: Interleukin 2: inception, impact, and implications, *Science* 240:1169, 1988.
76. Spits H, editor: *IL-4: structure and function,* Boca Raton, Fla., 1992, CRC Press.
77. Yokota T, Coffman RL, Hagiwara H et al: Isolation and characterization of lymphokine cDNA clones encoding mouse and human IgA enhancing factor and eosinophil colony-stimulating factor activities: relationship to IL-5, *Proc Natl Acad Sci USA* 84:7388, 1987.
78. Cox G, Gauldie J: Structure and function of IL-6. In Kunkel SL, Remick DG, editors: *Cytokines in health and disease,* New York, 1992, Marcel Dekker Inc.
79. Namen AE, Schmierer AE, March CJ et al: B-cell precursor growth promoting activity: purification and characterization of a growth factor active on lymphocyte precursors, *J Exp Med* 167:988, 1988.
80. Yang YC: Human interleukin-9: a new cytokine in hematopoiesis, *Leuk Lymphoma* 8:441, 1992.
81. Anderson KC, Morimoto C, Paul SR et al: Interleukin 11 promotes accessory cell-dependent B-cell differentiation in humans, *Blood* 80:2797, 1992.
82. Moore KW, O'Garra A, de Waal Malefyt R et al: Interleukin 10, *Annu Rev Immunol* 11:165, 1993.
83. Stern AS, Podlaski FJ, Hulmes JD et al: Purification to homogeneity and partial characterization of cytotoxic lymphocyte maturation factor from human B-lymphoblastoid cells, *Proc Natl Acad Sci USA* 87:6808, 1990.
84. Brown KD, Zurawski SM, Mosmann TR, Zurawski G: A family of small inducible proteins secreted by leukocytes are members of a new superfamily that includes leukocyte and fibroblast-derived inflammatory agents, growth factors, and indicators of various activation processes, *J Immunol* 142:679, 1989.
85. Golde DW, Baldwin GC: Myeloid growth factors. In Gallin JI, Goldstein IM, Snyderman R, editors: *Inflammation: basic principles and clinical correlates,* New York, 1992, Raven Press.
86. Beutler B, Cerami A: Cachectin and tumor necrosis factor as two sides of the same coin, *Nature* 320:584, 1986.
87. Gray PW, Aggarwal BB, Hilgers J et al: Cloning and expression of cDNA for human lymphotoxin, a lymphokine with tumor necrosis activity, *Nature* 312:721, 1984.
88. Baggiolini M, Dewald B, Walz A: Interleukin 8 and related chemotactic cytokines. In Gallin JI, Goldstein IM, Snyderman R, editors: *Inflammation: basic principles and clinical correlates,* New York, 1992, Raven Press.
89. Payan DG: Neuropeptides and inflammation: the role of substance P, *Annu Rev Med* 40:341, 1989.
90. Kovacs EJ: Fibrogenic cytokines: the role of immune mediators in the development of scar tissue, *Immunol Today* 12:17, 1991.
91. Shepard V: Cytokine receptors. In Kunkel SL, Remick DG, editors: *Cytokines in health and disease,* New York, 1992, Marcel Dekker Inc.
92. Yarden Y, Ullrich A: Growth factor receptor tyrosine kinases, *Annu Rev Biochem* 57: 443, 1988.

93. Sanborg R, Smolen J: Early biochemical events in leukocyte activation, *Lab Invest* 59:300, 1988.

Cellular and molecular events of inflammation

94. Cotran RS, Majno G: A light and electron microscopic analysis of vascular injury, *Ann NY Acad Sci* 116:750, 1964.
95. Bevilacqua MP: Endothelial-leukocyte adhesion molecules, *Annu Rev Immunol* 11:767, 1993.
96. Lasky LA, Rosen SD: The selectins: carbohydrate-binding adhesion molecules of the immune system. In Gallin JI, Goldstein IM, Snyderman R, editors: *Inflammation: basic principles and clinical correlates,* New York, 1992, Raven Press.
97. Kishimoto TK, Anderson DC: The role of integrins in inflammation. In Gallin JI, Goldstein IM, Snyderman R, editors: *Inflammation: basic principles and clinical correlates,* New York, 1992, Raven Press.
98. Zimmerman GA, Prescott SM, McIntyre TM: Endothelial cell interactions with granulocytes: tethering and signalling molecules, *Immunology Today* 13:93, 1992.
99. Shimuzu Y, Newman W, Tanaka Y, Shaw S: Lymphocyte interactions with endothelial cells, *Immunol Today* 13:106, 1992.
100. Holmes WE, Lee J, Kuang W-J et al: Structure and functional expression of a human interleukin 8 receptor, *Nature* 253:1278, 1991.
101. Gerard NP, Gerard C: The chemotactic receptor for human C5a anaphylatoxin, *Nature* 349:614, 1991.
102. Gardner JP, Melnick DA, Maleck HL: Characterization of the formyl peptide chemotactic receptor appearing at the phagocytic cell surface after exposure to phorbol myristate acetate, *J Immunol* 136:1400, 1986.
103. Snyderman R, Smith CD, Verghese MW: Model for leukocyte regulation by chemoattractant receptors: roles of guanine nucleotide regulatory protein and polyphosphoinositide metabolism, *J Leukoc Biol* 40:785, 1986.
104. Didsbury J, Weber RF, Bokoch GM et al: *Rac*, a novel *ras*-related family of proteins that are botulinum toxin substrates, *J Biol Chem* 265:5990, 1990.
105. Stossel TP: The mechanical responses of white blood cells. In Gallin JI, Goldstein IM, Snyderman R, editors: *Inflammation: basic principles and clinical correlates,* New York, 1992, Raven Press.
106. Wright SD: Receptors for complement and the biology of phagocytosis. In Gallin JI, Goldstein IM, Snyderman R, editors: *Inflammation: basic principles and clinical correlates,* New York, 1992, Raven Press.
107. Wolff SM, Dale DC, Clark RA et al: The Chediak-Higashi syndrome: studies of host defenses, *Ann Intern Med* 76:293, 1972.
108. Gallin JI: Neutrophil specific granule deficiency, *Annu Rev Med* 36:263, 1985.
109. Wright DG, Bralove DA, Gallin JI: The differential mobilization of human neutrophil granules effects of phorbol myristate acetate and ionophore A23187, *Am J Pathol* 87:273.
110. Fantone JC, Ward PA: Role of oxygen-derived free radicals and metabolites in leukocyte-dependent inflammatory reaction, *Am J Pathol* 107:397, 1982.
111. Klebanoff, SJ: Oxygen metabolites from phagocytes. In Gallin JI, Goldstein IM, Snyderman R, editors: *Inflammation: basic principles and clinical correlates,* New York, 1992, Raven Press.
112. Mandell GL: Bactericidal activity of aerobic and anaerobic polymorphonuclear neutrophils, *Infect Immunol* 9:337, 1974.
113. Bromberg Y, Pick E: Activation of NADPH-dependent superoxide production in a cell-free system by sodium dodecyl sulfate, *J Biol Chem* 260:13539, 1985.
114. Clark RA, Leidal KG, Pearson DW, Nauseef WM: NADPH oxidase of human neutrophils: subcellular localization and characterization of an arachidonate-activatable superoxide generation system, *J Biol Chem* 262:4065, 1987.
115. Tauber AI, Borregaard N, Simons E, Wright J: Chronic granulomatous disease: a syndrome of phagocyte oxidase deficiencies, *Medicine* 62:286, 1983.
116. Green SJ, Mellouk S, Hoffman SL et al: Cellular mechanisms of nonspecific immunity to intracellular infection: cytokine-induced synthesis of toxic nitrogen oxides from L-arginine by macrophages and hepatocytes, *Immunol Lett* 25:15, 1990.
117. Adams DO, Nathan CF: Molecular mechanisms of tumor cell killing by activated macrophages, *Immunol Today* 4:166, 1983.
118. Herberman RB: Cytotoxic activities of lymphocytes. In Gallin JI, Goldstein IM, Snyderman R, editors: *Inflammation: basic principles and clinical correlates,* New York, 1992, Raven Press.
119. Grimm EA, Mazumder A, Zhang HZ, Rosenberg SA: Lymphokine-activated killer cell phenomenon, lysis of natural killer cell resistant fresh solid tumor cells by interleukin 2–activated autologous human peripheral blood lymphocytes, *J Exp Med* 157:884, 1983.
120. Podack ER: The molecular mechanisms of lymphocytic-mediated tumor cell lysis, *Immunol Today* 6:21, 1985.

Regulation of inflammation

121. Killingsworth LM: Plasma protein patterns in health and disease, *CRC Crit Rev Clin Lab Sci* 3:1, 1979.
122. Koj A: Definition and classification of acute phase proteins in the acute phase response to injury and infection. In Gordon AH, Koj A, editors: *The acute-phase response to injury and infection,* Amsterdam, 1985, Elsevier.
123. Gauldie J, Baumann H: Cytokines and acute phase protein expression. In Kimball EH, editor: *Cytokines in inflammation,* West Caldwell, NJ, 1991, Telford Press.
124. Besedovsky H, Rey AD, Sorkin E, Dinarello CA: Immunoregulatory feedback between interleukin-1 and glucorticoid hormones, *Science* 233:652, 1986.
125. Goldstein RA, Bowen DL, Fauci AS: Adrenal corticosteroids. In Gallin JI, Goldstein IM, Snyderman R, editors: *Inflammation: basic principles and clinical correlates,* New York, 1992, Raven Press.
126. Wallner BP, Mattaliano RJ, Hession C et al: Clonining and expression of human lipocortin, a phopholipase A_2 inhibitor with potential anti-inflammatory activity, *Nature* 320:77, 1986.
127. Rubin LA, Nelson DL: The soluble interleukin 2 receptor: biology, function and clinical application, *Ann Intern Med* 113:619, 1990.
128. Aderka D, Wysenbeek A, Engelmann H et al: Correlation between serum levels of soluble tumor necrosis factor receptor and disease activity in systemic lupus erythematosus, *Arthritis Rheum* 36:1111, 1993.
129. Ulich TR, Yin S, Remick DG et al: Intratracheal administration of endotoxin and cytokines. IV. The soluble tumor necrosis factor receptor type I inhibits acute inflammation, *Am J Pathol* 142:1335, 1993.
130. Eisenberg SP, Evans RJ, Arend WP et al: Primary structure and functional expression from complementaray DNA of a human interleukin I receptor antagonist protein, *Nature* 343:341, 1990.
131. Wakabayashi G, Gelfand JA, Burke JR et al: A specific receptor antagonist for interleukin I prevents *Escherichia coli*–induced shock in rabbits, *Fed Am Soc Exp Biol* 5:338, 1991.
132. Chensue SW, Bienkowski M, Eessalu TE et al: Endogenous IL-1 receptor antagonist protein (IRAP) regulates schistosome egg granuloma formation and the regional lymphoid response, *J Immunol* 151:3654, 1993.
133. Dorf M, Benacerraf B: Suppressor cells and immunoregulation, *Annu Rev Immunol* 2:127, 1984.
134. Mosmann TR, Moore KW: The role of IL-10 in cross-regulation of Th1 and Th2 responses, *Immunol Today* 12:A49, 1991.
135. Mosmann TR, Cherwinski H, Bond W et al: Two types of murine helper T-cell clones, I. Definition according to profiles of lymphokine activities and secreted proteins, *J Immunol* 136:2348, 1986.
136. Locksley RM, Scott P: Helper T-cell subsets in mouse leishmaniasis: induction, expansion and effector function, *Immunol Today* 12:A58, 1991.
137. Rocklin RE: Modulation of cellular immune responses in vivo and in vitro by histamine receptor bearing lymphocytes, *J Clin Invest* 57:1051, 1976.
138. Wahl SM: The role of transforming growth factor beta (TGF β) in inflammation: a cause and a cure, *J Clin Immunol* 12:61, 1992.

19 Repair and Regeneration

Peter S. Amenta
Antonio Martínez-Hernández
Robert L. Trelstad

An organism's response to injury is composed of two major processes: limiting the extent of the injury—inflammation—and restoring function in the preexisting structure—repair and regeneration. The responses that lead to restoration of function represent the evolutionary accumulation, through millions of years, of multiple molecular and cellular mechanisms. Each new mechanism was added onto or integrated into the preexisting ones, modifying and to some extent improving on them. In that evolution is not a goal-oriented process but a random series of events, those mechanisms that confer no advantage (but result in no disadvantage) are preserved, adding to the overall complexity of biologic processes.

Some forms of repair and regeneration exist even in unicellular organisms. If the cell membrane of an ameba is punctured, the cytoplasmic proteins in the proximity of the puncture coagulate to form a solid plug. This plug allows the normal turnover of the cell membrane to fill the defect. Once the cell membrane defect is sealed the cytoplasmic plug is degraded in autophagic vacuoles and the lost protein and structure are restored as part of the normal turnover of the cell membrane. This apparently simple reaction expands and becomes more complex with progress up the phylogenetic scale, to become almost unrecognizable in higher organisms. Nevertheless, three basic elements remain central to almost all repair reactions: (1) a phase change—blood clotting in higher organisms for plugging the wound, (2) removal of damaged components—degradation, and (3) generation of components to replace lost ones—regeneration. Obviously, an organism that could regenerate all components potentially would be immortal. Organisms that could not regenerate any lost components would die during embryogenesis. In nature, there is a balance between these two extremes. In general, organisms lower in the phylogenetic scale tend to have greater regenerative capacity than those at the top. At first glance, it would seem that regeneration should be a highly desirable trait. However, for regeneration to occur, either existing differentiated cells undergo some degree of dedifferentiation before redifferentiation, or stem cells of that tissue undergo differentiation. If neurons were to regenerate, any dedifferentiation would result in the loss of the information associated with those neurons. In a similar vein, regeneration in the heart would require some myocardial cells to cease contracting. Viewed in this light, regeneration becomes a somewhat less desirable characteristic.

Repair and regeneration begin immediately after injury and, as such, overlap with the inflammatory response and thus form a continuum. It is primarily for didactic reasons that they are described separately.

Events common to all repair and regeneration reactions include changes in parenchymal cells, changes in vascular and neural elements, and changes in the supporting extracellular matrix.[1-3] The extracellular matrix and the cells characteristic of the injured tissue modify the reaction to injury to a significant extent. Chapter 18 describes the inflammatory response. In the present chapter we review the individual components of repair and regeneration reactions in general and then in specific organs.

COMPONENTS OF THE REPAIR AND REGENERATION REACTIONS

Extracellular matrix

The extracellular matrix (ECM) is a structural network of macromolecules surrounding stromal cells and underlying most endothelia and epithelia.[4] The ECM is not only a physical scaffold, but also a crucial modulator of biologic processes including differentiation, development, regeneration, tumor progression, and repair.[4-6] The ECM has effects on these diverse phenomena through solid-phase signals, released polypeptides, glycosaminoglycans, and selective binding and subsequent release of growth-regulating factors.

The ECM consists of four major macromolecular groups: the collagens, elastin, structural glycoproteins, and proteoglycans. The ECM of various tissues and organs is composed of the same groups of molecules and, in many cases, the same individual components. Different concentrations, ratios, and associations of these components result in an ECM that is tailored for the specific needs and functions of the respective tissue and organ. Therefore these ECM components can be viewed as basic building blocks used to build the matrix best suited to the unique needs of an individual organ. By combining into almost limitless combinations, the ECM supports a multitude of functions including homeostasis, differentiation, shape and size determination, and repair and regeneration.

The ability of the ECM to adapt to new stimuli is prominently displayed during repair and regeneration. Although there is similarity of healing reactions among various tissues, each has its own particular requirements, dictated in part by the composition of the respective ECM of the individual organs.

It is becoming clear that these matrices differ, not only in the relative ratios of the major macromolecular groups such as collagen, glycoproteins, and proteoglycans, but also in the heterogeneity of the respective proteins within each group. This heterogeneity was first appreciated in the collagens.

Collagens

The collagens were initially identified by electron microscopy as banded fibrils. Collagen is the most abundant protein in vertebrates. At present, at least 19 different collagens have been identified, the product of more than 30 genes.[7-11]

All collagen types have certain common characteristics in their chemistry, their helical folding, and their prominent structural properties. All collagens contain three polypeptide chains, called alpha (α) chains, with an amino acid sequence consisting in great part of Gly-X-Y repeats, where *X* and *Y* are often proline and hydroxyproline. The glycine in each third position results in segments of the molecule forming right-handed polyproline helices and the three α chains in turn form a left-handed, triple-helical molecule referred to as the collagenous domain, or COL (Fig. 19-1). At the amino and carboxy termini, the α chains do not have the Gly-X-Y sequence and do not form triple helices. These regions of the molecules are important for proper fibril assembly and subsequent cross-linking to yield biomechanically sound fibrils. The non–triple helical regions are often called noncollagenous domains, or NC, domains.

By convention, all collagens are designated by a roman numeral. Its constituent α chains are designated with arabic numerals (α1, α2, and so forth), followed by the roman numeral designating the collagen type in parentheses, such as α1(I) or α2(I). The last consideration in designating the entire molecule is the ratio of the various α chains. Collagen homotrimers would be designated $[\alpha 1(II)]_3$ and $[\alpha 1(III)]_3$ and heterotrimers would be $[\alpha 1(I)]_2[\alpha 2(I)]$ and $[\alpha 1(XI)\,\alpha 2(XI)\,\alpha 3(XI)]$.

Specific collagen forms in situ

In that collagen molecules can be heterotrimers and thus the product of more than one collagen gene, in some tissues collagen aggregates can also be heterotypic, and formed from mixtures of different collagen molecules.[12-15] Similarly, heterogeneity and complexity pertain to many other matrix components. Ascending the hierachy of the organization of fibril-forming collagens is as follows: collagen molecule → fibril → bundles → fascicles → tendons. With the discovery of the multitudes of collagens, several classification systems have been proposed. It has proven useful to subclassify the collagens either by their supramolecular organization or by their molecular size. The following subclasses reflect current terminology: fibrillar, fibril associated, network forming, filamentous, short chain, and long chain. Fig. 19-2 summarizes the salient features and attributes of the first 13 members of the collagen family.[8,11]

Fibrillar collagens

Type I, II, III, V, and XI collagens compose this subgroup. These collagens form cable-like fibrils and bundles and are credited with providing tensile strength to tissues, such as skin, bone, and ligaments. The transparency of the cornea is dependent on the

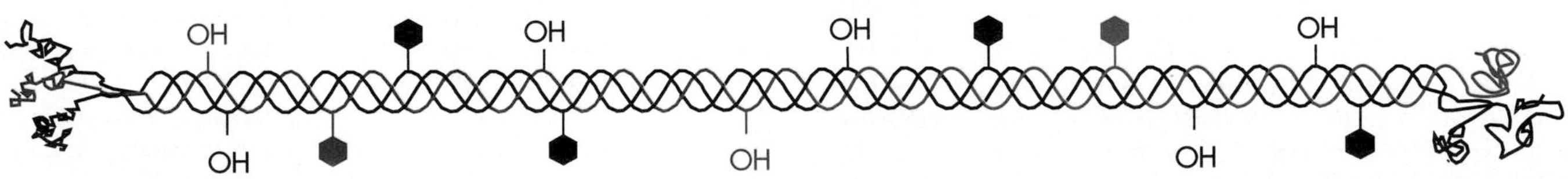

Fig. 19-1 Diagram of a procollagen molecule containing the N and C propeptides.

The Collagen Family

Type	Chains	Association	Aggregate	Tissue Disturbance
I	α 1(I), α 2(I)			Ubiquitous, most abundant protein in the body
II	α 1(II)			Major cartilage collagen
III	α 1(II)			Widely distributed; most abundant in pliable tissues: blood vessels, uterus, etc.
IV	α 1(IV) α 2(IV) α 3(IV) α 4(IV) α 5(IV) α 6(IV)			Component of all basement membranes
V	α 1(V) α 2(V) α 3(V)	???		Minor component; distribution similar to collagen Type I
VI	α 1(VI) α 2(VI) α 3(VI)			Abundant, present in most tissues
VII	α 1(VII)			Anchoring fibrils; binds basement membranes to other ECM components
VIII	α 1(VIII) α 2(VIII)	???		Secreted by some endothelia
IX	α 1(IX) α 2(IX) α3(IX)	???		Minor cartilage collagen
X	α 1(X)	???		Present in mineralizing cartilage
XI	α 1(XI) α 2(XI) α 3(XI)	???		Present in mineralizing cartilage
XII	α 1(XII)	???		Ligaments, perichondrium
XIII	α 1(XIII)	???		Tissue distribution undefined

Fig. 19-2 The collagen gene family. (Modified from Rubin E, Farber JL: *Pathology*, ed 2, Philadelphia, 1994, Lippincott.)

regularity of diameter and packing of fibrillar collagen. Most fibrils are mixtures of these different fibril-forming collagens and are thus heterotypic. Common mixtures include type I with type III (skin) and type I with type V in the cornea.[13-15]

Fibrillar collagens are cross-striated or banded when viewed by electron microscopy (Fig. 19-3) or x-ray diffraction. The 67 nm repeat banding pattern is based on the staggered arrangement of the individual collagen molecules (Fig. 19-4). Collagen molecules are approximately 4.4 times the length of the 67 nm period (D). A space is present between the amino terminus of one molecule and the carboxy terminus of the next molecule in line, and each molecule is laterally related to its neighbors in a 67 nm staggered manner. This pattern continues throughout the fibril, resulting in regions of overlaps of adjacent molecules and gaps. Any D period thus consists of a gap zone and an overlap zone, the former constituting approximately 60% of the unit and the latter 40%.

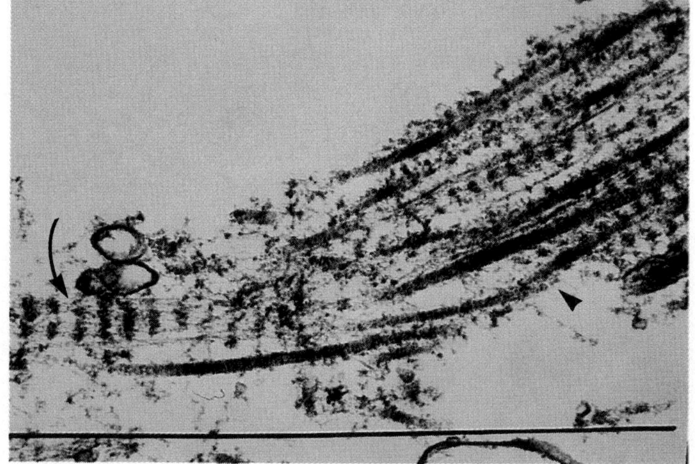

Fig. 19-3 Electron micrograph from a sarcoma demonstrating banded collagen fibers *(arrowhead)*. In addition, fibrous long-spaced fibers (Luse bodies) are also present *(curved arrow)*.

Network-forming collagens

This subfamily has type IV collagen as its major member. It is discussed in greater detail below in the section on basement membranes. Presently, there are six distinct α chains within the type IV collagen subfamily. A characteristic feature of the type IV α chains are interruptions in the Gly-X-Y sequence within the COL domains, yielding flex points along the molecule's axis, at which it can bend. These molecules, in part, form the complex network of structural support of basement membranes through lateral and end-to-end associations.

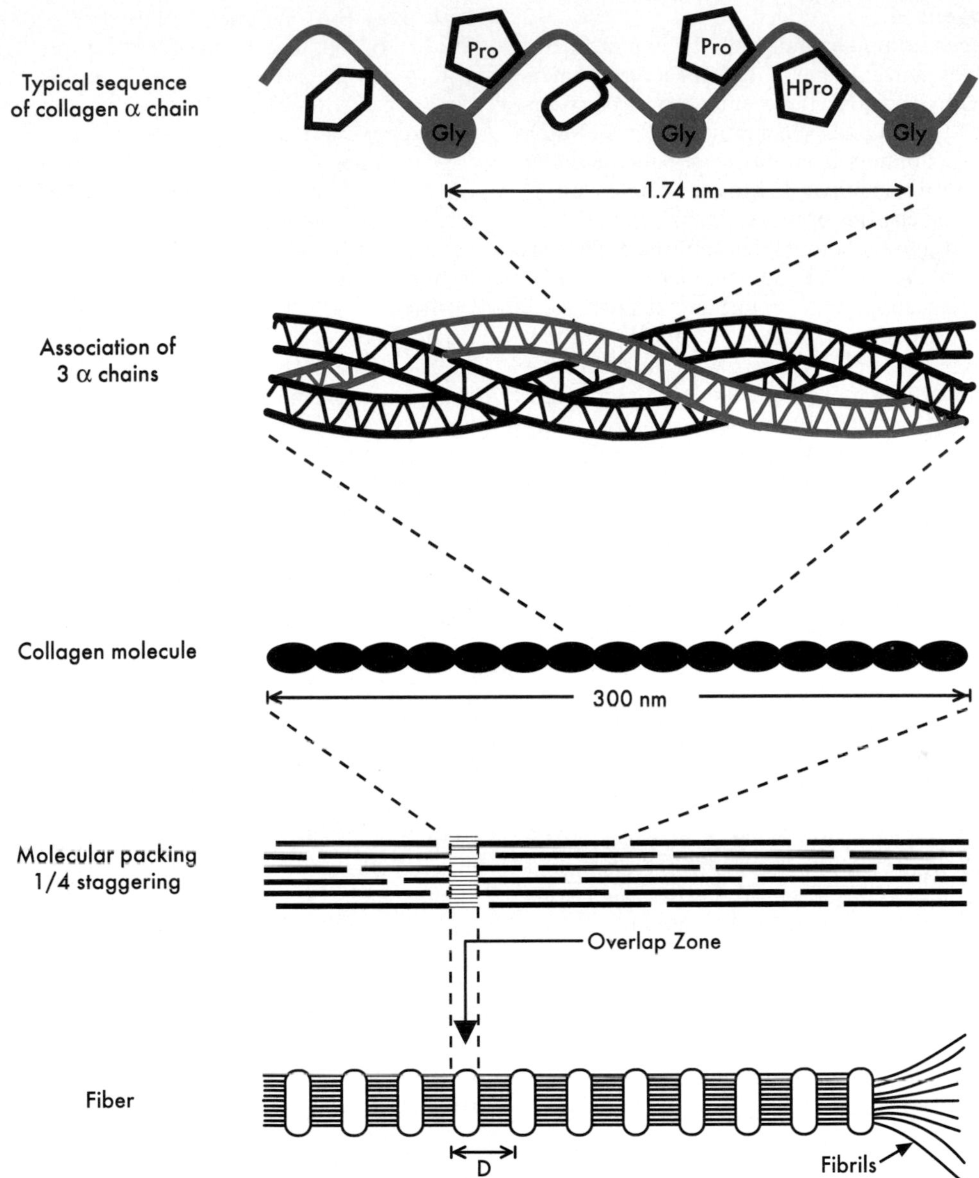

Fig. 19-4 Diagram of the assembly of a collagen α chain into fibrils. The α chains are characterized by a Gly-X-Y amino acid sequence. Glycine is the amino acid found in every third position; whereas proline is often present in the X position. The polypeptide chain rotates at the glycine molecule at an angle of approximately 120 degrees. Three glycine residues will complete the rotation. A collagen molecule forms from three α chains. The chains assemble in quarter-stagger array. The space between the ends of the individual molecules, the gap zone, permits penetration of metals, whereas the overlap zone excludes them. The characteristic cross-banding pattern observed by electron microscopy results (Fig. 19-3). *Bottom figure,* The assembly of molecules results in fibril formation.

Filamentous fibrils

The filamentous fibril subfamily contains only type VI collagen, a ubiquitous collagen present in most connective tissues. Type VI collagen is a heterotrimeric molecule with short triple-helical regions and large globular domains at each terminus. Two of these molecules align in a head-to-tail arrangement to form a dimer. The dimers then form tetramers, which associate to form 6 to 10 nm (in diameter) beaded fibrils. Type VI collagen is often in close association with other collagen types and has been proposed as a connecting protein. In cartilage, type VI collagen surrounds chondrocytes. The association of type VI collagen with other collagen types contributes to the heterogeneity of collagen bundles.[12]

Short-chain collagens

Short-chain collagens consist of individual molecules 150 nm long, or half the length of that of the fibrillar collagens. This subclass has as its only member type VIII collagen, first identified in endothelial cell cultures. Subsequently it has been identified in Descemet's membrane of the cornea. Similar structurally to type X collagen, it forms a hexagonal network in Descemet's membrane.

Long-chain collagens

The long-chain collagen group contains only the homotrimeric type VII collagen. The molecule has a 420 nm long, uninterrupted COL region with a large NC1 domain at the carboxy terminus and a smaller NC domain at the amino terminus (NC2). Type VII collagen forms dimers from molecules interacting at their amino terminuses in an antiparallel fashion and by disulfide bonding. Lateral associations of these dimers form anchoring fibrils, which insert into the lamina densa of the epidermal basement membrane, where the NC1 domain binds to type IV collagen. The dimer is nearly 1 μm long, and if each NC1 domain binds to the basement membrane, a loop is formed. Such loops act like one face of a "Velcro patch" to secure the epithelium to the stroma. When one NC1 domain binds to the basement membrane and the other to the unique matrix structures called "stromal anchoring plaques," the dimers anchor the epidermal basement membrane to the stroma.

Fibril-associated collagens with interrupted triple helices (FACITs)

Type IX, X, and XII collagens compose this group, which contains collagens that are associated with the surface of fibrils of the fibrillar subclass. They are characterized by triple-helical domains, with a single interruption by a non–triple helical domain, causing the molecule to kink. One portion of the triple-helical domain is responsible for lateral interactions with the banded collagen fibril, and the kink causes a second region of the triple helix to project off the surface of the fibril. At the end of the projecting segment is another non–triple helical globular domain, responsible for interactions with the adjacent matrix. Because of their location on the surface of large fibrils, the FACIT collagens modulate fibril assembly and affect binding to the adjacent ECM. Type IX collagen has a glycosaminoglycan (GAG) chain covalently linked at the kink region. This GAG chain has both steric influences on the molecular interactions of type IX collagen and is also involved in other GAG-related bindings and interactions (see the discussion of GAG on p. 428).

New collagens

Type XIII collagen, as with most of the more recently discovered collagen types, was identified by hybridization techniques and screening of cDNA libraries.[16] The homotrimeric type XIV collagen was extracted from fetal calf tendon and skin.[17] The molecule shows similarity to collagen type XII in its COL I domain (approximately 65% primary structure homology). The localization and functions of this collagen type have yet to be determined. Screening of a human-placenta cDNA library has yielded a unique collagen chain that has been provisionally named α1 XV collagen.[18]

Collagen genes

The chromosomal localization of more than 30 collagen genes has been established in humans. Designation of collagen genes is designated as follows: *COL* is followed by the arabic number of the collagen type, *A* for the α chain and the chain number. For example, the α1 chain gene of the type I collagen gene is as follows: COL1A1. Considering the structural similarity among collagen types, the similarity among their encoding genes is not surprising.[7,19] The helical COL regions of the fibrillar collagens are encoded for within approximately 44 exons. The majority of these exons are 54 base pairs (bp) in length, with some 108 bp and others 45, 99, or 162 bp. The exons for the triple-helical regions begin with a glycine codon and end with an amino acid for the Y position. These data indicate that the collagen genes may have a common ancestor.

The genes of the FACIT collagens lack the long, uninterrupted helical regions of the fibrillar collagens by virtue of the kink region. The triple-helical regions on either side of the kink have exons of 54 bp. This is apparently not the case at the amino terminus, where there is divergence from this exon length.

The short-chain collagen genes, in contrast to the other collagen genes, contain one exon of 2000 bp encoding both the triple-helical and carboxy globular domains. Type IV collagen genes also diverge from the 54 base-pair exon but have multiple small exons for encoding the triple-helical regions.

Available data indicate that transcriptional regulation of the collagen genes may be the principle means of controlling collagen production. Defining the factors that control transcription will be central to a better understanding of repair and regeneration and developing future therapies to modulate these processes.[20-22]

Collagen biosynthesis

The pathway of collagen biosynthesis is similar to that for all proteins targeted for export, with translation on membrane-bound ribosomes, transport into the cisternae of the rough endoplasmic reticulum, and movement to the Golgi complex and then to the extracellular space. Each collagen polypeptide chain has a signal sequence at the amino terminus, which is cleaved shortly after translation, resulting in the procollagen chain, which consists of three major regions: the nonhelical amino and carboxy termini and the central helical domain. While in the cisternae of the endoplasmic reticulum, the respective procollagen α chains aggregate to form the procollagen molecule, which will undergo additional posttranslational modifications such as hydroxylation of proline and lysine residues, glycation, and disulfide bonding for certain collagens. Procollagen hydroxylation is accomplished by three enzymes lysyl hydroxylase, prolyl-4-hydroxylase, and prolyl-3-hydroxylase, dependent on vitamin C or ascorbic acid, α-ketogluturate, ferrous ion, and O_2.[23,24] Procollagen glycation varies for each collagen type and includes both O-linked glycation of glucose and galactose to hydroxylysine and N-linked glycation of complex oligosaccharides to asparagine. After glycation, the procollagen chains are packaged in the Golgi complex into secretory vesicles, transported to the plasma membrane, and secreted into the extracellular environment.

Collagen fibrillogenesis in situ

The fibrillar collagens have been extensively studied in vitro where they self-assemble into D-periodic, or 67 nm, striated fibrils spontaneously. Many but not all of the principles derived from these in vitro studies apply to the process in vivo. At least three separate but overlapping phases of fibril assembly occur in fibroblasts: (1) a self-assembly phase, (2) a cell-mediated phase, and (3) a postdepositional phase. The self-assembly phase has as a prerequisite extracellular processing that occurs within a confined space formed by deep plasmalemmal invaginations, which are unique extracellular compartments[25,26] (Fig. 19-5). Before the molecules can effectively interact and self-assemble into D-periodic fibrils, the nonhelical ends of the procollagen molecule must be cleaved by extracellular amino-

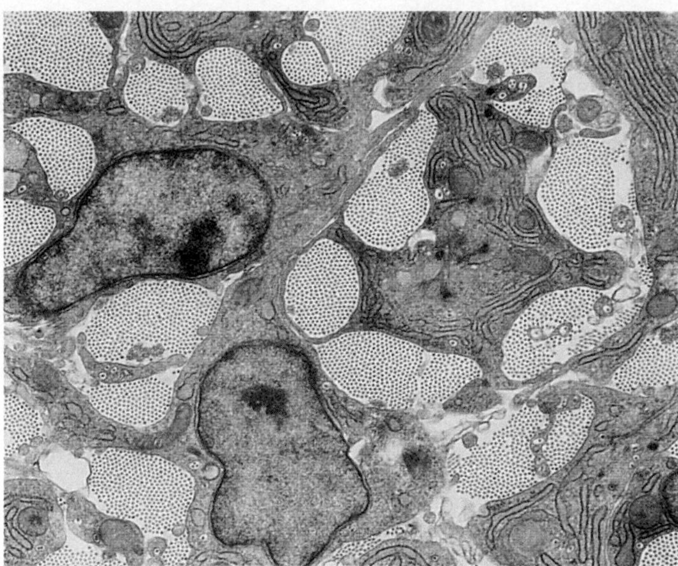

Fig. 19-5 Fibroblasts demonstrating fibril and bundle forming compartments. Fibroblasts are surrounded by well-formed bundles of collagen, around which there are cytoplasmic processes. The fibril segments are discharged into the bundle-forming compartments where the segments adhere linearly and laterally to form longer, thicker biomechanically stable structures. (Courtesy David Bird, Ph.D., Boston, Mass)

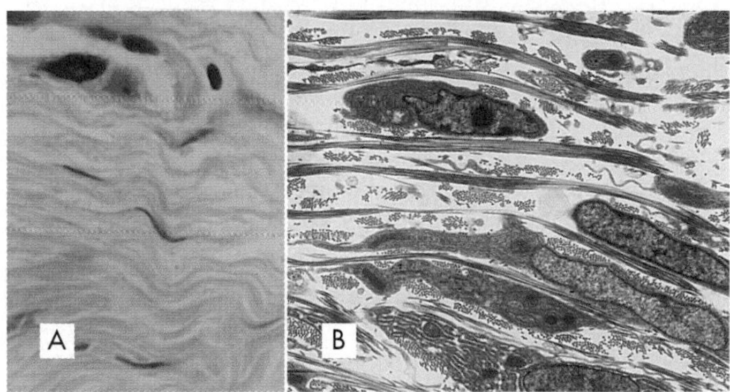

Fig. 19-6 **A**, Moderately dense connective tissue demonstrating fusiform fibroblasts located between undulating bundles of collagen. **B**, Notice the abundant rough endoplasmic reticulum in the fibroblasts. This relatively thick section (1.5 µm) reveals that the collagen is predominately present as bundles not as individual interlacing fibrils. (Courtesy David Bird and Plenum Press. **B** from Bird et al: *Matrix assembly in cell biology of extracellular matrix,* 1991.)

and carboxy-propeptidases. The processed molecules, now with 11 amino acid nonhelical extension peptides (telopeptides), associate through noncovalent interactions (Fig. 19-4) in a quarter-stagger array to form D-periodic fibril segments approximately 15 µm long. This self-assembly is modulated by the fibroblast, in that the cell controls in unknown ways, the rates of secretion, the sites of the extracellular compartments, and the environment (pH, ionic strength, enzymes) of these compartments (Fig. 19-5). Either within the fibril assembly compartment or in the larger bundle-forming compartment into which the segments are positioned by the cell, an essential covalent bonding occurs, which results in the cross-linking of collagen by means of lysine-derived aldehydes generated by lysyl oxidase. The resultant intermolecular and intramolecular bonds are necessary for the collagen fibril to reach its maximum tensile strength. One final step or set of steps occurs after deposition and involves an annealing of the fibril segments into longer and thicker fibrils. These postdepositional fusions and rearrangements occur at a macroscale, and their molecular mechanisms are poorly understood.

Functions of collagens

The tensile strength of collagen is attributable to the hierarchical association of molecules into fibrils and bundles, linked by intramolecular and intermolecular bonds (Fig. 19-4). The orientation of the collagen fibrils is critical to their function. In tendons (Fig. 19-6) the linear array of the type I collagen fibrils, bundles, and fascicles result in a resilient structure; in the cornea the arrangement of types I and V collagen fibrils into orthogonal lamellae leads to transparency. Thus, although type I collagen imparts great tensile strength or even transparency, type III collagen is associated with pliability, and type VII collagen is associated with anchorage of the epidermal basement membranes to the dermis. Anchoring functions have also been proposed for type VI collagen.[12,27]

In addition to the structural function at a biomechanical level, the fibrillar and nonfibrillar collagens are effective stimulants of platelet aggregation, substrates for cell attachment for purposes of stability or locomotion, and permselective filters for nutrients and water in the basement membrane, especially for the whole organism, in the glomeruli.

Pathology of collagen

A variety of conditions, affecting various stages of fibrillogenesis, result in defective collagen structures or stabilities.[8] Given the importance of copper as a cofactor for lysyl oxidase, thus collagen cross-linking, it is not suprising that copper chelation, or other abnormalities of copper metabolism, interfere with collagen fibrillogenesis. The Menkes syndrome is a sex-linked disorder characterized by abnormal copper absorption and, as a sequela, defective collagen fibril stability. Ehlers-Danlos syndrome (EDS) represents a group of heritable disorders of collagen and elastin processing, manifested by hyperelasticity, tissue fragility, bladder diverticula, joint hypermobility, and a hemorrhagic diathesis. In type VII Ehlers-Danlos syndrome, there is a deficiency of N-terminal procollagen peptidase, resulting in the retention of the nonhelical amino terminus on either the $\alpha1(I)$ or $\alpha2(I)$ chains and inhibition of normal collagen fibril, bundle, and fascicle formation. Type IX EDS is similar to the Menkes syndrome and is attributable to abnormal copper metabolism. Osteogenesis imperfecta (OI) is characterized by mutations in both α chains of type I collagen. Patients with these conditions have a cluster of abnormalities including brittle bones, defective hearing, and impaired wound healing. The mutations in OI can be at multiple points along the α chains, and the clinical syndrome varies significantly depending on where the loss of normal triple-helical structures occurs. There are more than 100 mutations that have been characterized in the COL1A1 and COL1A2 chains.[28] Diseases such as osteoporosis, osteoarthrosis, achondrogenesis, and aortic aneurysms have been associated with mutations of collagen genes. Mutations in the COL2A1 gene are causes of diseases such as achondrogenesis II, hypochondrogenesis, and other forms of achondrogenesis.[29]

Although the effect of local and systemic influences have a role in collagen deposition, little is known concerning the mechanisms by which they regulate collagen synthesis, secretion, deposition, and fibril diameter. For example, in many tumors, abnormal fibrils similar to fibrous long-spaced collagens fibrils, which can be obtained in vitro, occur in vivo. These fibrous long-spaced collagen fibers (Luse bodies) (Fig. 19-3) represent the result of abnormal collagen fibrillogenesis.

Although collagen synthesis and deposition is central to the normal repair and regeneration reactions, excessive collagen accumulation occurs in several conditions with consequent loss of structural and functional attributes. Such is seen in hypertrophic scars, keloids, progressive systemic sclerosis, hepatic cirrhosis, and interstitial pulmonary fibrosis. Homotrimeric type α1(I) collagen is deposited in some of these fibrotic conditions and has been postulated to have a role in the progression of conditions characterized by excessive fibrosis.[30]

Considerable effort has gone into the study of the factors regulating collagen gene expression in these processes. This information could provide a foundation for new, more rational therapeutic interventions to control the excessive collagen accumulation that characterizes these entities.[22,31-33]

Elastin

Elastin, true to its name, is an elastomer that when stretched will return to its original shape. Elastin plays a major role in providing for skin pliability and the recoil of distended, aerated tissues of the lung. Elastin is a hydrophobic, insoluble, nonglycated protein[34-36] found as the central core of a composite structure called the *elastic fiber*, of which the outer sheath is a microfibrillar component (including fibrillin, see below). Elastin polymerizes in the ECM to form either irregular fibers or lamellae. It is rich in glycine, proline, leucine, and the lysine-derived cross-linking derivatives known as desmosine and isodesmosine. The extensive cross-linking in elastin leads to its elastomeric capacities and incidentally to its pronounced insolubility. The precursor form of elastin, tropoelastin, was first identified from swine aorta and consists of a single polypeptide chain of approximately 800 amino acid residues (70 kD). Like silk and collagen, approximately one third of the amino acids are glycine. In contrast to collagen, elastin has only a small fraction of hydroxyproline and hydroxylysine residues, and glycine is randomly distributed in the molecule. The unique cross-linking of elastin occurs among four oxidized lysine molecules, forming pyridine nuclei.

The elastomeric action of elastin makes it ideal for tissue requiring pliability, such as lung and large arteries. Several theories have been proposed to explain this feature of the protein and include the random-chain arrangement and the hydrophobicity of elastin. The latter theory has as its foundation the stresses in the protein when the hydrophobic groups are exposed to water, leading to physical stretching and eventually recoil.

In humans, the elastin gene is located on chromosome 7. Approximately one third of the exons are alternatively spliced to produce several different tropoelastin molecules.

Elastic fibers

By light microscopy, elastic fibers appear as eosinophilic, wavy fibers or as sheets within the media of arteries. By electron microscopy, these fibers are composed of the central core (elastin) of the elastin polymer surrounded by a peripheral microfibrillar network, composed of fibrillin and other glycoproteins (Fig. 19-7).

Peripheral microfibrils

By electron microscopy, a system of 10 nm microfibrils is found in many ECM,[37] and elastic fibers are usually heavily surrounded by such a network. A 350 kD component of these peripheral microfibrils was identified from fibroblast cultures and named *fibrillin*.[38,39] Electron microscopy immunohistochemistry has localized this protein to the 10 nm microfibrils surrounding elastin and in other non–elastin-associated microfibrils. Immunohistochemical studies have localized other proteins to this system of microfibrils, and such a finding indicates a complex composition. The functions of the microfibrillar sheath range from an influence on elastin deposition during development to providing linkages to the surrounding ECM.

Biosynthesis of elastin

Several cell types, including smooth muscle cells, fibroblasts, and myofibroblasts, can synthesize elastin. Elastin is apparently synthesized in the classical pathway used by other secreted proteins and goes into the extracellular space as the soluble tropoelastin. It appears that tropoelastin polymerizes at specified areas in the extracellular space where there are cell membrane infoldings. The soluble, monomeric tropoelastin is deposited at the surface of the assembling elastic fiber, where it is cross-linked into the fiber by means of lysyl oxidase. The fiber assembly occurs adjacent to the cell surface, where microfibrils are the first evidence of elastin polymerization and formation of the elastic fibril complex. The central elastin core forms in the inner regions of microfibrillar aggregates, with the latter remaining at the periphery of the fiber. Initially, microfibrils are the predominant component, but as the fiber matures, the central core of elastin is predominant.

Inherited anomalies of elastin

Marfan's syndrome is characterized by structural abnormalities of the skeletal, cardiovascular, and ocular systems.[40-42] A neonatal form of the syndrome is also described and has additional features of cutis laxa, joint contractures, muscle

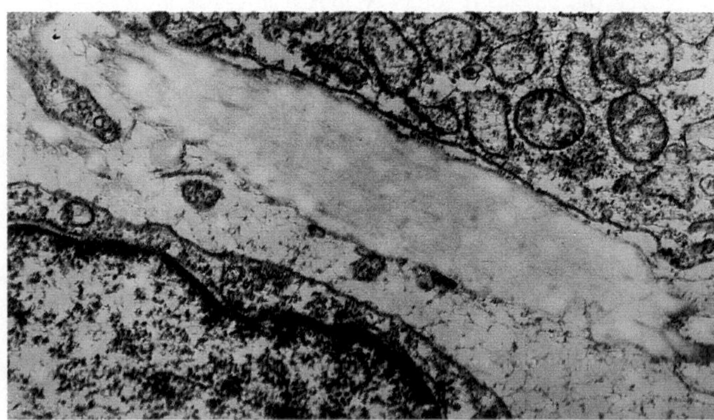

Fig. 19-7 Transmission electron microscopy of an elastic fiber (15-day rat embryo aorta). The fiber consists of an amorphous central fiber with numerous 6 to 10 nm microfibrils at the periphery. (Courtesy Joel Rosenbloom, Ph.D., Philadelphia, Penn)

hypoplasia, ear deformities, ocular anomalies, and pulmonary emphysema.[43] While Marfan's syndrome has many clinical features similar to those induced in animals by β-aminopropri-onitrile, an inhibitor of lysyl oxidase, it is now believed that a defect in microfibrils is central to the pathogenesis of this autosomal dominant disorder.

Recent studies have demonstrated that the Marfan's syndrome locus is present on chromosome 15 colocalizing with the fibrillin gene. Subsequently, fibrillin mutations have been identified in patients with Marfan's syndrome leading to decreased fibrillin mRNA levels and abnormal fibril morphology. Other disorders affecting the elastic fibers include: cutis laxa, an entity in which the dermis lacks elastin; proline dipeptidase deficiency, where the elastic fibers are decreased in size and number; and pseudoxanthoma elasticum, where elastic fibers are mineralized.

Basement membranes

Basement membranes (BM) are ubiquitous, specialized extracellular matrices, located at the boundary between cells and adjacent stroma.[44-47] BM separate epithelial cells of most organs, such as the gastrointestinal tract, glands, and epidermis from the adjacent connective tissues, as well as individually surrounding many mesenchymal cells, that is, lipocytes and skeletal, smooth, and cardiac muscle cells. They also separate epithelial and endothelial cells, as in the glomerulus and alveolus. The central nervous system has only vascular BM, whereas in the peripheral nervous system, Schwann cells are encased by a multilayered BM. All endothelial cells are lined by a continuous BM, except those of the sinusoids in the liver, spleen, lymph nodes, and bone marrow. Synovial cells, fibroblasts, and histiocytes either lack a BM or have only a fraction of their surface associated with one.

By light microscopy, BM appear as pale, eosinophilic structures that react with a variety of histochemical stains, including periodic acid–Schiff stain, reflecting their abundance of carbohydrates. By electron microscopy, most BM are approximately 60 to 90 nm in thickness and have two recognizable regions when stained with conventional heavy-metal stains. The region adjacent to the cell membrane is electron lucent and called the *lamina rara* or *lamina lucida*. The regions adjacent to the interstitium, characterized by higher electron density, is called the *lamina densa* (Fig. 19-8). There are exceptions to this general organization of the BM associated with thickening or fusion of BM. The BM of the lens capsule, for example, has a very thick lamina densa (over 1000 nm, or 1 μm). The glomerular BM and segments of the alveolar BM result from fusion of an endothelial and epithelial BM, with two 30 nm laminae rarae sandwiching the thick lamina densa. In humans the average thickness of this fused glomerular BM is approximately 1200 nm.

Components of basement membranes

Fig. 19-9 summarizes the properties of the major BM components.

Structural glycoproteins

Laminins represent a family of structural glycoproteins, first identified by Engelbreth-Holm and Swarm (EHS) in a tumor in the mouse, which has a morphology initially believed to represent a chondrogenic sarcoma. Additional studies have revealed this tumor to be a teratocarcinoma, in which the predominant ECM component is basement membrane.[48-51] EHS laminin was first characterized and consists of three chains formerly called *A*, *B1*, and *B2* folded into a cruciform molecule. Each chain contributes to the "long" and "short" arms of the folded protein in a complex intertwined manner. The A chain forms the axis of the long arm of the cross along with the carboxy termini of the B1 and B2 chains. The three short arms are formed from the B1, B2, and A chains. Globular domains are present along the three short arms and the end of the long arm. The A chain has two globular domains, one at or near the amino terminus, the other at the carboxy terminus. Laminin (Fig. 19-10) has been found in all basement membranes studied up to now.[12,52,53]

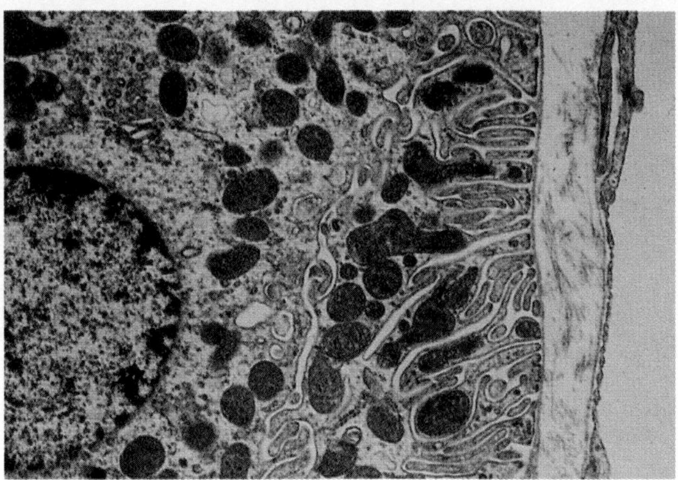

Fig. 19-8 The tubular epithelial basement membrane consists of a lamina rara and lamina densa separating the tubule from the adjacent interstitial connective tissue.

It is now known that the laminins compose a family of proteins with several isoforms. These isoforms include chains homologous to the EHS A chain, the M chain, and an s chain, homologous to the B1 chain. These chains aggregate to form the various laminin isoforms, such as merosin and s-laminin respectively. In addition, other related proteins such as kalinin, K-laminin, and epilegrin are present in anchoring filaments of epidermal BM.[54,55] The ability of laminin to bind to cells and to increase cell motility and migration led to the discovery of several cell-laminin and laminin-ECM interactions, including those for cells, heparin, entactin, and type IV collagen. The cell-attachment region is near the intersection of the three arms. Domains responsible for neurite (axon) outgrowth and heparin binding are present in the carboxy terminus of the A chain. Regions with homology to epidermal growth factor have been described on the B chains.

Recently, a new nomenclature for laminins has been proposed. The A, B1, and B2 designation for EHS laminin and its subsequently identified isoforms are replaced by α, β, and γ, respectively.[56] The isoforms of each chain class are further designated by an arabic number, based on their order of discovery. For example, EHS, or A,B1,B2, laminin, are designated $\alpha1\beta1\gamma1$, merosin $\alpha2\beta1\gamma1$, and s-laminin $\alpha1\beta2\gamma1$. In addition, the assembled forms will be designated as laminin-1, laminin-2, and laminin-3, respectively. The genes for the different chains are designated as LAMA1, LAMA2, LAMA3, LAMB1, and so forth.

COMPONENTS	CONSTITUENT CHAINS	MOLECULAR COMPOSITION	SUPRAMOLECULAR AGGREGATE	FUNCTION
COLLAGEN TYPE IV	α 1(IV) α 2(IV) α 3(IV) α 4(IV) α 5(IV)	3 α Chains	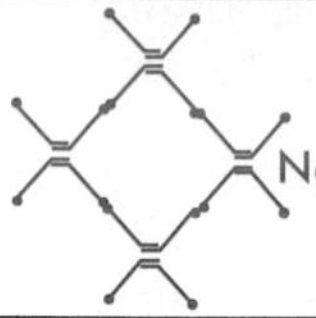 Network	Structural
LAMININ	A,MS,B1,B2	3 Chains Either A or M Either S or B1 and B2	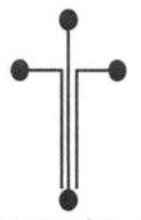 Cross-shaped	Cell Attachment Growth Promotor
ENTACTIN	Single Polypeptide Chain	Single Polypeptide Chain	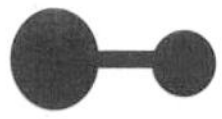 Globular	Unknown
HEPARAN SULFATE PROTEOGLYCAN	Polypeptide Chain Glycosaminoglycan Side Chains	Protein Core Glycosaminoglycan Side Chains	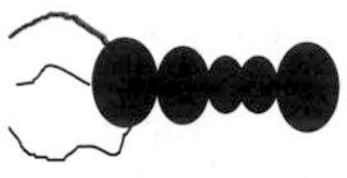	Electrostatic Charge

Fig. 19-9 Basement membrane components. (Modified from Rubin E, Farber JL: *Pathology,* ed 2, Philadelphia, 1994, Lippincott.)

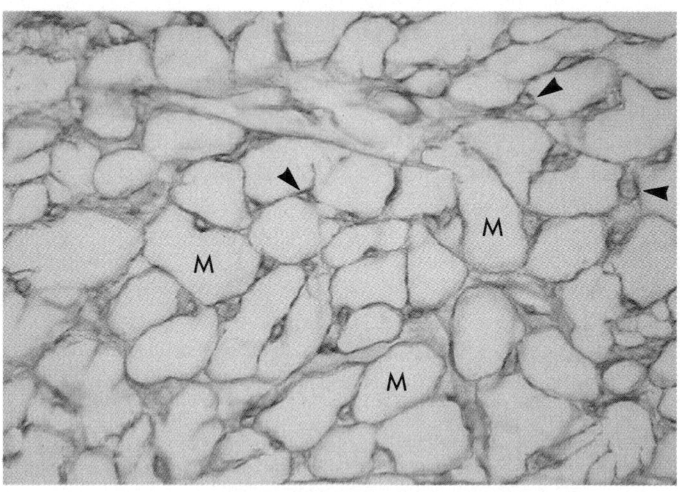

Fig. 19-10 Localization of laminin β1 chain in adult skeletal muscle. The laminin, in its localization to the basement membranes surrounding skeletal muscle fibers, *M* (myofibers), participates in the partitioning of the contractile myofibers into discrete units and to partition it from the vasculature. *Arrowheads,* Capillaries. (Courtesy Peter Yurchenco, M.D., Ph.D., Piscataway, N.J.)

Laminin functions are multiple, as judged by their spatial and temporal distribution and by extrapolation of in vitro data. For example, although M and s chains are expressed during hepatic ontogenesis and regeneration, this expression is downregulated with maturation of the liver and the completion of regenerative process, respectively.[57] Merosin in vitro has also been shown to modulate axon outgrowth in a manner similar to EHS laminin.[58]

Entactin, or nidogen

Entactin, another structural component of the BM, was also first identified in a mouse teratocarcinoma.[55,59] Also referred to as nidogen, entactin is a highly sulfated glycoprotein (relative molecular mass 150 kilodaltons) restricted to the BM. Recombinant studies have demonstrated three globular domains in the molecule. It interacts at one globular domain with the B1 chain near the center of the laminin multimer. The functions of entactin remain a mystery; however, some postulate that by its interaction with the cell attachment site of laminin, it modifies cell binding properties of laminin. Further, entactin may be a modulator of BM assembly because of its binding to laminin, type IV collagen, and perlecan.

Osteonectin (SPARC)

Osteonectin (also known as SPARC, or secreted protein acidic and rich in cysteine) is a glycoprotein (32 kD), first identified from guanidine extracts of mineralizing calf bone.[60,61] Osteonectin binds to type I collagen and hydroxyapatite. Its name reflects its binding to the mineral and collagen components of bone. It is also found in dentin but not in enamel or calcified cartilage. The bridging between ECM and hydroxyapatite by osteonectin has indicated an important function in initiating mineralization. Osteonectin is found immediately subjacent to the zone of calcified cartilage on new bone surfaces and on mineralized metaphyseal and subperiosteal trabeculas in long and membranous bones. Studies have also demonstrated the presence of osteonectin in nonosseous tissues rich in BM.

Type IV collagen

Collagen type IV[47,62-64] is composed of at least six different α chains—α1(IV) to α6(IV). The α1(IV) and α2(IV) genes have been localized to chromosome 13; the α3(IV) and α4(IV) chains to chromosome 2; and α5(IV) and α6(IV) chains to the X chromosome.

The most common form of type IV collagen molecule is the heterotrimer $[\alpha1(IV)]_2\,[\alpha2(IV)]$, which is ubiquitously distributed. In what fashion the remaining, so-called minor chains

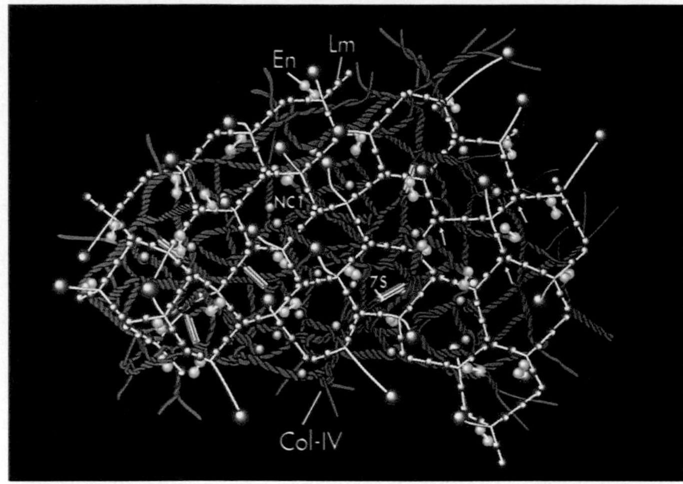

Fig. 19-11 Model of a BM scaffolding. Laminin *(red, Lm)* binds to itself through short-arm peripheral domains *(arrows* indicate binding sites*)* to form a quasihexagonal mesh. Independently, type IV collagen *(gray, Col-IV)* forms a network through lateral, N-terminal *(7S)* and C-terminal *(NC1)* interactions. The terminal bonds become covalently cross-linked through disulfide and lysyl oxidase–dependent interactions. Entactin/nidogen *(green, En/Nd),* which binds to the α1 chain of laminin, bridges many but not all laminin molecules to type IV collagen. (Courtesy Peter Yurchenco, M.D., Ph.D., Piscataway, NJ and Academic Press.)

are incorporated into collagen IV molecules is being elucidated.[65] Their tissue distribution is restricted when compared with the α1 and α2 chains. Study of the diseases associated with the BM will help unravel the distribution and function of the various components. For example, mutations in the α5 chain have been found to have a central role in the pathogenesis of Alport's syndrome,[66-69] an inherited (often X-linked) progressive renal disease[68] in which striated fibrils are present in the lamina densa.

Unlike the fibrillar collagens, collagen type IV molecules interact in a unique manner to form a complex network. The lateral interactions are not periodic, as in fibrillary collagens and involve twisting together of the interacting molecules, both laterally and at their ends. Disulfide bonds form between the carboxy termini of two molecules and among the amino termini of four molecules to generate a network. These end-to-end and side-to-side relationships result in a network that has tensile strength, pliability, and porosity. The other BM components bind to this structure to form the BM (Fig. 19-11). Type IV collagen also binds to cells. By means of its interactions with ECM components and cells, it mediates its effects on cell migration and differentiation.[69]

Perlecan

The negative charge characteristic of BM is attributable, in great part, to the presence of a high-molecular-weight, low-density, heparan sulfate proteoglycan called perlecan. The alignment of the globular domains in a manner reminiscent of a string of pearls underlies its name.[69-71] Perlecan is a large protein (500 to 600 kD) consisting of five or six globular domains. The multiple globular domains foreshortens the native structure to a length of approximately 270 nm. The importance of protein folding in the final structure of ECM components is well illustrated when one compares the mass and length of perlecan with a type I collagen α chain: 500-600 kD/80 nm for perlecan to 100 kD/300 nm for α1(I). Fig. 19-12 gives comparisons of mass and size of various ECM components. The core protein of perlecan has a molecular weight of 500 to 600 kD and glycosaminoglycan (GAG) chains of approximately 65 kD.[72] At the N terminus, three GAG chains of heparan sulfate are covalently linked, forming a *tailed* structure (see Fig. 19-9). The complete sequence of human perlecan has been determined, and the various domains have sequence homologies with a neural-cell adhesion molecule, laminin, epidermal growth factor, and low-density lipoprotein receptor.[70,73,74]

Perlecan interacts with numerous ECM molecules including laminin, collagen type IV, and itself, to form complex, multimolecular structures. In the BM, the GAG chains of perlecan probably form important permselective barriers for charged plasma filtrants. In addition to structural functions, perlecan binds to basic fibroblast growth factor and extracellular superoxide dismutase as well as to cells.

Biosynthesis of basement membrane components

BM components are synthesized and deposited by the cells that are coated by or in immediate contact with them, that is, epithelia, skeletal muscle, cardiac muscle, adipocytes, and endothelia. Recent studies have also indicated that fibroblasts may contribute to the synthesis of the BM that line the basal surface of epithelia, such as those of the intestine and epidermis. Presumably, the components contributed by the fibroblasts are capable of either diffusing to the epithelial basal surface or are being *plastered* against the epithelial basal surface by processes extending from the fibroblasts.[75,76]

Basement membrane assembly

The assembly of the BM occurs, in part, by a process of self-assembly. Type IV collagen interacts with itself by side-to-side and end-to-end associations, including disulfide-bonding, into a strong, three-dimensional network. Laminin self-assembles into a complex multimer independently of type IV collagen. This laminin polymer has as one arrangement, a planar configuration with all long arms directed similarly, yielding a polarized polymer. Heparan sulfate aggregates by protein-protein interactions at its N termini to form dimers and its GAG chains to form multimers. When mixed together in appropriate ratios, these components create a sheetlike BM structure (Fig. 19-11) with perlecan modulating the binding of the individual components to themselves and to one another.[47,77,78]

Basement membrane functions

Basement membranes are a cell surface coat, providing for mechanical stability, tissue pliability, cell attachment, and ultrafiltration of interstitial fluids. The tensile strength of BM largely rests on its collagenous network. The tensile support is evident in muscular contraction, whether in skeletal muscle, smooth muscle, or cardiac muscle. The ability of cells to proliferate and migrate along the BM is critical for epithelial regeneration, as in ulcerative lesions and organogenesis.

Ultrafiltration by means of the BM is appreciated in capillaries, especially those of the renal glomerulus. Although originally considered to act as a molecular sieve, excluding proteins based on their size and shape, BM filtration capacity depends, to a large extent, on the anionic charge imparted by perlecan.

A large volume of data concerning the role of the BM in modulating development has accumulated. Many of these

Matrix components: Solid phase Soluble phase Cell surface phase	GAG chain type	Core protein size (kD)	Size (nM) / 300 nM	Intermolecular interactions homotypic & heterotypic
Aggrecan	CS/KS	320		Types I, II, III, V, XI Type IV Type VI Type VII Type VIII Type XII
Betaglycan		90		
Biglycan	CS/DS	40		
CD44	CS*	85		
Cartilage matrix pr.		150		
Collagen I - III & V		310		
Collagen IV		525		
Collagen VI		300		
Collagen VII		590		
Collagen IX		225		
Collagen IX		225		
Collagen X		200		
Collagen XII		590		
Decorin	CS/DS	40		
Entactin/Nidogen		120		
Fibrillin		350		
Fibromodulin	CS/DS	60		
Fibronectin		500		
Glypican	HS	65		
Hyaluronan		0		
Intergrins		220		
Laminins		840		
Link		40		
Osteocalcin		6		
Osteopontin		35		
Perlecan	HS	600		
Serglycin	CS/DS	11		
Sparc/Osteonectin		40		
Syndecan	HS/CS	35		
Tenascin		320		
Thrombomodulin	CS*	90		
Thrombospondin	HS*	450		
Versican	CS/DS	250		
Vitronectin		50		

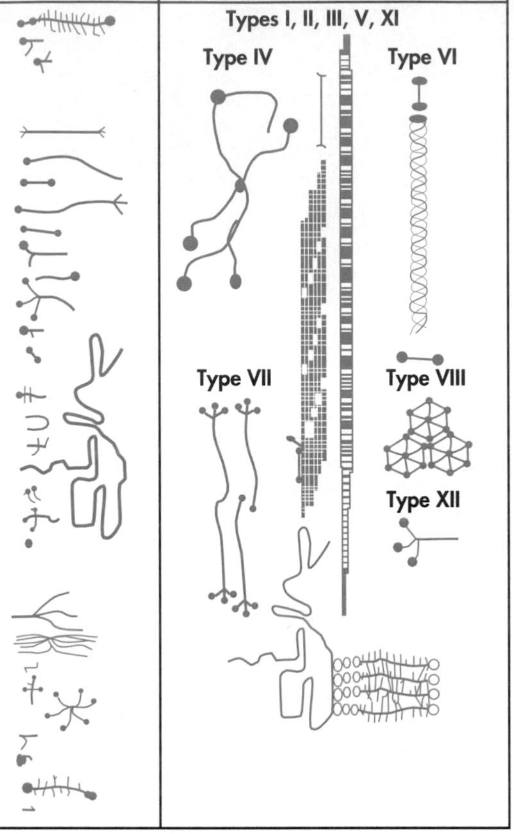

Fig. 19-12 The extracellular matrix is composed of various combinations of proteins, proteoglycans, and glycoproteins with unique functions and shapes. The shapes of these molecules are of critical importance to their various roles as solid-phase components such as the structural collagens; soluble-phase elements such as circulating fibronectin or hyaluronan; and integral cell surface components such as syndecans and integrins or non–integral cell surface components such as basement membranes composed of type IV collagen, laminin, decorin, and perlecan. The table presents the molecules drawn to scale based on electron microscopic studies. Notice that the size of a molecule in real space, measured in nanometers, is not readily predictable from its size in kilodaltons (kD) as measured by various techniques. The differences between apparent mass in kilodaltons and actual size depends on the extended configuration of the molecules in space. Notice that laminin is nearly three times the mass of type I collagen but half its length and that type VI collagen, with its globular domains at both ends has the same mass as type I collagen but is much shorter. Attached to many of the molecules are side chains composed of glycosaminoglycan chains (GAG). The GAG types are *CS,* chondroitin sulfate; *KS,* keratan sulfate; *DS,* dermatan sulfate; *HS,* heparan sulfate. Those molecules with intermittent GAG chains or "part-time" proteoglycans are indicated with an asterisk. All these molecules interact in a complex set of homotypic ("with each other") and heterotypic ("with others') modes. Some of the simplest examples are shown at the *right.* The hyaluronan-aggrecan heteropolymer at the lower right is the essential structure of articular cartilages. The type VII collagen homopolymers form anchoring fibrils essential for maintenance of epidermal integrity; the type VIII network is present in Descemet's membrane in the cornea; the types I, II, III, V, and XI striated fibrils are the essential warp and woof of the animal kingdom.

functions can be attributed to the functions of individual BM components.[6,79] Examples of such activity of the BM is the role of laminin in the transformation of renal mesenchyme to epithelia or in the loss of BM in the transformation of the urogenital ridge epithelium to mesenchyme.[80-85]

Pathology of basement membranes

The basement membrane has been the subject of interest since the earliest studies of histopathology because a frequent morphologic finding that is associated with various disorders is BM thickening, visible by light microscopy. This is a nonspecific change that is present in glomerulonephropathies, bronchiolar BM in asthma, and diffusely in diabetes, since synthesis and deposition of BM is a common response to injury. In asthma and chronic bronchitis the BM thickening is of little consequence. In contrast, in glomerular diseases, the BM changes represent a crucial pathogenetic event. Detailed reviews of the role of the BM in pathology are available.[44,46]

BM are involved in many disorders including neoplastic, genetic, metabolic, infectious, and immunologic disorders.

To metastasize, neoplasms must invade into vascular structures, a process that requires that the tumor cells attach or bind to and penetrate through a series of parenchymal and vascular BM.[86]

Diabetes mellitus is characterized by accelerated atherosclerosis (macroangiopathy) and a microangiopathy. A central feature of both entities is a thickening of the capillary BM in muscle, retina, skin, and kidney. In glomeruli, this is characterized as either diffuse or nodular (Kimmelstiel-Wilson) glomerulosclerosis (Chapter 65). The exact mechanism responsible for the BM abnormalities in diabetes is unclear, but a relative decrease in perlecan, abnormalities in proteoglycan glycation, and nonenzymatic glycation of BM components have been proposed.[87] These issues are covered in detail in Chapter 65.

Alport's syndrome is a hereditary glomerulopathy characterized by persistent microscopic hematuria, gross hematuria, and progressive renal failure.[68,69] The BM is characterized by pronounced thinning and discontinuity of the lamina densa, with the unexpected presence of striated fibrils. Epithelial and endothelial glomerular BM fail to fuse (splitting). It is believed that these morphologic BM abnormalities are attributable to mutations of the α5(IV) chain; making Alport's syndrome (in the sex-linked form) the first described genetic disease of BM. The α3 and α4 chains are mutated in the autosomal forms of the disease.

Immunologic diseases affecting the BM are characterized by immune complex deposition in the glomerular BM. In most types of glomerulonephritis, the BM is altered by filtration of and consequent nonspecific trapping of immune complexes and subsequent complement fixation. Anti-GBM disease, or Goodpasture's syndrome, is characterized by acute hemoptysis and hematuria and is attributable to antibodies directed against glomerular antigens including type IV collagen.[88,89] Epidermolysis bullosa is a blistering disease of the skin in which mild trauma to epidermis results in subepidermal cleavage.[8] This entity is associated with absence of type VII collagen or with antibodies directed against type VII collagen of the anchoring fibers. Recent studies have implicated a loss of the skeletal muscle BM laminin, called merosin, in the pathogenesis of a form of muscular dystrophy.[90]

Structural glycoproteins

This class of ECM glycoproteins plays a role in cell adhesion, cell-matrix ligands, solid-phase agonists, and modulators of cell behavior. As common features, they have epidermal growth factor–like domains, polymer-forming capacities, and amino acid sequences that interact with cellular receptors.

Fibronectins

The fibronectins (FN) represent a class of structural glycoproteins that exist in chemically and immunologically distinct, soluble (plasma) and insoluble (cellular) forms.[91-93] Soluble FN is present in many body fluids, including plasma, urine, amniotic, and cerebrospinal. FN consists of two polypeptide chains (250 kD), connected by disulfide bonds at the carboxy termini (Fig. 19-13). FN binds or interacts with many macromolecules, bacteria, other ECM components, and cells. These interactions occur through specific, globular domains located along the molecule, and this polyvalency gives FN a multiadhesive quality.

Although there are immunologic and structural differences between plasma and cellular FN, both are the products of a single gene located on human chromosome 2. DNA sequencing has demonstrated three distinct, partially homologous (25% to

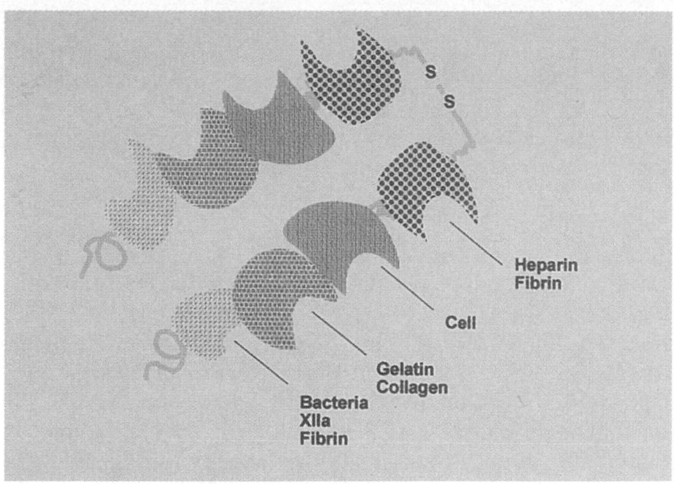

Fig. 19-13 Fibronectin is a polypeptide linked at the carboxy termini by disulfide bonds. Individual discrete globular domains with specific binding properties characterize this molecule and interact with cells, extracellular matrix, bacteria, and plasma components. (Modified from Leadbetter W, Gordon S, Buckwalter J: *Inflammation and healing of sports induced soft tissue injury,* Park Ridge, Ill, 1990, American Academy of Orthopaedic Surgeons.

50%), repeating units called types I, II, and III. These units are repeated throughout the FN polypeptide chains, having a greater or lesser frequency within certain domains. For example, the type I unit is repeated in the collagen- and fibrin-binding regions, whereas the type III unit is prevalent in cell- and heparin-binding regions. Cellular FN has an additional type III unit, the so-called extra-domain (ED) unit, absent from plasma FN. Genetically, plasma and cellular fibronectin genes are identical, but by means of alternative splicing, the two messages differ. Alternative splicing of mRNA can actually result in at least six different FN molecules, but the significance of this heterogeneity is not clearly understood. In addition, posttranslational modifications, including glycation are significant for maintaining the biologic activity of FN. For example, N-linked glycation is critical in protecting the collagen binding domain from proteolysis.

FN is ubiquitous in the ECM, where it forms either fine filaments or granular deposits. It is often found coating the surface of collagen fibers and is adjacent to but not within the BM.[12,52] FN is not found in mature cartilage, and only traces are found in tendons; however, it is abundant in the ECM of most soft tissues and skeletal muscle.

It has been shown that a fragment from a type III repeat of fibronectin induces fibronectin to bind to itself by means of disulfide cross-links. This results in fibronectin forming a multimeric structure forming fibrils and has been postulated to represent the tissue form of fibronectin. Its enhanced adhesive capabilities in cell culture has led to its being referred to as "superfibronectin."[92]

During development, FN is a prominent component of the fetal matrix surrounding mesenchymal cells. As the cells differentiate toward their definitive phenotype, they produce a more specialized ECM.[82,94]

In wound healing, plasma FN is a component of the initial clot. The glutamine in FN allows for its being cross-linked by transglutaminases to plasma and tissue components forming the initial, primitive matrix that will eventually be replaced by the definitive scar.[95-98]

The study of the cell-binding properties of FN led to the identification of the specific amino acid sequence responsible for this activity, that is, arginine-glycine-asparagine (RGD).[99] The RGD sequence is not unique to FN, and other proteins with cell-binding properties such as vitronectin, fibrinogen, laminin, and collagen also contain this sequence.

Tenascin

Tenascin (also known as cytotactin, J1, or hexabrachion) is a six-armed, spiderlike glycoprotein with a relative molecular mass of 1.9 kD (Fig. 19-14).[93,100-103] The subunits are similar, linked by interchain disulfide bonds, joined at the amino terminus, forming a central globular domain. Tenascin is often compared with thrombospondin and osteonectin (SPARC) in its functional capacity as a mediator of cell-matrix interactions.[61] Tenascin has both a binding capacity and the ability of inhibiting cell binding. It binds to fibronectin and some proteoglycans. Like laminin, tenascin arms have a series of EGF-like repeats in their amino termini, responsible for the antiadhesive activities. A cell adhesion site is present near the carboxy terminus, adjacent to a fibrinogen-like globule. Tenascin, like fibronectin, undergoes alternative splicing to form three variant molecules.

Tenascin[104] appears in a wound 48 hours after an injury and is primarily associated with fibroblasts. This deposition increases to form a network of tenascin at the wound site, which is intense by 5 days. Tenascin is absent from the mature scar.

Thrombospondin

Thrombospondin is a glycoprotein composed of three identical 140 kD arms, joined centrally by disulfide bonds.[61,93,105] Initially identified in the granules of platelets, it is synthesized by endothelial cells, smooth muscle cells, fibroblasts, keratinocytes, glial cells, and macrophages. Although initially characterized as an important modulator of platelet aggregation and clotting, it is now known to modulate cell-matrix interactions.

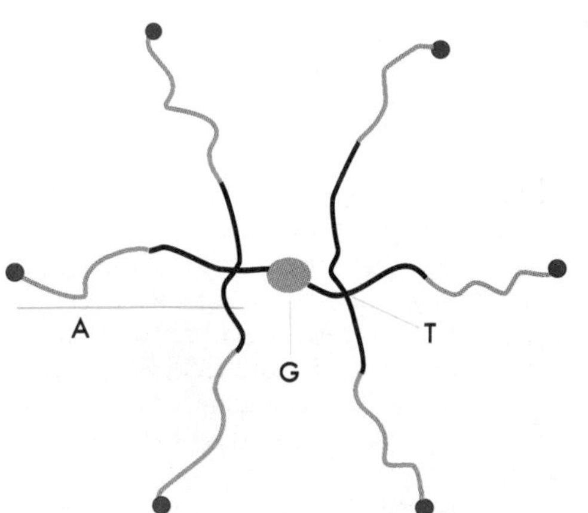

Fig. 19-14 This spiderlike molecule is tenascin. It is characterized by six identical arms. Each arm has a 30 nm long, thin, proximal component. The thicker terminal portions have a 55 nm and contain globular domains at their end. The three arms connect at a T-junction, and these two groups can then join at a central globular domain. (Modified from Leadbetter W, Gordon S, Buckwalter J: *Inflammation and healing of sports induced soft tissue injury,* Park Ridge, Ill, 1990, American Academy of Orthopaedic Surgeons.)

Each chain contains several functional domains. The amino terminus is a globular heparin binding domain. A type I procollagen domain, properdin-like repeats, EGF-like repeats, Ca^{++} binding domains, and a cell binding domain at the C terminus compose the remainder of the chain. As with other ECM components, isotypic forms of this molecule have been described.[105]

Thrombospondin binds with several other ECM components including cell surface heparan sulfate proteoglycans, collagen, and laminin. In addition it binds to integrins and sulfatides. It enhances cellular attachment and migration of some cells while inhibiting these events in others. For example, it functions as an adhesive protein for keratinocytes and platelets but impairs attachment of fibroblasts and endothelial cells to a fibronectin-rich matrix. By these modulatory roles it has profound effects on cell-matrix interactions in repair reactions. Further, thrombospondin bound to an ECM indirectly promotes angiogenesis and thus may stimulate this event in wound healing.[106] The synthesis of thrombospondin is stimulated by cytokines, transforming growth factor-β, and platelet-derived growth factor.

Pathology of glycoproteins

Studies of the distributions of fibronectin, laminin, and tenascin, as well as other structural glycoproteins in many pathologic processes are beginning to provide some insight into their roles in these entities.[97,107] For example, in cirrhosis fibronectin is believed to provide the initial matrix that potentiates the formation of fibrous tissue septa during the formation of the regenerative nodules. Similarly, fibronectin is deposited in the early stages of wound healing.[95] Therefore, FN appears to be an important component in forming the initial matrix in wound healing and providing the foundation to establish the scar. The catabolism of these proteins during the progression of repair often is associated with elevated serum concentrations and serves as some measure of repair and disease activity.[108]

Proteoglycans

Proteoglycans are a heterogeneous group of molecules containing a variable number (1 to 100) of glycosaminoglycan (GAG) side chains, covalently linked to a core protein.[72,109-112] They appear in the intracellular space, cell surface, and extracellular space. Although the respective core proteins are the product of unique genes, the GAGs are often the same and in the past imparted their name to the proteoglycan. For example, the major proteoglycan of cartilage was called *chondroitin sulfate proteoglycan.* However, when the same GAG is present on different core proteins, a modifier such as cell surface or BM should be used, as with heparan sulfate proteoglycan, that is, cell surface versus BM HSPG. A new nomenclature based on several features, including their morphology, distribution, and functions, is developing for these molecules. For example, in the case of heparan sulfate proteoglycans, the cell surface HSPG is called syndecan (from the Greek *syndein,* 'to bind together'), since it connects the cells to the ECM, and BM-HSPG is called *perlecan,* since it is composed of globular domains resembling a string of pearls.

Structure of proteoglycans

The morphology of proteoglycans is highly dependent on methods of preparation. Tissue dehydration results in collapse of the large hydrophilic domains; therefore the images obtained by electron microscopy represent only a fraction of the actual space occupied by the proteoglycans. In most tissues, ECM proteoglycans appear as convoluted filaments with abundant lateral projections. They are often found associated with collagen fibers, cell surfaces, and other ECM components.

Glycosaminoglycans

Glycosaminoglycans are defined as linear heteropolysaccharides characterized by a disaccharide repeat.[72] The disaccharide repeats contain an amino sugar with D-glucosamine or galactosamine and the second unit typically either D-glucuronic or iduronic acid and are variably N- and O-sulfated. There are seven major glycosaminoglycans: chondroitin sulfate, dermatan sulfate, heparan sulfate, keratan sulfate, hyaluronic acid, and heparin. All the GAGs listed, except heparin and hyaluronic acid, are linked to core proteins forming proteoglycans.

Hyaluronic acid

Hyaluronic acid consists of alternating polymers of *N*-acetylglucosamine and glucuronic acid and has a molecular mass up to 10 million daltons. It can associate with itself to form elaborate matrices. Hyaluronic acid synthesis does not appear to involve the Golgi complex.

Matrix-associated proteoglycans

Extracellular matrix proteoglycans can be divided into three major groups: large interstitial, small interstitial, and BM proteoglycans. Large interstitial proteoglycans include the cartilage proteoglycan, aggrecan, and that present in blood vessels, versican. Decorin, biglycan, and fibromodulin are two small interstitial proteoglycans. Heparan sulfate and chondroitin sulfate proteoglycans are associated with BM.

Cell surface–associated proteoglycans

Proteoglycans can be integral elements of the plasma membranes of cells.[109,113] This interaction occurs by intercalation of the core protein in its hydrophilic region, covalent linkage of the core protein with phosphatidylinositol, or noncovalent linkage to the plasma membrane binding proteins.

Syndecan is a HSPG primarily found in epithelial cells. Like other binding/receptor proteins, syndecan contains cytoplasmic, transmembrane, and extracellular domains. Syndecan interacts with collagen, fibronectin, and thrombospondin. Its intracellular domain is believed to interact with cytoskeletal elements.

Intracellular proteoglycans

Mast cells are rich in a proteoglycan called *serglycin*, a chondroitin sulfate proteoglycan. Heparin is present in mast cells, where it provides a cationic exchange matrix, allowing organization of basic molecules such as histamine in the granules of these cells.

Biosynthesis of proteoglycans

Synthesis of the proteoglycans occurs in the cisterns of the rough endoplasmic reticulum, where addition of N-linked oligosaccharides occurs. With transfer to the Golgi apparatus, the GAG side chains are extended on the protein core. Subsequently, those PG targeted for the ECM are secreted into the extracellular space where they aggregate and complex with other ECM components.

Function of proteoglycans

Proteoglycans, by the nature of their ability to retain water and become hydrated, act as excellent *shock absorbers*. The functions of proteoglycans can also be appreciated from their localization.[71] Membrane-intercalated proteoglycans typically act as receptors. Betaglycan acts as a receptor for transforming growth factor-β.[114] Syndecan binds cells to the ECM. Aggrecan, the major proteoglycan of cartilage, provides resilience to that tissue. Decorin coats collagen fibers and is believed to modulate fibrillogenesis. Other proteoglycans have roles in cell attachment and migration, such as versican for fibroblasts.

In addition, GAGs have a considerable role in modulating coagulation. This, in part, is responsible for the nonthrombogenic properties attributed to the endothelial cell surface. These activities occur by the deactivation of coagulation enzymes by means of antithrombin, the latter's activity being enhanced by GAGs.[115]

Pathology of proteoglycans

Diseases of the glycosaminoglycans and proteoglycans are usually the consequence of either their excessive production or insufficient degradation. The latter conditions are attributable to absence of key lysosomal enzymes and result in excessive accumulation of GAGs in the lysosomes. This heterogeneous group of diseases is discussed in detail in Chapter 12. The group of diseases classically associated with excessive degradation of proteoglycans are the arthritides. The arthritides are defined as an inflammatory process of the joints and synovium responsible for the production of proteases (including collagenases) and the breakdown of ECM, followed by deposition of ECM and cells in the form of a pannus. This is associated with an increase in synovial and serum concentrations of proteoglycan fragments.

Proteoglycans also have key roles in several other disease states. In some glomerular diseases characterized by proteinuria, such as, diabetes mellitus,[87] decreased proteoglycans and the concomitant loss of anionic charge of the GBM are central to the pathogenesis of these lesions. In the progression of malignant tumors, proteoglycans are degraded as tumor cells invade the adjacent BM and interstitium. Tumors such as Wilm's tumor, chondroblastoma, and mesothelioma have been associated with elevated serum levels of GAGs. Serum elevations such as these represent excessive breakdown of the ECM surrounding tumors or increased synthesis. Proteoglycan deposition has also been hypothesized as having a central role in the pathogenesis of Alzheimer's disease.[116]

Extracellular matrix degradation

In any active process such as ontogenesis and repair, there must be mechanisms for removal of cells and matrix as remodeling and reorganization of the tissue occurs. Failure of such would result in the excessive accumulation of ECM and loss of normal structural and functional characteristics of a tissue.

There are several mechanisms by which ECM is degraded, including specific proteases such as the collagenases, elastases, stromelysin, plasmin, polymorphonuclear serine proteases, and lysosomal phagocytic pathways. Mineralized matrices such as bone, cementum, and dentin are degraded by an osteoclastic pathway. The major mechanism of ECM degradation is mediated by the matrix metalloproteinase (MMP) family of enzymes.[117]

The MMP consist of four types of enzymes, the interstitial collagenases, stromelysins, gelatinases, and the broad category listed under the heading of putative metalloproteinases (PUMPS). The latter group includes stromelysin-3 and macrophage metalloelastase. The MMPs have as a common structural feature the presence of a five-domain modular structure. The collagenases that degrade interstitial collagens under native conditions do so at a specific site, approximately three fourths of the distance along the helix from the amino terminus. Tumor cells can secrete collagenases, including type IV collagenase, which enhance their capability to invade through BM.[86]

The phagocytic pathway of matrix degradation is the only one that is active in the intracellular environment, whereas the other enzyme systems noted above are active in the pericellular and extracellular environment. The plasmin pathway is particularly significant during the ECM remodeling that is associated with cell migration, tumor and trophoblastic invasion, and embryogenesis.

As with all enzymatic systems, an inhibitory regulatory system is associated with the MMPs. The tissue inhibitor metalloproteinases, or TIMPs, complex with the active form of MMPs or possibly interacting with the zymogen, thus regulating the activity of these enzymes.

ECM-cell interactions

The repair reaction relies on the ability of cells to interact with one another and with the ECM. When epithelial cells proliferate to replace a denuded surface, they migrate over the BM matrix. Similarly, inflammatory and stromal cells interact with matrix components as they migrate within a wound site.[118] These activities require that cells first are able to attach to the ECM. As indicated above, many ECM components contain the amino acid sequence Arginine-glycine-asparagine (RGD), which binds to a family of transmembrane receptors, the integrins.

Integrins

The integrin family[119-126] of cell receptors (Fig. 19-15) are functional in both cell-cell (discussed below) and ECM-cell binding, though they seem to be the primary mediators of the latter. Through the integrins, a route of communication exists for the ECM to influence cell behavior such as migration, growth, and differentiation and conversely for cells to interact with the ECM.[123]

The integrins consist of glycoprotein chains, with 11 α chains and six β chains having been identified. These α and β chains combine to form at least 16 different integrins. The α subunit is paired with several different β subunits (Fig. 19-16). ECM components binding to integrins include collagens, fibronectin, laminin, tenascin, thrombospondin, and vitronectin. The interaction of the intracellular domain with subplasmalemmal proteins, such as talin, are responsible for torsional effects on the cytoskeleton. By means of these cytoskeletal interactions and inductions of second-messenger systems, the ECM is capable of modulating cell behavior. The nature of the second messenger is yet to be defined.[127]

ECM soluble-phase agonists

The discovery of the ECM cell membrane receptors initiated an intense search for the domains of the ECM proteins responsible for cellular binding and subsequently identification of the domains of the molecules responsible for the biologic activities of these proteins. Eventually peptide sequences responsible for

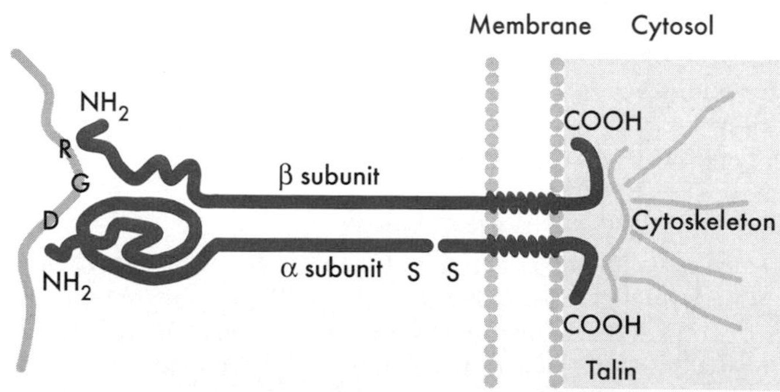

Fig. 19-15 The integrins are a family of cell surface transmembrane proteins characterized by two polypeptide chains, α and β chains. The α chain comprises subunits connected by disulfide bonds, whereas the β chain is a polypeptide chain. The integrins span the extracellular, intramembranous, and intracellular compartments. The N-terminus contains the matrix binding site, which typically recognizes the arginine-glycine-asparagine (RGD) sequence. Other sequences are bound to and by integrins. Interaction of integrins with subplasma membrane protein such as talin, which is also connected to cytoplasmic filaments, results in exchange of information between the extracellular matrix and the intracellular compartment. (Modified from Rubin E, Farber JL: *Pathology,* ed 2, Philadelphia, 1994, Lippincott.)

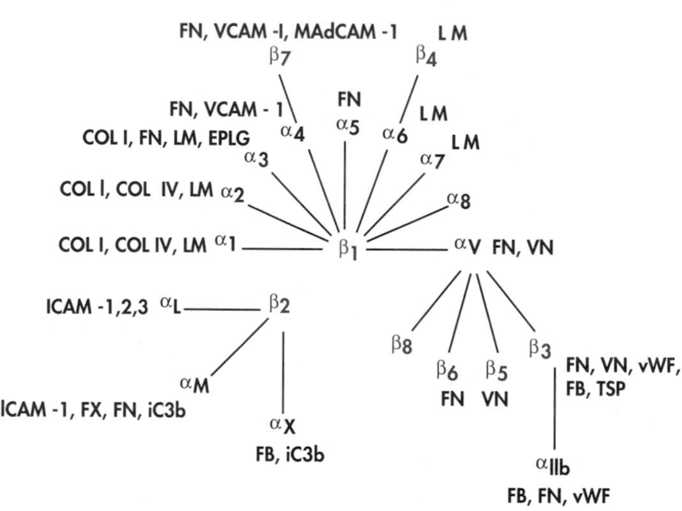

Fig. 19-16 The integrins are a family of heterodimeric transmembrane adhesion molecules composed of one α chain and one β chain. Up to now, 8 β chains and 13 α chains have been relatively well characterized. In their heterodimeric states they have varying affinities for components in the extracellular space. The binding of cells to the extracellular environment by means of the integrins has implications in wound healing, normal development, and immune functions. The diagram indicates the known interactions of various heterodimeric combinations. It is apparent from the listed ligands that overlap in specificity occurs among various combinations. It is also apparent that these adhesion molecules bind to both solid-phase matrix components such as collagen type I (COL I), to cell surface–phase molecules such as collagen type IV and laminin in basement membranes (COL IV and LM) or other adhesions molecules (ICAM or VCAM), and to soluble-phase elements such as the inactivated C3b component of complement (iC3b). *COL I,* Type I collagen; *COL IV,* type IV collagen; *EPLG,* epiligrin; *FN,* fibronectin; *LM,* laminin; *ICAM,* intercellular adhesion molecule; *VCAM,* vascular cell adhesion molecule; *FB,* fibrinogen; *vWF,* von Willebrand factor; *MAdCAM,* mucosal addressin cell adhesion molecule; *VN,* vitronectin; *iC3B,* inactivated complement component C3; *TSP,* thrombospondin.

these activities were isolated. The first and now classical sequence that binds with cells was the arginine-glycine-asparagine-serine peptide, now referred to as the RGD sequence. First identified in the cell binding domain of fibronectin, RGD has also been found in some other matrix components.

A few other signal peptides, such as another adhesive peptide of leucine-asparagine-valine (in fibronectin), have since been identified. Several such peptides have been identified in laminin. The sequence of tyrosine-isoleucine-glycine-serine-arginine (YIGSR) is postulated by some as an important mediator of cell migration. Other peptide sequences of laminin believed to have biologic activities are IKVAV and PDSGR.

Extracellular matrix in repair

The above discussion has illustrated the complex nature and functional capacity of the ECM. In summary, it is useful to consider the ECM as an integrated, dynamic functional unit composed of interconnected sheets, cables, and networks, coated by and embedded within a heterogeneous, biologically active protein matrix that is assembled to fit the unique needs of individual tissues. In a similar fashion, the matrix deposited throughout wound healing must be assembled to accommodate the particular needs of that tissue as it is repaired. This matrix needs to provide an environment to maintain structural integrity during repair and modulate cellular motility, activation, and differentiation, while often undergoing simultaneous deposition and degradation.

It should be evident that a system of checks and balances is provided by individual matrix components and their isoforms to help regulate the dynamic state of the matrix. For example, some ECM proteins enhance cellular migration, whereas others inhibit it. Tenascin, thrombospondin, and SPARC provide excellent examples of such modulatory proteins. Similarly, entactin modulates the ability of laminin to bind to cells. The ratios and temporal and spatial expression of these components during repair are as important to regulating repair and regeneration as they are in normal development and homeostasis.

CELLS OF THE REPAIR PROCESS

In addition to the cells specific to the injured tissue (epidermal cells, neurons, hepatocytes, and so forth), the stromal cells such as fibroblasts, smooth muscle, inflammatory cells, and endothelial cells, have a major role in repair. These cells are the source of ECM components, cytokines, and factors active in the repair process. All these cells have a common mesodermal lineage and share many properties.

A cell lineage defines a group or groups of cells derived from a common progenitor. For example, virtually all mesenchymal cells are derived from embryonic mesoderm, except in the head, where it derives from the neural crest. As depicted in Fig. 19-17, a common mesodermal progenitor cell gives rise to the majority of the mesenchymal cell lineages. Cells as diverse as cardiac myocytes and adipose cells thus have common ancestors and share some properties. For example, most adult mesenchymal cells contain vimentin or desmin as their major intermediate filament, whereas epithelial cells contain keratin. Further, many adult mesenchymal cells retain some proliferative capacity, and thus are typically stable cells and can synthesize ECM.

The major lineages of the mesodermal germ layer are the endothelial, hematopoietic, muscle (cardiac, skeletal, and smooth), bone, cartilage, fibroblastic, and adipocytes. Virtually all these cells are essential elements of the normal repair reaction by the nature of their phagocytic capabilities, synthesis of cytokines, chemotactic factors, and ECM production.

Endothelial cells

Endothelial cells are flattened squamous cells (Fig. 19-18), typically containing a prominent nucleus, a cytoplasm rich in biosynthetic organelles, and lined on the abluminal surface by a BM.[128-130] The Weibel-Palade body is a unique cytoplasmic structure that contains von Willebrand factor and a protein, GP 140, which is exposed on the cell's surface shortly after injury. The vascular endothelium provides the initial barrier between the blood and adjacent connective tissue. Their nonthrombogenic surface is essential for maintanance of normal blood flow and also acts as a permeability barrier.

Endothelial cells (Fig. 19-18) are critical mediators of the repair reaction. Their proliferation and organization into a vascular network at the wound site, as well as their biosynthetic

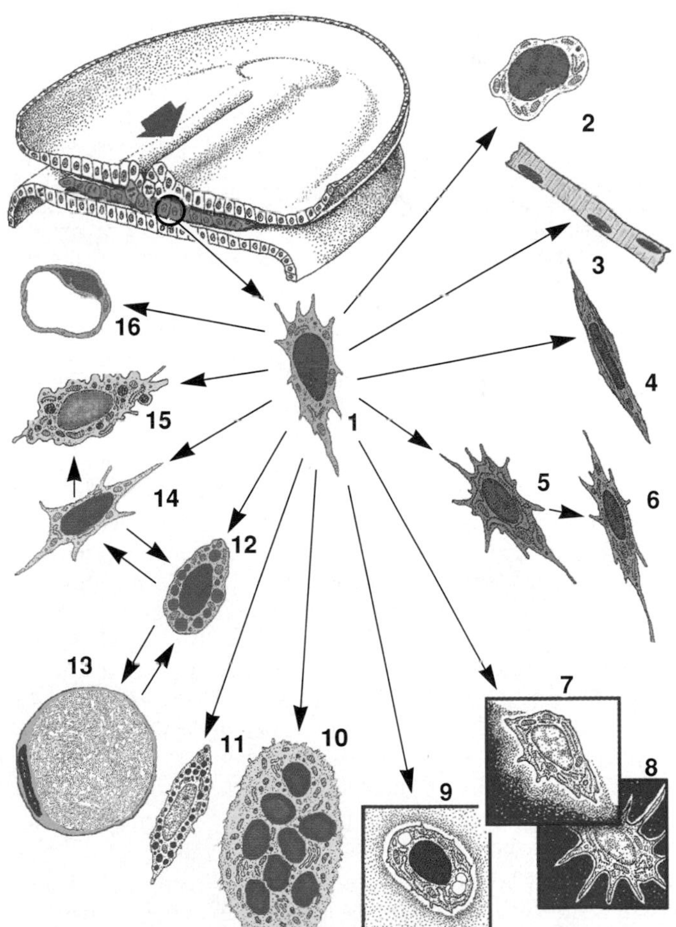

Fig. 19-17 Diagram illustrating the derivation of the various lineages from the mesoderm. (1) Primitive uncommitted mesenchymal cell, (2) monocyte, (3) skeletal muscle, (4) smooth muscle, (5) fibroblast, (6) fibrocyte, (7) osteoblast, (8) osteocyte, (9) chondrocytes, (10) megakaryocyte, (11) mast cell, (12) lipoblast, (13) lipocyte, (14) pericyte, (15) histiocyte, and (16) endothelial cell. Modified from Krstić, RC: *General histology of the mammalian*, Berlin, 1989, Springer Verlag.

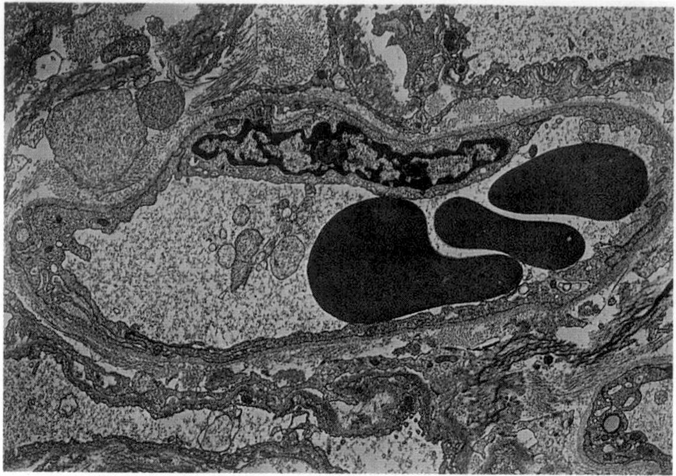

Fig. 19-18 A capillary with an endothelial cell, *E.*

capacity, are essential for the successful completion of repair.

Endothelial cells are an important source of ECM components and cellular mediators of repair. Endothelial cells of most capillaries and larger vessels synthesize and assemble a BM, whereas sinusoidal endothelial cells, though associated with deposits of some BM components, do not form a continuous BM. Endothelial cells also produce fibronectin, thrombospondin, elastin, collagen, and proteoglycans. Endothelia also synthesize numerous vasoactive substances that modify vascular diameter and permeability and cytokines. Angiogenesis is central to the granulation tissue formation and normal wound healing.[129]

Platelets

In addition to their prominent role in hemostasis, platelets also play an important role in repair in that they attach to the matrix, aggregate with other platelets, and release mediators that have chemoattractant, vasoactive, permeability, and mitogenic effects.[131] There are three major cytoplasmic granules in platelets: the α granule, the lysosome, and the dense granule. The α granule is the site of storage for cytokines, platelet-derived growth factor (PDGF), and the transforming growth factor family, including epidermal growth factor (EGF), transforming growth factor-β (TGF-β), and platelet factor 4. Lysosomes contain hydrolases, elastase, and collagenases, as well as permeability factors and cathepsins. Dense bodies contain serotonin, adenine nucleotides, calcium, and pyrophosphate.

The main functions of platelets during hemostasis consist in forming a cellular plug at the point of vascular injury and the release of mediators. The adherence of platelets to subendothelial collagen stimulates platelets to release their mediators, thus promoting additional aggregation and vasoconstriction (see Chapter 22).

In wound repair, platelets containing chemoattractant, vasoactive, permeability, and mitogenetic agents are potent elements in the initiation of the repair process. Therefore platelets contribute to initial matrix formation in areas of vascular damage by establishing a cellular plug or aggregate, releasing mitogens and chemoattractants, and stimulating smooth muscle proliferation and matrix deposition.

Smooth muscle cells

Smooth muscle cells are spindle-shaped, contractile cells rich in actin and myosin filaments that also secrete a number of ECM components including collagens, elastin, and proteoglycans. Each smooth muscle cell is ensheathed by a BM, which the cell produces. In atheromatous plaques smooth muscle cells are responsible for the production of the matrix components characteristic of these lesions. In addition to these ECM, smooth muscle cells produce several growth factors, including platelet-derived growth factor and fibroblast growth factor. The capacity to synthesize matrix components and cytokines underscores the important role these cells play within repair and regeneration.[132]

Fibroblasts

At present, there are no specific markers of fibroblasts; therefore their identification is one of exclusion. By light microscopy, the term *fibroblast* is often used to refer to histiocytes, matrix-secreting fibrocytes, contractile myofibroblasts, and probably reserve or stem cells. Fibroblasts of different organs, though having similar morphologies, are actually a large family of cells with different functional capacities. For example, fibroblasts in the heart have different functional capacities from those present in liver or gastrointestinal tract.[133]

Fibrocytes have an elongated cytoplasm, rich in endoplasmic reticulum, with a perinuclear Golgi complex. The surface area is enhanced by a system of elaborate cell compartments formed by cytoplasmic recesses. These compartments are the sites of fibril and bundle assembly.[125] Fibrocytes, in both normal and injured tissues, synthesize nearly all ECM components including elastin, collagens, fibronectin, and proteoglycans. The stochiometries of these various products, their spatiotemporal distributions, and rates and extents of degradation determines the phenotype that we call *scarring* or *wound healing* or *regeneration*. If matrix deposition in a skin wound is modest, it is described as well healed; if slightly excessive, a scar; if quite excessive, a hypertrophic scar; if virtually tumorous, a keloid. Accordingly, the factors that orchestrate expression of the products of fibrocytes (Fig. 19-19) qualitatively and quantitatively, temporally and spatially, and in stability dictate central aspects of the repair and regeneration process.[134] This same set of reactions is brought to play by injurious growths such as neoplasms. The type, extent, and stability of an ECM surrounding a tumor often helps differentiate between a benign and a malignant growth.

Myofibroblasts

Myofibroblasts by light microscopy are indistinguishable from fibrocytes, unless reacted with antibodies directed against muscle proteins, since myofibroblasts are rich in actin and myosin filaments.[135] Electron microscopy demonstrates the abundance of contractile elements in the peripheral cytoplasm. In addition, like the fibroblast, the cytoplasm of these cells is rich in rough endoplasmic reticulum and Golgi apparatus material. The nucleus is often indented, much like that of a smooth muscle cell. Myofibroblasts are often surrounded by an incomplete BM. These cells are involved in wound reactions, as discussed below. Myofibroblasts have been identified in healing wounds, hypertrophic scars, fibromatoses, and the stroma of numerous tumors.

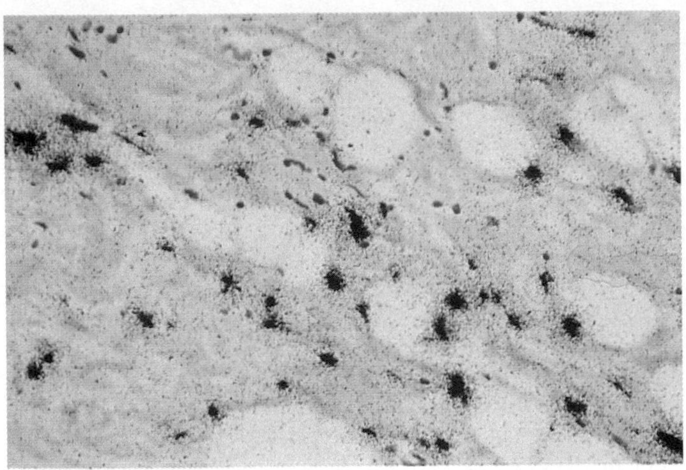

Fig. 19-19 In situ hybridization demonstrating message for collagen in fibrotic tissue hybridized with ^{35}S-labeled cDNA for procollagen type I. (Courtesy Irene Wapnir, M.D., New Brunswick NJ)

Mononuclear phagocytes

Circulating monocytes give rise to tissue macrophages, giant cells, and osteoclasts. Macrophages have a variety of morphologic appearances given their circumstance.[136,137] In areas of fat necrosis, they are often rich in cytoplasmic lipid vacuoles. In tissues with a foreign body, they have an eosinophilic cytoplasm containing the foreign debris and are multinuclear, having formed by fusion of multiple monocytes. In bone, the osteoclast is a highly specialized cell resulting from monocyte fusions, which has the capacity to demineralize and degrade bone. Macrophages play a key role in removing dead or damaged cellular debris, as well as ECM components. They also secrete growth factors that stimulate mitogenesis in several cell types and chemoattraction. Macrophages are thus more than scavengers, since they help orchestrate the complex set of interacting elements that constitute repair and regeneration.[138]

Mast cells

Mast cells are ovoid to spindle-shaped, ubiquitous connective tissue cells, rich in basophilic granules.[135] These metachromatic granules are easily detected by stains such as toluidine blue. They are typically distributed in perivascular and perineural regions. The granules are rich in heparin, and mucosal mast cells contain chondroitin sulfate proteoglycan and numerous enzymes including collagenases. These cells have been shown to enhance the deposition of collagen in vitro and are believed to play roles in the remodeling of ECM during wound healing, progression of rheumatoid arthritis, and the progression of fibrotic diseases such as interstitial pulmonary fibrosis, progressive systemic sclerosis, and retroperitoneal fibrosis.[135,139,140]

Cell-cell interactions

Cell-cell interactions play an important role in modulating and maintaining normal tissue morphogenesis and also play an important role in wound healing. Several adhesive molecules between cells have been identified and their roles in morphogenesis and repair have been described.[121,122] Cell adhesion molecules (CAMS) consist of three major groups: (1) immunoglobulin superfamily, (2) cadherins, and (3) the selectins (or Lec-CAMS). The IgG superfamily comprises ICAM-1, VCAM-1, and PCAM-1, which engage in intercellular adhesion, vascular cellular adhesion, and platelet endothelial cell adhesion respectively. ICAM has the widest distribution, being present on endothelial, epithelial, and hematopoietic cells, and fibroblasts. ICAM-1 is responsible for the adherence of neutrophils to endothelial cells and modulates migration of neutrophils to a wound site. VCAM-1 plays a similar role in leukocyte adherence to endothelial cells. PCAM present on endothelial cells and platelets has an important role in hemostasis and wound repair.

The cadherins (or calicum-dependent cell adhesion molecules) are subdivided into groups found on neural, muscular, placental, and epithelial cells.

The selectins, or Lec-CAMs, are so named because of their homology to the carbohydrate moieties on lectins. Two selectins, E-selectin and L-selectin, are associated with endothelial cells and lymphocytes respectively, and P-selectin is present on platelets. These proteins also function in leukocyte adhesion to endothelial cells.

The cell cycle and regenerative potential of tissue

The eventual outcome of the healing process repair with scarring or regeneration depends to a large extent on the potential for division of the cells forming the organ, and that potential relates to the cell cycle. The cell cycle is defined as the interval between two consecutive cell divisions.[141] It forms the basis for understanding and treating diseases ranging from tissue repair to neoplasia. The cell cycle varies for different cell types. For example, myocardial muscle and neurons lose their capacity to proliferate early in postnatal life, whereas the bowel epithelium replenishes itself weekly, and blood cells do so in a similar length of time.

The cell cycle is divided into two major phases, the interphase and the mitotic periods. Interphase is divided into three major phases, G_1, S, and G_2 and occupies 90% of the cell cycle. The G_1 phase (gap 1) is characterized by cellular synthetic and biologic activities specific to individual cells. The G_2 phase is characterized by cells having a tetraploid content of DNA, is shorter than the G_1 phase, and precedes mitosis (M). DNA synthesis occurs during the S (-synthesis) phase. Based on their cell cycle, cells are divided into one of three major groups: labile, stable, and permanent cells.

Labile cells

Labile cells are those that continuously traverse the cell cycle and consist of tissues in which greater than 1.5% of cells are in mitosis. Labile cells are typical in epithelia, including skin, gastrointestinal and genitourinary tracts, and bone marrow. In skin and mucosal surfaces, stem cells located either in the basal layers or in the base of glands are responsible for the replacement of their more mature or injured descendants. The daughter cells derived from the stem cells divide, with one remaining as the stem cell and the other differentiating to assume the mature phenotype. In many instances, this mature phenotype requires that the stem cells be pluripotent. For example, in the gastrointestinal tract, the stem cells give rise to absorptive enterocytes, goblet cells, Paneth cells, and neuroendocrine cells. Similarly, in the bone marrow the pluripotent hemocytoblast satisfies the need for the erythrocytic, granulocytic, and megakaryocytic progeny. It is not surprising that tissues composed of labile cells are those that often repair themselves by regeneration.

Stable cells

Stable cells are cells that, to varying degrees, proliferate or reenter the cell cycle if stimulated and are defined as tissues in which less than 1.5% of cells are in mitosis. A stimulus is needed to return these cells to the cell cycle. The liver, though having only rare cells in mitoses in the normal state, undergoes considerable proliferative activity during regeneration. Other tissues containing stable cells includes the parenchymal cells and the connective tissue cells of endocrine organs, liver, kidney, and pancreas and the dispersed connective tissues, including those of the skin, bone, tendons, and ligaments. Skeletal myocytes are often misplaced in the group of permanent cells (see below). However, regeneration occurs in skeletal muscle when satellite cells differentiate into skeletal muscle myoblasts, which in turn fuse to form multinucleated cells that differentiate into mature myocytes.

Permanent cells

Permanent cells lose their ability to divide soon after birth. This occurs in neurons, the crystalline-containing cells of the eye, and cardiac muscle. The reasons for this lost capacity differs. The posterior lens cells virtually lose their nuclei in a manner similar to what transpires with red blood cells. Neurons and cardiac myocytes, on the other hand, retain their nuclei, but their reactivation in humans does not occur. This is not the case in amphibians, for example, which have remarkable regenerative capacities.

Subsequent to injury, tissues rich in permanent cells repair either by scarring, that is, replacement by connective tissue cells and matrix, or in the case of the brain by the proliferation of glial cells to fill the spatial void caused by the death of neurons, a process called *gliosis*.

Cytokines

A variety of soluble factors that have modulatory effects on cell activation, proliferation, and migration are released by different cells.[142-148] These cytokines, or growth factors, have mitogenetic effects on their own (complete mitogens), require another substance to have a mitogenic effect (incomplete mitogen), or inhibit mitogenesis.[149]

Platelet-derived growth factor

Platelet-derived growth factor (PDGF) consists of two chains, A and B, which associate in a combination of one of three configurations.[150] PDGF is released from the alpha granules of activated platelets into the extracellular space. Molecules with homologies with PDGF are produced by endothelial and smooth muscle cells, macrophages, and some tumors. The primary effect of PDGF on cells such as smooth muscle, microglia, and fibroblasts is to stimulate mitogenesis. PDGF and other growth factors act via a cell surface receptor with tyrosine kinase activity. In addition to its mitogenic effects, PDGF influences both the immigration of cells into wounds and the replication of cells at injured sites.

Macrophage-derived growth factor

A factor (or group of factors) present in macrophages and monocytes stimulates the proliferation of fibroblasts.[151] These factors have been collectively named *macrophage-derived growth factor* (MDGF). MDGF, unlike PDGF, is secreted directly into the ECM. MDGF stimulates both endothelial and smooth muscle cell proliferation in vitro.

Epidermal growth factor

Epidermal growth factor (EGF), a 53-amino acid polypeptide, has a broad range of physiologic effects.[148] After binding to a transmembrane protein receptor common on epithelial cells, it becomes internalized and assumes tyrosine kinase activity. Cells then become mitotically active and somewhat less differentiated. Through these effects, EGF has an important role in healing of ulcers of several organ systems including the cornea, skin, and gastrointestinal tract by potentiating reepithelialization.

Fibroblast growth factor

Fibroblast growth factors exist as two distinct polypeptides differentiated as basic and acidic forms.[149] The basic form has approximately 10 times greater activity than the acidic form. Both are the gene product of single but separate genes on chromosome 4. Basic FGF is mitogenic for fibroblasts, endothelial cells, and smooth muscle cells and also has angiogenic properties. Acidic FGF is present strictly in neural tissues.

Transforming growth factors

Transforming growth factor-β is present in transformed cells, the α granules of platelets, and lymphocytes.[152,153,154] TGF-β acts by increasing the number of fibroblasts at a wound site, thus increasing collagen and other matrix components and enhancing fibrillogenesis and consequently regaining wound strength. It also acts as a chemoattractant for macrophages. TGF-α is homologous to EGF and functions in a similar capacity.

Hepatocyte growth factor

Hepatocyte growth factor, also known as hepatopoietin A (HPTA), is a powerful mitogen, as well as an inducer of hepatocyte hypertrophy.[149,155] Hepatopoietin A has homologous sequences with plasminogen and other coagulation proteins and binds to heparin. Its mitogenetic effect is lessened by both heparin and TGF-β. The receptor for HPTA is different from that of epidermal growth factor to which its effect is additive. Several other substances have been associated with HPTA and hepatocyte regeneration. These include basic fibroblast growth factor, hepatopoietin B, and hepatocyte stimulatory substance. HPTA has been identified in many tissues.[155]

Cell migration

Cells reach a wound site by migrating through the ECM and accomplish this movement by using a variety of guidance mechanisms. Movement per se is a function of the cell's cytoskeletal apparatus and contractile filamentous systems. Vectorial movement occurs because of chages in the cell's chemical, physical, and social environments. Cells are contact inhibited by each other such that they do not overgrow into each other's local sites, thereby assuring some kind of orderly disposition. In a wound, voids are caused by cell death, hemorrhage, edema, and the like resulting in loss of contact inhibition and consequent imigration of cells at the edge into the wound. Other factors causing directed migration are chemotactic agents and haptotactic surfaces. Chemotaxis is defined as the migration of cells toward a soluble chemoattractant. Haptotaxis is defined as the migratory activity of cells on a substratum along an adhesion gradient. In haptotaxis, cells extend processes randomly in search of the proper substratum. Those processes that reach such a substratum spread to cover it. Cells then migrate along this substratum and send out new cellular processes to continue this migratory activity.

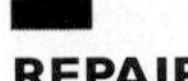

REPAIR

As an evolutionary survival response, organisms have developed mechanisms to replace the tissue lost by injury, and the major modes of this replacement or healing are repair or regeneration. Repair is the replacement of lost tissue by ECM and fibroblasts with resultant formation of scar tissue.

Phases of the repair reaction

In repair, tissue lost as a result of injury is replaced with a series of connective tissues, beginning with granulation tissue, which matures to form a scar. Injuries often induce inflammation, and in the immediate period (approximately 1 week) after an injury, inflammation and repair are coexistent. Overall, there are three major, overlapping phases in wound healing—the inflammatory, proliferative, and maturation phases (Fig. 19-20). These phases occur in a noncomplicated environment. In contrast, conditions such as infection, chemotherapy, or radiation alter the sequence of events as well as the length of time of each phase. For example, in some patients with radiation therapy, wounds will not heal in the patient's lifetime.

Inflammatory phase

The inflammatory phase of wound healing is characterized by hemorrhage or plasma exudation into the wound site. A fibrin clot forms as a result of the coagulation cascade being activated. Fibronectin is covalently cross-linked to fibrin, to itself, and to collagen by transglutaminase, including factor XIII. Deficiency in factor XIII results in poor wound healing. The presence of the clot and the cross-linking of plasma proteins with ECM molecules provides the initial tensile strength in a wound. This phase is also responsible for the initial degradation of the damaged tissue, including the ECM. The generation of plasmin by the coagulation casade, as well as the chemoattractants produced by neutrophils and macrophages are critical in this respect. Platelets and macrophages release growth factors which are both chemoattractants and mitogenetic, thus supportive of angiogenesis. In summary, the inflammatory phase is responsible for providing the initial tensile strength to a wound, the initiation of the removal of damaged tissue, and the beginnings of angiogenesis.

Proliferative phase

The proliferative phase is characterized by the development of an immature highly vascular connective tissue, which on gross examination was noted, even in ancient times, to have a granular appearance and hence has been called *granulation tissue* (Figs. 19-21 and 19-22). This tissue is typified by the accumulation of proliferating endothelial cells, myofibroblasts, fibroblasts, macrophages, and lymphocytes (Fig. 19-23). Several factors are responsible for the migration of these cells into the injured area, including cytokines derived from macrophages and platelets, as well as TGF-β. Low O_2 tension at the center of the wound is also a chemoattractant for these cells, as is fibronectin and other ECM breakdown products.

As the newly formed blood vessels enter into the wound site, they are accompanied by fibroblasts and myofibroblasts, which

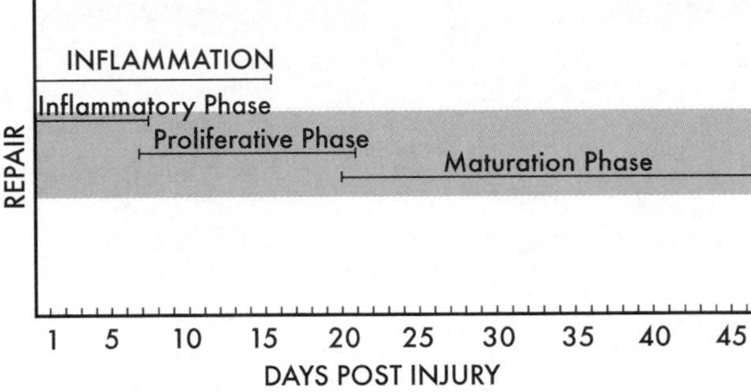

Fig. 19-20 Response to injury is characterized by inflammation and repair. The repair phase can be divided into three overlapping phases—the inflammatory phase, proliferative phase, and finally the maturation phase. As depicted in this figure, the inflammatory phase of the repair action will overlap the organism's inflammatory response. (Modified from Leadbetter W, Gordon S, Buckwalter J: *Inflammation and healing of sports induced soft tissue injury,* Park Ridge, Ill, 1990, American Academy of Orthopaedic Surgeons.)

typically arrange themselves in an orderly manner around adjacent blood vessels. The initial ECM of granulation tissue is rich in fibronectin and proteoglycan, with relatively little collagen. However, by the end of the first week, type III collagen begins to accumulate, a process that is associated with elevated serum levels of type III collagen amino-terminal propeptide in serum and wound fluid.[95,156] In another 5 days, type I collagen is secreted and becomes prominent, exceeding the concentrations of type III collagen. Tenascin is also prominent at this stage. With an increasing type I collagen concentration and consequent fibril formation, the tensile strength of the wound increases. In large wounds, with a large loss of surface tissue, regenerative epithelial replacement is difficult. The contraction of wounds because of this granulation tissue leads to a decrease in size, such that successful epithelial regeneration occurs.

Angiogenesis, the formation of new vessels, is a prominent event in the formation of granulation tissue.[130] In wounds the new vessels sprout from preexisting vessels. Sprouting results from proliferation of endothelial cells in the wall of preexisting vessels in conjunction with degradation of the vascular BM. The chemoattractant forces of the wound site, including the low O_2 tension, result in many of these sprouts to project toward the wound site. The capillaries that develop by sprouting have poorly formed intercellular attachments and are thus leaky vessels, leading to the considerable edema characteristic of granulation tissue (Fig. 19-22).

Maturation phase

The maturation phase is characterized by some level of restitution or restoration of the prior tissue with various degrees of replacement of that tissue by fibrous connective tissue or scar. The cellularity of the wound from cells including macrophages, inflammatory cells, myofibroblast, and fibroblasts decreases during this phase, with the accumulation of type I collagen and the formation of a definitive scar composed of dense collagen bundles. The cross-linking of the collagen fibers is essential to the proper acquisition of tensile strength. This phase may go on for months to years, and an exact dating of wounds is impossible. For example, scarring in the heart takes months after the initial infarction.

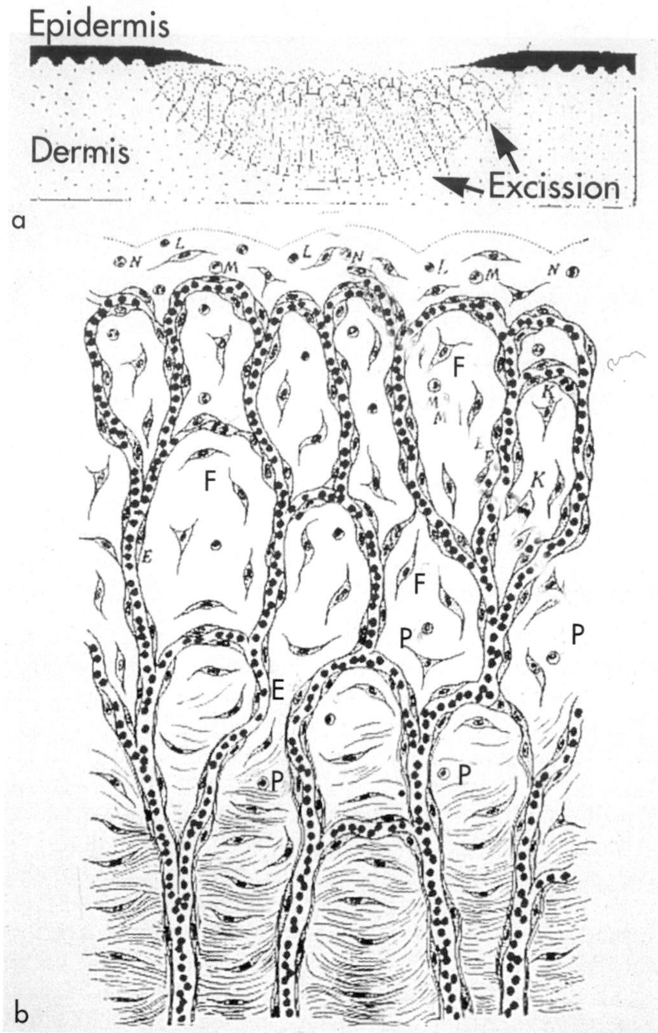

Fig. 19-21 Diagram of granulation tissue.

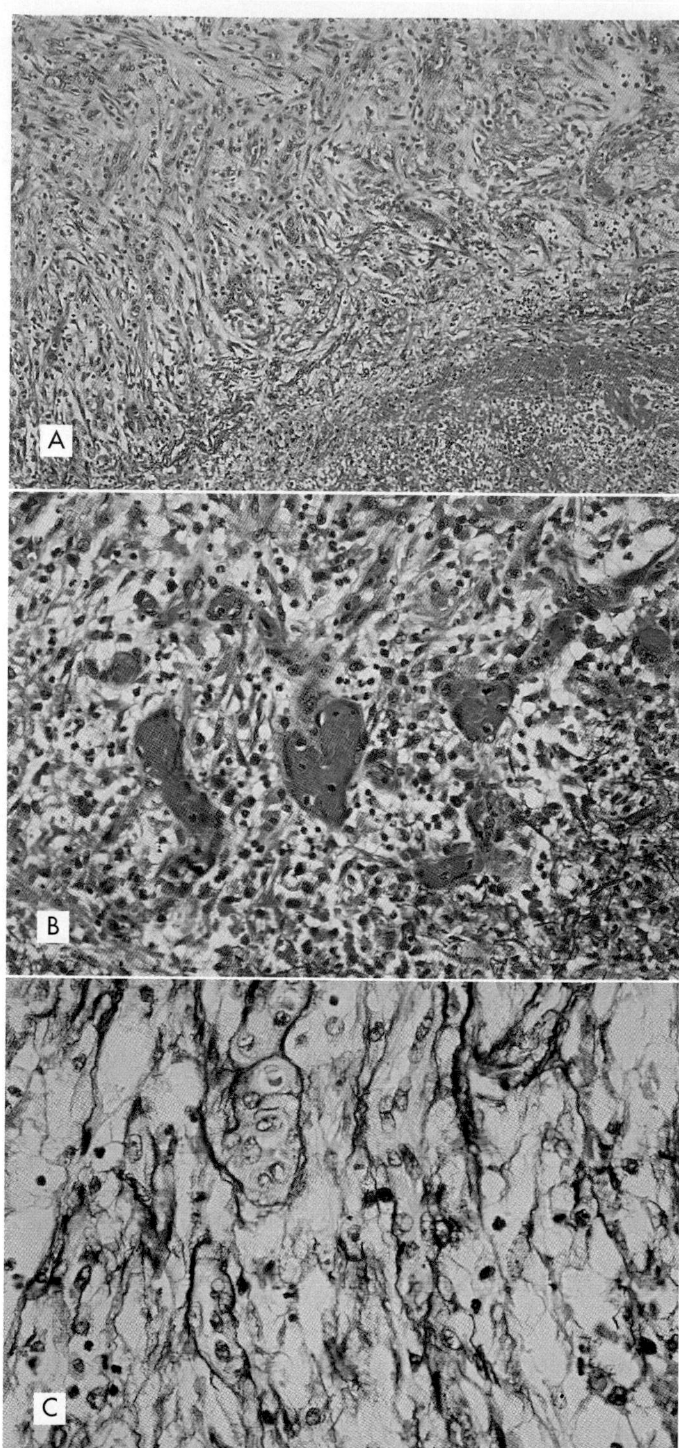

Fig. 19-22 Granulation tissue consists of prominent, proliferating, congested blood vessels surrounded by spindle-shaped cells, macrophages, and granulocytes, **A** and **B.** A reticulin stain, **C,** demonstrates the network of fibers associated with the cellular component.

Summary of the repair reaction

Subsequent to injury hemostasis is responsible for providing the initial plug to stop the wound from propagating (Fig. 19-24). With hemostasis, the presence of fibrin and fibronectin, along with tissue collagen and the cross-linking capacity of transglutaminases results in the polymerization of a meshwork of fibers to provide the initial tensile strength of a wound. Other factors contributed by the hemostatic response are the release of plasmin and the accumulation of platelets. Platelets activated by their binding with ECM components result in the release of PDGF and TGF-β. These two factors are responsible for chemotaxis of polymorphonuclear leukocytes and the monocyte-macrophage cell system, and proliferation of stromal cells including fibroblasts, endothelium, and smooth muscle cells. These cells are subsequently responsible for the production of additional cytokines, including PDGF, TGF-β and MDGF. With the production of matrix from the accumulating stromal cells and angiogenesis, granulation tissue forms. The exuberance of this response is controlled in part by the cytokine system, as well as the enzymes released by neutrophils, macrophages, and stromal cells. Collagenases and elastases and other matrix-degrading enzymes along with controlled matrix deposition and proteolysis results in remodeling of a wound and the formation of the definitive scar.

Scarring is often the outcome or result of injury in most tissues. Typically, there is a loss of parenchymal tissue, loss of functional capacity, and loss of evidence of the initiating injury. For example, interstitial pulmonary fibrosis, cirrhosis, and end-stage renal disease have the same morphology and loss of function regardless of the initiating injury. The mechanisms described above in the repair reaction all function as

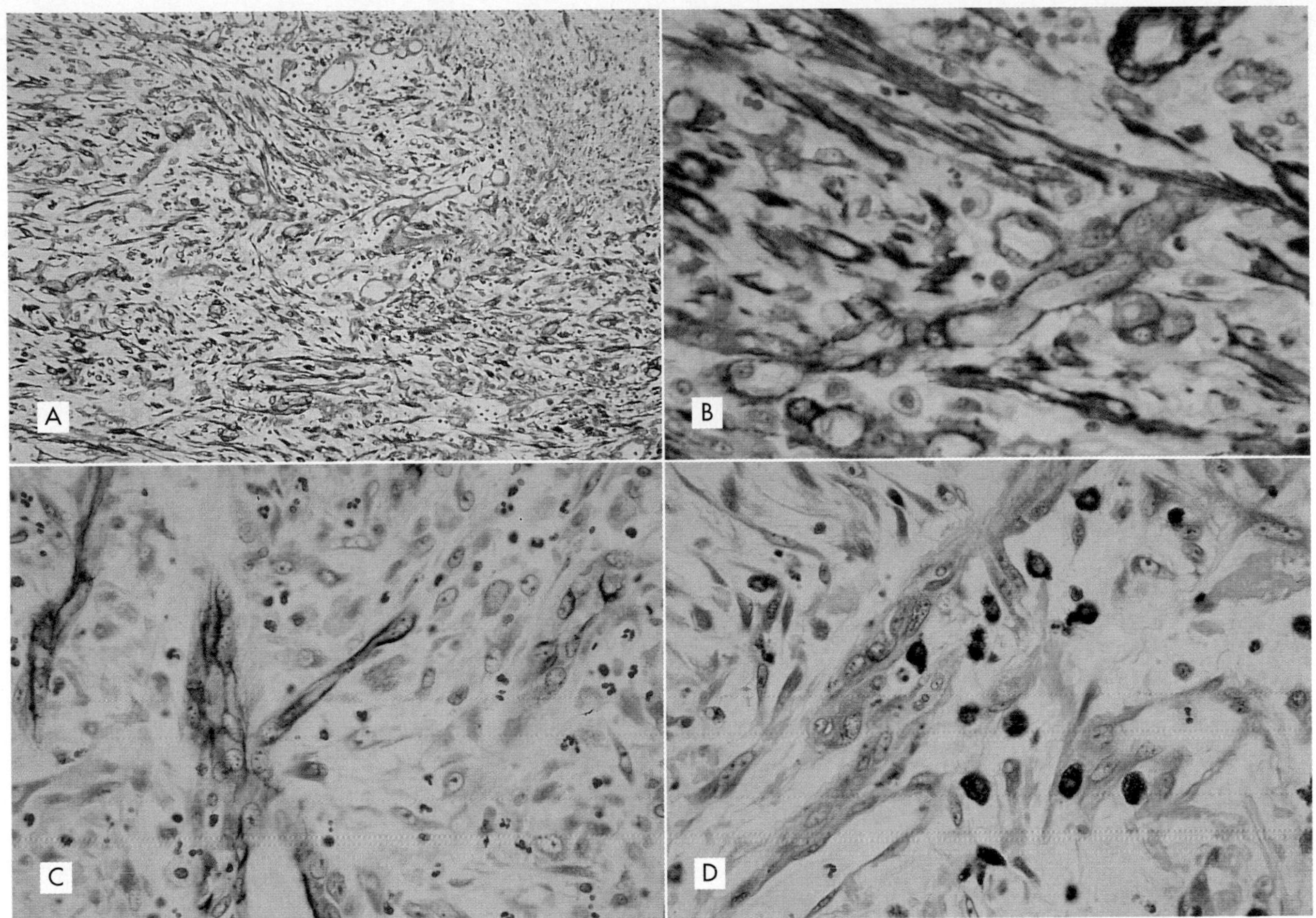

Fig. 19-23 Antibodies directed against muscle-specific actin, **A** and **B,** demonstrate the population of myofibroblasts. Endothelial cells react with antibodies to factor VIII and CD31, **C.** Macrophages also are present, **D.**

checks and balances, modulating the formation of the final product of the repair reaction, the scar.

Factors modifying repair

Factors that are critical in the control of wound healing are divided into local and systemic.

Local factors

The type, size, and the location of the wound have a considerable effect on the final outcome of an injury. For example, a clean, sharp surgical incision of the forehead would heal more efficiently and have fewer sequelae than a laceration brought about by blunt trauma. Wounds over large bones often result in poor wound healing because of tissue adhesion to that surface and impaired wound contraction.

The ability to vascularize a wound site is a critical event in the formation of granulation tissue. Therefore tissues that are better vascularized provide for a superior environment for wound healing than poorly vascularized tissue. Other complications such as infection, ionizing radiation, and foreign bodies result in delays in healing.

Systemic factors

Systemic factors and nutritional status play an important role in wound healing. Vitamin C (ascorbic acid) is an essential cofactor of collagen synthesis by being involved in prolyl hydroxylation. Patients with scurvy characteristically have poor wound healing and fragile vessels and suffer life-threatening hemorrhages. Before the eighteenth century, most sailors suffered scurvy on ocean voyages and generally half would die on each trip for this reason.

Hormonal imbalances also result in poor wound healing. Diabetic patients or those with Addison's disease are predisposed to infection. Glucocorticoids and other chemotherapeutic agents that depress protein synthesis will inhibit wound healing.[157] In contrast, studies have indicated that growth hormone in vitro stimulates the development of granulation tissue.[158]

Complications of the repair reaction

Deficient scar formation

Any abnormality of the initial phases of wound healing resulting in poor granulation tissue formation or inability to form an adequate ECM will result in poor scar formation. Diseases characterized by immunodeficiencies or cytopenias result in decreased levels of growth factors and thus deficiencies in chemotaxis, angiogenesis, and granulation tissue formation. A serious consequence of deficient scar formation is wound dehiscence or breakdown and separation of the edges of a closed wound.

Excessive scar formation

A major disadvantage to the repair reaction is the occasion when there is excessive scarring or fibrosis. Fibroblasts and

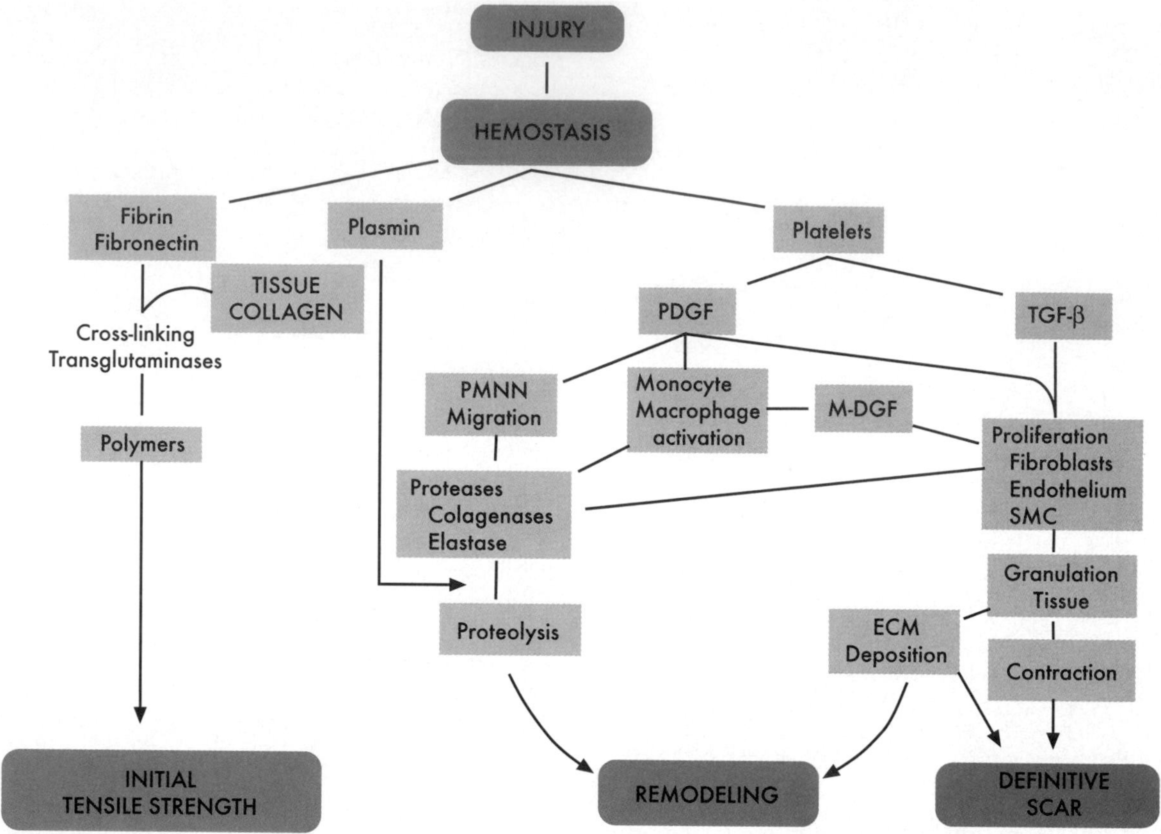

Fig. 19-24 Flow chart of potential interactions among components of hemostasis, extracellular matrix, growth factors, and cells that occur during repair. The relative interactions that occur after an individual injury and within an individual organ determine the outcome of the healing. (Modified from Rubin E, Farber JL: *Pathology,* ed 2, Philadelphia, 1994, Lippincott.)

myofibroblasts are key modulators of this process. In fibrosis, the scale tips in favor of factors responsible for matrix synthesis, deposition, and limited degradation, which result in the excessive accumulation of ECM.

Numerous conditions are characterized by excessive scarring, such as the classic systemic disease progressive systemic sclerosis. Sclerosis of the skin, or scleroderma, is the hallmark clinical attribute of the disease. In addition, systemic sclerosis involving the viscera (heart, lungs, alimentary tract, and kidneys) and joints may occur (see Chapter 26). Other so-called connective tissue diseases such as rheumatoid arthritis and ankylosing spondylitis may result in fibrosis of joints and viscera.

Other conditions, such as retroperitoneal fibrosis and peritoneal fibrosis may result in significant morbidity and mortality. Retroperitoneal fibrosis typically results in obstruction of the ureters and hydronephrosis. The drug methysergide maleate, used in the treatment of migraine headaches, has been associated with this condition.

A group of fibrotic conditions characterized by a tumorlike growth of connective tissue have been described. These lesions histologically at times may appear malignant but do not have the propensity for metastasis. These have been divided into three major groups: nodular fasciitis (and related entities), fibromatoses (superficial and deep), and proliferative lesions of infancy.[159]

Keloids are defined as tumorlike, protuberant accumulations of connective tissue (Fig. 19-25). Hypertrophic scars differ from keloids in that they remain confined to the borders of the initial wound. Other fibromatoses, such as Dupuytren's (palmar) contracture,[160] *Lederhosen* (German: 'leather breeches'), and Peyronie's disease, involve the palm, plantar surface, and cavernous tissue of the penis, respectively. Musculoaponeurotic fibromatoses (desmoid) in abdominal and extra-abdominal sites may result in disfigurement.

The cause of these diseases remains unknown; however, in many of these conditions there is increased collagen deposition, excessive collagen cross-linking, and an increased type III/type I collagen ratio. Recent studies have also demonstrated overexpression of fibronectin in keloids and hypertrophic scars.[161] Fibroblasts from keloids are refractory to the typical downregulation of collagen synthesis induced by glucocorticoids.[157] The latter observation indicates an arrest of the healing process, continued stimulation, or impaired regulatory mechanisms of matrix deposition.

Deficient contraction

Large scars form when wounds are overlying hard tissues. For example, those wounds adjacent to large bones have poor healing, since there is adhesion of the granulation tissue on the hard surface, wound edges cannot approximate, and granulation tissue continues to form. Because of the lack of approximation of the wound, there is deficient reepithelialization. When such instances occur, very often skin grafts are required to replace the lost tissue.

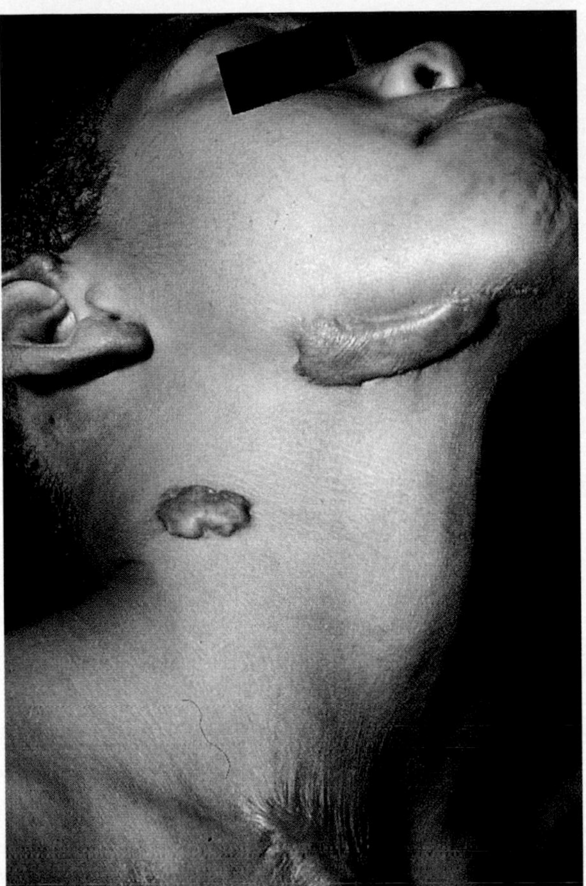

Fig. 19-25 Keloids.

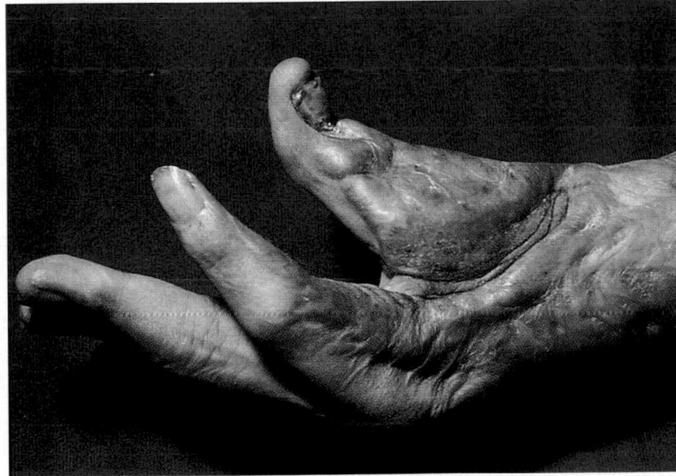

Fig. 19-26 Contracture of the hand after a burn.

Excessive contraction

Contracture results when there is exaggerated contraction of granulation tissue. This is also referred to as *cicatrization.* Again this is often seen in large wounds such as burns of the skin (Fig. 19-26) and ingestion of lye, which often results in constriction of the esophagus and dysphagia. Dupuytren's (palmar) contracture,[160] *Lederhosen,* and Peyronie's disease also often result in excessive contraction.

Calcification

Calcification of tissues occurs as either dystrophic calcification or metastatic calcification. In the latter type, calcification occurs in normal tissues in the presence of a high calcium or phosphate product in the blood. Calcification is also a common sequela of tissue injury. When calcification occurs in injured tissues, in the presence of normal calcium levels, it is referred to as dystrophic calcification. Osteogenesis may occur in sites of such calcification.

REGENERATION

Regeneration is the replacement of lost cells and tissues with those of identical function and morphology. This process is restricted to tissues composed of labile or stable cells. The injury to those tissues results in cell proliferation, migration and ECM formation, and finally differentiation to replace the lost tissue. A classic model of regeneration is that of the rabbit tracheal mucosa in which the epithelium is curetted from the tracheal wall.[162] The healing of the wound undergoes three stages of progression: (1) inflammation and clot formation, (2) epithelial regeneration, (3) differentiation. Initially, cells at the wound edge migrate over the wound surface to begin to cover the wound surface. Subsequently, stem cells and some ciliated cells present at the wound edge divide and migrate over the surface of the wound as a simple squamous epithelium. Within 4 days this squamous epithelium will differentiate into an adult respiratory epithelium consisting of mucous cells, respiratory epithelial cells, and neuroendocrine cells. The completion of this regeneration requires up to 6 weeks. This pattern of growth and repair can be seen in many organs. Subsequent to lobar pneumonia, resolution of the inflammation often occurs with return of totally normal architecture, and in the liver after hepatectomy, regeneration results in the return of a normal-sized liver and normal architecture. Although the stimuli necessary to induce regeneration are still being elucidated, the growth factors described above and the ECM are believed to play important roles in modulating these events.

HEALING IN SPECIFIC ORGANS

Fig. 19-27 diagrams the factors responsible for determining whether an injury in a specific organ heals by repair or by regeneration.

Skin

Skin wounds provide excellent models to study the factors that modulate the healing process. They have been divided into two major types: healing by first intention or primary union and those healing by second intention or secondary union (Fig. 19-28). It should be emphasized that the processes involved in healing by primary or secondary intention are identical. The only differences are the initial tissue loss and the outcome. In both cases, there is healing both by repair and by regeneration.

Healing by primary intention

Healing of skin wounds by primary intention is best illustrated by the healing of a clean, sharp surgical wound where

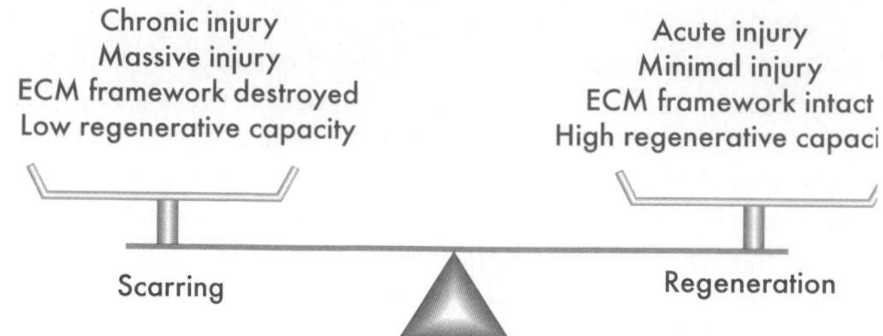

Fig. 19-27 Balance of factors at work that determine the mode of healing in a particular organ.

there is a minimal loss of tissue, no infection, and good approximation of the edges of the wound. With a surgical incision there is minimal loss of tissue including epithelial and mesenchymal tissue. The wound is formed under sterile conditions and is approximated by suture or adhesive tape. A fibrin clot forms at the incision line and, by its interactions with connective tissue proteins, including fibronectin, forms a matrix, which provides the initial tensile strength of the wound. The surface of this clot dries and is referred to as the *scab*. The sequence of events for the next 2 weeks varies by how closely met the above mentioned requirements of sterility and so forth are maintained. Within 24 hours of the injury, inflammatory cells, predominantly neutrophils, enter the wound site and begin to remove the dead and dying tissue. At the same time, proliferative activity (regenerative) activity of the epithelial surface begins with mitotic activity at the edge of the incision in stem cells, which begin to migrate over the wound surface as a simple squamous epithelium. Over the next several days, maturation of the cellular epithelium begins. In the middle of the first week, macrophages become the predominant cell within the wound site and cause the proliferation of fibroblasts, as well as performing their phagocytic and chemotactic functions. Subsequently, granulation tissue begins to form. The amount of granulation tissue is minimal in these wounds, as is the degree of contraction. With maturation there is a decrease in edema, leukocytic infiltrate, and vascularity. Over the next few months the scar becomes a pale structure with adnexal elements in the area of the damaged skin lost forever.

Healing by secondary intention

In the case of wounds with a large tissue defect, healing occurs by secondary intention. Lesions such as massive burns, lacerations, and stasis ulcerations heal by secondary intention. These wounds are characterized by considerable inflammation and necrosis and often exceed the capacity of epithelial cells to reepithelialize the wound without significant contraction. Therefore granulation tissue formation is an essential component of healing by secondary intention because it leads to wound contraction while simultaneously providing the necessary substratum for the epithelial ingrowth.

Fibroblasts apparently undergo a phenotypic change during wound healing of the skin. Fibroblasts in the adjacent tissue proliferate and migrate into the wound site by the fourth day after injury. Within the wound, the fibroblasts synthesize and excrete an ECM rich in type I collagen. By the end of the first week, the predominant cellular phenotype is myofibroblastic. These cells attach to the ECM components by pseudopodia

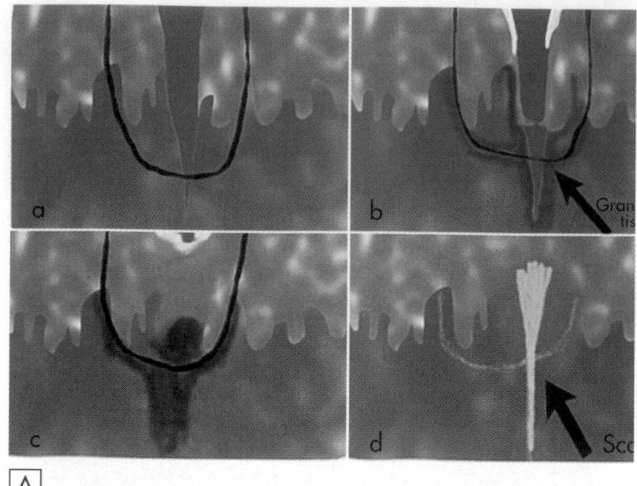

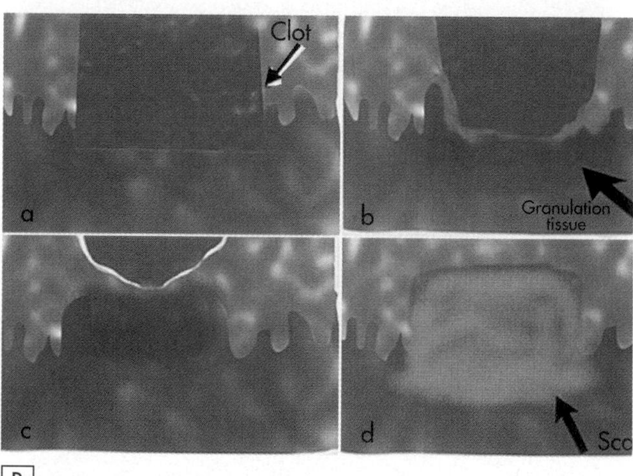

Fig. 19-28 **A**, *a*, Diagram of healing by *primary* intention. In this shallow, incised wound characterized by a minimal loss of tissue, a clot fills the incised region rapidly and a zone of necrosis surrounds the wound site. *b*, Inflammatory cells remove the necrotic debris, and granulation tissue begins to form. The epithelium begins to proliferate and migrate to cover the wound site. *c*, The epithelium begins to differentiate and assume the appearance of the mature epithelium. Granulation tissue–induced contraction occurs, and, *d*, the scar forms. **B,** In healing by *secondary* intention, many of the same events occur but on a larger scale with contraction being more prominent and the result being a larger scar.

and contract the wound. Subsequently, these cells undergo apoptosis, and the scar forms.[163]

Epithelial cells proliferate at the margin of the wound to replace those that migrate over the wound surface. In cases where the wound exceeds the capacity of this healing process, skin grafting is often necessary. This is a common mode of treatment in patients having burns covering large areas of their body. In large burns, the first stage of treatment involves débridement of the burn eschar, to a depth that reaches viable tissue. This exposed base forms the granulation bed, atop which is placed a split-thickness graft of skin from the patient (autologous), another human (heterologous), another species such as pig (xenograft) or an artificial matrix with or without epithelial cells.

There is a suprising difference in skin wound healing in thermal injury depending on whether the skin is subjected to a full-thickness burn or to full-thickness freeze. In the former, the healing by secondary intention proceeds as described. In the latter, the early phases with inflammation, degradation, scab formation, and granulation tissue outgrowth are greatly diminished or absent. As a consequence the necrotic skin remains relatively intact while all phases of repair commence beneath and undermine it. With less contraction and scarring, the wound heals in this modified manner with improved cosmetic results.[164]

Heart

Myocardium can heal only by repair, independent of the type of injury. The most common injury suffered by the myocardium is ischemic infarction. Within the first week subsequent to a myocardial infarction and the development of granulation tissue, the myocardium is susceptible to rupture. The replacement of contractile tissue by scar leads to impaired myocardial function by decreasing the effectiveness of myocardial contractility and to conduction abnormalities.

Cardiac valves, though normally avascular, become vascularized and scarred after injury. In rheumatic valvulitis the cardiac valves becomes thickened, fibrotic, and ineffective while the chordae tendineae become short, thickened, and fused. These valves are stenotic or regurgitant.

Endothelial and mesothelial cells of the pericardium can regenerate; however, because of the severity or chronicity of injuries, the pericardium and endocardium typically heal by scarring. In the latter cases endocardial and pericardial fibrosis results in restriction of normal cardiac motility. Auscultation reveals pericardial friction rubs, the hallmark of pericardial disease.

Arteries

An example of chronic injury is hypertension. The systemic arteries respond to this injury with predominant reaction characterized by atherosclerosis (see Chapter 47). The response to chronic injury occurs over many years and is a complex repair reaction within the vessel wall characterized by smooth muscle cell proliferation, ECM deposition, and cholesterol accumulation. Smooth muscle cells, macrophages, and platelets all play significant roles in the generation of these complex wounds by production of cytokines such as PDGF and ECM deposition.

Pulmonary arteries respond to hypertensive injury with medial hypertrophy and hyperplasia. Only at the end stage is there intimal proliferation and fibrosis of the aneurysmal dilatation, the so-called plexiform lesion. Recent studies indicate that smooth muscle cells actively synthesize matrix components in pulmonary vessels undergoing these changes[165] (Fig. 19-29). These different responses to hypertension by both the systemic and pulmonary arterial system illustrates the idiosyncratic nature of the repair reaction.

Lung

The lung is capable of healing with the result being complete resolution and the return of normal pulmonary structure and function, or by scarring. For example, pneumococcal pneumonia typically results in an acute inflammatory exudate within the alveoli, with accumulation of fluid and fibrin deposition. In the majority of cases, there is a complete resolution or disappearance of the exudate and a return to a normal structural and functional capacity. Pulmonary epithelial cells regenerate to cover the alveolar BM. In a similar manner, respiratory epithelium of the tracheobronchial tree is capable of regeneration. Occasionally, organization of the intra-alveolar exudate into granulation tissue and finally intraalveolar fibrosis can occur (Fig. 19-30).

In contrast, with a persistent infection or a massive injury in which the ECM structural framework is destroyed, the lung undergoes healing by repair and scarring. Interstitial pulmonary fibrosis is the common end point to numerous pulmonary diseases, including some cases of bacterial pneumonia.[153] Histologic features include a disruption of the pulmonary architecture with infiltration of inflammatory cells followed by proliferation of stromal cells and the excessive production and accumulation of ECM. Studies have indicated increased collagen and elastin content in animal models of interstitial pulmonary fibrosis, as well as a shift to a predominance of type I collagen production over type III collagen.[166,167] As in other examples of repair, type I collagen deposition is preceded by fibronectin and type III collagen deposition.

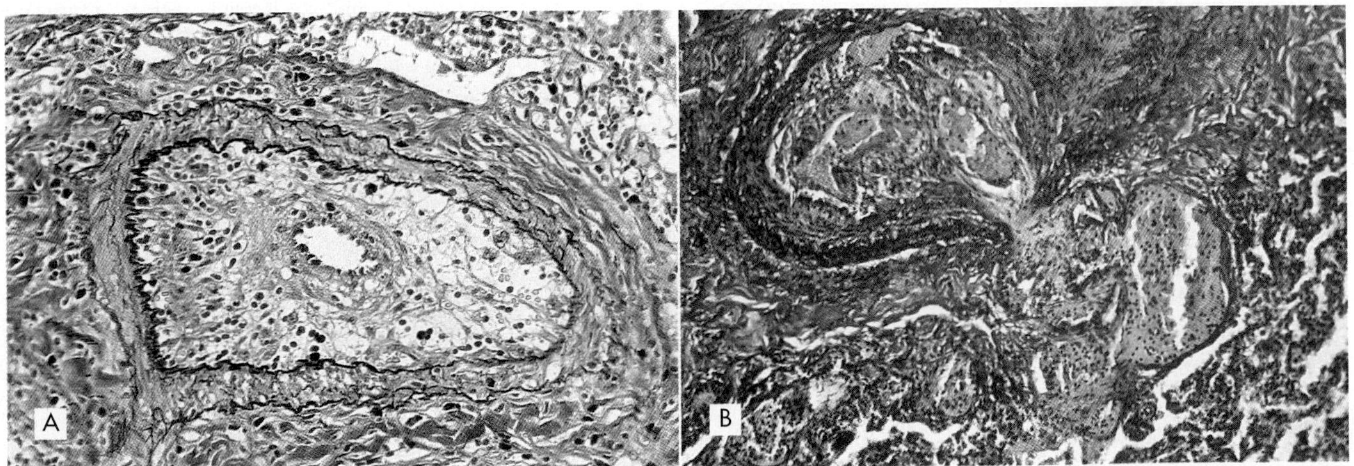

Fig. 19-29 **A,** Pulmonary artery with intimal fibrosis. **B,** Pulmonary arteriole in which a plexiform lesion has formed. (Verhoeff–van Gieson stain.)

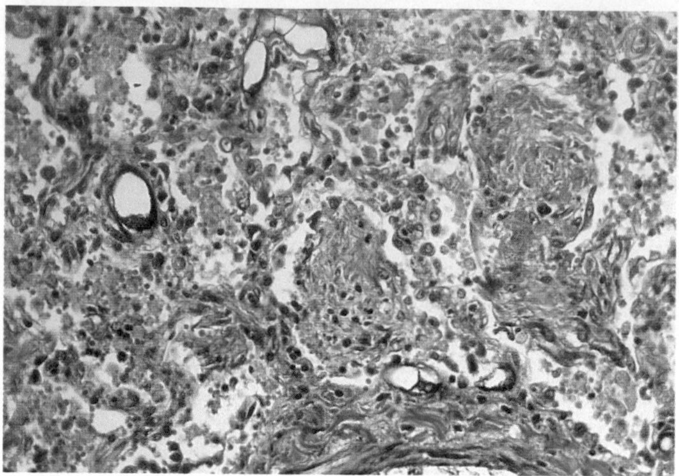

Fig. 19-30 Intraalveolar fibrosis of the lung. (Trichrome stain.)

Kidneys

The renal glomeruli are incapable of regenerative capacity and heal with the deposition of a connective tissue matrix rich in interstitial collagens and in some conditions BM material.[168,169] The mesangial cells are pericytelike cells, normally encased by a BM-like matrix containing some interstitial collagens. In addition, these cells also have phagocytic properties. These cells in culture and in repair secrete a complex matrix comprising both BM components and fibrillar collagens.[169] The diseases associated with this injury reaction in the glomerulus are classified as primary glomerular diseases (glomerulopathies), systemic diseases (such as, vasculitides), or hereditary disorders (see Chapter 65).

In contrast to the glomeruli, tubules can regenerate if the ECM framework is maintained. In a manner reminiscent of most epithelia, tubular epithelial cells adjacent to a site of injury and epithelial sloughing proliferate and cover the exposed BM. If the initial injury caused no significant destruction of the BM and adjacent matrix but led only to epithelial loss, there is no noticeable residuum of the tubular injury. However, if there is destruction of the BM, many of the tubules may be lost to fibrosis.

Gastrointestinal tract

The alimentary tract, as in other organs lined by a mucosa such as the urinary bladder and endometrium, heals by epithelial regeneration if there is no significant damage to the BM. Scarring of submucosal connective tissues occurs with stricture formation when there is repeated or deeply penetrating ulceration.

The prototypical lesion of the gastrointestinal tract is an ulcer. An ulcer is defined as a loss of epithelial and submucosal tissues, often extending to the muscle wall. The relative depth of an ulcer varies, with perforation of the external muscle layer being the most severe complication. In the process of erosion into the wall, blood vessels are injured, lose their integrity, and result in the common clinical finding of acute or chronic, clinical or subclinical blood loss.

In repair of ulcers, the epithelium must proliferate to cover the area of denudation and, when appropriate, differentiate into glandular elements. The epithelium at the edge of an ulcer bed proliferates and migrates over the surface of the ulcer as a simple squamous epithelium. These cells differentiate into the functional parenchymal cells of the corresponding organ, that is, stomach, duodenum, colon. In vitro studies have shown that EGF, TGF-β, and FGF enhance migration and restoration of the epithelial integrity to gastrointestinal mucosal defects.

Liver

The liver is capable of regeneration, with recovery of normal hepatic structure and function, or severe scarring, with loss of normal hepatic structure and function. Smaller wounds or areas of zonal necrosis heal by scarring.

In some cases of necrosis, where the overall architecture of the hepatic ECM is maintained, healing occurs by regeneration. The regenerative capacity of the liver was appreciated, at least intuitively, by the ancient Greeks, who presented us with the story of Prometheus. CCl_4-induced liver injury provides an excellent model for studying liver regeneration because a single sublethal injection will result in hepatic necrosis followed by regeneration. Similarly, a hepatectomy of greater than 30% results in regeneration. Early regeneration is characterized by an explosive proliferation of the hepatic parenchyma, with nodules of hepatocytes forming, resembling those of the early stages of hepatic development. However, within 2 weeks the normal hepatic plate–like architecture returns to the prehepatectomy size of the liver.

Epidermal growth factor-α, transforming growth factor-α, acidic fibroblast growth factor, the hepatocyte growth factor (hepatopoietin A), hepatopoietin B, and hepatic stimulatory substance are complete mitogens for hepatocytes. Substances including norepinephrine, estrogens, insulin, glucagon, vasopressin, angiotensin II, and angiotensin III are incomplete mitogens. In contrast, TGF-β, and interleukin-1β are inhibitory to hepatocyte mitogenesis. The interaction of these growth factors regulates the regenerative process.[149]

The ECM also has a role in modulating hepatic regeneration.[57,170] Laminin, a constituent of the fetal hepatic sinusoid, is reexpressed in the hepatic sinusoid of the regenerating liver (α2, β1, β2, and γ1 chains but not α1 chain).

In cases of massive hepatic necrosis where the ECM framework of the hepatic sinusoids is destroyed or in cases of repeated injury, the liver heals by scarring (cirrhosis). Cirrhosis includes broad scars and surrounding nodules of regenerating hepatocytes as its defining characteristics. Within the nodules there is often a loss of the normal hepatocyte/sinusoid relationship, with many sinusoidal vessels assuming a capillary phenotype with a continuous BM. These events have significant repercussions for normal hepatocyte function, including exchange of materials between hepatocytes and plasma and altering hepatic blood flow to hepatocytes.[171] The classic experimental model of cirrhosis uses repeated exposure to CCl_4. In this model, fibronectin deposition precedes that of collagen type I and other matrix components, both temporally and spatially during the formation of the fibrotic scars.

Ito cells are a major source of matrix components in the liver. The fat-storing cells are present in the subsinusoidal space and they contribute to the deposition of the matrix components in cirrhosis and also appear to be the source of laminin during regeneration.[96,172] Thus the Ito cell modifies its ECM biosynthetic profile to correspond with the repair taking place within the liver and resembles, in principle, the mesangial cell, able to synthesize both BM components and fibrillar collagens.[170,173]

Endocrine organs

Endocrine organs are composed of stable cells for the most part. The adrenal gland regenerates from the zona glomerulosa, dependent on those hormones produced by the gland. The thyroid gland has only minimal regenerative capacity. Similarly, there is minimal regeneration of the pituitary gland, and it typically heals with scarring. Pancreatectomy does not induce proliferation of islet cells, but residual islets can increase their output with maintenance of relatively normal organ function with fewer cells. This behavior underscores the reserve found in many cell types.

Skeletal muscle

Skeletal muscle cells are permanent cells and in the adult demonstrate no capacity to regenerate. However, adjacent to the skeletal muscle fibers and ensheathed or encased within their BM is a group of stem, or reserve cells, the satellite cells. Upon injury and death of the adult skeletal muscle fibers, these cells proliferate and differentiate to form new skeletal muscle cells. These cells proliferate in conditions such as muscular dystrophy, polymyositis, and infectious diseases. In severe muscle injury, associated with hematoma formation, calcification may occur within the scar.[174]

Tendons

The end product of tendon repair depends on several factors such as the degree of injury to the tendon, extent of damage to the vascular supply, type of tendon, and extent of immobilization. In the first several days subsequent to injury there is an inflammatory phase with migration of fibroblastic cells from the surrounding connective tissue and from connective tissue forming the epitendinous and endotendinous cells. These cells have phagocytic properties, but some develop into fibroblastic cells. Collagen synthesis becomes evident 7 to 10 days after injury. Approximately 2 weeks after the injury, fibroblasts become the predominant cell type. The next several months are characterized by remodeling of the collagen fibers, which are initially perpendicular to the longitudinal axis of the tendon. After 4 to 5 months of repair, the wound is completely healed and the tendon eventually acquires a relatively normal tensile strength.[175]

Cartilage

The repair reaction of cartilage suffers because of the avascular nature of the tissue. Therefore, arthroscopic surgical removal of torn cartilage is often a necessary therapeutic intervention. As a general rule, cartilage cells adjacent to the perichondrium or subchondral bone do have sufficient access to blood vessels to give rise to an inflammatory phase of healing. In this type of injury, healing proceeds with granulation tissue formation after an inflammatory response. Even though a relatively normal structure eventually returns to the cartilage, it has a low content of proteoglycans and becomes greatly attenuated as the result of subsequent wear and tear.[176]

Bone

Bone fractures repair by proceeding through a repair reaction that typically results in a complete resolution of the fracture with no trace of the injury. There are remarkable similarities between healing in bone and other tissues. Initially, a clot fills the fracture site, and inflammatory cells, including macrophages and neutrophils, enter the wound site. Neovascularization begins at the edge of the clot. Bone and cartilage is then deposited into this unique form of granulation tissue, referred to as callus. Over the next several weeks the closure of the fracture site by the callus occurs. The final stage of remodeling may take years; however, when remodeling is completed, detection of the fracture site may prove to be impossible. These phases correlate with ECM protein expression, that is, type III collagen is expressed in the inflammatory phase; type II collagen in the callus; and type I collagen in the ossification that characterizes remodeling.[177]

Nervous system

Neurons are incapable of regenerative activity, and therefore injuries to the CNS are subject to permanent loss of tissue and functional capacity. In contrast to the other tissues and organs discussed to this point, scar tissue with fibroblasts and type I collagen does not form. Subsequent to necrosis the affected region receives an influx of neutrophils and macrophages, resulting in a cystic cavity. Fibroblasts and the ECM components discussed above are present in the brain but only in a perivascular distribution. Therefore these components play no significant role in the repair of injury in the CNS. The reparative cell, the microglial cell, proliferates and seals the cystic infarction by a reactive gliosis. Gliosis occurs in regions surrounding abscesses and tumors.

Neurons of the peripheral nervous system resemble those in the CNS and, if lethally injured, are unable to regenerate. However, regeneration of nerve processes can occur if there is no injury to the body of the nerve cell proper. There are limitations to this regenerative capacity dependent on the local environment, such as extent of injury.

The description of nerve injury and the morphologic changes are described extensively in Chapter 77. Briefly, within 7 days after the injury, axons disintegrate and the myelin sheet surrounding them forms globules. Macrophages and inflammatory cells remove the damaged myelin, and Schwann cell proliferation is initiated. The axon at the point of injury swells with organelles and neurofilament protein, and the newly formed myelin sheets surround these axonal dilatations. As the axonal sprouts enter the region of Schwann cells, they become myelinated until connection with the end organ is reestablished. Nerve growth factor produced by Schwann cells stimulate the neurons to synthesize proteins necessary for this regeneration to occur. Recent studies have also implicated the ECM as playing a critical role in the regeneration of neurites. Using a glioma cell line it has been shown that laminin and fibronectin enhance neurite outgrowth. The neurite outgrowth activity on laminin has been mapped to the end of the long arm of the classic α1-chain of laminin, as well as the laminin isotype merosin.[58]

Fetal tissues

The healing of incisional skin wounds in adults is characterized by fibrosis, scarring, and potentially contracture. In contrast, studies of wound healing in the fetus have demonstrated considerable differences when compared with wound healing in the adult.[178-180] The rate of healing is greater in the fetus, where there is no scab formation, only minimal inflammation, rapid epithelialization, decreased angiogenesis, enhanced regeneration, and a lack of scarring. Fetal-wound ECM is rich in hyaluronic acid, whereas the ECM in adult wounds is rich in collagen. Other environmental factors of the fetal wounds play a crucial role in modulating their repair, including the surrounding amniotic fluid, increased temperatures, less differentiated tissues, a fetal immune system, and decreased oxygenation. An improved understanding of the factors modulating the scarless wound healing of the fetus may lead to the development of approaches to alleviate some of the untoward sequelae of healing in the adult.

REFERENCES

1. Clark RAF, Henson PM: *The molecular and cellular biology of wound repair,* New York, 1988, Plenum Press.
2. Falcone PA: Wound metabolism [Review], *Clin Plastic Surg,* 17:443, 1990.
3. Hammar H: Wound healing, *Int J Dermatopathol* 32:6, 1993.

Extracellular matrix

4. Hay, ED: *Cell biology of extracellular matrix,* New York, 1992, Plenum Press.
5. Adams JC, Watt FM: Regulation of development and differentiation by the extracellular matrix, *Development,* 117:1183, 1993.
6. Trelstad RL: *Extracellular matrix in development,* New York, 1984, Liss.
7. Cheah KS: Collagen genes and inherited connective tissue disease, *Biochem J* 229:287, 1985.
8. Kivirikko KI: Collagens and their abnormalities in a wide spectrum of diseases, *Ann Intern Med* 25:113, 1993.
9. Linsenmayer TF Collagen. In Hay E, editor: *Cell biology of extracellular matrix,* New York, 1991, Plenum Press.
10. van der Rest M, Bruckner P: Collagens: diversity at the molecular and supramolecular levels, *Curr Opin Struct Biol* 3:430, 1993.
11. van der Rest M, Garrone R: Collagen family of proteins, *FASEB J* 5:2814, 1991.
12. Amenta PS, Gay S, Vaheri A, Martínez-Hernández A: The extracellular matrix is an integrated unit: ultrastructural localization of collagen types I, III, IV, V, VI, fibronectin, and laminin in human term placenta, *Coll Relat Res* 6:125, 1986.
13. Birk DE, Fitch JM, Babiarz JP, Linsenmayer TF: Collagen type I and V are present in the same fibril in the avian corneal stroma, *J Cell Biol* 106:999, 1988.
14. Keene DR, Sakai LY, Bachinger HP, Burgeson RE: Type III collagen can be present on banded collagen fibrils regardless of fibril diameter, *J Cell Biol* 105:2393, 1987.
15. Linsenmayer TF, Fitch JM, Gross J, Mayne R: Are collagen fibrils in the developing avian cornea composed of two different collagen types? Evidence from monoclonal antibody studies, *Ann N Y Acad Sci* 460:232, 1985.
16. Pihlajaniemi T, Tamminen M: The $\alpha 1$ chain of type XIII collagen consists of three collagenous and four noncollagenous domains, and its primary transcript undergoes complex alternative splicing, *J Biol Chem* 265:16922, 1990.
17. Dublet B, van der Rest M: Type XIV collagen, a new homotrimeric molecule extracted from fetal bovine skin and tendon, with a triple helical disulfide-bonded domain homologous to type IX and type XII collagens, *J Biol Chem* 266:6853, 1991.
18. Myers JC, Kivirikko S, Gordon MK et al: Identification of a previously unknown human collagen chain, $\alpha 1$(XV), characterized by extensive interruptions in the triple-helical region, *Proc Natl Acad Sci USA* 89:10144, 1992.
19. Olson BR: Collagen biosynthesis. In Hay E, editor: *Cell biology of extracellular matrix,* New York, 1991, Plenum Press.
20. Brenner DA, Westwick J, Breindl M: Type I collagen gene regulation and the molecular pathogenesis of cirrhosis, *Gastrointest Liver Physiol* 27:G589, 1993.
21. Kadler KE: Learning how mutations in type I collagen genes cause connective tissue disease, *Int J Exp Pathol* 74:319, 1993.
22. Slack JL, Liska DJ, Bornstein P: Regulation of expression of the type I collagen genes, *Am J Med Genet* 45:140, 1993.
23. Kagan HM, Trackman PC: Properties and function of lysyl oxidase, *Am J Respir Cell Mol Biol* 5:206, 1991.
24. Shah MA, Scaman CH, Palcic MM, Kagan HM: Kinetics and stereospecificity of the lysyl oxidase reaction, *J Biol Chem* 268:11573, 1993.
25. Birk DE, Zycband EI, Winkelmann DA, Trelstad RL: Collagen fibrillogenesis *in situ:* discontinuous segmental assembly in extracellular compartments, *Ann N Y Acad Sci* 580:176, 1990.
26. Trelstad RL, Hayashi K: Tendon fibrillogenesis: intracellular collagen subassemblies and cell surface changes associated with fibril growth, *Dev Biol* 71:228, 1979.
27. Keene DR, Engvall E, Glanville RW: Ultrastructure of type VI collagen in human skin and cartilage suggests an anchoring function for this filamentous network, *J Cell Biol* 107:1995, 1988.
28. Prokup DJ: Mutations in collagen genes as a cause of connective tissue diseases, *N Engl J Med* 326:540, 1992.
29. Spranger J, Winkerpacht A, Zobel B: The type II collagenopathies: a spectrum of chondrodysplasias, *Eur J Pediatr* 153:56, 1994.
30. Rupard JH, Dimari SJ, Damjanov I, Haralson M: Synthesis of type I homotrimer collagen molecules by cultured human lung adenocarcinoma cells, *Am J Pathol* 133:316, 1988.
31. Brenner DA, Veloz L, Jaenisch R, Alcorn, JM: Stimulation of the collagen $\alpha 1$(I) endogenous gene and transgene in carbon tetrachloride–induced hepatic fibrosis, *Hepatology* 17:287, 1993.
32. Brenner DA, Westwick J, Brendl M: Type I collagen gene replication and the molecular pathogenesis of cirrhosis, *Gastrointest Liver Physiol* 27:G589, 1993.
33. Peltonen J, Kahari L, Uitto J, Jiménez SA: Increased expression of type VI collagen genes in systemic sclerosis, *Arthritis Rheum* 33:1829, 1990.
34. Mecham RP, Heuser JE: The elastic fiber. In Hay E editor: *Cell biology of extracellular matrix,* New York, 1991, Plenum Press.
35. Pasquali-Ronchetti I, Baccarani-Contri M, Fornieri C et al: Structure and composition of the elastin fibre in normal and pathological conditions, *Micron* 24:75, 1993.
36. Rosenbloom J, Abrams WR, Mecham R: Extracellular matrix 4: The elastic fiber, *FASEB J* 7:1208, 1993.
37. Cleary EG, Gibson MA: Elastin-associated microfibrils and microfibrillar proteins, *Int Rev Connect Tissue Res* 10:97, 1983.
38. Sakai LY, Keene DR, Engvall E: Fibrillin, a new 350-kD glycoprotein, is a component of extracellular microfibrils, *J Cell Biol* 103:2499, 1986.
39. Dahlbäck K, Ljungquist A, Löfberg H et al: Fibrillin immunoreactive fibers constitute a unique network in the human dermis: immunohistochemical comparison of the distributions of fibrillin, vitronectin, amyloid P component, and orcein stainable structures in normal skin and elastosis, *J Invest Dermatol* 94:284, 1990.
40. Dietz HC: Molecular biology of Marfan's syndrome, *J Vasc Surg* 15:927, 1992.
41. McGookey DM, Pyeritz RE, Crawford S, Byers PH: Marfan syndrome: defective synthesis, secretion, and extracellular matrix formation of fibrillin by cultured dermal fibroblasts, *J Clin Invest* 89:79, 1992.
42. McKusick VA: The defect in Marfan syndrome, *Nature* 352:279, 1991.
43. Superti-Furga A, Raghunath M, Willems PJ: Deficiencies of fibrillin and decorin in fibroblast cultures of a patient with neonatal Marfan syndrome, *J Med Genet* 29:875, 1992.
44. Martínez-Hernández A, Amenta PS: The basement membrane in pathology, *Lab Invest* 48:656, 1983.
45. Rohrbach D, Timpl R: *Molecular and cellular aspects of basement membranes,* Orlando, Fla, 1993, Academic Press.
46. Timpl R, Dziadek M: Structure, development and molecular pathology of the basement membrane, *Int Rev Exp Pathol* 29:1, 1986.
47. Yurchenco PD, Schittny JC: Molecular architecture of basement membranes, *FASEB J* 4:1577, 1990.
48. Chung AE, Freeman IL, Braginski JE: A novel extracellular membrane elaborated by a mouse embryonal carcinoma-derived cell line, *Biochem Biophys Res Commun* 79:859, 1977.
49. Kleinman HK, Cannon FB, Laurie GW *et al:* Biological activities of laminin, *J Cell Biochem* 27:317, 1985.
50. Martin GR, Timpl R: Laminin and other basement membrane components, *Annu Rev Cell Biol* 3:57, 1987.

51. Timpl R, Rohde H, Robey PG et al: Laminin—a glycoprotein from basement membranes, *J Biol Chem* 254:9933, 1979.
52. Amenta PS, Clark CC, Martínez-Hernández A: Deposition of fibronectin and laminin in the basement membrane of the rat parietal yolk sac: immunohistochemical and biosynthetic studies, *J Cell Biol* 96:104, 1983.
53. Martínez-Hernández A, Chung AE: The ultrastructural localization of two basement membrane components: entactin and laminin in rat tissues, *J Histochem Cytochem* 32:289, 1984.
54. Engvall E: Laminin variants: Why, where, and when? *Kidney Int* 43:2, 1993.
55. Uitto J: Cell-cell and cell-matrix interactions in the skin, *Lab Invest* 69:133, 1993.
56. Burgeson RB, Chiquet M, Deutzmann R et al.: A new nomenclature for the laminins, *Matrix Biol* 14:209, 1994.
57. Wewer UM, Engvall E, Paulsson M et al: Laminin A, B1, B2, S, and M subunits in the postnatal rat liver development and after partial hepatectomy, *Lab Invest* 66:378, 1992.
58. Engvall E, Earwicker D, Day A et al: Merosin promotes cell attachment and neurite outgrowth and is a component of the neurite promoting factor of RN 22 schwannoma cells, *Exp Cell Res* 198:115, 1992.
59. Carlin B, Jaffe R, Bender B, Chung AE: Entactin, a novel basal lamina–associated sulfated glycoprotein, *J Biol Chem* 256:5209, 1981.
60. Mason IJ, Taylor A, Williams JG et al: Evidence from molecular cloning that SPARC, a major product of mouse embryo parietal endoderm is related to an endothelial cell "culture shock" glycoprotein of M_r 43,000, *EMBO J* 5:1465, 1986.
61. Sage EH, Bornstein P: Extracellular proteins that modulate cell-matrix interactions, *J Biol Chem* 266:14831, 1991.
62. Crouch EC: Molecular diversity of basement membrane collagen: elucidation of the Goodpasture's epitope, *Am J Respir Cell Mol Biol* 5:99, 1991.
63. Hudson BG, Reeders ST, Tryggvason KT: Type IV collagen: Structure, gene organization, and role in human diseases: molecular basis of Goodpasture and Alport syndromes and diffuse leiomyomatosis, *J Biol Chem* 268:26033, 1993.
64. Kefalides NA: Isolation of collagen from basement membrane containing three identical alpha chains, *Biochem Biophys Res Comm* 45:226, 1971.
65. Johansson C, Butkowski R, Wieslander J: The structural organization of type IV collagen: identification of these NC1 populations in the glomerular basement membrane, *J Biol Chem* 267:24533, 1992.
66. Kashton CE, Kleppel MM, Butkowski RJ et al: Alport syndrome, basement membrane, and collagen, *Pediatr Nephrol* 4:523, 1990
67. Tryggvason K, Zhou J, Hostikka SL, Shows TB: Molecular genetics of Alport's syndrome, *Kidney Int* 43:38, 1993.
68. Nomura S, Osawa G, Sai T et al: A splicing mutation in the α5(IV) collagen gene of a family with Alport's syndrome, *Kidney Int* 43:1116, 1993
69. Timpl R: Structure and biological activity of basement membrane proteins, *Eur J Biochem* 180:487, 1989.
70. Cohen IR, Grassel S, Murdoch AD, Iozzo RV: Structural characterization of the complete human perlecan gene and its promoter, *Proc Natl Acad Sci USA* 90:10404, 1993.
71. Yanagishita M: Function of proteoglycans in the extracellular matrix, *Acta Pathol Jpn* 43:283, 1993.
72. Jackson RL, Busch SJ, Cardin AD: Glycosaminoglycans: molecular properties, protein interactions, and role in physiological processes, *Physiol Rev* 71:481, 1991.
73. Iozzo RV: Perlecan: a gem of a proteoglycan, *Matrix Biol* 14:203, 1994.
74. Murdoch AD, Liu B, Schwartz R et al: Widespread expression of perlecan proteoglycan in basement membranes and extracellular matrices of human tissues as detected by a novel monoclonal antibody against domain III and by *in-situ* hybridization, *J Histochem Cytochem* 42:239, 1994.
75. Marinkovich MP, Keene DR, Rimberg CS, Burgeson, RE: Cellular origin of the dermal-epidermal basement membrane, *Dev Dynam* 197:255, 1993.
76. Simon-Assmann P, Bouziges F, Freund JN et al: Type IV collagen mRNA accumulates in the mesenchymal compartment at early stages of murine developing intestine, *J Cell Biol* 110:849, 1991.
77. Yurchenco PD, Ruben GC: Basement membrane structure in situ: evidence for lateral associations in the type IV collagen, *J Cell Biol* 105:2559, 1987.
78. Yurchenco PD, Ruben GC: Type IV collagen lateral associations in the EHS tumor matrix: comparison with amniotic and in vitro networks, *Am J Pathol* 132:278, 1988.
79. Schuger L, O'Shea KS, Nelson BB, Varani J: Organotypic arrangement of mouse embryonic lung cells on a basement membrane extract: involvement of laminin, *Development* 110:1091, 1990.
80. Donahue PK, Hutson JM, Ikawa H et al: Molecular dissection of Müllerian duct regression. In Trelstad RL, editor: *Extracellular matrix in development*, New York, 1984, AR Liss.
81. Ekblom P: Formation of basement membranes in the embryonic kidney: an immunohistological study, *J Cell Biol* 91:1, 1981.
82. Ekblom P, Alitalo K, Vaheri A et al: Induction of a basement membrane glycoprotein in embryonic kidney: possible role of laminin in morphogenesis, *Proc Natl Acad Sci USA* 77:485, 1980.
83. Ishii N, Wadsworth WG, Stern BD et al: UNC-6, a laminin-related protein, guides cell and pioneer axon migrations in *C. elegans*, *Neuron* 9:873, 1992.
84. Klein G, Ekblom M, Fecker L et al: Differential expression of laminin A and B chains during development of embryonic mouse organs, *Development* 110:823, 1990.
85. Trelstad RL, Hayashi A, Hayashi K, Donahoe PK: The epithelial-mesenchymal interface of the male rat Müllerian duct: loss of basement membrane integrity and ductal regression, *Dev Biol* 92:27, 1982.
86. Stetler-Stevenson WG, Aznavoorian S, Liotta L: Tumor cell interactions with the extracellular matrix during invasion and metastasis, *Annu Rev Cell Biol* 9:541, 1993.
87. Mynderse LA, Hassell JR, Kleinman HK et al: Loss of heparan sulfate proteoglycan from glomerular basement membrane of nephrotic rats, *Lab Invest* 48:292, 1983.
88. Hudson BG, Kalluri R, Gunwar S et al: Molecular characteristics of the Goodpasture autoantigen, *Kidney Int* 43:135, 1993.
89. Kefalides NA, Ohno N, Wilson CB: Heterogeneity of antibodies in Goodpasture syndrome reacting with type IV collagen, *Kidney Int* 43:85, 1993.
90. Hayashi YK, Engvall E, Arikawa-Hirasawa E et al: Abnormal localization of laminin subunits in muscular dystrophies, *J Neurol Sci* 119:53, 1993.
91. Hynes RO, Schwarzbauer JE, Tamkun JW: Fibronectin: a versatile gene for a versatile protein, *Ciba Found Symp* 108:75, 1984.
92. Morla A, Zhang Z, Ruoslahti E: Superfibronectin is a functionally distinct form of fibronectin, *Nature* 367:193, 1994.
93. Yamada YM: Fibronectin and other cell interactive glycoproteins. In Hay E, editor: *Cell biology of extracellular matrix*, New York, 1991, Plenum Press.
94. Weiss RE, Reddi AH: Appearance of fibronectin during the differentiation of cartilage, bone, and bone marrow, *J Cell Biol* 88:630, 1981.
95. Kurkinen M, Vaheri A, Roberts PJ, Stenman S: Sequential appearance of fibronectin and collagen in experimental granulation tissue, *Lab Invest* 43:47, 1980.
96. Martínez-Hernández A: The hepatic extracellular matrix. II. Electron immunohistochemical studies in rats with CCl_4-induced cirrhosis, *Lab Invest* 53:166, 1985.
97. Sabet MD, Gordon SR: Ultrastructural immunocytochemical localization of fibronectin deposition during corneal wound repair: evidence for cytoskeletal involvement, *Biol Cell* 65:171, 1989.
98. Williams IF, McCullagh KG, Silver IA: The distribution of types I and III collagen and fibronectin in the healing equine tendon, *Connect Tissue Res* 12:211, 1984.
99. Ruoslahti E, Hayman EG, Kuusela P et al: Isolation of a tryptic fragment containing the collagen-binding site of plasma fibronectin, *J Biol Chem* 254:6054, 1979.
100. Chiquet R, Fambrough DM: Chick myotendinous antigen. 1. A monoclonal antibody as a marker for tendon and muscle morphogenesis, *J Cell Biol* 98:1926, 1984.
101. Erickson HP, Iglesias JL: A six-armed oligomer isolated from cell surface fibronectin preparations, *Nature* 311:267, 1984.
102. Mackie EJ, Thesleff I, Chiquet-Ehrismann R: Tenascin is associated with chondrogenic and osteogenic differentiation *in vivo* and promotes chondrogenesis *in vitro*, *J Cell Biol* 105:2569, 1987.
103. Sakakura T, Kusano I: Tenascin in tissue perturbation repair, *Acta Pathol Jpn* 41:247, 1991.

104. Betz P, Nerlich A, Tubel J et al: Localization of tenascin in human skin wounds: an immunohistochemical study, *Int J Legal Med* 105:325, 1993.
105. Iruela-Arispe ML, Liska DJ, Sage EH, Bornstein P: Differential expression of thrombospondin 1, 2, and 3 during murine development, *Dev Dynam* 197:40, 1993.
106. Nicosia RF, Tuszynski GP: Matrix-bound thrombospondin promotes angiogenesis in vitro, *J Cell Biol* 124:193, 1994.
107. Inuzuka S, Ueno T, Torimura T et al: Vitronectin in liver disorders: biochemical and immunohistochemical studies, *Hepatology* 15:629, 1992.
108. Collazos J, Diaz F: Serum laminin in patients with chronic active hepatitis and mild liver diseases, *Int Hepat Comm* 2:52, 1994.
109. David G: Integral membrane heparan sulfate proteoglycans, *FASEB J* 7:1023, 1993.
110. Iozzo RV: Proteoglycans: structure, function, and role in neoplasia, *Lab Invest* 53:373, 1985.
111. Ruoslahti E: Structure and biology of proteoglycans, *Ann Rev Cell Biol* 4:229, 1988.
112. Trelstad RL, Kemp PD: Matrix glycoprotein and proteoglycans. In Sledge CB, Ruddy S, Harris ED, Kelley WN, editors: *Arthritis surgery,* New York, 1994, Saunders.
113. Bernfield M, Kokenyesi R, Kato M et al: Biology of the syndecans: a family of transmembrane heparan sulfate proteoglycans, *Annu Rev Cell Biol* 8:365, 1992.
114. Ruoslahti E, Yamaguchi Y: Proteoglycans as modulators of growth factor activities, *Cell* 64:867, 1991.
115. Bourin M-C, Lindahl U: Glycosaminoglycans and the regulation of blood coagulation, *Biochem J* 289:313, 1993.
116. Celesia GG: Alzheimer's disease: the proteoglycan hypothesis, *Semin Thromb Hemost* 17:158, 1991.
117. Birkedal-Hansen H, Moore WGI, Bodden MK et al: Matrix metalloproteinases: a review, *Crit Rev Oral Biol Med* 4:197, 1993.
118. Walsh LJ, Murphy GF: Role of adhesion molecules in cutaneous inflammation and neoplasia, *J Cutan Pathol* 19:161, 1992.
119. Albelda SM: Role of integrins and other cell adhesion molecules in tumor progression and metastasis, *Lab Invest* 68:4, 1993.
120. Albelda SM, Buck CA: Integrins and other cell adhesion molecules, *FASEB J* 4:2868, 1990.
121. Benton LD, Khan M, Greco RS: Integrins, adhesion molecules and surgical research, *Surg Gynecol Obstet* 177:311, 1993.
122. Garrod DR: Cell to cell and cell to matrix adhesion, *Br Med J* 306:703, 1993.
123. Humphries MJ, Mould AP, Tuckwell DS: Dynamic aspects of adhesion receptor function: integrins both twist and shout, *BioEssays* 15:392, 1993.
124. Juliano R: Signal transduction by integrins and its role in the regulation ot tumor growth, *Cancer Metastasis Rev* 13:25, 1994.
125. Ruoslahti E: Integrins, *J Clin Invest* 87:1, 1991.
126. Ruoslahti E: Integrins as receptors for extracellular matrix. In Hay E, editor: *Cell biology of extracellular matrix,* New York, 1991, Plenum Press.
127. Wang N, Butler JP, Ingber DE: Mechanotransduction across the cell surface and through the cytoskeleton, *Science* 260:1124, 1993.

Cells of the repair process

128. Davies MG, Hagan PO: The vascular endothelium: a new horizon, *Ann Surg* 218:593, 1993.
129. Folkman J, Klagsburn M: Angiogenic factors, *Science* 235:442, 1987.
130. Madri JA, Bell L, Marx M et al: Effects of soluble factors and extracellular matrix components on vascular cell behavior *in vitro* and *in vivo:* models of deendothelialization and repair, *J Cell Biochem* 45:123, 1991.
131. Harrison P, Cramer EM: Platelet alpha-granules, *Blood Rev* 7:52, 1993.
132. Clowes AW, Reidy MA: Prevention of stenosis after vascular reconstruction: pharmacologic control of intimal hyperplasia, *J Vasc Surg* 13:885, 1991.
133. Doane KJ, Birk DE: Fibroblasts retain their tissue phenotype when grown in three-dimensional collagen gels, *Exp Cell Res* 195:432, 1991.
134. Grinnell F: Fibroblasts, myofibroblasts, and wound contraction, *J Cell Biol* 124:401, 1994.
135. Hebda PA, Collins MA, Tharp MD: Mast cell and myofibroblast in wound healing, *Dermatol Clin* 11:685, 1993.
136. Stein M, Keshav S: The versatility of macrophages, *Clin Exp Allergy* 22:19, 1992.
137. Wahl SM, McCartney-Francis N, Allen JB et al: Macrophage production of TGF-beta and regulation by TGF-beta, *Ann NY Acad Sci* 593:188, 1990.
138. Beekhuizen H, van Furth R: Monocyte adherence to human vascular endothelium, *J Leukoc Biol* 54:363, 1993.
139. Choi KL, Claman HN: Mast cells, fibroblasts, and fibrosis: new clues to the riddle of mast cells, *Immunol Res* 6:145, 1987.
140. Parwaresch MR, Horny HP, Lennert K: Tissue mast cells in health and disease, *Pathol Res Prac* 179:439, 1985.
141. Baserga R: The cell cycle, *N Engl J Med* 304:453, 1981.

Cytokines

142. Cromack DT: Current concepts in wound healing: growth factor and macrophage interaction, *J Trauma* 30:S129, 1990.
143. Evans SW, Whicher JT: The cytokines: physiological and pathophysiological aspects, *Adv Clin Chem* 30:1, 1993.
144. Herndon DN, Nguyen TT, Gilpin DA: Growth factors: local and systemic, *Arch Surg* 128:1227, 1993.
145. Kiritsy CP, Lynch AB, Lynch SE: Role of growth factors in cutaneous wound healing: a review, *Crit Rev Oral Biol Med* 4:729, 1993.
146. LeRoy EC, Trojanowska MI, Smith EA: Cytokines and human fibrosis, *Eur Cytokine Network* 1:215, 1990.
147. Lowry SF: Cytokine mediators of immunity and inflammation, *Arch Surg* 128:1235, 1993.
148. McKay IA, Leigh IM: Epiderman cytokines and their roles in cutaneous wound healing, *Br J Dermatol* 124:513, 1991.
149. Michalopoulos GK: Liver regeneration: molecular mechanisms of growth control, *FASEB J* 178:176, 1990.
150. Ross R, Bowen-Pope DF, Raines EW: Platelet-derived growth factor and its role in health and disease, *Philos Trans R Soc Lond, Series B [Biol]* 327:155, 1990.
151. Rappolee DA, Werb Z: Macrophage-derived growth factors, *Curr Top Microbiol Immunol* 181:87, 1992.
152. Davidson JM, Broadley KN: Manipulation of the wound-healing process with basic fibroblast growth factor, *Ann N Y Acad Sci* 638:306, 1991.
153. Khalil N, Greenberg AH: The role of TGF-beta in pulmonary fibrosis, *Ciba Found Symp* 157:194, 1991.
154. Wahl SM, McCartney-Francis N, Allen JB et al: Macrophage production of TGF-beta and regulation by TGF-beta. *Ann N Y Acad Sci* 593:188, 1990.
155. Wolf HK, Zarnegar R, Michalopoulos GK: Localization of hepatocyte growth factor in human and rat tissues: an immunohistochemical study, *Hepatology* 14:488, 1991.

Repair

156. Jensen LT, Garbarsch C, Horslev-Petersen K: Collagen metabolism during wound healing in rats: the aminoterminal propeptide of type III procollagen in serum and wound fluid in relation to formation of granulation tissue, *APMIS* (Copenhagen) 101:557, 1993.
157. Russell SB, Trupin KM, Myers JC et al: Differential glucocorticoid regulation of collagen mRNAs in human dermal fibroblasts, *J Biol Chem* 264:13730, 1989.
158. Rasmussen LH, Garbarsch C, Schuppan D et al: Influence of human growth hormone on granulation tissue formation, collagen deposition, and the amino-terminal propeptide of collagen type III in wound chambers in rats, *Wound Rep Reg* 2:31, 1994.
159. Enzinger FM, Weiss SW: *Soft tissue tumors,* ed 3, St. Louis, 1995, Mosby.
160. Murrell GAC, Francis MJO, Bromley L: The collagen changes of Dupuytren's contracture, *J Hand Surg* 16B:263, 1991.
161. Sible JC, Eriksson E, Smith SP, Oliver N: Fibronectin gene expression differs in normal and abnormal human wound healing, *Wound Rep Reg* 2:3, 1994.

Regeneration

162. Wilhelm DL: Regeneration of tracheal epithelium, *J Pathol Bacteriol* 67:361, 1954.

Healing in specific organs

163. Clark RA: Regulation of fibroplasia in cutaneous wound repair, *Am J Med Sci* 306:42, 1993.
164. Li KC, Ehrlich HP, Trelstad RL et al: Differences in healing of skin wounds caused by burn and freeze injuries, *Ann Surg* 191:244, 1980.
165. Botney MD, Liptay MJ, Kaiser LR et al: Active collagen synthesis by pulmonary arteries in human primary pulmonary hypertension, *Am J Pathol* 143:121, 1993.
166. Raghu G, Striker LJ, Hudson LD, Striker GE: Extracellular matrix in normal and fibrotic human lungs, *Am Rev Respir Dis* 131:281, 1985.
167. Torikata C, Villiger B, Kuhn C, McDonald JA: Ultrastructural distribution of fibronectin in normal and fibrotic human lung, *Lab Invest* 52:399, 1985.
168. Couchman JR, Beavan LA, McCarthy KJ: Glomerular matrix: Synthesis, turnover, will role over in mesangial expansion, *Kidney Int* 45:328, 1994.
169. Glick AD, Jacobson HR, Haralson MA: Mesangial deposition of type I collagen in human glomerulosclerosis, *Hum Pathol* 23:1373, 1992.
170. Martínez-Hernández A, Martínez-Delgado F, Amenta PS: The extracellular matrix in hepatic regeneration: Localization of collagen types I, III, IV, laminin, and fibronectin, *Lab Invest* 64:157, 1992.
171. Martínez-Hernández A, Martínez J: The role of capillarization in hepatic failure: studies in carbon tetrachloride–induced cirrhosis, *Hepatology* 14:864, 1991.
172. Friedman SL: Cellular sources of collagen and regulation of collagen production in liver, *Semin Liver Dis* 10:20, 1990.
173. Greenwel P, Schwartz M, Rosas M et al: Characterization of fat-storing cell lines derived from normal and CCl_4-cirrhotic livers: differences in the production of interleukin-6, *Lab Invest* 65:644, 1991.
174. Caplan A, Carlson B, Faulkner J et al: Skeletal muscle. In Woo SL-Y, Buckwalter JA, editors: *Injury and repair of musculoskeletal soft tissues,* Park Ridge, Ill, 1980, American Academy of Orthopaedic Surgeons.
175. Gelberman R, Goldberg V, An K-N et al: Tendon. In Woo SL-Y, Buckwalter JA, editors: *Injury and repair of musculoskeletal soft tissues,* Park Ridge, Ill, 1980, American Academy of Orthopedic Surgeons.
176. Buckwalter J, Rosenberg L, Coult R et al: Articular cartilage: injury and repair. In Woo SL-Y, Buckwalter JA, editors: *Injury and repair of musculoskeletal soft tissues,* Park Ridge, Ill, 1980, American Academy of Orthopedic Surgeons.
177. Hiltunen A, Aro HT, Vuorio E: Regulation of extracellular matrix genes during fracture healing in mice, *Clin Orthop* 297:23, 1993.
178. Adzick NS, Longaker MT: *Fetal wound healing,* New York, 1991, Elsevier.
179. Longaker MT, Chiu ES, Adzick S et al: Studies in fetal wound healing. V. A prolonged presence of hyaluronic acid characterizes fetal wound fluid, *Ann Surg* 213:4, 1991.
180. Longaker MT, Whitby DJ, Adzick NS et al: Studies in fetal wound healing. VI. Second and early third trimester fetal wounds demonstrate rapid collagen deposition without scar formation, *J Pediatr Surg* 25:63, 1990.

20 Amyloidosis

Robert Kisilevsky
Iain D. Young

The term *amyloidosis* encompasses a diverse group of diseases, each of which is characterized by the extracellular accumulation of fibrillar protein deposits. Virchow first used the term *amyloid,*[1] meaning 'starchlike,' to describe the deposits he observed in amyloidotic tissue stained with iodine solutions (Fig. 20-1). Although Virchow had correctly identified a carbohydrate moiety in amyloid, it was subsequently demonstrated that the principal constituent of the amyloid fibril is protein. Since about 1973 it has been determined that many disparate proteins may form amyloid under a wide variety of clinical circumstances. The tissue distribution of these different amyloids and the consequent clinical manifestations of different amyloidoses vary tremendously. Therefore it is important to recognize that *amyloidosis* refers to a pathologic process, not a specific disease, and that *amyloid* is the generic designation of the characteristic protein deposit, which is its defining feature.

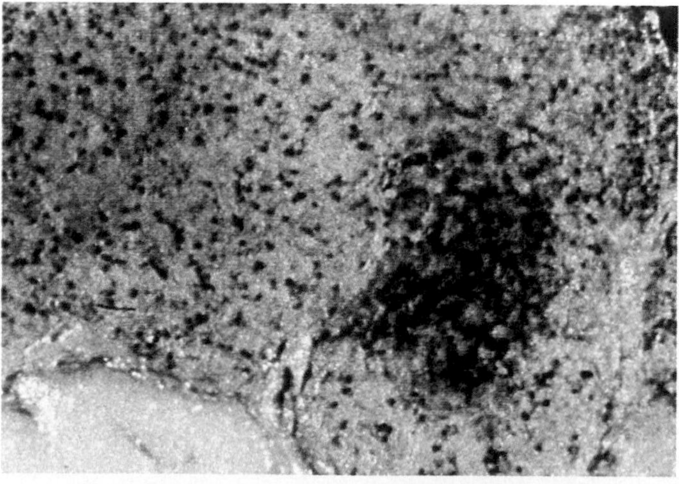

Fig. 20-1 The cut surface of an amyloidotic kidney treated with the iodine reaction originally used by Virchow to demonstrate the carbohydrate nature of these deposits. Notice the blue-black reaction in the medulla and the individual glomeruli in the cortex.

CLASSIFICATION

Despite a common appearance, staining, and structural properties, approximately 20 different proteins are responsible for amyloid deposits. Usually, each amyloid protein is found in a unique clinical disorder. When a single amyloid protein occurs in different clinical disorders, it reflects a common pathologic process (such as persistent acute inflammation) as a feature of the underlying disease. Attempts to identify homologous or consensus amino acid sequences in these varied proteins to explain their common amyloidogenic properties have not been fruitful. A complete classification of the various amyloids according to protein type is listed in Table 20-1, as modified from the WHO-IUIS Nomenclature Sub-Committee.[2] In addition, mutations in lysozyme and fibrinogen have also been reported to give rise to amyloid.[3,4]

AMYLOIDOGENESIS

It is now apparent that amyloidosis is not one disease. Where common pathogenetic mechanisms are involved, regardless of the specific disease (as in inflammatory states), the same protein forms the amyloid. Where different pathogenetic mechanisms are operative the genesis of different forms of amyloid arises from unique proteins.

Nevertheless, there is an underlying structure that is clearly common to all amyloid and begs the question how such diverse proteins manage to organize themselves into this common structure, which we call "amyloid." Many accept that an overall pathogenetic mechanism, or final common pathway, is operative in all cases. Amyloid precursor proteins when produced in excess have specific amino acid substitutions as a result of mutations, or are subjected to altered proteolytic cleavage, result in the generation of proteins or peptides that self-aggregate into fibrils. The characteristic feature of these fibrils is extensive of intracrossed or intercrossed beta-pleated sheeting that exists within or between peptide subunits. This view is

Table 20-1 Nomenclature and classification of amyloid and amyloidosis

Amyloid protein*†	Protein precursor	Protein type or variant	Clinical diagnosis
AA	apoSAA		Inflammation-associated amyloidosis Familial Mediterranean fever Familial amyloid nephropathy with urticaria and deafness (Muckle-Wells syndrome)
AL	κ or λ light chains		Idiopathic (primary) amyloidosis, associated with myeloma or macroglobulinemia or plasma cell dyscrasias
AH	IgG I (γI)		
ATTR	Transthyretin (TTR)	Various mutations Normal TTR	Familial amyloid polyneuropathy, several types Familial amyloid cardiomyopathy, Danish Systemic senile amyloidosis
AApoA-I	apoA-I	Arg 26‡	Familial amyloid polyneuropathy, Iowa
AGel	Gelsolin	Asn 187	Familial amyloidosis, Finnish
ACys	Cystatin C	Gln 68	Hereditary cerebral hemorrhage with amyloidosis, Icelandic
Aβ	β-protein precursor e.g. βPP 695§	Various mutations	Alzheimer's disease Down syndrome Hereditary cerebral hemorrhage with amyloidosis, Dutch
Aβ_2M	β_2-microglobulin		Associated with chronic dialysis
APrP	Prion protein precursor 33-35 kD cellular form	Prion protein 27-30 kD Several mutations	Creutzfeldt-Jakob disease, etc. Gerstmann-Sträussler-Scheinker syndrome
ACal	(Pro)calcitonin	(Pro)calcitonin	In medullary carcinomas of thyroid
AANF	Atrial natriuretic factor		Isolated atrial amyloid
AIAPP	Islet amyloid polypeptide (IAPP)		In islets of Langerhans Diabetes type II, insulinoma
AIns	Insulin		Islet amyloid in the degu (a rodent)
AApoA-II	apoA-II (murine)	Gln5	Amyloidosis in senescence-accelerated mice

* Nonfibrillar proteins, such as protein AP (amyloid P-component) excluded.
†*AA*, Amyloid A protein; *apo*, apolipoprotein; *H*, immunoglobulin heavy chain; *L*, immunoglobulin light chain; *SAA*, serum amyloid A protein.
‡Amino acid position in the mature precursor protein.
§ Number of amino acid residues.

based on information obtained from work that focused on (1) studies of the amino acid sequence and mutational variants of the amyloid precursor proteins, (2) factors that regulate the synthesis of these specific proteins, (3) attempts to understand the proteolytic mechanisms degrading these proteins and the cells believed to be responsible for the specific proteases, and (4) the mechanisms by which the proteins or peptides self-assemble into an amyloid fibril. Each of these areas has provided important information vis-à-vis amyloid formation, but they have also brought to light contradictions and confounding issues with our current view.

Primary structure and mutation

The significance of primary structure and the effects of mutation are best exemplified when one considers the amyloids related to transthyretin. Transthyretin is a plasma protein produced in the liver that transports thyroxin and, by virtue of its binding of retinol binding protein, also vitamin A.[5-7] Transthyretin is present in senile systemic amyloid, senile cardiac amyloid, and the majority of the familial amyloidotic polyneuropathies (FAP).

The early identification of a methionine for valine substitution at position 30 of transthyretin in one form of FAP[8] supported the idea that understanding the mutational variants of transthyretin would shed light on the mechanism of FAP amyloid formation. At present count, there are 40 different mutations associated with FAP.[9] These mutations are not found in any one region of transthyretin but are scattered throughout the molecule. With few exceptions, each mutation tends to give rise to a different "FAP syndrome" with differing ages of onset, speed of disease progression, and peripheral anatomic distributions.[10]

Similar observations are now being made with other amyloidogenic proteins. These include the beta-protein and its precursor in Alzheimer's disease,[11,12] the prion protein in Gerstmann-Sträussler syndrome and Creutzfeldt-Jakob disease,[13] and the light-chain amyloids associated with plasma cell dyscrasias.[14-16]

Synthetic polypeptides in which "mutations" have been manufactured by alteration of the amino acid sequence during the process of synthesis have been studied.[17,18] When used in appropriate in vitro conditions, such amino acid substitutions

metabolic coin. Viewed from one side, basement membrane protein binding to an amyloidogenic precursor may influence the precursor to initiate the process of amyloid deposition (as seen with perlecan and SAA, or sulfate ions and the beta-peptide). Viewed from the other, the amyloid precursor, on binding to basement membrane proteins that are not yet part of a basement membrane, precludes these basement membrane proteins from forming a structural basement membrane. This perspective ties together the earliest steps in the process of amyloidogenesis with disturbed basement membrane formation, a common feature of amyloid deposits.

Integrated view

Using the foregoing discussion as a guide, one can construct an integrated view that incorporates the various steps believed to be involved in amyloidogenesis (Fig. 20-2).

In all settings an adequate amyloid precursor pool must be present. In some, as in AA amyloidogenesis, inflammation induces the upregulation of the necessary genes for the process of acute-phase protein synthesis. This, however, occurs for physiologic purposes related to inflammation, not amyloid formation. In others, as with TTR, an upregulation of TTR gene expression is not required.

The localization of specific forms of amyloid is in part determined by the natural function of the amyloid protein precursor itself. In the case of SAA and AA amyloid, SAA may serve as an address, directing HDL to cells of the reticuloendothelial system for the purpose of cholesterol transport during inflammation. If SAA is mishandled, amyloid is subsequently deposited at these sites. Thus the affinity of a protein for specific cell types may determine where the precursor can be mishandled, and the specific anatomic sites of amyloid deposition associated with certain amyloidogenic proteins emerges as a natural consequence of the physiologic role of these proteins. Mutations may alter not only the amyloidogenic potential of a protein, but also its tissue affinities. This may explain why normal TTR is deposited systemically in senile systemic amyloid but mutant TTR with a methione for valine substitution tends to be deposited in the peripheral and autonomic nervous system. Furthermore, a mutation by introducing a change in the sequence of amino acids may convert a nonamyloidogenic protein into one that has a permissive but noncausative structure for amyloid formation.

An appropriate microenvironment is necessary for the permissive amyloid potential to be expressed. Alterations in the microenvironment at the sites of the precursor protein's physiologic affinity likely involve changes in basement membrane protein metabolism. The nature of the factors governing the alteration of basement membrane protein expression are only now being investigated. The observation that amyloids in general tend to be disorders associated with older people is suggestive that extracellular matrix protein expression changes with age. This may play a critical role in determining when amyloid deposition commences. It may also explain why, in familial forms of amyloid, depositions do not begin until much later in life. As shown in AA amyloidogenesis, amyloid deposition likely commences in association with specific components of the basement membrane involving specific regions of these basement membrane proteins.

AEF is likely operating temporally very close to the events concerned with basement membrane protein expression. Although neither the nature nor the mode of action of AEF has been determined, it has been suggested by several investigators that it acts as a nidus for amyloid deposition. This remains to be established.

Proteolysis of amyloid precursors in some forms of amyloidosis may occur as part of the processing or posttranslational modifications of these proteins. As such, these prefibrillogenic cleavage steps are generating a partially cleaved but normal product that may in appropriate conditions lead to amyloid deposition. Proteolysis of amyloid precursors as it relates to the size of amyloid peptides found in deposits is inferred to occur at a point beyond their incorporation into fibrils. The different complement of proteases from the various tissues will process the fibrils to a point where further proteolytic degradation becomes difficult. Thus several peptides of varying size may all be present in the same amyloid deposit, but a predominant species reflects the protease complement of the tissue concerned. This may differ from tissue to tissue. This process of fibril turnover is likely to be very slow. In the absence of continued amyloid deposition the slow proteolytic removal of amyloid implies that, with sufficient time, amyloid deposits can be mobilized, allowing the physiologic recovery of involved organs. Such cases have been reported both clinically and experimentally.[66-70] They hold promise for therapeutic approaches that, in preventing further amyloid deposition, may lead to physiologic recovery.

PATHOLOGY

Gross

The gross appearance of amyloidotic organs varies depending on the volume of amyloid present and, to a certain extent, the specific site of amyloid deposition within the tissue. Although amyloidotic tissue may be grossly unremarkable, significant visceral involvement is usually associated with organomegaly and a pale cut surface that has a waxy or greasy texture (Fig. 20-3). However, extensive vascular involvement, as in renal amyloidosis, may cause ischemic atrophy and a consequent reduction of organ size.

The spleen shows variable gross patterns of involvement. Predominant deposition in splenic sinusoids and red pulp produces broad interlacing trabeculas of pallor (Figure 20-3, *A*). Alternatively, amyloid may be localized principally within splenic follicles and produce multiple small pale nodules, the so-called sago spleen. Hepatic and adrenal amyloid accumulation follow the sinusoidal pattern of the organs and may be easily observed in advanced cases (Fig. 20-3, *B* and *C*).

Microscopic

Amyloid possesses unique structural and tinctorial properties. By light microscopy, it is an amorphous deposit that appears devoid of distinguishing features. However, ultrastructurally, amyloids are composed of a network of long, nonbranching fibrils having a diameter of 7 to 10 nm.[71,72] The amyloid fibrils may be randomly disposed in a haystack pattern or appear as parallel arrays and bundles (Fig. 20-4). Some types of amyloid fibrils show minor structural variations. For example, the neurofibillary tangle of Alzheimer's disease is composed of bundles of 18 nm paired helical filaments,[73,74] and the fibrils of β_2M amyloid show a propensity to be curvilinear.[75,76]

The typical amyloid fibril is a composite of parallel subunit filaments that twist one around the other. The filaments comprise aggregated protein subunits and possess extensive crossed beta-pleated sheet structure,[77] an organization that may serve to impart stability on the fibril. Although the beta-pleated sheet conformation is highly characteristic of amyloid, it may not be an absolute requirement for fibril formation. Other secondary structures have been identified in some experimentally produced amyloid fibrils.[78]

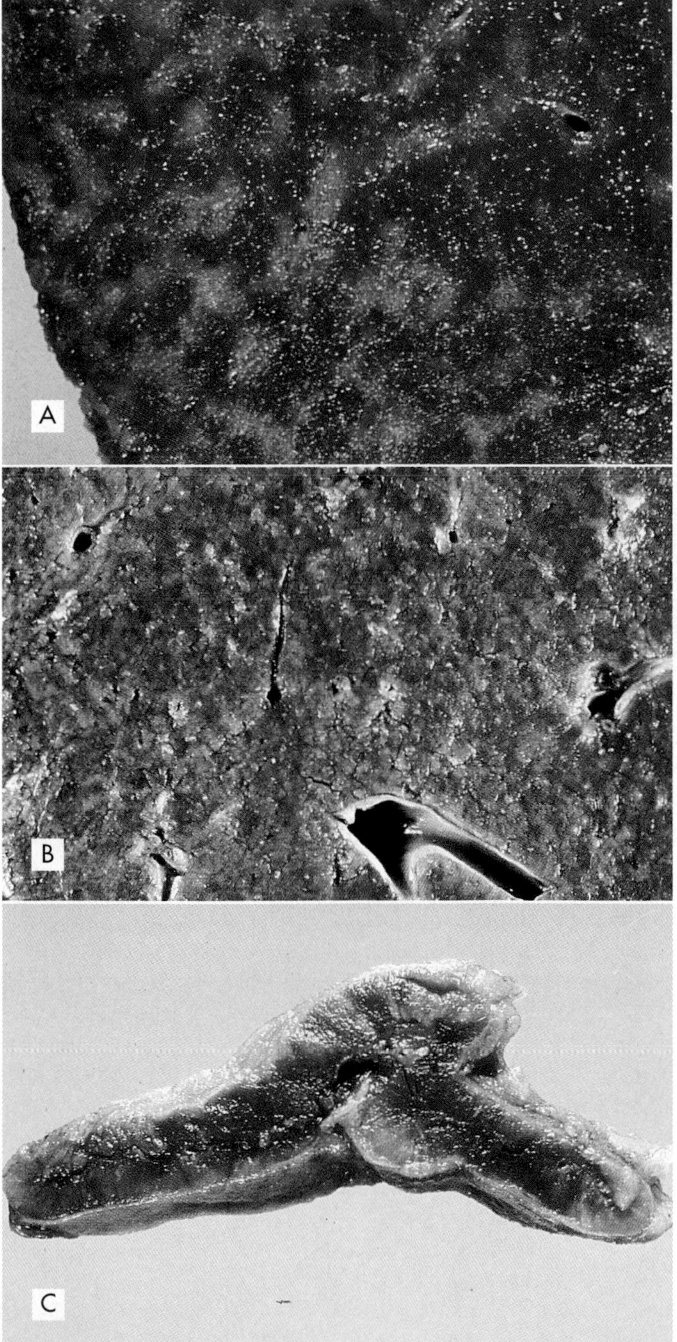

Fig. 20-3 **A,** Close-up view of the cut surface of a spleen with AA amyloid. *Pale areas,* Extensive deposition in the sinusoidal areas. **B,** The gross appearance of liver infiltrated with AA amyloid. Notice the pale, exaggeration of the sinusoidal architecture. **C,** Close-up view of the gross appearance of AA amyloid in the adrenal. Notice the loss of the characteristic yellow cortex and the pale infiltrate representing amyloid deposits.

Amyloid deposits include constituents other than the fibril protein. Amyloid-P component, a serum-derived protein, is present in all forms of amyloid.[49,79] Ultrastructurally, it is a pentagonal structure that is composed of five identical subunits and is organized into stacks oriented perpendicularly to the amyloid fibrils.[50,80] Highly sulfated glycosaminoglycans, principally heparan sulfate, represent the major amyloid-associated carbohydrate identified by Virchow.[81-83] Electron-dense dyes have been used to show that glycosaminoglycans, like amyloid-P component, are closely related structurally to the amyloid fibril.[84,85] The potential significance of these components is considered in greater detail in the discussion of amyloidogenesis.

Routine histochemical stains identify amyloid as a pink, acellular, hyaline deposit (Fig. 20-5, *A*). The characteristic tinctorial feature of amyloid, which also represents the definitive histochemical test for its presence, is its ability to bind the dye Congo red. With this stain, amyloid appears pink to orange-red and demonstrates the cardinal feature of green birefringence when viewed under polarized light (Fig. 20-6) The highly ordered binding of linear Congo red molecules in parallel array along the fibril axis appears to underly this optical property.[86]

Amyloids stain metachromatically with methyl violet and crystal violet. The binding of the dye thioflavine to amyloid and its fluorescence under ultraviolet radiation are very sensitive and are useful in screening for amyloid. However, positive results must be confirmed with Congo red because of the lack of specificity of the thioflavine stain. Sulfated Alcian blue can be useful to identify the glycosaminoglycan component of amyloid deposits (Fig. 20-5, *B*). The fibril protein (such as AA, light chain, procalcitonin) component of a variety of amyloids can be specifically identified by immunohistochemistry (Fig. 20-7) (Table 20-2).

Through a combination of structural and optical features, amyloid can be defined as an abnormal, generally extracellular protein deposit that exhibits the following properties: (1) an amorphous light microscopic appearance, (2) red-green birefringence under polarized light after Congo red staining, (3) a fibrillar ultrastructure with a fibril diameter of 7 to 10 nm, and (4) a predominant beta-pleated sheet secondary structure.

Microscopically, amyloid is located extracellularly, and deposits typically have a close topographic relationship with

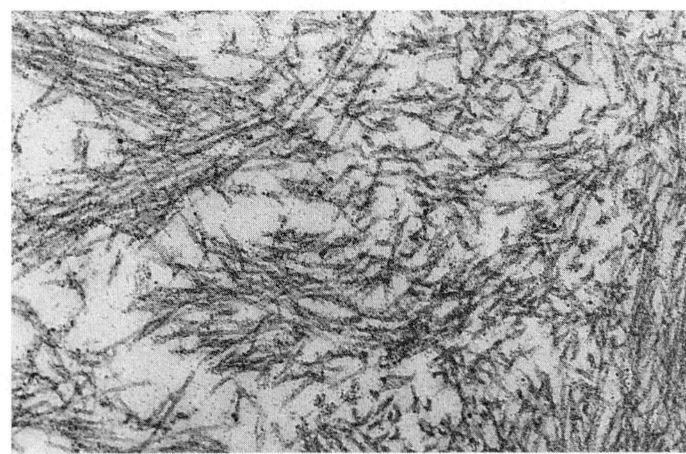

Fig. 20-4 Splenic AA amyloid fibrils showing their characteristic 7 to 10 nm diameter nonbranching nature and organization into occasional parallel bundles.

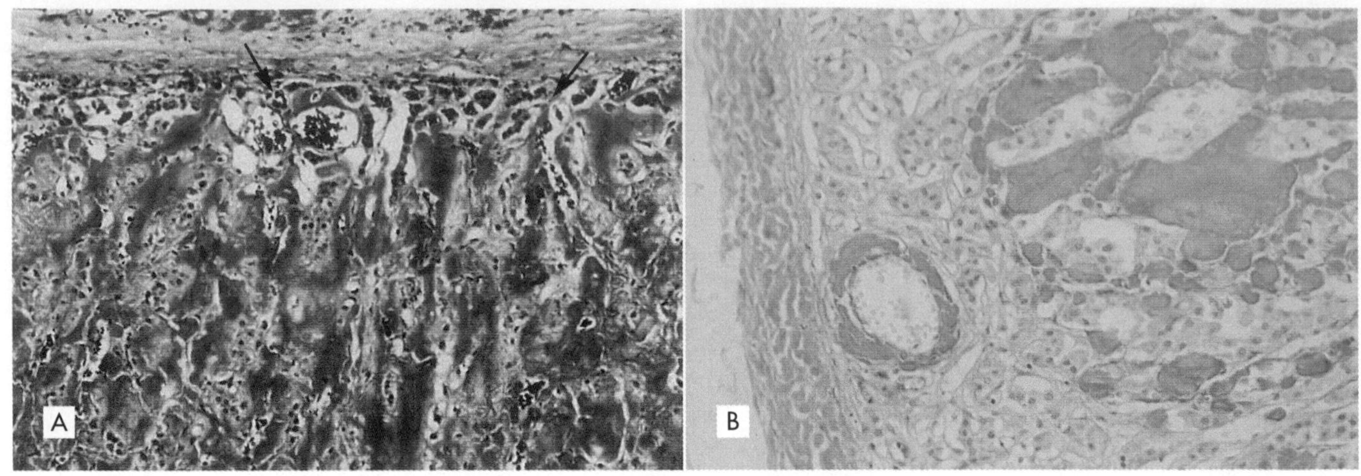

Fig. 20-5 **A,** Microscopic appearance of adrenal amyloid stained with hematoxylin, phloxine, and saffron. Notice the remnants of atrophic adrenocortical cells under the capsule *(arrows)* and replacement of essentially all the cortex by amorphous deposits of AA amyloid. **B,** A sulfated Alcian blue stain of adrenal amyloid illustrating the sulfated glycosaminoglycans present in all amyloid deposits.

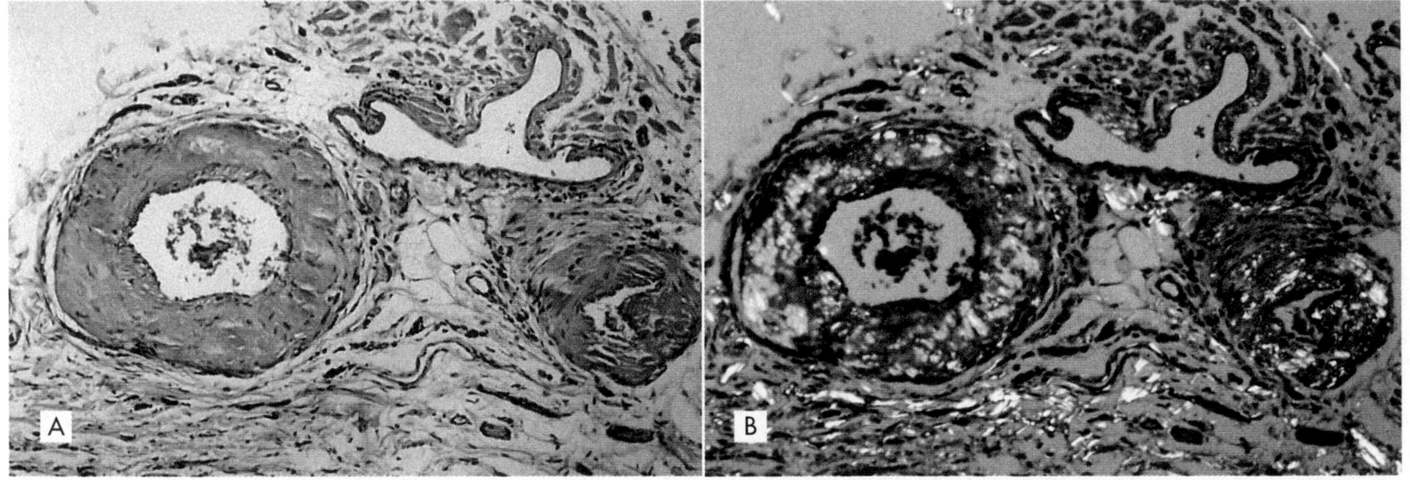

Fig. 20-6 **A,** Congo red staining of a sections of mesenteric blood vessels infiltrated with AL amyloid. **B,** Same sections as in **A,** but viewed in crossed polarized filters. Notice the red-green birefringence of amyloid and the silvery appearance of collagen.

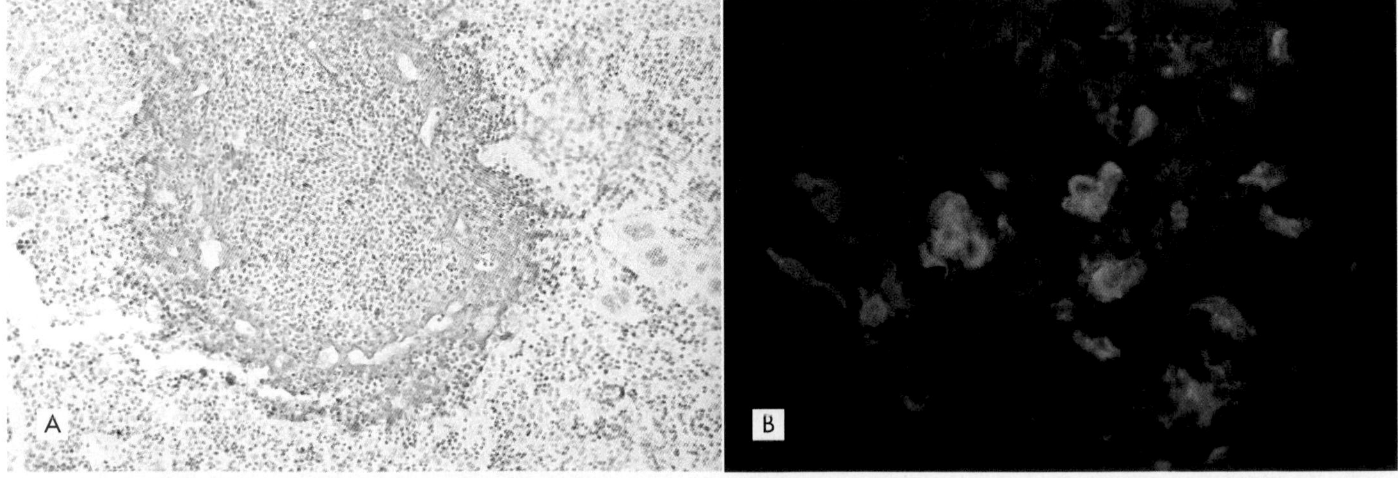

Fig. 20-7 **A,** Immunohistochemical demonstration of AA amyloid in murine spleen with the use of rabbit anti–murine AA antisera. Notice the perifollicular distribution of the deposit and the close topographic relationship of the deposit to capillaries in this area. **B,** Immunofluorescence of glomerular AL amyloid with anti–human lambda-light-chain antisera.

Table 20-2 Staining characteristics of amyloid

Stain	Appearance of amyloid	Diagnostic utility
H&E/HPS*	Pink, hyaline, amorphous	Nonspecific
Methyl violet or crystal violet	Metachromasia	Nonspecific
Thioflavine T or thioflavine S	Secondary fluorescence under ultraviolet radiation	Nonspecific but is the most sensitive screening test
Sulfated Alcian blue	Blue-green	Nonspecific but may be useful as a screening test
Congo red	Red-green birefringence under polarized light	Definitive diagnostic test
Immunohistochemistry using antibody specific for fibril protein	Positive immunoreactivity	Allows classification of type of amyloid

*Hematoxylin and eosin/hematoxylin, phloxine, and saffron.

basement membranes. Early amyloid deposits in the spleen are associated with capillaries and reticuloendothelial cells in the marginal zone of the lymphoid follicles. Hepatic deposits begin in the space of Disse of the centrilobular region. All compartments of the kidney may be involved in established cases of renal amyloidosis. Initial renal deposits appear to occur in the subendothelial zone of glomerular capillaries and the mesangium, but deposits are often also abundant in the peritubular basement membrane zone and parenchymal blood vessels. In the carpal tunnel syndrome associated with AL or Aβ_2M amyloids, deposits are present in the synovium, tendon sheaths, ligaments, and perineural tissue of the wrist. Interstitial deposition occurs in the heart where amyloid surrounds and isolates myofibers. Amyloid may deposit in cardiac valves as well as in both small intramyocardial and major coronary arteries.

In general, the progressive deposition of amyloid follows the stromal architecture of the involved organ. As it accumulates, amyloid isolates parenchymal cells and interferes with normal circulation, leading to striking atrophy in advanced cases (Fig. 20-5). Nonetheless, the volume of amyloid must be considerable before organ function is significantly impaired.

CLINICAL FEATURES

Amyloidosis is not an esoteric pathologic process. In aggregate, the amyloidoses are a significant cause of morbidity and mortality in Western countries. Alzheimer's disease is likely the most prevalent form of amyloidosis in North America and represents the fourth leading cause of death in the United States.[87,88] Cerebral congophilic angiopathy, in which beta-amyloid deposition is restricted to cerebral blood vessels, is a common cause of spontaneous intracerebral hemorrhage.[87,89,90] β_2-Microglobulin amyloidosis is a clinically important complication of chronic hemodialysis, the incidence of which approaches 100% in patients dialyzed for 15 to 20 years.[91-94] AL amyloidosis develops in 15% to 20% of patients with multiple myeloma, and AA amyloid deposition complicates numerous chronic inflammatory disorders, particularly the rheumatic diseases.[95-96]

Amyloid deposition is also a feature of several other extremely common chronic diseases, though the role amyloid may play in their pathogenesis remains uncertain. Examples include IAPP amyloid, which is deposited in the pancreatic islets of Langerhans in 90% to 95% of cases of type II diabetes mellitus,[97,98] the isolated atrial natriuretic factor amyloid deposits that are very common in the failing and aging heart,[99-101] and an as-yet undefined amyloid in the joints of individuals with osteoarthritis.[102]

Because of the variability in the tissue distribution and volume of amyloid deposits that occur between individuals, there are no signs and symptoms that are characteristic of amyloidosis. The clinical presentation of a single patient is determined by the principal sites of amyloid deposition in that individual.[103-105] Symptomatic cardiac amyloidosis typically manifests as congestive heart failure and a low-voltage electrocardiogram, though arrhythmias are significant complications.[106,107] Of clinical importance is the propensity of amyloid to sequester digoxin, which may predispose to digoxin toxicity despite low therapeutic doses.[108] Restrictive cardiomyopathy occurs uncommonly. The hallmark of renal amyloidosis is heavy proteinuria, which is often associated with the nephrotic syndrome,[109,110] but disease progression may cause chronic renal failure. Bence Jones proteinuria is a common feature of AL amyloidosis.[110] Nerve involvement produces peripheral and autonomic neuropathies,[111,112] and the carpal tunnel syndrome is an important manifestation of synovial amyloid deposition.[91-93,113] Malabsorption syndromes, motility disturbances, hemorrhage, and macroglossia may develop secondary to gastrointestinal involvement.[114,115] Hepatic amyloidosis causes organomegaly and may be associated with portal hypertension and jaundice.[116,117] Hyposplenism arises not uncommonly as a consequence of splenic amyloidosis.[110,117,118]

Although the clinical sequelae of the amyloidoses are variable, different forms of amyloidosis do demonstrate certain patterns of tissue involvement. For example, AA amyloid typically presents with renal manifestations and involvement of the spleen and liver.[119] Gastrointestinal involvement is also frequent in AA amyloid, whereas the heart and peripheral nerves are very rarely affected. In contrast, AL amyloid often involves the heart, peripheral nerves, and carpal tissue as well as the abdominal viscera.[104,120] In familial ATTR amyloid, peripheral and autonomic nervous system involvement predominates and carpal tunnel syndrome is common, whereas renal amyloidosis is infrequent and hepatic amyloidosis rare.[121,122] Aβ_2M amyloid affects principally the musculoskeletal system and manifests as carpal tunnel syndrome, spondyloarthopathies, and bone cysts, though gastrointestinal amyloid may occur.[91,92]

Isolated deposits of amyloid may rarely develop at virtually any site in the body. The best recognized form of localized amyloid is witnessed in the stroma of medullary carcinoma of the thyroid and is composed of procalcitonin.[123,124] Amyloid is an important diagnostic feature of this tumor (Chapter 61). However, the most common sites of localized amyloidosis are the lungs, genitourinary tract, and skin.[124-126] Such isolated amyloid deposits are often composed of immunoglobulin light chains yet are rarely a manifestation of systemic AL amyloidosis.

DIAGNOSIS

Although certain groupings of clinical signs and symptoms may be highly suggestive of amyloidosis in an individual patient, a definitive diagnosis requires the histologic identification of tissue deposits of amyloid, which demonstrate typical red-green birefringence after Congo red staining. It is important to recognize that small amounts of amorphous eosinophilic amyloid can be very difficult to detect in sections stained with hematoxylin and eosin. This is especially true in specimens such as tenosynovium in which the presence of amyloid may not be anticipated by the pathologist. Pertinent clinical information can be very useful in suggesting the diagnosis in such cases.

A biopsy of any involved tissue may be diagnostic. Renal and hepatic biopsies have a high positive yield in most forms of systemic amyloidosis.[127,128] However, hemorrhage is a significant complication of biopsy of amyloidotic visceral organs because of the propensity of amyloid to involve blood vessels and the frequent association of abnormalities in hemostasis with amyloidosis.[129] Consequently, although renal, cardiac, or hepatic biopsies may be required to make a diagnosis in specific cases, biopsies of more easily accessible sites by relatively noninvasive techniques should be used in the initial work-up of the patient with suspected amyloidosis.

Rectal biopsy is a widely implemented, sensitive technique for the diagnosis of systemic amyloidosis.[103,119,127,130] Needle aspiration of subcutaneous abdominal fat is also becoming a commonly used initial screening procedure. A diagnostic sensitivity that can approach that of rectal biopsy, high specificity, and positive predictive value, simplicity, and minimal invasiveness combine to make needle aspiration of subcutaneous fat a useful initial test.[131-134] However, the interpretation of these specimens is associated with certain caveats. For instance, the diagnostic sensitivity of rectal biopsy is dependent on the presence of submucosa. As well, numerous amyloids have limited distributions. For instance, extra-articular involvement in Aβ_2M amyloidosis is typically minor, and fat aspiration and rectal biopsy are consequently inadequately sensitive to make this diagnosis.[92,93] Similarly, AA amyloid caused by familial Mediterranean fever does not appear to form in subcutaneous fat.[135] Despite these shortcomings, these techniques will provide diagnostic material in the majority of cases. Other readily accessible sites that may provide diagnostic material in individual cases include bone marrow and labial salivary glands.[119,136]

The role of the pathologist does not end with the documentation of amyloid in a tissue biopsy. The identification of the specific type of amyloid is important because it may have significant prognostic and therapeutic ramifications. For example, systemic AL amyloidosis may be treated with chemotherapy, whereas the diagnosis of ATTR amyloidosis could result in the identification of a kindred of familial amyloidosis and the consequent need for genetic counseling.

Clinical information may indicate the type of amyloid present in a biopsy. A history of multiple myeloma is suggestive of AL amyloid; individuals receiving chronic hemodialysis are prone to Aβ_2M amyloid; and an intercurrent chronic inflammatory disease raises the possibility of AA amyloid. However, regardless of the clinical setting, the pathologist should attempt to classify the amyloid using ancillary techniques. Serum and urine immunoelectrophoresis should be recommended to search for an M protein, the presence of which would substantiate but not prove a diagnosis of AL amyloid. Congo red staining of certain amyloids is potassium permanganate sensitive, whereas others are resistant.[105] However, this characteristic is not specific and cannot be used reliably in a diagnostic setting. Whenever possible, the type of amyloid should be defined by immunohistochemistry using commercially available antibodies specific for a variety of fibril proteins including light chains, transthyretin, β_2-microglobulin, and the AA peptide.[120,137-139]

Diagnostic molecular genetics has become important in the clinical approach to kindreds of heritable amyloidoses such as the familial amyloidotic polyneuropathies.[140-143] In these autosomal dominant diseases, the underlying point mutations in the genes encoding the fibril proteins may be defined, and these data are used to allow genetic counseling and prenatal diagnosis in affected families. Although familial amyloidoses are rare, the diagnosis of ATTR amyloid in a tissue specimen should lead to a consideration of whether a molecular genetic work-up is warranted. These issues are also relevant to familial forms of Alzheimer's disease and hereditary cerebral amyloid angiopathy associated with cerebral hemorrhages.[144-147]

An emerging and potentially very important adjunct in amyloid diagnosis is ^{125}I-SAP scintigraphy.[53,148] In this nuclear medicine technique, the avid binding of SAP to amyloid deposits is exploited to allow identification of amyloidotic tissues in vivo in a noninvasive fashion. This technology may contribute to the diagnosis of amyloidosis and will facilitate the monitoring of the course of treated and untreated disease.

REFERENCES

1. Virchow R: Zur Cellulosefrage, *Virchows Arch Pathol Anat Physiol* 6:416, 1854.

Classification

2. Kazatchkine MD, Husby G, Araki S et al: Nomenclature of amyloid and amyloidosis—WHO-IUIS Nomenclature Sub-Committee, *Bull WHO* 71:105, 1993.
3. Pepys MB, Hawkins PN, Booth DR et al: Human lysozyme gene mutations cause hereditary systemic amyloidosis, *Nature* 362:553, 1993.
4. Benson MD, Liepnieks J, Uemichi T et al: Hereditary renal amyloidosis associated with a mutant fibrinogen alpha-chain, *Nat Genet* 3:252, 1993.

Amyloidogenesis

5. Kanda Y, Goodman DS, Canfield RE et al: The amino acid sequence of human plasma prealbumin, *J Biol Chem* 249:6796, 1974.
6. Robbins J, Rall JE: Proteins associated with the thyroid hormones, *Physiol Rev* 40:415, 1960.

7. Kanai M, Raz A, Goodman DS: Retinol-binding protein: the transport protein for vitamin A in human plasma, *J Clin Invest* 47:2025, 1968.
8. Saraiva MJM, Birken S, Costa PP et al: Amyloid fibril protein in familial amyloidotic polyneuropathy, Portuguese type: definition of molecular abnormality in transthyretin (prealbumin), *J Clin Invest* 74:104, 1984.
9. Araki S, Ikegawa S: Transthyretin and apoA-I amyloidosis. In Kisilevsky R, Benson MD, Frangione B et al, editors: *Amyloid and amyloidosis 1993,* Park Ridge, NJ, 1994, The Parthenon Publishing Group.
10. Benson MD: Inherited amyloidosis, *J Med Genet* 28:73, 1991.
11. Yoshioka K, Miki T, Katsuya T et al: The 717Val→Ile substitution in amyloid precursor protein is associated with familial Alzheimer's disease regardless of ethnic groups, *Biochem Biophys Res Commun* 178:1141, 1991.
12. Crawford F, Hardy J, Mullan M et al: Sequencing of exons 16 and 17 of the beta-amyloid precursor protein gene in 14 families with early onset Alzheimer's disease fails to reveal mutations in the beta-amyloid sequence, *Neurosci Lett* 133:1, 1991.
13. Gajdusek DC, Beyreuther K, Brown P et al: Regulation and genetic control of brain amyloid, *Brain Res Rev* 16:83, 1991.
14. Eulitz M, Breuer M, Linke RP: Is the formation of AL-type amyloid promoted by structural pecularities of immunoglobulin L-chains? Primary structure of an amyloidogenic alpha-L-chain, *Biol Chem Hoppe-Seyler* 368:863, 1987.
15. Liepnieks JJ, Dwulet FE, Benson MD: Amino acid sequence of a kappa-I primary (Al) amyloid protein (AND), *Mol Immunol* 27:481, 1990.
16. Kitajima Y, Hirata H, Kagawa Y et al: Partial amino acid sequence of an amyloid fibril protein from nodular primary cutaneous amyloidosis showing homology to lambda-immunoglobulin light chain of variable subgroup-III (A-lambda-III), *J Invest Dermatol* 95:301, 1990.
17. Goldfarb LG, Brown P, Haltia M et al: Synthetic peptides corresponding to different mutated regions of the amyloid gene in familial Creutzfeldt-Jakob disease show enhanced in vitro formation of morphologically different amyloid fibrils, *Proc Natl Acad Sci USA* 90:4451, 1993.
18. Maury CPJ, Rossi H, Nurmiaho-Lassila EL: Accelerated amyloid formation of peptides homologous to mutant ASN-187 or TYR-187 gelsolin. In Kisilevsky R, Benson MD, Frangione B, et al, editors: *Amyloid and amyloidosis 1993,* Park Ridge, NJ, 1994, The Parthenon Publishing Group.
19. Husby G, Araki S, Benditt EP et al: The 1990 guidelines for nomenclature and classification of amyloid and amyloidosis. In Natvig JB, Førre O, Husby G, et al, editors: *Amyloid and amyloidosis 1990,* Dordrecht, 1991, Kluwer Academic Publishers.
20. Lian JB, Skinner M, Benson MD et al: Fractionation of primary amyloid fibrils: characterization and chemical interaction of the subunits, *Biochim Biophys Acta* 491:167, 1977.
21. Ericsson LH, Eriksen N, Walsh KA et al: Primary structure of duck amyloid protein A: the form deposited in tissues may be identical to its serum precursor, *FEBS Lett* 218:11, 1987.
22. Perry G, Lipphardt S, Mulvihill P et al: Amyloid precursor protein in senile plaques of Alzheimer disease, *Lancet* 2:746, 1988.
23. Tagliavini F, Ghiso J, Timmers WF et al: Coexistence of Alzheimer's amyloid precursor protein and amyloid protein in cerebral vessel walls, *Lab Invest* 62:761, 1990.
24. Kirschner DA, Inouye H, Duffy LK et al: Synthetic peptide homologous to B protein from Alzheimer disease forms amyloid-like fibrils in vitro, *Proc Natl Acad Sci USA* 84:6953, 1987.
25. Connors LH, Shirahama T, Skinner M et al: In vitro formation of amyloid fibrils from intact beta-2–microglobulin, *Biochem Biophys Res Commun* 131:1063, 1985.
26. Mackiewicz A, Speroff T, Ganapathi MK et al: Effects of cytokine combinations on acute phase protein production in two human hepatoma cell lines, *J Immunol* 146:3032, 1991.
27. Ganapathi MK, Rzewnicki D, Samols D et al: Effect of combinations of cytokines and hormones on synthesis of serum amyloid-A and C-reactive protein in HEP 3B-cells, *J Immunol* 147:1261, 1991.
28. Edbrooke MR, Burt DW, Cheshire JK et al: Identification of *cis*-acting sequences responsible for phorbol ester induction of human serum amyloid A gene expression via a nuclear factor kB-like transcription factor, *Mol Cell Biol* 9:1908, 1989.
29. Li XX, Liao WSL: Cooperative effects of C/EBP-like and NFchiB-like binding sites on rat serum amyloid A1 gene expression in liver cells, *Nucl Acid Res* 20:4765, 1992.
30. Benditt EP, Eriksen N, Hanson RH: Amyloid protein SAA is an apoprotein of mouse plasma high density lipoprotein, *Proc Natl Acad Sci USA* 76:4092, 1979.
31. Westermark P, Sletten K, Johansson B et al: Fibril in senile systemic amyloidosis is derived from normal transthyretin, *Proc Natl Acad Sci USA* 87:2843, 1990.
32. McAdam KPWJ, Elin RJ, Sipe JD et al: Changes in human serum amyloid-A and C-reactive protein after etiocholanolone-induced inflammation, *J Clin Invest* 61:390, 1978.
33. Morrow JF, Stearman RS, Peltzman CG et al: Induction of hepatic synthesis of serum amyloid A protein and actin, *Proc Natl Acad Sci USA* 78:4718, 1981.
34. Kisilevsky R, Subrahmanyan L: Serum amyloid A changes high density lipoprotein's cellular affinity: a clue to serum amyloid A's principal function, *Lab Invest* 66:778, 1992.
35. Snow AD, Kisilevsky R: Temporal relationship between glycosaminoglycan accumulation and amyloid deposition during experimental amyloidosis: a histochemical study, *Lab Invest* 53:37, 1985.
36. Lyon AW, Narindrasorasak S, Young ID et al: Co-deposition of basement membrane components during the induction of murine splenic AA amyloid, *Lab Invest* 64:785, 1991.
37. Hardt F, Ranlov P: Transfer amyloidosis, *Int Rev Exp Pathol* 16:273, 1976.
38. Kisilevsky R, Axelrad MA, Corbett WEN, et al: The role of inflammatory cells in the pathogenesis of amyloidosis, *Lab Invest* 37:544, 1977.
39. Varga J, Flinn MS, Shirahama T et al: The induction of accelerated murine amyloid with human splenic extract: probable role of amyloid enhancing factor, *Virchows Arch [B]* 51:177, 1986.
40. Ali-Khan Z, Quirion R, Robitaille Y et al: Evidence for increased amyloid enhancing factor activity in Alzheimer brain extract, *Acta Neuropathol* 77:82, 1988.
41. Cathcart ES, Sipe JD, Gonnerman WA et al: Amyloid resistance in the CE/J mouse. In Kisilevsky R, Benson MD, Frangione B, et al, editors: *Amyloid and amyloidosis 1993,* Park Ridge, NJ, 1994, The Parthenon Publishing Group.
42. Axelrad MA, Kisilevsky R, Willmer J et al: Further characterization of amyloid enhancing factor, *Lab Invest* 47:139, 1982.
43. Niewold ThA, Hol PR, van Andel ACJ et al: Enhancement of amyloid induction by amyloid fibril fragments in hamster, *Lab Invest* 56:544, 1987.
44. Shirahama T, Abraham CR, Ju ST et al: Isolation of a 16kD fraction with extremely high AEF activity. In Natvig JB, Førre O, Husby G, et al, editors: *Amyloid and amyloidosis 1990,* Dordrecht, 1991, Kluwer Academic Publishers.
45. Le PT, Mortensen RF: In vitro induction of hepatocyte synthesis of the acute phase reactant mouse serum amyloid P component by macrophages and IL 1, *J Leukoc Biol* 35:587, 1984.
46. Pepys MB, Baltz M, Gomer K et al: Serum amyloid P component is an acute-phase reactant in the mouse, *Nature* 278:259, 1979.
47. Pepys MB, Baltz ML: Acute phase proteins with special reference to C-reactive protein and related proteins (pentaxins) and serum amyloid A protein, *Adv Immunol* 34:141, 1983.
48. Baltz ML, Caspi D, Evans DJ et al: Circulating amyloid P component is the precursor of amyloid P component in tissue amyloid deposits, *Clin Exp Immunol* 66:691, 1986.
49. Tape C, Tan R, Nesheim M et al: Direct evidence for circulating apoSAA as the precursor of tissue AA amyloid deposits, *Scand J Immunol* 28:317, 1988.
50. Bladen HA, Nylen MU, Glenner GG: The ultrastructure of human amyloid as revealed by the negative staining technique, *J Ultrastruct Res* 14:449, 1966.
51. Hamazaki H: Calcium-mediated hemagglutination by serum amyloid P component and the inhibition by specific glycosaminoglycans, *Biochem Biophys Res Commun* 150:212, 1988.
52. Hawkins PN, Myers MJ, Lavender JP et al: Diagnostic radionuclide imaging of amyloid: biological targeting by circulating human serum amyloid P component, *Lancet* 1:1413, 1988.

53. Hawkins PN, Lavender JP, Pepys MB: Evaluation of systemic amyloidosis by scintigraphy with I-123-labeled serum amyloid-P component, *N Engl J Med* 323:508, 1990.
54. Nelson SR, Hawkins PN, Richardson S et al: Imaging of haemodialysis-associated amyloidosis with I-123-serum amyloid-P component, *Lancet* 338:335, 1991.
55. Snow AD, Bramson R, Mar H et al: A temporal and ultrastructural relationship between heparan sulfate proteoglycans and AA amyloid in experimental amyloidosis, *J Histochem Cytochem* 39:1321, 1991.
56. Snow AD, Kisilevsky R: A close ultrastructural relationship between sulphated proteoglycans and AA amyloid fibrils, *Lab Invest* 57:687, 1988.
57. Schultz RT, Pintha JV, McDonald T et al: Ultrastructural studies of vascular lesions in experimental amyloidosis in mice, *Am J Pathol* 119:138, 1985.
58. Mooradian AD: Effects of aging on the blood brain barrier, *Neurobiol Aging* 9:31, 1988.
59. Horiguchi Y, Fine JD, Leigh IM et al: Lamina densa malformation involved in histogenesis of primary localized cutaneous amyloidosis, *J Invest Dermatol* 99:12, 1992.
60 Yamaguchi H, Yamazaki T, Lemere CA et al: Beta-amyloid is focally deposited within the outer basement membrane in the amyloid angiopathy of Alzheimer's disease: an immunoelectron microscopic study, *Am J Pathol* 141:249, 1992.
61. Schultz RT, Pintha J: Relation of the hepatic and splenic microcirculations to the development of lesions in experimental amyloidosis, *Am J Pathol* 119:127, 1985.
62. Niewold TA, Landeira JMF, Vandenheuvel LPWJ et al: Characterization of Proteoglycans and glycosaminoglycans in bovine renal AA-type amyloidosis, *Virchows Arch [B]* 60:321, 1991.
63. Kisilevsky R, Lyon AW, Young ID: A critical analysis of postulated pathogenetic mechanisms in amyloidogenesis, *Crit Rev Clin Lab Sci* 29:59, 1992.
64. Perlmutter LS, Barron E, Saperia D et al: Association between vascular basement membrane components and the lesions of Alzheimer's disease, *J Neurosci Res* 30:673, 1991.
65. Narindrasorasak S, Lowery DE, Altman RA et al: Characterization of high affinity binding between laminin and the Alzheimer's disease amyloid precursor proteins, *Lab Invest* 67:643, 1992.
66. Karsenty G, Ulmann A, Droz D et al: Clinical and histological resolution of systemic amyloidosis after renal cell carcinoma removal, *Kidney Int* 27:232, 1985.
67. Wegelius O: The resolution of amyloid substance, *Acta Med Scand* 212:273, 1982.
68. Tang AL, Davies DR, Wing AJ: Remission of nephrotic syndrome in amyloidosis associated with a hypernephroma, *Clin Nephrol* 32:225, 1989.
69. Edwards P, Cooper DA, Turner J et al: Resolution of amyloidosis (AA type) complicating chronic ulcerative colitis, *Gastroenterology* 95:810, 1988.
70. Shirahama T, Cohen AS: Redistribution of amyloid deposits, *Am J Pathol* 99:539, 1980.

Pathology

71. Cohen AS, Calkins E: Electron microscopic observations on fibrous component in amyloid of diverse origins, *Nature* 183:1202, 1959.
72. Shirahama T, Cohen AS: High resolution electron microscopic analysis of the amyloid fibril, *J Cell Biol* 33:679, 1967.
73. Gorevic PD, Goni F, Pons-Estel B et al: Isolation and partial characterization of neurofibrillary tangles and amyloid plaque core in Alzheimer's disease: immunohistological studies, *J Neuropathol Exp Neurol* 45:647, 1986.
74. Kidd M: Alzheimer's disease: an electron microscopical study, *Brain* 87:307, 1964.
75. Casey TT, Stone WW, DiRaimondo CR et al: Tumoral amyloidosis of bone of beta-2-microglobulin origin in association with long-term hemodialysis: a new type of amyloid disease, *Hum Pathol* 17:731, 1986.
76. Gorevic PD, Casey TT, Stone WJ et al: Beta-2 microglobulin is an amyloidogenic protein in man, *J Clin Invest* 76:2425, 1985.
77. Glenner GG: Amyloid deposits and amyloidosis: the B-fibrilloses. Parts I and II, *N Engl J Med* 302:1283, 1980.
78. Lansbury PT: In pursuit of the molecular structure of amyloid plaque—new technology provides unexpected and critical information, *Biochemistry* 31:6865, 1992.
79. Pepys, MB: Amyloid P-component: structure and properties. In Marrink J, Van Rijswijk MH, editors: *Amyloidosis*, Dordrecht, 1986, Martinus Nijhoff.
80. Pinteric L, Painter RH: Electron microscopy of serum amyloid protein in the presence of calcium: alternative forms of assembly of pentagonal molecules in two-dimensional lattices, *Can J Biochem* 57:727, 1979.
81. Snow AD, Willmer J, Kisilevsky R: Sulphated glycosaminoglycans: a common constituent of all amyloids? *Lab Invest* 56:120, 1987.
82. Snow AD, Willmer J, Kisilevsky R: Sulphated glycosaminoglycans in Alzheimer's disease, *Hum Pathol* 18:506, 1987.
83. Snow AD, Kisilevsky R, Willmer J et al: Sulfated glycosaminoglycans in amyloid plaques of prion diseases, *Acta Neuropathol* 77:337, 1989.
84. Young ID, Willmer JP, Kisilevsky R: The ultrastructural localization of sulfated proteoglycans is identical in the amyloids of Alzheimer's disease and AA, AL, senile cardiac and medullary carcinoma–associated amyloidosis, *Acta Neuropathol* 78:202, 1989.
85. Snow AD, Lara S, Nochlin D et al: Cationic dyes reveal proteoglycans structurally integrated within the characteristic lesions of Alzheimer's disease, *Acta Neuropathol* 78:113, 1989.
86. Glenner GG, Page DL: Amyloid, amyloidosis, and amyloidogenesis, *Int Rev Exp Pathol* 15:2, 1976.

Clinical features

87. Vinters HV, Miller BL, Pardridge WM: Brain amyloid and Alzheimer's disease, *Ann Intern Med* 109:41, 1988.
88. Mozar HN, Bal DG, Howard JT: Perspectives on the etiology of Alzheimer's disease, *JAMA* 257:1503, 1987.
89. Mandybur TI: Cerebral amyloid angiopathy: the vascular pathology and complications, *J Neuropathol Exp Neurol* 45:70, 1986.
90. Vinters HV: Cerebral amyloid angiopathy: a critical review, *Stroke* 18:311, 1987.
91. Gejyo F, Homma N, Arakawa M: Long-term complications of dialysis: pathogenic factors with special reference to amyloidosis, *Kidney Int* 43:S78, 1993.
92. Koch KM, Gennari FJ, Vanypersele C et al: Dialysis-related amyloidosis, *Kidney Int* 41:1416, 1992.
93. Floege J, Schaffer J, Koch KM et al: Dialysis related amyloidosis: a disease of chronic retention and inflammation, *Kidney Int* 42:S78, 1992.
94. Honkanen E, Grönhagen-Riska C, Teppo AM et al: Acute-phase proteins during hemodialysis: correlations with serum interleukin-1β levels and different dialysis membranes, *Nephron* 57:283, 1991.
95. Buxbaum J: Mechanisms of disease—monoclonal Immunoglobulin deposition—amyloidosis, light chain deposition disease, and light and heavy chain deposition disease, *Hematol Oncol Clin North Am* 6:323, 1992.
96. Dhillon V, Woo P, Isenberg D: Amyloidosis in the rheumatic diseases, *Ann Rheum Dis* 48:696, 1989.
97. Westermark P, Wilander E, Westermark GT et al: Islet amyloid polypeptide–like immunoreactivity in the islet B-cells of type-2 (non–insulin-dependent) diabetic and non-diabetic individuals, *Diabetologia* 30:887, 1987.
98. Westermark P, Johnson KH, Obrien TD et al: Islet amyloid polypeptide: a novel controversy in diabetes research, *Diabetologia* 35:297, 1992.
99. Gibbons G, Cornwell GG, Murdoch WL et al: Frequency and distribution of senile cardiovascular amyloid, *Am J Med* 75:618, 1983.
100. Hodkinson HM, Pomerance A: The clinical significance of senile cardiac amyloidosis: a prospective clinico-pathological study, *Q J Med* 46:381, 1977.
101. Steiner I: The prevalence of isolated atrial amyloid, *J Pathol* 153:395, 1987.
102. Egan MS, Goldenberg DL, Cohen AS et al: The association of amyloid deposits and osteoarthritis, *Arthritis Rheum* 25:204, 1982.
103. Kyle RA, Bayrd ED: Amyloidosis: a review of 236 cases, *Medicine* 54:271, 1975.

104. Kyle RA, Greipp PR: Amyloidosis (AL): clinical and laboratory features in 229 cases, *J Soc Med* 76:665, 1983.
105. Wright JR, Calkins E: Clinical-pathologic differentiation of common amyloid syndromes, *Medicine* 60:429, 1981.
106. Buja LM, Khoi NB, Roberts WC: Clinically significant cardiac amyloidosis: clinicopathologic findings in 15 patients, *Am J Cardiol* 26:394, 1970.
107. Roberts WC, Waller BF: Cardiac amyloidosis causing cardiac dysfunction: analysis of 54 necropsy patients, *Am J Cardiol* 52:137, 1983.
108. Rubinow A, Skinner M, Cohen AS: Digoxin sensitivity in amyloid cardiomypathy, *Circulation* 63:1285, 1981.
109. Triger DR, Joekes AM: Renal amyloidosis: a fourteen year follow-up, *Q J Med* 42:15, 1973.
110. Stone MJ, Frenkel EP: The clinical spectrum of light chain myeloma: a study of 35 patients with special reference to the occurrence of amyloidosis, *Am J Med* 58:601, 1975.
111. Kelley JJ, Kyle RA, O'Brien PC et al: The natural history of peripheral neuropathy in primary systemic amyloidosis, *Ann Neurol* 6:1, 1979.
112. Kyle RA, Kottke BA, Schirger A: Orthostatic hypotension as a clue to primary systemic amyloidosis, *Circulation* 34:883, 1966.
113. Kyle RA, Eilers SG, Linscheid RL et al: Amyloid localized to tenosynovium at carpal tunnel release, *Am J Clin Pathol* 91:393, 1989.
114. French JM, Hall G, Parish DJ et al: Peripheral and autonomic nerve involvement in primary amyloidosis associated with uncontrollable diarrhea and steatorrhea, *Am J Med* 39:277, 1965.
115. Battle WM, Rubin MR, Cohen S et al: Gastrointestinal motility dysfunction in systemic amyloidosis, *N Engl J Med* 301:24, 1979.
116. Levine RA: Amyloid disease of the liver: correlation of clinical, functional, and morphologic features in forty-seven patients, *Am J Med* 33:349, 1962.
117. Gertz MA, Kyle RA: Hepatic amyloidosis (primary [AL], immunoglobulin light chain): the natural history in 80 patients, *Am J Med* 85:73, 1988.
118. Gertz MA, Kyle RA, Greipp PR: Hyposplenism in primary systemic amyloidosis, *Ann Intern Med* 98:475, 1983.
119. Gertz MA: Secondary amyloidosis (AA), *J Intern Med* 232:517, 1992.
120. Kyle RA, Gertz MA, Linke RP: Amyloid localized to tenosynovium at carpal tunnel release immunohistochemical identification of amyloid type, *Am J Clin Pathol* 97:250, 1992.
121. Gertz MA, Kyle RA, Thibodeau SN: Familial amyloidosis: a study of 52 North American born patients examined during a 30-year period, *Mayo Clin Proc* 67:428, 1992.
122. Reilly MM, King RHM: Familial amyloid polyneuropathy, *Brain Pathol* 3:165, 1993.
123. Sletten K, Westermark P, Natvig JB: Characterization of amyloid fibril proteins from medullary carcinoma of the thyroid, *J Exp Med* 143:993, 1976.
124. Tariq SM, Morrison D, McConnochie K: Solitary bronchial amyloid presenting with haemoptysis, *Eur Respir J* 3:1230, 1990.
125. Ehara H, Deguchi T, Yanagihara M et al: Primary localized amyloidosis of the bladder: an immunohistochemical study of a case, *J Urol* 147:458, 1992.
126. Okuzono Y, Gondoh T, Kawano H et al: Histopathology of cutaneous amyloid: a comparative study on 144 cases of localized cutaneous amyloidosis and 20 cases of systemic amyloidosis. In Glenner GG, Osserman EF, Benditt EP, et al, editors: *Amyloidosis,* New York, 1986, Plenum Press.

Diagnosis

127. Blum A, Sohar E: The diagnosis of amyloidosis: ancillary procedures, *Lancet* 1:721, 1962.
128. Stauffer MH, Gross JB, Foulk WT et al: Amyloidosis: diagnosis with needle biopsy of the liver in 18 patients, *Gastroenterology* 41:92, 1961.
129. Yood RA, Skinner M, Rubinow A et al: Bleeding manifestations in 100 patients with amyloidosis, *JAMA* 249:1322, 1983.
130. Tribe CR, MacKenzie JC: *The kidney and rheumatic diseases,* London, 1982, Butterworth.
131. Duston MA, Skinner M, Meena RF et al: Sensitivity, specificity, and predictive value of abdominal fat pad aspiration for the diagnosis of amyloidosis, *Arthritis Rheum* 32:82, 1989.
132. Blumenfeld W, Hildebrandt RH: Fine needle aspiration of abdominal fat for the diagnosis of amyloidosis, *Acta Cytol* 37:170, 1993.
133. Libbey CA, Skinner M, Cohen AS: Use of abdominal fat tissue aspirate in the diagnosis of systemic amyloidosis, *Arch Intern Med* 143:1549, 1983.
134. Duston MA, Skinner M, Shirahama T et al: Diagnosis of amyloidosis by abdominal fat aspiration: analysis of four years' experience, *Am J Med* 82:412, 1987.
135. Tishler M, Pras M, Yaron M: Abdominal fat tissue aspirate in amyloidosis of familial Mediterranean fever, *Clin Exp Rheumatol* 6:395, 1988.
136. Delgado WA, Mosqueda A: A highly sensitive method for diagnosis of secondary amyloidosis by labial salivary gland biopsy, *J Oral Pathol* 18:310, 1989.
137. Ii K, Kyle RA, Dyck PJ: Immunohistochemical characterization of amyloid proteins in sural nerves and clinical associations in amyloid neuropathy, *Am J Pathol* 141:217, 1992.
138. Fitzmaurice RJ, Bartley C, McClure J et al: Immunohistological characterisation of amyloid deposits in renal biopsy specimens, *J Clin Pathol* 44:200, 1991.
139. Donini U, Casanova S, Zucchelli P et al: Immunoelectron microscopic classification of amyloid in renal biopsies, *J Histochem Cytochem* 37:1101, 1989.
140. Nordvåg BY, Husby G, Ranløv I et al: Molecular diagnosis of the transthyretin (TTR) Met111 mutation in familial amyloid cardiomyopathy of Danish origin, *Hum Genet* 89:459, 1992.
141. Nichols WC, Padilla LM, Benson MD: Prenatal detection of a gene for hereditary amyloidosis, *Am J Med Genet* 34:520, 1989.
142. Ii S, Minnerath S, Ii K et al: Two-tiered DNA-based diagnosis of transthyretin amyloidosis reveals two novel point mutations, *Neurology* 41:893, 1991.
143. Morris M, Nichols W, Benson M: Prenatal diagnosis of hereditary amyloidosis in a Portuguese family, *Am J Med Genet* 39:123, 1991.
144. Murrell J, Farlow M, Ghetti B et al: A mutation in the amyloid precursor protein associated with hereditary Alzheimer's disease, *Science* 254:97, 1991.
145. Goate A, Chartier-Harlin MC, Mullan M et al: Segregation of a missense mutation in the amyloid precursor protein gene with familial Alzheimer's disease, *Nature* 349:704, 1991.
146. Bakker E, van Broeckhoven C, Haan J et al: DNA diagnosis for hereditary cerebral hemorrhage with amyloidosis (Dutch type), *Am J Hum Genet* 49:518, 1991.
147. Jonsdottir S, Palsdottir A: Molecular diagnosis of hereditary cystatin-C amyloid angiopathy, *Biochem Med Metab Biol* 49:117, 1993.
148. Hawkins PN, Richardson S, Vigushin DM et al: Serum amyloid-P component scintigraphy and turnover studies for diagnosis and quantitative monitoring of AA-amyloidosis in juvenile rheumatoid arthritis, *Arthritis Rheum* 36:842, 1993.

21 Circulatory Disturbances

Jack L. Titus
Jesse E. Edwards

The circulation serves as a delivery system to the organs and tissues. The system provides substances required for cellular nutrition, respiration (oxygenation), water balance and hormonal regulation, and removal of waste products of cellular metabolism.

The basic requirements for normal function of the circulation are three: normal anatomic features, normal physiologic controls, and normal biochemical composition of the blood. All are needed to maintain normal blood flow and perfusion pressures to tissues. This chapter is a description of the morphologic abnormalities of the circulation and their functional consequences. Physiologic adjustments that lead to variations in cardiac output and vascular resistance to flow are covered concisely by Shepherd and Vanhoutte,[1] among others. Abnormalities of composition of the blood that may affect intravascular colloid osmotic pressure are not discussed in this chapter.

FETAL CIRCULATION

Some disturbances of the circulatory system may result from abnormalities of the fetal circulation and changes in it that occur after birth to constitute the postnatal circulation.

In the fetus, that portion of right atrial blood that is channeled through the tricuspid valve passes through the right ventricle into the pulmonary trunk. From the pulmonary trunk, the major portion of the right ventricular blood is directed through the *ductus arteriosus* to the descending aorta. Only a small amount of blood goes into the left and right pulmonary arteries, and therefore only a small volume of blood passes through the pulmonary vascular bed to reach the pulmonary veins and the left atrium[2] (Fig. 21-1).

The blood that reaches the aorta through the ductus arteriosus flows distally and, for the greater part, into the common iliac arteries and their external iliac arterial branches. Umbilical arteries arise from the homolateral external iliac arteries and proceed via the umbilical cord to the placenta. In the placenta, multiple branchings of the umbilical arteries lead to capillaries in the chorionic villi. At this level, substances are exchanged between the fetal blood within the capillaries of the chorionic villi and the maternal blood in the intervillous spaces of the placenta. Blood from the capillaries in the chorionic villi is then directed into tributaries of the umbilical vein, which enters the fetus at the umbilicus.

The umbilical vein passes from the umbilicus toward the hepatic hilum along a course that becomes the round ligament of the liver after birth. Near the hilum of the liver, the umbilical vein joins the inferior aspect of the left portal vein. Fetal blood crosses the left portal vein and passes into the *ductus venosus*. The ductus venosus connects to the left hepatic vein, thereby completing the route from the umbilical vein to the inferior vena cava and right atrium.

The major portion of the blood of the inferior vena cava is diverted from the right atrium into the left atrium through the foramen ovale. Only a small part of inferior vena caval blood reaches the right ventricle and pulmonary trunk.

Blood that enters the left atrium passes into the left ventricle and the ascending aorta and arch. Most of the blood reaching the aortic arch is distributed to the brain through the branches of the arch. Little flow occurs in the aortic segment between the left subclavian artery and the ductus arteriosus, the *aortic isthmus*.

Venous blood leaving the brain flows through the internal jugular veins to the superior vena cava. The superior vena caval blood is directed toward the tricuspid valve, forming a stream through the right atrium to the right ventricle and pulmonary trunk. As described previously, most of the blood in the pulmonary trunk passes through the ductus arteriosus to the aorta and ultimately to the placenta for reoxygenation.

POSTNATAL CIRCULATION

With birth and separation of the placenta, there is an immediate change in the site for oxygenation of blood from the placenta to the lung. With the first breath, the volume of pulmonary arterial blood flow increases. There follows a corresponding increase in flow of blood to the left atrium from the pulmonary veins. The increased left atrial pressure over the

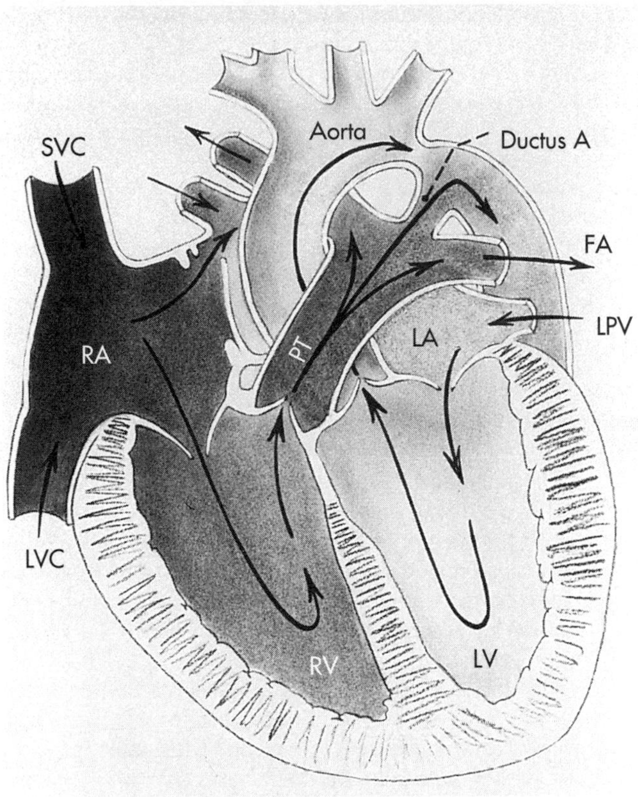

Fig. 21-1 Central circulation in fetus. Blood returning from the inferior vena cava crosses the foramen ovale into the left atrium and left ventricle and goes to the ascending aorta for major distribution through the branches of the aortic arch. Blood returning to the right atrium from the superior vena cava passes to the pulmonary trunk, from which the primary flow is into the ductus arteriosus and descending aorta, ultimately to the placenta for oxygenation. *Ductus A,* ductus arteriosus; *IVC,* inferior vena cava; *LA,* left atrium; *LPA,* left pulmonary artery; *LPV,* left pulmonary vein; *LV,* left ventricle; *RA,* right atrium; *RV,* right ventricle; *SVC,* superior vena cava.

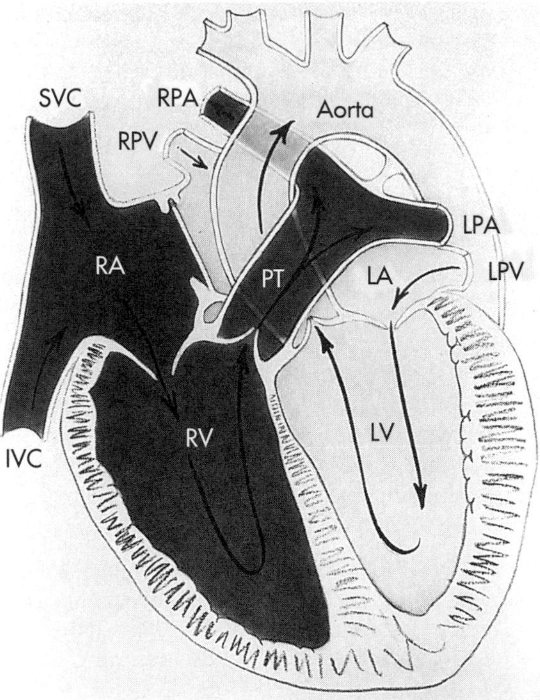

Fig. 21-2 Central circulation in the postnatal state. The foramen ovale is closed, and the ductus arteriosus is obliterated. Abbreviations as in Fig. 21-1.

right atrial pressure causes the flaplike valve of the foramen ovale to press against the atrial septum and prevent trans–atrial septum flow (Fig. 21-2).

In the early hours of postnatal life, the ductus arteriosus functionally closes.[3] In the weeks before birth, the intima of the ductus arteriosus develops multifocal intimal thickenings (ridges) that are cellular with intercellular deposits of mucoid material. These are distributed longitudinally along the intima. In cross section, these ridges appear as pads (Fig. 21-3). These pads participate in the early closure of the ductus, which results from spasm of its wall. By about a month after birth, the ductus has closed anatomically and becomes the *ligamentum arteriosum.*

Before closure of the ductus arteriosus, the systemic and pulmonary arterial pressures are essentially equal. With the initial closure of the ductus arteriosus, the pulmonary vascular resistance falls, as does the pulmonary arterial pressure, so that the normal postnatal differences between systemic and pulmonary arterial pressures develop.

The venous channels that had led from the placenta to the right atrium undergo significant changes postnatally. The umbilical vein, extending from the umbilicus to the left portal vein, undergoes closure by major addition of fibrous tissue to its adventitia. The ductus venosus, connecting the left portal and left hepatic veins, undergoes major intimal fibrous thickening, ultimately forming a fibrous cord, the *ligamentum venosum.*

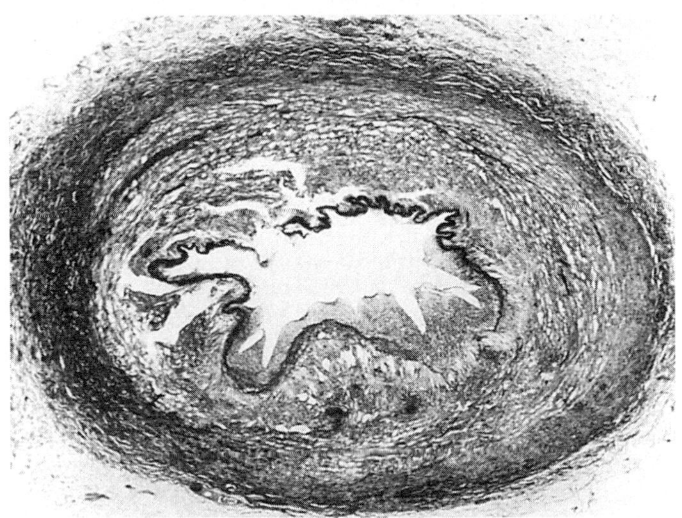

Fig. 21-3 Photomicrograph of ductus arteriosus in a fetus. The cross section shows some intimal accumulations of mucoid connective tissue, which create protrusions toward the lumen. Postnatally, mild contraction of the media is assisted in ductal closure by these protrusions. At a later stage, the lumen of the ductus arteriosus becomes obliterated anatomically.

As the pulmonary arterial pressure falls with closing of the ductus arteriosus, so does the right ventricular pressure. The fetal state in which the two ventricles are of near-equal thickness is followed by progressive, partly relative, thinning of the right ventricular wall. The usual postnatal differences in thickness between the two ventricles is established by about the third postnatal month.

ABNORMALITIES OF CIRCULATION

Normal function of the circulatory system requires the following characteristics:

- Closed systems
- Separation of greater (systemic) and lesser (pulmonic) systems
- Unobstructed pathways for blood flow
- Competent cardiac valves
- Adequate functioning myocardium (pump)
- Normal cardiac rhythm and rate

Deviations from or violation of the normal characteristics result in circulatory disturbances. The following sections show examples considered and consequences of violations of each of the normal characteristics resulting in disease states.

Disruption of closed system: hemorrhage, shock

Anatomic disruption of the closed state of the circulatory systems results in loss of blood from the system, that is, hemorrhage of some type.

Significant hemorrhage may be associated with rupture of large veins, arteries of any size, or cardiac chambers.

Various terms describe the gross morphologic appearance, or anatomic location, or size of hemorrhages confined to the body. *Hematoma* describes a localized collection of blood (*hemat-* 'blood', *oma-*'tumor') within a tissue. Hemorrhagic foci, usually on the skin, or mucus membranes, or serosal surfaces are termed *petechiae* if less than 1 to 2 mm in size, *purpura* for larger foci up to 1.5 cm in diameter, and *ecchymoses* if large, blotchy areas. When the hemorrhage extends into a body cavity, the terms *hemothorax, hemopericardium,* or *hemoperitoneum* designate the anatomic site in which blood accumulates.

Consequences

With hemorrhage, compensatory mechanisms occur to maintain blood pressure and perfusion of tissues. These mechanisms are (1) arteriolar vasoconstriction, which increases vascular resistance, and (2) increased heart rate as an attempt to deliver relatively greater volumes of blood into the circulation.

Blood pressure is the product of the volume of flow and the resistance to flow. Resistance, which is the inverse of capacity, is determined by the state of contraction of the medial muscle of the arterioles. For a given pressure, flow is inversely related to resistance. The same principles apply to cardiac chambers. In the heart, resistance to filling of chambers is attributable to the state of the ventricular wall during diastole. The term *compliance* as applied to the ventricular wall is the inverse of resistance. The greater the diastolic compliance, the less resistance to filling of the cardiac chamber. Ventricular compliance is similar to preload.

The compensatory mechanisms of peripheral vasoconstriction (increased peripheral resistance) may be sufficient to maintain blood pressure and perfusion of tissues, even though the total blood volume is reduced acutely by as much as 15%. With greater blood or fluid losses occurring over a short period of time, hypovolemic shock may occur.

Shock is circulatory collapse that leads to inadequate perfusion of tissues and cells because the effective circulating blood volume is reduced and compensatory mechanisms cannot maintain blood pressure. Shock resulting from decreased blood volume is *hypovolemic shock.* It may follow hemorrhage as described or massive loss of fluids as with major burns, severe diarrhea, or prolonged vomiting. *Cardiogenic shock* describes shock secondary to ineffective pumping of the heart as may result from large myocardial infarcts, cardiac rupture, obstruction to ventricular outflow (such as pulmonary embolism), cardiac arrhythmias, and pericardial tamponade. *Neurogenic shock* results from peripheral vasodilatation, which may accompany injuries to the central nervous system.

Septic shock, as may occur in gram-negative bacterial infections with endotoxin production or massive gram-positive infections, is not synonymous with shock because of hypotension from hypovolemia. In septic shock, endothelial cellular injury and disseminated intravascular coagulation occur. Both the development and progression of septic shock result from a complex array of biochemical substances,[4] which are not discussed in this chapter.

The consequences of shock with inadequate cellular perfusion causes cellular hypoxia and accumulation of metabolites. Initially, cellular injury is reversible, but with prolongation of shock, irreversible cellular injury occurs. The progression of the shock state is from a compensated state to a decompensated stage to an irreversible state, often with vasodilatation and death.

The morphologic abnormalities of shock are the result of cellular hypoxia leading ultimately to cellular death. The organs in which pathologic findings are characteristically present are heart, kidneys, lungs, brain, adrenals, and gastrointestinal tract. In the heart, the lesions related to shock, as opposed to myocardial infarct that may have caused shock, are focal subendocardial and subepicardial interstitial hemorrhage, often with cellular necroses, and small or large, scattered areas of contraction band change (necrosis) of myocardial cells. Acute tubular necrosis of the kidneys is a common finding. In the lungs, diffuse alveolar damage (adult respiratory distress syndrome) characterized by interstitial edema, plasma protein-rich edema fluid in alveoli, and variable degrees of desquamation of alveolar lining cells. Hypoxic encephalopathy may occur. The adrenals often manifest the findings of stress that include lipid depletion of cortical cells with scattered foci of necrosis. Foci of mucosal hemorrhage and cellular necrosis occur in the gastrointestinal tract. Liver cells may have fatty change, and central lobular necrosis may be present. It should be stressed that none of these morphologic abnormalities are entirely specific for shock.

Loss of separation of the greater and lesser circulations

Failure of maintenance of separation of the lesser (pulmonic) and greater (systemic) circulatory systems may be represented by a cardiac septal defect or abnormal communication between major vessels or between vessels and cardiac chambers.

The bases for lack of separation may be either congenital (see Chapter 46) or acquired in origin and either central or peripheral in location.

Acquired abnormal communications may be acute or chronic. Most are acute. Acquired central communications include such states as an aneurysm of the aorta rupturing into a chamber or vessel of the lesser (pulmonic) system. These conditions include rupture of an aortic sinus aneurysm, either congenital or acquired, leading to a communication between the aorta and the right atrium or the ventricle. Rupture of an aortic aneurysm into a pulmonary artery or into the superior vena cava are other examples. Another type of an acquired central communication is that of rupture of the ventricular septum, either traumatic or as a complication of acute myocardial infarction.

The chronic types of central communication include congenital atrial septal defect, ventricular septal defect, and communications of the pulmonary arterial system and the aorta, of which the most common type is patent ductus arteriosus.

Peripheral communications may occur in either the systemic or lesser circulations as communications between one or more arteries and veins of that system, creating pulmonary[5] or systemic[6] *arteriovenous fistulas* (Figs. 21-4).

Consequences

The consequences of the abnormal communication depend, in part, upon the width of the communication and whether it was present at birth. When a communication between the two systems exists, commonly a shunt results. The term *shunt* refers to direct flow of blood from one system to the other. Whether acute or chronic, there are two main types of shunt, depending on whether the flow is from the greater (systemic) into the lesser (pulmonic) system *(left-to-right shunt)* or from the lesser system into the greater *(right-to-left shunt)*. If the shunt is left to right, the flow of blood through the lungs is greater than the systemic flow is, and the lungs are congested. If the shunt is right to left, desaturated blood enters the systemic system and *cyanosis* may occur.

In atrial septal defect, the two atria may be considered to be one chamber with two outlets, namely, the tricuspid valve, leading to the right ventricle, and the mitral valve, leading to the left ventricle (Fig. 21-5). The major flow from the atria is into that ventricular chamber, offering less resistance to filling than the other ventricle. In the uncomplicated state, the right ventricle is thinner and more compliant than the left. Accordingly, with an atrial septal defect, more atrial blood enters the right ventricle than the left. The source for the greater flow into the right ventricle is the left atrium, hence the left-to-right shunt. If the right ventricle thickens, as with complicating pulmonary hypertension, the right ventricle may become less compliant than the left ventricle. Under this circumstance, there is a greater volume of flow from the atria into the left ventricle than into the right ventricle. The source for the greater flow into the left ventricle is the right atrium, hence the right-to-left shunt.

In dealing with communications between the ventricles or between the great arteries, the direction of shunt depends on relative resistance to flow into the systemic and pulmonic circulations. With an unobstructed ventricular septal defect, when there is no obstruction to pulmonary flow (Fig. 21-6), the shunt is left to right (from the left ventricle to the pulmonary arterial system). Obstruction to pulmonary flow may be present in the right ventricular outlet (Fig. 21-6, *center*) or in the pulmonary vascular bed (Fig. 21-6, *right*). When resistance to flow through the pulmonary vascular bed exceeds the resistance to flow through the systemic vascular bed, the shunt is right to left.

When there is an absolute barrier from a chamber or a vascular bed, a shunt is necessary for the flow of blood. Such a shunt is called an *obligatory shunt* (Fig. 21-7). Chambers or vessels carrying chronically shunted blood are enlarged in concert with the prevailing volume of blood entering that structure.

Cyanosis is an abnormal bluing of the skin or mucus membranes. Since cyanosis is an interpretation by the examiner, some variations in definition occur. Usually, when examiners agree on the presence of cyanosis, the circulating blood has at least 5 g of reduced hemoglobin per 100 ml. Among the borderline situations are the cases in which there is severe ane-

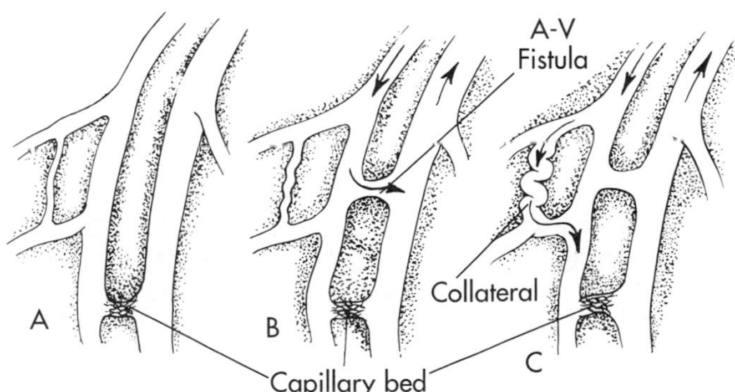

Fig. 21-4 Systemic arteriovenous fistula. **A,** An artery and a vein showing the major connection between the artery and the vein by way of a capillary network. **B,** An arteriovenous (A-V) fistula exists, representing a gross connection between the artery and the vein. Through this, a left-to-right shunt occurs, with a fall in blood pressure in the artery beyond the fistulous site. **C,** As a consequence of the fall in arterial blood pressure, a collateral system develops by dilatation of previously present connections between branches of the artery lying proximally and distally to the site of the fistula.

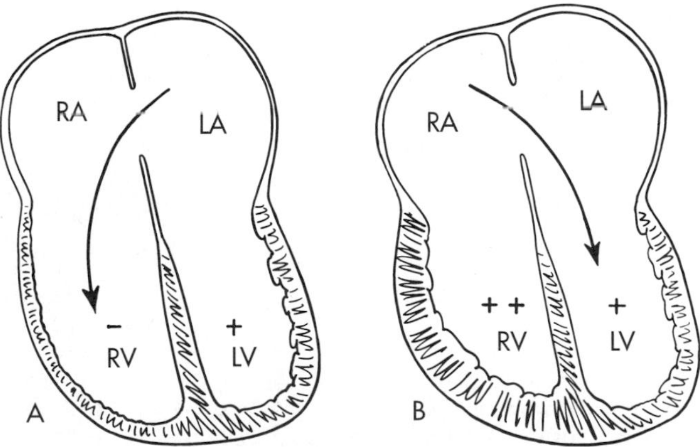

Fig. 21-5 Atrial septal defect. **A,** The right ventricular wall is thinner than the left ventricle, favoring a shunt from left atrium into the right side of the heart. **B,** Right ventricular hypertrophy causes the right ventricle to be more resistant (less compliant) than the left ventricle. The shunt through the atrial septal defect changes into a right-to-left direction.

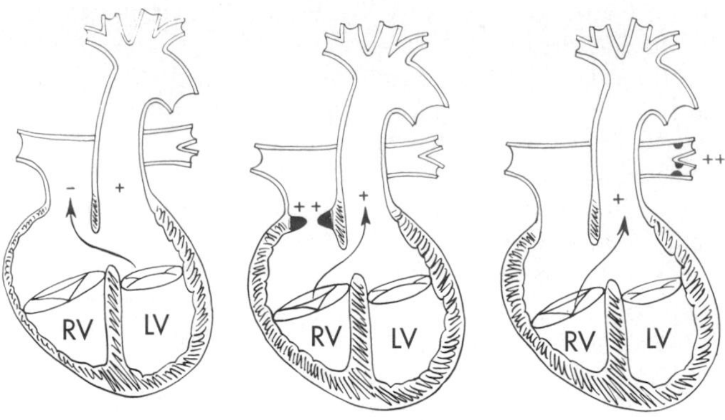

Fig. 21-6 Distribution of ventricular blood in ventricular septal defect. In each instance, the defect is unobstructed. *Left,* the pulmonary vascular resistance (shown as minus in the pulmonary artery) is less than the systemic vascular resistance (shown as plus) in the aorta. Major ventricular output is in the direction of the pulmonary artery. Contribution from the left ventricle constitutes a left-to-right shunt. *Center,* The resistance to pulmonary flow is increased by virtue of stenosis at the pulmonary valve, favoring a flow of blood into the aorta, constituting a right-to-left shunt. *Right,* Obstruction to pulmonary flow lies in the small pulmonary arterial branches. This raises the resistance to exit from the right ventricle in a manner functionally similar to pulmonary valvular stenosis, leading to a shunt in a right-to-left direction.

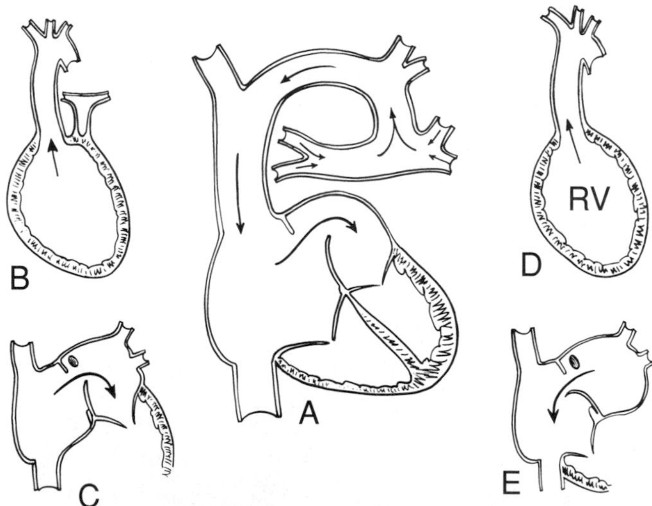

Fig. 21-7 Examples of causes of obligatory shunts. **A,** The entire pulmonary venous flow is into the systemic venous system, accounting for an obligatory, left-to-right shunt. Mixed blood is then shunted from the right atrium into the left. **B,** The ventricular system is connected to the aorta and pulmonary artery, but there is atresia of the pulmonary arterial system. Therefore an obligatory shunt from the right ventricle to the aorta occurs. **C,** Atresia of the tricuspid valve leads to an obligatory right-to-left shunt across the atrial septum. **D,** The situation is similar to that in **B.** In **B** the pulmonary valve was atretic, whereas in **D** no pulmonary artery is present. In each situation, the entire ventricular flow is into the aorta. **E,** Atresia of the mitral valve with obligatory shunt occurring in a left-to-right direction across the atrial septum.

mia. In such situations, despite high degrees of oxygen desaturation, the anemic state may preclude the presence of 5 g of reduced hemoglobin per 100 ml of blood needed for cyanosis to be appreciated. In individuals with dark skin, cyanosis may be appreciated best by examination of the mucus membranes.

Cyanosis may result from one of three factors, either alone or in combination. These are (1) right-to-left shunt, (2) poor oxygenation of blood by the lungs, and (3) cardiac failure with low cardiac output. In the latter instance, there is a greater than normal extraction of oxygen at the systemic capillary level, leading to increased arteriovenous oxygen differences and sufficient desaturation of the blood at the systemic capillary level for cyanosis to occur. Cyanosis on the basis of heart failure with low cardiac output may be termed *peripheral cyanosis.* Bluing of the skin or mucus membranes may be present for reasons other than the presence of reduced hemoglobin, such as methemoglobinemia.

In instances of chronic shunts occurring with systemic arteriovenous fistula, the left-to-right shunt is associated with development of *collateral channels.*[4] This occurs between the proximal and distal segments of the involved artery. The basis for the development of collateral channels is as follows. The connection or connections between the artery and vein serve to cause a fall in arterial pressure beyond the connection or connections. There are normally small connections between branches of given arteries. As the arterial pressure falls beyond the site of the fistula, blood flow increases across the normally occurring connections between segments of the involved artery at levels both proximal and distal to the arteriovenous fistula. Through such connections a system of collateral flow develops between the arterial segments proximal and distal to the fistulous site (Fig. 21-4).

Loss of unobstructed pathways

Obstruction of pathways may be inflow (that is, toward the heart) or outflow (that is, away from the heart) and occur either centrally or peripherally. Additionally, obstructions may occur acutely or be chronic.

Inflow obstructions (peripheral, central)

Examples of peripheral inflow obstruction are stenosis of pulmonary veins in the lesser circulation, or venous thrombosis in the major circulation (Fig. 21-8).

Central inflow obstruction may be caused by constrictive pericardial disease, including pericardial effusion (Fig. 21-9) and encasement of heart by solid tissue (such as fibrous tissue or tumor), atrioventricular valvular stenosis (Fig. 21-10), and restrictive ventricular disease. The last includes increased preload of ventricular failure or atrioventricular valvular insufficiency and restrictive cardiomyopathy. Other conditions related to decreased compliance of either or both ventricles, that is, increased preload, are ventricular or atrial space occupation by thrombus or tumor (Fig. 21-11). Increased preload also may result from ventricular hypertrophy, myocardial scarring, or ventricular failure.

Consequences

Inflow obstruction causes elevation of pressures proximal to the site of the obstruction resulting in *passive hyperemia (congestion)* and interstitial *edema* of the tissues. Passive hyperemia (congestion) reflects engorgement of the capillaries proximal to the obstruction. Passive hyperemia, as discussed

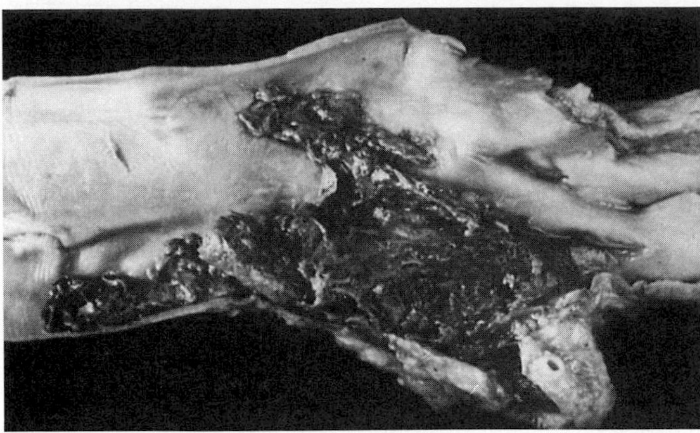

Fig. 21-8 Systemic venous obstruction by a thrombus in a major systemic vein.

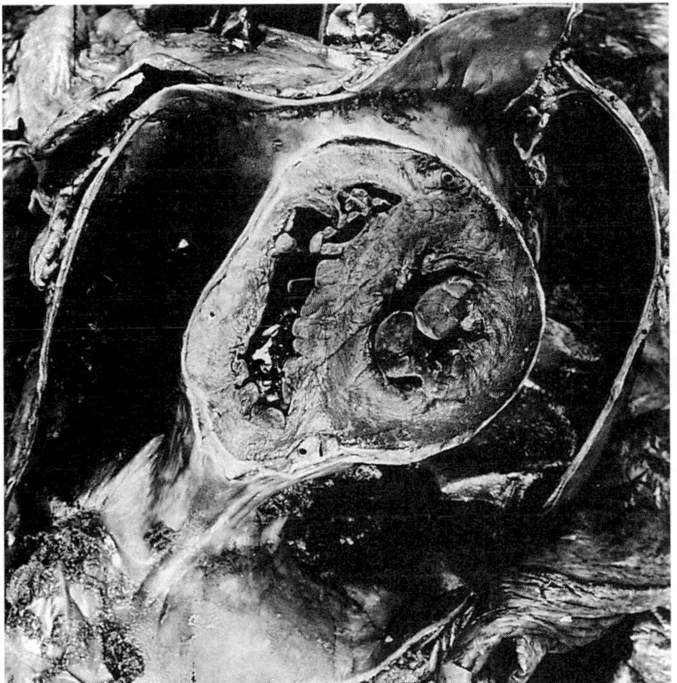

Fig. 21-9 Central inflow obstruction from chronic pericardial effusion, shown by a cross section of the heart and the parietal pericardium. Except for an adhesion between the heart and the parietal pericardium, there is a wide space that had contained fluid and caused significant compression of the heart, resulting in central inflow obstruction. (From Edwards JE: *An atlas of acquired diseases of the heart and great vessels,* Philadelphia, 1961, Saunders.

herein, is distinguished from *active hyperemia,* which is the congestion of tissue resulting from dilatation of arterioles and small arteries secondary to neurogenic activity or vasoactive amines.

Edema occurs when the intravascular hydrostatic pressure exceeds the combination of plasma oncotic pressure and the normal interstitial (intercellular) pressure. Lymphatic obstruction also causes interstitial edema. The edema fluid initially is primarily a transudate of plasma. With chronic obstructions, partly depending on the anatomic site of the inflow obstruction, fluid may accumulate in the pleural spaces *(hydrothorax),* the peritoneal cavity (*ascites*), or, to lesser degree, the pericardial sac (hydropericardium). The transudation of fluid into the interstitial spaces is partly overcome by an increased flow of lymph in the lymphatic channels.

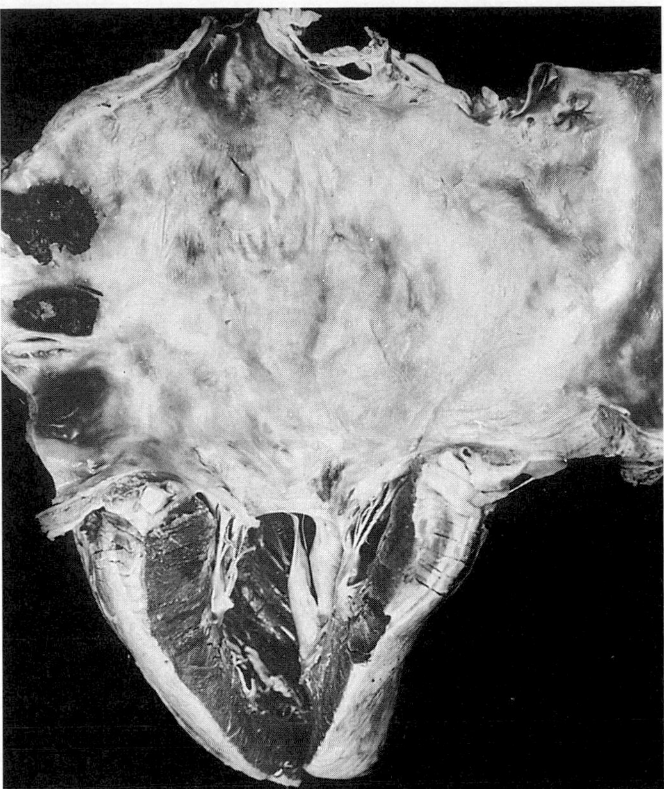

Fig. 21-10 Mitral stenosis as a site of central inflow obstruction into the left side of the heart. The left chambers are shown. There is a normal-sized left ventricle, whereas the left atrium is grossly dilated. On the left and in one of the pulmonary veins shown in the upper level, thrombi are present secondary to the stasis from inflow obstruction into the left ventricle.

Chronically congested organs may be enlarged. Enlargement of the liver (*hepatomegaly*) or of the spleen (*splenomegaly*) are commonly identified as consequences of central inflow obstruction resulting from increased systemic venous pressure.

In the systemic circulation, prolonged inflow obstruction may be complicated by systemic venous thrombosis (Fig. 21-12). Because the process of thrombosis is dependent partially on stasis of blood flow, there is a greater tendency for thrombosis in the longer rather than the shorter of the paired veins. Of the bilateral systemic veins, those on the left side are longer than the ones of the right, and the left veins are more susceptible to thrombosis than the right-sided veins are.

Fragmentation of systemic venous thrombi leads to thrombotic emboli. Thrombotic emboli originating from the systemic venous system usually lodge in pulmonary arteries as *pulmonary emboli* (Fig. 21-13). When an opening or a potential opening between the two sides of the heart is present, such as the commonly occurring valvular competent patent foramen ovale, emboli in the right side of the heart may cross into the left side. Such emboli are termed *paradoxical emboli.*[7]

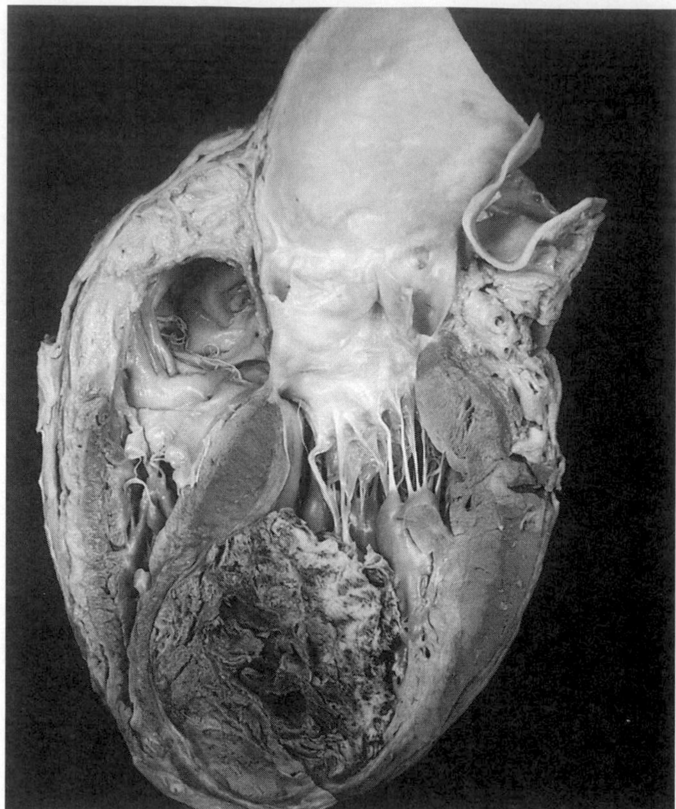

Fig. 21-11 In the left ventricle is a major thrombus causing major inflow obstruction.

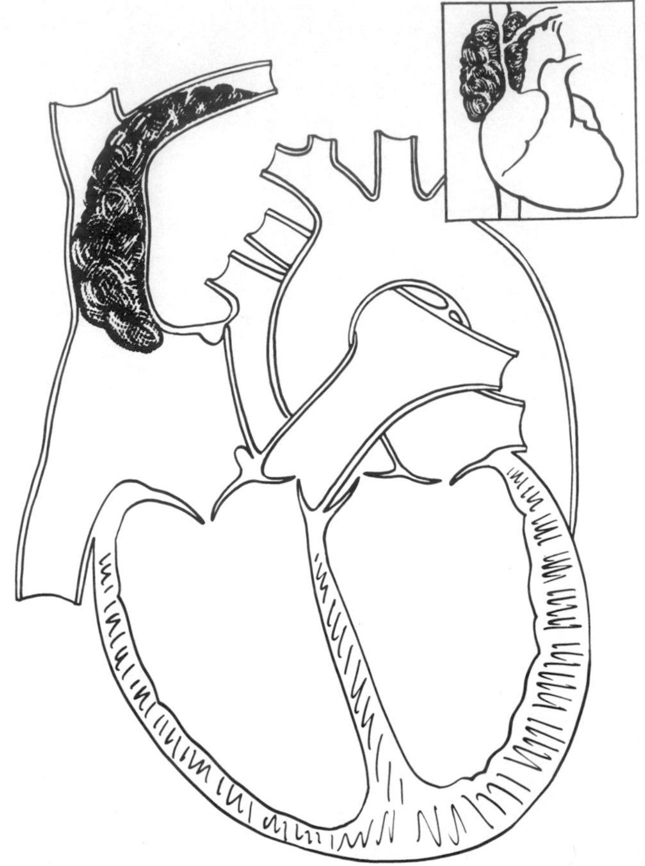

Fig. 21-12 Major systemic venous obstruction. The superior vena cava is obstructed by a mass, which may represent either tumor or thrombus. *Inset,* There is encasement of the superior vena cava system by mediastinal tumor. (From Edwards JE: *Cardiovasc Clin* 4(2):282, 1972.)

Although not specifically related to inflow obstruction, materials other than thrombotic types may gain access to the bloodstream and be carried to a site distant to their point of origin. Nonthrombotic emboli include fat, bone marrow, calcific fragments (such as those from cardiac valves), portions of atheromas, amniotic materials, air, and foreign bodies, such as oil, talc, cotton fibers, prostheses, and fragments of bullets. The consequences of these emboli depend on the vascular system involved, since all tend to lodge in a vessel of smaller luminal diameter than that of the vessel of origin.

Chronic localized obstruction of major veins favors the development of collateral channels from the venous compartment proximal to the site of obstruction to the segment central to the site of obstruction.

Outflow obstructions (peripheral, central)

Outflow obstruction, like inflow obstruction, also may be either peripheral or central. In both types, acute and chronic examples occur.

Peripheral outflow obstruction

In either circulation, the primary site of vascular control is at the precapillary, the arteriolar, level. The vascular resistance created at this level represents cardiac afterload. Peripheral causes of obstruction may be functional or anatomic. Vasoconstriction at the arteriolar level is a functional cause and is the most common type of peripheral outflow obstruction. Chronic obstruction in peripheral arteries and in coronary arteries commonly is atherosclerotic. Acute occlusion of peripheral or

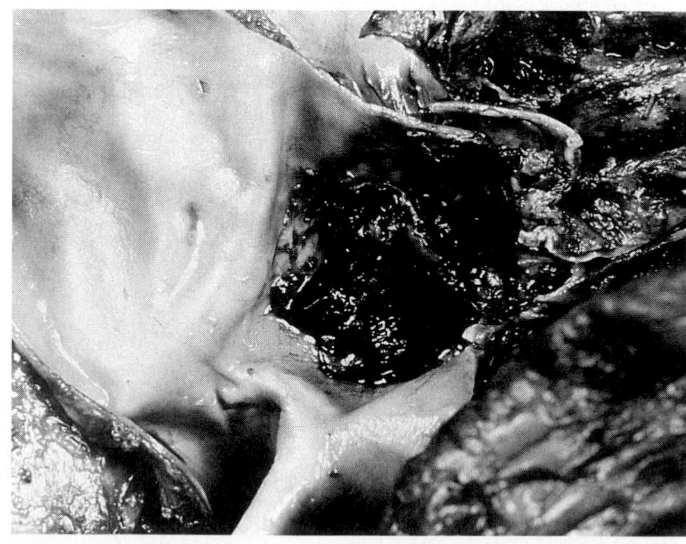

Fig. 21-13 Obstruction of major pulmonary arteries by emboli of thrombotic material originating in systemic veins.

coronary arteries usually is due to thrombotic occlusion, which often is associated with atherosclerosis at the site of the occlusion. In the peripheral arteries, acute occlusion often is caused by emboli originating from the left heart chambers or the aorta (Fig. 21-14).

Consequences

Since blood pressure results from volume of blood flow and resistance to flow, increase in resistance (afterload) may result in hypertension of the vascular system involved, whether lesser or greater circulations. When high peripheral vascular resistance is associated only with vasoconstriction and no anatomic stenosing lesions are present, with constant blood flow the resistance and consequently the blood pressure will vary with the degree of vasoconstriction. Chronic elevation of pressure may result in secondary intimal changes (disease) in the arterioles and small muscular arteries. Such changes may be anatomically obstructive and thus maintain high levels of peripheral resistance and of elevated blood pressure in addition to the contribution of vasoconstriction.

When a major artery is obstructed, the immediate potential is that of death of tissue from inadequate blood supply. In extremities, death from inadequate blood supply usually is termed *gangrene*. In organs, tissue death from this cause is termed *infarction*.

If obstruction of an artery is present chronically, collateral vessels bypass the level of arterial obstruction[8,9] and tend to minimize tissue injury from decreased arterial blood supply. In the extremities, the collateral system develops from the main arterial compartment proximal to the obstruction through branches connecting the proximal segment to segments distal to the obstruction. When the obstruction is in an artery arising centrally or located near the torso, the source of collateral supply is both the proximal segment of the artery and branches of the contralateral artery, the branches crossing the midline. For example, in obstruction within a subclavian artery, collateral supply comes not only from the proximal segment of the involved artery, but also from branches of contralateral subclavian artery, the latter connection crossing the midline. By such connections, obstruction in one subclavian artery may "steal" blood from the contralateral arterial system.[10]

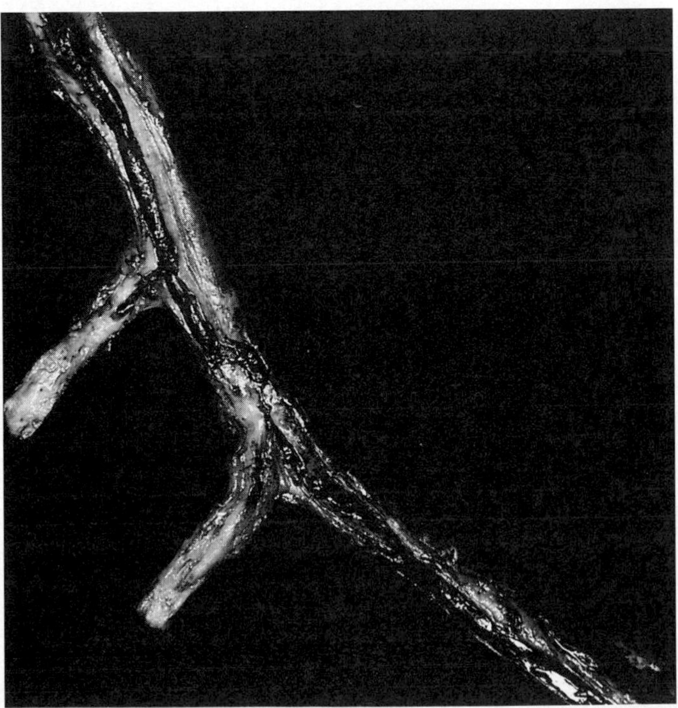

Fig. 21-14 Occlusion of an artery of a lower extremity by embolism from the left atrium.

Central outflow obstruction

Central obstruction occurs in or at the outlets from the ventricles or atria. On the left side, ventricular outflow obstruction may be at the left ventricular outlet or in the aorta. On the right side, comparable situations apply, that is, obstruction at the right ventricular outflow tract or the pulmonary artery. Causes of atrial outflow obstruction include stenosis at the atrioventricular valves, atrial tumors, and conditions that create increased preload such as decreased compliance of a ventricle. Pericardial constrictive disease also may cause atrial outflow obstruction.

Consequences

The primary effect of central outflow obstruction, whether atrial, ventricular, or in a major vessel, is that proximal to the site of obstruction the pressure rises whereas distal to the obstruction the pressure falls, creating a *pressure differential*. The elevation of pressure proximal to the obstruction causes an increase in velocity of blood flow across the obstructed site, which may permit a normal volume of flow.

Increased ventricular systolic pressure results in ventricular hypertrophy. Cardiac hypertrophy, that is, an increase in the mass of myocardial tissue, may involve the myocardium of one or more of the cardiac chambers in a given patient. When present, hypertrophy is most apparent in the ventricles and is commonly associated with an increase in cardiac weight. Two types of ventricular hypertrophy are recognized, concentric hypertrophy and eccentric hypertrophy.

Concentric hypertrophy is characterized by an increase in myocardial mass without noticeable dilatation of the involved chamber. The features of this condition are increased thickness of the wall of the involved chamber and an increase in the weight of the wall of that chamber and usually of the heart as a whole. In classical concentric hypertrophy, there may be reduction in the volume of the chamber as it is encroached upon by the increase in mass of muscle (Fig. 21-15).

The major causes of concentric hypertrophy are obstructions to the outlet from the involved chamber without failure of that chamber. In the right ventricle, concentric hypertrophy commonly is caused either by pulmonary hypertension or pulmonary valvular stenosis. Concentric hypertrophy of the left ventricle most commonly is associated with aortic valvular stenosis or systemic arterial hypertension. Most commonly, when hypertrophy of an atrial wall occurs, the hypertrophy is eccentric.

Eccentric hypertrophy is characterized by the involved chamber showing not only an increase in its myocardial mass, but also dilatation of the cavity. The size of a cardiac chamber as seen in an autopsy specimen reflects the prevailing diastolic volume in that chamber during life (Figs. 21-16 and 21-17). The increase in cavity size may have been derived from (1) regurgitation of blood through one or both valves related to that chamber, (2) failure of the myocardium of the chamber for

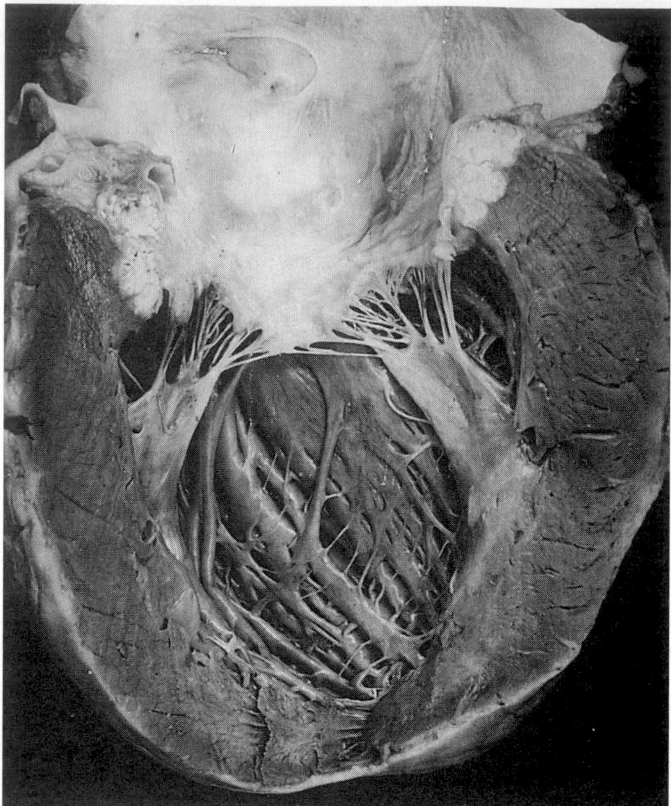

Fig. 21-15 Left atrium and left ventricle showing concentric hypertrophy of the left ventricle. The wall is greatly thickened, whereas the chamber remains relatively normal in size.

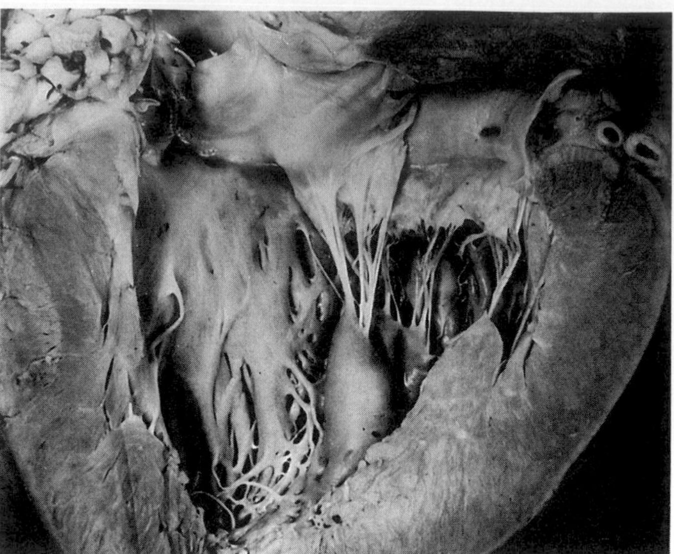

Fig. 21-16 Eccentric hypertrophy of the left ventricle as a result of left ventricular failure. The wall is thickened, whereas the chamber is enlarged.

any reason, resulting in a lowered *ejection fraction* during the emptying period and abnormal diastolic retention of blood, or (3) a combination of the two foregoing.

When there is significant obstruction between high-pressure and low-pressure systems, a narrow, high-velocity stream flows into the low-pressure system. When this stream strikes the wall of the low-pressure chamber or vessel, it causes a fibrous endocardial (or intimal) reaction, which may be termed a *jet lesion*.[11] Examples of jet lesions are those in the intima of the pulmonary arterial system in classical patent ductus arteriosus (Fig. 21-18), in the endocardium of the right ventricle in instances of small (restrictive) ventricular septal defect, and in the left atrium in some forms of mitral valvular regurgitation. The lesion is characterized by development of nonvascular laminated connective tissue, mostly collagen with lesser amounts of elastic tissue.

Loss of cardiac valvular competence

Incompetence (insufficiency, regurgitation) of valves may be congenital or acquired. Valvular incompetence may result from increased diameter of the valvular orifice as in ventricular failure, or from abnormality of any or all of the units of the valve, which include the leaflets, chordae tendineae, and papillary muscles.

Consequences

Since valvular incompetence is characterized by, in effect, some degree of a to-and-fro flow of blood across the involved valve, the related chambers and vessels involved are dilated. Ventricular chambers develop eccentric hypertrophy in which the increased mass of myocardium is overshadowed by dilatation of the involved chamber. The endocardium of the chambers may be uniformly thickened secondary to dilatation, and focal endocardial thickening may occur at the site of impact of the regurgitant stream as *jet lesions*[10] (Fig. 21-19). Jet lesions

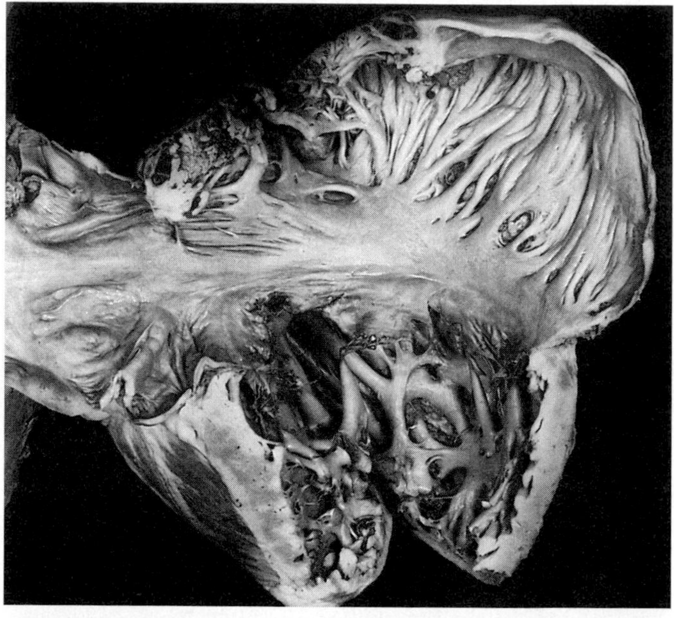

Fig. 21-17 Right atrium and right ventricle in a case of pulmonary hypertension with right ventricular failure. There is eccentric hypertrophy of the right ventricle, as well as major dilatation of the right atrium. The latter process may be considered secondary to obstruction imparted by the failing right ventricle, with elevated end-diastolic pressure.

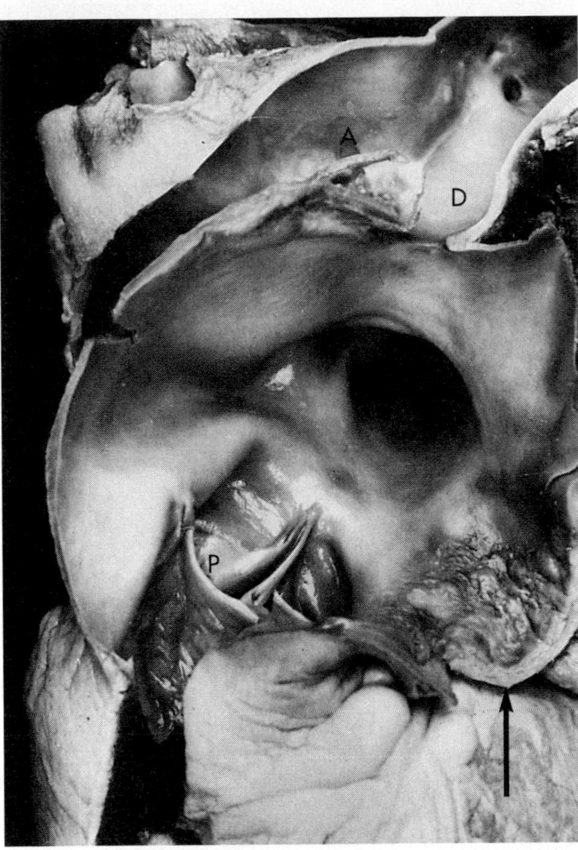

Fig. 21-18 Patent ductus arteriosus and related great arteries. The ductus arteriosus is of the classical type. The pulmonary arterial lining opposite the ductal opening is thickened and irregular *(arrow)* by virtue of jet lesions caused by a left-to-right shunt through the ductus arteriosus. *A,* Aorta; *P,* pulmonary valve.

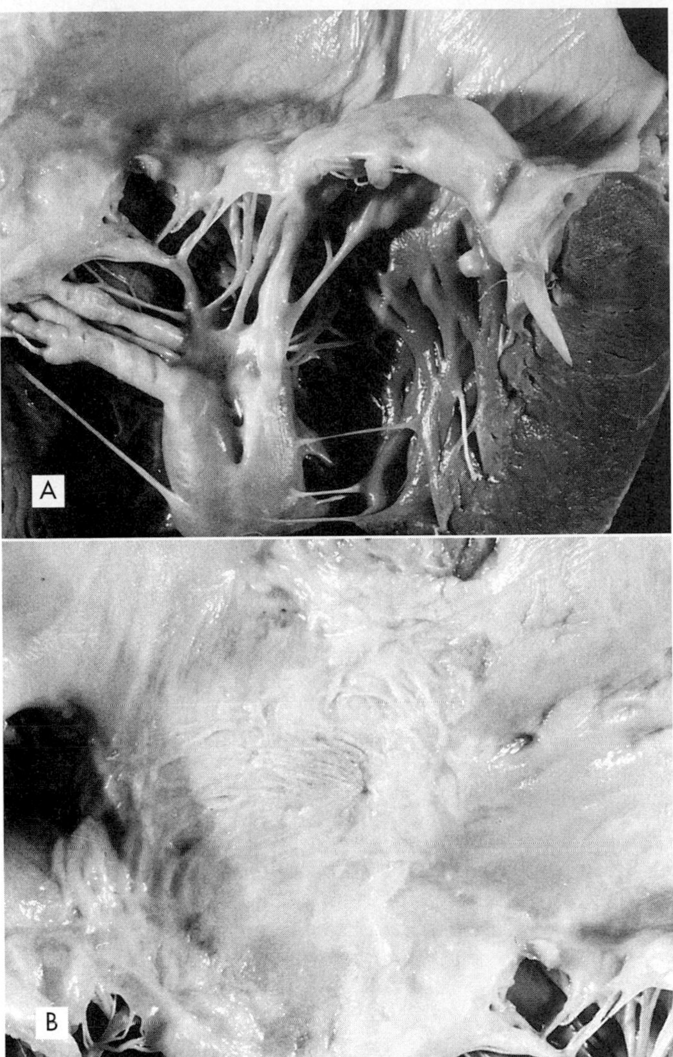

Fig. 21-19 **A,** A portion of the left atrium and mitral valve in a case with ruptured chordae to the mitral valve. The related portion of the valve shows major hooding from which blood is directed in the opposite direction toward the atrial septum. **B,** The atrial septum. The numerous, semicircular irregularities represent jet lesions from the impact of regurgitant blood directed across the atrium from the partially unsupported mitral valve.

in valvular incompetence also may be termed *regurgitant lesions,* usually characterized by a group of semicircular rows of endocardial thickening. Each row of thickening may protrude into the cavity and form a shallow, valvelike pocket. Under the aortic valve, left ventricular regurgitant lesions have been called *pockets of Zahn.*

The site of the jet impact is subject to the development of infection. For example, infection complicating classical patent ductus starts at the site of impact of the shunt. Infective endocarditis often causes valvular incompetence; in this situation, organisms from the infected valve are carried retrograde with the regurgitant blood and lead to infection at the site of impact as a *regurgitant infection.*

Loss of adequate functioning myocardium

Inadequate functioning myocardium refers to two situations, inadequate amount of myocardium and inadequate function of the myocardium, which may be of adequate mass. In either case, myocardial failure results. The failure may be most evident during the systolic or the diastolic phase of ventricular contraction. Frequently, when one is present, so is the other. Myocardial failure may be acute or chronic.

Acute myocardial failure commonly is due to acute myocardial infarction or ventricular arrhythmia. Acute hemodynamic challenges such as acutely developing shunts or valvular insufficiencies are rarer causes of acute myocardial failure. Each of the latter may be a complication of acute myocardial infarction, as rupture of the ventricular septum causing an acutely developing, interventricular shunt or rupture of a left ventricular papillary muscle resulting in acute mitral insufficiency.

Chronic myocardial failure has many causes. Among these are loss of myocardial tissue from prior myocardial infarction and active or healed myocarditis. Dilated (congestive) cardiomyopathy, causes of which are known in some cases but unknown in many, is characterized by chronic heart failure.

Conditions causing diastolic dysfunction include those conditions in which there is or appears to be failure of adequate relaxation of the myocardium during diastole. This decreased compliance of the myocardium creates increased resistance to ventricular filling, that is, increased preload.

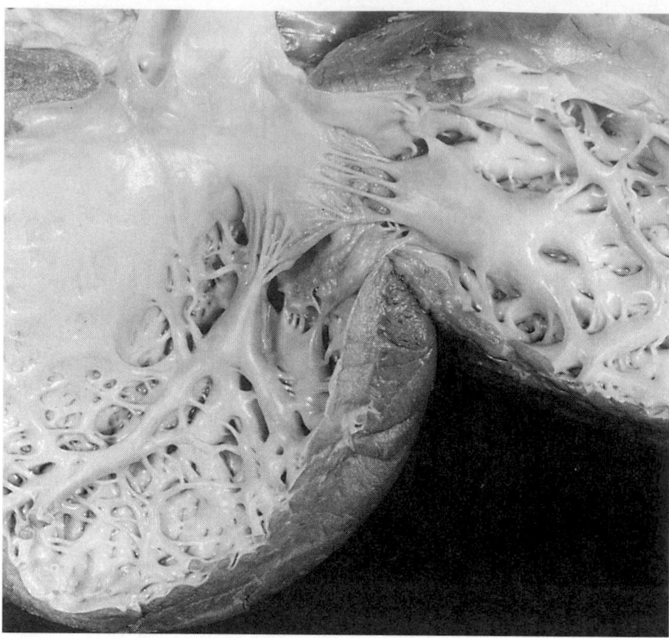

Fig. 21-20 Left ventricle from a case of so-called primary endocardial fibroelastosis. The mural endocardium is grossly thickened by pale connective tissue, giving major opacity to this layer.

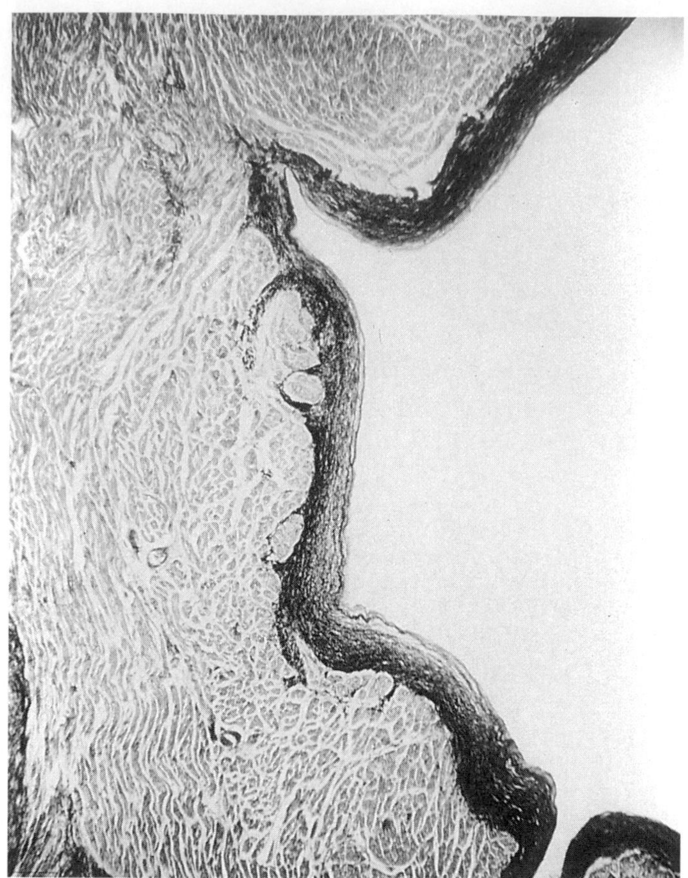

Fig. 21-21 Fibroelastosis. The endocardium is thickened by more or less parallel layers of elastic tissue and collagen. (Elastic tissue stain.)

Examples of conditions exhibiting diastolic dysfunction are infiltrative processes of the myocardium such as amyloid disease, interstitial fibrosis of the myocardium, asymmetric ventricular hypertrophy, concentric hypertrophy from various causes, and ventricular failure from conditions causing systolic dysfunction.

Consequences

Inadequate myocardial function reduces cardiac output, which may be measured in several ways, depending on the basic process. The low cardiac output in cases with acute systolic dysfunction may be easily identified as having a low systemic blood pressure as a consequence of significant reduction in the forward flow of blood.

In instances of chronic systolic dysfunction, the proportion of the ventricular blood volume ejected with each systole is reduced. Whereas in the normal person, the ventricle in systole ejects somewhat over 50% of its diastolic volume, when chronic systolic dysfunction is present, less than 50% of the diastolic volume is ejected. Myocardial systolic dysfunction also may be expressed as the volume of blood ejected by the ventricle (cardiac output) in comparison to body size. Normal values[1] for cardiac output are (1) in sedentary men 3.5 liters/square meter of body surface per minute at rest, (2) in athletes 3.8 L/m^2/min, and (3) in men during severe exercise 10.5 L/m^2/min. In states of low cardiac output, increased extraction of oxygen from the tissue may be of such degree as to be associated with peripheral cyanosis.

In chronic ventricular failure for any reason, the mural ventricular endocardium may be thickened (Fig. 21-20) by additional layers of collagen and elastic tissue to the mural endocardium, creating *acquired endocardial fibroelastosis* (Fig. 21-21). This process, at least in part, is secondary to stretching of the fibrous tissue of the mural endocardium. This concept is supported by the finding of localized endocardial fibroelastosis at the site of healed myocardial infarcts.

With systolic dysfunction, the decreased ejection of blood is associated with stasis of blood and an associated tendency for intracardiac thrombosis. In chronic low cardiac output syndromes, thrombosis may occur in any of the chambers. In the atria, the appendages are favored sites for thrombosis, whereas in the ventricles, the apices are more commonly thrombosed.

The specific effects of diastolic dysfunction include increased diastolic (filling) pressure of the ventricles and reduced cardiac output. The increased diastolic pressure is reflected as increased pressure in the venous and capillary system that faces the involved ventricle. This leads to the tendency for interstitial edema in the tissues drained by that venous compartment. Increased right ventricular diastolic pressure in the lesser circulation may be complicated by systemic venous thrombosis (Fig. 21-8).

Loss of normal cardiac rhythm or rate

Abnormal cardiac rate or rhythm may reduce the pumping effectiveness of the heart, creating decreased cardiac output and its consequences of inadequate perfusion of tissues. Diastolic filling of the ventricles is governed in part by cardiac rate. With tachycardia, the diastolic time interval shortens and the volume of blood that may be ejected is reduced. Tachycar-

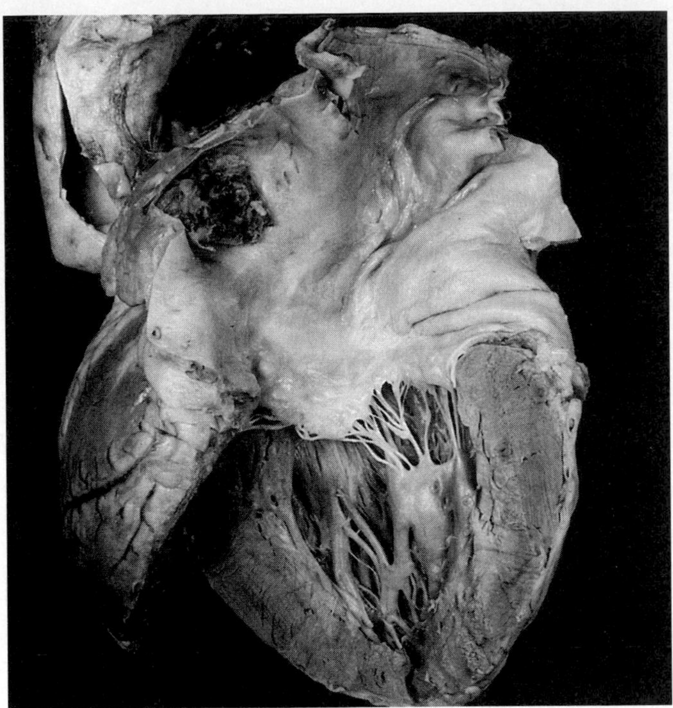

Fig. 21-22 Left atrium with thrombus in appendage.

dia may be associated with sinus rhythm or be an abnormal rhythm, such as ventricular tachycardia.

Among the various arrhythmias, reduction in delivery of blood to the tissues may come about in different ways. *Atrial fibrillation* may be associated with a reduction in cardiac output when *ventricular tachycardia* is associated. Atrial fibrillation is associated with mural thrombosis of atrial appendages (Fig. 21-22). *Ventricular fibrillation* is characterized by independent, noncoordinated contraction of the myriad of myocardial fibers. As a result, effective pumping function is lost. The result is *circulatory arrest,* which also occurs with asystole (lack of myocardial contraction).

Delayed contraction of either ventricle, as with *right or left bundle branch block,* usually has no significant hemodynamic effect. The same is true for minor degrees of delayed atrioventricular conduction. Major atrioventricular conduction defects, however, such as *complete heart block,* result in bradycardia. The associated decrease in pulse rate may result in periodic fainting, probably from cerebral anoxia. Such fainting attacks are named *Stokes-Adams syndrome.*

In instances of death occurring acutely or suddenly *(sudden cardiac death),* the underlying mechanism usually is ventricular fibrillation. Among such cases, there are two groups, one without pulmonary edema and one in which pulmonary edema is present. In cases without pulmonary edema, the usual mechanism is sudden onset of ventricular fibrillation, and less commonly cardiac asystole occurred. Pulmonary edema, which may develop within as little as 5 minutes after the onset of symptoms, probably reflects a short period of ventricular tachycardia, during which pulmonary edema occurred, and was followed either by asystole, or, more commonly, ventricular fibrillation and death. The pathologic findings in instances of fatal arrhythmia may reveal certain pathologic states.[12] Common in North America is the presence of coronary atherosclerosis, often with myocardial infarction that may be old or recent. Many cases have scars of old myocardial infarction with chronically obstructed coronary arteries but do not have acute changes in the myocardium or coronary arteries that can be demonstrated by morphologic changes. Other pathologic states causing sudden cardiac death include ventricular hypertrophy from diseases such as chronic valvular disease, particularly aortic stenosis or insufficiency. Active myocarditis or chronic cardiomyopathy are among the conditions found. In not all cases of fatal ventricular fibrillation is a reasonable anatomic cause found.

REFERENCES

1. Shepherd JT, Vanhoutte PM: *The human cardiovascular system: facts and concepts,* New York, 1979, Raven Press.
2. Marshall RJ, Shepherd JT: *Cardiac function in health and disease,* Philadelphia, 1968, Saunders.
3. Heymann MA, Rudolph AM: Control of the ductus arteriosus, *Physiol Rev* 55:62, 1975.
4. Zimmerman JJ, Dietrich KA: Current perspectives on septic shock, *Pediatr Clin North Am* 34:131, 1987.
5. Bosher LH Jr, Blake DA, Byrd BR: An analysis of the pathologic anatomy of pulmonary arteriovenous aneurysms with particular reference to the applicability of local excision, *Surgery* 45:91, 1959.
6. Holman E: Arteriovenous aneurysm: clinical evidence correlating size of fistula with changes in the heart and proximal vessels, *Ann Surg* 80:801, 1924.
7. Ingham DW: Paradoxical embolism, *Am J Med Sci* 196:201, 1938.
8. Winsor T, Payne JH, Rudy N, Beatty JO: Collateral circulation in health and disease, *Arch Surg* 74:20, 1957.
9. Siegel MB, Levinsky NG: Collateral circulation after renal artery occlusion in the rat, *Circ Res* 41:227, 1977.
10. Reivich M, Holling HE, Roberts B, Toole JF: Reversal of blood flow through the vertebral artery and its effect on cerebral circulation, *N Engl J Med* 265:878, 1961.
11. Edwards JE, Burchell HB: Endocardial and intimal lesions (jet impact) as possible sites of origin of murmurs. Second symposium on cardiovascular sound, *Circulation* 18:946, 1958.
12. Virmani R, Roberts WC: Sudden cardiac death, *Hum Pathol* 18:485, 1987.

22 Hemostasis and Thrombosis

Robert L. Reddick
Dwight A. Bellinger

NORMAL HEMOSTASIS

Hemostasis defines the arrest of bleeding, or the arrest of the circulation in a blood vessel. It is one aspect of a system that regulates the balance between coagulation and anticoagulation.[1,2] The physiologic mechanisms that underly hemostasis are complex and involve both the fluid and cellular components of the blood as well as the extracellular tissues. These compartments act mutually to achieve hemostasis after vascular injury. There are numerous checks and balances that enable bleeding to be arrested when necessary yet maintain blood fluidity. Blood coagulation begins through the initiation of a series of reactions in which inactive zymogen precursors are sequentially activated by limited proteolysis. The classical model of blood coagulation evokes a cascade system in which once initiated, a series of sequential reactions occurs and ends in the formation of a stable fibrin clot.

Two systems of hemostasis that differ by the mode of initiation are the intrinsic and extrinsic pathways[3] (Fig. 22-1). The *intrinsic pathway* is activated when factor XII (Hageman factor) is exposed to surfaces (which are usually negatively charged) that allow contact activation. Collagen, exposed by vascular injury, is assumed to be the usual surface that promotes activation, though other tissues may initiate coagulation. Prekallikrein and high-molecular-weight (HMW) kininogen are important contributors to this initial activation phase, resulting in the activation of factor XII to factor XIIa. Factor XIIa then activates XI to XIa. The *extrinsic system* is activated by the combined action of factor VII and tissue factor on factor X (Xase complex). Both the extrinsic and intrinsic systems converge at the final common pathway, activation of factor X (Stuart-Prower factor) to factor Xa. Calcium and phospholipids are necessary for many of these reactions to occur. In the final common pathway, both calcium and phospholipids act with factor Va to produce factor Xa. Through the common pathway, factor Xa and factor Va act on prothrombin to produce thrombin, which is responsible for the conversion of fibrinogen to fibrin. A more recently proposed system indicates that fibrinogen may be initially converted to fibrin monomers and eventually to fibrin polymers. The fibrin polymers are cross-linked and stabilized by activated factor XIII (fibrin-stabilizing factor). A series of feedback loops are believed to exist and indicate that thrombin may be responsible for the activation of blood clotting factors and thereby further

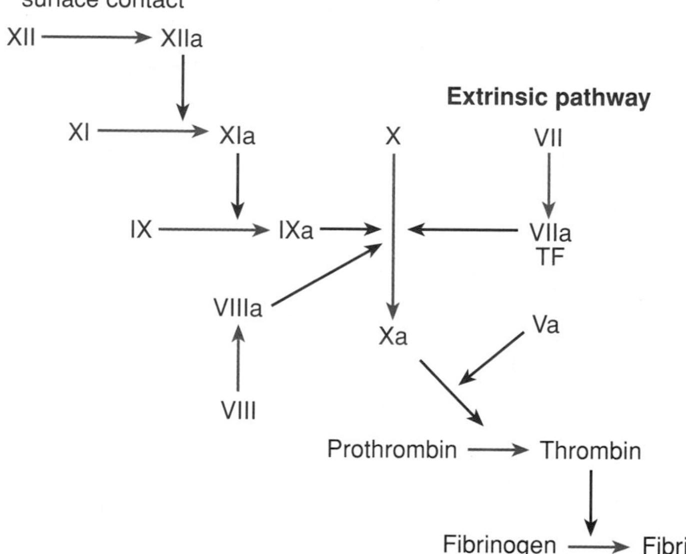

Fig. 22-1 The cascade/waterfall hypothesis of blood coagulation. There is a series of steps in which activation of either the intrinsic or extrinsic system results in activation of the final common pathway mediated through factor X. Calcium and phospholipids are required for many of these reactions to occur. Feedback loops exist for many of these steps. *HMW,* High molecular weight; *TF,* tissue factor.

promote the activation of the intrinsic pathway of blood coagulation. Regulatory mechanisms may modify this process. Antithrombin III (AT III) and the protein C casade are important in maintaining the hemostatic balance. Antithrombin III is one of several glycoprotein serine protease inhibitors and is an inhibitor of thrombin (IIa) and Xa. Protein C and AT III are discussed in further detail later in this chapter.

Table 22-1 summarizes proteins that participate in blood coagulation. Except for von Willebrand factor, all other coagulation factors, as well as protein S, protein C, and antithrombin III, are produced by the liver. The coagulation proteins II, VII, IX, and X are generally referred to as the vitamin K–dependent proteins because vitamin K is necessary for these proteins to achieve a functional state. Protein C and protein S are also vitamin K dependent. All the vitamin K–dependent proteins contain an epidermal growth factor domain, in addition to a Gla domain (calcium binding regions). von Willebrand factor is synthesized by the megakaryocyte and endothelial cells. The endothelial cell is the site of synthesis of thrombomodulin and the lipoprotein-associated coagulation inhibitor. Lipoprotein-associated coagulation inhibitor is also referred to as tissue factor pathway inhibitor (TFPI). The TFPI binds to and inactivates factor Xa as well as the VIIa-TF complex. In plasma, TFPI is bound largely to low-density lipoprotein and is present in high-density lipoproteins complexed to apolipoprotein II. Platelets also contain TFPI and is released after platelet aggregation. Tissue factor pathway inhibitor is believed to have an important role in a hypothesized coagulation system in which the VIIa-TF complex initiates coagulation. This system as proposed discounts the extrinsic and intrinsic coagulation pathways, provides for an explanation of normal hemostasis and accounts for the bleeding tendencies associated with factors VIII, IX, and XI.[4]

Table 22-1 Blood coagulation and coagulant proteins

Coagulation factor	Site of synthesis	Chromosomal location
Fibrinogen (I)	Hepatocyte	4
Prothrombin (II)	Hepatocyte	11
Tissue factor (III)	Different sites	1
Factor V	Hepatocyte	1
Factor VII	Hepatocyte	13
Factor VIII	Hepatocyte	X
Factor IX	Hepatocyte	X
Factor X	Hepatocyte	13
Factor XI	Hepatocyte	4
Factor XII	Hepatocyte	5
Factor XIII	Hepatocyte	1, 6
von Willebrand factor	Endothelial cell Megakaryocyte	12
Anticoagulant proteins		
Protein C	Hepatocyte	2
Protein S	Hepatocyte	3
Thrombomodulin	Endothelial cell	20
Antithrombin III	Hepatocyte	1
Lipoprotein-associated coagulation inhibitor	Endothelial cell	2

Platelets

The platelet has a central role in normal hemostasis. Platelets are produced by the megakaryocyte, being formed by endoreduplication and segmentation of the cytoplasm of the megakaryocyte. Platelets circulate in the blood as discoid bodies, with a life-span of 4 to 6 days. Under normal conditions, the blood contains 150,000 to 300,000 platelets per cubic millimeter. Platelet numbers may decrease (thrombocytopenia) as a result of bleeding, drug use, chemotherapy, sepsis, or viral infection (human immunodeficiency virus, adenovirus).[5-8] There are several autoimmune or neoplastic conditions that are associated with decreased production or increased destruction of platelets.[9] Failure of the bone marrow (see Chapter 41) may cause thrombocytopenia.

Platelet numbers may be increased (thrombocytosis) in certain conditions.[10] These include malignancies, such as metastatic carcinoma and Hodgkin's disease, chronic inflammatory diseases, after splenectomy, and in the recovery phase of thrombocytopenia. Platelet numbers may also be increased after acute bleeding and in patients with iron deficiency anemia. Thrombocytosis may be associated with increased platelet production or lack of platelet pooling in the spleen. A second condition referred to as *thrombocythemia* describes an increase in platelet production, usually because of an uncontrolled increase in numbers of megakaryocytes.[10] Causes include chronic myelogenous leukemia and polycythemia rubra vera or other myeloproliferative disorders.

Defects in platelet function causing abnormal hemostasis arise from genetic or acquired disorders.[11-13] The genetic defects may be subdivided into those based in abnormal platelet adhesion to foreign substances (Bernard-Soulier syndrome) or those that interfere with primary or secondary aggregation (Glanzmann's thrombasthenia, storage pool disease). Table 22-2 summarizes the more common platelet defects. A complete characterization of platelet disorders is beyond the scope of this chapter, though additional information may be found in standard textbooks of hematology.

Table 22-2 Platelet disorders important in hemostasis and thrombosis

Genetic, related to adhesion
Bernard-Soulier syndrome—absence of GP-Ib
Genetic, related to aggregation
Glanzmann's thrombasthenia—absence of GP-IIb/IIIc
Storage pool disease—abnormal response to agonists
Aspirinlike and release reaction defects—abnormal response to agonists
Genetic, coagulation factor related
Platelet factor 3 deficiency
Afibrinogenemia
Factor VIII:C and factor IX deficiencies
Acquired, associated with other disorders
Disseminated intravascular coagulation
Uremia
Diabetes
Liver disease
Drug induced
Cancer associated

GP, Glycoprotein.

The morphology of the normal platelet is important in understanding the role of platelets in normal hemostasis and thrombosis. Platelet granules contain adenosine diphosphate (ADP), serotonin (5-HT), lysosomal enzymes, platelet factor 4, and thromboxane A_2. The platelet alpha granules contain von Willebrand factor, and located on the membrane is a receptor for von Willebrand factor, the GPlb-IX receptor complex. In addition, membrane glycoprotein (MGP) receptors for fibrinogen (GPIb-IIIa) and a thrombin receptor, GP-V, are also present on the platelet surface. A system of canalicular channels that are important in regulating calcium flux exist within the platelet cytoplasm. The shape of the platelet is maintained by a subplasmalemmal collection of microtubules that are important for granule centralization in activated platelets during thrombus formation. For normal platelet function all of the above must exist and be responsive to external and internal stimuli.[14]

Once the platelet is activated by an agonist, such as thrombin, or by collagen after a blood vessel is injured, there occurs a series of reactions that lead to platelet secretion of additional agonists. This secretion triggers the recruitment of platelets and promotes additional platelet aggregation. The shape of platelets changes during their activation, the discoid shape is lost, granules are centralized, and pseudopods form. In concert with platelet activation and aggregation, the coagulation system is activated. The production of thrombin, a potent platelet agonist, produces further platelet aggregation and also promotes fibrin formation. Activated coagulation factor X, Xa, is bound to the platelet surface. In conjunction with factor Va, thrombin is formed and is responsible for the conversion of the fibrinogen to fibrin (Fig. 22-1). The polymerized fibrin, which becomes admixed with the platelets, serves to strengthen and consolidate the platelet thrombus. Leukocytes and red cells are also incorporated into the forming platelet thrombus. To control thrombus formation, the fibrinolytic system becomes activated.[15] *Plasmin,* the activated serine protease of plasminogen carries out thrombolysis. Activators of plasminogen include tissue plasminogen activator (t-PA) and urokinase. A feedback loop exists for control of the fibrinolytic system. These include alpha$_2$-antiplasmin, plasminogen activator inhibitor-1 (PAI-1). Thrombin production is regulated by antithrombin III. The delicate balance that exists between coagulation and anticoagulation is necessary for the maintenance of blood fluidity.

Endothelial cells

The role of the endothelial cell in hemostasis has achieved a new focus in the past few years[16] (Table 22-3). The endothelial cell is responsible for many of the initial events that control hemostasis, and their roles in the normal coagulant process are shown in Fig. 22-2. The endothelial cell synthesizes both coagulant and anticoagulant factors, and the formation of the hemostatic plug at sites of vascular injury is dependent on endothelial cell constituents. The balance of these activities is responsible for maintenance of blood fluidity. With injury, this balance is altered and may lead to thrombus formation if the coagulant functions dominate or to hemorrhage if anticoagulant functions are predominant. The endothelial cell synthesizes von Willebrand factor (vWF). The importance of vWF in platelet adherence to sites of vascular injury in both normal hemostasis and thrombosis is discussed later in this chapter.

Table 22-3 Endothelial cell functions important in hemostasis and thrombosis

Synthesis of anticoagulant protein and coagulation factors
- von Willebrand factor
- Fibronectin
- Thrombomodulin
- Tissue factor
- Protein S

Fibrinolysis
- Tissue type of plasminogen activator (t-PA)
- Urokinase-like plasminogen activator (u-PA)
- Plasminogen activator inhibitor (PAI)

Vasoconstrictor molecules
- Endothelin-1
- Angiotensin II

Inhibitors of platelet aggregation and secretion
- Endothelium-derived nitric oxide (EDNO)
- Prostacyclin (PGI_2)
- Heparin-like glycosaminoglycans

Other factors synthesized by the endothelial cell important in the regulation of platelet adhesion include endothelium-derived nitric oxide (EDNO), heparin-like antithrombins, and prostacyclin (PGI_2). Some of the functions of endothelial cells in hemostasis are mediated by the vasomotor functions of the cells. EDNO has been shown to be a potent vasodilator of both arteries and veins and to perform important processes in the initial phases of hemostasis. Vasoconstrictor molecules produced by the endothelium include endothelin, angiotensin II, and vasoconstrictor prostaglandins. EDNO is also believed to inhibit the proliferation of smooth muscle cells, in contrast to the proliferative effects that endothelin has on smooth muscle cells. Further, EDNO is an inhibitor of platelet aggregation and adhesion to endothelial surfaces. The vasomotor properties of the endothelium are affected by injury as in hypertension or altered integrity of the thromboresistant properties of the endothelium, which normally serve to prevent platelet adhesion and produce procoagulants on the endothelial cell surface. Endothelial cell function is compromised by the subsequent development of endothelial damage, fibrin deposition, and thrombus formation.

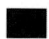

ABNORMAL HEMOSTASIS

There is an enormous diversity of hemostatic disorders, both hereditary[16] and acquired.[17] Evaluation of the patient with hemostatic disorder requires careful history, including drug use, physical evaluation, and laboratory testing, which further includes assessment of the complete blood count, platelet numbers, prothrombin time, activated partial thromboplastin time, and bleeding time (in some situations). A complete discussion of these disorders is outside the scope of this textbook and is more appropriately considered in textbooks of laboratory medicine or hematology. However, a relatively simple classification of hemostatic disorders recognizes four types of defects: vascular, platelet, coagulation proteins, and multifactorial. These are briefly discussed.

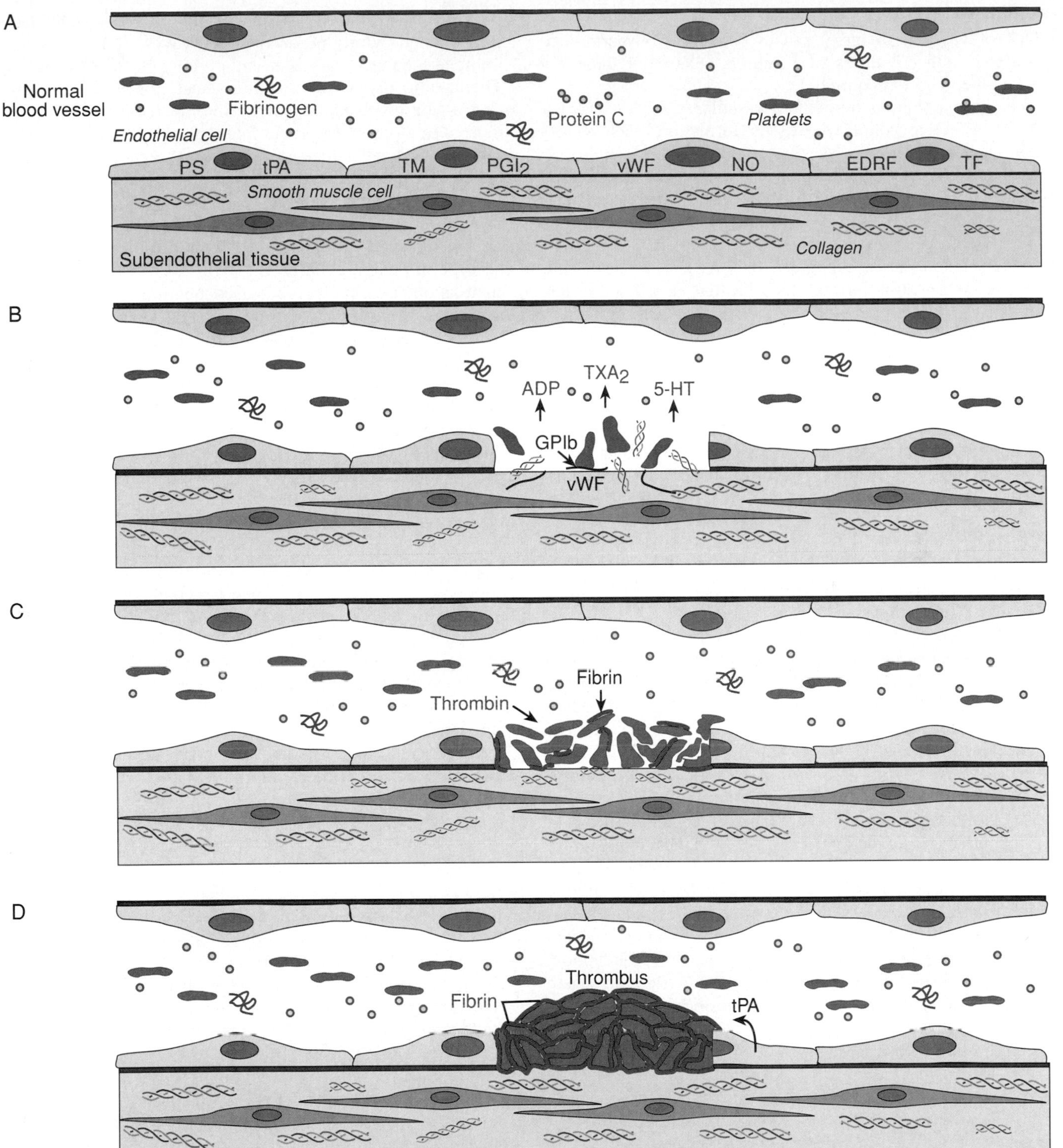

Fig. 22-2 **A,** Intact layer of endothelial cells separates the contents of the bloodstream from tissues of the blood vessel wall. After endothelial cell injury or removal, **B,** disruption of the endothelial layer exposes the flowing blood to subendothelial tissues. Platelets adhere to the area of injury. Platelet adhesion is mediated by vWF interaction with the platelet membrane glycoprotein Ib (GP-Ib). After activation, platelet-shape change occurs, and there is release of substances that induce further platelet activation and recruitment to the site of injury. **C,** Thrombin generation is responsible for fibrin production, which forms a scaffold for the growing platelet thrombus. GP-IIb/IIIa is important for platelet-fibrin interaction and platelet spread over the area of injury. The consolidated thrombus, **D,** consists of a tight meshwork of platelets and fibrin that completely covers the injured area. Erythrocytes and leukocytes also become incorporated into the growing thrombus. Resolution of the thrombus begins with the release of t-PA from the endothelial cell, and eventually endothelial regrowth occurs to cover the defect. *ADP,* Adenosine diphosphate; *EDRF,* endothelium-derived relaxation factor; *5-HT,* serotonin; *NO,* nitric oxide; *P,* platelet; *PGI*$_2$, prostaglandin I_2; *PS,* protein S; *SMC,* smooth muscle cell; *TF,* tissue factor; *TM,* thrombomodulin; *t-PA,* tissue plasminogen activator; *TXA*$_2$, thromboxane A_2; *vWF,* von Willebrand factor.

Vascular defects

A lack of vascular integrity causes petechiae, purpura, easy bruising, or other features of bleeding.[18] Vascular disorders may be hereditary or acquired.

The more common hereditary vascular disorders have a basis in defective connective tissue formation, such as the Ehlers-Danlos syndrome, Marfan syndrome, and pseudoxanthoma elasticum. Congenital hemangiomas of varying sizes may be related to hemostatic disorders.[19] The Kasabach-Merritt syndrome describes the association of giant cavernous hemangiomas and disseminated intervascular coagulation. Hereditary hemorrhagic telangiectasia, or Osler-Weber-Rendu syndrome, is a well-described disorder that, as a feature, has telangiectatic lesions that possibly represent an absence of elastic tissue in vascular walls.

Acquired vascular defects include defective metabolism, as occurs in Cushing's syndrome and diabetes mellitus; connective tissue diseases; systemic lupus erythematosus; and paraprotein disorders including amyloidosis[20] and can be drug induced. Although the pathophysiology of the vascular defect differs among these disorders, a common feature is compromise of the integrity of the vessel wall.

Platelet defects

Thrombocytopenia

Petechiae, easy bruising, and bleeding from mucosal surfaces after mild trauma are signs of defective platelet number or function. Reduced numbers of platelets may be related to impaired platelet production or maturation or increased destruction of platelets. Platelets are diminished in number in Fanconi's syndrome, Wiskott-Aldrich syndrome,[21] and May-Hegglin syndrome.[13] Each of these hereditary diseases has variable degrees of thrombocytopenia. Defective platelet production is often seen as a feature of aplastic anemia. Infiltration of the marrow by metastatic tumors may compromise platelet production. Thrombocytopenia often occurs after cancer chemotherapy, reflecting toxicity to megakaryocytic precursors. Thrombocytopenia may be caused by increased consumption or destruction of platelets. The hemolytic uremic syndrome (HUS)[22] discussed in Chapter 65 has platelet consumption as a feature. Thrombotic thrombocytopenic purpura (TTP) is an enigmatic condition associated with infection, pregnancy, and adverse drug reaction.[23] In this condition, there are widespread microthrombi in small arterioles and capillaries. These serve as the focal point for platelet aggregation, thus causing thrombocytopenia.

Hypersplenism is a cause of thrombocytopenia. Normally the spleen pools approximately one third of the platelet volume. With splenomegaly, or hypersplenism, pooling of platelets is increased. Hypersplenism may be caused by deposits of material within the spleen, such as amyloid and Gaucher's disease. Another cause is neoplastic disease involving the spleen, such as lymphoma and leukemia. Hypersplenism accompanies some autoimmune disorders, such as systemic lupus erythematosus and rheumatoid arthritis. An autoimmune disorder typified by increased platelet destruction is immune thrombocytopenic purpura (ITP).[9] This illness, which occurs predominantly in children after a viral illness, appears to be caused by the binding of immune complexes to glycoprotein receptors on platelet surface. These platelets are then removed by the reticuloendothelial system, notably the spleen. The chronic form of ITP differs from acute ITP. Chronic ITP occurs in adults and usually lacks a well-defined viral prodrome. However, this is also an immune-mediated disorder involving platelet bound IgG. Therapeutic drugs are a major cause for immune-mediated destruction of platelets. Among the mechanisms is the formation of a drug platelet complex that is recognized by the immune system as foreign. That result, again, is clearance of platelets from circulation.

Thrombocytosis and thrombocythemia

Thrombocytosis describes an increase in platelet count because of benign conditions.[10] This may be caused by drugs, such as epinephrine, or decreased pooling of platelets within the spleen. Thrombocythemia implies an increased platelet count because of a malignancy, such as the myeloproliferative syndromes.

In both thrombocytosis and thrombocythemia the platelet count may exceed $1,000,000/mm^3$. Paradoxically, many patients have a hemostatic disorder, with hemorrhage and thrombosis being common complications.

Defective platelet function

Platelet function defects may be attributable to defective adhesion, defective aggregation, or defective secondary aggregation. The Bernard-Soulier syndrome is an autosomal dominant trait that typifies abnormal platelet adhesion.[11] Surface glycoproteins are absent from the platelet membrane. The platelet is dysfunctional, and the clinical and laboratory features are similar to those of von Willebrand disease. Glanzmann's thrombasthenia is a rare disorder of defective primary platelet aggregation. Glycoprotein lb is missing from the platelet membrane, placing the patient at risk for petechiae and hemorrhage. Secondary platelet aggregation disorders are much more common than primary aggregation defects. The storage pool diseases are included in this category. The major laboratory manifestations are the absence of either epinephrine or an ADP-induced secondary aggregation. These patients have prolonged bleeding times. Included in these two disorders are the so-called isolated defect, the Hermansky-Pudlak syndrome, and platelet disorders associated with immune deficiency such as Chédiak-Higashi syndrome and Wiskott-Aldrich syndrome.

Aggregation defects may also be attributable to deficiencies of cyclooxygenase or thromboxane synthase. These "aspirin-like" defects are so named because of their similarity to therapeutic effects of aspirin.

Acquired platelet dysfunction may accompany myeloproliferative syndromes, uremia, paraprotein disorders, and drug therapy. In uremia, which is commonly complicated by platelet dysfunction, there is increased circulating guanidinosuccinic acid, which compromises platelet factor III activity. The most common acquired platelet defect is attributable to therapeutic drugs, such as aspirin, and related drugs that block the synthesis of prostaglandins.

Defects of coagulation proteins

Congenital deficiencies

Although congenital deficiencies of virtually all protein factors involved in the coagulation cascade are known, they are rare, except for von Willebrand syndrome.[16] Congenital abnormalities of fibrinogen include afibrinogenemia, characterized by low fibrinogen levels, or dysfibrinogenemia, where the fibrinogen molecule demonstrates abnormal polymerization. Disorders of prothrombin, factor X, factor V, and factor XIII have been described.

Disorders of the intrinsic pathway of factor X activation underlie several of the hemophilia syndromes.[24-26] A deficiency of factor VIII:C is termed *hemophilia A*. This recessive X-linked disease affects males at an incidence of approximately 20 per 100,000 people. The severity of the hemophilia is directly related to the factor VIII:C concentration in plasma, and the defective molecule is unable to catalyze the conversion of factor X to factor Xa. Patients with classic hemophilia are subject to joint hemarthrosis and muscle bleeding, easy bruising, and prolonged hemorrhage after injury.

Disorders of factor IX are responsible for hemophilia B, or Christmas disease. Clinically, hemophilia B is similar to hemophilia A.[26] Levels of factor IX activity in the plasma correlate with the severity of the clinical syndromes.

Defective clotting may also occur in the absence of appropriate regulatory factors, such as antithrombin III, protein C, alpha$_2$-antiplasmin, and protein S.[1,27] Finally, combined congenital coagulopathies are also well recognized.

von Willebrand disease

von Willebrand's disease, which affects both men and women, is attributable to abnormal interaction between platelets and endothelium.[28-31] Usually there is an insufficient amount of von Willebrand factor, a protein coded by chromosome 12. This glycoprotein molecule is produced by endothelial cells and megakaryocytes. von Willebrand factor on the platelet surface is important for the binding of the platelet to collagen and other substances in the subendothelium. von Willebrand factor is also important in platelet-to-platelet adhesion. Any of several genetic defects can give rise to von Willebrand disease. These variations are termed type I, type II, and type III, according to the amount and function of von Willebrand factor and the severity of the bleeding.

Acquired forms of von Willebrand disease have been described, and in some cases, they have been related to antibodies directed against von Willebrand factor.

Acquired defects

Because of the central role of the liver in the synthesis of coagulation proteins, vitamin K deficiency, cirrhosis, or other hepatocellular diseases may lead to abnormal hemostasis.[17]

Disseminated intravascular coagulation

Disseminated intravascular coagulation (DIC) is a paradox, in that widespread intravascular coagulation leads to uncontrolled bleeding.[32] Acute DIC is associated with obstetric procedures, intravascular hemolysis triggered by transfusion reaction, disseminated malignancy, burns and massive injury. Pathophysiologically, both thrombin and plasmin are in circulation, with concurrent activation of the complement cascade and kinin system. Microvascular thrombosis may cause renal failure, muscular damage, liver failure, and pulmonary failure.

The morphologic features of DIC are evident in the peripheral blood, principally through decreased platelet count and abnormal red blood cell fragments. Microthrombi may be present in various organs. Assessment of thrombin time, activated partial thromboplastin time, and tests for circulating fibrinogen degradation products are helpful. In general, a panel of laboratory tests are required.

THROMBOSIS

To understand the concept of thrombosis requires a working knowledge of the normal hemostatic process. Thrombosis, or thrombus formation, generally refers to a pathologic event that results from abnormal hemostasis and may impair blood flow to distant tissues. Under normal conditions, hemostasis refers to the mechanisms involved in the arrest of bleeding after injury. The normal hemostatic process involves a complex series of events that were previously described in this chapter. Normal hemostasis incorporates elements of the fluid and cellular components of the blood, as well as the extravascular matrix.[14] In the most simplified version of hemostasis, the important final elements are platelets and the accompanying fibrin matrix (Fig. 22-2). Exaggeration of the hemostatic process leads to thrombus formation. As a response to injury, the vessel wall undergoes a series of changes that initially consists of a vasoconstrictive response followed by the release of endothelial cell components that promote loss of the thromboresistant properties of the endothelial layer in the area of injury. The events important in the development of pathologic hemostasis or thrombosis is the focus of this portion of this chapter.

Under normal conditions, vascular injury is followed by the release of blood components into the extracellular matrix. Initially, the exposed collagen and extracellular matrix promote platelet deposition and induce blood coagulation. Both are important in this process, since fibrin formation serves as a scaffold for platelet adherence and stabilization in the site of injury. A limited microenvironment is set up where coagulation is initiated and culminates with the formation of a stable platelet-fibrin plug. Two important events in this stage of hemostasis are that blood flow from injured vessels is impeded and that the process is self-limited. Under normal conditions, there is resolution of the hemostatic thrombus with subsequent repair of the injury. This may involve neovascularization and increased collagen formation. Unless there are conditions that impair the arrest of the blood, repair occurs in a relatively short time.

vWF is important in primary hemostasis, through mediating platelet adhesion to the blood vessel wall. Under high shear conditions, such as those that exist in the microcirculation, vWF is necessary for platelet adherence to occur. Two primary compartments of vWF exist plasma and cellular. vWF is present in the subendothelium and within the extracellular matrix. After injury to a vessel wall, the initial adhesion of platelets to the subendothelium is mediated by plasma vWF by means of the collagen receptor or other domains within the vWF molecule. Plasma vWF then binds to the subendothelial matrix, and the subsequent interaction with GPlb-IX-V complex initiates platelet adhesion. This interaction results in the activation of GPIIb/IIIa, which is responsible for platelet spread over an area of injury. Both plasma and released cellular vWF foster additional recruitment of platelets to the site of injury. The VIII/vWF complex is necessary for this sequence of reactions and to produce a stable platelet-fibrin thrombus.

Mechanisms of thrombus formation

There are three conditions that are conducive to thrombus formation: (1) injury to the vascular system, (2) cessation of blood flow, and (3) localized activation of the coagulation sys-

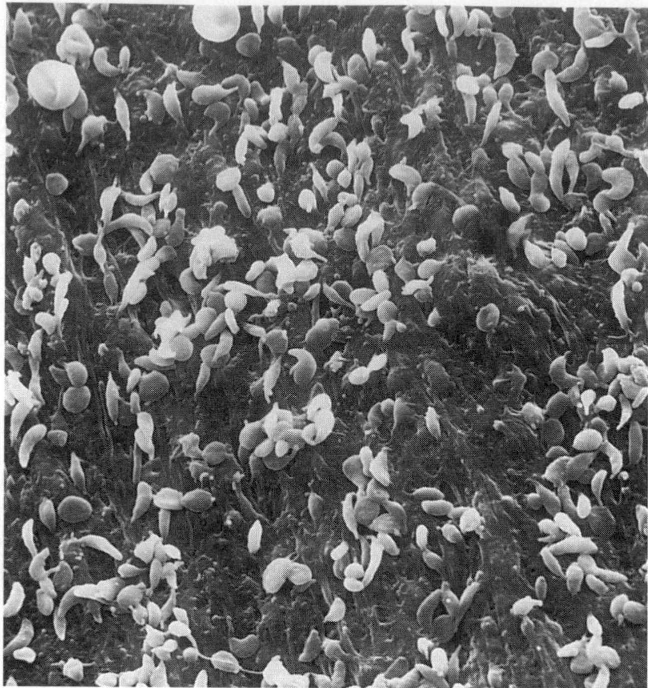

Fig. 22-3 After simple endothelial denudation, platelets adhere to the subendothelium in a monolayer fashion. This photograph corresponds to the diagram in Fig. 22-2, **B.**

tem.[14,16] In experimental models, superficial injury or removal of the endothelial layer of muscular arteries promotes platelet deposition without accompanying fibrin formation (Fig. 22-3). Platelets initially adhere to the denuded surface, but after a short period the surface becomes refractory to further platelet deposition. This process, termed *pacification,* describes a loss of platelet attractants or changes in the injury site that retard further platelet deposition. Over time, there is endothelial regrowth, and the area of injury is once again thromboresistant. With injury to the tunica media of the vessel or injury to atherosclerotic plaques, thrombus formation occurs (Fig. 22-4). In these areas, fibrin is incorporated into the thrombus, causing an increase in the size of the thrombus at the area of injury. Complete restitution of the thromboresistant surface of tissues or tears in atherosclerotic plaques, for unknown reasons, may not occur, and the plaques may exhibit a heightened tendency to thrombus formation (Fig. 22-5). Whether this tendency is attributable to loss of the normal thromboresistant properties of the local endothelial cells or changes in blood flow produced by the plaque is under investigation. Patients who have undergone angioplasty provide evidence that recurrent thrombosis is a continuing problem, presumably because of the thrombogenic properties of the vessel surface. Flow abnormalities and shear forces induced by the partial vascular obstruction may also be important in the increased tendency toward thrombus formation.

Tendencies toward thrombosis occur in many clinical settings where genetic abnormalities, atherosclerosis, cancer, or autoantibodies may promote abnormal hemostasis (Table 22-4). Common to all these conditions is either a subtle or direct injury to the endothelial cell. A discussion of these conditions follows.

ABNORMAL THROMBUS FORMATION

Conditions where genetic abnormalities promote thrombus formation include deficiency of antithrombin III, protein S, or protein C.[27,33,35] These natural inhibitors of intravascular coagulation are important in maintaining fluidity of the blood. When deficient, individuals may present clinically with unexplained and recurrent thromboses of both arterial and venous systems. Efforts to explain thrombosis in these patients has clarified our understanding of the regulatory mechanisms of these natural anticoagulants in hemostasis and thrombosis. For example, coagulation factors VIII, V, VII, and fibrinogen are important in thrombus generation and in hypercoagulable states. The regulation of these factors then are of importance in the maintenance of blood fluidity. In association with the increased tendency to thrombosis produced by these coagulation factors, the integrity of the endothelium and platelet factors are also of importance. Demonstration that von Willebrand factor is necessary for thrombosis to occur after injury to the vessel wall further substantiates the importance of endothelial injury and the vessel wall in thrombus formation. The relationship of vessel wall constituents, endothelium, intact coagulation system, and the blood cells, including platelets, is important in the elucidation of the events that occur with congenital defects in the regulatory mechanisms of thrombosis.

Protein S and protein C are vitamin K–dependent plasma proteins.[27] The function of protein S is to promote binding of activated protein C to membrane surfaces. The binding of protein S to protein C is important in producing the anticoagulant function of protein C. The series of steps that regulate protein C activation have become known as the protein C pathway.[34,35] The association of protein S and protein C with the vascular endothelium is important because injury to endothelial cells promotes platelet deposition and local hemostasis. In the protein C pathway, protein C is activated by thrombin through interactions with another important endothelial cell transmembrane protein—*thrombomodulin,*[36] which further promotes reduction of activated clotting factors in the microenvironment. The activated complex, PC/PS, inactivates factors Va and VIIIa and thereby reduces the thrombotic tendency.[16] As a result, protein C is of vital importance in the local regulation of clotting within the vascular space. Deficiency of protein S is also associated with thrombotic diseases.[37-39] A crucial role of the endothelial cell in this process is thrombin inactivation, which further decreases the thrombogenicity at the site of injury. A second and equally important function of the endothelial cells is to promote fibrinolytic activity by release of tPA.[40] Loss of this function results in the inability for clot lysis to occur. It has been suggested that this dual function of the endothelial cell is to limit the area of intravascular coagulation and to facilitate repair of the defect by controlled lysis of the hemostatic plug.

Antithrombin III (AT III) is a serine protease inhibitor that is produced in the liver and protects against spontaneous thrombus formation.[15] AT III inactivates thrombin and other serine proteases. The ability of AT III to prevent clotting through thrombin inactivation is augmented by heparin. Slight reductions in the serum concentration of AT III leads to thrombus formation by a mechanism related to a lack of inactivation

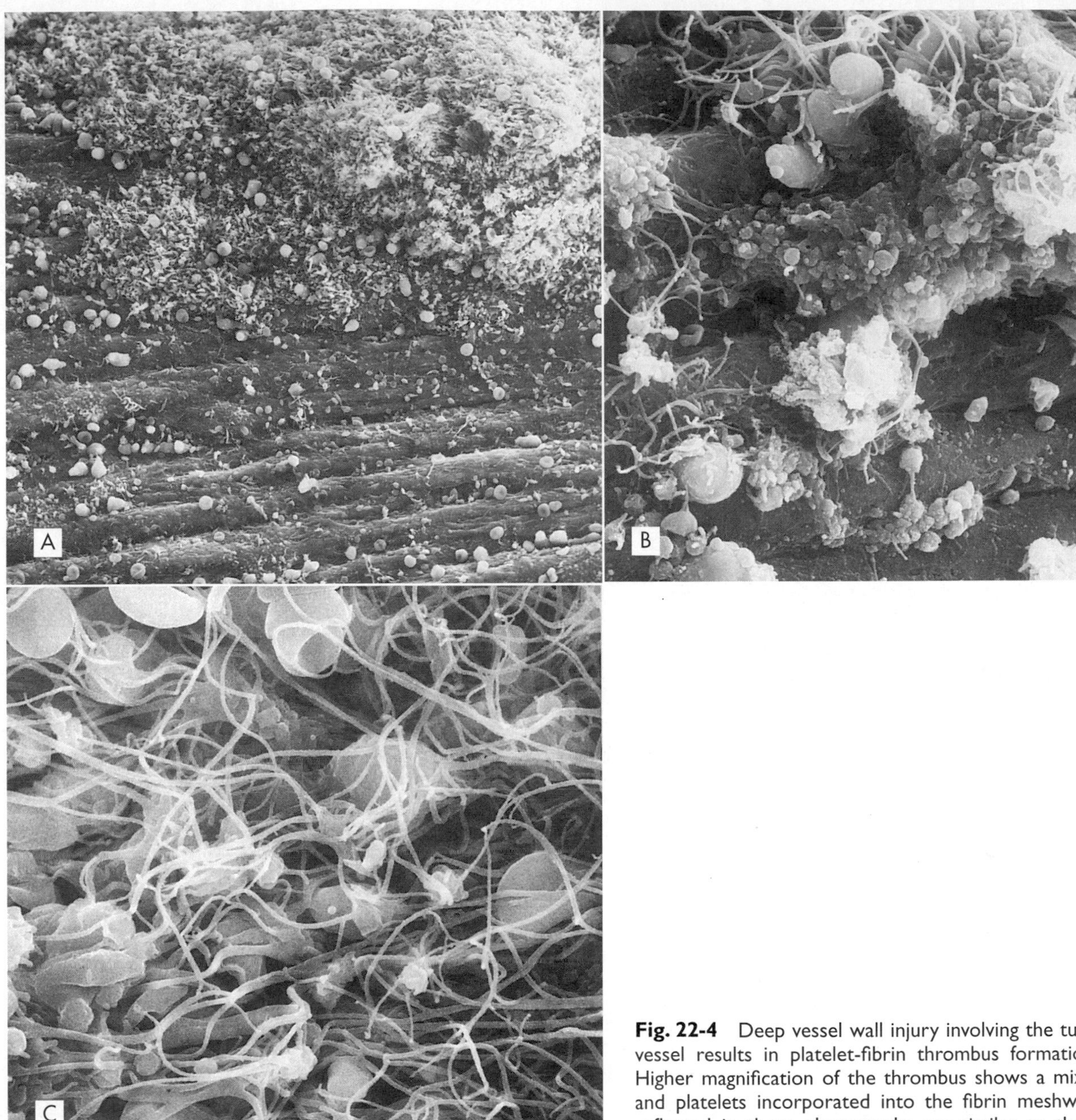

Fig. 22-4 Deep vessel wall injury involving the tunica media of the vessel results in platelet-fibrin thrombus formation, **A** and **B. C**, Higher magnification of the thrombus shows a mixture of red cells and platelets incorporated into the fibrin meshwork. The changes reflected in these photographs are similar to those diagramed in Fig. 22-2, **C** and **D.**

of factors Xa, IXa, XIa, and XIIa. Further, thrombin is not inactivated. In addition to the inherited deficiency of AT III, reduced levels of AT III have been described in patients with renal disease or disseminated intravascular coagulation, in use of oral contraceptives, and in liver disease. Individuals with AT III deficiency most commonly experience venous thrombotic events in the mesenteric and deep veins of the lower extremities and have a tendency to develop pulmonary emboli. These symptoms usually appear in affected individuals during their teenage years. There are two known forms of the deficiency. In some individuals, there is absence of normal, physiologically active AT III (CRM−) and others have a dysfunctional form (CRM+). Heterozygotes for AT III deficiency have also been described, and these individuals also exhibit thrombotic tendencies.

CANCER AND THROMBOSIS

Certain human malignancies cause systemic activation of the coagulation system, resulting in thrombotic complications.[41-47] The common examples are carcinomas of the pancreas, colon, lung, kidney, and promyelocytic leukemia. Different mechanisms have been proposed to explain the thrombotic tendencies of cancer patients. These include the production of a tumor procoagulant activity, macrophage activation of coagulation, endothelial cell injury, and platelet activation by their interaction with tumor cells. The serum concentration of coagulation factors such as V, VIII, VII, and fibrinogen is often elevated in patients with cancer. In mucinous colon cancer, activation of factor X occurs, presumably through an interaction

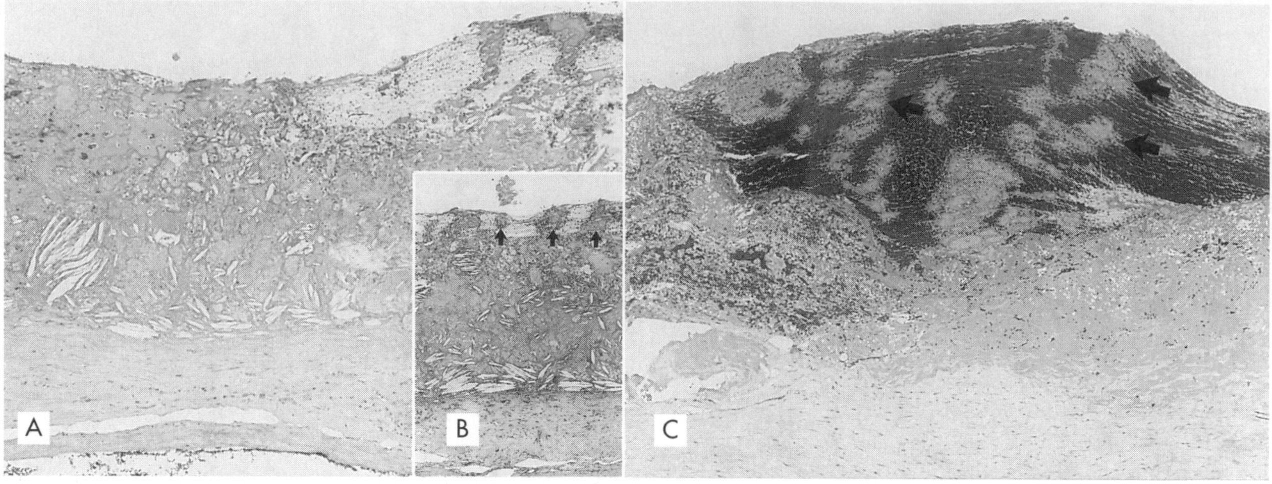

Fig. 22-5 Thrombus overlying atherosclerotic plaque. A large thrombus is present and contains cholesterol clefts at the base. The vessel wall is thinned and sclerotic, **A.** Columns of platelets *(arrows)* alternating with fibrin, erythrocytes, and leukocytes are shown in **B** and **C.**

Table 22-4 Thrombotic syndromes

Genetic tendencies to thrombosis
Protein S
Protein C
Antithrombin III deficiency
Acquired tendencies to thrombosis
Anticardiolipin
Thrombosis associated with disorders of lipoprotein Metabolism
Thrombosis in cancer
Thrombosis in atherogenesis

Table 22-5 Antiphospholipid syndrome: clinical and laboratory features

Clinical
Recurrent arterial and venous thrombosis
Recurrent fetal loss
Livedo reticularis
Neurologic dysfunction
Systemic and pulmonary hypertension
Myocardial infarction
Laboratory
Presence or absence of lupus anticoagulant
Positive anticardiolipin test (IgG or IgM)
False-positive VDRL test results
Thrombocytopenia
Prolonged activated partial thromboplastin time
Prolonged Russell's viper venom time
Possible alterations in protein S, protein C, thrombomodulin
AntiDNA antibodies

with a cysteine protease found in the mucin associated with these tumors. Activation of the other coagulation factors may occur. This may be especially true if there is extensive metastatic carcinoma.

A role of vessel wall injury with subsequent activation of the extrinsic coagulation system may partially explain the role of endothelial cell–tumor cell interaction and endothelial damage. A heightened thrombotic tendency under these conditions may be either a local process or may trigger disseminated intravascular coagulation (DIC).[32] Local aberrations exist in areas of vessel wall injury and also produce activation of factor X to Xa. In this situation, the resulting thrombi are platelet rich. von Willebrand factor most likely has a role in this process. It has been shown that high levels of circulating thrombomodulin are present in patients with hematologic malignancies, in those with liver disease, and in those with DIC. Similarity, t-PA is also elevated. These findings indicate that conditions that promote injury to the endothelium may be an important part of the process that promotes thrombosis in patients with malignancies because all of the changes described may be seen in situations in which endothelial injury is present. Thrombin generation may also have a role in this process because thrombin also produces activation of coagulation factors V and VIII and activates protein C, which inactivates Va and VIIIa. Thrombin, as mentioned, is regulated by AT III, alpha$_2$-macroglobulin, and heparin cofactor II.

Antiphospholipid syndrome

Antiphospholipid antibodies encompass a group of autoantibodies that interact with negatively charged phospholipids.[48-60] The most common are the anticardiolipin (aCL) antibody and the lupus anticoagulant. The possible relationship between thrombosis and the presence of a "lupus anticoagulant" was originally suggested in 1963. Since that time, it has been recognized that the antiphospholipid syndrome (APS), as it is now called, represents a grouping of clinical and laboratory findings (Table 22-5). Many of the patients with APS carry the diagnosis of systemic lupus erythematosus (SLE), whereas others with anticardiolipin antibodies do not have well-characterized autoimmune disorders. The syndrome, as currently recognized, is characterized by recurrent thrombosis in young people, recurrent spontaneous abortions, thrombocytopenia, and elevated levels of antiphospholipid antibodies.

These antibodies may be one of three idiotypes—IgG, IgM, or IgA.[50]

The most frequently detected antiphospholipids are the anticardiolipin antibody, the lupus anticoagulant, and the false-positive antibody found in the VDRL test for syphilis. Although individuals with APS have SLE, this syndrome may occur in individuals without associated autoimmune disorders.

Arterial thrombosis most commonly involves the intracerebral vessels[61] though thrombosis of decidual and placental vessels and placental infarction is found.[55] Fetal loss in the APS usually occurs in the second and third trimesters. An elevated IgG anticardiolipin level has been associated with an increased risk for myocardial infarction and unstable angina. Other studies have shown that IgG and IgM idiotypes, with or without the presence of the lupus anticoagulant, may be associated with occlusive vascular disease. IgG-anticardiolipin antibodies have also been found to be elevated in patients with cerebral and peripheral vascular disease. In some patients IgM-anticardiolipin antibodies are increased after percutaneous transluminal coronary angioplasty. Such patients are more likely to have early re-stenosis than those patients without anticardiolipin.[52] Not all studies have confirmed this relationship.

The paradoxical nature of this syndrome is illustrated by the in vitro laboratory findings of anticoagulation tendencies and the clinical findings of recurrent thromboses. The parallel to disseminated intravascular coagulation is striking because both anticoagulation and thrombosis are also present in DIC. The major difference, however, is the underlying cause of the hemorrhagic tendency and intravascular thrombosis. The mechanism by which antiphospholipids promote thrombosis is not completely understood (Table 22-6) and remain controversial. In the APS, in vitro, antiphospholipid antibodies are believed to inhibit clotting by interfering with the action of the prothrombin activator complex. Intravascular thrombosis may be related to interference with the natural inhibitors of coagulation, protein C, antithrombin III, and the fibrinolytic system. These activities are related to normal endothelial cell function, and in some unknown way, the antiphospholipids may alter the natural anticoagulant mechanisms of these cells. Further, the lupus anticoagulant may interfere with the activity of thrombomodulin in the protein C system. Platelet activation may also be initiated by the interaction of the antibody with the lipid on the platelet surface to initiate platelet aggregation.

Table 22-6 Mechanisms of action related to thrombogenesis in the antiphospholipid syndrome

Interaction of antiphospholipid antibodies with endothelial cells
Production of beta$_2$-glycoprotein I antibodies
Interaction with congenital deficiencies of proteins S and C
Inhibition of prostacyclin release
Inhibition of the catalytic activity of thrombomodulin
Decreased tissue plasminogen activator activity
Increased plasminogen activator inhibitor-1
Antiphospholipid antibody neutralization of phospholipids necessary for protein C activation
Increased platelet-activating factor
Inhibition of the function of antithrombin III

In combination, there is reduced fibrinolytic activity and an increased tendency to thrombus formation.

Individuals with the APS usually have antibodies to phosholipids in high titer. These antibodies are a heterogeneous assortment of immunoglobulins with binding affinity to negatively charged phospholipids. The laboratory detection of antiphospholipid antibodies (aPL) is by the lupus anticoagulant (LA) test and the anticardiolipin test.[62] Other lupus workups are also performed, since many of the patients who are diagnosed as having the APS also have lupus. In SLE, the frequency of aCL antibody ranges from 21% to 63% (normal controls 0 to 7.5%). In the absence of SLE, aCL is found in 4% to 87% of patients with the APS.[59,60] There is evidence to indicate that a strong relationship may exist between the presence of the lupus anticoagulant and anticardiolipin antibodies. Individuals who were found to have both LA and aCL antibodies are more likely to have an increased thrombotic tendency and thrombocytopenia.

Atherosclerosis and plasma lipoprotein–associated thrombosis

With the evidence that a possible relationship existed between lipoproteins, thrombosis, and atherosclerosis, the role of lipids in re-stenosis after coronary angioplasty, in thrombosis in genetic lipoprotein disorders, and cardiovascular diseases have been the focus of considerable attention.[63] Studies have linked a high-level plasma lipid composition with increased platelet responsiveness to agonists, and such a combination modifies the antithrombogenic properties of endothelial cells and coagulation factors. It has been shown that the lipid content and size of clots is increased in patients with coronary artery disease. These studies also showed that coagulation was accelerated and platelets were more activated with regard to adhesion and aggregation. In individuals with type III hyperlipoproteinemia, platelets have a shortened life-span and an increased rate of aggregation and release.

Rupture or fissuring of atherosclerotic plaques promotes thrombus formation. The acute coronary syndromes include unstable angina, acute myocardial infarction, and sudden cardiac death. The mechanism or mechanisms most commonly used to explain the cause of this syndrome are plaque fissuring and vasoconstriction, followed by coronary thrombosis. However, in areas of plaque fissuring, the smooth muscle cell layer is thinned and vasospasm may not play a significant role. Injury to atherosclerotic plaques with exposure of thrombogenic tissues such as collagen and smooth muscle cells promotes thrombus formation. This process is remarkably similar to what occurs after coronary angioplasty. Several factors may play a role in this process, including the level of serum cholesterol, local shear factors, exposure of thrombogenic surfaces, and vasoconstrictive effects. A cascade model has been proposed to explain restenosis occurring after angioplasty. In this model, cytokine expression produces a self-sustaining and continuing production of growth factors by various cell types leading to restenosis. In this model, restenosis would occur despite the use of antithrombotic agents and would indicate that thrombosis in these areas may be less important. However, it is clear that the degree of vascular stenosis and thrombus formation that occurs after plaque injury are important factors to explain the rapid vascular occlusion often present after angioplasty.

High concentration of plasma lipoprotein(a), Lp(a), is considered to be important in both thrombosis and ather-

Table 22-7 Presumptive mechanisms of thrombosis by Lp(a)

Competition with plasminogen and t-PA for fibrin binding
Reduction of plasminogen activation by increased synthesis of PAI-1
Binding to t-PA by apolipoprotein B-100/E receptor

osclerosis.[64-72] Lp(a), first reported in 1963, represents a class of lipoproteins that differ in size and density. Lp(a) consists of two protein moieties, apolipoprotein B-100 and apolipoprotein(a), linked by disulfide bonds. The apo(a) gene is present on chromosome 6. Lp(a) is structurally similar to low-density lipoprotein. The molecular mass of apo(a) varies between 400 and 700 kD, a range that may be a reflection of the protein:lipid ratio, apo B-100:apo(a) interaction and the size of the apo(a) isoform to which it is attached. Nineteen alleles, identified by pulsed-field gel electrophoresis and genetic blotting, have been described; however, this exceeds the 11 isoforms that have been identified using SDS-polyacrylamide gel electrophoresis. cDNA analysis has shown that Lp(a) has a considerable homology to plasminogen, a serine protease, the active form of which, plasmin, degrades fibrin. Sequence analysis shows that the 5′ coding region of apo(a) and plasminogen are identical for 95 base pairs. Apo(a) has been shown to contain a single serine protease domain and a variable number of lysine binding kringle domains. In contrast, plasminogen has five kringle regions considered to be important in fibrin binding. Despite this degree of homology, apo(a) does not have a role in fibrinolysis. This lack is believed to be attributable to the substitution of a single amino acid, arginine, for serine in plasminogen.

Lp(a) is considered to be an independent risk factor for coronary artery disease.[64] The increased susceptibility to arterial thrombosis may be attributable to the homology with plasminogen (Table 22-7). Lp(a) inhibits the active site binding of plasminogen to its activator site on endothelial surfaces. Lp(a) competes for the plasminogen receptor site, and plasminogen is therefore less susceptible to activation by t-PA. This allows Lp(a) to exhibit a prothrombotic role by reducing clot lysis. Additional roles of Lp(a) in thrombus promotion may be the result of the binding to fibrin thereby reducing the activation of plasminogen in the presence of fibrin. Lp(a) has also been shown to promote the synthesis and release of plasminogen activator inhibitor type 1 (PAI-1) from endothelial cells. This interaction with t-PA reduces plasminogen activation and thereby enhances thrombus formation.[71,73]

REFERENCES

1. Briet E, Engesser L, Brommer EJ: Regulation of blood coagulation and thrombosis, *Haemostasis* 15:228, 1985.
2. Alvin BM, Comp PC: Recent advances in understanding clotting and evaluating patients with recurrent thrombosis, *Am J Obstet Gynecol* 167:1184, 1992.
3. Roberts HR, Lozier JN: New perspectives on the coagulation cascade, *Hosp Pract* 27:97, 1992.
4. Broze GJ Jr: Tissue factor pathway inhibitor and the revised hypothesis of blood coagulation, *Trends Cardiovasc Med* 2:72, 1992.
5. Gardner F, Bessman JD: Thrombocytopenia due to defective platelet production, *Clin Haematol* 12:23, 1983.
6. Baranski B, Young N: Hematologic consequences of viral infections, *Hematol Oncol Clin North Am* 1:167, 1987.
7. Bick RL: Platelet defects. In *Disorders of hemostasis and thrombosis: a practical clinical appraoch,* New York, 1985, Thieme.
8. Mieschner PA, Graf J: Drug-induced thrombocytopenia, *Clin Haematol* 9:505, 1980.
9. Kelton JG, Gibbons S: Autoimmune platelet destruction: idiopathic thrombocytopenic purpura, *Semin Thromb Hemost* 8:83, 1982.
10. Murphy S: Thrombocytosis and thrombocythaemia, *Clin Haematol* 12:89, 1983.
11. Lusher JM, Barnhart MI: Congenital disorders affecting platelets, *Semin Thromb Hemost* 4:123, 1977.
12. Triplett DA: Platelet disorders. In Murano G, Bick RL, editors: *Basic concepts of hemostasis and thrombosis,* Boca Raton, Fla, 1980, CRC Press.
13. Godwin NA, Ginsburg AD: May-Hegglin anomaly: a defect in megakaryocyte fragmentation, *Br J Haematol* 26:117, 1974.
14. Bennett JS: Mechanisms of platelet adhesion and aggregation: an update, *Hosp Pract* 27:124, 1992.
15. Bick RL: Physiology of hemostasis. In *Disorders of thrombosis and hemostasis,* Chicago, 1992, ASCP Press.
16. Wu KK: Endothelial cells in hemostasis, thrombosis, and inflammation, Hosp Pract 27:145, 1992.
17. Lechner K, Niessner H, Thaler E: Coagulation abnormalities in liver disease, *Semin Thromb Hemost* 4:40, 1977.
18. Bick RL: Vascular disorders associated with thrombohemorrhagic phenomenon, *Semin Thromb Hemost* 5:167, 1979.
19. Kasabach HH, Merritt KK: Capillary hemangioma with extensive purpura, *Am J Dis Child* 59:1016, 1940.
20. Lachner H: Hemostatic abnormalities associated with paraprotein abnormalities, *Semin Hematol* 10:125, 1973.
21. Wolff JA: Wiskott-Aldrich syndrome: clinical, immunologic, and pathologic observations, *J Pediatr* 70:221, 1967.
22. Mosgrave JE et al: The hemolytic-uremic syndrome, *Clin Pediatr* 17:218, 1978.
23. Lian ECY: Pathogenesis of thrombotic thrombocytopenic purpura, *Semin Hematol* 24:82, 1987.
24. Pecorara M et al: Hemophilia A: carrier detection and prenatal diagnosis by DNA analysis, *Blood* 70:531, 1987.
25. Gitschier J et al: Mutations of factor VIII cleavage sites in hemophilia A, *Blood* 72:1022, 1988.
26. McGraw RA et al: Structure and function of factor IX: defects in haemophilia B, *Clin Haematol* 14:359, 1985.
27. Esmon CT: Protein S and protein C: biochemistry, physiology, and clinical manifestation of deficiencies, *Trends Cardiovasc Med* 2:214, 1992.
28. Holmberg L, Nilsson IM: von Willebrand disease. In Ruggeri ZM, editor: *Clinics in haematology: coagulation disorders,* London, 1985, Saunders.
29. Nichols WL, Fass DN: Bowie symposium on von Willebrand's disease: introduction, *Mayo Clin Proc* 66:503, 1991.
30. Ruggeri ZM, Ware J: von Willebrand factor, *FASEB J* 7:308, 1993.
31. Ginsburg D: The von Willebrand factor gene and genetics of von Willebrand's disease, *Mayo Clin Proc* 66:506, 1991.
32. Bick RL: Disseminated intravascular coagulation and related syndromes: a clinical review, *Semin Thromb Hemost* 14:299, 1988.
33. Mannucci PM, Tripodi A, Bottasso B et al: Markers of procoagulant imbalance in patients with inherited thrombophilic syndromes, *Thromb Haemost* 67:200, 1992.
34. Walker FJ, Fay PJ: Regulation of blood coagulation by the protein C system, *FASEB J* 6:2561, 1992.
35. Esmon CT, Johnson AE, Esmon NL: Initiation of the protein C pathway, *Ann NY Acad Sci* 614:30, 1991.
36. Dittman WA, Majerus PW: Structure and function of thrombomodulin: a natural anticoagulant, *Blood* 75:329, 1990.
37. Walker FJ: Protein S and thrombotic disease, *Proc Soc Exp Biol Med* 200:285, 1992.
38. Green D, Otoya J, Oriba H, Rovner R: Protein S deficiency in middle aged women with stroke, *Neurology* 45:1029, 1992.
39. Walker FJ: Protein S and thrombotic disease, *Proc Soc Exp Biol Med* 200:285, 1992.

40. Gertler JP, Abbott WM: Prothrombotic and fibrinolytic function of normal and perturbed endothelium, *J Surg Res* 52:89, 1992.
41. Patterson WP: Coagulation and cancer, *Semin Oncol* 17:137, 1990.
42. Zacharski LR, Wojtukiewicz MZ, Costantini V et al: Pathways of coagulation/fibrinolysis activation in malignancy, *Semin Thromb Hemost* 18:104, 1992.
43. Bick RL: Coagulation abnormalities in malignancy: a review, *Semin Thromb Hemost* 18:353, 1992.
44. McGregor BC, McGregor JL, Weiss LM et al: Presence of cytoadhesins (IIb-IIIa–like glycoproteins) on human metastatic melanomas but not on benign melanocytes, *Am J Clin Pathol* 92:495, 1989.
45. Ey FS, Goodnight SH: Bleeding disorders in cancer, *Semin Oncol* 17:187, 1990.
46. Riccio JA, Colley T, Cera PJ: Hepatic vein thrombosis (Budd-Chiari syndrome) in the microglandular variant of acute promyelocytic leukemia, *Am J Clin Pathol* 92:366, 1989.
47. Luzzatto G, Schafer AI: The prethrombotic state in cancer, *Semin Oncol* 17:147, 1990:
48. Triplett DA: Antiphospholipid antibodies and thrombosis: a consequence, coincidence, or cause, *Arch Pathol Lab* 117:78, 1993.
49. Bick RL, Baker WF: Anticardiolipin antibodies and thrombosis, *Hematol Oncol Clin North Am* 6:1287, 1992.
50. Cervera R, Font J, López-Soto A et al: Isotype distribution of anticardiolipin antibodies in systemic lupus erythematosus: prospective analysis of a series of 100 patients, *Ann Rheum Dis* 49:190, 1990.
51. Khamshta MA, Hughes GRV: Detection and importance of anticardiolipin antibodies, *J Clin Pathol* 46:104, 1993.
52. Eber B, Schumacher M, Auer-Grumbach P et al: Increased IgM-anticardiolipin antibodies in patients with restenosis after percutaneous transluminal coronary angioplasty, *Am J Cardiol*, 1225, 1992.
53. Harris EN: A reassessment of the antiphospholipid syndrome, *J Rheumatol* 17:733, 1990.
54. McGee GS, Pearce WH, Sharma L et al: Antiphospholipid antibodies and arterial thrombosis: case report and a review of the literature, *Arch Surg* 127:342, 1992.
55. Contractor S, Hiatt M, Kosmin M, Kim HC: Neonatal thrombosis with anticardiolipin antibody in baby and mother, *Am J Perinatol* 409, 1992.
56. López LR, Santos ME, Espinoza LR, LaRosa FG: Clinical significance of immunoglobulin A versus immunoglobulins G and M anti-cardiolipin antibodies in thrombocytopenia, and recurrent abortion, *Am J Clin Pathol*, 98:449, 1992.
57. Viard JP, Amoura Z, Bach JF: Association of anti–beta$_2$ glycoprotein I antibodies with lupus-type circulating anticoagulant and thrombosis in systemic lupus erythematosus, *Am J Med* 93:181, 1992.
58. Harrison RL, Alperin JB: Concurrent protein C deficiency and lupus anticoagulants, *Am J Hematol* 40:33, 1992.
59. Bick RL, Baker WF Jr: The antiphospholipid and thrombosis syndromes, *Med Clin North Am* 78:667, 1994.
60. Alarcón-Segovia D, Deleze M, Oria CV et al: Antiphospholipid antibodies and the antiphospholipid syndrome in systemic lupus erythematosus: a prospective analysis of 500 consecutive patients, *Medicine* 68:353, 1989.
61. Coull BM: Stroke in the young patient: coagulation disturbances, *Stroke: Clinical Updates* 1:117, 1990.
62. Khamashta MA, Hughes GRV: Detection and importance of anticardiolipin antibodies, *J Clin Pathol* 46:104, 1993.
63. Genest J Jr: Genetic lipid disorders in cardiovascular disease, *Trends Cardiovasc Med* 2:140, 1992.
64. Watts GF, Kearney EM, Taub NA, Slavin BM: Lipoprotein(a) as an independent risk factor for myocardial infractions in patients with common hypercholesterolemia, *J Clin Pathol* 46:267, 1993.
65. Malekpour A, Saber-Tehrani M, Radhad S: Lipoprotein(a): structure, properties, and clinical interest, *Lab Med* 24:31, 1993.
66. Scanu AM: Lipoprotein(a): its interitance and molecular basis of its atherothrombotic role, *Mol Cell Biochem* 113:127, 1992.
67. Hoff HF, Beck GJ, Skibinski CI et al: Serum Lp(a) level as a predictor of vein graft stenosis after coronary artery bypass surgery in patients, *Circulation* 77:1238, 1988.
68. Scanu AM: Genetic basis and pathophysiological implications of high Lp(a) levels, *J Intern Med* 231:679, 1992.
69. Ichinose A: Multiple members of the plasminogen-apolipoprotein(a) gene family associated with thrombosis, *Biochemistry* 31:3113, 1992.
70. Dahlen GH: Lipoprotein(a), atherosclerosis and thrombosis, *Prog Lipid Res* 30:189, 1991.
71. Rouy D, Grailhe P, Nigon F et al: Lipoprotein(a) impairs generation of plasmin by fibrin-bound tissue type plasminogen activator: in vitro studies in a plasma milieu, *Arterioscler Thromb* 11:629, 1991.
72. Miles LA, Fless GM, Levin EG et al: A potential basis for the thrombotic risks associated with lipoprotein(a), *Nature* 339:301, 1989.
73. Duerr RL, Ross RS: Acute myocardial infarction in a young man. Are there any risk factors? *Trends Cardiovasc Med* 3:44, 1993.

23 Radiation Injury

Robert E. Anderson
Morgan Berthrong
Luis F. Fajardo

INTRODUCTION

Under appropriate circumstances, all forms of radiation are potentially harmful to living organisms.

Life on earth has evolved in the presence of ionizing radiation. This natural, or background, radiation is derived from three major sources: cosmic rays from the sun and outer space, radium and other radioactive elements contained in the earth's crust, and potassium 40 and other naturally occurring radionuclides that are normally present in the body. Cosmic radiation varies with altitude. Residents of Albuquerque, New Mexico, for example, receive approximately twice the dose as the inhabitants of Boston, Massachusetts. Airline personnel and astronauts are also exposed to above-average doses of cosmic rays. Similarly, the radiation emitted by the earth's crust varies greatly by geographic region depending on variations in the content of radioactive materials in the soil and subterranean rock. Terrestrial radiation is of particular importance to miners who may be exposed to radioactive components of the earth's crust in aerosol form in the atmosphere of mines. Inhalation of these substances, when they are of appropriate size and shape, results in their deposition in the terminal air passages of the lungs where they may emit radioactivity for a prolonged time, much to the detriment of the host.

In addition to natural radiation, humans are exposed to radiation from man-made sources. The largest component of man-made radiation comes from exposures associated with medical diagnosis and treatment. Lesser contributions come from "technologically enhanced" sources (such as the use of radionuclide-containing minerals in phosphate fertilizers and building materials), fallout from atomic weapons, nuclear power production, and consumer products (faulty color television sets, smoke detectors, luminescent instruments and clock dials, and so on).

Table 23-1 shows the estimated annual exposure to various types of man-made and natural radiation. Table 23-2 shows how these doses compare with other whole-body exposures, the latter in logarithmic increments. Only somatic effects are included in this table, since the dose levels at which an increased incidence of genetic abnormalities may be expected in humans are still uncertain.

Basic to an understanding of radiation-induced tissue injury is an appreciation of the physics of radiation and the effects of radiation on individual cells and their subcellular components. A discussion of these general concepts is followed by a description of the morphologic and clinical features of radiation injury involving cells and tissues in vivo, with particular reference to the acute and delayed effects of whole-body or partial-body exposure of humans.

Table 23-1 Sources and average annual effective dose equivalent of ionizing radiation from the environment

Category (% total)	Source	Effective dose equivalent		
		mSv	(mrem)	% total
Natural (82%)	Radon	2.0	200	55
	Cosmic	0.27	27	8
	Terrestrial	0.28	28	8
	Internal	0.39	39	11
Artificial (18%)	Medical diagnosis	0.55	55	15
	Consumer products	0.10	10	3
	Occupational	<0.01	<1.0	<0.3
	Nuclear fuel cycle	<0.01	<1.0	<0.03
	Fallout	<0.01	<1.0	<0.03
	Miscellaneous	<0.01	<1.0	<0.03
TOTAL		3.6	360	100.0

Modified from Committee on the Biological Effects of Ionizing Radiations (BEIR V); Board on Radiation Effects Research, Commission on the Life Sciences, National Research Council, National Academy Press, 1990.
mSv, millisievert; *mrem,* milliroentgen equivalent man.

Table 23-2 Biologic consequences of a single whole-body exposure to indicated dose of radiation

Dose (rad)	Biologic response
0.01	No detectable somatic effects (this dose is approximately 10 times the average daily effective dose equivalent exposure)
0.1	No detectable somatic effects
1.0	No detectable somatic effects
10	Detectable morphologic and functional alterations in specific subpopulations of lymphocytes; probable chromosomal abnormalities
100	Mild radiation sickness in some persons with nausea and vomiting; decrease in mitotic index in hematopoietic cells; transient lymphopenia
1000	Severe necrosis of hematopoietic cells with consequent pancytopenia; extensive necrosis of gastrointestinal tract epithelial cells; severe radiation sickness; death within 2 weeks
10,000	Immediate disorientation or coma; death within hours
100,000	Acute necrosis of most cells; death within minutes
1,000,000	Death of most of the organisms that constitute the normal flora
10,000,000	Death of all living organisms; some denaturation of proteins

Modified from Warren S: *The pathology of ionizing radiation,* Springfield, Ill, 1961, Charles C Thomas.

Radiation will continue to increase in importance in the diagnosis and treatment of disease. For this reason, considerable emphasis is placed on the biologic basis for the use of radiation in the treatment of persons with malignant tumors and on the consequences to the host of radioisotopes administered therapeutically or diagnostically.[1-5]

ATTRIBUTES OF RADIATION

Radiation may be characterized by the mode its energy is emitted, propagated, or absorbed. With respect to propagation, radiation classically has been classified as electromagnetic or particulate.[6-8]

Electromagnetic radiation

Electromagnetic radiation represents energy propagated by wave motion. The penetrating power varies greatly depending on the wavelength, which varies along a continuous spectrum (Fig. 23-1). Microwaves and radio waves exhibit long wavelengths (up to several miles), but the number of waves emitted per unit of time is small. At the other end of the spectrum are gamma and roentgen (x) rays, which have short wavelengths and high frequencies. Intermediate between these extremes are infrared radiation, visible light, and ultraviolet radiation.

Short-wavelength and high-frequency electromagnetic radiation carries sufficient energy to ionize the materials that absorb them. In other words, on passage through matter, they produce ions and eject electrons.

For the purpose of these discussions, gamma rays and x-rays are identical. By convention, however, x-rays are produced artificially by a roentgen-ray tube, and gamma rays are emitted spontaneously by a radioactive substance. Gamma rays have defined energies characteristic of the atomic nucleus responsible for their emission, whereas the energies of x-rays depend on the energy characteristics of the source.

Particulate radiation

Particulate radiation, caused by the movement of subatomic particles, occurs naturally by the decay of radioactive substances, or artificially by accelerating electrons, protons, deuterons, or other subatomic particles to high speeds in an artificial device such as a cyclotron. Particulate radiation may be subclassified by the type of particles—alpha particles (helium nuclei), beta particles (emitted electrons), protons, neutrons, deuterons, or mesons. These particles differ in mass, charge, and angular momentum. The energy of these particles

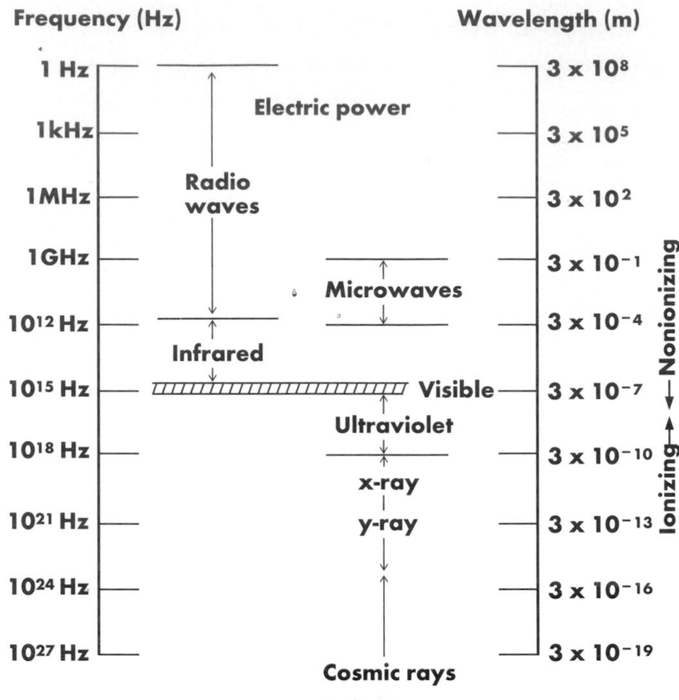

Fig. 23-1 Physical characteristics of ionizing and nonionizing radiation of electromagnetic spectrum. (From *Human health and the environment—some research needs*, DHEW Pub. No. NIH 77-1277, US Department of Health, Education and Welfare, 1977.)

depends on their rest mass and their velocity and is measured in electron volts or, more commonly, in million electron volts (MeV).

A substance is said to be radioactive when it possesses an unstable nucleus that spontaneously decays with the release of energy. This decay may involve naturally occurring atoms, such as radium or thorium, or atoms rendered radioactive by artificial means. Both natural and artificially produced radioactive substances are termed *radioisotopes*. These radioactive atoms, or nuclides, give off radiation as a result of the disintegration or decay of individual atoms. During radioactive decay, unstable daughter nuclei are often formed, which in turn undergo disintegration.

Radioactive decay

The three common types of decay are alpha emission, beta emission, and electron capture. Many nuclei with high atomic numbers decay by emission of alpha particles and thus are known as alpha (a) emitters. During decay, energy is released, which is transmitted as the kinetic energy of the alpha particles. Alpha particles from a specific nuclide are ejected with discrete energies. Additional energy may also be released as gamma radiation. The total energy released during the radioactive decay of a nucleus is termed the *transition energy*. For example, radium, with an atomic number of 88 and a mass number of 226, decays to radon ($^{222}_{86}Rn$) as follows:

$$^{226}_{88}Ra \rightarrow ^{222}_{86}Rn + ^{4}_{2}He + \text{gamma radiation}$$

Beta (β) emitters are the most abundant radioactive isotopes. β^- decay, or negatron decay, involves the transformation of a neutron into a proton. Energy is released as the kinetic energy of a neutrino (ν), energetic electrons (beta particles), and gamma rays. Neutrinos are uncharged particles with zero rest mass. β^+ decay, or positron decay, is somewhat more complicated but involves the transformation of a proton to a neutron followed by a variable series of steps that include the release of a neutrino and a positron. β^+ decay may also be accompanied by electron capture.

Beta decay leaves the nucleus lacking an electron. These holes, or vacancies, in the electron shell are promptly filled by electrons cascading from energy levels farther away from the nucleus. As these vacancies are filled, energy is released, usually in the form of electromagnetic radiation. The movement of an electron, usually from the innermost shell to the nucleus, with the release of a neutrino, is known as "electron capture."

Gamma rays are often emitted during the transition from the excited state to a stable energy level. However, no radioactive substance decays solely by gamma emission. Gamma transition is always preceded by either electron capture or emission of an alpha or a beta particle.

The rate of decay of a radioactive substance is referred to as the activity of the sample, and until recently the unit of measurement has been the curie (3.7×10^{10} disintegrations per second). Gradually, the curie (Ci) is being replaced by the international equivalent, the becquerel. The becquerel (Bq) is a reciprocal second and thus represents one disintegration per second; 1 Ci therefore equals 3.7×10^{10} Bq, and 1 Bq represents 2.7×10^{-11} Ci.

It is customary to express the activity in terms of half-life ($t_{1/2}$) or the time necessary to reduce the activity to one half of the initial value. The half-life periods of radioactive isotopes range from a fraction of a second to many centuries.

It is important to note that the becquerel and curie are not a measure of energy. In characterizing a radionuclide in terms of disintegrations per second, no indication is given as to the character of the radiation emitted.

In addition to the specific activities and the physical characteristics of the radiation emitted, the biologic consequences of exposure to a radionuclide depend on at least two other factors: (1) the distribution of the isotope within the host and the rate of excretion and (2) the half-life of the substance involved. The internal deposition of radium in humans illustrates the importance of these factors. Radium has a very long half-life (1638 years), is concentrated in the skeleton, and, together with its poorly soluble decay products, subjects the involved tissues to a continuous bombardment of alpha and beta particles and gamma rays throughout the life-span of the host. Thus, as little as 0.1 microcurie (3.7×10^3 Bq) of radium deposited in the human body is dangerous to the health of the recipient.

Measurement of radiation

Several units are employed to measure amounts of ionizing radiation. The oldest, the roentgen, is used for x-rays and gamma (γ) rays as the unit of the charge produced as these rays ionize a given volume of air. Thus the roentgen is a unit of exposure and not absorption. Furthermore, to encompass intensity, a time frame must also be indicated (such as roentgens per minute).

To represent particulate radiation in terms that can be related to x- and gamma rays, two other units—the rad and the gray—have been devised. These units are based on absorbed dose. One *rad* is the dose of radiation that will result in the absorption of 100 ergs of energy per gram of the absorbing substance. The energy absorbed by 1 gram of most tissues on exposure to 1 γ of roentgen rays is about 93 ergs, or almost the same as 1 rad. Therefore, in many discussions involving radiobiology, *rads* and *roentgens* are employed almost interchangeably. As with roentgens, the rad is a measure of quantity, and to convey intensity, an indication of time in the form of dose rate must also be introduced.

In *Système Internationale* (SI) units the *gray* (Gy) is the accepted measure of absorbed dose. One *gray* is the dose of any form of radiation resulting in the absorption of 1 joule of energy per kilogram of the absorbing material. Thus 1 gray corresponds to 100 rad.

One rad of particulate radiation generally causes more damage to a biologic system than 1 rad of x-rays or gamma rays does. For this reason, the *rem* was introduced to normalize the differences in biologic effects produced by different types of radiation. One *rem* is loosely defined as that dose of any type of radiation that produces a biologic effect equivalent to 1 rad of x or gamma rays. In situations where the rem is an inconveniently large unit of measure, the *millirem* (mrem), which is 1/1000 of a rem, is employed. The *sievert* is the accepted SI unit of dose equivalence. One sievert is that dose producing a biologic effect equivalent to 1 gray of x- or gamma rays. One sievert thus corresponds to 100 rem.

CELLULAR AND MOLECULAR RADIATION BIOLOGY

Much of our understanding of the effects of ionizing radiation in humans comes from studies that involve the exposure of cells grown in tissue culture. Such cells can be analyzed for (1) overt injury, such as cell death or loss of the ability to undergo cell division, and (2) occult injury, including nonlethal alterations of plasma membranes, enzymes, and even specific molecules.[9-11] In this section a portion of these data are discussed with particular reference to the mechanisms by which radiation injures and kills cells.

Reproductive death

After a population of cells is irradiated, a variable number become pyknotic, undergo lysis, or otherwise exhibit evidence of cell death.[12] The residual cells remain viable and are indistinguishable morphologically from their nonirradiated counterparts. However, despite the absence of recognizable morphologic alterations, many of the irradiated cells have lost their capacity to divide. The loss of a cell's ability to divide, known as reproductive death, is one of the most important effects of radiation on mammalian cells. On occasion, irradiated cells may continue to divide and grow but fail to separate. The resultant multinucleated giant cells are a morphologic hallmark of radiation injury.

Reproductive death is documented by the loss of the ability of irradiated cells to proliferate indefinitely. The ability of hematopoietic stem cells to form macroscopic colonies in the spleen after intravenous transfer to lethally irradiated mice of the same inbred strain is a frequently employed in vivo method to quantitate the reproductive capacity of stem cells. Because each colony is derived from a single stem cell that has divided innumerable times, irradiation of the bone marrow cells before transfer permits the development of a dose-response curve, which inversely relates radiation dose to the capacity of the irradiated cells to reproduce in their new environment.

Alternatively, the irradiated cells may be grown in tissue culture, and colony formation rate determined in vitro. In this setting, it is also known that each colony arises from a single viable cell because nonreproductive cells will not form colonies. Abortive colonies, containing subnormal numbers of cells, are not included in the calculation of the survival curves. Survival curves determined in vitro closely approximate those obtained in vivo for the same cell population.

The pathobiology of reproductive death is poorly understood but explained by two theories, the "target theory" and the "indirect-effects theory."

The *target theory* predicts that a biologic unit (such as a cell, a cell membrane, or a specific molecule) will undergo lethal damage after a minimum number of direct radiation "hits," or absorption events. The *indirect-effects theory* proposes inactivation of target molecules by free radicals produced by ionizing radiation. Water, a major constituent of all cells, provides an ample source of hydrogen and hydroxyl free radicals. Free radicals are extremely strong oxidizing or reducing agents. As such, they can react with water to form peroxides, or form cross-linkages with critical molecules such as DNA and RNA, or attach directly to key structures, such as plasma membranes, to impair their normal functions.[13-17]

Factors affecting radiation response

Physical, chemical, and biologic factors affect the degree of radiation injury of mammalian cells. Although discussed separately, their contributions usually overlap in both the experimental and the therapeutic settings.

Physical factors include the character of the radiation, the total amount administered, and the time within which this dose is given. The term *relative biologic effectiveness* (RBE) allows one to compare the effectiveness (in terms of absorbed dose) of two forms of radiation in producing the same biologic effect. The reference standard for this comparison is x-rays generated at 150 to 300 kiloelectron volts (keV) with a standard filter to remove extraneous energies. Fast neutrons are more effective than x-rays in producing most of the late somatic effects associated with radiation injury. Therefore, with these effects, fast neutrons have an RBE of greater than one.

Chemical factors may either protect against or potentiate the effects of ionizing radiation. Molecular oxygen is the most important substance in this regard. Bubbling oxygen into a cell suspension immediately before irradiation potentiates cell killing. The oxygen effect is especially pronounced with x rays and gamma rays. The oxygen likely serves as a substrate for production of free radicals by radiation; this is exploited in hyperbaric therapy of malignant tumors, which attempts to increase the oxygen tension in tumors before radiotherapy.

Another group of agents that have been used clinically to increase the radiosensitivity of cells is the halogenated pyrimidines. These analogs of DNA bases can increase severalfold the radiosensitivity of cells in culture. The mechanism, however, is not known.

Chemical agents also can protect against radiation-induced cell injury. Radioprotective agents include the sulfhydryl amines, such as cysteine and cystamine. The sulfhydryl groups of these molecules are oxidized by free radicals, thus protecting DNA from oxidation.

Biologic factors that influence the response of individual cells to radiation are exceedingly complex and poorly understood. Two important factors are the timing of the radiation exposure relative to the cell cycle and the repair of nonlethal injury. When synchronous cells in culture are studied, most are especially sensitive to radiation during G_2 and mitosis, less sensitive in G_1, and least sensitive toward the end of the S period. Therefore, rapidly dividing cells are generally more radiosensitive than slowly dividing cells, reflecting radiation-induced inhibition of DNA synthesis.

Repair of sublethal radiation injury appears to begin immediately after the damage is incurred. Repair is discussed in greater detail when radiation-induced injury to DNA is considered.

Radiation effects on macromolecules

Although radiation affects DNA, RNA, and many proteins, DNA is the "target" of greatest radiobiologic importance. For example, in experiments using microbeams of radiation, a cell was more likely to be killed if the nucleus, rather than the cytoplasm, was irradiated. In addition, the sensitivity of cells from different species to reproductive death is directly proportional to their DNA content. Finally, as will be seen subsequently, DNA alterations are implicated in many of the delayed effects of radiation exposure.

Both in vitro and in vivo, the effects of radiation on DNA are dependent on the dose, the quality or type of particle involved, and the stage of the cell cycle during which the irradiation occurs. In vitro, the irradiation of DNA may result in several possible outcomes: (l) breaking of hydrogen bonds, (2) nucleotide damage, (3) disruption of the sugar-phosphate backbone of the molecule, (4) impairment of the ability of DNA to act as a template for the synthesis of a new DNA strand, and (5) formation of cross-linkages between adjacent strands or closely apposed regions of the same strand. The last two phenomena have received particular attention recently.

Radiation can break one or both DNA strands, directly by ionization, or indirectly by activation of a specific DNAase. Most single-stranded breaks are rapidly repaired, with the intact strand serving as a template to direct the rejoining process. The majority of double-strain breaks are believed to be irreparable. The total loss of local structure and the formation of DNA fragments, which quickly become separated, are believed to produce a situation in which restoration of normal structure is extremely unlikely.

The exposure of rapidly dividing mammalian cells to doses in the order of 0.5 to 1.0 Gy (50 to 100 rad) generally results in a phenomenon known as "division delay." Typically, irradiated cells immediately cease cell division for a period proportional to the dose. After this delay, the cells resume their normal growth patterns for one or more generations. Cell death, when it occurs, usually takes place during the first postirradiation division, though damaged cells occasionally undergo several divisions before death. Less commonly, radiation can induce DNA synthesis outside the period of normal synthesis in the cell cycle. This phenomenon, which involves all phases of the cell cycle, is referred to as *unscheduled* DNA synthesis. Unscheduled synthesis can also be induced by ultraviolet rays and alkylating agents. The biologic implications of unscheduled synthesis are not entirely known, but the phenomenon is probably related to the repair process.

Experiments designed to evaluate the effects of radiation on RNA typically assessed RNA synthesis *in toto,* without species analysis (messenger RNA, ribosomal RNA). In addition, because RNA synthesis depends on DNA integrity, the relative contribution of these two effects upon radiation-induced cell injury has been difficult to differentiate experimentally. Despite these technical problems, however, RNA synthesis is believed to be less radiosensitive than DNA synthesis.

Large doses of radiation are required to destroy the function of most proteins. Several enzymes have been carefully investigated in this regard. The radioresistance of most proteins may be attributable to their relatively small size, particularly in comparison with such molecules as DNA and RNA.

RADIATION INJURY IN HUMANS

Although all mammalian cells are affected by ionizing radiation, moderate variability exists among different cell types and tissues with respect to their susceptibility to a specific effect such as cell death.[18-26] In general, rapidly dividing cells are more radiosensitive than slowly dividing cells. This difference presumably has to do with radiation-induced inhibition of DNA synthesis and interference with normal cell division. The consequences of these changes include chromosomal abnormalities, such as translocations, breaks, deletions, and the formation of fragments and rings. Such alterations are best appreciated by chromosome analysis. However, abnormal mitotic figures may be seen in tissue sections, often in association with the multinucleated giant cells that reflect the failure of dividing cells to separate physically.

Vascular changes are an extremely important consequence of irradiation and may be responsible for many of the acute and delayed effects of such exposure. Vascular abnormalities are seen after irradiation of both normal and neoplastic tissues. Endothelial cells are not especially radiosensitive, but with time, degenerative vascular abnormalities are almost always seen in association with an irradiated neoplasm. Furthermore, degenerative vascular changes are not confined to the tumor but also involve the adjacent normal parenchyma of the affected organ and other tissues that may be interposed between the source of the radiation and the tumor.

Vascular dilatation is responsible for the erythema of the skin that is frequently noted after irradiation. Similar dilatation of the blood vessels probably occurs in a variety of other sites and may account for the transient increase in function documented in some organs after exposure. Somewhat later and generally in association with high dose levels, regressive changes appear, including swelling and vacuolization of the endothelium, focal necrosis of the vessel wall, sometimes with hemorrhage, or, on occasion, even rupture. Months or years after exposure various degenerative abnormalities are apparent. They include (1) fibrosis of the subintimal region and media of small arteries and arterioles, which results in focal narrowing, (2) myointimal cell proliferation, which may narrow the lumen, and (3) decreased numbers of capillaries with considerable ectasia of those that persist.

From the above description, it is not difficult to visualize the alterations that might be expected in one irradiated several years previously. Grossly, the organ will be small because of necrosis and loss of radiosensitive parenchymal cells and the subsequent ischemia of less radiosensitive cells by a compromised circulation. Microscopically, atrophic or absent parenchymal cells will have been replaced by dense hyalinized connective tissue, which may contain pleomorphic, large fibroblasts. Multinucleated giant cells may be present except in organs populated by fixed postmitotic cells. Small arteries and arterioles will be lined by increased numbers of unusually prominent endothelial cells. Focally, the walls of these vessels will be thick and sclerotic and the lumen small or obliterated.

By convention, the early effects are those that produce signs and symptoms of radiation damage in humans from the time of exposure to 60 days. In humans, early effects occur only after relatively high doses (above about 0.5 Gy) delivered over a short period. Above this dose level, symptoms increase in severity with increasing dose. Although all major organs of the body probably are affected, acute symptoms reflect malfunction of rapidly proliferating tissues vital to homeostasis, including the bone marrow, lymphoid organs, and the epithelium of the alimentary tract.

Delayed or late effects appear many months or, more commonly, years after exposure. Radiation carcinogenesis is a well-known delayed effect. Other life-threatening delayed effects involve many organs, including heart, lungs, kidneys, and the central nervous system (Table 23-3). Surgical procedures are generally more difficult in tissues that were irradiated months or years previously. The increased amounts of dense connective tissue make dissection of vital structures more difficult than usual. Postoperatively, hypoperfusion of the area by abnormal blood vessels improves wound healing and also compromises local defense mechanisms. These types of delayed effects are more often associated with repeated (fractionated) local exposures than from a single whole-body exposure.

The effects of radiation injury can also be classified as stochastic or nonstochastic. A stochastic (random) effect varies in frequency but not in severity with dose and fails to exhibit a threshold, a dose below which no effect is seen. Examples of

Table 23-3 Relative radiosensitivity of various organs 5 years post exposure

Radio-sensitivity	Organ	Complication	Dose range* Gy	(rad)
Very high	Bone marrow	Hypoplasia	2.0-5.5	(200-550)
	Testes	Sterilization	2.0-6.5	(200-650)
	Optic lens	Cataract	5.0-12.0	(500-1200)
	Ovary	Sterilization	3.0-12.0	(300-1200)
	Breast (prepubescent)	Arrested development	10.0-15.0	(1000-1500)
	Growing cartilage	Arrested growth	10.0-30.0	(1000-3000)
High	Growing bone	Arrested growth	20.0-30.0	(2000-3000)
	Kidney	Nephrosclerosis	23.0-28.0	(2300-2800)
	Liver	Cirrhosis	35.0-45.0	(3500-4500)
	Lung	Fibrosis	40.0-60.0	(4000-6000)
	Heart	Pericarditis	40.0- >100.0	(4000- >10,000)
	Stomach	Ulcer	45.0-50.0	(4500-5000)
	Small intestine	Ulcer, stricture	45.0-65.0	(4599-6500)
	Colon	Ulcer, stricture	45.0-65.0	(4500-6500)
	Salivary gland	Xerostomia	50.0-70.0	(5000-7000)
	Thyroid	Hypothyroidism	45.0-150.0	(4500-15,000)
	Cornea	Keratitis	50.0- >60.0	(5000- >6000)
	Pituitary	Hypopituitarism	45.0-250.0	(4500-25,000)
	Growing muscle	Arrested growth	25.0-45.0	(2500-4500)
	Spinal cord	Necrosis (transverse myelitis)	50.0- >60.0	(5000- >6000)
	Brain	Necrosis	50.0- >60.0	(5000- >6000)
	Skin	Ulcer, fibrosis	55.0-70.0	(5500-7000)
	Rectum	Ulcer	55.0-80.0	(5500-8000)
Intermediate	Esophagus	Ulcer, stricture	60.0-75.0	(6000-7500)
	Oral mucosa	Ulcer	60.0-75.0	(6000-7500)
	Urinary bladder	Ulcer, contracture	60.0-80.0	(6000-8000)
	Adult bone	Osteonecrosis, fracture	60.0-150.0	(6000-15,000)
	Adult cartilage	Necrosis	60.0-100.0	(6000-10,000)
Low	Adrenal	Hypoadrenalism	>60.0	(>6000)
	Vagina	Ulcer, fistula	90.0- >100.0	(9000- >10,000)
	Uterus	Necrosis	100.0- >200.0	(10,000- >20,000)
	Pancreas	Stromal fibrosis	>60.0	(>6000)

Modified from Fajardo LM: *Pathology of radiation injury*, New York, 1982, Masson Publishing Inc, and Mettler FA, Moseley RD: *Medical effects of ionizing radiation*, New York, 1985, Grune & Stratton, Inc.

*Dose resulting in a rate of severe complications of 1 to 5% (first figure) to 25 to 50% (second figure) among patients treated in standard fashion.

stochastic effects are heritable effects on germ cells, teratogenic effects on the developing embryo, and some radiation-induced tumors. Nonstochastic effects vary in severity but not in frequency with dose and often exhibit a threshold. Many of the early effects of radiation injury are nonstochastic in nature.

Our understanding of radiation effects comes from persons accidentally or purposefully exposed to biologically significant amounts of ionizing radiation. Some of these populations are summarized in Table 23-4. Even among these carefully studied groups, direct comparisons are often complicated by differences in age, variability in the conditions of exposure (extent, magnitude, time, external versus internal emitters, and so on), and the presence or absence of known preexisting disease.

Somatic effects

Somatic effects of radiation injury may be early or delayed. Among the early effects, acute lethality is of prime concern. Some of the important delayed effects are carcinogenesis, abnormalities of growth and development, alterations in life-span, and a broad range of injuries to individual organs.

Early lethality

Key to an understanding of early lethality is an appreciation of the concept of lethal dose. In toxicology the lethal dose 50, or LD_{50}, is the amount of an agent that causes a 50% mortality in the experimental group. The same approach has been applied to radiation injury, especially injury associated with whole-body exposure. However, death after whole-body exposure is often delayed for days or even weeks, depending primarily on the magnitude of exposure. Therefore, with respect to radiation exposure, mortality is expressed in terms of a specific period of time, generally 30 days. The $LD_{50(30)}$ is defined as the dose associated with a 50% mortality within 30 days of exposure.

Table 23-4 Summary of irradiated populations

Population and years of exposure	Primary type of radiation	Region primarily irradiated	Sample size	Conditions with increased frequency
British adults irradiated for ankylosing spondylitis (1935-1954)	x-rays	Spine	14,106	Leukemia, chromosomal abnormality
Children irradiated for suspected enlarged thymus and other benign lesions of head, neck, and scalp (1910-1959)	x-rays	Mediastinum, scalp, tonsillar and nasopharyngeal regions	24,604*	Thyroid tumors, leukemia, lymphoma
American radiologists (1905-1949)	x-rays, radium	Partial to whole body	425 to 82,441*	Aplastic anemia, hematopoietic malignancy, skin and brain tumors, decreased life-span
Radium-dial painters and related workers; adults treated with radium (1905-1926; 1945-1955)	Gamma rays, alpha particles, beta particles (^{226}Ra, ^{228}Ra, ^{224}Ra)	Skeleton	4532†	Bone tumors
Thorium dioxide (1930-1951)	Alpha particles	Predominantly liver, spleen, bone marrow	16,074*	Hepatic and other neoplasms, cirrhosis, blood dyscrasias, and local granulomas at site of injection
Children irradiated in utero during diagnostic or therapeutic procedures involving the mother (1947-1954)	x-rays	Whole body	14,294	Congenital abnormalities, mental retardation, leukemia, and solid tumors
Marshall Islanders (1954)	Gamma rays and internally deposited radionuclides	Whole body but with disproportional irradiation of thyroid	7266*	Retardation of growth and development, benign and malignant thyroid tumors, chromosomal abnormalities, possible increased frequency of miscarriages and stillbirths
Japanese atomic bomb survivors (1945)	Gamma rays and neutrons	Whole body	120,312*	Developmental abnormalities, benign and malignant tumors, and degenerative changes

*Includes comparable group of nonexposed ("control") individuals; for the Japanese atomic bomb survivors, this group consists of 26,580 persons not in either city at the time of the bomb.

†Includes only American workers.

In humans the sequence of events after radiation injury is slower than that for experimental animals. For this reason, the frame of reference generally employed for humans is the $LD_{50(60)}$ or the amount of radiation that would be expected to kill 50% of a population within 60 days of exposure.

A quantitative dose-response relationship for early lethality in humans is not known. Several investigators have derived hypothetical dose-response curves based on experience with reactor accidents and the atomic explosions in Japan. From these observations, the $LD_{50(60)}$ for humans exposed to a single dose of highly penetrating electromagnetic radiation (x- or gamma rays) delivered over a period of less than 24 hours is believed to be in the 2.50 to 4.0 Gy (250 to 400 rad) range in the absence of medical intervention. The survivable dose is somewhat higher with intensive care and up to 10.5 Gy (1050 rad) with a bone marrow transplant.

Host and environmental factors influence the response of the individual to whole-body irradiation. In general, males are more radiosensitive than females. Middle-aged persons appear to exhibit a greater degree of tolerance to radiation than either the young or the old. The presence of infection sharply increases the mortality from whole-body exposure; often these infections are derived from the normal flora of the gastrointestinal tract.

If an area of the body is shielded, the effects of a constant amount of radiation are decreased, protecting an individual from an otherwise lethal exposure to ionizing radiation. Shielding of the bone marrow, spleen, and gastrointestinal tract is especially efficacious.

The relationship between survival time and magnitude of whole-body exposure in terms of mode of death is illustrated in Fig. 23-2 . The curve shows three distinct components. The first region covers the dose range of 4.0 to 12.0 Gy (400 to 1200 rad). This range is generally referred to as the region of *hematopoietic death* because bone marrow damage is the most prominent finding, both clinically and at autopsy. Other organs are also damaged, however, and necrosis of gastrointestinal tract mucosa and subsequent bacteremia contribute greatly to lethality in the hematopoietic range.

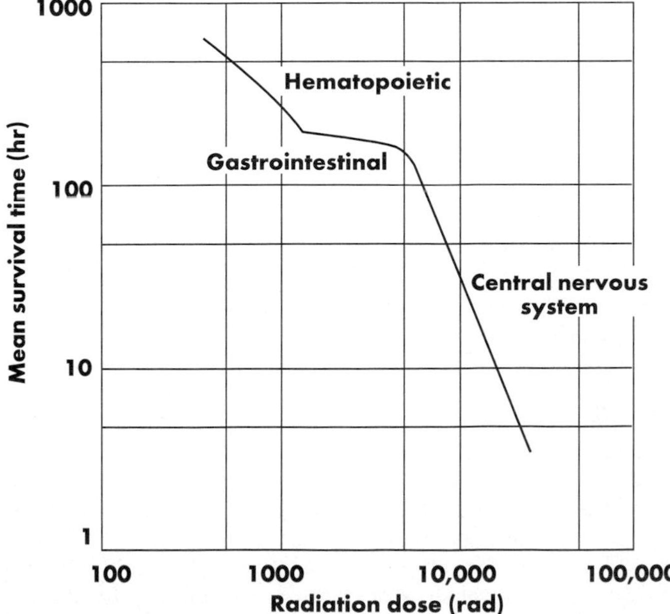

Fig. 23-2 Relationship between mean survival time, magnitude of whole-body exposure, and primary mode of death in humans. (After Langham WH et al: *Aerospace Med* 36:1, 1965.)

Throughout the dose range of 12.0 to 50.0 Gy (1200 to 5000 rad) there is a plateau in the mean survival curve (Fig. 23-2). This part of the dose-response curve is generally referred to as the region of *gastrointestinal death.* Again, this distinction is based on the most prominent clinical and morphologic findings. Morphologically there is a progressive loss of gastrointestinal mucosa secondary to impaired proliferation of the stem cell or renewal population. Necrosis of mucosal cells leads to ulceration, bacteremia, hemorrhage, and loss of fluids and electrolytes. In this dose range the bone marrow is totally aplastic, and numerous other tissues also show severe damage.

Above about 50.0 Gy (5000 rad), mean survival time again begins to decrease exponentially with increasing dose (Fig. 23-2), and death is characterized by a variety of central nervous system signs and symptoms. For this reason, the region of the survival curve associated with exposures in excess of 50.0 Gy (5000 rad) is referred to as the region of *central nervous system death.* Incapacitation occurs relatively rapidly and is characterized by confusion, convulsions, apathy, and coma, followed by death (Table 23-5).

Delayed somatic effects

Various somatic effects are the result of radiation injury, including carcinogenesis, abnormalities of growth and development, changes in life span, and degenerative lesions of most major organ systems. The last is discussed in a subsequent section.

Carcinogenesis. The carcinogenic effects of ionizing radiation have been recognized for almost a century. Pioneer radiation workers developed epidermoid and basal cell carcinomas of the hands, because of the focusing of equipment on the bones of their own hands, or positioning their patients with their unshielded hands while the equipment was in operation.

Despite the early recognition of this untoward effect of ionizing radiation, even today the mechanisms involved in radiation-induced neoplasia remain poorly understood, in part because of our incomplete understanding of carcinogenesis in general (Chapter 24). Considerable effort has been given to an attempt to define in mathematical terms the relationships between dose of irradiation and tumor incidence, especially at low dose levels. The latter are of particular importance in defining maximum permissible exposure levels for radiation workers. Unfortunately, the available data are insufficient to establish with confidence the shape of the dose-incidence curve at low doses. Hence, efforts to estimate the possible risks of low-level irradiation involve extrapolation from observations made at higher dose levels. These extrapolations, based upon assumptions yet to be proved, yield three types of curves: linear nonthreshold, linear threshold, and linear-quadratic. These curves are represented schematically in Fig. 23-3.

The concept of threshold is of critical importance in a consideration of the carcinogenic effects of radiation. As depicted in Fig. 23-3, threshold implies a "safe" dose of radiation below which there is no increased incidence of the disease in question. At present the available evidence fails to support or refute the concept of a threshold in relation to the carcinogenic effects of radiation. For this reason, most authorities have recommended that the linear, nonthreshold dose-incidence model be employed to derive risk estimates for the development of all tumors except leukemia among people exposed to low doses of radiation. This conservative approach assumes that any level of exposure is associated with some risk of harm. Major corollaries to this axiom are two: no exposure to radiation is justifiable if it is avoidable or fails to provide a benefit commensurate with the presumed risk, and every exposure, even when amply justified, must be kept as low as possible.

In contrast with low-dose effects, considerable data concerning the characteristics of the dose-incidence curve at intermediate and high exposure levels are available. In many instances the linear quadratic model (Fig. 23-3) appears to best describe stochastic effects at these dose levels. This model also best describes leukemia at low doses.

Under appropriate circumstances, most human tissues are believed to be susceptible to the carcinogenic effects of radiation. A well-recognized exception is the small lymphocyte. Thus chronic lymphocytic leukemia, a relatively common malignancy in Western populations, is not increased in frequency after whole-body or local irradiation. And even among susceptible organs, the dose of radiation required for tumorigenesis varies greatly. As a consequence, in an irradiated population, the relative risk (or the ratio between incidence in the irradiated group and that in the nonirradiated members of the population) differs greatly for various tumor types. Fig. 23-4 shows the relative risk for specific types of malignant tumors among Japanese atomic bomb survivors exposed to 1.0 Gy. Notice that this figure is based upon mortality data, hence the absence of neoplasms such as carcinoma of the thyroid known to be radiation-induced but of low potential for death.

Heredity also plays a major role in radiation carcinogenesis. In many inherited conditions in which individuals are prone to develop tumors, radiation appears to potentiate the risk of tumorigenesis. For example, children with one form of retinoblastoma occasionally also develop osteogenic sarcoma at various sites including especially the extremities; however, patients irradiated for retinoblastoma not infrequently develop osteogenic sarcomas in the field of therapy. This finding indicates a genetic predisposition to osteogenic sarcoma in these children that is made even more manifest by the action of radiation. Several children with the hereditary multiple basal cell nevus syndrome have developed basal cell nevi concentrated in the field of previous irradiation for medulloblastoma. Cells from cancer-prone persons (such as persons with ataxia telangiectasia, Fanconi's anemia, and the dysplastic nevus syndrome) exhibit an enhanced sensitivity to irradiation during the G_2 phase of the cell cycle as manifest by an increased frequence of chromatidic breaks and gaps.

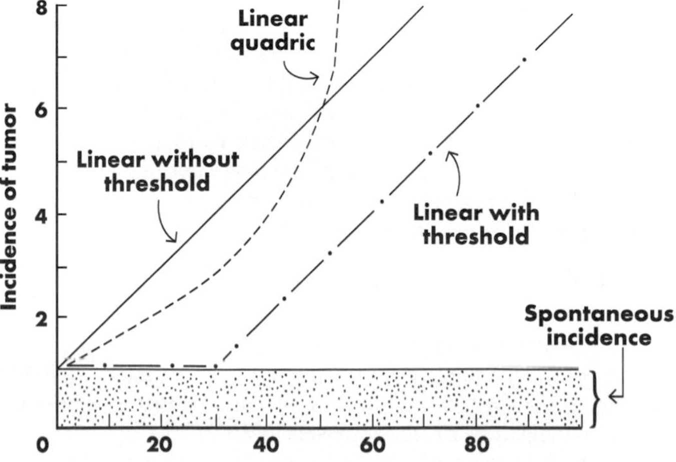

Fig. 23-3 Hypothetical dose-response curve for radiation carcinogenesis.

Abnormalities of growth and development. Radiation is especially injurious to rapidly dividing tissues. For this reason, the developing embryo and the preadolescent child are particularly susceptible to radiation-induced disorders of growth and development. In general, the character of the defect reflects those tissues that are undergoing the most rapid growth and differentiation at the time of exposure. From this standpoint it is convenient to divide radiation-related disorders of growth and development into four phases: the preimplantation period, the period of major organogenesis, the fetal period, and the postnatal period.

Irradiation shortly after conception is associated with one of two extremes; it is either lethal, or of no apparent significance to the preimplantation embryo, which therefore survives without evidence of abnormality. When the organism consists of only a few cells, radiation-induced damage to only one cell is likely to be fatal to the embryo. Under such circumstances, the mother is generally unaware that she has even conceived.

During the period of major organogenesis, which begins at the time of implantation (day 8 or 9) and extends through the initial 6 weeks of gestation, the developing fetus is maximally radiosensitive. Radiation exposure during this period of remarkable growth and differentiation is associated with one or more of a vast number of possible congenital malformations.

From the sixth week of gestation until the time of parturition, susceptibility to recognizable morphologic anomalies decreases. Most of the organ systems are structurally differentiated, and therefore exposure of the fetus would not be expected to result in gross congenital abnormalities. However, susceptibility to radiation-induced functional disabilities persists during this period. Such disturbances, which involve particularly the central nervous system and the gonads, are often difficult to recognize and identify, especially since development of these tissues continues until well after birth. Radiation during the fetal period apparently depletes the total number of functional nerve and reproductive cells. With respect to the central nervous system, such depletion may be manifest by a reduced intelligence quotient.

Radiation-induced abnormalities in the postnatal period, especially of bone, are associated with the exposure of infants and children before the cessation of physical growth and development. With respect to bone, the magnitude of impairment appears to depend on the rate of growth at the time of exposure. Other tissues that continue to develop in the postnatal period, such as the eye, the central nervous system, and the teeth, are also susceptible to radiation-induced abnormalities in growth and development.

On the basis of some of the preceding observations, many institutions have adopted a policy that limits elective diagnostic medical radiographic examinations among women of childbearing age to the first 10 days after the start of the last menses. This approach is designed to prevent exposure of an unsuspected conceptus.

Finally, it should be emphasized that the discussion in this section has focused especially upon exposure from external

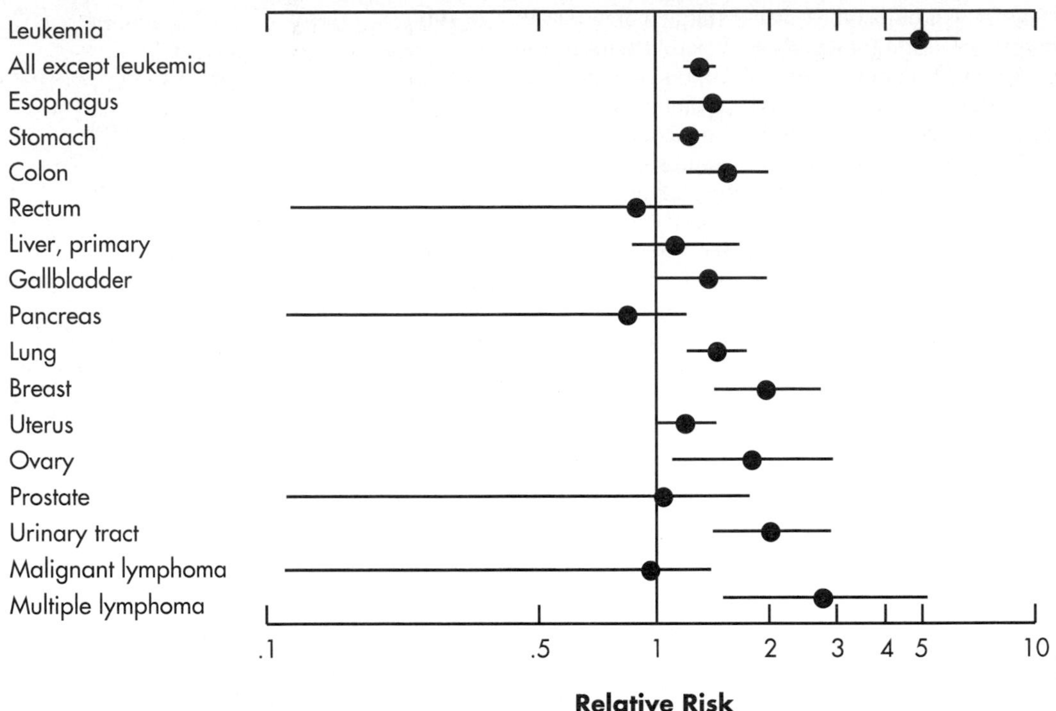

Fig. 23-4 Relative risk and 90% confidence intervals of site-specific cancer mortality from 1950 to 1985 among atomic-bomb survivors receiving 1.0 Gy (100 rad) in comparison with persons who were radiation free. (Modified from Shimizu Y, Kato H, Schull WJ: *Radiat Res* 121:120, 1990.)

sources. Fetal irradiation may also occur when radioactive isotopes are administered to the mother. Radioactive iodine, strontium, tritium, phosphorus, and plutonium are among the many isotopes that can cross the placenta to become incorporated into and thereby injure fetal tissues. For example, radioactive iodine administered late in pregnancy for maternal hyperthyroidism can be concentrated in the thyroid of the developing fetus and result in cretinism.

Life-span. Sublethal whole-body irradiation of rodents causes shortened life-span. This life shortening results from an increase in age-specific mortality and persists even when appropriate corrections are made for the early mortality associated with radiation sickness and the late deaths caused by radiation-induced neoplasms.

Up to now, however, experimental studies have not shown unequivocally that radiation truly accelerates the aging process. The possibility remains that radiation reduces life-span by some other mechanism. Autopsies of irradiated animals reveal that death is generally caused by the same diseases that kill their nonexposed contemporaries. In particular, radiation hastens the development of a variety of degenerative and neoplastic diseases as well as autoimmune phenomena. Not all age-dependent alterations, however, are temporally advanced by irradiation, and even for those that are advanced, the magnitude of change is not necessarily uniform.

Comparable data pertinent to humans are fragmentary. One of the first suggestions of a similar life-shortening effect came from the observation that pioneer American radiologists experienced a higher age-specific death rate than other specialists did. The increase in mortality was not attributable to a specific lesion and was interpreted as a nonspecific shortening of life-span from occupational exposure. Interestingly the excess mortality has progressively decreased in all but the oldest age groups, possibly because of improved shielding and other radiologic safety procedures. Recently, similar advancement of age-specific mortality from a variety of nonneoplastic diseases has been observed among the atomic bomb survivors.

Genetic effects

Ionizing radiation was the first mutagenic agent discovered. Radiation-induced mutations may affect either somatic cells, in which case the effects are limited to the irradiated individual, or germinal tissues, in which case the consequences may affect future generations. Mutations may also be classified as point mutations or chromosomal aberrations. Both may occur simultaneously within the same cell.

Point mutations. Point mutations, small alterations in the sequence of DNA bases, occur spontaneously at a low natural rate. Estimates indicate that approximately 10% may be attributable to the natural, or background, radiation that has always been a part of our environment; the remainder are believed to be caused by either mutagenic chemicals or the thermal movement of molecules.

Chromosomal aberrations. Chromosomal aberrations arise when radiation breaks a chromosome or a chromatid at one or more points along its length. Such an interruption may result in an alteration in the number of genes in the cell or in the linear sequence of the genes, or both. The broken ends of a chromosome may (1) rejoin with no resultant lesion, (2) heal without rejoining, (3) join with the broken ends of other chromosomes, or (4) fail to heal. It is estimated that 90% of individual chromosome breaks rejoin with no demonstrable lesion.

As might be expected, the frequency of nonviable chromosomal aberrations is greater than the frequency of nonviable gene (point) mutations. Chromosomes also exhibit increased stickiness just before or during metaphase when irradiated with doses of one Gy (100 rads) or more. This poorly understood phenomenon often causes individual chromosomes to stick together and to form loosely adherent clumps. At anaphase such clumps do not separate properly, and such aberrant separation results in an unequal distribution of genes to the daughter cells.

Dose-response effects. In general, the number of detectable point mutations increases linearly with increasing dose. No threshold effect is evident, so even doses as low as 0.01 Gy may cause damage. In common with point mutations, single chromosome breaks, also known as single-hit aberrations, bear a linear relationship to dose. Two-hit chromosome breaks are the result of two single aberrations that occur in proximity. As might be expected, two-hit breaks exhibit a threshold and then increase in frequency at a rate greater than the single power of the dose.

Geneticists are appropriately concerned about the hazards of the exposure of human beings to ionizing radiation, particularly with respect to the implications for future generations. Most radiation-induced mutations are transmitted as recessive traits; as such, they can be transmitted to large numbers of offspring, an occurrence that goes undetected until matings between carriers begin to occur. For this reason, deleterious recessive mutations, though not evident immediately, are more dangerous to a population than harmful dominant mutations are, particularly when the latter are damaging enough to prevent carriers from reproducing.

With respect to radiation exposure, geneticists are particularly concerned about radiology personnel, patients receiving radioactive isotopes, workers in nuclear installations, and patients exposed to x rays during diagnostic radiologic examinations. Diagnostic radiology is an indispensable part of medical practice, but physicians must be aware of the genetic effects of radiation to balance the benefits of a specific procedure against the possible hazards.

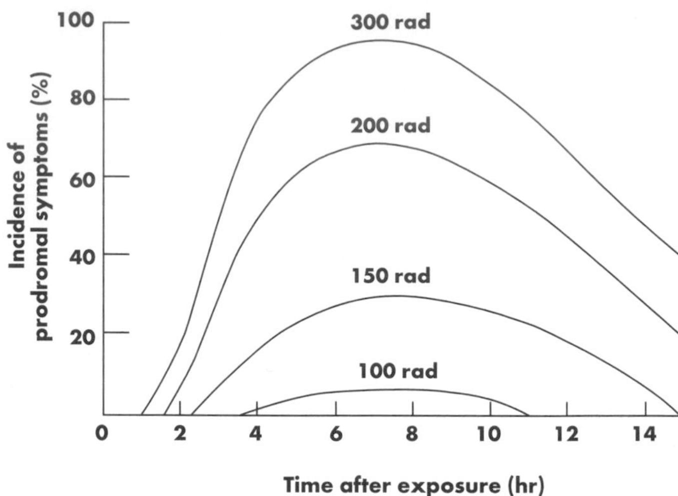

Fig. 23-5 Incidence and duration of prodromal symptoms as function of dose. (From Langham WH et al: *Aerospace Med* 36:1, 1965.)

Acute radiation syndrome

The clinical signs and symptoms produced by intensive exposure of the entire body to penetrating radiation are referred to as the "acute radiation syndrome," or radiation sickness.[63-66] This syndrome is characterized by three successive phases.

1. *A transient prodromal phase, which develops within a few hours of exposure to as little as 0.75 to 1.0 Gy (75 to 100 rad).* In humans this phase is characterized by apathy, anorexia, nausea, and vomiting. As shown in Fig. 23-5, the incidence and duration of prodromal symptoms are dose dependent and therefore provide a rough indication of the degree of irradiation in persons accidentally exposed to a dose of unknown magnitude. The prodromal phase rarely exceeds 24 hours except in very severe cases.

Table 23-5 Important features of the acute radiation syndrome

Subcategory	Clinical threshold dose*	Latent period	Primary morphologic manifestations	Characteristic signs and symptoms	Mechanism of death	Time of death after exposure (mean)
Hematopoietic syndrome	100	2-3 weeks	Hypoplasia of bone marrow with leukopenia, thrombocytopenia and (occasionally) anemia	Petechiae, purpura, hemorrhage, infection	Infection	3 weeks
Gastrointestinal syndrome	500	3-5 days	Depletion of epithelium of small intestine with ulceration	Fever, diarrhea, fluid-electrolyte disturbances, infection	Dehydration, infection, electrolyte loss	10-14 days
Central nervous system syndrome	2000	15 minutes to 3 hours	Edema, necrosis of neurons, vasculitis	Confusion, apathy, somnolence, tremor, ataxia, convulsions, coma	Increased central nervous system pressure	14-36 hours

*Air doses in roentgens.

2. *An ensuing asymptomatic latent period, which reflects the time required for the development of disturbances in specific organs.* As will be seen subsequently, this period generally reflects the time required for the depletion of cells in mitotically active tissues through interference with normal renewal mechanisms. As such, the duration of the latent period is also dose dependent.
3. *The principal phase of the illness.* As noted previously, the acute radiation syndrome can be divided into three major categories on the basis of the organ system most conspicuously involved; these are the hematopoietic, gastrointestinal, and central nervous system syndromes. In varying degrees, each syndrome is associated with death, and much of our understanding of the acute radiation syndrome has been gained from an evaluation of persons accidentally exposed during reactor accidents.

Some of the clinical and morphologic characteristics of the individual components of the acute radiation syndrome are summarized in Table 23-5. The most sensitive organ is the bone marrow, and symptoms relating to hematopoietic dysfunction are apparent after exposure to as little as 0.5 to 1.0 Gy (50 to 100 rad). Maximum expression of symptoms referable to the bone marrow is generally delayed until 2 to 3 weeks after exposure. At the other end of the range is the central nervous system (CNS) syndrome, which follows very large doses (10 Gy or more) and where the clinical manifestations are often apparent within minutes of exposure. Intermediate between these extremes is the gastrointestinal syndrome.

The cellular basis of the gastrointestinal and hematopoietic syndromes is directly related to the rate of cell turnover in these organs. The epithelial cells lining the digestive tract and the circulating leukocytes are short lived and therefore must be renewed at a rapid rate.

Except for lymphocytes, the mature elements of the peripheral blood are remarkably resistant to the effects of radiation. However, they have a finite life-span and cannot reproduce themselves. After whole-body exposure of sufficient magnitude, the majority of bone-marrow stem cells are damaged or dead and therefore are not available for division and maturation to replace those cells lost by natural attrition. The consequences of this situation, in order of appearance, are lymphopenia, thrombocytopenia, neutropenia, and anemia.

In the gastrointestinal tract, the stem cell population is located in the crypts of Lieberkühn. Irradiation of these cells inhibits division or, if the dose is sufficiently large, kills them outright. The mature cells at the tips of the villi undergo spontaneous aging at the usual rate and are sloughed into the lumen of the intestine. Meanwhile, partially mature cells continue to migrate toward the tips of the villi to replace these senescent cells, thus depleting the crypts even further. In the absence of appropriate replacements, the villi become denuded, and vital functions are compromised. In particular, loss of the normal mucosa permits fluid and electrolytes to escape from exposed tissue spaces and allows microorganisms, especially the normal intestinal flora, easy access to the bloodstream. Hemorrhage from exposed blood vessels may further complicate the clinical situation. If recovery is to occur, small foci of regenerating epithelium are generally evident by the end of the first week. This sequence of events is shown diagrammatically in Fig. 23-6.

The acute response of the stomach, colon, and rectum is similar to that of the small intestine. However, because cell turnover is highest in the small intestine, cell depletion occurs earlier there than elsewhere.

The pathogenesis of the CNS component of the acute radiation syndrome is not known. Current evidence indicates that injury to small blood vessels may be the initiating event. Vacuolization of capillary endothelial cells, perivascular foci of hemorrhage, and perivascular collections of inflammatory cells have been described. Vascular permeability is known to be increased, and cerebral edema is uniformly present among both persons exposed accidentally and animals exposed experimentally. It may well be that significant edema of other organs is associated with the high doses responsible for the CNS syndrome but that the rigid confines of the adult skull dictate that CNS symptoms precede those attributable to other organs. At extremely high dose levels, death may be caused by direct neuronal damage; the estimated intracerebral dose associated with this phenomenon is in excess of 1000 Gy (100,000 rad) for humans.

Ultimately, the severity of the acute radiation syndrome depends primarily on the number of surviving stem cells in

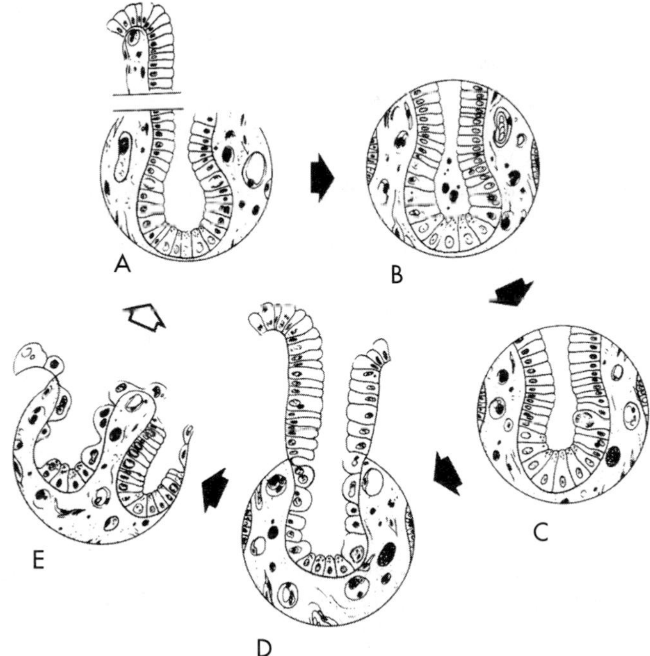

Fig. 23-6 Early radiation injury to epithelium of small intestine. **A,** Normal state. Crypt area consists of basally situated Paneth cells, zone of proliferating cells, and narrow band of differentiating cells immediately beneath gland neck. Villus is lined by mature, epithelial cells, which undergo continuous migration to cell-extrusion zone at villus tip. **B,** Six hours after irradiation. Notice inhibition of mitosis and pronounced necrosis of immature cells in proliferative zone. **C,** Twelve to 24 hours after irradiation. Inhibition of mitosis ceases with large number of abortive cell divisions, many of which are abnormal and result in death of involved cells or abnormal daughter cells. **D,** One to 6 days after irradiation. In absence of effective cell division, epithelial cell population continues to diminish, and many of residual cells are abnormally large and pleomorphic. Villi become progressively shortened, and residual abnormal cells spread out, possibly to preserve in part the integrity of the epithelial barrier. **E,** Six to 8 days after irradiation. If regeneration is to occur, small foci of regenerating epithelium are evident by end of first week. (Modified from White DC: *Atlas of radiation histopathology,* ERDA Report TID-26676, Washington, DC, 1975.)

mitotically active tissues. These cells constitute the only available source of the cells required for the restoration of tissue integrity.

Repair and regeneration

After whole-body exposure, recovery of damaged-cell populations occurs by two primary mechanisms: (1) repair of nonlethal injuries in individual cells and (2) proliferation of radioresistant or otherwise spared stem cells. The latter mechanism is of prime importance in the recovery of the bone marrow and the gastrointestinal tract after whole-body exposure. Stem cell proliferation begins almost immediately after irradiation, generally within 24 to 48 hours. In the bone marrow, recruitment of previously nondividing stem cells, which appear to serve as a reserve component for just such occasions, accelerates the process. Production of additional stem cells appears to have preference over the maturational phases. Some 2 to 3 weeks after exposure the absolute number of bone-marrow stem cells and other nucleated hematopoietic precursors exceeds preexposure levels. Over the subsequent several weeks this situation is reversed, and normal steady-state dynamics ensue.

MORPHOLOGY OF RADIATION INJURY

None of the morphologic abnormalities that result from radiation injury is unique (Table 23-6).[18-23] Each alteration encountered in irradiated cells may accompany other forms of injury, such as that caused by ischemia, heat, cold, microbiologic agents, or toxic substances. In fact, the effects of some alkylating agents so closely mimic those associated with ionizing radiation that they are often referred to as radiomimetic drugs.

Cells injured by radiation show changes involving both the nucleus and the cytoplasm. As noted previously, the nucleus of most cells appears to be more radiosensitive than the cytoplasm.

Nuclear changes

At low dose levels, the nuclear chromatin becomes somewhat clumped, and the nucleus is swollen and edematous. At moderate to high dose levels, the nucleus is often pyknotic and may show karyorrhexis. Swelling and focal loss of the nuclear membrane and fragmentation of the chromatin may be observed by electron microscopy. Multinucleation may occur.

The relationship between radiosensitivity and mitotic activity was first appreciated in 1906 by Bergonié and Tribondeau, and their names have been applied to what has become a key concept in radiobiology. They stated that:

> X-rays are more effective on cells which have greater reproductive activity; the effectiveness is greater on those cells that have a longer dividing future ahead, on those cells the morphology and the function of which are least fixed. From this law, it is easy to understand that roentgen radiation destroys tumors without destroying healthy tissues.[18]

These relationships, semiquantitated for normal cells in Table 23-3, have been paraphrased as follows: radiosensitive tissues are those with the greatest mitotic activity and the least degree of differentiation.

Cytoplasmic changes

The cytoplasmic changes after irradiation include edema, vacuolization, and alterations in the various components of the plasma membrane. Ultrastructurally, variable degrees of disintegration of the endoplasmic reticulum are also apparent. Mitochondria have been noted to be enlarged, and distorted forms are readily apparent; however, these changes may be secondary to metabolic and membrane alterations, since several studies have shown that mitochondria themselves are relatively radioresistant.

Vascular damage

Vascular damage is an extremely important consequence of irradiation, causing acute and delayed effects in both normal and neoplastic tissues. The steps involved in radiation injury are summarized in Fig. 23-7. Early after irradiation vascular dilatation may cause skin erythema or transient increase in organ function. Somewhat later, and generally in association with high dose levels, regressive changes appear, including swelling and vacuolization of the endothelium and focal necrosis of the vessel wall, sometimes with hemorrhage, or, on

Table 23-6 Morphologic hallmarks of acute and delayed radiation injury

	Acute	Delayed
Radiosensitive parenchymal and epithelial cells (intestinal epithelium, spinal cord axons, breast ductal epithelium, spermatogonia, splenic lymphocytes, and myeloid and erythroid precursors)	Necrosis	Atrophy and cell loss because of ischemia; ulceration; impaired stem cell reserves and reduced capacity to repopulate after a second insult (infection, trauma, re-irradiation); also hypertrophy, hyperplasia, metaplasia, atypia, dysplasia, neoplasea
Vessels	Dilatation, especially of arterioles and capillaries; necrosis of endothelial cells; increased vascular permeability	Sclerosis of small arteries and arterioles; capillary telangiectasia; hypertrophy of myoepithelial cells
Stroma	Edema	Fibrosis and collagen deposition; abnormal fibroblasts

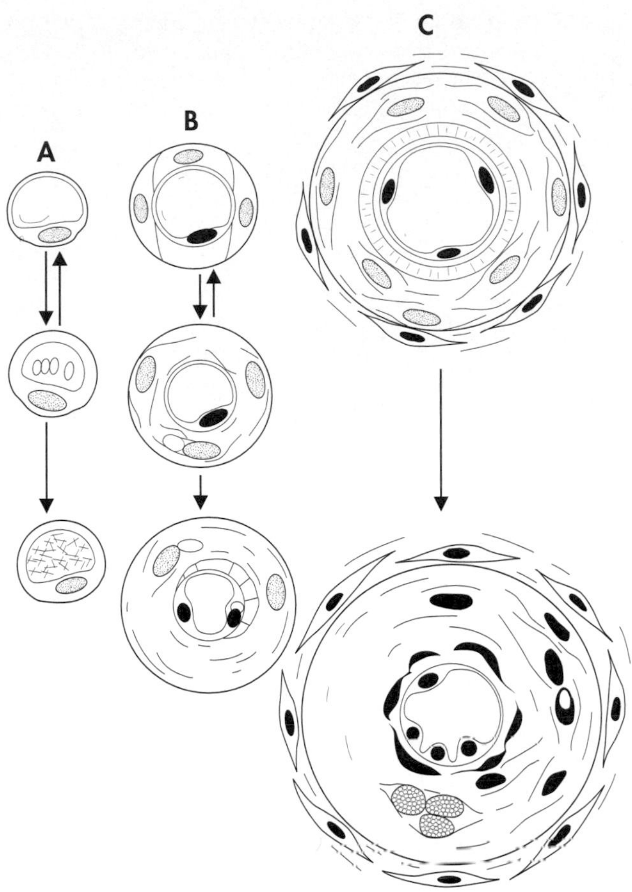

Fig 23-7 Radiation injury involving capillary, arteriole, and small artery. **A,** Capillary. Acute response of capillary is dilatation accompanied by increased permeability. This is followed by narrowing of lumen from swelling of endothelial cells and sclerosis of vessel wall. Later a thrombus may form and occlude lumen completely. **B,** Arteriole. Changes in arteriole are similar to those noted in capillary. Initial vasodilatation is followed by endothelial swelling and edema of smooth muscle, both of which serve to narrow lumen. Subsequent degenerative changes include endothelial proliferation, subendothelial deposition of hyalin-like substance, and thickening of vessel wall with focal destruction of smooth muscle cells. **C,** Small artery. Because small arteries are fairly rigid structures, early changes are less pronounced. With passage of time, however, progressive damage to endothelium and tunica media becomes evident. There is fragmentation and discontinuity of internal elastic lamella, degenerative changes in smooth muscle of media with large accumulations of hyalin-like substance, and fibrosis of the adventitia. (Modified from White DC: *Atlas of radiation histopathology,* ERDA Report TID-26676, Washington, DC, 1975.)

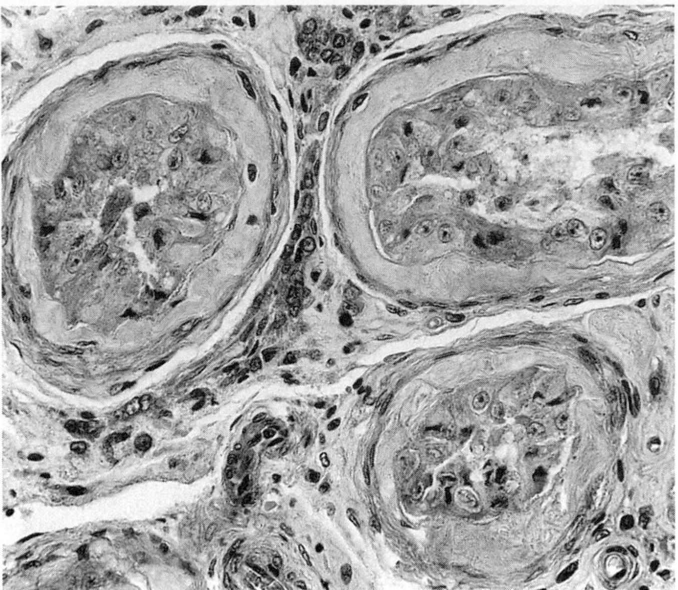

Fig. 23-8 Severe damage to the internal elastic lamina of this vessel is apparent in thyroid tissue adjacent to a papillary carcinoma. The patient was a child exposed to radiation after the Chernobyl disaster. (Courtesy Yuri Nikiforov, M.D.)

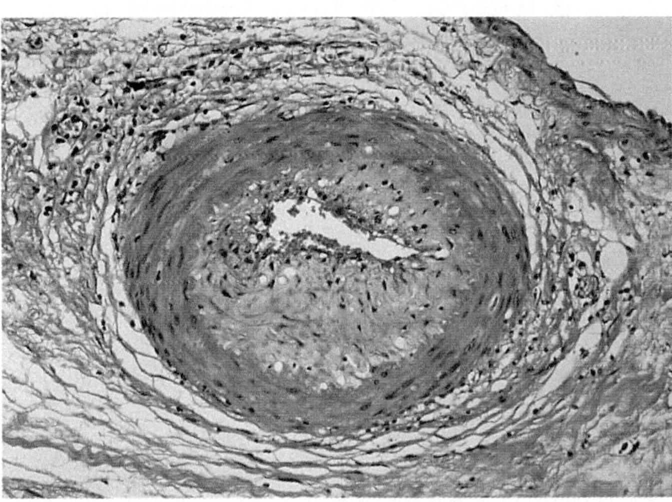

Fig. 23-9 Delayed radiation injury of small artery. This vessel in the gastric antrum was included in the treatment field of an individual who received 50.0 Gy (5000 rad) for carcinoma of common bile duct administered 1 year before death. Notice severe intimal fibrosis with complete occlusion of lumen.

occasion, even rupture (Fig. 23-8). Months or years after exposure various degenerative abnormalities are apparent. They include (1) fibrosis of the subintimal region and tunica media of small arteries and arterioles, which results in focal narrowing (Fig 23-9), (2) myoepithelial cell proliferation, which may partially obliterate the lumen (Fig. 23-10), and (3) decreased numbers of capillaries with considerable ectasia of those that persist (Table 23-7).

From the above description, it is not difficult to visualize the alterations that might be expected in an organ irradiated several years previously. Grossly, the organ will be small because of necrosis and loss of radiosensitive parenchymal cells and subsequent ischemia of less radiosensitive cells by a compromised circulation. Microscopically, atrophic or absent parenchymal cells will have been replaced by dense hyalinized connective tissue, which may contain pleomorphic, often very large, fibroblasts. (Fig 23-11). Multinucleated giant cells may be present except in organs populated by fixed postmitotic cells. Small arteries and arterioles will be lined by increased numbers of unusually prominent endothelial cells. Focally, the walls of these vessels will be thick and sclerotic and the lumen small or obliterated.

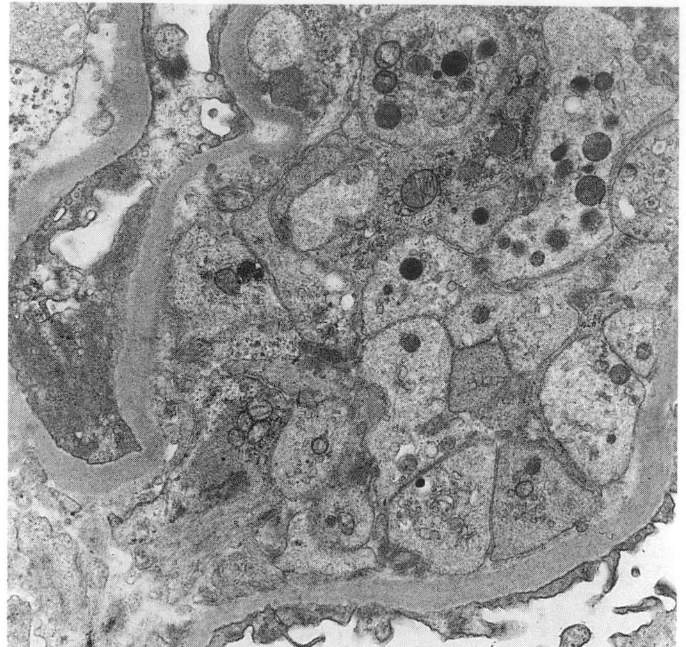

Fig. 23-10 Early radiation injury of glomerular capillary. Notice the entire lumen is obliterated by platelet thrombus with admixed erythrocytes. Nucleus of endothelial cell at lower right. (From Fajardo LF: *Pathology of radiation injury,* New York, 1982, Masson.)

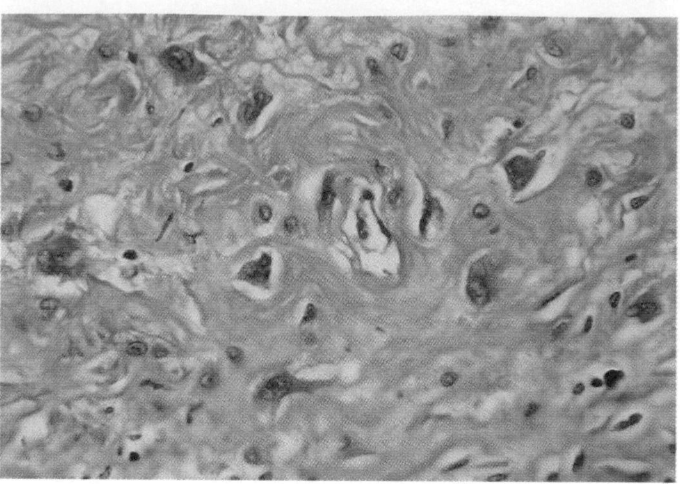

Fig. 23-11 Delayed stromal response to radiation injury. Notice hyalinized collagen and large atypical fibroblasts. This represents a generalized connective tissue response to radiation injury. The specimen could have been obtained from any one of several sites.

Table 23-7 Vascular injury: early and delayed morphologic and functional consequences in select organs

Organ (primarily vascular abnormalities)	Early (endothelial injury, vasodilatation, increased permeability)	Delayed (sclerosis/ischemia)
Skin	Erythema	Epidermal and adnexal atrophy, dermal fibrosis
Heart	Minimal	Interstitial fibrosis
Lung	Edema, hyaline membrane formation	Interstitial and intraalveolar fibrosis
Alimentary track	Edema, ulcer formation	Ulcer formation
Liver	Venoocclusive disease	Venoocclusive disease
Kidney	Vasodilatation, increased glomerular filtration rate	Cortical atrophy, interstitial fibrosis
Brain	Edema possibly resulting in acute incapacitation syndrome	Radionecrosis of white matter, gliosis
Spinal cord	Acute transient myelopathy	Transverse myelitis? (may relate to other influences)

RADIATION INJURY IN SPECIFIC TISSUES

The effects of radiation in most tissues are quantitatively related to dose.[67-88] But many factors influence the magnitude of organ dysfunction, including the number of cells irreparably damaged, the capacity of uninjured cells to undergo compensatory hypertrophy with or without hyperplasia, and the regenerative capability and reserve capacity of the irradiated tissue (Fig 23-12).

Most organs are composed of many interdependent cell types, each of which responds in a somewhat different fashion to radiation. Therefore, instead of referring to "radiation lung injury," for example, precise nomenclature is "radiation injury to the bronchial mucosa, to type I alveolar lining cells, or to capillary endothelial cells." Unfortunately, our knowledge of the response to radiation of the constituent cells of most organs is limited. Therefore, despite the inherent oversimplifications, the subsequent discussion is focused on the response of an entire organ rather than the effects on individual components.

As noted previously, radiation injury has early and delayed effects. Although somewhat artificial, this division underscores the differences in the pathogenesis of the host response. Both the early and the delayed consequences of irradiation affect parenchymal and epithelial cells, stroma, and blood vessels. However, the type and degree of involvement differs greatly as shown in Table 23-8. Early effects are most evident in rapidly dividing tissues such as hematopoietic stem cells, the germ cells of the testes, the epithelium of the alimentary tract, and an ever-changing range of tissues in the embryo. Early vascular injury is less specific, mainly vasodilatation and increased permeability. The early stromal changes are largely a consequence of vascular injury and are characterized by edema.

The delayed effects of radiation are dominated by degeneration and repair. They may involve any tissue or organ in the body. In part, this reflects widespread vascular injury,

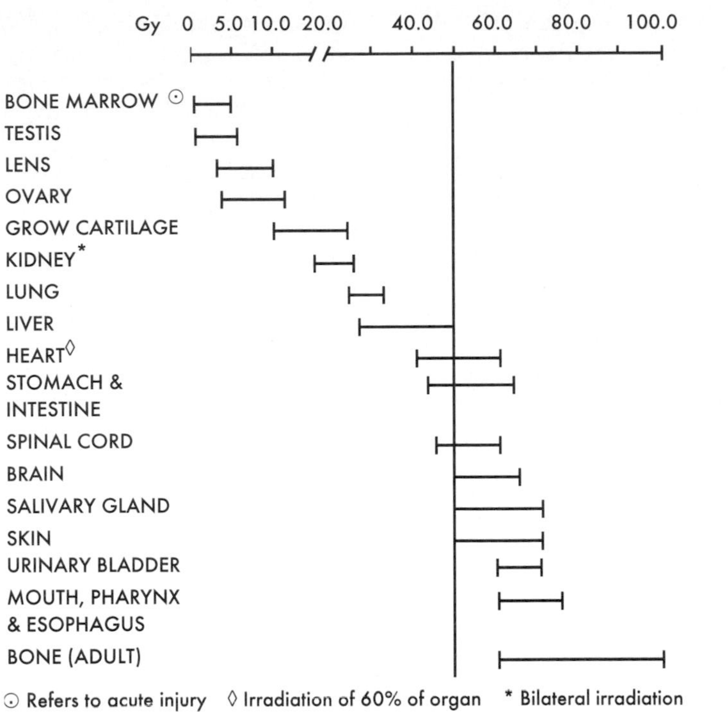

Fig. 23-12 Relative radiosensitivity of various normal cell types. The indicated ranges represent approximate doses associated with clinically severe complications in 5% to 50% *(bar on right)* of treated patients within 5 years of irradiation. Unless otherwise indicated, these estimates relate to delayed complications from therapeutic exposures administered as five fractions per week, 2.0 Gy (200 rad) per individual exposure. (From Fajardo LF: *Pathology of radiation injury*, New York, 1982 Masson.)

Table 23-8 **Select characteristics of early and delayed vascular injury.**

	Relative radiosensitivity	Morphologic manifestations	
		Early	Delayed
Capillaries/sinusoids	High	Strong evidence of endothelial injury with edema, rupture of plasma membrane, pycnosis, fragmentation of basement membrane	Considerable reduction in vessel number and luminal capacity; telangiectasia
Small arteries (<100 μm external diameter)	Intermediate	Endothelial injury with edema of cytoplasm and pycnosis of nucleus	Subintimal fibrosis; foamy macrophages in intima
Medium-sized arteries (100 to 500 μm)	Intermediate	Endothelial injury with edema of nucleus and cytoplasm	Myointimal fibrosis; foamy macrophages
Large arteries (> 500 μm)	Low	Endothelial injury	Myointimal fibrosis
Small veins	Intermediate	Endothelial injury	Thrombosis
Large veins	Very low	Usually absent	Usually absent

which may precede stromal fibrosis or accelerated atherosclerosis. Atrophy and necrosis secondary to ischemia may cause epithelial ulceration, an extremely painful and often intractable complication of irradiation. Other manifestations of delayed injury involving epithelial and parenchymal cells include hypertrophy, hyperplasia, metaplasia, atypia, dysplasia, and neoplasia.

Today, radiation injury involving normal tissues is encountered most frequently after radiotherapy for an adjacent neoplasm. This is especially important for delayed lesions where, as will be seen subsequently, the incidence of some types of complications is reduced by the fractionated kilorad exposures currently employed to treat many types of tumors.

Skin

The very first observed untoward consequences of irradiation involved the skin of the pioneer radiation workers. Shielding was unknown, and many of these individuals developed chronic radiation dermatitis from repeated exposures. In 1902 the first neoplasm attributed to radiation injury was reported, an epidermoid carcinoma of the hand of an x-ray tube maker, who tested his tubes by examining the bones of his hand.

Perhaps the best study of the relationship between radiation and skin cancer involves the children treated with epilating doses of 100 kVp x-rays to the scalp for tinea capitis. These persons absorbed an average dose of 4.5 Gy (450 rad) to the scalp. Tumors began to appear about 20 years after exposure and manifested primarily as basal cell carcinomas. Interestingly, these tumors were reported only in whites, most commonly in those areas most proximate to the exposure field not covered by hair or clothing. These observations are consistent with the hypothesis that the tumorigenic effects of x rays were enhanced by prior or subsequent exposures to ultraviolet radiation.

The sequence of early effects and the associated doses are summarized in Table 23-9. These effects are characterized by varying degrees of edema, necrosis, and inflammation and are sometimes collectively or individually referred to as "radiation dermatitis" despite the paucity of inflammation associated with most of the responses (Fig. 22-13). With cell death as an end point, the radiosensitivity of the involved components, in decreasing sensitivity, is as follows: sebaceous glands, hair follicles, epidermis, and sweat glands.

Whereas the early effects of irradiation are generally evident clinically, the delayed consequences may be less obvious, appearing only after a considerable time as (1) an atrophic dry parchment-like epidermis, with hyperkeratosis, telangiectasia, and both hyperpigmentation and hypopigmentation (poikiloderma); (2) susceptibility to injury by trauma, infection, additional irradiation or chemotherapy with poor healing capabilities and a strong propensity to ulcer formation; (3) dysplasia or malignancy (Figs. 23-12 to 23-15).

Cardiovascular

For a long time the heart was believed to be radioresistant. Recently, this supposition has been reexamined because of

Table 23-9 Sequence of early effects of skin irradiation

Manifestation	Time of appearance (after exposure)	Minimum dose implicated (Gy)	Etiology and pathogenesis
Erythema	5-7 days	4.0	Capillary dilatation, increased vascular permeability
Epilation	2-3 weeks	2.0	Necrosis of hair follicle cells
Dryness	3-4 weeks		Necrosis of sebaceous cells
Desquamation			
Dry	4-5 weeks	10.0	Loss of sebaceous glands (dryness), atrophy of epidermal cells, sclerosis of blood vessels, incontinence of pigment
Moist	3-4 weeks	40.0	As above as well as necrosis of epidemal cells, formation of bulli, ulceration, inflammation

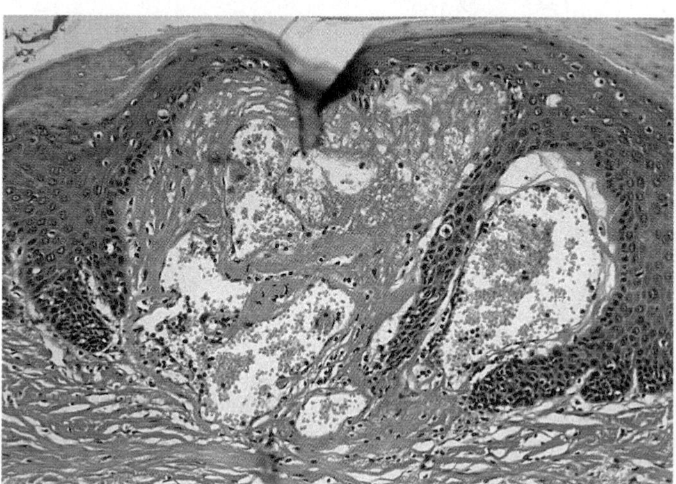

Fig. 23-13 Delayed radiation injury of skin. Notice hyperkeratosis, slight atypia of epidermal basal cells, telangiectasia, and pronounced sclerosis of dermal collagen.

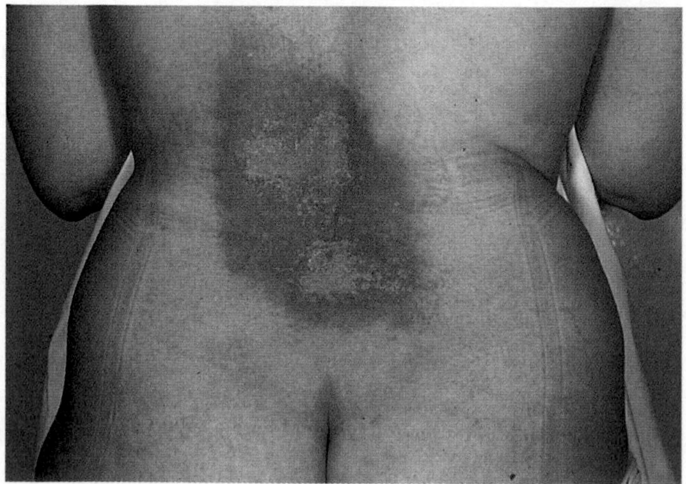

Fig. 23-14 Delayed radiation injury of skin. Pigmented area corresponds to posterior aspect of treatment field for carcinoma of uterus. Notice central atrophy and desquamation.

increased cardiac complications among persons who have received therapeutic radiation.

Radiation-induced heart disease affects 2% to 9% of patients irradiated to the mediastinum for malignant lymphoma and 3.4% of patients irradiated for carcinoma of the breast. The most common abnormality is fibrous pericarditis, often accompanied by an effusion, which may organize, constrict the heart, and necessitate pericardiectomy (Fig. 23-16). At present, irradiation constitutes one of the most common causes of constrictive pericarditis in the United States. Diffuse interstitial fibrosis of the myocardium occurs less often and is attributable to ischemia secondary to injury of capillaries. Radiation-induced coronary artery disease has received recent attention among people irradiated in childhood for Hodgkin's disease.

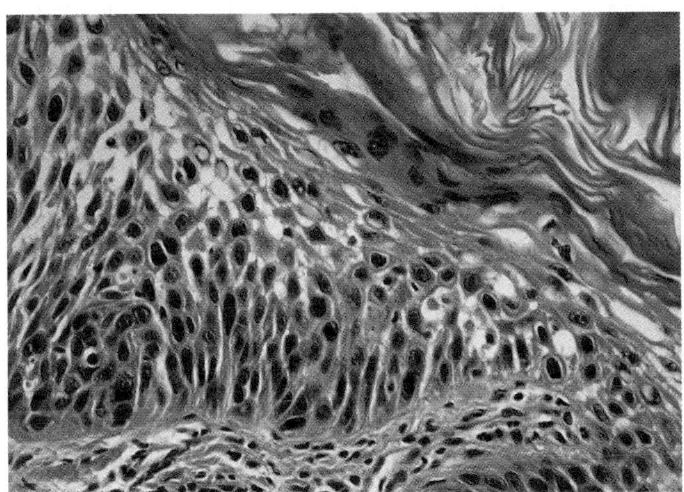

Fig. 23-15 Actinic keratosis attributable to chronic exposure to ultraviolet radiation. Notice pronounced parakeratosis, disorderly maturation, and considerable dysplasia. This lesion can be confused histologically with carcinoma *in situ*.

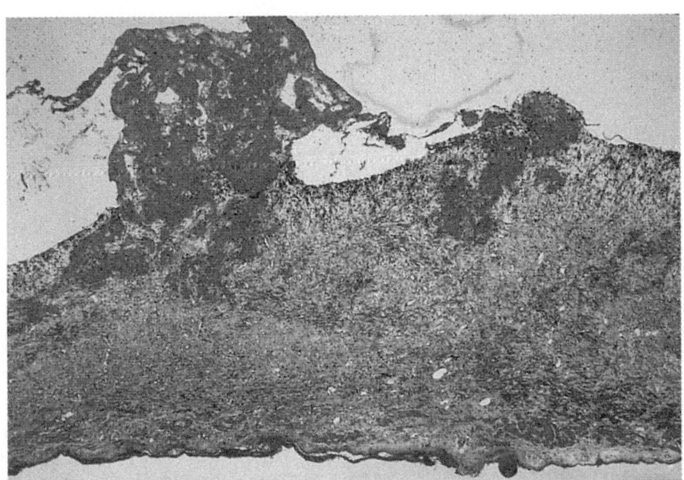

Fig. 23-16 Delayed radiation injury of pericardium. Tissue removed at surgery for constrictive pericarditis in a 37-year-old women irradiated therapeutically 5 years previously for Hodgkin's disease of mediastinum. Notice acute and chronic inflammation, recent fibrin deposition, and well-organized and partially organized fibrous connective tissue.

Patients who receive both radiation to the heart and doxorubicin (Adriamycin) are at risk of developing cardiotoxicity at lower doses considered safe than when either agent is employed singly.

Respiratory tract

Radiation injury of the lung most frequently follows radiotherapy for carcinoma of the lung, esophagus, or breast or for mediastinal tumors. The magnitude of the attendant effects is dependent not only on the usual physical factors (dose, dose rate, and so on), but also on the presence or absence of preexisting lung disease such as chronic obstructive pulmonary disease (COPD) or injury caused by prior cancer chemotherapy.

As might be expected with a highly vascular organ, the lung is extremely susceptible to both the early and delayed effects of irradiation. Some degree of damage probably occurs among virtually all patients who receive radiotherapy for thoracic tumors. Often, however, this injury is inapparent clinically, reflecting the tremendous reserve capacity of the lungs.

In persons without preexisting lung disease, the incidence of clinically evident radiation-induced pulmonary disease is related to the volume of lung exposed, the dose, and the dose rate. With total-lung or other large-volume external exposures in the therapeutic range (35 to 40 Gy administered in 30 to 40 fractions), roughly 10% to 15% of patients will develop signs and symptoms consistent with so-called radiation pneumonitis—deteriorated pulmonary function associated with dyspnea and a nonproductive chronic cough.

The earliest morphologic manifestations of radiation-induced lung injury are interstitial and intra-alveolar edema, associated with pronounced swelling of the endothelial cells of small blood vessels and increased capillary permeability (Fig. 23-17). Somewhat later, injury to both types of alveolar lining cells becomes evident and the manifestations include necrosis

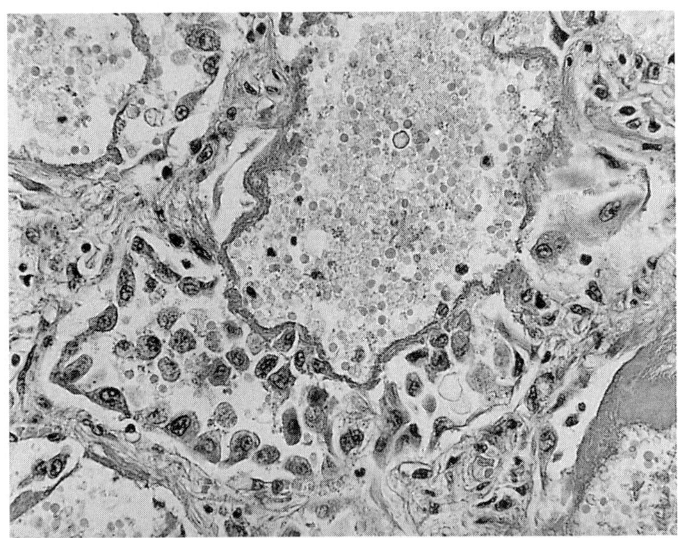

Fig. 23-17 Early radiation injury of lung. Specimen obtained at autopsy from 54-year-old man who received 45.0 Gy (4500 rad) to the mediastinum and supraclavicular region for Hodgkin's disease; 2 months after the completion of radiotherapy he developed adult respiratory distress syndrome. Notice enlarged alveolar lining cells and thin hyaline membrane lining alvoelar wall. (From Fajardo LF: *Pathology of radiation injury*, New York, 1982, Masson.)

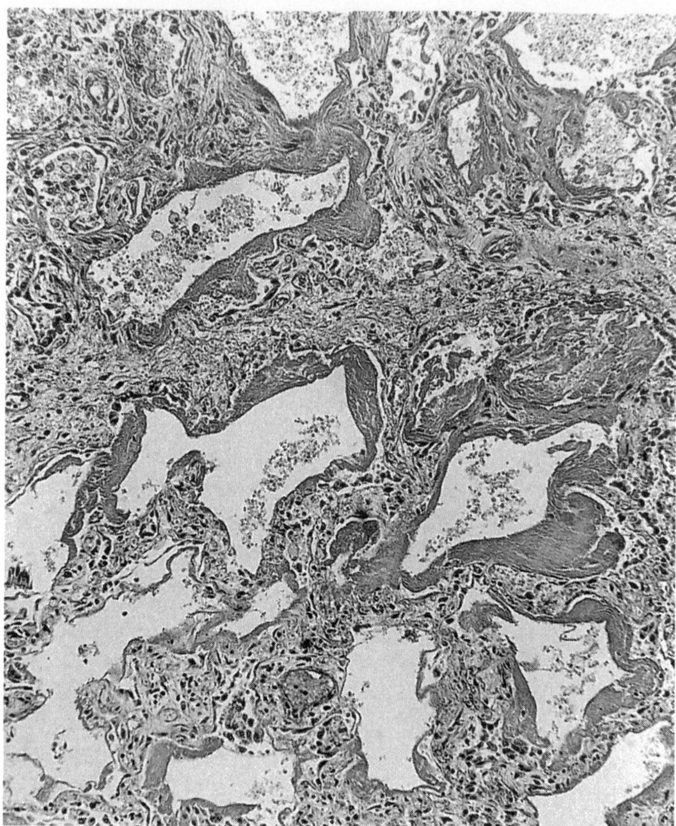

Fig. 23-18 Early radiation injury of lung. Same specimen as shown in Fig. 17. Notice hyaline membranes lining most alvoelar spaces and greatly thickened edematous alveolar septa with early organization by fibrous connective tissue.

(type I pneumocytes) and hypertrophy and hyperplasia (type II pneumocytes). Hyaline membrane formation (Fig. 23-18) is also an early finding. Thus, in sum, the histologic appearance of early radiation injury is indistinguishable from the acute alveolar injury (acute respiratory distress syndrome, or ARDS) occasioned by a myriad of agents.

Acute radiation pneumonitis (ARS) occurs 8 to 15 weeks after initiation of therapy. It is often followed by delayed fibrosis—usually localized to the exposed area—which may overlap with ARS or, more typically, develops beyond 16 weeks.

In contrast to external exposures, inhalation of radioactive substances in humans is usually associated with long-term low-dose-rate irradiation from internally deposited alpha emitters. Analysis of the exposed populations is confounded by the complexity of the attendant dosimetry of the radionuclides and in particular their disposition in the respiratory tract as well as the smoking habits of the individual.

Underground mines and especially uranium mines contain variable amounts of the gaseous radionuclide radon. Radon 222 (^{222}Rn) and its radioactive progeny attach to aerosol products in the environment. When inhaled, these aerosols are distributed throughout the tracheobronchial tree, primarily on the basis of particle size. The smaller particles, particularly those between 1.0 and 5.0 µm in diameter, reach the bronchioles and alveoli and remain trapped to deliver high-LET (linear energy transfer) radiation to the surrounding lung parenchyma. Recently, radon in the home has caused citizen concern in some regions of the United States and Canada.

Both external and internal irradiation are associated with an increased incidence of carcinoma of the lung in humans, especially when combined with other carcinogenic influences, such as smoking.

With external irradiation, the minimum latent period for tumorigenesis is approximately 9 years among the heavily irradiated spondylitics, and the incidence remained increased 20 years after first treatment. The influence of cigarette smoking has been studied in the Japanese atomic bomb survivors, and both a simple additive and a multiplicative model have been proposed to account for the increased additional risk attributable to smoking.

Inhalation of radioactive particles of a size and configuration known to reach alveoli results in a much higher incidence of pulmonary neoplasms than external irradiation does. In this connection, lung carcinoma is an occupational hazard among certain groups of miners. For example, in the period 1921 to 1926, 50% of the deaths among the miners in the Schneeberg region of Saxony were attributable to carcinoma of the lung. An increased mortality from lung cancer has also been reported among fluorspar miners in Newfoundland, iron ore miners in Britain, uranium miners of the Colorado Plateau of the United States, and tungsten, fluorspar, and lithium miners in former Czechoslovakia. In miners who develop carcinoma of the lung, the average duration of exposure is 15 to 20 years. Small cell undifferentiated carcinoma is the most frequent type of tumor. Among the uranium miners, and perhaps other mining populations as well, cigarette smoking appears to be a potent cocarcinogen.

Early and delayed radiation injury of the larynx is almost always associated with the therapeutic irradiation of this structure for carcinoma. Few clinically evident complications are evident at dose levels below 20.0 Gy (2000 rad). At higher doses complications have been documented in 23% of patients. Edema is the most prominent and bothersome early effect, whereas submucosal fibrosis characterizes delayed injury.

Cigarette smoke contains several chemical carcinogens. It has been suggested that one or more radionuclides in tobacco may also act as synergistic agents in cigarette-related carcinoma of the lung. Two radionuclides implicated in this regard are polonium 210 and lead 210. The former is an alpha emitter of the uranium series, which is present in trace amounts in most plants and foodstuffs. Lead 210 is also present in cigarette smoke in the form of insoluble particles of high specific activity that are derived from the combustion of trichromes in the tobacco leaf. The insoluble lead-210 particle, which is retained in the lung and has a physical half-life of 22 years, decays by beta emission to polonium 210.

Alimentary tract

The sequence of radiation-induced alterations in the mucous membranes of the mouth and upper digestive tract is similar to that of the skin, only the clinical evidence of injury appears sooner. After irradiation the salivary gland is noticeably swollen. Edema and then fibrous tissue replaces the normal structure of the gland (Fig 23-19). There may be an elevation in serum amylase and dryness of the mouth (xerostomia). Radiation injury of the oral mucosa and salivary glands is of particular importance because radiotherapy is the treatment of choice in many tumors of the head and neck. Dental caries constitutes an important complication of irradiation of the mouth.

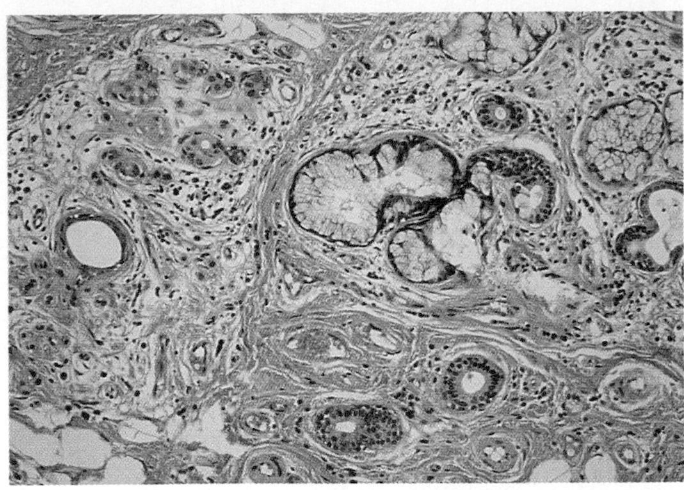

Fig. 23-19 Delayed radiation injury of salivary gland. Gland included in treatment field during radiation therapy for carcinoma of oral mucosa several years before death. Notice pronounced atrophy of acinar cells and fibrosis of stroma. Small ducts and mucin-producing cells are less radiosensitive and therefore show less change.

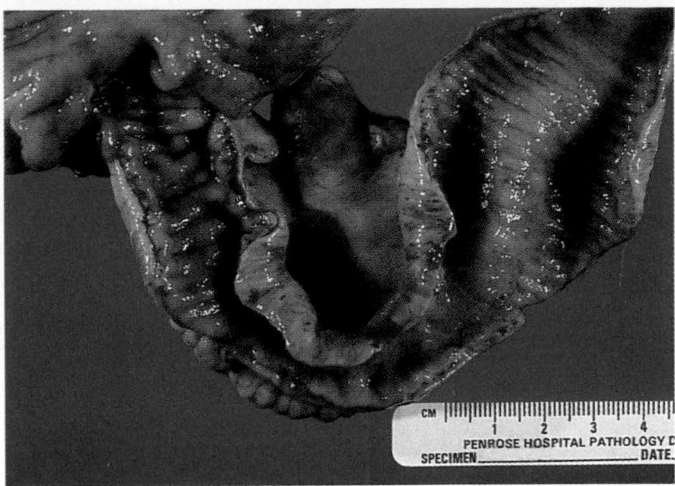

Fig. 23-20 Delayed radiation injury of small intestine. Segment of ileum removed surgically because of acute obstruction years after radiotherapy for carcinoma of ovary. Notice pronounced thickening of wall and distorted mucosal folds on left.

The onset of esophagitis, gastritis, enteritis, colitis, or proctitis occurs 1 to 3 weeks after exposure, depending primarily on how much of the gastrointestinal tract is irradiated and the exposure level. The morphologic and clinical manifestations result from the loss of the regenerative capacity of stem cells, precursors of the epithelial lining cells. With no pool of dividing stem cells and normal exfoliation of mature epithelial cells, the result is a denuded surface, which is exceedingly susceptible to infection and loss of fluid and electrolytes (Fig. 23-6). The attendant symptoms resemble those associated with other ulcerative disorders.

The delayed sequelae of gastrointestinal exposure include strictures, fistulas, chronic ulcers, and malignant tumors. Strictures are responsible for varying degrees of obstruction, whereas ulcers predispose to fistulas and less commonly perforation and hemorrhage. These delayed sequelae are most commonly located in the small intestine, colon, and rectum (Figs. 23-20 and 23-21). Radiation-induced injury to small blood vessels account for most late sequelae (Fig. 23-6). The resultant ischemia causes atrophy of the mucosa and reactive fibrosis. The atrophic mucosa is especially prone to ulcer formation. Corrective surgery is difficult because of radiation-induced vascular insufficiency, widespread peritoneal fibrosis, and poor healing of anastomotic sites.

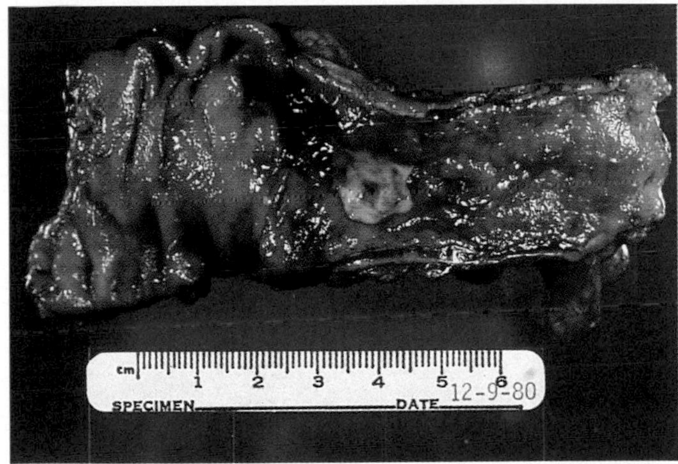

Fig. 23-21 Delayed radiation injury of large intestine. Segment of distal colon removed surgically many years after radiotherapy for carcinoma in situ. Notice ulcer, stricture, and pronounced edema of proximal mucosa.

Liver

The liver is of intermediate radiosensitivity. Most patients who receive 40.0 or more Gy (4000 rad) to the entire liver develop clinically significant hepatic dysfunction. Although still the subject of some controversy, the pathogenesis of this disorder appears related to injury of the endothelial cells of the small hepatic veins. Children are more susceptible than adults to radiation injury of the liver, also known as venoocclusive disease.

Venoocclusive disease usually appears within 90 days of radiation therapy and is therefore a subacute rather than a delayed lesion. The initial alterations involve the endothelium of centrilobular veins, the terminal portions of the afferent sinusoids, some sublobular veins, and an occasional small portal vein. There is precipitation of delicate fibrin strands within the lumen, followed by the deposition of collagen, which forms a fine network that traps erythrocytes and obstructs the lumen. Acute centrilobular congestion results with variable amounts of centrilobular congestion and necrosis.

A rare but dramatic example of hepatic injury by radiation occurred after the administration of thorium dioxide (Thorotrast) for diagnostic imaging in the 1950s. The alpha particle–emitting isotope, localized in the Kupffer cells, has been associated with cirrhosis, pronounced dilatation of sinusoids (peliosis), hepatic cell carcinoma, cholangiocarcinoma, and hemangioendothelioma. The latent period of Thorotrast-induced tumors is relatively long, ranging from 15 to more than 40 years.

Bone marrow

The bone marrow is extremely sensitive to both the acute and the delayed effects of ionizing radiation. Acute necrosis of hematopoietic stem cells causes panhypoplasia of the bone marrow and peripheral blood cytopenias (Fig 23-22). These are associated with whole-body exposures in excess of 0.5 to 1.0 Gy (50 to 100 rad). Whole-body exposures in the 1.0 to 6.0 Gy (100 to 600 rad) range result in the hematopoietic syndrome as discussed previously. However, with strong medical support, whole-body exposures as high as 12.0 Gy (1200 rad) in six equal fractions can be tolerated in association with marrow ablation before to bone marrow transplantation.

The recovery of normal peripheral blood cells after bone marrow irradiation depends on both the total dose and the proportion of marrow exposed. Shielding a portion of hematopoietically active marrow acts like a transplant, providing stem cells to irradiated sites. Other factors affecting recovery of the hematopoietic system after irradiation include the possible presence of space-occupying metastatic tumor in the marrow and the effects of others agents such as chemotherapeutic drugs.

The leukemogenic action of radiation was recognized in 1911 in a report of five instances of leukemia among radiation workers. Subsequently, well over 500 cases of leukemia have been attributed to occupational, therapeutic, or accidental exposure. Whole-body exposure is more leukemogenic than local irradiation. The type of leukemia depends primarily on the age at the time of exposure. Thus acute and chronic myelogenous leukemias are associated with irradiation in adult life, whereas acute lymphatic leukemia is more characteristic of the exposure of children. No data currently link the incidence of chronic lymphocytic leukemia with irradiation. Multiple myeloma is also increased among irradiation individuals.

In persons irradiated for ankylosing spondylitis and in the atomic bomb survivors, an increased incidence of leukemia first became evident 2 years after exposure, reached a peak 6 to 7 years after irradiation, and declined thereafter but has yet to reach background levels.

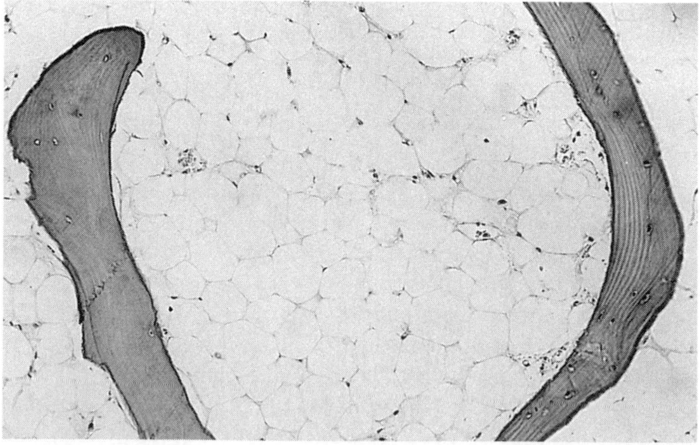

Fig. 23-22 Delayed radiation injury of bone marrow. Specimen obtained at autopsy from patient treated with high-dose radiotherapy. Notice pronounced hypoplasia of hematopoietic elements with replacement by adipose tissue. (From Fajardo LF: *Pathology of radiation injury*, New York, 1982, Masson.)

Lymphoid tissues

The response of lymphocytes to irradiation is unique in several ways. Both T-cells and B-cells are exquisitely radiosensitive, and both morphologic and functional abnormalities occur after exposure to as little as 0.1 Gy (10 rad). Second, lymphocytes have been shown to die immediately after irradiation, so-called interphase cell death. Third, membrane-associated properties such as tissue homing and recirculation are altered by small doses of radiation. And finally, despite morphologic similarity, at least at the light microscopic level, subpopulations of lymphocytes appear to differ in relative sensitivity.

The early consequences of lymphoid irradiation can be anticipated from the above comments. Even after doses in the 0.25 to 0.50 Gy (25 to 50 rad) range, pronounced but transient atrophy of the thymus, lymph nodes, and gastrointestinal tract–associated lymphoid tissue becomes apparent almost immediately. With whole body exposures, regeneration begins 10 to 14 days after irradiation and is essentially complete by day 30. However, residual effects persist and include an increased susceptibility to certain types of infection and possibly to neoplasia, the latter attributable to putative irreversible damage to the immune surveillance mechanism.

An increased occurrence of malignant lymphoma has been described among the pioneer American radiologists and persons irradiated for ankylosing spondylitis but not among the atomic bomb survivors.

Urinary tract

The kidney is moderately radiosensitive, but controversy continues with respect to the relative radiosensitivity of the various components and thus the pathogenesis of the early and delayed effects. Injury to the convoluted tubules or the glomerular capillaries has been most strongly implicated in this regard.

Acute radiation injury of the kidney is characterized by vasodilatation, interstitial edema, and proteinuria. After a variable asymptomatic latent period, progressive vascular and tubular changes develop quite regularly in both humans and experimental animals exposed to large doses. Usually, the sclerosis of the glomerular capillaries proceeds slowly, often accompanied by varying degrees of hypertension. The vascular lesions result in ischemia of nephrons with tubular atrophy. Hyalinization of glomeruli has been attributed to direct injury by irradiation or ischemia. With unilateral exposures, removal of the irradiated organ may alleviate the hypertension. Grossly the kidney of chronic radiation injury is small with a thin cortex and a finely irregular surface and may resemble the nondiagnostic kidney of end-stage renal disease.

In contrast with the kidney, where chronic effects are of paramount importance, the urinary bladder is highly susceptible to acute radiation injury. The bladder mucosa, a regenerative epithelium, is injured in the same fashion as the skin. The presence of urine, especially in association with a denuded mucosa, exacerbates the situation. Initial hyperemia is often followed by suppression of normal cell division, loss of mucosal cells, and erosion. Submucosal fibrosis, contracture, bleeding, infection, and carcinogenesis are other important delayed complications of radiation injury of the bladder (Fig. 23-23).

Radiation-induced tumors of the urinary bladder and, to a lesser extent, the kidney have been reported among the Japan-

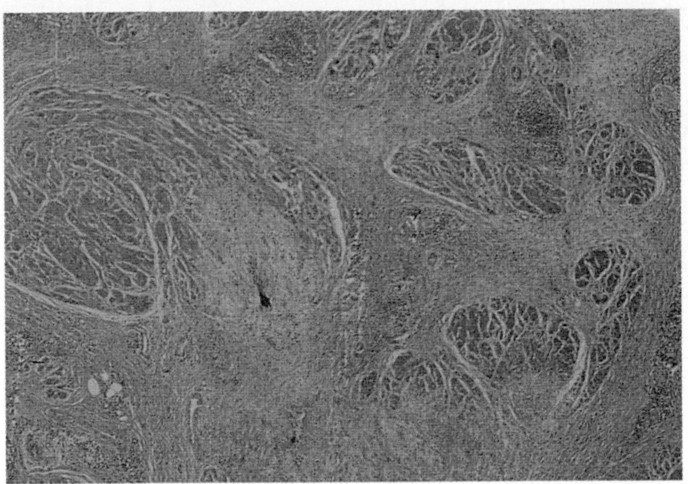

Fig. 23-23 Delayed radiation injury of urinary bladder. Specimen obtained at autopsy from person irradiated for transitional cell carcinoma of bladder; maximum filling capacity before death was 50 ml. Notice pronounced fibrosis with distortion of muscle bundles. Residual tumor cells present but difficult to identify at this magnification.

ese atomic bomb survivors. Women who received radiotherapy for benign gynecologic disorders also have shown an increased incidence of carcinoma of the bladder, as have women irradiated for carcinoma of the cervix. The latter population has additionally been shown to be at increased risk for malignant tumors of the kidney as well as the ureter. Bladder tumors are also increased in the male patients irradiated therapeutically for ankylosing spondylitis.

Cartilage and bone

The sensitivity of cartilage and bone to radiation injury differs between growing and mature tissues, with growing tissues being relatively radiosensitive.

Growth abnormalities of tumors may arise from radiation of bone and cartilage. A variety of malignant tumors have been documented among the radium-dial painters. The first reports, which concerned the development of osteogenic sarcoma, began to appear some 10 years after the initial exposure to this bone-seeking radionuclide.

Tumors other than osteogenic sarcomas occur after radium exposure. They include soft-tissue tumors, such as fibrosarcomas, and carcinomas of the paranasal sinuses, the mastoid air cells, the gingival tissues, and the nasopharynx. These epithelial cells, because of their proximity to the bones of the skull, were also exposed to significant amounts of radiation. Recently, an apparent increase in the prevalence of blood dyscrasias, multiple myeloma, and malignant tumors of the central nervous system has also been noted.

Endocrine glands

Thyroid tumors are closely associated with radiation exposure. Japanese atomic bomb survivors, the Marshall Islanders who were accidentally exposed to nuclear fallout, and children irradiated therapeutically have developed thyroid neoplasms. Papillary adenocarcinomas, adenomas, and hyperplastic nodules have been associated with these exposures. Most carcinomas found among the Hiroshima and Nagasaki survivors were first noted at autopsy. Some of the adenomas documented among the Marshall Islanders were associated with hypothyroidism.

Persons with prior thyroid irradiation should be carefully followed medically. In addition, patients with suspected thyroid tumors should be questioned carefully about possible prior irradiation of the head and neck region.

A relationship between iodine-131 administration for thyrotoxicosis and carcinoma of the thyroid has been postulated but not confirmed. If such a relationship exists, it must be rare. The reason for this may be the severe local destructive effect of the doses employed (50 to 500 Gy or more to the thyroid), which probably completely destroys the epithelial component of the gland.

Relation-related neoplasms, both benign and malignant, have been documented for virtually all endocrine organs. They are, however, much less common than tumors of the thyroid are.

Testes and ovary

The germinal epithelium of the testes is extremely radiosensitive. Even after low dose exposures, recovery is very slow and may never be complete. Acutely, radiation produces an immediate suppression of meiosis followed by necrosis of the germinal cells. Spermatogonia B are more sensitive than spermatocytes and spermatids. Persistent effects include sclerosis of seminiferous tubules and hyalinization of blood vessels. Intense irradiation may cause total tubular atrophy and hyalinization (Fig. 23-23). Sertoli cells and interstitial cells are relatively radioresistant and may appear especially prominent in an otherwise atrophic organ.

The ovary is also radiosensitive. Within several days after exposure to 3.0 Gy (300 rad), the human ovary shows a sharp increase in atretic follicles. However, a few primary primordial oocytes and their follicular epithelium are spared. Thus, about 6 months later, the cortex typically contains a few maturing follicles in an otherwise atrophic fibrous parenchyma.

Radiation is the treatment of choice for some types of carcinoma of the cervix and prostate. On occasion, the differential diagnosis between radiation effects and residual or recurrent tumor can be exceedingly difficult (Fig. 23-24).

Breast

A surprisingly large number of women have accidentally or therapeutically received significant amounts of ionizing radiation to the breast. Particularly common are women who received radiation as the sole modality of therapy for small mammary carcinomas. In the latter group especially, subsequent rebiopsy of the involved area of the breast can cause serious diagnostic problems for the surgical pathologist concerned with the histologic distinction between delayed radiation injury and recurrent tumor.

Analysis of the populations of women exposed to ionizing radiation referenced above indicate that the breast is extremely sensitive to radiation carcinogenesis. Each of these groups exhibit an increased prevalence approximately 10 years after exposure (latent period), with a peak incidence 15 to 20 years after irradiation. However, irrespective of age at exposure, radiation-related cancers are rarely seen before 25 years of age, which is about the same age that spontaneous carcinomas of the breast are first seen in the general population.

The delayed effects of irradiation of the female breast can mimic the morphologic abnormalities associated with neoplasia, more specifically those found with scirrhous adenocarci-

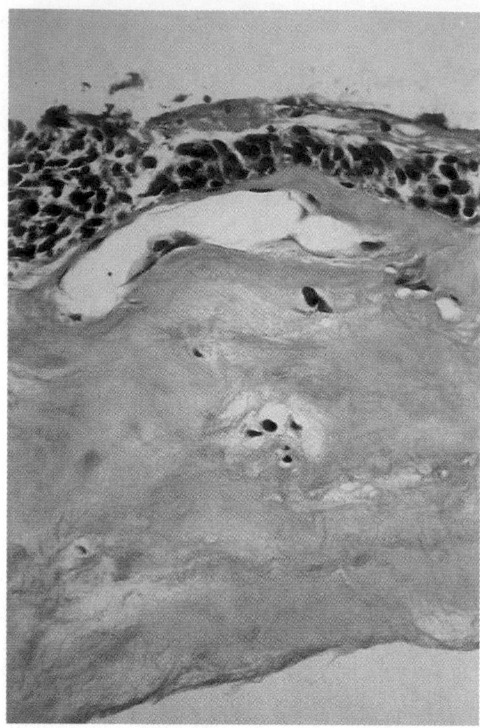

Fig. 23-24 Delayed radiation injury of uterine cervix. Biopsy specimen taken 12 years after radiotherapy for carcinoma in situ. Notice pronounced atypia of epithelial cells with hyperchromasia and disorderly maturation. Submucosal connective tissue is hyalinized with atypical fibroblasts and telangiectatic vessels.

nomas. The epithelial cells are pleomorphic and are embedded in dense fibrous connective tissue and often lack the normal acinar arrangement. Abnormal mitotic figures may be present in both circumstances. Above all, the critical nature of resolving this diagnostic dilemma accurately underscores the importance of obtaining a complete clinical history in women with suspicious lesions on biopsy. In the past, the unwary pathologist has occasionally been confronted with a history of prior irradiation after rendering a diagnosis of malignancy on a borderline case.

Central nervous system

The development of the brain may be severely disturbed by exposure to small amounts of radiation during early embryonic development. Mature nervous tissue is relatively resistant to acute morphologic changes though functional abnormalities are often encountered, especially after whole-body exposure to doses in excess of 50 Gy (5000 rad). Delayed morphologic abnormalities of the brain are not uncommon, however, especially after local exposures. They include focal or diffuse necrosis (Fig. 23-25) of the white matter, where it is associated with demyelinization.

Irradiation of the spinal cord can also lead to delayed or acute necrosis. The cord usually has been unavoidably included in the treatment field of a thoracic or abdominal tumor. Vascular injury and thrombosis of small blood vessels are believed to be responsible for the necrosis of the spinal cord, which in its most severe form may result in permanent paraplegia and a syndrome known as transverse myelitis (Fig. 23-26).

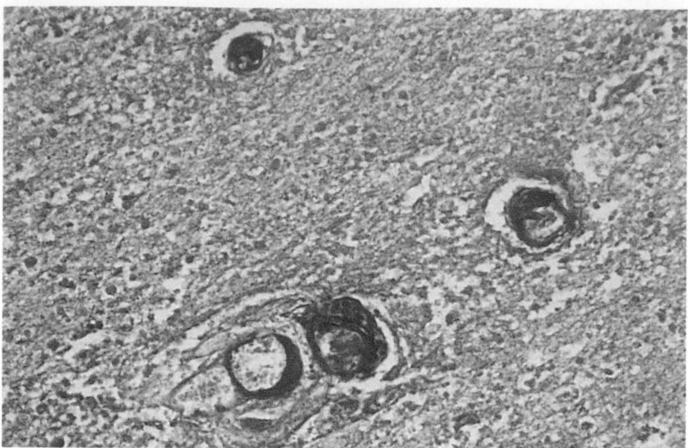

Fig. 23-25 Delayed radiation injury of brain. Autopsy specimen from a patient who received approximately 50.0 Gy (5000 rad) 2.5 years before death for a low-grade astrocytoma. Notice region of necrosis with adjacent arterioles that show irregular thickening and fibrinoid necrosis of the wall.

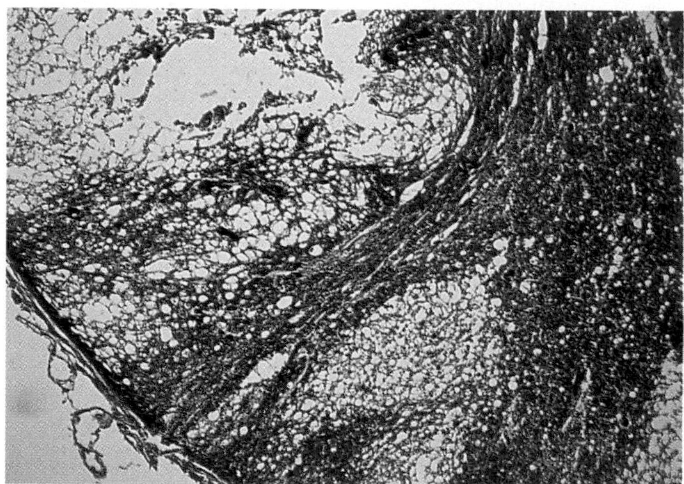

Fig. 23-26 Delayed radiation injury of spinal cord. Autopsy specimen from 55-year-old woman who received a therapeutic dose of radiation to the larynx for epidermoid carcinoma 2 years before death. After radiotherapy, patient developed a left paraplegia, a neurogenic bladder, and loss of pain and temperature sensation on her left side. Notice pronounced demyelinization involving predominately the posterior and lateral columns. In other sections of the cord, endothelial proliferation and hyaline thickening of the vessel wall was found (myelin stain).

Radiation increases the incidence of tumors of the central nervous system in both laboratory animals and humans. Children exposed to diagnostic x radiation in utero appear to be at particular risk. Both benign (meningiomas) and malignant (astrocytomas) have been implicated in the above regard.

Eye

The lens is susceptable to the formation of opacities, which may progress to clinically significant cataracts. Cataract formation depends on the magnitude of the dose and the character of the radiation; densely ionizing radiation is especially cataractogenic. A single acute exposure is more injurious and produces opacities sooner than the same dose administered in divided exposures. Recently ultraviolet light has also been implicated in this regard. Lesions of the retinal and ciliary arteries may also complicate therapeutic irradiation of the eye, such as that for retinoblastoma.

RADIOTHERAPY

Late in the nineteenth century, Wilhelm Konrad Roentgen's discovery of a "new kind of ray," coupled with the discovery of radium by Marie and Pierre Curie, launched a new era in medicine. Physicians quickly began to use x-rays and radium diagnostically and therapeutically. X-rays and radium became the treatment of choice for almost every type of illness imaginable. As a result, many tragic examples of radiation injury, of both patients and physicians, occurred and were subsequently documented. Unfortunately the untoward effects often were not manifest until many years later, and only relatively recently have stringent controls been adopted to protect patients, physicians, and technical personnel.

On the positive side, the therapeutic value of radiation was quickly recognized, and the complete eradication of otherwise fatal tumors was reported. A new discipline of medicine was soon launched, and today radiotherapy, singly or with surgery and chemotherapy, represents the treatment of choice for several types of neoplasms. Before a more detailed consideration of radiation as a therapeutic modality is presented, it is important to review a few aspects of the radiobiology of tumors.

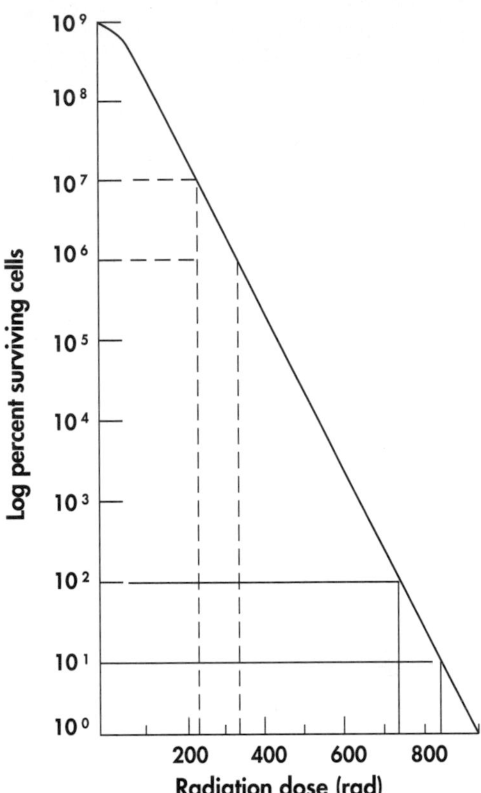

Fig. 23-27 Hypothetical survival curve for tumor cells.

Tumor radiobiology

Fig. 23-27 shows a hypothetical dose-response curve for tumor cells grown in tissue culture and irradiated. The narrow shoulder indicates that these cells are relatively poorly equipped to repair sublethal damage. The steep slope of the linear portion of the curve indicates that the tumor cells are relatively radiosensitive. The exponential character of the curve indicates that most cells are killed by small amounts of radiation but that a large dose is required to kill the last viable malignant cell. Put another way, it requires the same dose to reduce the number of viable cells from 10^7 to 10^6 (a reduction of 9 million cells) as from 10^2 to 10^1 (a reduction of 90 cells). The critical task of the radiotherapist in attempting to eradicate a malignant tumor is either to kill all tumor cells or to reduce the number to such a level that host defense mechanisms can complete the task. The radiotherapist must accomplish this without undue injury to adjacent normal tissues and intervening vital structures. In balancing these competing objectives, the radiotherapist is greatly assisted by the difference between normal and abnormal cells with respect to repair of radiation-induced injury. When radiation is given in fractionated doses, the injury created among the normal and abnormal cells by each individual exposure dose, or fraction, is the same. However, the interval (24 to 72 hours) between the completion of one radiation exposure and the start of the next provides a period for both the normal and abnormal cells to repair radiation-induced lesions. Since normal tissues generally possess a greater capability for repair than neoplastic cells do, a larger fraction of the former is present at the beginning of each subsequent treatment. For this reason, most radiation treatments are fractioned and protracted over a period of several weeks or months.

Fig. 23-28 depicts the effect of treatment, as a function of radiation dose, on normal and malignant cells. The optimal dose is the amount of radiation that will kill the greatest number of tumor cells while simultaneously injuring the smallest possible number of normal cells. Although a small amount of normal tissue destruction is acceptable, the dose must not be so large as to approach the linear portion of the "normal tissue damage" curve in Fig. 23-28.

Types of radiation generators

X- and gamma rays cover a broad range of wavelengths. Within this range, the shorter the wavelength, the greater the energy and penetrating power of the rays. For this reason long wavelengths generated at 30 to 80 keV are used for routine diagnostic procedures in radiology. Although most of the radiation is absorbed by the skin, enough energy reaches the underlying structures to provide a satisfactory roentgenographic or fluoroscopic image. In radiation therapy, shorter wavelengths are generally employed to deliver a greater proportion of the energy to deeper structures. Hence, x-ray machines designed for diagnostic purposes are not used for radiotherapy. It also follows that a given dose of x-rays from a diagnostic machine will produce greater skin damage and less injury to underlying tissues than the same dose delivered by a therapy machine.

On the basis of the foregoing discussion, it is evident that a variety of radiation energies must be available to treat patients with dissimilar tumors in optimal fashion. For example, energies in the lower ranges, 50 to 100 keV, are employed to treat some superficial skin tumors. Energies in the orthovoltage range, 200 to 400 keV, are used to treat larger or more aggres-

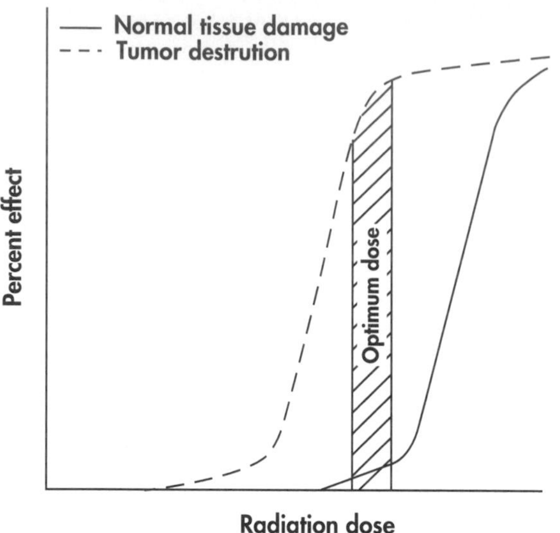

Fig. 23-28 Effect of treatment as function of dose with respect to normal and abnormal cells. Optimal dose for specific tumor-host system is amount of radiation that will cause greatest number of tumor cells to be destroyed in exchange for minimal amount of normal tissue damage. (Modified from Kligerman MM: Principles of radiation therapy. In Holland JF, Frei E, editors: *Cancer medicine,* Philadelphia, 1973, Lea & Febiger.)

sive skin tumors such as carcinomas of the lip. Energies in the supervoltage range, 2 MeV or greater, are important in the treatment of most deep-seated tumors.

X-rays are most commonly produced when electrons are accelerated to a variable degree and then are permitted to strike a tungsten target. Absorption of the energy by the target results in the production of electromagnetic radiation and heat. Depending on the energy imparted to the electrons, x-rays in the superficial orthovoltage or supervoltage range are produced. The Van de Graaff generator and the linear accelerator are two machines used to accelerate electrons. The latter is the most common supervoltage machine in use today.

Currently there is considerable interest in the use of neutrons and other high-LET particles in radiotherapy because of their ability to kill anoxic tumor cells. So much ionization is produced when heavy particles pass through tissues that little recovery is possible regardless of the presence or absence of oxygen. Therefore the relative advantage enjoyed by tumor cells, which are generally less well oxygenated than the surrounding normal tissues, is largely abolished. Although neutrons were first employed to treat malignant tumors in the late 1930s, the initial experience was marred by significant injury to adjacent normal tissues. At that time, the concept of relative biologic effectiveness (RBE) and the inhibition of normal tissue repair by heavy-particle irradiation had not yet been appreciated. Because of extensive injury to normal tissues and a variety of unfortunate complications, neutron therapy lost favor among radiotherapists until the past several years when interest again developed based upon a better understanding of the biologic effects of this particle and in particular how to take advantage of the high RBE to kill slowly cycling tumors.

Palliative and curative therapy

Radiation therapy may be employed to relieve symptoms of an inoperable tumor or to eradicate totally a malignant neoplasm. Radiation may be the treatment of choice for stage I and stage II malignant lymphomas, retinoblastoma, seminoma, epidermoid carcinomas of the laryngeal glottis, cervix, skin, lip, nasopharynx, and mouth, adenocarcinoma of the prostate, and select transitional cell carcinomas of the urinary bladder. Curative radiotherapy is also often employed with surgery in one of two ways: (1) prophylactically, when the surgeon believes that the tumor has been completely removed but cannot discount the possible presence of tumor cells in areas adjacent to the primary neoplasm such as the draining lymphatics or regional lymph nodes, and (2) therapeutically, when the surgeon is unable to resect the tumor totally because of adjacent vital structures.

Palliative radiotherapy attempts to relieve symptoms or to abort impending complications. An example of the latter is the irradiation of a tumor metastasis in the femoral neck that, if left untreated, might result in a pathologic fracture. Palliative radiotherapy is also used to relieve pain, which often occurs in association with bone tumor metastases, to relieve compression of a vital structure, such as the spinal cord, or to prevent ulceration by a subcutaneous or submucosal metastasis.

Radiotherapy employs kilodoses in the 40 to 70 Gy (4000 to 7000 rad) range administered in fractionated fashion. As with surgery, injury to normal tissues is an inevitable consequence of radiation therapy. One must include in the treatment field a margin of normal tissue adjacent to a treatable tumor to anticipate possible microscopic extension. Regional lymph nodes are often irradiated to eradicate possible metastases. Intervening tissues and structures are also injured by ionizations. The morphologic consequences of such injury in specific organs were previously discussed.

Radiation therapy can also cause radiation sickness or depress the number of circulating platelets and leukocytes. Radiation sickness is associated with treatment of the thorax or abdomen, most frequently the latter. The symptoms of radiation sickness (fatigue, anorexia, vomiting) are short lived and are usually controlled by small reductions in the daily dose. Leukopenia and thrombocytopenia can occur when large portions of the bone marrow are included in the treatment field and may dictate temporary interruption of treatment. Radiation may also increase dramatically the morphologic manifestations of malignancy in a tumor, presumably by the negative selection of a more malignant phenotype and, thereby, blur the distinction between possible residual radioresistant tumor cells and altered normal cells (Fig. 23-29).

A small but significant risk of inducing a new malignant tumor exists among therapeutically irradiated patients. Other complications of radiotherapy include actinic conjunctivitis; cataract formation, especially in children; sterility; transverse myelitis; asymmetric growth retardation in children after exposure of long bones; radiation injury of the lung or heart (pericarditis); and constriction of a hollow viscus (especially the intestine) by fibrous connective tissue.

Radioisotopes

It was noted in the previous discussion that certain naturally occurring substances such as radium, thorium, and actinium give off radiant energy spontaneously. In addition, unstable isotopes of most known elements can be produced artificially. Since the radioactive isotope of an element is essentially identical chemically to the nonradioactive form, these substances have found widespread diagnostic and therapeutic application.

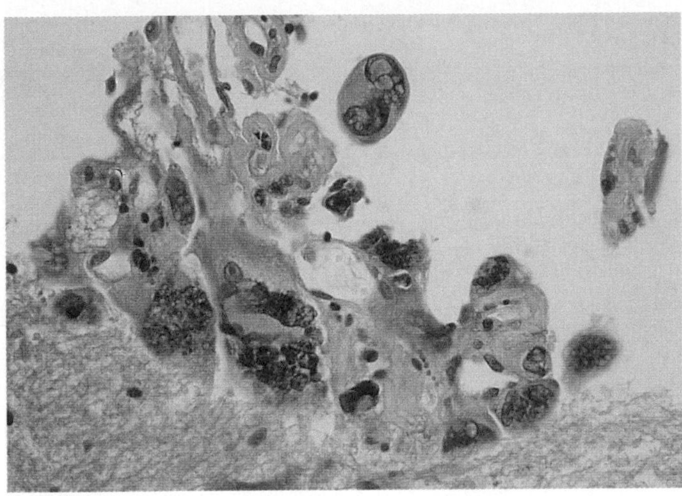

Fig. 23-29 Effects of radiation upon malignant tumor cells. Irradiation of this metastatic adenocarcinoma to the brain resulted in rapid increase of pleomorphism of tumor cells.

Diagnostic advantage is taken of the known propensity of organs to concentrate specific elements. For example, the thyroid gland concentrates iodine. By the administration of radioactive iodine, the physician can determine, with appropriate counting techniques, the capacity of this gland to concentrate iodine normally. More important, however, the organ can be scanned, and the relative distribution of the isotope throughout the gland can be quantitated. Failure of the radioactive iodine to be distributed evenly throughout the gland indicates the possible displacement of normal thyroid by nonfunctioning tissue, such as a cyst, an abscess, a nonfunctioning adenoma, or a carcinoma. Similar methods are used with other organs.

Radioisotopes are also used therapeutically. The administration of large doses of an isotope such as iodine 131, with a known propensity to concentrate in a specific organ, ensures the release of a significant amount of radioactivity within that organ. This approach may be employed to damage or destroy a malignant tumor or suppress a hyperfunctioning gland. In this connection, it is important to note that the selective concentration of most elements is not complete and therefore other tissues may be exposed, albeit to much smaller doses. This latter observation is of primary concern with the gonads and possible radiation-induced genetic effects.

Finally, it is important to remember that radiation may also be received by the fetus when a radioactive isotope is administered to the mother, who may or may not be aware that she is pregnant. Radioactive strontium, plutonium, phosphorus, tritium, iodine, and many other isotopes cross the placenta and can become incorporated into the fetus. Perhaps the most striking example is radioactive iodine, which, when administered to the mother late in pregnancy, is also concentrated in the fetal thyroid where the resultant radiation-induced injury can result in cretinism. Other examples have been documented experimentally in rodents and have been associated with malformations, neoplasms, and decreased life-span in the fetus.

INJURY FROM NONIONIZING RADIATION

Thus far tissue injury caused by ionizing radiation has represented the primary focus of this chapter.[89-92] In the past several years it has been recognized that tissues may also be injured by nonionizing forms of radiation. Table 23-10 lists some of the known deleterious effects of exposure to various types of nonionizing radiation. The industrial and medical applications of these forms of energy continue to increase dramatically. Therefore the potential for human injury from nonionizing radiation will also increase.

Numerous electronic devices represent potential sources of injury from nonionizing radiation. Currently, popular devices of this type include radar units, microwave ovens, and lasers. Despite the increasing use of these devices, surprisingly little attention has been paid to possible deleterious effects.

Microwaves represent a form of electromagnetic radiation in the frequency rate between ultrahigh frequency television and the infrared region of the spectrum. Potential sources of exposure to microwaves include microwave ovens and the high-output radar devices used in navigation and weather systems as well as burglar alarms. Animal experiments have shown that lens opacities and hematologic, endocrine, and possibly genetic effects can be caused by microwave radiations.

Microwave ovens appear to represent a particular health hazard for several reasons. In the first place, these ovens are becoming increasingly popular. Second, several surveys have documented detectable leakage around the door, especially with older models. And last, most owners and operators appear to be unaware of any radiation hazard.

The laser also represents a potential source of injury by nonionizing radiation. Because of the focusing characteristics of the lens of the eye, the retina is especially vulnerable to laser radiation. Even reflected beams represent a potential hazard. Pulsed lasers, which operate at very high power levels, can cause retina burns in 1 microsecond or less. The medical and industrial applications of lasers have increased dramatically in the past several years. Unfortunately, until relatively recently, occupational safety measures lagged behind the technologic advancements.

Finally, it is often forgotten that ultraviolet (UV) radiation is a carcinogen especially when absorbed with exogenous photosynthesizers such as 8-methoxypsoralin (8-MOP), a chemical employed with UV radiation to treat certain skin diseases. The evidence in support of UV radiation as a carcinogen in man includes the following observations: (1) human fibroblasts can be transformed in vitro after exposure to UV irradiation; (2) persons with certain genetic diseases, such as xeroderma pigmentosum and albinism, exhibit strong sensitivity to the effects of UV irradiation, which is matched by a sharp increase in the incidence of skin tumors that also tend to develop at an unusually early age; (3) persons who work outdoors have an increased frequency of skin tumors that preferentially develop on the exposed portions of the body; (4) in whites, the incidence of malignant melanoma is directly proportional to magnitude of sunlight exposure and again there is a strong predilection for these tumors to develop on the chronically exposed portion of the body. This body of human experience is buttressed by a large reservoir of data in rodents, where repeated UV irradiations also produce skin tumors as well as alterations in the proportion of several types of recirculating lymphocytes.

Radiation protection standards and the concept of relative risk

Recognition of some of the untoward effects of radiation occurred within months of Roentgen's discovery of x-rays in 1895. Beginning soon thereafter various national and interna-

Table 23-10 Types of injury caused by types of nonionizing radiation

Type of radiation	Sources	Populations at particular risk	Effects
Ultraviolet	Sun; sun lamps; welder's arcs; industrial and medical equipment	All mankind; sun worshippers; select occupational groups	Burns of skin and eye, malignant melanoma, benign skin tumors, senile keratoses
Visible light	Sun; artificial lights; lasers; communications; industrial and medical equipment	All mankind; occupational groups	Burns of retina, photosensitization
Infrared	Sun; industrial and military equipment	All mankind; occupational groups	Cataracts
Microwaves; radio waves	Ovens; radar, radio, and TV; industrial, military, and medical equipment	Much of mankind; occupational groups	Thermal effects at high power levels; cataracts;

Modified from DHEW Publ. No. NIH 77-1277, U.S. Department of Health, Education and Welfare.

tional committees developed radiation-protection standards. The efforts of these groups received significant impetus during the 1950s when large-scale testing of nuclear weapons led to widespread concern about the possible hazards of global contamination by radioactive fallout. More recently, the development of nuclear power as an energy source, in conjunction with our increasing knowledge of the risks associated with low-level exposure, has promoted a continuing assessment of radiation safety standards. Viewed in historical perspective, the evolution of these standards represents a movement toward progressively more cautious exposure limits both for the general public and for radiation workers.

As shown in Table 23-1, the average dose of radiation to the general public from medical and dental uses in medically advanced countries currently approaches that from natural background. Approaches for reducing the exposure to the patient include using radiography in preference to fluoroscopy whenever practical; proper installation and use of equipment; shielding tissues outside the area of interest, especially the gonads; using fast film to reduce the duration and intensity of exposure per radiograph; reducing the number of radiographs per procedure; limiting the size of the field to regions of prime interest; and the proper education of personnel working in the field.

Possible risks related to the nuclear power industry deserve special mention, especially in light of the American accident at Three Mile Island in 1979 and the Russian accident at Chernobyl in 1986. Both appear to have resulted from a combination of human error and technical problems. The release of radioactivity at Chernobyl was significant and resulted in at least 52 acute deaths. At the time of this writing, the size of the exposed population is not known but approximately 135,000 people were evacuated from the area, of whom 50 are believed to have received 0.5 or more Gy (50 rad); an additional 200, 1.0 or more Gy (100 rad); and 100, 3.0 or more Gy (300 rad). Roughly 24,000 persons received 40 or more mSv (40 rem). Thus it appears inevitable that a significant proportion of the survivors will develop malignant tumors. Beginning in 1990, a definite increase in thyroid cancer in children residing near the areas around the nuclear power station was noted. One report of 84 cases of thyroid carcinoma in children 5 to 14 years of age has appeared.[92]

The exposures at Three Mile Island were much smaller than Chernobyl, less than 1 mSv (100 mrem) maximum dose; at this dose level, roughly two persons with adverse health effects (fatal and nonfatal neoplasms and genetic effects) can be expected among the 2,000,000 people living within 50 miles of the facility.

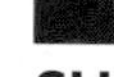

SUMMARY

If one takes into account the significant variability among individuals, the response of humans to irradiation is highly predictable. Anticipating the response of a person or a group of persons depends on the type of radiation, the dose, the dose rate and the age, sex, and general health of the recipient. Other factors to keep in mind are as follows:

- Rapidly dividing cells are more radiosensitive than slowly dividing ones (law of Bergonié and Tribondeau).
- Short of cell death, most forms of radiation injury are capable of repair; therefore, in the majority of circumstances, a given dose of radiation causes greater injury when administered as a single dose rather than in divided (fractionated) fashion.
- A given dose of external radiation causes greater injury when administered in whole body (as opposed to regional) fashion, but shielding a part of the host reduces the effects of radiation injury.
- Complex tissues (such as the lung or kidney) represent a montage of radiosensitivities with each component exhibiting its own specific response to the dose administered; therefore, both the acute and delayed effects tend to reflect injury of the most radiosensitive components.
- Because of the sensitivity of endothelium and the hydrodynamic characteristics of tubular structures such as blood vessels, vascular damage is responsible for a large proportion of the immediate and delayed effects of radiation injury.

- As with other insults, irradiation of the fetus is characterized by impairment of the tissues undergoing the most pronounced development at the time of exposure.
- In the absence of therapy, the $LD_{50(60)}$ for humans from a single dose of highly penetrating radiation is 2.50 to 4.0 Gy (250 to 400 rad).
- None of the morphologic alterations caused by irradiation are unique to this form of injury; there are, however, a combination of changes that should alert suspicion.
- In humans, damage from radionuclides depends on the physical and biologic properties of the radioactive material and especially its specific activity, decay characteristics, distribution in the host, and rate of excretion.
- Repair mechanisms in normal tissues are generally more efficient than those in tumors.
- All forms of radiation are carcinogenic.
- Under appropriate circumstances, radiation is a complete carcinogen.
- All tissues are susceptible to the carcinogenic effects of radiation but not equally so; in general, tissues that undergo rapid renewal are more susceptible than those that undergo limited or slow renewal.
- Radiation increases the incidence of tumors that are characteristic of the population at risk in terms of sex, age, up to the point of sterilization (saturation), and so on.
- The incidence of all radiation-induced tumors is proportional to dose, dose rate, the volume of tissue exposed, and the physical characteristics of the radiation source especially in terms of LET (linear energy transfer).
- There are no molecular or morphologic features that serve to distinguish radiation-induced tumors from the naturally occurring variety.

REFERENCES

General

1. Behrens CF, King ER, Carpender JWJ, editors: *Atomic medicine,* ed 5, Baltimore, 1969, Williams & Wilkins Co.
2. Hall EJ: *Radiobiology for the radiologist,* ed 3, Philadelphia, 1988, Lippincott.
3. *Ionizing radiation: sources and biological effects,* United Nations Scientific Committee on the Effects of Atomic Radiation 1982 Report to the General Assembly, New York, 1982, United Nations.
4. *Genetic and somatic effects of ionizing radiation,* United Nations Scientific Committee on the Effects of Atomic Radiation 1986 Report to the General Assembly, New York, 1986, United Nations.
5. Upton AC: *Radiation injury: effects, principles and perspectives,* Chicago, 1969, The University of Chicago Press.

Radiation spectrum; radioactive substances; radiation units

6. Hendee WR, Ritenour ER: *Medical imaging physics,* ed 3, St. Louis, 1992, Mosby.
7. Hendee WR: *Radiation therapy physics,* St. Louis, 1981, Mosby.
8. Johns HE, and Cunningham JR: *Physics of radiology,* ed. 4, Springfield, Ill, 1982, Charles C Thomas, Publisher.

Cellular and molecular radiation biology

9. Altman KL, Gerber GB, Okada S: *Radiation biochemistry,* vol 1, New York, 1970, Academic Press.
10. Bacq ZM, Alexander P: *Fundamentals of radiobiology,* ed 2, New York, 1971, Pergamon Press.
11. Cornforth MN, Bedford JS: X-ray-induced breakage and rejoining of human interphase chromosomes, *Science* 222:1141, 1983.
12. Elkind MM, Whitmore GF: *Radiobiology of cultured mammalian ceils,* New York, 1967, Gordon & Breach.
13. Gantt R, Parshad R, Price FM, Sanford KK: Biochemical evidence for deficient DNA repair leading to enhanced G2 chromatid radiosensitivity and susceptibility to cancer, *Radiat Res* 108:117, 1986.
14. Puck TT: Effect of radiation on mammalian cells. In Puck TT, editor: *The mammalian cell as a microorganism,* San Francisco, 1972, Holden-Day.
15. Puck TT, Marcus PI: Action of x-rays on mammalian cells, *J Exp Med* 103:653, 1956.
16. Sinclair WK: Cyclic x-ray responses in mammalian cells in vitro, *Radiat Res* 33:620, 1968.
17. Tili JE, McCullock EA: A direct measurement of the radiation sensitivity of normal mouse bone marrow cells, *Radiat Res* 14:213, 1961.

Morphology of radiation injury

18. Bergonié J, Tribondeau L: Interprétation de quelques résultats de la radiothérapie et essai de fixation d'une technique rationnelle, *Compt Rend Acad Sci* 143:983, 1906.
19. Fajardo LF: *Pathology of radiation injury,* New York, 1982, Masson.
20. Upton AC, Lushbaugh CC: The pathological anatomy of total-body irradiation. In Behrens DF, King ER, Carpender JWJ, editors: *Atomic Medicine,* ed 5, Baltimore, 1969, Williams & Wilkins.
21. Warren S: Effects of radiation on normal tissues, *Arch Pathol* 34:443, 562, 749, 917, 1070, 1942; 35:121, 304, 1943.
22. Warren S: Histopathology of radiation lesions, *Physiol Rev* 24:225, 1944.
23. White DC: *An atlas of radiation histopathology,* ERDA Rep TID-26676, Washington, DC, 1975, Technical Information Center, Office of Public Affairs, US Energy Research and Development Administration.

Radiation injury in humans

24. Advisory Committee on the Biological Effects of Ionizing Radiation: *The effects on populations of exposure to low levels of ionizing radiation* (BEIR Report), Washington, DC, 1990, National Academy of Sciences—National Research Council.
25. Anderson RE: The delayed consequences of exposure to ionizing radiation: pathology studies at the Atomic Bomb Casualty Commission, Hiroshima and Nagasaki, 1945-1970, *Hum Pathol* 2:469, 1971.
26. Andrews GA: Criticality accidents in Vinca, Yugoslavia, and Oak Ridge, Tennessee, *JAMA* 179:191, 1962.
27. Berthrong M, Fajardo LF: Radiation injury in surgical pathology. Part II. Alimentary tract, *Am J Surg Pathol* 5:153, 1981.
28. Boice JD, Fraumeni JF, editors: Radiation carcinogenesis: epidemiology and biological significance. In *Progress in cancer research and therapy,* vol 26, New York, 1984, Raven Press.
29. Borek C, Hall EJ: Effect of split doses of x-rays on neoplastic transformation of single cells, *Nature* 252:499, 1974.
30. Brent RL: Effects of radiation on the fetus, newborn and child. In Fry RJM et al, editors: *Late effects of radiation,* London, 1970, Taylor & Francis.
31. Darby SC, Dole R, Gill SK, Smith PB: Long term mortality after a single treatment course with x-rays in patients treated with ankylosing spondylitis, *Br J Cancer* 55:179, 1987.
32. Evans RD: The effect of skeletally deposited alpha-ray emitters in man, *Br J Radiol* 39:881, 1966.
33. Fajardo LF: Ionizing radiation and neoplasia. In Fenoglio-Preiser CM, Weinstein RS, Kaufman N, editors: *The International Academy of Pathology,* Baltimore, 1986, Williams & Wilkins.
34. Fajardo LF, Berthrong M: Radiation injury in surgical pathology. Part 1, *Am J Surg Pathol* 2:159, 1978.
35. Hachiya M: *Hiroshima diary—the journal of a Japanese physician, August 6–September 30, 1945,* Chapel Hill, 1955, The University of North Carolina Press.
36. Hamilton TE, van Belle G, LoGerfo JP: Thyroid neoplasia in Marshall Islanders exposed to nuclear fallout, *JAMA* 258:629, 1987.
37. Harvey EB, Boice JD, Jr, Honeyman, M, Flannery JT: Prenatal x-ray exposure and childhood cancer in twins, *N Engl J Med* 312:541, 1985.
38. Langham WH, Brooks PM, Grahn D: Radiation biology and space environmental parameters in manned spacecraft design and operations, *Aerospace Med* 36:1, 1965.
39. Langlois RE et al: Evidence for increased somatic cell mutations at the glycophorin A locus in atomic bomb survivors, *Science* 236:445, 1987.
40. Loewe WE, Mendelsohn E: Revised dose estimates at Hiroshima and Nagasaki, *Health Physics* 41:663, 1981.
41. Martland HS: Occupational poisoning in manufacture of luminous watch dials, *JAMA* 92:466, 1929.

42. Matanoski GM, Seltser R, Sartwell PE et al: The current mortality rates of radiologists and other physician specialists: deaths from all causes and from cancer, *Am J Epidemiol* 101:188, 1975.
43. Matanoski GM, Seltser R, Sartwell PE et al: The current mortality rates of radiologists and other physician specialists: specific causes of death, *Am J Epidemiol* 101:199, 1975.
44. Miller RW: Delayed radiation effects in atomic-bomb survivors, *Science* 166:569, 1969.
45. Neel JV, Kato H, Schull WJ: Mortality in the children of atomic bomb survivors and controls, *Genetics* 76:311, 1974.
46. Okada S et al: A review of thirty years study of Hiroshima and Nagasaki atomic bomb survivors, *Radiat Res* 16(suppl):1, 1975.
47. Otake M, Schull WJ: In utero exposure to A-bomb radiation and mental retardation: a reassessment, *Br J Radiol* 57:409, 1984.
48. Oughterson AW, Warren S: *Medical effects of the atomic bomb in Japan,* New York, 1956, McGraw-Hill.
49. Polednak AP, Stehney AF, Rowland RE: Mortality among women first employed before 1930 in the U.S. radium dial-painting industry, *J Epidemiol* 107:179, 1978.
50. Prentice RL, Thompson DJ: *Atomic bomb survivor data: utilization and analysis,* Proceedings of a conference sponsored by SIAM Institute for Mathematics and Society, Philadelphia, 1984, Society for Industrial and Applied Mathematics.
51. Roesch WC, editor: *Final report of U.S.–Japan reassessment of atomic bomb radiation dosimetry in Hiroshima and Nagasaki,* Hiroshima, 1987, Radiation Effects Research Foundation.
52. Setlow RB, Carrier WL: The disappearance of thymine dimers from D.N.A.: an error-correcting mechanism, *Proc Natl Acad Sci USA* 51:226, 1964.
53. Shimizu Y, Kato H, Schull WJ et al: Studies of the mortality of A-bomb survivors. 9. Mortality, 1950-1985: Part 1. Comparison of risk coefficients for site-specific cancer mortality based on the DS 86 and T65DR shielded kerma and organ doses, *Radiat Res* 118:502, 1989.
54. Shimizu Y, Kato H, Schull WJ: Studies of the mortality of A-bomb survivors. 9. Mortality, 1950-1985: Part 2. Cancer mortality based on the recently revised doses (DS 86), *Radiat Res* 121:120, 1990.
55. Shimizu Y, Kato H, Schull WJ, Hoel DG: Studies of the mortality of A-bomb survivors. 9. Mortality, 1950-1985: Part 3. Noncancer mortality based on the recently revised doses (DS 86), *Radiat Res* 130:249, 1992.
56. Shimizu Y, Schull WJ, Kato H: Results obtained for the period 1950-1985 and future studies of cancer mortality among atomic bomb survivors (RERF Life Span Study) *BIR Report 22: The future of human radiation Research,* 1991.
57. Shore RE, Albert RE, Reed M et al: Skin cancer incidence among children irradiated for ringworm of the scalp, *Radiat Res* 100:192, 1984.
58. Shore RE, Woodard E, Hildreth N et al: Thyroid tumors following thymus irradiation *J Natl Cancer Inst* 74:1177, 1985.
59. Smith PG, Doll R: Age and time-dependent changes in the rates of radiation-induced cancers in patients with ankylosing spondylitis following a single course of x-ray treatment. In *Late biological effects of ionizing radiation,* vol 1, Vienna, 1978, International Atomic Energy Agency.
60. Spiers FW, Lucas HF, Anast GA: Leukaemia incidence in the U.S. dial workers, *Health Physics* 44(suppl 1):65, 1983.
61. United States Department of Health, Education and Welfare: *Review of the use of ionizing radiation for treatment of benign diseases,* Washington, DC, 1977, US Government Printing office.
62. Upton AC: Physical carcinogenesis: radiation history and sources. In Becker FF, editor: *Cancer, a comprehensive treatise,* vol 1, New York, 1975, Plenum Press.

Acute radiation syndrome

63. Bond VP, Cronkite EP, Conard RA: Acute whole body radiation injury: pathogenesis, pre- and postradiation protection. In Behrens CF, King ER, Carpender JWJ, editors: *Atomic medicine,* ed 5, Baltimore, 1969, Williams & Wilkins.
64. Bond VP, Fliedner TM, Archambeau JO, editors: *Mammalian radiation lethality: a disturbance in cellular kinetics,* New York, 1965, Academic Press. (Cell turnover and acute radiation injury.)
65. Cerstner HB: Acute clinical effects of penetrating nuclear radiation, *JAMA* 168:381, 1958.
66. Hempelmann LH, Lisco H, Hoffman JC: The acute radiation syndrome: a study of nine cases and a review of the problem, *Ann Intern Med* 36:279, 1952.

Radiation injury of select tissues

67. Anderson RE, Nishiyama H, Ii Y et al: Pathogenesis of radiation-related leukemia and lymphoma, *Lancet* 1:1060, 1972.
68. Archambeau JO, Mathieu CR, Brenneis HJ et al: The response of the skin of swine to increasing single exposures of x-rays (250 kVp), *Radiat Res* 37:141, 1969.
69. Berthrong M: Radiologic changes secondary to radiation, *World J Surg* 10:155, 1986.
70. Cuzick J: Radiation-induced myelomatosis, *N Engl J Med* 304:204, 1981. (Multiple myeloma in irradiated populations.)
71. DeGroot L, Paloyan E: Thyroid carcinoma and radiation: a Chicago endemic, *JAMA* 225:487, 1973.
72. Fajardo LF: Pathology of radiation-induced heart disease. In Bricker JT, Green DM, D'Angio GJ, editors: *Cardiac toxicity after treatment for childhood cancer,* New York, 1993, Wiley-Liss.
73. Fajardo LF, Berthrong M: Vascular lesions following radiation, *Pathol Annu* 23:297, 1988.
74. Fajardo LF, Stewart JR: The pathogenesis of radiation-induced myocardial fibrosis, *Lab Invest* 29:244, 1973.
75. Haley TJ, Snider RS: *Response of the nervous system to ionizing radiation,* New York, 1962, Academic.
76. Hancock SL, Donaldson SS: Radiation-related cardiac disease: risks after treatment of Hodgkin's disease during childhood and adolescence. In: Bricker JT, Green DM, D'Angio GJ, editors: *Cardiac toxicity after treatment for childhood cancer,* New York, 1993, Wiley-Liss.
77. Hempelmann LH: Risk of thyroid neoplasms after irradiations in childhood, *Science* 160:159, 1968.
78. Ichimaru M, Ishimaru T: Leukemia and related disorders: a review of thirty years' study of Hiroshima and Nagasaki atomic bomb survivors. II. Biological effects, *J Radiat Res* 16(suppl):89, 1975.
79. Knowlton NP Jr et al: Beta ray burns of human skin, *JAMA* 141:239, 1949.
80. Land CE, Boice JD Jr, Shore RE et al: Breast cancer risk from low-dose exposures to ionizing radiation: results of parallel analysis of three exposed populations of women, *J Natl Cancer Inst* 65:353, 1980.
81. Nishiyama H, Anderson RE, Ishimaru T et al: The incidence of malignant lymphoma and multiple myeloma in Hiroshima and Nagasaki atomic bomb survivors, *Cancer* 32:1301, 1973.
82. Puck TT: Cellular aspects of the mammalian radiation syndrome, *Radiat Res* 27:272, 1966.
83. del Regato JA: Twenty years followup of patients with inoperable cancer of the prostate (stage C) treated by radiotherapy: report of a national cooperative study, *Int J Radiat Oncol Biol Phys* 26:197, 1993.
84. Saccomanno C, Archer VE, Auerbach O et al: Histologic types of lung cancer among uranium miners, *Cancer* 27:515, 1971.
85. Shore RE, Hildreth N, Woodard E et al: Breast cancer among women given X-ray therapy for acute postpartum mastitis, *J Natl Cancer Inst* 77:689, 1986.
86. Stewart JR, Fajardo LF: Radiation-induced heart disease: an update, *Prog Cardiovasc Dis* 27:173, 1984.
87. Stewart JR, Fajardo LF: Dose respondence in human and experimental radiation-induced heart disease: application of the nominal standard dose (NSD) concept, *Radiology* 99:403, 1971.
88. Yamamoto T, Kopecky KJ, Fujikura T et al: Lung cancer incidence among Japanese A-bomb survivors, 1950-80, *J Radiat Res* 28:156, 1987.

Injury from nonionizing radiation

89. Brill AB, Johnston RE: Exposure of man to radiation. In Fry RJM, et al, editors: *Late effects of radiation,* Proceedings of a colloquium, University of Chicago, 1969; London, 1970, Taylor & Francis.
90. Microwave hazards, *Lancet* 2:694, 1975. (Editorial.)
91. Peyton MF, editor: *Biological effects of microwave radiation,* New York, 1961, Plenum Press.
92. Nikiforov Y, Gnepp DR, Demidchik EP: *Pediatric thyroid cancer after the Chernobyl disaster: pathomorphological study of 84 recent cases (1991-1992) from the Republic of Belarus.*

24 Neoplasia

Michael W. Lieberman
Russell M. Lebovitz

Dramatic advances in the understanding of neoplasia continue to parallel the spectacular developments in cell and molecular biology. These include but are not limited to the characterization of oncogenes, chromosomal rearrangements, and tumor suppressor genes. Many developments are related to technical advances, such as the polymerase chain reaction (Chapter 11), yet the effect of these advances must be understood against a backdrop of observations in tumor biology, for it is the behavior of tumors, as they are observed microscopically, biochemically and clinically, that embodies neoplasia and defines many challenging questions.

Neoplasia, along with infectious and cardiovascular diseases, is a major cause of morbidity and mortality. In the United States in 1995 there were about 1.2 million new cases of cancer (exclusive of nonmelanotic skin cancer) and more than 500,000 deaths from cancer.[1]

DEFINITIONS

Neoplasia

Fundamental to a discussion of neoplasia is an understanding of certain concepts and terms. No completely satisfactory definition of neoplasia exists. The difficulty is that neoplastic growth shares many features with other disturbances in cell growth and even normal growth, and therefore is hard to distinguish from these semantically. Advances in our understanding of the regulation of cell growth, and differentiation have emphasized the similarities among different types of growth and have not as yet identified properties that unequivocally distinguish neoplastic growth, thus exacerbating the problem of definition. The definition of Willis, however, remains one of the most widely cited and useful: *"A neoplasm is an abnormal mass of tissue, the growth of which exceeds and is uncoordinated with that of the normal tissues and persists in the same excessive manner after cessation of the stimuli which evoked the change."*[2] In practice, the clinical behavior of a neoplasm and its microscopic appearance define neoplastic change operationally. For the experimentalist, the situation is more complicated; if cells suspected of being neoplastic are transplanted to a syngeneic host, for example, and they persist at the transplantation site, is the investigator observing a neoplastic mass, a homograft, or some combination of the two? The study of neoplasia, like much of biology, remains a descriptive enterprise in which description (however sophisticated or molecular) replaces definition.

Tissue regeneration and repair

In response to injury many tissues are capable of restoration of approximately normal structures. Thus an epidermis denuded by abrasion is replaced by new epidermis. Or, if part of the liver is lost through injury or partial hepatectomy, it regenerates to its preinjury mass. Restoration results from cell division and thus shares features with normal growth, with hyperplastic responses to injury and neoplasia. An essential feature of tissue repair, absent in neoplasia, is the cessation of growth after restoration.

Hyperplasia

An increase in the number of cells in a tissue or organ is termed *hyperplasia*. It follows that only cells and tissues that are capable of cell division undergo hyperplasia, and a stimulus or increased responsiveness to an existing stimulus must be present. Epidermal cells, for example, in response to abrasion or pressure, increase mitotic rate and increase in number. Experimentally, this process can be induced by the application of acetic acid or tumor-promoting chemicals (such as tetradecanoylphorbol acetate or benzoyl peroxide)[3] to the skin. Although the induction of hyperplasia by these agents is often associated with changes that might be expected to accompany proliferation of epidermal cells (such as increased ornithine decarboxylase activity and altered transcription of epidermis-specific keratins),[4,5] the molecular basis for these changes is unknown. In the prostate, hyperplasia of both glandular (epithelial) and stromal (fibromuscular) elements occurs with advancing age (Fig. 24-1). Prostatic hyperplasia is associated with increased conversion of androgens to dihydrotestosterone.[6,7] Administration of androgens or high levels of dihydrotestosterone to castrated dogs results in prostatic hyperplasia.[8] Dihydrotestosterone is also involved in prostatic hyperplasia in men, and agents that inhibit its formation (5α-reductase inhibitors) appear to arrest and partially reverse prostatic hyperplasia.[9] As with epidermal hyperplasia, the molecular basis of prostatic hyperplasia remains unknown. Prostatic hyperplasia is clinically important, of course, because it may cause urethral obstruction and urinary retention.

Hyperplasia in endocrine organs is often dramatic. Thyroid-stimulating hormone (TSH) and antibodies to the TSH receptor can cause thyroid hyperplasia and thyrotoxicosis. Likewise, hyperplasia of the adrenal cortex can result from increased levels of circulating adrenocorticotropic hormone (ACTH).

Compensatory hyperplasia may occur in response to loss of a paired organ. This phenomenon is seen after unilateral nephrectomy; the contralateral kidney responds by an increase in the cellularity, an increase in cell size, and thus gross hypertrophy visible to the naked eye.

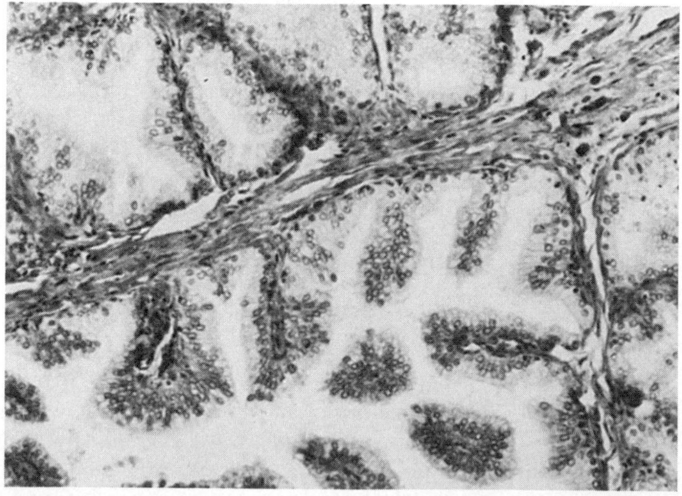

Fig. 24-1 Hyperplasia of prostate. In this example the process mainly involves epithelium, which because of an increased number of cells is arranged in fronds with a vascular stalk.

Hyperplasia can place an organ at increased risk for neoplasia, especially if there is chronic stimulation of cell division. An increased percentage of cells in the cell cycle increases the possibility of spontaneous chromosomal abnormalities, altering oncogene structure and function and inducing mutations, or rearrangements. It has been suggested, for example, that the hyperplastic response of epidermis to tumor promoters increases the pool of cells at risk for papilloma formation and that these, in turn, provide increased numbers of cells for malignant tumor (carcinoma) genesis.[3,10] Agents that damage liver cells (such as hepatitis viruses, alcohol, and other chemical toxins) cause a loss of hepatic mass followed by regeneration and local hyperplasia (hyperplastic nodules).[11] These stimuli, which are often chronic, increase the risk of hepatocellular carcinoma manyfold.

Hypertrophy

Organs or tissues that respond to stimuli by an increase in cellular mass, without an increase in cell number, are said to undergo hypertrophy. Often these are tissues in which regenerative capacity is limited. Thus, in response to increased work load resulting from cardiac valvular deformity, individual myocardial fibers thicken, and the heart hypertrophies. Exercise and anabolic steroids result in similar changes in skeletal muscle. A combination of hypertrophy and hyperplasia can occur simultaneously.

The degree to which repair, hyperplasia, and hypertrophy may share related features can be illustrated by considering responses to a growth factor termed *transforming growth factor-β* (TGF-β) (Table 24-6). This polypeptide, originally discovered in supernatants from cultures of tumor cells, stimulates proliferation of fibroblasts in cell culture and inhibits the proliferation of kidney and other types of cultured epithelial cells. TGF-β plays a key role in the repair of connective tissue in vivo by promoting fibroblastic growth, capillary formation, and collagen synthesis after wounding.[12,13] After wounding, platelets, macrophages, and lymphocytes are attracted to the wound. All of these are known to secrete TGF-β,[12,13] which stimulates the restoration of dermal structure. Two other growth factors, epidermal growth factor and platelet-derived growth factor, are considered not to be involved in this process,[1] but these and other growth factors and hormones, such as insulin-like growth factor and fibroblast growth factor, may play other roles in wound healing and in other examples cited later.[14,15]

It is instructive to consider related pathologic conditions that occur in different contexts. A hyperplastic response of skin to injury, termed *keloid formation*, results in extensive local overproduction of connective tissue with thick collagenous bands. Local oversecretion of TGF-β or heightened sensitivity to it may be in part responsible. A similar pattern of connective tissue proliferation, termed *desmoplasia*, is observed in association with the growth of several different tumors; common examples include the desmoplastic response seen in pancreatic cancer, colon cancer, and breast cancer (scirrhous carcinoma; Fig. 24-2).

Many neoplastic cells secrete TGF-β and it is reasonable to assume that this desmoplastic response results at least in part from TGF-β release. TGF-β may also play an important role in the growth of tumors derived from fibroblasts (that is, fibrosarcomas) through a mechanism known as autocrine

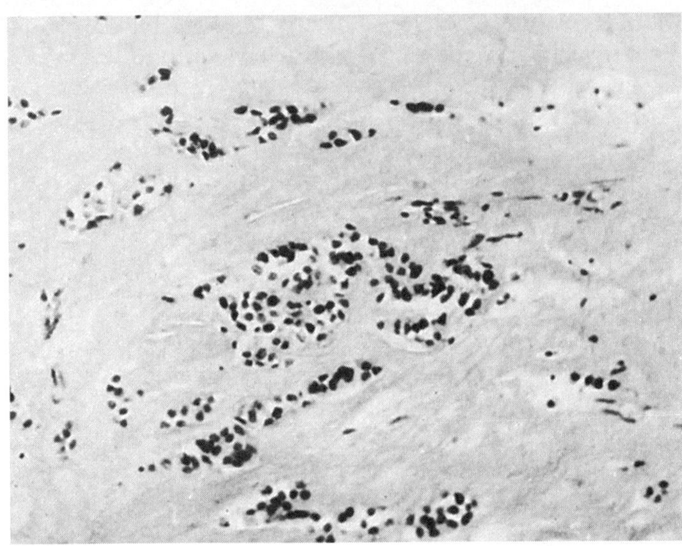

Fig. 24-2 Carcinoma of breast with extensive desmoplasia.

stimulation. However, as mentioned above, many epithelial cells are inhibited in cell culture by TGF-β, whereas their neoplastic counterparts are often resistant to the inhibitory effects of TGF-β. There is one example of escape from this regulatory control by loss of surface receptors for TGF-β; loss of TGF-β sensitivity correlates with a loss of receptors in a childhood tumor of retinal cells, retinoblastoma.[16] How other epithelial tumors escape regulation by TGF-β is not known, but it may involve the shutting off of a system that converts an inactive form of this growth factor to one that is active. The role or potential role of TGF-β in many phenomena illustrates how closely related seemingly different patterns of cell growth can be. Many apparently disparate phenomena may have a common molecular basis; undoubtedly, in the next few years other regulatory pathways will become better understood.

Atrophy

A diminution in the size of an organ is termed *atrophy*. This results from a reduction in cell size, cell number, or both. Thus, for example, through disuse, age, or loss of innervation, skeletal muscle fibers may lose bulk, secondary to a loss of positive trophic stimuli. Atrophy of the glandular elements of the breast and endometrial tissue after menopause represents a reduction in cell number, subsequent to loss of hormonal stimuli. Atrophy may also result from stimuli that actively cause regression. Programmed cell death as part of development may be viewed in this light, as discussed in Chapter 17.[17] Recently the gene for müllerian inhibiting substance (MIS) has been cloned.[18] The protein, secreted by the developing testis, causes involution of the müllerian duct, the embryonic origin of the uterus, fallopian tubes, and upper third of the vagina. The protein shows a partial amino acid identity with TGF-β, which, though stimulatory for fibroblastic cells, is inhibitory for many epithelial cells. Cachexia, or "wasting" (actually atrophy), which accompanies many chronic diseases, including cancer, is brought about in part by a protein known as *tumor necrosis factor (TNF)*, or *cachectin*.[19] Thus atrophy, like hyperplasia and hypertrophy, can be an active response to external stimuli as well as a response to loss of trophic factors.

Metaplasia

A change in cell type (usually resulting from a stimulus) is referred to as *metaplasia*. The most frequent example of metaplasia is among epithelial cells. Chronic airway irritation, including smoking, causes replacement of the normal pseudostratified columnar lining by squamous epithelium ("squamous metaplasia"). Metaplasia usually involves the loss or destruction of the normal cell population, and its replacement during "tissue repair" with another, usually derived from "reserve cells," or basal epithelial cells of an organ (such as bronchial epithelium). Metaplasia may be permanent without continued stimuli, or revert to the native cell if the stimulus is removed. Metaplasia is not necessarily a preneoplastic lesion, since the replacement cells are morphologically normal; however, in some instances it precedes neoplasia. For example, cigarette smoke–induced squamous metaplasia precedes carcinoma of the lung. It is likely that various stimuli result in different types of metaplasia. In cell culture it is possible to stimulate the conversion of one cell type into another. Several lines of mouse fibroblasts convert spontaneously to adipocytes, myocytes, or chondrocytes.[20] Agents that demethylate DNA (such as 5-azacytidine) and thus alter the regulation of gene expression greatly increase the percentage of converted cells.[20,21] Part of the process has been studied in detail and appears to be under the control of a gene known as *myo D*, the expression of which is sufficient to convert mouse fibroblasts to myoblasts.[22] Although this phenomenon has been viewed as a model for differentiation and development,[23] it is also reasonable to view it as a model for a metaplasia within a mesenchymal lineage, especially if metaplasia in vivo results from reserve cells that differentiate. At present, in vitro systems do not model all the complexities of in vivo change, but they provide a perspective for how the process might be studied.

Dysplasia

Morphologic atypia of cells (though generally less severe than malignant cells), with or without disorganized growth pattern, is dysplasia. Dysplastic cells are often *pleomorphic* (varying in size and shape) with hyperchromatic (darkly staining) nuclei and irregular chromatin distribution. The normal ratio of nuclear to cytoplasmic area and the number of mitoses may be increased. Dysplastic tissues often lack orderly maturation of their normal counterparts. Thus, in dysplastic squamous epithelium, mitoses are not confined to the basal cell layer, and progressive keratinization and nuclear dissolution are partially lost. Although, in theory, any disorganized, altered cells might be thought of as dysplastic, the term is usually confined to epithelial lesions. Dysplasia is often reversible, but it may also be a precancerous change, and distinguishing severe dysplasia from early malignant neoplasia or carcinoma in situ can be difficult (Fig. 24-3).

Although this distinction may be very important clinically, biologically one may view normal growth, dysplastic growth and neoplastic growth, as a continuum.

Anaplasia

The term *anaplasia* is used to describe malignant tumors that lack histologically identifiable features of a tissue of origin

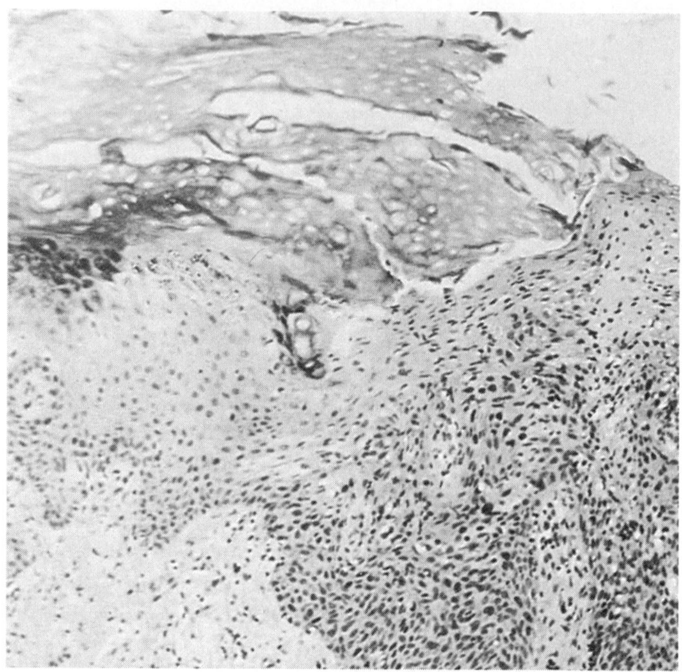

Fig. 24-3 Carcinoma arising in arsenical keratosis showing hyperkeratosis, dysplasia (atypical hyperplasia), and early carcinoma.

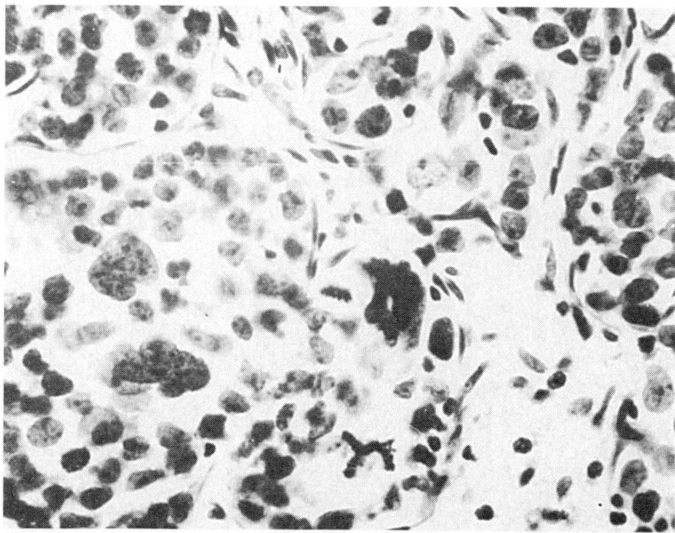

Fig. 24-4 Extremely anaplastic cancer showing abnormal mitoses, multinucleated tumor giant cells, and extensive pleomorphism.

(such as gland formation in epithelial cells or stainable fat in adipocytes). By definition, anaplastic tumors are dedifferentiated (Fig. 24-4); they are usually pleomorphic and usually exhibit rapid growth.

Hamartoma, or choristoma

Rarely, minor developmental anomalies may be confused with neoplasms. They fall into two classes: aberrant tissue foci (choristomas and ectopic foci) and hamartomas. The former probably have their origin in various developmental rests, which are the vestiges of cell migration and differentiation during embryogenesis. They are generally without significance, except that tumors may rarely arise from them (such as carcinomas in retrosternal thyroid tissue).

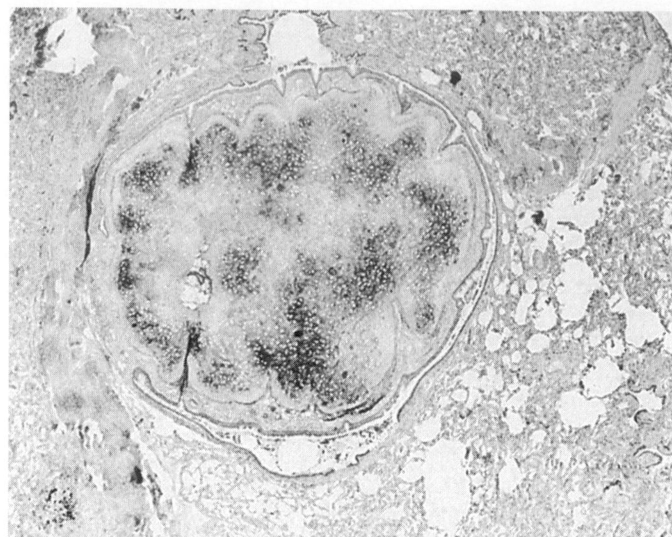

Fig. 24-5 Hamartoma of lung. Although overgrowth contains bronchial epithelium and mucous glands, its chief component is cartilage.

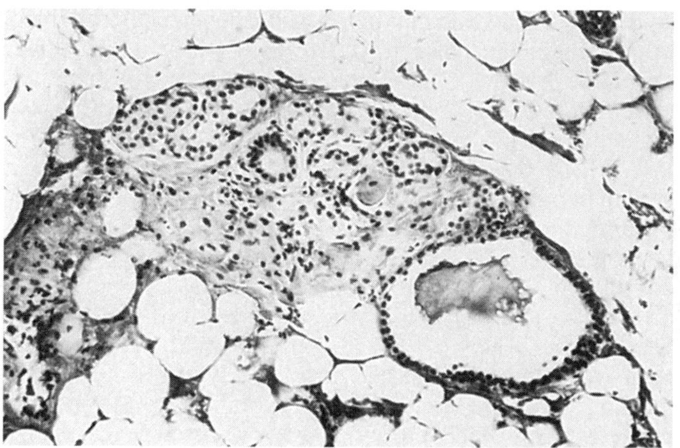

Fig. 24-6 Ectopic thyroid tissue in mediastinal fat.

Hamartomas occur in many organs and are composed of foci or nodules of tissues indigenous to these sites. In the lung, for example, it is not unusual to find discrete foci composed of mature cartilage and bronchial epithelium (Fig. 24-5), which represent a "pulmonary hamartoma."

The distinction between hamartomas and nonmalignant tumors (see nomenclature just below) is not always clear. For example, a focus of normal-appearing vascular tissue (thus a hamartoma) is referred to as an *angioma* (the designation for a benign tumor). A *choristoma* is similar to a hamartoma, except that the tissues of which it is composed are not normally present in the sites in which they are found; for example, benign chondromas of the skin may occur on the foot. The term *ectopic* is sometimes applied to normal-appearing tissue in an abnormal location. Thus, when a focus of apparently normal thyroid tissue is found in the mediastinal fat, it is referred to as ectopic thyroid tissue (Fig. 24-6); similarly adrenal gland tissue may be found in the urinary bladder.

Table 24-1 Nomenclature of tumors*

Cell or tissue of origin	Benign	Malignant
Tumors of epithelial origin		
Squamous cells	Squamous cell papilloma	Squamous cell carcinoma
Basal cells		Basal cell carcinoma
Glandular or ductal epithelium	Adenoma Papillary adenoma Cystadenoma	Adenocarcinoma Papillary adenocarcinoma Cystadenocarcinoma
Transitional cells	Transitional cell papilloma	Transitional cell carcinoma
Bile duct	Bile duct adenoma	Bile duct carcinoma (cholangiocarcinoma)
Islets of Langerhans	Islet cell adenoma	Islet cell carcinoma
Liver cells	Liver cell adenoma	Hepatocellular carcinoma (hepatoma)
Neuroectoderm	Melanocytic nevus	Malignant melanoma
Placental epithelium		Choriocarcinoma, hydatidiform mole
Renal epithelium	Renal tubular adenoma	Renal cell carcinoma (hypernephroma)
Respiratory tract		Bronchogenic carcinoma
Skin adnexal glands:		
Sweat glands	Syringoadenoma, sweat gland adenoma	Syringocarcinoma, sweat gland carcinoma
Sebaceous glands	Sebaceous gland adenoma	Sebaceous gland carcinoma
Germ cells (testis and ovary)		Seminoma (dysgerminoma) Embryonal carcinoma, yolk sac tumor
Tumors of mesenchymal origin		
Hematopoietic and lymphoid tissues		Leukemias Lymphomas Hodgkin's disease Multiple myeloma
Neural and retinal tissue		
Nerve sheath	Neurilemoma, neurofibroma	Malignant peripheral nerve sheath tumor
Nerve cells	Ganglioneuroma	Neuroblastoma
Retinal cells (cones)		Retinoblastoma
Connective tissue		
Fibrous tissue	Fibroma	Fibrosarcoma
Fat	Lipoma	Liposarcoma
Bone	Osteoma	Osteogenic sarcoma
Cartilage	Chondroma	Chondrosarcoma
Muscle		
Smooth muscle	Leiomyoma	Leiomyosarcoma
Striated muscle	Rhabdomyoma	Rhabdomyosarcoma
Endothelial and related tissues		
Blood vessels	Hemangioma	Angiosarcoma Kaposi's sarcoma
Lymph vessels	Lymphangioma	Lymphangiosarcoma
Mesothelium	Benign mesothelioma	Malignant mesothelioma
Meninges	Meningioma	Malignant meningioma
Uncertain origin		Ewing's tumor
Other origins		
Renal anlage		Wilms' tumor
Trophoblast		Choriocarcinoma, hydatidiform mole
Totipotential cells	Benign teratoma	Malignant teratoma

*No classification of tumors can be complete. Rather this list is intended to introduce a nomenclature scheme. As indicated in the text, the extant nomenclature is very mixed. More extensive classifications (with synonyms) may be found in the fascicles of the *Atlas of Tumor Pathology,* published by the Armed Forces Institute of Pathology, Washington, D.C., and in the *International Histologic Classification of Tumors,* published by the World Health Organization, Geneva.

TUMOR NOMENCLATURE

Tumor classification and nomenclature provide a convenient short way for communication among pathologists, clinicians, and researchers. Current usage is a hybrid of terms based on biologic behavior, function, histogenesis, embryogenesis, site of origin, and eponyms (Table 24-1).

Assessing the biologic behavior of tumors provides the single most important piece of information about them. Benign tumors are, in general, slow-growing, innocuous tumors (Table 24-2) that are usually of little consequence to the host unless they secrete bioactive molecules, undergo hemorrhage, or are anatomically placed to compromise vital organs (Fig. 24-7).

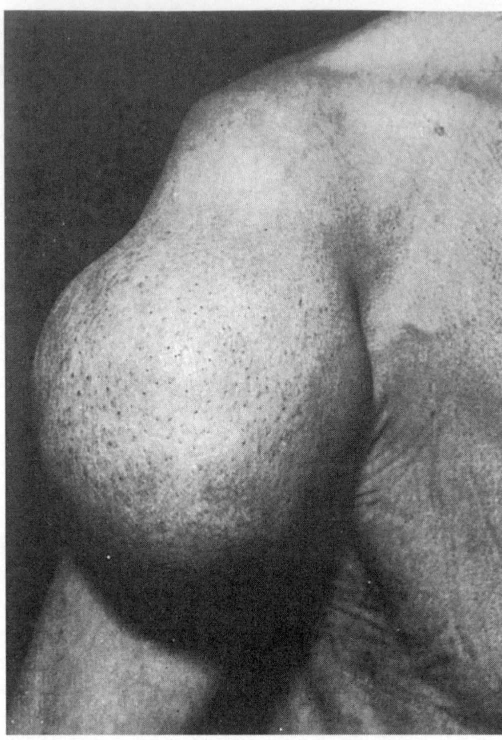

Fig. 24-7 Subcutaneous lipoma that had gradually increased in size over a period of 6 to 8 years in 70-year-old man. Notice stretching of skin as evidenced by widely separated pores.

Table 24-2 Some characteristics of typical benign and malignant tumors

	Benign	Malignant
Growth rate	Slow	Rapid
Mitoses	Few	Many
Nuclear chromatin	Normal	Increased
Differentiation	Good	Poor
Local growth	Expansive	Invasive
Encapsulation	Present	Absent
Destruction of tissue	Little	Much
Vessel invasion	None	Frequent
Metastases	None	Frequent
Effect on host	Often insignificant	Significant

For example, benign tumors of the beta cells of the islets of Langerhans (beta-cell tumors) can result in life-threatening hypoglycemia (Fig. 24-8), and ependymal tumors, which may obstruct the aqueduct of Sylvius, can result in hydrocephalus.

Malignant tumors have more rapid growth rates than benign tumors, invade and destroy adjacent tissue (Fig. 24-9), and metastasize to distant sites (Fig. 24-10).

A neoplasm ('new growth') may be benign or malignant. Epithelial tumors, which constitute a majority of both benign and malignant lesions, are derived from any of the three germ layers (see Table 24-1). Malignant tumors of epithelial or organ parenchymal derivation are referred to as *carcinomas*. If the cells are of glandular or ductular origin, they are referred to as *adenocarcinomas* (see Fig. 24-9). Alternatively, those of squamous cell origin, are referred to as *squamous cell* or *epidermoid* carcinomas (Fig. 24-11).

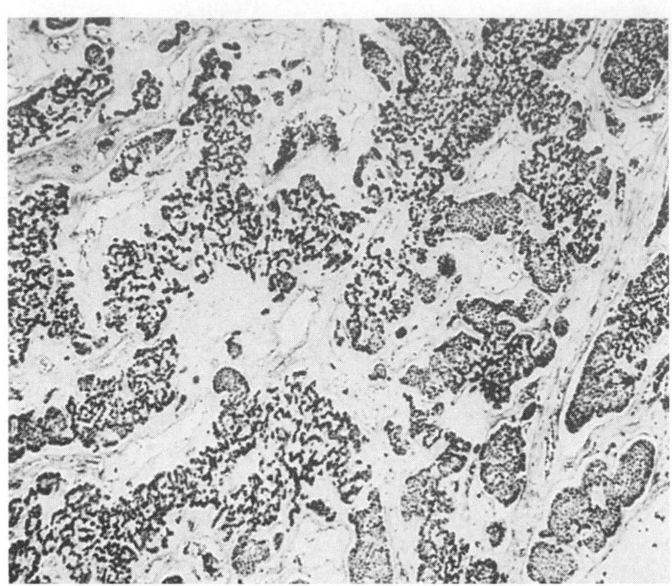

Fig. 24-8 Islet cell tumor. Solid clusters and ribbonlike growth are reminiscent of normal islets of Langerhans.

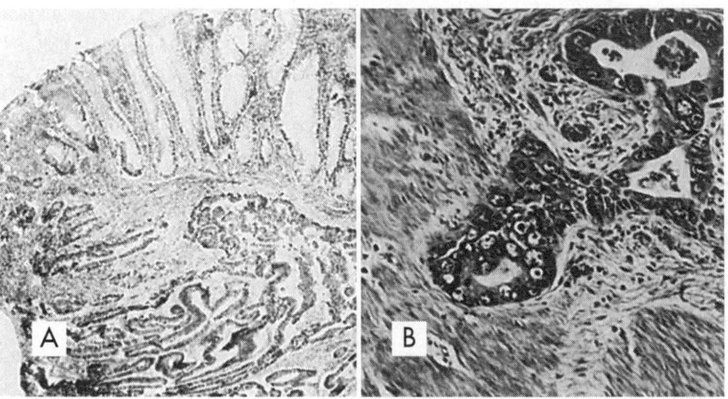

Fig. 24-9 A, Invasion of submucosa and muscularis by well-differentiated adenocarcinoma of colon. Notice glandular pattern typical of an adenocarcinoma. Some normal mucosa remains. **B,** Colonic adenocarcinoma invading muscularis.

The nomenclature for benign epithelial lesions is more varied, often causing confusion (see Table 24-1). Usually, the suffix *-oma* denotes a benign neoplasm. Thus a benign tumor of glandular epithelium is usually referred to as an *adenoma* (Fig. 24-12), whereas a benign tumor of squamous or transitional cell epithelium with a papillary conformation is referred to as a *papilloma*.

The nomenclature of tumors derived from specific types of epithelia is more direct, such as renal cell carcinoma and sweat gland carcinoma. Two important exceptions, *melanoma* and *hepatoma*, are malignant tumors of melanocytes and hepatocytes respectively and should be designated as *malignant melanoma* and *hepatocellular carcinoma*.

Malignant tumors of mesenchymal origin are *sarcomas*, whereas their benign counterparts simply bear the suffix *-oma*. A malignant tumor of fat cells, for example, is termed a *liposarcoma*, whereas the benign counterpart is *lipoma* (Fig. 24-13).

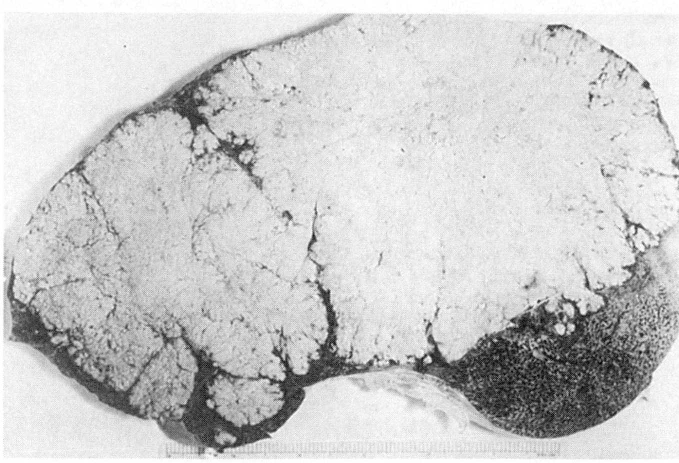

Fig. 24-10 Section of liver showing almost complete replacement of parenchyma by metastatic carcinoma. Primary tumor was in the colon.

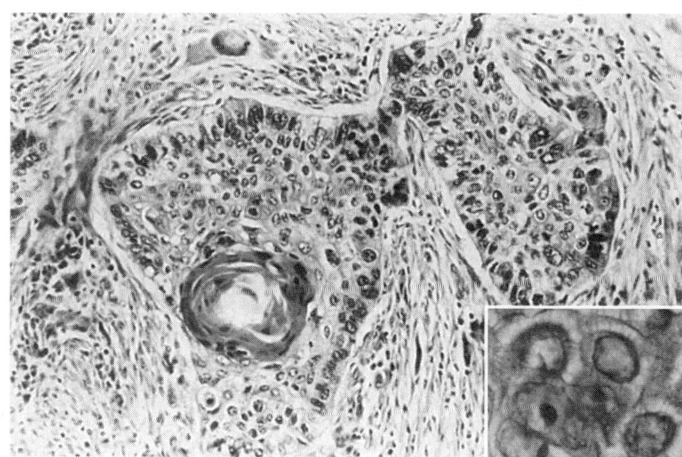

Fig. 24-11 Well-differentiated squamous cell carcinoma showing irregular margins, keratin pearls, and intercellular bridges (Courtesy Dr. Ibrahim Ramzy, Houston, Texas.)

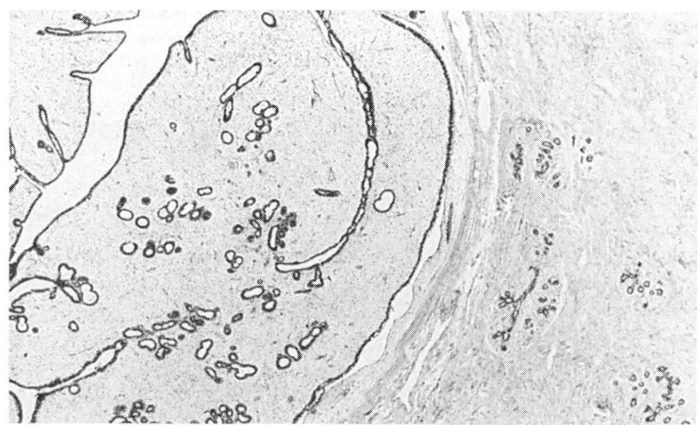

Fig. 24-12 Portion of adenofibroma of breast. Breast tissue at right is normal except for compression by tumor.

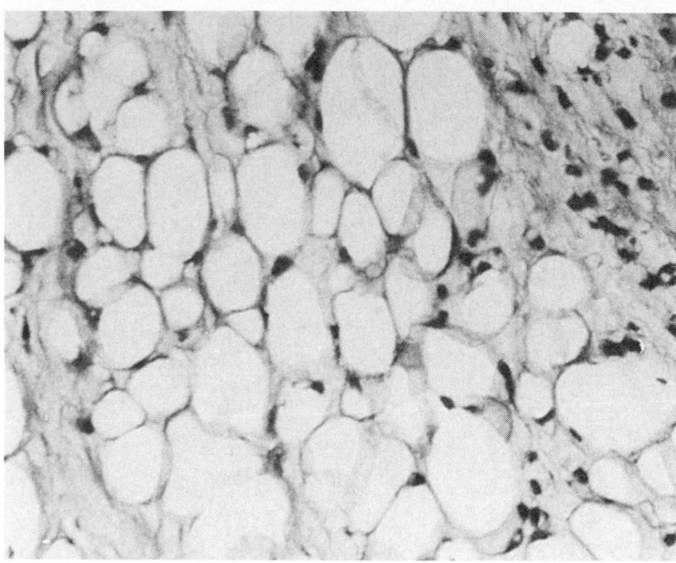

Fig. 24-13 Liposarcoma showing well-differentiated lipid-containing cells and more primitive cells. (Courtesy Dr. Ibrahim Ramzy, Houston, Tex.)

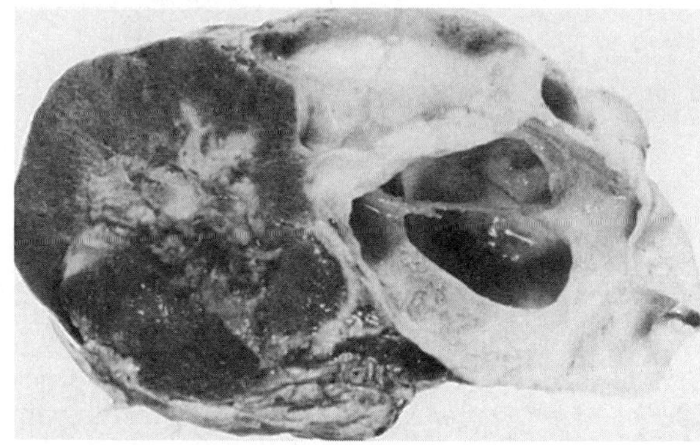

Fig. 24-14 Cystic teratoma of ovary. This benign neoplasm shows both solid and cystic foci. Microscopically, the tumor was composed of various types of tissue.

These so-called rules sometimes break down. A malignant tumor of mesothelium, the cells lining the pleural, pericardial, and peritoneal surfaces, is commonly referred to as a *mesothelioma*, though its precise designation should be *malignant mesothelioma*, to distinguish it from a benign counterpart (benign fibrous mesothelioma). Malignant tumors of the hematopoietic system are also unique. All leukemias are malignant and named according to their course (acute versus chronic) and the cell of origin, granulocytic (myeloid) or lymphocytic (discussed in Chapter 41). A remarkable number of classification schemes are used to describe the malignant lymphomas (Chapter 42).

Tumors that differentiate along all three germ layers (endoderm, ectoderm, and mesoderm) are designated *teratomas* and are classified as *mature* or *immature* (Figs. 24-14 and 24-15).

This basic scheme has several variations. A tumor of pancreatic β-cells, referred to previously as a *β-cell tumor*, can also be called an *insulinoma*, reflecting its function, and an *islet cell adenoma*, in reference to its anatomic origin (see

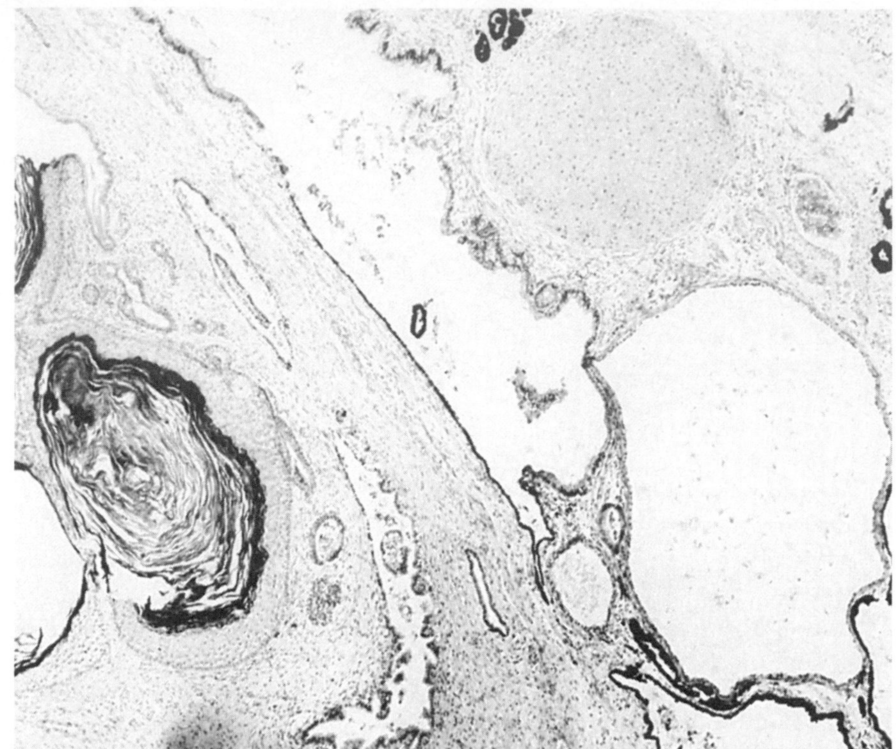

Fig. 24-15 Teratoma of testis. In addition to several types of glandular epithelium centrally, a nodule of cartilage is present in upper right and masses of keratinizing squamous epithelium at left.

Fig. 24-8). Another example of omission of the cell of origin in favor of the anatomic site of origin is the term *bronchogenic carcinoma*, encompassing several different histologic types that arise in the lung. Often, however, designations are prefaced and convey more complete information, as in *papillary adenocarcinoma*, which defines the growth pattern of the tumor, or *mucinous cystadenoma*, which provides explicit information about differentiation. The suffix *-blastoma* is used to designate tumors of embryonic origin. The terms medulloblastoma (brain), hepatoblastoma (liver), nephroblastoma (kidney), retinoblastoma (retina), and neuroblastoma (adrenal) are in common use. Time-honored eponyms remain. Some, like Hodgkin's disease, a malignant neoplasm possibly derived from dendritic reticulum cells, and Ewing's sarcoma, a malignant neoplasm of uncertain origin, have no semantic equivalent. Others, like Wilms' tumor, are eponyms for more precise designations (nephroblastoma). Other eponyms are vestiges from another era; a variant of renal cell carcinoma (*hypernephroma*) is occasionally referred to as a *Grawitz tumor*, and a benign tumor of the salivary gland with both epithelial and lymphoid elements (papillary cystadenoma lymphomatosum or adenolymphoma) is often designated a *Warthin tumor*.

CHARACTERISTICS OF NEOPLASTIC CELLS

In normal adults, some cells do not replicate (such as neurons, chondrocytes), others replicate only very slowly, at a rate sufficient to replace lost cells (such as hepatocytes, renal tubular cells), whereas others replicate more or less continuously to replace continuous cell loss (such as intestinal epithelial cells, hematopoietic cells). The proliferation and maturation of normal cells is controlled and results only in a net replacement of cells. In contrast, neoplastic cells escape regulation and accumulate to form a mass. Traditional distinctions between benign and malignant patterns of cell growth are presented in Table 24-2.

Growth rate and differentiation

In general, benign tumors tend to be slow growing and well differentiated, often resembling their tissue of origin to a remarkable degree. Thus a lipoma on microscopic examination may be composed of mature adipocytes, which are hardly distinguishable from normal fat cells. The only clue that the tissue is neoplastic may be that the mass has slowly increased in size over many years (see Fig. 24-7). In contrast, malignant tumors grow much more rapidly and may bear only slight resemblance to the parent tissue; hence an adenocarcinoma may grow rapidly, and the only clue to its origin may be the identification of occasional cells that stain positively for mucin.

The accumulation of tumor mass is dependent on several factors, including transit time through the cell cycle, the fraction of cells that remain in the cycle to proliferate rather than differentiate, and "spontaneous," intermittent growth arrest. Cell-cycle time is probably only a minor factor in tumor growth; normal cells actually traverse the cell cycle faster than some tumor cells do.[24] More important is the retention of cells in the cell cycle. Normally in the small intestine, for example, the division of every crypt cell is followed by a partition in which one daughter cell remains in the proliferating compartment and the other differentiates and migrates toward the luminal surface. In neoplasia this partition is altered, and too many cells remain in the proliferating compartment.

It is worth noting that, within tumors, cells often differentiate normally into mature postmitotic cells; a good example is the maturation seen in squamous and basal cell carcinomas of the skin (see Fig. 24-11). Occasionally neuroblastomas have been reported to differentiate into ganglioneuromas. A current goal of experimental cancer therapy is to devise ways to induce malignant cells to differentiate and leave from the cell cycle. Although there is little experimental work on intermittent, variable growth rates in tumors, clinical observations indicate that this phenomenon may not be infrequent. For example, recurrence may occur years after removal of a primary malignant melanoma. The erratic clinical course of many women with breast cancers may be another example of intermittent growth. Extrinsic factors (such as changes in serum concentration of hormones and growth factors) and intrinsic factors (such as changes in tumor cell-surface receptors) are probably involved. Thus, linear correlations between cell-doubling times and tumor mass are an idealized model of tumor growth, if one does not consider intermittent variations in tumor growth rate, "progression" (the acquisition of more aggressive characteristics), or necrosis.

Cytomorphology

As tumor cells acquire increased autonomy and aggressiveness, they may manifest bizarre, atypical features in either histologic tissue section, or cytologic preparations, discussed in detail in Chapter 4. Neoplastic cells that vary greatly in size and shape are said to be "pleomorphic" (Fig. 24-4). Nuclei of malignant cells may be large and deeply basophilic with hematoxylin-based stains. Such nuclear hyperchromicity is reflective of increased DNA content and alterations in chromatin structure.

Many malignant tumors have abnormalities of karyotype and DNA content. Although these changes are at best characterized in leukemias and lymphomas (see Chapter 42),[25] many examples are known in solid tumors and reflect molecular genetic abnormalities associated with malignancy (Tables 24-4 and 24-5). Mitotic figures are the morphologic expression of the increased rate of cell proliferation. The mitotic rate, usually expressed as the number of mitoses per 10 high-power fields (HPF), is important in the diagnosis of many malignancies, for example, the distinction between benign and malignant smooth muscle tumors of the uterus (see Chapter 68). One usually determines mitotic rate by counting the number of mitoses in 50 high-power fields of highly cellular areas and then dividing by 5. As an isolated feature, mitotic rate is not diagnostic of malignancy. Many benign, tissue-reparative reactions are mitotically active. More useful are abnormal mitoses, such as tripolar or quadrapolar (Fig. 24-16).

Nuclear and cell contours may vary sharply from the parental cell type, and the cytoplasm often becomes scant and somewhat hyperchromatic, reflective of increased ribosomal RNA and synthetic activity. Giant cells may develop. All these changes must be judged with reference to the cells of origin, since there is considerable variation among neoplasms. Pleomorphism is not an absolute criterion of malignancy.

Angiogenesis and stromal support

For tumors, whether benign or malignant, to expand beyond a small mass, vascularization and often the development of stromal support are necessary. Tumor cells secrete growth factors like TGF-β , which stimulate capillary ingrowth and fibroblastic growth.[12-15,26,27] These nonneoplastic tissue elements are present in most tumors but are particularly prominent in carcinomas. A tumor with intense fibroblastic response is said to be *desmoplastic* (Fig. 24-2). The development of vascular and stromal support is regulated by neoplastic cells, a phenomenon that may be more prevalent than suspected, and one that might offer a novel approach to therapy.

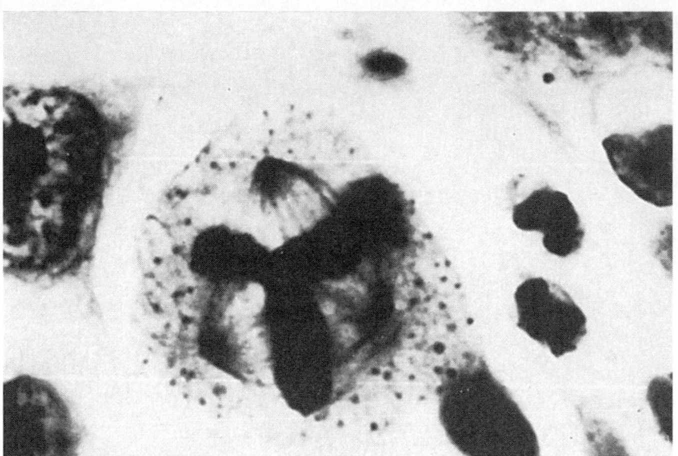

Fig. 24-16 Abnormal tripolar mitosis occurring in malignant melanoma. (Phosphotungstic acid–hematoxylin.)

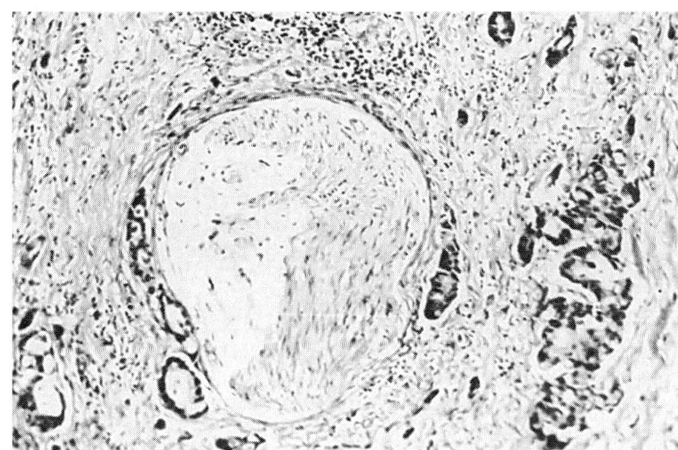

Fig. 24-17 Adenocarcinoma of lung with perineural invasion. Part of nerve shows degeneration.

Local growth

When benign tumors expand, they compress surrounding tissue (Fig. 24-12) and are often "encapsulated" (that is, surrounded by a rim of fibrous tissue). Local growth of malignant tumors is characterized by invasion of the surrounding tissue, often with extensive tissue destruction. Malignant tumors are unencapsulated, but, when malignant foci arise in benign tumors, capsular invasion may be seen. This invasiveness is well illustrated by thyroid carcinoma. Invasion and metastasis (spread to distant sites) are important characteristics to distinguish malignant from benign tumors (Figs. 24-9, 24-10, 24-17, and 24-18). However, similar phenomena are seen in some benign processes, such as the "invasion" that accompanies fibromatoses and the "metastasis" of endometriosis.

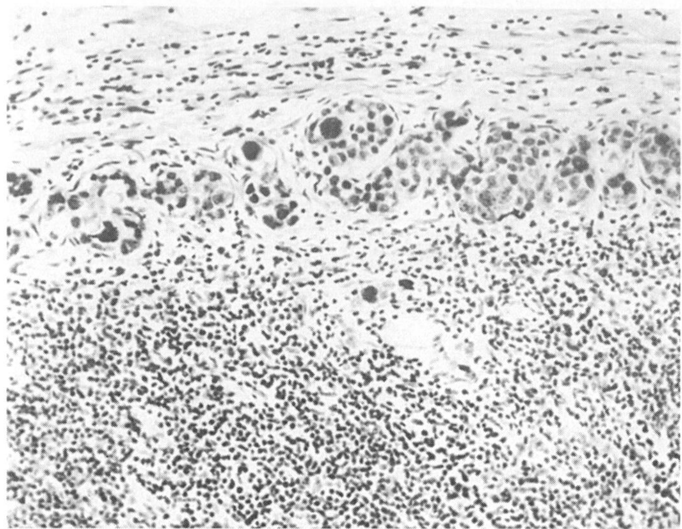

Fig. 24-18 Metastatic carcinoma in the peripheral sinus of inguinal lymph node. The tumor lies just beneath the capsule and is beginning to invade the cortex.

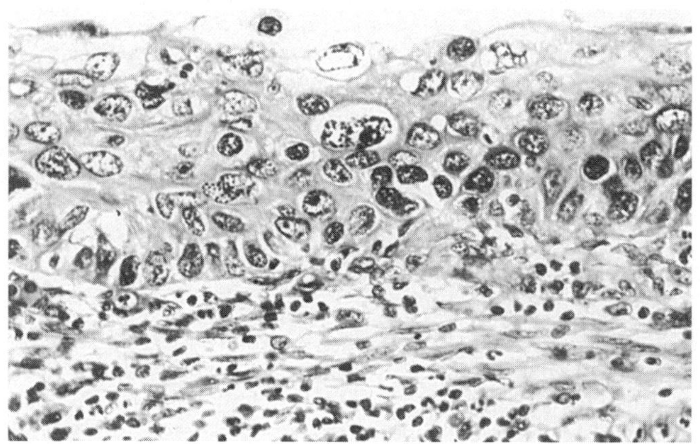

Fig. 24-19 Carcinoma in situ of the cervix. Notice the extreme atypicality of cells near the surface and that one cell has desquamated. From such desquamated cells, a cytologic diagnosis of cancer can be made.

Epithelial cells usually rest on a basement membrane. In carcinomas local invasion involves penetration of the basement membrane, followed by infiltration of deeper tissues. Carcinomas can acquire the morphologic characteristics of malignant tumors without showing invasion through the basement membrane. This lesion is referred to as *carcinoma in situ*, a process that is well described in the uterine cervix (Fig. 24-19).

Local invasion

Local invasion is a complicated balance between tissue destruction and the synthesis of vascular and stromal support. The ability of tumor cells to synthesize and secrete extracellular proteases is clearly a prerequisite for invasion.[28-30] Tumor cells secrete proteases, including transin (stromolysin) and collagenases. These can attack components of basement membranes and extracellular matrix (laminin, fibronectin, and collagen).[29,31-33] Other proteases, like fibrinolysin, also participate in invasion. These aid in destruction of extracellular matrix and probably destroy normal cells as well. As mentioned previously, TGF-β, which is secreted by many tumor cells (including epithelial tumors), stimulates fibroblastic growth and migration into an area but inhibits epithelial growth. Factors like TGF-β and müllerian inhibiting substance might promote the local spread of tumors by inhibiting the growth of normal cells and stimulating the development of stromal support. Presumably, epithelial tumors that secrete TGF-β are not inhibited by it. Although loss of TGF-β receptors has been implicated in one example of escape from TGF-β inhibition,[16] in most cases the mechanism of escape remains unknown. Frequently inflammation accompanies invasion. Since inflammatory cells secrete proteases as well as growth factors, it is likely that the contribution of inflammatory cells to both invasion and metastasis is substantial.

Yet invasiveness also involves recognition of extracellular matrices, and perhaps other cell types, by tumor cells; tissue destruction may provide access to new areas, but recognition of substratum and binding are necessary for most tumors to establish growth. Tumor cells attach more readily to laminin[34] than nontumor cells do, and this property (presumably related to increased numbers of laminin receptors or increased affinity of existing receptors) is probably in part responsible for increased tumor migration.[34,35] Similarly, fibronectin receptors may play a role in the migration of malignant cells.[36] TGF-β stimulates fibronectin synthesis and cell-adhesion-protein receptors (integrins), which may be involved in cell migration and the ability to grow in semisolid medium (a prominent in vitro property of tumor cells).[37] Also, the cytoskeleton of tumor cells differs greatly from that of their normal counterparts, and communication between cytoskeleton and extracellular matrix occurs at points of cell adherence.[37] Thus, local invasion requires a balance between the degradation of the local environment and preservation (or resynthesis) of a crucial molecular substratum. This balance appears to be achieved by a transmembrane feedback system involving the cytoskeleton, which itself is responsible for cell motility.

Integrins

As may be gathered from the preceding discussion, the cell surface plays a key role in invasion. It is largely through a series of integrin molecules that cell-cell adhesion, cell–basement membrane adhesion and cell–extracellular matrix adhesion are achieved.[38] Table 24-3 offers a simplified version of integrin structure and function. Integrins are heterodimers in which different members of the α and β subunit families can combine to form molecules with diverse interactions. Although extensive experimental detail is lacking, it seems that local invasion is accompanied by changes in cell-cell recognition molecules, which result in the "loosening of ties" to some cells and the identification and selection of others. Similarly, the binding to and recognition of new extracellular molecules but failure to recognize others must be crucial aspects of invasion. It is important to reemphasize that these binding reactions signal intracellular biochemical changes, which result in altered (invasive) cellular behavior.[39]

The degree to which all the aforementioned factors affect the behavior of individual tumors is extremely variable. Thus, for example, the need for some stromal support for tumor cells is more apparent in papillary carcinoma of the thyroid than in giant cell carcinoma of the thyroid, which grows with little apparent organization and with significant tissue destruction.

Table 24-3 Simplified classification of integrins based on binding characteristics

Subunit	Ligands
I. Integrins that function as cell-cell adhesion molecules	
α_L/β_2 (LFA-1)	ICAM-1
α_M/β_2 (MAC-1)	ICAM-1, C3bi, endotoxin
α_x/β_2 (gp150,95)	?
α_4/β_1	VCAM-1
II. Integrins that bind primarily to basement membrane proteins	
α_1/β_1	Laminin/collagen
α_2/β_1	Collagen/laminin
α_3/β_1	Laminin/collagen/fibronectin
α_6/β_1	Laminin
α_6/β_4	Laminin
III. Integrins that bind primarily to matrix proteins of inflammation, wound healing, and development	
α_4/β_1	Fibronectin (CSII site)
α_5/β_1	Fibronectin (RGD site)
α_v/β_1	Fibronectin
α_v/β_3	Vitronectin, fibrinogen thrombospondin, von Willebrand's factor
α_v/β_5	Vitronectin

From Albelda SM: *Lab Invest* 68:4, 1993.

CSII, Chondroitin sulfate II; *gp,* glycoprotein; *ICAM,* intercellular adhesion molecule; *LFA,* lymphocyte function–associated antigen; *MAC,* mucosal addressin cell adhesion molecule; *RGD,* arginine-glycine-asparagine; *VCAM,* vascular cell adhesion molecule.

Invasion can be very extensive, as evident in basal cell carcinomas of the skin and malignant tumors of the central nervous system, which do not metastasize but spread without vascular or lymphatic entry.

Regional extension

Tumors may breach the surface of an organ, particularly in colon and ovarian carcinomas, as well as in bronchogenic carcinomas. The result is tumor cell seeding of the serosal surface of the peritoneal cavity and its organs, or the pleural surfaces. If seeded to a hospitable site, the tumor cells may form nodules. In carcinomas of the gastrointestinal tract, for example, it is extremely rare to find colonial spread distal to a primary tumor within the lumen, even though the sloughing of viable tumor cells must be frequent. The movement of gastrointestinal contents, their destructive character, and the resistance of epithelium to intrusion prevent such spreading.

Metastasis

The spread of malignant tumors to distant sites (metastasis) occurs through the lymphatics or the bloodstream after the tumor acquires additional properties that are related to but somewhat independent of invasiveness. These include the ability to gain access to the vessel, to survive in the vasculature, and to exit and grow in a foreign organ. Usually carcinomas metastasize through lymphatic channels. Careful sampling of surgical pathologic specimens often reveals lymphatic invasion by carcinomas. This finding is prognostically significant in common tumors, such as those in the colon and breast. In some organs, such as the prostate and pancreas, the perineural space and the lymphatics are frequently involved. Fig. 24-17 shows this process in an adenocarcinoma of the lung. A consequence of lymphatic invasion is metastasis to regional lymph nodes and then to more distant sites. Sarcomas usually metastasize through venous and capillary channels, rarely affecting regional lymph nodes. Many important exceptions to these generalizations have been observed; renal cell carcinomas and hepatocellular carcinomas commonly invade the renal and hepatic veins respectively. Epithelioid sarcoma and synovial sarcoma frequently metastasize to lymph nodes. Careful inspection of routine surgical pathologic material may show vascular spread of carcinomas (Fig. 24-20).

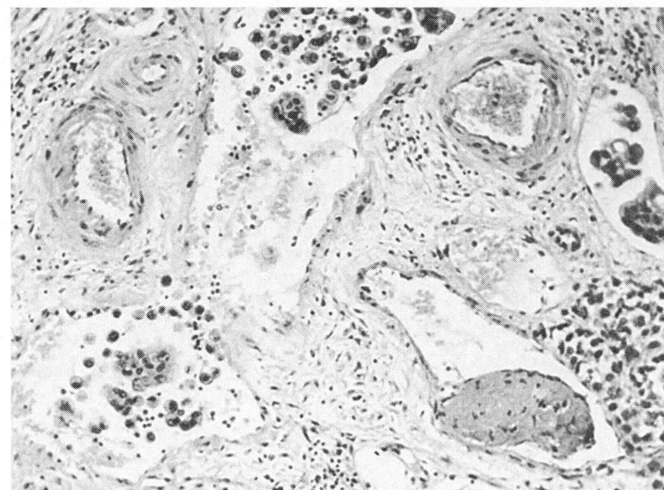

Fig. 24-20 Extensive blood vessel invasion by carcinoma of pancreas. Notice thrombus in one small vein (arrow).

The microvasculature of tumors is often more accessible to cancer cells than those vessels are in normal tissues.[40] Such observations indicate that many of our preconceived notions about invasion and metastasis based on normal tissues may not be directly applicable to tumor biology.

The acquisition of metastatic potential and the distribution of metastases have been the subject of many studies. Regardless of whether the initial entry is by the lymphatic or the venous system, many tumors gain access to larger veins and then to the microvasculature of the venous system in different organs. Particular types of tumors often show strong predilection for metastatic sites. Breast and bronchogenic carcinomas, for example, metastasize disproportionately frequently to the central nervous system and adrenal glands, whereas metastasis of carcinomas to the spleen is not common. An interaction between distant microvasculature and arriving tumor cells appears to be a critical factor in metastasis formation.[40] The inflammation resulting from damage caused by the lodging of foreign cells in the microvasculature leads to the release of proteases and growth factors, which enhance access to foreign tissues. A common experimental assay for metastatic potential involves analysis of colonization at distant sites. Tumor cells (carcinomas or sarcomas) are injected into the tail vein of a nude or syngeneic mouse, and the ability of cells to colonize tissues is scored several weeks or months later.[28] Although the assay only partially mimics the metastatic process, the assay represents a reasonable way to assess the metastatic potential of cells. Some aspects of organ specificity have been analyzed with this assay. If a murine "melanoma" cell line is injected into the tail vein, colonies are observed in many organs. If a colony is recovered from a given organ (such as lung or brain) and the cells are reinjected, the proportion of lung or brain colonies is much higher in the second set of mice.[28,41] Although the biochemical basis of this phenomenon is not yet known, recognition and specific binding of basement membrane and fibronectin (in the extracellular matrix), presumably by specific integrin molecules, appear to be critical to invasion and colony establishment in the lung, since these phenomena can be blocked by either antibodies to cellular laminin receptors or peptides, which compete with laminin and fibronectin for receptor binding.[34,35,42] There is some evidence that an "active" form of the *ras* oncogene predisposes to metastasis,[43,44] but it has been difficult to control these studies for other factors, like growth rate and local invasiveness.

Progression

The acquisition of increasingly aggressive characteristics by premalignant or malignant tumors is termed "progression." The changes manifest themselves most frequently by changes in morphology (from well-differentiated tumor cells that resemble normal cells to the more poorly-differentiated ones) or growth rate (from slower to faster).

The question whether benign tumors progress to malignant tumors often arises. Experimental evidence indicates that malignant tumors may arise from benign tumors but that malignant tumors sometimes appear to develop in the absence of an identifiable benign lesion (that is, de novo). For example, when mouse skin is treated with carcinogens, squamous cell carcinomas develop, both in benign papillomas (which themselves may regress fully) and in areas of skin that lack papillomas. In some human cancers (such as small cell undifferentiated carcinoma of the lung), benign precursors cannot be identified. Many benign lesions (such as lipomas, leiomyomas of the uterus and dermal nevi) are only rarely precursors for malignant lesions, whereas others, like tubular and villous adenomas of the colon, often precede adenocarcinomas. Thus, some benign tumors are clearly precursors for malignant tumors. Whether they are obligatory precursors cannot be determined with certainty; it is always possible to argue that the original benign lesion was very small or was destroyed by its malignant progeny.

ETIOLOGY OF NEOPLASIA

Molecular basis

Experimental and epidemiologic observations, beginning with Sir Percival Pott in 1775, have led to the suggestion that neoplasia is usually associated with somatic mutations induced by physical and chemical damage to DNA.[45] These observations have included (1) the correlation of specific chromosomal alterations with particular types of cancer,[25] (2) the transfer of the neoplastic phenotype between organisms by means of oncogenic viruses,[46] (3) the recognition that most chemical and physical carcinogens are also potent mutagens,[47] and (4) the association of increased cancer incidence with occupational exposure to a wide variety of chemical and physical agents, including high-energy electromagnetic energy (gamma irradiation and x-rays), radium in watch painters, radon-related products in miners, and benzene or vinyl chloride in chemical workers.[48] Until recently, the basis for these observations remained obscure. Investigators could measure only gross changes in total DNA or changes in chromosomal bands, and analysis of specific mutations affecting individual genes was technologically impossible. However, with rapid advances in molecular biology, it is now possible to isolate and characterize individual genes from as little as a single tumor cell and to identify mutations at the level of a single nucleotide.

With these tools firmly in hand, investigators have identified two classes of cancer genes: oncogenes[49] and tumor-suppressor genes.[50] Although our understanding of the role played by cancer genes and their products in the development and progression of human tumors is far from complete, general mechanisms have been recognized.[50] Both classes of cancer genes encode proteins that regulate transduction of growth and differentiation signals within a cell and between cells. In general, oncogenes encode positive regulators of cell proliferation, such as growth factors and growth factor receptors, which tend to activate intracellular growth pathways (Table 24-4). In contrast, tumor-suppressor genes whose actions are less understood at present encode negative regulators of growth (Table 24-5). The pathways regulating cell growth and differentiation are quite complex, and a surprisingly large number of different genes cause neoplastic transformation as a direct result of mutations or deletions.

Viral oncogenes

The first oncogenic virus to be described, the Rous sarcoma virus, was identified in 1911 as a filterable agent capable of transferring sarcomas among chickens.[51] Peyton Rous, an experimental pathologist at the Rockefeller Institute, won the 1968 Nobel Prize for these efforts, which led to speculation that many if not all human tumors might result from infection with oncogenic viruses. By preparing soluble extracts from each of the spontaneously occurring chicken sarcomas he encountered, Rous demonstrated that a cell-free filtrate from one of these extracts could induce similar sarcomas when injected into healthy chickens. Subsequent analysis revealed Rous sarcoma virus as an RNA-containing retrovirus capable of stably integrating its genome into that of its host. Many different oncogenic retroviruses were subsequently discovered in a variety of species, and each of these viruses was observed to induce a characteristic type of tumor (such as fibrosarcomas, myeloblastomas, osteosarcomas[52]). These observations also indicated that oncogenic retroviruses carry one or more "transforming" genes, or oncogenes, capable of inducing the neoplastic phenotype in stably infected host cells. However, identification of the transforming components of these viruses, as well as their mechanisms of action, awaited further advances in genetics and molecular biology.

In addition, several classes of DNA viruses including papovaviruses, adenoviruses, and herpesviruses can induce neoplastic transformation in vitro and to a lesser degree in vivo. Both DNA and RNA oncogenic viruses encode gene products that either mimic or alter the function of cellular proteins responsible for regulation of pathways related to cell growth and development.

Fittingly, the first viral transforming gene to be isolated and characterized was the *src* gene of Rous sarcoma virus, in 1976.[53] Since that time, more than 100 different viral oncogenes have been identified, some of which are listed in Table 24-4.

Table 24-4 Representative oncogenes

Gene	Associated cancer types	Putative cellular location	Mechanism of action	Origin	Chromosomal location
erbB2/neu (HER-2)	Amplified in some breast and ovarian cancers	Cell membrane	Cell surface receptor	Rat neuroglioblastoma	17qq11-12
fgr				Feline sarcoma retrovirus	1p1p36
L-*myc*	Lung carcinomas	Nucleus	Nuclear regulatory protein	Human lung carcinoma	1p32
N-*myc*	Amplified in more aggressive neuroblastomas	Nucleus	Nuclear regulatory protein	Human neuroblastoma	2p23-24
abl	Chronic myelogenous leukemia	Cytoplasm		Murine leukemia retrovirus	9p34
bcl1	B-cell lymphomas			Human B-cell tumor	11q13
bcl2	B-cell lymphomas	Mitochondria	Mitochondrial protein	Human B-cell tumor	18q21
c-*myc*	Burkitt's lymphoma, other carcinomas	Nucleus	Nuclear regulatory protein	Avian leukemia retrovirus	8q24
erbA		Nucleus	Thyroid hormone receptor	Avian erythroblastosis retrovirus	17q11-12
erbB1		Cell membrane	Epidermal growth factor receptor	Avian erythroblastosis retrovirus	7p11-12
ets				Avian leukemia retrovirus	21q22
fes				Feline sarcoma retrovirus	15q25-26
2fms		Cell membrane	Granulocyte and Macrophage–colony stimulating factor receptor	Feline sarcoma retrovirus	5q34
fos		Nucleus	Transcription factor	Murine sarcoma retrovirus	
H-*ras*	Pancreatic and other carcinomas	Inner cytoplasmic membrane	GTPase involved in signal transduction from surface receptors to nucleus	Rat sarcoma virus	6q16-22
int2				Mouse mammary tumor	11q13
jun		Nucleus	Transcription factor	Avian sarcoma retrovirus	
K-*ras*	Lung, colon, and other carcinomas	Inner cytoplasmic membrane	GTPase involved in signal transduction from surface receptors to nucleus	Murine sarcoma virus	6p11-12
met				Human osteosarcoma	7q22
mos				Murine sarcoma retrovirus	8q11-22
myb		Nucleus	Nuclear regulatory protein	Avian myeloblastosis retrovirus	6q22-24
pim	Mouse T-cell lymphomas			Mouse T-cell lymphoma	6p21-22
raf		Cytoplasm	Kinase involved in signal transduction from surface receptors to nucleus	Mouse sarcoma cell line	3p25
sis		Secreted protein	Closely related to platelet derived growth factor	Monkey sarcoma retrovirus	22q13
ski				Avian sarcoma retrovirus	1q22-24
src		Cytoplasm and inner surface of membrane	Tyrosine kinase involved in signal transduction from surface receptors to nucleus	Avian sarcoma retrovirus	20q13
yes		Cytoplasm and inner surface of membrane	Tyrosine kinase involved in signal transduction from surface receptors to nucleus	Avian sarcoma retrovirus	18q21
ret	Multiple endocrine neoplasia types 2A, 2B Familial medullary thyroid carcinoma	Transmembrane	Receptor and tyrosine kinase		10q11.2

Table 24-5 Tumor-suppressor genes

Gene	Associated cancer types	Putative cellular location	Mechanism of action	Hereditary syndromes	Chromosomal location
APC	Colon cancer	Cytoplasm	Unknown	Familial adenomatous polyposis	5q21
DCC	Colon cancer	Membrane	Cell adhesion	Unknown	18q21
NF1	Neurofibroma	Cytoplasm	GTPase activator	Neurofibromatosis type 1	17q11
NF2	Meningioma, schwannoma	Membrane, inner surface	Cytoskeleton-membrane link	Neurofibromatosis type 2	22q
p53	Colon, lung, breast cancer plus others	Nucleus	Transcription factor	Li-Fraumeni syndrome	17p13
Rb	Retinoblastoma	Nucleus	Transcription factor	Hereditary retinoblastoma	13q14
ret	Thyroid cancer pheochromocytoma	Membrane	Receptor tyrosine kinase	Multiple endocrine neoplasia type 2	10q11.2
VHL	Renal cancer	Membrane	Unknown	von Hippel-Lindau syndrome	3p25
WT1	Nephroblastoma	Nucleus	Transcription factor	Wilms' tumor	11p13

Cellular oncogenes as homologs of viral oncogenes

Although most of the viral oncogenes exhibit little structural homology with one another, each of the retrovirus-derived oncogenes (v-*onc* gene) is closely related to a homologous cellular gene (c-*onc* gene) present within the DNA of most eukaryotic organisms. These cellular homologs are referred to as *protooncogenes* or *cellular oncogenes*. The striking similarity between corresponding v-*onc* and c-*onc* genes strongly indicates that viral oncogenes may have been derived from cellular protooncogenes by viral transduction and subsequent mutation.[54] The normal c-*onc* gene products play important regulatory roles related to cellular proliferation and differentiation. However, when altered by point mutations, truncations, gene rearrangements, or other genetic insults, expressions of these genes may result in loss of growth control and, ultimately, neoplastic transformation. As such, c-*onc* genes probably represent the major targets for the actions of carcinogens.[55] More recent studies of genetic alterations in human cancers indicate that neoplastic transformation in vivo probably requires accumulation of mutations affecting multiple oncogenes and tumor suppressor genes (see below).

Somatic mutation

The role of mutated cellular oncogenes in human neoplasia has been dramatically underscored by an elegant series of experiments in which purified nuclear DNA from various human tumor-cell lines (such as T24 bladder carcinoma cells) was used to transform a second, morphologically normal cell line to the neoplastic phenotype.[56] In most experiments of this type, introduction of tumor cell DNA into normal, growth-regulated recipient cells leads to dramatic changes in the growth pattern of the recipient cells (fibroblasts), whereas introduction of DNA from normal cells has little or no detectable effect. The observed alterations in growth pattern include (1) the ability to grow at high cell densities, (2) the ability of "transformed" cells to grow directly on top of one another (that is, focus formation), and (3) the ability to grow in semisolid media (that is, anchorage-independent growth). The frequency of neoplastic transformation observed in these experiments indicates that a single copy of a mutant gene may be responsible for the initiation and maintenance of the neoplastic phenotype in T24 cells. Interestingly, the tumor-inducing gene present in T24 cells is a mutated form of the previously characterized cellular protooncogene known as c-Ha-*ras*. In this case, however, a single base change in codon 12 converts c-Ha-*ras* from a regulatory gene controlling growth and development to a "transforming" oncogene promoting uncontrolled growth.[56, 57]

Subsequent studies have demonstrated that cellular oncogenes may be activated by many different molecular mechanisms, including point mutations, gene rearrangements, and gene amplification.[52,54,58] Some cellular oncogenes, such as *ras*, can be activated by mutations within coding regions that enhance the specific activity of the oncogene products. Other oncogenes tend to be activated primarily by mutations within regulatory regions of the gene, leading to either increased or aberrant expression. Furthermore, most cellular oncogenes require multiple mutations or translocation in order to become activated.[54] For example, expression of the cellular oncogene, c-*fos*, is induced to very high levels by a variety of growth factors and hormones, and the *fos* gene product appears to stimulate both cell growth and DNA replication. However, the induction of c-*fos* by these factors is transient, and c-*fos* levels return to base-line values within 2 hours, even if the hormone remains present throughout the induction period. The transient nature of c-*fos* induction is tightly controlled by sequences at both the 5′ and 3′ ends of the gene.[59] If both of these regulatory sequences are inactivated concomitantly by somatic mutation, c-*fos* is expressed constitutively, and neoplastic transformation may result.[36]

Neoplastic transformation of some cell types requires the activation of more than one oncogene. For example expression of the mutated *ras* gene derived from T24 cells (*ras*T24) is sufficient to transform cultures of immortalized cell lines but insufficient for transformation of primary (that is, freshly isolated) cultures. However, when primary cultures are transformed simultaneously with activated *ras* and *myc* oncogenes, neoplastic transformation is readily observed.[60] These results are consistent with the idea that, in some cells, growth regulation must be overridden at two or more control points to cause neoplastic transformation. In this respect, the avian erythroblastosis viruses contain two different viral oncogenes, *erb*-A and *erb*-B, which are derived from separate regions of the host genome.[61] Recent studies based on both mathematical models of epidemiologic data[62] and molecular analysis of human tumors[63] indicate that most commonly occurring human cancers may require between 3 and 12 mutations.

Oncogene products

As a group, the cellular oncogenes encode polypeptides that are involved in the initiation and intracellular transduction of signals related to cell growth and differentiation.[64-66] Most of the cellular oncogenes identified at present fall into one of the following categories: (1) those encoding known or suspected trophic (growth) factors (such as c-*sis,* transforming growth factors α and β) (see below), (2) those encoding membrane-bound receptors for extracellular growth factors (such as c-*fms* and c-*erb*-b), (3) those encoding polypeptides associated with either the cytoplasm or the inner surface of the plasma membrane that transduce signals between membrane and cytoplasmic proteins (such as c-*src,* c-*ras,* c-*abl*), (4) those encoding soluble cytoplasmic receptors for hormones, such as steroids and thyroid hormones (such as c-*erb*-a), and (5) those encoding nuclear polypeptides that bind specifically to regulatory DNA regions and presumably modulate transcription and replication (such as c-*fos,* c-*myc,* c-*myb,* c-*jun*).

In addition to the growth-promoting effects of oncogenes, expression of activated oncogenes in some cell types results in cessation of cell division and the acquisition of differentiated phenotypes. For example, PC12 pheochromocytoma cells stop dividing and assume the shape of differentiated nerve cells in response to expression of an activated *ras* (*ras*T24) gene.[67,68] Nerve growth factor has an identical effect on PC12 cells. Similarly, expression of c-*fos* in myeloid precursor cells is associated with a decreased growth rate, as well as the induction of markers characteristic of monocytic differentiation.[69] It is difficult to understand how a single gene (such as *ras*T24) could have growth-stimulating effects in one cell type and growth-inhibitory effects in another. However, the overall data indicate that cellular oncogenes may form part of an intracellular communications network that is triggered by specific extracellular factors. These factors may have either growth-promoting or growth-inhibiting effects, depending on the target cell. The particular response of a cell to the binding of these factors depends on the developmental lineage of that cell, rather than on any inherent stimulatory or inhibitory properties of a particular oncogene or factor.[64] Two important corollaries of this model for oncogene action have implications for the diagnosis and treatment of cancer. The first predicts that because various cell types respond differently to any one oncogene, each cell type may be highly susceptible to neoplastic transformation by only a limited subset of cellular oncogenes. The strikingly consistent correlation of N-*myc* with neuroblastoma,[70] c-*abl* with chronic myelogenous leukemia,[71] and c-*myc* with B-cell lymphomas,[72,73] support this hypothesis. The second corollary predicts that, for a given cell type, different activated oncogenes or tumor-suppressor genes may induce neoplastic transformation by entirely different mechanisms. As a result, the prognosis, as well as the optimal therapy, for a tumor may be determined only after the mechanism of neoplastic transformation, that is, the activated oncogene or oncogenes or suppressor gene or genes (see right), has been identified. Past therapies have taken advantage of increased rates of cell division in tumor cells because this represents a final common pathway that is independent of the particular genes involved. However, future therapies directed toward the action of a particular oncogene may prove, in some cases, to be more effective. Recent studies have attempted to introduce either cytotoxic or tumor-suppressor genes directly into tumor cells in vivo using modified viral vectors. The results of these early forays into "gene therapy" appear promising.[74]

Tumor-suppressor genes

In addition to a well-substantiated role for activated cellular oncogenes in many human cancers, studies of familial cancer syndromes have identified a second, closely related mechanism of neoplastic transformation involving inactivation or deletion of tumor-suppressor genes, which serve to keep cellular growth in check.[50] Although the precise mechanisms through which tumor-suppressor genes function are not yet entirely clear, they appear to act as negative regulators of the same intracellular pathways that are activated by cellular oncogenes. Tumor-suppressor genes that have been identified at present include the retinoblastoma gene (Rb), p53, the Wilms' tumor gene (WT1) and others listed in Table 24-5. Tumor-suppressor genes are usually associated with neoplastic transformation only after both copies have been inactivated by mutation or deletion.[50,63,75,76] This leads to either sporadic, or familial forms of cancer, depending on whether the first mutation (Hit #1) occurred at the level of a somatic, or genus, cell. For example, individuals inheriting one active tumor-suppressor allele and one inactivated allele (germinal mutation) have substantially increased risk of cancer because only a single mutation in a single cell of the appropriate type is required for neoplastic transformation. In contrast, patients carrying two active copies of a given suppressor gene must undergo two rare and independent mutational events in the same cell. In patients with hereditary retinoblastoma, most children inheriting one normal and one mutant Rb allele develop multiple retinoblastomas by 1 year of age, and they pass this trait to 50% of their offspring.[77] In contrast, sporadic retinoblastoma requires two independent Rb somatic mutations in the same retinoblast, which occurs at very low frequency in the general population, usually results in only a single tumor, and is not passed to subsequent generations. Similar familial cancer syndromes have been associated with other tumor-suppressor genes including Li-Fraumeni syndrome[78] (p53 gene) and von Hippel-Lindau disease[79] (VHL gene). Familial cancer syndromes should be suspected whenever one or more of the following criteria are satisfied:

1. **Clustering of cancers within families.** Families may present a wide range of cancer types, as in Li-Fraumeni families,[80] or with a very limited range of cancers, as in hereditary colon or breast cancer families.[81]
2. **Onset of adult type cancers at unusually early ages.**
3. **Multiple independent cancers arising within individuals.**

It has been estimated that approximately 10% of colon, breast, and prostate cancers arise in association with predisposing genetic factors. Genetic lesions associated with familial predisposition to cancer include those involving oncogenes and tumor-suppressor genes, genes affecting the extent and fidelity of DNA repair,[82] and genes affecting processing of exogenous and endogenous carcinogens. In addition, it is conceivable that mutations affecting genes responsible for immune recognition and elimination of tumors might predispose individuals or families to cancer (see section on tumor surveillance).

Tumor-suppressor genes, therefore, play a prominent role in both sporadic and familial cancers. Recent evidence also indicates that oncogenic DNA viruses frequently induce neoplastic transformation by specific inhibition of tumor-suppressor gene products. As examples, both the oncogenic papovaviruses (SV40, polyoma, and some human papillomavirus serotypes[83]) and the oncogenic adenoviruses[84] encode proteins that sequester or inactivate the p53 and Rb gene products.

The role of oncogenes and tumor-suppressor genes in the evolution, prognosis, and treatment of human cancers is provided in these following three brief examples, which reflect current thinking.

Neuroblastoma. Human neuroblastoma represents both the first and the most successful application of molecular biology to clinical management of solid tumors up to now. Traditionally, the prognosis of patients with neuroblastoma parallels clinical stage, with 3-year survival rates varying from greater than 90% (stage I) to approximately 10% (stage IV).[85,86] However, approximately 10% to 30% of patients presenting initially with low-stage disease (stages I and II) subsequently experience rapid progression of their disease. These patients would benefit immeasurably from markers of the aggressive nature of their tumor at the time of initial diagnosis, thus facilitating active intervention at the earliest stages. Landmark studies have demonstrated, unequivocally, that amplification of the N-*myc* gene in neuroblastomas correlates with poor prognosis, irrespective of clinical stage at the time of initial presentation.[70,87,88] As a result of these studies, neuroblastomas with amplification of N-*myc* are generally treated as stage IV tumors regardless of clinical stage.[85,86] The degree of N-*myc* amplification within neuroblastomas ranges from 3 to 300 copies of N-*myc* per haploid genome.[85] It is important to emphasize that, although amplification of the N-*myc* gene (that is, increased number of gene copies) is frequently associated with unusually high levels of N-*myc* mRNA (that is, overexpression), amplification and overexpression are distinct entities. Overall, only 5% to 10% of low-stage neuroblastomas exhibit N-*myc* amplification, but almost all of these carry a rapidly progressive phenotype.

These findings raise important questions, the answers to which may provide critical insights into the mechanisms underlying the development of neuroblastoma or other solid tumors. These questions address the following concerns: (1) the role of possible rearrangements or point mutations within the amplified N-*myc* genes, (2) whether N-*myc* amplification can arise anew in stage I and II neuroblastomas, (3) the role of N-*myc* overexpression in neuroblastomas with no evidence of amplification, (4) the role of other oncogene-related products, which may facilitate or complement the transforming activities of N-*myc*. Although the definitive diagnostic test for N-*myc* amplification involves direct analysis of neuroblastoma DNA by Southern blotting, the amplified N-*myc* DNA can also be detected at the cytogenetic level as noncentromeric, double minute (DM) chromosomes, consisting of tandem arrays of N-*myc* genes, and homogeneous-staining regions (HSR), consisting of DM-DNA which has integrated randomly within the normal centromeric chromosomes.[89-91]

Most DNA studies of neuroblastoma show little or no evidence of rearrangement or point mutations within the amplified N-*myc* genes,[92] an indication that overexpression of the wild type of N-*myc*, rather than mutant N-*myc*, may be linked to the poor prognosis observed in these patients.[86] These findings are reinforced by independent studies that demonstrate a direct role for the nonmutated N-*myc* gene in tumorigenic transformation of established cell lines,[93] cooperation with activated *ras* in the transformation of primary rat fibroblasts,[94] and the rescue of primary fibroblast cultures from senescence.[95] In addition, increased expression of the wild type of N-*myc* plays an etiologic role in MuLV-dependent lymphomagenesis,[96] and the wild type of N-*myc* can directly induce lymphomas when overexpressed in transgenic mice.[97]

Colorectal carcinoma. Colorectal carcinoma presents a particularly accessible model for studying hyperplastic, dysplastic, and neoplastic changes, since a relatively large number of early tumors can be detected and snared during routine endoscopic examinations. Examination of a large series of adenomas and carcinomas using cytogenetics and restriction fragment length polymorphisms (RFLP) indicate that colorectal carcinomas usually arise by accumulation of multiple, independent somatic mutations involving both oncogenes and tumor-suppressor genes.[63,98] Three of the most frequently affected genes are (1) the *ras* proto-oncogene, which is mutated in the majority of colorectal carcinomas,[99,100] (2) the p53 tumor-suppressor gene, which may be deleted or mutated in these tumors,[99-102] and (3) the deleted-in-colorectal-carcinoma (DCC) gene, located on the long arm of chromosome 18 (18q) and missing in the majority of colorectal carcinomas[103]. A fourth locus, located on the long arm of chromosome 5 (5q21), contains two different genes, MCC and APC, which appear to be altered in a significant subset of colorectal carcinomas.[104-108] APC represents the genetic locus responsible for familial adenomatous polyposis, in which affected individuals develop literally thousands of adenomatous polyps by 30 years of age, and most develop colorectal carcinoma by 50 years. A fifth locus, the *hMSH2* gene located at 2p22–21, is mutated in both sporadic and familial nonpolyposis colon cancers.[82] Interestingly, the *hMSH2* gene is responsible for repair of DNA containing complementary-base mismatches, and mutations at this locus would be expected to increase the somatic mutation rate at many different loci.

Mutations in the K-*ras* gene have been detected in approximately 50% of colorectal carcinomas and adenomas.[98] Other *ras* genes appear to be affected much less frequently. Most of these mutations are single point mutations at codons 12, 13 or 61, all of which activate the *ras*-gene transforming potential.[109] Interestingly, similar mutations in the K-*ras* gene occur in approximately 50% of colorectal adenomas with no evidence of carcinoma, an indication that K-*ras* mutations are not sufficient to induce carcinoma, but they may play a critical role in the progression of adenomas. This hypothesis is supported by data indicating that the frequency of *ras* mutations decreases to approximately 10% in adenomas smaller than 1 cm.[98] In addition, *ras* gene mutations appear more frequently in adenomas with villous or tubulovillous patterns, both of which progress to carcinoma more frequently than those displaying only a tubular pattern.

MCC, a second gene from the 5q21 region also implicated in colorectal carcinogenesis, has been identified in non-FAP colorectal tumor cells, which carry a rearrangement of the 5q21 region.[107] At least 15% of sporadic colorectal carcinomas appear to carry alterations of the MCC locus.[108] The predicted

MCC polypeptide product exhibits little sequence homology with other products in either the protein or DNA data bases. Interestingly, the overall structure of the MCC product resembles myosins and intermediate filament proteins, such as vimentin, keratins, and nuclear lamins.[110]

Alterations in the structure of the p53 gene represent one of the most common genetic changes associated with human cancers.[111] Mutations, deletions, or rearrangements of the p53 gene occur in approximately 25% to 50% of malignant tumors involving the colon,[112] breast,[113] lung,[114] and CNS.[115] The most likely explanation underlying this pervasive role of p53 in human malignancies lies in the structure of the p53 protein and the unusual effect of missense mutations on its activity. Whereas single amino acid substitutions in most proteins result either in a decrease or complete loss of activity, single point mutations at specific sites of p53 may induce either increased activity or the appearance of new functions.[50,111] In the case of p53, this new activity may be highly oncogenic. Because oncogenicity can be elicited from the p53 gene after a single point mutation, the probability of p53 activation as a result of random mutations is much greater than that for other transforming genes, in which multiple, independent mutations may be necessary for oncogenic activation. Several mutational "hot spots" have been observed for the p53 gene, all of which occur within four blocks of highly conserved amino acid sequences. The most frequently observed mutations result in amino acid substitutions at residues 175, 248, and 273,[116] though at least 30 different mutation sites have been documented. This situation is somewhat analogous to that observed for the H- and K-*ras* genes, in which a single point mutation at codon 12, 13, or 61 dramatically increases the oncogenic potential of the *ras* gene product.[109] It is interesting to note in this regard that mutational activation of *ras* also occurs frequently in a variety of human tumors.

Recent evidence indicates that the p53 gene product serves as an important regulator of the cell cycle by inducing the synthesis of cell-cycle inhibitors such as p21, which inhibits the activity of one or more cyclin-dependent kinases. Initial findings indicate that the majority of cancers may carry mutations in either p53, p21, or p16, another cell-cycle inhibitor specific for cyclin-dependent kinase 4 (cdk4).[117-120]

Analysis of p53 alleles in colorectal carcinoma indicate that, in the majority of these tumors, both p53 alleles have undergone somatic mutations, frequently resulting in one mutant allele with increased oncogenic potential and one allele that has been deleted.[101,112] Presumably, these allelic mutations have occurred independently, and each confers a selective growth advantage on the affected tumor cells. Vogelstein and coworkers have proposed that in most cases the missense mutation precedes deletion of the remaining allele and have identified several "intermediate-stage" tumors in which one allele had undergone a substitution mutation, but the normal allele had not yet been deleted.[121]

Cytogenetic and linkage analyses indicate that the gene responsible for familial adenomatous polyposis (FAP), an autosomal-dominant genetic disease characterized by hundreds to thousands of benign adenomatous polyps, some of which eventually progress to carcinoma, lies in the vicinity of chromosome region 5q21.[122,123] A similar region of chromosome 5q is deleted in many adenomas and carcinomas from patients without evidence of FAP.[122,123] These findings indicate that one or more genes associated with 5q21 may control the proliferation of colonic epithelial cells and that deletions or inactivating mutations in these genes, whether somatic or germinal, may predispose to adenomatous proliferation of the epithelial cells. Somewhat surprisingly, the tumor-suppressor gene associated with FAP does not appear to require deletion or mutational inactivation of both alleles to express the FAP phenotype.[63] This contrasts directly with the retinoblastoma tumor-suppressor gene (Rb), in which predisposed individuals inherit only a single intact copy of the gene, and neoplasia results after spontaneous deletion or mutational inactivation of the remaining copy.[75,77] A putative candidate for the FAP-associated gene (referred to as APC) has recently been identified and characterized from FAP families carrying relatively small (100 to 260kilobase pair) deletions in the vicinity of 5q21.[104-106,108] The APC gene encodes two related mRNAs by alternative splicing of exon 9; the predicted polypeptide product of the smaller mRNA lacks 101 amino acids encoded by exon 9 but is otherwise identical to the putative product of the larger APC mRNA. The larger and more abundant APC mRNA encodes a predicted polypeptide of 2844 amino acids with a molecular weight of 311.8 kD. Comparisons with protein and DNA data bases revealed no genes or proteins with a high degree of sequence similarity, though short regions of similarity to myosins and keratins were noted. In addition, the putative APC product is compact in structure, predominantly hydrophilic, carries no recognizable signal peptides or hydrophobic membrane-anchoring regions and is therefore presumably located in the cytoplasm.

The DCC (for deleted in colorectal carcinoma) gene, which is located on the short arm of chromosome 18, has recently been cloned and characterized,[103] and it shares extensive homology with previously characterized cellular adhesion molecules. Approximately 70% of colorectal carcinomas carry deletions involving 18q and DCC, and these frequencies are similar to those observed for p53. If DCC represents a gastrointestinal tract–specific cellular adhesion molecule, the loss of a single allele, and the resultant 50% decrease in surface density, would be sufficient to reduce intercellular adhesion drastically.[124] Reduced adhesiveness, in turn, might increase the potential for local invasion and metastatic dissemination. Evaluation of DCC structure and expression therefore may have important prognostic value in the management of colorectal carcinomas. Other studies have demonstrated loss of heterozygosity at 18q in breast carcinomas, and these results indicate the possibility that DCC inactivation may be implicated in a variety of different tumors.[125]

Breast carcinoma. Carcinoma of the breast remains the leading cause of cancer in women. Estimates are that as many as 1 in 9 American women will be stricken with this disease during their lifetime.[126,127] It has recently been suggested that all women with carcinoma of the breast, including those without evidence of axillary nodal involvement (that is, axillary node negative, or ANN), could benefit from adjuvant chemotherapy or tamoxifen.[128] However, because both chemotherapy and antiestrogens carry a significant risk of morbidity, it would be advantageous to develop diagnostic or prognostic tools that could identify for treatment those ANN patients at highest risk for recurrent or rapidly progressive disease. Since as many as 30% of ANN patients with tumors less than 2 cm in diameter are expected to die of their disease within 20 years after initial diagnosis,[129] the value of an early prognostic marker for breast carcinoma cannot be underestimated.

Unfortunately, no single marker yet predicts reliably which ANN patients are most likely to experience recurrent disease. Instead, a composite profile of tumor characteristics consisting of size,[116,130] S-phase fraction,[131] ploidy,[132] and estrogen receptor status[133] appears to correlate both predictably and reliably with the probability of recurrence. In addition, two molecular markers that have only recently been identified, HER-2 and cathepsin D, greatly extend the efficacy of these composite indices. HER-2 (also referred to as *neu* or *erb*B2) encodes a 185 kD cell surface protein with extensive homology to the epidermal growth factor (EGF) receptor.[134,135] Like the EGF receptor, the HER-2 gene product exhibits tyrosine kinase activity. Although a single amino acid substitution appears sufficient to activate the transforming potential of the HER-2 gene, most primary human breast carcinomas, which have been subjected to molecular analysis, demonstrate amplification and overexpression of the wild type of HER-2 gene.[136] These findings are reminiscent of the relationship between N-*myc* and neuroblastomas, in which expression of a single copy (per haploid genome) N-*myc* gene does not affect the prognosis, but higher levels of expression from amplified N-*myc* is associated with rapidly progressive disease. The existence of a transformation threshold may apply to both HER-2 in breast carcinomas and N-*myc* in neuroblastomas. Approximately 25% to 30% of human breast carcinomas display evidence of HER-2 amplification, and virtually all these overexpress the HER-2 gene product.[136] The prognostic value of HER-2 amplification in breast carcinoma is somewhat ambiguous at present.

Growth factors

In a previous edition of this book it was possible to list representative growth factors, their structural characteristics, and their functions.[26] The field has expanded rapidly, and there are more than 100 members of growth factor families; the EGF family alone has at least 13 known members. Table 24-6 presents a simplified overview of growth factor families. It is not possible in this chapter on neoplasia to provide a comprehensive summary.

Table 24-6 Representative growth factor families

- Epidermal growth factor family (EGF, TGF-α, VVGF, AR, Cripto)
- Fibroblast growth factor family (aFGF, bFGF, *hst*-1, *hst*-2, FGF-5, *int*2, KGF)
- Platelet-derived growth factor family (PDGF, B-chain/c-sis)
- Platelet-derived endothelial cell growth factor
- Hepatocyte growth factor
- Insulin-like growth factor family (IGF-I, IGF-II)
- Colony-stimulating factor family (Multi-CSF, GM-CSF, G-CSF, M-CSF, KL)
- Erythropoietin
- Interleukin family (IL-1 to IL-12)
- Transforming growth factor-β family (TGF-sβs, bone morphogenetic protein [BMPs], inhibins, müllerian-inhibiting substance [MIS])
- Interferons (α, $β_1$, γ)
- Oncostatin M

Courtesy H. Moses, Nashville, Tenn, 1995 (personal communication).

Growth factors are polypeptides or small proteins that are released by cells into the local environment and exert powerful regulatory effects on nearby cells (*paracrine effects*) or on the secreting cells themselves (*autocrine effects*).[26]

They differ from polypeptide hormones in that they act locally and usually do not circulate, with few exceptions (for example, platelet-derived growth factor, PDGF, is released in the circulation during clotting). Growth factors bind specific receptors on the plasma membrane of the target cell, triggering receptors to "transduce" signals to cytoplasmic pathways (such as protein kinase–mediated effects) and then to the nucleus.[26,137] Recognition patterns are complex with several growth factors sharing the same receptor; thus within the EGF family, the EGF receptor can bind EGF, TGF-α, and four other members of this family.[138] Transduction occurs largely through receptor protein kinases;[139] for neoplasia, an important subset of these is a group of receptors known as mitogen-associated protein (MAP) kinases, which play an important role in the cell cycle.[140] The biologic effects of growth factors may result from increased levels of the growth factor, increased numbers of receptors, altered receptors (that is, they behave as if they were "occupied"), or altered pathways.

In cell culture, transformed cells have reduced or absent growth factor requirements; this is probably an important aspect of autonomous growth of tumors in vivo. Tumor cells respond in both an autocrine and paracrine manner. Their relative independence from exogenous factors represents phenomena such as increased rates of synthesis of growth factors or their receptors or the development of altered receptors. This view is supported by the previously mentioned relationship between oncogenes and growth factors and their receptors and hormones; thus the *erb*B oncogene encodes the cytoplasmic and transmembrane portion of the TGF-α/EGF receptor, the *sis* oncogene is similar to the B-chain of the PDGF, *erb*A encodes part of the thyroid hormone receptor, and the C-*fms* proto-oncogene encodes the receptor for colony-stimulating factor-1 (CSF-1). Cells are usually responsive to several different growth factors that may (TGF-α and EGF) or may not (TGF-α and FGF) share the same receptors. Because of this overlap, it is often difficult, even in vitro, to unravel regulatory interactions. One result of stimulation of growth factor pathways is cell proliferation. This phenomenon is well illustrated by the effects of IL-2 on T-lymphocyte proliferation or the effects of EGF on the growth of cultured cells. However, growth factors also produce changes in differentiation and maturation, as evidenced by nerve growth factor (NGF)–stimulated neurite (axon) outgrowth from PC12 cells and the stimulation of precocious eye-opening and tooth eruption by EGF. They sometimes have opposite effects in different cells; we have mentioned the stimulation of fibroblast lineages by TGF-β and its inhibition of many epithelial lines, and lymphotoxin not only inhibits the growth of many transformed cells, but also stimulates B-lymphocyte proliferation.[141] Thus, as part of the acquisition of the neoplastic phenotype, the escape from growth factor regulation may involve escape from inhibition, as well as loss of dependence on positive-stimulating factors.

The foregoing discussion has focused on how growth factors might be involved in the growth of tumor cells themselves. We have mentioned that for tumors to grow they often require stromal and vascular support and they frequently destroy or invade surrounding tissue. Part of these processes may be achieved by paracrine signaling to surrounding cells.

Thus TGF-α, TGF-β, FGF, EGF, PDGF, and endothelial cell growth factor (ECGF) stimulate angiogenesis or fibroblast growth, or both,[12-14,27,142] and TGF-β lymphotoxin, EGF, IL-2, and TNF-α can be cytostatic or cytotoxic.[26,141] As a result, growth factors may be powerful modulators of tumor biology by virtue of their paracrine effects on heterologous cells.

Chromosomal changes in cancer

A role for chromosomes in neoplastic transformation has been suspected since the early twentieth century. Boveri and von Hansemann postulated that the abnormal mitotic figures observed in stained tumor sections were directly related to the acquisition of the neoplastic phenotype.[143,144] An understanding of chromosomal abnormality was severely constrained until reproducible preparations of mammalian chromosomes were achieved in the late 1950s. Soon afterwards, in 1960, a specific chromosomal abnormality associated with a particular cancer was reported by Nowell and Hungerford.[145] This abnormality is manifest because of an unusually small G-group chromosome (later identified as 22), which has become known as the "Philadelphia chromosome." Subsequently, higher-resolution chromosome-banding methods, which allowed identification of relatively small and subtle structural abnormalities, fostered the field of cancer cytogenetics.

The resolution of chromosome analysis has been improved substantially by the recent introduction of fluorescent in situ hybridization (FISH). Fluorescent dye–coupled nucleotides are incorporated directly into cloned DNA fragments, and after in situ hybridization to chromosome spreads, the chromosomal location of a given gene can be easily determined and compared between neoplastic and nonneoplastic cells. In addition, application of the FISH technique to interphase cells allows amplifications, deletions, and rearrangements to be detected with greatly increased sensitivity. An example of gene localization by FISH is shown in Fig. 24-21 and is discussed extensively in Chapter 10.

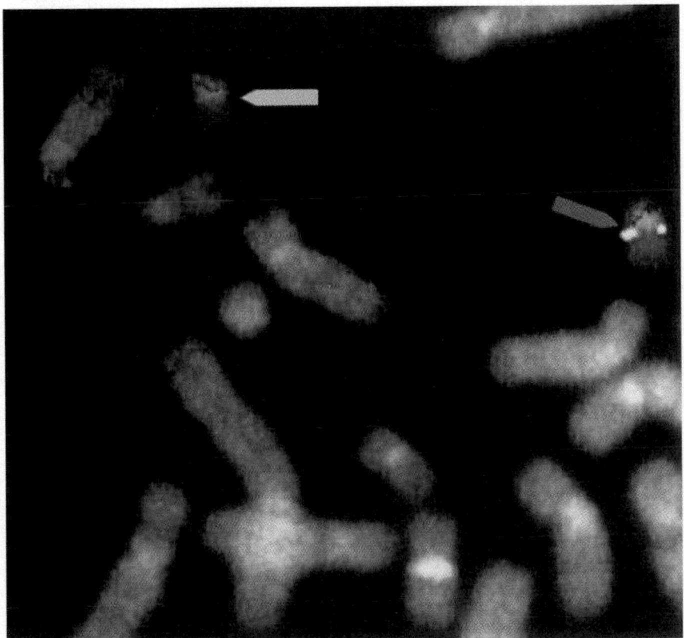

Fig. 24-21 Fluorescent in situ hybridization can be used to localize individual chromosomes

Chromosomal structure

The normal human karyotype contains 46 chromosomes, 22 pairs of autosomes and one pair of sex chromosomes (XX for females; XY for males). Genetic information is transmitted from parent to offspring as whole chromosomes; one member of each homologous chromosome pair is inherited from each parent. The analysis of chromosomes from a single tissue or individual usually requires the preparation of intact chromosomes from a suspension of growing cells. Chromosome preparations are produced by controlled osmotic lysis of mitotic cells, followed by specific staining techniques that produce, for each pair of homologous chromosomes, a unique and characteristic pattern of horizontal bands. An example of a banded preparation of normal human chromosomes is shown in Fig. 24-21. In many cases, the only indication of chromosomal abnormality is an alteration in the banding pattern for one or more chromosomes. Somatic changes in chromosomal structure, as seen with many tumors, usually occurs in only one member of a homologous chromosome pair. The precise mechanisms by which chromosome segments are broken and rejoined are not completely understood. However, it is clear that the frequency of these events can be increased by agents that damage DNA, such as radiation, chemical carcinogens, and viruses.[146]

One of the most provocative observations related to the origin of cancer cells has been the consistent association of specific chromosomal abnormalities with certain types of cancer. Subsequent to the discovery of the Philadelphia chromosome in chronic myelogenous leukemia (CML), investigators uncovered many other examples of this phenomenon. Often the specific chromosomal abnormality affects only the neoplastic cells, disappears with clinical remission, and reappears immediately before relapse.[25,146]

The rapid growth in cancer cytogenetics has resulted primarily from fortuitously coincidental advances in the molecular biology of neoplasia and the high-resolution analysis of chromosomal structure.[147] As discussed in a previous section, recent advances in molecular biology have led to the discovery and characterization of cellular oncogenes, tumor-suppressor genes, and their products. Simultaneous advances in cytogenetic analysis have permitted the chromosomal mapping of each cellular oncogene. DNA analysis of chromosomal breakpoint regions indicates that chromosomal rearrangements can activate cellular oncogenes by juxtaposition of inactive oncogenes within transcriptionally active chromosomal regions.[72,73,148,149] As such, chromosomal rearrangements are alternative mechanisms of somatic mutation, analogous to point mutations and deletions, but they are detectable at the karyotypic level. Since a single chromosomal band contains approximately 100 to 300 genes, only rearrangements involving very large fragments can be detected. A list of chromosomal abnormalities associated with specific human malignancies is presented in Tables 24-4 and 24-5. For a more detailed and comprehensive treatment of this subject, see reference 155.

Some cellular oncogenes are more likely than others to become activated by chromosomal rearrangements, and diseases associated with these particular oncogenes are more frequently associated with chromosomal translocation. In addition, most diseases associated with chromosomal rearrangements should also be associated with more localized gene rearrangements, since both mechanisms can generate similar changes in gene structure. Two examples illustrate this point clearly. Chronic myelogenous leukemia (CML) apparently results from inappropriate expression of the c-*abl* oncogene in immature hematopoietic cells.[71] In greater than 75% of patients with CML, c-*abl* is activated by a chromosomal translocation between chromosomes 9 and 22, in which the c-*abl* oncogene from chromosome 9 is fused to the control region of a gene, known as *bcr*, on chromosome 22.[148] One result of this translocation is a distinctively small remnant of chromosome 22 that is known as the Philadelphia chromosome.[145] The CML cases without this translocation are referred to as Philadelphia chromosome–negative CML. Recent experimental evidence, however, indicates that most cases of Philadelphia chromosome–negative CML contain a *bcr*/c-*abl* gene fusion, which is similar or identical to that observed in Philadelphia chromosome–positive CML.[150] These results demonstrate that the development of CML depends primarily on the formation of a *bcr*/c-*abl* fusion gene.

The second example concerns chromosomal alterations associated with the hereditary and sporadic forms of retinoblastoma. Approximately 5% of patients with hereditary retinoblastoma have a heterozygous deletion of band 13q14 within the long arm of chromosome 13.[25] This deletion, inherited at the time of conception, is present in every cell and is therefore referred to as a constitutional deletion. Subsequent studies have shown that the other 95% of patients with hereditary retinoblastoma also have a heterozygous deletion of genetic material from band 13ql4, but this deletion is too small to be visible karyotypically. As discussed in a previous section, retinoblastoma results when the remaining copy of the Rb gene, located at 13q14, is deleted or inactivated by a somatic mutation that may or may not be visible karyotypically. Thus, although karyotypically visible deletions are present only in a minor subpopulation of retinoblastoma patients, intensive study of these deletions has led to the isolation and characterization of a gene responsible for the majority of retinoblastomas.[75] In conclusion, both karyotypically detectable and nondetectable gene rearrangements may result in alterations in the activities of oncogenes and antioncogenes. Some cell types, such as lymphoid cells, contain specific DNA recombinases and may therefore be particularly susceptible to chromosomal rearrangements.[151]

Chemical and physical carcinogens

A majority of cancer in humans results from exposure to chemical and physical carcinogens.[1,87,152-154] In the United States about 30% of all cancer deaths have a single cause, the exposure to tobacco products.[1,152,153] In addition to the well-known link between lung cancer and tobacco use (Fig. 24-22), individuals who smoke or chew tobacco are at increased risk for the development of cancers of the oral cavity, larynx, esophagus (in heavy drinkers), pancreas, and urinary system.[155]

Epidemiologic studies indicate that other chemical carcinogens often act synergistically with tobacco. Thus, not only is asbestos a carcinogen for mesothelium and bronchial epithelium, but asbestos exposure in combination with smoking results in substantial incidence rates for bronchogenic carcinoma. Radon-gas exposure (uranium miners) also results in bronchogenic carcinoma and acts synergistically with tobacco smoke to increase cancer risk.

The most common cause of (nonfatal) cancers in the United States is exposure to solar radiation (primarily ultraviolet B, 290 to 330 nm), which results in hundreds of thousands of squamous and basal cell carcinomas on exposed areas of skin each year. It is also a major contributor to the incidence of malignant melanoma, which is now increasing in incidence faster than any other cancer in the United States (Fig. 24-23).

Although there is much discussion about industrial exposure to chemicals as a cause of cancer in the United States and there are several, well-described "cancer clusters," only a small percentage of human cancer is traceable to such exposure. Most of the increased risk of cancer from exposure to chemicals and radiation is a result of life-style and personal choice, not industrial or environmental exposure.[153] It is often easier, however, to identify occupational causes of cancer because of the clustering of cases and intense or protracted exposure (Fig. 24-24).

Chemical carcinogens

There are two major mechanisms of chemical carcinogenesis. The first, like radiation, produces covalent modification of cellular constituents, such as DNA. These carcinogens are some-

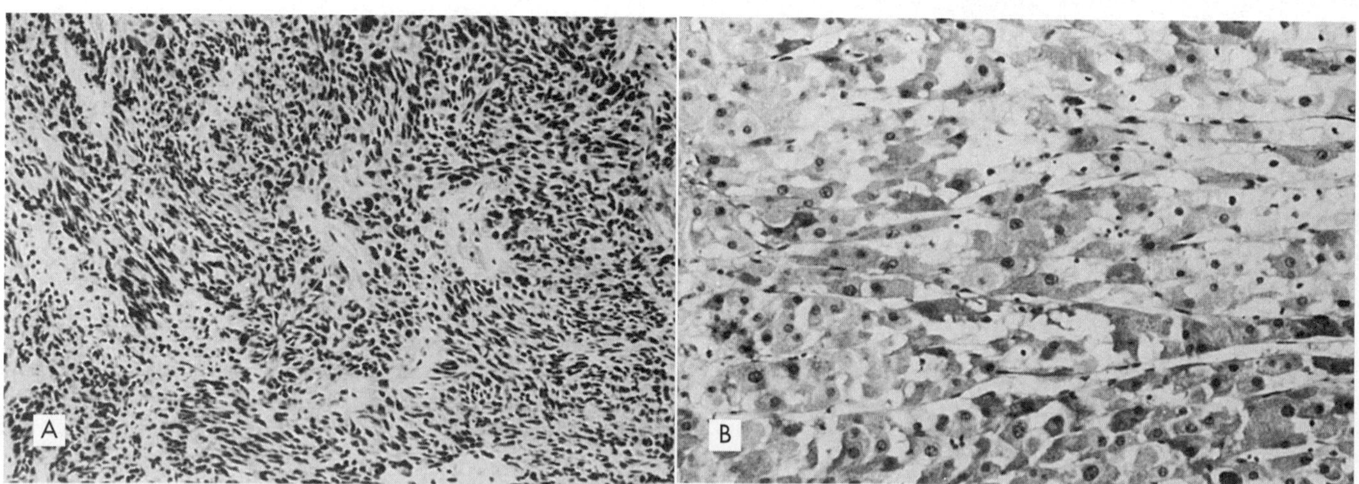

Fig. 24-22 A, Carcinoma of bronchus, small-cell type. Since tumor cells are often spindle shaped, cancer is sometimes called "oat cell." This tumor secreted excessive ACTH resulting in adrenocortical hyperplasia, **B,** and Cushing's syndrome.

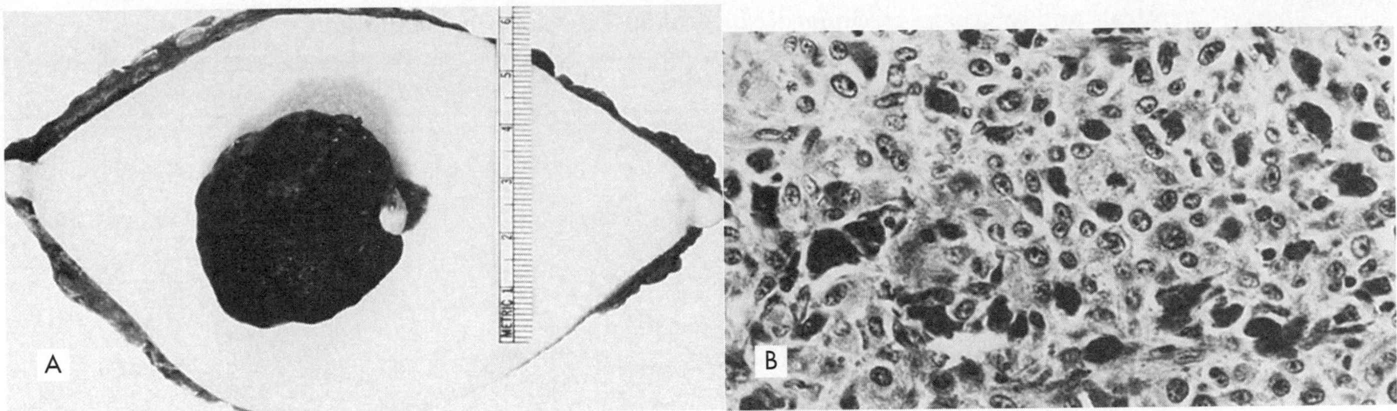

Fig. 24-23 Malignant melanoma of skin of back. **A,** Dark color is attributable to production of large amounts of melanin by tumor cells. **B,** Photomicrograph of same tumor as **A.** Dark tumor cells contain melanin pigment.

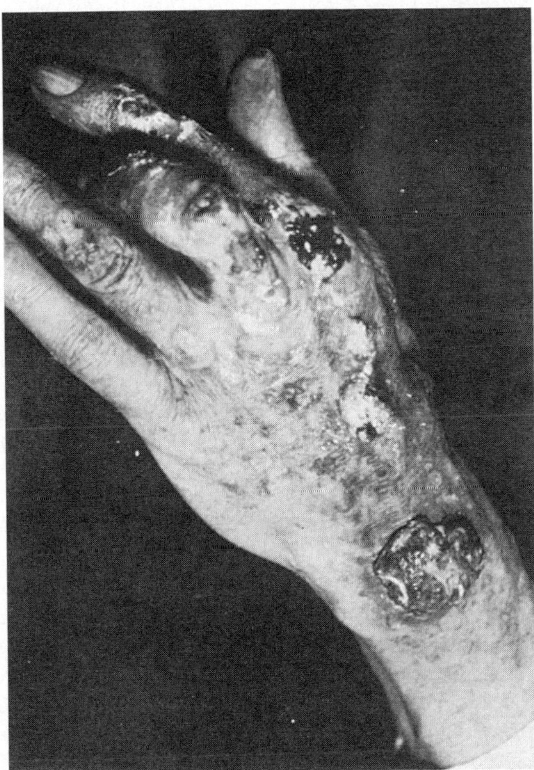

Fig. 24-24 X-ray dermatitis and multiple carcinomas of 5 years' duration in 83-year-old male physician after 15 years of repeated small exposure to x irradiation.

times referred to as *genotoxic carcinogens*; the second group, which does not produce covalent modification, is referred to as *nongenotoxic carcinogens*. The list of agents that are known animal carcinogens runs into the hundreds,[156] and a subset of these and related compounds are known to be human carcinogens (Table 24-7).

Chemical carcinogens that form covalent bonds with cellular constituents (genotypic carcinogens) either do so directly (direct-acting carcinogens) or are metabolized from precarcinogens to direct-acting intermediates (ultimate carcinogens).[10,157] The metabolism, termed *bio organic transformation*, usually occurs in mammalian cells but sometimes is the result of action by intestinal flora. The result is the generation of electrophilic intermediates or free radicals, which attack most cellular constituents, of which DNA is the most significant.

Chemical carcinogens are ubiquitous (Fig. 24-25). Many are natural products, including, for example, cycasin (present in the cycad fern), safrole (found in the sassafras tree and present in extracts that were once used in flavoring root beer), aflatoxin B_1(a mold product contaminating grains stored under moist conditions), and mitomycin C (a mold product used as an anticancer drug) (Fig. 24-25). Carcinogens like benzo [a] pyrene, 7,12-dimethylbenz [a] anthracene, and other polycyclic hydrocarbons are found among the combustion products of wood and fossil fuels.

Other carcinogens are the products of industrial activity. Nitrogen mustard is a direct-acting alkylating agent, synthesized as an anticancer agent, whereas bis(chloromethyl) ether is an industrial alkylating agent. The use of alkylating agents in treating human cancers results in a greatly increased risk of a second cancer.[158] Metabolism of precarcinogens to ultimate carcinogens is an unfortunate by-product of cellular attempts to detoxify organic xenobiotics and render them water soluble. Usually only a small percentage of total metabolites is carcinogenic; the rest are inactive and excreted. Many dietary compounds affect carcinogen metabolism and often can decrease the already small percentage of carcinogenic metabolites of precarcinogens; these agents are sometimes referred to as *anticarcinogens*.[159-161] Agents like these, along with those like retinoic acid, that modify differentiation and gene expression are under active investigation as protective agents against cancer.[151, 159-163]

Genotoxic carcinogens, as well as ultraviolet and ionizing radiation, damage cellular DNA in several ways, including formation of covalent adducts with the DNA bases and the phosphodiester backbone, single- and double-strand breaks, loss of purines and pyrimidines, and formation of photohydrates.[164,165] The importance of DNA repair in protection against carcinogenesis is illustrated by persons with the rare autosomal recessive disorder *xeroderma pigmentosum*. To varying degrees, these individuals lack the ability either to excise damaged regions or to bypass them during DNA replication. Severely affected individuals develop numerous carcinomas on skin exposed to sunlight in childhood.[165] However, two other syndromes associated with faulty DNA repair, Cockayne's syndrome and a photosensitive form of brittle-hair

Table 24-7 Chemicals and mixtures carcinogenic or probably carcinogenic in humans

Agent	Site
Life-style and personal choice exposure	
Tobacco	Lung, pancreas, oral cavity and pharynx, larynx, urinary tract
Tobacco quids and betel nut	Oral mucosa
Ethanol with smoking	Esophagus
Industrial exposure	
Arsenic compounds	Skin, lungs
p-Biphenylamine and *o*-nitrobiphenyl	Urinary bladder
Asbestos	Pleura, peritoneum, lung
Asbestos with cigarette smoking	Synergistic increase in lung
Benzidine (4,4′-diaminobiphenyl)	Urinary bladder
Bis(chloromethyl) ether	Lung
Bis(2-chloroethyl) sulfide	Respiratory tract
Chromium compounds	Lung
2(or β)-Naphthylamine	Urinary bladder
Nickel compounds	Lungs, nasal sinuses
Soots, tars, oils	Skin, lung
Vinyl chloride	Liver mesenchyme
Radon gas (radiation)	Lung
Radon gas with cigarette smoking	Synergistic increase in lung
Drugs and therapeutic exposure	
N,N-Bis(2-chloroethyl)-2-naphthylamine (Chlornaphazine)	Urinary bladder
Cancer chemotherapy regimens	Leukemias, lymphomas, solid tumors
Diethylstilbestrol	Vagina
Estrogen	Breast, uterus
Phenacetin	Renal pelvis
Psoralen with ultraviolet radiation	Skin

disease (PIDIBS), do not have elevated rates of cancer.[164] It is also of interest that repair genes are, in some cases at least, part of the transcriptional apparatus, perhaps helping to explain why transcribed genes are preferentially repaired.[164] It is now clear that repair occurs at different rates within a given gene.[166] Further, one group has shown that repair of pyrimidine dimers occurs more slowly at mutation hotspots in the p53 gene during skin cancer.[167] One set of important targets for chemical carcinogens and radiation is oncogenes and tumor-suppressor genes, and repair processes may protect against mutations in these genes. The fact that there is a variation in rates of repair within individual genes emphasizes that "hotspots" may result either from increased susceptibility to damage or from reduced rates of repair.

The consequences of unrepaired DNA damage are mutations, including point mutations (base substitution, insertions, or deletions), rearrangements, deletions, insertions, or amplifications. Although the importance of mutation in the mechanism of action of carcinogens has long been postulated, until recently genomic targets were unknown. It is now clear that an important mode of action of chemical carcinogens is the alteration of the structure or regulation of oncogenes. In experimental chemical carcinogenesis in rodents, breast, liver, and skin cancers may show point mutations in codon 12 or 61 of the c-H-*ras* oncogene.[109] Mutations in the p53 gene may also result from exposure to chemicals. Further, carcinogens may be involved in some of the rearrangements and amplifications now known to be associated with other forms of oncogene activation and tumor-suppressor gene inactivation in humans (see Tables 24-4 and 24-5), but few detailed model studies in animal systems are available. It cannot be stressed too strongly, however, that carcinogens may induce many changes in addition to oncogene modification. These include damage and modification of many genes besides the *known* oncogenes, the induction of metabolizing enzymes and repair systems, effects on DNA replication, and effects on noninitiated, surrounding parenchymal cells. Many or all of these may be crucial in the generation and progression of neoplastic change. Discussions of chemical carcinogens usually focus on individual well-defined compounds or groups of compounds that can be studied with great precision with respect to metabolism, DNA damage, and so forth. It is worth considering the role of dietary fat in colorectal cancer here because the problem is important epidemiologically and fats do not fit this neat paradigm. It is generally believed that diet plays a significant role in colorectal cancer, and many studies have implicated high-fat, low-fiber diets in the genesis of this lesion.[168-170] However, some studies have failed to confirm the relationship between fat intake and high risk of colon cancer, or have documented only a modest increase in risk.[168,171] Refinement of measurements such as the analysis of saturated versus unsaturated fat, intake of animal fat, or total energy intake have failed to clarify this situation. Diets are complex mixtures of hundreds of chemicals, which may have opposing effects. Most likely contradictory studies reflect multiple causation, with certain environmental and dietary factors being more important in some populations than in others. Molecular analysis of colon cancer indicates that progression to a fully malignant state is a multistep process that does not necessarily have to occur in a single sequence.[63] Thus, how dietary factors including fats alter neoplastic and malignant change is not at all clear; they may act as carcinogens (or anticarcinogens[161]) or promoters (see

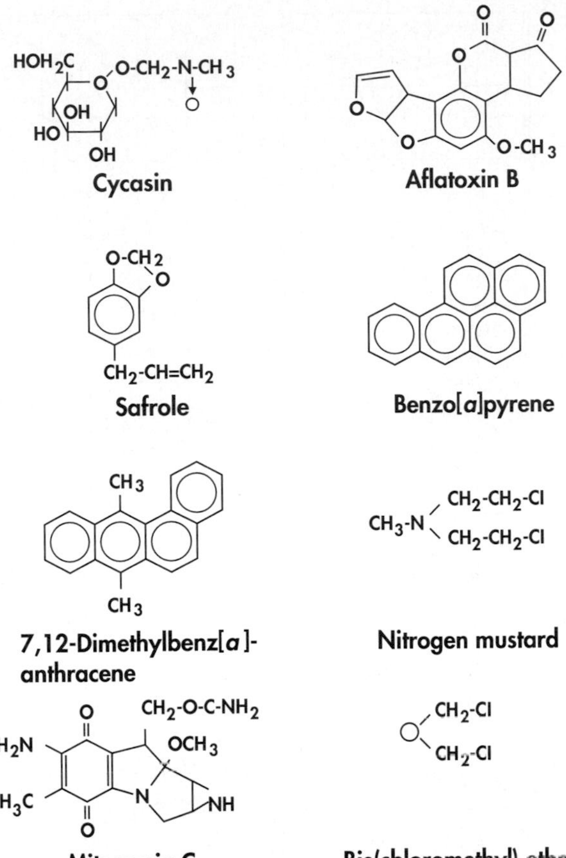

Fig. 24-25 Examples of chemical carcinogens. All these chemicals are genotoxic (form covalent bonds with DNA). Cycasin, aflatoxin B_1, safrole, benzo[*a*]pyrene, and 7,12–dimethylbenz[*a*]anthracene require metabolic activation, whereas the others are direct acting.

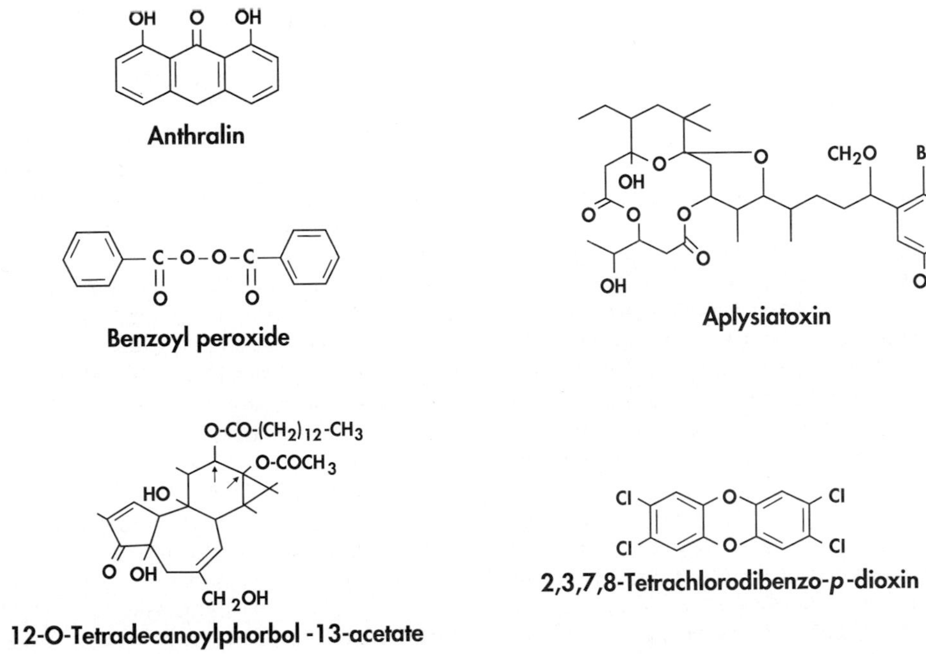

below) or simply be correlates of change without having a mechanistic role.

Promoters

Some agents known to be involved in carcinogenesis in either human or animal systems do not appear to form covalent bonds with cellular constituents; these include a variety of agents classified as nongenotoxic carcinogens and tumor promoters[172] (Fig. 24-26). Based on epidemiology from an industrial accident, one class of these agents (dioxins) is related to an increased risk of cancer in people.[173]

Promoters are not carcinogenic by themselves but greatly enhance the rapidity of onset or the yield of tumors (both benign and malignant) after carcinogen administration. The most potent promoters are the phorbol esters (such as tetradeconylphorbol acetate, TPA) and structurally unrelated compounds with a similar mode of action, such as teleocidins and aplysiatoxin.[10,172] Biochemical phorbol esters seem to act by the protein kinase C pathway,[10] to trigger the synthesis or activation of several transcription-regulating nuclear binding factors (AP-1 and AP-3), that regulate many cellular genes.[174] The molecular mechanism or mechanisms of action of other tumor promoters is not known in detail, but all tumor promoters stimulate cell division to some degree.

Carcinogens that do not appear to bind covalently to cellular DNA include estrogens, saccharin, inert plastic films, and asbestos. The molecular action of these agents is unclear, but like tumor promoters, most of these agents stimulate cell division. Examples include phorbol esters (mouse epidermal cells), estrogens (mouse breast parenchymal cells), saccharin (rat urothelium), plastic films (rat fibroblasts), and asbestos (mesothelial cells). The unifying feature may be an increased probability of mutation in a large mass of proliferating cells. Some agents, like the estrogens and TPA, probably alter the

Anthralin

Aplysiatoxin

Benzoyl peroxide

12-O-Tetradecanoylphorbol-13-acetate

2,3,7,8-Tetrachlorodibenzo-*p*-dioxin

Fig. 24-26 Chemical structures of skin tumor-promoting agents.
(From Yuspa SH: *J Am Acad Dermatol* 15:1031, 1986.)

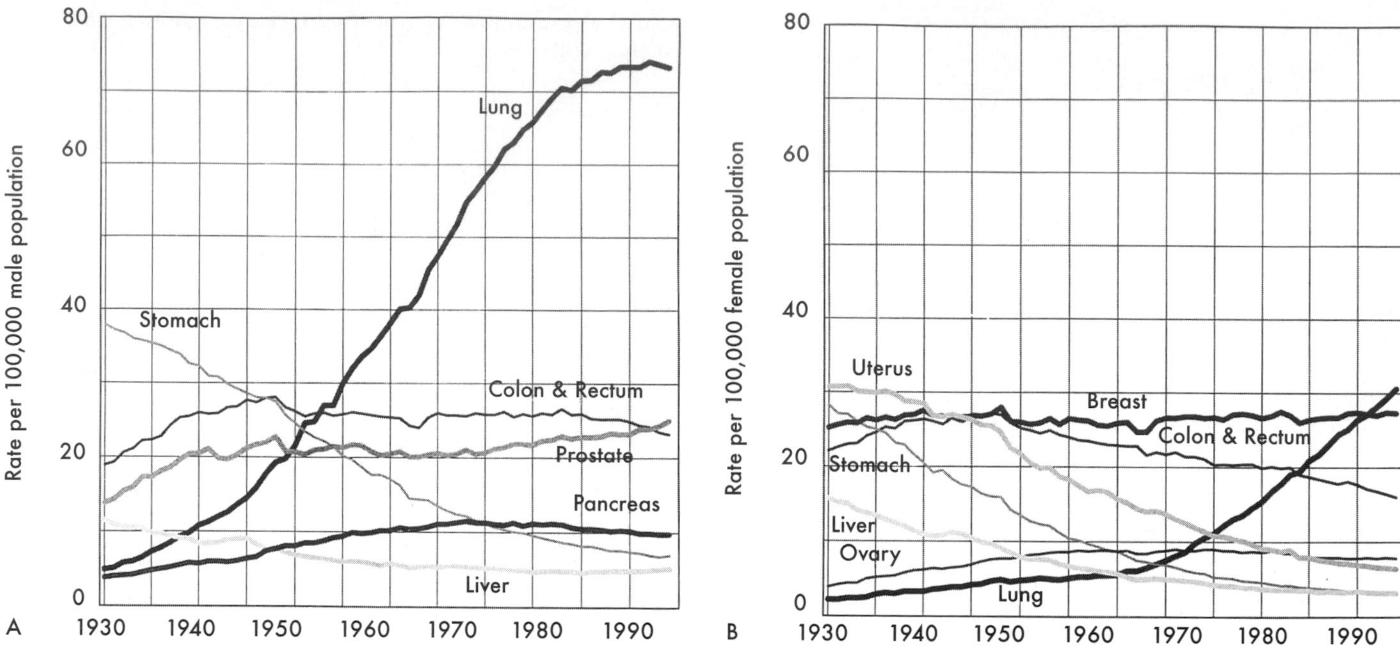

Fig. 24-27 Cancer death rates by site, United States, 1930-1989. **A,** Males. **B,** Females. Rates are adjusted to the 1970 U.S. census population. (From *Cancer facts and figures,* Atlanta, Ga, 1993, American Cancer Society.)

range of expressed genes during proliferation. There may be similarity in the mode of action of these agents and some viruses associated with neoplasia. As suggested elsewhere, one effect of hepatitis B virus on liver cells and HTLV-I on lymphoid cells may be an enlarged pool of proliferating cells. However, stimulation of proliferation alone is unlikely to account for the entire action of these chemicals or viruses. It may be that some of these agents also have other effects; asbestos, for example, may stimulate free-radical formation in macrophages and thus result in DNA damage.

Metals and metallic compounds including arsenic, beryllium, chromium (oxidation state IV), and nickel are carcinogenic in humans[175] (Table 24-7). Other metals may be cocarcinogenic, or inhibitors of carcinogenesis in animals. The effects of metals on biologic systems are diverse, including mutagenesis in short-term tests like the Ames' test and reduced fidelity of DNA synthesis; however, no comprehensive theory of metal carcinogenesis exists. In fact, several mechanisms, both genotoxic and nongenotoxic, are likely responsible for their carcinogenicity. Estimating risk from exposure to chemical carcinogens for the entire United States population is difficult because it involves extrapolating from high-dose animal experiments across species barriers or from relatively small numbers of humans exposed to high levels of carcinogens (often in the workplace).[176,177] Yet it is clear that, except for smoking-related cancers and malignant melanoma, the incidence rates for cancer have not climbed significantly, despite a large increase in the manufacture of chemicals since World War II (Fig. 24-27).

Prostate cancer, the incidence of which has risen rapidly, especially among blacks, in the last 15 to 18 years, represents another exception; however, much of this increase may represent better reporting and diagnostic methods. Although there are undeniable examples of industrially generated cancers (Fig. 24-27), the total number of known cases does not begin to approach the number of smoking-associated cancers in the United States in a year.[1,152,157] The reason for this observation is not that many industrial agents are not potent, since many are extremely effective experimental carcinogens, but rather, that thousands of workers exposed to varying levels of carcinogen, often for only a few years, do not develop as many cancers as millions of Americans smoking as many as two or more packs of cigarettes a day from an early age.

Many aspects of habit, diet, and environment alter the risk of developing cancer. Recently attempts have been made to assess this risk on the basis of both the potency of individual carcinogens and human exposure to them.[176] One may estimate daily exposure to agents like chloroform in municipal tap water (an unavoidable by-product of chlorination as protection against pathogenic bacteria), aflatoxin (in peanut butter), or formaldehyde (in mobile-home air) and the level of agent that produces tumors in 50% of exposed rodents. The possible implications are sobering; the amount of ethanol from a single glass of wine is many times more hazardous than the average American's daily exposure to polychlorinated biphenyls (PCBs), and the daily exposure to formaldehyde in mobile-home air is much more hazardous than exposure to the residue of ethylene dibromide on grain products consumed in an average day. An approach of this type should allow eventual elimination of unnecessary exposure to carcinogens and a better understanding of the trade offs when exposures are unavoidable. All of these comparisons are based on assumptions about extrapolation of risk. Data (especially animal data) are obtained from the exposure of a relatively small number of individuals to high levels of chemicals. We lack good ways to extrapolate risk at low levels of exposure from these types of data. There is some evidence that the dependence of risk from exposure for some agents may be exponential, and so a linear model would overestimate risk at low levels of exposure; however, regulators have adopted a conservative approach and have used linear extrapolation models.

We have already mentioned the importance of *progression* in the development of neoplasia. Two experimental systems, the development of skin cancer in mice and liver cancer in rats after the administration of tumor promoters and carcinogens, form the basis of much of our understanding of this process.[11,172] It is clear that cancer often develops as part of a selective process after the generation of papillomas (skin) or early nodules (liver) and that only a minority of these lesions progress to more aggressive lesions and finally to cancer. Experiments in which rats are exposed to carcinogen for a relatively brief period (2 to 3 weeks) indicate that, in liver at least, although the continued presence of carcinogen is not necessary, the development of frank hepatocellular carcinoma takes many months; also only a few carcinomas develop despite the presence of thousands of putative preneoplastic lesions.[11,178] There has been much speculation on how many steps are required to generate a malignant tumor and what the role of carcinogens is. However, it is also known that, after carcinogen administration, carcinomas in mouse skin or rat liver[179] can develop without identifiable preneoplastic lesions. These observations and present knowledge of oncogene function render these questions, as formulated, largely moot. Rather, it is more appropriate to ask what properties must be acquired by individual cell types to make them identifiable as neoplastic or malignant and, in molecular terms, how these properties are acquired. What is required to generate a central nervous system ependymal tumor, a locally invasive squamous cell carcinoma of the skin, and a potentially metastatic hepatocellular carcinoma may be very different. Like so many questions in biology, questions about the number of "steps" or number of "hits" involved in the production of cancer must be examined carefully in an appropriate context and on a case-by-case basis.

Viral carcinogens

In the past decade, both DNA and RNA viruses have been implicated in human cancers[180-182] (Table 24-8).

Although it has been known for over 75 years from work by Ellermann and Bang and by Rous that avian leukemias and sarcomas can be transmitted by filterable agents, only the careful epidemiology and molecular biology of many workers has established an unequivocal role for viruses in the cause of human cancer.[53,180,183] Unlike the original work on avian tumors and the investigation of the oncogenic action of active transforming retroviruses that grew out of it, analysis of human cancer has indicated that often only a small percentage of infected individuals develop cancer. The seminal observation, from which explanatory hypotheses have flowed, is the finding in the 1930s by Rous and his collaborators that a synergy existed between the Shope papillomavirus (CRPV) and chemical carcinogens in the development of cutaneous tumors. What has also become apparent with the advent of molecular biology is that viruses play a variety of different roles in the carcinogenic process, roles that differ substantially from tumor to tumor.

Strong epidemiologic evidence links hepatitis B virus (HBV) with hepatocellular carcinoma.[53,183] Although relatively rare in the United States, worldwide it is one of the most common tumors, and its geographic distribution parallels the prevalence of HBV carriers. Only a small percentage of those infected with HBV become chronic carriers of the virus (hepatitis B surface antigen positive), but the relative risk of developing hepatocellular carcinoma compared with noncarriers is about 200. Because of the long lag between infection and hepatocellular carcinoma (about 35 years) other events, in addition to the presence of the HBV genome, are necessary for tumor formation. Of interest in this regard is that no oncogene or growth factor–like functions have yet been identified for this small DNA virus. One model proposes that chronic destruction of the virus-infected hepatocytes causes continual hepatocyte proliferation, with replicating cells at risk for other events (such as mutation) that lead to neoplastic progression. One identifiable risk factor is the presence of aflatoxin (see Fig. 24-25), a powerful carcinogen in many species, in areas with a high incidence of hepatocellular carcinoma.[184,185] Because vaccination against HBV is available, hepatocellular carcinoma, like lung cancer and skin cancer, may be in large part preventable. Recent epidemologic evidence has also linked hepatitis C virus (HCV) with hepatocellular carcinoma.[186] This RNA virus is unrelated to hepatitis B virus; at present no gene product related to neoplastic change has been uncovered. It is generally believed that cycles of cellular damage and regeneration predispose to cancer in much the way that hepatitis B does.[186,187] In the United States approximately half of hepatocellular carcinomas are positive for HCV and negative for HBV.[188]

The relation between the Epstein-Barr virus (EBV) and Burkitt's lymphoma (a B-cell lymphoma) is similar in broad detail to the HBV story. Although EBV infects more than 90% of all people worldwide by adulthood, Burkitt's lymphoma occurs most frequently in equatorial East Africa, a region in which malaria is endemic. Since African Burkitt's lymphoma appears to be a monoclonal proliferation of EBV-positive cells, it has been hypothesized that somehow malarial infection stimulates the immune-cell proliferation from which these clones emerge or perhaps limits T-cell inhibition of B-cell growth. Whether two antigens encoded by EBV (EBNA and LYDMA) function as regulatory molecules remains to be seen (see Table 24-8). As mentioned earlier, the characteristic chromosomal translocation and *myc* activation may represent a late or final step in the process.[189,190] EBV-DNA is almost invariably found in biopsy specimens of nasopharyngeal carcinoma, and the incidence is especially high in Chinese.[191] This observation provides an interesting counterpoint to many demographic studies of cancer, in that these individuals, regardless of locale, seem to be at increased risk for this cancer. There is also an association between nasopharyngeal carcinoma and exposure to carcinogens or substances suspected of harboring carcinogens (nitrosamines, fumes, smoke), and like the Shope papilloma carcinogen model in rabbits, EBV and identifiable carcinogens may be synergistic in human nasopharyngeal carcinoma.

The human papillomaviruses (HPV) represent a family of over 50 related DNA viruses of intermediate size (8000 base pairs).[109] Papillomaviruses have been known to be oncogenic since the work of Shope in the 1930s.[109] Although there is a strong association between HPV-5 and HPV-6 and carcinomas that arise in the rare skin disease epidermoplasia verruciformis, the epidemiologic relationship of importance is between certain HPVs (especially HPV-16 and HPV-18) and genital cancers.[180,192] Normally HPV replicates episomally, but in several studies it has been found integrated into the tumor cell genome and transcribed, leading to relaxed expression of two presumed oncogenes, E6 and E7 proteins.[193] It is likely that, in part at least, the mechanism of action of E6 and E7 oncogenes involves binding and inactivation of the retinoblastoma (Rb) and p53 gene products.[83,194] As with

Table 24-8 Selected oncogenic viruses*

Viruses	Animal tumors	Human tumors	Active factor
Adenoviruses	Fibrosarcomas (hamsters)	None identified	E1A protein E1B protein
Hepadnaviruses			
Hepatitis B virus		Hepatocellular carcinoma	None identified
Woodchuck hepatitis virus	Hepatocellular carcinoma (woodchuck)		None identified
Hepatitis C virus		Hepatocellular carcinoma	None identified
Herpesviruses			
Epstein-Barr virus		Burkitt's lymphoma, nasopharyngeal carcinoma	?EBNA antigen ?LYDMA antigen
Frog herpesvirus	Renal adenocarcinoma (frog)		
Papillomaviruses			
Bovine papillomavirus	Dermal and esophageal papillomas and squamous cell carcinomas		
Human papillomavirus		Cutaneous and genital carcinomas (especially types 16 and 18)	E6 protein E7 protein
Polyomaviruses			
Polyomavirus of rodents	Mouse adenocarcinomas, fibrosarcomas	None identified	Large T, small t antigens
Simian virus 40 (SV40)	Fibrosarcomas (hamster), lymphomas, osteosarcomas	None identified	Large T, middle t, small t antigens
Poxviruses	Shope fibroma (rabbit)	None identified	Vaccinia growth factor (EGF-like)
Retroviruses (RNA)			
Acute leukemia and sarcoma viruses	Leukemias, sarcomas	None identified	Common oncogenes (*ras, sarc, myc,* etc.)
Chronic leukemia viruses	Leukemias	None identified	None
Transregulating viruses			Transregulator of fat
Bovine leukemia virus	B-cell leukemias		
HTLV-1		Some T-cell leukemias,	
HTLV-2		T-cell variant of hairy cell leukemia	

EBNA, Epstein–Barr nuclear antigen; *EGF,* endothelial growth factor; *HTLV,* human T-lymphocyte virus
LYDMA, lymphocyte determined membrane antigen.
*Many oncogenic retroviruses are listed in Table 24-4.

other human cancers, only a small portion of women with cervical infections develop neoplasia. The virus may be sexually transmitted, since in different geographical areas with differing cancer incidences, the incidence ratio between cervical carcinoma and penile carcinoma remains similar. The codependence of cancer development on papillomavirus infection and chemical carcinogens is seen in another example. In the Scottish Highlands, cattle exposed to bovine papillomavirus 4 (BPV4 or possibly other BPVs) show a high incidence of carcinomas of the esophagus and foregut only if they graze on bracken fern (known to contain several strongly carcinogenic pyrrolizidine alkaloids). Although this dependence on *known* chemical carcinogens is not obligatory, it may provide a partial paradigm for explaining why not all infected women and men develop genital cancer. It is of interest, for example, that the incidence of cervical carcinoma is higher in women who smoke than in those who do not. Since a large majority of women who develop cervical cancer have lesions that are HPV positive, it may be that carcinogens in vaginal fluids from cigarette smoke act synergistically with HPV.[180]

Two (RNA) retroviruses, HTLV-I and HTLV-II, are associated with two different human leukemias, adult T-cell leukemia and the T-cell variant of hairy cell leukemia, respectively. They are unusual in that their 3′ ends code for a transregulating factor, hence the designation, "transregulating retroviruses." These genes appear to enhance transcription from the viral promoter and possibly from cellular genes. What is at first examination surprising is that, of all the known oncogenic retroviruses, only this small subclass is associated with human cancer. This observation may in part be explained by the suggestion that most of the acute transforming retroviruses (that is, those that carry known oncogenes and produce tumors rapidly) are inadvertent laboratory artifacts.

At present, only a very small percentage of human leukemias are associated with a virus. HTLV-I may be transmitted through sexual contact (blood) and to infants during breast feeding. In areas where HTLV-I is endemic (as in

Japan), less than 1% of seropositive individuals develop leukemia and the latent period may be many years. Although sites of integration vary from individual to individual, there may be preferred sites that predispose to malignancy, but exactly how integration, transregulation, and host factors interact to lead to leukemia is unknown at present. Nontransregulating, chronic leukemia retroviruses appear to transform, at least in part, by a mechanism known as "promoter insertion," that is, by inserting a viral transcription start site in front of cellular genes with potential oncogenic properties such as oncogenes and growth factors. What role this mechanism plays in HTLV-I or HTLV-II oncogenesis remains unknown.

Some associations between viruses and human neoplasms are not causal. Rather, the transformation process allows these cells to serve as hosts for viral growth. A well-known example is the recovery of herpes simplex virus from some cervical cancers.

TUMOR-HOST INTERRELATIONSHIP

Local effects

Benign tumors usually affect the host by their size or location. For example, a tumor in the region of the ampulla of Vater may be less than 1 cm in diameter and still cause severe biliary obstruction, and an ependymal tumor near the Sylvian aqueduct may result in hydrocephalus. A large benign tumor may be only a nuisance or a cosmetic problem. Because benign tumors, especially the larger ones, often undergo retrogressive changes, such as infarction and hemorrhage, they may show a sudden increase in size, giving the false impression of rapid cellular growth. A small but important minority may have life-threatening effects through products they secrete.

Malignant neoplasms harm the host through mass effects and the destruction of normal tissues both locally and at distant sites. In addition, malignant neoplasms may release toxic metabolites or bioactive molecules after tissue destruction, or tumor necrosis; release hormones, growth factors, and regulatory molecules by the tumor; and cause psychosocial responses to cancer (anxiety, depression, listlessness). Another complication is the destruction of normal tissues during treatment (hematopoietic and lymphoid tissues and oral and gastrointestinal mucosae are particularly sensitive to chemotherapy and radiotherapy). Sometimes the molecular basis of symptoms is easily understood, as with endocrine tumors, the products of which are well characterized. In other cases, such as the action of tumor- or host-synthesized growth factors, we are nearing an understanding of effects in selected instances; the analysis of TGF-β and its effects is an example. However, it will probably be many years before all these factors are known and characterized and their host effects are fully appreciated (see the following section and Table 24-6).

Systemic effects

Some benign endocrine tumors, even when small, may produce excessive amounts of hormone and result in life-threatening symptoms. The production of insulin by some islet cell adenomas, with its resulting hypoglycemia, and the secretion of parathyroid hormone by parathyroid adenoma, with its resulting hypercalcemia, are two examples.

More complicated are conditions like anemia and cachexia, the generalized wasting seen in cancer patients mentioned earlier. Anemia may result from replacement of large portions of the marrow by metastatic tumor, destruction of hematopoietic cells by therapy or marrow shutdown resulting from synthesis of negative regulatory factors by tumors, and so on. Similarly cachexia probably results in part from the action of powerful inhibitors of cell growth (cachectin/tumor necrosis factor and other as yet undiscovered factors; it is worth noting again that TGF-β and müllerian-inhibiting substance have selective inhibitory actions) and, in part, from lack of appetite, anemia, infection as a result of the more general systemic effects of cancer, psychosocial factors, and cancer treatment. Another consequence of advanced disease is infection, and cancer patients frequently die of bronchopneumonia, often caused by opportunistic bacteria or fungi.

There are many other systemic effects termed *paraneoplastic epiphenomena* produced by tumors. Since the mechanisms of their development are poorly understood, only a few are mentioned as examples: dermatomyositis may develop in patients with various types of cancer; unexplained peripheral neuritis and degenerative brain changes may occur in cancer patients; and acanthosis nigricans (a hyperpigmented, keratotic skin lesion) indicates the likelihood of carcinoma, usually of the stomach. Many tumor effects are biochemical. For example, there may be a disturbed salt metabolism in some patients who have small-cell, undifferentiated carcinoma of the lung; there may be a diminution or elevation of various serum enzymes, such as acid phosphatase, that often is elevated in patients with prostatic cancer. Many changes in the blood, especially in serum proteins, have been reported in cancer patients, such as a deficiency in specific proteins or the presence of abnormal proteins. Since increased coagulability of the blood may complicate cancers, particularly those of the pancreas and stomach, the development of sudden, unexplained thrombotic episodes indicates the possibility of cancer of the upper abdomen.

An interesting challenge of clinical investigation is the analysis of paraneoplastic effects in molecular terms. There is also a large number of endocrine syndromes that result from ectopic hormone production by tumors. Thus tumors may secrete ACTH, vasoactive peptides, somatomedins, gastrin, parathyroid hormone–like polypeptides, serotonin, calcitonin, vasopressin (ADH), renin, glucocorticoids, sex hormones, glucagon, and insulin.

Tumor immunology

Many spontaneous and carcinogen-induced tumors express unique tumor-associated antigens, which may, under certain circumstances, provide specific targets for immunologic attack by lymphocytes and antibodies. The immunogenicity of tumor-associated antigens has led to the development of novel strategies for stimulating the immune response to these antigens as a means toward eliminating, or substantially reducing, the presence of residual tumor cells.[195] Studies of transplanted tumors between isogenic mice demonstrated that rejection of transplanted tumors occurred only in mice with functional T-lymphocytes. Both $CD4^+$ and $CD8^+$ T-cells appear to play important roles in immune recognition of transplanted tumors. In addition, natural killer (NK) cells and cytokine-activated macrophages also demonstrate substantial activity against tumor cells. Lymphokine-activated killer cells (LAK), derived from NK cells by stimulation with cytokines, including interferon-α and IL-2, have some therapeutic activity against some experimental and human tumors. In contrast to the antitumor activity exhibited by lymphocytes and macrophages, transfer of antibodies directed against tumor-associated antigens does not generally result in immune destruction of tumor cells.[195]

The immune surveillance theory proposes a critical role for the immune system in the recognition and destruction of early tumors, predominantly by cell-mediated immune mechanisms. Independent lines of evidence indicate that immunosuppression increases the susceptibility of both humans and experimental animals to development of tumors. First, neonatal thymectomy increases the susceptibility of experimental animals to tumors induced by oncogenic viruses. Second, organ transplant recipients receiving long-term immunosuppressive therapy have an increased incidence of lymphomas and lymphoproliferative diseases. Patients with the acquired immunodeficiency syndrome develop lymphoma, Kaposi's sarcoma, and epidermoid carcinomas at increased frequency. Despite anecdotal evidence supporting the concept of immune surveillance, numerous observations argue against the significance of immunosurveillance as a protective mechanism. Most of the tumors observed in immunosuppressed patients are lymphoproliferative diseases; the more common types of carcinomas are very rarely observed in these patients. Second, not all thymectomized animals exhibit increased tumor susceptibilities, and some exhibit decreased frequencies. It has been proposed that immune surveillance may be important for virus-induced and carcinogen-induced tumors, where immunogenic tumor-associated antigens are expressed at the cell surface.

Although the role of immune surveillance in protection from spontaneous tumors remains controversial, many investigators have attempted to stimulate immune responses against extant tumors by a variety of different strategies. Tumor vaccines, monoclonal antibodies against tumor-cell surface antigens, cytokine infusion, and gene therapy with cytokines and superantigens have been attempted in recent years with variable success. These approaches are likely to attract a great deal of attention in the near future.

COURSE AND TREATMENT

Benign tumors not only grow slowly, but also at times reach a point at which they seem to become dormant or even to regress. This is true, for example, with leiomyomas of the uterus, which often cease growing after menopause. Occasionally even malignant tumors enter a stage of dormancy, and in rare but well documented instances they may regress spontaneously. Spontaneous regression is defined as the complete or partial disappearance of cancer that cannot be attributed to treatment. The explanations for the phenomenon are inconclusive. Cancers of many different sites and types have shown such regression, the more common being renal cell carcinoma, neuroblastoma, choriocarcinoma, and malignant melanoma; however, complete spontaneous disappearance of a malignant tumor is extremely rare.

The usual course of untreated cancer is continuous local and metastatic extension with progressive systemic effects, all of which combine to weaken the host in diverse ways until cachexia and death from sepsis or bronchopneumonia, or both, ensue. About half of the deaths in cancer patients result from infection, the most common being bronchopneumonia, septicemia, and peritonitis. The majority of infections are caused by gram-negative bacilli or fungi. Other causes of death in these patients include organ failure, tumor infarction and hemorrhage, and carcinomatosis (widespread dissemination of the tumor). With treatment, many tumors, though not cured, may persist for years before ultimately causing death. Some patients live many years with cancer even without treatment. Daland studied 100 cases of untreated cancer of the breast and found that 22% of the patients were alive at the end of 5 years and 5% at the end of 10 years; the last surviving patients died 13 years after their first symptoms.

Although an extensive description[196] of cancer therapy is beyond the scope of this chapter, a few general principles should be kept in mind. First, no therapy should be initiated without a definitive diagnosis, including histopathologic or cytopathologic examination and appropriate grading and staging procedures. For some tumors, surgery remains the only effective treatment, and the extent to which surgical management of recurrences is possible will reflect survival. Thus, for adenocarcinoma of the colon or malignant melanoma, surgical treatment is essential, since there are no standard effective chemotherapies or radiotherapies for these diseases. However, in other cases, such as Hodgkin's disease, Wilms' tumor, choriocarcinoma, and acute lymphocytic leukemia, various combinations of chemotherapy, radiotherapy, and surgery often achieve cures. Most tumors show some response to chemotherapy or radiation therapy, and treatment sometimes results in cures and usually gives symptomatic relief (palliation). For example, the severe pain of carcinoma of the prostate from metastases to bone may be controlled for a time by the lowering of androgen levels, surgically or biochemically. Cancer of the breast in premenopausal women may respond favorably to antiestrogens (Tamoxifen), removal of estrogen (oophorectomy, adrenalectomy, hypophysectomy), or testosterone administration.

Anticancer drugs now in use, in addition to hormones and other steroid compounds, include alkylating agents (such as cisplatin), antimetabolites (such as 5-fluorouracil), and miscellaneous drugs, such as actinomycin D. In some instances chemotherapeutic drugs produce a favorable and even a prolonged response. Since such agents interfere with the synthesis of nucleic acids and proteins, not only tumor cells, but also normal cells, are often destroyed, and one of the elusive goals of drug development is identification of agents that have more selective anticancer effects. Standard practice is to rotate anticancer drugs as patients become refractory. Often, however, patients show cross-resistance of chemically unrelated drugs; this phenomenon, known as *multidrug resistance*, often results from amplification of the MDR1 gene, which codes for a P-glycoprotein responsible for more efficient drug efflux.[197,198] The basis of this process is the energy-dependent efflux of these agents mediated by a series of transporters (the ABC cassette superfamily).[199] Although only the MDR1 gene has been identified with certainty, the family is a large one, and cells can acquire multidrug resistance in the absence of MDR1 amplification.[199,200] In addition, in experiments with cultured cells long-term exposure to anticancer drugs results in an altered range of resistance.[201] Thus the phenomenon is complex, and other MDR genes or genes unrelated to the ABC cassette superfamily are likely identified in the near future.

Radiation therapy is often very effective because treatment can be delivered to precise areas without systemic effects. Thus, for example, in some series the survival rates for prostatic cancer after radiation therapy are comparable to surgery. Radiosensitivity refers to the responsiveness of a tumor to ionizing radiation, which, like alkylating agents, brings about cell death by damaging cellular targets (DNA, the mitotic apparatus, cell membranes). In general, poorly differentiated tumors respond to radiation well, and better differentiated tumors respond poorly. There are, however, major exceptions to this. It is important to remember that radiosensitivity and radiocurability are not synonymous. In fact, some of the most radiosensitive tumors are seldom cured by this treatment. This apparent paradox results from the fact that poorly differentiated tumors are often fast growing and have a high proportion of cells in drug-sensitive phases of the cell cycle (the S, M, and G_2), whereas slow-growing well-differentiated tumors may consist largely of G_0 and G_1 cells.

Recently agents referred to under the generic rubric of biologic response modifiers have been used in cancer therapy and chemoprevention. These include the tumor-specific antibodies, interferons, the interleukins, and autologous cells activated in vitro by these and similar factors. There is great enthusiasm among oncologists for the use of these biologic response modifiers, but judged against standard therapies, gains have been modest. Clinical trials are also underway to determine the effectiveness of vitamin A and retinoids in chemoprevention.[151,159-163] These agents presumably act by promoting differentiation.

DEMOGRAPHIC AND FAMILIAL ASPECTS OF CANCER

Demographic and geographic factors

In this section we examine demographic and geographic aspects of cancer and, where possible, relate them to cause. We have already mentioned that in 1995 more than 500,000 people will die of cancer in the United States. For all ages cancer was the second leading cause of death behind heart disease. Lung cancer is now estimated to be the leading cause of cancer death in both men and women (Table 24-9 and Fig. 24-27). In men, lung cancer as a cause of death is followed by prostate cancer, colon and rectal cancer, and leukemias and lymphomas, in that order. Death rates, however, tell only part of the story; for example, the incidence of clinically significant prostate cancer and lung cancer in men is equal, but prostate cancers tend to grow slowly and are more easily controlled, albeit with considerable morbidity. In women, after lung and breast cancer, colon and rectal cancer and leukemias and lymphomas are the leading causes of death.

Over the past 50 years there have been dramatic changes in death rates from some cancers. Lung-cancer death rates have increased more than tenfold in men and almost tenfold in women and probably reflect primarily increases in smoking during this period (see Fig. 24-27). Recently in men the rate of increase has slowed, and this change may reflect a decline in smoking that began in the 1970s. Other important trends include a long-term decline in death rates for gastric cancer in both men and women, a change in the death rates for cancer of the uterus, and a dramatic rise in deaths from malignant melanoma in men and women. The decline in gastric cancer is believed to relate to some change in life-style, perhaps diet, but no generally accepted explanation has emerged. Reduced death rates from uterine cancer probably reflect better diagnosis and treatment as well as changes in life-style. Increases in the incidences of malignant melanoma and other skin cancers reflect population shifts to the sun belt and a more outdoor life-style among Americans. The disease is rare among blacks. It is also instructive to look at death rates from cancer in different countries (Table 24-10).

Even when differences in reporting and diagnosis and treatment are allowed for, differences in death rates can be dramatic. The death rate in Japan from stomach cancer is about seven times that in the United States, whereas death rates from breast and prostatic cancer are about one fourth the United States rates. Worldwide, liver cancer (hepatocellular carcinoma) is one of the more common causes of death from cancer, yet in the Unites States only a small fraction of cancer deaths (about 1% to 2%) are the result of hepatocellular carcinoma.[1,183] In some parts of Africa cancer of the penis is very common, whereas it is rare in the United States.[202] Over the decades, investigators have learned much about the etiology of cancer from these observations. For example, an analysis of Americans of Japanese descent indicated that their death rates from gastric and colonic cancer reflected those of the United States population, not Japan's, thus ruling out a genetic component and suggesting an important role for life-style and environment. The distribution of liver cancer worldwide reflects the distribution of hepatitis B virus and, to some extent, aflatoxin contamination of foodstuffs and has implicated these agents as causes of hepatocellular carcinoma in humans.[185,183] Cancer of the penis is rare in circumcized men; its prevalence in some areas may reflect poor personal hygiene (and exposure to carcinogens and irritants) and endemic papillomavirus infections. Occasionally, there are strong regional trends within a country. In China, Linhsien in Hunan Province has an extremely high incidence of cancer of the esophagus, which appears to be related to nitrosamines consumed in local pickled vegetables. In Uganda, Burkitt's lymphoma is confined to the humid lowlands and is believed to be related to mosquito-borne malarial infections (superimposed upon EBV infection). The role of infection is unknown, but one may speculate that it stimulates cell proliferation in the immune system under circumstances that are favorable for translocations (see section on etiology and pathogenesis).

Familial and genetic factors

Analysis of inherited and familial patterns of cancer incidence have provided important clues to the causes and contributed to prevention. A large number of tumors of childhood and infancy have a familial form; these include retinoblastoma, Wilms' tumor, and hepatoblastoma and are frequently associated with chromosomal abnormalities.[203,204] In retinoblastoma, for example, tumors have been associated with deletions on chromosome 13 (most of which are detectable only by genetic probes).[203] It appears that most familial cases can be explained by the inheritance of a mutation in one copy of a gene and a somatic mutation in the second. It has been suggested that this gene functions to prevent the development of neoplasia (that is, as a tumor-suppressor gene), and its inactivation by mutation results in tumors. Recently the gene has been cloned and is now being studied.[205,206]

Another class of inherited disorders associated with an increased incidence of tumors includes syndromes associated with increased rates of mutation or chromosomal instability, or both. Xeroderma pigmentosum, ataxia telangiectasia, Fanconi's anemia, and Bloom's syndrome are members of this group. Xeroderma pigmentosum is associated with reduced rates of DNA repair and more than a thousandfold increased

Table 24-9 Estimated new cancer cases and deaths, United States—1995*

	Estimated new cases			Estimated deaths		
	Both sexes	Male	Female	Both sexes	Male	Female
All sites	1,252,000	677,000	575,000	547,000	289,000	258,000
Buccal cavity and pharynx (oral)	28,150	18,800	9,350	8,370	5,480	2,890
Lip	2,500	1,900	600	100	80	20
Tongue	5,550	3,600	1,950	1,870	1,200	670
Mouth	11,000	6,900	4,100	2,300	1,300	1,000
Pharynx	9,100	6,400	2,700	4,100	2,900	1,200
Digestive organs	223,000	118,000	105,000	124,330	66,130	58,200
Esophagus	12,100	8,800	3,300	10,900	8,200	2,700
Stomach	22,800	14,000	8,800	14,700	8,800	5,900
Small intestine	4,600	2,400	2,200	1,120	590	530
Large intestine (colon-rectum)	100,000	49,000	51,000	47,500	23,000	24,500
Rectum (colon-rectum)	38,200	21,700	16,500	7,800	4,200	3,600
Liver and biliary passages	18,500	9,800	8,700	14,200	7,700	6,500
Pancreas	24,000	11,000	13,000	27,000	13,200	13,800
Other and unspecified digestive	2,800	1,300	1,500	1,110	440	670
Respiratory system	186,300	108,400	77,900	162,950	99,470	63,480
Larynx	11,600	9,000	2,600	4,090	3,200	890
Lung	169,900	96,000	73,900	157,400	95,400	62,000
Other and unspecified respiratory	4,800	3,400	1,400	1,460	870	590
Bone	2,070	1,100	970	1,280	750	530
Connective tissue	6,000	3,300	2,700	3,600	1,800	1,800
Melanoma of skin	34,100	18,700	15,400	7,200	4,500	2,700
Breast	183,400	1,400	182,000	46,240	240	46,000
Genital organs	333,100	252,200	80,900	67,380	40,980	26,400
Cervix uteri (uterus)	15,800	—	13,800	4,800	—	4,800
Corpus & unspecified (uterus)	32,800	—	32,800	5,900	—	5,900
Ovary	26,600	—	26,600	14,500	—	14,500
Other and unspecified genital, female	5,700	—	5,700	1,200	—	1,200
Prostate	244,000	244,000	—	40,400	40,400	—
Testis	7,100	7,100	—	370	370	—
Other and unspecified genital, male	1,100	1,100	—	210	210	—
Urinary organs	79,300	54,400	24,900	22,900	14,600	8,300
Bladder	50,500	37,300	13,200	11,200	7,500	3,700
Kidney and other urinary	28,800	17,100	11,700	11,700	7,100	4,600
Eye	1,870	1,000	870	240	130	110

*Excludes basal and squamous cell skin cancers and in situ carcinomas except bladder. Carcinoma in situ of the uterine cervix accounts for about 65,000 new cases annually, carcinoma in situ of the female breast accounts for about 25,000 new cases annually, and melanoma carcinoma in situ accounts for about 10,000 new cases annually. Overall, about 120,000 new cases of carcinoma in situ of all sites of cancer are diagnosed each year.

Basal cell and squamous cell skin cancers account for more than 800,000 new cases annually. About 2,100 nonmelanoma skin cancer deaths will occur in 1995.

Incidence estimates are based on rates from NCI SEER program 1989-91.
From *Cancer Facts and Figures*, American Cancer Society, 1995.

(Continued)

risk of skin cancer on exposed skin surfaces.[164,207] Although the causes of the genetic instability are unknown in ataxia telangiectasia, Fanconi's anemia, and Bloom's syndrome, all show increased incidences of neoplasia. Patients with ataxia telangiectasia have an increase in leukemias and lymphomas as well as other cancers.[208,209] There is a large increase in leukemia rates in patients with Fanconi's anemia and in heterozygotic relatives and carriers.[210] Patients with Bloom's syndrome are particularly susceptible to the development of leukemia and to a lesser extent other cancers.[211] Because rearrangements are common in leukemias, cancer development may be related to the high rates of sister-chromatid exchange seen in this syndrome.

A variety of uncommon syndromes is also associated with an increased incidence of human cancer.[212] Two multiple endocrine adenomatosis syndromes predispose to pituitary, parathyroid, and islet cell adenomas (type 1) or to pheochromocytoma, medullary carcinoma of the thyroid and parathyroid hyperplasia/adenoma (type 2). Because the type and occurrence of tumors is so varied in the first of these syn-

Table 24-9 (continued)

	Estimated new cases			Estimated deaths		
	Both sexes	**Male**	**Female**	**Both sexes**	**Male**	**Female**
Brain and central nervous system	17,200	9,700	7,500	13,300	7,300	6,000
Endocrine glands	15,380	3,900	11,480	1,780	760	1,020
Thyroid	13,900	3,200	10,700	1,120	440	680
Other endocrine	1,480	700	780	660	320	340
Leukemia	25,700	14,700	11,000	20,400	11,100	9,300
Lymphocytic leukemia	11,000	6,700	4,300	6,400	3,500	2,900
Granulocytic leukemia	11,100	5,900	5,200	8,400	4,600	3,800
Other and unspecified leukemia	3,600	2,100	1,500	5,600	3,000	2,600
Other blood and lymph tissues	71,200	41,100	30,100	34,450	18,120	16,330
Hodgkin's disease	7,800	4,500	3,300	1,450	820	630
Non–Hodgkin's lymphoma	50,900	29,500	21,400	22,700	12,000	10,700
Multiple myeloma	12,500	7,100	5,400	10,300	5,300	5,000
All other and unspecified sites	45,230	30,300	14,930	32,580	17,640	14,940

Table 24-10 **Age–adjusted cancer death rates per 100,000 people in selected countries, 1988–1991**

	Colon and rectum		Stomach		Breast	Prostate	Leukemia	
Country	**Males**	**Females**	**Males**	**Females**	**Females**	**Males**	**Males**	**Females**
United States	16.7	11.4	5.2	2.3	22.4	16.6	6.3	3.4
Greece*	6.8	5.5	9.6	4.9	15.2	8.1	5.7	3.4
Japan*	15.1	9.7	34.9	15.5	6.3	3.8	4.3	2.8
Mexico*	3.3	3.1	10.5	7.6	8.1	10.6	3.8	3.0
Singapore*	19.1	14.0	20.3	10.6	12.9	4.2	4.2	3.0

From Boring CC, Squires TS, Tong T, Montgomery S: Cancer Statistics, 1994, American Cancer Society, *Ca-Cancer Journal Clin,* 44:7, 1994.
*1988-1990 only

dromes, it has been proposed that a mechanism similar to that described for retinoblastoma may be responsible, except that the gene is expressed in many tissues.[212] Type 2 is inherited in a dominant fashion. One of the genes involved has been localized to chromosome 10 and has been identified as the RET tumor-suppressor gene.[213,214] Neurofibromatosis (von Recklinghausen's disease) is a dominant condition that predisposes to neurofibroma (and sarcoma), pheochromocytoma, meningioma, and glioma. Different pedigrees appear to have different tumor distributions, a finding that may implicate different genes or different allelic variants. Basal cell nevus syndrome is dominantly inherited and results in a high frequency of basal cell carcinomas, as well as osseous, neurologic, and endocrine stigmas. The relation between a dominant mode of inheritance and the appearance of basal cell carcinomas during the second decade on skin exposed to solar radiation is not understood.[212]

Breast cancer, colon cancer, and renal cancer are known to be familial (though not necessarily inherited) to varying degrees. Female relatives of breast cancer patients have a two- to threefold increased risk of developing breast cancer.[215] There are also pedigrees in which cancer of both the female and male breast are inherited, thus demonstrating that genetic events are involved in at least some cases. Studies of changes in oncogene expression and loss of heterozygosity (see section on etiology and pathogenesis) should be helpful in unraveling the relation among hereditary factors, somatic cell mutation, and other factors (such as hormonal status, ethanol consumption, and fat consumption) in the cause of breast cancer. Although colon cancer is not strongly familial, in patients with multiple adenomatous polyposis (a dominantly inherited disorder), the incidence of colon cancer approaches 100%. This observation is significant because most colonic carcinomas are believed to arise in polyps, and prophylactic colectomy is warranted in patients with adenomatous polyposis. We have discussed the molecular changes related to colon cancer in detail in the section on the molecular basis. It is worth noting here that familial habits and cultural patterns expose individuals to fats, mutagens, and tumor promoters in ways that increase cancer rates (see Table 24-10 and Fig. 24-27). Finally, occa-

25 Immunopathologic Mechanisms

Stewart Sell
James L. Wisecarver

Immunity and immunopathology are opposite edges of the proverbial "double-edged sword." Whereas immunity is a state of protection from disease, immunopathology is the study of how immune reactions cause disease. One edge of the sword offers protection; the other edge potentially destroys tissues.

Specific immune reactions are unleashed by reaction of products generated as a result of an immune response. An immune response involves recognition of "foreign" antigens by specific receptors on immune cells, and such recognition triggers proliferation and differentiation of these cells. As a result of exposure to antigens, specific immune reactive cells are activated, leading to production of effector arms of the immune response, proteins (antibodies), and specifically reactive cells. These products have the capacity to recognize, react with, and eliminate the noxious agent or infecting organism. When an individual exhibits an adverse reaction to a previously innocuous exposure because of activation of an immune reaction, the reaction is called *hypersensitivity*. When an individual has no deleterious or minimal reaction to an agent that was previously toxic or destructive, the reaction is called *immunity*. *Allergy* is a term that has different meanings. Von Pirquet, in 1906, used "allergy" to mean altered reactivity because of previous exposure to an agent, without implying whether the altered reaction was beneficial or destructive. This same meaning is generally applied in Great Britain. In the United States *allergy* describes anaphylactic or atopic reactions (see later).

THE IMMUNE RESPONSE

The essence of the immune response is the production of antibody or cells *that protect the host from injury by an invading pathogen.*[1-16]

Antigenicity and immunogenicity

An immunogen is a substance that induces an immune response. Antigens are substances that can react with the products of an immune response. A complete antigen can both induce an immune response (that is, is immunogenic) and react with the products of an immune response. An incomplete antigen can react with immune products but not induce an immune response. *Haptens* are incomplete antigens that can become immunogenic if chemically joined to larger immunogenic molecules (carriers).

As a result of recognition and activation of the immune system to an antigen, the immune system acquires specific information and learns to respond differently to a second exposure to the same antigen. The *afferent phase* is the delivery of the antigen to specifically reactive cells, usually but not always, in lymph nodes. The *central phase* consists of the processing of the antigen by the reacting cells, culminating in proliferation and differentiation of cells producing antibodies or specifically sensitized cells that recognize and react with the antigen. The *efferent phase* is the delivery of the immune products to tissues that contain the antigen, where reaction of the immune products initiates an inflammatory reaction. Protection results if the antigen is an infecting organism or noxious material; the reaction may be destructive if the inflammatory reaction destroys normal tissue.

Immunoglobulins and antibodies

Antibodies belong to a group of structurally related proteins known collectively as "immunoglobulins" (Table 25-1). Four polypeptide chains, two light chains, and two heavy chains are joined by sulfhydral bonds to form Y-shaped immunoglobulins. The paired light chain and heavy chain form an antigen binding site, or *paratope,* located at the top of each arm of the Y. The stem of the Y is composed of the remaining part of the two heavy chains. When an antibody binds with an antigen, the antibody undergoes a change in its tertiary structure, so that the heavy chains that make up the stem of the Y can react with other molecules, such as the serum complement components (see Chapter 17), and activate inflammatory reactions. The manifestations of the reaction of antibodies with antigen in vivo depend on the class of immunoglobulin to which the antibody belongs, the nature of the antigen, and the site in the body where the reaction takes place.

The antigenic structure (determinant) recognized by an antibody is the *epitope*. The epitope of an antigen binds to the *paratope* of the antibody. The paratope is formed by folding of segments of the light and heavy chains at the ends of the Y of the immunoglobulin molecule called *hypervariable regions,* so that these regions fit over the epitope of the antigen in a way that align electrostatic charge, hydrogen bonds, and hydrophilic fields that bind the paratope to the epitope. Most antigens contain many epitopes; the composite reactivity of the epitopes of the antigen is the *epitype*.

Antibodies may serve as epitopes for other antibody molecules. The epitopes recognized by anti-antibodies are called *idiotopes* and the antibodies to them are *anti-idiotypes* (Fig. 25-1). The most important anti-idiotypic antibodies are those that react specifically with the paratope. The antigen binding site of the first antibody serves as the epitope for the second antibody. This is called *molecular mimicry* and has important implications for mechanisms that control the immune response and for autoimmune diseases.

Antibody-antigen reactions

A primary antibody-antigen reaction is the joining of the paratope (binding site) of an antibody to the epitope (antigenic determinant) of an antigen. The resultant antibody-antigen complex is an equilibrium reaction described by the equation:

$$Ag + Ab \rightleftharpoons AgAb.$$

The antibody-antigen complex may initiate different secondary reactions, depending on the antigen, the class of the antibody, and other accessory molecules, such as complement. If the antigen is soluble, the complex may become insoluble and precipitate. If the antigen is a larger particle, such as a blood cell or a microorganism, agglutination may result. Other secondary reactions include complement fixation, immobilization of mobile organisms, lysis of cells, and inactivation (neutralization) of biologically active molecules. A further consequence of secondary reactions is tissue damage.

Humoral versus cellular immune responses

Whereas antibodies play an important role in protecting the host from pathogenic microorganisms present in the blood-

Table 25-1 **Properties of immunoglobulin classes**

IgG		12	140,000	2	+	Major class, precipitating	Toxic complex neutralization, cytotoxic
IgA		2.5	160,000 to 320,000 (dimer)	4	–	Secretory	Toxic complex (rare)
IgM		1	900,000* (pentamer)	10	++	First formed, highly lytic, B cell surface	Cytotoxic
IgE		0.0005	180,000	2	–	Binds to mast cells	Anaphylactic
IgD		0.03	200,000*	2	–	B-cell surface	?

–, None; +, some; ++, more.
*μ and δ chains contain an N-derived polypeptide associated with B-cell membrane insertion.

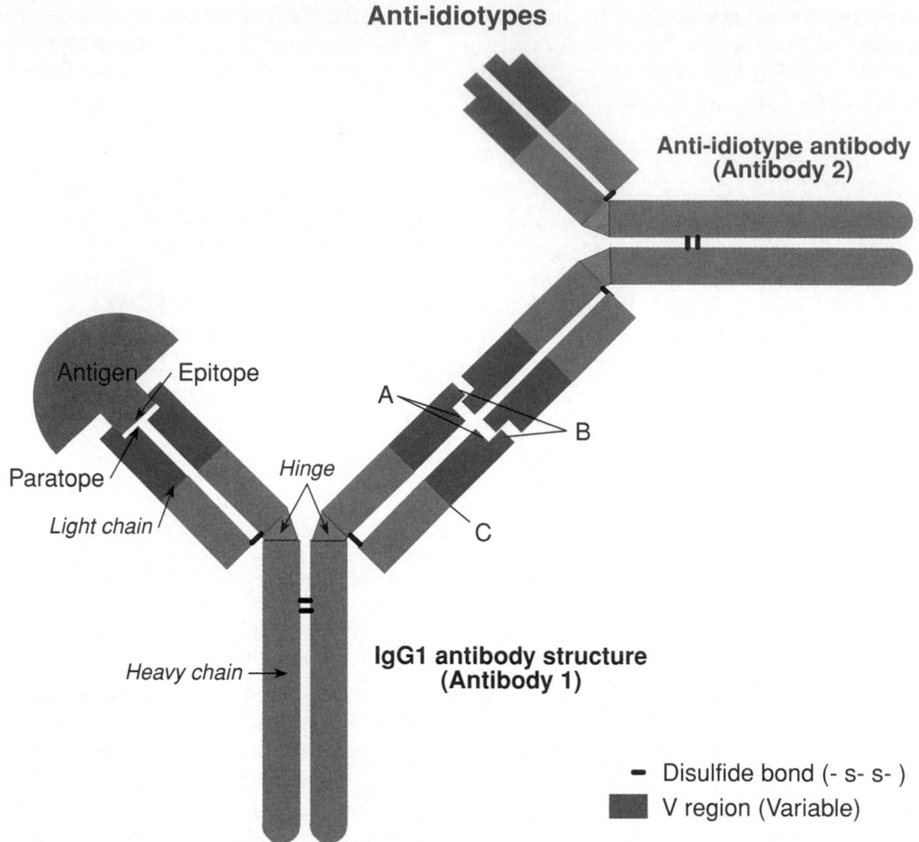

Fig. 25-1 Anti-idiotypic antibodies. Antibodies produced during the immune response to an antigen may in turn elicit an autoantibody response. This antiantibody is termed *anti-idiotype*. The original antibody is termed *antibody 1*; the anti-idiotypic antibody is called *antibody 2*. Anti-idiotypic antibodies (antibody 2) may react with the paratope of the first antibody (site A), with part of the paratope and part of the adjacent nonparatope variable region (site B), or with part of the variable region away from the paratope (site C). When an anti-idiotype antibody binds the paratope, it mimics the antigen (epitope) and provides an *internal image* of the antigen that will block the binding of the antigen to the antibody completely. Anti-idiotype antibody binding to site B will partially block, binding to site C may or may not block antigen binding, depending on the extent of alteration of the tertiary structure.

stream and body fluids, many microbial pathogens have evolved growth patterns that enable them to avoid encountering the antibody response of the host. These organisms enter and reside within the cells of the host, where the cell membrane protects them from circulating antibodies. The cellular immune system protects the host from intracellular pathogens by the recognition and elimination of infected cells. Both the humoral and the cellular immune responses are initiated and mediated by lymphocytes and specialized antigen processing and presenting cells (such as macrophages and dendritic reticulum cells). In most cases, these reactions are controlled to permit destruction and elimination of the invading pathogen. However, these processes may also cause tissue injury.

Cells of the immune system

Immunopathologic reactions are initiated when antibodies or differentiated lymphocytes bearing specific receptors on their surface membranes encounter the appropriate antigen. After specific recognition of antigen, nonspecific accessory cells such as polymorphonuclear leukocytes or macrophages may play critical roles for completion of the reaction (see the discussion of inflammation, Chapter 18). Cells with specific receptors for antigen recognition belong to two major classes of lymphocytes: B-cells and T-cells. B-cells differentiate into plasma cells that produce specific antibodies; specifically reactive T-cells proliferate after contact with antigen and disseminate throughout the body where they are responsible for specific cell-mediated immunity (CMI).

B-cells and T-cells are indistinguishable by light and electron microscopy but are easily identified by immunologic methods. B-cells have cell-surface immunoglobulin. After immune stimulation, B-cells proliferate and differentiate into plasma cells, which synthesize and secrete large amounts of specific antibodies (immunoglobulins). T-cells do not express immunoglobulin but have cell surface molecules expressed at different stages of T-cell development. These molecules are defined by monoclonal antibodies named according to "clusters of differentiation," or CDs (Table 25-2). Different T-cell subpopulations have different functions during induction of an immune response or in the effector stage of the immune response. Major effector lymphocyte populations are listed in Table 25-3. The two major lymphocyte subpopulations responsible for cell-mediated tissue reactions in vivo are the $CD4^+$ delayed-hypersensitivity cells or T_{DTH} cells and the $CD8^+$ cytotoxic T-cells, or T_{CTL}. Both of these types of T-cells recognize antigen through specific T-cell antigen receptors. For this

Table 25-2 Some important T-cell subsets identified by monoclonal antibodies

Cluster of differentiation	Subpopulation/function
CD1	Cortical thymocytes, Langerhans' cells
CD2	Pan T-cell, natural killer (NK) subset
CD2R	Activated T-cells
CD3	T-cell receptor complex
CD4	T-helper subset, MHC class II; HIV receptor
CD5	Mature T-cells, medullary thymocytes
CD8	T-suppressor subset; MHC class I receptor
CD25	IL-2 receptor
CD28	T subset, B7/BB1 antigen receptor
CD45	Common leukocyte antigen (phosphatase)
CD54	Activated T-cells; ICAM-1
CD56	NK and T subset; N-CAM
CD71	Proliferating cells; transferrin receptor

HIV, Human immunodeficiency virus; *ICAM*, intercellular adhesion molecule; *IL*, interleukin; *MHC*, major histocompatibility complex; *N-CAM*, neural cell adhesion molecule.

Table 25-3 Lymphocyte effector cells for cell-mediated immunity

Population	Phenotype	Functional activity
T_{CTL}	CD8	Specific cell-mediated cytotoxicity
T_{DTH}	CD4	Specific DTH, release lymphokines when activated, lymphokines attract and activate macrophages
NK	CD11, 45, 46, 57	Nonspecific, lyse tumor cells
K	Fc, Ig receptors	Antibody dependent cell mediated cytoxicity
TIL	Activated NK	Lyse cells more effectively than NK

CD, Cluster of differentiation; *CTL*, cytotoxic T lymphocyte; *DTH*, delayed-type hypersensitivity cells; *Fc*, fragment, crystallizable (of immunoglobulin); *Ig*, immunoglobulin; *K*, killer cells; *NK*, natural killer cells; *TIL*, tumor-infiltrating lymphocyte.

recognition to occur, the antigen must be delivered in combination with specialized antigen-presenting molecules on the surface of the host's tissues (antigen presentation). The human leukocyte antigens (HLA), encoded within the major histocompatibility complex, serve this function.

Other mononuclear cells participating in immunopathologic processes include natural killer cells (NK cells) and killer cells (K-cells). Although related to T-cells, they lack T-cell receptors for antigens. NK cells react with certain tissue cells in particular, tumor cells, causing their destruction. This activity can be increased by treatment of the cells with interleukin-2 in vitro, a product of activated T-cells, resulting in so-called lymphokine activated killer, or LAK cells. LAK cells are under active investigation for treatment of cancer. K-cells have receptors for the Fc regions of antibodies and are armed by uptake of specific immunoglobulin antibody, so-called antibody-dependent, cell-mediated cytotoxicity, or ADCC. ADCC may be responsible for some forms of human tissue destruction, such as autoimmune thyroiditis, but their immunopathologic function has not been clearly defined.

T-cell receptors

The T-cell receptor (TCR) consists of two major polypeptide chains (α and β), which have variable and constant regions similar to immunoglobulin, and distinct intramembranous and cytoplasmic domains. The variable (V) region of the TCR is connected to the constant region by means of a joining (J) segment. The TCR-β chain contains an additional diversity (D) segment. Immature lymphocytes have several different V-, J-, and, in the case of the β chain, D-segment genes that can be randomly selected and assembled during intrathymic lymphocyte maturation. This provides the necessary structural diversity at the antigen recognition site (Fig. 25-2). Additional junctional diversity occurs when the lymphocyte enzyme terminal deoxynucleotidyl transferase (TDT) randomly adds nonencoded nucleotides to the junctions between the V, D, and J regions before joining. These mechanisms for generating structural diversity result in the production of T-cells having receptors that are capable of recognizing and reacting with the large number of possible antigens that may be encountered. Activation of T-cells occurs when the TCR is able to recognize

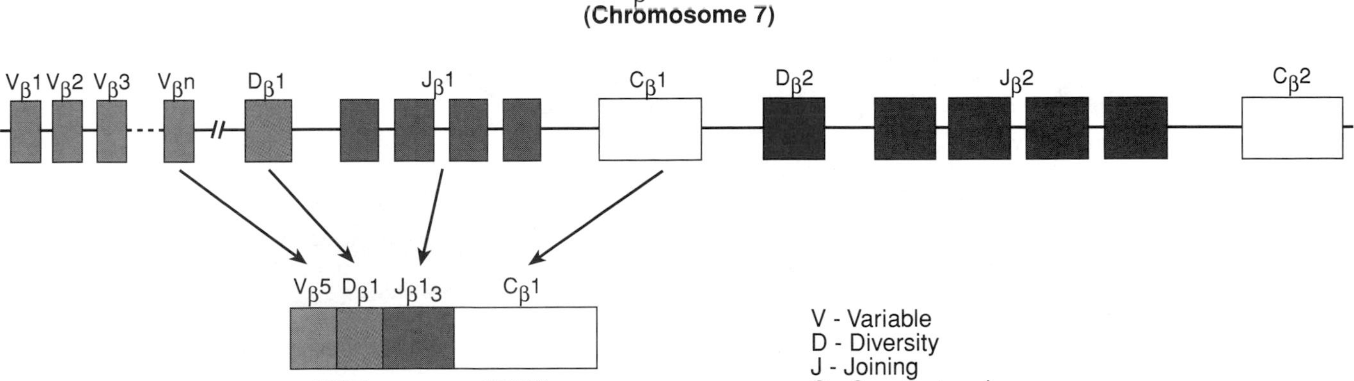

Fig. 25-2 Schema of TCR β chain gene (chromosome 7) rearrangement. One of several different variable regions, *V*, combines with a diversity, *D*, segment and one of several joining, *J*, region genes that then combines with a constant region gene, *C*.

chain. These class II invariant-chain complexes are transported to vesicles within the cytoplasm of the antigen-presenting cell, which fuse with endosomes containing material sampled from the surrounding environment. Within the acidic milieu of these endosomal vesicles, protein antigens gathered from the external environment are degraded into peptides by the action of lysosomal enzymes, and the invariant chain dissociates from the binding groove, permitting peptides of appropriate size and conformation to bind in the groove. These vesicles then fuse with the cell membrane, allowing the class II peptide complexes to be expressed on the surface of the antigen-presenting cell (Fig. 25-6). T-cell receptors on $CD4^+$ T-lymphocytes are configured to interact with the class II–peptide complex, and T-cell activation occurs once antigen recognition and binding occurs.

The differences in the distribution and synthesis between the two classes of MHC molecules is informative as to their role in the immune response. The class I molecules with their widespread distribution and ability to express intracytoplasmic peptides makes them useful in protection against invasion by intracellular parasites such as viruses. In addition to native host peptides, a virus-infected cell expresses viral peptides in the peptide-binding groove of the host cell's class I molecules and these are recognized by $CD8^+$ T-cells with TCRs capable of binding with the class I–peptide complex. This interaction between class I–peptide complex and the TCR results in activation of the $CD8^+$ T-cell with subsequent destruction of the infected cell.

The class II molecules, by virtue of the fact that the peptide-binding site is protected from native or host-cell peptide binding, primarily bind peptides that the antigen-processing cell has scavenged from the external environment. These class II–peptide complexes are recognized by the $CD4^+$ subset of T-lymphocytes. Once the class II–peptide complex recognition has occurred, the $CD4^+$ T-cell becomes activated. It has become apparent that there are differences in the way $CD4^+$ helper T- (T_H) cells respond once they become activated by exposure to antigen. In some instances, the activated $CD4^+$ T-cell also encounters proteins, such as interferon-α (IFN-α), interferon-γ (IFN-γ), and interleukin-12 (IL-12) that have been produced by other activated cells. Exposure to these "cytokines" induces production of a different group of cytokines from the activated T-cell, including interleukin-2 (IL-2), IFN-γ, and tumor necrosis factor β (TNF-β). This set of cytokines acts upon neighboring macrophages and phagocytic cells, triggering activation of intracellular enzyme systems that are effective in killing intracellular microorganisms such as *Mycobacterium* species. The IL-2 and other cytokines produced by these activated T-cells also act upon B-lymphocytes, previously activated by the same antigen, triggering the production of antibodies, predominantly IgM and IgG. Such cells belong to the $CD4^+$ subset known as TH_1.

If, on the other hand, the activated T-cell encounters interleukin-4, the T-cell begins to produce and secrete a different series of interleukins, IL-4, IL-10, and IL-13, that inhibit macrophage activation and instead stimulate B-lymphocytes to

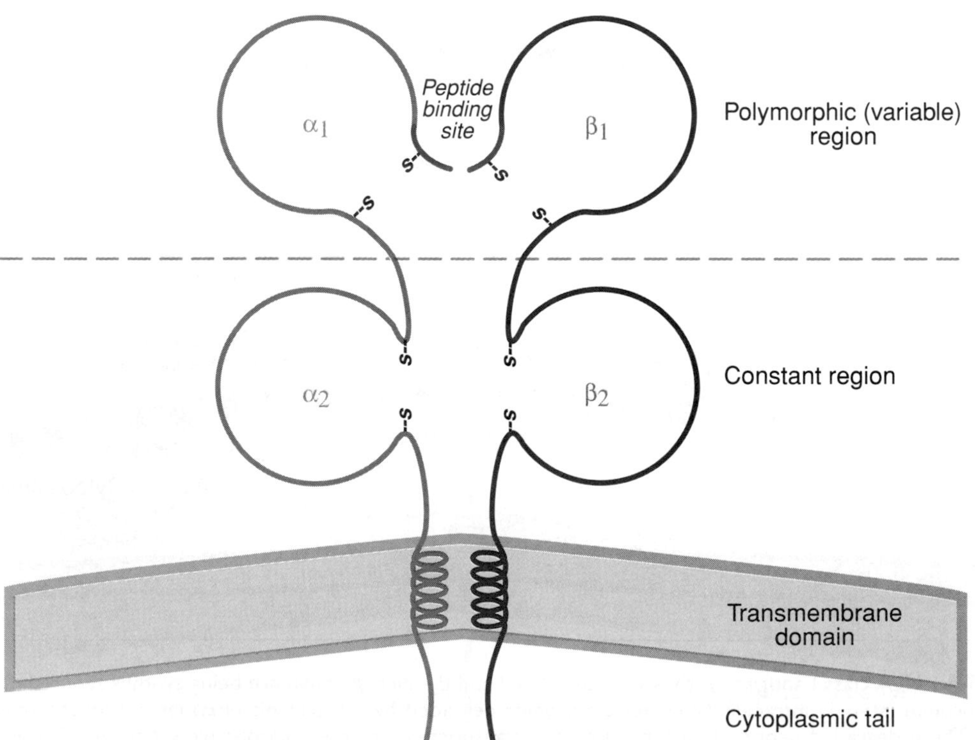

Fig. 25-5 Schema of HLA class II antigen structure. In contrast to the class I molecule, class II molecules are constructed from two noncovalently bound chains (α and β). The peptide-binding groove is located on the outer portion of the molecule, where the a1 and b1 domains are approximated.

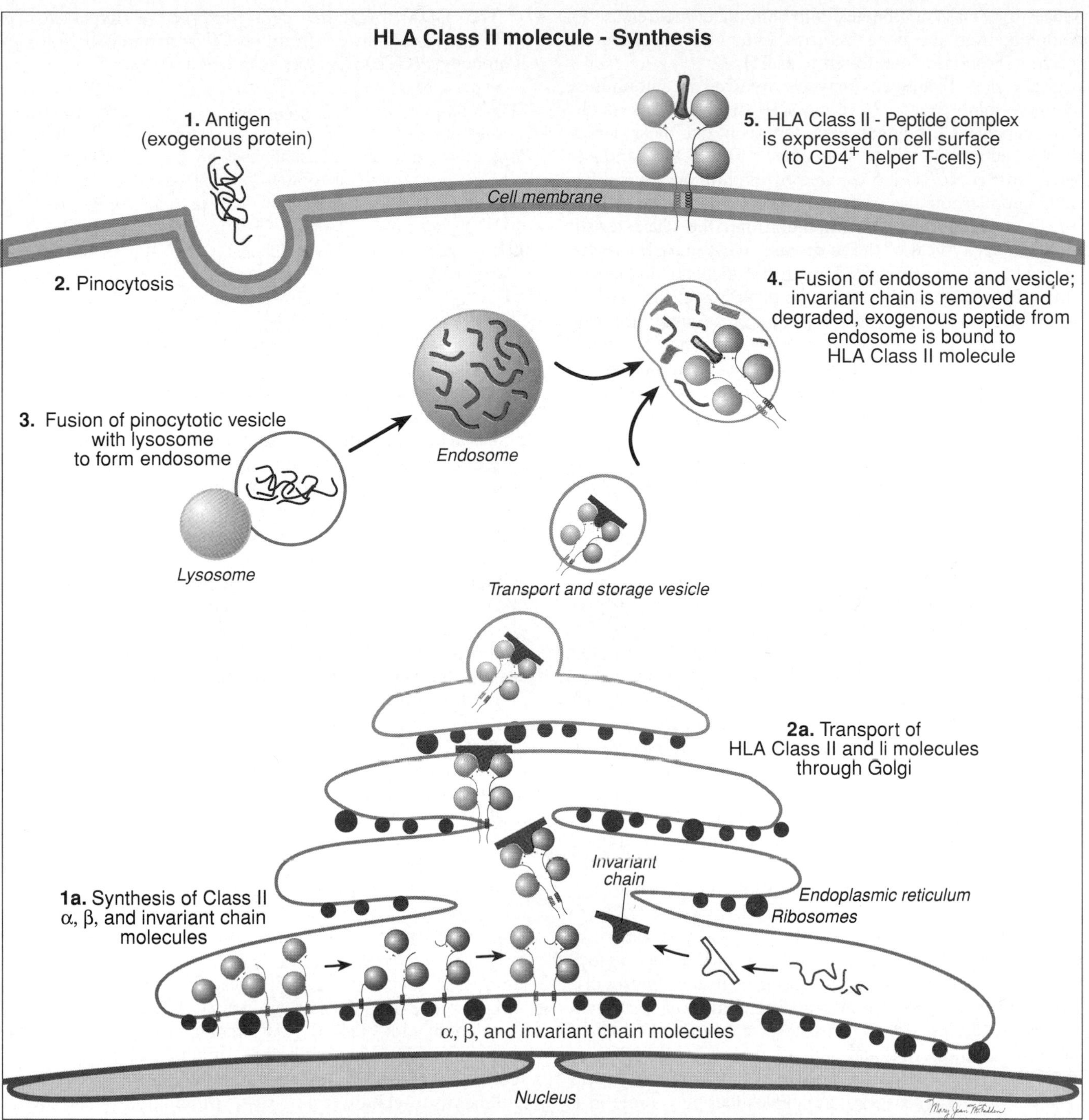

Fig. 25-6 HLA Class II antigen synthesis. Antigen processing and presenting cells (that is, macrophages, B-lymphocytes) are continuously sampling proteins from their immediate environment (steps 1 and 2). Once these have been internalized by pinocytosis, these vesicles then fuse with lysosomes, and the lysosomal enzymes are released into the vesicle, forming an endosome. Concurrently, class II molecules are being synthesized in the endoplasmic reticulum, with the peptide-binding pocket being protected by the invariant chain (step 1a). The newly synthesized class II molecules with the invariant chain attached are then transported to fuse with endsomes (step 2a) containing the exogenously derived proteins, which have been partially degraded by proteases from lysosomes. Within the acidic environment of the endosome, the invariant chain is removed, and a peptide fragment from the exogenously derived proteins is bound into the binding groove on the class II molecule (step 4). The class II–peptide complex then is fused with the cell surface membrane, where the MHC-peptide complex is available to be recognized by $CD4^+$ T-lymphocytes.

produce IgE class antibodies and stimulate the release of eosinophils from the bone marrow. Lymphocytes producing this type of response are referred to as TH_2.

Certain class II antigens may be involved in autoimmune responses. Some patients have class II MHC with a structure that is capable of binding peptides such that host T-cells become activated. For example, HLA-DQ antigens (DQα_1*0501,β_1*0201) are capable of binding and expressing gliadin peptides on the surface of their intestinal epithelial cells. This results in T-cell activation and the characteristic mucosal injury typical of celiac disease. HLA class II associations have also been reported in insulin-dependent diabetes mellitus and rheumatoid arthritis. In these cases, the patient's HLA molecules may bind host peptides, or possibly viral peptides with structural similarity to native tissue components but different enough to elicit a T-cell response. Regardless of the initiating event, the ensuing immune response produces damage to the patient's tissues resulting in autoimmune disease.

Activation of the immune system

The $CD8^+$ T-cell receptor is configured to recognize and interact with class I HLA molecules, whereas the $CD4^+$ TCR is configured to interact with HLA class II molecules. As part of thymic maturation, T-cells bearing receptors incapable of binding to the native HLA molecules are deleted, as are those bearing TCRs that bind and become activated when encountering HLA molecules containing native (self) peptides. The T-cells that survive thymic maturation include those that have specificity for host HLA molecules containing foreign (nonself) peptide epitopes. Once the TCR has recognized and bound to an HLA-peptide complex, several other accessory molecules help to anchor the cells together and to provide the additional signals necessary for T-cell activation. The most important signaling set of molecules is the CD3 complex, a cluster of proteins intimately associated with the TCR. The molecules making up the CD3 complex have long cytoplasmic domains that are responsible for providing the intracellular signals necessary for cell activation. Once TCR-HLA recognition and binding has occurred, tyrosine residues within these cytoplasmic domains are phosphorylated by tyrosine kinases. These phosphorylated domains then associate with these kinase systems resulting in further phosphorylation of other cellular enzymes and activation of membrane lipids. The resulting signals activate protein kinase C, which is involved in transcriptional activation and gene expression (Fig. 25-7).

There are several accessory molecules that play a role in T-cell activation; the CD28 molecule, residing on the T-cell, and its complementary ligand B7 present on the target cell. Antibodies having specificity for these cell surface molecules have been shown to prevent T-cell activation when an appropriate stimulus is provided. A variety of other accessory molecules have been described, but the role they may play is less clear, and discussion of these is beyond the scope of this text. Refer to the references listed at the end of this chapter for a more comprehensive discussion of this subject. In summary, there are several different signaling systems used by cells of the immune system to regulate the magnitude and type of response elicited by an antigen. Ultimately the activation of the T-cell results in cellular proliferation and production of lymphokines (Chapter 17) and other products that act on other white blood cells called *interleukins*.

The $CD4^+$ mediated delayed type of hypersensitivity (DTH) response differs from the $CD8^+$ mediated cytotoxic T-lymphocyte (CTL) response as indicted below:

Primary reaction		Secondary reaction		In vivo effect
T_{DTH} cell + Ag	→	Transcriptional activation Proliferation Lympholine release	→	Macrophage attraction and activation
T_{CTL} + Target cell Ag	→	Transcriptional activation Perforin Granzymes	→	Target cell killing

Activated T_{DTH} cells produce lymphokines that attract and activate macrophages. Activated macrophages are among the most potent killing machines, causing destruction of organisms or tissues at the direction of the specific T_{DTH} cells. T_{CTL} react with antigens on target cells and cause their destruction. This is defensive if the target cells are infected cells or allograft tissue but destructive if the target cells are normal tissue cells.

Whether the cellular or humoral arm of the immune system becomes activated depends on the type of infection or inflammatory reaction that is occurring. According to the present understanding of the immune response, the immunoglobulin class of antibody, or type of T-cell response (T_{DTH} or T_{CTL}), after contact with antigen depends on the route of antigen processing, the nature of the antigen-presenting cell, and the type of T-cell involved.

A brief working model of this process is presented in Fig. 25-8. The current paradigm proposes that the major factor in determining the class of antibody is the type of helper T-cell that is activated. TH_1 cells preferentially stimulate B-cells to produce IgM and IgG, whereas TH_2 cells stimulate IgE and IgA production.

For induction of cell-mediated immunity the additional influence of antigen processing must be considered. Endogenous processing by means of HLA class I delivers antigens to T_{CTL} precursors, which then proliferate and differentiate into cytotoxic T-cells, capable of destroying cells that express this antigen on their class I molecules. Exogenous (or classical) antigen processing delivers antigens to $CD4^+$ helper T-cells in association with class II MHC molecules. This theoretically could result in either antibody production or delayed hypersensitivity (T_{DTH}). Thus an additional event must separate antibody stimulation from T_{DTH} stimulation. This event is most likely antigen processing by different cells. Therefore, antigen processing by follicular dendritic cells in B cell zones of lymphatic tissue results in antibody production; antigen processing by interdigitating macrophages in the T-cell zones (such as paracortex of lymph node) leads to DTH.

Lymphoid tissue and the immune response

The immune response is associated with characteristic changes in the lymphoid tissues, such as lymph nodes, spleen, and mucosa-associated lymphoid tissues (MALT), gut-associated lymphoid tissue (GALT), bronchus-associated lymphoid tissues (BALT), and the secretory immune system or the salivary glands and breast. T-cells develop in the thymus and migrate to the so-called thymus-dependent or T-cell zones of the lymphoid organs. B-cells develop from yolk sack–derived organs (liver and gas-

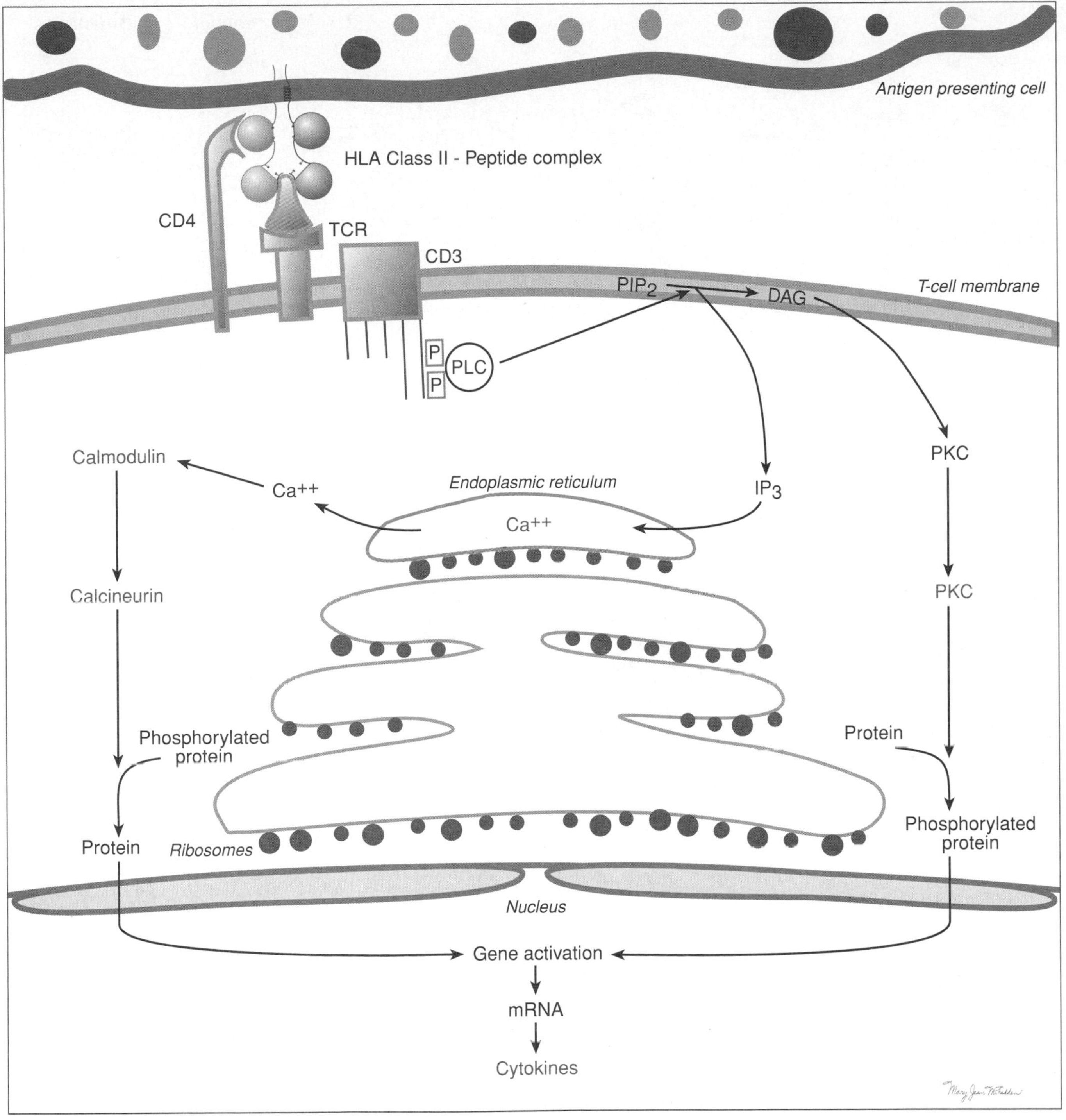

Fig. 25-7 Schema of the events involved in T-cell activation. After recognition and binding to the MHC-peptide complex, the CD3 complex associated with the T-cell receptor on the T-cell surface becomes phosphorylated resulting in cleavage and activation of membrane lipids (phosphatidylinositol biphosphate) to produce diacylglycerol (DAG) and inositol triphosphate (IP_3). Inositol triphosphate causes release of sequestered calcium into the cytoplasm, whereas diacylglycerol activates protein phosphorylation pathways. These mechanisms result in gene activation with the production of cytokines and T-cell proliferation.

trointestinal tract) and migrate to B-cell zones (see Chapter 26). In the lymph node the B-cell zone is represented by follicles; the T-cell zone by interfollicular or diffuse cortical areas.

The size and microscopic appearance of lymphoid organs depend on antigen stimulation. Lymph nodes enlarge and assume a different structure during immune response. Lymph nodes have an outer cortex and an inner medulla. Afferent lymphatics enter the lymph node through the cortex, collect together in the medulla, and leave through efferent lymphatics at the hilum of the node. The cortex is the site of T- and B-cell reactions during an immune response. The B-cells are organized into ball-like clusters in the cortex called follicles; the T-

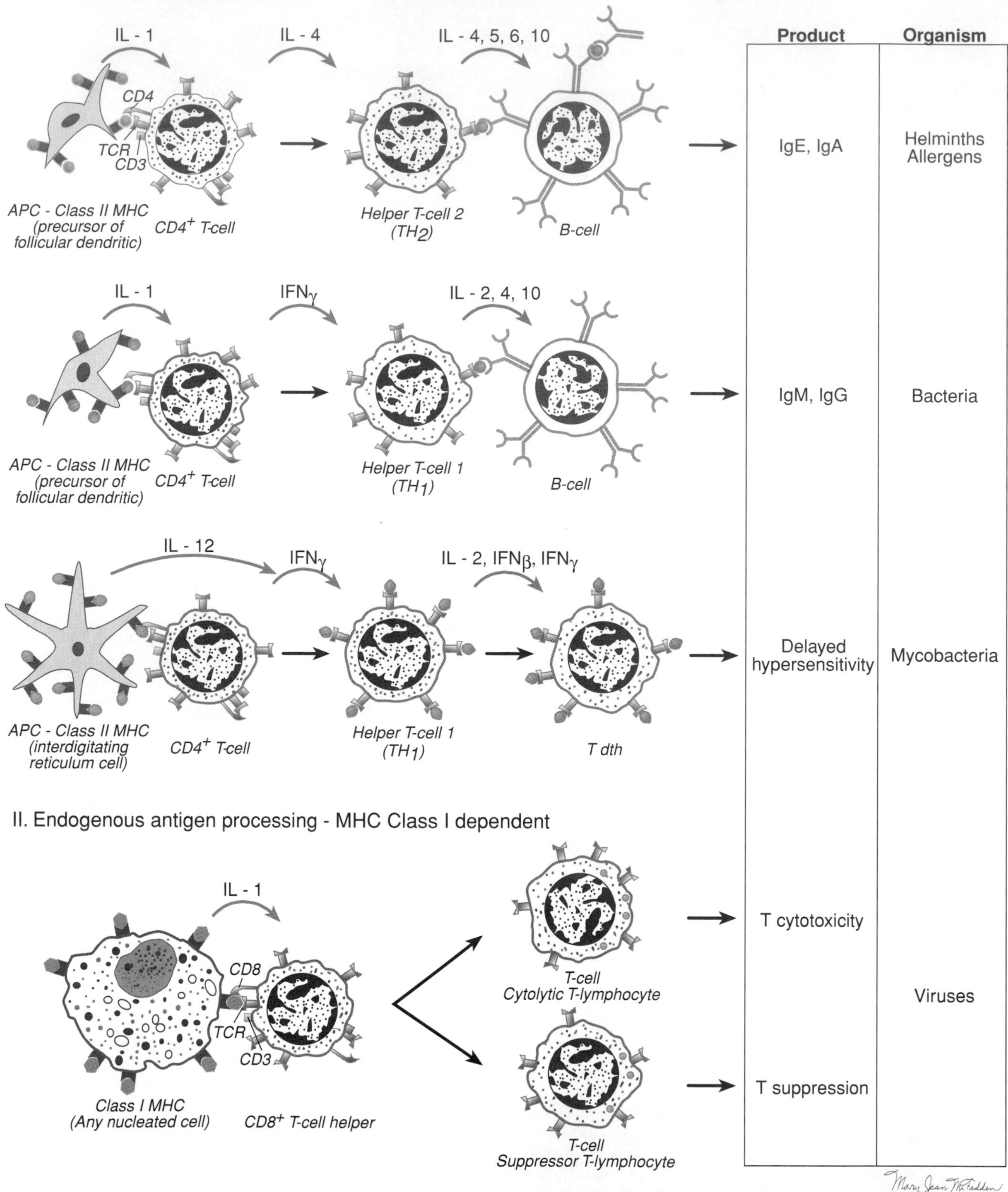

Fig. 25-8 Simplified diagram depicting the role of antigen processing and T-helper cell subsets in different types of immune responses. IgE, IgA, and some IgG subclasses of antibodies result from *exogenous* antigen processing by class II MHC+ dendritic follicular cells, presentation of antigen to $CD4^+$ helper T-cells, activation of TH_2 cells and differentiation of B-cells to produce IgE and IgA. IgM and IgG antibodies are produced by B-cells if *exogenous* processing involves the TH_1 subset of helper cells instead of TH_2. DTH also results from activation of TH_1 cells, but DTH may result from *exogenous* antigen processing by *interdigitating reticulum cells* in the T-cell zones of lymph nodes or spleen. Cytotoxic $CD8^+$ T-cells are produced after *endogenous* antigen processing by class I MHC^+ cells to $CD4^+$ helper cells. DTH cells are $CD4^+$; CTL cells are $CD8^+$.

cells are located in between the follicles. If the follicle is well formed, it has a less dense center surrounded by a dense rim of lymphocytes (secondary follicle). Follicles composed of densely packed lymphocytes without a less dense center are primary follicles.

The type of immune response (either antibody mediated or cell mediated) causes an increase in cell numbers in either the follicular (antibody) or interfollicular (T-cell) zones (Fig. 25-9). Induction of immunoglobulin production is associated with the development of enlarged secondary follicles (germinal centers). Germinal centers form around dendritic macrophages (follicular dendritic precursor cells) that contain antigen. Dendritic macrophages are elongated, spindle-shaped cells, which have cytoplasmic extensions that contact many lymphocytes in the cortex of the lymph node or the white pulp of the spleen. Presentation of antigen through the exogenous pathway by dendritic macrophages to helper T-cells leads to pronounced focal cell proliferation that pushes the nonreacting small lymphocytes to the edge of the spherical mass of proliferating cells. The result is a germinal center with a packed rim (marginal zone) of small lymphocytes (secondary follicle). Within 3 to 5 days after immunization, plasma cells appear below the germinal centers and then migrate into the medullary cords of the medulla where they produce and secrete antibody, which is released into the lymphatic vessels (medullary sinusoids). In addition, there are produced memory B-cells, which enable previously immunized individuals to produce large amounts of antibody more rapidly upon a repeat exposure to the antigen.

T-cells proliferate in the zones of the lymph node cortex between the follicles (paracortical zone) and in the periarteriolar zones of the spleen, which contain a specialized antigen-presenting cell, the interdigitating reticulum cell. A few days after introduction of antigen, "blast" cells with enlarged nuclei and mitotic cells are seen. Hyperplasia of small lymphocytes in this area precedes release of sensitized T-cells into the medullary sinusoids and circulation. Often, both antibody and specifically reactive T-cells are produced. However, the predominance of one type of immune response over another may determine whether there is a protective or a destructive outcome. Understanding these morphologic patterns of hyperplasia is important in the differential diagnosis of non-Hodgkin's lymphoma (Chapter 42).

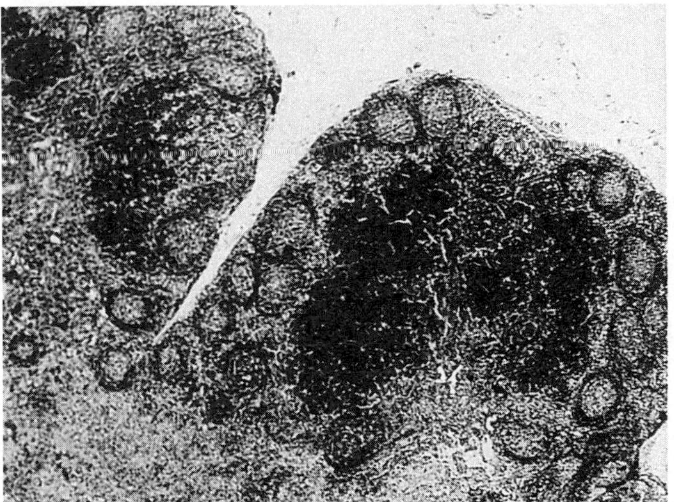

Fig. 25-9 Response of lymph nodes to antigenic stimulation. Induction of antibody formation is associated with prominent germinal center development in the cortex and plasma cell production in medullary cores; delayed hypersensitivity is accompanied by hyperplasia of paracortical zones.

Control of the immune response

Lymphocyte proliferation after antigen stimulation must be controlled, otherwise the individual would succumb to clinical symptoms of lymphoma. Patients who are immunosuppressed and lack T-cell control of B-cell proliferation develop polyclonal B-cell lymphomas similar to Burkitt's lymphoma. In addition, production of an immune response to self-antigens (autoimmunity) may result in immune-mediated injury to an individual's own tissues (Chapter 26).

Proposed mechanisms for controlling the immune responses are as follows: (1) The need for continued antigen exposure to drive the immune response (degradation of the antigen by reaction with antibody or T-cells removes the activation stimulus). (2) Specific circulating antibody provides a feedback signal to block further proliferation of B-cells. Once the antigen is degraded, excess antibody will turn off the response. (3) Specific T-cells (suppressor T-cells) are produced during an immune response that inhibit further proliferation of B-cells and T-cells. (4) Antibody to the specific antibody (anti-idiotype) is produced and acts to block further proliferation of cells through reaction with idiotypic epitopes on cells with receptors for the antigen. (5) Reactive T-cell and B-cell populations may have an inherent refractory period after stimulation.

The diversity of proposed mechanisms for control of the immune response indicates our poor understanding of this important phenomenon. Loss of control of proliferation may underlie the development of lymphocytic leukemia or lymphoma and certain autoimmune diseases.

Immune effector mechanisms

The immune response requires that, after production of specific antibody or of specifically reactive T-cell immunity, the immune individual reacts differently to subsequent exposure to the antigen. This altered reactivity is expressed by the activation of immune effector mechanisms either individually or in combinations of different mechanisms. Four immune effector (immunopathologic) mechanisms were proposed by Gell and Coombs in 1963, but an expanded classification identifying three additional mechanisms is used in this chapter (Table 25-4). The first four immune effector mechanisms listed in Table 25-4 are mediated by reaction of specific antibodies with antigen in vivo. T-cell cytotoxic and delayed hypersensitivity reactions are mediated by specifically sensitized lymphocytes. Granulomatous reactions may be initiated by either antibody

Table 25-4 Classification of immune mechanisms

Original classification, Gell and Coombs (1963)	Classification used in this chapter
—	1. Inactivation or activation
Type II	2. Cytolytic
Type III	3. Immune complex
Type I	4. Anaphylactic
—	5. Cell-mediated cytotoxicity
Type IV	6. Delayed hypersensitivity
—	7. Granulomatous reactions

Table 25-5 The "double-edged sword" of immune reactions

Immune effector mechanism	Protective function, or "immunity"	Destructive reaction, or "allergy"
Neutralization	Diphtheria, tetanus, cholera, endotoxin neutralization, blockade of virus receptors	Insulin resistance, pernicious anemia, myasthenia gravis, hyperthyroidism
Cytotoxic	Bacteriolysis, opsonization	Hemolysis, leukopenia, thrombocytopenia
Immune complex	Acute inflammation, polymorphonuclear leukocyte activation	Vasculitis, glomerulonephritis, serum sickness, rheumatoid diseases
Anaphylactic	Focal inflammation, increased vascular permeability, expulsion of intestinal parasites	Asthma, urticaria, anaphylactic shock, hay fever
Cell-mediated cytoxicity	Destruction of virus-infected cells, cancer cells	Contact dermatitis, autoallergies, viral exanthems, graft rejection
Delayed hypersensitivity	Destruction of infected macrophages, tuberculosis, syphilis, leprosy	Autoallergies, postvaccinial encephalomyelitis, multiple sclerosis
Granulomatous*	Leprosy, tuberculosis, helminths, fungi, isolation of organisms in granulomas	Berylliosis, sarcoidosis, tuberculosis, filariasis, schistosomiasis

Modified from Sell S: *Hum Pathol* 9:24, 1978.
*Granulomatous reactions, like other inflammatory lesions, may result from nonimmune stimuli as well as from an immune reaction inactivated by antibody or by sensitized cells.

or cells and have poorly degradable antigens as an essential feature.

Each immune effector mechanism has defensive and destructive capabilities (Table 25-5). Antibody-mediated effector mechanisms provide important protection against bacteria; cell-mediated reactions operate against viruses, mycobacteria, and fungi. Neutralization or inactivation of biologically active toxins released by infectious organisms is clearly beneficial, but inactivation of hormones or enzymes required for normal tissue function is pathologic. Antibody-mediated cytotoxic or lytic reactions are highly desirable when reacting against infecting organisms but not desirable when they react against blood cells. The acute inflammatory effects that result from release of mediators from mast cells during an atopic (allergic) reaction aid in defense against infecting organisms but also cause debilitating effects in asthmatics. Spasmodic contractions and massive diarrhea produced as a result of gastrointestinal anaphylaxis may serve to eliminate parasites but is not welcome as an allergic reaction to food allergens.

As a consequence of immune complex formation in vivo, inflammatory mediators are produced that increase vascular permeability, promote adherence of acute inflammatory cells to vascular endothelium, and activate polymorphonuclear leukocytes. Although providing defense against bacteria, the same inflammation caused by immune complex deposition in vessel walls causes destructive vasculitis or glomerulonephritis. T-cell cytotoxicity is effective against virus-infected cells and causes their destruction but also may kill normal cells in autoimmune diseases. Delayed hypersensitivity reactions mobilize and activate the macrophages against intracellular infections, such as tuberculosis and leprosy, but the same reaction may produce extensive tissue damage and loss of normal function. Granulomatous reactions function to isolate or localize insoluble toxic materials or microorganisms, but the collections of chronic inflammatory cells that result may replace normal tissue and eventually produce disease, as in chronic tuberculosis.

At the abnormal dose level used in the laboratory or in medical practice, or with the use of nonphysiologic routes of entry (intravenous injection), reactions that rarely occur naturally may result, such as anaphylactic shock, serum sickness, transfusion reactions, and graft rejections. Chemicals or drugs in medical practice can produce allergic drug reactions or iatrogenic diseases. There are also numerous naturally occurring immune-mediated diseases: hemolytic anemias, leukopenias, erythroblastosis fetalis, allergies, polyarteritis nodosa, glomerulonephritis, contact dermatitis, granulomatoses, and so on. For these diseases, infectious agents often do not appear to be the initiating cause.

INACTIVATION AND ACTIVATION OF BIOLOGICALLY ACTIVE MOLECULES

Antibodies to important biologic molecules (such as hormones, hormone receptors, blood clotting factors) may cause disease by inactivating the function of the molecule.[17-36] Alternatively, antibodies to cell receptors can activate the secretory function of the cell, producing disease by hyperactivity of the cells.

Antibodies may inactivate biologically active molecules or receptors by five major mechanisms (Fig. 25-10).

Steric hindrance. Antibody binding blocks interaction of hormone and receptor.

Conformational inactivation. Antibody binding to a hormone or receptor alters tertiary structure of the hormone so that it cannot bind to the receptor or alters the receptor so that it no longer is able to transduce an activation signal after binding to the hormone.

Immune elimination. Antibody binding to hormone produces aggregated Fc's of immunoglobulin, which binds to reticuloendothelial cells resulting in increased catabolism of the hormone. In some situations, such as insulin, binding of antibody to a hormone may prolong the blood half-life of the hormone. Paradoxically, this can increase serum concentrations of insulin while diminishing insulin function.

Receptor modulation. Antibodies to cell surface receptors may induce endocytosis of the receptor so that it is no longer available for reaction with a stimulating ligand.

Antibody-dependent cell-mediated cytotoxicity. Antibodies reacting with receptors may direct NK lymphocytes, which react with the aggregated Fc regions of the immunoglobulin bound to the cells and cause destruction of the receptor.

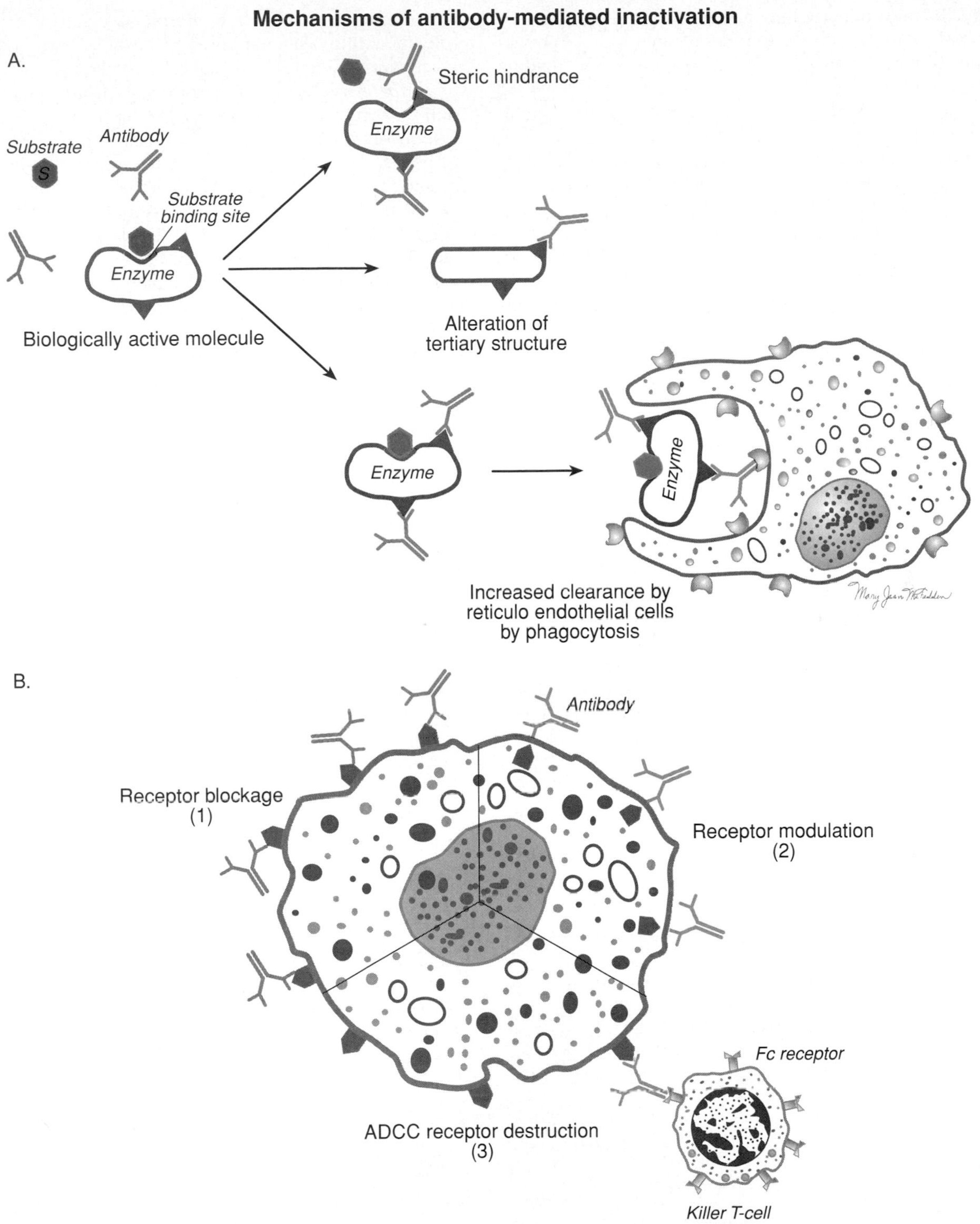

Mechanisms of antibody-mediated inactivation

Fig. 25-10 Different mechanisms effect the inactivation or activation of biologic molecules. **A,** Reaction of antibody with the binding site for a ligand for an enzyme or other biologically active molecule may result in loss of biologic function because of steric hindrance of binding of the substrate with its receptor. However, direct inactivation usually is attributable to alteration of the tertiary structure of the enzyme after reaction with antibody. This reaction affects the structure of the substrate binding site indirectly or inactivates the enzyme molecule. In vivo, increased catabolism of an enzyme-hormone complex may lead to decreased availability of the active molecule. **B,** Antibodies to cell surface receptors have several effects, as illustrated clockwise. They may block or stimulate the receptor *(1)*, or cause receptor modulation by endocytosis *(2)*, or trigger destruction of the cell by antibody-dependent cell-mediated cytotoxicity (ADCC) *(3)*.

Antibodies may enhance the biologic functions of enzymes or other molecules by binding to the molecule, or by mimicking the function of the biologically active molecule by binding directly with its receptor.

Conformational stabilization. Biologically active molecules may exist in inactive and active conformations. Antibodies to the active form of the enzyme β-galactosidase convert the inactive conformation of the enzyme to the active conformer, thus increasing enzyme activity.

Increased binding affinity. Divalent antibodies may increase binding between a ligand and a receptor. The activity of epidermal growth factor on the growth of fibroblasts in vitro may be increased by divalent antibodies but not by univalent fragments.

Receptor selection. Antibodies to one epitope on a hormone may block the ability of the hormone to react with one receptor and direct hormone binding from one receptor to another. Human growth hormone has at least four distinct epitopes defined by monoclonal antibodies. Antibodies to one of these epitopes blocks binding to target cells in vitro, but increases activity when injected into experimental animals.

Buffering. Most hormones are rapidly degraded by enzymes. Some antibodies prevent degradation of the hormone. "Superactive" forms of insulin are protected by binding to serum albumin; this "carrier" function may also be provided by antibodies to insulin. Enhanced effects of prolactin and TSH may also be produced by this mechanism.

Receptor activation. Antibodies with paratopes that mimic a hormone may directly bind to the hormone receptor, triggering the expected response of the receptor binding its natural ligand. A well-understood example are antibodies to thyroid epithelial cells.

Some specific antibodies to biologically active molecules are listed in Table 25-6. Diabetes mellitus and hypothyroidism are offered as examples of hormone inactivation; hyperthyroidism and myasthenia gravis are examples of activation and inactivation of cell receptors, respectively.

Diabetes mellitus. Diabetes results from impaired production or decreased utilization of insulin as a result of impaired insulin secretion, from a loss of insulin receptors or receptor response, or because of a blocking of insulin activity, each producing an increase in blood glucose and related abnormalities of metabolism (Table 25-7). About 20% of patients have "insulin-dependent," or type I, diabetes (that is, the insulin receptors or responsive cells are normal, but insulin availability is low); the remaining 80% have "insulin-independent," or type II, diabetes (insulin availability is normal, but the number of receptors is low).

At least four different antibodies are associated with diabetes mellitus: antibodies to insulin, to islet cell cytoplasm (glutamic acid decarboxylase), to islet cell surface antigen, and to insulin receptors. In type I diabetes there is a loss of beta cells in the pancreas as a result of immune attack early in life (juvenile diabetes), or there may be neutralizing antibodies to insulin. It is likely that the islet cells are destroyed by a T-cell mechanism and the loss of beta cells is associated with a lymphocytic infiltrate. Insulin-neutralizing antibodies develop after insulin-replacement therapy and are responsible for insulin resistance. In type II diabetes there may be loss of receptors secondary to antibody to receptors. However, most patients with type II diabetes have neither anti-insulin nor antireceptor antibodies.

Hypothyroidism and hyperthyroidism. Most of the common thyroid diseases other than cancer are immune in origin: hypothyroidism, hyperthyroidism, and thyroiditis. Autoantibodies to thyroid antigens are found in many individuals with normal thyroid function (particularly with aging) as well as associated with thyroid diseases. Antibodies to thy-

Table 25-6 Antibody-mediated diseases of immune inactivation/activation

Disease	Antigen
Diabetes mellitus	Insulin Insulin receptor Islet cell cytoplasm (glutamic acid decarboxylase) Islet cell surface
Thyroid disease	
Hyperthyroidism	Thyroid-stimulating hormone receptor
Hypothyroidism	Triiodothyronine
Pernicious anemia	
Atrophic gastritis	Parietal cells
Megaloblastic anemia	Intrinsic factor
Infertility (induced)	Chorionic gonadotropin estrogen, progesterone
Aplastic anemia	Erythropoietin
Chronic asthma	β-Adrenergic receptor
Myasthenia gravis	Acetylcholine receptor
Polyendocrinopathy	Multiple (adrenal, thyroid, parathyroid, gonads, pancreas, melanocytes)
Hemophilia, other blood diseases	Blood-clotting factors (multiple)

Table 25-7 Immunologic factors in diabetes mellitus

Type	Etiologic factor
Immune	
Type Ia juvenile onset	T-cell or ADCC-mediated destruction of beta cells, Early, but not late, anti–islet cell antibody; HLA-DR3, DR4 associated
Type Ib juvenile onset	T-cell or ADCC-mediated destruction of beta-cells, Both early and late islet cell antibody, associated with endocrinopathies
Insulin resistent	Anti-insulin antibodies in response to injection therapy
Insulin receptor (type II)	Autoimmune insulin receptor antibodies
Nonimmune	
Type II maturity onset	May develop insulin resistance
Secondary	Pancreatic disease (type III, hormonal (corticosteroid excess, etc.), drug induced

ADCC, Antibody-dependent cell-mediated cytotoxicity.

roid hormone or thyroid-stimulating hormone (TSH) may be responsible for hypothyroidism, whereas antibodies to the thyroid receptor for TSH may produce hyperthyroidism (Graves' disease). Antibody-dependent or cell-mediated immunity to thyroid antigens causes inflammation of the thyroid (thyroiditis) and may lead to destruction of the thyroid gland (Chapter 61).

Autoantibody to thyroid-stimulating hormone receptors that cause hyperthyroidism is termed *long-acting thyroid stimulator (LATS)*. LATS is an antibody that can, on the one hand, inhibit the binding of TSH to human thyroid membranes and, on the other hand, stimulate thyroid cyclic AMP and thyroid hormone release. Animals that are immunized with thyroid hormone not only produce blocking antibodies, but also may produce a thyroid-stimulating globulin as a result of an autoanti-idiotypic response (see below). Thus, either hyperthyroidism (Graves' disease) or hypothyroidism may result from an autoimmune response. Which result depends on the degree of tissue damage and the type and amount of autoantibody produced.

Myasthenia gravis. Myasthenia gravis is characterized by muscle weakness and easy fatigability; weakness is most prominent in the muscles of the face and throat. There is a functional abnormality of conduction of nerve impulses from the motor nerve to the muscle fiber. Neuromuscular transmission is mediated by acetylcholine (ACh) released from vesicles in the neuronal axon that bind to acetylcholine receptors (AChR) in the motor end plate. Immune-mediated myasthenia gravis is caused by antibodies that block or cause loss of acetylcholine receptors (Chapter 76).

CYTOLYTIC REACTIONS

Mechanisms

Cytotoxic or cytolytic reactions occur when antibody binds to the cell membrane and activates either of two complement-mediated pathways: (1) activation of the complete cascade with insertion of membrane attack complexes and lysis of the target cell, or (2) formation of aggregated immunoglobulin Fc or C3b binding producing "immune adherence" of antibody-coated cells to phagocytic cells resulting in phagocytosis (Fig. 25-11).[37-53] Destruction of affected blood cells occurs extravascularly by phagocytosis and destruction of antibody or complement-coated cells in the spleen and liver, but intravascular cell lysis may also occur. Blistering diseases of the skin are also mediated, in part, by cytolytic reactions (see Chapter 71).

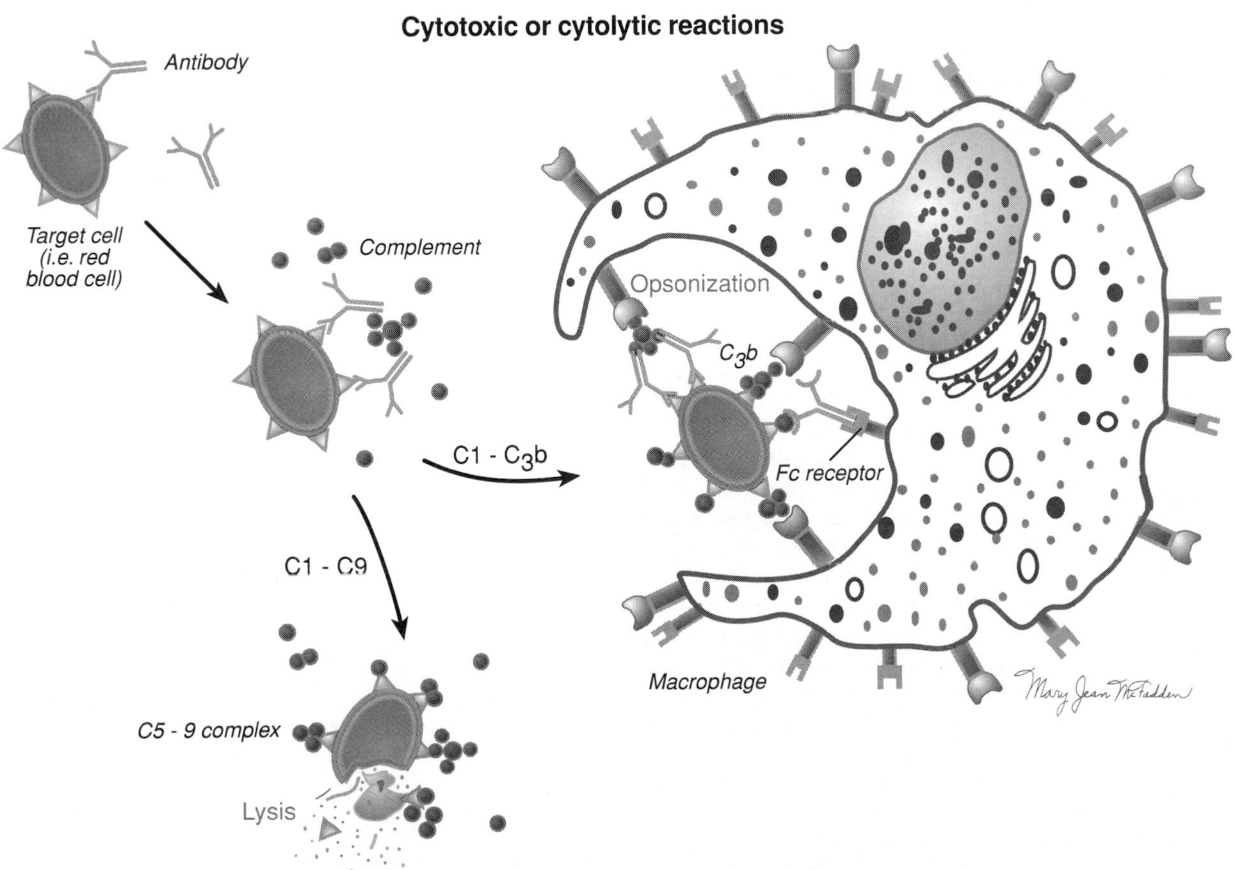

Fig. 25-11 Cytotoxic or cytolytic reactions. These reactions most often affect cellular elements in intimate contact with circulating plasma, such as erythrocytes, leukocytes, or platelets. Circulating humoral antibody reacts with antigens present on cell membranes. In vitro, through action of the complement system, the integrity of cell membrane is compromised and the cell is lysed. The osmotic difference in intracellular and extracellular fluids causes release of intracellular fluids. In vivo, the cells coated with immunoglobulin antibody or complement are subject to phagocytosis and sequestration in the spleen and liver.

Cytotoxic or cytolytic reactions are initiated by IgM or those IgG subclasses that activate complement. As discussed in Chapter 18, selected IgG subclasses bind complement better than others do; for example, IgG_3 and IgG_1 are more active than IgG_2 and IgG_4. IgM is the most efficient complement-fixing antibody. Because IgM is a pentamer, one IgM antibody molecule bound to a cell provides an aggregated heavy-chain structure that is sufficient to activate complement, whereas two IgG molecules in close apposition are required to produce an Fc aggregate. IgM antibodies are approximately 600 times more efficient in fixing complement than antibodies of the IgG class. IgG-coated erythrocytes are cleared predominantly in the spleen via Fc and C3b receptors, whereas IgM-coated cells are sequestered predominantly in the liver through C3b receptors. Clearance of IgM-coated cells is entirely complement dependent, whereas clearance of IgG-coated cells is not, since the clearing phagocytic cells have receptors for aggregated Fc regions of IgG_1.

The ultimate clinical effect depends on the type of cell involved, antibody characteristics, the number of antigen sites per cell, and the amount of antibody available. The cells usually affected are red blood cells (erythrocytes), white blood cells, and platelets. The resulting diseases are hemolytic anemia, agranulocytosis, and thrombocytopenia; they are grouped together as immunohematologic diseases.

Representative diseases

Several disease conditions result from the immune destruction of red blood cells. These disorders include transfusion reactions, erythroblastosis fetalis, acquired autoimmune hemolytic diseases, and hemolytic reactions to drugs (Fig. 25-12).

Transfusion reactions. A cytolytic reaction occurs when circulating antibody of host origin contacts erythrocytes from an incompatible donor. The red blood cells of an incompatible donor possess antigens not found on the recipient's cells. Blood group antigens are genetically controlled cell-surface structures present on blood cells. The major antigens belong to the ABO group. Isoantibodies are defined as antibodies to antigens within the same species. Individuals who lack an ABO blood group antigen produce isoantibodies to it. If a B-negative individual is transfused with type B blood, the anti-B antibodies coat the B erythrocytes. This coating sensitizes cells to lysis by complement or destruction by the spleen.

Over 14 human red blood cell antigen systems, which include over 60 different blood group factors, are known. The ABO and Rh systems are the most important to identify for transfusion because these represent the majority of antibodies implicated in clinical transfusion reactions. Transfusion reactions are usually predictable from blood group typing, serum screening for anti-erythrocyte antibodies, and cross-matching.

Erythroblastosis fetalis. The condition erythroblastosis fetalis, also termed *hemolytic disease of the newborn*, is caused by maternal antibodies that cross the placenta and attack fetal erythrocytes. The conditions for hemolytic disease exist when a pregnant woman who lacks Rh antigens (Rh^-) carries a fetus that has Rh^+ erythrocytes. An Rh^- mother may become sensitized to Rh^+ erythrocytes, produce antibody that crosses the placenta, and destroy the fetal erythrocytes. Destruction of fetal erythrocytes occurs by the action of antibody and complement or by an antibody-dependent, cell-mediated mechanism. Thus red blood cells (RBC) from infants with maternal anti-Rh may be coated with maternal antibody and killed by fetal lymphocytes or macrophages that react with the antibody on the RBC surface through Fc receptors (ADCC). The spleen and liver of an affected fetus exhibit extramedullary hematopoiesis, as an attempt to compensate for the destruction of fetal erythrocytes. Because of the severe destruction of red cells, high concentrations of one hemoglo-

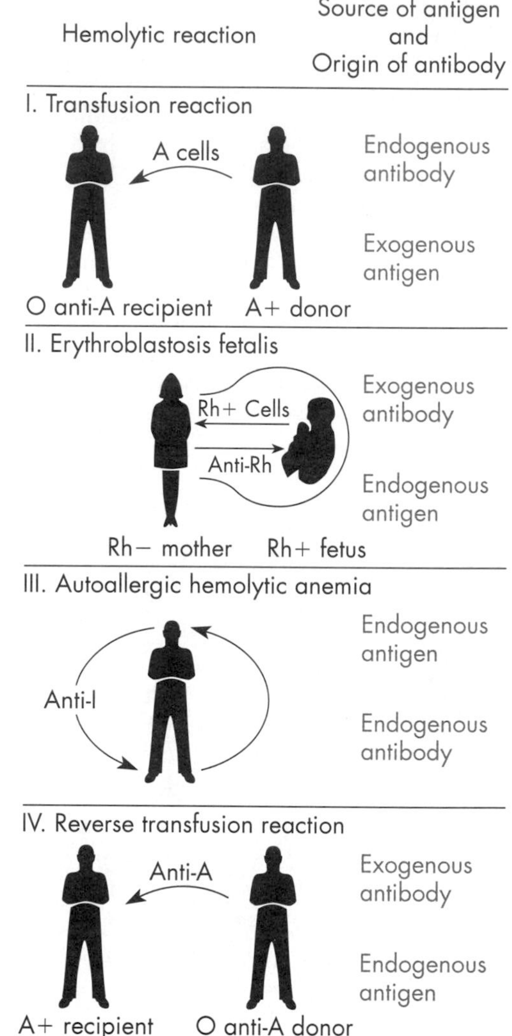

Fig. 25-12 Hemolytic reactions. Depicted are four types of hemolytic reactions caused by antibody-mediated complement activation classified by the source of the antibody and antigen. I. *Transfusion reaction.* Erythrocytes from a donor (A+) that contain antigens not present in the recipient whose serum contains antibody to the donor's blood group antigen (O anti-A) will be lysed immediately upon transfusion, resulting in release of hemoglobin from the lysed cells and a syndrome known as a transfusion reaction. **The origin of the antibody is exogenous; the source of the antigen is endogenous.** II. *Erythroblastosis fetalis.* Fetal erythrocytes containing Rhesus antigens (Rh+) cross the placenta and stimulate the production of maternal antibody to the Rh antigens if the mother is Rh–. These maternal antibodies may cross back through the placenta to attack fetal erythrocytes. **The origin of the antibody is exogenous; the antigen, endogenous.** III. *Autoimmune hemolytic anemia.* Autoantibodies react with self-antigens. **Endogenous antibody and antigen.** IV. *Reverse transfusion reaction.* Antibodies to recipient red blood cells are transfused from a donor. This passively transferred antibody causes lysis of the recipients cells. **Endogenous antigen and exogenous antibody.**

bin breakdown product, bilirubin, during the immediate neonatal period may lead to brain damage secondary to deposition of bilirubin in the brain (kernicterus).

In contrast, ABO hemolytic disease of the newborn is usually mild to minimal clinically, even if the mother's blood contains high titers of anti-A or anti-B antibodies and the fetus's blood is A, B, or AB. There are three possible explanations for this phenomenon: (1) anti-A antibodies and anti-B antibodies are usually IgM and therefore do not cross the placenta; (2) ABO blood group antigens are widely distributed in the fetal tissues and the placenta, and so the effect on fetal erythrocytes of any IgG anti-A or anti-B antibodies that may cross the placenta is diluted out in the sense that antibodies react with many other tissue sites, not just blood cells; and (3) ABO blood group carbohydrates are not fully expressed on fetal erythrocytes.

Acquired autoimmune hemolytic disorders. In the conditions of acquired autoimmune hemolytic disorders individuals form antibodies to antigens present on their own erythrocytes. Immune and congenital hemolytic diseases differ in that congenitally defective erythrocytes do not survive normally in either the patient or a "normal" individual.

Leukocytes (agranulocytosis)

Antibody effects similar to those described above for erythrocytes may also occur with polymorphonuclear leukocytes, resulting in loss of neutrophils (neutropenia or agranulocytosis). Most cases of agranulocytosis are secondary to a lack of proliferation of granulocytes in the bone marrow on a nonimmune basis, either congenital or drug induced. Autoimmune neutropenia (AIN), which may be primary or secondary, accounts for about 10% of clinically recognized neutropenia. Two major forms of AIN are primary and secondary. Primary AIN is seen in children before 3 years of age. Secondary AIN occurs with the highest frequency between 40 and 60 years of age, usually associated with autoimmune thrombocytopenia, connective tissue disease, or lymphoma. Antibodies to granulocytes in AIN are detected by immunofluorescence or agglutination. The bone marrow usually shows normal cellularity or hypercellularity, with a 50% reduction in mature neutrophils. The peripheral blood shows neutrophil counts around 250 cells/μl. Patients are affected by bacterial infections of the skin, upper respiratory tract, and middle ear. Treatment is usually symptomatic with antibiotics. Spontaneous remissions occur in most patients, and immune globulin or steroids may induce remission in prolonged cases. Low white cell counts in a neonate may be caused by destruction of fetal white blood cells coated by antibodies that cross the placenta from the mother after immunization of the mother to fetal leukocyte antigens. Destruction of a patient's own white blood cells may also be caused by autoantibodies or by antibodies to certain drugs that adhere to white blood cells and function as haptens. Sulfapyridine and aminopyrine are two of the drugs that have been implicated. The consequence of leukocyte destruction is a decreased ability to defend against infection.

Thrombocytopenia

Immune reactions to platelets may cause destruction of platelets with resulting purpura and other hemorrhagic manifestations. The word *purpura* ('purple') describes hemorrhage into the skin and is easily recognized by the red or purple discoloration produced by the presence of extravasated red blood cells. The color is first red but becomes darker (purple) and fades to a brownish yellow as the red blood cells are destroyed or cleared from the site of hemorrhage by macrophages. Since platelets function to prevent such hemorrhages, a loss of platelets permits purpuric lesions to develop. An antiplatelet antibody can be demonstrated in about 60% of the affected individuals. Recent studies reveal that, in some diseases, antigen-antibody complexes cause thrombocytopenia. Currently, sensitive immunoassays are being developed, and they should increase the sensitivity of antiplatelet antibody tests. Thrombocytopenia may also occur congenitally or secondarily because of an increased splenic function (hypersplenism) or other nonimmune platelet consumptive disorders. Neonatal thrombocytopenia and drug-induced autoimmune purpura occur as for other immunohematologic diseases.

Drug reactions

At least five mechanisms underlie cytotoxic reactions because of antibodies to drugs (Table 25-8). Drugs may attach to cell membranes where they function as haptens, forming a cell-drug complex that induces an immune reaction. The resulting antibody binds with the drug on the cell surface, causing lysis of the cell. Immune complexes of antibody and drugs found in the circulation may adhere to cell membranes, act to fix complement, and cause lysis of the cell. Such immune complexes may bind to other cells, causing destruction. In this case the red blood cell is an "innocent bystander" because it does not contain the antigen responsible for the hemolytic reaction.

Table 25-8 Examples of drug-induced hemolytic reactions

Type	Mechanism	Antibody producing direct antiglobulin test positivity	Examples of causative drugs
Hapten	Antibody reactions with drug on cell membrane	Anti-IgG	Penicillin
Immune complex	Antibody-drug complex binds to cells	Anticomplement (C3d)	Quinidine, stibophen
Neoantigen	Antibody reacts to new antigen (frequently Rh)	Anti-IgG	α-Methyldopa
Complement transfer	Complement binds to normal cells after antibody activation	Anticomplement (C3d)	Penicillin
Nonspecific	IgG attaches to altered membrane	Anit-IgG and anticomplement (C3d), or both	Cephalosporins

Drugs may induce structural changes in the carbohydrates expressed in developing cells so that the mature cells express a "new" antigen that is autoimmunogenic. The autoantibody reacts with the patient's own cells in the absence of the drug. Normal erythrocytes may also be destroyed by complement activated by reaction of antibody with another cell if the complement fragments are not inactivated rapidly or are produced in such large amounts that inactivation of all active components cannot be accomplished quickly. Some drugs alter the cell membrane so that some plasma proteins attach to the membrane. If immunoglobulin attaches and forms aggregated Fc regions, complement activation and hemolysis may occur.

IMMUNE COMPLEX REACTIONS

Mechanisms

Immune complex–mediated inflammation is caused by antibody reacting directly with tissue antigens (usually basement membrane antigens) or by antibody reacting with circulating antigen to form soluble antigen-antibody complexes that become deposited in tissues.[54-72] In addition, antibodies may react with movable cell surface antigens, which are then shed. If shedding occurs into the circulation, these complexes are removed by the reticuloendothelial system. However, if the complexes are shed into adjacent basement membrane, they may initiate immune complex inflammation. Despite different initiating events, the subsequent inflammatory reaction, mainly mediated by complement, is essentially the same (Fig. 25-13). IgG antibody reacting with tissue antigens accumulates to form aggregates of complement-fixing Fc regions in tissues. Soluble complexes, formed in the circulation by a single IgG molecule reacting with a soluble antigen, form aggregates of IgG when two or more complexes from the blood are deposited closely in tissue. Shed antibody-antigen complexes contain aggregated antibody molecules. These deposits of antigen-antibody complexes provide aggregations of Fc regions of immunoglobulin that fix complement with activation of the anaphylactic and chemotactic activities of C4a, C3a, and C5a. This results in the attraction and activation of neutrophilic polymorphonuclear leukocytes. Upon reaction with the aggregated immune complexes these neutrophils release lysosomal enzymes and reactive oxygen metabolites that cause destruction of the elastic lamina of arteries (serum sickness), basement membrane of the kidney glomerulus (glomerulonephritis), walls of small vessels (Arthus reaction), articular cartilage of joints (rheumatoid arthritis), or basement membrane of skin (pemphigoid).

The alternate pathway for complement activation, entered by activation of C3 (the C3 shunt), is active in the pathogenesis of some types of lesions that are similar to immune complex–mediated lesions. Activation of either the classical or alternate pathway results in formation of C3a and C5a, production of complement chemotactic factors (mostly C5a), accumulation of polymorphonuclear cells, and destruction of tissue. Complement mediators such as anaphylatoxin (C4a, C3a, and C5a) may induce endothelial cell contraction and open cell junctions so that soluble complexes can be deposited in basement membranes or inflammatory cells can enter into tissue spaces (see Chapter 17).

Arthus reaction

The Arthus reaction was first described by Marcus Aruthus in 1903 as a dermal inflammatory response caused by the reaction of a precipitating antibody with antigen placed in the skin. The deposition of antibody and antigen in the tissues may be compared to the double-diffusion precipitation in agar (Ouchterlony) reaction. The mechanism of this reaction is complement-mediated neutrophil attraction and activation after deposition of immune complexes in vessel walls.

The tissue reaction consists of edema, erythema, and hemorrhage, which develops over a few hours, reaching a maximum in 3 to 5 hours or even later if the reaction is severe. Gross necrosis is seen in reactions of high intensity when there is local thrombosis. Histologically there is polymorphonuclear leukocyte and platelet thrombosis, edema, hemorrhage, vascular fibrinoid necrosis, and massive diapedesis of neutrophils (Fig. 25-14). Neutrophils are seen within the vessel wall in early reactions and later lose their granules as they migrate perivascularly, giving rise to the term *leukocytoclastic vasculitis*. Damage to the vascular wall and thrombosis may lead to necrosis of the surrounding tissues. Immune complexes can be demonstrated within the wall of vessels (Fig. 25-15).

Serum sickness

Untoward systemic effects of the administration of xenogeneic serum were noted by von Bering in 1891, when hyperimmune horse serum was introduced for the treatment of children with diphtheria, and the syndrome of serum sickness was first described in detail by von Pirquet and Schick in 1905. Serum sickness manifests as fever, arthritis, glomerulonephritis, and vasculitis appearing 10 days to 2 weeks after passive immunization with horse serum (that is, horse antitetanus toxin). The disease is the result of the production of circulating antibody to the injected horse serum. The lesions of serum sickness directly correlate with the presence of soluble immune complexes. In experimental models, the lesions of serum sickness appear at the time of immune elimination when soluble complexes in antigen excess are present in the serum. Immune complexes in antibody excess or equivalence are cleared by the reticuloendothelial system (RES) because of the presence of aggregated Fc region of IgG or C3b. The phagocytic cells of the reticuloendothelial system have receptors for aggregated Fc regions and C3b. However, soluble complexes in antigen excess (toxic complexes) are not cleared efficiently by the reticuloendothelial system and deposit in vessels and glomeruli, where accumulation of complexes results in aggregation of Fc regions and complement activation.

Representative diseases

Glomerulonephritis

Immune complex disorders are the most common cause of glomerulonephritis (Fig. 25-16). Lesions are caused either by deposition of blood-borne antibody-antigen complexes, such as that seen in serum sickness, by direct reaction of antibody with glomerular basement membrane antigens, or by antibodies to renal epithelial cell surface antigens that shed and deposit in the glomerular basement membrane (Heymann nephritis). The critical feature of the glomerulus is that the capillary basement membrane is not completely covered by endothelial cells. This permits antibody to basement membrane, circulating soluble immune complexes, or shed cell sur-

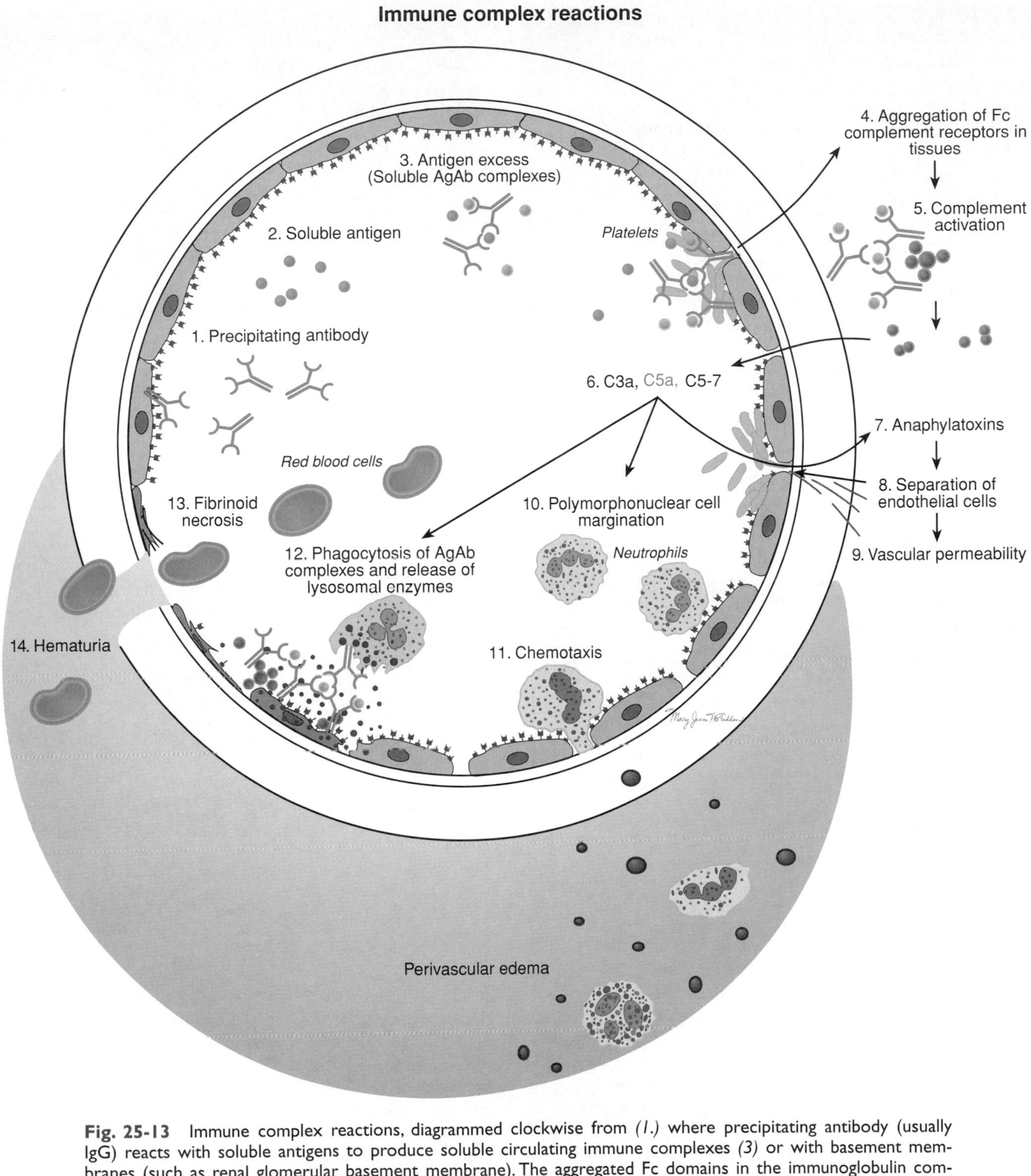

Immune complex reactions

1. Precipitating antibody
2. Soluble antigen
3. Antigen excess (Soluble AgAb complexes)
4. Aggregation of Fc complement receptors in tissues
5. Complement activation
6. C3a, C5a, C5-7
7. Anaphylatoxins
8. Separation of endothelial cells
9. Vascular permeability
10. Polymorphonuclear cell margination
11. Chemotaxis
12. Phagocytosis of AgAb complexes and release of lysosomal enzymes
13. Fibrinoid necrosis
14. Hematuria

Platelets

Red blood cells

Neutrophils

Perivascular edema

Fig. 25-13 Immune complex reactions, diagrammed clockwise from *(1.)* where precipitating antibody (usually IgG) reacts with soluble antigens to produce soluble circulating immune complexes *(3)* or with basement membranes (such as renal glomerular basement membrane). The aggregated Fc domains in the immunoglobulin complexes cause activation of complement *(4)* with formation of inflammatory (phlogistic) complement fragments. Fragments C3a, C4a, and C5a (anaphylatoxin) cause constriction of vascular endothelium resulting in increased vascular permeability *(7-9)*. C5a is also chemotactic for polymorphonuclear leukocytes, and C3b enhances phagocytosis *(10-12)*. Released lysosomal polymorphonuclear enzymes digest tissues, producing "fibrinoid" necrosis *(13)*. Fibrinoid means 'fibrinlike' and refers to the histologic appearance of the acellular amorphous areas produced by "digestion" of tissue by lysosomal enzymes, which resemble the appearance of fibrin in clotted blood.

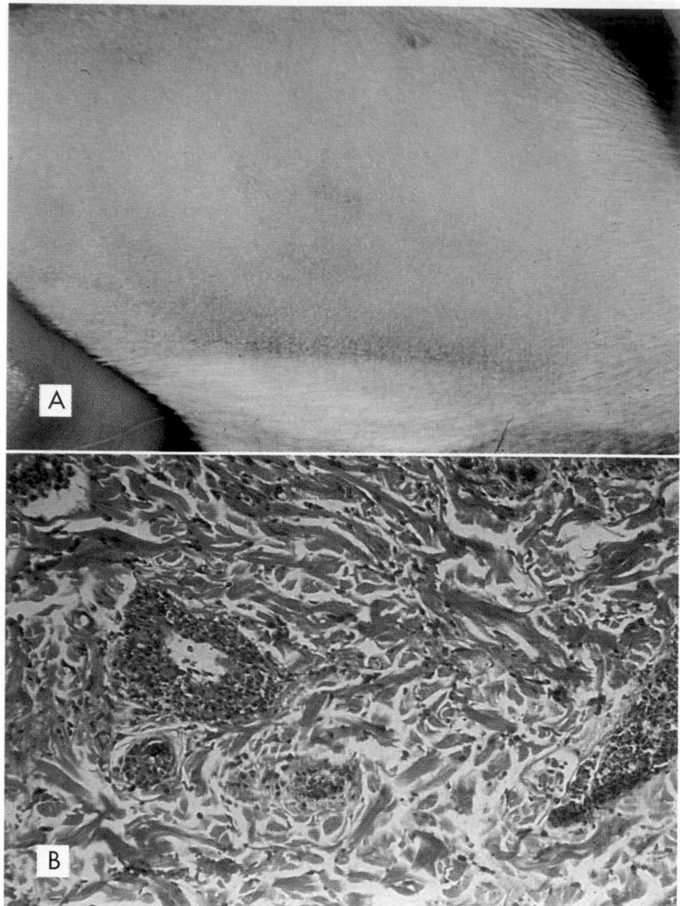

Fig. 25-14 Arthus skin reaction. **A,** Gross appearance of Arthus reactions 6 hours after intradermal injection of antigen into sensitized guinea pig. Dark color in center is caused by escape of red blood cells in sites where blood vessels have been severely damaged. **B,** Microscopic appearance. The blood vessel wall is infiltrated with polymorphonuclear neutrophils, and these induce focal fibrinoid necrosis. Vascular damage permits leakage of blood cells and fluid into the dermis, producing edema and erythema. If the reaction is severe, thrombosis of affected vessels occurs and there may be central necrosis of the lesion.

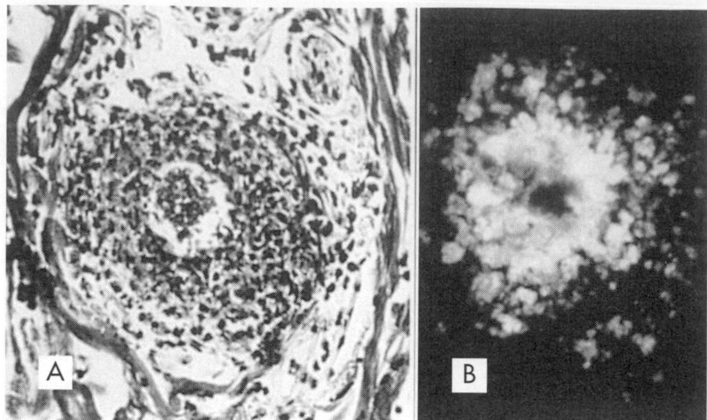

Fig. 25-15 Serum sickness vasculitis (coronary artery) induced in a rabbit after a single large dose of intravenous bovine serum albumin (BSA) as antigen. Photomicrographs of different sections of the same tissue block stained by hematoxylin and eosin, **A,** and fluorescent anti-BSA, **B,** showing localization of antigen in the vessel wall. Lesions occur at the time of antigen elimination from the serum. (Courtesy Frank J. Dixon, La Jolla, California.)

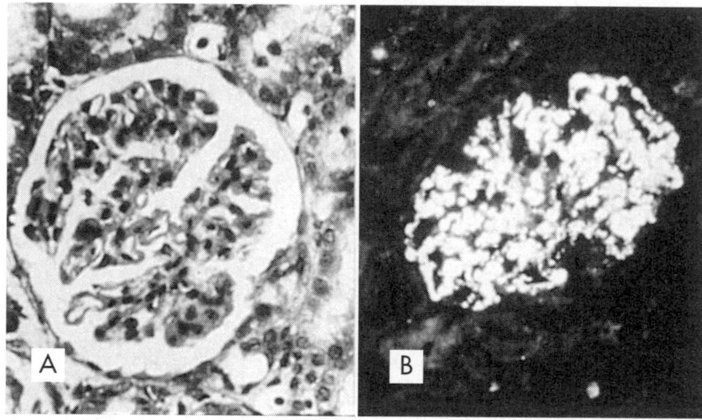

Fig. 25-16 Membranous glomerulonephritis in rabbits after small daily intravenous injections of bovine serum albumin (antigen). Photomicrographs of different sections of the same tissue block stained by hematoxylin and eosin, **A,** and fluorescent anti-BSA, **B.** (Courtesy Frank J. Dixon, La Jolla, California.)

face antigen-antibody complexes to filter into the basement membrane. Complement activation (anaphylatoxin) or mast cell mediators may produce further separation by causing contraction of endothelial cells and further exposure of the membrane. The deposition of aggregated Fc regions leads to inflammation and destruction of the basement membrane. In addition, the membrane attack complex of complement (MAC) may be deposited in the basement membrane. MAC deposits in the glomerular basement membrane are associated with a protein called *clusterin.* The exact pathologic role of MACs and clusterin in the glomerular basement membrane is not known, though lytically active MACs could contribute to glomerular damage and the MAC-clusterin deposits could contribute to membrane thickening. The pathology of glomerulonephritis is discussed in detail in Chapter 65.

Vasculitis

Inflammation of vessels is a primary feature of many immune complex–mediated diseases, including many of the manifestations of connective tissue diseases. The endothelial lining of the blood vessels usually repels white blood cells and has been called *Teflon-like*. This protective barrier becomes less effective when vasculitis develops, allowing the deposition of immune complexes on vascular endothelial surfaces, where they aggregate to fix complement, which in turn attracts and activates granulocytes. Often biopsies are performed on the lesions at a stage of development when the neutrophils have passed through the wall of the vessel and have partially disintegrated. This is referred to as *leukocytoclastic vasculitis.* Autoantineutrophil antibodies may form to proteases (C-ANCA, cytoplasmic immunofluorescence) or to myeloperoxidase (P-ANCA, perinuclear immunofluorescence) released from neutrophils and their presence in the sera aids the diagnosis of vasculitis.

Other immune complex lesions

Inflammation secondary to immune complex deposition is likely to occur in many human diseases that are poorly understood. *Cellular interstitial pneumonia* is an inflammatory disease of the alveolar walls associated with deposition of IgG and C3 and circulating soluble immune complexes. *Arthritis* and *vasculitis* frequently occur transiently during infections. *Uveitis* is associated with circulating immune complexes and immune complexes in the aqueous humor of the anterior chamber of the eye. Granular deposits of immune deposits are found in the basement membrane of thyroid follicles in certain forms of *thyroiditis*. *Orchitis* in men with certain forms of infertility also is associated with immune complex deposits in the basement membrane of the seminiferous tubules. In these diseases immune complexes may be secondary phenomena and not causative of lesions. Immune complex vasculitis and glomerulonephritis are components of *renal graft rejection* (see below).

ATOPIC AND ANAPHYLACTIC REACTIONS (ALLERGY)

The term *anaphylaxis* was coined by Portier and Richet in 1902 to indicate adverse reactions in dogs to a toxin derived from the sea anemone. They expected that repeated injections of the toxin would lead to antibody neutralization of the toxic effect, but instead elicited lethal responses after repeated doses of the toxin that were previously innocuous. Although the word "anaphylaxis" literally means 'without protection,' the term as used by Portier and Richet implied a reaction that is the opposite of prophylaxis, that is, a destructive rather than a protective reaction. Coca applied the term *atopy* in the 1920s for a variety of peculiar reactions in humans, at that time not yet described in other species. The origin of this term is from the Greek word *atopia*, meaning 'strangeness.' Although the association of seasonal allergic rhinitis *(Catarrhus aestivus)* with grass pollen in England and in the United States *(autumnal catarrh)* with ragweed was reported in 1872, a general name for this group of "diseases" was not forthcoming until much later. The word *allergy* was introduced by Pirquet in 1906 to designate "altered reactivity" as a result of previous exposure. Allergy is now mostly used for atopic or anaphylactic reactions, in particular for hay fever, but is also used indiscriminately as a general term for reactions of discomfort of unknown origin. Acute reactions (wheal and flare and systemic shock) are generally referred to as *anaphylactic*; chronic recurring reactions (hay fever) are referred to as *atopic*. However, this distinction is not always made, and there is considerable overlap in the use of the terms. An atopic individual is one who is prone to develop this type of allergic reaction.[73-101]

Mechanisms

The effects produced by allergic (atopic or anaphylactic) reactions are the result of a two-phase inflammatory system initiated by mediators that are released by the reaction of antigen with effector cells passively sensitized by IgE antibody (Fig. 25-17). Antigens that elicit these responses are also called *allergens*. The *mast cell* (tissue) or *basophil* (peripheral blood) is the major effector cell for acute reactions, whereas T-cells and eosinophils play important roles in persistent lesions (Fig. 25-18).

Acute phase mediators

After reaction with allergens, mast cells release several biologically active substances including histamine, heparin, and serotonin (early phase reaction), as well as arachidonic acid, which is converted by other cells into prostaglandins and leukotrienes responsible for the later-phase inflammation reactions (Fig. 25-19). The acute phase is characterized by immediate smooth muscle constriction or dilatation. On the one hand, the smooth muscle of arterioles is stimulated to dilate by reaction of histamine with H_2 receptors, causing increased blood flow locally (erythema) or shock systemically. On the other hand, the smooth muscle of pulmonary bronchi (asthma), gastrointestinal tract (cramps and diarrhea), and the genitourinary system, as well as endothelial cells (edema), are stimulated to contract by action of histamine on H_1 receptors (Table 25-9). The effects of these agents include contraction of smooth muscle, increased vascular permeability, early increase in vascular resistance followed by collapse (shock), and increased gastric, nasal, and lacrimal secretion. The type of lesion observed depends on the dose of antigen, the route of contact with antigen, the frequency of contact with antigen, the tendency for a given organ system to react (shock organ), and the degree of sensitivity of the involved individual. This final factor may be genetically controlled or may be altered by environmental conditions (temperature), unrelated inflammation (presence of a viral upper respiratory infection), or the emotional state of the individual. Some of the reactions seen clinically are anaphylaxis, urticaria (wheal and flare, hives), asthma, and hay fever.

Late-phase mediators

The later acting prostaglandins and leukotrienes cause infiltration of affected tissues with polymorphonuclear leukocytes, eosinophils, and other hallmarks of acute inflammation 6 to 12 hours after allergen exposure. Leukotriene E_4 (slow-reacting substance of anaphylaxis) causes later vasoreactions, whereas leukotriene B_4 is chemotactic for acute inflammatory cells. This late phase causes an indurated, erythematous, painful reaction in the skin or, in the lung, a more prolonged deterioration in airflow as compared with the rapidly appearing wheal-and-flare skin reaction or asthma characterized by rapidly reversible bronchoconstriction of the immediate or early phase.

Chronic reactions such as hay fever and persistent asthma are accompanied by a lowering of the threshold to atopic stimuli. This hyperreactivity is associated with chronic tissue infiltration with mast cells, macrophages, T-cells, B-cells, and eosinophils. The increased numbers of inflammatory cells, as well as smooth muscle hypertrophy, sets up conditions whereby lower levels of stimulation may trigger fits of sneezing or asthmatic attacks. One school of thought implicates TH_2 cell stimulation of eosinophil differentiation by IL-3, IL-5, and GM-CSF leading to platelet release of leukotrienes (LTC_4/LTD_4) and platelet-activating factors that contribute to the chronic inflammation in atopic conditions. However, the relative importance of this mechanism to those of the other possible mechanisms remains to be clarified. (For more details on inflammatory mediators see Chapter 17).

Reaginic antibody

Specific allergic reactions are mediated by the IgE class of antibodies, which have a special ability to bind to skin or other tissues. The term *atopic reagin* was adopted to refer to the "tissue-fixing" property of the antibody. The original use of the word *reagin* was to designate the reacting serum component responsible for the Wassermann reaction, the serologic

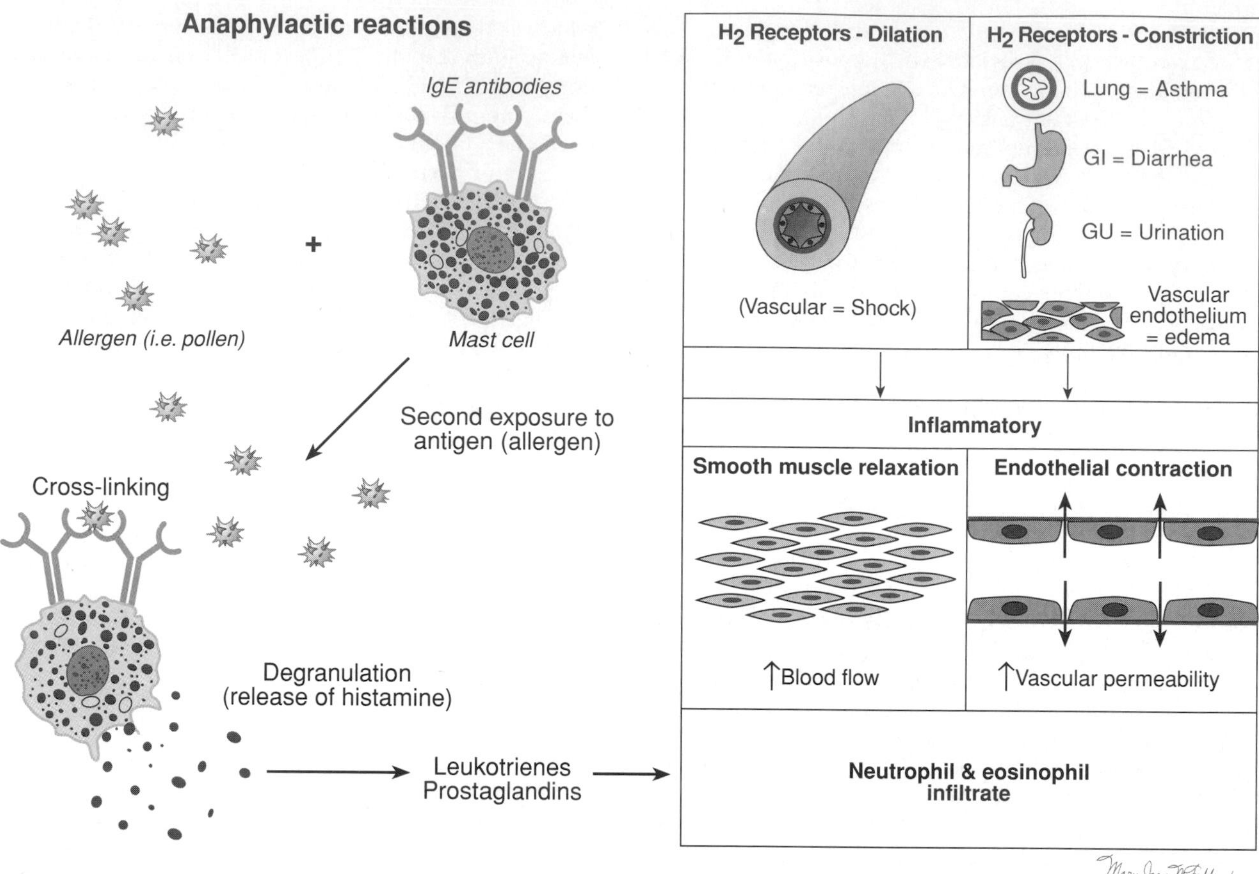

Fig. 25-17 Atopic or anaphylactic reactions. Reaction of antigen (allergen) with reaginic antibody (IgE) fixed to effector (mast) cells causes release of pharmacologically active agents stored in cytoplasmic granules (degranulation of mast cells). These released mediators, primarily histamine and serotonin, cause contraction of endothelial cells (edema), contraction of bronchial smooth muscle (asthma), and dilatation of vascular smooth muscle (systemic shock).

test for syphilis. The Wassermann reagin is a peculiar serum reactant found in individuals infected with syphilis. The Wassermann reagin is demonstrable by its ability to combine with an antigen extracted from ungulate heart muscle (cardiolipin) and has no relation to anaphylactic or atopic reactions. IgE antibody is termed *skin fixing* because it binds to mast cells in skin or basophils in the blood and "sensitizes" these cells to react to allergen. IgE anaphylactic antibodies have structures on the Fc piece of the molecule that fit receptors of the mast cell. There are two Fcγ receptors, FcγRI and FcγRII. FcγRI is the highest affinity Fc receptor known, is found only on mast cells and basophils, and is responsible for transmission of the mast cell degranulation signal upon reaction of Fc-bound IgE antibody with allergen. FcγRII is a low affinity receptor also found on macrophages, lymphocytes, eosinophils, and platelets. It is not well defined chemically and is believed to be involved in control of IgE synthesis and in ADCC-mediated parasite killing. The range of FcγRIs on a mast cell is estimated to be 10,000 to 40,000. The number of FcγRI cell-bound IgE antibody molecules determines the sensitivity of mast cells to an allergen. However, the amount of mediators released from a given cell depends on enzyme systems that regulate the biochemical mechanisms of mediator release. Allergen cross-linking two adjacent IgE molecules on the cell surface initiates events leading to mediator release. Mediator release may also be initiated by reaction of cross-linking IgE on the cell surface by antibodies to IgE. Cross-linking IgE leads to activation of phospholipase C and protein kinase C, followed by a series of further activation steps leading to mast cell degranulation.

Passive cutaneous anaphylaxis (Prausnitz-Küstner reaction)

The reaginic activity of an immunoglobulin is determined by its ability to fix to skin of the same species. If serum from a sensitive individual is passively transferred to the skin of a normal recipient, the classic wheal-and-flare reaction can be elicited at this site upon application of the antigen (Prausnitz-Küstner test) (Fig. 25-19). In 1921 Carl Prausnitz (the Herr Professor) and Heinz Küstner (a lowly medical student) reported the passive transfer of anaphylactic reactions both systemically and cutaneously by injection of serum from a patient sensitive to fish into a normal individual (Mr. Küstner). Because the antibody fixes to the skin, the transfer site may be tested up to 45 days later and still elicit a positive reaction. In contrast, with local passive transfer of nonreaginic antibody

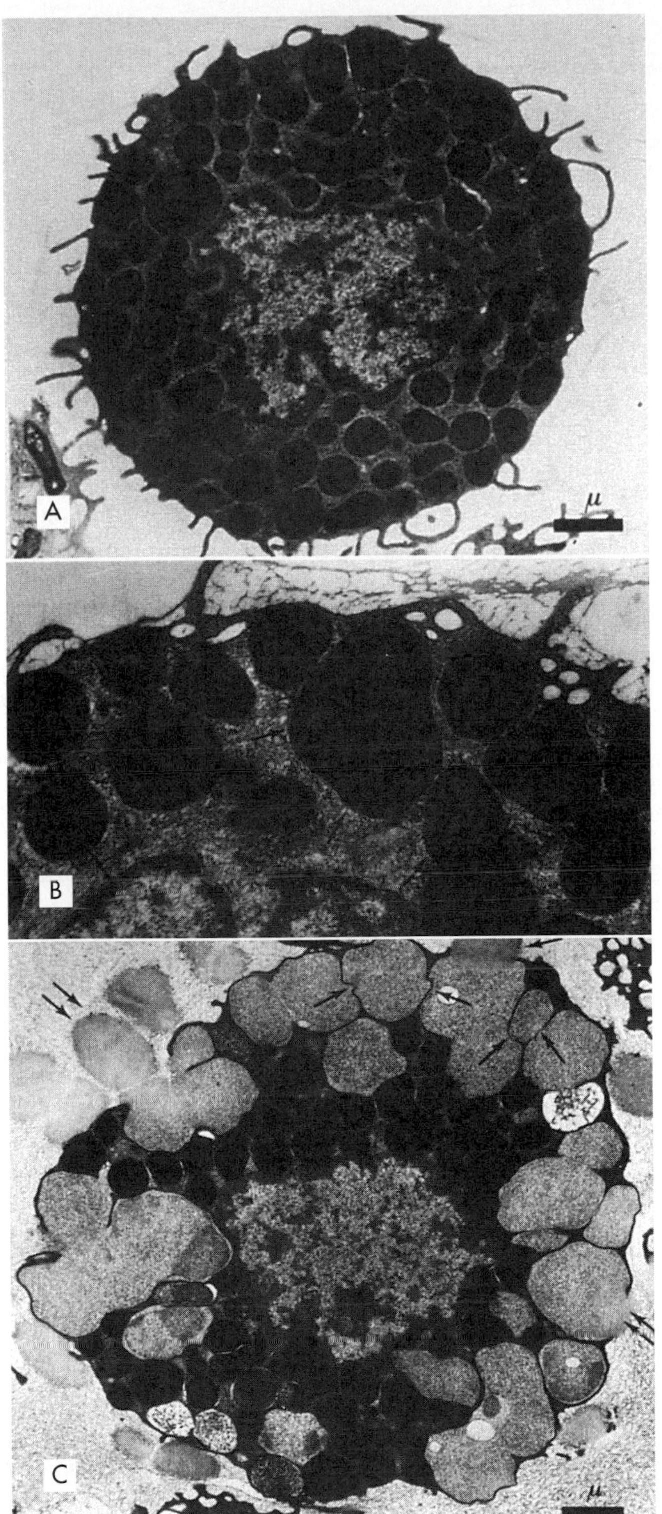

Fig. 25-18 Mast cell degranulation. **A,** Electron micrograph of rat mast cell. Many homogeneous, electron-dense granules are seen in the cytoplasm. **B,** Higher magnification of mast cell granules surrounded by perigranular membranes *(arrows)*. Human mast cell granules contain whorls of membranous structures. **C,** Degranulation of sensitized mast cell 60 seconds after exposure to allergen *(double arrows)*. (From Anderson P, Slorach SA, Uvnas B: *Acta Physiol Scand* 88:359, 1973; courtesy Borje Uvnas, Karolinska Institute, Stockholm, Sweden.)

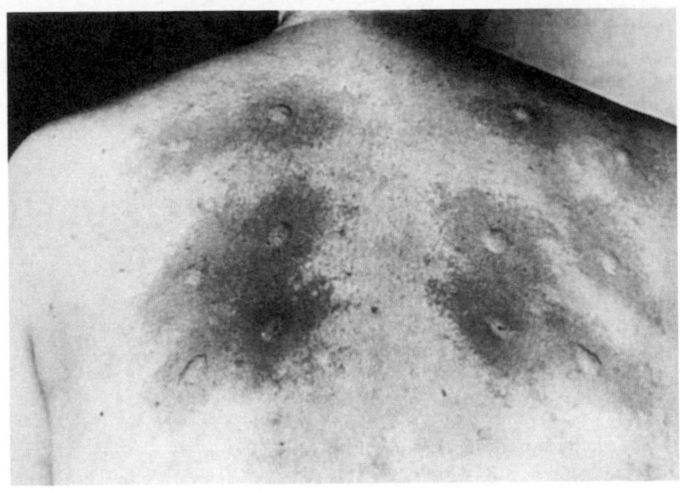

Fig. 25-19 Passive cutaneous anaphylaxis (Prausnitz-Küstner reaction). Cutaneous wheal-and-flare reactions after injection of horse-dandruff extract into skin sites on back of a nonreactive person who has had local inoculations of dilutions of sera from a person sensitive to horse dandruff. Central raised edematous area (wheal) is surrounded by flat erythematous rim (flare). (Courtesy Dr. Dennis Stanworth, University of Birmingham, England.)

(passive Arthus reaction), the skin site must be tested within a few hours in order to obtain a positive passive Arthus reaction before the non–skin fixing IgG antibody diffuses away.

Representative diseases

Anaphylaxis

Clinically, anaphylaxis is edema and congestion that may occur locally (cutaneous anaphylaxis) or a systemic shock reaction (systemic anaphylactic shock). *Cutaneous anaphylaxis* (urticaria, wheal and flare, hives) is elicited in a sensitive individual by a skin test (scratch or intradermal injection of antigen). Grossly visible manifestations are erythema, itching, a pale, soft, raised, wheal, pseudopods, and a spreading flare, reaching a maximum in 15 to 20 minutes and fading within an hour (Fig. 25-19). Early there is edema, with essentially no cellular infiltration until 12 to 18 hours. The mechanism is the same as in systemic anaphylaxis, but the reaction is localized because of antibody fixation in the skin and release of histamine or histamine-like substances into the skin with local changes in vascular permeability. Cutaneous anaphylaxis may be differentiated from the Arthus reaction in terms of both time of appearance and morphology of the reaction. Arthus reactions reach a maximum at 6 hours, are firmer, and feature neutrophilic vasculitis.

Systemic anaphylaxis or anaphylactic shock is a generalized reaction elicited in a sensitized animal by the intravenous injection of antigen or in a human by natural exposure or iatrogenic injection of an allergen. In humans, bronchial and gastrointestinal smooth muscle contraction is prominent, as well as increased permeability of small vessels, leukopenia, fall in temperature, hypotension, and slowing of the heart rate. Systemic anaphylaxis may be acutely fatal in severe reactions to insect stings or as a reaction to allergens in food (see below).

Table 25-9 Allergic symptoms: histamine receptors and organ systems

Histamine receptor	Reactive tissue	Constriction	Dilatation	Symptom
H_2	Vascular		×	Shock
H_1	Pulmonary	×		Asthma
	Gastrointestinal	×		Vomiting and diarrhea
	Genitourinary	×		Involuntary urination
	Endothelium	×		Edema

Atopic allergies

Atopic allergy is a term applied to a group of chronic human allergies to natural antigens, including asthma, hay fever, allergic rhinitis, urticaria (hives), eczema, serous otitis media, conjunctivitis, and food allergy. The mechanisms are essentially the same as those involved in systemic and cutaneous anaphylaxis. The *clinical features* of atopic allergy are itching and whealing, sneezing, and respiratory embarrassment. The pathologic features include edema, smooth muscle contraction, and leukopenia. The pharmacologic characteristics are repeated episodes of histamine release and partial protection by antihistamines as well as involvement of leukotrienes and prostaglandins. The type of reaction seen clinically depends on three factors:

1. *Route of access of antigen.* If contact occurs at the skin, hives (wheal and flare) predominate; if contact is at the respiratory mucous membranes, asthma and rhinitis occur; if contact occurs at the eyes, conjunctivitis will predominate, or if through the ears, serous otitis; if contact occurs at the gastrointestinal tract, food allergy, with cramps, nausea, vomiting, and diarrhea results.

2. *Dose of antigen.* The rarity of death from most atopic allergies, in contrast to anaphylaxis, is most likely because of the dose and route of access of the antigen. In systemic anaphylaxis, inadvertent large doses of antigen are usually given intravenously; in atopic allergy, the doses are low and contact is across mucous membranes. Such a conclusion is justified by the observation that anaphylactically sensitized guinea pigs exposed to small amounts of antigen by inhalation develop typical asthmatic symptoms. However, in highly sensitive individuals minute doses of allergen may elicit fatal reactions, and in sensitized individuals injected with relatively large doses of allergen in the form of drugs, severe, sometimes fatal, anaphylactic reactions may occur. In addition to foods and insect stings (see below) acute anaphylactic reactions have been elicited by exposure to hair spray, other cosmetics, and detergent additives and after intercourse by women who are allergic to seminal fluid. Animal and laboratory workers frequently develop allergies to animal dander. During the days of mounted cavalry as many as 20% of cavalrymen had to be assigned to different duty because of allergic reactions to horse dander. Documentation of allergic reactions of horses to humans has not been found.

3. *The shock organ.* Individual differences in reactivity depend on individual idiosyncrasy, pharmacologic abnormality of the target tissue (increased numbers of mast cells or increased H receptors on target organs), or increased susceptibility of a given organ because of nonspecific irritation or inflammation. Many affected individuals commonly have an atopic reaction involving one organ system (asthma) without involvement of other organs.

Asthma

The word *asthma* is Greek and means 'panting,' a general term for difficulty in breathing. Asthma presents as reversible acute respiratory distress from airway obstruction, presumably caused by constriction of the smooth muscles of the small bronchi and mucus secretion, after reaction of an inhaled allergen with IgE on bronchial mast cells. Osler described presentation of asthma "with a distressing sense of want of breath and a feeling of great oppression of the chest. Soon the respiratory efforts become violent, and all of the accessory muscles are brought into play. In a few minutes the patient is in a paroxysm of the most intense dyspnea."

Constriction of bronchial smooth muscle may be triggered by a variety of nonimmune mechanisms, including chemical irritation, change in temperature, physical activity, and emotional stress, as well as by a variety of respiratory infections. In cases of nonimmune forms of asthma no exogenous eliciting antigen can be identified, and no IgE antibodies may be demonstrated. One form is caused by exposure to aspirin and other nonsteroidal anti-inflammatory agents through blocking of the cyclooxygenase pathway for metabolism of arachidonic acid and increased production of leukotrienes, which cause chronic airway inflammation and bronchial constriction. Chronic inflammation with infiltration of the bronchial mucosa with inflammatory cells and hyperplasia of bronchial smooth muscle leads to a lowering of the threshold for a bronchospastic response to a variety of stimuli.

Numerous pathologic changes have been found in the lungs of patients with either allergic or "nonallergic" asthma. In the acute attack, which may be fatal because of acute asphyxiation, there is considerable constriction of the bronchi and occlusion of the bronchi with a particularly thick mucus secretion (mucus plugs). In chronic asthma the pulmonary changes are (1) pronounced thickening of the basement membrane of the bronchial mucosa, (2) hypertrophy of the bronchial smooth muscle, (3) hyperplasia of the bronchial mucous glands, (4) eosinophils, chronic inflammatory cells in the bronchial wall with a substantial increase over normal in the number of mast cells, and (5) the presence of mucus in the bronchi containing large numbers of eosinophilic leukocytes. In addition, T-cells are prominent in the lungs of chronic asthmatics. The thickened basement membrane may contain deposits of IgG or IgM, but IgE has not been detected often. Eosinophil degranulation may contribute to epithelial desquamation. Other stigmas of chronic inflammation and airway obstruction not specific for asthma, including focal fibrosis and scarring, emphysema, and atelectasis, may be found in the periphery of the lung. Since repeated asthma attacks are also associated with increased susceptibility to pulmonary infections, some of the pathologic changes may be attributable to repeated bronchopneumonia. The severity and duration of asthmatic attacks is greatly influenced by psychologic factors. Typical attacks are more frequent during periods of emotional stress.

Atopic reactions

Seasonal upper respiratory reactions to pollen are commonly referred to as hay fever or seasonal allergic rhinitis. Perennial allergic rhinitis is caused by animal dander, house dust, house dust mites, and molds that cause a reaction in the nasal passages and eyes of affected individuals. In temperate climates, seasonal allergic rhinitis is caused by nonflowering, wind-pollinated plants. Larger pollen particles (>10 μm) are efficiently filtered out by the nasal mucosa and cause rhinitis, whereas smaller particles, less than 1 to 2 μm, pass into the tracheobronchial tree and cause asthma. Hay fever symptoms include sneezing, nasal congestion, watery discharge from the eye, conjunctival itching, and cough with mild bronchoconstriction. Similar symptoms may be caused by vasomotor rhinitis caused by parasympathetic hyperactivity, a foreign body, and infection, in particular, the common cold. The diagnosis is usually made by history of nasal itching, sneezing, nasal discharge and difficulty breathing, particularly during the pollen season. Pathologic changes are not extensive. Usually there is edema of the submucosal tissue with an infiltration of eosinophils that is reversible. The degree of reaction and severity of symptoms are directly related to the amount of exposure to the allergen responsible. The lesion is caused by release of mediators from mast cells in the nasal mucosa: histamine, serotonin, eosinophil and neutrophil chemotactic factors, and mast cell proteases, as well as newly formed, membrane-derived lipid mediators such as prostaglandin D_2 and other arachidonic acid metabolites. These mediators produce vasodilatation, mucosal edema, mucus secretion, stimulation of itch receptors and reduction in the threshold for sneezing.

Nasal polyps are tumorlike masses that form in the nasal air passages, causing chronic airway obstruction and rendering nasal breathing very difficult or impossible. These masses can be removed surgically but usually recur promptly. The relationship between nasal polyps and allergic rhinitis is uncertain. Polyps are frequently found in patients with perennial rhinitis, and it has been suggested that persistent contact with small amounts of antigen leads to the characteristic picture. Nasal polyps characteristically show pronounced edema, swelling of hydrophilic ground substance, and scattered eosinophilic infiltration. Eosinophilic polymorphonuclear leukocytes are associated with severe persistent allergic rhinitis. The prolonged nature of the swelling may be explained by continued production of hydrophilic ground substance by tissue fibroblasts.

Food allergy

Ingestion of allergens may lead to remarkable gastrointestinal reactions known collectively as *food allergy.* Systemic anaphylaxis has been unleashed by ingestion of beans, rice, shrimp, fish, milk, cereal mixes, potatoes, Brazil nuts, and tangerines. The relationship of the gastrointestinal reaction to atopic sensitivity is not clear. Many individuals with positive skin reactions to an allergen do react to ingestion of the allergen, whereas individuals with repeated episodes of vomiting or diarrhea that occur on eating a given food may not produce a skin reaction to the food. Food allergens are most likely to be those that survive the process of digestion, or to drugs added to foods as preservatives. Food allergy may lead to hypoproteinemia from the loss of protein in the gastrointestinal tract and persistent diarrhea. Other manifestations of food allergy are extensive skin eruptions (urticaria or eczema) or systemic shock.

Insect allergy

Atopic or anaphylactic reactions to *insects* may be divided into three groups: inhalant or contact reactions to insect body parts or products, skin reactions (wheal and flare) to biting insects, and systemic shock reactions to stinging insects. This reaction is important clinically and individuals known to be "allergic" to insects should carry epinephrine for rapid injection when in situations where insect exposure is likely. The common mosquito bite is a cutaneous anaphylactic reaction. Asthmatic or hay fever–like reactions may occur after airborne exposure of a sensitive individual to large numbers of insects or their body parts. This happens outdoors with insects that periodically appear in large numbers, such as locusts or grasshoppers, and indoors, more chronically, to beetles, flies, and spiders. It is not clear what survival advantage these acute allergic reactions to insect bites and stings provide. The reaction does induce immediate avoidance behavior and may limit the exposure of a bitten individual to a dose of a toxic venom that could be even more damaging. On the other hand, a systemic anaphylactic reaction to an insect sting may be interpreted as an immune mechanism that should be protective but is instead deleterious and potentially fatal.

Urticaria

Urticaria is a condition of red or pale, itchy edematous swellings of the skin (hives), usually short lived; angioedema is a more extensive swelling of the subcutaneous tissues and mucous membranes. Urticaria and angioedema may coexist and are believed to have similar mechanisms. The types of urticaria and angioedema may be arbitrarily classified into physical (see the discussion of anaphylactoid reactions below), immunologic, hereditary, and idiopathic. Urticaria (hives) is usually attributable to release of mediators from mast cells as a result of allergen reacting with IgE bound antibody, by bites of insects, by physical trauma (dermatographia), or by exercise, heat, cold, sunlight, and so forth. *Angioedema* is a diffuse pale swelling of the skin or mucous membrane that may be associated with other forms of allergic reactions.

Anaphylactoid reactions

Any event causing histamine release may cause atopic symptoms that may be confused with a true allergic reaction. Anaphylactoid shock is produced in normal (nonimmune) animals by injection of a variety of agents capable of releasing histamine or activating arachidonic acid metabolism without the mediation of an antigen-antibody reaction. The resulting clinical, physiologic, and pathologic picture is virtually indistinguishable from true anaphylaxis but is not produced by immune reaction. Physical agents (heat, cold), trauma (dermatographia), emotional disturbances, or exercise may evoke pharmacologic mechanisms that mimic allergic reactions.

However, there are increasingly convincing data that most of these reactions are IgE mediated. "Dermatographia" literally means 'writing on the skin.' Stroking the skin results in whealing at the contact points of the stroke. Pressure urticaria is closely related. Swelling may occur at the wrists or ankles if tight clothing is worn, or over the buttocks if the individual sits for long periods of time. Dermatographia and pressure urticaria may be caused by the release of anaphylactic mediators from mast cells by a degree of physical trauma that does not induce a reaction in normal individuals.

Hereditary angioedema is a specific form of angioedema, first reported in 1882, that involves a defect in the ability to inactivate the first component of complement. Massive swellings may involve the eyelids, lips, tongue, and areas of the trunk. Involvement of the gastrointestinal tract may produce symptoms of acute abdominal distress, but the symptoms almost always disappear in a few days without surgical intervention. Biochemically, there is a deficiency of Cl esterase inhibitor (C1-INH) or Cl esterase inhibitor is present in an inactive form. Cl esterase is the active form of the first component of complement. If normal serum is incubated at 37° C, there is a gradual "spontaneous" loss of complement activity. In patients with angioedema this spontaneous decrease may not occur because of a lack of C1-INH.

Control of anaphylactic reactions

The severity of an anaphylactic reaction depends not only on the amount of allergen and reaginic antibody, but also on the reactivity of mast cells, the responsiveness of the end organ (such as smooth muscle cells), and the activation state of the autonomic nervous system (Fig. 25-20). Imbalances among these homeostatic control mechanisms may explain how exposure to various nonimmunologic stimuli, such as heat, cold, physical exercise, light, or psychologic stress, may

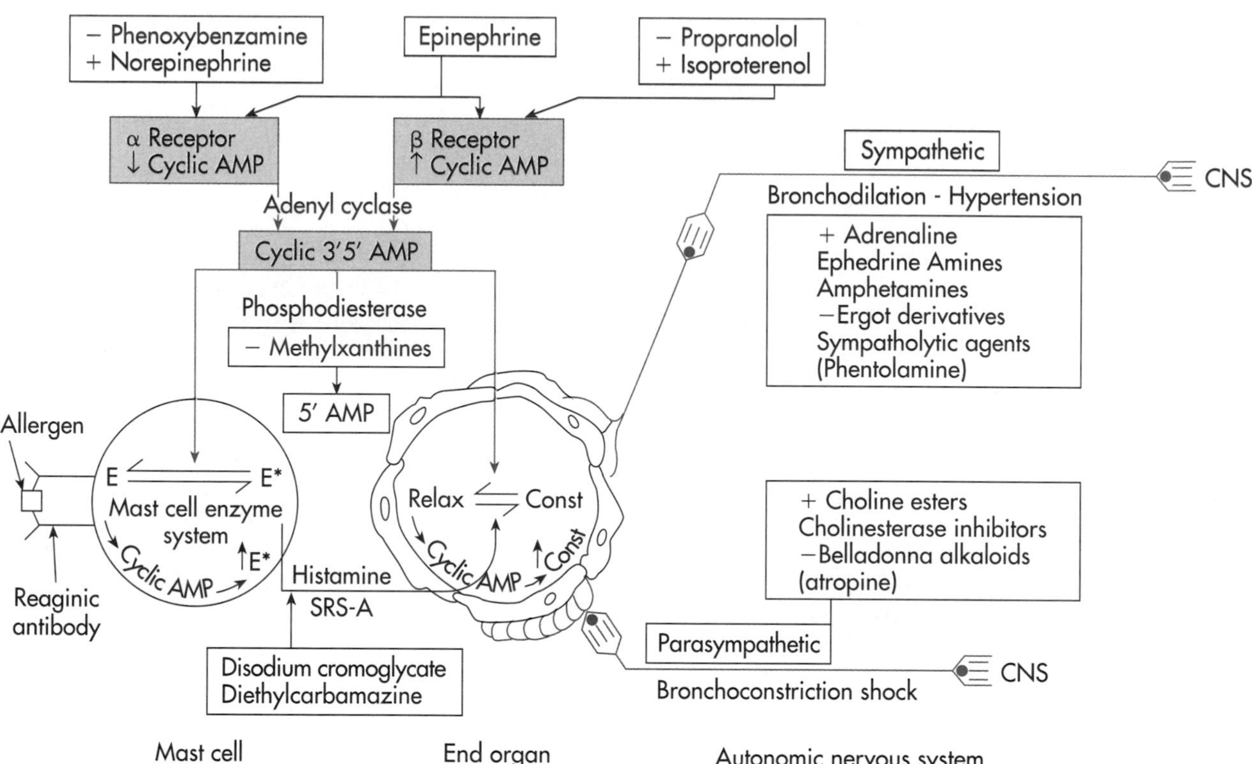

Fig. 25-20 Pharmacologic and neurologic control of anaphylactic reactions. The effects of atopic or anaphylactic reactions are mediated by biologically active mediators released by mast cells that act on smooth muscle or endothelial cells (end organs). Amount of mediators released by mast cells and reactivity of end organs are controlled by cellular messenger systems. Mast cell sensitivity depends on amount of reaginic antibody coating the cells and on intracellular level of cyclic AMP (cAMP). Cyclic AMP levels are controlled through adrenergic receptors. Stimulation of α-receptors decreases levels of cAMP and increases reactivity; stimulation of β-receptors activates adenyl cyclase, increases cAMP, and decreases reactivity. Adrenergic receptor–controlled levels of cAMP also determine reactivity of end-organ cells.

Degree of mast cell and end-organ excitability may be modified by pharmacologic agents that operate through adrenergic or autonomic systems. Cyclic AMP is broken down to 5′-AMP by phosphodiesterase, so that inhibition of phosphodiesterase activity by methylxanthines increases cAMP and decreases sensitivity of mast cells and end organs. Epinephrine stimulates both α- and β-receptors but predominantly reverses acute allergic reactions at the usual therapeutic dose. Disodium cromoglycate and diethylcarbamazine inhibit histamine release from mast cells. Excitability of end organs is also controlled by the autonomic nervous system. Parasympathetic effects are similar to anaphylactic effects (bronchial constriction, endothelial contraction, increased peristalsis, dilatation of bladder sphincter, and so forth), whereas sympathetic effects are the opposite. Emotional states may result in temporary imbalance of these systems and lower the threshold for an acute reaction, such as an asthmatic attack in an individual under stress (increased parasympathetic tone).

excite reactions that mimic allergic reactions, anaphylactoid reactions, or lower the threshold for allergen-mediated reactions. Pharmacologic treatment of atopic reactions may be effective at the level of the mast cell, end organ, or autonomic nervous system. Agents that stimulate beta receptors or sympathetic nerves, or drugs that block alpha receptors or the parasympathetic system may alleviate the effects of allergic reactions.

Protective role of IgE

The protective role of atopic or anaphylactic reactions has been the subject of considerable speculation. The most popular hypothesis is that anaphylactic reactions serve to open small blood vessels by means of endothelial cell contraction and permit the exudation of other immunoglobulin classes of antibodies or inflammatory cells into the tissue containing the offending antigen, the "gate-keeper effect." In immunized animals containing IgG antidiphtheria toxin antibodies, the simultaneous injection of ragweed antigen and diphtheria toxin into the skin results in an increase in toxin neutralization if the skin site is prepared by previous sensitization with reaginic antibody for the ragweed antigen. It is concluded that the increased toxin-neutralizing capacity of the local skin sites in passively immunized animals is attributable to increased transudation of serum IgG antibody into the skin test sites.

Anaphylactic reactions may also serve to protect the individual against intestinal parasites. Parasitic worm infestations are frequently associated with IgE antibody response. It has been postulated that gastrointestinal anaphylactic reactions may help expel intestinal parasites by acute severe diarrhea. Mechanisms of expulsion of intestinal parasites include primary expulsion of the first infection, which is associated with pronounced acute inflammation, and rapid expulsion, which is associated with increased intestinal motility, pronounced mucus secretion, hyperplasia of goblet cells, eosinophilic infiltrate, and mast cell hyperplasia. The histopathologic features of asthma and the rapid expulsion reaction share many similarities. It is also possible that the sneezing associated with acute asthma dislodges potential infectious agents from the lungs. Eosinophils may play a direct role in destruction of intestinal parasites through an ADCC mechanism. The major basic protein of eosinophils not only is cytotoxic for parasites, but also can activate mast cell degranulation.

Finally, acute anaphylactic reactions may force the sensitized individual to avoid further exposure to the offending allergen. By avoiding exposure to the antigens, more prolonged extensive immune-mediated damage may be prevented. Avoidance may prevent formation of immune complex disease or delayed hypersensitivity to the same antigen, since anaphylactic reactions may be elicited by extremely small doses of an antigen.

T-CELL–MEDIATED CYTOTOXICITY (CMC)

Mechanisms

Cell-mediated immunity: T_{CTL}, T_{DTH}, and NK cells

The term *cell-mediated immunity* (CMI) was first used to refer to the effects of specifically sensitized lymphocytes after reaction with antigen or target cells in vitro.[102-125] CMI has been extended to include two types of specific T-cell–mediated effects in vivo: T-cell killing (T_{CTL}) and T-cell–mediated delayed hypersensitivity (T_{DTH}) (Fig. 25-21), as well as other cellular effects (see Table 25-3). Cytotoxic T-cells (T_{CTL}) lyse, or "kill," target cells expressing specific antigens in vitro. Delayed hypersensitivity T-cells (T_{DTH}) release "lymphokines" with potent biologic activity after reaction with specific antigens in vitro. The full manifestations of DTH, which involves lymphokine attraction and activation of macrophages, can occur only in living tissues. T-cell killing is initiated by a $CD8^+$ subpopulation of specifically sensitized T_{CTL} that react with cell surface antigens in peptides associated with *MHC class I* molecules and destroy the target cells; DTH is a local inflammatory reaction caused by the release of lymphokines from a $CD4^+$ T_{DTH} cells that react with antigens associated with Class II MHC.

Upon reaction with antigens in association with class I MHC on tissue cells, T_{CTL} are activated to kill the target cell. T_{CTL}s contain multicomponent cytoplasmic granules containing cytolytic molecules such as perforin, proteoglycans, and serine proteases (granzymes), which, in the presence of calcium, mediate lysis of target cells. These enzymes are also active in NK cell–mediated killing, and the mechanisms of cell lysis by T_{CTL} and NK cells appear to be very similar. The effectiveness of T_{CTL} killing is related to the expression of cell adhesion molecules, such as H-CAM (CD44) and $\alpha 4\beta 1$-integrin (VLA-4), which determine the ability of the T_{CTL} to bind to target cells. The subset of CD4-8 T-cells, which make up 1% to 2% of circulating T-cells, may serve as an "early-warning" rapid response T_{CTL} system that acts to hold infections in check during the first few days after exposure. These cells are constitutively activated and can kill target cells in vitro without being activated by IL-2.

Delayed hypersensitivity (DTH) reactions are variations on a theme of chronic inflammation. Specific $CD4^+$ T-cells that initiate DTH reactions (T_{DTH} cells) are attracted to gradients of antigen release from tissues and interact with endothelial cells through reaction of lymphocyte receptors L-selectin (LAM-1), $\alpha 4\beta 1$-integrin (VLA-4), $\alpha L\beta 2$-integrin (LFA-1), and H-CAM (CD44), with E-selectin, VCAM-1, ICAM-1, and carbohydrates on endothelial cells. Upon reaction with antigens in association with class II MHC on dermal dendritic cells, sensitized T_{DTH} cells release lymphokines, such as TNF, IL-2, INF-γ, and other inflammatory initiating factors, which attract and activate macrophages. In turn, activated macrophages produce TNF, IL-1, IL-6, and PGE_2, which contribute to the late phase of the DTH reaction. However, the main function of activated macrophages is to phagocytose and digest cells and tissue debris. DTH reactions are particularly effective against intracellular parasites that can replicate within macrophages, such as mycobacteria and *Leishmania* species. The products of activated T_{DTH} cells enable infected macrophages to destroy the organisms they harbor. T_{DTH}-activated macrophages are also effective against extracellular infections, such as fungi and syphilis. However, these defensive specific DTH reactions may result in extensive tissue destruction and produce lesions (the "double-edged sword").

NK cells may also take part in what may be considered a mirror image of T_{CTL}-mediated cytolytic mechanisms. T_{CTL} recognize foreign peptides complexed to class I MHC and are activated to kill the cell; NK cells recognize class I MHC molecules complexed with self-protective peptides and do not kill the cells. Class I MHC expression by tissue cells protects

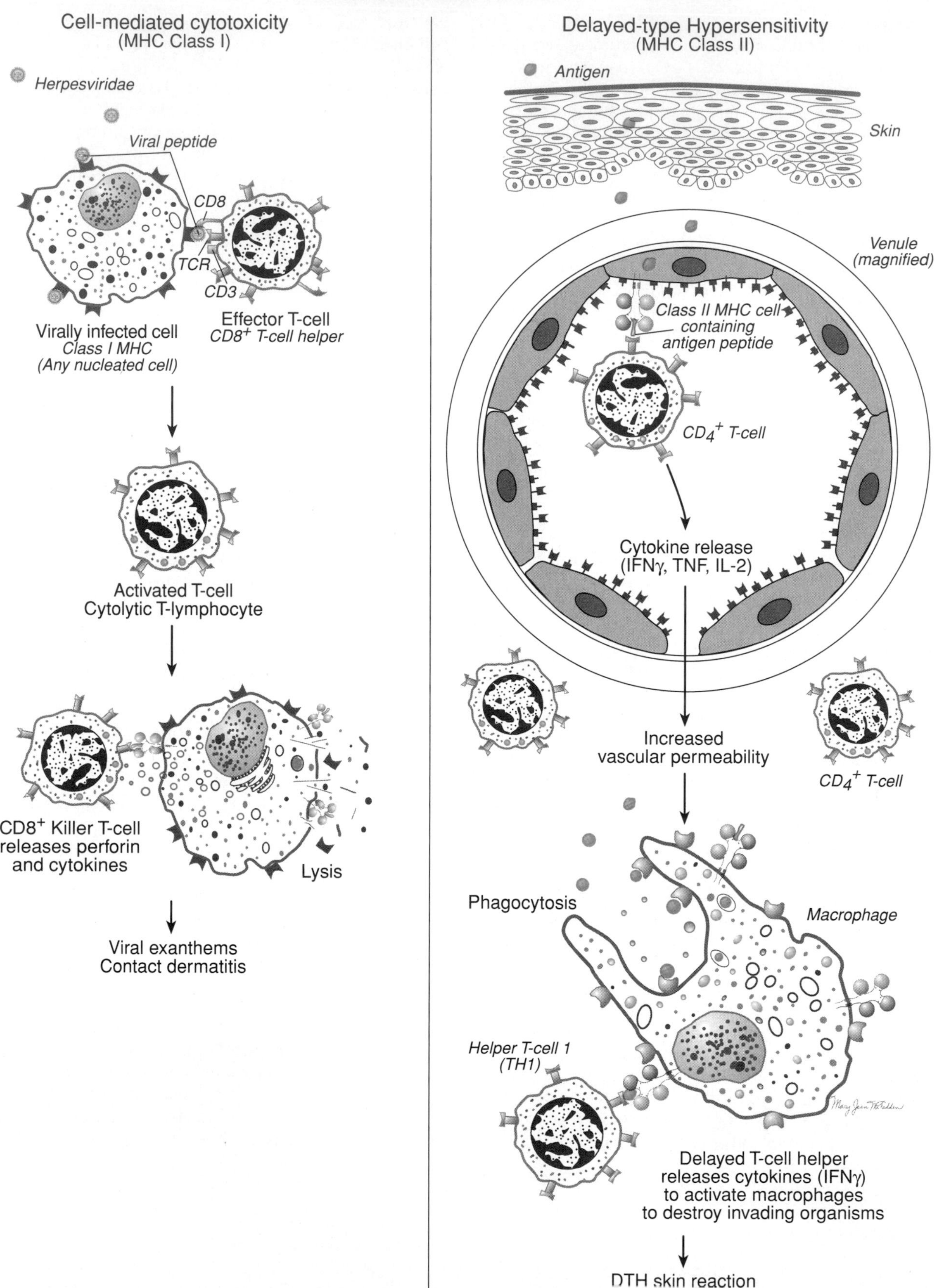

Fig. 25-21 Cell-mediated hypersensitivity reactions. In cell mediated cytotoxicity (left panel) there are T-lymphocytes with T-cell receptors that recognize antigen to initiate the reaction. T_{CTL} kill the target cells expressing the antigen. This contrasts delayed-type hypersensitivity (right panel) where T_{DTH} cells release mediators (cytokines) that act to influence other nonsensitive cells to participate in the reaction. This consists of recruiting additional lymphocytes as well as attracting and activating macrophages. The activated macrophage is a singularly effective killer cell and produces many "monokines" that contribute not only to late stages of delayed hypersensitivity reactions, but also to nonimmune chronic inflammation and healing.

against NK lysis by binding protective peptides, such as heat-shock protein, elongation factor 2, histone H_3, and ribosomal proteins that occupy the peptide-binding groove on the MHC molecules. Cells with abnormal MHC class I expression or insufficient protective peptide binding, such as tumor cells or virus-infected cells, are subject to lysis by NK cells. The conserved protective peptides appear to be similar to peptides encoded by infectious agents (such as viruses), but the peptides produced by infectious agents have critical amino acid substitutions that do not confer protection. Upon infection, peptides from the infectious agent compete with self-peptides for presentation by MHC molecules. Complexes of these peptides with MHC prevents self-recognition by the NK receptor, rendering an infected cell susceptible to NK lysis. Although there is considerable interest in the adaptation of NK cells for tumor immunotherapy, it is not clear what role NK cells play during naturally occurring immune responses in vivo.

It was not until the mid-1960s that most immunologists began to consider CMI as an important immune mechanism. It is now known that T-cell killing and delayed hypersensitivity constitute the major defense mechanism against many infectious diseases, as well as the effector mechanism in homograft rejections and many autoimmune diseases. It differs from the immune reactions mentioned previously in this text in that no humoral antibody is involved and reactivity cannot be transferred by serum, but only by cells; the time course of the development of the lesion is much prolonged; and the gross and microscopic appearance are different. Cell-mediated reactions feature infiltrations of tissues by mononuclear cells (lymphocytes and macrophages). The importance of CMI in infectious diseases has been brought to the forefront by the variety and number of opportunistic infections with viruses, protozoa, fungi, and mycobacteria in AIDS patients who have defective $CD4^+$ T-cell–mediated immunity.

T-cytotoxic reactions

T_{CTL} were first identified because they could "kill" specific target cells in vitro. An identical type of interaction between lymphocytes and target cells may occur in vivo in tissue reactions mediated by lymphocytes, such as the cell-mediated rejection of a renal allograft or development of experimental allergic thyroiditis. The T_{CTL} pass between the renal tubule cells or the thyroid follicular cells, causing them to separate from each other and from the basement membrane, eventually destroying the renal tubule or thyroid follicle cells. The basement membrane appears intact during the development of the lesion. Infiltration of mononuclear cells, with separation, isolation, and destruction of target cells, is seen in contact dermatitis and viral exanthems, as well as in many autoimmune diseases and during tissue graft rejections.

Representative diseases

Contact dermatitis

Contact allergy (contact eczema, dermatitis venenata) is exemplified by the common allergic reaction to poison ivy. It also occurs as an allergic response to a wide variety of simple chemicals in such things as ointments, clothing, cosmetics, dyes, and adhesive tape, as well as metals such as nickel in sewing thimbles. The antigens are usually highly reactive chemical compounds capable of combining with proteins; they are also lipid soluble and can penetrate the epidermis. The antigen often is an incomplete antigen (hapten) that combines with some constituent of the epidermis to form a complete antigen. Sensitization occurs by exposure of the skin once or repeatedly to sufficiently high concentrations of antigen to induce an immune response. Langerhans cells within the epidermis are believed to play an important role in antigen processing and delivery of the antigen to the draining lymph node where sensitization takes place. In addition, epidermal keratinocytes express MHC class I antigens and may be able to present antigen directly to MHC class I restricted T_{CTL} precursors.

The characteristic skin reaction is elicited in sensitized individuals by exposure of the skin to the antigen (natural exposure, patch tests). The reaction is a sharply delineated, superficial skin inflammation, beginning as early as 24 hours after exposure and reaching a maximum at 48 to 96 hours. It is characterized by redness, induration, and vesiculation. The reaction may take longer to reach a maximum than the tuberculin skin test (see below) because of the longer time required for the antigen to penetrate the epidermis and persist for longer times because of the time required to remove the antigen from the epidermis. Histologically the dermis shows perivenous accumulation of lymphocytes and monocytes and some edema. The epidermis is invaded by these cells and shows intraepidermal edema (spongiosis), which progresses to vesiculation and death of epidermal cells (Fig. 25-22). In lesions, there is upregulation of the cell adhesion molecule ICAM-1 on keratinocytes that are associated with LFA-1 positive lymphocytes. Thus, these cell adhesion molecules may play an important role in the T_{CTL} keratinocyte interaction.

The characteristics of the eliciting antigen determine the nature of the reaction. In poison ivy reactions, for example, because the lipid-soluble antigen is mainly present in the epidermis, it takes about 2 days for the reacting mononuclear cells (mainly lymphocytes but also macrophages) to invade

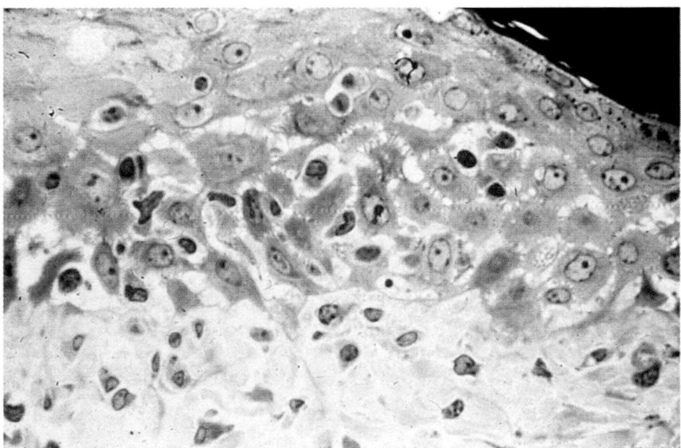

Fig. 25-22 Early lesion in experimental contact dermatitis. Mononuclear cells pass from venules in the dermis through the basement membrane into the epidermis, where they separate and detach the epidermal cells, producing small spaces (vesicles) that later coalesce to form larger vesicles seen grossly. Notice separation of epidermal cells as indicated by prominent intracellular bridges. Resolution is accomplished by regeneration of epidermal cells from the basal layer and sloughing of the upper epidermis. (Courtesy Martin Flax, Tufts University, Boston, Massachusetts.)

from the dermis and react with the antigen. As a result of this invasion and reaction, epidermal cells are destroyed and small foci (sterile microabscesses) are formed, eventually leading to vesicle formation, which can be seen on the skin as small, fluid-filled blebs. Since all of the hapten may not be degraded in the vesicles, rupture of the vesicles by scratching may spread the antigen to uninvolved areas of the skin and provoke new reactions. Proliferation of the basal epidermal cells results in eventual sloughing of the affected epidermal cells. This process may take up to a week to 10 days, depending on the amount of antigen present and the degree of sensitization of the individual. Poison ivy or poison oak oleoresin may remain stable in the dry state for long periods of time, and so indirect exposure may occur from touching clothes, tools, or animals that are contaminated with dried plant resins.

Tissue graft rejection

Classic tissue graft rejection is caused by cell-mediated immunity to alloantigens, but antibody to donor antigens can also initiate complement-mediated injury. Both direct killing of target cells by $CD8^+$ MHC class I restricted T_{CTL} and release of lymphokines from $CD4^+$ MHC class II restricted T_{DTH} cells that attract and activate macrophages, are involved in immune destruction of a tissue graft. In the absence of immunosuppressive therapy rejection of tissue grafts is associated with mononuclear cell infiltrate. For skin, kidney, and liver grafts, for example, the major target antigens are on differentiated epithelial cells: the squamous epithelium of the skin, the tubule lining cells of the kidney, and the bile duct cells of the liver. Early histologic signs of rejection feature the infiltration of lymphocytes across the basement membrane into and between the epithelial cells with killing of individual keratinocytes, tubule cells, or bile duct cells. The major cellular infiltrate in the epithelial cells is made up of $CD8^+$ cells; $CD4^+$ cells are seen in the interstitial connective tissues. Cell-mediated rejection of the kidney, for example, is characterized by tubulitis: the infiltration of lymphocytes into the renal tubules (Chapter 65). Interstitial infiltrates of mononuclear cells are not specific for graft rejection. Thus the major mechanism of rejection of solid organs in untreated recipients is attributable to the cytotoxicity of T_{CTL}s for epithelial cells.

Viral exanthems

Cell-mediated cytotoxic reactions to viral infections also illustrate the "double-edged sword" of protective and destructive effects of immunity. Cell-mediated immunity to viral antigens may be either protective by limiting viral infections or destructive by destroying functioning host cells that are expressing viral antigens. On the one hand, T_{CTL} cells are responsible for destruction of virus-infected cells and recovery from infections such as measles, herpes simplex, and smallpox. On the other hand, T_{CTL} cells reacting to viral antigens on vital host cells may lead to loss of tissue function, or viral infections may lead to reaction to self tissue antigens (autoimmunity).

An exanthem is a disease or fever associated with eruptive skin lesions. Pirquet in 1907 observed that the local lesion occurring after smallpox vaccination (vaccinia) consisted of a two-stage reaction. Early (first 8 days), there is a papular vesicular lesion because of the growth of the inoculated virus; later (8 to 14 days) an indurated erythematous reaction (a take) follows. The take reaction corresponds to the development of CMI and is interpreted as evidence that protective immunity has been established. Similar lesions appear at the same time on different parts of the body, even though the different areas are inoculated with the virus at different times. Animal experiments have shown that protection against the virus is associated with T_{CTL}, and that the infective virus disappears from the local lesion when systemic CMI is maximal. The same concept was considered valid by Pirquet for other viral exanthems (measles, varicella) in which multiple, disseminated lesions occur as a result of T_{CTL} reaction to viruses located at the sites of lesions. Some of the lesions of the viral exanthems may be modified by humoral antibody reacting with viral antigens to produce an Arthus-like reaction in the skin or delayed hypersensitivity reactions; however, T_{CTL}-mediated killing of virus infected cells is the major mechanism. Lesions are caused by destruction of infected epithelial cells.

Immunity to the smallpox virus is induced by stimulation of T_{CTL}. Vaccination against smallpox is accomplished by inoculation into the skin of a related virus (vaccinia) that usually produces only a local lesion. The local lesion, called a *take*, is produced by T-cytotoxic to vaccinia antigens, which are shared with the virulent smallpox virus. The *take* reaction is a focal necrotic reaction produced by infiltrating cytotoxic

Table 25-10 Cell-mediated experimental and clinical autoimmune diseases

		Histologically similar human disease	
Experimental disease	**Tissue involved**	**Acute monocyclic**	**Chronic relapsing**
Allergic encephalomyelitis	Myelin (central nervous system)	Postinfectious encephalomyelitis	Multiple sclerosis
Allergic neuritis	Myelin (peripheral nervous system)	Guillain-Barré polyneuritis	
Phacoanaphylactic endophthalmitis	Lens		Phacoanaphylactic endophthalmitis
Allergic uveitis	Uvea	Postinfectious iridocyclitis	Sympathetic ophthalmia
Allergic orchitis	Germinal epithelium	Mumps orchitis	Nonendocrine chronic infertility
Allergic thyroiditis	Thyroglobulin	Mumps thyroiditis	Subacute and chronic thyroiditis
Allergic sialadenitis	Glandular epithelium	Mumps parotitis	Sjögren's syndrome
Allergic adrenalitis	Cortical cells		Cytotoxic contraction of adrenal
Allergic gastritis	Gastric mucosa		Atrophic gastritis

Modified from Waksman BH: *Int Arch Allergy Appl Immunol* 14(suppl):1, 1959.

lymphocytes killing virus-infected epithelial cells, resulting in a lesion similar to contact dermatitis.

Autoimmune disease (Table 25-10)
Thyroiditis is one of the most extensively studied experimental autoimmune diseases and is mainly mediated by T_{CTL}. It occurs 6 to 14 days after immunization of an experimental animal with thyroid extract or thyroglobulin in complete Freund's adjuvant. The lesion begins as a perivenous infiltration of lymphocytes, and destruction of the thyroid follicular epithelium is accomplished by the invasion of specifically sensitized cells similar to the lesion of contact dermatitis. The major effector mechanism for the disease is T_{CTL}-mediated destruction of follicle cells. $CD4^+$ cells are active in passive transfer of the experimental disease, but $CD8^+$ cells are found in situ in the lesions and are able to kill follicular cells in vitro. In active lesions, secretion of INF-γ induces expression of ICAM-1 and class II MHC and ICAM-1 on thyroid cells. This may contribute to binding of T_{CTL} between ICAM-1 and $\alpha L\beta 2$-integrin (LFA-1) and maintenance of the inflammatory response to autoantigens on thyroid cells by DTH. Of interest is the finding that about 20% of cancer patients treated with IL-2 or INF-γ develop hypothyroid symptoms and evidence of autoimmune thyroiditis. The clinical and morphologic features of thyroiditis are further discussed in Chapter 61.

DELAYED HYPERSENSITIVITY

Delayed hypersensitivity[126-149] is an in vivo reaction, which cannot be duplicated in vitro. The delayed hypersensitivity reaction in tissue begins with a perivascular accumulation of lymphocytes and monocytes at the site where antigen is located. Only a few of the infiltrating cells are specifically sensitized. The reaction of these few sensitized cells with the antigen in the tissue causes increasing numbers of nonspecific inflammatory cells to infiltrate the area, with subsequent tissue destruction. Destruction of infecting organisms or tissue is caused by macrophages that are attracted to the site and activated by lymphokines released by T_{DTH} after reaction with antigen. Activated macrophages also release numerous cytokines that contribute to chronic inflammation. Specifically sensitized T_{DTH} cells are also activated to proliferate upon contact with antigen (blast transformation) resulting in an increased number of specifically sensitized cells, and mitogenic factors stimulate proliferation of nonsensitized cells.

The term *delayed* is applied because of the course of the inflammatory skin reaction that follows intradermal injection of antigen into an individual who has been sensitized. The reaction takes several days to peak, in contrast to cutaneous anaphylactic reactions, which reach their peak in a few minutes, and the Arthus reaction, which occurs in hours. The term *tuberculin type of hypersensitivity* is used because for many years the study of this type of immune response was essentially the study of the delayed-hypersensitivity immune response to tuberculin (proteins extracted from cultures of *Mycobacterium tuberculosis*) and infection with tubercle bacilli.

T_{DTH} activation and superantigens

A group of toxins produced by various strains of *Staphylococcus aureus* and related toxins (Table 25-11) produces food poisoning, and one of the toxins is responsible for tampon-related toxic shock. These toxins are also called *superantigens* because they directly activate class MHC II restricted T_{DTH} cells. These molecules are not processed to smaller peptides but bind to class II MHC molecules as whole molecules. The toxins, or superantigens, are intermediate-sized proteins that bind to the V region of the T-cell receptor in association with the class II DR protein, outside of the peptide binding cleft, and directly activate T-cells. The most likely pathogenesis of symptoms is that the toxins produce massive T-cell stimulation and consequent release of T-cell–derived lymphokines such as interleukin-2 and tumor necrosis factor. Large amounts of these lymphokines released into the body cause the food poisoning or toxic shock reaction. It is also possible that toxins could stimulate macrophages through class II MHC binding, but experimental studies in mice that lack T-cells but have normal macrophage activity indicate that activation of macrophages is not sufficient to produce disease. In addition, studies on human cells in vitro show not only that both monocytes and T-cells are required, but also that the monocytes and T-cells must be in contact with each other. Interleukin-1 (produced by macrophages) is elevated after toxin stimulation of human cells but may not be sufficient to produce shock by itself.

Delayed hypersensitivity skin reaction

The classic example of a delayed hypersensitivity skin test is the delayed type of tuberculin skin reaction. It is elicited in sensitive individuals by intradermal injection of tuberculoprotein antigens (PPD, OT). Delayed skin reactions to tubercle bacilli were first noted in 1890 by Koch, who injected live tubercle bacilli into guinea pigs previously infected with tuberculosis. Redness and swelling were seen 24 hours after injection. If severe, the lesion may progress to local tissue necrosis. This reaction was not observed in previously unin-

Table 25-11 Diseases caused by superantigens

Superantigen, or toxin	Source	Disease
Staphylococcal enterotoxins	*Staphylococcus aureus*	Food poisoning
Toxic-shock syndrome toxin (TSSTI)	*Staphylococcus aureus*	Toxic shock syndrome
Exfoliating toxins A and B	*Staphylococcus aureus*	Scalded-skin syndrome
Pyrogenic exotoxins A, B, and C	*Staphylococcus pyogenes*	Rheumatic fever, scarlet fever
Mycoplasma arthritidis supernatant	*M. arthritidis*	Arthritis, shock

Modified from Marrack P, Kappler J: *Science* 248:705, 1990.

fected animals but could be demonstrated in infected animals using killed bacilli or extracts of the bacilli. The extract originally used was called *old tuberculin* (*OT*), a crude extract of cultures of tubercle bacilli. This was replaced by a more purified protein derivative (PPD) of cultures. Because the reaction occurred in hypersensitive animals, not in nonsensitized animals, and appeared much later after testing than the Arthus reaction, it was called *delayed hypersensitivity*.

After injection of antigen into the skin of an individual sensitive in a delayed manner there is little or no reaction until after 4 to 6 hours. The grossly visible induration and swelling usually reach a maximum at 24 to 48 hours. Histologically there is accumulation of mononuclear cells around small veins. Later, mononuclear cells may be seen throughout the area of the reaction with extensive infiltration in the dermis (Fig. 25-23). Polymorphonuclear cells constitute fewer than one third of the cells at any time, and usually few are present at 24 hours or later unless the reaction is severe enough to cause necrosis. There may also be infiltration and degranulation of basophils, perhaps contributing to the increased vascular permeability and edema observed. The CD4 and CD8 subsets of T-cells in the perivascular areas are in the same ratio as in the peripheral blood, but the cells in the diffuse infiltrate in the dermis are predominately CD4 T-cells. The perivascular infiltrate may include nonspecifically attracted cells, whereas the diffuse infiltrate includes more specifically sensitized T_{DTH} cells. The degree of skin reactivity to tuberculin antigens is used as a measure of cellular immunity to tuberculosis.

The role of lymphocyte mediators in delayed hypersensitivity reactions may be summarized simply as follows: Upon contact with antigen, lymphocytes release migratory-inhibitory, skin-reactive, macrophage-specific chemotactic, and macrophage-activation factors, each of which serves to attract and hold macrophages in the reaction site. The number of specifically sensitized cells may be increased by lymphocyte-stimulating factors, which induces proliferation of lymphocytes. Cytotoxic factors may cause death of tissue cells in the reactive area; proliferative-inhibitory factor may inhibit nonlymphoid cell growth; and lymphocyte-permeability factor may increase the magnitude of the inflammatory reaction by causing more cells to accumulate.

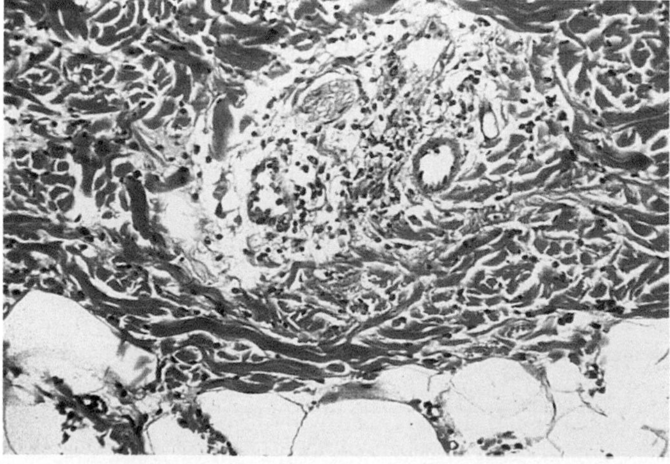

Fig. 25-23 Delayed hypersensitivity skin reaction in sensitized guinea pig. There is accumulation of mononuclear cells in and around small vessels; later these extend into the adjacent dermal tissue. Arterioles (primary site of involvement in Arthus reactions) are not involved, and there is no fibrinoid necrosis.

Cutaneous basophil hypersensitivity

The term *cutaneous basophil hypersensitivity* (CBH) is used to denote a group of lymphocyte-mediated, basophilic reactions that differ histologically from classic DTH reactions. Basophils may be found in a variety of cell-mediated reactions, including skin-graft rejection, tumor rejection, reactions to viral infections, and contact allergy. In contact dermatitis infiltration of lymphocytes precedes basophils by at least 12 hours, probably releasing a lymphokine responsible for attracting basophils. The function of the basophilic infiltrate is not known but might serve as a phagocytic cell that supplements the macrophage.

The term *Jones-Mote reaction* originally referred to the reappearance of a delayed type of sensitivity to serum proteins after the development and regression of an Arthus reaction, noted in humans by Jones and Mote in 1934. This term was extended to cover the transient form of delayed skin reaction to protein antigens occurring before antibody production in experimental animals, a finding also previously observed in humans. With a better appreciation of the basophilic nature of these reactions, the term *cutaneous basophil hypersensitivity* has been applied. As an immunologic reaction, the significance of CBH reactions remains unclear. Since the presence of basophils in varying numbers has been described in human tuberculin as well as in Jones-Mote reactions, it may be that basophils are not really a distinguishing feature but are a variable constituent of delayed-hypersensitivity reactions. Some experimental evidence indicates that tissue mast cells must be present in the dermis in order for antigens to elicit a DTH reaction. The mast cells may function to permit vasodilatation and increased vascular permeability. However typical DTH cutaneous reactions have been elicited in strains of mice lacking tissue mast cells.

Delayed hypersensitivity and infection

For many years the study of immunity was directed to the role of humoral antibody-mediated effects. During the 1960s the importance of CMI in defense against viral, fungal, protozoal, and parasitic diseases became increasingly recognized. The role of T_{CTL} in defense against viral infections of the skin (such as smallpox) was presented earlier in this chapter. The opportunistic infections seen in the acquired immunodeficiency syndrome (AIDS) have driven home the significance of cellular immunity. The major immune deficit in AIDS is a lack of functional CD4+ T-cells. Humoral antibody can prevent infections from first exposures, but once a virus infection has occurred, it will be combated by CMI. The effects of CMI in the pathogenesis of syphilis and viral infections (encephalomyelitis) will now be covered as an example of the "double-edged sword" of immunity. The role of T_{DTH} is also critical for the pathogenesis of tuberculosis (see p. 37).

Representative diseases

Syphilis

The role of the immune response in determining the outcome of an infection is illustrated by syphilis. The tissue-clearing mechanism resulting in the healing of primary (chancre) and secondary syphilis lesions is T_{DTH}-mediated delayed hypersensitivity. Four stages of syphilis are primary, secondary, latent, and tertiary disease, each of which is determined largely by the immune response of the host. The evolution of the primary lesion, the chancre, the first clinical manifestation of primary syphilis, follows closely the pattern of a delayed hypersensitivity reaction in the skin. It lasts from 1 to 5 weeks, is initiated by sensitized T-cells reacting with antigen, and is resolved by phagocytosis and digestion of organisms by macrophages (Fig. 25-24). Protection against reinfection may be partially mediated by antibody neutralization of organisms, but macrophages activated by a delayed-hypersensitivity reaction appear to be the most effective way of killing the organism. Immunity to infection (chancre immunity) is established only by active infection for at least 3 months.

The skin and mucous membrane lesions of secondary syphilis, which appear 2 weeks to 6 months after primary infection also appear to be a delayed-hypersensitivity reaction at sites of dissemination and replication of *Treponema pallidum.* The cellular reaction is similar to that of primary lesions. Although vasculitis has been described in secondary lesions, it is an exception to the rule. Thus there is little evidence for immune complex–mediated vasculitis in syphilitic lesions. The lesions heal spontaneously, and the patient is cured or enters a period of latency. It is hypothesized that individuals with a predominance of DTH will be cured, whereas those with predominant antibody response will remain infected.

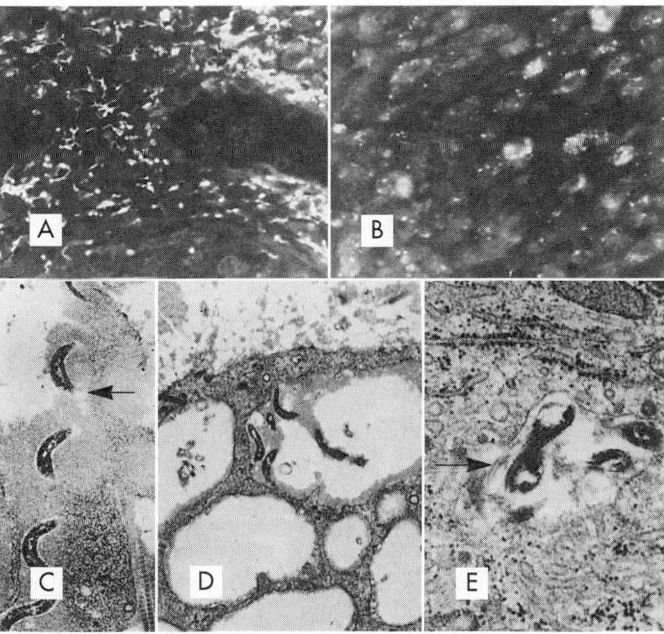

Fig. 25-24 Phagocytosis and digestion of *Treponema pallidum* in primary chancre of syphilis. **A,** Immunofluorescence of *T. pallidum* in experimental rabbit orchitis 10 days after infection. **B,** Immunofluorescence of *T. pallidum* 14 days after infection. **C,** Electron micrograph of intact *T. pallidum* in extracellular ground substance 10 days after infection. **D,** *T. pallidum* in phagocytic vacuoles of macrophage. **E,** Disintegration of *T. pallidum* in phagocytic vacuoles. Between 12 and 17 days after inoculation the organisms are cleared from the tissues by a delayed type of hypersensitivity, which produces phagocytosis and digestion of organisms by macrophages. *Arrows,* Characteristic periplasmic flagella (axial filaments) in intact, **C,** and disintegrating, **E,** organisms. (From Sell S, Baker-Zander S, Powell HC: *Lab Invest* 46:355, 1982.)

In latent syphilis there is no clinical evidence of infection. However, some *T. pallidum* survive the immune attack of the host and remain viable. There does not appear to be any abnormality of the immune system; indeed, persons with latent syphilis are resistant to reinfection; that is, they are immune yet are infected (concomitant immunity).

The destructive lesions characteristic of tertiary syphilis are granulomatous reactions (gummas), which occur in areas where spirochetes apparently persist during latency, as in brain, skin, bone, or viscera. Because no differences in immune potential distinguish patients who develop tertiary disease from those who do not, it is not known why some patients move from latency to tertiary disease. Development of tertiary lesions could result either from an increased state of hypersensitivity causing more intense inflammation or from a decreased state of reactivity permitting organisms to proliferate and initiate a destructive reaction.

T_{DTH}-mediated autoimmune disease

Several autoimmune diseases affecting solid tissues are the result of delayed hypersensitivity.

Experimental allergic encephalomyelitis (EAE) is produced by the injection of central nervous system tissue incorporated into complete Freund's adjuvant. In rats, hind-leg paralysis occurs after 2 to 3 weeks and is associated with a disseminated focal perivascular accumulation of inflammatory cells involving small veins or venules in the white matter of the nervous system. The inflammatory cells, which accumulate within the vessel wall and in the perivascular space, are usually mononuclear, but polymorphonuclear leukocytes may be prominent in very acute reactions. Demyelination occurs in intimate association with the focal vasculitis and most likely is a result of the action of macrophages activated by specifically sensitized T_{DTH} cells; toxic complex activation of polymorphonuclear neutrophils may be responsible for acute lesions. The antigen, encephalitogenic protein, has been studied extensively and the amino acid sequence determined. The major encephalitogenic determinant is a nonapeptide with the amino acid sequence Phe-Ser-Trp-Ala-Glu-Gly-Gln-Lys, the important amino acids being Trp and Gln. The astrocytes in the CNS and Schwann cells in peripheral nerves are able to present antigen to T-cells, and there is experimental evidence that endogenous myelin basic protein may be presented to autoreactive T-cells that constantly move through the nervous system. Study of T-cell clones that are active in passive transfer of EAE indicates that the T-cell receptors employed for EAE are highly restricted—using only two V, one Jα, two Vα, and two Jα gene segments and a highly conserved third hypervariable region, the Vβ gene segment. Reactivity of the encephalitogenic peptide with reactive T-cell clones can be blocked by anti-Vβ monoclonal antibody, and such blocking indicates that such an antibody may be used to treat demyelinating lesions. In the experimental model, immunization with the putative myelin basic protein peptide binding region of the T-cell receptor appears to result in the production of a cytotoxic T-cell that reacts with the TCR of the encephalitogenic T-cell and prevents reaction of the encephalitogenic T-cell with the myelin basic protein in vivo, blocking development of EAE.

Although the reaction of specifically sensitized cells with myelin antigen and subsequent attraction of macrophages is believed to be the major pathologic event (T-cells are required to transfer the disease and monoclonal antibodies to activated

T-cells block development of the disease in experimental animals), humoral antibody may also play an important effector role. The venules of the brain do not permit lymphocytes to pass through, as they do in other organs (blood-brain barrier). Humoral antibody may react with myelin antigens released from the brain normally or as the result of a viral infection. The antibody-antigen reaction may activate anaphylactic or complement mediators, causing contraction and separation of endothelial cells, thus permitting extravasation of lymphocytes into brain tissue. In addition, demyelination may occur secondary to upregulation of expression of MHC class I antigens on oligodendrocytes without involvement of antibody or T-cells.

The prominent tissue lesion is perivascular infiltration of the white matter of the brain and spinal cord with lymphocytes. Antigen reactive T_{DTH} may first recognize myelin antigens on vascular cells at the blood-brain interface and release cytokines that activate the CNS endothelium to express cell adhesion and chemoattractant molecules. Activated T-cells appear to be able to cross the blood-brain barrier. The phenotype of the cells in experimental lesions are mainly TCR^+, $CD4^+$ T-cells. T-cell infiltration is followed by migration of macrophages into tissue containing myelinated nerve fibers, and by stripping of myelinated fibers by macrophages, culminating in phagocytosis and digestion of the myelin. Toxic products of activated T_{DTH} appear to have a role as treatment of recipient mice with antibodies to lymphotoxin, and tumor necrosis factor-α prevents cell-mediated passive transfer of the disease.

The human disease takes three forms: acute hemorrhagic encephalomyelitis, acute disseminated encephalomyelitis, and multiple sclerosis (Chapter 77).

Graft rejection

The interplay of antibody and cell-mediated immunity is exemplified by solid tissue graft rejection. The solid tissue taken from one individual of a species transplanted to a genetically different individual of the same species will evoke a characteristic *allograft* (homograft) rejection. If transplantation is made from one part of the body of an individual to another part of the same individual *(autograft)* or between two genetically identical individuals *(syngraft)* such as monozygotic twins, a graft rejection reaction will not take place.

A graft rejection reaction is perhaps best illustrated by the rejection of two skin grafts from the same donor to the same recipient, with the second graft placed about 1 month after the first graft. Revascularization begins during the second or third day after the first grafting procedure and is complete by the sixth or seventh day. A similar response is observed in autografts, syngrafts, and allografts. However, after about 1 week, the first signs of rejection appear in the deep layers of an allograft. There occurs a perivascular (perivenular) accumulation of mononuclear cells that is similar to that seen in the early stages of a tuberculin skin reaction. The infiltration steadily intensifies, and the graft becomes grossly edematous. The lymphocytic infiltrate then extends into the epidermis, resulting in an appearance similar to that of contact dermatitis. Thrombosis of the dermal vessels then occurs with necrosis and sloughing of the graft. This entire process usually requires 11 to 14 days and is called a *first-set rejection.* A syngraft or autograft does not undergo this process but remains viable with little or no inflammatory reaction.

When a second graft from the same genetically unrelated donor who provided the first graft is transplanted, a more rapid and more vigorous rejection occurs *(second-set rejection).* During the first 3 days after the second transplant the second graft is handled in essentially the same way as the first graft. However, vascularization is abruptly halted at 4 to 5 days when thrombosis results in ischemic necrosis. Because the graft never becomes vascularized and the blood supply is cut off by the second-set rejection, there is little chance for cellular infiltration to occur. The primary target for the second-set rejection appears to be the capillaries taking part in vascularization. Although the first-set reaction is most consistent with a cell-mediated reaction, there is evidence that circulating antibody is involved in the vasculitis characteristic of second-set reactions. Similar events occur after grafting other solid organs such as heart or kidney. Clinical features of graft rejection and the related graft versus host disease are discussed and illustrated in Chapter 29.

GRANULOMATOUS REACTIONS

Granulomas are lesions consisting of focal collections of inflammatory cells, including macrophages, histiocytes, epithelioid cells, and giant cells as well as lymphocytes and plasma cells surrounded by varying amounts of fibrous tissue.[150-183] The epithelioid cell is derived from a macrophage and has a prominent eosinophilic amorphous cytoplasm and a large, oval, pale-staining nucleus with a sharp, thin nuclear membrane and large nucleoli. This characteristic pathologic appearance has been recognized for over 150 years. These cells have been called "epithelioid" because of their resemblance to epithelial cells. Granulomas may progress from highly cellular reactions to fibrous scars.

Mechanisms

The formation of a granuloma is a way that the body deals with substances that it finds difficult to eliminate by the usual process of phagocytosis and digestion by macrophages (Fig. 25-25). The fixed macrophages within tissues and the monocytes that infiltrate sites of inflammation are primarily scavenger cells that are able to break down most infectious agents, as well as foreign bodies and residua of inflammation, by an array of toxic effector molecules and hydrolytic enzymes. It is ironic that many infectious agents, including protozoa, bacteria, fungi, mycobacteria, and viruses actually preferentially infect and replicate within these same cells. Complex signals generated through the products of activated T-cells as well as other cytokines induce a state of activation in the infected macrophage, which kills the intracellular parasites. In addition, T_{CTL} that react with antigens of the infecting organisms expressed on macrophages may attack and kill infected cells, with subsequent destruction of the now extracellular organisms by phagocytosis and digestion by other activated macrophages. The major killing mechanism of activated macrophages may be through generation of nitrogen oxides derived from L-arginine. How cytokines activate the pathway of L-arginine conversion to L-citrulline with formation of nitrogen oxides remains unclear.

Granulomas form because of the sometimes massive load of organisms or poorly digestible products of the organisms. Activation of macrophages by cytokines prevents proliferation of the infecting organisms, and the infection may be cleared early on with little residual evidence in the tissues that infection ever occurred. Positive DTH skin tests provide evidence of previous infection in some individuals with no evidence of disease. However, if the infecting organisms are allowed to multiply, the macrophage system may be faced with an incredible clean-up job, and continued survival and multiplication of some organisms may continue even when there is massive destruction of most of the infecting agents. This results in a sometimes life-long life-and-death struggle between the host and the infection. Prolonged chemotherapy may hold replication of the organisms in check and allow the immune response to get the upper hand. However, if therapy is stopped too soon or the immune system is weakened by age, immunosuppressive drugs, or other infections, recurrence of active infection is the expected course.

The origin of the most characteristic cell of granulomatous hypersensitivity reaction—the epithelioid cell—is most likely from a phagocyte that has ingested foreign material but cannot digest or exocytose the material. Multinuclear giant cells form by fusion of macrophages or epithelioid cells (Fig. 25-26). Granulomatous hypersensitivity reactions may evolve in weeks or even months because of the persistent nature of the stimulus. Several T-cell factors that modulate granuloma formation have been identified: Interleukin-4 causes aggregation and fusion of macrophages, and interferon-γ causes inhibition of macrophage migration and fusion of monocytes. In addition, macrophage-derived factors, including interleukin-1, stimulate fibrosis and scarring in granulomas.

Representative diseases

Granulomatous hypersensitivity diseases include infectious diseases such as tuberculosis, leprosy, and parasitic infestations; responses to known antigens such as zirconium granuloma and berylliosis, and other diseases of unknown cause in which epithelioid granulomas are the primary lesion. Epithelioid granulomas occur in other diseases such as tertiary syphilis, fungus infections, and some foreign-body reactions (such as around urate deposits in gout). Granulomas are also a prominent feature of early asbestosis and silicosis.

Tuberculosis

Granulomas are the single most striking feature of tuberculosis. Tuberculosis is the classic example of mixed protective and pathogenic effects of immune and nonimmune inflammatory reactions to a single agent. Primary infection begins by inhalation of a droplet containing a viable bacillus and implantation in the lung, usually in a lower lobe, and, depending on the dose of infection and the strength of the host's immune response, may lead to progressive infection, arrested infection, or complete cure. In complete cure residual whorled scars may be found in the lung or hilar lymph nodes, which represent "healed granulomas." In arrested infection the granulomas may still retain the characteristic cellular appearance because there is continued stimulation of the granulomatous response. The center of the granuloma may become necrotic so that grossly it looks like cottage cheese. This is termed *caseous necrosis*. Viable organisms may survive for long periods of time in the center of a caseous granuloma, where they are protected from the immune response of the host. Progressive infection features multiple active cellular granulomas that eventually fill the lung and cause death because of insufficient normal lung for oxygenation of the blood.

The granulomatous "lesions" of tuberculosis are the result of the host-parasite immune interaction. Clearly a granulomatous reaction represents a defensive reaction that is not always successful. Nonspecific T γ/δ cytotoxic cells may be active during the first few days after infection and may be able to control low numbers of organisms. Continued infection results in induction of T_{DTH}, presumably by antigen processing by MHC class II interdigitating reticulum cells, as well as T_{CTL} through endogenous antigen presentation by MHC class I cells, presumably infected macrophages. Upon reaction with *M. tuberculosis* antigens, T_{DTH} cells secrete lymphokines that enable activated macrophages to limit dissemination of the organism. T_{CTL} are also activated and may kill infected macrophages. This may contribute to the necrosis seen but may cause release of organisms from protected sites in macrophages that are unable to be activated because of their infection. T_{CTL}-mediated destruction of infected macrophages allows T_{DTH}-activated macrophages to phagocytose and digest the organisms, thus clearing the intracellular infection. T_{DTH} reacting with antigens on the bacilli released from infected macrophages lysed by T_{CTL} release factors that attract and activate macrophages. If the infiltrating macrophages are not activated, reinfection of macrophages may be a weakness in the battle against tuberculosis, contributing to spread of the infection or resulting in the formation of granulomas. If extensive, this proliferation of macrophages and accumulation of granulomas as the result of ongoing chronic infection can lead to eventual loss of organ function as the normal tissue is replaced by granulomas.

Leprosy

The clinical features of leprosy depend on the immune reaction of the infected individual: DTH leads to arrested infection (tuberculoid leprosy), and antibody formation leads to progressive disease (lepromatous leprosy). The immune characteristics of different clinical classifications of leprosy are discussed in Chapter 34.

Zirconium granulomas

Some 6 months after the marketing of stick deodorants containing zirconium salts, individuals were observed with axillary granulomas. The injection of zirconium into the skin of such patients resulted in the delayed appearance of a typical epithelioid granuloma. Further studies have clearly implicated zirconium as the causative agent. Some type of hypersensitivity was suspected because only relatively few individuals who used such deodorants actually developed lesions. When the use of zirconium was discontinued, lesions no longer occurred.

Berylliosis

Two forms of lung disease are associated with inhalation of beryllium. An acute chemical inflammation caused by heavy exposure and a chronic progressive pulmonary disease after low exposure featuring multiple small noncaseating granulomas, first reported in 1946. The conclusion that a type of hypersensitivity is involved in the latter is based on the observations that only a small number of the exposed individuals actually develop the disease and that there may be a delay of months or years from the time of exposure to the development of berylliosis. Beryllium was once used for the manufacture of fluorescent light bulbs, and many exposed individuals

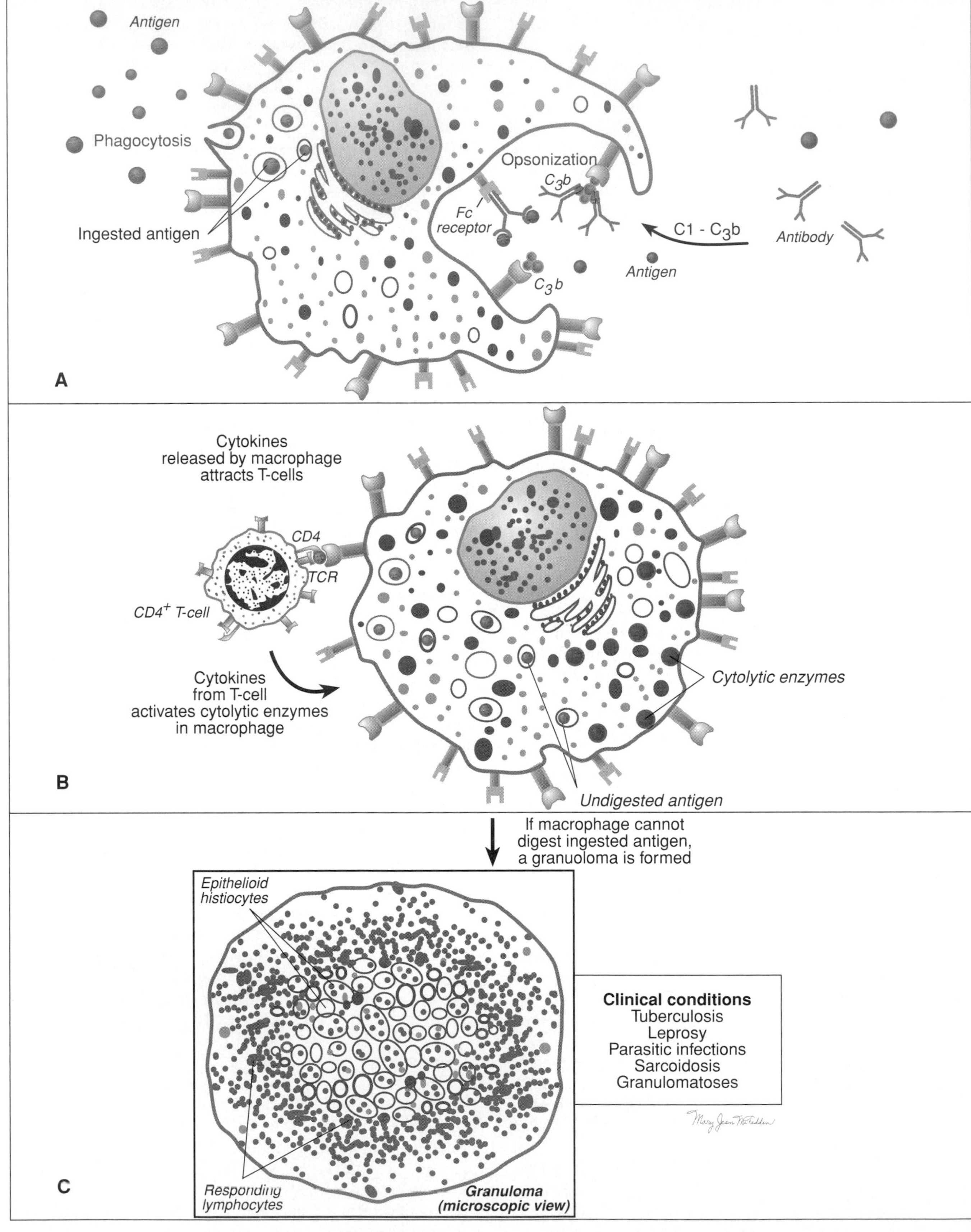
Antigen
Phagocytosis
Ingested antigen
Opsonization
C_3b
Fc receptor
C1 - C_3b
Antibody
Antigen
C_3b
A
Cytokines released by macrophage attracts T-cells
CD4
TCR
$CD4^+$ T-cell
Cytokines from T-cell activates cytolytic enzymes in macrophage
Cytolytic enzymes
Undigested antigen
B
If macrophage cannot digest ingested antigen, a granuoloma is formed
Epithelioid histiocytes
Clinical conditions
Tuberculosis
Leprosy
Parasitic infections
Sarcoidosis
Granulomatoses
Responding lymphocytes
Granuloma (microscopic view)
C

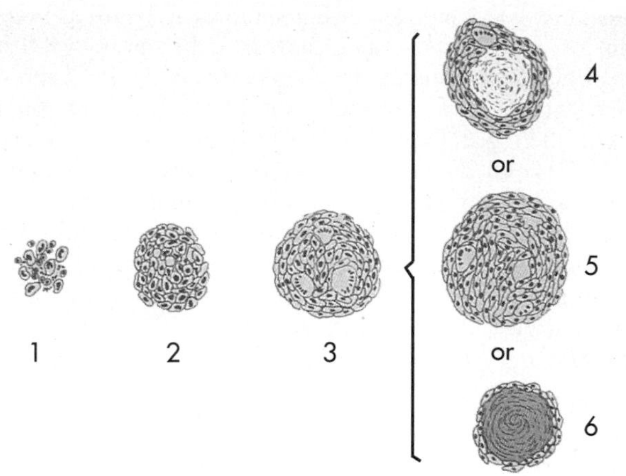

Fig. 25-26 Progression of granulomas. *1*, Granulomas begin as small collections of lymphocytes and macrophages that form around poorly degradable antigens. *2*, Macrophages change to epithelioid cells and become organized into a cluster of cells. *3*, Further progression results in ball-like clusters of cells and fusion of macrophages into giant cells. Further progression may include: *4*, development of necrosis in the center as characteristic of chronic tuberculosis; *5*, continued enlargement and replacement of normal tissue (progressive disease); or *6*, fibrosis with scar formation, characteristic of "healed" sarcoidosis.

remained symptomless. Beryllium is no longer used for this purpose, and the disease has been greatly reduced. Berylliosis has been reported more recently after low exposure in precious-metal refining, and beryllium is still used in the aircraft industry. Cases have been reported occurring after exposure to levels previously believed to be safe. The chronicity of the disease may also be attributable to the fact that beryllium tends to remain in the tissue indefinitely. It has been reported that patients with berylliosis give positive patch test reactions with the antigen, but the validity of this observation has been questioned. Further studies have shown that beryllium is an active inducer of contact sensitivity, and a beryllium patch test measures delayed hypersensitivity. A more relevant test is the production of a granuloma upon intradermal application of beryllium in patients with berylliosis. Application of beryllium in a patch test most likely does not stimulate a granulomatous reaction, which requires deposition of the eliciting antigen in tissues. The lymphocytes of patients with berylliosis will transform in vitro upon exposure to beryllium sulfate, further indicating that cellular sensitization to beryllium probably occurs. Zirconium as well as beryllium may bind serum proteins and function as a hapten in the production of contact sensitivity. However, the relation of this mechanism to the development of granulomas remains obscure. Berylliosis may be considered an example of hypersensitivity pneumonitis.

Granulomatous vasculitis

Vasculitis is a component of several granulomatous reactions. The lesions listed include several vascular and granulomatous reactions for which the exact mechanism is not known. However, polyarteritis nodosa is most likely an immune complex–mediated lesion, whereas eosinophilia granuloma is a granulomatous lesion. Allergic granulomatosis, or Churg-Strauss syndrome, includes necrotizing vasculitis, extravascular granulomas, and tissue infiltration, with eosinophils occurring in association with bronchial asthma. Such a combination of lesions may indicate the involvement of different immune effector mechanisms—such as immune complex, anaphylactic and granulomatous—in response to the same eliciting antigen.

Sarcoidosis

Boeck's sarcoidosis is a systemic noncaseating granulomatous process of unknown cause predominantly involving the lymph nodes, lungs, eyes, and skin, with lesions that may be indistinguishable from those of tuberculosis, fungus infections, or other granulomatous hypersensitivity reactions. The term *sarcoid* was coined by Caesar Boeck in 1899 for the skin lesions; systemic involvement was recognized by Schaumann in 1917. The clinical presentation of sarcoidosis may masquerade as acute rheumatoid arthritis, tuberculosis, erythema nodosum, or Crohn's disease, but usually appears as pulmonary masses and bilateral hilar adenopathy on a chest x-ray film of a young adult with dyspnea. An infectious agent is suspected, but as yet no specific agent has been identified. The characteristic noncaseating granuloma is not pathognomonic; identical histopathologic lesions may be seen with mycobacterial and fungal infections, brucellosis, mineral dust exposure, hypersensitivity pneumonitis, and Wegener's granulomatosis. The granuloma has a central zone with tightly packed cells, including epithelioid cells, macrophages, and giant cells, surrounded by a peripheral zone with more loosely arranged mononuclear cells. The giant cells may contain concentrically laminated basophilic structures (Schaumann bodies), and smaller spindle-shaped inclusions with radiating spines (asteroid bodies) may be found at the outer edge of the central zone of the granuloma. The granulomas ultimately resolve leaving no morphologic lesion or alternatively undergo fibrosis and contraction. The lesions are believed to be caused by T-cell activation leading to accumulation, fusion, and epithelioid changes in macrophages, but

---

Fig. 25-25 Mechanism of granuloma formation. The process begins when macrophages ingest infectious organisms or foreign material that they are incapable of digesting. These antigens persist within phagolysosomes in the macrophage cytoplasm (**A**). The macrophage breaks down some of the antigen and presents antigenic peptides to passing T-lymphocytes via cell surface MHC class II molecules. If a T-cell bearing receptors capable of recognizing the MHC-peptide complex is encountered, the T-cell becomes activated and releases cytokines (IFN-γ) capable of activating the cytoplasmic killing machinery of the macrophage (**B**). In most cases, this destroys the invading microbe or foreign material. Some microbes have developed resistance to killing by the macrophage, and the antigen may persist for prolonged periods within the cell. In such cases, the continuous expression of antigen and subsequent cytokine release from both macrophages and T-cells results in recruitment of additional macrophages and lymphocytes into the vicinity of the infection. This continued cell recruitment leads to the formation of what is recognized histologically as a granuloma (**C**).

the "antigen" responsible for the T-cell activation has not been identified. Patients with sarcoidosis generally exhibit a depression of delayed hypersensitivity and increased levels of circulating antibody. The relationship of these findings to the disease process remains unclear but is suggestive of an imbalance in the immune system, with a relatively incompetent T-cell system. This could be because of a redistribution of T-cells in the inflammatory process or to an inherent loss of T-cell activity. The reason for the polyclonal activation of B-cells is not known but may be secondary to production of interleukins by activation of T-helper cells during granuloma formation or to a form of immune deviation. Helper T-cells ($CD4^+$) predominate early in the disease, but suppressor T-cells ($CD8^+$) predominate during regression of the granulomas. T-cells have been reported to be elevated in the blood and lung of patients with sarcoidosis.

Wegener's granulomatosis

Wegener's granulomatosis is a triad of granulomatous arteritis, glomerulonephritis, and sinusitis that has been recognized as a distinct clinicopathologic entity for over 60 years. The glomerulonephritis may or may not be present, and the granulomas may be disseminated but are usually prominent in the lungs, nasal and oral cavities, and spleen. The granulomatous lesions are destructive and contain fibroblastic proliferation, necrosis, and prominent Langhans' giant cells. This disease may be related to polyarteritis nodosa, and some authors have called it "polyarteritis of the lungs," or a type of hypersensitivity angiitis. However, the lesions of Wegener's granulomatosis are distinctive enough to warrant a separate diagnosis. An unusual finding is granulomatous glomerulonephritis, believed to be caused by a reaction to fibrin mixed with immune complexes in gaps in Bowman's capsule, leading to destruction of Bowman's capsule and a surrounding granulomatous inflammation. The natural history of the disease is invariable rapid progression with destruction of the upper respiratory system. The relation of Wegener's granulomatosis to other necrotizing granulomatous processes, such as midline lethal granuloma of the face, is not clear. No infectious agent has been consistently isolated from patients with any of these diseases.

Antibodies to neutrophils, called *antineutrophil cytoplasmic antibodies* (ANCA), have been found in patients with Wegener's granulomatosis. Although a pathogenic role for ANCA is not established, it is possible that infections (such as pneumonitis) cause degranulation of neutrophils and release of lysosomal enzymes that elicit an autoimmune response. Excessive stimulation of neutrophils by ANCA and the proteolytic effects of released lysosomal enzymes may then cause endothelial damage and tissue necrosis.

Regional enteritis

Regional enteritis is a peculiar chronic inflammatory lesion of unknown cause related to ulcerative colitis. The primary feature is thickening and scarring of the intestinal wall that may occur at any level of the gastrointestinal tract but usually involves the terminal ileum. Histologically the inflammatory changes vary from those consistent with a delayed hypersensitivity reaction (dense infiltration of mononuclear lymphoid follicles often containing germinal centers) to those of granulomatous hypersensitivity (typical epithelioid granulomas with prominent giant cells, essentially identical to the pulmonary lesions of sarcoidosis). The lesions appear to begin as accumulations of lymphocytes and plasma cells around intestinal crypts. Later macrophages are seen associated with destruction of the crypt *(crypt abscess)* followed by formation of epithelial cells and then granulomas. The T-cell ratios in mature lesions are 2:1 $CD4^+/CD8^+$, about the same as in control tissues. The mononuclear inflammation of regional enteritis may be the result of the development of delayed hypersensitivity to soluble antigens in the diet, and the granulomatous inflammation may be attributable to the development of granulomatous hypersensitivity to insoluble antigens in the diet, but no causative antigen has yet been identified.

SUMMARY

Seven distinctive immunopathologic mechanisms may act to protect us from infection or to cause disease (see Table 25-2).

1. *Inactivation and activation reactions.* Circulating antibodies to biologically active molecules may effectively inactivate or neutralize the activity of these molecules and thus neutralize bacterial toxins or produce diseases because of the loss of a vital biologically active molecule. In some instances, autoantibodies may actually stimulate increased function by binding to and activating receptors. Biologically active molecules that may be affected by antibodies include hormones, enzymes, growth factors, clotting factors, and cell surface receptors. Inactivation may occur by alteration of tertiary structure, blocking of active sites, or modulation of cell surface receptors. Autoantibodies to endocrine glands, hormones, or hormone receptors are the best understood examples of these activation or inactivation reactions.

2. *Cytotoxic or cytolytic reactions.* Cytotoxic or cytolytic reactions are caused by circulating antibody to cell surface structures with subsequent complement fixation. This mechanism may kill invading microorganisms or vital cells. The cell surface antigens may be an integral part of the cell membrane or may be acquired by passive absorption. Reaction of antibody of the IgM or IgG class with the cell surface antigens results in activation of complement and destruction of the cell by complement-mediated lysis or by phagocytosis by macrophages with receptors for activated complement components or aggregated immunoglobulin. Cells in contact with the circulating blood are most often the target cells; these include red blood cells, white blood cells, and platelets. The disease states are the result of a loss of the function of the affected cells. Examples of such diseases are hemolytic anemia, agranulocytosis, and thrombocytopenic purpura. In addition, epithelial cells of the skin may be targets of cytotoxic reactions leading to blistering skin diseases.

3. *Immune complex reactions.* Immune complex reactions are caused by immunoglobulin antibody reacting with tissue antigens, by formation of antibody-antigen complexes that deposit in vessel walls or basement membrane of capillaries, or by antibodies that react with basement membrane antigens. This mechanism activates an acute inflammatory response that is effective in killing infecting organisms or host tissues. Tissue destruction is mediated by lysosomal enzymes released from polymorphonuclear leukocytes attracted and activated by complement components (C3a, C5a). Acute lesions feature tissue digestion by enzymes, whereas chronic lesions may be caused by deposition of large amounts of immune complexes

or scarring. Typical diseases caused by this mechanism include serum sickness, glomerulonephritis, vasculitis, collagen diseases, and many types of skin eruptions. The antigens involved may be host tissue antigens (autoimmune reaction) or foreign (bacterial, viral) antigens.

4. *Anaphylactic reactions.* Anaphylactic (acute) or atopic (chronic) reactions are caused by activation of mast cells by reaction of reaginic antibody fixed to the mast cell surface. Reaginic antibody belongs to a unique class of immunoglobulin, IgE, which has the capacity to bind, or "fix," to receptors on mast cells. Mast cells are stimulated by reaction with allergen to release pharmacologically agents stored in cytoplasmic granules (degranulation) such as histamine and serotonin, which produce acute reactions. In addition arachidonic acid from membrane phospholipids is converted to leukotrienes and prostaglandins, which produce or cause later inflammatory lesions. These released mediators act on smooth muscle cells and endothelial cells, causing constriction. This in turn produces clinical symptoms because of bronchoconstriction (asthma), loss of intravascular fluid (edema, cutaneous anaphylaxis, shock), or chronic accumulation of mucus (hay fever, nasal polyps).

Anaphylactic reactions may serve a protective role in providing rapid egress of other antibodies or cells into sites of antigen deposition by inducing endothelial cell separation. However, allergic reactions cause problems for a large number of people and constitute the basis for the practice of a major clinical specialty—the allergist.

5. *T-cell cytotoxicity.* Cell-mediated immune (CMI) reactions are initiated by reaction of specifically sensitized lymphocytes with antigen in tissues. Two major T lymphocyte populations are involved: T_{CTL} killing of antigen-bearing target cells and T_{DTH} (delayed hypersensitivity). Examples of T_{CTL}-mediated reactions presented in this chapter include contact dermatitis, viral exanthems (smallpox), tissue graft rejections, and autoimmune diseases, such as thyroiditis. Specifically sensitized T_{CTL} may kill infected cells and limit infection, or produce loss of vital functions of cells.

6. *Delayed hypersensitivity.* T_{DTH} cells release lymphocytic mediators when activated by antigen that produce tissue inflammation mainly by attracting and activating macrophages. Most of the tissue damage seen in vivo is mediated by macrophages. Delayed hypersensitivity reactions include the delayed type of skin test reactions (tuberculin), immune response to syphilis infection, and autoimmune encephalomyelitis. Both T_{CTL} and T_{DTH} activity are called into play in the intracellular infections with tuberculosis, but the inflammatory response that results from DTH reactions is very effective in destroying solid organs and is the major effector mechanism for some autoimmune diseases.

7. *Granulomatous reactions.* Granulomatous reactions are characterized by the accumulation of modified mononuclear cells in tissue. The typical tissue lesion contains large mononuclear cells that look like epithelial cells (epithelioid cells), multinucleated giant cells, lymphocytes, and plasma cells. Granulomatous reactions may be a variant of delayed hypersensitivity reactions to insoluble antigens but also frequently occur in association with vasculitis or in response to nonantigenic foreign bodies. It is likely that poorly degradable antigens or insoluble antibody-antigen complexes produce granulomas, whereas soluble complexes cause vasculitis or glomerulonephritis. The mechanism of granulomatous reactivity is not clear, but the inability of macrophages to digest antigens is believed to be a major pathogenic feature. Granulomatous tissue reactions serve to isolate infectious agents such as tubercle bacilli, leprosy bacilli, or parasites. Deleterious effects of these reactions occur because of the displacement of normal tissue by granulomas and healing by fibrosis, leading to a loss of normal function.

Immune mechanisms in disease. Emphasis in this chapter has been placed on the characteristics of different immunopathologic mechanisms. However, in many diseases more than one mechanism may be responsible for the lesions seen. For instance, in rheumatoid arthritis (see Chapter 75), the initial inflammatory reaction is believed to be caused by immune complexes, but the chronic progressive stage of the disease involves cell-mediated immunity. In many infectious diseases one type of immune effector mechanisms may be protective; the other, however, may not contribute to defense but even cause destructive lesions. For example in leprosy, DTH is protective and limits infection; antibody is not protective and is responsible for immune complex—mediated vasculitis. To comprehend the pathogenic progress in any given individual with an immune disease, it is necessary to be able to appreciate the contribution made by different immunopathologic mechanisms.

REFERENCES

The immune response

1. Bjorkman PJ, Saper MA, Samraoui B et al: Structure of the human class I histocompatibility antigen, HLA-A2, *Nature* 329:506, 1987.
2. Gell PGH, Coombs RRA: *Clinical aspects of immunology,* Oxford, 1963, Blackwell.
3. Jerne NK: Towards a network theory of the immune response, *Ann Immunol* (Paris) 5:125C, 373, 1974.
4. Jorgensen JL, Reay PA, Ehrich EW, Davis MM: Molecular components of T-cell recognition, *Annu Rev Immunol* 10:835, 1992.
5. Keegan AD, Paul WE: Multichain immune recognition receptors: similarities in structure and signaling pathways, *Immunol Today* 13:63, 1992.
6. Linsley PS, Ledbetter JL: The role of the CD28 receptor during T-cell responses to antigen, *Annu Rev Immunol* 11:191, 1993.
7. Montefort S, Holgate ST: Adhesion molecules and their role in inflammation, *Respir Med* 85:91, 1991.
8. Mosmann TR, Coffman RL: Heterogeneity of cytokine secretion patterns and functions of helper T-cells, *Adv Immunol* 46:111, 1989.
9. Paul WE, editor: *Fundamental immunology,* New York, 1989, Raven Press, p 1123.
10. Peltz G: A role for CD4+ T-cell subsets producing a selective pattern of lymphokines in the pathogenesis of human chronic inflammatory and allergic diseases, *Immunol Rev* 123:23, 1991.
11. Perelson A: Immune network theory, *Immunol Rev* 110:5, 1989.
12. Rose NR, De Macario EC, Fahey JL et al: *Manual of clinical laboratory immunology,* ed 4, Washington, DC, 1992, American Society for Microbiology, p 987.
13. Sell S: *Immunology, immunopathology, and immunity,* ed 4, New York, Amsterdam, 1987, Elsevier, p 852.
14. Shimizu Y, Shaw S: Lymphocyte interactions with extracellular matrix, *FASEB J* 5:2292, 1991.
15. Turk JL, Oort J: Germinal center activity in relation to delayed hypersensitivity. In Cottier J, Odartchenko N, Schindler R, Congden CC, editors: *Germinal centers in immune responses,* New York, 1967, Springer.
16. Weiss AT: T-cell antigen receptor signal transduction: a tale of tails and cytoplasmic protein-tyrosine kinases, *Cell* 73:209, 1993.

Inactivation and activation

17. Aston R, Cowden WB, Ada GL: Antibody-mediated enhancement of hormone activity, *Mol Immunol* 26:435, 1989.

18. Rotman MB, Celada F: Antibody-mediated activation of a defective β-D-galactosidase extracted from an *Escherichia coli* mutant, *Proc Natl Acad Sci USA* 60:660, 1968.
19. Faustman D: Mechanisms of autoimmunity in type I diabetes, *J Clin Immunol* 13:1, 1993.
20. MacLaren NK: Viral and immunologic basis of beta cell failure in insulin-dependent diabetes, *Am J Dis Child* 131:1149, 1977.
21. Obberghen EV, Kahn, CR: Autoantibodies and insulin receptor, *Mol Cell Endocrinol* 22:271, 1981.
22. Pope CC: The immunology of insulin, *Adv Immunol* 5:209, 1966.
23. Vardi P, Brik R, Barzilai D: Insulin autoantibodies: reflection of disturbed self-identification and their use in the predicition of type I diabetes, *Diabetes Metab Rev* 7:209, 1991.
24. Jacobsen DE, Gorman CA: Endocrine ophthalmopathy: current ideas concerning etiology, pathogenesis and treatment, *Endocrinol Rev* 5:200, 1984.
25. Karlsson FA, Wibell L, Wide L: Hypothyroidism due to thyroid-hormone-binding antibodies, *N Engl J Med* 296:1146, 1977.
26. Kohn LD, Kuppers RC: Thyrotropin receptor autoantibodies in thyroid autoimmune disease; epitopes and origin, *Clin Immunol* 12:169, 1992.
27. McKenzie JM, Zakarija M: LATS in Graves' disease, *Recent Prog Horm Res* 33:29, 1977.
28. Ochi Y, DeGroot LJ: Long acting thyroid stimulator of Graves' disease, *N Engl J Med* 278:718, 1968.
29. Levinson AI, Zweiman B, Lisak RP: Immunopathogenesis and treatment of myasthenia gravis, *J Clin Immunol* 7:187, 1987.
30. Lindstrom JM, Engel AG, Seybold ME et al: Pathological mechanisms in experimental autoimmune myasthenia gravis. II. Passive transfer of experimental autoimmune myasthenia gravis in rats with anti-acetylcholine receptor antibodies, *J Exp Med* 144:739, 1976.
31. Lindstrom J, Shelton D, Fujii Y: Myasthenia gravis, *Adv Immunol* 42:233, 1988.
32. Lopate G, Pestronk A: Autoimmune myasthenia gravis, *Hosp Pract* 28:55, 1993.
33. Dwyer DS, Vakil M, Kearney JF: Idiotypic network connectivity and a possible cause of myasthenia gravis, *J Exp Med* 164:1310, 1986.
34. Rodey GE: Anti-idiotypic antibodies and regulation of immune responses, *Transfusion* 32:361, 1992.
35. Shoelson SE, Marshall S, Horikoski H et al: Antiinsulin receptor antibodies in an insulin-dependent diabetic may arise as autoantiidiotypes, *J Clin Endocrinol Metab* 63:56, 1986.
36. Zanettu M, Bigazzi PE: Anti-idiotypic immunity and autoimmunity. I. In vitro and in vivo effects of anti-idiotypic antibodies to spontaneously occurring autoantibodies to rat thyroglobulin, *Eur J Immunol* 11:187, 1981.

Cytolytic reactions

37. Stec N, Shirey RS, Smith B et al: The efficacy of performing red cell elution studies in the pretransfusion testing of patients with positive direct antiglobulin tests, *Transfusion* 69:266, 1983
38. Schmidt PJ: Transfusion reaction: Status in 1982, *Clin Lab Med* 2:221, 1982.
39. Bowman JM: Fetomaternal ABO incompatibility and erythroblastosis fetalis, *Vox Sang* 50:104, 1986.
40. Clarke CA, Mollison PL: Deaths from Rh haemolytic disease of the fetus and newborn, 1877-1987, *J R Coll Physicians Lond* 23:181, 1989.
41. Levine P: The discovery of Rh hemolytic disease, *Vox Sang* 47:187, 1984.
42. Taylor JF: Sensitization of Rh-negative daughters by their Rh-positive mothers, *N Engl J Med* 276:547, 1967.
43. Atkinson JP, Frank MM: Studies on the in vivo effects of antibody: interaction of IgM antibody and complement in the immune clearance and destruction of erythrocytes in man, *J Clin Invest* 54:339, 1974.
44. Dacie JV, Wolledge SM: Autoimmune hemolytic anemia, *Prog Hematol* 6:1, 1969.
45. Müller-Eckardt C, Salama A: Drug-induced immune cytopenias: a unifying pathogenetic concept with special emphasis on the role of drug metabolites, *Trans Med Rev* 4:69, 1990.
46. Petz LD, Garraty G: *Acquired immune hemolytic anemias*, New York, 1980, Churchill Livingstone.
47. Poschmann A, Fisher K: Autoimmune hemolytic anemia: recent advances in pathogenesis, diagnosis and treatment, *Eur J Pediatr* 143:258, 1985.
48. Sokol RJ, Booker DJ, Stamps R: The pathology of autoimmune haemolytic anaemia, *J Clin Pathol* 45:1047, 1992.
49. Bux J, Kissel K, Nowak K et al: Autoimmune neutropenia: clinical and laboratory studies in 143 patients, *Ann Hematol* 61:249, 1991.
50. Madyastha PR, Glassman AB: Neutrophil antigens and antibodies in the diagnosis of immune neutropenias, *Ann Clin Lab Med Sci* 19:146, 1989.
51. Pisciotta AV: Immune and toxic mechanisms in drug induced agranulocytosis, *Semin Hematol* 10:279, 1973.
52. Kollar CA: Immune thrombocytopenia purpura, *Med Clin North Am* 64:761, 1980.
53. Skacel PO, Contreras M: Neonatal alloimmune thrombocytopenia, *Blood Rev* 3:174, 1989.

Immune complex reactions

54. Andres G, Brentjens JR, Caldwell PRB et al: Formation of immune deposits and disease, *Lab Invest* 55:510, 1986.
55. Cochrane CG, Koffler D: Immune complex disease in experimental animals and in man, *Adv Immunol* 16:185, 1973.
56. Dixon FJ: The role of antigen-antibody complexes in disease, *Harvey Lect* 58:21, 1962.
57. Arthus M: Injections répétées de sérum de cheval chez le lapin, *C R Soc Biol* (Paris) 55:817, 1903
58. Gell PGH, Hinde IT: Observations on the histology of the Arthus reaction and its relation to other known types of skin hypersensitivity, *Int Arch Allerg* 5:23, 1954.
59. Cochrane CG: Mediators of the Arthus and related reactions, *Prog Allergy* 11:1, 1967.
60. Crawford JP, Movat H, Ranadive NS, Hay JB: Pathways to inflammation induced by immune complexes: development of the Arthus reaction, *Fed Proc* 41:2583, 1982.
61. Dixon FJ, Vasquez JJ, Weigle WO, Cochrane CG: Pathogenesis of serum sickness, *Arch Pathol* 65:18, 1958.
62. Germuth FG: A comparative histologic and immunologic study on rabbits of induced hypersensitivity of serum sickness type, *J Exp Med* 97:257, 1953.
63. von Pirquet CF, Schick B: *Serum sickness, 1905,* translated by B Schick, Baltimore, 1951, Williams & Wilkins.
64. Adler S, Baker P, Pritzl P, Couser WG: Effects of alterations in glomerular charge on deposition of cationic and anionic antibodies to fixed glomerular antigens in the rat, *J Lab Clin Med* 106:1, 1985.
65. Brentjens JR, Andres G: Interaction of antibodies with renal cell surface antigens, *Kidney Int* 35:954, 1989.
66. Gauthier VJ, Mannik M: A small proportion of cationic antibodies in immune complexes is sufficient to mediate their deposition in glomeruli, *J Immunol* 145:3348, 1990.
67. Rifai A, Imai H, Oka D: IgA immune complexes and disease: an experimental perspective, *Pathol Immunopathol Res* 5:278, 1986.
68. Benoit FL, Rulon DB, Theil GB et al: Goodpasture's syndrome: a clinicopathologic entity, *Am J Med* 37:424, 1964.
69. Hudson BG, Wieslander J, Wisdom BJ, Noelken ME: Goodpasture syndrome: molecular architecture and function of basement membrane antigen, *Lab Invest* 61:256, 1989.
70. Churg A, Churg J, editors: *Systemic vasculitides,* New York, 1991, Igaku-Shoin.
71. Goeken JA: Antineutrophil cytoplasmic antibody: a useful serological marker for vasculitis, *J Clin Immunol* 11:161, 1991.
72. LeRoy EC, editor: *Systemic vasculitis: the biologic basis,* New York, 1992, Marcel Dekker.

Atopic and anaphylactic reactions

73. Bochner BS, Lichtenstein, LM: Current concept—anaphylaxis, *N Engl J Med* 324:1785, 1991.
74. Coca AF, Grove EF: Studies on hypersensitiveness. XIII. A study of the actopic reagins, *J Immunol* 10:445, 1925.
75. DeJarnatt AC, Grant JA: Basic mechanisms of anaphylaxis and anaphylactoid reactions, *Immunol Allergy Clin North Am* 12:501, 1992.

76. Portier RH, Richet C: De l'action anaphylactique de certains venins, *C R Soc Biol* 54:170, 1902.
77. Prausnitz C, Küstner H: Studies on sensitivity. *Zentralbl Bakteriol* (Orig) 86:160, 1921. English trans in Gell PGH, Coombs RRA: *Clinical aspects of immunology*, Philadelphia, 1963, Davis, p 808.
78. Quinke H: On acute localized edema of the skin, *Monatshefte Prakt Dermatol* 1:129, 1882.
79. Ishizaka K, Ishizaka T, Hornbrook MH: Physico-chemical properties of human reaginic antibody. IV. Presence of a unique immunoglobulin as a carrier of reaginic activity, *J Immunol* 97:75, 1966.
80. Block KS: The anaphylactic antibodies of mammals including man, *Prog Allergy* 10:84, 1967.
81. Metzger H: The receptor with high affinity for IgE, *Immunol Rev* 125:37, 1992.
82. Buist AS: Asthma mortality: what have we learned? *J Allergy Clin Immunol* 84:275, 1989.
83. Calderon E, Lockey RF: A possible role for adhesion molecules in asthma, *J Allergy Clin Immunol* 90:852, 1992.
84. Osler W: *The principles and practice of medicine*, New York, 1892, Appleton & Low, p 499.
85. While MV, Slater JE, Kaliner MA: Histamine and asthma, *Am Rev Respir Dis* 135:1165, 1987.
86. Raphael GD, Baraniuk JN, Kaliner MA: How and why the nose runs, *J Allergy Clin Immunol* 87:457, 1991.
87. Simmons FER: Allergic rhinitis: recent advances, *Pediatr Clin North Am* 35:1053, 1988.
88. Stechschulte DJ: Leukotrienes in asthma and allergic rhinitis, *N Engl J Med* 323:1769, 1990.
89. Wyman M: *Autumnal catarah; hay fever*, Cambridge, Mass, 1872, Hurd & Houghton.
90. Michaelsson G, Juhlin L: Urticaria induced by preservatives and dye additives in food and drugs, *Br J Dermatol* 88:525, 1973.
91. Rowe AH, Rowe A Jr: *Food allergy*, Springfield, Ill, 1972, Charles C Thomas.
92. Schmidt E, editor: *Food allergy*, (Nestle Nutrition Workshop Series, vol 17), New York, 1988, Vevey/Raven Press.
93. Frazier CA: Biting insect survey: a statistical report, *Ann Allergy* 32:200, 1974.
94. King TP: Insect venom allergy, *Monogr Allergy* 28:84, 1990.
95. Reisman RE: Insect sting anaphylaxis, *Immunol Allergy Clin North Am* 12:535, 1992.
96. Kaplan AP: Urticaria and angioedema. In Gallin JL, Goldstein IM, Snyderman R, editors: *Inflammation: basic principles and clinical conditions*, New York, 1988, Raven Press.
97. Ebken RK, Bauschard FA, Levin MI: Dermatographism: its definition, demonstration, and prevalence, *J Allergy* 41:338, 1968.
98. Moqbel R, Pritchard DI: Parasites and allergy: evidence for a "cause and effect" relationship, *Clin Exp Allergy* 20:611, 1990.
99. Rothwell TLW: Immune expulsion of parasitic nematodes from the alimentary tract, *Int J Parasitol* 19:139, 1989.
100. Stebbings JH Jr: Immediate hypersensitivity: a defense against arthropods, *Perspect Biol Med* 17:233, 1974.
101. Steinberg P, Ishizaka K, Norman PS: Possible role of IgE-mediated ractions in immunity, *J Allergy Clin Immunol* 54:359, 1974.

T-cell–mediated cytoxicity

102. Berke G, Rosen D, Ronen D: Mechanism of lymphocyte-mediated cytolysis: functional cytolytic T-cells lacking perforin and granzymes, *Immunology* 78:105, 1993.
103. Biberfield P, Holm G, Perlmann P: Morphologic observations on lymphocyte peripolesis and cytotoxic action in vitro, *Exp Cell Res* 52:672, 1968.
104. Henkert PA: Mechanisms of lymphocyte-mediated cytotoxicity, *Annu Rev Immunol* 3:31, 1985.
105. Rodrigues M, Nussenzweig RS, Romero P, Zavala F: The in vivo cytotoxic activity of CD8+ T-cell clones correlates with their levels of expression of adhesion molecules, *J Exp Med* 175:895, 1992.
106. Versteeg R: NK cells and T-cells: mirror images? *Immunol Today* 13:244, 1992.
107. Yewdell JW, Bennink JR: Cell biology of antigen processing and presentation to major histocompatibility complex class I molecule-restricted T lymphocytes, *Adv Immunol* 52:1-123, 1992.
108. Flax MH, Caulfield JB: Cellular and vascular components of allergic contact dermatitis, *Am J Pathol* 43:1031, 1963.
109. Kalish RS, Johnson KL: Enrichment and function of urushiol (poison ivy)–specific T lymphocytes in lesions of allergic contact dermatitis to urushiol, *J Immunol* 145:3706, 1990.
110. Kligman AM: Poison ivy *(Rhus)* dermatitis: experimental study, *Arch Dermatol* 77:149, 1958.
111. Willis CM, Stephens CJM, Wilkinson JD: Selective expression of immune-mediated surface antigens by keratinocytes in irritant contact dermatitis, *J Invest Dermatol* 96:505, 1991.
112. Corson JS: The pathologist and the kidney transplant, *Pathol Annu* New York, 1972, Appleton Century Crofts.
113. Mason DW, Morris PJ: Effector mechanisms in allograft rejection, *Annu Rev Immunol* 4:119, 1986.
114. Porter KA et al: Human renal transplants, *Lab Invest* 16:153, 1967.
115. Sibley RK: Pathology and immunopathology of solid graft rejection, *Transplant Proc* 21:14, 1989.
116. Stetson CD: The role of humoral antibody in the homograft rejection, *Adv Immunol* 3:97, 1963.
117. Behbehani AM: The small pox story: life and death of an old disease, *Microbiol Rev* 47:455, 1983.
118. Jenner E: *An inquiry into the causes and effects of the variolae vaccine*, London, 1798, Low.
119. von Pirquet CF: *Klinische Studien über Vakzination und vakzinale Allergie*, Leipzig, 1907, Deuticke.
120. Askanasy M: Pathologische-anatomische Beiträge zur Kenntnis des Morbus Basedowii, insbesondere über die dabei auftretende Muskelerkrankung, *Dtsch Arch Klin Med* 61:118-186, 1898.
121. Atkins MB, Mier JW, Parkinson DR et al: Hypothyroidism after treatment with interleukin-2 and lymphokine activated killer-cells, *N Engl J Med* 318:1557, 1988.
122. Flax MH: Experimental allergic thyroiditis in the guinea pig. II. Morphologic studies on the development of the disease, *Lab Invest* 12:119, 1963.
123. Hashimoto H: Zurkenntnis der lymphomatosen Veränderung der Schilddrüse (Struma lymphomatosa), *Arch Klin Chir* 97:219, 1912.
124. Roitt IM, Doniach D, Campbell PN, Hudson RV: Autoantibodies in Hashimoto's disease (lymphadenoid goitre), *Lancet* 2:820, 1956.
125. Witebsky E, Rose NR, Terplan K et al: Chronic thyroiditis and autoimmunization, *JAMA* 64:1439, 1957.

Delayed hypersensitivity

126. Cohen S: The role of cell-mediated immunity in the induction of inflammatory responses, *Am J Pathol* 88:502, 1977.
127. Dvorak HF, Galli SJ, Dvorak A: Cellular and vascular manifestations of cell mediated immunity, *Hum Pathol* 17:112, 1986.
128. Ferreri NR, Millet I, Paliwal V et al: Induction of macrophage TNF α, IL-1, IL-6, and PGE_2 production by DTH-initiating factors, *Cell Immunol* 137:389, 1991.
129. Gell PGH, Benacerraf B: Delayed hypersensitivity to simple protein antigens, *Adv Immunol* 1:319, 1961.
130. Lawrence HS: The delayed type of allergic inflammatory response, *Am J Med* 20:428, 1956.
131. Simon FA, Rackeman FF: The development of hypersensitiveness in man. I. Following intradermal injection of the antigen, *J Allergy* 5:439, 1934
132. Turk JL: *Delayed hypersensitivity*, New York, 1967, Wiley.
133. Uhr JW: Delayed hypersensitivity, *Physiol Rev* 46:359, 1966.
134. Waksman BH: Delayed hypersensitivity: a growing class of immunological phenomona, *J Allergy* 31:468, 1960.
135. Herman A, Kappler JW, Marrack P, Pullen AM: Superantigens: mechanism of T-cell stimulation and role in immune responses, *Annu Rev Immunol* 9:745, 1991.
136. See RH, Kum WWS, Chang AH, Goh SH, Chow AW: Induction of tumor necresis factor and interleukin-1 by purified staphlococcal toxic shock syndrome toxin 1 requires the presence of both monocytes and T lymphocytes, *Infect Immunity* 60:2612, 1992.

Cutaneous basophil hypersensitivity

137. Askanase PW, Atwood JE: Basophils in tuberculin and "Jones-Mote" delayed reactions of humans, *J Clin Invest* 58:1145, 1976.
138. Dvorak HF, Mihm MC Jr: Basophilic leukocytes in allergic contact dermatitis, *J Exp Med* 135:235, 1972.
139. Jones TD, Mote JR: The phases of foreign sensitization in human beings, *N Engl J Med* 210:120, 1934.
140. Richerson HB, Dvorak HF, Leskowitz S: Cutaneous basophil hypersensitivity: a new interpretation of the Jones-Mote reaction, *J Immunol* 103:1431, 1969.
141. Dennie CC: *A history of syphilis,* Springfield, Ill, 1962, Charles C Thomas.
142. Chesney AM: Immunity in syphilis, *Medicine* 5:463, 1926.
143. Sell S: The pathology of syphilis is determined by the level of delayed hypersensitivity. In Hook EW III, Lukehart SA, editors: *Syphilis,* Cambridge, Mass, Blackwell Scientific Pub, Inc. (In press.)
144. Sell S, Norris SJ: The biology, pathology, and immunology of syphilis, *Int Rev Exp Pathol* 24:203, 1983.
145. Turner TB, Hollander DH: *Biology of the treponematoses,* Geneva, 1957, World Health Organization.
146. Hickey WF: Migration of hematogenous cells through the blood-brain barrier and the initiation of CNS inflammation, *Brain Pathol* 1:97, 1991.
147. Martin R, McFarland HF, McFarlin DE: Immunological aspects of demyelinating diseases, *Annu Rev Immunol* 10:153, 1992.
148. Sobel RA, Kuchroo VK: The immunopathology of acute experimental allergic encephalomyelitis induced with myelin proteolipid protein: T-cell receptors in inflammatory lesions, *J Immunol* 149:1444, 1992.
149. Waksman BH: Experimental allergic encephalomyelitis and the "autoallergic" diseases, *Int Arch Allergy Appl Immunol* (suppl) 14, 1959.

Granulomatous reactions

150. Adams DO: The granulomatous inflammatory response, *Am J Pathol* 84:164-192, 1976.
151. Boros DL: *Basic and clinical aspects of granulomatous disease,* New York, 1981, Elsevier/North Holland.
152. Epstein WL: Granulomatous hypersensitivity, 11:36, 1967.
153. Kaufmann SHE: Immunity to intracellular bacteria, *Annu Rev Immunol* 11:129, 1993.
154. Langhans T: Ueber Riesenzellen mit manche ständigen Kernen in Tuberkeln und die fibrose Form des Tuberkels, *Virchows Arch Pathol Anat Physiol Kim Med* 42:382, 1868.
155. McInnes A, Rennick DM: Interleukin 4 induces cultured monocytes/macrophages to form giant multinuclear cells, *J Exp Med* 167:598, 1988.
156. Müller J: *Ueber den feineren Bauformen der krankhaften Geschwulste,* Berlin, 1838.
157. Spector WG, Heesom N: The production of granulomata by antigen-antibody complexes, *J Pathol* 98:31, 1969.
158. Turk JL: The role of delayed hypersensitivity in granuloma formation, *Res Monogr Immunol* 1:275, 1980.
159. Dannenberg AM: Delayed-type hypersensitivity and cell-mediated immunity in the pathogenesis of tuberculosis, *Immunol Today* 12:228, 1991.
160. Katz J, Kunofsky S, Krasnitz A: Variation in sensitivity to tuberculin, *Am Rev Respir Dis* 106:202, 1972.
161. Koch R: Weitere Mitteilungen über ein Heilmittel gegen Tuberculose, *Dtsch Med Wochenschr* 16:1029, 1890.
162. Lowrie DB: Is macrophage death on the field of battle essential to victory, or a tactical weakness in immunity against tuberculosis? *Clin Exp Immunol* 80:301, 1990.
163. Lurie MB: *Resistance to tuberculosis: experimental studies in native and acquired defensive mechanisms,* Cambridge, Mass, 1964, Harvard University Press.
164. Orme IM, Anderson P, Boom WH: T-cell response to *Mycobacterium tuberculosis* infection, *J Infect Dis* 167:1481, 1993.
165. Rich AR: *The pathogenesis of tuberculosis,* Springfield, Ill, 1951, Charles C Thomas.
166. Rook GAW, Attiyah R: Cytokines and the Kock phenomenon, *Tubercle* 72:13, 1991.
167. Youmans GP: Relation between delayed hypersensitivity and immunity in tuberculosis, *Am Rev Respir Dis* 111:109, 1975.
168. Arnoldi J, Gerdes J, Flad HD: Immunohistologic assessment of cytokine production of infiltrating cells in various forms of leprosy, *Am J Pathol* 137:749, 1990.
169. Kaufmann SHE: Immunology of leprosy: new findings, future perspectives, *Microb Pathog* 1:107, 1986.
170. Skinsnes OK: Immunopathology of leprosy: the century in review pathology, pathogenesis and the development of classification, *Int J Leprosy* 41:329, 1973.
171. Turk JL, Bryceson ADM: Immunological phenomena in leprosy and related disease, *Adv Immunol* 13:209, 1971.
172. Cullen MR, Kominsky JR, Rossman MD et al: Chronic beryllium disease in a precious metal refinery: clinical, epidemiologic and immunologic evidence for continuing risk from exposure to low level beryllium fume, *Am Rev Respir Dis* 135:201, 1987.
173. Hardy HL, Tabershaw IR: Delayed chemical pneumonitis occurring in workers exposed to beryllium compounds, *J Ind Hyg Toxicol* 28:2693, 1946.
174. Tepper LB, Hardy HL, Chamberlin RI: *Toxicity of beryllium compounds,* Amsterdam, 1961, Elsevier.
175. Balbi B, Moller DR, Kirby M et al: Increased numbers of T lymphocytes with $\gamma/\delta+$ antigen receptors in a subgroup of individuals with pulmonary sarcoidosis, *J Clin Invest* 85:1353, 1990.
176. Boeck C: Multiple benign sarkoid of the skin, *J Cutan Genit Urin Dis* 17:543, 1899.
177. James DG, Williams, WJ: *Sarcoidosis and other granulomatous disorders,* Philadelphia, 1985, Saunders.
178. Fahey JL, Leonard E, Churg J: Wegener's granulomatoses, *Am J Med* 17:168, 1954.
179. Fauci AS, Wolff SM: Wegener's granulomatosis: studies in eighteen patients and a review of the literature, *Medicine* 52:535, 1973.
180. Jennette JC, Falk RJ: Antineutrophil cytoplasmic autoantibodies and associated diseases: a review, *Am J Kidney Dis* 15:517, 1990.
181. Klinger H: Grenzformen der periarteritis nodosa, *Frankfurt Z Pathol* 42:455, 1931.
182. Crohn BB, Ginzburg L, Oppenheimer GD: Regional ileitis: a pathologic and clinical entity, *JAMA* 99:1323, 1932.
183. Janowitz HD, Sachar DB: New observations in Crohn's disease, *Annu Rev Med* 27:269, 1976.

26 Autoimmunity and Autoimmune Diseases

David J. Bylund
Howard S. Fox
Robert M. Nakamura

BACKGROUND

Autoimmunity can be defined as the failure of an organism to recognize its own healthy tissue as self and includes humoral (such as circulating autoantibodies) as well as cellular (such as delayed hypersensitivity) immune responses to the host's own tissue. Normally, each of us is endowed with an immune system that can distinguish self from nonself. However, many alterations of control mechanisms that regulate self-recognition can result in an autoimmune response. During the past several years, research advancements in immunology, molecular biology, and immunogenetics have revised current thinking related to the autoimmune response and autoimmune disease.

Natural autoimmunity

At the beginning of this century, Ehrlich postulated the concept of *horror autotoxicus,* wherein the body does not normally mount immune responses against itself.[1] It was believed that if an autoimmune response did occur it was harmful to the host. Thus, under "normal" conditions the host immune system is capable of responding to any foreign molecule but usually avoids adverse reactions against self antigens.

Today, we know that some autoimmune responses are normal and important in regulation of the immune system.[2,3] Self antigens may elicit a "natural" autoimmunity of the host without an accompanying autoimmune disease. Thus not all autoimmune responses are harmful or "forbidden." Currently, we believe autoimmunity is an event that can account for normal regulatory mechanisms such as physiologic clearance of dead cells or cell components, aging, and response to infections as well as the pathogenesis of such immune-mediated diseases as Goodpasture's syndrome or systemic lupus erythematosus (SLE).

Autoimmune diseases

Self-reactive T- or B-cells, or both types, are required for autoimmunity, but their mere presence is not indicative of autoimmunity. The term *autoimmune disease* describes a condition in which a host immune response against self components contributes to the pathogenesis of the disease. Thus, merely finding an autoantibody simultaneous with a disease state does not prove that such a disease is autoimmune. Such antibodies may be a convenient marker for the disease and may give insights into its pathogenesis. Autoantibodies will be referred to more frequently than autoreactive T-cells in descriptions of autoimmune diseases because of the relative ease of discovering and measuring humoral immune responses versus cell-mediated responses. Furthermore, it is likely that, in the majority of diseases involving autoantibodies, T-cell help is required for the production of those antibodies and disease expression. Autoantibodies remain the most effective markers to define and monitor disease states, but in many cases they remain as markers and have not been shown to be pathogenic.

Self-reactivity has many causes. Autoreactive antibodies and cells are normal in the immune system, such as low-affinity, naturally occurring antibodies that can react with self and foreign components.[4,5] Autoimmune reactions may arise through cross-reactivity after infection, as in acute rheumatic fever following group A streptococcal infections.[6] Non–immune mediated injury to tissue can induce an autoimmune response, such as anticardiac myosin antibodies produced after cardiac damage.[7] Finally, autoimmunity may arise without known initiating factors though the pathogenic agent of disease is suspected, such as anti–thyroid stimulating hormone (TSH) receptor antibodies in Graves' disease.[8]

How can we then identify an autoimmune disease? Currently, diseases with no other known cause are considered to be autoimmune if evidence for autoreactivity can be found.

Autoreactivity in the form of self-reactive antibodies or cells is sought, followed by an attempt to identify the antigen to which the immune attack is directed. The ultimate challenge is then to show that such self-reactivity is pathogenic. Nature has provided useful data, since transplacental transmission of autoantibodies can lead to disease in the fetus and newborn in many maternal conditions, including Graves' disease.[9] The pathogenicity of autoantibodies has been also observed by direct transfer experiments in idiopathic thrombocytopenia.[10]

Animal models, principally rodents, have provided insight into autoimmune disease. Animals offer genetic models of disease (such as the NOD mice for insulin-dependent diabetes mellitus, IDDM), immunization strategies with autoantigens (such as acetylcholine receptor for myasthenia gravis), passive transfer techniques like placing autoantibodies (from pemphigus patients) into newborn mice, or peripheral blood mononuclear cells (from SLE patients) into immunodeficient mice, all of which recreate various aspects of the human disease.[11-14] Yet in general, despite suggestive evidence that many diseases may be autoimmune in nature, formal proof is still lacking.

Tolerance

For an autoimmune disease to occur, there must be a basic defect in the immune system in the sense that tolerance, the mechanism preventing pathologic responses against self, has been broken. Factors leading to the breakdown of tolerance are likely complex and vary among diseases. Much current work focuses on how tolerance is initiated and largely examines two potential mechanisms: the *clonal deletion* theory of Burnet, in which self-reactive lymphoid cells are eliminated, and the *clonal anergy* theory of Nossal, in which self-reactive lymphoid cells become functionally inactivated; recently, *clonal ignorance* has been added to these nonexclusive categories.[15-17] Experiments utilizing transgenic mice, in which the genome has been modified with a bias toward the production of specific antibodies, T-cell receptors, foreign antigens, or immune modulating molecules, allowing the easier identification of self-reactive cells, have provided support for such theories and given us insight into tolerance and autoimmune mechanisms.

These studies indicated that tolerance arises through multiple pathways, acting on both B-cells and T-cells. Depending on the system, B-cells that are reactive against self can be eliminated; they may be present but are functionally inactivated, or they may be present and potentially functional but "ignore" the antigen, having not received the necessary signals to become activated. Timing of expression of the self antigen, amount of the self antigen, and degree of cross-linking of the B-cell antigen receptors may all play a role in determining whether a self-reactive cell is eliminated, is inactivated, or remains ignorant. Studies of transgenic mice have also revealed ways B-cells may escape tolerance. In mice that transgenically express an antierythrocyte antibody, the majority of such self-reactive B-cells are eliminated.[18] However, these self-reactive cells can be found in the peritoneal cavity, and if activated, the secreted antibody leads to hemolytic anemia.[19] Such cells either "escaped" to the peritoneum or developed within the peritoneum, where they are not normally exposed to their RBC self antigen and thus are not eliminated. Introduction of RBC into the peritoneal cavity can then trigger these self-reactive B-cells to undergo apoptotic death.

Similarly, self-reactive T-cells may be deleted, rendered anergic, or "ignorant." Much work has addressed the issue of *central* (thymic-mediated) versus *peripheral* (nonthymic) tolerance. In central tolerance, self antigens that are presented in the thymus during T-cell development largely induce deletion of self-reactive thymocytes. Tissue-specific antigens that are sequestered in organs are not presented in the thymus but rather induce peripheral tolerance by inducing anergy in the T-cells when the self antigen is encountered, or, if not rendered anergic, such cells merely don't respond to the antigen. In transgenic mice that ectopically expressed an antigen from lymphocytic choriomeningitis virus (LCMV) on the surface of the beta cells of the pancreas, self-reactive T-cells could be demonstrated in vitro, but autoimmunity was absent in vivo, even when an additional transgenic T-cell receptor reactive to LCMV was introduced into the mice. However, infection of these mice with LCMV was then shown to activate these self-reactive cytotoxic T-cells in vivo, overcoming their ignorance and resulting in autoimmunity.[20,21]

LCMV infection may overcome tolerance in these animals by supplying antigen in a more stimulating form to the immune system, possibly in an increased amount, through the use of "professional" antigen-presenting cells such as macrophages in conjunction with MHC class II molecules, or by inducing necessary costimulatory factors to induce immune activation. Indeed, support for the latter hypothesis has been obtained by inducing expression of the cytokine interferon-γ in the beta cells of the pancreas. In the transgenic mice used for these experiments, autoimmune diabetes results, and T-cells reactive with pancreatic islets can be demonstrated in vivo.[22,23]

Two other significant theories of tolerance induction have been studied, both of which involve active suppression of immune responses. Although the evidence for their relevance is inconclusive, this may in fact represent our experimental limitations. The *network theory,* proposed by Jerne, holds that a dynamic network of idiotype (the variable region of immunoglobulin and T-cell receptors) and self anti-idiotype reactivity can hold autoimmunity in check while allowing for immune responses to foreign antigens.[24] Specific *suppressor cells* remain attractive candidates for preventing autoimmune reactions, but we still await the identification of such cells.[25]

PATHOPHYSIOLOGY

Autoimmune diseases are frequently associated with genetic or viral factors that interact with the immune system and trigger abnormal responses of T- and B-cells, resulting in immune dysregulation. No single theory or mechanism explains all features of the many human autoimmune diseases. Both genetic and environmental factors contribute to regulation of the immune system and the development of autoimmunity.

Genetic factors in autoimmunity

The susceptibility to autoimmune diseases is multifactorial and polygenic.[26] Most autoimmune diseases are not inherited in a simple Mendelian segregation. Even with a proved susceptible genotype, not all individuals of that type develop autoimmunity. In the most concordant autoimmune diseases, such as rheumatoid arthritis (RA) and IDDM, approximately one in three monozygotic twins pairs are both affected by disease.[27,28] The genetic factors in autoimmunity provide a determinant of susceptibility.

Cells of the immune system normally recognize foreign antigens by any of three surface molecules: (1) B-cell immunoglobulins (Ig), (2) T-cell receptors (TcR), and (3) glycoprotein products of the major histocompatibility complex (MHC), known as the human leukocyte antigens (HLA). The first two types of recognition structures are found only on lymphocytes, whereas the MHC glycoproteins are present on the surface of nearly all nucleated cells of the body. Because of genomic DNA rearrangements and mutations, each mature lymphocyte (or clone of lymphocytes) expresses a unique Ig or TcR, whereas all cells of the body express a subset of the same MHC gene products.

Although some association has been claimed for specific Ig and TcR haplotypes and autoimmunity, substantial data support the role of specific MHC linkage to autoimmunity. The MHC molecules are highly polymorphic among individuals, with numerous alleles existing for each molecule. The two types of molecules, class I (HLA-A, B, C) and class II (HLA-DR, DQ, and DP), have different functions. Class I molecules are expressed on most nucleated cells and are recognized by the $CD8^+$ subset of mature T-cells. Class II molecules are restricted to antigen-presenting cells and are recognized by $CD4^+$ T-cells. The major function of MHC molecules is to present antigens to T-cells by acting as receptors for processed peptides. Intracellular antigens, such as intracellular viral antigens, are preferentially presented by class I molecules to cytotoxic $CD8^+$ T-cells. Such antigens are produced in the cytoplasm and actively transported to the endoplasmic reticulum for assembly and presentation. Class II molecules present external antigens, processed through the proteosomal system, to helper/inducer $CD4^+$ T-cells.

Autoimmune diseases have been associated with both class I and II MHC molecules. However, linkage to MHC loci does not prove autoimmune pathogenesis or even linkage to a specific antigen-presenting molecule. Genes other than those for class I and II molecules are located within the MHC complex on chromosome 6, such as genes encoding complement components (class III MHC), the cytokines tumor necrosis factor (TNF-α) and related lymphotoxins (LT-α and LT-α), several heat-shock proteins, some of the proteosome components, and the peptide transporter molecules, all of which have profound effects on the immune system.

There are strong correlations between autoimmune diseases and certain MHC class II genotypes.[29] Some HLA-DR alleles correlate with multiple diseases: IDDM, SLE, Sjögren's syndrome (SS), myasthenia gravis, dermatitis herpetiformis, celiac disease, and Graves' disease, all are linked to HLA-DR3; and IDDM, rheumatoid arthritis, and pemphigus vulgaris are linked to HLA-DR4. For HLA-DR2, there is a positive linkage to multiple sclerosis, SLE, and narcolepsy (the possible autoimmune nature of the latter disease is quite intriguing but not at all a certainty), whereas a negative correlation exists with IDDM. Correlations have also been reported for the HLA-DR alleles and other class II molecules, HLA-DQ and HLP-DP. Research using a molecular analysis of the different alleles at specific class II loci is currently refining these correlations.

Fewer correlations match class I or class III MHC molecules with specific diseases. The most notable are the strong correlation between HLA-B27 (class I) and ankylosing spondylitis and the deficiency of complement components C2 and C4 (class III) in patients with SLE.

Sex is also a major influence on autoimmunity. Most autoimmune diseases are female predominant; for disorders such as SLE, primary biliary cirrhosis, and Hashimoto's thyroiditis, women are afflicted approximately 10 times more frequently than men.[30,31] Sex steroid hormones are the major physiologic influence on autoimmune disorders. Most occur during the reproductive years, when it is likely that steroids play a major role. Notable exceptions are ankylosing spondylitis, which shows male predominance, and SS, which is strongly predominant in females (tenfold higher) but often arises postmenopausally.

Animal models support a role for sex steroids in autoimmunity. F_1 mice produced by crossing NZB and NZW mouse strains suffer from a disease resembling SLE. Female mice have more severe disease than males do, and estrogens have been shown to accelerate but androgens to ameliorate the disease.[32,33] Similarly, in the NOD strain, female mice have a higher incidence of diabetes than male mice do, and androgens can protect mice from this disease.[34,35] The mechanisms by which sex steroids affect the immune system is unknown, but their effects on immune-modulating cytokines have been reported.[36,37]

Environmental factors in autoimmunity

In regard to the body's external environment, infectious agents are often implicated as contributory, if not causative, of autoimmunity. Infections with many different pathogens have been linked to autoimmune diseases: *Klebsiella pneumoniae* with ankylosing spondylitis, coxsackievirus B with IDDM, and various bacteria with RA.[38-40] These agents may act by a variety of means, including T-cell bypass, molecular mimicry, release of sequestered antigens after tissue damage, and creation of new self determinants, as described below. However, the correlation between specific infectious agents and autoimmune diseases is weak. Recently there have been found microbial agents that may act as superantigens, which can activate large numbers of T-cells. The result may be pyrogenicity, depressed antibody production, and shock.[41] Superantigens may also participate in the induction of RA and multiple sclerosis, but convincing evidence remains to be gathered.[42]

Chemical agents, such as drugs, can lead to autoimmune reactions and autoimmune disease. For example, procainamide, hydralazine, quinine, mercury salts, gold salts, polyvinyl chloride, bleomycin, D-penicillamine, and possibly silicone can induce autoimmune responses.[43] Like viruses, they evidently act through various mechanisms.

General mechanisms of autoimmunity

In the initiation of autoimmune reactions, autologous ("self") antigen may be presented in a manner abnormal to either a normal or altered immune system.[2,44,45] That is,

1. Autologous antigen may be presented abnormally to a normal immune system.
2. Regulating mechanisms may be defective within the immune system itself.

Abnormal presentation or an immunologic imbalance may arise from any alteration or disturbance of the activities of regulating T-cells. As discussed above, genetic or environmental factors can modulate the immune system.

Several of the inductive mechanisms of autoimmunity are listed in Table 26-1. These mechanisms are not mutually exclusive, as certain basic reactions do overlap.

T-cell bypass mechanism

A T-cell bypass autoimmune reaction may occur when an immunocompetent B-cell is stimulated to produce autoantibody without the need for an immunocompetent specific T-cell. B-cells may be stimulated in this way by two general pathways:

1. Autoantigens or cross-reactive foreign antigens may form immunogenic units to initiate T-helper cell signals to stimulate immunocompetent B-cells. Stimuli for this pathway may be drugs, viruses, or bacteria.
2. Immunocompetent B-cells may be nonspecifically stimulated by viruses, adjuvants, or allogenic cells, initiating a graft-versus-host reaction with the production of autoantibodies. This phenomenon is referred to as *polyclonal activation of B-cells.*[46,47] Bacterial antigens, such as lipopolysaccharides, and viruses, such as Epstein-Barr virus (EBV), can initiate polyclonal B-cell activation, which may induce an autoimmune reaction.

Table 26-1 Inductive mechanisms of autoimmunity[44]

Mechanism
T-cell bypass
Alternative helper T-cell signal initiation
Polyclonal B-cell activation
Sequestered antigen release
Abnormal regulation
Suppressor activity
Cytokines
Molecular mimicry
Heat-shock proteins (hsp)
Idiotypic antibody

The T-cell bypass mechanism may play a role when there is (1) alteration of self antigen, (2) combination of self antigen with a foreign determinant antigen, or (3) presentation of self antigen with increased MHC class II expression of the antigen-presenting cells.

Environmental agents. Some drugs combined with host tissue may initiate a helper T-cell signal that stimulates competent B-cells to produce autoantibody (Fig. 26-1).[48,49] Similarly, certain viruses such as EBV may stimulate immunocompetent B-cells directly through polyclonal B-cell activation. Immunologic adjuvants are nonspecific stimulators of lymphocytes and can help initiate autoimmune responses. Additionally, lipopolysaccharides or purified protein derivatives of tuberculin are polyclonal B-cell activators. Finally, bacterial infections that liberate products with adjuvant activity, such as *Bordetella pertussis* infection, can also produce polyclonal lymphocyte activation and autoimmunity.[49] The need for a specific T-cell is thereby bypassed (Fig. 26-2).

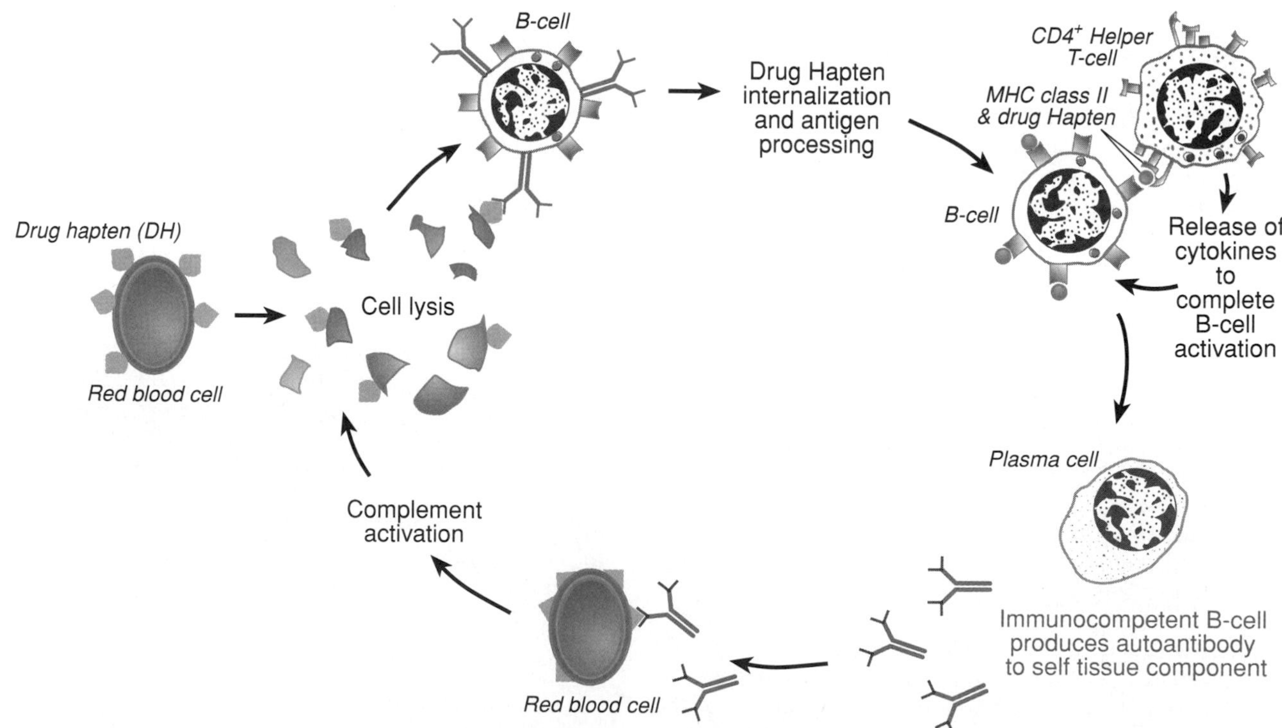

Fig. 26-1 Autoimmunity after drug administration. The drug (as a drug hapten) can combine with host tissue to form immunogenic units. The anti–drug hapten response of T-cells will initiate the T-cell helper effect without the intervention of specific T-cells and will eliminate the need for such cells. The immunocompetent B-cells are activated to produce autoantibodies. (Modified from Nakamura MC, Nakamura RM: *J Clin Lab Anal* 6:275, 1992.)

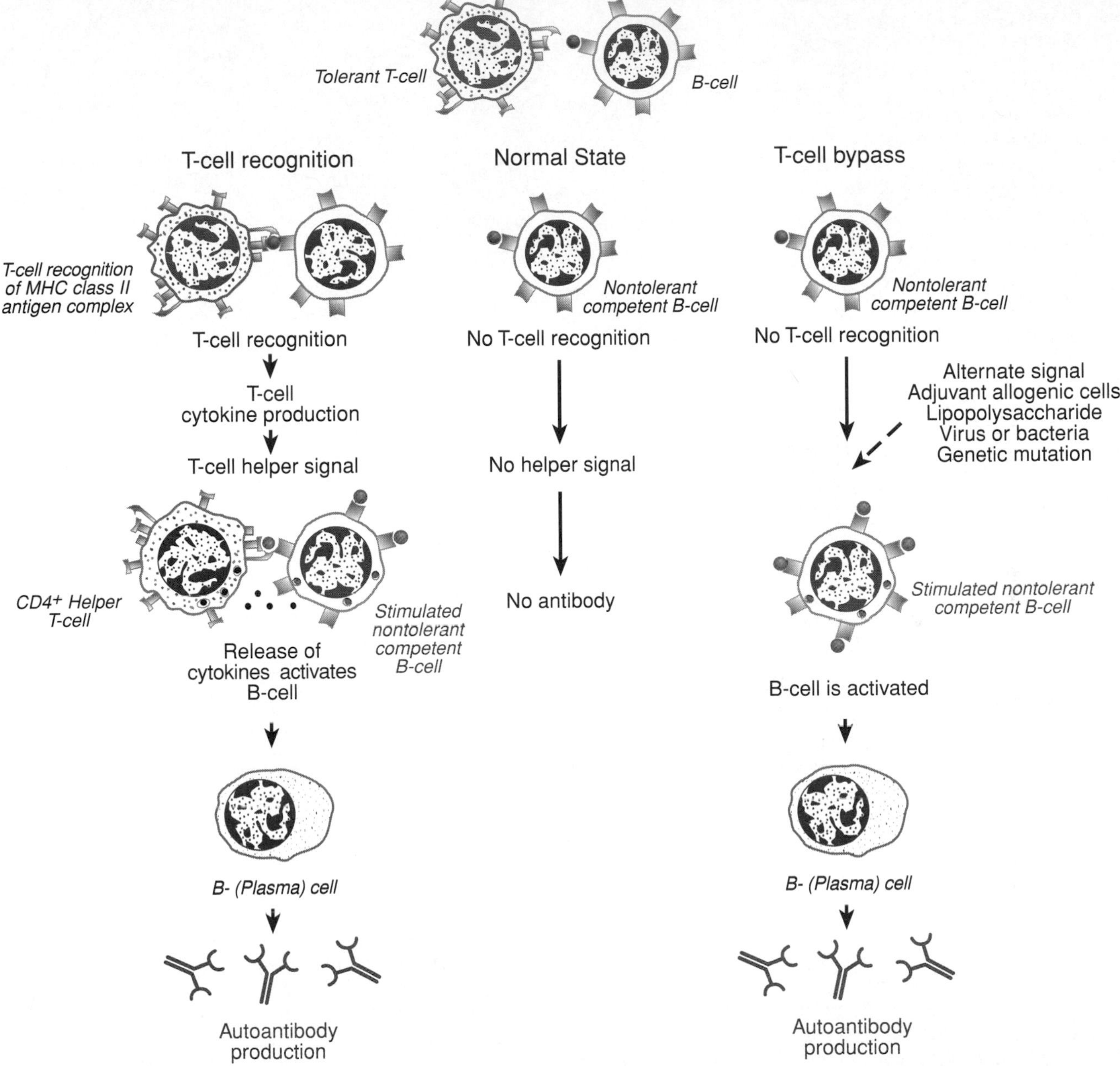

Fig. 26-2 Nonspecific stimulation by immunologic adjuvants in initiation of autoimmune reaction. Adjuvants can help initiate autoimmune reactions by bypassing the need for specific T-cells. The adjuvants nonspecifically stimulate T-cells to initiate a T-cell helper effect. In the case of lipopolysaccharides, direct activation with polyclonal stimulation of B-cells can occur with the production of auto-antibodies. (Modified from Nakamura MC, Nakamura RM: *J Clin Lab Anal* 6:275, 1992.)

Degradation and alteration of antigens. Tissue damage that alters host antigens may elicit an autoimmune reaction.[48,49] Even partial degradation of antigens can expose determinants that are not normally available, and these can react with T-lymphocytes to induce autoimmunity. Many bacterial, viral, and parasitic infections are associated with transient positive tests for rheumatoid factor, and among the underlying mechanisms are partial degradation or alteration of host antigens.

Allogeneic cells. When a nonhistocompatible donor's lymphocytes are introduced into an allogeneic recipient, a graft-versus-host reaction may occur.[48-50] To achieve this reaction, the donor T-cells stimulate the host B-cells nonspecifically and lead to the production of autoantibodies.

Sequestered antigen

An autoimmune response resulting from the release of sequestered antigen involves the interaction of competent T-cells or B-cells with self antigens that are normally confined to closed compartments of the body. Because the antigen was sequestered, no immune tolerance developed.[51,52] Some examples are sperm antigens, lens proteins, and myelin basic proteins. Their release and contact with the immune system can occur after tissue injury. Myelin basic protein (MBP), an anti-

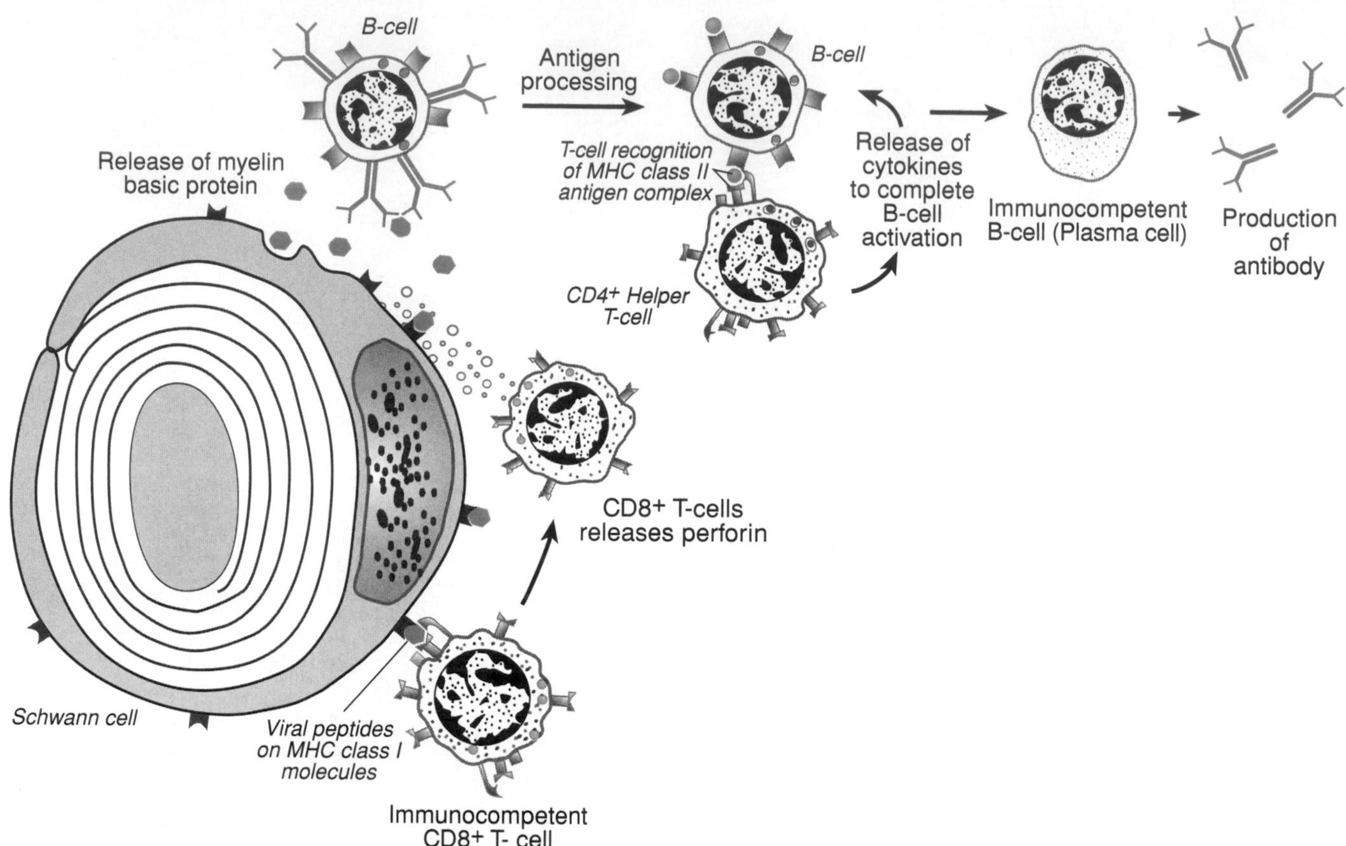

Fig. 26-3 Sequestered antigen release mechanisms of autoimmunity in experimental and postinfectious encephalitis. The sequestered antigen is myelin basic protein. When released by various means such as viral inflammation, it will stimulate both immunocompetent T-cells and B-cells. The primary mechanism of injury in experimental and post–viral encephalitis status is a cell-mediated injury. (Modified from Nakamura MC, Nakamura RM: *J Clin Lab Anal* 6:275, 1992.)

gen of the central nervous system (CNS), has been considered a sequestered antigen because of its confinement behind the blood-brain barrier. However, quiescent T- and B-cells that are immunocompetent in response to MBP exist normally (Fig. 26-3). This normal unresponsive state may be ascribed to the sequestered nature of antigen or to the lack of expression of class I or class II MHC molecules in the CNS. In many experimental animals, immunization with MBP leads to a disease that closely resembles multiple sclerosis.

Abnormal immune regulation

In the course of normal immune function, "suppressor T-cells" may block a self antigen from triggering a signal that activates helper T-cells.[52,53] In addition, such suppressors may block and thereby inhibit competent B-cells from producing autoantibody. Suppressor T-cells may be antigen-specific or nonspecific, but when this regulatory role fails in the immune system, autoimmune disease may follow.

Cytokines

Cytokines, which include the interleukins (IL), interferons (IFN), and related molecules, mediate interactions within the immune system and between the immune system and the host. Some cytokines can promote autoimmune reactions, whereas others may serve to suppress the development of autoimmunity. For example, in an experimental model of arthritis, tumor necrosis factor (TNF)-α stimulates the development of autoimmune disease, and TGF-β reduces disease.[54] Although the factors that regulate cytokine production are complex, subsets of $CD4^+$ T-cells have been defined (Th1 and Th2) based upon the profile of cytokines they produce.[55,56] The Th1 cells, which in general promote T-cell/ inflammatory immune interactions, produce such cytokines as IL-2, IFN-γ, TNF-α, and LT-α, which can promote autoimmunity and inhibit Th2 cells. In contrast, the Th2 cells, which promote humoral immunity, produce IL-4, IL-10, and TGF-β and inhibit the delayed type of hypersensitivity responses as well as Th1 cell functions. Defects in or abnormal regulation of the Th2 cells, which keep the autoimmune-stimulatory Th1 cells in check, may lead to the development of disease. Furthermore, infectious stimuli, with the induction of a Th1-biased response, may also contribute to the development of autoimmunity.

Molecular mimicry

Molecular mimicry describes a phenomenon in which similar structures are shared by molecular products from dissimilar genes.[57,58] That is, the amino acid sequence or conformational structure may be partially similar for molecules of different origins. Often a viral or bacterial structure mimics a similar structure in a normal host, resulting in an autoimmune reaction. This reaction probably occurs when microbe and host determinants are similar enough to induce a cross-reactive response and yet different enough to terminate T- or B-cell immunologic tolerance. An example is the cross-reaction of beta-hemolytic streptococcus and cardiac myosin in patients with poststreptococcal rheumatic heart disease. Molecular mimicry between microbes and self components of the host they infect is no longer considered a rarity.

Fujinami and Oldstone[59] injected hepatitis B virus polymerase peptide into rabbits and induced perivascular lymphocytic infiltrative lesions in the CNS similar to the lesions of allergic encephalitis induced by MBP. One region of this polymerase gene contains 6 of 10 amino acids also found in MBP, and immunization with this peptide produced an immune response against MBP. Also, Neu and associates[8] observed myocarditis and autoantibody to myosin in mice infected with coxsackievirus B3 infection. Subsequently, transfer of this specific antibody to normal mice induced myocarditis. After research established that a region of coxsackievirus B3 and myosin share 7 of 11 amino acids, inoculation of the shared peptide sequence induced myocarditis and autoantibody to myosin in mice.

Heat-shock protein and gamma-delta (γ /δ) T-cells

Heat-shock proteins (hsp) are highly conserved peptides found on prokaryotic and eukaryotic cells. On the basis of their approximate molecular mass, hsp can be divided into a number of families, such as hsp65, hsp70, and hsp90.

Bacterial hsp are major target antigens for cell-mediated immune effector mechanisms.[60,61] Although highly conserved, the bacterial hsp are sufficiently different from their mammalian homologs to be immunogenic and perceived by the host immune system as foreign. For example, hsp65 of *Mycobacterium tuberculosis* is approximately 50% identical with a human homolog in mitochondria and displays 20% conservative replacements. Mycobacterial hsp are immunoreactive with T-cells from rats with adjunct arthritis, and it has been suggested that hsp from microorganisms may be involved in RA.

Viruses differ from bacteria in that they do not carry hsp genes and can cause enhanced expression of endogenous host hsp, which in turn may stimulate a subset of T-cells, specifically, a subset of those expressing the γ/δ chain of the TcR (T-cell receptor). T-cells that bear the TcR may be reactive to self hsp and are part of the human immune system. The γ/δ T-cells differentiate in the thymus, possess surface markers, and mediate a variety of functions characteristic of T-lymphocytes but are distinct from the majority of T-cells, which express the α/β chain of the TcR.

The exact way in which hsp interacts with γ/δ T-cells remains to be elucidated. Doherty and associates[60] hypothesized that, after certain viral infections, there is increased expression of host hsp65, which is reactive with γ/δ T-cells. With respect to autoimmune disease, significant numbers of γ/δ T-cells have been found in lesions of human multiple sclerosis.[62,63] Although the exact pathogenic mechanism is unknown, the lymphokines secreted by the γ/δ T-cells may initiate an autoimmune reaction.

Idiotypes

Idiotypes are antigenic epitopes located in the antigen-binding regions of antibody molecules.[63,64] Autoimmunity may result from cross-reactions among separate idiotypes. Additionally, the idiotypes on autoantibody may cross-react with an antibody directed against a virus or bacteria.

Plotz[65] and Oldstone[58] presented evidence that autoantibodies may arise through a cross-reaction between the idiotype on an antiviral antibody and a cellular receptor for virus (the anti-idiotype is envisioned as an internal image of the virus).

Other studies support the theory that idiotypic/anti-idiotypic control mechanisms may play a role in human diseases.[63,64] In patients with SLE, anti-idiotypic responses specific for antibodies having anti-DNA reactivity evidently ameliorated the disease. Also, sera of patients with myasthenia gravis in remission contained apparent anti-idiotypic serum antibodies that reacted with the murine monoclonal anti–acetylcholine receptor antibody. This was the first demonstration of a receptor-specific anti–idiotypic response in a human disease.

As a brief example of the complex etiopathogenesis of autoimmunity, consider Hashimoto's thyroiditis (HT) and Graves' disease (GD). In both cases, women are affected at a five- to tenfold higher frequency than men are. Roles for cytokine-induced upregulation of HLA molecules, possibly secondary to viral infection, and subsequent self-antigen presentation to the immune system have been proposed for both diseases, and HT and GD are linked to HLA-DR but to different alleles. Both groups of patients have autoantibodies reactive with thyroid constituents, including thyroglobulin, thyroid peroxidase, and the TSH receptor, yet only the anti-TSH receptor antibodies in GD are known to be pathogenic in the disease. Given the massive inflammatory infiltrate in HT, a cell-mediated pathogenesis is likely. The similarities (thyroid, women, autoantibodies) and differences (HLA-DR alleles, humoral versus cell-mediated pathways) in these diseases illustrate some of the knowledge we have gained in studying autoimmune diseases and also reveal the deficiencies in our understanding.

CLASSIFICATION AND DIAGNOSIS OF AUTOIMMUNE DISEASES

The autoimmune disorders, listed in Table 26-2,[48-50] can be broadly separated as to whether they are organ-specific autoimmune diseases or systemic autoimmune diseases.

Organ-specific diseases

These disorders are characterized by chronic inflammation of and damage to a single organ. The autoantibodies in these diseases target antigens of the diseased organ; the best examples of this group are the organ-specific endocrine autoimmune diseases. Familial clustering of diseases within this group occurs with high frequency.

Diseases with non–organ specific autoantibodies with lesions restricted to one organ or a few organs combine the features of both organ-specific and systemic categories. Examples of this group are primary biliary cirrhosis and autoimmune hepatitis. These autoimmune liver disorders are characterized by the production of non–organ specific and non–species specific autoantibodies, such as antimitochondrial or anti–smooth muscle cell autoantibodies. Whether these autoantibodies bear any relationship to immune injury and tissue lesions is unknown, since amounts of the autoantibodies do not correlate with the severity or duration of disease. There

Table 26-2 Organ-specific and systemic autoimmune diseases

Disease	Antigen involved	Methods for detection of antibody
Endocrine		
Autoimmune thyroiditis, primary myxedema, thyrotoxicosis	Thyroglobulin	IFT—methanol-fixed human or monkey thyroid; passive hemagglutination; latex agglutination
	Cytoplasmic microsome	IFT—unfixed human hyper-plastic thyroid tissue; passive hemagglutination; complement fixation text
Graves' disease (diffuse toxic goiter)	TSI or anti-TSH antibody	Bioassay; measurement of adenyl cyclase activity after incubation of thyroid tissue with Ig from patient's serum; radioreceptor assay for antibodies competing with TSH for the receptor on thyroid membranes
Addison's disease	Adrenal cell cytoplasm	IFT (indirect) on unfixed monkey or human adrenal cortex
Parathyroid insufficiency	Parathyroid cytoplasmic antigen	IFT (indirect) on unfixed monkey or human parathyroid gland
Insulin-resistant diabetes associated with acanthosis nigricans	Anti-insulin receptor	Inhibition of ^{125}iodine-insulin binding to receptors on monocytes or adipocytes
Insulin-resistant diabetes associated with ataxia-telangiectasia	Anti-insulin receptor	Inhibition of ^{125}iodine-insulin binding to receptors on monocytes or adipocytes
Insulin-dependent diabetes (IDDM)	Antibodies to islet cells (cytoplasmic)	IFT on unfixed human or monkey pancreas
	Antibodies to glutamic acid decarboxylase (GAD)	RIA, immunoblotting, ELISA
Premature ovarian failure	Interstitial cells and corpus leuteum cells	IFT with human or monkey ovary
Systemic		
Lupus erythematosus	Nuclear antigens (DNA, histone, Sm, RNP, SS-A SS-B, nucleolar, etc.)	IFT on cells or tissue-section substrates, ELISA, immunoblotting, agglutination, immunoprecipitation
Mixed connective tissue disease	RNP	Immunoprecipitation, agglutination, ELISA, immunoblotting
Drug-induced lupus	Histones	IFT, ELISA
Sjögren's syndrome	Nuclear antigens (nucleolar, SS-A, (SS-B)	IFT on cells or tissue-section substrates, immunoprecipitation, ELISA, immunoblotting
Scleroderma/CREST syndrome	Nuclear antigen (nucleolar DNA, RNP, Scl-70) centromere	IFT on cells or tissue section substrates, immunoprecipitation, ELISA, immunoblotting
Dermatomyositis/polymyositis	Nuclear antigens (DNA, PM-1), Jo-1	IFT on cells or tissue section substrates, immunoprecipitation, ELISA, immunoblotting
Rheumatoid arthritis	Altered γ-globulin; rheumatoid arthritis–-associated nuclear antigen (RANA)	IFT, latex agglutination (rheumatoid factor), Rose test, sheep-cell agglutination, immunoprecipitation
Gastrointestinal		
Atrophic gastritis	Gastric cell microsomes	IFT (indirect)—human, monkey, mouse, or rat gastric mucosa substrate
Pernicious anemia	Intrinsic factor	Radioactive vitamin B_{12} binding assay
	Salivary duct-cells	IFT—unfixed human salivary gland
	Gastric parietal cells microsomes	IFT (indirect)—human, monkey, mouse, or rat gastric mucosa substrate
Ulcerative colitis	Colon, lipopolysaccharide	IFT—human or rat colon, hemagglutination
Crohn's disease	Reticulin, epithelial antibodies	IFT—mouse kidney or liver
Celiac disease	Reticulin; gluten or gliadin; endomysium of smooth muscle	IFT—mouse kidney or liver; EIA; IFT-IgA class endomysial antibodies on monkey esophagus

Table 26-2 Organ-specific and systemic autoimmune diseases—cont'd

Disease	Antigen involved	Methods for detection of antibody
Autoimmune chronic active hepatitis	Smooth muscle (contractile proteins)	IFT—mouse gastric mucosa or kidney; human cervical tissue; ELISA
Primary biliary cirrhosis	Mitochondrial	IFT—mouse kidney or HEp-2 cell, unfixed or fixed, ELISA
Skin		
Pemphigus vulgaris	Prickle cell desmosomes	IFT (direct on human skin biopsy specimen and indirect on monkey or guinea pig esophagus); peroxidase-labeled antibody
Bullous pemphigoid	Epithelial basement membrane	IFT (direct on human skin biopsy specimen and indirect on guinea pig or monkey esophagus); peroxidase-labeled antibody
Cicatricial pemphigoid	Epithelial basement membrane	IFT (direct on human skin biopsy specimen and indirect on guinea pig or monkey esophagus); peroxidase-labeled antibody
Dermatitis herpetiformis	Reticulin	IFT (indirect)—reticulin antibody detected on rat kidney or liver
	Endomysium of smooth muscle	Endomysium antibody of IgA class detected on monkey esophagus; IFT (direct)—staining for IgA deposits in dermal papillae
Other		
Myasthenia gravis	Anti-AChR	Immunoprecipitation of ^{125}iodine-α-bungarotoxin–conjugated AchR (human skeletal muscle); ELISA
Goodpasture's syndrome	Glomerular and lung basement membrane	IFT—biopsy of patient's kidney; IFT—patient's serum reacted on kidney substrate; radioimmunoassay performed on serum
Autoimmune hemolytic anemia	Red blood cell	Coombs' antiglobulin test (direct and indirect)
Demyelinating diseases (that is, multiple sclerosis)	Myelin, tubulin myelin, basic protein, myelin-associated glycoprotein	IFT—mammalian spinal cord; ELISA; immunoblotting
Spontaneous male infertility	Sperm	Agglutination and immobilization of spermatozoa

Modified from Nakamura RM, Binder WL: *Arch Pathol Lab Med* 112:869, 1988.
AchR, Acetylcholine receptor; *CREST*, calcinosis, Raynaud's phenomenon, esophageal dysmotility, sclerodactyly, and telangiectasia (syndrome); *EIA*, enzyme immunoassay; *ELISA*, enzyme-linked immunosorbent assay; *IFT*, immunofluorescence test; *IHYP*, iodohydroxybenzylpindolol; *HEp-2*, human epithelioid cells; *Jo-1*, (histidyl tRNA synthetase); *PM*, polymyositis; *RIA*, radioimmunoassay; *RNP*, ribonucleoprotein; *Scl*, scleroderma; *Sm*, Smith; *SS*, Sjögren's syndrome (A and B); *TSH*, thyroid-stimulating hormone; *TSI*, thyroid-stimulating immunoglobulin.

is evidence that the mechanisms of immunologic injury in liver disorders involve primarily a cellular immune mechanism by means of the suppressor and cytotoxic effector cell functions. In addition, humoral immunoregulatory factors modulate these cellular functions in the pathogenesis of immunologic liver disorders.

Systemic autoimmune diseases

These diseases cause widespread pathologic changes in many different organs and tissues throughout the body. Furthermore, the associated serum autoantibodies often lack organ or species specificity, and the lesions are not readily produced experimentally. However, similar diseases arise spontaneously in certain inbred animal strains.

Diagnosis

The patient's history, physical examination, and routine laboratory tests help both the clinician and the pathologist in the selection of further tests that may help in the evaluation of suspected autoimmune disease.

Laboratory assays that have proved useful in the routine initial evaluation of patients with suspected autoimmune disorders include those for (1) antinuclear antibodies (ANA), (2) rheumatoid factor, (3) immune complexes in serum, (4) concentrations of serum immunoglobulins and complement components, and (5) cryoglobulins.

The clinical laboratory assays most commonly ordered for patients with autoimmune diseases are those for detecting circulating autoantibodies. Tests of cellular immune function may help evaluate certain diseases, such as multiple sclerosis.[48] However, tests for cellular immune function are technically challenging and are not generally available in clinical laboratories.

A direct approach of assessing an affected organ is tissue biopsy for histologic study and, if needed, special studies. This approach is used often for patients with autoimmune diseases of the kidney or skin. The pathologist can evaluate the tissue injury pattern at those sites and document any immune-mediated mechanism by observing the immunofluorescent localization of immunoglobulin and complement components.

Immunofluorescence, enzyme-labeled antibody, and radioimmunoassay are methods that allow one to assess primary antigen-antibody binding and, because of their sensitivity, are preferred for the detection of circulating and tissue-bound autoantibodies and antigens.

Tests that involve secondary antigen-antibody preparations, such as complement fixation, agglutination, and precipitation in agar gel, may be less sensitive than immunofluorescence or radioimmunoassay in some circumstances but may be technically more suitable for the identification of certain autoantibodies.

Immunofluorescence tests

The indirect immunofluorescence test is the most comprehensive test used for screening autoantibodies in serum. The assay is performed by placing test serum onto a fixed and permeabilized cell monolayer or tissue section on a glass slide, washing to remove unbound autoantibodies, and then applying fluorescent-labeled anti–human immunoglobulin antibodies to label patient autoantibody attached to antigen on the substrate. Slides are then examined with a fluorescence microscope. Specific fluorescence is visualized as apple-green fluorescence of nuclear or cytoplasmic structures when one is using fluorescein isothiocyanate as conjugate. Antigen or antibody bound to tissue can be detected in a similar fashion.

The patterns that are usually seen in indirect immunofluorescence are neither specific nor diagnostic of a particular autoimmune disease. When available, confirmatory testing using a method specific for detecting the suspected autoantibody is advised. For example, the presence of a homogeneous immunofluorescent pattern indicates the need for follow-up testing using *Crithidia luciliae* or ELISA to confirm the presence of autoantibodies to native double-stranded DNA (Fig. 26-4).

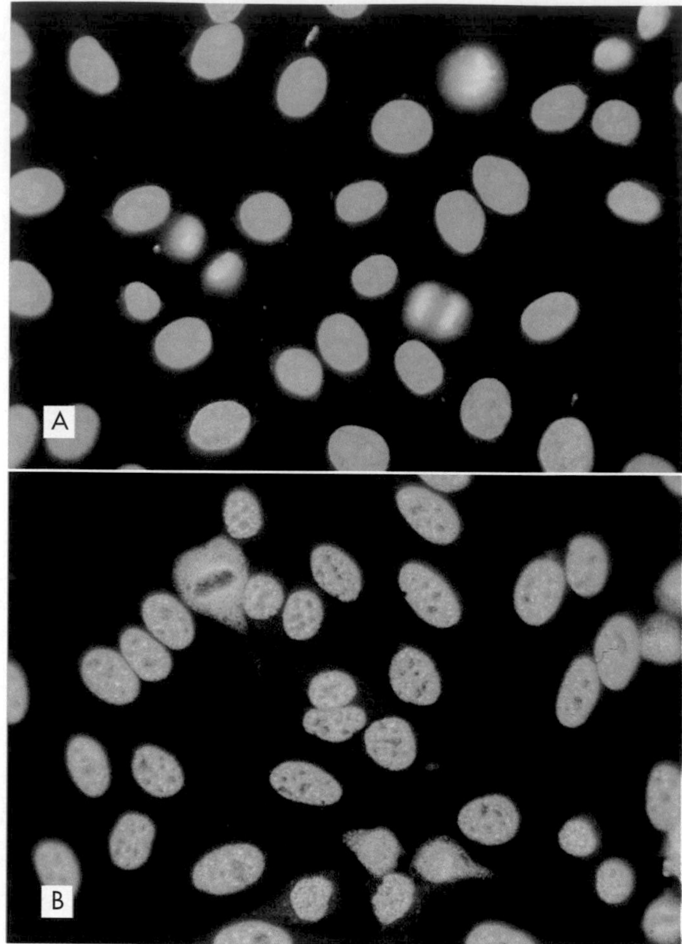

Fig. 26-4 Indirect immunofluorescence detection of antinuclear antibodies using commercial Hep-2 cell monolayer. **A,** Homogeneous nuclear staining pattern. **B,** Speckled nuclear staining pattern. Although both patterns are commonly seen when screening for serum autoantibodies, neither is disease specific, and so additional testing is required.

Interpretation of serum autoantibody levels in autoimmune disease

Caution is advised in the interpretation of positive autoantibody results. Patients with autoimmune disease tend to have high titers of autoantibody, whereas normal persons or patients with a wide variety of nonrheumatic conditions tend to have low titers of autoantibodies. Liver diseases, neoplasms, or infective disorders such as active tuberculosis or subacute bacterial endocarditis are examples of conditions that may have autoantibodies in serum.

A very high titer of autoantibody is a significant indicator of disease, though a low titer or lack of autoantibody does not rule out the possibility of an autoimmune disorder. For example, a negative antinuclear antibodies (ANA) on indirect immunofluorescence is generally considered strong evidence against the diagnosis of systemic lupus erythematosus. However, patients with so-called ANA-negative lupus often have autoantibody to the SS-A/Ro antigen that went undetected on screening, because of loss of the SS-A antigen during preparation of the substrate slides.

In severe active thyroiditis, the thyroid gland may act as an immunoadsorbent and remove circulating antibody. In addition, thyroglobulin may be released into the circulation during the acute stage and neutralize circulating autoantibody. Little or no autoantibody would be evident in either situation. In such circumstances, the titer of a given autoantibody must be interpreted in relation to the stage or treatment of the particular disease.

In contrast, levels of serum autoantibody to epidermal intercellular substance in pemphigus, anti–double stranded DNA in SLE, and antineutrophil cytoplasmic antibody in Wegener's granulomatosis correlate with the severity and course of the disease.

A small percentage of normal individuals, about 5% to 10%, will have a low titer (<1:320) of ANA. The incidence of this low-titer ANA in apparently normal individuals is increased in women and in older persons. The production of antiparietal cell and antithyroid autoantibodies shows similar age and sex dependence.

Other autoantibodies, such as anti–smooth muscle autoantibody and rheumatoid factor, do not show correlation with advancing age or female sex.

The most important principle to remember when interpreting any autoantibody result is to be aware of the patient information and to consider this laboratory finding in the clinical context.

REPRESENTATIVE SYSTEMIC AUTOIMMUNE DISEASES

The nosology of these diseases remains somewhat confusing, since immunologists and immunopathologists tend to refer to multiorgan autoimmune disorders as systemic autoimmune diseases, whereas clinicians often use the terms connective tissue, collagen vascular, or rheumatic diseases. We use the terms interchangeably in our discussion, which focuses on the diseases that involve multiple organ systems, including systemic lupus erythematosus (SLE), scleroderma (Scl), Sjögren's syndrome (SS), along with overlap syndromes. These diseases, as a group, compose a collection of systemic disorders characterized by protean clinical manifestations, autoantibodies, and putative autoimmune origin. Disorders with predominate organ-specific features, including rheumatoid arthritis, polymyositis/dermatomyositis, and systemic vasculitides,[66] are discussed in the chapters dealing with that respective organ system, particularly Chapter 75. Autoantibody tests useful in the evaluation of the diseases are given in Table 26-3.[67]

The multisystem autoimmune disorders share many epidemiologic features. Despite tremendous advances in the understanding of these disorders because of advances in cellular immunology and molecular pathology, their cause remains unknown. The role of interaction among genetic and environmental factors is not yet clearly defined and may be additive with disease expression modified by both endogenous and exogenous entities.[68] Although these diseases occur much more frequently in women and their association with HLA-DR4 is well documented, no single gene or group of genes, either MHC or non-MHC, is fully responsible for the clinical expression of disease.

Systemic lupus erythematosus

Systemic lupus erythematosus (SLE) is a clinical syndrome characterized by multisystem chronic inflammatory disease with demonstrable defects in both humoral and cellular immunity.[68,69] SLE is characterized by B-cell hyperactivity, a vast array of non–organ specific serum autoantibodies, especially antinuclear antibodies (ANA), and organ damage attributable to immune complexes.[68]

Epidemiology

The prevalence of SLE varies from 15 to 50 patients per 100,000 population.[70] Although SLE may occur at any age in either sex, this is primarily a disorder of women in their childbearing years, especially young black females.[68] The female-to-male ratio ranges from 3:1 to 8:1. In fact, clinical expression of the disease may vary depending on the age of presentation.[71] Younger patients tend to have more severe disease with involvement of the CNS or kidneys.[71,72] The disease occurs worldwide and in multiple populations at a prevalence ranging from 2.9/100,000 to 400/100,000.[73] Of Americans 18 to 65 years of age, the incidence is 1/1000 in white females and 1/250 in black females. Worldwide, the disease appears more commonly among blacks and other Asian populations.[69,74,75]

A genetic predisposition to SLE is suggested by familial, twin, and ethnic studies.[76] Ten percent of SLE patients have one or more first- or second-degree relatives with SLE.[77] The concordance of this disease among monozygotic twins exceeds that among dizygotic twins. Forty percent of individuals with a homozygous deficiency in components of the classical complement pathway, particularly C2 or C4 deficiency, have SLE.[77] The association with HLA-B8 and DR3 is strong but somewhat weaker with HLA-DR2 and DR3.[76,77]

Pathogenesis

Although the cause of SLE remains unknown, the disease is characterized by multiple immune defects. SLE is often presented as the classic immune complex disease. These immune complexes form either in situ or deposit by the circulation in numerous sites, particularly the renal glomeruli. The immune complexes activate complement, causing the release of anaphylatoxins and chemotactic factors, recruitment of neutrophils and T-lymphocytes, release of soluble mediators of

Table 26-3 Autoantibodies in systemic autoimmune disease

Antigen	Disease	Autoantibody frequency (%)
Double-stranded DNA	Systemic lupus erythematosus (SLE)	40
Sm	Systemic lupus erythematosus (SLE)	30
Histone (H2A-H2B)-DNA complex	Drug-induced lupus erythematosus	95
SS-A/Ro	SLE; Sjögren's syndrome	35
SS-B/La	Sjögren's syndrome	15
nRNP (u1-RNP)	MCTD	>95
Jo-1	Polymyositis/dermatomyositis	25
PM-Scl	Polymyositis/scleroderma overlap	8
Centromere	CREST	70-80

From Nakamura RM, Tan EM: *Clin Lab Med* 12:1, 1992.

CREST, Calcinosis, Raynaud's phenomenon, esophageal dysmotility, sclerodactyly, and telangiectasia (syndrome); *Jo-1,* histidyl tRNA synthetase; *MCTD,* mixed connective tissue disease; *nRNP,* nuclear ribonucleoprotein; *Sm,* Smith.

inflammation, and subsequent production of a localized, inflammatory lesion. Of primary importance in SLE are vasculitic lesions, which may be a key factor in its pathogenesis. The features of immune dysregulation in SLE include both B-cell and T-cell hyperactivity. Activated peripheral B-cells produce hypergammaglobulinemia.

Some T-cell alterations in active SLE include an increased number of T-cells with MHC class II surface molecules, increased secretion of B-cell stimulatory factors, decreased production of and responsiveness to interleukin-2, and depressed T-cell suppressor function. Natural killer cell activity is decreased.[76]

The interaction between T-cells and B-cells is altered, resulting in the excessive production of autoantibodies; 80% of these patients make lymphocytotoxic autoantibodies with specificities to HLA, non-HLA, T-lymphocyte, and tissue antigens. ANA of various specificities are characteristic, and the typical patient with SLE has three or more types. Many also have antibodies to plasma proteins and constituents of cell membranes.

The mononuclear phagocyte system's removal of immune complexes is decreased in active SLE. The mononuclear cells in patients with active SLE demonstrate diminished numbers of membrane receptors for C3, which play a major role in removing circulating immune complexes. This deficient clearance of immune complexes is usually prominent in those patients with active lupus nephritis.[78]

Pathology

There are no pathognomonic pathologic findings in SLE. Certain lesions presented in the literature as characteristic of SLE, such as hematoxylin bodies, Libman-Sacks verrucous endocarditis, or onionskin periarterial fibrosis in the spleen, are seldom seen in practice.[69] The range of pathologic lesions on light microscopy, however, includes inflammation with a mixture of cell types—lymphocytes, plasma cells, histiocytes, and some neutrophils; vasculopathy with or without thrombosis; basement membrane alterations in skin or kidney glomeruli; hematoxylin (basophilic) bodies; necrosis; and collagen sclerosis.[79] The pathologist must correlate the wide array of inflammatory findings in multiple organ systems with the clinical presentation to arrive at a differential diagnosis that includes SLE. Pathologic manifestations of SLE are seen in the skin and mucous membranes, kidneys, cardiovascular system, lungs, brain, musculoskeletal system, liver, and nonbiliary gastrointestinal tract. Involvement of either the kidneys or the brain portends a poor prognosis.[68]

The mucocutaneous lesions of SLE can be separated on the basis of clinical features into subgroups of chronic, subacute, or acute forms.[80] The characteristic histopathology of chronic cutaneous SLE includes hyperkeratosis, follicular plugging, liquefactive degeneration of the epidermal basal layer, telangiectasias, and superficial as well as deep perivascular-perifollicular inflammation consisting mainly of lymphocytes and histiocytes (Fig. 26-5). A PAS stain, after diastase predigestion, may reveal a thickened or discontinuous basement membrane zone (Fig. 26-6). Special stains, such as colloidal iron without and with hyaluronidase predigestion, show hyaluronic acid in the dermis (Fig. 26-7). Acute cutaneous lupus erythematosus (LE) shows epidermal liquefactive degeneration but will not demonstrate chronic epidermal changes, such as follicular plugging or hyperkeratosis. Subacute LE typically has "coat-sleeve" perivascular inflammation (Fig. 26-8) and anti-SSA (Ro) autoantibody in the patient's serum. This latter entity points out that although histopathology may be useful in separating cutaneous types of LE the clinical presentation correlated with laboratory findings remains the correct method for classifying cutaneous LE.

In the differential diagnosis of SLE, direct immunofluorescence can be useful to demonstrate continuous, granular, fluorescent bands (lupus band test) of immunoglobulins (IgG, IgA, IgM) and complement (C1q, C3) along the basement membrane zone of skin or oral mucosa (Fig. 26-9). Whereas in discoid lupus erythematosus deposition of immune complexes is limited to involved skin, patients with SLE have such deposits in both involved and uninvolved skin at sites exposed to the sun or not exposed. Although skin dIF may not be necessary in the rheumatologist's opinion, given the sensitivity and specificity of assays for ANA and the availability of other, easier

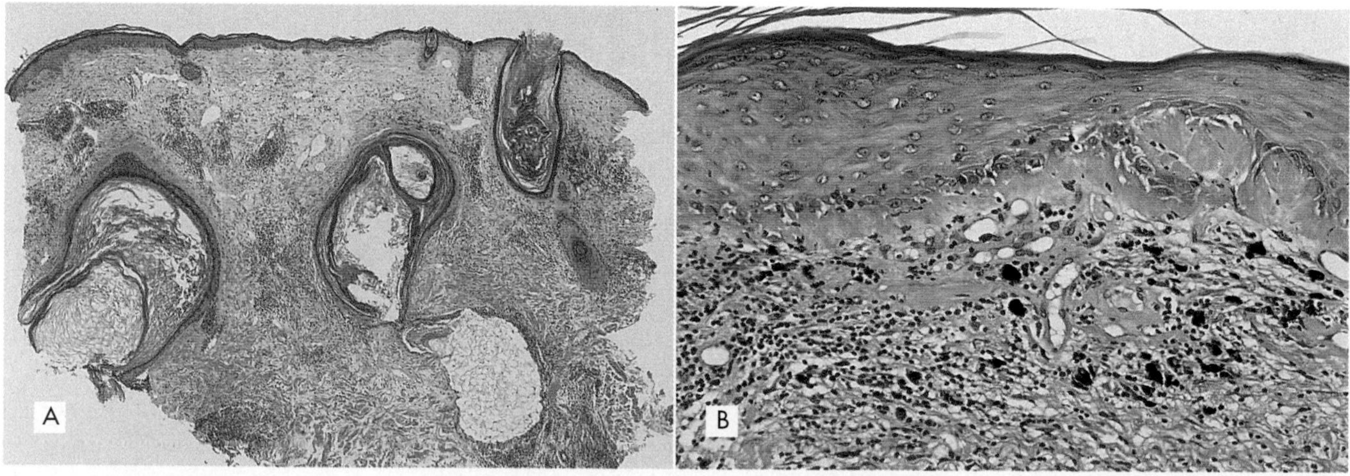

Fig. 26-5 Microscopic sections of chronic cutaneous lupus erythematosus. **A,** Low-power photomicrograph demonstrates superficial and deep perivascular chronic inflammation and follicular plugging. **B,** High-power view from a different case shows basal epidermal liquefactive degeneration, thickened basement membrane zone, telangiectasias, and dermal chronic inflammation.

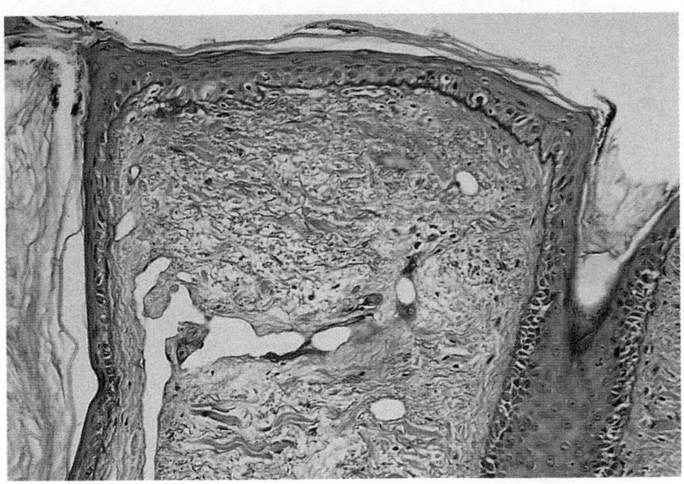

Fig. 26-6 dPAS stain demonstrates a wrinkled and slightly thickened basement membrane zone in chronic discoid lesion of systemic lupus erythematosus.

assays, direct immunofluorescence results may be diagnostic for cutaneous lupus erythematosus and therefore critical to resolving the dermatologist's differential diagnosis.

The microscopic differential diagnosis of cutaneous lupus erythematosus includes photoallergic eruptions, lupus-like drug eruptions, and polymorphous light eruptions. The special stains as noted above, and clinical correlation are useful in characterizing these lesions.

Lupus panniculitis (lupus profundus) is predominantly a lobular panniculitis with a peculiar pattern of hyalinized collagen replacing subcutaneous fat (Fig. 26-10). In many cases, septal inflammation is prominent. Identification of interstitial hyaluronic acid is a helpful diagnostic finding. Epidermal changes of lupus are present in about 25% of cases. Direct immunofluorescence, which can show immune deposits along the basement membrane zone as in clinical discoid lupus erythematosus, reveals intense staining of fibrin and fibrin precursor proteins, which give the peculiar hyalinized appearance to subcutaneous fat.

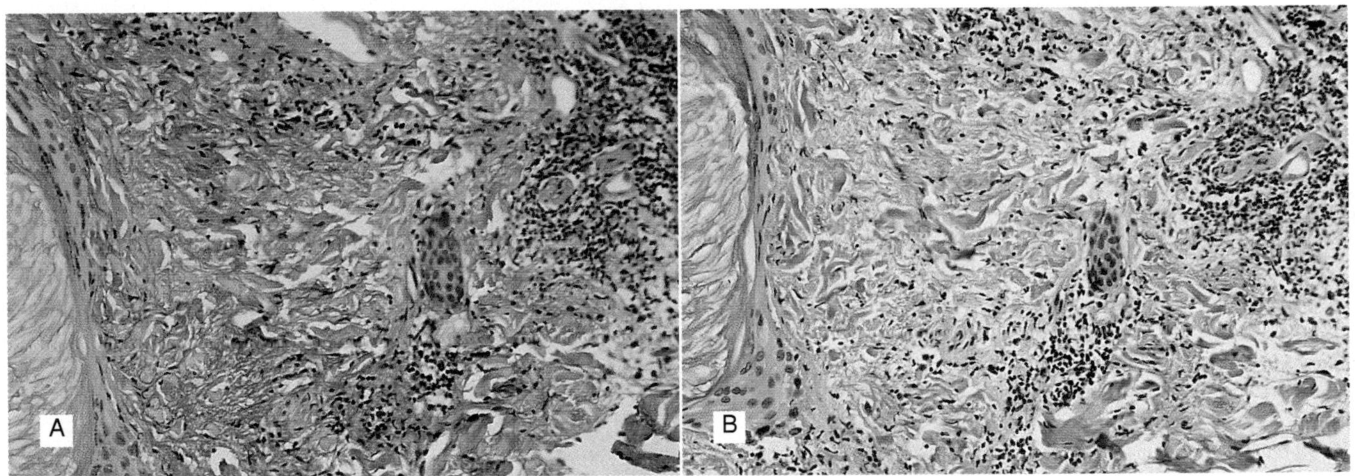

Fig. 26-7 Photomicrographs of a skin biopsy specimen from a case of systemic lupus erythematosus demonstrates abundant interstitial hyaluronic acid using the colloidal iron stain, **A,** without and, **B,** with hyaluronidase predigestion. The fibrillary blue interstitial material is hyaluronic acid. Notice the follicular keratotic plug at left.

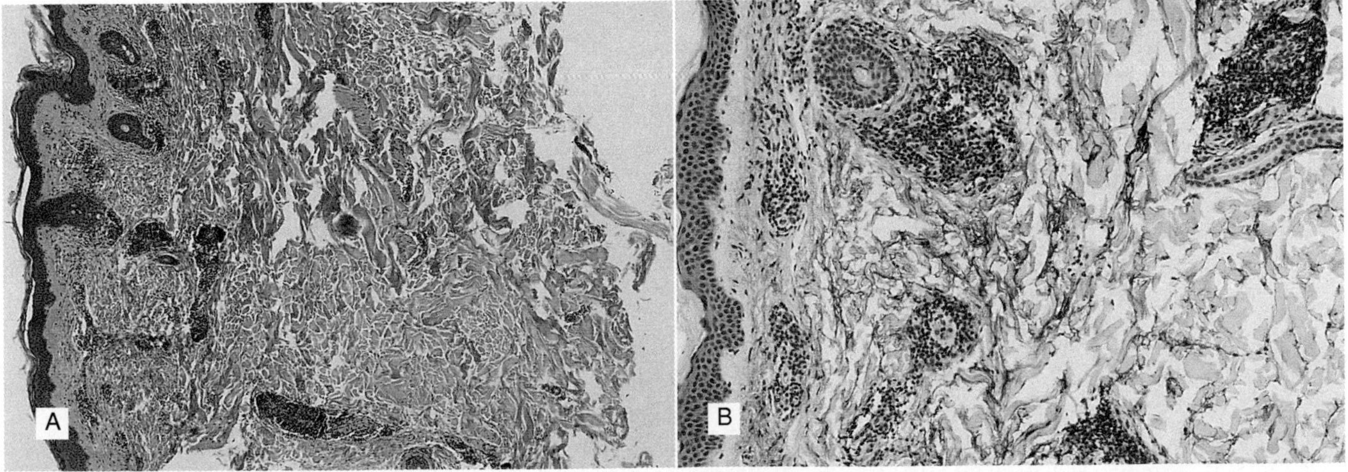

Fig. 26-8 **A,** Low-power photomicrograph of subacute lupus erythematosus showing prominent superficial and deep perivascular chronic inflammation without prominent epidermal changes or follicular plugging. Colloidal iron stain, **B,** dermal interstitial hyaluronic acid, a finding useful in the microscopic differential diagnosis.

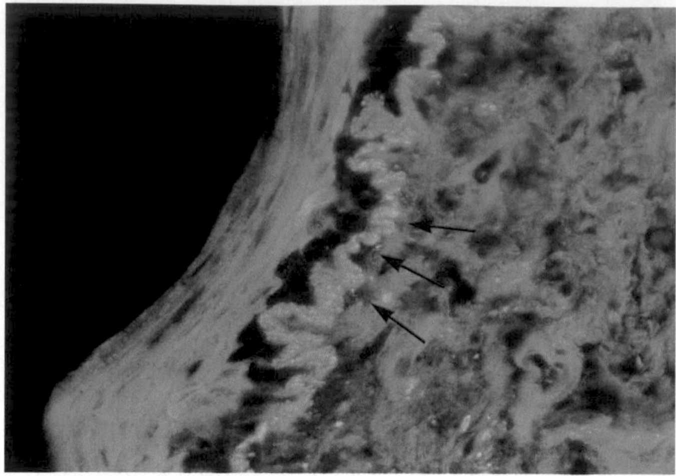

Fig. 26-9 High-power photomicrograph of direct immunofluorescence done on a skin biopsy specimen from a patient with systemic lupus erythematosus. There is continuous, granular, basement-membrane-zone immunofluorescence for immunoglobulins (IgG, IgA, and IgM) and complement (C1q, C3) (*arrows*).

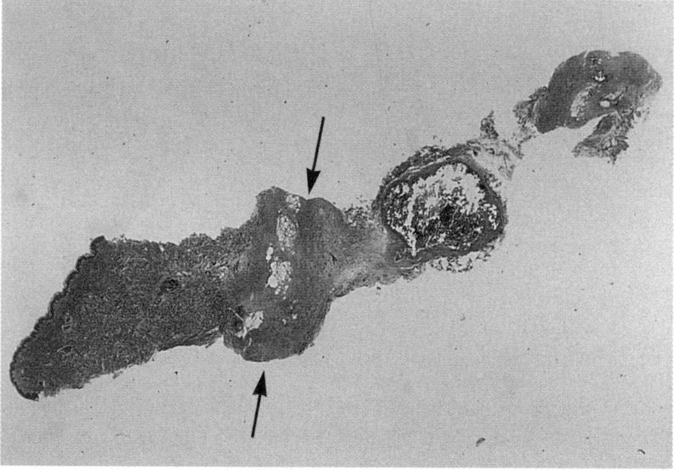

Fig. 26-10 Low-power photomicrograph of lupus panniculitis. Notice the zone of subcutaneous hyalinized collagen (*arrows*) and dystrophic calcification beneath a relatively unremarkable dermis.

Lymphocytic vasculitis with lymphocytes in the walls of dermal blood vessels can be seen in patients with SLE, SS, or other connective tissue disorders. Cutaneous vasculitis, however, when present, is most commonly leukocytoclastic vasculitis characterized by neutrophils in blood vessel walls, vessel wall necrosis, microthrombi, and extensive interstitial nuclear debris (Fig. 26-11). This presents clinically as palpable purpura or necrotic ulcers of the lower extremities. Although the clinician may proceed with therapy if a clinical diagnosis of palpable purpura is virtually certain, direct immunofluorescence of a skin sample may reveal immunoglobulins or C3 in vessel walls, depending on the time of biopsy related to the age of the lesion. These immunofluorescent findings, though characteristic of vasculitis, are not specific for leukocytoclastic vasculitis.

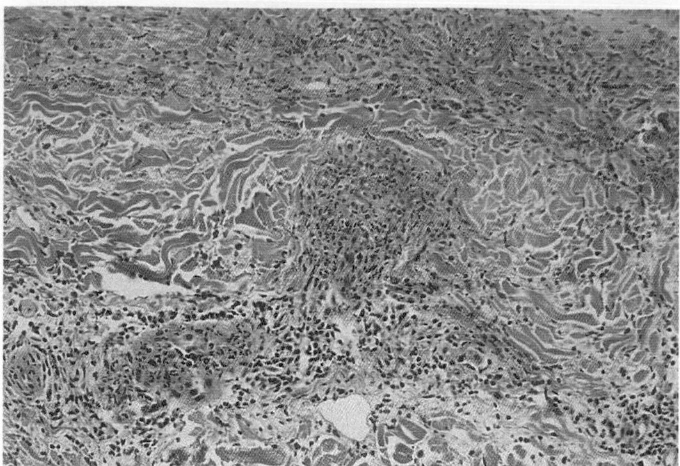

Fig. 26-11 Cutaneous leukocytoclastic vasculitis with purpura. There are extravasated red blood cells, neutrophils in blood vessel walls, and interstitial nuclear debris.

Kidneys. Lupus nephritis is often presented as the model for immune complex disease. Renal lesions in SLE may include those of glomeruli, renal tubules, or blood vessels. The range of renal disease in SLE is discussed in Chapter 65.

Cardiovascular system. Cardiac manifestations attributable to SLE, or the complications of SLE and its therapy, continue as clinical problems.[81] The principle histopathologic lesion in primary lupus carditis is one of mixed acute and chronic inflammation, in various stages of organization, involving the pericardium, myocardium, or valve leaflets.[81] However, the prevalence of histologic inflammation identified in postmortem material or surgical biopsy specimens exceeds the prevalence of symptomatic clinical carditis.

Pericarditis (Fig. 26-12) is the most common clinical manifestation of carditis,[81] occurring at some time in 30% to 50% of patients, presenting most frequently as pleuritic chest pain with or without a friction rub, less often as a pericardial effusion, and rarely as pericardial tamponade.

The classic lesion of lupus carditis is the endocardial, nonbacterial, verrucous valvulitis of Libman-Sacks. Mitral valve involvement predominates in most serial studies,[81] with lesions found on both surfaces of the valve leaflets (Fig. 26-13). This latter gross finding distinguishes this lesion from that of nonbacterial thrombotic endocarditis, and the absence of bacteria distinguishes lupus carditis from infective endocarditis. Transesophageal echocardiography is a very sensitive method to detect valvular vegetations or excrescences. Again, however, the prevalence of valve vegetations on transesophageal echo will exceed the prevalence of symptomatic clinical lupus valvulitis. Microscopic findings of lupus valvulitis include necrosis and fibrinoid change, hematoxylin bodies, and chronic inflammation with lymphocytes and plasma cells. Healing occurs with fibrosis and dystrophic microcalcifications, though valvular dysfunction is uncommon.

The occurrences of symptomatic myocarditis with ventricular dysfunction and arrhythmia is very uncommon.

Secondary heart disease may result from ischemic coronary artery disease, systemic hypertension, or, rarely, infective endocarditis.[81]

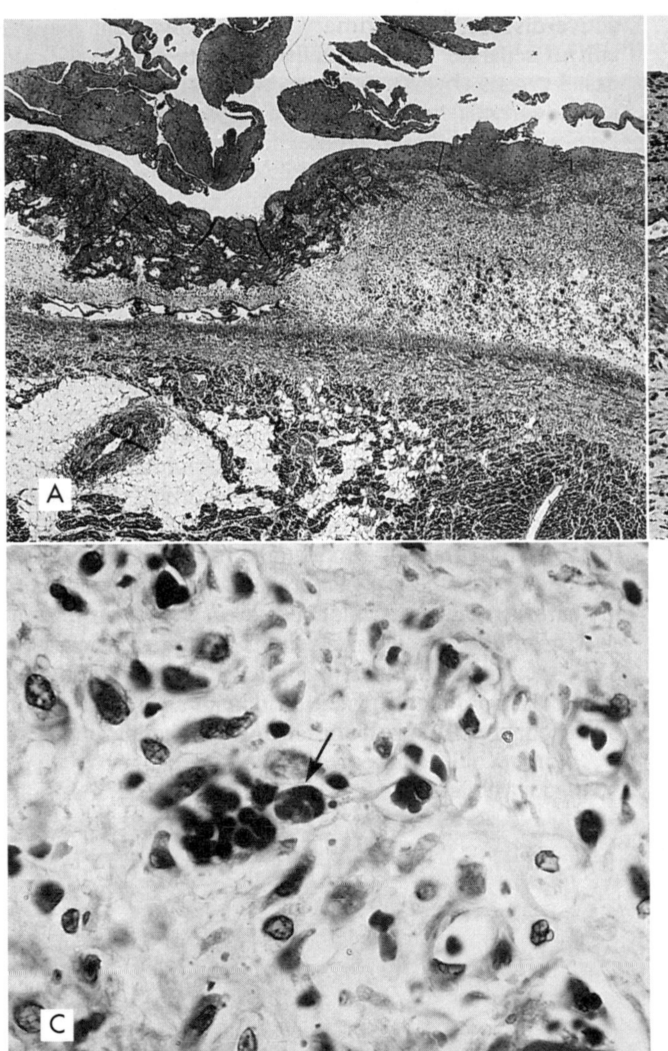

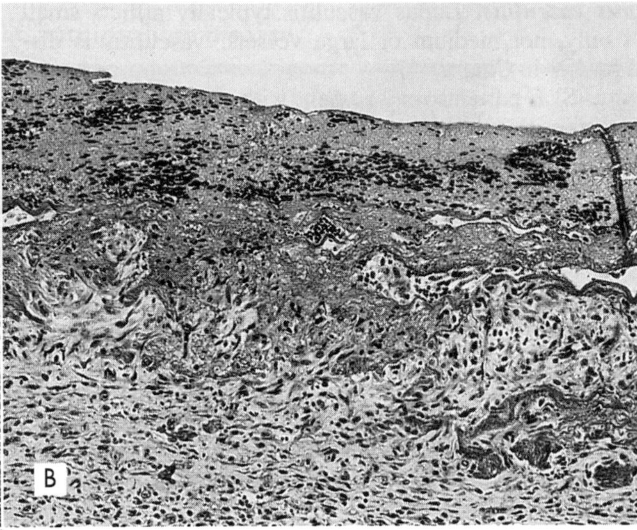

Fig. 26-12 Section of the myocardium and pericardium showing organizing fibrinous pericarditis in a 30-year-old woman with a 20-year history of systemic lupus erythematosus. **A,** Low-power view showing organizing fibrinous pericarditis. **B,** Higher power of the area of fibrin with underlying organization with neovascularization, inflammatory cells, and macrophages. **C,** Lupus erythematosus cell *(arrow)* within the area of granulation tissue. (Courtesy Drs. R. Virmani and T.T. Antonovych, Department of Cardiovascular Pathology, Armed Forces Institute of Pathology, Washington, D.C.)

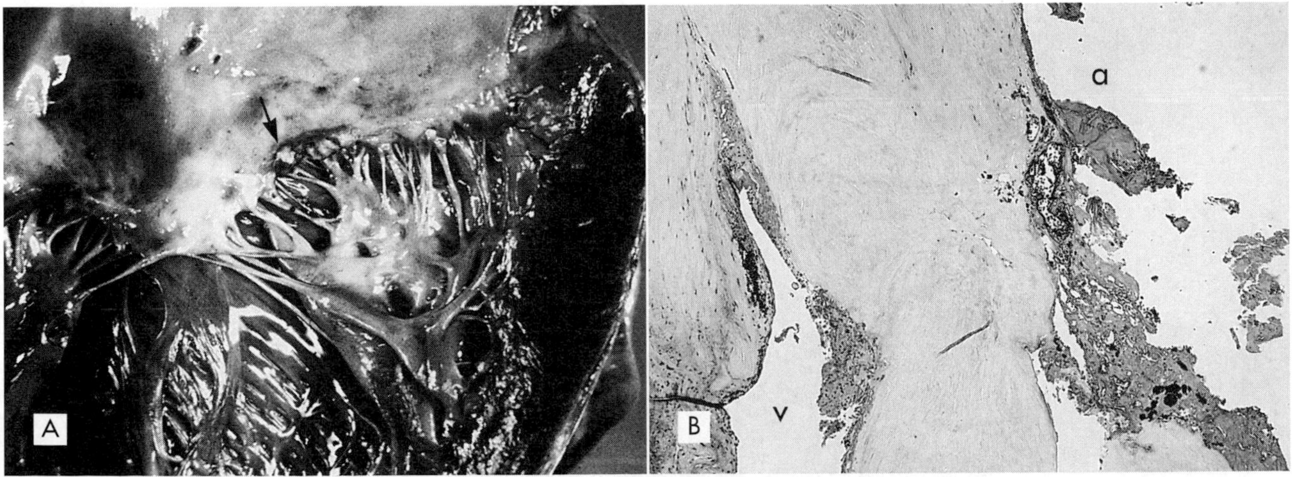

Fig. 26-13 Gross appearance of Libman-Sacks endocarditis *(arrowhead)* of the mitral valve. The vegetations are attached to the margin of the leaflet. **B,** Section of the mitral valve showing bland vegetations on the atrial and ventricular surface of the leaflet. *a,* Atrial surface; *v,* ventricular surface. (Courtesy Drs. R. Virmani and T.T. Antonovych, Department of Cardiovascular Pathology, Armed Forces Institute of Pathology, Washington, D.C.)

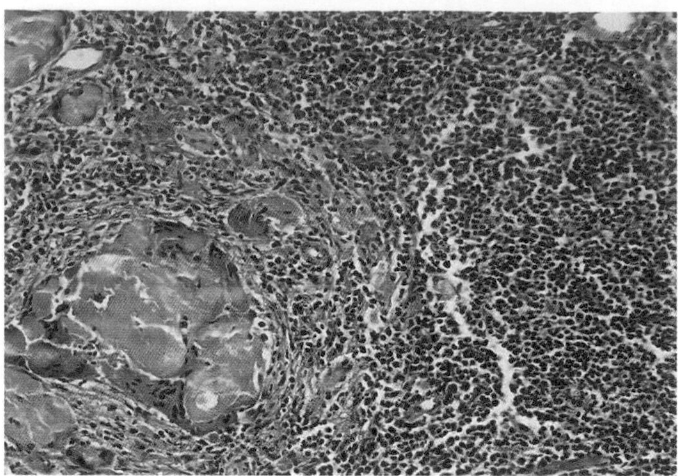

Fig. 26-18 Low-grade lymphoma with plasmacytoid features and amyloid deposits in the lungs of a patient with Sjögren's syndrome. (Courtesy T. Colby, Mayo Clinic, Rochester, Minn.)

hypertriglyceridemia, pancreatitis, alcoholism, and cirrhosis. HIV infection, viral hepatitis B or C, syphilis, and tuberculosis are infectious processes that can simulate SS. Anticholinergic drugs, used in a wide variety of clinical situations, usually will exacerbate the symptoms of dry eyes. Miscellaneous but important conditions that may mimic SS include graft-versus-host disease, sarcoidosis, post–radiation induced tissue injury, and endocrine disorders.

Laboratory findings include common nonspecific findings such as anemia, leukopenia, or elevated erythrocyte sedimentation rate. Serum immunoelectrophoresis shows polyclonal hypergammaglobulinemia in approximately 50% of SS patients, though some patients may have monoclonal IgM-κ; patients who become severely hypogammaglobulinemic and whose autoantibodies disappear should be carefully followed for the development of malignant lymphoma.[89]

Patients with SS may have high titers of RF (90%) and ANA (>1:640). Other autoantibodies often present include anti-SSA, anti-SSB, and anti–salivary duct antibodies. The presence of anti-SSB is considered relatively specific for primary SS. However, anti-SSA may be found in SS alone, in SLE, or in SLE with SS.

Treatment and prognosis

Treatment for SS is by moisture replacement for dry eyes and mouth, treatment of systemic autoimmune manifestations, and supportive management of nonspecific symptoms such as fatigue or depression. There is no curative treatment; however, the overall prognosis is generally good.

The development of a poorly differentiated carcinoma carries a poor prognosis because of the high risk for distant metastases, which ultimately causes the death of the patient in more than 33% of cases.[118]

RHEUMATOID ARTHRITIS

The pathologic and clinical manifestations of rheumatoid arthritis are discussed extensively in Chapter 75.

REFERENCES

1. Ehrlich P, Morgenroth J: In Himmelweit F, editor: *The collected papers of Paul Ehrlich—1990,* Oxford, 1956, Pergamon Press.
2. Theofilopoulos AN, Dixon FJ: Autoimmune diseases: immunopathology and etiopathogenesis, *Am J Pathol* 108:321, 1982.
3. Rose NR: Current concepts of autoimmune disease, *Transplant Proc* 20: 3, 1988.
4. Casali P, Prabhakar BS, Notkins AL: Characterization of multireactive autoantibodies and identification of Leu-1 B-lymphocytes as cells making antibodies binding multiple self and exogenous molecules, *Int Rev Immunol* 3:17, 1988.
5. Dighiero G, Lymberi P, Guilbert B et al: Natural autoantibodies constitute a substantial part of normal circulating immunoglobulins, *Ann N Y Acad Sci* 475:135, 1986.
6. Froude J et al: Cross-reactivity between streptococcus and human tissue: a model of molecular mimicry and autoimmunity, *Proc Natl Acad Sci USA* 145:5, 1989.
7. de Scheerder IK, de Buyzere ML, Delanghe JR et al: Anti-myosin humoral immune response following cardiac injury, *Autoimmunity* 4:51, 1989.
8. Neu N, Ploier B, Ofner C: Cardiac myosin-induced myocarditis. Heart autoantibodies are not involved in the induction of the disease, *J Immunol* 145:4094, 1990.
9. Davies T, DeBernardo E: *Thyroid autoantibodies and diseases: an overview in autoimmune endocrine disease,* New York, 1983, Wiley.
10. Harrington WJ, Minnich V, Hollingsworth JW et al: Demonstration of a thrombocytopenic factor in the blood of patients with thrombocytopenic purpura, *J Lab Clin Med* 115:636, 1990.
11. Kikutani H, Makino S: The murine autoimmune diabetes model: NOD and related strains, *Adv Immunol* 51:285, 1992.
12. Lindstrom J et al: Myasthenia gravis, *Adv Immunol* 42:233, 1988.
13. Anhalt GJ, Labib RS, Voorhees JJ et al: Induction of pemphigus in neonatal mice by passive transfer of IgG from patients with the disease, *N Engl J Med* 306:1189, 1982.
14. Duchosal MA, McConahey PJ, Robinson CA et al: Transfer of human systemic lupus erythematosus in severe combined immunodeficient (SCII) mice, *J Exp Med* 172:985, 1990.
15. Burnet FM: *The clonal selection theory of acquired immunity,* Cambridge, 1959, Cambridge University Press.
16. Nossal GJV: Cellular mechanisms of immunologic tolerance, *Annu Rev Immunol* 1:33, 1983.
17. Goodnow CC: Transgenic mice and analysis of B-cell tolerance, *Annu Rev Immunol* 10:489, 1992.
18. Okamoto M, Murakami M, Shimizu A et al: A transgenic model of autoimmune hemolytic anemia, *J Exp Med* 175:71, 1992.
19. Murakami M, Tsubata T, Okamoto M et al: Antigen-induced apoptotic death of Ly-1 B-cells responsible for autoimmune disease in transgenic mice, *Nature* 357:77, 1992.
20. Ohashi PS, Oehen S, Buerki K et al: Ablation of "tolerance" and induction of diabetes by virus infection in viral antigen transgenic mice, *Cell* 65:305, 1991.
21. Oldstone MBA, Nerenberg M, Southern P et al: Virus infection triggers insulin-dependent diabetes mellitus in a transgenic model: role of anti-self (virus) immune response, *Cell* 65:319, 1991.
22. Sarvetnick N, Liggitt D, Pitts SL et al: Insulin-dependent diabetes mellitus induced in transgenic mice by ectopic expression of class II MHC and interferon-gamma, *Cell* 52:773, 1988.
23. Sarvetnick N, Shizuru J, Liggitt D et al: Loss of pancreatic islet tolerance induced by beta-cell expression of IFN-γ, *Nature* 346:844, 1990.
24. Jerne NK: The natural selection theory of antibody formation, *Proc Natl Acad Sci USA* 41:849, 1955.
25. Diaz-Gallo, Moscovitch-Lopatin CM, Strom TB et al: An anergic, islet-infiltrating T-cell clone that suppresses murine diabetes secretes a factor that blocks interleukin 2/interleukin 4–dependent proliferation, *Proc Natl Acad Sci USA* 89:8656, 1992.

Pathophysiology

26. Sinha AA, Lopez MT, McDevitt HO: Autoimmune diseases: the failure of self tolerance, *Science* 248:1380, 1990.

27. Tattersall RB, Pyke DA: Diabetes in identical twins, *Lancet* 2:1120, 1972.
28. Aho K, Koskenvuo M, Tuominen J et al: Occurrence of rheumatoid arthritis in a nationwide series of twins, *J Rheumatol* 13:899, 1986.
29. Erlich HA, McDevitt HO, Lock CB: The role of the MHC in autoimmune disease. In Bona CA, Siminovitch KA, Zanetti M et al, editors: *The molecular pathology of autoimmune diseases,* Switzerland, 1993, Harwood Academic Publishers.
30. Ansar Ahmed S, Penhale WJ, Talal N: Sex hormones, immune responses, and autoimmune diseases, *Am J Pathol* 121:531, 1985.
31. Grossman CJ: Interactions between the gonadal steroids and the immune system, *Science* 227:257, 1985.
32. Roubinian JR, Papoian R, Talal N: Androgenic hormones modulate autoantibody responses and improve survival in murine lupus, *J Clin Invest* 59:1066, 1977.
33. Roubinian JR, Talal N, Greenspan JS et al: Effect of castration and sex hormone treatment on survival, anti-nucleic acid antibodies, and glomerulonephritis in NZB/NZW F_1, *J Exp Med* 147:1568, 1978.
34. Fox HS: Androgen treatment prevents diabetes in nonobese diabetic mice, *J Exp Med* 175:1409, 1992.
35. Fitzpatrick F, Lepault F, Homo-Delarch F et al: Influence of castration, alone or combined with thymectomy, on the development of diabetes in the nonobese diabetic mouse, *Endocrinology* 129:1382, 1991.
36. Fox HS, Bond BL, Parslow TG: The interferon-gamma promoter is regulated by estrogen, *J Immunol* 146:4362, 1991.
37. Araneo BA, Dowell T, Diegel M et al: Dihydrotestosterone exerts a depressive influence on the production of interleukin-4 (IL-4), IL-5, and gamma-interferon, but not IL-2 by activated murine T-cells, *Blood* 78:688, 1991.
38. Schwimmbeck PL, Oldstone MBA: *Klebsiella pneumoniae* and HLA B27–associated diseases of Reiter's syndrome and ankylosing spondylitis, *Curr Top Microbiol Immunol* 45:45, 1989.
39. Yoon JW et al: Virus-induced diabetes mellitus: Isolation of a virus from the pancreas of a child with diabetic ketoacidosis, *N Engl J Med* 300:1173, 1979.
40. Rock GAW, Lydyard PM, Standord JL: A reappraisal of the evidence that rheumatoid arthritis and several other idiopathic diseases are slow bacterial infections, *Ann Rheum Dis* 52(suppl 1):S30, 1993.
41. Taub DJ, Blank KJ: Superantigens and microbial pathogenesis, *Ann Intern Med* 119:89 1993.
42. Acha-Orbea H: Bacterial and viral superantigens: role in autoimmunity, *Ann Rheum Dis* 52:S6, 1993.
43. Goldman M, Druet P, Gleichmann E: T_H2 cells in systemic autoimmunity: insights from allogeneic diseases and chemically-induced autoimmunity, *Immunol Today* 12:223, 1991.
44. Talal N, editor: *Autoimmunity: genetic, immunologic, virologic, and clinical aspects,* New York, 1990, Academic Press.
45. Rose NR: Pathogenic mechanisms in autoimmune diseases, *Clin Immunol Immunopathol* 53:S7, 1989.
46. Goodman ME, Weigle WO: Role of polyclonal B-cell activities in self/non-self discrimination, *Immunol Today* 2:54, 1981.
47. Dziarski R: Autoimmunity: polyclonal activation or antigen induction, *Immunol Today* 9:340, 1988.
48. Nakamura RM, Binder WL: Current concepts and diagnostic evaluation of autoimmune disease, *Arch Pathol Lab Med* 112:869, 1988.
49. Nakamura MC, Nakamura RM: Contemporary concepts of autoimmunity and autoimmune diseases, *J Clin Lab Anal* 6:275, 1992.
50. Hokama Y, Nakamura RM: *Immunology and immunopathology: basic concepts,* Boston, 1982, Little, Brown & Co.
51. Weigle WO: Analysis of autoimmunity through experimental models of thyroiditis and allergic encephalomyelitis, *Adv Immunol* 30:159, 1980.
52. Miller A, Hafler DA, Weiner HL: Tolerance and suppressor mechanisms in experimental autoimmune encephalomyelitis: implications for immunotherapy of human autoimmune diseases, *FASEB J* 15:2560, 1991.
53. Miller KB, Schwartz RS: Autoimmunity and suppressor T-lymphocytes, *Adv Intern Med* 27:281, 1982.
54. Thorbecke GJ, Shah R, Leu CH et al: Involvement of endogenous tumor necrosis factor α and transforming growth factor β during induction of collagen type II arthritis in mice, *Proc Natl Acad Sci USA* 89:7375, 1992.
55. Mosmann TR, Coffmann RL: TH1 and TH2 cells: different patterns of lymphokine secretion lead to different functional properties, *Annu Rev Immunol* 7:145, 1989.
56. Powrie F, Coffman RL: Cytokine regulation of T-cell function: potential for therapeutic intervention, *Immunol Today* 14:270, 1993.
57. Oldstone MA: Molecular mimicry and autoimmune disease, *Cell* 50:819, 1987.
58. Oldstone MBA: Molecular mimcry as a mechanism for the cause and as a probe uncovering etiologic agent(s) of autoimmune disease, *Curr Top Microbiol Immunol* 45:127, 1989.
59. Fujinami RS, Oldstone MBA: Amino acid homology between the encephalitogenic site of myelin basic protein and virus: mechanism for autoimmunity, *Science* 230:1043, 1985.
60. Doherty PC, Allan W, Eichelberger M et al: Heat-shock proteins and the gamma-delta T-cell response in virus infections: implications for autoimmunity, *Springer Semin Immunopathol* 13:11, 1991.
61. Winfield JB, Jarnour WN: Stress proteins, autoimmunity and autoimmune disease, *Curr Top Microbiol Immunol* 167:161, 1991.
62. Wucherpfennig KW, Newcombe J, Li H et al: γ/δ T-cell receptor repertoire in acute multiple sclerosis lesions, *Proc Natl Acad Sci USA* 89: 4588, 1992.
63. Shimonkevitz R, Colburn C, Burnham JA et al: Clonal expansions of activated γ/δ T-cells in recent-onset multiple sclerosis, *Proc Natl Acad Sci USA* 90:923, 1993.
64. Male DK: Idiotypes and autoimmunity, *Clin Exp Immunol* 65:1, 1986.
65. Plotz PH: Autoantibodies are anti-idiotype antibodies to antiviral antibodies, *Lancet* 2:824, 1983.

Classification and diagnosis of autoimmune diseases

66. Schumacher HR Jr: Rheumatoid arthritis: classification of the rheumatic diseases. In Schumacher HR Jr, Klippel JH, Robinson DW, editors: *Primer on the rheumatic diseases,* Atlanta, 1993, The Arthritis Foundation.

Representative systemic autoimmune diseases

67. Nakamura RM, Tan EM: Update on autoantibodies to intracellular antigens in systemic rheumatic diseases, *Clin Lab Med* 12:1, 1992.
68. Ferrell PB, Tan EM: Systemic lupus erythematosus. In Rose NR, Mackay IR, editors: *The autoimmune diseases,* New York, 1985, Academic Press.

Systemic lupus erythematosus

69. Alarcón-Segovia D: Systemic lupus erythematosus: pathology and pathogenesis. In Schumacher HR Jr, Klippel JH, Robinson DR, editors: *Primer on the rheumatic diseases,* Atlanta, 1993, The Arthritis Foundation.
70. Hahn BH: Systemic lupus erythematosus. In Isselbacher KJ, Braunwald E, Wilson JD et al, editors: *Harrison's principles of internal medicine,* ed 13, New York, 1994, McGraw-Hill.
71. Cervera R, Khamashta MA, Font J et al: Systemic lupus erythematosus: clinical and immunologic patterns of disease expression in a cohort of 1,000 patients, *Medicine* 72:113, 1993.
72. Barron KS, Silverman ED, Gonzales J et al: Clinical, serologic, and immunogenetic studies in childhood-onset systemic lupus erythematosus, *Arthritis Rheum* 36:348, 1993.
73. Alarcón-Segovia D: Systemic lupus erythematosus. In Schumacher HR Jr, Klippel JH, Robinson DR, editors: *Primer on the rheumatic diseases,* Atlanta, 1988, The Arthritis Foundation.
74. Hochberg MC: Epidemiology of the rheumatic diseases. In Schumacher HR Jr, Klippel JH, Robinson DR, editors: *Primer on the rheumatic diseases,* Atlanta, 1988, The Arthritis Foundation.
75. Schur PH: Third International Conference on Systemic Lupus Erythematosus, *Arthritis Rheum* 35:1238, 1992.
76. Woods VL Jr: Pathogenesis of systemic lupus erythematosus. In Kelley WN, Harris ED Jr, Ruddy S et al, editors: *Textbook of rheumatology,* vol 1, ed 4, Philadelphia, 1993, Saunders.
77. Fessel WJ: Epidemiology of systemic lupus erythematosus, *Rheum Dis Clin North Am* 14:15, 1988.
78. Woods VL Jr: Human systemic lupus erythematosus. In Bona CA, Siminovitch KA, Zanetti M et al, editors: *The molecular pathology of autoimmune diseases,* Switzerland, 1993, Harwood Academic Publishers.

79. Gardner DL: Systemic lupus erythematosus. In *Pathological basis of the connective tissue diseases,* Philadelphia, 1992, Lea & Febiger.
80. Callen JP: Mucocutaneous changes in patients with lupus erythematosus: the relationship of these lesions to systemic disease, *Rheum Dis Clin North Am* 14:79, 1988.
81. Stevens MB: Systemic lupus erythematosus and the cardiovascular system: the heart. In Lahita RG, editor: *Systemic lupus erythematosus,* New York, 1992, Churchill Livingstone.
82. Palmaz JC, Windelar SA, Garcia F et al: Balloon expandable intraluminal grafting of atherosclerotic rabbit aortas, *Radiology* 160:723, 1986.
83. Colby TV, Lombard C, Yousem SA et al: *Atlas of pulmonary surgical pathology,* Philadelphia, 1991, Saunders.
84. McCallum RM, Haynes BF: Management of patients with pulmonary manifestations of collagen-vascular diseases. In Shelhamer J, Pizzo P, Parrillo J et al, editors: *Respiratory disease in the immunosuppressive host,* Philadelphia, 1991, Lippincott.
85. Bluestein HG: The central nervous system in systemic lupus erythematosus. In Lahita RG, editor: *Systemic lupus erythematosus,* New York, 1992, Churchill Livingstone.
86. Cronin ME: Musculoskeletal manifestations of systemic lupus erythematosus, *Rheum Dis Clin North Am* 14:99, 1988.
87. Matsumoto T, Yoshimine T, Shimouchi K et al: The liver in systemic lupus erythematosus: pathologic analysis of 52 cases and review of Japanese autopsy registry data, *Hum Pathol* 23:1151, 1992.
88. Schnitzer B: Reactive lymphadenopathies. In Knowles DM, editor: *Neoplastic hematopathology,* Baltimore, 1992, Williams & Wilkins.
89. Fye KH, Sack KE: Rheumatic diseases. In Stites DP, Terr AI, editors: *Basic and clinical immunology,* Norwalk, Conn, 1991, Appleton & Lange.
90. Sontheimer RD, Gilliam JN: Systemic lupus erythematosus and the skin. In Lahita RG, editor: *Systemic lupus erythematosus,* New York, 1992, Churchill Livingstone.
91. Hughson MD, McCarty GA, Sholer CM et al: Thrombotic cerebral arteriopathy in patients with the antiphospholipid syndrome, *Mod Pathol* 6:644, 1993.
92. Buyon JP: Neonatal lupus syndromes. In Lahita RG, editor: *Systemic lupus erythematosus,* New York, 1992, Churchill Livingstone.
93. Tan EM, Chan EKL, Sullivan KF et al: Antinuclear antibodies (ANAs): diagnostically specific immune markers and clues towards the understanding of systemic autoimmunity, *Clin Immunol Immunopathol* 47:121, 1988.
94. Rubin RL: Autoimmune reactions induced by procainamide and hydralazine. In Kammuller ME, Bloksma N, Seinen W, editors: *Autoimmunity and toxicology,* Amsterdam, 1989, Elsevier Science Publishers.
95. Burlingame RW, Rubin RL: Drug-induced anti-histone autoantibodies display two patterns of reactivity with substructures of chromatin, *J Clin Invest* 88:680, 1991.
96. Totoritis MC, Tan EM, McNally EM et al: Association of anti-histone (H2A-H2B) complex antibody with symptomatic procainamide-induced lupus, *N Engl J Med* 318:1431, 1988.

Scleroderma

97. Alarcón-Segovia D: Scleroderma. In Rose NR, Mackay IR, editors: *The autoimmune diseases,* New York, 1985, Academic Press.
98. Gilliland BC: Systemic sclerosis (scleroderma). In Wilson JD, Braunwald E, Isselbacher KJ et al, editors: *Harrison's principles of internal medicine,* ed 12, New York, 1991, McGraw-Hill.
99. Maddison PJ, Stephens C, Briggs D et al: Connective tissue disease and autoantibodies in the kindreds of 63 patients with systemic sclerosis, *Medicine* 72:103, 1993.
100. Medsger TA Jr: Systemic sclerosis and localized scleroderma. In Schumacher HR Jr, Klippel JH, Robinson DR, editors: *Primer on the rheumatic diseases,* Atlanta, 1993, The Arthritis Foundation.
101. Seibold JR: Scleroderma. In Kelley WN, Harris ED Jr, Ruddy S et al, editors: *Textbook of rheumatology,* Philadelphia, 1993, Saunders.
102. Frieri MA: Systemic sclerosis: the role of the masT-cell and cytokines, *Ann Allergy* 69:385, 1992.
103. Gardner DL: Systemic sclerosis and allied disorders. In *Pathological basis of the connective tissue diseases,* Philadelphia, 1992, Lea & Febiger.
104. Yousem SA: The pulmonary pathologic manifestations of the CREST syndrome, *Hum Pathol* 21:467, 1990.
105. LeRoy CE, Medsger TA Jr: The spectrum of scleroderma-related syndromes. In Schumacher HR Jr, Klippel JH, Robinson DR, editors: *Primer on the rheumatic diseases,* Atlanta, 1993, The Arthritis Foundation.
106. Gilliland BC: Systemic sclerosis (scleroderma). In Isselbacher KJ, Braunwald E, Wilson JD et al, editors. *Harrison's principles of internal medicine,* ed 13, New York, 1994, McGraw-Hill.

Sjögren's syndrome

107. Fox RI, Saito I: Criteria for diagnosis of Sjögren's syndrome, *Rheum Dis Clin North Am* 20:391, 1994.
108. Fox RI, Kang H-I: Sjögren's syndrome. In Kelley WN, Harris ED Jr, Ruddy S et al, editors: *Textbook of rheumatology,* vol 1, ed 4, Philadelphia, 1993, Saunders.
109. Talal N: Sjögren's syndrome. In Schumacher HR Jr, Klippel JH, Robinson DR, editors: *Primer on the rheumatic diseases,* Atlanta, 1993, The Arthritis Foundation.
110. Talal N: Sjögren's syndrome. In Rose NR, Mackay IR, editors: *The autoimmune diseases,* New York, 1985, Academic Press.
111. Vitali C, Bombardieri S, Moutsopoulos HM et al: Preliminary criteria for the classification of Sjögen's syndrome: results of a propective concerted action supported by the European Community, *Arthritis Rheum* 36:340, 1993.
112. Daniels TE: Labial salivary gland biopsy in Sjögren's syndrome, *Arthritis Rheum* 27:147, 1984.
113. Tarpley TM, Anderson LG, White CL: Minor salivary gland involvement in Sjögren's syndrome, *Oral Surg Oral Med Oral Pathol* 37:64, 1974.
114. Smith CA: Labial salivary gland histopathology and autoantibodies in Sjögren's syndrome and other connective tissue diseases (Letter to the Editor), *Arthritis Rheum* 35:367, 1992.
115. Leroy J-P, Pennec Y-L, Letoux G et al: Lymphocytic infiltration of salivary ducts: a histopathologic lesion specific for primary Sjögren's syndrome? *Arthritis Rheum* 35:481, 1992.
116. Burke JS: Extranodal lymphoid proliferations: general principles and differential diagnosis. In Knowles DM, editor: *Neoplastic hematopathology,* Baltimore, 1992, Williams & Wilkins.
117. Burke JS: Waldeyer's ring, sinonasal region, salivary gland, thyroid gland, central nervous system, and other extranodal lymphomas and lymphoid hyperplasias. In Knowles DM, editor: *Neoplastic hematopathology,* Baltimore, 1992, Williams & Wilkins.
118. Huvos AG: Salivary glands. In Sternberg SS, Antonioli DA, Carter D et al, editors: *Diagnostic surgical pathology,* vol 1, New York, 1989, Raven Press.

27 Primary Immunodeficiencies

Thomas A. Seemayer
Christian Nezelof

Between the descriptions in the early 1950s of what is now known as severe combined immunodeficiency (SCID) by Glanzmann and Riniker[1] and agammaglobulinemia by Bruton[2] and the most recent Primary Immunodeficiency Registry listing of the World Health Organization scientific group in 1992,[3] more than 70 types of primary immunodeficiency conditions have been delineated. In most instances, their genetic transmission, clinical expression, immunologic aberrations, and pathogenetic mechanisms have been elucidated. In little more than 40 years, the two conditions described initially have been characterized fully, and the responsible genes have been cloned. This explosive progress is a vivid reflection of the integration of work stemming from histopathology, clinical pediatrics, immunology, and molecular biology. Moreover, these "experiments of nature"[4] have led to seminal discoveries regarding the normal immune response, the dichotomy of T-cells and B-cells and the workings of the lymphoid and hematopoietic systems. Few areas of medicine can attest to such a golden childhood. Clearly, Robert A. Good stands out as a pivotal force in this period. On the one hand, he contributed to our understanding of the immune system through his own works. Perhaps more importantly, he trained legions of investigators who, inspired by his brilliance, drive, and honesty, left their mark in these annals, as cited by many references that follow.

Primary immunodeficiencies are usually diseases of infancy and childhood. Nearly 40% present within the first year of life; by 6 years of age, over 95% have declared themselves. Those cases presenting in adulthood are usually represented by common variable immunodeficiency. Most children with primary immunodeficiencies are males. Since many genes central to the immune system's function are believed to be located on the X-chromosome, this would explain this biased sex incidence.[5] Six X-linked immunodeficiencies have been described; five affect lymphocytes; one, phagocytes. Five of these six involved genes have been cloned (Fig. 27-1).

The incessant and troublesome recurrence of infections represents the hallmark of almost all immunodeficiencies. These infections are often generalized and attributable to banal agents, often designated as "opportunistic," such as *Candida,* cytomegalovirus, and *Pneumocystis carinii.* Even normally harmless live vaccines, such as Bacille Calmette-Guérin (BCG), can be lethal for the immunocompromised child.

In general, recurrent bacterial infections are suggestive of aberrations in the humoral (B-cell) immune response, phagocytic system, complement cascade, or leukocyte adhesion molecules. Alternatively, viral, fungal, and parasitic infections are suggestive of T-cell malfunction. Autoimmune and neoplastic phenotypes reflect, in general, T-cell defects. Not uncommonly, deficiencies of both B-cells and T-cells are present, offering a mixed and expanded clinical phenotype.

In the early halcyon days traditional histopathology played a pivotal role in the diagnosis of many immunodeficiencies. Its present role is now complementary to other more mechanistically oriented disciplines such as immunology and molecular biology. Nonetheless, modern techniques of pathology employing immunohistochemistry, monoclonal antibodies, cell separation by flow cytometry, and in situ hybridization can delineate defective receptor expression and lymphokine defects useful to define and classify the immunodeficiency condition. Two excellent reviews describe a practical and cost-effective approach to the laboratory evaluation of a child suspected to have a primary immunodeficiency.[6,7]

The increasing number and complexity of primary immunodeficiencies render impossible a coherent classification for these conditions. The classification employed in this text will

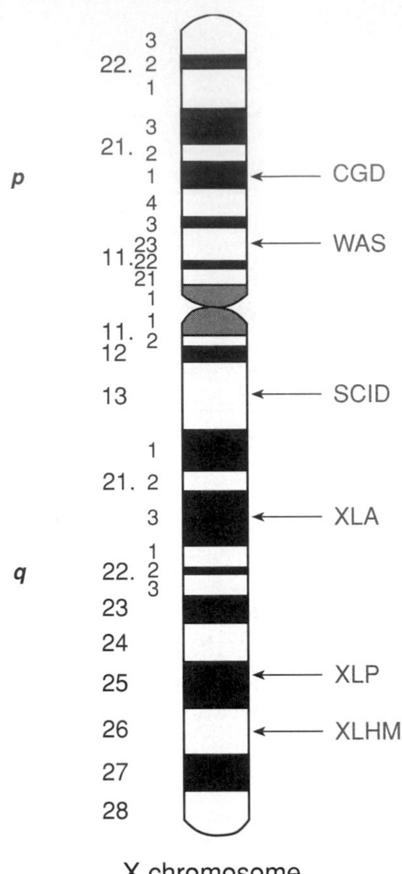

Fig. 27-1 Illustration of the X-chromosome depicting location of six X-linked immunodeficiency genes. *CGD,* Chronic granulomatous disease; *SCID,* severe combined immunodeficiency; *WAS,* Wiscott-Aldrich syndrome; *XLA,* X-linked agammaglobulinemia; *XLHM,* X-linked hypergammaglobulinemia IgM; *XLP,* X-linked lymphoproliferative disease.

be clinicopathologic with emphasis on "full-blown" defects affecting cellular or humoral immunity, selective defects, and, finally, more complex conditions.

SEVERE COMBINED IMMUNODEFICIENCY (SCID)

Severe combined immunodeficiency (SCID) represents the archetypical primary immunodeficiency, since it features impairment of both cellular and humoral responses. However, because normal T-cell function is a prerequisite for most normal B-cell function, SCID represents, in fact, a complex, heterogeneous, and lethal group of disorders, including not only the absence of a category of immunocompetent T-cells but also some specific defects in antigen presentation (HLA) and functional (receptors) immune molecules.

Autosomal recessive form (absence of T- and B-cells)

The *autosomal recessive (AR) variant* is the quintessential form of immune deficiency since both T-cell and B-cell functions are ablated. It is characterized by a near-complete absence of T- and B-cells, though some activated lymphoid cells, probably of maternal origin, can be found occasionally in the peripheral blood, liver, and spleen of patients.[8] Affected children feature a near absence of lymphoid tissue and plasma cells, a minute dysplastic thymus, a profound T-cell ($CD2^+$ and $CD3^+$) lymphopenia, yet sparing the natural killer ($CD16^+$, $CD36^+$) activity, a diminution of B (CD19) cells, and a severe agammaglobulinemia (Swiss type of agammaglobulinemia). Without bone marrow transplantation, death is rapid because of generalized viral infection or graft-versus-host (GVH) reactions after unirradiated blood transfusions. Unlike the murine SCID model in which a defective recombination of T-cell receptor genes has been demonstrated,[9] the responsible molecular mechanisms have not been elucidated in humans.

In one variant, however, the gene has been cloned, the Zap-70 gene, which codes for a tyrosine-kinase essential for the development of CD8(+) T-cells as well as T-cell receptor signal transduction.[87-91]

X-linked form (presence of B-cells)

The *X-linked variant* is probably the most common expression of SCID. The mutated gene, mapped to Xq13, has recently been found to be identical to the gene encoding the T-cell interleukin-2 receptor gamma chain.[10] This variant is characterized by a severe and progressive T-cell immunodeficiency. Although this feature can be occasionally also observed in the AR form, the B-cells are normal or elevated in number. These B-cells have a phenotype ($CD5^+$, $CD11c^+$) similar to that of neonatal B-cells. Generally, immunoglobulin production is impaired. But in some cases, immunoglobulins are quantitatively and qualitatively normal.This feature correlates with the presence of numerous tissue plasma cells and defines the Nezelof syndrome.[11] The report of this condition, as with the DiGeorge anomaly, was of seminal importance because it confirmed in humans the dichotomy of the T- and B-cell systems that had been established previously in birds, rabbits, and mice.[12-14] Although some antibodies are present, these immunoglobulins are usually nonfunctional and decrease with time. In addition to a dysplastic thymus, histologic examination reveals severe lymphoid depletion of the deep cortex (T zone) of lymph nodes, contrasting with the presence of cortical primary and rudimentary lymph follicles totally devoid of germinal center activity. In many ways, the Nezelof syndrome reproduces an immunologic situation similar to that of human AIDS and that seen in a species of laboratory mice termed *moth-eaten.*

Uncommon variants

In the framework of SCID, several separate conditions have been defined. *Reticular dysgenesis,* an autosomal recessive disorder, is characterized by an alymphocytosis and an absence of myeloid cells, suggestive of an impairment of hematopoietic precursor cells.[15] Death occurs early in the first year of life after overwhelming sepsis.

Combined immunodeficiency with eosinophilia (Omenn's syndrome) is characterized by generalized erythroderma, enlargement of the spleen and lymph nodes, and the presence of activated T-lymphocytes (possibly of maternal origin) in the blood, skin, and spleen, a condition akin to severe graft-versus-host disease.[16]

SCID may be associated with two conditions manifesting abnormalities in purine metabolism. *Adenosine deaminase (ADA) deficiency* results in the accumulation of deoxyadenosine, which is toxic for quiescent T- and B-cells and impairs endogenous DNA repair.[17] The condition is characterized by a profound T- and B-lymphopenia sometimes associated with chondrodysostosis, dystonia, or central blindness.[18] The mutated gene, now cloned, resides at 20q13ter.[19] Partial mutations allowing a residual ADA activity, sufficient to ensure a normal T-cell differentiation, have also been described.[17] ADA deficiency is opening the way for ADA replacement by blood transfusions[19] and specific gene therapy.[20]

Purine nucleoside phosphorylase (PNP) deficiency results in the accumulation of deoxyguanosine, which, like deoxyadenosine, is toxic and inhibits T-cell differentiation but spares B-cell function.[21] It reflects a condition resembling Nezelof's syndrome, albeit with frequent neurologic manifestations. The gene has been cloned and mapped to chromosome 14.[22]

SCID may rarely stem from the *defective expression of major histocompatibility complex (MHC) antigens (bare lymphocyte syndrome)*. This defect is characterized by a lack of synthesis of MHC class I and II antigens, probably linked to an impairment of transcription, since no abnormality has been defined in the MHC genes. In this deficiency there are normal numbers of T- and B-cells but impaired cellular and humoral responses to foreign antigens. In particular, class II molecule expression, as detected by monoclonal antibodies on the surface of macrophages or activated lymphoid cells, is absent or reduced, except in the medullary part of the thymus, which maintains a normal Hassallian differentiation.[23]

SCID, involving mainly T-cell function, has been also found associated with the *membrane expression of aberrant or defective T-cell receptors*. These abnormalities are characterized by a normal number of circulating lymphoid cells yet an impaired T-cell function. In one variant, the defect is probably linked to a block in intrathymic differentiation, as suggested by abnormalities in thymic epithelial differentiation.[24] In another, mutations in the gene encoding the CD3-γ subunit of the T-cell receptor–CD3 complex have been defined.[25]

Profound T-cell dysfunction can also result from *defective production of interleukin-2* (IL-2), either selectively or associated with other cytokines. The mechanisms responsible for this are presently unknown.[26]

The thymus in SCID

Besides the extensive atrophy of all peripheral lymphoid tissues, the thymic changes appear original and almost specific for severe T-cell immunodeficiency. They have been described under the generic term of *thymic dysplasia*.[27,28] The features of thymic dysplasia are a dramatic reduction in size (usually less than g 5), a rudimentary and foliated appearance of the gland, depletion of lymphoid cells, and a lack of maturation of epithelial cells which appear primitive and fail to differentiate into Hassall's corpuscles. According to the severity of these changes, four types have been described.[29] Thymic dysplasia is consonant with the thymic abnormalities consistently seen in immunodeficient animals, especially nude and SCID mice.[9] It substantiates the pivotal experimentally established role of the thymic epithelium in T-cell maturation and immunologic education. Thymic dysplasia is believed to represent a failure or an arrest in the embryologic development of the gland. But it is not known, as yet, whether it represents an intrinsic and primary disorder or a secondary phenomenon caused by the lack of migration or intrinsic lack of some cell receptor of a medullary T-cell precursor. Nonetheless, there is a symbiotic relationship between maturing thymic epithelial cells and developing lymphocytes;[30,31] moreover, the thymus is the first lymphoid tissue to be repopulated after a successful bone-marrow transplantation.[29]

Thymic dysplasia is present at birth. It should be distinguished from the profound atrophic if not destructive changes that occur after malnutrition,[32] severe and chronic infection, including AIDS,[33] graft-versus-host reaction,[34] and the effects of drugs, such as corticosteroids and cyclosporin A.[35] Severe atrophic changes are also observed in purine nucleoside phosphorylase deficiency, lack of expression of MHC antigens, abnormal expression of T-cell receptors and defective IL-2 production. Occasionally, the distinction between severe thymic atrophy and thymic dysplasia may be difficult. Some differential morphologic features are given in Table 27-1 and illustrated in Fig. 27-2 to Fig. 27-5.

Table 27-1 Comparison of thymic dysplasia with severe thymic atrophy

	Thymic dysplasia	Severe thymic atrophy
Weight of the gland	<5 g	>5 g
Foliated architecture	Well preserved	Blurred
Interlobular and perilobular tissue	Fatty	Fibroadipose with inflammatory cells
Size of the vessels	Small	Enlarged for the size of the lobules
Perivascular spaces	Empty	Fibrohyaline deposits
Thymic epithelial network	Maintained	Collapsed and disorganized
Epithelial maturation	Totally defective	Partially defective
Hassall's corpuscles	Absent	Absent/necrotic/calcified
Cytokeratin expression	Present	Often reduced
Class II MHC expression	Present	Present
Lymphoid cells		
CD1	Absent	Absent
CD2	Absent or rare	Some present
CD4	Absent	Some present
CD8	Absent	Some present
Plasma cells	Absent	Present, sometimes abundant

From Nezelof C: Thymic pathology in primary immunodeficiency, *Histopathology* 21:499, 1992.

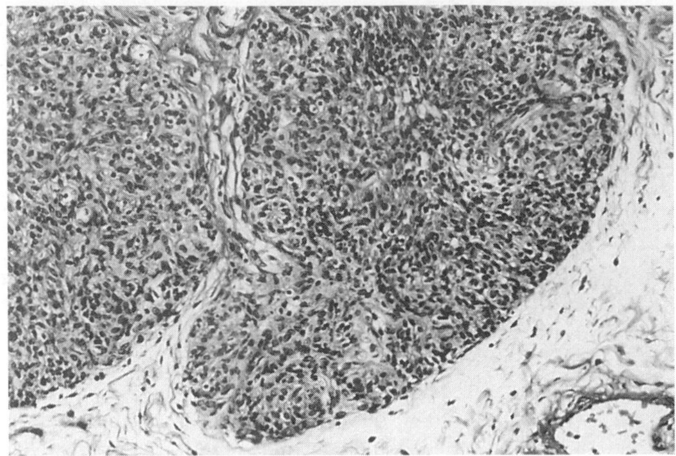

Fig. 27-2 Low-power photomicrograph of thymus from child with severe combined immunodeficiency illustrating an embryonic appearance of the gland.

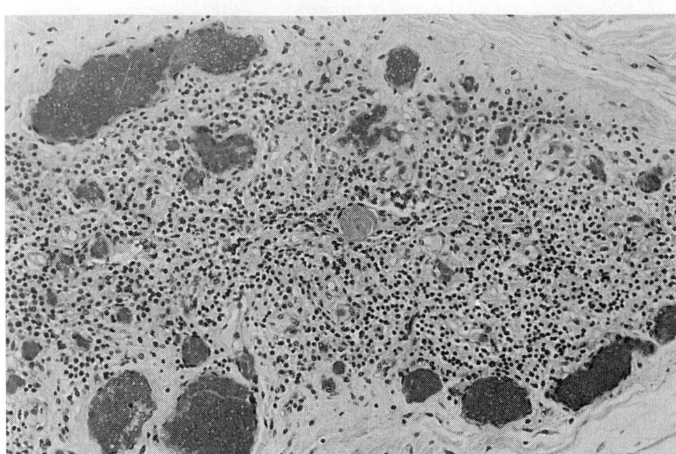

Fig. 27-4 Low-power photomicrograph of thymus from a 6-year-old boy with normal immune function after liver transplantation for fulminant hepatitis.

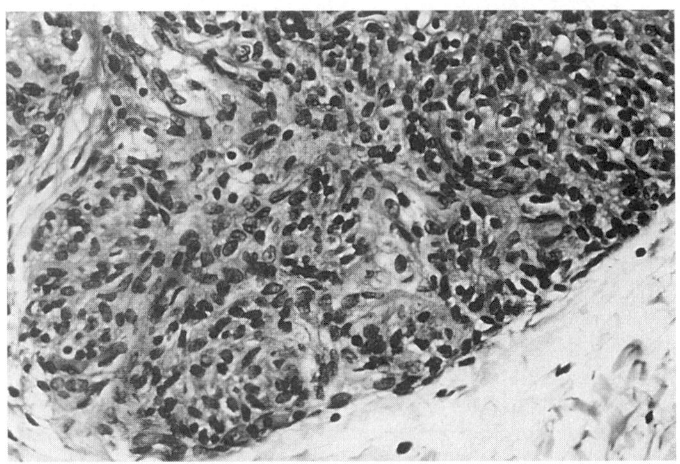

Fig. 27-3 Higher-power view of same gland from SCID child in Fig. 27-2.

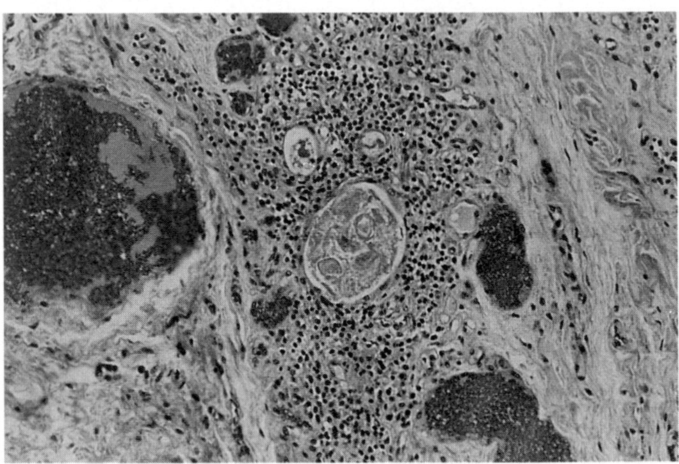

Fig. 27-5 Higher-power of same gland from child in Fig. 27-4 illustrating preserved Hassall's corpuscle.

SELECTED PRIMARY IMMUNODEFICIENCIES

Whereas SCID features profound T-cell abnormalities, the selected immunodeficiencies essentially involve the B-cell system as reflected by their defective immunoglobulin production.

Bruton's X-linked agammaglobulinemia (XLA)

Bruton's X-linked agammaglobulinemia, the subject of a case report in 1952,[2] illustrates beautifully the dissection of the immune system from phenotype to genotype. Over the course of some 4 years, a young boy suffered from repetitive episodes of bacterial sepsis, often caused by *Streptococcus pneumoniae* and other pyogenic organisms. In this condition, the sites of infection are generally respiratory, synovial, and meningeal. Chronic lung disease, the consequence of repetitive infections, often develops; with time, concurrent viral and protozoan infections are not infrequent.

The index patient was noted to have a severe reduction of serum gammaglobulin, hence the term *agammaglobulinemia*. Subsequently, boys have been shown to feature, in addition to low levels of all serum immunoglobulins (IgA, IgM, IgG), reduced numbers of circulating and marrow B-cells yet normal numbers of marrow pre-B-cells. Their lymphoid tissues (apart from the thymus, which is histologically normal) are sparse, devoid of plasma cells and germinal centers. Since T-cell numbers and function are normal, these boys feature a selective B-cell defect.

Molecular studies have pinpointed the defect. Firstly, an aberration in translocating Vh-region genes during B-cell ontogeny was described.[36] Not long thereafter, glucose-6-phosphate dehydrogenase (G6PD) activity, as determined in lysates from peripheral blood leukocytes of women heterozygous for XLA and the alleles of G6PD, showed that the defect is intrinsic to the B-cell lineage.[37] Restriction fragment length polymorphisms (RFLP) of genomic DNA employing restriction endonucleases sensitive to DNA methylation confirmed the intrinsic B-cell defect and also facilitated the detection of carriers.[38] More recently, the molecular defect at Xq22 has been identified[39] and shown to stem from mutations of the *src* proto-oncogene family of protein-tyrosine kinases.

Therapy, initiated years ago, monthly intravenous immunoglobulin, is of great benefit to these boys because it reduces the incidence and severity of infections.

Selective IgA deficiency

Selective IgA deficiency, first described in 1962,[40] is the most common primary immune deficiency diagnosed by laboratory techniques; about 1 out of 700 persons are deficient in serum and secretory IgA. Occasionally, there may be an associated IgE deficiency or, less commonly, IgG_2 and IgG_4 deficiencies. In several patients, deletions and ring chromosomes involving chromosomes 18 have been described. Their role, if any, in the pathogenesis of the deficiency is unexplained.

Curiously, most patients are asymptomatic, but a few incur allergies, repetitive infections (usually of mucosal surfaces), malabsorption (because of *Giardia* infestation or gluten-sensitive enteropathy), and diverse autoimmune conditions such as rheumatoid arthritis, systemic lupus erythematosus, and pernicious anemia. It is noteworthy that up to 44% of patients have antibodies to IgA in their serum. This requires that all transfused blood products received by such patients be devoid of IgA. A small number of patients, those with IgG subset deficiencies, may benefit from monthly immunoglobulin administration. This therapy must be administered cautiously because there is a risk of an anaphylactic response.

Common variable immunodeficiency

Common variable immunodeficiency is the most difficult to describe, if not define. The key word is *variable;* the disease is quite heterogeneous, reflected by variable degrees of impaired antibody responses in a setting of hypogammaglobulinemia.[41] Above all, it is the most common form of primary symptomatic immunodeficiency. As a rule, symptoms appear late, generally in the second or third decade of life. Thus, it is also known as *late-onset immunodeficiency.* Most cases are sporadic.

These patients feature very low serum concentration of IgG with variable degrees of IgA and IgM deficiency. Antibody production is invariably abnormal. Usually, circulating B-cells are normal in number yet functionally immature. Rarely, T-cells are reduced in number or dysfunctional by virtue of their suppression of B-cell function or an inadequacy in promoting B-cell differentiation. As a result, IL-2 production is deficient.[92]

The clinical symptoms are generally centered on two themes: recurrent, chronic infections, either sinopulmonary or gastrointestinal, and immune dysregulation as manifest by diverse "autoimmune" conditions affecting the gut (sprue-like enteropathy usually attributed to *Giardia lamblia* or nodular lymphoid hyperplasia), hematopoietic system (hemolytic anemia, thrombocytopenia, leukopenia, pernicious anemia) or collagen vascular diseases.

Treatment is monthly intravenous immunoglobulin or polyethylene glycol-conjugated IL-2.[93]

With extended survival, some patients (8%) have been found to develop malignancies, both lymphoid and gastrointestinal carcinomas, in middle life.

IMMUNODEFICIENCIES ASSOCIATED WITH "OTHER" DEFECTS

DiGeorge's syndrome

The description in 1965[42] by Angelo DiGeorge, an astute pediatric endocrinologist, of a polytypic defect, including dysmorphic facies with micrognathia, severe cardiovascular anomalies (truncus arteriosus), and thymic and parathyroid hypoplasia or aplasia, was of seminal importance because it linked an isolated cellular immunodeficiency to a definite thymic abnormality and reproduced in humans the immunologic abnormalities obtained by JFAP Miller in neonatally thymectomized mice.[12]

This anomaly reflects an abnormal embryogenesis of the third and fourth pharyngeal pouches, coinciding with cardiac formation occurring at about 4 to 6 weeks of gestation.

Complete absence of the thymus is a rare event. Most often, careful and painstaking dissection of the neck and upper mediastinum reveals tiny remnants of a normal or atrophic thymus in an ectopic or aberrant location. Death is more often related to congenital tetany or cardiac failure rather than recurrent bacterial, fungal, or viral infections that occur later. The B-cell system is generally intact. However, T-cells, notably $CD3^+$ cells, are decreased and often fail to respond to mitogens, antigens, and allogeneic cells. There is generally a close relation between the severity of the cellular immunodeficiency and the amount of thymic tissue. Contrary to patients with severe combined immunodeficiency, DiGeorge infants do not develop graft-versus-host disease after blood transfusions.

Although familial forms have been reported, the DiGeorge anomaly is usually sporadic and affects males and females equally. Many patients have a variable partial monosomy of 22q11ter or 10p. Treatment witnessed years ago the inauguration of fetal thymic transplants.[43,44] At this writing, the gene has not been cloned.

Ataxia-telangiectasia

Ataxia-telangiectasia, also known as the Louis-Bar syndrome, was initially described years ago in Europe[45,46] as one that featured progressive choreoathetosis or cerebellar ataxia and ocular or cutaneous telangiectasia. The definitive description came some 31 years later. Boder and Sedgwick coined the term *ataxia-telangiectasia* (AT), emphasizing the heredofamilial nature, oculocutaneous telangiectasia, the dominant neurologic feature (ataxia), and the great susceptibility to sinopulmonary infection.[47] Over the years, AT has been further characterized as an autosomal recessive disease with multisystem involvement featuring recurrent infections, an embryonic dysplastic thymus, selective cerebellar (Purkinje and granular cell) degeneration with atrophy, oculocutaneous telangiectasia, and, to a lesser extent, mental deficiency, endocrine disturbances, growth retardation, and progeric changes of hair and skin.[48] The presenting symptom usually is ataxia, generally by 1 year of age; recurrent infections and telangiectasia follow.

Laboratory studies reveal an unexplained elevated concentration of serum α-fetoprotein and carcinoembryonic antigen. The thymic abnormality translates to defective and decreased helper T-cell function and low serum concentration of IgA, IgE, and subclasses of IgG. This said, there is considerable heterogeneity in the immunologic profile.

These children are exquisitely sensitive to ionizing radiation, including sunlight (stemming from ineffective DNA repair mechanisms), and are subject to spontaneous chromosomal instability, particularly at sites of genes coding for T-cell (7p14 gamma chain, 7q35 beta chain, 14q12 alpha chain) receptors and the Ig heavy chain (14q32). They also feature generalized nucleomegaly and a high incidence (at least 33%) of malignancy, notably T-cell lymphoma, lymphocytic leukemia, and Hodgkin's disease.

Linkage analysis placed the gene (or genes) for AT at chromosome 11q23. Families have been assigned to five complementation groups based on a fibroblast assay. This differentiation indicates that either several AT genes exist or that multiple defects of a single gene are responsible for this pleiotropic disease.

Heterozygous carriers of an AT allele, about 1% of the United States population, are at risk to develop cancer; females are especially at risk for mammary carcinoma. They, too, are unduly susceptible to ionizing radiation.

Therapy has been by immunoglobulin transfusions, fetal thymus transplants, and injections of thymosin, a thymic hormone. Up to now, none has proved to be effective.

Wiskott-Aldrich syndrome

The Wiskott-Aldrich syndrome (WAS) is characterized by severe eczema, thrombocytopenia, and recurrent infections. WAS, an X-linked condition, affects roughly four infants per million live male births. Signs and symptoms, including bloody diarrhea and chronic otitis, appear in the first months of life. Survival beyond the teens is rare. Death is related to pyogenic as well as protozoan and viral infection and also to autoimmune complications and malignancies (12%). WAS patients have normal or elevated concentrations of immunoglobulins and respond normally to protein antigens yet fail to respond to polysaccharide antigens, especially to bacteria with polysaccharide capsules such as *Haemophilus influenzae* and pneumococci. For the same reason, they have low titers of serum isohemagglutinins.

The platelets are not only reduced in number, but more characteristically are small (average diameter 1.82 ± 0.1 μm compared with the normal 2.23 ± 0.1 μm).[49] More specifically, peripheral T-cells appear "bald" and devoid of microvilli, a scanning electron-microscopic finding that can serve as screening in the study of cord blood lymphocytes.[50] This feature seems to be linked to defective expression of sialophorin, a CD43, transmembrane, mucinlike molecule normally present on the surface of most circulating cells.[51] The latter is known to be necessary for cell-cell contacts and T-lymphocyte and monocyte activation and is believed to play a role in the regulation of T-lymphocyte senescence. Since the gene encoding sialophorin has been mapped to the short arm of chromosome 16, the CD43 abnormality cannot serve as the sole basis to characterize the syndrome. Indeed, the gene for WAS has been mapped to Xp11.22-11.3, cloned and found to encode a 501 amino acid protein pivotal to lymphocyte and platelet function.[94]

X-linked lymphoproliferative disease

X-linked lymphoproliferative disease (XLP) was described in 1975 by Purtilo et al.[52] He reported the death of three brothers and three maternally related cousins of the Duncan kindred after infection with the Epstein-Barr virus (EBV).[52] Since then, an international registry was established to promote research and offer clinical guidance in the management of these boys. At this writing, some 270 boys from 75 kindreds have been entered into the registry.[53]

The disease features three dominant phenotypes after EBV infection: (1) fulminant infectious mononucleosis (FIM), with death occurring from marrow and liver failure about 28 days after onset, (2) hypogammaglobulinemia, and (3) extranodal B-cell lymphomas containing EBV. Since the early days, additional (but far less common) phenotypes have emerged: necrotizing vasculitis, T-cell lymphoproliferation (lymphomatoid granulomatosis), and aplastic anemia. It must be noted that these phenotypes generally evolve *after EBV infection.* A small percentage of boys feature IgM hypergammaglobulinemia and IgG_1 and IgG_3 subclass deficiencies before EBV infection. Since the gene for IgM hypergammaglobulinopathy is not too distant from that for XLP,[54] these patients are of considerable interest.

The condition is highly lethal; some 77% of boys have died; no one has lived beyond 50 years of age. Clearly, the most virulent form of XLP is expressed in FIM, which often features diffuse histiocytic proliferation, akin to the virus-associated hemophagocytic syndrome (VAHS).[55]

A constitutional interstitial deletion placed the gene at Xq.25.[56] Work is in progress to clone this gene, which must be central to orchestrating an immune response to an ubiquitous DNA virus. In the meantime, families of XLP boys are studied by RFLP analysis utilizing informative loci that flank the gene to determine XLP status in unaffected male siblings and carrier status in female siblings.

Therapy, at present, is restricted to bone marrow transplantation[57,58] and, most recently, umbilical cord stem-cell transplantation.[59] Monthly intravenously administered immunoglobulins, rich in EBV antibodies, are administered because these boys are devoid of antibodies to the Epstein-Barr virus and often feature profound IgG subclass deficiencies.

IMMUNODEFICIENCIES ASSOCIATED WITH DEFECTIVE CHEMOTACTIC ACTIVITY

Recurrent infections can be related to some inherited defects in the migration and adherence of leukocytes. Some of these abnormalities, often associated with other manifestations, are established as syndromes.

Leukocyte adhesion defect

The leukocyte adhesion defect (LAD) represents an autosomal recessive disorder characterized by delayed cord dehiscence and scar formation, recurrent diarrheal and respiratory symptoms, and pronounced leukocytosis.[60,61] Contrasting with the peripheral blood leukocytosis, few granulocytes are present at sites of tissue inflammation. This discrepancy reflects the inability of phagocytic cells to adhere to endothelial cells and migrate to sites of infection. It has been established that the LAD is attributable to the mutation of a gene encoding the beta subunit (CD18) shared by three adhesive alpha heterodimers: LFA-1, (CD11a), MAC1, or CR3 (CD11b), and a p150.95, or C1 (CD11c).[62] An absent or abnormal CD18 leads to defective expression of the three other heterodimers. CD11a is normally expressed on all leukocytes, CD11b mostly on phagocytes and large granular lymphocytes, and CD11c on activated lymphocytes and cytolytic lymphoid cells. LAD lymphocytes respond poorly to low concentrations of lectins and anti-CD3 and have impaired cytotoxic activity and defective antibody production, despite normal or elevated blood levels of immunoglobulins. The beta-alpha union takes place in the Golgi system, and the glycoproteins are secondarily transported to the cell membrane. The CD18 has homology to the beta subunit of the fibronectin receptor and has been mapped to chromosome 21. Bone marrow transplantation is presently the only treatment available. Despite aggressive preconditioning, marrow engraftment is sometimes difficult to achieve.

Chédiak-Higashi syndrome

The Chédiak-Higashi syndrome is a rare autosomal disorder involving the cytoskeleton and lysosomal organization. It is characterized by abnormalities of pigmentation (believed to be related to impaired melanin migration); the presence of large primary granules in granulocytes, lymphocytes, and monocytes; defective NK-cell activity; and frequently a terminal lymphohistiocytic proliferative disorder.[63]

Job's syndrome

Job's syndrome, as initially described by Davis et al[64] and expanded by Buckley et al,[65] is characterized by "cold" visceral and cutaneous abscesses, chronic mucocutaneous candidiasis, pronounced blood and tissue eosinophilia, and hypergammaglobulinemia E (in excess of 2000 IU per milliliter), the most salient feature. The immunologic abnormality is not well understood. It has been shown that B-cells from these patients produce excessive amounts of IgE "in vitro." Both males and females are affected. A dominant transmission has been reported in some kindreds.

IMMUNODEFICIENCIES ASSOCIATED WITH DEFECTIVE BACTERICIDAL ACTIVITY

Chronic granulomatous disease

Chronic granulomatous disease (CGD), a rare condition (1 per one million newborns), has shed much light on the workings of the neutrophil/monocyte response to bacteria and fungi.[66] The defect resides in the inability of phagocytes to produce toxic reactive compounds such as superoxide and its derivatives, leading to an ineffective reduction of molecular oxygen by a phagocytic-specific membrane-bound NADPH oxidase, also called the *respiratory burst oxidase*. Over 90% of patients have levels of superoxide production less than 1% of normal, a feature that can be detected and measured by the nitroblue tetrazolium test.[67] This test is simple and provides both qualitative and semiquantitative information for the patients and carriers in the X-linked forms.

In fact, CGD is a heterogeneous disorder ascribed to defects in genes encoding any one of the four key protein components of NADPH oxidase. The X-linked form is related to a lack of neutrophil cell surface expression of cytochrome *b*, whereas autosomal recessive forms stem from mutations of the cytosolic and soluble fractions. The neutrophils of affected children have normal motility, phagocytosis, and degranulation but fail to express the respiratory burst associated with phagocytosis.

The prototypic infant develops chronic and recurrent infections involving the lung, liver, bone, skin, and lymph nodes, which are characterized by central necrosis and, more typically, a granulomatoid response, which may wrongly indicate cat-scratch disease, atypical mycobacterial infection, yersinosis, brucellosis, or even more rare infections. The presence of numerous pigmented macrophages, initially identified as a hallmark of familial pigmented reticulosis,[68] can offer a valuable morphological clue for the diagnosis. Causative organisms are many, particularly those (*Staphylococcus aureus* or Enterobacteriaceae) that produce catalase, which deprives the phagocytes of exogenous peroxide as an alternative microbicidal mechanism.

The X-linked gene was cloned in 1989[69] after reports of an interstitial deletion that localized the gene to Xp21.[70] Through subtraction analysis, a transcript, identified in normal phagocytes, was found to be absent in boys with the disease. Three autosomal recessive forms of CGD have been linked to chromosomes 1, 7, and 16. They appear to stem from mutations of genes that code for other membrane and cytosolic components central to the respiratory-burst oxidase.[71]

Therapy has included granulocyte infusions (for acute infectious emergencies), continuous antibiotics, bone marrow transplantation, and interferon-γ, the last an activator of phagocyte function.

Complement deficiencies

The complement system involves some 19 proteins: 11 for the classical pathway, 3 for the alternative pathway, and 5 regulatory proteins. The complement cascade, once activated, is central to setting the stage for the elimination of microorganisms, attracting and mobilizing an appropriate host response, the lysis of bacterial membranes, fixing antigen, and the clearance of immune complexes.

Aberrations in the complement system can produce disease ranging from autoimmunity to infection. Defects of both the classic and alternative pathways have demonstrated disease-associated conditions. Allowing for considerable overlap, autoimmune (immune complex) conditions affecting vessels and glomeruli dominate when genes central to the early classic pathway are mutated. Alternatively, pyogenic infections, especially those caused by *Neisseria* organisms, tend to develop when mutations ablate the function of genes related to the later complement components. Finally, deficiency of a regulatory protein, the C1 inhibitor, results in the autosomal dominant syndrome of hereditary angioneurotic edema, probably through the activation of vasoactive molecules (Table 27-2).

Table 27-2 Complement deficiencies

Condition	Disease
C1q	Systemic lupus erythematosus (SLE), glomerulonephritis
C1q dysfunction	SLE
C2 deficiency	SLE, chronic glomerulonephritis, membranoproliferative glomerulonephritis, Henoch-Schönlein purpura, septicemia
C3 deficiency	Severe bacteremia, SLE, membranoproliferative glomerulonephritis
C6, C7, C8, C9 deficiencies	Disseminated gonococcal/meningococcal infection
C1-inhibitor deficiency	Hereditary angioneurotic edema

OPPORTUNISTIC CANCERS IN IMMUNODEFICIENCY

In the early 1970s, Gatti and Good signaled the heightened incidence of malignancy in patients with primary immunodeficiencies.[72] Since then, a similar phenomenon has been described in organ transplant recipients and patients with cancer.

Three international registries were established to follow this phenomenon: The Immunodeficiency Cancer Registry,[73] The Cincinnati Transplant Tumor Registry,[74] and The X-Linked Lymphoproliferative Disease Registry.[53]

Among primary immunodeficiencies, patients with Wiskott-Aldrich syndrome, ataxia-telangiectasia, severe combined immunodeficiency, common variable immunodeficiency, and X-linked lymphoproliferative disease are at particular risk to develop a neoplasm.[75] In Wiskott-Aldrich syndrome and severe combined immunodeficiency, non-Hodgkin's lymphomas predominate; in ataxia-telangiectasia, T-cell lymphoma, leukemia, and Hodgkin's disease are common; in X-linked lymphoproliferative disease, extranodal B-cell lymphomas dominate. In contrast, adenocarcinomas and non-Hodgkin's lymphomas are seen in common variable immunodeficiency. In many but not all of the immunodeficiency settings, chromosomal aberrations occur at sites that code for genes vital to the immune system's normal function. Thus it is not difficult to accept the association of neoplasia arising in some of these conditions.

MOLECULAR GENETICS OF PRIMARY IMMUNODEFICIENCIES

In 1993 and 1994, five genes central to primary immunodeficiencies have been cloned.

The first was the gene mutated in Bruton's agammaglobulinemia.[39] Since this disease was the first immunoglobulin deficiency described, it was fitting. The gene, a resident of Xq21.3-Xq22 and member of the *src* oncogene family, encodes for the intracellular protein tyrosine kinase. Deletions and point mutations of this gene, which is normally expressed in B-cells, were detected in eight boys with X-linked agammaglobulinemia. The gene, "ATK" (agammaglobulinemia tyrosine kinase), is the first of the *src* family to encode for an intracellular, as opposed to cell membrane, tyrosine kinase. The lack of a protein product in boys with this condition is believed to be central to the inability of pre-B marrow cells to develop into mature circulating B-cells. The finding has been further explored in a murine model.[76,77]

The gene for hyper-IgM immunodeficiency was next cloned.[54] The disorder is rare, features recurrent bacterial infections, and is associated with elevated serum levels of IgM and IgD in association with decreased levels of IgA and IgG. Isotype switching involves the binding of a novel protein TRAP (TNF-related activation protein), which is expressed on T-cells with the CD40 ligand on B-cells.[95] Point mutations in TRAP result in an inability of T-cells and B-cells to interact, with ensuing failure of isotype switch.

The T-cell immune response is highly regulated by the production of interleukin-2 (IL-2) and its receptor (IL-2 receptor). A family of IL-2 receptors is known; they each have diverse affinities for IL-2 signaling. The gene for the gamma IL-2 receptor, situated at Xq13, was found to be mutated in three boys with X-linked severe combined immunodeficiency. The mutation, different in each of these three patients, provided a molecular basis for the X-linked form of this disease.[10] These were followed with cloning a gene for one form of AR-SCID [88-90] and that for Wiskoff-Aldrich syndrome.[94]

Four additional genes implicated in immunodeficiencies were previously cloned: X-linked CGD,[69] ADA-deficiency-SCID,[78] PNP-deficiency-SCID,[79] and LAD.[62]

THERAPY FOR PRIMARY IMMUNODEFICIENCIES

The treatment of primary immunodeficiencies is in itself a reflection of changing times. Since infection is generally a common problem, supportive therapy, largely in the form of antibiotics, has been given. Some children are treated by replacement therapy, that is, high-titer intravenous immunoglobulin infusions, adenosine deaminase (ADA)–rich red blood cell transfusions, polyethylene glycol–conjugated bovine ADA and IL-2, and granulocyte infusions. More definitive therapy has been performed with fetal thymic grafts,[42,43] cultured thymic epithelium,[80] bone marrow,[57,58,81,82] or umbilical cord stem-cell[59] transplants. The latter two have offered cure for many children, particularly since the risk of GVH disease attending allogeneic cell transfer is relatively low in the young child. However, definitive therapy would require that the mutated gene be replaced by a normal copy of that gene. Not long ago, the gene for ADA was inserted into a population of marrow[20] and umbilical cord stem cells and transfused to children with ADA-deficient severe combined immunodeficiency. As additional genes central to primary immunodeficiencies are cloned and methods of gene therapy are improved, more reports of such therapy are certain to follow.

EPICRISIS

This chapter, in the context of all of human pathology, occupies but a small portion of this textbook. This is fitting because the primary immunodeficiencies, in contrast to other conditions, are relatively rare. Yet, these disease states, when properly studied, have shed much light on the orchestration of the immune system.

Table 27-3 cites some of these immunologic milestones. In tabulating them, a pattern emerges. Quite often, a child or several children are described in a typical clinicopathologic presentation. This is then followed by bench work in the immunology laboratory, either with human or experimental material. In due course, clinical genetic linkage analysis and cytogenetic studies, the latter sometimes stemming from case reports, pinpoint the chromosomal region that is altered. Finally, molecular biologists home in, clone the normal gene, and define mutations central to the pathogenesis of the disease. If one takes the index report from Switzerland as a starting point, this remarkable sequence has evolved over 44 years. Above all, it illustrates that to understand human disease, the cross-fertilization of multiple disciplines and international cooperation are required.

In 1957, E. Donnall Thomas presented the results of the first bone marrow transplantation performed in humans.[83] This

Table 27-3 Immunologic milestones

1950	Swiss type of severe combined immunodeficiency[1]
1952	Bruton's agammaglobulinemia[2]
1954	Agammaglobulinemia and thymoma association[4]
1957	Definitive description of ataxia-telangiectasia [47]
1957	First bone marrow transplantations[83]
1958	Initial description of thymic dysplasia[27]
1961, 1962	Immunologic function of the thymus defined in animals[12,13]
1964	Nezelof syndrome[11]
1965	Delineation of the T- and B-cell systems[14]
1965	DiGeorge's syndrome [42]
1968	Bone marrow transplantation for severe combined immunodeficiency (SCID) syndrome and Wiskott-Aldrich syndrome[81,82]
1968	Fetal thymus transplantation for DiGeorge syndrome[43,44]
1971	Association of malignancy with immunodeficiency disease[72]
1972	Adenosine-deaminase deficiency and SCID[18]
1975	X-linked lymphoproliferative disease (XLP)[52]
1979	Peripheral stem-cell transplantation[85]
1989	Gene for X-linked chronic granulomatous disease cloned[69]
1990	Gene therapy for adenosine deaminase–deficient SCID initiated[20]
1992	Umbilical cord stem-cell transplantation for XLP[59]
1993	Gene for Bruton's agammaglobulinemia cloned[39]
1993	Gene for X-linked SCID cloned[10]
1993	Gene for hyper-IgM cloned[54]
1994	Gene for Wiskott-Aldrich syndrome cloned[95]
1994	Gene for AR-SCID cloned[88-90]

work, stemming from experiments designed and conducted by his own hands and those of others, demonstrated that it was feasible to envision bone marrow transplantation as a curative modality for diverse malignancies and potential radiation disasters. He showed that bone marrow, whether it be obtained from fetal or adult cadavers, could be preserved and eventually given safely to needy recipients. This report immediately inaugurated a new era in medicine, as witnessed by marrow transplantation in radiation victims in Belgrade[84] and a flurry of early attempts to eliminate and replace marrow ridden with leukemia. Since then, the field has evolved to embrace the isolation and subsequent transfusion of peripheral blood[85,86] and umbilical cord[59] stem cells as alternative treatments for diverse conditions. Not unjustly, E. Donnall Thomas shared the Nobel Prize in medicine and physiology in 1990.

In homeostasis, the immune system discretely eliminates infectious agents, foreign (allogeneic) cells, and possibly neoplastic cells. An excellent example of this elegant response occurs after infection with EBV. Most of us produce lifelong antibodies to the virus, yet only a small percentage is subject to the lethargy of clinical infectious mononucleosis. Still fewer are victims of the immunologic anarchy that occurs in those who inherit a mutated gene in the X-linked lymphoproliferative disease. In these boys, the thymus, lymph nodes, spleen, liver, and bone marrow are the site of a battlefield characterized by extensive destruction. Stemming from a gene defect, the normal immune response, akin to a Mozart divertimento (a matter of taste), is subverted to cacophony.

It is but a matter of time before additional genes central to primary immunodeficiencies are cloned. The identification of the normal protein product of these mutated genes should pave the way for a greater understanding of these rare diseases and the daily workings of the immune system. Human gene therapy came to fruition with one of these rare "experiments of nature."[20] A new era has begun.

REFERENCES

1. Glanzmann E, Riniker P: Essentielle Lymphocytophthise: ein neues Krankheitsbild aus der Säuglingspathologie, *Ann Paediatr* (Basel) 175:1, 1950.
2. Bruton OC: Agammaglobulinemia, *Pediatrics* 9:722, 1952.
3. Rosen FS, Wedgwood RJ, Eibl M et al: Primary immunodeficiency diseases: report of a WHO scientific group, *Immunodefic Rev* 3:195, 1992.
4. Good RA: Agammaglobulinemia—a provocative experiment of nature, *Bull Univ Minn Med Found* 26:1, 1954.
5. de Saint Basile G, Fischer A: X-linked immunodeficiencies: clues to genes involved in T-and B-cell differentiation, *Immunol Today* 12:456, 1991.
6. Buckley RH: Immunodeficiency diseases, *JAMA* 268:2797, 1992.
7. Stiehm ER: Immunodeficiency disorders: general considerations. In *Immunologic disorders in infants and children,* ed 3, Philadelphia, 1989, Saunders.
8. Fischer A: Severe combined immunodeficiencies, *Immunodefic Rev* 3:83, 1992.
9. Malynn BA, Blackwell TK, Fulop GM et al: The SCID defect affects the final step of the immunoglobulin VDJ recombinase mechanism, *Cell* 54:453, 1988.
10. Noguchi M, Yi H, Rosenblatt HM et al: Interleukin-2 receptor gamma chain mutation results in X-linked severe combined immunodeficiency in humans, *Cell* 73:147, 1993.
11. Nezelof C, Jammet ML, Lartholary P et al: L'hypoplasie héréditaire du thymus: sa place et sa résponsibilité dans une observation d'aplasie lymphocytaire, normoplasmocytaire et normoglobulinémique du nourisson, *Arch Fr Pediatr* 21:897, 1964.
12. Miller JFAP: Immunological function of the thymus, *Lancet* 2:748, 1961.
13. Good RA, Dalmasso AP, Martinez C et al: The role of the thymus in development of immunologic capacity in rabbits and mice, *J Exp Med* 116:773, 1962.
14. Cooper MD, Peterson RDA, Good RA: Delineation of the thymic and bursal lymphoid systems in the chicken, *Nature* 205:143, 1965.
15. De Vaal OM, Seynhaeue V: Reticular dysgenesis, *Lancet* 2:1123, 1959.
16. Jonan H, Le Deist F, Nezelof C: Omenn's syndrome: pathologic arguments in favor of a graft versus host pathogenesis: a report of nine cases, *Hum Pathol* 18:1101, 1987.
17. Hirschorn R: Genetic deficiencies of adenosine deaminase and purine nucleoside phosphorylase: overview, genetic heterogeneity and therapy, *Birth Defects* 19:74, 1983.
18. Giblett ER, Anderson JE, Cohen F et al: Adenosine-deaminase deficiency in two patients with severely impaired cellular immunity, *Lancet* 2:1067, 1972.
19. Hirschorn R: Adenosine deaminase deficiency, *Immunodefic Rev* 2:175, 1990.
20. Culver KW, Berger M, Miller AD et al: Lymphocyte gene therapy for adenosine deaminase deficiency, *Pediatr Res* 31:149A, 1992.
21. Giblett ER, Ammann AJ, Sandman R et al: Nucleoside phosphorylase deficiency in a child with severely defective T-cell immunity and normal B-cell immunity, *Lancet* 1:1013, 1975.
22. Markert ML: Purine nucleoside phosphorylase deficiency, *Immunodefic Rev* 3:45, 1991.
23. Touraine J: The bare-lymphocyte syndrome: report on the registry, *Lancet* 1:319, 1980.
24. Reinherz EL, Cooper MD, Schlossman SF: Abnormalities of T-cell maturation and regulation in human beings with immunodeficiency disorders, *J Clin Invest* 68:699, 1981.
25. Arnaiz-Villena A, Timon M, Corelli A et al: Brief report: primary immunodeficiency caused by mutations in the gene encoding the CD3-gamma subunit of the T-lymphocyte receptor, *N Engl J Med* 327:529, 1992.

26. Weinberg K, Parkman R: SCID due to a specific defect in the production of interleukin-2, *N Engl J Med* 327:1718, 1990.
27. Tobler R, Cottier H: Familiare Lymphopenia mit Agammaglobulinämia und schwerer Moniliasis, *Helv Paediatr Acta* 13:313, 1958.
28. Gitlin D, Vawter G, Craig JM: Thymic alymphoplasia and congenital aleukocytosis, *Pediatrics* 33:184, 1964.
29. Nezelof C: Thymic pathology in primary immunodeficiencies, *Histopathology* 21:499, 1992.
30. Haynes BF: Human thymic epithelium and T-cell development: current issues and future directions, *Thymus* 16:143, 1990.
31. Skares EW, Van Ewijk W, Singer A: Disorganization and restoration of thymic epithelial cells in T-cell receptor-negative SCID mice: evidence that receptor-bearing lymphocytes influence maturation of the thymic microenvironment, *Eur J Immunol* 21:1657, 1991.
32. Purtilo DT, Connor DH: Fatal infections in protein-caloric malnourished children with thymolymphatic atrophy, *Arch Dis Child* 50:149, 1975.
33. Seemayer TA, Laroche AC, Russo P et al: Precocious thymic involution manifest by epithelial injury in the acquired immune deficiency syndrome, *Hum Pathol* 15:469, 1984.
34. Seemayer TA: The graft-versus-host reaction: a pathogenetic mechanism of experimental and human disease. *Perspect Pediatr Pathol* 5:93, New York, 1979, Masson.
35. Beschorner WE, Nammoum JD, Hess AD et al: Cyclosporin A and the thymus: immunopathology, *Am J Pathol* 126:487, 1987.
36. Schwaber J, Molgaard H, Orkin SH et al: Early pre-B-cells from normal and X-linked agammaglobulinemia produce Cμ without an attached VH region, *Nature* 304:355, 1983.
37. Conley ME, Brown P, Pickard AR et al: Expression of the gene defect in X-linked agammaglobulinemia, *N Engl J Med* 315:564, 1986.
38. Fearon ER, Winkelstein JA, Civin CI et al: Carrier detection in X-linked agammaglobulinemia by analysis of X-chromosome inactivation, *N Engl J Med* 316:427, 1987.
39. Vitrie D, Vorechovský I, Sideras P et al: The gene involved in X-linked agammaglobulinemia is a member of the *src* family of protein-tyrosine kinases, *Nature* 361:226, 1993.
40. West CD, Hong R, Holland NH: Immunoglobulin levels from the newborn period to adulthood and in immunoglobulin deficiency states, *J Clin Invest* 41:2054, 1962.
41. Rosen FS, Janeway CA: The gammaglobulins. III. The antibody deficiency syndromes, *N Engl J Med* 275:709, 1966.
42. DiGeorge AM: A new concept of the cellular basis of immunity (discussion), *J Pediatr* 67:907, 1965.
43. August LS, Rosen FS, Filler RM et al: Implantation of a foetal thymus, restoring immunological competence in a patient with thymic aplasia (DiGeorge's syndrome), *Lancet* 2:1210, 1968.
44. Cleveland WW, Fogel BJ, Brown WT, Kay HEM: Foetal thymus transplant in a case of DiGeorge's syndrome, *Lancet* 2:1211, 1968.
45. Syllaba L, Henner K: Contribution à l'indépendance de l'athétose double idiopathique et congénitale, *Rev Neurol* 1:541, 1926.
46. Louis-Bar D: Sur un syndrome progressif comprenant des télangiectasies capillaires cutanées et conjonctivales symétriques, à disposition naevoïde et de troubles cérébelleux, *Confinia Neurol* (Basel) 4:32, 1941.
47. Boder E, Sedgwick RP: Ataxia-telangiectasia: a familial syndrome of progressive cerebellar ataxia, oculocutaneous telangiectasia and frequent pulmonary infection, *Univ South Calif Med Bull* 9:15, 1957.
48. Gatti RA, Boder E, Vinters HV et al: Ataxia-telangiectasia: an interdisciplinary approach to pathogenesis, *Medicine* 70:99, 1991.
49. Murphy S, Oski FA, Haimar JL et al: Platelet size and kinetics in hereditary and acquired thrombocytopenia, *N Engl J Med* 286:499, 1972.
50. Kenney DM, Cairns L, Remold-O'Donnell E et al: Morphological abnormalities in the lymphocytes of patients with the Wiskott-Aldrich syndrome, *Blood* 68:1329, 1986.
51. Parkman R, Kenney DM, Remold-O'Donnell et al: Surface protein abnormalities in lymphocytes and platelets from patients with Wiskott-Aldrich syndrome, *Lancet* 2:1387, 1981.
52. Purtilo DT, Yang JPS, Cassel CK, Harper R: X-linked recessive progressive combined variable immunodeficiency disease (Duncan's disease), *Lancet* 1:935, 1975.
53. Seemayer TA, Grierson H, Pirruccello SJ et al: X-linked lymphoproliferative disease, *Am J Dis Child* 147:1242, 1993.
54. Korthäuer U, Graf D, Mages HW et al: Defective expression of T-cell CD40 ligand causes X-linked immunodeficiency with hyper-IgM, *Nature* 361:539, 1993.
55. Risdall RJ, McKenna RW, Nesbit ME et al: Virus-associated hemophagocytic syndrome: a benign histiocytic proliferation distinct from malignant histiocytosis, *Cancer* 44:993, 1979.
56. Wyandt HE, Grierson HC, Sanger WG et al: Chromosomal deletion of Xq25 in an individual with X-linked lymphoproliferative disease, *Am J Med Genet* 33:426, 1989.
57. Williams LL, Rooney CM, Conley ME et al: Correction of Duncan's syndrome by allogeneic bone marrow transplantation, *Lancet* 2:587, 1993.
58. Pracher E, Panzer-Grümayer ER, Zoubek A et al: Successful bone marrow transplantation in a boy with X-linked lymphoproliferative syndrome and acute severe infectious mononucleosis, *Bone Marrow Transpl* 13:655, 1994.
59. Vowels MR, Lam-Po-Tang R, Berdoukos V et al: Brief report: Correction of X-linked lymphoproliferative disease by transplantation of cord-blood stem cells, *N Engl J Med* 329:1623, 1993.
60. Hayward AR, Harwey BAM, Leonard I et al: Delayed separation of the umbilical cord, widespread infections and defective neutrophil mobility, *Lancet* 2:1099, 1979.
61. Nezelof C: Chronic omphalitis in a 4 month-old girl, *Pathol Res Pract* 187:334, 1991.
62. Springer TA, Thompson WS, Miller LJ et al: Inherited deficiency of the Mac-1, LFA-1, p150,95 glycoprotein family and its molecular basis, *J Exp Med* 160:1901, 1984.
63. Root RK, Rosenthal AS, Balestra DJ: Abnormal bactericidal, metabolic, and lysosomal functions of Chediak-Higashi syndrome leukocytes, *J Clin Invest* 51:649, 1972.
64. Davis SD, Schaller J, Wedgwood RJ: Job's syndrome: recurrent "cold" staphylococcal abscesses, *Lancet* 1:1013, 1966.
65. Buckley RH, Wray BB, Belmaker EZ: Extreme hyper-immunoglobulin E and undue hypersensitivity to infection, *Pediatrics* 49:59, 1972.
66. Berendes H, Bridges RA, Good RA: A fatal granulomatosis of childhood: the clinical study of a new syndrome, *Minn Med* 40:309, 1957.
67. Baehner RL, Nathan DG: Quantitative nitroblue tetrozolium test in chronic granulomatous disease, *N Engl J Med* 278:971, 1968.
68. Landing BH, Shirkey HS: A syndrome of recurrent infection and infiltration of viscera by pigmented lipid histiocytes, *Pediatrics* 20:431, 1957.
69. Royer-Pokora B, Kunkel LM, Monaco AP et al: Cloning the gene for an inherited human disorder—chronic granulomatous disease—on the basis of its chromosomal location, *Nature* 322:32, 1986.
70. Francke U, Ochs HD, de Martinville B et al: Minor Xp21 chromosomal deletion in a male associated with expression of Duchenne muscular dystrophy, chronic granulomatous disease, retinitis pigmentosa and McLeod syndrome, *Am J Hum Genet* 37:250, 1985.
71. Hopkins PJ, Bemiller LS, Curnutte JT: Chronic granulomatous disease: diagnosis and classification at the molecular level, *Clin Lab Med* 12:277, 1992.
72. Gatti RA, Good RA: Occurrence of malignancy in immunodeficiency diseases: a literature review, *Cancer* 28:89, 1971.
73. Filipovich AH, Heinitz KJ, Robison LL, Frizzera G: The immunodeficiency cancer registry: a research resource, *Am J Pediatr Hematol Oncol* 9:183, 1987.
74. Penn I: Cancers complicating organ transplantation, *N Engl J Med* 323:1767, 1990.
75. Filipovich AH, Mathur A, Kamat D, Shapiro RS: Primary immunodeficiencies: genetic risk factors for lymphoma, *Cancer Res* 52:5465s, 1992.
76. Thomas JD, Sideras P, Edvard Smith CI et al: Colocalization of X-linked agammaglobulinemia and X-linked immunodeficiency genes, *Science* 261:355, 1993.
77. Rawlings DJ, Saffran DC, Tsukada S et al: Mutation of unique region of Bruton's tyrosine kinase in immunodeficient XID mice, *Science* 261:358, 1993.
78. Wiginton DA, Adrian GS, Hutton JJ: Sequence of human adenosine deaminase cDNA including the coding region and a small intron, *Nucleic Acids Res* 12:2439, 1984.

79. Williams SR, Goddard JM, Martin DW Jr: Human purine nucleoside phosphorylase cDNA sequence and genomic clone characterization, *Nucleic Acids Res* 12:5779, 1984.
80. Hong R, Santosham M, Schulte-Wisserman H et al: Reconstitution of B and T-lymphocyte function in severe combined immunodeficiency disease after transplantation with thymic epithelium, *Lancet* 2:1270, 1976.
81. Gatti RA, Meuwissen HJ, Allen HD et al: Immunological reconstitution of sex-linked lymphopenic immunological deficiency, *Lancet* 2:1366, 1968.
82. Bach FH, Albertini RJ, Anderson JL et al: Bone marrow transplantation in a patient with the Wiskott-Aldrich syndrome, *Lancet* 2:1364, 1968.
83. Thomas ED, Lochte HL Jr, Lu WC, Ferrebee JW: Intravenous infusion of bone marrow in patients receiving radiation and chemotherapy, *N Engl J Med* 257:491, 1957.
84. Mathé G, Jammet H, Pendic L et al: Transfusions et greffes de moelle osseuse homologue chez les humains irradiés à haut dose accidentellement, *Rev Fr Etudes Clin et Biol* 4:226, 1959.
85. Goldman JM, Catovsky D, Hows J et al: Cryopreserved peripheral blood cells functioning as autografts in patients with chronic granulocytic leukaemia in transformation, *Br Med J* 1:1310, 1979.
86. Kessinger A, Armitage JO, Landmark JD et al: Autologous peripheral hematopoietic stem cell transplantation restores hematopoietic function following marrow ablative therapy, *Blood* 71:723, 1988.
87. Roifman CM, Hummel D, Martinez-Valdez H et al: Depletion of CD8+ cells in human thymic medulla results in selective immune deficiency, *J Exp Med* 170:2177, 1989.
88. Arpaia E, Shahar M, Dadi H et al: Defective T-cell receptor signaling and CD8(+) thymic selection in humans lacking Zap-70 kinase, *Cell* 76:947, 1994.
89. Elder ME, Lin D, Clever J et al: Human severe combined immunodeficiency due to a defect in ZAP-70, a T-cell tyrosine kinase, *Science* 264:1599, 1994.
90. Chan AC, Kadlecek TA, Elder ME et al: ZAP-70 deficiency in an autosomal recessive form of severe combined immunodeficiency, *Science* 264:1599, 1994.
91. Perlmutter RM: Zapping T-cell responses, *Nature* 370:249, 1994.
92. Sneller MC, Strober W: Abnormalities of lymphokine gene expression in patients with common variable immunodeficiency, *J Immunol* 144:3762, 1990.
93. Cunningham-Rundles C, Kazbay K, Hassett J et al: Brief report: enhanced humoral immunity in common variable immunodeficiency after long-term treatment with polyethylene glycol-conjugated interleukin-2, *N Engl J Med* 331:918, 1994.
94. Derry JMJ, Ochs HD, Franke U: Isolation of a novel gene mutated in Wiskott-Aldrich syndrome, *Cell* 78:635, 1994.
95. Geha RS, Rosen FS: The genetic basis of immunoglobulin-class switching, *N Engl J Med* 330:1008, 1994.

28 Acquired Immunodeficiency Syndrome (AIDS)

Stephen A. Geller
Jonathan W. Said
Vijay V. Joshi

Epidemics have been known for as long as there has been written history. Terrible scourges have destroyed entire cities, decimated populations, and even changed the course of history.[1,2] For today's student of medicine the disorders that led to the deaths of literally millions of people are of only secondary interest because of their rarity in modern times: bubonic plague, typhus, smallpox, malaria, polio, and influenza. Especially dramatic was the epidemic of bubonic plague, or the "Black Death," described so well by Boccaccio in *The Decameron.* Caused by *Yersinia pestis,* bubonic plague raged across Europe for almost 30 years in the early fourteenth century, dramatically affecting society, including economic, political, and cultural endeavors. In our time the fatal condition *acquired immunodeficiency syndrome* (AIDS) has become the quintessential paradigm of a major disease that affects entire and diverse nations. The etiologic agent of AIDS, human immunodeficiency virus (HIV-1), is believed to have spread from the rural communities of Africa to the United States, Europe, Asia, and elsewhere.[3] It has been suggested that HIV was transmitted to human beings from African monkeys, though this theory has not been conclusively proved. The nonhuman primate lentivirus called *simian immunodeficiency virus* (SIV) is easily recovered in many parts of Africa, but only one of the SIV strains thus far characterized has been shown to be closely related to HIV-1, the virus responsible for almost all the AIDS cases in the United States. Unless otherwise specified in this chapter, *HIV infection* refers to the illness caused by HIV-1. HIV-2, which is rare in the United States but common in West Africa and parts of India, is closely related to SIV isolated from African *Rhesus* macaques.[4] Mathematical models have been developed to describe the evolution of the AIDS epidemic and to determine the length of time it may have taken for the virus to originate in one village, spread to neighboring villages, then increase to a recognizable level within Africa, and ultimately spread to the rest of the world.[5,6] The modeling has suggested that AIDS may have emerged as long as 100 years ago and also that the number of cases of HIV infection increases at a greater rate than expected with time.

It has been estimated that more than 1 million individuals in North America are infected with HIV, with as many as 8 million in the world. Of the infected people, there have already been at least 100,000 deaths in the United States and 1 million worldwide.[7] The annual number of men, women, and children in the United States diagnosed with AIDS continues to increase, with the probability that more than 75,000 new cases will occur each year.[8] By the year 2000, an estimated 40 million of the world's people will have been infected.

Since 1492, when Columbus bridged the seas, and since 1903, when the Wright brothers initiated the age of air travel, there has been increasing potential for dispersal of disease agents from one nation to the entire world. AIDS has exemplified that possibility and is literally a worldwide disease. Because of the ease of modern transportation and also because of the virtually instantaneous worldwide communication, there is remarkable awareness by the world community of this dreaded disorder. AIDS has affected mankind not only in terms of healthcare, but also throughout the fabric of society.

It is a disease that has dramatically affected the arts, leading to the illness and death of many of the great young talents of our time in the fields of music, dance, theater, painting, sculpture, literature, and film, while simultaneously contributing to new avenues of artistic expression as creative people attempt to understand and adapt to this scourge. Athletes, in the prime of their careers, have been affected. AIDS has made discussions of sexual practices a matter of importance in terms of public welfare and has transferred those discussions from the private to the public arena. AIDS has forced societies to look at the way laws are shaped and the effect of those laws on persons with disabilities of all kinds. There have been international issues raised in terms of immigration from countries in which HIV has become endemic. AIDS has shown us examples of shining courage and integrity as well as new avenues for the expression of ignorance and bigotry. AIDS has been a part of national debates, as it was in the 1992 presidential elections in the United States.

This chapter cannot devote itself to the many and complex social issues of AIDS, though knowledge of them is appropriate and necessary for the physician, who will surely at one time or another be called upon to assist in the care of a patient with this protean disorder or a family member or friend of someone with AIDS or someone in contact with an AIDS patient or perhaps a person just concerned about the disease. Indeed, AIDS has even led to a focused and sometimes acrimonious debate about the role and responsibilities of the physician who may be called upon to care for the patient with AIDS.[9-11]

EPIDEMIOLOGY

AIDS was virtually unknown until 1980, at which time two separate clusters of *Pneumocystis carinii* pneumonia (PCP) were noted in relatively young, homosexual males in Los Angeles and New York.[12-15] Until that time PCP was uncommon, occurring almost exclusively in individuals who were undergoing chemotherapy for malignant diseases, most often Hodgkin's disease and the non-Hodgkin's lymphomas. At about the same time, Kaposi's sarcoma (KS) was also recognized in young, homosexual males. In these patients, KS was a rapidly spreading, highly malignant disorder involving any skin surface, including the face and chest, as well as internal organs, such as the heart, lungs, intestinal tract, and liver. Previously, KS was a well-recognized, histologically malignant, but usually clinically indolent skin disorder afflicting mostly elderly men of Mediterranean origin and involving particularly the lower extremities.

Primarily on the basis of an enormous amount of research stimulated by these early observations, it became clear that AIDS was a novel immunodeficiency disease. For a few years, when AIDS was recognized principally as a disease of male homosexuals and AIDS was known as "gay-related immune deficiency (GRID)," it was suspected that some external chemical agent, unique to the homosexual culture, impaired the ability of the immune system to respond appropriately. We now understand that HIV-1 itself causes remarkable alteration in the human immune response and directly contributes to the development of the disease state.

AIDS can occur in all people, not just homosexual men. HIV-1 affects bisexual men, sexually active heterosexuals who have had many partners, spouses of HIV-infected individuals, intravenous drug users, and children born to women infected with or at risk for the development of AIDS. Recipients of blood and blood products (factor VIII used for the treatment of hemophilia was at one time a significant vehicle for HIV-1 transmission) and recipients of organ transplants were at considerable risk before March 1985, when clinical testing for antibodies to HIV became practical. The likelihood of being infected with HIV after any given exposure is not completely known; a single encounter may lead to transmission if the viral dose is significant; alternatively, there can be multiple encounters with an HIV-infected individual without transmission. The risk of transmission from an HIV-infected individual is probably greatest during a period of overt clinical illness, a time at which high numbers of virions are circulating. Individuals with genital ulcers have a heightened risk of contracting HIV infection.[16]

In the last few years an unexpectedly rapid increase in the number of women with HIV infection and AIDS has been documented and is attributable to a variety of social, economic, and family structure factors.[17,18] For example, transmission from a drug-using partner is particularly common.[18] Also, AIDS is most prevalent in African-American and Hispanic women, in contrast to AIDS in men, which is most often seen in whites.[19] In this regard, the HIV epidemic affects some of the most socially and medically vulnerable individuals, whose survival is already in jeopardy because of their minority status, their socioeconomic condition, in many cases their own drug addiction, and, not least, their relative lack of access to health care services. There is also increasing concern about the biologic differences in the way women respond to AIDS, since women and men present with different types of opportunistic infections. HIV appears to be more readily transmitted from men to women than from women to men,[20] and the survival time after diagnosis is shorter for women than for men.[17] More than 27,000 women have been diagnosed with AIDS in the United States.[18] HIV-related disease is expected to become one of the five leading causes of death in young women nationally.[21]

CLINICAL COURSE

HIV infection is a chronic disorder that has, as its major manifestation, the development of immunodeficiency. There remains the misconception that AIDS progresses rapidly from time of infection to death. It is now well understood that AIDS does not become manifest in the typical patient for about 10 years after the initial infection and that patients generally survive at least 2 years after the onset of clinical AIDS.[22] The term *AIDS-related complex* (ARC) has been used to describe patients with symptomatic HIV infection other than AIDS. The definition of ARC as used by different investigators has varied over time but generally includes symptom complexes of progressive, generalized lymphadenopathy, fever, fatigue, diarrhea, night sweats, and weight loss. Because of the lack of consensus as to what symptoms should be included in the definition of ARC, there is increasing agreement that the term is no longer useful and should be discarded. Although the definition of AIDS has also varied over time, the criteria for its definition have been outlined in detail in continuously updated reports by the Centers for Disease Control and Prevention (CDC), as described in Table 28-1 and discussed below.

Table 28-2 Key features of AIDS

Life-threatening opportunistic infections
Pneumocystis carinii
Candida albicans
Herpes simplex
Toxoplasma gondii
Cryptococcus neoformans
Cytomegalovirus
Mycobacterium avium-intracellulare complex
Generalized lymphadenopathy
Lymphoma
Kaposi's sarcoma
Wasting
Central nervous system dysfunction

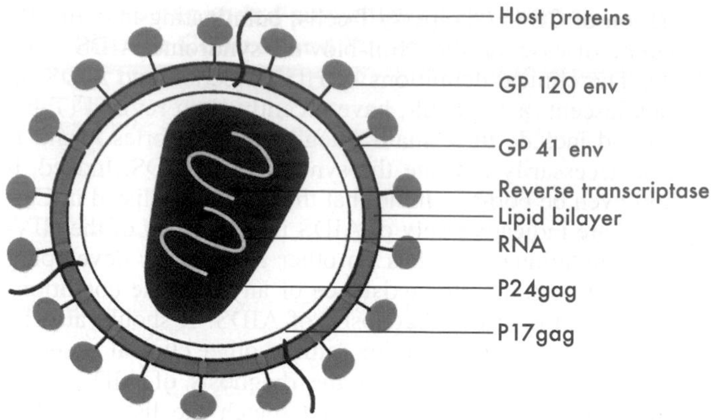

Fig. 28-2 Diagrammatic structure of HIV-1.

Structure

Particles of HIV appear as 100 nm spherules, with a central, truncated core (Fig. 28-2). Antibodies have been produced against several HIV proteins, including the core proteins, p17, p18 and p24, p25, and the surface glycoprotein, gp120, noncovalently bound to transmembrane protein, gp41. Some of these antibodies are used in immunodiagnostic tests for HIV infection. Virus-encoded surface glycoproteins appear ultrastructurally as spikes or knobs.[31] Viral coat protein, gp120, has a similar structure to class II major histocompatibility complex (MHC) proteins,[32] and gp120 bound to CD4 may trigger a long-term allogeneic immune response.[33]

The CD4 molecule acts as a receptor for HIV, explaining specific tropism of the virus for helper T-lymphocytes, monocytes, macrophages, and related cells such as the microglia of the brain, all of which have been shown to have CD4 receptors. HIV-1 transcripts have been identified in CNS endothelial cells, but infection of neuronal cells is not clearly established. However a neuron-specific 9.0 kilobase pair transcript, which shares homology with antisense transcripts of HIV-1 *gag* gene, has been identified in neurons from patients with or without HIV infection, and this may have an important role in the interactions of HIV with neuronal cells.[34]

After fusion with the host cell membrane, the virus particle uncoats, releasing two identical strands of RNA. These in turn act as a template for DNA synthesis using the viral enzyme, reverse transcriptase. Newly synthesized DNA is circularized and integrates into the host nucleus as a provirus, though much of the DNA remains unintegrated in the cell cytoplasm.

Immunopathogenesis

Mechanisms of $CD4^+$ cell destruction after infection have been shown to be the same for all $CD4^+$ cells and include replication and budding from infected cells damaging the cell membrane and fusion of viral envelope protein to the CD4 molecule on uninfected cells, forming a multinucleated syncytium. In addition to destruction of $CD4^+$ cells, the virus affects other aspects of the immune system. A segment of the HIV envelope mimics lymphokines that induce B-cell activation and hyperplasia. $CD8^+$ cells (predominantly suppressor T-cell subset) are increased in number and may contribute to suppression of immune function, and natural killer (NK) cell function is defective. In addition to acting as reservoirs and transporting the virus throughout the body, monocytes and macrophages release monokines, such as tumor necrosis factor and cachectin, which contribute to the severe fevers and wasting of chronically infected patients.[35]

The clinically latent phase of HIV infection lasts a median of 10 years. Although the viral burden in peripheral-blood mononuclear cells is low in the clinically latent period, the virus is disseminated throughout the body and propagates in lymphoid tissue.[22] Viral replication continues at these sites and is associated with progressive depletion of $CD4^+$ cells.

In the early phases of HIV infection, the germinal centers remain intact, but they contain numerous extracellular HIV virions. HIV, in turn, stimulates oligoclonal proliferation of follicular B-cells. Dendritic cells trap virus, but such trapping, although causing temporary curtailment of viremia, does not suppress viral replication. Virions can be demonstrated within germinal centers by electron microscopy (Fig. 28-3), immunohistochemistry, or in situ hybridization (Fig. 28-4).

HIV disease is active in lymphoid tissue throughout the period of so-called clinical latency, even when there is minimal circulating virus in the blood.[36] The term *clinical latency* is misleading, however, since there is gradual deterioration of the immune system with a fall in the $CD4^+$ T-cell count, and at no time after HIV infection is there absence of viral expression indicative of complete microbiologic latency.[22] HIV disease continues to progress during this so-called latent period, and zidovudine has become the standard treatment in the United States for asymptomatic HIV-infected patients with $CD4^+$ T-cell counts below 500 cells per cubic millimeter.[37] During the period of clinical latency the lymphoid organs function as reservoirs of HIV infection as HIV particles are progressively trapped within the network of dendritic cells. Eventually there is degeneration of dendritic cell processes and recirculation of HIV particles released from the constraints of lymph node entrapment.[22] The late stages of the disease, when there are less than 200 $CD4^+$ cells/mm^3, are characterized by high levels of viremia.

Laboratory tests

Immunoassays

Screening and confirmatory tests for HIV were first introduced into medical practice in March 1985. Their subsequent refinement, and universal utilization, has led to increasing confidence in the safety of the nation's blood supply for transfusion purposes. The tests most widely used to screen for HIV infec-

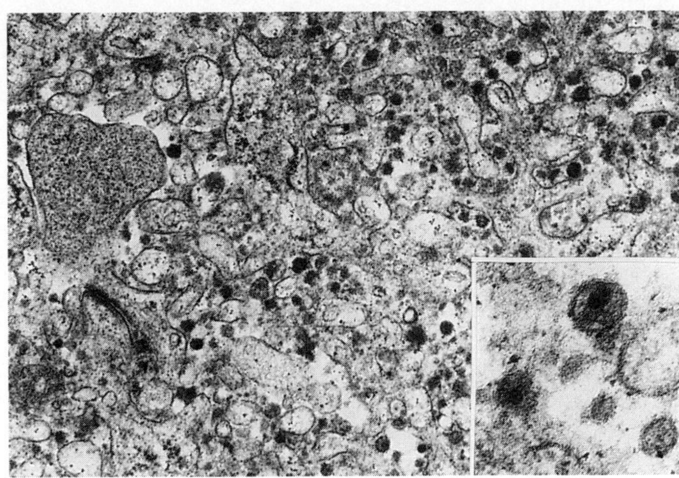

Fig. 28-3 Electron micrograph of follicle dendritic cell in a case of progressive generalized lymphadenopathy (PGL). Virions are extracellular in relation to the processes of dendritic histiocytes. *Inset,* Characteristic virion with central truncated core.

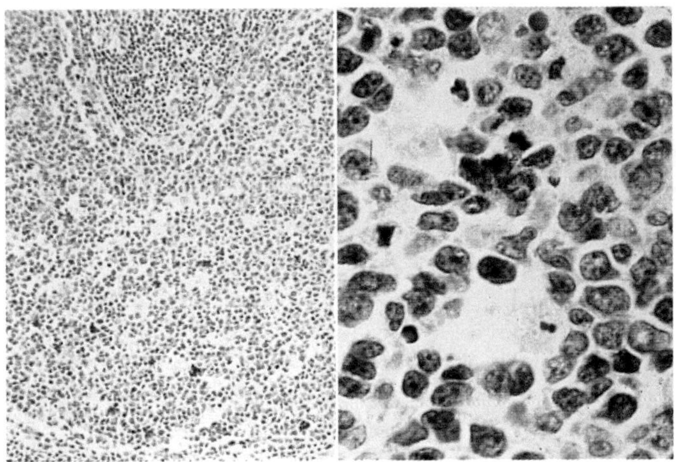

Fig. 28-4 Follicle from a case of PGL stained with antibody to HIV p24 antigen. Immunohistochemical staining is localized to follicular dendritic cells.

tion employ the techniques of enzyme immunoassay (EIA) and enzyme-linked immunosorbent assay (ELISA) to detect HIV antibodies. ELISA is the most common assay used to screen for HIV because of its low cost, standardized procedure, high reliability, and rapid time of performance.[38] Sensitivity of ELISA for HIV has been reported as being between 93% and 99%, [38] and specificity as 99%.[39] In the event of a positive result, the western blot assay is utilized, since false-positive results may be obtained with either EIA or ELISA.[40] The western blot assay can detect the presence of antibodies specific for a range of HIV proteins, including the outer glycoprotein, gp120, the transmembrane protein, p41, and the internal core protein, p24 (Fig. 28-5). The western blot assay is the most commonly used confirmatory test for the presence of HIV-specific antibodies. When these antibody tests are performed in a competent laboratory, false-positive results are exceedingly rare.[41]

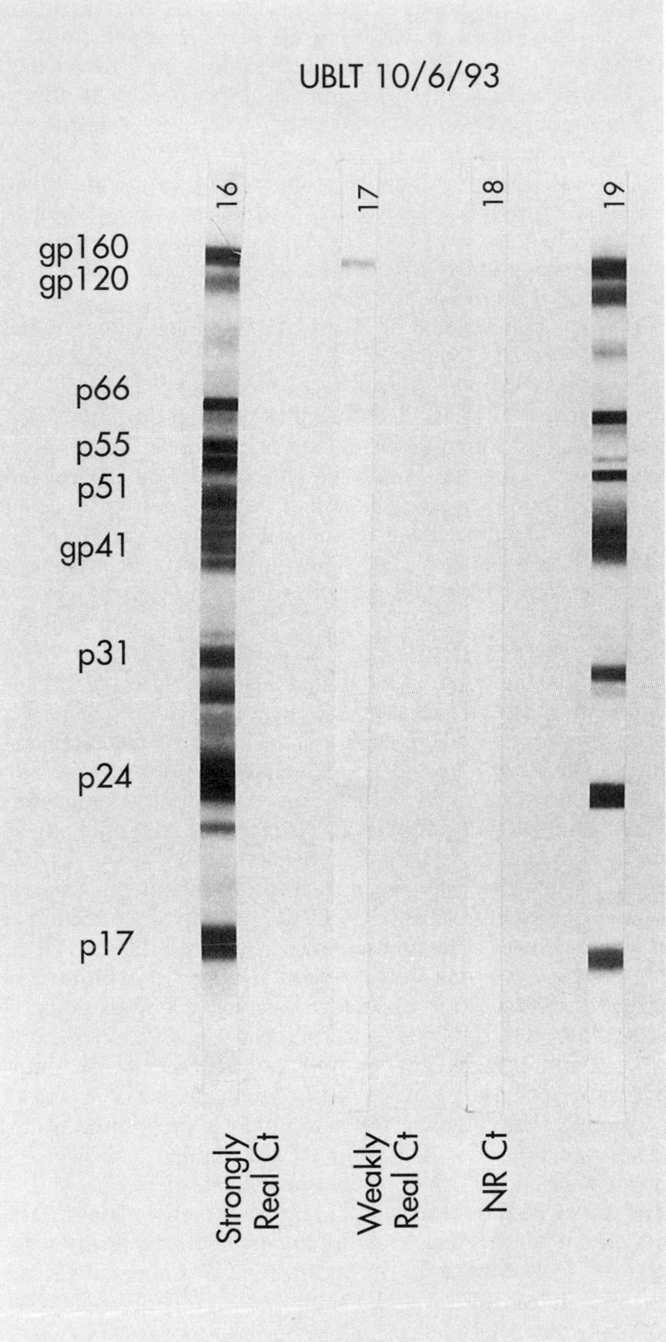

Fig. 28-5 Western blot assay confirming the diagnosis of HIV infection in a seropositive patient. Strip 16 is the strongly reactive control; strip 17 is the weakly reactive control; strip 18 is a nonreactive control; strip 19 is from the patient and shows reactivity to many surface glycoproteins *(gp)* and core proteins *(p)* of HIV.

Development of an antibody response ("seroconversion") may not occur for as long as 6 months after infection, and seronegative individuals are potentially infective. Blood donor center practices use specific interview questions, in addition to serologic testing, to identify individuals potentially at risk for HIV infection. HIV testing is also carried out as a part of the diagnostic evaluation for a patient manifesting signs and symptoms suggestive as AIDS. In some states, the law requires written documentation of informed consent before HIV testing is performed,[42] and the ways in which results of testing are released may be restricted. Informing individuals of an almost certainly fatal disorder requires the availability of sympathetic and knowledgeable staff who can provide appropriate counseling.

However, since in infants younger than 18 months of age tests for serum IgG antibody do not distinguish between infant antibody and maternal antibody, molecular biologic tests, viral culture, and clinical follow-up study are often necessary to determine if an infant has HIV infection. These tests are also done for demonstration of HIV or HIV components in tissues of fetuses of HIV-infected mothers.[43] The need for early diagnosis in newborns, to allow for treatment that can contribute to enhancement of the both the quality and the quantity of life, has prompted suggestions for and considerable debate about mandatory screening of newborns for HIV.[44] It is generally believed, however, that the legal, social, and psychologic problems preclude against such a program and that an approach of voluntary counseling and testing of women of child-bearing age could achieve the desired goal.

Molecular diagnostics

HIV can be identified in blood and tissues of affected individuals with the polymerase chain reaction (PCR) for amplification of portions of HIV nucleic acid or by specific HIV culture. PCR has proved to be an invaluable tool in molecular biology and has rapidly moved into the clinical arena as a diagnostic technique,[45] but these direct detection methods are rarely indicated in standard medical practice, since they are each technically difficult and labor intensive and thereby expensive and are generally available only in academic or research centers. The ability of PCR to screen directly for the presence of proviral DNA or viral RNA has permitted the detection of the virus before the development of antibodies.[46] Any PCR method intended for clinical use must demonstrate the maximum degree of specificity, achieved by the utmost avoidance of false-positive results, which can occur as a result of sample contamination when scrupulous attention to testing detail and specimen separation is not applied and also as a result of high background reactivity at the detection level.[47] The use of PCR or virus culture may, however, be beneficial in the case of the HIV-exposed infant, for the reasons discussed above.[38,48] Recently, reverse transcriptase–initiated PCR has been used to measure HIV-1 mRNA in peripheral blood mononuclear cells as a part of a long-term prospective study.[49] It was found that there were dramatic differences in HIV mRNA expression among individuals with otherwise similar clinical and laboratory findings and that this variation strongly correlated with the future course of the disease, an indication that PCR determination of HIV-1 mRNA could have significant clinical utility as a means of evaluating response to therapy and of determining prognosis.

Lymphocyte counts

The laboratory evaluation of the patient with confirmed HIV infection is based on continuous monitoring of the patient's lymphocytes (Fig. 28-1). As discussed previously, the helper T-cells in the peripheral blood bear surface CD4 molecule that serves as the cellular receptor for HIV gp120. In the healthy adult there are 500 to 1600 $CD4^+/mm^3$ in the peripheral blood, accounting for 32% to 56% of the total number. The number of helper T-lymphocytes in the peripheral blood falls ("lymphopenia") as HIV-disease progresses. There is reversal of the usual 2:1 ratio of $CD4^+$ to $CD8^+$ blood lymphocytes, depressed lymphocyte responses to mitogens, and impaired NK cell function in vitro. Individuals who have fewer than 200 $CD4^+$ cells/mm^3 are especially susceptible to the development of the many complications of AIDS, particularly opportunistic infections.

Instances of pronounced $CD4^+$ T-lymphocytopenia have been reported in patients who lack evidence of HIV infection.[50,51] The clinical condition of the patients and incidence of opportunistic infections in these individual case reports varies, but all share persistently low $CD4^+$ T-cell levels, no evidence of HIV type 1 or 2 infection by serology, culture, or PCR analysis, and no evidence of human T-cell lymphotropic virus (HTLV) types I or II.[52,53] Fewer than half of these patients have had risk factors for AIDS, and there are wide geographic and age distributions. Many patients have remained clinically stable, and there has been spontaneous reversal of the $CD4^+$ counts to normal.[52,54] Serum immunoglobulin concentration has been normal or decreased, compared to HIV-infected patients who usually have hypergammaglobulinemia.[55] There appears to be no clustering or common cause for this syndrome, and there is no epidemiologic evidence for a transmissible agent or association with exposure to blood components.[56] This rare syndrome may have a complex cause, which is yet poorly understood.[57,58]

SYSTEMIC MANIFESTATIONS

Lymphoid manifestations

HIV-related lymphoid hyperplasia

Persistent generalized lymphadenopathy (PGL) is defined as lymphadenopathy of two or more noncontiguous sites, of at least 3 months in duration, in the absence of intercurrent illness or drug use associated with lymphadenopathy. Associated constitutional symptoms include fever, headache, photophobia, night sweats, weight loss, and severe malaise. Other findings include hepatosplenomegaly, anemia, leukopenia, and hypergammaglobulinemia.

In the early stages of lymphadenopathy (Table 28-3) there is explosive follicular hyperplasia (Fig. 28-6). Expanded follicles may lose follicular mantles (so-called naked follicles), and there is infiltration of follicles by $CD8^+$ T-cells. Islets of mantle cells can also be found within follicular centers, and there may be intrafollicular hemorrhage.[59] Several abnormal immunohistochemical findings are found in PGL (Table 28-4). There is paracortical hyperplasia with increased immunoblasts and plasma cells and arborizing postcapillary venules with activated, cuboidal endothelial cells. Mutinucleated giant cells may be present in the medulla (Fig. 28-7), and they represent infected syncytia of T-cells.[60] In addition to sinus histiocytosis there are aggregates of monocytoid B-cells, and there are neutrophils, resembling the inflammation seen in toxoplasmosis (Fig. 28-8).

As PGL progresses, and in association with falling $CD4^+$ cell counts, follicular dissolution and disruption of germinal centers ensues. In the late stages there is lymphoid depletion (Fig. 28-9), absence of follicles or residual lymphoid-depleted follicles, and increased vasculature associated with immunoblasts and plasma cells. Lymph nodes with diffuse hyperplasia

Table 28-3 Morphology of persistent generalized lymphadenopathy

Early
Cortical hyperplasia
Expanded geographical follicles
Follicles extending through cortex and medulla
Aggregates of small lymphocytes within follicles
Hemorrhage in germinal centers
Paracortical hyperplasia
Small lymphocytes, immunoblasts, plasma cells
Polykaryocytes (multinucleated giant cells)
Arborizing postcapillary venules with high endothelium
Monocytoid B-lymphocytes
Sinus reticular hyperplasia
Intermediate (follicular fragmentation)
Follicular involution
Loss of demarcation between cortex and medulla
Increased plasma cells and immunoblasts
Late (follicular dissolution)
"Burnt-out" follicles
Hyaline vascular follicles
Hypocellularity and lymphoid depletion
Increased vascularity
Fibrosis

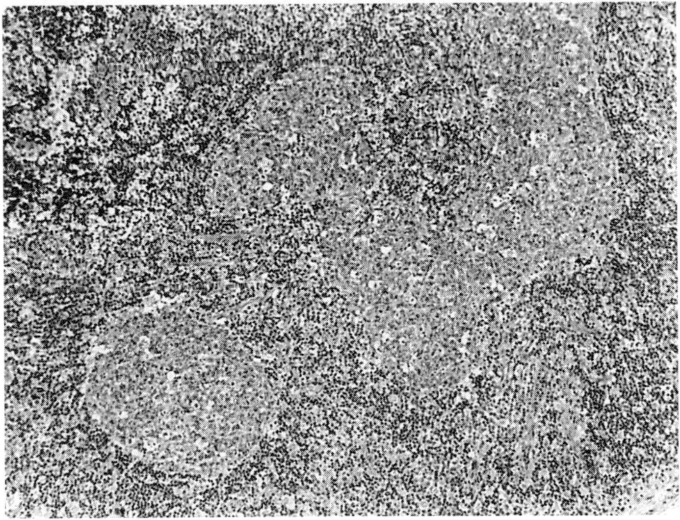

Fig. 28-6 Hyperplastic lymph node in the early phase of PGL with expanded geographical follicles.

can resemble other immunoproliferative disorders, including angioimmunoblastic lymphadenopathy, with prominent vessels and increased immunoblasts (Fig. 28-10). In some cases hyalinized vascular follicles, similar to those seen in Castleman's disease, may be present (Fig. 28-11); and this histologic subtype has been associated with an increased incidence of Kaposi's sarcoma.[61]

Although none of the features described above is specific for HIV infection, the grouping of features that comprise the clinical syndrome of PGL and histologic findings is highly characteristic of HIV-related lymphadenopathy. Monoclonal antibodies or in situ hybridization can localize HIV to the follicular processes of dendritic histiocytes, where viral immune complexes are trapped early in the course of HIV infection in immune complexes.[62] Antibodies useful to localize HIV in routinely processed tissue sections include antibodies to p24, p17, gp41, and gp120. Proteinase digestion increases sensitivity of staining to the envelope proteins.[63]

Table 28-4 Immunohistochemical findings in HIV-related lymphoid hyperplasia (PGL)

Polyclonal immunoglobulins in germinal centers (dendritic pattern)
Aggregates of small lymphocytes $CD8^+$ in germinal centers
$CD4^+$ polykaryocytes
Increased Ki67 staining in germinal centers
Antibody to dendritic cells (DRC-1) reveals fragmentation of the follicular framework (follicular lysis)
Antibodies to HIV-1 localized in the dendritic cell meshwork
Inversion of the normal CD4/$CD8^+$ cell ratio in the paracortex
Eventual depletion of $CD4^+$ cells
Increased polyclonal plasma cells
Immune complex deposition

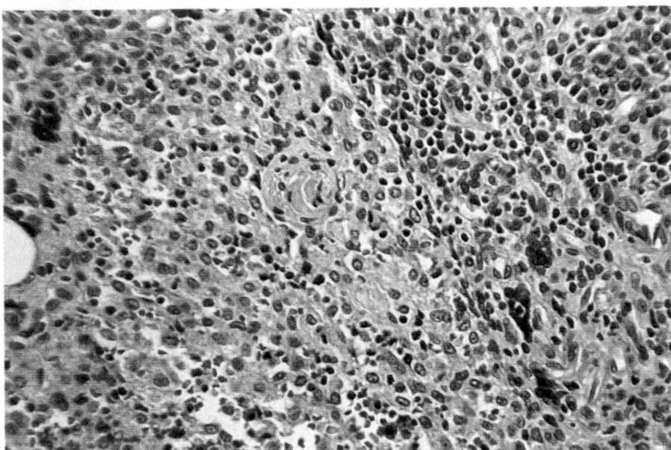

Fig. 28-7 Medullary region of a lymph node with PGL showing the presence of multinucleated polykaryocytes.

HIV particles can also be identified in extracellular locations by electron microscopy. Tubuloreticular inclusions similar to those found in systemic lupus erythematosus and other abnormal immune states are frequently present in vascular endothelium and lymphoid cells (Fig. 28-12). Epstein-Barr virus (EBV) has also been implicated in HIV-related lymphoid hyperplasia. Using in situ hybridization, EBV DNA has been localized predominately to interfollicular B-lymphocytes and rare T-lymphocytes in cases of PGL.[64]

Salivary lymphoid hyperplasia

Lymphoid hyperplasia in the parotid gland and surrounding lymph nodes is common in HIV-infected individuals. In the gland there may be ductal proliferations that resemble the myoepithelial islands characteristic of the benign lymphoepithelial lesion of Sjögren's syndrome.[65] Salivary ducts frequently become cystic, and the duct lining can undergo squa-

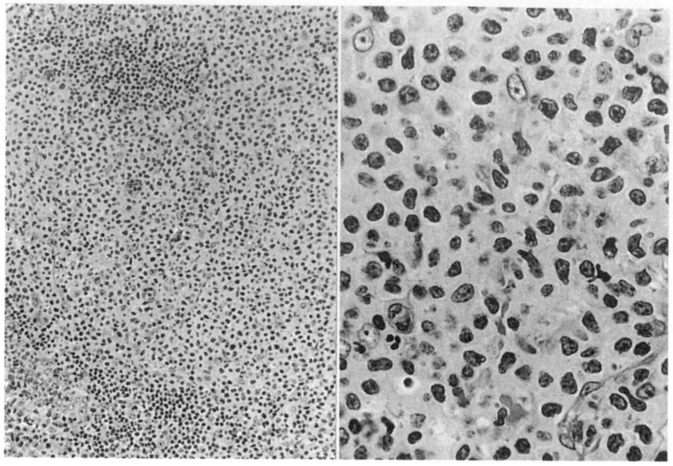

Fig. 28-8 Parasinusoidal proliferation of monocytoid lymphocytes. Higher magnification *(right)* reveals irregular nuclei and abundant clear cytoplasm.

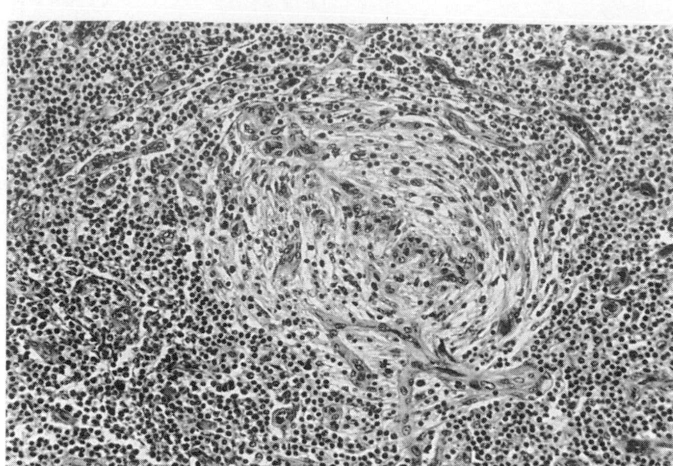

Fig. 28-11 Hyaline vascular lymphoid follicle.

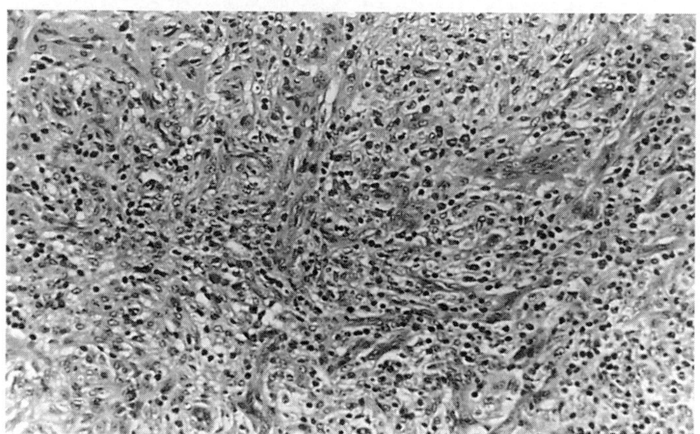

Fig. 28-9 In the late phase of HIV-1–related lymphoid hyperplasia, node is hypocellular with depletion of lymphoid follicles and prominent venules.

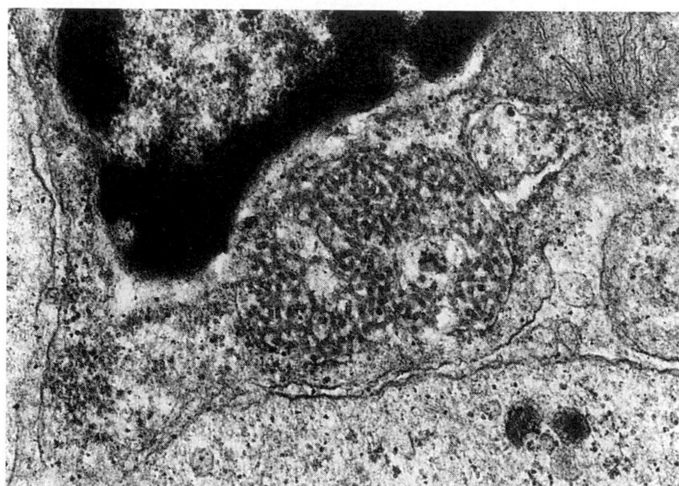

Fig. 28-12 Tubuloreticular structure characteristically numerous in lymphoid and endothelial cells in early HIV-1 infection. These "interferon footprints" are cytokine induced and not specific for the AIDS virus.

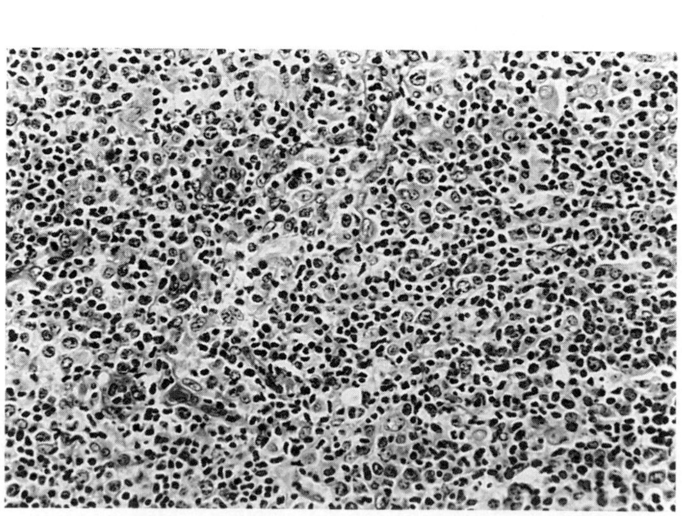

Fig. 28-10 Diffuse form of lymphoid hyperplasia with absence of follicles, increased vascularity, and scattered immunoblasts.

mous metaplasia (Fig. 28-13). Other features of Sjögren's syndrome, such as the presence of rheumatoid antibodies in the blood, are usually absent. The submandibular gland is less frequently involved. Follicular dendritic cells within the hyperplastic follicles are a site of active HIV-1 replication, and, in keeping with the benign reactive nature of this process, there is no clonal rearrangement of immunoglobulin genes or c-*myc*.[66]

Rarely, high-grade malignant lymphomas have been described in salivary gland–associated lymphoid tissue in patients with HIV infection, and EBV latent gene products have been localized in oral HIV-associated T-cell lymphomas.[67]

Other lymphadenopathies

Kaposi's sarcoma (KS) may involve lymph nodes in the absence of lesions in the skin. This lymphoma-like presenta-

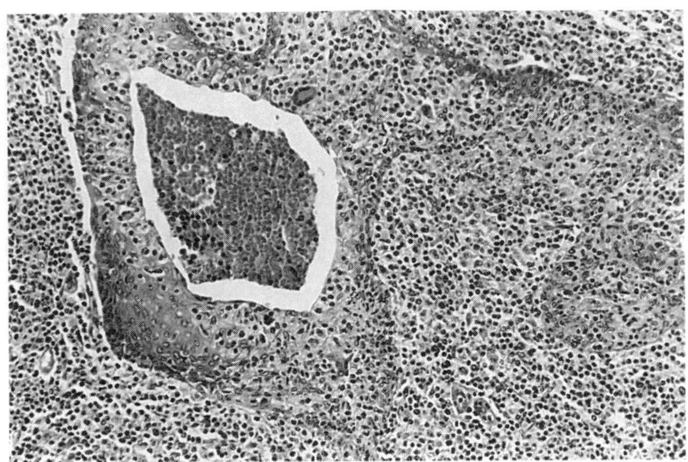

Fig. 28-13 Cystic salivary duct with myoepithelial proliferation surrounded by lymphoid hyperplasia.

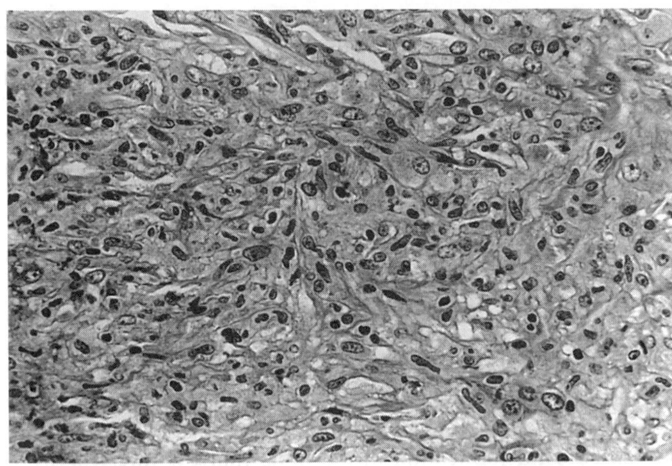

Fig. 28-14 Spindle cell proliferation (spindle cell pseudotumor) in lymph node infected with *Mycobacterium avium.*

tion of KS is associated with a highly vascular, follicular hyperplasia that is similar to Castleman's disease[68](Fig. 28-11). Histologically, lymph node involvement is characterized by peripheral and subcapsular dilated lymphatic and vascular channels, and central spindle cell nodules.

Vascular transformation of lymph node sinuses, which is characterized by conversion of lymph node sinuses into vascular channels, may be mistaken for KS. The distinguishing features are the sinusoidal distribution and lack of atypical spindle cells.[69]

Mycobacterial spindle-cell pseudotumor describes a process in lymph nodes where the parenchyma is replaced by spindle cells and macrophages containing mycobacteria[70] (Figs. 28-14, and 28-15). Mycobacterial pseudotumor occurs in other organs, including the liver and the lungs. *Pneumocystis carinii* may involve lymph nodes, bone marrow, or other organs. The morphology of extrapulmonary infection, including the characteristic foamy exudate, is similar to that seen in the lung.

Bacillary angiomatosis of lymph nodes must be differentiated from KS. In bacillary angiomatosis, the vascular proliferation is associated with eosinophilic interstitial edema, neutrophils, and leukocytoclasis[71] (Fig. 28-16). Clumps of bacteria can be demonstrated with silver impregnation methods such as the Warthin-Starry stain. By molecular diagnostic methods these bacteria have been classified as rickettsia-like organisms related to *Rochalimaea* species *(R. quintana* or *R. henselae)*[72-75] (see Chapter 35).

Hematologic manifestations

Peripheral blood

HIV infection may cause varied peripheral blood abnormalities, including anemia, granulocytopenia, and lymphopenia. Anemia in untreated cases is usually normochromic and normocytic, resembling the anemia of chronic disease. Iron stores are mostly increased, with low serum iron levels, low or normal total iron-binding capacity (TIBC), and increased ferritin. Macronormoblastic erythroid maturation may be prominent, particularly after antiretroviral therapy.[76]

Thrombocytopenia is common in asymptomatic HIV-infected individuals. Purpuric thrombocytopenia is not associ-

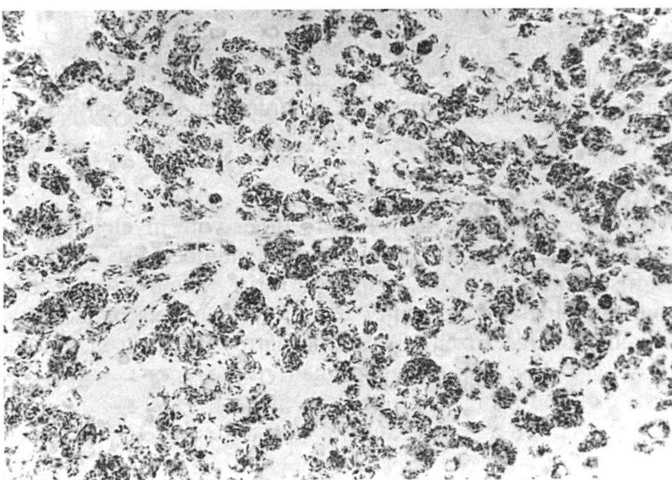

Fig. 28-15 Ziehl-Neelson stain reveals numerous atypical mycobacteria.

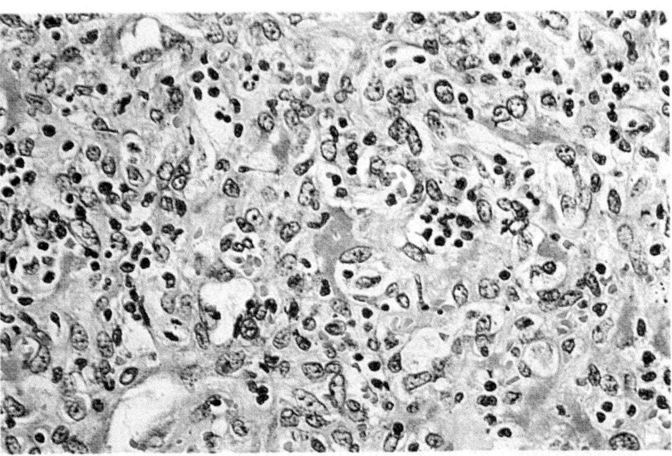

Fig. 28-16 Bacillary angiomatosis with prominent vasculature, interstitial edema, and inflammatory cells. Extracellular eosinophilic material corresponds to clusters of bacteria.

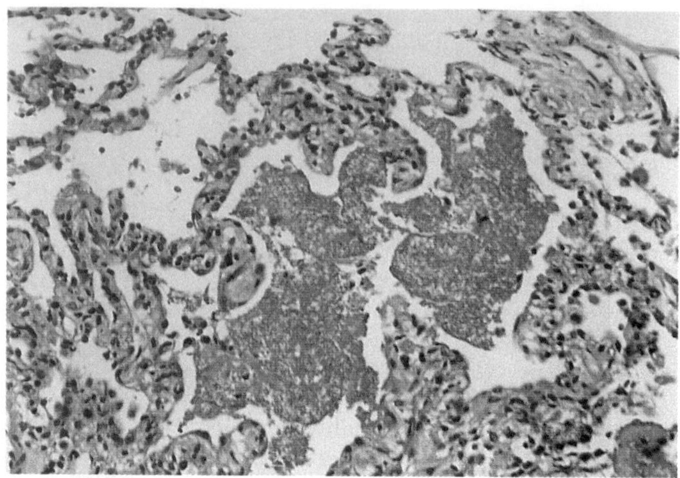

Fig. 28-22 Lung biopsy showing alveoli filled with a granular, eosinophilic, mostly acellular fibrinous exudate.

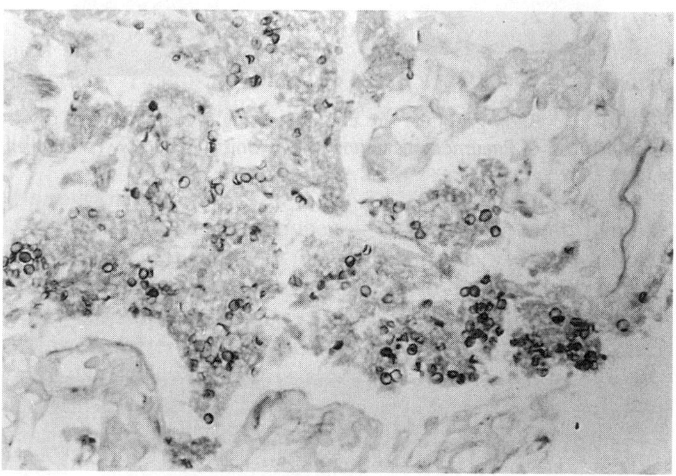

Fig. 28-23 Lung biopsy stained with Gomori's methenamine silver to demonstrate the partially collapsed cysts of *Pneumocystis carinii*.

Cytomegalovirus

In the AIDS patient, cytomegalovirus (CMV) affects many organs, with examples being the intestinal tract, pancreas, liver, kidney, genitourinary organs, lungs, adrenal glands, pituitary, brain, hematopoietic organs, and skin.[89-91] In the nervous system, CMV can cause an ascending, aggressive radiculomyelitis that clinically resembles Guillain-Barré syndrome. As many as 20% of AIDS patients develop CMV retinitis, which, when untreated, progresses relentlessly to blindness.[92] Often CMV is identified in multiple organs at autopsy, without necessarily causing specific clinical symptoms. However, CMV infection of the intestinal tract and lungs may be life threatening. CMV infection often appears as hemorrhagic foci, generally less than 1 cm in diameter, sometimes with central yellow zones indicative of necrosis on the pleural or serosal surfaces, as well as throughout the lung parenchyma.

Microscopically, the findings are cellular enlargement and a large intranuclear inclusion (Fig. 28-19) with or without granular cytoplasmic inclusions. Inclusions are typically found in epithelial cells but also in fibroblasts and endothelial cells. The resulting small vessel vasculitis causes ulceration in the intestinal tract, and perforation may occur. In general, cytoplasmic inclusions are not easily seen in AIDS patients, though they can be demonstrated by immunohistochemistry or in situ hybridization.[93] Antiviral agents, such as ganciclovir, have been successful in ameliorating infection in many patients.

Cryptosporidium parvum

Cryptosporidiosis is a well-recognized occupational hazard for veterinarians working with large animals such as sheep and cattle but was virtually unknown as a pathogen for other individuals until it became recognized in AIDS patients. Although cryptosporidiosis is not usually life threatening, it causes considerable morbidity. *C. parvum* typically inhabits the small and large intestine, causing protracted watery diarrhea, weight loss, malabsorption, bloating, and vague abdominal pain.[94] Patients may become severely dehydrated. The organisms appear as 1 to 2 μm spheres adherent to the mucosal surface, with only nonspecific reactive epithelial changes and a relatively mild, nonspecific inflammatory cell response[95] (Fig. 28-24). Ultrastructurally, the organism is tightly applied to the cell membrane, within the glycocalyx layer, with local injury to the cell membrane (Fig. 28-25). The infestation impairs the absorption ability of the enterocyte. Diagnosis can be established by identification of the organisms in a stool specimen stained with the Kinyoun modification of the acid-fast stain, in endoscopically obtained aspirates from either the small or large intestine, and in biopsy as well. There is no specific therapy. In some patients, the organisms migrate from the intestinal tract into the biliary tree, causing clinical signs and symptoms of cholecystitis or even biliary obstruction. The organism may affect the respiratory tract through the aspiration of infected gastroduodenal contents.

Toxoplasma gondii

Almost any organ, including lymph nodes, heart, liver, peripheral muscle, and others, may be infected by *Toxoplasma gondii*. Central nervous system involvement, however, is clinically the most important. Toxoplasmosis is the most common cause of an intracerebral mass lesion in the AIDS patient, and it may account for almost half the cases of neurologic disease in AIDS.[96-98] Typically, there are focal neurologic disturbances on a background of a global encephalopathy, often preceded by a prodrome of fever and malaise. Mild hemiparesis is common, and there may also be headaches, seizures and chorea. Computerized tomography classically demonstrates multiple "ring-enhancing" lesions with edema and mass effect, with a predilection for the basal ganglia and frontoparietal lobes. Biopsy is not always performed, and diagnosis is sometimes determined by response to empiric therapy.[99] Biopsy generally demonstrates the organism with a moderate chronic inflammatory cell response (Fig. 28-26).

Mycobacterium avium–Mytcobacterium intracellulare complex

Prior to the AIDS epidemic, organisms of the *Mycobacterium avium-intracellulare complex,* (MAC) complex were an uncommon cause of pneumonia in persons with chronic lung diseases.[100] The number of cases has dramatically increased, matching the AIDS epidemic. Acquisition is believed to occur through either the respiratory or, more often, the intestinal

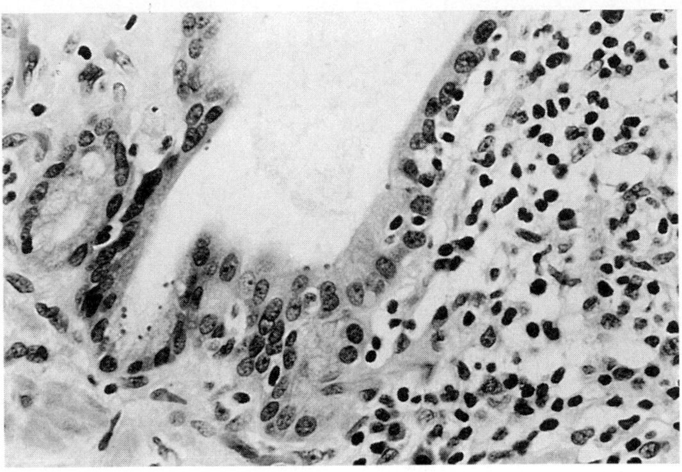

Fig. 28-24 Appendix from a 4-year-old girl, whose mother was an intravenous drug abuser, showing cryptosporidiosis at the surface of the epithelial cells. The child died a few months later of *Pneumocystis carinii* pneumonitis.

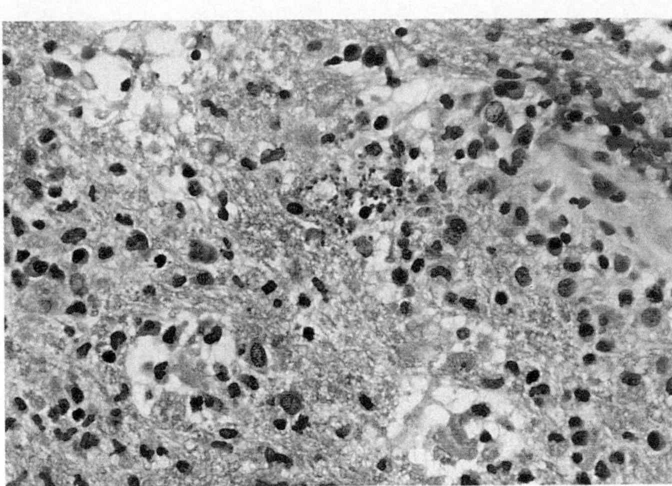

Fig. 28-26 Biopsy of the brain showing toxoplasmosis, with an acute and chronic inflammatory cell infiltrate and a cluster of *Toxoplasma* tachyzoites.

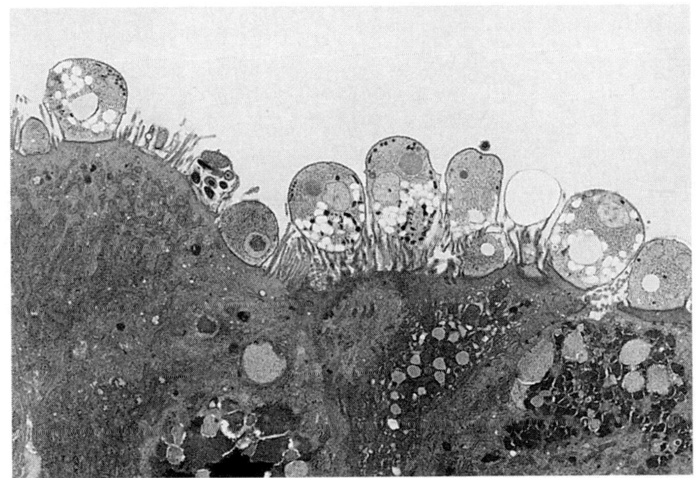

Fig. 28-25 Electron micrograph showing cryptosporidia attached to microvilli of enterocytes.

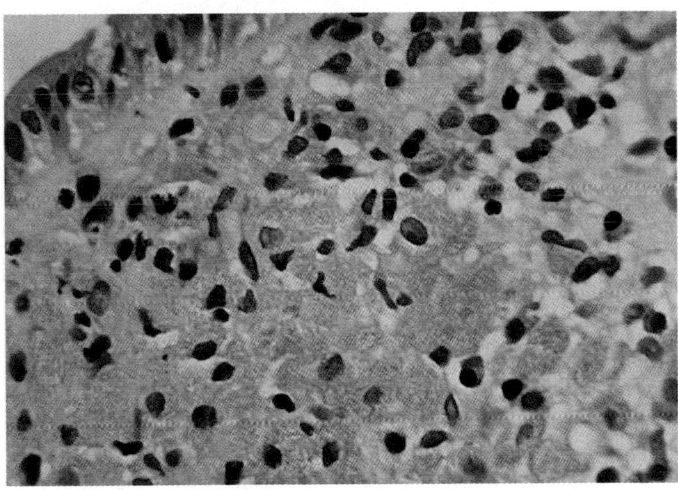

Fig. 28-27 Large intestine biopsy showing characteristic lamina propria histiocytic clusters of *Mycobacterium avium-intracellulare* complex. This patient also had *Giardia lamblia,* not seen in this photomicrograph.

tract.[101] In the immunocompetent individual colonization of the respiratory or gastrointestinal tract occurs without dissemination. In the HIV-infected patient, however, the organism can disseminate to any organ. Within affected tissues, macrophages with distended cytoplasm are numerous. Acid-fast stains will reveal innumerable acid-fast bacilli within the cytoplasm (Figs. 28-27 and 28-28). The infiltrate of macrophages in the lamina propria of the small intestine is remarkably similar to that of Whipple's disease.[102] In some patients, the inflammatory response to infection can form a tumor composed of spindle-shaped macrophages that resemble a fibroblastic proliferation.[103] The inflammatory cell response is generally modest, and granulomas are generally not seen or, when they do occur, are poorly formed. Death results, in many cases, from associated malnutrition and only rarely from specific organ compromise.[104]

Mycobacterium tuberculosis

There has been a resurgence of *Mycobacterium tuberculosis,* including highly virulent, antibiotic-resistant strains in the United States, affecting both immunocompetent individuals and those with AIDS. Initially, it was believed that *M. tuberculosis,* when it occurs in AIDS, arises from a previously contained focus of infection ("reactivation"), rather than from primary acquisition. As the number of cases of *M. tuberculosis* has increased, this theory is believed to be less tenable. The rising epidemic has been particularly conspicuous in New York City, where there were 50 cases per 100,000 people in 1991, compared to less than 25 cases per 100,000 people in 1984, but is thought likely to eventually involve most major urban areas. Overall, in the United States, the TB case rate in nonurban areas decreased from 1985 to 1992 while the rate in urban areas increased by 29%.[105] In general, the disease

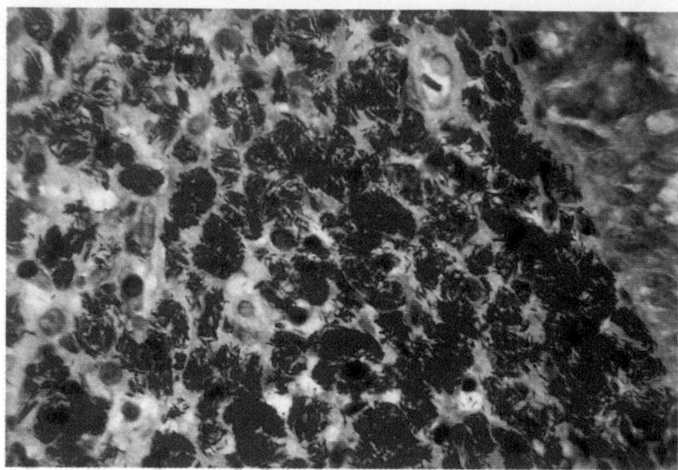

Fig. 28-28 Ziehl-Neelson stain to demonstrate the innumerable acid-fast bacilli.

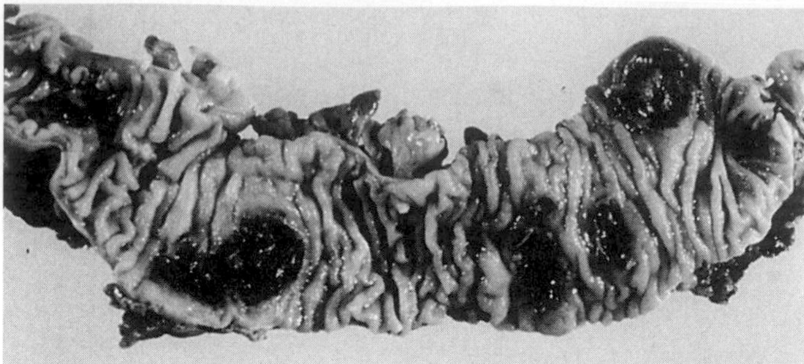

Fig. 28-29 Gross photograph of Burkitt-like lymphoma of the bowel with multiple ulcerated mass lesions.

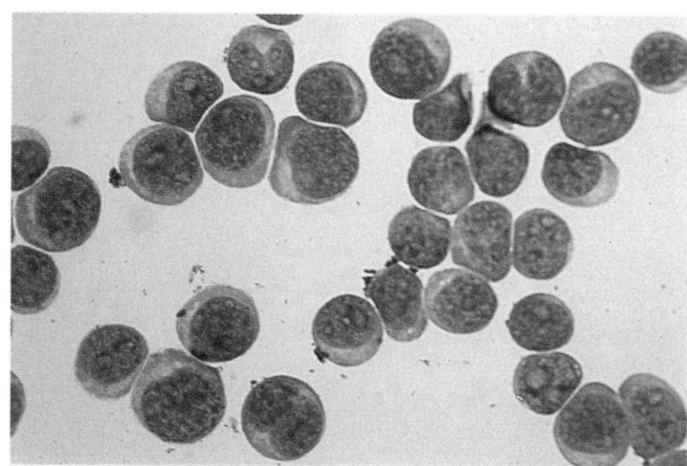

Fig. 28-30 Cytocentrifuge preparation from pleural cavity–based B-cell immunoblastic lymphoma reveals that the cells have a plasmacytoid appearance.

resembles classic tuberculosis and primarily affects the lungs but may also cause tuberculous lymphadenitis, enteritis, and encephalitis. Typical caseating granulomas may be seen, but poorly formed granulomas may also occur. In contrast to *M. avium,* acid-fast bacilli are not abundant. Drug-resistant strains of tuberculosis are an increasingly significant problem (see Chapter 33).

Candida

Infection with *Candida albicans* is common in the AIDS patient though not usually life threatening. Typically the patient will have esophageal or oropharyngeal candidiasis.[106] Other sites are less commonly affected. Rarely, *Candida* organisms may cause abscess formation and, in certain sites such as the brain or the lungs, may be potentially lethal.

Epstein-Barr virus

The Epstein-Barr virus (EBV) is responsible for several complications in the AIDS patient. EBV is associated with *oral hairy leukoplakia,* a distinctive condition, unique to AIDS, in which there are poorly demarcated, elevated, white, papilliform lesions on the tongue or the buccal mucosa.[107] Lesions may be single or multiple and are histologically characterized by hyperkeratosis, parakeratosis, papillomatosis, koilocytotic atypia, and a variety of other epithelial cytoplasmic changes. EBV has been demonstrated in these lesions by DNA in situ hybridization.[108] Oral hairy leukoplakia is considered an ominous prognostic sign in HIV-infected individuals, who are otherwise symptom free, because it heralds the full development of AIDS. Papillomavirus has been suggested as another, less common, cause for this lesion. EBV is also associated with non-Hodgkin's lymphoma in the AIDS patient, as is discussed subsequently.

NEOPLASIA

Non-Hodgkin's lymphoma

Lymphoma is a late complication of HIV infection.[109] Because patients with AIDS are surviving longer, with profound immunosuppression and $CD4^+$ cell depletion, the incidence of AIDS-related intermediate-grade and high-grade lymphomas is increasing.[110] Unlike Kaposi's sarcoma, which predominantly occurs in homosexual and bisexual males, malignant lymphoma affects all groups of the HIV-infected population, with similar clinical and pathologic features.[111]

Clinical

Disease is usually widespread at presentation and may involve multiple extranodal sites. Most commonly involved are the central nervous system, gastrointestinal tract (Fig. 28-29), bone marrow, and liver. Lymphoma may affect unusual sites, including the myocardium, soft tissues, and oral cavity. There may be extensive organ infiltration leading to organ failure, particularly in the bone marrow and liver. Lymphoma may also involve the pericardial space, pleura, or peritoneal cavity (Fig. 28-30).

Burkitt-like lymphoma is generally seen at a younger age than immunoblastic lymphoma is seen,[112] and it most often presents in peripheral sites or bone marrow.[109] It is often preceded by generalized reactive lymphadenopathy and occurs earlier in the course of the disease in patients with less severe immunodeficiency. It may respond better, at least initially, to chemotherapy.

Primary CNS lymphomas have predominantly an immunoblastic or large cell morphology.[109] The central nervous system is involved in about one third of AIDS patients by lymphoma, usually causing one or two deep-seated, mass lesions in the brain. An important differential diagnostic consideration is cerebral toxoplasmosis, though, in the latter condition, lesions are usually multiple and smaller. In children with AIDS primary lymphoma is the most common mass lesion in the brain.[113]

The emergence of lymphoma in an AIDS patient with a low $CD4^+$ cell count (<100/mm^3) portends poor prognosis, just as advanced stage disease and bone marrow involvement do. In addition to chemotherapy and radiation therapy, improved results may be obtained in combination with antiretroviral therapy and hematopoietic growth factor support, including GM-CSF, G-CSF, and erythropoietin.

Pathogenesis

The pathogenesis of lymphoma in patients with AIDS is not completely understood. Chronic antigenic stimulation and EBV infection, in association with impaired immune surveillance, can result in prolonged B-cell proliferation. Proliferating B-cells are at risk for genetic alterations and may finally undergo malignant transformation. In support of this multistep hypothesis, emergence of EBV-infected B-cell clones in patients with persistent generalized lymphadenopathy has been correlated with the subsequent development of lymphomas.[114,115]

Polyclonal and oligoclonal B-cell expansion frequently precedes the development of lymphoma in HIV-infected individuals.[116] Lymphomas may contain multiple copies of monomorphic EBV genomes, indicating that infection occurred before the clonal expansion in these tumors.[117] Two types of EBV that differ at the EBV nuclear antigen (EBNA) gene loci have been described. Healthy Western populations rarely harbor the B type of EBV, whereas patients infected with HIV, cardiac transplant recipients, and subjects from endemic Burkitt's lymphoma areas regularly carry the B type of EBV.[118,119] Lymphomas in HIV+ patients have been associated with both A and B types of EBV.[118,119]

EBV infection of neoplastic cells has been demonstrated in about 40% of cases of HIV-related lymphoma.[114,117,120] EBV is identified in a higher percentage of CNS lymphomas and cases with immunoblastic morphology (85% to 100%). Incidence of infection of tumor cells with EBV in small noncleaved or Burkitt-like lymphomas resembles sporadic rather than endemic cases.[116,121,122] The latent EBV nuclear antigen (EBNA-1) transcripts in HIV-related lymphomas are similar to those in Burkitt lymphomas, but HIV-related lymphomas also express transcripts for EBV latent membrane protein (LMP-1).[123]

Chromosomal translocations may result in activation of oncogenes including c-*myc* in about 42% of cases.[123] Less common genetic alterations[124] can involve *ras* oncogene, *bcl-2*, and point mutations of tumor suppressor gene, p53.[125] c-*myc* activation[126] and p53 inactivation occur more often in cases with Burkitt-like morphology. Molecular mechanisms of c-*myc* activation resemble those found in sporadic rather than endemic Burkitt's lymphoma.[124] HIV lymphomas are biologically heterogeneous, and three or four different clones have been described in the same neoplasm.[116]

Immunoglobulin gene rearrangement studies reveal monoclonal patterns in many cases of B-cell lymphoma, particularly Burkitt-like lymphomas. Immunoblastic lymphomas are more variable and may reveal multiple clonal B-cell expansions with multiple distinct genetic lesions within the same tumor.[116,127] Two or more immunoglobulin rearrangement bands may be present in addition to the germline band, and biopsy specimens from lymphomas at different anatomic sites may display distinct rearrangements, suggestive of having an origin from different clones. This situation is analogous to lymphomas arising in other immunosuppressed groups including transplant recipients. CNS lymphomas are more homogeneous monoclonal B-cell neoplasms, are positive for EBV, and lack c-*myc* rearrangement.[127]

Pathology

Approximately 70% to 90% of non-Hodgkin's lymphoma related to HIV infections have high-grade immunoblastic or small noncleaved (Burkitt-like) morphology.[109] Immunoblastic lymphomas are composed of large cells with a single central macronucleolus, or several nucleoli and amphophilic or plasmacytoid cytoplasm (Fig. 28-31). CNS lymphomas are usually immunoblastic, with characteristic perivascular localization of the neoplastic lymphoid cells (Fig. 28-32). Immunoblastic

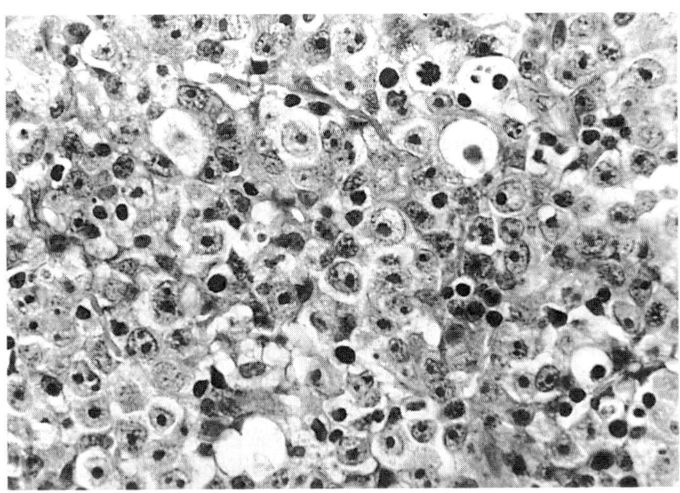

Fig. 28-31 B-cell immunoblastic lymphoma with characteristic large lymphoid cells with prominent central nucleoli, marginated chromatin, abundant cytoplasm, and frequent mitoses.

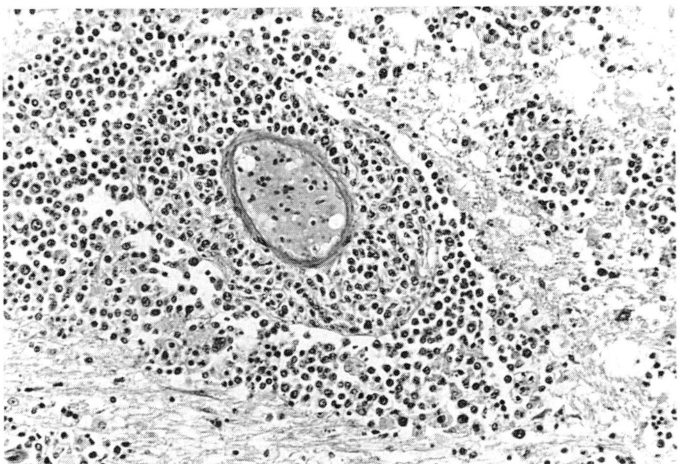

Fig. 28-32 B-cell immunoblastic lymphoma of the brain with characteristic perivascular infiltrates.

Table 28-7 Gastrointestinal tract disease in AIDS

Oral cavity and oropharynx
Herpes simplex infection
Candidiasis
Idiopathic aphthous ulcers
Kaposi's sarcoma
Esophagus
Candidiasis
Cytomegalovirus infection
Herpes simplex infection
Mycobacterium avium-intracellulare complex (MAC) infection
Histoplasmosis
Kaposi's sarcoma
Stomach
Cytomegalovirus infection
Kaposi's sarcoma
Candidiasis
Small intestine
Cryptosporidiosis
Cytomegalovirus infection
MAC infection
Microsporidiosis
Isospora belli infection
Giardia lamblia infection
Entamoeba histolytica infection
Cryptococcosis
Histoplasmosis
Coccidioidomycosis
Kaposi's sarcoma
Lymphoma
"AIDS enteropathy"
Appendix
Cryptosporidiosis
Cytomegalovirus infection
MAC infection
Mycobacterium tuberculosis infection
Isospora belli infection
Kaposi's sarcoma
Lymphoma
Large intestine
Cryptosporidiosis
Cytomegalovirus infection
MAC infection
Salmonellosis
Shigellosis
Campylobacter species infection
Clostridium difficile infection
Isospora belli infection
Entamoeba histolytica infection
Cryptococcosis
Histoplasmosis
Coccidioidomycosis
Kaposi's sarcoma
Lymphoma
Anorectum
Cytomegalovirus infection
Herpes simplex infection
Kaposi's sarcoma
Lymphoma

Table 28-8 Hepatobiliary disease in AIDS

Hepatic parenchymal disease
Cytomegalovirus infection
Mycobacterium avium-intracellulare complex (MAC)
Cryptococcosis
Candidiasis
Aspergillosis
Coccidioidomycosis
Hepatitis B virus infection
Hepatitis C virus infection
Drug toxicity
Kaposi's sarcoma
Lymphoma
Biliary disease
Cytomegalovirus cholangitis
Cryptosporidium cholangitis
Kaposi's sarcoma
Lymphoma

generalized process, such as cytomegalovirus, *MAC*, viral hepatitis, and lymphoma. Nonspecific findings, such as steatosis, sinusoidal abnormalities, and nondiagnostic granulomas are also seen. In some patients HIV antigenic material has been found in Kupffer cells and, rarely, hepatocytes.[181] The significance of this is not well understood.

Cardiovascular system

Cardiac dysfunction affects patients with AIDS, including cardiac tamponade, dilated cardiomyopathy (DCM), cardiac failure, refractory ventricular tachycardia, and sudden death. The histopathology of these lesions has been described and parallels that of non-AIDS cardiac disease.[182] Neoplasms, such as Kaposi's sarcoma and malignant lymphoma, also involve the heart.

Pericardium

Pericardial infections and nonspecific pericardial effusion can both result in cardiac tamponade. Pericardial involvement occurs in the presence of systemic infections caused by MAC, CMV, *Cryptococcus* neoformans, and other microbials. Nonspecific pericardial effusion may be associated with nonspecific pericarditis and DCM.

Myocardium

Myocardial complications in AIDS may include biventricular dilatation associated with DCM, myocardial infections, and idiopathic myocarditis. The heart is enlarged in DCM and microscopically demonstrates interstitial edema, interstitial fibrosis, and myofibrillar dropout. Myocarditis from infectious or idiopathic causes may be seen but need not be present. The pathogenesis of DCM is unknown. Infection, immunologic factors, anemia, and nutritional factors have been suggested to play a role in the pathogenesis of DCM, yet this remains unproved. The presence of T-cells, in contrast to the absence of B-cells, in the inflammatory infiltrate in idiopathic myocarditis, has been considered as indicative of cell-mediated autoimmune injury to the myocardium.[183] Among the nutritional factors, selenium deficiency is of interest. Selenium deficiency has been described in cardiomyopathy in patients with long-term total parenteral nutrition. Low selenium levels have been described in the cardiac tissue at autopsy from patients with AIDS.[184] DCM is associated with cardiac failure, which frequently results in death. Myocardial infections are usually secondary to systemic infections.

Toxoplasma gondii, Sarcosporidium spp, *C. neoformans, Candida* spp, CMV, and *Mycobacterium tuberculosis* and *M. avium-intracellulare* complex are the causative organisms. Focal myocardial infections, which are usually incidental findings at autopsy, may lead to cardiac dysfunction and arrhythmia in some cases. Idiopathic myocarditis in AIDS is defined by the following criteria: (1) degeneration or necrosis of myocardial fibers associated with an adjacent inflammatory infiltrate and, (2) lack of evidence of any infectious cause. This has been reported to occur in up to 40% of autopsy cases of AIDS in adults. In some cases, idiopathic myocarditis may be associated with DCM, cardiac arrhythmias, or sudden death.

Endocardium

The endocardium can be affected by inflammatory disease, including nonbacterial thrombotic endocarditis and infectious endocarditis. The former is related to the chronic debilitating nature of AIDS ("marantic endocarditis"). Both may be associated with embolic complications.

Conduction system

These lesions, which have most often been described in children with AIDS, include myocarditis and fibrosis of the sinoatrial (SA) node; fibrosis of the atrioventricular (AV) node, bundle of His, and left and right bundle branches; and degenerative changes, with myocarditis of the left bundle branch.[185] Thrombosis, adventitial or intimal fibrosis with or without luminal narrowing, and calcification of the tunica media were observed in the SA and AV nodal arteries and smaller arteries within the nodes. In one of the six children in a series of cases,[185] ECG showed left hemiblock, which correlated with the lesions of the left bundle branch. Although overwhelming opportunistic infection and malignancies are the commonest causes of death in patients with AIDS, sudden unexpected death is also seen in rare instances. Cardiac arrhythmia attributable to involvement of the cardiac conduction system may be a factor.

Arteriopathy

In children with AIDS an arteriopathy affects small and medium-sized arteries of many organs. There is intimal fibrosis, fragmentation of the elastic tissue, and fibrosis and calcification of the media with variable luminal narrowing. Fragmentation of elastic tissue appears to be the primary and the earliest change.[186] HIV antigens can be demonstrated in vessel walls by immunohistochemistry.[187] Aneurysms of the coronary artery and cerebral arteries have also been reported and may cause cerebrovascular accidents in pediatric AIDS.[188] Arterial lesions of the type seen in children have not been studied systematically in adults with AIDS, though similar lesions in renal and other arteries have been described in a few cases.

Pulmonary system

Infections

The lungs are involved, at some stage of the disease, in almost every patient with AIDS. Pulmonary insufficiency is the principal cause of death in many patients. Infection is the most common pulmonary complications of AIDS, and *Pneumocystis carinii* pneumonitis (Fig. 28-22) is the prototypical disorder. A host of other opportunistic infections can also be found, including viral pneumonia, mycobacteriosis, candidiasis, histoplasmosis, coccidiosis, cryptococcosis, aspergillosis, and toxoplasmosis. Interstitial pneumonias, for which specific organisms cannot be identified, also occur, as do Kaposi's sarcoma and non-Hodgkin's lymphomas.

Generally, spontaneously produced sputum has a low diagnostic yield, but induced sputum, using an aerosol of hypertonic saline, may permit the diagnosis of pneumocystosis. Bronchoalveolar lavage, performed during fiberoptic bronchoscopy, as well as transbronchial biopsy generally provide the diagnosis. In some cases, open lung biopsy may be required.

Lymphoid lesions

Pulmonary lymphoid lesions in children range from pulmonary lymphoid hyperplasia (PLH) to lymphoid interstitial pneumonitis (LIP).[189] In PLH there are lymphoid follicles, with or without germinal centers, around bronchioles. In LIP there is diffuse infiltration of alveolar septa by an admixture of lymphocytes, plasma cells, plasmacytoid lymphocytes, and a few immunoblasts (Fig. 28-41). These cells are polyclonal, as indicated by immunoperoxidase stains for the kappa and lambda light-chain immunoglobulins. Cell-marker studies on biopsy and bronchoalveolar lavage specimens have shown admixture of both B-cells and T-cells with a preponderance of $CD8^+$ suppressor cells among the latter. There may be a morphologic overlap between PLH and LIP, hence the designation *PLH-LIP complex*. There is neither involvement of blood vessels nor destruction of bronchi. Granulomas composed of pale mononuclear cells and multinucleated giant cells are seen in some cases. Sometimes there may be an intra-alveolar accumulation of mononuclear cells resembling desquamative interstitial pneumonitis[190] (Fig. 28-42). The PLH-LIP complex is associated with a characteristic linear-nodular pattern on chest roentgenograms. Children with AIDS who present with pulmonary disease related to PLH-LIP complex have a longer survival than those with opportunistic infection. There is evidence indicating that the interaction between EBV and HIV

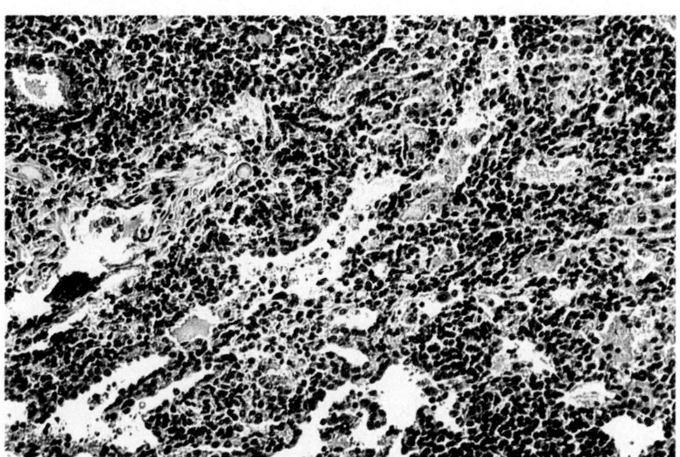

Fig. 28-41 Lymphoid interstitial pneumonitis characterized by dense chronic inflammatory cell infiltrate in the alveolar septa. Notice the occasional Russell bodies. (From Joshi VV, Oleske JM, Minnefor AB: *Hum Pathol* 16:241, 1985.)

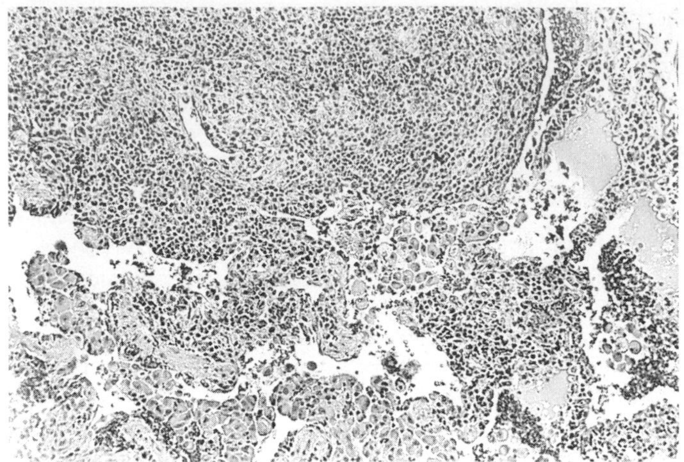

Fig. 28-42 Lymphoid nodule with extension of lymphoid infiltrate into the alveolar septa. Notice the clusters of mononuclear cells in the alveoli. (From Joshi VV, Oleske JM: Pathology of AIDS in children. In Wormser GP, Stahl RE, Bottone E, editors: *AIDS and other manifestations of HIV infection,* Park Ridge, NJ, 1987, Noyes Publications.)

Table 28-9 Clinicopathologic features of nonspecific interstitial pneumonitis (NIP) and lymphocytic interstitial pneumonitis (LIP) in adults with AIDS

Feature	NIP	LIP
Symptoms	Mild to moderate	Moderate to severe
Extrapulmonary involvement	Uncommon	Common
Lymphoid infiltrates (degree)	Mild to moderate	Severe
Lymphoid infiltrates (distribution)	Peribronchiolar, perivascular, pleural, interlobular, septal	In addition, alveolar, septal
Lymphoid follicles	Present	Present

Modified from Travis WD et al: *Hum Pathol* 23:529, 1992.

may be involved in the cause and pathogenesis of the PLH-LIP complex. EBV infection is present in most of these patients, and the EBV genome has been demonstrated in lung biopsy specimens. HIV has been demonstrated in the bronchoalveolar lavage fluid and lung biopsy specimens in only rare instances. HIV has been shown, however, to replicate in the EBV-transformed B-lymphocytes and alveolar macrophages.[191,192]

Lymphoid pneumonitis (LP) has been described in adults with AIDS.[193] Two patterns can be seen: (1) nonspecific interstitial pneumonitis (NIP) and (2) lymphoid interstitial pneumonites (LIP). The clinicopathologic features of NIP and LIP in adults with AIDS are outlined in Table 28-9. NIP and LIP in adults may correspond to PLH and LIP respectively, described in children with AIDS, since there are morphologic similarities between the corresponding lesions. However, EBV could not be demonstrated as an etiologic agent in LIP in adults.[193]

Thymic pathology

Pathologic lesions in the thymus are seen in the fetuses of HIV-infected mothers and in infants and children with AIDS. A variety of thymic changes have been described: infiltration by macrophages occurs in the cortex, medulla, Hassall's corpuscles, and lobular septa with large areas of lymphoid depletion noted in the cortex with sclerosis of the lobular septa.[194] Rare cells express HIV antigens and RNA, as demonstrated by immunofluorescence and in situ hybridization.

In infants and children, thymitis, precocious involution, and involution mimicking dysplasia ("dysinvolution") are seen in biopsy and autopsy specimens.[195,196] Thymitis, seen primarily in the thymic biopsy specimens, is characterized by (1) medullary lymphoid follicles with germinal centers, (2) multinucleated giant cells in the medulla (Fig. 28-43), or (3) diffuse lymphoplasmacytic or lymphomononuclear infiltrate in the cortex and medulla. Another lesion, the multilocular thymic cyst, which can be regarded as a part of the range of manifestation of thymitis, has been observed.[197] This lesion may be a sequel to reactive changes in the thymus. Precocious involution, defined as involution occurring prematurely and in excess of the amount of stress, is characterized by considerable depletion to virtual absence of lymphocytes, loss of corticomedullary differentiation, and microcystic dilatation of Hassall's corpuscles, which remain present in normal numbers. Dysinvolution is characterized by the same changes as in precocious involution, except that the Hassall's corpuscles are greatly reduced in number or virtually absent (Fig. 28-44). In many fatal cases severe hyalinization of the thymus is seen at autopsy.

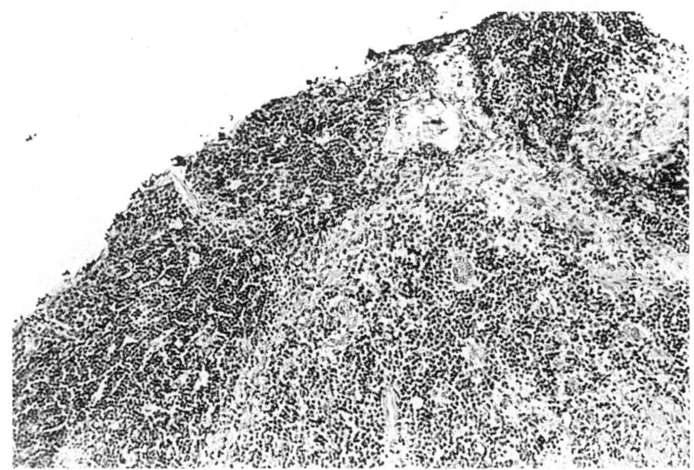

Fig. 28-43 Thymus showing multinucleated giant cell in the medulla. (From Joshi VV et al: *Arch Pathol Lab Med* 110:837, 1986.)

HIV infection of the thymus, as demonstrated by culture of HIV from thymic biopsy specimens and from fetal thymuses, as well as by the presence of HIV antigens and HIV RNA in the thymic cells, appears to play a major role in the pathogenesis of thymic injury. Both thymic epithelial cells and thymic lymphocytes are infected by HIV. It has been suggested that HIV infection of the thymus during early fetal life may lead to abnormal thymic development manifesting as the lesion described above as dysinvolution, whereas thymic injury occurring late in fetal life or after birth may result in thymitis followed by precocious involution.[198]

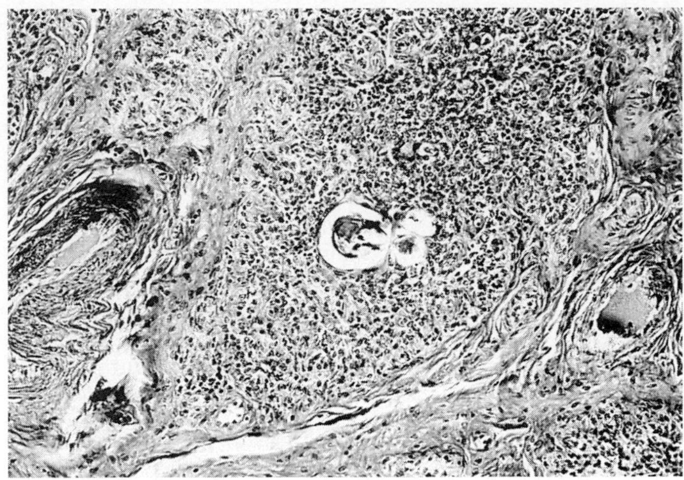

Fig. 28-44 Thymic lobule showing obscured corticomedullary differentiation and virtual absence of lymphocytes in the cortex and medulla. Only a single microcystic Hassall's corpuscle was found in one of the lobules in step-serial sections of the thymus.

Thymic injury apparently contributes significantly to the cellular immunodeficiency in children with AIDS. Thymic injury may also be a major impediment to the effectiveness of anti-HIV therapy in AIDS, since the thymic abnormalities are likely to be permanent and irreversible. Severe involutionary changes with thymic epithelial injury and thymitis with presence of lymphoid follicles or Castleman's disease-like changes have been reported in adults.[195,199,200] Thymic transplantation with variable results has been attempted in adults afflicted with AIDS in order to augment cell-mediated immunity. Such an attempt has not, thus far, been made in children.

Kidney

Nephropathy, which occurs in HIV-infected individuals with or without other manifestations of AIDS or ARC,[201] is occasionally the initial presentation of HIV infection. Signs of involvement of the kidney in HIV infection include heavy proteinuria, the nephrotic syndrome, or renal failure, usually with rapid evolution to end-stage renal disease.[202]

The features of HIV nephropathy are focal and segmental glomerulosclerosis, associated with tubulointerstitial disease. In the early stages the glomerular visceral epithelial cells are hyperplastic, with collapse of the underlying capillary walls and aggregates of lipid macrophages. This is followed by obliteration of capillaries, increase in mesangial matrix, and eventual segmental or global glomerulosclerosis.[201] The characteristic tubular lesion is microcystic dilatation with pale-staining casts containing plasma proteins.[203]

Immunofluorescence microscopy discloses segmental granular deposits of IgM and C3 at the site of segmental glomerulosclerosis. Associated ultrastructural findings include effacement of glomerular epithelial foot processes and endothelial cells containing numerous, 24 nm, tubuloreticular structures associated with the endoplasmic reticulum cisternae.[201,204] These "interferon footprints" can be induced in tissue culture on exposure to interferon -α.[201] They are seen in renal diseases unrelated to HIV but are most numerous in HIV nephropathy and systemic lupus erythematosus.

The entire gamut of renal disorders that affect non–HIV infected persons have a strong effect on HIV-infected patients.[205] Of these, diffuse mesangial hyperplasia is associated with HIV infection in children. Rarely, non-Hodgkin's lymphoma may be present in the kidney in patients with AIDS.[206]

PEDIATRIC AIDS

The lesions described above in terms of specific organ systems also occur in children with AIDS, though the incidence of the lesions may be different from that of adults. For example, KS is far less frequent in children than in adults, whereas arteriopathy occurs almost exclusively in children and is not seen in adults. Other lesions particularly pertinent to AIDS in the pediatric population are described below.

Perinatal pathology

Children can acquire HIV infection by (1) intrauterine or perinatal transmission from the mother, (2) breast milk, (3) transfusion of contaminated blood or blood products, or (4) sexual abuse. In a few cases, no route of transmission can be verified. Perinatal transmission accounts for most pediatric HIV infections. With the increasing frequency of heterosexual transmission of HIV, more women of child-bearing age are affected. At present, 1800 infants per year acquire HIV infection in the United States. The overall rate of vertical transmission in HIV-infected women is about 15%. The rate may be higher in women who have overt AIDS, with low CD4 cell counts.

HIV has been isolated from cervical tissue and secretions, placenta, amniotic fluid, and fetal tissues.[147] Villitis does not occur in the infected placenta, though HIV infects the Hofbauer cells and probably also trophoblastic cells, as demonstrated by immunoperoxidase stain and in situ hybridization for HIV antigens and RNA, respectively. It is not clear if the placenta plays a protective role in HIV transmission to the fetus. It is possible that such a protective action is compromised when other infections such as syphilis are present. A higher incidence of chorioamnionitis has also been reported in HIV-infected mothers; this lesion could enhance the possibility of HIV transmission. The pathologic changes in the tissues of HIV-infected aborted fetuses have not been studied systematically. The thymic lesion in the fetuses is described previously in the general discussion of thymic pathology in AIDS. There may be higher incidence of congenital heart disease in infants born to HIV-infected mothers. The brain of HIV-infected fetuses may be normal or may show one or more changes, including pronounced decrease in the number of neurons, generalized edema, and microglial proliferation.[207]

The timing of vertical transmission of HIV has been debated. Although transplacental intrauterine transmission of HIV does occur, the more frequent mode of infection appears to be related to the exposure of the traumatized skin and mucosal surfaces to maternal blood and cervical secretion during birth. The timing of infection is of importance, since early infection can interfere with normal development of the infected tissues and organs.

LABORATORY ISSUES

Universal precautions

AIDS is an infectious, fatal disease. Occupational exposure is well recognized, particularly through accidental puncture by needles or contamination of skin wounds or mucous membranes by infected blood and other body fluids.[208] The AIDS epidemic has led to wide implementation of "universal precautions" in health care settings such as hospitals and physicians' and dentists' offices.[209,210] There has also been attention paid to the design of laboratory instruments used for the study of patient material. For example, modern blood analyzers are designed so that laboratory personnel are not required to remove test-tube caps to obtain a sample.

AIDS autopsy considerations

Since the late 1960s, the number of autopsies performed in hospitals in the United States has dropped precipitously to the point that as few as 5% to 8% of people dying in hospitals are studied after death.[211] The justifiable concern for the potential risk of performing an autopsy on a patient who has died with AIDS has suggested to some that autopsies are not particularly useful in this population group. The carefully performed autopsy does not appear to be of significant risk to the prosector.[212,213] There has, thus far, been no evidence of work-place transmission of HIV, documented by either seroconversion or clinical AIDS, to a pathologist or autopsy assistant through blood-exposure autopsy.[208,209]

Those experienced in the performance of autopsies on AIDS patients recognize that no two patients behave similarly and that the range of disease varies considerably from patient to patient. Discrepancies between clinical diagnoses and actual autopsy findings may be higher in this group of patients than in any other. Individuals with AIDS may be afflicted with the same conditions that affect the population at large and can also die of potentially treatable diseases.[214-217] Many important lessons remain to be learned from the AIDS autopsy, and the value of the autopsy findings to the clinician who has dealt with the difficult and often confusing problems of the AIDS patient is inestimable. The autopsy continues to be a valuable source of information about the pathobiology of the many disorders that can affect the AIDS patient, and it will be critical to our understanding the usefulness and deleterious effects of newer therapies. Systematic autopsy studies can also serve a surveillance role in helping to identify new and thus far unrecognized complications of AIDS, when they occur.[218]

CONCLUSIONS

AIDS has had an unparalleled effect on our society while simultaneously providing extraordinary pressures on and opportunities for the scientific community. In only a few short years of experience with this virulent disorder, its cause has been established. At the same time, some of the pathogenetic mechanisms have been elucidated, and a diverse wealth of information about mechanisms of infectivity, retroviruses, the immune system, and cellular and molecular biology has been uncovered. The pandemic has led to new understandings about neoplasia. New and potentially useful drugs are being developed.[219,220] Infection with HIV has become the leading cause of death in young adults in the United States.[221] The grim nature of the disease has brought out some of the worst and most xenophobic responses of which our society is capable while also providing examples of shining courage, integrity, and hope.

The story is told that William Osler, almost a century ago, advised an assembled audience that "if you know all about diabetes mellitus, you know half of medicine." It is further said, perhaps apocryphally, that he then whispered under his breath, "And if you know all about syphilis, you know the other half." In our time, a modern Osler might very well use AIDS as the example of a disease whose manifestations may, at various times, be indistinguishable from those of the majority of the known disorders affecting humans. As a painfully acquired benefit of the many years of experience and experimentation that will be required before we are able to end the AIDS epidemic, we may well uncover a wealth of information equal to almost all that has gone before. The most basic mechanisms of infection, host response, immunity, and neoplasia are becoming revealed. It is reasonable to expect that ultimately this devastating disease will be eradicated, and the steps that lead to that desired goal will help us advance, both in terms of the control of present and future diseases and perhaps even in terms of the further development of the human spirit.

REFERENCES

1. Castiglioni A: *A history of medicine,* New York, 1947, Alfred A Knopf.
2. Krause RM: The origins of plagues: old and new, *Science* 257:1073, 1992.
3. Blattner WA: HIV epidemiology: past, present, and future, *FASEB J* 5:2340, 1991.
4. Johnson PR, Hirsch VM: SIV infection of macaques as a model for AIDS pathogenesis, *Int Rev Immunol* 8:55, 1992.
5. Anderson RM: Understanding the AIDS pandemic, *Sci Am* 266:58, 1992.
6. May RM, Anderson RM: The transmission dynamics of human immunodeficiency virus (HIV), *Philos Trans R Soc Lond [Biol]* 321:565, 1988.
7. Centers for Disease Control and Prevention: Update: mortality attributable to HIV infection/AIDS among persons aged 25-44 years—United States, 1990 and 1991, *MMWR* 42:481, 1993.
8. Centers for Disease Control and Prevention: Projections of the number of persons diagnosed with AIDS and the number of immunosuppressed HIV-infected persons—United States, 1992-1994, *MMWR* 41:1, 1992.
9. Emanuel EJ: Do physicians have an obligation to treat patients with AIDS? *N Engl J Med* 318:1686, 1988.
10. Pelligrino ED: The medical profession as a moral community, *Bull NY Acad Med* 66:221, 1990.
11. Eakin JM, Taylor KM: The psychosocial impact of AIDS on health workers, *AIDS* 4(suppl 1): S257, 1990.
12. Centers for Disease Control and Prevention: *Pneumocystis* pneumonia—Los Angeles, *MMWR* 30:250, 1981.
13. Centers for Disease Control: Kaposi's sarcoma and *Pneumocystis* pneumonia among homosexual men—New York City and California, *MMWR* 30:305, 1981.
14. Gottlieb MS, Schroff R, Schranker HE et al: *Pneumocystis carinii* pneumonia and mucosal candidiasis in previously healthy homosexual men, *N Engl J Med* 305:1425, 1981.
15. Masur H, Michelis MA, Greene JB et al: An outbreak of community-acquired *Pneumocystis carinii* pneumonia: initial manifestation of cellular immune dysfunction, *N Engl J Med* 305:1431, 1981.
16. Greenblatt RM, Lukehart SA, Plummer FA et al: Genital infection as a risk factor for human immunodeficiency virus infection, *AIDS* 2:47, 1988.
17. Ickovics JR, Rodin J: Women and AIDS in the United States: epidemiology, natural history, and mediating mechanisms, *Health Psychol* 11:1, 1992.
18. Legg JJ: Women and HIV, *J Am Board Fam Pract* 6:367, 1993.
19. Centers for Diseases Control and Prevention, Division of HIV/AIDS: US AIDS cases reported through December 1992, *HIV/AIDS Surveillance Report,* 1, Feb 1993.

20. Padian NS, Shiboski SC, Jewell NP: Female-to-male transmission of human immunodeficiency virus, *JAMA* 266:1664, 1991.
21. Chu SY, Buehler JW, Berkelman RL: Impact of the human immunodeficiency virus epidemic on mortality in women of reproductive age, United States, *JAMA* 264:225, 1990.

Clinical course

22. Pantaleo G, Graziosi C, Fauci AS: The immunopathogenesis of human immunodeficiency virus infection, *N Engl J Med* 328:327, 1993.
23. Daar ES, Moudgil T, Meyer RD, Ho DD: Transient high levels of viremia in patients with primary human immunodeficiency virus type I infection, *N Engl J Med* 324: 961, 1991.
24. Clarke SJ, Saag MS, Decker WD et al: High titers of cytopathic virus in plasma of patients with symptomatic primary HIV-1 infection, *N Engl J Med* 324: 954, 1991.
25. Abrams DI, Lewis BJ, Beckstead JH et al: Persistent diffuse lymphadenopathy in homosexual men: endpoint or prodrome? *Ann Intern Med* 100:801, 1984.
26. Fauci AS, Masur H, Gelmann EP et al: NIH conference: the acquired immunodeficiency syndrome: an update, *Ann Intern Med* 102:800, 1985.
27. Price RW, Brew B, Sidtis J et al: The brain in AIDS: central nervous sytem HIV-1 infection and AIDS dementia complex, *Science* 239:586, 1988.

HIV-1 and HIV-2

28. Erice A, Mayers DL, Strike DG et al: Brief report: Primary infection with zidovudine-resistant human immunodeficiency virus type 1, *N Engl J Med* 328:1163, 1993.
29. Centers for Disease Control and Prevention: Testing for antibodies to human immunodeficiency virus type 2 in the United States, *MMWR* 41:RR-12, 1-9, 1992.
30. Centers For Disease Control and Prevention: Seroconversion to simian immunodeficiency virus in two laboratory workers, *MMWR* 1992:678, 1992.
31. Hart TK, Klinkner AM, Ventre J, Bugelski PJ: Morphometric analysis of envelope glycoprotein gp120 distribution on HIV-1 virions, *J Histochem Cytochem* 41:235, 1993.
32. Maddox J: AIDS research turned upside down, *Nature* 353:297, 1991.
33. Kion TA, Hoffman GW: Anti-HIV and anti-anti-MHC antibodies in alloimmune and autoimmune mice, *Science* 253:1138, 1991.
34. Wu T-C, Kanayama MD, Hruban RH et al: Detection of a neuron-specific 9.0-kb transcript which shares homology with antisense transcripts of HIV-1 *gag* gene in patients with and without HIV-1 infection, *Am J Pathol* 142:25, 1993.
35. Lähdevirta J, Maury CP, Teppo AM, Repo H: Elevated levels of circulating cachectin/tumor necrosis factor in patients with acquired immunodeficiency syndrome, *Am J Med* 85:289, 1988.
36. Pantaleo G, Graziosi C, Demarast JF et al: HIV infection is active and progressive in lymphoid tissue during the clinically latent stage of disease, *Nature* 362:355, 1993.
37. Lenderking WR, Gelber RD, Cotton DJ et al: Evaluation of the quality of life associated with zidovudine treatment in asymptomatic human immunodeficiency virus infection, *N Engl J Med* 330:738, 1994.
38. Bylund DJ, Ziegner UHM, Hooper DG: Review of testing for human immunodeficiency virus, *Clin Lab Med* 12:305, 1992.
39. Centers for Disease Control and Prevention: Public Health Service guidelines for counseling and antibody testing to prevent HIV infection and AIDS, *MMWR* 36:509, 1967.
40. Centers for Disease Control and Prevention: Interpretation and use of the Western blot assay for serodiagnosis of human immunodeficiency virus type 1 infections, *MMWR* 38 (S-7):1, 1989.
41. Jackson JB, MacDonald KL, Cadwell J et al: Absence of HIV infection in blood donors with indeterminate Western blot tests for antibody to HIV-1, *N Engl J Med* 322:217, 1990.
42. Greenlaw PS: HIV antibody testing: legal considerations and sound hospital policy, *J Health Hosp Law* 25:80, 1992.
43. Rogers MF, Schochetman G, Hoff R: Advances in diagnosis of HIV infection in infants. In Pizzo PA, Wilfert CM, editors: *Pediatric AIDS: the challenge of HIV infection in infants, children and adolescents,* ed 2, Baltimore, 1994, Williams & Wilkins.
44. Fleischman AR, Post LF, Dubler NN: Mandatory newborn screening for human immunodeficiency virus, *Bull NY Acad Med* 71:4, 1994.
45. Erlich HA, Gelfand DH, Saiki RK: Specific DNA amplification, *Nature* (London) 331:461, 1988.
46. Hosburgh CR, Ou CY, Jason J: Duration of human immunodeficiency virus infection before detection of antibody, *Lancet* 1:637, 1989.
47. Whetsell AJ, Drew JB, Milman G et al: Comparison of three nonradioisotopic polymerase chain reaction–based methods for detection of human immunodeficiency virus type 1, *J Clin Microbiol* 30:845, 1992.
48. El-Sadr W, Oleske W, Agins BD et al: *Evaluation and management of early HIV infection,* Clinical Practice Guideline No. 7, AHCPR Publication No. 94-0572, Rockville, Md, Jan 1994, Agency for Health Care Policy and Research, Public Health Service, US Department of Health and Human Services, pp 82.
49. Saksela K, Stevens C, Rubinstein P, Baltimore D: Human immunodeficiency virus type 1 mRNA expression in peripheral blood cells predicts disease progression independently of the numbers of $CD4^+$ lymphocytes, *Proc Natl Acad Sci USA* 91:1104, 1994.
50. Kessler H, Duncan R, Blok T et al: Update: $CD4^+$ T-lymphocytopenia in persons without evident HIV infection—United States, *MMWR* 41:578, 1992.
51. Laurence J, Siegal FP, Schattner E et al: Acquired immunodeficiency without evidence of infection with human immunodeficiency virus types 1 and 2, *Lancet* 340:273, 1992.
52. Fauci AS: CD4+ T-lymphocytopenia without HIV infection—no lights, no camera, just facts, *N Engl J Med* 328:429, 1993.
53. Centers for Disease Control and Prevention: Unexplained $CD4^+$ T-lymphocyte depletion in persons without evident HIV infection—United States, *MMWR* 41:541, 1992.
54. Spira TJ, Jones BM, Nicholson JK et al: Idiopathic $CD4^+$ T-lymphocytopenia: an analysis of five patients with unexplained opportunistic infections, *N Engl J Med* 328:386, 1993.
55. Duncan RA, von Reyn CF, Alliegro GM et al: Idiopathic $CD4^+$ T-lymphocytopenia—four patients with opportunistic infections and no evidence of HIV infection, *N Engl J Med* 328:393, 1993.
56. Aledort LM, Operskalski EA, Dietrich SL et al: Low $CD4^+$ counts in a study of transfusion safety, *N Engl J Med* 328:441, 1993.
57. Smith DK, Neal JJ, Holmberg SD: Centers for Disease Control Idiopathic CD4+ T-lymphocytopenia Task Force: Unexplained opportunistic infections and $CD4^+$ T-lymphocytopenia without HIV infection, *N Engl J Med* 328:373, 1993.
58. Vermund SH, Hoover DR, Chen K: $CD4^+$ counts in seronegative homosexual men, *N Engl J Med* 328:442, 1993.

Systemic manifestations

59. Baroni CD, Uccini S: The lymphadenopathy of HIV infection, *Am J Clin Pathol* 99:397, 1993.
60. Kamel OW, LeBrun DP, Berry GJ et al: Warthin-Finkeldey polykaryocytes demonstrate a T-cell immunophenotype, *Am J Clin Pathol* 97:179, 1992.
61. Harris NL: Hypervascular follicular hyperplasia and Kaposi's sarcoma in patients at risk for AIDS, *N Engl J Med* 310:462, 1984.
62. Temin HM, Bolognesi DP: Where has HIV been hiding? *Nature* 362:292, 1993.
63. Nadasdy T, Hanson-Painton O, Davis LD et al: Conditions affecting the immunohistochemical detection of HIV in fixed and embedded renal and nonrenal tissues, *Mod Pathol* 5:283, 1992.
64. Arber DA, Shibata D, Chen Y-Y, Weiss LM: Characterization of the topography of Epstein-Barr virus infection in human immunodeficiency virus–associated lymphoid tissues, *Mod Pathol* 5:559, 1992.
65. Hyjek E, Smith WJ, Isaacson PG: Primary B-cell lymphoma of salivary glands and its relationship to myoepithelial sialadenitis, *Hum Pathol* 19:766, 1988.
66. Labouyrie E, Merlio JPH, Beylot-Barry M et al: Human immunodeficiency virus type 1 replication within cystic lymphoepithelial lesion of the salivary gland, *Am J Clin Pathol* 100:41, 1993.
67. Thomas A, Cotter F, Hanby AM et al: Epstein-Barr virus–related oral T-cell lymphoma associated with human immunodeficiency virus immunosuppression, *Blood* 81:3350, 1993.
68. Rywlin A, Recher L, Hofman EP: Lymphoma-like presentation of Kaposi's sarcoma, *Arch Dermatol* 93:554, 1966.

69. Chan JKC, Warnke RA, Dorfman R: Vascular transformation of sinuses in lymph nodes: a study of its morphological spectrum and distinction from Kaposi's sarcoma, *Am J Surg Pathol* 15:732, 1991.
70. Chen KTK: Mycobacterial spindle cell pseudotumor of lymph nodes, *Am J Surg Pathol* 16:276, 1992.
71. Chan JKC, Lewin KJ, Lombard CM et al: Histopathology of bacillary angiomatosis of lymph node, *Am J Surg Pathol* 15:430, 1991.
72. Relman DA, Louitit JS, Schmidt TM et al: The agent of bacillary angiomatosis: an approach to the identification of uncultured pathogens, *N Engl J Med* 323:1573, 1990.
73. Koehler JE, Quinn FD, Berger TG et al: Isolation of *Rochalimaea* species from cutaneous and osseous lesions of bacillary angiomatosis, *N Engl J Med* 327:1625, 1992.
74. Reed JA, Brigati DJ, Flynn SD et al: Immunocytochemical identification of *Rochalimaea henselae* in bacillary (epithelioid) angiomatosis, parenchymal bacillary peliosis, and persistent fever with bacteremia, *Am J Surg Pathol* 16:650, 1992.
75. Welch DF, Pickett DA, Slater LN et al: *Rochalimaea henselae* sp. nov., a cause of septicemia, bacillary angiomatosis, and parenchymal bacillary peliosis, *J Clin Microbiol* 30:275, 1992.
76. Snower DP, Weil SC: Changing etiology of macrocytosis, *Am J Clin Pathol* 99:57, 1993.
77. Stricker RB, Abrams DI, Corash L, Shuman MA: Target platelet antigen in homosexual men with immune thrombocytopenia, *N Engl J Med* 313: 1375, 1985.
78. Bauer S, Khan A, Klein A, Starasoler L: Naked megakaryocyte nuclei as an indicator of human immunodeficiency virus infection, *Arch Pathol Lab Med* 116:1025, 1992.
79. Zauli G, Re MC, Davis B et al: Impaired in vitro growth of purified (CD34+) hematopoietic progenitors in human immunodeficiency virus-1 seropositive thrombocytopenic individuals, *Blood* 79:2680, 1992.
80. Kitano K, Abboud CN, Ryan DH et al: Macrophage-active colony-stimulating factors enhance human immunodeficiency virus type 1 infection in bone marrow stem cells, *Blood* 77:1699, 1991.
81. Zucker-Franklin D, Jermin CS, Cooper MC: Structural changes in the megakaryocytes of patients infected with human immunodeficiency virus (HIV-1), *Am J Pathol* 134:1295, 1989.
82. Mehta K, Gascon P, Robboy S: The gelatinous bone marrow (serous atrophy) in patients with acquired immunodeficiency syndrome: evidence of excess sulfated glycosaminoglycan, *Arch Pathol Lab Med* 116: 504, 1992.
83. Karcher DS, Frost AR: The bone marrow in human immunodeficiency virus (HIV)–related disease, *Am J Clin Pathol* 95:63, 1991.
84. Murray JF, Mills J: Pulmonary infectious complications of human immunodeficiency virus infection, *Am Rev Respir Dis* 141:1356, 1582, 1990.
85. Kovacs JA, Hiemenz, JW, Macher AM et al: *Pneumocystis carinii* pneumonia: a comparison between patietns with the acquired immunodeficiency syndrome and patients with other immunodeficiencies, *Ann Intern Med* 100:663, 1984.
86. Travis WD, Pittaluga S, Lipschik GY et al: Atypical pathologic manifestations of *Pneumocystis carinii* pneumonia in the acquired immunodeficiency syndrome, *Am J Surg Pathol* 14:615, 1990.
87. Unger PD, Rosenblum M, Krown SE: Disseminated *Pneumocystis carinii* pneumonia in a patient with acquired immunodeficiency syndrome, *Hum Pathol* 19: 113, 1988.
88. DeRoux SJ, Adsay NV, Ioachim HL: Disseminated pneumocystosis without pulmonary involvement during prophylactic aerosolized pentamidine therapy in a patient with the acquired immunodeficiency syndrome, *Arch Pathol Lab Med* 115:1137, 1991.
89. Gehrz RC: Human cytomegalovirus: biology and clinical perspectives, *Adv Pediatr* 38:203, 1991.
90. Gold JWM, Armstrong D: Infectious complications of the acquired immune deficiency syndrome, *Ann NY Acad Sci* 437:383, 1984.
91. Drew WL: Cytomegalovirus infection in patients with AIDS, *Clin Infect Dis* 14:608, 1992.
92. Heinemann M-H: Characteristics of cytomegalovirus retinitis in patients with acquired immunodeficiency syndrome, *Am J Med* 92(suppl 2A):12S, 1992.
93. Wu G-D, Shintaku IP, Chien K, Geller SA: A comparison of routine light microscopy, immunohistochemistry, and in situ hybridization for the detection of cytomegalovirus in gastrointestinal biopsies, *Am J Gastroenterol* 84:1517, 1989.
94. García LS, Current WL: Cryptosporidiosis: clinical features and diagnosis, *Crit Rev Clin Lab Sci* 27:439, 1989.
95. Godwin TA: Cryptosporidiosis in the acquired immunodeficiency syndrome: a study of 15 autopsy cases, *Hum Pathol* 22:1215, 1991.
96. Luft BJ, Remington JS: Toxoplasmic encephalitis in AIDS, *Clin Infect Dis* 15:211, 1992.
97. Bishburg E, Eng RH, Slim J et al: Brain lesions in patients with the acquired immunodeficiency syndrome, *Arch Intern Med* 86:521, 1989.
98. Porter SB, Sande MA: Toxoplasmosis of the central nervous system in the acquired immunodeficiency syndrome, *N Engl J Med* 327:1643, 1992.
99. Luft BJ, Hafner R, Korzun AH et al: Toxoplasmic encephalitis in patients with the acquired immunodeficiency syndrome, *N Engl J Med* 329:995, 1993.
100. Horsburgh CR: *Mycobacterium avium* complex infection in the acquired immunodeficiency syndrome, *N Engl J Med* 324:1338, 1991.
101. Klatt EC, Jensen DF, Meyer PR: Pathology of *Mycobacterium avium-intracellulare* infection in acquired immunodeficiency syndrome, *Hum Pathol* 18:709, 1987.
102. Gillin JS, Urmacher C, West R et al: Disseminated *M. avium-intracellulare* infection in AIDS mimicking Whipple's disease, *Gastroenterology* 85:1187, 1983.
103. Wood C, Nikoloff BJ, Taylor NR: Pseudotumor resulting from atypical mycobacterial infection: histoid variety of *Mycobacterium avium-intracellulare* complex infection, *Am J Clin Pathol* 83: 524, 1985.
104. Wallace JM, Hannah JB: *Mycobacterium avium* complex infection in patients with the acquired immunodeficiency syndrome, *Chest* 93: 926, 1988.
105. Centers for Disease Control and Prevention: Tuberculosis mortality—United States, *MMWR* 42:696, 1992.
106. Saral R: *Candida* and *Aspergillus* infections in immunocompromised patients: an overview, *Rev Infect Dis* 13:487, 1991.
107. Reichert PA: Oral manifestations of recently described viral infections, including AIDS, *Curr Opin Dent* 1:377, 1991.
108. Ernberg I: Epstein-Barr virus and acquired immunodeficiency syndrome, *Adv Viral Oncol* 8:203, 1989.

Neoplasia

109. Levine AM: Acquired immunodeficiency syndrome–related lymphoma, *Blood* 80:8, 1992.
110. Pluda JM, Yarchoan R, Jaffe ES et al: Development of non-Hodgkin lymphoma in a cohort of patients with severe human immunodeficiency virus (HIV) infection on long-term antiretroviral therapy, *Ann Intern Med* 113:276, 1990.
111. Ragni MV, Belle SH, Jaffe RA et al: Acquired immunodeficiency syndrome–associated non-Hodgkin's lymphomas and other malignancies in patients with hemophilia, *Blood* 81:1889, 1993.
112. Beral V, Peterman T, Berkelman R, Jaffe H: AIDS-associated non-Hodgkin's lymphoma, *Lancet* 337:805, 1991.
113. Epstein LG, DiCarlo FJ, Joshi VV et al: Primary lymphoma of the central nervous system in children with acquired immunodeficiency syndrome, *Pediatrics* 82:355, 1988.
114. Shibata D, Weiss LM, Nathwani BN et al: Epstein-Barr virus in benign lymph node biopsies from individuals infected with the human immunodeficiency virus is associated with concurrent or subsequent development of non-Hodgkin's lymphoma, *Blood* 77:1527, 1991.
115. Weinberg RA: Oncogenes, antioncogenes and the molecular bases of multistep carcinogenesis, *Cancer Res* 49:3713, 1989.
116. Ballerini P, Gaidano G, Gong J et al: Molecular pathogenesis of HIV-associated lymphomas, *AIDS Res Hum Retroviruses* 8:731, 1992.
117. Neri A, Barriga F, Inghirami G et al: Epstein-Barr virus infection precedes clinical expansion in Burkitt's and acquired immunodeficiency syndrome–associated lymphoma, *Blood* 77:1092, 1991.
118. Boyle MJ, Sewell WA, Sculley TB et al: Subtypes of Epstein-Barr virus in human immunodeficiency virus–associated non-Hodgkin's lymphoma, *Blood* 78:3004, 1991.

119. Boyle MJ, Vasak E, Tschuchnigg M et al: Subtypes of Epstein-Barr virus (EBV) in Hodgkin's disease: association between B-type EBV and immunocompromise, *Blood* 81:468, 1993.
120. Subar M, Neri A, Inghirami G et al: Frequent c-*myc* oncogene activation and infrequent presence of Epstein-Barr virus genome in AIDS-associated lymphoma, *Blood* 72:667, 1988.
121. DeAngelis LM, Wong E, Rosenblum M, Furneaux H: Epstein-Barr virus in acquired immune deficiency syndrome (AIDS) and non-AIDS primary central nervous system lymphoma, *Cancer* 70:1607, 1992.
122. Chang KL, Flaris N, Hickey WF et al: Brain lymphomas of immunocompetent and immunocompromised patients: study of association with Epstein-Barr virus, *Mod Pathol* 6:427, 1993.
123. Shibata D, Weiss LM, Hernandez AM et al: Ebstein-Barr virus associated non-Hodgkin's lymphoma in patients infected with human immunodeficiency virus, *Blood* 81:2102, 1993.
124. Ballerini P, Gaidano G, Gong JZ et al: Multiple genetic lesions in acquired immunodeficiency syndrome–related non-Hodgkin's lymphoma, *Blood* 81:166, 1993.
125. Nakamura H, Said JW, Miller CW, Koeffler HP: Mutation and protein expression of p53 in acquired immunodeficiency syndrome–related lymphomas, *Blood* 82:920, 1993.
126. Delecluse HJ, Raphael M, Magaud JP et al: Variable morphology of human immunodeficiency virus–associated lymphomas with c-*myc* rearrangements, *Blood* 82:552, 1993.
127. Meeker TC, Shiramizu B, Kaplan L et al: Evidence for molecular subtypes of HIV-associated lymphoma: division into peripheral monoclonal, polyclonal and central nervous system lymphoma, *AIDS* 5:669, 1991.
128. Shiramizu B, Herndier B, Meeker T et al: Molecular and immunophenotypic characterization of AIDS-associated, Epstein Barr virus–negative, polyclonal lymphoma, *J Clin Oncol* 10:383, 1992.
129. González-Clemente JM, Ribera JM, Campo E et al: Ki-1 positive anaplastic large-cell lymphoma of T-cell origin in HIV-infected patient, *AIDS* 5:751, 1991.
130. Herndier BG, Shiramizu BT, Jewett NE et al: Acquired immunodeficiency syndrome–associated T-cell lymphoma: evidence for human immunodeficiency virus type 1–associated T-cell transformation, *Blood* 79:1768, 1992.
131. Hessol NA, Katz MH, Liu J et al: Increased incidence of Hodgkin disease in homosexual men with HIV infection, *Ann Intern Med* 117: 309, 1992.
132. Ames ED, Conjalka MS, Goldberg AF et al: Hodgkin's disease and AIDS: twenty-three new cases and a review of the literature, *Hematol Oncol Clin North Am* 5:343, 1991.
133. Uccini S, Monardo F, Stoppacciaro A et al: High frequency of Epstein-Barr virus genome in Hodgkin's disease of HIV-positive patients, *Int J Cancer* 46:581, 1990.
134. Audouin J, Diebold J, Pallesen G: Frequent expression of Epstein-Barr virus latent membrane protein-1 in tumour cells of Hodgkin's disease in HIV-positive patients, *J Pathol* 167:381, 1992.
135. Moran CA, Tuur S, Angritt P et al: Epstein-Barr virus in Hodgkin's disease from patients with human immunodeficiency virus infection, *Mod Pathol* 5:85, 1992.
136. Herndier BG, Sánchez HC, Chang KL et al: High prevalence of Epstein-Barr virus in the Reed-Sternberg cells of HIV-associated Hodgkin's disease, *Am J Pathol* 142:1073, 1993.
137. Pinkus GS, Lones M, Shintaku IP, Said JW: Immunohistochemical detection of Epstein-Barr virus encoded latent membrane protein in Reed-Sternberg cells and variants of Hodgkin's disease, *Mod Pathol,* 7:454, 1994.
138. Guarner J, del Rio C, Hendrix L, Unger ER: Composite Hodgkin's and non-Hodgkin's lymphoma in a patient with acquired immune deficiency syndrome, *Cancer* 66:796, 1990.
139. Boiocchi M, Dolcetti R, De Re V et al: Demonstration of a unique Epstein-Barr virus–positive cellular clone in metachronous multiple localizations of Hodgkin's disease, *Am J Pathol* 142:33, 1993.
140. Chang Y, Cesarman E, Pessin MS et al: Identification of herpesvirus-like DNA sequences in AIDS-associated Kaposi's sarcoma, *Science* 266:1865, 1994.
141. Niedt GW, Myskowski PL, Urmacher C et al: Histologic predictors of survival in acquired immunodeficiency syndrome–associated Kaposi's sarcoma, *Hum Pathol* 23:1419, 1992.
142. Northfelt DW, Kahn JO, Volberding PA: Treatment of AIDS-related Kaposi's sarcoma, *Hematol Oncol Clin North Am* 5:297, 1991.
143. Regezi JA, MacPhail LA, Daniels TE et al: Human immunodeficiency virus–associated oral Kaposi's sarcoma, *Am J Pathol* 143:240, 1993.
144. Gachupin-García A, Selwyn PA, Budner NS: Population-based study of malignancies and HIV infection among injecting drug users in a New York City methadone treatment program, 1985-1991, *AIDS* 6:843, 1992.
145. Jenkins JR, Sturzbecher H-W: The p53 oncogene. In Reddy EP, Skalka AM, Curran T, editor: *The oncogene handbook,* Amsterdam, 1988, Elsevier Science Publishers B.V. (Biomedical Division).
146. Centers for Disease Control: 1993 Revised classification system for HIV infection and expanded surveillance case definition for AIDS among adolescents and adults, *MMWR* 41:961, 1992.
147. Joshi VV: Pathology of AIDS in children: overview, update and future direction, *Ann NY Acad Sci* 693: 71, 1993.
148. Conner E, Boccon-Gibod L, Joshi VV et al: Cutaneious AIDS associated Kaposi's sarcoma in pediatric patients, *Arch Dermatol* 126:791, 1990.
149. Andiman WA, Eastman R, Martin K et al: Opportunistic lymphoproliferations associated with Epstein-Barr viral DNA in infants and children with *AIDS, Lancet* 2:1390, 1985.
150. Lee E, Dickman PS, Jaffe R et al: Post-transplant spindle cell tumor (PTST): an entity associated with Epstein-Barr virus, *Mod Pathol* 6:127A, 1993.

Specific organ systems

151. Berger JR, Moskowitz L, Fischl M et al: Neurologic disease as the presenting manifestation of acquired immunodeficiency syndrome, *South Med J* 80: 683, 1987.
152. Gray F, Gherardi R, Scaravilli F: The neuropathology of the acquired immune deficiency syndrome (AIDS), *Brain* 111:245, 1988.
153. Berger JR, Levy RM: The neurologic complications of human immunodeficiency virus infection, *Med Clin North Am* 77:1, 1993.
154. Navia BA, Jordan BD, Price RW: The AIDS dementia complex: II. neuropathology, *Ann Neurol* 19:525, 1986.
155. Price RW, Brew B, Sidtis J et al: The brain in AIDS: central nervous system HIV-1 infection and AIDS dementia complex, *Science* 239:586, 1988.
156. Weisberg LA, Ross W: AIDS dementia complex, *Postgrad Med* 86: 213, 1989.
157. Sharer LR, Epstein LG, Cho E-S et al: Pathologic features of AIDS encephalopathy in children: evidence for LAV/HTLV-III infection of brain, *Hum Pathol* 17:271, 1986.
158. Grafe MR, Wiley CA: Spinal cord and peripheral nerve pathology in AIDS: the role of cytomegalovirus and human immunodeficiency virus, *Ann Neurol* 25:561, 1989.
159. Cornblath DR, McArthur JC, Kennedy PGE et al: Inflammatory demyelinating peripheral neuropathies associated with human T-cell lymphocytotrophic virus type III infection, *Ann Neurol* 21:32, 1987.
160. Dalakas MC, Pezeshkpour GH, Gravell M et al: Polymyositis associated with AIDS retrovirus, *JAMA* 256:2381, 1986.
161. Dalakas MC, Illa I, Pezeshkpour GH et al: Mitochondrial myopathy caused by long-term zidovudine (AZT) therapy, *N Engl J Med* 328:1098, 1990.
162. Simpson DM, Citak KA, Godfrey E et al: Myopathies associated with human immunodeficiency virus and zidovudine: can their effects be distinguished? *Neurology* 43:971, 1993.
163. Chariot P, Monnet I, Gherardi R: Cytochrome *c* oxidase reaction improves histopathological assessment of zidovudine myopathy, *Ann Neurol* 34:561, 1993.
164. Berger JR, Kaszovitz B, Post MJD et al: Progressive multifocal leukoencephalopathy associated with human immunodeficiency virus infection, *Ann Intern Med* 107:78, 1987.
165. Einsiedel RWv, Fife TD, Aksamit AJ et al: Progressive multifocal leukoencephalopathy in AIDS: a clinicopathologic study and review of the literature, *J Neurol* 240:391, 1993.
166. Telenti A, Aksamit AJ, Proper J, Smith TF: Detection of JC virus DNA by polymerase chain reaction in patients with progressive multifocal leukoencephalopathy, *J Infect Dis* 162:858, 1990.

167. Aksamit AJ, Major EO, Ghatak NR et al: Diagnosis of progressive multifocal leukoencephalopathy by brain biopsy with biotin labeled DNA: DNA in situ hybridization, *J Neuropathol Exp Neurol* 46:556, 1987.
168. Vazuex R, Cumont M, Girard PM et al: Severe encephalitis resulting from coinfection with HIV and JC virus, *Neurology* 40:944, 1990.
169. Wiley CA, Grafe M, Kennedy C, Nelson JA: Human immunodeficiency virus (HIV) and JC virus in acquired immunodeficiency syndrome (AIDS) patients with progressive multifocal leukoencephalopathy, *Acta Neuropathol* 76:338, 1988.
170. Laughon BE, Druckman DA, Vernon A et al: Prevalence of enteric pathogens in homosexual men with and without acquired immunodeficiency syndrome, *Gastroenterology* 94:984, 1988.
171. Anthony MA, Brandt LJ, Klein RS et al: Infectious diarrhea in patients with AIDS, *Dig Dis Sci* 33:1141, 1988.
172. Rene E, Marche C, Regnier B et al: Intestinal infections in patients with acquired immunodeficiency syndrome: a prospective study in 132 patients, *Dig Dis Sci* 34:773, 1989.
173. Smith PD, Quinne TC, Strober W et al: Gastrointestinal infections in AIDS, *Ann Intern Med* 116:63, 1992.
174. Friedman SL: Gastrointestinal and hepatobiliary neoplasms in AIDS, *Gastroenterol Clin North Am* 17:465, 1988.
175. Schneiderman DJ: Hepatobiliary abnormalities of AIDS, *Gastroenterol Clin North Am* 17:615, 1988.
176. Comer GM, Mukherjee S, Scholes JV et al: Liver biopsies in the acquired immune deficiency syndrome: influence of endemic disease and drug abuse, *Am J Gastroenterol* 84:1525, 1989.
177. Cello JP: Acquired immunodeficiency syndrome cholangiopathy: spectrum of disease, *Am J Med* 86:539, 1989.
178. Bach N, Theise ND, Schaffner F: Hepatic histopathology in the acquired immunodeficiency syndrome, *Semin Liver Dis* 12:205, 1992.
179. Kahn E, Greco MA, Daum F et al: Hepatic pathology in pediatric acquired immunodeficiency syndrome, *Hum Pathol* 22: 1111, 1991.
180. Lebovics E, Thung SN, Schaffner F et al: The liver in the acquired immunodeficiency syndrome: a clinical and histologic study, *Hepatology* 5:293, 1985.
181. Hoda SA, White JE, Gerber MA: Immunohistochemical studies of human immunodeficiency virus-1 in liver tissues of patients with AIDS, *Mod Pathol* 4:578, 1991.
182. Anderson DW, Virmani R: Cardiac pathology of HIV disease. In Joshi VV, editor: *Pathology of AIDS and other manifestations of HIV infection,* New York, 1990, Igaku Shoin.
183. Beschorner WE, Baughman K, Turnicky RP et al: HIV-associated myocarditis: pathology and immunopathology, *Am J Pathol* 137:1365, 1990.
184. Dworkin BM, Antonecchia PP, Smith F et al: Reduced cardiac selenium content in the acquired immunodeficiency syndrome, *J Parenter Enteral Nutr* 13:644, 1989.
185. Bharati S, Joshi VV, Connor EM et al: The conduction system in children with AIDS, *Chest* 96:406, 1989.
186. Joshi VV, Pawel B, Connor E et al: Arteriopathy in children with AIDS, *Pediatr Pathol* 7:261, 1987.
187. Kure K, Park YD, Kim TS et al: Immunohistochemical localization of an HIV epitope in cerebral aneurysmal arteriopathy in pediatric acquired immunodeficiency syndrome (AIDS), *Pediatr Pathol* 9:655, 1989.
188. Park YD, Belman AL, Kim TS et al: Stroke in pediatric acquired immunodeficiency syndrome, *Ann Neurol* 28:303, 1990.
189. Joshi VV: Pathology of childhood AIDS, *Pediatr Clin North Am* 38:97, 1991.
190. Joshi VV, Oleske JM: Pulmonary lesions in children with acquired immunodeficiency syndrome: a reappraisal based on data in additional cases and follow-up study of previously reported cases, *Hum Pathol* 17:641, 1986.
191. Joshi VV: Pathologic findings associated with HIV infection in children. In Pizzo PA, Wilfert CM, editors: *Pediatric AIDS: the challenge of HIV infection in children and adolescents,* ed 2, Baltimore, 1994, Williams & Wilkins.
192. Joshi VV: Systemic lymphoproliferative lesions in children with AIDS, *Pediatr AIDS HIV Infect Fet Adoles* 1:44, 1990.
193. Travis WD, Fox CH, Devaney KO et al: Lymphoid pneumonitis in 50 adult patients infected with human immunodeficiency virus: lymphocytic interstitial pneumonitis versus nonspecific interstitial pneumonitis, *Hum Pathol* 23:529, 1992.
194. Papiernik M, Brossard Y, Mulliez N et al: Thymic abnormalities in fetuses aborted from human immunodeficiency virus type 1 seropositive women, *Pediatrics* 89:297, 1992.
195. Joshi VV, Oleske JM: Pathologic appraisal of the thymus gland in acquired immunodeficiency syndrome, *Arch Pathol Lab Med* 109:142, 1985.
196. Joshi VV, Oleske JM, Saad S et al: Thymus biopsy in children with acquired immunodeficiency syndrome, *Arch Pathol Lab Med* 110:837, 1986.
197. Baird DB, Joshi VV: Pathology of thymus. In Moran C, editor: *Synopsis of AIDS pathology in children,* Washington, DC, 1995, Armed Forces Institute of Pathology.
198. Joshi VV, Oleske JM, Connor EM: Morphologic findings in children with AIDS: pathogenesis and clinical implications, *Pediatr Pathol* 10:155, 1990.
199. Seemayer TA, Laroche AC, Russo P et al: Precocious thymic involution manifested by epithelial injury in AIDS, *Hum Pathol* 15:469, 1984.
200. Prevot S, Audouin J, André-Bougaran J et al: Thymic pseudotumorous enlargement due to follicular hyperplasia in a human immunodeficiency virus sero-positive patient: immunohistochemical and molecular biologic study of viral infected cells, *Am J Clin Pathol* 98:420, 1992.
201. D'Agati V, Suh J-I, Carbone L et al: Pathology of HIV-associated nephropathy: a detailed morphologic and comparative study, *Kidney Int* 35:1358, 1989.
202. Rao TKS, Friedman EA, Nicastri AD: The types of renal disease in the acquired immunodeficiency syndrome, *N Engl J Med* 316:1062, 1987.
203. Cohen AH, Nast CC: HIV-associated nephropathy: a unique combined glomerular, tubular, and interstitial lesion, *Mod Pathol* 1:87, 1988.
204. Chander P, Soni A, Suri A et al: Renal ultrastructural markers in AIDS-associated nephropathy, *Am J Pathol* 126:513, 1987.
205. Bourgoignie JJ, Pardo V: HIV associated nephropathies, *N Engl J Med* 327:729, 1992.
206. Tsang K, Kneafsey P, Gill MJ: Primary lymphoma of the kidney in the acquired immunodeficiency syndrome, *Arch Pathol Lab Med* 117:541, 1993.

Pediatric AIDS; laboratory issues

207. Lyman WD, Soelro R, Rahsbaum WK: HIV-1 infection of human fetal central nervous system tissue. In Kozlowski PB, Snider DA, Vietze PM, Wisniewski HIM, editors: *Brain in pediatric AIDS,* Basel, 1990, Karger.
208. Decker MD, Schaffner W: Risk of AIDS to health care workers, *JAMA* 256:3264, 1986.
209. Nelsing S, Nielsen TL, Nielsen JO: Occupational blood exposure among health care workers: II. Exposure mechanisms and universal precautions, *Scand J Infect Dis* 25:199, 1993.
210. Centers for Disease Control and Prevention: Guidelines for prevention of transmission of human immunodeficiency virus and hepatitis B virus to health-care and public-safety workers, *MMWR* 38 (S-6):1, 1989.
211. Geller SA: Autopsy, *Sci Am* 248:124, 1983.
212. Geller SA: The autopsy in acquired immunodeficiency syndrome: how and why, *Arch Pathol Lab Med* 114:324, 1990.
213. Geller SA, Gerber MA: Guidelines for high risk autopsy cases. In Peters HJ, Hutchins GM, editors: *Autopsy performance and reporting,* Skokie, Ill, 1990, College of American Pathologists.
214. Wilkes MS, Fortin AH, Felix JC et al: Value of necropsy in acquired immunodeficiency syndrome, *Lancet* 2:85, 1988.
215. Stein M, O'Sullivan P, Wachtel T et al: Causes of death in persons with human immunodeficiency virus infection, *Am J Med* 93:387, 1992.
216. Geller SA: HIV and the autopsy, *Am J Clin Pathol* 94:487, 1990.
217. Farizo KM, Buehler JW, Chamberland ME et al: Spectrum of disease in persons with human immunodeficiency virus infection in the United States, *JAMA* 267:1798, 1992.
218. Joshi VV: Pathologic surveillance of pediatic HIV infection: importance of biopsies and autopsies, *Pediatr AIDS HIV Infect Fet Adoles* 1: 9, 1990.
219. Hirsch MS, D'Aquila RT: Therapy for human immunodeficiency virus infection, *N Engl J Med* 328:1686, 1993.
220. Letvin NL: Vaccines against human immunodeficiency virus—progress and prospects, *N Engl J Med* 329:1400, 1993.
221. Selik RM, Chu SY, Buehler JW: HIV infection as leading cause of death among young adults in US cities and states, *JAMA* 269:2991, 1993.

29 Transplantation Pathology

George E. Sale
Dale C. Snover
Stanley J. Radio

BACKGROUND

Although successful organ transplantation was first accomplished in the 1950s, it was not until the past decade that transplantation became a major therapy for end-stage diseases. Improved methods of organ procurement and preservation, improved techniques for determining histocompatibility, and new immunosuppressive drugs to minimize allograft rejection have all fostered the growth of this field. The organs that are commonly transplanted are summarized in Table 29-1. The increased use of transplantation has fostered the development of organized networks to recruit organ donors, though unfortunately, for many diseases the availability of organs remains a limiting factor.

Information provided by the pathologist and laboratory is essential for a successful transplant program. During the initial patient evaluation a biopsy of the failing organ is essential to determine when and if transplantation is warranted. Next, the laboratory is essential in matching the blood types and, when appropriate, histocompatibility of tissues between donor and recipient. Before transplantation, many organs are histologically assessed to verify that the organ is viable and undamaged. Finally, after transplantation, ongoing histopathologic evaluation may be needed to monitor for rejection, as well as other complications such as infection, vascular insufficiency, drug toxicity, or recurrent disease.[1]

Several factors are common to all organ transplants, such as the genetics of transplantation, rejection, and other complications.[2] A discussion of these general processes follows.

Genetics of transplantation

Allograft rejection is a major limiting factor in transplantation. Basic to the discussion is the concept that the immune system plays a central role in distinguishing self from nonself tissues. The gene complex that is most involved in this process in humans is the major histocompatibility complex (MHC), part of the immunoglobulin supergene family on chromosome 6 that is involved in immune surveillance. The protein products of the MHC function as self-recognition molecules. These molecules trigger T-dependent immune response against foreign antigens, as discussed in Chapter 25. Three distinct classes of molecules are produced by the MHC. Class I molecules, designated HLA, HLA-B, and HLA-C, are present on all nucleated cells. Class II molecules are designated HLA-DR, HLA-DQ, and HLA-DP. The expression of class II is limited to B-cells, cells of the mononuclear/macrophage lineage, endothelial cells, and activated T-cells. Class II molecules can

Infection

The immunosuppression that makes transplantation possible also renders the recipient susceptible to bacterial, fungal, viral, and protozoal organisms. *Candida* spp., *Aspergillus* spp., cytomegalovirus, herpes simplex virus, and *Pneumocystis carinii* are among organisms that occur at high frequency in these patients. Virtually any organisms can be a pathogen in the immunocompromised individual; thus the term *opportunistic pathogen* is used descriptively.

SKIN GRAFTS

Skin grafting has been important for burn therapy and to provide insight into transplantation immunology.[6] The ability to grow confluent epidermal cell cultures with the help of epidermal growth factors provides new opportunities. Wounds have been covered with autologous epidermis grown in dishes. Studies of the basic biology of epidermal stem cells, hair follicles, and techniques such as skin explants and organotypic cultures containing both dermis and epidermis have injected new hope and vitality into the field. Understanding of how best to replace epidermal and adnexal stem cells after injury will flow from such research.

Full-thickness skin grafts contain the dermis and epidermis. Split-thickness grafts are shaved by a special instrument and contain only epidermis and papillary dermis for the most part with some of the hair follicular bulbs presumably left behind. Most experiments in rejection have been MHC-incompatible combinations. In these models the clear primary target of the most vigorous reaction has been the endothelial cells of the dermal vessels. If severe enough to obliterate the vessels, this reaction obviously is capable of causing an infarct as the vessels become coagulated. A clear secondary target, however, to which less attention has been paid, is the epidermal cell. Infiltrates of mononuclear cells certainly occur in both sites. Immunohistologic studies of these reactions have shown that the prominent lymphoid cell in endothelium is the $CD4^+$ lymphocyte whereas in the epidermis it is the $CD8^+$, or killer T-cell. This finding has great interest when the results compared to those of GVHD, where the pairing of donor and host is made much closer. There the endothelium may be a lesser or equal target compared to the epithelial cell, but the most frequently found T-cell type in the epidermis is the $CD8^+$, or killer, T-cell just as in skin graft rejection. Similarly, it is interesting to notice that just as in other areas such as bone marrow transplantation, the strong preference is for autologous grafting, whenever possible, because the whole problem of allograft reactions can be conveniently sidestepped in those clinical settings. In the usual skin graft situation, burn therapy, the commonest major clinical problems are related to infections and their sequelae.

KIDNEY TRANSPLANTATION

Background

On a numerical basis, kidney transplantation is the most common solid-organ transplant procedure in the United States. This reflects both the high incidence of end-stage renal disease, principally attributable to a common disease, diabetes mellitus, and the explosion of knowledge that has occurred in transplantation immunology.[7] Kidney transplantation, first performed in 1954,[8] served as an early model for understanding the immunopathologic mechanisms of allograft rejection and therapies that could prolong graft survival. The seminal work, both clinical and experimental, performed over many years, culminated in a Nobel Prize for Dr. Joseph E. Murray[9] in 1990 (shared with E.D. Thomas for his work in marrow transplantation). Most transplanted kidneys are derived from cadaveric donors (80%), whereas 20% are donated by relatives of the recipient.

The extent to which allograft biopsy has been used to monitor organ function or dysfunction has varied during different decades. In the 1970s and early 1980s, allograft biopsy was rarely performed because it was believed that laboratory tests could provide adequate monitoring of the graft without the potential complications of renal allograft biopsy. Current thinking, however, indicates that the information gained from allograft biopsy outweighs the potential complications, which are quite minimal, typically including hematuria or hemorrhage. A variety of tests of the urine or blood have been proposed to monitor the allograft, but none has proved as reliable or accurate as kidney biopsy.[10]

Cytologic methods of evaluating renal transplants include fine-needle renal aspiration and urinalysis to quantitate and characterize lymphocytes in the graft and urine. Although these methods are used to assess graft rejection at several transplant centers,[11] the majority of institutions rely on biopsy morphology.

The major indication for renal allograft biopsy is dysfunction of the allograft. Causes for allograft dysfunction are multiple and often depend on the interval after transplantation at which the dysfunction occurs. Soon after transplantation, the major causes of dysfunction are related to inadequate graft perfusion before transplantation, intraoperative or postoperative ischemia, both of which can cause acute tubular necrosis, or hyperacute rejection. Later on, acute or chronic allograft rejection, infections and immunosuppressive nephrotoxicity may necessitate biopsy in the weeks, months, or years that follow. Because the treatment for each of these conditions differs, renal biopsy provides valuable information in determining therapy.

Handling of the renal biopsy

Obtaining optimal information from a biopsy requires careful handling of the tissue, preserving appropriate portions for light microscopy, immunofluorescence, immunohistochemical examination, and, on occasion, electron microscopy. Ideally the biopsy is divided in such a way that glomerular tissue is available for each technique.

Hyperacute rejection

Hyperacute rejection, as its name implies, occurs soon after transplantation. The process is well understood from an immunopathologic view point, as preformed recipient circulating cytotoxic antibodies cause vascular injury to the graft with ensuing acute inflammation and necrosis. In the early history of transplantation, an association was noted between this lesion and antibodies against ABO antigens or HLA class I antigens of the donated organ.[12] More recently, recipient antibodies against graft vascular endothelial antigens may induce similar lesions.[13] Now, the incidence of hyperacute rejection has decreased considerably as pretransplant tissue typing has become standard practice.

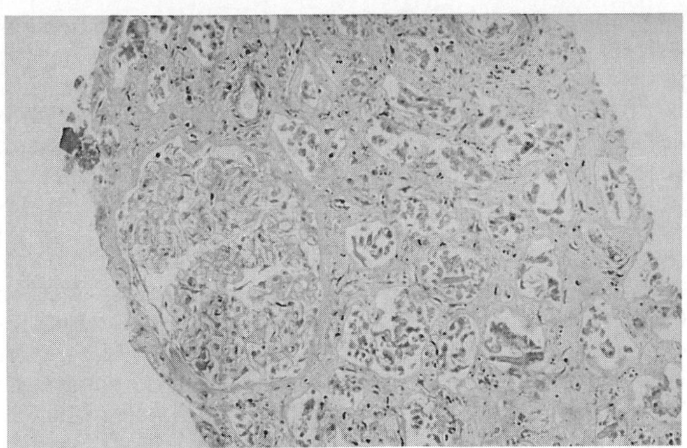

Fig. 29-1 Percutaneous renal biopsy illustrating cortical necrosis.

Clinical criteria

The manifestation of hyperacute rejection is the abrupt loss of renal function. Often, this will occur intraoperatively or within minutes, hours, or days after a vascular anastomosis has been established.

Histopathology

Immunofluorescent studies demonstrate fibrin and antibodies, usually IgM and complement, bound to glomeruli and vascular endothelial cells, the primary targets. Antibody, capable of fixing complement, results in an acute inflammatory reaction with a diffuse accumulation of polymorphonuclear cells within the graft. Activation of the coagulation cascade can also ensue, causing platelet and fibrin thrombi of glomeruli with hemorrhage and ischemic cortical necrosis (Fig. 29-1). Muscular arteries may feature thrombi or acute necrosis.

Because the clinical picture is quite characteristic, there are few diagnostic considerations. Perfusion injury, or acute infarction caused by vascular thrombosis, may cause microvascular thrombosis that resembles hyperacute rejection.

Acute rejection

Acute rejection is pathogenetically more complex than hyperacute rejection. Acute rejection may be mediated by either T-cell (acute cellular rejection) or humoral (acute vascular-humoral rejection) mechanisms, which respectively have a strong influence on the tubulointerstitium or vascular structures. The composition of its inflammatory infiltrate is diverse, generally an admixture of polymorphonuclear cells, lymphocytes, and plasma cells. The classification for acute rejection is provided in Table 29-2.

Clinical features

The clinical manifestations of acute rejection are protean, emerging from weeks to years after transplantation. Patients with acute rejection have a progressive or rapid decline in urine output and a rise in serum creatinine. The graft may be tender because of edema. Some patients have incurred acute rejection years after transplantation, consequential to cessation of immunosuppressive therapy.

Pathologic features

Acute cellular tubular rejection. The dominating feature of acute cellular tubular rejection, the most common form of rejection, is a tubulointerstitial infiltrate of mononuclear inflammatory cells. Within the interstitium, especially perivascularly, lymphocytes, transformed lymphocytes, plasma cells, and macrophages are present. The tubules are infiltrated by lymphocytes (tubulitis), a process termed *emperipolesis* (Fig. 29-2). This leads to tubular necrosis (Fig. 29-3) and, if the process is not arrested, the loss of tubular mass and interstitial fibrosis (Fig. 29-4). The degree of rejection may be quantitated as mild, moderate, or severe, with the latter showing severe tubulitis and perivascular aggregates.[14]

Table 29-2 Acute renal rejection

Acute vascular humoral rejection	Rare
Acute cellular tubular rejection	Common
Acute cellular interstitial rejection	Rare

There have been substantial efforts to correlate the nature of cellular infiltrates in acute cellular rejection with prognosis based on immunophenotyping. Studies have shown an absolute increase in the $CD8^+$ T-cells to be associated with acute cellular tubular rejection.[15]

Acute cellular interstitial rejection. A far less common type of acute rejection is termed *acute cellular interstitial rejection*. In this process there is an interstitial infiltrate dominated by $CD4^+$ lymphocytes and lesser numbers of polymorphonuclear leukocytes and eosinophils (Fig. 29-5). Because the infiltrate is purely interstitial, tubulitis is not a feature of this form of rejection.

Acute vascular rejection. The acute vascular type of rejection is an uncommon form of rejection, generally occurring 1 to 2 months after transplantation. Both antibody- and cell-mediated mechanisms are involved. The dominant feature is an endotheliitis and its extreme form, vasculitis, in which mononuclear cells infiltrate the vascular endothelium and walls of medium and large arteries. Mild cases are associated with endotheliitis in which both antibody and complement, as well as T-cells and macrophages, can be demonstrated in the endothelium (Figs. 29-6 and 29-7). In severe cases, fibrinoid necrosis or transmural destruction of the vascular wall by

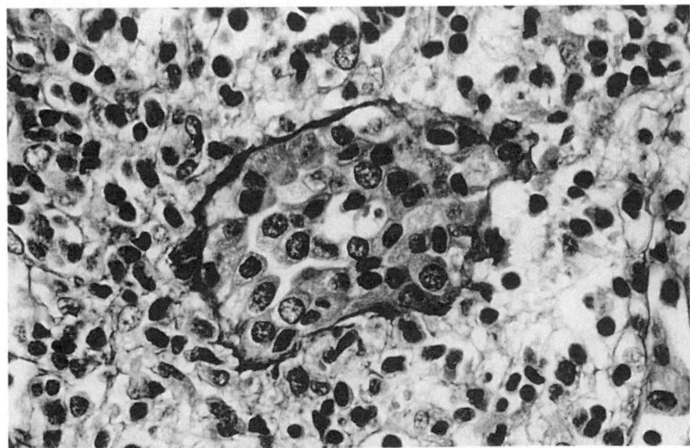

Fig. 29-2 Acute tubulitis featuring tubular infiltration by lymphocytes and intense interstitial mononuclear cell infiltration. (Jones silver stain.)

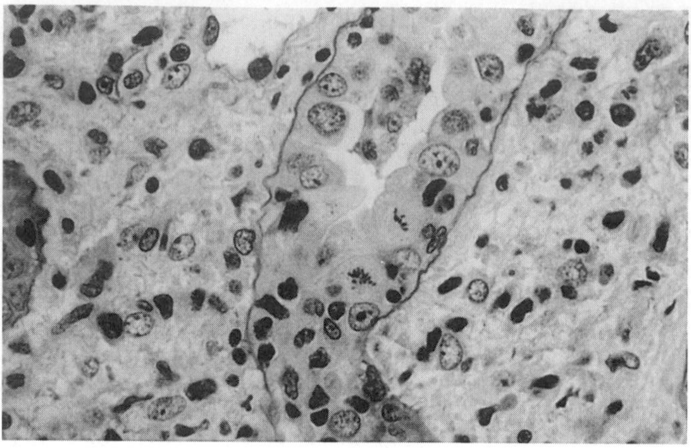

Fig. 29-3 Acute tubulitis with epithelial injury and attempted recovery manifest by mitoses. (PAS stain.)

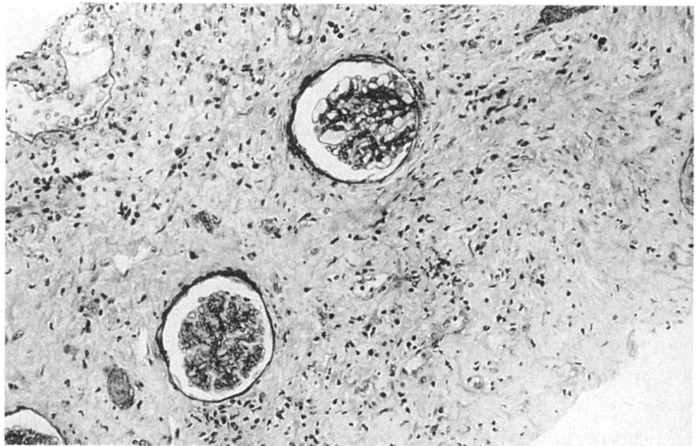

Fig. 29-4 Pronounced interstitial fibrosis, the consequence of the prolonged, cryptic renal tubular injury of acute cellular rejection. (PAS stain.)

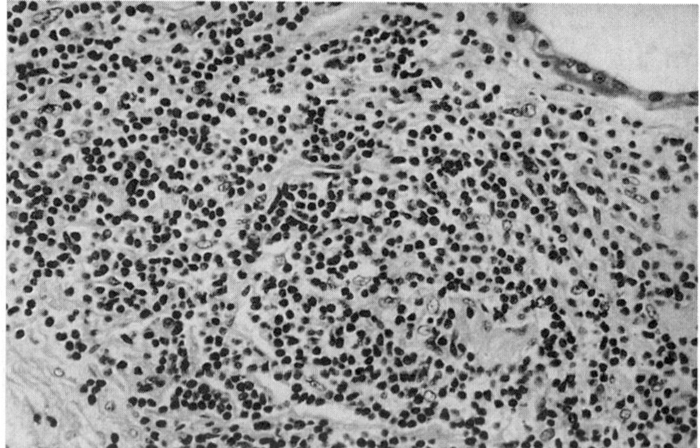

Fig. 29-5 Pronounced acute interstitial cellular renal rejection. (PAS stain.)

macrophages and neutrophils leads to vascular necrosis, a picture akin to polyarteritis nodosa or Wegener's granulomatosis (Fig. 29-8).

Complicating the evaluation of acute allograft rejection is the notion that each of the major types of acute rejection can occur independently, or in combination with each other. As well, tubular damage or ischemia (unrelated to rejection) may also occur in acute rejection, the extreme manifestation of which being frank acute tubular necrosis (Figs. 29-9 and 29-10). The glomeruli are not totally spared in acute rejection because they may rarely be infiltrated by inflammatory cells (glomerulitis) and undergo thrombosis or necrosis. If vascular lesions are extensive, glomeruli may incur ischemia and become contracted, with reduction of their capillary lumens and wrinkling of their basement membranes.

There are several considerations in the differential diagnosis of acute cellular rejection. A variety of drugs may trigger acute interstitial inflammation: infection by either cytomegalovirus or bacterial organisms can evoke inflammatory responses that resemble acute tubulointerstitial rejection.

Chronic rejection

A gradual and progressive decline of renal function in the absence of specific causes that develops over months to years after transplantation is termed *chronic rejection*. This form of rejection constitutes a significant form of late graft loss. Although its pathogenesis is unclear, diverse forms of injury to nephrons and vascular structures are probably crucial in its development.

Atrophic lesions are visited upon the glomeruli and tubules stemming from ischemia attributed to vascular fibrosis and narrowing. The vascular lesions are not dissimilar to idiopathic arteriosclerosis (Fig. 29-11) or even the atherosclerosis that accompanies venous homografts in coronary bypass surgery. Tubular loss is accompanied by interstitial fibrosis and a modest infiltrate of Ig^+ plasma cells. Most authors attribute its pathogenesis to repetitive, cryptic episodes of acute rejection.

Transplant glomerulopathy

Long-term surviving allografts may develop gradual dysfunction with heavy proteinuria. The histologic features of transplant glomerulopathy are glomerular enlargement, proliferation of mesangial and endothelial cells, and variable deposition of IgM, C3, and fibrinogen within glomerular basement membranes. The lesion simulates Type I membranoproliferative glomerulonephritis (Fig. 29-12). The cause of this disorder is unknown, though some authors suggest a linkage to chronic rejection.

Nonrejection complications

Cyclosporin A nephrotoxicity

Cyclosporin A causes dose-dependent nephrotoxicity, manifested by elevated serum creatinine and decreased creatinine clearance. Several different forms of cyclosporin A nephrotoxicity have been identified.[16] *Acute cyclosporin glomerulopathy,* though uncommon, occurs early after transplantation, causing both thrombocytopenia and acute renal failure. Glomeruli are congested by a thrombotic angiopathy akin to that seen in the hemolytic uremic syndrome (Fig. 29-13). Histologically, hyperacute rejection, perfusion injury, disseminated intravascular coagulation or other conditions enter into

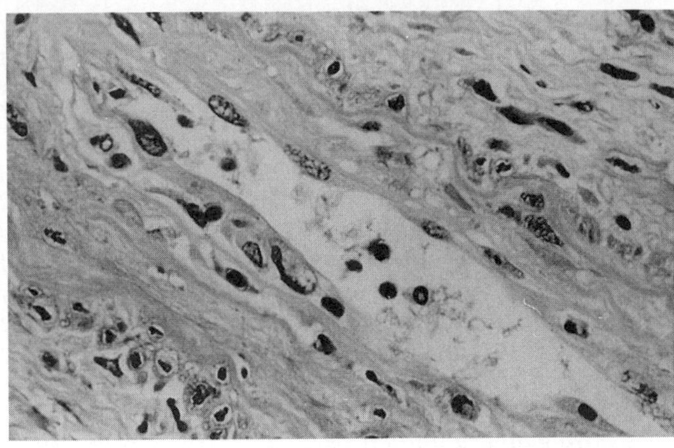

Fig. 29-6 Acute renal humoral rejection featuring subtle mononuclear cell infiltration of venule.

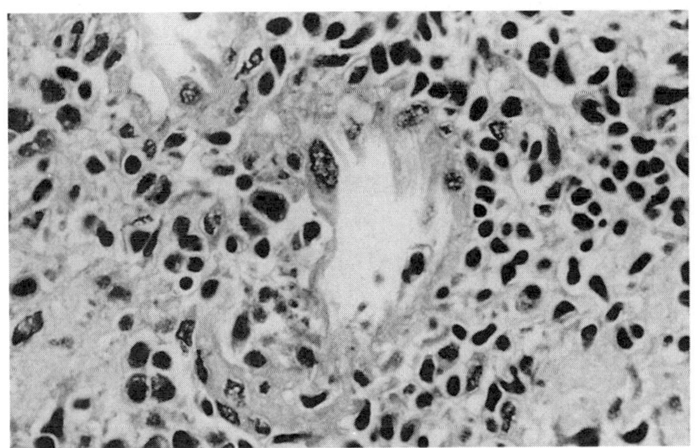

Fig. 29-7 Acute renal humoral rejection featuring intense mononuclear cell vascular infiltration and destruction.

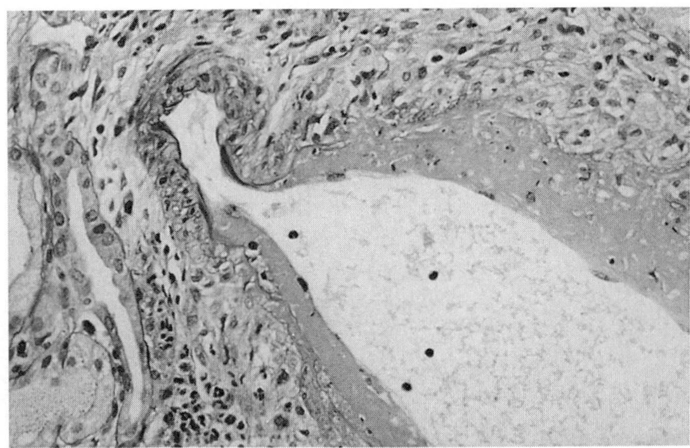

Fig. 29-8 Acute renal humoral rejection featuring fibrinoid necrosis of vessel wall. (PAS stain.)

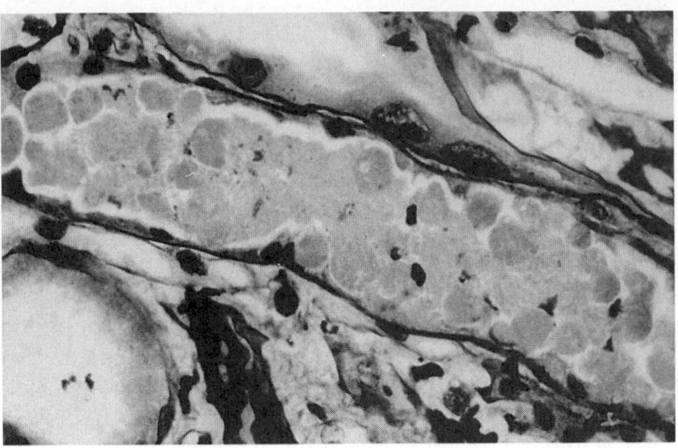

Fig. 29-9 Acute tubular necrosis illustrating tubular cast replete with necrotic cells. (Jones silver stain.)

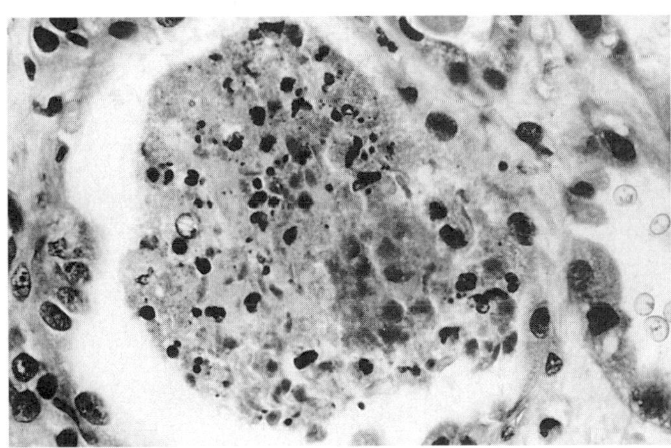

Fig. 29-10 Ectactic, severely injured renal tubule with cast of necrotic cells and debris.

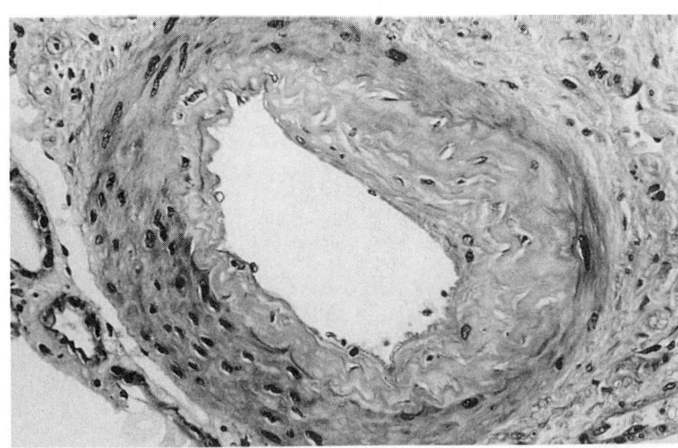

Fig. 29-11 Chronic renal rejection featuring extensive arterial subintimal and mural fibrosis.

the differential diagnosis. *Acute cyclosporin A tubulopathy with arteriolopathy* causes allograft dysfunction at any time after transplantation. Tubules (an infrequent target) are vacuolated and contain calcium crystals (tubulopathy); arterioles (a common target) feature luminal narrowings, myocyte necrosis, intramural protein (hyaline-like) deposits (Figs. 29-14 and 29-15), and even thrombi (arteriolopathy); there is patchy interstitial edema and an interstitial infiltrate of mononuclear cells. This infiltrate, along with an associated swelling of endothelial cells, makes acute cyclosporin A nephrotoxicity difficult to distinguish from acute rejection. The distinction is important, since the treatment for the two conditions is diametrically opposed: cessation or augmentation of cyclosporin A. Lastly, *chronic cyclosporin A nephropathology* features interstitial fibrosis, tubular atrophy, and a sparse mononuclear cell infiltration. The appearance resembles that of smoldering acute cellular rejection. Immunohistochemistry may be useful in discriminating acute cellular rejection from cyclosporin A toxicity. The former shows a predominance of $CD8^+$ T-lymphocytes. It is also possible to demonstrate cyclosporin A in the biopsy tissue by immunohistochemical labeling techniques.

Recurrent renal disease

Most patients who receive renal transplants do so for their chronic renal failure. In our experience, apart from diabetes mellitus, the underlying disease is frequently unknown. Diseases that are most common to recur in renal allografts are diabetic glomerulopathy, focal glomerular sclerosis, anti-GBM disease, membranoproliferative glomerulonephritis types I and II, IgA nephropathy, membranous glomerulonephritis, and hemolytic uremic syndrome. Curiously, the paradigm of autoimmune diseases systemic lupus erythematosus rarely recurs in the renal allograft. Possibly the immunosuppressive therapy given to stem allograft rejection affects the perturbed immunologic state of these patients.

De novo glomerulonephritis

Although any type of glomerulonephritis may develop de novo in the renal allograft, the most common to do so is membranous glomerulonephritis. Pathologically, the disease is identical to the primary idiopathic form by featuring the nephrotic syndrome, subepithelial deposits of IgG, IgM, and C3 and typical subepithelial electron-dense deposits on electron microscopy.

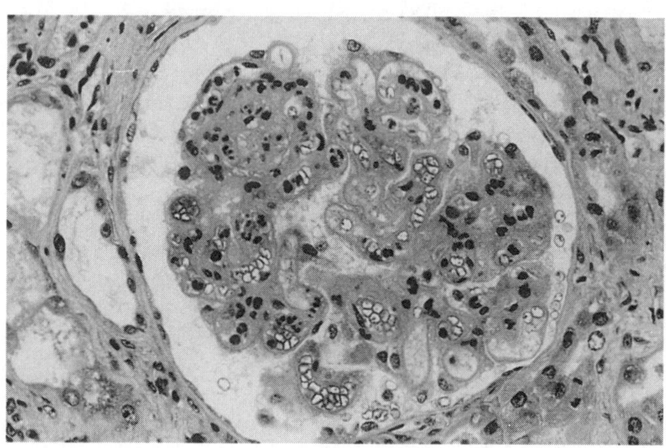

Fig. 29-12 Glomerulus featuring lobulation, mesangial and endocapillary proliferation, and thick basement membranes, reflecting transplant glomerulopathy.

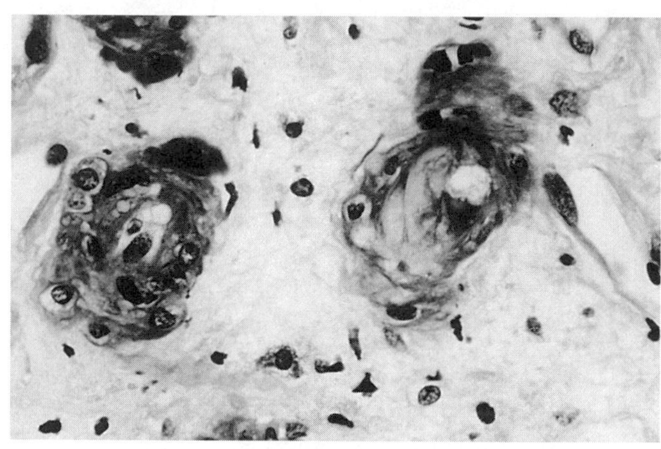

Fig. 29-14 Acute cyclosporin A nephrotoxicity, featuring arteriolar luminal narrowing and myocyte injury.

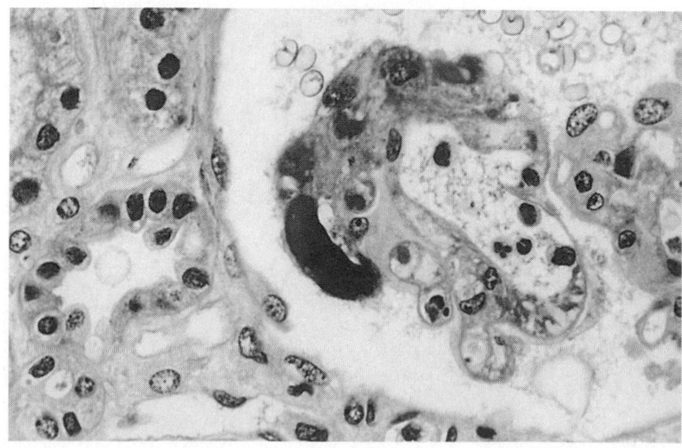

Fig. 29-13 Acute cyclosporin A toxicity, manifesting with glomerular thrombus formation.

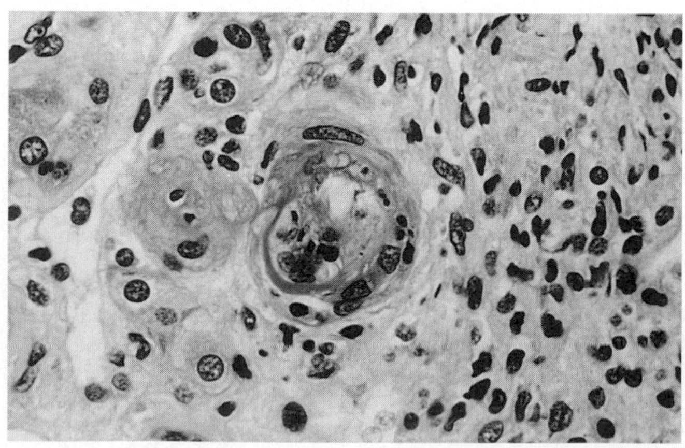

Fig. 29-15 Acute cyclosporin A toxicity, featuring arteriolar myocyte necrosis and hyaline replacement.

Infection

Among the many infections that may affect transplant recipients, cytomegalovirus (CMV) disease is among the most common. CMV may be acquired by a seronegative recipient receiving a new organ that harbors CMV. Alternatively, latent CMV may become reactivated in a seropositive individual. Whichever the case, diagnostic inclusions of cmv may sometimes be present in the renal biopsy.

LIVER TRANSPLANTATION

Nonrejection complications

Transplantation of the liver is one of the most complicated of all transplants. The transplanted organ is subject to technical complications, infections, drug reactions, and rejection[17-24] (Table 29-3).

Vascular anastomoses may be the source of complications, including *ischemia* related to thrombosis of the hepatic artery or portal vein anastomoses and *Budd-Chiari syndrome* related to obstruction at the suprahepatic inferior vena cava anastomosis. Biliary tract obstruction and biliary peritonitis and sepsis may follow stricture or breakdown of the bile duct anastomosis respectively. Although these complications tend to occur early after transplant, they may occur at virtually any time.

The transplanted liver is also prone to infections by the hepatotrophic viruses hepatitis B, C, and delta, opportunistic viruses (especially cytomegalovirus and Epstein-Barr virus), and fungi.[21] In addition, the liver is affected in bacterial sepsis, often causing cholestasis.[22,23]

Hepatotoxicity may result from the drugs routinely used in transplant patients.[24-29] These drugs, with their potential hepatotoxic effects, are listed in Table 29-4.

A potential complication of liver transplantation is recurrence of the disease that first necessitated transplantation. Diseases that may recur in the transplanted organ are listed in Table 29-5.

Hepatocellular carcinoma and cholangiocellular carcinoma recurs commonly. In some centers these diseases are a relative contraindication to transplantation.

The recurrence rate of certain diseases is controversial. The reported recurrence rate of primary biliary cirrhosis (PBC) varies substantially among transplant centers, with some reporting a high rate of recurrence, whereas others question if PBC ever recurs.[30,31] Overall, recurrent PBC is uncommon, though we do believe that it happens. Recent well-documented data would indicate a recurrence rate of 16%.[21a] However, accurate diagnosis of recurrence is hampered by the similarity of PBC to chronic rejection. Even those centers reporting a high incidence of recurrence do not indicate a high rate of graft loss because of this recurrence.

Hepatitis B and C recurs in approximately 80% to 100% of grafts in patients transplanted for chronic viral hepatitis–induced cirrhosis.[31,36] Hepatitis C seems not to carry a high risk of early graft loss, but recurrent hepatitis B causes graft loss in more than 25% of transplant recipients. A unique complication of recurrent hepatitis B is a subfulminant form of loss known as *fibrosing cholestatic hepatitis,* which is associated with a very heavy load of virus with the development of pericellular sinusoidal fibrosis (that is, fibrosis surrounding individual hepatocytes), cholestasis, and graft loss.[33,34] This type of hepatitis B has not been reported outside the context of liver transplantation. Other than this histologic pattern, recurrent hepatitis B or C appears morphologically similar to the disease in the nontransplanted livers.

Finally, rejection represents the unique pathologic state of the transplanted organ. The liver may manifest rejection in hyperacute, acute, or chronic form. There has been debate regarding the appropriateness of this terminology for the liver, with major criticism being made of the fact that these terms imply a temporal course of disease that may not be totally accurate. For example, acute rejection may occur several years after transplantation if the patient stops prophylactic immunosuppression. The alternative terms proposed include *humoral rejection* for hyperacute rejection, *cellular rejection* for acute rejection, and *ductopenic rejection* for chronic rejection. The first two of these terms are an attempt to apply terminology based on presumed mechanisms of rejection. Although accurate (at least for hyperacute rejection, which is by definition humorally mediated), these terms oversimplify the mechanisms, since there may well be a humoral mechanism to both acute and chronic rejection. This oversimplification renders the term *humoral rejection* ambiguous and the term *cellular rejection* somewhat misleading. Although ductopenic rejection describes one of the major histologic features of chronic rejection, it is neither a specific nor a definitional feature and hence offers no benefit over the term *chronic rejection,* with its

Table 29-3 Differential diagnosis of liver dysfunction after liver transplantation

Time period	Common diagnoses	Less likely diagnoses
First week	Technical problems (especially vascular anastomoses) Acute rejection Primary graft failure	Hyperacute rejection Drug reaction Opportunistic infection Chronic vascular rejection Vanishing bile duct syndrome
1 week to 2 months	Acute rejection Opportunistic infection Drug reaction Technical problems (especially biliary anastomosis)	
2 months and beyond	Chronic vascular rejection Vanishing bile duct syndrome Recurrence of original disease Transfusion-related viral infections (hepatitis B or C)	Acute rejection Drug reaction Opportunistic infection Technical problems

From Snover DC: The liver biopsy in transplantation. In Snover DC: *Biopsy diagnosis of liver disease*, Baltimore, 1992, Williams & Wilkins.

Table 29-4 Drugs commonly administered to transplant patients and their reported hepatotoxicity

Drug	Effect
Cyclosporin A	Cholestasis
Azathioprine	Cholestatic hepatitis Venoocclusive disease Peliosis hepatis
Corticosteroids	Fatty change Sinusoidal dilatation Nodular regenerative hyperplasia
Trimethoprim-sulfamethoxazole	Hepatitis Cholestatic hepatitis
Penicillin and derivatives	Hepatitis Cholestatic hepatitis
Cephalosporins	Hepatitis (uncommon) Cholestatic hepatitis (uncommon)
Amphotericin	Sinusoidal dilatation Nodular regenerative hyperplasia Hepatitis (uncommon)
Ketoconazole	Hepatitis Cholestatic hepatitis
Fluconazole	Rare hepatitis (one case)
Hyperalimentation preparations	Cholestatic hepatitis Portal fibrosis with obstructive features Central ballooning degeneration

From Snover DC: Drug-induced liver disease. In Snover DC: *Biopsy diagnosis of liver disease*, Baltimore, 1992, Williams & Wilkins.

implication of irreversibility. For consistency sake, the classical terms seem acceptable given that they are generally understood by clinicians and do not presuppose mechanisms or histologic features as part of the definition.

Management of rejection requires accurate diagnosis, which usually requires core needle biopsy of the organ. In many centers protocol liver biopsy specimens are taken at predetermined intervals after transplantation to identify rejection before its clinical symptoms. If such protocol biopsy specimens are used, the pathologist must follow stringent diagnostic criteria to avoid overdiagnosis of rejection and adverse effects caused by overexcessive immunosuppression. Alternatively, liver biopsy may be reserved for transplant patients showing signs of organ dysfunction. There are no data to support one approach over the other. Fine-needle aspiration biopsy has been recommended by some as useful in the diagnosis of rejection.[40-42] The utility of this approach remains to be determined.

Hyperacute rejection

Hyperacute rejection of the liver is uncommon, compared to the frequency of hyperacute rejection in other organs.[43,44] This is believed to be attributable to the size and functional reserve of the liver and to the sinusoidal architecture that limits ischemia in the face of focal thrombosis. Nevertheless, hyperacute rejection can occur in transplant recipients with preexisting antibodies. These patients manifest poor graft function immediately after transplantation, with eventual loss of graft caused by ischemic necrosis. The histologic features include arteritis and a neutrophilic infiltrate with zonal or diffuse hepatocellular necrosis. Several animal models exhibit a relatively bland, hemorrhagic necrosis as a manifestation.[45,46] Bland necrosis in the immediate postoperative period does occasionally occur in the human allograft. The exact cause is usually undetermined and therefore such cases are often diagnosed as *primary graft failure*.[47,48]

Table 29-5 Recurrence of disease after liver transplantation

Diseases that recur commonly
Viral hepatitis B, C, delta
Malignancy
Diseases that recur uncommonly
Primary biliary cirrhosis
Autoimmune hepatitis
Primary sclerosing cholangitis
Budd-Chiari syndrome

Acute rejection

Acute rejection is a potentially reversible form of cell-mediated rejection. The reported incidence varies from less than 50% to more than 90% of graft recipients.[17,49-51] The diagnosis of rejection may be based on biopsy morphology or combination of biopsy morphology and clinical symptoms. Lower incidence would be expected when both features are required for diagnosis, and the higher incidence when biopsy morphology is the only diagnostic criterion. The latter situation may lead to overimmunosuppression and increased problems with infection.

Clinical signs of acute rejection are nonspecific, such as fever, mental status changes, and decreased bile output. Although there are abnormalities of hepatic enzymes, no laboratory finding is a specific marker of rejection. Therefore the biopsy remains the standard for diagnosis. In general, treatment of acute rejection should not commence without biopsy confirmation of rejection, or at least of the absence of other significant pathologic conditions, which may be causing the liver dysfunction.

The targets of acute rejection are bile ducts and vascular endothelium[17,49-51] (Figs. 29-16 and 29-17). The diagnostic triad of acute rejection is a portal inflammatory lymphoid infiltrate, bile duct damage, and endotheliitis (inflammation of vascular endothelium). The infiltrate always contains lymphocytes, and eosinophils are nearly always present. Neutrophils may also be present, but plasma cells are usually absent. Hepatocellular necrosis and inflammation are not typical of rejection, though severe rejection may cause central ischemic necrosis. The severity of bile duct and vascular damage is variable.

Up to now, consensus has not been reached on a grading system for acute rejection. Most cases of acute rejection respond well to therapy, regardless of the degree of inflammation. Several grading systems have been proposed, though most have not been demonstrated to be reproducible or to have clinical significance. One system is based on the findings that loss of interlobular bile ducts, arteritis, or ischemic central necrosis are associated with a poor outcome and graft loss.[52] Therefore, these findings are indicative of severe acute rejec-

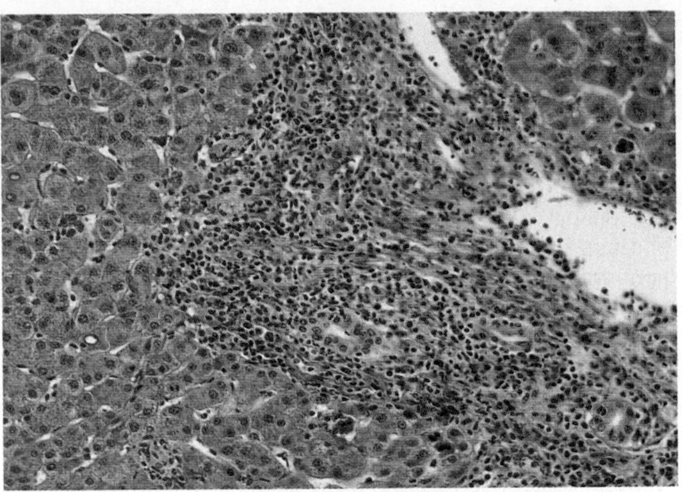

Fig. 29-16 Acute liver rejection portal changes.

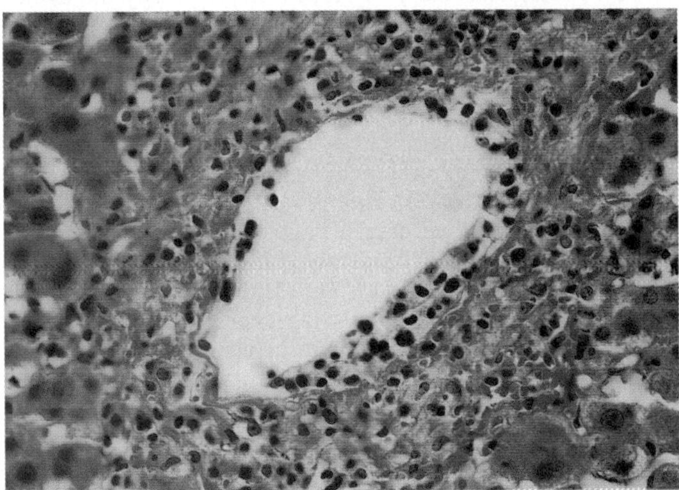

Fig. 29-17 Acute liver rejection with endotheliitis.

tion. Most other grading systems also use extensive necrosis as a marker of severe rejection.[49,53] Mild and moderate rejection are separated on the basis of degree of bile duct damage. One illustrative grading system is summarized in Table 29-6.[54]

As mentioned above, most cases of acute rejection respond well to increases in immunosuppression. However, some subsets develop extensive loss of interlobular bile ducts or progress to chronic vascular rejection. Monitoring of therapy by repeat biopsy is recommended to detect such progression, as well as to allow weaning of immunosuppression as rapidly as possible as improvement occurs.

Chronic rejection

Chronic rejection of the liver results in irreversible damage and organ failure. Although this definition is understandable, it is difficult to determine when liver damage is irreversible. There is no temporal significance to the term *chronic*, because histologic manifestations can appear as early as 1 month, or as long as years after transplantation. The incidence of chronic rejection ranges from 6% to 20% in different centers.[55] Synonyms for chronic rejection include *ductopenic rejection* and the *vanishing bile duct syndrome*,

Table 29-6 University of Minnesota grading system for liver rejection

Diagnosis	Histologic features
Consistent with, not diagnostic of rejection	Lymphocytic or mixed portal infiltrate, < 50% damaged bile ducts, no endotheliitis
Acute rejection, grade 1	As above, with endotheliitis
Acute rejection, grade 2	Lymphocytic or mixed portal infiltrate, > 50% damaged bile ducts, with or without endotheliitis
Acute rejection, grade 3	Acute rejection plus arteritis, paucity of bile ducts, or central hepatocellular ballooning with confluent dropout of hepatocytes

Modified from Snover, Freese DK, Sharp HL, *Am J Surg Pathol* 11:1, 1987.

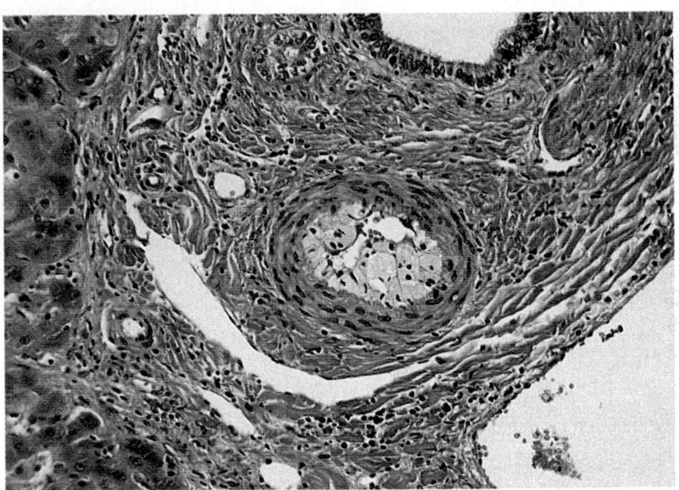

Fig. 29-18 Chronic vascular rejection of the liver vascular changes.

though neither term offers significant advantages over chronic rejection.

Two histologic patterns occur in chronic rejection, differing by the presence or absence of vascular obliteration.[56] In general there has not been a systematic attempt to separate these types, though in our experience they predict different clinical outcome.

Chronic vascular rejection has an obliterative endarteritis that is similar to that seen in many organ allografts[56-59] (Fig. 29-18). This arteritis, in turn, leads to ischemic damage of the liver and eventual liver failure. The specific immunopathologic mechanism of chronic rejection is unknown. Reported risk factors include previous acute rejection, CMV infection, positive crossmatch, and MHC matching at class II with mismatch at class I.[56,60,61] Of these, only prior acute rejection is the risk factor that is widely accepted. There is dispute regarding the role of HLA matching and CMV infection.[62] The significance of CMV infection is particularly intriguing, given its association with chronic cardiac rejection and atherosclerosis.[63,64]

The clinical manifestation of chronic vascular rejection is a gradual and inexorable deterioration of liver function charac-

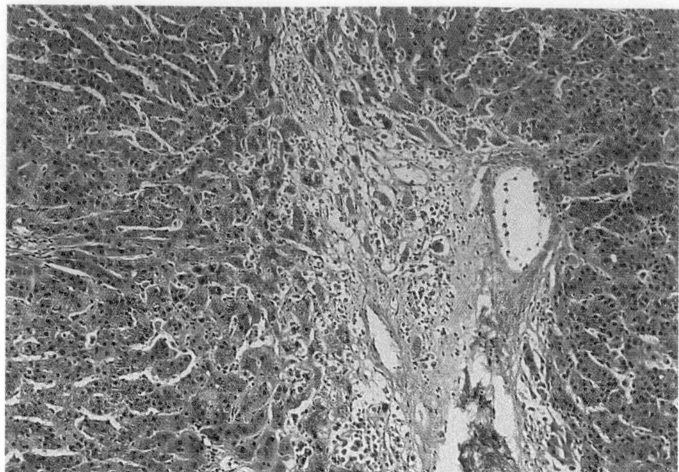

Fig. 29-19 Chronic vascular rejection, ischemic biopsy.

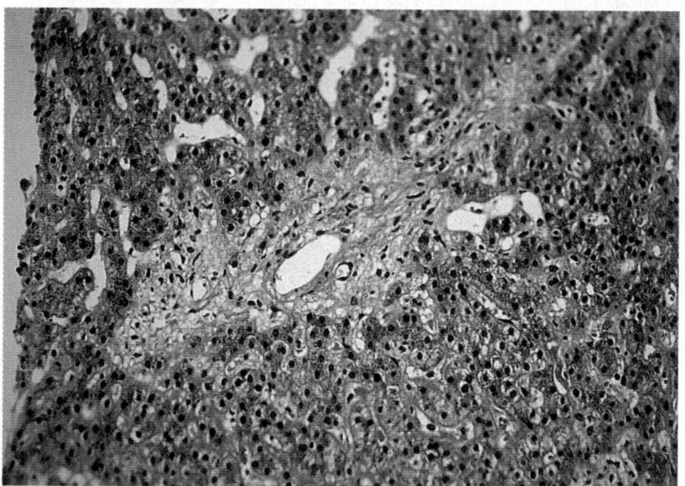

Fig. 29-20 Vanishing bile duct syndrome in hepatic rejection.

terized by increased serum concentration of hepatocellular and biliary enzymes and bilirubin. Terminally the liver fails to synthesize enzymes and other proteins. Death ensues unless retransplantation is performed. Biopsy features of chronic rejection are nonspecific and are manifest as central ischemic changes often associated with loss of interlobular bile ducts (Fig. 29-19). Since the arteries affected by the process are almost never seen in needle biopsy, the diagnosis always requires clinicopathologic correlation and evaluation for other technical causes of ischemic liver damage.

A second form of "chronic rejection" has been described, and it does not have a vascular component.[56,58] This form, which as been variously labeled as *pure vanishing bile duct* syndrome, or *progressive rejection with paucity of ducts*, is characterized by near-total loss of interlobular bile ducts, without the ischemic changes seen in the vascular form of chronic rejection (Fig. 29-20). The major clinical manifestation is elevated bilirubin. There is minimal elevation of hepatocellular enzymes and no loss of synthetic function. Despite the designation as "chronic rejection," many of these cases seem to be reversible, though the time to reversal may be as much as 1 year.[56,65,66] This type of rejection has not been so well recognized or characterized as the vascular form, but in some reports it does not seem to have the same association with CMV as the vascular form.[56]

HEART TRANSPLANTATION

Background

The operative procedure of heart transplantation is less complicated than liver transplantation, and so technical complications are relatively uncommon.

The major pathologic consideration is rejection, though infections with CMV or *Toxoplasma* organisms are a consideration. Recurrence of primary disease is rare, though, as described below, chronic rejection has some similarities to native atherosclerosis and has been termed by some authors as *accelerated atherosclerosis*.

Most centers performing heart transplants monitor the graft by protocol biopsies. This practice has derived from the belief that cardiac rejection is often clinically silent, necessitating biopsy to diagnosis early rejection. As previously mentioned, protocol biopsies require strict criteria to avoid overdiagnosis and overimmunosuppression. A somewhat philosophic discussion that has been debated in the heart literature is that of the histologic definition of rejection. Some contend that any infiltrate in the transplanted heart constitutes rejection, though not all cases of rejection by this definition require treatment. Others have argued that rejection should be diagnosed only if treatment is deemed necessary. Philosophical arguments aside, this debate has led to considerable differences in the reported incidence of acute rejection from less than 30% in some institutions to over 90% in others. In general, both philosophies appear to provide similar levels of patient care, since survival figures from most large centers are comparable.

Acute rejection

Acute cardiac rejection is generally thought of as a cell-mediated, potentially reversible condition. A form of acute rejection without a cellular infiltrate of the myocardium has been reported, though the frequency of this phenomenon is controversial.[73]

The clinical features of acute cellular rejection vary from subtle cardiac enlargement, electrocardiographic abnormalities, and decreased ejection fraction to frank cardiac failure. Because many of the findings are subtle or require radiologic study, protocol biopsy provides a useful monitor. With appropriate therapy, most cases of acute rejection resolve, though some patients will die from acute heart failure.

The diagnosis of acute rejection requires a heart biopsy. The rejecting heart contains an interstitial infiltrate of lymphocytes, with or without myocyte damage or necrosis (Fig. 29-21). Although this histologic picture is characteristic of rejection, it is nonspecific because it occurs in other types of myocarditis. As a practical matter, however, other forms of myocarditis are rarely, if ever, seen in the transplanted heart.

As previously discussed, some pathologists will diagnose rejection only when treatment is deemed appropriate, whereas others diagnose rejection at a more subtle state and treat only rejection, which they categorize as "moderate" rather than "mild." These philosophical differences aside, it is clear that not all inflammation of the heart requires augmented immunosuppression.[67-71] Therefore, some categorization of the degree of rejection is necessary to determine the need for therapy. In the past, numerous grading schemes have been proposed for this purpose; the most widely used in the United States was

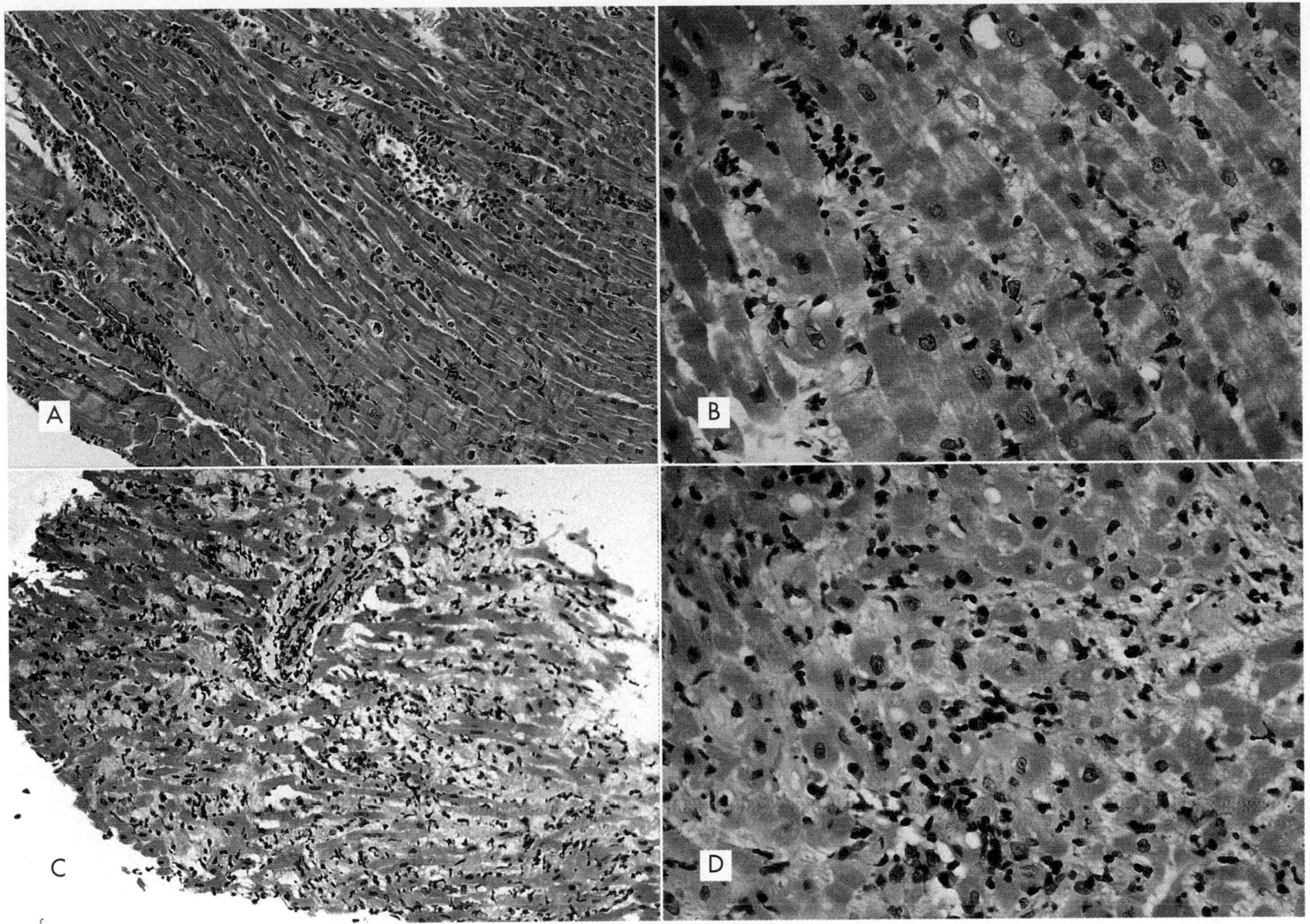

Fig. 29-21 Several views of acute heart rejection. **A,** Multifocal infiltrants of mononuclear cells are evident at low magnification. **B,** These cells are interposed between cardiac myocytes. **C,** At low magnification interstitial edema may also be evident. **D,** Necrosis of cardiac myocytes is evident in severe acute heart rejection.

devised by Margaret Billingham at Stanford University. Because of the need for transplant centers to compare data accurately, a consensus system for grading inflammation in a biopsy was proposed in 1990.[72] The details of this system are shown in Table 29-7.

In essence, the degree of inflammation is used to guide therapy. Focal mild (grade 1A) inflammation manifests as one or two foci of perivascular infiltrates, is usually inconsequential, and does not require increased immunosuppression. Many cases of grade 1B, 2, and perhaps even some 3A are also inconsequential, but these degrees of inflammation require close correlation with clinical parameters and evaluation of sequential biopsy specimens to evaluate progression or regression of inflammation. Most patients having biopsies with grade 3B and essentially all patients with grade 4 inflammation have cardiac dysfunction and require treatment.

A somewhat controversial type of acute rejection has been referred to as *acute humoral rejection*, to distinguish it from hyperacute rejection, which is also humorally mediated.[73] In acute humoral rejection a cellular infiltrate is not present in the endomyocardial biopsy. There may be some endothelial swelling and edema, though these changes are usually subtle. The diagnosis is made by the finding of immunoglobulin on the endothelial surfaces. In some series, up to 20% of hearts are reported to demonstrate humoral rejection, though many

Table 29-7 Acute cardiac rejection grading system

Grade	Description
0	No rejection
1A	Focal (perivascular or interstitial infiltrate) without necrosis
1B	Diffuse but sparse infiltrate without necrosis
2	One focus only with aggressive infiltration or focal myocyte damage, or both
3A	Multifocal aggressive infiltrates or myocyte damage, or both
3B	Diffuse inflammatory process with necrosis
4	Diffuse aggressive polymorphous infiltrate with myocyte necrosis, or edema, or hemorrhage, or vasculitis, or all signs

Modified from Billingham ME, Cary NRB, Hammond ME et al: *J Heart Transplant* 9:587, 1990.

centers have not reported this phenomenon. The death rate is high as well, requiring aggressive therapy. If heart failure occurs in a patient whose biopsy specimen is essentially unremarkable, additional tissue should be obtained for appropriate immunofluorescence studies.

Chronic rejection

Chronic rejection is an insidious process characterized by concentric narrowing of the coronary arteries[67,74-76] (Fig. 29-22). The intima may contain foamy histiocytes, smooth muscle cells, or fibroblasts. This arteriopathy differs from typical atherosclerosis because it is concentric, rather than eccentric, and it involves the artery in a continuous and diffuse rather than patchy or focal manner and affects the smallest branches of the artery. For these reasons, it is difficult to detect the development of this process on a single arteriogram. Therefore serial arteriograms are useful to allow comparison of the diameter of the vessels over time. Newer techniques such as intravascular ultrasound and coronary angioscopy hold considerable promise to provide earlier and more dependable detection of this transplant arteriopathy. The endomyocardial biopsy is of little use in detection of chronic rejection, though occasionally ischemic changes to the myocardium will be evident, and some authors suggest a correlation with thickening of intramural arterioles on biopsy and arteriopathy of epicardial arteries.

Clinically, patients with chronic rejection are often asymptomatic until sudden death as a result of a massive ischemic event. It is probable that denervation of the heart, as part of the routine transplant process, minimizes clinical symptoms at an earlier stage. If detected by serial arteriograms, retransplantation can be performed before this terminal event.

Technical problems

The major technical problems related to heart transplant pathology are those related to biopsy interpretation, rather than technical causes of dysfunction. Major among these are biopsy-site changes, perioperative ischemic events, and the Quilty effect.[67-69]

Because biopsy specimens are taken routinely from the ventricular septum and near the apex of the right ventricle and because the right ventricular cavity contour tends to guide the bioptome to the same region, over time there is an increased probability of sampling the site of a previous biopsy. Early on, these sites contain active fibroblastic proliferation associated with a mixed inflammatory infiltrate and later by dense fibrosis with a lymphocytic infiltrate (Fig. 29-23). Since biopsy sites are almost always *inflamed,* they are not appropriate tissue for evaluation of rejection and thus should be ignored in the evaluation process.

Ischemia after transplantation may result from perioperative ischemia, acute vascular (humoral) rejection, or chronic vascular rejection. In general, perioperative ischemia results in small areas of necrosis that may be mistaken for rejection though their focality and mixed nature of the associated infiltrate with a relative paucity of lymphocytes usually allows distinction.

The so-called *Quilty effect* is one of the most interesting aspects of heart transplantation in the cyclosporin A era. This phenomenon, named after the first patient in whom it was noted, manifests as a dense subendocardial accumulation of small lymphocytes (Fig. 29-24). Although it may be seen in conjunction with rejection, it is not in and of itself a form of treatable rejection that requires additional immunosuppression. Its appearance after the introduction of cyclosporin A was suggestive that it may represent a form of cyclosporin A

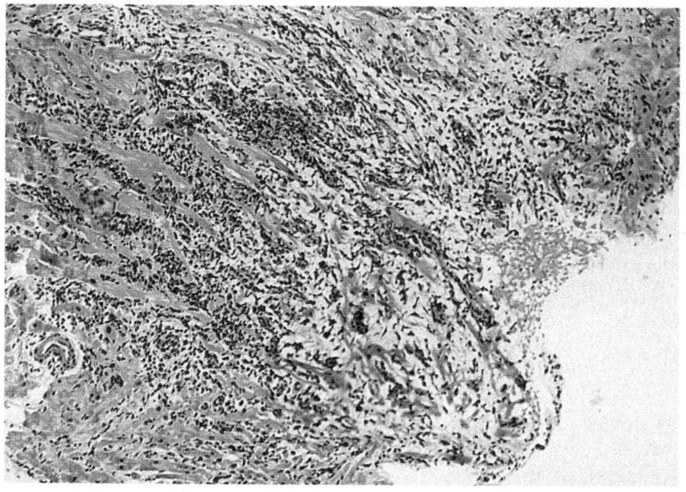

Fig. 29-23 A previous biopsy site showing inflammation in the heart.

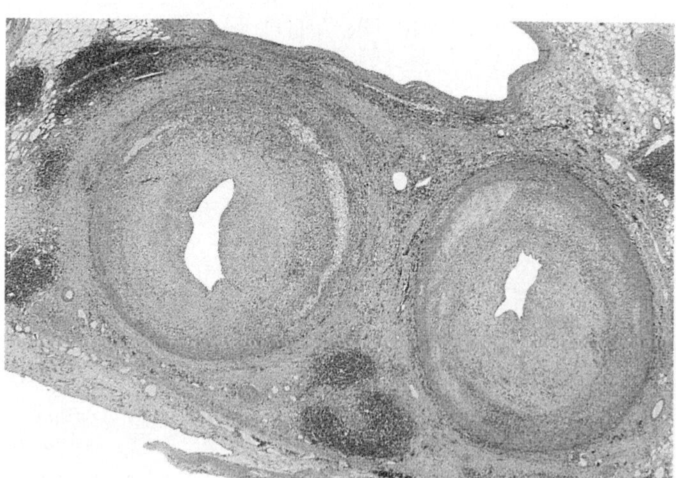

Fig. 29-22 Chronic vascular rejection of the heart.

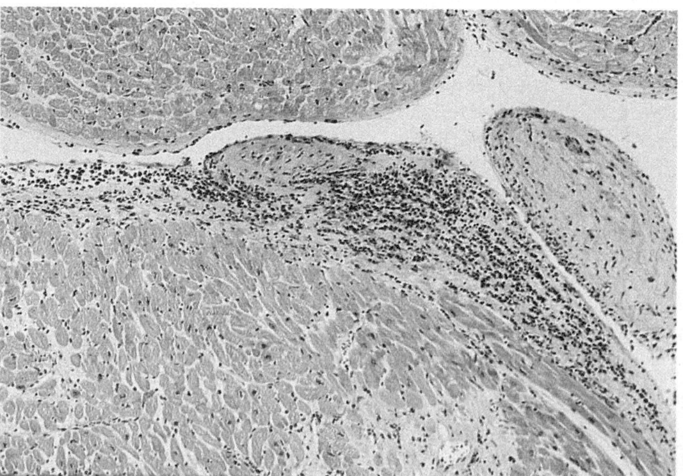

Fig. 29-24 Quilty effect manifested by dense subendocardial accumulation of small lymphocytes.

toxicity, though more recently the possibility that it represents a form of inhibited rejection has been raised.[70] Its major importance, however, is in not misinterpreting it as treatable rejection or as an immunoproliferative process.

Infections

Infections of the transplanted heart are unusual. Rarely CMV inclusions are encountered. Even more rarely, toxoplasmosis is identified by its characteristic intracytoplasmic organism. In both of these infections there is likely to be disseminated disease at the time the organism is noted in the heart.

LUNG AND HEART-LUNG TRANSPLANTATION

Background

Lung transplantation and combined heart-lung transplantation are relatively recent procedures. Although in the initial years the heart-lung transplant was preferred because of the simplicity of the procedure, the number of single and double lung transplants performed has been increasing.[77,78]

It was originally proposed that heart biopsy would be a useful tool to monitor the lung in combined heart-lung transplant. However, the lung appears to be more susceptible to rejection than the heart, necessitating transbronchial lung biopsy. Many institutions perform protocol lung biopsies, but since precise diagnostic criteria for lung rejection have not been developed, the diagnosis rests on a combination of clinical and histologic parameters. Other considerations in evaluation of the lung biopsy specimen include infection, especially with opportunistic viruses and *Pneumocystis carinii* (Chapter 49), procedure-related preservation damage and nonspecific interstitial inflammation.[79]

Acute rejection

Acute rejection affects 40% to 75% of lung transplant recipients. The symptoms of fever, dyspnea, and cough are often accompanied by bilateral infiltrates on chest x-ray film. Because these findings are nonspecific and are identical to those of pulmonary infection, lung biopsy is necessary to confirm the diagnosis.

The histology of acute rejection is a perivascular lymphocytic infiltrate that may extend into the adjacent interstitium as the disease progresses[77,80-82] (Fig. 29-25). A prerequisite for accurate diagnosis is the presence of vessels in the biopsy. Any specimen without adequate vessels is inadequate for diagnosis. In early acute rejection the infiltrate may be patchy and inconspicuous. During progression of rejection, the infiltrate becomes more intense and diffuse, eventually extending into the lung interstitium. Severe rejection is characterized by a more polymorphous infiltrate, which may be accompanied by hemorrhage and intra-alveolar fibrinous exudate. In addition to the perivascular infiltrate one may see infiltration of vascular endothelium (endotheliitis) and peribronchial inflammation.

A grading system for rejection similar to that developed for the heart has recently been devised.[83] The features of this system are shown in Table 29-8. The prognostic significance of this system has not yet been determined.

Chronic rejection

Chronic rejection of the lung affects approximately 25% to 70% of patients. Because the usual result is death, or loss of graft, it is a major impediment to lung transplantation.[77,84-86] The clinical

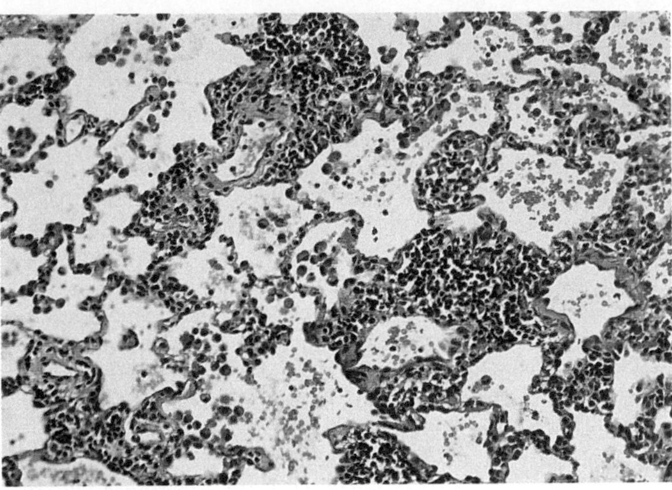

Fig. 29-25 Acute lung rejection

Table 29-8 Acute pulmonary rejection grading system

A. ACUTE REJECTION
0. GRADE 0—no significant abnormality
1. GRADE 1—Minimal (difficult to find perivenular mononuclear infiltrate)
   a. with bronchiolar inflammation
   b. without bronchiolar inflammation
   c. with large airway inflammation
   d. no bronchioles present
2. GRADE 2—Mild (easily found perivenular, predominantly mononuclear cell infiltrate)
   a. with bronchiolar inflammation
   b. without bronchiolar inflammation
   c. with large airway inflammation
   d. no bronchioles present
3. GRADE 3—Moderate (as grade 2 with interstitial infiltrates)
   a. with bronchiolar inflammation
   b. without bronchiolar inflammation
   c. with large airway inflammation
   d. no bronchioles present
4. GRADE 4—Severe (as grade 3 with alveolar injury—fibrin membranes, exudates)
   a. with bronchiolar inflammation
   b. without bronchiolar inflammation
   c. with large airway inflammation
   d. no bronchioles present

B. ACTIVE AIRWAY DAMAGE WITHOUT SCARRING (in the absence of pulmonary rejection)
1. Lymphocytic bronchitis
2. Lymphocytic bronchiolitis

C. CHRONIC AIRWAY REJECTION
1. Bronchiolitis obliterans, subtotal
   a. active
   b. inactive
2. Bronchiolitis obliterans, total
   a. active
   b. inactive

D. CHRONIC VASCULAR REJECTION

Modified from Yousem SA, Berry GJ, Brunt EM et al: *J Heart Transplant* 9:593,1990.

symptom is progressive shortness of breath. This reflects the characteristic pathologic feature of fibrous obliteration of small respiratory airways, a process known as *obliterative bronchiolitis* (Fig. 29-26). Because small airways are affected, the major findings on pulmonary function tests are those of reduced forced vital capacity and forced expiratory volume and flow.[85-87] The biopsy diagnosis is complicated by the patchy nature of the inflammation and by the difficulty in sampling distal airways by the transbronchial route. Nevertheless, given sufficient tissue and repeat biopsy, diagnosis is usually possible.

In addition to the bronchial changes, vascular obliteration similar to other transplanted organs may occur in chronic lung rejection. Because ischemia appears less important than airway obstruction, the vascular lesion is less often identified. We have not seen it on biopsy though it has been seen in resected lungs and at autopsy. In addition to the changes of chronic rejection, there are often changes of residual acute rejection as well. In general, bronchiolitis obliterans does not respond to therapy.

Technical problems

The major technical problems after lung transplantation are reimplantation response, perioperative hemorrhage, and dehiscence of the bronchial anastomoses.[77] The latter two complications require surgical intervention and are usually diagnosed clinically rather than by biopsy.

The *reimplantation response* refers to a decreased pulmonary function in the immediate postoperative period associated with impaired ventilation, decreased compliance, and edema. The histologic features are dilated lymphatics and edema, occasionally with a neutrophilic inflammation. This is believed to be the result of surgical trauma, ischemia, severing of lymphatics during the procedure, and possibly reperfusion injury.

Infections

More than most transplanted organs, transplanted lungs are susceptible to infections.[77,78] Bacteria account for 50% of infections, followed by viruses (especially CMV, HSV, and EBV), *Pneumocystis carinii,* and fungi. The general topic of pulmonary infection is covered in Chapter 49, but several comments regarding the differentiation of rejection from infection are in order. First, rejection and infection are not mutually exclusive diagnoses. They may occur simultaneously, or infection may affect a patient during increased immunosuppression for rejection. Second, some organisms, including cytomegalovirus and *P. carinii,* may cause mild perivascular infiltrates that will mimic mild rejection.[79] Therefore, caution must be exercised in diagnosing rejection if one of these infections is present. In general, mild rejection should be ignored in this context, at least until the infection is successfully treated.

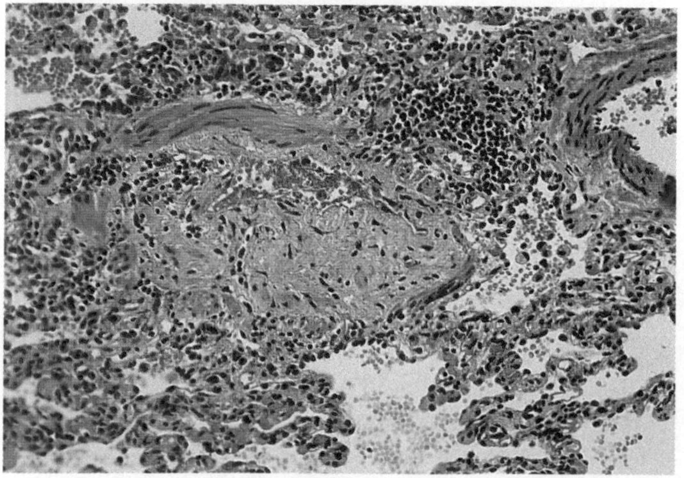

Fig. 29-26 Lung rejection in the form of obliterative bronchiolitis.

PANCREAS TRANSPLANTATION

Background

Diabetes mellitus afflicts approximately 5% of the general population and is currently the third most common disease and the eighth leading cause of death in the United States.[88] Pancreas transplantation offers effective therapy for diabetes mellitus by (1) achieving insulin independence by restoring normal insulin production, (2) gaining superior metabolic control by normalizing glucose homeostasis, and (3) preventing (and perhaps reversing) the progressive complications of diabetes mellitus.[89,90] The pancreas may be transplanted with a kidney (combined pancreas-kidney) or alone (solitary pancreas). Combined pancreas-kidney transplantation is a viable treatment of the type 1 diabetic patient with significant nephropathy who can tolerate the operation, postoperative immunosuppression, and possible associated complications. The specific selection criteria for solitary-pancreas transplantation are not yet established. Ideally, solitary-pancreas transplantation would precede the development of diabetic complications. However, reliable markers do not exist to predict when diabetic patients will develop such complications.

Since the first human pancreas transplant in December 1966, over 4000 pancreas transplants have been performed worldwide.[91] Approximately 70% of these have been combined pancreas-kidney transplants to address concurrent renal failure of diabetics, and the remaining 30% were equally divided among nonuremic diabetics receiving a solitary-pancreas transplant, and diabetics with a functioning kidney transplant who subsequently receive a pancreas allograft. Most North American transplant centers use *whole-organ vascularized pancreas transplantation*, with the duodenal segment draining into the urinary bladder. Alternative techniques include *whole-organ pancreaticoduodenal transplantation with enteric drainage, segmental-pancreas transplantation with pancreatic duct injection,* and *segmental-pancreas transplantation with either enteric or bladder drainage*. For the pathologist, the significance of these procedures lies in the options provided for assessment of graft-rejection and the associated complications that may require diagnostic evaluation.

Whole-organ pancreas transplantation has the advantages of a greater islet cell mass, a lower risk of thrombosis because of improved blood flow, and a reduced incidence of pancreatitis or fistulas. The major advantage of bladder drainage is direct access to exocrine secretions for monitoring of pancreas allograft function, whether by chemical tests of urine, urine sediment cytology tests, or cystoscopic needle biopsy. The disadvantages of bladder drainage include urologic problems (hematuria, urine leaks, cystitis, urethral stricture, or disruption, lower urinary tract infections, and stone formation), metabolic problems (dehydration, metabolic acidosis, and erythrocytosis), and reflux-associated hyperamylasemia, or pancreatitis.

Islet cell transplantation, though in its developmental stages, offers the potential advantages of a low-morbidity surgical procedure and in the future the potential to alter the antigenic potential of the islets so that they may be transplanted without immunosuppression. The most popular technique of islet cell transplantation is by intraportal injection through a cutdown of the falciform ligament with cannulization of the umbilical vein. Current roadblocks to successful islet cell transplantation include efficient isolation and purification, cell preservation, identification of the optimal site of transplantion, prevention and detection of rejection, recurrent autoimmune disease, or functional deterioration, and islet cell supply.[92]

Acute rejection

The susceptibility of pancreas allografts to rejection is unknown. Studies of rejection in recipients of combined pancreas-kidney transplant recipients indicate that the manifestations of renal allograft rejection usually precede those of pancreas rejection.[93-96] Rejection is probably initiated in parallel when both organs are from the same donor, but the clinical manifestations of kidney rejection are detected earlier. Whether this disparity in kidney and pancreas allograft rejection is attributable to inherent differences in organ susceptibility to rejection, anatomic differences in vascularization (lower blood flow in the pancreas), differential exocrine and endocrine sensitivity to rejection, or the accuracy of currently available tests of pancreatic function, is unknown. Among patients undergoing combined pancreas-kidney transplantation the overall patient and graft survival rates are 91% and 75% respectively.[91]

Table 29-9 Diagnosis of pancreas allograft rejection

Serologic parameters
Endocrine (glucose, insulin, C-peptide, glucagon, pancreatic polypeptide, provocative tests)
Exocrine (immunoreactive anodal trypsin, pancreatic specific protein, secretory trypsin inhibitor, amylase, lipase, bicarbonate, zinc)
Immune (β_2-microglobulin, interleukin-2 receptor, neopterin, immunoreactive thromboxane B_2, prostaglandin E_2, C-reactive protein, platelet-activating factor)
Pancreatic juice and urinary parameters
Endocrine (insulin)
Exocrine (amylase, lipase, pH, zinc, trypsinogen)
Immune (β_2-microglobulin, interleukin-2 receptor, neopterin, HLA-DR antigen, thromboxane B_2, prostaglandin E_2)
Nonivasive imaging
Ultrasonography
Radionucleide perfusion scan
Platelet-labeling scan
Nuclear magnetic resonance
Position-emission tomography
Histopathology
Open biopsy
Percutaneous needle core biopsy
Percutaneous fine-needle aspiration biopsy
Cystoscopically directed biopsy (bladder drainage)
Endoscopically directed biopsy (enteric drainage)
Cytology
Pancreatic juice
Urine (bladder drainage)
Fine-needle aspiration

Modified from Stratta RJ: *Transplant Pathology,* 1994, ASCP Press.

Unfortunately, patients receiving solitary-pancreas transplant experience irreversible pancreas allograft rejection at a much higher rate, leading to a 20% to 30% reduction in overall graft survival.[91] The prediction of rejection episodes in recipients of solitary-pancreas allografts remains difficult because measurement of concurrent renal rejection is not an option.[93-97]

Clinical criteria

Pancreas rejection is often subtle. During pancreas allograft rejection patients will often experience fever, leukocytosis, ileus, allograft swelling and tenderness, and abdominal pain. Differentiation from pancreatitis is difficult because none of these features are consistently present or pathognomonic of rejection.[93-96]

Several tests are being investigated as potential early markers of rejection (Table 29-9). Serologic assays of exocrine or metabolic function that may allow prediction of pancreas rejection are limited. In general, serum amylase concentrations do not correlate well with allograft rejection. Although hyperamylasemia is common early after pancreas transplantation, this is only rarely attributable to rejection.[97-100] Hyperglycemia is a valid but delayed and often the terminal indicator of pancreas allograft rejection, both experimentally and clinically. Because the exocrine pancreas is more sensitive to rejection than the endocrine pancreas, a reduction in exocrine function often precedes the onset of hyperglycemia. Measurement of serum anodal trypsinogen and pancreatic specific protein as early serologic markers for pancreas rejection have been encouraging.[101,102]

A theoretical advantage of pancreatic duct drainage into the urinary tract is the ability to monitor directly exocrine function such as urinary amylase concentrations. When expressed per unit of time, this value consistently decreases before hyperglycemia, though the dilutional effects associated with diuresis can occasionally interfere with the accurate diagnosis of rejection. Some investigators base the diagnosis of pancreas rejection on the decreased excretion of urinary amylase.[96]

Histopathology

Despite persistent efforts to develop reliable noninvasive markers for pancreas rejection, histopathologic examination of the pancreas remains the only definitive method of diagnosing rejection. When allograft dysfunction occurs, a specimen from an open biopsy readily distinguishes rejection from other causes of pancreas allograft dysfunction[96,103] (Table 29-10). In

Table 29-10 Differential diagnosis of pancreas allograft dysfunction

Rejection: acute or chronic
Vascular thrombosis or insufficiency
Pancreatitis
Ischemic injury
Immune mediated
Infection (CMV)
Reflux
Duct occlusion
Chronic
Exocrine leakage
Sepsis
Insufficient islet cell mass
Recurrent diabetes
Drug toxicity (diabetogenic effect)

Modified from Stratta RJ: In *Transplant Pathology,* 1994, ASCP Press.

Table 29-13 Comparison of findings in duodenal allografts and in jejunal tissue used in segmental pancreatic transplants

	Epithelial necrosis	Crypt loss	Reactive atypia	Intrepithelial inflammation	Villous atrophy	Nerve inflammation	Muscle inflammation
Jejunal tissue	2	0	1	3	0	1	2
Duodenal allograft	6	8	9	9	7	6	8
p value (χ^2)	0.31	0.0065	0.012	0.11	0.015	0.12	0.087

Modified from Nakhlen RE, Gruesner RWG, Tzardis PJ et al: *Clin Transplant* 5:242, 1991.

Table 29-14 Comparison of features in duodenal allograft tissue corresponding to pancreases with and without acute rejection

	Epithelial necrosis	Crypt loss	Reactive atypia	Intraepithelial inflammation	Villous atrophy	Nerve inflammation	Muscle inflammation
Duodenal tissue from pancreases with acute rejection ($n = 9$)	6	7	7	7	6	6	7
Duodenal tissue from pancreases *without* acute rejection ($n = 5$)	0	1	2	2	1	0	1
p value (χ^2)	0.064	0.13	0.41	0.41	0.26	0.064	0.13

Modified from Nakhlen RE, Gruesner RWG, Tzardis PJ et al: *Clin Transplant* 5:242, 1991.

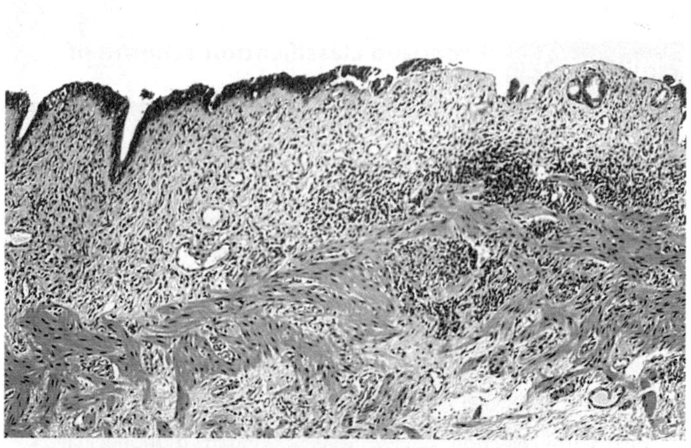

Fig. 29-29 Cystoscopic needle biopsy of duodenal mucosal cuff of pancreas allograft with features of acute rejection including mononuclear cell infiltrate, villous blunting, crypt cell necrosis, and endotheliitis.

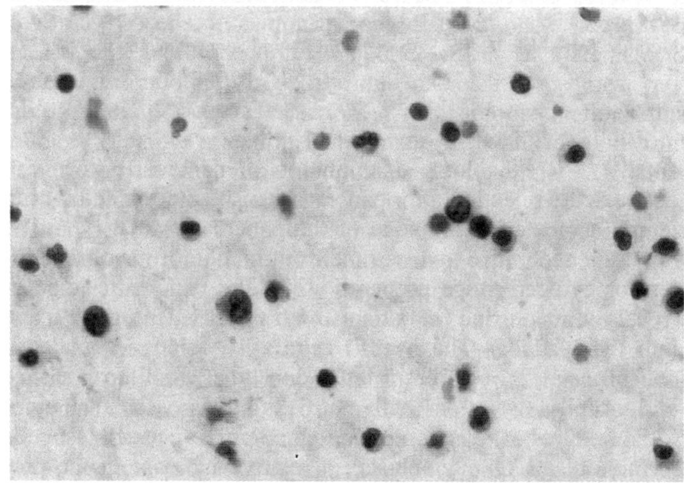

Fig. 29-30 Urine cytology from bladder-drained pancreas allograft with lymphocyturia including lymphoblasts representing acute rejection.

(because of lymphocyturia), respectively, the cytologic findings of rejection. In addition, stringent conditions of collection and handling are necessary to prevent cellular degeneration, which can limit proper evaluation. In both pancreas and renal transplant recipients urine cytology has little value in detecting chronic vascular rejection or acute cellular rejection that occurs late (greater than 6 months after transplantation).[119] Urine cytologic monitoring is a useful noninvasive method of detecting acute rejection as a sensitive screening test to indicate optimal timing for performing confirmatory cystoscope-directed core biopsies.

Chronic rejection

Chronic rejection manifests histologically as dense mononuclear cell infiltrates, acinar cell loss and fibrosis, and intimal hyperplasia and luminal narrowing of small to medium-sized arteries that often leads to thrombosis[103,107] (Fig. 29-32). To distinguish chronic rejection from chronic pancreatitis requires previously documented acute rejection or chronic vascular changes. The vascular changes in chronic pancreas rejection are morphologically similar to the transplant arteriopathy of cardiac, renal, and hepatic allografts. Medium-sized arteries have an intima thickened by lipids and proteoglycans, contain-

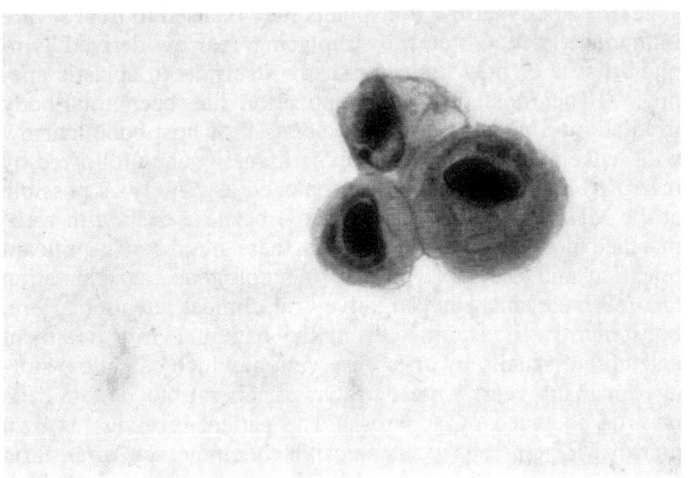

Fig. 29-31 Epithelial cells in urine cytology from bladder-drained pancreas allograft with large eosinophilic intranuclear inclusion and perinuclear clearing of cytomegalovirus (CMV) infection.

ing numerous foam cells, smooth muscle cells, and T-cells[120] (Figs. 29-33 and 29-34). Transplant arteriopathy is a common process that begins early after pancreas transplantation and probably contributes to the eventual graft failure.

Nonrejection complications

Besides rejection, pancreatic grafts may fail because of vascular thrombosis, pancreatitis, and infection. Additional surgical complications include urologic problems of cystitis, urethritis or urethral stricture.[96,121]

Vascular complications include hemorrhage, thrombosis, stenosis, pseudoaneurysm formation, and arteriovenous fistulas. These are a potentially devastating source of morbidity and a rare cause of mortality after pancreas transplant. Arterial or venous thrombosis is a dreaded complication that often results in graft loss. Early diagnosis is critical to graft salvage, but despite prompt surgical intervention, a high rate of graft loss may occur.[121]

Since many patients may have a neurogenic bladder from diabetes, reflux pancreatitis complicates transplantation. The symptoms include fever, lower abdominal pain, allograft swelling or tenderness, ileus, distention, or constipation. The diagnosis is grounded on clinical and radiographic findings, but hyperamylasemia is also a feature, as is direct evidence of pancreatitis at laparotomy with edema and saponification.[121] The combination of pancreatitis with subsequent liquefactive necrosis and possible bacterial contamination can lead to peripancreatic abcess formation, which often proves difficult to treat.

The major feature seen in biopsy specimens in patients with recurrent *diabetes mellitus* is an infiltration of mononuclear cells within and around the islets, with associated beta-cell destruction and islet disarray.[103]

Infections

Pancreas transplant recipients are prone to the same opportunistic infections as other solid organ transplant recipients. Of particular concern to pancreas allograft recipients are bacterial urinary tract infections related to bladder drainage and peripancreatic or intra-abdominal abcesses associated with the

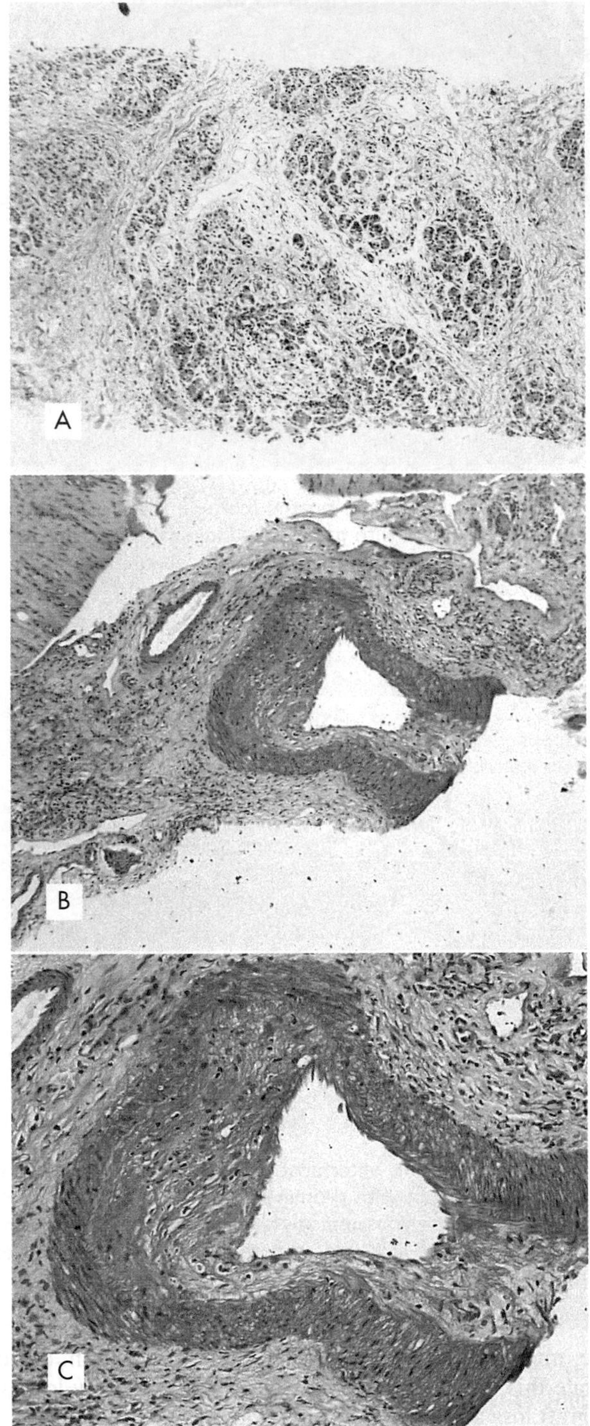

Fig. 29-32 Cytoscopic transduodenal needle biopsy specimen of pancreas allograft with features of chronic rejection including acinar cell loss and fibrosis (**A,** Movat's pentachrome) along with transplant arteriopathic changes of intimal thickening consisting of smooth muscle cells and fibrosis (**B** and **C**).

operative procedure. Many of the urinary tract infections are caused by organisms that do not commonly cause urinary tract infections, such as *Staphylococcus epidermidis, Citrobacter* spp., and *Enterococcus* spp. The combination of pancreatic enzyme activation, an alkaline environment, and immmunosuppression seems to predispose the bladder to infection by venocclusive disease must be interpreted in the milieu of considerable centrolobular congestion or hemorrhage and is associated early with endothelial damage to the central vein, subendothelial swelling and hemorrhage, with later fibrin and coagulant deposition and pericentral sinusoidal fibrosis. GVHD is a mild form of lobular and triadic hepatitis with a particular tendency to involve the small interlobular and intralobular small bile ducts.[141,142] Here the same lesion of apoptosis with lymphocytic infiltration characterizes the process as has been described in the skin and gut. The differential diagnosis between this process and viral hepatitis is never completely certain, especially early and very late after transplantation. Furthermore, the bile duct abnormalities may be particularly mimicked in hepatitis C, which is the most difficult differential diagnosis.

Chronic GVHD is a syndrome of lichenoid skin lesions, a sicca syndrome, with occasional scleroderma and hepatitis occurring 80 to 400 days after marrow transplantation and associated with prolonged immunodeficiency.[143-145] The manifestations are protean and provide an overlap syndrome resembling mixed connective tissue diseases. The skin lesions most closely resemble lichen planus, both histologically and clinically, just as the lesions of the mouth (cheeks, tongue, and palate) do (Fig. 29-38). However a flair of chronic GVHD, or de novo onset chronic GVHD, may resemble acute GVHD. This is seen frequently when discontinuing cyclosporin A or other immunosuppressive therapy. The skin lesions of chronic GVHD have the largest infiltrate of mononuclear cells at the dermoepidermal junction, as any stage of GVHD. Hyperkeratosis and acanthosis with parakeratosis may be prominent. Involvement of hair follicles and sweat ducts is more common in chronic GVHD (Fig. 29-39). Many patients have focal subclinical involvement of rete ridges or the hair follicle neck regions when biopsied at the day-100 follow-up examination. This feature indicates high risk for clinical disease and requires close follow-up study. Some patients develop, at various times, a panniculitis with associated sclerosis of the subcutaneous fat, which can be quite profuse and generalized (Fig. 29-40). A few of these patients develop a debilitating diffuse sclerodermatous picture, which may be associated with esophageal fibrosis but rarely with other visceral fibrosis. Preventing this is one of the goals of the long-term follow-up biopsies (Fig. 29-41).

Lip biopsies, at day 100 and 1 year after transplantation, serve similar long-term screening purposes.[146] The squamous epithelium of the lip can show damage similar to the epidermis, namely, apoptosis and satellitosis (Figs. 29-42 and 29-43). The lip biopsy specimen may also contain a lobule or two of minor salivary gland, which may be evaluated for duct

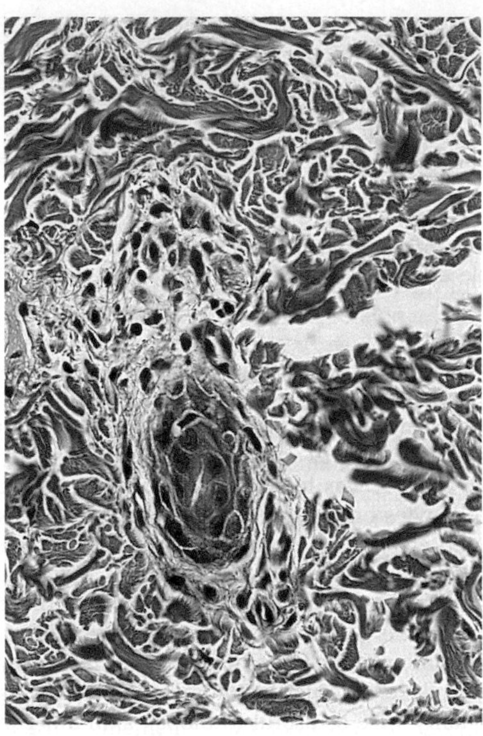

Fig. 29-39 Detail of sweat duct lesion in case of early chronic GVHD showing the periductal lymphocytic infiltrate and the sparse infiltration of lymphocytes into the duct with necrosis of duct epithelial cells.

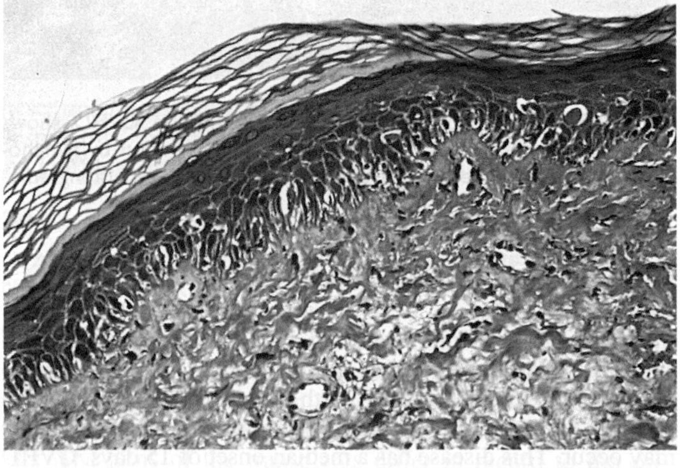

Fig. 29-38 Example of lichenoid phase of chronic GVHD of the skin with acanthosis and with a modest band of lyphocytes and plasma cell at junction.

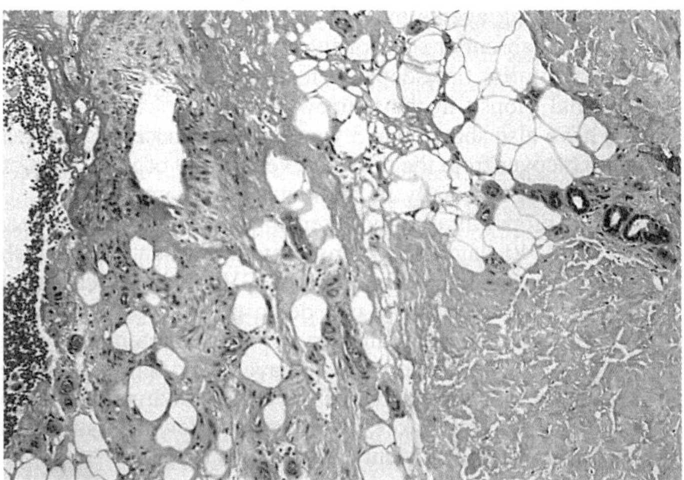

Fig. 29-40 Dermal subcutaneous fat junction in chronic GVHD shows a modest serous panniculitis characteristic of the early phase of collagenization of the subcutaneous tissue in chronic GVHD, which is the early phase of the scleroderma like type of GVHD.

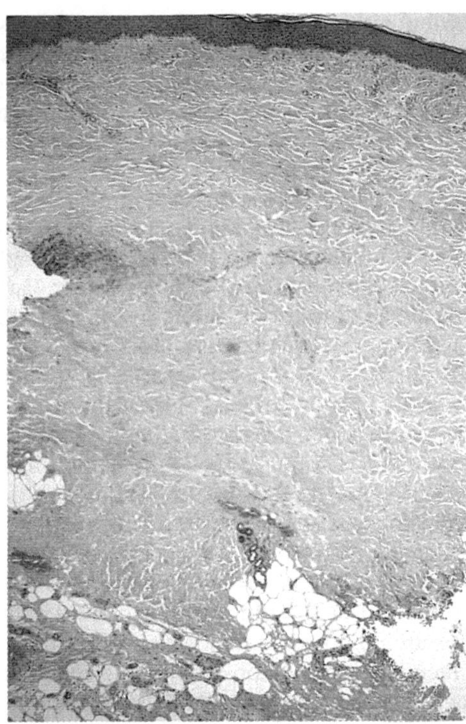

Fig. 29-41 Chronic GVHD with sclerodermatous features including extension of dense fibrosis into subcutis and loss of adnexae.

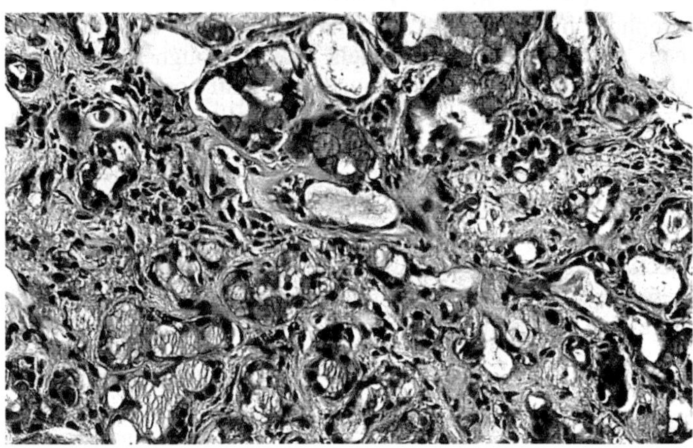

Fig. 29-42 Minor salivary gland from lip biopsy with infiltrate of lymphocytes into duct near center of photo (arrow) and general chronic inflammation of the gland. Patient with chronic GVHD on day 100 after transplantation.

damage, with secondary sialadenitis and fibrosis. These findings are very useful criteria for diagnosis and correlate well with Schirmer's test for tear production in the diagnosis of a sicca syndrome resembling Sjögren's syndrome. The lymphoid infiltrates are typically less prominent than that in classical Sjögren's syndrome, and there are occasional Langerhan's giant cells adjacent to degenerating ducts and acini. Acinous involvement is sometimes simultaneous with ductal. The tongue may have severe lichenoid lesions with obliteration of papillae and replacement by hyperkeratotic plaques or atrophy.

In some individuals, esophageal lesions are a complication of both acute and chronic GVHD. During the acute period fungal, viral, and reflux problems compete as diagnostic alternatives with acute GVHD in the lower third of the esophagus. Stomach and duodenal crypt lesions can be seen in association with chronic nausea and anorexia. In some chronic GVHD cases severe acute and chronic inflammation with fibrosis of multiple layers occurs in the proximal third of the esophagus, associated with web formation and extreme dysphagia. This can result in perforation.

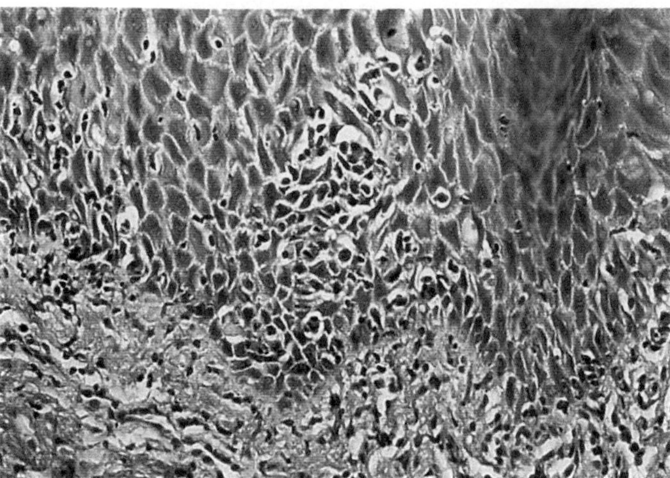

Fig. 29-43 Lip biopsy specimen from same patient as in Fig. 29-42 with invasion of squamous epithelium with the same type of infiltrate and similar individual cell death as seen in skin and esophagus in GVHD.

Chronic GVHD of the liver is indolent but can cause severe complications, including cirrhosis in a minority of cases. The major differential diagnostic considerations are chronic post-transplantation viral hepatitis, particularly C hepatitis, for which newer molecular, diagnostic, and serologic techniques are helpful. Ductopenia is a frequent finding in the triads of these patients.

The toxicity of radiation and chemotherapy is a major problem in marrow transplantation, in terms of both direct toxicity and in confusing the diagnosis of infectious diseases and GVHD. Venoocclusive disease of the liver, discussed previously, is a major dose limiting toxicity in this field (Fig. 29-44). Low-dose radiation toxicity to the lung is clearly a risk factor for the idiopathic interstitial pneumonias and diffuse alveolar damage of the lung so frequent in these patients. Marrow and gut toxicity are a constant concern as well. So many new drugs and their combinations are used that a high autopsy rate is ethically mandatory to look for both suspected and unsuspected toxic problems in the nonsurvivors.

Infections

Infections pose the greatest threat to marrow transplant recipients during the leukopenic period, between days 0 and 30. Between days 30 and 100 interstitial pneumonias attributable to viruses or of unknown cause show their peak incidence. After day 100 the major problems are with chronic GVHD patients who have severe immunodeficiency to gram-positive bacteria, to herpes zoster and herpes simplex, and to *Pneumocystis carinii*. Several advances in prophylaxis and treatment have helped these problems immensely including sulfonamides for the *Pneumocystis* and ganciclovir and immune

41. Lautenschlager I, Hockerstedt K, Salmela K et al: Fine needle aspiration biopsy in the monitoring of liver allografts, *Transplantation* 50:798, 1990.
42. Carbonnel F, Samuel D, Reynes M et al: Fine needle aspiration biopsy of human liver allografts, *Transplantation* 50:704, 1990.
43. Hanto DW, Snover DC, Noreen HJ et al: Hyperacute rejection of a human orthotopic liver allograft in a presensitized recipient, *Clin Transplant* 1:304, 1987.
44. Bird G, Friend P, Donaldson P et al: Hyperacute rejection in liver transplantation: a case report, *Transplant Proc* 21:3742, 1989.
45. Knechtle SJ, Kolbeck PC, Tsuchimoto S et al: Hepatic transplantation into sensitized recipients: demonstration of hyperacute rejection, *Transplantation* 43:8, 1987.
46. Gubernatis G, Lauchart W, Jonker M et al: Signs of hyperacute rejection of liver grafts in Rhesus monkeys after donor-specific presensitization, *Transplant Proc* 19:1082, 1987.
47. D'Alessandro AM, Kalayoglu M, Sollinger HW et al: The predictive value of donor liver biopsies for the development of primary nonfunction after orthotopic liver transplantation, *Transplantation* 51:157, 1991.
48. Ploeg RJ, D'Alessandro AM, Knechtle SJ et al: Risk factors for primary dysfunction after liver transplantation—a multivariate analysis, *Transplantation* 55:807, 1993.
49. Williams JW, Peters TG, Vera SP et al: Biopsy directed immunosuppression following hepatic transplantation in man, *Transplantation* 39:589, 1985.
50. Demetris AJ, Lasky S, Van Thiel DH et al: Pathology of hepatic transplantation: a review of 62 adult allograft recipients immunosuppressed with a cyclosporine/steroid regimen, *Am J Pathol* 118:151, 1985.
51. Hübscher SG: Histological findings in liver allograft rejection: new insights into the pathogenesis of hepatocellular damage in liver allografts, *Histopathology* 18:377, 1991.
52. Snover DC, Freese DK, Sharp HL et al: Liver allograft rejection: an analysis of the use of biopsy in determining outcome of rejection, *Am J Surg Pathol* 11:1, 1987.
53. Ludwig J, Gross JB Jr, Perkins JD et al: Persistent centrilobular necroses in hepatic allografts, *Hum Pathol* 21:656, 1990.
54. International working party, Terminology for hepatic allograft rejection, in press.
55. Wiesner RH, Ludwig J, Krom RA et al: Hepatic allograft rejection: new developments in terminology, diagnosis, prevention, and treatment, *Mayo Clin Proc* 68:69, 1993.
56. Freese DK, Snover DC, Sharp H et al: Chronic rejection after liver transplant: a study of clinical, histopathologic, and immunologic features, *Hepatology* 13:882, 1991.
57. van Hoek B, Weisner RH, Krom RAF et al: Severe ductopenic rejection following liver transplantation: incidence, time of onset, risk factors, treatment, and outcome, *Semin Liver Dis* 12:41, 1992.
58. Ludwig J, Weisner RH, Batts KP et al: The acute vanishing bile duct syndrome (acute irreversible rejection) after orthotopic liver transplantation, *Hepatology* 7:476, 1987.
59. Oguma S, Belle S, Starzl TE, Demetris AJ: A histometric analysis of chronically rejected human liver allografts: insights into the mechanisms of bile duct loss: direct immunologic and ischemic factors, *Hepatology* 9:204, 1989.
60. O'Grady JG, Alexander GJ, Sutherland S et al: Cytomegalovirus infection and donor/recipient HLA antigens: interdependent co-factors in pathogenesis of vanishing bile-duct syndrome after liver transplantation, *Lancet* 2:302, 1988.
61. Donaldson PT, Alexander GJ, O'Grady et al: Evidence for an immune response to HLA class I antigens in the vanishing-bile duct syndrome after liver transplantation, *Lancet* 1:945, 1987.
62. Batts KP, Moore SB, Perkins JD et al: Influence of positive lymphocyte crossmatch and HLA mismatching on vanishing bile duct syndrome in human liver allografts, *Transplantation* 45:376, 1988.
63. McDonald K, Rector TS, Braunlin EA et al: Association of coronary artery disease in cardiac transplant recipients with cytomegalovirus, *Am J Cardiol* 64:359, 1989.
64. Stovin PG, Sharples L, Hutter JA et al: Some prognostic factors for the development of transplant-related coronary artery disease in human cardiac allografts, *J Heart Lung Transplant* 10:38, 1991.
65. Noack KB, Weisner RH, Batts K et al: Severe ductopenic rejection with features of vanishing bile duct syndrome: clinical, biochemical, and histologic evidence for spontaneous resolution, *Transplant Proc* 23:1448, 1991.
66. Hübscher SG, Buckels JAC, Elias E et al: Vanishing bile duct syndrome following liver transplantation—is it reversible? *Transplantation* 51:1004, 1991.

Heart transplantation

67. Billingham ME: Pathology of the transplanted heart and lung, *Cardiovasc Clin* 20:71, 1990.
68. Kottke Marchant K, Ratliff NB: Endomyocardial biopsy: pathologic findings in cardiac transplant recipients, *Pathol Annu* 25:211, 1990.
69. Sibley RK, Olivari MT, Bolman RM et al: Endomyocardial biopsy in the cardiac allograft recipient, *Ann Surg* 203:177, 1986.
70. Forbes RD, Rowan RA, Billingham ME: Endocardial infiltrates in human heart transplants: a serial biopsy analysis comparing four immunosuppression protocols [see comments], *Hum Pathol* 21:850, 1990.
71. Laufer G, Laczkovics A, Wollenek G et al: The progression of mild acute cardiac rejection evaluated by risk factor analysis: the impact of maintenance steroids and serum creatinine, *Transplantation* 51:184, 1991.
72. Billingham ME, Cary NRB, Hammond ME et al: A working formulation for the standardization of nomenclature in the diagnosis of heart and lung rejection: Heart Rejection Study Group, *J Heart Transplant* 9:587, 1990.
73. Hammond EH, Yowel RL, Nunoda S et al: Vascular (humoral) rejection in heart transplantation: pathologic observations and clinical implications [see comments], *J Heart Transplant* 8:430, 1989.
74. Billingham ME: Histopathology of graft coronary disease, *J Heart Lung Transplant* 11:S38, 1992.
75. Valantine HA: Long-term management and results in heart transplant recipients, *Cardiol Clin* 8:141, 1990.
76. Cary NR: Diagnostic criteria of chronic rejection in transplanted hearts, *Transplant Proc* 25:2026, 1993.

Lung transplantation

77. Randhawa P, Yousem SA: The pathology of lung transplantation, *Pathol Annu* 27:247, 1992.
78. Egan TM, Cooper JD: Surgical aspects of single lung transplantation, *Clin Chest Med* 11:195, 1990.
79. Tazelaar HD: Perivascular inflammation in pulmonary infections: implications for the diagnosis of lung rejection, *J Heart Lung Transplant* 10:437, 1991.
80. Stewart S, Cary N: The pathology of heart and heart and lung transplantation—an update, *J Clin Pathol* 44:803, 1991.
81. Scott JP, Fradet G, Smyth RL et al: Prospective study of transbronchial biopsies in the management of heart-lung and single lung transplant patients, *J Heart Lung Transplant* 10:626, 1991.
82. Kirby TJ, Mehta A, Rice TW et al: Diagnosis and management of acute and chronic lung rejection, *Semin Thorac Cardiovasc Surg* 4:126, 1992.
83. Yousem SA, Berry GJ, Brunt EM et al: A working formulation for the standardization of nomenclature in the diagnosis of heart and lung rejection: lung rejection study group, *J Heart Transplant* 9:593, 1990.
84. Keenan RJ, Bruzzone P, Paradis IL et al: Similarity of pulmonary rejection patterns among heart-lung and double-lung transplant recipients, *Transplantation* 51:176, 1991.
85. Burke CM, Theodore J, Dawkins KD et al: Post-transplant obliterative bronchiolitis and other late lung sequelae in human heart-lung transplantation, *Chest* 86:824, 1984.
86. Scott JP, Sharples L, Mullins P et al: Further studies on the natural history of obliterative bronchiolitis following heart-lung transplantation, *Transplant Proc* 23:1201, 1991.
87. Otulana BA, Higenbottam TW, Scott JP: Pulmonary function monitoring allows diagnosis of rejection in heart-lung transplant recipients, *Transplant Proc* 21:2583, 1989.

Pancreas transplantation

88. Harris M, Hadden WC, Knowles WC, Bennett PH: Prevalence of diabetes and impaired glucose tolerance and plasma glucose levels in the U.S. population aged 20-74 years, *Diabetes* 36:523, 1987.
89. Sutherland DER: Pancreatic transplantation: an update, *Diabetes Rev* 1:152, 1993.
90. Lillehei RC, Simmons RL, Najarian JS et al: Current state of pancreatic allotransplantation, *Transplant Proc* 33:318, 1971.
91. Sutherland DER et al: International Pancreas Transplantation Registry analysis, *Transplant Proc* 22:571, 1990.
92. Robertson RP: Pancreatic and islet transplantation for diabetes—cures or curiosities? *N Engl J Med* 327:1861, 1992.
93. Baumgartner D, Largiader F, Uhlschmid G, Binswinger U: Rejection episodes in recipients of simultaneous pancreas and kidney transplants, *Transplant Proc* 15:1330, 1983.
94. Traeger J, Dubernard JM, Piatti PM et al: Clinical aspects of pancreatic rejection in pancreatic and pancreaticorenal transplants, *Transplant Proc* 16:718, 1984.
95. Stratta RJ, Sollinger HW, Perlman SB et al: Early diagnosis and treatment of pancreas allograft rejection, *Transplant Int* 1:6, 1988.
96. Stratta RJ, Radio SJ, Markin RS: Monitoring pancreas allograft rejection. In Kolbeck PC, McManus BM, Markin RS, editors: *Transplant pathology,* Chicago, 1994, ASCP Press.
97. Prieto M, Sutherland DER, Fernández-Cruz L et al: Experimental and clinical experience with urine amylase monitoring for early diagnosis of rejection in pancreas transplantation, *Transplantation* 43:73, 1987.
98. Munn SR, Engen DE, Barr D et al: Differential diagnosis of hypoamylasuria in pancreas allograft recipients with urinary exocrine drainage, *Transplantation* 49:359, 1990.
99. Lievens MM: Potential pitfalls in the determination of amylase activity in the urine of pancreas-transplanted patients with bladder drainage, *Transplantation* 50:526, 1990.
100. Stratta RJ, Sollinger HW, Groshek M et al: Differential diagnosis of hyperamylasemia in pancreas allograft recipients, *Transplant Proc* 22:675, 1990.
101. Marks WH, Borgström A, Sollinger HW et al: Serum anodal trypsinogen is a predictive biochemical marker of pancreas allograft rejection, *Transplant Proc* 22:673, 1990.
102. Powell CS, Lindsey NJ, Nolan MS et al: The value of urinary amylase as a marker of early pancreatic allograft rejection, *Transplantation* 43:921, 1987.
103. Marks WH, Borgström A, Sollinger H, Marks C: Serum immunoreactive anodal trypsinogen and urinary amylase as biochemical markers for rejection of clinical whole-organ pancreas allografts having exocrine drainage into the urinary bladder, *Transplantation* 49:112, 1990.
104. Sibley RK, Sutherland DER: Pancreas transplantation: immunohistologic and histopathologic examination of 100 grafts, *Am J Pathol* 128:151, 1987.
105. Sutherland DER, Casanova D, Sibley RK: Role of pancreas graft biopsies in the diagnosis and treatment of rejection after pancreas transplantation, *Transplant Proc* 19:2329, 1987.
106. Nakhleh RE, Gruesner RWG, Tzardis PJ et al: Pancreas transplant pathology: a morphologic, immunohistochemical, and electron microscopic comparison of allogenic grafts with rejection, syngeneic grafts, and chronic pancreatitis, *Am J Surg Pathol* 15:246, 1991.
107. Allen RDM, Grierson JM, Ekberg H et al: Longitudinal histopathologic assessment of rejection after bladder-drained canine pancreas allograft transplantation, *Am J Pathol* 138:303, 1991.
108. Nakhleh RE, Sutherland DER: Pancreas rejection: significance of histopathologic findings with implications for classification of rejection, *Am J Surg Pathol* 16:1098, 1992.
109. Allen RDM, Wilson TG, Grierson JM et al: Percutaneous biopsy of bladder-drained pancreas transplants, *Transplantation* 51:1213, 1991.
110. Carpenter HA, Engen DE, Munn SR et al: Histologic features of rejection in cystoscopically-directed needle biopsies of pancreaticoduodenal allografts in dogs and humans, *Transplant Proc* 22:707, 1990.
111. Carpenter HA, Barr D, Marsh CL et al: Sequential histopathologic changes in pancreaticoduodenal allograft rejection in dogs, *Transplantation* 48:764, 1989.
112. Tydén G, Reinholt F, Brattström C et al: Diagnosis of rejection in recipients of pancreatic grafts with enteric exocrine diversion by monitoring pancreatic juice, cytology, and amylase secretion, *Transplant Proc* 19:3892, 1987.
113. Binimelis J, Sutherland DER, Sibley RK et al: Phenotypes of in vivo activated T lymphocytes from a pancreas allograft, *Transplant Proc* 19:403, 1987.
114. Carpenter HA, Barr D, Marsh CL et al: Sequential histopathologic changes in pancreaticoduodenal allograft rejection in dogs, *Transplantation* 48:764, 1989.
115. Schuman GB, Burleson RL, Henry JB, Jones DB: Urinary cytodiagnosis of acute renal allograft rejection using the cytocentrifuge, *Am J Clin Pathol* 67:134, 1977.
116. Hayry P, von Willebrand E: Cytologic evaluation of in situ inflammatory response of rejection in human renal transplantation, *Transplant Proc* 13:81, 1981.
117. Simpson MA, Madras PN, Cornaby AJ et al: Sequential determinations of urinary cytology plasma and urinary lymphokines in the management of renal allograft recipients, *Transplantation* 47:218, 1989.
118. Kubota K, Reinholt FP, Tyden G et al: Cytologic patterns in juice from human pancreatic transplants: correlation with histologic findings in the graft, *Surgery* 109:507, 1991.
119. Dooper IMM, Jose M, Bogman T et al: Immunocytology of urinary sediments as a method of differentiating acute rejection from other causes of declining renal graft function, *Transplantation* 52:266, 1991.
120. Radio SJ, Stratta RJ, Taylor RJ, Linder J: Urine cytologic monitoring for rejection after vascularized pancreas transplantation, *Transplant Proc* 24:903, 1992.
121. Radio SJ, Stratta RJ, Taylor PJ, Linder J: The utility of urine cytology in the diagnosis of allograft rejection after combined pancreatic-kidney transplantation, *Transplantation* 55:509, 1993.
122. Radio SJ, Stratta RJ, Wisecarver JL et al: Transplant arteriopathy in pancreas allografts: an intimal proliferation contributing to early and late graft failure, *Mod Pathol* 6(1):113A, 1993.

Marrow and thymic transplantation

123. Thomas ED, Storb R, Clift RA et al: Bone marrow transplantation, *N Eng J Med* 292:832, 895, 1975.
124. Thomas ED: Marrow transplantation for malignant diseases, *J Clin Oncol* 1:517, 1983.
125. Storb R, Buckner CD: Human bone marrow transplantation, *Eur J Clin Invest* 20:119, 1990.
126. O'Reilly RJ: Allogeneic bone marrow transplantation: current status and future directions, *Blood* 62:941, 1983.
127. Hong R: Reconstitution of T-cell deficiency by thymic hormone or thymic transplantation therapy, *Clin Immunol Immunopathol* 40:136, 1986.
128. Storb R, Prentice RL, Buckner CD et al: Graft-versus-host disease and survival in patients with aplastic anemia treated by marrow grafts from HLA-identical siblings: beneficial effect of a protected environment, *N Engl J Med* 308:302, 1983.
129. Sale GE, Buckner CD: Pathology of bone marrow in transplant recipients, *Hematol Oncol Clin North Am* 2:735, 1988.
130. Sale GE, Shulman HM, Hackman RC: Bone marrow transplantation and graft-versus-host disease. In: Colvin R, Bhan A, McCluskey R, editors: *Diagnostic immunopathology, ed 2,* New York, 1994, Raven Press.
131. Sale GE, Shulman HM, Hackman RC: Pathology of bone marrow transplantation. In Forman SJ, Thomas ED, Blume KG, editors: *Bone marrow transplantation,* Cambridge, Mass., 1994, Blackwell Scientific Publications.
132. Sloan JP, Thomas JA, Imrie SF et al: Morphological and immunohistological changes in the skin in allogeneic bone marrow recipients, *Clin Pathol* 37:919, 1984.
133. Paller AS, Nelson A, Steffen L et al: T-lymphocyte subsets in the lesional skin of allogeneic and autologous bone marrow transplant patients, *Arch Dermatol* 124:1795, 1988.
134. Sviland L, Pearson ADJ, Eastham EJ et al: Histological features of skin and rectal biopsy specimens after autologous and allogeneic bone marrow transplantation, *J Clin Pathol* 41:148, 1988.

135. Snover DC, Weisdorf SA, Vercellotti GM et al: A histopathologic study of gastric and small intestinal graft-versus-host disease following allogeneic bone marrow transplantation, *Hum Pathol* 16:387, 1985.
136. Sviland L, Pearson ADJ, Green MA et al: Expression of MHC class I and II antigens by keratinocytes and enterocytes in acute graft-versus-host disease, *Bone Marrow Transplant* 4:233, 1989.
137. Sviland L, Pearson ADJ, Green MA et al: Immunopathology of early graft-versus-host disease: a prospective study of skin, rectum, and peripheral blood in allogeneic and autologous bone marrow transplant recipients, *Transplantation* 52:1029, 1991.
138. Sviland L, Pearson ADJ, Green MA et al: Prognostic importance of histological and immunopathological assessment of skin and rectal biopsies in patients with GVHD, *Bone Marrow Transplant* 11:215, 1993.
139. Beschorner WE: Destruction of the intestinal mucosa after bone marrow transplantation and graft-versus-host disease, *Surv Synth Pathol Res* 3:264, 1984.
140. Shulman HM, McDonald GB, Matthews D et al: An analysis of hepatic venocclusive disease and centrilobular hepatic degeneration following bone marrow transplantation, *Gastroenterology* 79:1178, 1980.
141. Shulman HM, Sharma P, Amos D et al: A coded histologic study of hepatic graft-versus-host disease after human bone marrow transplantation, *Hepatology* 8:463, 1988.
142. Snover DC, Weisdorf SA, Ramsey NK et al: Hepatic graft-versus-host disease: a study of the predictive value of liver biopsy in diagnosis, *Hepatology* 4:123, 1984.
143. Shulman HM, Sale GE, Lerner KG et al: Chronic cutaneous graft-versus-host disease in man, *Am J Pathol* 91:545, 1978.
144. Shulman HM, Sullivan KM, Weiden PL et al: Chronic graft-versus-host syndrome in man: a long-term clinicopathologic study of 20 Seattle patients, *Am J Med* 69:204, 1980.
145. Sullivan KM, Shulman HM, Storb R et al: Chronic graft-versus-host disease in 52 patients: adverse natural course and successful treatment with combination immunosuppression, *Blood* 57:267, 1981.
146. Sale GE, Shulman HM, Schubert MM et al: Oral and ophthalmic pathology of graft versus host disease in man: predictive value of the lip biopsy, *Hum Pathol* 12:1022, 1981.

Corneal transplantation

147. Sale GE, Chandler J: Pathology of corneal transplantation. In Sale GE, editor: *The pathology of organ transplantation,* Stoneham, Mass., and London, 1990, Butterworth.
148. Polack FM: The pathologic anatomy of corneal graft rejection, *Surv Ophthalmol* 11:391, 1966.

Intestinal transplantation

149. Madara JL: Intestinal transplantation. In Sale GE, editor: *The pathology of organ transplantation,* Stoneham, Mass., and London, 1990, Butterworth.
150. Langrehr JM, Banner B, Lee KKN et al: Clinical course, morphology, and treatment of chronically reflecting small bowel allografts, *Transplantation* 55:242, 1993.

30 Pathology of Prosthetic Materials and Devices

Stanley J. Radio
Bruce M. McManus

MATERIALS AND METHODS

The expanding field of biomaterials

Biomaterials are synthetic or modified biologic materials that are used in implants or extracorporeal medical devices that augment or replace abnormal body structures and provide a new level of function to otherwise disabled or diseased bodily components. Such biomaterials include polymers, metals, ceramics, carbons, processed collagen, and glutaraldehyde-preserved heart valves, blood vessels, pericardium, and tendons. The biomaterial and medical device industry has grown to a 100-billion-dollar worldwide venture involving inventors, physicists, chemists, biologists, and pathologists.[1-4]

It was estimated in the 1988 National Health Interview Survey[1] that no less than 15 million people in the United States have at least one artificial body part implanted or attached. Each year over 17 million dollars are spent by the federal government on prosthetics research. Manufacturing devices or materials with the aim of recapitulating tissues or organs, the functions of which have evolved to natural perfection over millions of years, is a daunting and expensive challenge.

Biomaterials describe materials that are used in medical devices, particularly in applications where the device for any period of time, as a whole or as a part of a system that treats, augments, or replaces any tissue, organ, or function of the body. Types of biomaterials include synthetic polymers, metals, ceramics, and natural macromolecules that are manufactured or processed to be suitable for use in or as a medical device.

The criteria for selection of a material or materials are mandated by the intended application of the device. For many devices several different materials are necessary to form a multicomponent structure with complex function. A device's particular size, form, expected implant duration, and specific mode of interface with the host will largely determine the required material properties. Some materials are available in specifically designated biomedical grades with a certification of their biocompatibility or more precisely their lack of cytotoxicity provided by the manufacturer. For other materials, special cleaning or extraction is necessary to make commercial-grade materials acceptable.[5,6]

Some selected specific properties that are of importance in selecting materials have been outlined by Helmus and Hubbell.[6]

Strength is required in applications such as aortic vascular grafts and heart valves, and these are provided by engineering plastics, fiber composites, and metals.

Modulus refers to the degree to which a material possesses stiffness or rigidity. The modulus can also be applied to torsion and flex, which are of interest in devices such as cardiac catheters. These catheters are torqued and pass through tortuous paths to reach their destination. The compliance of a material is the inverse of the modulus and refers to the ability of a material to elongate with little load. Indwelling catheters, cardiac and vascular patches, and vascular grafts, for example, require moderate or high compliance. Materials with moderate-to-high compliance (low modulus) include elastomers, especially silicone rubbers and many polyurethanes. High modulus (low compliance) is required in the structural components of such devices as heart valves. This is characteristic of such materials as engineering plastics (such as polyetherketones and polyimides) and, in most metals, ceramic and glassy carbons.

Creep resistance indicates a material's ability to maintain its configurational integrity under stress from constant loading without continuing elongation or shape change. Most engineering plastics and nearly all metals, ceramics, and carbons possess excellent creep resistance.

Fatigue resistance is the ability of the material to undergo cyclic stressing and relaxing without deleterious crack propagation. Failures have been observed in welded heart-valve struts and artificial heart bladders. Metals and engineering plastics are highly fatigue resistant.

Permeation rate is related to the diffusivity of a compound or substance of interest in the polymer and is a function of the thickness of the membrane. The permeation rate is determined by the molecular weight, its ability to partition itself into the polymer phase, and the glassiness of the polymer. Silicone rubbers and fluoropolymers are particularly permeable to oxygen, making them quite useful in some oxygenator configurations. Hydrogels and biologically derived materials and macromolecules are particularly permeable to water and water-soluble species. This is a desirable feature in drug-delivery systems and dialysis.

Water absorption occurs in materials with chemical moieties that allow hydrogen bonding. Physical properties such as strength, modulus, and creep and fatigue resistance can be significantly altered by relatively small amounts of water absorption.

Biostability refers to the ability of a material to maintain its properties in situ and resist such processes as polymer degradation and calcification. In the case of temporary implants such as sutures, controlled resorption without cytotoxicity is a desirable property. Bioresorbable materials can serve as carriers for drug delivery. *Bioactivity* is the ability of a material surface to participate in specific biologic reactions such as preventing thrombus formation or initiation clot lysis. Incorporation of broad-range antibiotics into a biomaterial such as orthopedic bone cement can impart an antimicrobial activity.

Preimplant analysis of biomaterials and devices

Bulk analysis

Bulk characterization of biomaterials, especially polymers, can confirm the material's identity as well as fillers, plasticizers, antioxidants, low-molecular-weight polymers, unreacted monomers, and so forth. In addition, possible toxic leachables can be suggested.[7] Polymers can be categorized into a few main groups according to structural properties: tensile and thermal properties; physical properties, such as density or porosity; and polymer-solvent interactions.

Surface analysis

The surface chemistry of synthetic materials in contact with biologic tissues is believed to be transmitted through structural or conformational changes in adsorbed conditioning-film macromolecules.[8] These conditioning-film macromolecules may include extracellular matrix, bacterial exopolymer, or components of the medium. Surface energy, surface charge, structure and chemical functionality, defects in structure, and degradation or corrosion potential are parameters of the substratum and may play a role in modifying the conditioning film.[8] The techniques that are available for surface analysis are outlined in Table 30-1.[9] The choice of which technique to employ will be dependent on their availability within a particular institution and the results of the initial exams.

Methods to examine prosthetic devices

Because of limited longevity of biomaterials, pathologists will encounter an increasing number of working and failed prosthetic implants on the surgical pathology desk and at autopsy. The most frequent devices are for orthopedic problems, artificial eye lenses, artificial joints (primarily hips and knees), earvent tubes for frequent otitis media, artificial heart valves, and heart pacemakers.[2] The survey of 122,000 individuals, extrapolated to the entire population, indicated a high frequency of structural or functional problems with implants, which often necessitates their removal, because of pathologic or materials defects.

The assessment of failed devices and prostheses in the clinical setting or in research protocols should follow guidelines determined by the nature of the adverse interaction. For example, thrombosis is a major issue with respect to cardiovascular materials and devices, whereas aseptic loosening remains a problem for orthopedic implants. Results of a thorough assessment directed toward the basis of device or material failure must be cast in light of interinstitutional differences, which may heavily influence their interpretation (Table 30-2.) The following discussion provides a framework for the evaluation of devices and materials that can be modified according to individual needs.

Implant retrieval

General considerations in implant retrieval have been summarized.[10-13] Objectives of retrieval are summarized in Table 30-3. Various modes of dysfunction must be anticipated for each device. Careful gross examination of implants and associated tissues (both local and more distant) is carried out at animal necropsy, during human postmortem examination, or on receipt of a specimen taken at reoperation. Irrespective of device type, a careful gross examination in situ is essential, since removal of the prosthesis from its physical context may destroy critical relationships. For example, artifactual dislodgment of thrombotic deposits may occur. Careful photography using various views of the key areas of a prosthesis provides important documentation; close-up photographs, often taken at several points in the dissection, can be extremely useful.[14] Diagrams of gross findings not only provide a systematic and standardized means to record pathologic data, but also may be used to denote sites and orientation of tissue sections processed for histology.[10,13]

Principles of retrieval strategies may be illustrated by a representative schema for analysis of mechanical and bioprosthetic cardiac valves and for cardiac assist devices.[10] Detailed analysis of replacement heart valves varies according to type and design.[10,15-18] For valves in development, the analysis is modified for novel structural features and anticipated complications of specific designs. Standardized data recording forms to be used for experimental studies of new valve configurations or for design modifications of existing valves, as well as the use of preselected standards for semiquantitative grading of pathologic features, are strongly encouraged.[10] Many such features are subjective and are greatly benefited by standardization. For specific valve types, special analyses and approaches may be appropriate, such as scanning electron microscopy (SEM) of critical surfaces and wear areas of mechanical valves,[5,16] dimensional and configurational analyses,[17-19] determination of tissue calcium concentrations, or

Table 30-1 Capabilities of and concerns with common methods to characterize biomaterial surfaces

Method	Principle	Depth analyzed	Spatial resolution	Analytical sensitivity
Contact angles	Liquid wetting of surfaces is used to estimate the energy of surfaces	0.3 to 2 nm	1 mm	Low or high depending on the chemistry
Electron spectroscopy for chemical analysis (ESCA)	X rays cause the emission of electrons of characteristic energy	1 to 25 nm	8 to 150 μm	0.1 atomic %
Auger electron spectroscopy[2]	A focused electron beam causes the emission of Auger electrons	5 to 100 nm	10 nm	0.1 atomic %
Secondary ion mass spectrometry (SIMS)	Ion bombardment leads to the emission of surface secondary ions	1 nm to 1 μm	50 nm	Very high
Attenuated total reflection infrared (ATR-IR) spectroscopy	Infrared radiation is absorbed in exciting molecular vibrations	1 to 5 μm	10 μm	1 mole %
Scanning tunneling microscopy (STM)[4]	Measurement of the quantum tunneling current between a metal tip and a conductive surface	0.5 nm	0.1 nm	Single atoms
Scanning electron microscopy (SEM)	Secondary electron emission caused by a focused electron beam is measured and spatially imaged	0.5 nm	4 nm typically	High; not quantitative

Modified from Ratner BD: Characterization of Biomaterial Surfaces. In Harker LA, Ratner BD. Didisheim P, editors: Cardiovascular biomaterials and biocompatibility: a guide to the study of blood-tissue-material interactions, *Cardiovasc Path* 2(suppl):875, 1993.

Table 30-2 Difficulty in comparing modes and mechanisms of prosthetic dysfunction from one institution to another

Patient selection
Prosthesis source, type, or handling
Surgical skill
Criteria for prosthetic failure
Likelihood of retrieval
Manner of evaluation
Statistical approaches

Table 30-3 Objectives of device retrieval analysis

Enhanced
- Patient management and recognition of complications
- Device selection criteria
- Patient to prosthesis matching

Elimination of complications by device development
Identification of subclinical patient-prosthesis interactions
Elucidation of mechanisms of interactions of tissue with biomaterials

transmission electron microscopy (TEM) of tissue valves.[20-22] In vitro postimplantation functional studies (such as study of heart valve prostheses in a pulse simulator device) can add important information in particular situations.

For vascular grafts, major issues relate to the extent of surface tissue coverage, cell morphology, and the thickness of ingrown or deposited layers.[23,24] For experimental specimens, preharvest injection with Evan's blue dye facilitates assessment of component endothelial cell coverage. Endothelialized surfaces having intact barrier function are not stained with Evan's blue, a dye that stains nonendothelialized surfaces. Consideration should be given to the possibility of fixation by physiologic pressure perfusion in vivo with glutaraldehyde-containing solutions. However, although pressure perfusion preserves fine structural detail for electron microscopy and morphometric studies, it precludes the preparation of unfixed specimens for immunohistochemical, genetic or biochemical analyses. The latter consideration particularly emphasizes the need for the development of a carefully designed protocol for specimen harvest and analysis that addresses the major pathobiologic issues most efficiently.[10]

For cardiac assist devices, systemic dissection of any patient who dies is particularly important for documentation of thrombotic or biomaterial embolism. Key features of a protocol for the analysis of temporary cardiac assist devices have been described.[13] Moreover, surface and bulk analysis of the implant is an important adjunct to device retrieval and analysis.[11,13,25] The latter analysis includes attention to inflow cannula, valve, and graft, inner housing, diaphragm, outflow valve and graft, compliance chamber, and the energy source and related components.

For orthopedic implants, particularly total joint arthroplasties, evaluation of the tissue interface membrane requires light microscopy and polarized-light microscopy to characterize the wear-particle debris. Light microscopy as well as enzyme histochemistry are needed to evaluate the nature of infiltrating cells as well as the presence of markers for activation (such as lysozyme and acid phosphatase). Tissue and cell culture allow for measurement of growth factors and other cellular products (such as collagenase and prostaglandins) in certain pathologic conditions. Undecalcified, methyl methacrylate embedding of bone allows for examination of the interface-bone histology. Backscatter electron microscopy is helpful in examining the interlock of porous ingrowth prostheses, and scanning electron microscopy is used for surface analysis in the evaluation of erosion and wear. Quantitative analysis of particle debris requires techniques such as energy dispersive analysis of x-rays and atomic absorption spectrophotometry.[10,26]

Tissue characterization

The various techniques used to study cells and tissues are summarized in Table 30-4. Light microscopy (histology) is the most frequently used to confirm gross findings and observe overall tissue architecture, diagnose infection and extent of healing, and characterize emboli (that is, whether thrombotic, septic, calcific, or biomaterial fragments).[27] Glycolmethacrylate (GMA) plastic-embedded tissue sections are generally superior from a morphologic standpoint to those in paraffin (especially to preserve interfaces of heterogeneous substances such as tissue to biomaterial or tissue to calcification). However, such sections take longer and are more expensive to produce and have limitations with respect to special staining techniques. Tissue-preparation techniques applicable to biomaterials and medical device investigation and their limitations have been discussed in detail.[10,27]

The specific approach to each material and device removed from the body at operation or at autopsy will continue to have a generic stepwise basis but will evolve as the devices and materials themselves change. Considering the necessity that

Table 30-4 Techniques in evaluation of explanted tissue and prosthetic devices

Technique	Purpose
Specimen harvest at animal surgery or necropsy or human surgery or postmortem examination	Obtain tissues; observe gross local and systemic pathologic states, including interactions with device
Microbiologic cultures	Diagnose the presence of infectious organisms
Radiographic examination	Determine the distribution of angiographic dyes, detect and localize mineral deposits, or identify bioprostheses
Enzyme histochemistry	Demonstrate the presence and location of enzymes in gross or histologic tissue sections (such as gross tetrazolium staining for myocardial necrosis, nonspecific esterase to identify monocytes)
Chemical and spectroscopic analysis	Assess the bulk concentration of mineral or other constituents
Biochemical assay	Determine the concentration of a molecular moiety
Angiography	Assess vascular patency and morphology of vessel lumens
Light microscopy (LM)	Study microscopic tissue architecture; special stains for collagen, elastin, other matrix components, organisms, mineral, etc., may be used
Transmission electron microscopy (TEM)	Study ultrastructure (that is, fine structure) and identify cells and their organelles and environment
Scanning electron microscopy (SEM)	Study the topography and structure of surfaces
Energy-dispersive x-ray analysis	Perform site-specific chemical analysis (such as Ca, P) on surfaces
Immunohistochemistry; immunofluorescence and immunoperoxidase (LM or TEM)	Identify and localize specific molecules, usually proteins, for which a specific antibody is available (such as factor VIII [vWF] antigen for endothelial cells; collagen subtypes)
Autoradiography (LM or TEM)	Localize the distribution of injected radioactive material introduced into biologic tissues
Morphometric studies (gross, LM, or TEM)	Quantitate the relative quantities, configuration, and distribution of specific structures
Functional studies	Assess device performance in vitro after in vivo service

Modified from Schoen FJ: *Interventional and surgical cardiovascular pathology: clinical correlations and basic principles,* Philadelphia, 1989, Saunders.

hospitals and manufacturers of medical devices report any product malfunction that causes death or serious injury to the Food and Drug Administration (Mandatory Device Reporting Regulations of 1984 and Medical Device Act of 1990), pathologists will continue to participate and play a vital role in this interesting and demanding field. The medicolegal interface will emerge many times more, and the need for expert consultation will be ever greater.

GENERAL PRINCIPLES UNDERLYING PROSTHESIS FAILURE

Design

Prosthetic devices must achieve biocompatibility with the host while meeting necessary functional requirements. Biocompatibility is the absence of particular unacceptable incompatibilities, with the acknowledgment that design often is established with incomplete knowledge of the factors that will affect the device over its lifetime. Design has been called a process of reconciling a "network of ideas" so that they work in concert to achieve a purpose optimally, with allowance for certain constraints.[28-30]

Modes of failure include undesirable effects of the device on the host or, conversely, adverse effects of the host on the implant. An example of the former is the destruction of erythrocytes and the adhesion and activation of platelets in the setting of supraphysiologic shear stress created by certain cardiovascular processes. Device-associated thrombosis typifies device-initiated thrombosis processes, the final outcome of which are determined by several device factors including flow characterics and surface chemistry, and the status of the host blood components (such as hypocoagulable or hypercoagulable).

Deleterious effects of the host on a device include mechanical failure because of rupture, cracking, or distortion of the implant. In cardiac valve prostheses the most common type of mechanical failure is fatigue related, attributable in part to the large number of flexures coinciding with the cardiac cycle. A particular model of the Björk-Shiley convexoconcave tilting disk valve, manufactured in the late 1970s, has experienced sudden failure of the outflow strut, whose cause is partly attributed to poor welding practices, prompting withdrawl of this valve from the market.[5,31]

Design of modern hip prostheses is in part governed by consideration of biomechanical factors, which may promote component fracture, cement fracture, interface loosening, and stress-related bone resorption and remodeling. Stresses at the hip joint depend on joint loading, joint configuration, material properties, and interface conditions. For example, the relative contributions of cement layer thickness, stem stiffness, stem length, and stem cross-sectional shape have been established and quantified through stress analysis studies.[32]

Processing

The processing of a biomaterial may determine its suitability in a particular device design, or it may underly its failure in the host. For example, certain cobalt-nickel-chromium-iron metallic alloys can be more easily drawn into fine wires, whereas other cobalt-chromium systems cannot. Sterilization is a universal process that may introduce unwanted effects on the biomaterial. Methods for sterilization include gaseous chemicals such as ethylene oxide, thermal processes, radiation from gamma rays or electron beams, and aqueous chemicals based on aldehydes and propylene oxide. Nucleophilic sites including material surfaces such as primary amines and primary hydroxyls can by altered by gas sterilization.

Contamination by bacteria, endotoxins, and particulate debris are controlled during processing by the manufacturer. Such alterations to a biomaterial could have profound effects on inflammatory responses to implants.

EFFECT OF THE HOST ON THE IMPLANT

Physical and mechanical effects

Abrasive wear

Surface wear is a possibility whenever there is relative movement between implant surfaces or implant-host surfaces. Four related processes may play a role: (1) Release of wear debris can expose subsurface materials with different properties, or increase the surface area of the device. (2) The wear debris in the surrounding tissue may be maintained locally or carried systemically to a variety of organs. The induction of host reaction will be dependent on the material type, size, shape, and quantity. (3)The wear-debris particles can further accelerate the wear process of the parent device. (4) Moderate to severe wear of the device can result in malfunction and fracture of implants.[33]

Fatigue

Failure of a device that results from fracture after cyclic loading is termed *fatigue*. The process often starts on the surface of a device in a region of tension, such as a surface imperfection, or a region of stress concentration. A small crack begins because of tensile stress and subsequently extends during cyclic loading. Thus candidate materials are evaluated for stress and cycling levels necessary to initiate and then propagate cracks.

Corrosion

Candidate metals and alloys for implant systems are usually evaluated initially by in vitro potentiostatic or potentiodynamic electrochemical test methods in 0.9% saline solutions to determine the metal's electrochemical corrosion properties.[34] Preimplantation and postimplantation surface analysis, including scanning electron microscopy and optical microscopy, can usually identify most corrosion phenomena such as pitting, crevices, and stress.

After implantation, the presence of metallic corrosion often discolors adjacent tissues: black stains are noted from titanium, blue-green from cobalt, and brown from iron-based alloys. Standard histologic and quantitative chemical analyses should be performed on adjacent tissue to correlate biodegradation to type and quantity of metallic debris.

Degeneration and dissolution

A general ranking of biodegradation characteristics shows the least biodegradable to be the ceramics and carbons, followed by metallic alloys and polymers. Hydrolytic degradation is an important process that affects ester and amide links. Certain cellulosic esters and nylons, for example, can lose up to 83% of their tensile strength in 2 years of exposure to water.[33]

Organic polymers are susceptible to autoxidation, through the autocatalytic reactions with oxygen. Autoxidation is usually initiated by abstraction of a hydrogen atom during device production involving heat and shear, such as pelletizing, compounding, extrusion, and injection molding. Normally the oxygen tension in the venous system and most tissue beds are low and not favorable for autoxidation; inflammation and the foreign body responses, however, result in the release of oxidants directly on the biomaterial surface.[35]

Biologic effect of absorption of substances from tissues

Lipid absorption can lead to the loss of properties and fragmentation in silicones and polyurethanes. Early models of caged-ball heart valve prostheses contained silicone elastomeric ball occluders that absorbed blood lipids, causing swelling, distortion, cracking, and eventually embolization of poppet material or abnormal poppet motion. Insudation of cholesterol has been described in porcine bioprosthetic valves in the mitral, tricuspid, and inferior vena cava positions though the presence of such lipid deposits were not the primary cause of prosthetic failure.[36]

COMPLICATIONS COMMON TO PROSTHETIC DEVICES

Infection

Infection is a serious complication of implanted devices. Although improvements in materials and operative techniques have decreased the incidence of infectious complications in prostheses implanted beneath the skin to a few percent (Fig. 30-1), the rate for temporary prostheses or for those only partially implanted beneath the skin are several times higher. Infections affecting orthopedic prosthesis cause considerable morbidity, usually resulting in functional device failure and necessitating surgical removal for cure of the infection.[37,38] The incidence of infections in total joint arthroplasties is approximately 1% to 2%, or lower in centers that utilize prophylactic antibiotics and ultraclean unidirectional airflow operating rooms.[37-42] Additional preventive measures include incorporation of antibiotics into acrylic bone cement.[40,41] The annual cost to treat infected joint prostheses exceeds 100 million dollars per year in the United States.[37,38] Prosthetic valve endocarditis occurs in 1% to 6% of valve replacements with a greater than 50% mortality.[43-45]

Deep sepsis after total hip arthroplasty has been divided into three clinical stages.[37-42] Stage 1 infections typically result from infected hematomas, which can often be successfully treated with immediate débridement and parenteral antibiotics. Stage 2 infections are characterized by persistent hip pain 6 to 24 months after surgery and are difficult to differentiate from aseptic loosening. In both conditions, routine radiography may reveal radiolucent lines adjacent to the bone-cement interface. Artifacts from metallic components render noninvasive modalities such as computerized assisted tomography and nuclear imaging nonapplicable. *Arthrography,* on the other hand, provides a method of obtaining joint aspirates for Gram stain and microbial culture that will enable isolation of the causal microorganism in two thirds. Scintigraphy with ^{111}In-labeled autologous leukocyte images can allow detection of infected arthroplasties and differentiate infection from aseptic loosening though these scans are reliable only after 6 to 8 months after surgery.[39] Patients with stage 3 infection present with acute onset of hip pain and fever, often more than 2 years after surgery, often after a remote infection or dental or genitourinary manipulations.

Prosthetic valve endocarditis (PVE) can also be classified as early (less than) or late (greater than) 60 days after valve replacement. Early PVE is commonly attributable to skin flora organisms, whereas late infections are more likely to be attrib-

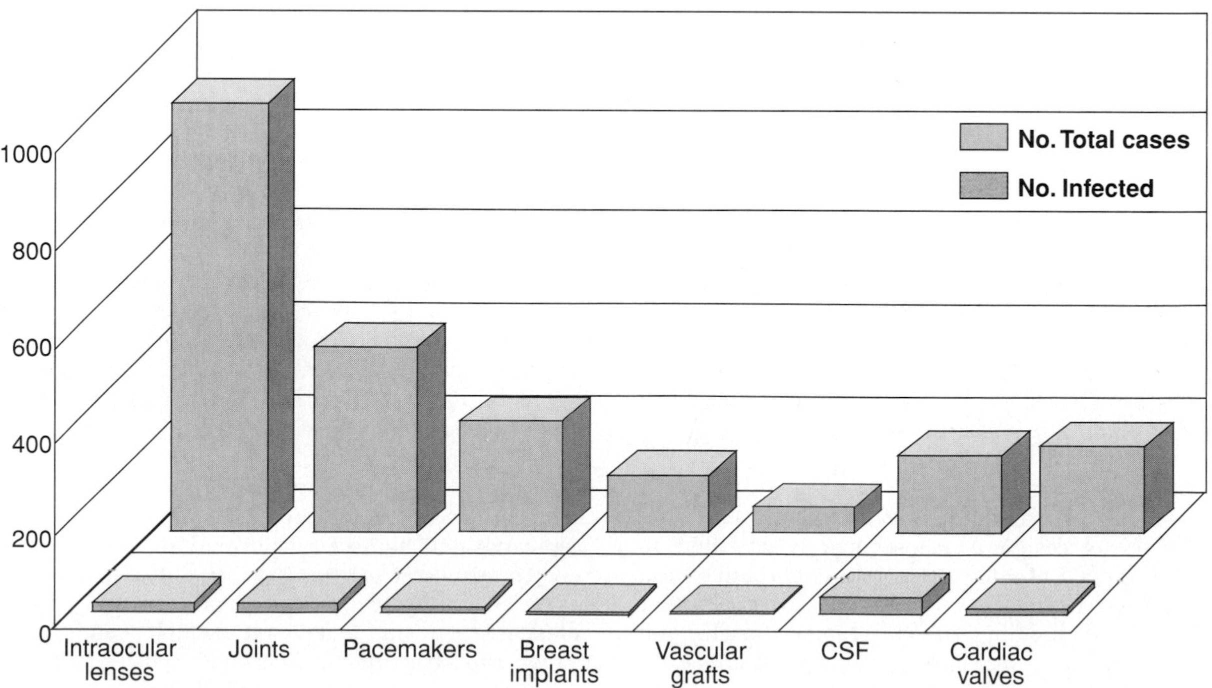

Fig. 30-1 Total number of implants and associated number of infected implants. (From Sugarman B, Young EJ: *Infect Dis Clin North Am* 3:187, 1989.)

utable to bacteremia associated with dental or surgical procedures. Streptococci, gram-negative bacilli, and fungi are also important pathogens in PVE.[43-45]

Infections after total knee arthroplasty are commonly associated with previous surgical incisions, multiple intra-articular corticosteroid injections, or previous septic arthritis. Additional risk factors associated with infected arthroplasty include systemic diseases such as rheumatoid arthritis and diabetes mellitus, obesity, and previously infected implants.[38,39]

Staphylococci are the most common isolate of infected orthopedic prostheses and early PVE. *Staphylococcus aureus* was initially the most frequently isolated organism, but more recently *Staphylococcus epidermidis* is the most frequently identified gram-positive organism.[39]

The diagnosis of deep orthopedic arthroplasty infection relies on the microbial culture and histologic appearance, with most authors stressing the usefulness of polymorphonuclear neutrophils (PMNs).[46,47] Mirra[46] showed that bacterial cultures were positive in 21 of 22 cases of failed prostheses in which more than five PMNs were present per high-power field (2+/3+) in the tissues (Fig. 30-2). In patients with cultures growing low virulence or contaminant organisms there was no PMN response. Acute inflammation was not seen in cases of excessive wear debris unless infection was also present. More recently, lymphocytes and mononuclear cells have been shown to be important components of infiltrating infected arthroplasty membranes. This is especially true in chronic infections.[48,49] While focal PMN accumulations can also be seen in patients with rheumatoid arthritis, accompanying features of rheumatoid disease such as synovial hyperplasia and lymphocytes and plasma cells are more common.

Because synthetic material are unable to support bacterial or fungal growth, infections of mechanical prostheses are almost always localized to the prosthesis-tissue interface at the sewing ring, producing a ring abscess. Destruction of the tissue adjacent to the valve prosthesis can cause dehiscence of the prosthesis and regurgitation around the prosthesis.

Endocarditis of bioprosthetic valves, in contrast, may involve only the cuspal tissue with resultant perforation or destruction and associated regurgitation.

The role of foreign bodies (implants) in potentiating infection has been recognized since the fourteenth century when the French surgeon Guy de Chauliac observed improvement of wound infection control with the removal of foreign bodies. Elek and Cohen in the 1950s showed that 10^6 *Staphylococcus pyogenes* organisms were required to produce a pus-forming clinical infection in human volunteers, but the addition of a foreign body reduced the bacteria inoculum necessary by 10^4.

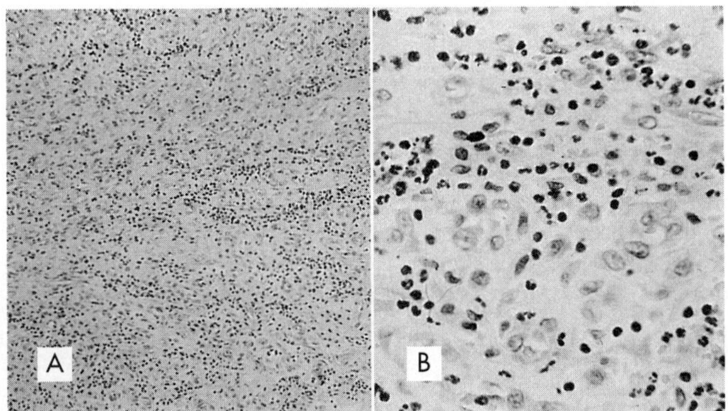

Fig. 30-2 Interface membrane from infected arthroplasty at low power, **A,** and high power, **B,** with prominent inflammatory infiltrate including large numbers of neutrophils and lymphocytes as well as neovascularity.

Several mechanisms have been postulated to play a role in prosthesis-associated infections. An implanted foreign body may result in tissue liquefaction and sterile abscess formation by inciting an acute inflammatory reaction, as demonstrated when reactive materials, such as cobalt or copper, are implanted into soft tissues.[50] Tissue damage can be exacerbated by the release of enzymes and oxygen-free radicals and other inflammatory mediators. Although contemporary biomaterials are selected for their inert characteristics, and thus expectantly limited foreign body–mediated tissue injury, tissue reactivity can be greatly increased by the production of particulate wear debris.[51-53] Implants may alter local host immune defenses by reducing the phagocytic and bactericidal ability of granulocytes. Infection may also be enhanced because of sequestration of bacteria from phagocytes in the early postoperative period.

Bacteria are dependent on adhesive colonization of substrata for survival, whether in osteomyelitis or in biomaterial-associated infections.[8,54] An important factor in microbial adhesion to implant surfaces is the production of bacterial glycocalyx, or extracellular slime (biofilm) substance that is produced by strains of *Staphylococcus epidermidis* that cause clinical and experimental device-associated infection (Fig. 30-3). Infection is not so common with strains that do not produce slime. In vitro properties of glycocalyx produced by *S. epidermidis* that may protect microorganisms (Fig. 30-4) from local host defenses include inhibition of neutrophil chemotaxis, phagocytosis and oxidative metabolism, suppression of mononuclear cell lymphoproliferative response, helper/suppressor T-cell ratios, natural killer cell cytotoxicity, and immunoglobulin synthesis. In addition to coagulase-negative staphylococcus, *Streptococcus viridans, Pseudomonas aeruginosa,* and *Staphylococcus aureus* are likewise capable of synthesizing slime.

Plasma proteins such as fibronectin, fibrinogen, collagen, and others also influence the adherence of bacteria as well as endogenous host cells to implanted materials.[8,54] Fibronectin and collagen appear to enhance adherence of *Staphylococcus aureus* and *Staphylococcus epidermidis* to foreign substances as well as promoting in vitro colonization of plastic vascular grafts by vascular endothelial cells. Albumin and other proteins not only may reduce bacterial adherence to high-molecular-weight polymers, but also may increase corrosion of cobalt, copper, and certain alloys as a result of the formation of soluble complexes.

The establishment of tissue integration of the implant or the development of bacterial colonization and subsequent device-associated infection is influenced by numerous host environmental and immune defense factors that interact with biomaterial properties in what has been termed by Gristina as the "race for the surface" of the interface.[8] Prosthesis design and prevention of implant-associated infection must include consideration for the interaction of the biomaterial with the host tissue and the contribution of each to the microenvironment.

Thrombosis and related blood-surface interactions

Absorption

Soon after exposure of a foreign material to circulating blood, plasma proteins are deposited on the interface of the mate-

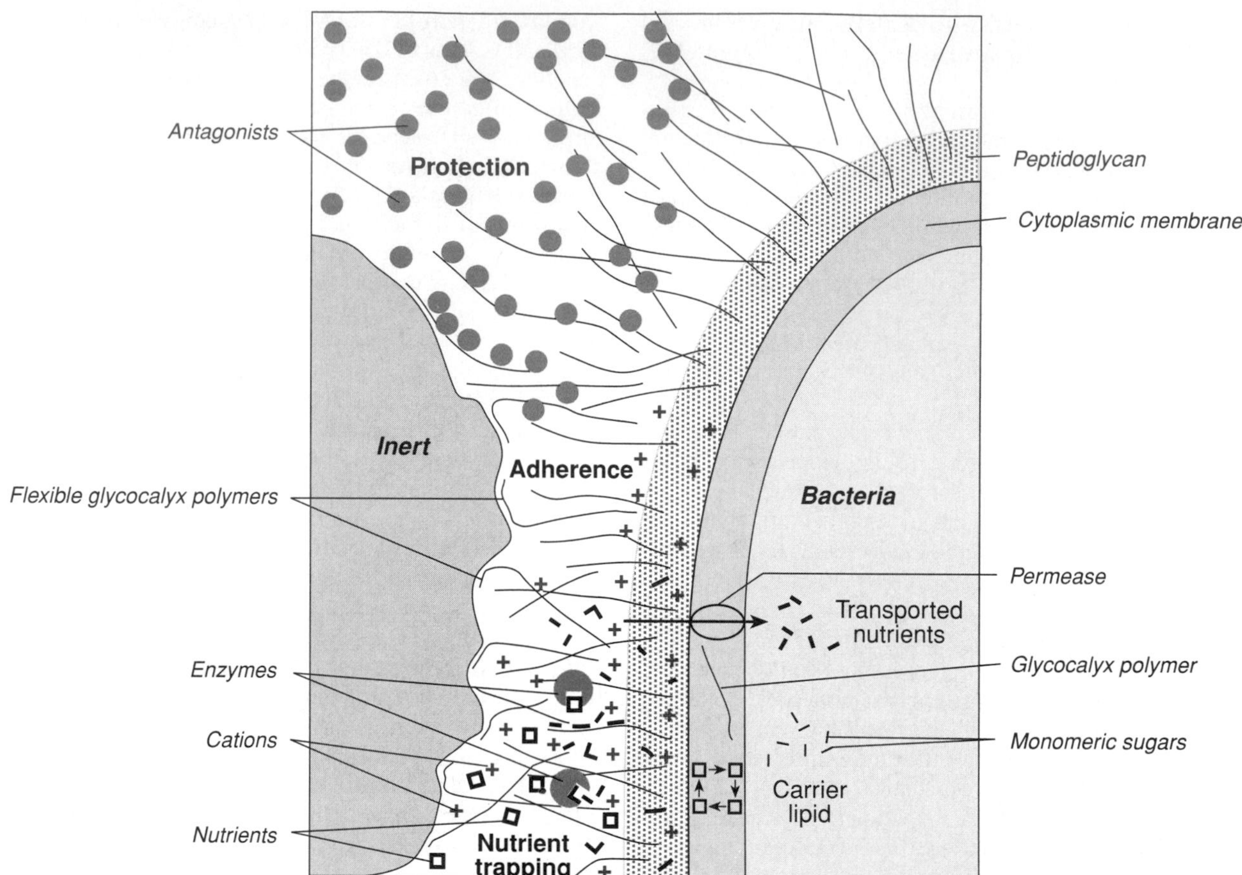

Fig. 30-3 The role of glycocalyx in implant-related infections. (Modified from Gristina AG, Costerton JW: *Orthop Clin North Am* 15:517, 1984.)

rial.[55,56] These plasma proteins will greatly alter the subsequent response of blood components to the surface. The type of implant surface as well as hemorheologic parameters influence the nature of protein absorption. This protein film is susceptible to enzymatic degradation, denaturation, or replacement by other proteins.[57]

Evaluation of the test surface after exposure to blood is accomplished by light microscopy to quantitate adherent erythrocytes, leukocytes, and platelets as well as to evaluate cell adhesion and spreading.[58] This can be further characterized by scanning electron microscopy for a three-dimensional perspective of the material surface and transmission electron microscopy for high-resolution pictures of that surface. Quantitation of the amount of protein on the material surface can be achieved by radiolabeling (with use of ^{125}I), fluorescence labeling, or attenuated total reflection Fourier-transform infrared (ATR/FT-IR) technique. X-ray photoelectron spectroscopy (XPS, ESCA) can also provide useful information.

Coagulation

The critical components and processes in thrombotic phenomena associated with cardiovascular materials and devices include a thrombogenic surface exposed to circulating blood, platelet adherence, aggregation and activation, thrombin generation and fibrin formation, and plasmin generation and fibrinolysis.[5] In order to maintain device patency a balance must be struck between the tendency to thrombus formation and the tendency to thrombus dissolution. The thrombotic milieu on the foreign surface of the prosthetic material appears primed by the deposition of albumin, globulins, and other proteins. The adherence of platelets to a nonendothelialized surface is followed by a series of interactive reactions prompting platelet aggregation, thrombus growth, and stabilization[11] (Fig. 30-4). Activation of both the intrinsic and extrinsic coagulation pathways occurs and the progression of thrombus formation can be offset only by the release of tissue plasminogen activator by endothelium and the catalytic conversion of plasminogen to plasmin. Plasmin, in turn, digests fibrin (fibrin degradation products).

In this dynamic interplay, thrombus may be formed and retained or may be formed and completely removed. Naturally or therapeutically activated fibrinolysis may protect against the retention of thrombus and the ultimate aberrant healing of such thrombus (which may lead to prosthetic valve dysfunction). Evidence that a prosthetic device is associated with protracted thrombus formation may be derived from measures of protein and lipid metabolites from the coagulation cascade including fragment 1.2 of prothrombin, thromboxane B_2, platelet factor 4, β-thromboglobulin, plasmin α_2-antiplasmin complex, fibrin degradation products, and fibrinopeptides A and B.[5,11]

The clinical problem of thrombosis associated with prosthetic materials and devices exposed to the bloodstream has not been solved despite many early approaches to make the surface of various prostheses less thrombogenic.[5]

The importance of anticoagulation therapy for mechanical prosthetic heart valves has long been appreciated. Currently, full anticoagulation with heparin or warfarin is recommended

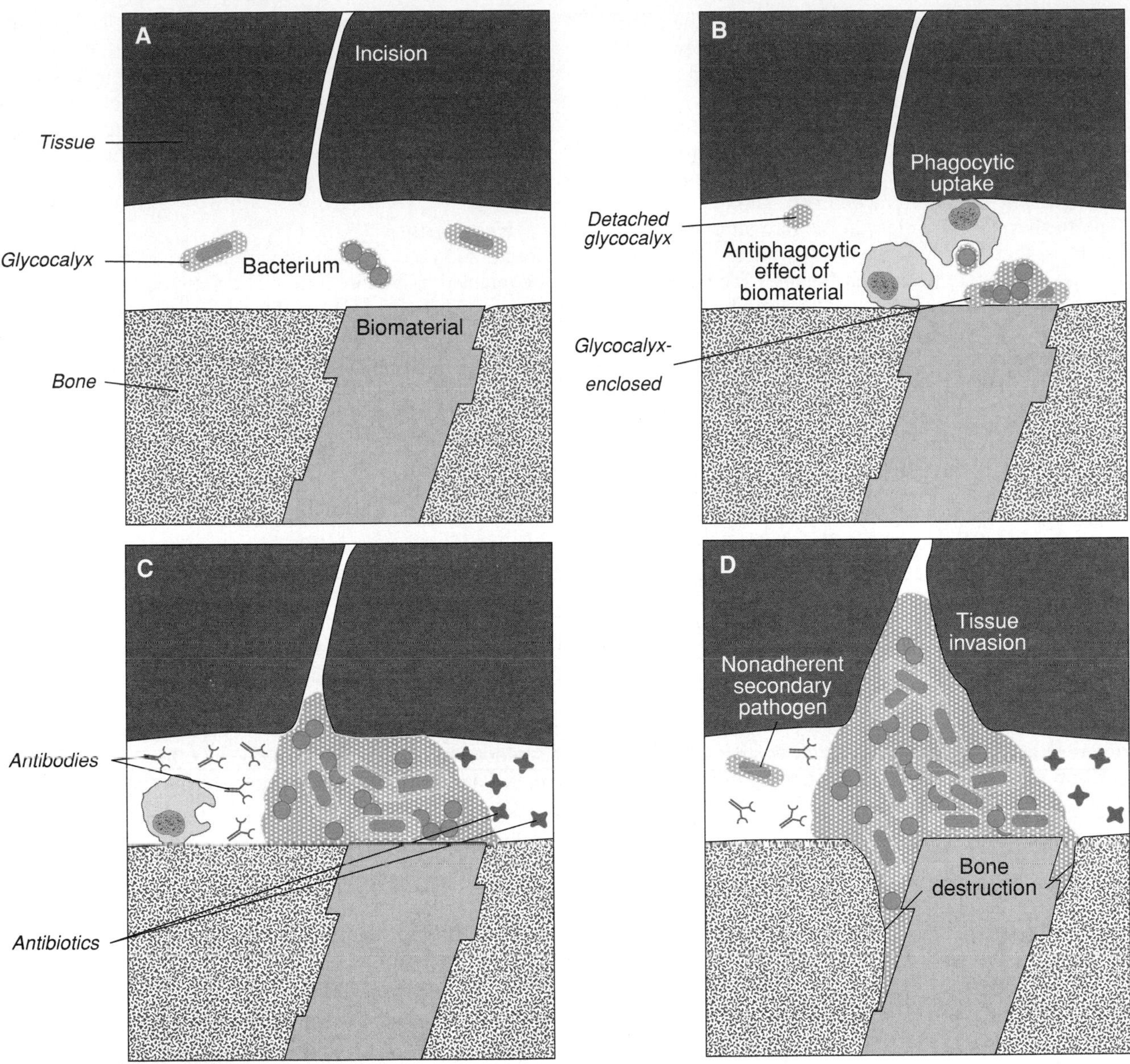

Fig. 30-4 Evolution of infection associated with biomaterial: **A,** adherence; **B,** biofilm that protects from phagocytosis; **C,** ion-exchange protects from antibiotics and antibodies; **D,** pathogens cause destruction, but less adherent secondary pathogens may dominate aspirates and confuse diagnosis. (Modified from Gristina AG, Costerton JW: *Orthop Clin North Am* 15:517, 1984.)

for patients with mechanical valves. Long-term warfarin therapy reduces the frequency and magnitude of embolic events. Other approaches to combat the development of thrombi include the use of agents like acetylsalicylic acid (aspirin) and thromboxane synthase inhibitors, which have significant antiplatelet actions.[59]

Special circumstances affect prosthetic heart valve failure when the valves are placed on the right side of the heart. The contribution of low flow and stasis may be important with respect to the tendency of valves of mechanical prosthetic valves in the tricuspid position to thrombose.[60] In this experience, 7 of 28 patients had thrombosis of the tricuspid Björk-Shiley tilting disk prosthesis. Treatment with streptokinase administered intravenously resulted in complete regression of all signs of thrombosis in the first 24 hours of therapy though rethrombosis occurred in three patients with initial successful response. No anticoagulants were used in the treatment of these patients. As the authors noted, the spontaneous resolution of immobility caused by a thrombus may reflect the capacity of native fibrinolytic activity to dissolve prosthesis-related thrombi over time.

Hereditary disorders involving the coagulation system, including antithrombin III deficiency, protein C deficiency, and familial plasminogen dysfunction, may place children at risk for thrombosis. Similarly, dehydration and sepsis may contribute. Fibrinolytic therapy has been successful in the reversal of shunt thrombosis,[61,62] emphasizing the critical role of thrombogenic surfaces. The reversal of thrombosis is most successful when it is delivered over several hours to a few days after thrombosis although this therapy may be successful up to several years after installation of the graft. The possibility of blood leakage through a polytetrafluoroethylene (PTFE) graft after thrombolytic therapy must be considered.[63] In addition to thrombolytic therapy, mechanical relief of modified Blalock-Taussig shunts can be achieved with balloon angioplasty. In such circumstances, the benefit may be more so for technically narrowed proximal or distal anastomoses or in those grafts where pseudointima and neointima have accumulated. One further consideration, in the rare situation of shunt thrombosis, is that the presence of a systemic or localized infection may contribute to graft thrombosis. Thus, obstructed shunts at operative removal or autopsy should be sampled histologically with a view toward possible infection.[64]

The thrombogenicity of PTFE, or Dacron, graft material in humans relates to the poor degree of endothelialization, as compared to animals.[65] Endothelial seeding of grafts implanted in humans has not been successful.[65] If a complete endothelialized neointima could be formed in these grafts and other hydrodynamic factors were normal, the frequency of thrombosis would be low. Residual surface fibrin is often unchanged for months or years after graft implant. Fortunately, this prosthetic surface is of low thrombogenicity. Only when grafts have less than a 5 mm internal diameter does the frequency of thrombosis rise unacceptably.[66] In the latter study, PTFE grafts in infants less than 3 months of age were closed in 84% of patients by 30 months after operation.

Fibrinolysis

Fibrinolysis is activated in concert with the coagulation system. As fibrin is formed, plasminogen binds to it and is incorporated into the thrombus. Tissue plasminogen activator (tPA) also binds to fibrin and converts plasminogen to plasmin. After formation of plasmin in plasma and in the absence of fibrin, it is inactivated by α_2-antiplasmin. In the physiologic setting of an intact endothelial surface, tPA is both activated and protected from inactivation by (PAI-1).[67] Biomaterial surfaces that lack an endothelium with its antithrombotic mechanisms tip the balance in favor of thrombosis. In addition, certain artificial surfaces have the potential to activate the contact coagulation system. Plasma proteins deposited on the biomaterial surface may promote platelet adhesion and activation.

Platelet adhesion and activation

As noted, the formation of a thrombus is the result of the balance between thrombogenic factors and protective mechanisms. After exposure to lethal and sublethal toxins or mechanical insult, endothelial cells may become thrombogenic. Such activated endothelial cells increase their synthesis of tissue factor and secretion of type 1 plasminogen activator inhibitor (PAI-1). If endothelial damage is more severe, platelets bind to the exposed subendothelium by interaction of platelet glycoprotein (GP) Ib with von Willebrand factor (vWF), which in turn binds to collagen. If the vascular injury and associate flow disturbances are great enough, platelets aggregate and are stabilized by fibrin to form mural thrombi.

When circulating blood is exposed to a biomaterial surface, the lack of an endothelium creates a thrombogenic environment. As platelets adhere and aggregate on biomaterial surfaces, they form thrombotic masses that obstruct blood flow and embolize to distal sites. Interaction with the material surface can also result in altered platelet survival or functional properties.[68,69]

Platelet adhesion measurements evaluate the overall retention of platelets on a surface, since platelet adhesion in vivo and in vitro is rapidly followed by platelet aggregation. Tests developed to measure platelet retention include biomaterial-bead columns, glass-bead columns, centrifugation test, bioluminescence measurement of platelet ATP, direct evaluation of platelet deposition, and scanning electron microscopy.[68,69]

Hemolysis

Red blood cells interacting with a surface can lyse or they can be retained in the circulation in an altered form.[67,68,70] The tendency of a biomaterial to induce red blood cell hemolysis can be evaluated in vitro under shearing conditions. In order for this evaluation to be accomplished, shear stress is induced as a blood sample is circulated between a pair of rotating parallel disks composed of a given biomaterial.[71]

Calcification

Pathologic or dystrophic calcification may be encountered as ectopic ossification in soft tissues surrounding an implant (such as total hip arthroplasty or cardiac valve replacement) or as biomaterial-associated mineralization occurring in prosthetic heart valves, vascular grafts, or ventricular assist devices.

Calcification of heart valves usually begins and is enhanced in areas of leaflet flexion where deformations are maximal, especially the cuspal commissures and bases in valves. However, the presence of similar-appearing calcification in subcutaneous implant models is suggestive that dynamic stress promotes but is not an absolute prerequisite for calcification.

Calcific degeneration of the bovine pericardial valves remains a major cause of failure in these devices (Fig. 30-5). The mechanism of calcification of these valves appears to be similar to that occurring in non–cross-linked valve substitutes

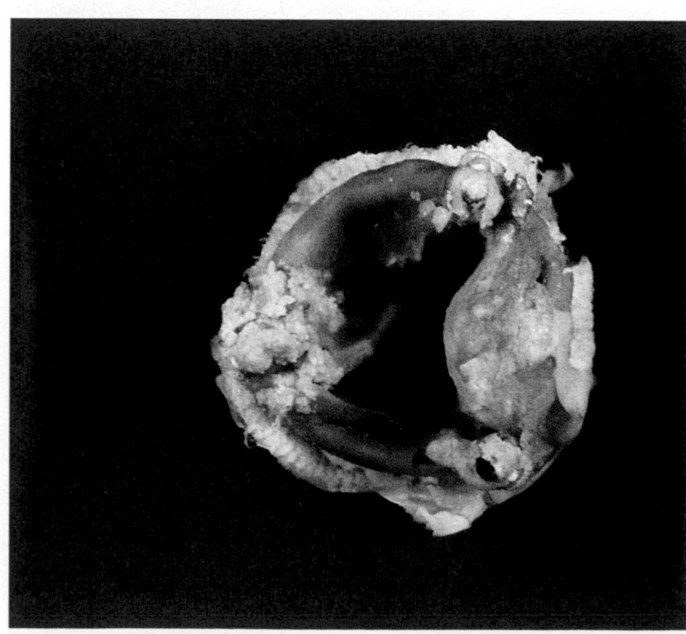

Fig. 30-5 Failed bovine bioprosthetic valve with extensive tears and parastent calcific deposits.

like cadaveric homografts, native dystrophic calcification, and physiologic bone mineralization. Thus mineralization of the bovine pericardial valve by hydroxyapatite (calcium phosphate) is not unique. It is observed in polymeric heart valves, and it is also seen on fabric coverings, various synthetic materials, heterografts and homografts, and pumping diaphragms and bladders of artificial hearts and ventricular assist devices in the pseudointima. The precise mechanisms by which calcification occurs in the glutaraldehyde-fixed and cross-linked pericardial valve cusps is unknown. It is believed that mineralization occurs after nucleation of calcium phosphate deposition of cellular debris and surface defects. Most calcification occurs within the collagen bundles and within the mesenchymal cells of the pericardial tissue, and occasional surface thrombi and vegetations may calcify and calcospherules may develop. Such deposits enlarge with time and progress to apatite. This mineralization ultimately results in stiffening and embrittlement of the implanted material.[72-76]

Schoen and colleagues[72-76] have hypothesized that calcification of glutaraldehye-preserved bioprosthetic valves is related to modification of physiologic ionic fluxes. Thus, although calcium influx into cells of the prosthetic valves persists, the energy-dependent mechanisms for calcium removal are no longer functional. Calcium and phosphorus levels are high at the sites of bioprosthetic mineralization in such membrane-bound organelles as mitochondria.

Although it is known that physiologic solutions such as plasma are saturated with hydroxyapatite, they escape spontaneous mineralization through macromolecule chelation of ions and the presence of inhibitors. Encouraging results are seen in prevention of mineralization of bioprosthetic valves through local administration of ethane-1-hydroxy-1,1-diphosphonate (etidronate, EHDP) adjacent to prosthetic tissue. Likewise experimental pretreatment of implant cuspal tissue with covalently bound aminopropane hydroxydiphosphonate reduces calcification. The proposed mechanisms and potential approaches for diminution of calcification are presented in Table 30-5.

Toxicity

A basic premise in the design and application of any biomedical device is to attain maximum benefit with a minimum of risk. To achieve this, toxicity testing is an essential component of any device development. The basic mechanisms of material toxicity are (1) biologically active leachables, (2) physical contact with the material, and (3) biodegradation of the material to alter its physical or compatibility properties or produce free bioactive molecules.[77]

For more than 60 years dental materials and subsequently various other medical materials have been tested for toxicity through subcutaneous, muscle, or abdominal cavity implantation utilizing rat, rabbit, or canine models. Since passage of the medical device amendments of 1967, all medical devices are classified into three broad categories by the United States Food and Drug Administration (FDA):

- Class I — Devices requiring only general control (the least dangerous devices, if dangerous at all)
- Class II — Devices requiring written performance standards and general controls (most devices appear to fall into this class and generally a require biologic test for safety)
- Class III — Devices requiring premarket approval (these devices are considered the most potentially dangerous items, and thus, testing similar to a new drug are required)

Several organizations issue guidelines for toxicity testing. The *United States Pharmacopeia* (USP) issues tests guidelines for plastic testing and extract media. The *Annual Book of American Society for Testing and Materials* (ASTM) *Standards* contains a section of biologic tests for medical devices. Protocols are provided in the American National Institute/American Dental Association's *Recommended Standard Practices for Biological Evaluation of Dental Materials*.[77]

The biologic reactivity of metals, ceramics, and polymers depends on the extraction and intracellular incorporation of low-molecular-weight chemicals and small particles. Biologic reactivity is most readily affected by low-molecular-weight substances that can permeate cell membranes. High-molecular-weight substances such as polymers of 500,000 daltons generally remain outside the cell and have no effect or depend on a cell surface receptor or endocytosis to affect the cell. Currently, many in vitro cell culture methods are available to detect toxic components of biomaterials. Such methods offer increased sensitivity as well as being much less expensive.[77]

Table 30-5 Calcification of bioprostheses

Putative mechanisms	Approaches to limit
Preservation by glutaraldehyde	Other preservatives (more rapid is better?)
Membranes of devitalized cells take up calcium in environment of phosphates	
Dynamic mechanical stress and strain	Improvements in design, maintenance of collagen crimps
Static mechanical deformation	
Surface defects	
De novo calcification (microcrystallization)	Quality control in handling antiplatelet therapy prevents overgrowth
Calcification of thrombi	
Ischemia in areas of pseudointimal	
Overgrowth	
Vitamin K-dependent calcium binding	
Proteins (with a-carboxyglutamic acid residue)	
Lack of natural inhibitors of calcification	Phosphocitrate (reflected in benefit of ethanehydroxydiphosphonate)

Tumorigenesis

The induction of malignant tumors in experimental animals has been observed with almost every type of solid material. However, only anecdotal reports describe malignant tumors associated with human implants despite the large number of implants. Tumors associated with human implants or induced experimentally are usually of mesenchymal origin and develop after a long latent period. Experimental data indicate that the phenomenon termed *solid-state carcinogenesis* is related to the following factors: (1) a continuous, smooth, impermeable surface, (2) the implant must be of a minimum size, (3) the implant must be in situ for a minimum period of time, and (4) the composition per se is of little importance in the absence of leachable carcinogens. Furthermore tumorigenicity is positively correlated with mature foreign body–reactive fibrous tissue encapsulation and negatively correlated with active cellular inflammation.

Some chemicals with demonstrated or suspected carcinogenic potential are employed in polymer synthesis. Several studies present conflicting results on the possible effect of biodegradation of polymers on carcinogenesis.[72,77]

Systemic reaction

Medical devices not only have interactions with the recipient at the site of the implant, but also can cause distant or systemic effects[2] (Table 30-6). Thrombotic occlusion and thromboemboli can occur with all currently utilized prosthetic valves and grafts, with a frequency of 1% to 4% per patient-year for cardiac valve prostheses and rates of greater than 50% for vein catheters. The function of prosthetic heart valves may be impaired by thrombi, or thromboemboli can migrate to distal arterial beds. The central nervous system is the most common site of clinically detectable involvement.[5] An uncommon but dramatic complication associated with intravascular prostheses (catheters, valves) is embolization of particles of the device material.

In animals and patients with either stainless-steel or cobalt-based orthopedic total joint replacement components, corrosion and wear may induce long-term changes in blood composition. These include elevations of both tissue metal content (at both local and remote sites) and of serum and urine metal ion concentrations. In patients with total joint replacements, large elevations in chromium concentration in serum occurs in the early postoperative period.[78] Moreover, significant elevations may persist for more than a decade, with accumulations of 10 to 100 times normal chromium and nickel content in tissues remote from an implanted hip.

"Metal allergy" is a well-recognized phenomenon, frequently associated in women with the use of cheap, high-nickel alloy costume jewelry or earrings. Allergy to nickel-containing mechanical heart valves has been reported.[79] Metal ions, by themselves, lack the structural complexity required to challenge the immune system. However, when combined with proteins, such as those available in the skin, connective tissues, and blood, a wide variety of metals induce immune responses and thus must be considered haptens. Cobalt, chromium, and nickel are included in this category, with nickel perhaps the most potent; at least 10% of a normal population will be sensitive by skin test to one or more of these metals at some threshold level. The most typical response of a metal-sensitized individual to a challenge is a type IV delayed hypersensitivity. Immune responses to polymers in clinical use have not been reliably reported, but there is some evidence for such a response to silicones.[80]

Device material migration to lymph nodes

The silicone gel contained in a breast prosthesis may migrate or "bleed" through a structurally intact solid silicone bag. Foreign-body reaction to the gel is commonly noted in tissues adjacent to the implants, especially in and around the encapsulating fibrous tissue. Once freed from the envelope, silicone gel tends to disperse in the soft tissues. Lymphatic migration of silicone material has been reported in prosthetic mammoplasty,[81] as well as in other circumstances, including finger prostheses and injections of silicone liquid for mammary augmentation. Although large lymph node deposits of silicone with associated sinus histiocytosis and foamy macrophages may be readily recognized by light microscopy, smaller particles can represent a challenge to identification.

Table 30-6 Fundamental host prosthetic interactions

Fundamental host prosthetic interactions
Effect of the implant on the host
Local
Aberrant healing
Exuberant encapsulation
Foreign-body reaction
Pannus formation
Aneurysm formation
Anastomotic intimal hyperplasia
Malposition
Blood–material surface interactions
Protein absorption and adsorption
Platelet adhesion, activation, and release
Coagulation
Fibrinolysis
Complement activation
Leukocyte adhesion and activation
Hemolysis
Foreign-body reaction
Infection
Toxicity
Tumorigenesis
Systemic and remote
Embolization
Thrombus
Vegetation
Biomaterial
Hypersensitivity
Elevation of unusual elements in blood
Lymphatic particle transport
Effect of the host on the implant
Physical and mechanical effects
Abrasive wear
Fatigue
Stress-corrosion cracking
Corrosion
Degeneration and dissolution
Biologic effects
Absorption of substances from tissues
Enzymatic degradation
Calcification

There is no known association of breast carcinoma with lymphatic migration of silicone from mammary prostheses. However, such cases are more likely to be evaluated as a suspicious lymphadenopathy in the setting of breast carcinoma to rule out recurrent cancer.

The clinically observed immunologic reponse to silicones from implant rupture and bleed is controversial. Some authors suggest that silicone predisposes some patients to conditions that mimic various rheumatologic diseases.[82-86] One theory proposed for such associated complications invokes a sequence of native protein denaturation by silicone, which then triggers an antibody-mediated reaction. A retrospective study of 749 women who received breast implants from 1964 through 1991 compared the incidence of connective-tissue disorders and other disorders to that of a cohort who did not receive implants. The authors found no significant increase of connective-tissue disorders associated with the implants.[87]

In a similar regard polyethylene, cement, and metal wear debris particles can be demonstrated in the tissue membrane surrounding hip and knee joint prostheses, and metal and polyethylene particles have been reported to migrate to inguinal lymph nodes.[88]

SPECIAL TYPES OF DEVICES

Orthopedic devices

Orthopedic hardware such as fixation plates, screws, rods, and pins will be removed and pass through the surgical pathology bench after a relatively short implantation period and thus they do not usually invoke significant device-associated complications. Total joint prostheses (hip, knee, shoulder, elbow) are designed to remain implanted and are associated with complications such as infection and aseptic loosening.

Total hip arthroplasty is an increasingly common procedure with approximately 150,000 performed annually.[32] The common causes for undergoing arthroplasty include osteoarthritis (60%), fracture dislocations (11%), rheumatoid arthritis (7%), aseptic bone necrosis (7%), and revision of previous hip operations (6%). Biomaterials used in current total hip replacement include alloys such as cobalt-chromium- and titanium-based systems, polymers such as poly(methyl methacrylate) and polyethylene, and ceramics. Systemic complications from total hip relacement are thromboembolic, such as venous thrombosis and, less commonly under appropriate prophylaxis, pulmonary thromboembolism. Infection occurs in 1% to 2% of patients undergoing total hip arthroplasty. Risk factors for arthroplasty infection include previous surgical incisions, multiple intra-articular steroid injections or previous septic arthritis, systemic disease such as rheumatoid arthritis or diabetes mellitus, obesity, and previous infected implants.

The most common cause of total arthroplasty failure is aseptic loosening, which occurs in approximately 10% of patients (Fig. 30-6). Although the exact sequence of events culminating in aseptic loosening of joint arthroplasties remains unknown, several factors may act in concert to lead to initial microscopic motion at the bone-cement interface: difference in elastic modulus of bone and cement, early bone necrosis from chemical or thermal trauma during surgery, or poor cement fixation. Obesity, increased physical activity, and improper stem position may increase stress on the joint and exacerbate these factors.

The histologic appearance of the tissue membrane from the bone-prosthesis interface from failed prostheses displays three distinct histologic zones:[89-94] (1) superficial layer of lining cells at the prosthesis surface, (2) midzone of histiocytes and giant cells, and (3) deep fibrous layer at the bone surface (Fig. 30-7).

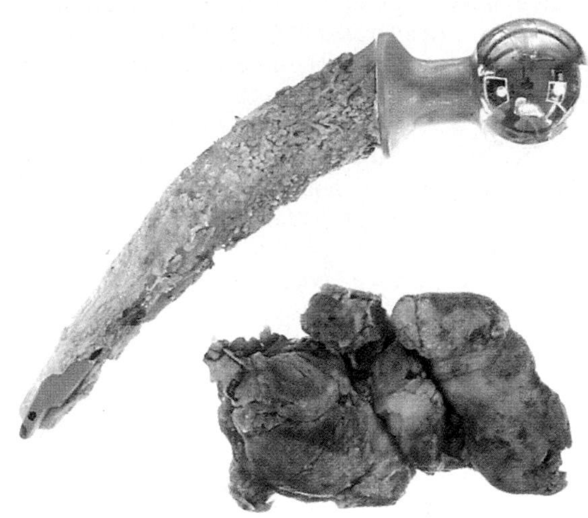

Fig. 30-6 Cobalt-chromium femoral prosthesis with acrylic cement adherent to stem along with removed prominent femoral canal interface tissue membrane.

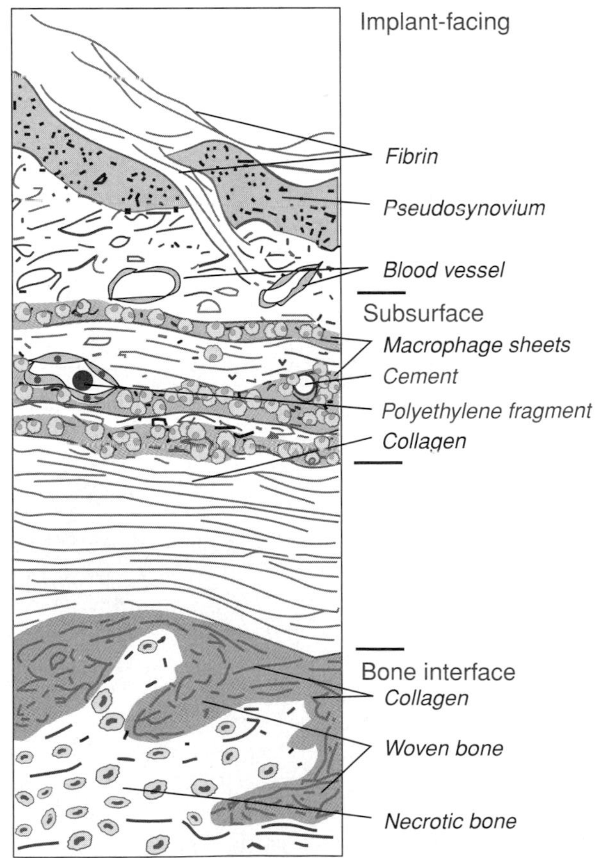

Fig. 30-7 Diagram of histologic regions of interface tissue membrane associated with orthopedic prostheses. (Modified from Lennox DW, Schofield BH, McDonald DF, Riley LH Jr: *Clin Orthop* 225:171, 1987.)

The cement surface is lined by a one- to two-cell thick layer of round to polygonal cells palisading at the superficial edge giving a "synovium-like" appearance (Fig. 30-8). Variable amounts of fibrin and necrosis are also present at the prosthesis surface. Deep to and contiguous with the lining cells is a loose fibrovascular stroma with scattered histiocytes and mononuclear cells. The middle zone is composed of fibrovascular tissue and sheets of granular histiocytes and mononuclear cells with interspersed giant cells. The deepest (bone surface) zone is composed primarily of dense collagen with occasional small vessels along with scattered fibroblasts.

It is widely held that wear debris not only is an indicator of abnormal prosthesis motion, but can also contribute to the pathogenesis of further loosening. Debris from total joint prostheses may be derived from ultrahigh-molecular-weight polyethylene (UHMWPE) debris from the acetabular or patellar components, poly(methyl methacrylate) debris from cement, and metal debris. Wear, creep, and oxidative degradation are accelerated by frictional heating during articulation of prostheses.

Micromotion at the implant (cement)–bone interface is believed to lead to the activation of macrophages directly and indirectly through debris formation. Several authors have demonstrated that activated macrophages produce acid phosphatase, collagenase, and prostaglandin E_2,[90,94] and more recently tumor necrosis factor;[94] all are implicated in bone lysis. Osteoclasts are also stimulated by motion, further promoting bone resorption. Bone loss results in macroscopic motion causing mechanized abrasion and wear products that will induce further histiocyte response with perpetuation of the process resulting in clinical loosening and pain.

According to Lennox,[92] membranes from failed biologic ingrowth uncemented prostheses rarely contain areas similar in appearance to the pseudosynovial lining seen with cemented prosthesis. More commonly, uncemented interface membranes contain macrophages and a loosely organized fibrous tissue with large active fibroblasts and areas of woven bone. In the absence of significant metallic debris particles, fewer macrophages, lymphocytes, and plasma cells are present than those in cemented membranes.

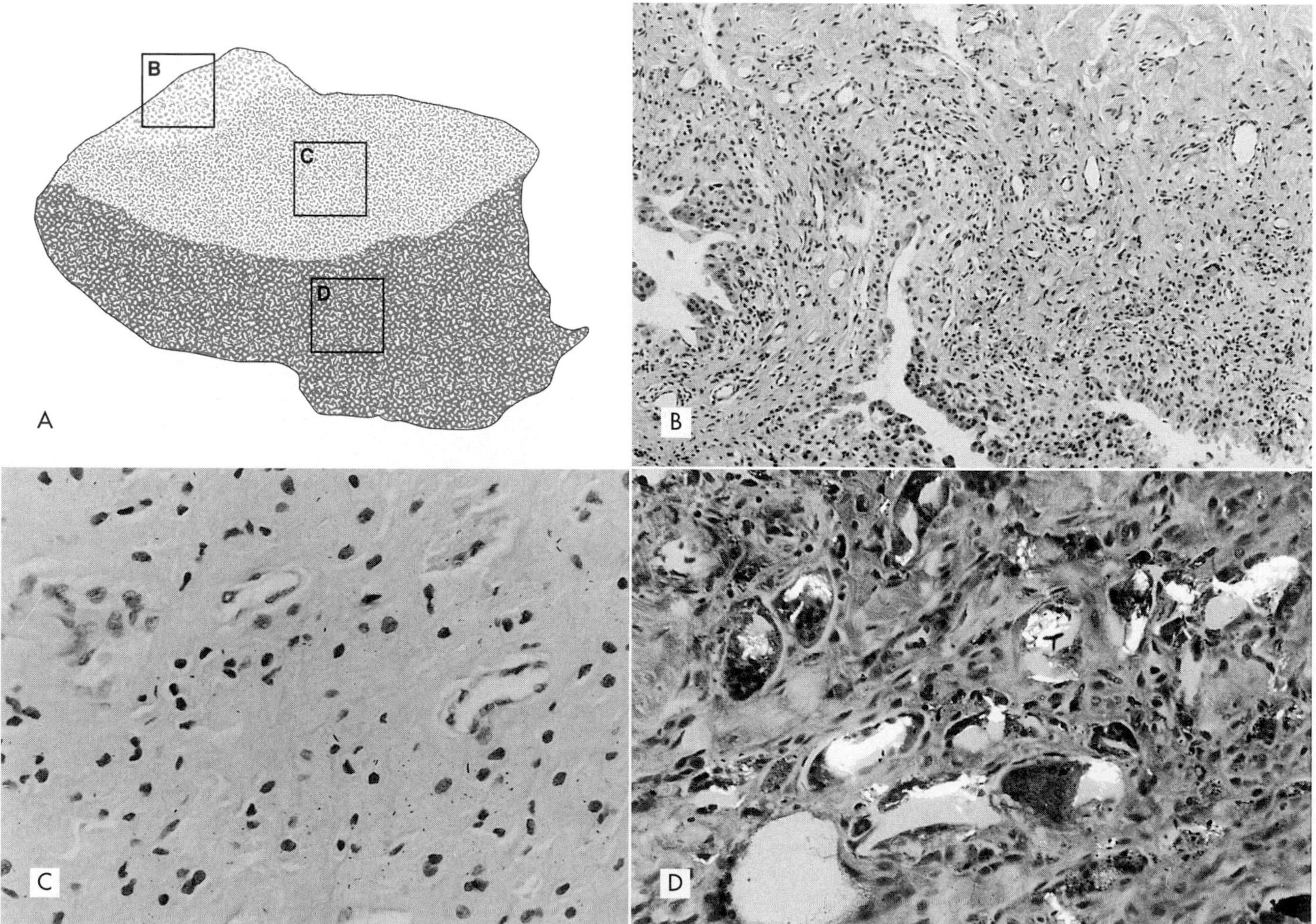

Fig. 30-8 **A,** Line drawing of gross tissue specimen from hip prosthesis removed for aseptic loosening. **B,** Superficial and middle zones of membrane tissue with palisading of "synovium-like" cells. Beneath this are numerous lymphocytes and histiocytes. **C,** Middle and deeper regions of tissue with histiocytes containing small black particles consistent with metallic debris. **D,** High-power view of superficial and middle zones containing histiocyte and giant cell response to refractile material consistent with polyethylene.

Aggressive granulomatous lesions after hip arthroplasty appear to represent a separate entity from the usual cases of loosening with a distinctive radiographic appearance of a large tumorlike ovoid lytic area without evidence of infection and a rapidly progressive course.[95] Histologically, these lesions consist of large sheets of histiocytes and giant cells, and immunohistopathologic studies have shown a paucity of activated fibroblasts as compared to the usual cases of aseptic loosening.[94,96] The usual progression from histiocyte infiltrate to fibroblast proliferation and synthesis of extracellular matrix by activated fibroblasts appears disrupted in these patients. Whether this is attributable to an imbalance between monokines that promote fibroblast proliferation (such as platelet-derived growth factor AB, transforming growth factor B1, interleukin-1B) and substances, such as PGE_2, that inhibit it has not been clarified.[94,97]

Biomaterials used in total joint replacement are selected for their mechanical and chemical compatibility. However, all foreign materials elicit some tissue reaction and in vivo wear at the articular surface and with time produce particulate debris that typically elicits a stronger tissue response. Examples of materials seen in tissue sections from failed prostheses are further demonstrated in Table 30-7. The ultimate nature and extent of tissue reaction to orthopedic prostheses depend on the chemical and physical characteristics of the implant, as well as the shape, size, and amount of wear debris. In vitro work indicates that titanium-alloy debris particles may be more likely to cause release of mediators that promote osteolysis than debris from cobalt-chromium.[98,99]

Cardiovascular devices

Cardiac valves

Heart valve prostheses have been successfully used for more than three decades. Currently, more than 100,000 prosthetic valves are implanted worldwide annually. The most serious problems and complications associated with heart valve prostheses have been and continue to be (1) thrombosis and thromboembolism, (2) anticoagulation-related hemorrhage, (3) tissue overgrowth, (4) infection, (5) perivalvular leaks attributable to healing defects, and (6) valve failure attributable to material

Table 30-7 Malignant neoplasms missed clinically: discovered at autopsy

Material	Ordinary light	Polarized light	Cellular reaction and other features
Metal	Black spheres or angular rods 1 to 1 μm in diameter	Moderately refractile about edges	1. Usually found within mononuclear histiocytes or extracellularly 2. Moderate to massive amounts found in multinucleated histiocytes and in association with chronic inflammation
Metal-like artifact			
Formalin pigment	Black rods 3 to 6 μm in length; aggregates are petal-like formations	Negative	Usually deposited on erythrocytes and not in histocytes
Hemosiderin pigment	Brownish red aggregates, globular 6 to 10 μm in diameter	Negative	
Polyethylene	Translucent fibers with smooth irregular edges 5 to 40 μm long, occasionally 100 μm or greater	Strongly refractile	1. Positive staining with Oil Red O performed on formalin-fixed paraffin-embedded tissue 2 Fibers <10 μm in mononuclear histiocytes 3. Fibers 10 to 40 μm in foreign-body giant cells or extracellularly 4. Fibers >40 μm surrounded by giant cells 5. >500 μm surrounded by scar tissue
Cotton fibers	Long slender fibers several hundred micrometers long, translucent	Strongly refractile	1. Out of plane of section 2. No tissue reaction 3. Haphazardly arrived, usually on edges of tissue
Starch	Moderately birefringent, Maltese cross pattern		
Extraneous materials	Variably opaque or translucent	Variable refractile	Usually out of plane of section, haphazardly oriented, no tissue reaction
Acrylic cement	1. Clear spaces (dissolved by xylene) 2. If barium sulfate added, 1 to 2 μm granules may be seen	1. Barium sulfate granules, moderately birefringent 2. Recrystallized needles, strongly birefringent	Globules of acrylic usually surrounded by fibrous histiocytes, multinucleated giant cells, or scar tissue

Modified from Mirra JM, Amstolz HC, Maddows M, Gold R: *Clin Orthop* 117:221, 1976.

fatigue or chemical change. The two general categories of valve prostheses are mechanical, made from synthetic components, and tissue, made, at least in part, of animal or human tissue.[100,101]

Basic types of mechanical valve prostheses include ball and cage, tilting disk, and bileaflet. Mechanical valves are manufactured from a variety of materials including pyrolytic carbon, titanium, Stellite, silicone rubber, elgiloy (cobalt-nickel alloy), Teflon, and Dacron. The components of a mechanical valve prosthesis include a rigid, mobile occluder (poppet) around which blood must flow, the cagelike superstructure that guides and restricts poppet motion, and the valve body or base. Current tilting-disk valve occluders are coated with pyrolytic carbon, which possesses high strength, high resistance to wear and fatigue, and high thromboresistance.[100,101]

Mechanical valves available in the United States include the Starr-Edwards cage Silastic ball (S-E), the Medtronic-Hall tilting disk (M-H), the Omni Science tilting disk (OS), and the St. Jude Medical bileaflet (SJM) valves.[101]

Because the S-E valve has an unacceptably large pressure gradient as well as considerable flow separation, turbulence, and increased hemolysis, it is rarely used. The Björk-Shiley (BS) valve and the Medtronic-Hall tilting disk valve (M-H) are among the more commonly used tilting disk valves. The BS valve has evolved in design, and in 1981 the valve ring of the BS valve was modified to have the valve ring and guide structure machined from a single piece of titanium (monostrut). Thus the current M-H tilting disk valve is a ring and strut combination machined from a single piece of titanium, and the strut is sigmoidal in shape.

Anticoagulation therapy is required for all mechanical valve patients; fortunately thromboembolism in valve thrombosis remain significant but infrequent occurrences.

The St. Jude Medical valve (SJM) is a pyrolytic carbon bileaflet valve first introduced in 1977. The in vitro fluid dynamic characteristics of bileaflet valves are somewhat more favorable than other mechanical valve design types. Although pressure gradients across these valves have been in general lower than either Starr-Edwards cage ball or Ionescu-Shiley pericardial valves, clinical data show no significant difference between pressure gradients of M-H tilting disk valve and SJM bileaflet valves.[101]

Valve thrombosis for SJM prostheses is lower than that in other mechanical valve designs, with a linearized rate of valve thrombosis causing obstruction of 0.28%/patient-year. The linearized rate of systemic embolism for the SJM valve is reported to be 2.09%/patient-year for the mitral position and 0.99%/patient-year for the aortic position.[101,102]

Some generalizations can be formulated when one compares the performance of mechanical valves in the published literature.[103,104] The tendency for thromboembolism to occur more frequently with mitral than with aortic valve replacement can be seen for the SE, SJM, and OS valves. The rate of prosthetic valve endocarditis is comparable for the SE, MH, and SJM valves.

Bioprosthetic valves are usually assembled from chemically preserved (cross-linked) animal tissue mounted on a prosthetic frame (stent). The other tissue valve in use is the human aortic allograft, which is processed but not cross-linked and implanted directly into the aortic root without a stent.[101] Generally, porcine valves have much fewer problems with thrombosis and do not require anticoagulation therapy. However, the durability of bioprostheses is inferior to that of mechanical valves. Pericardial valves, made from glutaraldehyde-treated bovine pericardium, were introduced clinically in 1967, and the design evolved to the Ionescu-Shiley (IS) valve in the 1970s.[101-113]

Early failures of porcine bioprostheses were followed by reports regarding the failure of bovine pericardial prostheses,[107-109] particularly in young children.[108] In the latter experience, a prominent overgrowth of collagenous tissue on the ventricular surface of the prostheses placed in the mitral position caused severe prosthetic dysfunction. Similar overgrowth of tissue on right-sided bioprosthetic valves has been observed. Thromboembolic phenomena related to the bovine pericardial valve are generally less than 0.5%/patient-year of implantation. The rate of thromboembolism may be lower than that for the porcine heterograft.

A significantly higher frequency of primary valve dysfunction and failure has been described for the gluteraldehyde-treated bovine pericardial valve (Ionescu-Shiley) than in porcine heterografts, particularly when implantation greater than 48 months was observed.[109-113] Both valve types had frequent cuspocalcific deposits and associated tears with connective tissue degeneration, and foci of inflammatory cells and occasional giant cell responses were observed, though the deterioration of the Ionescu-Shiley valve typically results in regurgitation. When calcification is diffuse, the cusps may become rigid, causing predominant stenosis, red blood cell hemolysis, and hemosiderosis.

A special feature of the Ionescu-Shiley bovine pericardial heart valve relates to the manner of alignment of the artificial prosthetic valve cusp. This is accomplished by placement of a suture at the commissure and results in a "tailoring" point that transmits undue stress to the valvular tissue, and, with time, larger and larger calcific deposits and cuspal tears occur. The pathogenetic sequence to these tears has been described by Walley and Keon[113] (Fig. 30-9).

Prosthetic valves or vascular grafts are subject to a variable amount of overgrowth of fibrous connective tissue from the adjacent supporting vascular wall or valve annulus. Although usually limited in degree, occasionally this "pannus" formation can be substantial enough to produce incomplete valve occluder opening or closure.[101] This pannus formation may exist with ongoing or intermittent nonocclusive thrombus formation (Fig. 30-10). Although the histologic distinction between healed or organized thrombus and pannus formation is not always possible, the former may include more glycosaminoglycan-rich areas whereas the latter tends to be predominantly more collagenized. The overlap in morphology indicates that both ingrowth and thrombotic processes may be at play in the evolution of valve immobilization.

Similar overgrowth of tissue on right-sided bioprosthetic valves has been observed by others. In the series of Murphy and colleagues,[36] connective tissue overgrowth resulted in retraction of leaflets, incorporation of bioprosthetic valve cusps in the valve ring itself, and prominent valvular regurgitation. The basis of this type of valve failure, which is characterized by pronounced valvular regurgitation is not known. The possibility that low flow, stasis, and turbulence lead to chronic incomplete excursion of the leaflets with concurrent surface microthrombus formation on struts, rings, and leaflets has been entertained.

Homograft/allograft aortic valves are utilized mostly in patients with pulmonary valve or pulmonary artery replace-

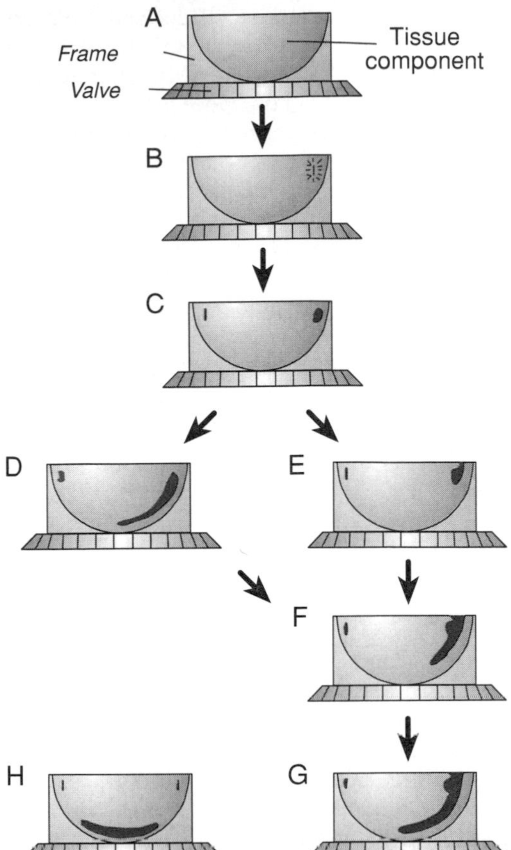

Fig. 30-9 Proposed pathogenesis of tears in Ionescu-Shiley standard bioprostheses. Normal valve, **A,** may undergo wear at the commissural suture or alignment stitch, **B,** at which site a hole may then develop, **C.** The free margin of the cusp may then tear, **E,** and the tear may propagate to varying lengths, **F** and **G.** Alternately, the hole, **C,** may cause a tear to start that runs to the base of the valve, **D.** The free margin of the cusp may tear later, producing tears of varying lengths, **F** and **G.** Occasional tears may originate at the cusp base, perhaps because of abrasion, **H,** and these may propagate to varying lengths in varying directions. (From Walley VM, Keon WJ: *Thorac Cardiovasc Surg* 93:925, 1987.)

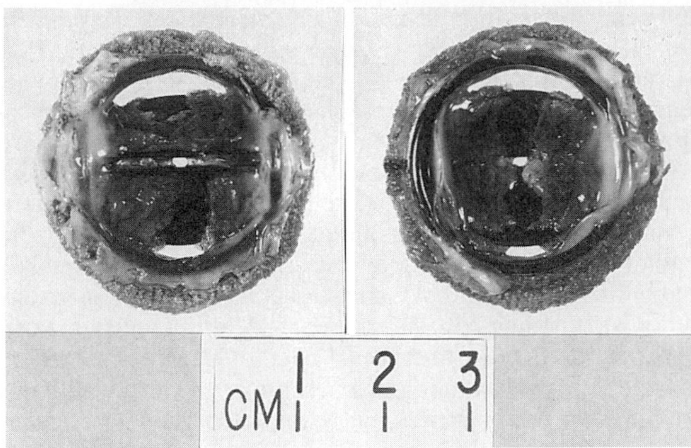

Fig. 30-10 Atrial, **A,** and ventricular, **B,** views of explanted St. Jude Medical prosthetic valve with recent (reddish) and healing (gray-white) thrombic material resulting in orifice occlusion and fixation of leaflets in semiopen position.

Table 30-8 Pathologic analysis of mechanical and bioprosthetic valves

Gross examination	Radiography	Histology
Tissue overgrowth	Valve identification	Vegetations and organisms
Thrombi	Calcification	Thrombi
Vegetations	Degree	Host cell interactions
Cuspal stiffness	Localization	Degeneration
Cuspal hematomas		Calcification
Calcification		Degree
Fenestration and tears		Morphology
		Location
Cuspal abrasion		Endothelialization
Cuspal stretching		
Strut relationships		
Mechanical dysfunction		
Extrinsic interference and damage		

From Schoen FJ, Levy RJ, Piehler HR: *Cardiovasc Pathol* 1:29, 1992.

ment for congenital heart disease or in patients with annular destruction or dilatation accompanying aortic valve disease. Allografts possess excellent hemodynamic properties as well as a low rate of thromboembolism. Unfortunately, they are subject to cuspal rupture, distortion with retraction, or perforations leading to valvular incompetence.[100] Explanted allografts are uniformly devoid of surface endothelium and deep connective tissue cells. Proximal intimal fibrous sheath, aortic wall calcification, and occasionally cuspal calcific deposits are seen in allografts with longer implantation duration.

Explant analysis in the routine hospital setting at autopsy or surgical removal begins with photography from all pertinent angles and examination for thrombi, vegetations, exuberant tissue overgrowth, and structural defects. Probing for paravalvular leaks should be done on autopsy specimens. Mechanical valves should be examined for functional adequacy including excursion and seating of poppets as well as signs of abrasive wear, asymmetries, and defects or fractures[100] (Table 30-8). Bioprostheses are examined to assess cuspal hematomas, calcific nodules, and central migration of struts (creep). Radiography may aid in identification of the prosthesis type as well as in semiquantitative assessment and location of valve calcifications. Histologic examination of the cross sections of bioprosthetic cusps is done to determine tissue-prosthesis interactions, cuspal degeneration, and the degree and specific morphology of calcific deposits.

Vascular grafts

Vascular graft performance depends primarily on graft type and location.[9,23,24,26,114,115] Dacron (polyethylene terephthalate, PET) grafts in current use generally perform well in large-diameter, high-flow, low-resistance locations such as the aorta and the iliac and proximal arteries of the lower extremities. The 10-year patency rate of Dacron prostheses is nearly 100% at the aortic bifurcation, approximately 75% to 80% in the aorta-femoral position, and 50% in the above-knee femoropopliteal position. In contrast, small-diameter fabric vascular grafts (<6-8 mm in diameter) have lower flow rates and generally perform less well. The most widely used small-vessel replacements are autogenous saphenous vein and expanded polytetrafluoroethylene (ePTFE). The patency of femoropopliteal autologous saphenous vein bypass grafts is approximately 50% at 10 years. Patency of above-knee grafts of ePTFE is nearly comparable to that of reversed autologous saphenous vein grafts, but more distal ePTFE bypass grafts have a 3- to 4-year patency rate of only 30% to 50%. Complications of vascular grafts that can occur in any site of implantation include thrombosis and thromboembolism, infection, periprosthetic fluid collection, pseudoaneurysm, and structural degeneration. The importance of each of these complications in large or small vascular grafts is summarized in Table 30-9.

The concept of providing increased blood flow to oligemic lungs by operative intervention led to the development of several systemic to pulmonary arterial shunt procedures beginning with the Blalock-Taussig anastomosis reported in 1945.[61] The original procedure using native arteries and an end-to-side anastomosis of the right or left subclavian arteries to their respective ipsilateral pulmonary artery branches was modified in the late 1970s by the interposition of synthetic graft material, polytetrafluoroethylene (PTFE).[60-64] The modified shunt is the generally preferred method to increase pulmonary blood flow in children with tetralogy of Fallot and pulmonic valve atresia.

Failure of the modified Blalock-Taussig shunt is related in part to the size mismatch of the growing pulmonary artery and the synthetic material site of anastomosis, in part by other causes of deformation along the course of the graft, including that caused by the inherent thrombogenic properties of the PTFE graft. Shunt failure, including thrombosis, has been reported in up to 14% of patients,[60-62] however, recent data from experience in 62 infants less than 3 months of age indicates that up to 27 out of 63 (43%) had shunt failure before 2 years of age.[62] Thrombosis of the shunt (Fig. 30-11) may occur early,[10,62] within hours to days after the procedure, or late.

Anastomotic intimal hyperplasia

The biologic surface lining the blood-contacting region of a vascular graft could hypothetically arise from either (1) host vessel–derived tissue growth across anastomotic sites, (2) trans–interstitial tissue migration, or (3) deposition of tissue from blood. However, healing of the inner capsule of contemporary vascular grafts is primarily derived from endothelial cells (EC) and smooth muscle cells (SMC), arising from the artery adjacent to the anastomosis. SMC migrate and proliferate in association with the endothelial growing edge.[5,9] In contrast, trans–interstitial tissue growth occurs only under special circumstances (such as high porosity), and there is no evidence to support the notion that there is deposition of cells from blood capable of differentiating into EC. Except under specialized circumstances, anastomotic overgrowth is generally restricted to a zone near and contiguous with the viable artery, often despite postoperative intervals of many years. Thus the ability of humans to endothelialize synthetic cardiovascular prostheses is limited, with EC ultimately extending only 10 to 15 mm or less across an anastomosis. The blood-contacting surface of the graft is perhaps best termed *neointima* if the surface is composed of any other biologic material, such as fibrin, collagen, platelets, or SMCs.

Intimal hyperplasia

Failure of small-diameter vascular prostheses is most frequently attributable to occlusion by thrombus formation or anastomotic or generalized intimal hyperplasia (IH). Although synthetic vascular prostheses develop IH predominantly at or near anastomoses, IH is often diffuse in vein grafts, leading to progressive stenosis of the entire graft.

IH is an exaggeration of the normal arterial healing response, arising from the intimal migration and proliferation of medial SMC derived from the host vessel with a synthetic vascular graft and from either host vessel or the graft itself when the graft has viable cells (such as an autogenous saphenous vein). There is a common mechanistic thread through the major clinical syndromes of IH, including not only vein-graft intimal fibrosis and synthetic-graft anastomotic hyperplasia, but also atherosclerosis, angioplasty restenosis, cardiac transplant vascular disease and other situations.[9,26,115-118] To a large extent, all such states represent the response to a vascular injury: intense SMC activity, manifested as proliferation in the media, migration to the intima, proliferation in the intima, increased cellular volume, and extracellular matrix prodution.[116-118]

The biologic, hemodynamic, and mechanical factors contributory to the initiation and progression of IH are not well understood (Table 30-10). A critical factor in IH is probably acute or ongoing injury to the endothelium (such as damage

Table 30-9 Major complications of vascular grafts

	Large Dacron graft	Small synthetic graft	Autogenous saphenous vein
Thrombus or thromboembolism		×	×
Infection	×	×	
Perigraft seroma		×	
Erosion into adjacent structure	×	×	
Anastomotic pseudoaneurysm	×	×	
Intimal fibrous hyperplasia		×	×
Degradation with fragmentation or dilatation		×	×

Modified from Schoen FJ: Interventional and surgical cardiovascular pathology: clinical correlations and basic principles, Philadelphia, 1989, Saunders.

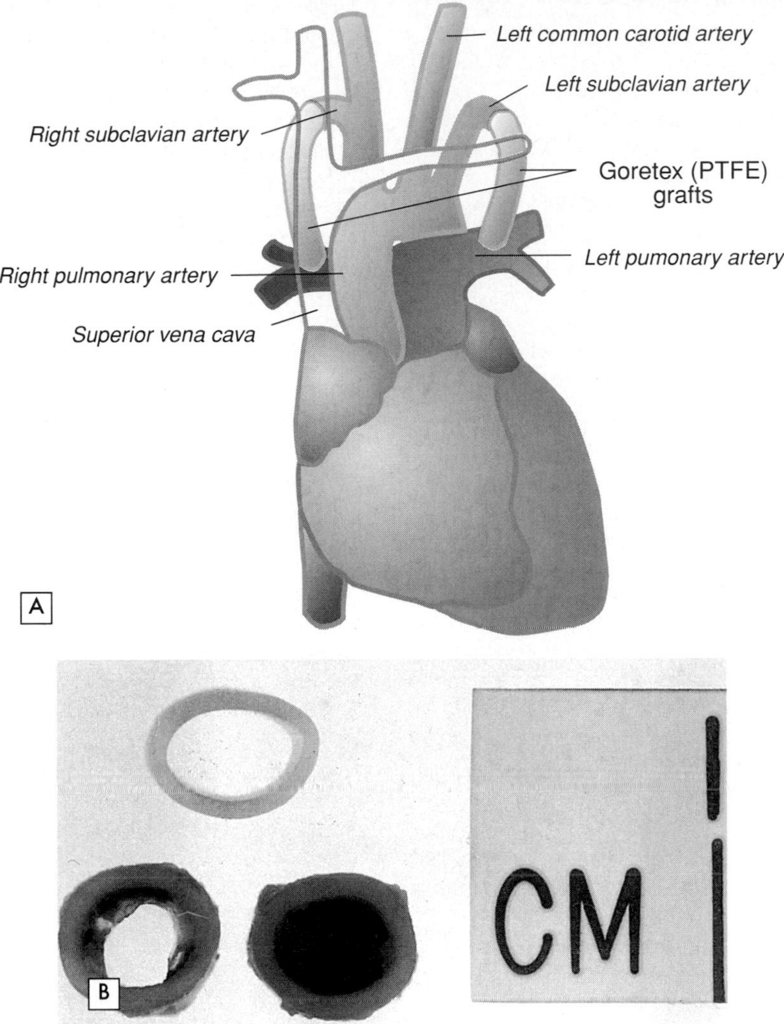

Fig. 30-11 **A,** Diagram of left and right modified Blalock-Taussig shunts. **B,** Transverse sections of open, partially occluded, and completely thrombosed segments of a 5 mm diameter PTFE Blalock-Taussig shunt.

that occurs during the harvesting and preparation of a vein graft, ongoing damage at an anastomosis, or wall injury as a result of arterial pressure within a vein). The SMC proliferation of IH in vascular grafts is considered similar to that which underlies restenosis after coronary or peripheral balloon angioplasty and heart transplant coronary disease. The latter processes are often called *accelerated atherosclerosis,* since intimal proliferation of SMCs is a critical component of typical atherosclerosis. Although typical atherosclerosis usually requires many years to develop, angioplasty restenosis or cardiac transplant vascular disease commonly occur over several months to a few years.[26]

An intense interest in modification of the fibroproliferative response is stimulated by the high rate of failure of vascular grafts and percutaneous transluminal angioplasty caused by IH (up to 40%), and of cardiac allografts.[9] Exciting areas for research focus on the pharmacologic inhibition of SMC proliferation are (1) endogenous SMC growth inhibitors (particularly heparin);[119,120] (2) exogenous pharmacologic agents (particularly angiotensin-converting enzyme inhibitors),[121] (3) growth factor–linked toxins specific for proliferating SMCs,[122] and (4) genetic engineering of vascular wall cells.[123]

Aneurysm formation

Mechanical failure at an anastomotic site or in the body of a prosthesis can lead to aneurysm (if vascular continuity remains intact) or false aneurysm (if rupture occurs). False aneurysms are not uncommon near an anastomosis, but false aneurysms in the graft body are unusual.[124-126]

Specific clinical situations may potentiate graft aneurysm or pseudoaneurysm. Since local infection can induce an acidic pH environment, infection could potentiate the degradation of polyester or other fabrics. Moreover, perigraft hematoma or pseudoaneurysm may occur within an interposed arteriovenous fistula used for hemodialysis access that is punctured frequently by needles and in which there are multiple coalescent holes.[127]

Aneurysm formation is an important problem associated with the operative repair of aortic coarcts. Olsson and colleagues[128] as well as Walter and colleagues[129] reported fre-

Table 30-10 Pathologic features of extracardiac conduits

- Aortic homografts
- Calcification
  - Intimal peel (neointima)
  - Endocarditis
  - Thrombosis
- Valved synthetic conduits
  - Bioprosthetic valve
    - Stenosis secondary to:
    - Calcification
    - Secondary thrombosis at commissures of valve stenosis
    - Fusion of cusps
    - Insufficiency secondary to:
    - Degeneration with cuspal tears
    - Thrombotic adhesions
    - Endocarditis
    - Fusion of cusps
  - Conduit
    - Fibrous peel (neointima)
    - Thrombosis
    - Pannus formation at anastomoses
- Nonvalved synthetic conduits
  - Fibrous peel (neointima)
  - Thrombosis

Modified from Virmani R, Atkinson JB, Forman MB: Aortocoronary bypass grafts and extracardiac conduits. In Silver M, editor: Cardiovascular pathology, ed 2, New York, 1991, Churchill Livingstone.[132]

quent occurrence of aneurysms at the site of Dacron patch grafting. Although patch repair is generally associated with a low frequency of reintervention for coarctation and operative death, compared to alternative procedures (end-to-end anastomosis, subclavian flap, or interposition graft) it clearly is the only repair procedure for coarctation associated with a significant frequency of aneurysm formation.[130,131]

Microscopic and macroscopic examination of these aneurysms typically reveals the operative suture lines to be intact and the Dacron to be unremarkable. The wall of the aorta at this point is considerably thinned and may have focal "eggshell" calcifications. There is often severe-to-complete degeneration, fragmentation and loss of elastin fibrils, a decrease in the number of medial smooth muscle cells with basketweave fibrosis of the media, and focal intimal thickening. The latter is often rich in cells and in glycosaminoglycans. No inflammatory cell infiltrate is typically present and a foreign-body giant-cell reaction is not seen. Adventitial vasa vasorum remain normal. The aneurysms are technically true anatomic aneurysms because all three layers of the aortic wall remain, but the severity of degeneration and destruction of the normal medial architecture in these aneurysms leads to a largely fibrous plaque, which could be construed as a variant of false aneurysm. It is easy to understand how confusion might exist regarding terminology in respect to this lesion.

The basis of this lesion is probably multifactorial but is in part related to resection and injury at the time of operation, in part related to hemodynamic factors, and in part to factors yet to be established. Several speculations have arisen regarding the basis of aneurysm formation including the influence of retention of the posterior wall to the coarct as well as the strong effect of resection of the coarct membrane.

Extracardiac conduits

Rastelli first described an extracardic conduit in 1965, and subsequently conduits have been used in the treatment of congenital obstructions of the aortic or pulmonary valve or left or right ventricular outflow tract.[9,132] Conduits are either valved or nonvalved and heterograft (Dacron) or aortic homograft. Pathologic changes may involve the bioprosthetic valve or the conduit (Table 30-10). The valvular changes are similar to those of intracardiac bioprosthetic valve with calcification, degeneration, and tears common along with cuspal fusion and thrombosis, especially in the young population. The conduits universally develop a luminal fibrous "peel," or neointima, of variable thickness, which may progress to obstruct the lumen (Fig. 30-12). Histologically, the neointima consists of a luminal region of dense collagen and a conduit portion of active granulation tissue, inflammation, and fibrosis[132] (Fig. 30-13). A varying amount of fresh or organized thrombotic material is usually present between the conduit wall and the neointima. Obstruction of the conduit may be attributable to valve stenosis, thick neointima, or thrombotic separation of the neointima.[133]

Cardiac patches

In addition to the forementioned blood-surface interactions, cardiovascular implants also possess a surface or surfaces that interface with areas of vascular wall and surrounding supporting tissues not directly exposed to the circulating blood. In these regions the biomaterial will induce a foreign-body reaction composed of foreign-body giant cells as well as granulation tissue. Depending on the topography and form of the implanted material this granulation tissue will be composed of varying amounts of fibroblasts, macrophages, and capillaries.

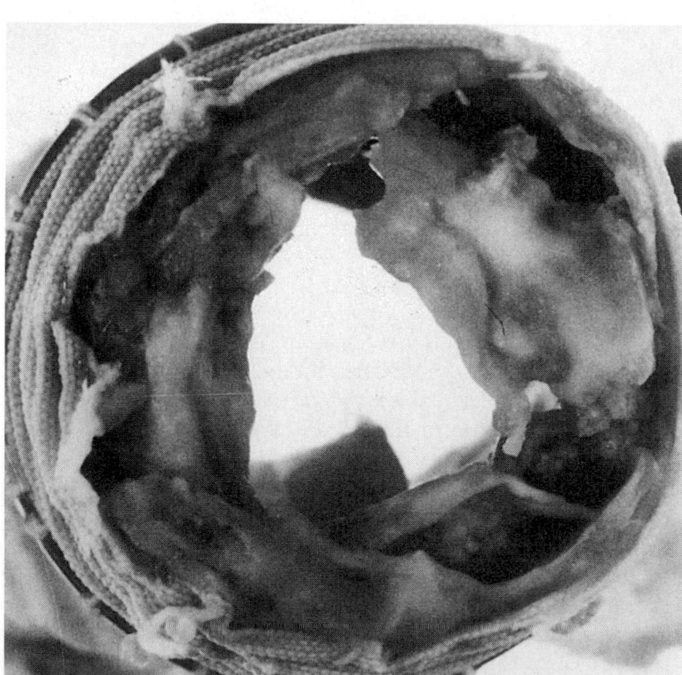

Fig. 30-12 Gross photograph of a narrowed Dacron conduit illustrating involvement of the porcine valve and the apparent poor adherence of the connective tissue to the Dacron *(upper left).*

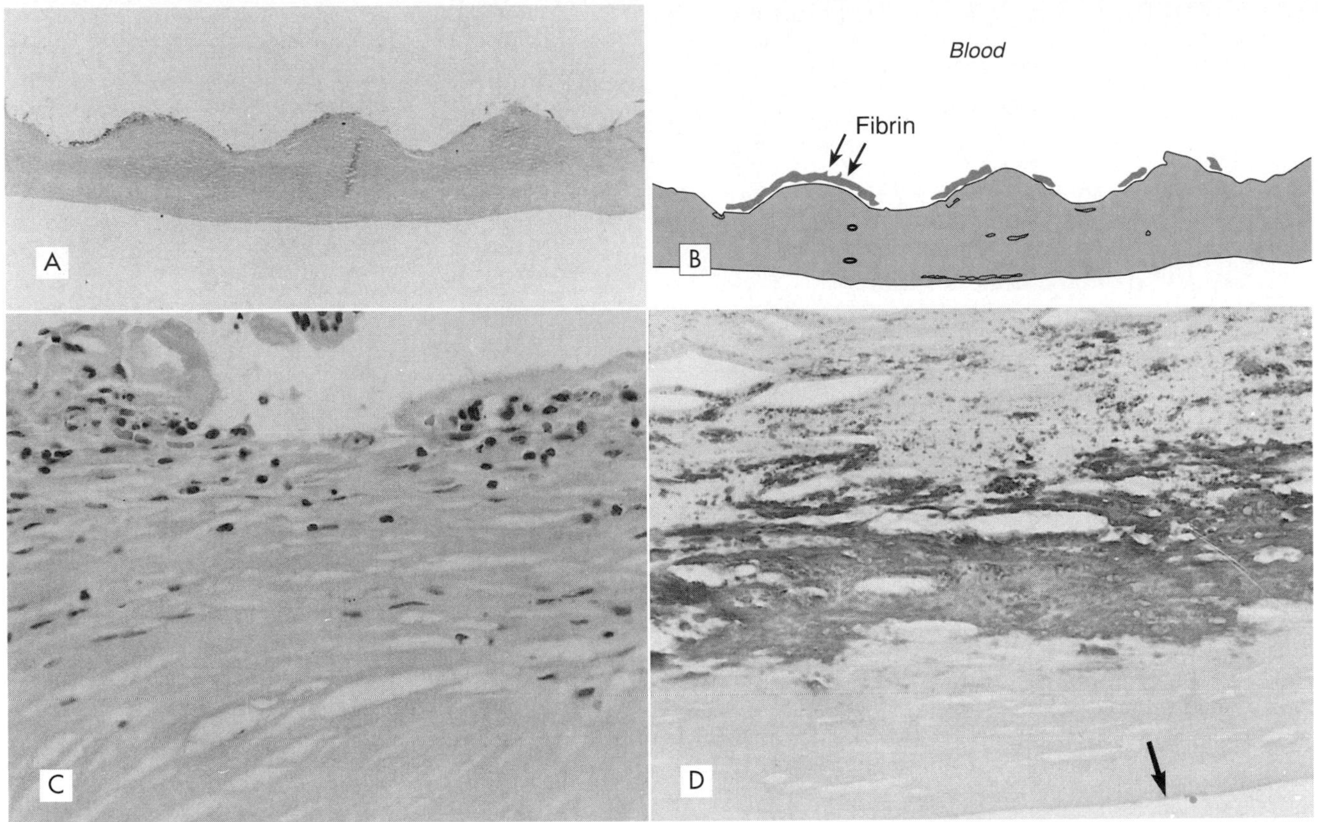

Fig. 30-13 Photographs (**A, C,** and **D**) and diagram **(B)** of a section of neopseudointima from the conduit in Fig. 30-12. The corrugated margin has areas of "activity" indicated by arrows, **B,** and illustrated in higher power in **C.** The basket weave collagen of the pseudointima has foci of dystrophic calcification, **D.** It is also evident that this membrane has no endothelium, **D,** *arrow.*

The foreign-body reaction may persist at the tissue-implant interface for the lifetime of the implant but is usually isolated from the local tissue environment by fibrous encapsulation.

An example of this type of implant is the recently developed atrial septal defect closure device. Closure of the atrial septum has traditionally been an operative challenge involving sutures or patches. Indeed, most of these patches have been synthetic material, either Dacron or PTFE. Nearly 20 years ago King and Mills demonstrated the feasibility of closure of atrial septal defects utilizing transvascular, nonoperative approaches.[134] Rashkind extended this early work by developing a slightly different device that required a smaller catheter (15 French versus 23 French). Their additional efforts to use the latest model of atrial septal defect closure device (a double-hinged "clamshell" umbrella) (Figs. 30-14 and 30-15) resulted in correct placement of 6 of 8 umbrellas with documentation of complete closure (functionally and anatomically) post mortem. Current concerns regarding even the latest device relate to the frequency of late embolization, thrombus formation, arrhythmogenesis, penetration of the metallic supports through cardiac tissues, and an altered risk for endocarditis. Limited pathologic information regarding the closure and healing of these devices is available. In preliminary studies,[135] the interaction of the polyurethane mesh of Rashkind occluders with blood constituents was studied grossly and histologically in five animals post mortem and in 2 children for whom the device was removed for inadequate closure of an atrial septal defect. Fibrin-platelet infiltration of the mesh occurred within 1 day of placement in both animals and humans. Between 3 and 10 days in the animals, organization of fibrin-platelet infiltrates ensued with patchy collagen deposition, ingrowth of surface endothelium, and a granulomatous giant cell response to the mesh (Fig. 30-16). Active fibrosis was most prominent at the mesh-endocardial interfaces. The new "clamshell" occluder is made of Dacron and may produce healing differently from one made of polyurethane.

In the most recent clinical experience with the double-hinged "clamshell" occluder, 32 of 34 carefully selected patients had successful occlusion of an atrial septal defect.[136] In imaging studies an average of 6.5 months after device placement, 12 of 19 patients had no residual atrial shunt (Fig. 30-5).[136] As this approach to closure of the atrial septal defect, ventricular septal defects, and other openings between the pulmonary and systemic circulations continues, further evaluation of the gross structural relationships of the devices and the cardiac chambers as well as the process of healing and immunologic or infectious complications will need study.

Cardiac pacemakers

Cardiac pacing is achieved through interconnected components consisting of a pulse generator, one or more electrically insulated conductors leading from the pulse generator to the heart, an electrode at the distal end in vitro, one or more of the conductors, and a tissue, or blood and tissue, interface

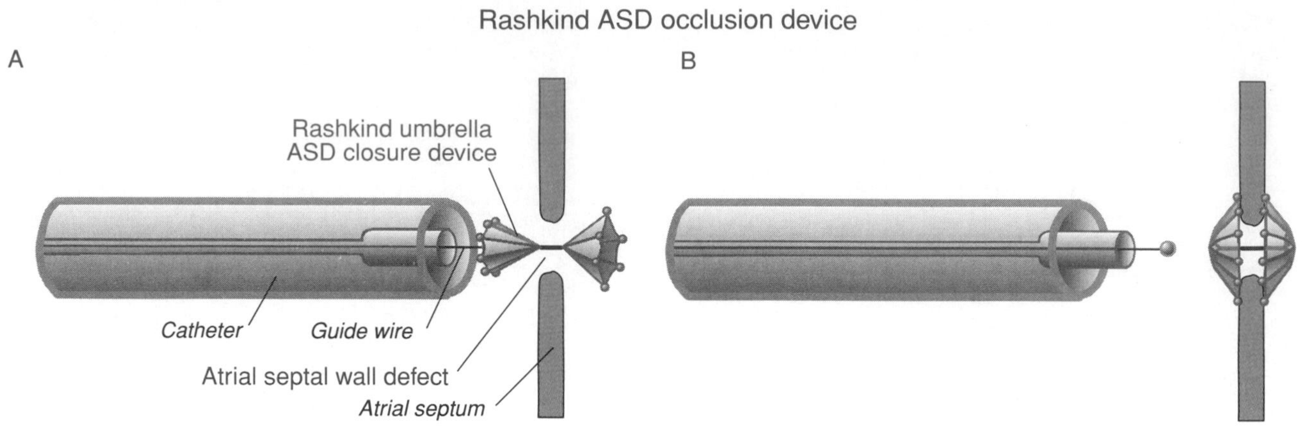

Rashkind ASD occlusion device

A

Rashkind umbrella
ASD closure device

Catheter

Guide wire

Atrial septal wall defect

Atrial septum

B

Fig. 30-14 Illustration on the process of implant *(left)* and final idealized position *(right)* of the "clamshell" occluder.

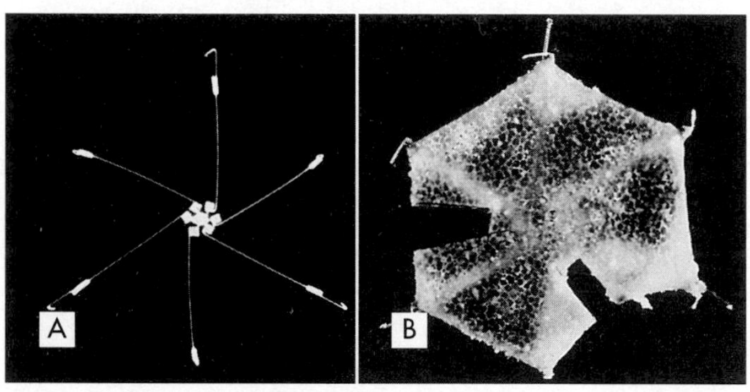

Fig. 30-15 X-ray film, **A,** and actual "first generation" atrial septal defect occluder device specimen, **B,** removed 1 day after implant. Noted are the six arms of the occluder and the three alternative arms with small hooks. The polyurethane foam is involved by fibrin, platelets, and red blood cells. Two tissue sections have been removed from the specimen.

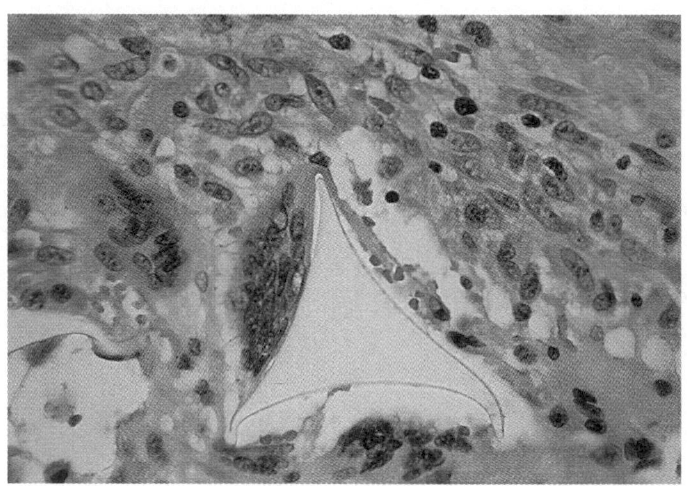

Fig. 30-16 Triangular polyurethane components of the atrial septal defect occluder device are evident, surrounded by fibrin, platelets, red blood cells, and monocyte-macrophages directly against the polyurethane.

between electrode and adjacent myocardium. In temporary cardiac pacing, a single pacing is usually placed transvenously into the right ventricle, and the pulse generator is located outside of the body. Temporary pacing may be applied during cardiac surgery by suturing insulated wires with bare ends contacting the surface the atrium or ventricles to the epicardial surface of the heart.[137]

Permanent cardiac pacing requires implantation of the pulse generator. The electrode tip is positioned against endocardium of the right atrium or right ventricle and the lead passes to the cephalic vein in the deltopectoral groove tunneled from the vein to a subcutaneous position. In children and patients with thin chest walls, pulse generators may be placed in an abdominal location.[138]

Currently the most common type of pacemaker is of the ventricle inhibited, or "demand," mode, in which stimulation is interrupted by any spontaneous cardiac activity. Thus, artificial pacing occurs as needed in response to intermittent failure of the patient's conduction. A three-letter (three-position) code is used to describe configurations of pacing sytems in which the first letter refers to the chamber paced: *V* (ventricle), *A* (atrium), *D* (both atrium and ventricle). The second letter designates the chamber, and the third letter refers to the response of the pacemaker to a sensed beat: *T* (triggered), *I* (inhibited), *D* (double) atrium triggered and ventricle inhibited.[137]

Complications of cardiac pacing can be classified as intraoperative, related to the pacemaker pack and site of implantation, related to pacing leads, or related to the pacing electrode (Table 30-11). The most dramatic of complications related to pacemakers is loss of the stimulus for pacing because of failure of an electronic component or battery depletion. Additional problems may be brought on by inappropriate resetting of the stimulation threshhold by electromagnetic interference from a spurious signal. Electromagnetic radiation can also damage the demand type of pacemakers by interfering with sensing of the cardiac electrogram. Battery depletion, electronic component failure, or "phantom" programming can be

Table 30-11 Factors potentially contributing to fibrous intimal hyperplasia in vascular replacement

Operative trauma
Surface thrombogenesis with organization or growth factor delivery by platelets
Degree of reendothelialization
Chronic endothelial injury
Growth factor production by graft-associated and adjacent endothelial and smooth muscle cells
Loss of growth-inhibitory interactions of endothelial and smooth muscle cells
Mechanical and hemodynamic factors
Configurational graft-to-artery mismatch

Modified from Schoen FJ: *Interventional and surgical cardiovascular pathology: clinical correlations and basic principles,* Philadelphia, 1989, Saunders.

detected by detailed electric examination of the pacemaker, and so pathologists at autopsies should collect and forward pacemaker components to the manufacturer.[137]

In examining cardiac pacemakers at autopsy, the pulse generator and lead including electrode tips should be exposed to careful dissection with minimal traction or bending of the lead. Evidence of infection of the generator pouch or thrombosis along the transvenous course of the lead should be evaluated. The course of transvenous leads through the heart as well as location of electrode insertion should be described. Histologic sections required should be oriented to permit evaluation of the thickness of nonstimulatable tissue separating the electrode from underlining myocytes. A practical approach to evaluation of the pulse generator and lead is to forward them to the manufacturer for examination.

The increasing number of patients surviving ventricular tachycardia and ventricular fibrillation has driven the development of alternative approaches to drug therapy or surgical resection. The automatic implantable cardioverter-defibrillator (AICD) is one such approach that uses a pair of epicardial patch electrodes for stimulation and a pair of screw-in epicardial electrodes for sensing. The AICD discharges when it senses a heart rate above a preset level or a probability density consistent with fibrillation. In addition to the usual complications of pacemakers, the AICD has the specific problem of false-positive discharges and interaction with pacemaker systems. New hybrid AICD/ventricular demand pacers will alleviate much of these problems.

Breast implants

Many unsuccessful efforts at breast augmentation ranging from free fat grafts to injectable silicone to polyvinyl alcohol sponge prostheses were attempted until the 1960s when silicone polymer implants was adopted into wide use. Most current breast prostheses consist of a shell made of silicone elastomer that is filled with silicone gel or saline solution. The elastomer shell surface may be smooth, textured by mold casting or molecular impact surface texturing, or textured by a polyurethane foam covering. Many implant developers believe that a textured surface allows some fibrous ingrowth and thus prevents formation of a contracting fibrous capsule. The use of polyurethane foam covering ended in 1991 when concerns developed over the possibility that the covering might degrade to form 2,4-toluene diamine, a carcinogen in laboratory animals.

The most common complication associated with breast implants is capsular contracture. Although some degree of scar formation is expected as a part of wound healing after the trauma of implantation of any device, the compressible nature of breast implants allows for greater contracture. The degree of contracture ranges from undetectable to severe breast deformation, causing hardness and pain.

When the components of an implant are much larger than the macrophage and thus not readily phagocytosed or degraded, as is the case with the silicone rubber surface of breast implants, fibrous scar tissue encapsulates and isolates the material. As this tissue capsule contracts, as part of the wound-healing process, in the case of rigid noncompressible implants such as hip prostheses, there is no deformation of the implant. However, fibrosis can deform breast implants in approximately 40% of patients, enough to force the pliable breast implant to conform, yielding varying degrees of roundness and an unnatural-appearing mass effect referred to as *capsular contracture*.[26]

Silicone gels and other fluids present within the breast implant can escape to the surrounding tissues through *device rupture* or by gel diffusion of these lower-molecular-weight substances through the semipermeable silicone envelope known as *bleed*. The tissue capsule associated with silicone breast implants is characterized grossly by a fibrous scar and histologically by a variable mixture of dense collagen, fibroblasts, macrophages, giant cells, lymphocytes, and, in some cases, plasma cells (Fig. 30-17). Devices coated with a layer of polyurethane foam tend to exhibit a similar pattern of inflammation, though giant cells tend to be more prevalent with fewer numbers of lymphocytes and plasma cells.[139]

Other

A discussion of the vast array of prosthetic devices in use in neurosurgery, plastic surgery, abdominal wound and hernia repair, and urology is beyond the scope of this chapter. The universal use of catheters across many disciplines certainly warrants a brief discussion. Catheters are essential for intravenous, intra-arterial, and intraperitoneal delivery of drugs or intravenous fluids, diagnostic pressure monitoring, or imaging.

Depending on the site and intended use, a catheter must possess enough stiffness or rigidity to resist kinking but so much as to induce unacceptable trauma to the endothelium and promote thrombosis. The most common biomaterials that have been used in catheters are polyvinylchloride, polyethylene, polytetrafluoroethylene (Teflon), polyurethane, and silicone elastomer.[26] Polyvinylchloride (PVC) is used extensively in central vein access and diagnostic arteriography and venography, where its stiffness and rigidity is necessary to allow manipulation of the catheter. Polyethylene is widely used in short-term intravenous and intra-arterial monitoring catheters, but its long-term use is limited by release of wear particles into the soft tissues, which produce an inflammatory response. Silicone elastomer (Silastic) is the most commonly used material used for chronic indwelling devices such as central-line catheters, shunts for the treatment of hydrocephalus, and chronic ambulatory peritoneal dialysis (CAPD) catheters. The softness, elasticity, and hydrophobic surface of Silastic are features that allow it to remain indwelling for longer periods of time.

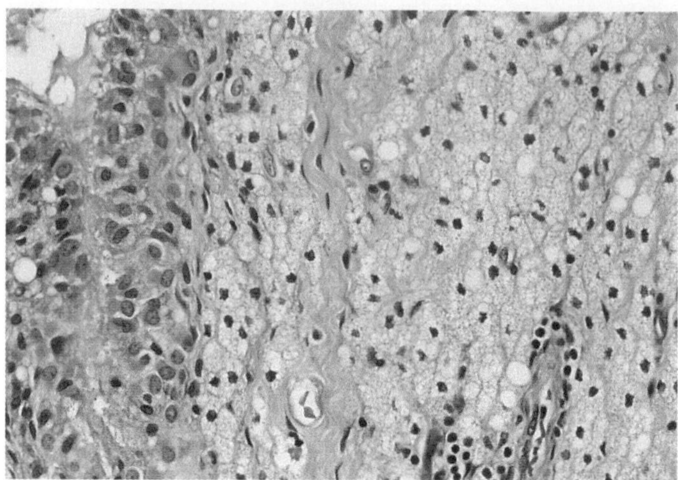

Fig. 30-17 Tissue capsule associated with silicone gel breast implant, here with palisading cells along the superficialmost surface in the so-called synovial metaplasia pattern. Numerous foamy histiocytes and occasional lymphocytes are present in the deeper areas.

Infections are the most common and most serious complication associated with catheters. The microorganisms that colonize catheters may originate from skin flora at the entry or exit site, from contaminated infusions, or from hematogenous spread. Numerous studies have demonstrated adherence of glycocalyx-forming microorganisms to the surface of catheters. As with other foreign implants, the microorganisms within the biofilm are protected from antibiotics. Factors that determine when colonization becomes clinical catheter infection are not fully known, but bacterial factors such as ability to produce slime, biomaterial difference in adhesion (PVC greater than Teflon greater than silicone elastomer) and host immune status are important.[26]

CURRENT DEVELOPMENTS AND SPECIAL ISSUES

Tremendous strides have been made in the past several decades in utilizing biomaterials in components of numerous medical devices. Early problems related to mechanical function of devices or bulk properties of biomaterials have largely been conquered and no longer represent significant problems to the patient or the developers of bioprosthetics. Persistent challenges encountered with implants focus on the cellular interactions between foreign surfaces and the host tissues, whether they are bone, soft tissue, or blood. The most important challenges currently facing the use of implanted prosthetics are (1) thrombosis or thromboembolism, (2) anticoagulant-related hemorrhage, (3) infection, (4) device dysfunction related to host reaction, including intimal hyperplasia, (5) structural dysfunction related to biodegradation, including calcification, and (6) wear and its associated host reaction. Numerous recent and ongoing developments hold promise to help solve these problems, as is briefly outlined.

Various strategies depend on surface modification techniques and pharmacologic alteration or activation of biomaterial surfaces, which modify growth factors and cytokines involved in vascular lesion formation and inhibit platelet function and thrombus formation.[140-146]

Novel approaches to the problem of devising a vascular device with a near-natural endothelial lining include endothelial cell seeding of prosthetic arterial grafts and gene-transfer modification of endothelial cells.[143-146]

In vascular grafts, one new theory is leaning toward developing resorbable vascular grafts that would reorganize through natural repair processes if the scaffold of a vascular graft were made of a slowly disappearing polymer fabric.

Characterization of functional domains within adhesive proteins such as fibronectin, laminin, and type IV collagen, as well as the elucidation of their interactions with specific cell-surface receptors will aid in the development of hybrid biomaterials that promote cell type–specific adhesion, spreading, and motility.[26,141]

REFERENCES

1. National Center for Health Statistics: Vital and Health Statistics: *Current estimates from the National Health Interview Survey, 1988,* series 10, no 173, pp 166, Oct 1989.
2. Vital and Health Statistics of the National Center for Health Statistics: *Advance data: use of selected medical device implants in the United States, 1988,* no 191, Feb 26, 1991.
3. Hench LL: Biomaterials, *Science* 208:826, 1980.
4. Barenberg SA: Abridged report of the Committee to Survey the Needs and Opportunities for the Biomaterials Industry, *J Biomed Mater Res* 22:1267, 1988.
5. Harker LA, Ratner BD, Didisheim P, editors: Cardiovascular biomaterials and biocompatibility: a guide to the study of blood-tissue-material interactions, *Cardiovascular Pathology* 2(suppl): 3S, 1993.
6. Helmus MN, Hubbell JA: Materials selection. In Harker LA, Ratner BD, Didisheim P, editors: Cardiovascular biomaterials and biocompatibility: a guide to the study of blood-tissue-material interactions, *Cardiovascular Pathology* 2(suppl): 53S, 1993.
7. Hergenrother RW, Silver JH, Kardos JL, Cooper SL: Bulk characterization. In Harker LA, Ratner BD, Didisheim P, editors: Cardiovascular biomaterials and biocompatibility: a guide to the study of blood-tissue-material interactions, *Cardiovascular Pathology* 2(suppl): 73S, 1993.
8. Gristina AG: Biomaterial-center infection: microbial adhesion versus tissue integration, *Science* 237:1588, 1987.
9. Gardella JA, Vargo TG, Hook TJ et al: In Ratner BD, editor: *Surface characterization of biomaterials,* Amsterdam, 1988, Elsevier Science Publishers.
10. Schoen FJ: *Interventional and surgical cardiovascular pathology: clinical correlations and basic principles,* Philadelphia, 1989, Saunders.
11. Anderson JM: Implant retrieval and evaluation. In Ratner BD, Hoffman AS, Lemons JE, Schoen FJ, editors: *Biomaterials science: an introductory text,* San Diego, Calif, 1994, Academic Press.
12. US Department of Health and Human Services, Public Health Service, NIH: *Guidelines for blood-material interactions,* NIH Pub no 85-12185, 1985.
13. Schoen FJ, Anderson JM, Didisheim P et al: Ventricular assist device (VAD) pathology analyses: Guidelines for clinical studies. *J Appl Biomat* 1:49, 1990.
14. Edwards WD: Photography of medical specimens: experiences from teaching cardiovascular pathology, *Mayo Clin Proc* 63:42, 1988.
15. Schoen FJ: Surgical pathology of removed natural and prosthetic heart valves, *Hum Pathol* 18:558, 1987.
16. Schoen FJ, Titus JL, Lawrie GM: Durability of pyrolytic carbon-containing heart valve prostheses, *J Biomed Mater Res* 16:559, 1982.
17. Schoen FJ, Goodenough SH, Ionescu MI, Braunwald NS: Implications of late morphology of Braunwald-Cutter mitral heart valve prostheses, *J Thorac Cardiovasc Surg* 88:208, 1984.
18. Schoen FJ, Schulman LJ, Cohn LH: Quantitative anatomic analysis of "stent creep" of explanted Hancock standard porcine bioprostheses used for cardiac valve replacement, *Am J Cardiol* 56:110, 1985.

19. Broom ND, Thomson FJ: Influence of fixation conditions on the performance of glutaraldehyde-treated porcine aortic valves: towards a more scientific basis, *Thorax* 34:166, 1979.
20. Schoen FJ, Kujovich JL, Webb CL, Levy RL: Chemically determined mineral content of explanted porcine aortic valve bioprostheses: correlation with radiographic assessment of calcification and clinical data, *Circulation* 76:1061, 1987.
21. Schoen FJ, Levy RJ, Nelson AC et al: Onset and progression of experimental bioprosthetic heart valve calcification, *Lab Invest* 52:523, 1985.
22. Schoen FJ, Tsao JW, Levy RL: Calcification of bovine pericardium used in cardiac valve bioprostheses, *Am J Pathol* 123:134, 1986.
23. Anderson JM: Procedures in the retrieval and evaluation of vascular grafts. In Kambic H, Kantrowitz A, Sung P, editors: *Vascular graft update: safety and performance,* ASTM STP 898, Philadelphia, 1986, Am Soc Testing and Materials.
24. Zacharias RK, Kirkman TR, Clowes AW: Mechanisms of healing in synthetic grafts, *J Vasc Surg* 6:429, 1987.
25. Ratner BD, Johnston AB, Lenk TJ: Biomaterial surfaces, *J Biomed Mater Res: Appl Biomat* 21(A1):59, 1987.
26. Greco RS, editor: *Implantation biology: the host response and biomedical devices,* Boca Raton, Fla, 1994, CRC Press.
27. Schoen FJ: Tissue organization and histology. In Ratner BD, Hoffman AS, Lemons JE, Schoen FJ, editors: *Biomaterials science: an introductory text,* San Diego, Calif, 1994, Academic Press.
28. Lenonard EF: Principles of cardiovascular device design. In Harker LA, Ratner BD, Didisheim P, editors: Cardiovascular biomaterials and biocompatibility: a guide to the study of blood-tissue-material interactions, *Cardiovascular Pathology* 2(suppl): 3S, 1993.
29. Pahl G, Beitz W: *Engineering design* (English Ed.), London, 1984, The Design Council.
30. Boretos JW, Eden M, editors: *Contemporary biomaterials, material and host response, clinical applications, new technology and legal aspects,* Park Ridge, N.J., 1984, Noyes Publications.
31. Bain WH, Pollack JCS, Rodger RA: Five years experience of the Björk-Shiley monostrate prosthesis: valve-related events and hemodynamic performance, *J Cardiovasc Surg* 29:5, 1988 (abstract).
32. Wilson PD, Gordon SL, editors: Proceedings of the NIH Consensus Development Conference—Total Hip Joint Replacement, *J Orthop Res* 1:189, 1983.
33. Clarke IC, McKellop HA: Wear testing. In von Recum AF, editor: *Handbook of biomaterials evaluation: scientific, technical, and clinical testing of implant materials,* New York, 1986, Macmillan.
34. Lemon JE: Corrosion and biodegradation. In von Recum AF, editor: *Handbook of biomaterials evaluation: scientific, technical, and clinical testing of implant materials,* New York, 1986, Macmillan.
35. Stokes K: Biodegradation. In: Harker LA, Ratner BD, Didisheim P, editors: Cardiovascular biomaterials and biocompatibility: a guide to the study of blood-tissue-material interactions, *Cardiovascular Pathology* 2(suppl): 111S, 1993.
36. Murphy SK, Fleming WH, Rogler WC, McManus BM: Retraction of bioprosthetic heart valve cusps into valve rings: a cause of wide-open regurgitation in right-sided heart valves, *Hum Pathol* 19:140, 1988.
37. Sugarman B, Young EJ: Infection associated with prosthetic devices: magnitude of the problem, *Infect Dis Clin North Am* 3:187, 1989.
38. Dougherty S, Simmons RL: Endogenous factors contributing to prosthetic device infections, *Infect Dis Clin North Am* 3:199, 1989.
39. Fitzgerald RH: Infections of hip prostheses and artificial joints, *Infect Dis Clin North Am* 3:329, 1989.
40. Buchholz HW, Elson RA, Engelbrecht TE et al: Management of deep infection of total hip replacement, *J Bone Joint Surg* 63B:342, 1981.
41. Schutzer SF, Harris WH: Deep wound infection of total hip replacement under contemporary aseptic conditions, *J Bone Joint Surg* 70A:724, 1988.
42. Salvati EA, Robinson RP, Zeno SM et al: Infection rates after 3,175 total hip and total knee replacements performed with and without a horizontal unidirectional filtered airflow system, *J Bone Joint Surg* 64A:525, 1982.
43. Wilson WR, Danielson GK, Giuliani ER, Geraci JE. Prosthetic valve endocarditis, *Mayo Clin Proc* 57:155, 1982.
44. Ivert TSA, Dismukes WE, Cobbs CG et al: Prosthetic valve endocarditis, *Circulation* 69:223, 1984.
45. Calderwood SB, Swinski LA, Waternaux CM et al: Risk factors for the development of prosthetic valve endocarditis, *Circulation* 72:31, 1985.
46. Mirra JM, Marder RA, Amstutz HC: The pathology of failed total joint arthroplasty, *Clin Orthop* 170:175, 1982.
47. Gristina AG, Kolkin J: Current concepts review: total joint replacement and sepsis. *J Bone Joint Surg* 65(A):128, 1983.
48. Antti-Poika I, Josefson G, Konttinen Y et al: Hip arthroplasty infection, *Acta Orthop Scand* 61:163, 1990.
49. Merritt K, Panigutti MA, Kraay MJ, Brown SA: Incidence of infection and analysis of contributing factors in revision joint arthroplasty over a two-year period, *J Appl Biomater* 5:103, 1994.
50. MacNamara A, Williams DF: Response to intramuscular implantation of pure metal, *Biomaterials* 2:33, 1981.
51. Aginis HJ, Alcock NW, Bansal M et al: Metallic wear in failed titanium-alloy total hip replacement: a histologic and quantitative analysis, *J Bone Joint Surg* 70:347, 1988.
52. Poss R, Thornhill TS, Ewald FC et al: Factors influencing the incidence and outcome of infection following total joint arthroplasty, *Clin Orthop* 182:117, 1984.
53. Jones EC, Insall JN, Inglis AE, Ranawat CS: GUEPAR knee arthroplasty results and late complications, *Clin Orthop* 140:145, 1979.
54. Gristina AG, Costerton JW: Bacterial adherence in the glycocalyx and their role in musculoskeletal infection, *Orthop Clin North Am* 15:517, 1984.
55. Dutton, DC, Webber, AJ, Johnson AS et al: Microstructure of initial thrombus formation on foreign materials, *J Biomed Mater Res* 3:13, 1969.
56. Vroman L, Adams AL: Identification of rapid changes at plasma-solid interfaces, *J Biomed Mater Res* 3:43, 1969.
57. Bruck SD: Interactions of synthetic and natural surfaces with blood in the physiologic environment, *J Biomed Res Symp* 8:1, 1977.
58. Kusserrow BK: The use of pathologic techniques in the evaluation of emboli from prosthetic devices, *Bull NY Acad Med* 48:468, 1972.
59. Gerrard JM: Platelet aggregation: cellular regulation and physiologic role, *Hosp Pract* 23:89, 1988.
60. Boskovic D, Elezovic I, Boskovic D et al: Late thrombosis of the Björk-Shiley tilting disc valve in the tricuspid position, *J Thorac Cardiovasc Surg* 91:1, 1986.
61. Blalock A, Taussig HB: The surgical treatment of malformations of the heart in which there is pulmonary stenosis or pulmonary atresia, *JAMA* 128:189, 1945.
62. Rajani RM, Dalvi BV, Kulkarni HL, Kale PA: Acutely blocked Blalock-Taussig shunt following cardiac catheterization: successful recanalization with intravenous streptokinase, *Am Heart J* 120:1238, 1990.
63. Rabe FE, Becker GJ, Richmond BD et al: Contrast extravasation through Dacron™ grafts: a sequela of low dose streptokinase therapy, *Am J Radiol* 138:917, 1982.
64. Carvalho JS, Belcher P, Knight WB: Infection of modified Blalock shunts, *Br Heart J* 58:287, 1987.
65. Pasquinelli G, Freyrie A, Preda P et al: Healing of prosthetic arterial grafts, *Scanning Microsc* 4:351, 1990.
66. Tamisier D, Vouhe PR, Vernant F et al: Modified Blalock-Taussig shunts: results in infants less than 3 months of age, *Ann Thorac Surg* 49:797, 1990.
67. Salzman EW, Merrill EW: Interactions of blood with artificial surfaces. In Coleman RW, Hirsch J, Marder VJ, Salzman EW, editors: *Hemostasis and thrombosis,* Philadelphia, 1982, Lippincott.
68. Moroff G: Methods for evaluating alteration in platelet and red cell properties. In von Recum AF, editor: *Handbook of biomaterials evaluation: scientific, technical, and clinical testing of implant materials,* New York, 1986, Macmillan,
69. Bernstein EF, Marzec UM: Effect of wall interactions, shear stress and osmotic injury on erythrocyte adenosine triphosphate concentration, 2,3-diphosphoglycerate concentration, and the oxyhemoglobin dissociation curve, *Trans Am Soc Artif Intern* Organs 20:47, 1974.
70. Colman RW: Mechanisms of thrombus formation and dissolution. In Harker LA, Ratner BD, Didisheim P, editors: Cardiovascular biomaterials and biocompatibility: a guide to the study of blood-tissue-material interactions, *Cardiovascular Pathology* 2(suppl): 23S, 1993.

71. Offeman RD, Williams MC: Material effects in shear-induced hemolysis, *Biomater Med Dev Artif Organs* 7:359, 1979.
72. Schoen FJ: Biomaterial-associated infection, neoplasia and calcification: clinicopathologic features and pathophysiologic concepts, *Trans Am Soc Artif Organs* 33:8, 1987.
73. Schoen FJ, Tsao JW, Levy RJ: Calcification of bovine pericardium used in cardiac valve bioprostheses: implications for the mechanisms of bioprosthetic tissue mineralization, *Am J Pathol* 123:134, 1986.
74. Golomb G, Schoen FJ, Smith MS et al: The role of glutaraldehyde-induced crosslinks in calcification of bovine pericardium used in cardiac valve bioprostheses, *Am J Pathol* 127:122, 1987.
75. Levy RJ, Schoen FJ, Lund SA et al: Prevention of leaflet calcification of bioprosthetic heart valves with diphosphonate injection therapy: experimental studies of optimal dosages and therapeutic duractions. *J Thorac Cardiovasc Surg* 94:551, 1987.
76. Levy RJ, Wolfrum J, Schoen FJ et al: Inhibition of calcification of bioprosthetic heart valves by local controlled-release diphosphonate, *Science* 228:190, 1985.
77. Lawrence WH: Perspectives of toxicity testing; and Northup SJ: Mammalian cell culture models. In von Recum AF, editor: *Handbook of biomaterials evaluation: scientific, technical and clinical testing of implant materials,* New York, 1986, Macmillan.
78. Black J: *Orthopedic biomaterials in research and practice,* New York, 1988, Churchill Livingstone.
79. Lyell S, Bain WH, Thomsom RM: Repeated failure of nickel-containing prosthetic heart valves in a patient allergic to nickel, *Lancet,* pp 657, Sept 23, 1978.
80. Kossovsky N, Heggers JP, Robson MC: The bioreactivity of silicone. In Williams DF, editor: *CRC Critical reviews in biocompatibility* 3:53, Boca Raton, Fla, 1987, CRC Press.
81. Hausner HJ, Schoen FJ, Fernández-Méndez MA et al: Migration of silicone gel to axillary lymph nodes after prosthetic mammoplasty, *Arch Pathol Lab Med* 105:371, 1981.
82. Yoshida S, Gershwin ME: Autoimmunity and selected environmental factors of disease induction, *Semin Arthritis Rheum* 22:399, 1993.
83. Kossovsky N, Freiman CJ: Silicone breast implant pathology: clinical data and immunologic consequences, *Arch Pathol Lab Med* 118:686, 1994.
84. Brody GS, Conway DP, Deapen DM et al: Consensus statement on the relationship of breast implant to connective-tissue disorders, *Plast Reconstr Surg* 90:1102, 1992.
85. Council on Scientific Affairs, American Medical Association: Silicone gel breast implants, *JAMA* 270:2602, 1993.
86. Kossovsky N, Papasian N: Clinical reviews: mammary implants, *J Appl Biomater* 3:239, 1992.
87. Gabriel SE, O'Fallon WM, Kurland LT et al: Risk of connective-tissue diseases and other disorders after breast implantation, *N Engl J Med* 330:1697, 1994.
88. Albores-Saavedra J, Vuitch F, Delgado R et al: Sinus histiocytosis of pelvic lymph nodes after hip replacement: a histiocytic proliferation induced by cobalt-chromium and titanium, *Am J Surg Pathol* 18:83, 1994.
89. Anderson JM: Inflammatory response to implants, *Am Soc Artif Intern Organs* 11:101, 1988.
90. Mirra JM, Amstoltz HC, Maddows M, Gold R: Pathology of joint tissues and its clinical relevance in prostheses failure, *Clin Orthop* 117:221, 1976.
91. Goldring SR, Schiller AL, Roelke M et al: The synovial-like membrane at the bone-cement interface in loose total hip replacements and its proposed role in bone lysis, *J Bone Joint Surg* 65A:575, 1983.
92. Lennox DW, Schonefeld BH, McDonald DF, Reilly LH: The histologic comparison of aseptic loosening of cemented, press-fit and biologic ingrowth prostheses, *Clin Orthop* 225:171, 1987.
93. Bullough PG, DiCarlo EF, Hansraj KK, Naves MC: Pathologic studies of total joint replacement, *Orthop Clin North Am* 19:611, 1988.
94. Santavirta S, Konttinen Y, Bergroth V et al: Aggressive granulomatous lesions associated with hip arthroplasty: Immunopathological studies, *J Bone Joint Surg* 72A:252, 1990.
95. Harris WH, Schiller AL, Scholler J-M et al: Extensive localized bone resorption in the femur following total hip replacement, *J Bone Joint Surg* 58-A:612, 1976.
96. Tallroth K, Eskola A, Santavirta S et al: Aggressive granulomatous lesions after hip arthroplasty, *J Bone Joint Surg* 71B:571, 1989.
97. Linder L, Lindberg L, Carlsson A: Aseptic loosening of hip prostheses: a histologic enzyme histochemical study, *Clin Orthop* 175:93, 1983.
98. Haynes DR, Rogers SD, Hay S et al: The differences in toxicity and release of bone-resorbing mediators induced by titanium and cobalt-chromium-alloy wear particles, *J Bone Joint Surg* 75A:825, 1993.
99. Horowitz SM, Doty SB, Lane JM, Burstein AH: Studies of the mechanism by which the mechanical failure of polymethylmethacrylate leads to bone resorption, *J Bone Joint Surg* 75A:802, 1993.
100. Schoen FJ, Levy RJ, Piehler HR: Pathological considerations in replacement cardiac valves, *Cardiovasc Pathol* 1:29, 1992.
101. Giddens DP, Yoganathan AP, Schoen FJ: Prosthetic cardiac valves. In Harker LA, Ratner BD, Didisheim P, editors: Cardiovascular biomaterials and biocompatibility: a guide to the study of blood-tissue-material interactions, *Cardiovascular Pathology* 2(suppl):23S, 1993.
102. Armenti F, Stephenson LW, Edmunds LH Jr: Simultaneous implantation of St. Jude Medical aortic and mitral prostheses, *J Thorac Cardiovasc Surg* 94:733, 1987.
103. Vogt S, Hoffmann A, Roth J et al: Heart valve replacement with the Björk-Shiley and St. Jude Medical prostheses: a randomized comparison in 178 patients, *Eur Heart J* 11:583, 1990.
104. Antunes MJ: Clinical performance of St. Jude and Medtronic-Hall prostheses: a randomized comparative study, *Ann Thorac Surg* 50:743, 1990.
105. Cohn LH, Collins JJ Jr, DiSesa VJ et al: Fifteen-year experience with 1678 Hancock porcine bioprosthetic heart valve replacements, *Ann Surg* 210:435, 1989.
106. Hammermeister KE, Henderson WG, Burchfiel CM et al and Participants in the Veterans Administration Cooperative Study on Valvular Heart Disease: Comparison of outcome after valve replacement with a bioprosthesis versus a mechanical prosthesis: initial 5 year results of a randomized trial, *J Am Coll Cardiol* 10:719, 1987.
107. García-Bengochea JB, Siebert MF, Carreno CI et al: Clinical experience with the Ionescu-Shiley xenograft valve: four to five-year follow-up, *Tex Heart Inst J* 9:285, 1982.
108. Galioto FM, Midgley FM, Kapur S et al: Early failure of Ionescu-Shiley bioprosthesis after mitral valve replacement in children, *J Thorac Cardiovasc Surg* 83:306, 1982.
109. Schoen FJ, Titus JL, Lawrie GM: Autopsy-determined causes of death after cardiac valve replacement, *JAMA* 249:899, 1983.
110. Schoen FJ, Levy RJ. Bioprosthetic heart valve failure, *Cardiol Clin,* 2:717, 1984.
111. Spencer FC, Baumann FG, Grossi EA et al: Experiences with 1643 porcine prosthetic valves in 1492 patients, *Ann Surg* 203:691, 1986.
112. Schoen FJ, Fernandez J, Gonzalez-Lavin L, Cernaianu A: Causes of failure and pathologic findings in surgically removed Ionescu-Shiley standard bovine pericardial heart valve bioprostheses: emphasis on progressive structural deterioration, *Circulation* 76:618, 1987.
113. Walley VM, Keon WM: Patterns of failure in Ionescu-Shiley bovine pericardial bioprosthetic valves, *J Thorac Cardiovasc Surg* 93:925, 1987.
114. Snyder RW, Tenney B, Guidoin R: Strength and endurance of vascular grafts. In Kambic HE, Kantrowitz A, Sung P, editors: *Vascular graft update: safety and performance,* ASTM STP 898, Philadelphia, 1986, American Society for Testing and Materials.
115. Clowes AW, Gown AM, Hanson SR, Reidy MA: Mechanism of arterial graft failure. I. Role of cellular proliferation in early healing of PTFE prostheses, *Am J Pathol* 118:43, 1985.
116. Anderson JM: Mechanisms of inflammation and infection with implanted devices. In Harker LA, Ratner BD, Didisheim P, editors: Cardiovascular biomaterials and biocompatibility: a guide to the study of blood-tissue-material interactions, *Cardiovascular Pathology* 2(suppl): 33S, 1993.
117. Ip JH, Fuster V et al: Syndromes of accelerated atherosclerosis: role of vascular injury and smooth muscle proliferation, *J Am Coll Cardiol* 15:1667, 1990.
118. Clowes AW, Clowes MM, Fingerle J, Reidy MA: Regulation of smooth muscle cell growth in injured artery, *J Cardiovasc Pharmacol* 14:S12, 1989.

119. Castellot JJ, Wright TC, Karnovsky MJ: Regulation of vascular smooth muscle cell growth by heparin and heparin sulfates, *Semin Thromb Hemost*, 13:489, 1987.
120. Castellot JJ: Heparin sulfates: physiologic regulators of smooth muscle cell proliferation? *Am J Respir Cell Mol Biol* 2:11, 1990.
121. Powell JS, Clozel JP, Müller RKM et al: Inhibitors of angiotensin-converting enzyme prevent myointimal proliferation after vascular injury, *Science* 245:186, 1989.
122. Lindner V, Lappl DA, Baird A et al: Role of fibroblast growth factor in vascular lesion formation, *Circ Res* 68:106, 1991.
123. Dichek DA, Neville RF, Zwiebel JA et al: Seeding of intravascular stents with genetically engineered endothelial cells, *Circulation* 80:1347, 1989.
124. Clagett GP, Salander JM, Eddleman WL et al: Dilation of knitted Dacron™ aortic prostheses and anastomotic false aneurysms: etiologic considerations, *Surgery* 93:9, 1983.
125. Watanabe T, Kusaba A, Kuma H et al: Failure of Dacron™ arterial prostheses caused by structural defects, *J Cardiovasc Surg* 24:95, 1983.
126. Nucho RC, Gryboski WA: Aneurysms of a double velour aortic graft, *Arch Surg* 119:1182, 1984.
127. Anderson JM, Hering TM, Ansel, AT, Johnson JM: Nosocomial graft fragmentation and healing response to an ePTFE angioaccess graft, *J Biomed Mater Res Appl Biomater* 21:153, 1987.
128. Olsson P, Soderlund S, Dubiel WT, Ovenfors CO: Patch grafts or tubular grafts in the repair of coarctation of the aorta, *Scand J Thorac Cardiovasc Surg* 10:139, 1976.
129. Walter P, Flameng W, Hehrlein FW: Early and late complications due to direct and indirect aortic-isthmus-plastic, *ThoraxchirVask Chir* 24:369, 1976.
130. Bergdahl L, Ljungqvist A: Long-term results after repair of coarctation of the aorta by patch grafting, *J Thorac Cardiovasc Surg* 80:177, 1980.
131. Hehrlein FW, Mulch J, Rautenburg HW et al: Incidence and pathogenesis of late aneurysms after patch graft aortoplasty for coarctation, *J Thorac Cardiovasc Surg* 92:226, 1986.
132. Virmani R, Atkinson JB, Forman MB: Aortocoronary bypass grafts and extracardiac conduits. In Silver M, Editor: *Cardiovascular pathology*, ed 2, New York, 1991, Churchill Livingstone.
133. King TD, Mills NL: Secundum atrial septal defect: nonoperative closure during cardiac catheterization, *JAMA* 235:2506, 1976.
134. Edwards WD, Agarwal KC, Feldt RH et al: Surgical pathology of obstructed, right-sided, porcine-valved extracardiac conduits, *Arch Pathol Lab Med* 107:400, 1983.
135. Latson LA, Sobczyk, WL, Kilzer KL, McManus BM: Closure of atrial septal defects with the Rashkind occluder: rapid loss of permeability, *Circulation* 76:265, 1987.
136. Lock JE, Rome JJ, Davis R et al: Transcatheter closure of atrial septal defects: experimental studies, *Circulation* 79:1091, 1989.
137. Meere D, Lesperance J: Surgical techniques in cardiac pacing. In Thalen HJ, Meere C, editor: *Developments in cardiovascular medicine*. vol 3: *Fundamentals of cardiac pacing*, Boston, 1979, Martinus Nijhoff.
138. Wilson GJ: The pathology of cardiac pacing. In Silver MD, editor: *Cardiovascular pathology*, ed 2, New York, 1991, Churchill Livingstone.
139. Cocke WM, Leathers HK, Lynch JB: Foreign body reactions to polyurethane covers of some breast prostheses, *Plast Reconstr Surg* 56:527, 1975.
140. Hoffman AS: Biomedical applications of plasma gas discharge processes, *J Appl Polymer Sci;Appl Polymer Symp* 42:251, 1988.
141. Jozefonvicz J, Jozefowicz, M: Interactions of biospecific functional polymers with blood proteins and cells, *Intern Biomater Sci Polym Ed* 1:147, 1990.
142. Hubbell JA: Pharmacologic modification materials. In Harker LA, Ratner BD, Didisheim P, editors: Cardiovascular biomaterials and biocompatibility: a guide to the study of blood-tissue-material interactions, *Cardiovascular Pathology* 2(suppl): 121S, 1993.
143. Plautz G, Nabel EG, Nabel FG: Introduction of vascular smooth muscle cells expressing recombinant genes in vivo, *Circulation* 83:578, 1991.
144. Wilson JM, Birinyi LK, Salomon RN et al: Implantation of vascular grafts lined with genetically modified endothelial cells, *Science* 244:1344, 1986.
145. Nabel EG, Plautz G, Nagel GJ: Site-specific gene expression in vivo by direct gene transfer into the arterial wall, *Science* 249:1285, 1990.

Acknowledgment: Certain materials developed for this chapter were organized for a United States and Canadian Academy of Pathology short course on host-prosthetic interactions. The contributions of Dr. Frederick Schoen to that effort are greatly appreciated.

31 Nutritional Deprivation Diseases

Herschel Sidransky
Nathan D. Bills

The role of nutrition in the pathogenesis of disease has been of great concern to scientists and physicians for many years. The importance of nutrition to well-being has been understood by civilized societies for centuries. Indeed, the state of nutrition in a society has usually correlated well with its socioeconomic development and advancement. Thus humans have been greatly concerned with the availability of adequate and balanced diets. Diseases that are consequences of inadequate diets have long plagued humankind. Unfortunately, they remain with us today and most probably will be with us for years to come.

Historically, nutrition gained eminence as a medical science with the discoveries that the absence of essential nutrients, such as single vitamins, induced a variety of important and specific nutritional deficiency diseases. These monumental findings led to a clearer understanding of how essential nutrients play vital roles in the normal functioning of cells, tissues, and organs of animals and humans.

In recent years, as knowledge has rapidly expanded in many areas of biologic and medical science, it has become apparent that the nutritional intake and utilization by any host, animal or human, are important not only in the prevention of deficiency states but also in the host's adaptation and responses to environmental stresses and strains. This chapter reviews how malnutrition and deficiency diseases develop, the manifestations of certain deficiency states, nutritional imbalances, and the way nutritional alterations may influence the host's responses to certain environmental manifestations.

As an introduction to malnutrition and deficiency diseases, it is essential to mention briefly the dietary components involved in normal and adequate nutrition. The human body requires some 50 to 60 organic and inorganic compounds in quantities ranging from micrograms to grams.[1-3] These are included in six basic groups: proteins, carbohydrates, fats, vitamins, minerals, and water. Proteins are made up of amino acids, eight of which must be supplied by dietary intake because they cannot be synthesized by the body in the amounts needed. These are isoleucine, leucine, lysine, methionine, phenylalanine, threonine, tryptophan, and valine. In addition, an exogenous supply of histidine is needed for early growth and development and therefore may be considered essential. Carbohydrates in themselves are not essential, but they provide needed dietary calories. Fats, or their constituent fatty acids, also provide calories. However, three fatty acids, linolenic, arachidonic, and especially linoleic, are currently considered essential. Vitamins, certain minerals, and water are indispensable dietary components.

In an attempt to characterize the various types of malnutrition or deficiency diseases as they affect individuals, one may consider them as (1) single deficiency states, (2) multiple deficiency states, (3) imbalances, and (4) excesses. The term *single deficiency states* implies that the disease results from the absence of a single essential or indispensable compound. Much of the information regarding such deficiency states has been derived from animal experimentation in which the variables were carefully monitored. Single vitamin deficiencies are the best examples. *Multiple deficiency states* develop when more than one necessary component is lacking in the diet. In humans, multiple deficiencies occur frequently, because a diet deficient in one component is usually deficient in others. Thus the pathologic changes may reflect each deficiency to some degree. *Nutritional imbalances* occur when the proportion of one dietary component to another or others is such that pathologic changes occur. Nutritional imbalances can occur under a variety of conditions. One example is the disease kwashiorkor, in which there is a protein deficiency in the presence of adequate or even high caloric intake. In contrast, marasmus occurs when there is a deficiency of total food intake (protein and all other components). Experimentally, amino acid imbalances have been demonstrated to induce a variety of pathologic changes.[4] The concept of nutritional imbalances has been gaining recognition and stresses that the quantity of intake of each dietary component in relation to other components is of great importance. *Nutritional excesses,* single or multiple, are becoming increasingly important, especially in affluent society. Obesity caused by excessive intake, particularly of calories (often lipids), is a common condition. Hypervitaminosis occurs when specific vitamins are given in excessive amounts and can have serious pathologic manifestations.

PRIMARY AND SECONDARY NUTRITIONAL INADEQUACY

A nutritional deficiency disease develops when the amounts of essential nutrients provided to the cells are inadequate for their normal metabolic functions. The deficiency may be primary or secondary in origin. A *primary nutritional inadequacy* is induced by a poor diet, one that lacks essential nutrients in either kind or amount or that provides an imbalance of nutrients. A *secondary nutritional inadequacy* is related to factors that interfere with the ingestion, absorption, or utilization of nutrients, as well as from metabolic or functional conditions that increase the requirement for nutrients or cause unusual destruction or abnormal excretion of nutrients.

Fig. 31-1 diagrams the pathogenesis of nutritional deficiency diseases. After a nutritional inadequacy (primary or secondary) begins, there is a time lapse before the onset of a nutritional deficiency disease. The time interval may depend on the degree of nutritional inadequacy and the level of nutrient reserves. An important safety factor is the nutrient reserves on which the tissues may draw during temporary lapses in the supply of nutrients. These reserves may be large or small, depending on the specific nutrient and the overall state of the reserve tissues. Tissue depletion follows the exhaustion of nutrient reserves and may occur rapidly or slowly, depending on the degree of nutritional inadequacy, the amount of nutrient reserves, and the requirement of the body for essential nutrients.

Biochemical lesions develop as a consequence of tissue depletion. Such lesions can best be illustrated by deficiencies of vitamins that are involved with enzyme systems dealing with the release of energy and other metabolic reactions. Biochemical alterations develop and may result in the accumulation of certain metabolites and in the altered metabolism of others. Functional changes in tissues and organs may then occur. Anatomic lesions develop and often are specific for or related to the missing nutritional component or components. Although this sequence has been presented in a stepwise manner, no one step in the chain of events from nutritional inadequacy to anatomic lesions need necessarily be complete before the next begins.

Primary nutritional inadequacy is caused by a diet that lacks essential nutrients in either kind or amount or that provides an imbalance of nutrients. Such inadequacy has always existed at one time or another in some parts of the world. It has been especially prevalent during and after wars, after crop failures, and in relation to poverty, ignorance, faddism, and cultural taboos. Throughout the world today, protein-calorie malnutrition is the most prominent example of this form of nutritional inadequacy. This is reviewed in a subsequent section.

Although malnutrition and nutritional deficiency diseases are usually considered to arise solely from an inadequate diet, under certain circumstances these may occur in the presence of dietary adequacy. Secondary nutritional inadequacy is caused by a variety of factors other than a poor diet. This type of nutritional inadequacy is of special importance in affluent societies as in the United states. Factors that may be involved are as follows:

Interference with ingestion: gastrointestinal disorders (acute gastroenteritis, gallbladder disease, peptic ulcers, diarrheal diseases, obstructive lesions of the bowel), neuropsychiatric disorders (neurasthenia, psychoneurosis, migraine), anorexia (alcoholism, congestive heart failure, cancer therapy, infectious diseases), food allergy, loss of teeth, pregnancy

Increased nutritive requirement: abnormal activity, abnormal environmental factors, fever, hyperthyroidism, pregnancy, lactation

Interference with absorption: gastrointestinal diseases (associated with hypermobility or reduction of absorbing surfaces), achlorhydria, biliary diseases

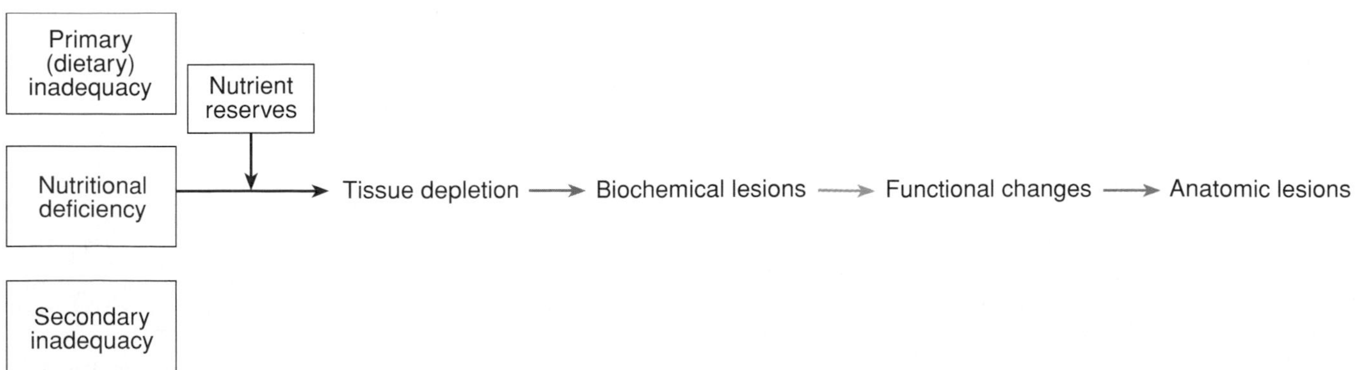

Fig. 31-1 Pathogenesis of nutritional deficiency diseases.

Interference with utilization: hepatic dysfunction, hypothyroidism, malignancy
Increased excretion: polyuria, lactation, excessive perspiration
Increased destruction: achlorhydria

From the listings under the above six factors, it becomes apparent that certain specific diseases, such as alcoholism, diabetes, and acute gastroenteritis, as well as iatrogenic causes from commonly used therapeutic agents, such as sulfonamides, antibiotics, alkalis, and diuretics, may under some circumstances be responsible for the development of secondary nutritional inadequacy. An important disease in which secondary nutritional inadequacy plays a major role is acquired immunodeficiency syndrome (AIDS). The wasting syndrome is one of the most devastating aspects of AIDS. The complexity of this wasting syndrome is related to the metabolic disturbances induced by the HIV infection itself as well as by a secondary infection or infections and induced anorexia, which all contribute to debilitation and weight loss. Malabsorption may also decrease the availability of nutrients. Failure to recuperate fully from episodes of weight loss lead to progressive debilitation and wasting.[5] The above examples stress the importance that physicians be aware of the possibilities of secondary nutritional inadequacies developing in patients and, if possible, attempt to prevent their occurrence or, if already existing, attempt to rectify the consequences.

TYPES OF MALNUTRITION

Starvation

Starvation occurs in individuals of all ages. Much information about this condition was gained from postmortem studies in prison camps during World War II.[6] In general, the overall pathologic changes are minimal; atrophy is the main feature. The changes caused by inanition include great loss of weight, serous atrophy of fat throughout the body, reduced amounts of lymphoid tissue, and pronounced atrophy of testes or ovaries, cardiac and skeletal muscle, thymus, and liver. Hemosiderosis of the spleen and lipid depletion of adrenal glands are also common findings.

Protein-calorie malnutrition

The most prevalent form of primary nutritional deficiency disease is protein-calorie malnutrition.[7-9] According to the World Health Organization (WHO), protein-calorie malnutrition is rampant throughout the world. The two diseases associated with this malnutrition, marasmus and kwashiorkor, affect pre–school aged children in the developing countries of the world. Marasmus is a form of childhood starvation caused by inadequate total food intake. Its manifestations are those of starvation in which pathologic changes are minimal.[8,10,11] Kwashiorkor, the most important and widespread nutritional deficiency disease in the world today (affecting more than 100 million children) according to WHO, has long been attributed to protein deficiency. In the 1950s, it was established that kwashiorkor is caused by a combination of protein deficiency and relatively high carbohydrate intake.[12,13] Such a nutritionally deficient and imbalanced diet leads rapidly to pathologic changes in several organs.[14] Many children throughout the world die from this disease. In addition, it is speculated that children who survive may later develop an enhanced susceptibility to hepatic injury caused by viruses, toxins, or chemical carcinogens and, as adults, may have an increased incidence of cirrhosis and primary liver cancer. In recent years, some authors have reported that protein-calorie malnutrition is being recognized with increasing frequency in hospitalized patients as well as in the geriatric population.[15-17] Also, in nursing home populations there have been reported to be cases of protein-calorie malnutrition.[18] These considerations relating to the occurrence of protein-calorie malnutrition are derived from evaluations based upon biochemical and anthropometric measurements. Whether these parameters correlate with morphologic findings characteristic or diagnostic of protein-calorie malnutrition still needs to be established.

Marasmus

Marasmus (Fig. 31-2) is a form of starvation that occurs during childhood. It results from an overall deficit in food intake, including all dietary components (protein, carbohydrate, lipid, vitamins, salts). Therefore it has often been referred to as "balanced starvation."

Marasmus occurs most commonly during the first year of life and is found in most developing countries. A common cause is early cessation of breast feeding with lack of food intake. The clinical features and findings in marasmus are growth failure (low weight and height, prominent ribs, mon-

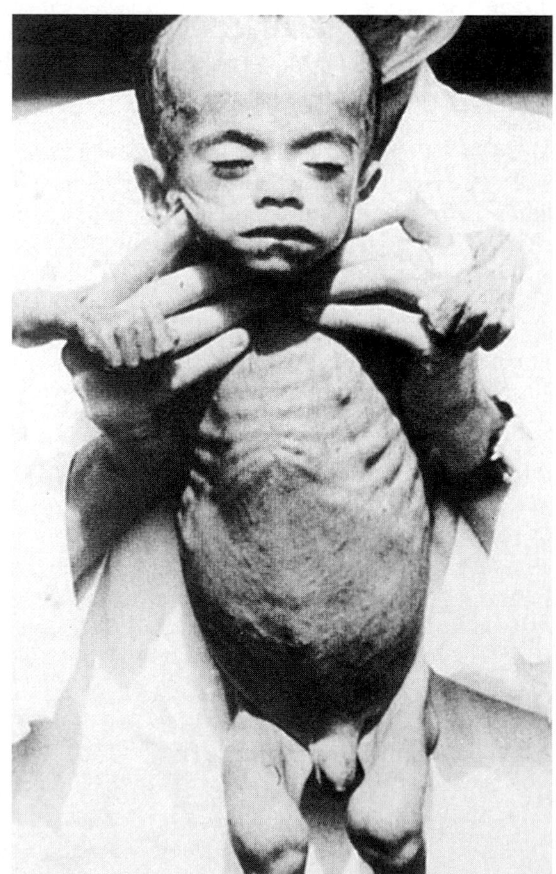

Fig. 31-2 Marasmus. Extreme wasting in a child from the Netherlands during World War II. (From Latham MD et al: *Scope manual on nutrition,* Kalamazoo, Mich, 1972, The Upjohn Co.)

key-like face, protuberant abdomen, thin limbs), muscle wasting and loss of subcutaneous fat, anemia, and diarrhea (common but not a constant feature). Edema is absent, mental changes are uncommon, and appetite is good. Serum protein levels are reduced. Other than the small size or atrophy of organs, no specific gross or microscopic (pathologic) changes are present. The liver is not fatty.

Kwashiorkor

Kwashiorkor[9,12-14] (Fig. 31-3) has been recognized for centuries and has been referred to by many names throughout the world. In the Ghanaian Ga language it means 'condition seen in the displaced child.' In 1936, Dr. Cicely Williams of the Gold Coast of Africa first presented a detailed description of kwashiorkor. Since that time, kwashiorkor has gained notoriety as the most widespread and important dietary deficiency disease in the world.

Although at first kwashiorkor was considered to result from protein deficiency alone, the cause is now recognized to be related to a nutritional imbalance attributable to protein deficiency and adequate or high carbohydrate intake. The disease occurs mainly in children 6 months to 3 years of age. It usually follows weaning when the infant is fed the poor and limited foods of the area (corn, cassava, or other grains and vegetables), which are relatively high in carbohydrates but contain inadequate amounts of proteins, which are often of poor quality.

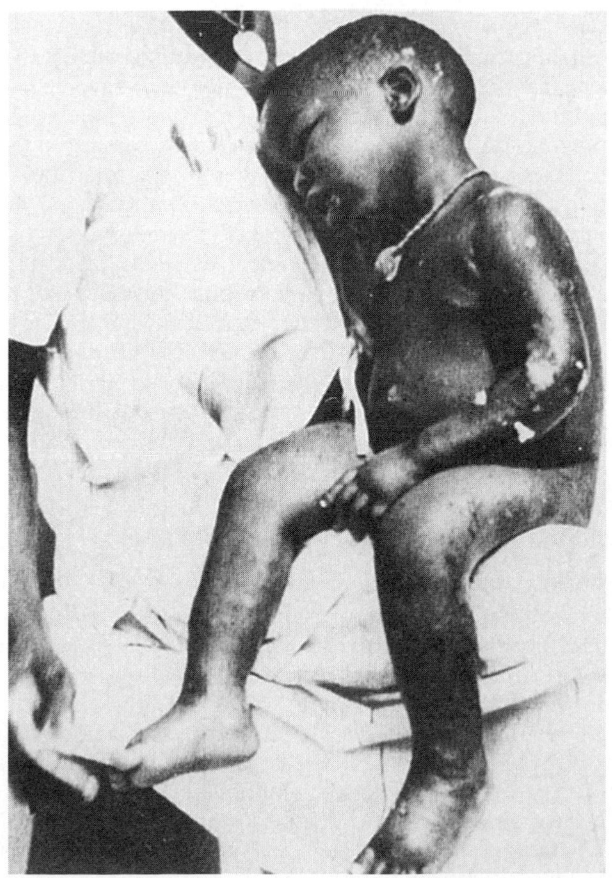

Fig. 31-3 Kwashiorkor. African child showing edema and dermatosis. (From Latham MC et al: *Scope manual on nutrition,* Kalamazoo, Mich, 1972, The Upjohn Co.)

The clinical features and findings in kwashiorkor are growth failure; wasting of muscles of arms and legs but preservation of subcutaneous fat; edema; mental changes, such as apathy, irritability, and lack of interest in surroundings; changes in hair color, texture, and strength; depigmentation of skin; hepatomegaly; diarrhea; and anemia. The main pathologic findings manifest as an enlarged, fatty liver with periportal distribution of lipid and atrophy of the pancreas, salivary glands, small intestine glands, and skeletal muscles.

Consequences of kwashiorkor

Although many children die from kwashiorkor, others survive as a consequence of mild involvement and treatment with a well-balanced diet containing adequate and good-quality proteins. Thus, in the developing countries many adults have had this nutritional deficiency disease during childhood. In the past, epidemiologists have suggested that the fatty liver of kwashiorkor could progress directly to nutritionally induced cirrhosis in adult life. Such adults were believed to have a higher than normal predilection for primary hepatocellular carcinoma. More current views indicate that the liver damage resulting from kwashiorkor may render these individuals more susceptible to injury by hepatotoxic agents (such as viruses or aflatoxin), which may then in later life progress to cirrhosis and in some cases to primary liver cancer.

Much interest exists in the possibility that stunted mental development may occur as a consequence of kwashiorkor during childhood. In several studies, children who had kwashiorkor during early childhood scored lower on IQ tests than did their siblings who did not have kwashiorkor.[19,20]

Although the conclusions from the preceding examples are still speculative, they involve important and significant problems that may be consequences of malnutrition during childhood. Absolute proof that these associations are valid is difficult to document. Therefore many investigators have attempted to use experimental kwashiorkor-like models[21-25] in animals to probe into the pathogenesis of the induced lesions and thereby determine the possible consequences of these alterations in later life. Such studies have provided valuable information relating to nutritional deficiencies and imbalances and their effects both on specific organs and on the whole organism.

Experimental kwashiorkor-like models

Several investigators have developed experimental models of kwashiorkor. This has been approached by feeding diets deficient in amino acids or protein to experimental animals. The experimental model that probably most closely resembles the pathologic changes reported in infants dying from kwashiorkor[14] is one in which animals were force-fed by stomach-tube purified diets devoid of single essential amino acids.[24] Lesions developed within 3 to 10 days in these force-feeding experiments and resembled those described in children with kwashiorkor. The morphologic changes manifested as periportal fatty liver, excess hepatic glycogen, and atrophy of the pancreas, submaxillary gland, stomach, spleen, and thymus. Major conclusions based on these experimental studies are the following:

1. Both total intake and caloric intake of a deficient diet must be adequate to induce pathologic changes. Rats fed a deficient diet ad libitum eat little and develop a maras-

mus-like rather than a kwashiorkor-like condition. This explains the need to maintain an adequate intake by force-feeding the deficient or imbalanced diet to induce the pathologic changes.
2. Overall, the pathologic changes are similar regardless of which single essential amino acid is eliminated from the diet. Also, poor-quality plant proteins as the sole source of protein with adequate amounts of all other components in force-feeding experiments induce the pathologic changes. This indicates that protein deficiency rather than deficiency of a single essential amino acid is important in inducing the disease.
3. The pathologic changes are not directly mediated through adrenal or pituitary hormonal stimulation.
4. Loss of skeletal muscle protein occurs early and is important. Although muscle protein synthesis is decreased, hepatic protein synthesis is maintained at a high level. Pronounced alterations in hepatic lipid and glycogen metabolism occur.
5. Treatment with a complete, balanced, purified diet rapidly reverses the condition.

Secondary protein-calorie malnutrition

Involuntary weight loss or wasting indicative of severe protein-energy malnutrition is a frequent complication of AIDS and may significantly contribute to the progression of AIDS, including death. The magnitude of tissue depletion and losses in lean body cell mass is related to the mortality from wasting. The mechanism or mechanisms of weight loss in AIDS have not been clearly elucidated. The cause appears to be multifactorial, resulting from interactions between decreased caloric intake, malabsorption, and altered energy utilization or expenditure secondary to infection, hormonal, or metabolic abnormalities. In AIDS wasting syndrome, evidence exists for alterations in lipid metabolism, cytokine response, and energy/nitrogen balance, as well as for gastrointestinal dysfunction caused by infection or inflammatory cytokines.

New nutrition-related diseases

Since 1981, two new nutritionally related diseases have occurred. These two entities are described mainly to stress the importance of their unexpected occurrences and that physicians should be alerted to similar new conditions, that may surface in the future.

Toxic oil syndrome

Although there have been numerous past reports of mass poisonings by various forms of toxic oils, the epidemic caused by the consumption of adulterated rapeseed oil in Spain in 1981 and known as the toxic oil syndrome was one of the largest intoxications ever recorded, resulting in 20,000 cases and over 300 deaths.[26] Initially, clinical findings pertaining to the respiratory system were particularly prominent. However, other organs, including skin, gastrointestinal tract, spleen, and liver, were involved. Eosinophilia was a striking finding. The most prominent pathologic feature was a peculiar nonnecrotizing vasculitis that affected mainly the intima and involved vessels of every type and size in practically every organ.[27] Although epidemiologic and analytic chemical studies have clearly linked the toxic oil syndrome to the ingestion of oil mixtures containing rapeseed oil denatured with aniline, the precise identity of the etiologic agent in the oil has not been determined.

Eosinophilia-myalgia syndrome

In the fall of 1989, a newly recognized illness manifesting predominantly as connective tissue disease and eosinophilia was first reported and named the "eosinophilia-myalgia syndrome."[28] Based upon epidemiologic findings, it was rapidly concluded that the disease was related to the ingestion of L-tryptophan, an indispensable amino acid, which, probably because it is a precursor to the neurotransmitter serotonin, has been widely used as a natural agent for relieving insomnia, pain, depression, hyperactivity, and eating disorders. The implicated L-tryptophan has been traced to a single Japanese manufacturer who had modified its production process. This L-tryptophan contained minute amounts of impurities or contaminants.[29]

The pathologic lesions in patients with the eosinophilia-myalgia syndrome have consisted of widespread inflammatory cells (monocytes, lymphocytes, macrophages, plasma cells), mainly scattered in skin, muscle, and connective tissue. Endothelial cells reveal swelling, degeneration, and necrosis. Fibroblast proliferation and fibrosis are frequent findings. In many patients, the condition became a chronic process. Therapy has been mainly directed toward treatment of symptoms.

The cause and pathogenesis of the eosinophilia-myalgia syndrome is unclear. The FDA stopped the distribution of L-tryptophan, and no new cases have subsequently been reported. Speculation as to how this disease arises and progresses indicates that it may be related to an autoimmune response. However, in the absence of an experimental model of the disease in animals, its cause and pathogenesis remain a puzzle.

In light of the two new diseases, comparisons between the clinical manifestations of the two syndromes have revealed several interesting similarities.[30,31] Many manifestations of the eosinophilia-myalgia syndrome are strikingly similar to those of the intermediate and chronic stages of the toxic oil syndrome. These include severe and persistent myalgia, skin lesions, eosinophilia, and elevated liver enzyme levels.

The preceding two relatively new epidemic diseases are cited as examples of toxicologic nutritional diseases that may in part be related to rapid technologic developments in our present society. Based upon their occurrences, it is likely that similar new nutritionally related diseases will arise in the future. Physicians need to be aware of such possibilities and their implications.

CONSEQUENCES OF MALNUTRITION

Brain function

In an earlier section, the possibility that stunted mental development occurs secondarily to kwashiorkor was mentioned. Indeed, several studies have shown that many types of malnutrition retard the development of the human brain and adversely affect the patterns of learning and behavior in early life.[32-36] Whether the deficiency is in total calories, total protein, specific amino acids, micronutrients, or combinations of these factors, the result too often is a brain that is far below average size for the age of the child. When the underprivileged are better nourished (and viral and other infections of the central nervous system better controlled), the accepted level of human performance will be raised, and the problems of the social scientist will be considerably simplified.

Cancer

Much attention has been given to the possible association between nutrition and cancer (Chapter 24). Of the many environmental factors considered to be influential in the induction of cancer, diet and nutrition have gained much notoriety. This association has been derived mainly from diverse epidemiologic data but also from limited experimental studies with animals.[37-49]

In relating dietary factors and cancer, one must consider the following:

1. Food additives or contaminants, as well as the nutrients themselves, may act as carcinogens, cocarcinogens, promoters, or combinations of these.
2. Nutritional deficiencies or imbalances may lead to biochemical abnormalities that in turn promote neoplastic processes.
3. Excessive intake of certain nutrients may produce metabolic abnormalities that promote neoplasms.

A few of the suspected carcinogenic food contaminants are mycotoxins (specifically aflatoxin) and nitrosamines. Studies have revealed that the charred parts of broiled meat and fish contain a series of new heterocyclic amines in the pyrolyzate of amino acids and proteins, which are mutagenic, and that two amines from tryptophan pyrolyzates—3-amino-1,4-dimethyl-5*H*-pyrido(4,3-*b*)indole and 3-amino-1-methyl-5*H*-pyrido(4,3-*b*)indole—are carcinogenic in animals.[50]

Also, the amounts and type of fiber in the diet have been considered to be influential in the induction of bowel cancer in experimental animals.[40,44,51] Deficiencies of iron, iodine, riboflavin, vitamin A, pyridoxine, folates, and choline have been considered to play a role in the induction of certain types of neoplasms. Based on epidemiologic data and also on animal studies, high dietary fat intake has been reported to increase breast cancer incidence in females.[52,53] In general, it is believed that the dietary effects occur mainly in relation to promotion, the second stage of the process of carcinogenesis.

Several experimental studies have revealed that diet or dietary components may act to prevent the induction of certain cancers.[54] Certain dietary components have been demonstrated to induce enzyme systems that detoxify chemical carcinogens. Also, some food additives, which are antioxidants, act to inhibit chemical carcinogenesis. Studies with vitamin A treatment in animals have also indicated an inhibitory effect, particularly in relation to changes in cell differentiation, on the induction of certain types of cancers. Several experimental studies revealed that selenium supplementation protects against certain neoplasms induced by carcinogens.[40]

Recently, much interest has centered on the role of antioxidant nutrients in relation to cancer. The antioxidant vitamins (vitamin E, β-carotene, and vitamin C) have been considered to be of importance in association with the occurrence of cancers at various sites. A recent FDA conference on antioxidant nutrients and cancer has reviewed current developments and knowledge in this area.[55] All panelists agreed that proper intake of antioxidant vitamins through adequate dietary ingestion of fresh fruits and vegetables is beneficial to health as well as possibly effective in reducing the incidence of chronic diseases, especially cancer. The mechanism or mechanisms by which the protective effect occurs remain unknown (speculation persists but conclusive data are not yet available).

Overall, the present state of basic knowledge of the association between nutrition and cancer is limited. Further information is needed before a clear understanding of their association is clearly utilized in the prevention and treatment of cancer in humans.

VITAMINS

All metabolic functions require transformations of compounds that are mediated through enzymes. In many cases these enzymes require cofactors for their catalytic action that the organism cannot produce by reason of an evolutionary loss of synthetic ability. One aspect of "vitamins'" function is serving as enzyme cofactors. It must be recognized that vitamins are often species-specific: for example, vitamin C is a vitamin only for primates, guinea pigs, passeriform birds, and most fish, whereas other animals have retained the enzyme gulonolactone oxidase necessary to synthesize vitamin C from D-glucose.[56,57] Vitamins are required in small amounts (from 2 μg to 90 mg/day)[55] and must be obtained from the diet or from supplements. Table 31-1 details the important attributes of the vitamins.

Historically, certain pathologic lesions were determined to be caused by specific nutrient deficiencies. Unfortunately, the dramatic recoveries from pathologic processes attributable to deficiencies that were accomplished with simple vitamin therapy led to the erroneous belief that vitamins were wonder drugs capable of curing many diseases, especially when consumed in large quantities. This dangerous paradigm has resulted in the development of an enormous quasi-scientific supplement industry. One wonders why many of the public would readily accept that an order of magnitude greater intake of, for example, water (an intake of 60 rather than 6 glasses, 8 ounces, per day) would not improve health or well-being, yet they may readily accept this specious logic (10,000 retinol equivalents of vitamin A rather than 1000 retinol equivalents, a potentially toxic dose) as promoting health. This is not to disparage the rational use of high-dose vitamins as potential pharmacologic agents or their potential role as antioxidants in cancer chemoprevention. However, the pharmacologic activity of high-dose vitamins does not always coincide with their normal biologic function, and the potential toxicity of these compounds at high doses should be a concern.

RDA

Recommended dietary allowances (RDA) for nutrients have been prepared regularly since 1941 by the Food and Nutrition Board. These recommendations are based on the following:

1. Studies of subjects maintained on diets containing low or deficient levels of a nutrient, followed by correction of the deficit with measured amounts of the nutrient
2. Nutrient balance studies that measure nutrient status in relation to intake
3. Biochemical measurements of tissue saturation or adequacy of molecular function in relation to nutrient intake
4. Nutrient intakes of fully breastfed infants and of apparently healthy people from their food supply
5. Epidemiological observations of nutrient status in population in relation to intake
6. In some cases, extrapolation of data from animal experiments[55]

Table 31-1 Nutrients—their chemical forms, functions, and effects of deficiency

Nutrient	Chemical forms	Function	Deficiency
Calories Protein Carbohydrates Lipids Ethanol (not essential)		Growth Tissue structure Metabolic substrates	Marasmus caloric deficit Growth failure Anemia Atrophy Skeletal muscle Thymus, lymph nodes Subcutaneous fat absent
Protein Essential amino acids isoleucine leucine lysine methionine phenylalanine threonine tryptophan valine histidine (children)		Growth Structure Protein constituents Precursors to many bioactive compounds	Kwashiorkor Primarily protein deficit Growth failure Peripheral edema Mental changes Fragile hair Dermatosis Poor appetite Anemia Fatty (periportal) liver Hepatomegaly Subcutaneous fat present Atrophy Skeletal muscle Thymus, lymph nodes
Vitamin A Retinol	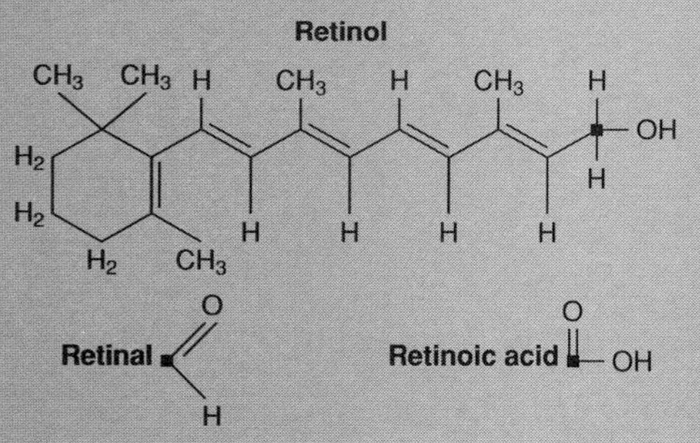 Retinol CH_3 CH_3 H CH_3 H CH_3 H —OH; H_2 H_2 H_2 CH_3 H H H H H Retinal (=O, H) Retinoic acid (=O, —OH)	Vision rhodopsin Ephithelial integrity chondroitin sulfate Differentiation Growth Reproduction	Night blindness Xerosis of conjunctiva and cornea Bitot's spots Xerophthalmia Blindness Follicular hyperkeratosis Susceptibility to infection Stunting

Table 31-1 Nutrients—their chemical forms, functions, and effects of deficiency—cont'd

Nutrient	Chemical forms	Function	Deficiency
Vitamin D	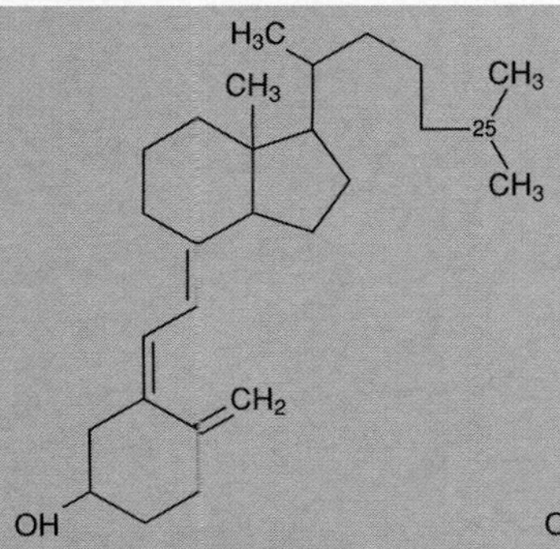 Vitamin D_3 Cholecalciferol; 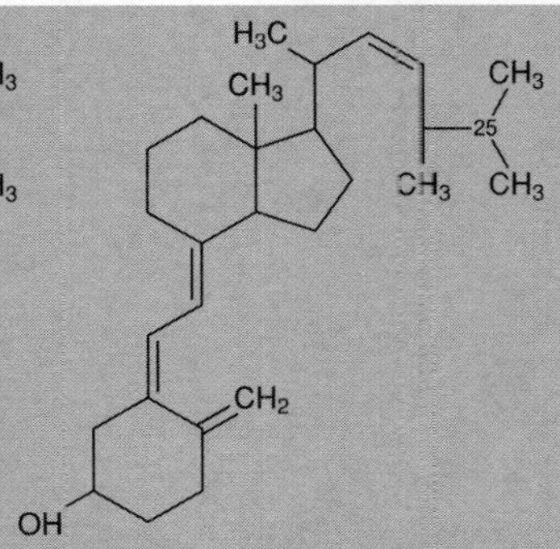 Vitamin D_2 Ergocalciferol	Blood calcium regulation Absorption of calcium and phosphorus Bone calcification Activates alkaline phosphatase	Rickets (children) Osteomalacia (adults)
Vitamin E	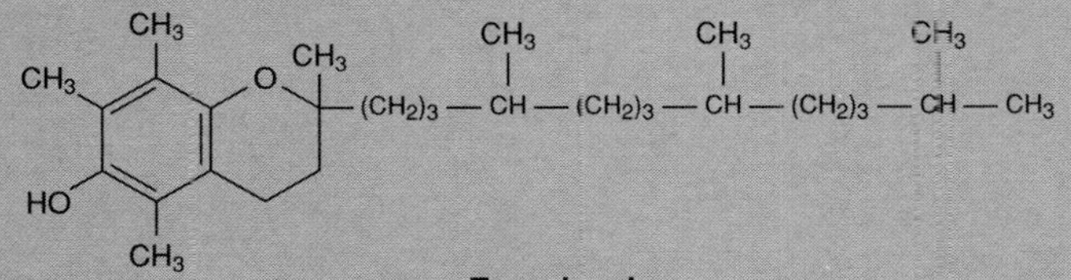 α-Tocopherol	Antioxidant for polyunsaturated fatty acids Quenches free radicals Cellular membrane integrity	Hemolytic anemia (infants) Rare deficiency in adults Possible spinocerebellar degeneration Possible skeletal muscle abnormalities
Vitamin K	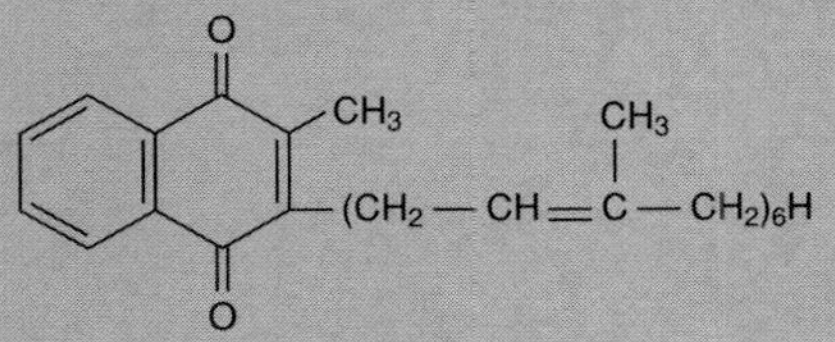 Vitamin K_2 (menaquinone)	Blood clotting prothrombin Factors II, VII, IX, and X Proteins C, S, and Z	Hemorrhage (particularly neonates)

(continued)

Table 31-1 Nutrients—their chemical forms, functions, and effects of deficiency—cont'd

Nutrient	Chemical forms	Function	Deficiency
Thiamin, thiamine, Vitamin B_1	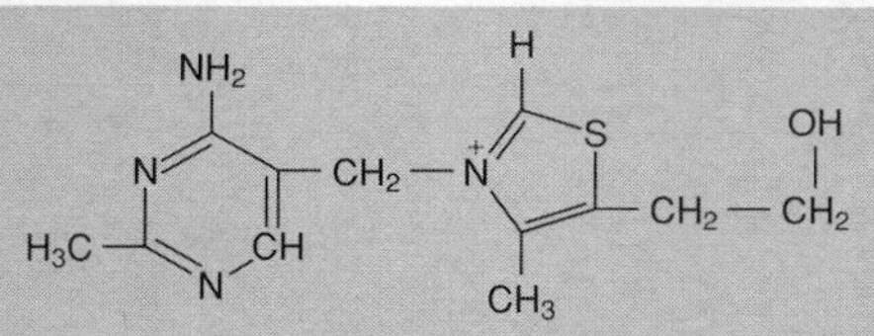 Thiamin (vitamin B_1) 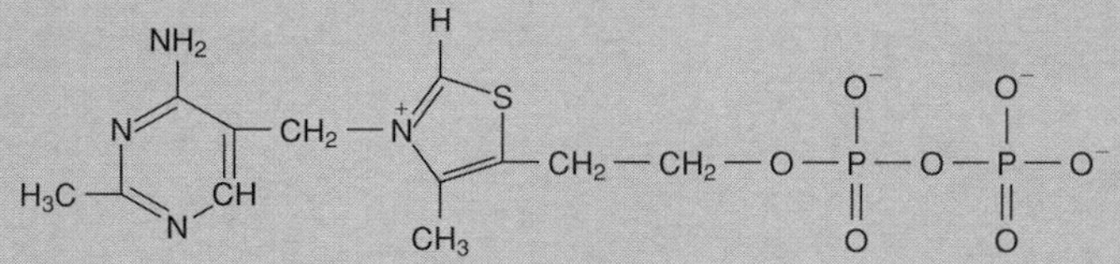 Thiamin pyrophosphate 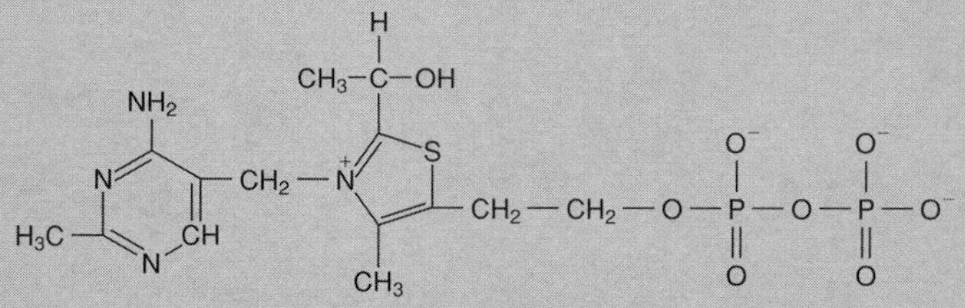 α-Hydroxyethylthiamine pyrophosphate	Intermediary metabolism Decarboxylations Pyruvic acid→Acetyl CoA Transketolations Hexose monophosphate shunt	Beriberi Polyneuritis Peripheral edema Heart failure Wernicke's encephalopathy

Table 31-1 Nutrients—their chemical forms, functions, and effects of deficiency—cont'd

Nutrient	Chemical forms	Function	Deficiency
Riboflavin Vitamin B_2 (term not often used)	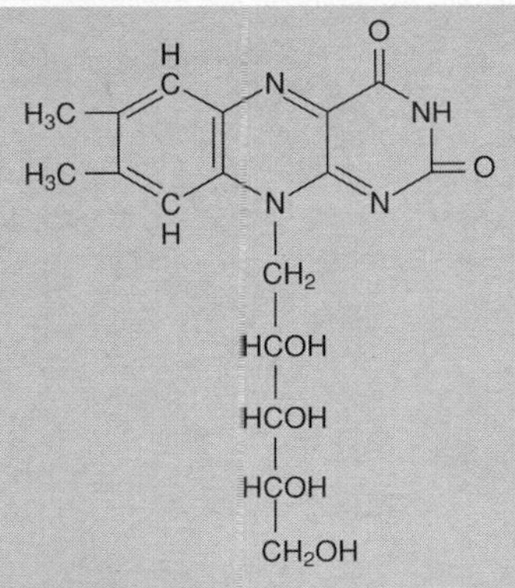 Riboflavin 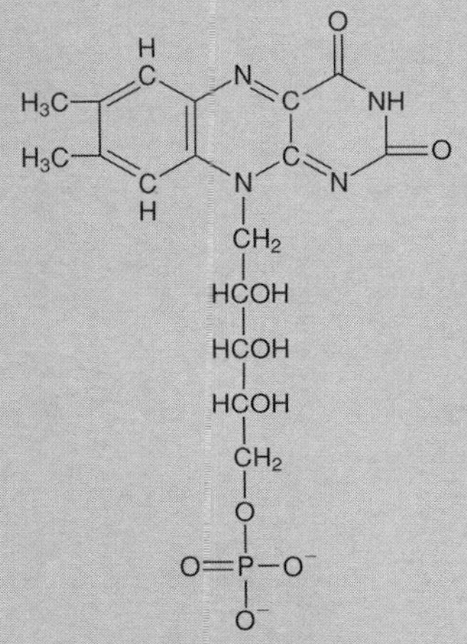 Flavin mononucleotide (FMN) 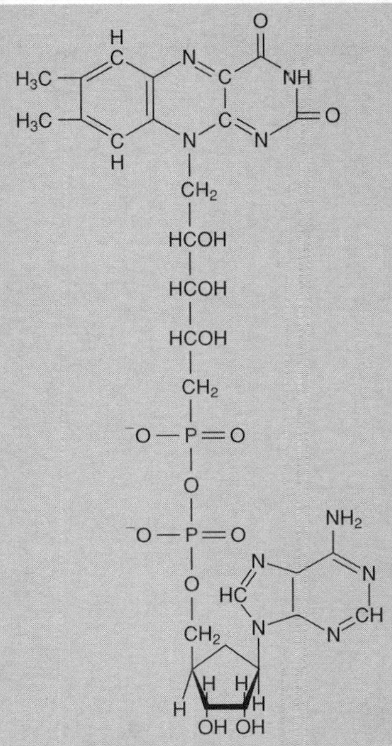 Flavin adenine dinucleotide	Flavoproteins Flavin mononucleotide Flavin adenine dinucleotide Fatty-acid synthesis β-Oxidation of fatty acids Deamination of amino acids ATP production-respiratory chain Pyruvic acid→Acetyl CoA	Deficiencies rare Cheilosis Dermatitis Glossitis Corneal vascularization

(continued)

Table 31-1 Nutrients—their chemical forms, functions, and effects of deficiency—cont'd

Nutrient	Chemical forms	Function	Deficiency
Niacin	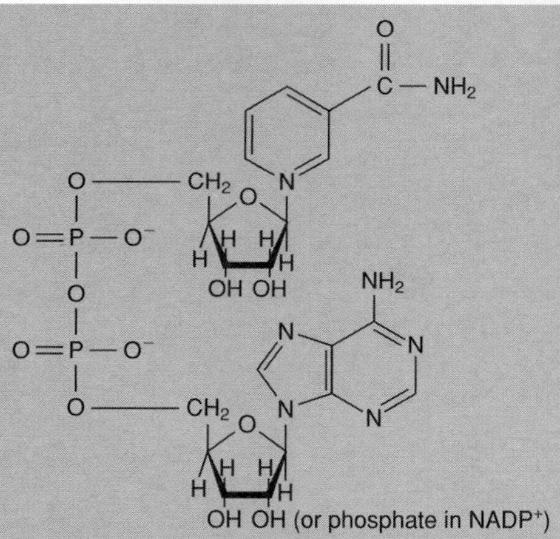 Nicotinamide adenine dinucleotide 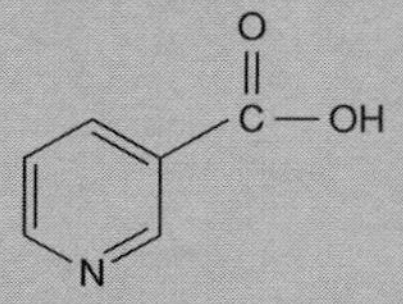 (OH OH (or phosphate in $NADP^+$)) Nicotinic acid 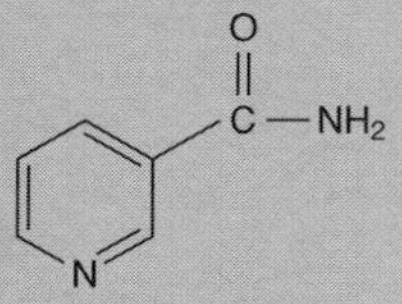 Nicotinamide	NAD^+, NADP Glycolysis Pyruvic acid→Acetyl CoA Respiratory chain Hexose monophosphate shunt Deamination Fatty-acid synthesis β-Oxidation of fatty acids Steroid synthesis	Pellagra 3 *D's* Diarrhea Dermatitis Dementia
Vitamin B_6, pyridoxine, pyridoxal, pyridoxamine	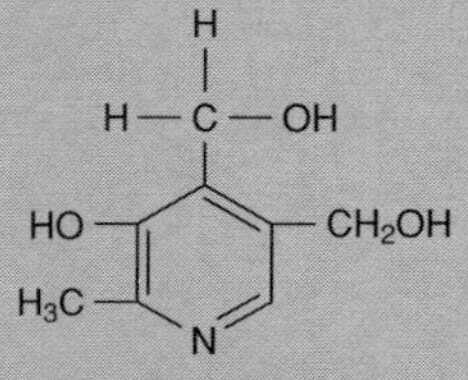 Pyridoxine 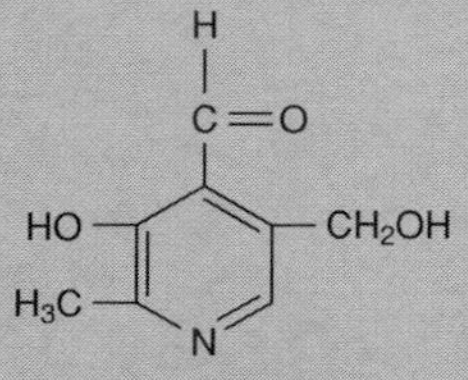 Pyridoxal 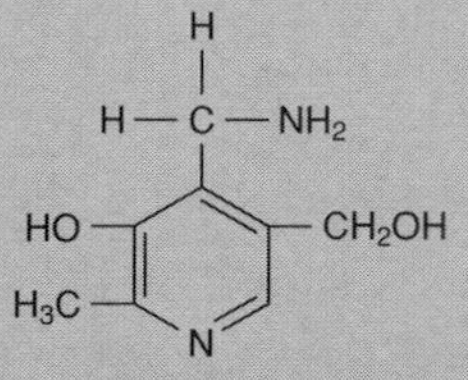 Pyridoxamine	NH_2 transport/exchange Amination Deamination Transamination Sulfur transferases Nonoxidative decarboxylations Amino acid absorption and transport Amino acid metabolism Tryptophan→Niacin Linoleic acid→Arachidonic acid Serotonin, GABA, heme Norepinephrine, histamine Bile acids, acetylcholine Folic acid metabolism	Seizures Depression Neuropathy Lymphocyte depression

Table 31-1 Nutrients—their chemical forms, functions, and effects of deficiency—cont'd

Nutrient	Chemical forms	Function	Deficiency
Pantothenic acid	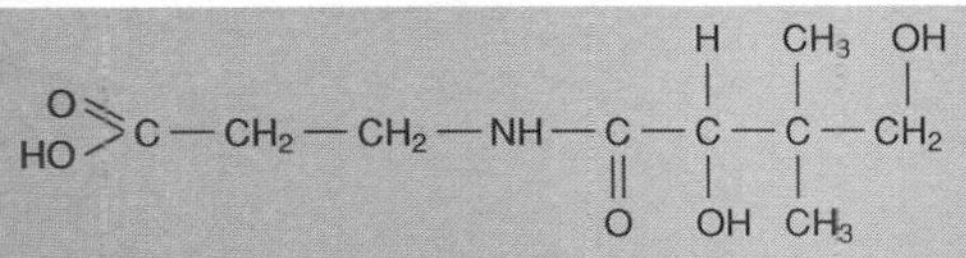 $HOOC-CH_2-CH_2-NH-C(=O)-CH(OH)-C(CH_3)_2-CH_2OH$ **Pantothenic acid**	Pyruvic acid→Acetyl CoA β-Oxidation of fatty acids Ketogenic amino acid catabolism Fatty acid synthesis Steroid synthesis Acetylcholine synthesis Porphyrin synthesis	None documented
Biotin	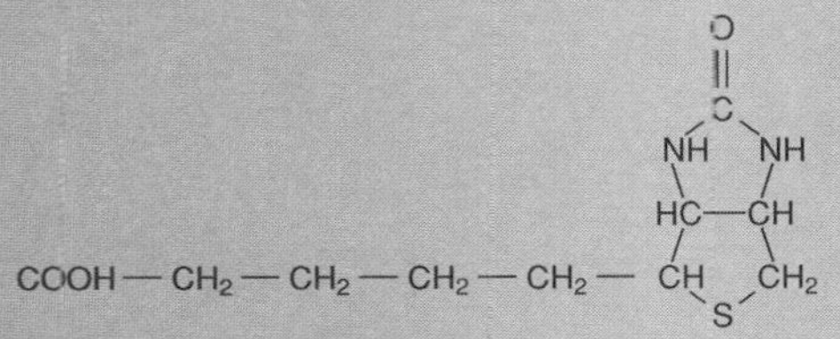 $COOH-CH_2-CH_2-CH_2-CH_2-$ (ring: CH, HC—CH, NH, C=O, NH, S, CH_2) **Biotin**	Carboxylations Pyruvate→Oxaloacetate Fatty acid synthesis	Dematitis Anorexia Lethargy depression Muscle pain Anemia Hypercholesterolemia (rare—associated with antivitamin in raw egg white)
Choline	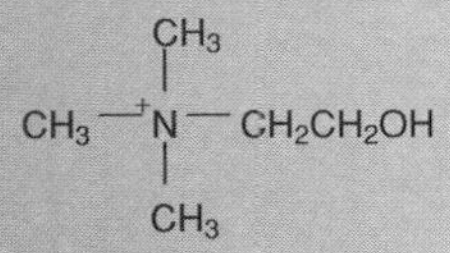 $CH_3-N^+(CH_3)_2-CH_2CH_2OH$ **Choline**	Methyl group donor Lipotrope Lecithin Acetylcholine Sphingomyelin	Fatty liver (not documented in humans)

(continued)

Table 31-1 Nutrients—their chemical forms, functions, and effects of deficiency—cont'd

Nutrient	Chemical forms	Function	Deficiency
Folic acid	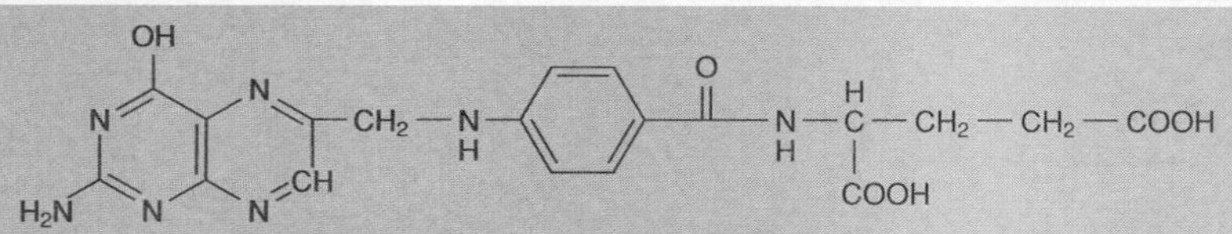 Folic acid 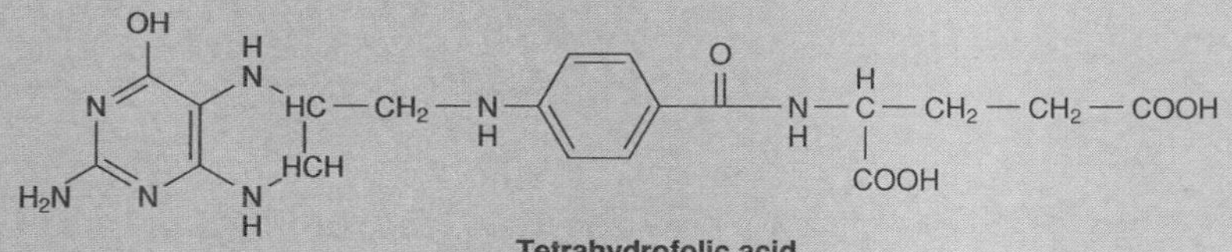 Tetrahydrofolic acid 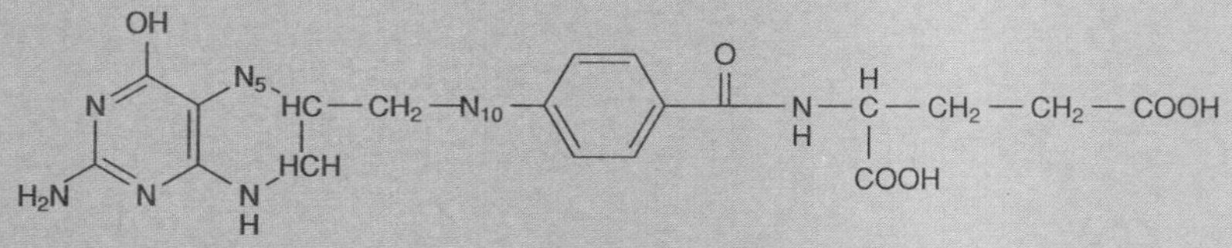 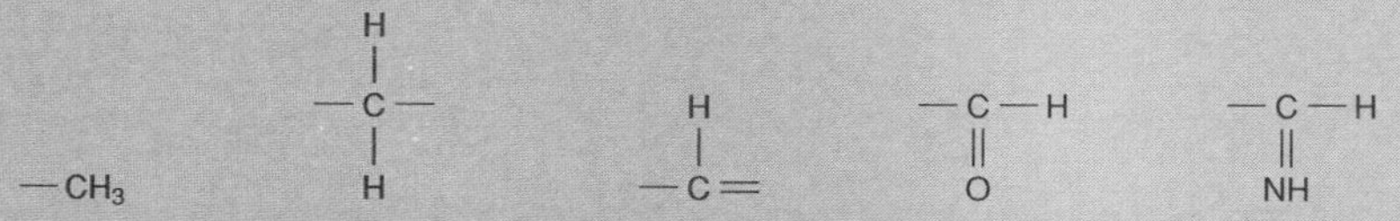 $-CH_3$ Methyl; Methylene; Methenyl; Formyl; Formimino 1-carbon N^5 or N^{10} or N^5-N^{10} substitutions	Nucleic acid synthesis Methylation reactions Amino acid interconversions Cellular reproduction Hematopoiesis Synthesis of: methione serine histidine choline	Megaloblastic anemia Possible perinatal neural tube defects

Table 31-1 Nutrients—their chemical forms, functions, and effects of deficiency—cont'd

Nutrient	Chemical forms	Function	Deficiency
Vitamin B_{12}, cobalamin	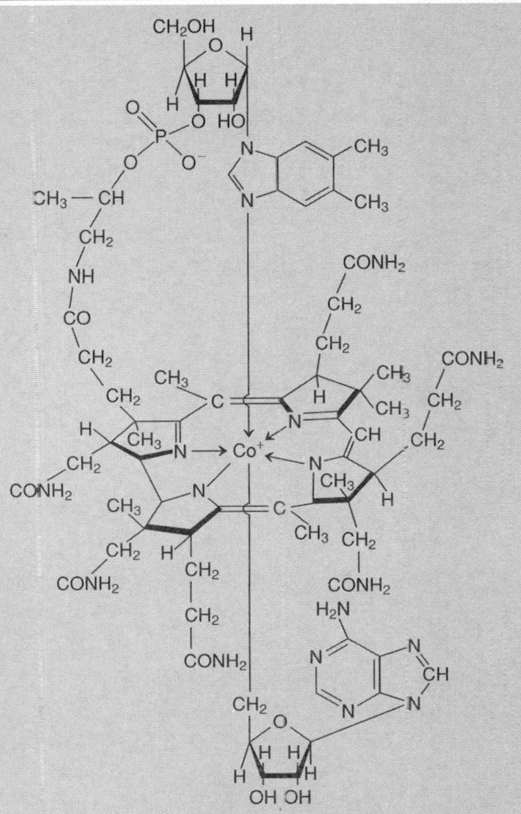 5'-Deoxyadenosylcobalamin	Nucleic acid synthesis Purine metabolism Folic acid metabolism Methione synthesis Hematopoiesis Protein synthesis Nerve tissue maintenance	Pernicious anemia (megaloblastic anemia with neural sequelae)
Vitamin C, ascorbic acid	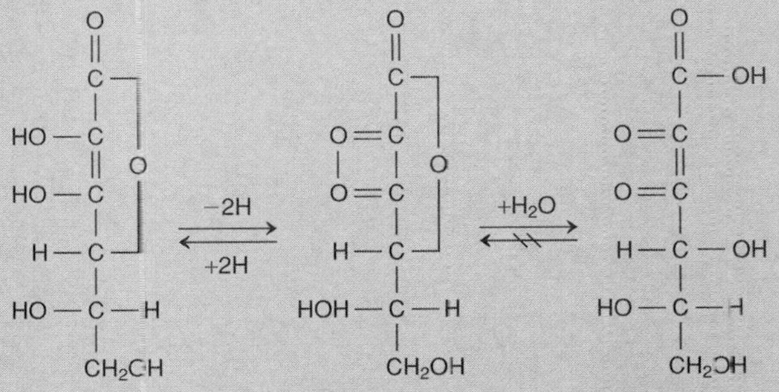 L-Ascorbic acid ⇌ (−2H / +2H) L-Dehyroascorbic acid → (+H_2O) Diketogulonic acid	Oxidation reduction Tyrosine metabolism Folacin activation Iron reduction and storage Synthesis of: collagen serotonin norepinephrine thyroxine corticosteroids	Scurvy Poor wound healing Perifollicular petechiae Anemia Hysteria, depression, anxiety Gingivitis Bone deformities (children) Fatigue, weakness, apathy Loosened teeth

(continued)

Table 31-1 Nutrients—their chemical forms, functions, and effects of deficiency—cont'd

Nutrient	Chemical forms	Function	Deficiency
Calcium	Multiple	Structural mineral Bones Teeth Intracellular signaling Muscle contaction-relaxation Enzyme activation Prothrombin→Thrombin	Osteomalacia (adults) Rickets (children)
Iron	Multiple	Oxygen transport Hemoglobin Myoglobin Cytochromes	Simple anemia
Zinc	Multiple	Ligand Energy metabolism Collagen synthesis Sexual maturation Amino acid metabolism	Growth retardation Dwarfism Hypogonadism Poor wound healing Loss of taste and smell acuity Skin inflammation
Selenium	Multiple	Antioxidant Glutathione peroxidase catalyzes hydroperoxide breakdown	Possible Keshan's disease Probable enterovirus involvement
Copper	Multiple	Hemoglobin formation Respiratory chain Phospholipid synthesis Collagen synthesis Melanin synthesis	Anemia
Iodine	Multiple	Thyroid hormones Thyroxine Triiodothyronine Diodotyrosine	Goiter Myxedema Cretinism (prenatal)
Fluoride	Multiple	Replaces hydroxyapatite with fluorapatite Stronger Teeth Bones	*Not* essential Dental caries Osteoporosis

The RDA recommendations take into account average physiologic requirements. They are then adjusted to compensate for both bioavailability and differences among individuals. Thus these recommendations already include a safety factor and exceed the requirements for most individuals.

Mechanism of action

Vitamins, though not used as energy sources themselves, are required for the metabolic transformations of foodstuffs. As the disciplines of biochemistry and nutrition advanced, specific enzymatic biologic functions were ascribed to the various vitamins. Although some vitamins act as cofactors for intracellular enzyme systems, others, such as vitamin D, act much like hormones. The essential difference between hormones and vitamins is that the former are synthesized endogenously for activities local or distant, whereas the latter must be obtained from an exogenous source. In some instances, defects in enzyme systems caused by genetic errors can be overcome with high doses of necessary vitamin cofactors.

Sources

Vitamins are usually obtained from the diet by ingestion of foods derived from plants and animals that either synthesized them for their own biochemical functions or ingested them. Therapeutically, to correct a deficiency, or to prevent a deficiency pharmacologically or prophylactically, vitamins can be taken orally or injected parenterally. The requirements for vitamins have been fairly accurately determined. Vitamins can be classified according to their solubility in either aqueous or lipid solutions. It is rare for water-soluble vitamins to cause toxicity (except for vitamin B_6) because they are readily excreted after exceeding renal thresholds. Fat-soluble vitamins, on the other hand, because lipids are highly conserved and because of the relative absence of lipid excretion pathways, can readily accumulate to toxic levels after excessive intake.

Vitamin function

The consequences of vitamin deficiencies were observed as puzzling disease entities (scurvy, beriberi, pellagra) that were amenable to treatment with certain diets or foods. During the first half of the twentieth century there was a flurry of research involving chemical fractionation of foods to determine the specific chemical entities responsible for curing these diseases. Studies using chemical extracts of foods removed or added to diets fed to animals elucidated the various essential nutrients and the pathologic effects of deficiency. Later, biochemists determined specific biochemical roles for these nutrients and, in many cases, were able to correlate pathologic changes with defective biochemistry caused by lack of certain nutrients. Most vitamins function in several biochemical roles, yet many additional functions for nutrients are still being discovered.

Classical vitamin nomenclature had its origin in the chemical fractionation of foodstuffs to discover biologic effects. Thus fat-soluble fraction A contained vitamin A, water-soluble fraction B contained the B-complex vitamins, and so forth. All the well-recognized vitamins are included under the following headings: vitamin A, vitamin B complex (many specific factors), vitamin C, vitamin D, vitamin E, and vitamin K. More recently, chemical names for the vitamins have replaced some of these classical names. Many of these vitamins are composed of several active related chemical entities called either *congeners* or *vitamers*.

The pathologic features of vitamin deficiencies can be classified into primary and secondary effects. Primary changes result from physiologic metabolic disturbances caused directly by lack of a specific vitamin, whereas secondary changes such as inanition, organ atrophy, and growth arrest can be observed upon prolonged deficiency.

Chemical compounds that are structurally closely related to vitamins may in some cases be used to analyze their functions because these compounds can compete with or block active sites where vitamins function. Some of these compounds have been found to be therapeutically useful in certain diseases, such as isoniazid[58] (an analog of niacin used to treat tuberculosis) and methotrexate[59] (an analog of folic acid useful as a chemotherapeutic agent). There are also naturally occurring substances that can block the absorption or function of vitamins. Examples of these include avidin,[60] a component of raw egg yolk that binds tightly to biotin, and thiaminase,[61] a compound found in certain species of fish that destroys thiamin.

Bioavailability

Bioavailability is defined as the fraction of the chemical form of the vitamin found in foods or supplements that is absorbed, transported, and available for metabolic function. Food sources vary greatly in the bioavailability of specific components, with iron bioavailability being especially relevant to health.[62,63] In the case of iron, vegetable sources are very poorly absorbed, whereas animal sources are efficiently absorbed. However, simultaneous ingestion of vitamin C with iron results in greatly increased iron bioavailability.

FAT-SOLUBLE VITAMINS

The fat-soluble vitamins differ from water soluble vitamins in that toxic amounts are easier to accumulate (see above) and because their deficiencies are often caused by fat malabsorption. Pancreatic disease, hepatobiliary disorders, and prolonged diarrhea (or steatorrhea) interfere with the absorption of fat-soluble vitamins. However, because of the storage of vitamin A and D in the liver, deficiencies may not develop for several months after malabsorption begins.

Vitamin A, retinoids, and carotenoids

Chemically, vitamin A is an alcohol called *retinol* containing a ring structure and a hydrocarbon chain containing all *trans* double bonds.[52] Vitamin A is necessary for vision (primarily night vision), epithelial integrity, growth, reproduction, and normal cellular differentiation.[64] Two related forms of vitamin A are the aldehyde, called *retinal*, and the acid, called *retinoic acid*. Retinal is the active form of vitamin A involved in vision;[65] retinoic acid will support growth but not vision or reproduction.[66,67] Although retinal and retinol are interconvertible, neither compound can be produced from retinoic acid. These three compounds together with a large number of synthetic analogs are called *retinoids* and have varying degrees of vitamin A activity.[68]

Dietary sources of vitamin A include preformed vitamin A (usually as retinyl ester), which is generally found in animal sources (fish oil is an excellent source), and a variety of carotenoids, which are primarily of vegetable origin. Carotenoids are essentially two retinoid molecules joined together and then cleaved to form two molecules of retinoids either in the intestinal mucosa or in the liver. The strict structural requirements for vitamin A biologic activity mean that carotenoids vary greatly in their pre–vitamin A activity,[69] with β-carotene being the most important biologic precursor as well as the most significant dietary source of vitamin A activity. The RDA for adult females and males are 800 and 1000 μg retinol equivalents per day, respectively.[55]

Absorption

Vitamin A esters are hydrolyzed in the small intestine and then are reesterified in intestinal mucosal cells (primarily to palmitic acid) and, along with uncleaved carotenoids, are carried in chylomicrons to the liver and adipose where they are stored as retinyl esters. (Retinoids derived from carotenoids that are cleaved in the intestinal mucosal cells follow the same pathway.) Retinol is transported in the blood as a complex with retinol-binding protein and transthyretin.[70,71] The pro–vitamin A activity of carotenoids in dark green or yellow-orange vegetables varies widely. In the United States diet the main sources of vitamin A are liver, carrots, eggs, vegetable soups, and milk products.[72]

Function

Vitamin A functions to:

1. Maintain structure and function of certain specialized forms of epithelium.
2. Form rhodopsin, a visual pigment of the visual rods. Briefly, retinol is converted to retinal and then to *cis*-retinal, which binds to opsin to form rhodopsin. Retinal is split off of rhodopsin by a quantum of light, which triggers a nerve impulse to the brain. Most of the retinal is then regenerated in the dark reaction. Thus shortage of vitamin A leads to poor night vision.
3. Maintain skeletal growth.
4. Enable normal cellular membrane function.
5. Lead to cellular differentiation and development. In the absence of vitamin A, mucus-secreting cells become keratinizing cells; adding vitamin A to such cells in tissue culture reverses this process.[73,74]

Toxicity and overdoses

Toxicity may be caused by sustained doses of preformed vitamin A at about 10 times the RDA or by very large single doses.[75] Symptoms include headache, vomiting, diplopia, alopecia, dry mucous membranes, desquamation, bone abnormalities, and liver damage. In addition, teratogenic effects, which induce spontaneous abortion, and birth defects, such as learning disabilities, occur from overconsumption during early pregnancy.[76] Overconsumption of carotenoids does not produce hypervitaminosis A but does result in the benign condition of hypercarotenosis characterized by carotenoderma, where jaundice-appearing skin is evident in the nasolabial folds and the fat pads of the palms of the hands and the soles of the feet.[55] Hypercarotenosis can be differentiated from jaundice by the fact that the sclerae of the eyes are clear in hypercarotenosis.

Deficiency

The most characteristic effects of experimental vitamin A deficiency are in epithelia. Epithelia of the salivary glands, respiratory tract, genitourinary tract, pancreatic ducts, skin, conjunctivae, and enamel organs of the teeth undergo atrophy, proliferation of the basal layer, and replacement of original structure by stratified keratinizing epithelium. Correction of the deficiency results in autolysis of the keratinizing cells and replacement of the affected epithelium by differentiation of the persisting basal layer.[74]

Pathology

Vitamin A deficiency leads to retarded growth in children and emaciation of persons of all ages. Atrophy of skeletal and lymphatic tissue and moderate anemia, probably attributable to bone marrow atrophy, are observed.

Night blindness is often observed in vitamin A deficiency. The lack of retinol and therefore retinal for combination with opsin to form rhodopsin or visual purple (which functions in the black-and-white vision retinal rods) is responsible for this effect.

A more serious result of vitamin A deficiency is xerophthalmia, which has caused permanent blindness to millions of victims worldwide. More than a million children worldwide go blind every year because of vitamin A deficiency.[77] Xerophthalmia can be observed with prolonged deficiency and is evidenced by progressive degeneration of the conjunctiva and cornea. Keratomalacia is the term used for the corneal ulceration and loss of aqueous humor. Punctuate keratopathy is seen during the early stages of corneal degeneration. Triangular grayish areas in the scleral conjunctiva (Bitot's spots) represent accumulations of keratinized epithelium. This lesion may be seen in cases of prolonged, mild deficiency.

Follicular hyperkeratosis is an often observed skin lesion. Multiple firm papules, 1 to 5 mm in diameter, which may be almost confluent, develop as a result of the formation of keratin plugs in the sebaceous glands, giving a characteristic phrynoderma ('toad-skin') appearance. The skin is dry and scaly, and furuncles are also commonly present.

Squamous metaplasia is seen in the trachea, bronchi, renal pelvises, uterus, pancreatic ducts, and certain other epithelial structures. Obstruction of pancreatic ducts by keratotic plugs may lead to cystic dilatation of the ducts and acini. The consequence of long-standing squamous metaplasia with possible progression to anaplasia has been considered in the pathogenesis of some neoplasms.[78]

Although renal calculi are common in vitamin A–deficient animals, there is no evidence that this deficiency causes nephrolithiasis in humans.

Clinically vitamin A deficiency may be diagnosed by the speed of adaptation of vision in weak light. Serum or plasma vitamin A concentrations are diagnostic of deficiency when very low (<100 μg/L) and of hypervitaminosis when very high (>1000 μg/L).[79,80]

The finding of keratinized epithelial cells in the urine, vaginal secretions, and corneal and nasal scrapings may be helpful in diagnosis. Deficiency occurs at all ages but has a higher morbidity and mortality in infants. Papulocutaneous lesions, most often seen in adults, are most numerous on the thighs and forearms and may also involve the shoulders, chest, back, and buttocks. Acnelike lesions may appear on the face; however, an etiologic relationship between vitamin A deficiency and acne vulgaris has not been demonstrated.

The increased susceptibility to bacterial infections, most notably conjunctivitis, furunculosis, bronchopneumonia, and pyelonephritis, is probably attributable to the lack of protective epithelial secretions rather than to a direct effect of vitamin A deficiency on the immune response.

In cirrhosis of the liver (both naturally occurring and experimentally produced), there is a decreased conversion of carotene to vitamin A. Serum vitamin A drops sharply, and in humans the result is often night blindness. Other types of liver damage may produce similar effects.

Vitamin E

Vitamin E consists of two groups of compounds found in plants. These include the tocopherols of which alpha-tocopherol is the most active and abundant form. Tocotrienols have less activity than the tocopherols.[52] The activity of the various compounds with vitamin E activity is calculated from animal experiments. A complicated nomenclature exists to differentiate the various racemic isomers of the various vitamers. From 20% to 80% of ingested vitamin E is absorbed along with fat and is transported similarly to that of retinol in chylomicrons to the liver, where it is packaged into lipoproteins for transport to cellular membranes.[81] The biologic function of vitamin E is to protect membrane integrity by serving as an antioxidant. It neutralizes "free radicals" produced by unsaturated fatty acids and is converted to other metabolic products in the process.[82] Therefore the requirement for vitamin E is proportional to the dietary intake of unsaturated fats. The RDA for adult women and men is 8 and 10 mg alpha-tocopherol equivalents per day, respectively.[56]

The striking findings observed in deficiencies of experimental animals has led to the erroneous conclusion that many human diseases with similar pathologic features are curable with vitamin E. Animals deficient in vitamin E cease growing, have nutritional "muscular dystrophy" (guinea pigs and rabbits), become sterile, and have myocardial necrosis and fibrosis.[83] Human correlates to these abnormalities have not been found and vitamin E has not been shown to be effective as a treatment for muscular dystrophy or heart disease.[84]

Human vitamin E deficiency is seen in premature infants of very low birth weight where hemolytic anemia and possible hemorrhage is found.[85] Patients with enteropathies causing chronic steatorrhea have low serum tocopherol levels.[86] In particular, patients with cystic fibrosis have been studied, and although no frank hemolytic anemia has been observed, studies have shown a shortening of the half-life of circulating erythrocytes. There is some evidence that patients with abetalipoproteinemia have axonal dystrophy leading to degeneration of the posterior column.[87] Also deposits of ceroid, a lipopigment that is found deposited in fat tissue in vitamin E–deficient animals has been found in the small intestines from these patients. Although no toxic effects have been found for doses of up to 800 mg/day of vitamin E, the knowledge that it is a fat-soluble vitamin and the lack of evidence of benefits for higher doses cautions against excessive intake of this vitamin.

Vitamin K

Vitamin K is an exception to the historical derivation of vitamin nomenclature in that its name does not derive from the chemical fractionation of foodstuffs but rather from its function: the designation "K" is from the German word *Koagulationsvitamin*. This vitamin was discovered by the Danish biochemist C.P.H. Dam in 1934 as a result of careful study of a hemorrhagic disease that he observed in chickens.[88] Later it was isolated by Doisy and associates.[89] Vitamin K designates a group of closely related forms with the essential active moiety 2-methyl-1,4-naphthoquinone. Although vitamin K is fat soluble, certain water-soluble derivatives of menadione, a synthetic analog of vitamin K, are alkylated in the liver to compounds that have vitamin K activity.

Functionally, vitamin K is essential for the posttranslational carboxylation of glutamic acid to form gamma-carboxyglutamic acid. This modified amino acid is required for the function of prothrombin (factor II), and five other factors (VII, IX, X, protein C, and protein S) that are essential for blood clotting. Without this modification these proteins are synthesized but the clotting mechanism is ineffective. As with other fat-soluble vitamins, vitamin K is transported primarily in chylomicrons. The body pool of vitamin K is small (on the order of 50 to 100 µg). The RDA for vitamin K is 65 and 80 µg/day for women and men, respectively.

Clinically vitamin K is important in preventing hemorrhagic disease in newborns. Simple deficiency is rare in adults because of its relative abundance in the diet (particularly in leafy vegetables but also in dairy products, meat, eggs, cereals, and fruits) and because the bacterial flora of the jejunum and ileum synthesize vitamin K. From 40% to 70% of dietary vitamin K is absorbed (bioavailable).[55]

Deficiency can occur because of a variety of causes including dietary inadequacy, such as low-fat diets or with protein-energy malnutrition .[90,91] Other causes include biliary obstruction (gallstones, strictures, fistulas), any syndrome where fat is malabsorbed (that is, cystic fibrosis, sprue, celiac disease, ulcerative colitis, short bowel syndrome, regional ileitis), and liver disease, since both bile acids and pancreatic juice are required for normal absorption.

Drug therapy can cause vitamin K deficiency. Anticoagulants that function by interfering with vitamin K metabolism, such as coumarin and warfarin, are often causes.[92] Antibiotics that interfere with normal intestinal bacterial synthesis of vitamin K can cause deficiency.[93] Overdoses of vitamin E or A can cause a vitamin K–responsive condition, particularly in patients being treated with anticoagulants.[94,95]

Although toxic effects of overdoses of vitamin K itself have not been observed, excessive doses of menadione can cause hemolytic anemia, hyperbilirubinemia, and kernicterus in newborns.[96]

WATER-SOLUBLE VITAMINS

Vitamins of the B group

The name *vitamin B* was originally applied to the substance that cured experimental beriberi and that Funk isolated from rice polishings in 1911.[97] Although not chemically pure, it is now known that thiamin was the main bioactive factor that cured beriberi. Concentrates derived from yeast, wheat germ, rice polishings, and other sources contain several factors that collectively are known as the *vitamin B complex*. This complex is a group of essential compounds that are chemically unrelated but occur together in foods, such as liver, milk, and leafy green vegetables. This is not surprising, since most of these compounds are involved in the intermediary metabolism of proteins, carbohydrates, and lipids. Vitamin B_{12} and folic acid are important vitamins in nucleic acid synthesis and metabolism and in hematopoiesis.

Our knowledge of the specific effects of single-vitamin deficiencies was originally derived from studies that used experimental animals. In humans, deficiency of several of these factors usually occurs simultaneously; however, specific disease entities are known to be caused by specific single nutrient deficiencies, probably exacerbated by concomitant multiple deficiencies. Thus, no specific disease is recognized as being attributable to lack of the entire B complex. Individual deficiency states are addressed under the section of each vitamin of this complex.

Thiamin

For many years, beriberi, a peripheral nervous system disease, has been recognized. The Dutch physician Eijkman noted that fowl fed diets consisting of polished rice had symptoms similar to those seen in beriberi. These symptoms could be reversed by the addition of rice polishings to the diet. Thiamin is found in the thermolabile portion of the B complex, whereas the other members of the B complex are thermostable. Funk, at the Lister Institute in London, isolated thiamin and coined the word *vitamine* because he incorrectly believed that all such substances were chemically amines.[97] Thiamin was the first vitamin to have its biochemical function elucidated. The foundations of metabolic and nutritional biochemistry and of neurochemistry were established in the process of elucidating its mechanisms of action.

Thiamin consists of pyrimidine and thiazole rings linked by a methylene bridge. The active form is the diphosphate, called *thiamin pyrophosphate*, which acts as a coenzyme in several alpha-ketoacid decarboxylations and ketolations important in intermediary metabolism.[52] Deficiency interrupts carbohydrate metabolism at the pyruvic acid stage, and pyruvic acid accumulates in the tissues and the blood. In addition, thiamin has a yet undetermined role in central nervous system transmission. Thiamin is actively absorbed in the duodenum and proximal jejunum. This absorption is impaired in alcoholics. Thiamin is transported in the plasma mostly bound to albumin. The RDA for thiamin is 1.1 and 1.5 mg/day for women and men, respectively.[55]

Deficiency

Thiamin is not stored in the body in large amounts. The depletion period before the onset of deficiency symptoms is variable, depending on the metabolic rate and unknown factors.[98] Deficiency occurs where diets are mainly unenriched milled grains.[99] Also, deficiency is found in areas where low thiamin diets are accompanied by the ingestion of raw fish with associated (fish intestinal) microbial thiaminase activity.[100]

Important syndromes associated with thiamin deficiency are chronic peripheral neuritis (dry beriberi), wet beriberi (including symptoms of edema tachycardia and congestive heart failure),[101] and the Wernicke-Korsakoff syndrome.[102,103]

Nerve degeneration is characteristic of the dry or chronic form of beriberi, which occurs chiefly in adults. This syndrome is seen with deficiency accompanied by decreased caloric intake and physical output. Myelin degeneration and, in severe cases, fragmentation of the axis cylinders are seen in the affected nerves, which may be those of the extremities, the vagi, or the cranial nerves. In thiamin-deficient pigeons, axis cylinder degeneration begins distally and progresses until the neurons are involved. If thiamin is given before neuron death, regeneration of axis cylinders occurs at the usual normal rate. In dogs similar degenerative changes have been described in the central nervous system. "Wet" beriberi is a result of deficiency accompanied by high dietary (carbohydrate) intake and physical exertion.

The most common gross lesions of beriberi are muscle atrophy, dilatation (with or without hypertrophy) of the right side of the heart, generalized edema, serous effusions, and chronic passive congestion of the viscera, along with emaciation. Death may be caused by high-output cardiac failure, acute pulmonary edema, or pneumonia or other infections. The edema is caused by cardiac failure, but hypoproteinemia and sodium and water retention are probably contributory factors in many cases.

A thiamin-deficiency disease more likely to be encountered in industrialized countries related to chronic ethanol abuse is the Wernicke-Korsakoff syndrome.[104] The confused state of Korsakoff's psychosis, characterized by confabulation and loss of recent memory, is an early stage in the development of Wernicke's disease, which is characterized by nystagmus and extraocular palsy. Ganglion cell degeneration and focal demyelinating lesions and hemorrhage in the nuclei surrounding the ventricles and aqueduct are found, particularly in the nuclei of the extrinsic muscles of the eye. Adding thiamin to the diet causes prompt clearing of the neurologic symptoms; however, Korsakoff's psychosis improves more slowly and underlying psychotic elements often remain.

The mechanism by which thiamin deficiency produces its characteristic lesions is still not clear. It appears that the coenzyme function of thiamin in carbohydrate function may not be related to the neurologic lesions caused by deficiency, since those regions of the brain with the highest thiamin content and yet the lowest rate of carbohydrate metabolism are the most susceptible to lesions. However, since the metabolism of the nervous system is almost totally dependent on carbohydrate metabolism, it is possible that the degenerative changes in the peripheral nerves and central nervous system are the result of interrupted carbohydrate metabolism. Cardiac symptoms may also be explained by the deficient carbohydrate metabolism and reduced oxygen uptake in thiamin deficiency.[105,106]

A diet composed largely of carbohydrate is an important contributing factor in the development of thiamin deficiency, since thiamin requirements are proportional to carbohydrate intake. Symptoms of peripheral neuritis and mental confusion are explained on the basis of nervous tissue degeneration or anoxia (dry beriberi), and cardiorespiratory symptoms such as tachycardia, edema, cyanosis, and pulmonary congestion are partially explained by similar considerations (wet beriberi). In infantile beriberi, vomiting, cyanosis, and tachycardia may be followed by death (probably from pulmonary edema) within 24 to 36 hours. The mortality of beriberi varies from 5% to 50%, depending on the severity of symptoms and on the promptness and adequacy of treatment.

Riboflavin

The word *flavus*, Latin for 'yellow', characterizes this vitamin. The chemical identity for riboflavin is 6,7-dimethyl-9-(d,l-ribityl)isoalloxazine. In 1932 Warburg and Christian isolated an enzyme complex that they dissociated into an apoenzyme and a protein.[107] The structure was verified by synthesis in 1935.[108,109] Historically, riboflavin was the first vitamin to be identified as a constituent of an enzyme system.

Absorption

Large amounts of relatively free riboflavin are found in milk and eggs carried by binding proteins. In most other foods flavins are bound to enzymes with 60% to 90% as flavin adenine dinucleotide. Phosphatases in the intestinal lumen, especially nucleotide diphosphatase, yield free riboflavin. This is absorbed in the proximal small intestine by a sodium-dependent saturable mechanism.[52] The RDA for riboflavin is 1.3 and 1.7 mg/day for women and men, respectively.[55]

Function

Flavin coenzymes function as electron carriers in a variety of oxidation and reduction reactions including the electron-transport chain of mitochondria. The two primary cofactors are flavin mononucleotide (FMN) and flavin adenine dinucleotide (FAD). These cofactors work with enzymes important as hydrogen carriers in fatty acid synthesis, β-oxidation of fatty acids, and deamination of amino acids and in the essential metabolic step of pyruvic acid to acetyl CoA, all enzyme systems of particular importance to cellular respiration.

Toxicity

Riboflavin is relatively insoluble in water and is absorbed by an active-transport mechanism. This probably explains why no cases of toxicity have been reported in humans.[110]

Deficiency

In humans ariboflavinosis is characterized by cheilosis (fissure formation and crusts at the angles of the mouth) and by redness and irritation of the lips and tongue with smooth, purple-tinged glossitis. Of less common occurrence are circumoral pallor and seborrheic dermatitis of the nasolabial folds and ears[111] (Fig. 31-4). Rarely the dermatitis has a more generalized distribution characterized by areas of dryness and greasy scaling. Vascularization of the cornea by capillary sprouts from the limbic plexus (Fig. 31-5) was first noted in riboflavin-deficient rats and later was recognized as an important and early sign of deficiency of the vitamin in humans.[112-114] In the later stages conjunctivitis develops. The ingrowth of capillaries into the normally avascular cornea probably is an attempt to compensate for the breakdown of oxidation processes in the corneal cells. Eyes are sensitive to light and burn and fatigue easily. The ocular lesions in humans and experimental animals progress to the formation of keratitis and ulceration of the cornea. Depression and hysteria may result from deficiency in nerve tissue. Deficiency in infants and children causes growth retardation, and prenatal deficiency can result in fetal handicaps and malformations. Riboflavin deficiency sometimes occurs in a pure form but more often in patients with pellagra or various multiple deficiencies.

Niacin

The classic pellagra syndrome of the three *D*'s, dermatitis, diarrhea, and dementia, followed by the fourth *D*, death, was a scourge early in the present century in the southeastern United States. The manner by which the U.S. Public Health Service, led by Dr. Goldberger, proved that pellagra was a deficiency disease, not caused by an infectious or contagious agent, is a fascinating account of medical detective work. At one point Dr. Goldberger and his associates voluntarily ingested skin scrapings, urine, and feces (swallowed in capsules) to prove that they would not become infected.[115]

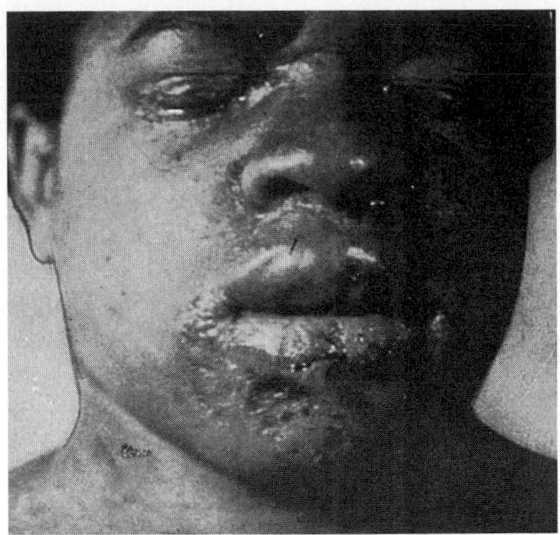

Fig. 31-4 Ariboflavinosis. Cheilosis, nasolabial lesion, and blepharospasm. (From Sydenstriker VP et al: *JAMA* 114:2437, 1940.)

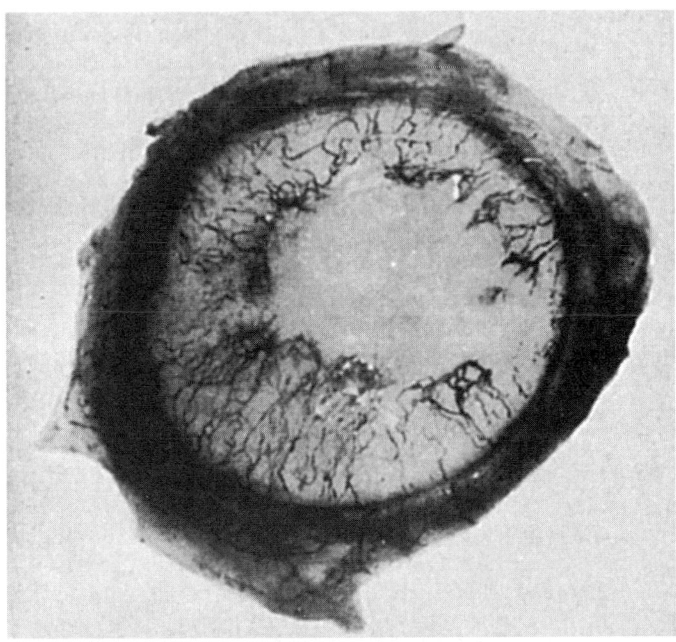

Fig. 31-5 Vascularization of cornea caused by riboflavin deficiency. Rat eye injected with india ink to demonstrate plexus of newly formed blood vessels. (From Eckardt RE, Johnson LV: *Arch Ophthalmol* 21:315, 1939.)

Chemically, niacin (nicotinic acid) can be prepared by the oxidation of the alkaloid nicotine. The familiar oxidation-reduction coenzymes NAD (nicotinamide adenine dinucleotide) and NADP (nicotinamide adenine dinucleotide phosphate) contain niacin and function in more than 50 metabolic reactions. The requirement for niacin is 19 and 15 niacin equivalents per day for males and females, respectively.[55]

Tryptophan to niacin

Strictly speaking, niacin might not be a vitamin, since it can be synthesized from the amino acid tryptophan. Tryptophan is converted to niacin at a ratio of about 60:1, that is, 60 mg of tryptophan in the diet is converted to 1 mg of niacin. Tryptophan is used preferentially as an amino acid for protein synthesis so that when it is limited in the diet niacin deficiency occurs. The tryptophan-to-niacin pathway requires pyridoxine (vitamin B_6) as a cofactor.[116]

Absorption

Animal food sources of niacin are largely composed of nicotinamide, whereas cereals contain niacytin, which has limited bioavailability. In some cultures cereals are treated with alkali before consumption, and this treatment releases the nicotinic acid. This method explains why pellagra is rare in Mexico because the corn flour of tortillas is soaked overnight in lime before preparation. Niacin is absorbed from the small intestine by a sodium-dependent, saturable process. The best sources are grains, legumes, and seed oils. Meat has less niacin than these sources; however, the availability of tryptophan in meat-containing diets in quantities that are generally greater than are needed for protein synthesis leaves excess available for niacin synthesis.[117]

Function

Both NADP and NADPH function as hydrogen carriers in glycolysis, in the alternative pathway the hexose monophosphate shunt, in the transformation of pyruvic acid to acetyl CoA, in the citric acid cycle, and in the respiratory chain. It also functions in deamination, fatty acid synthesis, β-oxidation of fatty acids, and steroid synthesis. Thus it is essential for energy production and the metabolism of all three energy substrates, carbohydrates, proteins, and lipids.[52]

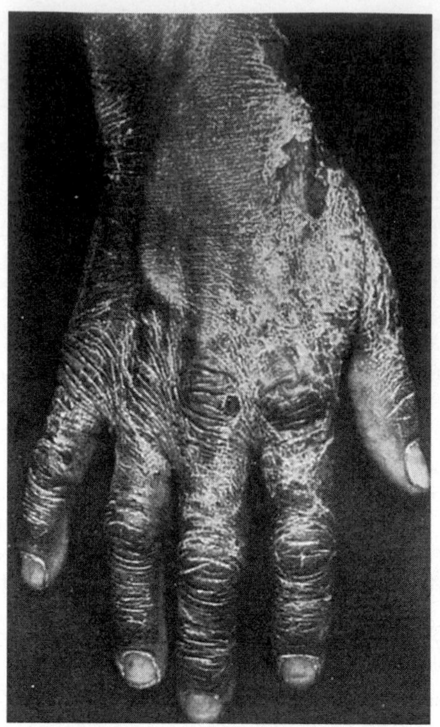

Fig. 31-6 Pellagra. Dermatitis and pigmentation on back of hand. (Courtesy Dr Grover W Wende; from Sutton RL Jr: *Diseases of the skin,* ed 11, St Louis, 1956, Mosby.)

Pellagra

In animals, niacin deficiency results in anorexia, stunting, and inflammation of the oral tract. Niacin deficiency (or pellagra, which literally means 'rough skin') is now rarely seen in first-world countries except for that caused by alcoholism, but it is still endemic in areas of India, China, and Africa.[118] Lesions of deficiency typically include a dermatitis characterized by scaly, dark pigmentation in areas that are exposed to the sun (Fig. 31-6). These generally have clearly demarcated margins and are hyperkeratotic and scaly. Microscopically, congestion of the papillary blood vessels and edema of the papillae are seen. There is moderate lymphocytic infiltration in the corium. Most striking is the noticeable thickening of the keratinized layer of the epidermis. Diarrhea and vomiting result from changes in the gastrointestinal tract. The tongue, buccal membranes, gums, and palate become swollen and red and eventually ulcerate. Infection with Vincent's organisms often causes a gray membrane to form. Intestinal symptoms are exacerbated by achlorhydria, resulting in reduced bacteriostatic activity. The wall of the colon is thickened with edema and lymphocytic infiltration. Membranous enteritis, with or without ulceration, is often seen. Cystic dilatation and atrophy of the crypts of Lieberkühn are characteristic (Fig. 31-7).

Symptoms of dementia include anxiety and insomnia progressing to disorientation and delusions. These neurologic and even psychotic manifestations are common and clear up rapidly if niacin is administered early. They may be the only manifestations of the deficiency. Pathologic lesions in the nervous system appear late in the course of the disease. Demyelinization of the posterior and lateral columns of the spinal cord and focal demyelinization and ganglion cell degen-

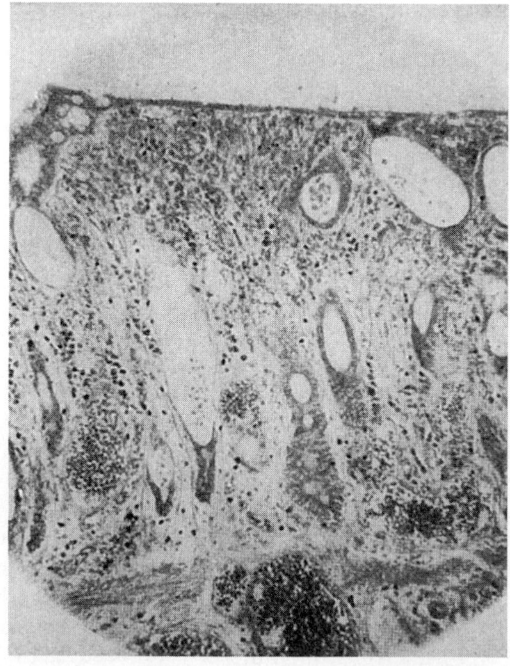

Fig. 31-7 Lesion in colon from patient with pellagra. Specimen (from collection of Dr. James Denton) illustrating cystic glands characteristically found in pellagra, sprue, and possibly other related deficiency diseases. Lesion was formerly known as "colitis cystica superficialis" and is associated with malnutrition. (From Eddy WH, Dalldorf G: *The avitaminoses,* ed 3, Baltimore, Md, 1944, Williams & Wilkins.)

eration in the cerebrum have been described.[119] On postmortem examination, nonspecific changes may include general emaciation, visceral atrophy, fatty infiltration and focal necrosis of the liver, and terminal bronchopneumonia.

It is important to realize that simultaneous lesions of beriberi or ariboflavinosis or other concomitant deficiencies may occur and will respond only to appropriate treatment.

Pellagra can also be caused by a diet low in tryptophan, or in diets that contain an excess of leucine (an amino acid that is high in millet), which inhibits the conversion of tryptophan to niacin.[120-122] It is also found occasionally in alcoholics eating a multiply deficient diet and in tuberculosis and in cancer. Iatrogenic causes include treatment with drugs such as isoniazid and 6-mercaptopurine.[123,124] In the carcinoid syndrome serotonin is produced from its precursor tryptophan, which can deplete the body of this niacin precursor and ultimately niacin. Diseases of absorption, such as chronic diarrhea, and Hartnup's disease, where several amino acids are poorly absorbed, can also lead to pellagra.

Pyridoxine (vitamin B_6)

Pyridoxine was first identified in 1934 as a relatively heat-stable, water-soluble yeast extract that cured or prevented a scaly symmetric peripheral dermatitis (rat acrodynia).[125] The paws, snout, and ears become hyperemic and swollen, with eventual desquamation and ulceration. Although the dermatitis has been described as "acrodynia-like," there is no evidence that human acrodynia is caused by pyridoxine deficiency. Within 4 years the active chemical was isolated by Lepkovsky[126] and by at least three other groups. The structure was determined within a year[127] to be a pyridine derivative with the empiric formula $C_8H_{11}NO_3$.

Vitamin B_6 refers collectively to three naturally occurring ring substances: pyridoxine, pyridoxal, and pyridoxamine, which are substituents on the 4 position of 3-hydroxy-5-hydroxymethyl-2-methylpyridine of the alcohol, the aldehyde, and the amine respectively. All three are converted to the active coenzyme forms, pyridoxal 5′-phosphate or pyridoxamine 5′-phosphate. The recommended dietary allowance for vitamin B_6 is 2.0 and 1.6 mg per day for adult males and females respectively.[55]

Absorption

Vitamin B_6 is primarily absorbed by a nonsaturable passive process mostly in the jejunum. Phosphorylated forms are dephosphorylated by alkaline phosphatase and absorbed where they are metabolically trapped as the phosphate forms. Food sources of vitamin B_6 are generally greater than 75% bioavailable. Availability may be limited by the existence of glucosides and other bound forms such as 6-hydroxypyridoxine. Processing in extreme heat can form unavailable epsilon-pyridoxylysine. The lack of bioavailability of this compound is probably responsible for the occurrence of vitamin B_6–responsive seizures in infants receiving commercial unfortified formula.[128] After absorption vitamin B_6 is transported primarily in plasma bound to albumin and in red blood cells bound to hemoglobin.

Function

The major functions of vitamin B_6 are in amino acid metabolism. Pyridoxine is involved in transaminations, decarboxylations, transmethylation of methionine, metabolism of tryptophan to niacin and 5-hydoxytryptophan, and formation of melanin. It is an essential coenzyme for glycogen phosphorylase, the first step in the transformation of glycogen to glucose. More than 100 enzymatic reactions use pyridoxal phosphate as a cofactor. Vitamin B_6 is also involved in the formation of serotonin, gamma-aminobutyric acid, heme, norepinephrine, histamine, bile acids, and acetylcholine as well as in folic acid metabolism and hematopoiesis.

Toxicity

High-dose pyridoxine has been used as an experimental therapy for premenstrual syndrome and neurologic disorders such as carpal tunnel syndrome. This has resulted in several cases of neurotoxicity and photosensitivity.[129,130] Doses between 2 and 250 mg/day appear to be nontoxic.

Deficiency

In several experimental animals, including pigs, prolonged pyridoxine deficiency causes severe microcytic anemia, which is improved by the administration of pyridoxine. Other lesions found in experimentally induced deficiency in animals are demyelination of peripheral nerves, dorsal root ganglia, and dorsal columns of the spinal cord and fatty infiltration and hemosiderosis of the liver.

Clinical symptoms of vitamin B_6 deficiency are usually seen only in tandem with other deficiencies. Certain residual symptoms in persons with pellagra occasionally respond to pyridoxine administration, apparently because it is a coenzyme for the conversion of tryptophan to niacin. Hyperirritability and convulsions in infants, without other discoverable cause, have been associated with pyridoxine deficiency in a commercial formula.[128]

Experimental pyridoxine deficiency has been induced in humans by administration of the antivitamin deoxypyridoxine. The lesions noted include seborrheic dermatitis of nasolabial folds, cheilosis, and glossitis, as well as a mild normochromic hypoplastic anemia. Thus several of the lesions appear to overlap with those ascribed to riboflavin and niacin deficiency.

The treatment of tuberculosis with isoniazid sometimes results in an iatrogenic pyridoxine deficiency, with cheilosis and peripheral neuritis. These lesions are resolved by the administration of pyridoxine. Also, pyridoxine deficiency has been reported in patients receiving antihypertensive drugs, patients with Parkinson's disease being treated with L-dopa, and women taking oral contraceptives. However, the perceived deficiency in patients taking oral contraceptives (and during pregnancy) is probably attributable to a normal physiologic shift of vitamer concentrations in the plasma.

Several vitamin B_6-dependency syndromes have been described. They respond only to pyridoxine in very large doses, 200 to 6000 mg of pyridoxine HCl per day, in contrast to the normal requirement of 1.5 to 2 mg per day. These syndromes are as follows:

1. Convulsions in infants who have become dependent because their mothers were given large doses of the vitamin for hyperemesis gravidarum
2. Hypersideritis anemia with deposition of hemosiderin in the marrow and liver
3. Xanthurenic aciduria
4. Cystothionuria
5. Homocysteinura

The last four conditions usually are related to an inherited enzymatic defect and are examples of genetically conditioned deficiencies.

Pantothenic acid

Pantothenic acid[52,55,131] is composed of carboxylic acid attached to β-alanine. It is the functional moiety of coenzyme A. It is widely distributed in foodstuffs, thus its name derives from the Greek 'from everywhere.' Pantothenic acid is present in most animal tissues and in yeast, and evidence indicates that it may be a growth-promoting substance of almost universal importance. Since it is found almost everywhere, uncomplicated deficiency is never found. Estimated safe and adequate intake ranges from 4 to 7 mg/day.[55] It is involved in the transformation of pyruvic acid to acetyl CoA, β-oxidation of fatty acids, the catabolism of ketogenic amino acids, the synthesis of fatty acids, steroids, and acetylcholine, and it is a component of porphyrins. Pantothenic acid was discovered because it prevents or cures a type of dermatitis peculiar to chickens. In rats, deficiency of this compound causes a dermatitis, intestinal ulceration, and hemorrhagic necrosis of the adrenal cortex. There is evidence indicating that pantothenic acid may be of importance in preventing the graying of hair that occurs in certain laboratory animals with nutritional deficiencies. The pantothenate level of the blood is below normal in pellagra, beriberi, and ariboflavinosis. Experimental pantothenic acid deficiency in humans causes malaise, headache, insomnia, and nausea but no significant interference with adrenal function. Despite the physiologic importance of this vitamin, evidence for spontaneous occurrence of lesions resulting from deficiency remains inconclusive.

Biotin

Biotin[52,55,132] (vitamin H or coenzyme R) is a compound essential for the respiration of certain lower organisms and probably of all cells. It combines with avidin, a substance present in uncooked egg white, to form a compound that is not absorbed in the intestines (formation of avidin-biotin complexes are important in diagnostic pathology). Our present knowledge of biotin deficiency has been gained largely through observations of animals or humans who have ingested large amounts of raw egg white. In human volunteers fed a diet in which egg white furnished 39% of the total caloric intake, a fine "branny" cutaneous desquamation developed in 3 to 4 weeks. Later, anemia, dryness of the skin, lassitude, mental depression, muscle pains, and other symptoms appeared. Biotin works as a coenzyme in carboxylation reactions and is essential for transformation of pyruvate to oxaloacetate and for fatty acid synthesis. Estimated safe and adequate intake for adults ranges from 100 to 200 μg/day.[55]

Choline

Choline[52,55,133] is a dietary requirement for dogs, cats, rats, and guinea pigs. In humans it can be synthesized from dietary methionine. It functions as a methyl donor and is an important factor in fat metabolism. Many experimental studies have been concerned with the mechanisms by which it acts. It is an essential component of lecithin, a phospholipid that is a constituent of all cells. Lecithin is probably formed in the liver as a preliminary step in the oxidation of fatty acids. Choline deficiency in experimental animals (dogs, rats, and rabbits), particularly when combined with a high intake of fats with saturated fatty acids, reduces the oxidation of fats in the liver and leads to the accumulation of fat in the liver cells (central lobular distribution) and eventually to cirrhosis. Recent experimental studies have suggested that a choline-deficient diet may act as a promoter in liver carcinogenesis induced by chemical carcinogens. In young rats, in addition to fatty livers, hemorrhagic cortical necrosis of the kidneys, hemorrhages in other organs, and involution of the thymus are found. Cystine-rich diets intensify the liver and kidney lesions, whereas methionine, like choline, reverses the process. Choline deficiency has not been demonstrated in humans, and whether choline is an essential dietary factor for humans is not known.

Folic acid and vitamin B_{12}

Both folic acid and vitamin B_{12} deficiencies cause megaloblastic anemia, and it was in the search for the cure to this anemia that they were discovered. Both vitamins are essential for the synthesis of nucleic acids, and cells that are rapidly dividing become abnormal when they are limiting. Thus during deficiency megaloblasts are observed primarily in the hematopoietic cells and in mucosal cells of the gastrointestinal tract.

Although both folic acid and vitamin B_{12} cause megaloblastic anemia, and either vitamin will correct hematologic megaloblastosis, only B_{12} will cure symptoms of pernicious anemia, which has a neurologic as well as a hematologic influence. Minot and Murphey in 1926 found that pernicious anemia responded to the feeding of liver.[134] William Castle and associates were able to demonstrate that there was an "intrinsic factor" found in gastric juice that combined with an "extrinsic factor" found in animal protein that resulted in the absorption of a substance that cured pernicious anemia.[135] Wills and associates were able to reproduce symptoms of megaloblastic anemia in monkeys and found that crude but not purified liver extracts cured the disease.[136]

Chemically, vitamin B_{12} (cyanocobalamin) is composed of a planar corrin nucleus and 5,6-dimethylbenzimidazole attached to the corrin nucleus by D-1-amino-2-propanol and also attached to ribose. Although cyanocobalamin, the cyano derivative of cobalamins, is the compound designated by the term vitamin B_{12}, coenzyme B_{12} (5-deoxyadenosylcobalamin) and methylcobalamin are the active forms in metabolism. The RDA for vitamin B_{12} is 2 μg/day for both men and women.[55]

Folic acid refers to pteroylglutamic acid, the oxidized form of folate. It consists of a pteridine moiety, linked to *para*-aminobenzoic acid linked to glutamic acid. The folate family consists of multiple congeners characterized by changes in oxidation state of the pteridine ring (either fully oxidized or the reduced forms 7,8-dihydrofolate or 5,6,7,8-tetrahydrofolate), various one-carbon adducts on the 5 and 10 positions of the molecule and by one to eight glutamic acid residues linked to one another by gamma-amino bonds except for the requisite β-linked initial glutamic acid. The RDA for folic acid is 180 and 200 μg/day for women and men, respectively.[55]

Absorption

Absorption of vitamin B_{12} requires both an "intrinsic factor" found in gastrointestinal secretions and the "extrinsic factor" vitamin B_{12} itself. Pernicious anemia can develop when either factor is missing. Food vitamin B_{12} is freed from peptide linkages by gastric acid and digestive enzymes. Next the B_{12} binds to salivary R binder polypeptide. This binder protein is digested by pancreatic trypsin, and the free B_{12} binds to intrinsic factor. This complex (a dimer of two molecules of intrinsic factor and two molecules of B_{12}) is absorbed in the ileum by means of specific receptors. In addition, about 1% of free vitamin B_{12} is absorbed by diffusion. The absorbed vitamin is then transported by transcobalamins I, II, and III in the serum.[137,138]

Since food folate is primarily in the form of polyglutamates, these must be split off before absorption primarily in the proximal small bowel. The enzyme responsible is pteroylpolyglutamate hydrolase, which is found on the brush border. This hydrolase is significantly inhibited by food factors found in beans and yeast in vitro, but this effect has not been verified in vivo. The deficiency seen in alcoholics may be the result of a reduced intake exacerbated by reduced absorption attributable to inactivation of brush-border hydrolases. Folates are transported in plasma either free or bound to low- or high-affinity binders.[139]

Function

Cobalamin functions in the transfer of methyl groups. Important reactions include the synthesis of methionine, folic acid metabolism, and nucleic acid synthesis. It is therefore important in cellular reproduction and protein synthesis. Although the specific mechanism of its action has not been elucidated, it is also important for maintenance of nerve tissue.

Folates have overlapping functions with cobalamin in nucleic acid synthesis. Folates are important in one-carbon metabolism including methylation reactions, interconversions of amino acids. It is essential for the synthesis of the amino acids methionine, serine, and histidine as well as in the synthesis of choline.[52]

Toxicity

Like that of other water-soluble vitamins, excessive doses of these two vitamins that exceed the binding capacity of carrier proteins and the renal threshold are simply excreted. Extremely high doses of folic acid compete with carrier proteins for anticonvulsant drugs and may have contributed to one or more instances of seizures in epileptics who were orally given therapeutic doses of folic acid.[140,141]

Deficiency

Symptoms of deficiency include weakness, tiredness, dyspnea, sore tongue, diarrhea (particularly in folate deficiency), anorexia, syncope, headache, palpitation, fever, icterus plus pallor, glossitis, and vitiligo. Symptoms specific to vitamin B_{12} deficiency include damaged myelin resulting in impaired positional sense, ataxia, and diminished vibration sense. However, irritability and forgetfulness are seen primarily in folate deficiency.

Folic acid deficiency in monkeys causes a nutritional anemia, with reversal of the lymphocyte-neutrophil ratio. In humans, folic acid is useful in the treatment of sprue and megaloblastic nutritional anemia. It brings about hematologic remission in pernicious anemia but, unlike vitamin B_{12}, does not prevent or improve the degenerative lesions in the spinal cord.[52]

Vitamin C (ascorbic acid)

Although James Lind is erroneously credited with discovering that dietary citrus cured scurvy, his early clinical nutrition experiment with six pairs of scorbutic sailors treated with six different dietary supplements did prove the efficacy of citrus in treatments. Scurvy continued to be a scourge on both land and sea, with scurvy occurring during the American Civil War, during the California gold rush, and during the Great Potato Famine in Europe. It was Albert Szent-Györgyí and Glen King who independently isolated pure ascorbic acid.[142,143] By 1933 a chemical synthesis from glucose was developed. Only a few species have lost the synthetic pathway to convert D-glucose to ascorbic acid; these include humans and monkeys, guinea pigs, the Indian fruit bat, and the red-vented bulbul bird of India. This ability was presumably lost because of the availability of abundant dietary ascorbate to these species.[56,57] Ascorbic acid exists in natural sources chiefly in the form of L-ascorbic acid, a six-carbon compound closely related to glucose. In this form, it readily loses two hydrogen atoms to become dehydroascorbic acid, which is reversibly reduced in the body. The physiologic action of vitamin C therefore depends on its ability to carry out oxidation-reduction reactions. The RDA for vitamin C is 60 mg/day for both men and women.[55]

Absorption

Ascorbic acid is absorbed in the small intestine by an energy-dependent active saturable transport mechanism. Thus physiologic intakes less than 180 mg/day are absorbed completely, whereas pharmaceutical doses of multiple grams are only 50% absorbed.[144] Being a small molecule, ascorbate is believed to be transported by solubilization in serum and extracellular fluids. Intracellular concentration of ascorbate varies widely and is especially high in pituitary, adrenals, leukocytes, and the brain. These high concentrations indicate that an active energy-driven transport mechanism may be involved in cellular uptake.[52]

Function

Ascorbate[52] can provide reducing equivalents through its reversible transformation to dehydroascorbic acid. During collagen synthesis, vitamin C is a cofactor for posttranslational hydroxylation of proline and lysine, thus allowing the cross-linking that stabilizes tropocollagen. It is the lack of ascorbate for these reactions that causes the characteristic symptoms of scurvy. Ascorbate is required for carnitine biosynthesis and the formation of norepinephrine from dopamine as well as the hydroxylation of tryptophan to form serotonin. In addition, ascorbate is important to the mixed-function oxygenase system and the microsomal hydroxylation of cholesterol. There is good evidence that it maintains certain important sulfhydryl enzymes in the active state. It is clear that ascorbic acid is necessary for the production and maintenance of several intercellular substances, notably collagen, osseomucin, chondromucin, and dentin. Considerable attention has been given to the antioxidant function of ascorbic acid in neutralizing extracellular reactive oxidants produced during phagocytic activity and in protecting cell membranes from free-radical damage.

Toxicity

Exceptional health claims for the intake of high levels of ascorbic acid have been promoted by some scientists and the lay press.[145] It is not therefore surprising that potential adverse effects of these pharmacologic doses have been investigated. The only adverse effects that have been observed are those relating to the osmotic effects of megadoses causing nausea and diarrhea.[144] Concern is expressed that oxalic acid, a metabolite of ascorbic acid, may contribute to hyperoxaluria and kidney stones.[146] Ascorbate is excreted largely intact, however, and this risk is probably exaggerated.[147] There is danger that excessive intakes of ascorbate can interfere with laboratory tests for glycosuria and fecal occult blood. In addition, cholesterol, glucose, and ceruloplasmin oxidase assays are affected by ascorbate.[148] Coumarin or heparin anticoagulant therapy is interfered with by high doses of ascorbate.

Deficiency

Symptoms of scurvy include fatigue, apathy, hysteria, depression and anxiety, painful joints, anemia, loosened teeth, bleeding gums and gingivitis, impaired wound healing, ocular hemorrhages, perifollicular petechiae, dry itchy skin, and increased susceptibility to infection.[149] Early symptoms include petechiae surrounded by a classical red hemorrhagic halo. These symptoms progress to oral symptoms, impaired wound healing, and infectious disease. In infants and young children chest deformities are observed to be caused by faulty bone ossification. Frank scurvy is rarely observed, though it is occasionally observed in alcoholics and drug abusers subsisting on a substandard diet. Subacute deficiency as a result of an inadequate diet may occur in institutionalized or homebound populations of the elderly.

MINERALS

In addition to carbon, hydrogen, oxygen, and nitrogen, 16 elements are considered essential for life: calcium, magnesium, potassium, sodium, sulfur, phosphorus, chlorine, iron, copper, cobalt, manganese, zinc, iodine, selenium, molybdenum, and probably fluorine. Minerals make up about 4% of body weight and are classified as major minerals (those that compose more that 0.01% of body weight) and trace minerals (those that compose less than 0.01% of body weight). Major minerals include calcium, phosphorus, potassium, sulfur, sodium, chlorine, and magnesium. Trace minerals include iron, zinc, manganese, selenium, copper, iodine, cobalt, molybdenum, chromium, fluoride, silicon, vanadium, nickel, tin, and arsenic. The above do not include all minerals found in the body and may exclude some that may later prove to be essential. Because of their ubiquitous presence in foods, deficiencies of potassium, sulfur, sodium, chlorine, magnesium, manganese, cobalt, molybdenum, chromium, silicon, vanadium, nickel, tin, and arsenic have not been seen in man (exceptions include certain inborn errors of metabolism) and are not discussed here.

Features common to most of the minerals include homeostasis within rather narrow limits controlled by absorption, utilization, storage, and excretion.

Calcium

Although calcium[150] composes 1.5% to 2.2% of body weight and the process of bone mineral deposition and mobilization is dynamic, plasma calcium is closely modulated at 10 mg/dl. Ninety-nine percent of the 1200 g of calcium in the adult is found in bony material. Bones are constantly being resorbed and reformed, with the process of calcium homeostasis being accomplished by mechanisms involving several hormones including PTH from the parathyroid gland and vitamin D metabolism, which are discussed in detail elsewhere. Extracellular calcium is important in blood clotting, membrane permeability, muscle contraction, and nerve conduction. Insufficient ionized extracellular calcium results in hypocalcemic tetany from continuous excitation. Intracellular calcium is important in signal transduction and in ATP hydrolysis. The importance of calcium and phosphorus in rickets and osteomalacia are discussed elsewhere in the chapter on bone. Adequate bone mineralization is dependent on adequate calcium intake, especially among adolescent females, the importance of an adequate intake for individuals of these age groups cannot be overstressed. The RDA for calcium is 1200 mg/day for adult males and for females from 11 to 24 years of age; females from 25 to 50 years of age should ingest 800 mg/day.[55]

Iron

Total iron content of the body averages from 2 to 6 g depending on an individual's size.[151] The amount of iron is closely regulated by changes in absorption efficiency. Food iron varies greatly in bioavailability, and this combined with its limited dietary availability makes deficiency a frequent event.

Absorption

Depending on its chemical form, iron is absorbed by two different mechanisms. Dietary iron consists of either heme or nonheme iron. About 40% of iron in meat is heme, and about 25% of this heme iron is bioavailable The remainder of the iron in meats and the iron in vegetable products is nonheme iron, which is about 2% bioavailable. Availability of nonheme iron can be greatly enhanced by dietary factors, the most important of which are meat products themselves and ascorbic acid (vitamin C). Monsen and colleagues[63] have generated equations with which to calculate the availability of iron in a given diet using these factors. Iron is transported in the blood bound to transferrin. The Recommended Dietary Allowance for iron is 10 and 15 mg/day for adult males and females, respectively.[55]

Function

Iron functions to transport oxygen in erythrocytes and in the respiratory chain. It is a component of hemoglobin, myoglobin, cytochromes, and several enzymes.

Toxicity

Hemosiderosis is the result of excessive iron intake, such that the iron-carrying capacity of transferrin is overloaded, resulting in deposition of iron in tissues. About 2000 cases of iron poisoning are observed in the United States annually, usually from the accidental intake of supplements by children. Only 3 g of iron are lethal for a 2 year old. Causes of iron overload include hemochromatosis, an inborn error of metabolism resulting in increased iron absorption, siderosis caused by the ingestion of food and alcoholic beverages prepared in iron or steel vessels, alcoholic cirrhosis, pancreatic insufficiency, shunt hemochromatosis from shunts between portal and systemic veins (usually to treat esophageal varices), prolonged iron therapy, and severe chronic anemias treated with iron supplements or transfusions.

Deficiency

Iron-deficiency anemia is often called simple or nutritional anemia. Deficiency results from an imbalance between intake, utilization, and loss and can be caused by inadequate absorption or intake, an increased requirement not offset by increased intake or by chronic blood loss. Red blood cells become microcytic and hypochromic. Tissues become hypoxic and the heart becomes enlarged. Heart enlargement is usually reversible with iron supplementation. Nails may become spoon shaped (koilonychia). Fatigue, weakness, pallor, dyspnea on exertion, palpitation, and paresthesia of the hands and feet are found. Glossitis with varying degrees of papillary atrophy, angular stomatitis, dysphagia, and decreased neutrophils and lymphocytes may be seen.

Zinc

Two to 3 g of zinc are found in the average adult.[152] Zinc has a multitude of functions in metabolism as a coenzyme in most major metabolic pathways, in gene expression, in alcohol detoxification, and in elimination of carbon dioxide through its role in carbonic anhydrase. Zinc deficiency in rats causes corneal vascularization, alopecia, skin and esophageal keratinization, and death. Human deficiency has been observed in Egypt and Iran among individuals consuming high phytate (high whole grain, vegetarian) diets. Symptoms of human deficiency include growth retardation, hypogonadism, hypospermia and delayed sexual maturation, alopecia, night blindness, acrodermatitis enteropathica, anorexia with diarrhea, poor wound healing, and loss of taste and smell acuity. The RDA for zinc is 15 and 12 mg/day for men and women respectively.[55] It is questionable whether subclinical zinc deficiency occurs in the United States. Several studies have indicated that among certain populations zinc supplementation increases the rate of wound healing and improves poor appetite and impaired taste acuity. Symptoms of toxicity include gastrointestinal irritation and vomiting. Neutropenia and hypocupremia have been observed in patients given 10 to 30 times the RDA for several months.

Selenium

Selenium functions as an antioxidant through its association with glutathione peroxide.[153] In this it functions similarly to vitamin E but in different cellular compartments. In some measure vitamin E and selenium can substitute for each other. It is well known that there are areas in the world where soils have low or high selenium and that these are associated with either deficiency or toxicity in livestock. Rats fed a selenium-deficient diet develop hair loss, growth retardation, and reproductive failure. Keshan (pronounced /kə-shán/) disease is a cardiomyopathy endemic in low-selenium areas in a belt running from northeastern (with Keshan in Heilongjiang Province) to southwestern China. Histopathologically, it presents as multifocal necrosis, myocytolysis, and fibrous replacement of the myocardium. It appears that Keshan disease is preventable by selenium supplementation, but it appears that a cardiotoxic virus may also be involved in its etiology. Toxicity symptoms include hair loss, fragile nails, fatigue, and nausea and vomiting. The RDA for selenium is 70 and 55 μg/day for men and women, respectively.[55]

Copper

Copper is an essential part of lysyl oxidase, an enzyme responsible for cross-linking of collagen and elastin.[154] It is also important in hematopoiesis. In all species tested, deficiency results in anemia, neutropenia, and osteoporosis. Most disorders of copper metabolism result from inborn errors of metabolism. Menke's disease is a fatal X-linked copper metabolism disorder with symptoms of mental retardation, kinked hair, and maldistribution of copper. Wilson's disease is an autosomal recessive disease. Copper accumulates in the liver, brain, and the cornea of the eye. Copper deficiency has also been observed in total parenteral nutrition and in premature infants fed exclusively on milk formulas (milk is low in copper). There is no RDA for copper, but the National Academy of Sciences Food and Nutrition Board recommends estimated safe and adequate daily dietary intakes of 1.5 to 3.0 mg/day.[55]

Iodine

Goiter can be prevented but not cured by adequate iodine intake.[155] A discussion of iodine and thyroid function will be found in another chapter. Toxicity is found at intakes of between 200 to 500 mg/kg per day. Iodized salt is an effective public health measure for the elimination of goiter. The recommended dietary allowances is 150 μg/day.[55]

Fluorine

No conclusive evidence that fluorine is an essential element has been presented.[55] Its established role in preventing tooth decay and its possible role in preventing osteoporosis and osteomalacia have stressed its importance in nutrition. Consequences of "deficiency" therefore are increased incidence of dental caries and possible fractures. Symptoms of toxicity are fluorosis and disorders in kidney function. To produce these symptoms the intake must be in the range of 20 to 80 mg/day for years. Water supplemented at 1.0 mg/liter is an effective public health measure to greatly reduce the incidence of dental caries. The estimated safe and adequate daily dietary intake is between 1.5 and 4.0 mg/day.[55]

This chapter has been limited to selected topics dealing with how altered nutrition may induce and influence disease states. It has not covered many important areas dealing with nutrition and its interrelationships, such as those with obesity,[156] heart and vessel diseases,[157] infection and the immune system,[158-161] aging,[49,162,163] and drugs.[164-167]

REFERENCES

1. American Academy of Pediatrics, Committee on Nutrition: Commentary on breast-feeding and infant formulas, including proposed standards for formulas, *Pediatrics* 57:278, 1976.
2. Irwin MI: *Nutritional requirements of man: a conspectus of research,* New York, 1980, The Nutrition Foundation, Inc.
3. National Academy of Science, NRC, Food and Nutrition Board: *Recommended dietary allowances,* ed 8, Washington, DC, 1980, US Government Printing Office.
4. Harper AE, Benevenga NJ, Wohlhueter RM: Effects of ingestion of disproportionate amounts of amino acids, *Physiol Rev* 50:428, 1970.
5. Grunfeld C, Feingold KR: Metabolic disturbances and wasting in the acquired immunodeficiency syndrome, *N Engl J Med* 327:329, 1992.

Types of malnutrition

6. Keys A: *The biology of human starvation,* Minneapolis, 1950, University of Minnesota Press.
7. Blix G: *Mild-moderate forms of protein-calorie malnutrition,* Uppsala, 1963, Almquist & Wiksells.
8. Bhattacharyya AK: Protein-energy malnutrition kwashiorkor-marasmus syndrome: terminology, classification and evolution, *World Rev Nutr Diet* 47:80, 1986.
9. Olson RE: *Protein-calorie malnutrition,* New York, 1975, Academic Press.
10. Jeliffe DD, Welbourn HF: Clinical signs of mild-moderate protein-calorie malnutrition of early childhood. In Blix G, editor: *Mild-moderate forms of protein-calorie malnutrition,* Uppsala, 1963, Almqvist & Wiksell.

11. Latham MC: *Human nutrition in tropical Africa,* Rome, 1965, Food and Agriculture Organization of the United Nations.
12. Brock JF, Autret M: Kwashiorkor in Africa, *WHO Monogr Ser* 8:36, 1952.
13. Davies JNP: Nutrition and nutritional diseases, *Annu Rev Med* 3:99, 1952.
14. Trowell HC, Davies JNP, Dean, RFA: *Kwashiorkor,* New York, 1982, Academic Press.
15. Bistrian BR, Blackburn GL, Hallowell E, Heddle R: Protein status of general surgical patients, *JAMA* 230:858, 1974.
16. Bistrian BR, Blackburn GL, Vitale J et al: Prevalence of malnutrition in general medical patients, *JAMA* 235:1567, 1976.
17. Smith JL, Wickiser AA, Korth LL et al: Nutritional status of an institutionalized aged population, *J Am Coll Nutr* 3:13, 1984.
18. Pinchcofsky-Devin, GD, Kaminski MV Jr: Incidence of protein calorie malnutrition in the nursing home population, *J Am Coll Nutr* 6:109, 1987.
19. Birch GE, Pineiro C, Alcalde E et al: Relation of kwashiorkor in early childhood and intelligence at school age, *Pediatr Res* 5:579, 1971.
20. Lloyd-Still JD: Clinical studies on the effects of malnutrition during infancy and subsequent physical and intellectual development. In Lloyd-Still JD, editor: *Malnutrition and intellectual development,* Littleton, Mass, 1976, Publishing Sciences Group.
21. David H: *Die Leber bei Nahrungsmangel und Mangelernahrung,* Berlin, 1961, Akademie-Verlag.
22. Follis RHJ: *Deficiency disease,* Springfield, Ill, 1958, Charles C Thomas.
23. Platt BS, Heard CRC, Stewart RJC: Experimental protein-calorie deficiency. In Munro HN, Allison JB, editors: *Mammalian protein metabolism,* New York, 1964, Academic Press.
24. Sidransky H: Chemical and cellular pathology of experimental acute amino acid deficiency, *Methods Achiev Exp Pathol* 6:1, 1972.
25. Sos J: *Die Pathologie der Eiweissernahrung,* Budapest, 1964, Verlag der Ungarischen Akademie der Wissenschaften.
26. Kilbourne EM, Rigau-Pérez JG, Heath CW Jr et al: Clinical epidemiology of toxic-oil syndrome, *N Engl J Med* 309:1408, 1983.
27. Martinex-Tello J, Navas-Palacios JJ, Ricoy JR et al: Pathology of a new toxic syndrome caused by ingestion and adulterated oil in Spain, *Virchows Arch Pathol Anat* 397:261, 1982.
28. Varga J, Jiménez SA, Uitto J: L-Tryptophan and the eosinophilia-myalgia syndrome: current understanding of the etiology and pathogenesis, *J Invest Dermatol* 100:975, 1993.
29. Hille RH Jr, Caudill SP: Contaminants in L-tryptophan associated with eosinophilia-myalgia syndrome, *Arch Environ Contam Toxicol* 25:134, 1993.
30. Kilbourne EM, Delpaz MP, Borda IA et al: Toxic oil syndrome—a current clinical and epidemiologic summary, including comparisons with the eosinophilia-myalgia syndrome, *J Am Coll Cardiol* 18:711, 1991.
31. Philen RM, Hill RH Jr: 3-(Phenylamino)alanine: a link between eosinophilia-myalgia syndrome and toxic oil syndrome? *Mayo Clin Proc* 68:197, 1993. (Comments: 67:1134, 1992; 68:823, 1993).

Consequences of malnutrition

32. Cravioto J, DeLicardie ER: Nutrition and behavior and learning, *World Rev Nutr Diet* 16:80, 1973.
33. Latham MC: Protein-calorie malnutrition in children and its relations to psychological development and behavior, *Physiol Rev* 54:541, 1974.
34. Morgan BLG, Winick M.: Pathological effects of malnutrition on the central nervous system. In Sidransky H, editor: *Nutritional pathology,* New York, 1985, Marcel Dekker.
35. Read MS: Behavioral correlation of malnutrition. In Brazier MAB, editor: *Growth and development of the brain,* New York, 1975, Raven Press.
36. Scrimshaw NS, Gordon JE, editors: *Malnutrition, learning and behavior,* Cambridge, Mass, 1968, MIT Press.
37. Calories and energy expenditure in carcinogenesis, *Am J Clin Nutr* 45:149, 1987.
38. Conference on nutrition and cancer, *Cancer Res* 37(7, pt.2):2322, 1977.
39. Assembly of Life Sciences, National Research Council, *Diet, nutrition, and cancer,* Washington, DC, 1982, National Academy Press.
40. Newell GR, Ellison NM: Nutrition and cancer: etiology and treatment, *Prog Cancer Res Ther* 17:1, 1981.
41. Reddy, BS: Nutrition and its relationship to cancer, *Adv Cancer Res* 32:238, 1980.
42. Poirier LA, Boutwell RK: Current problems in nutrition and cancer, *Fed Proc* 35:1307, 1976.
43. Symposium on nutrition in the causation of cancer, *Cancer Res* 35:3231, 1975.
44. Winick, M: Nutrition and cancer, current concepts (*Current Concepts in Nutrition,* vol 6), New York, 1977, John Wiley & Sons.
45. American Cancer Society, Workshop conference on nutrition in cancer causation and prevention, *Cancer Res* 43:2385, 1983.
46. Cohen LA: Diet and cancer, *Sci Am* 257:42, 1987.
47. Mettlin CJ, Aoki K: Recent progress in research on nutrition and cancer, *Prog Clin Biol Res* 346:1, 1990.
48. Weisburger JH: Nutritional approaches to cover prevention with emphasis on vitamins, antioxidants, and carotenoids, *Am J Clin Nutr* 53:2265, 1991.
49. Kritchevsky D: Diet, lipid metabolism, and aging, *Fed Proc* 38:2001, 1978.
50. Matsukura N, Kawachi T, Morino K et al: Carcinogenicity in mice of mutagenic compounds from a tryptophan pyrolyzate, *Science* 213:346, 1981.
51. Vahouny GV: Dietary fibers. In Sidransky H, editor: *Nutritional pathology,* New York, 1985, Marcel Dekker.
52. Workshop on fat and cancer, *Cancer Res* 41:3677, 1981.
53. Carroll KK: Dietary fat and cancer. In Horisberger M, Bracco US, editors: *Lipids in modern nutrition,* New York, 1987, Raven Press.
54. Wattenberg LW: Inhibitors of chemical carcinogenesis, *Adv Cancer Res* 26:197, 1978.
55. Proceedings of the FDA Public Conference on Antioxidants, Nutrients, and Cancer and Cardiovascular Disease, Nov. 1-3, 1993, Washington, DC.

Vitamins

56. Chaudhuri CR, Chatterjee IB: L-Ascorbic acid synthesis in birds: phylogenetic trend, *Science* 164:435, 1969.
57. Chatterjee IB: Biosynthesis of L-ascorbic in animals. In McCormick DD, Wright LD, editors: *Methods in enzymology,* New York, 1970, Academic Press.
58. Biehl JP, Vilter RW: Effects of isoniazid on pyridoxine metabolism, *JAMA* 156:1549, 1954.
59. Burchenal JH: Folic acid antagonists, *Am J Clin Nutr* 3:311, 1955.
60. Green NM: Evidence for a genetic relationship between avidins and lysozymes, *Nature* 217:254, 1968.
61. Green R, Carlson WE, Evans CA: The inactivation of vitamin B_1 in diets containing whole fish, *J Nutr* 23:165, 1942.
62. Monsen ER: Iron, nutrition and absorbtion: dietary factors which impact iron bioavailability, *J Am Diet Assoc* 88:786, 1988.
63. Monsen ER: Estimation of available dietary iron, *Am J Clin Nutr* 31:134, 1978.

Fat-soluble vitamins

64. Wolfe G: Multiple functions of vitamin A, *Physiol Rev* 64:873, 1984.
65. Wald G: Molecular basis of visual excitation, *Science* 162:230, 1968.
66. De Luca HF: Retinoic acid metabolism, *Fed Proc* 38:2519, 1979.
67. Appling DR, Chytil F: Evidence for a role of retinoic acid, vitamin A-acid, in the maintenance of testosterone production in male rats, *Endocrinology* 108:2120, 1981.
68. Olson JA: Vitamin A. In Machlin LJ, editor: *The handbook of vitamins,* New York, 1984, Marcel Dekker.
69. Sharma RV, Mathur SN, Ganguly J: Studies on the relative biopotencies and intestinal absorption of different apo-β carotenoids in rats and chickens, *Biochem J* 158:377, 1976.
70. Blomhoff R, Green MH, Berg T, Norum KR: Transport and storage of vitamin A, *Science* 250:399, 1990.
71. Goodman DS: Vitamin A and retinoids in health and disease, *N Engl J Med* 310:1023, 1984.
72. Block G, Dresser CM, Hartman AM, Carol MD: Nutrient sources in the American diet: quantitative data from the NHANES II survey. I vitamins and minerals, *Am J Epidemiol* 122:13, 1985.
73. Sporn MB, Roberts AB: Role of retinoids and differentiation in carcinogenesis, *Cancer Res* 43:3034, 1983.

74. Siegenthaler G, Saurat JH, Ponec M: Retinol and retinal metabolism: relationship to the state of differentiation of cultured human keratinocytes, *Biochem J* 268:371, 1990.
75. Bauernfeind JC: *The safe use of vitamin A,* Washington, DC, 1980, The Nutrition Foundation.
76. Lammer EJ, Chen DT, Hoar RM et al: Retinoic acid embryopathy, *N Engl J Med* 313:837, 1985.
77. Tielsch JM, Sommer A: The epidemiology of vitamin A deficiency and xerophthalmia, *Annu Rev Nutr* 4:183, 1984.
78. Lippman SM, Kessler JF, Meyskens FL Jr: Retinoids as preventive and therapeutic anti-cancer agents, Part I, *Cancer Treat Rep* 71:391, 1987.
79. Olson JA: Metabolism of vitamin A, *Biochem Soc Trans* 14:928, 1986.
80. Olson JA: Recommended dietary intakes RDI of vitamin A in humans, *Am J Clin Nutr* 45:704, 1987.
81. Traber MG, Ingold KU, Burton GW, Kayden HJ: Absorption and transport of deuterium substituted 2R,4′R,8′R-alpha-tocopherol in human lipoproteins, *Lipids* 23:791, 1988.
82. Burton GW, Ingold KU: Auto-oxidation of biological molecules: I. The antioxidant activity of vitamin E and related chain breaking phenolic antioxidants *in vitro, J Am Chem Soc* 103:6472, 1981.
83. Combs GF: Assessment of vitamin E status in animals and men, *Proc Nutr Soc* 40:187, 1981.
84. Bieri JG: Medical uses of vitamin E, *N Engl J Med* 308:1063, 1983.
85. Ehrenkranz, RA: Vitamin E and the neonate, *Am J Dis Child* 134:1157, 1980.
86. MacMahon MT, Neal G: The absorption of alpha tocopherol in control subjects and in patients with intestinal maladsorption, *Clin Sci* 38:197, 1970.
87. Muller, DPR: Vitamin E, Its role in neurological function, *Postgrad Med J* 62:107, 1986.
88. Dam H: The antihaemorrhagic vitamin of the chick: occurrence and chemical nature, *Nature* 135:652, 1935.
89. McKee RW, Binkley S, Thayer SA et al: Isolation of vitamin K_2, *J Biol Chem* 131:327, 1939.
90. Kark R, Lozner EL: Nutritional deficiency of vitamin K in man, *Lancet* 237:1162, 1939.
91. Aggler PM, Lucia SP, Fishbon HM: Purpura due to vitamin K deficiency in anorexia nervosa, *Am J Dig Dis* 9:227, 1942.
92. McGehee WG, Klotz TA, Epstein DJ et al: Coumarin necrosis associated with hereditary Protein C deficiency, *Ann Intern Med* 101:59, 1984.
93. Allison PM, Mummah-Schendel LL, Kindberg CG et al: Effects of a vitamin K deficient diet and antibiotics in normal human volunteers, *J Lab Clin Med* 110:180, 1987.
94. Smith FR, Goodman DW: Vitamin A transport in human vitamin A toxicity, *N Engl J Med* 294:805, 1976.
95. Corrigan JJ, Marcus FI: Coagulopathy associated with vitamin E ingestion, *JAMA* 230:1300, 1974.
96. Owen CAJ: Pharmacology and toxicology of the vitamin K group. In Sebrell WH, Harris RS, editors: *The vitamins,* New York, 1971, Academic Press.

Water-soluble vitamins

97. Funk C: The etiology of the deficiency diseases, *J State Med* 20:341, 1912.
98. Ziporin ZZ, Nunes WT, Powell RC et al: Thiamine requirement in the adult human as measured by urinary excretion of thiamine metabolites, *J Nutr* 85:297, 1965.
99. Anderson SH, Vickery CA, Nicol AD: Adult thiamin requirements and the continuing need to fortify processed cereals, *Lancet* 2:85, 1986.
100. Edwin EE, Jackman R: Thiaminase I in the development of cerebrocortical necrosis in sheep and cattle, *Nature* 228:772, 1970.
101. Inouye K, Katsura E: Etiology and pathology of beriberi. In Shimazono N, Katsura E, editors: *Review of Japanese literature on beriberi and thiamine, Vitamin B Research Committee of Japan,* Tokyo, 1965, Igaku Shoin.
102. Wood B, Currie J, Breen K: Wernicke's encephalopathy in a metropolitan hospital, *Med J Aust* 144:12, 1986.
103. Harper CG, Giles M, Finlay-Jones R: Clinical signs in the Wernicke-Korsakoff complex: a retrospective analysis of 131 cases diagnosed at necropsy, *J Neurol Neurosurg Psychiatry* 49:341, 1986.
104. Leevy CM, Baker H: Vitamins and alcoholism, *Am J Clin Nutr* 21:1325, 1968.
105. Williams RD, Mason HL, Smith BF, Wilder RM: Induced thiamin vitamin B_1 deficiency and the thiamin requirement of man: further observations, *Arch Intern Med* 69:721, 1942.
106. Hawk PD, Oser BL, Summerson WH: Vitamins and deficiency diseases. In Hawk PD, Oser BL, Summerson WH, editors: *Practical physiological chemistry,* New York, 1954, Blakiston.
107. Warburg O, Christian W: Über das gelbe Ferment und seine Wirkungen, *Biochem Z* 266:377, 1933.
108. Kühn R, Reinemund K, Weygan F, Strobele R: Über die Synthese des Lactoflavins Vitamin B_2, *Chem Ber* 68:1765, 1935.
109. Karrer P, Schopp K, Benz F: Synthesis von Flavinen IV, *Helv Chim Acta* 18:426, 1935.
110. McCormick DB: Riboflavin In Shils ME, Olson JA, Shike M, editors: *Modern nutrition in health and disease,* ed 8, Philadelphia, 1988, Lea & Febiger.
111. Lakshmi AV, Bamji MS: Tissue pyridoxal phosphate concentration and pyridoxamine phosphate oxidase activity in riboflavin deficiency in rats and man, *Br J Nutr* 32:249, 1974.
112. Bessey W, Wolbach SB: Vascularization of the cornea of the rat in riboflavin deficiency with a note on corneal vascularization in vitamin A deficiency, *J Exp Med* 69:1, 1939.
113. Spies TD, Vilter RW, Ashe WF: Pellagra, beriberi and riboflavin deficiency in human beings, *JAMA* 113:931, 1939.
114. Tisdall FF, McCreary JF, Pearce H: The effect of riboflavin on corneal vascularization and symptoms of eye fatigue in R.C.A.F. personnel, *Can Med Assoc J* 49:5, 1943.
115. Jukes TH, Sebrell WH, Roe D et al: Conquest of pellagra, *Fed Proc* 40:1519, 1980.
116. Horwitt MK, Harvey CC, Rothwell WS et al: Tryptophan-niacin relationship in man, *J Nutr* 60 (suppl 1):1, 1956.
117. Mason JB, Gibson N, Kodicek E: The chemical nature of the bound nicotinic acid of wheat bran: studies of nicotinic acid containing macromolecules, *Br J Nutr* 30:297, 1973.
118. Swenseid ME, Jacob RA: Niacin. In Shils ME, Olson JA, Shike M, editors: *Modern nutrition in health and disease,* Philadelphia, 1994, Lea & Febiger.
119. Youmans JB: *Nutritional deficiencies, diagnosis and treatment,* Philadelphia, 1941, Lippincott.
120. Bender DA: Effects of a dietary excess of leucine on the metabolism of tryptophan in the rat: a mechanism for the pellagragenic action of leucine, *Br J Nutr* 50:25, 1983.
121. Bender DA: Effects of dietary excess leucine and of the addition of leucine and 2-oxo-isocaproate on the metabolism of tryptophan in isolated rat liver cells, *Br J Nutr* 61:629, 1989.
122. Salter M, Bender DA, Pogson CI: Leucine and tryptophan metabolism in rats, *Biochem J* 225:277, 1985.
123. Bender DA: Inhibition in vitro of the enzymes of the oxidative pathway of tryptophan metabolism and nicotinamide nucleotide synthesis by Benserazide, Cabidopa and isoniazid, *Biochem Pharm* 29:707, 1980.
124. Bender DA: Effects of Benserazide, Carbidopa and isoniazid administration on tryptophan-nicotinamide nucleotide metabolism in the rat, *Biochem Pharm* 29:2099, 1980.
125. György P, Eckhardt RE: Vitamin B_6 and skin lesions in rats, *Nature* 144:512, 1939.
126. Lepkovsky S: Crystalline factor I, *Science* 87:169, 1938.
127. György P: Developments leading to the metabolic role of vitamin B_6, *Am J Clin Nutr* 24:1250, 1971.
128. Coursin DB: Convulsive seizure in infants with pyridoxine deficient diet, *JAMA* 154:406, 1954.
129. Shaumburg H, Kaplan J, Windebank A et al: Sensory neuropathy from pyridoxine abuse, *N Engl J Med* 309:445, 1983.
130. Leklem JE: Vitamin B_6. In Machilin LJ, editor: *Handbook of vitamins,* New York, 1991, Marcel Dekker.
131. Plesofsky-Vig N: Pantothenic acid and coenzyme A. In Shils ME, Olson JA, Shike M, editors: *Modern nutrition in health and disease,* ed 8, Malvern, Penn, 1994, Lea & Febiger.

132. Krishnamurti D: Biotin. In Shils ME, Olson JA, Shike M, editors: *Modern nutrition in health and disease,* ed 8, Malvern, Penn, 1994, Lea & Febiger.
133. Zeisel SH: Choline. In Shils ME, Olson JA, Shike M, editors: *Modern nutrition in health and disease,* ed 8, Malvern, Penn, 1994, Lea & Febiger.
134. Minot GR, Murphy WP: Treatment of pernicious anemia by a special diet, *JAMA* 87:470, 1926.
135. Castle WB: Observation on the etiologic relationship of achylia gastrica to pernicious anemia, *Am J Med Sci* 178:748, 1929.
136. Wills L, Cluterbuch PW, Evans BDF: A new factor in the production and cure of macrocytic anaemias and its relation to other haemopoietic principles curative in pernicious anaemia, *Biochem J* 31:2136, 1937.
137. Kapadia CR, Donaldson RM Jr: Disorders of cobalamin vitamin B_{12} absorption and transport, *Annu Rev Med* 36:93, 1985.
138. Seetharam B, Alpers DH: Absorption and transport of cobalamin vitamin B_{12}, *Annu Rev Nutr* 2:343, 1982.
139. Halsted CH: Intestinal absorption of dietary folates. In Picciano, MF, Stokstad ELR, Gregory JF III, editors: *Folic acid metabolism in health and disease,* New York, 1990, Wiley-Liss.
140. Colman N, Herbert V: Folate metabolism in brain. In Kumar S, editor: *Biochemistry of brain,* Oxford, 1979, Pergamon Press.
141. Colman NH, Herbert V: Folates and the nervous system. In Blakley RL, editor: *Folates and pterin,* New York, 1986, McGraw-Hill.
142. Jukes TH: The identification of vitamin C, and historical summary, *J Nutr* 118:1290, 1988.
143. Carpenter KJ: *The history of scurvy and vitamin C,* New York, 1986, Cambridge University Press.
144. Rivers JM: Safety of high-level vitamin C ingestion, *Ann N Y Acad Sci* 498:445, 1987.
145. Pauling L: Evolution and the need for vitamin C, *Proc Natl Acad Sci USA* 67:1643, 1970.
146. Chalmers AH, Cowley DM, Brown JM: A possible etiological role for ascorbate in calculi fromation, *Clin Chem* 32:333, 1986.
147. Schmidt KH, Hagmaier V, Hornig DH et al: Urinary oxalate excretion after large intakes of ascorbic acid in man, *Am J Clin Nutr* 34:305, 1981.
148. Mayson JS, Schumaker O, Nakamura RM: False negative tests for urine glucose, *Lancet* 1:780, 1973.
149. Jacob RA: Vitamin C. In Shils ME, Olson JA, Shike M, editors: *Modern nutrition in health and disease,* ed 8, Malvern, Penn, 1994, Lea & Febiger.

Minerals

150. Allen LH, Wood RJ: Calcium and phosphorus. In Shils ME, Olson JA, Shike M, editors: *Modern nutrition in health and disease,* ed 8, Malvern, Penn, 1994, Lea & Febiger.
151. Fairbanks VF: Iron in medicine and nutrition. In Shils ME, Olson JA, Shike M, editors: *Modern nutrition in health and disease,* ed 8, Malvern, Penn, 1994, Lea & Febiger.
152. King JC, Keen CL: Zinc. In Shils ME, Olson JA, Shike M, editors: *Modern nutrition in health and disease,* ed 8, Malvern, Penn, 1994, Lea & Febiger.
153. Levander OA, Burk RF: Selenium. In Shils ME, Olson JA, Shike M, editors: *Modern nutrition in health and disease,* ed 8, Malvern, Penn, 1994, Lea & Febiger.
154. Turnland JR: Copper. In Shils ME, Olson JA, Shike M, editors: *Modern nutrition in health and disease* ed 8, Malvern, Penn, 1994, Lea & Febiger.
155. Hetzel BS, Clugston GA: Iodine. In Shils ME, Olson JA, Shike M, editors: *Modern nutrition in health and disease,* ed 8, Malvern, Penn, 1994, Lea & Febiger.
156. Van Itallie TB: Obesity: adverse effects on health and longevity, *Am J Clin Nutr* 32:2723, 1979.
157. Kritchevsky D: Nutrition and cardiovascular disease. In Sidransky H, editor: *Nutritional pathology,* New York, 1985, Marcel Dekker.
158. Chandra PK: Interactions of nutrition, infection and immune response: immunocompetence in nutritional deficiency, methodological considerations and intervention strategies, *Acta Paediatr Scand* 68:137, 1979.
159. Ross RL, Newberne PM: Role of nutrition in immunologic function, *Physiol Rev* 60:188, 1980.
160. Mata L: The malnutrition-infection complex and its environment factors, *Proc Nutr Soc* 38:29, 1979.
161. Watson RS: *Nutrition, disease resistance, immune function,* New York, 1984, Marcel Dekker.
162. Hutchinson ML, Munro H: *Nutrition and aging,* New York, 1986, Academic Press.
163. Young VR: Diet as a modulator of aging and longevity, *Fed Proc* 38:1994, 1979.
164. Hathcock JN, Coon J: *Nutrition and drug interrelations,* New York, 1978, Academic Press.
165. McDanell REM, McLean AEM: Role of nutritional status in drug metabolism and toxicity. In Sidransky H, editor: *Nutritional pathology,* New York, 1985, Mercel Dekker.
166. Roe DA: Pathological changes associated with drug-induced malnutrition. In Sidransky H, editor: *Nutritional pathology,* New York, 1985, Marcel Dekker.
167. Roe DA: *Drug-induced nutritional deficiencies,* Westport, Conn, 1978, AVI Publishing.

32 Pathology of Obesity

Ivan Damjanov

Obesity is a major health problem of Western civilization.[1-4] Up to 35 million adults are obese in the United States. Obesity is, however, not limited to industrialized countries, and a recent increase in the prevalence of obesity has been reported in the developing countries. Hence, one may consider obesity a worldwide problem and a major determinant of morbidity and mortality in diverse human populations.

Definition. Obesity, or adiposity, is a systemic disorder that results in excessive accumulation of body fat. As with many other multifactorial disorders, obesity is arbitrarily defined by empirical criteria derived from population studies. The most often used charts are tables of average weights periodically published by the National Health and Nutrition Examination Surveys (NHANES).

Ideal weight tables have been compiled by insurance companies, such as table of heights and weights compiled by the Metropolitan Life Insurance Company (Table 32-1).

Measures of obesity. The fat content of the body can be measured or estimated. The most often used method for estimating the fat content of the body is based on the weight-to-height ratio, which can be used to determine the body mass index (BMI). The empirical formula for BMI is:

$$BMI = W/H^2$$

The weight (W) for this formula must be expressed in kilograms and the height (H) in meters. If the weight is expressed in pounds and the height in inches, the result must be multiplied by 703.1. A BMI of 25 is normal; 25 to 29.9 denotes overweight, and over 30 obesity. Severe obesity is a weight that exceeds twice desirable weight.

Other approaches for estimating body fat contents include densitometry, total body water estimates, total body potassium measurement, skin-fold measurements, wrist-to-hip ratio. The data obtained with these measurements generally correlate with the BMI.[3]

Prevalence of obesity. Epidemiologic studies of obesity are fraught with problems.[5,6] The results depend on the definition of obesity used and on the populations surveyed. Furthermore, since obesity is not always included in health reports and statistics, most data are imprecise. Estimates are that one third of the adult population in the USA is either overweight or obese. Differences in obesity of various groups stratified by sex, ethnic background, race, social status, and education have been reported.[5,6]

PATHOGENESIS OF OBESITY

The pathogenesis of obesity is controversial yet relatively simple: it occurs when the caloric intake exceeds caloric expenditure.[7] The causes of obesity are thus either overeating or decreased activity. Increased intake is in most instances attributable to overeating, which is related to psychologic and social

Table 32-1 Acceptable weights from the 1983 height and weight tables of the Metropolitan Life Insurance Company

Height		Women Acceptable range		Men Acceptable range	
cm	Inches	kg	Pounds	kg	Pounds
147	58	46-60	102-131	—	—
150	59	46-61	103-134	—	—
152	60	47-62	104-137	—	—
155	61	48-64	106-140	—	—
157	62	49-65	108-143	58-68	128-150
160	63	50-67	111-147	59-70	130-153
163	64	52-69	114-151	60-71	132-156
165	65	53-70	117-155	61-73	134-160
168	66	54-72	120-159	62-75	136-164
170	67	56-74	123-163	63-76	138-168
173	68	57-76	126-167	64-78	140-172
175	69	59-77	129-170	65-80	142-176
178	70	60-79	132-173	65-82	144-180
180	71	61-80	135-176	66-84	146-184
183	72	63-81	138-179	68-85	149-188
185	73	—	—	69-87	152-192
188	74	—	—	70-90	155-197
190	75	—	—	72-92	158-202
193	76	—	—	74-94	162-207

Modified from Metropolitan Life Insurance Company from tables published in *Metropolitan Life Foundation Statistical Bulletin* 64:2, Jan.-June 1983; raw data from Build Study, 1979, Schaumburg, Ill, and Springfield, Mass, 1980, Society of Actuaries and Association of Life Insurance Medical Directors of America.

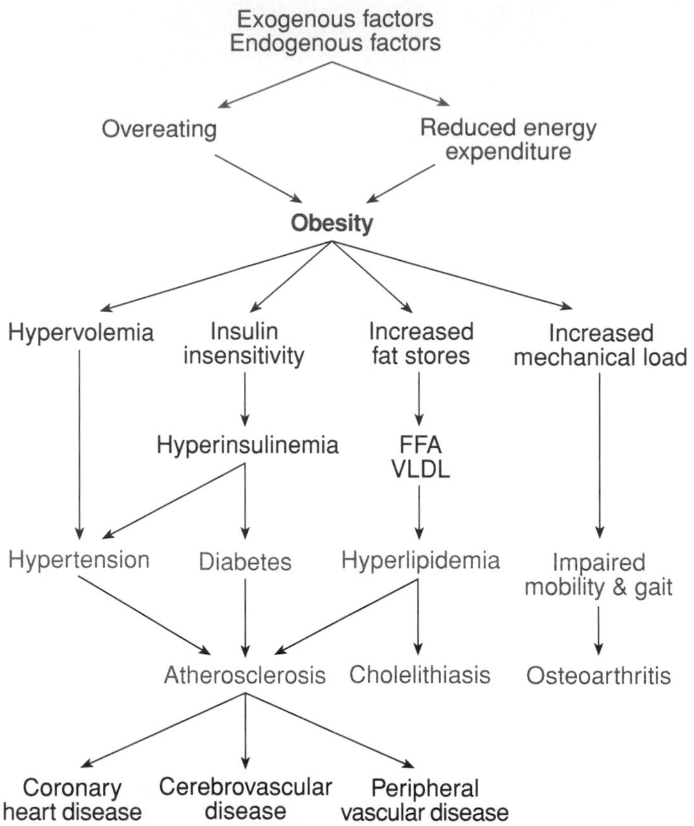

Fig. 32-1 Pathogenesis of complications of obesity.

Table 32-2 Classification of overweight and obesity

Primary
Overweight
Obesity
Morbid obesity
Secondary
Hypothalamic disorders
Froehlich's syndrome
Lawrence-Moon-Biedl syndrome
Prader-Willi syndrome
Craniopharyngioma
Hypothyroidism
Cushing's syndrome
Polycystic ovary syndrome

influences. Medical causes of obesity are rare[8] and are usually secondary to diseases affecting the hypothalamus or the endocrine glands (Table 32-2).

Fat cells. In contrast to carbohydrates and proteins that require water for storage, fat can be stored in cells without additional water. Most of the body fat is stored in fat cells (adipocytes), distributed in many sites throughout the human body. Major fat stores are in the subcutaneous tissues, retroperitoneum, omentum. Additional fat cells occur in the muscles and internal organs. The number of fat cells increases proportionally to the size of the body during childhood and puberty.[9,10] After the cessation of body growth, the number of fat cells appears to remain constant.

Experimental studies in genetically obese rodents have lead to the concept that obesity can occur because of a numerical increase of fat cells *(fat cell hyperplasia)* and an increased size of fat cells *(fat cell hypertrophy)*. The number of fat cells in the human body increases during the early years of life. In part, the number of cells is genetically predetermined; in part, it can be stimulated by overeating.[11-14] After puberty, concomitantly with the cessation of body growth, the fat cells stop multiplying. Accordingly, postpubertal obesity is mostly the result of fat cell hypertrophy and massive accumulation of fat in preexisting adipocytes. In severe obesity there is also recruitment of new adipocytes that are formed from preadipocytes, that is, undifferentiated mesenchymal cells that have a capacity for storing fat under extreme circumstances. Weight loss can be achieved by reduction of the body content of fat. The number of adipocytes cannot be reduced by dieting.

Experimental models of obesity

There are several models of obesity in laboratory animals, the most important of which are the genetically obese mice and rats.[15-17] One can also induce overeating in rodents by inflicting mechanical injury to the ventromedial area of the hypothalamus.[18] Five single gene mutations leading to obesity have been described in inbred mice, the best known of which is the *ob* gene. Mice, homozygous for the *ob* gene, develop severe obesity and diabetes as part of a syndrome that resembles morbid obesity in humans.

The *ob* gene, believed to be the primary cause of genetic obesity in mice, has been isolated recently.[17] The gene encodes a small protein produced by fat cells. It was proposed that this protein is the putative "satiety factor" that acts on hypothalamic control centers regulating the intake of food. Adipocytes of mice homozygous for the *ob* gene do not synthesize this satiety factor, which results in overeating and obesity. It remains to be shown whether this fat cell-derived protein is secreted into the circulation or acts on regulatory centers of hypothalamus, or interacts with insulin and other hormones. It is also possible that the action of this protein may be impeded by a defect in a putative receptor, the existence of which has been suggested by the data on *db/db* mice.[16] This mutation causes rejection of food and death because of starvation. Further studies of *db/db* mice may lead to the recognition of the receptor for the protein encoded by the *ob* gene.

Animal models of obesity appear to be most relevant for the understanding of severe (morbid) obesity in humans. The *ob* gene is phylogenetically conserved among various vertebrate species, and the cloning of a homologous human gene could be anticipated in the near future. Animal experiments also provide correlates for the rare hypothalamic forms of human obesity, such as those encountered in patients with craniopharyngioma or surgically induced hypothalamic lesions. The relevance of these animal models for the common variety of obesity is less apparent.

Although there is no doubt that genetic and hypothalamic factors contribute to human obesity, it would be too simplistic to explain this obviously multifactorial disease with a single gene defect. As pointed out in the review of Bouchard and Perusse,[12] the human obesity genotypes are multigene systems interacting with environmental influences. Single gene mutations might play a role in such systems, but their effect cannot be discovered readily.

METABOLIC ASPECTS OF OBESITY

Obesity is accompanied by significant alterations in the metabolism of lipids, carbohydrates, and proteins (Table 32-3). Although it is not known which of these metabolic disturbances has the primary role in the pathogenesis of adiposity and which is secondary, the most important and the most constant are the changes related to the action of insulin, and the turnover of lipids.

Hyperinsulinemia is one of the most common features of obesity. In normal individuals, insulin secretion decreases to a low basal level during fasting, whereas eating usually triggers insulin release. Basal insulin levels are elevated in obese persons. This hyperinsulinemia is secondary to relative insulin resistance of tissues that normally express insulin receptors.[19] The postreceptor mechanisms of transduction of signals of insulin bound to the insulin receptor seems to be intact and function normally inside the cell cytoplasm in all except the extremely obese persons. Insulin resistance is probably the most important reason for the increased incidence of diabetes mellitus in obese persons. Hyperinsulinemia also contributes to hyperlipidemia, by stimulating the hepatic production of very-low-density lipoproteins (VLDL).

Hyperlipoproteinemia is a constant feature of obesity.[20,21] There is hypertriglyceridemia, which is typically associated with elevated serum levels of VLDL. The liver secretes increased amounts of VLDL, which could be related to stimulation by insulin and the availability of free fatty acids (FFA). The serum levels of cholesterol are variable, and although there is a greater than normal turnover of cholesterol, cholesterol excretion in bile is high. This leads to hypersaturation of bile and an increased incidence of cholesterol gallstones.

Hyperlipoproteinemia may be reduced by dieting and weight loss, but the changes of the plasma lipid response to an energy-restricted low-fat diet vary depending on the type of obesity.[22]

MEDICAL COMPLICATIONS OF OBESITY

Obesity is accompanied by increased morbidity and mortality.[23,24] The most important diseases related to or aggravated by obesity are listed in Table 32-4.

Diabetes mellitus is a common complication of obesity. Although fewer than 10% of obese persons ultimately develop diabetes mellitus, more than 85% of all those with insulin-independent diabetes mellitus are obese. Diabetes develops because of relative insulin resistance of tissues in obese persons. Diabetes is most strongly associated with an upper body fat distribution.

Hypertension is a common complication of obesity. The reason for the occurrence of hypertension is unknown, though empirical data shows that nevertheless the association of obesity and hypertension is not fortuitous; it is approximately four to five times more common than that in nonobese persons. A genetic link between obesity and hypertension has been suggested.

Cardiovascular diseases are the most common cause of morbidity in obese persons. Increased incidence of atherosclerosis, coronary heart disease, and strokes has been related to the combined effects of hyperinsulinemia, hyperlipidemia, and hypertension.

Table 32-3 Serum abnormalities in obesity

Cholesterol	N
Triglycerides	+
High-density lipoprotein	N
Low-density lipoprotein	N
Very-low-density lipoprotein	++
Insulin	++
T_3	N or +
T_4	N
TSH	N
ACTH	N
Cortisol	N

N, Normal

Table 32-4 Complications of obesity

Diabetes mellitus
Hypertension
Atherosclerosis
Cholelithiasis
Osteoarthritis
Pickwickian syndrome
Intertrigo

Osteoarthritis affecting the hip and knee joints is directly related to overweight and the abnormal gait of obese persons.

Cholelithiasis is a common complication of obesity, especially in women. It is related to increased excretion of cholesterol in bile.

Pickwickian syndrome, named after the obese boy, Joe, described by Charles Dickens in his *Pickwick Papers,* is a rare but important complication of severe obesity. Because of excess of fat tissue compressing the thorax and impeding the normal respiration, these patients hyperventilate and develop carbon dioxide retention. Excess CO_2 acts on the central nervous system, suppressing the respiratory centers with consequent somnolence and periods of nighttime apnea.

Intertriginous dermatitis develops as a result of increased moisture caused by sweat accumulating in the folds of skin in the groin, lower abdomen, and pendulous breasts.

Fatty infiltration of internal organs is common in obesity. Fat cells appear enlarged in normal fat depots but also in subepicardial fat tissue, in the hilum of many lymph nodes, in the pancreas, and in interstitial spaces of striated muscles. The liver cells contain cytoplasmic vacuoles and often show considerable nuclear clearing with accumulation of glycogen. These histologic findings are not diagnostic of obesity and are also found in diabetic patients.[25]

COMPLICATIONS OF WEIGHT LOSS

The treatment of obesity is often unsuccessful, and weight regain is a common occurrence. Furthermore, all therapeutic approaches have been accompanied by some possible medical complications. These poor therapeutic results have spawned an entire industry, and a variety of drastic and often dangerous techniques of weight reduction have been introduced.

Gradual weight loss by controlling the intake of food is the safest method of treatment and produces few side effects. A *very low calorie diet* administered under medical control is also safe if administered for a limited period, usually not more than 16 weeks. Side effects of this diet are usually functional and include fatigue, menstrual irregularities, and syncopes. An increased incidence of cholecystitis and pancreatitis has been reported.[2] *Drug therapy* aimed at suppressing the appetite may result in addiction and psychosocial and psychosomatic disorders.

Surgical treatment used previously in the treatment of morbid obesity has been abandoned because of numerous complications. The complications of jejunoileal bypass surgery include chronic diarrhea, electrolyte loss, hepatic functional and histologic changes, and formation of oxalate kidney stones.

REFERENCES

General references

1. Pi-Sunyer X: Obesity. In Wyngaarden JB, Smith LH Jr, editors: *Cecil textbook of medicine,* ed 19, Philadelphia, 1992, Saunders.
2. Olefsky JM: Obesity. In Isselbacher KJ, Braunwald E, Wilson JD et al, editors: *Harrison's principles of internal medicine,* ed 13, New York, 1994, McGraw-Hill.
3. Foster D: Eating disorders: obesity, anorexia nervosa and bulimia nervosa. In Wilson JD, Foster DW, editors: *Williams' textbook of endocrinology,* ed 8, Philadelphia, 1992, Saunders.
4. Hirsch J et al: A biological basis of human obesity, *J Clin Endocrinol Metab* 73:1153, 1991.

Epidemiology

5. Stallones RA: Epidemiologic studies of obesity, *Ann Intern Med* 103:1003, 1985.
6. Hodge AM, Zimmet PZ: The epidemiology of obesity, *Bailliere's Clin Endocrinol Metab* 8:577, 1994.

Pathophysiology

7. Ravussin E, Swinburn BA: Pathophysiology of obesity, *Lancet* 340:404, 1992.
8. Kopelman PG: Hormones and obesity, *Balliere's Clin Endocrinol Metab* 8:549, 1994.
9. Ailhaud G, Grimaldi P, Negrel R: Cellular and molecular aspects of adipose tissue development, *Annu Rev Nutr* 12:207, 1992.
10. Dietz WH: Critical periods in childhood for the development of obesity, *Am J Clin Nutr* 59:955, 1994.
11. Tucker LA, Kano NJ: Dietary and body fat: a multivariate study of 205 adult females, *Am J Clin Nutr* 56:616, 1992.
12. Bouchard C, Perusse L: Genetics of obesity, *Annu Rev Nutr* 13:337, 1993.
13. Borecki IB, Bonney GE, Rice T et al: Influence of genotype-dependent effects of covariants on the outcome of aggregation analysis of the body mass index, *Am J Hum Genet* 53:656, 1993.
14. Carmelli D, Cardon LR, Fabsitz R: Clustering of hypertension, diabetes, and obesity in adult male twins: same genes or same environments? *Am J Hum Genet* 55:566, 1994.
15. Proietto J, Thorburn AW: Animal models of obesity: theories and etiology, *Bailliere's Clin Endocrinol Metab* 8:509, 1994.
16. Rink TJ: In search of a satiety factor, *Nature* 372:406, 1994.
17. Zhang Y, Proenca R, Maffei M et al: Positional cloning of the mouse obese gene and its human homologue, *Nature* 372:425, 1994.
18. Jeanrenaud B: Central nervous system and peripheral abnormalities: clues to the understanding of obesity and NIDDM, *Diabetologia* 37:5170, 1994.
19. Caro JF: Insulin resistance in obese and non-obese men, *J Clin Endocrinol Metab* 73:691, 1991.

Metabolic changes in obesity

20. Despres JP: Dyslipidemia and obesity, *Bailliere's Clin Endocrinol Metab* 8:629, 1994.
21. Stone JN: Secondary causes of hyperlipidemia, *Med Clin North Am* 78:117, 1994.
22. Roust LR, Kottke BA, Jensen MD: Serum lipid responses to a eucaloric high-complex carbohydrate diet in different obesity phenotypes, *Mayo Clin Proc* 69:930, 1994.

Complications of obesity

23. Bray GA: Complications of obesity, *Ann Intern Med* 103:1052, 1985.
24. Pi-Sunyer FX: Medical hazards of obesity, *Ann Intern Med* 119:655, 1993.
25. Abraham S, Furth EE: Receiver operating characteristic analysis of glycogenated nuclei in liver biopsy specimens: quantitative evaluation of their relationship with diabetes and obesity, *Hum Pathol* 25:1053, 1994.

Part Three

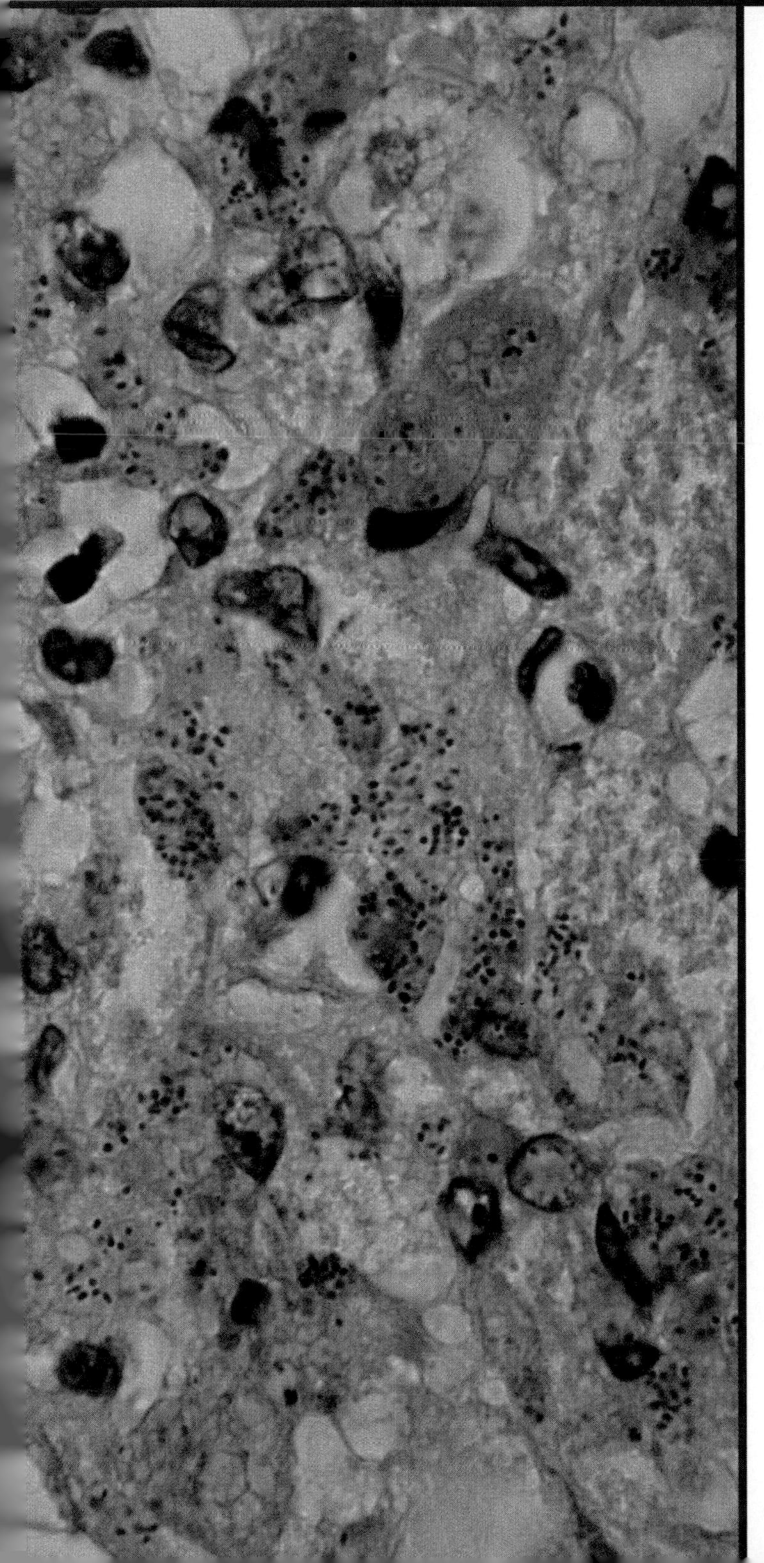

INFECTIOUS DISEASES

33 Bacterial Diseases

Washington C. Winn, Jr.
John M. Kissane

BACTERIA AND THEIR HOSTS

Long before human beings sought domination over the earth, long before the dinosaurs roamed the land, microbes had developed their varied life cycles and established their complex interrelationships. If it is a possibility that bacteria and viruses may be progenitors of parts of our genes or cellular machinery, it is a certainty that we have had to learn to coexist with these ubiquitous neighbors. Cedric Mims has mapped relationships in his masterful and extremely readable book *The Pathogenesis of Infectious Disease*.[1] In this chapter we provide an introduction to the fascinating complexities that face the pathologist who enters the field of infectious disease.

There is a complex ecologic interrelationship inherent in our coexistence with infectious agents, encompassing inanimate nature, plants and other animals, and even interactions among different types of microbes. A traditional diagram of these relationships includes spheres for the host (in our anthropocentric world, a human being), the microbe, and the environment. Establishing our individual ecosystems begins immediately after birth. It is clear that the external environment is not a required factor after that event, but it is such a frequent participant that it must be factored into any equation.

There is no single event, function, or characteristic that determines the onset of an infection. One can view the results of ongoing interactions as a balancing act, much like a scale, between defense mechanisms of the host and virulence factors possessed by the microbes. Environmental considerations may also affect the balance between the two sides and tilt the scales toward an infectious episode. To understand where the balance falls, therefore, one must be able to analyze and synthesize aggressive factors, defensive mechanisms, and conditions that facilitate their interaction.

The ideal relationship between microbe and host is peaceful coexistence. When an infectious agent establishes residence on a body surface, be it cutaneous ectoderm or mucosal endoderm, a state of colonization is established. Once these anatomic barriers have been breached, invasion of normally sterile tissues and fluids follows.

If each party derives benefits from the association, the relationship is described as symbiotic. When one party profits without doing damage to the other, a commensal state has been achieved. A saprophytic organism (saprobe) is one that feeds off decaying vegetable matter and thus it is not strictly an agent in human biology; the term *saprophyte* is often used more loosely, however, to describe organisms that are, in truth, commensal. From the viewpoint of both the host and the microbe, commensalism and symbiosis are preferred states because the continued coexistence of the partners is assured. If the relationship benefits one partner at the expense of the other, the phenomenon is called *parasitism*. Sublethal injury is compatible with survival of the parasite and may even facilitate propagation if host defenses are diminished. Lethal damage, however, is not in the best interest of either parasite or victim. If lethality is produced faster than the susceptible population can be replenished and there is no means of access to new populations, survival of the parasite is also in jeopardy. Some semantic confusion results from the use of the term *parasite* to describe eukaryotic infectious agents as well as to define a functional relationship between microbe and host. The principal interactions between bacteria and their chosen hosts are summarized in Table 33-1.

There is a range of interactions once a parasitic relationship has been established. An infection occurs when peaceful coexistence is replaced by aggressive behavior, no matter how restrained. The features that define the initiation of an infectious state include:

1. Penetration from a mucosal or skin surface into a normally sterile body tissue or fluid
2. Elicitation of an immunologic response
3. Elicitation of an inflammatory response
4. Production of tissue damage

A major exception to these generalizations is when a colonizing bacterium produces a potent exotoxin without actually invading tissue. In this case the aggressive behavior manifests itself as an intoxication, rather than an infection.

Aggressive bacterial behavior often results in disease, but this eventuality is not preordained. Disease is manifested by the last three events above—development of an inflammatory response, an immune response, immunopathologic damage, or destruction of tissue mediated by the bacteria themselves. Clinical symptoms develop if the damage is sufficiently extensive to impair function or if the inflammatory response can be perceived or measured. Those infections in which minimal damage does not produce symptoms are described as subclinical. The asymptomatic incubation period of many encounters that eventually result in disease may be viewed as a temporary state of subclinical infection. The importance of this concept lies in the frequent communicability of the microbe in that critical period before host defenses are activated to suppress the organism and before symptoms have alerted medical personnel to initiate offensive (therapy) and defensive (isolation) control measures.

The borderline between colonization and invasion is not always well delineated because the anatomic point at which tissues become sterile is not always rigidly defined. As a consequence, certain transitional states may be viewed as either colonization or subclinical infection. An example is colonization of the upper respiratory tract with bacteria and viruses. The lower respiratory tract is often viewed as sterile, though transient entry of infectious agents into the airspaces may well be common. As experience with *Pneumocystis carinii* infection expanded during the AIDS epidemic, earlier reports that this infectious agent was frequently a resident of the lower respiratory tract in the absence of any disease were confirmed and emphasized. Most individuals have developed an antibody to this agent by 2½ years of age and the organism can occasionally be fortuitously demonstrated in the lung of asymptomatic individuals.[2] Does this condition represent a colonization state for the airspaces, previously considered as sterile sites? Or is this a subclinical infection? The frequent presence of antibody to *Pneumocystis carinii* in normal populations speaks for subclinical infection as the best characterization of the phenomenon. It can be argued that unrecognized primary tuberculosis presents a similar situation when it is successfully contained. The cutaneous reactivity to tuberculin documents the immunologic response, and the primary complex in lung and lymph node, which may be calcified, is the morphologic testament to the encounter. Although no symptoms have been experienced, viable tubercle bacilli may lie dormant in the granulomas, patiently waiting for a chance to continue the infection.

The relationship between host and microbe is a dynamic process, influenced by many variables. Each member of *Homo sapiens* is different, just as each strain of a microbial species is different. Furthermore, individuals change over time, influenced by the environment, aging, or previous interactions with other microbes. For example, strains of *Corynebacterium diphtheriae* that do not produce toxin may inhabit the upper respiratory tract as part of the indigenous flora in a state of colonization. Once strains are infected with a bacteriophage that contains the toxin gene, however, a severe, even lethal infection may be produced, representing a change from the saprophytic to the parasitic state.[3] Similarly, addition of a foreign body or prosthesis facilitates the transmogrification of *Staphylococcus epidermidis* from a commensal organism on the skin to an infectious agent that can produce extensive morbidity.[4]

The scales of infection: microbial factors

Bacteria are unicellular organisms without a nucleus that is separate from the cytoplasm (prokaryotic). Bacteria divide asexually by binary fission and are bounded by at least one

Table 33-1 Relationships between bacteria and humans

Condition or process	Definition	Example
Colonization	Presence of an infectious agent on a surface membrane without damage to the host	*Staphylococcus epidermidis* on the surface of the skin or in the accessory glands and follicles; *viridans* streptococci in the throat
Saprobe (saprophyte)	Relationship in which one partner benefits and the other is not affected	*Staphylococcus epidermidis* on skin in normal state
Commensal	Relationship in which both parties benefit from the interaction	*Viridans* streptococci in throat, which inhibit growth of pathogens; enteric flora that facilitate digestion of food; *Lactobacillus* spp. in vagina, which maintain acid pH and inhibit proliferation of pathogens
Parasite	Relationship in which one part benefits and the other is damaged	Pneumococcal pneumonia; *Bordetella pertussis* production of whooping cough, bronchiolitis, and pneumonia

Table 33-2 Systems of classification of bacterial infections

Classification	Examples	Combination	Examples
Etiologic	*Staphylococcus aureus* *Escherichia coli*	Anatomic	*Staphylococcus aureus* Pneumonia *Escherichia coli* Pyelonephritis
Pathologic*	Acute (pyogenic) Chronic (mononuclear) Granulomatous Abscess	Etiologic and anatomic	Pyogenic *Staphylococcus aureus* pneumonia Granulomatous *Yersinia* lymphadenitis
Clinical†	Septicemia Endocarditis	Etiologic	*Escherichia coli* septicemia Streptococcal endocarditis

*Based on morphology of tissue obtained at biopsy.
†Based on signs, symptoms, and imaging techniques.

cell membrane and a cell wall that contains diaminopimelic acid. The bacterial domain is extremely diverse, ranging from free-living forms to obligate intracellular parasites. Species that are pathogenic for humans compose only a small portion of the total bacterial population. A variety of scientific and empiric classifications may be used to make sense of bacteria and bacterial infections (Table 33-2). Most bacterial pathogens and their diseases are considered in this chapter. Certain specialized bacteria, such as *Chlamydia, Rickettsia,* and *Mycoplasma* (Chapter 35), and *Mycobacterium* (Chapter 34) are discussed elsewhere.

Bacterial virulence factors

Virulence factors are those characteristics that enhance the ability of an organism to produce an infection, as opposed to colonization. Virulence is a quantitative term that describes the relative ability of a microbe to produce an infectious disease, with all other factors being held constant. At one end of the virulence scale are organisms that produce disease, even in immunocompetent hosts; such microbes are referred to as *pathogens* and are considered to be of high virulence. Pathogenesis refers to the process and mechanisms by which pathogens produce disease. *Pathogenicity,* a term sometimes used to describe the capacity of microbes as pathogens, is the product of virulence mechanisms they possess.

At the other end of the scale are microbes that produce infections in only the most debilitated hosts; these infectious agents are referred to as *saprobes* and are of low virulence. Between these extremes is a continuum of organisms with increasing capacity for producing infection and disease. These microbes are often described as potential pathogens or opportunistic pathogens.

The factors that contribute to virulence are enormously varied and may be situation specific, depending on the potential host. Any characteristic that favors entry into the host and survival in the face of defense mechanisms is by definition a virulence mechanism (Table 33-3). It is difficult to define virulence mechanisms that are instrumental in human disease. Occasionally the data suffice, as in the conversion of nontoxigenic *Corynebacterium diphtheriae* to a virulent state by infection with a bacteriophage.[3] Such interpretations, however, should be made most cautiously. Demonstration of a particular activity in vitro does not establish that the material has an analogous activity in vivo, and the limitations of animal models make the translation of conclusions between species problematic. An example of the complexity that requires very sophisticated analysis is provided by *Legionella pneumophila.* Investigators identified a major secretory protein that elicited a cellular and humoral immune response in experimental animals, which were subsequently protected from reinfection.[5] The temptation to ascribe a role in virulence to this clearly protective molecule was tempered by the appreciation that strains lacking the protein were still fully virulent.[6]

The most basic virulence factors are those that facilitate attachment of bacteria to cells of cutaneous or mucosal surfaces. Without the ability of the bacterial invader to latch on to a surface, it will be swept away by bathing, the mucociliary escalator of the respiratory tract, and the flowing secretions in the gastrointestinal (GI) or urinary tracts. In gram-negative bacteria the most common attachment mechanisms are specialized appendages, called *fimbriae,* or *pili,* but there are also binding molecules in the outer membrane proteins. Pili and fimbriae are less prominent in gram-positive bacteria, though they are present on some streptococcal strains. This particular virulence mechanism facilitates subsequent interactions with a host and therefore is a likely prerequisite either for colonization or for invasive disease. Attachment is not, however, sufficient of itself to produce infection and disease; additional virulence mechanisms are required.[7] It has even been suggested that loss of pili or other attachment mechanisms is necessary for production of invasive disease; phase variation with loss of pili has been demonstrated in vitro and in vivo. For example, in one study many but not all strains of *Haemophilus influenzae* that colonized the nasopharynx possessed pili and adhered to buccal epithelial cells, but none of the invasive isolates from cerebrospinal fluid, paired from the same patients, possessed pili or adhered to epithelial cells.[8]

The surface components of gram-positive organisms are equally important. Surface constituents, such as lipoteichoic acids, are important for the attachment of many gram-positive organisms.[9] The M-proteins embedded in the peptidoglycan wall of *Streptococcus pyogenes* are determinants of virulence by mechanisms that have not yet been completely elucidated; M-proteins may also function as adherence factors to certain cell types.

Different streptococcal species of the *viridans* group associate with different areas of the oral cavity at least partially because of differing adherence factors on the streptococcal surface. *Streptococcus salivarius* is found primarily in the saliva and on the buccal surfaces but is rarely found on the

Table 33-3 Virulence factors of bacteria

Class of factor	Mechanism	Example
Attachment to cells and artifical surfaces	Pili or fimbriae	Interaction of gram-negative bacilli and epithelial cells
	Outer membrane proteins	*Neisseria gonorrhoeae* and epithelial cells
	Cell-associated polysaccharides	Streptococcal dextrans and tooth surfaces or fibrin clots
		Staphylococcal slime and plastic catheters
Interference with humoral response	Destruction of immunoglobulins on mucosal surfaces	IgA protease of *Neisseria gonorrhoeae*
	Resistance to bactericidal effect of serum	Serum resistance in *Neisseria gonorrhoeae*
Interference with inflammatory response	Destruction of leukocytes	Staphylococcal leukocidins; streptoccal DNA-ases
Induction of tissue ischemia	Activation of clotting system	Gram-negative endotoxin induction of disseminated intravascular coagulation
Interference with cellular physiology		
Destruction of cells and tissue	Cytotoxin production	
Competition with host for nutrients	Siderophore-mediated utilization of iron	*Yersinia pestis, Neisseria gonorrhoeae* siderophores
Resistance to host defenses	Resistance to bactericidal activity of phagocytes	Various facultative intracellular bacterial pathogens
Resistance to adverse environmental factors	Resistance to desiccation	Long-term survival of anthrax spores
	Resistance to disinfectants	*Pseudomonas aeruginosa* and *Burkholderia cepacia*
	Resistance to antibiotics	Selective advantage over indigenous flora

surfaces of teeth and has not been implicated in the pathogenesis of dental caries. In contrast, *Streptococcus mutans,* rich in dextrans, adheres preferentially to dental surfaces, where it produces plaque and participates in the formation of dental caries. Not only does dextran facilitate the initial adherence of *S. mutans* to dental surfaces, but bacterial production of large amounts of extracellular dextrans from exogenous sucrose further enhances the association.

The importance of these dextrans in establishing tropism extends beyond attachment at the initial contact point. Although many oral streptococci enter the bloodstream transiently after such oral trauma as tooth brushing, certain species are disproportionately represented as causes of bacterial endocarditis. Two of the most common endocardial pathogens, *Streptococcus mutans* and *Streptococcus sanguis,* produce extracellular dextrans that facilitate adherence to fibrinous clots on the surfaces of damaged heart valves, much as they facilitate adherence to the surfaces of teeth. Those streptococcal species that are most commonly isolated from the blood of patients with bacterial endocarditis adhere to fibrin-platelet clots in vitro more efficiently than strains uncommonly found in endocarditis do.[10] Experimentally, it is possible to demonstrate a similar adherence to fibrin clots that have been induced by trauma to the aortic valve of experimental animals; pretreatment of bacterial inocula with dextranase diminishes the ability of the bacteria to produce endocarditis.[11]

The critical initial attachment of bacteria to cells is determined in some cases by the host as well as the microbe. An example is the surprisingly rapid alterations of bacterial flora of the upper respiratory tract in certain hospitalized patients. Within 24 hours after hospitalization, particularly for patients who are in intensive care units, the normal gram-positive flora of the oropharynx is often replaced by gram-negative bacilli.[12] The mechanism for this switch is a change in the surface structures of the epithelial cells in which receptors for gram-positive organisms are replaced by compounds with an affinity for Enterobacteriaceae and pseudomonads. The presence of fibronectin on the surface of cells is one of the components that defines the normal oropharyngeal flora as predominantly gram positive.[13] Fibronectin inhibits the adherence of gram-negative bacteria to epithelial cells, and loss of fibronectin after hospitalization facilitates adherence of *Pseudomonas aeruginosa,* which then becomes the colonizing flora. The consequence of this shift is that the etiologic agents of pneumonia in severely ill, hospitalized patients tend to become gram-negative bacilli rather than gram-positive cocci. Additionally, the development of specific antibody to infecting organisms may block the ability of those strains to continue their association with epithelium.[14] Adherence of bacteria to cell surfaces may also be influenced by medical intervention. A variety of virulence mechanisms, including the factors responsible for adherence to epithelium, may be altered by concentrations of antibiotics that are too small to inhibit bacterial growth.[15] Some potential virulence mechanisms must await the development of technologic advances for their significance to be appreciated. The complex extracellular polysaccharide slime produced by *Staphylococcus epidermidis* is responsible for the ability of this species to stick to plastic surfaces.[4] Such a facility was of little import in human disease until the advent of modern invasive technology, when the introduction of intravascular tubes and cerebrospinal fluid shunts conducted this species into a major role as a nosocomial (hospital-acquired) infection.

Attachment mechanisms may also partially define the niches of the colonizing flora and the association of bacterial species with host species. The association of particular microbes with specific cells or tissues is referred to as *tropism. Neisseria gonorrhoeae* attaches to fallopian tube epithelium of humans and of chimpanzees, which are apes, but not of baboons, which are monkeys.[16] Pili of this sexually transmitted pathogen mediate attachment to the columnar epithelium. Experimentally attachment is optimal to cells of the squamocolumnar transition zone, the primary site of gonococcal infection. In contrast, attachment to vaginal squamous epithelium occurs very poorly.[17] As a result gonococcal infection may affect the uterine cervix, fallopian tubes, urethra, rectum, or oropharynx, but not the squamous mucosa of the vagina, mouth, or anus. The specificity of this interaction is further illustrated by the observation that vaginal infection may be produced in a prepubertal girl before the epithelium becomes cornified. The definition of the normal flora, beginning with the newborn infant, also appears to be influenced by attachment mechanisms.[18]

After a microbe has attached itself to an epidermal or mucosal surface, the process may stop (colonization), or it may proceed to the development of local or disseminated infection. This dichotomy does not imply benign or serious disease because local infection may be fatal whereas disseminated infection may be self-limited. The site of the original invasive infection is referred to as *primary,* usually designated by the name of the organ and the suffix *-itis* because of the inflammatory nature of the process. Thus infection of the kidney is pyelonephritis; of the bladder, cystitis; and of the bone and bone marrow, osteomyelitis. Infection of the lung, however, is usually designated by the historical name *pneumonia,* rather than *pneumonitis.* When the pathogen invades the blood or lymphatic systems, disseminated infection may result. The secondary site of infection is described as *metastatic.* The simple presence of bacteria in the bloodstream is called *bacteremia.* Bacteremia may be transient, often after trauma to a mucosal surface by maneuvers as simple as brushing one's teeth or chewing. Fortunately, clearance mechanisms of the body are so efficient that the shower of bacteria may be removed in a single pass through the blood system. Episodic bacteremia is associated with periodic spillover from a deep-seated source of infection, such as an abdominal abscess. Sharp elevations of body temperature ("spikes") follow the bacteremic episode within 30 to 60 minutes because bacterial endotoxin stimulates the release of pyrogenic cytokines[19] from a variety of cells, primarily monocytes and macrophages. This sequence of events has led to the facetious recommendation that blood cultures for documentation of bacteremia should be collected one-half hour before the onset of fever. The first pyrogen to be characterized was interleukin-1, but subsequent studies have implicated interleukin-6, tumor necrosis factor, and interferon-α. Continuous bacteremia is suggestive of an intravascular source of infection, such as the cardiac endocardium, an aortic aneurysm, or an intravascular catheter. An infection of the vascular wall frequently results in partial or complete destruction of the arterial wall, a process called by convention a *mycotic aneurysm* without regard to the nature of the infecting organism.

Virulence factors produced by bacteria may be encoded by chromosomal DNA or may be present on round or ovoid pieces of DNA within the bacterial cell that are called *plasmids.* The genetic code may be continuously transcribed into messenger RNA and translated into cytoplasmic proteins, in which case the factor is always present and is described as *constitutive.* Alternatively expression of the genetic material may be repressed until it is stimulated by changes in the external or internal environment. Under these conditions production of the factor is not detectable in the basal state, though the genetic potential is present. Given the appropriate stimulus, however, production of the inducible factor will be geared up. If this complexity is not enough, free passage of genetic material among bacterial strains is possible by several mechanisms:[20]

Transformation. Transformation is the transfer of portions of DNA molecules directly from one bacterium to another. The principle was discovered inadvertently during studies of pneumococcal virulence and the identity of the material as DNA by Avery, Macleod, and McCarty.[21] The enormity of their identification of the genetic material was not appreciated, however, for many years.

Transduction. Transduction is the transfer of portions of DNA from a virus (bacteriophage) into a susceptible bacterium. The result is similar to transformation, but the process is more easily controlled and more reproducible.

Conjugation. Conjugation is the ability to transfer genetic material by sexual mating, using a conjugative plasmid in the male donor cell. The sexual transfer can be accomplished by sex pili or by transposons. Large amounts of genetic material can be transferred by this method.

Toxins

An important virulence mechanism is the production of a toxin. There are two basic types of bacterial toxins. Exotoxins, which are produced predominantly by gram-positive bacteria, are secreted from the bacterial cell and may be found free in the surrounding environment. They are usually protein in nature and are often inactivated by heat, a fact that has been utilized by manufacturers of vaccines. Structurally, most toxins consist of two components, one responsible for binding to a target cell membrane and a second for effecting the biologic activity. For instance, cholera toxin consists of five "B" subunits that are responsible for binding of the toxin to G_{M1}-ganglioside receptors on cells. These receptor subunits are bound by a linking subunit "A1" to the active subunit "A2," which actually initiates fluid secretion by cells.[22]

A toxin may in some cases accumulate in the extracellular environment so that the toxin, rather than the parent bacterium, is responsible for disease. The most straightforward bacterial diseases are, in fact, intoxications rather than infections in a strict sense and include staphylococcal food poisoning, botulism, and diphtheria.

The toxin may be produced by bacteria that produce an asymptomatic local infection, an isolated infectious disease, or a systemic infection. The purest form of intoxication occurs when the toxin producer is a colonizer without invasion of tissue, or contaminates food that will be the vehicle for ingestion of the toxin. In the latter case there may not even be any multiplication of the pathogenic microbe in vivo.

Endotoxins

The family of compounds called *endotoxins* are integral to the bacterial cell wall and are not secreted freely into the external environment. Endotoxins are associated with gram-negative bacteria.[23] Classical endotoxin, as found in members of the Enterobacteriaceae, consists of a highly conserved lipid core (lipid A) that is firmly anchored in the cell membrane, a transmembrane stable polysaccharide segment, and a highly variable carbohydrate segment that is accessible on the outer cell membrane and determines the "O" (somatic) antigenic specificity of the bacterium. The biologic effects of endotoxin are diverse and powerful. The most clinically devastating effects are on the peripheral circulatory system, where endotoxin mediates the septic shock found in overwhelming bacterial infection. The biologic effects of endotoxin can be detected simply and with great sensitivity by measurement of the gelling of an amebocyte lysate from the horseshoe crab *(Limulus)* or by immunologic methods. The importance of endotoxin in lethal gram-negative sepsis is suggested by the therapeutic potential of antibodies against conserved segments of the endotoxin molecule. Unfortunately, this promise has been difficult to realize, perhaps because of the complexity of the biologic interactions and the multiplicity of factors that are responsible for septicemia.

The sepsis syndrome occasionally complicates infections with gram-positive organisms. Gram-positive bacteria do not contain endotoxin; other components of the gram-positive cell wall may be involved. Recent investigations of streptococcal and staphylococcal toxic shock syndrome have characterized *superantigens,* which elicit multitudinous biologic effects, including the production of tumor necrosis factor,[24] recognized to be one of the effectors in sepsis mediated by lipopolysaccharide (endotoxin).

Enzymes

The distinction between enzymes and toxins blurs in some instances because the former term is defined chemically whereas the latter is an operational designation. Thus some compounds that have traditionally been considered toxins actually function chemically as enzymes. Bacterial enzymes may function to promote infection and disease in a variety of ways:

Enzymatic inactivation of host defenses. Bacterial enzymes may destroy defensive factors at several stages in the pathogenesis of an infectious disease. Elaboration of proteases that destroy immunoglobulins or leukocytes, such as the leukocidins of staphylococci, helps to counter the cellular inflammatory response. Streptococci also possess leukocidins, which kill polymorphonuclear neutrophilic leukocytes by inducing intracytoplasmic rupture of the leukocytic granules.[25] The complexity of the biologic interactions is, however, demonstrated by the further findings that the neutrophilic leukocytes are still capable of killing the toxic streptococci, and possession of the leukocidin does not, of itself, impart virulence to the streptococcal strain.[26]

Enzymes that inactivate antibiotics. Bacterial enzymes that inactivate or bypass virtually every class of antibiotic have been discovered. The most important enzymes inactivate aminoglycosides or destroy the β-lactam ring of penicillins and cephalosporins through the action of β-lactamases. Enzymatic defenses may have developed to fend off damaging substances in the environment or even to prevent suicide by the bacterium that produced the antibiotic.[27] In this regard it is interesting to note that enzymes capable of inactivating penicillin were identified before common therapeutic use of the antibiotic.[28] The bacterial enzymes may be constitutive or inducible. The β-lactamases of gram-negative bacilli are located in the periplasmic space between the cell membrane and the outer membrane, where they inactivate antibiotics in the process of traversing the membrane; the enzymes, therefore, provide protection only for the bacterial cell that produced them. In contrast, staphylococcal β-lactamases are freely secreted into the extracellular environment. These extracellular β-lactamases can then inactivate β-lactam antibiotics in the immediate vicinity, thus protecting not only the bacterial cell of origin, but in a mixed infection also facilitating replication of other species that do not produce the enzymes.[29,30] Resistance to β-lactam antimicrobial agents has become a major complication to the therapy of serious infections.

Enzymes that destroy host tissues. Many bacterial enzymes facilitate the spread of infection, producing structural damage in the process. For example, experimental studies have demonstrated a role for catalase in the virulence of *Staphylococcus aureus,* but superoxide dismutase, which theoretically would have a similar protective effect against aggressive neutrophils, did not correlate with lethality for mice.[31] Spread of *Streptococcus pyogenes* through tissue planes may be facilitated by the collagenases and hyaluronidases. Some of the enzymes, such as the coagulases of staphylococci, produce thrombosis, whereas others, such as the streptokinases of streptococci, have a thrombolytic effect. Another class of enzymes destroys structural components. For instance, exotoxins and proteases, including elastase of *Pseudomonas aeruginosa,* have been demonstrated to be important virulence factors in animal models[32] and may be responsible in part for the propensity of this organism to interrupt vascular structures and produce hemorrhagic disease. The myonecrosis produced by *Clostridium perfringens* in classical gas gangrene results from a variety of extracellular enzymes, especially lecithinase, which destroys cell membranes.[33] Similarly, the necrotizing nature of infections produced by *Clostridium septicum* and *Vibrio vulnificus* may derive from destructive enzymes produced by the bacteria. Necrotizing fasciitis as a component of group A streptococcal infections is significantly associated with a streptococcal protease.[34]

Bacterial surface structures

In addition to mediating adherence to host cells, many of the major surface structures of important pathogens have an antiphagocytic effect. For example, the capsular polysaccharide of *Streptococcus pneumoniae,* or *Haemophilus influenzae* type B, or *Neisseria meningitidis* can thwart the potent phagocytic response of macrophages or polymorphonuclear neutrophils in naïve hosts.[35] Also, deficient production of antibody to capsular polysaccharide facilitates recurrent infection.[36] The capsule of *Bacteroides fragilis* is an important virulence factor;[37] although *B. fragilis* is a minority member of the normal anaerobic GI flora, this single species is responsible for a disproportionate number of serious infections.

Adequate testimony to the potency of capsular polysaccharides as a virulence mechanism is provided by the effectiveness of vaccines directed specifically against them. Once again, host characteristics must be entered into the equation along with bacterial factors. Pneumococcal vaccines, which must be directed at many individual serotypes and are aimed primarily at an elderly population in which production of antibody is less efficient, have been moderately successful. In contrast, once properly constructed, vaccines against the capsular polysaccharide of *Haemophilus influenzae* type B have virtually eliminated this important pathogen as a cause of severe morbidity and mortality in young children.[38] Other surface structures that also serve as antiphagocytic factors include pili and the M-proteins of *Streptococcus pyogenes.*

Bactericidal activity of normal human serum is presumably a defense against invasion by organisms that have colonized mucosal surfaces. Some strains of pathogenic species, such as *Neisseria gonorrhoeae,* have developed resistance to this lethal defense and may be more likely to produce bacteremic, disseminated infection.[39] In the case of *N. gonorrhoeae*, resistant strains have distinctive physiologic profiles[39] and outer membrane proteins appear to play a role in evasion of bactericidal activity.[40]

Other factors

Resistance to adverse environmental conditions provides a mechanism for survival of the bacteria and a selective advantage in comparison with indigenous flora. The spores of *Bacillus* species and *Clostridium* species assure survival in nature for long periods even when desiccation, which is lethal to most bacteria, is extreme. Spores of *Bacillus anthracis* were still detectable on a Scottish island 35 years after the soil was intentionally contaminated.[41] Some *Pseudomonas* species survive and even thrive in solutions commonly used as disinfectants, providing a survival advantage in hospitals.[42] Many pathogenic bacterial species derive a competitive advantage from resistance to antimicrobial agents. *Clostridium difficile* produces disease almost exclusively in the setting of prior antimicrobial therapy.

Bacteria have developed other mechanisms for evading host defenses[43] or competing for nutrients. Siderophores are bacterial compounds that bind iron compounds, which are important in the physiology of many bacterial species.[44] *Legionella pneumophila,* which does not contain siderophores, but requires iron compounds for optimal growth, has developed an alternative pathway for acquisition of iron.[45] The ability to compete for iron stores is potentially important for invasive infection but is probably not sufficient, of itself, to establish virulence. Resistance to the bactericidal activity of phagocytes is a particular virulence factor for faculative intracellular bacteria.[43,46]

Medical practices may elevate protective mechanisms that were presumably developed for other purposes to a new level of importance. For instance, *Yersinia enterocolitica* and *Pseudomonas fluorescens* have the characteristics of psychrophiles because they are able to grow at 4° C. This characteristic allows the bacteria to replicate in refrigerated blood, and these species appear prominently in bacterial sepsis after transfusion.[47] The cold adaptation of *Yersinia enterocolitica* also permits replication of bacteria in refrigerated food, even after pasteurization.[48] Other bacteria that grow best at higher temperatures, such as *Klebsiella oxytoca, Citrobacter freundii, Proteus vulgaris, Providencia rettgeri, Serratia marcescens,* and enterococci, may also replicate under refrigeration,[49] enhancing their ability to contaminate refrigerated reagents.

The ability of bacterial species to replicate in solutions prepared for intravenous use may provide an opportunity for these organisms to produce serious infections. A nationwide epidemic of sepsis caused by contamination of intravenous fluid bottles with *Klebsiella species, Enterobacter species and Serratia species* was precipitated by defects in the design of the bottles[50] and by the ability of these species to replicate in solutions that contained dextrose and water but lacked other nutrients.[51]

The human equation

Physical defenses

The first lines of defense against bacterial infection are the cutaneous and mucosal barriers that serve as the primary portals of entry for pathogens. The physical defenses fall into three main categories:

Mechanical barriers. The epidermis with its superficial keratin layer is an extremely effective block to the entry of most pathogens. Few organisms can enter through intact skin because most require an abrasion or minor cut. The importance of these structural defenses is clearly illustrated by the frequency and severity of infections when disease or injury disrupts the barrier, such as full-thickness thermal burns and ulcerative or exudative skin disease.

Structural clearance systems. The ciliary escalator of the lower respiratory tract serves an important function since the name implies sweeping cells and particulate material from the distal respiratory tract through the bronchi and larynx into the upper airway.[52] The ciliated columnar epithelium of the nasopharynx and sinuses serve similar functions. In the genitourinary tract the cilia of the fallopian tubes, which are designed to facilitate passage of ova, also serve a cleansing function. Genetic abnormalities in cilia or acquired damage to normal cilia increase the risk for infection. Damage may come from inflammatory or neoplastic disease or less commonly from toxins directed specifically at cilia.[53] (Figs. 33-1 and 33-2). As an illustration of the interdependence of defense mechanisms, the ciliary clearance system of the lower respiratory tract removes particulate materials, such as bacteria, but also depends on alveolar macrophages to remove phagocytized bacterial cells.[54]

Hydrostatic clearance systems. The unobstructed flow of fluid through tubular structures, such as the biliary and urinary tracts or the ducts of exocrine glands, has an important anti-infective effect. Normal anatomic variation or sex-related structural differences may also play significant roles. Any acquired abnormality that compromises flow, such as formation of calculi or stenosis from inflammation or neoplasia, increases the risk of infection.

Much as in a plumbing system, diverticuli and surgically created blind loops lead to stagnation and may be sources of bacterial overgrowth and perhaps subsequent infection.

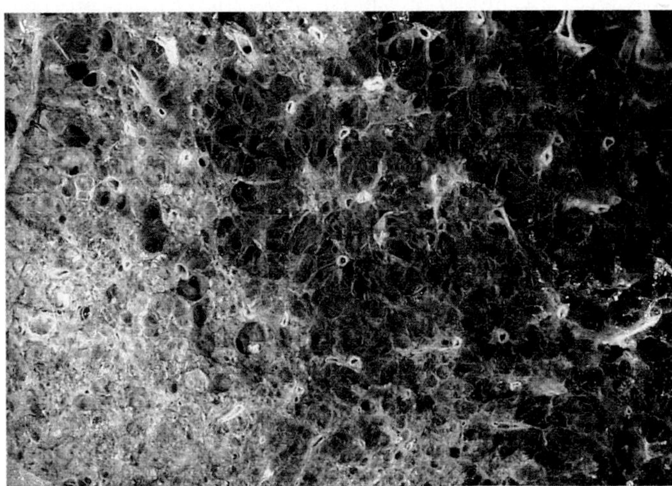

Fig. 33-1 Pneumococcal pneumonia in a smoker with severe emphysema. A fibrinopurulent exudate fills the enlarged airspaces. interference with clearance of bacteria from the damaged lung predisposes to infection with a wide variety of bacteria. *Streptococcus pneumoniae* isolated in pure culture from lung. Lung section floated on water.

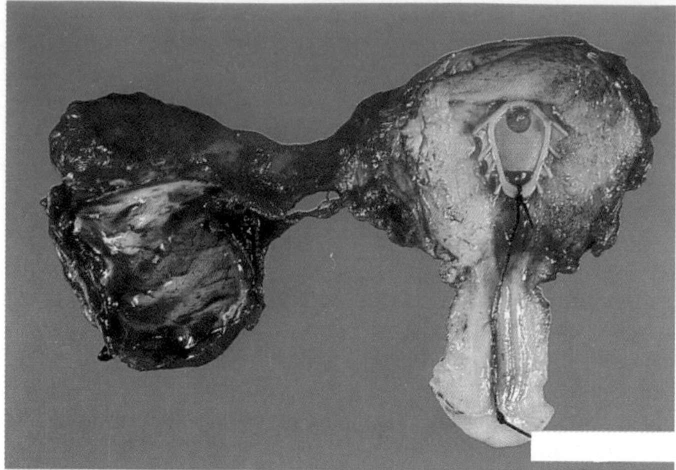

Fig. 33-2 Tuboovarian abscess in a patient who used an intrauterine device, which facilitated the entrance of bacteria from the vagina into the normally sterile uterus and ultimately the tubes and ovaries, bypassing a normal protective mechanism.

Obstruction to physical flow may exacerbate problems with ciliary function, as in the distorted bronchial system of bronchiectasis or the encroachment of carcinoma on the bronchial lumens.

The urinary tract provides an excellent primer on the range of defects that may have infectious consequences. Infant males are at higher risk for urinary infection than girls are, and circumcision may have some protective effect.[55] In older childhood and young adult life, however, the short female urethra facilitates the ascent of bacteria from the perineum to the bladder, where infections may result. With the onset of sexual activity, intercourse provides additional trauma to the urethra, leading to the sobriquet "honeymoon cystitis," a disingenuous description from a more innocent age.[56] Infections are uncommon in young boys, but even a single episode may indicate a structural or functional problem, such as vesicoureteral reflux. The tables are turned in old age when the onset of prostatic hyperplasia narrows the urethra and impinges on the neck of the bladder. Bacteriuria and urinary tract infection are equal-opportunity scourges of the elderly. Women are at higher risk of bacteriuria than men are, but males are at significant risk for the first time since infancy. At any age in either sex, compromise of urine flow by denervation of the bladder or by obstruction from tumor or urinary calculi increases the risk of ascending infection,[57] as does introduction of a foreign body, such as an indwelling catheter.[58]

Humoral defenses

Nonimmunologically specific. Chemical and physical characteristics of some body fluids are inimical or inhibitory to many bacteria, such as the acidity of gastric secretions or the hypertonicity of the vitreous humor of the eye. Although the upper GI tract is not sterile, the bacterial population of the stomach and duodenum is generally less than 100 per milliter. Patients with achlorhydria, however, have greater numbers of bacteria in their gastric contents and are at greater risk from GI pathogens.[59] A species that has adapted to the acidic environment is *Helicobacter pylori,* which successfully uses the gastric mucin for protection, and may cause peptic ulcer disease.

Chemical compounds secreted into body fluids or onto mucosal surfaces have demonstrable antibacterial activity in vitro and may be partially protective in vivo. Examples of these substances include lysozyme in ocular secretions and lactoferrin on a variety of mucosal surfaces. Lactoferrin may also have a role to play in systemic infection by competing with invading bacteria for the iron stores that are important for replication of many bacterial species.[60]

One of the most important nonspecific components of the humoral defenses is the complement system, which is activated by many pathogens at the initial stages of infection before antibody has been produced (Chapter 18). In the absence of immunoglobulins, the alternative pathway is most commonly used by infectious agents, but some bacterial antigens are capable of activating the classical pathway.[61] The early components, particularly C3b, serve as opsonins, linking the bacteria to complement receptors on the cell membranes of phagocytes. Once the membrane has been stimulated by attachment, phagocytosis and subsequent killing can procede. The early and intermediate components, especially C3a and C5a, serve a phlogistic function as powerful chemoattractants for the all-important polymorphonuclear neutrophils. The terminal complement components, C7 to C9, have a direct bactericidal activity for certain organisms, such as meningococci, by punching holes in the bacterial membrane.[62] Up-regulation of complement receptors on the surfaces of phagocytes has been demonstrated in human inflammatory processes in vivo.[63] Other nonimmunologically specific compounds such as fibronectin (opsonic glycoprotein)[64] or surfactant[65] may also facilitate phagocytosis before specific immunoglobulins are produced in response to an infection.

Immunologically specific. The immunologically specific humoral defenses are the B-lymphocytes and the antibodies they produce (see Chapters 25 and 27). Secretory IgA plays an important role in the initial host defenses on mucosal surfaces. Antibodies initially of the IgM class and subsequently of IgG specificity serve directly as important opsonins, activate the complement system by the classical method,[66] and participate in antibody-dependent cellular cytotoxicity. Opsonization occurs by means of receptors for the nonimmunologically specific Fc portion of the immunoglobulin molecule.[67] Complement fixation and activation varies by antibody class and subclass. Interestingly, secretory IgA has the effect of blocking opsonization by IgG and IgM in some clinical situations.[68]

Cellular defenses

Nonimmunologically specific. The lynchpin of the nonspecific cellular defenses is the mononuclear phagocyte system. Its two components, circulating (monocytes) and fixed (macrophages or histiocytes), are diffusely distributed throughout the body. The components of the fixed system, referred to in the aggregate as the reticuloendothelial system, are derived from circulating monocytes.[69] Cells of this system have specific names in certain organs, such as Kupffer cells in the sinusoids of the liver, microglia in the brain, and alveolar macrophages in the airspaces of the lung. The dendritic cells of the lymphoid system and Langerhans cells of the skin, though not phagocytic, are related. The pathway of differentiation from circulating to fixed phagocytes is unidirectional, but limited division and differentiation of fixed cells may occur.[70] The function of the mononuclear phagocytic system is dual. Macrophages phagocytize and kill many bacterial pathogens. They often serve as the front-line defense because they are resident in the peripheral tissues and need not be recruited from the blood. Interactions with the nonimmunologically specific (complement) and specific (immunoglobulin)[71] systems are important for function of the reticuloendothelial system. In addition, macrophages serve the second important function of processing antigen and presenting it to lymphocytes for activation of the specific immune system.

One of the central themes of macrophage biology is the concept of activation, first promulgated by Mackaness in the 1960s.[72] The state of activation is defined operationally as enhancement of a variety of functions, including microbicidal and tumoricidal activity, chemotaxis, phagocytosis, and antigen-presenting activity.[46] The multinucleated giant cells that are an integral part of the cell-mediated immune response, as manifested by granulomas, function as activated macrophages.[73] The critical role of T-lymphocytes in the activation processs was established early by studies in which these cells were ablated with anti-lymphocyte globulin. Macrophages can be activated, however, by chemical mediators in the absence of lymphocytes.[74] Furthermore, experimental studies emphasize the function of macrophages and the reticuloendothelial system at a stage of infection when immunologically specific responses have not yet been triggered.[75]

It is now recognized that the primary mechanism for activation of macrophages by lymphocytes is interferon-γ.[76-78] Tumor necrosis factor (TNF) is an additional cytokine that can activate macrophages.[79] The complexity of the process is emphasized by the recognition that IL-2 may also participate, either directly,[76] or by facilitating production of interferon γ. by macrophages.[80] The mediators for the enhanced microbicidal activity include generation of toxic oxygen derivatives in an acidic phagolysosome and non–oxygen dependent mechanisms. In some systems the generation of nitrous oxide in the phagosome appears to be the effector mechanism.[81] In other systems restriction of access to iron compounds needed for growth is an important factor.[82]

The interactions between bacteria and macrophages exhibit considerable variation. Some important pathogens, such as staphylococci, are effectively phagocytized and killed by resting macrophages;[83] the clearance of these bacterial species from the lung is correspondingly efficient.[84] For organisms that are obligate or facultative intracellular pathogens, effective microbicidal activity is dependent on generation of the activated state. Even among this group of pathogens there is considerable variation in the outcome of the interaction. Although bacteriostatic activity can be demonstrated in many situations, it has been much more difficult to document bactericidal activity. For instance *Legionella pneumophila* is inhibited but not killed by activated monocytes and macrophages, even in the presence of effective antibiotics.[85]

The second major component of cellular defenses is the polymorphonuclear neutrophilic leukocyte (PMNL).[86] Together with the macrophages these cells are sometimes referred to as *professional phagocytes*. Produced in the bone marrow in large numbers they circulate comparatively briefly through the blood, into and out of organs and tissues, attracted to sites of injury in a one-way flow. Inflammatory chemoattractants, such as activated complement components and leukotriene products of arachidonic acid metabolism,[87] cause circulating leukocytes to adhere to endothelial surfaces and migrate through the vascular wall into the site of inflammation (Chapter 18).[88] Those chemotactic influences are energized in active bacterial infections.[89] Synergistic activity between monocytes and neutrophils is provided by chemotactic substances for each cell type produced by the other.[90]

PMNL actively phagocytize bacteria that have attached to the cell membrane by means of IgG or complement receptors.[67] Matrix proteins on biologic surfaces, such as fibronectin, vimentin, laminin, vitronectin, and type IV collagen also appear to activate PMNL and enhance neutrophilic killing of *Staphylococcus aureus*.[91]

Phagocytosis is accompanied by an oxidative burst.[43] Subsequent fusion of the phagosome with neutrophilic lysosomal granules produces bactericidal activity both by oxygen-dependent and oxygen-independent mechanisms. The myeloperoxidase-peroxide-halide system generates peroxide, hydroxyl radical, singlet oxygen, and hypochlorous acid, all potent bactericidal compounds.[92] Oxygen-independent mechanisms include lactoferrin, lysozyme, and a variety of cationic proteins.

Immunologically specific. The thymus-derived (T) lymphocytes constitute the immunologically specific cellular immune system.[93] With increasing sophistication the molecular details of both human and murine cellular immune systems have been elucidated. The elegance and complexity of the system becomes increasingly evident (see Chapter 25 for details). Tragically the plague of human immunodeficiency virus, (HIV), which has a tropism for the CD4 T-lymphocyte, and patients with congenital absence of CD4 cells[94] dramatically emphasize the critical central role of this cell as the conductor of the immunologic orchestra. CD4 lymphocytes are the core of immunologic memory and serve helper function for other T-cells.[95] They also regulate the response of B cells to many antigens.[96] Other T-lymphocytes of the CD8 specificity are directly cytotoxic to tumor cells and virus-infected cells and also suppress B-lymphocyte activity.[97] Natural killer (NK) cells,[98] which do not require presensitization for cytotoxic activity, acquire greater effectiveness and immunologic specificity by interaction with specific antibody that has bound to targets (antibody-dependent cellular cytotoxicity).[99] The cellular immune system exerts antibacterial effects in two ways: first, by direct cytotoxicity against the microbe; second, by activation or regulation of humoral and effector cell defenses. Cell-mediated immunity is particularly important for obligate and facultative intracellular pathogens, but it is also critical for some extracellular pathogens, such as *Bacteroides fragilis,*[100] perhaps through its control over the humoral immune system.

Defects in humoral and cellular defenses may have catastrophic consequences for the affected host. In general defects in humoral immunity result in recurrent infections by encapsulated pathogens, such as *Streptococcus pneumoniae, Haemophilus influenzae,* and *Neisseria meningitidis*. These infections are often concentrated in the sinuses and lower respiratory tract. Selective IgA deficiency is the most common humoral immune deficiency. Most patients with IgA deficiency experience no adverse consequences, but some patients are afflicted with recurrent sinopulmonary infections.[101] Selective deficiencies of IgG or its subclasses are uncommon but are also associated with recurrent infections of the respiratory tract caused primarily by bacteria with polysaccharide capsules.[36] Complications of the more common nonselective immunoglobulin deficiencies are similar.

Patients who are deficient in components of the complement system are also at increased risk for developing infection with encapsulated bacteria.[102] Interestingly, although patients who are deficient in complement components, especially the terminal attack complex, are at greater risk of developing meningococcal infections, those deficient patients who are infected tend to have less severe infections than their normal counterparts have.[103] The mechanism for the milder disease may be that the harmful effects on the patient of complement-mediated inflammatory responses are also diminished. Certain patients who are asplenic are another group at increased risk for life-threatening infections with encapsulated bacteria.[104] Those at risk include children who have had splenectomies for congenital hemolytic anemia or Hodgkin's disease,[105] certain adults who have had incidental or post-traumatic splenectomies in the first years after the operation, and patients with sickle cell disease[106] in whom an in vivo splenectomy has resulted from recurrent thrombosis and infarction. The defects resulting from splenectomy result from a combination of decreased ability to opsonize encapsulated pathogens and compromise to the cellular phagocytes of this important reticuloendothelial organ. As a result particulates, such as bacteria or deformed erythrocytes, are removed from the circulation less efficiently.[107]

Defects in cellular immunity may be developmental[108] or may accompany neoplasia, particularly of the lymphoid system. They are also an unwanted consequence of vigorous chemotherapy for neoplasia or for suppression of the immune response in recipients of transplants. HIV is the most notorious viral infection associated with depression of cellular immunity, but other viral agents, including Epstein-Barr virus,[109] also produce a transient immunosuppression. In many situations the immunologic defects include humoral immunity and phagocytic function, as well as cellular immunity. The immunosuppression that occurs during measles may be responsible for the increased frequency of secondary bacteremia associated with that viral infection.[110]

The most common defects in PMNLs are numerical deficiencies caused by diseases that ablate myelocytic precursors and by toxins that are encountered accidentally or received intentionally in therapy of neoplastic disease. Even small numbers of PMNLs are recruited to sites of infection, and so overwhelming disease occurs only when severe neutropenia develops.[111] The risk of infection increases as the neutrophil count drops below the lower limit of normal, 1500 to 2000 cells per mm^3. The risk of infection increases dramatically when less than 500 leukocytes per mm^3 are present. The pathogens most commonly seen in severe, prolonged neutropenia are staphylococci, gram-negative bacilli, and fungi.

Functional defects in PMNLs range from impaired locomotion and chemotaxis[112] to defective microbicidal activity.[113] Most are uncommon and are characterized by recurrent bacterial infections, again primarily caused by staphylococci and gram-negative bacilli.

A particularly instructive defect is the absence of an oxidative burst after phagocytosis that characterizes chronic granulomatous disease.[114] This condition may be X-linked or autosomal and varies from partial to complete loss of oxidative killing mechanisms. The pathogens most commonly encountered are *Staphylococcus aureus, Nocardia asteroides, Aspergillus species,* and gram-negative bacilli, particularly *Serratia marcescens, Salmonella* species, *Citrobacter* species, *Pseudomonas aeruginosa,* and *Pseudomonas cepacia.* All these pathogens elicit an acute inflammatory response with a predominance of PMNLs in normal hosts. The tissue reaction to these same pathogens in patients with chronic granulomatous disease is dominated by macrophages and eosinophils. Granulomas with palisading macrophages may be accompanied by central necrosis and are indistinguishable from those usually associated with mycobacterial or fungal infection.[115] Therapy with interferon-γ augments the function of these defective neutrophils.[116] Transient defects in the function of neutrophils may also be produced by a concurrent infection.

Too much of a good thing can be as much a problem as too little. Patients who have iron overload because of therapy or underlying disease are at increased risk of more severe infection by several bacterial pathogens, such as *Vibrio vulnificus*[117] and *Yersinia enterocolitica.*[118] One of the mechanisms for the increased risk may be decreased function of PMNLs,[119] but coexisting liver disease may also play a role.

The inflammatory response

Relationship of pathogens to inflammatory cells. Most bacteria, which replicate in vitro and in vivo in the extracellular environment, are extracellular pathogens. For these microbes phagocytosis by a PMNL or macrophage is the first step in a losing battle with host defenses. Staphylococci, streptococci, enterococci, most enteric gram-negative bacilli, pseudomonads, mycoplasmas, *Haemophilus* species, and *Neisseria* species are among the many examples of this group of organisms. The typical host response to these pathogens is acute inflammation, dominated by the PMNL.

A smaller group of pathogens has developed mechanisms for survival within monocytes and resident macrophages. These microbes, which can also grow on the surface of agar, are referred to as *facultative intracellular pathogens.* The pathogenesis of infection with these organisms may involve multiplication in mononuclear phagocytes, which serve as a breeding ground rather than a burial place. As mentioned above, the onset of specific cellular immunity and activation of the macrophages results in enhanced bactericidal or bacteriostatic activity, but control of bacterial growth may still be incomplete. *Mycobacterium* spp., *Legionella* spp., some *Salmonella* spp., and *Listeria monocytogenes* fall into this group. Some fungi and parasites also exhibit these characteristics. The hallmark of host response to facultative intracellular pathogens, as exemplified by *Mycobacterium tuberculosis,* is the granuloma, but a purulent response is also commonly produced by some of these pathogens.

Most obligate intracellular pathogens are viruses, but a few bacterial genera that are deficient in the ability to generate energy share the need to infect cells. *Chlamydia* spp., *Rickettsia* spp., *Coxiella burnetti,* and *Erlichia* spp. not surprisingly produce infections that differ in many ways from most other bacterial infections. Cell-mediated immunity is critical for control of these pathogens also (Chapter 27).

Classes of inflammatory response

The tissue reaction to bacterial infections may take a variety of forms. Although the physiologic alterations are profound, there may be little or no morphologic changes if the pathogenesis of the disease is mediated by alterations in biochemical pathways. A good example of a potentially fatal disease in which there are no anatomic disturbances is the intense fluid secretion into the gastrointestinal tract produced by *Vibrio cholerae.*

The response to most bacterial infections is dominated initially by the accumulation of PMNLs and accompanying

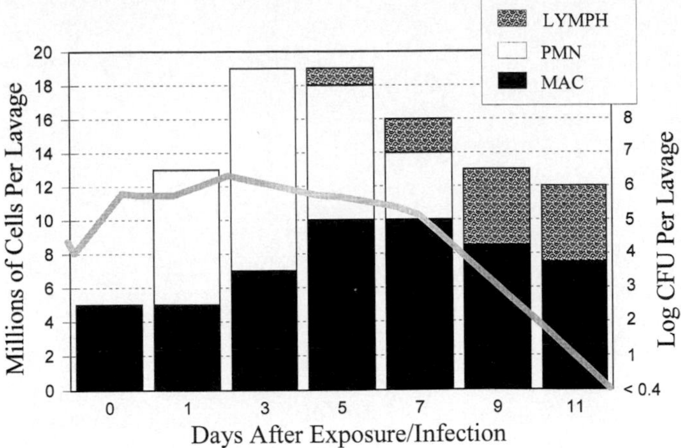

Fig 33-3 The inflammatory response to a bacterial infection. Guinea pigs were infected by aerosols of *Legionella pneumophila* serogroup I. The resultant bacterial growth and inflammatory response are depicted. Resident alveolar macrophages, present at the time of infection, are joined by recruited polymorphonuclear neutrophils, monocyte/macrophages, and lymphocytes.

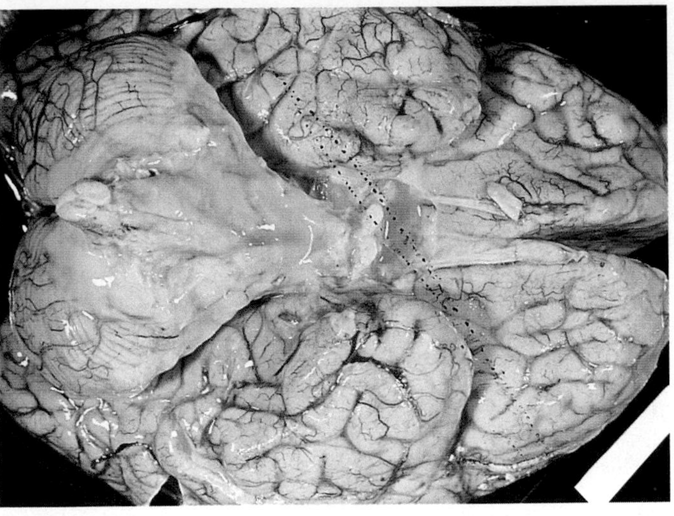

Fig. 33-4 Purulent meningitis. The characteristics of pus are dramatically demonstrated in the thick greenish-yellow exudate at the base of the brain in this case of gram-negative meningitis.

humoral factors,[120] followed by the recruitment of monocytes or macrophages.[121] The sequential events are illustrated in Fig. 33-3, which depicts the inflammatory events in experimental *Legionella pneumophila* pneumonia.[122] In this case the airspaces have been sampled by bronchoalveolar lavage to document the cellular response to an aerosol infection. The initial cellular response manifests, therefore, as the resident alveolar macrophages. Within 12 to 24 hours, however, there is a dramatic influx of PMNLs preceded by fluid exudation from the now leaky capillaries into the interstitium and airspaces. The invasion of PMNLs quickly dwarfs the resident macrophage population, but the generation of chemoattractants for mononuclear cells results in an augmentation of macrophages 48 to 72 hours after infection. Approximately 5 days after infection an increase in lymphocytes can be detected and the cellular phase of immunity is in full swing. As bacterial proliferation is controlled, the stimulus for further recruitment of phagocytes is diminished. Neutrophils disappear from the exudate first because they have the shortest life-span. Macrophages and lymphocytes disappear slowly or even remain at the site of the skirmish.

Pyogenic. The accumulation of inflammatory cells, bacteria, and proteinaceous exudate results in a thick, acidic yellow-green fluid called pus (Fig. 33-4). The bacteria that result in a large amount of pus are referred to as *pyogenic*. It should be emphasized that this most common inflammatory reaction to bacterial infection is shared by certain species that exhibit characteristics of facultative intracellular pathogens in vitro. For example, both *Legionella pneumophila* pneumonia and *Listeria monocytogenes* meningitis are characterized by a predominant neutrophilic inflammatory response in most human cases.

Hemorrhagic and coagulative. Some degree of coagulative necrosis and hemorrhage characterizes many infections, but certain pathogens produce enzymes that directly damage the walls of blood vessels, producing an excessively hemorrhagic lesion. On occasion the vascular effects dominate in the histologic picture, and the appearance is that of an infarct rather than a purulent infection. The best documented example is the infiltration of *Pseudomonas aeruginosa* through the walls of small vessels, producing distal infarction.[123]

Hemorrhagic lesions occur also when bacteria or their products interact with the clotting system. Classically, disseminated meningococcal infection precipitates disseminated intravascular coagulation, resulting in purpura and extensive ecchymoses, the Waterhouse-Friderichsen syndrome.[124] Similar pathologic complications may accompany infections with other bacteria, such as *Streptococcus pneumoniae, Haemophilus influenzae,*[124,125] and *Capnocytophaga canimorsus.*[126] Endotoxin is considered to be a prime mediator of the hypercoagulable state, and the presence of incomplete endotoxin molecules in anaerobic bacteria, such as *Bacteroides fragilis,* may account for the infrequency of intravascular coagulation in anaerobic infections.[127]

Gas-forming. Gas formation in tissues is classically associated with clostridial cellulitis or myonecrosis (gas gangrene), most commonly caused by *Clostridium perfringens.* (Figs. 33-5 and 33-6).[128] Other species of *Clostridium*[129] and even other genera, such as *Fusobacterium,*[130] *Aeromonas,*[131] and *Peptostreptococcus,*[132] can produce disease that is similar clinically. On occasion enteric gram-negative bacilli, staphylococci, streptococci, and enterococci may produce abundant gas in tissue, particularly in diabetic patients.[133]

Abscess forming/necrotizing. The combined result of the potent extracellular enzymes produced by many bacterial pathogens is often a necrotizing infection with tissue necrosis. When a localized lesion is produced, the combination of pus and tissue necrosis is referred to as an abscess (Fig. 33-7). An inflammatory response results from any injury, but an injury sufficiently intense to produce pus is usually caused by bacteria or fungi, and abscesses are virtually pathognomonic of infection by these groups of pathogens. Aggressive microbial factors favor the formation of abscesses,[134] including production of proteolytic enzymes[135] and capsules that inhibit phagocytosis.[136] Host factors also play an important role, including the presence of immune response,[136] the ability to generate chemotactic substances,[137] and proper function of the reticu-

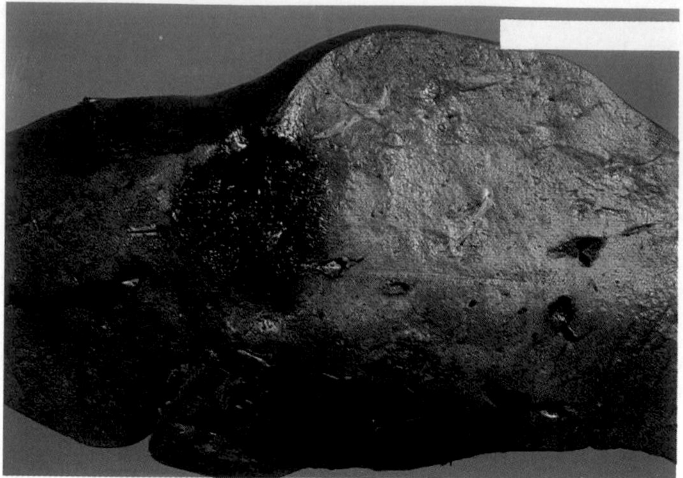

Fig. 33-5 Clostridial abscess. This single, large liver abscess is hemorrhagic. The liver tissue is distorted by the production of large amounts of gas. *Clostridium perfringens* was isolated from tissue.

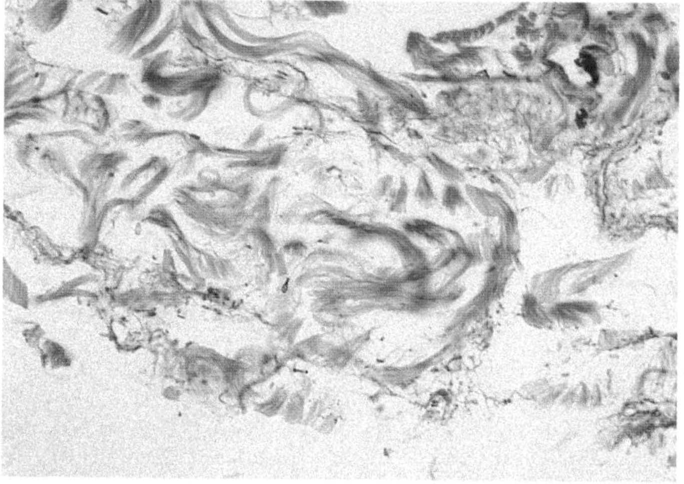

Fig. 33-6 Clostridial myonecrosis. Bacilli are demonstrated in the interstitium of muscle tissue. The clear swellings in the bacteria represent spores. *Clostridium septicum* was isolated from tissue. The bacilli of *Clostridium perfringens* are larger and more regular (boxcar shaped) and do not usually contain demonstrable spores in vitro or in vivo. Both species may decolorize easily and appear gram negative. (Periodic acid–Schiff technique.) (Case contributed by Stephen Allen, MD).

loendothelial system.[138] Interestingly, bacterial characteristics may also play a role in minimizing tissue destruction. *Streptococcus pneumoniae,* the most common cause of bacterial pneumonia, characteristically elicits an acute inflammatory response but only rarely produces necrotizing pneumonia. Recent experimental studies have demonstrated that the pneumococcus, which does not itself produce proteases, can inhibit the function of neutrophilic elastase in vitro.[139] In contrast, *Pseudomonas aeruginosa, Klebsiella pneumoniae,* and *Staphylococcus aureus,* all organisms that cause necrotizing infection or abscesses and the source of their own destructive enzymes, did little to reduce neutrophilic elastase. In these latter infections, therefore, there are two sources of enzymes that can damage tissue.

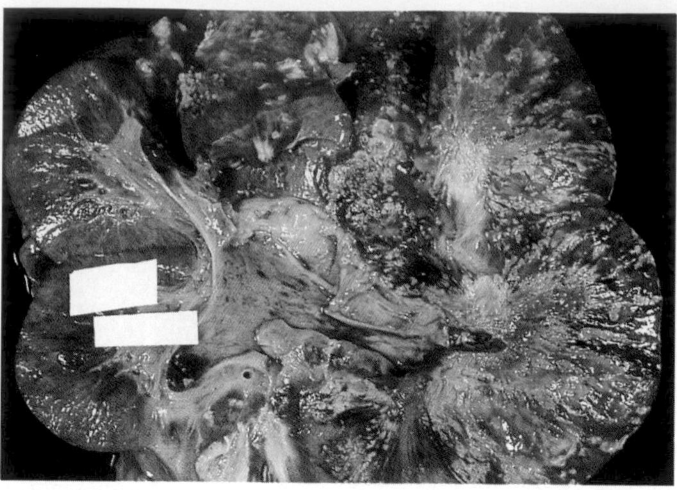

Fig. 33-7 Confluent necrotizing pyelonephritis with abscess formation. The necrotic yellow lesions are accentuated by the hyperemic tissue. *Pseudomonas aeruginosa* isolated from tissue.

Once established, characteristics of the abscess tend to vitiate normal host defenses and therapeutic intervention. The anaerobic atmosphere and low pH in abscesses decrease the efficiency of both PMNLs[140] and antibiotics.[141]

The term *abscess* is sometimes applied to variant lesions such as *cold abscesses* in patients who have defects in neutrophilic function or have been infected with *Mycobacterium tuberculosis.* Amebic "abscesses" are destructive lesions but are not usually associated with a purulent inflammatory response of the magnitude found in bacterial infection. Necrotizing infection may occur when the destructive process is not contained or circumscribed. Gangrenous lesions produced by mixtures of anaerobic or aerobic and anaerobic bacteria are classic examples of devastating necrotizing infections.

Sepsis. When the bacteremia is accompanied by systemic symptoms, including fever, chills, hypotension, and circulatory collapse, the process is septicemia or sepsis. The pathogenesis of sepsis includes a complex mixture of bacterial factors (such as endotoxin) and host factors, such as cytokines, produced in response to infection (such as TNF and interleukin-1).[142] A septic response to bacterial infection indicates a poor prognosis, but both the underlying status of host defenses[111] and the nature of the microbe[143] may be important variables in determining the outcome.

Granulomatous. Granulomas are, in their simplest form, localized, organized collections of activated macrophages. The classical lesion contains epithelioid macrophages arranged around a central core of amorphous (caseous) necrotic tissue, multinucleated giant cells, and a peripheral mantle of lymphocytes and proliferating fibroblasts (Fig. 33-8). Granulomas are the morphologic correlate of active cellular immunity[144] and are predominantly reactions to facultative intracellular pathogens. Some facultative intracellular bacteria, such as *Legionella* species, however, do not elicit a granulomatous response. The granulomas may have no necrosis, classic central caseation necrosis, or stellate necrosis. In the stellate or suppurative granuloma typical features, such as macrophages and palisading of epithelioid macrophages are present, but the central necrotic area contains ghosts and fragments of macrophages and PMNLs, rather than the eosinophilic coagu-

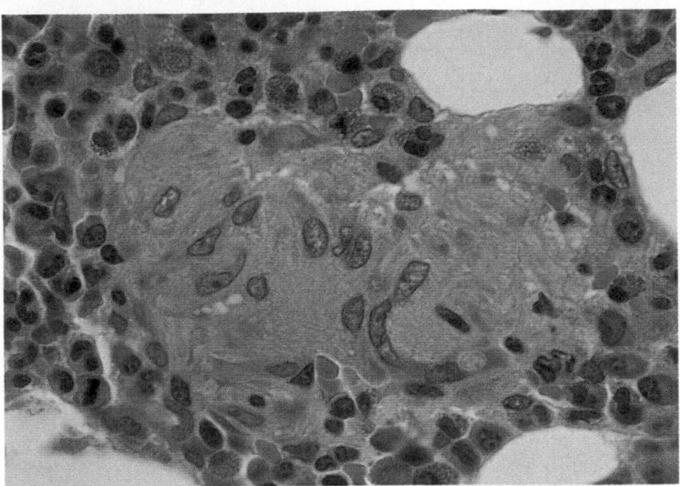

Fig. 33-8 Undulant fever. Noncaseating granulomas in the bone marrow consist of aggregated activated macrophages with formation of multinucleated giant cells. *Brucella suis* was isolated from blood. The patient had worked in an abattoir approximately 30 years earlier. (Case contributed by Barbara Tindle, MD, Burlington, Vt.)

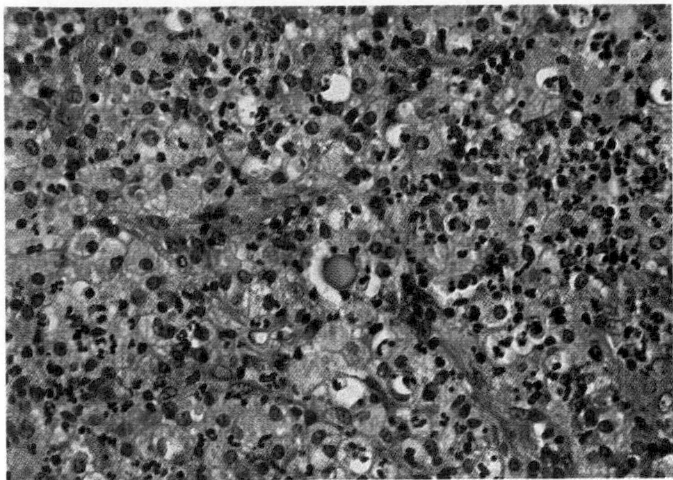

Fig. 33-10 Malakoplakia. A dense collection of foamy macrophages in the submucosa of the bladder is infiltrated by acute inflammatory cells. A Russell body is evident, but the characteristic intracellular Michaelis-Gutmann bodies are not seen. (Case contributed by Robert McDowel, MD.)

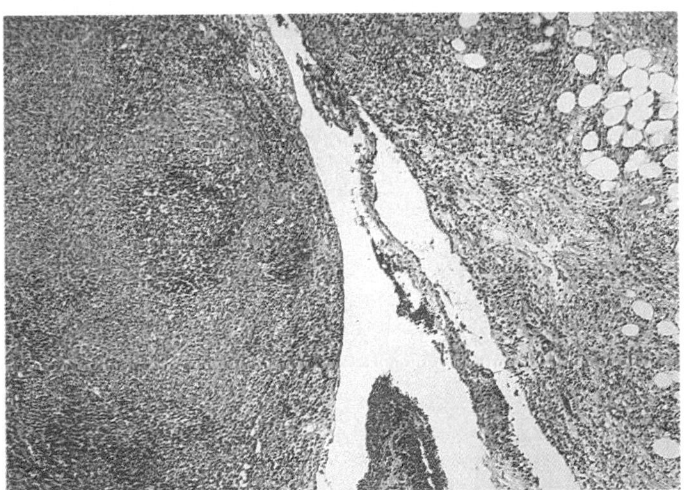

Fig. 33-9 *Yersinia* mesenteric lymphadenitis. A large stellate granuloma is present in the lymph node. The inflammatory response has extended through the capsule and into the mesenteric fat. *Yersinia pseudotuberculosis* isolated in pure culture from lymph nodes.

lum of caseous necrosis. The outlines of the granulomas and their necrotic centers is irregular, giving rise to the designation *stellate* (Fig. 33-9). Both stellate and caseous granulomas may coexist in the same lesion. The differential diagnosis of the bacterial causes of granulomas includes *Treponema pallidum, Brucella* spp., *Salmonella* spp., *Yersinia* spp., *Franciscella tularensis, Tropheryma whippelii* (the recently classified etiologic agent of Whipple's disease), *Bartonella henselae,* and *Afipia felis* (the last two species recently recognized as the causes of cat-scratch disease) (see Chapter 35).

Lymphocytic inflammation. Although primarily associated with the response to viral infections, a minority of bacterial infections elicit a lymphocytic response. In some cases, such as *Bordetella pertussis,* the usual response manifests as lymphocytes, both in the affected tissue and as a lymphocytosis in the peripheral blood. In other cases, the mononuclear response represents an atypical response to a chronic infection by a pathogen that usually produces an acute inflammatory response. A good example of the chronic presentation of disease caused by a pyogenic pathogen is Brodie's abscess, a localized bone lesion caused by *Staphylococcus aureus.* The lesions are usually single, located near the metaphysis, most commonly of the distal tibia, and characterized by lymphocytes and macrophages.[145]

Malakoplakia. Malakoplakia is an unusual chronic inflammatory response to bacterial infection and is characterized by collections of macrophages that may have a foamy appearance (Fig. 33-10). Intracellular bacteria are stained by the periodic acid–Schiff (PAS) technique. A distinctive cytoplasmic inclusion, the Michaelis-Gutmann body, is laminated and basophilic in hematoxylin-and-eosin stains. The laminated inclusions stain by the von Kossa method, an indication that they contain calcium. Malakoplakia occurs most commonly in the bladder[146] but can be found in other organs.[147]

Determinants of the inflammatory response

The nature of the inflammatory response is determined both by bacterial factors and host factors. A typical scenario can be defined for representative strains of a particular species that is infecting a normal host. The further either factor diverges from the norm, the more unpredictable becomes the inflammatory response. In patients who are severely immunosuppressed, such as those who are infected with HIV, pathologists must be prepared for any histologic response or even no response.

THE ENVIRONMENT: INTERFACE BETWEEN MICROBE AND HUMAN HOST

Endogenous infections. Within hours after birth, colonization of most body surfaces begins, both internally and externally. Many bacterial infections arise from the indigenous flora of the body without the necessity for an external source. These infections may be community acquired or acquired in the hospital (nosocomial). The "normal" flora of the body is influenced considerably by the local environment. For instance, the colonizing flora of the upper respiratory tract consists predominantly of gram-positive organisms, *Haemophilus* species, and gram-negative cocci, including *Moraxella catarrhalis*. As a result most cases of community-acquired pneumonia are caused by these colonizing organisms.[148] Very soon after admission to the hospital the colonizing flora of the upper airways undergoes a major shift to gram-negative bacilli, including prominently members of the Enterobacteriaceae and pseudomonads.[12]

Other factors that may affect the colonizing flora significantly include prolonged antimicrobial therapy, especially with broad-range antibiotics. These effects may be manifest in two ways: first, suppressing susceptible species and allowing overgrowth of others; second, antimicrobial therapy may select for resistant variants.

Although the proximate source of these endogenous infections is colonizing flora, the original source may have been in the environment or in another infected patient. Cross-infection from patient to patient on the hands of medical personnel has been well recognized since the pioneering studies of Semmelweis in nineteenth-century Vienna.[149] Unfortunately, the medical community has found it very difficult to effect the simple control measures, such as handwashing.[150]

Exogenous infections. As free-living organisms, most bacterial species exist either in the inanimate environment or in nonhuman animals. Infection of humans requires proximity to a "contaminated" source and transmission from that source to a susceptible individual. Examples of transfer from the inanimate environment include inhalation (or possibly aspiration) of *Legionella* spp. from contaminated cooling towers or potable-water supplies[151] or *Clostridium botulinum* from contaminated honey in infant botulism.[152] Transfer of an infectious inoculum from the environment requires an efficient method of disseminating an aerosol, such as a cooling tower or nebulizer.

Some pathogens exist in nature as colonizers or pathogens of animals. These animals may be entirely asymptomatic. Domestic animals are the primary source of infections,[153] but game animals are a risk, and some exotic species may be unexpected transmitters of infectious agents.[154] Investigators who study infectious diseases in experimental animals are also at risk.[155] Some examples are shown in Table 33-4. *Franciscella tularensis* is a particularly instructive example of how knowledge of the full biology of the microbe can make sense of epidemiologic and clinical data. In some parts of the United States tularemia has a biphasic seasonal incidence.[156] One peak occurs during the summer months, reflecting transmission of the infection through the bites of infected arthropod vectors. A second peak occurs during the winter, representing contact with infected game animals, particularly rabbits. Some pathogens, such as *Salmonella* spp.[157] and *Campylobacter* spp.,[158] are frequent fecal flora of poultry and to a lesser extent cattle and may be transmitted to humans by meat that has become contaminated during processing. Alternatively, milk or egg shells may be contaminated from fecal sources. In addition, a less common

Table 33-4 Zoonotic transmission of bacterial infections

Bacterium	Animal host	Mode of transmission
Franciscella tularensis	Small rodents, especially rabbits and muskrats	Contact with infected animal; bite of tick, deerfly, or mosquito vector
Brucella abortus	Cattle	Contact with animals; infected unpasteurized milk or cheese
Brucella melitensis	Goats	Contact with animals; infected unpasteurized milk or cheese
Brucella suis	Swine	Contact with infected animals
Salmonella spp. (other than *S. typhi*)	Poultry, cattle	Infected animals; infected eggs or unpasteurized milk
Campylobacter jejun/coli	Poultry,cattle	Infected animals; unpasteurized milk
Listeria monocytogenes	Cattle	Infected milk
Escherichia coli O157:H7	Cattle	Undercooked contaminated hamburger
Yersinia pestis	Rats, groundhogs, and many others	Direct contact with infected animals or from bites of flea vectors
Yersinia enterocolitica	Rodents, cattle, swine, cats, dogs	Direct contact with infected animals or excretions; ingestion of contaminated milk
Bacillus anthracis	Cattle, goats	Contaminated hides, wool, bristles, soil
Leptospira interrogans	Dogs, cattle, rodents, wild mammals, cats	Contaminated water
Borrelia spp. (tick borne)	Rodents	Bite of soft ticks *(Ornithodoros)*
Borrelia burgdorferi	Mice, deer	Bite of hard ticks *(Ixodes* and *Amblyomma)*
Pasteurella multocida	Dogs, cats	Bite
Capnocytophaga canimorsus	Dogs	Bite or scratch
Bartonella henselae	Cats, especially kittens	Bite or scratch
Afipia felis	Cats	Bite or scratch
Bordetella bronchiseptica	Dogs, cats, others	Association weak
Spirillum minus	Rats, other small mammals	Bite
Streptobacillus moniliformis	Rats, other small mammals	Bite
Pseudomonas mallei	Horses, donkeys, mules	Direct contact
Citrobacter diversus	Alligators	Bite
Aeromonas hydrophilia	Alligators	Bite

Table 33-5 Portals of entry of bacterial pathogens

Portal of entry	Pathogen	Examples	Vehicle
Gastrointestinal tract	Gastrointestinal pathogens	*Salmonella, Shigella, Campylobacter, Vibrio*	Infected food or water
	Enteric flora	Enteric bacilli, anaerobes, enterococci	Migration through bowel wall or defect in bowel
Respiratory tract	Exogenous respiratory pathogens	*Legionella* spp., *Bordetella pertussis*	Inhalation or contact with contaminated water or secretions
	Endogenous respiratory pathogens	*Streptococcus pneumoniae, Haemophilus influenzae*	Aspiration
Urinary tract	Uropathogens	Enteric bacilli, Pseudomonads, enterococci, staphylococci	Ascending infection from perineum
Genital tract	Sexually transmitted pathogens	*Neisseria gonorrhoeae, Treponema pallidum, Haemophilus ducreyi, Calymmatobacterium granulomatosis*	Contact with infected genital secretions
Skin and subcutaneous tissue	Primary pathogens	*Staphylococcus aureus, Streptococcus pyogenes*	Wounds greatly increase the list of possible pathogens
	Environmental pathogens	*Franciscella tularensis* *Bacillus anthracis*	Through abrasions or lacerations
	Zoonotic pathogens	*Franciscella tularensis* *Bartonella henselae*	Through bites or scratches
Mucous membranes	Sexually transmitted pathogens	*Treponema pallidum* *Neisseria gonorrhoeae*	Through abrasions or ulcerations
Blood (natural)	Endogenous flora	*Streptococcus* spp., enterococci, *Staphylococcus aureus*	Bacteremia after manipulation of oral or genitourinary sites; source unknown
Blood (nosocomial)	Bacteremic pathogens, skin flora, psychrophilic bacteria	Various	Fortuitous bacteremia in donor; contamination of units, through intravascular catheters

mechanism for infection of the egg itself is before hatching. Both *Salmonella* spp.[159] and *Yersinia enterocolitica*[48] have produced epidemics traced to pasteurized milk in which no defect in the manufacturing process could be demonstrated. Pasteurization and thorough cooking are normally sufficient to kill all these pathogens even if food has been contaminated. If a few bacteria escape the pasteurization process, however, the ability of *Yersinia* species to multiply at 4° C makes subsequent infection possible. Faulty technique may lead to contamination of foods, such as lettuce, that will subsequently be eaten uncooked. The exposure to the infected animal source may be remote, even decades previously, in the case of diseases such as brucellosis, which may be latent or chronic, or spores that may remain dormant in soil for decades.

Maintenance in nature. All infectious agents must have some mechanism for maintenance in nature. The cycle may occur entirely within the inanimate environment or may involve animal hosts. If an arthropod vector is a part of the process, there is often a cycle of transmission among wild animals with humans being the incidental hosts. Some pathogens infect only humans. Examples include *Borrelia recurrentis* (louse-borne relapsing fever), *Treponema pallidum, Salmonella typhi,* and *Bordetella pertussis*. Between infections or epidemics *Borrelia recurrentis* can survive in its arthropod vector.[160] *Salmonella typhi* can multiply in environmental water supplies, producing epidemic disease.[161] *Treponema pallidum* cannot survive outside of the infected human host, but it can produce chronic, latent infection as a means of prolonged survival.[162] *Bordetella pertussis,* however, would appear to occupy an extremely vulnerable niche. Over the past decade it has become clear that this pathogen, which produces severe infection in young children and infants, can circulate within families, producing mild or subclinical disease in older children and adults who are partially or completely immune.[163]

Portal of entry. The portal of entry for infectious agents depends on the environmental biology of the microbe, the mechanism of transmission, and the characteristics of the host. Most bacteria that enter through the skin or mucous membranes do so at the site of a cut or abrasion. Some agents are able to enter through intact mucous membranes *(Treponema pallidum)* or skin *(Franciscella tularensis).* Others avoid the difficulty of entry altogether by enlisting the help of an obliging arthropod or medical facility, which can introduce the agent through a bite or a transfusion. Fortunately the former is uncommon and the latter increasingly rare. Of course, the portal of entry is predetermined for endogenous pathogens by their site of colonization. Portals of entry and associated vehicles are summarized in Table 33-5.

DIAGNOSIS OF BACTERIAL INFECTIONS

The etiologic diagnosis of a bacterial infection is best made by recovery of the causative agent in culture. Immunologic methods provide a second method for making a specific diagnosis. Detection of a serologic response is extremely valuable for infections caused by microbes that are difficult to culture, such as *Brucella* spp. or *Bartonella henselae,* or dangerous to culture, such as *Franciscella tularensis.* The two drawbacks of serologic diagnosis are the frequent presence of immunologic cross-reactions and the necessity in most instances to wait for a convalescent serum specimen to demonstrate a rising titer of antibodies. Direct immunologic detection of bacterial antigens in clinical specimens has a major advantage in providing a rapid, specific diagnosis, but the problem of immunologic cross-reactions is troublesome, especially when specimens that may be colonized by indigenous flora are tested. In a few instances detection of a bacterial product correlates better with the presence of disease than recovery of the organism itself in culture does. For example, nontoxigenic strains of *Clostridium difficile* are recovered frequently from stool specimens of asymptomatic individuals,[164] and so detection of the toxin directly in stool or testing of isolated strains for toxin production provides a more accurate diagnosis.

The molecular age has added important new tools to the diagnostic armamentarium.[165] Hybridization techniques, including Southern blots and in situ hybridization, and amplification procedures, such as the polymerase chain reaction, have been used in two ways. First, these methods have been used successfully to elucidate the etiology of conditions that were recognized clinically or pathologically,[166] such as bacillary angiomatosis *(Bartonella henselae)*[167] and Whipple's disease *(Tropheryma whippelii).*[168] Although still experimental for most bacterial infections, the techniques are now being applied to diagnosis of infections caused by previously characterized agents. Use of broad-based primers in amplification assays can obviate the difficulties encountered in immunologic searches, where it is necessary to know the likely answer before the question can be asked. We will undoubtedly see an increase in molecular approaches during the coming decade, but it is unlikely that cultural approaches will become obsolete. Determination of antimicrobial susceptibility profiles and characterization of strains for epidemiologic purposes are still best performed on isolated bacteria.

Although nonspecific, histochemical bacterial stains furnish a useful adjunct to rapid diagnostic techniques. In the appropriate clinical and pathologic setting the morphology of the bacteria may provide a solid *presumptive* diagnosis. For example, the presence of large irregularly gram-positive bacilli without spores in an acellular exudate from a patient with gaseous myonecrosis provides a presumptive diagnosis of *Clostridium* and on statistical grounds of *Clostridium perfringens.* Small, curved bacilli beneath the gastric mucus in a patient with chronic antral gastritis and reactive lymphoid follicles are virtually diagnostic of *Helicobacter pylori* infection. In most cases an attempt to isolate the causative bacterium in culture should be made, but morphologic diagnosis may suffice for clinical management in selected situations.

The morphology of the bacteria and the clinical setting must be factored into the equation along with the color of the microbes. The battle-tried microbiologist might select as an epitaph: "Remember to your dying day: Not all cocci are round and not all rods are short!" *Streptococcus pneumoniae* is classically elongated or "lancet shaped"; some forms in a heavy infection may become quite elongated. *Streptococcus mutans* derives its name from its variable cellular morphology: coccobacilli when grown aerobically and uniform cocci when cultivated in an anaerobic environment. Many clostridial species decolorize easily and may appear either totally gram-negative or gram-negative with gram-positive inclusions. In particular, *Clostridium perfringens* often stains pink when Gram stain is applied to necrotic muscle. One species, *Clostridium clostridioforme,* stains gram-negatively reliably. More than one unwary microbiologist or clinician has fallen into the morphologic trap of mistaking the short gram-negative coccobacilli of *Acinetobacter* for the gram-negative cocci of *Neisseria gonorrhoeae* or *Neisseria meningitidis.*

Additionally, it must be remembered that the appearance of bacteria may be altered in an inflammatory exudate. Bacteria may appear "chewed up," and gram-positive bacteria may stain irregularly or even gram-negatively. One must always be alert to the presence of artifacts, such as stain debris and nuclear fragments that can resemble gram-positive bacteria, or background material, such as fibrin strands that can resemble gram-negative bacilli. As if that were not enough, antimicrobial therapy, particularly with antibiotics that interfere with the formation of cell membranes, will produce aberrant and distorted forms.[169] Finally, it is important to remember the possibility that reagents (including water for stains or for floating histologic sections) may be contaminated with microorganisms (Fig. 33-11). More than one pseudoepidemic has resulted from these unwanted visitors. After all these caveats it is ironic to note that the Clinical Laboratories Improvement Amendments of 1988 regulations initially classified Gram stain only as a moderately complex test, much to the dismay of many clinicians who objected to any standards for this "simple" test.

The nonspecificity of histochemical stains may on occasion be an advantage because one need not know the probable

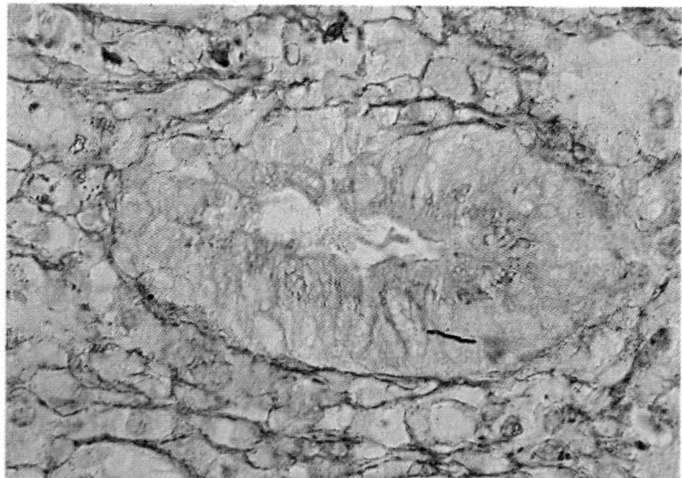

Fig. 33-11 False-positive silver impregnation stain. A single bacillus sits astride a colonic gland, unaccompanied by cellular disease or an inflammatory response. Similar bacteria were present on the glass adjacent to the section and probably represent saprophytic bacteria that were picked up with the section from the water bath. The sensitivity of the silver stains accentuates this problem. (Dieterle method.)

Table 33-6 Histochemical stains for demonstration of bacteria

Function	Stain	Primary use	Advantages	Disadvantages
Primary	Hematoxylin and eosin	General tissue stain	If sufficient numbers of bacteria are present, they may be visible without special stains	This stain is insensitive and the Gram reaction cannot be determined
Primary	Brown and Brenn	Tissue Gram stain	Stain of choice if gram-positive organisms are suspected, such as actinomycetes	Suboptimal for delineation of gram-negative bacteria
Primary	Brown-Hopps	Tissue Gram stain	If properly performed, optimal detection of gram-negative organisms	Difficult stain; gram-negative results may be stained magenta rather than pink or red
Primary	Warthin-Starry, Steiner, Dieterle	Interchangeable silver impregnation stains	Very sensitive for detection of all bacteria	Cannot determine gram reaction; silver deposition distorts bacterial morphology
Ancillary	Giemsa	General stain	Similar to hematoxylin and eosin	Difficult stain to perform
Ancillary	Periodic acid–Schiff technique	Used with diastase to reveal fungal forms Bacterial detection secondary	Many bacteria stain positively	Gram reaction cannot be determined.
Ancillary	Gomori silver methenamine	Used to reveal fungal forms Bacterial detection secondary	Sensitive method for detection of *Actinomyces* spp. and *Nocardia* spp.	Gram reaction cannot be determined; may color other bacteria, including *Mycobacterium* spp., especially if overstained
Ancillary	Ziehl-Neelsen	Tissue acid-fast stain	Useful for detection of *Rhodococcus equi* and *Legionella micdadei* as well as mycobacteria.	May not color some isolates
Ancillary	Auramine-rhodamine	Fluorescent stain for mycobacteria	More sensitive than Ziehl-Neelsen Easier to screen large areas of tissue	Requires fluorescent microscope; careful attention to morphology essential to maintain specificity
Ancillary	Fite or Putt modifications	Acid-fast stain with gentle decolorization	Necessary for demonstration of *Nocardia* spp.; may be required for *Rhodococcus* spp. *Legionella* spp.	Putt modification may color some non–acid fast organisms, such as *Actinomyces* spp.[173]

Data from Robboy SJ, Vickery AL: *N Engl J Med* 282:593, 1970.

identity of the pathogen to select the appropriate reagent. The agent or agents of cat-scratch disease[170] and *Helicobacter pylori* were originally detected by application of silver impregnation methods to histologic sections.[171]

The most common histochemical stains for diagnosis of bacterial infections are summarized in Table 33-6. Refer to standard textbooks of diagnostic microbiology for details on diagnostic techniques.[172]

The choice of a histochemical stain depends to a considerable extent on the capabilities of the histology laboratory. Many of these stains are finicky, requiring those sleight-of-hand techniques that go beyond recipes in a manual. If the laboratory is proficient in a particular version of a categorical stain (such as silver impregnation stains), that version should be the stain of choice.

It is important that appropriate controls be performed and examined on each day of use. The common practice of using colonic tissue to capture the diverse GI flora should be discouraged because it is difficult to detect subtle defects in the staining procedure. It is preferable to use separate pieces of tissue from gram-positive and gram-negative infections, which may be mounted in the same block. The gram-negative organism should be one that stains faintly, such as *Legionella pneumophila,* to provide an adequate challenge for the stain.

GRAM-POSITIVE COCCI

Staphylococci

Staphylococci are representatives of the family *Micrococcaceae. Staphylococcus aureus* (coagulase positive), the most important pathogen, developed increased significance in the 1970s with the acquisition of resistance to the penicillinase-resistant penicillins, which were the mainstay of therapy. Coagulase-negative staphylococci,[4] especially *S. epidermidis,* have become increasingly important as nosocomial and iatrogenic pathogens. *S. saprophyticus* is a common cause of urinary tract infections in young women.

Staphylococci are gram-positive organisms 0.7 to 1.2 μm in diameter with a tendency to grow in clusters. Cluster formation is evident and of diagnostic utility in smears and sections of infected material. After isolation in the laboratory, examination of young broth cultures is the most reliable method for determining morphology because an erroneous impression of clumping may be produced by streptococci when taken from the surface of agar plates. Staphylococci that have been phagocytosed by PMNLs may be only weakly gram-positive or even gram-negative in smears or sections.

Staphylococci can survive many unfavorable environmental conditions. They can be cultured from dried surfaces after several months, are relatively heat resistant, and can survive high salt concentrations.

Staphylococcus aureus

Pathogenesis. *Staphylococcus aureus* produces and secretes a large array of enzymes and toxins that are critical for the organism's pathogenesis.[174]

Catalase. All staphylococcal strains produce catalase, which converts hydrogen peroxide to oxygen and water. It has been suggested that catalase contributes to pathogenicity of staphylococci by splitting toxic oxygen radicals important in killing phagocytosed bacteria.[31]

Coagulase. Both cell-bound and soluble coagulases mediate coagulation by steps that differ from those that participate in normal thrombosis.

Hyaluronidase. Hyaluronidase hydrolyzes hyaluronic acids, acid mucopolysaccharides in the extracellular matrix of connective tissue.

β-Lactamases. β-Lactamases hydrolyze β-lactam antibiotics.

Others. Staphylococcus aureus produces a phosphodiesterase with a hydrolytic action on DNA that is used for taxonomic studies. *S. aureus* also produces several lipases.

α-Toxin. Among five toxins that damage cell membranes this electrophoretically heterogeneous protein acts on erythrocytes, leukocytes, platelets, fibroblasts, and HeLa cells but not bacterial cell membranes. α-toxin is dermonecrotic when injected subcutaneously.

β-Toxin. β-Toxin degrades sphingomyelin, an important component of cell membranes.

γ-Toxin. *γ*-Toxin lyses erythrocytes of many species including human beings.

δ-Toxin. The electrophoretically heterogeneous *δ*-toxin disrupts surface membranes by a detergent-like action and also stimulates cAMP production in rabbit and guinea pig ileum, an action that may play a role in the pathogenesis of diarrhea associated with staphylococcal infections.

Leukocidin. Leukotoxin produces a prominent reversible granulocytopenia when injected into rabbits or human beings probably by forming pores in the membranes of granulocytes allowing entry of cations.

Exfoliatins. Exfoliatins are a group of proteins responsible for dermatologic features of several staphylococcal diseases including staphylococcal scalded skin syndrome (see Chapter 71) and toxic shock syndrome (TSS; see below).

Enterotoxins. About half of all strains of *S. aureus* produce one or more enterotoxins, of which six (A to F) have been demonstrated. Enterotoxin F is identical to the TSS toxin, now named TSST-1.

Epidemiology. Shortly after birth staphylococci from the contiguous human environment colonize the infant's umbilical stump, skin, perineum, and sometimes the GI tract.[175] Older children and adults become staphylococcal carriers either transiently or more persistently. The most common site of such carriage is the anterior nasal vestibule. The nasal carrier rate in randomly cultured adults is between 20% and 40% depending on seasonal and other factors. Over time about 30% of adults have a prolonged course, and about 50% are intermittent carriers, whereas about 20% are never colonized. The fact that approximately 10% of premenopausal women have staphylococci in vaginal secretions, with more present during menstrual periods,[176] is important in the pathogenesis of TSS.

Some groups have staphylococcal carrier rates higher than the general population. Physicians, nurses, and hospital attendants are particularly prone to staphylococcal colonization.[177] Diabetic patients receiving insulin injections, patients receiving dialysis, and intravenous drug abusers more frequently harbor staphylococci than members of the general population do. There is no significant nonhuman reservoir.

Pathology. From its primary focus in the anterior nasal cavity or on the cutaneous surface, *S. aureus* readily gains access to subcutaneous tissues either of the carrier himself or of another person when the protective barrier of the skin is breached, whether inadvertently or deliberately. In the subcutaneous tissue or another site that it has reached by direct implantation or by the blood or lymphatic streams, the staphylococcus evokes a typical acute inflammatory reaction of which the major cellular component is the polymorphonuclear leukocyte. More than this, the staphylococcus is the quintessential pyogen (pus former) that early and characteristically produces a localized area of acute inflammation surrounding a focus of necrosis, that is, an abscess.

Clinical features

Organ infections. S. aureus produces a variety of cutaneous and subcutaneous lesions conveniently divided between localized infectious lesions, collectively referred to as *staphylococcal pyodermas* (Fig. 33-12), and localized lesions associated with a diffuse skin rash having characteristic histologic features (Fig. 33-13). It is a major cause of purulent infections of wounds and may cause septicemia without an identified focus of infection.[178] *S. aureus* is an important pathogen in a variety of organ infections, including endocarditis, osteomyelitis, arthritis, intracranial suppuration, and pneumonia. *S. aureus* is a major pathogen in the early stages of cystic fibrosis, later joined by *Haemophilus influenzae* and *Pseudomonas aeruginosa.*[179]

Toxic shock syndrome. In 1978, Todd and associates described in seven children and adolescents a syndrome characterized by fever, shock, diarrhea, renal failure, mental confusion, and erythroderma.[180] One of the patients died. Five were colonized with phage group I *S. aureus.* In 1980 the disease emerged as a multisystem disorder, mainly of menstruating women. Recently developed hyperabsorptive vaginal tampons probably contributed to the dramatic increase in frequency.[181] Langmuir and associates have suggested[182] that the mysterious "plague of Athens" that killed Pericles in the fifth century B.C.

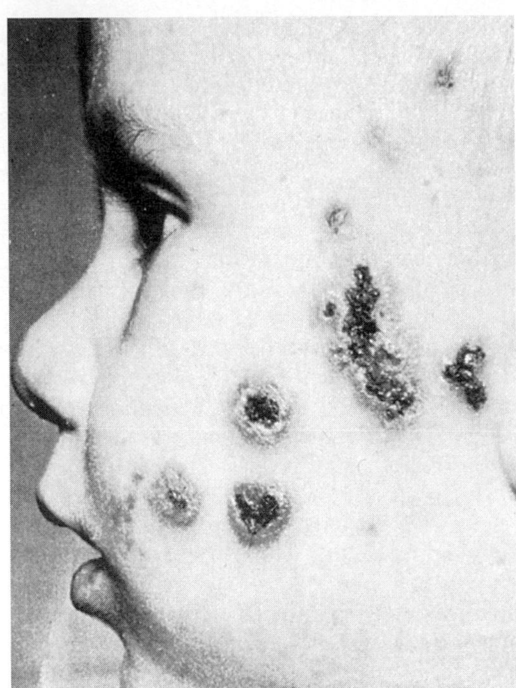

Fig. 33-12 Impetigo. Older lesions are dark and encrusted. (From Wehrle PF, Top FH: *Communicable and infectious diseases*, ed 9, St. Louis, 1981, Mosby.)

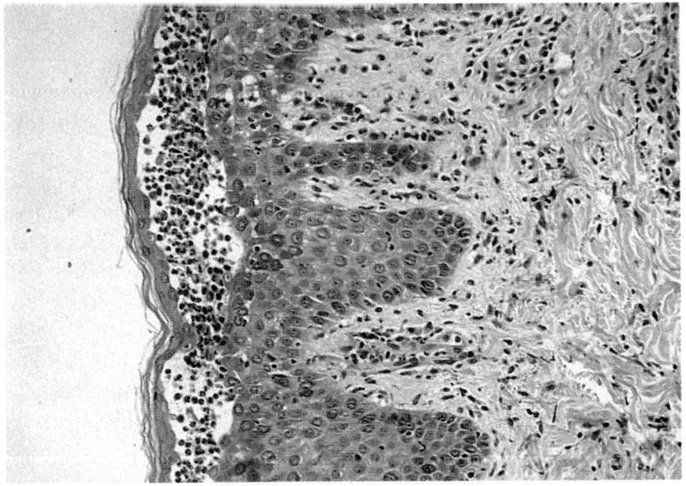

Fig. 33-13 Staphylococcal pyoderma. An intraepidermal abscess is the microscopic counterpart of the clinical pustule. There is dermal edema and inflammation.

may have been a toxic shock–like syndrome associated with staphylococcal postinfluenzal pneumonia. Whether this suggestion is true or not, it is good to have a description by Thucydides, who himself contracted the disease but survived. At any rate viral infection, including influenza[183] and varicella-zoster infection,[184] predispose to staphylococcal infection with attendant TSS. Chronic, recalcitrant, desquamating skin lesions in patients with acquired immunodeficiency syndrome have been associated with staphylococcal toxic shock toxin.[185]

TSS is rare in men and nonmenstruating women[186] but may be associated with staphylococcal infections of any site, including cryptogenic locations, such as the sinuses. The mortality is currently about 3%.[187] *S. aureus* is cultured from vaginal secretion of 98% of menstruating women with TSS and from other sites in all nonmenstruating cases.[188] An identical syndrome may rarely be associated with *Streptococcus pyogenes* (group A) infection,[189,190] and similar cases have been attributed to *Streptococcus agalactiae* (group B).[191] The disease has been ascribed to enterotoxin F or exotoxin type C (probably the same compound) produced by phage group I *Staphylococcus aureus,* usually of type 29 or 52.[192] The syndrome has been described in patients who were infected with strains lacking these toxins, and so there are likely multiple mechanisms.[193] Antibody appears to be protective, but many patients with TSS develop serum antibody slowly and at low titer.[194] Patients who are poor responders may in fact be at increased risk of developing the syndrome, and recurrent infections are common, especially in patients who have not been treated with antistaphylococcal antibiotics.[195] "Staphylococcal scarlatina" is best viewed as a *forme fruste* of TSS.

The cutaneous lesion early shows dermal perivasculitis. Sloughing later occurs at the dermoepidermal junction. Cervicovaginal mucosa may be focally inflamed and ulcerated. Changes in the kidneys, liver, lungs, lymphoid tissue, and central nervous system are nonspecific.[196]

S. aureus *food poisoning.* Staphylococcal food poisoning is not the result of an infection but results from ingestion of one or another of the heat-stable staphylococcal enterotoxins (A to F). About half of all isolates of *S. aureus* produce one or another enterotoxin. This disorder results from ingestion of food contaminated by enterotoxin-producing staphylococci, often from the hands of food handlers with staphylococcal cutaneous lesions. Staphylococci proliferate and elaborate toxin under conditions of inadequate refrigeration, and the preformed toxin is ingested. Creamed foods or salads are often responsible in the United States but meats, fish, or poultry more commonly in Great Britain.

Vomiting begins within a few hours after ingestion of toxin-laden food. There is occasionally diarrhea without blood or pus. The disorder is almost always self-limited, and recovery ensues within 24 to 48 hours.[197]

Miscellaneous infections. S. aureus is an important cause of perinatal pneumonia[198] that rapidly progresses to lung abscess or, more accurately, staphylococcal pyopneumatocele. Perinatal breast abscess, usually staphylococcal,[199] is as common in young boys as in girls. Manipulation of the breasts in a folk-medicine inspired effort to avert secretion of witch's milk (colostrum-like milk in newborns) is a common mechanism.

Botryomycosis. Botryomycosis[200] is a disorder in which solitary or multiple abscesses contain basophilic granules set in an acellular eosinophilic matrix rich in immunoglobulins. Rarely granules can be seen grossly. Botryomycotic abscesses are most common in deep subcutaneous tissue but also occur in liver, kidneys, lung, prostate, and lymph nodes. Trauma or foreign bodies are occasionally inciting factors. Pulmonary botryomycosis has been identified in patients with cystic fibrosis.[201] Most commonly *S. aureus* is isolated from botryomycotic abscesses (Fig. 33-14), but other organisms, such as *Pseudomonas aeruginosa,* may be responsible. Although abnormal responses to infection have been suggested as pathogenic mechanisms, no specific mechanism has been identified. The major differential diagnosis is a variety of deep mycotic infections that can be distinguished from botryomy-

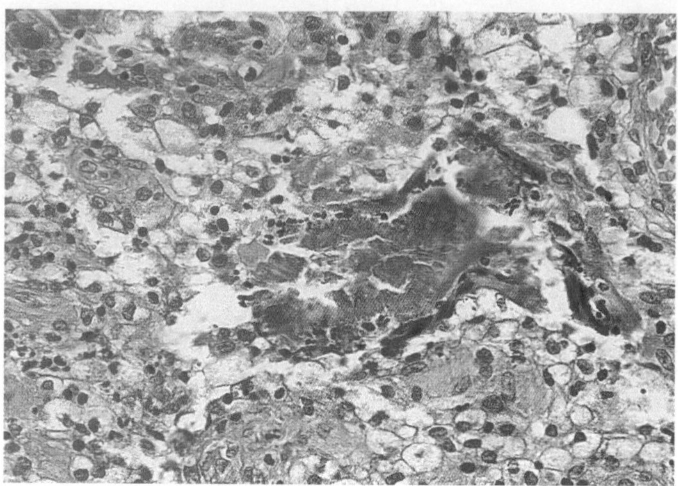

Fig. 33-14 Botryomycosis. An amorphous granule is surrounded by an acute and chronic inflammatory response. The most common cause of this infection is *Staphylococcus aureus*. *Pseudomonas aeruginosa* was isolated repetitively from this tissue.

cosis by culture or by demonstration of the organism (see Chapter 37).

Coagulase-negative staphylococci

Previously regarded as culture contaminants, coagulase-negative staphylococci are assuming importance as agents of human infections.[4,202]

Coagulase-negative staphylococci are natural inhabitants of the human skin. *Staphylococcus epidermidis* is the most prevalent of these. Most infections by *S. epidermidis* are hospital acquired. A common thread is the presence of implanted medical devices, such as orthopedic, valvular, vascular, breast, or ocular prostheses; intravascular, cerebrospinal fluid, or peritoneal dialysis catheters; pacemakers or power packs.[203] A distinctive glomerulonephritis, *shunt nephritis,* may complicate infection of cerebrovenous shunts.[204] Some strains of *S. epidermidis* elaborate an extracellular eosinophilic material known as "slime" that enmeshes organisms in contact with plastic or vitreous materials.[205] These "slimes" may contribute to the pathogenicity of these organisms related to implanted foreign materials.[206]

Coagulase-negative staphylococci have been described as agents of staphylococcal food poisoning.[207] *S. saprophyticus,* which is occasionally found in the genitourinary tract or on the skin, causes urinary tract infections in sexually active women outside the hospital.[208]

Streptococci

Streptococcus species are spherical or ovoid organisms that occur in short chains in clinical material and in chains of variable length in liquid media enriched with blood or serum. The classic morphology of *Streptococcus pneumoniae* is a pair of elongated cocci with somewhat pointed ends, described as "lancet shaped." Certain alpha-hemolytic streptococci, such as *Streptococcus mitis,* produce long, tangled chains in broth media.

Streptococci are gram-positive, nonsporulating, catalase-negative, usually nonmotile facultative anaerobes. Many species, including *S. pneumoniae* and *S. pyogenes,* prefer anaerobic conditions for primary isolation. Some alpha-hemolytic species require coaxing to grow in air, even with enrichment by CO_2, and may appear as anaerobic streptococci on primary isolation. Strains of some species require nutritional supplementation of commonly used agar media; they are referred to as nutritionally variant (or deficient) streptococci, thiol-dependent, or pyridoxal-dependent streptococci. They are important as causes of endocarditis, but the infections do not differ from those produced by less fastidious strains.

Hemolysis produced by streptococci growing on blood agar is described as beta-hemolysis (total lysis of cells with clearing of media), alpha-hemolysis (leaching of hemoglobin from damaged erythrocytes with greening of media), and gamma-hemolysis (no hemolysis and better designated *nonhemolytic*). The Lancefield designation identifies the cell wall carbohydrate. Groups A to H and K to U are identified. Groups A, B, C, D, F, and G are most commonly isolated from human beings; groups E, L, M, P, and U are rarely if ever isolated from human beings. The salt-and bile-tolerant streptococci that possess the group D antigen have been reclassified to their own genus, *Enterococcus*.

Streptococcus pneumoniae *(pneumococcus)*

Pathogenesis. *Streptococcus pneumoniae* is an important human pathogen.[209] Osler dubbed the lobar pneumonia primarily caused by this pathogen the "captain of the men of death." Despite a temporary setback with the introduction of penicillin, the emergence of resistance to multiple antibiotics has given the organism new vigor.[210]

The major virulence factor in *S. pneumoniae* is capsular polysaccharide, a complex hydrophilic polymer that forms on the cell surface. Organisms that produce capsular polysaccharide, formerly known as SSS (soluble specific substance), form smooth, even mucoid colonies on solid media and are pathogenic for humans or experimental animals, whereas those that do not produce such a substance grow in rough colonies and are nonpathogenic. Capsular polysaccharides are antigenically specific and constitute the primary basis for the typing of *S. pneumoniae;* some 84 antigenically distinct types are currently recognizable. Pathogenicity differs among the various capsular types, with types 1, 2, 3, 4, 7, 8, 12, and 14 being more pathogenic than others. The demonstration of conversion of capsular type by heat-killed organisms (the transforming principle) was the beginning of microbial genetics when the component responsible for capsular conversion was shown to be deoxyribonucleic acid.[21] Pneumococci also produce C substance, or C polysaccharide, as a component of the cell wall.[211] Precipitation of this substance by a serum β-globulin (C-reactive protein) in the presence of calcium is an indicator of acute inflammatory disease. Type-specific M-protein and an R-protein from rough pneumococci have been demonstrated but do not appear to contribute to pathogenesis.

Pathogenicity of *S. pneumoniae* resides in its ability to invade tissue successfully because of antiphagocytic properties of capsular polysaccharide.[212] Antibody induced by immunization with a polyvalent pool of purified capsular polysaccharide is protective,[213] though unfortunately the immune response in some of the important populations at risk is suboptimal.[214] Pneumococci produce a variety of other factors that may have toxic or toxinlike properties. These include pneumolysin, a purpura-producing factor, and a neuraminidase.

S. pneumoniae reside in the respiratory tracts of 5% to 70% of normal individuals. The distribution of capsular types depends on many factors that include age (more frequent in the young), season of the year, presence of children in the household, and presence of respiratory disease in the community.[215]

Pathology

S. pneumoniae, like other gram-positive cocci, is a classic extracellular pathogen that evokes an acute polymorphonuclear inflammatory response in the host. The distribution of capsular types shows that six types (8, 4, 1, 14, 3, and 7) contribute 50% of cases of pneumococcal diseases. Important among these are pneumococcal pneumonia[216] and its complications: empyema,[217] lung abscess, and purulent pericarditis (Fig. 33-15). Abscesses are uncommon and have been particularly associated with heavily encapsulated type 3 strains. In children, the pneumococcus is the most common cause of purulent otitis and acute inflammation of paranasal sinuses and mastoid.[218] The pneumococcus is the second most common cause of bacterial meningitis. About half of all patients with meningitis have underlying pneumonia; others have pneumococcal sinusitis, mastoiditis, or otitis media. Pneumococci are a cause of primary purulent peritonitis, defined as peritonitis without perforation of a viscus, especially in patients with ascites attributable to cirrhosis[219] or the nephrotic syndrome. An uncommon but important cause of bacterial endocarditis, the pneumococcus may form luxuriant mural vegetations as well as the more typical valvular lesions. Pneumococcal infections are more common after splenectomy[220] and in other conditions in which host responses are impaired, such as hemoglobinopathy, certain hematologic diseases, alcoholism, hypogammaglobulinemia, neutropenic states, and diabetes mellitus. Complement deficiencies also predispose to pneumococcal infection.[102] Typing of pneumococci that have been isolated in disease states had become relatively neglected but has resumed importance with the availability of polyvalent pneumococcal vaccines. Pathologic features of organ-specific pneumococcal infections are considered in discussions of the various organ systems.

Streptococcus pyogenes (group A beta-hemolytic streptococcus)

Pathogenesis. *Streptococcus pyogenes* is separated into at least 70 serotypes on the basis of immunologic differences in M-protein of their cell walls. Lipoteichoic acid[221] appears to be more important than M-protein[222] in attaching streptococci to pharyngeal epithelial cells.

Group A beta-hemolytic streptococci elaborate a variety of extracellular products. Besides two hemolysins, several enzymes theoretically facilitate spreading of organisms. Among these are four deoxyribonucleic acid hydrolases, DNA-ases A to D, a hyaluronidase, streptokinase, and several other incompletely characterized hydrolases.

Clinical features and pathology. As its name implies, *S. pyogenes* forms pus. In point of fact, the inflammatory response evoked by streptococci is more spreading than that evoked by the staphylococcus, and abscesses are less frequently formed. Of great clinical importance is the association of streptococcal infection with nonsuppurative tissue reactions,[223] acute rheumatic fever,[224] and acute glomerulonephritis,[225] which are considered in appropriate chapters. The resurgence of rheumatic fever in the past decade is particularly notable.[224]

Erysipelas. Erysipelas[226] is an acute infection of the skin caused by group A streptococci (rarely group C). The disease occurs predominantly in infants and in adults over 50 years of age. The disease most often involves the face, in which case there is often a history of antecedent streptococcal tonsillopharyngitis. Erysipelas of the trunk or extremities most often results from infection of a wound, either surgical or accidental. The cutaneous lesion begins as a patch of erythema and swelling that expands rapidly with elevated red margins and often central clearing.

Microscopically, the dermis is expanded by edema that soon become fibrinopurulent, though, particularly early, there may be surprisingly few PMNLs (Fig. 33-16). There is a loosely palisaded perivascular accumulation of histiocytes, lymphocytes, and PMNLs. The dermal expansion may be sufficiently pronounced to form a dermoepidermal cleavage plane with the development of vesicles or even small bullae. The epidermis shows nonspecific spongiosis. Streptococci are ordinarily easily seen in Gram-stained sections.

S. pyogenes may produce a variety of pyodermas including impetigo,[227] a more deeply ulcerating pyoderma known as ecthyma,[228] and clinically nondescript infections of wounds or burns. Streptococcal cellulitis (spreading infection of cellular connective tissue) may complicate postmastectomy lym-

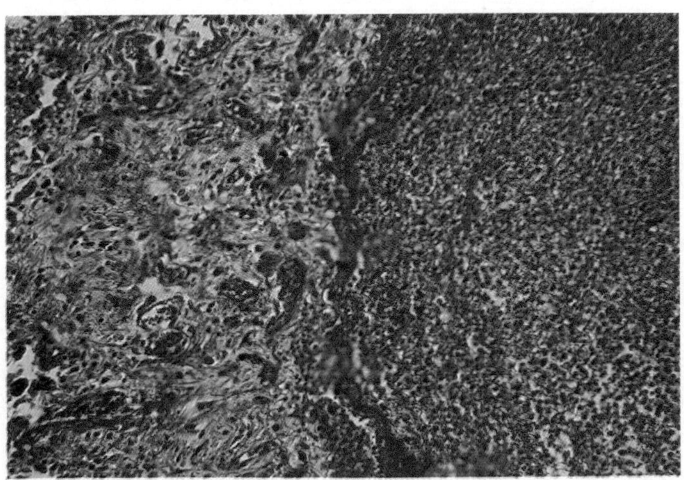

Fig. 33-15 Pneumococcal empyema. An acute polymorphonuclear infiltrate overlies a layer of granulation tissue on the pleura.

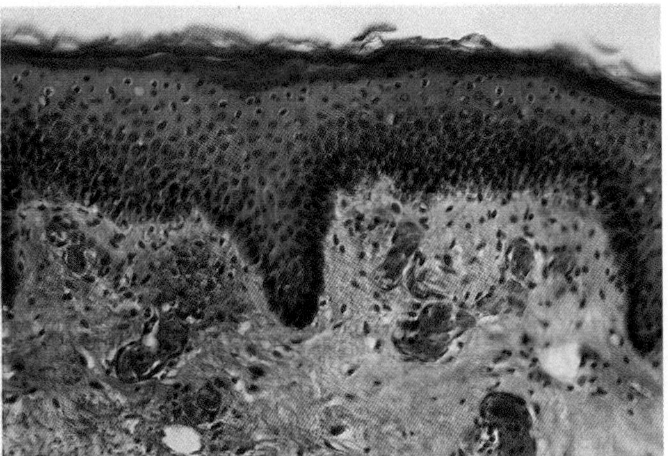

Fig. 33-16 Erysipelas. There is dermal edema, hyperemia, extravasation of erythrocytes, and focal inflammation.

phedema or filariasis. Cellulitis, presumed to be streptococcal because of its response to penicillin, may occur in lower extremities that have been donor sites of saphenous vein coronary arterial bypass grafts.

Tonsillopharyngitis. Group A streptococcus is the most common cause of bacterial tonsillopharyngitis, one of the most common bacterial infections of humans.[229] Although it can occur at any age, the disease is most frequent in children between 4 and 6 years of age. The infection involves epithelial crypts embedded in lymphoid tissue, such as the faucial tonsils. Exudation of serofibrinopurulent material from the crypts produces the familiar "crypt abscesses" that stud the tonsillar surfaces. Adjacent lymph nodes undergo acute hyperplasia and, if bacteria reach them through afferent lymphatic channels, may suppurate. Spread of infection to peritonsillar tissues results in peritonsillar abscess.[230] These lesions are pathologically undifferentiated acute purulent inflammations.

Spread of infection from the throat may involve paranasal sinuses or the middle ear. If the cribriform plate is traversed, epidural abscess, subdural empyema, purulent meningitis, dural sinus thrombosis, or brain abscess may result.

Scarlatina. Scarlatina (scarlet fever) is produced by scarlatinal toxin elaborated by some strains of group A streptococci infected by a temperate bacteriophage. Experimentally, erythrogenic toxin is pyrogenic and cytotoxic and enhances the action of endotoxin. Four serologically distinct forms (toxins A to D), each capable of inhibition by specific antibody, are recognized.

Scarlatina usually accompanies tonsillopharyngitis though it may result from pyoderma or endometritis produced by toxigenic streptococci.

The cutaneous lesion of scarlatina is rarely examined microscopically. The dermis is edematous and hyperemic. There is a scanty perivascular dermal infiltrate of lymphocytes and other mononuclear cells. In the epidermis, keratinization is accelerated in the middle layer (pseudokeratosis), and desquamation occurs through this plane (Fig. 33-17). The differential diagnosis includes viral exanthemas, drug or other allergies, toxic shock syndrome, and Kawasaki disease.

Toxic shock syndrome. Rare cases of TSS have been associated with streptococcal rather than staphylococcal infection.[189] In approximately half of these, necrotizing fasciitis is a prominent clinical feature.[189] The case mortality is 10% to 20%.

Systemic infection. Although *S. pyogenes* remains susceptible to penicillin, its essential virulence has reasserted itself with a vengeance (Fig. 33-18). The return of severe, even fatal scarlet fever and TSS has been paralleled by increasingly frequent overwhelming sepsis and pneumonia, of which Jim Henson, creator of the Muppets, died.[231]

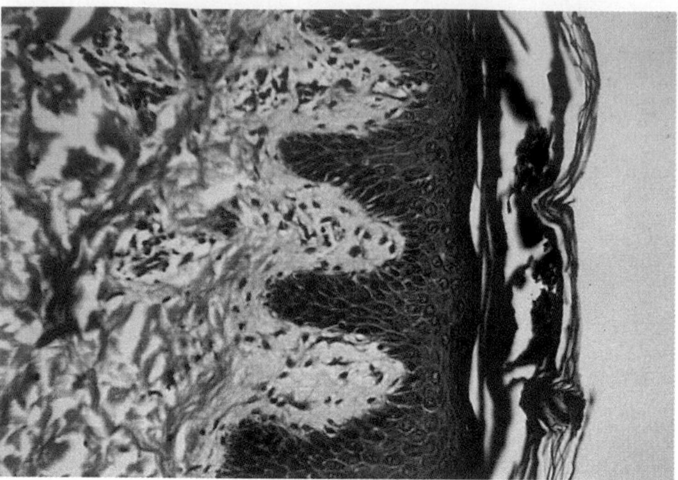

Fig. 33-17 Scarlet fever. There is keratinization in the middle of the epidermis. A superficial keratinous scale will eventually desquamate.

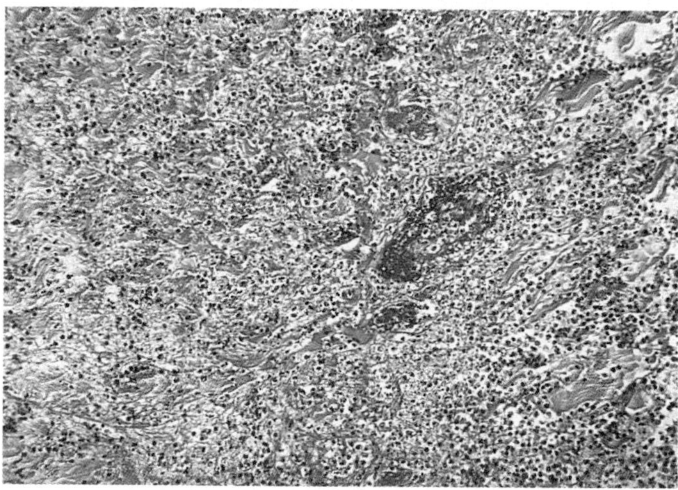

Fig. 33-18 Group A beta-hemolytic streptococcal gangrene. Hemorrhage, edema, and necrosis are accompanied by a mixed inflammatory infiltrate. In other sections the inflammatory exudate dissected along connective tissue planes. *Streptococcus pyogenes* isolated in pure culture.

Streptococcus agalactiae *(group B beta-hemolytic streptococcus)*

Clinical features and pathology. The group B streptococcus is a common cause of postpartum endometritis. Prolonged rupture of membranes, prolonged or instrumental delivery, and septic abortion are factors. The response is an undifferentiated acute purulent inflammation. The frequency of infected parametrial thrombophlebitis contributes to infected pulmonary infarcts.

The streptococcus is also an important cause of pneumonia or sepsis without organ localization in newborn infants. The group B streptococcus is the common agent.[232] In 20% to 40% of adult women the lower reproductive tract is colonized by group B streptococci. Pregnancy does not itself affect the incidence of colonization. Streptococci reach the infant either during labor or during passage through the birth canal. Nosocomial transmission by nursery personnel, as may occur at times of overcrowding, is less common. Both asymptomatic colonization and clinical infection are increased in preterm infants and in infants born after prolonged or instrumental delivery or after premature rupture of fetal membranes.

Congenital pneumonia results from contamination of amniotic fluid after premature rupture of membranes or during prolonged labor. Congenital pneumonia is often of lobar distribution because the lungs of the fetus are partially expanded with fluid. Microscopically, congenital pneumonia is an acute polymorphonuclear inflammation that lacks fibrin because of fibrinolytic properties of amniotic fluid. Squamous debris and other elements of meconium are increased. Interstitial participation in the inflammation is important in distinguishing true congenital pneumonia from the lungs of a newborn infant who "drowns in pus" (because of purulent chorioamnionitis).

Intranatally acquired streptococcal infections are divided into early (from birth to 7 days) and late infections. The mortality is much higher, and maternal factors such as prolonged labor or instrumental delivery are more common in early infections than in late-onset disease. In perinatal streptococcal pneumonia, intra-alveolar fibrin hyaline membranes are often conspicuous.[233] Distinction from noninfectious neonatal hyaline membrane disease is important and can usually be made by the recognition of a more pronounced polymorphonuclear exudate in perinatal pneumonia and by the presence of gram-positive cocci, usually in large numbers in the hyaline membranes.

Purulent meningitis is often present in fatal cases of perinatal streptococcal infection with the group B streptococcus, which ties with *Escherichia coli* for first place among bacterial causes of neonatal meningitis.

Alpha-hemolytic streptococci (viridans streptococci)

Streptococci other than pneumococci that produce partial hemolysis of erythrocytes are often designated "viridans," or 'greening,' streptococci. "Viridans" is a descriptive term, not a taxonomic name, and so italics are not appropriate.[234] The viridans streptococci are important components of the oropharyngeal flora and may also be found in the urogenital tract, in the alimentary tract, and on the skin. Viridans streptococci have been isolated from many types of infection, often in combination with other facultative bacteria and strictly anaerobic species. These infections are commonly adjacent to the mucosal surfaces, which the streptococci inhabit. Viridans and nonhemolytic streptococci accordingly participate in infections related to the oral cavity, including aspiration pneumonia, and in infections of the urogenital system. The most important diseases for which viridans streptococci are primary pathogens include dental plaque and caries, infective endocarditis, and abscesses in multiple organs.

Certain oral species, particularly *S. mutans* and *S. sanguis,* participate in the formation of dental plaque and subsequently caries by virtue of their ability to elaborate complex glycans from fructose. From these sites the streptococci may enter the bloodstream where they may produce intravascular infections if the endothelium has been damaged.

The ability to produce solitary or multiple abscesses is a lesser known capability of certain species. In the British nomenclature one group of etiologic agents is usually designated *Streptococcus milleri.* This name has no official taxonomic standing, but it has become entrenched by frequent usage and is the most common designation. *Streptococcus milleri* encompasses strains from several species in the American nomenclature, particularly *Streptococcus constellatus* and *Streptococcus intermedius.* The current recommendation for these strains is that they be included in the species *Streptococcus anginosus.*[234] The isolates may carry the Lancefield group F antigen, though application of the Lancefield typing system to isolates that are not beta-hemolytic is problematic. The abscesses may occur in any organ or in soft tissue,[235] including the liver,[236] brain, and lung involved.[237] Empyema and meningitis have been described. *S. anginosus* is a cause of primary bacteremia and bacterial endocarditis but less frequently than *S. mutans* or *S. sanguis.* It is of interest that abscesses of the myocardium figure prominently when endocarditis does occur.[238] Pathologically, they are undifferentiated acute inflammatory reactions.

The other viridans streptococcal species of particular note is *Streptococcus bovis.* This species, which shares the group D antigen with *Enterococcus* species, is a member of the fecal flora.[239] *S. bovis* is prominently associated with bacteremia and endocarditis.[240] Some strains have had decreased susceptibility to penicillin, including resistance to lethal antimicrobial effect. Meningitis, osteomyelitis, and visceral abscesses are less frequent manifestations. The pathologic characteristics of *S. bovis* infection cannot be differentiated from those of other streptococcal infections, but the clinical association with diseases of the GI tract is recurrent and impressive. Carcinoma of the colon figures most prominently,[241] but villous adenoma,[242] radiation damage, and inflammatory bowel disease have all been associated with *S. bovis* infection of various manifestations. Fecal carriage of this species, in the absence of bacteremia, has also been suggested as a risk factor for premalignant polyps.[243]

Serious disease, including endocarditis and abscesses, can be caused by other viridans streptococci. A specific identification is not provided by most clinical laboratories and that degree of microbiologic sophistication is not usually required for therapeutic guidance. Nutritionally deficient streptococci present a challenge to the microbiologist but are not differentiated in their clinical or pathologic presentations.[244]

Enterococcus species

Enterococcus species are part of the normal flora of the alimentary canal[239] and the urogenital system. The most common human pathogen is *Enterococcus faecalis,* with *Enterococcus faecium* a distant second. Other enterococcal species may occasionally cause human infection. Most clinical laboratories do not identify isolates beyond the genus level, though increasing resistance to antimicrobial agents has prompted some microbiologists to delineate *E. faecium* from other species. In the past decade enterococci have become increasingly prominent as human pathogens, perhaps in part because of their resistance to many antibiotics that are effective against other gram-positive cocci.[245] It is of particular significance that enterococci are intrinsically resistant to the commonly used cephalosporins, including the third-generation agents.

Enterococci adhere well to damaged cardiac valves[246] and are responsible for approximately 15% of cases of bacterial endocarditis.[245,247] Enterococci appear to interact with cardiac valves to initiate a local coagulative process, which can then serve as a nidus for attachment of additional bacteria.[248] The sources for enterococcal infection are the urinary or GI tracts; they are commonly nosocomial and may be derived from intravascular catheters. One of the major advances in medical therapeutics was the recognition of synergistic activity between penicillin and streptomycin against enterococci, but this advance has been compromised by bacterial acquisition of high-level resistance to aminoglycosides. The intrinsic resistance of enterococci to β-lactam antibiotics has been supplemented by β-lactamases that impart complete resistance. To make matters still worse, resistance has emerged to vancomycin, the major therapeutic backstop available. The other major site of enterococcal infections is the urinary tract. The infections are almost exclusively nosocomial, often associated with indwelling urinary catheters. Again selective pressure of antibiotics against other pathogens has been suggested as an explanation for the increased incidence of enterococcal infections.[249] Suppurative complications in adjacent organs have also been reported.[250]

Enterococci participate in abdominal infections, but the frequency is not so great as one might expect from their prevalence in the feces.[251] Meningitis and abscesses of the liver and genital tract have been reported. Enterococci are not frequent colonizers of the upper respiratory tract, and infection of the lung is correspondingly uncommon. Enterococcal pneumonia is usually a nosocomial infection and has been associated with enteral feeding in patients who were receiving broad-spectrum antimicrobial therapy.

Peptostreptococcus species and *Peptococcus* species

Among anaerobic bacteria, a group of anaerobic gram-positive cocci follows *Bacteroides* spp. in clinical importance. Chief among these are *Peptostreptococcus* spp., particularly *Peptostreptococcus magnus* and *Peptostreptococcus anaerobius.* Reclassification has left only a single species, rarely pathogenic for humans, in the genus *Peptococcus. Peptostreptococcus* spp. composed approximately 20% of the anaerobic isolates at Indiana University Medical Center.[172]

A *Peptostreptococcus* species is usually isolated from surgical wounds that follow operations for malignancies, inflammatory bowel disease, or hysterectomies.[252] Approximately 90% of these infections are by mixed agents.

Anaerobic pleuropulmonary infections by anaerobic cocci are common in individuals with poor oral hygiene, impaired consciousness, or reduced gag reflex or in those with intrabronchial obstruction particularly by foreign bodies.[253] Aspiration pneumonia progresses rapidly to putrid lung abscess or pulmonary gangrene, foul-smelling, sparsely cellular pulmonary consolidations that soon liquefy. Infections by these organisms are often mixed.

Skin and muscle infections are a major source of anaerobic cocci.[254] *Synergistic necrotizing cellulitis* is usually a mixed aerobic and anaerobic infection. *Anaerobic cellulitis* with crepitance must be differentiated from clostridial cellulitis or gas gangrene (myonecrosis).[255] Diabetic foot ulcers are usually mixed infections that include both aerobic and anaerobic flora.

GRAM-POSITIVE BACILLI WITH A DIPHTHEROID MORPHOLOGY

Corynebacterium and *Propionibacterium* species

Corynebacterium species are facultatively anaerobic, nonsporeforming, gram-positive bacilli or coccobacilli that grow slowly in culture. Most strains produce catalase and are susceptible to β-lactam antibiotics. Some species require special attention for successful isolation from clinical specimens. The morphology varies from coccal to bacillary; in classic configuration there are palisading arrangements of bacilli with swollen ends, producing a "Chinese-character" appearance. The morphology is sometimes referred to as "diphtheroidal" and describes several genera other than *Corynebacterium* and *Propionibacterium.* Metachromatic granules may be demonstrated in some strains with methylene blue but have no practical diagnostic value. Some strains may have rudimentary branching but never produce the highly developed branches of *Actinomyces*, *Arachnia*, and *Nocardia* species.

Corynebacterium diphtheriae

Epidemiology. Diphtheria is a historically important infectious disease that persists. The etiology was explicated more than a century ago by Loeffler.[256] Despite the development of an effective vaccine against the primary etiologic agent, *Corynebacterium diphtheriae,* epidemic and endemic disease continues to occur in populations that escape surveillance and immunization. Such populations include those disadvantaged by war and famine,[257] or those citizens of wealthy countries who are homeless or addicted to drugs, or debilitated by alcoholism.[258-261]

The common denominator in the populations at increased risk is probably lack of immunization, though alcoholism may contribute additional risks.[262,263] Immunization may affect clinical presentation as well as morbidity and mortality; membranes are less often present or are less extensive in patients who have received immunizations.[264] At the time of this writing an ongoing epidemic has affected more than 12,000 apparently immunized citizens of the Russian Federation.[265] Other risk factors may include the biotype of bacterium and certainly include the presence of the diphtheria toxin. Despite the epidemic in Seattle, cases of diphtheria in the United States have been reduced to a very low level.[266]

Microbiology and pathogenesis. Isolation of *C. diphtheriae* requires inoculation of an enriched blood agar; a serum-containing medium, such as Loeffler's medium; and a tellurite-containing medium, such as Tinsdale agar. Biotypes *gravis, intermedius,* and *mitis* have been recognized.[267] Some authorities believe that more serious disease is produced by *gravis* biotypes, but the correlation is inexact.[268] The three biotypes may coexist in the same geographic area.[269]

The most important microbiologic characteristic is the infection of bacterial strains by a corynebacteriophage that carries the diphtheria toxin.[3] The toxin consists of a subunit, A, that is responsible for biologic activity and a subunit, B, that mediates binding of the parent molecule to the target cell membrane. After proteolytic cleavage from the parent molecule, subunit A enters the cell, where it catalyzes the inactivation of transfer RNA translocase, also known as *elongation factor-2*. Without RNA translocase, which is present in mammalian cells but not in bacterial cells, transfer RNA cannot interact with messenger RNA, and so protein synthesis is effectively stopped.[270] This enzymatic toxin affects cells throughout the body with such a potency that concentrations of 0.1 μ/kg will kill susceptible animals.[271] The primary effects are on the myocardium with conduction abnormalities and on the nervous system, where the toxin produces demyelination of both central and peripheral nervous systems, yielding cranial nerve palsies and peripheral neuritis. The laboratory evaluation of *C. diphtheriae* is incomplete without a test for production of toxin. Formerly accomplished by subcutaneous inoculation of guinea pigs, the procedure is more easily accomplished by immunodiffusion or in cell culture.[267]

Toxigenic and nontoxigenic strains may coexist in the same environment.[272] Infection and invasive disease, including endocarditis, may occasionally result from nontoxigenic strains,[273] but most serious infections are a result of toxin production. Severe or even fatal disease may then result from rather mild local infection. Virulence in *C. diphtheriae* can be viewed as a two-stage process. A toxin that is apparently identical to that produced by *C. diphtheriae* has been associated with *Corynebacterium ulcerans.*[274]

The only reservoir for *C. diphtheriae* is the human host. Communicability is assumed to derive from close physical contact. A primary defense is therefore immunization against diphtheria toxin. Carriers are frequently found in populations where the disease is epidemic. The bacteria persist longer in skin lesions than in the respiratory tract[275]; ulcerative cutaneous lesions also serve as more efficient disseminators of bacteria to contacts than the respiratory system is.[276] In populations that are free of diphtheria asymptomatic carriage of the bacterium is uncommon.[277]

Clinical features and pathology. *C. diphtheriae* affects the respiratory tract and skin as primary targets.[278,279] The respiratory tract may be affected from the anterior nares to the tonsils and oropharynx, through the larynx, and into the trachea and bronchi, with the severity of the infection increasing as the disease moves centrally. The diphtheritic membrane is a thick, gray tenacious exudate that adheres tightly to the underlying submucosa (Fig. 33-19). The classical membrane is often tinged with green[280] and causes bleeding when stripped away. The differential diagnosis includes other infectious causes of pharyngitis with exudate, such as *Streptococcus pyogenes* and Epstein-Barr virus. A membrane that resembled the diphtheritic membrane was noted after ingestion of paraquat.[281]

A substantial proportion of cases may not have obvious membranes. Symptoms vary from mild to severe malaise, weakness, and respiratory difficulty. Sore throat and dysphagia are common symptoms. Cervical adenopathy and edema may produce a swelling, so-called bull neck.

In the skin *C. diphtheriae* produces chronic ulcers, which may also be covered with a tenacious gray membrane. *Streptococcus pyogenes* and *Staphylococcus aureus* are frequent coinfecting agents. The bacilli responsible for cutaneous infection often produce toxin, but the infection is usually protracted and indolent without symptoms of intoxication. The epidemic in Seattle manifested primarily as cutaneous diphtheria. In addition to the skin the cornea may be infected, producing ulcers with attendant membrane.[274]

Septicemia with disseminated abscesses has been caused by nontoxigenic *C. diphtheriae,*[282] again demonstrating the dissociation of the two virulence capabilities. Complications include toxin-induced myocarditis and neuritis. Rarely, hematologic complications may result in excessive bleeding, with or without thrombocytopenia, so-called hemorrhagic diphtheria.[283] Hemolytic uremic syndrome has been reported in a child with diphtheria.[284]

Diphtheria-pertussis-tetanus immunization has been complicated by localized cutaneous abscesses caused by *Streptococcus pyogenes,* but invasive disease has not been documented.

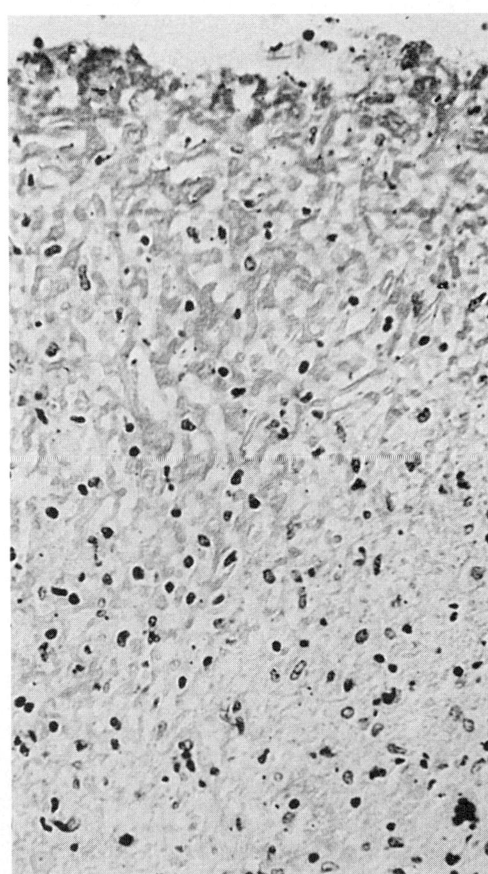

Fig. 33-19 Diphtheria. Membrane that overlies tonsil consists of a feltwork of fibrin, necrotic debris, and sparse leukocytes. (From Kissane JM: *Pathology of infancy and childhood*, ed 2, St. Louis, 1975, Mosby)

Corynebacterium jeikeium

For many years corynebacteria other than *C. diphtheriae* have been recognized as occasional pathogens, particularly of compromised hosts and those in hospitals.[285] In the 1970s an important group of these diphtheroid bacilli were delineated as group "JK bacilli." In his initial report Hande noted the characteristic metallic sheen of the colonies on blood agar and the clinically significant resistance to most antibiotics except vancomycin.[286] The group has now been assigned the name *Corynebacterium jeikeium.* These bacteria are common colonizers of the skin and cause disease in two groups of patients.[287] There have been two clinical situations in which this species has produced infection. The first are those who are severely immunosuppressed by virtue of disease or therapy.[285] Pneumonia, which may be cavitary or necrotizing, is a common manifestation of infection (Fig. 33-20). Neutrophilic infiltrates may not be prominent in patients who are profoundly

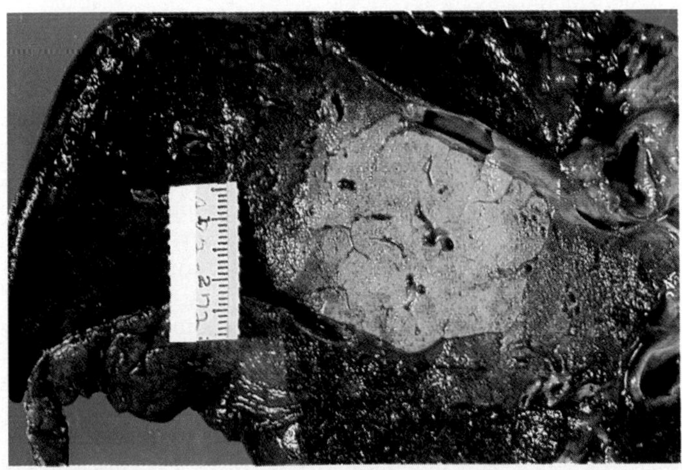

Fig. 33-20 Large, necrotizing, nodular lesion produced by *Corynebacterium jaykeium.* The patient was profoundly neutropenic.[288] (Courtesy Brenda Waters.)

neutropenic.[289] Generalized macular and papular skin lesions have been described in a patient who was receiving chemotherapy for a relapse of acute lymphocytic leukemia;[289] the dermal follicles were necrotic and effaced by proliferating bacilli. Severe infections with this bacterium of relatively low intrinsic virulence tend to occur late in the course of the disease or at the nadir of host resistance, and so the mortality from the infections is unfortunately high.

The second group of patients at increased risk for this infection are those who have prosthetic devices.[290] Infections of cerebrospinal fluid in patients with ventricular shunts and of peritoneal fluid in those undergoing peritoneal dialysis have been noteworthy. Cardiac infections have occurred in the presence of hardware, but endocarditis on native valves has also been reported;[291] in that case a myocardial abscess subsequently developed despite therapy with vancomycin.

Arcanobacterium hemolyticum

Arcanobacterium hemolyticum, which was formerly classified as *Corynebacterium hemolyticum,* has been recently emphasized as a cause of bacterial pharyngitis that may resemble *Streptococcus pyogenes* infection, but the syndrome was described as much as 20 years ago.[292] Approximately half the cases are accompanied by a scarlatiniform rash,[293] which is erythematous and macular with a rough, finely papular texture.[294] The rash occurs on the extremities and trunk. In contradistinction to *S. pyogenes* infection, which predominantly affects young children, *Arcanobacterium hemolyticum* causes disease in older children and adolescents. This species is beta-hemolytic and does not produce catalase, and so it may be confused with *Streptococcus pyogenes* if Gram stain is not performed.

A. hemolyticum has also caused endocarditis on a native valve and a probable case of mitral valve endocarditis with neurologic complications in a drug addict.

Actinomyces species and *Nocardia* species

Actinomyces israelii and *Nocardia* species produce chronic, suppurative lesions in many organs and tissues. *Actinomyces israelii* is a member of the normal oropharyngeal flora, and the infections are therefore endogenous. *Nocardia* species are soil organisms, and the infections are exogenous. These infections are considered in Chapter 37.

Listeria monocytogenes

Microbiology. *Listeria monocytogenes* is a small gram-positive, non–sporeforming, nonencapsulated coccobacillus that is motile at room temperature. In clinical material or in tissue, this organism may appear as pairs of cocci resembling *S. pneumoniae.* If overdecolorized, it may mimic *Haemophilus influenzae.* The bacteria have a morphology that resembles *Corynebacterium* and *Propionibacterium* species, microbes that are often encountered as contaminating skin flora. Too cavalier an approach to diagnosis may result in dismissing this important pathogen as extraneous.

Epidemiology. *Listeria* organisms are widely distributed in nature, being found in water, sewage, soil, and dust, as well as in at least 40 mammalian species, including horses, cattle, dogs, and cats, and in birds, several species of insects, and crustaceans. *Listeria* organisms can be recovered from the stools of about 1% of asymptomatic people. Eleven serotypes are identifiable, but three cause 70% of human infections. There is an epidemiologically important geographic variation in the distribution of serotypes.[295]

The portal of entry into a potential host is usually inapparent. *Listeria* organisms can enter the body through the skin or conjunctiva. Human cases rarely develop a pneumonia,[296] and so the respiratory tract is not considered to be the usual portal of entry. Food-borne outbreaks have occurred.[297-298] In view of the organism's wide distribution, the rarity of clinical cases is surprising. There seems to be a predisposition for the infection to occur in pregnant women.[299] Many older adult patients have malignant diseases, especially lymphoma, or are otherwise immunosuppressed.

Human infection may have several consequences, the most common of which is probably an asymptomatic carrier state after a subliminal or trivial illness. Sepsis of unknown origin is clinically undifferentiated,[300] except for the uncommon occurrence of a circulating monocytosis (greater than 8%), which may be suggestive of an infectious mononucleosis. When infection occurs in a pregnant woman, usually in the first trimester, it produces fever, often with chills that usually subside. The fetus may be aborted, born prematurely, born ill, or go to normal term.[301]

Prenatal infection, granulomatosis infantiseptica, produces a distinctive syndrome in the newborn period. Most affected infants are very ill; a few are merely listless and feed poorly. Infected infants have or develop within days abscesses of many organs, including skin, lungs, liver, kidneys, brain, bones, and soft tissues. Placenta and fetal membranes are almost always infected and in suspected cases should be examined and cultured, as should the mother's reproductive tract (Fig. 33-21). The lesions microscopically are undifferentiated acute abscesses that become mononuclear only in late stages. True epithelioid granulomas are not seen. The mortality is high.

Listeria species cause an acute leptomeningitis, usually in infants or in older adults, who often have malignant disease. Organisms may be few in cerebrospinal fluid and may be misinterpreted as contaminants. Other organ-specific infections, which may follow or accompany sepsis, include osteomyelitis, arthritis, endocarditis, empyema, cholecystitis, and wound

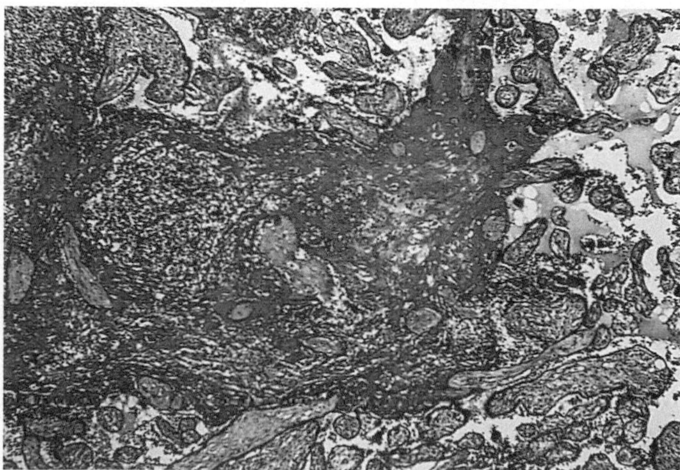

Fig. 33-21 Listeriosis. Acute placentitis is characterized by polymorphonuclear inflammation of the placental villi and an area of abscess formation.

infections. These lesions are pathologically nonspecific acute inflammations.

Erysipelothrix rhusiopathiae

Erysipeloid, an occupational disease of human beings, is caused by *Erysipelothrix rhusiopathiae,* a slender, nonmotile, nonencapsulated, nonsporeforming, gram-positive rod that infects many animal species of economic importance such as swine ("diamond skin") and sheep ("joint ill").[302] The organism is widely distributed throughout the world and is believed to have a free-living existence in soil and water that has been contaminated with dead or decaying organic matter.

Erysipeloid occurs in handlers of fish, especially shellfish, meat, or poultry, and in fishermen, farmers, veterinarians, and housewives. Rarely, there is no such contact. The organism enters the skin, almost always that of a finger, through a minor abrasion or scratch and causes a painful swollen expanding reddish lesion that clears centrally. Spread to the hand, wrist, or forearm occurs in about 20% of cases, but lymphangitis and regional lymphadenopathy are less prominent than in erysipelas caused by pyogenic cocci, particularly streptococci.[302] The cutaneous lesion of erysipeloid may be vesicular but does not suppurate unless superinfected.

A biopsy specimen shows acute inflammation of the epidermis with infiltration of the dermis by lymphocytes, histiocytes, and mast cells. In contrast to erysipelas, organisms can rarely be stained; formal culture of a full-thickness biopsy specimen is usually necessary for a specific diagnosis.[303]

The cutaneous lesion is usually self-limited after 1 to 2 weeks. A more chronic regional or generalized form, with or without a history of a primary cutaneous lesion occurs but is also usually self-limited. Approximately 40 cases of sepsis due to *E. rhusiopathiae* have been reported. Roughly half of the cases are in turn complicated by infectious endocarditis, often on a previously normal valve, usually the aortic valve and less commonly the mitral valve. Endocarditis is sufficiently common that it must always be considered in cases of *Erysipelothrix* sepsis. The lesion is an undifferentiated acute infective endocarditis that usually responds promptly to large doses of penicillin.

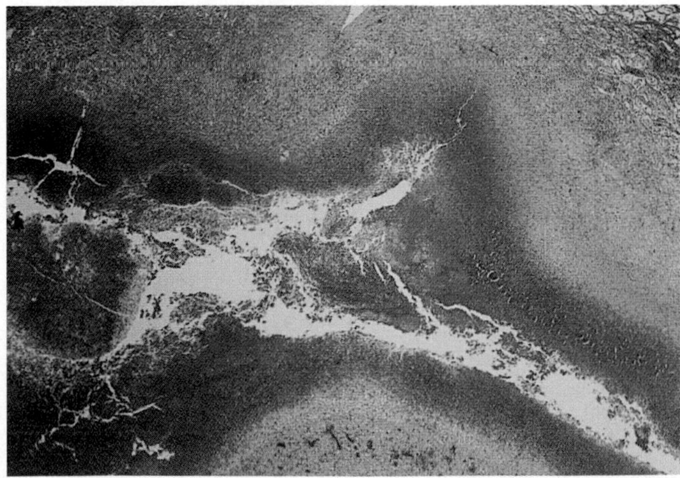

Fig. 33-22 Necrotizing, granulomatous, cavitary lesion in a patient with acquired immunodeficiency syndrome. *Rhodococcus equi* isolated from lung tissue. (Courtesy David Walker, MD, Galveston, Tex.)

Rhodococcus equi

Rhodococcus species are nonsporeforming, gram-positive bacilli that are members of the aerobic actinomycetes. *Rhodococcus equi,* the species most frequently encountered, is partially acid fast. It has also been known as *Corynebacterium equi* or *Mycobacterium rhodochrous.* The colonies of the isolated bacterium often have a distinctive salmon color. *R. equi* is commonly found in soil and is a pathogen of animals,[304] frequently of horses, as the name implies. It produces infections predominantly in immunosuppressed patients,[304] who have had exposure to animals. The portal of entry is believed to be the respiratory tract. Pneumonia, which may be cavitary,[305] is a common presentation, and the infection is difficult to treat (Fig. 33-22). Lymphadenitis, subcutaneous abscesses, brain abscesses, and endophthalmitis have been reported.

Plasmids that encode genes that correlate with virulence for mice have been identified.[306] Virulence is, however, relative and may be species-specific; this species is clearly of low virulence for humans. *R. equi* has some characteristics of a facultative intracellular pathogen, including the apparent participation of interferon-λ and tumor necrosis factor in defense against experimental infection.[79] Recurrent infections with *R. equi* have been described in immunosuppressed patients, suggestive of the pattern seen with other facultative intracellular pathogens.[307] The histologic response to this opportunistic pathogen may be acute, neutrophilic inflammation or may be granulomatous, suggestive of a mycobacterial or nocardial infection (Figs. 33-23 and 33-24).

Gardnerella vaginalis

Gardnerella vaginalis, formerly known as both *Corynebacterium vaginale* and *Haemophilus vaginalis,* is a nonsporulating, facultatively anaerobic bacillus that is commonly found in the female genital tract. Its morphology in Gram stains is best described as gram-variable coccobacilli, the ultimate hedge! This variability partially explains its erratic course through both gram-positive and gram-negative genera. *G. vaginalis*

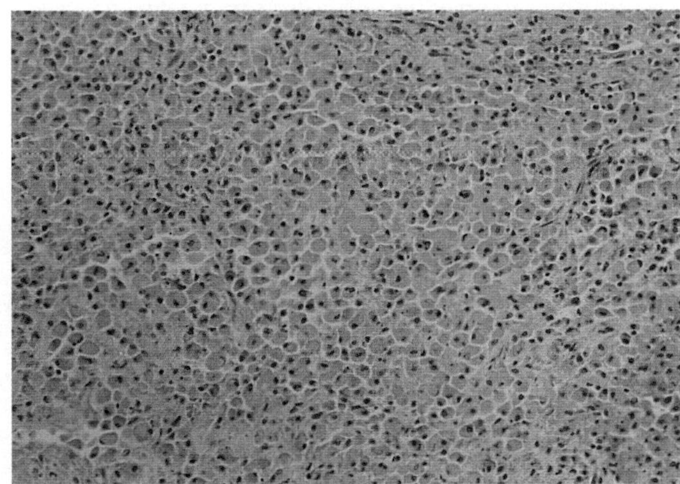

Fig. 33-23 *Rhodococcus* pneumonia. Extensive collections of foamy macrophages characterize the inflammatory response, resembling infection with other facultative or obligate intracellular pathogens, such as *Tropheryma whippelii, Mycobacterium leprae, mycobacterium avium–intracellulare. Rhodococcus equi* isolated from tissue. (Courtesy David Walker, MD, Galveston, Tex.)

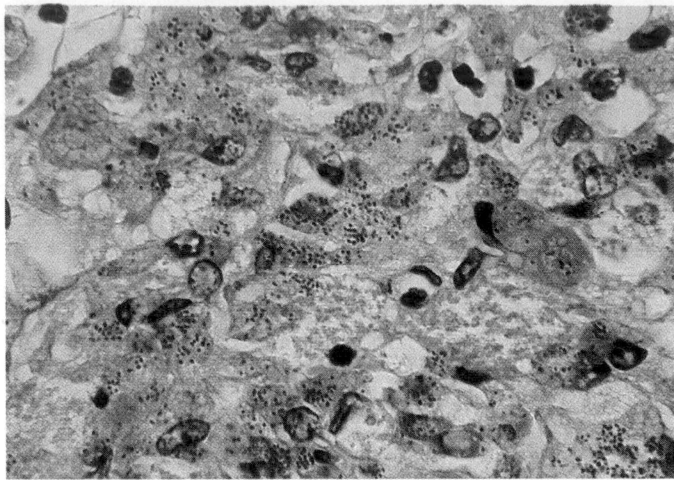

Fig. 33-24 *Rhodococcus* pneumonia. Numerous small gram-positive coccobacilli are present within macrophages in the cases illustrated in Fig. 33-23. Some strains of *Rhodococcus equi* are acid-fast in tissue (Brown-Hopps stain.) (Courtesy David Walker, MD, Galveston, Tex.)

causes nonspecific vaginitis, along with *Mycoplasma hominis*, *Mobiluncus* species, and a variety of anaerobic bacteria.[308] The infection is best diagnosed clinically or by Gram stain of vaginal secretions[309]; culture plays little role in the diagnosis. Clue cells, vaginal epithelial cells coated with *Gardnerella*, are reasonably specific but are an insensitive method of diagnosis. The infection may be transmitted sexually, but the bacteria are also common rectal and vaginal flora.[310]

Gardnerella vaginalis has been implicated as a cause of urinary tract infection in women,[311] but most isolates from the urine cannot be associated with clinical disease or an inflammatory response.[312] Bacteremia occurs circumpartum in both mother and neonate as a reflection of chorioamnionitis but usually resolves without complication. There are no pathologic data on *Gardnerella* infection.

SPOREFORMING GRAM-POSITIVE BACILLI

Clostridia

Clostridium perfringens

Microbiology. Clostridia are strictly anaerobic, sporeforming, gram-positive bacilli that produce a variety of extracellular enzymes and toxins important for human disease. *Clostridium perfringens*, the most commonly isolated species, grows well in common laboratory media. It produces large amounts of gas, a characteristic double-zone hemolysis on sheep blood agar, lecithinase that can be detected on egg yolk agar media, and stormy fermentation of milk. *C. perfringens* is nonmotile; morphologically it is a large boxcar-shaped bacillus, and spores are usually not demonstrable in clinical specimens or on most agar media.

C. perfringens produces 12 types of toxins, of which four major toxins form the basis for subclassification into five types (A to E).[313]

α-Toxin: phospholipase C, lecithinase; responsible for hemolysis in vitro and in vivo
β-Toxin: a toxin that is necrotizing and lethal for mice
ε-Toxin: a lethal, necrotizing toxin for mice; causes increased vascular permeability and peripheral vasoconstriction
ι-Toxin: a lethal toxin for mice
δ-Toxin: hemolysin; lethal for mice
θ-Toxin: an oxygen-labile hemolysin that is lethal for mice
κ-Toxin: gelatinase, collagenase; necrotizing and lethal for mice
λ-Toxin: a protease
μ-Toxin: hyaluronidase
ν-Toxin: deoxyribonuclease, leukocidin, hemolysin; necrotizing and lethal for mice
Enterotoxin: cytotoxic in ileal loop assays
Neuraminidase

Epidemiology. *C. perfringens* is widely distributed in soils and is a part of the normal intestinal flora of humans. Infections can be acquired both endogenously or exogenously, usually from contaminated soil or foodstuffs.[314,315] The most common foods are meats, stews, and gravies that have been cooked slowly and stored at ambient temperatures. *C.* perfringens gastroenteritis usually occurs in epidemic form and is one of the most common causes of food poisoning in the United States. An outbreak at a banquet in New York affected 900 of the 1800 attendees.[316]

Pathogenesis. The toxin most commonly incriminated in severe disseminated infection with intravascular hemolysis is the α-toxin.[317] The ability to hydrolyze phosphatidylcholine is associated with the N-terminus sequence of the toxin, whereas the C-terminus, which resembles the sequence of the inflammatory molecule arachidonate 5-lipoxygenase, is responsible for hemolysis and sphingomyelinase activity.[318] Phospholipase C also induces platelet aggregation in vitro.[319] The θ-toxin has properties that may contribute to myonecrois.[320] At low concentrations it stimulates endothelial cells to produce platelet-activating factor and induces degranulation of PMNLs; at higher concentrations it is cytotoxic. This toxin also participates in the hemolysis observed in agar media and induces shock in experimental animals. Clostridial collagenase inactivates complement component C1q in vitro. The enterotoxin produces fluid accumulation in the rabbit ileal loop by inducing cytoskeletal collapse and increased membrane permeability.[321] Enterotoxin can be detected in the stool and antienterotoxin antibodies in the serum of individuals who have had clostridial food poisoning but not in controls.[322] It has been suggested that some cases of sporadic diarrhea, in which clostridial enterotoxin can be detected, may be caused by *C. perfringens* in the absence of obvious food contamination; it is difficult to eliminate the possibility that the responsible food was not recognized. Gastroenteritis is produced by germination in the GI tract of spores that are not killed by cooking of foods.

The pathogenesis of *C. perfringens* infections is poorly understood despite the extensive knowledge of potentially important bacterial toxins. Colonizing strains contain the same potential virulence factors as isolates that have been incriminated in serious infection.

Clinical features

Food poisoning. The incubation period is 7 to 15 hours, after which profuse diarrhea and abdominal pain develop. Nausea and vomiting are unusual, and the disease usually resolves spontaneously within 24 hours. The pathologic features of the infection are unknown.

Enteritis necroticans. A more severe intestinal infection is produced by the β-toxin of *C. perfringens* type C in malnourished individuals.[323] Nausea, vomiting, and abdominal pain may be accompanied by the passage of bloody stools. The illness ranges from mild disease to rapidly fatal infection.

Enteritis necroticans was first recognized at the end of World War II in Germany, where it was named *Darmbrand,* meaning 'intestines on fire.'[323] In the 1960s a similar disease was recognized as an endemic infection in the highlands of New Guinea, where it was known as Pig Bel.[324] The pathologic changes range from focal mucosal erosions to extensive full-thickness necrosis, which may lead to perforation of the intestine.[325] A similar disease caused by several *Clostridium* species has been described in infants.[326]

Clostridial cellulitis and gas gangrene. Most infections caused by *C. perfringens* are polymicrobial and do not differ in characteristics from typical anaerobic infections. Rarely, gas-forming infections of soft tissues or viscera result. *Clostridial cellulitis* is defined as a localized or extensive soft-tissue infection with extensive gas formation and crepitance but few systemic symptoms.[327] There is a profuse, watery, foul-smelling seropurulent discharge from the affected tissue. Gas is not present in muscle. In contrast, gas gangrene involves the muscle and is associated with severe systemic symptoms, including shock and circulatory collapse.[128,327] There is less crepitance than in clostridial cellulitis. *Clostridial myonecrosis* is a better name because gas formation may be entirely absent. Gas gangrene also occurs in viscera. Necrotizing endometritis is a well-recognized complication of septic abortion but also complicates attended deliveries.[328] Approximately 5% of acute cholecystitis is caused by *C. perfringens,* which may produce gas gangrene or radiographically visible gas (emphysematous cholecystitis).[329] The septic picture may be accompanied by bacteremia and massive intravascular hemolysis that is rapidly fatal.[317] Bacteremia and massive hemolysis may also occur from an intestinal source, particularly in patients with neoplastic disease[330] or in the absence of an obvious primary infection. Massive hemolysis is a rare but devastating complication of uncomplicated biliary surgery, causing some surgeons to test for clostridia with intraoperative Gram stain of gallbladder mucosa (Fig. 33-25). Gas gangrene may be caused by other *Clostridium* species, particularly *Clostridium septicum, Clostridium novyi A,* and *Clostridium histolyticum.* The histologic findings in gas gangrene include extensive necrosis, proteinaceous exudate, typical boxcar-shaped gram-positive bacilli, and an exudate that is often scant.

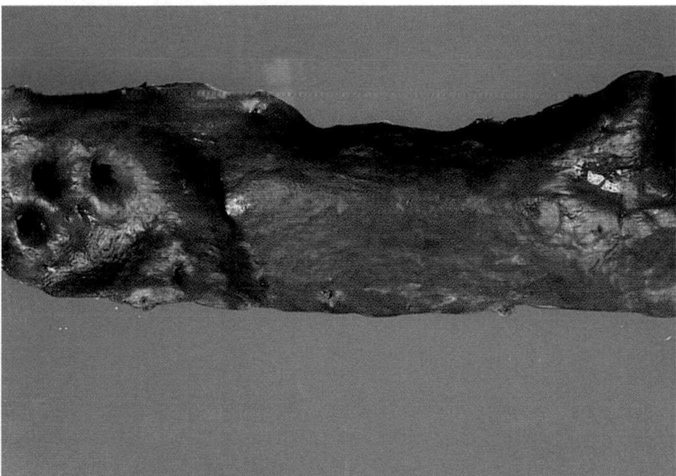

Fig. 33-25 Clostridial hemolysis. The intima of the aorta is stained deeply red by devastating hemolysis after an apparently uneventful cholecystectomy. *Clostridium perfringens* isolated from blood ante mortem.

Other infections. Necrotizing pneumonia and empyema are produced infrequently by *C. perfringens.* Infections of the central nervous system occur rarely.

Clostridium tetani

Tetanus is a severe neurologic disease produced by *Clostridium tetani.* This species is the only major pathogen among the species that have terminal spores. Its extensive motility produces swarming on the surface of agar plates. *C. tetani* is widely distributed in nature and is introduced into physically induced wounds, where the spores germinate and elaborate toxin. Neonatal tetanus, which is extremely rare in the United States, is acquired when inadequately immunized mothers deliver babies under conditions of poor hygiene.[331] Application of nonsterile creams or soil to the umbilicus has been associated with neonatal infection. Tetanus after a human bite[332] and after an anorectal infection[333] have been reported. The incubation period ranges from 2 weeks to several months.

Tetanus is a rare disease in the United States, of decreasing incidence.[334] Disease occurs at the extremes of age, and mortality exceeds 50% in the elderly.

The clinical disease is produced by a potent exotoxin called "tetanospasmin," which binds to neural gangliosides, especially at the myoneural junctions of alpha motor neurons.[335] Rarely, the central nervous system may be affected, and transverse myelitis has resulted. Muscle spasm is the hallmark of tetanus, resulting in weakness, stiffness, or cramping. Trismus from increased tone of the masseter muscle is often an early sign, providing the colloquial name of "lockjaw." Difficulty in mastication and dysphagia are also common presenting symptoms.[336] Impairment of respiratory function is a critical manifestation that requires expert intensive care.[337] Involvement of the autonomic nervous system may produce cardiac arrest.[337] Most survivors recover complete function, but some patients experience chronic ill-defined problems.[338]

Clostridium botulinum

Microbiology. The exotoxin of *Clostridium botulinum* is responsible for the clinical disease known as "botulism."[33,339] There are seven antigenic types (A to G) of botulinal toxin, but types A, B, and E produce most human infection. Spores of *C. botulinum* are resistant to heat, surviving even 100° C for several hours. Botulinus toxin, which is one of the most potent toxins known, exerts its effects by interference with acetylcholine transmission at neuromuscular junctions, producing a flaccid, descending paralysis.[339] A neurotoxin that is closely related to type F botulinus toxin is produced by *Clostridium baratii,*[340] and type E toxin has been associated with *Clostridium butyricum.*[341]

Epidemiology and pathogenesis. Three epidemiologic and clinical types of botulism are recognized, food-borne infection, wound botulism, and infant botulism.

Botulism is the king of food poisoning, the most common means by which the intoxication is acquired. The appearance of botulism as a medical problem parallels the development of techniques for canning in the early part of this century. If all the clostridial spores are not killed in the process of preparing food, the spores may germinate under a reduced oxygen environment (strictly anaerobic conditions are not required for this process to be initiated). Most cases result from home-prepared food.[342] The potential for widespread epidemic disease exists when commercial canneries or restaurants are the source. Type E botulism has been associated with various fish products.[343,344]

Wound botulism occurs after germination of spores that have been inoculated in wounds, which may be otherwise insignificant.[345] Not surprisingly, the increased prevalence of intravenous and subcutaneous injection of illicit drugs has provided an additional source for wound botulism.[346] Botulism has also been described as a complication of intestinal surgery.[347]

Infant botulism is the most recently recognized epidemiologic type. Food-borne infection is an exogenous infection. Wound botulism results from toxin production in local lesions. Infant botulism occurs after replication of vegetative cells in the GI tract.[348] The source of the spores is diverse, but honey has been prominently incriminated as the source for the infection.[349]

Clinical features and pathology. The symptoms of botulism are suggestive of a neurologic disease rather than an infectious process.[345,350] Symmetric, descending paralysis begins with the cranial nerves and may involve the bulbar centers of life support. Ocular abnormalities, which include ptosis, extraocular paralysis, and dilated, fixed pupils, are common.[351] If the epidemiologic association with food is not appreciated by the patient or family, the nature of the intoxication may not be appreciated, and specific antitoxin may not be made available. Schaffner suggests the following grouping of signs as clues to the presence of botulism:[339]

1. Unexplained orthostatic hypotension
2. Dilated, unreactive pupils
3. Dry mucous membranes
4. Descending paralysis with respiratory insufficiency
5. Absence of fever

The most lethal complication of botulism is respiratory paralysis. Recovery of function may take many months in survivors.[352]

Infant botulism manifests as hypotonia with poor feeding, weak sucking reflexes, and constipation.[353] Outpatients may be labeled "failure to thrive." Ocular abnormalities and respiratory insufficiency are features of disease in infants as well as adults. Several studies have suggested that infant botulism may be a rare cause of sudden infant death syndrome.[354]

Botulism is a result of physiologic neuronal dysfunction. There are no histologic correlates of functional damage.

Clostridium difficile

Epidemiology and pathogenesis. *Clostridium difficile* is a recent addition to the list of toxigenic clostridial pathogens. It is the primary cause of pseudomembranous colitis and secondarily of antibiotic-associated diarrhea. The cause of pseudomembranous colitis had eluded investigators for many years. During the 1950s it was associated with staphylococcal infection, but by the 1970s it was clear that staphylococci were not the primary causes of this severe infection. The disease was associated with toxigenic clostridia in the mid-1970s.[355] Initially *Clostridium sordellii* was suspected, but it was soon realized that *C. difficile* was the real culprit.

C. difficile is a member of the fecal flora. Both bacterium and toxin are detected frequently in the stool of neonates.[356] In adults carriage is uncommon unless antibiotics have been administered. *C. difficile* can be recovered from as many as 20% of adults who have recently received antibiotics, but toxin is detected in the stool infrequently.[357] Two toxins are produced.[358] Toxin A is an enterotoxin that elicits fluid secretion in isolated rabbit ileal loops and is lethal for hamsters. In contrast to the enterotoxins of *Vibrio cholerae* and *Escherichia coli,* toxin A appears to exert its effects through cytotoxicity and a resultant inflammatory response.[359] Toxin B, a potent cytotoxin, is less clearly implicated in disease, but detection of this toxin in stool specimens remains the best single laboratory test for *C. difficile* disease.[360] Toxin B cross-reacts with the toxin of *C. sordellii,* which was initially implicated as the cause of pseudomembranous colitis.[361] Both toxigenic and nontoxigenic strains coexist in the human intestine.[362] Recovery of the bacterium in culture is useful for demonstrating carriage in epidemiologic studies but is not sufficiently specific for use as a diagnostic test in human disease.[363]

C. difficile colonization and disease are nosocomial problems[364] because of their association with antimicrobial therapy. Pseudomembranous colitis has even occurred after administration of the antibiotics that are recommended for treatment of the infection.[365] The bacteria become widely distributed on environmental surfaces and on the hands of medical personnel.[364] It has been suggested that the organisms are often introduced into the hospital by newly admitted patients.[366] It should be remembered that chemotherapeutic agents with activity against indigenous stool flora include antineoplastic chemotherapeutic agents as well as traditional antibiotics.[367] Infection occurs rarely in the absence of administration of antimicrobial agents.[368]

Clinical features and pathology. Early in the course of illness pseudomembranous enterocolitis is characterized by fever, leukocytosis, and abdominal pain[369] that can mimic acute peritonitis.[370] The diarrhea is profuse, watery or mucoid, and foul smelling. Fecal leukocytes are present in approximately half of cases. The typical endoscopic appearance of the lesions is multiple small aphthous ulcerations (Fig. 33-26); the pseudomembranes may be overlooked when the ulcers are very small.[369] Microscopically the lesions are characterized by acute or chronic inflammatory exudate in the mucosa with overlying mucosal erosion but without true ulceration.[370] The

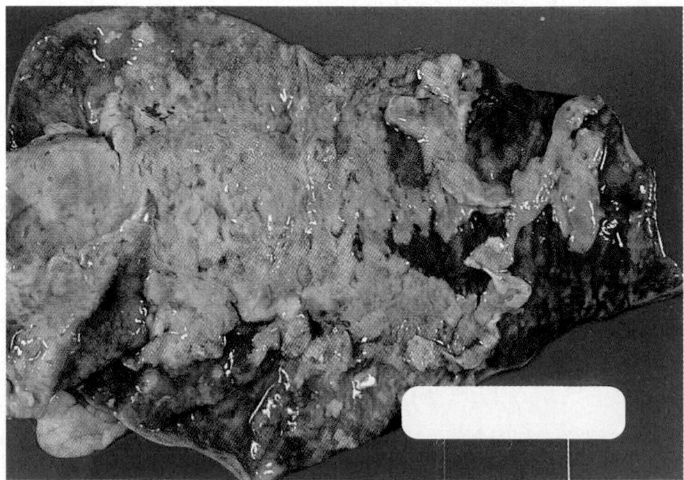

Fig. 33-26 Pseudomembranous colitis. Confluent, tenacious, yellow pseudomembranes cover the surface of the colon, which is dilated. (Courtesy Brenda Waters, MD.)

most characteristic feature is an eruptive pseudomembrane that spews from the inflamed mucosa like a fountain. Pseudomembranes may not be observed in biopsy specimens, however, even when they were visualized at endoscopy.[370] Crypt abscesses and vasculitis are not features of the disease. Massive edema of the intestinal wall has been described in a case of severe infection.[371] The differential diagnosis includes other inflammatory diseases of the intestine, particularly if the characteristic pseudomembranes are not present.[372] Chemical solutions used in cleaning endoscopes have produced mucosal ulcerations that mimicked pseudomembranous colitis.[373]

Relapses occur frequently in *C. difficile* gastroenteritis,[374] even after administration of the recommended therapy.[375] Extraintestinal infection is uncommon, but visceral abscesses have been reported.

Clostridium septicum

Clostridium septicum is a histotoxic *Clostridium* that has been increasingly recognized as a cause of severe, life-threatening disease. The infection may be acquired exogenously as a result of trauma[376] or after an injection.[377] More commonly, the source of a bacteremia is the GI tract, particularly in patients with neoplastic disease.[378] Diabetes and neutropenia are also risk factors. Metastatic, nontraumatic gas gangrene is a frequently lethal result of the bacteremia.[378] Bacteremia can result in other severe consequences, such as osteomyelitis, arthritis, endocarditis, pericarditis, mycotic aneurysm, and visceral abscesses. *C. septicum* is also a cause of necrotizing enterocolitis in neutropenic patients.[379] The pathologic hallmarks are gas production, tissue necrosis, and an inflammatory response that may be minimal (Figs. 33-27 and 33-28).

Bacillus species

Bacillus anthracis

Microbiology. *Bacillus anthracis*, a sporeforming, gram-positive bacillus, is the etiologic agent of anthrax. It is distinguished from other pathogenic *Bacillus* species by absence of motility and hemolysis, gelatine hydrolysis, and salicin fermentation.[172] *B. anthracis* contains two critically important virulence factors, both encoded by plasmids: a poly-D-glutamic acid capsule and a toxin that contains three components (protective antigen, edema factor, and lethal factor). Strains of *B. anthracis* that lack the gene for capsule formation have been recognized by phenotypic characteristics and confirmed by genetic analysis.[172]

Epidemiology and history. Anthrax is always an exogenous infection, contracted by contact with soil or animal products that are contaminated with spores. Simple contamination of soil is not sufficient for transmission of infection. Germination of spores with subsequent dissemination of spores appears to be important. It has been noted that particular microenvironments appear to harbor spores in a form that favors transmission to animals and potentially thereafter to humans. The resistance of anthrax spores to adverse environments and subsequent persistence in nature is illustrated by the story of Gruinard Island in Scotland.[41] During World War II the British, concerned about potential German germ warfare initiatives, exploded small bombs containing anthrax spores over an isolated island off the west coast of Scotland. Aerosols were observed passing over flocks of sheep that had been tethered downwind, and samples of soil had to be diluted for accurate counting of *B. anthracis* colonies on agar plates. The island was quarantined and monitored; by 1979, 36 years after contamination, the residual spores were still too numerous to use the island safely. Decontamination was finally attempted in the mid-1980s, and the island was finally declared free of anthrax in 1990.

Anthrax occurs in cutaneous, inhalational, and gastrointestinal forms. Cutaneous disease is by far the most common; inhalational and GI forms are rare. Humans are incidental hosts, infected by contact with contaminated animal materials. Direct contact with infected animals is the prime route for GI disease and is also a common means for transmission of spores to the skin. In addition, animal products, such as wool and hides, are frequently incriminated as sources of cutaneous anthrax, leading to the designation "bongo-drum disease."

Inhalational anthrax, a rapidly fatal infection in most cases, is the most dreaded form of the disease. Pulmonary anthrax, first recognized in industrial England during the nineteenth

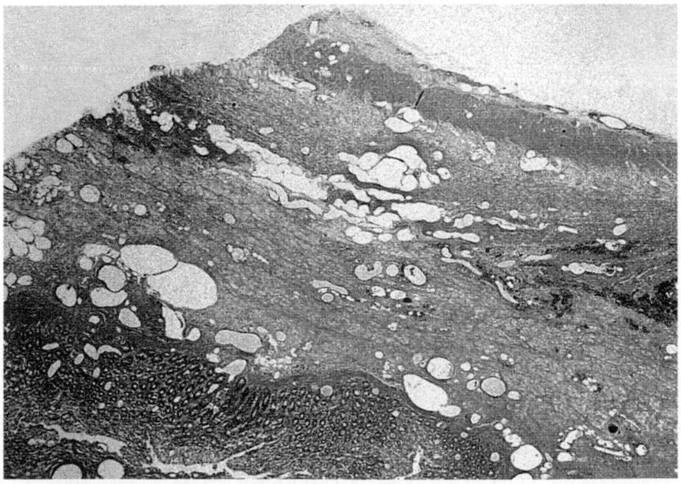

Fig. 33-27 Enteritis necroticans. This low-power view demonstrates extensive necrosis of the bowel wall, diffuse inflammation and edema, and dramatic formation of gas in the bowel wall. *Clostridium septicum* isolated from tissue. (Courtesy Stephen Allen, MD.)

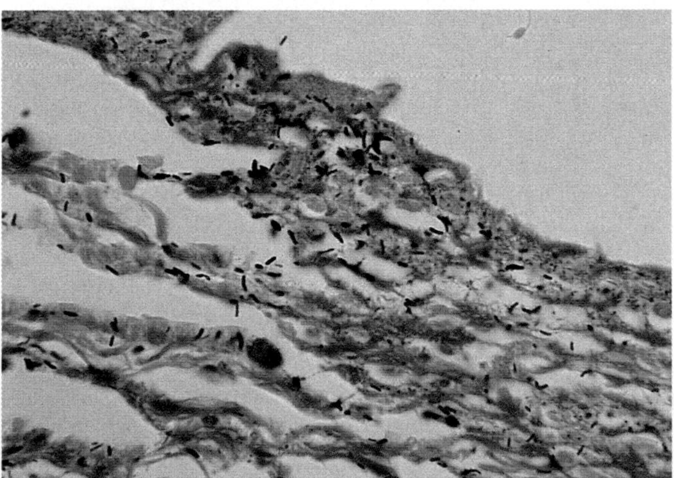

Fig. 33-28 Enteritis necroticans. Numerous gram-positive bacilli are evident in the serosal exudate of the lesion depicted in Fig. 33-38. (Brown-Hopps technique.) (Courtesy Stephen Allen, MD.)

century as an occupational disease of workers who processed contaminated wool, was named "woolsorters' disease."[380] Although rare, wool and fiber products continue to be risk factors for inhalational disease.[381] The last epidemic of inhalational anthrax in the United States occurred in workers who were indirectly exposed to contaminated wool.[382] The nefarious potential of the intrusion of governments into biology was illustrated by an epidemic of inhalational anthrax caused by an accident in a Russian germ warfare facility that did not officially exist.[383] After first denying the reports, the Russian government maintained that anthrax in Ekaterinburg (formerly Sverdlovsk and before that Ekaterinburg–microbiologic nomenclature is not the only unstable commodity!), a restricted security area, was gastrointestinal disease obtained by eating contaminated meat. It was not until after the dismantling of the Soviet Union that a team of Russian and American scientists was able to document the characteristic lesions of inhalational anthrax in pathologic specimens that had escaped destruction by the Soviet authorities.[384] Much of the modern knowledge of the pathogenesis of anthrax was born out of fear of the military uses of this bacterium.

Transmission of *B. anthracis* by flies and mosquitoes has been demonstrated in the laboratory, using experimental animals.[385] The importance of this method for transmission of infection has not been documented in nature. In the United States cutaneous anthrax is indigenous;[386] inhalational anthrax is extremely rare, and GI disease does not occur.

Pathogenesis. The pathogenesis of anthrax has engaged some of the best minds of science. Koch's recognition of the etiologic agent[387] led to his promulgation of the criteria for establishing a causal relationship between a microbe and a disease process that is now known as Koch's postulates.[388] Pasteur demonstrated the toxic basis of the infection.[389] Somewhat later Metchnikoff studied the relationship between the anthrax bacillus and macrophages.[390]

Strains of inbred mice differ in their susceptibility to the lethal toxin.[391] Part of the basis for susceptibility or resistance appears to reside in the interactions of anthrax bacillus with inflammatory cells. Delayed accumulation of PMNLs and macrophages, but not phagocytosis and killing of bacilli, was correlated with susceptibility to the Sterne vaccine strain in experimental animals.[392] The characteristics of the recruited macrophages also appear to be important. Purified toxin is lethal for macrophages from susceptible strains of inbred mice but not for macrophages from resistant strains.[393] Macrophages may also play a role in the expression of bacterial toxicity. The activity of lethal toxin in experimental animals is eliminated by reticuloendothelial blockade with silica and reconstituted by infusion of susceptible macrophages. Production of interleukin-1 but not tumor necrosis factor by the macrophages correlated with toxicity.[394]

A combination of protective antigen and edema factor (components of the anthrax toxin) suppresses the function of human PMNLs in vitro.[395] In experimental animals complement deficiency is associated with susceptibility to infection by the Sterne vaccine strain.[396]

The portal of entry for spores corresponds to the type of disease: cutaneous, pulmonary, or gastrointestinal. Bacteria may be introduced to the lips or eyebrows by rubbing with hands that are contaminated with spores.[397] The pathogenesis of anthrax includes spread of the bacteria from the portal of entry to regional lymph nodes through lymphatics. The role of macrophages in this process has been demonstrated experimentally.[398] Proliferation of bacilli in lymphatics and small blood vessels, thrombosis, edema, and necrosis — all features of human infection — have been documented as features of anthrax in experimental animals.[399]

Immunity to anthrax requires antibodies to the components of the toxin complex.[400] An immunologic response to the bacterial capsule does not appear to be necessary for immunity.

Clinical features and pathology. The characteristic features of anthrax are hemorrhage, edema, and necrosis at the portal of entry, in the regional lymph nodes, and in metastatic foci.[401] A "vasculitis" characterized by acellular proliferation of bacilli in the walls of blood vessels and luminal thrombosis is often observed. Aggregations of bacilli in lymphatics may be difficult to distinguish from vascular involvement of arterioles and venules.[397] Neutrophilic infiltration of the lesions is usually inconspicuous. Cutaneous anthrax in humans assumes two forms. The first is a necrotic sore that is caused by vascular thrombosis, hemorrhage, and acellular necrosis. The lesion often heals spontaneously without a scar. The second form begins as a blister, resembling a thermal burn, and is followed by extensive edema and tissue necrosis. Microscopically, there is massive edema of the epidermis, upper dermis, and interstitium. Collagen fibers are dramatically separated. Thrombosis of blood vessels is not accompanied by a prominent inflammatory response. The cutaneous lesions are sometimes described as carbuncles, (Fig. 33-29), but they in no way resemble true carbuncles, which are aggregations of abscesses.[397] Involvement of the eyes may result in corneal scarring.[402] Extension of the bacteria through the lymphatics results in regional lymphadenopathy with

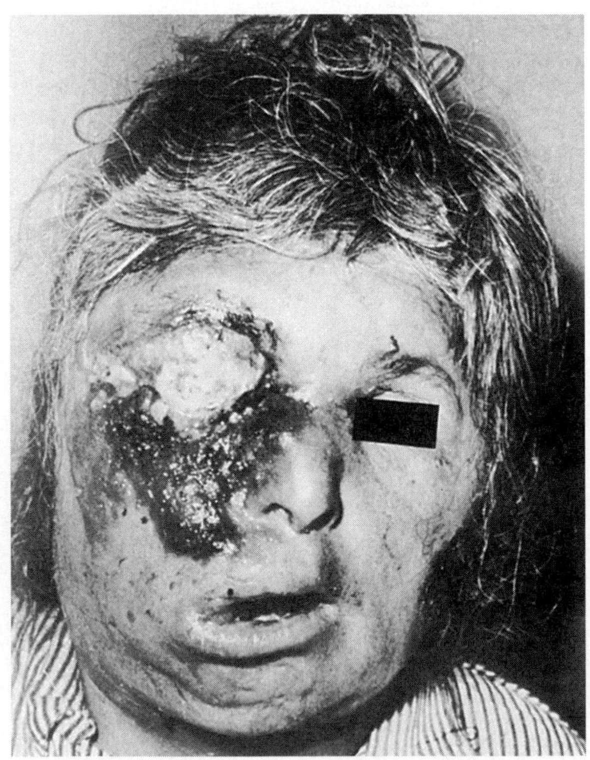

Fig. 33-29 Anthrax. Severe malignant pustule. (From Dutz W: *Int Pathol* 8:38, 1967.)

extensive hemorrhagic lymphadenitis. The differential diagnosis of necrotic cutaneous lesions after exposure to animals includes cowpox[403] and orf.[404]

Pulmonary anthrax results from inhalation of infectious aerosols. The bacteria are rapidly transmitted to the mediastinum, where a hemorrhagic exudate occurs in soft tissue and lymph nodes. At one time massive pulmonary hemorrhage and edema were considered secondary to mediastinal disease,[397] but recent observations on cases from the Sverdlovsk epidemic indicate that primary focal, necrotizing pneumonia may be common.[384]

Gastrointestinal anthrax is characterized by mucosal edema with numerous small necrotic ulcers and massive fluid loss.[405] Hemorrhagic lymphadenitis in the mesenteric lymph nodes results from spread of the bacilli through regional lymphatics.[397]

An unusual variant of anthrax involving the tongue, nasopharynx, and tonsil has been described.[406] A primary erosion, which may covered by a membrane, is followed by regional edema and hemorrhagic lymphadenopathy. Edema of the neck and anterior chest may be massive.[407]

Septicemia may follow any type of primary infection but is most common after inhalational anthrax. The most serious complication is anthrax meningitis, which is also manifested by hemorrhage, rather than cellular inflammation[384] (Fig. 33-30). Multiple erosions of the GI tract may result after dissemination from a pulmonary focus.[384]

Bacillus cereus

Microbiology. *Bacillus cereus* is a sporeforming gram-positive bacillus that is motile and produces hemolysis on sheep blood agar. Definitive identification of *Bacillus* species is difficult. The tendency of *Bacillus* species to decolorize easily leads to confusion with nonfermentative gram-negative bacilli.[408] The organism produces an enterotoxin, an emetic toxin, protease, and hemolysins.[409] The role of the enterotoxin and emetic toxin in human disease is better delineated than is the contribution of the other factors.

Epidemiology. *B. cereus* does not have the historic fearfulness of the anthrax bacillus, but its frequent presence in the environment and among the fecal flora[410] makes it a more common pathogen than *B. anthracis* in the developed world. It has been suggested that the intestinal carriage is transient and related to ingestion of bacilli or spores in foodstuffs.[411] Gastrointestinal disease is associated with ingestion of contaminated foods, which include meats, dairy products, and vegetables.[412] Traumatic infections, which are particularly common in the eye, result from introduction of environmental spores.[413] Nosocomial infections associated with medical devices probably have an exogenous source.[414] Intravenous inoculation of spores by users of illicit drugs or contaminated intravenous catheters represent another route for environmental spores to gain access to tissues. The portal of entry for many infections is unclear, with the gastrointestinal tract being a likely source. Bacteremia results in metastatic disease in many organs. Patients with neoplastic disease or neutropenia are at increased risk of serious infection.[415] Recovery from bacteremic infection has correlated temporally with recovery of neutrophils in addition to appropriate antimicrobial therapy.[416]

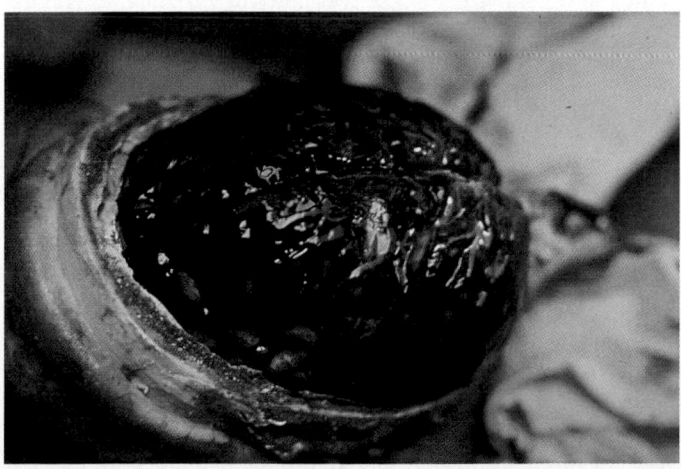

Fig. 33-30 Inhalation anthrax with dissemination. Extensive cerebral hemorrhage is evident after removal of the cranium. Case from the Sverdlovsk outbreak. (Courtesy David Walker, MD, Galveston, Tex.)

Clinical features and pathology. *B. cereus* food poisoning is usually a mild and self-limited disease.[417] The emetic form, which is particularly associated with contaminated fried rice,[418] has an incubation period of 1 to 6 hours, resembling staphylococcal food poisoning. The diarrheal form has an incubation period of 10 to 12 hours and resembles *Clostridium perfringens* gastroenteritis.

Invasive infections are characterized by a fulminant course, extensive destruction of tissue, and high mortality. The clinical syndrome of gas gangrene (myonecrosis) produced by *B. cereus* resembles clostridial infection, including the presence of gram-positive bacilli in the lesions.[419] Primary vesicular or pustular lesions of the skin have been reported in neutropenic children who were being treated for neoplastic disease.[415] Endophthalmitis is characterized by extensive destruction, sometimes with gas formation, and frequent loss of visual acuity.[413] Pneumonia may be accompanied by massive hemoptysis or cavitation.[420]

Bacteremia results in endovascular infection on native or prosthetic valves[421] and metastatic disease, including meningitis and osteomyelitis. The mortality of disseminated infection is high. Severe pneumonia and meningoencephalitis have been described in the neonatal period.[422]

Bacillus *subtilis*

Bacillus subtilis infections are of two basic types. The first, disseminated infection with or without metastatic disease is similar to the infections produced by *B. cereus.* Septicemia may be followed by endocarditis, meningitis, or osteomyelitis. The second form is a hypersensitivity pneumonitis as a reaction to vegetative and spore forms of the bacterium.[423]

Lactobacillus *species*

Lactobacilli are thin, nonsporulating, gram-positive bacilli that often form chains in broth culture. They are normal constituents of the mouth, intestine, and vagina, where it is the predominant genus.[424] Infections are most commonly related to the female genital tract, including chorioamnionitis and postpartum bacteremia.[425] Invasive infection also occurs adjacent to the oral cavity, often as a mixed infection.[426] The bacteremia is usually transient or responsive to commonly used antibiotics. Occasionally, however, visceral infection may result and serious neonatal infection, such as meningitis, is a rare complication.

GRAM-NEGATIVE COCCI

Neisseria *species*

Neisseria species are aerobic gram-negative diplococci that are nutritionally fastidious and require additional CO_2 for growth.[172] Primates are the only reservoir for the bacteria, and so neither the animate nor the inanimate environment plays a substantial role in maintenance or transmission. The two most important species in the genus are *Neisseria meningitidis* (meningococcus) and *Neisseria gonorrhoeae* (gonococcus). Both species are damaged by cold, and specimens should not be refrigerated before processing. They are also lethally damaged by desiccation. The gonococcus is an important cause of morbidity but rarely causes lethal infection, whereas meningococci cause disease uncommonly in developed countries but can produce devastating infection. The preferred medium is enriched chocolate agar. When specimens from mucosal surfaces are cultured, a selective medium with antibiotics should be inoculated to suppress growth of faster growing commensal flora. Some strains of *N. gonorrhoeae* are susceptible to vancomycin, which is commonly employed, and so inoculation of both selective and nonselective media is recommended.

Many of the pathogenetic mechanisms and virulence factors have already been discussed. The subject has been well reviewed by Brittigan and colleagues.[427] In summary, the important features include adherence to epithelium and inflammatory cells, resistance to phagocytosis, lipopolysaccharide (endotoxin), and resistance to the bactericidal activity of serum. The ability of pili to mediate adherence of gonococci to motile sperm[428] provides a vehicle for delivery of bacteria to multiple sites. The capsular serogroup and serotype have been associated with virulence in some studies;[429] unencapsulated meningococcal strains are rarely incriminated in disease. Pathogenic species of Neisseria produce IgA protease,[430] though the pathogenetic importance of this enzyme has been challenged. A major iron-regulated protein found in pathogenic species may also be important in the pathogenesis of infection.[431]

The initial phases of infection (as opposed to colonization) are characterized by local inflammation and mucosal damage.[432] The serious consequences of bacteremic infection, including shock and disseminated intravascular coagulation, derive from the action of bacterial lipopolysaccharide.[433]

Neisseria meningitidis

Epidemiology and pathogenesis. *N. meningitidis* is serologically defined by the capsular polysaccharide, the most important being groups A to C, X to Z, and W135. Meningococcal disease can occur sporadically or in epidemics. Infection is worldwide, but disease is concentrated in certain geographic areas, particularly in developing countries.[434] Individuals with complement deficiency,[62] and some patients with anatomic or functional asplenia[106] are at increased risk of infection. Physical crowding and close contact of susceptible individuals is a risk factor for both infection and epidemic disease.[435] A major factor appears to be the presence of serum bactericidal antibody; ironically nonbactericidal IgA antibodies may block the beneficial effect of coexisting bactericidal antibody.[436] Griffiss has proposed an interesting hypothetical model of epidemic meningococcal infection.[437] He suggests that enteric bacteria elicit an IgA antibody response that cross-reacts with *N. meningitidis* after transient colonization of the bowel. If an individual with predominantly IgM antibody encounters a meningococcal strain while IgA antibody circulates, the bactericidal activity of the IgM antibody is blocked and bacteremic infection results. Although most meningococcal infections are acquired in the community, nosocomial[438] or laboratory acquired[439] infections have been described.

The carrier state is an important factor in the epidemiology of meningococcal infections.[440] The rate of nasopharyngeal carriage is higher in close contacts of patients with meningococcal disease than in individuals with casual contact,[441] supporting the concept that transmission of the bacteria in nature is maintained through close association with colonized individuals. Although acquisition of an epidemic strain by a susceptible individual may increase the risk of infection, acquisition of a nonepidemic strain at other times may elicit antibodies, which may provide protection against subsequent encounters with pathogenic strains.[442] *N. meningitidis* has been isolated rarely from the uterus and cervix.[443]

Clinical features and pathology. Clinical disease that has been associated with *N. meningitidis* covers the range from subclinical infection to rapidly fatal septicemia.[435]

Bacteremia without sepsis or meningitis presents as a clinically undifferentiated febrile illness or may be dominated by symptoms referable to a nonneural organ. Bacteremia may be protracted.[444] Disease may be mild and may even resolve without antimicrobial therapy.[445] Isolation of meningococci from blood is often a surprise for everyone involved. Primary meningococcal pneumonia is indistinguishable from other bacterial pneumonias. Isolation of meningococci from the sputum must be evaluated critically because of the carriage state. The presence of a typable (encapsulated) strain increases the likelihood that there is an etiologic association. Group Y strains have been particularly associated with pneumonia. Meningococcal cardiac disease presents most commonly as pericarditis, sometimes complicated by tamponade. It has been suggested that group C strains are especially likely to produce this syndrome.[446] Meningococcal endocarditis has also been described. Septic arthritis may be a feature of more complicated meningococcal infection but also occurs as an isolated clinical problem. The disease is usually monoarticular with the knee joint most commonly involved. A maculopapular rash may accompany the arthritis, producing a clinical disease that is indistinguishable from disseminated gonococcal infection with arthritis.[447] When the source of the meningococci is the uterine cervix, the presumed cause may be disseminated gonococcal infection until final identification of the isolates is made in the microbiology laboratory.[443] It has been suggested that the relative frequency of arthritis caused by these two species is shifting. Rarely, meningococci may produce symptomatic disease of the urogenital system.[448]

Meningococcemia with sepsis is a frightening disease because of the rapidity of progression, the severity of sepsis, and the dramatic presentation of widespread hemorrhage (purpura fulminans). It has been suggested that the pathogenesis of the lesions are twofold: direct bacterial damage to the endothelium, resulting in fibrin, leukocyte and platelet thrombi, and disseminated intravascular coagulation from activation of the clotting system.[449] Mortality remains greater than 50% even with modern medical techniques.[450] Poor prognosis is related to the presence of fibrin split products in the circulation, the degree to which fibrinogen and protein C are depressed,[451] and minimal leukocytosis in the spinal fluid.[450] It has been suggested that the severity of infection in young children is related to the immaturity of the protein C system.[451] Widespread microvascular coagulation may result in coagulative necrosis of tissue, including necrosis of skin and autoamputation of digits[451] (Figs. 33-31 and 33-32). Similar necrotic lesions in the adrenal cortex in combination with sepsis produce the Waterhouse-Friderichsen syndrome.[452] Although this dramatic result is uncommon and has been deemphasized, adrenal necrosis continues to complicate meningococcal sepsis.[453] The Waterhouse-Friderichsen syndrome is not specific for meningococcal infection, having been reported in pneumococcal[454] and *Haemophilus influenzae* sepsis.[124] Bilateral renal cortical necrosis, reminiscent of the generalized Shwartzman

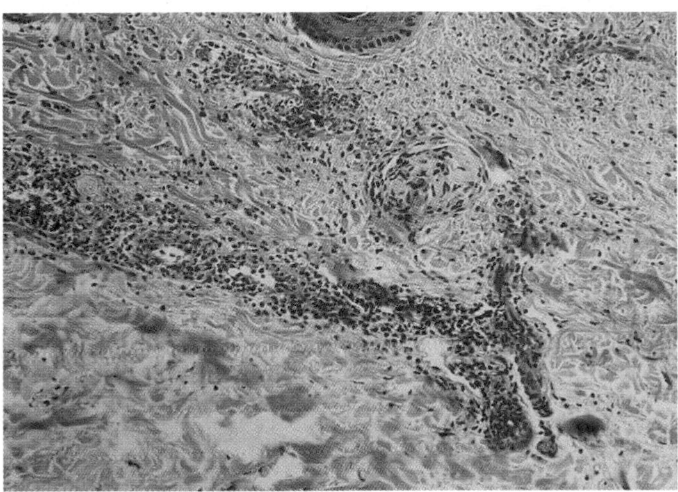

Fig. 33-31 Meningococcal vasculitis. Small blood vessels in the skin are infiltrated by an acute inflammatory exudate. Fibrin thrombi were present in other arterioles. The intravascular coagulation may result both from gram-negative endotoxin in the bacteria and from local endothelial damage. *Neisseria meningitidis* isolated from blood.

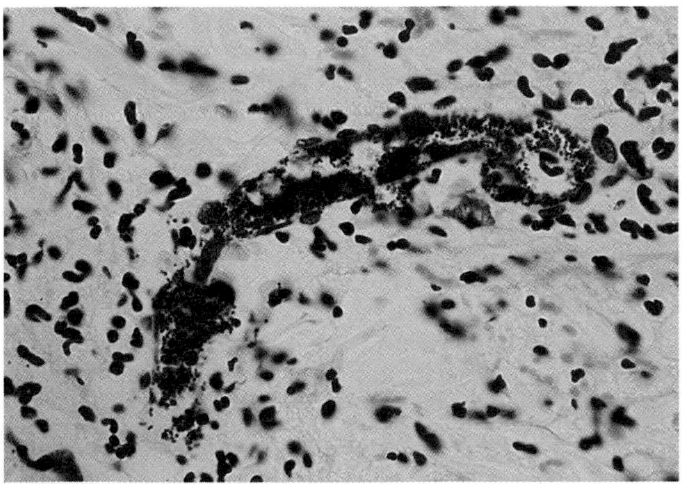

Fig. 33-32 Meningococcal vasculitis. Gram-negative diplococci are demonstrated in the arteriolar lesion illustrated in Fig. 33-31. (Brown-Hopps technique.)

reaction,[455] and splenic rupture have also been reported as complications.

Meningitis, which may occur with or without sepsis, is the second dreaded complication of bacteremia.[456] Spinal fluid pleocytosis may be delayed, and the first sample examined may contain viable bacteria in the absence of inflammatory cells. The prognosis is considerably worsened when parenchymal damage from vasculitis or thrombosis occurs.

The clinical presentation of meningococcal disease may be distinctive when purpura fulminans occurs. The pathologic findings are similarly distinctive but not diagnostic. Additional causes of vasculitis must be considered. Inflammatory lesions other than vasculitis are undifferentiated.

Neisseria gonorrhoeae

Epidemiology. Gonorrhea is a sexually transmitted infection. Without a reservoir in the animate or inanimate environment and without prolonged colonization of extragenital sites, the epidemiology is dominated by contact with genital secretions.[457] Although some of the risk factors that pertain to meningococcal infection, such as complement deficiency, pertain to gonorrhea also, the number of sexual partners and frequency of intercourse are much more important. Gonococcal infections are correspondingly concentrated in sexually active adolescents and young adults of any sexual preference. Immunity to infection appears to be specific for the infecting strain,[458] and repeat infections are common in patients who have preexisting antibody from a previous infection.[459] The tragic innocent victims in the scenario are children who have been sexually abused and the fetus or neonate who is infected during the birth process.

The potential reservoirs of bacteria and sites for new infection are defined by the presence of columnar epithelium. Transmission of infection, the portal of entry, and the site of initial infection are defined by the nature of the contact with secretions. Thus the most common manifestation of infection is cervicitis in the female and urethritis in either sex. The rectum and pharynx can be infected in either sex after rectal or oral intercourse.

Asymptomatic infection has been recognized in the female patient for years, but appreciation of asymptomatic urethral infection in the male has come more recently.[460] These individuals are the primary source for new infections, perhaps because symptomatic individuals are more likely to modify their sexual practices.[460] After a single sexual contact with an infected partner the risk of acquiring genital gonorrhea has been estimated to be 20% in men and up to 50% in women.[461] After multiple contacts the risk approaches 80%to 90% in both sexes.

Clinical features and pathology. The most common lesions in gonococcal infection are acute urethritis accompanied by dysuria, pyuria, and frequency (the acute urethral syndrome) and cervicitis. A neutrophilic exudate can be expressed from the urethra. In the male the presence of neutrophils with *intracellular* gram-negative diplococci in a urethral exudate is diagnostic of *N. gonorrhoeae* infection. The cervical infection is characterized by neutrophilic, lymphocytic, and plasmacytic inflammation, often mild, in the lumen, epithelium, or submucosa of the squamocolumnar junction.[462] Focal epithelial necrosis and reactive cellular atypia are present. The differential diagnosis includes other cervical pathogens, primarily *Chlamydia trachomatis* and herpes simplex virus. Reactive lymphoid follicles are more common in chlamydial infection, and mucosal ulceration is more characteristic of herpes infection than of gonorrhea.[462] Anorectal infection is more common in homosexual men than in women. The histologic features are entirely nonspecific, manifesting as acute and chronic inflammation.[463]

Infection of the upper genital tract is a complication in both sexes but particularly in women (pelvic inflammatory disease).[464] Endometritis and salpingitis carry the potentially serious consequence of tubo-ovarian abscess, usually caused by a mixture of aerobic and anaerobic vaginal bacteria. Damage to the ciliated epithelium of the fallopian tube may result in infertility or ectopic tubal pregnancy. In the young, sexually active man acute epididymitis is the corresponding complication.[465] A less common complication of upper tract infection is infection of the hepatic capsule (perihepatitis, or Fitz-Hugh–Curtis syndrome).[466] This syndrome is usually seen in women but has been documented in men.[467] The major differential diagnosis of upper tract infections is *Chlamydia trachomatis* infection.

Pharyngeal infection with *N. gonorrhoeae* occurs in both females and homosexual males and is correlated with the practice of fellatio.[468] Interestingly, clinical pharyngitis is also correlated with fellatio but not with gonococcal infection of the pharynx, an indication that other sexually transmitted pathogens might be involved. It has also been suggested that "French kissing" may transmit gonococcal infection, but the data are inconclusive.[469]

Pediatric infection is primarily manifested as gonococcal ophthalmia neonatorum,[470] which has been virtually eliminated with routine use of antimicrobial therapy to the eyes of newborn infants. A variety of other bacteria may produce neonatal ocular infection, but the primary concern is *Chlamydia trachomatis*. Erythromycin prophylaxis has been instituted as a means of controlling both chlamydial and gonococcal infection.[471] Rarely, ocular infection may occur in adults.[472] The inflammatory response is similar to that in the genital tract—neutrophilic exudate with intracellular gram-negative diplococci, but infection with minimal inflammation has also been described.[473]

Disseminated gonococcal infection is uncommon.[474] Paradoxically, disseminated infection usually occurs in patients without genital symptoms; in women dissemination occurs more commonly during pregnancy or the menstrual period than at other times, an indication of the importance of hormonal influences. The strains encountered in disseminated infection are resistant to the bactericidal action of human serum, whereas those that produce localized genital infection are susceptible.[39] Phagocytosis and bactericidal action by PMNLs is also less effective against serum-resistant strains than their susceptible counterparts.[475] Serum resistance is correlated with the presence of outer membrane protein-1 and the presence of certain physiologic characteristics (auxotypes).[39] The circle of correlations between auxotypes and clinical disease is completed when one notes that strains with similar physiologic profiles are more common in asymptomatic than in symptomatic men[476,477] and that these auxotypes are uncommonly found in homosexual men, who also have a decreased frequency of disseminated infection.[478]

The most frequent consequence of gonococcal dissemination is arthritis, which occurs in two clinical forms.[479] One group of patients experiences fever and chills, polyarticular arthritis or arthralgias, usually in small joints, that may be accompanied by tenosynovitis, and cutaneous lesions. The characteristic skin lesion is an erythematous papule surmounted by a hemorrhagic or vesiculopustular lesion. Gonococci are frequently isolated from blood but not from skin or joints. Gram-negative diplococci and PMNLs are present in the skin lesions. Isolation of cell wall–deficient gonococci from "sterile" skin lesions has been reported.[474] The second group of patients experience asymptomatic bacteremia followed by monoarticular arthritis, usually in large joints. The arthritis is accompanied by effusion, and gonococci can often be isolated from the acutely inflamed synovial fluid. Both types of clinical presentation may occur in the same patient,[474] and the presentation may include both pharyngitis and arthritis.[480] A syndrome of arthritis and skin rash that mimics disseminated gonococcal infection may be produced by *N. meningitidis*.[448] Additional complications of disseminated infection include meningitis, myocarditis, pericarditis, and endocarditis.[474] Gonococcal endocarditis is uncommon but is frequently accompanied by abscesses and destruction of the involved valve.[481]

Moraxella catarrhalis

Moraxella catarrhalis is a gram-negative diplococcus that was formerly classified as *Branhamella catarrhalis* and still earlier as *Neisseria catarrhalis*. Some strains share potential virulence characteristics with the pathogenic *Neisseria* species.[482] This organism colonizes the oropharynx, particularly in children and the elderly, and it produces infection most commonly in the respiratory tract. *M. catarrhalis* has been added to the list of pathogens that cause otitis media[483] and sinusitis. Lower respiratory infection may be manifested as tracheitis or pneumonia,[484] which can be acquired in the community or in the hospital. Localized infection may result in bacteremic disease.[485] Although systemic infection occurs in normal people, it has been suggested that immunosuppression may be a risk factor for dissemination.[486] Neonatal conjunctivitis mimicking gonococcal ophthalmia has been reported.[487]

GRAM-NEGATIVE BACILLI

Enterobacteriaceae

Members of the Enterobacteriaceae are a diverse group of organisms that are genetically related and share certain characteristics: plump gram-negative bacilli of short-to-moderate length, fermentation of glucose, reduction of nitrate to nitrite, and absence of cytochrome oxidase.[172] The family is divided into tribes, genera, and species (Table 33-7).

Members of the family are facultative anaerobes and grow rapidly on the surface of enriched media and agars that are selective for gram-negative bacilli. The identification of isolates is made primarily when one defines the biochemical profile, but serologic analysis is also important for identification of *Salmonella* species and *Shigella* species. In addition, characterization of the antigenic profile may be useful for other genera, particularly *Yersinia*.

Escherichia coli

The most important pathogen in the genus Escherichia is *E. coli*, for many years the only member of the genus. Other species are encountered rarely in clinical materials.

Epidemiology. *E. coli* is the member of the Enterobacteriaceae that is most commonly isolated from patients in devel-

Table 33-7 Enterobacteriaceae

Tribe	Genera
Escherichiae	Escherichia, Shigella
Edwardsiellae	Edwardsiella
Salmonellae	Salmonella
Citrobactereae	Citrobacter
Klebsielleae	Klebsiella
	Enterobacter
	Pantoea
	Hafnia
	Serratia
Proteeae	Proteus
	Morganella
	Providencia
Yersinieae	Yersina
Erwinieae	Erwinia

oped countries. Its predominance among gram-negative bacilli as a pathogen is reflected in the old classification, in which *E. coli* was designated the colon bacillus and other members of the family were paracolon bacilli. As the name implies, *E. coli* is a part of the normal intestinal flora and may also be found in the genitourinary system. Colonization of mucosal surfaces begins soon after birth, with strains coming both from the GI tract of the mother and from the environment.[488]

E. coli produces infections with contrasting characteristics: nosocomial versus community acquired and endogenous versus exogenous. Any combination of patterns may occur.

Community-acquired infections are primarily urogenital or gastrointestinal. The source of the pathogen for the urinary tract infections is usually endogenous, with the portal of entry being from colonizing flora in the vagina or on the perineum with subsequent migration up the urethra.[489]

The source of GI infections is almost always contaminated food or water.[490,491] Cases may be sporadic or part of an epidemic. Enterotoxigenic strains are particularly prevalent in developing countries and a common cause of traveler's diarrhea.[492] Colorful vernacular names have been applied to this discomforting condition, such as "Montezuma's revenge," *"La tourista,"* or "Delhi belly." Sporadic infections have been described in some populations in the United States, and epidemic disease associated with contaminated water has also occurred.[491] Enteropathogenic and enteroinvasive disease is likewise found frequently in developing countries but also afflicts individuals in developed countries.

The reservoir for the verotoxin-producing strains that cause hemorrhagic diarrhea and hemolytic-uremic syndrome (HUS) appears to be cattle.[493] National attention was drawn to the disease by an epidemic in Washington state that was associated with undercooked hamburgers.[494] Infection has been frequently associated with hamburger, which is prepared from multiple animals, but epidemics have not been associated with unground beef. The association with beef is not absolute, however, because outbreaks have been associated with freshly pressed apple cider.[495] Subsequently, it was recognized that sporadic infection by these verotoxin-producing strains was also common, at least in some geographic areas.[496] Children are at higher risk than adults of developing HUS, a potentially fatal complication,[497] but fatal disease has also been described in the elderly.[498]

Serious systemic infections, other than pyelonephritis, occur in neonates and infants, manifested primarily by meningitis,[499] and in patients of any age who have compromised host defenses. Underlying conditions include HIV infection, neoplasia, and infections of the abdomen and urinary tract. Individuals who have mucocutaneous defects at the site of a primary infection are at increased risk, as are those who have serious underlying conditions, such as alcoholism or diabetes.[500] Iatrogenic infection may result from instrumentation or insertion of medical devices or from transfusion of contaminated blood products.[501] Patients at risk of pyelonephritis are a subset of those who are likely to develop infections in the lower urinary tract.[57] The prognosis in patients with bacteremia is better if the source of the infection is the urinary tract than other sources.[502] Recovery is less likely if the patient is neutropenic or septicemic.[502,503]

Pathogenesis. Virulence factors in *E. coli* vary with the clinical setting.[504] Factors that promote adhesion to host cells are important in the GI tract[505] and in the urinary system.[506] Adhesins include type 1 fimbriae (inhibited by mannose) and P fimbriae (resistant to mannose). Antigenic variants of type 1 pili mediate the attachment of enteropathogenic and enterotoxigenic strains.[507] The adherence factor for verotoxin-producing strains is a surface structure other than fimbriae;[508] the cell receptor is globotriosylceramide and galabiosylceramide.[509]

The P fimbriae are clearly important for adherence to uroepithelial cells[510] but not for adherence in the GI tract.[508] Mannose-resistant adhesins are represented with significantly increased frequency in strains that have produced pyelonephritis in comparison with fecal strains.[510] The P designation derives from the adherence of the pili to erythrocytes that contain the human P blood group. The receptor for P fimbriae is galactose α1-4–galactose β.[511]

Outer membrane protein, lipopolysaccharide (O), flagellar (H), and capsular (K) antigens are important in the pathogenesis of *E. coli* infections. Certain of the capsular types cross-react with the capsular polysaccharide of *Neisseria meningitidis*[512,513] and *Haemophilus influenzae*.[514] The K1 capsular antigen appears to be an important virulence factor for strains that produce meningitis and septicemia in neonates.[515] This capsular type is also a common cause of invasive infections in adults,[516] but in one study K1 antigen was associated with a decreased likelihood of fatal infection.[517] An antigen related to the Vi capsular antigen of *Salmonella typhi* has been found in strains of *E. coli* that caused an epidemic of infantile diarrhea.[518] The association of certain enteropathogenic strains of *E. coli* with O antigens is correlated, at least in part, with adhesins that are determined by plasmid genes.[519]

A diverse group of enterotoxins is critical in the pathogenesis of GI disease; the characteristics of the toxin play a major role in defining the clinical features of the infection. There is a genetic relationship between strains that produce infantile diarrhea without the production of toxins and toxin-producing strains that cause hemorrhagic diarrhea, an indication that acquisition of additional virulence factors (toxins) may have enhanced the pathogenicity of already virulent strains.[520] Enterotoxins are primarily associated with GI infection, but they have been demonstrated also in bacteremic isolates.[521]

Other factors that have been suggested to be important in virulence of *E. coli* include iron-binding compounds (aerobactins) and resistance to the lethal activity of serum. The serum resistance appears to be related to the expression of K1 antigen in those strains.[522] The presence of aerobactin correlated with the presence of P fimbriae in one study, highlighting the difficulty of assigning a causative role to individual virulence factors in a complex biologic system.[523] The variety of mechanisms that this versatile pathogen employs in the production of GI disease are described as enterotoxic, enteropathogenic (enteroadherent), enteroinvasive, and enteroaggregative.

Enterotoxic Escherichia coli (ETEC) strains exert their effects primarily through the production of two types of toxins.[22] Heat-labile toxins (LT) are similar in mechanism of action to the toxin of *Vibrio cholerae,* exerting their effects on the GI tract by activation of adenylate and guanylate cyclases. LT can be demonstrated by the morphologic changes that they elicit in certain tissue culture cells in vitro or by the fluid secretion that they promote in isolated segments of rabbit ileum in vivo. A second class of enterotoxins is heat stable (ST) and exerts its effects through the guanidylate cyclase system in enterocytes.[524] Individual strains may secrete either toxin or both together. The net effect of the secreted toxins is to stimulate the secretion of water and sodium from the small intestine, producing a watery, noninflammatory diarrhea similar to that seen in cholera. These toxins are carried on plasmids that can be passed from one strain to another. Similar toxins have been found in *Klebsiella*[525] and *Citrobacter.*[526]

Enteropathogenic or *enteroadherent Escherichia coli* (EPEC),[505] which have defined serologic profiles (based on cell wall, flagellar, and capsular antigens), were identified as causes of epidemic gastroenteritis, primarily causing disease in newborn infants. These strains adhere to HeLa or HEp-2 cells with a localized or diffuse pattern.[527] The genetic material for the adherence-and-effacement phenomenon is located on bacterial plasmids.

Enteroinvasive Escherichia coli (EIEC)[528] are not content to produce their damage on the epithelial cell surface. Rather they invade and migrate through the epithelial cell, much as *Shigella* species do. The resultant acute inflammatory process including PMNLs may be associated with deep tissue invasion and bacteremia. These strains are also associated with certain serotypes. The invasive potential can be demonstrated by the Sereny test,[529] in which a bacterial suspension is instilled into the eye of a rabbit, with the other eye serving as a control. EPEC or ETEC will produce no visible effect, but EIEC strains will invade the conjunctival epithelial cells and produce an acute inflammatory response, which subsequently resolves. The genetic material for these traits is contained both on the bacterial chromosome and on plasmids.

Enterohemorrhagic Escherichia coli (EHEC) strains produce two toxins, which resemble the shigatoxin of *Shigella dysenteriae* (*Shigella*-like toxins, SLT1 and SLT2).[530] The toxins damage the intestinal mucosa and result in an inflammatory diarrhea, which is often hemorrhagic. These enterotoxins produce morphologic changes in certain continuous cell lines, such as HeLa and Vero, and are sometimes referred to as "verotoxins." The production of SLT1 and SLT2 is primarily associated with serotype O157:H7, the serotype responsible for illness attributable to undercooked hamburger,[531] but toxin is also produced by nonmotile O157 strains and by other serotypes.[532] *Shigella*-like toxins have also been described in *Citrobacter freundii* isolated from both humans and beef.[533] A strain of *C. freundii* that shared the O157 antigen has also been described.[534] Fortunately, the predominant O157:H7 strains of *E. coli* fail to ferment sorbitol, an unusual biochemical profile that provides a convenient screening test in the microbiology laboratory.[535] Direct detection of toxin in stool has the advantage that it is not limited to a single serotype,[532] but the technique is not widely available.

Enteroaggregative Escherichia coli (EAggEC) cause aggregation of masses of bacteria to the surfaces of cells or glass.[505] Persistent diarrhea has been associated with enteroaggregative strains,[536] but their position as pathogens is still unclear.

Clinical features and pathology. The clinical presentation and pathology of systemic and urinary *E. coli* infections are nonspecific. Apart from the clinical setting there are no distinguishing features. Infections of individual organs are covered in those respective chapters. It is interesting to note that strains of *E. coli* that are isolated from patients with cystic fibrosis may have the mucoid characteristics normally associated with *Pseudomonas aeruginosa.*[537] The features of GI infection depend on the operative pathogenic mechanisms. As expected, the enterotoxigenic strains produce a watery outpouring of fluid into the GI tract, and the clinical presentation can mimic cholera. The pathologic lesion is rarely seen, but the ileum of rabbits used for toxin assay demonstrates no morphologic abnormalities. The presentation of infection with enteropathogenic strains is similar. The cellular lesion in these infections is an effacement of the cell surface with a flattening of the absorptive microvilli, but the morphology is rarely visualized. The clinical features of enteroinvasive infection were delineated during an outbreak of *E. coli* dysentery associated with consumption of French Camembert cheese.[538] Patients experienced moderate fever, tenesmus, and cramping. The diarrhea was watery, though increased numbers of PMNLs were observed microscopically. Bloody stools were decidedly unusual, even in patients who had been instructed to look for this feature. Tissue for pathologic examination was not available, but the Sereny test was positive. In addition, fluid accumulation in isolated rabbit ileal loops was demonstrated after inoculation of isolates, corresponding to the watery character of the diarrhea in the patients.

In contrast, the enterohemorrhagic strains produce a profuse diarrhea that is bloody in at least 75% of patients.[498] In contrast to shigellosis, fever is an uncommon sign in hemorrhagic *E. coli* gastroenteritis.[496] The pathologic lesion produced by verotoxin-producing *E. coli* varies from mild, nonspecific inflammation to severe colitis, similar to that produced by *Shigella, Salmonella,* or *Campylobacter* species.[539] The right colon was most severely affected by patchy mucosal ulceration, hemorrhage, neutrophilic inflammation, and microvascular thrombi. Pseudomembranes similar to those produced by *Clostridium difficile* are present, but inconspicuous. Resolving lesions are characterized by plasmacytic infiltration of the submucosa and regeneration of the surface epithelium.[539]

Verotoxin-producing *E. coli* share with *Shigella* species the dubious distinction of causing HUS and thrombotic thrombocytopenic purpura. These severe, often fatal complications are primarily associated with serotype O157:H7,[531] but other serotypes have been implicated.[497] The pathologic features of the GI lesions resemble those seen in patients with bloody diarrhea alone.[540] A single case of hemorrhagic cystitis and balanitis caused by verotoxin-producing *E. coli* has been described.[541]

Shigella *species*

Microbiology. Bacilli of the genus *Shigella* cause bacillary dysentery, a worldwide disease that is included with infections by campylobacters, salmonellae, and *Escherichia coli* among the most common causes of bacterial diarrhea. A most important military problem, bacillary dysentery has, throughout history, caused more deaths in military personnel than enemy action has.[542]

Shigellae are gram-negative, nonmotile bacilli separated on the bases of serologic and fermentative properties into group A *(S. dysenteriae),* group B *(S. flexneri),* group C *(S. boydii),* and group D *(S. sonnei). S. sonnei* causes from 60% to 80% of cases in the United States. During the documented past, predominance of one or another group has changed about every 20 years, an indication that herd immunity allows a generation of immunologically naïve, susceptible individuals to accumulate in such periods.

Shigellae, exclusively human pathogens, occur throughout the world, but clinical disease is more common in the tropics than elsewhere.[543] The incidence of bacillary dysentery increases greatly under circumstances of substandard sanitation, impaired sewage disposal, and breakdown of provision of safe water. Outbreaks in emerged countries are often institutional, in orphanages, day care centers, nursing homes, or outdoor gatherings.[544] Single-source outbreaks have occurred in recreational swimmers[545] and rafters on the Colorado River.[546] This specific observation leads to the general admonition that surface waters in recreationally attractive areas of the United States, even as remote as the floor of the Grand Canyon, are not potable unless properly treated.

Food-borne outbreaks occur but are less a factor than in salmonellosis.[547] Fecal contamination of flies, fomites, and hands and fingers is an important factor for contagion. Person-to-person transmission is important and accounts for the frequency of multiple cases in a household. Shigellosis occurs in populations of homosexual men and is a risk in patients with AIDS.[548] Recurrent shigellosis has occurred in an HIV-positive man.[549]

Pathogenesis. The range of *Shigella* infections includes asymptomatic intestinal colonization, watery diarrhea, severe dysentery with fever and chills, tenesmus, and passage of frequent bloody mucoid stools.[550]

Shigella organisms are the most highly infectious bacterial agents of diarrheal illnesses. As few as 20 to 50 ingested organisms can cause disease.[551] This inoculum compares with 10^8 or 10^9 bacilli of *Salmonella* species or *Vibrio* species. The major mechanism for production of the disease is invasion of the epithelium of the colon. Microbial proliferation occurs there, and in the lamina propria,[552] where an acute inflammatory process occurs.

Different factors are essential for pathogenicity:[553] *lipopolysaccharide endotoxin,* which is essential for virulence; the *heat-labile Shiga* toxin,[554] long known to be neurotoxic and lethal in rabbits and mice; the same toxin is also cytotoxic in several in vitro systems[555] and produces secretion in the isolated rabbit ileal segment.[556] Varying amounts of Shiga toxin appear to be synthesized by all virulent strains of *Shigella* under complex interrelationships of chromosomal loci[557] and loci on a 180-to 230-kilobase virulence plasmid.[558] Shiga toxin may be responsible for the watery, cholera-like diarrhea early in the course of clinically apparent shigellosis. Its cytotoxicity is a consequence of inhibited protein synthesis by host cells. Shiga toxin does not immunologically resemble cholera toxin[559] and is more slow acting than cholera toxin in the isolated rabbit ileal loop,[560] in which it does not produce histologic changes. Effects of Shiga toxin and cholera toxin are additive and may share one or more rate-limiting steps.[561] Finally, the organism must have the ability to enter intestinal epithelial cells, particularly of the colon.[562]

Invasion beyond the lamina propria of the intestine is very unusual. Patients with bacillary dysentery actually less often have *Shigella* cultured from their bloodstream than other organisms.[563] Invasion of the bloodstream by *Shigella* may be more common in individuals with AIDS than in others.[564] In immunologically competent individuals, a long-term carrier state is unusual.[565]

Clinical features and pathology. Lesions of *Shigella* infection are confined to the intestine and are much more pronounced in the colon than in the small intestine. Early bacterial invasion of the epithelium is followed by an acute polymorphonuclear exudation, more severe in the crypts than over surface epithelium (Fig. 33-33). The lamina propria is hyperemic and hypercellular, including polymorphonuclear cells. Soon patches of epithelium ulcerate, and these ulcers become confluent, characteristically arranged transversely in the colon. Penetration through the wall is uncommon, and colonic perforation is correspondingly rare.

Shigella meningitis is very rare; most reported cases have been infants.[566] A neuropathy manifested by meningismus or convulsions and a peripheral neuropathy are rare complications.[567] Both are of uncertain pathogenesis. Shigellae may cause purulent ocular infections, usually in children, attributed to the patient rubbing his or her eyes with contaminated fingers.[568] *Shigella* may cause vaginitis, usually in prepubertal girls who may, rarely, have no history of diarrhea.[569] A splenic abscess from which *Shigella* organisms and *Bacteroides fragilis* were cultured has been reported in a diabetic man who had frequently visited Mexico.[570]

Reactive arthritis sometimes with complete Reiter's syndrome is a recognized complication of shigellosis, especially in patients of HLA-27 haplotype. The uncommon association of HUS with shigellosis[571] is provocative because of the recognized association of that syndrome with infections by enterotoxigenic *E. coli,* especially serotype O157:H7, which produce toxins that are similar to Shiga toxin.

With antibiotic and supportive therapy the death rate from shigellosis in otherwise healthy individuals is of the order of a few percent.[572]

Salmonella *species*

From a public health standpoint *Salmonella* is probably the most important genus among pathogenic Enterobacteriaceae. Not only are the human and animal diseases they cause of great clinical and economic importance, but the genus also exemplifies many features of Enterobacteriaceae: (1) an adjustment to intracellular parasitism exemplified by great species specificity, (2) complex ecologic and epidemiologic features, (3) elaborate antigenicity that leads to highly complex pathogenic mechanisms,[573,574] (4) multifaceted morpho-

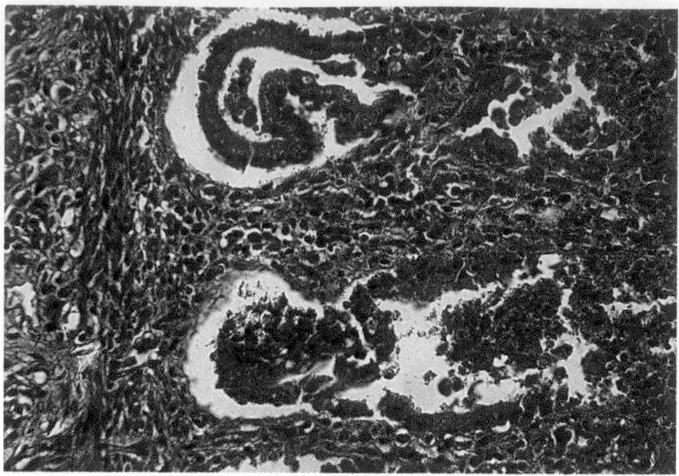

Fig. 33-33 Shigellosis. The surface of the colon in bacillary dysentery contains an inflammatory exudate and is focally ulcerated. There is acute inflammation in colonic crypts and in the lamina propria.

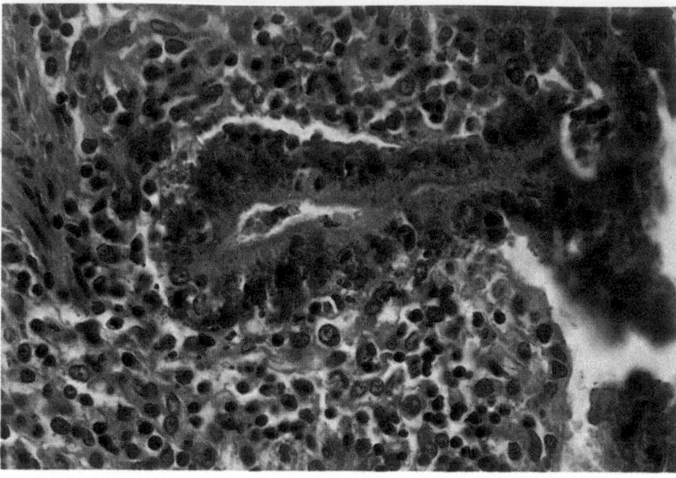

Fig. 33-34 Salmonellosis. Acute inflammation in the depths of a crypt in the ileum.

logic expressions of infection[575] resulting in a montage that includes acute exudative inflammatory reactions on the surface of the intestine or in solid viscera, even with abscess formation, mononuclear expressions of cellular immunity typified by granuloma formation, and proliferation of certain of the host's cells (Fig. 33-34).

Microbiology. Samonellae are gram-negative, nonsporeforming bacilli. All but *S. gallinarum-pullorum* are motile. Approximately 60 lipopolysaccharide (O) antigens are distinguishable as a component of the cell wall. Several hundred proteins form serologically distinct flagellar (H) antigens. Many salmonellae elaborate a capsular Vi antigen, a polymer of *N*-acetylgalactosaminuronic acid, which may block agglutination by anti-O serum. The Kauffmann-White schema groups salmonellae by their reactions with anti-O and anti-H sera.

The taxonomy of salmonellae has become bewilderingly complicated as the number of species increases. Currently each serotype is considered an individual species, such as *S. choleraesuis*.

Pathogenesis. Many salmonellae are strongly host adapted. *S. typhi,* for example, occurs spontaneously only in humans though nonhuman species can be experimentally infected. Few serotypes are specifically adapted to animals. Chickens, for example, are the major reservoir of *S. gallinarum-pullorum.* Most salmonellae, however, can infect both animals and humans.

The relationship of salmonellae to the host may exemplify various degrees of intimacy in the association of host and parasite. At one end of the continuum, asymptomatic bacterial colonization represents virtually a saprophitic relationship. Next in degree of intimacy is a predominantly surface infection with localized clinical manifestations, such as occurs in *Salmonella* enterocolitis. Systemic invasion and establishment of widespread inflammatory foci after bacteremia is a still more intimate relationship. In the case of *S. typhi* the association is intracellular. Finally, in the asymptomatic chronic carrier state, bacteria reside in a sanctuary, often a chronically inflamed gallbladder that houses calculi, to sally forth periodically into the intestine with epidemiologic consequences for the spread of infection.

Salmonellae are sensitive, as are vibrios, to gastric acidity.[59] Unless gastric acidity is impaired by a surgical procedure or antacid, ingestion of about 1000 bacteria causes symptoms in only about a fourth of volunteers.

After ingestion of an infectious bolus, bacteria enter the apical cytoplasm of intestinal epithelial cells, chiefly in the distal ileum, in membrane-bound vacuoles. In the first few hours the bacteria proliferate there[576] while the degenerated brush borders of the enterocytes reconstitutes.[577] There is recent evidence that the M-cells, specialized epithelial cells that surmount domes of lymphoid tissue in the intestine, are particular sites for penetration of salmonellae,[578] as they probably are for shigellae[579] as well.

Traversing the cytoplasm of enterocytes (or M-cells), the bacteria enter a space between the epithelial layer and the subjacent lymphoid tissue or into the lamina propria, where they are phagocytized by PMNLs and more importantly by macrophages in which further proliferation occurs.[580] A human volunteer who was given chloramphenicol one day after oral administration of an infectious dose of *S. typhi* developed typhoid fever 9 days later. Apparently the bacilli had found a sanctuary in the reticuloendothelial tissues within 24 hours.[574]

During an incubation period of 10 to 14 days organisms are transported throughout the body, most importantly reaching elements of the reticuloendothelial system—the spleen, liver, bone marrow, and lymph nodes—where further proliferation occurs (Fig. 33-35). After this stage, there is a secondary bacteremia during which organisms may lodge in any organ and establish inflammatory foci, which may form abscesses. The inflammatory foci in the reticuloendothelial system remain mononuclear, and when the immunologic reaction, chiefly of T-lymphocytes, occurs, the foci may become granulomatous. At this stage, the "fastigium" of traditional nomenclature, hepatosplenomegaly is present. Abdominal pain and diarrhea may appear and fever is practically continuous. Rarely the spleen may rupture and Peyer's patches may perforate. Satellite acute inflammatory foci may dominate the clinical picture. After 2 to 4 weeks, the fever resolves by lysis and resolution of inflammatory foci occurs, usually without scarring.

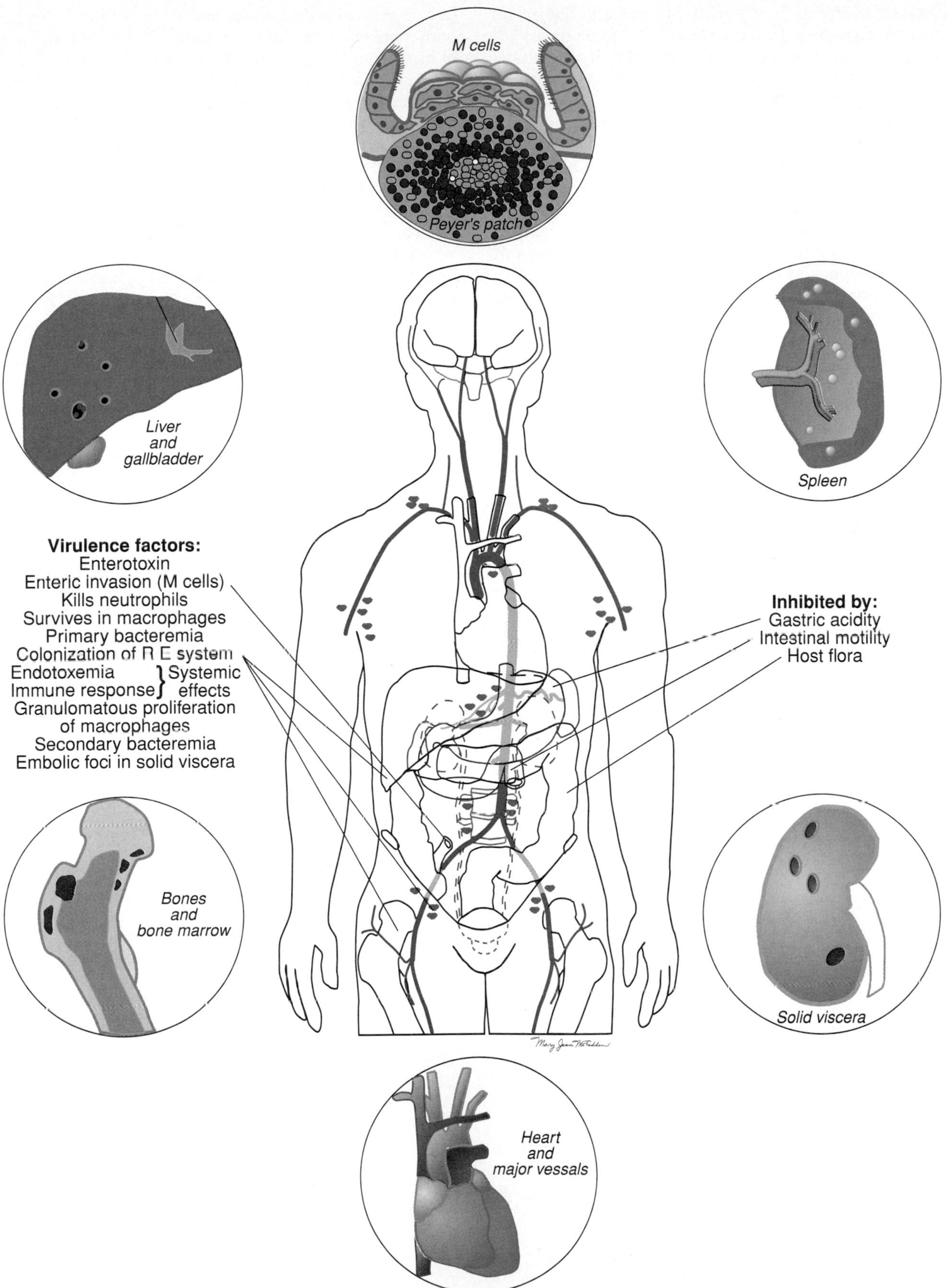

Fig. 33-35 The effects of salmonella can be manifested in multiple organs as abscesses, granulomatous inflammation, and lymphoid hyperplasia.

This series of events is a stereotypic scenario subject to interruption at any stage. Infection by enterotoxogenic salmonellae ordinarily stops at the stage of intestinal colonization, and the toxin may give rise to a watery cholera-like diarrhea without systemic symptoms or lesions.

Enteroinvasive salmonellae produce an enterocolitis, and particularly aggressive members of this group, such as *S. choleraesuis* and *S. typhimurium,* are especially prone to produce hematogenous abscesses in various viscera, ordinarily without the systemic manifestations that characterize typhoid fever. Finally, establishment of the chronic carrier state is much more commonly an end stage of typhoid fever than of infection by nontyphoidal salmonellae.

About one third of cases of infection by *Salmonella* have significant other diseases.[581] Hemoglobinopathy increases susceptibility by multiple mechanisms, including inhibition of the alternative complement pathway and "autosplenectomy" by multiple splenic infarcts.[582] Other hemolytic states, such as malaria and conditions in which hemophagocytosis occurs in the reticuloendothelial system, increase susceptibility to *Salmonella* infections by inhibiting further phagocytosis by macrophages.[583] Schistosomiasis, both *S. haematobium* and *S. mansoni* infections, predisposes to chronic bacteremic salmonellosis by actual parasitization of schistosomes by *Salmonella.*[584] Chronic or recurrent *Salmonella* bacteremia may occur in patients with leukemia or lymphoma or AIDS. Sexual transmission has been reported in homosexual men.[585]

Clinical syndromes. *Typhoid fever* is an acute systemic illness usually caused by *S. typhi, S. paratyphi* A, *S. schottmuelleri* (*S. paratyphi* B) and rarely *S. hirschfeldii* (*paratyphi* C) can cause a systemic illness ordinarily less severe than that cause by *S. typhi.* Because of this etiologic heterogeneity, some prefer the designation *enteric fever,* though the disease may not be "enteric." *Typhoid fever* is probably the best term, being widely understood.

Typhoid is an important disease. Although only a few hundred cases occur annually in medically advanced countries, the disease more commonly affects emerging countries, particularly when control of water and sewage breaks down. Food-borne outbreaks are less common.[586] The peak age incidence is in the midtwenties, and men are more often affected than women. Most cases in medically advanced countries are acquired abroad.[587] Most American cases originate in Mexico, Central America, or South America[588] and most British cases in India or Pakistan. It should be pointed out that large indigenous outbreaks occurred in Zermatt, Switzerland (water-borne),[589] Aberdeen, Scotland (originally imported from Argentina in canned corned beef),[586] and Dade County, Florida (water-borne).[590] But how does one characterize an outbreak on an intercontinental cruise liner?[591]

Signs and symptoms, which are very general, include fever, chills, anorexia, myalgia, headache, bradycardia, and leukopenia. Most adults have constipation early and diarrhea only later. Similarly varied complications include meningitis, endocarditis, empyema, myocarditis, osteomyelitis, abscess of virtually any organ, splenic rupture, and intestinal perforation.[592] Atheroma or atherosclerotic aneurysms may be colonized.[593] The gallbladder is frequently colonized and is the nidus for most examples of the carrier state, usually in older adult women with biliary tract disease.

Chloramphenicol has been the mainstay of antimicrobial therapy. However, a major outbreak of typhoid fever caused by chloramphenicol-resistant *S. typhi* occurred in Mexico in 1972 and involved at least 80 Americans travelers. The mortality is approximately 5%. Paradoxically, that from extraintestinal, nontyphoidal salmonellosis is somewhat higher.

Pathology. Changes of typhoid fever are described by clinical stage, though these may develop asynchronously or be otherwise atypical (Fig. 33-36). During the incubation stage, lymphoid tissue generally becomes hyperplastic, featuring predominantly large macrophages. A scanty mononuclear enterocolitis may be recognizable. The disease thereafter is characterized more by proliferation than by necrosis of lymphoid tissue in lymph nodes, spleen, and GI tract. Inflammatory foci in solid viscera, liver, and less commonly lungs, myocardium, skeletal muscle, or kidneys are predominantly mononuclear even in the presence of necrosis (Fig. 33-37).

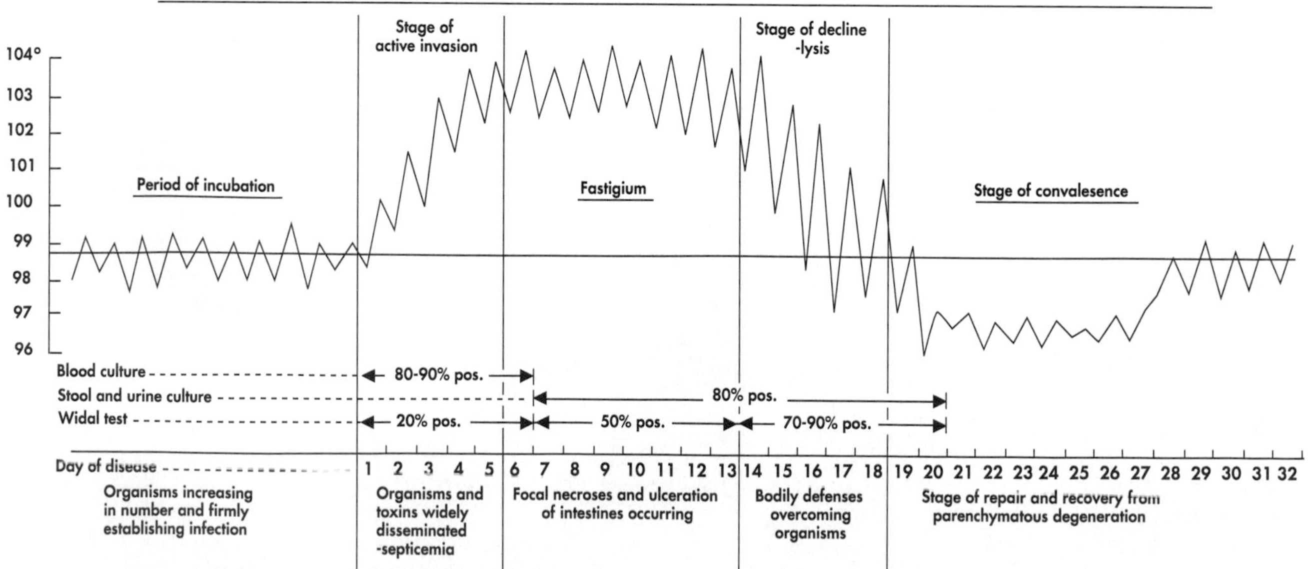

Fig. 33-36 Typhoid fever. Clinicopathologic correlation.

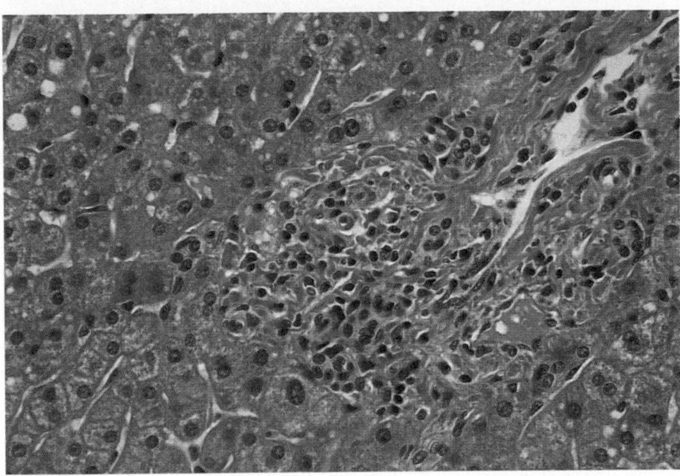

Fig. 33-37 Typhoid nodule. An aggregate of macrophages and lymphocytes in the liver is part of the response to dissemination of *Salmonella typhi* through the vascular system.

During the stage of invasion, when bacteremia is virtually invariable, lymphoid aggregates, as in lymph nodes, Peyer's patches in the small intestine, and malphigian bodies in the spleen, become swollen and pink. Microscopically this tissue features Mallory cells in granulomatous aggregates. These phagocytes are large mononuclear or binuclear cells with phagocytized erythrocytes and degenerating lymphocytes in their cytoplasm. Similar foci may be seen in solid viscera such as liver, myocardium, and lungs. During the "fastigium," systemic effects of endotoxin are prominent, and necrotic foci in lymphoid tissue may almost appear caseous. Peyer's patches may perforate, giving rise to peritonitis (Fig. 33-38). With lysis, proliferated lymphoid tissue sloughs or is slowly resorbed, and involved tissues return to normal. Splenic abscesses occur, and splenic rupture may occur either spontaneously or during physical examination.

In skeletal muscle, myocytes are hypereosinophilic and show so-called Zenker's hyaline degeneration.

Nontyphoidal salmonellosis

Unlike typhoid fever, nontyphoidal salmonellosis is overwhelmingly a disease of children, usually younger than 5 years, is more a problem in medically advanced than in emerging countries, and is much more commonly food related than water borne. Eggs are a particularly common source, but virtually any animal, poultry, or animal product has been documented as a vehicle. Pet turtles were a surprisingly important source of salmonellosis until regulated.[594] An outbreak was attributed to marijuana grown in heavily manured plots. Medical biologicals have been associated with various outbreaks: carmine dye (insect derived), hormones, pancreatin, and rattlesnake venom. The disease has been called "salmonella food poisoning," because of the predominantly intestinal manifestations, despite the fact that the disease is a "poisoning" only in the most general sense. Included among the differential diagnoses is staphylococcal food poisoning (a true exotoxicosis with a shorter incubation period), but far more common as a differential consideration is *Campylobacter*-related disease, and no one calls that "*Campylobacter* food poisoning." Ten serotypes of *Salmonella* account for three fourths of all cases.

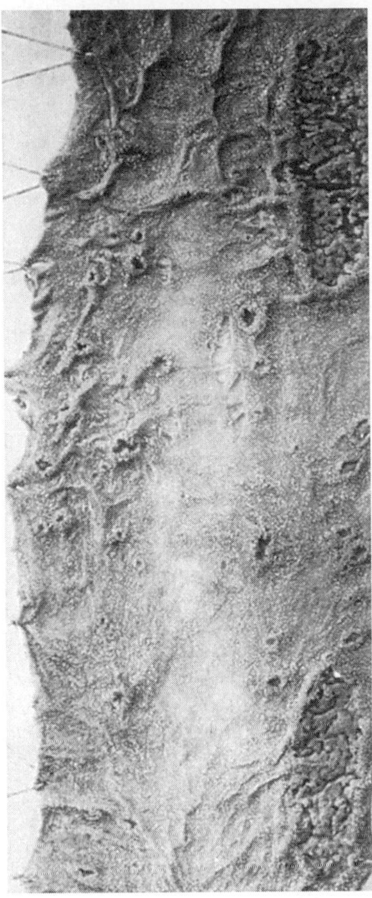

Fig. 33-38 Typhoid fever. Ulcerative lesions in the ileum correspond in location to lymphoid follicles and Peyer's patches. Where they occur in Peyer's patches, the long axis of their oval shape is parallel to that of the intestine. (AFIP 2803.)

Presently in the United States *Salmonella typhimurium* and *Salmonella enteritidis* are the most prevalent serotypes.

Diarrhea is usually the only clinical manifestation and is almost always self-limited. Antimicrobial treatment is not indicated in most cases and therapy may prolong the carrier state. Sepsis and metastatic abscesses are rare.[595] When tissue is studied (usually in more severe or clinically perplexing cases), colonic involvement is common, as well as the expected small intestinal lesion.[372,596]

Klebsiella *species*

Members of the genus *Klebsiella* are nonmotile, nonspore-forming, gram-negative bacilli. The most important species is *Klebsiella pneumoniae*. In recent years strains that produce indole from tryptophan have been reclassified as *Klebsiella oxytoca;* the clinical and pathologic characteristics of these strains do not differ significantly from those of *K. pneumoniae*. Two other species, *Klebsiella rhinoscleromatis* (rhinoscleroma) and *Klebsiella ozaenae* (ozena) are now believed to represent biochemically inert variants of *K. pneumoniae*.

Klebsiella pneumoniae. *K. pneumoniae* shares with *Streptococcus pneumoniae* a classic role as a cause of lobar pneumonia.[597] *K. pneumoniae* is a member of the oropharyngeal flora, and it produces pulmonary infection in the community.[598] It is also a part of the normal stool flora.[599] The classic pneumonia described by Friedländer is a lobar or sublobar pneumonia, distinguished from pneumococcal pneumonia by the tendency to abscess formation (Fig. 33-39). A mucoid appearance may be imparted to the cut surface of the lung by the large polysaccharide capsule produced by this species. The capsule may impart a mucoid appearance to the expectorated sputum, described as resembling currant jelly. *Klebsiella* capsules share antigenic determinants with the polysaccharides of other encapsulated bacteria, but their role in virulence is unclear. Specific virulence factors, other than resistance to antimicrobial agents, have not been identified.

The classic lobar presentation of pneumonia is unusual, however, and most pulmonary infections are focal pneumonias that have been acquired in the hospital. *K. pneumoniae* also causes urinary tract infection on occasion. The portal of entry for bacteremic infection is usually either the urinary or the respiratory tract.[600] Acquisition of resistance to multiple antimicrobial agents has compounded the difficulty of treating these nosocomially acquired infections.[601] Patients with bacteremia have been treated with antimicrobial agents that select for this pathogen.[602] *K. pneumoniae* is also an occasional bacteremic pathogen in children.[603] This species was one of the pathogens that caused a nationwide epidemic of septicemia after defective bottles of intravenous fluid were contaminated.[51]

Metastatic infection may occur in a variety of organs. The inflammatory response to infection is purulent and nonspecific.

A heat-stable enterotoxin related to that produced by *E. coli* has been described in *K. pneumoniae*,[525] which has been suggested as a cause of gastroenteritis.[604] Infections may be accompanied by gas production,[605] sometimes with crepitance and even myonecrosis. *K. pneumoniae* may cause false-positive serologic test results for infectious mononucleosis, rheumatoid factor, and cryptococcal antigen.

Klebsiella rhinoscleromatis. Rhinoscleroma is a chronic infection of the upper respiratory tract, particularly of the nasal cavities, produced by *K. rhinoscleromatis*.[606] The disease is common in some areas of the tropical world,[607] but the infection appears to be poorly communicable. Changing patterns of immigration to the United States have resulted in an increased frequency of rhinoscleroma in this country.[608] A chronic inflammatory response is dominated by lymphocytes, plasma cells, and macrophages, including large vacuolated cells with an eccentric nucleus and many intracellular bacilli (Mikulicz cells).[609] These cells are reminiscent of the bacteria-laden macrophages found in infections caused by *Mycobacterium leprae* (lepra cells), *Mycobacterium avium–intracellulare* (in patients with AIDS), and *Tropheryma whippelii* (Whipple's disease). The intracellular bacteria are demonstrated well by the PAS reaction and by the Hotchkiss-McManus stains; Brown and Brenn, Brown-Hopps, and Dieterle stains were less efficient means of demonstrating the bacteria.[610] The bacilli are not acid fast. By electron microscopy the PAS-positive material was strands extending from the intracellular bacilli. The number of Mikulicz cells in the lesions varies from few to many, and an immunoperoxidase test for bacterial antigen may be necessary to demonstrate small numbers of bacteria. Well-formed tuberculoid granulomas are not seen, and the lymphocyte subsets in the lesions resemble those in lepromatous leprosy. Lymphocytes of helper and suppressor phenotype are scattered diffusely throughout the macrophages without the presence of a peripheral mantle of lymphocytes.[611] The overlying mucosa may be thinned and atrophic, resembling the lesion of ozena, or may show pseudoepitheliomatous hyperplasia.[610]

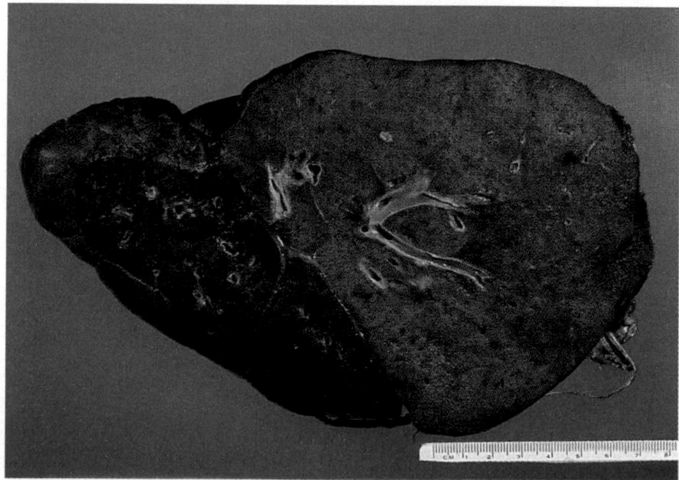

Fig. 33-39 Friedländer's pneumonia. Dense lobar consolidation is evident in the lung of this alcoholic patient who was infected with *Klebsiella pneumoniae* type 1. The lesion resembles pneumococcal pneumonia, but abscesses are more commonly found.

Complications of the infection are usually caused by bony erosion as the inflammatory mass extends locally. Extension through the sinus into the orbit, producing exophthalmus has been described.[612] Rarely, disseminated infection, characterized by Mikulicz cells in several organs, occurs.[613]

Enterobacter *species*

Enterobacter species conform to the definition of Enterobacteriaceae. They resemble *Klebsiella* species but are motile and produce less luxuriant capsules. *Enterobacter* species are normal flora of the GI tract, and almost all infections are endogenous or nosocomial, or both.[614] Intrinsic and acquired resistance to antimicrobial agents have increased the concern about these opportunists.[615] Other specific virulence mechanisms have not been defined. The species most commonly encountered is *Enterobacter cloacae*. *Enterobacter* species, particularly *Pantoeae agglomerans* (formerly *Enterobacter agglomerans* and before that *Erwinia herbicola),* figured prominently in an epidemic of septicemia associated with contaminated intravenous infusion bottles.[51]

Serratia *species*

The genus *Serratia* is composed of facultatively anaerobic, nonsporeforming, gram-negative bacilli that share the characteristics of the Enterobacteriaceae. *Serratia marcescens,* the most common pathogen of the genus, was formerly known as *Bacillus prodigiosus*. A minority of strains produce a distinctive red pigment known as "prodigiosin." The pigment has a long and fascinating history but is not known to be a virulence factor. *S. marcescens* has a predilection for growth on foodstuffs, especially those that contain starch.[616] It has been argued that production of red pigment after growth of *S. marcescens* on sacramental bread is responsible for the medieval "miracles," in which the blood of Christ appeared on consecrated wafers, as memorialized by Raphael in his fresco *The Mass of Bolsena*. In modern times the pigment has been used intentionally as a biologic marker. In the early part of the twentieth century *Serratia* organism were sprayed into the throats of soldiers, after which the pigmented bacteria were demonstrated on eating utensils. In the early 1950s the United States army released the bacterium into the ocean, after which it was blown over San Francisco, after which infections with this unusual bacterium were recognized in local hospitals. As late as the 1970s medical students were required to rub their hands in a bacterial suspension in order to demonstrate person-to-person transfer of infectious agents, and bacterial suspensions were sprayed in hospitals to study the dispersion of bacterial aerosols.

As suggested by these experiments, this species is an opportunistic pathogen. Most of the unwilling or unsuspecting recipients of the bacterial inoculum (including one of the authors) were unharmed by the exposure. Only a few cases of *Serratia* infection had been reported as recently as the late 1960s, but by the 1970s the importance of this bacterium as a nosocomial pathogen had been clearly recognized.[617] The sentinel characteristics of infections by this bacterium are nosocomial acquisition and frequent association with a common source, usually a medical device or fluid.[618] The problem continues in the 1990s.[619] *Serratia marcescens* is capable of replication under refrigeration[49] and has caused transfusion-associated sepsis.[620]

Serratia infections produce undifferentiated acute inflammation, frequently accompanied by abscesses.[621] Virulence factors are poorly defined, but a metalloprotease activates Hageman factor and prekallikrein.[622] The red pigment may even be evident in clinical infections, producing a pink or red exudate.[623] A particularly interesting situation was the "Case of the red diaper," for which an inborn error of metabolism was hypothesized until *S. marcescens* was found to be the predominant colonic flora of the infant.[624]

Citrobacter *species*

Citrobacter species are members of the Enterobacteriaceae that are opportunistic pathogens. They are part of the normal flora in the intestinal tract and may be found in the urinary and biliary tracts. *Citrobacter* infection occurs rarely, almost exclusively in compromised hosts, including neonates.[625,626] The two most commonly isolated species are *Citrobacter diversus* and *Citrobacter freundii*. In one study, infections with *C. diversus* tended to arise from the urinary tract, whereas the biliary system was the source for *C. freundii* infections.[625] The infections may be endogenous but are frequently transferred to patients on the hands of medical personnel.[627] Simple infection control measures, including handwashing and restriction of colonized care givers, are the most effective prevention.

Virulence factors in *Citrobacter* species are unclear, but it has been suggested from studies in human patients and experimental animals that a 32,000-dalton minor outer membrane protein may be a marker for virulence.[628] Some strains of *Citrobacter* possess a heat-stable enterotoxin similar to that found in *E. coli*.[526] Other strains possess a Shiga 2–like toxin[533] and the O157[534] lipopolysaccharide antigen that characterize enterohemorrhagic strains of *E. coli*. *C. freundii* has been suggested as a possible cause of infectious gastroenteritis,[629] but the data are inconclusive.

Citrobacter species produce a variety of infections, including sepsis[625,630] and endocarditis. Nosocomial infections of the urinary tract figure prominently in the catalog of infections, but the most dramatic and most lethal infections are meningitis and brain abscess in neonates.[631] *Citrobacter diversus* is the most common species implicated. Similar infections have been described in adults.[632]

Proteus, Providencia, *and* Morganella *species*

The protei are typical members of the Enterobacteriaceae, distinguished by the abundant production of urease. *Morganella morganii* and *Providencia rettgeri* were formerly classified in the genus *Proteus*. *Proteus mirabilis* and *Proteus vulgaris* remain as representatives of the genus. Of these *P. mirabilis* is the most common pathogen of humans. The genus *Proteus* is named after the minor sea god in *The Odyssey,* who constantly changed shape as he wrestled with Ulysses. This designation is derived from the vigorous motility of the species, which causes them to "swarm" across the surface of agar plates.

These species are members of the GI flora.[633,634] Most infections are inextricably linked to the urinary tract, with *P. mirabilis* being the most common isolate[635] and the only species commonly associated with community-acquired infections. The infrequency of *P. vulgaris* in the GI tract has been suggested as an explanation for the infrequency of this species in urinary tract infection.[636] The route to the urinary tract is from the feces with interim colonization of the perineum.[637] *Providencia stuartii* possesses uncharacterized adhesins that mediate adherence to uroepithelial cells.[638] Catheterization of the urinary tract is a common predisposing factor for urinary tract infection.[639] The ability of *Proteus* and *Morganella* species to encrust the catheter surface may contribute to their prevalence.[640] Condom catheters have also been shown to be a reservoir for *Providencia stuartii*.[641] IgA protease has been demonstrated in *Proteus* species, but its role in virulence is unknown.[642] The vigorous motility in *P. mirabilis* contributes to the ability of this species to migrate up the urinary tract in experimental animals.[643]

Urease plays a pathogenetic role beyond encrusting of the catheter. Urinary stone formation is enhanced in infections caused by these species because of the urea-splitting activity.[644] Furthermore, hyperammonemia is a complication of systemic *Proteus* infection and has been associated with coma in a patient without underlying liver disease.[645]

All the species are associated with nosocomial infections, which may be clustered.[641] Systemic disease usually occurs in patients with serious underlying disease, and the portal of entry is usually the urinary tract.[635] *Providencia stuartii* infections have been a particular problem in patients with thermal burns, aggravated by the intrinsic resistance of this species to multiple antibiotics.[646] Pneumonia is a well-recognized systemic manifestation of *Proteus infection*.[647] *Proteus meningitis* and cerebral abscess have been reported in a neonate.

Yersinia *species*

Yersinia pestis. The causal agent of plague, *Yersinia* (formerly *Bacillum* or *Pasteurella*) *pestis* is a small gram-negative, bipolar-staining coccobacillus that grows readily on most culture media. Unlike other *Yersinia* species, *Y. pestis* is nonmotile either at 24° or 37° C. Specific fluoresceinated antisera are available for direct identification of the bacilli in clinical specimens.

History and epidemiology. A disease with apocalyptic overtones, plague is of the greatest antiquity. Some identify as plague the description in the First Book of Samuel from the fourteenth century B.C. of "emerods in their secret parts" that occurred among Philistines who had misappropriated the Ark of the Lord. Others find this description more accurately suggestive of hemorrhoids complicating bacillary dysentery. At one point, plague virtually decimated the Roman army, and it is said that plague and malaria, more than the Goths, conquered Rome.[648] In the seventh century A.D. plague is said to have killed 5000 to 10,000 citizens of Constantinople daily. Largely quiescent in transalpine Europe until the Middle Ages, plague emerged again in the fifteenth century to kill 25 million individuals, a figure that may actually be conservative. Plague is said to have killed half a million in England in 1665.[649] Abruptly after 1743 these awesome figures declined until 1841 when, last among Western countries, Turkey became plague free. Reasons for this abrupt decline have provoked debate for years. Konkala attributes it to introduction of arsenic as a rat poison.[650]

Plague erupted again in Canton at the end of the nineteenth century, escaped to the world's sea lanes from the free port of Hong Kong, and reached San Francisco, Seattle, and New Orleans early in this century.[651] Suppressive laws were imposed in San Francisco and suspended only after civil rights litigation.[652] Currently, the world over, Vietnam has the most cases[653] followed by Tanzania and Madagascar. In 1994, an outbreak in India, killing hundreds of people, reminded the world of the continued presence of the organism.

Plague is a zoonosis (sylvatic plague) that involves primarily rats, both wild and domestic. Under appropriate circumstances the disease occurs in about 60 species of rodents and lagomorphs, including ground squirrels, rabbits, hares, moles, skunks, and raccoons. The sequence rat-flea-rat is basic to perpetuation of the disease but is subject to almost innumerable variations, in most of which human beings can intercede. Carnivores, both wild and domestic, may acquire infection from eating infected rodents, after which they can then become important vectors of the human disease. Currently about 3% of human cases result from contact with infected cats, including recently a wild bobcat.[654]

Three primal reservoirs of sylvatic plague are central Asia, central Africa, and the western United States. It seems ironic that a disease that was concentrated historically in congested urban areas is now relegated to the semiarid and sparsely populated outposts of steppe, veldt, and high plains. Meyer and others believe that the American reservoir antedates the importation of cases of human and rodent plague into the West Coast ports and possibly dates back to aboriginal migration over the land bridge between Asia and North America.[651]

Pathogenesis. Virulence of the organism is attributable to many factors, including pesticin,[655] lipopolysaccharide endotoxin,[656] envelope factors, V and W antigens that facilitate intracellular survival, and several metabolic factors. V and W antigens are plasmid mediated, the others are chromosomal.[657] Organisms proliferating in the proventriculus of a flea soon obstruct ingestion and lead to regurgitation of large numbers of bacteria into the bloodstream of the host, where they are phagocytized by both polymorphonuclear cells and macrophages. *Y. pestis* resists lysis by macrophages and elaborates an envelope antigen that renders the organism resistant to subsequent phagocytosis. About 10 cases a year currently occur in the United States, and approximately half of the patients die. Most of the infections occur in the summer; winter cases are rare.[658] Currently 60% of American patients are younger than 20 years. Native Americans, particularly children, account for a disproportionate number of cases.[659] Most infections occur within 1 mile of the home, but a few involve travelers who may not become symptomatic until they are hundreds, even thousands of miles away.[660] In recent years, almost all American infections have originated west of the 100th meridian,[661] but cases are spreading slowly eastward. Enzootic plague has already crossed the 100th parallel with detection of *Y. pestis* in wild rodents in Dallas, Texas.[662]

Clinical features. After the bacilli enter the bloodstream or are inhaled in aerosols, they are carried in cells to the first echelon of draining lymph nodes, where they escape from phagocytic cells and proliferate enormously. The resulting inflammatory response gives rise to tender lymphadenopathy (buboes). This sequence, which occurs within 24 to 48 hours, is accompanied by fever, myalgia, and prostration. Disseminated intravascular coagulation is common[663] and contributes to cutaneous ecchymoses, even gangrene (hence "black death"). Multiple organ failure progresses to circulatory collapse with death resulting in about half of all cases.

Bacteremia without regional adenopathy (typhoidal plague) and inhalation of infectious material (primary pneumonic plague) are other clinical forms. Sixty percent to 85% of cases are bubonic; 10% to 15% represent each of the other forms.

The patient and his fluids are highly infectious and constitute a distinct risk of secondary cases, which may be transmitted not only by arthropods, but also by direct person-to-person contact or by transmission in the laboratory. Veterinarians are at special risk.[664] A vaccine is available for those occupationally exposed or otherwise at high risk. Broad spectrum antibiotics are effective but must be put into use promptly and in adequate dosage.

Pathology. In bubonic plague there is rarely a lesion at the site of inoculation, though slightly tender nodules may rapidly develop along tracts of lymphatic drainage between that site and the first echelon of lymph nodes. Nodes rapidly enlarge and may become several centimeters in diameter within days. They are tender, soon become fluctuant, and occasionally discharge through sinuses to the overlying skin. Microscopically the process is an acute hemorrhagic lymphadenitis and cellulitis, conspicuously mononuclear, in which plague bacilli teem. An amphophilic, mucoid-appearing cloud of bacilli in sinusoids of the lymph nodes and in surrounding tissue produces a characteristic microscopic appearance (Fig. 33-40).

In typhoidal plague, that is, forms without recognizable portal of entry, necrotic foci occur in visceral lymphoid tissues and parenchymatous viscera. The dreaded pneumonic plague, primary or secondary, is a conspicuously mononuclear bronchopneumonia that rapidly gives rise to microabscesses. Four aspects of plague that have not previously been emphasized have recently emerged from Southeast Asia and from American experience: (1) the occurrence of isolated localized adenopathy without systemic features, pestis minor,[665] (2) the occurrence of minimally symptomatic pharyngeal plague, a potential source of an outbreak[665]; (3) the occurrence of "plague carbuncle,"[666] an indolent cutaneous ulcer with contiguous lymphangitis and lymphadenopathy, rather like farcy or the malignant pustule of anthrax; (4) GI manifestations of plague. Half of the cases in a recent outbreak in Southeast Asia had diarrhea, and many had abdominal pain. An Ameri-

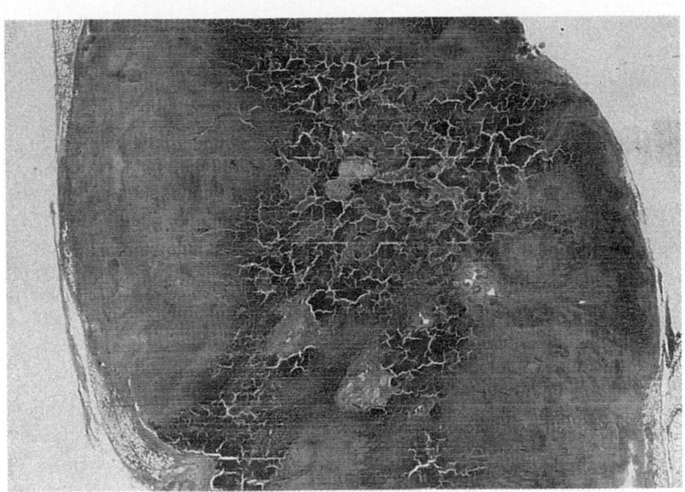

Fig. 33-40 Bubonic plague. Multiple necrotizing granulomas in a lymph node efface the architecture. The extensive dark blue areas are masses of proliferating bacilli.

can serviceman returning from Vietnam developed a tender inguinal mass that was diagnosed as an incarcerated hernia. It was a lymph node with lymphadenitis caused by *Y. pestis.*

Yersinia pseudotuberculosis *and* Yersinia enterocolitica. *Y. pseudotuberculosis* is a relatively large plump gram-negative bacillus that may show bipolar staining with methylene blue. *Y. enterocolitica* is smaller and does not show bipolar staining. Both species can be isolated on common laboratory media, but selective and differential media have also been developed.[172] The optimal temperature for growth is 32° C. Incubation of plates at room temperature may facilitate isolation; cold enrichment by storage of an inoculated broth at 4° C may be useful for detection of carriers and convalescent cases. Strains of *Y. enterocolitica* can be typed serologically by their somatic (O) antigens, providing a useful tool for epidemiologic studies.

History and epidemiology. Mallasey and Vignal in 1883 described a bacillus that produced in guinea pigs a disease that somewhat resembled tuberculosis.[667] Subsequently, several descriptions of infections likely caused by this organism were reported.[668-673]

Schleifstein and Coleman, who examined organisms cultured from human cases of diarrhea in which neither *Salmonella* nor *Shigella* could be identified, named the organism *B. enterocoliticum.*[674] Also known at one time as *Pasteurella X,* the bacterium is now classified as *Yersinia enterocolitica.*[675] Infections by *Y. enterocolitica* and *Y. pseudotuberculosis* are referred to collectively as "yersiniosis." Of the two, infection with *Y. enterocolitica* is much more common, and most clinical details refer to this species.

Y. enterocolitica is usually associated with an enterocolitis, whereas *Y. pseudotuberculosis* most typically produces a terminal ileitis with acute inflammation of regional mesenteric lymph nodes,[676] but there is considerable clinical and pathologic overlap between cases caused by these two organisms.

Y. pseudotuberculosis and *Y. enterocolitica* have been cultured from many animals.[677] In some animals, granulomatous lesions occur in the spleen, liver, and lymph nodes,[678] but the animals may not be ill and may represent a presumed reservoir. Swine, in particular, have been suggested as an important source of human yersiniosis.[679] Geese, ducks, turkeys, pheasants, and several nonedible species of birds may carry the organism. Humans may themselves be important reservoirs, but fewer than 1% of asymptomatic individuals excrete the bacteria.[680]

Clinical yersinosis occurs throughout the world.[681] Serotypes O3 and O9 of *Y. enterocolitica* cause most European cases, and serotype O3 predominates in Canada.[682] In the United States serotype O8 has predominated, though the prevalence of serotype O3 cases has increased in New York City.[683] Clinical cases may be more common in the winter months than in the summer. Most cases occur in children.[684] Hematologic disorders, especially thalassemia, seem to predispose to infection.[685] Blood products have been incriminated in human cases,[686] an association that is fostered by the ability of these bacteria to proliferate under refrigeration. Epidemics of infection by *Y. enterocolitica* have been attributed to dairy products and other refrigerated foods, illustrating the cold adaptation of these species.[687,688] In sizable outbreaks in two schools in Japan,[689] secondary cases were uncommon in families of students, an indication that person-to-person transmission may be less important than in some other enteric infections, such as shigellosis. Nosocomial outbreaks have occurred.[690] Several family outbreaks in some of which sick dogs were a feature, have been described.[691,692]

Pathogenesis. Y. enterocolitica produces a low molecular weight enterotoxin somewhat similar to *E. coli* enterotoxin.[693] An adhesin that attaches the organism to cultured cells has been identified.[694] *Y. pseudotuberculosis* produces a substance that is toxic to murine macrophages and resident peritoneal macrophages and depends on the presence of a 75 kilo–base pair plasmid.[695] Phagocytosis by neutrophils from patients receiving hemodialysis who have iron overload is less efficient against *Y. enerocolitica* than that of leukocytes of normal individuals or those receiving dialysis who are not iron overloaded.[119]

Clinical features and pathology. A crampy, mucus-diarrhea is a common clinical symptom. Abdominal pain in the right lower quadrant is often conspicuous. Frequently the clinical diagnosis is acute appendicitis.[696]

The most common lesion produced by *Y. enterocolitica* is a nonspecific enterocolitis,[680] but often this process is sharply localized to the terminal ileum. Hemorrhagic or membrane-coated ulcers may be longitudinally arrayed[697]; intestinal perforation is rare. The mucosa of the appendix may be normal, focally ulcerated, or, rarely, diffusely eroded. Regional lymph nodes are enlarged and acutely inflamed.[698] Typically they contain microabscesses in germinal centers with PMNLs stuffing peripheral sinuses. The lesions are described as necrotizing granulomas with stellate necrosis (Fig. 33-41). Inflammation and fibrosis may extend through the capsule into the surrounding soft tissue. A similar histologic appearance may be found in some appendiceal lesions. Organisms are occasionally demonstrated by histochemical stains (Fig. 33-42). Although this process is nonspecific, the anatomic location should raise the possibility of yersiniosis. Several patients have had pharyngitis that was very severe.[699]

Complications of *Y. enterocolitica* infection are very rare in children. Gastrointestinal symptoms may be prolonged. Bacteremia and meningitis have occurred. Visceral abscesses, as in the liver, are rare. Mycotic aneurysms and infectious endocarditis are very rare. An erysipelas-like cutaneous lesion

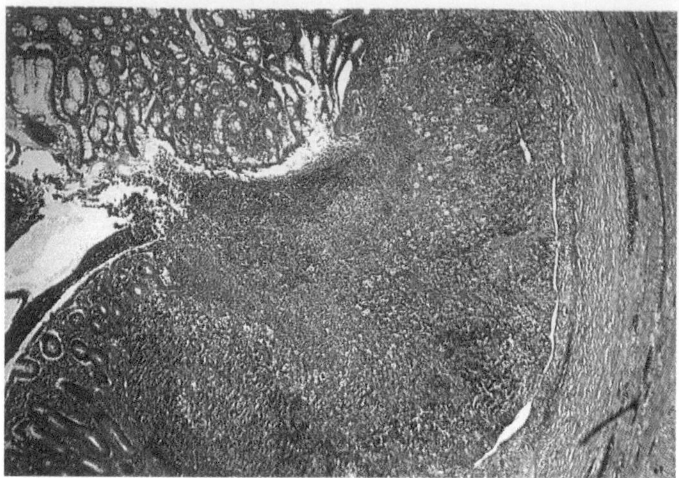

Fig. 33-41 Yersiniosis. Acute appendicitis is characterized by an ulcerative lesion with necrotizing granulomas that extend into and are concentrated in the submucosal lymphoid tissue, producing a histologic appearance that is differentiated from the common lesion of acute appendicitis. *Yersinia enterocolitica* was isolated from stool.

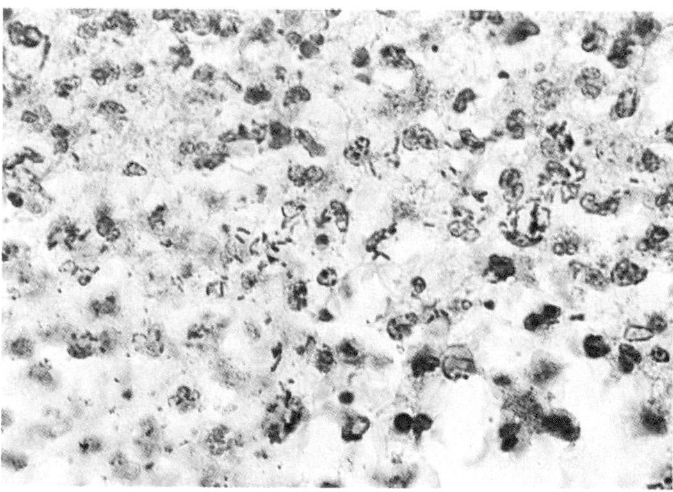

Fig. 33-42 Yersiniosis. Numerous bacilli are demonstrated by a silver impregnation stain in the necrotizing lesion illustrated in Fig. 33-42. Gram-negative bacilli were demonstrated in a section stained at the Armed Forces Institute of Pathology, using a modification of the Brown-Hopps technique. (Dieterle method.)

and other cutaneous lesions have been described, including a scarlatina-like syndrome with systemic toxemia. Patients with a variety of thyroid lesions may have antibodies against *Yersinia* spp. Hemolytic anemia and other hematologic disorders have been reported. More frequently in Europe than in North America, patients, especially adults, with *Y. enterocolitica* infection develop a reactive polyarthritis,[700] frequently with urethritis and conjunctivitis (Reiter's syndrome), especially in those of HLA-27 haplotype.[701] Erythema nodosum is common.[702] Septic arthritis also may occur.[703] Some patients have features that are suggestive of acute rheumatic fever,[704] other collagen-vascular diseases, or Kawasaki disease,[705] but a long follow-up study of patients who had recovered from yersiniosis did not show an increased incidence of systemic collagen-vascular diseases.[706] The patient described by Pile and co-workers had a necrotizing arteritis.[707] The pathologic process in infections by *Y. pseudotuberculosis* is similar but may include granulomas in mesenteric lymph nodes with giant cells, said not to occur in infections by *Y. enterocolitica*.[708] The differential diagnosis occasionally includes Crohn's disease.

Curved gram-negative bacilli

Vibrionaceae

Vibrio species are small, curved, gram-negative bacilli.[172] In contrast to members of the Enterobacteriaceae, they are oxidase positive, a feature that provides a useful screening test for colonies isolated on blood agar plates. *Vibrio* species are intensely motile by means of polar flagella. Many species other than *V. cholerae* require or are stimulated by NaCl in culture media (halophilic vibrios). Selective media are available for enhanced isolation, but most species also grow well on enriched media, such as sheep blood agar.

Vibrio cholerae

History and epidemiology. Cholera is of enormous importance historically, medically, socially, and politically.[709] It is probably the first infectious disease in which the etiologic microorganism was seen microscopically; it is the first disease for which treatment by intravenously administered fluids was proposed and desultorily tried; it is the first human bacterial disease for which vaccination was systematically tried.[710] The complement system, agglutination reaction, and precipitin reactions were all first discovered in studies of experimental infections by cholera vibrios. Public health administration prepared by disciples of Jeremy Bentham first emerged in Western societies in efforts to combat cholera. Active public health measures directed toward sanitary disposal of sewage and providing safe water supplies were first directed against *Vibrio cholerae*. This campaign culminated in Snow's persuasion of the town council of St. James Parish in Soho to remove the handle from the Broad Street pump, arresting the spread of cholera.[711]

Cholera smoldered in the Indian subcontinent throughout recorded history, perpetuated by religious fairs and regional pilgrimages. Portuguese traders recognized the disease in the sixteenth century. It is doubtful that cholera, at least in its quintessential epidemic form, occurred in Europe before the nineteenth century. It is epidemiologically important that there was no word for the disease "cholera" in Arabic in 1821. That the name "cholera" has been derived from the Greek words *cholē* ('bile') and 'flow', is probably wrong,[712] for the distinctive flux of the disease is not bilious. Some suggest an origin from Greek intestine or even χολέρα, 'eaves' or 'roof gutter.'[713]

Early in the nineteenth century, cholera erupted from its historic home in the delta of the Ganges and spread throughout much of the world in a succession of pandemics from 1816 to 1899.[715-717]

The strong effect of the second pandemic on the central United States has been neglected by medical historians.[714] In the epidemic of 1849 at least 10% of the inhabitants of St. Louis died, including several physicians and the patriarch of the founding family of the city.[718] The monumental bibliography assembled by Billings and co-workers, with excerpts from prior pandemics, is readily accessible in repositories of public documents.[719]

The Gulf Coast of the United States participates at a low level in the seventh pandemic, which began in 1961.[720] Recently, a new serotype, *V. cholerae* O:139 has been responsible for epidemic disease.

Pathogenesis. The disease is caused almost invariably by ingestion of water, water-freshened food products, or shellfish contaminated by excreta from human cases of cholera.[721] Within pandemics, miniature food-borne clusters of cases[722] and even transmission in bottled water occur.[723] Fomites, even soiled *saris,* may play a role.[724] *V. cholerae* survives in freshwater only for days, and in salt water for only a few weeks in conventionally cultivable form. The infectious dose, established in human volunteers without histories of gastric surgery and not taking antacids, is about 10^8 or 10^9 viable organisms per milliliter,[725] the same concentration of viable organisms that are observed in freshly evacuated choleric stool. This dose is theoretically possible in ambient water during hyperendemic periods. The source of organisms between epidemics is not known. There is no known nonhuman reservoir; subclinical cases are less common than in other well-studied diseases transmitted by the fecal-oral route. The carrier state, either convalescent or asymptomatic, is distinctly uncommon.[726]

The ecology of *V. cholerae* is poorly understood. It has been suggested that the organism may exist in an unculturable but viable state on plankton at subinfectious levels[727] and undergo mutation or become concentrated by salt-water shellfish[721] which filter hundreds of gallons of water daily, thereby occasionally achieving pathogenic levels in their tissues.

There are serologically distinct somatic O antigens, Inaba and Ogawa, each governed by a genetic locus. An uncommon sertotype is termed Hikojima. In 1905, a vibrio was identified at autopsy in six named pilgrims who did not have cholera at a quarantine station on the route from Mecca.[728] This station was named "el-tor" (officially now in Arabic Aṭ-Ṭūr, 'the-Mountain,' in the Sinai) for a nearby landform, and the relevant vibrio has since come to be known as the "El Tor" biotype.

After a period during which the disease caused by the *eltor* biotype was called "paracholera," it now emerges that the disease is indistinguishable from and can be every bit as severe as that attributed to "classical" (nonhemolytic) *V. cholerae. Eltor* survives in surface water longer than the classical vibrio does. The frequency of subclinical or nonclinical infections may be approximately one in 30 rather than one in six found in infections by "classical" vibrios. *Eltor* was the agent of only occasional cases of cholera outside India in the fifth and sixth pan demics, but in the recent (seventh) pandemic it has superseded classical vibrio[729] (after some rearrangement of O serogroups), except in Bangladesh where the "classical" vibrio has reemerged.[730] Other features unique to the present, seventh, pandemic are that it originated not in the primordial cradle of the disease, the Ganges Delta, but in the Indonesian island Sulawesi (Celebes).[716] It now involves in a major way West Africa and Latin America south of Mexico, an area that was infected from the United States in previous pandemics.

Cholera is a topical infection of the surface of the intestine. Clinical manifestations and the threat to life of the disease are the result of prodigious stimulation of secretion by the infected intestine in response to a potent exotoxin produced by cholera vibrios.

V. cholerae is very sensitive to acidity. It is rapidly lysed below pH 2.3, a level of acidity that is readily attained in normal gastric juice. It is well established that cholera is prone to occur in those whose gastric acidity is impaired by surgery, age, or medication. This barrier can be vitiated by achlorhydria whether as a result of gastric surgery, age, or ingestion of antacids.[731] In the outbreak of cholera in Jerusalem in 1969, 20% of those affected had prior gastric surgery for peptic ulcer disease, and in the 1972 outbreak in Bari, Italy, one third had either gastrectomy or vagotomy and pyloroplasty.[732]

Gastric and intestinal mucus is a more purely mechanical barrier to vibrios. There is an interesting suggestion that the cystic fibrosis heterozygote may be protected from cholera.[733] Indigenous intestinal flora provide another barrier to cholera vibrios, importantly by the production of bacteriotoxic fatty acids.

After vibrios have passed these defense mechanisms of the host, they must attach to intestinal epithelial cells to produce toxin.[734] The mechanism of attachment involves the flagella of the vibrios,[735] although motility per se is neither essential nor sufficient for attachment. Highly specific receptors are located in the flagella that bind to the brush border of intestinal epithelial cells. Cholera toxin is an 84,000-dalton protein with three components: two enzymatically active A subunits, each of 11,600 D molecular weight. The A1 subunit is bound to an A2 unit, which is in turn connected to a ring of B subunits by disulfide bonds. Cholera toxin has been in large part sequenced and has been visualized.[736]

Cholera toxin is active against virtually every cell system in which it has been examined. After binding of the B subunit to G_{M1} gangliosides in the intestinal brush border, the A2 subunit enters the cell to come into contact with the adenylate cyclase complex on the lateral membrane of the enterocyte. There the cyclase catalytic unit (A1) is maintained in an activated state, resulting in the elevation of intracellular cAMP, which in turn activates the secretory pathway for electrolytes through a series of protein kinases. The result is an outpouring of fluid into the intestinal lumen.[737] The intestinal flux in cholera is virtually isotonic with plasma, almost protein free, and odorless or faintly fishy smelling. The description "rice-water stools" describes flecks of mucin floating in this watery effusion.

Pathology. Sloughing of intestinal epithelium has been historically described in cholera, with the loss of fluid in intestinal discharges being attributed to oozing from the denuded surfaces with a magnitude equivalent to that seen in cutaneous burns. There is no question now that the small intestinal epithelium is intact in cholera and that denudation is a postmortem artifact. There is only slightly increased cellularity and vascular congestion in the lamina propria. Lymphoid follicles and Peyer's patches are slightly hyperplastic.[738] Acute renal tubular necrosis, myocardial degeneration, pulmonary edema with or without hyaline membranes, or bronchopneumonia are agonal complications or nonspecific features of extreme dehydration to which hypokalemia may contribute.

Historically one third to two thirds of patients with cholera died, often within hours. Rarely patients with ileus died without having passed a choleric stool—"dumb" or "mute cholera." With the introduction of modern fluid and electrolyte therapy, the mortality figures fell to about 5%. Currently with prompt, nonprofessionally administered oral therapy in patients outside hospitals, the mortality should not exceed 1%.

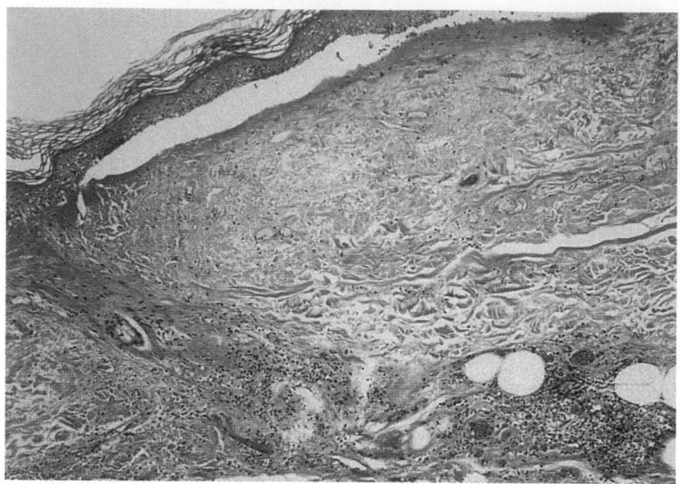

Fig. 33-43 Noncholera vibriosis. A large intraepidermal bullus is accompanied by an intense, necrotizing inflammatory response in the dermis and subcutaneous tissue. *Vibrio parahaemolyticus* isolated from tissue. (Case contributed by David Walker, MD, Galveston, Tex.)

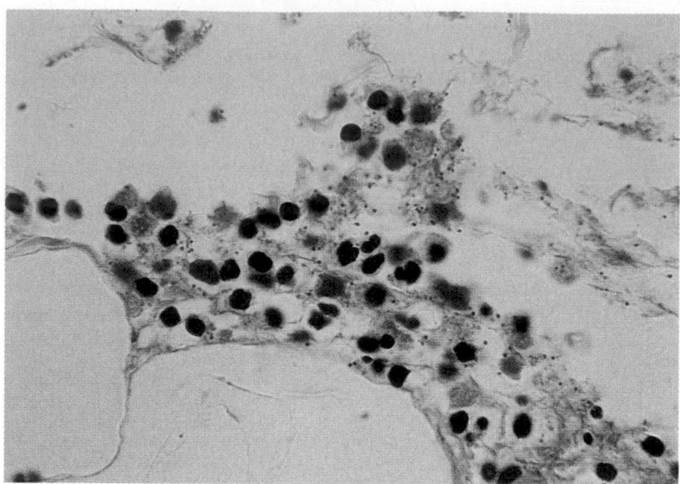

Fig. 33-44 Noncholera vibriosis. Numerous small gram-negative bacilli are demonstrated in the inflammatory exudate demonstrated in Fig. 33-43. The curved morphology of the bacilli is difficult to appreciate in the tissue sections. As is often true in tissue sections, the bacilli have a color that is more magenta than the pink of Gram's stain as performed on smears. In contrast gram-positive organisms are usually colored intensely blue. Brown-Hopps technique. (Case contributed by David Walker, MD, Galveston, Tex.)

Other vibrios

Some isolates of *V. cholerae* are of serotypes other than O1. Many of these are isolated from stools of patients with a severe cholera-like diarrhea,[739] a few from bacteremia, still fewer from wound infections and cases of otitis. Some of these strains produce an enterotoxin very similar to if not identical with cholera toxin itself. Many however, lack the gene sequence associated with production of cholera toxin. These strains have been shown to produce a variety of other toxins: an enterotoxin and a hemolysin that is toxic to cultured cells and lethal in mice.

Non-O1 *V. cholerae* is found in estuarine and riverine waters and in shellfish on the Gulf Coast of the United States. Patients with extraintestinal infections often have a history of exposure to seawater. Some clinical infections were in recent returnees from Mexico. Vibrios other than *V. cholerae* are rare causes of human infections,[740,741] but the wound infections may be devastating, causing bullous skin lesions (Figs. 33-43 and 33-44). The habitat of some of these species has been established to be aquatic, but others are either clearly not aquatic or are unknown. Unlike *V. cholerae,* these vibrios are truly invasive. Some of these agents, the lesions that have been associated with them, and comments on their epidemiology are included in Table 33-8. The most frequently encountered species have been *V. parahaemolyticus* and *V. vulnificus.*

Campylobacter *species*

Microbiology and taxonomy. Members of the genus *Campylobacter* (Gr. *kampylo-* 'curved', *bactron* 'rod') are a very common cause of bacterial diarrheal illness the world over.[742] Much less commonly, they cause human systemic disease. The genus consists of motile, nonsporulating, comma-shaped, gram-negative bacilli.[172] These organisms survive for weeks in milk or water at 4° C, an added factor in their pathogenicity. *Campylobacter* species are microaerophilic. Growth may occur in air enriched with 5% CO_2, but optimal growth occurs in an atmosphere of approximately 6% O_2. Growth of *Campylobacter jejuni* and *Campylobacter coli,* the most frequently encountered pathogens in the genus, is enhanced at 42° C, a temperature that also serves to inhibit most other intestinal flora. Selective media that incorporate antibiotics have also been developed for isolation of these species. If other species of *Campylobacter* are sought, however, incubation at 37° C on nonselective media must be performed. A membrane filter enrichment procedure takes advantage of the vigorous motility of these thin bacilli. Drying, freezing, pasteurization, and conventional chlorination of water supplies destroy them.

Campylobacters were initially described as causing septic abortion in cattle and sheep and were, on morphologic grounds, grouped with vibrios. Metabolic and genetic considerations have justified a genus distinct from *Vibrio.*[743]

The taxonomy of campylobacters is in a state of flux. European writers often use the nomenclature of Véron and Châtelain[744] rather than that of Bergey. These organisms do not metabolize carbohydrates, and so a relatively simple dimension of classification is not available. Currently there are 14 species, not all of which are widely accepted. *C. jejuni* and *C. coli* are so similar in metabolism and their pathogenicity for human beings is so similar that they can appropriately be considered together. Other species are very rare or uncertain human pathogens, often in selected patient populations.[745]

Epidemiology. Campylobacters are very widely distributed in the GI tracts of many animal species, wild and domestic, sick and well, including poultry (chickens, turkey, ducks, and pigeons), cattle, horses, swine, sheep, dogs, cats, and rodents but not, in contrast to salmonellae, reptiles.[746] Exotic species, including felines and ungulates, have low rates of infection by *C. jejuni.* Primates that are used either for exhibition or in the laboratory are frequently colonized.

Human infections by *Campylobacter* are grossly underreported, and so their overall frequency can only be approximated. In diagnostic laboratories, stool cultures positive for *Campylobacter* are equivalent to or more common than those

Table 33-8 Comparison of *Vibrio* species

Organism	Disease	Mode of acquisition	Mechanism	Distribution
V. cholerae 01	Cholera	Oral-fecal-oral; shellfish, vegetables, etc	CT	Worldwide since 1961 (seventh pandemic) including West Africa, Latin America, United States. Eltor biotype except in Bangladesh; Inaba serotype in New World; Ogawa serotype in Old World
Non-O1 *V. cholerae*	Diarrhea; wound infections; sepsis; meningitis	As *V. cholerae;* also raw shellfish, esp. oysters; underlying diseases; trauma	CLT; OT	Worldwide as above
V. parahaemolyticus	Diarrhea; ocular infection; otitis; sepsis	Raw seafood, esp. shellfish	OT; positive Kanagawa phenomenon;* variable isolated ileum	West Pacific rim, esp. Japan; three coasts of USA; Togo in West Africa; estuarine and brackish water; freshwater in India
V. mimicus	Diarrhea; otitis	Undercooked seafood, esp. shrimp; exposure to seawater	CLT; OT	Seawater
V. vulnificus	Diarrhea; wound infections; otitis; sepsis	Raw shellfish, esp. oysters; contact with seawater; liver disease; alcoholism; iron overload	I	Chesapeake Bay, Gulf Coast, NE coast, NW coast
V. fluvialis	Diarrhea	Seafood	CLT;OT	Bangladesh, Indonesia, United States, Brazil, England
V. alginolyticus	Wound infections; otitis; conjunctivitis; sepsis; diarrhea in Delhi	Contact with seawater	I	Spoiled mackerel
V. damscla	Wound infection (some very severe)	Exposure to seawater, shellfish; wounds from cleaning fish	U	Damselfish
V. fumissi	Gastroenteritis; one infant with diarrhea	Food related	CLT	Shellfish and estuarine waters
V. hollisae	Diarrhea; sepsis in liver disease	Raw seafood	OT	Marine environment; Gulf Coast, Chesapeake Bay
V. metschnikovii	One blood culture in patient with cholecystitis	U	U	Worldwide in fresh and brackish waters; shellfish
V. cincinnatiensis	Meningitis; sepsis (one case)	U	U	U
V. carchariae	Wound infection (one case)	Shark bite	U	Pathogenic in sharks; human infection in South Carolina

CT, cholera toxin; *CLT,* Choleralike toxin; *OT,* other toxins; *I,* invasion; *U,* unknown.
*Hemolytic on Wagatsuma agar (associated with pathogenicity).

positive for *Salmonella;* they are much more frequent than isolates of *Shigella.*[747] Both water-borne and food-borne outbreaks occur. Many milk-borne outbreaks have been attributed to unpasteurized (raw) milk.[748] Several thousand cases were documented in a large outbreak in Vermont that was traced to a municipal water system.[749] A school outbreak in Great Britain was attributed to contamination of drinking water by bird or bat excreta.[750] Contacts with animals, birds, or their products may be established,[751] but in view of the ubiquity of the organisms, such associations are neither common nor necessary for diagnosis. Person-to-person transmission is unusual, but both asymptomatic fecal excretion and proctitis caused by *Campylobacter* species occur in homosexual men.[752] Although infections by *Campylobacter* organisms occur at all ages, they are most common in children younger than 5 years[753] and are said to be least common between that age and puberty. Women infected during pregnancy may abort or go to term.[754] Infections occur in infants born to women with *Campylobacter*-related illness or asymptomatic carriers.

Asymptomatic bloody diarrhea may be a feature in newborn infants.[751] When *Campylobacter* infections occur in the elderly, they tend to involve those with underlying diseases. It should also be noted that campylobacters are a common cause of traveler's diarrhea.[755] Somewhat oddly, a prospective study of physicians' families traveling to Mexico does not mention *Campylobacter.*[492]

Pathogenesis. Campylobacters are highly infectious. A few hundred ingested organisms can cause disease,[756] an infectious dose larger than that necessary to cause shigellosis but far less than the inoculum required for salmonellosis, *Vib-*

rio-related disease, or yersiniosis. Several products of *Campylobacter* contribute to pathogenicity.[757] These include factors that protect the organism within the stomach, a cholera-like enterotoxin,[758] and a cytotoxin.[759]

Campylobacter spp. lack fimbriae but pathogenic strains possess factors that encourage adhesion to whole cells.[760] Organisms selectively traverse M-cells in rabbit ileum[761] and can survive in macrophages.[762]

Clinical features and pathology. Diseases caused by *Campylobacter* fall into five groups, sometimes with overlap:

1. A secretory diarrhea with explosive passage of watery stool, similar to cholera
2. An enteritis with crampy, mild abdominal pain, occasionally fever, and semiliquid, mucus-containing stools
3. A colitis with lower abdominal pain, tenesmus, and bloody or pus-containing stools
4. "Translocation syndrome"—organ-localized inflammatory foci in patients who may or may not have had gastrointestinal symptoms
5. Sepsis

Of these, enteritis is by far the most common. There is some correlation between clinical expression and pathogenic factors demonstrable in vitro .[763]

Tissue from human cases is infrequently available for examination, but the lesion in the small intestine of animals is a nonspecific acute inflammation of the intestinal surface and lamina propria usually with only microscopic mucosal erosions.[764] Human patients who are subjected to endoscopic examination and biopsy show colonic lesions.[765] Focal, occasionally hemorrhagic erosions microscopically reveal acute surface inflammation and inflammation of intestinal crypts, even with crypt abscesses quite suggestive of those in idiopathic ulcerative colitis. (Fig. 33-45)

The GI manifestations may be severe with as many as 10 stools per day. Fever, clinically significant fluid and electrolyte depletion, and toxic megacolon may occur.[766] The intestinal disease is usually self-limited, however, even without antibiotic treatment. Persistence longer than a week is uncommon and relapses even less common. Distinction between relapse and reinfection may be impossible. Deaths from GI disease alone are rare but have been reported.[767]

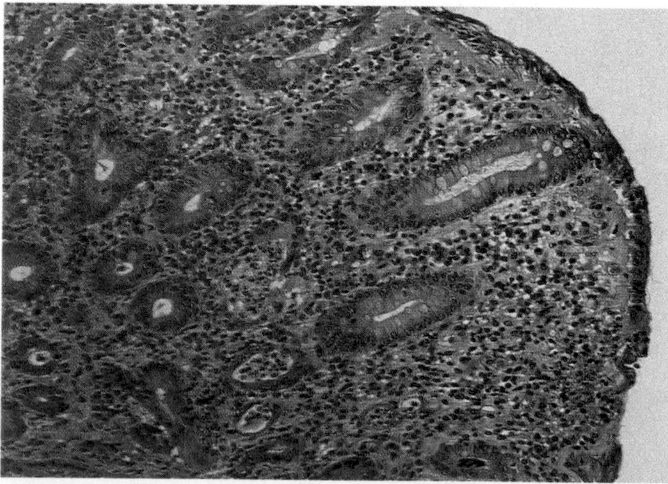

Fig. 33-45 *Campylobacter* colitis. The mucosa is endematous and inflamed. Acute inflammatory cells are evident in the lumens of glands (crypt abscesses) and partially destroyed glands are evident. *Campylobacter jejuni* was isolated from stool.

Complicating inflammatory processes are rare but occur both in patients with histories of GI disease and without.[768] These include urinary tract infections, cholecystitis, salpingitis, meningitis, appendicitis, pancreatitis, abscesses of various organs or soft tissues, endocarditis, arthritis both purulent and reactive, and peritonitis. Morphologic features are nonspecific.

Helicobacter pylori

The spiral bacterium *Helicobacter pylori* was originally recognized by application of silver-impregnation techniques to tissue from patients with gastritis. The organism, originally classified as *Campylobacter pylori* or *Campylobacter pyloridis,* was placed in the new genus based on analysis of genetic relationships.[769] A distinguishing feature of this species is the rapid and vigorous production of urease, which has been utilized as a clinical diagnostic test,[770] as well as for identification of the isolated bacterium. The ecologic niche of this microbe is the gastric mucus, where it is protected from the acidic environment of the stomach; it is also associated with intercellular junctions of gastric epithelial cells.[771] It has been suggested that the spiral form and rapid motility provide a selective advantage for movement through the viscous gel of the gastric mucus.

H. pylori causes chronic gastritis,[772] which may be accompanied by ulceration, primarily in the antrum of the stomach.[773] Bacteria with similar morphology also affect metaplastic gastric tissue in Barrett's esophagus[774] but not in Meckel's diverticulum.[775] The pathogenic role of these organisms is unknown. It has also been suggested that *H. pylori* is etiologically associated with gastric carcinoma[776] and primary lymphoma (MALT lymphoma).[777] It is now recognized that the spiral bacteria visualized in gastric tissue are a diverse group, including other species, such as *Helicobacter mustelae,* and other genera, such as *Gastrospirillum hominis.*

Other glucose-fermenting gram-negative bacilli

Aeromonas *species*

Members of the genus *Aeromonas* are gram-negative, fermentative bacilli that are easily confused with *E. coli* and *Enterobacter* species. *Aeromonas* is usually part of a mixture of infectious agents but appears to have been the primary pathogen in intra-abdominal infections; infection of skin, muscle, and soft tissue; meningitis; endocarditis; and sepsis in healthy as well as compromised individuals.[778] Human infections are often associated with exposure to water.[779] Some investigators believe that *A. hydrophila* and *A. sobria* can cause gastroenteritis, both in adults and in children, by production of an enterotoxin,[780,781] but there remains some controversy.

Plesiomonas shigelloides

The single member of the genus *Plesiomonas, P. shigelloides* has been previously referred to as *Pseudomonas shigelloides, Aeromonas shigelloides,* or *Vibrio shigelloides.* The organism possesses somatic O antigens closely related to those of *Shigella sonnei.* The natural habitat of the organism is surface water or mud.

Although *P. shigelloides* has not produced disease in human volunteers and does not produce an enterotoxin active in isolated rabbit ileum, the organism has been isolated in the absence of other bacterial pathogens from cases of a benign, self-limited gastroenteritis.[782] Cellulitis and even fatal septicemia have been rarely described.

Fastidious and non-glucose-fermenting gram-negative bacilli

Haemophilus influenzae

Microbiology. *Haemophilus* species are thin, aerobic gram-negative bacilli or coccobacilli that require nutritional supplements and added CO_2 for growth on agar surfaces. *Haemophilus influenzae,* the most important pathogen in the genus requires NAD (V factor) and hemin (X factor) for growth. Certain strains have a polysaccharide capsule, of which serotype b is the most significant clinically. The biologic characteristics of encapsulated strains and that of nonencapsulated strains of *H. influenzae* differ greatly. *Haemophilus aegyptius* (the Koch-Weeks bacillus) is now recognized as a biotype of *H. influenzae*.

Epidemiology. When selective media are employed, *H. influenzae* can be demonstrated in virtually 100% of children.[783] Most strains do not have detectable polysaccharide capsule (untypeable), but as many as 70% of toddlers in a day-care center were colonized at some time with type b strains.[784] Most colonized individuals do not develop either local or systemic infection. Risk factors for invasive infection include absence of protective antibody and living conditions that foster transmission of pathogenic strains. Humans are the reservoir for infections, and intrafamily spread of type b infections has been documented.[785] Attendance at day-care centers, presence of siblings, and crowded households are risk factors for invasive disease. Of these, family contact is more important than day care.[786] Encapsulated strains produce infection primarily in young children with relative sparing of neonates and infants, but disseminated disease occurs also in adults.[787] Nonencapsulated strains produce disease in all age groups, but the clinical presentation varies with age. Children develop upper and lower respiratory tract disease,[788] whereas infection in adults is mainly in the lower respiratory tract. *Haemophilus* disease is usually sporadic; although infections may occur in clusters, the epidemic disease associated with meningococci is not evident. Risk factors for invasive disease with encapsulated strains include immunoglobulin deficiency,[36] complement deficiency, and functional asplenia, as exemplified by sickle cell disease.[106] For strains with or without capsules the anatomy of the nasopharynx and eustachian tube may be an important factor in pediatric otitis media, whereas patients with chronic obstructive lung disease are at increased risk of lower respiratory infection in later life.[789]

Pathogenesis. The extensive studies of *H. influenzae* demonstrate the complexity of analyzing virulence factors and the danger of facile conclusions and assumptions. Adherence to epithelial cells is clearly important for colonization. The primary mediator of adherence is pili,[790] but other, incompletely characterized bacterial factors are also involved.[791] It is less clear, however, that adherence to epithelium is necessary for production of infection and disease. Porras and associates were unable to correlate the presence of adherence in vitro with the occurrence of otitis media in children.[7] Adherence actually appears to be negatively associated with encapsulation and invasive disease.[8] Although type b strains do colonize the nasopharynx in selected populations, nontypable strains adhere better to epithelial cells in vitro than encapsulated strains do.[792] The complexity of the interactions is illustrated by one experimental study in which inoculation of adherent, piliated bacteria into the nasopharynx of infant rats resulted in disseminated disease from which nonpiliated, nonadherent bacteria were isolated.[793]

The ability to produce local cell damage is probably important for both typable and nontypable bacteria. Invasion beyond the mucosa, however, is primarily associated with the presence of a polysaccharide capsule, particularly type b.[794] Thus pneumonia in adults is caused by strains of either type, but bacteremic infection is almost exclusively caused by type b strains.[787] As for other encapsulated bacteria the polysaccharide serves to diminish phagocytosis and bactericidal action of phagocytes until specific antibody is produced. A recently introduced conjugate vaccine against the type b polysaccharide has virtually eliminated invasive disease in pediatric populations,[38] providing testimony to the importance of this virulence factor.

Bacterial lipopolysaccharide (endotoxin) is important for generation of an inflammatory response and for producing the clinical picture of sepsis.[795] Generation of TNF has been documented as a marker for severe bacteremic infection. Outer membrane proteins may also cause tissue damage by interrupting the vascular endothelium.

A 25 mD plasmid and 72 kD minor outer membrane protein[796] are characteristically present in the *aegyptius* biotype that produces Brazilian purpuric fever. Lipopolysaccharide appeared to be related to virulence in an animal model.[797] These strains were cytotoxic for vascular endothelial cells in vitro, whereas strains from nonpurpuric infection were not.[798]

The role of immunity in *Haemophilus* infections is complicated. Bacterial polysaccharide produces a T-independent immune response, but some patients, who do not respond to polysaccharide vaccine with anticapsular antibodies, are at risk of developing invasive disease. Conjugation of the polysaccharide to an immunogenic protein carrier results in an additional T-dependent immunologic response, in which primed memory B-cells are produced. These conjugate vaccines have been remarkably successful in eliciting an antibody response, even in young children, and protecting the recipients against serious disease.[799] It has been suggested that antibodies to outer membrane proteins also play a protective role.[800]

The role of IgA in the pathogenesis of *Haemophilus* infections is unclear.[801] The bacteria produce an IgA protease, which could potentially inactivate one of the mucosal defense mechanisms. On the other hand, IgA in respiratory secretions has the effect of blocking the effect of bactericidal and opsonic antibody of other classes.[68]

Clinical features and pathology. Unencapsulated strains produce acute inflammatory disease of the upper airways (otitis media and sinusitis), the conjunctiva including ophthalmia neonatorum, and the lower respiratory tract (tracheitis, bronchitis, and pneumonia). *H. influenzae* joins *Staphylococcus aureus* and *Pseudomonas aeruginosa* as an important pathogen in the lower respiratory tract of patients with cystic fibrosis.[802] The *aegyptius* biotype has classically been associated with acute conjunctivitis, but most clinical laboratories do not make this sophisticated differentiation.

Type b *H. influenzae* produces bacteremic infection, which may be manifest by infection in one or more organs.[803] The most common diseases are epiglottitis, uvulitis, pneumonia, meningitis, pericarditis, cellulitis, and arthritis. In older children and adults *Haemophilus* species is a minor contributor to the cause of these infections; in young children it was the most common pathogen before the introduction of effective vaccines. The bacteremia may be accompanied by sepsis;[804] both purpura fulminans[805] and Waterhouse-Friderichsen syndrome[125] have been reported. Infection of the genitourinary tract and peritoneal cavity is occasional. Endocarditis is conspicuously missing from the list of associated diseases. Strains with polysaccharide capsules other than type b produce the same continuum of disease but are much less commonly encountered.

The inflammatory responses are neutrophilic and resemble other pyogenic bacteria. Abscesses are distinctly uncommon.[806] An unusual and characteristic clinical presentation is associated with type b facial cellulitis, which often imparts a blue color to the inflamed skin. This discoloration has been noted less frequently in adults.[807] A devastating manifestation of *H. influenzae* biotype *aegyptius* was recognized a decade ago in Brazil. Acute conjunctivitis is followed by the abrupt onset of fever, abdominal pain, vomiting, shock, and extensive cutaneous purpura.[796] Meningitis is conspicuously absent, but the mortality is very high. The infection was designated "Brazilian purpuric fever," but cases have now been described in Australia and Austria. Pathologically, there were hemorrhages in the skin, mucous membranes, and adrenal glands as well as edema of the lungs and brain.

Haemophilus parainfluenzae

Haemophilus parainfluenzae requires supplementation of media with hemin but not with NAD. It is also a member of the normal oropharyngeal flora.[783] It is an occasional pathogen, producing disease that resembles both encapsulated and unencapsulated strains of *H. influenzae*. Respiratory infections in patients with chronic obstructive lung disease[789] have been reported. Genitourinary tract disease may result in neonatal infection. More serious systemic diseases, including endocarditis, osteomyelitis, hepatic abscess, meningitis, and epiglottitis are rare manifestations of infection.

Haemophilus aphrophilus *and* Haemophilus paraphrophilus

These two species derived their name from the Greek word for 'foam,' *aphros,* referring to the high concentrations of CO_2 needed for growth. They are the only members of the genus that do not require hemin for growth under all conditions. NAD is necessary for growth of *H. paraphrophilus.*[172] These gram-negative coccobacilli produce infection rarely in humans, but serious disease can result. Endocarditis, osteomyelitis, and cerebral abscesses have been described. The vegetations produced during endovascular infections are often large, and embolic phenomena are relatively frequent.[808]

Haemophilus actinomycetemcomitans *(formerly* Actinobacillus actinomycetemcomitans)

Haemophilus actinomycetemcomitans is a small gram-negative, nonmotile, slow-growing coccobacillus that is part of the normal human oral flora.[809] There is a curious association with actinomycetes. The organism occurs in a rapidly destructive periodontal disease of adolescents (juvenile periodontitis).[810] *H. actinomycetemcomitans* elaborates a substance that impairs phagocytic function of polymorphonuclear leukocytes.[811]

The organism has infected both native and prosthetic cardiac valves,[812] particularly after dental procedures or in patients with severe periodontal disease. Morbidity and mortality have been high, perhaps because slow growth of the organism under aerobic conditions has delayed the diagnosis. Brain abscess, thyroid abscess, urinary tract infections, pneumonia, and vertebral osteomyelitis have been reported.[813] Infection of a congenital atrioventricular fistula has also been noted.

Haemophilus ducreyi

Haemophilus ducreyi is the etiologic agent of chancroid. It is a faintly staining, gram-negative coccobacillus that requires hemin but not NAD for growth.[172] The difficulty of isolating this species makes interpretation of clinical data on unconfirmed cases suspect, though methods for laboratory diagnosis have been improved in recent years. Chancroid is a sexually transmitted disease and is recognized primarily in nonwhite, uncircumcized men, perhaps because of the difficulty of recognizing the lesions in the female genital tract. The disease has a worldwide distribution, and the frequency has recently increased in the United States.[814] It is believed that this infection is significantly underreported.[815] The lesions are usually limited to the genital region,[816] where the bacterium produces intensely painful, nonindurated, ragged, and undermined ulcer (soft chancre) (Fig. 33-46). After experimental inoculation of human volunteers there is erosion of the epithelium and collections of PMNLs in epidermal pustules. The dermis contains a predominantly perivascular mononuclear infiltrate and proliferating endothelial cells. Inguinal lymphadenopathy often occurs, resulting in a fluctuant bubo, which may rupture if untreated. The lesions may be confused with ulcers produced by *Treponema pallidum,* herpes simplex virus, or *Chlamydia trachomatis* (lymphogranuloma venereum serovars).

Legionella *species*

Microbiology. Legionella species are thin, aerobic, motile, nonsporulating, gram-negative bacilli.[172] They require cysteine for initial isolation on agar media, and growth is stimulated by iron salts. Members of the genus are biochemically variable or inert. *Legionella micdadei* is weakly acid fast in clinical specimens but not after isolation on agar media. Presumptive identification of the species and serogroup is provided by

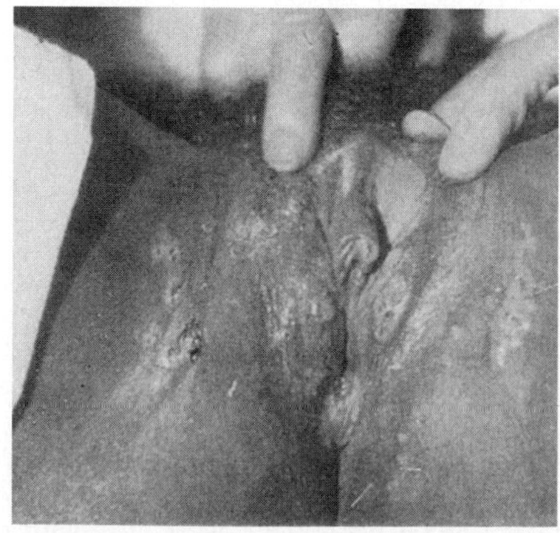

Fig. 33-46 Chancroid. Multiple ulcers on vulva, perineum, and thighs.

immunologic techniques, most commonly immunofluorescence. Definitive identification may require genetic analysis. The diagnosis of human infections is best made by recovery of the bacteria on agar media. Serodiagnosis plays an adjunctive role and direct detection of bacterial antigen is commercially available for *Legionella pneumophila* serogroup 1.

History and epidemiology. Legionella species were isolated from clinical specimens as long ago as 1943, but the significance of the isolates was not appreciated.[817] An epidemic of pneumonia at a convention of the Pennsylvania American Legion in Philadelphia in 1976 provided sufficient publicity to stimulate a successful effort to identify the etiologic agent,[818,819] which was named *Legionella pneumophila*. Although many scientists contributed their efforts and talents, the mystery was unraveled because of the persistence of one individual, Joseph McDade.[151] Shortly thereafter, an acid-fast bacillus associated with acute pneumonia in Pittsburgh was recovered on agar media, using techniques that had been developed for *L. pneumophila*.[820,821] The new agent was subsequently named *Legionella micdadei* in honor of Joseph McDade. Currently the number of *Legionella* species and serogroup numbers in the thirties with no end in sight. Most human infections, however, are caused by *L. pneumophila* serogroup 1.[822] With the addition of *L. pneumophila* serogroup 6, *L. micdadei,* and *Legionella dumoffii*, approximately 90% of infections are accounted for.

Legionella infections are acquired in the community and in hospitals. In both cases they cause approximately 1% to 6% of pneumonias.[823,824] The bacteria are opportunistic pathogens. Risk factors for severe infection include severe underlying disease, such as chronic cardiovascular disease and neoplasia, and immunosuppressive regimens, particularly corticosteroid therapy.[825] In addition, there must be an environmental source of bacteria.[826] Neutropenia is not a risk factor, and patients who are infected with HIV are surprisingly unaffected by these pathogens.[827]

Legionella species are aquatic bacteria in nature. They have been isolated from moist potting soil but never from dry earth.[828] The interactions between Legionella and other environmental microbes are complex. A particularly close association with free-living amebas has been repeatedly demonstrated.[829] Isolation of *Legionella* from environmental sources correlates with the presence of amebas and is sometimes accomplished only if the samples are preincubated with amebas before being plated onto agar media.[830,831] Colonization of humans rarely if ever occurs, and person-to-person transmission of infection has not been demonstrated.[832]

The portal of entry is almost always the respiratory tract after aerosolization of bacteria. The two major environmental sources of bacteria are potable water,[833] particularly hot-water systems,[834] and cooling towers.[835] The mechanism by which bacteria are disseminated is clear in the case of cooling towers, where bacterial suspensions are aerosolized in the drift from the tower. If individuals or air-intake vents in buildings are downwind, the bacteria may be inhaled in sufficient numbers to produce symptomatic infection. Aerosols of potable water are produced by nebulizers and showerheads, but the mechanism for dissemination is not recognized in most cases. An outbreak of *L. pneumophila* infection associated with a misting machine in the produce department of a grocery store emphasizes the degree to which we are surrounded by aerosols in daily life.[836] Rarely, legionellae in potable water may be introduced directly into open wounds.[837]

Pathogenesis. Legionella species are facultative intracellular pathogens with a particular affinity for monocytes and macrophages.[838] They attach to macrophages by means of complement receptors, after which they are phagocytized.[839] A peculiar, coiling type of phagocytosis has been demonstrated with some strains.[840] Conventional phagocytosis that is inhibited by cytochalasin also occurs.[841] After phagocytosis by naïve macrophages phagolysosomal fusion is blocked[842] and acidification of the phagosome is blocked.[843] Serum is not required for phagocytosis, but enhances the process. Polymorphonuclear neutrophils phagocytize the bacteria in the presence of opsonins, but bacterial replication does not result.[844]

After activation by cytokines monocytes and macrophages no longer support intracellular replication of *Legionella*. Interferon-γ appears to be the primary cytokine responsible for bacteriostasis.[845] One of the mechanisms by which replication is inhibited is restriction of bacterial access to intracellular iron, which is needed for growth.[82] Iron chelators reverse the effect. *Legionella*[846] infection in both humans and experimental animals elicits both a humoral and a cellular immune response; the latter appears to be more important. Infected animals are immune to reinfection,[847] and recurrent human disease has not been documented with certainty. A 24 kD outer membrane protein (macrophage infectivity protein, mip) enhances bacterial replication in macrophages,[848] and alteration of the encoding gene reduces infectivity for macrophages, but the mip is not required for virulence. The major secretory protein,[5] a porin, and a 65 kD outer membrane heat-shock protein induce protective immunity,[849] but again these proteins are not essential for virulence.[6] The cellular and humoral immune response elicited by the major outer membrane protein protects against cross-reacting *Legionella* species and serogroups.[850] The role of humoral antibody in protection against *Legionella* infection is less clear.[851]

A metalloprotease, similar to the elastase of *Pseudomonas aeruginosa*,[852] is produced by *L. pneumophila*.[853] A role for this enzyme in production of tissue necrosis has been hypothesized but not proved.

After deposition of *L. pneumophila* aerosols into the lungs of guinea pigs, bacterial replication in resident alveolar macrophages begins almost immediately[122](see Fig. 33-4). Shortly afterwards PMNLs are recuited in large numbers, and fluid exudation into the airspaces begins. Later circulating monocytes and lymphocytes appear in the airspaces. Viable bacteria are associated with the mononuclear cell fraction of lavaged alveolar fluid. Dissemination of bacteria occurs through the bloodstream. *Legionella* organisms are found in many extrapulmonary organs,[854] and extrapulmonary disease occurs occasionally.

Clinical features and pathology. *Legionella* species may produce four types of disease: asymptomatic infection, Pontiac fever, pneumonia, and extrapulmonary infection.

Asymptomatic infection can be inferred from the discordance between high prevalence of antibody and lower frequency of overt disease. Although some of the residual antibodies may represent cross-reactions with other bacteria, it is difficult to accept that explanation as the whole story. More definitive evidence accrues from studies of transplant recipients.[855] Even these immunocompromised, closely monitored patients develop antibody to *Legionella* in the absence of clinically obvious disease.

Pontiac fever was first recognized when an epidemic of acute respiratory disease afflicted almost all individuals in a public health department in Pontiac, Michigan. The disease is characterized by a very high attack rate (greater than 95%), a short incubation period (4 to 16 hours), and the absence of radiographic evidence of pneumonia. Affected individuals develop a flu-like syndrome with fever, malaise, myalgias, and nonproductive cough. Recovery occurs spontaneously. At the time of the original epidemic a faulty air-conditioning system was pinpointed as the source of the infection.[856] Guinea pigs developed a nodular pneumonia after they were exposed to air in the building and after they were exposed to an aerosol of water from the system back in Atlanta.[857] The investigators got agonizingly close to the answer, recognizing the presence of a bacterium in the guinea pig tissues, but were unable to isolate the organism in culture. The answer would not be forthcoming for another 10 years, when *L. pneumophila* serogroup 1 was recovered from frozen guinea pig lung. Attempts to demonstrate a serologic response in human sera from the outbreak against the guinea pig organism were unsuccessful initially but for still unexplained reasons were successful when repeated 10 years later.

Subsequently outbreaks of Pontiac fever have been linked to *Legionella feeleii, Legionella anisa,* and *Legionella micdadei.* A steam turbine condenser, a cooling tower, an automotive assembly line, and a whirlpool spa have been incriminated as sources for the bacteria.[151] Sporadic cases of nonpneumonic *L. pneumophila* infection differ from Pontiac fever only in their solitary occurrence.[835] As a self-limited nonfatal illness there are no pathologic studies of Pontiac fever.

Isolates of *L. pneumophila* serogroup 1 recovered from pneumonic and nonpneumonic disease are identical within the limits of the available techniques. Several hypotheses have been advanced to explain the differing clinical syndromes, but none explains all the facts. The most common manifestation of *Legionella* infection is acute pneumonia. Most of the published information pertains to the two most commonly encountered species, *L. pneumophila*[819,858] and *L. micdadei,*[821,859] but descriptions of disease caused by other species indicate that there may be no substantial differences among the species. *L. pneumophila* pneumonia was originally known as Legionnaires' disease, whereas Pittsburgh pneumonia was the original designation for *L. micdadei* infections.

The incubation period is 2 to 10 days, after which fever and respiratory distress abruptly ensue. Cough is prominent but minimally productive of sputum. Expectorated or aspirated secretions typically contain polymorphonuclear leukocytes, but bacteria are not usually demonstrable. Acid-fast bacilli have been observed in a few cases of *L. micdadei* pneumonia. The infiltrates are usually focal, but over several days they spread to involve the whole lobe or portions of multiple lobes. In some series rounded, pleura-based opacities were observed, suggesting the possibility of septic pulmonary emboli.[860] Cavitation is rarely demonstrated radiographically.

The pathologic lesion is a focal consolidative pneumonia that is distinctly lobular, but extension of the inflammatory process usually results in confluent lobular pneumonia, which may involve most of a lobe.[861] A distribution that is indistinguishable from lobar pneumonia has been described. After fixation the fibrinous character of the pneumonia imparts a dry, granular appearance to the cut surface, making it easy to scrape the exudate from the surface with a scalpel. Despite the rarity of clinically evident abscesses, they are observed in as many as 20% of pathologic specimens. The rounded opacities observed in radiographs are also distinctive macroscopic features. Pleural effusions are usually minimal, but empyema has been reported.

The histologic picture is dominated by extensive exudate in the airspaces. The cellular component may be predominantly mononuclear, predominantly polymorphonuclear, or most commonly a mixture of the two cell types. A case of plasma cell pneumonia in a lung from which *L. pneumophila* serogroup 1 was isolated has been described, but a causal relationship is conjectural.[862] Fibrin is prominent. Erythrocytes are frequently present, but the process is not primarily hemorrhagic. A characteristic but not diagnostic feature of the exudate is focal lysis of the inflammatory cells, extensive karyorrhectic nuclear debris imparting a dusty appearance that resembles leukocytoclastic vasculitis in the skin (Fig. 33-47). Areas of coagulative necrosis may be present, perhaps related to a focal vasculitis. In contrast to *Pseudomonas aeruginosa* pneumonia, bacteria are not concentrated in the inflamed blood vessels.

Less common histologic features include a bluish, mucoid redundant, relatively acellular exudate[863] and hyaline membranes,[864] which cannot always be explained by other potential causes of diffuse alveolar damage.

Bacteria are occasionally demonstrable in hematoxylin-eosin stains. A modification of the Brown and Hopps stain colors the bacteria effectively, and the Giemsa stain has been used successfully. Any of the silver impregnation stains, such as the Dieterle, Steiner, or Warthin-Starry methods, facilitate detection of the bacteria by the deposition of silver salts on the organisms, distorting the morphology in the process (Fig. 33-48). The stain of choice is the one that is performed best by the local histology laboratory. The simplest method for demonstrating the bacteria, however, is to stain an impression smear made from the cut surface of the lung with Gram's stain as performed in the microbiology laboratory (Fig. 33-49). The serogroup-specific and species-specific antigens sur-

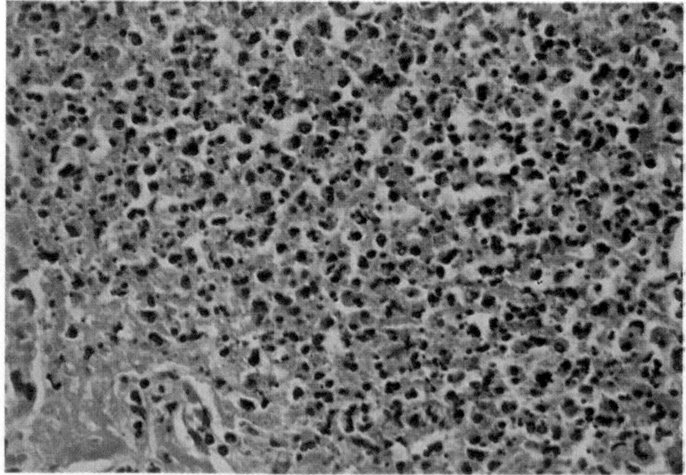

Fig. 33-47 Legionnaires' disease. The inflammatory infiltrate of neutrophils and macrophages is undergoing extensive lysis, producing a characteristic but nondiagnostic dusty appearance.

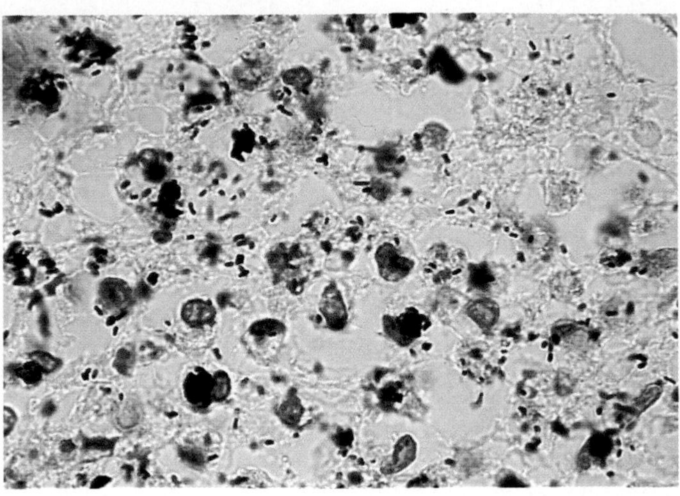

Fig. 33-48 Legionnaires' disease. Bacteria may be demonstrated with variable success using the Brown and Hopps or Brown-Brenn techniques. Silver impregnation methods are more sensitive. Large numbers of intracellular and extracellular bacteria are present. Same case as in Fig. 33-47. (Dieterle method.)

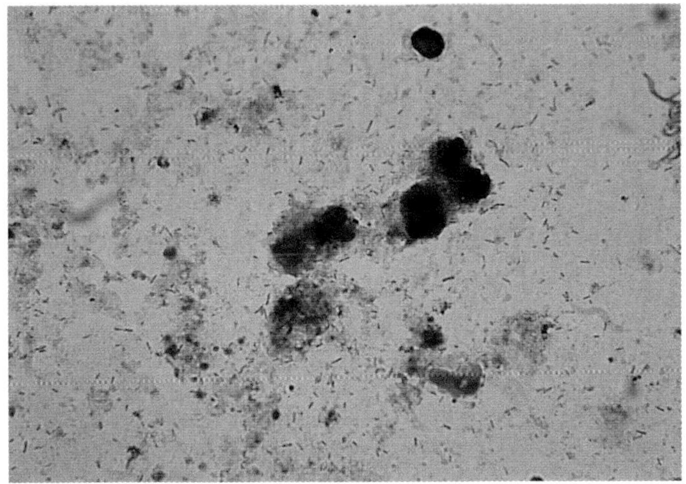

Fig. 33-49 Legionnaires' disease. Imprint smear of lung demonstrates numerous thin gram-negative bacilli. The sensitivity and ease of interpretation with this technique are far greater than with versions of Gram's stain adapted to tissue sections. *Legionella pneumophila* serogroup I isolated in pure culture from the lung. Gram's technique with 0.05% basic fuchsin (the dye employed in the Giménez stain) added to the safranin counterstain.

vive formalin fixation and subsequent processing, and so either immunofluorescence[865] or immunoenzyme[866] techniques may be used to provide a more specific diagnosis. Ziehl-Neelsen or modified acid-fast stains, such as the Fite stain, will reveal the cells of *L. micdadei*[821] (Fig. 33-50).

Histologically and ultrastructurally bacteria are present in the extracellular spaces and in phagocytic cells, especially macrophages. An unusual association of phagocytized bacteria with phagosomes that are lined by ribosomes was first demonstrated in well-fixed lung biopsy specimens[867] but are also characteristic of infected monocytes and macrophages obtained from humans[868] and experimental animals.[122] The role of the ribosomes is unknown.

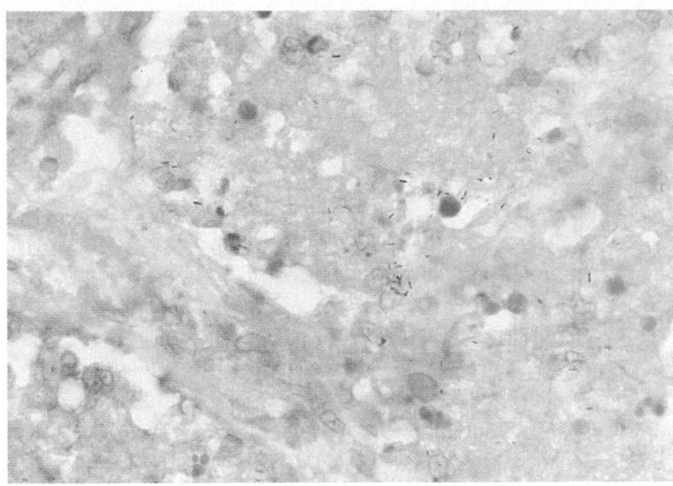

Fig. 33-50 Pittsburgh pneumonia. The acid-fastness of *Legionella micdadei* is demonstrated in tissue sections, but the bacteria lose this property after isolation on agar. (Ziehl-Neelsen method.) (Case courtesy Richard Myerowitz, MD.)

The radiographic lesions resolve slowly in survivors,[869] and the inflammatory exudate presumably resolves, but chronic inflammation and scarring have been demonstrated in well-documented cases of *L. pneumophila* pneumonia.[870]

Extrapulmonary infection occurs most commonly after a primary pneumonia.[151] Purulent inflammation, sometimes accompanied by abscesses, is usually present. Pericarditis could result from direct extension. Distant metastatic lesions, which result from bacteremia, include pyelonephritis, endocarditis, hemodialysis shunt infections, hepatic abscesses, cellulitis and perirectal abscesses. Rarely, extrapulmonary lesions occur without clinically evident pneumonia.[871] Sternal wound infection caused by *L. dumoffii* occurred after contaminated tap water was used to wash postoperative patients and clean their wounds.[837] Metastatic foci are far more common after infection with *L. pneumophila* than with other species.

Pseudomonadaceae

Microbiology. Pseudomonads are thin, aerobic, gram-negative bacilli that utilize glucose oxidatively and are motile by means of polar flagella. Most species produce cytochrome oxidase, some weakly. *Pseudomonas maltophilia* has been transferred into a new genus, *Xanthomonas. Burkholderia* is a new genus that was created for seven *Pseudomonas* species, including *P. cepacia, P. mallei,* and *P. pseudomallei. Burkholderia cepacia* is the type species.

Epidemiology and general virulence mechanisms. Pseudomonads are environmental organisms, usually found in aquatic habitats, but they may also be found as part of the human oropharyngeal and intestinal flora, particularly in hospitalized patients. All the species are opportunistic pathogens, but modern medicine has produced conditions that allow them to thrive in hospitals, where they now number among our most formidable foes. Widespread resistance to many antimicrobial agents, both intrinsic and acquired, has produced a selective advantage that has allowed pseudomonads to flourish where antibiotics are freely used. Infections may be endogenous, arising from the altered flora in sick patients, or exogenously transferred from the environment. Although a direct connection between an environmental site and the patient may occur, an equally or more important scenario is transfer of colonizing bacteria from one patient to another on the hands of medical personnel. The source of the infection may be a transiently contaminated individual who has not adequately practiced infection control techniques, but prolonged colonization, resistant to elimination by handwashing, has been demonstrated on the skin of nurses. Several species are also resistant to commonly used disinfectants, such as chlorhexidine. As a result these bacteria have even produced infection after the patient was exposed to a disinfectant solution.

The risk factors for *Pseudomonas* infection are factors that increase the likelihood of colonization, exposure to contaminated medical devices, and underlying conditions that reduce the ability to generate inflammatory or specific immunologic responses.[872] Severe neutropenia is a particularly important risk factor. Patients with neoplastic disease who have been treated with chemotherapeutic agents frequently have defects in both specific and nonspecific defense mechanisms.

Pseudomonas aeruginosa

Pathogenesis. Receptors that are exposed when fibronectin on the surface of cells is diminished in hospitalized patients allow *Pseudomonas aeruginosa* to establish residence on mucosal surfaces, from which an invasive infection can be launched. The adhesion is mediated by pili and in some situations by bacterial polysaccharide. The number and versatility of the virulence factors expressed by this species make one wonder why it is not a more significant pathogen in normal hosts. It is likely that some or all the potential virulence factors are active in human infections, and the effects may be additive.

Alginate (slime). Some strains of *P. aeruginosa* produce an extracellular polysaccharide capsule that is composed of alginate.[873] Copious production of this compound is closely correlated with cystic fibrosis, though the association is not exclusive. The resulting colonies are extremely mucoid when isolated on agar plates and may contribute to the tenacious sputum produced by patients with cystic fibrosis. This slime exerts an antiphagocytic effect[874] and also interferes with the function of neutrophils and lymphocytes.[875] The slime produces a biofilm on the surface of the tracheobronchial epithelium, in which the bacteria are trapped. It thus serves as a mechanism for adherence and persistence of bacteria and may be partially responsible for the intractable nature of pulmonary colonization and infection in patients with cystic fibrosis.[873]

Exotoxin A. Exotoxin A, which is closely related to diphtheria toxin,[876] is a heat-labile single-chain polypeptide that acts as a proenzyme. It inhibits protein synthesis by inhibiting elongation factor 2, an enzyme that normally catalyzes the assembly of polypeptides on the ribosome.[877]

Endotoxin. P. aeruginosa contains a lipopolysaccharide that resembles the endotoxin of the Enterobacteriaceae. This compound plays a major role in the production of sepsis and disseminated intravascular coagulation, which are a prominent part of bacteremic infection.

Elastase and other proteases.[32] Elastase, a serine protease, is the best studied exoenzyme produced by many strains of *P. aeruginosa. Pseudomonas* elastase is biochemically similar to the metalloproteinase produced by *L. pneumophila.*[852] Elastase and the alginate slime are coregulated, providing a means of assuring concurrent activity by two important virulence factors. The activities of the proteases that have potential pathogenetic import are legion, and their presence in the lungs of patients with cystic fibrosis who are infected with various *Pseudomonas* species has been documented as follows.[135]

DAMAGE TO EPITHELIUM. Elastase decreases the barrier function of cell monolayers, even without physical disruption of cell membranes.[878] Human neutrophil and *Pseudomonas aeruginosa* elastase act in a similar fashion to disrupt human ciliated nasal epithelium and reduce the frequency of ciliary beating in vitro. Elastase and alkaline protease both have been demonstrated to disrupt cilia physically in experimental animals.[879] The combined effect of these mechanisms is to diminish clearance of particulate matter, including bacteria, from the lungs in vivo.[880] Experimental studies have also demonstrated disruption of intercellular junctions of epithelial cells with a resultant increase in epithelial permeability.[881]

FACILITATION OF BACTERIAL ADHERENCE TO CELLS. Elastase strips fibronectin from the surface of epithelial cells and connective tissue cells,[882] promoting bacterial adherence to the altered cell surfaces. An alternative mechanism for enhancing adherence of bacteria may be by enzymatic damage to the epithelium, followed by bacterial adherence to underlying damaged mucosa and extruded mucus.[883]

EFFECTS ON THE COAGULATION AND COMPLEMENT SYSTEMS. Proteases, including elastase, activate the complement system, including the initiating components of the classical (C1q) and alternative (C3) pathways.[884] Activation of the kinin system by elastase is mediated by Hageman factor, and the effect on vascular permeability has been demonstrated experimentally.[885]

ACCENTUATION OF TISSUE DAMAGE. In conjunction with other proteases, especially neutrophil elastase, *Pseudomonas* elastase modifies transferrin and potentially increases the destructive activity of hydroxyl radicals generated in the inflammatory process.[886] The enzyme cleaves types III and IV collagen, which are components of the connective tissue stroma.[887] Destruction of basement membranes from several organs has been documented experimentally,[888] perhaps mediated by cleavage of both soluble and basement membrane–associated laminin.[889]

REDUCTION OF PHAGOCYTOSIS AND PHAGOCYTIC CELL FUNCTION. Elastase strips CR1, the complement receptor on the surface of neutrophils, and also C3bi from the surface of opsonized bacterial cells. In addition, neutrophils treated with bacterial elastase inhibits generation of superoxide by neutrophils and diminishes bacterial killing.[890] Purified elastase destroys human interferon-γ and tumor necrosis factor-α, both compounds that participate in the bactericidal activity of phagocytes or production of the sepsis syndrome.[891] Enzymatic degradation of basement membranes by *Pseudomonas aeruginosa* elastase may contribute to the vascular injury that characterizes these infections.[888]

INTERFERENCE WITH THE IMMUNE SYSTEM. Elastase degrades both serum IgA[892] and IgG[893] in vitro. The sputum of patients with permanent tracheostomies who were colonized with *P. aeruginosa* had higher levels of elastase and lower levels of IgA and produced greater binding of bacteria to epithelial cells than that from uncolonized patients.[894] The receptors on the surface of NK lymphocytes that mediate binding to target cells are destroyed by P. elastase reducing the effectiveness of these cells.[895] Nonspecific defense factors, such as lysozyme, are also degraded by these enzymes.[896]

Clinical features and pathology. Primary infections of the skin, urinary tract, or lungs are the most common sources of bacteremia,[897] which is associated with a mortality as high as 78%. Patients with extensive thermal burns are at high risk of developing skin infection complicated by sepsis. In one study, *P. aeruginosa* bacteremia was statistically predictive of a fatal outcome.[143] Endocarditis on both normal and damaged heart valves is an uncommon complication;[898] in abusers of intravenous drugs the tricuspid valve is frequently involved.[899] Infection is severe and often accompanied by sepsis, but is usually undifferentiated clinically unless characteristic necrotizing skin lesions (ecthyma gangrenosum) develop.[900]

The pathologic characteristics of *P. aeruginosa* infections derive from the virulence factors described above, particularly those that relate to destruction of basement membranes, connective tissue, and cells. Neutrophilic inflammation is often accompanied by abscess formation. More distinctive pathologic features are the presence of a septic vasculitis, which may be complicated by thrombosis and coagulative necrosis. Hemorrhage is a frequent feature of the lesions, even in the absence of infarcts. In neutropenic patients the cellular response may be considerably dampened. Experimentally, the *Pseudomonas* vasculitic lesion is characterized by relatively noninflammatory proliferation of bacteria in the adventitia of blood vessels.[123] These characteristics may occasionally be seen in human tissue, but in our experience the lesion is more discussed than observed.

Virtually any organ may be infected.[901] *P. aeruginosa* is a cause of malignant external otitis and participates prominently in chronic infections of the upper respiratory system, such as chronic suppurative otitis (swimmer's ear). Keratitis, endophthalmitis, and meningitis may be primary or secondary to bacteremic infection. Urinary tract infections are usually nosocomial. *P. aeruginosa* has replaced *Staphylococcus aureus* as the predominant cause of lower respiratory infection in patients with cystic fibrosis.[179] In addition to the metastatic cutaneous lesions that complicate bacteremia *P. aeruginosa* produces a primary dermatitis that is associated with exposure to contaminated water, such as whirlpools.[902]

Burkholderia (Pseudomonas) cepacia

Burkholderia cepacia (formerly *Pseudomonas cepacia* and before that *Pseudomonas multivorans,* or EO-1) shares many of the characteristics displayed by *P. aeruginosa.* It has been recently transferred into a new genus *(Burkholderia)* as the type species. The clinical and pathologic features are similar. Bacteremic infection occurs in immunocompromised patients as nosocomial infections.[903] This species has become a difficult clinical problem because of its propensity for causing infection in patients with cystic fibrosis,[904] even after lung transplantation.[905] Nosocomial transmission of the bacteria has been traced to respiratory therapy equipment and solutions used in therapy of these patients.[906] The interactions of host and bacterium range from colonization to necrotizing pneumonia with abscess formation.[904]

Xanthomonas (Pseudomonas) maltophilia

Xanthomonas maltophilia produces protease and elastase, similar to *P. aeruginosa.*[907] It has recently been transferred to a new genus, strentrophomones. This species is an opportunistic pathogen that is associated with hospitals, particularly intensive care units, prior antimicrobial therapy, and serious underlying disease.[908] The portal of entry is usually the lung, the urinary tract, or the skin. Bacteremic disease is associated with high morbidity and mortality. Ecthyma gangrenosum has been associated with the production of proteases.[907]

Burkholderia (Pseudomonas) mallei

Glanders is an infection of Equidae—horses, mules, and donkeys.[909] It is caused by a gram-negative, nonmotile, terminally granulated bacillus, *Burkholderia mallei.* Cattle and dogs are said to be highly resistant. The Danish veterinarian Viborg transmitted the disease by injecting matter from farcy buds into healthy animals.[910] Human glanders occurs almost exclusively in individuals who have been occupationally exposed to animals or their secretion: stable men, grooms, and knackers. Laboratory infections in those handling the organism are common, and serologic evidence of exposure approaches 40% in appropriate laboratory workers. It has not been described as a spontaneous disease in the United States since 1938. In Great Britain, the model "Glanders and Farcy Order" of 1894, revised in 1907, compensated slaughter of glandered animals and regulated disposal of their carcasses after which the human disease virtually disappeared.

Glanders occurs as farcy, a chronic septicemia that is characterized by many abscesses (farcy buds), often subcutaneous, with a chronic draining lymphangitis, and glanders itself characterized by one or a few abscesses in solid viscera with or without cutaneous lesions. Abscesses may appear caseous and may calcify.[911]

The human disease has a high mortality. The disease in animals responds to sulfonamides. Antibiotic or chemotherapy has not been standardized because of the rarity of the disease. Resistance can develop to sulfonamides.[912]

Burkholderia (Pseudomonas) pseudomallei

Epidemiology. Melioidosis was first recognized in Rangoon in morphine addicts on the Brahmaputra river front.[913] The name "melioidosis," which means 'resembling the distemper of asses,' was selected because of its resemblance to glanders. The disease is caused by a small irregularly staining gram-negative bacillus now classified as *Burkholderia pseudomallei.* The organism is distributed throughout the tropics in sufficient number that it is occasionally encountered as a laboratory contaminant.

P. pseudomallei resembles *B. mallei,* and the lesions of melioidosis morphologically resemble glanders,[914] but the epidemiology of the two diseases differs greatly. Recognition of melioidosis in an environment infested with rats led to a misguided preoccupation with an animal reservoir.[915] The organism can be found in rats, dogs, cats, cattle, sheep, and goats[916] and can experimentally infect insects, but its occurrence in water and soil is more important for the epidemiology of human cases than an animal reservoir or insect vector is. Practically all human cases can be attributed to contamination of wounds or by nontraumatic exposure to soil or water. Person-to-person transmission, including that by sexual contact, occurs but is very unusual.[917] A puzzling neonatal case has been reported.[918]

Human melioidosis occurs in the tropics,[919] especially in Southeast Asia, Indonesia, the Philippines, tropical Australia, Guam, and tropical Africa. The disease is very rare in the Western hemisphere, though cases have occurred in the Canal Zone and in at least two individuals who had never been outside the continental United States.[920] Laboratory infections have occurred but are uncommon.

French forces in Viet Nam experienced about 100 cases,[921] and American personnel during involvement in Southeast Asia sustained more than 300 cases with 43 deaths.[917] Approximately 10% of personnel with a year or more of experience in Viet Nam have serum antibodies against *B. pseudomallei,*[922] an implication that more than 100,000 Americans have been exposed to the organism. In view of that widespread exposure and the infrequency of clinical disease, the bacterium must be of very low virulence. In clinical cases there may be a history of war wounds, burns,[923] or immersion,[924] but often there is no obvious predisposing event.

Clinical features and pathology. Clinical melioidosis occurs in an acute septicemic form with abscesses just as glanders does. A more chronic form may be a prolongation of acute illness or develop insidiously sometimes many years (as many as 26 years)[925] later. Occasionally, recrudescent melioidosis is associated with diabetes, injury, surgical procedures, or malignancy.[925]

The lesion of melioidosis is an abscess with central coagulative necrosis and laminated with a mantle of acute inflammation and a more peripheral zone of mononuclear cells and granulation tissue (necrotizing granulomas with stellate necrosis).[926] Abscesses occur in virtually any organ, perhaps most importantly the lungs, often in upper lobes, sometimes with cavitation.[927] Additional sites include the liver, spleen (Fig. 33-51), bone, central nervous system, prostate, and myocardium. Isolated myocardial lesions have led to sudden death diagnosed as myocardial infarction.[928] Broad-spectrum antibiotics have lowered the mortality to 3% to 10% in diagnosed cases, but the mortality is higher among inhabitants of third-world countries. Diagnosis requires a high index of suspicion when confronted by a patient with appropriate exposure, even years before.

Acinetobacter *species*

The two most important species are *Acinetobacter calcoaceticus* (formerly *A. lwoffi* or *Mima*) and *Acinetobacter baumannii* (formerly *A. anitratum* or *Herrelea*). The bacteria are gram-negative coccobacilli that may assume a coccal form that causes confusion with *Neisseria* species. These species are opportunistic pathogens in compromised patients, particularly in the hospital. Bacteremic disease may be transient and accompanied by few symptoms,[929] but the serious potential of these pathogens has received more attention.[930] Infection of virtually any organ system may result. The resultant inflammatory response is acute, undifferentiated, and often accompanied by abscesses.

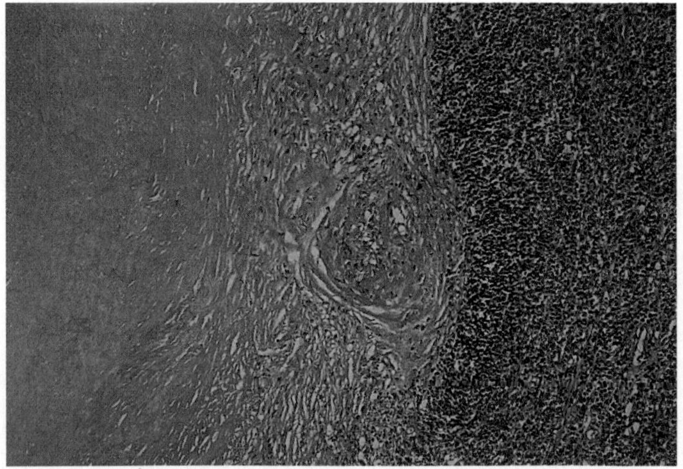

Fig. 33-51 Melioidosis. Large granuloma in the spleen of a patient with recrudescent disease. (Courtesy Robin Cooke, MD.)

Franciscella tularensis

History and epidemiology. In 1911 McCoy recognized a "plague-like disease of rodents" in Tulare County, California, while studying plague bacillus in indigenous wild rodents after the occurrence of human plague in San Francisco. In 1912 McCoy and Chapin cultivated the organism from rodents and named it *Bacterium tularense.*[931] Subsequently the bacterium was classified as *Pasteurella tularensis.* A human disease of unknown cause had been designated "deer-fly fever" by Pierce in Utah[932] and described in correspondence by Martin, an Arizona ophthalmologist.[933] Francis soon recognized the unity of these processes, which he termed "tularemia."[934] Genetic studies documented the differentiation of the etiologic agent from the genus *Pasteurella,* and the organism was finally (one hopes) renamed *Franciscella tularensis* in honor of Dr. Francis.

Tularemia is an infection of numerous species of wild rodents. The disease is propagated among rodents or lagomorphs, leading to the designation "rabbit fever,"[935] by hemophagous arthropods of many species,[936] most importantly the rat flea *Xenopsilla cheopis,* the Western deerfly, *Chrysops discalis,* and ticks of the same species that transmit Rocky Mountain spotted fever (RMSF). Tularemia has occurred in 200 species of animals[937] including wild muskrats.[938] Pond water may be sufficiently contaminated to be transiently infectious. With the infrequent exception of exposure to water and to isolated bacteria in the laboratory, human cases result from interposition of humans in the chain of infection. As a result the disease occurs chiefly in hikers, backpackers, rabbit hunters, and others who spend considerable time outdoors. The seasonal incidence has a bimodal pattern with peaks during summers (July and August), representing arthropod transmission, and in winters (December and January), representing exposure of hunters and trappers.[156] Cases have occurred in all 50 American states, most frequently in Arkansas, Texas, Missouri, and Oklahoma, and in many other countries, all in the Northern Hemisphere. As is the case for RMSF, another arthropod-borne disease, tularemia occurs in odd pockets, such as Cape Cod and Martha's Vineyard.[939] In Scandinavia, the disease is largely mosquito borne[940] or occurs in farmers during storage of hay that has been contaminated by the feces of rats.[941] Karpoff and Antonoff summarize the Russian experience, largely occupational.[942] There is considerable risk among laboratory personnel exposed to the agent.[936,943] Dr. Parker, director of the Public Health Service Laboratory, Hamilton, Montana, acquired tularemia in field studies of RMSF, and there were deaths from tularemia during those studies. Human tularemia has slowly decreased in incidence in the United States since the 1970s.

Clinical features. Six clinical forms have been described: ulceroglandular, oculoglandular, lymphadenoid, typhoidal, oropharyngeal, and pulmonic. This system seems overly refined and anatomically self-explanatory.[944] More significant to pathogenesis is that the portal of entry is usually obvious, followed rapidly by lymphangitis and involvement of regional lymph nodes.

Lymphadenopathy without a clear portal of entry or sepsis without obvious organ involvement is less common, and inhalation of highly infectious aerosols while one is handling sick rodents, dressing game animals, or performing laboratory procedures account for dangerous examples of pulmonic tularemia.[945] Pleural involvement without pneumonia occurs but is rare.[946] The mortality is appreciable, especially in tularemic pneumonia, but an outbreak of about 600 cases of inhalation tularemia, diagnosed by serologic analysis, occurred in northern Sweden without mortality.[941] Some observers believe that bacterial variants with greatly differing virulence account for the discrepancies.

Pathogenesis and pathology. The major factor in pathogenesis is proliferation of bacilli. From 10 to 50 organisms are pathogenic intradermally or by inhalation, whereas 10^8 organisms are required for infection after ingestion. Bacteria are said to be capable of penetrating intact skin, but at such a level of infectivity distinction between intact and minimally disrupted skin becomes academic. Technically, the organism in rodents and presumably in the human host is an intracellular parasite[947] and spreads widely through the lymphoreticular system,[934] but the local lesion, cutaneous, oropharyngeal, or ocular, is a simple pustule that only eventually becomes granulomatous (Fig. 33-52). In lymphoid tissue, lesions are polymorphonuclear with central necrosis mantled by lymphocytes. The necrosis may be caseous, and giant cells may occur. The isolated or confluent lesions, characterized as stellate necrosis, are not recognizably different from cat-scratch disease, plague, or the acute stage of lymphogranuloma venereum. Tularemic pneumonia is a distinctly necrotizing confluent bronchopneumonia with, nevertheless, considerable contribution of mononuclear cells.

Brucella *species*

Microbiology. *Brucella* species are very small coccobacilli that stain very faintly with Gram's stain. Growth on enriched media is slow, and the bacteria are relatively inactive biochemically. Identification is made by growth characteristics, morphology, limited biochemical tests, and serologic identification.[172] Serologic testing plays an important role in the diagnosis of this infection because of the difficulty of isolating the etiologic agent.

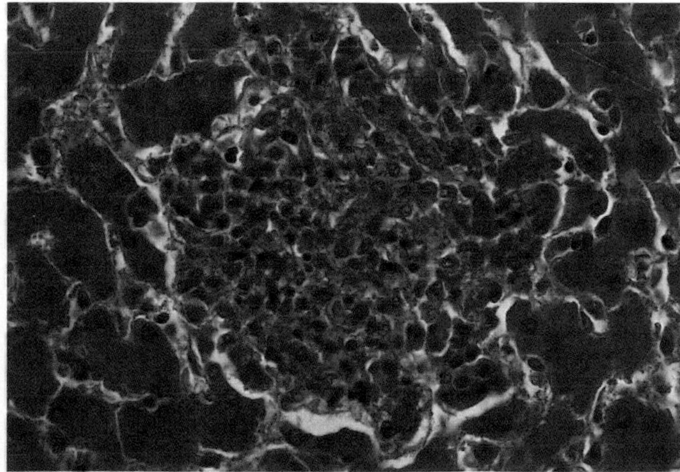

Fig. 33-52 Tularemia. A noncaseating granuloma in the liver is a manifestation of dissemination of the infection, which may occur as a complication of localized disease or as part of typhoidal disease.

History and epidemiology. Bacilli of the genus *Brucella* cause a family of zoonoses in appropriate species. Cattle are infected with *B. abortus,* swine with *B. suis,* and goats with *B. melitensis.* A bacillus was identified in cases of "Malta fever" (including his own infection) by Bruce in 1888,[948] and a similar organism was isolated from examples of economically significant abortions in pregnant cows by Bang in 1897.[949] Human examples of infection by any of the three species result from consumption of milk or other products of infected animals. Alternatively, occupational contact with infected animals in slaughterhouses may be the source of infection. In medically advanced countries, *B. abortus* has been historically the most common cause of human brucellosis. Recently *B. abortus* has lost primacy to *B. suis* because *B. abortus* infections in animals have been eradicated in several countries. *B. melitensis* infections in animals are said to have been eradicated in the United States,[950] but human cases continue to occur from ingestion of home-made goat cheeses introduced from Mexico.[951] *B. melitensis* remains an important public health problem in the Middle East, and sizable experiences with human cases, largely attributable to ingestion of unpasteurized milk, have accumulated.[952] Otherwise, in medically advanced countries, cases continue to occur in individuals occupationally exposed to infected animals:[953] butchers, meat cutters, veterinarians, laboratory workers, and shepherds. Brucellosis has occurred in newborn infants of mothers with clinical brucellosis.[953] A few human cases have been attributed to *B. canis* in owners of pet dogs.

Study of the pathologic anatomy of human brucellosis is limited by the low mortality of systemic forms (1% to 2% in the preantibiotic era,[954] virtually zero now) and rare access to material from organ-specific infections. The portal of entry is usually clinically silent, a phenomenon that is unusual for an infection that is so often acquired through the alimentary route. Brucellosis is to that extent always "typhoidal," but there are exceptions. An ileocecal enterocolitis was described endoscopically and histologically in a young woman who when visiting Portugal drank unpasteurized goat's milk and ate goat cheese.[955] A radiographically demonstrated segmental ileitis occurred in a young Hispanic girl who ate goat cheese; the lesion subsided after antibiotic therapy.[956] A septic patient with high levels of anti-*Brucella* antibodies had abdominal pain, hyperamylasemia, and, presumably, acute pancreatitis that subsided with antibiotic treatment.[957]

Hepatosplenomegaly is present in half of all cases seen clinically. At autopsy, the spleen averages approximately 500 g in weight. Lymph nodes are moderately enlarged but may not be accessible to clinical palpation.

Microscopically, spleen and lymph nodes show lymphoid hyperplasia. Often there are lymphohistiocytic aggregates sufficiently discrete to merit the characterization "granulomas," sometimes even resembling tubercles (see Fig. 33-9). Although progression to cirrhosis has occurred,[958] the inflammatory reaction is usually functionally unimportant in the liver.[959] In the bone marrow and spleen, the inflammatory foci may become large enough to be recognized grossly or radiographically if they become confluent[960] (Fig. 33-53). Pulmonary involvement is rare. Organ-specific lesions are not microscopically specific; etiologic diagnosis requires culture.

A considerable proportion of cases have neurologic manifestations. A nonspecific purulent meningitis certainly occurs but is less common than sterile encephaloneuropathies, often

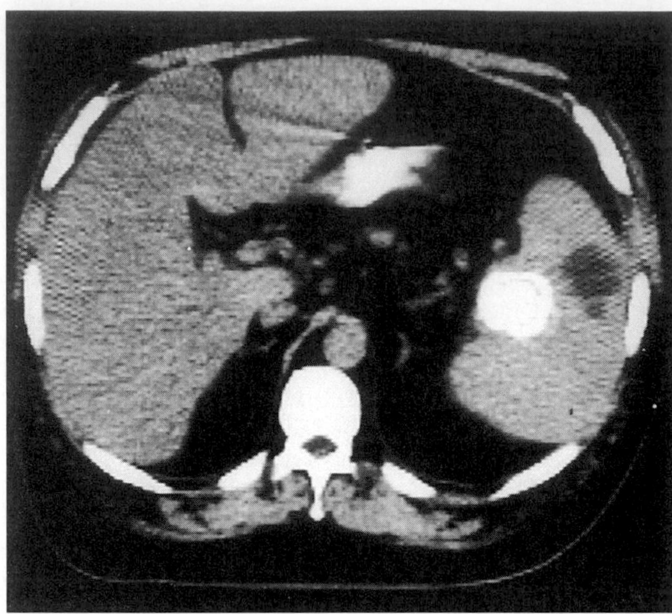

Fig. 33-53 Calcified *Brucella* granuloma. A large calcified lesion is demonstrated by computerized tomography in the spleen of the case depicted in Fig. 33-9. The lucent lesions in the adjacent tissue may represent active granulomas produced in the recrudescent infection. *Brucella suis* was isolated from blood.

clinically very bizarre. The manifestations include cerebellar and brainstem encephalopathies, peripheral neuropathies, psychoses, and neuroses.

Bacterial endocarditis is rare but important.[961] The infection may involve previously normal valves, congenital anomalies, acquired valvular lesions, or prosthetic valves. The lesions of *Brucella* endocarditis are nonspecific.[962] Clinical manifestations of brucellosis in children may mimic rheumatic fever.[963] Of interest is the uncommon isolation of *Brucella* species from severely atheroslerotic aortas or arteriosclerotic aortic aneurysms, sometimes in patients not at risk of brucellosis but who presumably sustain lodgment in mural thrombi or arterial lesions of bacilli during clinically silent episodes of bacteremia.

Approximately 20% of fatal cases have a nonspecific myocarditis. An epididymo-orchitis has occurred in fatal brucellosis.[964] Pregnant women with systemic brucellosis may abort, but inflammatory lesions in the genital tract or fetal membranes have not been described in human beings. Presumably they are the same as in animals.

A considerable number of patients with systemic brucellosis have arthralgias, usually migratory and involving several joints, thereby mimicking acute rheumatic fever. The joint lesions in brucellosis are usually sterile and may be reactive.[965] Once an important cause of uveitis, ocular involvement by brucellae is now largely historical.[966]

Bordetella *species*

Microbiology. Three species of the genus *Bordetella* are associated with human disease: *Bordetella pertussis* causes whooping cough (pertussis); *Bordetella parapertussis* causes a pertussis-like syndrome; and *Bordetella bronchiseptica,* originally described in a child with whooping cough, causes respiratory disease in patients with chronic lung disease. *B. pertussis* and *B. parapertussis* are small coccobacillary organisms that stain very faintly with Gram stain, are nonmotile, and do not grow on sheep blood agar. *B. bronchiseptica* is uniformly bacillary, stains more intensely, is motile, and grows well on sheep blood agar. Isolates of *B. pertussis* are best made on Bordet-Gengou agar or on a charcoal-containing medium developed by Regan and Lowe.[172] The preferred specimen is a nasopharyngeal swab, which has replaced the traditional cough plate. Immunofluorescence has been used for direct identification of *B. pertussis* and *B. parapertussis* in clinical specimens, but performance of the test has been erratic. *Bordetella* species were originally classified in the genus *Haemophilus,* but these organisms require neither X nor V factors for growth and since 1954 have been placed in the new genus.

Bordetella pertussis

History and epidemiology. *B. pertussis* is worldwide in distribution, and whooping cough as such occurs only in humans. Long recognized as "kink" ('spasm') in Scotland, the disease was probably first described by Baillou, the "Sydenham of France," in 1570.[967] Historically very common, pertussis has become less so in the past several decades. The disease has been reportable in the United States since 1922, and 265,269 cases, still the record for a single year, were reported in 1934. The greatest number of deaths was 9269, reported in 1923.[968] The decline both in incidence and mortality seems to have begun before widespread use of pertussis vaccine began in 1947. Pertussis caused 1748 deaths in a total population of 500,000 in Mauritius in 1948. As recently as 1968, pertussis ranked fifth as a cause of death in Kenya.[969]

Vaccination against pertussis, usually combined with that against diphtheria and tetanus as "DPT," is said to be about 60% effective.[970] Immunization is no longer compulsory in Sweden. Eradication of the disease is claimed in several European countries and is theoretically attainable in many others but has not yet been accomplished in the United States for several reasons.[971] Epidemics continue in populations that resist immunization for religious reasons.[972] The disease occurs in epidemic outbreaks approximately every 3 years at any time of year, though there is some tendency for epidemics to occur in late summer or early fall.

The reservoir of organisms during interepidemic periods has been a matter of controversy. There is no known nonhuman host. Some authorities deny a role of asymptomatic carriers,[973] and organisms were isolated only from contacts with overt infection in one well-designed study.[974] The organism is, however, notoriously difficult to culture and isolate, and it has been suggested that it may exist in forms not detectable by routine methods.[974] Recent studies that employed sophisticated serologic techniques have documented the spread of infection through family members, some of whom were asymptomatic.[163] Because there are no known nonhuman sources for pertussis, it is quite likely that low-level transmission among adults is the reservoir for infection. Immunization of susceptible individuals to reduce the population at risk is the primary strategy for interruption of epidemics,[975] but prophylactic treatment of close contacts may also help to break the cycle.[976]

Clinically apparent disease is not only more common, but also more severe in infants than in older children, and virtually all deaths now occur in patients younger than 1 year.[968] The newborn infant is protected only if its mother has been immunized late in pregnancy. Congenital cases probably do not occur, but peripartal transmission from infected mothers to babies has been documented.[977] There have been examples of spread of the disease by hospital personnel.[978] *B. pertussis* has been isolated unexpectedly from the lower respiratory tracts of patients infected with human immunodeficiency virus.[979]

Pathogenesis. *B. pertussis* is highly infectious; at least 80% of nonimmune individuals exposed to the agent acquire disease.[980] This sequence in the interactions between *B. pertussis* and its host entails thorough attachment, evasion of host defenses, and local tissue damage until there is systemic manifestation of disease.

B. pertussis is known to elaborate a host of factors.[981] These factors and certain of their activities that may contribute to virulence are summarized in Table 33-9.

Clinical features and pathology. Classically pertussis is characterized by three stages, each about 2 weeks long:

1. A prodomal stage indistinguishable from innumerable other illnesses—coryza, malaise, myalgia, undifferentiated cough, and sore throat with or without fever
2. A paroxysmal stage characterized by prolonged series of explosive coughs in as many as 40 episodes a day (or night!), characteristically terminating in the inspiratory whoop with vomiting. This stage is often characterized by a circulating lymphocytosis
3. A convalescent stage

Atypical cases are common, particularly in older children and adults,[982] only half of whom may have the whoop. The primary manifestation of the infection in adults may be a chronic cough. The disease is transmitted in respiratory microdroplets, and the portal of entry is the respiratory epithelial surface. Organisms attach specifically to the ciliated surface of epithelial cells,[983] where they proliferate and induce patchy desquamation of cilia and even death of cells. Lymphocytes predominate in the resulting endotracheitis, bronchitis, and bronchiolitis (Fig. 33-54).[984] *B. pertussis* is virtually noninvasive and remains confined to the epithelial surface, where organisms may be stained and seen enmeshed in cilia.[985] With acquisition of immunity, the inflammatory process subsides and damaged respiratory mucosa regenerates. Persistent patches of squamous metaplasia formed during recovery[986] may account for the chronic cough, often weeks in duration after the acute disease subsides.

The most common complication of pertussis is bacterial or viral superinfection with production of focal pneumonia. *B. pertussis* can certainly cause airspace disease,[986] but pneumonia is now more frequently a secondary complication. Interstitial, mediastinal, and subcutaneous emphysema and pneumothorax may occur from paroxysms of coughing. Subconjunctival hemorrhages are likewise probably of hemodynamic origin. In medically advanced countries with prompt antibiotic therapy of infectious complications and respiratory support facilities, the most common cause of death is encephalopathy of uncertain pathogenesis.[987] Besides an infec-

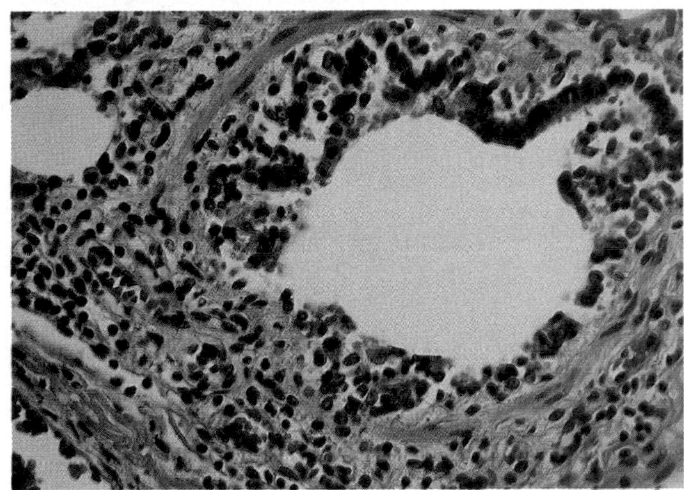

Fig. 33-54 Whooping cough. A prominent peribronchiolar and interstitial lymphocytic infiltrate characterizes the pulmonary inflammatory response in this child who was not immunized for religious reasons. Desquamated epithelial cells are present in the lumen. *Bordetella pertussis* was isolated from the lung in pure culture. (Case contributed by Paul Morrow.)

Table 33-9 Virulence factors of *Bordetella pertussis*

Name	Size	Clinical stage	Possible role in disease
Agglutinogen	22kD	A	Unknown (fimbriae); no clear evidence of a role in attachment
Adenylate cyclase toxin	Enzyme 70 kD Toxin, 190 kD	D,L,S	Catalyzes product of cAMP; inhibits immune effector cells
Dermonecrotic toxic	102 kD	L,S	Unknown
Filamentous hemagglutinin (hemolysis)	Unknown	L	Unknown
Lipopolysaccharide	Unknown	L,S	Unknown
Pertussis toxin	117 kD	A,D,L,S	ADP-ribosylation of guanine nucleotide-binding proteins; may act synergistically with adenylate cyclase toxin; may act with filamentous hemagglutinin to promote attachment to ciliated cells (inhibits response of immune effector cells; systemic features
Tracheal cytotoxin	<1.8 kD	D,L	Specifically toxic to ciliated cells Inhibition of DNA synthesis in ciliated cells

Modified from Weiss A, Hewlett EL: *Annu Rev Microbiol* 40:661, 1986.
A, Attachment; *D,* evasion of host defenses; *L,* local damage; *S,* systemic disease.

tious or parainfectious relationship to *B. pertussis* or to pertussis vaccine, anoxia, passive hyperemia, hemorrhage, even air embolism, have been suggested as factors in the production of encephalopathy.[988]

Other causes of the pertussis syndrome. *B. parapertussis* causes between 5% and 30% of cases of whooping cough, usually less severe than that caused by *B. pertussis* but otherwise indistinguishable from it.[989] Adenoviruses 12 and 5 have been identified in children with whooping cough indistinguishable (even, in some, to the presence of lymphocytosis) from the bacillary disease.[990] The etiologic role of adenoviruses, which may be isolated from asymptomatic individuals, remains controversial. An alternative explanation is that the fastidious *B. pertussis* was not successfully isolated; the phenomenon requires confirmation, using modern culture and serologic techniques. Protection from *B. parapertussis* and of course from viruses is not afforded by vaccines prepared against *B. pertussis*.

Bordetella bronchiseptica. *Bordetella bronchiseptica,* a common commensal in the mouths of small mammals, such as dogs, rabbits, swine, and mice, has been associated with a clinically nonspecific respiratory illness with some features of pertussis.[991,992] *B. bronchiseptica* also occurs as an opportunistic infection, usually of the respiratory system and usually in immunocompromised adults, those receiving chronic dialysis, or in patients receiving steroid therapy. About half the reported cases have had (sometimes tenuous) contact with animals. Pathologic features have been nonspecific.

The HACEK group of bacteria

The HACEK collection of fastidious gram-negative bacilli is linked by their association with bacterial endocarditis. The group is composed of *Haemophilus aphrophilus, Haemophilus (Actinobacillus) actinomycetemcomitans, Cardiobacterium hominis, Eikenella corrodens,* and *Kingella kingae*. To one degree or another they are all slow growing and are difficult to isolate. *Haemophilus aphrophilus, Haemophilus paraphrophilus,* and *Haemophilus (Actinobacillus) actinomycetemcomitans* are discussed elsewhere.

Cardiobacterium hominis. The slow growing, somewhat pleomorphic gram-variable, nonmotile rod called *Cardiobacterium hominis* is a resident of the upper respiratory tract and feces. It has been reported to infect previously damaged or prosthetic cardiac valves.[993] Cerebral emboli have been common in series of reported cases,[994] one with a mycotic aneurysm.[995]

Eikenella corrodens. *Eikenella corrodens* is a small, straight, gram-negative rod that may be pleomorphic. Eikenellae are nonmotile, nonsporeforming, nonencapsulated organisms that do not metabolize carbohydrates. The organism is part of the normal flora of the oral cavity and other body surfaces. Bacterial colonies have a distinctive "fried egg" appearance on the surface of agar and gives off the aroma of household bleach.[172]

Usually cultured with a variety of other organisms, both facultative and anaerobic, *Eikenella* species have been associated with abscesses that occur after surgery, accidental injury, manipulations, or drug abuse.[996] It has been the sole isolate in occasional examples of endocarditis, meningitis, subdural empyema, septic arthritis, and osteomyelitis.[997] Most infections that involve *Eikenella* are indolent and occur longer than a week after the responsible injury.[998]

Kingella kingae. *Kingella kingae* is a plump, gram-negative, nonfermentative bacillus that is a normal resident of the oropharynx. It has been isolated rarely from serious systemic infections, most commonly endocarditis, osteomyelitis, and arthritis.[999]

Pasteurella *species*

Epidemiology. Pasteurellae are small, nonmotile, bipolar-staining, gram-negative coccobacilli. These organisms are primarily animal pathogens. They cause sporadic and epidemic pneumonia and hemorrhagic septicemia in cattle, sheep, and swine. Fowl cholera results in chickens, turkeys, and ducks. Occasionally *Pasteurella* organisms cause focal infections, septicemia, or endocarditis in human beings. These infections fall into three groups:

1. Infection after animal bites or scratches
2. Infections in individuals exposed to animals but with no history of animal-related injury
3. Cases with no ascertainable contact with animals, with most of these having serious coexistent disease, often pulmonary

P. multocida (formerly *septica*), the type species, is the most common human pathogen. It is commonly found in the mouths and gastrointestinal tracts of many animal species: dogs, cats, swine, cattle, sheep, and birds—chickens, turkeys, and ducks. Some exotic species such as lions, a lynx, panthers, opossums, buffaloes, and reindeer have been related to human infections.[1000] Laboratory rodents commonly harbor this organism.

Pet owners, livestock handlers, veterinary students, food processors, and others who are habitually or occupationally exposed to animals may harbor *P. multocida* asymptomatically in their throats.[1001]

From 7% to 17% of patients who present in hospital emergency rooms, having been scratched by cats or bitten by pet dogs or cats, are infected by *P. multocida*.[1002] Infection is more frequent after injuries by cats than by dogs, and most injuries are on the hand or arm. One man sustained infection after bites by the same cat 33 months apart.[1003]

Clinical features. The wound becomes swollen and erythematous and exudes turbid yellow-gray fluid. Lymphangitis and regional lymphadenopathy occur in one third of cases. Complications include tenosynovitis, arthritis, and osteomyelitis. These infections progress rapidly and are often followed by disability.[1004] They require prompt, vigorous treatment.

P. multocida also causes infections in those occupationally or otherwise exposed to animals but who have no history of injury by an animal. These infections often involve the respiratory system (pneumonia and empyema or lung abscess)[1005] or meninges.[1006] A unique case of *Pasteurella* epiglottitis has been reported. Cerebellar abscess has followed otitis media. *Pasteurella* meningitis has a high mortality as has bacteremia without organ localization.[1007] Perinatal infections, often fatal, have occurred,[1008] sometimes in children of farm couples. *Pasteurella* appendicitis with localized peritonitis has responded to appendectomy.[1009]

This infection has rarely been identified in individuals without exposure to animals.[1010] Often there is previous pulmonary disease, such as bronchiectasis or emphysema. Primary peritonitis is particularly likely to occur in individuals with cirrhosis. A unique nosocomial outbreak has been reported in seriously ill hospital patients.[1011] Other *Pasteurella* species rarely cause human disease.

Flavobacterium *species*

Of uncertain status in *Bergey's Manual of Determinative Bacteriology,*[1012] this genus is recognized in clinical microbiology. At least five species are described, of which *Flavobacterium meningosepticum* is the best documented. This genus includes long, slender, nonmotile, gram-negative bacilli with swollen ends.

Most infections are reported in neonates, in whom meningitis is common.[1013] Adults have usually been subjected to operative or manipulative procedures[1014] or have been exposed to contaminated instruments or environment.[1015] Endocarditis in a drug abuser has been described. Adult infections are generally mild, and colonization of the respiratory tract may be asymptomatic.

Alcaligenes *species*

Members of the genus *Alcaligenes* are gram-negative, somewhat pleomorphic bacilli that are motile by virtue of peritrichous flagellae. Members of the genus are normal components of human feces and can colonize other surfaces.[1016] *A. faecalis* has been isolated from soil and water and from medical apparatus, such as respirators, hemodialysis equipment, and intravenous solutions. There are reports of septicemia in which *A. faecalis* was the sole isolate.[1017]

Chromobacterium *species*

Organisms of this genus are gram-negative pigmented, oxidative, or fermentative bacilli that resemble *Pseudomonas* species. Bergey recognizes *C. violaceum* (produce a violet pigment) and *C. lividum* (dark blue pigment).[1012] Some recognize *C. typhiflavium,* which produces a yellow pigment. Most examples of infection by this genus are from warm climates and involve recreational exposure to water.[1018] The organism may gain entry through cutaneous wounds[1019] or through the GI tract and may be associated with diarrhea. Rare examples of sepsis and liver abscesses have a high mortality.[1020] Patients with chronic granulomatous disease are particularly susceptible.[1021]

Achromobacter *species*

Not recognized in Bergey's manual,[1012] *Achromobacter xylosoxidans* is described in the clinical microbiologic literature as a gram-negative, glucose-oxidative, oxidase-producing, motile rod.[172] Two other strains are referred to as Vd biotypes 1 and 2. These organisms have been cultured from hospital water supplies and wash basins.[1022] Meningitis, infection of a cardiac valvular prosthesis, and a pancreatic abscess have been described.

Anaerobic gram-negative bacilli

Bacteroides *species*

The most important group of anaerobic bacteria in human disease is the various members of the genus *Bacteroides,* particularly members of the *Bacteroides fragilis* and pigmented *Bacteroides* groups. The former subspecies of *B. fragilis* (*Bacteroides fragilis, Bacteroides vulgatus, Bacteroides ovatus,* and *Bacteroides thetaiotaomicron*) have been elevated to species status. The black-pigmented group, formerly *Bacteroides melaninogenicus,* is now divided between the genera *Prevotella* and *Porphyromonas.* Identification to the level of species is often not required for clinical management of patients. These species are nonsporulating, strictly anaerobic bacteria with a coccobacillary morphology that closely resembles *Haemophilus.* The *B. fragilis* group is distinguished by stimulated growth in the presence of bile. The pigmented group is characterized by brick-red fluorescence under a long-wavelength ultraviolet lamp (Wood's light).[172]

Bacteroides fragilis. *B. fragilis* and its related species are normal flora of the gastrointestinal[1023] and genitourinary tracts.[424] Although it is quantitatively the least frequent species in the gut, *B. fragilis* is the most common human pathogen, reflecting its virulence factors. The other species are represented in human disease roughly in proportion to their population of the lower intestine.[1023] The primary virulence mechanism of *B. fragilis* is its polysaccharide capsule.[37,127] The immune response to the *B. fragilis* polysaccharide includes both the humoral and cellular immune systems.[100,1024]

Bacteroides infections occur adjacent to colonized mucosal surfaces and usually occur as a part of a polymicrobial infection, most commonly in the abdominal cavity.[251] In the genital tract *B. fragilis* participates in the syndrome of bacterial vaginosis[308] and is a common part of the polymicrobial flora in tubo-ovarian abscess and endometritis,[1025] including infection associated with intrauterine contraceptive devices. An anomaly is the participation of *B. fragilis* in 15% to 20% of necrotizing aspiration pneumonia, lung abscess, and empyema, though this species is infrequently cultured from the upper respiratory tract.[253]

The hallmark of *Bacteroides* infections is the production of abscesses. In an experimental model the two bacterial species that produced abscesses when mixed with sterile cecal contents were *Staphylococcus aureus* and *B. fragilis.*[134] In an animal model of mixed abdominal infection, *B. fragilis* was associated with the formation of abscesses, whereas *Escherichia coli* caused bacteremic infection and was more closely associated with increased mortality.[1026]

Bacteremia occurs occasionally and endocarditis has been described.[1027] The portal of entry is usually the GI tract, and neoplastic disease, diabetes mellitus, or trauma is commonly present.[1028,1029] Although disseminated intravascular coagulation has been described in *B. fragilis* bacteremia,[1030] the lipopolysaccharide does not produce the typical effects of gram-negative endotoxin[127] and septic shock is distinctly unusual.[1029] Perhaps because of associated diseases, the mortality is high in bacteremic infection.

Metastatic disease can occur in virtually any organ. Meningitis and brain abscesses may be metastatic or may arise from an adjacent focus in the middle ear or sinuses.[1031]

Other Bacteroides *species*. *Prevotella* species and *Porphyromonas* species are normal inhabitants of the upper respiratory tract. They are most commonly found as part of a polymicrobial infection in the lower respiratory tract, in chronic otitis and sinusitis, and in infections of the central nervous system related to adjacent disease. *B. bivius* and *B. disiens* are resistant to penicillin, like the *B. fragilis* group, and are found primarily in infections of the female genital tract.[1032]

Fusobacterium *species*

The common pathogens in this genus are *Fusobacterium nucleatum,* which is a thin, needle-shaped, gram-negative bacillus, and *Fusobacterium necrophorum,* which has a pleomorphic morphology. Fusobacteria are normal flora in the upper respiratory tract. They participate in polymicrobial infections of many organs but are primarily related to the respiratory tract.[1033] Diseases include peritonsillar abscess, chronic otitis media and sinusitis, necrotizing pneumonia, and empyema. Bacteremia may result in destructive endocarditis or abscesses in organs, such as the liver and brain. Septic thrombophlebitis and arterial thrombosis are recognized complications of fusobacterial infection, especially in the head and neck region.[1034]

SPIROCHETES

Treponema species

Microbiology

Treponema pallidum comprises three subspecies: pallidum, pertenue, and endemicum. The subspecies produce diseases with some clinical similarities but very different epidemiology and severity. The salient features are summarized in Table 33-10. Despite the differences among the species, *T. pallidum* subsp. pallidum and subsp. pertenue have a genetic code that is virtually identical, and antigens from all three are cross-reactive. Clinical immunity also appears to be cross-reactive; syphilis is uncommon in areas where yaws is endemic.[1035]

Treponema species are tightly coiled, spiral, gram-negative, microaerophilic bacteria that measure 0.1 to 0.2 μm wide and 6 to 20 μm long.[1036] Their motility is a characteristic rapid rotation about their long axis with flexing and bending of the spirochete. *T. pallidum* infects only humans in nature. A limited number of experimental animals, such as chimpanzees, rabbits, and hamsters, can be infected. Pathogenic treponemes cannot be cultured, and only laboratory-adapted strains survive for more than brief periods in vitro.[1037]

Treponema pallidum subsp. pallidum

Epidemiology and history. The agent of venereal syphilis has excited fear, and its victims have suffered for over 500 years. Some have claimed that Columbus brought the disease home with him as a present from the New World;[1038] in light of the plagues later brought to the Americas it can be argued that the invaders still came out ahead. There is abundant evidence of bone changes that resemble syphilis in New World skeletons, but the similarity of pathologic changes produced by the various species and by *Mycobacterium leprae* makes definitive conclusions impossible. Morphologic changes compatible with syphilis have been demonstrated in an 11,500-year-old bear unearthed in North America.[1039] At any rate syphilis was not a prominent part of European life until the sixteenth century. Pathologic lesions compatible with syphilis have been demonstrated in a mummy from the Italian Renaissance, and spirochetes were demonstrated by electron microscopy and immunofluorescence.[1040] The disease spread rapidly, however, and each country ascribed the origin of the infection to its enemy. In France it was the English or Italian disease, whereas the English considered it the French pox. By the end of the seventeenth century James Boswell, as avid a womanizer as biographer, noted in his diary: "I have got a disease from which I suffer severly. . . . I am patient under it, as a just retribution for my licentiousness."[1041] The connection between disease and sexual activity had clearly been made. At the end of the nineteenth century the protean manifestations had been sufficiently characterized for Sir William Osler to dub syphilis the "great imitator." Shortly thereafter Metchnikoff succeeded in transferring the infection to a chimpanzee, and Paul Ehrlich introduced arsenicals as the first "magic bullet."

The distribution of syphilis is the same as human sexual activity: worldwide, but concentrated where promiscuity or ignorance of preventive measures prevail. We have witnessed an unfortunate resurgence of syphilis in the past 20 years[1042] among male homosexuals, prostitutes, and abusers of cocaine.[1043] Similar risk factors have been demonstrated in pregnant women,[1044] resulting in a tragic increase in congenital infection. The extension of the epidemic into the teen and preteen years is particularly unfortunate. In one study of incarcerated adolescents in New York infection rates for gonorrhea among boys and girls were 3% and 18.3% respectively; the rates for syphilis were 0.63% and 2.5%.[1045] Syphilis and HIV are transmitted by similar mechanisms, and complex interactions between the two agents may occur. It has been suggested that genital sores, such as the chancre, are a risk factor for acquisition of the even more deadly virus.[1046] In addition to venereal transmission *T. pallidum* subsp. pallidum can be transmitted in the early stages by contact with infectious lesions on the skin or mucous membranes, through the placenta, by blood transfusion,[1045] and by accidental or intentional inoculation.[1047] The eighteenth-century English surgeon, John Hunter, infected himself with both *Neisseria gonorrhoeae* and *Treponema pallidum* subsp. pallidum in a successful but ill-fated attempt to demonstrate the transmissibility of venereal secretions.

Pathogenesis. Little is known about virulence factors in pathogenic treponemes because they have not been successfully cultivated. Receptor binding proteins for human cells have been demonstrated in *T. pallidum* subsp. pallidum,[1048] and binding to fibronectin has been documented.[1049] The

Table 33-10 Characteristics of *Treponema* species and associated infections

Species and subspecies	Geographic distribution	Disease	Invasiveness
T. pallidum subsp. pallidum	Worldwide	Venereal syphilis	Very invasive
T. pallidum subsp. pertenue	Tropical Asia, Africa, South and Central America	Yaws	Moderately invasive
T. pallidum subsp. endemicum	Africa, Southeast Asia, Middle East, Yugoslavia	Endemic, nonvenereal syphilis	Moderately invasive
T. carateum	Central and South America	Pinta	Minimally invasive
"*T. pallidum*"-like oral spirochetes	Worldwide	Necrotizing gingivitis	Minimally invasive

spirochete adheres to vascular endothelial cells and invades through intercellular junctions in vitro.[1050] A lipid component was found to be essential for macrophage activation by a polypeptide immunogen in experimental animals.[1051] Activation of complement has been postulated as the mechanism for the Jarisch-Herxheimer reaction that occurs occasionally after treatment of early syphilis,[1052] but classical gram-negative endotoxin does not appear to be involved in the pathogenesis of this complication.[1053]

The immune response to syphilis is both humoral and cellular. Antibodies of both IgG and IgM classes are elicited with waning of the response as infection progresses.[1054] IgG subclasses IgG_1 and IgG_3 account for most of the 7S antibodies.[1055] The antigens responsible for the immunoglobulin response have been characterized, and antigens that are relatively specific for syphilis have been identified.[1056] In addition to specific antibodies, immunoglobulins directed against phospholipids, such as cardiolipin, were identified in the early part of this century (reaginic antibodies), and they form the basis of the nontreponemal serologic tests, such as the VDRL and RPR tests.[1057] These reaginic antibodies are similar to those produced in systemic lupus erythematosus, the principal cause of persistent biologic false-positive nontreponemal antibody tests.[1058] Extensive cross-reactions with other spirochetes occur, complicating serologic diagnosis of disease in areas where multiple spirochetal infections coexist.[1059] The role of antibodies in pathogenesis and immunity is not entirely clear. Passive transfer of antibody into experimental guinea pigs delayed and ameliorated the development of primary lesions but did not prevent dissemination of the spirochetes to regional lymph nodes.[1060] Immunoglobulins serve as opsonins for *Treponema pallidum* in vitro, an activity that is beneficial only if the phagocytic cell can exert bactericidal activity.[1061] Immune complexes are demonstrable in early syphilis and clearly play a role in the development of glomerular disease and possibly other manifestations.[1062]

Adoptive immunity to syphilis can be transferred adoptively in experimental animals by injection of T-lymphocytes.[1063] In humans there is considerable evidence of depression of various aspects of the T-lymphocyte response at during the infection,[1064] possibly mediated by a serum factor.[1065] Suppression of NK cell activity has also been described, again related in part to a serum factor.[1066]

Immunity in syphilis is gradually acquired and is incomplete. Experimental studies on human volunteers demonstrated the development of primary lesions that contained treponemes in 9 of 11 men who had previously treated early syphilis, in 10 of 26 men with previously treated late latent syphilis, and in 4 of 5 individuals who had treated congenital syphilis.[1047] Fiumara and colleagues have described individuals who were reinfected after venereally[1067] or congenitally acquired primary infection.[1068]

The minimal inoculum for transmission of *T. pallidum* subsp. pallidum through the skin or mucous membranes is as few as 10 spirochetes.[1047] The 50% infectious dose was only 57 organisms, a figure that was considered to be a probable overestimate. Because only approximately one half of individuals who are exposed to an infected partner develop syphilis, the number of bacteria transmitted during a sexual contact must be quite small. A concentration of approximately 10^4 spirochetes per milliliter is required for demonstration of organisms with the dark-field technique! From the initial lesion the spirochetes spread to regional nodes and then throughout the body through the bloodstream. Once the immune phase of the infection begins, the spirochetes may be sequestered in lesions or in protected sites. Spirochetes have been demonstrated in ocular tissues and as viable organisms recovered from those tissues by inoculation of rabbits many years after the primary infection.[1069] Some of these patients with late syphilis no longer had demonstrable serum antibody.

Clinical features and pathology. The course of syphilis is conceptually divided into early and late stages:

- Early syphilis
  - Incubation period
  - Primary syphilis (chancre)
- Secondary syphilis (dissemination)
  - Early latent syphilis
- Late syphilis
  - Late latent syphilis
  - Tertiary syphilis

After inoculation of spirochetes local multiplication occurs, producing an incubation period of 3 to 90 days with a mean of 3 weeks. A transient erythematous papule marks the inoculation site.[1047] The primary phase is characterized by an ulcerated, indurated, painless lesion called a *chancre,* which develops at the inoculation site. Regional lymphadenopathy may accompany the chancre. Some patients do not develop a chancre or have a nonspecific lesion that is overlooked. A primary lesion is not present when the spirochetes are transmitted across the placenta or through blood transfusions. Pathologically, the chancre is characterized by lymphocytic and plasmacytic subepithelial inflammation, concentric proliferation of the endothelium, and an obliterative endarteritis (Fig. 33-55). The diagnosis can be made by visualization of the spirochetes in a patient with serologic evidence of syphilis or presumptively by suggestive histologic abnormalities with positive serologic test results. With or without treatment the chancre regresses within a month or two, leaving no residual or a minimal scar.

Approximately 25% of untreated individuals will develop secondary syphilis within 2 to 8 weeks after the regression of the primary lesion. The treponemes have been disseminated throughout the body, and an effective immunologic response has not yet been assembled. Virtually any organ may be involved. The most visible manifestations of disseminated syphilis are in the skin, where a rash of virtually any type except vesicular appears, characteristically involving the palms of the hands and soles of the feet.[162] A proliferative epithelial lesion on moist skin and mucous membranes is known as a condyloma lata and must be differentiated from a condyloma acuminata caused by human papillomaviruses, also venereally transmitted.[1070] Flat lesions on mucosal surfaces are known as "mucous patches." All these lesions, which are teeming with spirochetes, are infectious.

Invasion of the central nervous system during the secondary stage is more common than previously believed; *T. pallidum* subsp. pallidum was isolated from 40% of patients with untreated primary or secondary syphilis in a recent study.[1071] The presence of concurrent human immunodeficiency virus infection does not increase the likelihood of meningeal infection, but relapses despite recommended antimicrobial therapy do appear to be more common in those patients.[1072] In the secondary stage aseptic meningitis, sometimes with involvement of cranial nerves, is the most common manifestation.

Immune complex glomerulonephritis occurs at this stage.[1073] Hepatitis is a more common feature of secondary syphilis than originally appreciated.[1074,1075] Arthritis may represent the initial symptom of disseminated infection.[1076]

An occasional problem in primary or disseminated syphilis is a systemic reaction to the release of spirochetal products after therapy, the Jarisch-Herxheimer reaction.[1077] The syndrome includes pyrexia, leukocytosis, lymphopenia, and systemic hypotension. A similar phenomenon has been observed in other spirochetal infections, particularly louse-borne relapsing fever.

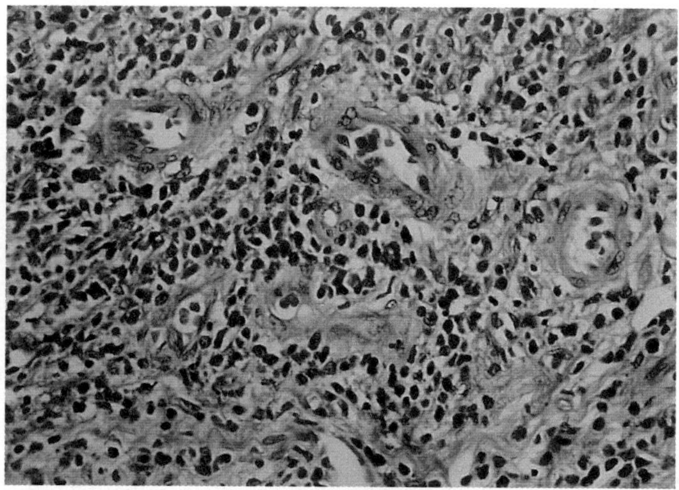

Fig. 33-55 Early syphilis. The subepithelial infiltrate is mononuclear with a prominent component of plasma cells. A proliferation of small blood vessels with plump endothelial produces an arborizing pattern. (Case contributed by Thomas Trainer, MD, Burlington, Vt.)

After the subsidence of the symptoms of disseminated infection a latent period ensues. Latency is divided somewhat arbitrarily into an early and a late segment. The early latent period, 4 years long, may be punctuated by clinical relapses. As time progresses, exacerbations become increasingly infrequent. The late latent period lasts until the onset of tertiary disease, which is recognized clinically in 30% to 40% of untreated patients. Anatomic evidence of syphilitic infection can be found at autopsy in a still higher percentage.

Tertiary syphilis is dominated by cardiovascular disease, neurosyphilis, and gummas in various organs. Cardiovascular syphilis, which occurs in approximately 10% of untreated patients, is characterized by obliterative endarteritis of the vasa vasorum, producing necrosis and scarring of the tunica media. The result is aneurysmal dilatation of the weakened aorta, particularly in the ascending portion (Fig. 33-56). If the aortic root is involved, the dilatation may produce functional regurgitation, though the valve leaflets themselves are undamaged.

Asymptomatic neurosyphilis develops in between 8% and 40% of untreated patients. Symptomatic disease occurs in a subset of these, but the protean and often nonspecific manifestations make definitive diagnosis problematic in many instances:[1078]

1. Meningovascular syphilis, caused by endarteritis that results in multiple small cerebral infarcts
2. Parenchymatous neurosyphilis, characterized by neuronal atrophy and disappearance
   a. "Paresis," a mnemonic for personality changes (emotional lability or paranoia), alterations of affect, hyperactive reflexes, alterations in eye function (Argyll-Robertson pupil), changes in sensorium (illusions, delusions, hallucinations), decreased intellect, and slurred speech.
   b. Tabes dorsalis, resulting from demyelination of the posterior column of the spinal cord, the dorsal roots, and dorsal root ganglia, resulting in ataxia, gait dis-

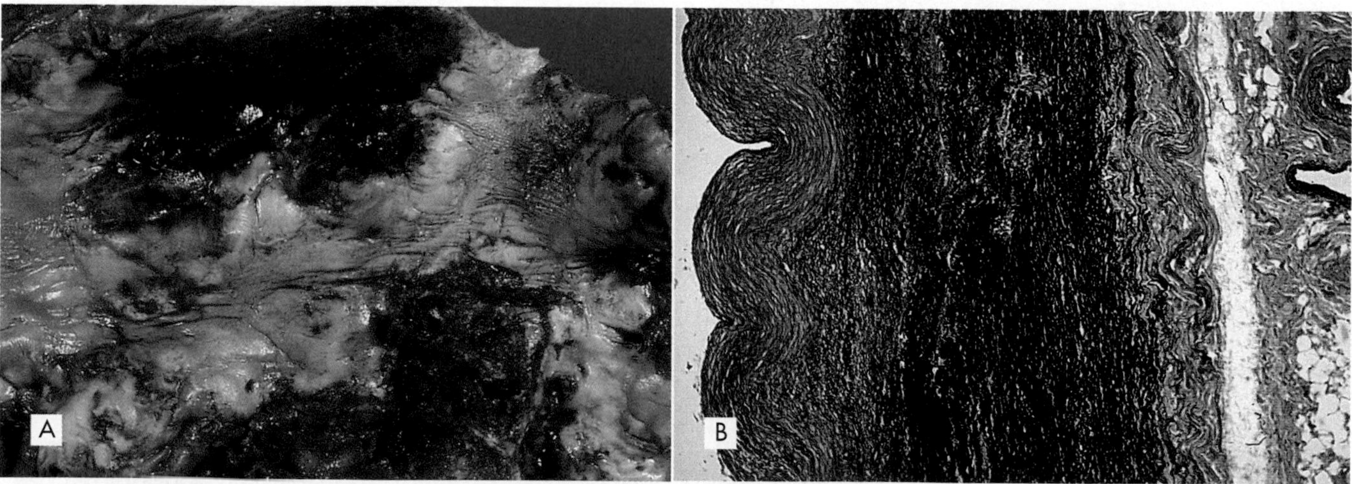

Fig. 33-56 Syphilitic aortitis. **A,** The scarred thoracic aorta is characterized by linear folds in the intima (tree barking). Superimposed atherosclerosis contributes to weakening of the aorta, which is predisposed to aneurysmal dilatation and widening of the aortic ring with resultant regurgitation through the aortic valve. **B,** There is disruption of the medial elastic fibrils *(black)*. The adventitia contains foci of mononuclear inflammatory cells around small blood vessels. The intima is proliferated. (Verhoeff–van Gieson stain.)

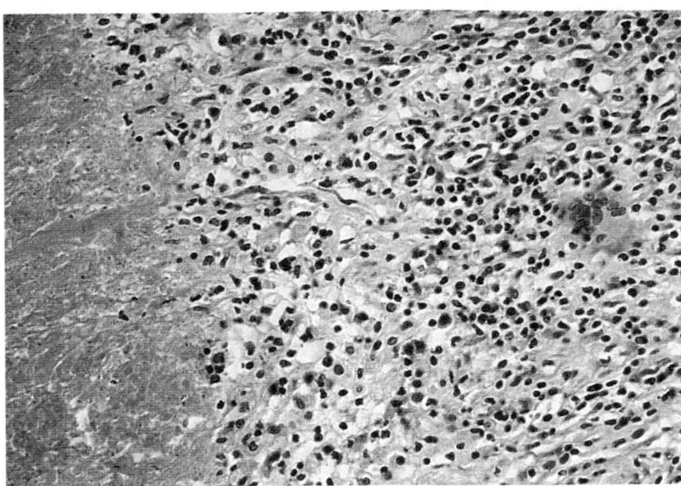

Fig. 33-57 Gumma. This mass lesion of tertiary syphilis consists of central necrosis surrounded by macrophages, lymphocytes, and fibroblasts.

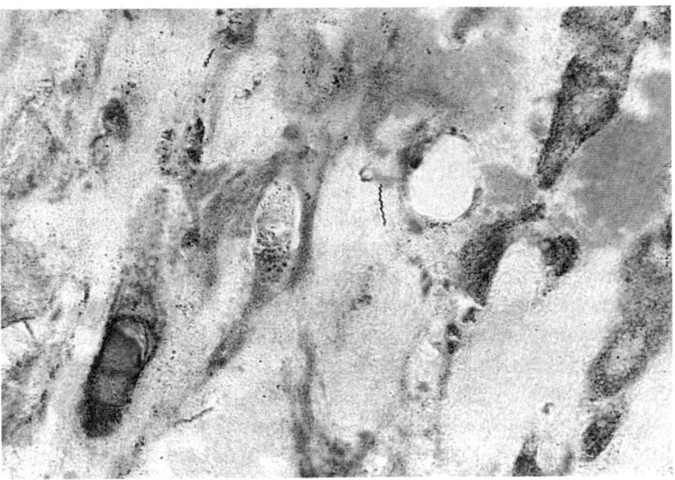

Fig. 33-58 Tightly coiled spirochetes of *Treponema pallidum* subsp. *pallidum* are present in a hydropic placenta. The clinical setting and morphology of the spirochetes establish a diagnosis of congenital syphilis for practical purposes. Serologic confirmation should be attempted. (Warthin-Starry method.)

turbances, incontinence of feces and urine, degenerative joint changes (Charcot joints), and ulcerations as a result of decreased sensory input

3. Cranial nerve neuropathy, particularly of the seventh and eighth nerves
4. Otitis, causing tinnitus and deafness; hydrops secondary to obliteration of the endolymphatic duct
5. Ocular defects, such as optic nerve atrophy and ptosis

The final type of tertiary lesion is the gumma (late benign syphilis), which may occur in any organ. Gummas are granulomatous, space-occupying lesions that may be mistaken for neoplasms until histologic examination is performed (Fig. 33-57).[1079] The necrotic process is initiated once again by obliterative endarteritis.

Congenital syphilis. Congenital and neonatal syphilis are acquired after maternal bacteremia and passage of the spirochetes across the placenta. The placenta shows typical but nondiagnostic changes that include acute or chronic inflammation of the villi, relative immaturity of the villi, endovascular proliferation, and plasmacytic inflammation in the decidua.[1080] The diagnosis is confirmed by demonstration of the spirochete in the placenta (Fig. 33-58).

The most severely affected infants are stillborn, and the only clues to an infectious cause may be hepatospenomegaly, chorioamnionitis, and nucleated erythrocytes in villous capillaries.[1081] The hallmarks of congenital syphilis are hepatosplenomegaly, generalized lymphadenopathy, skin rashes, interference with epiphyseal growth plates, rhinitis (sniffles), periostitis, and immaturity or inflammation in many organs.[1082,1083] Thrombocytopenia and anemia may be present. The primary differential diagnosis is with other congenital infections, such as toxoplasmosis, rubella, and cytomegalovirus. The Jarisch-Herxheimer reaction is common after antimicrobial therapy. Chronic sequelae include recurrent arthropathy with bilateral knee effusions (Clutton's joints), maldevelopment of the nose (saddle nose) and tibia (sabre shin), and notched, widely spaced incisors (Hutchinson's teeth).

Other Treponema *species*[162]

T. pallidum subsp. pertenue produces yaws, which is acquired nonvenereally in childhood. The histologic lesions and many of the clinical features resemble venereal syphilis. Cutaneous and osseous disease predominate.

T. pallidum subsp. endemicum causes endemic syphilis, or bejel, also acquired by nonvenereal contact with infected secretions. The clinical presentation and histologic features are indistinguishable from venereal syphilis, and the diagnosis is made by correlation of clinical history and epidemiology.

T. carateum is the etiologic agent of pinta. Lesions are limited to the skin, but the process can result in considerable cosmetic damage.

Leptospira interrogans

Microbiology. *Leptospira* organisms are motile, long, tightly coiled spirochetes with curved or hooked ends. Unlike most other spirochetes, they grow in appropriate laboratory media.

Before 1967 *Leptospira icterohaemorrhagiae* was regarded as the type species and the cause of Weil's disease.[1084] About 150 other serotypes were recognized, regarded as species and as causes of specific diseases, such as Fort Bragg fever attributed to *L. pomona*[1085] and "pretibial fever" attributed to *L. hebdomadis*. Since that time, it is recognized that any of the types can cause the severe hepatorenal disease characterized as Weil's disease. A single species, *L. interrogans,* is now recognized, with the variants designated as serovars, such as *L. interrogans* serovar *cunicola*. A free-living aquatic form is sometimes designated *L. biflexa*.

Epidemiology. Leptospirosis is a zoonosis of worldwide distribution that affects many species of wild and domestic animals. The world over, rats are the most common reservoir of human infection.[1086] In the United States, however, dogs, livestock, rodents, wild mammals, and cats are the sources of human infection in that descending order. Human infection is a dead-end phenomenon of parasitism because person-to-per-

thema annulare centrifugum and erythema marginatum by the presence of plasma cells and mast cells. Spirochetes are seen most often in the papillary dermis but may be present also in the reticular dermis. Fever and regional lymphadenopathy may accompany the rash, which regresses spontaneously but may recur. If the characteristic skin lesion is not present, the clinical presentation of fever and lymphadenopathy may be suggestive of a viral illness.[1140] Conjunctivitis has been noted during the acute phase. An immunologic response is often not detectable in the early stage,[1141] which has the characteristics of an infectious process. A Jarisch-Herxheimer reaction to therapy of acute infections, similar to that seen in other spirochetal infections, has been reported.[1142]

In the disseminated phase the spirochetes may localize in many organs, and the process has both infectious and immunopathologic features. Symptoms are primarily related to the skin, where erythematous lesions may reappear, the nervous system, the musculoskeletal system, and the heart. Involvement of the nervous system results in lymphocytic meningitis and neuropathies of both cranial and peripheral nerves (Bannwarths's syndrome).[1143] Encephalitis is uncommon and neurologic disease may occur in the absence of previous cutaneous disease. The inflammatory infiltrate in the meninges is mononuclear.[1138,1143] A lymphocytic infiltrate permeates the cerebral ganglia and interstitium of the peripheral nerves, and the small blood vessels are cuffed with lymphocytes. Microscopic documentation of encephalitis is scant, but microglial nodules have been observed. Spirochetes have been demonstrated in a case of clinical myositis; the muscle tissue was characterized by fiber atrophy and an interstitial infiltrate of lymphocytes and plasma cells.[1144] Subsequently the inflammatory component disappears, but angulated fibers mark the residual of denervation.[1145] Iritis progressing to panophthalmitis and blindness in one patient was accompanied by neutrophilic and lymphocytic inflammation; spirochetes were demonstrated by silver stain in the necrotic debris.[1146]

Cardiac involvement occurs in approximately 4% to 8% of patients several weeks after onset of the disease.[1112] The most common clinical presentation is heart block. Limited histologic studies of endomyocardial biopsy specimens has demonstrated myonecrosis and a lymphocytic-plasmacytic infiltrate in the endocardium or myocardium.[1147]

After intermittent episodes of migratory arthralgias and an unexplained delay of as long as 2 years, approximately 60% of the patients in the United States develop brief attacks of acute, asymmetric pauciarticular arthritis, primarily affecting the knee.[1112] White cell counts in the synovial fluid range from 500 to 110,000 cells per cubic millimeter, predominantly polymorphonuclear neutrophils. Many other organs may be involved rarely.

Persistent disease occurs in some patients. Recurrent attacks of arthritis may continue for years, decreasing in frequency each year in untreated patients.[1148] The synovial lesions of the persistent phase resemble those of rheumatoid arthritis.[1138] Common features include synovial villous hypertrophy, synovial cell hyperplasia, microvascular proliferation, fibrin deposits, plasma cell infiltrates, and lymphoid follicles. T-lymphocytes, primarily of the helper/inducer subset, are distributed diffusely throughout the tissue, and the nodular aggregates contain a mixture of T- and B-cells.[1149] Obliterative endarteritis, occasionally with an onionskin appearance, may be accompanied by demonstrable spirochetes in a perivascular distribution.[1150] Granulomas, necrosis, multinucleated giant cells, and eosinophils are not seen in *Borrelia* infection.[1138]

The central nervous system is the other organ that is characteristically involved in persistent disease. The most dramatic presentation is a progressive encephalitis,[1151] but most presentations are more subtle and the continuum of disease has not been clearly delineated. Keratitis may occur years after the initial infection.

Disseminated and persistent infection have features that are suggestive of both direct infectious damage and immunopathologic disease. Activation of B-cells[1152] and T-cells[1153] can be demonstrated in tissue. Local production of specific antibodies has been demonstrated in inflamed cerebrospinal fluid.[1154] The activated cells react not only with *Borrelia* antigens, but also with autoantigens.[1153] Rheumatoid factor and antibodies reactive with a variety of substances, including cardiolipin, have been demonstrated. Early in the infection IgM antibodies are accompanied by increased activity of suppressor cells; during the later stages suppressor cells are less active, potentially increasing the likelihood of tissue damage.[1155] Other features of Lyme disease that are suggestive of an immunologic component include the reproducible finding of immune complexes in serum early in the course and in synovial fluid later,[1156] documentation of reactivity of *Borrelia* antibodies with host cell tissue,[1157] and association of arthritis with certain HLA types.[1149] Some experimental data, however, indicate that immunopathologic damage may not be the whole story. Inoculation of NIH-3 mice, which are deficient in T-cells, B-cells, and NK cells, results in a progressive mononuclear inflammatory infiltrate in multiple sites, including the myocardium and synovium.[1158] Similar observations have been observed in the severe combined immunodeficiency mouse.[1159] Immunization with a 31 kD outer surface protein (OspA) inhibits adherence of spirochetes to endothelium in vitro[1160] and protects against infection in experimental mice,[1161] an indication that the spirochetes themselves play a direct role in the pathogenesis of infection. It is likely that both pathologic mechanisms are operative.

MISCELLANEOUS BACTERIA

Capnocytophaga canimorsus

Capnocytophaga canimorsus is a slow-growing, gram-negative bacillus originally designated DF-2 (dysgonic fermenter) because of its limited fermentative capacity.[1162] Its demand for carbon dioxide enrichment has led to its inclusion in the genus *Capnocytophaga* ('a cell that eats carbon dioxide'). The species was designated *canimorsus* ('dog bite') because of the very striking association of infection with dog bites,[1163] which occur in approximately one half the reported cases. The organism appears to be part of the normal flora of the mouths of dogs. Previous splenectomy, alcoholism, and lymphomas predispose to infection by this organism. Fulminating human infections are often accompanied by thrombophlebitis sometimes with symmetrical gangrene.[126] Meningitis is common. Infection does occur in uncompromised individuals, but fatality is not limited to those with underlying conditions. It has been recommended that splenectomized individuals who are bitten by a dog routinely be administered prophylactic penicillin.[1164] It has even been suggested that such individuals ought not to own dogs (or cats).

Capnocytophaga ochracea

The organism *Capnocytophaga ochracea* was previously designated DF-1 (dysgonic fermenter) by the Centers for Disease Control and Prevention and has a history of other aliases. It is a slender, somewhat fusiform, gram-negative bacillus that demonstrates gliding motility and requires enrichment of its atmosphere with carbon dioxide. This bacterium is associated with periodontal disease.[1165] Approximately 50 examples of infection have been described, both in immunocompetent individuals[1166] and in individuals who have been immunocompromised, usually by leukemia or other malignancies.[1165] Very conspicuous is the association of infection, sepsis, or endocarditis with leukopenia and significant oral pathologic conditions, such as ulcers or periodontal disease.[1167] In the immunocompetent individual, pulmonary infections have predominated,[1166] but wound infections, abscesses, and osteomyelitis have occurred. The organism has been shown to elaborate both a leukocytotoxic agent[1168] and a fibroblast-inhibiting factor.[1169]

Calymmatobacterium granulomatis

The etiologic agent of granuloma inguinale is a small gram-negative bacillus that has been isolated by inoculation of chicken egg yolk but does not grow on agar media. The organism was originally placed in the genus *Donovania,* and the disease was known as donovaniosis.

Ultrastructurally a cell membrane is surrounded by a cell wall and a capsule but no flagella.[1170] The bacteria are found in phagocytic vacuoles in macrophages (Donovan bodies), but only rarely in polymorphonuclear neutrophils.[1170] The bacteria proliferate intracellularly until the macrophage is disrupted. The Giemsa technique is most commonly used to demonstrate the bacteria, but they are also stained by the Papanicolau method.[1171] Little is known about virulence factors of the bacterium because of the lack of cultivated strains.

The infection is common in India, Australia, New Guinea, and the Caribbean. It is uncommon in the United States, but an outbreak of 20 cases occurred in Texas.[1172] Transmission is by sexual contact, and initial lesions occur on the genitalia, perineum, and perirectal area. The initial presentation of the infection is single or multiple cutaneous nodules. The dermis contains macrophages and plasma cells, but few PMNLs.[1173] Small dermal blood vessels show dilatation and proliferation. The epidermis may contain clusters of PMNLs, and pseudoepitheliomatous hyperplasia occurs in some cases. The histologic appearance may simulate granulation tissue.[1174]

As the lesions progress, fibrosis develops, and elephantiasis of the external genitalia may result.[1175] Extension of the inflammatory lesions may result in mutilating destruction of the external genitalia.[1176] Vaginal bleeding has been described as a complication. Granulomatous inflammation in the upper female genital tract and ureters occurs rarely, producing ureteral obstruction and hydronephrosis.[1177]

Very similar primary lesions may be produced by infection with *Haemophilus ducreyi.*[1178] As granuloma inguinale progresses, large nodules may simulate a neoplasm of soft tissue[1179] or cervical carcinoma.[1180]

Extragenital lesions, most commonly in the head and neck region,[1181] and disseminated disease[1182] have been described. In the absence of microbiologic or immunologic confirmation, reports of unusual disease in unusual locations must be considered provisional.

Streptobacillus moniliformis and *Spirillum minus*

Rat-bite fever is an acute febrile systemic illness that occurs worldwide. Cohen has described historic aspects of the disease.[1183] Two different organisms cause rat-bite fever. *Streptobacillus moniliformis* causes most cases in the United States, whereas *Spirillum minus* causes most cases elsewhere, particularly, *sokōnetsu* in Japan. The organisms are not similar, and there are obvious differences in clinical features between streptobacilliary and spirillar rat-bite fever. The two diseases really share only the epidemiologic association with bites of rats or other small rodents[1184] or other animals.[1185] Even here, both forms occur in cases in which there is no history of a bite by an appropriate animal. An outbreak of such cases occurred in Haverhill, Massachusetts (hence Haverhill fever), attributed to contamination of raw milk by rat excreta.[1186] The responsible organism, called *Haverhillia multiformis,* is presumably the same as *S. moniliformis.*[1187] A sizable outbreak at a girls' school in England was attributed to water transmission, though the school dispensed raw milk.[1188] In the United States, the disease usually occurs in children.[1189]

S. moniliformis is a pleomorphic, nonmotile, gram-negative bacillus that may form long beaded filaments, chains of bacilli, or coccobacillary forms. The organism occurs in the mouths of as many as 50% of wild and domestic rats and mice, both sick and healthy. It is also found in other species, notably guinea pigs and turkeys. Systemic features of streptobacillary rat-bite fever usually begin abruptly after the responsible bite (if any) has healed. Chills, fever, headache, myalgia, and a generalized morbilliform or petechial rash are the clinical features. Arthritis is common. The disease runs its course in a week or two but, if untreated, frequently relapses or gives rise to complications such as pneumonia, abscesses in various organs,[1190] or infective endocarditis, of which the mortality, if untreated, approaches 10%. Amnionitis has occurred in a pregnant woman.[1184]

Spirillum minus has not been cultured on artificial media but can be identified by dark-field examination of fluid from the site of the bite, lymph-node aspirates, or blood. It is a tightly coiled spiral organism with polar flagella. Spirillar rat-bite fever is often more gradual in onset than the streptobacillary type. Lymphangitis and lymphadenopathy are usual and occur proximally to the site of the bite, which may not have healed. The rash is more macular than that of the streptobacillary disease and may even be a urticaria. Arthritis is rare. The disease is usually self-limited but may relapse and remit even for years. Meningitis, myocarditis, nephritis, and hepatitis are rare complications. Endocarditis occurs; oddly, no patient with spirillar endocarditis has had a history of a bite.

Neither form of rat-bite fever displays specific pathologic manifestation. Diagnosis depends on culture of the streptobacillus or dark-field recognition of *S. minus* either directly or after mouse or guinea pig inoculation.

UNCULTURED BACTERIA

The application of molecular techniques to infectious diseases has resulted in the identification of bacterial pathogens in several disease that were previously assumed to be cause by infectious agents. *Bartonella (*formerly *Rochalimaea) henselae,* the etiologic agent of bacillary angiomatosis and primary cause of cat-scratch disease is discussed in Chapter 35. Concurrently this bacterium was successfully isolated in the laboratory. Next to fall was the problem of Whipple's disease, long assumed to be infectious because of the demonstration of intracellular bacteria by light and electron microscopy. The genetic structure of the etiologic agent, which has still not been isolated, has been characterized and the name *Tropheryma whippelii* assigned.[168] Phylogenetic analysis indicates that the bacterium is an aerobic actinomycete, more closely related to *Rhodococcus* and *Streptomyces* than to *Mycobacterium*.[168] Little is known about virulence mechanisms or pathogenesis because isolated bacteria have not been available for analysis.

The grouping of Whipple's disease comprises migratory polyarthritis, usually involving the large joints, followed, sometimes after the passage of months or years, by diarrhea, steatorrhea, and malabsorption. The typical patient is a middle-aged white man. Extremely varied neurologic abnormalities, cardiac disease including endocarditis, pigmentation of the skin, and lymphadenopathy are common.[1191] Much is known about the illness,[1992-1196] as discussed in chapter 54.

The extraintestinal lesions in Whipple's disease contain similar bacilli or macrophages that stain with the PAS technique. Sarcoid-like granulomas have been described in both intestinal[1197] and extraintestinal lesions.[1198] The epithelioid macrophages do not stain with the PAS technique, but intracellular bacilli have been observed.[1198] Pathologic descriptions of the arthritis are few in number. In one case the synovial membrane was infiltrated with characteristic macrophages and bacilli as well as large numbers of polymorphonuclear neutrophils.[1199] Aggregations of typical foamy macrophages are observed in lymphoid tissue, the central nervous system, and the heart. All layers of the heart may be affected, and endocardial infection may result in large, verrucous vegetations.[1200]

REFERENCES

Bacteria and their hosts

1. Mims CA: *The pathogenesis of infectious disease,* ed 3, London, 1987, Academic Press.
2. Dee P, Winn W, McKee K: *Pneumocystis carinii* infection of the lung: radiologic and pathologic correlation, *Am J Roentgenol* 132:741, 1979.
3. Groman NB: Conversion by corynephages and its role in the natural history of diphtheria, *Hygiene* 93:405, 1984.
4. Rupp ME, Archer GL: Coagulase-negative staphylococci: pathogens associated with medical progress, *Clin Infect Dis* 19:231, 1994.

The scales of infection: microbial factors

5. Blander SJ, Horwitz MA: Vaccination with the major secretory protein of *Legionella pneumophila* induces cell-mediated and protective immunity in a guinea pig model of Legionnaires' disease, *J Exp Med* 169:691, 1989.
6. Blander SJ, Szeto L, Shuman HA, Horwitz MA: An immunoprotective molecule, the major secretory protein of *Legionella pneumophila,* is not a virulence factor in a guinea pig model of Legionnaires' disease, *J Clin Invest* 86:817, 1990.
7. Porras O, Dillon HC Jr, Gray BM, Svanborg-Edén C: Lack of correlation of in vitro adherence of *Haemophilus influenzae* to epithelial cells with frequent occurrence of otitis media, *Pediatr Infect Dis J* 6:41, 1987.
8. Mason EO Jr, Kaplan SL, Wiedermann BL et al: Frequency and properties of naturally occurring adherent piliated strains of *Haemophilus influenzae* type b, *Infect Immun* 49:98, 1985.
9. Courtney HS, von Hunolstein C, Dale JB et al: Lipoteichoic acid and M protein: dual adhesins of group A streptococci, *Microb Pathog* 12:199, 1992.
10. Crawford I, Russell C: Comparative adhesion of seven species of streptococci isolated from the blood of patients with sub-acute bacterial endocarditis to fibrin-platelet clots in vitro, *J Appl Bacteriol* 60:127, 1986.
11. Scheld WM, Valone JA, Sande MA: Bacterial adherence in the pathogenesis of endocarditis: interaction of bacterial dextran, platelets, and fibrin, *J Clin Invest* 61:1394, 1978.
12. Johanson WG Jr, Pierce AK, Sanford JP: Changing pharyngeal bacterial flora of hospitalized patients: emergence of gram-negative bacilli, *N Engl J Med* 281:1137, 1969.
13. Stanislawski L, Simpson WA, Hasty D et al: Role of fibronectin in attachment of *Streptococcus pyogenes* and *Escherichia coli* to human cell lines and isolated oral epithelial cells, *Infect Immun* 48:257, 1985.
14. Tramont EC: Inhibition of adherence of *Neisseria gonorrhoeae* by human genital secretions, *J Clin Invest* 59:117, 1977.
15. Shibl AM: Effect of antibiotics on adherence of microorganisms to epithelial cell surfaces, *Rev Infect Dis* 7:51, 1985.
16. McGee ZA, Gregg CR, Johnson AP et al: The evolutionary watershed of susceptibility to gonococcal infection, *Microb Pathog* 9:131, 1990.
17. Draper DL, Donegan EA, James JF, Sweet RL, Brooks GF: Scanning electron microscopy of attachment of *Neisseria gonorrhoeae* colony phenotypes to surfaces of human genital epithelia, *Am J Obstet Gynecol* 138:818, 1980.
18. Long SS, Swenson RM: Determinants of the developing oral flora in normal newborns, *Appl Environ Microbiol* 32:494, 1976.
19. Dinarello CA, Cannon JG, Wolff SM: New concepts on the pathogenesis of fever, *Rev Infect Dis* 10:168, 1988.
20. Davis BD: Gene variation and transfer. In Davis BD, Dulbecco R, Eisen HN, Ginsberg HS, editors: *Microbiology,* ed 4, Philadelphia, 1990, Lippincott.
21. Avery OT, MacLeod CM, McCarty M: Transformation of pneumoccal types induced by a deoxyribonucleic acid fraction isolated from *Pneumococcus* type III, *J Exp Med* 79:137, 1944.
22. Guerrant RL: Lessons from diarrheal diseases: demography to molecular pharmacology, *J Infect Dis* 169:1206, 1994.
23. Wolff SM: Biological effects of bacterial endotoxins in man, *J Infect Dis* 128(suppl):259, 1973.
24. Schlievert PM: Role of superantigens in human disease, *J Infect Dis* 167:997, 1993.
25. Sullivan GW, Mandell GL: Role of neutrophil degranulation in streptococcal leukotoxicity, *Infect Immun* 33:267, 1981.
26. Sullivan GW, Mandell GL: Interactions of human neutrophils with leukotoxic streptococci, *Infect Immun* 30:272, 1980.
27. Medeiros AA: β-Lactamases, *Br Med Bull* 40:18, 1984.
28. Abraham EP, Chain E: An enzyme from bacteria able to destroy penicillin, *Nature* 146:837, 1940.
29. Drelichman V, Cushing RD, Bawdon RE, Lerner AM: Possible pseudoresistance of *Streptococcus pneumoniae* to penicillin G in a patient with a mixed pneumococcus–*Staphylococcus aureus* pneumonia, *Am J Med Sci* 287:39, 1984.
30. Brook I, Gilmore JD: Evaluation of bacterial interference and beta-lactamase production in management of experimental infection with group A beta-hemolytic streptococci, *Antimicrob Agents Chemother* 37:1452, 1993.
31. Mandell GL: Catalase, superoxide dismutase, and virulence of *Staphylococcus aureus:* in vitro and in vivo studies with emphasis on staphylococcal–leukocyte interaction, *J Clin Invest* 55:561, 1975.
32. Nicas TI, Iglewski BH: The contribution of exoproducts to virulence of *Pseudomonas aeruginosa, Can J Microbiol* 31:387, 1985.
33. Hatheway CL: Toxigenic clostridia, *Clin Microbiol Rev* 3:66, 1990.
34. Talkington DF, Schwartz B, Black CM et al: Association of phenotypic and genetic characteristics of invasive *Streptococcus pyogenes* isolates with components of streptococcal toxic shock syndrome, *Infect Immun* 61:3369, 1993.
35. Vitharsson G, Jónsdóttir I, Jónsson S, Valdimarsson H: Opsonization and antibodies to capsular and cell wall polysaccharides of *Streptococcus pneumoniae, J Infect Dis* 170:592, 1994.
36. Umetsu DT, Ambrosino DM, Quinti I et al: Recurrent sinopulmonary infection and impaired antibody response to bacterial capsular polysaccharide antigen in children with selective IgG-subclass deficiency, *N Engl J Med* 313:1247, 1985.

37. Onderdonk AB, Kasper DL, Cisneros RL, Bartlett JG: The capsular polysaccharide of *Bacteroides fragilis* as a virulence factor: comparison of the pathogenic potential of encapsulated and unencapsulated strains, *J Infect Dis* 136:82, 1977.
38. Peltola H, Kilpi T, Anttila M: Rapid disappearance of *Haemophilus influenzae* type b meningitis after routine childhood immunisation with conjugate vaccines, *Lancet* 340:592, 1992.
39. Schoolnik GK, Buchanan TM, Holmes KK: Gonococci causing disseminated gonococcal infection are resistant to the bactericidal action of normal human sera, *J Clin Invest* 58:1163, 1976.
40. Rice PA: Molecular basis for serum resistance in *Neisseria gonorrhoeae*, *Clin Microbiol Rev* 2(suppl):S112, 1989.
41. Manchee RJ, Broster MG, Melling J et al: *Bacillus anthracis* on Gruinard Island, *Nature* 294:254, 1981.
42. Nakahara H, Kozukue H: Isolation of chlorhexidine-resistant *Pseudomonas aeruginosa* from clinical lesions, *J Clin Microbiol* 15:166, 1982.
43. Densen P, Mandell GL: Phagocyte strategy vs. microbial tactics, *Rev Infect Dis* 2:817, 1980.
44. Martínez JL, Delgado-Iribarren A, Baquero F: Mechanisms of iron acquisition and bacterial virulence, *FEMS Microbiol Rev* 6:45, 1990.
45. Johnson W, Varner L, Poch M: Acquisition of iron by *Legionella pneumophila:* role of iron reductase, *Infect Immun* 59:2376, 1991.
46. Collins FM: Cellular antimicrobial immunity, *CRC Crit Rev Microbiol* 7:27, 1979.
47. Wagner SJ, Friedman LI, Dodd RY: Transfusion-associated bacterial sepsis, *Clin Microbiol Rev* 7:290, 1994.
48. Tacket CO, Narain JP, Sattin R et al: A multistate outbreak of infections caused by *Yersinia enterocolitica* transmitted by pasteurized milk, *JAMA* 251:483, 1984.
49. Flournoy DJ: Growth of clinical isolates in the cold, *Med Microbiol Immunol* (Berl) 173:45, 1984.
50. Mackel DC, Maki DG, Anderson RL, Rhame FS, Bennett JV: Nationwide epidemic of septicemia caused by contaminated intravenous products: mechanisms of intrinsic contamination, *J Clin Microbiol* 2:486, 1975.
51. Maki DG, Martin WT: Nationwide epidemic of septicemia caused by contaminated infusion products. IV. Growth of microbial pathogens in fluids for intravenous infusions, *J Infect Dis* 131:267, 1975.

The human equation

52. Green GM, Jakab GJ, Low RB, Davis GS: Defense mechanisms of the respiratory membrane, *Am Rev Respir Dis* 115:479, 1977.
53. Wilson R, Cole PJ: The effect of bacterial products on ciliary function, *Am Rev Respir Dis* 138:S49, 1988.
54. Green GM, Kass EH: The role of the alveolar macrophage in the clearance of bacteria from the lung, *J Exp Med* 119:167, 1964.
55. Crain EF, Gershel JC: Urinary tract infections in febrile infants younger than 8 weeks of age, *Pediatrics* 86:363, 1990.
56. Strom BL, Collins M, West SL et al: Sexual activity, contraceptive use, and other risk factors for symptomatic and asymptomatic bacteriuria: a case-control study, *Ann Intern Med* 107:816, 1987.
57. Ronald AR, Pattullo AL. The natural history of urinary infection in adults, *Med Clin North Am* 75:299, 1991.
58. Garibaldi RA, Burke JP, Dickman ML, Smith CB: Factors predisposing to bacteriuria during indwelling urethral catheterization, *N Engl J Med* 291:215, 1974.
59. Giannella RA, Broitman SA, Zamcheck N: Salmonella enteritis. I. Role of reduced gastric secretion in pathogenesis, *Am J Dig Dis* 16:1000, 1971.
60. Yamauchi K, Tomita M, Giehl TJ, Ellison RT: Antibacterial activity of lactoferrin and a pepsin-derived lactoferrin peptide fragment, *Infect Immun* 61:719, 1993.
61. Alberti S, Marques G, Camprubi S et al: C1q binding and activation of the complement classical pathway by *Klebsiella pneumoniae* outer membrane proteins, *Infect Immun* 61:852, 1993.
62. Densen P: Interaction of complement with *Neisseria meningitidis* and *Neisseria gonorrhoeae, Clin Microbiol Rev* 2(suppl):S11, 1989.
63. Berger M, Sorensen RU, Tosi MF, Dearborn DG, Doring G: Complement receptor expression on neutrophils at an inflammatory site, the *Pseudomonas*-infected lung in cystic fibrosis, *J Clin Invest* 84:1302, 1989.
64. Yang KD, Bohnsack JF, Hill HR: Fibronectin in host defense: implications in the diagnosis, prophylaxis and therapy of infectious diseases, *Pediatr Infect Dis J* 12:234, 1993.
65. Jalowayski AA, Giammona ST: The interaction of bacteria with pulmonary surfactant, *Am Rev Respir Dis* 105:236, 1972.
66. Verbrugh HA, Lee DA, Elliott GR et al: Opsonization of *Legionella pneumophila* in human serum: key roles for specific antibodies and the classical complement pathway, *Immunology* 54:643, 1985.
67. Noya FJ, Baker CJ, Edwards MS: Neutrophil Fc receptor participation in phagocytosis of type III group B streptococci, *Infect Immun* 61:1415, 1993.
68. Musher DM, Goree A, Baughn RE, Birdsall HH: Immunoglobulin A from bronchopulmonary secretions blocks bactericidal and opsonizing effects of antibody to nontypable *Haemophilus influenzae, Infect Immun* 45:36, 1984.
69. McIntyre PA: The reticuloendothelial system: organization and physiology, *Johns Hopkins Med J* 130:61, 1972.
70. Velo GP, Spector WG: The origin and turnover of alveolar macrophages in experimental pneumonia, *J Pathol* 109:7, 1973.
71. Brown EJ, Hosea SW, Frank MM: The role of antibody and complement in the reticuloendothelial clearance of pneumococci from the bloodstream, *Rev Infect Dis* 5(suppl 4):S797, 1983.
72. Mackaness GB: The influence of immunologically committed lymphoid cells on macrophage activity in vivo, *J Exp Med* 129:973, 1969.
73. Enelow RI, Sullivan GW, Carper HT, Mandell GL: Cytokine-induced human multinucleated giant cells have enhanced candidacidal activity and oxidative capacity compared with macrophages, *J Infect Dis* 166:664, 1992.
74. Rajagopalan P, Dournon E, Vilde JL, Pocidalo JJ: Direct activation of human monocyte-derived macrophages by a bacterial glycoprotein extract inhibits the intracellular multiplication of virulent *Legionella pneumophila* serogroup 1, *Infect Immun* 55:2234, 1987.
75. Hormaeche CE, Mastroeni P, Arena A, Uddin J, Joysey HS: T cells do not mediate the initial suppression of a *Salmonella* infection in the RES, *Immunology* 70:247, 1990.
76. Jiang X, Baldwin CL: Effects of cytokines on intracellular growth of *Brucella abortus, Infect Immun* 61:124, 1993.
77. Murray HW: The interferons, macrophage activation, and host defense against nonviral pathogens, *J Interferon Res* 12:319, 1992.
78. Jensen WA, Rose RM, Wasserman AS et al: In vitro activation of the antibacterial activity of human pulmonary macrophages by recombinant gamma interferon, *J Infect Dis* 155:574, 1987.
79. Nordmann P, Ronco E, Guenounou M: Involvement of interferon-gamma and tumor necrosis factor-alpha in host defense against *Rhodococcus equi, J Infect Dis* 167:1456, 1993.
80. Blanchard DK, Djeu JY, Klein TW et al: Interferon-gamma induction by lipopolysaccharide: dependence on interleukin 2 and macrophages, *J Immunol* 136:963, 1986.
81. Mayer J, Woods ML, Vavrin Z, Hibbs JB Jr: Gamma interferon–induced nitric oxide production reduces *Chlamydia trachomatis* infectivity in McCoy cells, *Infect Immun* 61:491, 1993.
82. Byrd TF, Horwitz MA: Interferon gamma–activated human monocytes downregulate transferrin receptors and inhibit the intracellular multiplication of *Legionella pneumophila* by limiting the availability of iron, *J Clin Invest* 83:1457, 1989.
83. Green LH, Green GM: Differential suppression of pulmonary antibacterial activity as the mechanism of selection of a pathogen in mixed bacterial infection of the lung, *Am Rev Respir Dis* 98:819, 1968.
84. Green GM, Kass EH: The influence of bacterial species on pulmonary resistance to infection in mice subjected to hypoxia, cold stress, and ethanolic intoxication, *Br J Exp Pathol* 43:360, 1965.
85. Bhardwaj N, Horwitz MA: Interferon-gamma and antibiotics fail to act synergistically to kill *Legionella pneumophila* in human monocytes, *J Interferon Res* 8:283, 1988.
86. Wade BH, Mandell GL: Polymorphonuclear leukocytes: dedicated professional phagocytes, *Am J Med* 74:686, 1983.
87. Reynolds HY: Lung inflammation: role of endogenous chemotactic factors attracting polymorphonuclear granulocytes, *Am Rev Respir Dis* 127:S16, 1983.

88. Downey GP, Worthen GS, Henson PM, Hyde DM: Neutrophil sequestration and migration in localized pulmonary inflammation: capillary localization and migration across the interalveolar septum, *Am Rev Respir Dis* 147:168, 1993.
89. Hill HR, Gerrard JM, Hogan NA, Quie PG: Hyperactivity of neutrophil leukotactic responses during active bacterial infection, *J Clin Invest* 53:996, 1974.
90. Doherty DE, Downey GP, Worthen G et al: Monocyte retention and migration in pulmonary inflammation: requirement for neutrophils, *Lab Invest* 59:200, 1988.
91. Hermann M, Jaconi ME, Dahlgren C et al: Neutrophil bactericidal activity against *Staphylococcus aureus* adherent on biological surfaces: surface-bound extracellular matrix proteins activate intracellular killing by oxygen-dependent and -independent mechanisms, *J Clin Invest* 86:942, 1990.
92. Klebanoff SJ: Antimicrobial mechanisms in neutrophilic polymorphonuclear leukocytes, *Semin Hematol* 12:112, 1975.
93. Schweitzer AN: CD4+ T-cell dynamics and host predisposition to infection, *Infect Immun* 61:1516, 1993.
94. Spira TJ, Jones BM, Nicholson JKA et al: Idiopathic CD4+ T-lymphocytopenia: an analysis of five patients with unexplained opportunistic infections, *N Engl J Med* 328:386-392., 1993.
95. Noelle RJ, Snow EC: Cognate interactions between helper T cells and B cells, *Immunol Today* 11:361, 1990.
96. Noelle RJ, Snow EC: T helper cell–dependent B cell activation, *FASEB J* 5:2770, 1991.
97. Lynch RG: Immunoglobulin-specific suppressor T cells, *Adv Immunol* 40:135, 1987.
98. Moretta L, Ciccone E, Pende D et al: Human natural killer cells: clonally distributed specific functions and triggering surface molecules, *Lab Invest* 66:138, 1992.
99. Santoni A, Herberman RB, Holden HT: Correlation between natural and antibody-dependent cell-mediated cytotoxicity against tumor targets in the mouse. II. Characterization of the effector cells, *J Natl Cancer Inst* 63:995, 1979.
100. Onderdonk AB, Markham RB, Zaleznik DF et al: Evidence for T cell–dependent immunity to *Bacteroides fragilis* in an intraabdominal abscess model, *J Clin Invest* 69:9, 1982.
101. Ammann AJ, Hong R: Selective IgA deficiency: presentation of 30 cases and a review of the literature, *Medicine (Baltimore)* 50:223, 1971.
102. Figueroa JE, Densen P: Infectious diseases associated with complement deficiencies, *Clin Microbiol Rev* 4:359, 1991.
103. Platonov AE, Beloborodov VB, Vershinina IV: Meningococcal disease in patients with late complement component deficiency: studies in the U.S.S.R., *Medicine (Baltimore)* 72:374, 1993.
104. Holdsworth RJ, Irving AD, Cuschieri A: Postsplenectomy sepsis and its mortality rate: actual versus perceived risks, *Br J Surg* 78:1031, 1991.
105. Green DM, Stutzman L, Blumenson LE et al: The incidence of postsplenectomy sepsis and herpes zoster in children and adolescents with Hodgkin disease, *Med Pediatr Oncol* 7:285, 1979.
106. Pearson HA: Sickle cell anemia and severe infections due to encapsulated bacteria, *J Infect Dis* 136(Suppl):S25, 1977.
107. Traub A, Giebink GS, Smith C et al: Splenic reticuloendothelial function after splenectomy, spleen repair, and spleen autotransplantation, *N Engl J Med* 317:1559, 1987.
108. Rosen FS, Cooper MD, Wedgwood RJP: The primary immunodeficiencies (second of two parts), *N Engl J Med* 311:300, 1984.
109. Cohen JI: Epstein-Barr virus lymphoproliferative disease associated with acquired immunodeficiency, *Medicine* (Baltimore) 70:137, 1991.
110. Hussey G, Simpson J: Nosocomial bacteremias in measles, *Pediatr Infect Dis J* 9:715, 1990.
111. Bodey GP, Buckley M, Sathe YS, Freireich EJ: Quantitative relationships between circulating leukocytes and infection in patients with acute leukemia, *Ann Intern Med* 64:328, 1966.
112. Quie PG, Cates KL: Clinical conditions associated with defective polymorphonuclear leukocyte chemotaxis, *Am J Pathol* 88:711, 1977.
113. Rotrosen D, Gallin JI: Disorders of phagocyte function, *Annu Rev Immunol* 5:127, 1987.
114. Clark RA, Malech HL, Gallin JI et al: Genetic variants of chronic granulomatous disease: prevalence of deficiencies of two cytosolic components of the NADPH oxidase system, *N Engl J Med* 321:647, 1989.
115. Nakhleh RE, Glock M, Snover DC: Hepatic pathology of chronic granulomatous disease of childhood, *Arch Pathol Lab Med* 116:71, 1992.
116. Gallin JI: Interferon-gamma in the treatment of the chronic granulomatous diseases of childhood, *Clin Immunol Immunopathol* 61:S100, 1991.
117. Bullen JJ, Spalding PB, Ward CG, Gutteridge JM: Hemochromatosis, iron and septicemia caused by *Vibrio vulnificus*, *Arch Intern Med* 151:1606, 1991.
118. Chiu HY, Flynn DM, Hoffbrand AV, Politis D: Infection with Yersinia *enterocolitica* in patients with iron overload, *Br Med J (Clin Res Ed)* 292:97, 1986.
119. Cantinieaux B, Boelaert J, Hariga C, Fondu P: Impaired neutrophil defense against *Yersinia enterocolitica* in patients with iron overload who are undergoing dialysis, *J Lab Clin Med* 111:524, 1988.
120. Kuhns DB, DeCarlo E, Hawk DM, Gallin JI: Dynamics of the cellular and humoral components of the inflammatory response elicited in skin blisters in humans, *J Clin Invest* 89:1734, 1992.
121. Verweij WR, Namavar F, Schouten WF, Maclaren DM: Early events after intra-abdominal infection with *Bacteroides fragilis* and *Escherichia coli*, *J Med Microbiol* 35:18, 1991.
122. Davis GS, Winn WC Jr, Gump DW, Beaty HN: The kinetics of early inflammatory events during experimental pneumonia due to *Legionella pneumophila* in guinea pigs, *J Infect Dis* 148:823, 1983.
123. Teplitz C: Pathogenesis of *Pseudomonas* vasculitis and septic lesions, *Arch Pathol* 80:297, 1965.
124. Jacobs RF, Hsi S, Wilson CB et al: Apparent meningococcemia: clinical features of disease due to *Haemophilus influenzae* and *Neisseria meningitidis*, *Pediatrics* 72:469, 1983.
125. McKinney WP, Agner RC: Waterhouse-Friderichsen syndrome caused by *Haemophilus influenzae* type b in an immunocompetent young adult, *South Med J* 82:1571, 1989.
126. Kullberg BJ, Westendorp RG, van't Wout JW, Meinders AE: Purpura fulminans and symmetrical peripheral gangrene caused by *Capnocytophaga canimorsus* (formerly DF-2) septicemia: a complication of dog bite, *Medicine* (Baltimore) 70:287, 1991.
127. Kasper DL, Onderdonk AB, Polk BF, Bartlett JG: Surface antigens as virulence factors in infection with *Bacteroides fragilis*, *Rev Infect Dis* 1:278, 1979.
128. Caplan ES, Kluge RM: Gas gangrene: review of 34 cases, *Arch Intern Med* 136:788, 1976.
129. Collier PE, Diamond DL, Young JC: Nontraumatic *Clostridium septicum* gangrenous myonecrosis, *Dis Colon Rectum* 26:703, 1983.
130. Taguchi Y, Sato J, Nakamura N: Gas-containing brain abscess due to *Fusobacterium nucleatum*, *Surg Neurol* 16:408, 1981.
131. Heckerling PS, Stine TM, Pottage JC Jr et al: *Aeromonas hydrophila* myonecrosis and gas gangrene in a nonimmunocompromised host, *Arch Intern Med* 143:2005, 1983.
132. Darke SG, King AM, Slack WK: Gas gangrene and related infection: classification, clinical features and aetiology, management and mortality: a report of 88 cases, *Br J Surg* 64:104, 1977.
133. Bird D, Giddings AE, Jones SM: Non-clostridial gas gangrene in the diabetic lower limb, *Diabetologia* 13:373, 1977.
134. Joiner KA, Onderdonk AB, Gelfand JA et al: A quantitative model for subcutaneous abscess formation in mice, *Br J Exp Pathol* 61:97, 1980.
135. Bruce MC, Poncz L, Klinger JD et al: Biochemical and pathologic evidence for proteolytic destruction of lung connective tissue in cystic fibrosis, *Am Rev Respir Dis* 132:529, 1985.
136. Onderdonk AB, Shapiro ME, Finberg RW et al: Use of a model of intraabdominal sepsis for studies of the pathogenicity of *Bacteroides fragilis*, *Rev Infect Dis* 6(suppl 1):S91, 1984.
137. Joiner KA, Gelfand JA, Onderdonk AB et al: Host factors in the formation of abscesses, *J Infect Dis* 142:40, 1980.
138. Minuk GY, Nicole LE, Sherman T: Cryptogenic abscess of the liver: evidence of underlying reticuloendothelial cell dysfunction, *Arch Surg* 122:906, 1987.
139. Dal Nogare AR, Vial WC, Toews GB: Bacterial species–dependent inhibition of human granulocyte elastase, *Am Rev Respir Dis* 137:907, 1988.

140. Hays RC, Mandell GL: pO_2, pH, and redox potential of experimental abscesses, *Proc Soc Exp Biol Med* 147:29, 1974.
141. Verklin RM Jr, Mandell GL: Alteration of effectiveness of antibiotics by anaerobiosis, *J Lab Clin Med* 89:65, 1977.
142. Dinarello CA, Gelfand JA, Wolff SM: Anticytokine strategies in the treatment of the systemic inflammatory response syndrome, *JAMA* 269:1829, 1993.
143. Miller PJ, Wenzel RP: Etiologic organisms as independent predictors of death and morbidity associated with bloodstream infections, *J Infect Dis* 156:471, 1987.
144. Kunkel SL, Strieter RM, Lukacs N, Chensue SW: Initiation and maintenance of the granulomatous response, *Chest* 103:135S, 1993.
145. Gillespie WJ, Moore TE, Mayo KM: Subacute pyogenic osteomyelitis, *Orthopedics* 9:1565, 1986.
146. McClurg FV, D'Agostino AN, Martin JH, Race GJ: Ultrastructural demonstration of intracellular bacteria in three cases of malakoplakia of the bladder, *Am J Clin Pathol* 60:780, 1973.

The environment: interface between microbe and human host

147. Moore WM, Stokes TL, Cabanas VY: Malakoplakia of the skin: report of a case, *Am J Clin Pathol* 60:218, 1973.
148. Holmberg H: Aetiology of community-acquired pneumonia in hospital treated patients, *Scand J Infect Dis* 19:491, 1987.
149. Carter KC, Tate GS: Texts and documents: the earliest-known account of Semmelweis's initiation of disinfection at Vienna's Allgemeines Krankenhaus, *Bull Hist Med* 65:252, 1991.
150. Doebbeling BN, Stanley GL, Sheetz CT et al: Comparative efficacy of alternative hand-washing agents in reducing nosocomial infections in intensive care units, *N Engl J Med* 327:88, 1992.
151. Winn WC Jr: Legionnaires disease: historical perspective, *Clin Microbiol Rev* 1:60, 1988.
152. Chin J, Arnon SS, Midura TF: Food and environmental aspects of infant botulism in California, *Rev Infect Dis* 1:693, 1979.
153. Weber DJ, Hansen AR: Infections resulting from animal bites, *Infect Dis Clin North Am* 5:663, 1991.
154. Flandry F, Lisecki EJ, Domingue GJ et al: Initial antibiotic therapy for alligator bites: characterization of the oral flora of *Alligator mississippiensis, South Med* J 82:262, 1989.
155. Hall CJ, Richmond SJ, Caul EO et al: Laboratory outbreak of Q fever acquired from sheep, *Lancet* 1:1004, 1982.
156. Guerrant RL, Humphries MK Jr, Butler JE, Jackson RS: Tickborne oculoglandular tularemia: case report and review of seasonal and vectorial associations in 106 cases, *Arch Intern Med* 136:811, 1976.
157. Holmberg SD, Osterholm MT, Senger KA, Cohen ML: Drug-resistant salmonella from animals fed antimicrobials, *N Engl J Med* 311:617, 1984.
158. Munroe DL, Prescott JF, Penner JL: *Campylobacter jejuni* and *Campylobacter coli* serotypes isolated from chickens, cattle, and pigs, *J Clin Microbiol* 18:877, 1983.
159. Ryan CA, Nickels MK, Hargrett-Bean NT et al: Massive outbreak of antimicrobial-resistant salmonellosis traced to pasteurized milk, *JAMA* 258:3269, 1987.
160. Felsenfed O: Borreliae, human relapsing fever and parasite-vector-host relationships, *Bacteriol Rev* 29:46, 1965.
161. Feldman RE, Baine WB, Nitzkin JL et al: Epidemiology of *Salmonella typhi* infection in a migrant labor camp in Dade County, Florida, *J Infect Dis* 130:335, 1974.
162. Tramont EC: *Treponema pallidum* (syphilis). In Mandell GL, Douglas RG Jr, Bennett JE, editors: *Principles and practice of infectious diseases,* ed 3, New York, 1990, Churchill Livingstone.
163. Long SS, Welkon CJ, Clark JL: Widespread silent transmission of pertussis in families: antibody correlates of infection and symptomatology, *J Infect Dis* 161:480, 1990.

Diagnosis of bacterial infections

164. McFarland LV, Surawicz CM, Stamm WE: Risk factors for *Clostridium difficile* carriage and *C. difficile*–associated diarrhea in a cohort of hospitalized patients, *J Infect Dis* 162:678, 1990.
165. Tenover FC: Diagnostic deoxyribonucleic acid probes for infectious diseases, *Clin Microbiol Rev* 1:82, 1988.
166. Relman DA: The identification of uncultured microbial pathogens, *J Infect Dis* 168:1, 1993.
167. Relman DA, Loutit JS, Schmidt TM et al: The agent of bacillary angiomatosis: an approach to the identification of uncultured pathogens, *N Engl J Med* 323:1573, 1990.
168. Relman DA, Schmidt TM, MacDermott RP, Falkow S: Identification of the uncultured bacillus of Whipple's disease, *N Engl J Med* 327:293, 1992.
169. Lorian V, Atkinson B: Abnormal forms of bacteria produced by antibiotics, *Am J Clin Pathol* 64:678, 1975.
170. Wear DJ, Margileth AM, Hadfield TL et al: Cat scratch disease: a bacterial infection, *Science* 221:1403, 1983.
171. Marshall BJ: Unidentified curved bacilli on gastric epithelium in active chronic gastritis, *Lancet* 2:1273, 1983.
172. Koneman EW, Allen SD, Janda WM et al: *Color atlas and textbook of diagnostic microbiology,* ed 4, Philadelphia, 1992, Lippincott.
173. Robboy SJ, Vickery AL: Tinctorial and morphologic properties distinguishing actinomycosis and nocardiosis, *N Engl J Med* 282:593, 1970.

Gram-positive cocci

Staphylococci

174. Kaplan MH, Tenenbaum MJ: *Staphylococcus aureus:* celluar biology and clinical application, *Am J Med* 72:248, 1982.
175. Fekety FR Jr: The epidemiology and prevention of staphylococcal infection, *Medicine* 42:593, 1964.
176. Martin RR, Buttram V, Besch P et al: Nasal and vaginal *Staphylococcus aureus* in young women: quantitative studies, *Ann Intern Med* 96:951, 1982.
177. Godfrey MI, Smith IM: Hospital hazards of staphylococcal sepsis, *JAMA* 166:1197, 1958.
178. Eykyn SJ: Staphylococcal sepsis: the changing pattern of disease and therapy, *Lancet* 1:100, 1988.
179. Stutman HR, Marks MI: Pulmonary infections in children with cystic fibrosis, *Semin Respir Infect* 2:166, 1987.
180. Todd J, Fishout M: Toxic-shock syndrome associated with phage-group-I staphylococci, *Lancet* 2:1116, 1978.
181. Chesney PJ, Davis JP, Purdy WK et al: Clinical manifestations of toxic shock syndrome, *JAMA* 246:741, 1981.
182. Langmuir AD, Worthen TD, Solomon J, Ray CG, Pertersen E: The Thucydides syndrome: a new hypothesis for the cause of the plague of Athens, *N Engl J Med* 313:1027, 1985.
183. MacDonald KL, Osterholm MT, Hedberg CW et al: Toxic shock syndrome: a newly recognized complication of influenza and influenzalike illness, *JAMA* 257:1053, 1987.
184. Jacobson JA, Burke JP, Benowitz BA, Clark PV: Varicella zoster and staphylococcal toxic shock syndrome in a young man, *JAMA* 249:922, 1983.
185. Cone LA, Woodard DR, Byrd RG et al: A recalcitrant, erythematous, desquamating disorder associated with toxin-producing staphylococci in patients with AIDS, *J Infect Dis* 165:638, 1992.
186. Osterholm MT, Davis JP, Gibson RW et al: Tri-state toxic-shock syndrome study. I. Epidemiologic findings, *J Infect Dis* 145:431, 1982.
187. Larkin SM, Williams DN, Osterholm MT et al: Toxic shock syndrome: clinical, laboratory and pathologic findings in non fatal cases, *Ann Intern Med* 96:858, 1982.
188. Davis JP, Osterholm MT, Helms CM et al: Tri-state toxic-shock syndrome study. II. Chemical and laboratory findings, *J Infect Dis* 145:441, 1982.
189. Stevens DL, Tanner MH, Winship J et al: Severe group A streptococcal infections associated with a toxic shock-like syndrome and scarlet fever toxin A, *N Engl J Med* 321:1, 1989.
190. Hoge CW, Schwartz B, Talkington DF et al: The changing epidemiology of invasive group A streptococcal infections and the emergence of streptococcal toxic shock-like syndrome: a retrospective population-based study, *JAMA* 269:384, 1993.
191. Schlievert PM, Gocke JE, Deringer JR: Group B streptococcal toxic shock-like syndrome: report of a case and purification of an associated pyrogenic toxin, *Clin Infect Dis* 17:26, 1993.

934. Francis E: Tularaemia IX tularaemia in the Washington (D.C.) market, *Public Health Rep* 38:1391, 1923.
935. Burroughs AL, Holdenried R, Longenecker DS, Meyer KF: A field study of latent tularemia in rodents with a list of all known naturally infected vertebrates, *J Infect Dis* 76:115, 1945.
936. Boyce JM: Recent trends in the epidemiology of tularemia in the United States, *J Infect Dis* 131:197, 1975.
937. Preiksaitis JK, Crawshaw GJ, Nayar GP, Stiver HG: Human tularemia in an urban zoo, *Can Med Assoc J* 121:1097, 1979.
938. Brooks GF, Buchanan TM: Tularemia in the United States: epidemiologic aspects in the 1960's and follow-up of the outbreak of tularemia in Vermont, *J Infect Dis* 121:357, 1970.
939. Teutsch SM, Martone WJ, Brink EW et al: Pneumonic tularemia on Martha's vineyard, *N Engl J Med* 301:826, 1979.
940. Uhari M, Syrjälä H, Salminen A: Tularemia in children caused by *Francisella tularensis* biovar *palaearctica*, *Pediatr Infect Dis* 9:80, 1990.
941. Dahlstrand S, Ringertz O, Zetterberg B: Airborne tularemia in Sweden, *Scand J Infect Dis* 3:7, 1971.
942. Karpoff SP, Antonoff N: The spread of tularemia through water, as a new factor in its epidemiology, *J Bacteriol* 32:243, 1936.
943. Overholt EL, Tigertt WD, Kadull PJ et al: An analysis of forty-two cases of laboratory-acquired tularemia: treatment with broad spectrum antibiotics, *Am J Med* 30:785, 1961.
944. Evans ME, Gregory DW, Schaffner W, McGee ZA: Tularemia: a 30 year experience with 88 cases, *Medicine* 64:251, 1985.
945. Miller RP, Bates JM: Pleuropulmonary tularemia: a review of 29 cases, *Am Rev Respir Dis* 99:31, 1969.
946. Funk LM, Simpson SQ, Mertz G, Boyd J: Tularemia presenting as an isolated pleural effusion, *West J Med* 156:415, 1992.
947. Kostiala AAI, McGregory DD, Logie PS: Tularemia in the rat. I. The cellular basis of host resistance to infection, *Immunology* 28:855, 1975.

BRUCELLA SPECIES

948. Bruce D: The micrococcus of Malta fever, *Pract* 40:241, 1888.
949. Bang B: The etiology of epizootic abortion, *J Comp Pathol Ther* 10:125, 1897.
950. Wise RI: Brucellosis in the United States: past, present and future, *JAMA* 244:2318, 1980.
951. Young EJ: Human brucellosis, *Rev Infect Dis* 5:821, 1983.
952. Al-Eissa YA, Kambal AM, Al-Nasser MN et al: Childhood brucellosis: a study of 102 cases, *Pediatr Infect Dis* 9:74, 1990.
953. Schirger A, Nichols DR, Martin WJ et al: Brucellosis: experience with 224 patients, *Ann Intern Med* 52:827, 1960.
954. Sharp WB: Pathology of undulant fever, *Arch Pathol* 18:72, 1934.
955. Jorens PG, Michielsen PP, van den Enden EJ et al: A rare cause of colitis—*Brucella melitensis*—report of a case, *Dis Colon Rectum* 34:194, 1991.
956. Petrella R, Young EJ: Acute brucella ileitis, *Am J Gastroenterol* 83:80, 1988.
957. Al-Awadhi NZ, Ashkenani F, Khalaf ES: Acute pancreatitis associated with brucellosis, *Am J Gastroenterol* 84:1570, 1989.
958. Hunt AC, Bothwell PW: Histological findings in human brucellosis, *J Clin Pathol* 20:267, 1967.
959. Spink WW, Hoffbauer FW, Walker WW, Green RA: Histopathology of the liver in human brucellosis, *J Lab Clin Med* 34:40, 1949.
960. Gedalia A, Howard C, Einhorn M: Brucellosis induced avascular necrosis of the femoral head in a 7 year old child, *Ann Rheum Dis* 51:404, 1992.
961. Flugelman MY, Galun E, Ben-Chetrit E et al: Brucellosis in patients with heart disease—When should endocarditis be diagnosed? *Cardiology* 77:313, 1990.
962. Peery TM, Belter LF: Brucellosis and heart disease. II. Fatal brucellosis: a review of the literature and report of new cases, *Am J Pathol* 36:673, 1960.
963. Lubani MM, Sharda DC, Helin I: Cardiac manifestations of brucellosis in children, *Arch Dis Child* 61:596, 1986.
964. Simpson WM: Undulant fever (brucellosis): a clinicopathologic study of ninety cases occurring in and about Dayton, Ohio, *Ann Intern Med* 4:238, 1930.
965. Khateeb MI, Araj GF, Majeed SA, Lulu AR: *Brucella* arthritis: a study of 96 cases in Kuwait, *Ann Rheum Dis* 49:994, 1990.
966. Walker J, Sheoma OP, Rao NA: Brucellosis and uveitis, *Am J Ophthalmol* 114:374, 1992.

BORDETELLA SPECIES

967. Cone TE Jr: Whooping cough is first described as a disease sui generis by Baillou in 1640, *Pediatrics* 46:522, 1970.
968. Brooks GF, Buchanan TM: Pertussis in the United States, *J Infect Dis* 122:123, 1970.
969. Brooksaler F, Nelson JD: Pertussis: a reappraisal and report of 190 confirmed cases, *Am J Dis Child* 114:389, 1967.
970. Cherry JD: The epidemiology of pertussis and pertussis immunization in the United Kingdom and the United States: a comparative study, *Curr Probl Pediatr.* 14:1, 1984.
971. Fine PEM: Epidemiological considerations for whooping cough eradication. In Wardlow AC, Parton R; editors: *Pathogenesis and immunity in pertussis*, Chichester, New York, Brisbane, Toronto, Singapore, 1988, Wiley.
972. Etkind P, Lett SM, Macdonald PD, Silva E, Peppe J: Pertussis outbreaks in groups claiming religious exemptions to vaccinations, *Am J Dis Child* 146:173, 1992.
973. Cherry JD, Brunell PA, Golden GS, Karzon DT: Report of the task force on pertussis and pertussis immunization—1988, *Pediatrics* 81 (suppl):939, 1988.
974. Linnemann CC Jr, Bass JW, Smith MHD: The carrier state in pertussis, *Am J Epidemiol* 88:422, 1968.
975. Nkowane BM, Wassilak SG, McKee PA et al: Pertussis epidemic in Oklahoma: difficulties in preventing transmission, *Am J Dis Child* 140:433, 1986.
976. Sprauer MA, Cochi SL, Zell ER et al: Prevention of secondary transmission of pertussis in households with early use of erythromycin, *Am J Dis Child* 146:177, 1992.
977. Beiter A, Lewis K, Pineda EF, Cherry JD: Unrecognized maternal peripartum pertussis with subsequent fatal neonatal pertussis, *Obstet Gynecol* 82:691, 1993.
978. Kurt TL, Yeager AS, Guenette S, Dunlop S: Spread of pertussis by hospital staff, *JAMA* 221:264, 1972.
979. Ng VL, York M, Hadley WK: Unexpected isolation of *Bordetella pertussis* from patients with acquired immunodeficiency syndrome, *J Clin Microbiol* 27:337, 1989.
980. Steketee RW, Wassilak SG, Adkins WN Jr et al: Evidence for a high attack rate and efficacy of erythromycin prophylaxis in a pertussis outbreak in a facility for the developmentally disabled, *J Infect Dis* 157:434, 1988.
981. Weiss A, Hewlett EL: Virulence factors of *Bordetella pertussis*, *Annu Rev Microbiol* 40:661, 1986.
982. Morse SI: Pertussis in adults, *Ann Intern Med* 68:953, 1968.
983. Linnemann CC Jr: Host-parasite interactions in pertussis. In *International Symposium on Pertussis*, Washington, DC, US Government Printing Office, 1979, Dept. of Health, Education and Welfare publ no (NIM) 79-1830, p 3.
984. Rich AR: On the etiology and pathogenesis of whooping cough, *Bull John Hopkins Hosp* 51:346, 1932.
985. Mallory FB, Hornor AA: Pertussis: the histological lesion in the respiratory tract, *J Med Res* 27:115, 1912.
986. Smith LW: The pathologic anatomy of pertussis with a special reference to pneumonia caused by the pertussis bacillus, *Arch Pathol* 4:732, 1927.
987. Davis LE, Burstyn DG, Manclark CR: Pertussis encephalopathy with a normal brain biopsy and elevated lymphocytosis-promoting factor antibodies, *Pediatr Infect Dis* 3:448, 1984.
988. Woolf AL, Caplin H: Whooping cough encephalitis, *Arch Dis Child* 31:87, 1956.
989. Linnemann CC Jr, Berry EB: *Bordetella parapertussis:* recent experience and a review of the literature, *Am J Dis Child* 131:560, 1977.
990. Connor JD: Evidence for an etiologic role of adenovirus infection in pertussis syndrome, *N Engl J Med* 128:390, 1970.
991. Ghosh HK, Tranter J: *Bordetella bronchicanis (bronchiseptica)* infection in man: review and case report, *J Clin Pathol* 32:546, 1979.
992. Brown JH: Bacillus bronchisepticus infection in a child with symptoms of pertussis, *Bull John Hopkins Hosp* 38:147, 1926.

THE HACEK GROUP OF BACTERIA

993. Geraci JE, Greipp PR, Wilkowske CJ et al: *Cardiobacterium hominis* endocarditis: four cases with clinical and laboratory observations, *Mayo Clin Proc* 53:49, 1978.
994. Francioli PB, Roussianos D, Glauser MP: *Cardiobacterium hominis* endocarditis manifesting as bacterial meningitis, *Arch Intern Med* 143:1483, 1983.
995. Laguna J, Derby BM, Chase R: *Cardiobacterium hominis* endocarditis with cerebral mycotic aneurysm, *Arch Neurol* 32:638, 1975.
996. Brooks GF, O'Donaghue JM, Rissing JP et al: *Eikenella corrodens,* a recently recognized pathogen: infections in medical-surgical patients and in associated with methylphenidate abuse, *Medicine* 53:325, 1974.
997. Dorff G, Jackson LJ, Rytel MW: *Eikenella corrodens:* a newly recognized human pathogen, *Ann Intern Med* 80:305, 1974.
998. Marsden HB, Hyde WA: Isolation of *Bacteroides corrodens* from infections in children, *J Clin Pathol* 24:117, 1971.
999. Woolfrey BF, Lally RT, Faville RJ: Intervertebral diskitis caused by *Kingella kingae, Am J Clin Pathol* 85:745, 1986.

PASTEURELLA SPECIES

1000. Weber DJ, Wolfson JS, Swartz MN, Hooper DC: *Pasteurella multocida* infections: report of 34 cases and review of the literature, *Medicine* 63:133, 1984.
1001. Jones FL Jr, Smull CE: Infection in man due to *Pasteurella multocida, Pa Med* 76:41, 1973.
1002. Francis DP, Holmes MA, Brandon G: Pasteurella multocida: infection after domestic animal bites and scratches, *JAMA* 233:42, 1975.
1003. Hansmann GH, Tully M: Cat bite and scratch wounds with consequent *Pasteurella* infection of man, *Am J Clin Pathol* 15:312, 1945.
1004. Arons MS, Fernando I, Polayes IM: *Pasteurella multocida:* the major cause of hand infection following domestic animal bites, *J Hand Surg* 7:47, 1982.
1005. Starkebaum GA, Plorde JJ: *Pasteurella* pneumonia: report of a case and review of the literature, *J Clin Microbiol* 5:332, 1977.
1006. Clapp DW, Kleiman MB, Reynolds JK, Allen SD: *Pasteurella multocida* meningitis in infancy: an avoidable infection, *Am J Dis Child* 140:444, 1986.
1007. Raffi F, Barrier J, Baron D et al: *Pasteurella multocida* bacteremia: report of thirteen cases over twelve years and review of the literature, *Scand J Infect Dis* 19:385, 1987.
1008. Strand CL, Helfman L: *Pasteurella multocida* chorioamnionitis associated with premature delivery and neonatal spepsis and death, *Am J Clin Pathol* 55:713, 1971.
1009. Raffi F, David A, Mouzard A et al: *Pasteurella multocida* appendiceal peritonitis: report of three cases and review of the literature, *Pediatr Infect Dis* 5:695, 1986.
1010. Hubbert WT, Rosen MN: *Pasteurella multocida* infections. II. *Pasteurella multocida* infection in man unrelated to animal bite, *Am J Public Health* 60:1109, 1970.
1011. Itoh M, Tierno PM Jr, Milstoc M, Berger AR: A unique outbreak of *Pasteurella multocida* in a chronic disease hospital, *Am J Public Health* 70:1170, 1980.

FLAVOBACTERIUM SPECIES

1012. Holmes B, Owen RJ, McMeekin TA: Flavobacterium. In Krieg NR, Holt JG, editors: *Bergey's manual of systematic bacteriology,* ed 8, Baltimore, 1984, Williams & Wilkins, p 353.
1013. Plotkin SA, McKitrick JC: Nosocomial meningitis of the newborn caused by a *Flavobacterium, JAMA* 198:662, 1966.
1014. Stamm WE, Colella JJ, Anderson RL, Dixon RE: Indwelling arterial catheters as a source of nosocomial bacteremia: an outbreak cause by *Flavobacterium* species, *N Engl J Med* 292:1099, 1975.
1015. Coyle-Gilchrist MM, Crewe P, Roberts G: *Flavobacterium meningosepticum* in the hospital environment species, *J. Clin Pathol* 29:824, 1976.

ALCALIGENES SPECIES

1016. DuPont HL, Spink WW: Infections due to gram-negative organisms: an analysis of 860 patients with bacteremia at the University of Minnesota Medical Centers 1958–1966, *Medicine* 48:307, 1969.
1017. Gardner P, Griffin W, Swartz M: Non-fermentative gram-negative bacilli of nosocomial interest, *Am J Med* 48:735, 1970.

CHROMOBACTERIUM SPECIES

1018. Centers for Disease Control: Epidemiologic notes and reports—chromobacteriosis—Florida, *MMWR* 29:613, 1981.
1019. Tucker RE, Winter WG, Wilson HD: Osteomyelitis associated with *Chromobacterium violaceum* sepsis: a case report, *J Bone Joint Surg* 61A:949, 1979.
1020. Johnson WM, DiSalvo AF, Steuer RR: Fatal *Chromobacterium violaceum* septicemia, *Am J Clin Pathol* 56:400, 1971.
1021. Macher AM, Casale TB, Fauci AS: Chronic granulomatous disease of childhood and *Chromobacterium violaceum* infections in the southeastern United States, *Ann Intern Med* 97:51, 1982.

ACHROMOBACTER SPECIES

1022. Igra-Siegman Y, Chmel H, Cobbs C: Clinical and laboratory characteristics of *Achromobacter xylosoxidans* infection, *J Clin Microbiol* 11:141, 1980.

Anaerobic gram-negative bacilli

BACTEROIDES SPECIES

1023. Polk BF, Kasper DL: *Bacteroides fragilis* subspecies in clinical isolates, *Ann Intern Med* 86:569, 1977.
1024. Kasper DL, Onderdonk AB, Bartlett JG: Quantitative determination of the antibody response to the capsular polysaccharide of *Bacteroides fragilis* in an animal model of intraabdominal abscess formation, *J Infect Dis* 136:789, 1977.
1025. Williams CM, Okada DM, Marshall JR, Chow AW: Clinical and microbiologic risk evaluation for post-cesarean section endometritis by multivariate discriminant analysis: role of intraoperative mycoplasma, aerobes, and anaerobes, *Am J Obstet Gynecol* 156:967, 1987.
1026. Onderdonk AB, Bartlett JG, Louie T et al: Microbial synergy in experimental intra-abdominal abscess, *Infect Immun* 13:22, 1976.
1027. Chow AW, Guze LB: Bacteroidaceae bacteremia: clinical experience with 112 patients, *Medicine* (Baltimore) 53:93, 1971.
1028. Felner JM, Dowell VR Jr: "*Bacteroides*" bacteremia, *Am J Med* 50:787, 1971.
1029. Sinkovics JG, Smith JP: Septicemia with *Bacteroides* in patients with malignant disease, *Cancer* 25:663, 1970.
1030. Yoshikawa TT, Chow AW, Guze LB: Bacteroidaceae bacteremia with disseminated intravascular coagulation, *Am J Med* 56:725, 1974.
1031. Heerema MS, Ein ME, Musher DM et al: Anaerobic bacterial meningitis, *Am J Med* 67:219, 1979.
1032. Snydman DR, Tally FP, Knuppel R et al: *Bacteroides bivius* and *Bacteroides disiens* in obstetrical patients: clinical findings and antimicrobial susceptibilities, *J Antimicrob Chemother* 6:519, 1980.

FUSOBACTERIUM SPECIES

1033. Brook I: Recovery of anaerobic bacteria from clinical specimens in 12 years at two military hospitals, *J Clin Microbiol* 26:1181, 1988.
1034. Sinave CP, Hardy GJ, Fardy PW: The Lemierre syndrome: suppurative thrombophlebitis of the internal jugular vein secondary to oropharyngeal infection, *Medicine* (Baltimore) 68:85, 1989.

Spirochetes

Treponema species

1035. Fitzgerald TJ: Treponema. In Balows A, Hausler WJ Jr, Herrmann KL et al, editors: *Manual of clinical microbiology,* ed 5, Washington, DC, 1991, American Society for Microbiology.
1036. Smibert RM: *Treponema* Schaudinn 1905. In Krieg NR, Holt JG, editors: *Bergey's manual of systematic bacteriology,* Baltimore, 1984, Williams & Wilkins.
1037. Prpic JK, Trewartha F, Graves SR: Enhanced retention of motility and virulence of *Treponema pallidum* (Nichols strain) in vitro by the addition of gelatin to anaerobic medium, *Sex Transm Dis* 8:1, 1981.
1038. Benditt J: The syphilized world, *Sci Am* 260:30, 1989.
1039. Rothschild BM: On the antiquity of treponemal infection, *Med Hypotheses* 28:181, 1989.
1040. Fornaciari G, Castagna M, Tognetti A et al: Syphilis in a Renaissance Italian mummy, *Lancet* 2:614, 1989.
1041. Pottle FA: *James Boswell: the earlier years, 1740-1769,* New York, 1966, McGraw-Hill, p 336.

1042. Rolfs RT, Nakashima AK: Epidemiology of primary and secondary syphilis in the United States, 1981 through 1989, *JAMA* 264:1432, 1990.
1043. Rolfs RT, Goldberg M, Sharrar RG: Risk factors for syphilis: cocaine use and prostitution, *Am J Public Health* 80:853, 1990.
1044. Nanda D, Feldman J, Delke I et al: Syphilis among parturients at an inner city hospital: association with cocaine use and implications for congenital syphilis rates, *NY State J Med* 90:488, 1990.
1045. Alexander-Rodríguez T, Vermund SH: Gonorrhea and syphilis in incarcerated urban adolescents: prevalence and physical signs, *Pediatrics* 80:561, 1987.
1046. Hook EW: Syphilis and HIV infection, *J Infect Dis* 160:530, 1989.
1047. Magnuson HJ, Thomas EW, Olansky S et al: Inoculation syphilis in human volunteers, *Medicine* 35:33, 1956.
1048. Baseman JB, Hayes EC: Molecular characterization of receptor binding proteins and immunogens of virulent *Treponema pallidum, J Exp Med* 151:573, 1980.
1049. Baughn RE: Role of fibronectin in the pathogenesis of syphilis, *Rev Infect Dis* 9(suppl 4):S372, 1987.
1050. Thomas DD, Navab M, Haake DA et al: *Treponema pallidum* invades intercellular junctions of endothelial cell monolayers, *Proc Natl Acad Sci USA* 85:3608, 1988.
1051. Akins DR, Purcell BK, Mitra MM et al: Lipid modification of the 17-kilodalton membrane immunogen of *Treponema pallidum* determines macrophage activation as well as amphiphilicity, *Infect Immun* 61:1202, 1993.
1052. Fulford KW, Johnson N, Loveday C et al: Changes in intra-vascular complement and anti-treponemal antibody titres preceding the Jarisch-Herxheimer reaction in secondary syphilis, *Clin Exp Immunol* 24:483, 1976.
1053. Young EJ, Weingarten NM, Baughn RE, Duncan WC: Studies on the pathogenesis of the Jarisch-Herxheimer reaction: development of an animal model and evidence against a role for classical endotoxin, *J Infect Dis* 146:606, 1982.
1054. Baker-Zander SA, Hook EWIII, Bonin P et al: Antigens of *Treponema pallidum* recognized by IgG and IgM antibodies during syphilis in humans, *J Infect Dis* 151:264, 1985.
1055. Baughn RE, Jorizzo JL, Adams CB, Musher DM: Ig class and IgG subclass responses to *Treponema pallidum* in patients with syphilis, *J Clin Immunol* 8:128, 1988.
1056. Dobson SR, Taber LH, Baughn RE: Recognition of *Treponema pallidum* antigens by IgM and IgG antibodies in congenitally infected newborns and their mothers, *J Infect Dis* 157:903, 1988.
1057. Larsen SA, Hunter EF, Kraus SJ: *Manual of tests for syphilis,* ed 8, Washington, DC, 1990, American Public Health Association.
1058. Levy RA, Gharavi AE, Sammaritano LR et al: Characteristics of IgG antiphospholipid antibodies in patients with systemic lupus erythematosus and syphilis, *J Rheumatol* 17:1036, 1990.
1059. Fohn MJ, Wignall S, Baker-Zander SA, Lukehart SA: Specificity of antibodies from patients with pinta for antigens of *Treponema pallidum* subspecies *pallidum, J Infect Dis* 157:32, 1988.
1060. Pavia CS, Niederbuhl CJ: Acquired resistance and expression of a protective humoral immune response in guinea pigs infected with *Treponema pallidum* Nichols, *Infect Immun* 50:66, 1985.
1061. Shaffer JM, Baker-Zander SA, Lukehart SA: Opsonization of *Treponema pallidum* is mediated by immunoglobulin G antibodies induced only by pathogenic treponemes, *Infect Immun* 61:781, 1993.
1062. Jorizzo JL, McNeely MC, Baughn RE et al: Role of circulating immune complexes in human secondary syphilis, *J Infect Dis* 153:1014, 1986.
1063. Pavia CS, Niederbuhl CJ: Adoptive transfer of anti-syphilis immunity with lymphocytes from *Treponema pallidum*–infected guinea pigs, *J Immunol* 135:2829, 1985.
1064. Jensen JR, From E: Alterations in T lymphocytes and T-lymphocyte subpopulations in patients with syphilis, *Br J Vener Dis* 58:18, 1982.
1065. Levene GM, Turk JL, Wright DJ, Grimble AG: Reduced lymphocyte transformation due to a plasma factor in patients with active syphilis, *Lancet* 2:246, 1969.
1066. Jensen JR, Jørgensen AS, Thestrup-Pedersen K: Depression of natural killer cell activity by syphilitic serum and immune complexes, *Br J Vener Dis* 58:298, 1982.
1067. Fiumara NJ: Reinfection primary, secondary, and latent syphilis: the serologic response after treatment, *Sex Transm Dis* 7:111, 1980.
1068. Fiumara NJ: Acquired syphilis in three patients with congenital syphilis, *N Engl J Med* 290:1119, 1974.
1069. Smith JL, Israel CW: Treponemes in aqueous humor in late seronegative syphilis, *Trans Acad Ophthalmol Otolaryngol* 72:63, 1968.
1070. Goldenring JM: Secondary syphilis in a prepubertal child: differentiating condylomata lata from condylomata acuminata, *NY State J Med* 89:180, 1989.
1071. Lukehart SA, Hook EW, Baker-Zander SA et al: Invasion of the central nervous system by *Treponema pallidum:* implications for diagnosis and treatment, *Ann Intern Med* 109:855, 1988.
1072. Musher DM, Hamill RJ, Baughn RE: Effect of human immunodeficiency virus (HIV) infection on the course of syphilis and on the response to treatment, *Ann Intern Med* 113:872, 1990.
1073. Gamble CN, Reardan JB: Immunopathogenesis of syphilitic glomerulonephritis: elution of antitreponemal antibody from glomerular immune-complex depositis, *N Engl J Med* 292:449, 1975.
1074. Baker AL, Kaplan MM, Wolfe HJ, McGowan JA: Liver disease associated with early syphilis, *N Engl J Med* 284:1422, 1971.
1075. Lee RV, Thornton GF, Conn HO: Liver disease associated with secondary syphilis, *N Engl J Med* 284:1423, 1971.
1076. Kazlow PG, Beyer B, Brandeis G: Polyarthritis as the initial symptom of secondary syphilis: case report and review, *Mt Sinai J Med* 56:65, 1989.
1077. Warrell DA, Perine PL, Bryceson ADM et al: Physiologic changes during the Jarisch-Herxheimer reaction in early syphilis: a comparison with louse-borne relapsing fever, *Am J Med* 51:176, 1971.
1078. Hooshmand H, Escobar MR, Kopf SW: Neurosyphilis: a study of 241 patients, *JAMA* 219:726, 1972.
1079. Rodríguez S, Teich DL, Weinman MD et al: Gummatous syphilis: a reminder, *J Infect Dis* 157:606, 1988.
1080. Qureshi F, Jacques SM, Reyes MP: Placental histopathology in syphilis, *Hum Pathol* 24:779, 1993.
1081. Young SA, Crocker DW: Occult congenital syphilis in macerated stillborn fetuses, *Arch Pathol Lab Med* 118:44, 1994.
1082. Oppenheimer EH, Hardy JB: Congenital syphilis in the newborn infant: clinical and pathological observations in recent cases, *Johns Hopkins Med J* 129:63, 1971.
1083. Dorfman DH, Glaser JH: Congenital syphilis presenting in infants after the newborn period, *N Engl J Med* 323:1299, 1990.

Leptospira interrogans

1084. Arean VM: The pathologic anatomy and pathogenesis of fatal human leptospirosis (Weil's disease), *Am J Pathol* 40:393, 1962.
1085. Fraser DW, Glosser JW, Francis DP et al: Leptospirosis caused by serotype Fort-Bragg: a suburban outbreak, *Ann Intern Med* 79:786, 1973.
1086. Feigan RD, Anderson DC: Human leptospirosis, *CRC Crit Rev Clin Lab Sci* 5:413, 1975.
1087. Heath CW Jr, Alexander AD, Galton MM: Leptospirosis in the United States: analysis of 483 cases in man, *N Engl J Med* 273:857, 1965.
1088. Edwards GA, Domm BM: Human leptospiras, *Medicine* 39:117, 1960.
1089. Feigan RD, Lobes LA Jr, Anderson D, Pickeveng L: Human leptospirosis from immunized dogs, *Ann Intern Med* 79:777, 1973.
1090. Alexander A, Baer A, Fair JR et al: Leptospiral uveitis: report of bacteriologically verified case, *Am Arch Ophthalmol* 48:292, 1952.
1091. Ramog-Morales F, Díaz-Rivera RS, Cintrón-Rivera AA et al: The pathogenesis of leptospiral jaundice, *Ann Intern Med* 51:861, 1959.
1092. Bhamarapravati N, Boonyapaknavig V, Viranuvatti V et al: Liver changes in leptospirosis: a study of needle biopsies in twenty-two cases, *Am J Proctol* 17:480, 1966.
1093. DeBrito T, Marcondes Machado M, Montans SD et al: Liver biopsy in human leptospirosis: a light and electron microscopic study, *Arch Pathol Anat* 342:61, 1967.
1094. Sitprija V: Renal involvement in human leptospirosis, *Br Med J* 2:656, 1968.
1095. Lai KN, Aaron I, Woodroffe AJ, Clarkson AR: Renal lesions in leptospirosis, *Aus NZ J Med* 12:4, 276, 1982.

Borrelia species

1096. Mekesha A: Louse-borne relapsing fever in children, *J Trop Med Hyg* 95:206, 1992.

1097. Burgdorfer W: The enlarging spectrum of tick-borne spirochetosis—Parker memorial address, *Rev Infect Dis* 8:932, 1986.
1098. Horton JM, Blaser MJ: The spectrum of relapsing fever in the Rocky Mountains, *Arch Intern Med* 145:871, 1985.
1099. Fihn S, Larson EB: Tick-borne relapsing fever in the Pacific Northwest: an underdiagnosed illness, *West J Med* 133:203, 1980.
1100. Thompson RS, Burgdorfer W, Russel R, Francis BJ: Outbreak of tick-borne relapsing fever in Spokane county, Washington, *JAMA* 210:1045, 1969.
1101. Fuchs PC, Oyama AA: Neonatal relapsing fever due to transplacental transmission of *Borrelia, JAMA* 208:690, 1969.
1102. Le CT: Tick-borne relapsing fever in children, *Pediatrics* 66:963, 1980.
1103. Stoenner HG, Dodd T, Larsen C: Antigenic variation of *Borrelia hermsii, J Exp Med* 156:1297, 1982.
1104. Bryceson ADM, Parry EHO, Perine PL et al: Louse-borne relapsing fever: a clinical and laboratory study of 62 cases in Ethiopia and reconsideration of the literature, *Q J Med* 39:129, 1970.
1105. Galloway RE, Leven J, Butler T et al: Activation of protein mediators of inflammation and evidence for endotoxemia in *Borrelia recurrentis* infection, *Am J Med* 63:933, 1977.
1106. Southern P, Sanford JP: Relapsing fever: a clinical and microbiological review, *Medicine* 48:129, 1969.
1107. Judge DM, Samuel I, Perine PL, Vukotic D: Louse-borne relapsing fever in man, *Arch Pathol* 97:136, 1974.
1108. Davis RD, Burke JP, Wright LJ: Relapsing fever associated with AIDS in a parturient women: a case report and review of the literature, *Chest* 102:630, 1992.
1109. Steere AC, Malawista SE, Snydman DR et al: Lyme arthritis: an epidemic of oligoarticular arthritis in children and adults in three Connecticut communities, *Arthritis Rheum* 20:7, 1977.
1110. Burgdorfer W, Barbour AG, Hayes SF et al: Lyme disease: a tick-borne spirochetosis, *Science* 216:1317, 1982.
1111. Steere AC, Grodzicki RL, Kornblatt AN et al: The spirochetal etiology of Lyme disease, *N Engl J Med* 308:733, 1983.
1112. Steere AC: Lyme disease, *N Engl J Med* 321:586, 1989.
1113. Anderson JF: Epizootiology of *Borrelia* in *Ixodes* tick vectors and reservoir hosts, *Rev Infect Dis* 11(suppl 6):S1451, 1989.
1114. Levine JF, Wilson ML, Spielman A: Mice as reservoirs of the Lyme disease spirochete, *Am J Trop Med Hyg* 34:355, 1985.
1115. Wilson ML, Adler GH, Spielman A: Correlation between abundance of white-tailed deer and that of the deer tick (Acari: Ixodidae), *Ann Entomol Soc Am* 172, 1986.
1116. Wilson ML, Telford SR III, Piesman J, Spielman A: Reduced abundance of immature (Acari: Ixodidae) following elimination of deer, *J Med Entomol* 25:224, 1988.
1117. Wilson ML, Spielman A: Seasonal activity of immature *Ixodes dammini* (Acari: Ixodidae), *J Med Entomol* 22:404, 1985.
1118. Ribeiro JM, Mather TN, Piesman J, Spielman A: Dissemination and salivary delivery of Lyme disease spirochetes in vector ticks (Acari: Ixodidae), *J Med Entomol* 24:201, 1987.
1119. Piesman J, Mather TN, Sinsky RJ, Spielman A: Duration of tick attachment and *Borrelia burgdorferi* transmission, *J Clin Microbiol* 25:557, 1987.
1120. Bosler EM, Ormiston BG, Coleman JL et al: Prevalence of the Lyme disease spirochete in populations of white-tailed deer and white-footed mice, *Yale J Biol Med* 57:651, 1984.
1121. Schmid GP: The global distribution of Lyme disease, *Rev Infect Dis* 7:41, 1985.
1122. Steere AC, Malawista SE: Cases of Lyme disease in the United States: locations correlated with distribution of *Ixodes dammini, Ann Intern Med* 91:730, 1979.
1123. Lastavica CC, Wilson ML, Berardi VP et al: Rapid emergence of a focal epidemic of Lyme disease in coastal Massachusetts, *N Engl J Med* 320:133, 1989.
1124. Barbour AG: Isolation and cultivation of Lyme disease spirochetes, *Yale J Biol Med* 57:521, 1984.
1125. Steere AC, Grodzicki RL, Craft JE et al: Recovery of Lyme disease spirochetes from patients, *Yale J Biol Med* 57:557, 1984.
1126. Kaeli AT, Volkman DJ, Gorevic PD et al: Positive Lyme serology in subacute bacterial endocarditis: a study of four patients, *JAMA* 264:2916, 1990.
1127. Steere AC, Taylor E, McHugh GL, Logigian EL: The overdiagnosis of Lyme disease, *JAMA* 269:1812, 1993.
1128. Duray PH, Ryan J: Demonstration of the Lyme disease spirochete by a modified Dieterle stain method, *Lab Med* 16:685, 1985.
1129. Dattwyler RJ, Volkman DJ, Luft BJ et al: Seronegative Lyme disease: dissociation of specific T- and B-lymphocyte responses to *Borrelia burgdorferi, N Engl J Med* 319:1441, 1988.
1130. Wilske B, Preac Mursic V, Schierz G et al: Antigenic variability of *Borrelia burgdorferi, Ann NY Acad Sci* 539:126, 1988.
1131. Craft JE, Fischer DK, Shimamoto GT, Steere AC: Antigens of *Borrelia burgdorferi* recognized during Lyme disease: appearance of a new immunoglobulin M response and expansion of the immunoglobulin G response late in the illness, *J Clin Invest* 78:934, 1986.
1132. Beck G, Habicht GS, Benach JL, Coleman JL: Chemical and biologic characterization of a lipopolysaccharide extracted from the Lyme disease spirochete *(Borrelia burgdorferi), J Infect Dis* 152:108, 1985.
1133. Benach JL, Fleit HB, Habicht GS et al: Interactions of phagocytes with the Lyme disease spirochete: role of the Fc receptor, *J Infect Dis* 150:497, 1984.
1134. Peterson PK, Clawson CC, Lee DA et al: Human phagocyte interactions with the Lyme disease spirochete, *Infect Immun* 46:608, 1984.
1135. Habicht GS, Beck G, Benach JL et al: Lyme disease spirochetes induce human and murine interleukin 1 production, *J Immunol* 134:3147, 1985.
1136. Stechenberg BW: Lyme disease: the latest great imitator, *Pediatr Infect Dis J* 7:402, 1988.
1137. Asbrink E, Hovmark A: Early and late cutaneous manifestations in *Ixodes*-borne borreliosis (erythema migrans borreliosis, Lyme borreliosis), *Ann NY Acad Sci* 539:4, 1988.
1138. Duray PH: The surgical pathology of human Lyme disease: an enlarging picture, *Am J Surg Pathol* 11(suppl 1):47, 1987.
1139. Berger BW: Erythema chronicum migrans of Lyme disease, *Arch Dermatol* 120:1017, 1984.
1140. Feder HM Jr, Gerber MA, Krause PJ et al: Early Lyme disease: a flu-like illness without erythema migrans, *Pediatrics* 91:456, 1993.
1141. Steere AC, Bartenhagen NH, Craft JE et al: The early clinical manifestations of Lyme disease, *Ann Intern Med* 99:76, 1983.
1142. Moore JA: Jarisch-Herxheimer reaction in Lyme disease, *Cutis* 39:397, 1987.
1143. Pachner AR, Steere AC: The triad of neurologic manifestations of Lyme disease: meningitis, cranial neuritis, and radiculoneuritis, *Neurology* 35:47, 1985.
1144. Atlas E, Novak SN, Duray PH, Steere AC: Lyme myositis: muscle invasion by *Borrelia burgdorferi, Ann Intern Med* 109:245, 1988.
1145. Schmutzhard E, Willeit J, Gerstenbrand F: Meningopolyneuritis Bannwarth with focal nodular myositis. A new aspect in Lyme borreliosis, *Klin Wochenschr* 64:1204, 1986.
1146. Steere AC, Duray PH, Kauffmann DJ, Wormser GP: Unilateral blindness caused by infection with the Lyme disease spirochete, *Borrelia burgdorferi, Ann Intern Med* 103:382, 1985.
1147. Reznick JW, Braunstein DB, Walsh RL et al: Lyme carditis: electrophysiologic and histopathologic study, *Am J Med* 81:923, 1986.
1148. Szer IS, Taylor E, Steere AC: The long-term course of Lyme arthritis in children, *N Engl J Med* 325:159, 1991.
1149. Steere AC, Duray PH, Butcher EC: Spirochetal antigens and lymphoid cell surface markers in Lyme synovitis: comparison with rheumatoid synovium and tonsillar lymphoid tissue, *Arthritis Rheum* 31:487, 1988.
1150. Johnston YE, Duray PH, Steere AC et al: Lyme arthritis: spirochetes found in synovial microangiopathic lesions, *Am J Pathol* 118:26, 1985.
1151. Ackerman R, Rehse-Kupper B, Golmer E, Schmidt R: Chronic neurologic manifestations of erythema migrans borelliosis, *Ann NY Acad Sci* 539:16, 1988.
1152. Sigal LH, Steere AC, Dwyer JM: In vivo and in vitro evidence of B cell hyperactivity during Lyme disease, *J Rheumatol* 15:648, 1988.
1153. Martin R, Ortlauf J, Sticht Groh V, Mertens HG: Isolation and characterization of *Borrelia burgdorferi*–specific and autoreactive T-cell lines from

the cerebrospinal fluid of patients with Lyme meningoradiculomyelitis, *Ann NY Acad Sci* 540:449, 1988.

1154. Wilske B, Schierz G, Preac Mursic V et al: Intrathecal production of specific antibodies against *Borrelia burgdorferi* in patients with lymphocytic meningoradiculitis (Bannwarth's syndrome), *J Infect Dis* 153:304, 1986.

1155. Moffat CM, Sigal LH, Steere AC et al: Cellular immune findings in Lyme disease: correlation with serum IgM and disease activity, *Am J Med* 77:625, 1984.

1156. Hardin JA, Steere AC, Malawista SE: The pathogenesis of arthritis in Lyme disease: humoral immune responses and the role of intra-articular immune complexes, *Yale J Biol Med* 57:589, 1984.

1157. Sigal LH, Tatum AH: Lyme disease patients' serum contains IgM antibodies to *Borrelia burgdorferi* that cross-react with neuronal antigens, *Neurology* 38:1439, 1988.

1158. Defosse DL, Duray PH, Johnson RC: The NIH-3 immunodeficient mouse is a model for Lyme borreliosis myositis and carditis, *Am J Pathol* 141:3, 1992.

1159. Schaible UE, Gay S, Museteanu C et al: Lyme borreliosis in the severe combined immunodeficiency (scid) mouse manifests predominantly in the joints, heart, and liver, *Am J Pathol* 137:811, 1990.

1160. Comstock LE, Fikrig E, Shoberg RJ et al: A monoclonal antibody to OspA inhibits association of *Borrelia burgdorferi* with human endothelial cells, *Infect Immun* 61:423, 1993.

1161. Fikrig E, Barthold SW, Kantor FS, Flavell RA: Protection of mice against the Lyme disease agent by immunizing with recombinant OspA, *Science* 250:553, 1990.

Miscellaneous bacteria

1162. Zumla A, Lipscomb G, Corbett M, McCarthy M: Dysgonic fermenter—type 2: an emerging zoonosis: report of two cases and review, *Q J Med* 68:741, 1988.

1163. Bobo RA, Newton EJ: A previously undescribed gram-negative bacillus causing septicemia and meningitis, *Am J Clin Pathol* 65:564, 1976.

1164. Kicklin H, Verghese A, Alvarez S: Dysgonic fermenter 2 septicemia, *Rev Infect Dis* 9:884, 1987.

1165. Applebaum PC, Ballard JO, Eyster ME: Septicemia due to *Capnocytophaga (Bacteroides ochracens)* in Hodgkin's disease, *Ann Intern Med* 90:716, 1979.

1166. Parenti DM, Snydman DR: *Capnocytophaga* species: infections in nonimmunocompromised and immunocompromised hosts, *J Infect Dis* 151:140, 1985.

1167. Buu-Hoi AY, Joundy S, Acar JF: Endocarditis caused by *Capnocytophaga ochracea*, *J Clin Microbiol* 26:1061, 1988.

1168. Shurin SB, Socransky SS, Sweeney E, Stossel TP: A neutrophil disorder induced by *Capnocytophaga*, a dental microorganism, *N Engl J Med* 301:849, 1979.

1169. Stevens RH, Sela MN, Shapira J, Hammond BF: Detection of a fibroblast proliferation inhibitory factor from *Capnocytophaga sputigena*, *Infect Immun* 27:271, 1980.

1170. Kuberski T, Papadimitriou JM, Phillips P: Ultrastructure of *Calymmatobacterium granulomatis* in lesions of granuloma inguinale, *J Infect Dis* 142:744, 1980.

1171. de Boer AL, de Boer F, Van der Merwe JV: Cytologic identification of Donovan bodies in granuloma inguinale, *Acta Cytol* 28:126, 1984.

1172. Rosen T, Tschen JA, Ramsdell W, et al: Granuloma inguinale, *J Am Acad Dermatol* 11:433, 1984.

1173. Sehgal VN, Shyamprasad AL, Beohar PC: The histopathological diagnosis of donovanosis, *Br J Vener Dis* 60:45, 1984.

1174. Mitchell KM, Roberts AN, Williams VM, Schneider J: Donovanosis in western Australia, *Genitourin Med* 62:191, 1986.

1175. Leung YC, McCartney AJ: Unusual gynaecological presentations of donovanosis as pseudo-elephantiasis and carcinoma of the cervix, *Aust NZJ Obstet Gynaecol* 30:172, 1990.

1176. Fritz GS, Hubler WR Jr, Dodson RF, Rudolph A: Multilating granuloma inguinale, *Arch Dermatol* 111:1464, 1975.

1177. Scrimgeour EM, Sengupta SK, McGoldrick IA: Primary endometrial and endocervical granuloma inguinale (donovanosis): case report, *Br J Vener Dis* 59:198, 1983.

1178. Verdich J: *Haemophilus ducreyi* infection resembling granuloma inguinale, *Acta Derm Venereol* (Stockh) 64:452, 1984.

1179. Barnes R, Masood S, Lammert N, Young RH: Extragenital granuloma inguinale mimicking a soft-tissue neoplasm: a case report and review of the literature, *Hum Pathol* 21:559, 1990.

1180. Jofre ME, Webling DD, James ST: Granuloma inguinale simulating advanced pelvic cancer, *Med J Aust* 2:869, 1976.

1181. Brigden M, Guard R: Extragenital granuloma inguinale in North Queensland, *Med J Aust* 2:565, 1980.

1182. Rajam RV, Rangiah PN, Anguli VC: Disseminated donovaniosis, *Br J Vener Dis* 30:73, 1954.

1183. Cohen H: Rat-bite fever: contributions to its history and war significance, *Bull Hist Med* 16:108, 1944.

1184. Dick GF, Tunnecliff R: A streptothrix isolated from the blood of a patient bitten by a weasel *(Streptothrix pertorii)*, *J Infect Dis* 23:183, 1918.

1185. Ripley HS, van Sant HM: Rat-bite fever acquired from a dog, *JAMA* 102:1917, 1934.

1186. Parker F Jr, Hudson NP: The etiology of Haverhill fever (erythema arthriticum epidemicum), *Am J Pathol* 2:357, 1926.

1187. Allbretten FF, Sheely RF, Jeffers WA: Haverhillan multiformis septicemia: its etiologic and clinical relationship to Haverhill and rat-bite fevers, *JAMA* 114:2360, 1940.

1188. McEvoy MB, Noah ND, Pitsworth R: Outbreak of fever caused by *Streptobacillus moniliformis*, *Lancet* 2:1361, 1967.

1189. Raffin BJ, Freemark M: Streptobacillary rat-bite fever: a pediatric problem, *Pediatrics* 64:214, 1979.

1190. Oeding P, Alarson H: *Streptothrix muris–ratti (Streptobacillus moniliformis)* isolated from a brain abscess, *Acta Pathol Microbiol Scand* 27:436, 1950.

Uncultured bacteria

1191. Dobbins WO III: Whipple's disease. In Mandell GL, Douglas RG Jr, Bennett JE, editors: *Principles and practice of infectious diseases*, ed 3, New York, 1990, Churchill Livingstone.

1192. Volpicelli NA, Salyer WR, Milligan FD et al: The endoscopic appearance of the duodenum in Whipple's disease, *Johns Hopkins Med J* 138:19, 1976.

1193. Geboes K, Ectors N, Heidbuchel H et al: Whipple's disease: endoscopic aspects before and after therapy, *Gastrointest Endosc* 36:247, 1990.

1194. Denholm RB, Mills PR, More IA: Electron microscopy in the long-term follow-up of Whipple's disease: effect of antibiotics, *Am J Surg Pathol* 5:507, 1981.

1195. Silva MT, Macedo PM, Moura Nunes JF: Ultrastructure of bacilli and the bacillary origin of the macrophagic inclusions in Whipple's disease, *J Gen Microbiol* 131:1001, 1985.

1196. Maliha GM, Hepps KS, Maia DM et al: Whipple's disease can mimic chronic AIDS enteropathy, *Am J Gastroenterol* 86:79, 1991.

1197. Babaryka I, Thorn L, Langer E: Epithelioid cell granulomata in the mucosa of the small intestine in Whipple's disease, *Virchows Arch [A] Pathol Anat Histol* 382:227, 1979.

1198. Wilcox GM, Tronic BS, Schecter DJ et al: Periodic acid–Schiff–negative granulomatous lymphadenopathy in patients with Whipple's disease: localization of the Whipple bacillus to noncaseating granulomas by electron microscopy, *Am J Med* 83:165, 1987.

1199. Rubinow A, Canoso JJ, Goldenberg DL et al: Arthritis in Whipple's disease, *Isr J Med Sci* 17:445, 1981.

1200. Lie JT, Davis JS: Pancarditis in Whipple's disease: electronmicroscopic demonstration of intracardiac bacillary bodies, *Am J Clin Pathol* 66:22, 1976.

34 Mycobacterial Diseases

Gail L. Woods
Wayne M. Meyers

Paleopathologic findings provide presumptive evidence for the extreme antiquity of mycobacterial infections in humans.[1,2] Bartels[3] described, for example, collapse of the fourth and fifth vertebrae and fusion with the sixth vertebra in a Neolithic skeleton (*ca.* tenth millennium B.C.) found near Heidelberg, Germany, and Ruffer[4] noted Pott's disease associated with a psoas abscess in the remains of an Egyptian priest of Ammon of the twenty-first dynasty (*ca.* 1100 B.C.). The origin of tuberculosis in humans is unknown; however, Morse et al.[5] suggest that the domestication of animals that began in the Neolithic Period promoted transmission of a "mutant variety" of the tubercle bacillus from livestock to humans.

Hippocrates (fifth century B.C.) recognized lesions of tuberculosis and called them "phthisis," or a 'wasting away.' Sylvius in the seventeenth century applied the name "tubercle" to nodules of tuberculosis, and Laënnec in the early nineteenth century proposed a common, albeit obscure, genesis of the various forms of the disease. Schönlein, in 1839, was perhaps the first to employ the word "tuberculosis" (see Grange[6]). Around 1868, Villemin, a French military physician, established the communicability and specificity of tuberculosis by inducing tuberculosis in rabbits through experimental inoculation of tissue from patients.

In 1873, Hansen identified the leprosy bacillus—not only the first mycobacterium, but indeed the first described etiologic agent of a chronic disease.[7] This seminal discovery in the annals of microbiology antedated by 9 years Koch's recovery of the tubercle bacillus in culture from humans. By priority of cultivation, the tubercle bacillus became the so-called typical mycobacterium.

Mycobacteria are slowly growing, aerobic, non–spore forming bacilli. The high lipid content in their cell wall confers upon them the distinctive property of acid-fastness. *Mycobacterium tuberculosis, Mycobacterium bovis,* and *Mycobacterium africanum* are the human pathogens that are included in the *Mycobacterium tuberculosis* complex (MTBC). These organisms, the "tubercle bacilli," are the etiologic agents of human tuberculosis. Mycobacteria other than the MTBC have been called "atypical" because they differ from the tubercle bacilli. The terms *nontuberculous mycobacteria* and *mycobacteria other than tubercle bacilli (MOTT)*, however, are preferred because these organisms are not atypical but simply have characteristics distinct from those of *M. tuberculosis*.

One of the earliest classifications of the nontuberculous mycobacteria was proposed by Runyon, who recognized four groups[8] (Table 34-1). However, limitations to this classification system exist. For example, *Mycobacterium kansasii* most often is a photochromogen but may be a nonphotochromogen or a scotochromogen. Members of the *Mycobacterium avium–intracellulare* complex are classified in Runyon's group III, but isolates may be slightly pigmented, potentially causing incorrect classification as a scotochromogen. *Mycobacterium szulgai* is a scotochromogen at 37° C and a photochromogen at 25° C. A clinically relevant classification of the nontuberculous mycobacteria based on their pathogenicity in humans is used here: potential pathogens and rarely pathogenic mycobacteria.[9]

Table 34-1 Runyon's classification of the nontuberculous mycobacteria

	Group	Description of colonies
I	Photochromogens	Pigmented only when exposed to light
II	Scotochromogens	Pigmented in light and in dark
III	Nonphotochromogens	Not pigmented in light or in dark
IV	Rapid growers	Grow in 7 days or less

LABORATORY DIAGNOSTIC TECHNIQUES

Skin testing

The tuberculin skin test is useful for identifying persons infected with MTBC, but it does not differentiate active disease from infection. Persons infected with MTBC develop a hypersensitivity reaction to proteins of the bacilli, which are the major constituents of the skin test reagent—PPD (purified protein derivative). The preferred method of skin testing is the Mantoux test, performed by intracutaneous injection of 0.1 ml of intermediate strength (5 tuberculin units [TU]) PPD-S. For children, first strength (1 TU) PPD-S should be used. The reaction is interpreted after 48 to 72 hours by measurement of the diameter of induration in millimeters.[10] Induration of 5 mm or more is a positive result in persons infected with human immunodeficiency virus (HIV), those who have had recent close contact with someone who has infectious tuberculosis, and those who have chest x-ray findings consistent with old healed tuberculosis. A reaction of 10 mm or more is positive in persons who do not meet the above criteria but who have other risk factors for tuberculosis. Included in this group are persons born in Asia, Africa, or Latin America where the prevalence of tuberculosis is high; intravenous drug users; medically underserved, low-income populations, especially racial or ethnic minorities; residents of long-term care facilities; and persons who have a medical condition associated with an increased risk of tuberculosis (such as silicosis, gastrectomy, jejunoileal bypass, 10% or more below ideal body weight, chronic renal failure, diabetes mellitus, treatment with high-dose corticosteroids or with other immunosuppressive drugs, and malignancies). A reaction of 15 mm or more is positive in all other persons.

False-positive PPD reactions result from infection with nontuberculous mycobacteria. False-negative reactions may be attributable to poor technique, such as injecting into the deep layers of the skin, or improper storage of the reagent. If the test is administered appropriately, false-negative reactions are uncommon in relatively healthy people but occur in up to 20% of individuals with known tuberculosis when they are first tested. Most of these false-negative reactions are attributed to the general illness and revert to positive after 2 to 3 weeks of therapy when health is restored. Factors causing a state of general anergy, such as protein malnutrition, concurrent viral infection, sarcoidosis, malignancy (especially lymphoma), immunosuppressive or corticosteroid therapy, and infection with HIV, also may cause a false-negative tuberculin reaction. To determine whether an individual is anergic, skin testing with mumps and candidal antigens should be performed simultaneously with the Mantoux test.

The Mantoux test generally remains positive as long as viable bacilli persist in quiescent foci. However, the reaction may wane below positive with increasing age, a phenomenon that occurs most frequently in those over 55 years of age. In these individuals the reaction will be boosted (or become positive) if retesting is performed as early as 1 week after the first test, a reaction termed the *booster effect*.

Skin test reagents prepared from nontuberculous mycobacteria include PPD-A *(Mycobacterium avium)*, PPD-B *(Mycobacterium intracellulare)*, PPD-F *(Mycobacterium fortuitum)*, PPD-G *(Mycobacterium scrofulaceum)*, and PPD-Y *(Mycobacterium kansasii)*. In the United States, these reagents once were available from the Centers for Disease Control and Prevention (CDC); however this service was discontinued because the antigens were not standardized and the skin reactions were difficult to interpret.

There is no diagnostic skin test for leprosy. Individual defense against *Mycobacterium leprae* is assessed by the size of induration (lepromin reaction) at the site of an intradermal injection of a standardized dose of a suspension of killed whole *M. leprae* (lepromin). These suspensions formerly employed tissue from lepromatous patients but now usually utilize tissue from experimentally infected nine-banded armadillos.[11] Lepromin reactions are biphasic: early responses are read at 48 hours ("Fernandez reaction"), and late responses at 3 to 4 weeks ("Mitsuda reaction").[12] These reactions are not diagnostic because 90% to 95% of most adult populations are positive, even those from areas nonendemic for leprosy.[13] Lepromin responses, especially the Mitsuda reaction, aid in classification of disease and hence are useful for prognosis.[14]

Skin tests for *Mycobacterium ulcerans* infections, employing a "New Tuberculin" preparation called *burulin*, have not proved useful for diagnosis of Buruli ulcer. During the active phase of ulceration burulin tests are usually negative but become positive in the healing granulomatous phase.[15]

Microbial stains

In smears stained with the Gram stain, most mycobacteria appear as slender, poorly stained, beaded gram-positive bacilli, but sometimes the bacilli do not take up the crystal violet or safranin and appear "gram neutral" or as "gram ghosts" (Fig. 34-1). Similar ghost images of bacilli are found in macrophages in Diff-Quik-stained cytologic materials (Fig. 34-2). All specimens collected from persons with suspected mycobacterial infection should be examined microscopically for acid-fast bacilli (AFB)—purple to red, slightly curved, short or long rods (2 to 8 μm), occasionally beaded or banded (Fig. 34-3, *A*). In general, the appearance of an acid-fast bacillus does not provide a species identification; however, cells of certain species have features that may be useful diagnostically. For example, cells of *M. kansasii* often appear as cross-barred bacilli (Fig. 34-3, *B*), larger than *M. tuberculosis*. Cells of *M. avium–intracellulare* complex typically are pleomorphic, occasionally coccobacillary, and stain positively with the periodic acid–Schiff (PAS) stain, a unique feature among mycobacteria. Cells of *Mycobacterium marinum* typically are longer and broader than those of *M. tuberculosis* and often show cross-banding.

Two types of stains are used for detection of AFB: carbol fuchsin stains (the classic Ziehl-Neelsen stain, which requires heating, and the cold Kinyoun's stain) and the fluorochromic auramine-rhodamine and rhodamine stains. Smears stained

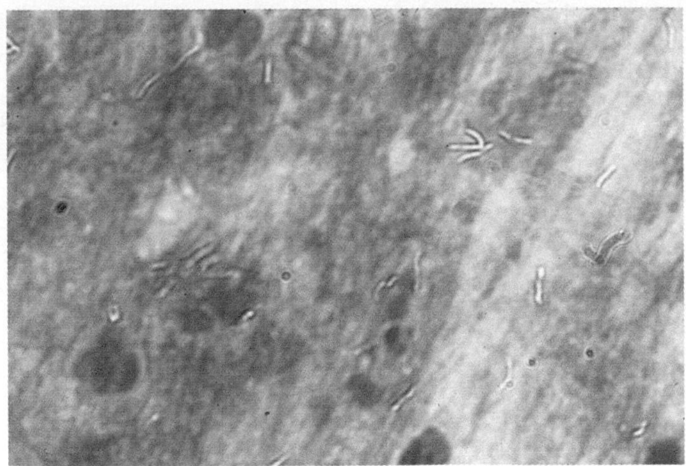

Fig. 34-1 Sputum specimen stained with the Gram stain shows nonstaining bacilli, or "Gram ghosts." A Kinyoun stain of this specimen was positive for acid-fast bacilli, and culture grew *Mycobacterium tuberculosis*.

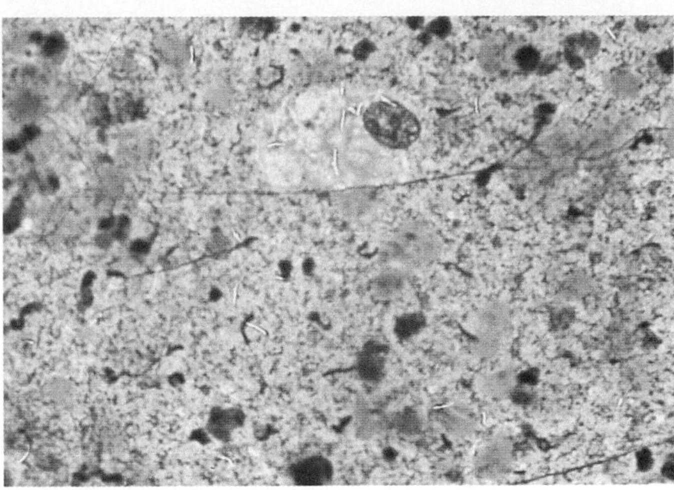

Fig. 34-2 Smear of a sputum specimen stained with Diff-Quik. Numerous acid-fast bacilli are evident as negative images within a macrophage.

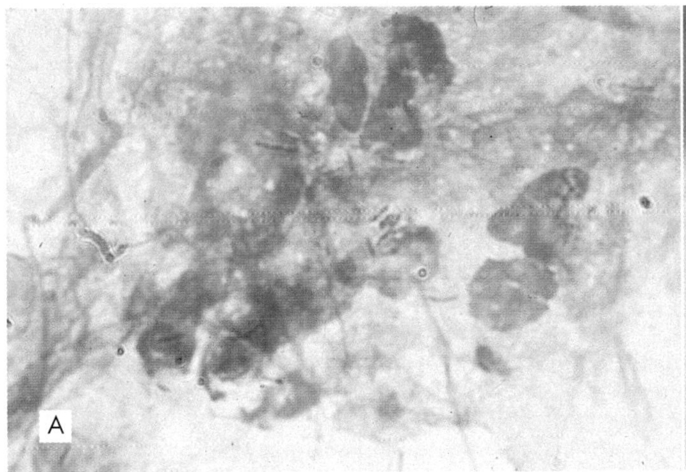

Fig. 34-3a Colonies of *Mycobacterium tuberculosis* on Löwenstein-Jensen medium. (Courtesy Cathy Looby, M.D., Medical College of Pennsylvania, Philadelphia. From Woods GL, Gutierrez Y: *Diagnostic pathology of infectious diseases,* Philadelphia, 1993, Lea & Febiger.)

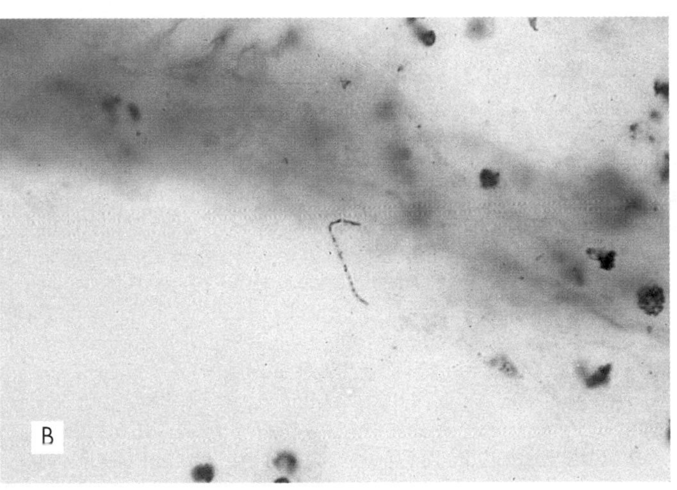

Fig. 34-3b Smear of an aspirate from a cervical lymph node stained with Kinyoun stain shows large, cross-barred acid-fast bacilli. Culture grew *Mycobacterium kansasii.* (Courtesy Vicki Schnadig, M.D., University of Texas Medical Branch at Galveston, Galveston, Tex.)

with a carbol fuchsin stain should be examined at 800× to 1000× (under oil immersion) and reported after viewing 100 fields, indicating whether the smear was prepared directly from the specimen or after concentration. Smears stained with a fluorochrome stain are examined at lower magnifications (250× and 400×), allowing visualization of more fields in less time. Cells of the *Mycobacterium fortuitum–-chelonae* complex, however, stain poorly with fluorochromic stains and may not be detected; therefore, when the latter organisms are suspected pathogens (as in postsurgical wound infections), restaining negative fluorescent smears with a carbol fuchsin stain is recommended.

The specificity of the acid-fast stain typically is 99% or more. False-positive results (positive stain, negative culture) may be caused by nonviable organisms; prolonged decontamination, killing mycobacteria as well as contaminating bacteria; or cross-contamination during the staining procedure. Sensitivity ranges from about 25% to about 75%.[16-18] Factors influencing results include (1) patient population (persons with cavitary lesions on chest x-ray film are more likely than those without cavities to have a smear-positive sputum), (2) specimen type (respiratory specimens are more likely than other types of specimens to be positive), (3) the number of specimens examined (the likelihood of a positive result increases with the number of specimens examined), (4) number of AFB in the sample (about 10^4 organisms per milliliter of specimen are needed for a positive result), (5) the species present (*M. tuberculosis* is more likely to be positive than the nontuberculous mycobacteria are), (6) observer experience, and (7) stain used. Fluorochromic stains are more sensitive and easier to read than carbol fuchsin stains and are recommended by the CDC.[19,20] To address the increasing incidence of tuberculosis in the United States, the CDC also recommends that results of stained smears be reported within 24 hours of specimen receipt, a requirement that means daily processing of contaminated specimens such as sputum.

The acid-fastness of *M. leprae,* though weaker than for most mycobacteria, is related, as in other mycobacteria, to mycolic acids in the cell wall.[21] In skin smears, the Ziehl-Neelsen technique stains *M. leprae* adequately, but in tissue sections, only the Fite-Faraco method demonstrates *M. leprae* optimally.[22] Viable organisms stain solidly, but degenerating bacilli first stain irregularly, then become granular, and eventually lose acid-fastness completely. The Gomori methenamine-silver method reveals non–acid fast carcasses of *M. leprae.*[23] Fluorochromic procedures stain *M. leprae;* however, they seldom offer significant advantages over classic methods and are not useful for morphologic evaluations.

Culture techniques

Several commercial systems based on solid or broth media are available or in the development or evaluation stages. For conventional mycobacterial culture two types of media are available: egg-based such as Lowenstein-Jensen and agar-based such as Middlebrook 7H10 and 7H11. If conventional culture is the only method used to recover mycobacteria, inoculation of at least one of each type of medium is recommended. For specimens such as sputum that are contaminated with normal bacterial flora, a selective medium containing antimicrobial agents also should be inoculated. Sterile body fluids (cerebrospinal fluid, joint fluid, pleural fluid, and peritoneal fluid) should be inoculated to solid media and a broth medium for enrichment. Specimens from cutaneous lesions should be inoculated to one egg-based and one agar-based medium, and to assure recovery of *Mycobacterium haemophilum* (discussed later) they also should be plated on chocolate agar, 5% sheep blood Columbia agar, Mueller-Hinton agar with Fildes supplement, or Lowenstein-Jensen containing 2% ferric ammonium citrate. All cultures should be incubated 8 weeks in 5% to 10% CO_2 at 35° to 37° C, and for specimens from cutaneous sites a second set of cultures should be incubated at 30° C because some mycobacteria that cause skin lesions—*M. marinum* and *M. haemophilum*—grow optimally at the lower temperature.

The major advantage of conventional culture is that colony morphology and pigmentation may be useful diagnostically, especially for distinguishing colonies of *M. tuberculosis* from those of some of the nontuberculous mycobacteria. The colony appearance and growth characteristics of the commonly encountered mycobacteria are outlined in Table 34-2. The primary disadvantage of conventional culture is the long incubation period; colonies often are not visible on tubed solid media for 3 to 4 weeks or more. Inoculation of agar plates, which then are examined under the microscope, allows more rapid detection of colonies, but this procedure is labor intensive, thus prohibiting its use in many clinical laboratories.[24]

A commercial radiometric system utilizes broth media (one for blood and another for all other specimen types) that contain ^{14}C-labeled palmitic acid substrate. Each specimen is inoculated into a separate vial, and bottles are incubated in ambient air at 37° C for at least 6 weeks. To ensure recovery of *Mycobacterium genavense,* blood cultures (especially those collected from patients with the acquired immunodeficiency syndrome [AIDS]) should be incubated 8 to 10 weeks. Bacilli multiply in the broth and utilize the labeled substrate, releasing $^{14}CO_2$ into the head space above the broth. The amount of $^{14}CO_2$ is measured by an instrument, and a growth index is calculated. A growth index greater than 10 indicates that mycobacteria may be present, and when the growth index reaches 50 to 100, a smear of the broth should be stained with an acid-fast stain. Vials containing AFB should be subcultured to a solid medium, and direct tests for identification (discussed in the following section) may be performed. For positive mycobacterial blood cultures from patients with AIDS, measures allowing recovery of *M. genavense* (subculture to Middlebrook 7H11 containing 2 mg/ml of mycobactin J) should be taken if initial subcultures from the broth show no growth, or the positive broth should be sent to a reference laboratory prepared to do the appropriate tests.

Advantages of radiometric detection are: (1) rapid detection of mycobacterial growth (time to detection is decreased to an average of 5 to 12 days), (2) detection of more positive cultures, (3) the ability to distinguish MTBC from other mycobacterial species (discussed below under the subject of tests for identification), and (4) rapid susceptibility testing of isolates of *M. tuberculosis* (described under the subject of susceptibility testing.[25-28] For optimal detection of mycobacteria in specimens other than blood, inoculation of one radiometric vial and one solid medium is recommended.[27] Brath systems, which are an alternative to radiometric detection have a similar rate of recovery of mycobacteria.[29,30]

Given the resurgence of tuberculosis in the United States, current recommendations favor both a broth system and a solid medium for culture of mycobacteria, such that mycobacterial growth will be detected within 14 days of specimen receipt.[19,20,31]

All reports of successful in vitro cultivation of *M. leprae* remain unconfirmed.[32] In the absence of in vitro cultivation,

Table 34-2 Colony morphology and growth characteristics of the mycobacteria commonly encountered in the clinical laboratory

Species	Colony morphology	Pigment	Growth rate*
M. tuberculosis	Rough	N (buff)	Slow
MAC	Smooth (rarely rough); transparent or opaque	N; lightly pigmented	Slow; up to 8 weeks
M. kansasii	Rough; beta-carotene crystals	P (rarely N or S)	Slow
M. fortuitum–chelonae	Smooth or rough	N (buff)	Rapid
M. gordonae	Smooth	S; orange	Slow

MAC, M. avium–intracellulare complex; *N,* nonphotochromogen; *S,* scotochromogen; *P,* photochromogen.
*Average growth rate on solid medium (does not apply to growth in liquid media): slow, 4 to 6 weeks; rapid, 5 to 7 days.

identification of *M. leprae* depends on the following alternate criteria: (1) failure to grow on currently available mycobacteriologic media; (2) infection of normal mouse footpads in a characteristic growth pattern;[33] (3) destruction of acid-fastness by exposure to pyridine;[34] (4) invasion of nerves in vivo; (5) production of a characteristic pattern of clinical responses to suspensions of killed bacilli when inoculated into the skin of patients (the lepromin reaction) with the various forms of leprosy; (6) production of a species-specific antigen, phenolic glycolipid-I,[35] and (7) specific DNA probes.[36,37]

M. ulcerans is strongly acid fast, stains well with Ziehl-Neelsen stains, and has an optimal growth temperature of 30° to 32° C on routine mycobacteriologic media. Primary isolation often requires incubation for 6 to 12 weeks or longer.

Tests for identification

Traditionally, identification of mycobacteria has been based on rate of growth on conventional media, colony morphology, pigmentation with and without exposure to light, and results of biochemical tests. Although most species will be identified in this way, results usually are not available for several weeks to months after colonies appear on solid media. More rapid methods of identification, to allow identification of MTBC within 21 days of specimen receipt, are recommended.[19,20]

The *para*-nitro-α-acetylamino-β-hydroxypropiophenone (NAP) test allows differentiation of members of the MTBC from nontuberculous mycobacteria within 4 to 5 days after AFB are detectable in a radiometric vial.[25] A volume of broth from the positive vial is injected into two fresh bottles of medium, one containing NAP. An increase in the growth index in the bottle without NAP and no increase in the growth index in the bottle containing NAP indicates that the isolate is a member of MTBC because only those species are susceptible to NAP.

Chemiluminescent DNA probes allow identification of a few species of mycobacteria within 1 to 2 hours after sufficient growth is present on a solid medium or in a vial.[32-35] Commercial probes specific for MTBC, *M. avium–intracellulare, M. avium, M. intracellulare, Mycobacterium gordonae,* and *M. kansasii* currently are available. The major advantage of these probes is rapid identification. Disadvantages include cost, the requirement for equipment (luminometer, sonicator, and heating block), failure to identify a small percentage (3% to 5%) of isolates of *M. avium–intracellulare,* rare false-positive results with the MTBC probe, and low sensitivity of the *M. kansasii* probe.[33,36]

Gas-liquid chromatography, high-performance liquid chromatography, and thin-layer chromatography allow identification of mycobacterial colonies on a solid medium in 2 to 4 hours. These techniques, which are technically complex and require expensive equipment, are performed predominantly in research and large reference laboratories.

Rarely, a mycobacterial isolate cannot be identified by any of the methods described above. An example is *M. genavense,* the identification of which has required sequence determinations of the hypervariable regions of the 16S ribosomal RNA gene.[37] This highly sophistocated test is performed only in specialized research or reference laboratories.

In the future, nucleic acid amplification methods, such as the polymerase chain reaction (PCR), may prove useful for detection of mycobacteria directly in clinical material. PCR has been evaluated in research laboratories for direct detection of MTBC and *M. avium–intracellulare* in clinical specimens, and commercial kits currently are being developed.[38,39] It is hoped that with these amplification techniques a result of positive or negative for the organism being sought will be available within 24 hours of specimen receipt.

Specific DNA probes with PCR technology seem promising for detection of *M. leprae* in tissue sections and skin or nasal smears. Prolonged formalin fixation degrades DNA of *M. leprae,* but fixation in 70% ethanol preserves DNA for PCR analysis. These methods seem capable of detecting a single *M. leprae* bacillus in suspension. Diagnosis of leprosy by PCR would seem inadvisable, especially in skin or nasal smears taken in an endemic area, as the risk of contamination of specimens by one or very few *M. leprae* of no clinical importance in such surroundings is potentially high.

Susceptibility testing

Currently, standardized guidelines for susceptibility testing of mycobacteria have been developed only for isolates of *M. tuberculosis*. Traditionally, the proportion method, a modified agar dilution test, has been used to evaluate susceptibility of isolates of *M. tuberculosis* to antituberculosis agents. With this method isolates showing greater than 1% resistance are considered resistant to that concentration of the drug. Results are available 21 days after plates are inoculated. The commercial radiometric system also may be used for susceptibility testing of MTBC and provides results 5 to 7 days after there is sufficient growth in a culture vial. Given the concern regarding multidrug resistant *M. tuberculosis,* systems that determine drug susceptibility within 28 days of specimen receipt are favored.[19,20]

Susceptibility testing may be performed on isolates of the nontuberculous mycobacteria; however, for some species, there may be no correlation between susceptibility test results and clinical response to drug therapy. Moreover, a standardized reference method has not been developed for testing these organisms. Methods that have been used are the proportion method, radiometric assays, and broth microdilution.[40,41] For isolates of *M. fortuitum–chelonae* complex disk diffusion and agar disk elution also have been evaluated.[42]

Lacking in vitro cultivation of *M. leprae,* growth in mouse footpads provides the only currently acceptable assay for viability and drug susceptibility of leprosy bacilli. A variety of other in vitro tests for determining *M. leprae* drug sensitivity are under development.[43-45]

MYCOBACTERIUM TUBERCULOSIS COMPLEX

Mycobacterium tuberculosis

Tuberculosis was a major problem in the seventeenth and eighteenth centuries, when it was responsible for about 25% of deaths in adults. In 1882, Koch discovered the tubercle bacillus and fulfilled his criteria ("Koch's postulates") for identification of the etiologic agent of an infectious disease: (1) The organism is found in the lesions of the disease regularly. (2) It can be isolated in pure culture on artificial media. (3) Inoculating the culture of the organism into animals produces a similar disease. (4) The organism can be recovered from lesions in the animals.

Currently, an estimated 8 to 10 million new cases of tuberculosis and 2 to 3 million deaths attributable to tuberculosis occur in the world each year, most caused by *M. tuberculosis.* In some parts of Africa, Asia, and Oceania and in persons immigrating to the United States from Asia during the first year after their arrival, the annual incidence may exceed 300 per 100,000 population.

In the United States the number of reported cases of tuberculosis steadily declined from about 84,300 in 1953, when national reporting of tuberculosis began, to 22,200 in 1985.[46] Almost 22,800 new cases of tuberculosis were reported to the CDC in 1986, the first year since 1953 that an increase in the number of cases occurred. From 1985 to 1991, the reported number of cases of tuberculosis increased by 18%; there were about 39,000 more cases than would have been expected had the decline continued.[47,48] In all age groups, the number of cases increased among blacks and Hispanics but decreased among whites, Asians/Pacific Islanders, and American Indians/Alaskan natives. Of the metropolitan areas, the steepest rise was reported in New York City. Factors contributing to the excess number of cases include the epidemic spread of HIV, a deterioration in the health-care infrastructure, and increases in the number of cases among the homeless, prisoners, migrant farm workers, immigrants, and elderly persons living in nursing homes.[49]

During the past few years, multidrug-resistant tuberculosis (MDR-TB), defined as disease caused by *M. tuberculosis* that is resistant to two or more primary antimycobacterial agents used in the United States to treat tuberculosis has become of increasing concern.[47,48] Several outbreaks of MDR-TB, involving over 200 cases, have occurred in hospitals and correctional facilities in New York State and Florida.[50-54] Most involved patients were infected with HIV, and many—72% to 89% in different outbreaks—died, often within 4 to 16 weeks after diagnosis. Moreover, occupational transmission of MDR-TB to health-care workers and others has been documented; some have developed active MDR-TB and a few have died.

M. tuberculosis is transmitted primarily by inhalation of dried residues of small infected droplets (1 to 10 μm in diameter). The most important source of infection is an undiagnosed person with cavitary (and sputum smear-positive) tuberculosis. The minimum infective dose for humans is unknown, but data indicate that infection may occur after inhaling one or two viable organisms.[55] Despite a high susceptibility to infection with *M. tuberculosis,* most infected individuals do not develop active disease. The risk of active pulmonary disease is low after a single exposure to the organism but increases under conditions of stress or in a confined environment where repeated exposures to the organism occur. *M. tuberculosis* also may be transmitted by direct inoculation of abraded skin, an event most likely to occur when pathologists or other laboratory personnel handle infected tissues.

The specific structures, antigens, and mechanisms responsible for the virulence of *M. tuberculosis* are unknown; however, two properties are associated with the ability of virulent strains to produce disease: cord factor and sulfatides. In vitro, cord factor is responsible for the morphologic appearance of *M. tuberculosis*—serpentine cords consisting of bacilli in close parallel arrangements. This growth pattern correlates with the presence in the bacillus of trehalose-6,6′-dimycolate, a glycolipid that when injected into mice inhibits neutrophil migration, elicits granuloma formation, and stimulates protection against virulent infection. Despite these activities in animals, the specific role of cord factor in the pathogenesis of human tuberculosis remains unknown. Sulfatides are peripherally located glycolipids that inhibit fusion of secondary lysosomes with bacilli-containing phagosomes within a macrophage, possibly promoting intracellular survival of the organism.

The usual host response to infection with *M. tuberculosis* is activation of the cell-mediated immune system. During primary (initial) infection, bacilli are inhaled, reach the alveolar spaces, and are ingested by resident macrophages. These macrophages cannot kill the mycobacteria, which multiply intracellularly during the first several days after infection. Infected macrophages migrate to regional tracheobronchial lymph nodes and present the sensitizing antigen or antigens to immunocompetent T-cells or enter the lymphatics and blood and travel back to the lungs (primarily the apices) and to distant organs (especially the lymph nodes, kidneys, epiphyseal areas of the long bones, vertebral bodies, and meninges), where bacilli continue to multiply until the cellular immune response is activated. Immunocompetent T-cells migrate from regional lymph nodes back to the site of infection in the lung and release chemotactic, migration-inhibitory, and mitogenic cytokines, resulting in recruitment of blood-derived monocytes and lymphocytes, in macrophage and lymphocyte division, and in macrophage activation. The activated macrophages have enhanced microbicidal activity and produce cytokines that stimulate or regulate other components of the immune system, properties that help limit the infection. However, the cytokines (interleukin-1, interferon-γ, and tumor necrosis factor) and lytic enzymes released by the macrophages also contribute to the concomitant local tissue destruction. With time, the activated T-cell population declines and is replaced by long-lived memory immune T-cells, which protect against reinfection with *M. tuberculosis* and provide some cross-protection against infection with other mycobacteria.

In approximately 90% of infected individuals, the initial infection becomes quiescent once the cellular immune system is activated and symptoms resolve. The lesion heals by fibrosis and eventually calcifies. In very young or immunocompromised hosts incapable of mounting the necessary immune response, the primary infection may disseminate, producing miliary disease, or progress and spread by contiguity or erosion into bronchi, resulting in cavity formation or large areas of consolidation (tuberculous pneumonia).

Despite the limitation of further mycobacterial multiplication in primary and metastatic foci by the activated macrophages and memory T-cells, a residual nidus of infection remains indefinitely in the lung (most frequently in the apex, where the oxygen tension is high) and less often in distant sites. Therefore, the potential exists for reactivation of disease in these quiescent foci during periods of immunosuppression. Most often foci of reactivation are localized and eventually heal by fibrosis. However, if the infection erodes into a bronchiole, the lesion transforms into a cavity, and miliary disease may occur if organisms enter the lymphatics and bloodstream, seeding distant organs. Localized extrapulmonary tuberculosis also is possible in distant sites such as the meninges, kidneys, adrenals, bones, fallopian tubes, and epididymis.

The primary focus of pulmonary infection (termed the *Gohn lesion*) most often is subjacent to the pleura in the lower part of the upper lobes or the upper part of the lower lobes of one lung, corresponding to areas of the lung receiving the greatest volume flow of inspired air. Lesions (tubercles) are well-circumscribed areas of grayish-white consolidation, 1 to 2 cm in diameter, with soft to necrotic centers (Fig. 34-4). Similar-appearing tubercles generally are found in the regional tracheobronchial lymph nodes, and these along with the primary lung lesion are termed the *Gohn complex*. Microscopically, tubercles are composed of well-circumscribed aggregates of histiocytes, lymphocytes, and epithelioid histiocytes with or without Langhans' giant cells, surrounded by proliferating fibroblasts (Fig. 34-5). Central caseation necrosis may or may not be present, and organisms may be seen in tissue sections stained with an acid-fast stain. With time these lesions are replaced by hyalinized fibrous tissue and eventually calcify. Cavitary lesions of variable size, most often located in the apices, commonly are traversed by thrombosed arteries. The lesions of miliary tuberculosis are small (one to several millimeters in diameter), distinct, yellow-white areas of consolidation without gross caseation that histologically resemble tubercles. The ability to form granulomas depends on the immunocompetence of the host. Individuals with AIDS, for example, may have extensive mycobacterial infection without well-formed granulomas. This is particularly true for *M. avium–intracellulare* infection.

In the United States pulmonary tuberculosis accounts for about 85% of cases of active disease. Manifestations of primary pulmonary disease vary in different age groups. Infants and young children most often are symptomatic, with fever, lassitude, and frequently cough. If the infection drains into a bronchus, pneumonia results. Many adults are asymptomatic, but some experience malaise, fatigue, and low-grade fever. Infrequently the infection progresses to pneumonia, occasionally with pleural involvement.

Chronic pulmonary tuberculosis in adults usually begins as a focus of pneumonitis in the subapical posterior aspect of an upper lobe. Symptoms include anorexia, weight loss, chilly sensations, afternoon remittent fever, night sweats, and cough productive of purulent sputum. Mild hemoptysis and chest pain (resulting from extension of the inflammatory process to the parietal pleura) may develop late in the disease.

Extrapulmonary tuberculosis may be localized but more commonly involves multiple organs with or without concurrent lung infection. Multiorgan tuberculosis, historically a disease of infants and young children, currently predominates among the elderly and immunocompromised individuals, especially those infected with both HIV and *M. tuberculosis*.[56-58] The clinical manifestations associated with extrapulmonary disease are summarized in Table 34-3.

Mycobacterium bovis

An association between tuberculous cervical adenitis (scrofula) in humans and drinking milk from diseased cows was recognized in 1846.[59] Robert Koch isolated the tubercle bacillus from human and bovine sources in 1882, a time when 20% to 40% of cattle in many European countries had tuberculosis.[60] *M. bovis* has one of the broadest host ranges of all known pathogens. The organism may be transmitted from cattle to humans by consumption of contaminated raw milk or by respiratory exposure to live infected cattle or their carcasses, from person to person by respiratory exposure, from humans to cattle by exposure to urine from persons with urinary tract infections caused by *M. bovis*, and from cattle to cattle probably by respiratory secretions. Moreover, *M. bovis* may be transmitted to cattle from wild animal reservoirs such

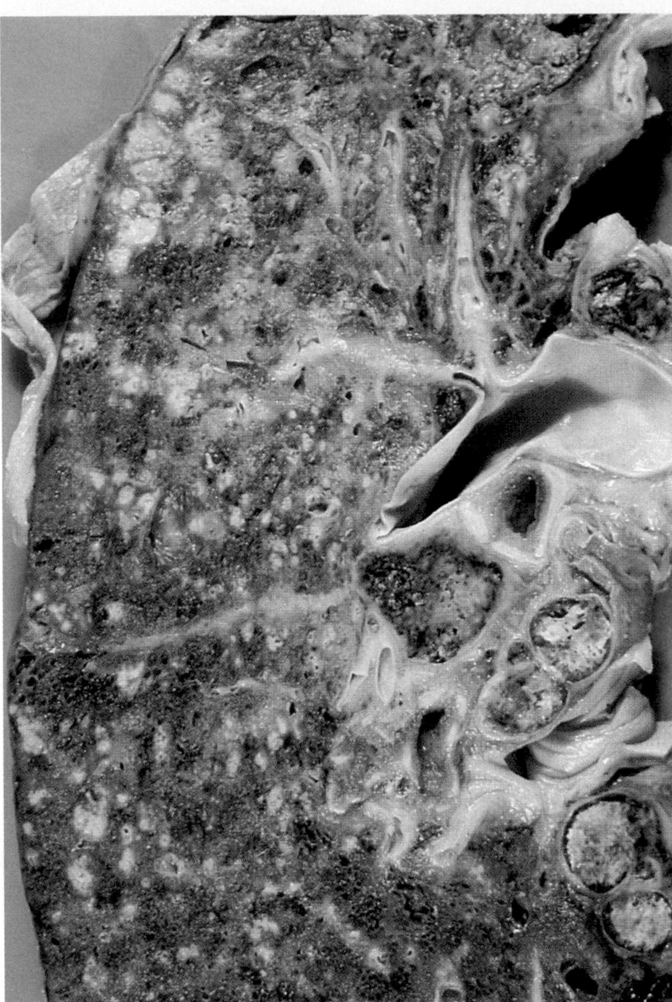

Fig. 34-4 Lung from a patient with pulmonary tuberculosis shows multiple tubercles. (Courtesy Cathy Looby, M.D., Medical College of Pennsylvania, Philadelphia. From Woods GL, Gutierrez Y: *Diagnostic pathology of infectious diseases*, Philadelphia, 1993, Lea & Febiger.)

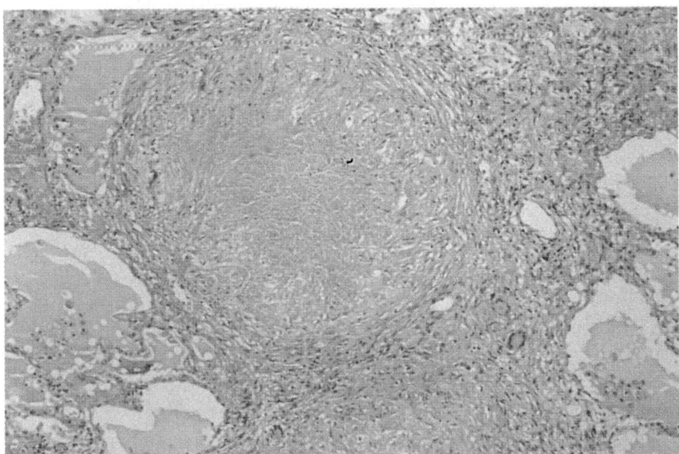

Fig. 34-5 Micrograph of lung tissue from a patient with tuberculosis shows granulomatous inflammation with caseous necrosis.

Table 34-3 Extrapulmonary manifestations of tuberculosis

Site	Clinical manifestations
Central nervous system	
Meninges	Acute or chronic meningitis (basal infiltrate)
Cerebral cortex	Tuberculoma—headache, seizures
Pericardium	Acute pericarditis (fever, chest pain); chronic pericarditis (cardiovascular compromise)
Skeletal	Osteomyelitis, arthritis
Genitourinary tract	
Renal	Dysuria, flank pain
Male genital	Tender scrotal mass, draining sinus
Female genital	Menstrual disorders, abdominal pain
Gastrointestinal tract	
Oral cavity	Nonhealing ulcer of tongue or oropharynx
Esophagus	Stricture, tracheoesophageal fistula
Stomach	Ulcer, diffuse thickening
Small intestine	Perforation, obstruction, enteroenteric or enterocutaneous fistula, hemorrhage, malabsorption
Large intestine	Abdominal pain, anorexia, diarrhea, obstruction, hemorrhage
Anus	Ulcer, fistula, abscess
Liver	Granulomatous hepatitis
Peritoneal cavity	Peritonitis (insidious or acute onset)
Lymph nodes	Lymphadenitis (draining cervical or supraclavicular nodes)
Skin	Ulcers, nodules, abscesses
Larynx	Erythema, ulcers, exophytic masses

as the bush-tailed possum in New Zealand and possibly the badger in Switzerland and Great Britain.[61]

Between 1900 and 1930, *M. bovis* was isolated from 6% to 30% of persons with tuberculosis in the United States and the United Kingdom.[61,62] Declining rates of human tuberculosis caused by *M. bovis* have been associated with milk pasteurization and with cattle-inspection programs.[61-63] Since 1950, *M. bovis* has accounted for fewer than 1% of cases of human tuberculosis in North America. Most infections are extrapulmonary (involving cervical and mesenteric lymph nodes, the intestines, bones, and kidneys), and some have been fatal.[64] Uncommonly infection follows intravesical instillation of bacille Calmette-Guérin (BCG) for treatment of superficial bladder carcinoma.[65]

Mycobacterium africanum

Mycobacterium africanum, the "African" tubercle bacillus, was first recovered from persons in West Africa in 1968.[66] Although *M. africanum* has been isolated primarily from individuals in Africa, the prevalence of infection with this organism worldwide is difficult to assess because it is not recognized in many laboratories or is misidentified as *M. bovis*. The modes of transmission, pathogenesis, and clinical manifestations of disease caused by *M. africanum* are the same as those associated with *M. tuberculosis*.

NONTUBERCULOUS MYCOBACTERIA

In general, very little is known about the antigens associated with the virulence of the nontuberculous mycobacteria; however, such antigens presumably are responsible for persistence of the organisms within the monocyte-macrophage system of the host. The immune response to infection with these mycobacteria also is poorly understood.

Mycobacterium avium–Mycobacterium intracellulare complex (MAC)

Mycobacterium avium and *M. intracellulare,* initially differentiated on the basis of their virulence in chickens and rabbits, have such similar growth characteristics and biochemical reactions that they often are not distinguished in the clinical microbiology laboratory; isolates of both species are reported as MAC. The MAC contains 28 serovars, identified by seroagglutination according to antigens located on the cell surface or thin-layer chromatography.

Overall, MAC is the second most frequently isolated set of mycobacteria in the United States, following *M. tuberculosis*. Since the epidemic of AIDS, the percentage of isolates of MAC has increased, equaling or even surpassing the number of isolates of *M. tuberculosis* in some parts of the country.

MAC bacilli are ubiquitous in the environment. They have been isolated from water, soil, food, house dust, and several animals, but the specific environmental sources responsible for human infection are not known.[67] The most likely portal of entry is the gastrointestinal tract, though entrance through the respiratory tract also is possible.[68] From sites of colonization, organisms enter the bloodstream and infect many organs, especially those of the monocyte-macrophage system.

Pulmonary disease caused by MAC previously occurred in elderly white men who had underlying chronic lung disease or who had undergone gastrectomy, but it has become more common in persons without predisposing factors, and in one study, disease among older individuals was more frequent in women than in men.[69] Disseminated MAC occurs almost exclusively in immunosuppressed individuals, and the numbers of such cases have increased considerably since the epidemic of AIDS. MAC is the most common cause of systemic bacterial infection in patients with AIDS in the United States. Disseminated MAC is diagnosed antemortem in 15% to 27% of persons infected with HIV and is found at autopsy in about 50%.[68,70] The degree of immune dysfunction, indicated by the $CD4^+$ lymphocyte count, is the major risk factor for disseminated MAC, which rarely occurs if the $CD4^+$ count is over 100/ml.

In the United States, serotypes 4 and 8 of *M. avium* are isolated primarily from blood and are recovered most commonly from persons with AIDS. In one study of isolates from persons with AIDS, serotype 4 predominated in New York City, all of the eastern states as a region, and San Francisco; serotype 8 predominated in Los Angeles; and serotypes 4 and 8 were almost evenly distributed in the western states as a region.[53] Serotypes of *M. intracellulare* accounted for a very small percentage of isolates of MAC from persons with AIDS and were recovered primarily from sputum and infrequently from blood, an indication that they rarely cause disseminated disease in these individuals.[71,72]

MAC bacilli generally have low virulence and often colonize an individual without causing disease. Risk factors for disease include preexisting pulmonary damage and cellular immune deficiency, such as occurs in AIDS or with steroid therapy.

The histologic findings of lesions caused by MAC vary: caseating granulomas with AFB, indistinguishable from tuberculosis; pulmonary interstitial fibrosis with organizing pneumonia; necrotizing granulomatous vasculitis resembling Wegener's granulomatosis; and, especially in persons with AIDS, aggregates of foamy macrophages (Fig. 34-6) containing many intracellular AFB which can be seen. In sections of gastrointestinal lesions stained with hematoxylin and eosin, such lesions mimic Whipple's disease.

Manifestations of disease caused by MAC vary depending on the site of infection. Pulmonary infection may be asymptomatic, or it may resemble tuberculosis. Disseminated disease in persons without AIDS is manifested by fever, weight loss, bone pain, lymphadenopathy, hepatosplenomegaly, and skin lesions. In those with AIDS, persistent fever, weight loss, and diarrhea are most common; anorexia, weakness, lymphadenopathy, or hepatomegaly also may occur.[68,72] Significant laboratory abnormalities are anemia and elevated alkaline phosphatase. Cervical lymphadenitis caused by MAC most often affects children but also occurs in adults. Other manifestations of infection with MAC are synovitis, genitourinary tract disease, cutaneous lesions, deep infections of the hand, osteomyelitis, meningitis, ulcers of the colon, and pericarditis.[73-77]

Mycobacterium scrofulaceum

Mycobacterium scrofulaceum was named in 1956, after cases of mycobacterial cervical lymphadenitis were reported in children.[78] The organism is antigenically similar to MAC; and because occasional isolates identified as *M. scrofulaceum* by biochemical tests serotype as MAC and vice versa, *M. scrofulaceum* sometimes is classified with the MAC as *M. avium–intracellulare–scrofulaceum* complex.

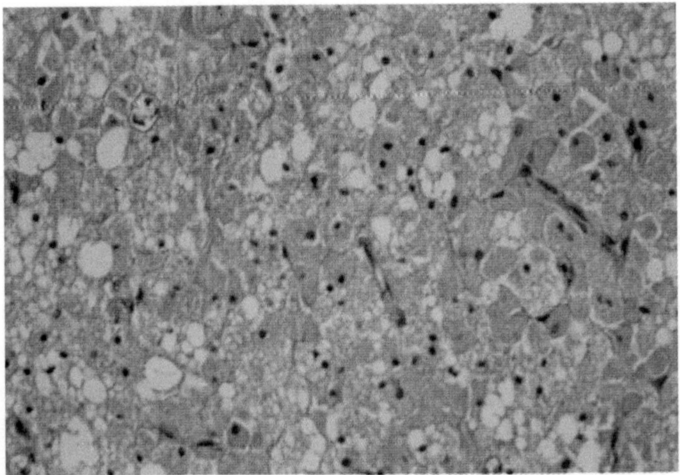

Fig. 34-6 Micrograph of a lymph node from a patient with AIDS shows aggregates of foamy histiocytes. Culture grew *Mycobacterium avium–intracellulare.*

M. scrofulaceum has been isolated from raw milk and other dairy products, pooled oysters, soil, and water.[76] These organisms most commonly cause cervical lymphadenitis in children 1 to 5 years of age, presumably entering the body through breaks in the skin or mucous membranes of the oral cavity. The disease usually is unilateral, involving lymph nodes high in the neck and close to the mandible. Affected children generally appear healthy, are afebrile, and complain of minimal if any pain and tenderness. With disease progression, the nodes soften and drain but occasionally heal by fibrosis and calcification. Extranodal manifestations of infection with *M. scrofulaceum* include pulmonary disease, disseminated disease, and rarely conjunctivitis, osteomyelitis, meningitis, and granulomatous hepatitis.[77] Lesions of *M. scrofulaceum* are histologically indistinguishable from those caused by *M. tuberculosis.*

Mycobacterium kansasii

Mycobacterium kansasii was first described in 1953 as the "yellow bacillus."[79] It accounted for 3% of mycobacterial isolates in the United States in 1979 and 1980, with the highest numbers being reported from California, Texas, Louisiana, Illinois, and Florida.[80] The natural reservoir of *M. kansasii* is unknown; however, it has been cultured from water samples.[76] Pulmonary disease is most common in males 50 to 60 years of age living in urban areas, among certain occupational groups (miners, welders, sandblasters, and painters), and among individuals with pneumoconioses and chronic obstructive pulmonary disease. Disseminated disease generally affects persons with impaired cellular immunity.

The histologic findings of lesions caused by *M. kansasii* vary. Lung and lymph node tissue often show caseating granulomas. Noncaseating granulomas have been seen in synovial tissue, and skin lesions may show granulomas with areas of necrosis or foci of acute and chronic inflammation without well-formed granulomas.[77] AFB are common in lung and lymph node tissue but are seen less frequently in tissue from other sites.

The most common manifestation of disease caused by *M. kansasii* is chronic cavitary pulmonary disease, usually involving the upper lobes. Extrapulmonary manifestations include cervical lymphadenitis in children; cutaneous disease resembling pyogenic abscesses, cellulitis, or sporotrichosis; musculoskeletal involvement (carpal tunnel syndrome, synovitis, arthritis, tendonitis and fascitis, or osteomyelitis); disseminated disease; isolated genitourinary tract disease; and pericarditis.[77]

Mycobacterium fortuitum–Mycobacterium chelonae complex

Mycobacterium fortuitum and *M. chelonae* are rapidly growing mycobacteria, forming visible colonies on solid media in 7 days or less.

M. fortuitum has been isolated from soil, water, and dust, and *M. chelonae,* from soil, water, and sewage. Most persons infected with these organisms give a history of a penetrating injury (trauma or surgical procedure) with possible soil or water contamination. Outbreaks of infection with *M. chelonae* have been associated with administration of diphtheria-pertussis-tetanus-polio vaccines, histamine injections, lidocaine administration using a jet injector, contaminated water in persons receiving intermittent peritoneal dialysis, contaminated hemodialyzers in persons treated with hemodialysis, and placement of contaminated porcine heterograft valves.[77,81-84]

Lesions produced by *M. fortuitum* and *M. chelonae* are characterized histologically by necrosis with minimal caseation, an infiltrate of neutrophils, and granulomas with foreign body or Langhans' giant cells; lipid-laden macrophages are seen occasionally. Clumps of extracellular AFB are found within aggregates of neutrophils in less than a third of cases. In lung tissue, foamy macrophages are frequent, a pattern resembling lipoid pneumonia.

Primary cutaneous disease—localized cellulitis, draining abscesses, or minimally tender nodules—caused by *M. fortuitum* or *M. chelonae* occurs 3 weeks to 12 months (most often 4 to 6 weeks) after a penetrating injury in persons with an intact immune system. Osteomyelitis is an occasional complication, especially after puncture wounds to the feet. Postoperative infections are characterized by a nonhealing wound or breakdown of a healed wound with serous drainage in a person with few systemic symptoms. They generally develop 3 weeks to 3 months after the procedure, especially median sternotomy, augmentation mammaplasty, or insertion of a percutaneous catheter.[85] Disseminated disease, which typically occurs in immunocompromised adults, is manifested by multiple, recurrent skin and soft-tissue abscesses with no evident primary source of infection. Chronic pulmonary disease resembles that caused by *M. kansasii* or MAC, except that cavitation is uncommon. Endocarditis involving a prosthetic valve usually becomes manifest 4 to 12 weeks after surgery. *M. fortuitum* and *M. chelonae* are rare causes of keratitis and corneal ulceration after trauma and of cervical lymphadenitis in all age groups.

Mycobacterium xenopi

Mycobacterium xenopi, first isolated from a toad in 1957, was recognized as a human pathogen in 1965.[86] It has been cultured from hot- and cold-water taps, hospital hot-water generators and storage tanks, and other environmental sources. In Great Britain, *M. xenopi* is found more often in coastal than in inland areas, and birds are a possible natural reservoir. Most pulmonary infections caused by *M. xenopi* have been reported from Europe and Great Britain. In the United States, *M. xenopi* accounted for only 0.2% of mycobacterial isolates reported to the CDC in 1980, and half were reported from Connecticut, Wisconsin, and California.[80] Disease has occurred only in adults, more frequently in males than in females. Most persons have preexisting lung damage or another predisposing condition, such as an extrapulmonary malignancy, alcoholism, diabetes mellitus, or immunosuppressive therapy. Nosocomial disease has been reported.[68] Disseminated disease is uncommon, and only a few such cases have occurred in persons with AIDS.[87,88]

Descriptions of the histologic findings of lesions caused by *M. xenopi* are limited but include nonspecific granulation tissue, epithelioid macrophages, Langhans' giant cells, and caseating granulomas containing AFB.

Pulmonary disease caused by *M. xenopi* may be chronic, subacute, or acute, producing symptoms indistinguishable from those caused by *M. kansasii* or MAC. Extrapulmonary infections—osteomyelitis, arthritis, lymphadenitis, and disseminated disease—are uncommon.[76]

Mycobacterium szulgai

Mycobacterium szulgai, first recognized in 1972, is an infrequent human pathogen found worldwide, but its natural reservoir is unknown.[89] The most common manifestation of infection is chronic pulmonary disease, which occurs predominantly in middle-aged males. The few reported cases of extrapulmonary disease include infections of the olecranon bursa associated with repeated trauma or with cortisone injections, extensive cutaneous disease in persons receiving corticosteroids, osteomyelitis, tenosynovitis with carpal tunnel syndrome, cervical lymphadenitis, and disseminated disease.[77] Microscopically, lesions caused by *M. szulgai* show noncaseating granulomas and granulation tissue with or without AFB.

Mycobacterium malmoense

Mycobacterium malmoense was reported as a new species in 1977, but its natural reservoir remains unknown.[90] Most human infections have been reported from England, Wales, and Sweden. *M. malmoense* has been isolated in various parts of the United States, but well-documented disease in humans is rare. The most common manifestation of infection with *M. malmoense* is chronic pulmonary disease, typically occurring in middle-aged men with pneumoconiosis, and cervical lymphadenitis in children has been described.[91,92]

Mycobacterium simiae

Mycobacterium simiae was first isolated from monkeys from India in 1965.[93] *M. simiae* is found in monkeys and has been recovered from tap water in hospitals. An uncommon human pathogen, *M. simiae* has been associated with chronic pulmonary disease, osteomyelitis, and disseminated disease.[77] Microscopically, lesions show caseating granulomas with AFB.

Mycobacterium marinum

Mycobacterium marinum, first described in 1926, was recognized as a human pathogen in 1951.[94,95] Human infection with *M. marinum* is acquired by trauma to the skin during contact with contaminated nonchlorinated freshwater or saltwater, trauma unassociated with water contact, or contact with water in the absence of preceding trauma. Typically, a single papulonodular lesion appears 2 to 3 weeks after inoculation, most commonly on the elbow, knee, foot, toe, or finger, and often becomes verrucous or ulcerated. Occasionally, an abscess forms at the site of inoculation, and several secondary nodules develop and progress centrally along the lymphatics, resembling sporotrichosis. Rarely, in immunocompromised persons, cutaneous lesions become disseminated.[96] Extracutaneous manifestations are uncommon and include synovitis, osteomyelitis, and ocular and laryngeal lesions.[97-99]

Histologic examination of an early skin lesion shows neutrophil aggregates surrounded by histiocytes. Later, lymphocytes, epithelioid histiocytes, occasional Langhans' giant cells, and foci of fibrinoid necrosis are seen; and in lesions present for over 6 months, aggregates of lymphocytes are found in the dermis, often surrounding blood vessels or skin appendages. Acid-fast stains usually are negative, but AFB may be seen within histiocytes.

Mycobacterium haemophilum

Mycobacterium haemophilum first was described in 1978 but probably was the noncultivable acid-fast bacillus recognized in skin ulcers in 1972 and 1974.[100-102] The organism is unique among the mycobacteria in its growth requirement for hemoglobin or hemin. Human infections caused by *M. haemophilum* are uncommon; fewer than 50 cases have been reported from Australia, the United States, Europe, and Canada.[103-105] Most infected persons have an underlying immunodeficiency, such as lymphoma, exogenous immunosuppression after organ transplantation, or AIDS, but a few cases of lymphadenitis have been reported in otherwise healthy children. Disease most commonly is manifested by multiple cutaneous nodules, ulcers, or painful swellings, usually involving the extremities, that increase in size and occasionally become abscesses and open fistulas draining purulent material. Microscopically, lesions show foci of necrosis without caseation surrounded by a polymorphous inflammatory infiltrate with occasional Langerhans' giant cells in the lower dermis. AFB are seen singly or in small clusters, often within cells.

Mycobacterium genavense

Mycobacterium genavense is a newly proposed species of *Mycobacterium* that has been recovered primarily from blood cultures but also from spleen and bone marrow of patients with AIDS.[37,106] Almost all patients had fever and malaise, and some had abdominal symptoms as well. Several patients were infected with another potential pathogen, such as MAC; therefore, it has been difficult to determine the role of *M. genavense* in the disease process.

Mycobacterium ulcerans infection (Buruli ulcer)

Mycobacterium ulcerans causes indolent, necrotizing, relatively nonpainful ulcers known commonly as *Buruli ulcer*.[107] *M. ulcerans* infections prevail in riverine or swampy terrain of warm countries, especially in lowlands subject to seasonal flooding in Africa, Mexico, India, and many other countries. After tuberculosis and leprosy, Buruli ulcer is probably the third most important mycobacterial infection of humans.

Incubation periods seem highly variable. In a group of 180 patients in Zaïre,[108] lesions developed in 14 patients at sites of trauma to the skin, 2 weeks to 3 years after the trauma. In 10 of these patients, ulcers appeared within 3 months after the trauma.

The earliest lesion is a firm, well-circumscribed, slowly enlarging nodule in the subcutaneous tissue and dermis, usually asymptomatic except for itching. As the lesion enlarges, necrosis erodes through the epidermis, discharging an oily liquid. This edema gradually subsides, leaving a zone of desquamation and hyperpigmentation at the periphery of the ulcer. Ulcers usually gradually enlarge but may remain small (1 to 2 cm), even though extensive necrosis continues to spread widely in the subcutaneous tissue.

Ulcers may persist for months to years and frequently become aggressive, destroying or maiming important structures such as eyes (Fig. 34-7) and genitalia in their path.

Microscopically, the preulcerative lesion is a circumscribed area of necrosis containing numerous AFB, largely confined to the center of the lesion. The lesion is symmetrical, with contiguous necrosis of the deep dermis and panniculus and sometimes fascia. Necrosis extends well beyond the areas containing bacilli. At the edge of the necrotic area there is interstitial

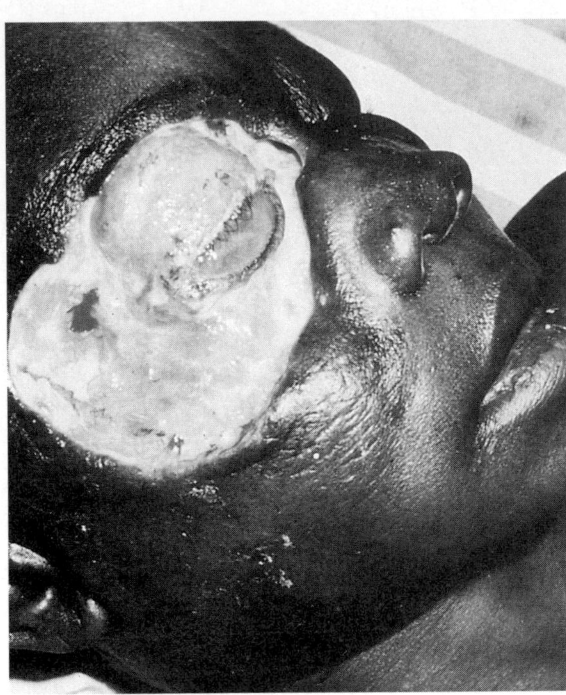

Fig. 34-7 *Mycobacterium ulcerans* infection in Zaïrian woman. Destruction of lids necessitated enucleation. (AFIP 76-11034-6.)

edema but little or no inflammatory exudate. Conspicuously, fat cells enlarge and die but retain their ghost outlines for variable periods. Capillaries and larger vessels are destroyed or damaged, perhaps contributing to the striking necrosis of fat. In fact, Hayman[109] attributes the fat necrosis more to infarction than to a direct effect of toxin; however, even in minimal lesions, necrosis of fat seems to be a primary event and reasonably assignable to a direct effect of bacterial toxin. The entire process, as lesions advance, could represent the combined effect of a cytotoxin and infarction, which in the panniculus leads to wide undermining of the overlying skin. Necrosis of the dermis and damage to the epidermis eventually lead to ulceration, beginning most often at the center of the lesion. AFB in Ziehl-Neelsen–stained sections are almost exclusively confined to necrotic slough in the bed of the ulcer and in necrotic fat. Surrounding tissue and dermis seldom reveal large numbers of AFB, if any.

As the ulcer enlarges, undermining proceeds most actively in the panniculus with at least partial sparing of the overlying dermis. This overhanging flap often reaches 10 cm or more and gradually reepithelializes, with granulation tissue developing in the base of the ulcer. Hypersensitivity granulomas, probably stimulated by mycobacterial antigens, and possibly granulomas responding to necrotic fat develop in the dermis and tissues surrounding the lesions. Healing occurs after this granulomatous phase (Fig. 34-8). Eventually most ulcers heal spontaneously, though often with disastrous deformity.

Rarely pathogenic mycobacteria

Mycobacteria that are rare human pathogens and the diseases with which they have been associated are outlined in Table 34-4.[110-121]

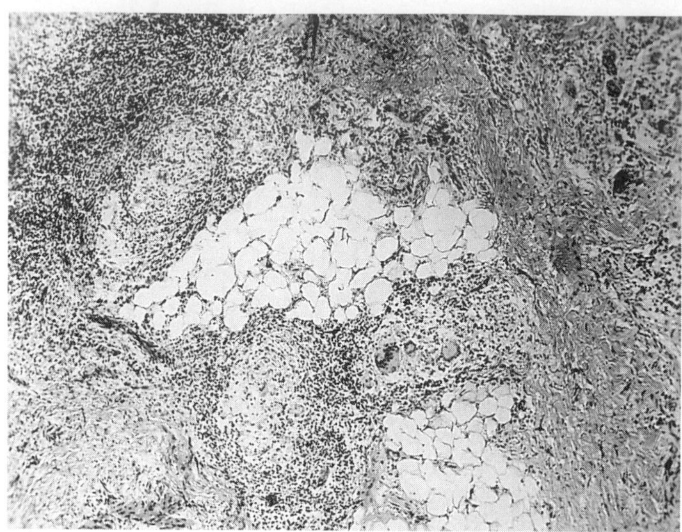

Fig. 34-8 Healing *Mycobacterium ulcerans* infection. Granulomas and fibrosis are replacing necrotic dermis and subcutis, eventually producing a depressed and potentially deforming scar. (AFIP 64-5096.)

Table 34-4 Diseases caused by rarely pathogenic mycobacteria

Species	Diseases
M. gordonae	Meningitis, hepatorenal disease, peritonitis, prosthetic valve endocarditis, cutaneous lesions, disseminated disease, pulmonary disease (?)
M. asiaticum	Pulmonary disease
M. thermoresistible	Pulmonary disease, cutaneous lesions
M. terrae–triviale complex	Septic arthritis, synovitis, osteomyelitis, disseminated disease (?)
M. nonchromogenicum	Pulmonary disease
M. flavescens	Pulmonary disease
M. shimoidei	Pulmonary disease
M. smegmatis	Skin and soft-tissue infections
M. neoaurum	Bacteremia
M. paratuberculosis	Crohn's disease (?)

?, Possible association but not proved unequivocally.

LEPROSY

Leprosy is a chronic infection caused by *Mycobacterium leprae* affecting primarily the cooler parts of the body: skin, upper respiratory tract, anterior segment of the eye, superficial portions of peripheral nerves, and testes.

Although often equated with leprosy, biblical descriptions of what is termed *tsara'ath* and translated *leprosy* in the Old Testament portray none of the diagnostic clinical features of *M. leprae* infection. Wycliffe, translating from the Vulgate in 1384, rendered *lepra* as *leprosy* in the first English Bible. This probably reflected popular images of leprosy in the Middle Ages, then a common disease in Europe and the British Isles, as an unholy or loathsome affliction.[122] Today, many prefer *Hansen's disease,* or *HD,* as synonyms for leprosy. Because of persisting social implications, pathologists should render a diagnosis of leprosy only with utmost caution and confidentiality.

Traditionally, most authorities did not consider leprosy contagious. Around 1870, however, Hansen became convinced of a specific transmissible etiologic agent from his study of 69 families with leprosy in western Norway.

Even from the time of Hansen's original discovery of the leprosy bacillus in 1873, investigators recognized that the nasal mucosa harbored massive numbers of organisms. Although many postulated modes of transmission remain uncertain, there is little doubt that the human nasorespiratory tract is the most common route of exit and entry of *M. leprae.*[123] DeWit and colleagues,[124] using PCR detected *M. leprae* DNA in nasal mucosal swabs of 19% of occupational contacts of leprosy patients and 12% of other inhabitants in endemic areas of leprosy. Skin-to-skin contact undoubtedly transmits leprosy[125] but is probably uncommon.

Human patients have long been considered the only reservoir of *M. leprae.* In 1974, however, Walsh and colleagues[126] found newly captured armadillos in Louisiana with advanced lepromatous disease, and recent estimates indicate that 5% to 25% of wild armadillos in Louisiana and eastern Texas may have naturally acquired leprosy.[127-129] Epidemiologic data support the argument that wild infected armadillos in these states transmit leprosy to humans, perhaps by direct contact or fomites.[130,131]

The World Health Organization (WHO) estimates that there are 5.5 million leprosy patients in the world, with highest prevalences in tropical Africa, South America, India, southeast Asia, the Philippines, and some South Pacific islands.[132] In the United States in 1992 there were 6098 registered leprosy patients, and in 1993 170 new patients, down from an annual high in modern times of 361 in 1985.[133] Although immigrants account for approximately 90% of new cases annually in the United States, leprosy remains indigenous in Hawaii, Louisiana, and Texas. There is no evidence of secondary transmission from imported cases in the United States; thus immigrants with leprosy present no health risk to the United States population.

Clinical features

Few diseases present as wide a range of clinical and pathologic forms as leprosy. The International Leprosy Congress in Madrid in 1953 adopted a system of classification that, with some refinements, has gained wide acceptance.[134] The Madrid Classification divides leprosy into two polar groups, tuberculoid and lepromatous, with all other forms classified as either indeterminate or borderline. In 1966, Ridley and Jopling[135] divided the range into 5 groups based on immunologic, pathologic, and clinical features. These groups are tuberculoid (TT), borderline-tuberculoid (BT), midborderline (BB), borderline-lepromatous (BL), and lepromatous (LL). Indeterminate and pure neural forms fall outside this classification.

For field workers, the WHO devised a simplified classification.[136] Patients with skin smears negative for AFB are termed *paucibacillary* (PB), and those with positive skin smears *multibacillary* (MB).

Incubation periods vary up to as long as 30 years but usually are 2 to 5 years. Because there are no detectable strain variations in *M. leprae,* except for drug sensitivity, the range of clinical forms is best attributable to the immune response of

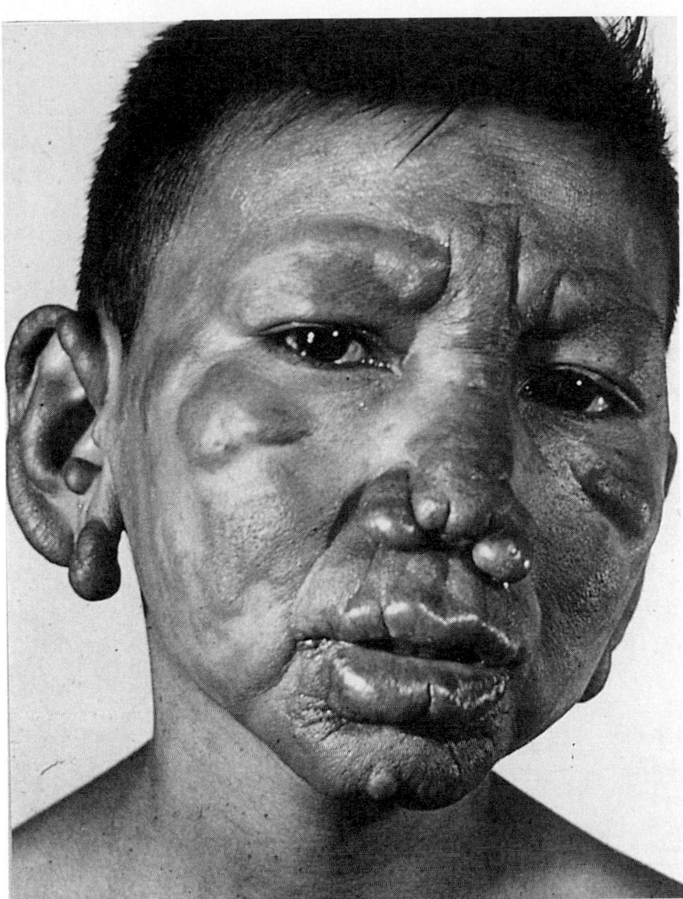

Fig. 34-9 Lepromatous leprosy. Notice madarosis and diffuse infiltration with nodules and plaques over central face and ears. (AFIP 77-9359-2.)

the patient.[137] If cutaneous sensory changes are included, nearly all leprosy patients have peripheral neuropathy. One in four patients has significant deformity.

Cardinal signs of leprosy are hypoesthetic skin lesions, enlarged peripheral nerves, and AFB in skin smears. In the absence of another obvious diagnosis, any one of these signs usually indicates leprosy (Fig. 34-9).

Pathogenesis

M. leprae causes disease by surviving and multiplying within macrophages, and interactions between this redoubtable parasite and the immune responses of its host determine the course of the pathogenesis of leprosy.

Compared with most other pathogenic bacteria, the cell wall of *M. leprae* is robust, requiring phagocytosis for destruction. Although knowledge of host responses has increased remarkably over the last decade, understanding of innate and acquired resistance to *M. leprae* remains ambiguous.[138]

Nonspecific or innate factors participate in defenses against *M. leprae*. For example, complement promotes phagocytosis of the leprosy bacillus,[139] and after phagocytosis, there is phagolysosomal fusion and intracellular killing, perhaps by the oxygen-independent system.[140]

Complex specific or acquired responses to *M. leprae* determine in large measure the form of leprosy that develops. Macrophages of leprosy patients may be innately inefficient in recognizing and presenting mycobacterial antigens.[141] In susceptible individuals, antigens of *M. leprae* may inhibit adherence of *M. leprae*, or abolish presentation by macrophages of *M. leprae* antigens to T-cells.[142,143]

Macrophage subpopulations, as identified by monoclonal antibodies in dermal infiltrates, vary in the different forms of leprosy, but their specific functions remain vague.[144,145] *M. leprae* produces several antigens similar to stress-induced proteins, which may protect the bacillus in an intracellular environment. These proteins may participate in the pathogenesis of leprosy and could serve as targets for immunoprophylaxis.[146,147]

Perturbations in the lymphocyte-macrophage interaction appear closely related to defective cell-mediated immunity (CMI) in leprosy. Peripheral blood leukocytes from active patients show decreasing sensitivity to *M. leprae,* proceeding downward from TT to LL.[148] Total numbers of circulating T-lymphocytes decrease as LL advances[149] but without consistent helper-to-suppressor T-lymphocyte subset ratios.[150] At the lesion level, however, T-lymphocyte subsets vary greatly in the different forms of leprosy.[151,152] In TT, helper cells abound in the central epithelioid cell-rich area, and suppressor cells selectively inhabit the peripheral mantle of the granuloma. In LL, lymphocytes admix with macrophages, with suppressor cells prevailing. One or more unique *M. leprae* antigens may directly suppress T-helper function or enhance suppressor T-cell activity.[153] Some investigators believe that lepromin and phenolic glycolipid-I (PGL-I) generate suppressor cell activity in vitro in peripheral leukocytes of LL but not of TT,[154,155] however, this point is controversial.[156,157]

Suppressor and helper T-lymphocytes recognize foreign antigens displayed by antigen-presenting cells respectively in association with class 1 and class 2 major histocompatibility molecules. Antigen recognition normally leads to interleukin-2 (IL-2) production by helper T-cells, which in turn increases interferon-gamma (IFN-γ) release and activation of macrophages. LL patients fail to produce IL-2, probably decreasing IFN-γ levels and diminishing macrophage activation. IFN-γ production is restored by the addition of IL-2 in vitro.[158] IL-2–bearing lymphocytes are greatly reduced in LL cellular infiltrations,[159] an indication that suppressor T-cells may influence IL-2 production in situ, reducing proliferation of specifically sensitized T-cells, suppressing release of IFN-γ, and inhibiting macrophage activation. Intradermal injection of IFN-γ into LL lesions causes an influx of helper T-cells with the stimulation of epithelioid and giant cell formation and reductions in the bacillary load.[160] Blockade of T-cell–dependent areas of lymph nodes by *M. leprae*–laden macrophages may cause secondary immunosuppression in advanced LL.[161]

Viable and nonviable *M. leprae* impede phagolysosomal fusion, but coating of *M. leprae* with specific antisera promotes fusion in vitro,[162] an indication that resistance to leprosy could involve an *M. leprae*–specific antibody that promotes phagolysosomal fusion and bacterial killing. In LL, the bacterial overload of macrophages could interfere with phagocytic activity and cause secondary disturbances of enzymatic activities in phagocytic vacuoles, leading to alterations in the production of oxygen radicals.

Monocytes from LL patients show increased production of superoxide, compared with monocytes from TT patients and from normal individuals.[163] PGL-I in vitro interferes with monocyte oxidative processes, but the role of this activity in regulating phagocytosis remains unclear.[164]

Although hyperinfection strongyloidiasis is a potentially serious complication in LL patients,[165] the course of most opportunistic infections in LL, including pulmonary tuberculosis, is similar to that in nonleprosy patients.[166]

Cutaneous pathology

Because of the stigma of leprosy, pathologists must guard against ambiguous diagnoses such as "consistent with leprosy." Thorough clinicopathologic correlations are important, especially when definitive histopathologic criteria are lacking. Most problems arise with the classification of indeterminate lesions.[167,168]

Ridley and Jopling[135,169] devised the histopathologic classification of leprosy in skin and nerves presented here, based on the following criteria: quality of granulomas, bacterial load, numbers of lymphocytes, damage to nerves, cellular infiltrations of the subepidermal zone, and epidermal changes.

The immunologic potential of the patient vis-à-vis leprosy is not obvious in indeterminate lesions. Nerves are intact and only small lymphocytic infiltrations surround some neurovascular bundles and appendages (Fig. 34-10). If leprosy is suspected, the search for AFB should first center on the nerves and subepidermal area. Occasionally AFB appear only in arrectores pilorum muscles but carry the same diagnostic significance as in nerves. A firm diagnosis of indeterminate leprosy without demonstrating AFB is risky, especially without correlations with a clinician experienced in leprosy.

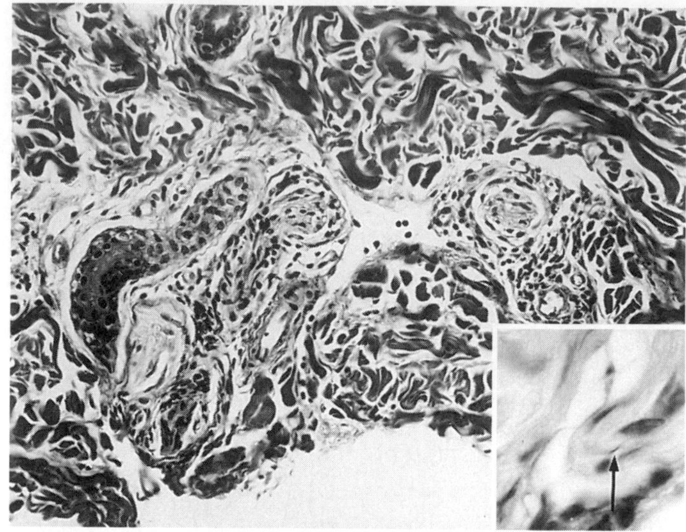

Fig. 34-10 Indeterminate leprosy showing small lymphocytic infiltrates around neurovascular channels in lower dermis. Nerves are well preserved. *Inset,* Single acid-fast bacillus *(arrow)* in otherwise normal nerve in parallel section. (AFIP 84-7138 and 84-7140.)

Tuberculoid lesions demonstrate high levels of CMI to *M. leprae.* Epithelioid cell granulomas in the dermis or subcutaneous tissue are compact and have mantles of varying numbers of lymphocytes (Figs. 34-11). Langerhans' giant cells may be present. If granulomas invade the subepidermal area, they frequently penetrate the deeper epidermal layers and sometimes ulcerate the epidermis. Damage to nerves is usually extensive, and in older lesions, granulomas may destroy cutaneous nerves beyond recognition. Staining for S-100 protein may reveal neural remnants in such granulomas.[170] Bacilli are rare, but examination of multiple sections usually reveals AFB. The most productive areas to search are, in descending order, nerves or nerve remnants, subepidermal zone, and arrectores pilorum muscles. Cellular exudates seldom contain AFB (Fig. 34-12).

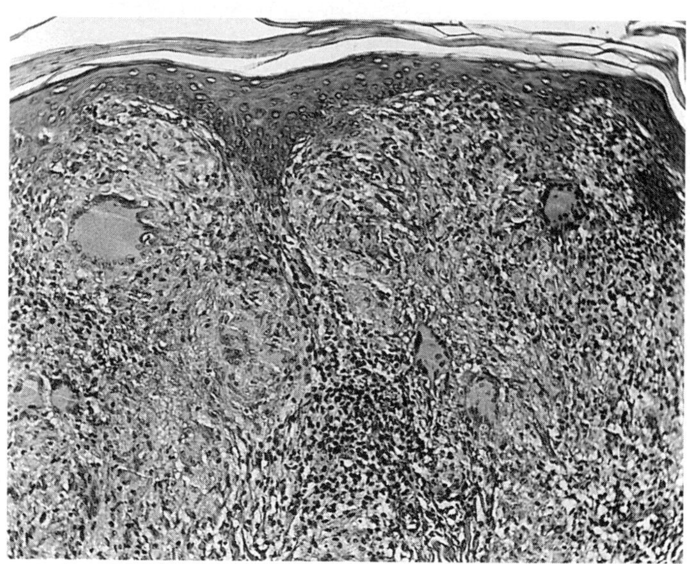

Fig. 34-11 Polar tubercluoid leprosy. Granulomas composed of epithelioid cells, giant cells, and lymphocytes focally invade the epidermis without leaving a subepidermal clear zone. (AFIP 72-12465.)

Granulomatous inflammation can destroy entire major nerve trunks, sometimes with massive caseous necrosis. Necrotic areas in these nerves provide the best hunting ground for AFB.

Borderline leprosy comprises a broad range of histopathologic patterns. In BT, cellular infiltrations differ from TT only slightly. Granulomas do not invade the epidermis, nerves are usually identifiable, and AFB are slightly more plentiful than those in TT (Fig. 34-13). In BB, fewer lymphocytes surround granulomas, and giant cells are uncommon. Nerves are more readily identifiable and have thickened perineuria. AFB are easily found, sometimes in small clusters, and tend to concentrate in nerves. Some histopathologists prefer to eliminate BB as an entity because of its instability and because a study of sufficient sections of most lesions usually reveals changes of BT or BL. In BL, histiocytes and irregularly distributed lymphocytes compose most granulomas. Lymphocytes are sometimes numerous, perineuria often considerably thickened, and nerves are easily identified. AFB are numerous and often found in clumps in nerves and histiocytes.

In its earliest stages, LL shows only a few macrophages around neurovascular bundles and appendages, with few AFB. As lesions age, two distinct patterns of cellular exudates may develop: polar lepromatous (LLp), or subpolar lepromatous (LLs). In LLs, infiltrations of histiocytes intermix with few-to-moderate numbers of lymphocytes of both T-helper and T-suppressor subsets.[171] Characteristically, nerves in LLs have greatly thickened, laminated perineuria. In older lesions, histiocytes accumulate lipid and become vacuolated. AFB abound in histiocytes, nerves, blood vessel walls[172] (Fig. 34-14), and arrectores pilorum muscles, with many in clumps and globi. Only a few leprosy bacilli invade dermal lymphatics, and such invasion indi-

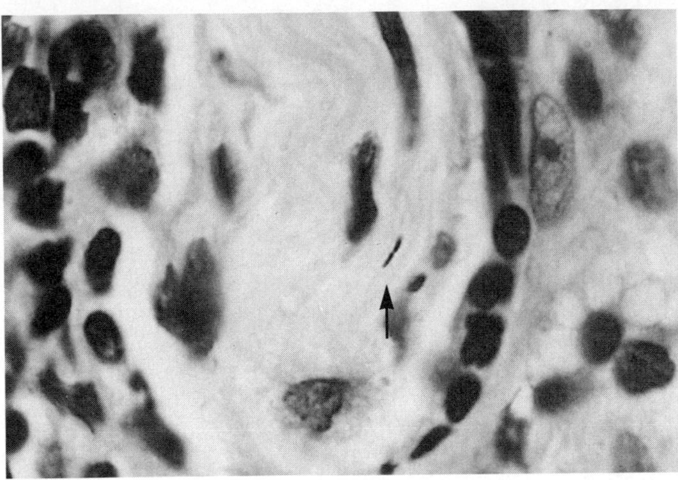

Fig. 34-12 Tuberculoid leprosy showing a pair of acid-fast bacilli *(arrow)* in a dermal nerve minimally invaded by epithelioid cells. (AFIP 84-8048.)

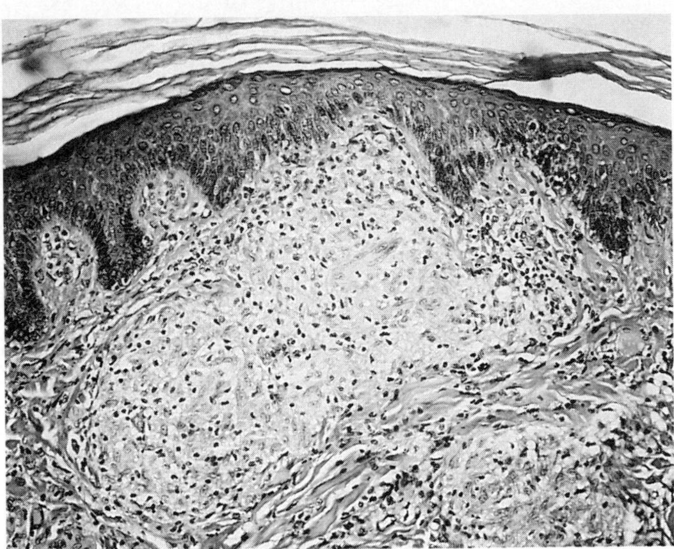

Fig. 34-13 Borderline-tuberculoid leprosy. Granulomas composed of epithelioid cells, giant cells, and lymphocytes replace upper dermis but leave a narrow subepidermal clear zone. (AFIP 87-5252.)

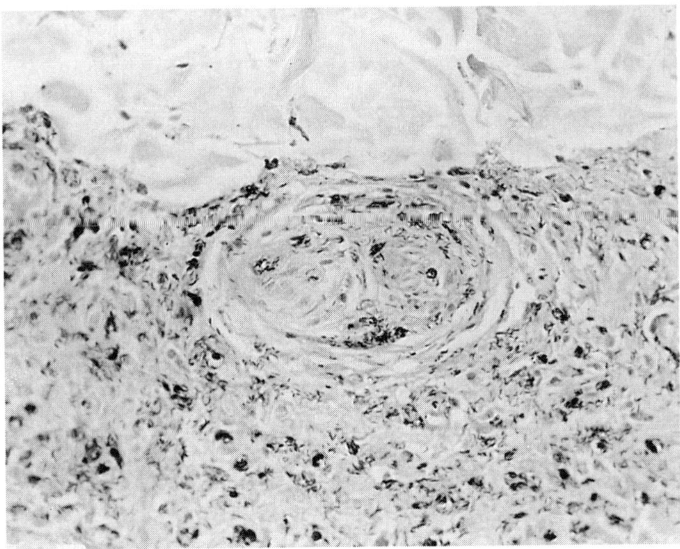

Fig. 34-14 Subpolar lepromatous leprosy showing lamellar thickening of the perineurium of a dermal nerve. The nerve and surrounding histiocytes contain many acid-fast bacilli.(AFIP 73-7532.)

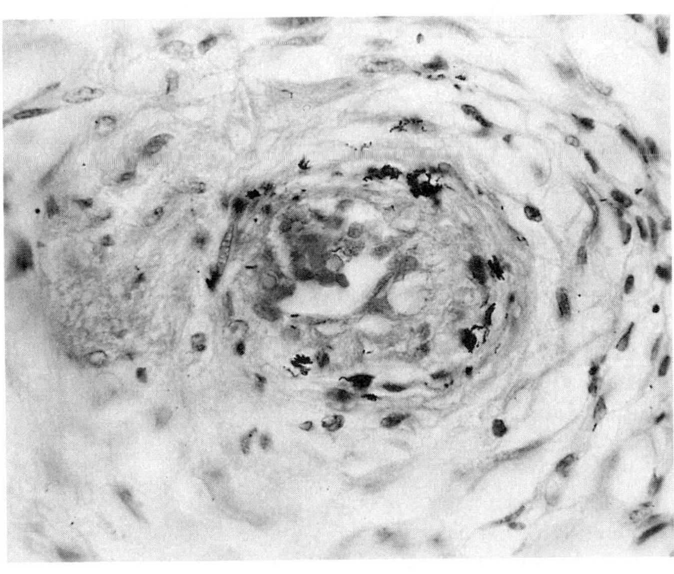

Fig. 34-15 Lucio form of lepromatous leprosy. Endothelial cell proliferation virtually obstructs lumen of a dermal blood vessel. Acid-fast bacilli colonize the endothelial cells. (AFIP 57-9794-1.)

cates that lymphatic channels play a less prominent role than blood vessels do in the dissemination of *M. leprae.*[173] Lymphatic routes, however, seem to clear lipids from bacilliferous lepromatous lesions, especially after initiating antileprosy treatment. LLp leprosy differs from LLs primarily in the scantiness of lymphocytes throughout the histiocytic infiltrations and lack of thickening of perineuria of dermal nerves.

Lucio leprosy is a subtype of LLp, with heavy colonization of endothelial cells of dermal blood vessels by *M. leprae* (Fig. 34-15). Frequently, endothelial cell proliferation obstructs blood vessels, producing infarction and ulceration ("Lucio phenomenon"). Immune complexes of antigens of *M. leprae* in blood vessel walls and perivascular areas probably contribute to the pathogenesis of this serious complication.[174]

The well-circumscribed elevated nodules of histoid lesions are composed mainly of spindle-shaped histiocytes laden with AFB (Fig. 34-16). AFB usually lie parallel to the long axis of cells.[175] The spindled histiocytes resemble fibrocytes, giving the lesion the appearance of dermatofibromas or even neurofibromas. In their most active form, histoid nodules expand rapidly, producing pseudocapsules of compressed collagen at their periphery. These nodules often have central liquefactive necrosis with massive bacillary proliferation and neutrophilic infiltrations, characteristic of the unique entity known as *local exacerbation reaction.* Some clinicians associate histoid leprosy with sulfone resistance;[176] however, such lesions most often contain sulfone-sensitive *M. leprae.*

Leprosy causes pathologic changes in many tissues and organs other than skin and nerves. Specimens from these locations seldom appear in most pathology services but deserve

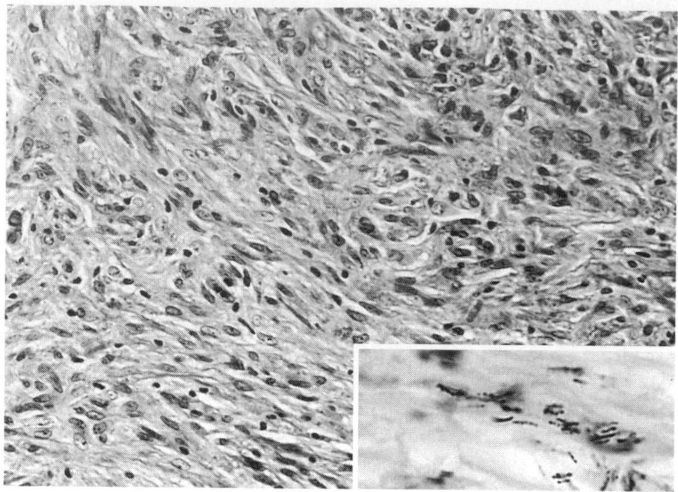

Fig. 34-16 Histoid form of lepromatous leprosy showing whorls of spindle-shaped histiocytes. *Inset,* Tendency for acid-fast bacilli to align with long axis of histiocytes. (AFIP 87-5248 and 87-5263.)

special mention because lesions at these sites contribute significantly to the morbidity of leprosy.

Peripheral blood monocytes contain leprosy bacilli in advanced untreated LL patients and disseminate *M. leprae* to every organ in the body. Temperature at central body sites is probably the most important factor inhibiting development of prominent lesions in, for example, the viscera and central nervous system. Ordinarily, reticuloendothelial cells of the liver and spleen phagocytose circulating bacilli, producing small aggregates of intracellular AFB in these organs. Such lesions usually do not progress, even though they may contain viable bacilli.

In LL patients, specific infiltrates invade the testes (leprous orchitis). Longstanding involvement of the testes leads to hyalinization of seminiferous tubules and replacement of lumens of the tubules and interstitial tissues by lepromatous infiltrates. Such patients experience sterility and impotence.

Osteitis and periostitis often damage bones of the hands and feet in LL patients and cause characteristic collapse of the nose and absorption of the central area of the maxilla. Trabeculas are atrophic with osteoid formation. Intratrabecular spaces contain macrophages and frequently foreign body giant cells, laden with AFB. Bone marrow aspirates from LL patients usually show macrophages containing bacilli. Proliferative periostitis may involve bones of the hands and feet and long bones. Synovia are sometimes thickened by leprous infiltrates, especially in patients with erythema nodosum leprosum (ENL).

In LL, *M. leprae* proliferate in the upper respiratory passages from the nares to the larynx, with extensive infiltrations of *M. leprae*–laden histiocytes in the submucosa. Before effective chemotherapy and use of anti-inflammatory agents, asphyxiation by laryngeal obstruction was common, most often in patients in reaction with ENL.

Sight-threatening complications frequently afflict patients, with leprosy ranking as the world's third leading cause of blindness.[177,178] Damage to the zygomatic and temporal branches of the facial nerve leads to paresis of the orbicularis muscle and lagophthalmos. Patients undergoing upgrading reversal reactions are most at risk. Exposure keratopathy complicates such patients, most prominently in patients with anesthesia of the cornea. LL patients may experience scleritis and iritis, particularly during ENL; however, few new lesions seem to appear in the eye after initiation of MDT.[179,180]

Lymph nodes draining the skin and hepatic portal areas in LL patients often show capsular thickening and replacement of paracortical regions by bacilli-laden macrophages. In ENL, lymph nodes sometimes suppurate. In TT, epithelioid cell granulomas may invade lymph nodes that drain affected skin. Granulomas in these nodes resemble those of sarcoidosis.[181,182]

Reactions

Approximately one half of all leprosy patients undergo acute inflammatory episodes called *reactions*. These episodes fall into two classic immunologic forms: type 1, a reversal reaction that complicates borderline leprosy, and type 2, erythema nodosum leprosum (ENL), which often occurs after chemotherapy but can occur in nontreated patients. The most characteristic features of type 1 reactions are edema, vascular dilatation, and necrosis. Type 2 reactions show endothelial swelling, vascular ectasia, and influx of neutrophils followed by lymphocytes (Fig. 34-17). To achieve optimal histopathologic evaluations of lesions in reaction, baseline biopsy specimens taken when the patient is not in reaction are helpful for comparison. Reactions in leprosy constitute a medical emergency, and rapid histologic confirmation may assist the clinician in therapy.[183-184]

Leprosy and HIV infection

The increased susceptibility of HIV-infected patients to tuberculosis indicates that leprosy may follow the same pattern. Only several dozen patients coinfected with *M. leprae* and HIV have been described in some detail, including five in the files of the Leprosy Registry at the AFIP.[185-187] No convincing

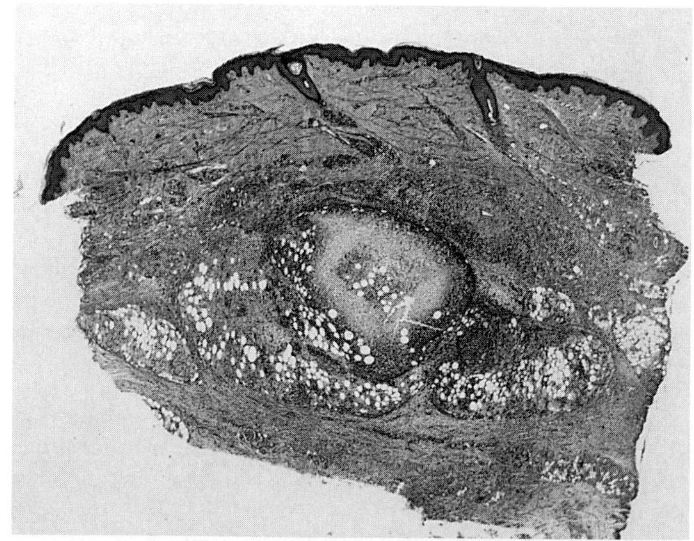

Fig. 34-17 Skin in lepromatous leprosy with erythema nodosum leprosum, showing severe panniculitis and abscess in center. (AFIP 87-5459.)

clinical evidence emerges from these patients, all of whom were receiving antileprosy therapy, to show that HIV adversely influences the course of leprosy. A few studies, however, suggest that rates of HIV seropositivity in leprosy patients are elevated, and HIV infection may lead to deterioration of leprosy.[188,189] One study in India, where HIV infections were then rare, suggests that there are cross-reactive antibodies for HIV and *M. leprae* in leprosy patients,[190] and the report by Kashala and colleagues[191] on leprosy patients in Zaïre and reports from elsewhere in Africa[192] are in agreement.

Although there seems to be no well-established association of HIV and leprosy, no prospective data are available. If ultimately no association of these two diseases can be established, some of the current concepts of the role of CMI in the immunopathogenesis of leprosy will need rethinking.[193]

Leprosy in animals

On discovering the leprosy bacillus, Hansen attempted unsuccessfully to transmit the disease to rabbits. During the next 80 years, many other trials in a large variety of animals were equally unsuccessful.[194] On the basis of observations made in the nineteenth century by Virchow, Binford in 1956 postulated that the leprosy bacillus grew best in the cooler parts of the body and that inoculation of ears, footpads, and testes of animals may prove fruitful approaches in the search for animal models of leprosy.[195] This led to the establishment of reproducible but limited growth of *M. leprae* in the mouse footpad by Shepard in 1960,[33,196] and ultimately to Storrs' introduction of the nine-banded armadillo, based on its cool body temperature (32° to 35° C), as the first useful model of disseminated MB leprosy.[197] In addition to normal mice, experimental leprosy has been established in three species of armadillos, in neonatally thymectomized rats and nude mice, and in immunologically intact sooty mangabey, rhesus, and African green monkeys.[198-200] As many as 80% of nine-banded armadillos, 67% of sooty mangabeys, 21% of rhesus monkeys, and 19% of African green monkeys develop disseminated leprosy (BL-LL) after experimental inoculation of *M. leprae*. Approximately one half of all monkeys with progressive disease develop neuropathic sequelae, including paralytic deformities. Serologic responses to PGL-I and other antigens, including neural antigens, in the sooty mangabey are similar to those in humans with MB leprosy.[201,202] Coinfection with *M. leprae* and simian immunodeficiency virus seems to enhance susceptibility of rhesus monkeys to leprosy.[203,204]

The prevalence of leprosy in recently captured armadillos in Louisiana establishes leprosy as a zoonosis.[126,127,205] As noted previously, evidence for the transmission of leprosy to humans from armadillos in Louisiana and Texas seems convincing; however, the importance of nonhuman primates as a reservoir of infection in endemic areas is not known.

Leininger and colleagues (1980) were the first to observe naturally acquired leprosy in a chimpanzee. This animal was imported into the USA from Sierra Leone.[206] Gormus and colleagues[207] reported naturally acquired leprosy in two additional chimpanzees housed in primate centers in Texas. Naturally acquired leprosy in a sooty mangabey monkey from West Africa was reported in 1985[208] with possible natural transmission to a cagemate.[209] The etiologic agent in all three species of these naturally infected animals satisfies all criteria for identification as *M. leprae*.

Klatser and associates,[210] using PCR techniques, detected *M. leprae* in nasal smears of 7.8% of 1217 individuals without leprosy in areas endemic for leprosy and, from their data, postulated the existence of reservoirs of leprosy in other than MB patients. Epidemiologic data derived from many leprosy-control programs show that treatment rapidly reduces prevalence, but incidence levels persist in the long-term in most areas. These observations indicate that nonhuman sources of *M. leprae* may play a role in the transmisson of leprosy.[211] The most likely nonhuman sources are animals and soil,[212,213] and continued relevant observations in endemic areas of leprosy seem warranted. Because of the high susceptibility of the sooty mangabey monkey in experimental studies, surveys in the habitat of this species in West Africa appear particularly appropriate.

TREATMENT AND PREVENTION

Treatment

Tuberculosis

The CDC recommends that initial isolates of *M. tuberculosis* from all patients with tuberculosis be tested for susceptibility to the primary antituberculosis agents—isoniazid, rifampin, pyrazinamide, streptomycin, and ethambutol—and that susceptibility be repeated if the patient continues to produce culture-positive sputum after 3 months of therapy.[20] Moreover, susceptibility to secondary drugs (ethionamide, kanamycin, capreomycin, ciprofloxacin, and cycloserine) also should be tested if resistance to more than one primary agent is suspected. The chemotherapeutic regimen currently recommended for treatment of tuberculosis (Table 34-5) should be initiated before susceptibility test results are available, but treatment should be changed based on those results if an isolate is found to be resistant.[20] Regimens commonly used to treat infections caused by the most frequently seen nontuberculous mycobacteria also are listed in Table 34-5. For many nontuberculous mycobacteria the optimal duration of therapy is unknown, but the interval indicated in the table has been successful in some cases.[68,76,77,214,215]

Leprosy

Sulfones, introduced in 1941,[216] remained the mainstay of the chemotherapy for leprosy until around 1973 when primary sulfone-resistance became a major concern.[217,218] Multidrug therapy (MDT), introduced in 1973,[219-221] proved highly effective and greatly reduced the numbers of registered patients. WHO adopted MDT recommendations in 1982,[136] based on efficacy, practical administrative constraints under field conditions, and cost.

Prevention

Mycobacterium tuberculosis

Four general strategies for controlling tuberculosis exist.[222] The most important is early identification and treatment of persons with infectious tuberculosis. This renders the infected person noncontagious within a few weeks and eventually results in a cure. To accomplish this, the mycobacteriology laboratory must provide rapid service, as discussed under Laboratory Diagnostic Techniques. Second, identification and treatment of individuals with noncontagious tuberculosis (extrapulmonary disease, primary pulmonary disease in children, bacteriologically unconfirmed pulmonary disease, and

Table 34-5 Therapy for infections with pathogenic mycobacteria

Species	Therapy	Duration (months)*
M. tuberculosis	INH, RIF, PZA, and ETH†	6§
MAC		
lymphadenitis	Surgery	
pulmonary	INH, RIF, ETH, and STREP‡ +/– surgery	18-24
disseminated	CLARI, ETH, and RFB	(24-48), nonAIDS
	(or CIPRO)	indefinite, AIDS
M. kansasii	INH, RIF, and ETH	18
M. fortuitum-chelonae	Surgery	
	AM and TET	1-2 after
response		
	(or CFX or RIF)	
M. marinum	RIF (or TET) alone or RIF and EMB; +/– surgery	18 or 1-2 after lesion resolves
M. ulcerans	Surgery, IRIF	
M. leprae	DAP, CLF, and RIF	6 to life‖

AM, Amikacin; *CFX*, cefoxitin; *CIPRO*, ciprofloxacin; *CLARI*, clarithromycin; *CLF*, clofazamine; *DAP*, dapsone; *ETH*, ethambutol; *INH*, isoniazid; *MAC*, *Mycobacterium avium–intracelluare* complex; *PZA*, pyrazinamide; *RFB*, rifabutin; *RIF*, rifampin; *STREP*, streptomycin; *TET*, tetracycline; +/–, may or may not be useful.
*Values in parentheses are suggested, but optimal interval is not established.
†STREP may be substituted for ETH; either is given until susceptibility to INH and RIF is documented. PZA is given only for the first 2 months.
§Therapy is given for 3 months after cultures convert to negative. For HIV-infected patients, therapy is given for 9 months and at least 6 months beyond culture conversion to negative.
‡Many experts currently believe that INH no longer has a role in MAC pulmonary disease.
‖See Pritze S, editor: *Criteria to determine the exact end of multidrug therapy in leprosy: a workshop*, Wurzburg, Germany, 1988, Armauer Hansen Institut; and Becx-Bleuminck M: Operational aspects of multidrug therapy, *Int J Lepr* 57:540, 1989.

infection with *M. tuberculosis* not yet causing disease) may prevent infectious cases. In countries, such as the United States, where the overall risk of new infection is still low, preventing progression of infection to active disease is especially useful.

The third strategy concerns creating a safe environment where the risk of transmitting infection is high, as in mycobacteriology laboratories, autopsy suites, sputum-induction cubicles, chest clinic waiting areas, and some shelters for the homeless. To accomplish this one must address several issues.[223] Rooms housing infectious patients or in which potentially infectious specimens are handled must be under negative pressure, and air likely to be contaminated with infectious droplet nuclei should be exhausted to the outside. A single-pass ventilation system (best accomplished by locating air-supply at the ceiling level and exhaust near the floor) and a minimum of six air changes per hour (12 exchanges per hour for autopsy suites) are recommended. Universal Precautions must be followed when handling all specimens, and both specimens and cultures must be handled in a certified, class II biologic safety cabinet. Moreover, a particulate respirator that filters out particles 1 to 5 μm in diameter should be worn (the standard surgical mask is not adequate), and personnel should be trained in a respirator program.

The fourth strategy involves the use of the BCG vaccine, an attenuated vaccine derived from a strain of *M. bovis* by Calmette and Guérin in France. The BCG vaccine was administered to humans first in 1921, and different preparations used in controlled trials conducted before 1955 yielded estimated efficacies of 56% to 80%.[224] Fifteen-year follow-up results of a large controlled trial in India begun in 1969 showed that the risk of sputum-positive tuberculosis in persons vaccinated with BCG was not lower than in persons given placebo.[225] However, observational studies, which are less reliable than controlled studies, have shown that the prevalence of tuberculous meningitis and miliary tuberculosis is 52% to 100% lower and that the prevalence of pulmonary disease is 2% to 80% lower in vaccinated children under 15 years of age than in unvaccinated controls.[222]

In the United States, the BCG vaccine is recommended only for infants and children who have negative tuberculin skin tests and who belong to selected population groups:[222] (1) those at high risk of intimate and prolonged exposure to persistently untreated or ineffectively treated persons with infectious pulmonary tuberculosis, who cannot be removed from the source of exposure, and for whom long-term preventive therapy is not possible; (2) those exposed continuously to persons with tuberculosis who have organisms resistant to isoniazid and rifampin; and (3) those in groups in which the rate of new infections is greater than 1% per year and for whom the usual surveillance and treatment programs have been attempted but are not feasible. The BCG vaccine was once recommended for health-care workers in the United States, but this has changed. The current recommendation for protection of health-care workers is adequate surveillance, which includes periodic (at least yearly) tuberculin skin testing and isoniazid preventive therapy for persons who have recently converted from tuberculin skin test negative to positive and for persons who are tuberculin skin test positive and who are close contacts of individuals with tuberculosis or who have medical conditions such as diabetes, renal failure, or immunosuppression associated with therapy or disease.[222]

The BCG vaccine should not be given to immunocompromised persons and should be given with caution to those at risk of infection with HIV. Disseminated *M. bovis* in a patient with AIDS and *M. bovis* lymphadenitis in symptomatic HIV-infected infants have been reported occurring after BCG vaccination.[226,227] However, disseminated *M. bovis* has not been reported in asymptomatic persons infected with HIV. In populations where the risk of tuberculosis is high, the World Health Organization recommends that the BCG vaccine be given to HIV-infected children at birth or as soon as possible thereafter but should not be given to children with symptomatic HIV infection; and in populations where the risk of tuberculosis is low, the BCG vaccine should not be given to persons known or suspected to be infected with HIV.[228]

Leprosy

Most patients probably acquire leprosy through the nasorespiratory tract;[123,124] thus, proximity to unidentified, untreated, multibacillary patients is most likely the highest risk factor. Given this mode of transmission, protection of general populations against exposure in the ambiance of most endemic regions is virtually impossible. With current technology, only control of leprosy by early detection and treatment of multibacillary patients can reduce risk of contagion. Chemoprophylaxis with antileprotics is practical only for highly motivated individuals.

In view of an apparent lack of infection immunity in leprosy in humans, the concept of a successful mass vaccination scheme is widely viewed with skepticism.

REFERENCES

1. Moodie RL: *Paleopathology: an introduction to the study of ancient evidences of disease,* Urbana, 1923, University of Illinois Press.
2. Ortner DJ, Putschar WGJ: *Identification of pathological conditions in human skeletal remains,* Washington, D.C., 1981, Smithsonian Institution Press.
3. Bartels P: Tuberkulose in der Jüngeren Steinzeit, *Archiv für Anthropologie* 6:243, 1907.
4. Ruffer MA: Pott'sche Krankheit an einer ägyptischen Mumie aus der Zeit der 21 Dynastie (um 1000 v. Chr.), *Zur historischen Biol Krankheitserreger* 3:9, 1910.
5. Morse D, Brothwell DR, Ucko PJ: Tuberculosis in ancient Egypt, *Am Rev Respir Dis* 90:524, 1964.
6. Grange JM: Mycobacterial disease in the world. In Ratledge C, Stanford J, Grange JM, editors: *The biology of the mycobacteria,* London, 1989, Academic Press, vol 3.
7. Harboe M: The work and concepts of Armaur Hansen: how do they stand today? *Ethiop Med J* 21:123, 1983.
8. Runyon EH: Anonymous mycobacteria in pulmonary disease, *Med Clin North Am* 43:273, 1959.
9. Woods GL: Mycobacteria. In Woods GL, Gutierrez Y: *Diagnostic pathology of infectious diseases,* Philadelphia, 1993, Lea & Febiger.

Laboratory diagnostic techniques

10. American Thoracic Society: Diagnostic standards and classification of tuberculosis, *Am Rev Respir Dis* 142:725, 1990.
11. Meyers WM, Kvernes S, Binford CH: Comparison of reactions to human and armadillo lepromins in leprosy, *Int J Lepr* 43:218, 1975.
12. Mitsuda K: On the value of a skin reaction to a suspension of leprous nodules, *Int J Lepr* 21:347, 1953.
13. Guinto RS, Doull JA, Mabalay EB: The Mitsuda reaction in persons with and without household exposure to leprosy, *Int J Lepr* 23:135, 1955.
14. Convit J, Avila JL, Goihman M, Pinardi ME: A test for the determination of competency in clearing bacilli in leprosy patients, *Bull WHO* 46:821, 1972.
15. Stanford JL: Immunologically important constituents of mycobacteria: antigens. In Ratledge C, Stanford JL, editors: *The biology of the mycobacteria,* vol 2, New York, 1983, Academic Press.
16. Strumpf IJ, Tsang AY, Sayre JW: Re-evaluation of sputum staining for the diagnosis of pulmonary tuberculosis, *Am Rev Respir Dis* 119:599, 1979.
17. Murray PR, Elmore C, Krogstad D: The acid-fast stain: a specific and predictive test for mycobacterial disease, *Ann Intern Med* 92:512, 1980.
18. Rickman TW, Moyer NP: Increased sensitivity of acid-fast smears, *J Clin Microbiol* 11:618, 1980.
19. Centers for Disease Control and Prevention: Meeting the challenge of multidrug-resistant tuberculosis: summary of a conference, *MMWR* 41(RR-11):51, 1992.
20. Tenover FC, Crawford JT, Huebner RE et al: The resurgence of tuberculosis: Is your laboratory ready? *J Clin Microbiol* 31:767, 1993.
21. Barksdale L, Kim KS: Mycobacterium, *Bacteriol Rev* 41:217, 1977.
22. Job CK, Chacko CJG: A modification of Fite's stain for demonstration of *M. leprae* in tissue sections, *Indian J Lepr* 58:17, 1986.
23. Wabitsch KR, Meyers WM: Histopathologic observations on the persistence of *Mycobacterium leprae* in the skin of multibacillary leprosy patients under chemotherapy, *Lepr Rev* 59:341, 1988.
24. Welch DF, Guruswamy AP, Sides SJ et al: Timely culture for mycobacteria which utilizes a microcolony method, *J Clin Microbiol* 31:2178, 1993.
25. Gross WM, Hawkins JE: Radiometric selective inhibition tests for differentiation of *Mycobacterium tuberculosis, Mycobacterium bovis,* and other mycobacteria, *J Clin Microbiol* 21:565, 1985.
26. Anargyros P, Astill DSJ, Lim ISL: Comparison of improved BACTEC and Lowenstein-Jensen media for culture of mycobacteria from clinical specimens, *J Clin Microbiol* 28:1288, 1990.
27. Stager CE, Libonati JP, Siddiqi SH et al: Role of solid media when used in conjunction with the BACTEC system for mycobacterial isolation and identification, *J Clin Microbiol* 29:154, 1991.
28. Abe C, Hosojima S, Fukasawa Y et al: Comparison of MB-Check, BACTEC, and egg-based media for recovery of mycobacteria, *J Clin Microbiol* 30:878, 1992.
29. Isenberg HD, D'Amato RF, Heifets L et al: Collaborative feasibility study of a biphasic system (Roche Septi-Chek AFB) for rapid detection and isolation of mycobacteria, *J Clin Microbiol* 29:1719, 1991.
30. D'Amato RF, Isenberg HD, Hochstein L et al: Evaluation of the Roche Septi-Chek AFB system for recovery of mycobacteria, *J Clin Microbiol* 29:2906, 1991.
31. Anhalt JP, Witebsky FG, Woods GL: College of American Pathologists position statement regarding rapid detection of *Mycobacterium tuberculosis, Arch Pathol Lab Med* 117(9):873, 876, 1993.
32. Kato L: Leprosy associated mycobacteria: implications, *Acta Leprol* 7:1, 1989.
33. Shepard CC: The experimental disease that follows the injection of human leprosy bacilli into foot pads of mice, *J Exp Med* 112:445, 1960.
34. Convit J, Pinardi ME: A simple method for the differentiation of *Mycobacterium leprae* from other mycobacteria through routine staining technics, *Int J Lepr* 40:130, 1972.
35. Gaylord H, Brennan PJ: Leprosy and the leprosy bacillus: recent developments in characterization of antigens and immunology of the disease, *Annu Rev Microbiol* 41:645, 1987.
36. Clark-Curtiss JE, Docherty MA: A species-specific repetitive sequence in *Mycobacterium leprae* DNA, *J Infect Dis* 159:7, 1989.
37. Williams DL, Gillis TP, Booth RJ et al: The use of a specific DNA probe and polymerase chain reaction for the detection of *Mycobacterium leprae, J Infect Dis* 162:193, 1990.
38. Iralu J, Sritharan V, Pieciak W et al: Diagnosis of *Mycobacterium avium* bacteremia by polymerase chain reaction [abstract no. U-56]. In *Abstracts of the 93rd General Meeting of the American Society for Microbiology,* Washington, D.C., 1993, American Society for Microbiology.
39. Tevere V, Hocknell P, Taurence J et al: Direct detection of mycobacteria in sputum using the PCR and species identification by a colorimetric microwell plate assay [abstract no. C-116]. In *Abstracts of the 93rd General Meeting of the American Society for Microbiology,* Washington, D.C., 1993, American Society for Microbiology.
40. Inderlied CB, Young LS, Yamada JK: Determination of in vitro susceptibility of *Mycobacterium avium* complex isolates to antimycobacterial agents by various methods, *Antimicrob Agents Chemother* 31:1697, 1987.
41. Heifets L: MIC as a quantitative measurement of the susceptibility of *Mycobacterium avium* strains to seven antituberculosis drugs, *Antimicrob Agents Chemother* 32:1131, 1988.
42. Wallace RJ Jr, Swenson JM, Silcox VA: The rapidly growing mycobacteria: characterization and susceptibility testing, *Antimicrobic Newsletter* 2:85, 1985.
43. Mittal A, Seshadri PS, Conalty ML et al: Rapid radiometric in vitro assay for the evaluation of the anti-leprosy activity of clofazimine and its analogues, *Lepr Rev* 56:99, 1985.
44. Ramasesh N, Hastings RC, Krahenbuhl JL: The metabolism of *Mycobacterium leprae* in macrophages, *Infect Immun* 55:1203, 1987.
45. Patel BKR, Banerjee DK, Butcher PD: Determination of *Mycobacterium leprae* viability by polymerase chain reaction amplification of 71-kDa heat-shock protein mRNA, *J Infect Dis* 168:799, 1993.

Mycobacterium tuberculosis complex

46. Rieder HL, Cauthen GM, Kelly GD et al: Tuberculosis in the United States, *JAMA* 262:385, 1989.

47. Centers for Disease Control and Prevention: National action plan to combat multidrug-resistant tuberculosis: recommendations of the CDC Task Force, *MMWR* 41(RR-11):1, 1992.
48. Centers for Disease Control and Prevention: Initial therapy for tuberculosis in the era of multidrug resistance: recommendations of the Advisory Council for the Elimination of Tuberculosis, *MMWR* 42(RR-7):1, 1993.
49. Stead WW, Lofgren JP, Warren E, Thomas C: Tuberculosis as an epidemic and nosocomial infection among the elderly in nursing homes, *N Engl J Med* 312:1483, 1985.
50. Centers for Disease Control and Prevention: Nosocomial transmission of multidrug-resistant tuberculosis to health-care workers and HIV-infected patients in an urban hospital—Florida, *MMWR* 40:718, 1991.
51. Centers for Disease Control and Prevention: Nosocomial transmission of multidrug-resistant tuberculosis among HIV-infected persons—Florida and New York, 1988-1991, *MMWR* 40:585, 1991.
52. Centers for Disease Control and Prevention: Transmission of multidrug-resistant tuberculosis among immunocompromised persons in a correctional system—New York, *MMWR* 41:507, 1992.
53. Fischl MA, Daikos GL, Uttamchandani RB et al: Clinical presentation and outcome of patients with HIV infection and tuberculosis caused by multiple-drug-resistant bacilli, *Ann Intern Med* 117:184, 1992.
54. Edlin BR, Tokars JI, Grieco MH et al: An outbreak of multidrug-resistant tuberculosis among hospitalized patients with the acquired immunodeficiency syndrome, *N Engl J Med* 326:1514, 1992.
55. Des Prez RM, Heim CR: *Mycobacterium tuberculosis*. In Mandell GL, Douglas RG Jr, Bennett JE, editors: *Principles and practice of infectious diseases*, ed 3, New York, 1990, Churchill Livingstone.
56. Chaisson RE, Schecter GF, Theuer CP et al: Tuberculosis in patients with the acquired immunodeficiency syndrome: clinical features, response to therapy, and survival, *Am Rev Respir Dis* 136:570, 1987.
57. Pitchenik AE, Fertel D, Bloch AB: Mycobacterial disease: epidemiology, diagnosis, treatment, and prevention, *Clin Chest Med* 9:425, 1988.
58. Kim JH, Langston AA, Gallis HA: Miliary tuberculosis: epidemiology, clinical manifestations, diagnosis, and outcome, *Rev Infect Dis* 12:583, 1990.
59. Moore VA: *Bovine tuberculosis and its control*, New York, 1913, Carpenter.
60. Francis J: *Bovine tuberculosis*, London, 1947, Staples.
61. Grange JM, Collins CH: Bovine tubercle bacilli and disease in animals and man, *Epidemiol Infect* 92:221, 1987.
62. Karlson AG, Carr DT: Tuberculosis caused by *Mycobacterium bovis*, *Ann Intern Med* 73:979, 1970.
63. Sjoegren I, Sutherland I: Studies of tuberculosis in man in relation to infection in cattle, *Tubercle* 56:113, 1974.
64. Habib NI, Warring FC: A fatal case of infection due to *Mycobacterium bovis*, *Am Rev Respir Dis* 93:804, 1966.
65. Kristjansson M, Green P, Manning HL et al: Molecular confirmation of bacillus Calmette-Guérin as the cause of pulmonary infection following urinary tract instillation, *Clin Infect Dis* 17:228, 1993.

Nontuberculous mycobacteria

66. Castets M, Boisvert H, Grumback F et al: Les bacilles tuberculeux de type africaine, *Rev Tuberc Pneumol* 32:179, 1968.
67. Meissner PS, Falkinham JO III: Plasmid DNA profiles as epidemiological markers for clinical and environmental isolates of *Mycobacterium avium*, *Mycobacterium intracellulare*, and *Mycobacterium scrofulaceum*, *J Infect Dis* 153:325, 1986.
68. Inderlied CB, Kemper CA, Bermudez LEM: The *Mycobacterium avium* complex, *Clin Microbiol Rev* 6:266, 1993.
69. Prince DS: Infection with *Mycobacterium avium* complex in patients without predisposing conditions, *N Engl J Med* 321:863, 1989.
70. Horsburgh CR Jr: *Mycobacterium avium* complex infection in the acquired immunodeficiency syndrome, *N Engl J Med* 324:1332, 1991.
71. Yakrus MA, Good RC: Geographic distribution, frequency, and specimen source of *Mycobacterium avium* complex serotypes isolated from patients with acquired immunodeficiency syndrome, *J Clin Microbiol* 28:926, 1990.
72. Guthertz LS, Damsker B, Bottone EJ et al: *Mycobacterium avium* and *Mycobacterium intracellulare* infections in patients with and without AIDS, *J Infect Dis* 160:1037, 1989.
73. Lincoln EM, Gilber LA: Disease in children due to mycobacteria other than *Mycobacterium tuberculosis*, *Am Rev Respir Dis* 105:683, 1972.
74. Sutker WL, Lankford LL, Tompsett R: Granulomatous synovitis: the role of atypical mycobacteria, *Rev Infect Dis* 1:729, 1979.
75. Pergament M, González R, Fraley EE: Atypical mycobacteriosis of the urinary tract: a case report of extensive disease caused by the Battey bacillus, *JAMA* 229:816, 1974.
76. Wolinsky E: Nontuberculous mycobacteria and associated diseases, *Am Rev Respir Dis* 119:107, 1979.
77. Woods GL, Washington JA II: Mycobacteria other than *Mycobacterium tuberculosis*: review of microbiologic and clinical aspects, *Rev Infect Dis* 9:275, 1987.
78. Prissick FH, Mason AM: Cervical lymphadenitis in children caused by chromogenic mycobacteria, *Can Med Assoc J* 75:798, 1956.
79. Buhler VB, Pollak A: Human infection with atypical acid-fast organisms, *Am J Clin Pathol* 23:363, 1953.
80. Good RC, Snider DE Jr: Isolation of nontuberculous mycobacteria in the United States, *J Infect Dis* 146:829, 1982.
81. Wenger JD, Spika JS, Smithwick RW et al: Outbreak of *Mycobacterium chelonae* infection associated with use of jet injectors, *JAMA* 264:373, 1990.
82. Band JD, Ward JI, Fraser DW: Peritonitis due to a *Mycobacterium chelonei*–like organism associated with intermittent chronic peritoneal dialysis, *J Infect Dis* 145:9, 1982.
83. Bolan G, Reingold AL, Carson LA: Infections with *Mycobacterium chelonei* in patients receiving dialysis and using processed hemodialyzers, *J Infect Dis* 152:1013, 1985.
84. Laskowski LF, Marr JJ, Spernoga JF et al: Fastidious mycobacteria grown from porcine prosthetic heart-valve cultures, *N Engl J Med* 297:101, 1977.
85. Wallace RJ Jr, Swenson JM, Silcox VA et al: Spectrum of disease due to rapidly growing mycobacteria, *Rev Infect Dis* 5:657, 1983.
86. Costrinia AM, Mahler DA, Gross WM et al: Clinical and roentgenographic features of nosocomial pulmonary disease due to *Mycobacterium xenopi*, *Am Rev Respir Dis* 123:104, 1981.
87. Damsker B, Bottone EJ, Deligdisch L: *Mycobacterium xenopi*: infection in an immunocompromised host, *Hum Pathol* 13:866, 1982.
88. Tecson-Tumang FT, Bright JL: *Mycobacterium xenopi* and the acquired immunodeficiency syndrome, *Chest* 86:145, 1984.
89. Marks J, Jenkins PA, Isukamura M: *Mycobacterium szulgai*—a new pathogen, *Tubercle* 53:210, 1972.
90. Schröder KH, Juhlin I: *Mycobacterium malmoense* sp. nov, *Int J Syst Bacteriol* 27:241, 1977.
91. Warren NG, Body BA, Silcox VA, Matthews JH: Pulmonary disease due to *Mycobacterium malmoense*, *J Clin Microbiol* 20:245, 1984.
92. Jenkins PA, Tsukamura M: Infections with *Mycobacterium malmoense* in England and Wales, *Tubercle* 60:71, 1979.
93. Karassova V, Weissfeiler J, Krasznay E: Occurrence of atypical mycobacteria in *Macacus rhesus*, *Acta Microbiol Acad Sci Hung* 12:275, 1965.
94. Aronson JD: Spontaneous tuberculosis in salt water fish, *J Infect Dis* 39:315, 1926.
95. Norden A, Linell F: A new type of pathogenic *Mycobacterium*, *Nature* 168:826, 1951.
96. Gombert ME, Goldstein EJC, Corrado ML et al: Disseminated *Mycobacterium marinum* infection after renal transplantation, *Ann Intern Med* 94:486, 1981.
97. Travis WD, Travis LB, Roberts GD et al: The histopathologic spectrum in *Mycobacterium marinum* infection, *Arch Pathol Lab Med* 109:1109, 1985.
98. Gould WM, McMeekin DR, Bright RD: *Mycobacterium marinum (balnei)* infection: report of a case with cutaneous and laryngeal lesions, *Arch Dermatol* 97:159, 1968.
99. Schönherr U, Naumann GOH, Lang GK, Bialasiewicz AA: Sclerokeratitis caused by *Mycobacterium marinum*, *Am J Ophthamol* 108:607, 1989.

100. Sompolinsky D, Lagziel A, Naveh D, Yankilevitz T: *Mycobacterium haemophilum* sp. nov., a new pathogen of humans, *Int J Syst Bacteriol* 28:67, 1978.
101. Lomvardias S, Madge GE: Chaetoconidium and atypical acid-fast bacilli in skin ulcers, *Arch Dermatol* 106:875, 1972.
102. Feldman RA, Hershfield E: Mycobacterial skin infection by an unidentified species: a report of 29 patients, *Ann Intern Med* 80:445, 1974.
103. Dawson DJ, Blacklock ZM, Kane DW: *Mycobacterium haemophilum* causing lymphadenitis in an otherwise healthy child, *Med J Aust* 2:289, 1981.
104. Gouby A, Branger B, Oules R, Ramuz M: Two cases of *Mycobacterium haemophilum* infection in a renal-dialysis unit, *J Med Microbiol* 25:299, 1988.
105. Centers for Disease Control and Prevention: *Mycobacterium haemophilum* infection—New York City Metropolitan Area, 1990-1991, *MMWR* 40:636, 1991.
106. Wald A, Coyle MB, Carlson LC et al: Infection with a fastidious mycobacterium resembling *Mycobacterium simiae* in seven patients with AIDS, *Ann Intern Med* 117:586, 1992.
107. Dodge OG, Lunn HF: Buruli ulcer: a mycobacterial skin ulcer in a Uganda child, *J Trop Med Hyg* 65:139, 1962.
108. Meyers WM, Shelly WM, Connor DH, Meyers EK: Human *Mycobacterium ulcerans* infections developing at sites of trauma to skin, *Am J Trop Med Hyg* 23:919, 1974.
109. Hayman J: Out of Africa: observations on the histopathology of *Mycobacterium ulcerans* infection, *J Clin Pathol* 46:5, 1993.
110. Weinberger M, Berg SL, Feuerstein IM et al: Disseminated infection with *Mycobacterium gordonae*: report of a case and critical review of the literature, *Clin Infect Dis* 14:1229, 1992.
111. Kurnik PB, Padmanabh U, Bonatsos C, Cynamon MH: *Mycobacterium gordonae* as a human hepato-peritoneal pathogen, with a review of the literature, *Am J Med Sci* 285:45, 1983.
112. Lohr DC, Goeken JA, Doty DB, Donta ST: *Mycobacterium gordonae* infection of a prosthetic aortic valve, *JAMA* 239:1528, 1978.
113. Blacklock ZM, Dawson DJ, Kane DW, McEvoy D: *Mycobacterium asiaticum* as a potential pulmonary pathogen for humans: a clinical and bacteriologic review of five cases, *Am Rev Respir Dis* 127:241, 1983.
114. Weitzman I, Osadczyi D, Corrado ML, Karp D: *Mycobacterium thermoresistibile*: a new pathogen for humans, *J Clin Microbiol* 14:593, 1981.
115. Dechairo DC, Kittredge D, Meyers A, Corrales J: Septic arthritis due to *Mycobacterium triviale*, *Am Rev Respir Dis* 108:1224, 1973.
116. Edwards MS, Huber TW, Baker CJ: *Mycobacterium terrae* synovitis and osteomyelitis, *Am Rev Respir Dis* 117:161, 1978.
117. Tsukamura M, Kita N, Otsuka W, Shimoide H: A study of the taxonomy of the *Mycobacterium nonchromogenicum* complex and report of six cases of lung infection due to *Mycobacterium nonchromogenicum*, *Microbiol Immunol* 27:219, 1983.
118. Casimir MT, Fainstein V, Papadopolous N: Cavitary lung infection caused by *Mycobacterium flavescens*, *South Med J* 75:253, 1982.
119. Wallace RJ Jr, Nash DR, Tsukamura M et al: Human disease due to *Mycobacterium smegmatis*, *J Infect Dis* 158:52, 1988.
120. Davison MB, McCormack JG, Blacklock ZM et al: Bacteremia caused by *Mycobacterium neoaurum*, *J Clin Microbiol* 26:762, 1988.
121. Chiodini RJ: Crohn's disease and the mycobacterioses: a review and comparison of two disease entities, *Clin Microbiol Rev* 2:90, 1989.

Leprosy

122. Brody SJ: *The disease of the soul: leprosy in medieval literature*, Ithaca, NY, 1974, Cornell University Press.
123. Rees RJW, McDougall AC: Airborne infection with *Mycobacterium leprae* in mice, *J Med Microbiol* 10:63, 1977.
124. de Wit MYL, Douglas JT, McFadden J, Klatser PR: Polymerase chain reaction for detection of *Mycobacterium leprae* in nasal swab specimens, *J Clin Microbiol* 31:502, 1993.
125. Leiker DL: On the mode of transmission of *Mycobacterium leprae*, *Lepr Rev* 48:9, 1977.
126. Walsh GP, Storrs EE, Burchfield HP et al: Leprosy-like disease occurring naturally in armadillos, *J Reticuloendothelial Soc* 18:347, 1975.
127. Smith JH, Folse DS, Long EG et al: Leprosy in wild armadillos *(Dasypus novemcinctus)* of the Texas Gulf Coast: epidemiology and mycobacteriology, *J Reticuloendothel Soc* 34:75, 1983.
128. Walsh GP, Meyers WM, Binford CH et al: Leprosy as a zoonosis: an update, *Acta Leprol* 6:51, 1988.
129. Truman RW, Kumaresan JA, McDonough CM et al: Seasonal and spatial trends in the detectability of leprosy in wild armadillos, *Epidemiol Infect* 106:549, 1991.
130. Lumpkin LR, Cox GF, Wolf JE: Leprosy in five armadillo handlers, *J Am Acad Dermatol* 9:899, 1983.
131. West BC, Todd JR, Lary CH et al: Leprosy in six isolated residents of northern Louisiana: time-clustered cases in an essentially nonendemic area, *Arch Intern Med* 148:1987, 1988.
132. Noordeen SK: Epidemiology and control of leprosy—a review of progress over the last 30 years, *Trans R Soc Trop Med Hyg* 87:515, 1993.
133. *MMWR*, US Department of Health & Human Services, Centers for Disease Control and Prevention, HHS Publ CDC 93-8017, Jan 7, 1994, p 1002.
134. Wade HW, Prieto JG, Vegas M et al: Technical resolution on classification at the VI International Congress of Leprosy, Madrid, 1953, *Int J Lepr* 21:504, 1953.
135. Ridley DS, Jopling WH: Classification of leprosy according to immunity: a five-group system, *Int J Lepr* 34:255, 1966.
136. WHO Expert Committee on Leprosy: *Chemotherapy of leprosy for control programmes*, Geneva, 1982, WHO Tech Rep ser no 675.
137. Williams DL, Gillis TP: A study of relatedness of *Mycobacterium leprae* isolates using restriction fragment length polymorphism analysis, *Acta Leprol* 7(suppl 1):226, 1989.
138. Britton WJ: Leprosy 1962-1992: immunology of leprosy, *Trans R Soc Trop Med Hyg* 87:508, 1993.
139. Schlesinger LS, Horwitz MA: Complement receptors and complement component C3 mediate phagocytosis of *Mycobacterium tuberculosis* and *Mycobacterium leprae*, *Int J Lepr* 58:200, 1990.
140. Rojas-Espinosa O: Macrophages, myeloperoxidase, and *Mycobacterium lepraemurium*, *J Leukoc Biol* 43:468, 1988.
141. Lad SJ, Mahadevan PR: Adherence of *Mycobacterium leprae* to macrophage as an indicator of pathogen induced membrane changes, *Indian J Med Res* 76:804, 1982.
142. Birdi TJ, Mistry NF, Mahadevan PR, Antia NH: Alterations in the membrane of macrophages from leprosy patients, *Infect Immun* 41:121, 1983.
143. Salgame PR, Mahadevan PR, Antia NH: Mechanism of immunosuppression in leprosy: presence of suppressor factor(s) from macrophages of lepromatous patients, *Infect Immun* 40:1119, 1983.
144. Collings LA, Waters MFR, Poulter LW: The involvement of dendritic cells in the cutaneous lesions associated with tuberculoid and lepromatous leprosy, *Clin Exp Immunol* 62:458, 1985.
145. Munro CS, Campbell DA, Collings LA, Poulter LW: Monoclonal antibodies distinguish macrophages and epithelioid cells in sarcoidosis and leprosy, *Clin Exp Immunol* 68:282, 1987.
146. Nerland AH, Mustafa AS, Sweetser D et al: A protein antigen of *Mycobacterium leprae* is related to a family of small heat shock proteins, *J Bacteriol* 170:5919, 1988.
147. Young D, Lathigra R, Hendrix R et al: Stress proteins are immune targets in leprosy and tuberculosis, *Proc Natl Acad Sci USA* 85:4267, 1988.
148. Myrvang B, Godal T, Ridley DS et al: Immune responsiveness to *Mycobacterium leprae* and other mycobacterial antigens throughout the clinical and histopathological spectrum of leprosy, *Clin Exp Immunol* 14:541, 1973.
149. Dwyer JM, Bullock WE, Fields JP: Disturbances of the blood T:B lymphocyte ratio in lepromatous leprosy, *N Engl J Med* 288:1036, 1973.
150. Rea TH, Bakke AC, Parker JW et al: Peripheral blood T-lymphocyte subsets in leprosy, *Int J Lepr* 52:311, 1984.
151. Modlin RL, Gebhard JF, Taylor CR, Rea TH: *In situ* characterization of T-lymphocyte subsets in the reactional states of leprosy, *Clin Exp Immunol* 53:17, 1983a.
152. Modlin RL, Hofman FM, Taylor CR, Rea TH: T-lymphocyte subsets in the skin lesions of patients with leprosy, *J Am Acad Dermatol* 8:181, 1983b.

153. Mohagheghpour N, Gelber RR, Engleman EG: T-cell defect in lepromatous leprosy is reversible in vitro in the absence of exogenous growth factors, *J Immunol* 138:570, 1987.
154. Mehra V, Mason LH, Rothman W et al: Delineation of a human T-cell subset responsible for lepromin-induced suppression in leprosy patients, *J Immunol* 125:1183, 1980.
155. Mehra V, Brennan PJ, Rada E et al: Lymphocyte suppression in leprosy induced by unique *M. leprae* glycolipid, *Nature* 308:194, 1984.
156. Kaplan G, Sampaio EP, Walsh GP et al: Influence of *Mycobacterium leprae* and its soluble products on the cutaneous responsiveness of leprosy patients to antigen and recombinant interleukin-2, *Proc Natl Acad Sci USA* 86:6269, 1989.
157. Prasad HK, Mishra RS, Nath I: Phenolic glycolipid-I of *Mycobacterium leprae* induces general suppression of in vitro concanavalin A responses unrelated to leprosy type, *J Exp Med* 165:239, 1987.
158. Nogueira N, Kaplan G, Levy E et al: Defective γ-interferon production in leprosy: reversal with antigen and interleukin-2, *J Exp Med* 158:2165, 1983.
159. Modlin RL, Melancon-Kaplan J, Young SMM et al: Learning from lesions: patterns of tissue inflammation in leprosy, *Proc Natl Acad Sci USA* 85:1213, 1988.
160. Kaplan G, Mathur NK, Job CK et al: Effect of multiple interferon injections on the disposal of *Mycobacterium leprae, Proc Natl Acad Sci USA* 86:8073, 1989a.
161. Turk JL: Cell-mediated immunological processes in leprosy, *Lepr Rev* 41:207, 1970.
162. Frehel C, Rastogi N: *Mycobacterium leprae* surface components intervene in the early phagosome-lysosome fusion inhibition event, *Infect Immun* 55:2916, 1987.
163. Hokama Y, Dayaon E, Iwamoto L et al: Significant enhanced superoxide anion (O_2^-) production in vitro by peripheral blood monocytes of lepromatous leprosy patients stimulated with liposome and suppression by C-reactive protein (CRP), *J Med Clin Exp Theor* 17:299, 1986.
164. Holzer TJ, Arnold JJ, Vachula M, Andersen BR: Phenolic glycolipid-I of *Mycobacterium leprae* induces altered monocyte oxidative responses *in vitro, Int J Lepr* 55:784, 1987.
165. Purtilo DT, Meyers WM, Connor DH: Fatal strongyloidiasis in immunosuppressed patients, *Am J Med* 56:488, 1974.
166. Hastings RC, Gillis TP, Krahenbuhl JL, Franzblau SG: Leprosy, *Clin Microbiol Rev* 1:330, 1988.
167. Fine PEM, Job CK, McDougall AC et al: Comparability among histopathologists in the diagnosis and classification of lesions suspected of leprosy in Malawi, *Int J Lepr* 54:614, 1986.
168. Fine PEM, Job CK, Lucas SB et al: Extent, origin, and implications of observer variation in the histopathological diagnosis of suspected leprosy, *Int J Lepr* 61:270, 1993.
169. Ridley DS: *Skin biopsy in leprosy,* ed 3, Basle, 1990, CIBA-Geigy.
170. Fleury RN, Bacchi CE: S-100 protein and immunoperoxidase technique as an aid in the histopathologic diagnosis of leprosy, *Int J Lepr* 55:338, 1987.
171. Wallach D, Flageul B, Bach M, Cottenot F: The cellular content of dermal leprous granulomas: an immuno-histological approach, *Int J Lepr* 52:318, 1984.
172. Mukherjee A, Meyers WM: Endothelial cell bacillation in lepromatous leprosy: a case report, *Lepr Rev* 58:419, 1987.
173. Mukherjee A, Misra SR, Meyers WMM: An electron microscopy study of lymphatics in the dermal lesions of human biopsy, *Int J Lepr* 57:506, 1989.
174. Quismorio FP, Rea T, Chandor S et al: Lucio's phenomenon: an immune complex deposition syndrome in leprosy, *Clin Immunol Immunopathol* 9:184, 1978.
175. Ridley MJ, Ridley DS: Histoid leprosy: an ultrastructural observation, *Int J Lepr* 48:135, 1980.
176. Rodriguez JN: The histoid leproma: its characteristics and significance, *Int J Lepr* 37:1, 1969.
177. Anonymous: Ocular complications of leprosy (Editorial), *Lancet* 340:642, 1992.
178. Johnstone PAS, George AD, Meyers WM: Ocular lesions in leprosy, *Ann Ophthalmol* 23:297, 1991.
179. ffytche TJ, McDougall AC: Leprosy and the eye: a review, *J R Soc Med* 78:397, 1985.
180. Rajan MA: Eye in multidrug therapy, *Indian J Lepr* 62:33, 1990.
181. Lowe J: Tuberculoid changes in lymph nodes in leprosy, *Int J Lepr* 7:73, 1939.
182. Sharma KD, Shrivastav JB: Lymph nodes in leprosy, *Int J Lepr* 40:41, 1958.
183. Malin AS, Waters MFR, Shehade SA, Roberts MM: Leprosy in reaction: a medical emergency, *Br Med J* 302:1324, 1991.
184. Naafs B: Reactions in leprosy. In Ratledge C, Stanford J, Grange JM, editors. *The biology of the mycobacteria*, vol 3, London, 1989, Academic Press.
185. Janssen F, Wallach D, Khuong MA et al: Association de maladie de Hansen et d'infection par le virus de l'immuno-déficience humaine: deux observations, *Presse Méd* 17:1652, 1988.
186. Lamfers EJP, Bastiaans AH, Mravunac M, Rampen FHJ: Leprosy in the acquired immunodeficiency syndrome, *Ann Intern Med* 107:111, 1987.
187. Moran CA, Nelson AM, Tuur SM et al: Leprosy in five HIV infected patients. *Mod Pathol* 8:662, 1995.
188. Meeran K: Prevalence of HIV infection among patients with leprosy and tuberculosis in rural Zambia, *Br Med J* 298:364, 1989.
189. Péan C, Pape JW, Deschamps MM, Dambreville M: Prévalence et évolution de l'infection au virus humain d'immunodéficience chez les lépreux en Haïti, *Int J Lepr* 57:306, 1989.
190. ShivRaj L, Patil SA, Girdhar A et al: Antibodies to HIV-1 in sera from patients with mycobacterial infections, *Int J Lepr* 56:546, 1988.
191. Kashala O, Marlink R, Ilunga M et al: Infection with human immunodeficiency virus type 1 (HIV-1), human T cell lymphotropic virus type 1 (HTLV-1), and type 2 (HTLV-2) among leprosy (patients) and their contacts: correlation between HIV-1 cross-reactivity and antibodies to lipoarabinomannan (LAM), *J Infect Dis.* 169:296, 1994.
192. Williams AD: *AIDS: an African perspective,* Boca Raton, Fla, 1991, CRC Press, pp 100, 239.
193. Lucas SB: Human immunodeficiency virus and leprosy, *Lepr Rev* 64:97, 1993.
194. Johnstone PAS: The search for animal models of leprosy, *Int J Lepr* 55:535, 1987.
195. Binford CH: Comprehensive program for inoculation of human leprosy into laboratory animals, *Public Health Rep* 71:955, 1956.
196. Meyers WM, Gormus BJ, Walsh GP: Experimental leprosy. In Hastings RC, editor: *Leprosy* (Medicine in the Tropics Series), ed 2, Edinburgh, 1994, Churchill Livingstone.
197. Storrs EE: The nine-banded armadillo: a model for leprosy and other biomedical research, *Int J Lepr* 39:703, 1971.
198. Colston MJ, Hilson GRF: Growth of *Mycobacterium leprae* and *M. marinum* in congenitally athymic (nude) mice, *Nature* 262:399, 1976.
199. Meyers WM, Binford CH, Walsh GP et al: Animal models of leprosy. In *Microbiology—1984,* Washington, DC, 1984, American Society for Microbiology.
200. Wolf RH, Gormus BJ, Martin LN et al: Experimental leprosy in three species of monkeys, *Science* 227:529, 1985.
201. Cho S-N, Gormus BJ, Xu K et al: Serologic responses to nerve antigens in sooty mangabey monkeys with experimental leprosy, *Int J Lepr* 61:236, 1993.
202. Gormus BJ, Ohashi DK, Ohkawa S et al: Serologic responses to *Mycobacterium leprae*–specific phenolic glycolipid-I antigen in sooty mangabey monkeys with experimental leprosy, *Int J Lepr* 56:537, 1988.
203. Baskin GB, Gormus BJ, Martin LN et al: Pathology of dual *Mycobacterium leprae* and simian immunodeficiency virus infection in rhesus monkeys, *Int J Lepr Other Mycobact Dis* 58:358, 1990.
204. Gormus BJ, Murphey-Corb M, Martin LN et al: Interactions between simian immunodeficiency virus and *Mycobacterium leprae* in experimentally inoculated rhesus monkeys, *J Infect Dis* 160:405, 1989.
205. Truman RW, Job CK, Hastings RC: Antibodies to the phenolic glycolipid-I antigen for epidemiologic investigations of enzootic leprosy in armadillos (*Dasypus novemcinctus*), *Lepr Rev* 61:19, 1990.
206. Leininger JR, Donham KJ, Meyers WM: Leprosy in a chimpanzee: postmortem lesions, *Int J Lepr* 48:414, 1980.
207. Gormus BJ, Xu K, Alford PL et al: A serologic study of naturally-acquired leprosy in chimpanzees, *Int J Lepr* 59:450, 1991.

208. Meyers WM, Walsh GP, Brown HL et al: Leprosy in a mangabey monkey—naturally acquired infection, *Int J Lepr* 53:1, 1985.
209. Gormus BJ, Wolf RH, Baskin GB et al: A second sooty mangabey monkey with naturally acquired leprosy: first reported possible monkey-to-monkey transmissio, *Int J Lepr* 56:61, 1988.
210. Klatser PR, van Beers S, Madjid B et al: Detection of *Mycobacterium leprae* nasal carriers in populations for which leprosy is endemic, *J Clin Microbiol* 31:2947, 1993.
211. Meyers WM, Gormus BJ, Walsh GP: Nonhuman sources of leprosy, *Int J Lepr* 60:477, 1992.
212. Kazda J, Irgens LM, Müller K: Isolation of non-cultivable acid-fast bacilli in sphagnum moss vegetation by foot pad technique in mice, *Int J Lepr* 48:1, 1980.
213. Kazda J, Irgens LM, Kolk AHJ: Acid-fast bacilli found in sphagnum vegetation of coastal Norway containing *Mycobacterium leprae*–specific phenolic glycolipid-1, *Int J Lep* 58:353, 1990.

Treatment and prevention

214. American Thoracic Society: Diagnosis and treatment of disease caused by nontuberculous mycobacteria, *Am Rev Respir Dis* 142:940, 1990.
215. Sanders WE Jr, Horowitz EA: Other *Mycobacterium* species. In Mandell GL, Douglas RG Jr, Bennett JE, editors: *Principles and practice of infectious diseases*, ed 3, New York, 1990, Churchill Livingstone.
216. Faget GH, Pogge RC, Johansen FA et al: The Promin treatment of leprosy: a progress report, *Pub Hlth Rep* 58:1729, 1943.
217. Pettit JHS, Rees RJW: Sulphone resistance in leprosy: an experimental and clinical study, *Lancet* 2:673, 1964.
218. Pearson JMH: The problem of dapsone-resistant leprosy, *Int J Lepr* 49:417, 1981.
219. Depasquale G: Rifampicin and isoprodian in combination in the treatment of leprosy, *Lepr Rev* 46(suppl):179, 1975.
220. Freerksen E: Preliminary experience with combined therapy using rifampicin and isoprodian (L73A), *Lepr Rev* 46(suppl):161, 1975.
221. Waters MFR: Chemotherapy of leprosy: current status and future prospects, *Trans R Soc Trop Med Hyg* 87:500, 1993.
222. Centers for Disease Control and Prevention: Use of BCG vaccines in the control of tuberculosis: a joint statement by the ACIP and the Advisory Committee for the Elimination of Tuberculosis, *MMWR* 37:663, 1988.
223. Barenfanger J: Making your lab safe against multi-drug-resistant *Mycobacterium tuberculosis*, *Clin Microbiol Newslett* 15:76, 1993.
224. Clemens JD, Chuong JJH, Feinsten AR: The BCG controversy: a methodological and statistical reappraisal, *JAMA* 249:2362, 1983.
225. Tripathy SP: Fifteen-year follow-up of the Indian BCG prevention trial. In International Union Against Tuberculosis, editors: *Proceedings of the XXVIth IUAT World Conference on Tuberculosis and Respiratory Diseases*, Singapore, Japan, 1987, Professional Postgraduate Services International.
226. Centers for Disease Control and Prevention: Disseminated *Mycobacterium bovis* infection from BCG vaccination of a patient with acquired immunodeficiency syndrome, *MMWR* 34:227, 1985.
227. Blanche S, LeDeist F, Fischer A: Longitudinal study of 18 children with perinatal LAV/HTLV III infection: attempt at prognostic evaluation, *J Pediatr* 109:965, 1986.
228. World Health Organization: Special Programme on AIDS and Expanded Programme on Immunization—joint statement: consultation on human immunodeficiency virus (HIV) and routine childhood immunization, *Wkly Epidemiol Rep* 62:297, 1987.
229. Stewart-Tull DES: Vaccines against leprosy, *Adv Biotechnol Processes* 13:201, 1990.

35 Rickettsial and Chlamydial Diseases

David H. Walker
J. Stephen Dumler

Rickettsiae and chlamydiae, including members of the genera *Rickettsia, Coxiella, Ehrlichia,* and *Chlamydia,* are obligate intracellular gram-negative bacteria. These microorganisms have never been cultivated outside of eukaryotic cells and thus occupy an interesting ecologic niche. Intracellular parasitism is necessary for their survival in nature.[1] It should be recognized that bacterial interactions with human cells form a range from free-living bacteria, such as *Pseudomonas aeruginosa,* to obligately intracellular rickettsiae and chlamydiae. Intermediate positions in the range of bacterium-host cell interaction include facultative intracellular bacteria (such as, *Mycobacterium, Legionella, Brucella, Listeria, and Salmonella),* which may grow within or outside of host cells, and extracellular organisms, such as *Bartonella (Rochalimaea),* which appear to grow best attached to the outside of the host cell.

Although superficially sharing a relationship to their host cells, these bacteria have evolved into a variety of phenotypes with a wide range of genetic relatedness (Table 35-1). *Rickettsia* species of the spotted fever and typhus groups are closely related to one another and have evolved only a short distance from *Ehrlichia, Bartonella,* the plant pathogen, *Agrobacter tumefaciens,* and mitochondria.[2] In contrast, *Chlamydia* and *Coxiella* have evolved great distances from *Rickettsia* and from one another. *Coxiella* is actually more closely related to *Legionella* than to any of the obligately intracellular bacteria. *Rickettsia tsutsugamushi,* a unique bacterium, deserves an independent genus. Many of these obligately intracellular and related bacteria cause zoonoses, a disease that is spread to humans from a reservoir in other animals. *Chlamydia psittaci* is spread to poultry workers from infected turkeys and other fowl and to those who own and sell infected pet birds. *Coxiella burnetii* is transmitted mainly in aerosol from infected ruminants, especially from the placentas of infected sheep, goats, and cattle. Rickettsiae are transmitted to humans from infected ticks, mites, chiggers, lice, and fleas.[3,4] As a group the zoonoses exist independently of humans, who are infected only accidentally and who only rarely shed the organism back into nature. *Chlamydia trachomatis* and *C. pneumoniae* are the only obligately intracellular bacteria that are routinely transmitted directly from one person to another.

Because these bacteria are cultivated with much more difficulty[5] and, in some instances, with more danger than other bacteria,[6] diagnosis is less often documented by isolation of the agent. More often a tentative diagnosis is made on clinical grounds, and later, acute and convalescent sera are tested to demonstrate the appearance or rise in titer of specific antibodies.[7] In contrast, cultivation of *C. trachomatis* has become a routine procedure in many hospital laboratories. Clinically useful diagnostic tools have been developed to demonstrate specific rickettsial and chlamydial antigens and nucleic acids in specimens from the patient.[8-12]

RICKETTSIAL DISEASES

Rickettsiae are small, obligately intracellular bacteria that reside in an arthropod host at least in part as their ecologic niche. The fact that the diverse organisms *Rickettsia, Ehrlichia, Bartonella (Rochalimaea),* and *Coxiella* have been considered as rickettsiae indicates that the concept itself may be outmoded. Organisms of *Bartonella* are not even obligately intracellular, having been cultivated in cell-free media. The different target cells of *Rickettsia, Ehrlichia,* and *Coxiella* result in diverse pathologic lesions and clinical manifestations (Table 35-2).

Spotted fever group rickettsioses

Rocky Mountain spotted fever

Etiology. *Rickettsia rickettsii* and R. prowazekii, the etiologic agents of Rocky Mountain spotted fever and louse-borne epidemic typhus fever, respectively, are prototype examples of the more than 20 *Rickettsia* species of the spotted fever and typhus groups. These organisms, including numerous nonpathogenic species, have 40% to 94% DNA homology. Species identification is determined by surface antigens, either proteins or lipopolysaccharides, and by genetic analysis. These thin

Table 35-1 Host interactions and phenotypic properties of obligately intracellular and related bacteria

Taxonomic group	Target cell	Location	Cell-free cultivation	ATP energy source	Cell wall		Developmental cycle	Plasmid
					LPS	Peptidoglycan		
Rickettsia (spotted fever and typhus groups)	Endothelium	Cytosol	n	Independent synthesis and parasitism	+	+	n	n
Rickettsia tsutsugamushi	Poorly documented	Cytosol	n	Independent synthesis	n	n	n	n
Ehrlichia	Mononuclear and polymorphonuclear phagocytes	Endosome	n	Independent synthesis	n	+	n	n
Coxiella	Mononuclear phagocytes	Phagolysosome	n	Independent synthesis	+	+	Proposed	+
Chlamydia	Respiratory, conjunctival, and genital epithelium and mononuclear phagocytes	Endosome	n	Obligate parasitism	+	n	+	+
Bartonella (or *Rochalimaea*)	Extracellular	Epicellular	+	Independent synthesis	+	+	n	+

LPS, lipopolysaccharide, *n*, none.

(0.3 μm by 1 to 2 μm) bacilli are highly adapted to the environment of the host endothelial cell cytosol from which they obtain ATP, ADP, AMP, nicotinamide adenine dinucleotide, lysine, proline, other amino acids, and uridine 5′-diphosphoglucose by specific carrier-mediated membrane transport systems.[13]

Epidemiology. With a 20% mortality for previously healthy, active persons in the preantibiotic era, Rocky Mountain spotted fever (RMSF) was among the most severe of infectious diseases.[14,15] The geographic distribution and seasonal variation are determined by human encounter with infected ticks, *Dermacentor variabilis* in the eastern two thirds of the United States, *D. andersoni* in the Rocky Mountains, *Rhipicephalus sanguineus* in Mexico, and *Amblyomma cajennense* in Mexico and Central and South America. Rickettsiae are maintained in nature primarily by vertical transmission from one generation of ticks to the next through infected ova.[16] Even in the parts of the United States with the highest incidence of Rocky Mountain spotted fever, fewer than 0.1% of vector species carry *R. rickettsii*.[4] Originally named because of its recognition in Idaho and Montana and a high incidence in western states, Rocky Mountain spotted fever has declined in the west and is diagnosed in nearly every state, with the highest incidence in southeastern and south-central states. Most cases occur between May and September. The incidence is highest among children and other tick-exposed persons. Long cycles of fluctuation of the incidence and changes in geographic distribution presumably are related to the tick population and tick-rickettsia interactions. Severity of illness is related to host factors and delayed antirickettsial treatment. The fatality-to-case ratio is significantly higher for blacks, males, and patients older than 30 years. Early treatment with doxycycline, tetracycline, or chloramphenicol cures most patients; however, late diagnosis and inappropriate treatment result in an overall mortality of 3%.[17-19]

Clinical features. After an incubation period of 2 to 12 days, the patient develops severe headache, fever, and frequently nausea, vomiting, or abdominal pain. In most cases, a maculopapular rash appears on the wrists and ankles 2 to 5 days later, usually spreads to involve the trunk, palms, and soles and may become petechial.[20,21] Nevertheless, delay or absence of rash and frequent lack of a history of tick bite make misdiagnosis and fatality a genuine problem.[18] In severe cases the patient may manifest signs of meningoencephalitis, noncardiogenic pulmonary edema, skin necrosis, coagulopathy with bleeding, acute renal failure, jaundice, and hypovolemic shock.[19,22] In fatal cases death usually ensues 7 to 15 days after onset of symptoms. There is a fulminant form of Rocky Mountain spotted fever observed most often in glucose-6-phosphate dehydrogenase–deficient black males in which the patient may die before the fifth day of illness.[15]

Pathology. Rickettsial infection injures endothelial cells and some vascular smooth muscle cells of the vasculature in virtually all organs (Fig. 35-1). However, swollen and necrotic endothelium is often difficult to detect in necropsy specimens. In patients who die after a rapid course of illness, vascular damage may be observed without any host response. The

Table 35-2 Rickettsial diseases of humans

Disease	Etiologic agent	Transmission	Pathologic lesion	Geographic distribution
Spotted fever group				
Rocky Mountain spotted fever	*Rickettsia rickettsii*	Tick bite	Microvascular injury involving skin, brain, lungs, and other organs	North and South America
Rickettsialpox	*Rickettsia akari*	Mite bite	Microvascular injury with rash and eschar	U.S.A., Europe, Korea
Boutonneuse fever	*Rickettsia conorii*	Tick bite	Microvascular injury with rash and eschar	Mediterranean and Black Sea basin, Africa, Indian subcontinent
North Asian tick typhus	*Rickettsia sibirica*	Tick bite	Microvascular injury with rash and eschar	Asiatic Russia, China, Mongolia
Queensland tick typhus	*Rickettsia australis*	Tick bite	Microvascular injury with rash and eschar	Australia
Oriental spotted fever	*Rickettsia japonica*	Tick bite	Microvascular injury with rash and eschar	Japan
Typhus group				
Epidemic typhus	*Rickettsia prowazekii*	Louse feces	Microvascular injury involving skin, brain, and other organs	Potentially worldwide, recently in Africa, South America, Central America, Mexico, Asia
Brill-Zinsser disease	*Rickettsia prowazekii*	Reactivation of latent infection	Microvascular injury involving skin, brain, and other organs	Potentially worldwide, including U.S.A., Canada, and eastern Europe
Flying squirrel typhus	*Rickettsia prowazekii*	Ectoparasite of flying squirrel	Microvascular injury involving skin, brain, and other organs	U.S.A.
Murine typhus	*Rickettsia typhi*	Flea feces	Microvascular injury involving skin, brain, and other organs	Worldwide
Scrubtyphus group	*Rickettsia tsutsugamushi*	Chigger bite	Microvascular injury involving skin, brain, lungs, and other organs	Southern Asia, Japan, western Pacific, Indonesia, Australia, Korea, Asiatic Russia, Indian subcontinent, Sri Lanka, China
Ehrlichioses				
Human monocytic ehrlichiosis	*Ehrlichia chaffeensis*	Tick bite	Perivasculitis; granulomas	U.S.A., Europe, Africa, possibly worldwide
Human granulocytic ehrlichiosis	*Ehrlichia* sp. closely related to *E. phagocytophila*	Tick bite	Unknown	U.S.A.
Sennetsu ehrlichiosis	*Ehrlichia sennetsu*	Unknown	Lymphoid hyperplasia	Japan, Malaysia
Q fever	*Coxiella burnetii*	Inhalation of aerosol from infected animals	Pneumonia; granulomas of liver, spleen, and bone marrow; endocarditis	Worldwide
Bartonella infections				
Oroya fever, verruga peruana	Bartonella *bacilliformis*	Sandfly bite	Acute hemolytic anemia; chronic cutaneous angiomas	Western South America
Trench fever	*Bartonella quintana*	Louse feces	Unknown	North America, Europe, probably worldwide
Cat-scratch disease, bacillary angiomatosis and peliosis	*Bartonella henselae*	Kitten scratch or bite	Granulomas, bacillary angiomas, bacillary peliosis of liver and spleen	U.S.A. and Europe, probably worldwide

microscopic lesions that are recognized by pathologists are focal hemorrhages (Fig. 35-2), and the later host response to rickettsial infection is characterized by intramural and perivascular lymphocytes and macrophages (Fig. 35-3). Polymorphonuclear leukocytes (PMNs) are inconspicuous. A very small proportion of infected blood vessels contain thrombi that, if present, are usually eccentric and nonocclusive. Most infected foci compose a large network of contiguous, infected endothelium of the microcirculation. In the skin these foci are located principally in the dermis. In the brain the lesions assume a characteristic appearance, so-called typhus nodules, found most frequently in the brainstem (Fig. 35-4). These perivascular accumulations of mononuclear cells, which measure 100 to 180 μm in diameter, indicate a probable rickettsial infection, though they are not pathognomonic. Other neuropathologic lesions include microinfarcts of white matter and a mild, mononuclear cell–rich leptomeningitis. Lungs are congested and heavy.[23] Microscopic pulmonary lesions include mononuclear interstitial pneumonia and interstitial and alveolar edema and hemorrhages (Fig 35-5).

The heart is grossly normal, except for epicardial or endocardial petechiae, but usually has a mild mononuclear intersti-

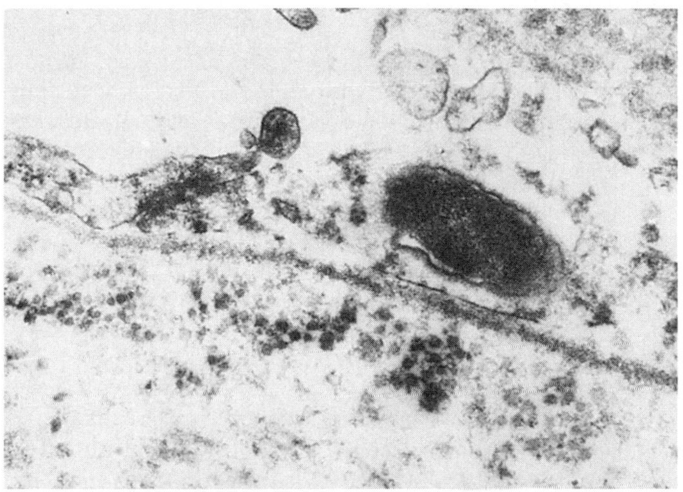

Fig. 35-1 Electron photomicrograph of *Rickettsia rickettsii* in the cytoplasm of an endothelial cell from a patient with Rocky Mountain spotted fever. (From Walker DH: Rickettsial diseases: an update. In Majno G, Cotran R, editors: *The inflammatory process and infectious diseases,* Baltimore, 1981, Williams and Wilkins.)

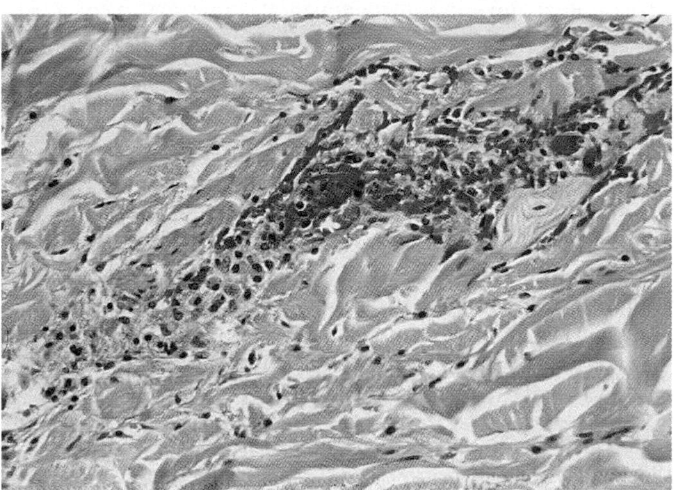

Fig. 35-2 Photomicrograph of dermis from a patient with RMSF and a petechial rash shows perivascular hemorrhage and mild lymphohistiocytic infiltrate. This type of lesion is more apparent to the pathologist than infected endothelium or perivascular edema early in the course of infection.

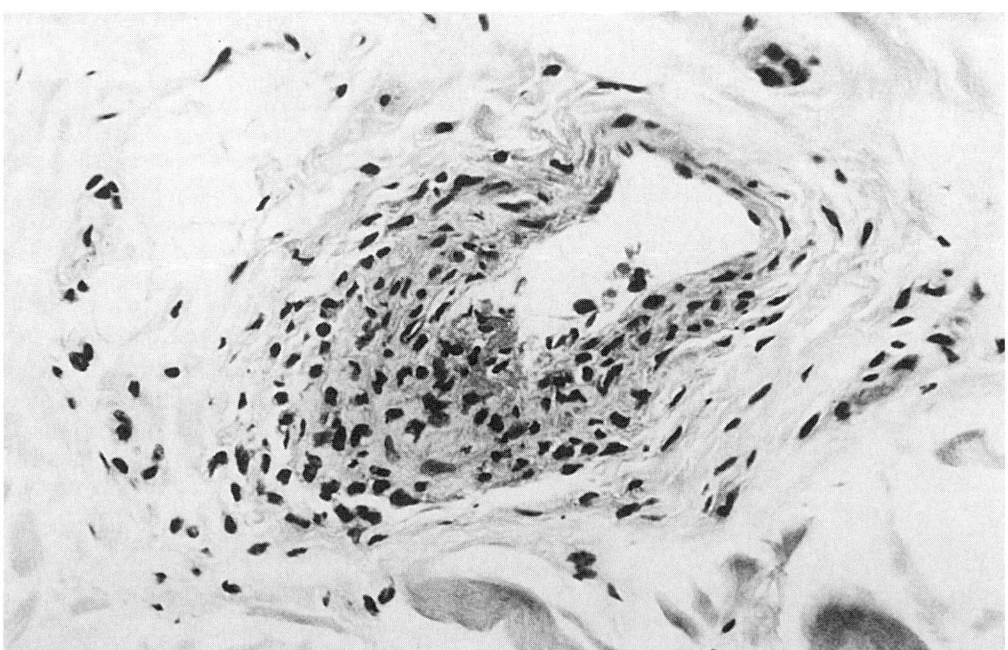

Fig. 35-3 Blood vessel from hemorrahagic skin lesion of patient with Rocky Mountain spotted fever shows characteristic rickettsial vasculitis with infiltration of blood vessel wall and perivascular tissue by mononuclear cells and with small, focal, nonocclusive thrombus. (From Green WR, Walker DH, Cain GG: *Am J Med* 64:523, 1978.)

tial myocarditis on microscopic examination[24-26] (Fig. 35-6). The liver shows portal triaditis and focal hepatic necrosis. Because rickettsiae grow best at temperatures of 32° to 35° C, classical vascular lesions are frequently detected in cooler parts of the body such as the testis and epididymis. Erythrophagocytosis occurs in hepatic Kupffer cells and macrophages within lymph nodes and spleen. In fulminant RMSF there are more thrombi and fewer intramural and perivascular lymphocytes and macrophages in the foci of vascular injury.[27]

Clinicopathologic correlations. Disseminated rickettsial infection[9,28] and microvascular injury results in leakage of intravascular fluid into the interstitial space with consequent edema and hypovolemia.[29] Consumption of platelets and coagulation factors in thrombi at the sites of injury can cause thrombocytopenia and, rarely, more severe coagulopathy. Secretion of antidiuretic hormone in response to the hypovolemic state frequently results in hyponatremia.[30] Focal lesions in the skin are the cause of the rash. Vasodilatation and petechiae are the basis of the cutaneous, erythematous macules and central "spots" respectively. Increased vascular permeability of the infected pulmonary microcirculation may result in noncardiogenic pulmonary edema.[23,31] Myocardial injury is not a significant pathophysiologic factor, though conduction disturbances result in arrhythmias.[26,31,32] Central nervous system lesions are the cause of cerebrospinal fluid (CSF) pleocytosis, coma, seizures, multifocal neurologic signs, and probably cardiorespiratory arrest.[33] Jaundice correlates with hemolysis and portal triad inflammation.[34] Acute renal failure results from hypovolemic, prerenal azotemia or, in more severe cases, acute tubular necrosis.[35] Vasculitis in the gastrointestinal tract and pancreas is the apparent pathologic basis for nausea, vomiting, and abdominal pain and tenderness.[36]

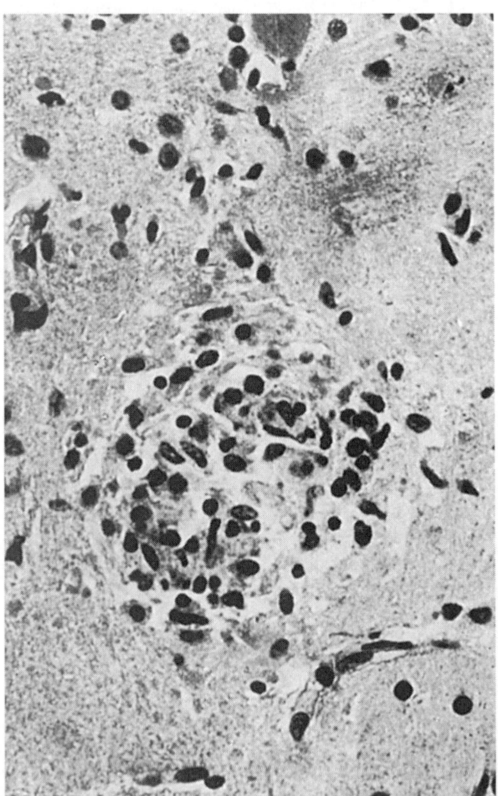

Fig. 35-4 Typhus nodules in gray matter of brain are generally considered to be adjacent to a blood vessel, though the vessel may not always be visible. Histologic components of these inflammatory foci are predominantly macrophages and lymphocytes. (AFIP 78556.)

Pathogenesis. After an attached tick has fed for 6 to 10 hours, rickettsiae released from tick salivary glandular cells are inoculated into the dermis. Rickettsial virulence is reactivated by the warmth of the skin and possibly some constituents of the blood during tick feeding. Rickettsiae apparently spread from the skin through lymphatic and blood vessels to the systemic and pulmonary circulation. Rickettsiae attach to the endothelial cell membrane by a rickettsial surface protein,[37] induce phagocytosis,[38] escape from the phagosome presumably by phospholipase A_2 activity,[39,40] and replicate in the cytosol by binary fission.[8] Rickettsiae escape from the host cell through the ends of long, thin cell projections propelled by host cell actin polymerization[8,41] and enter the bloodstream or adjacent endothelial cells. Rickettsiae kill heavily infected cells directly with prominent injury to the host cell membrane, which becomes increasingly permeable.[8,42] Injury has been associated with free radical–induced membrane damage, phospholipase A_2 activity, and protease activity.[43-45] There are no convincing data to support endotoxin, exotoxin, or immunopathology as pathogenic mechanisms, though interleukin-1 (IL-1), IL-6, and tumor necrosis factor-α (TNF-α) probably play roles in fever, and the acute-phase response and the kallikrein-kinin system may be activated.[46,47] Coagulation is generally appropriately regulated to effect deposition of hemostatic plugs in foci of endothelial necrosis without triggering true disseminated intravascular coagulation. Perivascular T-lymphocytes and macrophages mediate immune destruction of intracellular rickettsiae by secretion of interferon-γ (IFN-γ) and TNF-α, which stimulate target cell synthesis of rickettsicidal nitric oxide.[48,49]

Laboratory diagnosis. Clinical diagnosis is often difficult. The triad of fever, rash, and history of tick bite is present in only 3% of patients during the first 3 days of illness.[50] Nonspecific symptoms and signs often indicate a viral syndrome. Multisystem involvement with prominent manifestations in a particular organ system can lead to misdiagnosis of gastroenteritis, acute surgical abdomen, meningoencephalitis, or pneumonia.[33,34,36,50] Even onset of rash leaves an extensive differential diagnosis including toxic shock syndrome, meningococcemia, secondary syphilis, disseminated gonococcal infection, rubella, measles, infectious mononucleosis, enteroviral exanthema, idiopathic thrombocytopenic purpura, thrombotic thrombocytopenic purpura, and immune complex vasculitis.

Rickettsiae are seldom isolated because of the technical challenge and biohazard concerns. Immunohistologic demonstration of rickettsiae in cutaneous biopsy specimens or necropsy specimens is a specific, relatively sensitive approach to diagnosis[9,28,51] (Fig. 35-7). Although polymerase chain reaction (PCR) on blood samples does not appear to be sufficiently sensitive, except in the late stage of fatal illness, it is likely that PCR examination of rash lesions with *Rickettsia*-specific primers would yield sensitive, specific, and timely results. Serologic diagnosis should not be relied upon during the acute stage of illness when therapeutic decisions are being made.[7,45] However, demonstration of seroconversion by titration of acute and convalescent sera for the presence of antibodies to antigens of *R. rickettsii* (as by indirect fluorescent antibody assay) confirms the diagnosis.

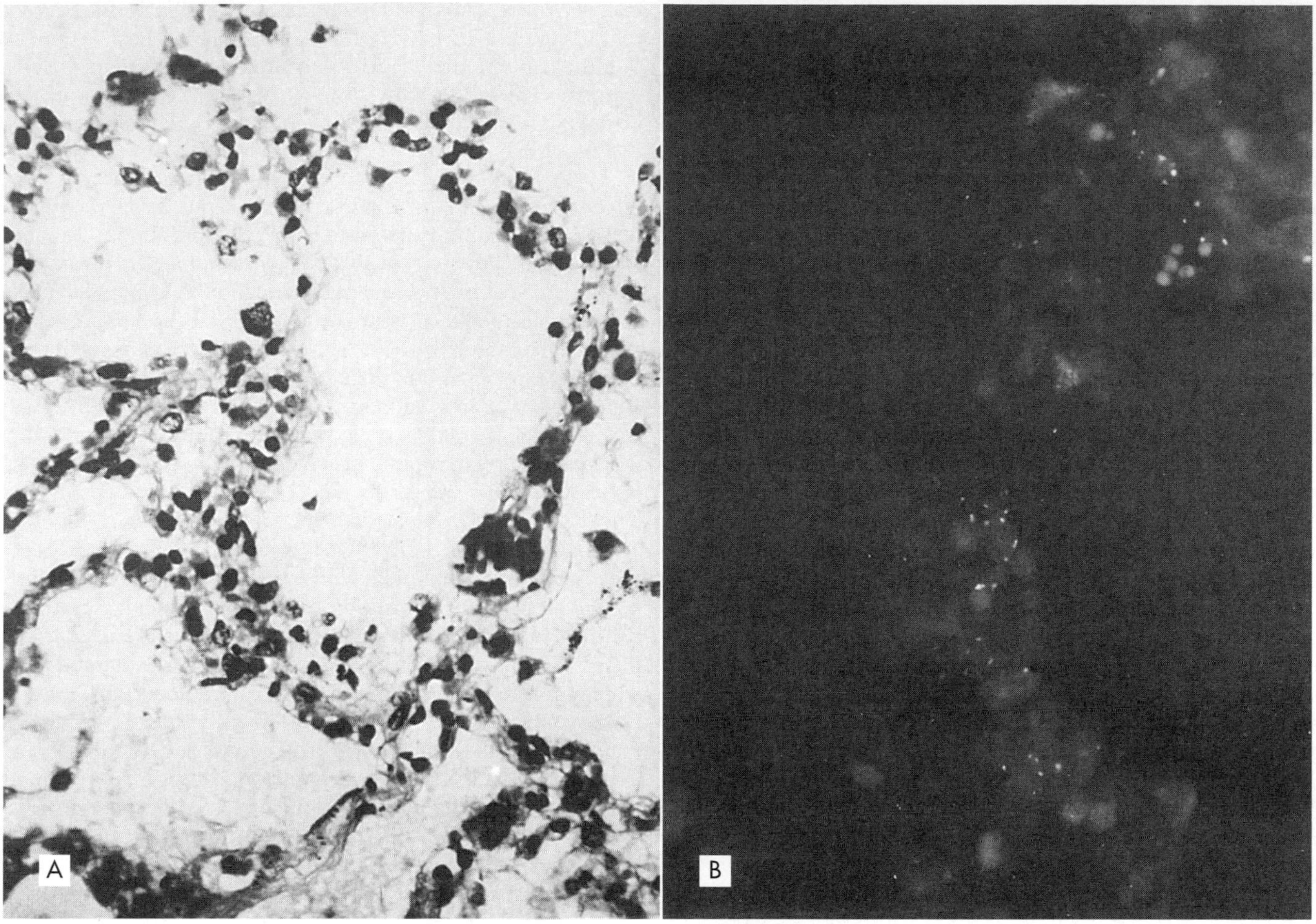

Fig. 35-5 **A,** Interstitial pneumonia of Rocky Mountain spotted fever with mononuclear infiltration of alveolar septa and proteinaceous edema fluid in alveolar spaces. **B,** Immunofluorescent *Rickettsia rickettsii* in thickened alveolar septum is the cause of noncardiogenic pulmonary edema in Rocky Mountain spotted fever. (From Walker DH, Mattern WD: *Am Heart J* 100:896, 1980.)

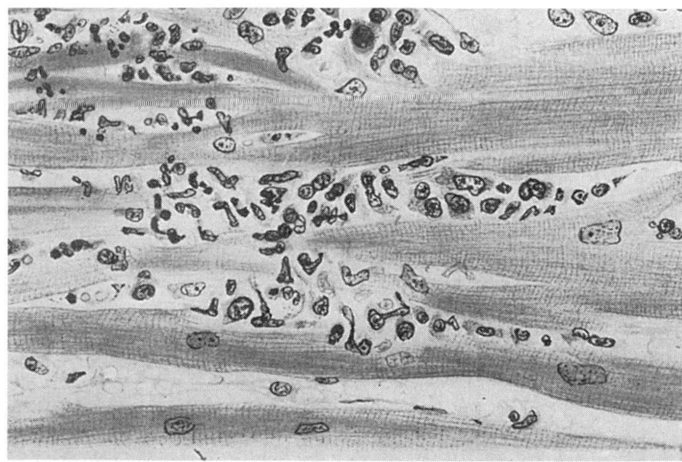

Fig. 35-6 Myocarditis in typhus fever. Infiltration of mononuclear cells and neutrophils between muscle fibers. (From Wolbach SB, Todd JL, Palfrey FW: *The etiology and pathology of typhus,* Cambridge, Mass, 1922, Harvard University Press.)

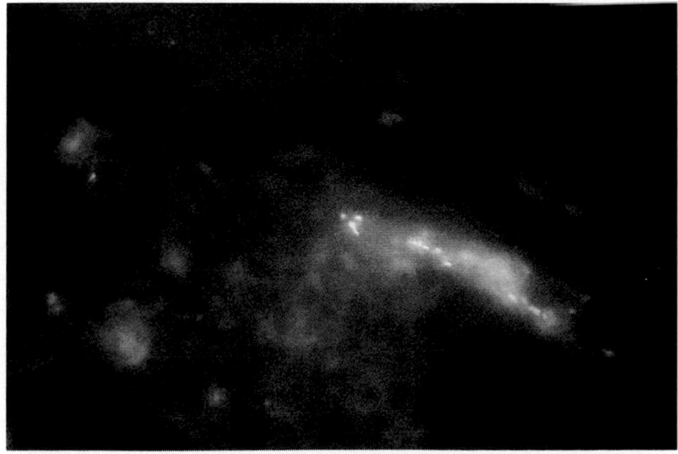

Fig. 35-7 Direct immunofluorescence staining of skin biopsy specimens with anti-*Rickettsia* antibodies facilitates rapid diagnosis. Rickettsiae are present in the vessel wall.

Other spotted fever group rickettsioses

In many parts of the world, spotted fever group rickettsioses are prevalent diseases[52-55] (Table 35-2). Although generally less severe than Rocky Mountain spotted fever, boutonneuse fever, Israeli spotted fever, and Queensland tick typhus have the potential of a fatal outcome.[56,57] Travelers frequently return from the Mediterranean region or Africa with *R. conorii* infections.[58] Boutonneuse fever, North Asian tick typhus, Queensland tick typhus, Oriental spotted fever, and rickettsialpox are usually characterized by the presence of an eschar at the site of the vector bite.[59] This lesion consists of epidermal and dermal necrosis surrounded by a network of blood vessels with infected endothelial cells and perivascular edema.[60-62] Vascular injury and perivascular T-lymphocyte– and macrophage-rich host response are characteristic.[63] Thrombi are seldom a prominent feature.[61] Autopsies of fatal cases of boutonneuse fever show widespread rickettsial vascular endothelial infection and injury involving the brain, kidneys, lungs, gastrointestinal tract, liver, pancreas, heart, and skin.[64,65] Hepatic biopsy specimens reveal multifocal hepatocellular necrosis and lymphohistiocytic response.[66]

Diagnosis of boutonneuse fever can be achieved by shell vial cell culture, immunohistologic demonstration of rickettsiae in biopsy specimens of the rash or eschar, and PCR amplification of rickettsial DNA from tissue samples of lesions.[67] *Rickettsia conorii* can also be detected by immunocytologic examination of circulating damaged endothelial cells captured by immunomagnetic beads coated with a monoclonal antibody to human endothelial cells.[68] Demonstration of seroconversion confirms the diagnosis in convalescence.

Typhus group rickettsioses

Louse-borne typhus fever

Epidemic louse-borne typhus fever is one of the classic scourges of mankind. In times of war, famine, and other disasters, louse infestation, crowding, and malnutrition join forces with *R. prowazekii* to cause explosive epidemics of typhus. It has been postulated that more wars have been lost as a result of epidemic typhus than have been won by battlefield victories. During and just after World War I, 15 million persons suffered from typhus, and more than 3 million died. Infections by *R. prowazekii* occur in the United States as a zoonosis with a reservoir in flying squirrels and their fleas and lice.[69-72] A milder, clinical type of typhus fever, known as Brill-Zinsser disease, occurs as recrudescence of an infection with *R. prowazekii* that has remained latent after acute typhus fever many years previously.[73-75] The reason for the recrudescence is not known.

Organisms of *R. prowazekii* proliferate in the intestinal epithelial cells of the human louse, are shed in its feces, and eventually kill the louse. After entry through human skin, the pathogenic events of typhus parallel those of RMSF and the other rickettsioses with spread through the bloodstream to skin, brain, and other organs. In contrast to RMSF, *R. prowazekii* infection involves only endothelial cells, and the rash begins on the trunk between days 4 and 8 of illness and spreads centrifugally to involve the arms and legs.[76] Pathologic lesions manifest as disseminated mononuclear vasculitis of skin, typhus nodules of brain (Fig. 35-4), interstitial myocarditis (Fig. 35-6), mild interstitial pneumonia, perivascular interstitial nephritis, and portal triaditis. Biopsy specimens of skin of patients with epidemic typhus in Poland at the end of World War I were examined by Wolbach, thus providing a sequence of pathologic lesions. The earliest lesion was swelling of endothelial cells parasitized by rickettsiae. Subsequently, leukocytic infiltration of the vessel wall was observed. The pathophysiology of typhus fever is similar to that of RMSF.[77]

Typhus rickettsiae contain a lipopolysaccharide that is relatively nontoxic.[78,79] In vitro experiments have shown that cell-membrane injury is associated with phospholipase activity.[80,81] The bursting of heavily infected cells is an overt cytolytic effect of *R. prowazekii* infection.[82] In vitro evidence for immune-mediated lysis of infected cells and expression of rickettsial antigens on the surface of infected cells indicate that there may be an undetermined but presumably minor contribution of immunopathologic mechanisms to the disease state.[83-86] Host contributions to the pathophysiologic derangements have been proposed, but their clinical importance is not established.[87]

Murine typhus

Flea-borne infections with *Rickettsia typhi* are likely the most prevalent rickettsiosis around the world, particularly in tropical and subtropical areas.[88] The former occurrence of more than 5000 annual cases of murine typhus in the United States was diminished by the effect of the insecticide DDT on fleas and by rat control. Currently murine typhus is recognized mainly in Texas and California, though throughout the world it is highly prevalent and usually undiagnosed. *R. typhi* is maintained in nature mainly by horizontal transmission in a rat-flea-rat cycle, though other flea species and cycles, such as an opossum–cat flea–opossum cycle, contribute to the epidemiology of murine typhus.[88-90] Humans are usually infected with these agents by scratching rickettsiae-laden flea feces into the skin. After an incubation period of 1 to 2 weeks, widespread endothelial infection results in fever, severe headache, myalgia, and nausea.[91] Rash is detected in only 18% at initial presentation and in 50% over the entire course of illness. Ten percent of patients are ill enough to require admission to an intensive care unit, and 1% die. Vascular infection, injury, and lymphohistiocytic infiltration (Fig. 35-8) may affect any organ, resulting in lesions such as interstitial pneumonia, meningomyeloencephalitis, interstitial myocarditis, interstitial nephritis, and portal triaditis.[92] A novel *Rickettsia* species, maintained transovarially in cat fleas, also appears to cause a similar human disease.[93]

Scrub typhus

Considerable genetic and antigenic differences between scrub typhus rickettsiae and rickettsiae of the spotted fever and typhus groups have led to a proposal to remove *R. tsutsugamushi* to its own independent genus.[94] Organisms of *R. tsutsugamushi* (from Japanese 'dangerous mite') are transmitted to humans by a feeding larval trombiculid mite.[95-97] Transovarian infection of chiggers accounts for the maintenance of *R. tsutsugamushi* in nature.[98] These rickettsiae have great diversity with many antigenically and genetically diverse strains that do not necessarily confer cross-protection, and prior infection does not confer long-term protection against reinfection.[99] Scrub typhus occurs in southern and eastern Asia, Japan, Indonesia, northern Australia, and the islands of the western Pacific. The disease was of military importance during World War II and the Vietnam War with loss of manpower to the morbidity of the infection.[95,96]

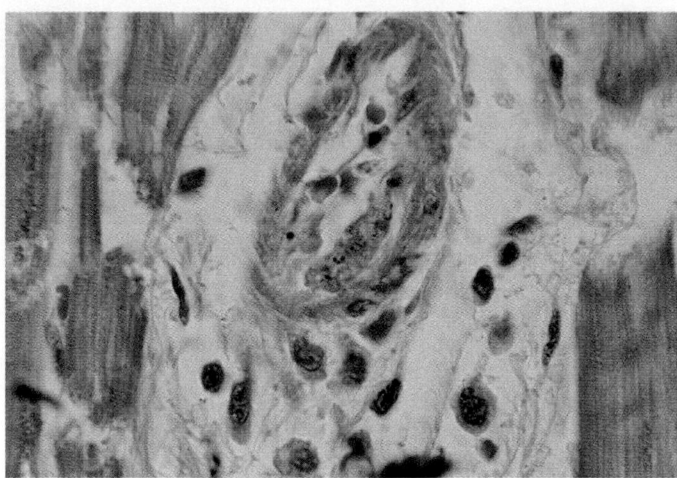

Fig. 35-8 Heart from a patient with murine typhus. Immunoperoxidase stain reveals *Rickettsia typhi* in a blood vessel with an eccentric, nonocclusive thrombus.

The severity of scrub typhus varies from mild to fatal in 7% of untreated patients and has not been correlated with particularly virulent strains or to defined rickettsial virulence traits. After an incubation period of 6 to 21 days, the onset of illness is characterized by fever, headache, and sometimes myalgia, cough, and gastrointestinal symptoms. An eschar appears at the site of chigger feeding in fewer than 50% of patients, usually before the onset of fever. Beginning as a papule, this focus of dermal and epidermal necrosis develops a 2 to 15 mm black crust surrounded by a 5 mm zone of erythema. Regional or generalized lymphadenopathy occurs frequently. A maculopapular rash is observed in fewer than half of the cases and typically appears after 4 to 6 days of illness. Signs and symptoms of interstitial pneumonia and encephalitis are particularly prominent in severe cases.[96]

Vascular injury and perivascular inflammation are observed in the eschar, skin rash, encephalitis, interstitial pneumonia, myocarditis, gastrointestinal tract, pancreas, and kidney.[100] Genuine demonstration of rickettsiae in tissues has rarely been accomplished, and mast cell granules are frequently misinterpreted as rickettsiae. Diagnosis by rickettsial isolation, PCR, and specific serology are technically feasible but are seldom achieved.

EHRLICHIAL DISEASES

At least three species of the genus *Ehrlichia* cause human infection. *Ehrlichia chaffeensis* causes monocytic ehrlichiosis, first described in the United States in 1987[101-103] (Fig. 35-9). *Ehrlichia sennetsu* (from Japanese 'glandular fever') causes an infrequently recognized mononucleosis-like illness in Japan and possibly in other regions of the Far East. An organism closely related to *E. phagocytophila* infects circulating granulocytes in febrile patients with pancytopenia and tick bite.

Characteristics of the agents

Ehrlichiae are obligately intracellular bacteria that infect specific hematopoietic cells.[104] *Ehrlichia chaffeensis* has been identified in ticks, the likely vectors of the disease.[105] Ehrlichiae of veterinary or human importance may be classified based upon (1) tropism for a particular target cell, such as mononuclear phagocytes *(E. chaffeensis, E. canis, E. sennetsu, E. risticii),* granulocytic phagocytes *(E. phagocytophila, E. equi, E. ewingii),* or platelets *(E. platys);* (2) similarities among 16S ribosomal DNA sequences; and (3) serologic cross-reactivity. Infection begins with phagocytosis of the organism after attachment to host cell surface ligands.[106] Ehrlichiae actively inhibit the ehrlichicidal event, phagosome-lysosome fusion.[107] These small, pleomorphic bacteria replicate by binary fission until a membrane-bound cluster, called a *morula*, because of its mulberry appearance, is observed.

In cell culture, infected cells die from cytolysis; however, the mechanism of tissue injury in vivo has not been clarified. Ehrlichiae lack detectable endotoxin components, and an immunopathologic mechanism has been suggested, since few organisms can be demonstrated in blood or tissues of infected, immune competent individuals. Fatal, overwhelming *E. chaffeensis* infection has been observed in two patients, one with human immunodeficiency virus (HIV) infection and a low CD4 count[108] and the other in a patient treated with high-dose corticosteroids,[109] an indication that immune suppression may be a risk factor for severe disease. In both, numerous morulas could be observed in a large percentage of infiltrating and fixed mononuclear phagocytes in hemaloxylin and eosin–stained tissues. Other fatal cases, often dying of opportunistic infections, have contained sparse quantities of ehrlichiae. Patients with ehrlichioses recover after a shortened course of illness when treated early in the course of illness with tetracycline or doxycycline.

Human monocytic ehrlichiosis

The clinical presentation of human ehrlichiosis in the United States often simulates Rocky Mountain spotted fever, except that skin rash is less frequent; leukopenia, thrombocytopenia, and hepatic injury are often present.[110,111] *Ehrlichia chaffeensis* infection varies from subclinical to fatal.[112] Infection is acquired after tick bite, and the ehrlichiae disseminate in blood to infect mononuclear phagocytes. Infection of fixed mononuclear phagocytes elicits a mild-to-moderate inflammatory cell response rich in mononuclear phagocytes and usually characterized by small, noncaseating granulomas, poorly formed histiocytic aggregates, or foamy, histiocytic infiltrates.[108,113]

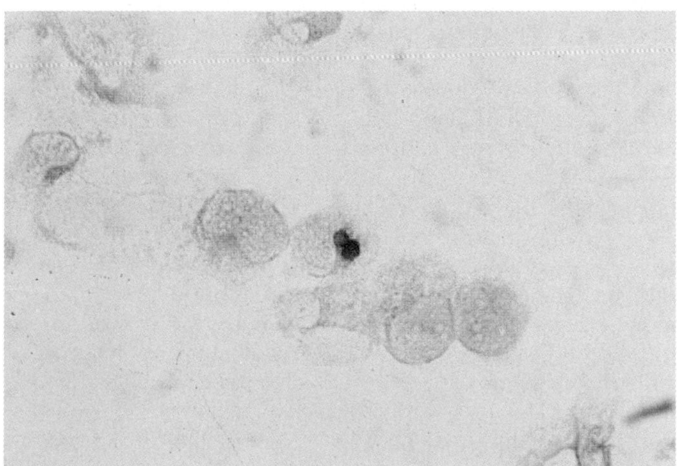

Fig. 35-9 Cells from the cerebrospinal fluid of a patient severely ill with human monocytic ehrlichiosis. Morulas (cytoplasmic vacuoles containing *Ehrlichia chaffeensis*) are stained red by an immunoenzyme method.

Aside from the stereotyped finding of perivascular lymphohistiocytic infiltrates in many tissues, other frequent observations include bone marrow hyperplasia, granulomas in bone marrow and liver, focal hepatocyte necroses with mild Kupffer cell hyperplasia, and hyperplasia of mononuclear phagocytes in spleen and lymph node. In severe cases, necrosis and leukocytoclasis may be observed in many organs.[109] Acute cholangitis with bile stasis has been observed in one case.[114] A mild, chronic, interstitial pneumonia or histiocyte-rich intra-alveolar infiltrate may be observed. In some patients, the meninges and brain have perivascular mononuclear cell infiltrates, and a mononuclear pleocytosis has been observed in the CSF.[109,115] Rarely, morulas may be observed in Wright-stained peripheral blood, bone marrow, or CSF mononuclear cells.[116] The diagnosis can be confirmed by specific serologic assays, immunohistologic demonstration of the organisms,[102, 113, 115, 117-119] and demonstration of ehrlichial nucleic acids in clinical samples.[109,117]

Sennetsu ehrlichiosis

Although first considered a member of the genus *Rickettsia, Erhlichia sennetsu* has been reclassified to reflect its intraphagosomal niche and its serologic cross-reactions with some other ehrlichiae. Both *E. sennetsu* and *E. chaffeensis* are bacterial parasites of mononuclear phagocytes, but the disparity in 16S rDNA sequences indicates that substantial evolutionary distance separates these two human pathogens.[117] Fatal *sennetsu* ehrlichiosis has never been reported. A vector has never been clearly identified, and thus the mode of transmission is unknown. The pathology is not well studied, but reports indicate that lymph nodes, spleen, liver, and bone marrow have diffuse and focal increases in mononuclear phagocytes, similar to findings in some cases of human ehrlichiosis.[120]

Human granulocytic ehrlichiosis

The strongest candidates for the etiologic agent of human granulocytic ehrlichiosis, a newly identified, potentially fatal ehrlichial disease of humans, include *E. phagocytophila* and *E. equi,* granulocytic ehrlichiae of bovines and ovines in Europe and horses in North America respectively.[118] Clinical findings are similar to human ehrlichiosis caused by *E. chaffeensis.* Fever, headache, and myalgias are prominent, and leukopenia, thrombocytopenia, and anemia are present in the majority of patients.[121] Diagnosis is made by the observation of the characteristic morulas in granulocytes in Wright-stained peripheral blood smears only during the acute illness (Fig. 35-10). Unlike *E. chaffeensis* infection, the agent of human granulocytic ehrlichiosis achieves substantial levels of morula-containing cells in the peripheral blood. Definitive identification has been made only by molecular analysis of the bacterial DNA extracted from clinical samples because granulocytic ehrlichiae have never been cultivated in vitro. The pathologic findings in one fatal case are similar to those of *E. chaffeensis* infection, except that morulas were more readily appreciated by tissue Giemsa stains. Secondary infection by nosocomial and opportunistic pathogens has also been observed in two fatal cases. The discovery of this new human ehrlichial infection by molecular methods is another example of our incomplete understanding of infections caused by noncultivable infectious agents and how technologic advances further our ability to identify and eventually treat previously undiagnosed conditions.

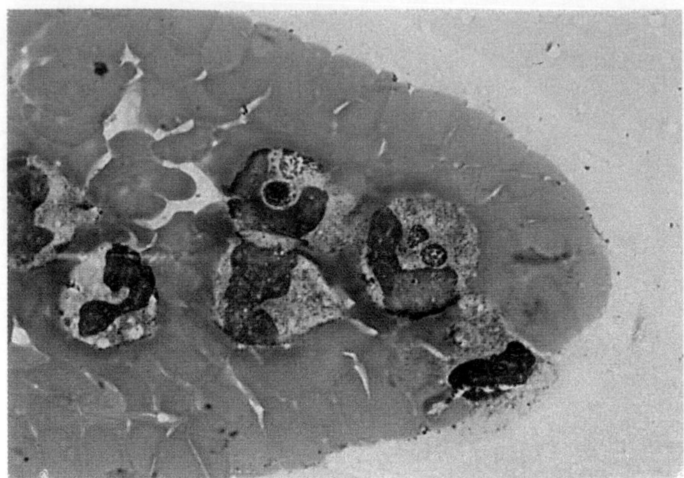

Fig 35-10 Peripheral blood smear of a patient with human granulocytic ehrlichiosis contains immature granulocytes with cytoplasmic vacuoles filled with ehrlichiae closely related to *E. phagocytophila.*

Q FEVER

Etiology. The causative agent of Q ('query') fever, *Coxiella burnetii,* occurs worldwide and is among the most highly infectious of all bacteria. Despite perceived similarities with *Rickettsia* species, *C. burnetii* is genetically unique. Surface lipopolysaccharide (LPS) changes from smooth to rough after serial cultivation outside of animal hosts and serologic responses to these phase I or phase II LPSs correlate with chronic and acute Q fever. The full-thickness phase I LPS probably helps to protect the bacterium from intracellular killing, inflammatory damage, and immune injury. With exposure of the cell wall proteins associated with the truncated LPS of phase II mutation, the organisms are effectively killed.[122] Electron microscopy reveals different structures, which indicate a probable developmental cycle and sporulation, attractive explanations for the latency and environmental stability of *C. burnetii.*[123] In fact, *C. burnetii* thrives in the acidic environment of the phagolysosome of mononuclear phagocytes as a result of specialized evolutionary adaptations. Particular plasmid and chromosomal DNA sequences and LPS types have not been convincingly associated with acute or chronic disease, and host factors may be the critical determinants of the course of infection.[124,125]

Epidemiology. Unlike arthropod-borne rickettsiae, *C. burnetii* is transmitted by aerosol or by ingestion of contaminated dairy products.[126,127] Infections are associated with abattoirs, parturient cows, sheep, goats, some household pets, and wild animals, including rabbits and deer.[126-128] Many patients with chronic Q fever are urban dwellers without significant exposure risks.[126] Although infrequently identified, it is estimated that for each case of Q fever diagnosed, 20 to 50 infections are not.[127] Seropositive rates may be as high as 30% in some randomly selected populations.[127] The relative risk is greatest in the elderly.[126,127] Moreover, persistence of viable organisms indicates that some hosts are at great risk for reactivation and chronic infection.[126] Thus Q fever is a major global infectious health risk.[127]

Clinical illness. Q fever comprises a variety of clinical conditions, including nonspecific fever, pneumonia, hepatitis, and endocarditis. Illness with Q fever is categorized by serology; acute Q fever is less severe, easily treated, and defined by high antibody titers to phase II *C. burnetii* antigens. Chronic Q fever is more severe, persistent, refractory to therapy, and diagnosed by high phase I antibody titers.[129] Recently infected patients may be asymptomatic or acutely ill with undifferentiated fever, an influenza-like illness, pneumonia, or granulomatous hepatitis,[127] which often subsides spontaneously. It is presumed that a persistent, subclinical infection may develop, and manifestations of chronic Q fever, including endocarditis, osteomyelitis, meningoencephalitis, or infection of prosthetic devices may supervene.[126,130] Tetracycline is the drug of choice for therapy.

Pathology. Pneumonia is a manifestation of acute Q fever, which is infrequently proved. Severe pneumonia is characterized by both interstitial lymphohistiocytic inflammation and intra-alveolar exudates with fibrin and abundant macrophages[127,131] (Fig. 35-11). The infection probably begins in the alveoli with infection of resident macrophages resulting in focal necrosis and influx of more macrophages. Spread to the terminal bronchioles leads to necrosis and regenerative changes in the bronchiolar epithelium. Bronchiolitis obliterans and organizing pneumonia may follow.[131,132] The inflammation, if focal, may cause a radiographic or gross pathologic impression of neoplasia.[132]

Next to fever, hepatic involvement is the most common clinical manifestation of Q fever in many investigations.[127] The serologic and clinical response is that of acute Q fever. Although not pathognomic, "fibrin-ring" granulomas in hepatic biopsy specimens are strongly suggestive of Q fever[133] (Fig. 35-12). Experimental infection shows that granulomas form within 8 days and may persist for years,[134] but *C. burnetii* are rarely found in these lesions. The "fibrin-ring" granuloma consists of deposition of fibrin within an aggregate of epithelioid histiocytes mixed with a few lymphocytes, occasional Langerhans' giant cells, and rare neutrophils, all of which surround a central, clear zone. Prominent Kupffer cells, lymphohistiocytic infiltration of the portal regions, focal hepatocellular necroses (Councilman-like bodies), and steatosis are also seen.[135,136] A link to progressive hepatic fibrosis and cirrhosis has been suggested.[137]

The most prominent finding in the bone marrow is a granuloma similar to that seen in the liver.[138] Prominent histiocytes and hemophagocytosis have been reported, and other nonspecific findings may include hyperplasia or abundant plasma cells. Marrow necrosis and fibrin deposition are rare findings.

Perhaps the most devastating of all the clinical syndromes is chronic Q fever endocarditis. Endocarditis in Q fever carries a particularly grave prognosis, with a case fatality rate as high as 60%.[126] Endocarditis usually develops on previously damaged valves; aortic and mitral valves are affected with equal frequency. Vegetations may be large, small, or microscopic and are composed of platelets and fibrin on an inflamed and focally necrotic valve. The inflammatory components are variable, and nonspecific chronic inflammation or mixed acute and chronic inflammation is frequent.[130,139,140] Microabscesses may be encountered. Scattered to numerous macrophages may be present, some epithelioid in appearance and others large and foamy. Granulomas are not present. Calcifications, foreign material, and fibrosis accompany most cases and may be related to the preexisting valvular lesion. The inflammation and necrosis may extend to involve adjacent myocardium, the valve ring, or the valvular sinuses.[140] Ultrastructural and immunohistologic studies show that most *C. burnetii* are present within macrophages. There are few extracellular organisms that localize to regions of degenerated cells.[127,141]

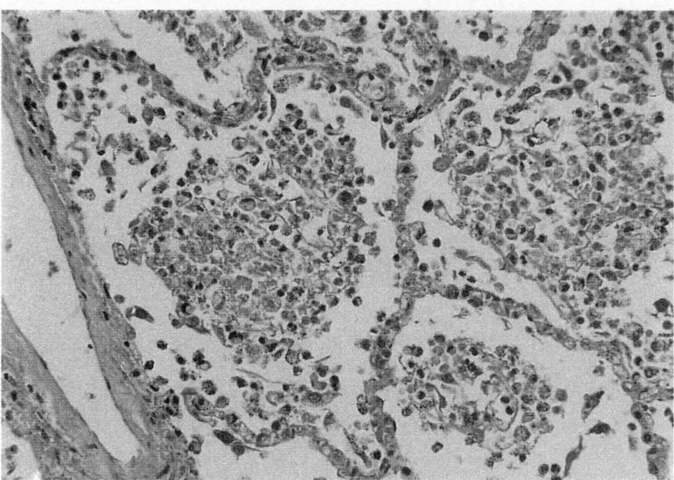

Fig. 35-11 Photomicrograph of lung from a patient with acute Q fever pneumonia shows numerous intraalveolar macrophages admixed with fibrin and a few polymorphonuclear neutrophils.

Other reported pathologic findings include Q fever associated with vascular prostheses, aneurysms, osteomyelitis,[126] immune complex vasculitis in skin biopsy specimens, postinfectious mesangioproliferative glomerulonephritis with immune complex deposition,[142] myocarditis with myocyte necrosis,[139] and "placentitis."

Pathogenesis. Various roles for host and bacterial factors have been suggested in the pathogenesis of Q fever.[124,125,143] Strains associated with chronic endocarditis seem to have evolved the ability not to stimulate a vigorous host response. In contrast, acute Q fever strains are more infectious and stimulate a host response with orders of magnitude fewer organisms. Thus persistent infection is in part related to bacterial factors. Clearly, after *C. burnetii* enters the host, the organisms infect macrophages and disseminate through the blood and perhaps lymphatics. The virulent, phase I LPS-containing organisms, with or without plasmids, are engulfed, resist killing, and divide within the acidified phagolysosome. These vacuoles may become grossly distended with hundreds of organisms and lyse. A progressive inflammatory reaction and a systemic acute phase response then ensue.[144,145] In most individuals, whether asymptomatic or ill, effective T-cell immunity, mediated by IFN-γ is established, thus reducing the burden of *C. burnetii* and leading to clinical recovery. Likewise, granulomas, in which *C. burnetii* cannot be detected, correlate with intact T-cell immunity, whereas chronic Q fever endocarditis patients, in whom *C. burnetii* are easily identified, fail to form granulomas, and their T-cells often do not respond to *C. burnetii* antigens. These findings help to explain the clinical persistence and poor outcome of chronic Q fever.[146]

Laboratory diagnosis. Acute Q fever is often mild and nonspecific, and the diagnosis is often missed.[127] On the other hand, the severity of chronic infection usually stimulates an extensive etiologic search. Diagnosis is usually based upon

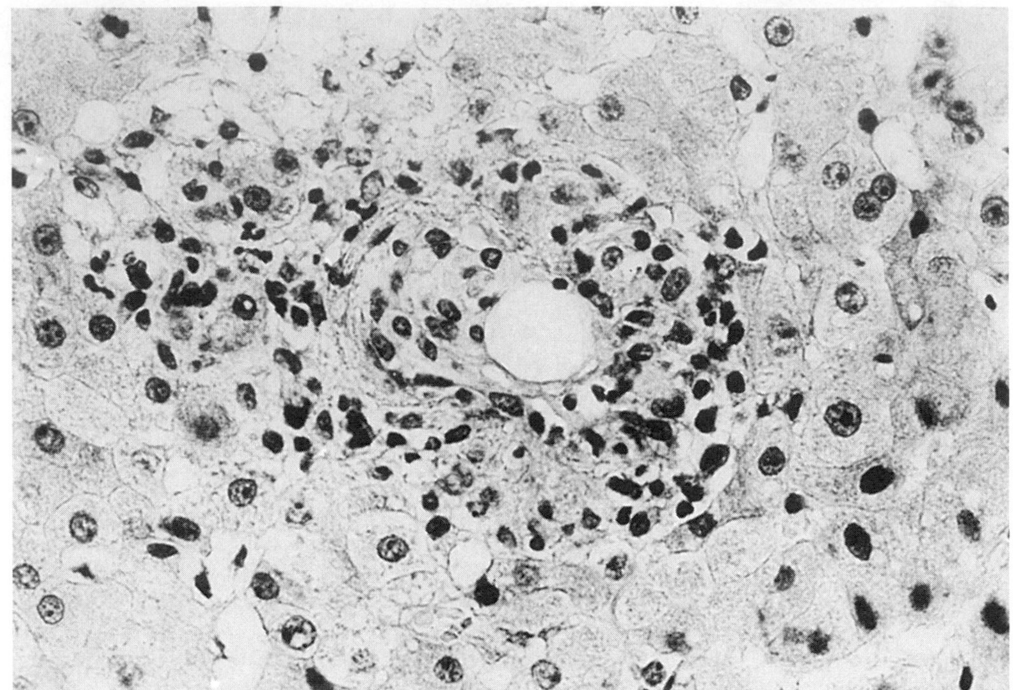

Fig. 35-12 Hepatic granuloma of Q fever with peripheral epithelioid macrophages and lymphocytes and characteristic central "doughnut" hole.

serology,[129,147] but demonstration of *C. burnetii* antigens or nucleic acids in clinical specimens is also diagnostic. Microbiologic isolation may be readily achieved but is only available in a few research facilities.

BARTONELLA (ROCHALIMAEA) INFECTIONS

Bartonellosis, also called Carrion's disease, is found only in South America on the western slopes of the Andes mountains where the vector *Lutzomyia verrucarum,* a bloodsucking sandfly, is found.[148] The etiologic agent is *Bartonella bacilliformis,* a small, gram-negative bacterium that invades erythrocytes and elicits tumorlike vascular proliferations. The disease may occur in outbreaks that involve numerous victims.[149] The organisms are inoculated into the blood, attach to, and penetrate erythrocytes to cause a febrile hemolytic anemia with a high mortality if untreated (Oroya fever). As recovery begins, proliferations of capillaries lined by plump endothelial cells form dermal nodules, called *verruga peruana* ('Peruvian wart').[150] Focal necrosis precedes neutrophilic infiltration, which is then replaced by lymphohistiocytic infiltrates before resolution. Giemsa stains may reveal intracytoplasmic bacterial clusters (previously called *chlamydozoa*) and extracellular aggregates of bacteria in early, florid lesions.[148] The pathologic picture is similar to that seen in bacillary angiomatosis, and, in fact, the agents of bacillary angiomatosis have been reclassified recently into the genus *Bartonella* by 16S rDNA sequence phylogeny.[151]

Trench fever

The name *trench fever* emphasizes its association with the close quarters occupied by affected military personnel during World War I. The infection is transmitted by lice and is caused by a bacterium that is capable of extracellular growth, *Bartonella (Rochalimaea) quintana*. Because axenic culture of this louse-borne agent was for decades unsuccessful, *B. quintana* was classified as a rickettsia. In fact, phylogenetic analysis indicates a relatively close relationship to species in the genus *Rickettsia*.[2,152] The illness is rarely fatal, and little is known concerning pathologic changes.

Other *Bartonella* infections

Trench fever was all but forgotten when the HIV became a serious threat. At risk for various opportunistic infections, some HIV-infected patients develop nonneoplastic, vascular nodules in skin and visceral organs, particularly the liver and spleen,[153,154] which may regress after antimicrobial therapy. Examination of sections of these lesions stained with a silver impregnation method reveals numerous bacilli in the interstitium. The identification of the causative agent, now designated *Bartonella (Rochalimaea) henselae,* was made simultaneously by amplification of the 16S ribosomal DNA from organisms in human tissues[152] and by isolation from the blood of febrile patients, one of whom was HIV infected.[155]

Bartonella (Rochalimaea) henselae and B. quintana are now proved agents of bacillary angiomatosis and visceral bacillary peliosis and may elicit vascular lesions in nearly any organ or tissue, including lymph node, brain, and bone.[153,156] Both can cause febrile bacteremia, in the absence of vascular proliferations, in immunocompromised or immunocompetent patients.[155] Epidemiologic investigation has revealed a close association of bacillary angiomatosis and peliosis with cat bites or scratches.[150] *Bartonella* species cause a periendothelial infection where they attach, elicit vascular proliferation, and cause tissue injury.

Lesions of bacillary angiomatosis consist of a lobular arrangement of capillaries with large, plump endothelial cells, often infiltrated by neutrophils, and containing interstitial leukocytoclastic debris and granular material[153] (Fig. 35-13). This latter finding corresponds to aggregates of bacteria, which may be visualized by silver stain, immunohistologic methods, or electron microscopy[157] (Fig. 35-14). Similar lesions may be seen in other tissues; however, infection in spleen and liver evolve into peliosis, a lesion that consists of multiple, thin-walled blood-filled cysts lined with endothelial cells and surrounded by myxoid stroma in which the clumps of bacteria may be identified.[154] The initial interpretations of silver stains in bacillary angiomatosis lesions indicated at least similar morphology to the bacilli seen on silver stains in cat-scratch lymphadenitis. Considerable controversy concerning the specific etiologic agent or agents responsible for cat scratch disease evolved; however, mounting evidence indicates that a substantial proportion of these cases may result from infection by *B. henselae* or an antigenically related bacterium.[158,159]

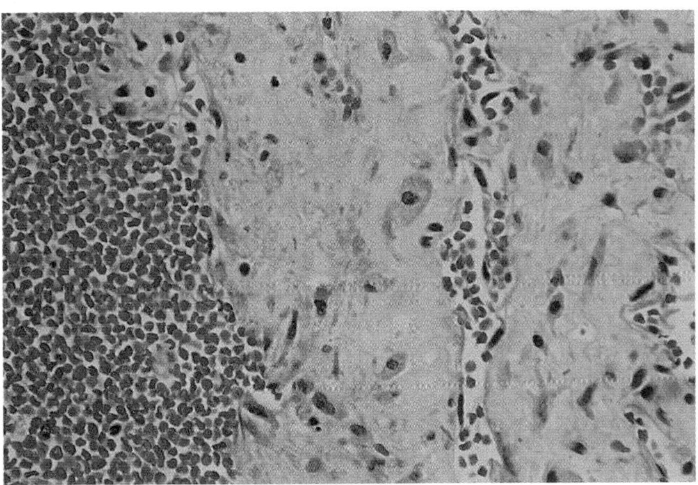

Fig. 35-13 Photomicrograph of bacillary peliosis hepatis in an immunocompromised patient. The amorphous, granular interstitial material represents clusters of *Bartonella (Rochalimaea)* organisms.

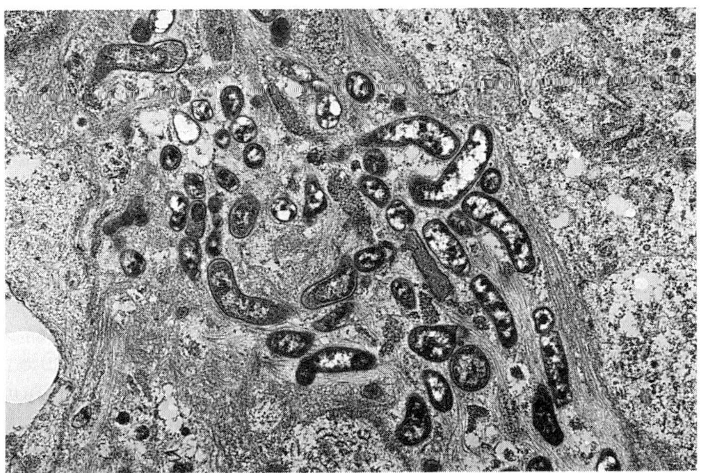

Fig. 35-14 Electron photomicrograph of a cluster of interstitial *Bartonella (Rochalimaea)* in a patient with cutaneous bacillary angiomatosis.

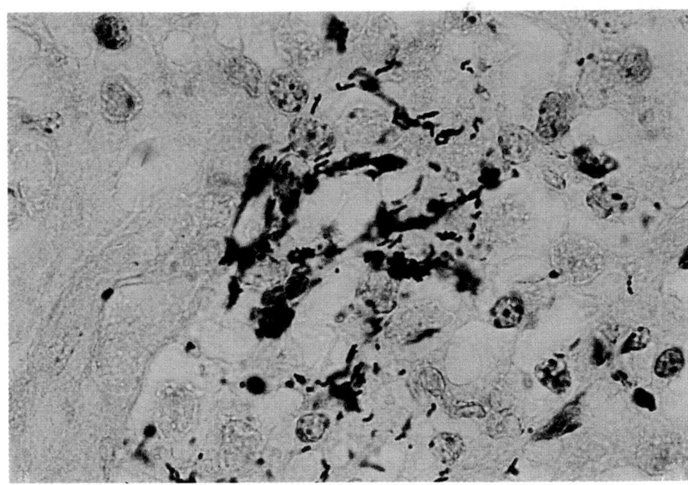

Fig. 35-15 Bacilli stained by the modified Warthin-Starry method in a lymph node of a patient with cat-scratch disease.

The syndrome of cat-scratch disease sometimes initiates as a papule at the site of inoculation within 4 to 6 days. Regional lymphadenopathy develops within weeks to months, and patients may be otherwise asymptomatic.[158] The adenopathy generally resolves after 2 to 4 months. Many atypical presentations have been documented, including hepatitis and meningoencephalitis, but the most frequent is Parinaud's oculoglandular syndrome, the combination of preauricular adenopathy with granulomatous conjunctivitis.[159] Serologic assays have identified that a preponderance of patients with suspected cat-scratch disease have antibodies to *B. henselae*, whereas few have antibodies to *Afipia felis*,[160] the original bacterium isolated from lymph nodes of patients with cat-scratch disease. The epidemiologic associations of the disease are evident from its name; however, kitten scratches and bites are most strongly linked to disease because mature cats are more likely to be immune. The possibility of flea and tick vectors has also been suggested.[161]

The characteristic pathologic appearance of cat-scratch lymphadenitis is the stellate abscess within a necrotizing granuloma. The distinctive feature is the presence of a rim of epithelioid histiocytes with occasional Langerhans' giant cells arranged peripherally around a suppurative core. Early lesions may lack abundant necrosis and neutrophilic infiltration. The pathologic appearance is nonspecific and may be observed with a variety of other infections, including lymphogranuloma venereum (*Chlamydia trachomatis* LGV strains), tularemia, and yersiniosis, among others. The most distinctive characteristic in silver-stained sections is the presence of bacillary organisms within the suppurative and necrotic foci[162] (Fig. 35-15). Recent immunohistologic studies have shown that, in cat-scratch lymphadenitis, these organisms stain positively with a *B. henselae*–specific polyclonal antibody, further strengthening the etiologic link.[163] The demonstration of these bacilli provides a presumptive diagnosis of *B. henselae* lymphadenitis, and definitive identification of the etiologic agent has been demonstrated by in vitro cultivation.[164] Diagnosis will probably require microbiologic cultivation of the agent, demonstration of its specific antigens or nucleic acids, or seroconversion using *B. henselae* antigens.

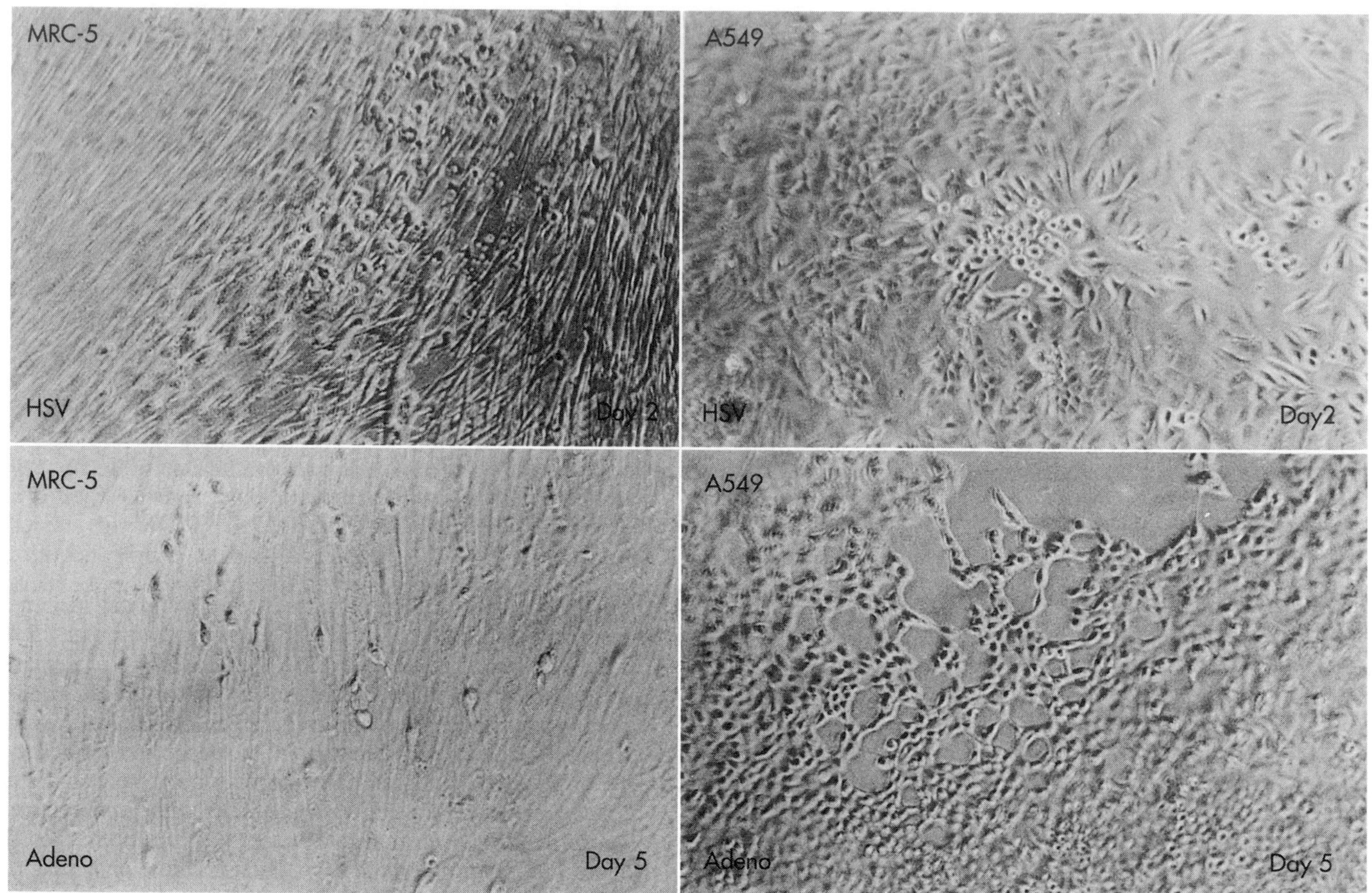

Fig. 36-4 Comparative cytopathic effects of adenovirus and herpes simplex virus in tissue culture.

Table 36-2 Cell lines used to identify viruses by cytopathic effect (CPE)

Virus	Cell lines			
	A549	MRC-5	PMK	Hep2
HSV	++	++	+/–	
VZV	+	+	–	–
CMV	–	+	–	–
Adeno	++	++	+/–	+++
Influenza	–	–	+	
Parainfluenza	–	–	H	
RSV	–	++	+/–	++
Entero	+	+	+	
Rhino	–	+	–	

+, CPE usually detected; ++ extensive CPE detected;
+/–, CPE variable; *H*, hemadsorption used for identification.

compound. This is also the key principle behind one such test for cytomegalovirus, the CMV pp65 antigen test. Early and immediate early proteins are the first to be produced after infection and are present before the virus enters replicative stages. Thus, CMV can be detected within 18 hours of culture, whereas in classical culture procedures virus may not be detected for days. Another confirmatory method is that of the agglutination of RBCs by viral antigens.

The hemagglutination inhibition test (HAI) is the most frequently used test for typing influenza virus and employs the use of a panel of antibodies against known influenza serotypes. Binding of antisera known to be specific for a certain serotype to the appropriate viral hemagglutinin interferes with its ability to attach to RBCs and therefore prevents hemagglutination.

Serology

The adaptation of tests from a complement-fixation (CF) format or indirect immunofluoresence assay to that of direct antibody capture techniques utilized in enzyme-linked immunoassays (ELISA) has made viral serology available to even small hospitals and clinics. Serologic procedures are extremely valuable for the screening of populations for detection of exposure to specific viruses, or for confirmation of infection by certain viruses in the recent or distant past. One classic example is the heterophile test for the detection of an acute antibody response that typically occurs in infectious mononucleosis.[9] The heterophile antibodies are not specific to EBV antigens but are rather antibodies that recognize epitopes on erythrocytes. A differential absorption procedure (Paul-Bunnell-Davidsohn) detects IgM heterophile antibodies that are differentiated from other antibodies by their absorption to bovine erythrocytes but not guinea pig kidney cells. Modifications of the procedure have resulted in rapid slide latex agglutination tests that incorporate horse RBCs as the target (Monospot test). In the slide test, nonspecific antibodies are first absorbed with guinea pig cells followed by detection of agglutination of horse RBCs. A negative test does not rule out the possibility of acute EBV infection, but a positive test is helpful, since infection by CMV, or other viruses that cause the infectious mononucleosis syndrome, do not result in production of the heterophile antibody. Heterophile antibody production is age dependent and is less useful in children than in adolescents and adults.

One of the important considerations for the interpretation of viral serologic test results is the effect of disease prevalence. In a population with a very low disease prevalence, even a test with good sensitivity and specificity may give an unacceptably high number of false-positive results. Enzyme immunosorbent assays (EIA or ELISA) have broad application for the detection of antibodies to viruses. Some versions of EIA tests employ disrupted whole virus preparations that are used to coat the microtiter plate well. Subsequent generations of tests, such as those for HIV, have used specific recombinant proteins with improvement in specificity. However, as in the case of EIA tests for HIV, confirmatory procedures such as IFA, western blot, or antigen detection assays are commonly needed. On the other hand, wide exposure or high prevalence may influence the interpretation of the result of an antibody titer level, such as those for influenzavirus. A second serum sample may be needed to demonstrate a rise in antibody levels over a 4- to 6-week period after the onset of symptoms, particularly when the opportunity for detecting IgM has passed. The importance of clinical history and physical findings cannot be overemphasized in the interpretation of serologic results. In some situations a single positive test for antibodies to St. Louis encephalitis virus, for example, will be accepted as sufficient evidence for causation of acute neurologic symptoms associated with typical symptoms and history, though paired sera are optimal. In other cases, such as those for HSV and CMV, tests for specific IgG can be combined with assays detecting IgM levels.

Since the various structural and regulatory proteins of many viruses have been identified, it is possible to search for specific antiviral antibodies as well as for viral antigens and develop detailed panels that can delineate between acute and past infection as well as the state of reactivation of a latent virus, such as Epstein-Barr virus (Fig. 36-5) or hepatitis-B virus (Fig. 36-6). Figs. 36-5 and 36-6 demonstrate the typical times during which either antibodies or antigens can be detected in the serum of infected individuals. The hepatitis B surface antigen (HBsAg) is detectable within weeks after exposure and before the development of symptoms closely followed by the appearance of e antigen. The timing of the appearance of *antibodies* to HBV antigens corresponds with development of clinical symptoms, and the levels of antibody can be shown to increase during a recovery phase. As antibody production increases, more of the virus is incorporated into antigen-antibody complexes and removed from circulation. The continuing detection of HBsAg in the serum is an indication of persistent infection. For EBV, the type of the antibody (either IgM or IgG), its specificity (whether against capsid or nuclear antigen), and the relative concentration of antibody detected are useful in the characteri-

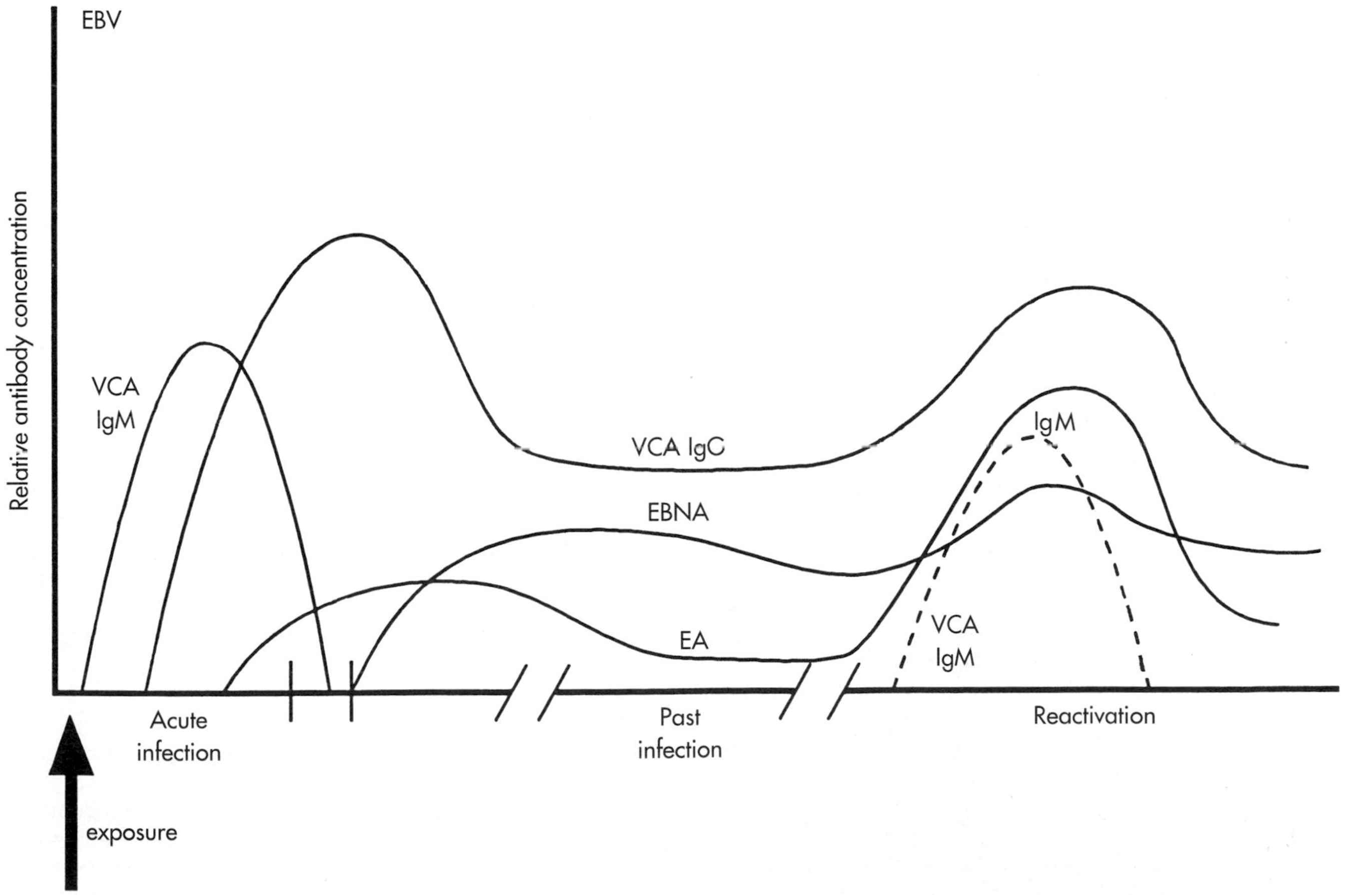

Fig. 36-5 Epstein-Barr virus serology. *VCA,* Viral capsid antigen; *EBNA,* Epstein-Barr nuclear antigen; *EA,* early antigen.

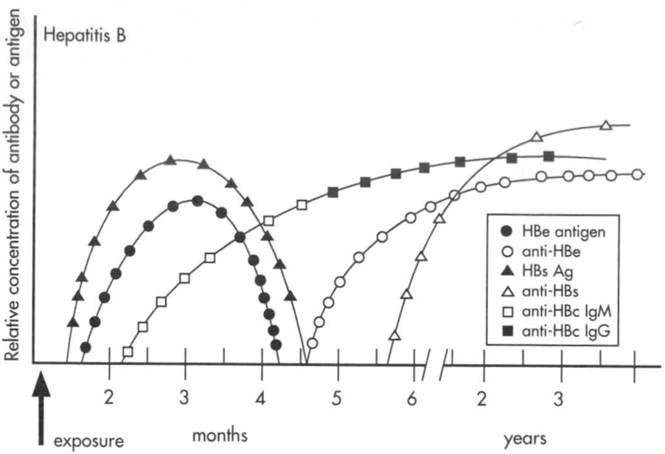

Fig. 36-6 Hepatitis B virus serology. IgM levels may fall below detection limits after 1–3 months.

zation of either primary infection, past infection, or reactivation of latent infection (Fig. 36-5). These multiple component tests are particularly helpful in identifying individuals who are in transition from acute infection to a convalescent state.

The great sensitivity of EIA screening tests when applied on a national scale (such as blood donor screening) results in a significant number of tests that are presumptively positive until confirmed.[10] Immunoblot assays (western blot) have been utilized for confirmation of EIA tests for either HIV or HTLV-I and II. Western blot procedures include the extraction of viral proteins from the complete virion and then electrophoresis through denaturing gels to separate the proteins by size. Subsequently, the proteins are transferred from the gel to a membrane that can be cut into strips and incubated with patient sera. Patient antibodies that bind to viral bands are detected by means of conjugated secondary antibodies that provide for a color reaction and the presence of a discrete band that corresponds to known viral proteins. Their particular utility results from being able to visualize the specific pattern of antigens detected in an infected patient's serum and identify those cases where reactivity on EIA is attributable to a nonspecific reaction.

On rare occasions the migration of a cellular antigen will be nearly identical to the migration of a viral antigen, resulting in a band at that location on the western blot. A p24 band on Western blot is typically the first to appear in newly HIV-infected patients. However, non–HIV infected multiparous females have also been shown to develop antibodies to antigens that comigrate with the viral p24. Repeated testing resolves the difficulty in very few cases.[11] Other nonviral bands or only one of three expected bands may be detected in other situations. These findings result in an interpretation of "indeterminant" or "inconclusive" by western blot, bringing great consternation to the patient, physician, and laboratory and require repeated testing after 6 to 8 weeks to document the lack of progression to a pattern diagnostic of HIV infection. The use of recombinant proteins for immunoblotting is expected to eliminate the cross-reactivity of antibodies to cellular proteins.[12]

Antigen detection

Antigen detection assays rely on the ability of specific antibodies to capture or detect viral proteins in a format adaptable to the clinical laboratory. Collection of vesicle fluid from herpetic lesions may be used for direct antigen detection using fluoroscein-conjugated antibodies with results available within an hour. Similarly, procedures have been used for detecting influenza B antigen from respiratory fluids.[13] Research procedures have utilized immunoprecipitation of viral proteins to concentrate antigen followed by detection by a second method such as western blotting. Alternatively, ELISA-based tests are widely used for the detection of antigen and employ the use of an antibody attached to the bottom of a well to capture the virus or viral antigen. Subsequently, a second antibody that may be conjugated with a chromogenic substrate or enzyme is utilized for quantitating the amount of virus captured. The format of these tests usually require their use in laboratories with significant patient volume. New test designs have resulted in kits that can be used for individual patients as needed such as that for rotavirus or influenza A and B. In these tests a color change is visually detected by the operator, and little equipment or machinery is required.

Molecular techniques

Molecular techniques are useful for the demonstration of virus in a variety of clinical specimens, principally when rapid detection is critical or when genome integration or viral latency are important questions.[14] Refer to Chapter 11 for details in the application of DNA or RNA probing or PCR. Theoretically, any virus may be detected through molecular techniques; DNA virus detection is particularly straightforward. The complication of using PCR for RNA viruses is that of conversion of viral RNA to DNA (by reverse transcriptase) before amplification.

The development of nonculture laboratory techniques has allowed for the rapid and specific diagnosis of viral infection that rivals or exceeds that available for the diagnosis of bacterial infections. These diagnostic procedures can support, replace, or complement the traditional morphologic and culture approach to viral diagnosis. However, several limitations exist, the most significant being the uncertain clinical significance of virus detection by molecular techniques, such as those with HPV and cervical lesions.

Electron microscopy

Ultrastructural morphology plays a key role in viral identification.[15] Clinically, its utility is limited by cost but in certain situations will provide useful information in a timely manner. Electron microscopy for diagnostic purposes is most commonly applied to the evaluation of stool or urine but can also be helpful in selected cases such as progressive multifocal leukoencephalopathy (PML). Many enteric viruses cannot be grown routinely, such as *Calicivirus* or *Coronavirus,* and electron microscopy is one of the few methods for detection. In research applications, the structural morphology contributes to viral classification, the important determinant being whether the virus has a naked capsid or an enveloped capsid.

VIRAL MECHANISMS AND PATHOGENESIS

Acute infection by a virus occurs when a virion from a contaminated fomite or fluid from an infected host is able to penetrate a new host cell followed by the production of new virions. Acute infection may result in either cell damage or cell death, referred to as a *lytic infection,* or may result in persistent infection without immediate cell death. Most contacts between viruses and host cells actually do not result in significant disease, and in many cases even a true infection may be asymptomatic. Thus a distinction must be drawn between infection and disease. A second distinction must be made between lytic infection and persistent infection.

Epidemiologic studies indicate that the majority of virus exposure and primary infection occurs in childhood, and for many viruses this infection does not appear to cause significant symptoms and may pass unnoticed. Thus infection does not always cause clinically apparent disease. Should an individual pass through childhood without exposure, it is possible that infection in adulthood will result in severe disease as occurs with varicella, mumps, hepatitis A, and Epstein-Barr viruses. The explanation for this difference in outcome of virus infection is believed to relate to the maturity of the immune system and the nature of the cells involved in the response.

Recovery from acute infection corresponds to clearance of the virus from the bloodstream or from entry of the virus into a dormant state. If the virus infection is cleared and the host develops immunity, subsequent encounters with the virus may result in abortive infection. During an abortive infection, the virion comes into contact with host cells but is not successful in the penetration of the cell or in completing replicative cycles. If the immune protection is incomplete or the virus alters its immunogenic determinants, subsequent reinfection is possible, though partial protection may result. For example, infection by influenzavirus A (Beijing type) with hemagglutinin H3 and neuraminidase N2, usually produces immunity against a repeat infection by the same virus type in that year's influenza season and may offer partial protection against a related strain in a subsequent year but will provide no protection against influenza B infection or influenza A with a different hemagglutinin or neuraminidase.

Each virus has a typical means of transmission. Contaminated water, food, or inhalation of virus in aerosolized droplets are common methods of transmitting viruses. Alternatively, transmission of virus may occur through the transfer of infected cells from one host to another through sexual contact, blood transfusion, or the transplantation of a donated organ.

Potential signs and symptoms of disease from acute viral infection may include cough, fever, rhinorrhea, and pharyngitis. These findings are nonspecific and are referred to as symptoms of a viral syndrome. On the other hand, the pattern of skin rash and its progression may be characteristic of a certain virus such as VZV and chicken pox.

How a cell becomes infected and whether progeny viruses are produced is determined by host cellular factors as well as viral factors. Cell types differ in their capability for supporting new virus production or replication. These determinants include extracellular and intracellular processes that define the concept of tissue tropism. Tissue tropism is the restriction of specific viruses to selected cell types for successful replication and may be determined by portal of entry, cell surface interactions, immune status of the host, and cellular processes. Intracellular processes that determine tissue tropism include growth phase of the cell (cell cycle), transactivation, nuclear transport mechanisms, integration of the viral genome into host genome, and the potential for establishing latency.

The portal of entry where viruses first circumvent host defensive barriers is usually limited in nature by anatomic and physical determinants. These determinants may be bypassed in experimental systems. The consequences of virus infection through a natural portal of entry may differ from those resulting from experimental or accidental injection of a virus into another site. In such situations, viral genes may demonstrate unexpected oncogenic potential that is not encountered as a result of natural infection. Adenovirus has not been associated with carcinoma in humans, yet adenoviruses can induce neoplastic changes when introduced into cells or animals through experimental procedures.

The portal of entry or initial site of infection may also not be the site of major disease. Enteroviruses such as coxsackievirus B enter the body through the respiratory or gastrointestinal mucosa with few accompanying symptoms until after spread of virus through the bloodstream (viremia) there results an infection of cells in a major organ, such as cardiac myocytes.

The physical properties of a virus contribute to the range of tissues involved in disease and have also been used in classification. Viruses that infect through the GI tract must survive the acidic pH of the stomach as well as the detergent action of bile salts and proteolytic digestion by enzymes. Therefore, enteric viruses (with the notable exception of coronaviruses) typically lack a lipid-containing envelope, whereas viruses of the respiratory tract that must penetrate mucus and do not encounter digestive processes typically are enveloped.

The steps involved in virus infection of a cell have been named in recognition of the common nature of the processes involved and include attachment to the cellular receptor, penetration of, or fusion with the cellular membrane, uncoating of the virus envelope or capsid, and transportation to cytoplasm or nuclear compartments before replication. Many of these steps have been extensively studied for some viruses such as adenoviruses, picornoviruses, herpesviruses, and HIV, whereas very little is known about other viruses. Cellular receptors for viral attachment and viral ligands that bind to cell receptors are a major determinant for tissue tropism, and their identification is a goal of research for most viruses[16] (Table 36-3). Virus attachment to a cellular receptor is followed by a biologic response leading to infection of the cell. For example, HIV attaches to CD4, a molecule on the surface of lymphocytes and macrophages, through a component of the virus envelope gp 120 (for the HIV glycoprotein of 120-kilodalton molecular weight).[17] Efficient infection of a T-cell by free or non–cell associated HIV occurs through attachment of the virion to the CD4 receptor. Sialic acids or sialyloligosaccharides are common attachment molecules for many viruses and also provide the basis for hemagglutination with RBCs. Specific RBC antigens have been identified as the receptor for *Parvovirus* B19.[18] Membrane fusion may occur after attachment as in HIV, influenzavirus, and other enveloped viruses. Paramyxoviruses have a specific fusion protein. The delta protein of reoviruses mediates cellular attachment, followed by receptor-mediated endocytosis.[19]

Cell receptors are not the exclusive means for a virus to gain entry into a cell; cell-to-cell spread may occur through direct contact and fusion. Viruses may also adhere nonspecifically to the cell surface and in some cases bind to an intermediate molecule that has the capability of attaching to the cell, such as those for CMV and β_2-microglobulin. Cell-surface heparin sulfate proteoglycans have been shown to be the initial attachment molecules for herpes simplex as well as CMV, whereas additional proteins, such as CD13, are involved in membrane fusion or mediate infection of the target cell.[20,20a] Since the internalization of chemicals and receptors through

clear fluid over 1 to 3 days. These lesions are painful, perhaps because of an associated radiculitis. Histologically, a vesicle shows cell death or necrosis as well as inflammatory effects. Evidence of direct viral antigen effect includes cell ballooning as well as a ground-glass appearance of the nucleus or inclusion bodies of the Cowdry type A. Infected cells are enlarged but not to the degree seen in CMV-infected cells. Multinucleated giant cells may be present. Spongiform degeneration precedes keratinocyte cell death within the parabasal and intermediate cells of the epithelium followed by vesicle formation. The vesicle contains predominantly clear serous fluid, cell debris, inflammatory cells, and infectious virions. The lesions aquire a cloudy or pustular appearance because of an increased number of inflammatory cells within the fluid. The lesions then rupture, releasing up to a million infectious particles. After rupture and acute ulceration the lesions form an escar over the shallow ulcers, which heal spontaneously. In immunocompetent hosts, lesions usually persist for 7 to 14 days in primary disease and for 3 to 5 days for recurrent disease.

HSV is relatively hardy and not tightly cell associated, and so HSV is easily isolated from swab specimens of lesions. HSV in routine cell culture is usually apparent within 24 to 72 hours of inoculation, but shell-vial methods lower detection time to less than 24 hours. Direct staining with monoclonal antibodies of cells scraped from the base of vesicular lesions is diagnostic within 1 to 2 hours and can distinguish vesicular lesions of VZV from those of HSV. The traditional Tzanck smear of scrapings from skin lesions is of less value because it lacks specificity, and the diagnostic giant cells (polykaryons) formed by cell fusion and cellular inclusions are not always seen even with definite herpesvirus infection. Cowdry type A inclusions, Lipschütz bodies, are not specific for either HSV-1 or HSV-2 and may be found in cells infected by any herpesvirus.

HSV infection causes greatly different clinical entities appearing in a wide range of age groups. Gingivostomatitis is the most common presentation of primary HSV-1 infection, but many HSV-1 primary infections are asymptomatic. The incubation period is 2 to 12 days with an illness lasting 1 to 2 weeks. Signs include fever, malaise, friable vesiculoulcerative lesions (on the palate, tongue, gingivae, and lips), local adenopathy, and fetor oris. Mucous membrane lesions become ulcers more rapidly than those on skin and have a irregular white to gray base often with scalloped edges. Lesions may spread to the chin and neck. Autoinoculation of other sites is common. In recurrent infection, intraoral lesions are rare, and vesicles occur first along the vermillion border. Generally, only supportive treatment is necessary; however, in severe primary or recurrent infections, acyclovir will decrease morbidity.

Herpes encephalitis is believed to occur through retrograde travel by neural routes.[58] Herpes encephalitis accounts for 5% to 20% of viral encephalitis and may be attributable to primary infection or reactivation of HSV. Herpes encephalitis usually begins with a nonspecific febrile illness followed by CNS signs and symptoms of altered mentation. Meningeal signs are uncommon. The electroencephalogram is usually abnormal, and temporal lobe localized findings appear very early in the disease. CT-scan abnormalities are usually a late finding, and MRI has become the neuroimaging procedure of choice. CSF pleocytosis with mostly lymphocytes may occur, but early in infection polymorphonuclear cells may predominate. CSF glucose concentration may be normal or low; CSF protein content is generally elevated. Red blood cells in CSF are supportive of HSV, reflecting hemorrhagic necrosis. Very rarely the CSF remains normal with repeated analysis. CSF culture is usually negative. Brain biopsy is the only definitive tool for diagnosis of herpes encephalitis but is being used less than in the past, except on experimental protocols. Although not solely diagnostic, the histologic finding of hemorrhagic necrosis is typically encountered on biopsy of focal lesions of the gray matter. Adjacent vascular structures show a perivascular cuff of lymphocytes. Antibodies to HSV can be employed on frozen-section material or touch preparations of brain tissue and make a conclusive diagnosis possible before culture results are available. DNA hybridization or amplification (such as polymerase chain reaction [PCR]) of DNA extracted from brain tissue or CSF are also useful for confirming a clinical diagnosis but if negative do not rule out the presence of virus. PCR of CSF-derived DNA using HSV primers has recently been shown to be 95% sensitive and nearly 100% specific in diagnosis of herpes simplex encephalitis.[59]

Genital HSV may also occur as either primary or recurrent infections, and both HSV-1 and HSV-2 can cause genital HSV.[60] HSV-1 has a predilection to *recur* in sites above the umbilicus, whereas HSV-2 recurs more frequently below the umbilicus. This led to the incorrect notion that all genital disease was attributable to HSV-2 and all oral disease was attributable to HSV-1. Primary disease can occur at any site with either serotype, but recurrent infections appear to segregate in location. This may relate to the ability of type 2 to establish latency better in lumbosacral ganglia, whereas type 1 establishes latency better in trigeminal ganglia. In primary genital infection, the symptoms appear about 2 to 7 days after exposure, peak within 1 to 2 weeks, and subside by 2 to 3 weeks. In recurrent genital HSV, the symptoms are usually less severe and more localized, and the lesions heal in 1 to 1 1/2 weeks. A self-limited meningitis occurs in 11% to 35% of primary genital HSV infections during the second week but is infrequent in recurrent disease. In 3% of cases, HSV can be isolated from the CSF. CNS symptoms generally resolve in 2 to 7 days. Other complications of genital HSV include transverse myelitis, extra-genital lesions, and secondary *Candida* infection.

HSV is no longer considered to be an etiologic agent of neoplasia of the genital tract, though for many years an association with cervical cancer was investigated.

Intrauterine HSV infection is rare but may present as low birth weight, small size for gestational age, diffuse brain damage, microcephaly, intracranial calcification, microphthalmia, cataracts, or retinal dysplasia. Neonatal HSV is usually acquired at delivery, but postnatal acquisition may occur by direct exposure to maternal lesions involving family members, nursery personnel, or other infected babies. In natally acquired HSV, 60% to 80% of mothers had no evidence of genital herpes at delivery.[60] Although most (~85%) neonatal HSV is attributable to HSV-2, the outcome from HSV-1 or HSV-2 is equally severe. Signs of neonatal HSV usually first appear 1 and 2 weeks after birth, but can be delayed up to 1 month of age. Signs may include skin vesicles, mouth ulcers, chorioretinitis, keratoconjunctivitis, a sepsis-like picture, pneumonitis, hepatitis, temperature instability, or signs of meningoencephalitis (bulging fontanelle, seizures, flaccidity, spasticity, opisthotonos, or coma).

Neonatal HSV may be localized to skin, eye, mouth, or mucocutaneous structures but may also disseminate. Disseminated disease associated with viremia can involve multiple organs (lung, liver, adrenals, and so on) with or without involvement of the skin, eyes, mouth, or the CNS. Isolated CNS disease also occurs. The frequency of skin vesicles found with CNS and disseminated infection has recently decreased, and therefore their absence at autopsy or in life does not rule out the possibility of HSV infection. Although infection of the skin, eyes, or mouth alone is rarely fatal, 70% of babies presenting with skin, eye, and mouth lesions progress to either encephalitis or disseminated disease. After the neonatal period, 96% of all herpes encephalitis cases are caused by HSV-1.

Ocular HSV is usually attributable to HSV-1 and appears as vesicles on the conjunctivae and lid margins (blepharitis) or may involve cornea, stroma, uvea, or retina. HSV infections of the eye are the most common cause of blindness in developed countries. HSV keratitis is believed to be an immmunomediated disease because of release of cytokines by infiltrating inflammatory cells. Keratoconjunctivitis manifests as ocular pain, photophobia, excess lacrimation, chemosis, blurred vision, lid edema, and corneal opacities or ulcers (typically dendritic).[61]

Whitlow is a suppurative HSV infection of the tip of a digit caused by autoinoculation (thumb-sucking in children with gingivostomatitis) or unprotected handling of infected secretions. Disseminated cutaneous HSV occurs with widespread herpetic involvement of the skin in patients with thermal or chemical burns. A subtype is Kaposi's varicelliform eruption (eczema herpeticum), an extensive cutaneous HSV infection of atopic dermatitis that extends to normal skin.

Varicella-zoster virus (HHV-3)

The varicella-zoster virus (VZV) virion has physical characteristics similar to those of HSV and is classified as an alphaherpesvirus.[62] The envelope contains at least five glycoproteins designated as gpI through gpV. These are homologs of the HSV glycoproteins E, B, H, I, and C. The viral glycoprotein B, important as an attachment factor, is also a candidate for a subunit vaccine. A thymidine kinase and DNA polymerase are virus specific. Many immediate early gene products appear homologous to HSV products. Antibody cross-reactivity with HSV has been detected.

VZV is highly contagious and is usually acquired through inhalation of aerosolized microdroplets containing virus. After local nasopharyngeal replication there is a primary viremia. Subsequently there is a 1- to 2-week incubation period followed by a secondary viremia. Varicella causes rash and fever. Infection is usually self-limited except in immunosuppressed individuals who may develop pneumonia and encephalitis. About 95% of adults have serologic evidence of previous infection by VZV, and approximately 15% of seropositive individuals may experience reactivation as zoster in later life.

Laboratory testing is needed to differentiate VZV from HSV-1 or HSV-2 or when exposure of nonimmune pregnant females or immunocompromised patients occurs. The infrequent congenital malformations occurring after maternal chickenpox infection usually occur after infection in the first half of pregnancy (Table 36-7). Gross features include cicatricial cutaneous lesions, musculoskeletal, neurologic, and ocular abnormalities. Antiviral treatment of pregnant women with chickenpox does not prevent congenital VZV and is not recommended unless maternal illness itself is severe enough to warrant treatment. Neonatal varicella may occur after maternal chickenpox during the last 3 weeks of pregnancy in approximately 25% of cases. The severity in the infant depends on the time of onset of maternal chickenpox in relation to delivery. If maternal chickenpox begins more than 5 days before delivery or the neonate becomes ill after the first 14 days of life, the disease is usually mild, probably because of protective transplacental antibody. If maternal chickenpox begins within 4 days before or 2 days after delivery and neonatal varicella begins at 5 to 10 days of age, disseminated disease (hepatitis, pneumonitis, encephalitis, and death) occurs in approximately 30% of cases.

Chickenpox can be severe in adults, causing pneumonia, with cough, fever, and respiratory distress usually appearing 3 to 5 days into the illness. VZV encephalitis occurs in 0.1% to 0.2% of cases and is characterized by headache, altered mentation, vomiting, and seizures. Mortality is 5% to 20% and neurologic sequelae occur in up to 15%. Varicella in the immunocompromised can be fatal, presents with more lesions than in immunocompetent hosts that may be hemorrhagic, lasts longer, and has greater risk for bacterial superinfection. The risk of developing disseminated VZV, malignant chickenpox, or purpura fulminans is also greater.

Varicella is highly cell associated but can be found by electron microscopy in clear vesicle fluid. VZV is difficult to isolate in cell culture, and care must be taken to aspirate fluid only from clear vesicles because culture of cloudy vesicles or crusted lesions rarely result in positive cultures. This difficulty in culture is paradoxical because VZV can be transmitted simply by sharing air with a varicella patient in the same room or via ducts to different rooms. In hospital, varicella patients require strict isolation.

Herpes zoster (shingles) is the condition resulting from reactivation of latent VZV infection from dorsal root ganglia originally acquired as chickenpox. The connection between shingles and VZV was first recognized when cases of chickenpox were noted in households where shingles in adults had appeared several weeks earlier. Therefore the latent condition likely represents one manner in which the virus remains in an immune population before infecting subsequent generations. Patients with zoster rarely are contagious by the airborne route. Direct contact is usually necessary for zoster to be infectious to another host. The frequency of shingles increases with age and corresponds with a decrease in immune function. The passage of virus from a dorsal root ganglion through sensory nerves results in a localized vesicular eruption in a dermatomal distribution. The lesions are similar to that of chickenpox but may be more clustered and are associated with intense pain. Neuralgia within a dermatome may occur 3 or 4 days before the vesicular eruption and may be associated with regional adenopathy. Fever, headache, malaise, and motor paralysis may occur. The preeruptive neuralgia may last for weeks and may not be followed by eruption at all. The eruptive stage usually lasts 2 weeks, but postherpetic neuralgia may persist for months. Involvement of the geniculate ganglion may result in facial paralysis.

Immunosuppressed VZV seropositive patients (such as chemotherapy or AIDS patients) are at risk for development of herpes zoster. New lesions may erupt for 2 to 3 weeks, and crusting may not occur until 3 to 4 weeks later. Mortality of VZV infection in children with leukemia is reported to be 7%. Chronic zoster (such that new lesions form with nonhealing of old vesicles) may occur, particularly in AIDS patients. Dis-

Table 36-7 Viruses associated with increased gestational risk

Virus	Frequency of maternal infection resulting in affected fetus	Possible effect on infant with acquired disease in utero	% seropositive women of child-bearing age	Delayed effects after asymptomatic fetal infection
Rubella (German measles)	After symptomatic infection Weeks of gestation: 0-12: 80-100% 12-16: 35-66% 16-24: 25% >24: ~0%	1. Cataracts, glaucoma, microphthalmia 2. Heart defects, patent ductus arteriosus, PAS, septal defects 3. Deafness 4. Meningoencephalitis 5. Anemia 6. Thrombocytopenia	75% to 94% (Currently, child-bearing-age U.S. women are rubella-immune by immunization, not disease)	Progressive encephalitis Up to a third of cases develop diabetes mellitus type I in second decade of life
Cytomegalovirus	Primary maternal infection: Transplacental infection rate 35%, with 10% clinically symptomatic at birth Reactivation of maternal "infection": Transplacental infection <3%, 0% to 1% clinically symptomatic	1. Microcephaly 2. Intracerebral calcifications 3. Chorioretinitis 4. Jaundice 5. Organomegaly 6. Thrombocytopenia 7. Low birth weight	Upper socioeconomic group 55% Lower socioeconomic group 85%	*Hearing loss:* Up to 50% (primary) 5% to 15% (reactivation) *Intellectual (IQ <70)/ motor impairment:* 5% to 15% (primary infection) and 0% to 1% (reactivation)
Parvovirus B-19 (erythema infectiosum)	Transplacental infection rate 33% with 1.2% to 2.5% fetal loss (Both rates drop with acquisition later in gestation)	Hydrops fetalis anemia	50%	
HIV	12% to 45%, highest rate early or late in maternal illness (when maternal blood-viral load is high)	Immune alteration, growth retardation	<2%	Pediatric AIDS
Enterovirus	Undefined but follows maternal symptoms in last week of gestation	Febrile illness and hepatitis, possibly meningitis, myocarditis	Variable	None defined in survivors
VZV	Late gestation: Rare (observed when maternal varicella rash onset is 5 days before or after delivery) Early gestation: Rare	*Late:* Severe, complicated, and potentially fatal varicella *Early:* Cicatrization of skin, cataracts, CNS injury	85% to 90%	

PAS, Pulmonary artery stenosis.

seminated zoster (involvement of the lungs, liver, or CNS) is seen almost exclusively in immunocompromised hosts, usually 6 to 10 days into the eruption. Postherpetic neuralgia is common in immunocompromised patients.

Whereas other viruses appear within the first months after bone marrow transplant, herpes zoster may not develop for 6 months or more, an indication of the importance of a particular subset of the immune system. Herpes zoster in these patients may lead to visceral involvement and in particular a hepatitis with hepatocellular necrosis and significant elevation in liver enzymes, which may be life threatening if not treated.

Congenital embryopathy has not been substantiated in women with herpes zoster occurring during gestation. Zoster in the neonate can occur if the mother acquired varicella early in pregnancy.

Epstein-Barr virus (HHV-4)

The Epstein-Barr virus was first identified by Epstein, Achong, and Barr during their studies of patients with African Burkitt's lymphoma.[63] An infectious cause for endemic African lymphoma in children had been sought by Dr. Denis Burkitt and others because of the characteristic epidemiologic features of the disease. Subsequently, EBV was associated with nasopharygeal carcinoma,[64] and the current spectrum of disease connected with EBV is broad and varied.

Infection by EBV typically occurs in childhood through the sharing of virally contaminated saliva and is largely asymptomatic.[65] In economically developed countries, exposure to EBV may not occur until adolescence or adulthood though the increased use of daycare situations for children may be reducing the number of EBV-seronegative individuals. The major route of transmission of EBV is through the saliva, though infected cells in blood products and transplanted organs or bone marrow may also transmit the virus. The intermittent presence of EBV in saliva is the result of reactivation of latent infection of oropharynx and salivary gland epithelial cells. Epithelial cells in the oral and nasal pharynx possess the receptor for EBV (CD21, or CR2), which is similar to the glycoprotein component of complement receptor (C3d) found on lymphocytes.[66] Binding to the cellular receptor by virus occurs through interaction with the virus envelope glycoproteins gp350 and gp220, which are the ligands for CD21. During a productive "lytic" infection of the epithelium the virus is able to infect adjacent B-lymphocytes through the same complement receptor. Infection of B-lymphocytes results in either a latent infection or a lytic infection.

Paul and Bunnell had associated the presence of a heterophile antibody with the clinical condition of infectious mononucleosis (IM) in the 1930s, but it was not until 1967 that an association was made between Epstein-Barr virus and infectious mononucleosis by the Henles.[9] EBV-induced IM is typically a self-limited lymphoproliferative disease classically characterized by pharyngitis, lymphadenopathy, and peripheral blood lymphocytosis with atypical lymphocytes. The atypical lymphocytes seen in the peripheral blood of patients with EBV mononucleosis are larger than normal lymphocytes and have a vacuolated cytoplasm. These atypical lymphocytes can be distinguished from those found in malignant diseases by their heterogeneous appearance and polyclonality. However, the clinical presentation and large number of atypical lymphocytes may mimic features of leukemia precipitating detailed evaluation and rarely a tissue biopsy. Although the atypical cells in very early acute infection are of either B-cell or T-cell lineage, by the time of clinical symptoms, EBV-containing B-cells have been removed from circulation and only cytotoxic T-cells remain as the predominant atypical cell of mononucleosis. These CTL are responsible for the destruction of infected B-lymphocytes and epithelial cells as well as the multifocal areas of hepatic cell death. Splenomegaly occurs in approximately 50% of patients with IM, and hepatitis with elevation of transaminases is common. The splenic enlargement and potential involvement of the liver are cited as reasons for avoiding blunt trauma to the abdomen. IM typically resolves after a 6 to 12-week period of prolonged fatigue and low-grade fever, with splenic rupture or bacterial pneumonia being rare complications.

Differentiation from streptococcal pharyngitis is important because of the common findings of severe throat pain, petechial hemorrhages, and pharyngeal exudate. In addition to the characteristic hematologic finding of atypical lymphocytes, the detection of nonspecific heterophile (Paul-Bunnell) antibodies with a test modified to exclude cross-reactivity with Forsmann antibody such as the slide Monospot test is helpful. However, up to 10% of adults and the majority of children under 4 years of age (80%) do not have detectable heterophile antibody. In these different groups diagnosis depends on the presence of antibodies against EBV-specific proteins.

The EBV genome is large, approximately 172,000 base pairs and exists in a linear form in virions. As with other herpesviruses the genome has a short unique region followed by an internal repeat sequence and then a long unique region. There are multiple terminal repeats that allow for the formation of a circular genome. After infection of permissive cells, the genome circularizes, and amplification of episomal virion DNA may occur. Integration into the host genome is random and is not common, with the genome remaining in an episomal form in most latent infections. The portion of the genome where circularization occurs is unique for each infection cycle and may therefore may be identified by molecular techniques. Two strains of EBV have been described, and their association with specific disease remains a subject of debate. The EBNA proteins appear to represent much of the difference between the two types of EBV, designated as EBV-1, or A, and EBV-2, or B. Proteins of diagnostic significance or involved in characterized mechanistic pathways include the viral capsid antigens (VCA), early antigen (EA), latent membrane proteins (LMP), nuclear antigens (EBNA 1-6), ZEBRA (or BZLF-1) and BCRF-1. LMP-1 is expressed during latency, is commonly detected in nasopharygeal carcinoma, and has been shown to upregulate *bcl*-2.[64] Although relatively few transcripts may be produced in infected cells during viral latency, as many as 50 viral proteins may be present during the virus replication cycle.

EBNA proteins play a key role in several aspects of the EBV life cycle. EBNA-1 has been shown to have transforming activity in animal systems and is expressed in all infected cells. It is the only protein expressed in Burkitt's lymphoma-derived cells that does not enter a lytic cycle, and thus EBNA-1 is considered to be an important latent protein. Three separate pathways leading to activation have been proposed.[67] In some pathways the induction of the lytic cycle involved expression of LMP proteins, whereas in other situations, LMP expression is associated with latency. One important marker of the switch from latency into lytic infection is the expression of ZEBRA.

The abundant EBV *e*ncoded small *R*NAs (EBER) are also transcribed during latency, but their function is unknown. Since EBERs are present in greater numbers than the viral DNA as well as most other RNAs, they are a convenient target for in situ hybridization in tissues suspected of being latently infected with EBV.

The incubation period for EBV after experimental transmission is 3 to 7 weeks. The appearance of antibodies to EBV proteins after infection follows a characteristic pattern (see Fig. 36-5). However, variations occur among individuals, and interpretation of EBV serologic test results may be complicated and require clinical correlation. The main complication is distinguishing the transition stage after acute infection from reactivation disease. Confirmation of acute infection and a positive heterophile antibody may be made by detection of IgM antibody to EBV antigens with low levels of IgG VCA antibodies. As with other herpesviruses, IgM antibodies may be detectable in cases of reactivation or chronic EBV infection though the literature contains various opinions on this issue. The detection of IgG VCA antibodies and the presence of IgG anti-EBNA antibodies are evidence of a past infection. EBNA antibodies are typically not found during the acute phase of infection but may appear during the transitional or early convalescent stage. Antibodies to the EAs are highly suggestive of EBV reactivation when present at significant titer levels, usually equal to or greater than 1:40 by immunofluorescence. EA antibodies may also be detected during the convalescent stage of IM as well as with chronic EBV infection, though at lower levels than that seen with reactivation disease. Both diffuse (EA-D) and restricted (EA-R) components of EA have been described. EA(D) is methanol resistant and typically found in

IM and in patients with nasopharyngeal carcinoma. Interestingly, antibody to EA(R) is principally found in patients with Burkitt's lymphoma. In the case of heterophile antibody negative IM or suspected cases of X-linked lymphoproliferative disease, Wiskott-Aldrich syndrome or ataxia telangiectasia, testing for antibodies to EBV capsid antigens, nuclear antigens, and early antigens provides important supportive evidence for the diagnosis.[68]

The mechanism of viral pathogenicity for EBV involves acute processes as well as those involved in proliferation and transformation. In primary EBV infection there occurs a cell-mediated response that is responsible for the "atypical lymphocytes" in the peripheral blood. By the second week of illness the majority of atypical lymphocytes are T-cells of the cytotoxic type. Therefore the CD4/CD8 ratio may be reversed in acute EBV infection for up to 2 months. NK cells are responsible for destruction of a portion of the EBV-infected B-lymphocytes, though antibody-dependent cell-mediated cytotoxicity may also play a role.

Since EBV is a polyclonal stimulator of B-cells, the progression to lymphoma is a potential outcome of this proliferation. Several factors play a role, including immunosuppression, lymphoid growth factors, and the maintenance of sufficient numbers of cytotoxic T-cell numbers with EBV-specific activity. For example, some Burkitt's lymphoma cells are partially resistant to cytotoxic T-lymphocytes. Recently, it has been shown that the EBV protein BCRF-1 is highly homologous to IL-10, an interleukin that downregulates synthesis of IFN-gamma and suppresses T-cell proliferation. The production of BCRF-1 leads to downregulation of IFN-gamma, limiting the cells' ability to fight infection and yet enhancing B-cell proliferation.[69,70]

The role of EBV in neoplasia has received considerable attention, since the recognition by Denis Burkitt and others of lymphomas with characteristic morphologic features. In addition to the presence of EBV antibodies in all children with African Burkitt's lymphoma, EBV DNA and protein were found in virtually all Burkitt's lymphomas. However, since EBV could be found in only 15% to 20% of Burkitt's lymphomas in the United States, the association was not convincing. Later, the finding of EBV in neoplasias arising in immunosuppressed individuals provided important insights.

It is now recognized that neoplasia results from a multistep process, and explanations for the apparent differences between African and non-African Burkitt's lymphoma have incorporated this concept. EBV genes are capable of immortalizing B-cells, but additional steps are needed for development of a full malignant phenotype, and correspondingly pathways other than EBV exist for the development of lymphoma.[71] The discovery of a characteristic chromosomal translocation in Burkitt's lymphoma with either detectable or undetectable EBV DNA provided key evidence for this hypothesis. The translocation of the c-*myc* gene from chromosome 8 to chromosome 14 results in increased c-*myc* expression with a subsequent additional effect on cell proliferation possibly completing the malignant transformation. Multiple processes may place the cell at risk for developing the 8 to 14 translocation, of which one is infection by EBV. Therefore, although EBV accounts for the majority of Burkitt's lymphoma cases in Africa, in the United States multiple other common pathways exist for the development of lymphoma. This variability emphasizes that the presence of characteristic morphologic features does not necessarily indicate a specific mechanistic process leading to malignancy.

The different rate of lymphoma occurring in EBV antibody–positive individuals in Africa versus North America has been postulated to be attributable to the great influence of malaria on the underlying condition established by persistence of EBV infection of B-lymphocytes.[65] Continual or repeated challenge of the immune system can result in the reactivation of latent EBV infection and subsequent stimulation of B-cell proliferation, increasing the chance for a translocation event.

The biology of nasopharyngeal carcinoma is equally complex as that of lymphoma, and it is expected that much more will be learned about the role of EBV and the mechanism involved with this cancer. The link between EBV and nasopharyngeal carcinoma is based on epidemiology as well as molecular studies. As discussed earlier, the nasopharyngeal epithelium is a site of EBV infection and therefore the finding of EBV in tumors from this site might be expected; however it is nasopharyngeal carcinoma and not squamous cell carcinoma that was found to contain EBV. In comparison with Burkitt's lymphoma, 100% of nasopharyngeal carcinomas from widely separated parts of the world contain EBV proteins or DNA. Most significantly, nasopharyngeal carcinoma tumor cells have been shown to be clonally derived as determined by the nature of the EBV genome within tumor cells.[72] The detection of EBV within metastatic lesions of undifferentiated carcinoma is useful in the identification of nasopharyngeal carcinoma. Typically EBV is detected by immunohistochemical staining with antibodies to EBV antigens or by in situ hybridization to detect EBER. Patients with nasopharyngeal carcinoma also have high levels of antibody to EBV capsid antigens (VCA), but serologic test results alone are not convincing, since 90% of adults are seropositive.

In addition to the well-known associations between EBV and Burkitt's lymphoma and nasopharyngeal carcinoma, many other conditions are influenced or caused by EBV. A partial list of the most common conditions includes posttransplantion lymphoproliferative disorders (PTLD), Hodgkin's lymphoma,[73] Richter's transformation of chronic lymphatic leukemia (CLL),[74,75] aplastic anemia, and numerous conditions associated with iatrogenic or aquired immunodeficiencies summarized in Table 36-8.[68] Three categories of patients with PTLD have been described, those with an IM-like picture with

Table 36-8 Disease entities associated with Epstein-Barr virus

Infectious mononucleosis
Immunoblastic lymphoma
Hairy leukoplakia
Gastric carcinoma
Posttransplantation lymphoproliferative disease
Hodgkin's lymphoma (other than being lymphocyte predominant)
AIDS-associated lymphomas
Richter's syndrome
Burkitt's lymphoma
Nasopharyngeal carcinoma
X-linked lymphoproliferative disease
B- or T-cell lymphomas

resolution after reduction of immunosuppression, those with a progressive fatal IM illness with involvement of visceral organs, and those that develop lymphomas in the CNS or GI tract. The maintenance of lower serum concentrations of cyclosporin A than in the past in transplant individuals has significantly reduced the occurrence of lymphoma. The prevalence of PTLD in transplant patients varies from 1% to 2.5% for kidney or liver transplants, approximately 5% in heart transplants and 9% in heart and lung transplants.

A lymphoproliferative disorder discovered in related males was first described by David Purtilo and associates and termed *X-linked lymphoproliferative disease* (XLP).[68] XLP is characterized by the development of symptoms of IM and acquired agammaglobulinemia with the subsequent proliferation of B and T-lymphocytes leading to non-Hodgkin's lymphoma. Young males with the syndrome demonstrate a defect in cytotoxic T-lymphocytes that renders their immune system unable to clear the virus and therefore B-cells remain under continual virus stimulation. Nearly two thirds of XLP patients die of complications of IM after primary infection with EBV, and all males die by 40 years of age.

The demonstration of EBV within mucosal epithelium in cases of oral hairy leukoplakia offer insight into the cause of the lesion.[77] Bone marrow failure with pancytopenia is receiving considerable attention in relation to EBV infection, with interstitial pneumonitis, malabsorption, uveitis, or neurologic abnormalities being less commonly reported.[76]

The association of EBV with such a wide variety of disorders has led many to wonder whether it could be responsible for other entities without a clear cut cause. One such proposed ill ness is the *chronic fatigue syndrome,* a term that has been used to categorize a wide variety of complaints, including debilitating fatigue, pharyngitis, low-grade fever, headaches, and depression. A unifying case definition of chronic fatigue has been proposed and may facilitate our understanding of the disorder. Evidence exists for the presence of EBV in many of these patients, but its pattern or frequency is not different from that of asymptomatic control patients.[78] It is equally likely that the underlying immune alteration leading to the development of chronic fatigue could lead to EBV reactivation as well as impaired immune function. Most such patients lack objective physical findings or lymphocytosis though they may have serologic profiles consistent with EBV infection and perhaps other subtle immunologic abnormalities. However, in patients with chronic fatigue syndrome from the Lake Tahoe outbreak, antibody profiles between chronic fatigue patients and control subjects were similar. Recent evidence indicates excess immune activation in many definition cases of chronic fatigue.

Treatment of EBV infections is usually limited to supportive measures, but corticosteroids can be lifesaving if acute airway obstruction is impending because of tonsillar enlargement and for treatment of hemolytic anemia or severe thrombocytopenia. Corticosteroids are hazardous because of their suppressive effects on T-cells, which are necessary to terminate the EBV-induced proliferation of B-cells that otherwise can result in lymphomas later in life. Therapy for complicated EBV infection in immunosuppressed patients is also controversial, particularly regarding the use of acyclovir and interferons.[79] Encouraging results have been seen with the use of interferon-alpha, but long-term experience is needed before this modality is widely used. Chronic immunoglobulin therapy is used in XLP patients.

Cytomegalovirus (HHV-5)

Cytomegalovirus (CMV) is a "slow-growing" beta-herpesvirus. CMV was first designated the *salivary gland virus* and later named *cytomegalovirus* based on the characteristic cytopathic effect on cells (cytomegalia). In tissues as well as in culture the infected cells become enlarged with a characteristic inclusion.[80] Disease caused by CMV was first described before the turn of the century in affected newborns with congenital infection. In addition to congenital disease, CMV causes a variety of other illnesses including non–EBV associated mononucleosis, but the overwhelming majority of CMV infections produce only mild self-limited illnesses. The potential severity of disease as a result of congenital CMV and transfusion-related infection remain as concerns; however the severe immunosuppression of organ transplantation and recently AIDS has greatly extended the types of CMV pathogenesis in the 1990s. Nearly 100% of HIV-infected individuals have antibodies to CMV and it is often the cause of life-threatening disease. In addition over 20% of AIDS patients have CMV retinopathy.[81]

CMV is a relatively large virus with a 240 kb DNA genome.[82] The replication cycle requires at least 24 hours (3 to 6 times longer than herpes simplex). As with other herpesviruses, the cascade of dozens of viral products necessary for replication include immediate early proteins (IE, < 4 hours after infection) and early antigens (EA), which appear after IE but before late antigens (LA) and do not require DNA replication. The structural antigens (LA) generally appear more than 24 hours after infection. Surface membrane–embedded glycoproteins (glycoprotein B, the major membrane immunogen), immediate early glycoproteins, a few internal phosphoproteins (pp65 used in detection assays), and the DNA polymerase (the focus of antivirals such as ganciclovir) have been studied in greatest detail.[83]

CMV differs from HSV and VZV in being species-specific; for example, human CMV will not replicate in animal models and animal CMVs do not replicate in humans. Animal and human CMVs share substantial DNA homology but have important differences in antiviral susceptibility and pathogenesis.[84] Congenital CMV infection in humans is a significant problem, but mouse CMV does not cause a congenital infection because of the nearly complete barrier effect of the mouse placenta.

The CMV virion is typical of all herpesviruses.[85] It has a DNA genome within an icosahedral capsid surrounded by tegument (also known as the matrix) and a lipid bilayer envelope containing glycoprotein spikes. CMV virions have a half-life of 1 hour at 37° C, are resistant to trypsin, but are inactivated by heparin. CMV does not encode a virus-specific thymidine kinase, and therefore acyclovir is less effective than ganciclovir.

Replication in vitro results in many more defective than infectious particles. Defective particles can be either dense bodies (virions lacking capsids) or noninfectious enveloped particles that lack only the DNA core. Both entities contain the tegument protein pp65. It is the major tegument protein and localizes almost immediately to the nucleus after infection thereby presenting a target for rapid diagnostic assays.

Over 30 viral polypeptides are constituents of the capsid, tegument, and envelope, with eight in the envelope and 20 in the tegument.[85] The major capsid protein (U_L 80) shares homology with VP-5 of HSV-1. Other capsid proteins include the minor capsid protein U_L 46 and the structural assembly protein U_L 80. Glycoprotein B (gB) is the major target of neutralizing antibody[83] and functions to promote virus penetration and the spread of virus from cell to cell and for syncytial formation.[20]

CMV is most frequently transmitted by direct contact between fresh infected secretions (saliva, urine, blood, semen, breast milk, vaginocervical secretions) and skin breaks or mucous membranes. Thus CMV may be spread by sexual contact.[86] Less often, transfusion with CMV containing blood products or organ transplantation from CMV-infected donors is the source.[87] Two major peaks of nonperinatal acquisition occur: in the pre–school aged children, especially day care attendees, and in adolescence.[88] Both ages are notable for frequent contact with fresh exogenous body secretions.

CMV infections are not seasonal. CMV is not spread by aerosols and is difficult to acquire by fomites, despite being quite stable in urine. Infection requires membrane fusion between the virion and the host cell. Thus agents that damage virion lipid membranes reduce infectivity. Washing with soap effectively prevents transmission by body surfaces. CMV is also inactivated by exposure to UV radiation, alcohol, formalin, detergents, heat (>56° C), room temperature, low pH, ether, and by freeze-thawing. Although a commonly encountered concern, the risk of transmission of CMV to seronegative pregnant women is low[89] (see Table 36-7 and Fig. 36-11).

CMV acquired via cutaneous or mucous membrane portals first replicates locally, spreads to the vascular compartment (viremia), and thereby can seed nearly any organ. In the primary viremic stage it associates principally with neutrophils but later is found latent in mononuclear blood cells. The detection of CMV in neutrophils is the basis of newer antigenemia tests. It can be weeks before the urine becomes a site of excretion, whereas blood and respiratory secretions are early sites of replicating virus. The host protein β_2-microglobulin has an affinity for CMV virions and may contribute to reduction in the recovery of viruses from urine specimens. Common targets of CMV include liver, spleen, adrenals, and lungs. Lymph nodes also become involved. The classic pathologic lesion is a type A Cowdry inclusion (Fig. 36-10) with mononuclear cell infiltrate locally and sufficient inflammation that tissue destruction occurs locally.[90] In contrast to HSV, CMV-infected cells may have both cytoplasmic and nuclear inclusion. Unlike in vitro replication, which involves mostly fibroblasts, CMV infection in vivo involves mostly epithelial cells of solid organs (Figure 36-10). Detection of CMV DNA by in situ hybridization in tissue without associated cellular infiltrate is common in nondiseased organs such as liver and kidney and may be explained by the presence of latent CMV. Detection of RNA transcripts or viral proteins, however, indicates replicating virus and is strongly suggestive that CMV is etiologic in local disease.

The extent of CMV's prevalence was not recognized until population-based serologic studies were performed in the 1960s and 1970s.[90] Data from blood donors and seroprevalence studies indicate that more than 50% of adults have been infected, with active excretion in about 10%. CMV primary infections are rarely diagnosed and usually produce mild if any signs and symptoms. The developing fetus is susceptible to severe disease from transplacental infection when mothers first acquire CMV in the first half of pregnancy.[91] However,

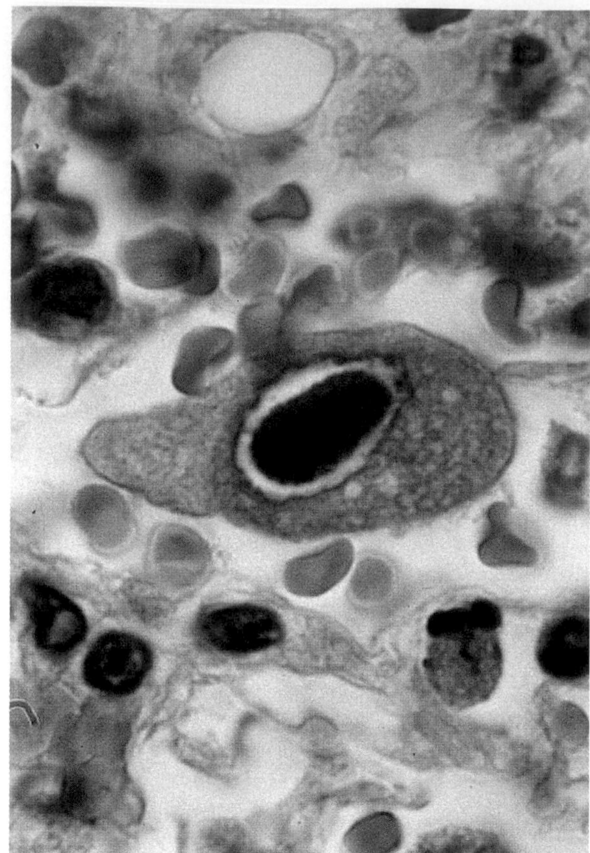

Fig. 36-10 Cytomegalovirus-infected cell with both intranuclear and cytoplasmic inclusions. (Courtesy James Newland, Omaha, Neb.)

less than 10% of CMV infections occur during the fetal and immediate neonatal periods. It is estimated that 37,000 congenitally CMV-infected infants are born each year, involving about 1.5% of all live births. These infants may exhibit dramatic signs and symptoms, consistent with cytomegalic inclusion disease (CID) (Fig. 36-11). Mortality during the first year of life ranges from 10% to 50% in CID infants. However, infants with CID represent less than 10% of all congenitally CMV-infected cases. Only 30% of mothers with primary gestational infection transmit to their infants and only 10% to 25% of these infants have CID-like disease. Most congenital infections are mildly symptomatic or even asymptomatic.[92] Seropositive mothers frequently (25% to 60%) reactivate CMV predominantly in cervical secretions or urine during pregnancy, but viremia is unusual in the presence of preexisting maternal immunity, and so placental exposure is not common. Thus reactivation infection during pregnancy results in a very low transmission rate (<1%) and even lower rates of symptomatic fetal infection. Congenitally infected infants may shed CMV particularly in their urine for up to 5 years. Older immunocompetent hosts who acquire CMV generally shed CMV for approximately 6 months after initial acquisition.

Perinatal infection by maternal blood, vaginal secretions, or breast milk also occur but are rarely symptomatic except in premature infants. A recurrent hepatitis/pneumonitis syndrome in infants has been described[93] but generally ceases to be a problem late in the second year of life.

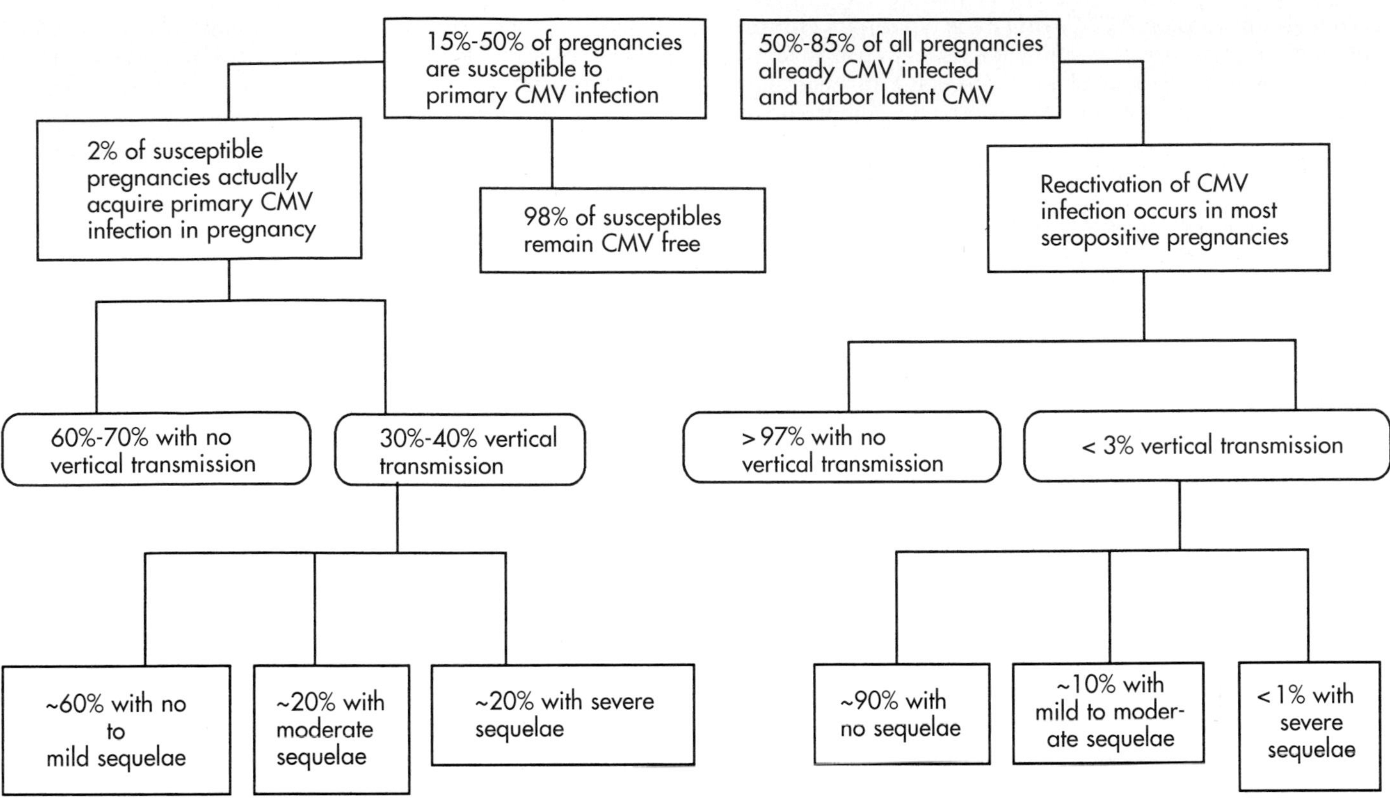

Fig. 36-11 Outcome of cytomegalovirus infection in pregnancy.

The most commonly detected illness attributable to CMV in the immunocompetent nonneonatal population is an EBV-negative mononucleosis.[94] The distinguishing clinical feature is the absence of sore throat during CMV mononucleosis, with the remaining signs and symptoms being virtually indistinguishable from EBV-induced mononucleosis. Fever for weeks, fatigue, adenopathy, and perhaps organomegaly are common findings. Peripheral lymphocytosis with atypical lymphocytes is common in the second to third week of infection. Liver enzyme elevations and thrombocytopenia are not infrequent. Distinction of CMV from EBV by laboratory techniques requires either an EBV-negative serologic profile or absence of EBV reactivation markers such as antibodies to EBV early antigen. CMV serologic features can be a Pandora's box, rarely being definitive for primary infection. This difficulty arises because up to 15% of reactivation infections result in IgM production, though at lower titers than with primary infection. The detection of IgM increases with age perhaps because of changes in immune function, with 63% of individuals over 60 found to be positive. Fourfold rises in IgG titers may also occur with reactivation. Thus it can be very difficult to attribute any current illness to CMV based on serology alone. Only seroconversion, seronegative to seropositive, confirms primary infection. Because CMV serology tests are currently performed with kits that do not permit titering, much of our older data have become even less useful in attempting to define primary CMV infection by means of serology testing.

Human CMV grows only in human cells, with fibroblasts being most permissive for culture. Detection in conventional cell culture can require up to 2 weeks; however, newer shell-vial centrifugation methods allow detection in as little as 24 hours. Mixtures of antibodies to IE, EA, or tegument proteins are currently used for rapid detection of CMV in patient samples. Direct antigen detection assays have also been developed for demonstration of virus in peripheral blood leukocytes.

Prototypic lab strains include AD169, Towne, and Davis. True serotypes have not been described, but restriction site differences are well described for clinical isolates. The genome is sufficiently diverse that cutting the genome with batteries of restriction enzymes can provide patterns that identify epidemiologically linked isolates. Geographic areas may have predominant strains, and in any given patient the restriction pattern remains relatively stable unless superinfection with new CMV strains occurs.

As with other herpesviruses, cell-mediated immune responses are most responsible for limiting primary CMV replication, for maintaining the immune surveillance that limits CMV to a latent state, and for preventing reactivation. Antibody responses appear capable of prophylactically modifying disease and perhaps clearing viremia, but antibody alone is unable to change existing disease (such as CMV pneumonia) in immunocompromised hosts. Antivirals do not cure CMV disease in that CMV excretion usually resumes soon after cessation of drug unless the host's immune capacity has become more effective in the interim. In immunocompromised hosts, transplant recipients, or HIV-infected patients, CMV can be devastating, with disease ranging from chronic fevers, hepatitis, retinitis, or thrombocytopenia to organ rejection, enhanced graft-versus-host disease, or fatal interstitial pneumonitis. Screening of blood donors for antibody to CMV has been used to decrease the transmission of CMV to immunocompromised individuals or neonates.[95] CMV disease is typically seen 5 to 6 weeks after transplantation. Even with aggressive treatment of CMV pneumonitis in transplant recipients with ganciclovir and immunoglobulin, the mortality is 40%, as compared with 85% if untreated. CMV retinitis may require chronic ganciclovir treatment to limit loss of vision in AIDS patients.[96]

Human herpesvirus type 6 (HHV-6)

HHV-6 was first described in 1986 after isolation from the blood of 6 patients with lymphoproliferative disorders and called "human B-lymphotrophic virus" (HBLV).[97] The virus was found to have typical herpesvirus virion characteristics under electron microscopy, though small DNA fragments did not cross-hybridize with any of the previously described herpesviruses. It was then found to infect T-cells frequently rather than B-cells and was given its current name. HHV-6 is now known to be the etiologic agent of the childhood exanthema, roseola, or exanthema subitum, for which an infectious agent had long been sought. HHV-6 has been proposed as an agent of interstitial pneumonitis[98] and bone marrow failure after transplantation.[99] In addition HHV-6 is being investigated as a cause of encephalitis, chronic fever, hepatitis, or pneumonitis in AIDS and transplant patients, and these possible associations remain a focus of continuing investigation.[100] No conclusive evidence has linked HHV-6 as a cause of chronic fatigue syndrome.

HHV-6 virions have the typical characteristics of all herpesviruses, and its genome is approximately 170 kb in length. HHV-6 is more closely related to CMV than to the other herpesviruses and has been classified as a beta-herpesvirus. This was determined by cross-hybridization of large DNA fragments with CMV and confirmed by examination of protein constituents. Antibodies to CMV glycoprotein B have been shown to cross-react with a putative glycoprotein B of HHV-6.[101] Homologies to HSV proteins and genes, DNA polymerase, and major capsid proteins have also been identified.

The mechanism of HHV-6 pathogenesis is only currently being defined. It is known that HHV-6 infection inhibits host DNA replication soon after viral DNA replication begins.

Seroprevalence studies showed that greater than 50% of children are infected by 10 months of life.[102] Acquisition is most common in early childhood, with the illness being roseola or simply high fever without localizing symptoms. During the febrile phase of primary infection, the virus can be isolated from the blood of virtually all patients but is detectable in only approximately 20% after 7 days. Antibody is first detectable soon after the onset of the rash or defervescence. HHV-6 cannot be isolated from healthy seropositive subjects but is readily isolated from saliva in patients with rash. A proportion of EBV-negative mononucleosis syndromes have been shown to be attributable to HHV-6.

HHV-6 appears to spread by the respiratory route, similar to VZV. Reactivation of latent HHV-6 has been observed on acquisition of other herpesviruses, such as CMV or EBV. HIV and HHV-6 can infect the same lymphocyte, but no definitive alteration in clinical disease has been described in HIV-infected patients. Transplant patients frequently reactivate HHV-6 when immunosuppression becomes moderately severe.

Similar to EBV, diagnosis of HHV-6 is more difficult than other herpesviruses because commercial assays are not widely available and it is difficult to isolate in cell culture. DNA hybridization and PCR methods for diagnosis are available in medical centers and can be used on DNA extracted from blood, secretions, tissues, or cell-rich fluids such as bronchial alveolar lavage. There are several strains of HHV-6, designated as GS, AJ, U1102, or Z29, differentiated by restriction enzyme cleavage sites and antigenic specificity.[103] Most roseola isolates are Z29, whereas isolates from AIDS patients are either Z29 or U1102.

In vitro susceptibility to available antivirals reveals that HHV-6 is resistant to acyclovir and zidovudine but is inhibited by in vivo achievable concentrations of ganciclovir and foscarnet.

Human herpesvirus type 7 (HHV-7)

Little is known other than the basic herpesvirus virion structure of the newest member of the herpesvirus family human herpesvirus type 7. It has been classified as a beta-herpesvirus with some homology to HHV-6 and CMV. Intense investigation has begun into possible clinical disease or syndromes associated with this potential pathogen. HHV-7 was first isolated from peripheral blood cells of healthy donors during attempts to isolate HIV-1. It produces CPE in culture that is similar to HHV-6. No definitive data are available on antiviral susceptibilities at present. Both HHV-7 and HIV-1 appear to utilize the CD4 molecule as a receptor, but confirmation is needed.

Viruses causing childhood illnesses or dermatologic manifestations

Many viral infections are first recognized on the basis of their dermatologic manifestations, which may be vesicular, macular, papular, or petechial. Typically infection occurs in childhood, though serologic evidence indicates that many adults have escaped infection. Viruses responsible for enanthems, or exanthems commonly appearing in childhood are presented here including measles, mumps virus, and rubella virus. The etiologic agents of roseola (HHV-6) and fifth disease *(Parvovirus)* are also presented. Vesicular lesions may be caused by HSV, VZV, coxsackieviruses, and other enteroviruses. Poxvirus, molluscum virus, and *Papillomavirus* cause pustular or proliferative lesions.

Measles

Measles virus is notable for being the most communicable respiratory virus. An individual may become infected by contact with coughed or sneezed droplets directly from the infected person, or even by a person transiently colonized but immune. Strict isolation is necessary to prevent spread, since infection can occur through contact with infected aerosol over a considerable distance. Attack rates among susceptibles are very high, being over 90% within families and closed populations. Patients are contagious for at least 7 days after symptom onset.

Currently the incidence of measles in the postvaccine era is 2 per 100,000 population. However, the outbreaks of modified and atypical measles on college campuses were rude awakenings for the medical community that considered measles under control and close to being eradicated. It has since become clear that a single immunization in infancy, even with live attenuated vaccine, produces inadequate immunity and a repeat immunization is necessary after infancy.[104] It remains to be determined whether an additional series of vaccine will be needed.

The nearly 16,000 nucleotide rubeola virus genome codes for six major proteins.[105] The virion contains functional groups similar to many other enveloped viruses. There is a fusion protein (F), a hemagglutinin (H), and a matrix protein associated with the envelope but no neuraminidase. There is also a nucleoprotein (N), a phosphoprotein, and a large (L) protein complexed to the RNA genome. The F and H proteins project from the virion membrane and allow virion attachment and membrane fusion with host cells for capsid entry.

Typical measles is diagnosed by the three *C*s (conjunctivitis, cough, coryza) coupled with a febrile morbilliform rash that begins on the head (approximately 14 days after exposure) and spreads centrally and downward, becoming more confluent with time. There is usually a 3- to 5-day febrile upper respiratory infection–like prodrome. The rash usually begins at the peak of respiratory symptoms and fever and is usually most confluent on the face. Infection typically begins in the upper respiratory tract, where it first replicates followed by a primary viremia and systemic spread of the virus and infection of T-lymphocytes and endothelial cells. Examination of lymphoid tissue after primary viremia may show Warthin-Finkeldy giant cells.[106,107] A pathognomonic enanthem, Koplik's spots, is an evanescent and transient collection of small whitish spots on the buccal mucosa but is present only early in the illness. Koplik's spots and the rash show similar histopathologic features reflecting infection of endothelial cells leading to hyperemia, edema, and lymphocytic infiltration.[108] Generalized adenopathy or splenomegaly are not uncommon. A relative leukopenia occurs with a more dramatic drop in lymphocytes than neutrophils. Symptoms usually begin to subside 3 to 5 days after the onset of rash, though the rash may persist for a week and the cough may last for 2 weeks.

Measles has a multitude of complications including encephalitis, severe pneumonia, and subacute sclerosing panencephalitis (SSPE).[109] Bacterial superinfections occur in nearly one third of measles patients. Common superinfecting pathogens include all the bacterial respiratory pathogens. Appendicitis may occur because of measles involvement of the appendix or secondary to the induced mesenteric adenitis. Progressive fatal measles giant cell pneumonia occurs in immunocompromised hosts or in nutritionally deficient hosts in developing countries. Measles giant cell pneumonia is a characteristic pulmonary lesion observed in hosts unable to mount an adequate immune response to the virus. Histologically, pulmonary parenchyma shows pronounced consolidation with massive formation of syncytial giant cells showing the characteristic intranuclear eosinophilic inclusions surrounded by a halo and intracytoplasmic inclusion bodies (Fig 36-12). Transient myocarditis occurs frequently, but long-term cardiac consequences are rare.

Clinically evident encephalitis occurs in about 0.1% of normal hosts with measles, usually within 8 days of the onset of symptoms. Mortality from encephalitis may reach 40% (usually 5% to 20%), and 20% to 40% of those recovering from measles encephalitis have sequelae. Measles may persist in the CNS after apparent clinical resolution, subsequently manifesting SSPE. Progressive fatal encephalitis also occurs in immunocompromised individuals. The risk of SSPE after natural measles infection is approximately 0.001%, with a higher risk if measles is acquired at an early age. The incubation for SSPE averages 7 years. Vaccines have an SSPE risk of about 0.0001%, but the incubation period averages 3.3 years.[110] Onset is insidious with gradual CNS deterioration extending over a 2- to 3-year period, often with speech and visual disturbances progressing to complex seizures and coma. Measles titers in serum are very high in SSPE, and measles antibodies can be detected in CSF.

SSPE is a rare complication of measles characterized by a progressive inflammatory brain disease of children and young adults. It was first described by Dawson in 1934, who suspected that it was a viral disease because of the inflammatory character of the lesions and the presence of intranuclear inclusion bodies in adjacent cells. These inclusion bodies are mainly found in neuroglial cells but also can be seen in neurons. Cytoplasmic inclusions are less numerous but can be found. The virus recovered from specimens from cerebral

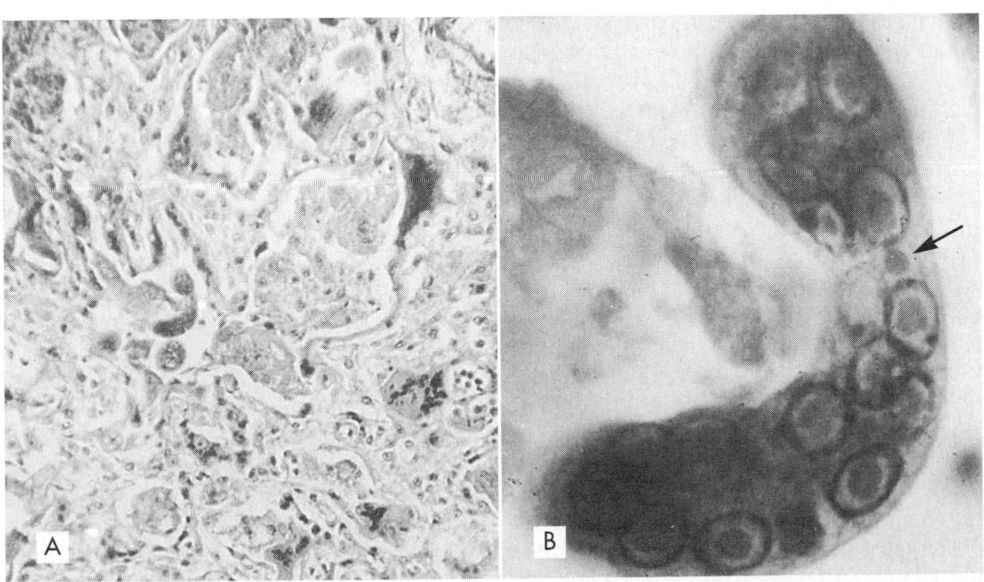

Fig. 36-12 Measles giant cell pneumonia. **A,** Low-power view showing syncytial giant cells lining alveoli and thickening of alveolar walls. **B,** High-power view of one giant cell seen in **A** showing many nuclear inclusions and one cytoplasmic inclusion *(arrow)*.

biopsies and lymph node biopsies of patients with SSPE represents a defective measles virus with a biochemical lesion that interferes with completion of the viral maturation process in the infected cell. The pathologic findings in SSPE are those of a subacute encephalitis involving both the white matter and gray matter of the cerebral hemispheres and the brainstem. There are perivascular lymphocytic infiltrates with evidence of neuronal loss. In later stages diffuse proliferations of glial cells and degeneration of myelin occur. By electron microscopy the inclusions are seen to contain tubular paramyxovirus-like nucleocapsids. Measles virus antigen can be demonstrated in the nuclei and cytoplasm of infected neurons and glial cells.

Atypical measles occurs in patients that received killed vaccine (no longer available in the United States) and results from subsequent infection by the wild type of measles virus. The incubation is the same as in typical measles, but coryza and conjunctivitis are not prominent, and Koplik spots are rare. The rash proceeds in a manner opposite to that of typical measles (from the extremities to the trunk). It may be confused with Rocky Mountain spotted fever rash.

Modified measles occurs in partially immune hosts resulting from incomplete vaccine-induced immunity, passive immunoglobulin administration, or occasionally in infants less than 9 months old with persistent maternal antibody. It proceeds similarly to typical measles, but symptoms are milder and of shorter duration.

Measles itself is immunosuppressive and can temporarily suppress the delayed type of hypersensitivity, as in the response to PPD skin tests. IL-2, interferon-alpha, and C reactive protein are elevated, whereas neutrophil, CD4, and natural killer cell function is reduced.

Rubella

Rubella virus is an RNA-enveloped virus composed of three major proteins, E1, E2, and C. E1 and E2 are glycosylated membrane proteins. The C protein and genome make up the nucleocapsid.[111]

In the prevaccine era, rubella (also called German measles, black measles, or 3-day measles) was the most common cause of congenital malformations. Thus rubella was greatly feared, and women often went into seclusion, or terminated employment during early pregnancy if they were not sure that they had rubella as a child. Rubella serology remains an important part of early prenatal care during pregnancy in the 1990s. Chances of rubella-näive pregnancies occurring in the future are expected to be further reduced by the inclusion of a second immunization after 5 years of age.[112] Universal vaccine used in childhood after 1969 has reduced the incidence of this disease at any age to a rarity in the United States.

Rubella virus typically produces a mild self-limiting exanthematous disease except in the early developing fetus. Because it has a direct effect on cell replication, fetal infections in the first trimester with this teratogenic agent can be devastating. Congenital rubella now occurs in less than 1 per 1,000,000 live births. However, among susceptibles attack rates of 50% to 90% occur upon exposure. Virus is shed in large quantities in respiratory secretions of infected persons for 5 days before and 6 days after onset of rash and is believed to be transmitted by aerosol and respiratory route. Man is the only naturally infected host. Winter and spring rates in the prevaccine era exceeded summer and fall rates.

On entry to the host, rubella virus initially replicates in the nasopharynx followed by a viremia with enhanced respiratory shedding just before onset of exanthem. In children, a prodrome of coryza or diarrhea often occurs after a variable incubation period of 14 to 21 days. In adults prodrome occurs more frequently and manifests as eye pain, headache, adenopathy, sore throat, cough, and fever. Posterior cervical and suboccipital lymphadenopathy is quite prominent in most infected children and adults, lasting longer than a week. Fever is generally mild and less than 38.5° C. The rash typically first appears on the face and spreads down and out over 24 hours finishing last on the hands and feet. The rash generally subsides 72 hours after onset. The rash is maculopapular and nonconfluent with discrete individual lesions. Nearly 25% of childhood rubella infections appear to be subclinical without apparent rash.

Arthritis is a common complication of rubella, ranging from 20% in children to over 70% in adults. Females have a higher incidence of arthritis than males. Fingers, wrists, and knees are most often involved. Encephalitis occurs usually 2 to 7 days after the onset of rash in about 1 per 5,000 cases of natural infection and is less severe than that caused by measles. Most patients recover without sequelae though death rates have appeared high in some outbreaks.

Congenitally infected infants excrete virus, sometimes for years. Defects in infants from first-trimester maternal infections primarily involve the inner ear, eye, and heart, but almost any organ or system can be involved.[113,114] Intrauterine growth retardation, meningoencephalitis, cataracts, sensorineural hearing loss, and congenital heart disease each occur in a notable proportion of congenitally infected infants. Mental retardation, hepatitis, hepatosplenomegaly, thrombocytopenia, and radiolucent lesions in long bones also occur not infrequently. Sequelae are reduced in incidence the later in pregnancy that maternal infection occurs. However, immunodeficiency can also occur in congenitally infected infants whose mothers become infected in late pregnancy.

No specific therapy exists, and prevention is the best "treatment." Screening of all pregnant females is recommended. Vaccine complications are uncommon.

Roseola infantum

Roseola, also called "exanthema subitum" ('sudden outflowering'), "baby measles," is the third common childhood exanthem. Yamanishi was the first to recognize the causative relationship between HHV-6 and the well-known roseola syndrome, though HHV-6 itself was first described in 1986.[115,116] For details on the virus see also HHV-6 in the herpesvirus section. It is nonseasonal and rarely is conferred to siblings. The incubation period appears to be 9 to 15 days. It is a generally benign, highly febrile (fevers of 39° C for 3 to 5 days are not uncommon) syndrome seen almost exclusively in infancy (6 months to 3 years of age). The rash begins on the trunk with later spread to neck and extremities. Roseola begins as discrete pink macules several millimeters in diameter which blanch with pressure and last from a few hours to several days. It resolves by "crisis" with defervescence appearing just after or in concert with the classic morbilliform rash. As such it leads to much anxiety among physicians and parents during the febrile preexanthem stage where other more serious illnesses must be considered. Up to 12% of emergency-department visits at some hospitals have been attributed to HHV-6 as well as many other less classic in presentation febrile illnesses. In the first days of fever, a leukocytosis is not uncommon, followed commonly by a leukopenia as the rash appears. Natural disease appears to confer permanent immunity. CSF findings are nearly always normal. Otitis media may follow roseola. No specific therapy is currently available.

Varicella

Varicella, or chickenpox, is the fourth common generalized childhood exanthem. Chickenpox, though usually benign in children, is a more serious illness in adolescents and adults with more frequent pneumonitis and a higher mortality. It is caused by varicella-zoster virus, the third member of the herpesvirus family. For more details on the virus and diseases other than varicella, refer to the section on VZV in the herpesvirus section of this chapter. The incidence of chickenpox is expected to decrease drastically following the release of OKA vaccine for use in children.[117] Boosters for this vaccine will probably be necessary to prevent outbreaks of serious cases of chickenpox among young adults because duration of vaccine-induced immunity is limited. Alternatively, the vaccine will be used in immunocompromised individuals in whom reactivation may be fatal.[118]

Varicella is highly contagious and can be spread by entering rooms previously occupied by a patient with varicella or even sharing air by means of heating and air conditioning systems. VZV DNA has been detected in air sampled from rooms having varicella patients. Face-to-face contact is not necessary for acquisition. Patients with varicella become contagious approximately 48 hours before the onset of rash and are believed to be contagious until the last vesicle has crusted over.

Chickenpox is generally a self-limited illness with a 7- to 21-day incubation and a 7- to 14-day course of exanthem. Fever and respiratory symptoms may be present for several days before the onset of exanthem. The exanthem generally begins on the head or in the scalp with gradual spread over 3 to 7 days to the rest of the body with the greatest density centrally on the body. The fever generally subsides 3 to 6 days after onset of the extremely pruritic rash.

The classic lesion begins as a blanching macule 2 to 4 mm in diameter and then becomes a papule and then a clear vesicle. Lesions larger than 5 mm should raise suspicion of an alternative cause or secondary bacterial infection. Vesicular fluid contains viable virus, and VZV can be detected by direct fluorescence of cell scraping from the base of vesicles using monoclonal antibodies against VZV. VZV can also be isolated in cell culture from clear vesicle fluid, but the virus is labile, and best results occur with bedside inoculation of vesicle fluid to cell cultures. DNA has been detected in nasopharynx and blood by PCR amplification techniques. Treatment with acyclovir is generally reserved for patients with a high probability of complications. Varicella-zoster immune globulin (VZIG) is used prophylactically and can successfully modify illness if given within 72 hours of known exposure to VZV.

Patients with impaired CMI frequently develop complicated varicella, mortality as high as 45% can occur in these populations. VZV is associated with a life-threatening dissemination or hepatitis in patients receiving chemotherapy or in bone marrow transplant patients if not recognized and treated. Even in immunocompetent hosts hepatitis and pneumonitis attributable to VZV may occur and may be life threatening. Encephalitis is a rare complication. Hemorrhagic varicella may be complicated by disseminated intravascular coagulopathy (DIC) and a fatal outcome. Pregnant women who develop chickenpox within 5 days before or after delivery transmit VZV to their infants perinatally, a malignant form of varicella with a high mortality frequently ensues. Congenital infection resulting from maternal varicella in early pregnancy is rare but can produce cicatrization lesions of the skin as well as CNS problems.

Erythema infectiosum

Parvovirus B19 ('small virus' in Latin) is the smallest DNA virus identified. The virus itself has no envelope and consists mainly of two capsid proteins, VP-1 and VP-2, surrounding a single-stranded DNA genome that is unique because the terminal sequences fold back on the middle portions to form a hairpin structure. Parvoviruses have been found in other animals such as dogs but have been shown to be species specific. Human parvoviruses include the prototype B19 (named from one of the original isolates) and the related adeno-associated virus (AAV).[119]

Erythema infectiosum (EI), also known as *fifth disease,* or *slapped cheek disease,* is the best known and most commonly diagnosed disease caused by parvovirus B19. The clinical manifestations are probably attributable to immune complexes, occurring after cessation of viral replication in most cases. The clinical syndrome of EI was described first in the late 1890s, and parvoviruses were discovered decades later in the 1970s. It was not until 1983-1984 that Anderson and colleagues described the association of parvovirus B19 with an outbreak of EI.[120] This disease is known as fifth disease because it is fifth on the list of "normal childhood exanthems" after measles, rubella, chickenpox, and roseola. It derived its third name, slapped cheek disease, from the prominent bilateral facial erythema that is part of the classic symptom complex. In most cases of primary infection, symptoms are minimal, and infection passes without notice. Over 50% of adults are seropositive.

Parvovirus is also the inciting agent for aplastic crises in patients with chronic hemolytic anemias.[121] In culture systems, the virus has shown strong tissue specificity and has been limited to growth in erythroid precursor cell lines. The mechanism for anemia is therefore likely to be a direct result of infection of a precursor in the erythrocyte lineage consistent with the finding that the cellular receptor is the erythrocyte P antigen.[18] The ability to affect erythrocyte precursors is also evidenced by an association of B19 with aplastic anemia. Platelets and neutrophils are rarely affected but have been reported to decrease occasionally.[122] Immunodeficient hosts, bone marrow transplants, HIV-infected patients, and chemotherapy recipients also may suffer severe or chronic anemias because of persistent lysis of RBC precursors from chronic parvovirus viremia and may exhibit persistent IgM antibodies to parvovirus.

More recently B19 has been associated with increased fetal wastage in women acquiring B19 in early pregnancy.[123] This results from direct infection of the placenta and fetus. Congenital anomalies have not been convincingly associated with this agent. The major fetal finding is hydrops fetalis, probably the result of an anemia induced by infection of erythrocyte precursors and perhaps a myocarditis.

Acquired arthritis has been commonly associated with B19 in adults and has been suggested to be an immune postinfectious syndrome. It is generally a self-limited symmetrical polyarthritis of wrists, hands, knees, and ankles occurring 2 to 4 weeks after initial infection. A more chronic arthritis of up to 13 months in duration that is clinically indistinguishable from juvenile rheumatoid arthritis has recently been reported in children.[124] The acute onset of symptoms resembles those seen after infection with *Borrelia burgdorferi*, and therefore Lyme disease should be considered in the differential diagnosis.

The incubation period is usually from 7 to 14 days with an overall attack rate of about 25% in susceptibles. Transmission is by contact with infectious material usually as aerosolized droplets via the respiratory tract. This generally requires close contact with the person during the period of viral shedding. Virus first infects the respiratory epithelium leading to a very high titered viremia (>10^{10} virions/ml). It is during this intense viremia that the reticulocytopenia occurs, thus producing a crisis in patients with chronic hemolysis who exhibit an extraordinary need for replenishing RBCs. Virus is excreted for at least a week.

Classic EI is a biphasic illness with a 2- to 3-day nonspecific febrile illness during initial respiratory tract replication preceding onset of the rash by 1 week. There are three stages to the rash beginning with a red area on each cheek followed by involvement of the trunk, arms, and legs and then a variable recurrence of the rash. On biopsy of this rash there is an epidermal edema with perivascular mononuclear cell infiltrate. The rash is uncommonly pruritic in children as opposed to adults and almost never involves palms and soles. Rash exacerbations are frequently related to exposure to direct sunlight or with taking hot baths or doing physical exercise.

Pregnant women believed to have acquired B19 can be monitored for changes in alpha-fetoprotein, which are suggestive of intrauterine hemolysis in the fetus. In utero transfusions have been used to treat hydrops fetalis attributable to such hemolysis, sometimes with apparent success. Intravenously administered immunoglobulin has been successful in affecting the anemia in immunodeficient hosts probably by modification of the persistent viremia by means of neutralizing antibody. No specific antiviral drugs exist.

Because the most infectious period is before the onset of the classical symptom complex, many pregnant women require counseling because of the anxiety produced on inadvertent exposure to children who subsequently exhibit EI. Although the diagnosis of EI is generally a clinical one, serologic or DNA amplification procedures may be helpful. Arthropathy, aplastic crises, and fetal infections are typically confirmed serologically because culture procedures for parvovirus are not adaptable for routine laboratory use. This difficulty arises from the absolute dependence on certain cell functions found only in dividing host cells in late S phase. Although human bone marrow cell lines and human fetal liver cells are permissive for in vitro growth, they are not used commonly for culture outside of specialized research laboratories. IgM appears by the second week after exposure and IgG by the third week of infection. IgM concentrations peak within 4 weeks and thereafter decline to below detectable levels. IgG has been dectected for several years after infection. Nucleic acid amplification and DNA hybridization may be useful in the testing of bone marrow and are available through reference laboratories.

Long-term sequelae outside of the chronic viremia/anemia in immunocompromised hosts are rare, though the arthritis in adults may persist for months.

Herpangina and hand-foot-and-mouth disease

Enteroviruses are the cause of two specific clinical entities that affect oral surfaces or the skin—herpangina and hand-foot-and-mouth disease.[24] Echoviruses can cause summertime epidemics of fever and maculopapular rashes in children under 10 years of age. Herpangina occurs most frequently in children but may also be seen in adults and typically results from infection by coxsackieviruses type A. It is recognized histologically as an inflammation of the mucosa and the muscularis. Clinically it presents as abrupt onset of fever and intense sore throat with the presence of small vesicles in the posterior area of the nasopharynx, soft palate, and tongue that progress to shallow ulcers and then resolve.

Hand-foot-and-mouth disease is characterized by moderately painful vesicular or nodular lesions on the soles and palms preceded by a vesicular exanthem of the buccal mucosa. Vesiculinodular lesions have also been observed on the buttocks and posterior area of the thighs. Herpangina may accompany hand-foot-and-mouth disease.

Mumps

Mumps is a febrile, usually self-limited disease caused by a member of the *Paramyxovirus* family and is most frequently diagnosed when associated with parotitis. Mumps infections in children and adolescents often produce only nonspecific signs and symptoms such as fever, malaise, and headache with parotid swelling not being present in the majority of cases. However, viremia occurs with mumps, and systemic signs may be present. Some mumps cases may present with swelling of only nonparotid salivary glands (<10% of cases). The relatively infrequent rate of parotid involvement is confirmed by prevaccine studies in which 88% of adults with no history of parotitis had mumps antibody.[125]

Transmission is by direct contact of respiratory mucous membranes with infected secretions of respiratory origin or contaminated fomites. The incubation period ranges from 12 to 22 days. Mumps is seen most frequently in late winter and early spring and in the prevaccine era major outbreaks occurred at 3- to 4-year cycles. Patients are considered noninfectious 7 days after the onset of parotid swelling. Fever persists for 3 to 5 days and is part of the nonspecific prodrome. When present, parotid swelling may be unilateral (25%) or bilateral (75%). The key diagnostic sign of acute parotitis is purulence in the opening of Stensen's duct.

Since 1980 widespread mumps immunization at 15 months of age has drastically altered the prevalence of this infection (more than a 90% decrease in incidence). It previously appeared predominantly in school-aged children (5 to 14 years old). Many physicians now practicing have never seen a confirmed case of mumps. The clinical diagnosis of mumps is often applied inappropriately to all cases of parotitis, leading to overdiagnosis, which is damaging to the public's confidence in a very efficacious vaccine. However there are true vaccine failures (4% to 8%), or infection after waning immunity in adolescence or young adulthood (up to 30% over 16 years of age). Other viruses capable of causing acute parotitis include influenza, parainfluenza, CMV, and enteroviruses. Drugs (phenylbutazone, thiouracil, iodides, and phenothiazines), diabetes mellitus, sarcoidosis, and Sjögren's syndrome can also produce nontender parotitis.

Since the advent of the vaccine and the major drop in incidence, serologic diagnosis of suspected mumps cases is encouraged. Confirmation of the diagnosis of mumps is also important for tracking true vaccine failures and notifying contacts. Mumps still appears periodically, and closed communities still occasionally experience outbreaks.[126] Mumps remains endemic in many foreign countries, and mumps immunization and reimmunization should be documented before travel to endemic areas.

Myocarditis caused by mumps virus is more frequent in adults than in children (up to 13% may have S-T changes). Intrauterine cardiac fibroelastosis may be the result of interstitial myocarditis with persistent left ventricular dilatation, relative mitral valvular insufficiency, and increased endocardial tension leading to compensatory hypertrophy. This in turn causes the accumulation of the thick layer of collagen and elastic tissue beneath the endocardial lining resulting in the development of endocardial fibroelastosis. However, this mechanism could be operational in myocarditis caused by a variety of viral agents.

A fourfold rise in antibody to mumps at 3 to 5 weeks by complement fixation (CF), hemagglutination inhibition assay, or neutralizing assay confirms the diagnosis. Mumps virus can also be isolated from the saliva from 6 days before to 9 days after the onset of symptoms, from the CSF during the initial 3 days of meningeal signs, from urine for 2 weeks, and from blood for the first 2 days of symptoms, but culture is rarely attempted except in the most ill patients. Amplification of nucleic acids after reverse transcription of RNA has been reported to be useful and may become important for diagnosis.

Males, especially if postpubertal, are at risk of orchitis (20% to 30%). Orchitis usually follows the onset of parotitis but resolves in concert with parotitis. Cases of isolated orchitis have been observed. Testicular atrophy may result in up to 50% of orchitis patients and infertility in about 13%. With bilateral orchitis, complete sterility is infrequent (2% to 6% incidence). Up to 5% of postpubertal women also may exhibit an oophoritis.

A twice-normal spontaneous abortion rate occurs in pregnant women who develop mumps. No congenital malformations have been convincingly linked to intragestational mumps, but endocardial fibroelastosis has been associated the most frequently.

Mumps is nearly always a self-limited disease of approximately 2 weeks in duration; however it appears to have a predilection for the nervous system. In the prevaccine era, it was the most common cause of acquired sensorineural hearing loss in children producing transient high-frequency deficits in 4% of patients and permanent unilateral deafness in 1 of 15,000 cases. Currently congenital CMV infection has supplanted mumps as the most common cause of acquired sensorineural hearing loss. Up to 6% of patients are hospitalized. Clinical meningitis occur in up to 17% of mumps cases, but as many as 50% have the characteristic CSF lymphocytic pleocytosis when tested.[127] Hypoglycorrhachia may also occur. Uneventful recovery is expected from the aseptic meningitis. Encephalitis is a rare but more serious CNS complication that sometimes occurs including prolonged coma and having a 1.4% mortality. Death is more likely in adults.

Pancreatitis occurs in up to 25% and is evidenced by epigastric pain and vomiting. Without these symptoms pancreatitis can easily be overdiagnosed biochemically because many patients with parotitis exhibit a rise in amylase released from the inflamed parotid gland. Therefore elevated serum lipase may be a more reliable indicator of pancreatic involvement. Epidemiology data indicates that mumps may be involved in juvenile-onset insulin-dependent diabetes, since these individuals of a certain HLA type show abnormal immunoreactivity against mumps virus antigen.

A polyarticular, salicylate-resistant arthritis occurs rarely with mumps, usually in males as the parotitis is waning, a complication that may persist up to 6 months but usually lasts only a few weeks.

Only supportive therapy (antipyretics and cold packs) is available for mumps. Immunoglobulin does not affect disease once present or prevent orchitis.

Poxviruses and molluscum virus

The poxviruses of mammals are a complex group of agents that produce vesicular skin lesions. They are the largest animal viruses, containing a double-stranded DNA genome. Poxviruses are very resistant to chemical and physical inactivation. They multiply in the cytoplasm of cells, and the virions mature in cytoplasmic foci, or "viral factories," a capability that is unique among DNA viruses. Some of the important poxviruses are the etiologic agents for vaccinia, variola, ectromelia, monkeypox, and molluscum contagiosum. As a result of the successful campaign sponsored by the World Health Organization (WHO), smallpox (variola) has been eradicated worldwide, with the last nonlaboratory case appearing in 1977 in Somalia. Two additional cases appeared in laboratory workers in England in 1978, but the outbreak was quickly controlled.[128] Molluscum virus has since become the most common poxvirus to infect humans. Monkeypox remains in West Africa, and although the pathogenesis is similar to smallpox, no eradication program is in effect. Lymphadenopathy is more pronounced in cases of monkeypox than in smallpox but has lower transmissibility.

Variola infection was limited to humans, and study of the virus has been limited because of the laboratory hazards. The clinical disease produced by smallpox has a severity that ranges from the very mild to the very severe and often fatal form. There are at least two strains of variola virus; the most virulent caused variola major with a mortality of 20% to 50%. Variola minor, or alastrim, has a mortality of less than 1%. Variola virus is transmitted by close contact and is spread through the air, gaining entrance to the respiratory tract where it multiplies in the epithelium and regional lymph nodes. This first replicative period is followed by viremia with dissemination of the virus to the reticuloendothelial system. There follows a second replicative phase, in which a second viremia spreads to the skin, lymphatics, and internal organs. This secondary viremia marks the beginning of clinical symptoms. Clinically smallpox is characterized by fever followed a few days later by a centrifugal papular rash that appears first on the face and the skull and spreads to the back, chest, arms, and legs. The macules become papules, vesicles, and finally pustules, which resolve and eventually leave a scar.

The cutaneous lesions in the papular stage have a diameter of 2 to 4 mm and are partially buried in the skin. Microscopically the cutaneous lesions first show vascular congestion with mononuclear cell infiltrate in the dermis. The epidermal cells show ballooning degeneration with formation of an intraepidermal vesicle. There is involvement of the adnexal elements. Cells with cytoplasmic inclusion bodies (Guarneri bodies) can be found in early vesicles and disappear with healing. These inclusion bodies are variable in size, granular, eosinophilic, round to oval, and surrounded by a halo. In fatal cases, pneumonia of the interstitial type is often seen.

The present vaccinia virus was probably derived from the cowpox virus by the process of person-to-person vaccination. In 1798, Jenner was the first to observe that pustular material from the lesions of cowpox protected humans from infection with smallpox. Jenner's observations formed the basis for vaccination. Vaccination results in a modified swelling at the site of vaccination and regional lymphadenopathy. Primary vaccination sites develop a vesicle within 3 to 5 days that will become pustular and reach maximum size after approximately 3 days. The lesion forms an eschar and leaves a circular scar approximately 1 cm in diameter. Complications that result from vaccination are postvaccination encephalitis, vaccinia gangrenosa seen in patients with T-cell immunodeficiencies, eczema vaccinatum seen in patients with atopic dermatitis, generalized vaccinia, and erythematous urticarial lesions.

The vaccinia virus now serves a valuable purpose as an expression vector capable of the production of foreign genes cloned into the genome, which remains replication competent.

Molluscum contagiosum

Molluscum contagiosum is a virus of worldwide distribution and is a benign skin disease characterized by raised, umbilicated, waxy, cutaneous nodules.[129] Although the lesions may be found on any body surface, typically they are found on perineal skin, and transmission through sexual contact is likely. Outbreaks occur in childcare situations. The lesions may be multiple or solitary. Histologically molluscum contagiosum is a proliferative lesion that is elevated above the adjacent skin and is composed of epidermal keratinocytes. The infected cells contain large intracytoplasmic eosinophilic inclusion bodies, termed *molluscum bodies* (Fig. 36-13). Since the lesion has a characteristic appearance, diagnosis is frequently made clinically, but in many cases the central umbilication is not obvious and a biopsy or cultures are taken. An interesting phenomenon occurs in culture, in that molluscum CPE is nearly identical to that of herpes simplex, and since the site cultured may be consistent with this impression, an erroneous report of nontypable herpes simplex may be made. Distinction can be made by determination of whether the virus can be passed to subsequent cultures because this is successful for herpes but not for molluscum.

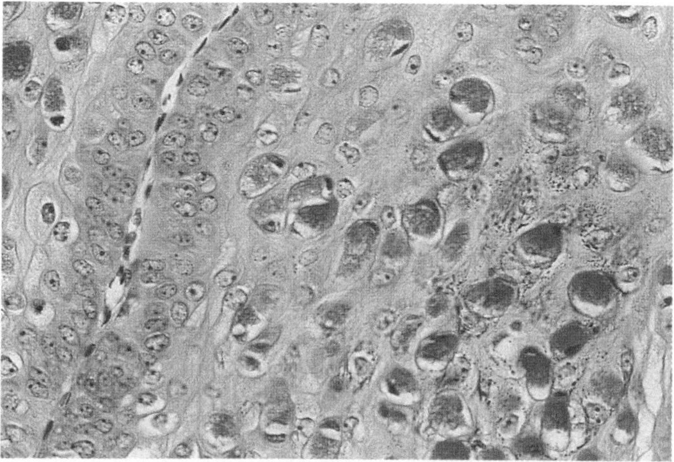

Fig. 36-13 Molluscum contagiosum with intracytoplasmic inclusions, "molluscum bodies."

Two additional poxviruses that cause disease in humans are the paravaccinia virus of cattle, which produces milker's nodules, and orf virus of sheep, which causes contagious pustular dermatitis.

Papovaviruses

The name *papova* is an acronym derived from *pa*pilloma, *po*lyoma, and simian *va*cuolating virus. This family of viruses can be divided in two genera, *Polyomavirus* and *Papillomavirus*. Papillomaviruses and polyomaviruses replicate in the nuclei of mammalian cells and form nonenveloped nucleocapsids, 30 to 50 nm in diameter, containing the DNA genome. The viruses remain in the nucleus until the cell dies and is lysed Papillomaviruses are distinguished from the polyoma group by the size of their capsid (55 nm in diameter) and their genome.[130]

Viruses of the papovavirus family have received extensive study by molecular biologists because they caused tumors in experimental animals and have been found in human transformed cells lines.[2] One papovavirus, simian vacuolating virus 40 (SV40) infects monkeys and contains a gene product capable of immortalizing cells in culture and hence was called the T (for 'tumor') antigen. Simian virus 40 is also notable for being a contaminant of the first inactivated and oral poliovirus vaccines. This initially led to concern for increased risk of cancer in vaccinated patients; however this is now known to be unwarranted.

Polyomaviruses

The relevant members of the *Polyomavirus* genus that infect humans are JC and BK viruses, named from the initials of the patients from whom they were first isolated.[131] Infection, by either virus, typically occurs in childhood, and up to 80% of adults have antibodies to JC and BK. Both viruses may latently infect the host. Acute infection by BK and JC virus in children is typically unrecognized; however, a mild respiratory illness has been noted in children with recent BK virus seroconversion. The mode of transmission has not been established but is likely to be respiratory. For both BK and JC virus, the kidney and uroepithelium, as well as mononuclear cells, have been shown to contain DNA sequences and are considered sites for viral latency. JCV has been detected in 50% of normal brains examined at autopsy and therefore the brain also appears to be a site of latency. BK and JC reactivation occurs in chronic illness and during immunosuppression as well as in pregnancy.

With the increased number of patients who are immunosuppressed it has become increasingly apparent that JC and BK cause specific disease in humans. JC virus causes progressive multifocal leukoencephalopathy (PML), and BK is associated with hemorrhagic cystitis.

BK virus was first isolated by Gardner and co-workers from the urine of a renal allograft recipient of immunosuppressive therapy.[131] It has also been isolated from the urine of patients with Wiskott-Aldrich syndrome and from a biopsy specimen of a cerebral lymphoma in a child with Wiskott-Aldrich syndrome. In immunosuppressed patients urinary cytologic tests may show cells with intranuclear inclusions that have been shown by electron microscopy to contain papovavirus capsids. The identification of these cells in urinary cytologic preparations has been correlated with reactivation of BK. Studies by Arthur and Shah described the association of BK virus in the urine with hemorrhagic cystitis occurring in bone marrow transplant patients. This correlation was challenged because many patients treated with chemotherapy develop bladder symptoms and the presence of BK may only reflect their immunosuppressed state and not be the cause of hemorrhage. DNA-amplification assays have been able to differentiate BK and JC, and it has now been shown that BK virus is much more frequent than JC in urine from bone marrow transplant patients.[132]

The diagnosis of PML and JC virus is made by clinical history and characteristic morphologic lesions on CT scans. PML is a neurologic disease that in the past primarily affected adults between 50 and 70 years of age usually with an underlying defect in cell-mediated immunity. In the 1990s PML is most often seen in immunocompromised hosts, especially in patients with AIDS, leukemia, lymphoma, Hodgkin's disease, diffuse carcinomatosis, sarcoidosis, or tuberculosis. It has also been reported in patients with congenital immunodeficiencies. PML is found in up to 24% of individuals infected by HIV. The neurologic manifestations of the disease indicate diffuse asymmetric involvement of the cerebral hemispheres. The duration from onset of symptoms to death is usually less than 6 months. The pathologic diagnosis of PML is usually established at postmortem examination, but it can be made on brain biopsy. At autopsy the gross lesions appear most often in the cerebrum, beneath the cortical ribbon, and resemble small necrotic areas. They tend to coalesce to form larger foci of demyelination. When several months old, the lesions appear as retracted foci grossly resembling a cerebral infarct. The distribution in the central nervous system is variable, with the cerebrum being the most frequently affected site.

Histopathologically, the hallmark of the disease is the presence of oligodendrocytes with enlarged nuclei containing basophilic intranuclear inclusion bodies. JC viral antigens can be shown to be present in the abnormal oligodendrocytes by immunohistochemical techniques, and ultrastructural examination reveals the presence of viruses often in a paracrystallinarray. Overall, the morphologic appearance is that of multifocal areas of demyelination without inflammation. This is consistent with the in vitro tropism for oligodendrocytes with the cytocidal effect leading to demyelination. Replication of JCV is low in established cell lines, and fetal brain cell cultures are required. No cytologic abnormalities are seen in neurons, ependymal cells, endothelial cells, or macrophages. The disease has not been transmitted to experimental animals, but monkeys have a pathologic lesion identical to PML that has been shown to be caused by the SV40 virus, the *Polyomavirus* of the monkey.

Considerable effort has been made, with little supporting evidence, to determine whether these viruses are associated with human cancer. However, it has been shown that selected tumors in children (choroid plexus papillomas) contain sequences that are related to the T antigen of SV40. Interestingly, these are the same tumors appearing in hamsters injected with SV40.

Papillomaviruses

Human *Papillomavirus,* or human wart virus, constitute the second family of human Papovaviridae of which more than 60 types have been identified. Papillomaviruses are highly species specific and tissue specific. They are noted for their capability for inducing epithelial and mesenchymal proliferative lesions in a variety of animals. In the human the papillomaviruses are epitheliotropic and replicate in the nucleus of squamous cells. Infection by HPV has reached epidemic proportions in certain age groups and has become one of the most common sexually transmitted diseases.

The various types of human papillomavirus are classed into groups, and the DNA of members cross-hybridize with no significant homology to other groups when tested under stringent conditions.[130] Serology plays little role in the taxonomy of this group of viruses. The genetic organization of *Papillomavirus* differs from *Polyomavirus,* for which separate DNA strands code for vegetative functions and structural proteins whereas in papillomaviruses there is only one coding strand. The genomes of HPV contain approximately 10 genes, including early genes, E1 through E7, and late genes, L1 and L2. The late genes are expressed only in productively infected cells.

A characteristic feature of HPV is the ability to induce epithelial cell proliferation. Cutaneous warts (verruca vulgaris) may be found anywhere on the skin. They are circumscribed nodular growths having a hyperkeratotic surface. Histologically the lesions appear papillary with thickening of the epithelium overlying a vascularized connective tissue core (hence papilloma) (Fig. 36-14). On non–pressure bearing surfaces, the lesion extends above the adjacent skin, whereas on the sole of the foot (plantar warts) the lesion extends inward displacing the underlying tissue. In addition to the digitated appearance, lesions show prominant keratohyalin granules, and individual cells may be surrounded by a clear halo. Cells with vacuolated or clear cytoplasm are called *koilocytes,* and by electron microscopy and immunocytochemistry have been shown to contain HPV particles or antigens.

One of the most significant observations in viral oncology was the finding in anogenital tissues that certain types of HPV are associated with benign lesions whereas other subtypes are found most commonly in high-grade lesions, thus the concept of low-risk and high-risk HPV. Low-risk HPV types are 6 and 11, whereas high-risk HPV are 16, 18, 31, 33, and 35. The evidence for associating HPV with human cervical cancer is con-

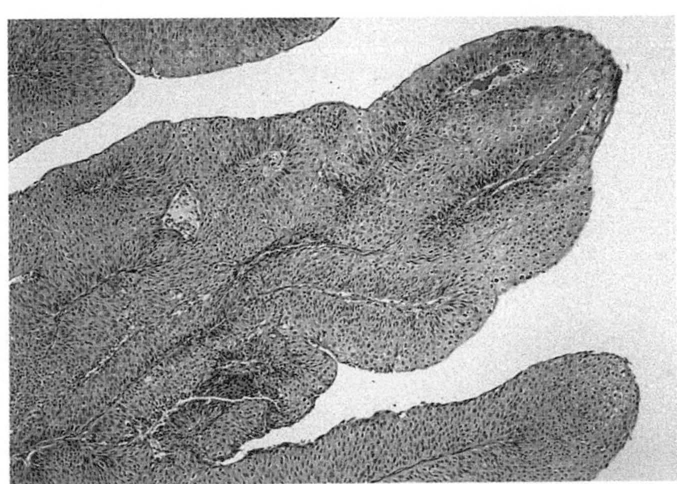

Fig. 36-14 Papilloma lesion, demonstrating the digitated or papillary appearance.

siderable and includes the finding that over 80% of cervical cancer tissues contain HPV genomes. The viral genome is found in an episomal form in benign or preneoplastic lesions, whereas the genome is integrated in the host chromosome in cell lines derived from epidermoid carcinoma of the cervix. Expression of integrated viral genome or genomes is most likely necessary for the maintenance of the malignant state. Specific genes of high-risk viruses are able to transform keratinocytes.[133] More than one virus type can infect a tissue simultaneously, and this may explain situations where a low-risk HPV type is found in a carcinoma.[134] Considerable information regarding the mechanism of neoplastic transformation has been obtained through in vitro experiments showing that the HPV gene E6 plays a role in decreasing levels of the dominant acting p53 gene.[135] It is believed that one of the major differences between high-risk and low-risk HPV types is their respective ability to complex with p53 and target it for degradation through the ubiquitin system.[136]

Skin warts and mucosal papillomas may regress spontaneously, and at least two thirds of the cases do so. There is a high incidence of papillomas in immunosuppressed patients or patients with congenital immune deficiencies. Malignant transformation of cutaneous warts does not occur except in some patients with epidermodysplasia verruciformis. Carcinomas can develop in long-lasting epidermodysplasia verruciformis lesions when additional factors such as ultraviolet rays act on HPV-infected cells. Multiple laryngeal papillomas occurring during infancy and childhood are commonly caused by papillomaviruses type 11 and are believed to be acquired at birth from exposure to an HPV-infected genital tract. HPV has been associated with several lesions in humans such as inverting papilloma, characterized by irregular folds of thickened mucosal epithelium. Other HPV-associated lesions are listed in Table 36-9. Although the morphology of keratoacanthoma is also suggestive of HPV, the association has not been fully studied.

Condylomata acuminata are verruciform anogenital lesions that are venereally transmitted and are not associated with skin warts. As a general rule, HPV types that infect skin do not also infect mucosa. Some of the condylomas may become very large. Verrucous carcinoma may also be seen in large condylomatous lesions.

Although papillomaviruses are found in many different species, no evidence exists for the transmission of the bovine, murine, or caprine papillomaviruses to humans (or toads). The so-called butcher's warts found in the skin of meat packers has been shown to be of the HPV 11 type.

Table 36-9 Lesions associated with human papillomavirus

HPV type	Disease associations
1	Plantar warts
2, 4, 7	Common skin warts
11	Butcher's warts
5, 8, 9, 12, 14, 15 17, 19-25, 28, 29	Epidermodysplasia verruciformis
5, 8, 14	Squamous cancer epidermodysplasia verruciformis
6, 11	Anogenital papillomas, laryngeal papillomas Cervical dysplasia
42	Vulvar papilloma
16, 18, 31, 33, 35, 39	Cervical neoplasia
18	Endocervical adenocarcinoma
30, 40	Laryngeal cancer
6	Inverted papilloma

Respiratory viruses

Many viruses can cause either upper or lower respiratory tract symptoms, the most common site of infectious disease affecting humans. The common cold caused by human rhinoviruses and influenza caused by orthomyxoviruses account for the majority of respiratory illnesses each year. *Flu* is a term frequently used by the public to describe a wide range of symptoms affecting the respiratory system or the GI tract. From a medical viewpoint, influenza refers to illness caused by influenzaviruses or parainfluenzaviruses in the Orthomyxoviridae or Paramyxoviridae family. Other significant viral causes of respiratory disease include adenoviruses, echoviruses, coronaviruses and herpesviruses; measles, mumps, rubella, and lymphocytic choriomeningitis viruses are less frequent causes. Even more uncommon is a potentially fatal influenza-like illness caused by hantaviruses.

Influenza

Influenza is usually diagnosed clinically in respiratory virus season (late fall to early spring) when symptoms are highly suggestive. Because therapy is available, and disease is usually more severe for influenza A than for influenza B, prompt and early diagnosis is important. The Orthomyxoviridae family includes influenza viruses A, B, and C and are differentiated on the basis of a soluble antigen (S antigen) associated with the internal ribonucleoprotien of the virion.[137] The viruses are further differentiated on the basis of the biologic properties of filamentous spikes extending from the glycoprotein envelope. These spikes convey both hemagglutinating and neuraminidase activity. Influenza A has three strains, categorized by their mix of 1 of 3 hemagglutinin (H) antigens and 1 of 2 neuraminidase (N) antigens, such as H1N1 or H3N2. Major changes in composition of either or both of the H or N antigens occur with influenza A alone and are referred to as *antigenic shift.* Shifts can produce widespread, more severe clinical disease than minor changes (antigenic drift) do. Drift can occur with either influenza A or B and is determined by a reduction in reactivity of immune serum against the prior year's strains carrying the H and N antigens with the same number. Cross protection between different variants of the same type are therefore incomplete. Natural infection conveys almost 4 years of type-specific protection in adults (probably less in children), whereas immunization cannot be counted on for more than 1 year's protection. Mild flu seasons occur when strains remain stable in consecutive years or the same strain recirculates after only a short hiatus.

Matrix, or membrane (M), proteins and nucleoproteins have been implicated as immunogenic targets for cellular responses. Neutralizing antibody is partially protective, but viral clearance depends on developing cytotoxic T-cell memory for the infecting strain. Symptoms vary with the serotype and with the degree of preexisting immunity.

Functionally, the H and N antigens have different properties.[138] Hemagglutinin binds to sialic acid–containing receptors on respiratory and nasopharyngeal epithelial cells. Viral hemagglutinin incorporated into host cell membranes or as a component of the virus envelope accounts for the binding of red blood cells to the surface of infected cells (hemadsorption) and the agglutination of RBCs, a property used to confirm isolation of the virus in the laboratory. The inhibition of this reaction by specific antisera provides the basis for tests providing serotype identification of these viruses. Except for RSV, all myxoviruses (influenza and parainfluenza) induce the synthesis and incorporation of viral hemagglutinin into the host cell plasma membrane and are therefore considered "hemadsorbing" viruses. The action of neuraminidase facilitates penetration of mucus and induces release of new virions.

At the molecular level, the influenza genome is segmented into eight separate pieces of RNA and undergoes rearrangement by a process termed *reassortment mutation* resulting in the generation of new subtypes (Table 36-10). Major antigenic shifts usually herald pandemics (worldwide epidemics) and are likely to result from genetic recombination of viruses that have replicated in nonhuman reservoirs. Continual shifting of RNA segments between animal and human influenza viruses allows for the emergence of new antigenic types that infect the human population.[139] Swine, ducks, and geese are natural reservoirs of the virus in which new antigenic types may arise. Once a new strain emerges it may be at a selective advantage, since there is a high level of immunity in the human population to the old strain but a lack of immunity to the new strain.

Influenza was considered the "last great plague" until the discovery of AIDS. Epidemics of influenza have been recorded for the past 400 years and before vaccination programs occurred every 2 to 3 years. The catastrophic pandemic of 1918 led to about 500,000 deaths in the United States alone and may have contributed to the early end of World War I.[140,141] Even in the 1990s, periods of excessive mortality particularly among the elderly and in patients with underlying chronic illness coincide with the influenza season. During flu season, nearly 50% of all febrile illnesses can be attributed to infection by influenza viruses. These seasonal outbreaks in communities occur on an annual basis often beginning in the fall of each year. Outbreaks are attributable to a limited number of defined strains and are commonly named for the site of first isolation, such as Hong Kong flu, Russian flu, Beijing flu.

Table 36-10 Influenza gene segments and their products

Gene segment	Product	Function	Immunity
1	PB2	Synthesis of RNA	Unknown
2	PB1	Synthesis of RNA	Unknown
3	PA	Synthesis of RNA	Unknown
4	H	Cell membrane attachment	Subtype specific
5	N	Virus progeny release	Subtype specific
6	NP	Synthesis of RNA	Type specific
7	M1, M2	Matrix (structural)	Type specific
8	NS1, NS2	Nonstructural unknown	

A worldwide surveillance program is in effect to identify the most likely strains for inclusion in the annual flu vaccine.

Influenza viruses are transmitted primarily in the air with subsequent infection of upper respiratory epithelium. Completion of replication in epithelial cells results in cell death, edema, and inflammation. The incubation period for influenza is typically 2 to 3 days. Large amounts of virus are present in secretions (10^6 particles/ml) accounting for the short incubation and explosive onset with minimal prodrome. Infected humans are the most common vector, and contact with infected secretions by means of fomites or hand to hand and self-inoculation of respiratory mucosa are the most frequent modes of spread. Most efficient spread occurs in crowded living conditions such as military barracks, dormitories, daycare facilities, and nursing homes. Influenza A is usually shed for 7 to 10 days, whereas influenza B can be shed for 2 to 3 weeks. In immunocompromised host, shedding can persist for months.[142]

Sudden onset of headache, myalgias, fever, and chills are classic symptoms of most influenza-induced illness. Although sore throat and dry cough are common, they are rarely self-reported because of the overwhelming systemic symptoms, which predominate. Influenza produces such a rapid onset of high fever that febrile seizures are frequently triggered in children. Influenza A produces more severe disease than influenza B does, and respiratory signs and symptoms predominate. With influenza B, milder symptoms that frequently have strong gastrointestinal components in addition to respiratory disease may be followed by a transient myositis especially in calf muscles. Gastrointestinal symptoms are more common in children than in adults (a five- to tenfold increase in incidence) and are also more common with influenza B.[143] Ocular burning and pain with eye movement are quite characteristic of influenza B. Adenovirus, enterovirus, and streptococcal diseases may be confused with influenza based on purely clinical grounds.

Morphologic features of acute influenza virus infection include desquamation of the ciliated and columnar epithelium of the nasopharynx, nasal cavity, and bronchi. Individual cells show pyknosis of the nuclei and loss of cilia. If the infection progresses to pneumonia, the bronchial epithelium may slough with intra-alveolar hemorrhage and hyaline membrane formation. The inflammatory infiltrate is sparse unless accompanied by a comcomitant bacterial infection.

Unless complications such as pneumonia or bacterial superinfection occur, prognosis is good in patients who are not elderly or in high-risk categories. Progressive viral pneumonia may occur in high-risk patients and is one of the reasons for recommending immunization annually for high-risk patients and aggressive treatment even of "ordinary" influenza in these populations. Reye's syndrome was an infrequent but consistent complication of influenza in the past but has nearly disappeared since aspirin use has been avoided for symptomatic therapy of influenza.[144] Guillain-Barré syndrome, transverse myelitis, acute glomerulonephritis, pericarditis, myocarditis, and aseptic meningitis are rare complications of influenza. Influenza C is not considered a major clinical pathogen of man and is not included in annual influenza vaccines.

Intrafamily spread of influenza is almost certain in the absence of vaccination. Thus, when one person in a family is diagnosed with influenza A, amantadine may be useful for treatment of the index case and as prophylaxis of family contacts.

Parainfluenza viruses

The Paramyxoviridae family includes the parainfluenza viruses, measles virus, and respiratory syncytial virus (RSV). The *Paramyxovirus* genus includes mumps virus, Newcastle disease virus, and four types of parainfluenza virus.[145] The viruses have a common mode of transmission, with hand fomite spread being the principle means of acquisition by macrodroplet aerosolization. Infection begins with replication in upper respiratory epithelium with entry via specific receptors involving both fusion and phagocytosis.[146] Infected material must contact respiratory mucosa, preferably conjunctiva for effective infection. Animal reservoirs are believed to be important, including cows, dogs, rabbits, and rodents; however, cows and monkeys also have their own parainfluenza viruses. The only natural hosts for RSV are humans, chimpanzees, and cows.

There are four types of parainfluenza in addition to the originally discovered Sendai virus, each causing seasonal outbreaks of respiratory disease. Three of these types were discovered before recognition of their relatedness and were given names based on tissue culture or clinical characteristics. Type 1 is also known as hemadsorbing virus 2 (HA-2) because cell layers infected with it were noted to hemadsorb guinea pig erythrocytes. Type 2 is known as croup-associated (CA) virus because it was first isolated by Chanock's group from croup patients and often cocirculates with parainfluenza 1 virus, which appears to produce croup outbreaks in the fall of odd-numbered years. It characteristically produces syncytia in cell culture. Type 3 is frequently associated with the pediatric croup and bronchiolitis syndromes diagnosed most frequently in the spring of each year after influenza season. Type 3 is the second most common cause of bronchiolitis after RSV and can also mimic mumps by producing parotitis. Types 1 to 3 are also found in guinea pigs, rabbits, and monkeys. Type 4 occurs only in humans and comprises 2 subtypes, A and B, producing common cold–like syndromes.

Similar to influenza, parainfluenzas have spikes of two glycoproteins extending from the virion surface. Unlike influenza viruses, which require endocytosis to enter cells, a fusion protein (F) of parainfluenza mediates infectivity and provides for fusion of the virus with a target cell. A protein dimer termed the *hemagglutinin-neuraminidase* (HN) mediates binding to sialic acid–containing receptors on cells and has an associated enzymatic activity. Antibodies that inhibit hemagglutination and those that neutralize bind to different parts of the HN molecule. There are at least six structural proteins as well. The nonglycosylated membrane (M) protein makes up the inner membrane. There is also a nucleoprotein (NP), a phosphoprotein (P), and a large protein with the catchy name "large" protein (L), which may be the polymerase. As with other RNA viruses, parainfluenza replicates in the cytoplasm. Virus is released by cell surface membrane budding; thus infected cells also have viral glycoprotein spikes on their surface, which mediate hemadsorption. There are no known shifts or drifts in antigenicity of parainfluenza viruses. There is no antigen common to all parainfluenzas, but there is a heterotypic antibody response among parainfluenza 1, 2, and 3 and mumps virus.[144]

The croup syndrome characteristically associated with parainfluenza viruses manifests as a dry seal bark–like cough that increases in severity over 3 to 5 days and clears over a similar time. Less than 5% of parainfluenza infections require hospitalization, since it is primarily a self-limited disease of 5 to 10 days in duration. Fever is usually mild if present at all. The most striking illnesses occur in young children with nightly exacerbations of the cough leading, rarely, to severe respiratory distress, which if untreated may result in sudden death. An anteroposterior radiograph of the soft tissues of the larynx frequently may reveal a pencil-tip or church-steeple shape to the dark air-containing subglottic area. Fever is usually mild if present at all. The major site of the disease is usually the upper respiratory tract, predominantly in the subglottic area with some involvement of the lower respiratory tract mucosa. The subglottic edema is responsible for the narrowing of the airway, which can become critical. Nearly all croup patients have some involvement of the lower tract with variable alveolar involvement. Parainfluenza-infected children who develop the croup syndrome have delayed cell-mediated immune responses as compared with parainfluenza-infected children who experience only coldlike symptoms. Adults usually have only upper tract symptoms (the common cold syndrome) but may also experience hoarseness or laryngitis symptoms. Elderly patients may develop frank bronchopneumonia. Reinfection is common but is usually milder than the initial infection with any given strain except in immunocompromised hosts (AIDS, severe combined immunodeficiency, or transplant recipients), who can develop fatal progressive giant cell pneumonia.[147]

Parainfluenza is usually diagnosed clinically in season when symptoms are highly suggestive. Because specific antiviral therapy is not available, cultures are not always collected. Disease is usually not severe, with resolution within 5 to 10 days, and less than 5% cases require hospitalization. The principle life-threatening risk is to the very young, the very elderly, and those with immumodeficiencies. Severe cases may respond to aerosolized ribavirin, but effectiveness is not consistent.

Sendai virus type 1, also known as murine parainfluenza virus, is a cause of respiratory illnesses in laboratory mice, whereas Sendai virus type 2 infects dogs. Newcastle's disease virus infects chickens and is a significant veterinary pathogen but is not transmitted to humans.

Respiratory syncytial virus

RSV is the most common cause of lower respiratory tract infection in young children (up to 40%) and particularly of bronchiolitis (up to 90%).[148] Transplacentally acquired maternal antibody is not protective, resulting in the most severe forms of pneumonia in infants infected during their first months of life. Attack rates as high as 98% occur in day care settings, and 5% of RSV infections may result in hospitalization. The mortality of RSV in previously healthy children is approximately 1 of 1,000 cases; however, in hospitalized children it can be as high as 3%.[149]

Spread of the virus occurs through aerosolization or directly through contaminated hand contact with conjuctiva or mucosa.[150] The incubation period for RSV averages 5 days. Infected patients usually shed for 8 to 10 days, but young infants and immunosuppressed hosts can excrete virus for up to 4 weeks. RSV produces annual outbreaks lasting 2 to 5 months usually in late winter, but infection may occur during any time of the year. Although the RSV season may overlap influenza season, it generally precedes it. Pediatric hospital admissions consistently increase during outbreaks with nearly 100,000 children hospitalized annually with RSV disease. In urban children's hospitals, hundreds of patients with RSV are seen per day during peak season, often leading to double-digit admissions per day for this condition. Repeated infections are common, but initial infection is generally more severe than reinfection.[149]

The viral genome is composed of RNA that produces at least 10 products, the seven largest being structural proteins and four of these being envelope proteins.[148] Two small proteins are nonstructural. The virus envelope is studded with glycoprotein spikes primarily composed of fusion protein (F) and the attachment protein (G) (Table 36-11). The F protein is responsible for the typical syncytial formation observed after 2 to 7 days in cell culture. There is a nucleocapsid protein (N), a phosphoprotein (P), and a polymerase (L). There are two strains A and B differing mostly at the G protein. Antibody to F protein cross-reacts between strains. There are conflicting data on whether infections attributable to RSV of the group A variety are more severe than those attributable to group B.

Infection rapidly causes ventilation and perfusion inequalities with resulting hypoxemia and generation of tissue injury, which may require weeks for resolution. Small airways are the initial target in the lower respiratory tract, and sloughing of the respiratory epithelium is followed by plugged lumens and subsequent air-trapping or atelectasis. A lymphocytic peribronchiolar infiltrate is observed with notable tissue eosinophilia.[151] The entire respiratory tract is involved but most severely in medium-to-small airways (bronchioles). Injury is partially mediated by direct viral injury and partially by the host's own immune system by means of cytotoxic T-cells and released inflammatory mediators such as virus-specific IgE, histamine, eosinophil cationic protein (ECP), and leukotrienes, such as B_4.[152] Secondary IgE-mediated histamine and leukotriene release adds to the bronchospasm, air-trapping, and airway edema. As a result, RSV is the major cause of wheezing pneumonia in children. It can sometimes be difficult to distinguish bronchiolitis because of RSV from the first attack of asthma or reactive airway disease. The potential clinical efficacy of treatment with ribavirin is not great even if it were immediately to eliminate all infectious virus because respiratory tract injury occurs rapidly and before most patients seek medical care.

Typically, the younger the host, the more severe is the clinical disease. Breast feeding for more than 1 month provides some protection, indicating that mucosal antibody may be more important than circulating antibody. Maternal smoking appears to increase the risk and severity of disease in infants, which may be the result of secondary or passive smoke effects in the infant. Typical bronchiolitis and the degree of hypoxia correlate with high concentrations (50 ng/ml) of ECP in respiratory secretions (the result of eosinophil degranulation). Although RSV infection and reinfection is common throughout childhood, bronchiolitis is rare after 12 months of age. Children with underlying heart (particularly with right-to-left shunting), lung, or immune disease are susceptible to more severe and even life-threatening disease beyond the newborn period. Because adults and older children with previous RSV infection generally develop only upper respiratory symptoms or mild bronchitis-like symptoms, they may be the source of nosocomial infections or bring the infection home to young infants.

RSV is readily recognized in cultured cells by its characteristic CPE, the production of syncytia in cell culture.[7] Replication of RSV is best in nearly confluent cell layers. For the detection of RSV, nasal wash specimens are preferred over nasal swabs because the viruses are most commonly intracellular. A high percentage of negative results in patients with symptoms consistent with RSV can be explained by the lack of cells in the specimen. Rapid commercial assays can produce results in as little as 1 hour, allowing early institution of infection control measures in hospitalized patients and specific antiviral treatment with ribavirin in severe cases.[153] Results from viral culture may not be available for 5 to 7 days unless special shell-vial techniques are used. The latter reduce the time to these results to a range of 24 to 72 hours.

Table 36-11 Key aspects of respiratory syncytial virus

- G glycoprotein mediates attachment to cell surface and usually requires 2 hours.
- F glycoprotein causes fusion with cell and results in typical syncytia in vitro.
- Replication occurs in cytoplasm.
- Virions begin to bud from cell surface after 12 hours *and* spread cell-to-cell (fusion) with logarithmic replication for another 10 hours.

Rhinoviruses (common cold virus)

Rhinoviruses are members of the Picornaviridae family and include more than 100 serotypes.[154] Much is known about the structure and function of the *Rhinovirus* virion and this information has been applied to the understanding of the entire picornavirus family. Some rhinoviruses are closely related at the sequence level to members of the poliovirus and enterovirus groups; however there is little functional antibody cross-reactivity even among *Rhinovirus* strains.

Rhinoviruses are the major cause of the common cold syndrome and can be readily isolated with routine culture techniques. Although common colds typically affect the upper respiratory tract, rhinoviruses may also infect the lower respiratory tract. It has been shown that rhinoviruses replicate well in the laboratory at temperatures (33° C) equivalent to those encountered in the respiratory tract. Molecular aspects of these viruses have been studied in an effort to answer the pleas of the general public to develop a cure for the common cold through various protective strategies. The classic vaccine strategy has been unsuccessful because of the multitude of serotypes and their antigenic variations. The large number of serotypes also explains the ability of rhinoviruses to cause frequent recurrences of the common cold. In addition, rhinoviruses are poorly immunogenic with as many as 50% of natural infections producing only low levels of antibody. Reinfection frequently fails to produce the classic fourfold increase in specific antibody. Antigenic drift also occurs. Chimpanzees and humans are natural hosts for human rhinoviruses.

Cold season lasts from September to May each year but predominates early and very late in that time of the year. Rhinovirus has also been responsible for outbreaks of "summer colds." Several serotypes may cocirculate in the community in any year, but individual serotypes rarely reoccur regularly from year to year. Rapid spread has been documented in grouped populations such as children within a classroom or day-care facility. Interestingly, attack rates from a child index case within families is low, revealing the difficulty of person-to-person transmission. Spread between spouses however is common (nearly 40%). It has been postulated that this is attributable to the amount of time spent in proximity not only to the infected person, but also to heavily contaminated environmental fomites. Ideal infection route appears to occur with self-inoculation of nose or conjunctiva from one's own hands contaminated by environmental fomites or shaking hands with an infected person.

In adults, rhinorrhea, nasal congestion, sore throat, cough, and hoarseness are common symptoms, with only 20% exhibiting fever. In young children up to 60% are febrile and over 50% exhibit lower respiratory symptoms (croup or bronchopneumonia). In addition symptoms are not only more severe, but also persist longer in young children. A bronchiolitis syndrome has also been observed to result from rhinovirus infection in infants.

Otitis media is a common sequel to rhinovirus infection in children younger than 5 years of age, and concurrent rhinovirus is predictive of increased failure of antibacterial therapy for acute otitis media.[155] Sinusitis is another known sequel to rhinovirus particularly in adults. Exacerbations of reactive airway disease occur in asthmatic patients with rhinovirus.

There is no specific effective antiviral therapy currently available for rhinoviruses.

Respiratory adenoviruses

Adenoviruses are agents of respiratory, neurologic, ocular, urinary tract, and gastrointestinal illnesses. There are 42 serotypes (Table 36-12) that have been subgrouped either by hemagglutinating capability (I through IV) or by guanine/cytosine content of the genome (groups A through F). This section is a discussion of the respiratory adenoviruses.

Adenoviruses are responsible for up to 5% of all respiratory illnesses. In children the rate can be as high as 24%.[156] They produce syndromes ranging from febrile common colds, pharyngoconjunctival infections with fever, and exudative tonsillitis to bronchiolitis or even fatal pneumonias.[157] A pertussis-like syndrome can also occur. Adenovirus type 7 is a common cause of so-called swimming pool conjunctivitis. Pharyngoconjunctivitis, where the conjunctivitis is nonpurulent, is most often caused by adenovirus. The differential diagnosis of adenoviral upper and lower respiratory disease includes group A streptococcus and mycoplasma, and EBV and enterovirus also are causes of similar upper respiratory illnesses. Frequently, adenovirus produces clinical signs and symptoms indistinguishable from group A streptococcal pharyngitis, including high fever, exudative tonsillitis, tender anterior cervical adenopathy, headache, myalgias, and even palatal petechiae.[158] High fever may persist for more than a week. Cough is common with adenovirus and rare with group A streptococcus. In adults and military recruits, an atypical pneumonia syndrome is not uncommon. Maculopapular rashes mimicking rubella or even rubeola (measles) have been observed early in adenovirus illnesses. A true latent state with later reactivation appears possible with adenoviruses.

Table 36-12 Adenovirus serotypes associated with disease

Serotypes	Disease
3, 4, 7	Respiratory
8	Respiratory and conjunctivitis
1, 2, 3, 5, 6, 7	Acute pharyngitis, infants and children
8, 19, 37	Epidemic keratoconjunctivitis
11, 21	Acute hemorrhagic cystitis
3, 4, 6, 7, 7A, 12	Meningoencephalitis
40, 41	Diarrhea, enteritis

At least 12 structural polypeptide products are produced by the DNA genome.[159] Structurally the virus is made of 252 capsomeres arranged around a nucleoprotein core with the genome and 2 to 4 internal proteins. Capsomere arrangement leads to vertices at five conjoining tips, resulting in a *penton,* which contains a base plate and a projecting "fiber." Nonvertex capsomeres are grouped in sixes and form *hexons,* which contain the adenovirus common complement-fixing antigen (also known as the hexon antigen, or alpha-antigen). The epsilon component exists within hexons and contains neutralizing epitopes. Fiber-related antigen also contains neutralizing epitopes. Although respiratory adenoviruses are readily isolated in culture using human diploid cell lines, most infections are not specifically diagnosed because of the self-limiting nature of the majority of adenovirus illnesses.

The CPE in tissue culture is characteristic, often showing grapelike clusters of infected cells. A minor antigen, cell-detaching factor, induces the rounding clumped CPE in tissue culture. Adenovirus attachment to host cells is slow (6 hours), but capsid entry is rapid and is followed by uncoating (2 hours). Adenovirus replicates in the nucleus like other DNA viruses. Histologically recognizable effects on cells appear as early as 8 hours after infection and two inclusion types may occur—an early eosinophilic and a later larger basophilic inclusion, which by EM can be shown to contain virus (Fig. 36-15).

Transplacentally acquired maternal antibody appears protective, and disease is uncommon in term infants less than 6 months old. Peak incidence of disease occurs between 6 months and 5 years of age, but notable rates of infection occur up to adolescence. Serotypes 1, 2, 3, 5, 6, and 7 are most frequently implicated in childhood disease. Seasonal patterns are not consistent and vary with serotype and populations. Close contact appears to be necessary for infection to spread. Transmission is by aerosolized droplets that reach respiratory mucous membranes. Excretion may persist for up to 30 days.

Adenovirus exhibits a predilection for infants and children under 5 years of age in day care. Day-care facilities, swimming pools, resident schools, and military barracks (particularly in the first 8 weeks of basic training) have served as points for outbreaks. Serious nosocomial outbreaks have been reported. Immunocompromised hosts appear more susceptible to fatal disseminated or pulmonary adenovirus disease. Neonates or immunocompromised hosts are at higher risk for severe pneumonia or disseminated infections, which are frequently fatal.[160] However the overwhelming majority of adenovirus respiratory infections are self-limited.

No specific therapy is currently available, but IV immunoglobulin has been used anecdotally with mixed success just as inhaled ribaviron has been.

Respiratory coronaviruses

There are two major groups of illnesses caused by coronaviruses, respiratory illnesses and gastrointestinal illnesses. This section considers the respiratory coronaviruses.

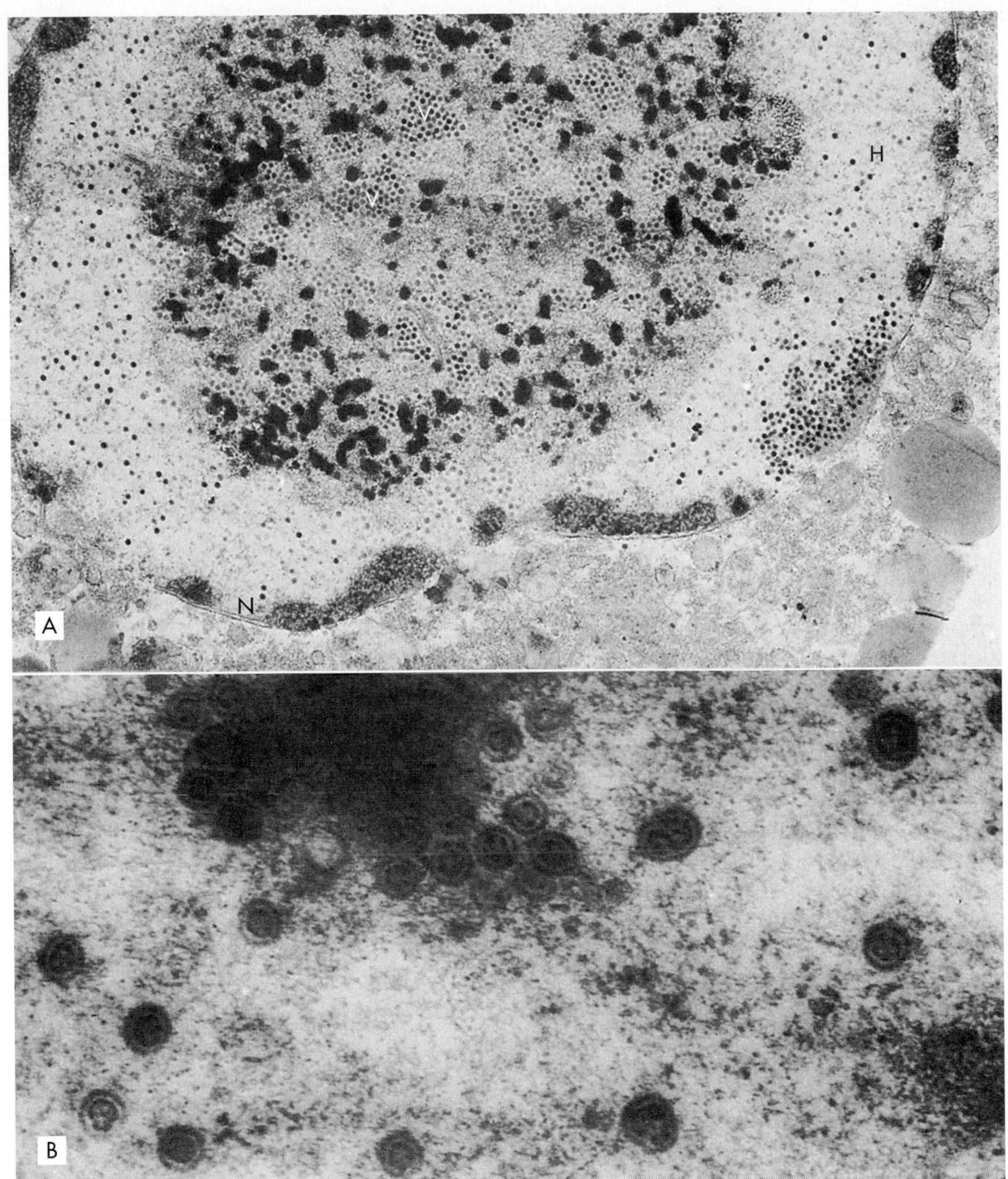

Fig. 36-15 Electron micrograph showing adenovirus inclusion body in cultured KB cell. Inclusion is composed of virions *(V)*, chromatin, and dense bodies of unknown nature. Between inclusion body and nuclear membrane *(N)* is halo *(H)*, **A.** At higher magnification virions are evident, **B.**

Coronaviruses are estimated to be responsible for nearly 20% of common cold syndromes and 8% of lower response infections. Colds caused by coronaviruses appear to produce excessive rhinorrhea compared to rhinovirus. Approximately 20% of cases exhibit fever.[161] *Coronavirus* has been documented as a cause of exacerbations of reactive airway disease and can induce bronchiolitis-like symptoms. The incidence of infection appears to be twice as high in winter compared with summer months, and there is no known age predilection, though ELISA antibodies have been detected in 90% to 100% of adults, indicating previous infection. The incubation period is 2 or 3 days, with cold symptoms lasting usually 7 to 10, but as long as 21 days. In family studies of known coronavirus outbreaks, two thirds of infected patients have URI symptoms, and the remainder exhibit lower response infection symptoms with cough, wheezing, and pleuritic chest pain.[162] In general the coronaviruses are not believed to be of major clinical significance.

Studies using human fetal cells for culture have shown that there are two prototype serologic types, OC43 and 229E.[163] The 229E strain may be isolated by cell culture, but the OC43 strain is not readily isolated in routine tissue culture, and thus our knowledge regarding the disease associations may be incomplete. Interestingly, the presence of neutralizing antibody to laboratory strains may not protect from clinical disease during reinfection, an indication that a change in certain epitopes may occur.

The name *coronavirus* is derived from the widely spaced, petal-shaped projections from the envelope surface of the virion having the appearance of crown. The helical capsid is composed of the nucleoprotein (NP), which is encoiled around the RNA genome. There are three glycoproteins embedded in the virion membrane: a matrix (M) protein, also termed E1; the petal-shaped surface protein (S), also known as E2; and a hemagglutinin (HE), also known as E3 (found in group II viruses). Cellular attachment of *Coronavirus* virions occurs by means of the HE protein or the S protein. After membrane fusion the capsid is endocytosed, and cellular enzymes strip the NP from the genome. One large polyprotein containing the polymerase is produced, and replication proceeds in the cytoplasm. Envelope proteins are acquired from cytoplasmic membranes. Eventually virion progeny are released by cell lysis or budding from cell membranes.

Outbreaks of respiratory symptoms caused by coronaviruses have occurred in military recruits. No specific therapy exists, leaving only symptomatic or supportive measures. Patients appear to recover in nearly all cases without long-term sequelae.

Hantavirus

Hantaviruses compose a distinct genus of six or more viruses within the Bunyaviridae family responsible for development of a respiratory illness presenting with influenza-like symptoms. These viruses have a worldwide distribution and cause similar diseases but are typically spread by different rodent vectors, such as rat, deer mouse, or field mouse. The virus is spread by aerosolization of contaminated rodent excreta. Outbreaks of a newly identified *Hantavirus,* called *Sin Nombre* virus, have occurred in the Four Corners region of the southwestern United States and elsewhere with a 67% mortality rate.[164] Clinical symptoms include the rapid development of pulmonary distress after the onset of fever, myalgia, nausea, and vomiting. Shortness of breath and hypoxia coincide with progressive bilateral pulmonary infiltrates. Diagnosis is made by serologic testing or the demonstration of viral antigen in lung tissue or by detection of viral RNA by means of amplification procedures with specific primers (PCR). Related hantaviruses are associated with hemorrhagic fever viruses, discussed later.

Viruses associated with gastroenteritis

The clinical symptoms collectively referred to as gastroenteritis, including diarrhea, cramping abdominal pain, nausea, and fever can be caused by a variety of viruses (Table 36-13). The mode of spread is typically by the fecal-to-anal route. A distinction should be made between those viruses that replicate in the gastrointestinal (GI) mucosal epithelium causing injury and inflammation (hence true gastroenteritis) from those viruses for which the GI tract is the portal of entry. Enteroviruses, for example, are not a significant cause of gastroenteritis, contrary to what their name may suggest. In such cases the GI tract or the nasopharynx serves as a point of entry with limited replication and subsequent dissemination of the virus after a primary viremia.

Table 36-13 Viruses associated with gastroenteritis

Rotavirus (Reoviridae family)
Norwalk virus group
Enteric adenovirus serotypes 40 and 41
Calicivirus
Astrovirus
Coronavirus

The public may refer to nausea and vomiting with fever as the "flu," and as such the name is a misnomer if it implies that influenza viruses are pathogenic for the GI tract. Much of the data collected for viruses that cause diarrhea have been generated from review of hospital admissions, which in turn implies significant disease. However, cases with significant short-term morbidity occur without hospitalization and are therefore underrepresented in hospital case studies.

The viruses that cause gastroenteritis are interesting in that their morphology can be used as an aid in identification, since culture is generally not attempted and negatively stained preparations for electron microscopy are readily performed. For example, the term *rotavirus* comes from the Latin word *rota,* meaning 'wheel' and describes its characteristic spoke and rim appearance. The term *calicivirus* denotes its resemblance to a chalice, whereas the astroviruses are star shaped, and the circumferential projections from coronaviruses resemble a crown. Serologic procedures are valuable diagnostically. Rotavirus antigen detection assays are now able to establish the presence of infection rapidly and with minimal expense. Conclusive evidence for enteric viruses causing gastroenteritis, other than rotavirus and Norwalk virus, has been difficult because these agents may be found in the stool of asymptomatic individuals.

Although biopsies for histologic review are not typically attempted for diagnosis of viral gastroenteritis, the histologic features associated with either rotavirus or Norwalk agents show many similarities to other inflammatory conditions, including shortening or blunting of the villae and a mononuclear cell infiltrate.

Rotaviruses

Rotaviruses belong to the reovirus family (Reoviridae). Their RNA genome is composed of 10 linear double-stranded segments with an icosahedral capsid surrounding the genome and an inner protein shell. The capsid is involved in many critical viral functions including attachment, penetration, progeny virus assembly, and protection of the genome during passage through the intestinal tract.[165]

Rotaviruses are considered to be the most frequent cause of gastroenteritis in children less than 2 years of age. Over 50% of family contacts may subsequently become infected, but infection in adults is commonly asymptomatic. Five human serotypes can be identified through neutralization assays, and serotype 2 is most frequently associated with clinical symptoms in children. Although serologic procedures can document past infection, serum antibodies are not completely protective since mucosal antibody is most important for immune defense. Passive immunization with maternal antibody appears to provide some protection, since non–breast fed infants are at higher risk for infection. Vaccines have been considered for use in children in the group under 6 months of age but are not presently available because of limited efficacy in large clinical trials.

A distinction can be made in the epidemiology of rotavirus infection in individuals living in tropical climates versus temperate climates. In tropical climates the infection may occur year round and account for nearly half of all acute diarrhea. In temperate climates rotavirus may account for an even greater percentage of acute diarrhea, especially those occurring in the cool winter months when infection is more common.

Rotavirus has an incubation period of 1 to 3 days. Fever and vomiting precede the onset of watery diarrhea, which is typically nonbloody and may persist for up to 1 week. The treatment is conservative with fluid replacement. Since the transmission is through a fecal-oral route and occasionally through water, good hygienic practices can limit the spread of infection. Commercial assays are available for testing of stool specimen and are in widespread use. Typically, culture and electron microscopy are reserved as research tools.

In immunocompromised hosts, oral administration of immunoglobulin has been used for chronic diarrhea with some success.

Enteric adenoviruses

Enteric adenoviruses are the second most common cause of gastroenteritis in young children. The enteric adenoviruses are also referred to as fastidious, since they do not grow in cell lines typically used to detect the other adenoviruses. These have been categorized as serotype numbers 40 and 41 and are significant for being the only DNA virus to cause a notable percentage of cases of gastroenteritis. It is now possible to isolate the enteric adenoviruses with a specific HEK cell line. A rapid antigen capture assay is commercialy available. Viral serotypes 1 to 39 are associated with respiratory symptoms. Although the adenoviruses account for a lower percentage of hospitalization of children with gastroenteritis, the infection is important because it is prolonged and diarrhea may persist for an average of 9 days. Electron microscopy cannot distinguish the respiratory adenoviruses from those causing enteric symptoms, and therefore reference procedures typically employ variations of an immunoassay.

Coronaviruses

Coronaviruses have been linked to gastroenteritis as well as necrotizing enterocolitis, though their overall prevalence has not been determined. Viral particles with this morphology are frequently encountered in the stool from individuals without symptoms and therefore a clear association with disease has not been possible. A more convincing association has been made with upper respiratory tract illnesses with symptoms in adults resembling the common cold symptoms.

Caliciviruses

Caliciviruses, one of the groups of viruses previously incorporated into the Picornaviridae, has now been established as the separate Caliciviridae family. These are single-stranded RNA viruses with a capsid and are cultivatable in human cell lines. Three strains of caliciviruses have been associated with community outbreaks of gastroenteritis. Further support for their etiologic role has been the development of specific IgM antibodies. In contrast with coronaviruses, *Calicivirus* particles are typically not seen in asymptomatic patients but are found in patients with gastrointestinal symptoms.

The clinical features of calicivirus infection have many similarities to those seen with infection by other enteric viruses; however, the vomiting and diarrhea appear to be less severe, lasting 3 or 4 days. The age of patients infected is also similar to that seen with rotaviruses. Diagnosis is by electron microscopy and serology.

Norwalk viruses

The Norwalk group of viruses demonstrate several features similar to the Caliciviruses including morphology and the presence of a single structural protein. However, some immunologic differences exist, and currrently the group is unclassified.[166] The Norwalk viruses are associated with epidemic viral gastroenteritis that occurs in families, communities, or institutions during any time of the year. One such outbreak occurred in Norwalk, Ohio, in 1968 and established the precedent for naming of related viruses, as well as the prototypic virus of this group.

Whereas young children are principally affected by rotaviruses, Norwalk viruses account for a significant percentage of gastroenteritis in young adults. One study demonstrated that 42% of nonbacterial gastroenteritis occurring between 1976 and 1980 was caused by the Norwalk agent[167] (Fig. 36-16). It is believed to be one of the most likely causes of the very severe and acute episodes of gastroenteritis lasting 1 or 2 days, symptoms frequently considered by the public to be food poisoning. The list of Norwalk agent–related viruses has been expanded by isolates from many different locations and

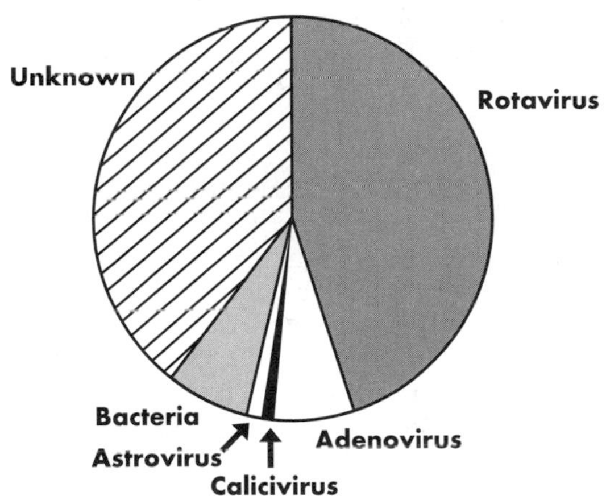

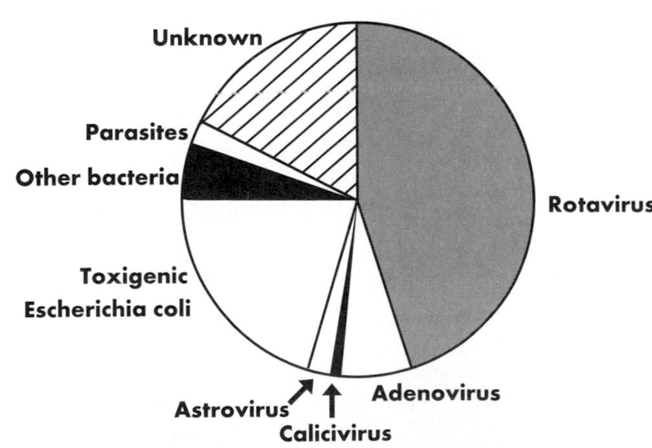

Fig. 36-16 Percentage of cases of gastroenteritis caused by Norwalk viruses in young adults as compared to cases caused by bacteria. (Courtesy Kapikan: JAMA 269:6278, 1993.)

countries. The Snow Mountain and Marin County agents have been definitely grouped with the Norwalk virus, whereas other viruses including the Hawaii, Wollon, Ditching, Cockle, and Paramatta agents are considered likely members of the Norwalk group.

Infection is spread by a fecal-oral route with fecal contamination of drinking water a likely source of common infection for a contained outbreak, not linked to food processing. The incubation period of Norwalk viruses ranges from 2 to 4 days with the subsequent symptoms occurring abruptly but lasting for a relatively short period of 2 days. Conservative therapy including fluid replacement is usually instituted for patients unable to maintain fluid requirements.

Although the typical presentation of an individual infected with Norwalk virus can be recognized, a confident diagnosis cannot be made on clinical grounds until the symptoms diminish as rapidly as they developed. Diagnostic tests of immune status are not useful, since antibodies within the blood are not protective. Diagnosis of Norwalk agent is typically performed by reference laboratories or government laboratories and includes immunoelectronmicroscopy, ELISA, or RIA.

Astroviruses

Astroviruses are an infrequent though important cause of gastroenteritis.[168] It is notable that astroviruses, as well as coronaviruses and rotaviruses, have been found in a wide range of animals, including pigs, calves, sheep, dogs, and monkeys. Therefore, evidence of the ability for astroviruses to cause diarrhea in animals has also been used as circumstantial evidence of their role in humans.

Five serotypes of astrovirus currently are recognized. The age group affected is slightly older than that seen for rotavirus with children up to 7 years of age experiencing infection. Clinically, astrovirus has a short incubation period of 1 or 2 days with symptoms resembling those seen with rotavirus, however, again with less severity but a slightly longer duration of 4 days.

Viruses associated with hepatitis

Numerous viruses are able to cause hepatocellular dysfunction, and the phrase viral hepatitis is nonspecific, though it commonly refers to infection of the liver by the hepatotropic hepatitis A, B, C, delta (or D), and E viruses presented in this section. Non-A, non-B hepatitis is also a general term originally used to describe characteristic clinical features of hepatitis for which a viral cause was suspected but could not be determined with serologic makers. The clinical features of hepatitis with elevated serum levels of liver enzymes may occur during the course of infection by many viruses (summarized in Table 36-14) such as that commonly seen with infection by EBV. EBV may also be associated with hepatocytic injury in cases of posttransplantation lymphoproliferative disease.[169] Measles is a well-known cause of hepatitis, and the sporadically encountered histologic diagnosis of syncytial giant-cell hepatitis has also been proposed to be caused by a *Paramyxovirus*.[170] Taken together, these viruses are a more frequent cause of hepatitis than alcohol, hepatotoxins, drugs, or other nonviral infectious agents including *Leptospira,* Q fever, or *Echinococcus* organisms.

Table 36-14 Viruses other than hepatitis A to E that cause hepatitis

Epstein-Barr virus
Cytomegalovirus
Varicella virus
Rubella virus
Adenovirus
Enterovirus
Measles virus

Hepatitis A

Hepatitis A virus (HAV) is a member of the picornavirus family. As its grouping with other enteroviruses would indicate, HAV is an enteric virus, transmitted predominantly by the fecal-oral route and is a common cause of acute hepatitis.[171] Widespread infection is typically associated with poor sanitation practices, and the incidence is increasing in intravenous drug abusers. The transmission of HAV in food, shellfish, and water is perhaps increased by its comparative heat stability; it can survive temperatures up to 60° C for up to 1 hour. HAV is classically remembered as short-incubation, infectious hepatitis.

Infection in children is believed to be largely asymptomatic, and up to 50% of infections in adults are also asymptomatic. The clinical importance of HAV lies in cases of acute severe hepatitis as well as in epidemics of the enterically transmitted disease.[172] Epidemics commonly occur in developed countries among nonimmune adults but may also be encountered in school and day-care settings. Symptoms that may be present in acute infections include puritus, fever, myalgia, nausea, and vomiting. Adults frequently develop jaundice, with a peak serum bilirubin of 10 mg/dl, which typically persists for approximately 4 weeks. Before the onset of jaundice, stools may become acholic and bilirubin is present in the urine. HAV differs from other viruses causing acute hepatitis by a relatively short incubation period (14 to 50 days) and its inability to develop a chronic state of hepatitis. Although it is not associated with chronic hepatitis, the initial infection may be prolonged, lasting up to 200 days with a concurrent elevation of IgM antibodies. Replication begins in the oropharynx followed by penetration of the intestinal epithelium and infection of the liver. Typically the incubation period is between 15 and 50 days, at which time flu-like symptoms herald the development of anorexia, hepatomegaly, and icterus when bilirubin exceeds 3 mg%. A preicteric stage is characterized by elevations in serum transaminases, ALT, and AST. Cholestatic patients usually show aminotransferase levels below 500 IU/L. Symptoms typically persist for 2 weeks, but fecal shedding of virus diminishes rapidly within days of the onset of symptoms and corresponds to the rise of antibodies. Corticosteroids may be used to shorten the cholestatic period but if tapered rapidly have been associated with relapse of cholestasis.

IgM antibodies to HAV are typically present at the onset of symptoms and may persist for as long as 1 year (typically 3 to 6 months). IgG antibodies also appear early in the course of infection and may persist for life. The diagnosis is largely made by epidemiologic features, history, physical findings, and serologic testing, and only rarely is a liver biopsy performed. Biopsy specimens typically show centrilobular cholestasis with some portal inflammation, which may suggest the diagnosis of chronic hepatitis if the serologic information is not available; however, progression to chronic hepatitis has never been documented with HAV. Complications of HAV do occur and include relapse of symptoms after an apparent recovery from primary infection. This biphasic or relapsing form of hepatitis A occurs in 6% to 10% of cases and may be recognized by the return of symptoms first seen in acute infection with aminotransferase levels less that 1000 IU/L. Also significant but rare are the extrahepatic manifestations of HAV infection, which include vasculitis and arthritis as well as induction of autoimmunity. The dermal vasculitis and arthritis may be attributable to circulating cryoglobulins, which have been shown to contain IgM to HAV. Affected patients have been shown to have defects in T-cell suppressor-inducer cells. This finding is consistent with the accepted mechanism for cell death in typical HAV hepatitis with cell injury not attributable to direct lysis of the cell, but rather a T-cell–dependent killing of infected cells.

HAV is a public health concern because outbreaks may be encountered in public situations and are associated with infected food handlers. By the time jaundice appears, viral shedding in the stool becomes low; therefore, when the disease is clinically apparent, contagion is no longer a major concern, since transmission to susceptible individuals has already occurred in the late incubation period. Prophylactic intramuscular immune serum globulin is indicated in known exposures and family members of infected patients. A new vaccine is expected to reduce outbreaks significantly in the future.

Hepatitis B

Hepatitis B virus (HBV) is an enveloped DNA virus that is reported to infect 300 million humans worldwide. As with hepatitis A, most acute cases of hepatitis B may progress undiscovered, and in many cases even patients with chronic hepatitis B viral infection have few or no symptoms and no physical abnormalities.[173] It has been concluded that an immune response results in the eradication of virus before extensive liver damage can occur. In contrast to hepatitis A, symptomatic hepatitis B infection in children frequently leads to chronic infection. In children infection by HBV is commonly anicteric but in adults is commonly icteric and progresses to chronic infection in less than 7% of the cases. The comparatively lower frequency of chronic infection and icterus are significant for distinguishing HBV from hepatitis C and E viruses. The epidemiology of the disease and the distinctive pathogenesis in children and adults also indicate that the immune system plays an important role in tissue injury. Chronic infection typically beginning in childhood is a major risk factor for hepatocellular carcinoma.

The incubation period for HBV ranges from 2 to 26 weeks with a mean of about 12 weeks. The mode of transmission has been considered to be through blood, but evidence of transmission is best established for saliva and semen. Thus the sexual partners of infected individuals are considered to be at high risk as are hemophiliacs, drug addicts, prostitutes, and sexually promiscuous individuals.

The complete HBV virion measures 42 nm and is termed the "Dane particle," but other forms may be seen on electron microscopy including long cylindrical structures with a 22 nm diameter composed entirely of envelope or surface antigen (HBsAg) proteins. Additional envelope proteins are termed *pre-*S_1 and *pre-*S_2. The nucleocapsid consists of core antigen (HBcAg) surrounding a partially double-stranded circular genome. A third antigen of diagnostic significance is the e antigen (HBeAg), which is produced from the same sequence as the HBcAg, the precore gene product.

The HBV genome is small, containing approximately 3200 base pairs, and its structure is unique with one complete circular strand and a second, incomplete strand.[174] The genome contains four open reading frames (ORF); pre-S_1/pre-S_2/S encoding envelope proteins, C gene encoding capsid and e antigen, a third ORF encoding a combined reverse transcriptase and DNA polymerase, and a fourth ORF encoding X or the *trans*-activating protein. Thus these four ORFs are capable of producing seven different translational products that may be further modified to result in additional protein diversity. This capability for diversity may explain the multiple clinical syndromes associated with HBV. The DNA virus genome is replicated using an RNA intermediate and the virally encoded reverse transcriptase, analogous to the mechanism for retroviruses.

Morphologic evidence for the presence of HBV includes the classical "ground-glass" hepatocyte, which on electron microscopy can be shown to correlate with the presence of abundant surface antigen. Immunohistochemical procedures utilizing antibody to HBsAg may also be utilized.

Patients with HBV infections demonstrate characteristic patterns of antibodies and antigens that are detected by clinical assays. In acute disease, HBsAg, HBeAg, and antibody to HBc can be found 2 to 4 weeks before symptoms appear (Fig. 36-6). The interval between disappearance of HBsAg and the appearance of anti-HBs is commonly termed the "window period." Although 149 amino acids of HBcAg and HBeAg are identical, antibodies directed against one of them do not show cross-reactivity with the other. The presence of HBeAg in the serum is an important clinical marker of viral replication and is associated with significant liver damage. Individuals who are chronically infected with HBV characteristically have HBeAg in the serum. Seroconversion from an HBeAg-positive/HBeAg antibody–negative status to HBeAg antibody–positive status is correlated with remission of clinical disease and likely corresponds with abrogation of viral replication. As with other viruses, once specific antibody is produced, the level of detectable antigen quickly decreases.

Persistence of HBV infection is commonly referred to as a carrier state and is characterized by the ability to detect HBsAg for more than 6 months.[175] It is now known that HBV may exist at very low levels in an infected individual, and typical serologic methods may be falsely negative in cases where HBV is detectable by DNA amplification techniques. Chronic HBV infection is characterized by repeated exacerbations of hepatitis analogous to the reactivations of EBV. Chronic carriers of HBV frequently have impaired cell-mediated immunity to the virus. Reactivation of HBV may be seen in HBeAg-negative, anti-HBe–positive individuals in addition to HBeAg–positive, HBsAg-chronic carriers of HBV.[176] Virus may persist in one of two states—either (1) integrated into the liver cell genome with only low-level viral replication, or (2) nonintegrated into host DNA with high levels of viral replication. Reactivation may also occur because of chemicals, drugs, or superinfection by other hepatropic viruses, but reinfection by a second strain of HBV is not common. Replication-incompetent viruses, in which mutations affect the essential core regions or the polymerase gene, may also be generated.

A distinct subset of chronically infected patients who do not have detectable HBeAg has been identified. This group of individuals is important for the rapidly progressive nature of hepatitis leading to cirrhosis as well for the understanding of the underlying biology that this situation provided. An explanation for the clinical situations where loss of HBeAg corresponds to recovery and the contrasting situation where HBeAg loss, even with comparable levels of HBeAg antibodies, corresponds with chronic infection is that there are certain HBV variants in which mutations occurred in the precore DNA sequences. These mutations result in the loss of capability for the production of HBeAg but apparently do not significantly decrease the ability of the virus to replicate.[177] Frequent mutational changes in the genome are an expected finding because the viral reverse transcriptase enzyme does not have the proofreading capability of polymerases from other DNA viruses. The mutant viruses remain replication competent and severe liver damage and chronic infection ensues. This is only one of several mechanisms allowing for persistence of the virus.

The epidemiologic linkage between HBV and hepatocellular carcinoma has led to multiple theoretical explanations for a mechanism.[178] If infected cells contain unstable integrated HBV, repeated cell division may increase the risk of an insertional mutation leading to malignancy, such as the inactivation of p53. Alternatively, continued viral replication and cell damage through activity of the immune system may also lead to increased risk for neoplasia through random cellular mutations. One region of HBV, termed the *X gene*, encodes a protein that has been shown to have transactivation capability. Transgenic animals expressing the X gene have developed hepatocellular carcinoma.[179] However, other transgenic mice expressing only surface antigen also develop liver tumors.[180] Although the specific events leading to neoplasia remain to be determined, it is clear that with the high incidence of HBV in densely populated areas of the world, hepatocellular carcinoma is one of the most common cancers in the world.

It is important to recognize that HBV may affect tissues and organs other than liver. Arthralgias are common as may be an erythematous macular skin rash in patients with acute hepatitis, and they both appear secondary to immune complex disease. Polyarteritis and membranous glomerulonephritis are associated with chronic hepatitis. Some cases of fulminent liver failure caused by viruses may also be accompanied by acute bone marrow failure.[181]

Detection of hepatitis B e-antigen greatly increases the likelihood of transmission of HBV to the infant who in turn has at least an 80% chance of becoming a chronic carrier. Transmission of HBV through blood products is also a concern but has been minimized by the screening of blood donors. The risk to health care workers by HBV is considerable, and recommendations have been made for the immunization of all health care workers against HBV. Additionally, universal childhood immunization against HBV has recently been recommended. HBV immunoglobulin is advised along with vaccine for infants born to HBsAg-positive mothers and others with known blood exposures to HBV.

A second agent, designated the *hepatitis delta virus* (HDV), also has a direct correlation with progression to severe chronic active hepatitis in patients infected with HBV.[182] HDV is an RNA virus that is defective in the sense that it requires the presence of HBV for replication.[183] The cooperation between HBV and HDV is remarkable, since the internal protein antigen of HDV is covered by the surface antigen of HBV. It is therefore reasonable to search for the presence of HDV only in patients infected with HBV. The transmission of HDV is similar to that of HBV with sexual partners of infected individuals at greatest risk as well as children born to HBsAg-positive women.

Hepatitis C

The presence of a viral agent able to cause hepatitis and yet distinct from HAV or HBV had been clinically apparent for many years. The large majority of these non-A, non-B hepatitis cases, also referred to as *posttransfusion hepatitis* cases, are now known to be caused by hepatitis C.[184] HCV is a small 50 to 60 nm enveloped RNA virus that has similarities to the flaviviruses and pestiviruses. Transmission follows the pattern of HBV though the incubation period may be somewhat shorter (means of 8 weeks versus 12 weeks). The infection may be subclinical without evidence of icterus in both children and adults. The symptoms of acute infection are not well characterized but appear to be milder than those seen with HBV. Less than a third of patients develop jaundice. The major difference between HCV and HBV is the high percentage of cases that go on to develop chronic hepatitis (50%) and also cirrhosis (20% to 25%). The risk for sexually related transmission also appears to be lower for HCV than for HBV.

Whereas up to 30% of blood transfusion recipients developed non-A, non-B hepatitis as recently as 1968, the institution of targeted screening procedures and now serologic procedures to detect antibodies to HCV has reduced the incidence of posttransfusion hepatitis to less than 3%.[185]

Initial studies with an ELISA procedure to detect antibodies to a nonstructural protein of HCV showed a high (70% to 85%) frequency of antibodies in patients with posttransfusion non-A, non-B hepatitis. Unfortunately, a high frequency of antibodies also appeared to be present in individuals without a history of blood transfusion as well as those with elevated gamma-globulin levels, and subsequently the need for a more specific test was recognized. With the use of assays employing multiple recombinant antigens the sensitivity and the specificity of the anti-HCV test has considerably improved.[186] Other tests include RNA-amplification procedures as well as antigen-detection tests.

Since many infected patients go on to develop chronic hepatitis, the use of interferon-alpha has been explored as a potential therapy. In addition, the use of gamma-globulin is recommended for individuals exposed to sources of non-A, non-B hepatitis, though no convincing evidence exists for its efficacy.

Hepatitis E

An enteric form of non-A, non-B hepatitis has been apparent since the 1950s when fecal contamination of drinking water led to epidemic hepatitis without evidence of antibodies to either HAV or HBV. Recently, isolation was made of a nonenveloped virus with morphologic and molecular similarities to the Caliciviridae family of viruses. Infection with hepatitis E has many similarities to that of hepatitis A virus infection and is frequently seen in areas with poor sanitation and inadequately treated drinking water.[187] The incubation period is longer than that for HAV. Although it has a self-limited course that may be prolonged, it does not appear to progress to chronicity. Currently diagnosis is by exclusion, through serologic evidence of lack of antibodies to hepatitis A, B, and C.

Viruses causing encephalitis, meningitis, or hemorrhagic fever

Viruses transmitted to humans through insects or animals can cause a variety of diseases including encephalitis, respiratory illnesses, and disorders grouped under the term *hemorrhagic fevers*. Viruses transmitted from person to person or from animal to human by means of arthropods were originally classified as *ar*thropod-*bo*rne animal viruses, or arboviruses. New information indicates that many different virus families were included under the original designation and that some members of those families were actually not transmitted by arthropod vectors. Therefore a reorganization was made and viruses transmitted by arthropod vectors are now classified according to their genome and morphology under either the Bunyaviridae, Togaviridae, Reoviridae, or Rhabdoviridae families. Two genera of the Reoviridae family cause significant disease in humans, the *Orbivirus* and the *Rotaviruses*. The disease associated with the rotaviruses is presented under the gastroenteritis section. Encephalitis or meningoencephalitis can be caused by viruses within the Arenaviridae, Bunyaviridae, Rhabdoviridae, or Togaviridae families, and little distinction may be possible on clinical grounds except for contact with certain animals, as in the case of rabies.

Hemorrhagic fevers are caused by viruses of the Arenaviridae, Flaviviridae, Reoviridae, Filoviridae, and Bunyaviridae families; key representative viruses are listed in Table 36-15. It is valuable to consider these viruses under one clinical heading to address the differential diagnosis and provide recommendations regarding appropriate serologic studies. Flaviviruses that are associated principally with hemorrhagic fevers include the yellow fever virus and dengue virus. Five hemorrhagic fever syndromes caused by arenaviruses include Lassa fever and Argentine, Bolivian, Venezuelan, and Brazilian hemorrhagic fever.

Rhabdoviruses

The rhabdoviruses are RNA viruses that infect vertebrates, insects, and plants. The most important rhabdoviruses in humans are rabies virus and vesicular stomatitis virus; however, others include the Mokola virus, the Lagos bat virus, the Obodhiang virus, and the Katonkan virus.

Rabies is one of the oldest known and most feared of human diseases.[188] It is primarily a disease of animals, and the epidemiology of human rabies closely parallels the epizoology of animal rabies. Where domestic animal rabies has not been controlled, dog or cat bites account for 90% of the reported human cases. In areas where the domestic animal rabies is well controlled, most exposures are the consequence of wild animal bites such as wolf, coyote, skunk, and raccoon bites. It is likely that rabies maintains itself as an endemic illness in each of these species. Rabies is transmitted to humans practically always as a result of a bite from a rabid domestic or wild animal. The disease has also rarely been transmitted through corneal transplants. Clinically the initial symptoms of the disease are nonspecific, such as malaise, fatigue, and headache followed by a period of acute neurologic symptoms including hyperactivity, disorientation, hallucinations, seizures, and bizarre behavior, followed by coma and death. All rabies exposure cases are to be reported to local health authorities. Combined immune serum and human-derived vaccine are the recommended postexposure prophylaxis of the disease in the United States. Specific chemotherapy for clinical rabies is not available. Treatment consists of intensive supportive care.

The rabies virus multiplies at the site of the local bite and travels to the CNS through the peripheral nerves. Once in the CNS it replicates within the neurons.[189] Postexposure prophylaxis must occur during the period before the virus enters the CNS. The closer the bite is to the CNS, the shorter the period for response and treatment. The degree of tissue damage and the corresponding amount of innoculum also influence the window of time for response. Grossly the brain and spinal cord show edema and petechial hemorrhages. Involvement of the spinal cord is most conspicuous when the portal of entry is on the lower part of the body. Microscopically the predominant inflammatory lesion consists of lymphocytic perivascular cuffing within the parenchyma of the nervous system. Little meningeal reaction is seen. Nodules of glial cells termed "Babeş nodes" are often present and consist of nonspecific glial aggregates. In about 75% of cases Negri bodies can be seen on hematoxylin and eosin–stained sections. These cytoplasmic inclusion bodies in the neurons are practically pathognomonic for rabies and are an important diagnostic finding.[190] They are most consistently present in the Purkinje cells of the cerebellum and in the large neurons of the hippocampus. They are found in intact neurons as round to oval eosinophilic bodies measuring 2 to 10 μm in diameter. Ultrastructural studies have shown that the Negri body consists of a mass of nucleocapsids surrounded by viral particles budding from intracytoplasmic membranes.[191,192] Those bodies can be seen in axons, and it is in this way that the virus spreads from the CNS to many organs of the body. Because Negri bodies are usually seen in intact neurons, they are found away from the inflammatory, nonspecific lesions (Fig. 36-17). Rabies viral antigens can be demonstrated in infected cells by means of fluorescent antibody techniques. Antigens can be shown to be present in cells in the absence of Negri bodies, and hence this technique is much more sensitive than the search of sections of brain for the pathognomonic cytoplasmic inclusions. Antemortem diagnosis can also be made by antigen detection in skin biopsy specimens from the nape of the neck.

Vesicular stomatitis virus (VSV) is capable of infecting a broad range of hosts, including horses, cattle, swine, small animals, and humans, but is limited to the Western Hemisphere in distribution.[193] Other related viruses, include Piry, Chandipura, and Isfahan virus. VSV causes mild influenza-like symptoms followed by the development of vesicular lesions that resemble herpetic vesicles of the mouth in about one fourth of patients. The lesions may be more widespread than in HSV and include the pharynx, tongue, buccal mucosa, and gums. The disease is uncommon in humans, and laboratory accidents account for more reports of disease than naturally occurring cases. It may be confused with hand-foot-and-mouth disease caused by enteroviruses and in veterinary practice with foot-and-mouth virus. The illness is short lived and lasts from 2 to 7 days with no sequelae.

Bunyavirus

The Bunyaviridae family is composed of over 150 individual viruses of which 14 constitute the California encephalitis

Table 36-15 Hemorrhagic fever viruses

Virus	Disease	Miscellaneous
Arenaviridae family		
Arenavirus genus	Pathogenesis due primarily to endothelial dysfunction.	No insect vectors; entry by abrasions/respiratory tract; biosafety level 4 pathogen.
Argentine (Junín) fever virus	Argentine hemorrhagic fever (AHF)	Rodent reservoir; live attenuated vaccine available (Junín only)
Lassa fever virus	Hemorrhagic fever	Person-to-person transmission; vaccine in development
Bunyaviridae family		
Nairovirus genus		Usually transmitted by ticks
Crimean-Congo hemorrhagic fever virus	Fever, prostration; usually severe hemorrhages.	Mortality in 10%; can be nosocomially acquired
Hantavirus genus		
Hantaan virus	"Korean hemorrhagic fever" (hemorrhagic fever with renal syndrome).	Usually transmitted by aerosolized rodent excreta; ribavirin of benefit
Phleborvirus genus		
Rift Valley fever virus	Fever, arthralgia; <5% more serious; hemorrhagic with liver necrosis; retinitis, or meningoencephalitis	Transmitted by sandflies and mosquitoes; maintained enzootically, usually in domestic animals (Africa); epizootics in distant areas
Filoviridae family		
Filovirus genus		Predominantly in sub-Saharan Africa; transmitted by close human contact; biosafety level 4 pathogen
Marburg virus	Severe hemorrhagic fever	Sporadic and rare cases in Africa; believed disease of monkeys and endemic in bats; virus may persist in semen
Ebola virus	Severe hemorrhagic fever	Reservoir unknown; there are Sudan and Zaïre subtypes
Flaviviridae family		
Flavivirus genus		Old "group B" arboviruses
Yellow fever virus (mosquito-borne)	Hemorrhagic fever, hepatitis, nephritis	In tropical America and Africa; live vaccine available
Dengue fever antigenic subgroup (mosquito-borne)	Fever, myalgia, hypotension, hemorrhages	Endemic in Southeast Asia; sporadic in Caribbean
Kyasanur Forest disease virus (tick-borne)	Fever, myalgia, hypotension, hemorrhages	Originally isolated in India and gradually spreading; maintained in vertebrates, including monkeys
Omsk hemorrhagic fever virus (tick-borne)	Like Kyasanur Forest, but frequent sequelae	Originally isolated in U.S.S.R.; transmission believed by insect from rodent dust
Togaviridae family		
Alphavirus genus		Old "group A" arboviruses; mosquito-borne
Chikungunya virus	Fever and polyarthritis; bleeding from gums but no significant hemorrhaging	Endemic in monkeys; predominantly in Africa; epidemics in Asia, India, Far East, and possibly southern U.S.

group and others form the recently reemphasized *Hantavirus* group. The virions are enveloped spherical particles approximately 100 nm in diameter, and they contain a three-part segmented genome of single-stranded RNA segments. As with influenza virus this segmented genome may allow for genetic recombination or reassortment to occur.

Since the original isolation of the prototype virus of the California encephalitis group, California encephalitis virus, few cases have been seen in California.[194] In contrast, California encephalitis virus has been found to be a common cause of aseptic meningitis in other regions of the United States, such as Ohio. A separate member of the group, the La Crosse (LAC) virus has emerged as a significant pathogen. The La Crosse virus is endemic to the midwestern United States and is transmitted to humans by *Aedes triseriatus*, a forest-dwelling mosquito of the north central and northeastern United States.

Infection of humans may result in a mild febrile illness or sometimes a severe encephalitis. Most patients appear to

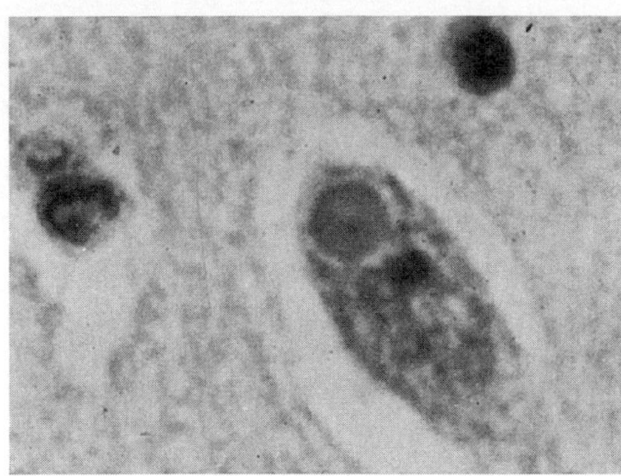

Fig. 36-17 Negri bodies of rabies.

recover completely, though personality changes and learning disorders have been reported as sequelae.

Togavirus

Two genera of Togaviridae have been described, the alphaviruses and the flaviviruses.[195] Togaviruses are spherical, enveloped virions measuring 40 to 90 nm in diameter with a nuclear capsid that exhibits cubic symmetry. Some members of the Togaviridae may be transmitted by means of arthropod vectors and are the etiologic agents of encephalitis, hemorrhagic fevers, and arthritis. As discussed previously, hepatitis A is also a member of the *Flavivirus* genus.

Alphavirus. The *Alphavirus* genus includes over 20 viruses that cause either encephalitis or acute arthropathy. They are enveloped spherical virions containing a single-stranded RNA genome. Eastern, western, and Venezuelan equine encephalitis are the three significant diseases caused by these viruses in humans. They are initiated by inoculation of the virus by a mosquito bite. In the laboratory, alphaviruses can be transmitted by aerosol and have caused numerous infections in laboratory workers. After inoculation, the virus multiplies in the nonneuronal tissues causing a febrile illness. The infection may be eliminated by the host defense mechanisms after a subclinical infection or a benign febrile illness, or the virus may invade the CNS, giving rise to an encephalitis. Alphaviruses replicate in the CNS, causing cell destruction and a severe inflammatory response. The mortality for western equine encephalitis is approximately 10% and for eastern equine encephalitis 70%. Total recovery is uncommon, and patients are left with sequelae that include mental retardation, behavioral changes, and convulsive disorders. The mortality resulting from Venezuelan equine encephalitis is generally low, though a more severe form of the disease has been recognized and is probably caused by the lymphocytolytic effect of the virus.

Gross examination of the brain in fatal cases of eastern equine encephalitis shows edema. Microscopically, there is a noticeable meningoencephalitis with a conspicuous, acute, neutrophilic infiltrate and an acute vasculitis with fibrinoid necrosis of the vessel wall. Neuronal necrosis and neuronophagia are very common. At later stages glial nodules and perivascular cuffing become prominent. The lesions involve all regions of the brain, but the brainstem and basal ganglia may be the most severely involved regions.

In western equine encephalitis the inflammatory response is less intense and composed of mononuclear cells. The greatest damage is seen in the basal ganglia and in the white matter of the cerebral hemispheres. Cystic degeneration of the white matter has been described in patients under 1 year of age.

Little is known about the pathology of Venezuelan equine encephalitis, since the mortality is low. The encephalomyelitis is milder than the other types and morphologically consists mostly of the perivascular cuffing and microglial nodules. The inflammatory lesions may be most prominent in the putamen and cerebral white matter.

Establishing the diagnosis of *Alphavirus* infection depends on clinical and epidemiologic information and obtaining the appropriate specimens for biologic and serologic tests. In fatal cases of encephalitis the virus may be isolated from the CNS tissues obtained at autopsy. As a rule, virus is not present in the CSF.

Flaviviruses associated with encephalitis. Flaviviruses are immunologically distinguishable from alphaviruses. They are enveloped, spherical, and slightly smaller than alphaviruses, measuring 40 to 50 nm. All flaviviruses except for dengue have complex primary cycles of transmission involving arthropod vectors, wild birds, and mammals. In many cases humans are an accidental end host because the levels of viremia produced are insufficient to infect vectors. Flaviviruses cause St. Louis encephalitis, Japanese encephalitis, tick-borne encephalitis, dengue (breakbone fever), and yellow fever.

St. Louis encephalitis was recognized in 1933 when an epidemic occurred in southern Illinois and in the area of St. Louis, Missouri. The virus was recovered from brain tissue at autopsy from persons who died of the disease during the 1933 epidemic. The St. Louis encephalitis virus replicates at the site of inoculation and probably gains access to the central nervous system through viremia. In fatal cases of St. Louis encephalitis the brain may appear normal at gross examination. The histologic features are those of a meningoencephalitis, with leptomeningeal mononuclear cell infiltration and parenchymal lesions consisting of perivascular cuffing and reactive microglial nodules. The lesions are more intense in the substantia nigra and thalamic nuclei.

Severe epidemics of encephalitis have occurred in Japan since 1871. The mortality in acute cases is between 30% and 40%, and epidemics are caused by the Japanese encephalitis virus transmitted by an arthropod. Cases have been reported in Japan, Korea, China, Southeast Asia, and India. Pathologically the meningoencephalitis involves especially the subcortical zone of the white matter. In long-term survivors, the lesions may become heavily calcified. Neuronophagia is commonly seen in the ventral horns of the spinal cord.

Tick-borne encephalitis virus, central Europe encephalitis virus (CEE), and Russian spring-summer encephalitis virus are responsible for epidemics of encephalitis in the confederation of Independent States, central Europe, and Scandinavia. The viruses are maintained between ticks and various warm-blooded mammals. Most clinical cases occur in people exposed to infections in forests or in the laboratory. The clinical disease ranges from meningeal irritation to frank meningoencephalitis with paralysis. In fatal cases there is congestion of the brain; microscopically lesions are found in the gray matter of the precentral cortex, basal ganglia, brainstem, cerebellum, and spinal cord. In the spinal cord the lesions are more severe in the cervical and lower lumbar segments.

Flaviviruses associated with hemorrhagic shock. In addition to the flaviviruses, which cause encephalitis, other members cause yellow fever and dengue. Yellow fever is an acute illness manifested by abrupt onset of chills and fever, conjunctival injection, leukopenia, a brief period of remission, and then reappearance of fever with jaundice, punctate hemorrhages of the soft palate, epistaxis, and gingival and gastrointestinal bleeding (black vomit).[195] Approximately 50% of the patients develop relative bradycardia in relation to the degree of fever. The yellow fever virus is viscerotropic, causing the most damage in the liver, kidney, heart, and gastrointestinal tract. The gross features in fatal cases are not specific. The heart when involved is flabby and pale with scattered pericardial and petechial hemorrhages. Microscopically there is degeneration of myocardial fibers and accumulation of fat. The kidneys may show edema; microscopically the features are those seen in cases of acute tubular necrosis. Hemoglobin casts may be seen.

The most characteristic pathologic changes are found in the liver.[196] The appearance of the lesions is typical between the seventh and ninth day of the illness. The liver is grossly normal in size but is pale and yellow because of fatty metamorphosis. Microscopically there is extensive midzonal necrosis, which in severe cases may extend to become panlobular. Intracellular condensations of cytoplasm that appear as round to oval, well-demarcated, eosinophilic inclusions are termed *Councilman bodies*. These are also found in the cytoplasm of Kupffer cells. These inclusions are not composed of virus particles and are nonspecific for the disease. They are periodic acid–Schiff (PAS) positive. A hallmark of the hepatitis caused by yellow fever virus is the absence of an inflammatory component. Also distinctive of the lesion is the fact that, despite massive necrosis, the overall framework of the hepatic lobule is preserved. Fatty metamorphosis of the microvesicular type is invariably seen.

Dengue virus has a human-mosquito-human cycle and is a worldwide health problem with epidemics occurring in tropical areas of Asia, Africa, and America.[195] It causes a syndrome initially similar to influenza but progresses to rash with muscle, joint, and bone pain (breakbone fever) or arthralgias. It also can cause severe and potentially fatal hemorrhagic disorders, dengue hemorrhagic fever (DHF), and dengue shock syndrome. There are four serotypes as determined by neutralization tests, and each serotype can cause either dengue or DHF. Diagnosis is based on clinical history of travel in an endemic area and serologic evidence of a rise in specific antibodies. Children develop DHF more commonly than adults, and it occurs principally after prior infection with a different dengue virus serotype. Dengue fever in adults is a self-limited disease after resolution of the high fever, which may persist for up to 1 week. As with yellow fever, initial symptoms may diminish after 2 or 3 days followed by a return of fever and rash. Biopsy studies of the rash seen in nonfatal dengue fever show a lymphocytic vasculitis in the dermis. In cases of fatal dengue hemorrhagic fever, the gross findings are petechial hemorrhages in the skin and hemorrhagic effusions in the plural, pericardial, and abdominal cavities. Hemorrhage and congestion is present in many organs, and histologic studies show hemorrhage, perivascular edema, and focal necrosis but no vasculitis or endothelial lesions. It is believed that most of the morphologic abnormalities seen result from disseminated intravascular coagulation and shock.

Orbivirus

Orbiviruses constitute a genus of viruses with several members that are significant pathogens of humans and animals. Human pathogens include Colorado tick fever virus (CTF), Changuinola, Kemerovo, Lebombo, and Orungo. Each virus appears to have an insect vector. The most common vector of CTF is the tick *Dermacentor andersoni*. CTF occurs in inhabitants or visitors to the forests of the North American Rocky Mountains. The association with a tick bite led to confusion with Rocky Mountain spotted fever. It differs in that rash is not a prominent feature but there are many influenza-like symptoms. A fever with biphasic pattern is common. Diagnosis is made through recognition of symptoms and serologic test results, but cultivation is possible in suckling mice. Since transmission by an insect vector is associated with abundant infectious particles in the blood, antigen can be detected in erythrocytes of infected patients. A low incidence of CNS involvement with meningitis and hemorrhagic fever may occur. Acute illness lasts 5 to 10 days with only supportive therapy used in most cases.

Arenaviruses

Arenaviruses are round, oval, or pleomorphic with a range in size between 100 and 130 nm. They are enveloped particles, and the envelope contains club-shaped projections at its surface. Electron-dense granules are found in variable numbers in the interior of the virions. These granules are 20 to 25 nm in diameter and represent host ribosomes. The sand-like granules gave the name to this group of viruses (*arena*, Latin for 'sand'). The genome of arenaviruses consists of four segments of single-stranded RNA and several smaller pieces of RNA, some of which may be of host origin. Rodents are the natural host of arenaviruses, and humans are accidentally infected when they come into contact with infected urine. Person-to-person spread is unusual except for Lassa virus. The relevant members of the Arenaviridae family are lymphocytic choriomeningitis virus (LCMV), Lassa virus, Junín virus, Machupo virus, Guanarito virus, and Sabia virus.

LCMV infection may be present throughout the world but has been rigorously documented only in North America and Europe. Four outbreaks of LCMV infection have occurred in the United States from 1965 to 1989, and either hamsters or mice experimentally infected were identified as vectors as transmission to humans.[197] The mode of spread of LCMV in most sporadic human cases is unknown, but studies suggest direct contact with rodents or spread by infected aerosols. Infection should be suspected in anyone with rodent exposure. The clinical disease produced by LCMV is a meningitis, a meningoencephalitis, or a self-limited febrile illness. Arthritis, parotiditis, orchitis, and myopericarditis have also been reported. Fatal cases in humans are extremely rare. In monkeys infected by inhalation, virus can be recovered from the lungs and hilar lymph nodes 2 days after infection. Lymphocytic meningitis is often the most conspicuous lesion, but hemorrhagic necrosis may also be seen in liver, kidney, heart, adrenal gland, and other organs. The spleen and the lymph nodes show hyperplasia.

Lassa fever is a disease that ranges in severity from mild and perhaps even subclinical infection to an inexorably progressive, multisystem failure with a mortality of over 45%.[198,199] The early symptoms of Lassa fever are nonspecific. The diagnosis may be made serologically or by isolation of the virus from serum, throat washings, pleural or ascitic fluid, or urine. Attempts to isolate the virus should be made only in a maximum containment laboratory.

Junín, Machupo, Guanarito, and Sabia viruses are the etiologic agents of the Argentine, Bolivian, Venezuelan, and Bolivian hemorrhagic fevers.[200] These fevers have similar clinical features, which result from involvement of the hematopoietic, cardiovascular, and central nervous systems, but differ in attack rates and mortality. Mortality from Junín and Machupo virus infection ranges from 10% to 20%. The illness begins with fever, malaise, pronounced myalgia, retro-orbital headache, and cutaneous hyperesthesia. As the illness progresses, there is hypertension, diaphoresis, and neurologic manifestations ranging from irritability to seizures and terminally hepatorenal failure and shock. The diagnosis is established by isolation of the virus or by demonstration of significant rises in neutralizing antibody in the serum of the patient. Recently, molecular tests based on homology found in the capsid genes of the arenaviruses have been developed.[201] Virus can be recovered from blood, throat, and less commonly urine.

The pathologic characteristics of hemorrhagic fevers disease caused by arenaviruses are variable.[7-9] The reticuloendothelial system appears activated, and phagocytic activity in Kupffer cells is a common finding. Interstitial pneumonitis, sometimes with hyaline membrane disease, is prominent. Autopsy findings include pulmonary edema and hemorrhage, acute tubular necrosis of the kidneys, and extensive hemorrhagic necrosis of the gastrointestinal tract. Morphologic evidence of encephalitis is unusual even though the clinical picture may include encephalopathy and other CNS symptoms. In all hemorrhagic fever diseases there are focal areas of central and pericentral hepatic necrosis. Eosinophilic or acidophilic bodies similar to Councilman bodies are present in the hepatocytes and Kupffer cells. The fatty metamorphosis observed in almost all cases of yellow fever is not present in Lassa fever.

Filoviruses

Two members of the Filoviridae family, Marburg virus and Ebola virus, are responsible for an extensive hemorrhagic shock syndrome with a high mortality, approaching 90% in an epidemic occurring in Zaïre in 1976. As their name suggests, the viruses have a unique filamentous appearance with an infectious unit length between 800 and 1000 nm and a diameter of 80 nm. The natural host or reservoir of these viruses is unknown; however, infections have resulted after the handling of tissues of African green monkeys. New outbreaks have occurred through the use of contaminated medical supplies by hospital personnel. Endemic areas for Marburg virus and Ebola virus are central and eastern Africa. Infection results in extensive visceral hemorrhagic necrosis affecting primarily the liver but also the kidneys and lymph nodes. The clinical symptoms include a typical viral syndrome followed by diarrhea and abdominal pain. Bleeding from the gastrointestinal tract typically begins 3 days after the onset of symptoms. Diagnosis is made by serologic testing. No specific therapy is available.

Bunyaviridae associated with hemorrhagic fever

In addition to members of the Bunyaviridae family that cause encephalitis, others members are the agents of hemorrhagic fevers with mild to severe clinical illness. Sandfly fever virus and Rift Valley fever virus *(Phlebovirus)* are capable of epidemic infections in humans and produce influenza-like symptoms with sudden high fevers but have a minimal risk of death. *Nairovirus,* or specifically Crimean-Congo Hemorrhagic fever virus, presents with similar symptoms but may progress to hemorhagic manifestations involving the skin and intestinal tract as well as hepatitis.

A separate genus, *Hantavirus* is composed of several viruses (such as Hantaan virus, Seoul virus, Sin Nombre virus, and Puumula virus) that have a worldwide distribution and cause diseases referred to as hemorrhagic fever with renal syndrome, Korean hemorrhagic fever, epidemic hemorrhagic fever, and nephropathia epidemica. The clinical presentation is similar to influenza, with high fever, myalgias, headache, and malaise, of which approximately one third of cases go on to develop petechial hemorrhages with hypotension and hemorrhagic shock. Such a condition was encountered by United Nations troops during the Korean War and termed *Korean hemorrhagic fever.* Involvement of the kidneys is variable, but, when present, necrosis of renal tubules is common. Hantaan virus infection has a 5% to 10% mortality, but Puumula virus and Seoul virus infections appear less severe.

Hantaviruses cause persistent infections in rodents and are spread by inhalation of aerosolized excreta to humans. Such a mode of transmission was recognized as the method for spread of the "Four Corners disease" in the southwestern United States. *Hantavirus* infection likely persists at some low level in its rodent vector at all times with outbreaks dependent on human contact with the predominant rodent vector population. Before the outbreak in the southwestern United States, screening studies detected antibodies to hantaviruses in 3 of 270 individuals tested. Infectious virus is excreted in saliva, feces, and particularly urine in experimental animals. There is currently no evidence of human-to-human spread. Therapy with ribavirin has been tried without success in the Four Corners outbreak.

Picornaviridae

The family Picornaviridae are nonenveloped, single-stranded RNA viruses with icosahedral capsids. They are associated with several different diseases including the common cold, poliomyelitis, myocarditis, and encephalitis. Genera of picornaviruses that commonly infect humans are enteroviruses, which have at least 67 recognized immunologic types, and the rhinoviruses, with more than 100 types infecting humans, including HAV. The single strand of picornavirus RNA (positive polarity) directly serves as a template for a large polypeptide that is cleaved by viral proteases. Four viral proteins, VP-1, 2, 3, and 4 unite to form a protomer, and 60 identical protomers subsequently assemble into icosahedral capsids. Structural studies with x-ray crystallography have provided images of the overall appearance of the virus with a proposed site of viral binding to cellular receptors within an antigenic "canyon."[202] The importance of this concept was that such a "canyon" could allow binding but because of its small size could exclude neutralization by circulating antibodies. The basic pentameric organization, or five-point axis of symmetry, of the virion containing the canyon was a seminal observation. The cellular receptor for the major group of rhinoviruses has been shown to be ICAM-1, a naturally occurring adhesion molecule, and low-density lipoprotein receptor for the minor group of rhinoviruses.[203,204] Integrin, VLA-2 has been identified as the receptor for echovirus 1.[205] It has been suggested, particularly for coxsackievirus B, that different structural features of the virus capsid are responsible for the wide variety of organs and tissues that may be infected by these viruses.[26]

Enteroviruses have been subdivided on the basis of antigenic relationships and differences in host range into polioviruses (3 serotypes), coxsackieviruses, groups A (23 serotypes) and B (6 serotypes), and echoviruses (31 serotypes). Currently such a distinction is no longer made for new isolates, and classification identifies viruses by serologic type within the enterovirus genus.

Poliovirus. The immunotypes of enteroviruses are distinguished on the basis of neutralization tests.[24] Most paralytic disease in the prevaccine era was caused by poliovirus type 1. Humans are the only natural host and reservoir of polioviruses, though in the laboratory polioviruses infect other primates. Early after infection in humans the virus replicates in the gut and adjacent lymphoid tissues, spreading to the regional lymph nodes. Subsequently, there is a minor viremia that disseminates the virus to all susceptible reticuloendothelial tissues. A developing immunologic antibody response may then limit the infection, which remains subclinical. In some cases extensive viral replication in the reticuloendothelial system gives rise to a second major viremia, which corresponds with the clinical minor illness or abortive poliomyelitis. These viremias may result in meningitis. It is probably through viremia that the viruses reach the CNS and replicate in the neurons of the gray matter, destroying them.

Before the late 1800s paralytic poliomyelitis was predominantly sporadic. Poliovirus infection undoubtedly occurred, but before good hygenic practices were routine it was an infection in infants that rarely resulted in paralytic disease. The institution of improved hygiene resulted in a change in the natural history of infection, shifting infection to later in life, with subsequent disease. Early in the nineteenth century epidemics were recognized in Scandinavia and western Europe, and in the first half of the twentieth century epidemics of the disease occurred in developed countries. In the early 1950s about 20,000 cases of paralytic disease were being reported annually in the United States. The introduction of inactivated vaccines in 1955 and attenuated oral vaccines in 1962 brought dramatic reduction in the incidence of paralytic poliomyelitis in the developed countries of the world. In the postvaccine era an increasing proportion of cases (though with dramatically lower numbers overall) of paralytic poliomyelitis in the United States are associated with the use of oral poliovaccines.[206] This vaccine-associated disease is seen not only in the recipients of the vaccine but occasionally in their contacts. The estimated risk of vaccine-associated disease is 1 recipient case and 2 contact cases per 10 million doses of trivalent oral polioviruses distributed. This has led to a proposal to use killed vaccine for the initial series and live vaccine only for boosters.

The manifestations of infection by polioviruses are extremely variable. The varieties of illness are inapparent infection; abortive, nonparalytic, spinal paralytic, or bulbar poliomyelitis; and encephalitis. Several risk factors are known to influence the likelihood that an individual will develop paralysis once infected with poliovirus. Boys are more commonly paralyzed than girls, and exercise, trauma, tonsillectomy, and pregnancy all increase the risk of paralytic forms of the disease. Tonsillectomized persons have a risk of acquiring bulbar poliomyelitis that is approximately eight times that in those with intact tonsils. The risk is true not only for those with onset of infection shortly before or after tonsillectomy but also when tonsillectomy is remote.

The gross pathologic condition in both acute and chronic cases of poliomyelitis infection may be inconspicuous. The most severe lesions are usually found in the anterior two thirds of the gray matter of the spinal cord. They vary from level to level and might be asymmetric in the same section of spinal cord. The ventral horns and the base of the dorsal horns are infiltrated by lymphocytes and hypertrophied microglial cells. Polymorphonuclear leukocytes are often numerous in the neuronophagic nodules that are seen in the early stages of the disease. The leptomeninges show a varying degree of infiltration with inflammatory cells. The earliest lesion in neurons is loss of Nissl substance in the cytoplasm. There is subsequent progression to eosinophilic necrosis with presence of type B intranuclear inclusions. Death of the neuron is followed by neuronophagia. The perivascular infiltration with lymphocytes and plasma cells in the leptomeninges and parenchyma may persist for weeks or even months. In cases that come to autopsy long after onset of paralysis the most obvious change is loss of neurons in the ventral horns. The axons of the neurons that have been destroyed undergo wallerian degeneration, and the affected muscle shows the typical features of denervation atrophy. Lesions outside the nervous system are less striking. In patients dying in the acute stage of the disease there is generalized lymph node enlargement with disseminated petechial hemorrhages.

Enteroviruses associated with meningitis and myocarditis. Aseptic meningitis was first noted during outbreaks of poliomyelitis in the early 1900s. Discovery of cell-culture methodology allowed detection of the ECHO viruses (enteric cytopathogenic human orphan viruses, or echoviruses) and coxsackieviruses as etiologic agents of meningoencephalitis and aseptic meningitis. Since the introduction of mumps vaccine, enteroviruses have become the most common cause of aseptic meningitis with peak incidence in late summer and early autumn. Etiologic agents can be detected in most cases classically termed *aseptic meningitis,* with 85% being enteroviruses.

Coxsackieviruses, like most members of the *Enterovirus* genus, are transmitted predominantly by the fecal-oral route rather than by respiratory secretions. Coxsackieviruses were first isolated in suckling mice from the feces of two children suffering from a poliomyelitis-like syndrome in the town of Coxsackie, New York. When additional agents of the same group were isolated, it was recognized that viruses classified as group A produced generalized myositis and flaccid paralysis in the mice used for isolation. Others, classified as group B, produced a focal myositis but also affected the myocardium, brown fat, pancreas, and CNS. Damage to the CNS results in spastic paralysis.

Coxsackieviruses cause myocarditis and pleurodynia (the "grippe") in adults and children.[24] Pleurodynia is characterized clinically by the acute onset of paroxysmal pain over the lower chest or upper abdomen. The pain is recurring but resolves over a period of weeks. Tropism for muscle cells is a particular feature of enterovirus infections usually resulting only in myalgia, but in some cases inflammation and necrosis of myocytes result from infection. Coxsackievirus B is most often associated with myocarditis, potentially rapidly fatal in infants, but myocarditis may be caused by group A viruses as well as echoviruses. A chronic myocarditis necessitating heart transplantation may occur in patients aquiring coxsackievirus B3 after infancy. Evidence for the association of coxsackievirus with myocarditis is the detection of virus in myocardium as well as endocardium and pericardial fluid and the appearance of IgM antibodies in cases of acute myocarditis.[207] However, viral antigen may not be detectable in biopsy specimens of patients with acute myocarditis and dilated cardiomyopathy even in the presence of histologic evidence of muscle damage. Therefore, molecular techniques have been used for the detection of virus RNA by in situ hybridization or amplification with specific primers after generation of DNA with reverse transcriptase.

The echoviruses were originally isolated from fecal specimens of healthy children. They produce cytopathic effects in primate cell cultures, but at isolation they were nonpathogenic for suckling mice or primates. They are immunologically distinct from polioviruses and have been associated with a variety of diseases including nonspecific febrile illnesses with or without respiratory symptoms, aseptic meningitis, paralysis and encephalitis, exanthema, generalized disease of the newborn, and neonatal diarrhea. They also have been associated with chronic, potentially fatal meningoencephalitis in agammaglobulinemic patients.

The onset of enteroviral meningitis is usually sudden with fever and headache, frequently frontal or retro-orbital. Fever, often biphasic in pattern, appears to vary by age with the highest and most prolonged fever in children who may suffer febrile seizures. Irritability is prominent just as myalgias and lethargy may be. During the first days of illness, photophobia is not uncommon, and vomiting occurs more frequently than diarrhea. Meningeal signs develop usually several days into the febrile course. Stiff neck and positive Brudzinski and Kernig signs occur in patients more than 9 months of age, whereas young infants may exhibit only fever and irritability. If still open, the fontanelle may become full or bulging in infants with meningitis.

Cerebrospinal fluid examination reveals leukocytosis, usually less than 500/mm^3, with lymphocytes predominating after a potential initial CSF neutrophilia. Usually the CSF protein is only mildly elevated and the glucose is normal; however, hypoglycorrhachia may occur, especially with echo viruses in infants. Diagnosis can be made by culture of the CSF or by serologic evidence of infection. More recently, the use of nucleic acid amplification techniques have proved capable of identifying the virus in a timely manner.

Symptoms persist for 7 to 14 days, sometimes with the headache and vomiting becoming so severe that therapeutic lumbar punctures are performed to relieve symptoms at intervals during the illness. Recovery is usually complete without sequelae except in some cases where enteroviral meningitis occurs in young infants who have been reported to exhibit neurologic signs as they grow into the second to the fifth year of life.

Retroviruses

Human T-cell leukemia virus (HTLV-I) was identified in 1981 by researchers in the United States and Japan, thereby becoming the first retrovirus to be associated with human disease. A second HTLV was identified in a cell line from a patient with hairy cell leukemia (HTLV-II). Molecular analysis indicates that these human retroviruses belong to the same class as the bovine leukemia virus within the oncovirus subfamily of Retroviridae. A third human retrovirus isolated from peripheral blood lymphocytes was subsequently shown to be distinctive from the previously isolated human retroviruses and renamed the human immunodeficiency virus (HIV), now classified in the Lentivirus subfamily. Another member of this group has been reported (HTLV-V), but confirmatory isolates have not appeared.

Human T-cell leukemia virus

HTLV-I is endemic to southern areas of Japan, particularly Kyushu, the southeastern United States, as well as tropical areas of Africa, Central America, and the Caribbean islands.[208,209] The virus was identified in established cells lines from a patient with adult T-cell leukemia (ATL) and a second patient with T-cell lymphoma of the skin. Although no longer perferred, the virus was also referred to as *human T-lymphotropic virus,* since it was found to infect CD4 T-cells. Electron microscopic studies of these cultures demonstrated the typical type C retrovirus morphology, which in combination with molecular studies led to classification within the Oncovirinae subfamily of retroviruses. Subsequent to the identification of a link between ATL and HTLV-I, additional associations were made between infection with HTLV-I and a distinct clinical entity termed *tropical spastic paraparesis* (TSP) or *HTLV-I associated myelopathy* (HAM).[210,211] HTLV-II was isolated from a patient with hairy cell leukemia, and additional isolates have been obtained from individuals with atypical forms of hairy cell leukemia,[212] but the typical form is not associated with infection by HTLV-II.

Evidence for HTLV-I being the etiologic agent of ATL and other disorders is based on serologic and epidemiologic data as well as in vitro studies.[213,214] Regions in the world endemic for HTVL are also areas where ATL and TSP/HAM are commonly diagnosed. Cocultivation of irradiated HTLV-I–containing cells and primary peripheral blood lymphocytes (PBL) results in transformation of the PBL and the production of reverse transcriptase, the viral enzyme responsible for conversion of retroviral RNA into DNA.[215] Leukemic cells have been shown to be monoclonal relative to the integration site of HTLV-I; however, the site of integration is different from one individual to another.[216] Although these observations support the conclusion that HTLV is the etiologic agent of ATL, they do not address the issue of mechanism critical to understanding the disease process. In addition, there are several puzzling issues, the most important of which being: Why do less than 1% of HTLV-I antibody–positive individuals develop ATL and only after a long incubation period extending to 30 years?[217] During this period an infected individual may have few if any symptoms, though atypical lymphocytes with the multilobated nucleus typical of ATL can be detected in the peripheral blood, a condition termed *chronic ATL.* Several biologic properties of HTLV likely contribute to the slow rate of disease progression, including the rate of viral replication, the level of viral gene expression, and the mechanism of viral spread. Infected cells demonstrate relatively low rates of viral replication as compared to other viruses. Since virus infection primarily occurs through cell-to-cell contact, the efficiency of transmission is much lower than that of a virus principally infecting cells through free virus attachment.

HTLV-I is not expected to activate the same oncogene consistently through site-specific integration (as with mouse mammary tumor virus and the Win I gene locus), but rather induce neoplasia through the activity of one of its own gene products.

Candidates for this function included the nonstructural proteins Tax and Rex, which regulate viral and cellular gene transcription. Since non–virus producing cell lines express the viral Tax protein, Tax was believed to act like an oncogene, but no cellular homolog was found. It now appears that expression of the Tax gene plays a critical role in the progression to neoplasia by increasing the level of essential growth-controlling genes. Tax is capable of increasing the expression of numerous cellular genes, many of which play a role in cell proliferation, including interleukin-2 receptor and granulocyte monocyte cell growth factor (GM-CSF).[41] This issue was investigated directly through the introduction of the Tax gene into mice. All transgenic mice expressing the Tax gene develop tumors of mesenchymal origin. The level of Tax gene expression is variable between different transformed T-cell lines; therefore other events also play a role in the development of diseases. HTLV-I is distinct from other oncoviruses in that nonstructural genes important for transformation are not homologs of human proto-oncogenes.

The envelope protein of HTLV-I gp46 may also play a role in the proliferation of lymphocytes from HTLV-I–infected individuals.[218] However, Tax alone is not able to transform cells, and gp46 blockade does not inhibit cell activation. It has also been proposed that infection by other organisms, including parasites, affects the progression to malignancy. It appears that each of these various processes play a part in the development of ATL, in that direct cell contact is required, a specific receptor is needed, and cellular gene expression increases to propel a smoldering ATL to the fully malignant phenotype.

Diagnosis of infection is made through a variety of available procedures, including ELISA with confirmation by western blot as well as recognition of neoplastic convoluted or multilobed lymphocytes. The leukemic cells in ATL are CD4 positive, show monoclonal rearrangement of the T-cell receptor beta gene and express elevated levels of the interleukin-2 receptor. Absolute lymphocyte counts during the chronic phase may be only slightly elevated but may exceed $100,000/mm^3$ during the acute stages. The leukemic disorder is particularly aggressive, with a median survival of 8 months after entry into the acute phase of disease. Hypercalcemia is a common finding, and patients may have lytic lesions of bone.

The investigation into other HTLV-I–induced entities such as pulmonary lymphocytosis, ocular uveitis, and TSP continues. The clinical findings in TSP/HAM include hyperreflexia and spasticity of the extremities.[219] Although the atypical lymphocytes of ATL are not usually present in the peripheral blood of TSP patients, antibodies to HTLV-I are present, and the CSF frequently contains elevated numbers of lymphocytes with bizarre nuclear lobulation. The lymphocytes in cases of TSP have a polyclonal pattern of HTLV integration. A second major difference between ATL and TSP is the relatively short interval between infection and the appearance of clinical symptoms.

Transmission of HTLV-I and II may occur in several ways, from mother to child through either infected lymphocytes in breast milk or transplacentally, through sexual intercourse, or intravenously through blood products or infected instruments. Although the incidence of infection by HTLV-I or II is low in the United States, the incidence appears to be increasing, particularly among drug users. Therefore screening of blood donors has been instituted to limit spread of the virus through this means.

HIV

HIV is the causative agent of the acquired immunodeficiency syndrome (AIDS) in which illness and death usually results because of the inability of the immune system to defend against opportunistic pathogens. The first descriptions of AIDS in bisexual and homosexual men were reported[220,221] in 1981. Subsequently a human retrovirus was isolated by three different research groups and given the separate names *lymphadenopathy-associated virus, human T-cell leukemia virus type III*, and *AIDS-associated retrovirus* (LAV, HTLV-III, and ARV).[222-224] In 1986, on recommendation by the International Committee on Taxonomy of viruses, the name *human immunodeficiency virus* (HIV) was adopted. In that same year a subtype of HIV was isolated and identified as HIV-2.[225] This virus was determined to have more sequence similarity to simian immunodeficiency virus (SIV) than to the former virus, now called HIV-1. Accordingly, antibodies to HIV-2 envelope glycoproteins generally cross-react with SIV but not the antibodies of HIV-1.[226] Immunodeficiency syndrome attributable to HIV-2 infection manifests more gastrointestinal and central nervous system symptoms than disease attributable to HIV-1.

The genome of HIV exists within infectious virions as RNA of approximately 9800 nucleotides in length. The life cycle of HIV is typical of a retrovirus and is depicted in Fig. 36-7. After infection of a permissive cell, a DNA copy of the genome is produced in the nucleus by viral reverse transcriptase. Circular forms of the virus may be produced in the nucleus but are not a prerequisite for integration, and their function has not been determined. Integration allows for subsequent transcription of viral RNAs of varying lengths. The viral genome contains coding sequences for genes including-group associated antigen proteins (Gag), polymerase (including reverse transcriptase and integrase) and envelope proteins, in addition to the long terminal repeats (LTR) found at both ends of the genome. Early in infection, viral transcripts that are multiply spliced or shortened and code for regulatory proteins are produced; the two most understood are Tat (*trans*-activator) and Rev. Tat enhances LTR-directed transcription and is required for high-level expression of viral proteins. It mediates this effect by interaction with cellular proteins at the *trans*-activator–responsive (TAR) region in RNA transcripts. Later in infection, viral structural genes are transcribed through the production of primarily full-length unspliced RNAs. The switch from production of regulatory proteins to structural proteins is mediated through the activity of rev proteins, which define the fate of the transcript. In the absence of rev, full-length transcripts remain in the nucleus and short, doubly spliced transcripts accumulate in the cytoplasm. After the accumulation of structural proteins around full-length viral RNA, they are then packaged into budding virions at the cell outer membrane. Other HIV genes include Vif, Nef, Vpr, and Vpu. HIV proteins that are detectable by the serum of infected individuals are depicted when analyzed by the western blot procedure. The glycosylation of proteins gp120, gp160, and gp40 accounts for the slight variation in size and the associated thickened band observed on western blot.

The body of evidence supporting the conclusion that HIV is the causative agent of AIDS is extensive. The critical issue is whether some other infectious agent could be responsible for the cluster of findings in patients with AIDS. First, AIDS is associated with a depletion of CD4 cells in humans, and it is this same subset of cells that can be infected by HIV in culture. Second, HIV-1 and HIV-2 are related at the molecular level to SIV, a retrovirus that has fulfilled Koch's postulates by the introduction into monkeys with subsequent generation of an illness resembling human AIDS. Third, there have occurred laboratory accidents in which purified virus or virus-containing liquids have come into contact with workers who have subsequently developed AIDS. The isolated strain was shown to match the laboratory strain in these workers, who were HIV negative before exposure. Fourth, serologic conversion from negative to positive for antibodies to HIV correlates with the subsequent development of AIDS, and, fifth, in twins born to an HIV-positive mother with AIDS, the infant who was HIV positive developed AIDS whereas the twin who remained HIV negative did not develop AIDS.

HIV is acquired by sexual or parenteral contact with blood or blood products of infected individuals or perinatally either by the swallowing of infected amniotic fluid, by contact with maternal blood during the birth process, or via breast milk. The site of primary infection is believed to be the activated T-cell, resident macrophage, and mucosal cells in bowel or uterine cavity. Although $CD4^+$-cells are most efficiently infected, HIV may also enter some cells by a CD4-independent mechanism as well as by cell-to-cell contact.[227] After primary infection, individuals may develop high titers of infectious virus (>5000 infectious particles/ml) in the blood.[228,229] Subsequently, individuals may manifest symptoms of a generalized virus infection and within 1 to 3 weeks the $CD4^+$ lymphocyte count falls. Eventually the viremia is suppressed by the functioning immune system and $CD4^+$ cell counts return to near-normal levels by 3 months. Although individuals then harbor HIV in peripheral blood mononuclear cells (PBMCs), they may remain asymptomatic for 14 years or longer.[230] During this time, however, virus is replicating in lymph nodes and PBMCs, and the $CD4^+$ count is progressively decreasing as the HIV titer in the blood rises. The mechanism of $CD4^+$ depletion during this time may reflect increased cytopathic effect of the HIV isolates generated in later stages of infection. The more cytopathic HIV isolates are believed to be cleared quickly by an adequately functioning immune system, allowing persistence of the relatively noncytopathic variants during the asymptomatic stage of HIV infection. However, during the period of immune function decline, HIV variants that are more cytopathic continue to replicate at high efficiency and are believed to surpass noncytopathic variants. Although later HIV isolates from AIDS individuals vary greatly in their in vitro replication characteristics as compared with earlier isolates within an individual, whether this characteristic correlates with increased pathogenicity in vivo remains to be verified in primates. When $CD4^+$ cell numbers fall below 300 cells/μl, symptoms of immune deficiency appear, and there is a second release of HIV in the blood. The free virus titer in blood remains high, and $CD4^+$ cell numbers continue to drop until death ensues, usually because of an uncontrollable opportunistic infection.

The hallmark of clinical disease is a profound $CD4^+$ lymphocyte depletion, eventually resulting in the inability to mount an effectual immune response against opportunistic pathogens. The specific mechanism by which the $CD4^+$ cell count is depleted has not yet been elucidated but may be the result of direct cytotoxicity of HIV proteins; apoptosis of $CD4^+$ cells initiated by HIV itself, by one of its components or by immune response it generates, or by immune cell-mediated killing. There are no data demonstrating that syncytium induction plays a role in cell death in vivo.

Soon after the association of HIV with AIDS it was noted that the length of time from infection to disease varied between individuals, even between members of the same cohort. This may be explained by the genetic susceptibility of the individual's immune system to infection as well as by the degree to which individuals are infected by other agents. Infections, viral products, or cytokines activate T-cells and facilitate increased replication of HIV and continued progression of disease.[231] Indeed it has been demonstrated that HIV may remain latent and unintegrated for several days within quiescent lymphocytes and might not be integrated into the host cell genome and actively expressed until the lymphocytes are activated. Specific examples of how virus infections may act as cofactors for HIV diseases progression are the induction of Fc receptors on cells by herpesviruses, allowing entry of HIV complexed with antibody; also, some strains of HHV-6 induce CD4 on the surface of $CD8^+$ cells, thereby permitting HIV infection.[232]

A property that distinguishes the *Lentivirus* HIV from the onco-retroviruses is its ability to infect nondividing cells[233] such as macrophages and microglia. Indeed it is the macrophage that is believed to be the major reservoir of HIV infection and the vehicle that transports HIV to tissue sites such as the brain. Neurologic disorders are a common cause of morbidity in HIV seropositive individuals and have a direct HIV cause as well as an opportunistic mode of neuropathogenesis.

As basic research elucidates HIV biologic characteristics, targets for antiretroviral agents are being identified. Because of the rapidity with which HIV mutates (estimated at one nucleotide change per viral genome replication), successful future therapy will require a combination of agents targeted at more than one stage of the retroviral life cycle. For example, the combination of a protease inhibitor and two reverse transcriptase inhibitors targeted at different epitopes may make the simultaneous development of compensatory mutations impossible. A cure for AIDS is not likely in the near future though initiation of the multiple-agents approach soon after infection is recognized may be successful in turning the diagnosis of HIV seropositivity from a death sentence into that of a manageable chronic condition.

A complete discussion of the pathologic findings in AIDS is presented in Chapter 28.

Slow viruses

Historically, the spongiform encephalopathies kuru and Creutzfeldt-Jakob disease (CJD) and scrapie, the prototypic disease of animals, have been described as "slow virus" diseases because of the filterable nature of the etiologic agent and the usually long incubation period between exposure to the agent and the onset of disease. The agent consistently found in the diseases kuru and CJD is termed a *prion*. Prion-related diseases are discussed in Chapter 40.[234-243]

VIRUS THERAPEUTICS

Antiviral agents

Viruses have no cell walls and no capability for independent protein synthesis. Therefore classical antibacterials are not effective antiviral agents and alternative strategies are necessary.[244] Antiviral agents may be either chemical compounds (such as nucleic acid analogs or enzyme inhibitors) or naturally occurring preparations such as interferon, compounds that induce immune responses or concentrated antibody preparations with specific viral activity. Thus several strategies are now in common use in addition to vaccines. New synthetic compounds with antiviral activity are being developed as specific biologic targets involved in viral replication are identified. Immunologic interventions are also being further refined as specific immune mechanisms of protection and viral clearance are understood for many viruses. As more information becomes available regarding the interaction between viruses and the cell, it is likely that agents that block viral attachment will also be developed.[16]

The list of potential antivirals has expanded and contracted as new strategies for inhibiting viral replication have been conceived and then tested. These strategies evolved as a result of the discovery of essential viral and cellular processes. Despite many promising candidates, few drugs have survived the evaluation process for use in clinical medicine because of problems of toxicity in vivo or rapid induction of resistance. It may be no surprise that as new antiviral agents are used, resistant strains appear, resulting in the expanding spiral so common to antibiotics and bacteria. The essential problem in the development of antiviral drugs is that viruses lack common targets that are present in other microorganisms such as the translational machinery for generating proteins. However, viruses are unique in other ways, such as the presence of an RNA-dependent RNA polymerase, which open the door for therapeutic strategies. One such opportunity is the presence of the unique thymidine kinase of herpesviruses types 1 and 2 targeted by the synthetic purine nucleoside, an acycloguanosine (acyclovir). It was discovered that host cellular thymidine kinase could not use acyclovir as a substrate, but viral thymidine kinase would effectively convert acyclovir into acyclovir monophosphate.[245] Subsequently cellular enzymes convert the monophosphate into diphosphate and triphosphate nucleotides. Acycloguanosine triphosphate interferes with herpes simplex virus DNA polymerase and results in premature DNA chain termination. In addition, it is preferentially taken up by virus-infected cells. However, utilization is limited because some viruses in the Herpesviridae family, notably CMV, lack the unique thymidine kinase. In distinction to HSV infection, the use of acyclovir to treat EBV infection has not clearly been shown to be effective.

Acyclovir is now recognized as the most effective agent for the treatment of herpes encephalitis. Acyclovir is also used for the treatment of recurrent orofacial HSV, genital HSV, or whitlow. Chronic suppressive therapy with acyclovir is helpful in patients with frequently recurring herpetic lesions and greatly reduces the frequency and severity of recurrences in genital HSV.

Acyclovir was approved for treatment of chickenpox in 1992 but, because of its marginal efficacy in routine VZV, is reserved for cases with a high probability of complications. These patients include any immunocompromised host, adults, newborns, patients exhibiting more than 200 virions in the first 24 hours and perhaps second cases within families. Only supportive therapy is indicated for uncomplicated chickenpox in children. Acyclovir therapy of uncomplicated varicella may be unwise because there is some concern that such treatment predisposes to earlier and more frequent zoster.

CMV lacks the thymidine kinase present in HSV 1 and 2, and therefore a greater effect on viral DNA polymerase was achieved through the development of a different acyclic nucleoside analog, Ganciclovir. The mechanism for reduction of viral replication with a nucleoside analog such as Ganciclovir is dependent on the formation of the nucleotide triphosphate, which is a strong inhibitor of viral DNA polymerases. In comparison with acyclovir, Ganciclovir has considerably greater activity against CMV. Since cellular polymerase alpha may also be inhibited at high doses, a dose limit exists. Long-term (months) prophylaxis with Ganciclovir or high-dose acyclovir plus immunoglobulin is needed when immune systems are severely compromised, but toxicity may become a limiting factor in the use of Ganciclovir.[246] Since cellular immunity is more important than humoral immune function in long-term control of CMV, eventually T-cell function must be reestablished. The most common side effect of Ganciclovir is bone marrow suppression, which may predispose patients to other infectious agents or suppress engraftment of hematopoietic stem cells. In addition, Ganciclovir-resistant strains of CMV have appeared, and they require use of an alternative drug (foscarnet). The mechanism of resistance is due to a mutation in the viral gene (UL97) responsible for the initial phosphorylation of Ganciclovir to a monophosphate.[246a]

Trisodium phosphonoformate (Foscarnet) is currently used for TK and DNA polymerase mutants of HSV, VZV, and CMV resistant to standard acyclovir or Ganciclovir therapy. It also has activity against hepatitis B virus polymerase and retrovirus reverse transcriptase. It reduces activity of the viral polymerase by noncompetitive inhibition of the pyrophosphate binding site on the enzyme. Typical protocols require the isolation of CMV and demonstration in vitro of resistance to Ganciclovir and acyclovir before foscarnet is started. Foscarnet has a high toxicity profile with bone marrow suppression being a common side effect in addition to renal toxicity and potentially severe electrolyte disturbances. Foscarnet can be administered only intravenously.

Adenine arabinoside (vidarabine, or ara-A) is a purine nucleoside analog with activity against all members of the herpesvirus family. Ara-A has multiple methods of activity, with inhibition of viral DNA polymerase being most signficant. It is licensed for use in neonatal HSV. The efficacy of ara-A is similar to ACV, but acyclovir is generally preferred because of its safety and ease of administration.

Amantadine and rimantadine are virustatic agents effective in the treatment of influenza A when initiated within 72 hours of the onset of symptoms.[247] Both agents are complex symmetrical amines. Their method of action is in the inhibition of viral RNA release into the host cell either through inhibition of penetration or uncoating. Amantadine is also useful prophylactically in patients or caregivers likely to be exposed and not previously immunized. Side effects of amantidine can be limiting factors and correlate to serum concentrations, which in turn correlate with CNS concentrations. Amantadine is estimated to be 70% effective. With both amantidine and rimantadine, resistant mutants have been recovered but appear more frequent with rimantidine. When one person in a family is diagnosed with influenza A, amantadine may be useful for treatment of the index case and as prophylaxis of family contacts. No similar effective strategy exists for treatment or prophylaxis of influenza B. Severe influenza B may respond to aerosolized ribavirin, but data are mostly anecdotal. Yearly immunization is the only effective preventive strategy for influenza A and B.

Ribavirin is a synthetic purine analog that resembles guanosine. It is sequentially phosphorylated to a triphosphate form with both monophospate and triphosphate forms having effects through decreasing intracellular GTP and inhibiting RNA polymerase respectively. Ribavirin is administered through aerosol and has been shown to provide statistically significant benefit with improved clinical scores and oxygen saturation in patients infected with RSV. Although statistically significant, these benefits are of limited clinical significance except in the most severe cases or patients with underlying disease that place them at high risk of the need for ventilation.[248] Thus who and when to treat is still debated. There are anecdotal reports of clinical improvement with ribavirin treatment of patients with adenoviral pneumonia, but no widely accepted treatment currently exists for the treatment of adenovirus infection. Vitamin A and ribavirin have been used to treat severe measles pneumonia with varied results.[249]

Currently, the majority of experience with anti-HIV compounds has concentrated on drugs that target the HIV reverse transcriptase. These agents are classified as either nucleoside analogs, such as AZT, ddI, and ddC, or nonnucleoside analogs, such as the TIBO agents. Unfortunately both classes of compounds have side effects and readily allow the development of resistant strains. Although combined therapy of nucleoside and nonnucleoside analogs may thwart appearance of double mutants, the combination of anti–reverse transcriptase compounds with inhibitors of other HIV molecules may be more efficacious. For example, the combination of anti–reverse transcriptase with protease inhibitor are being actively investigated.

Interferons are being shown to have effectiveness for the treatment of several viral diseases, and numerous clinical trials are ongoing. HPV, HBV, and herpesviruses have shown reasonable clinical response. Results of a recent study of topical IFN-alpha for recurrent genital herpes are encouraging.

Immunoglobulin is utilized in several situations for the treatment of viral infection or to interrupt a possible infection during the incubation period. Such therapy usually is dependent on the previous demonstration of a high titer of virus-specific antibodies in the immunoglobulin preparation if made from pooled donors, as is the case with varicella-zoster immune globulin (VZIG). VZIG can successfully modify illness if given within 72 hours of known exposure to VZV, and candidates for therapy include immunocompromised seronegative patients and newborns born to mothers with active infection. There is also a potential role for high-dose intravenous immunoglobulin in modifying VZV disease in transplant recipients. Hyperimmune antibody preparations against CMV are in clinical trials for use in selected viral infections or to limit infection in organ transplant recipients.

A proposed therapeutic modality for the treatment of CMV or EBV is the use of $CD8^+$ cytotoxic lymphocytes, which have specific activity against CMV.

Vaccines

Vaccines continue to provide the first line of the human-engineered defense against viruses. Virtually every human virus that causes significant morbidity is a candidate for vaccine development. Vaccines have been successful in eliminating the smallpox virus, which, until its eradication, had decimated previously isolated populations of the world. Vaccine programs for the control of viral childhood illnesses and specifically polio have been very successful when fully implemented.[250] The requirement for documentation of all recommended vaccinations before school matriculation can be credited with its success; however, in many urban populations in the United States, the failure to obtain vaccination on a timely basis has reopened the window for viral disease in the pre–school aged child. The essential goal of vaccine programs is to obtain immunity to viral infection in sufficient numbers so as to prevent epidemic spread of the contagious agent. This level of protection typically occurs when approximately 80% of the entire population is immune, providing the so-called herd immunity.

The essential question facing health officials is the risk to an individual from any vaccine in comparison with the benefit to the individual and to society, since there are well recognized risks associated with the administration of vaccines. The Oka vaccine approved for VZV causes lesions in newly vaccinated children with leukemia and has been associated with reactivation and herpes zoster.[251] Although the debate about the use of vaccines is not new (Thomas Jefferson was personally involved in smallpox vaccine campaigns in the colonies), the development of molecular techniques for the production of specific viral peptides as immunogen has reduced the risk for bad outcomes from vaccine administration. Nonetheless, some viruses such as influenza are only partially amenable to this approach and require production in cell lines or other means.

Various methods are available for vaccine production, and several common terms are essential knowledge. Table 36-16 lists the most commonly used vaccine types and summarizes the essential technique. Inactivation of whole virus is accomplished by a variety of means including heat or chemicals. A split or subunit vaccine is created by disruption of a whole virus by agents such as detergents followed by fractionation of selected components for inclusion into the vaccine. One generates live attenuated vaccines by creating or selecting a virus incapable of replication but capable of eliciting an immune response. Nucleotide changes can be introduced in a manner predicted to result in attenuation, or mutations may be selected through growth of the virus at reduced temperatures such as the cold-adapted *Influenzavirus* strain. Alternatively, attenuation can be accomplished through introduction of a short genetic sequence that disrupts a gene critical for virus activity, such as neuraminidase.[252] Up to now most successful vaccines have provided protection by stimulation of antibody production in the recipient. Newer vaccines are being designed to enhance CMI with the goal of protecting against pathogens that have proved difficult to control, such as VZV.[251] For better vaccine design, knowledge of which CMI responses to enhance is essential.

Immunization of elderly and high-risk patients is the cornerstone to prevention of excess mortality associated with influenza outbreaks. High-risk patients include ex-premature infants with bronchopulmonary dysplasia, transplant recipients, and patients with congenital or chronic heart disease, reactive airway disease, cystic fibrosis, HIV infection, neuromuscular disease, neoplasms, diabetes mellitus, and chronic renal or chronic lung disease.[250] Influenza vaccine usually

Specific viruses and associated diseases

Latency

47. Mocarski ES Jr: Cytomegalovirus biology and replication. In Roizman B, Whitley RJ, Lopez C: *The human herpesviruses,* New York, 1993, Raven Press.
48. Stevens JG, Haar GL, Porter D et al: Prominence of the HSV latency-associated transcript in trigeminal ganglia from sero-positive humans, *J Infect Dis* 158:117, 1988.
49. Gershon AA, LaRussa PL: Varicella-zoster virus infections. In Krugman S, Katz SL, Gershon AA, and Wilfert CM, editors: *Infectious diseases of children,* St. Louis, 1992, Mosby.

Herpesviruses

50. Roizman B: Herpesviridae: a brief introduction. In *Virology,* ed 2, Fields BN, Knipe DM, editors: New York, 1990, Raven Press.
51. Whitley RJ, Gnann JW Jr: The epidemiology and clinical manifestations of herpes simplex virus infections. In Roizman B, Whitley RJ, Lopez C, editors: *The human herpesviruses,* New York, 1993, Raven Press.
52. Honess RW, Roizman B: Regulation of herpesvirus macromolecular synthesis I. Cascade regulation of the synthesis of three groups of viral proteins, *J Virol* 14:8, 1974.
53. Linneman CC, Buchman TG, Light IJ et al: Transmission of herpes simplex virus II in a nursery for the newborn; identification of viral isolates by DNA fingerprinting, *Lancet* 1:964, 1978.
54. Nahmais AJ, Roizman B: Infection with herpes simplex virus I and II, *N Engl J Med* 289:667, 719, 781, 1973.
55. Bernstein DI, Bryson WJ, Lovett MA: Antibody response to type-common and type-unique epitopes of herpes simplex virus polypeptides, *J Med Virol* 15:251, 1985.
56. Wagner EK, editor: *Herpes virus transcription and its regulation,* Boca Raton, Fla, 1991, CRC Press.
57. Heine JW, Honess RW, Cassai E, Roizman B: Proteins specified by herpes simplex virus XII: The polypeptides of type I strains, *J Virol* 14:640, 1974.
58. Whitley RJ: Herpes simplex viruses. In Fields BN, Knipe DM, editors: *Virology,* ed 2, New York, 1990, Raven Press.
59. Aurelius E, Johansson B et al: Rapid diagnosis of herpes simplex encephalitis by nested polymerase chain reaction assay of cerebrospinal fluid, *Lancet* 337:189, 1991.
60. Reeves WC, Corey L, Adams HG et al: Risk of recurrence after first episodes of genital herpes: relation to HSV type and antibody response, *N Engl J Med* 305:315, 1981.
61. Doymaz MZ, Rouse, BT: Herpetic stromal keratitis: an immunopathologic disease mediated by CD4 T-lymphocytes, *Invest Ophthalmol Vis Sci* 33:2165, 1992.
62. Gelb LD: Varicella-zoster virus. In Fields BN, Knipe DM, editors: *Virology,* ed 2, New York, 1990, Raven Press.
63. Epstein MA, Achong BG: Discovery and general biology of the virus. In Epstein MA, Achong BG, editors: *The Epstein-Barr virus,* Berlin, 1979, Springer-Verlag.
64. Raub-Traub N: Epstein-Barr virus and nasopharyngeal carcinoma, *Semin Cancer Biol* 3:297, 1992.
65. Miller G: Epstein-Barr virus: biology, pathogenesis, and medical aspects. In Fields BN, Knipe DM, editors: *Virology,* ed 2, New York, 1990, Raven Press.
66. Fingeroth JD, Weiss JJ, Tedder TF et al: Epstein-Barr virus receptor of human B lymphocytes is the C3d receptor CR2, *Proc Natl Acad Sci USA* 81:4510, 1984.
67. Rowe M, Lear AL et al: Three pathways of Epstein-Barr virus gene activation from EBNA1-positive latency in B lymphocytes, *J Virol* 66:122, 1992.
68. Purtilo DT, Strobach RS, Okano M, Davis JR: Biology of disease, Epstein-Barr virus-associated lymphoproliferative disorders, *Lab Invest* 67:5, 1992.
69. Griffin BE, Smith PR: Strategies of the Epstein-Barr virus. In Doerfler W, Bohm P, editors: *Virus strategies molecular biology and pathogenesis,* New York, 1989, VCH.
70. Burdin N, Peronne C, Banchereau J, Rousset F: Epstein-Barr virus transformation induces B lymphocytes to produce human interleukin 10, *J Exp Med* 177:295, 1993.
71. Klein G: Lymphoma development in mice and humans: diversity of initiation is followed by convergent cytogenetic evolution, *Proc Natl Acad Sci USA* 76:2442, 1979.
72. Raab-Traub N, Flynn N, Pearson K et al: The differentiated form of nasopharyngeal carcinoma contains Epstein-Barr virus DNA, *Int J Cancer* 39:25, 1987.
73. Herbst H, Niedobitek G, Kneba M et al: High incidence of Epstein-Barr virus genomes in Hodgkin's disease, *Am J Pathol* 137:13, 1990.
74. Momose H, Jaffe ES et al: Chronic lymphocytic leukemia/small Reed-Sternberg–like cells and possible transformation to Hodgkin's disease, *Am J Surg Pathol* 16(9):859, 1992.
75. Rubin D, Hudnall D et al: Richter's transformation of chronic lymphocytic leukemia with Hodgkin's-like cells is associated with Epstein-Barr virus infection, *Mod Pathol* 7:91, 1994.
76. Baranski B, Armstrong G, Truman JT et al: Epstein-Barr virus in the bone marrow of patients with aplastic anemia, *Ann Intern Med* 109:695, 1988.
77. Greenspan JS, Greenspan D, Lennet ET et al: Replication of Epstein-Barr virus within the epithelial cells of oral hairy leukoplakia, an AIDS associated lesion, *N Engl J Med* 313:1564, 1985
78. Schluederberg A, Straus SE, Phillip P et al: NIH Conference chronic fatigue syndrome research, *Ann Intern Med* 117:325, 1992.
79. Straus SE, moderator, NIH Conference: Epstein-Barr virus infections: biology, pathogenesis and management, *Ann Intern Med* 118:45, 1993.
80. Hanshaw JB: Congenital CMV infection, *Pediatr Ann* 23:124, 1994.
81. Drew L: Cytomegalovirus infection in patients with AIDS, *J Infect Dis* 158: 4449, 1988.
82. Huang ES, Chen ST, Pagano JS: Human cytomegalovirus. I. Purification and characterization of viral DNA, *J Virol* 12:1473, 1973.
83. Britt WJ, Vugler L, Butfiloski EJ, Stephens EB: Cell surface expression of human cytomegalovirus (HCMV) gp55-116 (gB): use of HCMV-recombinant vaccinia virus-infected cells in analysis of the human neutralizing antibody response, *J Virol* 64:1079, 1990.
84. Storz J, Ehlers B, Todd WJ, Ludwig H: Bovine cytomegaloviruses: identification and differential properties, *J Gen Virol* 65:697, 1984.
85. Mocarski ES Jr: Cytomegalovirus biology and replication. In Roizman B, Whitley RJ, Lopez C, editors: *The human herpesvirus,* New York, 1993, Raven Press.
86. Demmler CJ, O'Neil GW, O'Neil JH et al: Transmission of cytomegalovirus from husband to wife, *J Infect Dis* 154:545, 1986.
87. Toplin MD, Stewart JA, Warren D et al: Transfusion transmission confirmed by restriction endonuclease analysis, *J Pediatr* 107:953, 1985.
88. Jones LA, Duke-Duncan PM, Yeager AS: Cytomegaloviral infections in infant-toddler centers: centers for the developmentally delayed versus regular day care, *J Infect Dis* 151:953, 1985.
89. Adlser SP: Cytomegalovirus and child day-care: Risk factors for maternal infection, *Pediatr Infect Dis J* 10:590, 1991.
90. Ho M: Cytomegalovirus: biology and infection. In Greenough WB, Merigan TC, editors: New York, 1982, Plenum Publishing Corp.
91. Stagno S, Pass RF, Dworsky ME et al: Congenital cytomegalovirus infection: the relative importance of primary and recurrent maternal infection, *N Engl J Med* 306:945, 1982.
92. Fowler KB et al: The outcome of congenital CMV infection in relation to maternal antibody status, *N Engl J Med* 326:663, 1992.
93. Harrison CJ, Waner JL: Natural killer cell activity in infants and children excreting cytomegalovirus, *J Infect Dis* 1521(2):301, 1985.
94. Zaia JA: Epidemiology and pathogenesis of cytomegalovirus disease, *Semin Hematol* 27:1, 1990.
95. Rodriguez GE, McVoy MA, Adler SP: Cytomegalovirus infections in seropositive patients after transfusion: immunoglobulin G subclass responses and the effect of red cell storage and volume, *Transfusion* 30:528, 1990.
96. Felsenstein E, D'Amico DJ, Hirsch MS et al: Treatment of cytomegalovirus retinitis with 9-[2-hydroxyl-1-(hydroxymethyl)ethoxymethyl]guanine, *Ann Intern Med* 103:377, 1985.
97. Lopez C, Honess RW: Human herpesvirus-6. In Fields BN, Knipe DM, editors: *Virology,* ed 2, New York, 1990, Raven Press.
98. Russler SK, Tapper MA et al: Pneumonitis associated with coinfection by human herpesvirus 6 and *Legionella* in an immunocompetent adult, *Am J Pathol* 138:1405, 1991.

99. Drobyski WR, Dunne WM, Burd EM et al: Human herpesvirus-6 (HHV-6) infection in allogeneic bone marrow transplant recipients: I. Evidence of a marrow suppressive role for HHV-6 in vivo, *J Infect Dis* 167:735, 1993.
100. Drobyski WR, Knox KK, Majewski D, Carrigan DR: Brief report: fatal encephalitis due to variant B human herpesvirus 6 infection in a bone marrow transplant recipient, *N Engl J Med* 330:1356, 1994.
101. Adler SP, McVoy M, Chou S et al: Antibodies induced by a primary cytomegalovirus infection react with human herpesvirus 6 proteins, *J Infect Dis* 168:1119, 1993.
102. Briggs EM, Fox JD, Tedder RS: Human herpesvirus 6. In Zuckerman AJ, Banatvala JE, Pattison JR, editors: *Principles and practice of clinical virology,* ed 2, Chichester, England, 1990, John Wiley & Sons.
103. Drobyski WR, Eberle M et al: Prevalence of human herpesvirus 6 variant A and B: infections in bone marrow transplant recipients as determined by polymerase chain reaction and sequence specific oligonucleotide probe hybridization, *J Clin Microbiol* 31:1515, 1993.

Viruses causing childhood illnesses or dermatologic manifestations

104. Rand KH, Emmons RW, Merigan TC: Measles in adults: an unforeseen consequence of immunization, *JAMA* 236:1028-1031, 1976.
105. Norrby E, Oxman MN: Measles virus. In Fields BN, Knipe DM, editors: *Virology,* ed 2, New York, 1990, Raven Press.
106. Solinga DWR, Ban LJ, Ackerman AB: Role of measles virus in skin lesions and Koplick spots, *N Engl J Med* 283:1139, 1970.
107. Finkeldev W: Über Riesenzellbefunde in den Gaumenmandeln, zugleich ein Beitrag zur Histopathologie der Mandelveränderungen im Maserninkubationsstadium, *Virchows Arch* 281:323, 1931.
108. Warthin AS: Occurrence of numerous large giant cells in tonsils and pharyngeal mucosa in prodromal stage of measles: report of four cases, *Arch Pathol* 11:864, 1931.
109. Siegel MM, Walter TK, Ablin AR: Measles pneumonia in childhood leukemia, *Pediatrics* 60:38, 1977.
110. Modlin JF, Jabbour JT, Witte JJ et al: Epidemiologic studies of measles, measles vaccine, and subacute sclerosing panencephalitis, *Pediatrics* 59:505, 1977.
111. Wolinsky JS: Rubella. In Fields BN, Knipe DM, editors, *Virology,* ed 2, New York, 1990, Raven Press.
112. Centers for Disease Control: Rubella prevention: recommendations of the Immunization Practices Advisory Committee (ACIP), *MMWR* 39:RR-15, 1990.
113. Esterlev JR, Oppenheimer EH: Intrauterine rubella infection. In Rosenberg HS, Bolande RP, editors: *Perspectives in pediatric pathology,* vol 1, St. Louis, 1973, Mosby.
114. Driscoll SC: Histopathology of gestational rubella, *Am J Dis Child* 118:19, 1969.
115. Yamanishi K, Okuno T, Shiraki K et al: Identification of human herpes virus 6 as the causal agent for exanthem subitum, *Lancet* 1:1065, 1988.
116. Salahuddin SZ, Ablashi DV, Markham PD et al: Isolation of a new virus, HBLV, in patients with lymphoproliferative disorders, *Science* 234:596, 1986.
117. Takahashi M, Otsuka T, Okuno Y et al: Live vaccine used to prevent the spread of varicella in children in hospital, *Lancet* 2:1288, 1974.
118. André FE: Worldwide experience with the Oka-strain live varicella vaccine, *Postgrad Med J* 61:1113, 1985.
119. Shade RO, Blundell MC et al: Nucleotide sequence and genome organization of human parvovirus B19 isolated from the serum of a child during aplastic crisis, *J Virol* 58:921, 1986.
120. Anderson MJ, Lewis E, Kidd IM et al: An outbreak of erythema infectiosum associated with human parvovirus infection, *J Hyg* 93:85, 1984.
121. Pattison JR: Parvoviruses. In Fields BN, Knipe DM, editors: *Virology,* ed 2, New York, 1990, Raven Press.
122. Anderson MJ, Higgins PG, Davis LR et al: Experimental parvovirus infection in man, *J Infect Dis* 152:257, 1985.
123. Knott PD, Welply GAC et al: Serologically proved intrauterine infection with parvovirus, *Br Med J* 289:1660, 1984.
124. Nocton JJ, Miller LC, Tucker LB, Schaller JG: Human parvovirus B19–associated arthritis in children, *J Pediatr* 122:186, 1993.
125. Brickman A, Brunell PA: Susceptibility of medical students to mumps: comparison of serum neutralizing antibody and skin test, *Pediatrics* 48:447, 1971.
126. Sullivan KM, Halpin TJ, Marks JS, Kim-Farley R: Effectiveness of mumps vaccine in a school outbreak, *Am J Dis Child* 139:909, 1985.
127. Sosin DM, Cochi SL, Gunn RA et al: Changing epidemiology of mumps and its impact on university campuses, *Pediatrics* 84:779, 1989.
128. Baxby D: Poxviruses. In Zuckerman AJ, Banatvala JE, Pattison JR, editors: *Principles and practice of clinical virology,* ed 2, Chichester, England, 1990, John Wiley & Sons.
129. McFadden G, Pace WE et al: Biogenesis of poxviruses: transitory expression of Molluscum contagiosum early functions, *Virology* 94:297, 1979.

Papovaviruses

130. Zur Hausen H, Schneider A: The papillomaviruses. In Salzman NP, Howley PM, editors: *The Papovaviridae,* vol 2, New York, 1987, Plenum Press.
131. Shah KV: Polyomaviruses. In Fields BN, Knipe DM, editors: *Virology,* ed 2, New York, 1990, Raven Press.
132. Markowitz RB, Thompson HC, Mueller JF et al: Incidence of BK virus and JC virus viruria in human immunodeficiency virus-infected and uninfected subjects, *J Infect Dis* 167:13, 1993.
133. Munger K, Phelps W, Bubb V et al: The E6 and E7 genes of the human papillomavirus type 16 together are necessary and sufficient for transformation of primary human keratinocytes, *J Virol* 63:4417, 1989.
134. Nuovo GJ, Darfler MM, Impraim CC et al: Occurrence of multiple types of human papillomavirus in genital tract lesions, *Am J Pathol* 138:53, 1991.
135. Werness B, Levine A, Howley P: Association of human papilloma-virus types 16 and 18 E6 proteins with p53, *Science* 248:76, 1990.
136. Hubbert NL, Sedman SA, Schiller JT: Human papillomavirus type 16 increases the degradation of p53 in human keratinocytes, *J Virol* 66:3547, 1992.

Respiratory viruses

137. Murphy BR, Webster RM: Orthomyxoviruses. In Fields BN, Knipe DM, editors: *Virology,* ed 2, New York, 1990, Raven Press.
138. Schulze, IT: The structure of influenza virus. I. The polypeptides of the virion, *Virology* 42:890, 1970.
139. Webster RC, Campbell CH, Granoff A: In vivo production of new influenza A viruses. I. Genetic recombination between avian and mammalian influenza viruses, *Virology* 44:317, 1971.
140. Bollet AJ: Wilson and the influenza epidemic, *Resident & Staff Phys* Feb 1983.
141. Sartin JS: Infectious diseases during the Civil War: the triumph of the "Third Army," *Clin Infect Dis* 16:580, 1993.
142. Harrison CJ, Jenski L, Cox N et al: Onset of cell-mediated immune function after bone marrow transplantation coincides with cessation of chronic shedding of influenza A virus. In Kendal A, Patriarca P, editors: *Options for the control of influenza,* New York, 1985, Alan R Liss.
143. Glezen WP: Serious morbidity associated with major respiratory viruses, *Pediatr Ann* 19:535, 1990.
144. Corey L, Rubin RJ, Thompson TR et al: Influenza B associated Reye's syndrome: incidence in Michigan and potential for prevention, *J Infect Dis* 135: 398, 1977.
145. Orvell C, Norrby E: Antigenic structure of paramyxoviruses. In Van Regenmortel EMHV, Neurath AR, editors: *Immunochemistry of viruses: the basis for serodiagnosis and vaccines,* Amsterdam, 1985, Elsevier Science.
146. Wolinsky JS, Gilden DH: In vivo studies of parainfluenza 1 (6/94) virus: mononuclear cell interactions, *Arch Virol* 49:25, 1975.
147. Delage G, Brochu P, Pelletier M et al: Giant cell pneumonia caused by parainfluenza virus, *J Pediatr* 94:426, 1979.
148. Hall CB: Respiratory syncytial virus. In Feigin RD, Cherry JD, editors: *Textbook of pediatric infectious diseases,* ed 3, Philadelphia, 1992, Saunders.
149. Glezen WP, Tabe LH, Frank AL et al: Risk of primary infection and reinfection with respiratory syncytial virus, *Am J Dis Child* 140:543, 1986.
150. Hall CB, Douglas RG Jr, Geiman JM: Possible transmission by fomites of respiratory syncytial virus, *J Infect Dis* 141:98, 1980.

151. Garofalo R, Kimpen JL, Welliver RC, Ogra PL: Eosinophil degranulation in the respiratory tract during naturally aquired respiratory syncytial virus infection, *J Pediatr* 120:28, 1992.
152. Henderson FW, Clyde WA Jr, Collier AM et al: The etiologic and epidemiologic spectrum of bronchiolitis in pediatric practice, *J Pediatr* 95:183, 1979.
153. Falsey AR: Noninfluenza respiratory virus infection in long-term care facilities, *Infect Control Hosp Epidemiol* 12:602, 1991.
154. Couch RB. Rhinoviruses. In Fields BN, Knipe DM, editors: *Virology*, ed 2, New York, 1990, Raven Press.
155. Sung BS, Chonmaitree T, Broemeling LD et al: Association of rhinovirus infection with poor bacteriologic outcome of bacterial-viral otitis media, *Clin Infect Dis* 17:38, 1993.
156. Maletzky AJ, Cooney MK, Luce R et al: Epidemiology of viral and mycoplasmal agents associated with childhood lower respiratory illness in a civilian population, *J Pediatr* 78:407, 1971.
157. Abzug MJ, Levin MJ: Neonatal adenovirus infection: four patients and review of the literature, *Pediatrics* 87:890, 1991
158. Edwards KM, Thompson J, Paolini J et al: Adenovirus infections in young children, *Pediatrics* 76:420, 1985.
159. Horowitz MS: Adenoviruses. In Fields BN, Knipe DM, editors: *Virology*, ed 2, New York, 1990, Raven Press.
160. Krilov LR, Rubin LG, Frogel M: Disseminated adenovirus infection with hepatic necrosis in patients with human immunodeficiency virus infection and other immunodeficiency states, *Rev Infect Dis* 12:303, 1990.
161. Bradburne AF, Somerset BA: Coronavirus antibody titres in sera of healthy adults and experimentally infected volunteers, *J Hyg* (Camb) 70:235, 1972.
162. Cavallaro JJ, Monto AS: Community wide outbreak of infection with a 229E-like coronavirus in Tecumseh, Michigan, *J Infect Dis* 122:272, 1970.
163. Macnaughton MR: Coronaviruses. In Zuckerman AJ, Banatvala JE, Pattison JR, editors: *Principles and practice of clinical virology,* ed 2, Chichester, England, 1990, John Wiley & Sons.
164. Arnold R, Kaizek T, Peters CJ: Update: outbreak of hantavirus infection–southwestern U.S., 1993, *MMWR* 42:23, 1993.

Viruses associated with gastroenteritis

165. Estes MK: Rotaviruses and their replication. In Fields BN, Knipe DM, editors: *Virology*, ed 2, New York, 1990, Raven Press.
166. Kapikian AZ, Chanock RM: Caliciviridae: Norwalk group of viruses. In Fields BN, Knipe DM, editors: *Virology,* ed 2, New York, 1990, Raven Press.
167. Kapikian AZ: Viral gastroenteritis, *JAMA* 269:6278, 1993.
168. Herrman JE, Taylor DN et al: Astroviruses as a cause of gastroenteritis in children, *N Engl J Med* 324:1757, 1991.
169. Randhawa PS, Jaffe R, Demetris AJ et al: Expression of Epstein-Barr virus–encoded small RNA (by the EBER-1 gene)in liver specimens from transplant recipients with post-transplantation lymphoproliferative disease, *N Engl J Med* 327:1710, 1992.
170. Phillips JM, Blendis LM, Poucell S et al: Syncytial giant-cell hepatitis, *N Engl J Med* 324:455, 1991.
171. Hollinger FB, Ticehurst J: Hepatitis A virus. In Fields BN, Knipe DM, editors: *Virology*, ed 2, New York, 1990, Raven Press.
172. Carey WD, Patel G: Viral hepatitis in the 1999s, part I: current principles of management, *Cleve Clin J Med* 59:317, 1992.
173. Raney AK, McLachlan A: The biology of hepatitis B virus. In: McLachlan A, editor: *Molecular biology of the hepatitis B virus,* Boca Raton, Fla, 1991, CRC Press.
174. Hollinger FB: Hepatitis B virus. In Fields BN, Knipe DM, editors: *Virology,* New York, 1990, Raven Press.
175. Wands JR, Liang TJ, Blum H, Shafritz DA: Molecular pathogenesis of liver disease during persistent hepatitis B virus infection, *Semin Liver Dis* 12:252, 1992.
176. Hadziyannis SJ, Lieberman HM, Karvountzis GG, Shafritz DA: Analysis of liver disease, nuclear HBcAg, viral replication, and hepatitis B virus DNA in liver and serum of HBeAg vs. anti-HBe positive carriers of hepatitis B virus, *Hepatology* 3:656, 1983.
177. Okamoto H, Yotsumoto S, Akahane Y et al: Hepatitis B viruses with precore region defects prevail in persistently infected hosts along with seroconversion to antibody against e antigen, *J Virol* 64:1298, 1990.
178. Hayashi PH, Zeldis JB: Molecular biology of viral hepatitis and hepatocellular carcinoma, *Comprehensive Therapy* 19:188, 1993.
179. Kim C-M, Koike K, Saito I et al: HBx gene of hepatitis B virus induces liver cancer in transgenic mice, *Nature* 351:317, 1991.
180. Chisari FV, Ferrari C, Mondelli MW: Hepatitis B virus structure and biology, *Microbiol Pathog* 6:311, 1989.
181. Bouffard P, Zeldis JB: Hepatitis viruses and bone marrow depression. In Young NS, editor: *Viruses and bone marrow,* New York, 1993, Marcel Dekker.
182. Carey WD, Patel G: Viral hepatitis in the 1990s, part II: hepatitis B and delta virus, *Cleve Clin J Med* 59:393, 1992.
183. Purcel RH, Gerin JL: Hepatitis delta virus. In Fields BN, Knipe DM, editors: *Virology*, ed 2, New York, 1990, Raven Press.
184. Bradley DW: Virology, molecular bioloogy, and serology of hepatitis C virus, *Transfus Med Rev* 6:93, 1992.
185. Zhang HY, Kuramoto IK et al: Hepatitis C virus in blood of volunteer donors, *J Clin Microbiol* 31:606, 1993.
186. Gish RG, Warmerdam MT et al: Variation in antibody reactivity to the hepatitis C virus by comparative immunoscreening and enzyme immunoassay, *Viral Immunol* 6:49, 1993.
187. Reyes GR, Baroudy BM: Molecular biology of non-A, non-B hepatitis agents: hepatitis C and hepatitis E viruses, *Adv Virus Res* 40:57, 1991.

Viruses causing encephalitis, meningitis, or hemorrhagic fever

188. Baer GM, editor: *The natural history of rabies,* New York, 1975, Academic Press.
189. Murphy FA, Harrison AK, Winn WC, Bauer SP: Comparative pathogenesis of rabies and rabies-like viruses, *Lab Invest* 29:1, 1973.
190. Dupont JR, Earle KM: Human rabies encephalitis: a study of 49 fatal cases with a review of the literature, *Neurology* (Minneap) 15:1023, 1965.
191. Negri A: Beitrag zum Studium der Aetiologie der Tollwuth, *Z. Hyg Infektionskrankh* 43:507, 1903.
192. Sung JH, Hayano M, Mastri AR, Okagaki T: A case of human rabies and ultrastructure of the Negri body, *J Neuropathol Exp Neurol* 35:541, 1976.
193. Baer GM, Bellini WJ, Fishbein : Rhabdoviruses. In Fields BN, Knipe DM, editors: *Virology*, ed 2, New York, 1990, Raven Press.
194. Gonzalez-Scarano F, Nathanson N: Bunyaviridae. In Fields BN, Knipe DM, editors: *Virology*, ed 2, New York, 1990, Raven Press.
195. Monath TP: Flaviviruses. In Fields BN, Knipe DM, editors: *Virology,* New York, 1990, Raven Press.
196. Smetana HF: The histopathology of experimental yellow fever, *Virchows Arch [Pathol Anat]* 335:111, 1962.
197. Dykewicz CA, Dato VM, Fisher-Hoch SP et al: Lymphocytic choriomeningitis outbreak associated with nude mice in a research institute, *JAMA* 267:1349, 1992.
198. Walker DH, Wulff H, Lane JV, Murphy FA: Comparative pathology of Lassa virus infection in monkeys, guinea pigs, and *Mastomys natalensis, Bull WHO* 52:523, 1975.
199. Wind WC Jr, and Walker DH: Pathology of human Lassa fever, *Bull WHO* 52:535 1975.
200. Tesh RB, Jahrling PB, Salas R, Shope RE: Description of Guanarito virus (Arenaviridae: *Arenavirus*), the etiologic agent of Venezuelan hemorrhagic fever, *Am J Trop Med Hyg* 50:452, 1994.
201. Griffiths CM, Wilson SM, Clegg JCS: Sequence of the nucleocapsid protein gene of Machupo virus: close relationship with another South American pathogenic arenavirus, *Junin Arch Virol* 124:371, 1992.
202. Rossmann MG: The canyon hypothesis: hiding the host cell receptor attachment site on the viral surface from immune surveillance, *J Biol Chem* 264:14587, 1989.
203. Hofer F, Gruenberger M, Kowalski H et al: Members of the low density lipoprotein receptor family mediate cell entry of a minor group common cold virus, *Proc Natl Acad Sci USA* 91:1839, 1994.

204. Greve JM, Davis G, Meyer AM et al: The major human rhinovirus receptor is ICAM-1, *Cell* 56: 839, 1989.
205. Bergelson JM, Shepley MP, Chan BMC et al: Identification of the integrin VLA-2 as a receptor for echovirus 1, *Science* 255:1718.
206. Nkowane BM, Wassilak SGF, Orenstein WA et al: Vaccine-associated paralytic poliomyelitis. United States: 1973 through 1984, *JAMA* 257:1335, 1987.
207. Archard LC, Bowles NE et al: Molecular probes for detection of persisting enterovirus infection of human heart and their prognostic value, *Eur Heart J* 12(supl D):56, 1991.

Retroviruses

208. Blattner WA, Blayney DW et al: Epidemiology of human T-cell leukemia/lymphoma virus, *J Infect Dis* 147:406, 1983.
209. Fleming AF, Maharajan R et al: Antibodies to HTLV-I in Nigerian blood-donors, their relatives and patients with leukemias, lymphomas, and other diseases, *Int J Cancer* 33:809, 1986.
210. Gessain A, Barin R et al: Antibodies to the human T-lymphotropic virus type I in patients with tropical spastic paraparesis, *Lancet* 2:407, 1985.
211. Osame M, Usuku K et al: HTLV-I associated myelopathy, a new clinical entity, *Lancet* 1:1031, 1986.
212. Rosenblatt JD, Gasson JC et al: Relationship between HTLV-II and atypical hairy cell leukemia: a serologic study of hairy-cell leukemia patients, *Leukemia* 1:397, 1987.
213. Gallo RC, Kalyanaraman VS et al: Association of the human type C retrovirus with a subset of adult T-cell cancers, *Cancer Res* 43:3892, 1983.
214. Hinuma Y, Komoda H et al: Antibodies to adult T-cell leukemia virus associated antigen (ATLA) in sera from patients with ATL and controls in Japan: a nationwide sero-edidemiologic study, *Int J Cancer* 29:631, 1982.
215. Hollsberg P, Wucherpfennig KW et al: Characterization of HTLV I *in vivo* infected T-cell clones, IL2 independent growth of non-transformed T-cells, *J Immunol* 148:3256, 1992.
216. Cann AJ, Chen ISW: Human T-cell leukemia virus types I and II. In Fields BN, Knipe DM, editors: *Virology*, ed 2, New York, 1990, Raven Press.
217. Gallo RC: The first human retrovirus, *Sci Am* 256:88, 1987.
218. Jaffe ES, Blattner WA et al: The pathological spectrum of adult T-cell leukemia/lymphoma in the United States, *Am J Surg Pathol* 8:263, 1984.
219. Wu E, Dickson DW et al: Neuroaxonal dystrophy in HTLV-1-associated myelopathy tropical spastic paraparesis–neuropathologic and neuroimmunologic correlations, *Acta Neuropathol* 86:224, 1993.
220. Gottlieb MS, Schroff R, Schanker H et al: *Pneumocystis carinii* pneumonia and mucosal candidiasis in previously healthy homosexual men, *N Engl J Med* 305:1425, 1981.
221. Masur H, Michelis MA, Greene JB: An outbreak of community-acquired *Pneumocystis carinii* pneumonia, *N Engl J Med* 305:1431, 1981.
222. Barre-Sinoussi F, Chermann J-C, Rey F et al: Isolation of a T-lymphotropic retrovirus from a patient at risk for acquired immune deficiency syndrome (AIDS), *Science* 220:868, 1983.
223. Gallo RC, Sarin PS, Gelmann EP et al: Isolation of human T-cell leukemia virus in acquired immune deficiency syndrome (AIDS), *Science* 220:865, 1983.
224. Levy JA, Hoffman AD, Kramer SM et al: Isolation of lymphocytopathic retroviruses from San Francisco patients with AIDS, *Science* 225:840, 1984.
225. Clavel F, Guétard D, Brun-Vézinet F et al: Isolation of a new human retrovirus from West African patients with AIDS, *Science* 233:343, 1986.
226. Clavel F, Mansinho K, Chamaret S et al: Human immunodeficiency virus type 2 infection associated with AIDS in West Africa, *N Engl J Med* 316:1180, 1987.
227. Sato H, Orenstein J, Dimitrov D, Martin M: Cell-to-cell spread of HIV-1 occurs within minutes and may not involve the participation of virus particles, *Virology* 186:712, 1992.
228. Clark SJ, Saag MS, Decker WD et al: High titers of cytopathic virus in plasma of patients with symptomatic primary HIV-1 infection, *N Engl J Med* 324:954, 1991.
229. Daar ES, Moudgil T, Meyer RD, Ho DD: Transient high levels of viremia in patients with primary human immunodeficiency virus type 1 infection, *N Engl J Med* 32:961, 1991.
230. Lifson AR, Buchbinder SP, Sheppard HW et al: Long-term human immunodeficiency virus infection in asymptomatic homosexual and bisexual men with normal CD4+ lymphocyte counts: immunologic and virologic characteristics, *J Infect Dis* 163:959, 1991.
231. Bukrinsky MI, Stanwick TL, Dempsey MP, Stevenson M: Quiescent T lymphocytes as an inducible virus reservoir in HIV-1 infection, *Science* 254:423, 1991.
232. Lusso P, DeMaria A, Malnati M, Lori F: Induction of CD4 and susceptibility to HIV-1 infection in human CD8+ T lymphocytes by human herpesvirus-6, *Nature* (London) 349:533, 1991.
233. Bukrinsky MI, Haggerty S, Dempsey MP et al: A nuclear localization signal within HIV-1 matrix protein that governs infection of non-dividing cells, *Nature* 365:666, 1993.

Slow viruses

234. Prusiner SB: Novel proteinaceous infectious particles cause scrapie, *Science* 216:136, 1982.
235. Borchelt DR, Scott M, Taraboulos A et al: Scrapie and cellular prion proteins differ in their kinetics of synthesis and topology in cultured cells, *J Cell Biol* 110:743, 1990.
236. Basler K, Oesch B, Scott M et al: Scrapie and cellular PrP isoforms are encoded by the same chromosomal gene, *Cell* 46:417, 1986.
237. Lugaresi E, Medori R, Montagna P et al: Fatal familial insomnia and dysautonomia with selective degeneration of thalamic nuclei, *N Engl J Med* 315:997, 1986.
238. Poulter M, Baker HF, Frith CD et al: Inherited prion disease with 144 base pair gene insertion. 1. Genealogical and molecular studies, *Brain* 115:675, 1992.
239. Owen F, Poulter M, Collinge J et al: A dementing illness associated with a novel insertion in the prion protein gene, *Mol Brain Res* 13:155, 1992
240. Stahl N, Baldwin MA, Teplow D et al: pp 369-379 in Prusiner SB, Collinge J, Powell J, Anderton B, editors: *Prion diseases of humans and animals*, London, 1992, Ellis Horwood.
241. Prusiner SB, Scott M, Foster D et al: Transgenetic studies implicate interactions between homologous PrP isoforms in scrapie prion replication, *Cell* 63:673, 1990.
242. Bueler H, Fischer M, Lang Y et al: Normal development and behavior of mice lacking the neuronal cell-surface PrP protein, *Nature* 356:577, 1992.
243. Bosque PJ, Vnencak-Jones CL, Johnson MD et al: A PrP gene codon 178 base substitution and a 24 bp interstitial deletion in familial Creutzfeldt-Jakob disease, *Neurology* 42:1864, 1992.

Viral therapeutics

244. Galasso GJ, Whitley RJ, Merigan TC, editors: *Antiviral agents and viral diseases of man*, New York, 1990, Raven Press.
245. Hirsch MS, Kaplan JC: Antiviral agents. In Fields BN, Knipe DM, editors: *Virology*, ed 2, New York, 1990, Raven Press.
246. Goodrich JM, Motomi M, Gleaves CA et al: Early treatment with ganciclovir to prevent cytomegalovirus disease after allogeneic bone marrow transplantation, *N Engl J Med* 325:1601, 1991.
246a. Littler E, Stuart AD, Chee MS: Human cytomegalovirus UL97 open reading frame encodes a protein that phosphorylates the antiviral nucleoside analogue ganciclovir, *Nature* 358:160, 1992.
247. Wingfield WL, Pollack D, Grunert RR: Therapeutic efficacy of amantadine HCl and rimantadine HCl in naturally occurring influenza A2 respiratory illness in man, *N Eng J Med* 281:579, 1969.
248. McIntosh K, Kurachek SC, Cairns LM et al: Treatment of respiratory viral infection in an immunodeficient infant with ribavirin aerosol, *Am J Dis Child* 138:305, 1984.
249. Hussey GD, Klein M: A randomized trial of vitamin A in children with severe measles, *N Engl J Med* 323:160, 1990.
250. Dennehy PH, Jost EE, Peter G: Active immunizing agents. In Feigin RD, Cherry JD, editors: *Pediatric infectious diseases*, Philadelphia, 1992, Saunders.

251. Gershon AA, Steinberg SP and NIAID: Varicella Vaccine Collaborative Study Group: Persistence of immunity to varicella in children with leukemia immunized with live varicella vaccine, *N Eng J Med* 320:892, 1989.

252. Castrucci MR, Bilsel P, Kawaoka Y: Attenuation of influenza A virus by insertion of a foreign epitope into the neuraminidase, *J Virol* 66:4647, 1992.

253. Kapikian AZ, Mitchell RH, Chanock RM et al: An epidemiologic study of altered clinical reactivity to respiratory syncytial virus infection in children previously vaccinated with an unactivated RSV virus vaccine, *Am J Epidemiol* 89:405, 1969.

254. Centers for Disease Control: Rubella vaccination during pregnancy—United States, 1971-1988, *MMWR* 38:289, 1989.

255. Brunell PA, Novelli VM, Lipton SV, Pollock B: Combined vaccine against measles, mumps, rubella and varicella, *Pediatrics* 81:779, 1988.

256. Stanberry LR, Harrison CJ, Bernstein DI et al: Herpes simplex virus glycoprotein immunotherapy of recurrent genital herpes factors influencing efficacy, *Antiviral Res* 11:203, 1989.

37 Fungal Diseases

Francis W. Chandler
John C. Watts

GENERAL CHARACTERISTICS

Fungi are eukaryotic, unicellular, or filamentous organisms that are ubiquitous in nature. Most are saprophytes that live in organic debris or in soil enriched with organic matter. Of more than 100,000 fungal species, only about 150 are pathogenic for humans. Their ability to cause disease depends on the virulence and dose of the agent, the route of infection, and the immunologic status of the host. Fungal diseases are grouped arbitrarily into three broad categories based on the predominant location of infection within the body: superficial, cutaneous and subcutaneous, and systemic. The staining qualities and histopathologic features of the more common mycoses (fungal diseases) in each of these categories are summarized in Tables 37-1 through 37-5.

The *superficial mycoses* (Table 37-2) are those in which the fungus is usually confined to the keratinized layer of the skin and its appendages. Because fungal growth is superficial, there is little or no inflammatory response. These infections are the more common of the mycoses, cause minor discomfort, and are primarily of cosmetic importance. They are rarely encountered by the histopathologist. The *cutaneous and subcutaneous mycoses* (Table 37-3) are a polymorphic group of diseases caused by a wide variety of fungi. These fungi enter the skin and subcutaneous tissue as a result of traumatic implantation or contamination of open wounds. Although infections usually remain localized, they occasionally spread by the lymphatics to involve other sites. The *systemic mycoses* (Table 37-4) usually have a pulmonary inception, from where they may disseminate to other organs. The gastrointestinal (GI) tract is occasionally a primary focus of infection, and primary cutaneous forms of the systemic mycoses rarely occur as a result of direct inoculation of an agent after injury. In some patients, systemic infections are asymptomatic. In others they produce severe disease that can be fatal if not promptly diagnosed and treated.

Traditionally, the diseases actinomycosis and nocardiosis have fallen within the province of medical mycology and are therefore included in this chapter, though their etiologic agents are filamentous bacteria in the order Actinomycetales and not true fungi (Table 37-5). Diseases caused by the *Prototheca* spp. are also included, though these agents are considered by most taxonomists to be achloric mutants of green algae. For further information on the taxonomy of the fungi and classification of mycotic diseases, several references are recommended.[1-4]

Except for tinea versicolor, dermatophytosis, and candidiasis in the newborn, there is no clear-cut evidence that the mycoses are communicable. Most mycoses are contracted by exposure to environmental sources. A few, such as actinomycosis and candidiasis, are endogenous. The agents of these endogenous infections occur as commensals on the skin and mucous membranes and in the GI tract.

Mycologic terminology

arthroconidium Conidium formed by mycelial disarticulation

bud (blastoconidium) Conidium produced by lateral outgrowth from a parent cell: buds may be single or multiple

chlamydoconidium Thick-walled, rounded, resistant conidium formed by direct differentiation of the mycelium

conidium Asexual spore formed on but easily detached from a conidiophore

conidiophore Specialized hypha that produces and bears conidia

dematiaceous Naturally pigmented, usually brown or black

dimorphic Term applied to fungi that grow as hyphae in vitro at 25° C and as budding yeastlike cells or spherules in infected tissues or in vitro at 37° C on special media

endospore Asexual spore formed within a closed structure such as a spherule

germ tube Tubelike process, produced by a germinating conidium, that eventually develops into a hypha

granule (grain) Compact aggregate of organized mycelium that may be embedded in a cementlike substance; formed in actinomycosis, and in actinomycotic and eumycotic mycetomas; also formed by nonfilamentous bacteria in botryomycosis

hypha Filament that forms the thallus or body of most fungi

mycelium Mass of intertwined and branched hyphae

pseudohypha Short hyphal-like filament produced by the successive buds of a yeast that elongate and fail to separate

septate Having cross-walls

spherule Closed, thick-walled, spherical structure within which asexal endospores are produced by progressive cytoplasmic cleavage

Splendore-Hoeppli material Eosinophilic, refractile substance that surrounds some fungi and represents a localized antigen-antibody reaction in the hypersensitized host

yeast Spherical to oval unicellular fungus that reproduces by budding

RISK FACTORS

Although some of the systemic mycoses, such as coccidioidomycosis and histoplasmosis, are caused by fungi that are familiar pathogens, many others are caused by "opportunistic" fungi. These opportunists are saprophytes that are usually innocuous and assume the role of pathogens only when conditions render a host abnormally susceptible to infection.[5-7] They rarely infect the noncompromised, healthy person. During the past two decades, there has been an alarming increase in the incidence of opportunistic infections, particularly candidiasis, aspergillosis, cryptococcosis, zygomycosis, and nocardiosis. Contributing to this increased incidence is the widespread use of modern medical treatments that predispose patients to infection, such as cancer chemotherapeutic agents, irradiation, immunosuppressive agents, hyperalimentation, and the prolonged and frequent use of broad-spectrum antibiotics. Persons with malignancies (especially leukemia and lymphoma), burns, organ transplants, metabolic diseases, malnutrition, the acquired immunodeficiency syndrome (AIDS), or inborn immunologic deficiencies, and those who have undergone abdominal or cardiac surgery or who have received repeated intravenous injections are at special risk for mycotic infections. Some of the basic alterations believed to be responsible for this increased susceptibility are leukopenia, suppression of humoral and cellular immunity, suppression of the acute inflammatory response, neutrophil or mononuclear phagocyte dysfunction, disruption of mucosal and cutaneous barriers, and reduction of the bacterial flora of the body that normally inhibit fungal overgrowth. Other factors contributing to the increased incidence of certain mycoses include migration of susceptible persons into highly endemic areas, aging of the population, and greater awareness of fungal infections in compromised hosts. In the future, "new" opportunists will surely be recognized as agents of disease in the compromised host.

DIAGNOSIS

There are four basic approaches to the diagnosis of mycotic diseases: (1) clinical, (2) mycologic, (3) immunologic, and (4) pathologic.[2-4, 8-13] The *clinical* diagnosis of fungal infection is sometimes aided by the appearance of the lesion (such as tinea cruris) or travel history. The *mycologic* identification of fungi is valuable for those organisms (such as *Aspergillus* and *Fusarium*) that are morphologically similar in tissue sections or in rare situations where fungal drug sensitivity testing is desired.

Diseases caused by fungi may be difficult to distinguish, both clinically and pathologically, from those caused by other microbial agents. Because serologic tests have certain limitations and have not been developed for some fungal diseases, a definitive diagnosis of a mycotic disease often rests on direct microscopic demonstration of a fungus in tissues and exudates, or on isolating and identifying it in culture. Histopathology should not be a substitute for mycologic culture; rather the two should complement each other whenever possible. A variety of specimens are suitable for mycologic culture, including scrapings, body fluids, and tissue biopsy specimens. Sometimes fungal culture is not possible, as when only fixed tissues are available. Nevertheless, the histopathologist can provide a presumptive or specific diagnosis of a mycotic disease if the agent can be detected in a tissue section and can be accurately identified. The agents of some mycoses, such as lobomycosis and rhinosporidiosis, have not yet been isolated in culture on synthetic media, and the only means of establishing a diagnosis is by direct microscopic examination of tissue or exudate. Although certain inflammatory patterns are suggestive of the presence of a fungus, the diagnosis of a mycotic infection can never be based on the inflammatory reaction alone.[1,8,9,14,15]

Histopathologic evaluation provides indisputable evidence of tissue invasion and therefore can confirm the pathogenic significance of a cultural isolate that belongs to the normal body flora or that is usually encountered as an environmental contaminant in culture. Histopathology can also confirm the presence of coexisting infections by other fungi, bacteria, viruses, and protozoans, thus guiding the clinician in selecting the most appropriate therapy and management for the patient. No other diagnostic approach can assess whether the host response signifies tissue invasion or a purely allergic reaction, such as invasive versus allergic aspergillosis.

Although most fungi can be isolated from clinical materials, the cultivation and characterization of an isolate may take weeks, and the clinician usually cannot wait to begin therapy. Because the management of one mycosis may be entirely different from that of another, the pathologist must often play a key role in recognizing the mycoses and identifying their etiologic agents. In attempting to identify fungi using conventional histologic methods, it is helpful to remember that these microbes appear in tissue either as hyphae, yeastlike cells, or endosporulating spherules, or as a combination of these forms. Based on the morphologic distinctiveness of their etiologic agents in tissue, the mycoses can be grouped as follows[1,9]:

1. *Those caused by fungi that can be identified because they have a distinctive morphology in tissue.* If typical forms are observed, a specific diagnosis can be made (such as adiaspiromycosis, blastomycosis, coccidioidomycosis, cryptococcosis, histoplasmosis capsulati, histoplasmosis duboisii, lobomycosis, paracoccidioidomycosis, protothecosis, rhinosporidiosis, and sporotrichosis).

2. *Those caused by any one of several species of a genus that are morphologically "similar" and therefore can be identified only to the genus level.* Nevertheless, the diseases they cause can be diagnosed generically (such as aspergillosis, candidiasis, and nocardiosis).

3. *Those caused by any of a number of fungi belonging to various genera that appear similar if not identical to one another in tissue.* Although the agent cannot be specifically identified, the mycosis can still be diagnosed (such as actinomycosis, chromoblastomycosis, dermatophytosis, phaeohyphomycosis, and zygomycosis).

4. *Mycetomas, which are special cases that constitute a group by themselves.* Because most agents of mycetoma form their own distinctive type of granule, the etiologic agent can be identified by the size, shape, architecture (morphology of mycelial elements and their arrangement), and color of a granule. It can be determined whether the granule is composed of an actinomycete (filamentous bacterium) or a eumycete (true fungus), and whether it is hyaline (white grain) or dematiaceous (black grain).

Although some fungi and related pathogens can be detected in hematoxylin and eosin–stained tissue sections, special histologic stains are usually necessary to demonstrate their morphology in detail. Table 37-1 lists these stains and their diagnostic applications.

Increasingly, cytologic materials, rather than tissue biopsy, are obtained for the diagnosis of fungal infections. Fungi can be adequately detected in cytologic specimens obtained by fine-needle aspiration biopsy, brushing, washing, or scraping. In large part, the cytomorphology of the organisms is identical to that seen in tissue biopsy specimens. A drawback of cytologic specimens, however, may be the inability to distinguish invasive fungal infection from fungal colonization.

Table 37-1 Useful stains for demonstrating fungi and related pathogens in tissue sections

Stains	Diagnostic applications
Hematoxylin and eosin (H&E)	Demonstrates tissue response and some fungi, including those that are naturally pigmented; stains nuclei of some yeastlike cells
Special stains for fungi Gomori's methenamine - silver (GMS) Periodic acid–Schiff Gridley's fungus GMS with H&E counterstain (GMS/H&E)	Excellent for detecting fungi and studying their morphology in detail; GMS is best for screening purposes and also stains the actinomycetes and some other microbial pathogens; GMS/H&E demonstrates fungi and tissue components simultaneously
Mucin stains Mayer's mucicarmine Southgate's mucicarmine Alcian blue	Demonstrate mucoid capsule of *Cryptococcus neoformans,* thus differentiating this fungus from others of similar morphology
Modified Gram stains Brown and Brenn Brown-Hopps	Demonstrate gram-positive filaments of the actinomycetes and nonfilamentous bacteria of botryomycosis; some fungi, especially *Torulopsis glabrata* and the *Candida* spp., are gram positive
Modified acid-fast stains Fite's Kinyoun Ziehl-Neelsen	Demonstrate filaments of the *Nocardia* spp., most of which are weakly acid fast; fungal cell walls and the agents of actinomycosis are not acid fast
Giemsa stains May-Grünwald Wolbach's	Demonstrate kinetoplast of leishmanial forms and intracystic sporozoites of *Pneumocystis carinii;* both are protozoans that can be mistaken for yeastlike fungi
Melanin stain Fontana-Masson	Confirms and accentuates the presence of melanin or melanin-like substances in the lightly pigmented agents of phaeohyphomycosis; stains the cell wall of *Cryptococcus neoformans,* which contains melanin-like substances that reduce silver

Immunohistology, such as direct fluorescent antibody (DFA) staining of tissue sections, is a valuable adjunct procedure that can be used to confirm a presumptive histopathologic diagnosis.[1,9,12,16] Formalin-fixed, paraffin-embedded tissues are adequate for DFA studies of fungi because the polysaccharide antigens in fungal cell walls are not destroyed by formalin fixation. Because of the added dimension of serologic specificity, DFA can greatly increase the accuracy of conventional histologic evaluation, especially when only atypical forms of a fungus are present. A broad battery of sensitive and specific fluorescent antibody (FA) reagents is available for detecting and identifying many of the common pathogenic fungi, actinomycetes, and protothecae in tissue sections.[12,16] Only a few specialized diagnostic centers can presently perform these tests. However, a variety of immunohistochemical reagents are now available commercially. Molecular diagnostic tests are in use in the mycology laboratory to characterize fungal colonies, but direct DNA- or RNA-based identification of fungi in tissue is not yet being performed for diagnosis.

SUPERFICIAL MYCOSES

The superficial mycoses are fungal diseases that are usually confined to the outermost layers of the skin or its appendages.[17,18] Two of these diseases, black piedra and white piedra, involve the hair exclusively, and histopathology is not ordinarily used for their diagnosis. The agents of tinea nigra and tinea versicolor grow in the stratum corneum and rarely invade the deeper skin layers. The histopathologist seldom encounters these infections unless the lesions are atypical and the clinician suspects another disease (tinea nigra has been mistaken for junctional nevus or malignant melanoma). The histologic features of these mycoses are summarized in Table 37-2. For more detailed information, several texts are recommended.[2,4,17,18]

Dermatophytosis

The most important superficial mycosis is dermatophytosis, a clinical entity caused by any of 28 recognized species of pathogenic and taxonomically related fungi (dermatophytes) of the genera *Epidermophyton, Microsporum,* and *Trichophyton.*[19] This mycosis involves the skin, hair, and nails to a greater degree than do the other superficial mycoses. Diseases produced by the dermatophytes occur worldwide and are known as tineas, or ringworm. The more common tineas include (1) tinea capitis of the scalp, eyebrows, and eyelashes (2) tinea corporis of the body, (3) tinea cruris of the groin, (4) tinea pedis of the feet, and (5) tinea unguium of the nails (onychomycosis). Tineas of the hairy skin often present as circular or ring-shaped patches of alopecia with erythema and scaling, or as more diffusely distributed papules, pustules, vesicles, and kerions. Ringworm of the glabrous skin also commonly appears as erythematous and scaling patches, but more severe forms of tinea corporis may resemble other dermatologic disorders. Tinea unguium appears as thickening, discoloration, and deformity of the nails.

Histopathologic features of dermatophytosis are summarized in Table 37-2. Tissue forms of the dermatophytes are similar to one another. They usually stain with hematoxylin and eosin but are best demonstrated with special stains for fungi. Hyphae and arthroconidia invade the stratum corneum, hair follicles, and hair shafts (Fig. 37-1). The pattern of hair invasion is that of either an ectothrix, an endothrix, an endoectothrix, or a favus, depending on the etiologic agent.[17-19] Occasionally, rupture of a hair follicle and release of fungal elements into the dermis elicits acute suppurative inflammation that eventually becomes granulomatous.[20] The term *Majocchi's granuloma* refers to nodular, granulomatous lesions in the dermis that contain individual dermatophyte hyphae (Fig. 37-2, *A*). Aggregates of hyphae embedded in and surrounded by abundant Splendore-Hoeppli material in the dermis and subcutaneous tissues have been misinterpreted by some inves-

Table 37-2 Histologic features of the superficial mycoses

Disease	Biologic agent(s)	Typical morphology in tissue	Usual host reaction
Black piedra	*Piedraia hortai*	Pigmented, closely septate hyphae, 4-6 μmD, organized as nodules surrounding hair shaft; asci containing ascospores may also be present	None; involves the hair exclusively
Tinea nigra	*Phaeoannellomyces werneckii, Stenella araguata*	Pigmented, branched, septate hyphae, 1-3 μmD; elongated budding cells, 1-5 μmD	Mild to moderate hyperkeratosis; little or no dermatitis
Tinea versicolor	*Malassezia furfur*	Short, curved, and bent, hyaline hyphae, 2-4 μmD; clusters of oval or spherical, thick-walled cells (phialoconidia), 3-8 μmD	Like tinea nigra
White piedra	*Trichosporon beigelii*	Hyaline hyphae, 2-4 μmD; arthroconidia and blasto-conidia organized as nodules surrounding hair shaft; invades and destroys hair	Like black piedra
Dermatophytosis	Pathogenic members of the genera *Epidermophyton, Microsporum,* and *Trichophyton*	Hyaline, septate hyphae that break up into chains of arthroconidia	Hyperkeratosis, acanthosis, and mild mononuclear infiltrate in dermis; rarely, suppurative or granulomatous

D, Diameter

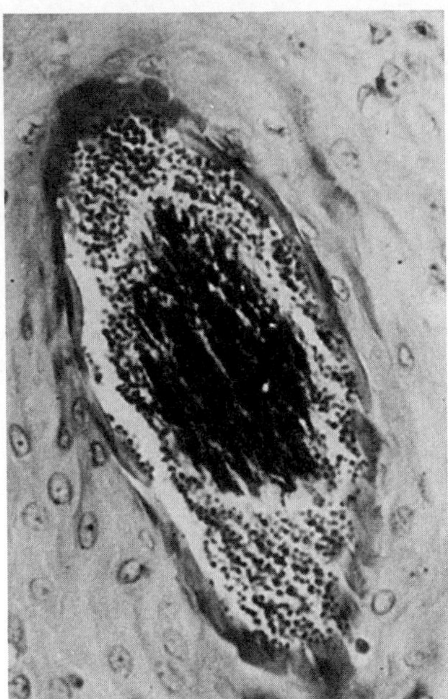

Fig. 37-1 Arthroconidia of *Microsporum canis* surrounding a partially degenerated hair.

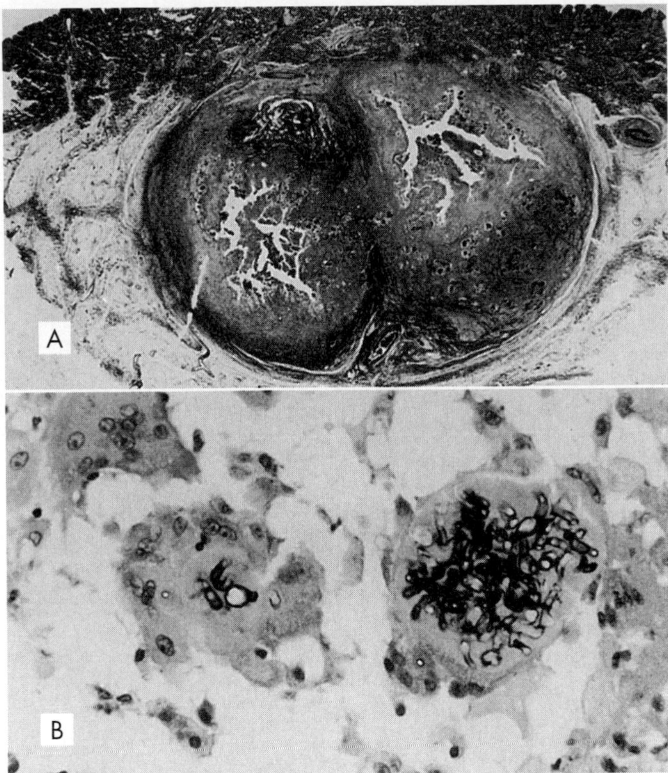

Fig. 37-2 Deep dermatophytic granuloma caused by *Microsporum canis*. **A,** Dermis and subcutaneous tissue contain multiple hyphal aggregates (pseudogranules) that stimulate an intense granulomatous reaction. **B,** Aggregates of dermatophytic hyphae (pseudogranules) ensheathed by Splendore-Hoeppli material. (**A,** periodic acid–Schiff; **B,** Gomori's methenamine silver/hematoxylin and eosin.)

tigators as being grains or granules, and therefore the infection has been mistaken for a mycetoma. These aggregates consist of clustered dermatophyte hyphae, each ensheathed by Splendore-Hoeppli material, and are actually pseudogranules (Fig. 37-2, *B*). Their microscopic appearance is strikingly similar from case to case, regardless of the dermatophytic agent.[1,9,21]

Agents of the superficial mycoses are routinely demonstrated by direct microscopic examination of skin scrapings or hair in 10% potassium hydroxide. Culture is required for their definitive identification.[3,4,19]

CUTANEOUS AND SUBCUTANEOUS MYCOSES

Certain fungi that commonly infect internal organs may also involve the skin and mucous membranes. The cutaneous and subcutaneous manifestations of these mycoses are discussed separately under their respective disease headings. Included here are those diseases that involve the skin and subcutaneous tissue predominantly or exclusively (Table 37-3).

Chromoblastomycosis

Chromoblastomycosis is an indolent cutaneous infection caused by any of several related dematiaceous (pigmented) fungi.[22] The six recognized agents are *Botryomyces caespitosus, Cladosporium carrionii, Fonsecaea compacta, F. pedrosoi, Phialophora verrucosa,* and *Rhinocladiella aquaspersa;* of these, *F. pedrosoi* is the most frequent agent.[2,23,24] The disease is cosmopolitan, but most cases are encountered in tropical or subtropical regions. A locally spreading verrucous plaque or solid nodule develops in the skin at the site of traumatic implantation of the fungus, usually on an extremity.[25] Satellite lesions may develop as a consequence of regional lymphatic spread or autoinoculation, but internal dissemination is rare.[23,24]

Although the agents of chromoblastomycosis can be distinguished from one another in culture, their tissue forms are identical. Round, thick-walled, dark brown muriform cells (*sclerotic bodies*), 5 to 12 μm in diameter, are grouped within the dermis, where they elicit a granulomatous and suppurative inflammatory reaction.[25] These cells reproduce by septation in one or two planes (Fig. 37-3). Nonseptate cells and, rarely, septate hyphae are also observed in the lesions. Associated epidermal changes include hyperkeratotic pseudoepitheliomatous hyperplasia with keratolytic microabscesses, and transepidermal elimination of the pigmented sclerotic bodies may be observed.[26]

Lobomycosis

Lobomycosis is a cutaneous mycosis that occurs in South America, especially in Brazil and Surinam, and in parts of Central America. Natural infection occurs only in humans and dolphins[27] and produces locally enlarging cutaneous nodules that become verrucous.[28] These lesions are best treated by surgical excision. *Loboa loboi,* the etiologic agent, does not grow in culture.

The yeastlike cells of *L. loboi* are abundant in the dermis of the cutaneous nodules. These thick-walled cells, 6 to 12 μm in diameter, are remarkably uniform in size and shape. They reproduce by progressive budding in chains, three to eight cells in length, each of which resembles a "string of pearls"

Table 37-3 Histologic features of the cutaneous and subcutaneous mycoses

Disease	Biologic agent(s)	Typical morphology in tissue	Usual host reaction
Chromoblastomycosis	*Botryomyces caespitosus, Cladosporium carrionii, Fonsecaea compacta, F. pedrosoi, Phialophora verrucosa,* Rhinocladiella *aquaspersa*	Large, 6-12 µmD, spherical to polyhedral, thick-walled, dark brown muriform cells (sclerotic bodies) with septations along one or two planes; pigmented hyphae sometimes present	Mixed suppurative and granulomatous
Lobomycosis	*Loboa loboi*	Spherical, budding yeastlike cells, 5-12 µmD, that form chains of cells connected by tubelike isthmuses; secondary budding may be present	Granulomatous
Mycetoma (actinomycotic)	*Actinomadura madurae, A. pelletieri, Streptomyces somaliensis, Nocardia* spp., and others	Granules, 0.1 to several mmD, composed of delicate filaments (about 1µm wide) that are often branched and beaded	Like actinomycosis
Mycetoma (eumycotic)	*Pseudallescheria boydii, Madurella grisea, M. mycetomatis, Curvularia geniculata, Exophiala jeanselmei, Leptosphaeria senegalensis,* and others	Granules, 0.2 to several mmD, composed of broad (2-6 µm), hyaline (white to yellow granules) or dematiaceous (black granules), septate hyphae that often branch and form chlamydoconidia	Like actinomycosis
Phaeohyphomycosis (subcutaneous)	*Exophiala jeanselmei, Phialophora parasitica, P. richardsiae, Wangiella dermatitidis,* and others	Pigmented (brown) hyphae, 2-6 µm wide, that may be branched and are often constricted at their frequent and prominent septations; yeast forms and chlamydoconidia sometimes present	Subcutaneous cystic or dispersed granulomas; overlying epidermis rarely affected
Rhinosporidiosis	*Rhinosporidium seeberi*	Large sporangia, 100-350 µmD, with thin walls (3-5 µm) that enclose numerous sporangiospores, 6-8 µmD	Nonspecific chronic inflammatory or granulomatous
Sporotrichosis	*Sporothrix schenckii*	Pleomorphic, spherical to oval and, at times, cigar-shaped yeastlike cells, 2-10 µmD, that produce single and, rarely, multiple buds	Mixed suppurative and granulomatous; Splendore-Hoeppli material surrounds fungus in some cases (asteroid body)
Zygomycosis (subcutaneous entomophthoromycosis)	*Basidiobolus ranarum, Conidiobolus coronatus*	Short, poorly stained hyphal fragments, 6-25 µm wide, with nonparallel sides, infrequent septa, and random branches	Eosinophilic abscesses and granulation tissue; hyphal fragments bordered by prominent Splendore-Hoeppli material

D, Diameter

(Fig. 37-4). Adjacent cells are connected to one another by tubelike isthmuses, and secondary budding may be observed. Nonbudding and single-budding cells are also present. The surrounding dermis contains a dispersed epithelioid and giant cell granulomatous inflammatory reaction.

Mycetoma (Madura foot, maduromycosis)

Mycetomas are tumorous lesions of the subcutaneous tissues and bone caused by a wide variety of geophilic actinomycetes and fungi that form granules (compact mycelial aggregates) within tissue.[29,30] Patients are infected when these exogenous organisms are introduced into some part of the body, usually the lower extremities or the trunk, as the result of trauma. Most cases of mycetoma occur in tropical regions such as Asia, Africa, and Central and South America; the disease is rarely encountered in the United States.[31,32] There are two distinct types of mycetomas: actinomycotic and eumycotic. Their principal agents are listed in Table 37-3.[1]

Accurate histologic differentiation between the granules formed by actinomycetes and fungi is crucial in determining the form of treatment and the prognosis of mycetoma. Actinomycotic mycetomas usually respond to antibiotics or sulfonamides, but eumycotic mycetomas do not. Treatment of the latter is limited primarily to surgical excision and débridement.[33,34]

Special stains for bacteria and fungi (Table 37-1) may be needed to determine whether a granule is actinomycotic or eumycotic. Granules of actinomycotic mycetomas contain delicate, gram-positive, branched, bacterial filaments, about 1 µm in width, whereas those of eumycotic mycetomas contain

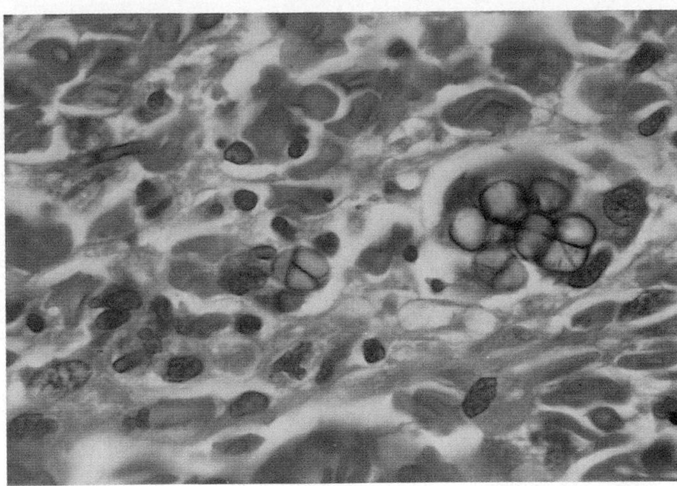

Fig. 37-3 Cutaneous chromoblastomycosis. Pigmented sclerotic bodies in the superficial dermis. Notice septation in one or two planes.

broad, septate, fungal hyphae, 2 to 6 μm or more in width[35,36] (Fig. 37-5). Chlamydoconidia are sometimes found near the periphery of eumycotic granules. Granules may be pigmented (black grain) or hyaline (white grain) and may contain an amorphous cementlike substance, depending on the etiologic agent. Because many granules have a characteristic architecture, presumptive etiologic identification can often be made histologically. However, culture is needed for definitive identification. Immunofluorescence reagents are available for detecting *Pseudallescheria boydii,* the most common agent of eumycotic mycetoma in the United States.

The inflammatory reaction in mycetoma is similar regardless of the causative agent.[29,35,36] Lesions contain multiple sinus tracts that usually discharge serosanguinous fluid and, occasionally, grossly visible granules of various colors, sizes, and degrees of hardness depending on the agent involved. Histologically, the dermis and subcutaneous tissue contain localized abscesses, each with one or more granules in its center. Eosinophilic, clublike Splendore-Hoeppli material may border the granules. Between abscesses, there is extensive granulation tissue, which results in tumefaction and deformity that is often severe enough to be mistaken clinically for a neoplasm. Mycetomas are insidious, localized infections, but they do not respect tissue planes. Infections often involve contiguous bone, resulting in destructive osteomyelitis. Lymphatic or hematogenous dissemination from the primary subcutaneous lesion rarely occurs.

Phaeohyphomycosis (subcutaneous and systemic)

Phaeohyphomycosis comprises those subcutaneous and systemic diseases caused by opportunistic naturally pigmented fungi that develop in tissue as dark-walled (brown), septate hyphae.[22,25,37,38] The inclusive name *phaeohyphomycosis* replaces the misleading and inappropriate terms *phaeosporotrichosis* and *chromomycosis* formerly applied to such infections. Phaeohyphomycosis can be caused by a wide variety of polymorphous fungi that are saprophytes of soil and wood, for example, *Exophiala (Phialophora) jeanselmei, Phialophora* spp., *Xylohypha (Cladosporium) bantiana,* and *Bipolaris (Drechslera)* spp. Infections are encountered in healthy persons, but those who are immunocompromised or chronically debilitated are at increased risk.

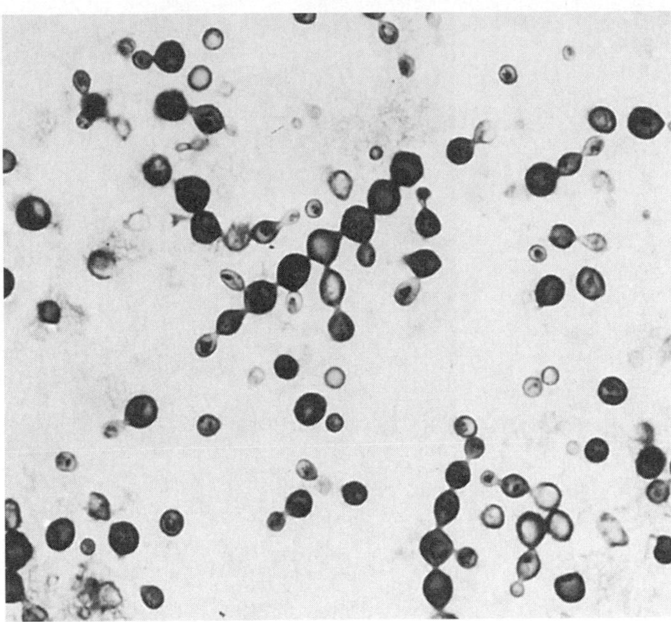

Fig. 37-4 Lobomycosis. Chains of budding cells with secondary budding. Nonbudding and single-budding cells are also present. (Gridley's stain.)

Phaeohyphomycosis has two main clinical forms: subcutaneous and systemic. The subcutaneous form (phaeomycotic cyst) usually occurs as a single, firm to fluctuant, painless abscess, up to 7 cm in diameter, in the deep dermis or subcutaneous tissue.[39-41] Lesions occur on exposed parts of the body after penetrating injury by a wood splinter or other foreign object, which acts as a vehicle of infection. Infection remains localized, and lymphangitis is uncommon. Microscopically, the overlying skin is usually unaffected. The subcutis contains a large, cystic granuloma composed of compact multinucleated giant cells and epithelioid histiocytes enclosed by granulation tissue or a well-defined, fibrotic capsule.[42] The centrally located abscess or cyst contains cellular debris, fibrin, polymorphonuclear leukocytes, and, at times, plant fibers or other foreign material.[43,44] Short, closely septate hyphae, 2 to 6 μm in width, and chains of budding yeastlike cells are present in the wall of the abscess and amidst the centrally located exudate. These moniliform fungi appear light brown when stained with hematoxylin and eosin, and they are well demonstrated with melanin stains and special stains for fungi (Table 37-1). However, special stains mask their natural brown color. *Phialophora* and *Exophiala* spp. are most often found in cystic lesions, whereas other genera, such as *Wangiella* and *Bipolaris,* are usually associated with a dispersed granulomatous reaction that may contain small, stellate abscesses.[45] Subcutaneous phaeohyphomycosis is cured by complete surgical excision.

In the systemic form (cerebral phaeohyphomycosis), infection generally occurs by way of the respiratory tract, and the most commonly encountered agent is *Xylohypha (Cladosporium) bantiana.*[46-48] This fungus is extremely neurotropic, and most infections are confined to the brain and meninges; the

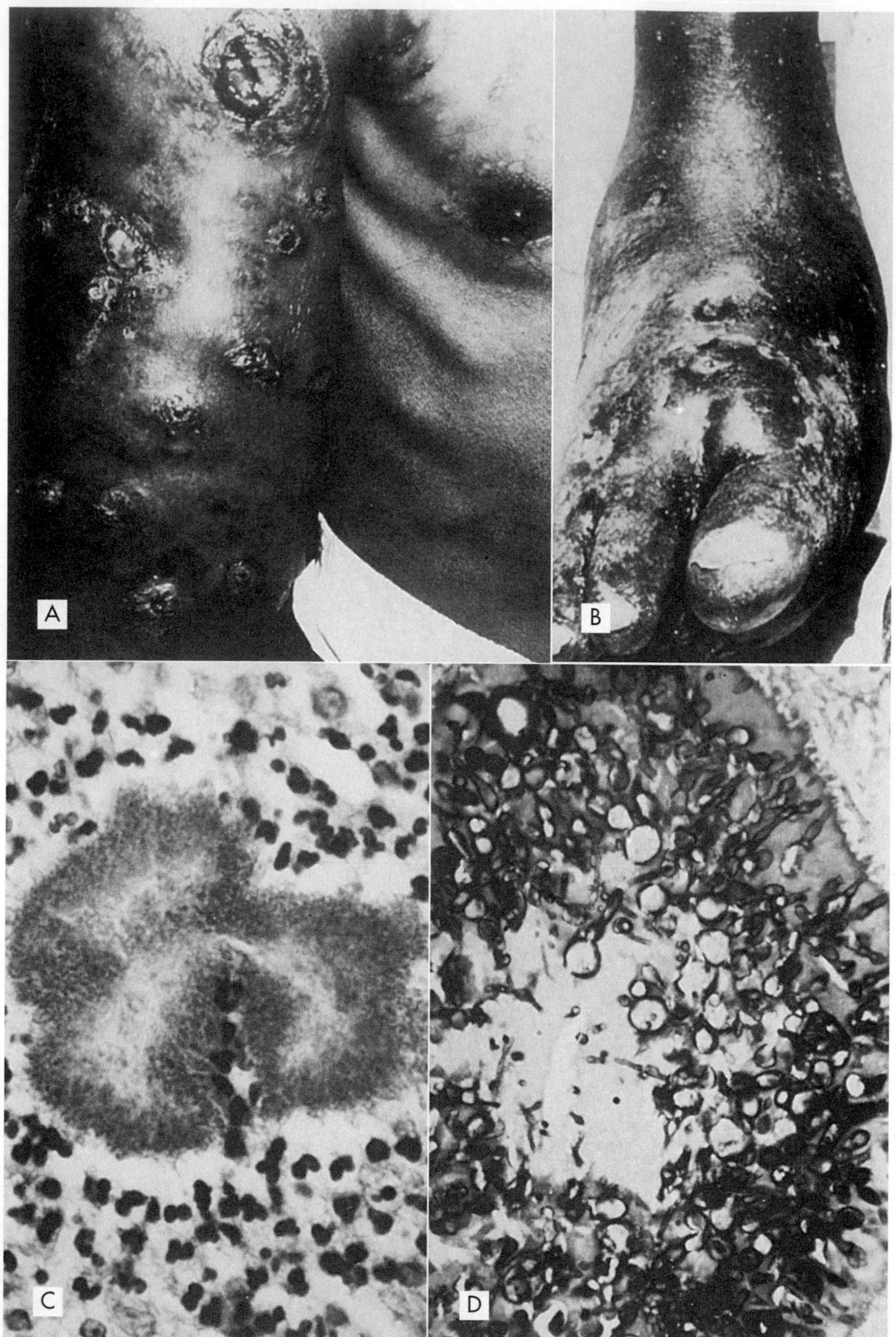

Fig. 37-5 **A,** Mycetoma of upper arm caused by *Nocardia brasiliensis.* Notice tumefaction and multiple openings of draining sinuses. **B,** Mycetoma (Madura foot). **C,** Granule of *N. brasiliensis* in biopsy specimen of lesion shown in **A.** **D,** Granule of *Madurella mycetomatis* bordered by Splendore-Hoeppli material. Radially oriented hyphae and vesicular chlamydoconidia form the granule. (***D,*** Periodic acid-Schiff.)

lungs and other organs are rarely involved. Cerebral lesions appear as encapsulated abscesses or generalized inflammatory infiltrates (Fig. 37-6, *A*). Symptoms include headache, nausea, vomiting, fever, and nuchal rigidity. The inflammatory reaction is similar to that seen in subcutaneous lesions. Treatment includes surgical excision of localized abscesses supplemented by systemic antifungal chemotherapy.

The agents of phaeohyphomycosis are morphologically and tinctorially similar in tissue sections, where they cannot be differentiated from each other. However, a disease diagnosis can

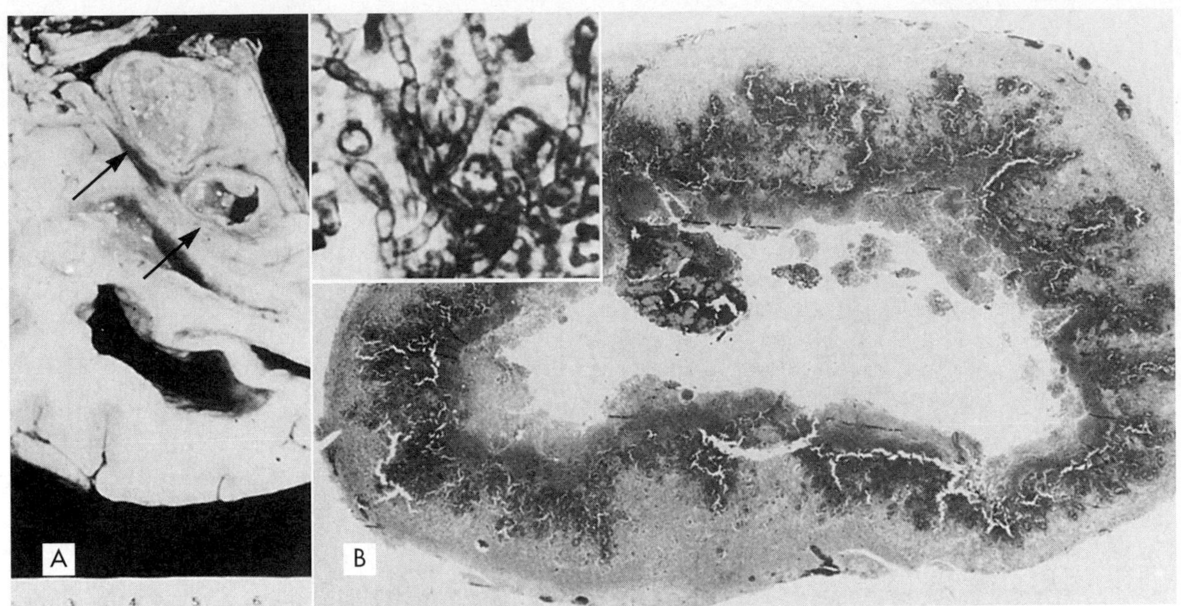

Fig. 37-6 Systemic (cerebral) phaeohyphomycosis. **A,** Two sharply circumscribed, encapsulated abscesses *(arrows)* caused by *Xylohypha bantiana* in brain of adult. **B,** Abscess caused by *X. bantiana* enucleated from left frontal lobe. The suppurative and necrotic center was lost during processing. (AFIP 62-5502; courtesy Dr. C.H. Binford, Armed Forces Institute of Pathology, Washington, DC.) *Inset,* Dematiaceous hyphae in wall of abscess are branched and constricted at their prominent septations.

be based on the natural brown color of morphologically typical fungi (Fig. 37-6, *B*). Culture is needed for specific identification of the etiologic agents.

Rhinosporidiosis

Rhinosporidiosis is a mucosal and cutaneous mycosis caused by *Rhinosporidium seeberi.* The disease is endemic in India, Sri Lanka, and parts of Africa, but sporadic cases occur in the Western Hemisphere, including the United States.[49] Infection produces bulky, friable mucosal polyps in the nasal cavity and nasopharynx and on the palate. The conjunctivae, larynx, genitalia, rectum, and skin are involved less commonly.[50] Lesions are treated by surgical excision.

R. seeberi cannot be isolated on synthetic media, though it will grow in cell culture.[51] Therefore, routine diagnosis of the disease depends on recognition of the distinctive morphology of the etiologic agent in tissue sections. The sporangia of *R. seeberi* are located predominantly in the stroma of the mucosal polyps. Spherical, uninucleate trophic forms (immature sporangia), 10 to 100 μm in diameter, develop into mature sporangia, 100 to 350 μm in diameter, by a process of progressive enlargement and endosporulation.[52] Sporangiospores are uninucleate, and the larger, mature sporangiospores contain globular eosinophilic inclusions. Maturation and zonation of sporangiospores within the sporangium are frequently observed.[53]

Cylindrical cell papillomas of the paranasal sinuses and nasal cavity that contain numerous intraepithelial mucous cysts can be mistaken for rhinosporidial polyps,[54] as discussed in Chapter 48.

Sporotrichosis

Sporotrichosis is a subacute or chronic disease caused by the dimorphic fungus, *Sporothrix schenckii.* The disease occurs worldwide, but most reported cases have originated from the United States, South Africa, Mexico, and South America. Infection usually results from the traumatic implantation of the fungus, growing in soil or on plant materials, into the skin and subcutaneous tissue. In rare instances, a primary cutaneous infection may disseminate to the bones, joints, lungs, and other organs.[55,56] Even more rarely, inhalation of the fungus results in primary pulmonary infection that may disseminate.[57-59] Sporotrichosis is not contagious, but infection can result from contamination of skin wounds with exudates from humans or animals with sporotrichosis. There is no evidence that underlying disease or immunosuppression predispose a person to infection.

The most common form of sporotrichosis is the lymphocutaneous form.[60,61] Clinically, this form is manifested as a chain of subcutaneous nodules along the course of lymphatics draining a primary skin lesion that may be nodular and ulcerated. Lymphocutaneous lesions develop 7 to 90 days or more after penetrating injury to an exposed part of the body, such as the hand, arm, neck, or foot. Eventually, the subcutaneous nodules soften, ulcerate, and discharge pus. Solitary, ulcerated, and verrucous lesions of the skin without lymphatic involvement also occur. They are sometimes mistaken for a neoplasm and excised surgically. The treatment of choice for sporotrichosis is potassium iodide, especially for lymphocutaneous infection. Amphotericin B and other antifungal agents may also be useful in systemic infection.[55,56] If untreated, the infection may persist for years.

S. schenckii usually elicits a mixed suppurative and granulomatous inflammatory reaction accompanied by microabscess formation and fibrosis[60,62,63] (Fig. 37-7, *A*). This type of inflammation is typical of all forms of the disease, but it is not specific. In tissue sections, *S. schenckii* appears as spherical, oval, or elongated (cigar-shaped) yeastlike cells, 2 to 6

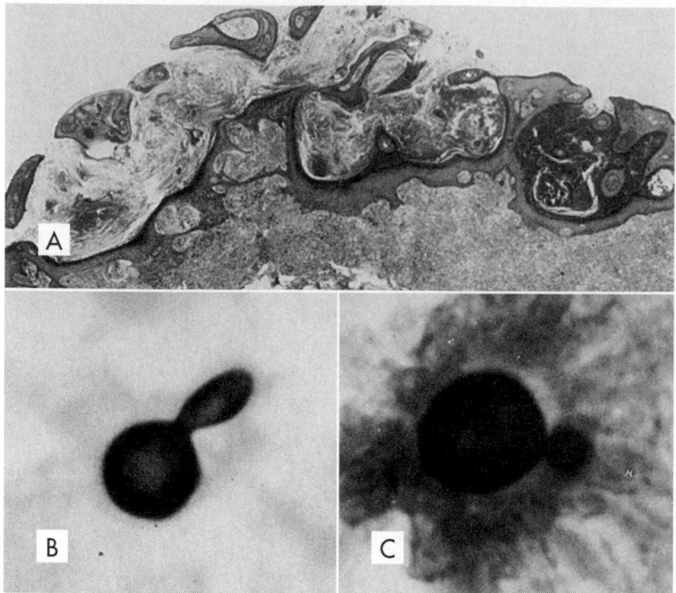

Fig. 37-7 Cutaneous sporotrichosis. **A,** Hyperplasia of epidermis and mixed suppurative and granulomatous inflammation in dermis. **B,** Single yeastlike cell of *Sporothrix schenckii* with elongated bud in dermal granuloma. **C,** Asteroid body consisting of a fungal cell surrounded by irregular spicules of Splendore-Hoeppli material. (**B,** Gomori's methenamine silver; **C,** Gomori's methenamine silver/hematoxylin and eosin.)

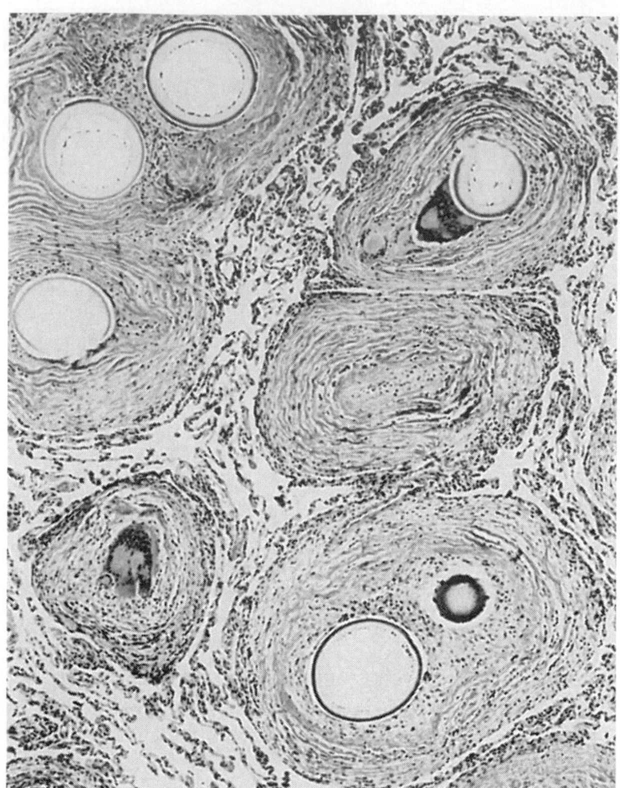

Fig. 37-8 Adiaspiromycosis. Fibrotic pulmonary granulomas contain large, thick-walled adiaconidia of *Chrysosporium parvum* var. *crescens*. Outer portion of each adiaconidial wall is eosinophilic; inner portion is hyaline.

µm or more in diameter. The fungal cells often bear elongated buds with narrow-based attachments to the parent cells (Fig. 37-7, *B*). Multiple budding is seen rarely. Although considered by some to be the classic tissue form of the fungus, cigar-shaped organisms are uncommon. When present, they occur in disseminated lesions. Hyphae are rarely formed in tissue.

The presence of asteroid bodies (fungal cells surrounded by Splendore-Hoeppli material) within microabscesses is helpful in making a presumptive histologic diagnosis of sporotrichosis[60,62] (Fig. 37-7, *C*). However, the asteroid body is not pathognomonic for this disease. Splendore-Hoeppli material may surround parasite ova, actinomycotic granules, eumycotic granules, foreign objects such as silk sutures, and other species of fungi, especially *Coccidioides immitis*, the *Aspergillus* spp., the *Candida* spp., and the agents of entomophthoromycosis.[64] In many cases of sporotrichosis, asteroid bodies cannot be detected. Generally, few *S. schenckii* cells are found in cutaneous lesions, and special stains for fungi, complemented by immunohistochemical staining,[65] are needed to identify the fungus in fixed tissues. When immunohistologic tests are not available, microbiologic culture or mouse inoculation is essential for an accurate diagnosis.

SYSTEMIC MYCOSES

Adiaspiromycosis

Adiaspiromycosis is an uncommon pulmonary mycosis caused by *Chrysosporium parvum* var. *crescens (Emmonsia crescens)*. With rare exception,[66] human infection is usually asymptomatic, self-limited, and confined to the lungs.[67,68] The inhaled conidia of *C. parvum* var. *crescens*, 2 to 4 µm in diameter, progressively enlarge within the lungs to a diameter of 200 to 400 µm at maturity, with chitinous walls 20 to 30 µm or more in thickness[68,69] (Fig. 37-8). No other fungus of medical importance has a wall this thick. Each mature adiaconidium is enclosed within a fibrotic granuloma that compresses the surrounding lung tissue. Since C. *parvum* var. *crescens* does not replicate within the human host, the degree of impairment of pulmonary function is related to the number of conidia inhaled and the frequency of exposure.[69]

Aspergillosis

The broad range of disease caused by fungi of the genus *Aspergillus* includes the following: allergic bronchopulmonary disease; colonization of pulmonary cavities; indolent superficial infection of the skin and mucosal surfaces; chronic, progressive pulmonary infection in mildly compromised hosts; and fulminant, invasive pulmonary infection with systemic dissemination in severely immunosuppressed patients. Aspergillosis is the second most common opportunistic mycosis among patients with malignant diseases, accounting for up to 30% of fungal infections found at autopsy in these patients.[70] *A. fumigatus* is the species most frequently isolated from patients with invasive or disseminated infections,[71] but *A. flavus, A. niger,* and other *Aspergillus* spp. can also cause disease.[72] Since the conidia of the aspergilli are ubiquitous in the environment, isolation of an *Aspergillus* sp. in microbiologic culture must be interpreted cautiously.[73] Its etiologic role in infection is best confirmed by demonstration of characteristic hyphae in tissue sections. A detailed account of the mycology of the aspergilli is provided by Raper and Fennell.[74]

Typical hyphae of the *Aspergillus* spp. have a characteristic appearance in tissue sections (Fig. 37-9, *A*). The hyphae are uniform, narrow (3 to 6 μm in width), tubular, and regularly septate. Branching is regular, progressive, and dichotomous. Hyphal branches tend to arise at acute angles from parent hyphae. Viable hyphae may be deeply basophilic, whereas degenerated or necrotic hyphae are often hyaline or eosinophilic. Hyphal morphology is demonstrated better with the special stains for fungi than with hematoxylin and eosin.

Under certain circumstances, the hyphae of the aspergilli may have an unusual or bizarre appearance in tissue sections. Degenerated hyphae encountered in pulmonary fungus balls and in indolent, granulomatous lesions assume bizarre shapes with globose varicosities and inconspicuous septa (Fig. 37-9, *B*). Such hyphae may be mistaken for those of the zygomycetes.[73] Conidial (fruiting) heads may be produced in lesions exposed to air, as in pulmonary fungus balls and in superficial infections involving the skin and bronchial mucosa (Fig. 37-9, *C*). Calcium oxalate crystals may accumulate within the mycelium of fungus balls in the lungs or paranasal sinuses.[75] Hyphal fragments in chronic granulomatous lesions are often coated with eosinophilic Splendore-Hoeppli material.

The clinical course and pathologic manifestations of aspergillosis are determined, for the most part, by the integrity of host defense mechanisms. In the hypersensitized host, the aspergilli can stimulate a variety of allergic pulmonary reactions that includes the syndromes of allergic bronchopulmonary aspergillosis, chronic eosinophilic pneumonia, mucoid impaction of proximal bronchi, bronchocentric granulomatosis with asthma, and microgranulomatous hypersensitivity pneumonitis.[76,77] There is considerable clinical and pathologic overlap among these allergic reactions, which seldom occur in pure form. Pathologic findings include mucus hypersecretion,

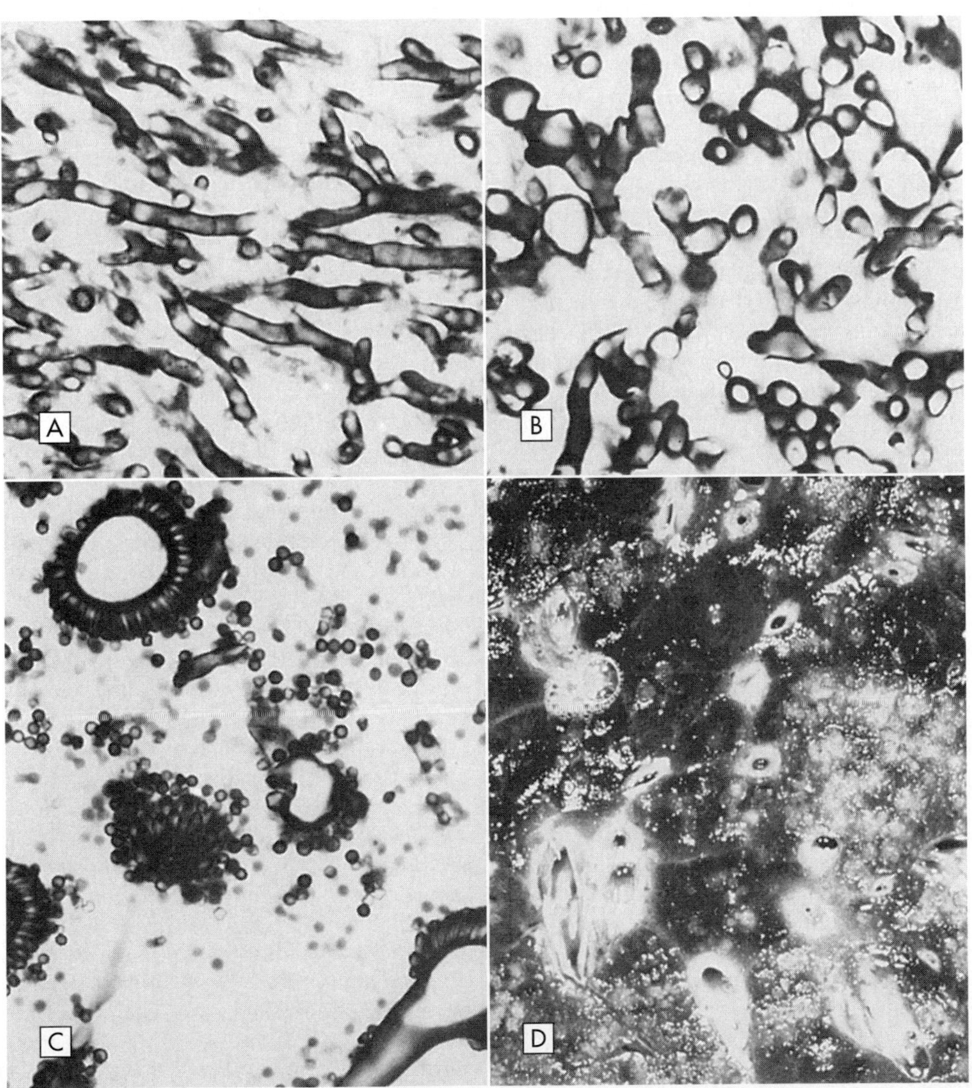

Fig. 37-9 Aspergillosis. **A,** Typical hyphae are uniform and septate and branch dichotomously. **B,** Bizarre, varicose hyphae in a pulmonary fungus ball. **C,** Conidial heads and conidia in a pulmonary cavity. **D,** The tendency for aspergillus to invade blood vessels may cause a characteristic targetoid lesion around blood vessels in the lung. (**A** to **C,** Gomori's methenamine silver.)

eosinophil infiltration with Charcot-Leyden crystals, bronchiolitis, and destructive granulomatous lesions of the airways.[76] Hyphae, which are difficult to find in these lesions, are fragmented and degenerated and do not invade adjacent pulmonary parenchyma or blood vessels.

The colonizing form of aspergillosis is typified by the pulmonary aspergilloma, or fungus ball. This is a compact mass of hyphae that forms within a preexisting, usually tuberculous, pulmonary cavity. The clinical diagnosis of aspergilloma is suggested by radiographic demonstration of an intracavitary mass, hemoptysis, and a positive serum precipitin reaction to *Aspergillus* antigens.[78] The mycelial ball measures up to 5 cm in diameter and is composed of tangled, often bizarre hyphae that may produce conidial heads. Erosion of the cavity wall by the mobile fungus ball results in recurrent or life-threatening hemoptysis, which may necessitate surgical resection of the cavity or involved pulmonary lobe. Because the aspergilli in these lesions are noninvasive colonizers that are confined within the cavity by host defenses, antifungal chemotherapy is not required. Fungus balls are occasionally produced by other fungi, notably *Coccidioides immitis* and *Pseudallescheria boydii*.

Another form of pulmonary aspergillosis, termed *chronic necrotizing pulmonary aspergillosis*,[79] or *semiinvasive pulmonary aspergillosis*,[80] shares some features of both the colonizing and invasive forms of aspergillosis. It is a locally progressive and destructive infection that occurs in mildly compromised patients who have underlying noncavitary structural lung disease, many of whom are being treated with low doses of corticosteroids.[81] Chest radiographs disclose parenchymal infiltrates and thick-walled cavities, about 40% of which contain intracavitary fungus balls. The pathologic features of chronic necrotizing pulmonary aspergillosis have not yet been described in detail. Major findings include large cavities that contain fungus balls or amorphous mycelial aggregates, and limited invasion and destruction of adjacent noncavitary lung tissue.

Invasive pulmonary aspergillosis is a fulminant opportunistic infection that occurs almost exclusively in patients whose defense mechanisms are severely compromised by hematologic malignancy, corticosteroids, cytotoxic chemotherapy, or granulocytopenia.[72,82] Clinical findings are nonspecific, and sputum cultures yield growth in only about one third of cases. Hyphae proliferate within the bronchial tree, invade through the walls of distal airways, and extend into adjacent arteries and veins. Vascular invasion and thrombotic occlusion result in characteristic nodular infarcts, several millimeters to 3 cm or more in diameter, that may replace much of a lobe (Fig. 37-9, *D*). Each of these nodules is composed of a central zone of ischemic necrosis, an intermediate zone of fibrinous exudate, and a peripheral zone of parenchymal hemorrhage.[83] Hyphae radiate throughout these nodules from a central, occluded blood vessel. Hyphal invasion and occlusion of larger, proximal arteries and veins result in large, wedge-shaped hemorrhagic infarcts. Suppurative bronchopneumonia may occur in nongranulocytopenic patients.[83]

Disseminated infection develops in about 25% of patients with invasive pulmonary aspergillosis. The GI tract, central nervous system (CNS), heart, kidneys, and liver are frequently involved, but lesions may be found in any organ.[72,82,84] The systemic lesions are infarctive, less often suppurative or granulomatous. Endocarditis of native or prosthetic cardiac valves results in bulky, friable vegetations and is usually accompanied by myocardial lesions.[85] Amphotericin B is the drug of choice for the treatment of invasive and disseminated aspergillosis.

The aspergilli cause a variety of indolent, superficial infections in mildly compromised hosts. Localized granulomatous infections can occur in the lungs, subcutaneous tissue, paranasal sinuses, and orbit of diabetics or patients treated with corticosteroids. Cutaneous lesions may result from disseminated infection or can occur primarily in burn patients. The aspergilli also cause superficial infections of the external ear canal and nails. Aspergillosis is a late and infrequent complication of AIDS.[86]

Other pathogenic fungi that form branched, septate hyphae can be mistaken for the aspergilli in tissue sections. These fungi include *Pseudallescheria boydii,* the *Fusarium* spp. and other opportunistic hyalohyphomycetes, and, on occasion, the *Candida* spp. Recognition of subtle differences in the morphology of these fungi may enable one to distinguish them from the aspergilli. However, unless typical conidial heads are observed, a histopathologic diagnosis of aspergillosis must be considered presumptive unless confirmed by immunohistochemistry[87] or by microbiologic isolation of an *Aspergillus* sp. from the lesion.

Blastomycosis

Blastomycosis is a chronic granulomatous and suppurative infection caused by the dimorphic fungus, *Blastomyces dermatitidis*.[88-90] This mycosis was long believed to be restricted to North America, but autochthonous cases are now known to occur in the Middle East and in several African countries. Although clinical and epidemiologic evidence indicates that blastomycosis is contracted from sources in nature such as soil, the natural habitat of *B. dermatitidis* has not yet been discovered. Most infections result from inhalation of the conidia of the saprophytic fungus, and thus the disease usually has a pulmonary inception.

Blastomycosis has two clinical forms: systemic and cutaneous.[91-93] Infection is often confined to the lungs in the systemic form or may spread through the bloodstream to other organs, especially the skin, bones, joints, male genital tract,[94] urinary bladder, brain, and spinal cord.[95-97] Pulmonary lesions are occasionally inapparent. Cutaneous blastomycosis appears as indolent, ulcerated or verrucous, granulomatous lesions that generally occur on exposed surfaces. Both forms of the disease are best treated with amphotericin B; 2-hydroxystilbamidine has also been effective.[98,99]

In tissue, *B. dermatitidis* appears as spherical, single-budding, yeastlike cells, 8 to 15 μm in diameter, with thick, "doubly contoured" walls.[91,95] Several basophilic nuclei may be visible when optimally fixed tissues are stained with hematoxylin and eosin. The broad-based budding of this fungus is diagnostic and aids in differentiating it from other yeast forms of similar size, such as *Histoplasma capsulatum* var. *duboisii* and *Cryptococcus neoformans*. These agents can also be distinguished from each other by direct immunofluorescence. Occasionally, small but morphologically typical forms of *B. dermatitidis*, 2-4 μm in diameter, are found in the lesions of blastomycosis, but they are always present as part of a continuous series of sizes ranging from the unusually small to the larger yeast forms characteristic of the fungus.[91] This mixture of small and typical forms should not be mistaken for coexisting mycoses. Giant yeast forms of *B. der-*

matitidis up to 40 μm in diameter are also occasionally encountered in blastomycosis.[100] Hyphae are rarely formed in tissue.

B. dermatitidis usually elicits a mixed suppurative and granulomatous inflammatory reaction.[91,95] Early lesions are predominantly suppurative, whereas older ones tend to be granulomatous, with central abscess formation and caseation. Although diffuse fibrosis is common in chronic infections, solitary fibrocaseous nodules, as seen in residual histoplasmosis capsulati, are extremely rare in blastomycosis. Florid pseudoepitheliomatous hyperplasia of skin lesions can mimic squamous cell carcinoma.

Candidiasis

Candidiasis is a superficial, mucocutaneous, or systemic mycosis most often caused by the endogenous species, *Candida albicans. C. tropicalis* is the next most frequently isolated pathogen in this genus, and occasional human infections are caused by other saprophytic species, including *C. guilliermondii, C. krusei, C. lusitaniae, C. parapsilosis,* and *C. pseudotropicalis.*[101-104] Although *Torulopsis glabrata* was tentatively merged with the genus *Candida* as *C. glabrata,* it is now considered taxonomically distinct and is discussed separately.

C. albicans is found in the normal flora of the oral cavity, upper respiratory tract, digestive tract, and vagina. The other *Candida* spp. are saprophytes or commensals that can be isolated from both human and environmental sources. Infection caused by the *Candida* spp. is almost always preceded by compromised host defense mechanisms. Factors that predispose to infection by these fungi include the following: disruption of cutaneous barriers caused by trauma, burns, surgery, or indwelling vascular catheters; genitourinary or GI mucosal ulceration; prolonged broad-spectrum antibiotic therapy that alters the normal balance of endogenous microflora; and impairment of cellular or humoral immunity as a result of underlying disease or its therapy, as occurs in diabetes mellitus, acute leukemia, granulocytopenia, corticosteroid therapy, and cytotoxic chemotherapy.[102,103,105-107] Candidiasis is the most frequent opportunistic mycosis in the United States, accounting for more than 75% of fungal infections in patients with neoplastic diseases.[102]

Superficial candidal infections involve the skin and the mucosal surfaces of the oral cavity and vagina. Intertriginous cutaneous infections occur in obese, diabetic, and alcoholic persons. Maceration of the skin caused by prolonged, repeated immersion in water may predispose to cutaneous candidiasis, paronychia, and onychomycosis. Vulvovaginal candidiasis occurs in patients with diabetes mellitus and during pregnancy. Infection of the oral cavity (thrush) is encountered in newborns, in patients treated with broad-spectrum antibiotics, and as a complication of diabetes mellitus, AIDS, or other debilitating diseases. Thrush manifests as soft, friable, white patches on the tongue and oral mucosa. These patches are composed of yeastlike cells, pseudohyphae, and hyphae enmeshed in an inflammatory pseudomembrane. Invasion of submucosal tissue does not ordinarily occur.

Chronic mucocutaneous candidiasis, a protracted superficial infection of the skin, nails, oral cavity, oropharynx, and vagina, usually afflicts patients who have underlying defects in cell-mediated immunity.[108] Five clinically distinct forms are recognized, one of which is associated with endocrine abnormalities, most commonly hypoparathyroidism and adrenal failure.[109] Mucocutaneous infection begins early in life and is particularly resistant to topical or parenteral antifungal chemotherapy. About 25% of patients with chronic mucocutaneous candidiasis have no demonstrable abnormality of cell-mediated immunity. Defective neutrophil chemotaxis can be demonstrated in some cases. The mucosal lesions of chronic mucocutaneous candidiasis resemble those of thrush. Disfiguring cutaneous lesions, termed *candida granulomas,* are warty, hyperkeratotic papules and plaques within which the fungal elements remain confined to the superficial epidermis.

Systemic candidiasis is an opportunistic mycosis that usually involves the GI tract, kidneys, heart, and CNS but can involve almost any organ.[102,107] Within the GI tract, the distal esophagus and stomach are involved most frequently.[110] The *Candida* spp. often colonize preexisting ulcers without giving rise to disseminated infection.[111] However, once invasion into underlying viable tissue occurs, the risk of vascular invasion and hematogenous dissemination increases, particularly in patients who are immunosuppressed.[112] Invasive GI lesions consist of punctate mucosal erosions or diffuse mucosal ulcers covered by friable inflammatory pseudomembranes that contain yeastlike cells and mycelial elements (Fig. 37-10, *A*). The fungal elements invade into the submucosa and submucosal blood vessels.

Primary infection of the urinary tract by the *Candida* spp. results in cystitis and ascending pyelonephritis that is often complicated by papillary necrosis. Sloughed necrotic papillae containing fungal elements form "fungus balls" that can cause ureteropelvic obstruction with secondary hydronephrosis. Infection of the kidneys during hematogenous dissemination results in bilateral miliary lesions, either abscesses or necrotic nodules, that contain abundant yeastlike cells and mycelial elements.

Cerebral candidiasis is the most frequent mycosis of the CNS, accounting for about one half of such infections encountered at autopsy.[113] It is a late complication of disseminated candidiasis in patients with cardiac and renal involvement. Cerebral lesions consist of multifocal microabscesses sometimes accompanied by noncaseating granulomas and localized meningitis.[114] Diffuse leptomeningitis does not occur.

The pathologic features of pulmonary candidiasis are largely determined by the route of infection.[115-118] Aspiration of *Candida* spp. from the oral cavity or upper respiratory tract results in asymmetrically distributed, nodular areas of bronchopneumonia involving the lower lobes predominantly.[119] This form of pulmonary infection, termed *endobronchial* or *primary pulmonary* candidiasis, is not commonly associated with disseminated candidiasis. Hematogenous pulmonary candidiasis is characterized by round, hemorrhagic, grayish-tan necrotic nodules, 2 to 4 mm in diameter, distributed randomly but symmetrically throughout both lungs.[115] Endobronchial and respiratory mucosal involvemet is uncommon in this form of pulmonary infection, whereas extrapulmonary involvement is frequently found in the esophagus, stomach, liver, spleen, and kidneys. A third form, embolic pulmonary candidiasis, occurs in children who have indwelling venous catheters.[116] Occlusion of small and medium-sized pulmonary arteries by mycotic emboli results in hemorrhagic pulmonary infarcts.

The *Candida* spp. are the most frequent etiologic agents of cardiac fungal infection.[120] Microabscesses or necrotic nod-

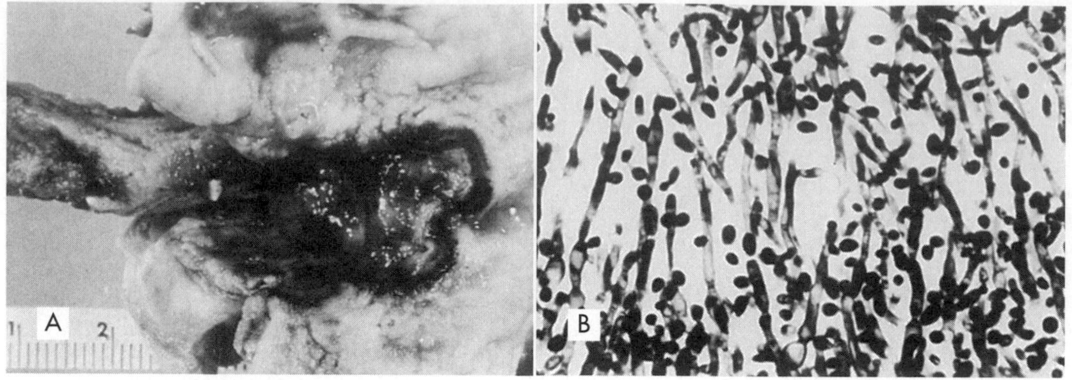

Fig. 37-10 Candidiasis. **A,** Ulcer at esophagogastric junction caused by *Candida albicans*. The 5-year-old patient was pancytopenic as a result of treatment for acute lymphocytic leukemia. At autopsy, the lungs, liver, and spleen contained friable, yellow, necrotic nodules. **B,** Yeastlike cells, pseudohyphae, and hyphae of *C. albicans*. (**B,** Gomori's methenamine silver.)

ules involving the myocardium are a sequela of disseminated candidiasis and may coexist with endocardial vegetations.[121] The latter are typically bulky and friable and may give rise to arterial emboli. Preexisting valvular deformity is not a necessary prerequisite for candidal endocarditis, which can also develop in immunosuppressed patients, drug addicts, and patients with indwelling central venous catheters whose valves are otherwise normal. Candidal infection of prosthetic cardiac valves develops on neoendocardium that grows onto the sewing cloth and struts of the prostheses, and systemic arterial emboli are a frequent complication.[122]

In noncompromised patients, the treatment of candidemia may require little more than removal of vascular catheters. Superficial infections may respond well to fluconazole. However, systemic candidiasis in the compromised host requires intensive antifungal chemotherapy with amphotericin B and flucytosine.[123]

The lesions of invasive candidiasis contain yeastlike cells and mycelial elements (Fig. 37-10, *B*). The oval yeastlike cells, 2 to 6 μm in diameter, reproduce by budding. The mycelial elements consist of both pseudohyphae and true hyphae. Pseudohyphae are formed by progressive budding of yeastlike cells that elongate and remain attached to one another in chains. There are segmental constrictions in these chains where adjacent cells remain apposed (Fig. 37-11). The branched, septate, tubular hyphae are narrower than the pseudohyphae and do not have conspicuous constrictions at sites of septation. An inflammatory response is minimal within superficial mucosal ulcers and in mucocutaneous lesions where the *Candida* spp. are colonizers or do not deeply invade viable tissue. The inflammatory response to invasive candidiasis in the nongranulocytopenic host is typically suppurative, but it may be both granulomatous and suppurative in chronic, indolent infections. Disseminated candidiasis in the granulocytopenic host produces nodular infarcts, a result of invasion and occlusion of small blood vessels.[115] Occlusion of large blood vessels and parenchymal infarction, which typify the lesions of aspergillosis and zygomycosis, are found infrequently in disseminated candidiasis.

On occasion, the *Candida* spp. can be mistaken for other fungal pathogens in tissue sections, notably the *Trichosporon* spp. and weakly pigmented agents of phaeohyphomycosis. If

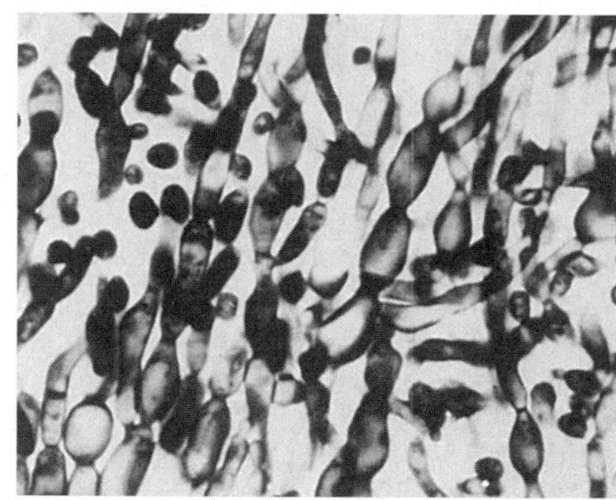

Fig. 37-11 Yeastlike cells and pseudohyphae of *Candida albicans*. There are constrictions between adjacent cells that form the pseudohyphae. (Gomori's methenamine silver.)

microbiologic culture is not available, the *Candida* spp. can be identified generically in tissue sections by immunofluorescence or immunohistochemistry.[124] The individual species are not morphologically distinguishable from each other in tissue sections.

Coccidioidomycosis

Coccidioidomycosis is a pulmonary infection caused by the dimorphic pathogen *Coccidioides immitis*. The disease is endemic in semiarid regions of the southwestern United States, northern and central Mexico, and in parts of Central and South America, where the mycelial form of *C. immitis* resides in desert soil.[125] Infection is acquired by inhalation of airborne arthroconidia.

The epidemiology and clinical aspects of coccidioidomycosis have been extensively reviewed elsewhere.[126-129] About 60% of patients who have primary pulmonary coccidioidomycosis are asymptomatic; the other 40% develop a mild influenza-like illness that resolves spontaneously in most cases. Symptoms or radiographic abnormalities persist beyond 6 to 8 weeks in a few patients, who may require treatment with amphotericin B. Chronic progressive coccidioidal pneumonia, an indolent but destructive fibrocavitary disease, occurs in about 1% of patients, and miliary pulmonary infection develops in about 4% of patients. Both forms require systemic antifungal chemotherapy. Benign residual pulmonary nodules, or coccidioidomas, are a late manifestation of pulmonary infection by *C. immitis* that do not ordinarily require antifungal chemotherapy. Disseminated coccidioidomycosis develops in less than 1% of patients with symptomatic primary pulmonary infection. Risk factors for the development of disseminated infection include pregnancy, extremes of age, race (blacks, Filipinos, and American Indians are more at risk), and immunosuppression, including AIDS.[128,130-132] Frequent sites of dissemination include the skin and subcutaneous tissue, bones, joints, lymph nodes, spleen, liver, kidneys, and meninges,[133,134] and the mortality is high. Primary extrapulmonary (cutaneous) coccidioidomycosis is exceedingly rare; most patients with skin lesions have disseminated infection from an inapparent pulmonary focus.

Primary pulmonary coccidioidomycosis is an acute suppurative and granulomatous pneumonitis. Diagnostic tissue forms of *C. immitis,* usually abundant in active lesions, consist of thin-walled, mature spherules, 30 to 200 μm in diameter (Fig. 37-12, *A*). Rupture of the spherules releases packets of endospores into the surrounding tissue[135] (Fig. 37-12, *B*), where they enlarge progressively to become immature spherules and, after endosporulation, mature spherules. The ultrastructure and developmental sequence of *C. immitis* in tissue have been reported by Donnelly and Yunis.[136]

The residual pulmonary coccidioidal nodule, or coccidioidoma, is a peripheral, sharply circumscribed and centrally necrotic granuloma that measures up to 3.5 cm in diameter.[137] About 25% of these nodules are centrally cavitated. Diagnostic endosporulating spherules are found in only about half the nodules, and a specific histopathologic or cytopathologic[138] diagnosis may require confirmation by direct immunofluorescence[139] or culture. Mycelium and arthroconidia are occasionally produced in cavitary lesions that communicate with the bronchial tree.[140] The lesions of disseminated coccidioidomycosis are granulomatous, or suppurative and granulomatous.[134,141]

Characteristic endosporulating spherules of *C. immitis* can be reliably distinguished from the sporangia of *Rhinosporidium seeberi* and the adiaconidia of *Chrysosporium parvum* var. *crescens* in tissue sections on the basis of size, wall thickness, and morphology of endospores (Table 37-4). The *parent bodies* and *endobodies* found in myospherulosis, a pseudomycosis of the upper respiratory tract and middle ear,[142] are similar in both size and morphology to the spherules and endospores of *C. immitis* but are distinguished by their inherent brown color. The structures of myospherulosis are derived from altered erythrocytes.[143]

Cryptococcosis

Cryptococcosis begins as a pulmonary disease that is usually acquired by inhalation of the soil-inhabiting yeast, *Cryptococcus neoformans.*[144-146] This saprophytic fungus is ubiquitous in nature and cosmopolitan in distribution. It is most abundant in avian habitats, particularly those that are heavily contaminated by pigeon excreta. Cryptococcosis is not contagious. Although the disease occurs in apparently healthy persons, those with defective cellular immunity and severe underlying diseases are particularly at risk.[144,145] Important predisposing factors in opportunistic cryptococcosis include hematologic malignancies (especially Hodgkin's disease), AIDS, and other conditions that impair cell-mediated immunity.[147-149]

Clinically, two forms predominate: pulmonary cryptococcosis[144,150,151] and, by hematogenous dissemination from a pulmonary focus, cerebromeningeal cryptococcosis.[145,146] Dissemination from a primary pulmonary infection less often results in cutaneous, mucocutaneous, osseous, and visceral forms. In disseminated cryptococcosis, primary lung infection is frequently undetected, and the incubation period is unknown. A primary pulmonary–lymph node complex develops in approximately 1% of the cases of first-infection cryptococcosis.[152] Rarely, cutaneous infection results from direct inoculation of the skin.[153,154]

For reasons that are poorly understood, *C. neoformans* is extremely neurotropic.[146,148] The clinical course of cerebromeningeal cryptococcosis varies from a few days to 20 years or more. However, it is usually fulminant and, if untreated, is almost invariably fatal. A diagnosis can be made by demonstration of *C. neoformans* cells in cerebrospinal fluid (CSF) or tissue, by isolation of the fungus in culture, or by demonstration of cryptococcal polysaccharide antigen in the

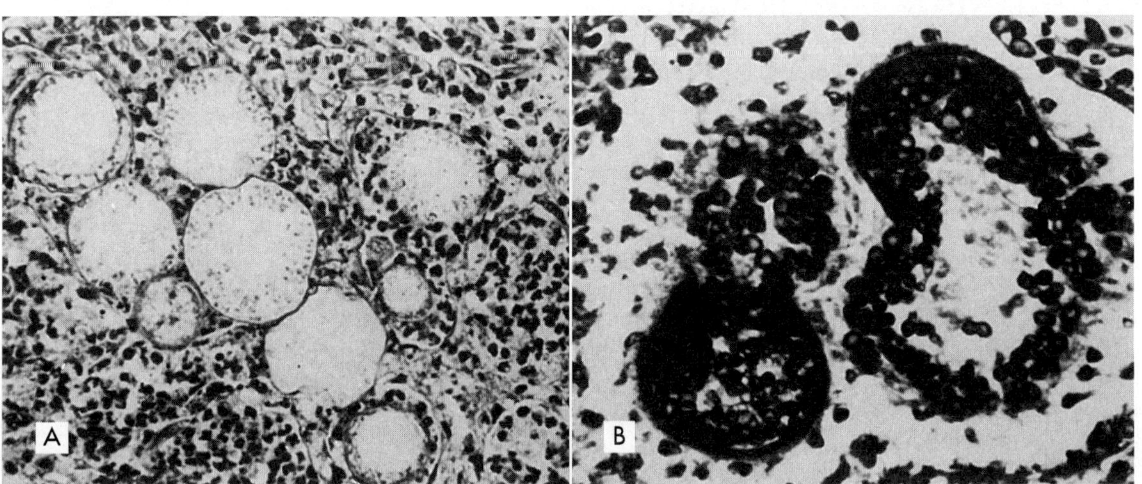

Fig. 37-12 Coccidioidomycosis. **A,** Endosporulating spherules in primary pulmonary coccidioidomycosis. **B,** Endospores released after rupture of spherules. (**B,** Gomori's methenamine silver/hematoxylin and eosin.)

Table 37-4 Histologic features of the systemic mycoses

Disease	Biologic agent(s)	Typical morphology in tissue	Usual host reaction
Adiaspiromycosis	*Chrysosporium (Emmonsia) parvum* var. *crescens*	Large adiaconidia 200-400 µmD, with thick (20-70 µm) walls	Granulomatous, fibrotic, and noncaseating
Aspergillosis	*Aspergillus fumigatus* group, *A. flavus* group, *A. niger* group, and other aspergilli	Septate, dichotomously branched hyphae of uniform width (3-6 µm); conidial heads may be formed in cavitary lesions	Nodular infarcts; rarely granulomatous or suppurative; tendency for angioinvasion
Blastomycosis	*Blastomyces dermatitidis*	Spherical, multinucleated yeastlike cells, 8-15 µmD, with thick walls and single, broad-based buds	Mixed suppurative and granulomatous
Candidiasis	*Candida albicans, C. tropicalis, C. parapsilosis, C. krusei, C. pseudotropicalis, C. guilliermondii, C. stellatoidea,* and others	Oval, budding yeastlike cells, 2-6 µmD, and pseudohyphae; septate hyphae may also be present	Suppurative, less commonly granulomatous or infarctive; minimal inflammation in preterminal infections; tendency for angioinvasion
Coccidioidomycosis	*Coccidioides immitis*	Spherical, thick-walled, endosporulating spherules, 30-200 µmD; mature spherules contain small (2-5 µmD), uninucleate endospores; arthroconidia and hyphae may be formed in cavitary lesions	Mixed suppurative and granulomatous
Cryptococcosis	*Cryptococcus neoformans*; rarely, other *Cryptococcus* spp.	Pleomorphic yeast-like cells, 2-20 µmD, with gelatinous, carminophilic capsules and single or multiple narrow-based buds; some strains are capsule deficient and may not be carminophilic	Varies from minimal reaction ("cystic" or "mucoid" lesion) to granulomatous
Fusariosis	*Fusarium moniliforme, F. napiforme, F. oxysporum, F. proliferatum, F. solani*	Septate hyphae that are uniform in width (3-8 µm) and branch at right angles	Like aspergillosis
Geotrichosis	*Geotrichum candidum*	Septate, infrequently branched hyphae, 3-6 µm wide; spherical yeastlike cells; and rectangular or oval arthroconidia, 4-10 µm wide, with rounded or squared ends	Varies from minimal reaction to acute suppurative inflammation and necrosis
Histoplasmosis capsulati	*Histoplasma capsulatum* var. *capsulatum*	Spherical to oval, budding, yeastlike cells, 2-4 µmD; often clustered because of growth within mononuclear phagocytes (reticulo-endothelial mycosis)	Granulomatous, caseating or noncaseating; parasitization of histiocytes may cause bland necrosis
Histoplasmosis duboisii	*Histoplasma capsulatum* var. *duboisii*	Spherical to oval, uninucleate, thick-walled yeast-like cells, 8-15 µmD, that bud by a narrow base, creating typical "hourglass" or "figure-eight" forms	Granulomatous; many fungi in cytoplasm of huge multinucleated giant cells
Malasseziasis (systemic)	*Malassezia furfur*	Spherical to oval, thick-walled, budding yeastlike cells (phialoconidia), 3-8 µmD, that often have a unipolar phialidic collarette	Varies from minimal reaction to suppurative and necrotizing

(continued)

CSF by the latex agglutination test. About 25% of patients with cerebromeningeal infection undergo exploratory surgery before the disease is detected. These patients are usually afebrile and have an expanding intracranial lesion that mimics a brain tumor. The combination of amphotericin B and 5-fluorocytosine is the treatment of choice for the disseminated and progressive pulmonary forms of cryptococcosis.[150,155] Fluconazole, a triazole antifungal agent, is also effective and routinely used as suppressive therapy for disseminated cryptococcosis in AIDS patients.[156]

In tissue sections, *C. neoformans* is a spherical, oval, or elliptical yeastlike fungus that ranges from 5 to 20 µm in diameter.[157] The cell walls of cryptococci are lightly basophilic when stained with hematoxylin and eosin, but they are demonstrated better with the special stains for fungi. Typically, a clear zone of varying width surrounds each fungal cell, representing the space occupied by a mucoid capsule before fixation and processing of the tissue. When stained with mucicarmine, the clear zone can be shown to contain carminophilic material that often has a spinous appearance because of irregular shrinkage of the mucopolysaccharide capsule during fixation (Fig. 37-13, *A*). Budding cells are numerous in lesions that contain abundant, rapidly proliferating cryptococci. Cryptococci usually have single buds that are attached to parent cells by narrow bases, and multiple buds are occasionally seen. Pseudohyphae and, rarely, true hyphae may be formed in tissue.

Because *C. neoformans* is unusually pleomorphic and its encapsulated forms are not always conspicuous, cryptococco-

Table 37-4 Histologic features of the systemic mycoses—cont'd

Disease	Biologic agent(s)	Typical morphology in tissue	Usual host reaction
Paracoccidioidomycosis	*Paracoccidioides brasiliensis*	Large spherical yeastlike cells, 5-60 μmD, with multiple buds attached by narrow necks ("steering wheel" forms)	Mixed suppurative and granulomatous; like blastomycosis
Penicilliosis marneffei	*Penicillium marneffei*	Spherical to oval yeastlike cells, 2.5-5 μmD, with a single transverse septum; short hyphal forms and elongated, curved "sausage" forms with one or more septa may be formed in necrotic and cavitary lesions	Like histoplasmosis capsulati
Phaeohyphomycosis (systemic)	*Xylohypha bantiana, Bipolaris hawaiiensis,* and others	Pigmented (brown) yeastlike cells and hyphae, 2-6 μm wide, that may be branched and are often constricted at their frequent and prominent septations	Mixed suppurative and granulomatous; large abscesses surrounded by giant cells
Pseudallescheriasis	*Pseudallescheria boydii*	Septate, randomly branched hyphae, 2-5 μm wide; conidia of scedosporium type may be formed in cavitary lesions	Like aspergillosis
Torulopsosis	*Torulopsis glabrata*	Spherical to oval yeastlike cells, 2-5 μmD	Varies from minimal reaction to suppurative and granulomatous
Trichosporonosis	*Trichosporon beigelii, T. capitatum (Blastoschizomyces capitatus)*	Blastoconidia, 3-8 μmD, septate hyphae, and arthroconidia	Like candidiasis
Zygomycosis (mucormycosis)	*Absidia corymbifera, Apophysomyces elegans, Cunninghamella bertholletiae, Mucor ramosissimus, Rhizomucor pusillus, Rhizopus oryzae, R. rhizopodiformis, Saksenaea vasiformis,* and others	Broad, thin-walled, infrequently septate hyphae, 6-25 μm wide, with nonparallel sides and randomly spaced branches	Suppurative necrosis, less commonly granulomatous; tendency for angioinvasion and infarction

D, Diameter.

sis should be considered in the differential histologic diagnosis of virtually any yeast infection.[158] When the capsules of typical cryptococci are carminophilic, a histopathologic diagnosis of cryptococcosis can be made with confidence. Capsule-deficient cryptococci or those with attenuated capsules produced by the so-called dry variants can be specifically identified in histologic and cytologic preparations by direct immunofluorescence. In most instances, however, at least some cryptococci will have capsules that are detectable with stains for mucin.[158,159] Because cryptococcal cell walls contain silver-reducing substances that react positively with melanin stains, a modified Fontana-Masson procedure can be used to identify capsule-deficient cryptococci in histologic sections.[160] Positive staining does not depend on the presence of capsular mucopolysaccharide.

There is a wide range in the inflammatory response to *C. neoformans,* and it varies from little or no inflammation to a purely granulomatous reaction. At times, particularly in terminal or disseminated infections, cryptococci multiply profusely with no apparent host response (Fig. 37-13, *A*). Yeastlike cells displace normal parenchyma and form "cystic" lesions filled with myriad, compact cryptococci whose wide mucoid capsules impart a glistening appearance and slimy consistency to lesions on gross examination. Generally, capsule-deficient cryptococci elicit granulomatous inflammation in which numerous yeastlike cells without conspicuous capsules are seen within huge multinucleated giant cells and epithelioid histiocytes[159,161] (Fig. 37-13, *B*).

Pulmonary infection by *C. neoformans* may occasionally result in solitary or multiple fibrocaseous granulomas (cryptococcomas) that, in hematoxylin and eosin–stained sections, are indistinguishable from those caused by infection with *Histoplasma capsulatum* var. *capsulatum* and *Coccidioides immitis.*[145,151] In these cryptococcomas, the yeastlike cells are usually atypical and fragmented and stain poorly with the special stains for fungi (Fig. 37-14). Their capsules may not be carminophilic, and it is often difficult to culture cryptococci from these lesions. Immunofluorescence staining is a valuable diagnostic tool in these cases.

Fusariosis

The *Fusarium* spp. are responsible for a variety of ocular, cutaneous, and invasive opportunistic fungal infections. These fungi have recently emerged as opportunists among patients with cutaneous burns[162] and patients whose systemic defense mechanisms are compromised by malignancy or its therapy.[163-168] The three major pathogens in this genus are *F. moniliforme, F. oxysporum,* and *F. solani,*[162] but human infection is occasionally caused by *F. napiforme* and *F. proliferatum.*

Disseminated fusariosis is usually preceded or accompanied by cutaneous infection in the form of burn wound colonization or painful, erythematous, and necrotic nodules. Local

of histoplasmosis capsulati is seen primarily in adults, and it may become clinically apparent only after a long dormancy.[178] Radiographs usually reveal unilateral cavities in the upper lung lobes that resemble those seen in tuberculosis. Sclerosing mediastinitis may complicate chronic infection.[192]

In tissue, the yeastlike cells of *H. capsulatum* var. *capsulatum* are spherical to oval, 2 to 4 μm in diameter, and reproduce by single budding.[177,193,194] In active lesions, fungal cells are readily detected with hematoxylin and eosin. Their basophilic cytoplasm is retracted from the rigid but thin, poorly stained cell wall, creating a clear space, or "halo," that gives the false impression of an unstained capsule (Fig. 37-17, *A*). Cell walls stain deeply with the special stains for fungi, and the "halo" is not evident (Fig. 37-17, *B*). Pseudohyphae are occasionally seen, and hyphae have been rarely observed near the surface of valvular vegetations in patients with endocarditis.[195]

In the disseminated form of the disease, numerous yeastlike cells replicate within mononuclear phagocytes in the nonimmune or compromised host,[180,184,189,196] whereas the fungus elicits an epithelioid and giant cell granulomatous reaction in the immune host.[177,194] Necrotic lesions may calcify, and epithelioid cell granulomas resemble those seen in sarcoidosis and tuberculosis.[177,193,194] Because of their intracellular confinement, fungal cells occur in prominent clusters.

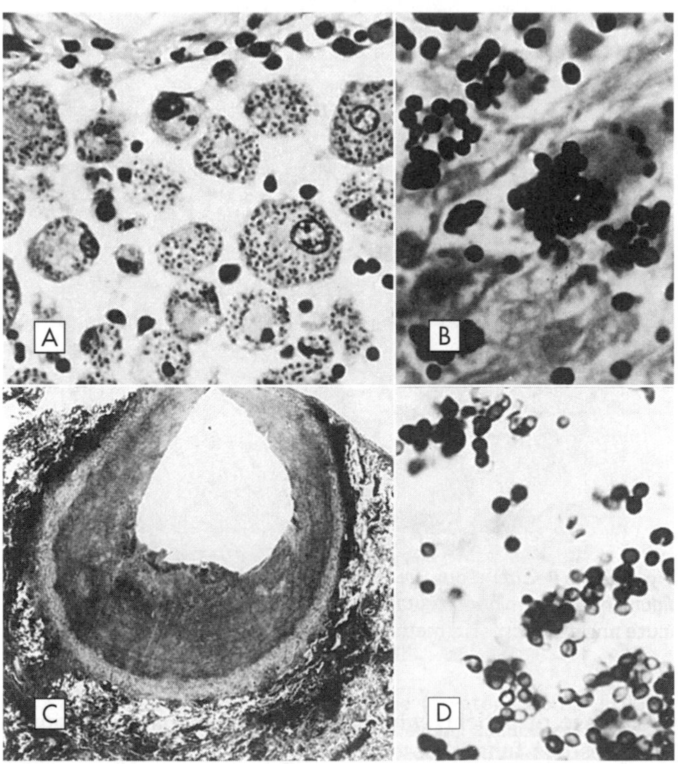

Fig. 37-17 Histoplasmosis capsulati. **A,** Acute pulmonary form. Alveolar macrophages are filled with small yeast forms, 2 to 4 μm in diameter, the dark cytoplasm of which is retracted, creating a clear space, or "halo." **B,** Disseminated form in adrenal gland. Notice clustering of fungal cells. There is no "halo" effect when special stains for fungi are used. **C,** Subpleural solitary nodule (histoplasmoma) in lung of adult man. **D,** Replicate section of nodule in **C** demonstrates distorted, poorly stained histoplasma cells in central caseous material. (**B** and **D,** Gomori's methenamine silver.)

Asymptomatic disease may not be detected until old fibrocaseous nodules are found incidentally at autopsy[178,193] or are suspected of being neoplasms on the basis of chest radiographs and are resected. Microscopically, these nodules (histoplasmomas) consist of a large central zone of caseous necrosis surrounded by a thick wall of dense collagenous connective tissue that may contain epithelioid and multinucleated giant cells (Fig. 37-17, *C*). In the caseous portion, small numbers of distorted and unevenly stained yeastlike cells are usually demonstrated with the Gomori methenamine silver stain (Fig. 37-17, *D*). The Gridley, periodic acid–Schiff (PAS), and hematoxylin and eosin stains do not reliably demonstrate the yeast cells in these lesions, and attempts to culture the fungus are usually unsuccessful. The organisms can be specifically identified in tissue sections by immunofluorescence staining.[177]

Poorly encapsulated cryptococci and small tissue forms of *Blastomyces dermatitidis* can resemble yeast forms of *H. capsulatum* var. *capsulatum*. However, cryptococci are usually carminophilic, and *B. dermatitidis* cells are multinucleated, have thick walls, and bud by a broad base. When these differentiating features are equivocal, immunofluorescence staining is invaluable. In hematoxylin and eosin–stained sections, intracellular forms of the *Leishmania* spp. and *Trypanosoma* spp. can mimic histoplasmas. The distinguishing bar-shaped kinetoplast of these two protozoans can sometimes be seen under an oil-immersion objective but is best demonstrated by Giemsa and Wilder's reticulum stains. Cells of *Toxoplasma gondii,* which can also be confused with histoplasmas, are smaller, stain entirely with hematoxylin and eosin, and are usually not found within phagocytes. The *Leishmania* spp., *Trypanosoma* spp., and *Toxoplasma gondii* are not reliably stained with the special stains for fungi.

African histoplasmosis

Histoplasmosis duboisii is a pulmonary disease with a pronounced tropism for bones and skin.[197-203] It is caused by the large-celled form or *duboisii* variety of *H. capsulatum*. When grown in vitro, mycelial and yeast forms of this fungus are indistinguishable from those of the classical, small-celled form or *capsulatum* variety of this species. The two can be distinguished only when one observes the size of the yeastlike cells that develop in tissue. Diseases caused by the two varieties of *H. capsulatum* are clinically and pathologically distinct.

Other than one autochthonous case from Japan, natural infection caused by *H. capsulatum* var. *duboisii* has been reported only in humans and nonhuman primates from Africa. The disease is rarely seen in the United States in persons who previously lived or traveled in Africa.[200,202] Clinically, patients usually present with one or more of the following: lymphadenopathy; mucocutaneous lesions that may be abscessed and ulcerated; and insidious osteolytic lesions, particularly of the ribs, long bones, and cranium. Disseminated disease may also involve the lungs, liver, spleen, and intestines. Amphotericin B and excision of isolated skin lesions are treatments of choice for disseminated and localized infections, respectively.

Lesions typically contain a dispersed granulomatous inflammatory reaction in which large numbers of yeastlike cells are seen within the cytoplasm of histiocytes and huge multinucleated giant cells[197,203] (Fig. 37-18, *A*), The spherical to oval fungal cells are uninucleate and 8 to 15 μm in diameter, have thick walls, and bud by a relatively narrow base. Classical "hour-

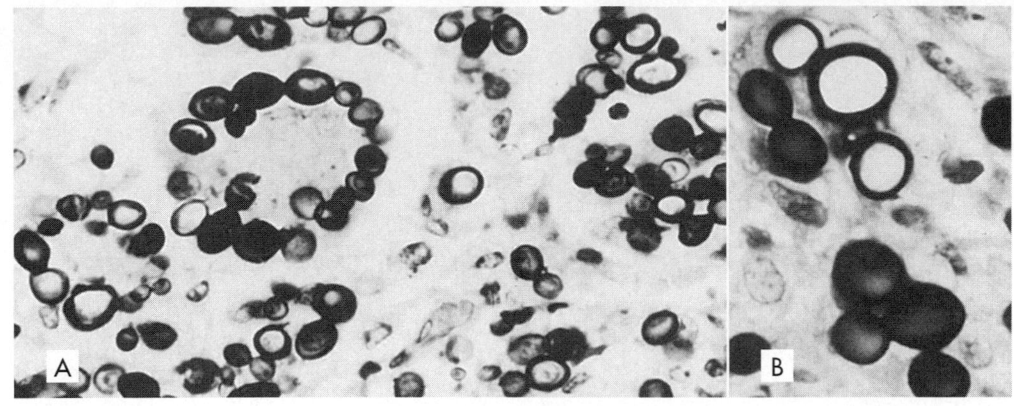

Fig. 37-18 Cutaneous histoplasmosis duboisii. **A,** Single and budding yeast forms within histiocytes and large multinucleated giant cells in dermis. **B,** Detail of classical "hourglass" or "double-cell" yeast forms, 8 to 15 μm in diameter, with narrow-based buds and thick cell walls. (Gomori's methenamine silver/hematoxylin and eosin.)

glass" and "double-cell" forms are created when budding daughter cells enlarge until they equal the size of the parent cells, to which they remain connected by a narrow base (Fig. 37-18, *B*). Tissue forms of *H. capsulatum* var. *duboisii* and *B. dermatitidis* are of similar size and shape and thus may be mistaken for each other. However, the latter buds by a broader base and is multinucleated. Histoplasmosis capsulati also occurs in Africa, but its causative agent is much smaller (2 to 4 μm) in tissue than the large-celled *duboisii* variety.

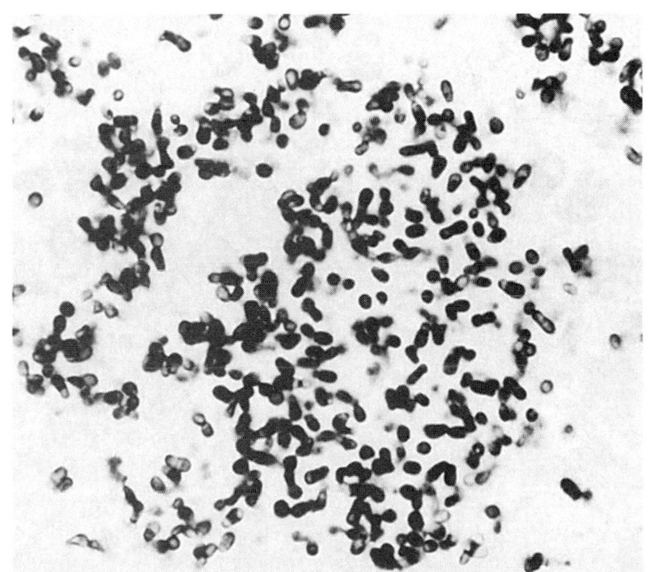

Fig. 37-19 Systemic malasseziasis in an infant. A pulmonary thromboembolus contains numerous yeastlike cells of *Malassezia furfur,* 3 to 8 μm in diameter, with single buds (phialoconidia). (Gomori's methenamine silver.)

Malasseziasis (systemic)

Malassezia furfur is usually encountered as the etiologic agent of tinea versicolor, a common superficial mycosis that occurs worldwide and is primarily of cosmetic importance. In rare instances, however, this lipophilic and lipid-dependent fungus can cause fungemia and systemic infection that is usually a specific complication of prolonged intralipid infusion through central venous catheters.[204,205] Most systemic infections have occurred in infants less than 14 weeks of age and in older patients with severe, chronic GI disease.[206,207] Although patients may be asymptomatic, they usually have fever and signs and symptoms of sepsis and thrombocytopenia. The lungs are most frequently involved, apparently because of increased lipid deposition in the walls of pulmonary blood vessels.[208]

In deep infections, elements of *M. furfur* appear as spherical or oval, thick-walled, budding yeastlike cells, 3 to 8 μm in diameter, that are considered to be phialoconidia (Fig. 37-19). Often, a small, unipolar, phialidic collarette can be seen at the point where a conidium (bud) was extruded from a parent cell; short, curved hyphae are rarely produced in deep infections. Fungal elements are either basophilic or amphophilic in hematoxylin and eosin–stained tissue sections but are best demonstrated with the special stains for fungi.

Prompt removal of colonized vascular catheters may be the only treatment necessary for *M. furfur* fungemia. Severe systemic infections have been treated successfully with miconazole and amphotericin B after catheter removal.[206,207]

Paracoccidioidomycosis (South American blastomycosis)

Paracoccidioidomycosis is a progressive pulmonary infection caused by the single dimorphic species *Paracoccidioides brasiliensis.*[209] The disease is highly endemic in South America, particularly in Brazil, Colombia, and Venezuela. Autochthonous cases have also been reported from Central America and Mexico, but cases discovered in the United States have all been acquired within endemic areas of Latin America.[210]

Paracoccidioidomycosis is predominantly a disease of rural adult males.[211] The primary focus of infection occurs in the lungs, but pulmonary involvement may be overshadowed clinically by manifestations of limited or widespread lymphatic and hematogenous dissemination.[212] Paracoccidioidomycosis of childhood is an acute, progressive pulmonary infection that rapidly disseminates to lymph nodes, liver, and spleen.[213] In adults, the infection pursues a more chronic course with variable periods of clinical latency.[212,214,215] Pulmonary and disseminated infections are treated with ketoconazole or amphotericin B. Excellent clinical responses with low rates of relapse have been achieved with itraconazole.[216]

Acute progressive pulmonary paracoccidioidomycosis is an acute suppurative pneumonitis that contains scattered multinucleated giant cells and yeast forms of *P. brasiliensis*. The chronic progressive form is characterized by granulomatous inflammation with extensive interstitial and conglomerate fibrosis, necrosis, and arterial intimal fibrosis leading to cor pulmonale[217,218] At autopsy, disseminated lesions are found in extrathoracic sites in the majority of patients, chiefly the oropharyngeal mucosa, larynx, trachea, skin, lymph nodes, liver, spleen, adrenal glands, intestines, and kidneys.[217,218] These disseminated lesions are granulomatous, or suppurative and granulomatous. Cutaneous and mucosal lesions also exhibit pseudoepitheliomatous hyperplasia similar to that typically found in the lesions of blastomycosis and sporotrichosis.

In tissue sections, *P. brasiliensis* occurs predominantly as pleomorphic yeastlike cells, 5 to 60 µm in diameter, that reproduce by budding. Small yeast forms and hyphae are occasionally found.[219] Thick-walled, effete "mosaic" cells with fractured walls are often numerous in chronic pulmonary lesions. A definitive histopathologic diagnosis of paracoccidioidomycosis requires identification of characteristic multiple-budding cells that resemble a ship's steering wheel (Fig. 37-20). The blastoconidia produced by these cells have an oval, tubular, or teardrop configuration and are attached to parent cells by narrow necks.

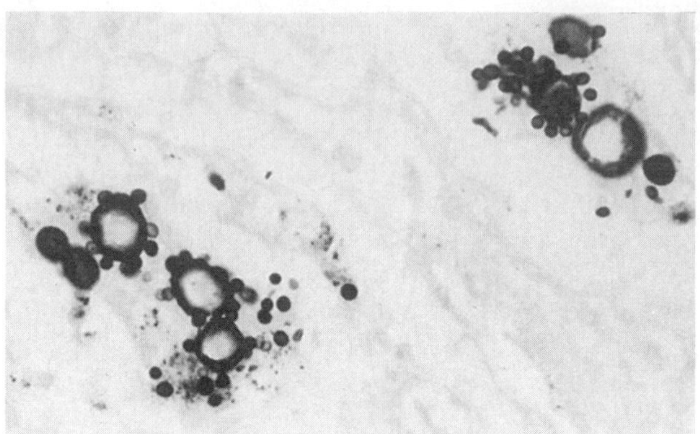

Fig. 37-20 Paracoccidioidomycosis. Several thick-walled cells have produced multiple blastoconidia. (Gomori's methenamine silver.)

Penicilliosis marneffei

Penicilliosis marneffei is a rare progressive and disseminated mycosis caused by *Penicillium marneffei,* a ubiquitous saprophyte of soil and decomposing organic matter.[220] Of the more than 150 recognized species of *Penicillium,* only *P. marneffei* is known to be dimorphic and to cause invasive infection. This mycosis is endemic in Southeast Asia and the Far East, and most human infections probably have a pulmonary inception after inhalation of airborne infectious conidia of *P. marneffei* produced in the environment.[221-224] Persons who are debilitated or immunocompromised, including those with HIV infection, appear to be at increased risk of infection.[225,226]

Patients with disseminated penicilliosis marneffei often present with chronic productive cough, mucoid sputum, chest pain, generalized lymphadenopathy, hepatosplenomegaly, draining skin ulcers, subcutaneous abscesses, osteolytic lesions, anemia, leukocytosis, and a history of weight loss and prolonged intermittent fever.[221] The course of the disease can range from 2 months to 3 years or more. Organs most frequently involved include the lungs, liver, intestines, lymph nodes, tonsils, skin, bone marrow, kidneys, and spleen.[221,223]

The host response in penicilliosis marneffei is similar to that seen in histoplasmosis capsulati, where numerous small yeastlike cells proliferate within histiocytes and distend them (Fig. 37-21). Slowly evolving pulmonary abscesses and granulomas can lead to fibrosis and cavitation, but calcification has not been reported. In histologic sections, the cells of *P. marneffei* are spherical to oval, 2.5 to 5 µm in diameter, and resemble those of *H. capsulatum* var. *capsulatum* (Fig. 37-21). However, unlike *H. capsulatum* spp. and other invasive yeastlike fungi, *P. marneffei* does not bud. Reproduction is by fission (schizogony) with the formation of a single transverse septum that stains more intensely with the special stains for fungi and is thicker than the external wall (Fig. 37-21, *inset*). Short hyphal forms and elongated, curved "sausage" forms with rounded ends and one or more septa are also occasionally produced, especially in necrotic and cavitary lesions.

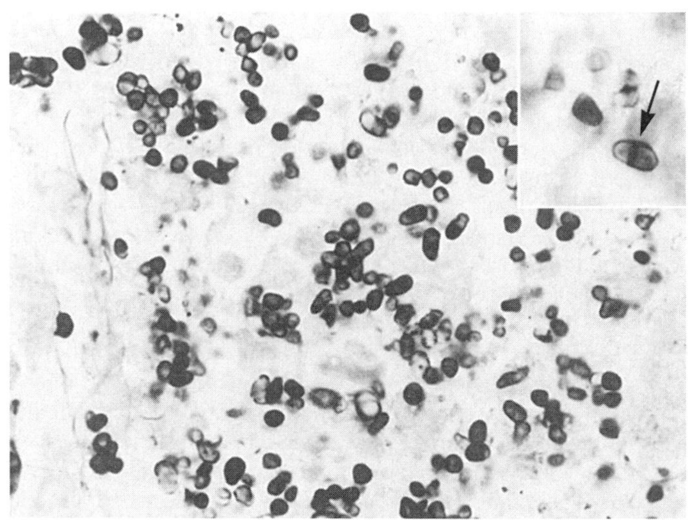

Fig. 37-21 Disseminated penicilliosis marneffei. Hepatic abscess contains individual and clustered yeastlike cells of *Penicillium marneffei,* 2.5 to 5 µm in diameter. *Inset, P. marneffei* cell with single, wide, transverse septum *(arrow)* and rounded ends. (Gomori's methenamine silver/hematoxylin and eosin.)

A definitive diagnosis of penicilliosis marneffei can be made by demonstration of typical yeastlike cells in clinical specimens and by microbiologic culture on standard mycologic media. The mycosis must be aggressively treated with amphotericin B, 5-fluorocytosine, or ketoconazole. Because relapse is common, antifungals should be given for several months.

Pseudallescheriasis

Pseudallescheria boydii is the most frequent etiologic agent of eumycotic mycetoma in the United States and is an occasional agent of otomycosis, keratitis, endophthalmitis, meningitis, brain abscess, and osteomyelitis.[227] This fungus can be isolated from clinical specimens in either of two forms: the asexual (anamorphic) form, designated *Scedosporium* (formerly *Monosporium) apiospermum,* and the sexual (teleomorphic) form, designated *Pseudallescheria* (formerly *Allescheria* and

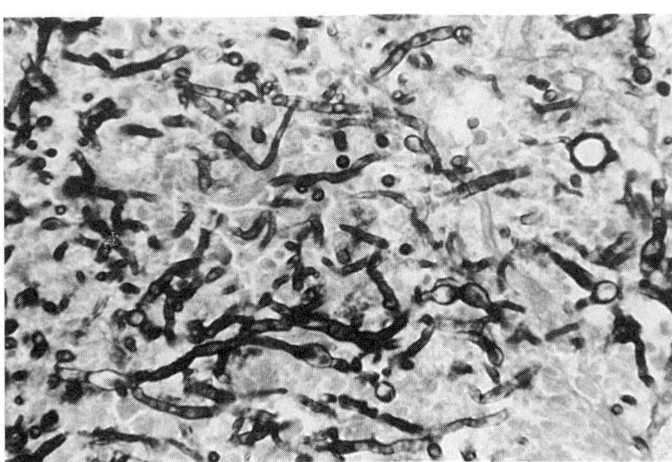

Fig. 37-22 Disseminated pseudallescheriasis. Slender hyphae of *Pseudallescheria boydii* are segmentally vesicular. A thick-walled, terminal chlamydoconidium is visible at upper right. (Gomori's methenamine silver.)

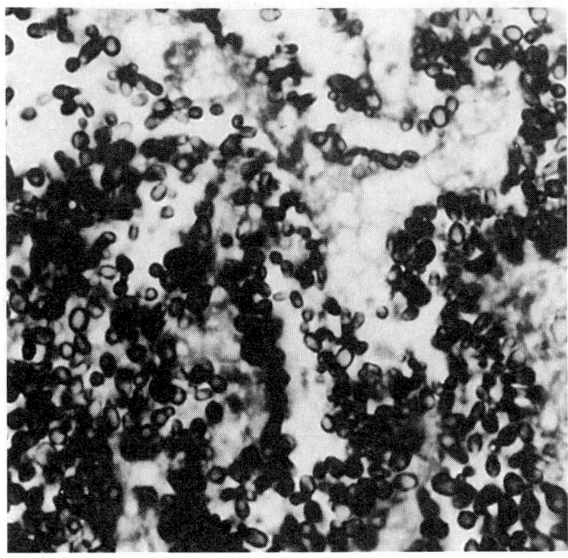

Fig. 37-23 Torulopsosis. Numerous single and budding yeastlike cells of *Torulopsis glabrata,* 2 to 5 μm in diameter, are embedded in an arterial thrombus. (Gomori's methenamine silver.)

Petriellidium) boydii. By convention, the disease is named for the sexual form.

P. boydii can colonize preexisting pulmonary cavities and form intracavitary fungus balls that resemble those produced by the *Aspergillus* spp.[228] The intracavitary mycelium consists of amorphous hyphal aggregates or of compact, concentrically laminated and intertwined hyphae. Invasive pulmonary and disseminated pseudallescheriasis are rare opportunistic infections that occur preferentially in patients treated for acute leukemia who are granulocytopenic.[229-231] Invasive lesions are infarctive as a consequence of mycelial invasion of blood vessels, but abscesses have also been reported.[230] Disseminated pseudallescheriasis frequently involves the brain,[232] thyroid gland, heart, and kidneys. Currently, miconazole is the drug of choice for treatment of invasive and disseminated pseudallescheriasis; the fungus is often resistant to amphotericin B.[123]

In tissue sections, the hyphae of *P. boydii* resemble those of the *Aspergillus* spp. The septate hyphae, 2 to 5 μm wide, branch in a dichotomous but haphazard pattern and may produce vesicles, truncated terminal conidia, and terminal or intercalated chlamydoconidia (Fig. 37-22). Hyphal vascular invasion is conspicuous in the invasive and disseminated lesions. Because the pathologic features of pulmonary and disseminated pseudallescheriasis, and the morphologic features of the hyphae in tissue sections, closely resemble those of aspergillosis, the diagnosis is best confirmed by culture or immunofluorescence.

Torulopsosis

Torulopsosis is a rare opportunistic mycosis caused by the small (2 to 5 μm), budding, spherical to oval, yeastlike fungus *Torulopsis glabrata,* a dominant member of the human natural flora.[233,234] Fungemia, the most common form of *T. glabrata* infection, has been associated with prolonged intravenous alimentation, severe abdominal trauma, and appendiceal abscesses.[235-238] Often, the source of fungemia is unexplained. Tissue invasion by *T. glabrata* is uncommon. When it occurs, the endocardium, kidneys, lungs, and CNS are sites most frequently involved with suppurative or, rarely, granulomatous inflammation.[235,236] The morphologic features of *T. glabrata* are similar to those of *Histoplasma capsulatum* var. *capsulatum,* especially when cells of the former are clustered within histiocytes (Fig. 37-23). However, unlike those of *Histoplasma,* the yeastlike cells of *T. glabrata* are amphophilic and stain entirely with hematoxylin and eosin; a "halo" or pseudocapsular effect is not evident. Culture or immunofluorescence is needed for definitive identification.

Trichosporonosis

The *Trichosporon* spp., like the agents of fusariosis, have recently emerged as significant systemic pathogens in compromised patients. These yeastlike fungi are soil saprophytes that also form a minor component of normal skin flora. Only two species are known to cause disseminated opportunistic infection. *T. beigelii (T. cutaneum),* the more frequent pathogen, is better known as the agent of white piedra, a nodule-forming trichomycosis. The other species, *T. capitatum,* has only rarely been implicated as an agent of disseminated infection[239] and has been reclassified into the genus *Blastoschizomyces* as *B. capitatus.*[240]

Disseminated trichosporonosis occurs principally in patients who are neutropenic as a result of treatment for acute leukemia, lymphoma, or solid tumors,[241-243] but it has also been reported in immunosuppressed transplant recipients. Purpuric cutaneous nodules are a frequent clinical manifestation, and the lungs, kidneys, myocardium, liver, spleen, and bone marrow are also frequently involved. Systemic lesions consist of abscesses,[244] granulomas,[245] or nodular infarcts,[246] the last a consequence of mycotic vascular invasion and occlusion.

In tissue sections, the *Trichosporon* spp. produce pleomorphic blastoconidia, 3 to 8 μm in diameter, septate hyphae, and arthroconidia that result from fragmentation of hyphal segments (Fig. 37-24). These fungi may be difficult to distinguish from some other opportunistic pathogens, such

Table 37-5 Histologic features of infections that resemble mycoses

Disease	Biologic agent(s)	Typical morphology in tissue	Usual host reaction
Actinomycosis	*Actinomyces israelii, A. naeslundii, A. viscosus, A. odontolyticus, A. bovis, Arachnia propionica, Rothia dentocariosa*	Organized aggregates (granules) composed of delicate, branched filaments about 1 µm wide; entire granules 30-3000 µmD*	Suppurative with multiple abscesses, extensive fibrosis, and formation of sinus tracts; Splendore-Hoeppli material usually borders granules
Botryomycosis	*Pseudomonas aeruginosa, Staphylococcus aureus, Escherichia coli, Streptococcus* spp., *Proteus* spp., and other bacteria	Organized aggregates (granules) composed of nonfilamentous gram-positive or gram-negative bacteria	Like actinomycosis
Nocardiosis	*Nocardia asteroides, N. brasiliensis, N. otitidiscaviarum (caviae)*	Long, delicate (about 1 µm wide), branched filaments that are gram positive, weakly acid-fast, and often beaded	Suppurative
Protothecosis	*Prototheca wickerhamii, P. zopfii*	Spherical, oval, or polyhedral sporangia, 2-25 µmD, that, when mature contain 2-20-sporangiospores	Varies from little or no reaction to granulomatous

D, Diameter.

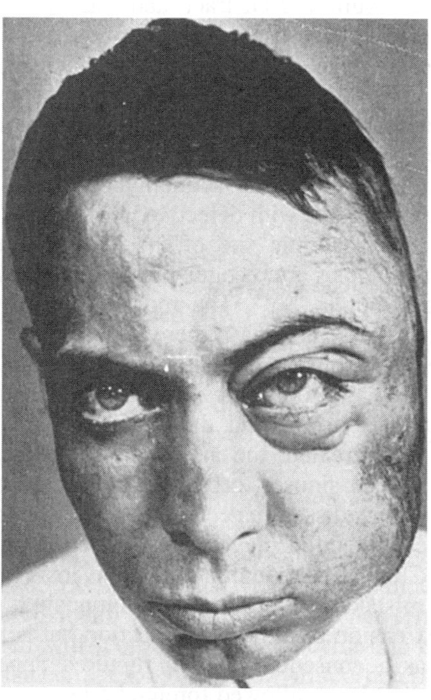

Fig. 37-27 Cervicofacial actinomycosis. Note swelling and openings of draining sinuses. (Courtesy Dr. Antonio González-Ochoa, Mexico City.)

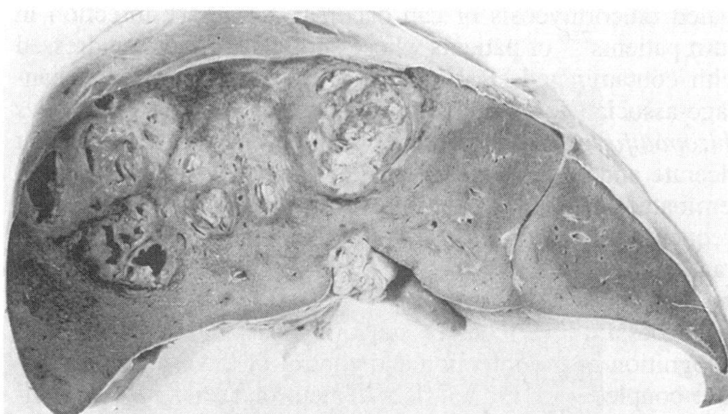

Fig. 37-28 Abdominal actinomycosis. Multiple abscesses in liver caused by *Actinomyces israelii*. Primary infection in cecum or appendix resulted in retrocecal abscess that extended to skin surface in right inguinal region. (Courtesy Dr. Roger D. Baker, Silver Spring, Md.)

toxylin and eosin, periodic acid–Schiff, and Gridley stains. Specific identification requires culture or immunofluorescence staining because, in tissue sections, the agents of actinomycosis cannot be distinguished from each other. Both gram-positive and gram-negative bacilli and cocci may be found in close association with actinomycetal filaments within a granule, but it is generally believed that these bacteria are secondary pathogens.

Penicillin is the drug of choice for treating actinomycosis.[266,267] It is speculated that fewer cases are seen today because of the widespread use of antibacterial antibiotics for treating minor, unrelated infections.

Botryomycosis (bacterial pseudomycosis)

Botryomycosis is a chronic, localized infection of the skin and subcutaneous tissue or viscera caused by nonfilamentous bacteria that form granules.[277,278] Disseminated infection is rare.[279,280] In hematoxylin and eosin–stained tissue sections, the granules can be mistaken for those of actinomycosis and actinomycotic mycetoma. The bacteria most commonly implicated include *Pseudomonas aeruginosa, Staphylococcus aureus, Escherichia coli,* and species of *Streptococcus* and *Proteus*. Botryomycotic granules and those of actinomycosis and mycetoma (see discussion of mycetomas) can be distinguished from each other if appropriate bacterial and fungal stains are used. This distinction is important because each of these diseases is managed differently.

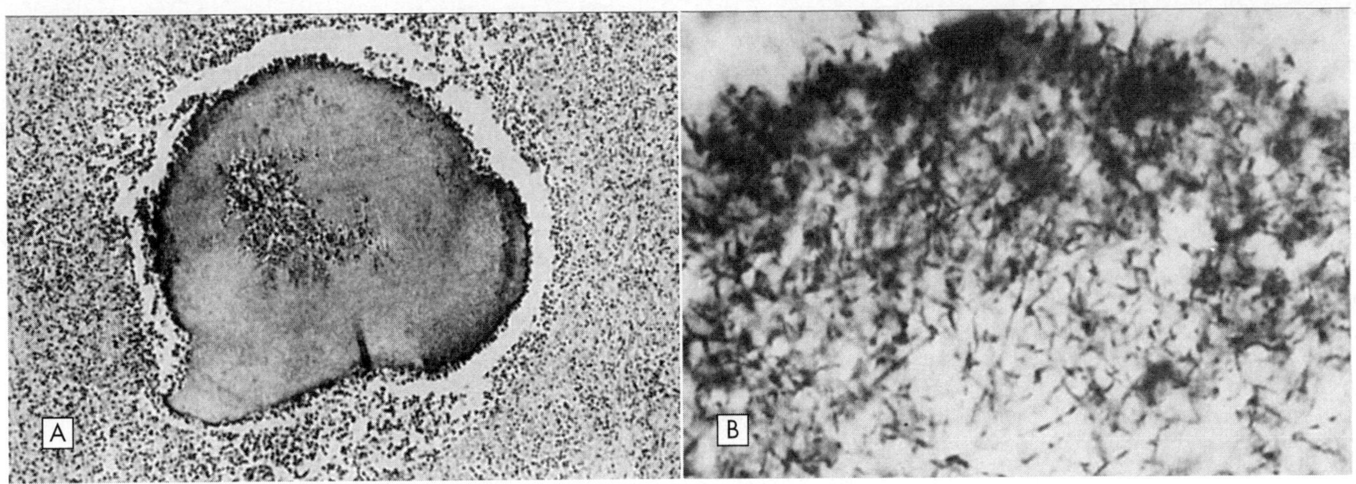

Fig. 37-29 Actinomycosis. **A,** Granule of *Actinomyces israelii* in hepatic abscess. **B,** Gram-positive, branched filaments and coccoid elements, about 1 µm in diameter, in replicate section of same granule as in **A.** (**B,** Brown and Brenn.)

Nocardiosis

Between 500 and 1000 new cases of nocardiosis, a subacute or chronic bacterial infection, are diagnosed annually in the United States.[281,282] In about 85% of these cases, infection is caused by *Nocardia asteroides*. The remaining 15% are caused by *N. brasiliensis* or *N. otitidis-caviarum (caviae)*.[282-284] Infections by these aerobic, filamentous bacteria of the order Actinomycetales occur worldwide and are usually seen in persons with underlying immunologic deficiency.[285] Well-recognized conditions that predispose patients to nocardial infection include lymphoma, Hodgkin's disease, chronic granulomatous disease of childhood, pulmonary alveolar proteinosis, and AIDS.[285-288] Unlike actinomycosis, nocardiosis is an exogenous disease, and infections are usually contracted by inhalation of nocardiae that live as saprophytes in nature. The disease is not contagious.

The clinical manifestations of nocardiosis are extremely variable.[282,286,289,290] All three *Nocardia* species may cause mycetoma, (discussed earlier in this chapter). More commonly, the disease is systemic with a pulmonary inception. Lung lesions may occur as large cavitating abscesses or as a diffuse fibrinosuppurative pneumonia similar to that caused by certain nonfilamentous bacteria. Fibrosis is usually minimal. There may be hematogenous dissemination to other body sites from a primary focus in the lungs. About 20% of patients with pulmonary nocardiosis have CNS involvement, usually in the form of cerebral abscesses.[282,284,291] Meningitis, a rare complication, results from rupture of an intracerebral abscess or from direct extension of nocardial osteomyelitis. Nocardiosis may also present as solitary or multiple subcutaneous lesions that are a result of either traumatic implantation or systemic infection.[283,292,293] These localized lesions, with chains of nodules leading from a primary skin ulcer, can mimic those of cutaneous sporotrichosis.[282] This entity is known as the sporotrichoid form of nocardiosis. Sulfonamides and trimethoprim-sulfamethoxazole are useful for treating all forms of the disease.[282,294,295] Because of a strong tendency for the disease to relapse, prolonged therapy may be required.

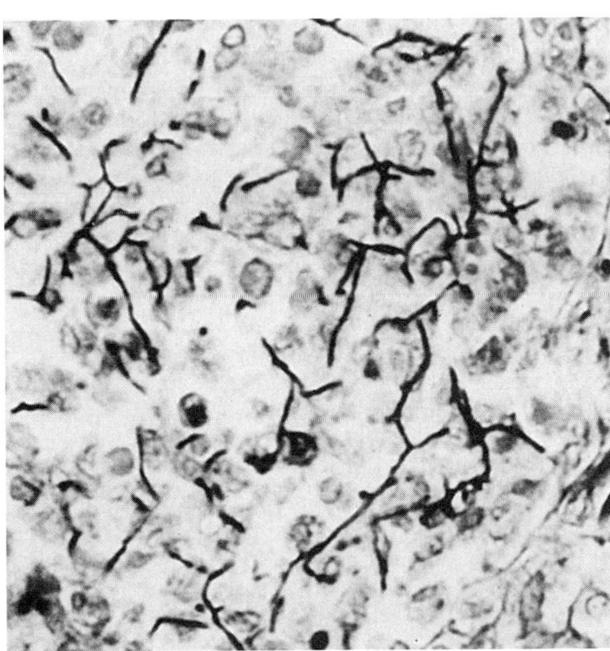

Fig. 37-30 Pulmonary nocardiosis. Delicate filaments that branch at approximately right angles are embedded in fibrinosuppurative, alveolar exudate. (Gomori's methenamine silver/hematoxylin and eosin.)

In systemic infections, the *Nocardia* spp. almost never form granules (organized filamentous aggregates). Rather, these organisms occur as individual, gram-positive, beaded filaments, about 1 µm in width, that branch at approximately right angles (Fig. 37-30). The delicate filaments are not stained by the hematoxylin and eosin, periodic acid–Schiff, or Gridley stains. They are, however, readily demonstrated with the Gomori methenamine silver and tissue Gram stains. All three *Nocardia* spp. are often partially acid fast in tissue sections when stained with modified acid-fast procedures using a weak decolorizing agent. They lose their acid fastness when cultured on artificial media. Usually, the agents of actinomycosis are not acid fast.

Protothecosis

Protothecosis is an infection caused by achlorophyllous algae of the genus *Prototheca.* Although they do not contain chloroplasts, these saprophytic algae are believed to be related to green algae of the genus *Chlorella.*[296] Three species of protothecae are recognized, of which two, *P. wickerhamii* and *P. zopfii,* are known to cause disease. Almost all authenticated cases of human protothecosis have been caused by *P. wickerhamii.*[297] Human infections are cosmopolitan in distribution, but most have occurred in the United States.[297] The source of infection is often not apparent but can be related to penetrating injury in some cases.

Two clinically distinct forms of protothecosis are recognized: cutaneous infection and olecranon bursitis. Cutaneous protothecosis, which occurs preferentially in debilitated or compromised patients, presents as spreading papulonodular or verrucous lesions, usually involving the distal extremities or head.[298] Infection may extend into the subcutaneous tissue and rarely spreads to regional lymph nodes.[298,299] Olecranon bursitis, which occurs in otherwise healthy hosts, presents as a subcutaneous nodule adjacent to the elbow.[298,300] Bursectomy is the treatment of choice. Chemotherapy alone cannot effectively eradicate localized infection in most cases. Two cases of disseminated human protothecosis have been reported. In the first case, disease occurred in a patient with transient depression of specific cell-mediated immunity to prototheca.[301] In the second, the patient had no known immunologic defect.[302] Both recovered after therapy with amphotericin B.

The protothecae are found in tissue sections in the form of endosporulating sporangia. Their asexual reproductive cycle in tissue is similar to that of the endosporulating fungi. Small, uninucleate, immature sporangia undergo nuclear division followed or accompanied by progressive cytoplasmic cleavage to produce mature sporangia that contain sporangiospores. Characteristically, the sporangiospores are polygonal or wedge shaped, fill the parent cell, and may be radially arranged around a central sporangiospore, producing the distinctive "morula" form (Fig. 37-31, *A*). The sporangia of the two pathogenic protothecae differ in size but are otherwise similar in morphology. Sporangia of the small form, *P. wickerhamii,* measure 2 to 12 µm in diameter, whereas those of *P. zopfii* measure 10 to 25 µm in diameter. Morula forms are uncommon in infections caused by *P. zopfii*. Endosporulating cells of *P. zopfii* are oval, and their larger nuclei are more conspicuous than those of *P. wickerhamii* (Fig. 37-31, *B*).

The cell walls of both the sporangia and the sporangiospores are stained with the special stains for fungi. With hematoxylin and eosin, these cells are hyaline, but their contents may be eosinophilic or basophilic. The two species are more reliably distinguished from one another in tissue sections by direct immunofluorescence and in culture by their patterns of carbohydrate assimilation.

Cutaneous lesions often show hyperkeratosis, parakeratosis, and acanthosis, and they may be ulcerated. Algal cells are abundant in the dermis and may also be found in the epidermis and keratin layer as a result of transepidermal elimination. An inflammatory reaction, when present, may be granulomatous or may consist of a mixture of acute and chronic inflammatory cells. Infection of the olecranon bursa produces necrotizing granulomatous inflammation. The bursal lining consists of a stellate zone of necrotic debris, neutrophils, and fibrin that is surrounded by palisaded epithelioid histiocytes and multinucleated giant cells. The adjacent soft tissue contains granulation tissue, acute and chronic inflammatory cells, and small granulomas. Prototheca cells are difficult to find in these lesions, which can be mistaken for rheumatoid nodules if special stains are not used to detect the algae. Endosporulating fungi such as *Coccidioides immitis* and *Rhinosporidium seeberi* are distinguished from the protothecae in tissue sections on the basis of their size and distinctive morphology.

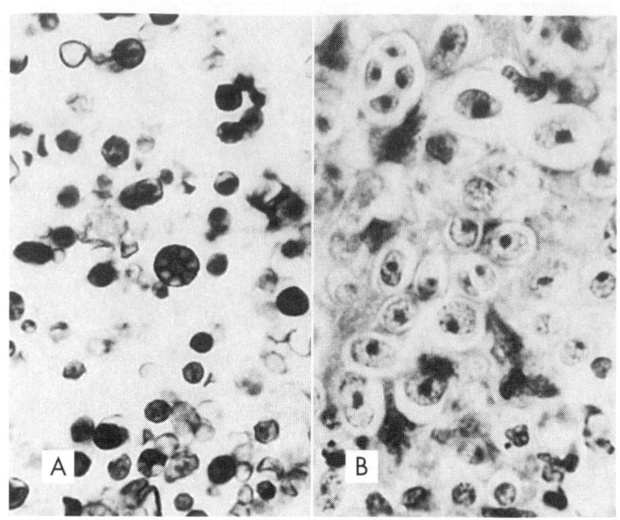

Fig. 37-31 Protothecosis. **A,** Distinctive endosporulating cell ("morula form") of *Prototheca wickerhamii (center).* **B,** Oval cells of *P. zopfii.* Nuclei are visible in most cells. One endosporulating cell is present *(top left).* (**A,** Gridley's stain.)

Green algae of the genus *Chlorella* cause cutaneous and systemic infections in animals, but human green algal infection has been recognized only recently.[303] In tissue sections, the cells of *Chlorella,* 6 to 14 µm in diameter, appear similar to those of *P. zopfii*. However, infections caused by the two algae can be differentiated by other criteria.[304] The protothecae can be distinguished from each other and from *Chlorella* in tissue sections by direct immunofluorescence.

REFERENCES

General

1. Chandler FW, Kaplan W, Ajello L: *Color atlas and text of the histopathology of mycotic diseases,* St. Louis, 1980, Mosby.
2. Kwon-Chung KJ, Bennett JE: *Medical mycology,* Philadelphia, 1992, Lea & Febiger.
3. McGinnis MR: *Laboratory handbook of medical mycology,* New York, 1980, Academic Press.
4. Rippon JW: *Medical mycology: the pathogenic fungi and the pathogenic actinomycetes,* ed 3, Philadelphia, 1988, Saunders.
5. Baker RD, Chick EW: Proceedings of International Symposium on Opportunistic Fungus Infections, *Lab Invest* 11:1017, 1962.
6. Grieco MH, editor: *Infections in the abnormal host,* New York, 1980, Yorke Medical Books.

7. Warnock DW, Richardson MD, editors: *Fungal infection in the compromised patient,* New York, 1982, John Wiley & Sons.
8. Baker RD, senior editor: *The pathologic anatomy of mycoses: human infection with fungi, actinomycetes and algae,* New York, 1971, Springer-Verlag.
9. Chandler FW, Watts JC: *Pathologic diagnosis of fungal infections,* Chicago, 1987, American Society of Clinical Pathologists Press.
10. Chandler FW, Watts JC: Fungal infections. In Dail DH, Hammar SP, editors: *Pulmonary pathology,* New York, 1993, Springer-Verlag.
11. Conant NF et al: *Manual of clinical mycology,* ed 3, Philadelphia, 1971, Saunders.
12. Palmer DF et al: *Serodiagnosis of mycotic diseases,* Springfield, Ill., 1977, Charles C Thomas.
13. Roberts SOB, Hay RJ, Mackenzie DWR: *A clinician's guide to fungal disease,* New York, 1984, Marcel Dekker.
14. Binford CH, Connor DH, editors: *Pathology of tropical and extraordinary diseases,* Washington, DC, 1976, Armed Forces Institute of Pathology.
15. Schwarz J: The diagnosis of deep mycoses by morphologic methods, *Hum Pathol* 13:519, 1982.
16. Kaplan W, Kraft DE: Demonstration of pathogenic fungi in formalin-fixed tissues by immunofluorescence, *Am J Clin Pathol* 52:420, 1969.

Mycoses

Superficial mycoses

17. Roscoe J, Farmer ER: Diseases caused by fungi. In Farmer ER, Hood AF, editors: *Pathology of the skin,* Norwalk, Conn, 1990, Appleton & Lange.
18. Graham JH, Barroso-Tobila C: Dermal pathology of superficial fungus infections. In Baker RD, editor: *The pathologic anatomy of mycoses: human infection with fungi, actinomycetes and algae,* New York, 1971, Springer-Verlag.

Dermatophytosis

19. Rebell G, Taplin D: *Dermatophytes: their recognition and identification,* ed 2, Coral Gables, Fla, 1970, University of Miami Press.
20. Alteras I et al: Unusual aspects of granulomatous dermatophytosis, *Mycopathologia* 86:93, 1984.
21. West BC, Kwon-Chung KJ: Mycetoma caused by *Microsporum audouinii:* first reported case, *Am J Clin Pathol* 73:447, 1980.

Chromoblastomycosis

22. Fader RC, McGinnis MR: Infections caused by dematiaceous fungi: chromoblastomycosis and phaeohyphomycosis, *Infect Dis Clin North Am* 2:925, 1988.
23. Carrion AL: Chromoblastomycosis and related infections, *Int J Dermatol* 14:27, 1975.
24. Vollum DI: Chromomycosis: a review, *Br J Dermatol* 96:454, 1977.
25. McGinnis MR: Chromoblastomycosis and phaeohyphomycosis: new concepts, diagnosis, and mycology, *J Am Acad Dermatol* 8:1, 1983.
26. Batres E et al: Transepithelial elimination of cutaneous chromomycosis, *Arch Dermatol* 114:1231, 1978.

Lobomycosis

27. Caldwell DK et al: Lobomycosis as a disease of the Atlantic bottle-nosed dolphin, *Am J Trop Med Hyg* 24:105, 1975.
28. Wiersema JP: Lobo's disease (keloidal blastomycosis). In Baker RD, editor: *The pathologic anatomy of mycoses: human infection with fungi, actinomycetes and algae,* New York, 1971, Springer-Verlag.

Mycetoma

29. Magana M: Mycetoma, *Int J Dermatol* 23:221, 1984.
30. McGinnis MR, Fader RC: Mycetoma: a contemporary concept. *Infect Dis Clin North Am* 2:939, 1988.
31. Green WO, Adams TE: Mycetoma in the United States: a review and report of seven additional cases, *Am J Clin Pathol* 42:75, 1964.
32. Tight RR, Bartlett MS: Actinomycetoma in the United States, *Rev Infect Dis* 3:1139, 1981.
33. Mahgoub ES: Medical management of mycetoma, *Bull WHO* 54:303, 1976.
34. Mahgoub ES, Murray IG: *Mycetoma,* London, 1973, William Heinemann Medical Books.
35. Cameron HM, Gatei D, Bremner AD: The deep mycoses in Kenya: a histopathological study. 1. Mycetoma, *East Afr Med J* 50:382, 1973.
36. Winslow DJ, Steen FG: Considerations in the histologic diagnosis of mycetoma, *Am J Clin Pathol* 42:164, 1964.

Phaeohyphomycosis (subcutaneous and systemic)

37. Ajello L: Phaeohyphomycosis: definitions and etiology. In *Mycoses,* Scientific publ no 304, Washington, DC, 1975, Pan American Health Organization, p. 126.
38. McGinnis MR: Human pathogenic species of *Exophiala, Phialophora* and *Wangiella.* In *The black and white yeasts,* Scientific publ no 356, Washington, DC, 1978, Pan American Health Organization, p 37.
39. Bambirra EA et al: Phaeohyphomycotic cyst: a clinicopathologic study of the first four cases described from Brazil, *Am J Trop Med Hyg* 32:794, 1983.
40. Moskowitz LB et al: *Phialophora richardsiae* in a lesion appearing as a giant cell tumor of the tendon sheath, *Arch Pathol Lab Med* 107:374, 1983.
41. Ziefer A, Connor DH: Phaeomycotic cyst: a clinicopathologic study of twenty-five patients, *Am J Trop Med Hyg* 29:901, 1980.
42. O'Donnell PJ, Hutt MSR: Subcutaneous phaeohyphomycosis: a histopathological study of nine cases from Malawi, *J Clin Pathol* 38:288-292, 1985.
43. Iwatsu T, Miyaji M: Phaeomycotic cyst: a case with a lesion containing a wooden splinter, *Arch Dermatol* 120:1209, 1984.
44. Ronan SG et al: Primary cutaneous phaeohyphomycosis: report of seven cases, *J Cutan Pathol* 20:223, 1993.
45. Estes SA Merz WG, Maxwell LG: Primary cutaneous phaeohyphomycosis caused by *Drechslera spicifera, Arch Dermatol* 113:813, 1977.
46. Crichlow DK, Enrile FT, Memon MY: Cerebellar abscess due to *Cladosporium trichoides (bantianum):* case report, *Am J Clin Pathol* 60:416, 1973.
47. Maslni T et al: Cerebral phaeohyphomycosis, *Clin Neuropathol* 4:246, 1985.
48. Riley O Jr, Mann SH: Brain abscess caused by *Cladosporium trichoides:* review of three cases and report of fourth case, *Am J Clin Pathol* 33:525, 1960.

Rhinosporidiosis

49. Jimenez JF, Young DE, Hough AJ Jr: Rhinosporidiosis: a report of two cases from Arkansas, *Am J Clin Pathol* 82:611, 1984.
50. Karunaratne WAE: *Rhinosporidiosis in man,* London, 1964, Athlone Press.
51. Levy MG, Meuten DJ, Breitschwerdt EB: Cultivation of *Rhinosporidium seeberi* in vitro: interaction with epithelial cells, *Science* 234:474, 1986.
52. Kannan-Kutty M, Teh EC: *Rhinosporidium seeberi:* an electron microscopic study of its life cycle, *Pathology* 6:63, 1974.
53. Bader G, Grueber HLE: Histochemical studies of *Rhinosporidium seeberi, Virchows Arch [A] (Pathol Anat)* 350:76, 1970.
54. Hyams VJ: Papillomas of the nasal cavity and paranasal sinuses, *Ann Otol Rhinol Laryngol* 80:192, 1971.

Sporotrichosis

55. Lynch PJ, Voorhees JJ, Harrell ER: Systemic sporotrichosis, *Ann Intern Med* 73:23, 1970.
56. Smith PW et al: Disseminated cutaneous sporotrichosis: three illustrative cases. *Arch Dermatol* 117:143, 1981.
57. Berson SD, Brandt FA: Primary pulmonary sporotrichosis with unusual fungal morphology, *Thorax* 32:505, 1977.
58. England DM, Hochholzer L: Primary pulmonary sporotrichosis: report of eight cases with clinicopathologic review, *Am J Surg Pathol* 9:193, 1985.
59. Watts JC, Chandler FW: Primary pulmonary sporotrichosis, *Arch Pathol Lab Med* 111:215, 1987.
60. Bullpitt P, Weedon D: Sporotrichosis: a review of 39 cases, *Pathology* 10:249, 1978.
61. Sperling LC, Read SI: Localized cutaneous sporotrichosis, *Int J Dermatol* 22:525, 1983.

62. Lurie HI: Histopathology of sporotrichosis, *Arch Pathol* 75:92, 1963.
63. Marrocco GR et al: Granulomatous synovitis and osteitis caused by *Sporothrix schenckii*, *Am J Clin Pathol* 64:345, 1975.
64. Liber AF, Choi HS: Splendore-Hoeppli phenomenon about silk sutures in tissue, *Arch Pathol* 95:217, 1973.
65. Marques MEA et al: Comparison between histochemical and immunohistochemical methods for diagnosis of sporotrichosis, *J Clin Pathol* 45:1089, 1992.

Adiaspiromycosis

66. Barbas Filho JV et al: Respiratory failure caused by adiaspiromycosis, *Chest* 97:1171, 1990.
67. Kodousek R et al: Pulmonary adiaspiromycosis in man caused by *Emmonsia crescens:* report of a unique case, *Am J Clin Pathol* 56:394, 1971.
68. Schwarz J: Adiaspiromycosis *Pathol Annu* 13:41, 1978.
69. Watts JC et al: Human pulmonary adiaspiromycosis, *Arch Pathol* 99:11, 1975.

Aspergillosis

70. Cho SY, Choi HY: Opportunistic fungal infection among cancer patients, *Am J Clin Pathol* 72:617, 1979.
71. Young RC, Jennings A, Bennett JE: Species identification of invasive aspergillosis in man, *Am J Clin Pathol* 58:554, 1972.
72. Young RC et al: Aspergillosis: the spectrum of disease in 98 patients, *Medicine* (*Baltimore*) 49:147, 1970.
73. Schwarz J: Aspergillosis, *Pathol Annu* 8:81, 1973.
74. Raper KB, Fennell DI: *The genus aspergillus,* Baltimore, 1965, Williams & Wilkins.
75. Kurrein F, Green GH, Rowles SL: Localized deposition of calcium oxalate around a pulmonary *Aspergillus niger* fungus ball, *Am J Clin Pathol* 64:556, 1975.
76. Katzenstein AL, Liebow AA, Friedman PJ: Bronchocentric granulomatosis, mucoid impaction, and hypersensitivity reactions to fungi, *Am Rev Respir Dis* 111:497, 1975.
77. Warnock ML, Fennessy J, Rippon J: Chronic eosinophilic pneumonia, a manifestation of allergic aspergillosis, *Am J Clin Pathol* 62:73, 1974.
78. Glimp RA, Bayer AS: Pulmonary aspergilloma: diagnostic and therapeutic considerations, *Arch Intern Med* 143:303, 1983.
79. Binder RE et al: Chronic necrotizing pulmonary aspergillosis: a discrete clinical entity, *Medicine* (Baltimore) 61:109, 1982.
80. Gefter WB et al: "Semi-invasive" pulmonary aspergillosis: a new look at the spectrum of aspergillus infections of the lung, *Radiology* 140:313, 1981.
81. Palmer LB, Greenberg HE, Schiff MJ: Corticosteroid treatment as a risk factor for invasive aspergillosis in patients with lung disease, *Thorax* 46:15, 1991.
82. Meyer RD et al: Aspergillosis complicating neoplastic disease, *Am J Med* 54:6, 1973.
83. Orr DP, Myerowitz RL, Dubois PJ: Patho-radiologic correlation of invasive pulmonary aspergillosis in the compromised host, *Cancer* 41:2028, 1978.
84. Boon AP, O'Brien D, Adams DH: Ten year review of invasive aspergillosis detected at necropsy, *J Clin Pathol* 44:452, 1991.
85. Atkinson JB et al: Cardiac fungal infections: review of autopsy findings in 60 patients, *Hum Pathol* 15:935, 1984.
86. Denning DW et al: Pulmonary aspergillosis in the acquired immunodeficiency syndrome, *N Engl J Med* 324:654, 1991.
87. Phillips P, Weiner MH: Invasive aspergillosis diagnosed by immunohistochemistry with monoclonal and polyclonal reagents, *Hum Pathol* 18:1015, 1987.

Blastomycosis

88. Drake RG Jr: North American blastomycosis: a review, *J Ky Med Assoc* 83:77, 1985.
89. Sarosi GA, Davies SF: Blastomycosis, *Am Rev Respir Dis* 120:911, 1979.
90. Tenenbaum MJ, Greenspan J, Kerkering TM: Blastomycosis, *CRC Crit Rev Microbiol* 9:139, 1982.
91. Chandler FW, Watts JC: Pathologic features of blastomycosis. In Al-Doory Y, DiSalvo AF, editors: *Blastomycosis,* New York, 1992, Plenum Press.
92. Cush R, Light RW, George RB: Clinical and roentgenographic manifestations of acute and chronic blastomycosis, *Chest* 69:345, 1976.
93. Recht LD et al: Blastomycosis in immunosuppressed patients, *Am Rev Respir Dis* 125:359, 1982.
94. Inoshita T et al: Blastomycosis presenting with prostatic involvement: report of 2 cases and review of the literature, *J Urol* 130:160, 1983.
95. Schwarz J, Salfelder K: Blastomycosis: a review of 152 cases, *Curr Top Pathol* 65:165, 1977.
96. Vanek J, Schwarz J, Haken S: North American blastomycosis, *Am J Clin Pathol* 54:384, 1970.
97. Witorach P, Utz JP: North American blastomycosis: a study of 40 patients, *Medicine* (*Baltimore*) 47:169, 1968.
98. Bradsher RW: Prognosis and therapy of blastomycosis. In Al-Doory Y, DiSalvo AF, editors: *Blastomycosis,* New York, 1992, Plenum Press.
99. Lockwood WR et al: The treatment of North American blastomycosis: ten years' experience, *Am Rev Respir Dis* 100:314, 1969.
100. Watts JC et al: Giant forms of *Blastomyces dermatitidis* in the pulmonary lesions of blastomycosis: potential confusion with *Coccidioides immitis*, *Am J Clin Pathol* 93:119, 1990.

Candidiasis

101. Hughes WT: Systemic candidiasis: a study of 109 fatal cases, *Pediatr Infect Dis* 1:11, 1982.
102. Maksymiuk AW et al: Systemic candidiasis in cancer patients, *Am J Med* 77(4D):20, 1984.
103. Myerowitz RL, Pazin GJ, Allen CM: Disseminated candidiasis: changes in incidence, underlying diseases, and pathology, *Am J Clin Pathol* 68:29, 1977.
104. Odds FC: *Candida and candidosis,* ed 2, London, 1988, Baillière Tindall.
105. Bodey GP, Fainstein V: Systemic candidiasis. In Bodey GP, Fainstein V, editors: *Candidiasis,* New York, 1985, Raven Press.
106. Bross J et al: Risk factors for nosocomial candidemia: a case-control study in adults without leukemia, *Am J Med* 87:614, 1989.
107. Parker JC Jr, McCloskey JJ, Knauer KA: Pathologic features of human candidiasis: a common deep mycosis of the brain, heart, and kidney in the altered host, *Am J Clin Pathol* 65:991, 1976.
108. Aronson IK, Soltani K: Chronic mucocutaneous candidosis: a review, *Mycopathologia* 60:17, 1976.
109. Dwyer JM: Chronic mucocutaneous candidiasis, *Annu Rev Med* 32:491, 1981.
110. Eras P, Goldstein MJ, Sherlock P: *Candida* infection of the gastrointestinal tract, *Medicine* (*Baltimore*) 51:367, 1972.
111. Katzenstein ALA, Maksem J: Candidal infection of gastric ulcers: histology, incidence, and clinical significance, *Am J Clin Pathol* 71:137, 1979.
112. Johnson TL et al: Candida hepatitis: histopathologic diagnosis, *Am J Surg Pathol* 12:716, 1988.
113. Parker JC Jr, McCloskey JJ, Lee RS: The emergence of candidosis: the dominant postmortem cerebral mycosis, *Am J Clin Pathol* 70:31, 1978.
114. Parker JC Jr, McCloskey JJ, Lee RS: Human cerebral candidosis: a postmortem evaluation of 19 patients, *Hum Pathol* 12:23, 1981.
115. Dubois PJ, Myerowitz RL, Allen CM: Pathoradiologic correlation of pulmonary candidiasis in immunosuppressed patients, *Cancer* 40:1026, 1977.
116. Kassner EG et al: Pulmonary candidiasis in infants: clinical, radiologic, and pathologic features, *AJR* 137:707, 1981.
117. Masur H, Rosen PP, Armstrong D: Pulmonary disease caused by *Candida* species, *Am J Med* 63:914, 1977.
118. Rose HD, Sheth NK: Pulmonary candidiasis: a clinical and pathological correlation, *Arch Intern Med* 138:964, 1978.
119. Haron E et al: Primary *Candida* pneumonia, *Medicine* (*Baltimore*) 72:137, 1993.
120. Walsh TJ et al: Fungal infections of the heart: analysis of 51 autopsy cases, *Am J Cardiol* 45:357, 1980.
121. Parker JC Jr: The potentially lethal problem of cardiac candidosis, *Am J Clin Pathol* 73:356, 1980.
122. Robboy SJ, Kaiser J: Pathogenesis of fungal infection on heart valve prostheses, *Hum Pathol* 6:711, 1975.
123. Terrell CL, Hughes CE: Antifungal agents used for deep-seated mycotic infections, *Mayo Clin Proc* 67:69, 1992.
124. Humphrey DM, Weiner MH: Candidal antigen detection in pulmonary candidiasis, *Am J Med* 74:630, 1983.

Coccidioidomycosis

125. Drutz DJ, Catanzaro A: Coccidioidomycosis: part I, *Am Rev Respir Dis* 117:559, 1978.
126. Bayer AS: Fungal pneumonias: pulmonary coccidioidal syndromes. I. Primary and progressive primary coccidioidal pneumonias: diagnostic, therapeutic, and prognostic considerations, *Chest* 79:575, 1981.
127. Bayer AS: Fungal pneumonias: pulmonary coccidioidal syndromes. II. Miliary, nodular, and cavitary pulmonary coccidioidomycosis: chemotherapeutic and surgical considerations, *Chest* 79:686, 1981.
128. Drutz DJ, Catanzaro A: Coccidioidomycosis: part II, *Am Rev Respir Dis* 117:727, 1978.
129. Stevens DA, editor: *Coccidioidomycosis: a text,* New York, 1980, Plenum Medical Book Co.
130. Ampel NM, Dols CL, Galgiani JN: Coccidioidomycosis during human immunodeficiency virus infection, *Am J Med* 94:235, 1993.
131. Deresinski SC, Stevens DA: Coccidioidomycosis in compromised hosts, *Medicine (Baltimore)* 54:377, 1974.
132. Graham AR et al: Quantitative pathology of coccidioidomycosis in acquired immunodeficiency syndrome, *Hum Pathol* 19:800, 1988.
133. Bouza E et al: Coccidioidal meningitis: an analysis of thirty-one cases and review of the literature, *Medicine (Baltimore)* 60:139, 1981.
134. Huntington RW et al: Pathologic and clinical observations on 142 cases of fatal coccidioidomycosis with necropsy. In Ajello L, editor: *Coccidioidomycosis,* Tucson, 1967, University of Arizona Press.
135. Drutz DJ, Huppert M: Coccidioidomycosis: factors affecting the host-parasite interaction, *J Infect Dis* 147:372, 1983.
136. Donnelly WH, Yunis EJ: The ultrastructure of *Coccidioides immitis, Arch Pathol* 98:227, 1974.
137. Deppisch LM, Donowho EM: Pulmonary coccidioidomycosis, *Am J Clin Pathol* 58:489, 1972.
138. Raab SS, Silverman JF, Zimmerman KG: Fine-needle aspiration biopsy of pulmonary coccidioidomycosis: spectrum of cytologic findings in 73 patients, *Am J Clin Pathol* 99:582, 1993.
139. Kaplan W: Application of the fluorescent antibody technique to the diagnosis and study of coccidioidomycosis. In Ajello L, editor: *Coccidioidomycosis,* Tucson, 1967, University of Arizona Press.
140. Meyer PR, Hui AN, Biddle M: *Coccidioides immitis* meningitis with arthroconidia in the cerebrospinal fluid: report of the first case and review of the arthroconidia literature, *Hum Pathol* 13:1136, 1982.
141. Sobel RA et al: Central nervous system coccidioidomycosis: a clinicopathologic study of treatment with and without amphotericin B, *Hum Pathol* 15:980, 1984.
142. Kyriakos M: Myospherulosis of the paranasal sinuses, nose, and middle ear: a possible iatrogenic disease, *Am J Clin Pathol* 67:118, 1977.
143. Rosai J: The nature of myospherulosis of the upper respiratory tract, *Am J Clin Pathol* 69:475, 1978.

Cryptococcosis

144. Diamond RD: *Cryptococcus neoformans* pneumonia. In Pennington JE, editor: *Respiratory infections: diagnosis and management,* New York, 1983, Raven Press.
145. Lewis JL, Rabinovich S: The wide spectrum of cryptococcal infections, *Am J Med* 53:315, 1972.
146. Littman ML, Walter JE: Cryptococcosis: current status, *Am J Med* 45:922, 1968.
147. Chechani V, Kamholz SL: Pulmonary manifestations of disseminated cryptococcosis in patients with AIDS, *Chest* 98:1060, 1990.
148. Clark RA et al: Spectrum of *Cryptococcus neoformans* infection in 68 patients infected with human immunodeficiency virus, *Rev Infect Dis* 12:768, 1990.
149. Gal AA et al: The pathology of pulmonary cryptococcal infections in the acquired immunodeficiency syndrome, *Arch Pathol Lab Med* 110:502, 1986.
150. Hammerman KJ et al: Pulmonary cryptococcosis: clinical forms and treatment: a Center for Disease Control cooperative mycoses study, *Am Rev Respir Dis* 108:1116, 1973.
151. McDonnell JM, Hutchins GM: Pulmonary cryptococcosis, *Hum Pathol* 16:121, 1985.
152. Baker RD: The primary pulmonary lymph node complex of cryptococcosis, *Am J Clin Pathol* 65:83, 1976.
153. Chu AC, Hay RJ, MacDonald DM: Cutaneous cryptococcosis, *Br J Dermatol* 103:95, 1980.
154. Noble RC, Fajardo LF: Primary cutaneous cryptococcosis: review and morphologic study, *Am J Clin Pathol* 57:13, 1972.
155. Larsen RA, Leal MAE, Chan LS: Fluconazole compared with amphotericin B plus flucytosine for cryptococcal meningitis in AIDS: a randomized trial, *Ann Intern Med* 113:183, 1990.
156. Sugar AM, Saunders C: Oral fluconazole as suppressive therapy of disseminated cryptococcosis in patients with acquired immunodeficiency syndrome, *Am J Med* 85:481, 1988.
157. Stoetzner H, Kemmer C: The morphology of *Cryptococcus neoformans* in human cryptococcosis: a light-, phase-contrast and electron-microscopic study, *Mycopathol Mycol Appl* 45:327, 1971.
158. Gutierrez F, Fu YS, Lurie HI: Cryptococcus histologically resembling histoplasmosis: a light and electron microscopical study, *Arch Pathol* 99:347, 1975.
159. Harding SA et al: Pulmonary infection with capsule-deficient *Cryptococcus neoformans, Virch Arch [B] (Pathol Anat)* 382:113, 1979.
160. Ro JY, Lee SS, Ayala AG: Advantage of Fontana-Masson stain in capsule-deficient cryptococcal infection, *Arch Pathol Lab Med* 111:53, 1987.
161. Farmer SG, Komorowski RA: Histologic response to capsule-deficient *Cryptococcus neoformans, Arch Pathol* 96:383, 1973.

Fusariosis

162. Wheeler MS et al: *Fusarium* infection in burned patients, *Am J Clin Pathol* 75:304, 1981.
163. Anaissie E et al: *Fusarium:* a newly recognized fungal pathogen in immunosuppressed patients, *Cancer* 57:2141, 1986.
164. Anaissie E et al: The emerging role of *Fusarium* infections in patients with cancer, *Medicine* (Baltimore) 67:77, 1988.
165. Blazar BR et al: Invasive *Fusarium* infections in bone marrow transplant patients, *Am J Med* 77:645, 1984.
166. Richardson SE et al: Disseminated fusarial infection in the immunocompromised host, *Rev Infect Dis* 10:1171, 1988.
167. Venditti M et al: Invasive *Fusarium solani* infections in patients with acute leukemia, *Rev Infect Dis* 10:653, 1988.
168. Young NA et al: Disseminated infection by *Fusarium moniliforme* during treatment for malignant lymphoma, *J Clin Microbiol* 7:589, 1978.

Geotrichosis

169. Sheehy TW, Honeycutt BK, Spency JT: *Geotrichum* septicemia, *J Am Med Assoc* 235:1035, 1976.
170. Fishbach RS, White ML, Finegold SM: Bronchopulmonary geotrichosis, *Am Rev Respir Dis* 108:1388, 1973.
171. Ghamande AR, Landis FB, Snider GL: Bronchial geotrichosis with fungemia complicating bronchial carcinoma, *Chest* 59:98, 1971.
172. Chang WWL, Buerger L: Disseminated geotrichosis, *Arch Intern Med* 113:356, 1964.
173. Jagirdar J, Geller SA, Bottone EJ: *Geotrichum candidum* as a tissue invasive human pathogen, *Hum Pathol* 12:668, 1981.
174. Kassamali H et al: Disseminated *Geotrichum candidum* infection, *J Clin Microbiol* 25:1782, 1987.

Histoplasmosis capsulati

175. Domer JE, Moser SA: Histoplasmosis: a review, *Rev Med Vet Mycol* 15:159, 1980.
176. Goodwin RA Jr, Des Prez RM: Histoplasmosis: state of the art, *Am Rev Respir Dis* 117:929, 1978.
177. Schwarz J: *Histoplasmosis,* New York, 1981, Praeger Publishers.
178. Sarosi GA, Davies SF: *Histoplasma capsulatum* pneumonia. In Pennington JE, editor: *Respiratory infections: diagnosis and management,* New York, 1983, Raven Press.
179. Vanek J, Schwarz J: The gamut of histoplasmosis, *Am J Med* 50:89, 1971.
180. Kauffman CA et al: Histoplasmosis in immunosuppressed patients, *Am J Med* 64:923, 1978.
181. Miller RL et al: Localized oral histoplasmosis: a regional manifestation of mild chronic disseminated histoplasmosis, *Oral Surg* 53:367, 1982.
182. Goodwin RA Jr et al: Chronic pulmonary histoplasmosis, *Medicine (Baltimore)* 55:413, 1976.

183. Straus SE, Jacobson ES: The spectrum of histoplasmosis in a general hospital: a review of 55 cases diagnosed at Barnes Hospital between 1966 and 1977, *Am J Med Sci* 279:147, 1980.
184. Walsh TJ, Catchatourian R, Cohen H: Disseminated histoplasmosis complicating bone marrow transplantation, *Am J Clin Pathol* 79:509, 1983.
185. Bonner JR et al: Disseminated histoplasmosis in patients with the acquired immune deficiency syndrome, *Arch Intern Med* 144:2178, 1984.
186. Case records of the Massachusetts General Hospital: A 27-year-old man with AIDS, a cough, fever, and pulmonary infiltrates, *N Engl J Med* 325:1228, 1991.
187. Kurtin PL et al: Histoplasmosis in patients with the acquired immunodeficiency syndrome: hematologic and bone marrow manifestations, *Am J Clin Pathol* 93:367, 1990.
188. Mandell W, Goldberg DM, Neu HC: Histoplasmosis in patients with the acquired immune deficiency syndrome, *Am J Med* 81:974, 1986.
189. Wheat LJ, Slama TG, Zeckel ML: Histoplasmosis in the acquired immune deficiency syndrome, *Am J Med* 78:203, 1985.
190. Johnson P, Sarosi G: Current therapy of major fungal diseases of the lung, *Infect Dis Clin North Am* 5:635, 1991.
191. Slama TG: Treatment of disseminated and progressive cavitary histoplasmosis with ketoconazole. Proceedings of a symposium on new developments in therapy for the mycoses, *Am J Med* 74:70, 1983.
192. Eggleston JC: Sclerosing mediastinitis, *Progr Surg Pathol* 2:1, 1980.
193. Baker RD: Histoplasmosis in routine autopsies, *Am J Clin Pathol* 41:457, 1964.
194. Binford CH: Histoplasmosis: tissue reactions and morphologic variations of the fungus, *Am J Clin Pathol* 25:25, 1955.
195. Hutton JP et al: Hyphal forms of *Histoplasma capsulatum:* a common manifestation of intravascular infections, *Arch Pathol Lab Med* 109:330, 1985.
196. Henochowicz S et al: Histoplasmosis diagnosed on peripheral blood smear from a patient with AIDS, *JAMA* 253:3148, 1985.

Histoplasmosis duboisii

197. Clark BM, Greenwood BM: Pulmonary lesions in African histoplasmosis, *J Trop Med Hyg* 71:4, 1968.
198. Cockshott WP, Lucas AO: Histoplasmosis duboisii, *Q J Med* 33:223, 1964.
199. Lanceley JL, Lunn HF, Wilson AMM: Histoplasmosis in an African child, *J Pediatr* 59:756, 1961.
200. Lobdell DH, Cappiello MA, Riccio FJ: African histoplasmosis in Connecticut, *Conn Med* 46:187, 1982.
201. Lunn HF: A case of histoplasmosis of bone in East Africa, *J Trop Med Hyg* 63:175, 1960.
202. Shore RN et al: African histoplasmosis in the United States, *JAMA* 245:734, 1981.
203. Williams AO, Lawson EA, Lucas AO: African histoplasmosis due to *Histoplasma duboisii*, *Arch Pathol* 92:306, 1971.

Malasseziasis (systemic)

204. Dankner WM et al: *Malassezia* fungemia in neonates and adults: complication of hyperalimentation, *Rev Infect Dis* 9:743, 1987.
205. Shek YH et al: *Malassezia furfur:* disseminated infection in premature infants, *Am J Clin Pathol* 92:595, 1989.
206. Marcon MJ, Powell DA: Epidemiology, diagnosis, and management of *Malassezia furfur* systemic infection, *Diagn Microbiol Infect Dis* 7:161, 1987.
207. Marcon MJ, Powell DA: Human infections due to *Malassezia* spp, *Clin Microbiol Rev* 5:101, 1992.
208. Redline RW et al: Systemic *Malassezia furfur* infections in patients receiving intralipid therapy, *Hum Pathol* 16:815, 1985.

Paracoccidioidomycosis

209. San-Blas G.: Paracoccidioidomycosis and its etiologic agent *Paracoccidioides brasiliensis*, *J Med Vet Mycol* 31:99, 1993.
210. Murray HW, Littman ML, Roberts RB: Disseminated paracoccidioidomycosis (South American blastomycosis) in the United States, *Am J Med* 56:209, 1974.
211. Restrepo A et al: Paracoccidioidomycosis (South American blastomycosis): a study of 39 cases observed in Medellín, Colombia, *Am J Trop Med Hyg* 19:68, 1970.
212. Giraldo R et al: Pathogenesis of paracoccidioidomycosis: a model based on the study of 46 patients, *Mycopathologia* 58:63, 1976.
213. Londero AT, Melo IS: Paracoccidioidomycosis in childhood: a critical review, *Mycopathologia* 82:49, 1983.
214. Londero AT, Ramos CD, Lopes JOS: Progressive pulmonary paracoccidioidomycosis: a study of 34 cases observed in Rio Grande do Sul (Brazil), *Mycopathologia* 63:53, 1978.
215. Londero AT, Severo LC: The gamut of progressive pulmonary paracoccidioidomycosis, *Mycopathologia* 75:65, 1981.
216. Brummer E, Castañeda E, Restrepo A: Paracoccidioidomycosis: an update, *Clin Microbiol Rev* 6:89, 1993.
217. Salfelder K, Doehnert G, Doehnert HR: Paracoccidioidomycosis: anatomic study with complete autopsies, *Virchows Arch [A] (Pathol Anat)* 348:51, 1969.
218. Tuder RM et al: Pathology of the human pulmonary paracoccidioidomycosis, *Mycopathologia* 92:179, 1985.
219. Londero AT, Severo LC, Ramos CD: Small forms and hyphae of *Paracoccidioides brasiliensis* in human tissue, *Mycopathologia* 72:17, 1980.

Penicilliosis marneffei

220. Pitt JI: *The genus Penicillium and its teleomorphic states Eupenicillium and Talaromyces*, New York, 1979, Academic Press.
221. Deng Z, Connor DH: Progressive disseminated penicilliosis caused by *Penicillium marneffei:* report of eight cases and differentiation of the causative organism from *Histoplasma capsulatum*, *Am J Clin Pathol* 84:323, 1985.
222. DiSalvo AF, Fickling AM, Ajello L: Infection caused by *Penicillium marneffei:* description of first natural infection in man, *Am J Clin Pathol* 60:259, 1973.
223. Jayanetra P et al: Penicilliosis marneffei in Thailand: report of five human cases, *Am J Trop Med Hyg* 33:637, 1984.
224. Pautler KB, Padhye AA, Ajello L: Imported penicilliosis marneffei in the United States: report of a second human infection, *Sabouraudia* 22:433, 1984.
225. So S et al: A case of invasive penicilliosis in Hong Kong with immunologic evaluation, *Am Rev Respir Dis* 131:662, 1985.
226. Tsui WMS, Tsang DNC: Disseminated *Penicillium marneffei* infection in HIV-infected subjects, *Histopathology* 20:287, 1992.

Pseudallescheriasis

227. Travis LB, Roberts GD, Wilson WR: Clinical significance of *Pseudallescheria boydii:* a review of 10 years' experience, *Mayo Clin Proc* 60:531, 1985.
228. Schwartz DA: Organ-specific variation in the morphology of the fungomas (fungus balls) of *Pseudallescheria boydii*, *Arch Pathol Lab Med* 113:476, 1989.
229. DeMent SH et al: Pulmonary, cardiac, and thyroid involvement in disseminated *Pseudallescheria boydii*, *Arch Pathol Lab Med* 108:859, 1984.
230. Enggano IL et al: *Pseudallescheria boydii* in a patient with acute lymphoblastic leukemia, *Arch Pathol Lab Med* 108:619, 1984.
231. Smith AG et al: Systemic pseudallescheriasis in a patient with acute myelocytic leukemia, *Mycopathologia* 90:85, 1985.
232. Dworzack DL et al: *Pseudallescheria boydii* brain abscess: association with near-drowning and efficacy of high-dose, prolonged miconazole therapy in patients with multiple abscesses, *Medicine* (Baltimore) 68:218, 1989.

Torulopsosis

233. Aisner J et al: *Torulopsis glabrata* infections in patients with cancer: increasing incidence and relationship to colonization, *Am J Med* 61:23, 1976.
234. Grimley PM, Wright LD, Jennings AE: *Torulopsis glabrata* infection in man, *Am J Clin Pathol* 43:216, 1965.
235. Heffner DK, Franklin WA: Endocarditis caused by *Torulopsis glabrata*, *Am J Clin Pathol* 70:420, 1978.
236. Hickey WF, Sommerville LH, Schoen FJ: Disseminated *Candida glabrata:* report of a uniquely severe infection and a literature review, *Am J Clin Pathol* 80:724, 1983.

237. Rodriguez R et al: *Torulopsis glabrata* fungemia during prolonged intravenous alimentation, *N Engl J Med* 284:540, 1971.
238. Valdivieso M et al: Fungemia due to *Torulopsis glabrata* in the compromised host, *Cancer* 38:1750, 1976.

Trichosporonosis

239. Winston DJ et al: Disseminated *Trichosporon capitatum* infection in an immunosuppressed host, *Arch Intern Med* 137:1192, 1977.
240. Martino P et al: *Blastoschizomyces capitatus:* an emerging cause of invasive fungal disease in leukemia pataients, *Rev Infect Dis* 12:570, 1990.
241. Hoy J et al: *Trichosporon beigelii* infection: a review, *Rev Infect Dis* 8:959, 1986.
242. Walling DM, McGraw DJ, Merz WG et al: Disseminated infection with *Trichosporon beigelii, Rev Infect Dis* 9:1013, 1987.
243. Walsh TJ et al: Trichosporonosis in patients with neoplastic disease, *Medicine* (Baltimore) 65:268, 1986.
244. Leblond V et al: Systemic infections with *Trichosporon beigelii (cutaneum):* report of three new cases, *Cancer* 58:2399, 1986.
245. Evans HL et al: Systemic mycosis due to *Trichosporon cutaneum:* a report of two additional cases, *Cancer* 45:367, 1980.
246. Gold JWM et al: Systemic infection with *Trichosporon cutaneum* in a patient with acute leukemia, *Cancer* 48:2163, 1981.
247. Kobayashi M et al: Immunohistochemical identification of *Trichosporon beigelii* in histologic sections by immunoperoxidase method, *Am J Clin Pathol* 89:100, 1988.

Zygomycosis

248. Lehrer RI, moderator: Mucormycosis, *Ann Intern Med* 93 (pt 1): 93, 1980.
249. Meyer RD, Rosen P, Armstrong D: Phycomycosis complicating leukemia and lymphoma, *Ann Intern Med* 77:871, 1972.
250. Chandler FW et al: Zygomycosis: report of four cases with formation of chlamydoconidia in tissue, *Am J Clin Pathol* 84:99, 1985.
251. Straatsma BR, Zimmerman LE, Gass JDM: Phycomycosis: a clinicopathologic study of fifty-one cases, *Lab Invest* 11:963, 1962.
252. Ingram CW et al: Disseminated zygomycosis: report of four cases and review, *Rev Infect Dis* 11:741, 1989.
253. Bigby TD et al: Clinical spectrum of pulmonary mucormycosis, *Chest* 89:435, 1986.
254. Lyon DT et al: Phycomycosis of the gastrointestinal tract, *Am J Gastroenterol* 72:379, 1979.
255. Neame P, Rayner D: Mucormycosis: a report on twenty-two cases, *Arch Pathol* 70:261, 1960.
256. Baker RD, Seabury JH, Schneidau JD: Subcutaneous and cutaneous mucormycosis and subcutaneous phycomycosis, *Lab Invest* 11:1091, 1962.
257. Gartenberg G et al: Hospital acquired mucormycosis *(Rhizopus rhizopodiformis)* of skin and subcutaneous tissue: epidemiology, mycology, and treatment, *N Engl J Med* 299:1115, 1978.
258. Marchevsky AM et al: The changing spectrum of disease, etiology, and diagnosis of mucromycosis, *Hum Pathol* 11:457, 1980.
259. Virmani R, Connor DH, McAllister HA: Cardiac mucormycosis: a report of five patients and review of 14 previously reported cases, *Am J Clin Pathol* 78:42, 1982.
260. Parfrey NA: Improved diagnosis and prognosis of mucromycosis: a clinicopathologic study of 33 cases, *Medicine (Baltimore)* 65:113, 1986.
261. Baker RD: The phycomycoses, *Ann NY Acad Sci* 174:592, 1970.
262. Williams AO: Pathology of phycomycosis due to *Entomophthora* and *Basidiobolus* species, *Arch Pathol* 87:13, 1969.
263. Joe LK, Eng NIT: Subcutaneous phycomycosis: a new disease found in Indonesia, *Ann NY Acad Sci* 89:4, 1960.
264. Gilbert EF, Khoury GH, Pore RS: Histopathological identification of *Entomophthora* phycomycosis: deep mycotic infection in an infant, *Arch Pathol* 90:583, 1970.

Infections that resemble mycoses

Actinomycosis

265. Brown JR: Human actinomycosis: a study of 181 subjects, *Hum Pathol* 4:319, 1973.
266. Causey WA: Actinomycosis. Part 3 of *Infections of the nervous system, Handbook of clinical neurology*, vol. 35, Amsterdam, 1978, North Holland Publishing.
267. Bennhoff DF: Actinomycosis: diagnostic and therapeutic considerations and a review of 32 cases, *Laryngoscope* 94:1198, 1984.
268. Kanya KJ: Cervico-facial actinomycosis (a case report), *J Oral Med* 40:166, 1985.
269. Suzuki JB, Delisle AL: Pulmonary actinomycosis of periodontal origin, *J Periodontol* 55:581, 1984.
270. Berardi RS: Abdominal actinomycosis, *Surg Gynecol Obstet* 149:257. 1979.
271. Bhagavan BS, Gupta PK: Genital actinomycosis and intrauterine contraceptive devices, *Hum Pathol* 9:567, 1978.
272. Gupta PK: Intrauterine contraceptive devices: vaginal cytology, pathologic changes and clinical implications, *Acta Cytol* 26:571, 1982.
273. Nayar M et al: Incidence of actinomycetes infection in women using intrauterine contraceptive devices, *Acta Cytol* 29:111, 1985.
274. Hotchi M, Schwarz J.: Characterization of actinomycotic granules by architecture and staining methods, *Arch Pathol* 93:392, 1972.
275. Oddo D, González S: Actinomycosis and nocardiosis: a morphologic study of 17 cases, *Pathol Res Pract* 181:320, 1986.
276. Robboy SJ, Vickery AL: Tinctorial and morphologic properties distinguishing actinomycosis and nocardiosis, *N Engl J Med* 282:593, 1970.

Botryomycosis

277. Richmond I, Mene A: Renal botryomycosis, *Histopathology* 20:67, 1992.
278. Winslow DJ: Botryomycosis, *Am J Pathol* 35:153, 1959.
279. Toth IR, Kazal HL: Botryomycosis in acquired immunodeficiency syndrome, *Arch Pathol Lab Med* 111:246, 1987.
280. Winslow DJ, Chamblin SA: Disseminated visceral botryomycosis: report of a fatal case probably caused by *Pseudomonas aeruginosa, Am J Clin Pathol* 33:43, 1960.

Nocardiosis

281. Beaman BL et al: Nocardia infections in the United States, 1972-1974, *J Infect Dis* 134:286, 1976.
282. Causey WA, Lee R: Vinken PJ, Bruyn GW, editors: Nocardiosis. In *Handbook of clinical neurology*, Amsterdam, 1978, North Holland Publishing Co.
283. Berd D: *Nocardia brasiliensis* infection in the United States: a report of nine cases and a review of the literature, *Am J Clin Pathol* 60:254, 1973.
284. Bradsher RW, Monson TP, Steele, RW: Brain abscess due to *Nocardia caviae:* report of a fatal outcome associataed with abnormal phagocyte function, *Am J Clin Pathol* 78:124, 1982.
285. Simpson GL et al: Nocardial infections in the immunocompromised host: a detailed study in a defined population, *Rev Infect Dis* 3:492, 1981.
286. Curry WA: Human nocardiosis: a clinical review with selected case reports, *Arch Intern Med* 140:818, 1980.
287. Jonsson S et al: Recurrent *Nocardia* pneumonia in an adult with chronic granulomatous disease, *Am Rev Respir Dis* 133:932, 1986.
288. Young LS et al: *Nocardia asteroides* infection complicating neoplastic disease, *Am J Med* 50:356, 1971.
289. Frazier AR, Rosenow EC III, Roberts GD: Nocardiosis: a review of 25 cases occurring during 24 months, *Mayo Clin Proc* 50:657, 1975.
290. Stevens DA: Clinical and clinical laboratory aspects of nocardial infection, *J Hyg* 91:377, 1983.
291. Pizzolato P et al: Nocardiosis of the brain: report of three cases, *Am J Clin Pathol* 36:151, 1961.
292. Boudoulas O, Camisa C: *Nocardia asteroides* infection with dissemination to skin and joints, *Arch Dermatol* 121:898, 1985.
293. Kalb RE, Kaplan MH, Grossman ME: Cutaneous nocardiosis: case reports and review, *J Am Acad Dermatol* 13:125, 1985.
294. Adams HG et al: Synergistic action of trimethoprim and sulfamethoxazole for *Nocardia asteroides:* efficacious therapy in five patients, *Am J Med Sci* 287:8, 1984.
295. Palmer DL, Harvey RL, Wheeler JK: Diagnostic and therapeutic considerations in *Nocardia asteroides* infection, *Medicine (Baltimore)* 53:391, 1974.

Protothecosis

296. Sudman MS: Protothecosis: a critical review, *Am J Clin Pathol* 61:10, 1974.
297. Connor DH, Gibson DW, Ziefer A: Diagnostic features of three unusual infections: micronemiasis, pheomycotic cyst, and protothecosis. In Majno G, Cotran RS, Kaufman N, editors: *Current topics in inflammation and infection,* International Academy of Pathology monogr no 23, Baltimore, 1982, Williams & Wilkins.
298. Tindall JP, Fetter BF: Infections caused by achloric algae (protothecosis), *Arch Dermatol* 104:490, 1971.
299. Davies RR, Wilkinson JL: Human protothecosis: supplementary studies, *Ann Trop Med Parasitol* 61:112, 1967.
300. Nosanchuk JS, Greenberg RD: Protothecosis of the olecranon bursa caused by achloric algae, *Am J Clin Pathol* 59:567, 1973.
301. Cox GE, Wilson JD, Brown P: Protothecosis: a case of disseminated algal infection, *Lancet* 2:379, 1974.
302. Chan JC et al: Visceral protothecosis mimicking sclerosing cholangitis in an immunocompetent host: successful antifungal therapy, *Rev Infect Dis* 12:802, 1990.
303. Jones JW et al: Green algal infection in a human, *Am J Clin Pathol* 80:102, 1983.
304. Chandler FW, Kaplan W, Callaway CS: Differentiation between *Prototheca* and morphologically similar green algae in tissue, *Arch Pathol Lab Med* 102:353, 1978.

38 Protozoal Diseases

Yezid Gutierrez
Franz von Lichtenberg

The Protozoa belong to the animal kingdom because they have organelles, such as a eukaryotic nucleus, Golgi apparatus, mitochondria, endoplasmic reticulum, and others, which make their cell structure similar to that of multicellular animals (Metazoa). This is in contrast to other infectious organisms that lack most of these organelles, making them more primitive phylogenetically. Infections by animal parasites (Protozoa and Metazoa) are commonly referred to as *parasitic infections*, but this term is technically a misnomer because other infectious agents (bacteria, viruses, fungi, rickettsiae, spirochetes, etc) are also "parasites," since they behave in the host in a similar manner. The phenomena of parasitism are wide in the scope in the morbidity they produce in humans.

The parasites classified as Protozoa are composed of a single cell that carries all the functions of feeding, locomotion, and multiplication. The size of a protozoan often requires magnifications of 1000 times or more for proper visualization and study. Like bacteria, the protozoa have the capability to increase their numbers in the host by sexual or asexual multiplication. The Metazoa comprise the "worms" and the "arthropods," and they vary widely in size from hardly visible with the naked eye to many feet in length. The Metazoa generally do not multiply (increase their numbers) in the host. Thus they produce limited infections. Also, the immunologic reactions that they elicit in the host are allergic in type, causing eosinophilia. The intensity of the eosinophilia is related to the degree of interaction between the parasite and the host tissue: metazoa with a migratory phase through the tissues, or residing in the tissues, produce the highest peripheral eosinophil counts.

In this chapter the main protozoa that infect humans are discussed. In the following chapter the metazoan parasites, including the most important arthropods, are studied.

LABORATORY DIAGNOSTIC TECHNIQUES

The diagnosis of parasitic infections is made in the laboratory, almost exclusively by the recognition of the organisms, or their eggs, or their larval stages, based on their morphologic characteristics. In the clinical parasitology laboratory only rarely are cultures performed for diagnosis of infections. Cultures are used in some instances for research purposes or for harvesting large numbers of parasites for preparation of antigens used in serologic diagnosis, or delayed hypersensitivity testing on the skin. A variety of samples are useful in the diagnosis of parasitic infection, as discussed subsequently.

Stools

Parasites in the gastrointestinal tract, the lungs, biliary tree, and portal system manifest themselves in the stools, where the trophozoites and cysts of protozoa, and eggs, larvae, or adult metazoa are routinely searched for and identified under direct microscopic examination. The techniques for collection, preservation, and handling of stool samples are well known, and they should be followed each time a parasitic infection is suspected clinically in a patient, necessitating confirmation by the laboratory. The techniques used for finding and identifying parasites in the stools are the wet preparations and the concentration of stools. These techniques are simple and were described and perfected many years ago, but they are still in use today. Wet stool preparations on microscope slides made by diluting a small amount of stools either in saline solution or in iodine solution for direct observation under the microscope. The saline solution allows study of protozoa or larvae under living conditions, permitting observations of movement and other characteristics necessary for diagnosis. The iodine preparations usually destroy the vegetative forms of the protozoan, but stain its cysts and the eggs and larvae of the metazoan. The concentration of parasitic stages in the stools are made by different techniques, such as sedimentation, formalin ethyl acetate, and others, the use of which permits the recovery of low numbers of organisms. Special methods for staining different protozoa are available and are used routinely in the laboratory: the trichrome stain for intestinal protozoa, or the Ziehl-Neelsen/Kinyoun stain for *Cryptosporidium* organisms. Finally, in some instances the antigens of the parasite may be investigated in the stools, but these technologies have not become routine in the clinical laboratory.

Blood

Blood samples are used for the identification of protozoa inhabiting the blood or the tissues and of some metazoa, such as filarial worms. The most important organisms diagnosed in blood are the malarial parasites, the trypanosomes, and some of the filarids (see below). Fresh, unclotted blood is the preferred sample, which in the laboratory is used for preparation of regular smears, or thick smears (a large drop of blood in a 1 cm square of the glass slide), which are stained with Giemsa or other blood stain and examined under the microscope. The microfilariae of the filarids can be concentrated by the use of the Knott technique (2 ml of blood in 8 ml of 1% formalin; shake well, centrifuge, and examine the sediment), by which smears for staining can be prepared.

Serum

Every serologic technique known has been adapted to the diagnosis of parasitic infections, but often with unsatisfactory results, because of the expense, the lack of sensitivity and specificity, or both. Moreover in most parasitic infections an abnormal serologic finding can be the only indication of the infection, requiring confirmation by the recovery of the parasite. Serologic techniques may provide some help for the clinician needing to make therapeutic decisions. The best use of serology in parasitology is for seroepidemiology where the discovery of the extent of infection in a community is valuable information. In the clinical laboratory today, serology is often used to determine prior exposure to *Toxoplasma* organisms in an individual who has been found positive for the human immunodeficiency virus, or in a woman who becomes pregnant in areas of the world where transmission of *Toxoplasma* organisms is high. Occasionally, the diagnosis of visceral larva migrans, schistosomiasis, or other parasitic infections requires serologic tests for the clinical management of the patient.

Other fluids

Parasites are searched for in spinal fluid, pleural and peritoneal effusions, urine, vaginal secretions, pus from abscesses or fistulas, saliva, and duodenal contents, using the classic techniques of direct visualization under the microscope in fresh or stain preparations.

Tissue sections

Biopsy specimens and tissues recovered during the autopsy are frequently studied for the diagnosis of parasitic infections in humans and animals. In these instances the pathologist is required to identify either protozoan or metazoan organisms, which because of their larger size are seen in longitudinal, oblique, or cross sections. Some of these findings are incidental in autopsy specimens or in biopsy specimens taken for reasons other than the diagnosis of a parasitic infection. The use of biopsies for the diagnosis of parasites is most frequently resorted to for trichinosis, schistosomiasis, visceral and cutaneous leishmaniasis, some cases of toxoplasmosis, and filariasis.

PROTOZOA

The Protozoa are a large and diverse subkingdom of unicellular animals living as free organisms in the environment or as parasites on other animals or on plants. Some of these organisms are parasitic in humans, producing morbidity and some mortality in many areas of the world; the morbidity caused by malaria, African trypanosomiasis, and leishmaniasis is legendary. In recent years some protozoan infections have become a significant clinical management problems in patients with the acquired immunodeficiency syndrome (AIDS), and new protozoan species have been discovered in these individuals, challenging both the clinician and the pathologist to learn about their diagnosis, treatment, and management.

The Protozoa are classified into many groups, but those of medical importance fall into five groups generally referred to as the flagellates, the amebas, the ciliated, apicomplexan, and microsporidian and related organisms.[1] Their life cycles may be either direct or indirect using a biologic vector such as a blood-sucking arthropod in which a necessary part of the development of the organism takes place. A clear understanding of protozoan infections and their diagnosis in humans requires knowledge of their morphologic characteristics, as well as their geographic distribution. The student of pathology needs many hours of work at the microscope to become familiar with the host reaction to parasites and their cytologic characteristics.[2] The techniques of serology and immunohistochemistry are also helpful but are not yet widely available outside specialized laboratories.

FLAGELLATES

The pathogenic flagellates of humans are *Giardia lamblia, Trichomonas vaginalis,* the *Trypanosoma brucei* group, *T. cruzi,* and the large number of species of *Leishmania,* producing both visceral and mucocutaneous diseases. In addition, other nonpathogenic flagellates are commonly found as commensals in healthy individuals and need to be recognized to be differentiated from pathogens. The nonpathogenic protozoa include *Trichomonas tenax* in the mouth and *T. hominis, Chilomastix mesnili,* and *Retortamonas intestinalis* in the intestine. *Dientamoeba fragilis* considered for many years as belonging to the amebas, is now known to be a flagellated organism, and its lack of pathogenicity is now in question.

Giardia lamblia

Giardia lamblia inhabits the duodenum, where the trophozoites are attached to the surface of the enterocytes. The parasite is pear shaped and has two nuclei and four pairs of flagella. It is flattened dorsoventrally, and on the anterior portion of the ventral surface it has an attachment disk, an organelle seen better with the electron microscope (Fig. 38-1, *A*). In the duodenum the parasites multiply by longitudinal division and begin forming cysts, which are evacuated with the feces. The cysts endure adverse environmental conditions and when ingested with food and water by the appropriate host produce the infection.[2] Contaminated water is the most important source of infections and results in local epidemics, some of which have occurred in the United States.[3,4] The role of animals in the transmission of *Giardia* was recognized when it was determined that the species of *Giardia* in animals and humans were the same.[5] *Giardia* is the most commonly diagnosed protozoan in the United States, and its prevalence is increasing.[6]

Clinical findings

Giardiasis in underdeveloped areas is an infection of children.[7] The infection usually results in a mild to severe diarrhea characterized by bulky, foamy stools containing undigested food and large amounts of lipids; if chronic, it resembles sprue. After the first bout of symptoms the patient usually becomes resistant to the parasite, and subsequent reinfections do not produce symptoms. This explains the large number of asymptomatic cyst carriers (up to 60%) in some areas of the world. In developed countries where the prevalence of the infection is very low, most of the population is susceptible to the disease, and symptomatic cases are found not only in children but also in adults. The clinical manifestations in adults are varied, with diarrhea or with symptoms suggestive of a peptic ulcer.[2,8] The mechanism for the production of symptoms in humans by *Giardia* is not known.

Pathology

The tissue pathology caused by giardiasis is variable and does not correlate with the symptoms of the patient. In duodenal biopsy specimens the appearance ranges from normal (Fig. 38-1, *B*) to severe distortion and fusion of the villi, inflammatory infiltration specially by mononuclear cells (lymphocytes and plasma cells), and increased mitotic index. The picture is nonspecific, and only the presence of the parasites allows a definitive diagnosis. In tissue sections trophozoites of Giardia are found in the lumen (Fig. 38-1, *B*), sometimes attached to the epithelial cells, but not in the tissues. The shape of the organisms varies with the orientation of the section, from elongated to rounded or semilunar. The presence of organelles inside the parasites, such as nuclei, axostile, and flagellar rests, should always be recognized for proper identification; special stains are not helpful, and electron microscopy is not necessary.[2] Taking duodenal biopsy specimens for the sole purpose of diagnosing giardiasis is not indicated. But the anatomic pathologist may encounter such specimens if the clinical symptoms dictate a biopsy. Usually, stool samples are preferred for diagnosis because the recognition of cysts and trophozoites in stools is a simple procedure.[8] Three samples of stool taken at intervals of 1 to 2 days usually suffice. If the first sample is positive, the patient should be instructed to disregard collecting the other. If the three samples are negative and it is still suspected that the patient has the infection, the collection of samples should be repeated 10 days to 2 weeks later because elimination of *Giardia* cysts in the stools is sometimes cyclical. The "string test" is no more effective than the stool examination (the patient swallows a capsule with a string after the end of the string has been taped to the cheek; the capsule reaches the duodenum where it is left for 24 hours, retrieved, and sent to the laboratory for examination). Testing for anti-*Giardia* antibodies in serum, or for Giardia antigen in the stools, are methods too expensive for the routine laboratory.[8] Brushing of the duodenal mucosa, followed by prepara-

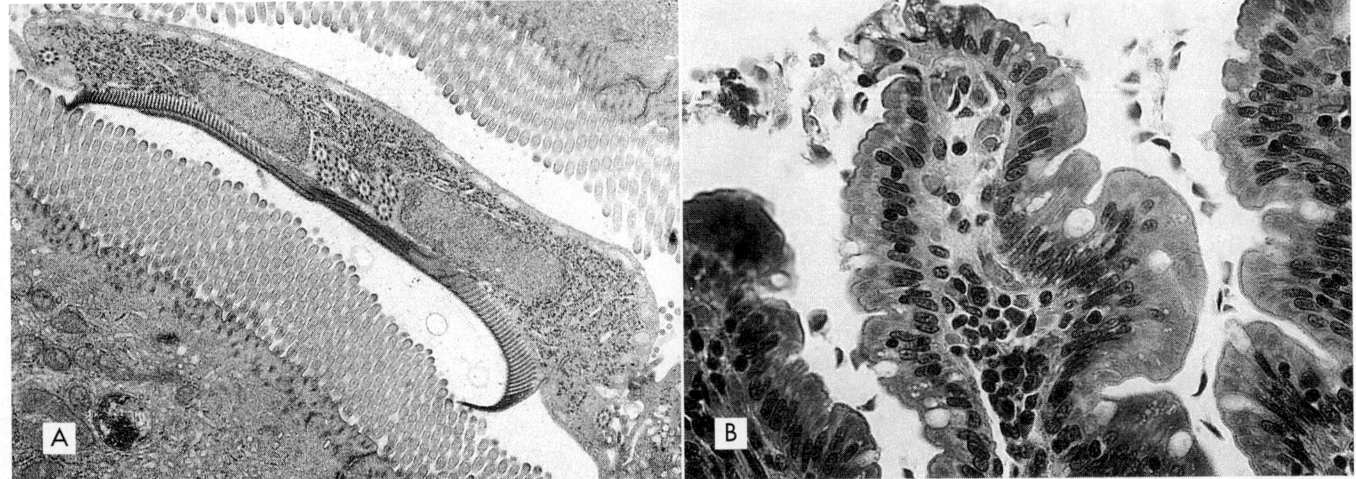

Fig. 38-1 *Giardia lamblia* in duodenum. **A,** Transmission electron microscopy photomicrograph, showing a transverse section of the parasite, demonstrating the attachment disk. Notice the lack of changes in the brush border. **B,** Histologic section demonstrating the organisms in the lumen. Their separation from the surface is artifactual because of fixation and processing.

tion of cytologic preparations, is sometimes attempted for diagnosis.

Trichomonas vaginalis

Trichomonas vaginalis is a flagellated organism with a direct life cycle, in which a cystic stage is lacking. The trophozoites are passed directly from one host to another most often during sexual intercourse. The prevalence of *Trichomonas* infection in the general population is unknown but was found to be high in surveys among women consulting for vaginal discharges, for sexually transmitted infections, or for other gynecologic problems. Surveys among lesbians are lacking, and the prevalence in males is also unknown and often underestimated or denied.

Clinical findings

Most commonly, trichomoniasis in women is an asymptomatic infection, found in 2% to 3% of healthy women having routine annual checkups. Some women present with a moderate vaginal discharge, but others may have vaginitis characterized by leukorrhea, pruritus, and burning sensation of the vagina and vulva; in the worst forms of vulvitis, erythema extending to the inguinal area is present. Symptoms are usually heightened during the estrogenic phase of the menstrual cycle. The vaginal discharge is greenish, frothy in character, or purulent, sometimes accompanied by dysuria.[9]

In males *Trichomonas organisms* can colonize the urethra and the prostate gland, producing urethritis and prostatitis, and colonize the preputial sac producing balanitis. The parasites can be recovered from prostatic secretions, spontaneous urethral discharges, and urine. The presenting symptom is usually a nongonococcal discharge of 4 or more weeks in duration, and the diagnosis is made by recovery of the parasites in the discharge fluid.[10] The histopathology anatomy of trichomoniasis in males is unknown.[2]

Pathology

The histologic changes in trichomoniasis are rarely documented but manifest as nonspecific cervicitis and vaginitis, with focal erosions of the mucosa. A reddened mucosa with punctate exudate (strawberry mucosa) is rarely seen. The epithelial surface is covered by coagulated material, mucus, erythrocytes, and white blood cells where the flagellates can be identified. The symptoms and the nature of the discharge often indicate a clinical diagnosis but should be confirmed by the microscopic study of a wet mount of vaginal fluid or by Papanicolaou smears.

The *Trypanosoma brucei* group

African trypanosomiasis is produced by trypanosomes of the *T. brucei* group, which infect both humans and animals exclusively in the tropical areas of the African continent. All members of the *brucei* group are indistinguishable on morphologic grounds, and are referred to as *T. brucei* when found in animals, and as *T. gambiense* or as *T. rhodesiense* when found in humans. Depending on their clinical manifestations and geographic location, these parasites are called *T. gambiense* (if chronic and in West Africa), or *T. rhodesiense* (if acute and in East Africa).[11]

Trypanosomes are flagellates living in the circulatory system, where they multiply by binary fission. They have a slender, elongated body with an undulating membrane supported by a single flagellum arising in the basal body in the posterior end of the body (Fig. 38-2). Next to the basal body is the kinetoplast seen as a dark granule in blood preparations; these stages, circulating in blood, are known as "trypomastigotes." The trypomastigotes of the *brucei* group are polymorphic, and at least three different morphologic types, slender, stout and intermediate, are recognized. The biologic vectors of the *brucei* group are flies belonging to the genus *Glossina* (tsetse flies), which ingest blood. If the blood contains trypomastigotes, the flagellates multiply in the intestine of the fly, invade the salivary glands, and become infective for the next host bitten by the fly.[1] As stated above, the trypomastigotes multiply in the blood of the host, where they survive by periodically changing their antigenic make-up. One antigenic type survives until antibodies are produced, at which time the trypomastigotes begin diminishing in numbers. At this moment another antigenic type arises, probably attributable to selection, and a new cycle begins. This phenomenon causes cyclic parasitemias.

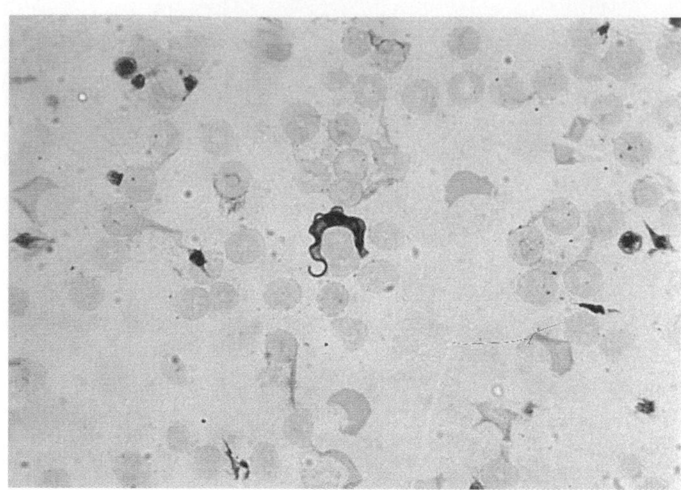

Fig. 38-2 *Trypanosoma brucei* in a blood smear. Trypomastigote. Notice the undulating membrane and the small kinetoplast. (Giemsa stain.)

African trypanosomiasis, or sleeping sickness, often begins with an inoculation chancre, at the site where the fly bites.[12] This lesion is seen more often in individuals from nonendemic areas who travel to Africa and become infected; it is also more common in infections with *T. rhodesiense*. After the initial bite the site becomes erythematous, indurated, and tender. The lesion may last 2 to 3 weeks, during which there is redness, desquamation, and often a central ulceration. After the inoculation chancre subsides, the infection with *T. rhodesiense* follows an acute, rapid course terminating with death. Infections with *T. gambiense* follow a more chronic course, in most cases, with central nervous system symptoms of encephalitis, with lethargy, ataxia, incontinence, lack of propioceptive reflexes, and coma.

The diagnosis of the infection is usually made by the finding of trypomastigotes in blood, spinal fluid sediment, or aspirates of enlarged lymph nodes.[13] Histologic sections of brain show a pronounced meningoencephalitis with meningeal and perivascular mononuclear cell infiltrate specially by lymphocytes and plasma cells (Fig. 38-3).

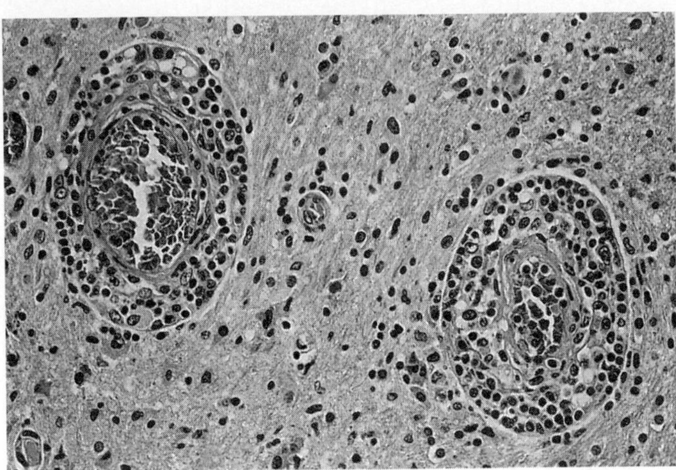

Fig. 38-3 *Trypanosoma brucei.* Section of brain demonstrating the pronounced, nonspecific encephalitis with perivascular mononuclear cell infiltrate.

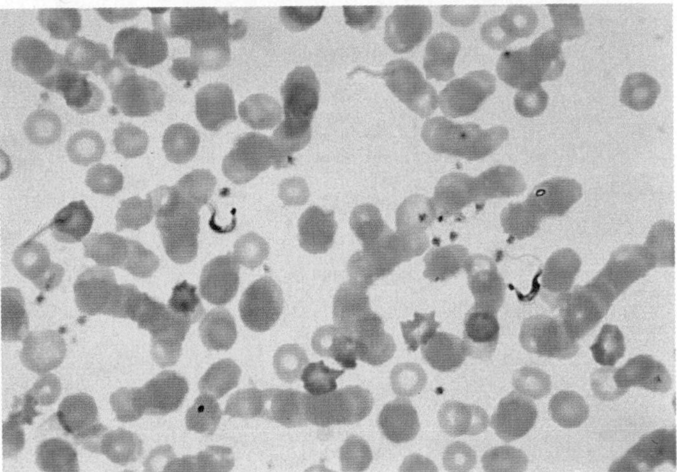

Fig. 38-4 *Trypanosoma cruzi* in a blood smear. Trypomastigote showing the lower number of folds of the undulating membrane and the large kinetoplast. (Giemsa stain.)

Trypanosoma cruzi

The agent of Chagas' disease, or American trypanosomiasis, is *T. cruzi*, a flagellated protozoan living intracellularly in the tissues and extracellularly in the blood of humans and animals. The geographic distribution of *T. cruzi* is restricted to the American continent, from the southern part of the United States to the northern part of Argentina and Chile.[1,2] The vector is a hematophagous reduviid (kissing bug) living in the forest and in poorly constructed, thatched houses. Over 100 different species of reduviids belonging to several genera, *Rhodnius, Triatoma*, and *Panstrongylus*, are good vectors of *T. cruzi*. Because of these ecologic characteristics, the prevalence of Chagas' disease is mostly restricted to areas of rural Latin America, where about 35 million people are infected.

Similarly to the African trypanosomes, the trypomastigotes inhabit the circulating blood, but they do not multiply in blood (Fig. 38-4). The reduviid bug ingests the trypomastigotes at the time of its meal, and the flagellates colonize the intestine of the insect, where they multiply. Infective, metacyclical trypomastigotes develop in the distal part of the intestine and are evacuated with the feces of the insect at the time of its meal. The infected feces of the insect are usually deposited on the skin of the host, from where the flagellates penetrate through lacerated skin, or through normal mucosae, transported by the fingers of the individual, after scratching the site of the bite. In the body, the parasites are capable of entering any type of cell, where they transform into aflagellates known as amastigotes and begin division. The cell harbors the amastigotes within the cytoplasm outside a parasitophorous vacuole, a mechanism that allows the flagellate to escape cellular killing mechanisms.[2] After the cell is filled with amastigotes, the amastigotes begin their transformation into trypomastigotes, at which time the cell is destroyed and the parasites are spilled into the circulation. Trypomastigotes in circulation travel to enter other cells and initiate the cycle again.

Clinical findings

Once an individual is infected with *T. cruzi*, he or she will remain infected, and the consequences of the infection can be lifelong.[14] The initial infection is also characterized by an inoculation chancre in the site of the bite or in the mucosae of the lips, or the mouth, sometimes in the conjunctiva, producing a unilateral conjunctivitis, known as "Romaña's sign." The manifestations of the acute infection vary. Children are most severely affected, often by a myocarditis resulting in a 10% mortality (Fig. 38-5). Adults in endemic areas have fewer or no symptoms, but immigrants or travelers from nonendemic areas may suffer a disease similar to that of children. Chagas' disease has affected individuals with AIDS, causing encephalitis and acute myocarditis.[14]

The chronic phase of the infection is more important. It follows the acute disease and manifests itself in different manners, including the destruction of the effector cells of the parasympathetic nervous system[15] and of the conduction system of the heart, resulting in a variety of defects of transmission of the electric impulses seen in electrocardiographic tracings such as right bundle branch or A-V block, T-wave changes, and low QRS voltages.[15] The destruction of the effector cells of the esophagus results in achalasia and megaesophagus; the destruction of those cells in the colon result in megacolon, similar to the congenital form of aganglionosis, or Hirschsprung's disease. These syndromes are seen mainly in Brazil.

Pathology

The pathologic anatomy of acute American trypanosomiasis is that of a generalized infection with areas of inflammation in all organs, produced by the multiplication of amastigotes and the destruction of the cells. Histologically, nests of intracellular amastigotes are the hallmark of the infection. In chronic infections, the changes are particularly pronounced in the heart, where the destruction of the muscle cells is attributed to formation of autoantibodies against the myocytes.[16] The inflammatory reaction is characterized by mononuclear cells, mostly lymphocytes and plasma cells, with few polymorphonuclear cells. The diagnosis of the infection is done usually in routine, or in thick blood smears.[13] In chronic cases blood cultures are better for recovery of the organisms, which are present in lower and lower numbers as time passes. Serologic tests are excellent because of their specificity and often are the

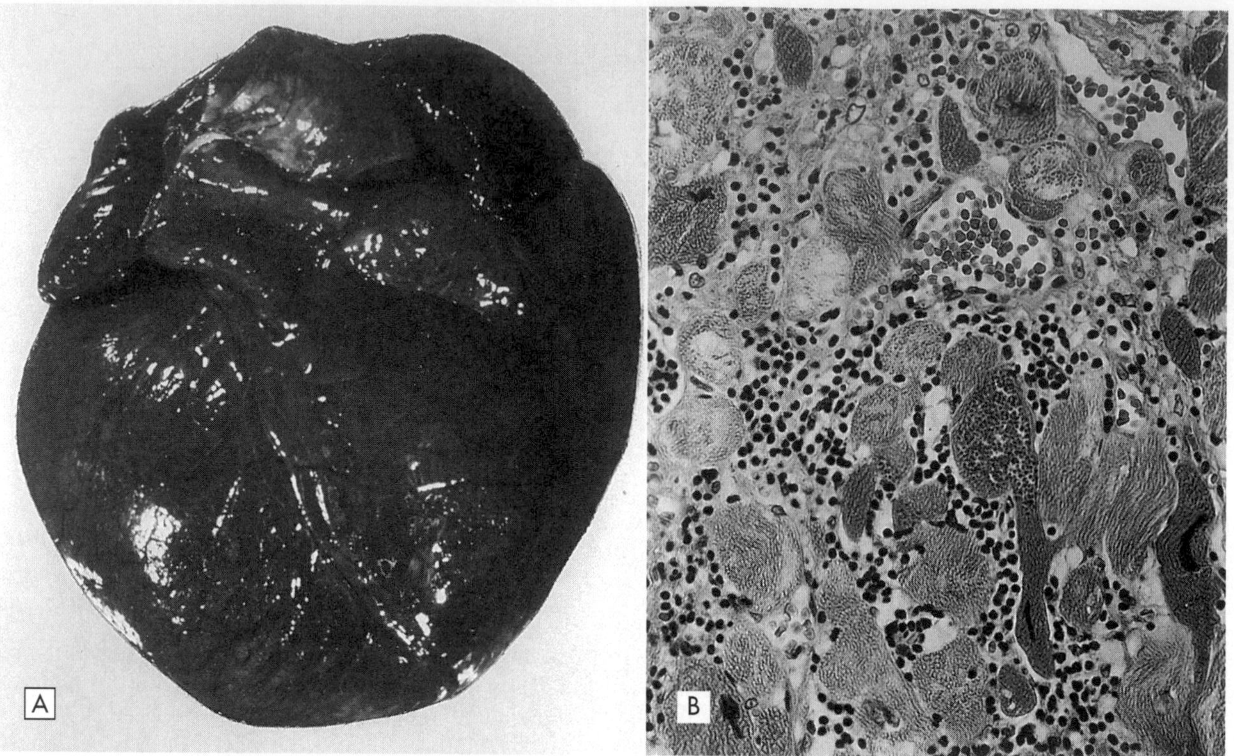

Fig. 38-5 *Trypanosoma cruzi* acute myocarditis. **A,** Gross specimen of heart, illustrating the globose, flabby appearance. **B,** Microscopic section showing destruction of the myocytes, the mononuclear infiltrate, and a nest of parasites tightly packed inside a myocardial fiber.

only manner by which one can diagnose the chronic phase of the infection.[2,13]

Because the infection produced by *T. cruzi* is lifelong, the parasites are always present in blood but unrecoverable by normal laboratory procedures. The contamination of the blood bank supply and congenital infections are real concerns, both in the United States where a large immigrant population of individuals from Central America and South America are living, and especially in these same endemic areas.[17,18]

Visceral leishmaniasis

Visceral leishmaniasis, or kala azar, is an infection produced by several species of leishmaniae, which are flagellates found in cells of the monocyte-macrophage lineage. The infection is prevalent among the poor living in certain parts of India, China, Latin America, the Middle East, southwestern Asia, and Africa. It is also endemic in the Mediterranean area, especially southern France, Italy, Spain, Greece, and other countries, which report sporadic cases.

The three species *Leishmania donovani, L. infantum,* and *L. chagasi* produce infections in the Indian subcontinent, the Mediterranean, and Latin America, respectively. The features of the infection they produce depends on the species, but in southwestern Asia, the Mediterranean, and in the Americas they are mostly infections of children 1 to 4 years of age, or new arrivals to an area.

The leishmaniae that produce visceral infections are mostly zoonotic, with life cycles occurring normally between wild or domestic animals and their vectors, and accidentally infecting humans. However, in some places in India the parasite has been urbanized with transmission occurring in a human-insect-human cycle. The vectors of the parasite are sand flies, belonging to the genus *Lutzomia* in the American continent and to *Phlebotomus* in the Old World. When a vector ingests the amastigotes by feeding on the vertebrate, amastigotes transform rapidly into flagellates (monomastigotes) in the intestinal tract of the fly. When their numbers increase sufficiently to obstruct the anterior part of the intestine, the insect regurgitates the infective organisms into the next vertebrate when it is feeding. The flagellates soon find their way into the macrophages, where they again transform into amastigotes (aflagellates) and begin multiplication.[1,2] In the macrophages, the parasites are contained within a parasitophorous vacuole, where they survive the killing mechanism of the cell by neutralizing the lysosomal enzymes discharged into the vacuole. Another mechanism of survival, directed to the manipulation of the phagocyte, consists in recruitment of immature monocytes, with lesser killing properties, to the infection site.[19]

Clinical findings

Epidemiologic studies indicate that subclinical infections are common. In endemic areas the most commonly affected individuals are the new arrivals and, as stated, the children. Visceral leishmaniasis also has the tendency to occur in epidemics especially after some natural calamity such as famine, floods, or displacement of populations.[20] In individuals with AIDS, the infection has been described as a rapid progressive acute disease.[21,22] The clinical infection is characterized by chronic fever, anorexia, and weight loss. At first, an indurated area in the skin at the site of inoculation is present, followed by ten-

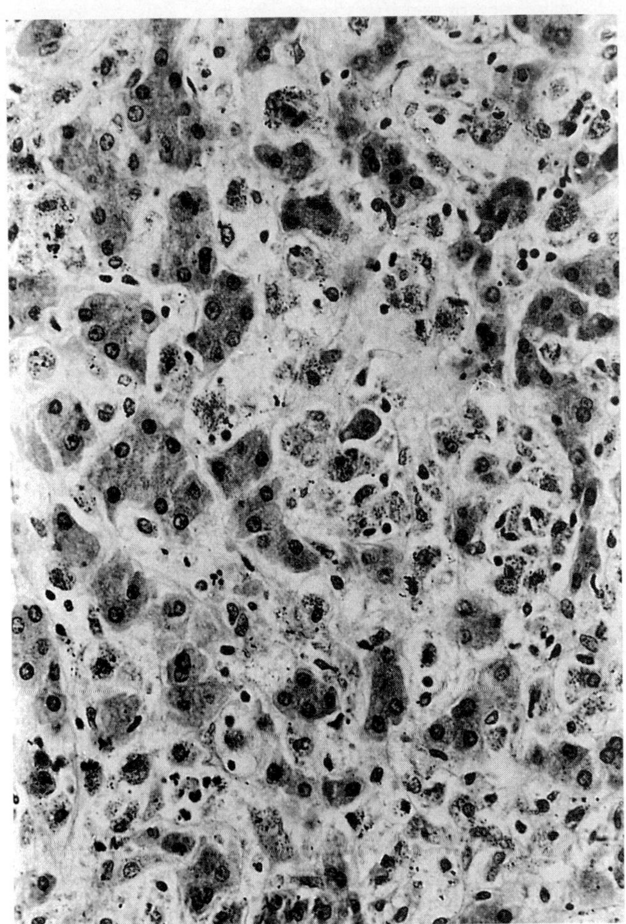

Fig. 38-6 *Leishmania donovani*. Section of liver demonstrating the typical massive infiltrate of the sinusoids by macrophages containing the parasites. At this magnification parasites are hardly visible.

derness of the left abdominal flank, with slight enlargement of the spleen. These changes are followed by symptoms of chronic disease with relentless enlargement of the spleen and the liver.

Pathology

Grossly and microscopically, the infection is characterized by a massive infiltration of macrophages into the viscera, many of which are filled by amastigotes (Fig. 38-6). Infiltration by lymphocytes and plasma cells varies from scanty to moderate. The organs affected are mainly the liver, spleen, and bone marrow, from which diagnostic samples can be obtained. In smears of bone marrow, or in imprints of the liver and spleen, the parasites are easily recognized as 2 to 4 μm oval structures with a pale blue cytoplasm and a rather large dark nucleus and the characteristic kinetoplast (Fig. 38-7). In tissue sections the parasites are seen as 1 to 2 μm granules inside the macrophages. The organelles (nucleus and kinetoplast) are difficult to visualize, but if an oil-immersion objective is used and they are seen, they are diagnostic. The difficulty often arises when infections with *Histoplasma capsulatum*, another organism inhabiting the macrophages, needs to be ruled out. Methenamine silver and periodic acid–Schiff (PAS) stains highlight *Histoplasma* organisms but not those of *Leishmania*.[2]

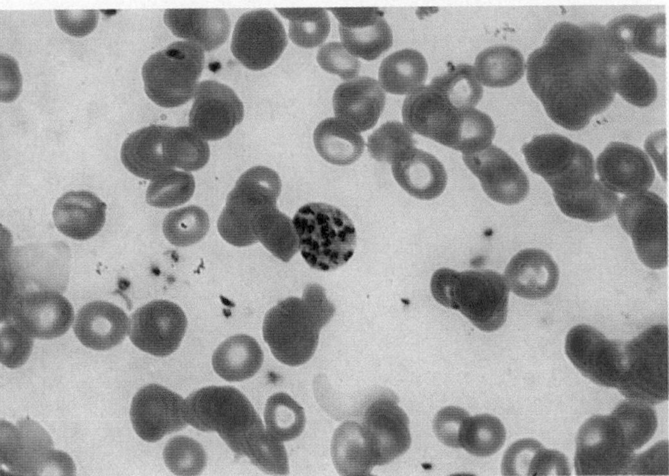

Fig. 38-7 *Leishmania donovani* in bone marrow. Notice the amastigotes within a cell, as well as those artifactually found outside. (Giemsa stain.)

Cutaneous leishmaniasis

Classically, the cutaneous disease caused by leishmaniae is divided into Old World and New World cutaneous leishmaniasis, but Latin American workers prefer the terms *tegumentary*, or *mucocutaneous*, leishmaniasis to include the lesions produced in the skin, the mucosae, or both, more commonly found in infections with the species of the American continent. Different species producing cutaneous leishmaniasis are found in different geographic locations.

The Old World Leishmaniae

At least three species, *Leishmania tropica*, *L. major*, and *L. aethiopica*, have been implicated as the etiologic agents of the cutaneous leishmaniasis of the Old World. The geographic distribution of the Old World cutaneous leishmaniae involves parts of Africa, the Middle East, extending to Pakistan and western India, and the southern region of the European continent. The lesions produced by these organisms are similar to those produced by the species of the American continent (see below). *Leishmania tropica* is usually urban in distribution and produces painless dry ulcerations with a tendency to large scars; *L. major* is mostly zoonotic, with a primarily rural distribution, producing wet ulcerations with a proclivity to coalesce and form painless ulcers, easily infected secondarily; *L. aethiopica* produces variable lesions if the immunologic conditions of the host are altered, including mucosal and dermal disseminated disease.

The New World Leishmaniae

The geographic distribution of the American cutaneous leishmaniae is mostly Central America and South America. A focus in northern Mexico extends to southern Texas, with cases being reported around the San Antonio area. The different species mentioned above overlap but tend to occur with more frequency in certain areas.

The species of cutaneous leishmaniae of the New World are more numerous and more difficult to classify and produce diseases that are more chronic than those of the Old World. *Leishmania braziliensis* produces chronic, single or multiple

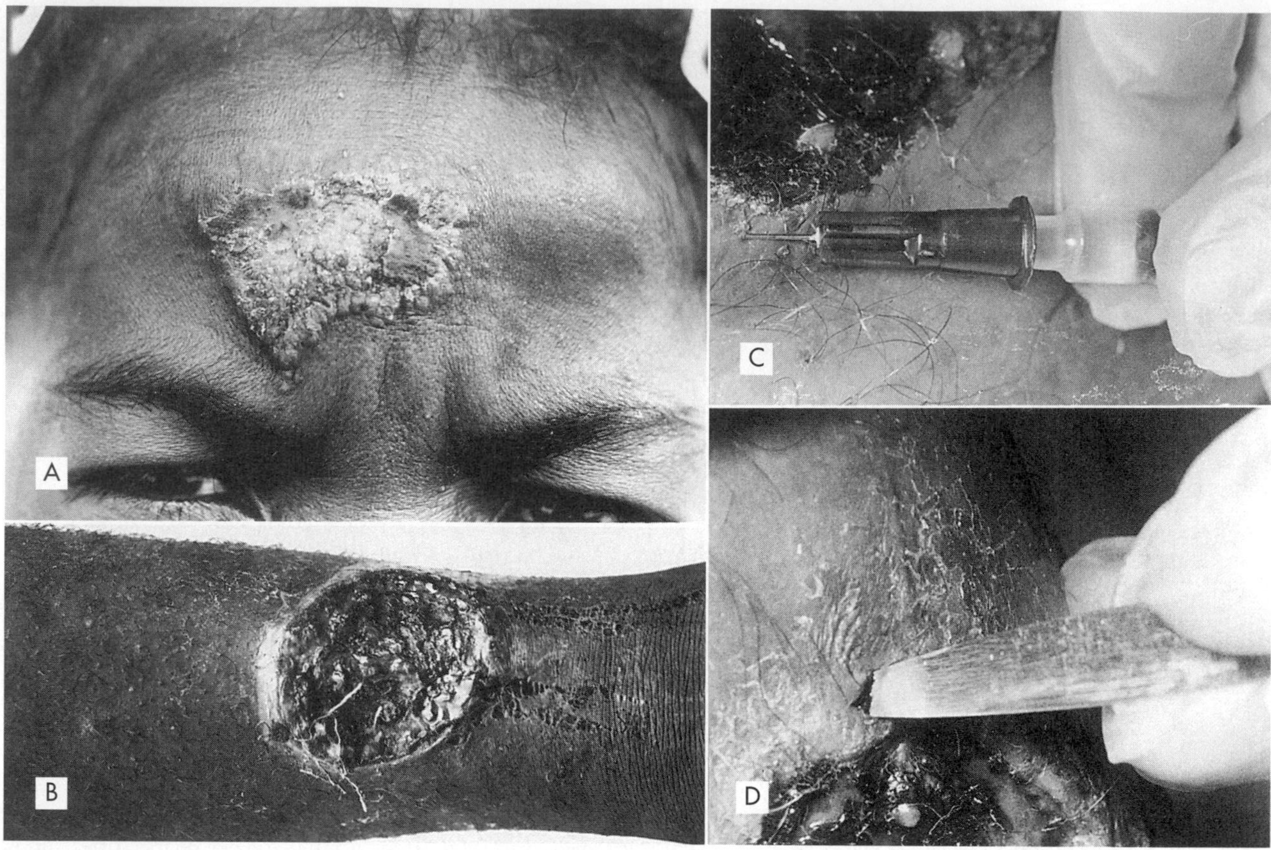

Fig. 38-8 Cutaneous leishmaniasis. **A** and **B,** Typical lesions in patients with American cutaneous leishmaniae. **C** and **D,** Proper methods of taking samples for diagnosis. (From Palma G, Gutierrez Y: *Clin Lab Med* 11:909, 1991.)

ulcers, with regional lymph node involvement, followed by ulcers of the oronasopharyngeal region with destruction of cartilages, causing the infection known as "espundia." Infections with *L. guayanensis* result in dry painless tumor nodules with regional lymph node involvement and satellite ulcerations, sometimes in several parts of the body. *Leishmania panamensis* produces persistent, chronic disease characterized by wet ulcerations and lymphatic involvement and metastasis to the oronasopharyngeal region. *Leishmania mexicana* is associated with "bay sores" or with "chiclero's ulcers" and causes single lesions often involving the ear, resulting in destruction of the helix. *Leishmania amazonensis* causes chronic ulcers that do not heal easily spontaneously. *Leishmania venezuelensis* produces single nodular lesions. These last three species are capable of producing disseminated dermal leishmaniasis, a disease seen in anergic hosts, characterized by the formation of multiple dermal nodules all over the body and resembling lepromatous leprosy. The nodules are collections of histiocytes (histiocytomas) filled with the parasites inside large vacuoles and with negligible or no inflammatory infiltration. *Leishmania peruviana* in the Andes of Peru causes a disease in children that heals spontaneously in about 4 months. Finally, other species have been recently characterized but are not mentioned here for reasons of brevity.

In simplest terms, the dermal leishmaniae share many characteristics with the visceral leishmaniae regarding life cycles, their behavior in the monocyte-macrophage system, and epidemiologically in terms of the populations affected. The differences are that generally the cutaneous leishmaniae are restricted to the skin and that their lesions are immunologically modulated and clinically polymorphous. Moreover, sometimes visceral leishmaniae can dermalize, and cutaneous leishmaniae can visceralize.[23-26]

Pathology

Morphologically and histologically the cutaneous leishmaniae of the Old and the New Worlds are similar; however, the American species tend to produce more aggressive and chronic disease. In general terms, the cutaneous leishmaniae produce a benign, limited disease in the exposed parts of the skin (Figs. 38-8, *A* and *B*), with a tendency to heal spontaneously and leave the host with resistance to reinfection by the same species, sometimes with cross resistance to other related species. The infection begins as a reddish papule at the site of the bite by the infected sandfly, progressing to induration and ulceration. It sometimes expands rapidly, centrifugally, resulting in an ulcer of several centimeters in diameter, characterized by sharp elevated borders, and if not superinfected by bacteria or fungi, it shows a clean reddish bottom covered with granulation tissue. In some instances dissemination to the regional lymphatics occurs, manifested as indurations,[24] rarely as satellite lesions. Most individuals infected with cutaneous leishmaniae develop a strong delayed hypersensitivity reaction to leishmanial antigens (the Montenegro skin test),[27] and low antibody titers.

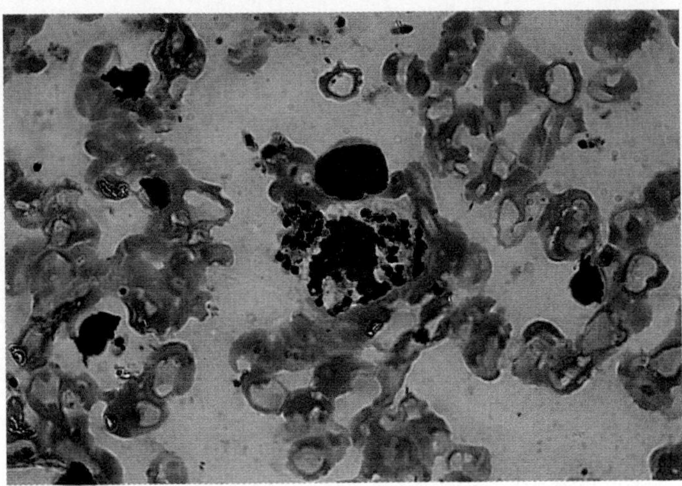

Fig. 38-9 Cutaneous leishmaniae. Smear from border of ulcer showing amastigotes inside a macrophage and outside because of breakage of the cell. (Giemsa stain.)

The diagnosis of cutaneous leishmaniae is made usually on clinical grounds by those in endemic areas knowledgeable of the clinical presentation and the origin of the patient. These parameters should help physicians in nonendemic areas, with the provision that they understand that traveling of the patient refers to travel to the forested areas of the country visited, the places where these zoonoses are acquired. A history of having visited exclusively the large metropolitan areas of a given country where leishmaniasis is endemic, almost rules out the diagnosis.[2,28]

The success of the diagnosis of cutaneous leishmaniae in the clinical laboratory rests on the proper collection of the samples for microscopic examination. Sometimes the pathologist collects the samples but more often directs the clinician as to how to collect them, and thus the pathologist should be acquainted with the proper procedures.[28] Smears are prepared from materials aspirated with a syringe or collected as scrapings of the bottom of an ulcer (Fig. 38-8, *C* and *D*). Cultures are optional and are not required for diagnosis unless the laboratory has the culture media, or the species infecting the patient needs to be identified by isoenzyme typing or DNA blotting. The smears should be stained with Giemsa stain or similar stains and examined under oil immersion.[28] The identification of the parasites is based on morphologic characteristics identical[2] to those described for the visceral leishmaniae (Fig. 38-9) (see above).

AMEBAS

The amebas belong to the Rhizopoda, unicellular organisms with locomotion by pseudopodia. The class Rhizopoda has numerous orders, genera, and species both free living and parasitic in humans and animals.[1] Most amebas parasitizing humans have direct life cycles, in which a trophozoite, the vegetative stage, forms cysts, the resistant stages necessary for transmission to the new host.

Two groups of amebas, the intestinal and the free-living, are discussed in the following paragraphs. The intestinal amebas are usually nonpathogenic organisms inhabiting the mouth and the colon. These amebas are of interest mainly to the clinical laboratory where their identification in fecal samples is carried out, based on their morphologic characteristics in wet mounts and in stained preparations. Three genera, *Entamoeba, Endolimax*, and *Iodamoeba*—with the following species: *Entamoeba histolytica, E. gingivalis, E. hartmanni, E. coli, E. polecki, Endolimax nana*, and *Iodamoeba buetschlii*—affect humans. *Entamoeba histolytica* is the most important because it has pathogenic strains that produce morbidity and mortality. Recent work on *E. histolytica* has resulted in the separation of two morphologically identical species: *E. dispar*[29] a nonpathogen, and *E. histolytica*, the pathogen. These two species can infect people alone, or as a mixed infection. *Entamoeba gingivalis* inhabits the mouth and lacks a cystic stage, with transmission occurring through passage of trophozoites by saliva droplets or during kissing.

The second group, the free-living amebas, comprises parasites living in water and moist soil, organisms that under certain circumstances become parasitic both in humans and animals. *Naegleria fowleri* is an ameboflagellate, converting to flagellate forms under appropriate conditions of temperature and culture. It causes primary amebic meningoencephalitis. Infections with one of several species of *Acanthamoeba* results in granulomatous amebic encephalitis in the brain as well as other lesions in various organs, including the eye.[2]

Entamoeba histolytica

The term *amebiasis* generally implies infection by *Entamoeba histolytica*, which is usually asymptomatic because the parasite has a low virulence. When it does not produce disease, it behaves in the intestine as any other commensal amebas do.[30] The term *symptomatic amebiasis* has been used to denote infection with clinical manifestations, indicating that the parasite has become a tissue dweller; *luminal amebiasis* has been used for the asymptomatic infections. The rates of prevalence of *E. histolytica* are now unknown because of the separation of the species *E. dispar*.[31] In underdeveloped countries, rates of prevalence of what should now be called *E. histolytica*–like amebas can reach 50%; in developed areas the prevalence is unknown, but sporadic infections in individuals without a traveling history do occur. Therefore, *E. histolytica* is cosmopolitan but more common in the tropics than in the subtropics. In 1981 estimates suggested that 480 million people in the world were infected with *E. histolytica* in the world, of whom 36 million developed amebic colitis or other disease and at least 40,000 died.[32] In developed countries the prevalence of *E. histolytica* in homosexual males is similar to that of the populations of underdeveloped countries.[33,34]

E. histolytica is acquired through ingestion, usually with food or water, of cysts passed in the feces of infected persons. Transmission by water results in epidemics, especially when the source of drinking water for a large number of people is contaminated. The cysts release the parasites in the intestine, which colonize the cecum and ascending colon. The preferred location of the organisms, in their trophozoite stage, is near the epithelium, within the mucus layer covering the colon. This area is known as the biotic zone, where the amebas multiply. Some trophozoites then begin to encyst and are shed with the fecal mass into the environment to infect another host. The trophozoites are about 20 μm in diameter and have a cytoplasm containing bacteria and other particulate matter within numerous vacuoles. The nucleus is relatively small, about 5 μm, and characteristically has a layer of uniform chromatin granules attached to the inner wall of the nuclear membrane and a single centrally placed karyosome. The mature cysts are about 10 to 15 μm in diameter and have four nuclei identical to those in the trophozoite.

Clinical findings

When *Entamoeba hystolytica* is virulent, it invades the tissues, but the stimulus or stimuli responsible for this behavior are unknown. Erosion of the colonic mucosa ensues, accompanied by inflammatory changes, hyperemia, and microscopic hemorrhages, progressing to deeper ulcers, reaching the submucosa (Fig. 38-10, *A*). The ulcers are described as typically being narrower at the level of the muscularis mucosae, that is, flask-shaped (Fig. 38-10, *B*), but this is not always the case. The ulcers are filled with necrotic debris and infiltrated with polymorphonuclear cells and lymphocytes at their base and margins. Except in the severest cases, the rest of the colonic mucosa may appear normal. The parasites vary in numbers and are usually located at the interface of necrotic and viable tissue. The trophozoites in invasive amebiasis have been described as being larger, 35 to 45 μm, than those of the lumen, with active movements, and have red blood cells in the vacuoles. It was believed that the pathogenic properties of *E. histolytica* were related to these morphologic changes, but with the separation of the species *dispar* from *histolytica*, this idea is now untenable.[29]

Once the parasites enter the tissues and lesions form, the patient is liable to have symptoms, and in most cases bouts of diarrhea alternating with constipation may progress to painful dysentery with numerous liquid bowel movements containing mucus and blood.[35] In these instances the colonic mucosa is edematous and hyperemic, with ulcerations measuring up to 3 cm in diameter. The course is usually subacute or chronic, but in some individuals, the disease presents in fulminant form, usually fatal despite diagnosis and institution of proper treatment; the mucosa is thin and friable with pronounced inflammation of the serosa. Amebic colitis is clinically indistinguishable from other forms of colitis, and fulminant amebiasis is clinically indistinguishable from toxic inflammatory bowel disease.[35] Thus their diagnosis is made only in the laboratory with the proper identification of the parasites in stool samples or tissue sections.[36] The morphologic characteristics of the amebas, described above, suffice for identification, but they should be applied rigorously to differentiate the parasite from resident tissue macrophages.[2]

The invasion of the colonic mucosae by *E. histolytica* may lead to dissemination of the organisms to other organs, a condition known as extraintestinal amebiasis.[37] Colonization of the blood vessels with formation of infected thrombi results in embolization and seeding of the liver when branches of the portal system are involved. Anastomosing veins between the portal system and vena cava of the lower sigmoid and rectum produce thrombi that embolize to the lungs. From the liver, or the lungs, secondary invasion to other organs is possible. Colonization of any organ by *E. histolytica* usually results in formation of abscesses, referred to as amebic liver abscess, amebic brain abscess, and so forth.

Amebic liver abscesses are more common in the right lobe, but those in the left lobe are more important because of the possibility of rupture to the pericardium. The lesions are characteristic grossly because they consist of a liquefaction of the liver parenchyma with a chocolate-like color and a foul smell. In 50% of the cases, these abscesses occur without a history of diarrhea or dysentery, are more common in males, and are usually fatal in children under 5 years of age. Rupture of the liver abscess from the diaphragm into the lungs and major bronchi results in expectoration of copious chocolate-like material, which is diagnostic clinically; they may also rupture into the pericardium, a fatal complication unless timely treatment is given, or to the skin. The second most important abscess site is the lung, where abscesses may form via the bloodstream or by extension from the liver.[37] The gross appearance of amebic lung abscesses is nonspecific, but microscopic examination reveals the cause of the infection.

Another important but less common site for infection by *E. histolytica* is the skin. Possible affected areas include the thorax and abdomen by fistulization or by extension of visceral disease to the perianal skin and sexual organs.[38] Ulcerations of sharp borders with clean bottoms around the anus or penis should be investigated for amebas, especially in homosexual

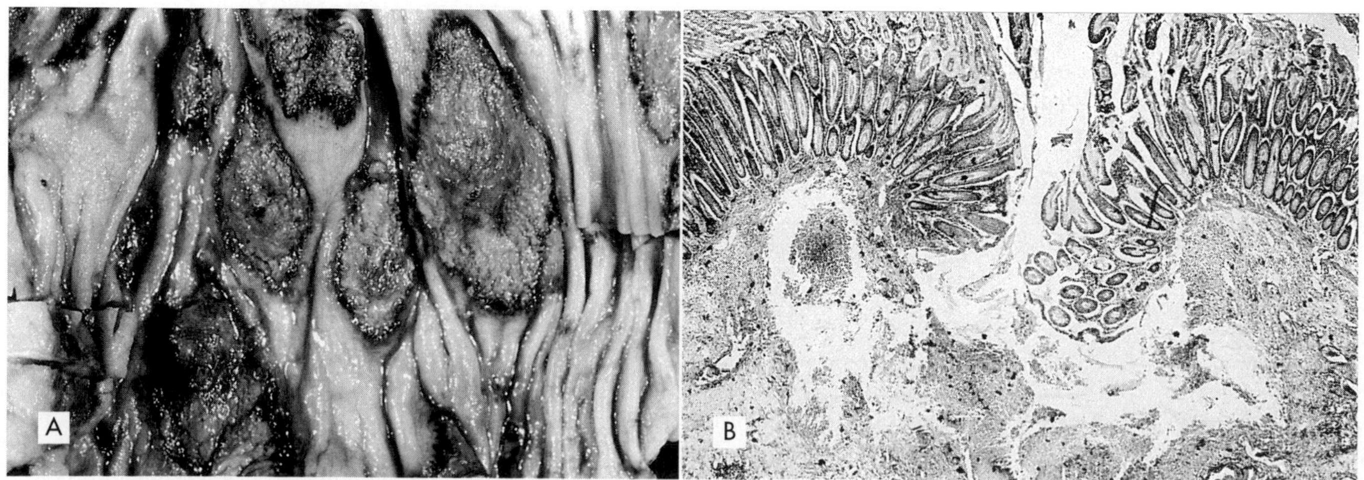

Fig. 38-10 *Entamoeba histolytica* lesions of the colon. **A,** Ulcerations in amebic colitis. **B,** Section of colon demonstrating the typical flask-shaped ulcer.

males. In women, cervical amebiasis may simulate an ulcerated carcinoma of the cervix, which has to be excluded later, after treatment, if only amebic infection is found in the samples studied.[2,39] *Entamoeba gingivalis* has recently been identified in lesions of the cervix, identical to those ascribed to *E. histolytica*. The significance of these findings are not understood at present.[40]

Naegleria fowleri

Naegleria fowleri is the agent of *primary amebic meningoencephalitis*, an infection reported in several countries and suspected to occur worldwide. The reported cases are clustered to the areas where the infection has received more attention because physicians and pathologists suspect and recognize the disease. Primary amebic meningoencephalitis is generally a fatal infection in those who acquire the infection while swimming in stagnant and warm freshwater.[41]

Naegleria is an ameboflagellate with both trophozoites and cysts in its life cycle but under in vitro conditions may form flagellated stages. The infection is acquired by humans while diving or swimming if water with the parasites enters nose. Colonization of the nasal mucosa is rapid. The organisms reach the olfactory mucosa and enter the nerve endings of the olfactory tract, passing through the cribriform plate to the base of the brain, where they invade the meninges (Fig. 38-11, *A*). From the meninges, following the perivascular spaces, the amebas enter the brain tissue.[1,2]

The symptoms and signs of the infection develop rapidly. At first, signs of a rhinitis are followed by headache and nausea. Within a week the patient is usually hospitalized with a clinical picture of meningitis, encephalitis, or both. The death of the patient usually occurs in less than 2 weeks and the diagnosis is often made at the autopsy table.[41] Diagnosis made ante mortem has resulted in institution of therapies that are rarely successful.

At autopsy, the brain shows meningeal hemorrhages, especially at its base. Microscopically, the parasites are found in abundance in both meninges and brain tissue, together with a lymphocytic infiltrate, few polymorphonuclear cells, and little or no necrosis.[2,41] The organisms are the hallmark of the lesion and require proper identification for diagnosis. Only the trophozoites are seen, measuring about 10 to 12 μm, with a vacuolated pale cytoplasm and a nucleus consisting of a thin nuclear membrane and a large, rounded, central nucleolus (Figs. 38-11, *B*, and 38-12). The parasites can also be seen in the spinal fluid sediment and, if fresh, can be resuspended in distilled water where in about 1 hour they began transforming into flagellates.[2] Cultures in nonnutrient agar overlaid with *Escherichia coli*, become positive at room temperature within a few days.[42]

Acanthamebas

Acanthamebas and related organisms occur worldwide in water and dirt and on plants and undergo life-cycle alterations between cysts and trophozoites. The trophozoites are about 25 μm in diameter, have a vacuolated cytoplasm with spinelike extensions of the membrane (the acanthopodia), and in fresh smears show a vacuole periodically filling slowly with fluid and suddenly being emptied to the outside by collapse of the vacuole. The nucleus has a thin, hardly visible membrane and contains a large, round nucleolus, and the cytoplasm has numerous perinuclear vacuoles of different sizes. The cysts measure 12 to 14 μm in diameter and have a thick irregular wall (ectocyst) containing a uninuclear organism (endocyst), which resembles a small trophozoite.[1,2] Cysts are formed during adverse conditions, such as desiccation, are light, and are easily transported with the wind. Because of these reasons, it is believed that infections of both animals and humans occur through the upper respiratory tract. Indeed, species of *Hartmanella*, related organisms also infecting humans, have been recovered in tissue cell cultures of the upper respiratory tract of healthy individuals.[43,44]

Infections with *Acanthamoeba* organisms have been found in many places, with the parasite being worldwide in distribution. An important patient group is those with AIDS, in whom the parasite is an opportunistic organism.[45] In these individuals the central nervous system is preferentially involved, but most other organs can be affected. Infections of the viscera are born from a primary focus such as a skin lesion or the marrow but more often from the upper respiratory tract, where the parasite is a saprophitic commensal. The lesions of individuals dying with acanthamebiasis consist of areas of cerebral necrosis resembling infarcts, usually less than 3 cm in diameter, and randomly distributed. In other parts of the body, they appear as abscesses (Fig 38-13). Microscopically, these lesions have granulomatous inflammation with many parasites present and

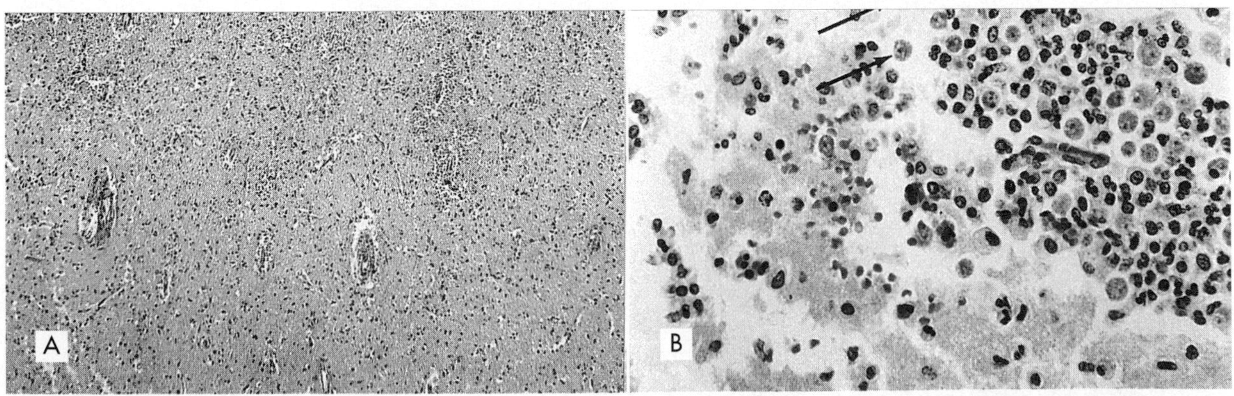

Fig. 38-11 *Naegleria fowleri* in brain producing amebic meningoencephalitis. **A,** Low magnification of section of brain, showing pronounced meningeal infection. **B,** Higher magnification, showing the infiltrate and the parasites *(arrows)*.

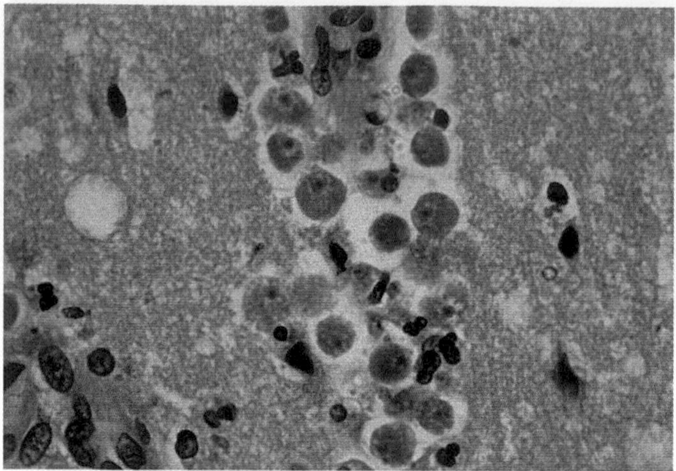

Fig. 38-12 *Naegleria fowleri* in brain producing amebic meningoencephalitis. Notice the parasites with typical nuclei and their relatively small size, not much larger than that of surrounding lymphocytes.

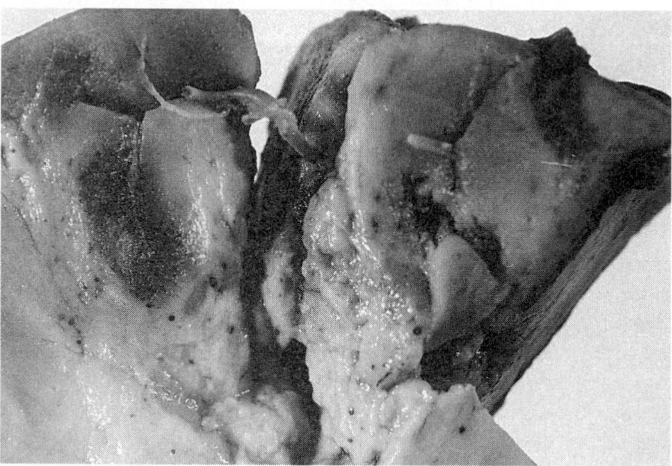

Fig. 38-13 *Acanthamoeba* organisms producing in brain of an individual with acquired immunodeficiency syndrome. Notice the areas of necrosis.

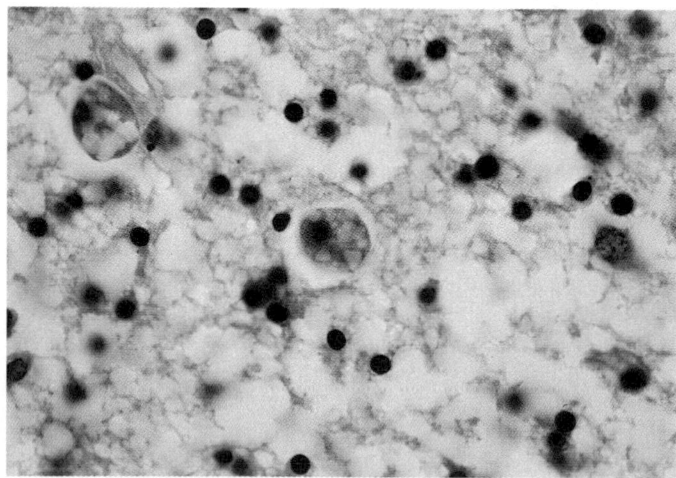

Fig. 38-14 *Acanthamoeba* organisms in brain illustrating the morphologic characteristics of the ameba.

with the formation of cysts. The finding of cysts in these lesions confirms the diagnosis of *Acanthamoeba* or *leptomyxid* amoeba because these are the only amebas of humans that form cysts in tissues,[2] but their cysts must be differentiated from the larger yeast forms of deep fungi, which they superficially resemble under the microscope.

In immune competent hosts *Acanthamoeba* is responsible for other infections such as granulomatous skin lesions, osteomyelitis mainly of the jaw,[46] otitis media, keratitis, and keratoconjunctivitis, most often observed in individuals wearing soft contact lenses worn for long periods.[47] The initial lesion in keratitis is ulceration of the superficial epithelium progressing to a very noticeable inflammation and destruction of the cornea, sometimes requiring corneal transplants for treatment. Microscopic examination of corneal biopsy specimens show the lesion and the amebas, often with cysts in the corneal matrix. Cultures are easily taken in a similar manner to those of *Naegleria* (see the previous page).[42]

Morphologic identification of the parasite species is not possible in tissue sections or cultures. Thus an ameba measuring 20 to 25 μm with the characteristic nucleus, acanthopods, vacuolated cytoplasm, and forming cysts in tissues may be an *Acanthamoeba*, or a *Hartmanella,* or a *leptomyxid* ameba (Fig. 38-14). Identification of the species is made after one harvests a large number of organisms from cultures and studies them in specialized laboratories.[2,42]

CILIATES

The distinguishing feature of this family are cilia that cover their cell membrane. Only one species has been found in humans, *Balantidium coli*, the largest protozon, measuring up to 200 μm in diameter, having a mouth, or cytostome, and two nuclei, the macronucleus and the micronucleus. The life cycle involves a trophozoite and a cyst, the infective stage.[2]

Balantidium coli is an inhabitant of the large intestine, where it is usually a lumen dweller resulting in asymptomatic infections. The parasite occurs naturally in pigs, and in humans it has often been recorded in people handling pigs. In some areas the prevalence rate is up to 28%[48]; in the United States the infection is sporadic. Like *Entamoeba histolytica, Balantidium* can be found in the tissues producing shallow ulcers involving the mucosa (Fig. 38-15, *A*), less frequently the submucosa, and rarely producing perforation and peritoneal invasion, or liver abscesses.[49,50] The symptoms are clinically indistinguishable from those seen in intestinal amebiasis with colitis and dysentery. The diagnosis of balantidiasis is made by the recognition of the organisms, trophozoites, and cysts in stool samples and trophozoites only in tissue sections. The size of the parasite, the presence of cilia, and the macronucleus, are diagnostic (Fig. 38-15, *B*); serologic tests are not available.[2]

APICOMPLEXANS

The phylum Apicomplexa comprises some of the most important protozoa parasitic in humans, producing diseases that result in important morbidity and mortality such as malaria, toxoplasmosis, and cryptosporidiosis. The common characteristics of the apicomplexan are a required intracellular develop-

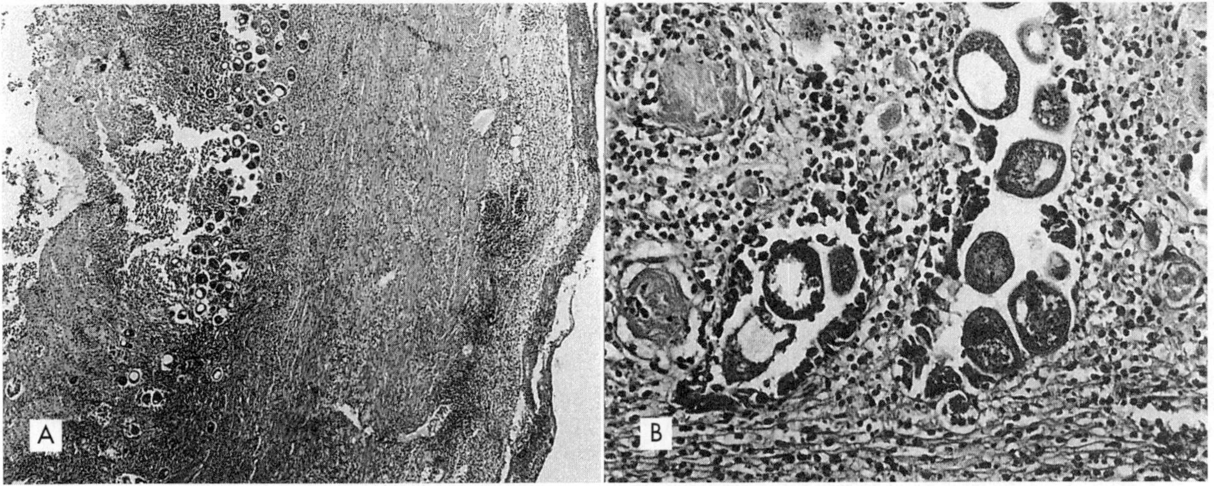

Fig. 38-15 *Balantidium coli* in large intestine. **A,** Low-power view of ulcer involving the mucosa and submucosa. Compare this shallow ulceration with that produced by *Entamoeba histolytica* (see Fig. 38-10, *B*). **B,** Higher magnification demonstrating the morphologic characteristics of the parasites, which have a large vacuole filled with fluid and a macronucleus visible in some sections.

ment for some stages of its life cycles, the existence of a sexual phase of reproduction, and the presence of ultrastructural organelles, the apical complex, which enable the parasite to enter host cells.[1,2]

The life cycles of the Apicomplexa are variable, some being monoxenous (one host), others heteroxenous (two hosts), but as stated above all require a phase of intracellular development.[1] Human infections are very common in most parts of the world, though some, such as malaria, have become geographically restricted. Certain apicomplexans elicit effective defense mechanisms in the host, which make these infections self-limited or latent in the immunocompetent host. However, when these defense mechanisms become deranged by AIDS or severe immunosuppression, apicomplexan opportunistic infections may become progressive or fatal. In the following paragraphs we examine the most important apicomplexan parasites found in humans.

Cryptosporidium parvum

Cryptosporidium infection of animals has been known for many years, but only since the mid 1970s has it been recognized as a parasite of the gastrointestinal tract of humans, colonizing both the small and large intestines.[51,52] Similar to the coccidia *Isospora* and *Sarcocystis, Cryptosporidium* divides in the intestinal epithelium. *Cryptosporidium* is transmitted by the fecal oral route and therefore produces infections worldwide.[2] The life cycle can be completed in a single host and starts after the ingestion of stages found in the feces of infected individuals. These stages, the oocysts, are 4 μm in diameter and contain four sporozoites, which are released in the intestine to invade the epithelial cells and locate within the brush border (Figs. 38-16 and 38-17). Once inside the cell the parasite begin multiplying asexually to form merozoites, rupture the cell, and enter other cells to repeat the cycle.[53] At some point some merozoites differentiate into the sexual stages, the male and female gametocytes, which after coupling develop into oocysts in the brush border. The oocysts are of two types: thin-walled and thick-walled oocysts, both maturing to infectivity within the intestine.

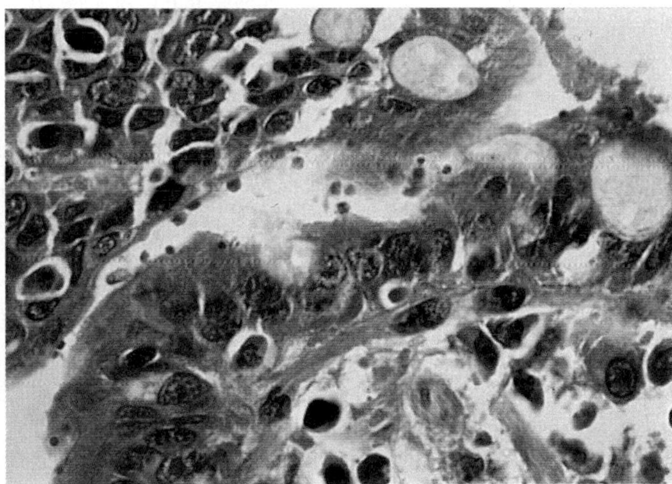

Fig. 38-16 *Cryptosporidium parvum* in duodenum. Photograph taken with oil immersion demonstrating the small organisms in the brush border of the cell.

Thin-walled oocysts break and liberate the sporozoites to infect other cells; the thick-walled oocysts are destined to be evacuated with the feces to infect other hosts.[53] Several species of *Cryptosporidium* infect animals and humans; the species apparently responsible for infections in humans is *Cryptosporidium parvum*.

Clinical findings

Infection with *Cryptosporidium* is worldwide, but prevalence rates in the general population vary geographically.[53] In the United States the prevalence has been estimated to be just over 4%, and Europe about 2%. In South American countries the rates are as high as 20%,[53] which make cryptosporidiosis the most significant parasitic infection producing diarrhea.[53] Outbreaks because of contaminated water have been described.[54] In nondeveloped areas with high infection rates, disease occurs principally in small children, the most susceptible pop-

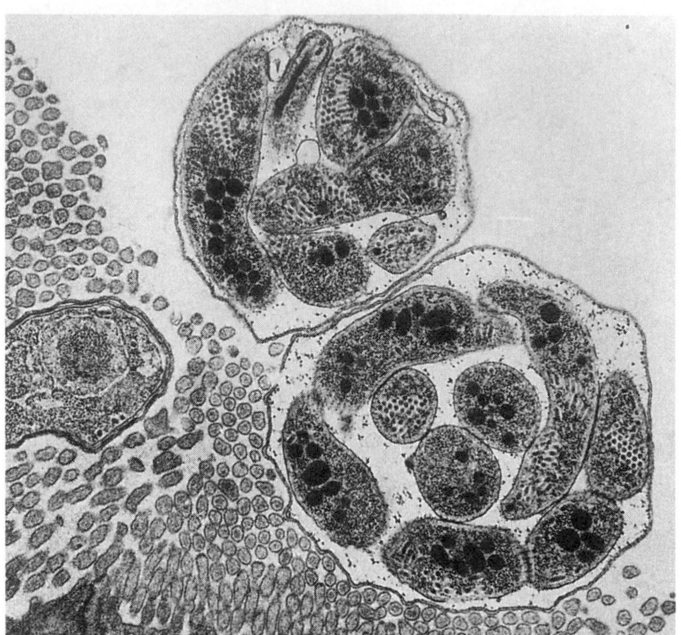

Fig. 38-17 *Cryptosporidium parvum* in duodenum. Transmission electron photomicrograph showing two parasites at the completion of the asexual cycle *(top)* with several merozoites inside each.

ulation. *Cryptosporidium* is also an important cause of traveler's diarrhea.[55] In immunocompetent hosts cryptosporidiosis is a self-limited infection that lasts about 2 weeks and is characterized by low fever, anorexia, borborygmus, watery diarrhea, abdominal pain, and loss of weight, sometimes of up to 10 pounds.[56] The parasites in the intestine may disappear with the symptoms, or they may persist sometimes for up to 3 months, with the patient becoming a symptomless carrier of the infection.[55]

In the immunocompromised individual, especially those with AIDS, the infection has symptoms identical to those described above, except that they do not abate spontaneously. Because no effective treatment is known for cryptosporidiosis, the infection continues symptomatically until the patient dies.[53,57] In the AIDS patient, *Cryptosporidium* organisms have been found in other organs besides the gastrointestinal tract, such as the pancreatic and biliary ducts,[58-60] and the pulmonary epithelium.[61] It has been postulated that in the biliary ducts *Cryptosporidium* organisms are responsible for eliciting sclerosing cholangitis and hepatitis.[58-60]

Pathology

No tissues from immunocompetent individuals with cryptosporidiosis have been examined to date. The lesions of the gut mucosa seen in individuals with AIDS are variable and

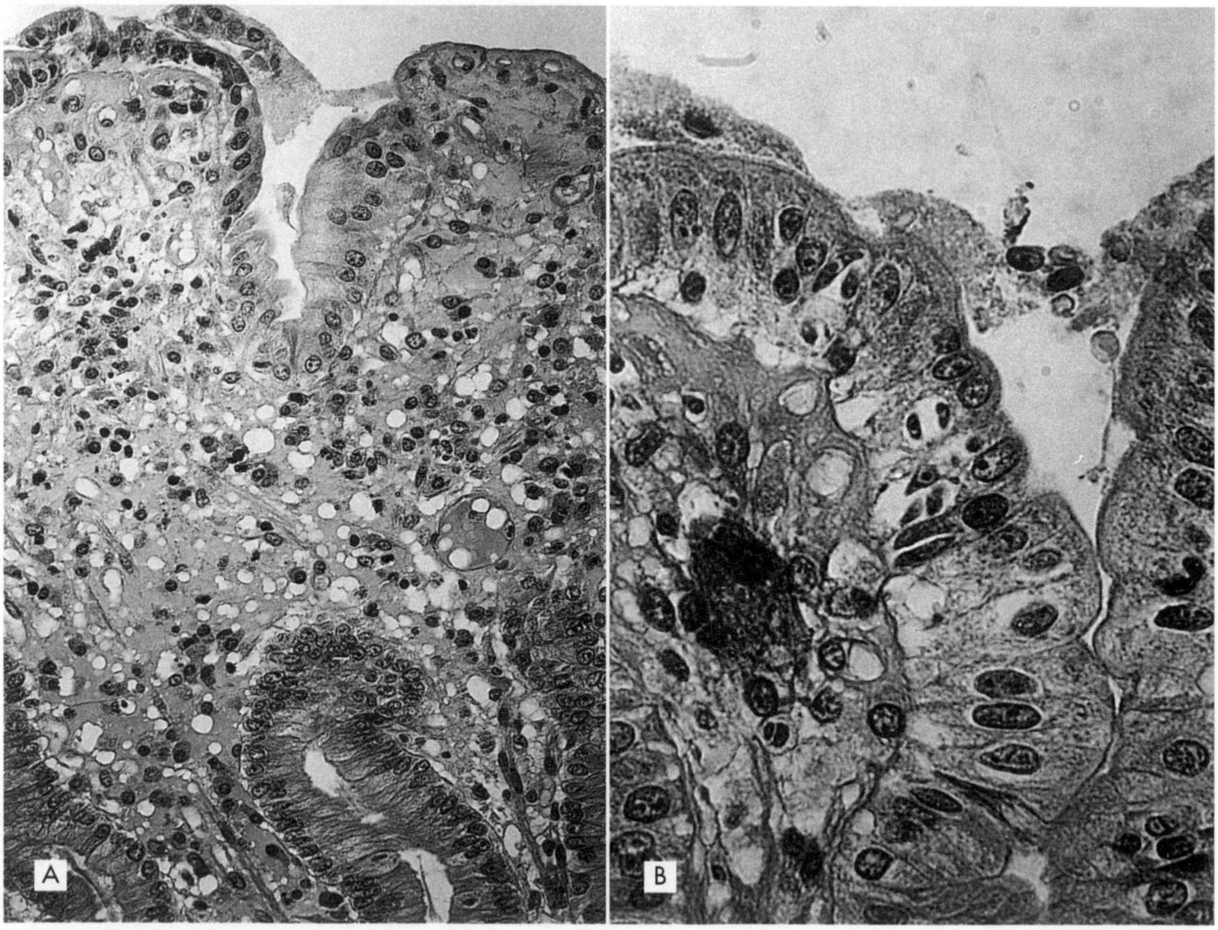

Fig. 38-18 *Isospora belli* in small intestine of an individual with AIDS. **A,** Lower-power magnification showing edema, and inflammatory infiltrate of the mucosa. Notice the damaged epithelial cells. **B,** Higher magnification of the parasites within the enterocytes.

nonspecific, and other infections cannot be excluded as their cause. Distortion of the architecture of the mucosa with pronounced inflammatory infiltrate by lymphocytes, plasma cells, and polymorphonuclear cells has been observed. Crypt abscesses are common, but the hallmark of the infection is the presence of parasites exclusively located within the brush border of the enterocytes[2,53] (Figs. 38-16 and 38-17). The organisms are about 4 μm or less and do not require more than hematoxylin and eosin stain for their identification (Fig. 38-16). In thin sections of the intestine examined with the light microscope, some stages of the cycle are recognizable, but the best manner to see them is with transmission electron microscopy (Fig. 38-17). However, the use of this technique is not necessary for routine diagnostic work.

The most effective diagnostic tool for diagnosis of cryptosporidiosis is examination of stool prepared with saline or iodine solution. Stained fecal smears with a modified acid-fast bacilli stain (Kinyoun stain) is the best for finding and identifying the parasites.

Isospora belli

Infections with *Isospora* species have been known for many years as a benign infection rarely producing symptoms in humans. The life cycle is similar to that of *Cryptosporidium* species with several important exceptions, which help to explain its epidemiology. The mature oocysts are ingested with food or water, and in the intestine release eight sporozoites contained in two sporocysts, and these sporozoites enter the epithelial cells of the upper part of the small intestine. The parasites are located within the cytoplasm of the cell (Fig. 38-18, *B*). Asexual reproduction resulting in the formation of several merozoites takes place, and the freed merozoites infect other cells to repeat the cycle. Some merozoites develop into gametocytes, which after joining produced immature oocysts, 20 to 33 μm by 10 to 19 μm in size, to be evacuated in the feces.[1,2] The oocysts require about 1 week to become infective (sporulate) in the environment. This delay explains why *Isospora* is not a common infection in developed areas of the world because it is not transmitted by the oral-fecal route but is common in underdeveloped ones, where there is contamination of the environment with human waste.[1,62]

Clinical findings

The clinical symptoms of isosporiasis in the general population have rarely been studied. Some infected individuals have no symptoms; others may have a mild diarrhea with abdominal discomfort and low-grade fever.[63] Oocysts usually are evacuated in the feces up to 20 days after the symptoms have ended. In the immune suppressed, *Isospora* organisms cause chronic diarrhea, diffuse abdominal crampy pain, nausea, and weight loss. In some, malabsorption with steatorrhea, similar to tropical sprue with enterocolitis and nonspecific jejunitis, has been described.[64] There may be peripheral blood eosinophilia, up to 25%, a feature not seen in other human protozoan infections.

Pathology

The histopathology caused by *Isospora* infection of immunocompetent hosts is poorly documented. In individuals with AIDS, the changes are nonspecific inflammation, clubbing of intestinal villi, which may flatten out in severe cases[2,65] (Fig. 38-18, *A*). The diagnosis is made when one finds and identifies the unsporulated oocysts in stool samples. When examined after delay, the oocysts are characteristically binucleate. Direct smears in saline solution or stained with iodine produce good results. In tissue sections the parasites need to be carefully searched for inside the cells and identified, based on their morphologic characteristics[1,2] (Fig. 38-18, *B*).

Sarcocystosis

Sarcocystosis is the most innocuous infection produced by the intestinal coccidia of humans. The parasite is heteroxenous, having two hosts in their life cycle, cattle for *Sarcocystis hominis* and pigs for *S. suihominis*. Infections occur worldwide but are seldom reported by the clinical laboratory because they are asymptomatic.[66] Infection occurs by the ingestion of uncooked or poorly cooked beef or pork, containing the infective stages (sarcocysts) within the muscle cells. The sarcocysts are filled with zoites, which are liberated when the sarcocyst is ruptured in the intestine, after which rupturing they enter an unknown cell located below the enterocytes and the muscularis mucosa. In these cells the zoites develop directly into male and female gametocytes and join to form an oocyst that matures within the cell. During maturation of the oocyst, two sporocysts are formed and are evacuated with the feces of the host; the sporocysts of *S. hominis* are 15 by 9 μm and those of *S. suihominis* 13 by 10 μm, each containing four sporozoites. The intermediate host becomes infected by ingestion of sporocysts passed in the feces; the sporozoites enter the intestinal wall and develop asexually in the endothelial cells of small and medium-sized arteries of most organs. This development occurs several times, to increase the number of organisms considerably, until finally the parasites invade the muscle cells to develop into sarcocysts.[1,2]

The principal lesion of *Sarcocystis* organisms in humans is the infection produced in the muscles after humans ingest sporocysts passed in the feces of animals infected with species of *Sarcocystis* native to these animals. In these instances humans behave as intermediate hosts, developing sarcocysts in the skeletal muscles or in the heart. Most cases reported are from the tropics, but some are from the temperate zone, especially the United States and Europe.[68]

Infections in humans, as stated above, are largely asymptomatic.[66] However, in a series of cases reported from Thailand, the infection resulted in a segmental eosinophilic enteritis in which the patients required surgical removal of the affected small intestine.[67]

Toxoplasma gondii

Toxoplasma gondii is an intestinal coccidian parasite of cats, with a life cycle similar to that of *Isospora* but with important differences, which are described here (Fig. 38-19). The intestinal cycle occurs only in felines; hosts other than cats, including humans, if infected with *Toxoplasma*, develop infections in the tissues, where the parasite multiplies only asexually within the cells. Two stages of development are found in the tissues of these hosts: the trophozoites, or tachyzoites, and the cysts, or bradyzoites. The tachyzoites multiply rapidly asexually and form numerous organisms known as *merozoites*, which destroy the cell. Freed merozoites invade other cells to repeat the cycle, but some develop slowly into cysts, or bradyzoites, which become dormant in the tissues and can infect other hosts if ingested. These two forms of development (one in cats and one in other animals) mean that *Toxoplasma* organisms have a direct cycle and an indirect cycle using an intermediate host. This also means that infections with *Toxoplasma*, in both cats and other hosts, occur in either one of two ways: ingestion of mature oocysts evacuated with the feces of cats, or ingestion of cysts in uncooked or poorly cooked meat.[1,2] One should also keep in mind that oocysts evacuated in cats are immature at the time of evacuation, and require maturation (sporulation) for a few days in the environment.

Toxoplasmosis is a common, worldwide infection in humans. The prevalence differs among geographic areas and the age of the population. In the United States the college group has about a 20% positivity for *Toxoplasma* antibodies, and the general population has about 50%;[69] older groups have even higher positivity. This indicates that infections with *Toxoplasma* occur at all times and that the number of antibody positives in any population is constantly increasing until theoretically it would reach 100%. All individuals with positive serologic results for *Toxoplasma* must have cysts in their tissues in numbers so low that they are practically undetectable by routine methods. The importance of this fact is that *Toxoplasma* is an opportunistic pathogen of individuals with AIDS or other immunologic defects. Usually, these infections are the result of reactivation, meaning the rupture of a cyst in the tissues, freeing the zoites, which begin a new infection.[70] As stated above, infections in humans are acquired by ingestion of mature oocysts evacuated with the feces of cats, or by ingestion of cysts in meat. However, other manners of infection occur: transplacentally, if the mother becomes infected during pregnancy;[71] with contaminated blood, if the donor has active infection at the time of donating the blood; and by receiving a transplanted organ from a seropositive donor.

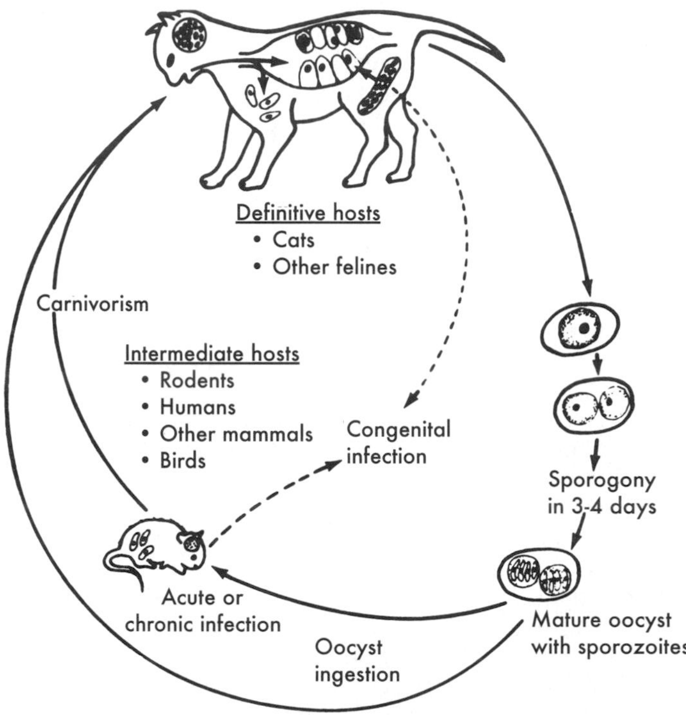

Fig. 38-19 *Toxoplasma gondii* life cycle. (From Gutierrez Y: *Diagnostic pathology of parasitic infections, with clinical correlations*, Philadelphia, 1990, Lea & Febiger.)

Acquired Toxoplasmosis

Toxoplasma infections in humans can be acquired or congenital, and disease manifestations vary depending on the immunologic status of the host, the extent of involvement, and the organs compromised. In immunocompetent hosts the majority of infections are asymptomatic or produce only flu-like symptoms.[2] A few individuals may develop cervical lymphadenopathy, low-grade fever, and weight loss, usually lasting a few weeks. *Toxoplasma* lymphadenitis is clinically characterized by nontender, mobile, enlarged lymph nodes and histologically by a histiocytic reaction with focal aggregates of enlarged, activated lymphocytes and poorly formed granulomas in the lymphoid tissue (Figs. 38-20, *A* and *B*). Finding the parasites in the lymph nodes is difficult, but if cultured in tissue cell cultures, they may be recovered. In case of questionable diagnosis, serology is helpful; the use of the polymerase chain reaction for detection of *Toxoplasma* organisms in lymph nodes has not been fruitful.[72]

Another important disease produced by *Toxoplasma* in the immunocompetent individual is a unilateral granulomatous

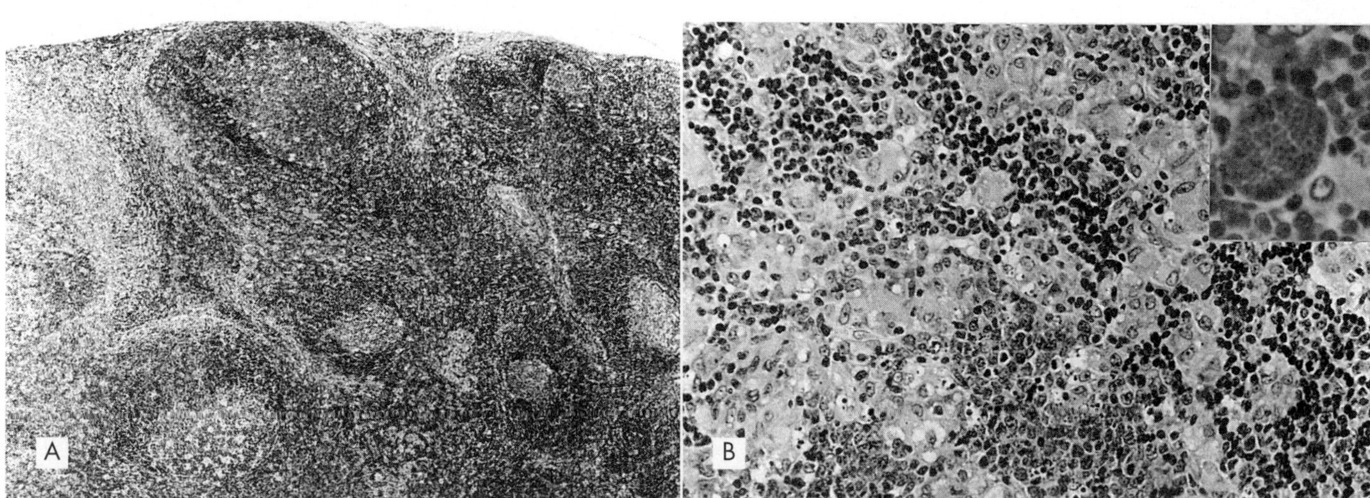

Fig. 38-20 *Toxoplasma gondii* in lymph node. **A,** Low-power view of lymph node showing a reactive lymphadenitis. **B,** Higher magnification demonstrating the histiocytic infiltrate, grouped as poorly formed granulomas. *Inset,* A cyst.

retinitis, which can result in loss of vision. It is believed to be a reactivation of a previous infection that left a residual cyst in the retina, which ruptures for unknown reasons and restarts an infection within the retinal cells only. This diagnosis is made usually by history and ophthalmologic examination. Serologic tests can demonstrate local production of specific immunoglobulins to *Toxoplasma* species in the vitreous.[73]

The bulk of the morbidity and mortality produced by *Toxoplasma* organisms occurs in immunosuppressed individuals. Persons suffering from the acquired immunodeficiency syndrome, or receiving immunosuppressive therapy organ transplants, lymphomas, or carcinomas, may undergo reactivation of an old infection; or they may acquire the primary infection (ingestion of oocysts, cysts in meat, infected transplanted organ, or blood transfusion) while immunosuppressed. In both cases they suffer a disease that, if not diagnosed and properly treated, is usually fatal. The fetus, also an immunosuppressed host, can acquire severe infection transplacentally (see below).

Toxoplasmosis in the immunosuppressed host is a protean disease because it may involve any organ.[74] However, the most salient lesions are those of the brain and the heart because in these two organs *Toxoplasma* organisms produce important morbidity and mortality. It is estimated that up to 10% of all individuals with the acquired immunodeficiency syndrome in the United States will develop toxoplasmosis of the central nervous system.[75] Clinically, the infection is different in children and in adults but usually manifests as encephalitis, headache, disorientation, and drowsiness.[76,77] If damage of brain tissue is extensive, the symptoms of a space-occupying lesion predominate, with intracerebral pressure, papilledema, and coma; if the motor cortex is involved, hemiparesis or seizures may be the presenting symptoms. Sometimes craneal neural involvement or spinal cord symptoms may occur. Psychotic symptoms are often associated with toxoplasmosis in individuals with AIDS but are more likely produced by the human immunodeficiency virus itself because they are not common in toxoplasmosis complicating other forms of immunosuppression.[2] The gross pathologic anatomy of toxoplasmosis in the central nervous system is that of multiple hemorrhagic or nonhemorrhagic necrotic lesions varying up to 4 cm in diameter, without any particular distribution (Fig. 38-21). Some of these lesions may cross the sulci to involve adjacent cortical tissue. If the patient dies of intracraneal pressure, the typical lesions of herniation will be found. Microscopically, the lesions are seen as necrotic areas with variable, sometimes sparse infiltration by inflammatory cells, both mononuclear and polymorphonuclear. The parasites are usually more abundant in the periphery than in the center of the lesion. Tachyzoites are seen as blue dots, 1 to 2 μm, difficult to outline in normal histologic sections but easier if 2 μm sections are made. When cells are filled with tachyzoites, they are often irregular and are called *pseudocysts*. True cysts in brain tissue are rounded, about 30 μm in diameter, and filled with tightly packed zoites, and have a wall 1 μm thick. Tachyzoites and bradyzoites have granules that stain positively with periodic acid–Schiff stain.[2]

Toxoplasmosis causes myocarditis when the parasite invades and then multiplies within the myocytes. Cyst rupture produces an inflammatory reaction, characterized by mononuclear cell infiltrate.[78] The heart is grossly globose and flabby and microscopically shows different degrees of tissue damage. The hallmark of cardiac infection are parasites in either pseudocysts or cysts.[2,78] In muscle fibers the cysts of *Toxoplasma* often take the shape of an elongated fiber.[2] One aspect of these lesions, important for the diagnostician pathologist, is the interpretation of the presence of nests of parasites within the cardiac myocytes, without an inflammatory reaction. If the sample is one obtained post mortem, one should speculate that if the patient had lived a few more days a myocarditis could have developed. In a myocardial biopsy specimen, the same finding is more difficult to interpret because of the small size of the sample, which usually shows only one or two nests of parasites.

Toxoplasmal myocarditis can complicate cardiac transplantation. In the United States and in England a transplant recipient seronegative for *Toxoplasma* has a 17% chance of receiving a heart from a seropositive person. Half of these individuals develop myocarditis, which is indistinguishable clinically and histologically (if parasites are not seen or identified) from rejection. This complication is often fatal if not treated.[79,80]

As previously stated, *Toxoplasma* causes other lesions in immunodeficient hosts, usually diagnosed at the autopsy table, rarely clinically. Pneumonitis,[74] pancreatitis, enteritis,[74] orchitis, and acute retinitis with necrosis[81] are just a few of those seen. In cases of acute retinal necrosis in the immunosuppressed, the polymerase chain reaction for detection of *Toxoplasma* organisms in the vitreous has been successful.[82]

Congenital toxoplasmosis

As a rule, congenital toxoplasmosis is most prevalent where transmission of *Toxoplasma* is most frequent, as in some parts of Latin America.[71] In France, a country with high endemicity,

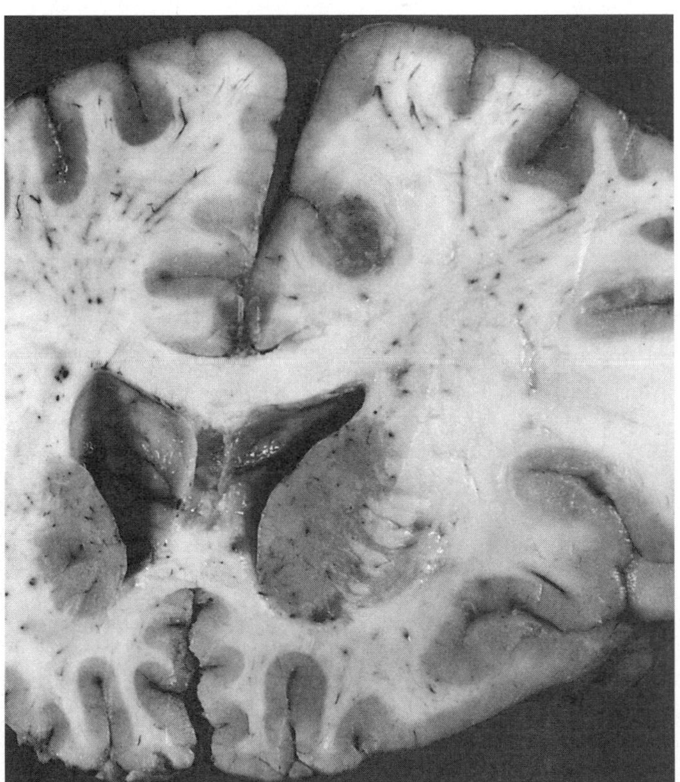

Fig. 38-21 *Toxoplasma gondii* in brain of an individual with AIDS. Notice the areas of necrosis.

congenital toxoplasmosis is low because of preventive measures. Transmission occurs transplacentally during the time the mother suffers a primary infection, even if she is asymptomatic.[71] The reason is that parasitemia in toxoplasmosis occurs only for a short period during primary infection when seeding of the placenta and the fetus is possible. At this time the blood is infectious, and if donated, it will also transmit the infection. This mechanism explains why a woman, or a blood donor, transmits the infection only once. Successive pregnancies or donated blood pose no danger of infection. The effects of *Toxoplasma* to the fetus depends on when during gestation the infection is acquired. If acquired during the first half, the fetus has signs of chronic infection. Infections acquired during the second half of the gestational period result in infants who, if delivered alive, have manifestations that vary from subclinical to severe disease with abnormalities such as hydrocephalus, microphthalmia, brain calcifications, enlarged liver, and icterus.[71] Patients with subclinical effects may survive to adulthood, sometimes showing mental deficits.

Grossly and microscopically the effects of infection are most apparent in the central nervous system. Necrosis, chronic inflammation, and calcifications of the brain substance are the prominent findings. An enlarged ventricular system is the rule in all cases of hydrocephalus because of destruction of brain tissue (Fig. 38-22, *A*). Foci of infection with the characteristic parasites are found in the placenta (Fig. 38-22, *B*), the umbilical cord, and every fetal organ studied microscopically.[71] Infants in whom the infection is suspected clinically may be diagnosed serologically in samples taken from both the mother and the infant.[73]

The clinical diagnosis of toxoplasmosis is difficult. The laboratory diagnosis of eye, heart, and brain, or in congenital infection is sometimes made by the study of sera, vitreous, and cerebrospinal fluid. Determination of specific IgG and IgM antibodies against *Toxoplasma* usually require acute and convalescent samples.[73] Measurement of local production of antibodies (CSF, vitreous) may be necessary before a diagnosis is made.[73] Tissue samples, especially large biopsy specimens, offer the best chance for specific diagnosis, whereas small biopsy specimens, when negative, provide little information. Biopsy specimens are processed by routine histologic methods, but before fixation they should be used to make imprints. Aspiration biopsy specimens, as smears of fluids or lesions, must be fixed in absolute alcohol and stained with Giemsa or other similar stains. The typical tachyzoites in smears are about 3 to 4 μm long by 1 to 2 μm wide, slightly curved, and with a central nucleus. The cytoplasm stains pale blue and the nucleus darkly. The cysts are rounded structures with numerous zoites, similar to the tachyzoites. Many cells may have the parasites in their cytoplasm, but many are extracellular, an artifact produced when the smears are made. Immune stains are very specific, especially in small biopsy samples.[2] In a few instances the parasite has been recovered from blood samples,[83] but this is not a recommended method for diagnosis because of low yields.[84]

Malaria

Human malaria is caused by apicomplexan protozoa of the genus *Plasmodium*, which live in the red blood cells of the host and require mosquitos of the genus *Anopheles* for transmission. Malaria transmission has been controlled in the developed countries of the world since the second half of this century but persists in many countries of the tropical belt and in some of the northern subtropics.[85] Therefore, although campaigns against malaria have been successful in many places, its incidence is still rising, making malaria one of the most important infectious diseases in the world today, producing about 200 million new cases each year, with a 2% mortality. It has been estimated that in Africa alone, the infection kills between 500,000[86] and one million children yearly. In the United States most cases of malaria seen are imported,[87] though clusters of reintroduced malaria have been recorded.[88,89]

The plasmodia of humans are classified into four species known as *P. falciparum, P. vivax, P. malariae,* and *P. ovale*.

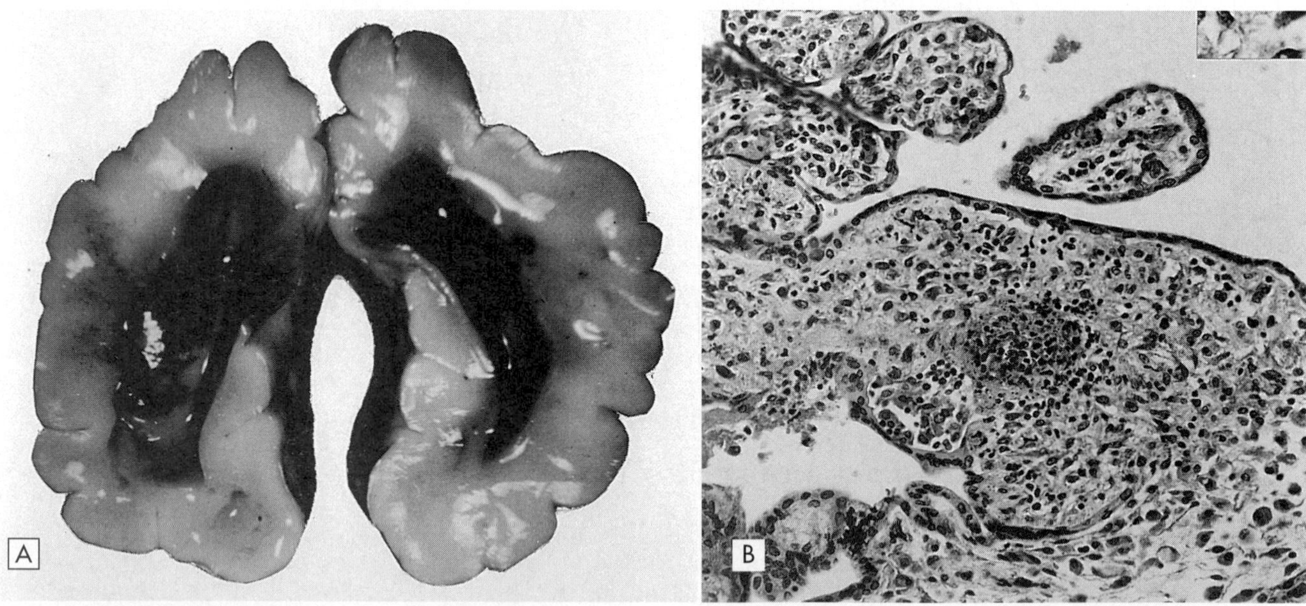

Fig. 38-22 *Toxoplasma gondii* in a newborn. **A,** Coronal section of brain demonstrating the hydrocephalus. **B,** Section of placenta showing the pronounced placentitis with a focus of necrosis. *Inset,* Pseudocyst of the parasite.

The disease they produce depends on the species involved, with *P. falciparum* being the one responsible for most fatal infections.[1,85] *Plasmodium malariae* produces the nephrotic syndrome, especially in African children, some resulting in deaths. The plasmodia have complicated life cycles, the knowledge of which is necessary to understand the epidemiology of the parasite, the human disease, and the concepts on which the modern ideas for a malaria vaccine are based. Fortunately for the student of pathology, the life cycles of malarial parasites are very similar.[1,2] Malarial parasites are inoculated into the bloodstream by the female *Anopheles* mosquito while it is feeding. The stages inoculated are known as "sporozoites," stored in the salivary glands of the insect. Once in the bloodstream the sporozoites travel to the liver where they enter the hepatocytes, to develop for a period of about 7 to 14 days, depending on the species. This is a silent, asexual phase of development that produces no inflammation or destruction of tissue and results in the production of thousands of stages called *merozoites*, which spill into the hepatic sinusoids and hence into the bloodstream.

Merozoites in the bloodstream make contact with and rapidly enter the erythrocytes, an active process directed by the parasite, which results in the formation of a parasitophorous vacuole; the merozoites divide asexually to generate more merozoites, the numbers of which are variable in accordance with the species of plasmodia. This part of the cycle is called the *erythrocytic cycle* and is completed more or less in synchrony (all merozoites grow into schizonts, which give rise to more merozoites, finishing their multiplication at the same time), in either 48 or 72 hours, depending on the species in question. The importance of this fact is that malaria is a disease characterized by episodes of intense fever occurring every 48 or every 72 hours, coinciding with the completion of the erythrocytic life cycle. Of the four species mentioned above, *P. malariae* is the only one with a 72-hour cycle. Thus the disease has been known as either tertian (occurs each third day) or quartan (each fourth day) malaria. Some of the merozoites produced in the red blood cells develop into gametocytes, male and female. These gametocytes are ingested by the mosquito and undergo a sexual development through a series of steps that culminate in the production of sporozoites which locate in the salivary glands of the mosquito, completing the life cycle.[1,2]

The above life cycle has a step in the liver, with important differences in the four plasmodia of humans. For example, in *P. falciparum* and *P. malariae*, all the sporozoites inoculated by the mosquito develop at once;[1] in *P. vivax* and *P. ovale*, which are more economic, only a portion of the inoculated sporozoites develop, with the rest remaining dormant in the hepatocytes.[1] This population of dormant stages is responsible for seeding the blood at different times, producing relapses of malaria. Since this part of the life cycle is known as the exoerythrocytic life cycle, it follows that *P. falciparum* and *P. malariae* do not maintain an exoerythrocytic life cycle but *P. vivax* and *P. ovale* do.[1,2] The infection produced by *P. falciparum* differs in many aspects from that produced by the other three plasmodia and is discussed separately.[2]

Plasmodium falciparum

Plasmodium falciparum is the only plasmodium of humans that produces acute fatal infections and completes its erythrocytic cycle in 48 hours; therefore the infection is known as *malignant tertian* malaria. *P. malariae* infections may also result in death from nephrotic syndrome, but not in an acute fashion (see below). As stated before, all sporozoites of *P. falciparum* mature in the liver at once, leaving no dormant forms to seed the peripheral circulation at a later time; this means that *P. falciparum* does not produce relapses. The natural duration of the infection in untreated individuals who survive it is about 18 months, including periods free of symptoms with the parasites undetectable in routine blood samples but still present in low numbers. A new bout of symptoms attributable to a surge of parasitemia is known as a *recrudescence*. Another important characteristic of *P. falciparum* is that the erythrocytic part of the life cycle, also known as *sporogony*, occurs hidden in the deep visceral capillaries. Soon after the merozoite enters the erythrocyte, it begins its development and division of the nuclear chromatin. This development is accompanied by changes, elicited by the parasites, on the red blood cell membrane; these changes are the formation of knobs (electron-dense structures) with surface molecules that allow the parasitized red blood cell to bind to receptors on the endothelial cells of the capillaries throughout the body.[90,91] The attachment usually occurs at the time the first nuclear division occurs and lasts until the completion of the sporogonic cycle, with the rupture of the red blood cell.[85] During this period the blood has few or no organisms circulating. This means that *P. falciparum* has in the peripheral circulation only early red blood cell stages known as trophozoites or ring forms and mature gametocytes. The other plasmodia have all stages of the erythrocytic life cycle in circulation. The advantage to the parasite of attachment to the endothelial cells is that infected erythrocytes do not pass through the spleen where they would be readily retained and destroyed; thus this advantage can be interpreted as a defense mechanism for *P. falciparum*.[92-94] The disadvantage to the host is the uncontrolled proliferation of parasites, resulting in fatal infections.

Initially, an uncomplicated infection with *P. falciparum* is clinically similar to that produced by the other plasmodia. It begins after an incubation period of 1 to 2 weeks, with prodromal symptoms of bone aches, headache, chills, nausea, and sometimes diarrhea. The typical malarial attack by *falciparum* malaria begins with low fever, headache, bone and muscle pain, sometimes anxiety and mental confusion, followed by an increase in temperature lasting for several hours, followed by profuse sweating. The fever is irregular, without periodicity, at the beginning of the infection but tends to become regular later, with a 3-day pattern, in which case the individual becomes asymptomatic between the attacks. Complicated, or pernicious, malaria presents clinically in many forms, depending on the main organ system involved. The sufferer with cerebral malaria presents with rapid development of coma and death and even with meningismus, paresis, mental changes, and epileptiform attacks. These later manifestations are not specific, and other causes should be ruled out even in individuals with circulating *falciparum* parasites,[2] especially when parasitemias are consistently low. One form of malaria seen in endemic areas is hemoglobinuric renal failure after massive erythrocytic hemolysis especially after primaquin or other oxidant drugs are administered to individuals with glucose-6-phosphatase (G6PD) deficiency. Hemoglobinuria develops rapidly, followed by shock and rapid renal failure.

Malignant or pernicious malaria occurs primarily in children and in recent immigrants or travelers to the endemic area because both lack immunity to the parasites, but newborns are somewhat protected by antibodies passed from the mother to the child, antibodies that disappear in a few months. Immunity to *falciparum* malaria is strain specific, and since in a given endemic area there may be many strains of the parasite producing infections, building an immunity requires many exposures until, theoretically, infections with all parasite strains have occurred. Also, immunity does not abolish the infection but suppresses the disease, and so infections with strains to which immunity exists can still occur but are asymptomatic. In endemic areas for *falciparum* malaria it is frequent to find parasitemic individuals without any symptoms. Thus the immune status of the host explains at least partially the high susceptibility of infants[95] and newcomers to the endemic areas, as well as the resistance of the adult population. It has been shown that individuals with AIDS do not appear to be more affected by malaria, though they have lower humoral responses to the parasite.[96]

The pathologic anatomy of *P. falciparum* infections is very striking. The organs are congested, with a gray or black pigmentation as a result of the accumulation of a by-product of the metabolism of hemoglobin by the parasite, known as "malarial pigment." Malarial pigment is a molecule consisting of iron and a protein moiety; it is a pigment that is phagocytized and processed by the macrophages. Accumulation of these macrophages in the tissues gives the dark pigmentation to the organs, a pigmentation that becomes deeper the longer the infection persists. Microscopically, in acute malaria there is pronounced hyperemia, with dilatation of all capillaries, showing numerous parasitized erythrocytes attached to the endothelial surface of the vessel (Fig. 38-23). Accompanying this are macrophages laden with pigment, especially in the liver, spleen, and bone marrow. The pigment is seen as crystalline clumps of dark green material that polarizes under polarizing light, a characteristic helpful in the differential diagnosis. In cerebral malaria the brain is swollen, and all vessels are dilated and riddled with pigment and contain red blood cells with parasites.[2]

P. vivax, P. malariae, and *P. ovale*

The three plasmodia *P. vivax, P. malariae,* and *P. ovale* produce malarial attacks occurring every 48 hours for *vivax* and *ovale* and every 72 hours for *malariae*. The natural history of untreated *vivax* infections is about 3.5 years, and that of *malariae* up to 60 years. The duration of *ovale* infections is unknown. *Plasmodium malariae* does not have an exoerythrocytic life cycle and thus can remain in circulation during all these years, making infections with it important in transmission of malaria through blood. Also, *P. vivax* and *P. ovale* have exoerythrocytic life cycles, a condition that means that treatment of the infection has to address the liver stages, requiring a different therapeutic regimen from that needed for *falciparum* and *malariae*. The anatomic pathologic state of acute malarial infections produced by *vivax* and *ovale* is minimal because no deaths occur and no lesions have been described.[2] *P. malariae* commonly produces nephrotic syndrome, a chronic complication attributable to antigen-antibody complexes, especially in West African children, resulting in deaths.

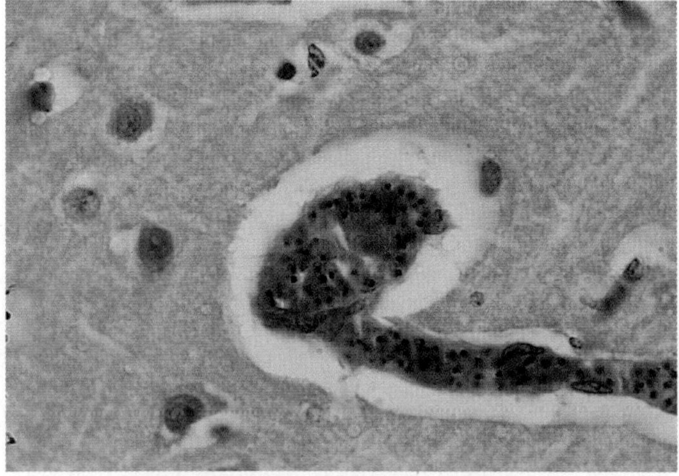

Fig. 38-23 *Plasmodium falciparum* in brain, illustrating the dilatation of the blood vessels and the presence of parasitized red blood cells, next to the endothelial cells.

Identification of malarial parasites is done in the clinical laboratory by the study of thick and thin blood smears. Two problems are encountered: finding the parasites and identifying them, both requiring excellent preparations of fresh blood, stained properly, preferably with Giemsa stain though other similar stains are more frequently used today. The morphology of the parasites found usually allows a specific diagnosis in experienced hands.[2] Quantitative counts are important in determining and monitoring treatment. Repeat smears at 12- or at 24-hour intervals, may help in understanding the behavior of the parasites and help with the identification of the species when this was not immediately possible. No special techniques are available to speciate malarial parasites. A variety of serologic and molecular methods are used mainly for epidemiologic studies, but old-fashioned microscopy remains the cornerstone of malaria diagnosis even today.

Babesiosis

Babesiae are common organisms, occurring in animals and sporadically in humans in most regions of the world.[1,2] They are intraerythrocytic parasites, resembling the plasmodia. The main differences between malarial parasites and the babesiae are the following: its trophozoites are small and solid and usually piriform and are arranged in pairs or tetrads within the cell resembling sometimes a maltese cross, and they do not produce pigment during the erythrocytic cycle, which is the main zoologic difference between the genera *Babesia* and *Plasmodium*.[1] As stated, many species of *Babesia* are known in animals where they produce babesiosis or pyroplasmosis, an acute, often fatal infection characterized by profound hemolyzis resulting in renal failure. Only four or five species of *Babesia* have been isolated from humans, but serologic data indicate that the infection may be more common than previously believed[97] and that several species may be involved in human infections.

Babesiae are transmitted by ticks, in which the sexual cycle occurs, producing sporozoites, which locate in the salivary glands. Ticks may also transmit the infection transovarially to their offspring, increasing the number of arthropods infected in a given area. In the vertebrate host, including humans, the inoculated sporozoites develop asexually in the red blood cells into four merozoites, which lyse the erythrocyte and once freed infect other red blood cells. Gametocytes develop and in the tick undergo the sexual part of the cycle.[1]

Babesia microti is the species known to produce most infections in humans and occurs in the New England area, where it is transmitted by *Ixodes scapularis* var. *dammini,* the same tick vector of Lyme disease; *B. equi* has been found in California; *B. divergens* in Ireland; and *B. bovis* in the former Yugoslavia.[1,2] The extent of human infections is unknown. The disease in humans is characterized by a hemolytic anemia, with gradual onset of malaise, fatigue, anorexia, and fever with profuse sweating and muscle and joint pains. In the worst cases, nausea, shaking chills, and vomiting occur. The temperature may be up to 40° C and slight splenomegaly may be palpated. Laboratory data show a steady decrease in the hemoglobin and an increase in reticulocytes, bilirubinemia, and normal white blood cell counts. Some patients have necessitated transfusions, and fatal infections have been recorded only in splenectomized individuals.

The clinical diagnosis of babesiosis is difficult, but often suspected by alert physicians in areas where the infection has been recognized.[98] Confirmation of the diagnosis is made in the laboratory by the identification of the parasites in blood smears taken under similar conditions, and with the same care as for the diagnosis of malaria. The typical morphologic characteristics of the organisms and the lack of pigment are diagnostic.[1,2]

MICROSPORIDIA

The Microsporidia are a large phylum of obligate intracellular protozoan organisms that only recently have been conclusively identified as producing disease in humans, especially in patients with the acquired immunodeficiency syndrome.[99] The basic classification, life cycle, and zoologic relationships of this group still need much additional work.[100]

Microsporidia are parasitic organisms found primarily in invertebrates. Until recently *Encephalitozoon* was the only genus found in several groups of vertebrates and humans, but more recently, several other species have been identified.[101] Their life cycles are not well known, but infections may occur either by inhalation, by contact of the organisms with a mucosa (conjunctiva), or by ingestion of the minute stages, which appear to be responsible for the transmission, known as "spores." The main stages of the life cycle known in vertebrates are the spores, oval structures that in most of the species described in humans are about 1 μm. In tissues stained with hematoxylin and eosin stain, the spores are intracellular and hardly visible, and with silver stains, the wall of the spore stains darkly; they are also darkly stained in plastic-embedded sections for electron microscopy. In electron micrographs, the spores are composed of a thick wall, a sporoplast, a nucleus, an attachment disk, and a microtubule arising from the attachment disk (Fig. 38-24, *A*). The microtubule curves into several loops (coils) around the sporoplast to give a characteristic look to the organism under the electron microscope (Fig. 38-24, *B*). Mature spores within the cell uncoil their microtubule and extrude it to the outside of the cell, reach a neighboring cell, and inject the sporoplast through the tubule to the new cell (Fig. 38-24, *A*). Infection then starts in the new cell, with the growth of the parasite to a plasmodial stage (Fig. 38-25, *B*), which soon begins dividing to produce spores.[100]

Microsporidiosis

Encephalitozoon

The characteristic of *Encephalitozoon* species is that they occur within vacuoles inside the cell. The species *E. cuniculi* is the best known, and at least one report of a central nervous infection in a child was recorded but disregarded later based on compelling evidence because of the faulty manner in which the diagnosis was made. Other cases of *E. cuniculi* compromising other organs have been reported but need further confirmation of the species.[102] *Encephalitozoon hellem* has been implicated in keratoconjunctivitis in immunocompetent individuals, producing superficial ulcerations[103] (Figs. 38-24), either devoid of inflammatory infiltrate, or with pronounced histiocytic and polymorphonuclear cells. This parasite is capable of dissemination in immunocompromised hosts, producing infections in macrophages and epithelial cells, resulting in nephritis, or bronchiolitis.[104] An *Encephalitozoon*-like organism, named *Septata intestinalis*, has recently been described[105] in the intestine of individuals with AIDS, producing infections similar to *E. bieneusi* (see below).[108]

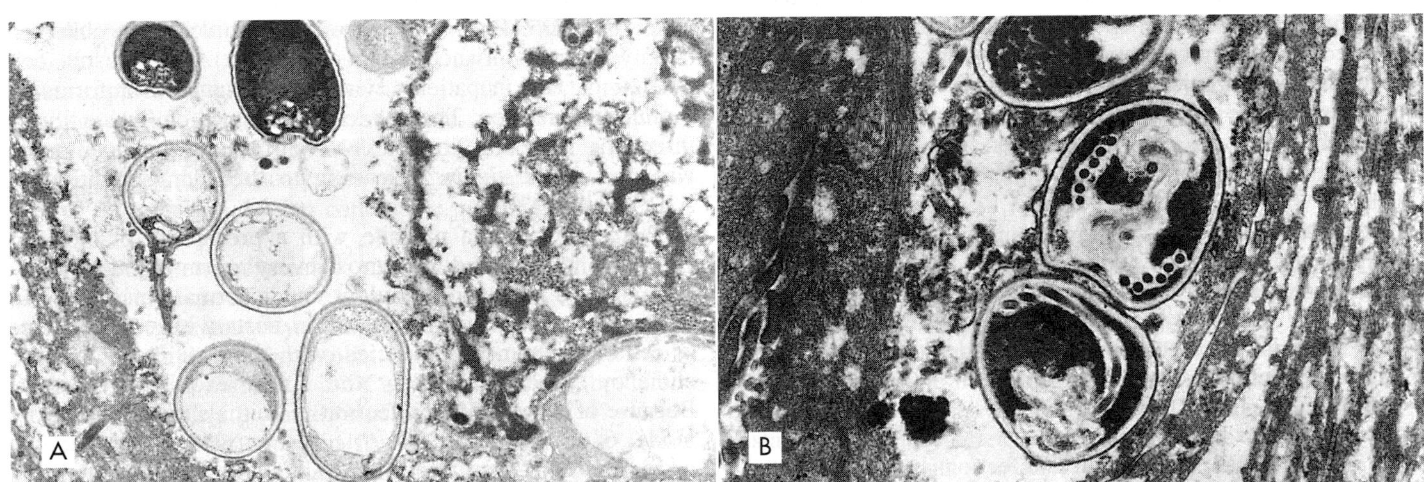

Fig. 38-24 *Encephalitozoon hellem* in electron micrographs of sections of cornea. **A,** The spores are within a vacuole, some of which are empty because they have already injected the sporoplasm to other cells. One spore at left shows a small part of the everted microtubule. **B,** Spores showing the typical coiled microtubule, the main characteristic of the group.

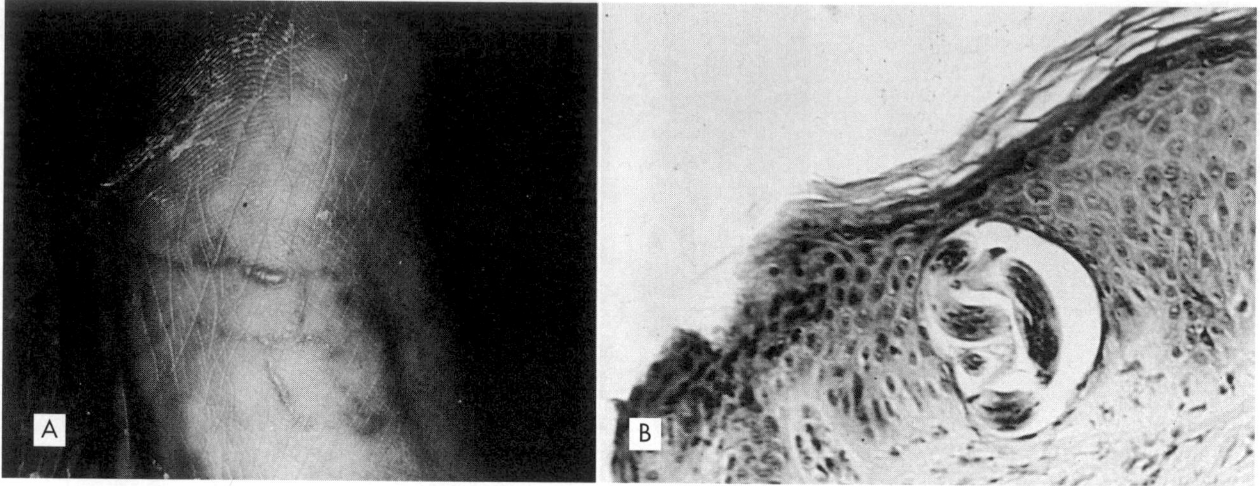

Fig. 39-11 Cutaneous larva migrans. **A,** Gross lesions in the foot, showing the typical tracts produced by the migrating parasites. **B,** Histologic appearance of the lesion demonstrating the location of the larva in the epidermis. (Courtesy H. Blank, MD, Miami School of Medicine, Miami, Fla. In Gutierrez Y: *Diagnostic pathology of parasitic infections with clinical correlations,* Philadelphia, 1990, Lea & Febiger.)

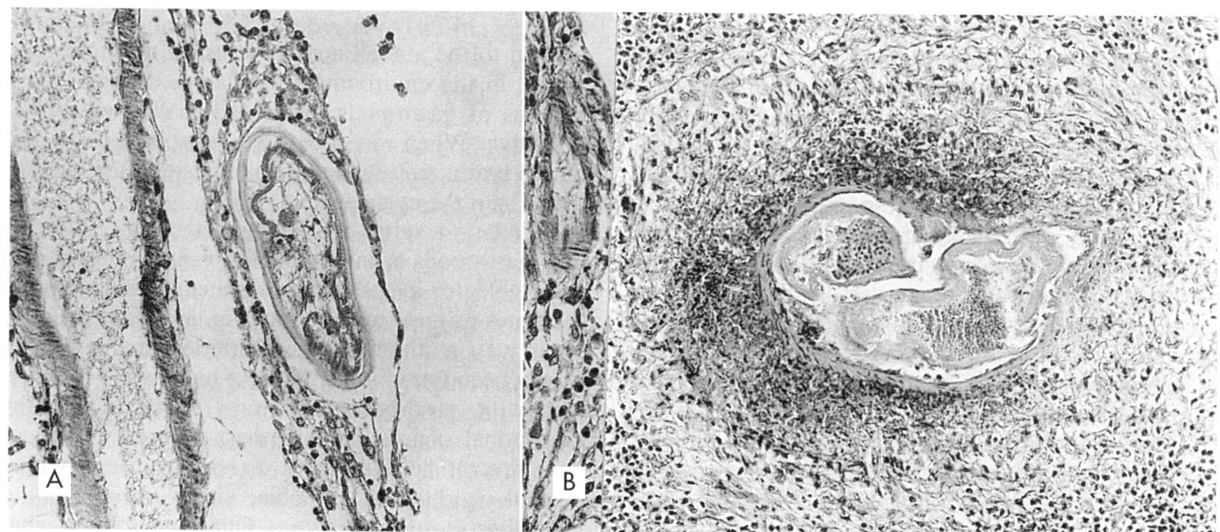

Fig. 39-12 *Angiostrongylus* in humans. **A,** Cross section of *A. cantonensis* in the meninges of a patient with eosinophilic meningitis. **B,** *A. costaricensis* in the wall of the cecum of a child with abdominal angiostrongylosis. Notice the worm within an area of arteritis.

Angiostrongylus costaricensis, produces abdominal angiostrongylosis, especially in Central America and South America.[2,3] The life cycle of *A. costaricensis* is similar to that of *A. cantonensis,* except that the worms mature in the splanchnic lymph nodes and the adults locate in the arteries feeding the terminal ileum, the ileocecal valve, and the appendix. The infection occurs mostly in children, and its presentation is often pain in the right iliac fossa, anorexia, vomiting, constipation, and abdominal rigidity. On palpation a mass is often felt in the right lower quadrant, and the temperature is slightly increased; the clinical diagnosis is often mild appendicitis. In most cases surgical intervention results in removal of a portion of the ileum.[49]

Grossly, the segment of ileum removed is inflamed, the wall is thickened, it has a serositis, and on section the wall shows small granulomas. In addition, the regional lymph nodes are enlarged. Microscopically the lesion consists of an overwhelming inflammation with granulomas sometimes containing larvae, and the inflammatory infiltrate is composed of mononuclear and polymorphonuclear cells, especially eosinophils. The adult worms are found in the lumen of the small-sized arteries[48,49] (Fig. 39-12, *B*). The diagnosis is clinically difficult outside the endemic areas, and the larvae, which are easily recovered in the stools of the natural hosts, are seldom found in the stools of humans.[3] Worms should be identified based on their morphologic characteristics for proper diagnosis of the infection.

Trichinelliasis, or trichinosis

Trichinelliasis is an infection both of the intestinal tract and the skeletal musculature produced by *Trichinella spiralis,* a nematode occurring widely in the temperate zones and to a lesser extent in other areas.[2,3] The parasite is naturally found in many domestic and wild animals, of which pigs play the most important role in transmission to humans. The infection is common in Eastern European countries and the former Soviet Union. In the United States the prevalence of the infection has steadily declined from over 400 cases reported yearly in the 1940s, to less than 100 today; one third of these cases are acquired by ingestion of meat from wild animals.[3]

The adult worms are about 2 mm in length and live in the small intestine, deep in the crypts, buried in the mucosa in a fashion similar to that of *Trichuris*.[50,51] Here, adults lay larvae, which enter the circulation and reach the skeletal muscles to encapsulate and become infective. The adults remain in the intestine for about 4 weeks, the time necessary for the body to mount an inflammatory reaction, which dislodges the worms from the duodenal mucosa, to be lost in the feces. From this description it follows that the clinical manifestations of trichinosis relate to the intestine and to the skeletal musculature. Infections occur usually in clusters because members of a family or a group of friends share the infective meal, usually poorly cooked pork. Symptoms of malaise, vomiting, diarrhea, nausea, and abdominal cramps commence soon after the infective meal and depend on the dose of larvae ingested. The clinical diagnosis at this stage is often food poisoning. After the intestinal symptoms subside, generalized manifestations become apparent, such as muscle aches, edema of the face (sometimes periorbital) and hands, and generalized weakness, or weakness of groups of muscles, progressing to difficulties in swallowing, chewing, and breathing. A generalized myositis with a strikingly high peripheral eosinophilia is the hallmark of the disease. In some cases myocarditis[52,53] or encephalitis[54] are fatal complications. Ten years after the acute disease, no sequelae have been found.[55]

The morphologic manifestations of the infection depend on the organ studied. The intestinal mucosa may look grossly normal but microscopically shows inflammation, with a large number of eosinophils infiltrating the wall, and sections of the worms may be seen deep in the crypts. These changes are rarely seen in humans because intestinal biopsy specimens are not taken for diagnosis. In the skeletal muscles larvae exist in different stages of encapsulation depending on when the sample is taken.[3] Larvae may be observed inside the muscle cell without changes (recently arrived larvae) or fully encapsulated (after 5 weeks), or in between these two extremes. Encapsulated larvae are coiled inside a translucent, hyalinized, oval, thick wall, with the poles slightly extended (Fig. 39-13). In early stages the larvae elicit a myositis because they destroy the skeletal muscle fibers, and an inflammatory infiltrate dominated by eosinophils is apparent. The myositis is more acute at the time of migration and encapsulation of the larvae and slowly subsides and disappears completely after encapsulation. Larvae in the muscles eventually die and sometimes calcify. The inflammatory infiltrates in the heart are similar to those in the muscles and result in myocarditis, but larvae are rarely found because they do not encapsulate in the myocardium. In heavy infections a fatal encephalitis and meningitis may occur because of the migration of larvae through the brain tissue producing multiple microscopic areas of necrosis with infiltration by eosinophils; larvae are difficult to demonstrate in tissue sections of brain because they do not encapsulate in the central nervous system.[2,3]

The diagnosis of trichinosis is often made clinically but requires confirmation by identification of the larvae in the skeletal muscles. The examination of the infectious meal, if available, can reveal the larvae. A biopsy of the deltoid muscle is customary and, if positive, reveals larvae in different stages of encapsulation and various degrees of myositis. Several serologic tests are available for diagnosis.

Intestinal capillariasis

Intestinal capillariasis is an acute disease characterized by watery diarrhea that does not respond to customary treatment and develops into a sprue-like syndrome with a weight loss as a result of vitamin, protein, and carbohydrate malabsorption.[56] The disease occurs in the Philippines and other Southeast Asian countries. The life cycle of the parasite involves small freshwater fish as their intermediate hosts, which are the source of infection for humans. In the small intestine the ingested infective larvae develop to adults, buried in the mucosal crypts. Some females lay eggs that rapidly develop into infective larvae in the intestine, and the larvae reenter the mucosa to grow to adults producing internal autoinfection. Other females lay eggs that are evacuated with the feces into the environment to infect the intermediate hosts.[57]

Human infections with *Capillaria philippinensis* are invariably fatal if not treated. In these cases the examination of the

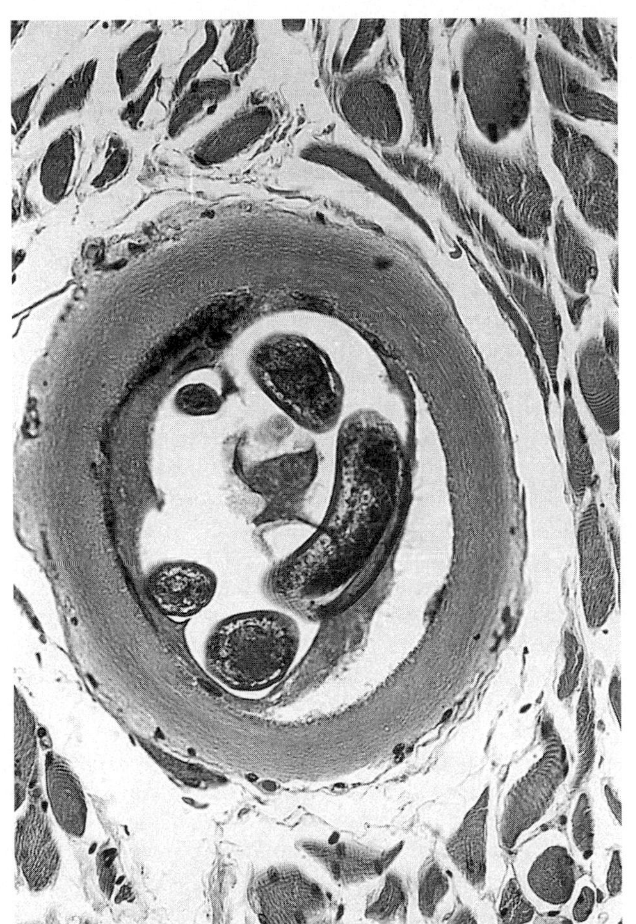

Fig. 39-13 *Trichinella spiralis* encapsulated in skeletal muscle. The section is a transverse one and thus there is a round appearance. There is a complete lack of inflammatory reaction because the infection is dormant at this stage.

small intestine shows changes varying from atrophy of the mucosa to thickening of the wall and superficial ulcerations. Microscopically, the main finding is the worms in the mucosa, sometimes seen with only scant inflammatory infiltrate.[58,59] The diagnosis is made usually on clinical grounds in endemic areas and is confirmed in the clinical laboratory by identification of the typical eggs in the stools.

Filariasis

Filarids are nematodes measuring from 2 to 30 cm in length, depending on the species. In the tissues of the host they produce progeny known as *microfilariae.* Microfilariae occur either in the skin or in circulating blood. Although their movements resemble those of a larva, microfilariae developmentally are immature stages between an egg and a larva. Because microfilariae are readily recovered from blood and possess morphologic characteristics that allow their speciation, they are the stages commonly used for the diagnosis of filarial infections[60] (Fig. 39-14). Filarial worms produce morbidity and mortality that is a major public health problem in some areas. In general, two groups of filarial infections are known: (1) The ones endemic in wide geographic areas produce large numbers of infections and usually lack an animal reservoir; (2) a less important group of filarids of worldwide distribution are those in wild and domestic animals that sporadically infect humans, producing relatively low morbidity and resulting in challenging diagnostic problems for the pathologist. The life cycle of filarial worms is complicated but can be simplified as follows: The adult worms in the tissues produce microfilariae, which enter the blood and are ingested by hematophagous arthropods; within the intermediate host they develop to infective larvae to be passed into the next definitive host. Infective larvae enter through the skin and develop to adults in the tissues specific for each species.[2,3] Humans are parasitized by about 25 species of filarids, a few of which are reviewed.

Elephantiasis

Elephantiasis is a chronic disease seen in certain tropical and subtropical areas of the world and produced by the infection of the lymphatic system with filarial worms belonging to the genera *Wuchereria* and *Brugia.* The life cycle of lymphatic filariae is identical to that described above, with mosquitoes of the genera *Culex, Anopheles, Aedes,* and *Mansonia* serving as the intermediate hosts.[2] The microfilariae circulate in blood between 10 P.M. and 2 A.M. and during the remaining part of the day reside in the pulmonary capillary bed. This phenomenon is known as *periodicity* and, in the case of lymphatic filariae, *nocturnal periodicity.* The distribution of elephantiasis is the tropical African belt, eastern India, Southeast Asia, parts of China, and in the New World Brazil and some of the Caribbean islands.[2,3]

The natural history of lymphatic filariasis is best understood in individuals who visit one of the endemic areas and become infected.[61] Beginning about 8 months after their visit, these individuals start suffering bouts of lymphadenitis and lymphangitis manifesting as enlargement of the inguinal and popliteal lymph nodes. The nodes are mobile and nontender, with signs of inflammation of the lymph channels. These bouts of lymphangitis and lymphadenitis last for about 18 months, interspersed with asymptomatic intervals. The lymph nodes of these individuals contain dead adult worms that have provoked a granulomatous inflammation admixed with eosinophils. Samples of blood do not contain microfilariae; this syndrome is referred to as *filariasis without microfilaremia.*[61,62] In individuals living in the endemic areas who sustain continued infection and reinfection by the parasite, the early clinical manifestations are similar. However, the bouts of lymphangitis and lymphadenitis become increasingly worse with severe funiculitis, epididymitis, and orchitis in males.[63] There is continuous inflammation of the lymphatic system not fully countered by its reparative process, resulting in blockage of lymph egress/outflow, chronic lymphedema, and eventually elephantiasis of the lower limbs (Fig. 39-14), the scrotum, the breast, or the arms.[63] The lymph nodes show more extensive fibrosis and calcification. Identification of the parasites is based on their morphologic characteristics on cross sections. Blood samples taken at midnight reveal the typical microfilariae of *W. bancrofti* or one of several species of *Brugia* (Fig. 39-15), often in very low numbers.[20,60]

Infections with lymphatic filariae are responsible for other diseases such as *tropical eosinophilia* and the *Meyers-Kouwenaar syndrome.* Tropical eosinophilia occurs in people from India or of Indian descent and manifests as chronic symptoms of asthmatic episodes at night, accompanied by high peripheral eosinophilia and pulmonary infiltrates, symptoms that recede with antifilarial treatment.[64] The Meyers-Kouwenaar syndrome is common in Southeast Asia and the Pacific Islands and manifests as enlargement of the spleen, or lymph nodes, or both, because of a granulomatous inflammation elicited by dead microfilariae. The disease follows a benign course and histologically is characterized by a lymphadenitis with granulomas and microabscesses containing large numbers of eosinophils. Two characteristics of both tropical eosinophilia and the Meyers-Kouwenaar syndrome are that microfilariae are not found in circulation and that the adult worms have not been recovered from these patients.[61]

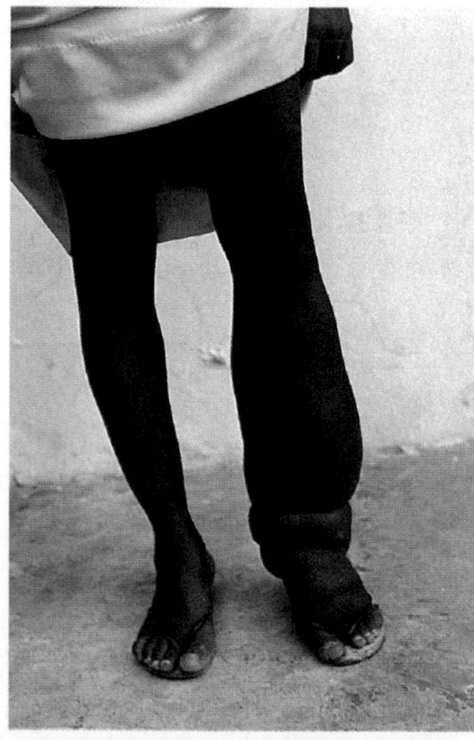

Fig. 39-14 *Wuchereria bancrofti,* causes elephantiasis as illustrated in the left leg of this patient.

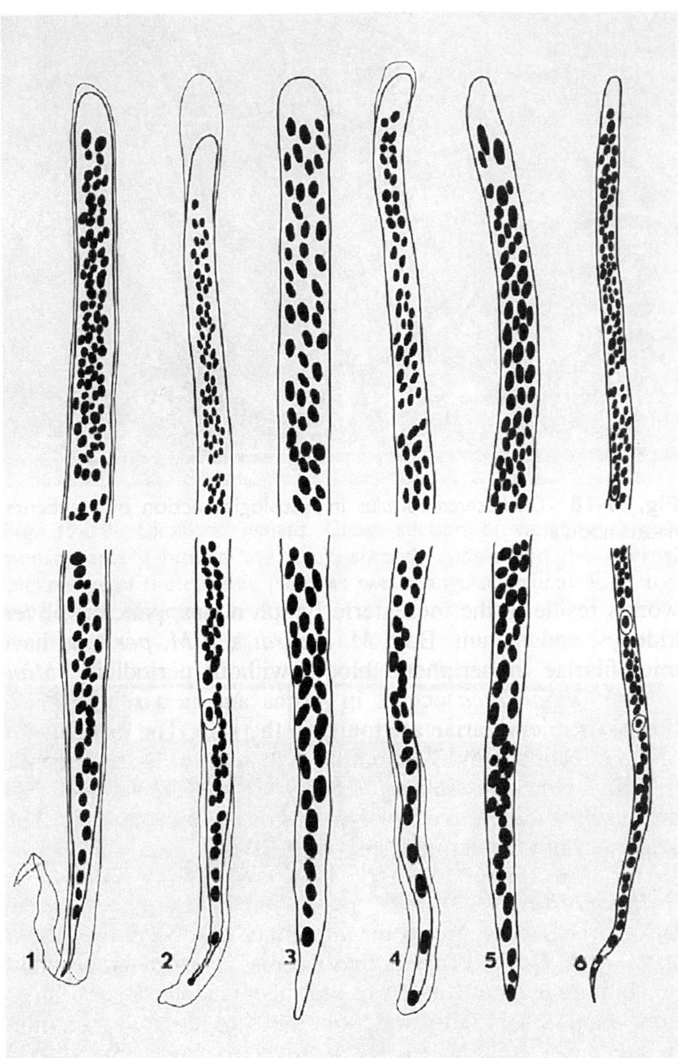

Fig. 39-15 Schema of diagnostic features of the main microfilariae found in humans. Notice both the presence or absence of a sheath and the nuclei at the tip of the tail. *1, Wuchereria bancrofti; 2, Brugia malayi; 3, Onchocerca volvulus; 4, Loa loa; 5, Mansonella perstans; 6, M. ozzardi.* (From Smith JW, Gutierrez Y: Medical parasitology. In Henry JB, editor: *Clinical diagnosis and management by laboratory methods,* ed 18, Philadelphia, 1991, Saunders.

Several species of *Brugia* from animals produce a sporadic granulomatous inflammation in patients from countries where the parasites are not endemic in humans. The majority of the cases have been recorded in the northeastern United States, diagnosed in lymph nodes removed because of inflammation, where the parasite has been identified. The histologic lesion is identical to that described for other *Brugia* infections[65,66] (Fig. 39-16).

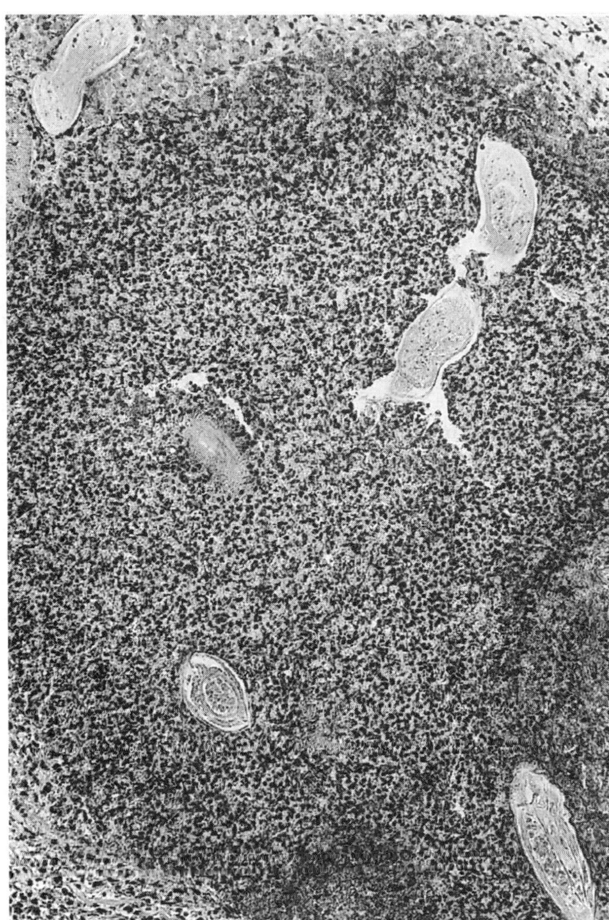

Fig. 39-16 *Brugia* species, one that caused lymphadenitis acquired in the northeastern United States. Notice the dead parasites within an abscess in the lymph node.

Onchocerciasis

Onchocerciasis, or river blindness, is an infection of the subcutaneous tissues and the dermis, caused by *Onchocerca volvulus,* a parasite found exclusively in humans living in the tropical African belt and in some places of the tropical American continents.[67] The adult worms live in the subcutaneous tissues, eliciting a fibrous reaction resulting in the formation of nodules up to 4 cm in diameter (Fig. 39-17). The nodules are painless and hard, located mainly in the upper part of the body of individuals living in the American continents, and in the lower part of the body of those from Africa. The life cycle of *Onchocerca* worms is similar to that of other filaria, except that the vector is a black fly (Simulium) and that the microfilariae reside in the skin.[68] The vectors of *Onchocerca* are distributed along the rivers, accounting for the geographic distribution of the disease. Since one of the main manifestations of onchocerciasis is blindness, the disease has been called "river blindness."[67,69]

The main clinical manifestations of onchocerciasis are subcutaneous nodules and an intermittent pruritic dermatitis with urticaria. The dermatitis may become permanent, producing lack of sleep, and secondary inflammations caused by scratching.[70] These symptoms are attributable to inflammation elicited by dead microfilariae in the skin. The chronic dermal insult results in different types of dermatitis with distinct characteristics depending on the geographic area.[70,71] One important lesion produced by the microfilariae of *Onchocerca* occurs in the eye. Microfilariae in the conjunctiva move through the cornea into the anterior and posterior chambers of the eye, eliciting inflammatory changes resulting in blindness.[63]

The clinical diagnosis of onchocerciasis is not difficult in the endemic areas but requires confirmation by the microscopic identification of microfilariae in fresh and stained skin samples (skin snips)[20,60] (Fig. 39-15). Microfilariae of

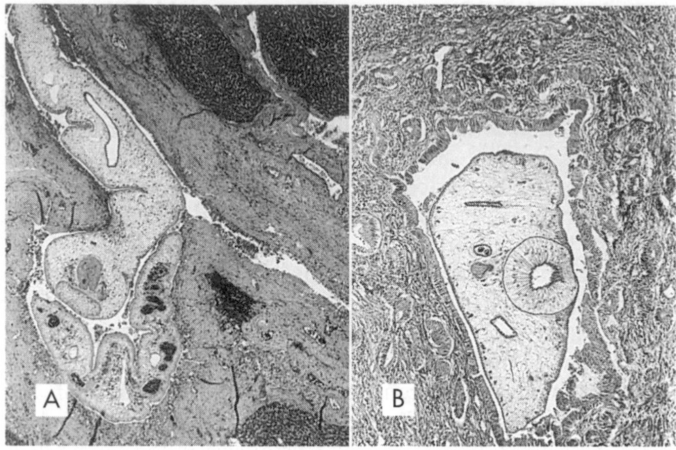

Fig. 39-25 *Clonorchis* in liver. **A,** Low-power view of a greatly fibrosed bile duct containing oblique sections of two parasites. **B,** Higher-power magnification illustrating the adenomatous proliferation of the bile duct epithelium.

The infection is usually asymptomatic, and in many endemic areas the prevalence is 100%. A few heavily infected individuals complain of biliary obstruction, often because dead parasites, eggs, or both, serve as the niduses for deposition of bile salts and formation of calculi. Symptoms are more commonly seen in individuals from nonendemic areas who become infected, and such symptoms manifest as general malaise, fever, slight jaundice, and enlargement of the liver. Eosinophils may account for up to 90% of the differential cell count. Long-term residence of the flukes in the bile ducts results in proliferation of the epithelium leading to adenomatous hyperplasia (Figs. 39-25, *B*). Individuals infected in endemic areas have a statistically significant higher incidence of cholangiocarcinomas.[93,94] The diagnosis of clonorchiasis and opisthorchiasis is made in the clinical laboratory with the identification of the typical eggs in the stools. The eggs cannot be speciated; thus the laboratory has to report the finding as eggs of *Clonorchis* or of *Opisthorchis*.[10,20] In symptomatic patients, imaging of the biliary tree shows obstruction and sometimes the parasites. The anatomic pathologists may find these organisms at autopsy or during examination of histologic sections, where the worms are seen inside the bile ducts (Figs. 39-25), which may have mild to moderate inflammation and consist of mononuclear cells and eosinophils. A pronounced fibrosis of the bile ducts is commonly found (Figs. 39-25, *A*).

Pulmonary trematodes

Paragonimiasis

Paragonimiasis is a chronic pulmonary disease, sometimes resembling tuberculosis clinically and radiologically, produced by several species of trematodes belonging to the genus *Paragonimus*. The infection is primarily seen in Korea, Japan, and Taiwan, but clusters of isolated cases have been reported from China, Vietnam, the Philippines, Thailand, Malaysia, India, some islands in the South Pacific, and certain countries of Africa, and Central America and South America.[2,3] In the United States autochthonous infections have been reported sporadically, but most cases are in Southeast Asian refugees and military personnel who have served in Korea.[95]

The life cycle of *Paragonimus* involves two intermediate hosts, the first a snail and the second a crustacean (crayfish and crabs), in which the infective stages develop. After ingestion of a raw crustacean, the larvae are freed in the intestine and pass into the peritoneal cavity, where they migrate to the lungs through the diaphragm. In the lung parenchyma, the juvenile worms grow in pairs or triplets, to attain a size of up to 1.5 by 0.7 by 0.6 cm. As the worms grow, the host's inflammatory reaction mounts and the destruction of tissue results in the formation of a cavity where the worms reside[2] (Fig. 39-26, *A*). This cavity may communicate with a bronchus, allowing the passage of eggs into the respiratory tree.[96]

The clinical manifestations of paragonimiasis are benign[97] because only one or two pairs of worms are found in most infected individuals. Infections among 10- to 25-year-olds are common, but severe infections are more common in the older population. The main manifestations are chronic cough with blood-tinged sputum and peripheral eosinophilia varying from 10% to 25%. The infection sometimes resembles chronic pulmonary tuberculosis, with chest radiographs showing cavitated lesions of up to 4 cm in diameter, sometimes with calcification. The pathologic anatomy produced by the disease is rather uniform, consisting grossly of firm, fibrotic pulmonary nodules of variable size, some with a cavity filled with necrotic debris. Recent lesions in humans and lesions in animals contain worms, but typically worms in humans die, leaving the cavity empty. Histologically, the lesion consists of different degrees of fibrosis and chronic granulomatous inflammation around the cavity. The granulomas are a response to eggs trapped in the tissues and are seen in the surrounding pulmonary parenchyma (Fig. 39-26, *B*). The inflammatory infiltrate is composed mostly of lymphocytes, plasma cells, and eosinophils. Operculated eggs are diagnostic of the genus *Paragonimus,* and the eggs should be identified in tissue sections by careful study of its morphologic characteristics, especially their size.[3] Since more than 20 different species of paragonimids have been found infecting humans, the specific identification of the parasites on the eggs alone is not possible. The most common species found in humans is *P. westermani,* and thus most textbooks refer only to this species.[2,3]

The migratory pathway followed by the worms from the intestine to the lungs results in ectopic locations in almost any other tissue in the body, where they produce unusual symptoms mimicking different diseases. The brain is the most important ectopic location because the symptoms resemble those of a brain tumor (Fig. 39-26, *C*). In the peritoneal cavity, nodules about 2 cm in diameter, with necrotic worms, or only masses of eggs are commonly found during autopsies or during abdominal surgery. Similarly, nodules produced by ectopic worms have been described in the heart, breast, and subcutaneous tissues.[3]

Schistosomiasis

Schistosomiasis is a group of chronic diseases produced by several species of trematodes belonging to the genus *Schistosoma* (blood flukes), which parasitize the portal system and the veins of the urinary tract. The main manifestations of the infection are hepatic fibrosis (Fig. 39-27), with portal and pulmonary arterial hypertension, and several types of uropathies. The schistosomes are the most important of the trematodes that infect humans, not only because of the morbidity and the mortality they produce, but also because of the sheer number of infected people worldwide.[2,98] Moreover, despite numerous campaigns to control the parasites, the disease is spreading in many areas because of the construction of hydroelectric and

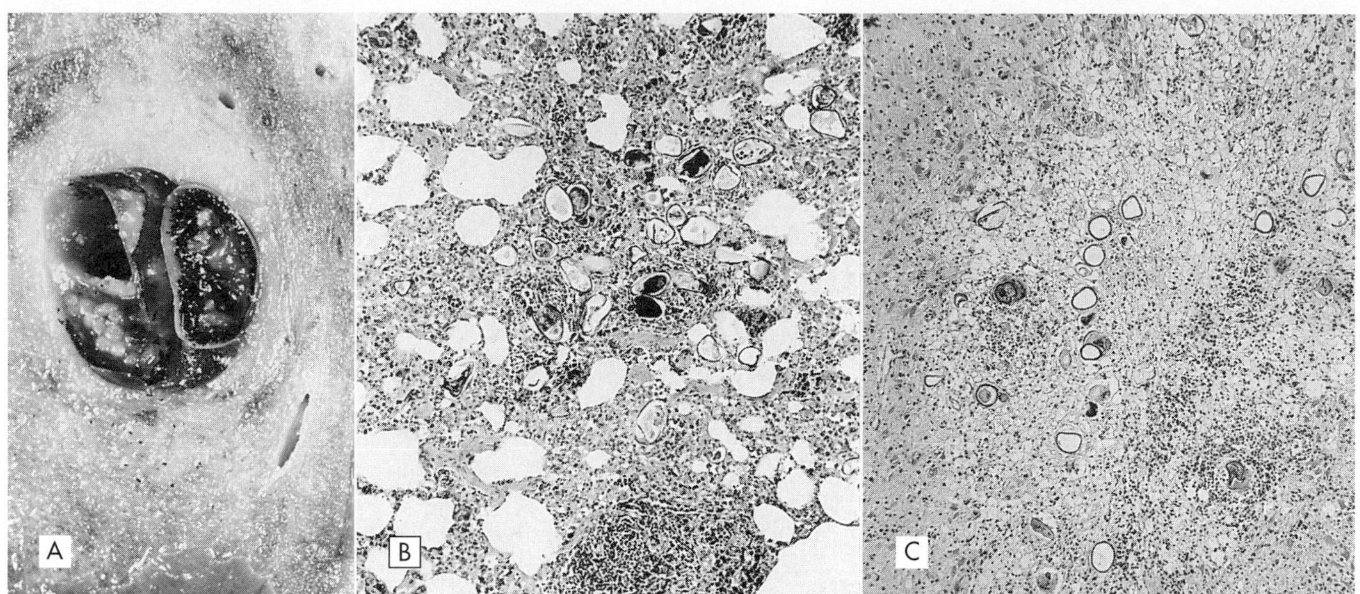

Fig. 39-26 *Paragonimus* lesions. **A,** Gross appearance of pulmonary lesion in an experimentally infected animal. **B,** Granulomatous inflammation in the lung. **C,** Lesion in brain showing numerous eggs among the reparative process.

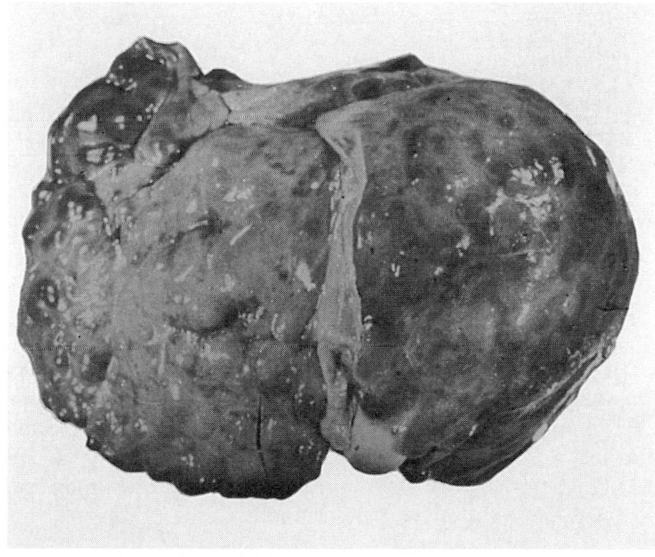

Fig. 39-27 *Schistosoma mansoni.* Gross appearance of liver in case of portal hypertension.

irrigation projects for agricultural purposes, which expand the habitat of the snails, their intermediate hosts.

Schistosomes are the exception to the rule that all trematodes are hermaphrodites; they have two sexes, but the worms remain paired for their entire adult lives. The worms are up to 1.6 cm long and the male folds its body longitudinally to form the gynecophoral canal, a tube where the female is located[2] (Fig. 39-28, *A*).

The species of schistosomes parasitizing humans are *Schistosoma mansoni, S. japonicum,* and *S. haematobium.* Other species of less importance are *S. mekongi* and *S. malayi,* described during the post–Vietnam War era, and some animal schistosomes similar to *S. haematobium,* which sporadically are found in people.[3] All schistosomes have similar life cycles: eggs are laid in veins, pass through the walls of the hollow viscera to be excreted with the feces or the urine of the infected host. In freshwater the egg frees a larva, the miracidium, which enters the snail, in which they develop into cercariae. The cercariae are released into the water from the snail, and they find an appropriate definitive host, enter through its unbroken skin, and via blood travel to the lungs and then to the liver where they mature and migrate to the smaller branches of the portal or pelvic venous systems.[2] *Schistosoma mansoni* and *S. japonicum* colonize the portal system. The *S. haematobium* group colonizes the venules of the pelvic venous plexes draining the urinary bladder, less commonly the female genital system, and the veins of the lower sigmoid and rectum. In these vessels the fully mature worms begin oviposition, an activity continuing for the life of the worms, which average 3 to 7 years but may extend to 47 years.[99]

The acute manifestations of schistosomiasis begin with the penetration of the cercariae in the skin; a localized urticarial rash with wheals and edema is common. When the worms reach their final location and oviposition commences, the symptoms of systemic allergic manifestations ensue. "Kataygama fever" symptoms depend on the species of *Schistosoma* involved, the number of worms, and the susceptibility of the individual; asymptomatic infections are common in many areas. The intestinal manifestations begin 4 weeks after the initial infection; they last about 2 months and are diarrhea, sometimes dysentery, fever, abdominal pain, anorexia, and loss of weight. Tenderness of the hepatic and splenic areas are easily elicited on examination, and peripheral white blood cell counts are high with large numbers of eosinophils. These acute manifestations subside and are followed by an asymptomatic phase during which oviposition continues relentlessly for many years.

From the above discussion, one has to visualize that the eggs of the schistosomes are released within the blood vessels but are excreted to the environment in the feces or the urine. The mechanism involved in the passage of eggs from the blood vessels to the lumen of the viscera explains the pathophysiology of the chronic manifestations of schistosomiasis in humans and animals.[3] The adult worms in the portal system do

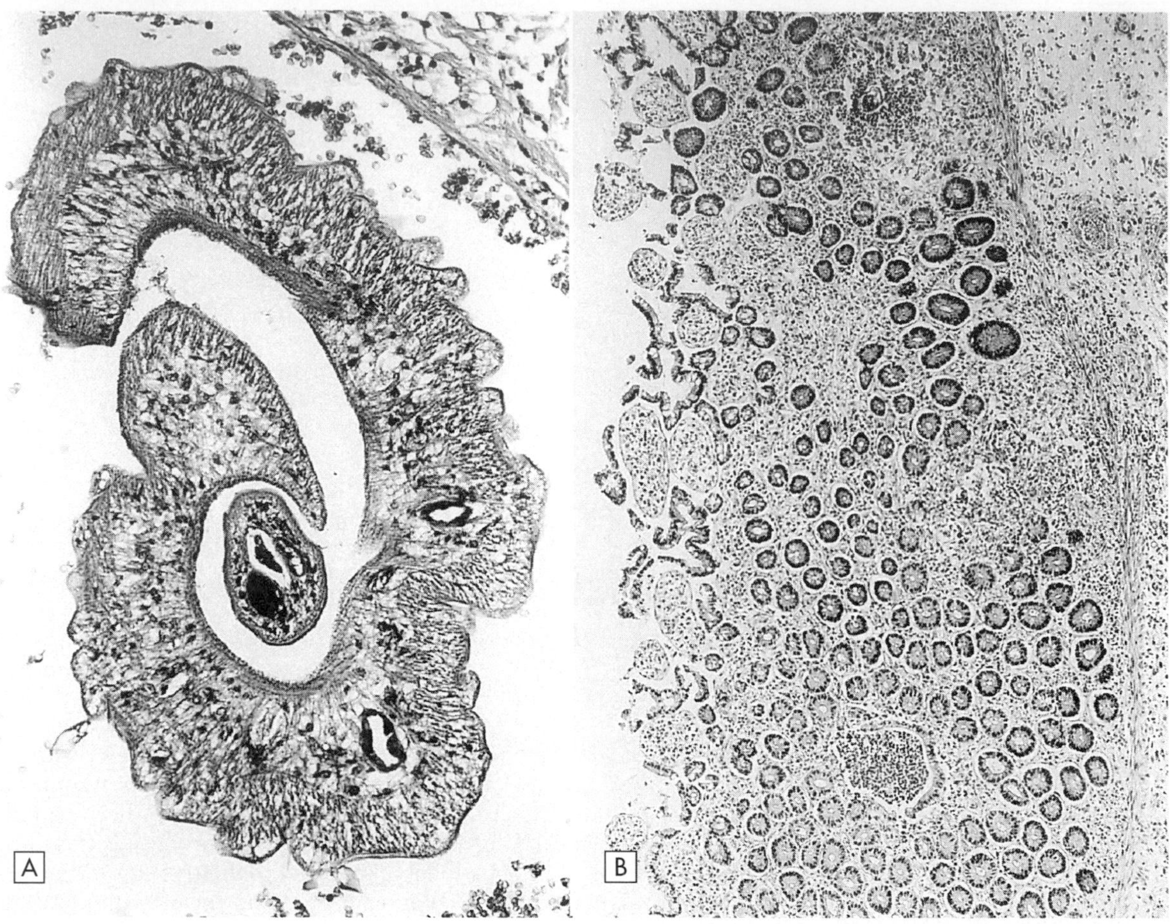

Fig. 39-28 *Schistosoma.* ***A,*** Cross section of adult *S. haematobium* worms to illustrate the folding of the male and the location of the female at the center of the gynecophoral canal. **B,** Section of colonic mucosa from patient with *S. mansoni* infection to show the granulomata elicited by the eggs and of how they are extruded to the lumen of the viscus.

not elicit an effective immunologic reaction because they have the ability to cover themselves with host proteins, rendering them unrecognizable by the immune system[100] (Fig. 39-28, *A*). Yet the immune response to new cercarial invasion results in significant attrition of the new invaders (concomitant immunity). The eggs laid in the blood vessels are different from the adult worms because they elicit a powerful T-cell dependent reaction, manifesting as granulomata (Fig. 39-28, *B*), which allow the egg to move to the lumen of the viscus. The mechanism for extrusion of eggs through the tissues works well at first, but as time passes, some eggs trapped in the colonic wall by the fibrosis of previous lesions interfere with the process. Alternately, newly laid eggs may be carried by the blood flow into the portal vein, and lodge in the liver. The chronic accumulation of eggs in the portal areas of the liver and the granulomatous inflammation they produce lead to fibrosis and portal vein obliteration with portal hypertension[2,3] (Fig. 39-27). Since the gross distribution of the fibrosis in the liver concentrates around portal areas, it is referred to as *Symmer's,* or *clay-pipestem, fibrosis*. Portal hypertension results in a clinicopathologic syndrome and pulmonary hypertension may result from eggs embolized through the collateral circulation into the smaller branches of the pulmonary artery. One interesting aspect of schistosomiasis is that of the manifestations produced by the ectopic locations of the worms, accompanied by oviposition at the site and producing local granulomatous inflammation responsible for unusual clinical manifestations in the brain or in the spinal cord (transverse myelitis).[101] Some differences in the morphology, geographic distribution, and other characteristics of the main schistosomes of humans are described in the following paragraphs.

Schistosoma mansoni

The geographic distribution of *Schistosama mansoni* is central Africa, the Nile Delta, South Yemen, Brazil, Venezuela, and Puerto Rico, making this parasite not an unusual finding among the Puerto Ricans living in the continental United States, though the number of cases is decreasing steadily.[2] The location of *S. mansoni* in the smaller venules of the colon produces both the acute and chronic manifestations of the infection by the mechanism explained above. In the intestine the most common lesions are thickening of the wall with fibrosis and inflammatory polyps of the mucosa which can result in anemia and hypoalbuminemia due to blood loss. The liver is fibrotic and smaller than normal, especially during the terminal stages of the infection,[103] and the spleen has changes of chronic passive congestion. Patients with heavy infections have all the symptoms and signs of portal and pulmonary hypertension. The liver, colon, and lungs have granulomas around the eggs; the granulomas are in different stages.

Patients may develop chronic glomerulonephritis. The presence of characteristic eggs in the granuloma are diagnostic of the lesions (see below).

The diagnosis of the infection is made clinically, especially in endemic areas. Laboratory confirmation of infection is by the finding of eggs, in the stools or in tissues, these eggs measure 114 to 175 μm in length by 45 to 68 μm in width, with a typical *lateral spine* (Figs. 39-29 and 39-30, *A*). Eggs are embryonated (have a miracidium) at the time of oviposition, seen easily moving within the egg in wet preparations of unfixed stools.[10,20] Diagnosis in biopsy specimens or other tissue samples are made also based on the recognition of the eggs.[3] A rapid method consists in taking a 2 to 3 cubic millimeter sample of fresh tissue, placing it between two microscope glass slides, and applying gentle pressure until the tissue has extended sufficiently to allow examination under the microscope under low power (Fig. 39-29). The preparation is immediately examined with the condenser of the microscope in a low position to augment the light contrast and to allow one to see the eggs in the tissue.[3] Several immunologic methods for diagnosis of the infection have been described.[102]

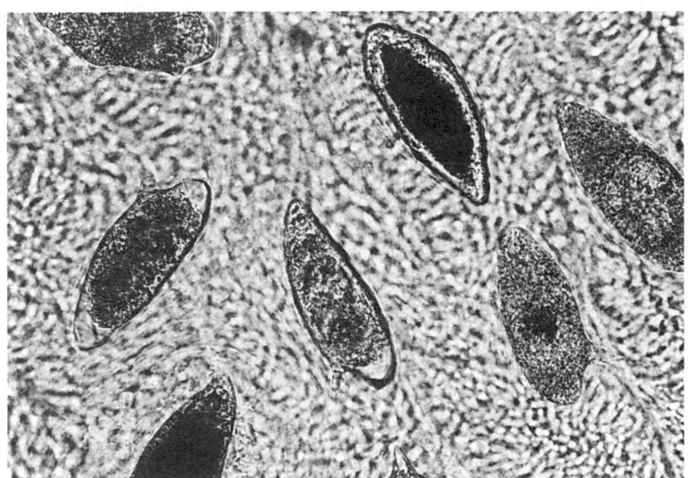

Fig. 39-29 *Schistosoma mansoni* in unstained squashed tissue preparation for rapid diagnosis. Notice the lateral spine in some of the eggs.

Schistosoma japonicum

The geographic distribution of *S. japonicum* is China, the Philippines, and Japan. The closely related species *S. mekongi* and *S. malayi* occur mainly in northern Thailand, Laos, and northern Cambodia. The disease produced by *S. japonicum* is similar to that of *S. mansoni,* and the diagnosis is made in a similar manner in stool and tissue samples. In sections of colon the eggs are clustered in large groups producing "composite" granulomas around masses of eggs, in contrast to *S. mansoni,* which deposits its eggs singly, eliciting "unioval" granulomas. The eggs of *S. japonicum* are less elongated, measure 70 to 100 μm by 50 to 65 μm, and have a minute, hardly visible spine on the side (Fig. 39-30, *C*); the eggs of *S. mekongi* are smaller; otherwise they look similar to those of *S. japonicum.*[10,20] One important aspect of infection by *S. japonicum* is the association between the infection and carcinoma of the colon.

Schistosoma haematobium

The geographic range of *Schistoma haematobium* is most of Africa, Madagascar, Saudi Arabia, and other Middle Eastern countries.[2] The diseases produced by *S. haematobium* are mainly related to the genitourtinary system.[3,104] The symptoms are seen in children and young adults and manifest as hematuria and terminal dysuria. As the infection becomes chronic, schistosomal polyposis of the urinary bladder, calcific sandy patches, schistosomal bladder ulcers, schistosomal contraction of the urinary bladder, and, most importantly, schistosomal obstructive uropathy (hydroureter and hydronephrosis)

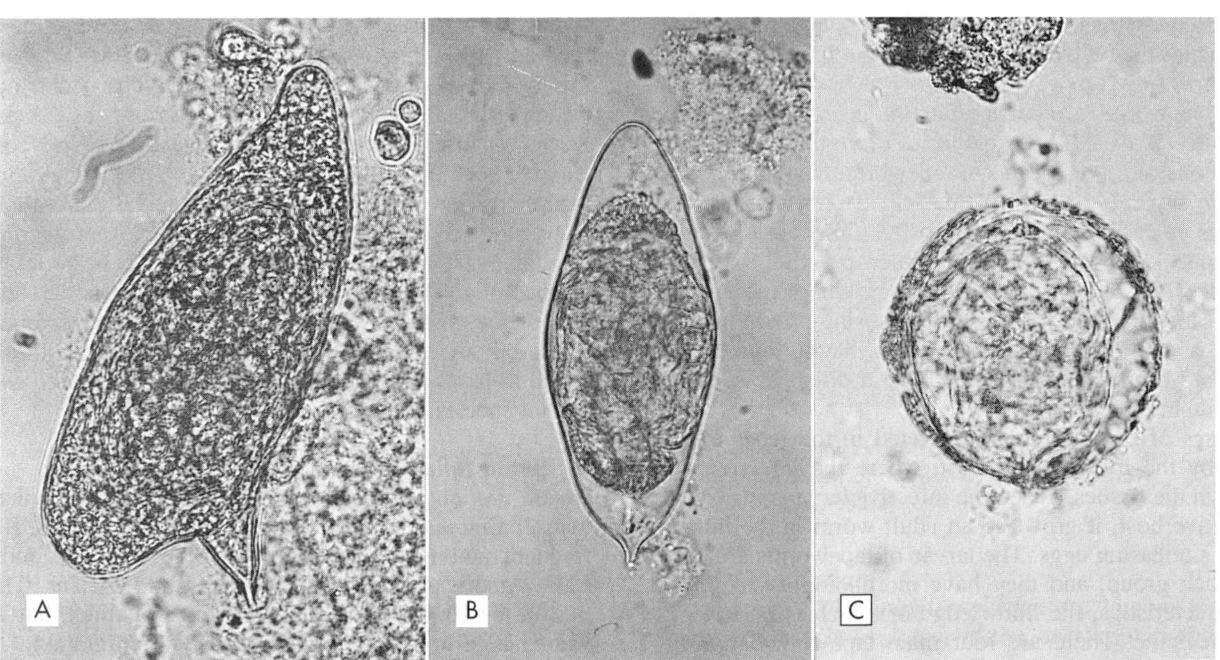

Fig. 39-30 *Schistosoma* eggs in the stools and urine, unstained. ***A,*** *S. mansoni.* ***B,*** *S. haematobium.* ***C,*** *S. japonicum.*

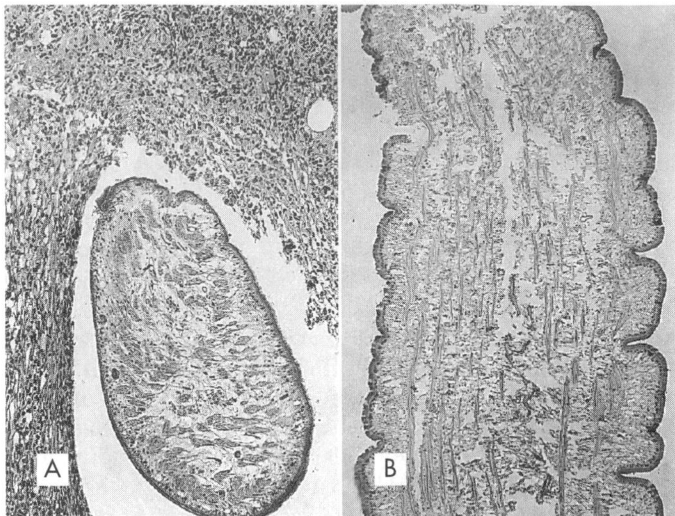

Fig. 39-33 Sparganum (or plerocercoid) larva in subcutaneous tissues. **A,** Transverse section of larva showing the characteristic longitudinal muscles *(arrows).* **B,** Longitudinal sections of the worm illustrating the orientation of the muscles *(arrows).*

length and passes eggs that are excreted with the feces, reach freshwater, where a crustacean, the first intermediate host ingests an egg, which develops into a *procercoid* larva; the crustacean with its procercoid larva is then ingested by a fish, in which the parasite develops into a *plerocercoid,* or *sparganum,* larva in the muscles. Ingestion of raw fish with the plerocercoid larva results in an infection with the adult worm. The disease is common in central Europe, Finland, Lithuania, and Sweden, where the highest rates of infection occur; it is also common in northern Russia, central Siberia, Manchuria, and Japan. In Canada *Diphyllobothrium* is the most common tapeworm reported and in the United States occurs in several foci, the best known in northern Minnesota. *Diphyllobothrium latum* is a parasite of many wild carnivores, which maintain the parasite in nature.[2]

The manifestations of the infection vary from asymptomatic to epigastric pain and diarrhea, or acute intestinal obstruction as a result of the mass of the worm. Infected individuals may pass periodically large portions of their worm in the feces, but the most dramatic symptoms result from a deficiency of vitamin B_{12} produced because the worm absorbs and stores in its body all the vitamin B_{12} ingested by the host. This complication of the infection is seen more commonly in northern European countries, rarely in other places where the parasite is endemic.

Larval cestodes

Cysticercosis

As stated above, some larval stages of cestodes produce infections in humans, of which the cysticercus of *T. solium* causes cysticercosis and neurocysticercosis, important diseases in endemic areas.[106] The infection results from ingestion of eggs with food or water contaminated with human excreta or retrograde peristalsis of eggs or proglottids into the stomach of a patient harboring adult *T. solium.* Once ingested, the eggs release in the intestine embryos no larger than a macrophage, and they penetrate the intestinal mucosa and via blood travel to the tissues where they begin to grow slowly, until they attain their normal size of about 1 cm in diameter[3,106] (Fig. 39-31, *A*). The tissues preferred by the cysticercus of *T. solium* are the subcutaneous tissues, the skeletal muscles and their fascia, the brain, and the eye. The growth of the parasites and their survival in tissues depends on the species of host and probably the tissue where they are located. If the cysticerci are not ingested by the appropriate final host within a certain time, their fate is to die in the tissues and undergo histologic changes that determine the clinical course of the infection.[3] Cysticerci may die and be resorbed without leaving traces; they may die and become fibrosed and calcified; or more importantly they may die and produce an inflammatory reaction. In the first two cases the infection is usually asymptomatic, but in the third instance symptoms occur with manifestations that depend on the site where the parasite is located.[3,106-107]

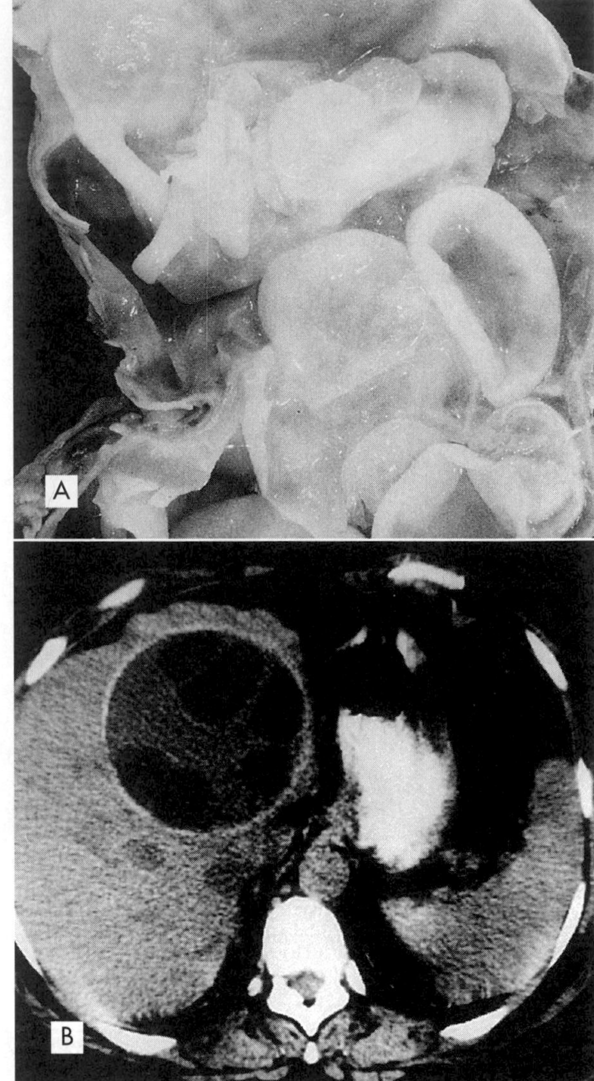

Fig. 39-34 *Echinococcus granulosus* cysts. **A,** Gross specimen showing the white acellular lamellated membrane and the daughter cysts. **B,** Liver scan illustrating the typical appearance of the cyst. The dense spaces are the daughter cysts.

In the skeletal muscle, the fascia, and the subcutaneous tissues, cysticerci produce few symptoms. Cysticerci located in

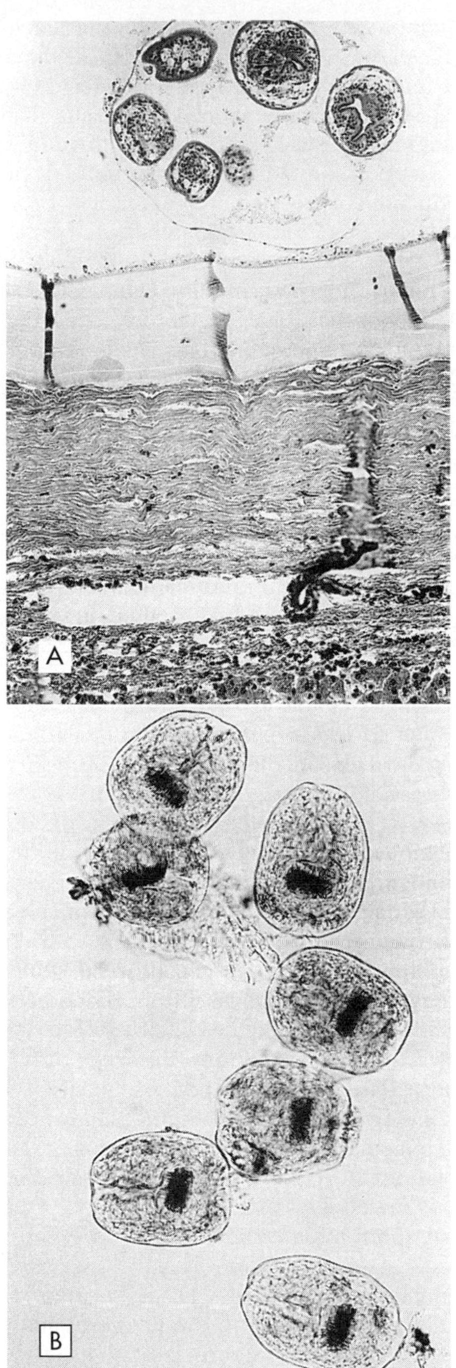

Fig. 39-35 *Echinococcus granulosus* microscopic appearance. **A,** Section through the cyst wall illustrating the different layers. At bottom is the normal liver tissue with little or no inflammatory infiltrate. Next is the fibrous capsule, followed by the thick lamellated membrane. The lamellated membrane is covered by the thin germinal membrane from where a brood capsule with six protoscolices are arising. **B,** Protoscolices in hydatid fluid, wet preparation, unstained.

the subcutaneous tissues are felt as a painless small nodule, but no particular significance is given to the finding, unless it is located near the eye, the lips, the breasts, or the genital organs. If the nodule is removed, it shows grossly and histologically a living cysticercus (Fig. 39-31, *B*). If the parasite dies and produces an inflammatory reaction, the nodule changes in size, and if it is removed at this time, grossly and histologically the larva is found in an abscess.[3]

In the central nervous system cysticerci behave in a manner identical to that described above: living cysticerci are asymptomatic and often invisible to the regular imaging techniques, but if they die and become inflamed, they produce symptoms[3] (Figs. 39-32). Neurocysticercosis, as this infection is known, has varied clinical manifestations depending on the location of the cyst in the brain and produces significant morbidity and mortality in the endemic areas. Most cases of cysticercosis and neurocysticercosis in the United States are imported, but recently the infection has been found with more frequency in Americans without a history of travel. Both infections with *T. solium* and cysticercosis are frequent among Latin Americans living in the United States.[105,108-110]

The incubation period of neurocysticercosis is variable because the larvae may remain alive in the brain for long periods. In some instance the symptoms have manifested 30 years after the infection, but in most cases they develop within 7 years. The main presentation of the infection is usually related to intracranial pressure, such as headache, nausea, vomiting, papilledema, changes of mental status, and cranial nerve palsies. Seizures occur in one half of the cases and are focal, generalized, jacksonian, or any combination of these.[106,111] Arachnoiditis with secondary hydrocephalus is a complication, often fatal. The clinical diagnosis is usually based on several of the radiologic imaging techniques available.[3,106,112] The morphologic finding at this stage manifests as an abscess approximately 1 to 2 cm in diameter, with a necrotic center containing the parasite. Microscopically the inflammatory reaction extends to the surrounding brain tissue, and the larva is often seen as pale staining, necrotic, or with polymorphonuclear cells attached to the tegument of the parasite, all signs of a dead organism.[3]

Sparganosis

Sparganosis is an infection of the subcutaneous tissues produced by the plerocercoid, or sparganum, larva of *Spirometra,* a genus of tapeworms of dogs and cats closely related to *Diphyllobothrium.* The infection occurs sporadically in most countries, but it is reported with more frequency in certain places such as Korea, Japan, the Philippines, and other Far Eastern countries. The life cycles of the known species of *Spirometra* are similar to those of *Diphyllobothrium,* and thus infections are acquired by humans through the ingestion of larvae in the intermediate hosts, usually snakes, frogs, and fish.[3] It has been established that the sparganum larva may occur in pigs and that ingestion of raw pork may be an important source of infection for humans.[113]

In the United States sparganosis is found mainly in the southeastern part of the country, where clinicians and pathologists encounter the disease not uncommonly.[3] The clinical presentation and the gross and microscopic features of the disease are identical to those of subcutaneous cysticercosis, but the sparganum larva has morphologic characteristics that make its identification possible grossly and microscopically (Figs. 39-33). The larva measures up to 20 cm in length by 2 to 3 mm in width. It is delicate, white, and somewhat flattened. In sections it shows characteristic longitudinal muscles.[3] In rare instances sparganum larvae have been found in other organs, such as the brain, lungs, intestinal wall, and peritoneal cavity, producing unusual symptoms. Moreover, fatal infections with proliferating cestode larvae have been described as "proliferating sparganosis."[114]

Coenurosis

Coenurosis is an uncommon infection of the subcutaneous tissues, the eye, and the brain, produced by the larva of certain tapeworms of wild and domestic dogs. The intermediate hosts of these parasites are sheep, goats, cattle, rabbits, hares, and accidentally humans. The infection has been described in the North American continent, Africa, France, England, and Brazil. The clinical presentation is variable depending on the location of the cyst, and the diagnosis is made by its removal and by the identification of the larva based on its morphologic characteristics; cysts may measure up to 10 cm in diameter.[2,3]

Echinococcosis

Echinococcosis is the infection produced by the larval stages of tapeworms belonging to the genus *Echinococcus,* parasites of animals.[2,3,115] This infection produces the important cestode disease in humans, not only because of the number of people infected around the world, but also because of the resulting morbidity and mortality. Four species of *Echinococcus* are recognized in nature, with adult worms measuring up to 6 mm in length, parasitizing the intestine of wild and domestic dogs and cats and having many intermediate hosts, ranging from sheep, goats, cattle, horses to medium-sized and small rodents, depending on the species.[3] The life cycle of these tapeworms is similar to that described above, and their larvae, the hydatid cyst, has gross and histologic characteristics that allow identification of the species of *Echinococcus.* One aspect of hydatidosis in humans not often stressed is that humans are abnormal hosts, and thus the pattern of growth of the larva is often different from that seen in the normal intermediate hosts. These differences explain some of the pathologic manifestations of the infection.[115]

Unilocular hydatid disease. *Echinococcus granulosis* produces the most common form of hydatidosis in humans, referred to as "unilocular hydatid disease." It is found in sheep- and cattle-raising areas of most of Europe, the former Soviet Union, China, the Middle East, southern Australia, New Zealand, the southern half of South America, and the northern and southern parts of Africa. Unilocular hydatid disease occurs in Canada and in the United States, especially Alaska, and in small foci in California and Utah.[2,3] Two life cycles of the parasite occur in nature: one, a life cycle among wild animals (wolves, the definitive hosts, and elk, deer, caribou, and moose, the intermediate hosts), an ecologic circumstance that results in sporadic infections of low virulence in humans; the other, a pastoral life cycle between domestic dogs and sheep, resulting in a greater number of human cases and greater morbidity.[3]

Infections with *E. granulosus* are acquired by the ingestion of eggs passed in the feces of dogs; the eggs release an embryo into the intestinal lumen which enters the wall and via blood travels to the tissues, where it begins growing at a rate depending on the host and the organ. In humans the cyst grows about 1 cm per year, and the organs most commonly affected are the liver (75%) (Fig. 39-34, *B*), lungs (9%), and muscles (5%), but cysts can be found in any organ or tissue.[3,115] The symptoms produced are those of a space-occupying lesion, growing slowly, and they depend on the organ and adjacent structures compromised. Cysts in the liver produce commonly ill-defined hepatic or biliary symptoms; if the cysts grow toward the lungs, pulmonary symptoms occur, whereas if it grows toward the abdominal cavity, it may attain an enormous size, producing epigastric pain, abdominal fullness, or compression of the portal system with symptoms of portal hypertension.[3]

The morphology of the cysts is characteristic. Grossly the cyst varies in size and appearance depending on its viability, but usually three distinct layers are apparent: the outer is a *fibrous* reaction of the tissues to the cyst and varies in thickness depending on the age and the organ where the cyst is located. The second, the *acellular* or *lamellated* layer, is produced by the parasite and is the most characteristic because it is white, with a rather uniform thickness, made of a friable substance resembling the albumin of a boiled egg (Fig. 39-34, *A*). The third is the *germinal* layer, seen better in viable cysts as a thin, semitransparent membrane from which the larvae *(protoscolices)* grow (Fig. 39-35, *A*). The protoscolices differentiate from the germinal membrane in bunches called *broods,* which break into the fluid filling the cyst and continue growing to form *daughter cysts.* The combination of the three layers described and the daughter cysts is what makes the hydatid characteristic. The fluid filling the cyst is like clear water, if it is not secondarily infected, and contains numerous protoscolices and brood capsules in suspension, known as the *hydatid sand*[3,115] (Fig. 39-35, *B*). Microscopically, the cyst has the same three layers described grossly and a slight to moderate chronic inflammatory infiltrate around the fibrous layer. The acellular membrane is composed of multiple lamella and stains positive with the periodic acid–Schiff stain. The germinal layer is one cell thick and has attached multiple protoscolices and brood capsules. The protoscolices have two rows of hooklets, which are diagnostic, and are often the only recognizable structure found in degenerated cysts.[3,115]

Alveolar hydatid disease. *Echinococcus multilocularis* has a geographic distribution in the northern temperate and arctic regions; in Europe it is known in Germany and parts of France, Switzerland, and Austria. In the former Soviet Union the parasite is widely distributed in the tundra, extending south to Turkey, northern India, China, and Japan.[3,116] In the American continents it is present in Alaska[117] and most of central Canada, extending south to the Dakotas, Illinois, Nebraska, and other adjacent states.[118,119] The life cycle involves Arctic foxes, domestic dogs and cats as definitive hosts, and small rodents as the intermediate hosts; in some places the life cycle is maintained in nature by household mice.[120]

Alveolar hydatid disease is usually a fatal infection because the larva in abnormal hosts, such as humans, grows as an infiltrating, disorganized mass, capable of producing metastasis to distant organs.[3,115] The symptoms are variable but usually refer to the liver because this is the usual location of the cyst. The patient usually dies within a year of the diagnosis,[121] though nonfatal infections have been reported in Alaska because the parasite fails to develop.[122] Grossly, the cysts consist of a mass of fibrous tissue with numerous small cavities filled with a gelatinous fluid; histologically, abundant fibrous tissue is present among delicate, collapsed layers of a thin acellular membrane with a disorganized germinal membrane sending prolongations into the fibrous layer. If these prolongations enter the blood vessels and break, they produce distant metastases.[115] Calcification of the cyst occurs early, and its pattern, consisting of small calcified rings of less than 0.5 cm in diameter, in plain radiographs, is often diagnostic. The ELISA test is good for indirect diagnosis.[123] The histologic diagnosis of a sarcoma has often been made in these lesions by inexperienced pathologists.[3]

Polycystic hydatid disease. The geographic distribution of *Echinococcus vogeli* is Central America and South America, the adult worms occur in wild dogs, and the larva in large rodents. The infection in humans is mostly benign, manifested as a cystic mass originating in the liver and extending into the peritoneal cavity, where it grows to an enormous size.[124,125] The growth of the larva in humans is by endogenous and exogenous proliferation, forming cysts varying between 0.2 and 8.0 cm in diameter.[125]

DISEASES CAUSED BY ARTHROPODS

Arthropods are important in human medicine for two reasons: First, many species serve as mechanical or more often as biologic vectors of important pathogens of humans. A mechanical vector is, for example, a house fly that transports pathogens to food, where they multiply in sufficient numbers to cause infection. A biologic vector is a specific required host for the parasite (virus, bacterium, rickettsia, protozoon, helminth), where the parasite undergoes some form of development to become infective. The second reason why arthropods are important is that they may produce infections (enter the tissues), or infestations (remain on the outside of the body), sometimes resulting in serious morbidity. In the following paragraphs the most common arthropods of humans are discussed.

Myiasis

Myiasis is the infection produced by the larval stages of flies, a large group of insects, with many known species occurring worldwide.[2,3] Flies have a life cycle similar to that of many other arthropods: adults, eggs, larvae, and pupae, which develop into adults. Flies may lay eggs, or larvae known as maggots, which need strict conditions for their development. Some fly larvae use animal or human tissues to develop, producing myiasis; others need decaying bodies, wounds, or feces. Larvae requiring living tissues produce *obligatory* myiasis, those in wounds *semispecific* myiasis, and those in dead bodies or feces *accidental* myiasis. The myiasis in humans are divided into several groups depending on the organ involved.

1. *Cutaneous myiasis* is the most commonly reported myiasis and is produced by a large number of species of *Gasterophilus* flies with larvae occurring in the epidermis, producing cutaneous larva migrans (see above), or in both the epidermis and the dermis such as *Hypoderma, Dermatobia, Cordylobia,* and *Wohlfahrtia,* producing a large abscess containing the developing parasite. The larvae of these flies arrive in the skin in different manners, some as eggs or as larvae laid by the fly directly on the skin; others are transported by a mosquito and passed to the skin when the mosquito is feeding. In each case, the larva burrows into the skin and begins feeding and growing.
2. *Ocular myiasis* is not a rare encounter in human medicine. It is produced by species of the same genera seen in cutaneous myiasis, as well as *Sarcophaga* and *Oestrus* among others. The infection may result in considerable damage of the eye.
3. *Intestinal myiasis* is an infection of the gastrointestinal tract produced by species of *Gasterophilus.*
4. *Urogenital myiasis* is produced by species of *Chrysomia.* These last two groups are difficult to document, and many spurious cases are reported.
5. Another group of myiasis commonly seen by pathologists is in *wounds, ulcers,* or *decaying bodies.* Maggots, often recovered from a dead person, a patient in a coma at the hospital, or at home, or from other similar circumstances, are submitted for diagnosis. The specific diagnosis based on the entire organism, not on sections of the larva, is done by the specialist.[2,3]

Tungiasis

Tunga penetrans is a flea with a life cycle in which the female is parasitic of glabrous skin in order to develop her eggs, producing tungiasis. The female *Tunga* is located within the squamous layer with its posterior end at the surface, allowing the eggs to reach the soil, where they complete their development. The infection is common in the poor areas of tropical Africa and America.[2,3] In the United States dermatologists and pathologists encounter the infection in individuals who traveled to endemic areas and walked barefooted or with sandals on dirt. It is often a diagnostic problem if neither the clinician nor the pathologist is familiar with the disease.[3]

Clinically the infection occurs in the foot and begins as a small insect bite–like lesion that grows slowly, with intense itching, to about 0.5 cm in diameter. At this stage a small indurated nodule with a small black center is seen (Fig. 39-36, *A*). The treatment is removal of the parasite by shelling of the flea from the edge of the lesion until the entire parasite is extracted. If a biopsy specimen is taken (not necessary), the organism is seen microscopically within the epidermis[3] (Fig. 39-36, *B*).

Demodicidosis

Demodex folliculorum and *D. brevis* are two species of mites found in the sebaceous glands of the face of every human, especially around the nose and the forehead. The mites are seen in sections of skin biopsy specimens or skin removed with tumors from the areas mentioned. No disease has been conclusively attributed to any of these organisms.[3]

Scabies

A large number of small mites living in the epidermis produce mange in animals and scabies in humans[126,127] (Fig. 39-37, *A*). The infecting mite burrows a tunnel in the upper layers of the epidermis, where it feeds on cells and juices oozing from chewed cells. The female lays eggs in the tunnel, where they develop, hatch, and grow to adults in about 7 to 8 days (Fig. 39-37). The tunnel made by the female reaches several centimeters in length during its life-span of 6 to 8 weeks.[2,3] The lesions produced by *Sarcoptes scabiei* are located in 60% of the cases in the skin of the hands and wrists, followed by 10%

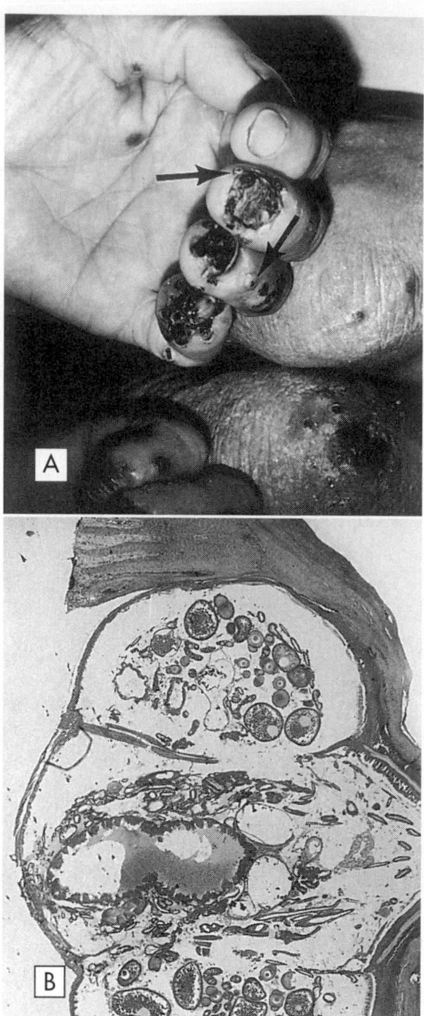

Fig. 39-36 *Tunga penetrans.* **A,** Massive tungiasis illustrating the character of the lesion *(arrows).* **B,** Section of female flea, showing its location within the epidermis and the opening *(right)* in the skin through which the eggs are laid.

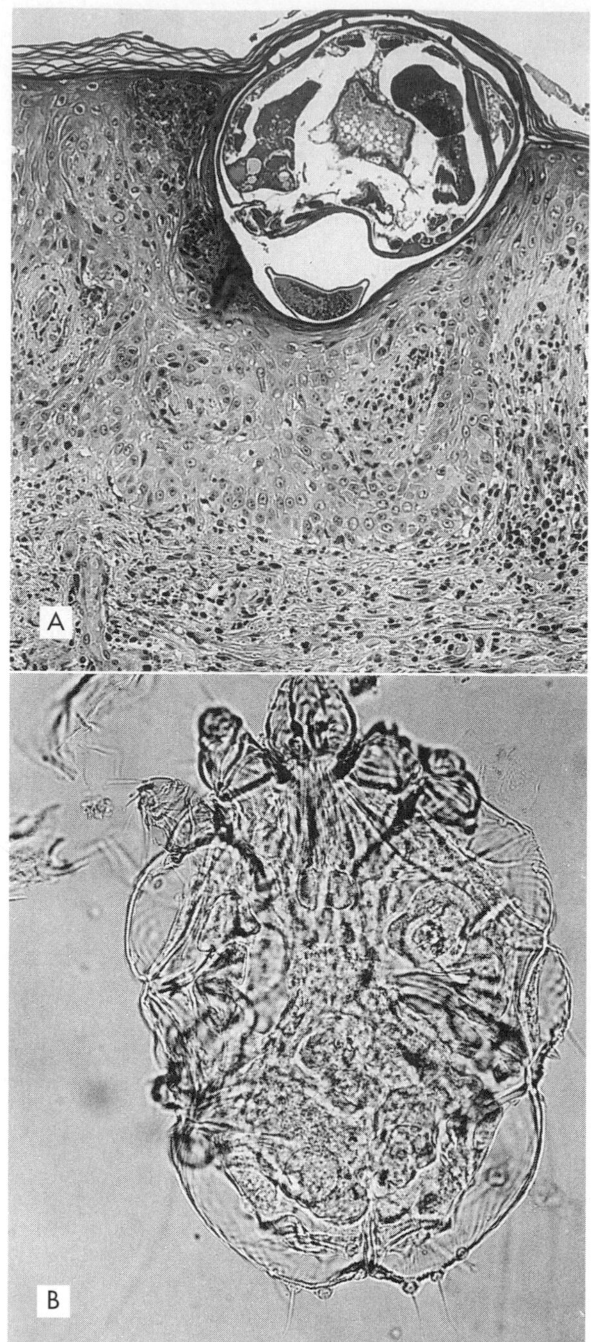

Fig. 39-37 *Sarcoptes scabiei.* **A,** Section of skin showing the female mite in the burrow within the epidermis. **B,** Adult female in scraping of skin, unstained.

to 12% in the elbows, feet, penis, scrotum, buttocks, and axillae. In over 50% of clinical cases of scabies between only one and five adult female mites are present, and in 20% between five and 10 mites.[126] Percentages of infections with more than 10 mites decrease rapidly. Scabies is a worldwide infection, but prevalence figures are scarce. In the United States the infection is well known and is rising, with transmission occurring by close contact between people, most commonly during sexual intercourse.[128]

The main clinical manifestations of scabies is symmetric itching of the skin of the finger webs and the wrists, extending to other parts of the body. The most common lesion is the tract produced by the burrowing mites, seen grossly as a wavy line on the epidermis, resembling cutaneous larva migrans. Continuous scratching of the lesions produce secondary infections, which complicate the clinical picture. Massive infections in individuals with AIDS or other forms of immunosuppression are clinically referred to as *Norwegian scabies* and are characterized by a large number of mites with numerous exfoliating scales over large areas or the entire body. These patients should be handled with care because the infection at this stage is easily transmitted.[126,129]

The histologic changes of scabies affect the entire dermis (Fig. 39-37, *A*) and sometimes the subcutaneous tissues.[3,126] The tunnels produced by the migrant female are seen histologically as empty spaces, rarely with the mite inside. The roof of the burrow is covered by orthokeratotic or parakeratotic cells, and the dermis may show an inflammatory infiltrate of variable character and intensity. Lymphocytes, histiocytes, and eosinophils are the most common infiltrating cells. Often a lymphoplasmocytic infiltrate in the dermis has been misdiagnosed as reticulosis and similar infiltrate extending down to the subcutaneous tissues has been diagnosed as cutaneous lymphoma.[126] Scabies is a clinical diagnosis, based on the appearance and distribution of the lesions: rarely the mites are recovered by scarification of the end of the tunnel and the recognition of the mite under microscopic examination. Rarely the mites are seen in skin biopsy specimens.[3,126] Norwegian scabies is easily diagnosed in skin scrapings and biopsy specimens because of the large number of mites present.[3,106]

REFERENCES

1. Cook GC: Gastrointestinal helminth infections, *Trans R Soc Trop Med Hyg* 80:675, 1986.
2. Beaver PC, Jung RC, Cupp EW: *Clinical parasitology,* ed 9, Philadelphia, 1984, Lea & Febiger.
3. Gutierrez Y: *Diagnostic pathology of parasitic infections with clinical correlations,* Philadelphia, 1990, Lea & Febiger.
4. Gilman RH, Marquis GS, Miranda E: Prevalence and symptoms of *Enterobius vermicularis* infection in a Peruvian shanty town, *Trans R Soc Trop Med Hyg* 85:761, 1991.
5. Wagner ED, Eby WC: Pinworm prevalence in California elementary school children, and diagnostic, methods. *Am J Trop Med Hyg* 32:998, 1983.
6. Sinniah B, Leopairut J, Neafie RC et al: Enterobiasis: a histopathological study of 259 patients, *Ann Trop Med Parasitol* 85:625, 1991.
7. Broadbent V: Children's worms (Letter), *Br Med J* 2:89, 1975
8. Simon RD: Pinworm infestation and urinary tract infection in young girls, *Am J Dis Child* 128:21, 1974.
9. Mattia AR: Perianal mass and recurrent cellulitis due to *Enterobius vermicularis, Am J Trop Med Hyg* 47:811, 1992.
10. Smith JW, Gutierrez Y: Medical parasitology, In Henry JB, editor: *Clinical diagnosis and management by laboratory methods,* ed 18, Philadelphia, 1991, Saunders.
11. Bundy DAP, Cooper S: *Trichuris* and trichuriasis in humans, *Adv Parasitol* 28:107, 1989.
12. Gilman RH, Chong YH, Davis C et al: The adverse consequences of heavy *Trichiuris* infection, *Trans R Soc Trop Med Hyg* 77:432, 1983.
13. Stephenson LS: The contribution of *Ascaris lumbricoides* to malnutrition in children, *Parasitology* 81:221, 1980.
14. Crompton DWT: Ascariasis and childhood malnutrition, *Trans R Soc Trop Med Hyg* 86:577, 1992.
15. Chaco DD: Intestinal parasites and asthma, *N Engl J Med* 283:101, 1970.
16. Loeffler W: Transient lung infiltration with blood eosinophilia, *Int Arch Allergy* 8:54, 1956.
17. Gelpi AP, Mustafa A: Seasonal pneumonitis with eosinophilia: a study of larval ascariasis in Saudi Arabs, *Am J Trop Med Hyg* 16:646, 967.
18. Odaibo SK, Awogun IA: Small intestinal perforation by *Ascaris lumbricoides, Trans R Soc Trop Med Hyg* 82:154, 1988.
19. Choi MH, Park IA, Hong IK et al: A case of biliary ascariasis accompanied by cholelithiasis, *Korean J Parasitol* 31:71, 1993.
20. Woods GL, Gutierrez Y: *Diagnostic pathology of infectious diseases,* Philadelphia, 1993, Lea & Febiger.
21. Ishikura H, Namiki M, editors: *Gastric anisakiasis in Japan: epidemiology, diagnosis, treatment,* New York, 1989, Springer-Verlag.
22. Ishikura H, Kikuchi K, editors: *Intestinal anisakiasis in Japan: infected fish, sero-immunological diagnosis, and prevention,* New York, 1990, Springer-Verlag.
23. Huff DS, Neafie RC, Binder MJ et al: The first fatal *Baylisascaris* infection in humans: an infant with eosinophilic meningoencephalitis, *Pediatr Pathol* 2:345, 1984.
24. Fox AS, Kasacos KR, Gould NS et al: Fatal eosinophilic meningoencephalitis and visceral larva migrans caused by the raccoon ascarid *Baylisascaris, N Engl J Med* 312:1619, 1985.
25. Kalkofen UP: Attachment and feeding behavior of *Ancylostoma caninum, Z Parasitenkd* 33:339, 1970.
26. Gill GV, Bell DR: Long-standing tropical infections among former war prisoners of the Japanese, *Lancet* 1:958, 1982.
27. Genta RM: Dysregulation of strongyloidiasis: a new hypothesis, *Clin Microbiol Rev* 5:345, 1992.
28. Lucas SB: Missing infections in AIDS, *Trans R Soc Trop Med Hyg* 84:34, 1990.
29. Brasitus TA, Gold RP, Kay RH et al: Intestinal strongyloidiasis: a case report and review of the literature, *Am J Gastroenterol* 73:65, 1980.
30. Tham KT: *Strongyloides* gastritis: report of a case, *J Trop Med Hyg* 82:21, 1979.
31. Couland JP, Deluol AM, Cenac J et al: L'Albendazole dans le traitement de la strongyloïdose: à propos de 66 observations, *Bull Soc Pathol Exot Filiales* 75:530, 1982.
32. Berger R, Kraman S, Paciotti M: Pulmonary strongyloidiasis complicating therapy with corticosteroids: report of a case with secondary bacterial infection, *Am J Trop Med Hyg* 29:31, 1980.
33. Barnish G, Ashford RW: *Strongyloides* cf. *fuelleborni* and hookworm in Papua New Guinea: patterns of infection within the community, *Trans R Soc Trop Med Hyg* 83:684, 1989.
34. Ashford RW, Barnish G, Viney ME: *Strongyloides fuelleborni:* infection and disease in Papua New Guinea, *Parasitol Today* 8:314, 1992.
35. Beshear JR, Hendley JO: Severe pulmonary involvement in visceral larva migrans, *Am J Dis Child* 125:599, 1973.
36. Beaver PC: The nature of visceral larva migrans, *J Parasitol* 55:3, 1969.
37. Vargo TA, Singer DB, Gillete PC et al: Myocarditis due to visceral larva migrans (Correspondence), *J Pediatr* 90:322, 1977.
38. Anderson DC, Greenwood R, Fishman M et al: Acute infantile hemiplegia with cerebrospinal fluid eosinophilic pleocytosis: an unusual case of visceral larva migrans, *J Pediatr* 86:247, 1975.
39. Molk R: Ocular toxocariasis: a review of the literature, *Ann Ophthalmol* 15:216, 1983.
40. Sorr EM: Meandering ocular toxocariasis, *Retina* 4:90, 1984.
41. Brumpt L-C, Sang HT: Larva currens seul signe pathognomonique de la strongyloïdose, *Ann Parasitol Hum Comp* 48:319, 1973.
42. Kliks, MM, Kroenke K, Hardman JM: Eosinophilic radiculomyeloencephalitis: an angiostrongyloidiasis outbreak in American Samoa related to ingestion of *Achatina fulica* snails, *Am J Trop Med Hyg* 31:1114, 1982.
43. Yii CY, Chen CY, Fresh JW et al: Human angiostrongyloidiasis involving the lungs, *Chin J Microbiol* 1:148, 1968.
44. Sonakul D: Pathological findings in four cases of human angiostrongyliasis, *Southeast Asian J Trop Med Public Health* 9:220, 1978.
45. Bunang T, Benjapong W, Noeypatimanond S et al: The recovery of *Angiostrongylus cantonensis* in the cerebrospinal fluid of a case of eosinophilic meningitis, *J Med Assoc Thai* 52:665, 1969.
46. Kuberski T, Bart RD, Briley JM et al: Recovery of *Angiostrongylus cantonensis* from cerebrospinal fluid of a child with eosinophilic meningitis, *J Clin Microbiol* 9:629, 1979.
47. Widagdo, Sunardi, Lokollo DM et al: Ocular angiostrongyliasis in Semarang, Central Java, *Am J Trop Med Hyg* 26:72, 1977.
48. Céspedes-Fonseca R, Salas J, Makbel S et al: Granulomas entéricos y linfáticos con intensa eosinofilia tisular producidos por un estrongiloideo (strongylata). I. Patología, *Acta Med Cost* 10:235, 1967.
49. Loría-Cortés R, Lobo-Sanahuja JF : Clinical abdominal angiostrongylosis: a study of 116 children with intestinal eosinophilic granuloma caused by *Angiostrongylus costaricensis, Am J Trop Med Hyg* 29:538, 1980.
50. Gardiner CH: Habitat and reproductive behavior of *Trichinella spiralis, J Parasitol* 62:865, 1976.
51. Wright KA: *Trichinella spiralis:* an intracellular parasite in the intestinal phase, *J Parasitol* 65:441, 1979.
52. Metzler MH, Sahgal KK, Wolf GS: Second degree atrioventricular block in acute trichinosis, *Am J Dis Child* 124:598, 1972.
53. Kirschberg GJ: Trichinosis presenting as acute myocardial infarction, *Can Med Assoc J* 106:898, 1972.
54. Ryczak M, Sorber WA, Kandora TF et al: Difficulties in diagnosing *Trichinella* encephalitis, *Am J Trop Med Hyg* 36:573, 1987.
55. Harms G, Binz P, Feldmeier H et al: Trichinosis: a prospective controlled study of patients ten years after acute infection, *Clin Infect Dis* 17:637, 1993.
56. Watten RH, Beckner WM, Cross JH et al: Clinical studies of capillariasis philippinensis, *Trans R Soc Trop Med Hyg* 66:828, 1972.

57. Cross JH, Banson T, Clarke MD et al: Studies on the experimental transmission of *Capillaria philippinensis* in monkeys, *Trans R Soc Trop Med Hyg* 66:819, 1972.
58. Canlas BD Jr, Cabrera BD, Dauz U: Human intestinal capillariasis. II. Pathological features, *Acta Med Philipp* 4:84, 1967.
59. Fresh JW, Cross JH, Reyes V et al: Necropsy findings in intestinal capillariasis, *Am J Trop Med Hyg* 21:169, 1972.
60. Eberhard ML, Lammie PJ: Laboratory diagnosis of filariasis. In Gutierrez Y, Little MD, editors: Diagnosis of important parasitic infections, *Clin Lab Med* 11:977, 1991.
61. Beaver PC: Filariasis without microfilaremia, *Am J Trop Med Hyg* 19:181, 1970.
62. Ball JD: Tropical pulmonary eosinophilia, *Trans R Soc Trop Med Hyg* 44:237, 1950.
63. WHO: *Lymphatic filariasis,* Tech Rep Ser No 702, Geneva, 1984, World Health Organization.
64. Danaraj TJ, Pacheco G, Shanmugaratnam K et al: The etiology and pathology of eosinophilic lung (tropical eosinophilia), *Am J Trop Med Hyg* 15:183, 1966.
65. Gutierrez Y, Petras RE: *Brugia* infection in northern Ohio, *Am J Trop Med Hyg* 31:1128, 1982.
66. Gutierrez Y: Diagnostic features of zoonotic filariae in tissue sections, *Hum Pathol* 15:514, 1984.
67. WHO: *WHO Expert Committee on Onchocerciasis,* third report, Tech Rep Series No 752, Geneva, World Health Organization.
68. Nelson GS: Human onchocerciasis: notes on the history, the parasite and the life cycle, *Ann Trop Med Parasitol* 85:83, 1991.
69. Marshal TF de C, Anderson J, Fuglsang H: The incidence of eye lesions and visual impairment in onchocerciasis in relationship to the intensity of the infection, *Trans R Soc Trop Med Hyg* 80:426, 1986.
70. Connor DH, Gibson DW, Neafie RC et al: Sowda: onchocerciasis in North Yemen: a clinicopathologic study of 18 patients, *Am J Trop Med Hyg* 32:123, 1983.
71. Connor DH, Morrison NE, Kerdel-Vargas F et al: Onchocerciasis: onchocercal dermatitis, lymphadenitis, and elephantiasis in the Ubangi territory, *Hum Pathol* 1:553, 1970.
72. Nelson GS: Filarial infections as zoonosis, *J Helminthol* 39:229, 1965.
73. Rakita RM, White AC Jr, Kielhofner MA: *Loa loa* infection as a cause of migratory angioedema: report of tree cases from the Texas Medical Center, *Clin Infect Dis* 17:691, 1993.
74. Little MD: Laboratory diagnosis of worms and miscellaneous specimens. In Gutierrez Y, Little MD, editors: Diagnosis of important parasitic infections, *Clin Lab Med* 11:977, 1991.
75. Oriole TC, Eberhard ML: *Mansonella ozzardi:* a redescription with comments on its taxonomic relationships, *Am J Trop Med Hyg* 31:1142, 1982.
76. Meyers WM, Connor DH, Harman LE et al: Human streptocerciasis: a clinico-pathologic study of 40 Africans (Zaïrians) including identification of the adult filaria, *Am J Trop Med Hyg* 21:528, 1972.
77. Ciferri F: Human pulmonary dirofilariasis in the United States: a critical review, *Am J Trop Med Hyg* 31:302, 1982.
78. Ro JY, Tsakalakis J, White VA et al: Pulmonary dirofilariasis: the great imitator of metastatic lung tumor. A clinico-pathologic analysis of seven cases and a review of the literature, *Hum Pathol* 20:6976, 1989.
79. Beaver PC, Orihel TC: Human infections with filariae of animals in the United States, *Am J Trop Med Hyg* 14:1010, 1965.
80. Beaver PC, Wolfson JS, Waldron MA et al: *Dirofilaria ursi*–like parasites acquired by humans in the northern United States and Canada: report of two cases, *Am J Trop Med Hyg* 37:357, 1987.
81. Müller R: Guinea worm eradication: four more years to go, *Parasitol Today* 8:387, 1992.
82. Ilegbodu VA, Kale OO, Wise RA et al: Impact of guinea worm disease on children in Nigeria, *Am J Trop Med Hyg* 35:962, 1986.
83. McLaughlin GE, Utsinger PD, Trakat WF et al: Rheumatic syndromes secondary to guinea worm infestation, *Arthritis Rheum* 27:694, 1984.
84. el Garf A: Parasitic rheumatism: rheumatic manifestations associated with calcified guinea worm, *J Rheumatol* 12:976, 1985.
85. Rahman KM, Idris MD, Azad Khan AK: A study of fasciolopsiasis in Bangladesh, *J Trop Med Hyg* 84:81, 1981.
86. Eastburn RL, Fritsche TR, Terhune CA Jr: Human intestinal infection with *Nanophyetus salmincola* from salmonid fishes, *Am J Trop Med Hyg* 36:586, 1987.
87. Wong RKH, Peura DA, Mutter ML et al: Hemobilia and liver flukes in a patient from Thailand, *Gastroenterology* 88:1958, 1985.
88. Hillyer GV, Soler de Galanes M, Rodríguez-Pérez, J et al: Use of the Falcon assay screening test–enzyme-linked immunosorbent assay (FAST-ELISA) and the enzyme-linked immunoelectrotransfer blot (EITB) to determine the prevalence of human fascioliasis in the Bolivian altiplano, *Am J Trop Med Hyg* 46:603, 1992.
89. Youssef FG, Mansour NS, Aziz AG: Early diagnosis by detection of coproantigens using counterimmunoelectrophoresis, *Trans R Soc Trop Med Hyg* 85:383, 1991.
90. Acosta-Ferreira W, Varcelli-Reta J, Falconi LM: *Fasciola hepatica* human infection: histopathological study of sixteen cases, *Virchows Arch [Pathol Anat]* 383:319, 1979.
91. Antón Aranda E, García Carasusán M, Celador Almaraz A et al: Fascioliasis hepática: revisión de 5 casos, *Rev Clin Esp* 176:410, 1985.
92. Park CI, Kim H, Ro JY, Gutierrez Y: Human ectopic fascioliasis in the cecum, *Am J Surg Pathol* 8:73, 1984.
93. Elkins DB, Haswell-Elkins MR, Mairiang E et al: A high frequency of hepatobiliary disease and suspected cholangiocarcinoma associated with heavy *Opisthorchis viverrini* infection in a small community in north-east Thailand, *Trans R Soc Trop Med Hyg* 84:715, 1990.
94. Kurathong S, Lerdverasirikul O, Wongpaitoon V et al: *Opisthorchis viverrini* infection and cholangiocarcinoma: a prospective case-controlled study, *Gastroenterology* 89:151, 1985.
95. Centers for Disease Control: Paragonimiasis in Hmong refugees—Minnesota, *MMWR* 30:176, 1981.
96. Diaconitǎ G, Goldis G: Investigations on pathomorphology and pathogenesis of pulmonary paragonimiasis, *Acta Tuberc Scand* 44:51, 1964.
97. Singh TS, Mutum SS, Razaque MA: Pulmonary paragonimiasis: clinical features, diagnosis and treatment of 39 cases in Manipur, *Trans R Soc Trop Med Hyg* 80:967, 1986.
98. WHO: *Epidemiology and control of schistosomiasis,* Tech Rep Ser No 643, Geneva, World Health Organization.
99. Hall HS, Kehoe EL: Prolonged survival of *Schistosoma japonicum, Calif Med* 113:75, 1970.
100. Wright MD, Davern KM, Mitchel GF: The functional and immunological significance of some schistosome surface molecules, *Parasitol Today* 7:56, 1891.
101. Pammenter MD, Haribhai HC, Epstein SR et al: The value of immunological approaches to the diagnosis of schistosomal myelopathy, *Am J Trop Med Hyg* 44:329, 1991.
102. Immunodiagnosis of schistosomiasis. In Gutierrez Y, Little MD, editors: Diagnosis of important parasitic infections, *Clin Lab Med* 11:1029, 1991.
103. Cheever AW: A quantitative postmortem study of schistosomiasis mansoni in man. *Am J Trop Med Hyg* 17:38, 1968.
104. Smith JH, von Lichtenberg F, Lehman JS: Parasitic diseases of the genitourinary system, In Walsh PC, Retik AB, Stamey TA, Vaughan EO, editors: *Campbell's Urology,* ed 6, Philadelphia, 1992, Saunders.
105. Sorvillo FJ, Waterman SH, Richards FO et al: Cysticercosis surveillance: locally acquired and travel-related infections and detection of intestinal tapeworm carriers in Los Angeles county, *Am J Trop Med Hyg* 47:365, 1992.
106. Richards Jr F: Diagnosis and treatment of neurocysticercosis, *IM* 7: 363, 1990.
107. Richards FO, Schantz PM, Ruiz-Tiben E et al: Cysticercosis in Los Angeles county, *JAMA* 254:3444, 1985.
108. Schultz TS, Ascherl JF Jr: Cerebral cysticercosis: occurrence in the immigrant population, *Neurosurgery* 3:164, 1978.
109. Schantz PM, Moore AC, Muñoz JL et al: Neurocysticercosis in an orthodox Jewish community in New York City, *N Engl J Med* 327:692, 1992.
110. Kruskal BA, Moths L, Teele DW: Neurocysticercosis in a child with no history of travel outside the continental United States, *Clin Infect Dis* 16:290, 1993.

111. Case records of the Massachusetts General Hospital: Case 20-1990, *N Engl J Med* 322:1446, 1990.
112. Shraberg D, Weisberg, L, de Urrutia JR et al: Cysticercosis cerebri: evolution of central nervous system involvement as visualized by computed tomography, *Comput Tomogr* 4:261, 1980.
113. Corkum KC: Sparganosis in some vertebrates of Louisiana and observations on a human infection, *J Parasitol* 52:444, 1966.
114. Beaver PC, Rolon FA: Proliferating larval cestode in a man in Paraguay: a case report and review, *Am J Trop Med Hyg* 30:625, 1981.
115. Thompson RCA, editor: *The biology of Echinococcus and hydatid disease,* Boston, 1986, George Allen & Unwin.
116. Gottstein B: *Echinococcus multilocularis* infection: immunology and immunodiagnosis, *Adv Parasitol* 31:321, 1992.
117. Wilson JF, Rausch RL: Alveolar hydatid disease: a review of clinical features of 33 indigenous cases of *Echinococcus multilocularis* infection in Alaskan Eskimos, *Am J Trop Med Hyg* 29:1340, 1980.
118. Storandt, ST, Kazacos KR: *Echinococcus multilocularis* identified in Indiana, Ohio, and east-central Illinois, *J Parasitol* 79:301, 1993.
119. Gamble WG, Segal M, Schantz PM, Rausch RL: Alveolar hydatid disease in Minnesota: first human case acquired in the contiguous United States, *JAMA* 241:904, 1979.
120. Pétavy AF, Deblock S, Walbaum S: The house mouse: a potential intermediate host for *Echinococcus multilocularis* in France, *Trans R Soc Trop Med Hyg* 84:571, 1990.
121. Mossiman F: Is the alveolar hydatid disease of the liver incurable? *Ann Surg* 192:118, 1980.
122. Rausch RL, Wilson JF, Schantz, PM: Spontaneous death of *Echinococcus multilocularis:* cases diagnosed serologically (by EM_2 ELISA) and clinical significance, *Am J Trop Med Hyg* 36:576, 1987.
123. Gottstein B, Eckert J, Fey H: Serological differentiation between *Echinococcus granulosus* and *E. multilocularis* infections in man, *Z Parasitenkd* 69:347, 1983.
124. Rausch RL, D'Alessandro A, Rausch VR: Characteristics of the larval *Echinococcus vogeli* Rausch and Bernstein, 1972 in the natural intermediate host, the paca, *Cuniculus paca* L. (Rodentia: Dasyproctidae), *Am J Trop Med Hyg* 30:1043, 1981.
125. D'Alessandro A, Rausch RL, Cuello C et al: *Echinococcus vogeli* in man, with a review of polycystic hydatid disease in Colombia and neighboring countries, *Am J Trop Med Hyg* 28:303, 1979.
126. Orkin M, Maibach HI, editors: *Cutaneous infestations and insect bites,* New York, 1985, Marcel Dekker.
127. Burgess I: *Sarcoptes scabiei* and scabies, *Adv Parasitol* 33:235, 1994.
128. Mellamby K: Biology of the parasite. In Orkin M, Maibach HI, editors: *Cutaneous infestations and insect bites,* New York, 1985, Marcel Dekker.
129. Glover R, Young L, Goltz RW: Norwegian scabies in acquired immunodeficiency syndrome: report of a case resulting in death from associated sepsis, *J Am Acad Dermatol* 16:396, 1987.

40 Prions

Stephen J. DeArmond
Stanley B. Prusiner

Prion diseases compose a group of human and animal neurodegenerative disorders that are classified together because their etiology and pathogenesis involve abnormalities of *prion protein* (PrP) metabolism. Prion diseases are similar to other neurodegenerative diseases because they encompass both sporadic and dominantly inherited (genetic) cases, but they are also unique because they are infectious. The particle that transmits these diseases among mammals has been designated a "prion" (prion: ***pro***teinaceous and ***in***fect***io***us) to distinguish it from conventional infectious agents, such as viruses. Despite intensive searches for nucleic acids over the past three decades, none have been found within prions; however, a modified isoform of *host-encoded* PrP is found in all infectious preparations. Furthermore, extensive experimental data argue that the sole functional component of prions is abnormal PrP.

The most common human prion disorder is sporadic *Creutzfeldt-Jakob disease* (CJD), which accounts for about 85% to 90% of the total cases. By definition, sporadic prion diseases are those with neither an infectious nor a genetic cause. Dominantly inherited genetic forms account for about 10% to 15% and have been linked to mutations in the PrP gene. These include familial CJD (FCJD), Gerstmann-Sträussler-Scheinker syndrome (GSS), GSS with neurofibrillary tangles (GSS-nft), and fatal familial insomnia (FFI). Eleven different pathogenic mutations of the human PrP gene have been reported.

Although prion diseases can be infectious, there is no evidence that they are contagious. There is a relatively small number of documented cases of human prion disease that were acquired by infection (1% or less of cases); and extraordinary methods are required to transmit these diseases to humans. The most infamous infectious prion disease is kuru, which was transmitted among the Fore people of New Guinea by ritualistic cannibalism. The only proved cases of infectious prion disease in the "civilized" world have been a small number transmitted by invasive medical procedures, which have been designated *iatrogenic Creutzfeldt-Jakob disease.*

Scrapie (Sc) of sheep and goats is the most common natural prion disease of animals. Animal feed prepared from scrapie-infected sheep is believed to be responsible for the current epidemic of bovine spongiform encephalopathy (BSE) in Great Britain. The epidemic followed a change in the procedures used to prepare meat and bone meal, which failed to deactivate the prion particle. Since 1986 when the epidemic was first recognized, more than 130,000 head of cattle have died of BSE, resulting in substantial economic loss. The epidemic has triggered an intense public health concern about the potential for spread of BSE to humans. Subsequently, strict regulations about the preparation and marketing of animal by-products have been put into place.

The neuropathologic features common to all prion diseases are *spongiform* (vacuolar) *degeneration* of neurons and their processes, neuronal loss and reactive astrocytic gliosis. There is no inflammation, and there are no viral inclusions. Variable amyloid plaque formation occurs within gray matter. The amyloid plaques are, as a general rule, not surrounded by a halo of dystrophic neurites and therefore differ from the neuritic (senile) plaques of Alzheimer's disease. The only exception is the amyloid plaques of GSS-nft. The plaques in prion diseases contain protease-resistant PrP.

The cause and pathogenesis of prion diseases appear to be related solely to abnormalities of PrP. Skepticism about the preeminent role of PrP was originally based on the absence of a precedent for a proteinaceous infectious agent. However, our current understanding is based on a large mass of varied and consistent data, with no objective evidence for a conventional infectious agent. Recent studies with transgenic (Tg) mice

Abbreviations

PrP	Prion protein
CJD	Creutzfeldt-Jakob disease
FCJD	Familial Creutzfeldt-Jakob disease
GSS	Gerstmann-Sträussler-Scheinker syndrome
GSS-nft	Gerstmann-Stäussler-Scheinker syndrome with neurofibrillary tangles
BSE	Bovine spongiform encephalopathy
Tg	Transgenic
PrP^{CJD}	Pathologic prion protein synthesized in humans
PrP^{Sc}	Pathologic prion protein in animals
PrP^{C}	Cellular prion protein isoform synthesized normally by humans and animals
ΔPrP	Mutated, pathologic prion protein
PRNP	Human prion protein maps to the short arm of chromosome 20
Prn-p	Designation for murine gene that encodes prion protein and maps to chromosome 2
FFI	Fatal familial insomnia
EEG	Electroencephalogram
hGH	Human growth hormone
CSF	Cerebrospinal fluid
FCJD	Familial Creutzfeldt-Jakob disease

expressing different forms of PrP have corroborated the central role of PrP. These have verified that genetic forms of prion diseases are linked to mutations of the PrP gene; that the host species barrier and different clinico-neuropathologic subtypes of prion disease are determined by the structure of PrP; and that the parameters which define prion isolates ("strains"), including incubation time and the distribution of spongiform degeneration in the brain, can be manipulated when one changes the amino acid sequence of PrP.

Prions differ from all known infectious pathogens in several respects. First, prions do not contain a nucleic acid genome that encodes for their progeny unlike viruses, viroids, bacteria, fungi, and parasites. Second, the only known component of the prion is the PrP^{CJD} protein in humans, or PrP^{Sc} in animals, both of which are encoded by a chromosomal gene. Third, in scrapie the accumulation of nascent PrP^{Sc} in the brain also appears to cause the clinically relevant neuropathology. More is known about the etiology and pathogenesis of CJD and related diseases than other neurodegenerative disorders because scrapie has been an accurate animal model and because the diseases can duplicated and manipulated in Tg mice.

The nomenclature to designate many aspects of prion disease is evolving. A provisional, simplified nomenclature designates PrP^{C} as the normal cellular isoform synthesized constitutively by humans and animals. PrP^{Sc} designates protease-resistant, pathogenic PrP in any prion-infected animal whether its synthesis was initiated by inoculation with human or animal prions. PrP^{CJD} designates protease-resistant, pathogenic PrP that is synthesized in and accumulates in humans, irrespective of whether the human prion disorder is sporadic or acquired by prion infection. Limited proteolysis of PrP^{CJD} and PrP^{Sc} digests about 67 amino acids from the N-terminus, yielding a 27 to 30 kDa peptide designated "PrP 27-30." Scrapie prions composed of PrP^{Sc}, or PrP 27-30, are equally infectious. Mutated (Δ), pathogenic PrP, which has been genetically linked to familial prion diseases when expressed in Tg mice, has been found to have protease resistance, which is less than that of PrP^{Sc}, but more than that of PrP^{C} and is therefore designated "ΔPrP."

The human PrP gene maps to the short arm of chromosome 20 and is designated "PRNP." The mouse PrP gene maps to the homologous chromosome 2 and is designated *"Prn-p."*[1] Tg mice expressing foreign or mutant PrP genes are labeled with the transgene in parentheses. For example, Tg mice harboring a mouse (Mo) PrP gene, which mimics the codon 102 mutation of human GSS, which results in the substitution of a leucine for proline, is designated "Tg(MoPrP-P101L)" (with codon 101 in mouse being homologous to codon 102 in humans).

HISTORICAL PERSPECTIVE

Scrapie

Sheep scrapie was the first prion disorder recognized. It was described in the records of the British Parliament in the early 1700s because of its strong effect on the wool industry. The clinical signs of scrapie include ataxia, tremor, weakness, wasting, excessive thirst, and a tendency to scrape off wool by rubbing the body against fixed objects. The importance of scrapie is that its clinical and neuropathologic features accurately imitate those in human prion disorders.

There is no epidemiologic evidence that scrapie from sheep has been transmitted to humans including sheep ranchers, veterinarians, and abattoir workers either by preparation or by ingestion of scrapie-infected food. However, scrapie has been transmitted to other animals through sheep scrapie-contaminated feed.

Characteristics

Scrapie is a transmissible disease with a long incubation time. The first experimental transmission of sheep scrapie to other sheep and to goats was by Cuillé and Chelle in 1936 by intraocular inoculation of scrapie-infected spinal cord.[2] Subsequent studies, carried out mostly in the United Kingdom, revealed several characteristics of the scrapie agent. Typically, the time to clinical signs after intracerebral inoculation of sheep or goats was 1 to 2 years. Incubation time was a function of the dose and the route of infection. With a single scrapie agent isolate, clinical signs and death occurred most rapidly after intracerebral inoculation, less rapidly after subcutaneous inoculation and slowest by the oral route.

Pattison and Millson[3] were the first to recognize that there are distinct clinical patterns of scrapie in sheep and goats and that these can be transmitted faithfully to other host animals. They reported that "the type of clinical syndrome produced by experimental inoculation will resemble the syndrome exhibited by the animal from which the material for inoculation was obtained." Subsequently, different scrapie isolates ("strains") were identified,[4] and they could be distinguished by scrapie incubation time, the distribution and intensity of spongiform degeneration in the central nervous system, and whether cerebral amyloid plaques formed in rodents. These characteristics are preserved during multiple, sequential passages of a given scrapie isolate within a single inbred mouse strain but vary greatly or even fail to occur when transferred to a different animal species or inbred mouse strain.

The term *species barrier* has been used to designate failure of transmission of scrapie or the prolongation of scrapie incubation time when a scrapie prion isolate is transferred from one animal strain or species to another. The molecular mechanism underlying the species barrier appears to be a lack of sufficient homology between PrP^{Sc} in the prion and PrP^{C} of the host animal.

Classic genetic analysis of short and long incubation times in sheep and then in mice indicated that scrapie incubation time was determined in part by the infecting prion isolate and in part by a host gene. The host gene was designated the scrapie incubation time, or *sinc,* gene.[5] The molecular mechanisms governing the complex interaction of incubation time genes with different prion isolates are better understood today as the result of two studies. After the discovery of the PrP gene it was found that long incubation times in I/LnJ mice and short incubation times in NZW mice were linked to two amino acid differences, which distinguished the PrP in these two inbred mouse strains.[6] The tight linkage of short and long incubation times to the two PrP alleles suggested that the PrP gene and the sinc gene are either very close together or one and the same. In a subsequent study, the influence of the PrP gene on scrapie incubation time was demonstrated in Tg mouse lines, which express different numbers of Syrian hamster (SHa) PrP transgenes, since incubation times were inversely proportional to the PrP mRNA level.[7] The complexity of the relationship between different prion isolates and PrP gene alleles appears to be attributable to differential affinity of PrP^{Sc} of the infecting prion isolate with PrP^{C} allotype in the host. In a PrP-homozygous host expressing a PrP^{C} with a high affinity for the PrP^{Sc} of the prion, a short incubation time occurs. At the other extreme, when there is little or no affinity of PrP^{Sc} for a PrP^{C} allotype, there is a host barrier to scrapie infection.[8] The structural factors within PrP^{Sc} and PrP^{C} molecules, which determine affinity, appear to reside in part in the amino acid sequence of PrP^{Sc} and PrP^{C} and in part by secondary and tertiary structures in PrP^{Sc}.

Human prion diseases and scrapie

Although the first description of a human prion disease, Creutzfeldt-Jakob disease, is attributed to Creutzfeldt's case report in 1920 of a 23-year-old woman with sensory, motor, and psychiatric disturbances, it is generally believed that this was not a genuine case of CJD, nor were three of the additional five cases reported by Jakob in 1921 and 1923. Only two of the latter cases had both the clinical features and spongiform degeneration accepted today as characteristic of the disease.[9] In 1936, the clinical and neuropathologic features of GSS were described;[10] however, its relationship to CJD was not established until recently.[11] Kuru, a neurodegenerative disease resembling CJD and scrapie that was confined to the Fore people of New Guinea, was described in the late 1950s (for personal observations and history see Gajdusek, 1979[12]). The clinical and neuropathologic features of kuru were largely those of cerebellar degeneration, sometimes with evidence of a progressive dementia.[13] *Kuru* is a word from the Fore language that connotes trembling associated with fear or cold. The epidemiology of kuru indicates that it may be an infectious disorder and that it was probably spread among the Fore people by ritualistic cannibalism. Some clinical cases of CJD present primarily with cerebellar signs; however, the clinical range of CJD is more varied, with dementia, basal ganglia signs, and lower motor neuron signs. The clinical and neuropathologic similarities of kuru to scrapie were first recognized by the veterinary pathologist Dr. William Hadlow and led to the comprehensive attempts to transmit human neurodegenerative diseases to animals at the National Institutes of Health by Gajdusek, Gibbs, and their colleagues. These studies revealed that kuru,[14] sporadic, infectious, and familial CJD,[15,16] and one other familial cerebral amyloidosis, GSS,[11] but not Alzheimer's disease or other more common neurodegenerative diseases, are transmissible to subhuman primates and other animal species.

The prion concept

With the successful transmission of scrapie and later kuru and CJD to animals, the hypothesis that they were caused by a "filterable" virus became popular. Although the neuropathology of scrapie and kuru were atypical of a viral infection (that is, no inflammation and no viral inclusions), it was not until Tikvah Alper and her colleagues showed that scrapie infectivity resists inactivation by ultraviolet (UV) and ionizing radiation[17,18] that a myriad of hypotheses on the chemical nature of the scrapie agent emerged. Other nonviral characteristics of the scrapie agent included its resistance to nondenaturing detergents, nucleases, proteases, glycosylases, and formalin fixation.[19-22]

Many attempts to purify the scrapie agent over several decades were unsuccessful. This was attributable in a large part to the cumbersome and tedious bioassays of scrapie infectivity titer in sheep and later in mice. It was difficult to develop an effective purification protocol when the interval between execution of the experiment and availability of the results was nearly a year! A more rapid and economical bioassay for scrapie infectivity titer was developed[23,24] after the discovery that scrapie incubation times were about 70 days in the Syrian hamster.

Consequent to this advance, infectivity of partially purified preparations of the scrapie agent from Syrian hamster brains was found to be attenuated by prolonged exposure to proteases but was unaffected by exposure to nucleases, psoralens, hydroxylamine, and UV irradiation. Based on these findings, the term *prion* was introduced to distinguish the scrapie agent from viruses and viroids.[25] Later, a 3000-fold purification of the scrapie agent from Syrian hamster brains was achieved, and it revealed that the main component of these highly enriched fractions was a 27 to 30 kDa protein, designated "PrP 27-30." The purification procedure included treatment with nuclease to hydrolyze nucleic acids and limited proteolysis with proteinase K. Proteinase K–resistant PrP 27-30 was not found in identical preparations from normal, uninfected control brains. Subsequently, a partial amino acid sequence of PrP 27-30 was obtained and used to synthesize oligonucleotide probes, which allowed retrieval of cDNA clones encoding PrP from a library.[26-28] This led to the discovery that PrP 27-30 is derived from a larger 33 to 35 kDa protein, designated PrP^{Sc}, by limited proteolysis with proteinase K without loss of infectivity (Fig. 40-1). In addition, it was discovered that there is a normal, constitutively expressed cellular form of the prion protein that is 33 to 35 kDa and proteinase K sensitive, designated "PrP^{C}."

Both PrP^{C} and PrP^{Sc} are synthesized from a single-copy chromosomal gene in which the entire open reading frame is contained in a single exon. The highest levels of PrP messenger RNA (mRNA) are expressed in neurons.[29,30] The level of PrP mRNA expression remains constant throughout scrapie and is identical to the level in normal, uninfected animals.

Search for a scrapie-specific nucleic acid

The search for a scrapie-specific nucleic acid has been intense, thorough, and comprehensive, yet it has been unrewarding. Highly purified scrapie prion fractions were analyzed for a scrapie-specific nucleic acid by a specially developed technique designated *return refocusing gel electrophoresis*, but no candidate polynucleotides above 80 bases in length were found.[31,32] Small, heterogeneous nucleic acid fragments, most of which ranged in size from 40 to 80 nucleotides, were found. Whether these small nucleic acids are contaminants or are essential for infectivity or for determining the strainlike behavior of different prion isolates is uncertain. To test the relevance of these nucleic acids, two different hamster prion isolates were exposed to UV radiation; however, neither scrapie infectivity nor the strainlike characteristics of the two isolates were changed (unpublished data). These findings extend the argument that the nucleic acid fragments are not necessary functional components of prions.

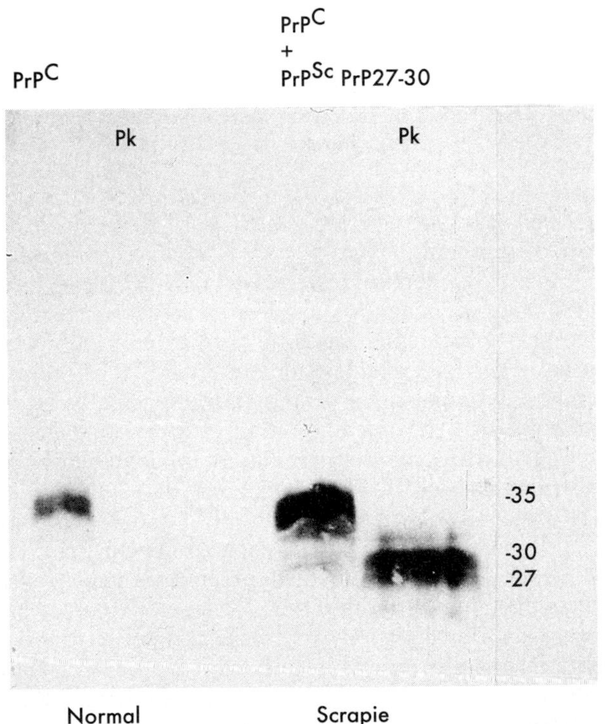

Fig. 40-1 PrP^{C} is completely digested by proteinase K (Pk), whereas PrP^{Sc} is partially digested, yielding PrP 27-30. PrP isoform bands, after electrophoresis in a polyacrylamide gel, are identified by their molecular weights and susceptibility to Pk digestion on a western transfer blot test. Their location is revealed by immunostaining with PrP-specific antibodies. PrP^{C} in a whole homogenate of normal Syrian hamster brain *(far left lane)* has a molecular weight of 33 to 35 kDa (Normal). The adjacent lane is from the same normal brain homogenate treated with Pk. Both PrP^{C} and PrP^{Sc} in a brain homogenate from a Syrian hamster terminally ill with scrapie (Scrapie) migrate at 33 to 35 kDa. There is from 10 to 100 times more PrP^{Sc} than PrP^{C} in the scrapie-infected brain, which accounts for the larger size and more intense staining of the 33 to 35 kDa band in scrapie, relative to normal. *Far right lane,* The scrapie brain homogenate was exposed to Pk, which digested all the PrP^{C} and partially digested PrP^{Sc} to PrP 27-30.

Search for a chemical modification

The discovery that the entire open reading frame of the PrP gene is contained within a single exon argued that PrP^{Sc} is not generated by alternate splicing.[33,34] This prompted the search for a posttranslational chemical modification to explain the differences in the properties of the two PrP isoforms.[35] Neither mass spectrometry nor Edman sequencing revealed amino acid substitutions or posttranslational chemical modifications that might differentiate PrP^{C} from PrP^{Sc}. These findings raised the possibility that conformation alone distinguishes the two PrP isoforms.

To test whether conformational changes feature in PrP^{Sc} synthesis, both PrP^{C} and PrP^{Sc} were purified by the use of nondenaturing procedures.[36] Fourier transform infrared (FTIR) spectroscopy and circular dichroism (CD) measurements showed that PrP^{C} has a high α-helix content (42%) and little or no β-sheet (3%). In contrast, the β sheet content of PrP^{Sc} is 43% and that of the α-helix 30%. PrP 27-30, which is derived from PrP^{Sc} by limited proteolysis, has an even higher β-sheet content (54%) and a lower α-helix content (21%).[37,38] Since PrP^{Sc} appears to be the only functional component of "infectious" prion particles, it is likely that this conformational transition is the fundamental event in the propagation of prions. In support of this is the finding that denaturation of PrP 27-30 under conditions that decrease β-sheet content reduces scrapie infectivity.[38]

MOLECULAR PATHOGENESIS OF PRION DISEASES

Our understanding of the pathogenesis of prion diseases has been greatly aided by two advances. First, Tg mice expressing different PrP transgenes have shown that the amino acid sequence of PrP profoundly influences the behavior of prion isolates. Second, a new, highly sensitive and specific technique termed *histoblotting* has been developed to localize and quantify PrP^{CJD} and PrP^{Sc}.[39,40] Immunohistochemical staining of histoblots yields a far more intense, specific, and reproducible PrP signal than can be achieved by immunohistochemistry on standard tissue sections (Fig. 40-2).

Origin of PrP^{Sc} from PrP^{C}

Most of the PrP^{C} that is synthesized appears to become attached to the outer surface of cells by a glycolipid (GPI) anchor.[41] Protein-turnover studies in cell lines chronically and stably infected with scrapie indicate that PrP^{Sc} is derived from preexisting PrP^{C}.[42-44] Thus it appears that PrP^{Sc}, either from an exogenous source of prions or produced endogenously as the

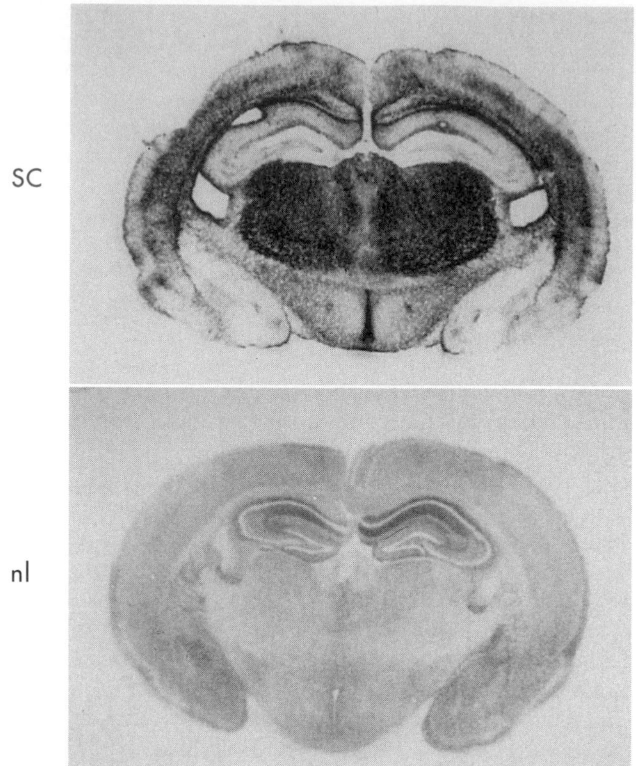

Fig. 40-2 Histoblots of coronal sections of Syrian hamster brain showing the location of PrP^{Sc} in the terminal stages of scrapie (sc) and of PrP^{C} in a normal, unifected animal (nl). The scrapie-infected animal had been inoculated in the thalamus with the Sc237 prion isolate 65 days earlier. The higher signal intensity of PrP^{Sc} in the thalamus is consistent with a 10- to 100-fold higher concentration, relative to PrP^{C} in normal animals.

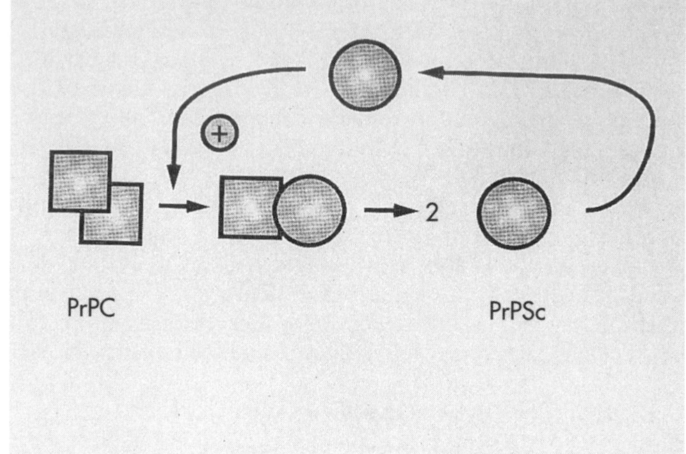

Fig. 40-3 Model of prion replication. The model is based on the experimental evidence that indicates that PrP^{Sc} is the sole functional component of prions and that PrP^{Sc} is derived from preexisting PrP^{C}. PrP^{Sc} is represented by *circles* and PrP^{C} by *squares*. Within a cell, PrP^{Sc}, either from inoculated prions or formed endogenously, binds to PrP^{C} and forms a heterodimer. Subsequently, PrP^{C} is converted into a nascent PrP^{Sc} molecule. The conversion involves increasing the β-sheet content of PrP^{C} and decreasing its α- helix content. The process becomes self-perpetuating, since the nascent PrP^{Sc} can bind to other PrP^{C} molecules and initiate their conversion to PrP^{Sc}.

result of preexisting scrapie infection, forms a transient complex with PrP^{C} (such as a heterodimer) and that this interaction leads to the conversion of PrP^{C} to nascent PrP^{Sc} (Fig. 40-3). The cellular compartments in which the heterodimer is formed and in which the structural transformation of PrP^{C} to PrP^{Sc} occurs are not known. Like other GPI-anchored proteins, PrP^{C} appears to reenter the cell through a subcellular compartment bounded by cholesterol-rich, detergent-insoluble membranes where PrP^{C} appears to be converted into PrP^{Sc}.[45] Subsequently, PrP^{Sc} is transported to lysosomes where some of it is stored.[46] The interaction of PrP^{Sc} with host PrP^{C} is selective and depends on amino acid homology between PrP^{Sc} and PrP^{C}. Various studies argue that the interaction between PrP^{Sc} and PrP^{C} is homophilic and that the interaction is governed by the amine acid sequence of the two molecules. The selectivity and specificity of the interaction between PrP^{Sc} and PrP^{C} may provide a molecular explanation for the species barrier to prior infection and for the clinical neuropathologic difference that distinguish scrapie isolates.[7,47,48]

Amyloid in prion diseases

The first evidence that PrP^{CJD} and PrP^{Sc} are pathogenic was the finding that the amyloid plaques in human and animal prion diseases react specifically with PrP antibodies[40,49-52] (Fig. 40-4). However, amyloid plaques are not a constant feature of prion diseases. They are detected by standard hematoxylin and eosin stain, periodic acid–Schiff reaction, or Congo red dye stain in only 5% to 10% of CJD and 50% to 70% of kuru cases.[11] By definition, all cases of GSS have amyloid plaques, since the diagnosis requires the triad of cerebellar or corticospinal tract degeneration, dementia, and cerebral amyloidosis.[10] Amyloid plaques are not found in all forms of experimental scrapie in rodents. Amyloidogenicity is determined in part by the infecting prion isolate and, in fact, has been one of the characteristics used to define differences among prion isolates[53-56] (Fig. 40-5).

The amyloidogenic potential of PrP^{Sc}, and presumably of PrP^{CJD}, is probably inherent in its high content of β-sheet, since all amyloids are composed of proteins in a β-pleated sheet configuration. PrP^{Sc} and PrP^{CJD} extracted from the brains of cases with or without amyloid plaques do not spontaneously form into amyloid rods in vitro; however, after proteinase K digestion and exposure to detergents, the resulting PrP 27-30 polymerizes into rods that bind Congo red dye and show green birefringence in polarized light.[57-59] The greater propensity of PrP 27-30 to polymerize into amyloid rods may be the result of its higher β-sheet content than that of PrP^{Sc}. The extraction of PrP rods from human brains has been used to identify and verify cases of CJD.[60,61] Some investigators believe that "scrapie-associated fibrils" (SAFs) are synonymous with prion rods and are composed of PrP; however, although this may be true, SAFs can be distinguished from PrP rods by their ultrastructure and failure to bind Congo red dye.[62,63]

PrP^{Sc} and brain dysfunction

There are multiple lines of evidence to indicate that accumulation of PrP^{CJD} and PrP^{Sc} in the gray matter causes spongiform degeneration and nerve cell loss. First, PrP^{CJD} and PrP^{Sc} are found only in human and animal prion diseases, respectively[40,60,61,64,65] (Fig. 40-2). Second, the highest concentrations

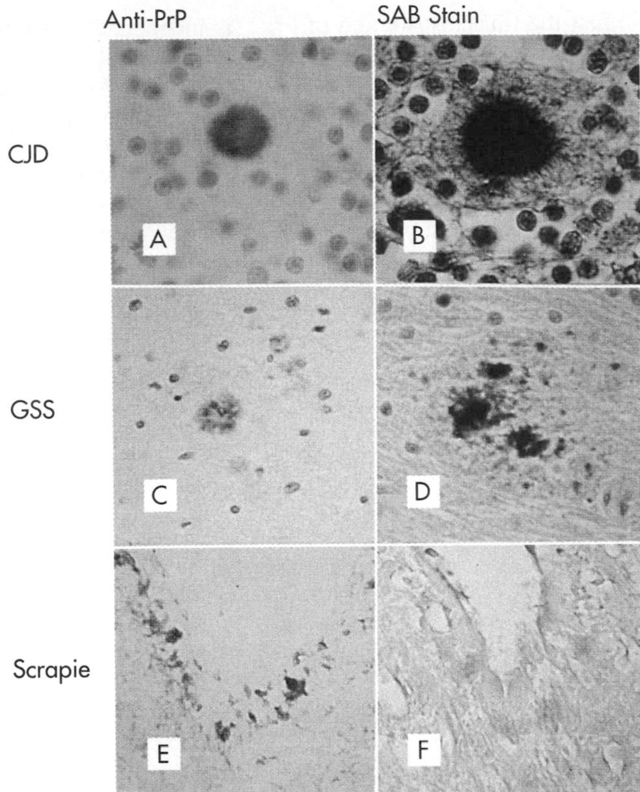

Fig. 40-4 Kuru type of amyloid plaques in Creutzfeldt-Jakob disease (CJD) **(A** and **B),** multicentric amyloid plaques in Gerstmann-Sträussler-Scheinker syndrome (GSS) **(C** and **D),** and primitive amyloid plaques in Syrian hamster scrapie **(E** and **F)** contain protease-resistant PrP by peroxidase immunohistochemistry with PrP antibodies (anti-PrP). Like all amyloids, they also contain sulfated glycosaminoglycans, as revealed by the sulfated Alcian blue histochemical method (SAB stain).[52] The primitive subependymal amyloid plaques in scrapie are strongly PrP immunopositive, **E,** but weakly SAB-positive, *F*. e, Ependyma.

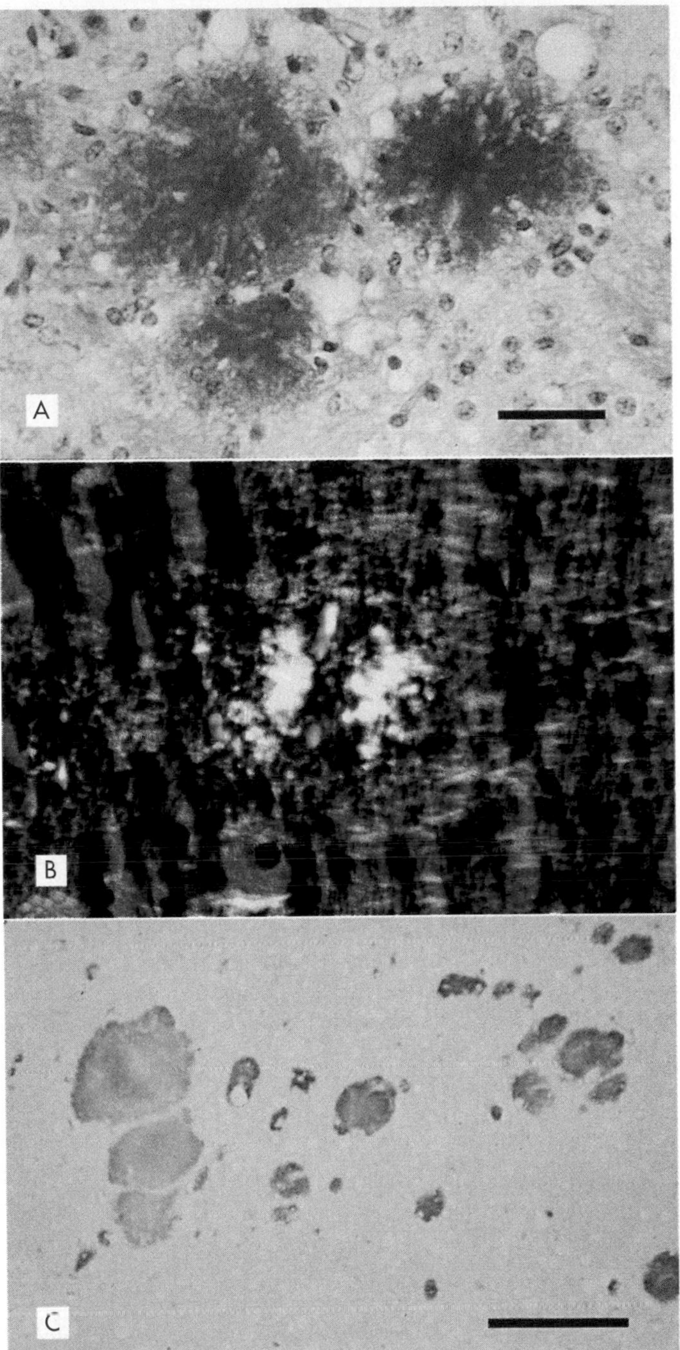

Fig. 40-5 PrP amyloid plaques develop spontaneously in transgenic mice expressing a PrP transgene mimicking the codon 102 mutation linked to human GSS(P102L). The plaques were most numerous in the caudate nucleus. They stained strongly by the periodic acid–Schiff reaction **(A),** showed green birefringence in polarized light following staining with Congo red dye **(B),** and were strongly PrP immunopositive **(C).** Bar for **A** and **B** is 50 µm. Bar in **C** is 50 µm.

of PrP^{Sc} are found in the brain.[27] Third, there is a temporal relationship between the accumulation of PrP^{Sc} in scrapie and the development of neuropathology, since spongiform degeneration and reactive astrocytic gliosis occur after PrP^{Sc} accumulation in that region.[29] Fourth, there is a precise collocalization of sites of PrP^{Sc} accumulation, spongiform degeneration, and reactive astrocytic gliosis in scrapie.[40,48,66,67] Other evidence that abnormal PrP is amyloidogenic and causes the clinically relevant neuropathologic features is the molecular genetic findings that have linked mutations in the human PrP gene to FCJD, GSS, GSS-nft, and FFI and the corroborative study, which followed, that Tg mice that express MoPrP mimicking the PRNP codon 102 mutation of GSS develop a neurodegenerative disorder spontaneously characterized by spongiform degeneration of gray matter and PrP amyloid plaque formation[56,68] (Fig. 40-5).

Mice designated *Prn-p*$^{\%}$ in which the PrP gene has been deleted seem to have normal life-spans without any structural or behavioral abnormalities.[69] *Prn-p*$^{\%}$ mice do not develop neuropathologic or clinical features and do not propagate prions after inoculation with prions. When a SHaPrP transgene, but not a MoPrP gene, was introduced into *Prn-p*$^{\%}$ mice by crossing them with Tg(SHaPrP) mice, which express $SHaPrP^{C}$, the resulting mice became susceptible to SHa prions but not to Mo prions.[70,71] These findings indicate that the absence of PrP^{C} expression is not the cause of disease, and they support the view that accumulation of PrP^{Sc} does. Furthermore, they indicate that prions require PrP^{C} expression for formation of new prions and for development of neuropathologic features.

PrP^{Sc} spread in the brain

Neurons appear to be the main source of PrP^{CJD}/PrP^{Sc} in the brain, since they express by far the highest levels of PrP mRNA[27,30] (Fig. 40-6) and since PrP^{C} can be detected within them.[40] However, the possibility that glia or other organs, particularly lymphatic organs, contribute to the pathogenesis of prion diseases in some humans and in some animal species cannot be excluded. The mechanisms of disease spread in the brain after inoculation of scrapie prions has been examined in Syrian hamsters and in Tg mice expressing different PrP constructs. Two mechanisms based on patterns of PrP^{Sc} accumulation have been identified.[72] In part, the disease spreads along neuroanatomic pathways that interconnect neuron populations. Presumably, PrP^{Sc} is carried by axonal transport mechanisms to synapses, where it is released and can infect the postsynaptic neuron if the latter is susceptible. The disease also spreads between regions that are not neuroanatomically interconnected through release of PrP^{Sc} into the CNS extracellular space, where it diffuses rapidly to target susceptible neuron populations. The fact that extracellular deposits of protease-resistant PrP characteristically occur as PrP amyloid plaques in prion diseases indicate that a significant proportion of PrP^{Sc} is released from sites of synthesis into the CNS extracellular space.

Selective vulnerability of neurons

CJD in humans and scrapie in animals has diverse clinical features. The concept that "strains" of scrapie agent account for this diversity arose when it was found that a set of clinical features could be transmitted faithfully among animals of the same genotype. Furthermore, the early studies of scrapie in inbred mouse strains showed that clinical diversity was associated with distinct distributions of spongiform degeneration in the brain. Thus each prion isolate appeared to cause degeneration of different nerve cell populations.[67,72] (Fig. 40-7).

Evidence indicates that prion isolates may target different nerve cell populations for conversion of PrP^{C} to nascent PrP^{Sc} and that the final distribution of PrP^{Sc} is independent of incubation time.[8,66,67] It also follows that since the local accumulation of PrP^{Sc} appears to cause neuronal degeneration, the distribution of PrP^{Sc} is the main determinant of the clinical and neuropathologic differences that distinguish prion isolates. Although the selectivity of prion isolates for different neuron populations was evident from these studies, the results also showed that the same brain regions were often targeted by one or more prion isolate. Whether this overlap is attributable to infection of different subpopulations of neurons in a brain region or a specific nerve cell type can synthesize different prion isolates is not known.

Prion diversity

All the experimental data argue for the unifying hypothesis that PrP^{Sc} is both the preeminent component of the infectious agent of scrapie and its accumulation in the brain cause the clinically relevant neuropathologic condition. The apparent

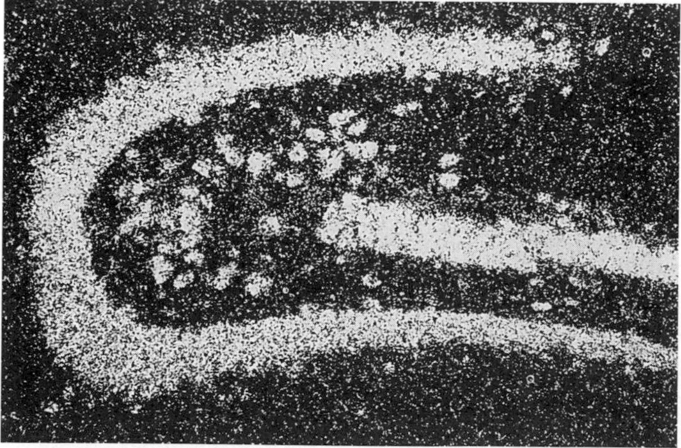

Fig. 40-6 Dark-field microscopy of tritiated PrP cDNA probe applied to cryostat section of hamster brain. The highest PrP mRNA copy numbers are consistently found in CNS neurons by in situ hybridization.[30] Above background numbers of silver grains exclusively overlay nerve cell bodies of the dentate gyrus and Ammon's horn in the hippocampus section depicted, whereas only background levels overlay astrocytes and other nonneuronal cells.

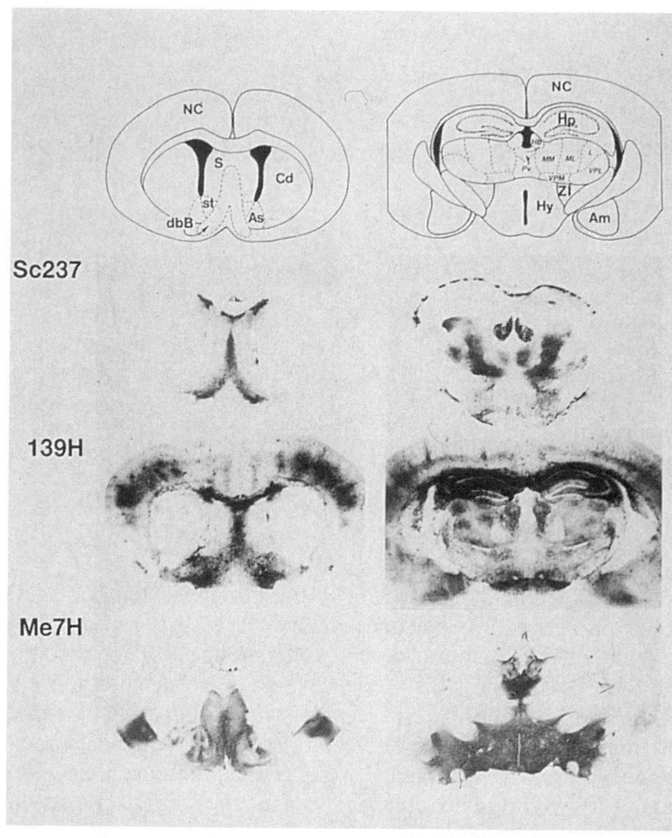

Fig. 40-7 The neuroanatomic distribution of PrP^{Sc} in the terminal stages of scrapie revealed by histoblots is unique for each prion isolate. In this study, Tg(SHaPrP) mice, which express high levels of $SHaPrP^{C}$, were inoculated in the thalamus with either the Sc237, 139H, or Me7H hamster-passaged prion isolate. Clinical signs of scrapie developed about 50 days after inoculation with the Sc237 and 139H isolates and about 185 days with the Me7H isolate. The same two brain regions are shown for each isolate. *Am,* Amygdala; *As,* accumbens septi; *Cd,* caudate nucleus; *dbB,* diagonal band of Broca; *Hp,* hippocampus; *Hy,* hypothalamus; *NC,* neocortex; *S,* septal nuclei; *st,* interstitial nucleus of the stria terminalis; *ZI,* zona incerta. *Thalamic nuclei in italics:* Hb, habenula; *L,* lateral; *ML,* medial, pars lateralis; *MM,* medial, pars medialis; *Pv,* paraventricular; *VPL,* ventral posterior lateral; *VPM,* ventral posterior medial.

inseparability of the infectious agent from the pathogenic effects in the brain argues further that the molecular and cellular mechanisms that determine selective vulnerability of neurons in prion diseases (such as selective targeting of different neuron populations by prion isolates) and the origin of prion isolate diversity are interrelated and inseparable. The fact that each animal species can synthesize multiple prion isolates with strainlike characteristics implies that specific information is transferred from PrP^{Sc} to PrP^{C} during its conversion to nascent PrP^{Sc}. Furthermore, it is assumed that the information must be "coded" by specific, stable structural configurations of PrP^{Sc}, given the constraints of experimental data that indicate that PrP^{Sc} is the sole functional component of prions.

Three possible mechanisms have been suggested to explain how PrP^{Sc} can attain multiple stable structural states. First, it has been proposed that an accessory cellular RNA, called a *co-prion,* can modify the properties of PrP^{Sc};[73] however, there is no physical or chemical evidence for a necessary second prion molecule.

An alternative hypothesis is that transferable information is stored exclusively in prion protein molecules. It is possible that the structural characteristics that give the PrP^{Sc} molecule strainlike properties are determined in part by the cells in which it is produced. One cell-specific molecular mechanism that could result in PrP^{Sc} diversity is cell-determined diversity of PrP^{C} structure, since PrP^{Sc} is derived from PrP^{C}. For example, each neuron population may synthesize different PrP^{C} isoforms with the same amino acid sequence but different carbohydrate side chains. This possibility is supported by ample evidence that there is variation in the glycosylation patterns of PrP^{Sc}.[74] Furthermore, cells potentially possess distinct repertoires of glycosyltransferases, which could result in synthesis of PrP^{C}'s with diverse carbohydrate structures. In this model of prion propagation, selective targeting of neuron populations for synthesis of PrP^{Sc} would be facilitated by neuron-determined structural homology between PrP^{Sc} and PrP^{C} residing in their carbohydrate trees.

A third possible cell-determined mechanism to account for prion isolate and neuropathologic diversity is indicated by the evidence that PrP^{Sc} has a high degree of β-sheet content whereas PrP^{C} is largely α-helical.[36] This argues that conversion of α-helices to β-sheets underlies the formation of both PrP^{Sc} and infectious prions. There are four potential α-helix domains in the PrP molecule, based on a comparison with amino acid sequences of other proteins.[75,76] (Fig. 40-8) Interestingly, the algorithm used to predict structural domains of PrP indicated that the putative α-helical domains showed both strong α-helix and strong β-sheet preferences.[75] Peptides corresponding to these putative α-helical regions were synthesized, and, contrary to predictions, three of the four spontaneously aggregated into amyloid rods, which were composed largely of β-sheet by infrared spectroscopy and showed green birefringence when stained with Congo red dye. These findings indicate that the conversion of PrP^{C} to PrP^{Sc} may involve transition of one or more putative α-helices into β-sheets. Furthermore, they indicate that different combinations and permutations of α-helices and β-sheets could account for the structural variations of PrP^{Sc} required to explain the diversity of prion isolates.

Whether cell-specific foldases, chaperonins, or other molecules play a role in the conversion of the PrP^{C}/PrP^{Sc} heterodimer into two molecules of PrP^{Sc} and account for the different patterns of PrP^{Sc} accumulation in the brain that characterize different prion isolates remains to be determined. In reality, it may be that a combination of cell-determined mechanisms influence the structure of PrP^{C} and cause the conformational differences which give PrP^{Sc} its properties.

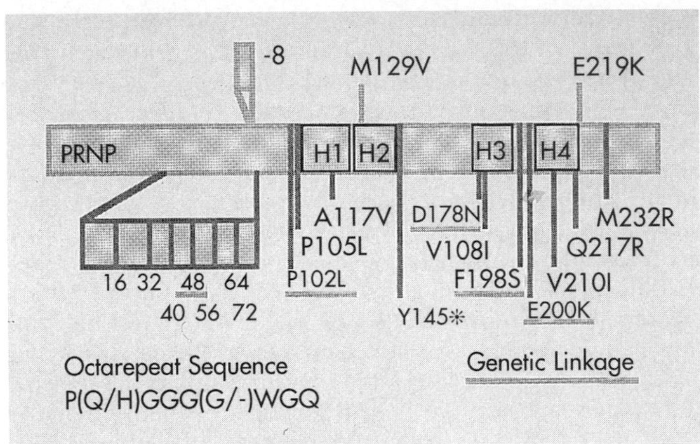

Fig. 40-8 Predicted α-helical regions (H1 through H4) of the prion protein and their relationship to known pathogenic mutations of the human PrP gene (PRNP). The locations of the α-helical regions are depicted in the bar representing the PrP open-reading frame. The H1 region extends from codon 109-122, H2 from 129-140, H3 from 178-191, and H4 from 202-218. Three nonpathogenic polymorphisms are shown above the bar and include an octapeptide deletion from the repeat region of the molecule (–8) and the Met/Val polymorphism at codon 129. Below the bar are the mutations identified in familial prion diseases. The mutations for which genetic linkage has been established are underlined. For octapeptide repeat insertions, genetic linkage has been determined only for the 48 amino acid insertion. The *asterisk* marks a mutation forming a stop codon, which leads to a truncated PrP molecule in one pedigree. Notice that most of the pathogenic mutations are in the region of the putative α-helices.

PrP OVEREXPRESSION NEUROMYOPATHY

Uninfected Tg mice that expressed the wild type of PrP^{C} developed a generalized paresis spontaneously that was more severe in the hindlimbs.[77] There was minimal vacuolation in the hippocampus and insufficient anterior horn cell loss in the spinal cord to account for the degree of weakness. The main pathologic condition that correlated with the clinical signs was found in skeletal muscle. It manifested as a necrotizing myopathy with multiple degenerating muscle fibers, phagocytosis of muscle fibers by macrophages, considerable variation in muscle fiber size, and endomysial fibrosis. The pathosis was most severe in the quadriceps femoris but was present to lesser degrees in all other skeletal muscles. Smooth and cardiac muscle appeared to be unaffected. In addition to the myopathic features, there was fiber type grouping of the type seen with neurogenic disorders. This correlated with a demyelinating peripheral neuropathy associated with axonal loss. Single muscle fiber necrosis, in the absence of neurogenic changes, was identified at as early as 90 days of age, which indicated that the myopathy preceded the peripheral neuropathy. PrP mRNA and PrP^{C} levels were significantly increased in skeletal muscle. No protease-resistant PrP was detected in either the brain or the skeletal muscle.

The skeletal muscle lesions in transgenic mice expressing high levels of PrP^C are very similar to the generalized myopathy reported in natural scrapie of sheep.[78-80] The incidence in scrapie-infected sheep varied from less than 5% of cases to almost 100%, depending on the study. Myopathy was reported in the propositus of an unusual CJD kindred.[81] Subsequently it was shown that this patient was descended from a British GSS pedigree carrying the codon P102L mutation (see below)[54] It is noteworthy that the codon E200K mutation, linked to FCJD, can also present with a neuropathy.[82] However, it may be that the PrP overexpression myopathy is a model for the common age-related muscle disease of humans, inclusion body myositis. Immunohistochemical studies indicate that both PrP and Aβ peptide (found in Alzheimer's disease) collocalize in the intracellular "amyloid" filaments that characterize this myopathy.[83]

HUMAN PRION DISEASES

Inherited forms

Familial prion diseases, which are far rarer than sporadic CJD, account for about 10% of human prion diseases, with an incidence of about 1 per 10 million. However, linking the dominantly inherited occurrence of neuropathosis, clinical signs, and spontaneous formation of prions to mutations of the PRNP gene and duplication of one of these disorders in Tg mice expressing a mouse PrP homolog of a human PrP gene mutation has been one of the strongest arguments for the preeminent role of the prion protein in the cause and pathogenesis of all forms of prion disease. Until recently, only two familial forms of human prion disease, FCJD[16] and GSS,[11] were recognized, based on dominant inheritance, on transmissibility to animals, and on the neuropathosis. With the discovery of the prion protein and sequencing of the human PrP gene,[84] molecular genetic studies verified that FCJD and GSS are PrP disorders and led to the discovery of new familial PrP disorders.

PrP mutations and genetic linkage

GSS cases in which ataxia predominates (ataxic-GSS) were the first to be linked to a mutation in the PRNP gene.[54] This mutation leads to the substitution of a Leu for a Pro at codon 102 denoted as P102L, which has been found in 10 different families in nine different countries.[85-88] The cause and effect relationship between the P102L mutation and prion disease was verified in Tg mice expressing a mouse (Mo) PrP transgene mimicking the mutation Tg(MoPrP-P101L) mice.[55,56] A primarily dementing form of GSS (telencephalic GSS) has been found to segregate with a PRNP gene codon 117 mutation resulting in the substitution of a Val for an Ala.[85,89] In Japan, GSS segregates with a PrP codon 105 mutation causing a substitution of Leu for Pro.[90]

A codon 200 mutation, which leads the substitution of Lys for Glu, denoted "E200K," has been identified in some familial CJD pedigrees.[91-93] This mutation among Libyan Jews represents the largest focus of CJD in the world with an incidence about 100 times greater than the worldwide incidence.[94,95] The E200K mutation has also been found in Slovaks originating from Orava,[91] in a cluster of familial cases in Chile,[96] and in a large German family living in the United States.[97] It is likely that the E200K mutation has arisen independently multiple times.[54,93] Mutation at PrP codon 210 leads to a Val-to-Ile substitution and produces CJD with classic symptoms and signs.[98,99]

In addition to point mutations in the PRNP gene, octapeptide repeat insertions have been identified in other families with CJD.[100-105] This mutation must have arisen through a complex series of events, since the human PrP gene contains only 5 octarepeats, indicating that a single recombination event could not have created the insert. Genealogic investigations have shown that all four families in southern England with this insertion are related, arguing for a single founder more than two centuries ago.[106]

Molecular genetics has led to the discovery of new prion disorders. PRNP gene codon 198 and 217 mutations[107,108] occur in a unique form of GSS, in which Alzheimer's disease–like neuropathologic changes, including neuritic plaques and neurofibrillary tangles, are associated with deposition of PrP amyloid plaques and not the Aβ peptide.[109-111] These unique pedigrees raise questions about the relationship of the Aβ peptide deposition to neuritic plaques in Alzheimer's disease and indicate that there is an overlap of pathogenic mechanisms in Alzheimer's disease and prion diseases.

A codon 178 mutation[112-114] has been found in families with fatal familial insomnia;[115] however, the same codon 178 mutation has also been described in some familial CJD pedigrees without features of insomnia.[112,116-118] Although the mutation at codon 178 results in the substitution of an Asp for an Asn in both FFI with D178N and FCJD with D178N, the two diseases differ in clinical presentation and distribution of lesions. In FFI, neuropathologic changes are confined largely to the mediodorsal and anterior ventral nuclei of the thalamus, whereas they are widespread in cerebral cortical and subcortical regions in 178-FCJD. Subsequently, it was discovered that the 178 mutation in FFI is also associated with a Met polymorphism at codon 129.[112] Thus the PRNP gene allele in FFI, which carries the codon 178 mutation, also codes for a Met at codon 129, and therefore the FFI mutation is designated "D178N, M129." In contrast, cases of FCJD with the D178N mutation code for Val at codon 129, and their mutation is designated "D178N, V129." When both PrP alleles contained a Met at codon 129 (Met homozygosity) in FFI, a more severe form of FFI resulted. Similarly, Val homozygosity at codon 129 resulted in a more severe form of FCJD(D178N).

It is probably not a coincidence that virtually all the pathogenic point mutations of the PRNP gene occur in and around domains coding for putative α-helical regions (Fig. 40-8). The mutations in these locations may destabilize α-helices or facilitate β-sheet formation.

Infectious forms

The only known cases of infectious prion disease in humans have been kuru, transmitted, one would assume, by ritualistic cannibalism in New Guinea and, in the "civilized" world, iatrogenic CJD, which appears to have been transmitted by invasive medical procedures.[119] The causes of iatrogenic CJD include the following: (1) Depth-recording EEG electrodes sterilized with 70% ethanol and formaldehyde vapors (two cases). Although the sterilization procedure used was effective for viruses, prions require exposure to 2N NaOH to denature PrP^{CJD}. (2) A corneal transplant in which brain extracts from the donor transmitted CJD to a chimpanzee. (3) Cadaveric dura homografts, implicated in 11 cases of CJD. Five of the 11 dura specimens came from a single manufacturer, where they had been treated with 10% hydrogen peroxide and ionizing radiation. They are now treated for 1 hour with 1N NaOH. (4) A pericardial homograft replacement of a tympanic membrane implicated in one case of CJD. (5) Human gonadotropin injections associated with CJD in four Australian women. (6) Injections of human growth hormone (hGH) prepared from pituitary glands harvested at autopsy. This last cause has been the most devastating in terms of numbers of CJD cases. As of this writing, more than 45 cases of CJD have been related to hGH therapy.[120-130] These patients received injections of hGH every 2 to 4 days for 4 to 12 years. The hGH-treated patients with CJD ranged from 10 to 41 years of age. The estimated risk of CJD in the hGH population is about 1 per 200, which is in considerable contrast to the risk of CJD in the general population under 40 years of age, which is about 1 per 20 million.[131] Interestingly, most of the patients presented with cerebellar syndromes that progressed over 6 to 18 months. Some of the patients became demented during the terminal phase of the illness. The clinical course of patients with early ataxia and late dementia resembled kuru more than ataxic CJD.[132] The possible incubation periods ranged from 4 to 30 years.[119] Many patients had received injections from several common lots of hGH at various times during their prolonged therapies. In the past, hGH was prepared from autopsy-derived pools of as many as 10,000 pituitary glands. It is estimated that about 1 per 10,000 people who died each year had CJD, which means that it is not improbable that a hGH lot may have been contaminated. How many lots of hGH may have been contaminated with prions is unknown. hGH is now prepared by recombinant DNA methods.

Seventeen of those who developed CJD after hGH inoculations did not have any known pathogenic mutations of the PRNP gene; however, 4 of 7 patients in the United Kingdom were homozygous for Val at PRNP codon 129.[133] In France and the United States, 4 of 9 patients were homozygous for Val, and four others were homozygous for Met.[119] One of the nine was heterozygous Met/Val. The normal distribution of the codon 129 polymorphism in the United States, United Kingdom, and France is virtually identical: Met/Val = 51%, Met/Met = 38%, and Val/Val = 11%. These results indicate that homozygosity at codon 129 is not necessary for development of infectious CJD, but they do indicate that it is associated with an increased susceptibility. Interestingly, 2 of 3 kuru patients are reported to be homozygous for Val at codon 129.

Sporadic Creutzfeldt-Jakob disease

A major unresolved problem concerns the cause of sporadic forms of CJD, which account for about 85% of human prion diseases. By definition, neither an infectious nor a familial cause can be demonstrated. Some cases may be caused by an age-related acquired mutation of the PRNP gene, since multiple mutations result in synthesis of pathogenic ΔPrP; other cases may be caused by spontaneous conversion of PrP^C to PrP^{CJD}, that is, PrP overexpression disease. Sporadic CJD is an age-related disorder with a peak onset at about 60 years of age. If the conversion of PrP^C to PrP^{CJD} occurs even in a single neuron, the experience from infectious scrapie indicates that an autocatalytic reaction could result, leading to the spread of disease to other susceptible neurons. This hypothesis predicts that any neuron or cell type could be the source of pathogenic PrP. In the context of the hypothesis that neurons determine prion isolates through an inherent control of PrP structure, the fact that sporadic CJD manifests as multiple, distinct clinico-neuropathologic syndromes is consistent with the somatic mutation or the spontaneous conversion hypotheses.

Homozygosity of the polymorphism at PRNP gene codon 129 appears to play a role in the pathogenesis of sporadic CJD. Because of the association of homozygosity at codon 129 with iatrogenic CJD and kuru, the possibility of homozygosity in cases of sporadic CJD was tested.[134] In one study, 95% of sporadic cases were homozygous (16 cases Met/Met, 5 cases Val/Val, and 1 case Met/Val). The one heterozygous patient in this group may not have been a true case of sporadic CJD, since his father died of dementia. In another group of CJD cases suspected to be sporadic, 11 were Met/Met, 6 Val/Val, and 4 Met/Val. Other examples of the importance of homozygosity at codon 129 are its association with more severe forms of familial prion diseases, such as FFI(D178N, M129) and FCJD(D178N, V129), described above. It may be that the homozygous state at codon 129 fosters spontaneous conversion of PrP^C to PrP^{CJD}, or 129 homozygosity may increase the risk of developing CJD from a putative environmental factor.

The influence of codon 129 homozygosity on the severity and rapidity of prion diseases may shed light on the mechanism of PrP^C transformation to PrP^{CJD}, in which it is believed that formation of a transient heterodimer is an essential step. It raises the possibility that the interaction of PrP^{CJD} with PrP^C requires formation of a complex composed of a dimer of PrP^{CJD} and a dimer of PrP^C. Putative PrP^C dimerization would possibly be favored when the amino acids at codon 129 are the same.

DIAGNOSTIC CRITERIA FOR HUMAN PRION DISEASES

Creutzfeldt-Jakob disease

Clinical

Those disorders we classify as CJD because of common clinical and neuropathologic features are the most complicated of prion diseases because they can have familial, infectious, or sporadic (idiopathic) causes. In many ways, CJD is not a single disease; rather it is a syndrome with multiple molecular, clinical, and neuropathologic features. CJD has a worldwide incidence of about 1 per 10^6 per year.[135,136] Males and females are affected in equal numbers. The peak incidence is about 60 years of age, with a range from 40 to 90 years, though a case of sporadic CJD at as early as 20 years of age has been reported.[137] As a general rule, the disease runs a relatively rapid course, leading to death within 4 to 12 months from start of signs and symptoms; however, cases with a chronic course, lasting 2 to 5 years, are not uncommon.[138,139] FCJD cases tend to present at an earlier age than sporadic CJD. For example, FCJD(E200K) has an onset at 55 ±8 years of age, which progresses to death in an average of 8 months, and FCJD(D178N, V129) has on onset at 46 ±7 years of age, with death occurring in an average of 22 months.[140] FCJD linked to octapeptide inserts presents at 23 to 35 years of age, followed by a particularly long progression to death in 4 to 13 years. The early onset of iatrogenic CJD in patients who received hGH (onset between 20 and 40 years of age) clearly differentiates it from sporadic CJD and most forms of FCJD. Clinical features that are suggestive of the diagnosis of CJD are often preceded by a prodromal period in which there are nonspecific clinical, signs including fatigue, sleep disturbances, memory disturbances, behavioral changes, vertigo, and ataxia. However, the most characteristic clinical features include rapid progression of mental deterioration with dementia, myoclonus, a broad range of motor disturbances (extrapyramidal, cerebellar, pyramidal, or anterior horn cell) and an electroencephalogram (EEG) showing periodic short-wave activity. When the quartet of dementia, myoclonus, periodic EEG activity and rapid progression are seen in a patient, the diagnosis of CJD is relatively certain.

In contrast to kuru, in which the clinical and neuropathologic features were relatively uniform, sporadic CJD has diverse clinical features that are matched by an equally wide range of intensity and distribution of pathologic lesions.[141] Beck and colleagues[142] split CJD into 16 subtypes. Malamud[138] preferred to subclassify CJD into six clinico-neuropathologic categories: cortical, corticostriatal with or without visual loss, corticostriatocerebellar, corticospinal, and corticonigral. About 15% of sporadic CJD cases develop ataxia as an early sign, followed by dementia.[143] In contrast, the majority of the patients who developed CJD after hGH injections presented with cerebellar syndromes that progressed over 6 to 18 months. The CJD subtypes with visual disturbances and a severe occipital cortex pathologic state have been designated the "Heidenhain variant." Because of the variability of clinical features and the temporal sequence in which they occur during the course of the CJD, the differential diagnosis is Alzheimer's disease, the parkinsonisms, cerebellar disorders, and amyotrophic lateral sclerosis.

Pathology

The gross appearance of the brain in CJD is variable and not diagnostic. In some cases, no recognizable abnormalities are seen, whereas others show varying degrees of cerebral cortical atrophy with widening of cerebral sulci, hydrocephalus *ex vacuo,* and brain weights as low as 850 g (normal range is 1200 to 1500 g).

The neurohistologic hallmarks of CJD are spongiform degeneration of neurons and their processes, neuronal loss, intense reactive astrocytic gliosis, and amyloid plaque formation; however, these vary considerably from case to case. In some cases, the only histologic clue is delicate vacuolization in the neuropil between nerve cell bodies with minimal or no detectable nerve cell loss or reactive astrocytic gliosis (Fig. 40-9). The vacuoles that produce spongiform degeneration are located in the neuropil between nerve cell bodies and should not be confused with spaces around nerve cell bodies and blood vessels, which are artifacts of formalin fixation and paraffin embedding. The vacuoles tend to be round to oval and vary in diameter from 5 to 25 μm. In other cases, there is extensive nerve cell loss, intense reactive astrocytic gliosis and so-called status spongiosus. The latter consists of larger vacuoles, as much as 100 μm in diameter, surrounded by a dense meshwork of reactive astrocytic processes (Figs. 40-10 and 40-11). By electron microscopy, spongiform degeneration is a manifestation of focal swelling of neuritic processes, both axonal and dendritic, and synapses with loss of internal organelles and accumulation of lacy abnormal membranes.[144-146] (Fig. 40-12) The relative disappearance of spongiform degeneration with progressive nerve cell loss is therefore consistent with the hypothesis that vacuolation is mostly confined to nerve cell processes. Vacuolation of some nerve cell bodies has also been reported. In CJD, spongiform degeneration can be found in the cerebral neocortex, subiculum of the hippocampus, putamen, caudate nucleus, thalamus, and molecular layer of the cerebellar cortex. It is usually minimal or absent in the globus pallidus, Ammon's horn, and dentate gyrus of the hippocampus, brainstem, and spinal cord.[138,139,141] Spongiform degeneration of the cerebral cortex occurs in virtually all cases regardless of the clinical presentation. In the cerebral cortex, the amount of vacuolation can vary considerably from region to region even within the same cortical section. It can be diffusely distributed to all cortical layers or have a pseudolaminar appearance.

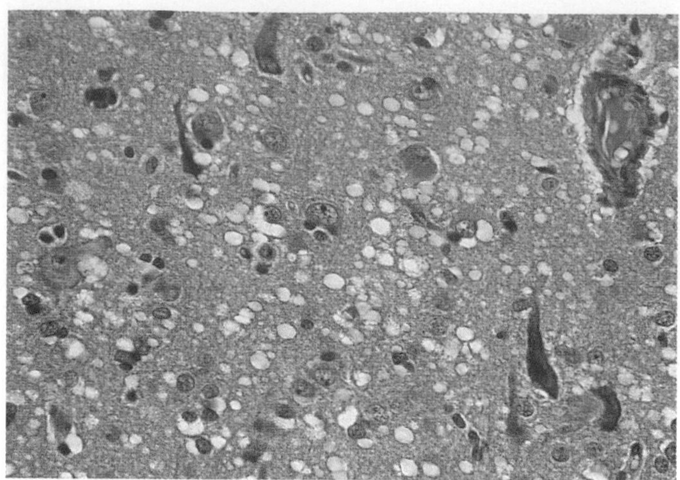

Fig. 40-9 The most characteristic neuropathologic feature of CJD and other prion diseases is spongiform (vacuolar) degeneration of the gray matter neuropil between nerve cell bodies. The section is from the cerebral cortex of a patient with CJD. The vacuoles in this case range in size from 5 to 20 μm in diameter. There is little or no reactive astrocytic gliosis and a mild degree of nerve cell loss.

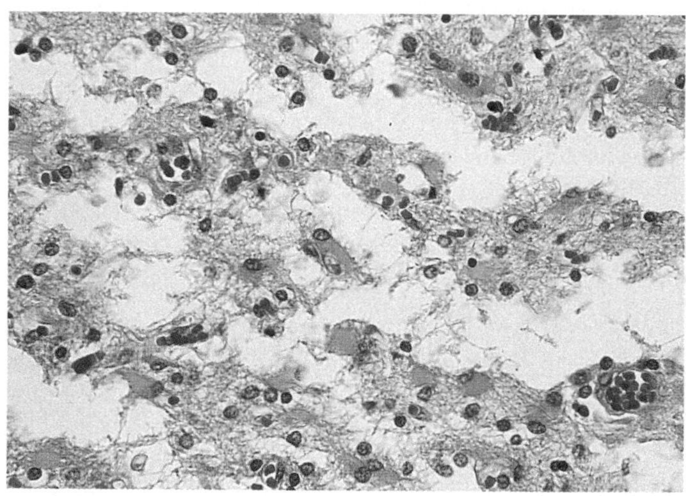

Fig. 40-10 Severe vacuolization of the cerebral cortex (status spongiosus)[139] with considerable loss of nerve cells and intense reactive astrocytic gliosis is an extreme form of spongiform degeneration in CJD. The gray matter vacuoles in this case are as large as 150 μm. The gray matter tissue surrounding the vacuoles is largely composed of reactive astrocytes and their processes (see Fig. 40-11).

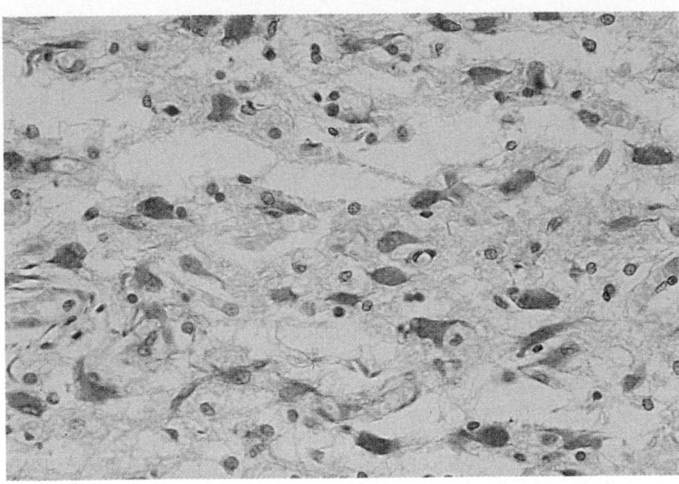

Fig. 40-11 The tissue surrounding the large gray matter vacuoles in the "status spongiosus" stage of CJD contains reactive astrocytes. Shown here is a serial section from the case in Fig. 40-10 stained by the perioxidase-immunohistochemical method for glial fibrillary acidic protein (GFAP) and counterstained with hematoxylin. The cell bodies of reactive astrocytes are strongly GFAP immunopositive.

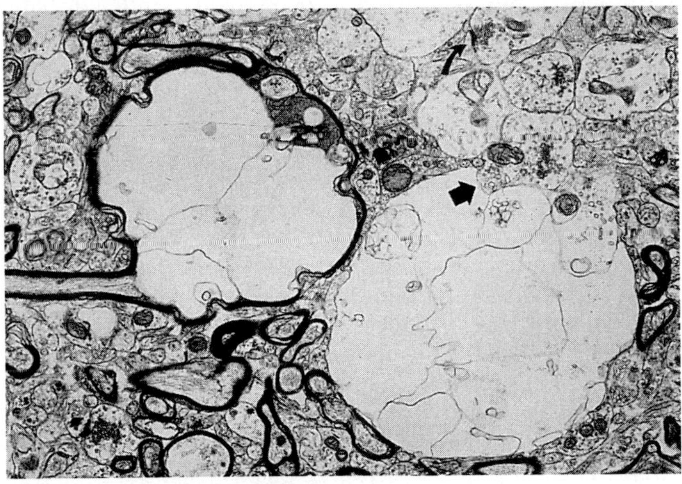

Fig. 40-12 Electron microscopy of cerebral cortical spongiform degeneration in a case of CJD with vacuolation similar to that in Fig. 40-9. Typically, there is swelling of neuritic processes with loss of internal organelles and formation of lacy, abnormal membranes within the space. *Left,* A myelinated axon showing focal swelling; *Right,* a swollen process in contact with synaptic boutons *(large arrow),* which may represent a dendritic process or swollen synaptic boutons. Clusters of enlarged, abnormal synaptic vessicles surrounded by a membrane in the region of the large arrow probably represent a swollen bouton. *Smaller arrow,* A synaptic density adjacent to swollen synaptic boutons.

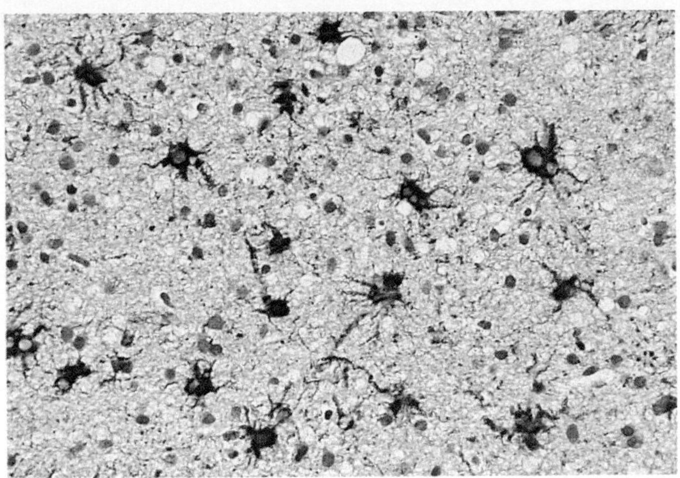

Fig. 40-13 Reactive astrocytic gliosis can be very intense (hypergliotic) in many but not all CJD cases. The section is from the cerebral cortex and was stained by the immunoperoxidase method for glial fibrillary acid protein to visualize astrocytes.

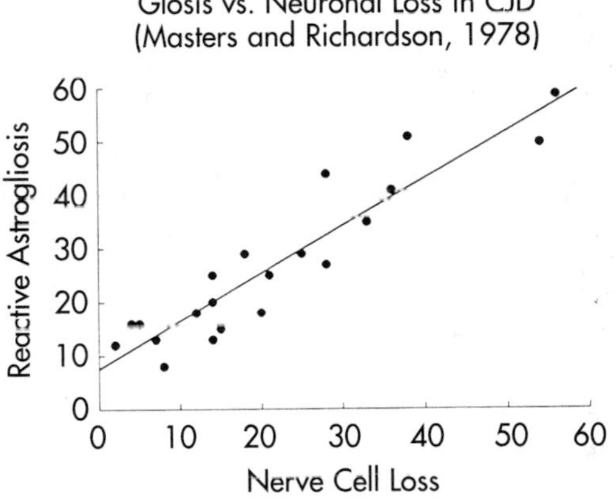

Fig. 40-14 The degree of reactive astrocytic gliosis in CJD is directly proportional to the degree of nerve cell loss. The graph was constructed from individual case neuronal loss and astrocytic gliosis scores published by Masters and Richardson (1978).[139]

It is generally agreed that when reactive astrocytic gliosis occurs in CJD and in scrapie, it is *hypergliotic,* an indication that it may be more intense than would be predicted by the degree of nerve cell loss.[147,148] (Fig. 40-13) In a morphometric study of 21 CJD cases, Masters and Richardson[139] found that the degree of reactive astrocytic gliosis correlated well with the degree of nerve cell loss (Fig. 40-14). PrP 27-30 in the form of prion rods has been found to stimulate astrocyte proliferation in vitro,[149] which may in part account for the very intense astrocyte reaction in prion diseases.

Generally, lesions in the white matter in CJD and other prion diseases are secondary to neuronal loss. However, a vacuolar myelopathy is found in some CJD cases, particularly in Japan.[150] Vacuolar myelopathy is a characteristic of scrapie in mice inoculated with the Rocky Mountain Laboratory (RML) and the Chandler scrapie prion isolates[6,7] and has been reported in mice after being inoculated with human CJD prions.[151] Electron microscopy in the latter study revealed vacuoles within the myelin sheath and occasional intraaxonal vacuoles.

Amyloid plaques are found in only 5% to 10% of CJD cases. As described above, they are immunoreactive with anti-PrP antibodies (Fig. 40-4). The plaques in CJD consist of discrete, eosinophilic spherical masses with radiating amyloid spicules at their periphery. Because this spiked ball–like amyloid plaque was emphasized as a neuropathologic characteristic of kuru, some investigators refer to them in CJD, scrapie, and other prion diseases as *kuru plaques.* In kuru and CJD, they are found most often in the granule cell layer of the cerebellar cortex but can occasionally be found in other brain regions, such as the cerebral cortex, basal ganglia, and thalamus.[13] Their presence is diagnostic of CJD. Most but not all patients in which ataxia is prominent have the kuru type of plaques in their cerebellum.[152] These patients exhibit a protracted clinical course, which may last up to 3 years. Kuru is another ataxic form of prion disease in which most patients developed amyloid plaques in the cerebellum.[13,141] Amyloid angiopathy has also been found in some cases of CJD; however, the vascular amyloid in these cases is composed of the Aβ peptide and not of PrP.[153]

More cases of CJD may be found to contain PrP plaques as a result of an improved technique for their detection by immunohistochemistry.[154] Before being immunostained, glass-mounted histologic sections of brain are immersed in 1.3 mM HCl and autoclaved for 10 minutes. This not only results in intense staining of kuru plaques, but also reveals numerous primitive PrP plaques in CJD (Fig. 40-15). Primitive PrP plaques stain poorly by the periodic acid–Schiff reaction and do not generally show green birefringence with Congo red dye.

The definitive diagnosis of CJD can be made at autopsy if the quartet of clinical signs and symptoms were present during life, and typical spongiform degeneration of gray matter is found in the absence of other confounding pathologic states. The definitive diagnosis can also be made if PrP amyloid plaques are found in the cerebellum. Otherwise, one must make the diagnosis by demonstrating transmission to animals, which may take more than a year, or rapidly now by the histoblot technique.[39] For the latter, a fresh frozen biopsy of cerebral cortex is sufficient for diagnosis in living patients. Since PrP^{CJD} is protease resistant, it is our experience that it can readily be demonstrated in brain tissue taken at autopsy (Fig. 40-16).

Gerstmann-Sträussler-Scheinker syndrome (GSS)

GSS is one of the rarest neurodegenerative diseases, with an incidence of 2 to 5 per 100 million.[155] The diagnosis of GSS requires dominant inheritance, a mixture of cognitive and motor disturbances, and multicentric amyloid plaques, but,

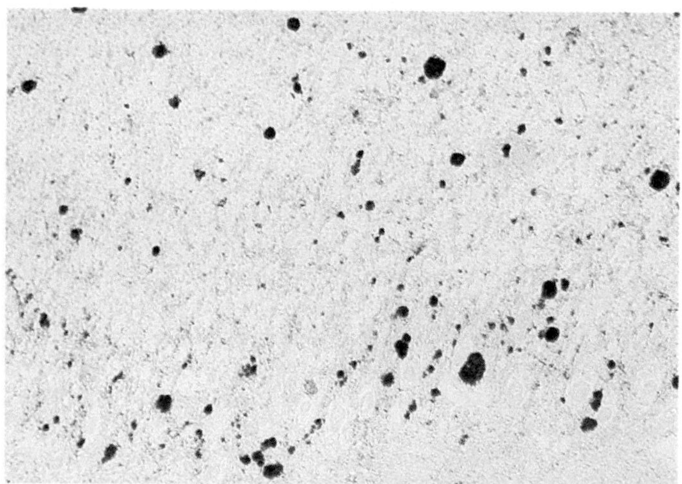

Fig. 40-15 Kuru type of amyloid plaques, as well as multiple primitive amyloid plaques not identified by routine histologic methods, can be seen in the granule cell layer of the cerebellum of some CJD cases when the slide is pretreated by the HCl-autoclaving method,[154] followed by PrP immunohistochemistry. The largest PrP plaques in the figure are of the kuru type and measure about 30 mm in diameter.

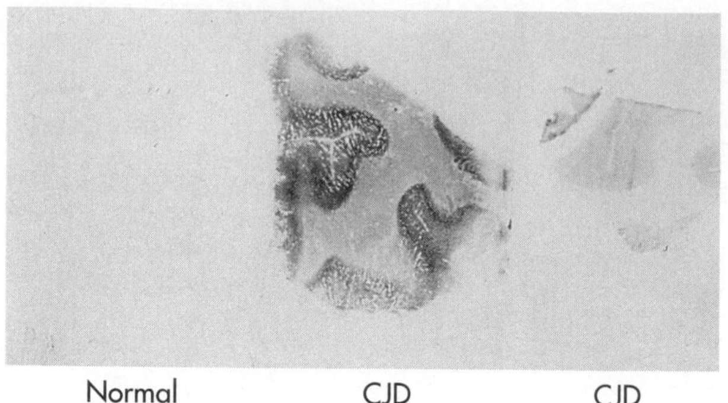

Normal CJD CJD

Fig. 40-16 Detection of protease-resistant PrP^{CJD} by the histoblot method is an efficient adjunct to the neuropathologic diagnosis of CJD. Frozen sections of unfixed cerebral cortex from two CJD cases and one normal control subject obtained at autopsy were blotted to nitrocellulose paper, exposed to proteinase K (100 mg/ml for 2 hours) to eliminate PrP^{C}, exposed to 3 M guanidinium thiocyanate to denature PrP^{CJD} and to enhance its antigenicity, and immunostained using PrP-specific antibodies. PrP^{CJD} is identified in the cerebral cortex of the two CJD cases but not in the normal control.

like CJD, GSS is not a single disease. There are three dominantly inherited disorders to which this name has been given. Each has a different clinical presentation, different neuropathologic features. and linkage to different mutations of the PrP gene. The unifying feature of these three diseases is the presence of GSS-type, multicentric PrP amyloid plaques (Fig. 40-4). The differential diagnosis includes Huntington's chorea, spinocerebellar degeneration, Alzheimer's disease, and multiple sclerosis.

Ataxic GSS (P102L)

Ataxic GSS resembles the disease first described by the neurologists Gerstmann and Sträussler and the neuropathologist Scheinker in 1936.[10] Seitelberger[156] defined it as a "spinocerebellar ataxia with dementia and plaque-like deposits." The codon 102 mutation has been found in American, British, German, Japanese, and Austrian families with ataxic GSS (see above). The clinical manifestations of GSS (P102L) vary, even within the same pedigree.[11] The weighted composite of clinical features include difficulty walking and unsteadiness and sometimes leg pains and paresthesias in the early stages, followed in the later stages by mental and behavioral deterioration. Neurologic examination reveals cerebellar ataxia, dysarthria, ocular dysmetria, hyporeflexia and Babinski's sign. Features of amyotrophy with muscle fasciculations and fibrillations have been reported.[88] Masters and colleagues[11] reported that 3 of 7 GSS cases were transmitted to nonhuman primates.

The pathologic hallmark of ataxic GSS is multicentric amyloid plaques (GSS plaques), which are most numerous in the molecular layer of the cerebellar cortex (Figs. 40-4 and 40-17) but are also found in the cerebral cortex (Fig. 40-18). These often consist of a larger central mass of amyloid surrounded by smaller satellite masses. Additionally, the molecular layer of the cerebellum, in some cases, contains numerous "amorphous" or "primitive" plaques, which are 150 to 200 μm in diameter.[157] (Fig. 40-19) These do not fulfill the criteria for mature amyloid, since they are weakly PAS positive and rarely show green birefringence with the Congo red stain. Unicentric kuru type plaques can also be found. The GSS plaques, kuru plaques, and primitive plaques immunostain specifically with

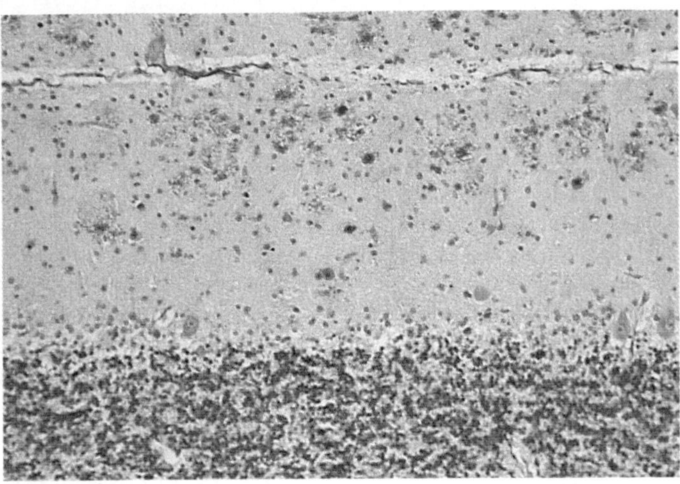

Fig. 40-17 In this case of GSS numerous, multicentric amyloid plaques (GSS-plaques) are found in the molecular layer of the cerebellar cortex. The section is from a case of ataxic GSS and is stained by the periodic acid–Schiff reaction.

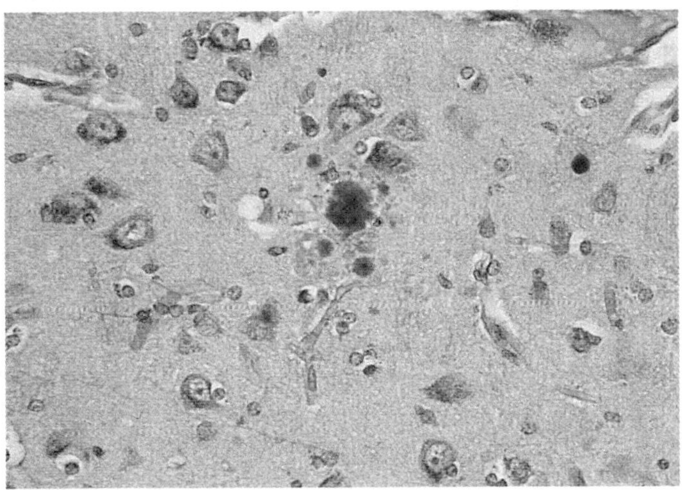

Fig. 40-18 In GSS, multicentric amyloid plaques of the GSS type can also be found in the cerebral cortex. (Periodic acid–Schiff reaction).

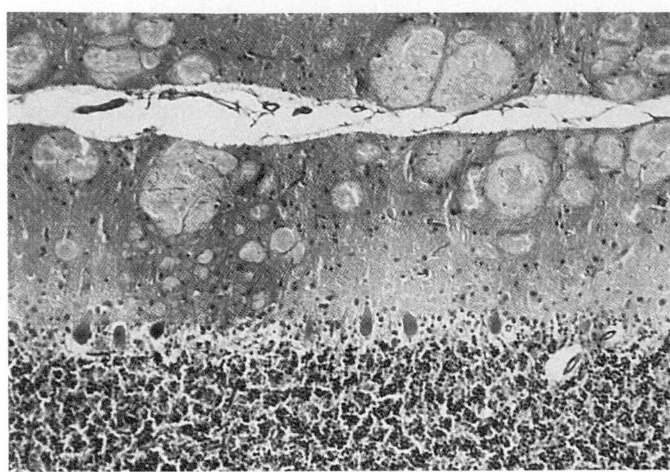

Fig. 40-19 In some GSS cases, large primitive amyloid plaques, which stain poorly by the periodic acid–Schiff reaction and with Congo red dye, are found in the cerebellar molecular layer.

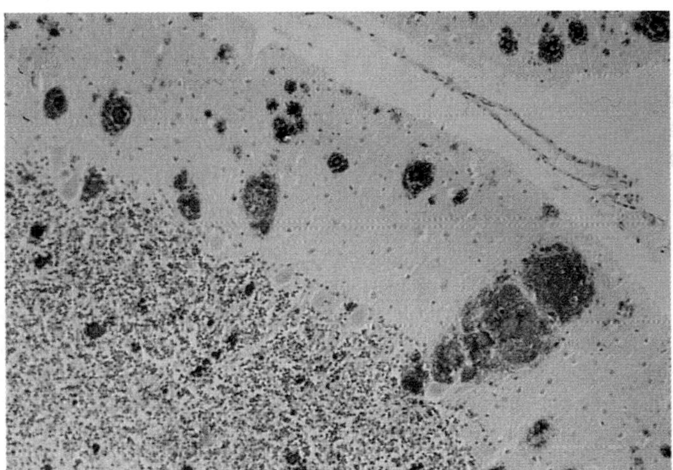

Fig. 40-20 Primitive amyloid plaques in GSS are strongly PrP immunopositive. (Courtesy Dr. Jeanne Bell, University of Edinburgh.)

PrP antibodies.[50,52,158] Immunostaining is facilitated by pretreatment of the glass-mounted formalin-fixed paraffin-embedded tissue section by the HCl-autoclave technique.[154] (Fig. 40-20). White matter degeneration resembling that of other systems degenerations, such as Friedreich's ataxia, is a prominent feature in most cases.[156] Neuronal loss is scattered throughout the brain and spinal cord. Spongiform degeneration is variable in degree and extent and can be difficult to detect. Neurofibrillary tangles, if present, are usually found in numbers and in locations consistent with the patient's age.

Telencephalic GSS (Q217R)

The clinical and pathological features of telencephalic GSS (Q217R) are best represented by those in the GCSA pedigree.[159] The main clinical features include progressive dementia, usually associated with dysarthria, rigidity, tremor, and hyperreflexia. Masked facies in several individuals, as well as tremor and rigidity, is suggestive of Parkinsonism. Ataxia and myoclonus are uncommon.

The most striking neuropathologic feature is widespread amyloid plaque formation of which four morphological types were identified.[159] First, there were multiple, multicentric GSS type of plaques consisting of four to more than 10 amyloid masses. The entire cluster of amyloid masses was 150 to 500 μm in diameter. These were located in the neocortex, hippocampus, caudate nucleus, and putamen. Some were also present in the subcortical white matter. Second, there were typical kuru type of amyloid plaques. These were 20 to 70 μm in diameter and located principally in the white matter. Third, there were 50 to 150 μm, unicentric amyloid plaques, without radiating spicules at their periphery, that resemble the cores of the senile plaques of Alzheimer's disease; however, they did not have a halo of dystrophic neurites surrounding them. These were found in the neocortex, hippocampus, caudate nucleus, and putamen. Fourth, there were "amorphous," or "primitive," plaques, which were 150 to 200 μm in diameter, similar to those seen in some ataxic GSS cases, and were located in the deep cerebral cortical layers. All the plaques immunostained specifically with PrP antibodies but not with antibodies to Alzheimer precursor protein.

There was no spongiform degeneration in cortical or subcortical gray matter. Astrocytic gliosis was primarily associated with amyloid plaques in the neocortex. The caudate nucleus, putamen, globus pallidus, and thalamus showed severe neuronal loss with astrocytic gliosis. There was mild neuronal loss in the substantia nigra. Unlike ataxic GSS, there were no amyloid plaques or other neuropathologic changes in the cerebellum.

GSS (F198S) with neurofibrillary tangles

The clinical features of the familial PrP disorder GSS (F198S) with neurofibullary tangles are exemplified by those in a large pedigree, designated the "Indiana kindred.[160] Individuals carrying the mutation are normal until their mid-30s to early 60s. The presenting symptoms are gradual loss of short-term memory and progressive clumsiness, which may be exaggerated when the individual is under stress or tired. The symptoms can progress rapidly over a period of a year or slowly over 5 years. Rigidity and bradykinesia generally occur late in the disease, at which time dementia also worsens. There is little or no tremor. The rigidity and bradykinesia improves with L-dopa analogs. Without treatment of the parkinsonism, the patient succumbs in about 1 year and, with treatment, succumbs to intercurrent illness in 2 to 3 years. Magnetic resonance imaging scans show iron accumulation in the globus pallidus and substantia nigra, which develop simultaneously with the parkinsonism. Prominent cerebellar atrophy is also seen.

Although the neuropathologic features of all forms of GSS center on the amyloid plaques, one population of amyloid plaques in GSS-nft are truly remarkable because they lead to the argument that there is overlap in the pathogenesis of Alzheimer's disease and this PrP disease. As with other forms of GSS, large numbers of multicentric GSS type of plaques and unicentric plaques were located throughout the cerebral and cerebellar cortex similar to ataxic GSS.[109] In addition, there were typical neuritic plaques with amyloid cores found in most areas of the cerebral cortex and hippocampus of the type found in Alzheimer's disease. The dystrophic neurites surrounding the core of amyloid immunostained with tau antibodies, as in Alzheimer's disease; however, the amyloid cores of neuritic and nonneuritic plaques immunostained with PrP antibodies but not with antibodies to the Aβ peptide of Alzheimer's disease. Another similarity to Alzheimer's disease was the presence of nerve cell bodies filled with neurofibrillary tangles in multiple cortical regions, particularly in the parahippocampal gyrus. Nerve cell loss occurred in almost all cerebral cortical regions. It was most severe in the cerebellar cortex where there was pronounced loss of Purkinje cells. Neuronal loss was also prominent in a variety of nuclei, including the substantia nigra, red nucleus, inferior olive and dentate nucleus. Spongiform degeneration was minimal and focal when it occurred.

Fatal familial insomnia (D178N, M129)

Fatal familial insomnia (D178N, M129), a dominantly inherited form of PrP disease, is an example of the relationship between the amino acid sequence of PrP and selective targeting of neurons for degeneration. Specifically, in FFI, a D178N mutation occurs on an allele that encodes a Met at position 129, and the major lesion is limited to the thalamus. In contrast, the pathologic changes are widespread in FCJD (D178N, V129) but do not include the thalamus, and the D178N mutation occurs on an allele that encodes Val at position 129.[161]

The clinical and neuropathologic data have been obtained from studies of two large kindreds with FFI.[113,115] The age of onset is between 35 and 61 years. FFI progresses relatively rapidly, with a course ranging from 7 to 36 months. The primary sleep-wake disturbances are progressive insomnia, followed by complex hallucinations and then stupor and coma. In addition, there are autonomic disturbances, including hyperhidrosis, pyrexia, tachycardia, hypertension, and irregular breathing. The principal motor findings are ataxia, spontaneous and evoked myoclonus, dysarthria, and pyramidal signs. In contrast, patients with FCJD (D178N, V129) present with dementia, but not insomnia.

In FFI, the most severe neuropathy occurred in the anterior ventral and medial dorsal nuclei of the thalamus, where there was over 50% loss of neurons with reactive astrocytic gliosis. The cerebral cortex was minimally affected with minimal to mild, patchy astrocytic gliosis. Mild spongiform degeneration of the cerebral cortex was largely confined to layers 2 to 4 in one case. In the cerebellum, there was swelling of the proximal axon (torpedoes) of many Purkinje cells, and there was mild loss of Purkinje cells and granule cells. There were no amyloid plaques. There was a greater than 50% loss of neurons from the inferior olives.

RISK OF PRION DISEASE TO HEALTH CARE GIVERS

There is concern that care of patients with the diagnosis of CJD may be inferior. It is not uncommon for diagnostic procedures, such as biopsies, as well as other invasive procedures, to be denied to such patients. It is also not uncommon for the pathologist to refuse to perform an autopsy. Aside from the medical and ethical questions, the epidemiologic data elicit the argument that CJD is not a significant health risk to medical personnel or to family and friends of patients to warrant such drastic measures.[162,163] There are reports of about 24 health care workers with CJD, including 6 physicians, 2 neurosurgeons, a pathologist, 3 dentists, a dental surgeon, 9 nurses, 3 nursing assistants, and 2 histopathology technicians.[164] Nevertheless, the incidence of CJD among health care workers seems to be the same as the general population.[119]

There is no evidence that increased risk is associated with exposure to breath, saliva, nasopharyngeal secretions, urine, or feces of a patients with CJD.[162] Although blood should be considered a potential source of infection, there is no epidemiologic evidence that blood transfusions are a risk for CJD.[165] Cerebrospinal fluid (CSF) is reported to contain CJD prions and should therefore be considered a potential source of infection.[166] The highest concentration of prions are found in the brain and spinal cord. Guidelines for handling surgical and autopsy tissues in patients suspected of having CJD are updated periodically.[162,167]

In handling surgical and autopsy specimens from CJD cases, one should take caution to avoid percutaneous exposure to blood, CSF, or tissues, particularly the brain and spinal cord. The success of transmission of a prion disease is affected significantly by the route of infection. For example, the effectiveness of transferring scrapie to animals using scrapie-infected brain tissue was highest for intracerebral inoculation, was reduced by a factor of 10^5 for intraperitoneal inoculation, and was reduced by a factor of 10^9 for oral exposure.[168]

Formalin fixation does not destroy prion infectivity,[169] Formalin fixation, followed by paraffin embedding, reduces the prion infectivity titer from $10^{9.6}$ to $10^{6.8}$ ID_{50} units/g of tissue.[170] A relatively simple method to eliminate virtually all residual infectivity of CJD and scrapie prions in formalin-fixed tissue blocks can be achieved by immersion of the fixed block of tissue for 1 hour in formic acid, followed by further fixation in formalin.[171] Histology or immunohistochemistry results are not significantly affected by formic acid treatment; however, in our experience the tissues become brittle.

EPILOGUE

Human prion diseases are the only neurodegenerative disorders that present as sporadic, genetic, and infectious variants. Investigations of these disorders described in this chapter have uncovered a new disease mechanism. There are two key elements in this mechanism. First, the prion protein can exist in a cell in two or more structurally stable states, of which one state performs an as yet unknown, normal cellular function and the other is pathogenic. The second key element in the pathogenesis of these disorders is that a normal cellular metabolic pathway converts the normal PrP into abnormal PrP, when abnormal PrP is presented to the cell, either as exogenously or endogenously derived prion particles (template hypothesis). Once begun, the process becomes self-perpetuating, and the conversion of normal to abnormal PrP in the presence of preexisting, abnormal PrP spreads from one susceptible neuron population to another. The biochemical pathway and cellular compartment in which this occurs and the factors that tend to drive the reaction toward accumulation of abnormal PrP remain to be determined. The relative inertness of abnormal PrP may explain the directional preference of the reaction. Another important pathogenic question to be resolved concerns the molecular and cellular mechanisms by which abnormal PrP accumulation and even excessive accumulation of normal PrP (PrP overexpression neuromyopathy) cause nerve and muscle dysfunction. And although prion diseases are relatively uncommon, it may be that variants of their pathogenic mechanisms play key roles in the pathogenesis of other diseases, such as cerebral amyloidosis and Alzheimer's disease.

REFERENCES

General concepts

1. Sparkes RS, Simon M, Cohn VH et al: Assignment of the human and mouse prion protein genes to homologous chromosomes, *Proc Natl Acad Sci USA* 83:7358, 1986.
2. Cuillé J, Chelle PL: Experimental transmission of trembling to the goat, *CR Séances Acad Sci* 208:1058, 1939.
3. Pattison IH, Millson GC: Scrapie produced experimentally in goats with special reference to the clinical syndrome, *J Comp Pathol* 71:101, 1961.
4. Bruce ME, Fraser H: Scrapie strain variation and its implications, *Curr Top Microbiol Immunol* 172:125, 1991.
5. Dickinson AG, Meikle VMH: Host-genotype and agent effects in scrapie incubation: change in allelic interaction with different strains of agent, *Mol Gen Genet* 112:73, 1971.
6. Carlson GA, Kingsbury DT, Goodman PA et al: Linkage of prion protein and scrapie incubation time genes, *Cell* 46:503, 1986.
7. Prusiner SB, Scott M, Foster D et al: Transgenetic studies implicate interactions between homologous PrP isoforms in scrapie prion replication, *Cell* 63:673, 1990.
8. Carlson GA, Ebeling C, Yang S-L et al: Prion isolate specified allotypic interactions between the cellular and scrapie prion proteins in congenic and transgenic mice, *Proc Natl Acad Sci USA* 91:5690, 1994.
9. Masters CL, Gajdusek DC: The spectrum of Creutzfeldt-Jakob disease and virus-induced subacute spongiform encephalopathies, *Recent Adv Neuropathol* 2:139, 1982.
10. Gerstmann J, Sträussler E, Scheinker I: Über eine eigenartige hereditär-familiäre Erkrankung des Zentralnervensystems zugleich ein Beitrag zur Frage des vorzeitigen lokalen Alterns, *Z Neurol* 154:736, 1936.
11. Masters CL, Gajdusek DC, Gibbs CJ Jr.: Creutzfeldt-Jakob disease virus isolations from the Gerstmann-Sträussler syndrome, *Brain* 104:559, 1981.
12. Gajdusek DC: Observations on the early history of kuru investigations. In Prusiner SB, Hadlow WJ, Prusiner SB, Hadlow WJ: *Slow transmissible diseases of the nervous system,* vol 1, New York, 1979, Academic Press.
13. Klatzo I, Gajdusek DC, Zigas V: Pathology of kuru, *Lab Invest* 8:799, 1959.
14. Gajdusek DC, Gibbs CJ Jr, Alpers M: Experimental transmission of a kuru-like syndrome to chimpanzees, *Nature* 209:794, 1966.
15. Gibbs CJ Jr, Gajdusek DC, Asher DM et al: Creutzfeldt-Jakob disease (spongiform encephalopathy): transmission to the chimpanzee, *Science* 161:388, 1968.
16. Masters CL, Gajdusek DC, Gibbs CJ Jr.: The familial occurrence of Creutzfeldt-Jakob disease and Alzheimer's disease, *Brain* 104:535, 1981.
17. Alper T, Haig DA, Clarke MC: The exceptionally small size of the scrapie agent, *Biochem Biophys Res Commun* 22:278, 1966.
18. Alper T, Cramp WA, Haig DA et al: Does the agent of scrapie replicate without nucleic acid? *Nature* 214:764, 1967.
19. Hunter GD, Millson GC: Attempts to release the scrapie agent from tissue debris, *J Comp Pathol* 77:301, 1967.
20. Hunter GD, Millson GC: Studies on the heat stability and chromatographic behavior of the scrapie agent, *J Gen Microbiol* 37:251, 1964.
21. Hunter GD, Gibbons RA, Kimberlin RH et al: Further studies of the infectivity and stability of extracts and homogenates derived from scrapie-affected mouse brains, *J Comp Pathol* 79:101, 1969.
22. Millson GC, Hunter GD, Kimberlin RH: The physico-chemical nature of the scrapie agent. In Kimberlin RH, Kimberlin RHS: *Slow virus diseases of animals and man,* New York, 1976, American Elsevier.
23. Prusiner SB, Groth DF, Cochran SP et al: Molecular properties, partial purification, and assay by incubation period measurements of the hamster scrapie agent, *Biochemistry* 19:4883, 1980.
24. Prusiner SB, Cochran SP, Groth DF et al: Measurement of the scrapie agent using an incubation time interval assay, *Ann Neurol* 11:353, 1982.
25. Prusiner SB: Novel proteinaceous infectious particles cause scrapie, *Science* 216:136, 1982.
26. Chesebro B, Race R, Wehrly K et al: Identification of scrapie prion protein-specific mRNA in scrapie-infected and uninfected brain, *Nature* 315:331, 1985.
27. Oesch B, Westaway D, Wälchli M et al: A cellular gene encodes scrapie PrP 27-30 protein, *Cell* 40:735, 1985.
28. Prusiner SB, Groth DF, Bolton DC et al: Purification and structural studies of a major scrapie prion protein, *Cell* 38:127, 1984.
29. Jendroska K, Heinzel FP, Torchia M et al: Proteinase-resistant prion protein accumulation in Syrian hamster brain correlates with regional pathology and scrapie infectivity, *Neurology* 41:1482, 1991.
30. Kretzschmar HA, Prusiner SB, Stowring LE et al: Scrapie prion proteins are synthesized in neurons, *Am J Pathol* 122:1, 1986.
31. Meyer N, Rosenbaum V, Schmidt B et al: Search for a putative scrapie genome in purified prion fractions reveals a paucity of nucleic acids, *J Gen Virol* 72:37, 1991.
32. Kellings K, Meyer N, Mirenda C et al: Further analysis of nucleic acids in purified scrapie prion preparations by improved return refocussing gel electrophoresis (RRGE), *J Gen Virol* 73:1025, 1992.
33. Basler K, Oesch B, Scott M et al: Scrapie and cellular PrP isoforms are encoded by the same chromosomal gene, *Cell* 46:417, 1986.

34. Westaway D, Cooper C, Turner S et al: Structure and polymorphism of the mouse prion protein gene, *Proc Natl Acad Sci USA* 91:6418, 1994.
35. Stahl N, Baldwin MA, Teplow DB et al: Structural analysis of the scrapie prion protein using mass spectrometry and amino acid sequencing, *Biochemistry* 32:1991, 1993.
36. Pan K-M, Baldwin M, Nguyen J et al: Conversion of α-helices into β-sheets features in the formation of the scrapie prion proteins, *Proc Natl Acad Sci USA* 90:10962, 1993.
37. Caughey BW, Dong A, Bhat KS et al: Secondary structure analysis of the scrapie-associated protein PrP 27-30 in water by infrared spectroscopy, *Biochemistry* 30:7672, 1991.
38. Gasset M, Baldwin MA, Fletterick RJ et al: Perturbation of the secondary structure of the scrapie prion protein under conditions associated with changes in infectivity, *Proc Natl Acad Sci USA* 90:1, 1993.

Molecular pathogenesis

39. Taraboulos A, Jendroska K, Serban D et al: Regional mapping of prion proteins in brains, *Proc Natl Acad Sci USA* 89:7620, 1992.
40. DeArmond SJ, Mobley WC, DeMott DL et al: Changes in the localization of brain prion proteins during scrapie infection, *Neurology* 37:1271, 1987.
41. Stahl N, Borchelt DR, Hsiao K et al: Scrapie prion protein contains a phosphatidylinositol glycolipid, *Cell* 51:229, 1987.
42. Borchelt DR, Scott M, Taraboulos A et al: Scrapie and cellular prion proteins differ in their kinetics of synthesis and topology in cultured cells, *J Cell Biol* 110:743, 1990.
43. Caughey B, Raymond GJ: The scrapie-associated form of PrP is made from a cell surface precursor that is both protease- and phospholipase-sensitive, *J Biol Chem* 266:18217, 1991.
44. Taraboulos A, Raeber AJ, Borchelt DR et al: Synthesis and trafficking of prion proteins in cultured cells, *Mol Biol Cell* 3:851, 1992.
45. Taraboulos A, Scott M, Semenov A et al: Cholesterol depletion and targeting to clathrin coated pits inhibit formation of the scrapie prion protein, *J Cell Biol* 129:121, 1995.
46. McKinley MP, Taraboulos A, Kenaga L et al: Ultrastructural localization of scrapie prion proteins in secondary lysosomes of infected cultured cells, *J Cell Biol* 111:316, 1990.
47. Scott M, Foster D, Mirenda C et al: Transgenic mice expressing hamster prion protein produce species-specific scrapie infectivity and amyloid plaques, *Cell* 59:847, 1989.
48. Scott M, Groth D, Foster D et al: Propagation of prions with artificial properties in transgenic mice expressing chimeric PrP genes, *Cell* 73:979, 1993.
49. DeArmond SJ, McKinley MP, Barry RA et al: Identification of prion amyloid filaments in scrapie-infected brain, *Cell* 41:221, 1985.
50. Kitamoto T, Tateishi J, Tashima I et al: Amyloid plaques in Creutzfeldt-Jakob disease stain with prion protein antibodies, *Ann Neurol* 20:204, 1986.
51. Roberts GW, Lofthouse R, Allsop D et al: CNS amyloid proteins in neurodegenerative diseases, *Neurology* 38:1534, 1988.
52. Snow AD, Kisilevsky R, Willmer J et al: Sulfated glycosaminoglycans in amyloid plaques of prion diseases, *Acta Neuropathol* (Berl) 77:337, 1989.
53. Bruce ME, Dickinson AG, Fraser H: Cerebral amyloidosis in scrapie in the mouse: effect of agent strain and mouse genotype, *Neuropathol Appl Neurobiol* 2:471, 1976.
54. Hsiao K, Baker HF, Crow TJ et al: Linkage of a prion protein missense variant to Gerstmann-Sträussler syndrome, *Nature* 338:342, 1989.
55. Hsiao KK, Scott M, Foster D et al: Spontaneous neurodegeneration in transgenic mice with mutant prion protein, *Science* 250:1587, 1990.
56. Hsiao KK, Groth D, Scott M et al: Serial transmission in rodents of neurologic disease from transgenic mice expressing mutant prion protein. (In preparation 1994.)
57. McKinley MP, Meyer R, Kenaga L et al: Scrapie prion rod formation *in vitro* requires both detergent extraction and limited proteolysis, *J Virol* 65:1440, 1991.
58. Prusiner SB, Bolton DC, Groth DF et al: Further purification and characterization of scrapie prions, *Biochemistry* 21:6942, 1982.
59. Prusiner SB, McKinley MP, Bowman KA et al: Scrapie prions aggregate to form amyloid-like birefringent rods, *Cell* 35:349, 1983.
60. Bockman JM, Kingsbury DT, McKinley MP et al: Creutzfeldt-Jakob disease prion proteins in human brains, *N Engl J Med* 312:73, 1985.
61. Brown P, Coker-Vann M, Pomeroy K et al: Diagnosis of Creutzfeldt-Jakob disease by western blot identification of marker protein in human brain tissue, *N Engl J Med* 314:547, 1986.
62. Merz PA, Rohwer RG, Kascsak R et al: Infection-specific particle from the unconventional slow virus diseases, *Science* 225:437, 1984.
63. Kimberlin RH: Scrapie and possible relationships with viroids, *Semin Virol* 1:153, 1990.
64. Prusiner SB, DeArmond SJ: Biology of disease: prions causing nervous system degeneration, *Lab Invest* 56:349, 1987.
65. Serban D, Taraboulos A, DeArmond SJ et al: Rapid detection of Creutzfeldt-Jakob disease and scrapie prion proteins, *Neurology* 40:110, 1990.
66. DeArmond SJ, Yang S-L, Lee A et al: Three scrapie prion isolates exhibit different accumulation patterns of the prion protein scrapie isoform, *Proc Natl Acad Sci USA* 90:6449, 1993.
67. Hecker R, Taraboulos A, Scott M et al: Replication of distinct prion isolates is region specific in brains of transgenic mice and hamsters, *Genes Dev* 6:1213, 1992.
68. Hsiao K, Scott M, Foster D et al: Spontaneous neurodegeneration in transgenic mice with prion protein codon 101 proline—leucine substitution, Ann *NY Acad Sci* 640:166, 1991.
69. Büeler H, Fischer M, Lang Y et al: Normal development and behaviour of mice lacking the neuronal cell–surface PrP protein, *Nature* 356:577, 1992 (comments: 356:560, 1992).
70. Büeler H, Aguzzi A, Sailer A et al: Mice devoid of PrP are resistant to scrapie, *Cell* 73:1339, 1993.
71. Prusiner SB, Groth D, Serban A et al: Ablation of the prion protein (PrP) gene in mice prevents scrapie and facilitates production of anti-PrP antibodies, *Proc Natl Acad Sci USA* 90:10608, 1993.
72. DeArmond SJ, Prusiner SB: The neurochemistry of prion diseases, *J Neurochem* 61:1589, 1993.
73. Weissmann C: A "unified theory" of prion propagation, *Nature* 352:679, 1991.
74. Bolton DC, Meyer RK, Prusiner SB: Scrapie PrP 27-30 is a sialoglycoprotein, J *Virol* 53:596, 1985.
75. Gasset M, Baldwin MA, Lloyd D et al: Predicted α-helical regions of the prion protein when synthesized as peptides form amyloid, *Proc Natl Acad Sci USA* 89:10940, 1992.
76. Huang Z, Gabriel JM, Baldwin MA et al: Proposed three-dimensional structure for the cellular prion protein, *Proc Natl Acad Sci USA* 91:7139, 1994.

PrP neuromyopathy

77. Westaway D, DeArmond SJ, Cayetano-Canlas J et al: Degeneration of skeletal muscle, peripheral nerves, and the central nervous system in transgenic mice overexpressing wild-type prion proteins, *Cell* 76:117, 1994.
78. Beck E, Daniel PM, Parry HB: Degeneration of the cerebellar and hypothalamo-neurohypophysial systems in sheep with scrapie; and its relationship to human system degenerations, *Brain* 87:153, 1964.
79. Bosanquet FD, Daniel PM, Parry HB: Myopathy in sheep: its relationship to scrapie and to dermatomyositis and muscular dystrophy, *Lancet* 2:737, 1956.
80. Hulland TJ: The skeletal muscle of sheep affected with scrapie, *J Comp Pathol Therap* 68:264, 1958.
81. Rosenthal NP, Keesey J, Crandall B et al: Familial neurological disease associated with spongiform encephalopathy, *Arch Neurol* 33:252, 1976.
82. Neufeld MY, Josiphov J, Korczyn AD: Demyelinating peripheral neuropathy in Creutzfeldt-Jakob disease, *Muscle Nerve* 15:1234, 1992.
83. Askanas V, Bilak M, Engel WK et al: Prion protein is abnormally accumulated in inclusion-body myositis, *NeuroReport* 5:25, 1993.

Inherited human prion disease

84. Kretzschmar HA, Stowring LE, Westaway D et al: Molecular cloning of a human prion protein cDNA, *DNA* 5:315, 1986.
85. Doh-ura K, Tateishi J, Sasaki H et al: Pro→Leu change at position 102 of prion protein is the most common but not the sole mutation related to

Gerstmann-Sträussler syndrome, *Biochem Biophys Res Commun* 163:974, 1989.

86. Goldgaber D, Goldfarb LG, Brown P et al: Mutations in familial Creutzfeldt-Jakob disease and Gerstmann-Sträussler-Scheinker's syndrome, *Exp Neurol* 106:204, 1989.
87. Kretzschmar HA, Honold G, Seitelberger F et al: Prion protein mutation in family first reported by Gerstmann, Straussler, and Scheinker, *Lancet* 337:1160, 1991.
88. Kretzschmar HA, Kufer P, Riethmüller G et al: Prion protein mutation at codon 102 in an Italian family with Gerstmann-Sträussler-Scheinker syndrome, *Neurology* 42:809, 1992.
89. Hsiao KK, Cass C, Schellenberg GD et al: A prion protein variant in a family with the telencephalic form of Gerstmann-Sträussler-Scheinker syndrome, *Neurology* 41:681, 1991.
90. Kitamoto T, Ohta M, Doh-ura K et al: Novel missense variants of prion protein in Creutzfeldt-Jakob disease or Gerstmann-Sträussler syndrome, *Biochem Biophys Res Commun* 191:709, 1993.
91. Goldfarb LG, Mitrova E, Brown P et al: Mutation in codon 200 of scrapie amyloid protein gene in two clusters of Creutzfeldt-Jakob disease in Slovakia, *Lancet* 336:514, 1990.
92. Gabizon R, Meiner Z, Cass C et al: Prion protein gene mutation in Libyan Jews with Creutzfeldt-Jakob disease, *Neurology* 41:160, 1991.
93. Hsiao K, Meiner Z, Kahana E et al: Mutation of the prion protein in Libyan Jews with Creutzfeldt-Jakob disease, *N Engl J Med* 324:1091, 1991.
94. Gabizon R, Rosenmann H, Meiner Z et al: Mutation and polymorphism of the prion protein gene in Libyan Jews with Creutzfeldt-Jakob disease, *Am J Hum Genet* 33:828, 1993.
95. Neugut RH, Neugut AI, Kahana E et al: Creutzfeldt-Jakob disease: familial clustering among Libyan-born Israelis, *Neurology* 29:225, 1979.
96. Goldfarb LG, Brown P, Mitrova E et al: Creutzfeldt-Jacob disease associated with the PRNP codon 200^{Lys} mutation: an analysis of 45 families, *Eur J Epidemiol* 7:477, 1991.
97. Bertoni JM, Brown P, Goldfarb L et al: Familial Creutzfeldt-Jakob disease with the PRNP codon 200^{lys} mutation and supranuclear palsy but without myoclonus or periodic EEG complexes, *Neurology* 42 (no 4, suppl 3):350, 1992.
98. Pocchiari M, Salvatore M, Cutruzzola F et al: A new point mutation of the prion protein gene in familial and sporadic cases of Creutzfeldt-Jakob disease, *Ann Neurol* 34:802, 1993.
99. Ripoll L, Laplanche J-L, Salzmann M et al: A new point mutation in the prion protein gene at codon 210 in Creutzfeldt-Jakob disease, *Neurology* 43:1934, 1993.
100. Owen F, Poulter M, Lofthouse R et al: Insertion in prion protein gene in familial Creutzfeldt-Jakob disease, *Lancet* 1:51, 1989.
101. Owen F, Poulter M, Shah T et al: An in-frame insertion in the prion protein gene in familial Creutzfeldt-Jakob disease, *Mol Brain Res* 7:273, 1990.
102. Collinge J, Brown J, Hardy J et al: Inherited prion disease with 144 base pair gene insertion. 2. Clinical and pathological features, *Brain* 115:687, 1992.
103. Goldfarb LG, Brown P, McCombie WR et al: Transmissible familial Creutzfeldt-Jakob disease associated with five, seven, and eight extra octapeptide coding repeats in the *PRNP* gene, *Proc Natl Acad Sci USA* 88:10926, 1991.
104. Owen F, Poulter M, Collinge J et al: A dementing illness associated with a novel insertion in the prion protein gene, *Mol Brain Res* 13:155, 1992.
105. Brown P: The clinico-pathological features of transmissible human spongiform encephalopathy, with a discussion of recognized risk factors and preventive strategies. [Abstr.] International Meeting on Transmissible Spongiform Encephalopathies, Impact on Animal and Human Health, Heidelberg, Germany, June 23-24, 1992, International Association of Biological Standardization.
106. Poulter M, Baker HF, Frith CD et al: Inherited prion disease with 144 base pair gene insertion. 1. Genealogical and molecular studies, *Brain* 115:675, 1992.
107. Dlouhy SR, Hsiao K, Farlow MR et al: Linkage of the Indiana kindred of Gerstmann-Sträussler-Scheinker disease to the prion protein gene, *Nature Genet* 1:64, 1992.
108. Hsiao K, Dlouhy S, Farlow MR et al: Mutant prion proteins in Gerstmann-Sträussler-Scheinker disease with neurofibrillary tangles, *Nature Genet* 1:68, 1992.
109. Ghetti B, Tagliavini F, Masters CL et al: Gerstmann-Sträussler-Scheinker disease. II. Neurofibrillary tangles and plaques with PrP-amyloid coexist in an affected family, *Neurology* 39:1453, 1989.
110. Giaccone G, Tagliavini F, Verga L et al: Neurofibrillary tangles of the Indiana kindred of Gerstmann-Sträussler-Scheinker disease share antigenic determinants with those of Alzheimer disease, *Brain Res* 530:325, 1990.
111. Tagliavini F, Prelli F, Ghisto J et al: Amyloid protein of Gerstmann-Sträussler-Scheinker disease (Indiana kindred) is an 11-kD fragment of prion protein with an N-terminal glycine at codon 58, *EMBO J* 10:513, 1991.
112. Goldfarb LG, Brown P, Haltia M et al: Creutzfeldt-Jakob disease cosegregates with the codon 178^{Asn} *PRNP* mutation in families of European origin, *Ann Neurol* 31:274, 1992.
113. Medori R, Montagna P, Tritschler HJ et al: Fatal familial insomnia: a second kindred with mutation of prion protein gene at codon 178, *Neurology* 42:669, 1992.
114. Medori R, Tritschler H-J, LeBlanc A et al: Fatal familial insomnia, a prion disease with a mutation at codon 178 of the prion protein gene, *N Engl J Med* 326:444, 1992.
115. Manetto V, Medori R, Cortelli P et al: Fatal familial insomnia: clinical and pathological study of five new cases., *Neurology* 42:312, 1992.
116. Brown P, Goldfarb LG, Kovanen J et al: Phenotypic characteristics of familial Creutzfeldt-Jakob disease associated with the codon 178^{Asn} *PRNP* mutation, *Ann Neurol* 31:282, 1992.
117. Goldfarb LG, Haltia M, Brown P et al: New mutation in scrapie amyloid precursor gene (at codon 178) in Finnish Creutzfeldt-Jakob kindred, *Lancet* 337:425, 1991.
118. Haltia M, Kovanen J, Goldfarb LG et al: Familial Creutzfeldt-Jakob disease in Finland: Epidemiological, clinical, pathological and molecular genetic studies, *Eur J Epidemiol* 7:494, 1991.

Infectious prion disease

119. Brown P, Preece MA, Will RG: "Friendly fire " in medicine: hormones, homografts, and Creutzfeldt-Jakob disease, *Lancet* 340:24, 1992.
120. Gibbs CJ Jr, Joy A, Heffner R et al: Clinical and pathological features and laboratory confirmation of Creutzfeldt-Jakob disease in a recipient of pituitary-derived human growth hormone, *N Engl J Med* 313:734, 1985.
121. Koch TK, Berg BO, DeArmond SJ et al: Creutzfeldt-Jakob disease in a young adult with idiopathic hypopituitarism. Possible relation to the administration of cadaveric human growth hormone, *N Engl J Med* 313:731, 1985.
122. Powell-Jackson J, Weller RO, Kennedy P et al: Creutzfeldt-Jakob disease after administration of human growth hormone, *Lancet* 2:244, 1985.
123. Titner R, Brown P, Hedley-Whyte ET et al: Neuropathologic verification of Creutzfeldt-Jakob disease in the exhumed American recipient of human pituitary growth hormone: epidemiologic and pathogenetic implications, *Neurology* 36:932, 1986.
124. Croxson M, Brown P, Synek B et al: A new case of Creutzfeldt-Jakob disease associated with human growth hormone therapy in New Zealand, *Neurology* 38:1128, 1988.
125. New MI, Brown P, Temeck JW et al: Preclinical Creutzfeldt-Jakob disease discovered at autopsy in a human growth hormone recipient, *Neurology* 38:1133, 1988.
126. Marzewski DJ, Towfighi J, Harrington MG et al: Creutzfeldt-Jakob disease following pituitary-derived human growth hormone therapy: a new American case, *Neurology* 38:1131, 1988.
127. Anderson JR, Allen CMC, Weller RO: Creutzfeldt-Jakob disease following human pituitary-derived growth hormone administration, *Br Neuropatholog Soc Proc* 16:543, 1990.
128. Billette de Villemeur TB, Beauvais P, Gourmelen M et al: Creutzfeldt-Jakob disease in children treated with growth hormone, *Lancet* 337:864, 1991.
129. Macario ME, Vaisman M, Buescu A et al: Pituitary growth hormone and Creutzfeldt-Jakob disease, *Br Med J* 302:1149, 1991.
130. Ellis CJ, Katifi H, Weller RO: A further British case of growth hormone induced Creutzfeldt-Jakob disease, *J Neurol Neurosurg Psychiatry* 55:1200, 1992.

131. Fradkin JE, Schonberger LB, Mills JL et al: Creutzfeldt-Jakob disease in pituitary growth hormone recipients in the United States, *JAMA* 265:880, 1991.
132. Prusiner SB, Gajdusek DC, Alpers MP: Kuru with incubation periods exceeding two decades, *Ann Neurol* 12:1, 1982.
133. Collinge J, Palmer MS, Dryden A: Molecular genetics of inherited, sporadic and iatrogenic prion disease. In Prusiner S, Collinge J, Powell J, Anderton B: *Prion Diseases in Humans and Animals*, New York, 1992, Ellis Howard, 96-119.
134. Palmer MS, Dryden AJ, Hughes JT et al: Homozygous prion protein genotype predisposes to sporadic Creutzfeldt-Jakob disease, *Nature* 352:340, 1991.
135. Masters CL, Gajdusek DC, Gibbs CJ Jr et al: Familial Creutzfeldt-Jakob disease and other familial dementias: an inquiry into possible models of virus-induced familial diseases. In Prusiner SB, Hadlow WJ, Prusiner SB, Hadlow WJS: *Slow transmissible diseases of the nervous system,* vol 1, New York, 1979, Academic Press.
136. Brown P, Cathala F, Raubertas RF et al: The epidemiology of Creutzfeldt-Jakob disease: conclusion of 15-year investigation in France and review of the world literature, *Neurology* 37:895, 1987.
137. Brown P: Virus sterility for human growth hormone, *Lancet* 2:729, 1985.

Clinical features of Creutzfeldt-Jakob disease

138. Malamud N: Creutzfeldt-Jakob's disease: a clincopathologic study. In Prusiner SB, Hadlow WJ, Prusiner SB, Hadlow WJS: *Slow transmissible diseases of the nervous system,* vol 1, New York, 1979, Academic Press.
139. Masters CL, Richardson EP Jr: Subacute spongiform encephalopathy Creutzfeldt-Jakob disease: the nature and progression of spongiform change, *Brain* 101:333, 1978.
140. Brown P, Goldfarb LG, Gibbs CJJ et al: The phenotypic expression of different mutations in transmissible familial Creutzfeldt-Jakob disease, *Eur J Epidemiol* 7:469, 1991.
141. Beck E, Daniel PM: Kuru and Creutzfeldt-Jakob disease; neuropathological lesions and their significance. In Prusiner SB, Hadlow WJ, Prusiner SB, Hadlow WJS: *Slow transmissible diseases of the nervous system,* vol 1, New York, 1979, Academic Press.
142. Beck E, Daniel PM, Matthews WB et al: Creutzfeldt-Jakob disease: the neuropathology of a transmission experiment, *Brain* 92:699, 1969.
143. Brown P, Rodgers-Johnson P, Cathala F et al: Creutzfeldt-Jakob disease of long duration: clinicopathological characteristics, transmissibility, and differential diagnosis, *Ann Neurol* 16:295, 1984.

Pathology of Creutzfeldt-Jakob disease

144. Beck E, Daniel PM, Davey AJ et al: The pathogenesis of transmissible spongiform encephalopathy: an ultrastructural study, *Brain* 105:755, 1982.
145. Chou SM, Payne WN, Gibbs CJ Jr et al: Transmission and scanning electron microscopy of spongiform change in Creutzfeldt-Jakob disease, *Brain* 103:885, 1980.
146. Lampert PW, Gajdusek DC, Gibbs CJ Jr: Subacute spongiform virus encephalopathies: scrapie, kuru and Creutzfeldt-Jakob disease: a review, *Am J Pathol* 68:626, 1972.
147. Dormont D, Delpech A, Courcel M-N et al: Hyperproduction de protéine glio-fibrillaire acide (GFA) au cours de l'évolution de la tremblante de la souris, *CR Acad Sci* (Paris) 293:53, 1981.
148. Mackenzie A: Immunohistochemical demonstration of glial fibrillary acidic protein in scrapie, *J Comp Pathol* 93:251, 1983.
149. DeArmond SJ, Kristensson K, Bowler RP: PrP^{Sc} causes nerve cell death and stimulates astrocyte proliferation: a paradox. In Yu ACH, Hertz L, Norenberg MD, et al: *Progress in brain research,* vol 94, Amsterdam, 1992, Elsevier Science Publishers.
150. Tateishi J, Doi H, Sato Y et al: Experimental transmission of human subacute spongiform encephalopathy to small rodents. III. Further transmission from three patients and distribution patterns of lesions in mice, *Acta Neuropathol* (Berl) 53:161, 1981.
151. Liberski PP, Yanagihara R, Gibbs CJJ et al: White matter ultrastructural pathology of experimental Creutzfeldt-Jakob disease in mice, *Acta Neuropathol* (Berl) 79:1, 1989.
152. Pearlman RL, Towfighi J, Pezeshkpour GH et al: Clinical significance of types of cerebellar amyloid plaques in human spongiform encephalopathies, *Neurology* 38:1249, 1988.
153. Tateishi J, Kitamoto T, Doh-ura K et al: Creutzfeldt-Jakob disease with amyloid angiopathy: diagnosis by immunological analyses and transmission experiments, *Acta Neuropathol* 83:559, 1992.
154. Muramoto T, Kitamoto T, Tateishi J et al: The sequential development of abnormal prion protein accumulation in mice with Creutzfeldt-Jakob disease, *Am J Pathol* 140:1411, 1992.

Gerstmann-Sträussler-Scheinker disease

155. Hsiao K, Prusiner SB: Molecular genetics and transgenic model of Gerstmann-Sträussler-Scheinker disease, *Alzheimer Dis Assoc Disord* 5:155, 1991.
156. Seitelberger F: Spinocerebellar ataxia with dementia and plaque-like deposits (Sträussler's disease). In Vinken PJ, Bruyn GW, Vinken PJ, Bruyn GWS. *Handbook of clinical neurology,* vol 42, Amsterdam, 1981, North-Holland.
157. Kuzuhara S, Kanazawa I, Sasaki H et al: Gerstmann-Sträussler-Scheinker's disease, *Ann Neurol* 14:216, 1983.
158. Roberts GW, Lofthouse R, Brown R et al: Prion-protein immunoreactivity in human transmissible dementias, *N Engl J Med* 315:1231, 1986.
159. Nochlin D, Sumi SM, Bird TD et al: Familial dementia with PrP-positive amyloid plaques: a variant of Gerstmann-Sträussler syndrome, *Neurology* 39:910, 1989.
160. Farlow MR, Yee RD, Dlouhy SR et al: Gerstmann-Sträussler-Scheinker disease. I. Extending the clinical spectrum, *Neurology* 39:1446, 1989.
161. Goldfarb LG, Petersen RB, Tabaton M et al: Fatal familial insomnia and familial Creutzfeldt-Jakob disease: disease phenotype determined by a DNA polymorphism, *Science* 258:806, 1992.

Laboratory considerations

162. Gajdusek DC, Gibbs CJ Jr, Asher DM et al: Precautions in medical care of and in handling materials from patients with transmissible virus dementia (CJD), *N Engl J Med* 297:1253, 1977.
163. Webb RM, Leech RW, Brumback RA: Spongiform encephalopathies: the physician's responsibility, *South Med J* 83:141, 1990.
164. Berger JR, David NJ: Creutzfeldt-Jakob disease in a physician: a review of the disorder in health care workers, *Neurology* 43:205, 1993.
165. Esmonde TFG, Will RG, Slattery JM et al: Creutzfeldt-Jakob disease and blood transfusion, *Lancet* 341:205, 1993.
166. Brown P: An epidemiologic critique of Creutzfeldt-Jakob disease, *Epidemiol Rev* 2:113, 1980.
167. Rosenberg RN, White LL III, Brown P et al: Precautions in handling tissues, fluids, and other contaminated materials from patients with documented or suspected Creutzfeldt-Jakob disease, *Ann Neurol* 19:75, 1986.
168. Prusiner SB, Cochran SP, Alpers MP: Transmission of scrapie in hamsters, *J Infect Dis* 152:971, 1985.
169. Pattison IH: Resistance of the scrapie agent to formalin, *J Comp Pathol* 75:159, 1965.
170. Brown P, Rohwer RG, Green EM et al: Effect of chemicals, heat, and histopathologic processing on high-infectivity hamster-adapted scrapie virus, *J Infect Dis* 145:683, 1982.
171. Brown P, Wolff A, Gajdusek CD: A simple and effective method for inactivating virus infectivity in formalin-fixed tissue samples from patients with Creutzfeldt-Jakob disease, *Neurology* 40:887, 1990.

Part Four

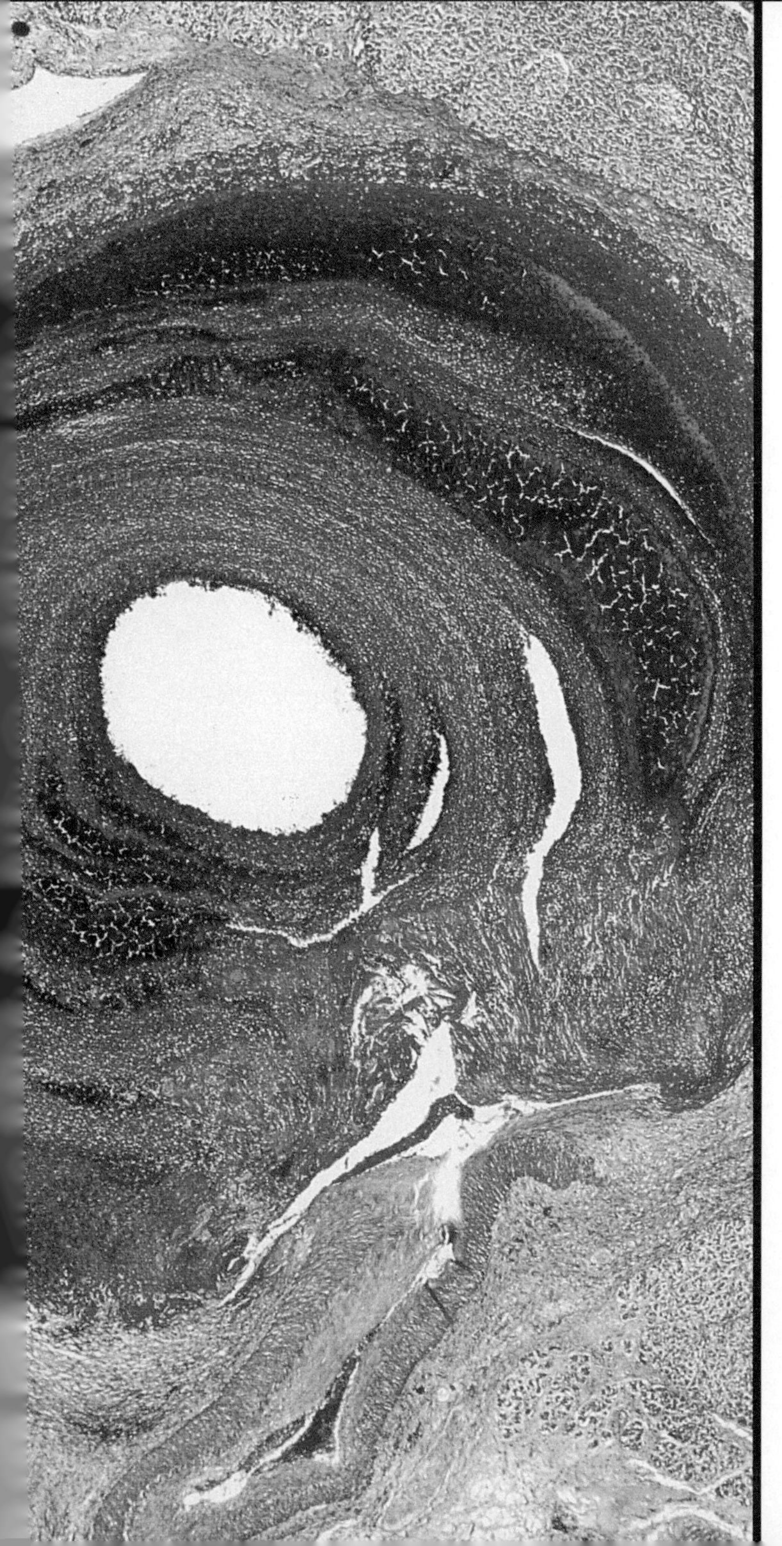

DISEASES OF THE BLOOD, HEART, AND LUNGS

41 Blood and Bone Marrow

Craig E. Litz
John S. McClure
Richard D. Brunning

NORMAL HEMATOPOIESIS

The hematopoietic system comprises the cells in the blood, the precursors of these cells in the bone marrow, and the hematopoietic cells in the lymph nodes, spleen, and other lymphatic tissue throughout the body. These cells are extraordinarily diverse both morphologically and functionally. The system is divided into two major components: myeloid and lymphocytic, both of which originate from a pluripotential stem cell that is assumed to be of bone marrow origin. The myeloid cells include neutrophils, eosinophils, and basophils (collectively referred to as granulocytes) and monocytes, erythroid cells, and megakaryocytes. Postnatal myelopoiesis occurs primarily in the bone marrow, which in aggregate amount is 1200 to 1500 g. Lymphoid cells include both T-cells and B-cells, which arise in the marrow and mature in several different sites, including lymph nodes, spleen, thymus, extranodal lymphatic tissue, and bone marrow.

Embryogenesis

The initial phase of hematopoiesis, the mesoblastic phase, occurs in the yolk sac of the embryo and consists principally of mesenchyme-derived primitive erythroblasts (Fig. 41-1). The second phase of hematopoiesis, the hepatic stage, commences in the second month of fetal life with the appearance of granulocytes and megakaryocytes in the sinusoids of the liver. The liver is the major site of hematopoiesis from 4 to 6 months of gestation. Hepatic and splenic hematopoiesis subside by the end of fetal life; bone marrow hematopoiesis commences around 5 months of fetal life and is the principal site of hematopoiesis at birth.[1,2] Myeloid hematopoiesis in the first year of postnatal life is present in both the axial and radial skeleton. There is gradual regression of hematopoietic tissue in the long bones. Beginning at about 15 years of age, the flat bones of the axial skeleton are the exclusive site of myelopoiesis.

Marrow morphology

The marrow consists of bone trabeculas and the medullary space, which includes hematopoietic cells, adipose tissue, and stroma. The stroma is composed of a delicate framework of connective tissue and vascular structures.[1,3-5] The principal vascular supply is derived from a nutrient artery that branches throughout the marrow space. The arterioles of the nutrient artery branch into capillaries, which are continuous with a system of thin-walled sinusoids. The structure of the sinusoids consists of an inner layer of endothelial cells and an outer layer of adventitial reticular cells. The fat cells of the marrow are derived from the adventitial cells.

Normal marrow consists of myeloid cells at all stages of maturation and a relatively small number of well-differenti-

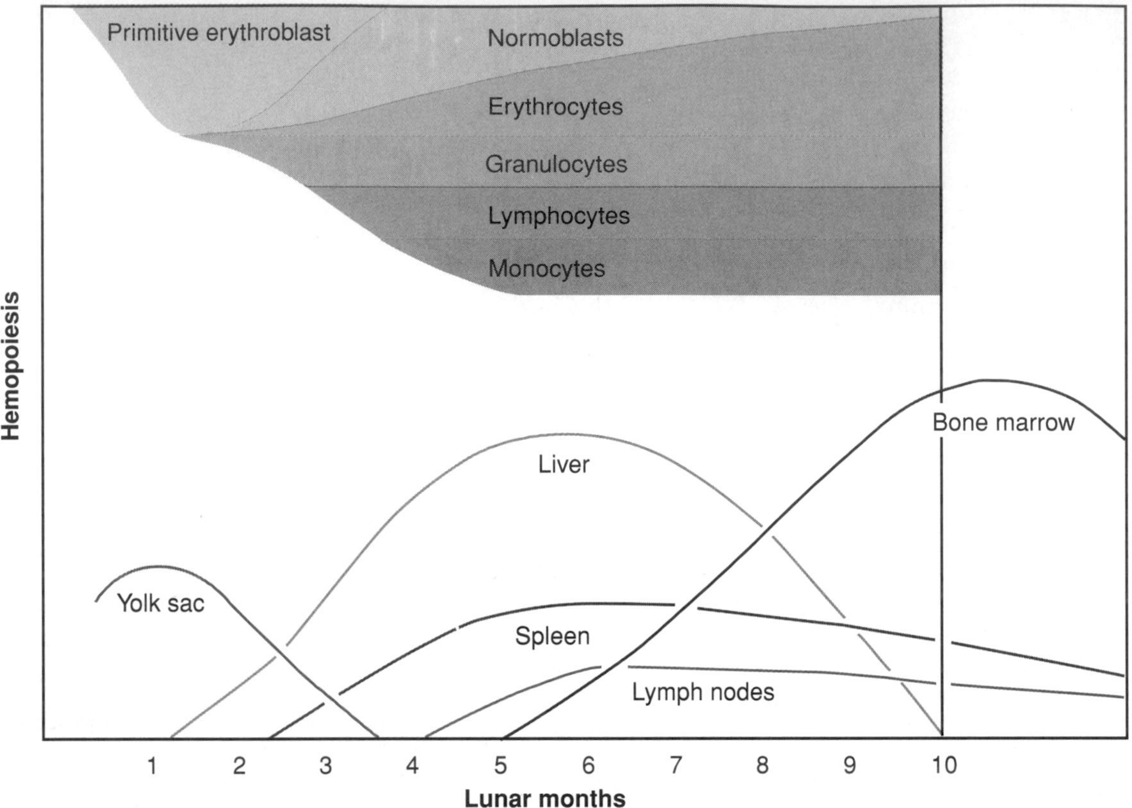

Fig. 41-1 Diagrammatic representation of embryonic hematopoiesis. The initial mesoblastic phase is in the yolk sac. Bone marrow hematopoiesis begins in mid embryonic life and is the only site of myeloid hematopoiesis at birth.

ated lymphocytes, plasma cells, and histiocytes. Approximately 60% to 65% of marrow cells are granulocytes and 20% are erythroid precursors. Lymphocytes constitute approximately 10% to 15% of the marrow cells. The granulocytes are principally neutrophils at all stages of maturation with a predominance of more mature cells. The predominant erythroid precursors are at the polychromatic stage of maturation. Megakaryocytes constitute approximately 2% to 5% of marrow cellularity.

Myeloid hematopoiesis, or myelopoiesis, includes the differentiation and maturation of the granulocytes, monocytes, erythroid cells, and megakaryocytes (Fig. 41-2). These cells have a common origin in a myeloid stem cell that is derived from the pluripotential hematopoietic stem cell. The process of differentiation involves the acquisition of characteristics that determine the lineage to which a cell is assigned. Maturation involves changes in nuclear and cytoplasmic features. The earliest morphologically identifiable cell for each of the major myeloid cell lineages is the proerythroblast, the megakaryoblast, the monoblast, and the myeloblast, which is the precursor of the granulocytes. In general, maturation in all cell lines is characterized by a decreasing nuclear-to-cytoplasmic ratio and acquisition of cytoplasmic constituents that reflect the functional capacity of the cells. Cytoplasmic maturation in the granulocytes is characterized by lineage-specific granule production and the loss of basophilia and erythroid maturation by hemoglobin synthesis (Fig. 41-3). The functional end cells of the granulocyte and monocyte series have lobated nuclei and characteristic granules. The functional product of the megakaryocyte is the platelet, a cytoplasmic fragment with granules. The functional cell of the erythroid series is the anucleate red cell.

There are no distinct morphologic stages in normal lymphocyte development that parallel the maturational stages of the myeloid cells. The lymphoblast and prolymphocyte are lymphocytes with morphologic features generally associated with immaturity such as dispersed or fine chromatin and nucleoli. These cells are present in leukemic proliferations and are not found in normal marrow and blood.

Other marrow cells related to the hematopoietic system are the tissue mast cell and the plasma cell. The tissue mast cell morphologically closely resembles the basophil and appears to be derived from the myeloid system. The plasma cell is derived from the lymphocyte system and is viewed as the most "immunologically advanced" B-cell. Marrow histiocytes are derived from monocytes.[6]

Osteoblasts and osteoclasts are cells involved in osteogenesis. The osteoblast is associated with bone production, and the osteoclast, which appears to be derived from the monocyte-macrophage system, is associated with bone resorption (Figs. 41-4 and 41-5).

Cytokines

The differentiation and maturation of myelopoietic cells are regulated by endogenously produced glycoproteins known as cytokines, or growth factors.[7,8] The three most well-characterized myeloid growth factors are erythropoietin (EPO), granulocyte colony stimulating factor (G-CSF), and granulocyte-

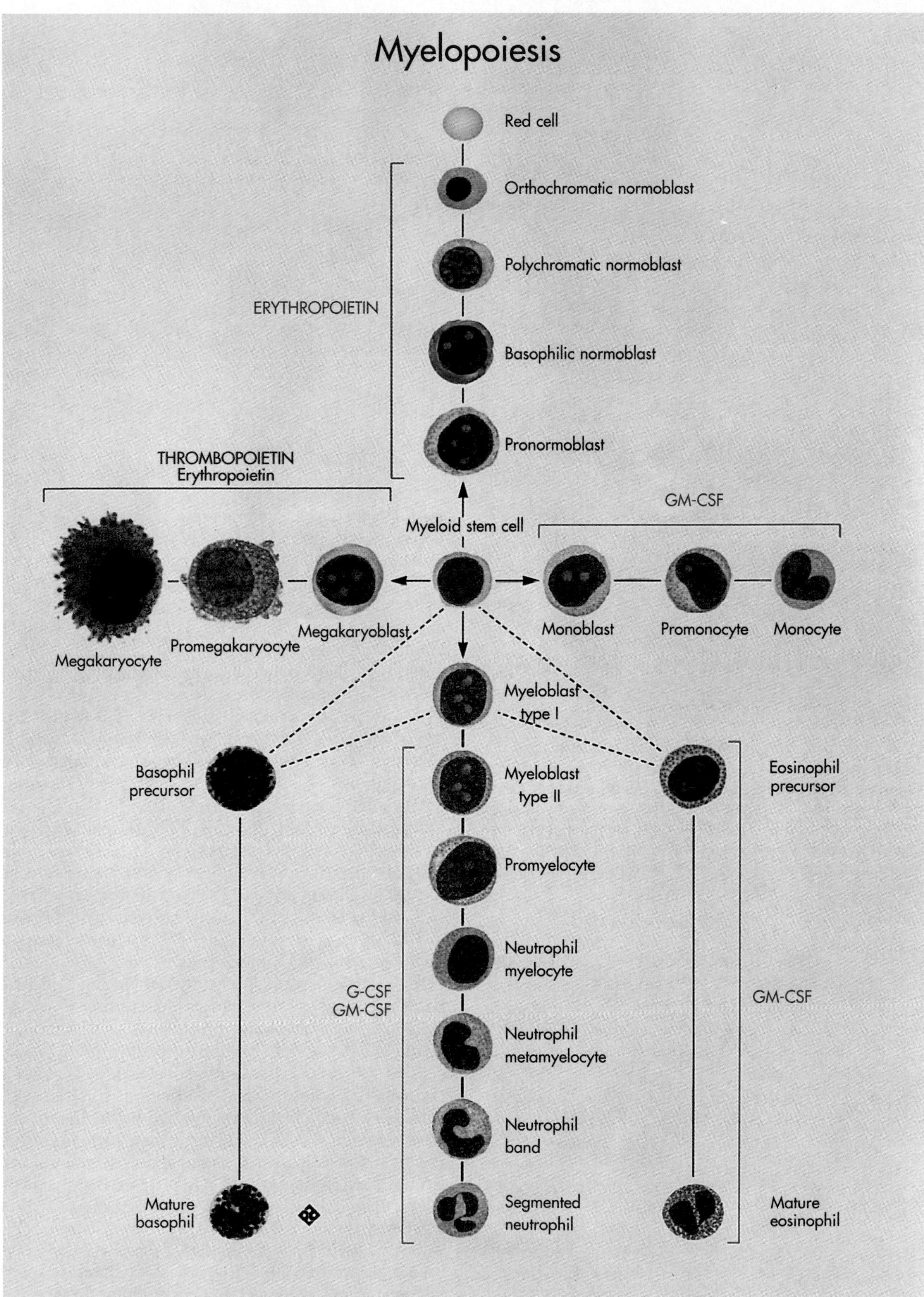

Fig. 41-2 Schematic representation of myeloid hematopoiesis and growth factor specificities. *GM-CSF,* Granulocyte/macrophage colony stimulating factor; *G-CSF,* granulocyte colony stimulating factor. (Modified from Brunning RD, McKenna RW: *Tumors of the bone marrow,* Armed Forces Institute of Pathology, Washington, D.C., 1994).

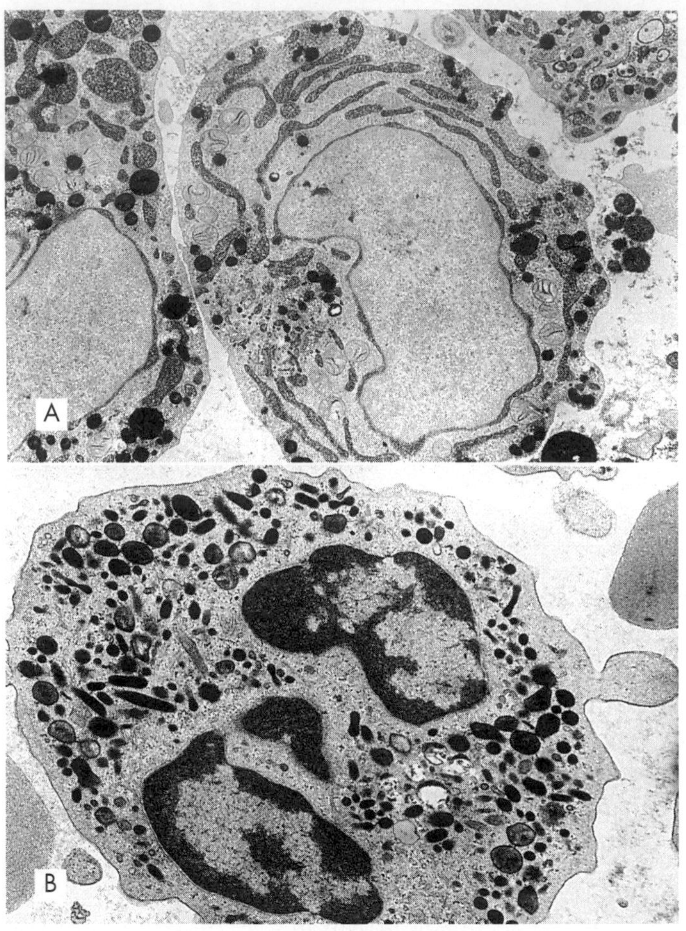

Fig. 41-3 A, Electron micrograph of a promyelocyte reacted for peroxidase. The dark positively reacting granules that are widely dispersed in the cytoplasm arise from the Golgi. These granules correspond to the azurophilic granules in the cytoplasm in light microscopy. (Lead citrate). **B,** Electron micrograph of a segmented neutrophil with numerous granules scattered throughout the cytoplasm. The granules show marked variation in size and shape (Uranyl acetate, lead citrate).

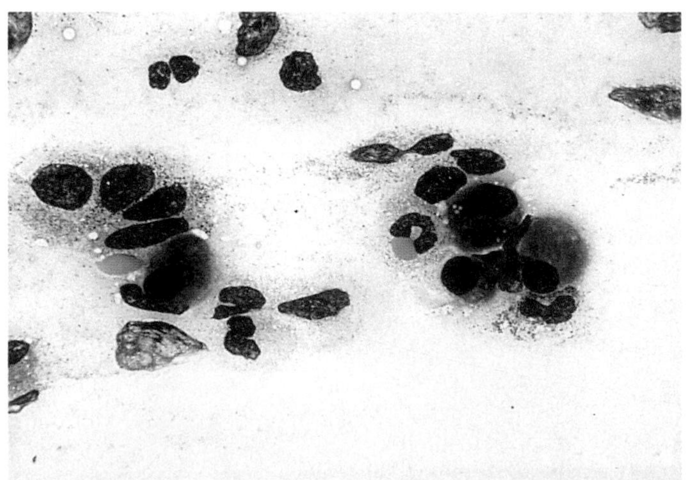

Fig. 41-4 Marrow aspirate showing four osteoblasts. The cells are larger than neutrophils with an eccentrically placed, round nucleus and abundant deep blue cytoplasm (Wright-Giemsa).

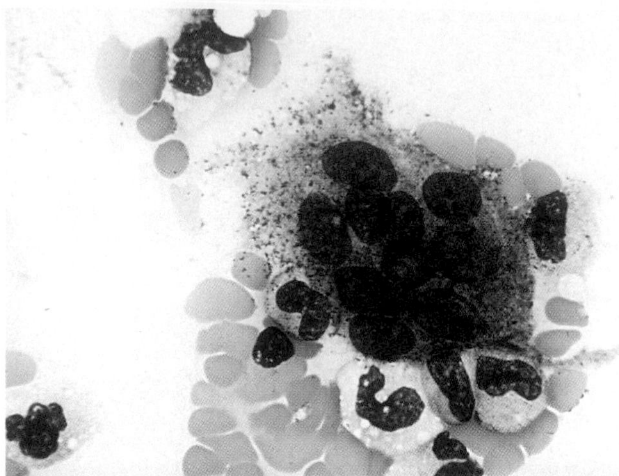

Fig. 41-5 Marrow aspirate showing an osteoclast. The cells are very large with abundant purplish granular cytoplasm and multiple round to oval nuclei (Wright-Giemsa).

macrophage colony stimulating factor (GM-CSF). Thrombopoietin, the primary regulatory factor for the development of megakaryocytes and platelets, has not been fully characterized because of the lack of adequate in vitro assays; however, a candidate glycoprotein with a molecular weight of 15,000 daltons has been described.[9] The myeloid cytokines act by binding to target cell surface protein receptors.[7,8] Intracellular portions of these bound receptors initiate cell events that are specific for the cell type and the receptor involved (see Fig. 41-2). The receptors for G-CSF, GM-CSF, and EPO belong to the hematopoietic cytokine growth factor receptor family, a subset of the immunoglobulin gene superfamily. The genes encoding many of the receptors and growth factors are clustered on the long arm of chromosome 5 (Fig. 41-6); included in this group are GM-CSF, M-CSF (macrophage colony stimulating factor) and the receptors for M-CSF. The genes for G-CSF, erythropoietin, and the erythropoietin receptor are located on chromosomes 17, 7, and 19, respectively.

Erythropoietin (EPO), a glycoprotein of molecular weight 46,000 daltons, is produced by cells of the renal proximal tubule and hepatic Kupffer cells.[7,10] The physiologic basis of EPO regulation appears to be arterial oxygen content. Erythropoietin receptors are present on the surface of erythroid stem cells and megakaryocytic precursors. These receptors, when bound to EPO, initiate the transformation of the erythroid stem cells to proerythroblasts and activate the genes necessary for erythroid proliferation and maturation. EPO acts in concert with thrombopoietin to promote the production of megakaryocytes in vitro.[11] Anemia stimulates increased endogenous production of EPO except in anephric patients, in whom there is a production defect of EPO. Patients with renal disease in which there is significant parenchymal damage will also have decreased amounts of EPO.[12]

Granulocyte colony stimulating factor (G-CSF) is produced by monocytes and bone marrow stromal cells. G-CSF receptors are present on segmented neutrophils and their precursors; the receptor density increases with maturation .[7,8] A small subset of monocytic cells binds low levels of G-CSF. The G-CSF receptors are not present on erythroid cells or megakaryocytes. Binding of G-CSF to receptors on neutrophils stimulates cellu-

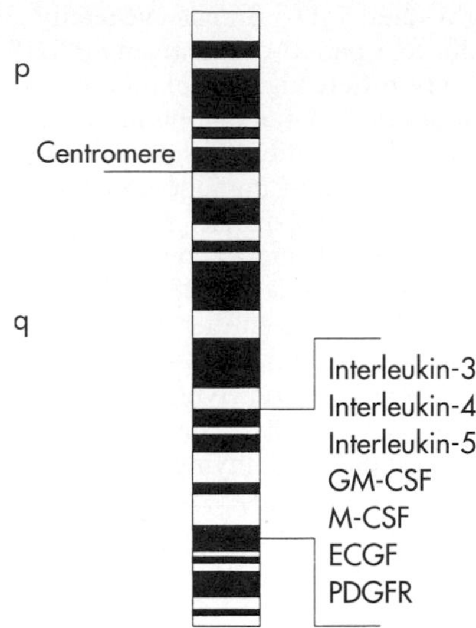

Fig. 41-6 Idiogram of chromosome 5 with location of growth factor genes identified. *ECGF,* Endothelial cell growth factor; *PDGFR,* platelet derived growth factor receptor. (Modified from Bagby GC, Segal GM: Growth factors and the control of hematopoiesis. In Hoffman R et al, editors: *Hematology: basic principles and practice,* New York, 1991, Churchill-Livingstone.)

lar production and activation. G-CSF production is greatly increased during infections and immediately after bone marrow transplantation and occasionally with solid tumors.

The endogenous sources of granulocyte-macrophage colony stimulating factor (GM-CSF) include T-lymphocytes, endothelial cells, macrophages, bone marrow stromal cells, and fibroblasts. The GM-CSF receptor is present on monocytes and eosinophils in addition to neutrophils. GM-CSF stimulates cell production and enhances the cytotoxicity of monocytes.

Recombinant G-CSF and GM-CSF have been used primarily to mitigate the neutropenia associated with myeloablative cancer therapy. These factors have also been administered to patients with congenital neutropenia and neutropenias associated with aplastic anemia and acquired immunodeficiency syndrome (AIDS).[13] Administration of G-CSF and GM-CSF produces morphologic and quantitative changes in neutrophil development that are similar to those manifest in patients with inflammatory processes (Fig. 41-7 and Table 41-1).

Immunology of hematopoiesis

Concurrent with morphologic development of the hematopoietic system, there are sequential changes in cell surface antigen expression. These antigens are classified by the cluster of differentiation (CD) nomenclature.[14] Each CD designation defines a cell surface or cytoplasmic antigen that is recognized by one or more antibodies. Based on functional characteristics and the antigenic determinants, the lymphocyte system is separated into two major components: B-cell and T-cell. Myeloid-specific antigens have also been identified.

The immunologic characteristics of hematopoietic cells have particular importance in the diagnosis and classification of the acute and chronic lymphocytic leukemias. The immunologic characteristics of lymphoid malignancies including surface and cytoplasmic immunoglobulin and CD profile combined with

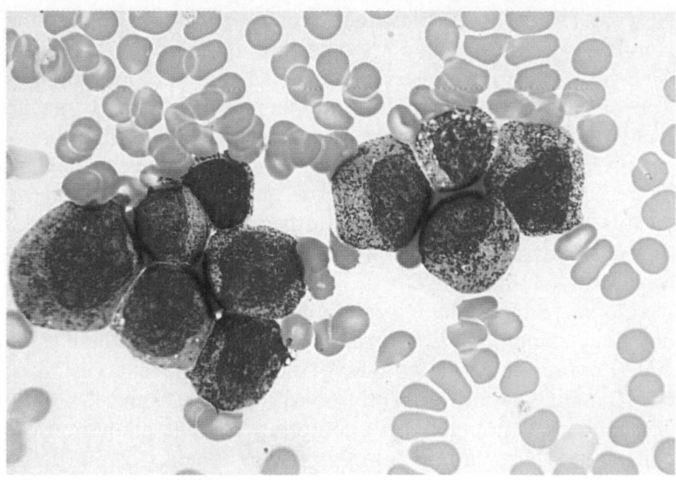

Fig. 41-7 Morphologic effects of growth factor. Marrow aspirate from a patient on G-CSF showing an early neutrophil response. There is a marked shift toward immaturity in the neutrophils with the majority at the promyelocyte and early myelocyte stages of maturation (Wright-Giemsa). (Courtesy Laura L. Schmitz, M.D., Hennepin County Medical Center, Minneapolis, Minn).

Table 41-1 Morphologic changes in the blood and marrow associated with G-CSF and GM-CSF therapy

Blood
Neutrophilic leukocytosis
Neutrophils: morphologic changes
Shift to immaturity (myeloblasts <3%)
Increased azurophilic granulation and Dohle bodies
Nuclear cytoplasmic dyssynchrony
Nuclear hyposegmentation and hypersegmentation
Leukoerythroblastosis
Marrow
Early changes (corresponding to a period when the absolute neutrophil count is less than 0.5 × 10⁹/L)
Relative neutrophilic hyperplasia with large increase in promyelocytes and early myelocytes
Large promyelocytes and myelocytes with increased azurophilic granulation
Late changes (corresponding to peak blood neutrophil count)
Neutrophilic hyperplasia; predominance of mature segmented neutrophils with increased azurophilic granulation

Modified from Schmitz LL et al: Morphologic and quantitative changes in blood and marrow cells following growth factor therapy, *Am J Clin Pathol* 101:67, 1994.

morphologic features and nuclear terminal deoxynucleotidyl-transferase lead to enhanced recognition of clinical pathologic groups with more predictable biologic courses. Because acute leukemias frequently represent proliferations of morphologically poorly differentiated blasts, assignment of a process as lymphocytic or myeloid may be possible only with the identification of surface or cytoplasmic antigens. In occasional instances, the antigenic profile of the blast will indicate proliferation involving both the myeloid and lymphoid lineages.

B-cell development is classified into maturational stages based on the expression of surface antigens, the nuclear enzyme terminal deoxynucleotidyltransferase (TdT) and the synthesis of surface and cytoplasmic immunoglobulin. Fig. 41-8 illustrates a proposed sequence of immunologic maturation based on studies of immunophenotypes from B-lineage leukemias and normal bone marrow cells.[15] The membrane surface antigens CD34, HLA-DR, CD19, and nuclear TdT are expressed at the earliest stage of B-lymphocyte development. At this stage, the immunoglobulin heavy-chain genes undergo the initial rearrangment step, D-J rearrangement, which is followed by V-D rearrangement.[16] CD10 appears early in B-cell development but is not expressed at the stage of normal B-cell ontogeny when surface immunoglobulin is expressed.[15,17] CD20 expression follows CD19 and CD10. Coexpression of CD10 and CD20 is frequently observed in fetal and leukemic B-lymphocyte populations but not in normal adult marrow cells.[15,18,19] The synthesis of cytoplasmic μ heavy chain (μHC) defines the pre–B-cell stage of maturation. Late in the pre–B-cell stage, μHC associates with surrogate light-chain molecules (ψLC) and is expressed on the cell surface in conjunction with the remaining two components of the B-cell antigen receptor, Iga and Igb.[20,21] After rearrangement of the immunoglobulin light-chain genes, κ or λ light chain is produced, and the intact B-cell receptor (IgM-κ or λ + Iga/Igb) is expressed on the cell surface.[16,21] The expression of surface immunoglobulin and the loss of TdT define the transition from the B-cell precursor to the immunologically mature B-cell. IgM alone is the initially expressed surface immunoglobulin followed by IgM and IgD. B-cells generally lose surface immunoglobulin and pan–B-cell antigens (CD19 and CD20) as they terminally differentiate to plasma cells. Plasma cells synthesize cytoplasmic immunoglobulin and express surface antigens CD38 and "specific" plasma cell antigens such as PCA-1.[19,22] The secretion of immunoglobulin by plasma cells is essential to the immune response.

T-cells are defined by the expression of lineage-specific surface antigens such as CD2, CD3, CD5, and CD7. Functional subsets of T-cells are further defined by characteristic antigen expression, CD4 on helper/inducer T-lymphocytes and CD8 on suppressor/cytotoxic lymphocytes. T-lymphocytes originate from progenitor cells in the bone marrow; the major site of their maturation is the thymus. Thymocyte maturation begins in the cortex and progresses as the precursors migrate to the medulla. The immunophenotypic sequence of T-cell ontogeny is illustrated in Fig. 41-9. The earliest cell-surface marker of T lineage is CD7, which is expressed throughout normal T-cell ontogeny.[23,24] CD3 is expressed early but is present initially only within the cytoplasm. During this early phase of development, the δ, γ, and β T-cell surface receptor genes undergo rearrangement. CD1 is expressed at a limited stage of T-cell development, the common thymocyte stage. During this stage, most T-cells express both the helper/inducer subset marker, CD4, and the cytotoxic/suppressor subset marker, CD8. As thymocytes enter the mature thymocyte stage, the α T-cell receptor gene undergoes rearrangement,

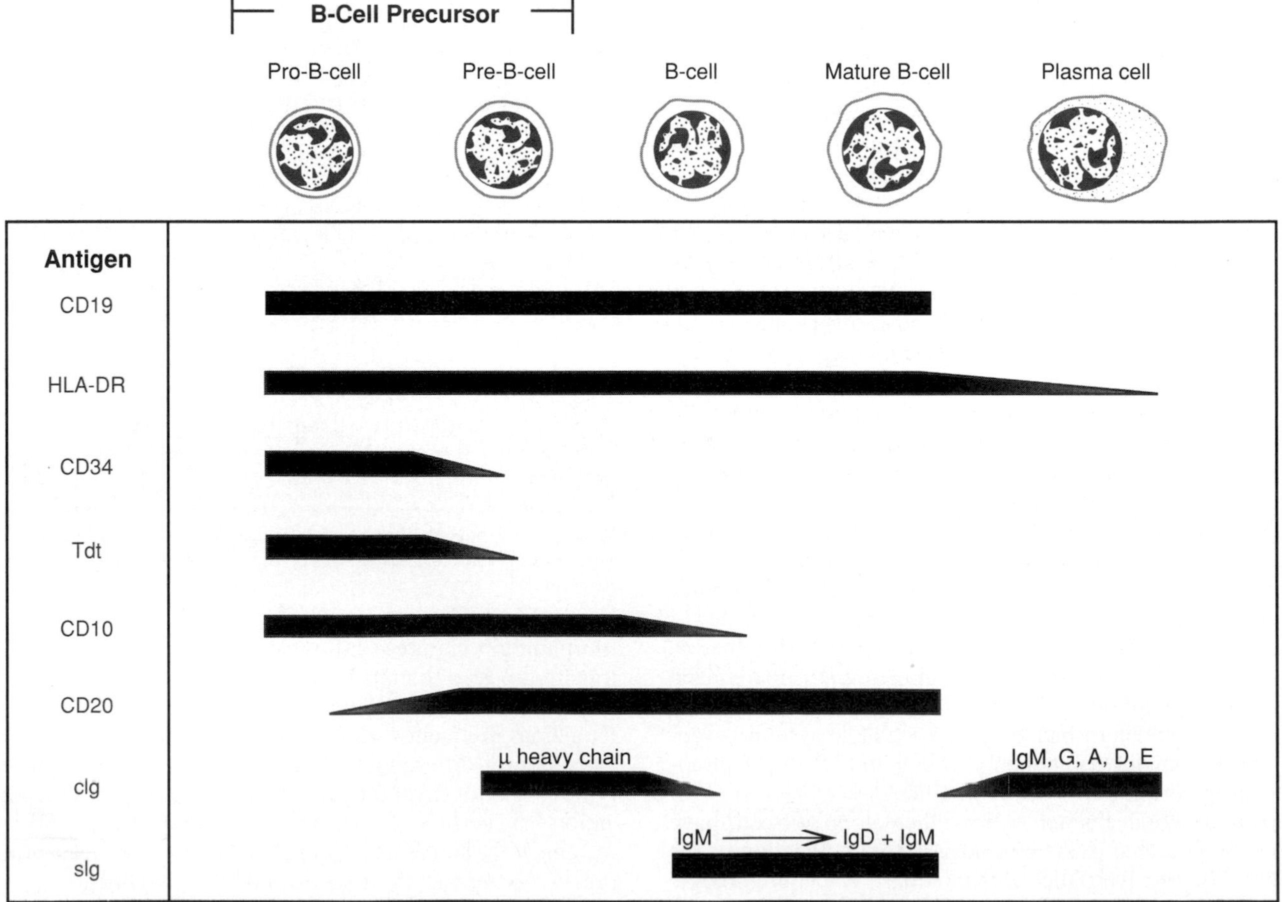

Fig. 41-8 Sequential pattern of antigen expression in B-cell ontogeny.

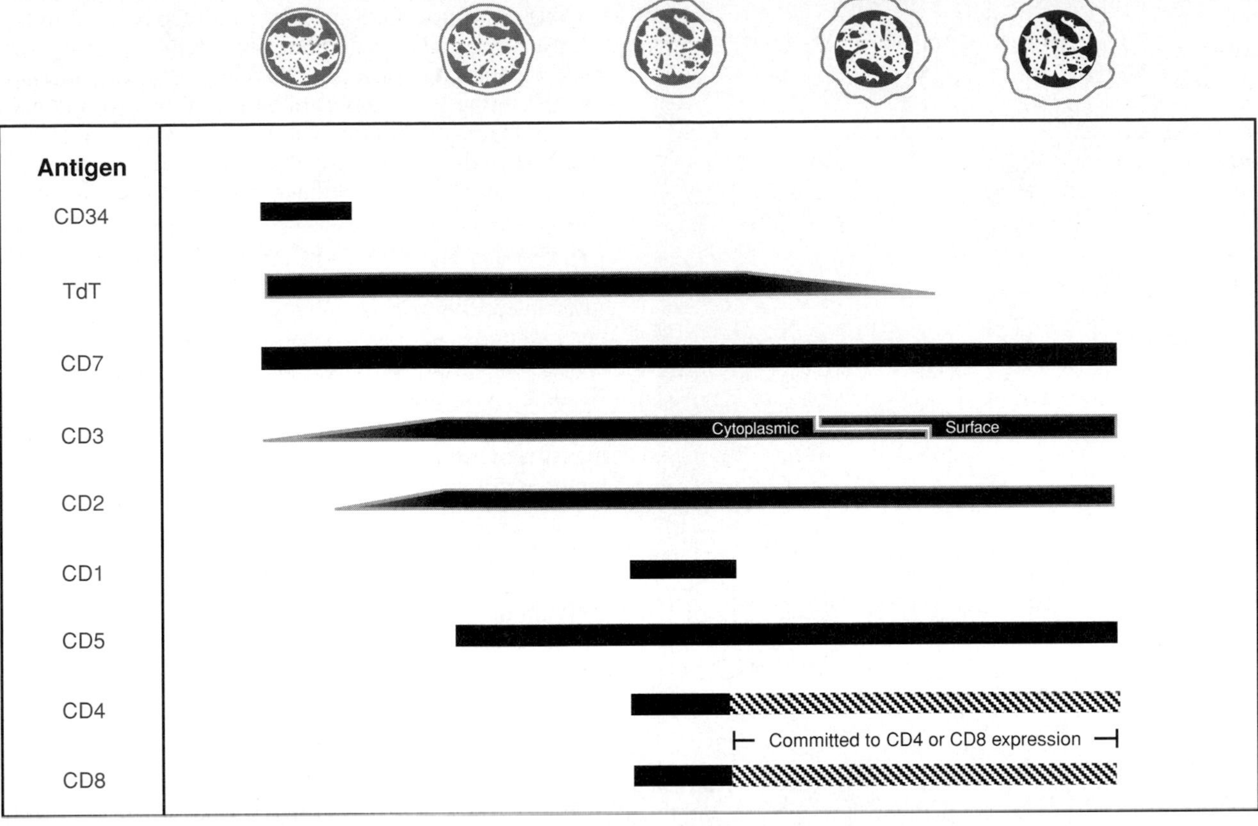

Fig. 41-9 Sequential pattern of antigen expression in T-cell ontogeny.

nuclear TdT expression is lost, and CD3 appears on the cell surface in noncovalent association with one of the T-cell receptor heterodimers, α/β or γ/δ.[18] The mature thymocyte stage is characterized by commitment to one of the major subsets with expression of either CD4 or CD8.[18,25] The post-thymic T-lymphocyte phenotype is characterized by surface CD3 expression, CD4 or CD8 expression, and the absence of cytoplasmic CD3 and nuclear TdT.

Many antigens have relatively restricted expression within the myeloid cell lines; however, no single antigen is sufficiently specific to allow one unequivocally to assign lineage. CD13 and CD33 are expressed on neutrophil and monocytic precursors at several stages of maturation. Antibodies that recognize CD41 and CD61, the platelet glycoprotein IIb and IIIa molecules, show relative specificity for megakaryocytes. Anti–glycophorin A is highly specific for erythroid cells. CD68 and CD14 show relative specificity for monocytes. CD14 expression has also been observed on cells of B lineage.[26]

Early committed granulocytic precursors express CD34, CD33, and the human leukocyte antigen HLA-DR. Subsequently, myeloblasts, the earliest morphologically recognizable stage of granulocyte development, lose expression of CD34 and acquire CD15 and CD13. CD13 is expressed throughout the remainder of neutrophil maturation. The promyelocyte stage is characterized by the loss of HLA-DR expression and increased density of CD15.[27] Cells at the myelocyte stage show a further increase in CD15 density and begin to express CD11b. Progression to the mature neutrophil is associated with progressive loss of CD33 and the expression of CD16.[27]

Marrow cellularity

Marrow cellularity refers to the amount of hematopoietic tissue (hematopoietic cells) per unit area and is inversely related to the amount of adipose tissue. The proportion of hematopoietic cells to fat cells is highest at birth and gradually decreases with age (Fig. 41-10). In the first decade of life, approximately 80% of the marrow is hematopoietic cells.[28] At the end of the third decade, the amount of hematopoietic tissue and fat cells is approximately equal; from the fourth to the seventh decades, the ratio is relatively stable. Thereafter, there is a gradual decrease in hematopoietic cells, and the mean cellularity is approximately 30% in the eighth decade.

Alterations in marrow cellularity result from increases or decreases in the amount of hematopoietic cells with corresponding decreases or increases in the number of fat cells. Hypercellular marrow may occur as a result of proliferation of normal myeloid cells, such as erythroid hyperplasia after increased red blood cell destruction in hemolytic anemias (Fig. 41-11) or may be the result of proliferation of abnormal hematopoietic cells as occurs in leukemia. In some hematologic disorders, such as the megaloblastic anemias, in which there is abnormal maturation of myeloid cells, the hypercellularity is associated with an increased rate of intramedullary destruction of the cells, ineffective hematopoiesis. The most well-characterized component of this process is ineffective erythropoiesis, which can be assessed by quantitation of the

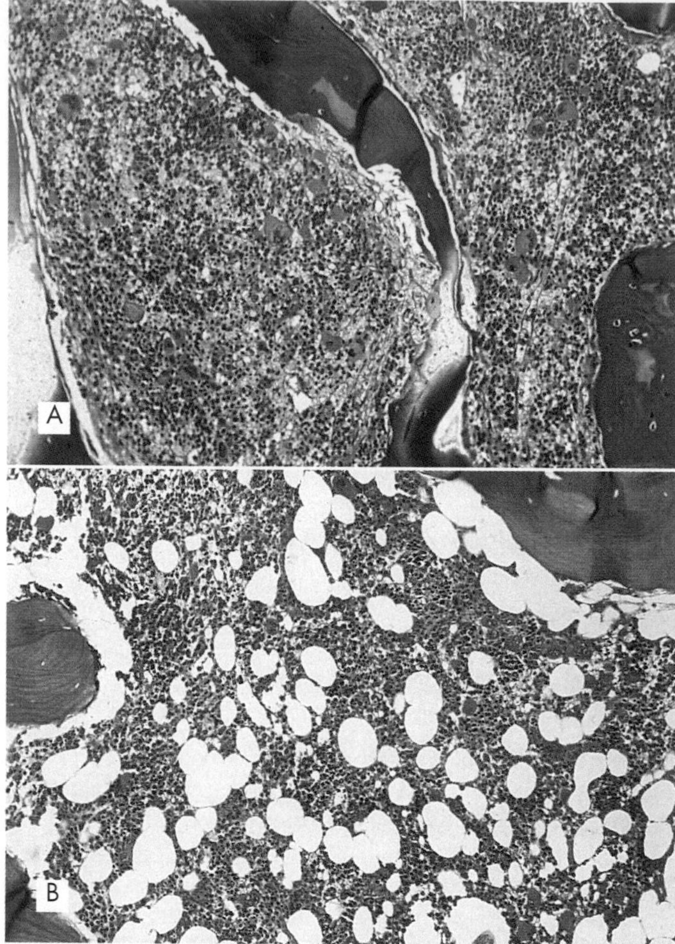

Fig. 41-10 Normal bone marrow. **A,** Child. Hypercellular bone marrow from a 6-month-old child with neurologic deterioration and normal hematologic findings. This degree of hypercellularity is a normal finding in the first year of life. **B,** Adult. Bone marrow from a 67-year-old adult being evaluated for marrow involvement by lymphoma. Hematopoietic cells constitute approximately 40% of marrow cellularity, which is within the normal range for an individual of this age.

products of hemoglobin catabolism resulting from increased intramedullary destruction of erythroid precursors.

Marrow hypocellularity may result from exposure to drugs, chemicals, ionizing radiation, or infectious agents, or it may be idiopathic. Aplastic anemia describes pronounced marrow hypoplasia with decreased numbers of all myeloid cells. This process is reflected in the blood by pancytopenia: anemia, neutropenia, and thrombocytopenia. In the most severe form of aplastic anemia, the medullary portion of the marrow consists almost exclusively of fat cells with scattered lymphocytes, plasma cells, and tissue mast cells (Fig. 41-12). In less severe forms, there may be small, scattered foci of myeloid cells.

Isolated hypoplasia of individual myeloid cell lines is uncommon. Erythroid hypoplasia or aplasia may present as a congenital disorder, erythrogenesis imperfecta (Diamond-Blackfan syndrome), or as an acquired abnormality. The causes of acquired erythroid hypoplasia are multiple, including parvovirus B-19 infection, spindle cell thymoma, and lymphoproliferative disorders (Fig. 41-13).[29,30] Granulocytic

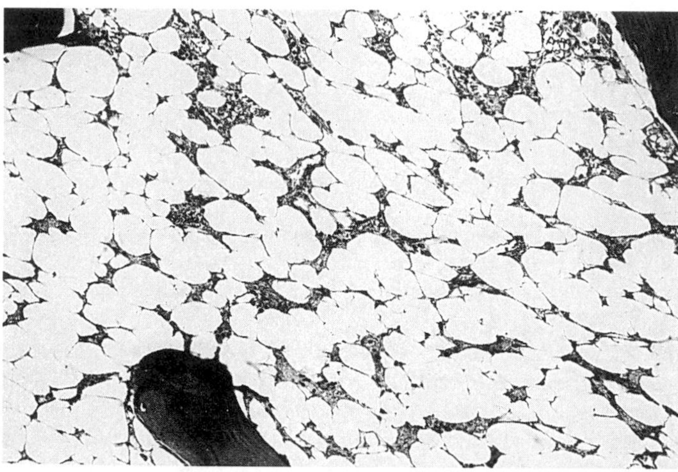

Fig. 41-12 Bone marrow biopsy from a 6-year-old child with aplastic anemia after viral hepatitis. There is a marked reduction in hematopoietic cells with expansion of fat cells.

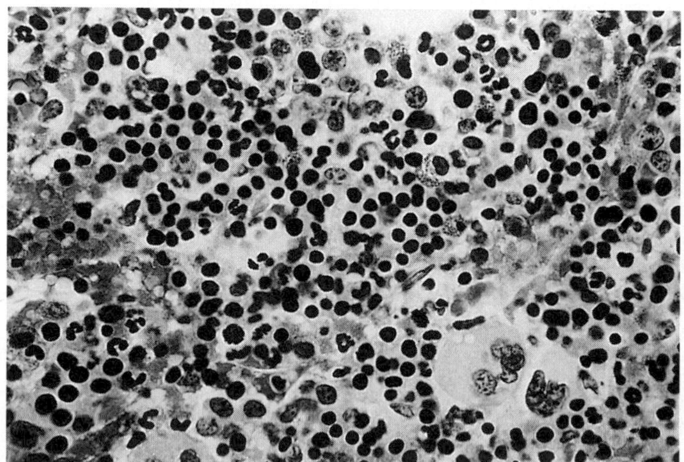

Fig. 41-11 Erythroid hyperplasia. Markedly hypercellular bone marrow from a patient with hemolytic anemia. The hypercellularity is due principally to an increase in erythroid precursors. Megakaryocytes and granulocytes at all stages of maturation are present.

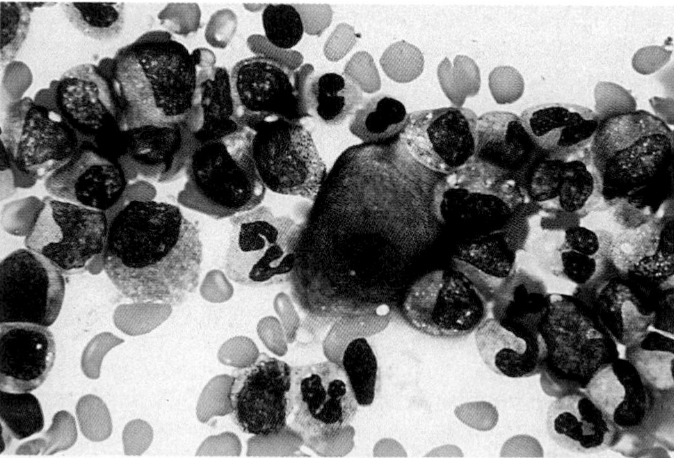

Fig. 41-13 Giant proerythroblast in a bone marrow smear from a 17-year-old boy with marked red cell hypoplasia and parvovirus B19 infection. There is a prominent intranuclear viral inclusion (Wright-Giemsa).

hypoplasia may occur as a congenital disorder as in the Kostmann syndrome, which is an autosomal recessive form of neutropenia with neutrophil counts less than 0.2×10^9/L, or as an acquired abnormality associated with drugs or toxic insults. Selective megakaryocytic hypoplasia as a congenital disorder is extremely rare and is uncommon as an acquired disorder. Megakaryocytic hypoplasia is usually associated with generalized marrow failure.

Serous or gelatinous atrophy of the marrow is a type of marrow hypoplasia usually associated with severe malnutrition.[31] The changes in the marrow are usually focal but may involve large areas. There is accumulation of a lightly eosinophil-staining substance, consisting primarily of hyaluronic acid, in the marrow interstitium with an associated atrophy of the fat cells and diminished hematopoietic tissue. Fat tissue in other areas of the body may show similar alterations.[31]

Myelophthisis denotes the replacement of normal marrow hematopoietic cells by abnormal cells, such as metastatic tumor, lymphoma, or abnormal macrophages as occurs in some of the lipid storage diseases such as Gaucher and Niemann-Pick. In a myelophthisic process the marrow is usually anatomically hypercellular, but there is a decreased number of normal and functional hematopoietic cells. This is usually accompanied by a leukoerythroblastic reaction in the blood, defined as the presence of red blood cell precursors and immature neutrophils.[32] Extensive myelophthisis may lead to marrow failure with pancytopenia.

Variations in blood cell number

Variations in the number of blood cells may result from abnormalities in the hematopoietic system or from pathologic processes occurring in other organ systems. *Leukocytosis,* an increased number of white blood cells, is most frequently caused by infectious agents; neutrophilic and monocytic leukocytosis usually accompanies bacterial infection, whereas lymphocytic leukocytosis is seen with viral infection. Pronounced lymphocytic leukocytosis is rare. The lymphocyte count uncommonly exceeds 20×10^9/L in infectious mononucleosis.[33] Eosinophilic leukocytosis frequently accompanies allergic reactions, parasitic infections, or metastatic malignancies. A frequent cause of basophilic leukocytosis is the myeloproliferative disorders, most notably chronic myeloid leukemia. The causes of thrombocytosis include myeloproliferative disorders, iron deficiency, splenectomy, and tumors. Erythrocytosis may result from decreased arterial oxygen saturation with decreased pulmonary function or congenital heart disease and is the principal finding in polycythemia vera, a chronic myeloproliferative disorder.

Cytopenias are usually related to intrinsic abnormalities of the hematopoietic system or extrinsic factors that lead to an increased rate of destruction of hematopoietic cells. The cytopenias may manifest in one cell line or all myeloid cells, pancytopenia. Pancytopenia may be transitory as observed in some viral infections; in other instances it persists in the absence of correction of the underlying defect. The causes of marrow failure resulting in pancytopenia include marrow aplasia or hypoplasia, myelophthisic processes, and metabolic deficiencies such as megaloblastic anemia caused by vitamin B_{12} or folate deficiency. Pancytopenia can also result from immune-mediated cell destruction or hypersplenism. In these instances the marrow is hypercellular.

Although marrow aplasia always results in marrow failure, marrow failure may occur with hypercellular marrows when the hypercellularity is a function of abnormal hematopoiesis; an example is a leukemic proliferation. The hypercellularity that occurs in the megaloblastic anemias is an example of a benign disorder in which there is a dissociation between marrow cellularity and marrow function. In this process there is an increased rate of intramedullary destruction of hematopoietic precursors, ineffective hematopoiesis, resulting in hyperplasia of the granulocyte and erythroid precursors.

A *leukemoid reaction* describes a pronounced neutrophilic leukocytosis with some shift to immaturity including myelocytes and occasional promyelocytes. The finding is usually associated with bacterial infection but may be related to other causes including tumor necrosis. The neutrophils usually have increased azurophilic granulation and Döhle bodies. Neutrophils with hypersegmented nuclei and cytoplasmic vacuoles may also be present.

PROCESSING OF BONE MARROW SPECIMENS

Most bone marrow examinations are performed on aspirate smears or particle crush preparations and trephine biopsy specimens obtained from the posterior iliac spine. The biopsy specimen should be at least 1 cm in length for adequate evaluation. Biopsy specimens of 2 to 3 cm are preferable when marrow biopsies are performed to determine involvement by lymphoma or other malignancies.

Approximately 1 ml marrow aspirate should be obtained for the preparation of marrow smears and particle crush preparations. Ideally, the aspirate should be obtained after the trephine biopsy. Smears can be made directly from the syringe immediately after the aspiration. In addition, a portion of the aspirate can be anticoagulated with powdered disodium EDTA, 1 mg/ml of fluid marrow, or other appropriate anticoagulant and buffy coat smears made in the laboratory.

There are several fixatives that can be used for marrow biopsy specimens including neutral buffered formalin, Zenker's, B5, and the zinc-based agents.[34] For routine histology and preservation of antigens for immunoreactivity, B5 is the preferred fixative. The optimal fixation time for B5 is 2 to 4 hours. After 4 hours the specimen becomes hard and brittle and is difficult to cut. After fixation the biopsy specimen is placed in a rapid acid decalcifier for approximately 1 to 2 hours. There are several decalcifying agents commercially available: decalcification periods vary slightly depending on specimen size. After decalcification, the specimen is washed in deionized water for 60 to 90 minutes. After the wash, the specimen can be placed in an automated tissue processor. For routine biopsies, paraffin is preferable to plastic embedding because of the ease of handling and the more easily performed immunohistochemical procedures. Hematoxylin and eosin is the most satisfactory routine stain.

Immunocytochemistry is increasingly utilized in the evaluation of marrow specimens. The technique can be applied to biopsy sections and air-dried smears and cytospin preparations. The development of antibodies reactive in paraffin-embedded sections and kits incorporating components of the avidin-biotin complex (ABC) and peroxidase-antiperoxidase (PAP) techniques have facilitated the application of immunohistochemistry to bone marrow sections. The immunoalkaline phosphatase technique can also be used with bone marrow sections; this method is preferred for immunocytochemistry on cytospin or smear preparations.

Several antibodies reactive in paraffin-embedded specimens are available. Polyclonal antimyeloperoxidase is an excellent antibody for identifying neutrophils at different stages of maturation including myeloblasts. A monoclonal antibody, L26, recognizes CD20, and polyclonal anti-CD3 marks T-cell proliferations; anti–hemoglobin A can be used for red blood cell identification.

INFLAMMATION

Granulomatous reactions are the most commonly recognized inflammatory processes in the bone marrow. Acute inflammatory reactions, as they occur in most other tissues, are rarely recognized. The etiologic bases for the granulomatous disorders are the same as for other organs and include fungi, *Mycobacterium tuberculosis, Mycobacterium avium–intracellulare,* and sarcoidosis. Granulomatous inflammation may also accompany viral infections, lymphomas, and immune disorders.

Granulomas in the marrow are morphologically similar to those in other tissues[35] (Fig. 41-14). The number varies from one to numerous to confluent lesions. Granulomas in patients with mycobacterial infections may be accompanied by a loosely structured, fibrinous necrosis of adjacent marrow. Fungi are usually identified with the periodic acid–Schiff or methenamine silver stains. An unusual type of granuloma, referred to as *ring,* or *donut granuloma,* has been associated with Q fever; however, the finding lacks specificity.[36] The descriptive term relates to a central clear area in the granuloma. In some instances these lesions appear to represent a form of vasculitis. Lipid granulomas are composed of aggregates of lipid-laden macrophages and are frequently associated with well-differentiated lymphocytes. As in other tissues, they have no diagnostic specificity, and their etiologic basis is unknown.

In patients with AIDS, a range of opportunistic pathogens may involve the marrow without causing granuloma formation. In these instances, organisms may be identified in macrophages scattered throughout the marrow interstitium.

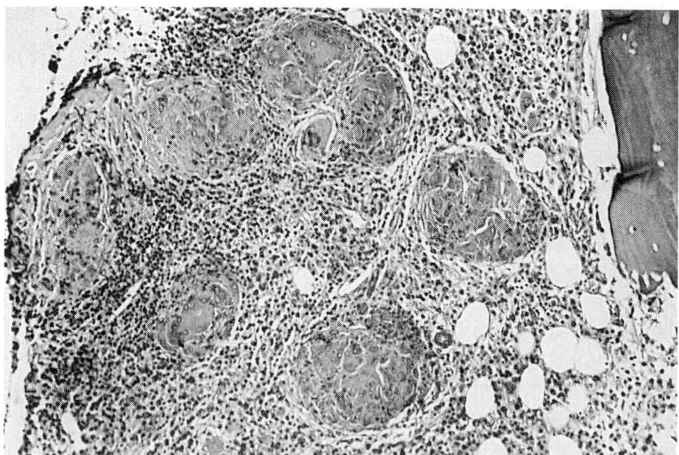

Fig. 41-14 Several confluent granulomas in a marrow biopsy from a patient with sarcoidosis.

A particularly noteworthy manifestation of an infectious process in the marrow is the presence of giant erythroblasts and erythroid hypoplasia in parvovirus B19 infection[29] (see Fig. 41-13). The parvovirus has a predilection for rapidly dividing cells. Infected proerythroblasts may show intranuclear inclusions. Transient erythroid hypoplasia, with which this virus is associated, may lead to a rapid hemoglobin decrease in patients with concurrent hemolytic anemia.

ANEMIAS

Anemias are defined as decreases in the hemoglobin concentration in the blood, which result in decreased oxygen-carrying capacity. The anemias may be classified by the morphologic characteristics of the red blood cells, or the pathophysiologic mechanisms resulting in the anemia. The morphologic classification takes into account both the size and the hemoglobin content of the erythrocytes. The pathophysiologic classification of anemia is a recognition of the basic defect or mechanism leading to anemia. With this classification the anemias can be broadly grouped into those attributable to (1) impaired production of erythrocytes, (2) inherited quantitative and structural abnormalities of hemoglobin synthesis, (3) increased rate of erythrocyte destruction, that is, hemolytic anemias, and (4) acute blood loss. Those attributable to impaired production may be normocytic, microcytic hypochromic, or macrocytic depending on the causative factor. The anemias attributable to an increased rate of destruction or acute blood loss are generally normochromic and normocytic.

Frequently, anemia has more than one cause. Patients with a hemolytic process may develop folic acid deficiency because of increased erythropoiesis and increased folic acid requirements. Anemia in severely ill patients is commonly multifactorial. Patients receiving chemotherapeutic drugs for neoplastic proliferations may have anemia as a result of marrow hypoplasia and abnormal myelopoiesis. The multifactorial nature of anemia is illustrated by the so-called aplastic crisis that occurs in patients with hemolytic anemias who develop parvovirus B19 infections; this viral infection may be associated with severe red blood cell hypoplasia. The combination of an increased rate of red cell destruction and decreased production results in a greatly decreased hemoglobin.

The reticulocyte is a stage of red blood cell maturation normally present in both the marrow and the blood. It is essentially the birth stage of the anucleate red cell and is identified by supravital dyes such as brilliant cresyl blue and new methylene blue, which stain a filamentous network of ribosomes and mitochondria. Reticulocytes account for approximately 1% of red blood cells in hematologically normal individuals. Variations in the number of reticulocytes are a reflection of the marrow response to anemia. The number of reticulocytes is increased in hemolytic anemias and acute blood loss. In the aregenerative anemias, a term frequently used for anemias caused by impaired production, the number of reticulocytes is inappropriately low for the degree of anemia. The number of reticulocytes in the blood after specific hematinic therapy, such as vitamin B_{12} replacement in pernicious anemia, is a measure of bone marrow response to the therapy. The response generally peaks several days after initiation of therapy, and the magnitude of the reticulocytosis is generally proportional to the severity of the anemia.

Anemias caused by impaired production

Decreased production of red blood cells may be attributable to several pathophysiologic mechanisms with marrow cellularity ranging from hypocellular to hypercellular. The major mechanisms are listed in Table 41-2. Some of the inherited anemias, with impaired production resulting from quantitative or structural abnormalities of hemoglobin synthesis such as the thalassemias, also have a hemolytic component. These are described under the category of quantitative and structural abnormalities of hemoglobin synthesis.

Aplastic anemia

Aplastic anemia describes those pancytopenias resulting from marrow hypocellularity where there is a marked decrease or depletion of all the major myeloid cell lines: erythroid precursors, granulocytes, monocytes, and megakaryocytes (see Fig. 41-12). Anemia is only one component of generalized marrow failure. Proposed criteria for aplastic anemia include a hypocellular bone marrow in individuals not being treated with marrow ablative agents or radiation therapy and two of three findings: leukocyte count less than 3.5×10^9/L, platelet count less than 50×10^9 /L, and hemoglobin less than 10g/dL with an absolute reticulocyte count of 30,000/mm^3 or less.[37]

Although aplastic anemia is primarily an acquired disorder, there are rare familial forms, such as Fanconi's anemia and Schwachman syndrome.[38-40] *Fanconi's anemia* is an autosomal recessive disorder in which marrow aplasia usually manifests between 5 and 10 years of age. The disorder may be associated with low birth weight, growth retardation, and cutaneous, skeletal and genitourinary tract abnormalities.[38] Chromosomal studies of the hematopoietic cells show an increased incidence of spontaneous cytogenetic abnormalities, including breakage and endoreduplication; the abnormalities may be accentuated in cells cultured with mitomycin C or diepoxybutane. Patients with Fanconi's anemia are at increased risk for developing acute myeloid leukemia.

Schwachman syndrome is a rare, autosomal recessive disorder characterized by exocrine pancreatic deficiency and various combinations of cytopenias and marrow hypocellularity.[40] Dysplastic changes may be present in myeloid cells with an increase in fetal hemoglobin in some patients. Patients with Schwachman syndrome are usually small physically and have recurrent pulmonary infections, steatorrhea, and failure to thrive.

The reported annual incidence of acquired aplastic anemia varies from an overall rate of 2.2 per million individuals in several European countries and Israel to 7.3 per million nonwhite females in Baltimore.[37,41] The incidence increases over age forty. Acquired aplastic anemias are idiopathic or secondary. The majority of cases are idiopathic because no etiologic basis is identified. In the secondary type, an underlying causative factor such as ionizing radiation, drugs, chemicals, or viral infection is identified. Several viruses have been implicated in aplastic anemia, including the Epstein-Barr virus and all three types of hepatitis virus.[39,42] The response of some patients with idiopathic aplastic anemia to anti-thymocyte globulin indicates a role for the T-lymphocytes in the pathogenesis of some cases. An aplastic marrow phase has been observed with paroxysmal nocturnal hemoglobinuria.

Although several causative factors have been related to the development of marrow aplasia, the common biologic event probably results from damage to the hematopoietic stem cell or the stromal cells of the marrow microenvironment that are integral to hematopoiesis. The success of bone marrow transplantation is evidence that the damaged cells can be replaced. Some patients undergo spontaneous recovery. The reported two year survival rate in 1985 was 49%.[41] The reported survival in 1994 with bone marrow transplantation is 90% to 95%.[43]

Table 41-2 Anemias resulting from impaired production

Aplastic anemia
Pure red blood cell aplasia
Nuclear maturation defects
Cytoplasmic maturation defects
Anemia of chronic disorders

Pure red blood cell aplasia

Pure red blood cell aplasia or hypoplasia is an uncommon cause of anemia which may occur as congenital or acquired disorders.[44] Congenital red cell aplasia, the Diamond Blackfan syndrome, manifests in the first year of life. Approximately 80% of cases are sporadic; the disease also occurs with an autosomal recessive or dominant pattern of inheritance. The anemia is macrocytic; there is a reticulocytopenia. Platelets and leukocytes are usually normal. The marrow shows marked erythroid hypoplasia or aplasia. Erythropoietin levels are increased. The basic defect appears to be due to a failure of response of erythroid precursors to inducers of erythroid proliferation and differentiation.

Transient erythroblastopenia of childhood is a form of red cell hypoplasia in children 1 to 4 years of age without evidence of an underlying cause; it is frequently preceded by a viral-like illness. The disorder is self limited.

A transient erythroid hypoplasia may occur with parvovirus B19 infection and is a frequent cause of "aplastic crisis" in patients with chronic hemolytic anemia. The virus appears to have a predilection for erythroid precursors. The marrow shows marked erythroid hypoplasia with giant proerythroblasts which may show viral inclusions. The period of hypoplasia is usually brief although occasional cases have a chronic course.

Chronic erythroid aplasia/hypoplasia occurs primarily in adults but may also present in children. Causative factors include thymoma, usually of spindle cell type, immune related disorders, and drugs. Thymectomy is usually curative in the thymoma associated cases.

Nuclear maturation defects

The principal nuclear maturation defects are the megaloblastic anemias due to vitamin B_{12} or folic acid deficiency.[45-47] Megaloblastic changes are primarily manifest as asynchronous nuclear and cytoplasmic maturation resulting from inadequate DNA synthesis for nuclear maturation and impaired cell division. Cytoplasmic maturation proceeds unimpaired. The dyssynchronous changes are manifest in all myeloid cells; the changes are exemplified in the red cell series by a large cell, the megaloblast (Fig. 41-15). Although most evident in hematopoietic cells, the impaired DNA synthesis affects dividing cells in every tissue of the body.

Vitamin B_{12}, a member of the cobalamin family, acts as a coenzyme with folic acid in the biochemical pathway for DNA

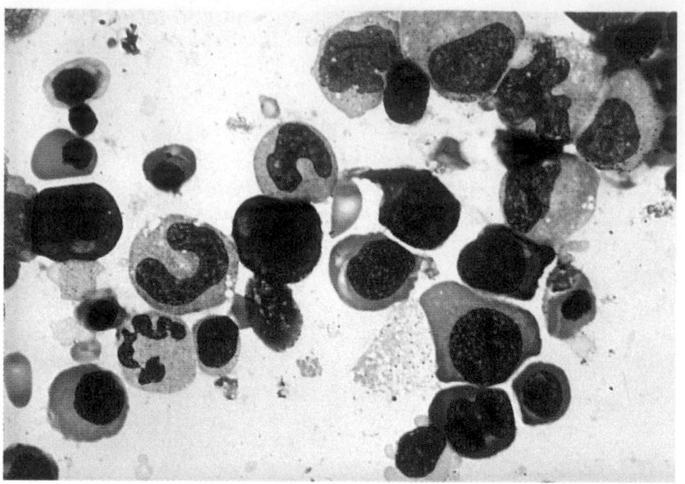

Fig. 41-15 Bone marrow aspirate smear from a patient with pernicious anemia with megaloblastic red cell precursors and giant metamyelocytes. The chromatin in the red blood cell nuclei is more dispersed than in normal red cell precursors at comparable stages of maturation; the giant metamyelocytes have dispersed nuclear chromatin in contrast to a normal metamyelocyte which has condensed chromatin (Wright-Giemsa).

synthesis.[45-47] There is no endogenous production of B_{12} in humans; the major source is the ingestion of animal foodstuffs. The cobalamin is separated from food by peptic digestion at acid pH, following which it binds to R protein (cobalophilin). The cobalamin is separated from the R protein in the duodenum by action of pancreatic enzymes. It then binds to intrinsic factor which is produced by the parietal cells of the cardia and fundus of the stomach. The cobalamin-intrinsic factor complex is absorbed via a specific receptor in the distal ileum. After absorption, the cobalamin is dissociated from intrinsic factor. Ninety percent of the absorbed cobalamin binds to transcobolamin II which transports it to cells throughout the body. Vitamin B_{12} in mammalian cells participates in the synthesis of methionine from homocysteine. Impairment of this reaction leads to decreased amounts of methylene tetrahydrofolate which is a requisite folate coenzyme for the synthesis of DNA. The primary storage sites of vitamin B_{12} are the liver and kidney. Body stores are sufficient to satisfy metabolic requirements for 5 to 7 years.

Folic acid is a pteroylglutamic acid which is present principally in a polyglutamate form in a variety of foods including vegetables, fruit, dairy products and cereals. It is absorbed primarily in the jejunum following conversion of the polyglutamate form to monoglutamate by folate hydrolase.[45-47] Folic acid in serum is principally in the form of methyltetrahydrofolate. Cellular uptake appears to be related to a high affinity binding protein on the cell membrane. Intracellular folate is in the polyglutamate form. Tetrahydrofolate, in its reduced form, participates in one carbon metabolism by coupling one carbon fragments. Methylene tetrahydrofolate which results from this process is required for the conversion of deoxyuridylate to thymidylate which appears to be a rate-limiting reaction in DNA synthesis. The liver is a major site of folate storage. In contrast to vitamin B_{12}, in which stores are sufficient to meet metabolic requirements for 5 to 7 years, body stores of folic acid are sufficient to meet metabolic requirements for only a few months.

Pernicious anemia (PA) is the prototypic megaloblastic anemia related to B_{12} deficiency. It is generally a disease of middle age or older individuals, and although it may occur in all racial groups, is more common in those of northern European ancestry. Pernicious anemia is associated with deficient gastric secretions due to gastric mucosal atrophy, atrophic gastritis. The gastric atrophy involves the parietal cells which are the source of intrinsic factor. Autoimmunity appears to have a major role in the pathogenesis of the disorder. Approximately 60% to 90% of patients with PA have serum parietal cell antibodies; 50% to 70% have antibodies to intrinsic factor in the serum or in gastric secretion or both. Pernicious anemia may occur in association with other autoimmune disorders such as thyroid disease, vitiligo, and diabetes mellitus. It is associated with an increased incidence of gastric cancer.

B_{12} deficiency can result from surgical procedures such as resection of the parietal cell–containing areas of the stomach and small bowel resection involving the terminal ileum. Other disease processes involving these anatomic sites may also be causative factors. Because B_{12} deficiency may develop gradually, over an extended period, the patient may adjust physiologically to very low hemoglobin levels.

An important clinical feature of pernicious anemia is the neurologic syndrome of subacute combined degeneration of the spinal cord, a demyelination process involving the dorsal and lateral columns of the cord. Gait disturbances and diminished proprioception result. Some patients have difficulties in mentation; occasional patients present with psychiatric disturbances. The hematologic and neurologic abnormalities are reversed with vitamin B_{12} therapy.

Juvenile pernicious anemia manifests in the first to fifth year of life and is marked by megaloblastic anemia, retarded growth, and neurologic abnormalities. Unlike PA in adults, the gastric mucosa is normal and there are no antibodies to intrinsic factor. The underlying abnormality in juvenile PA includes both failure to produce intrinsic factor and the production of functionally inactive intrinsic factor.[48]

Inherited disorders of cobolamin transport and metabolism are rare causes of megaloblastic anemia. These may be associated with retarded growth and neurologic abnormalities.[48] Macrocytic anemia and megaloblastosis are also a component of hereditary orotic aciduria and hypoxanthine phosphoribosyltransferase deficiency (Lesch-Nyhan syndrome), which are rare disorders of purine and pyrimidine metabolism.[49]

Megaloblastic anemia due to folic acid deficiency is usually the result of severe nutritional deprivation, but may also result from defects in intestinal absorption, such as may occur with sprue syndromes.[45-47] Surgical resection of the jejunum may also lead to deficiency of this vitamin.

The megaloblastic anemias are basically panmyelopathies and abnormalities are present in the erythroid cells, neutrophils, and megakaryocytes. In addition to anemia, patients with uncomplicated megaloblastic anemia usually have neutropenia and thrombocytopenia; marked pancytopenia may be present. The anemia may be severe, with hemoglobin levels of 3-4g/dL, and is macrocytic with a mean corpuscular volume (MCV) usually in the range of 100 to 140 μm^3. Varying degrees of red blood cell anisopoikilocytosis are present with macroovalocytes and dacryocytes; basophilic stippling and Howell-Jolly bodies may be present in erythrocytes in the blood smear. In severe anemia, megaloblasts may be present in the blood. Large neutrophils with hypersegmented nuclei, frequently six to eight lobes, referred to as macropolycytes, are also present.

In megaloblastic anemia the erythroid cells are large with nuclear chromatin that is more dispersed than appropriate for the level of cytoplasmic maturation, i.e., nuclear cytoplasmic asynchrony (Fig. 41-15). The changes are present at all levels of maturation, but are most obvious in the polychromatic and orthochromatic stages. Nuclear lobation and karyorrhexis may be present. The characteristic neutrophil change is the giant metamyelocyte, a large neutrophil precursor with a somewhat horseshoe-shaped nucleus which has a more dispersed chromatin than a normal metamyelocyte (Fig. 41-15). The marrow is markedly hypercellular. The megakaryocytes are frequently hyperlobated and large in size.

The distinction between B_{12} and folate deficiency is based on the determination of B_{12} and folic acid. In pernicious anemia, the serum B_{12} level is reduced. In folic acid deficiency both the serum and red blood cell folate concentrations are reduced. Because of intramedullary destruction of erythroid precursors, ineffective erythropoiesis, the serum bilirubin is elevated as are other indicators of increased red cell destruction. Serum levels of lactic acid dehydrogenase are frequently markedly elevated due principally to an increase in lactic acid dehydrogenase isoenzymes 1 and 2.[45,47] Methylmalonic acid is markedly increased in vitamin B_{12} deficiency.

In the uncomplicated cases of B_{12} or folic acid deficiency, the hematologic abnormalities normalize with appropriate therapy. Patients with vitamin B_{12} deficiency will respond hematologically to pharmacologic doses of folic acid; however, the neurologic abnormalities persist emphasizing the importance of appropriate diagnosis.

Cytoplasmic maturation defect

Cytoplasmic maturation defects of the red blood cells have as an unifying feature decreased synthesis of hemoglobin. This may result from decreased polypeptide chain production, as occurs in the thalassemia syndromes, or from disturbances in the production of the heme portion of the hemoglobin molecule. A frequent cause of decreased heme synthesis is iron deficiency. Less common are the disorders collectively referred to as the sideroblastic anemias, which are discussed in the section on myelodysplastic syndromes.

Iron deficiency anemia. The normal body iron stores are approximately 4 to 5 g in adult males (50 mg/kg body weight) and 2.5 to 3 g in adult females (35 mg/kg); approximately 80% of this iron is present in the hemoglobin molecule.[46,50] The remaining iron is in storage form in hepatocytes and the monocyte/macrophage system of the spleen, liver, and bone marrow. Approximately half of the storage iron is in the form of ferritin, a protein-iron complex; the remainder is stored as hemosiderin. Small amounts of iron are present in heme enzymes and attached to the transport protein, transferrin.

Dietary intake of iron is approximately 10 to 18 mg per day. Ten percent is absorbed, approximately 0.6 to 1.0 mg/day in males and 1 to 2 mg per day in females. Total body iron in normal individuals is maintained at constant levels by regulating iron absorption to parallel iron loss. Iron is absorbed in the proximal duodenum in the ferrous form and then transported to the erythroid precursors in the marrow and storage sites by the transport protein, transferrin, a beta globulin synthesized by the liver. Transferrin has two binding sites to which the iron is tightly attached. After transfer across the red blood cell membrane, iron combines with protoporphyrin 9 to form heme, which then combines with two alpha polypeptide chains and two beta polypeptide chains to form hemoglobin.

Iron deficiency anemia is the most common form of anemia worldwide. The incidence varies in different geographic areas and generally correlates with nutritional deprivation. In countries with adequate food supplies, the incidence is relatively low, with most cases occurring in women of child-bearing age due to inadequate intake and excessive menstrual blood loss. In men and postmenopausal women, iron deficiency usually reflects blood loss from abnormal bleeding sites such as ulcers, polyps, or carcinoma in the genitourinary and gastrointestinal tracts.

Iron deficiency is a continuum of negative iron balance. The initial manifestation is transfer of iron from the storage sites to satisfy daily metabolic requirements; with continuing loss, iron stores are depleted, leading to the next stage, iron-deficient erythropoiesis. The end result of continued negative iron balance is microcytic, hypochromic anemia.

The laboratory parameters of iron deficiency include low concentration of serum iron and ferritin, increased iron-binding protein, transferrin, which has a low percent saturation, usually less than 16%, and elevated free erythrocyte protoporphyrin. The status of the body iron stores can be assessed directly by bone marrow biopsy and staining for iron, or by the serum ferritin, which indirectly reflects the body iron stores. Ferritin levels of less than 12 ng/ml are indicative of iron deficiency. The bone marrow shows no storage iron and decreased numbers of sideroblasts, less than 20% of the nucleated red blood cells. Red blood cell precursors are normal or slightly increased in number.

Anemia of chronic disease

Anemia of chronic disease (ACD) is an acquired anemia occurring in patients with infectious, inflammatory, or malignant diseases and is associated with a decrease in serum iron and an increase in reticuloendothelial storage iron.[51,52] The pathogenesis of ACD is complex; erythrocyte survival is slightly decreased, but there is inadequate erythroid response in the marrow. The etiology of bone marrow dysfunction is uncertain; diminished erythropoietin production, impaired marrow response to erythropoietin, and inadequate transfer of iron from the reticulendothelial cells to developing erythrocytes have all been implicated.[53,54] The anemia is usually mild and normochromic, normocytic; more severe anemia with a hematocrit less than 25%, microcytosis, and hypochromasia may occur.[55] The serum iron and iron-binding protein, transferrin, are both decreased; the percent saturation of transferrin is frequently between 15 and 20, which is a threshold value between normal and decreased. This differs from iron deficiency anemia in which the decreased serum iron is accompanied by increased iron-binding protein. Serum ferritin is frequently elevated in ACD. Iron stains of bone marrow aspirates show increased deposition of iron in histiocytes and a decreased number of sideroblasts, less than 20% of nucleated red blood cell precursors.

Anemias caused by inherited disorders of hemoglobin synthesis

Inherited disorders of hemoglobin synthesis include the quantitative abnormalities in globin chain production, which are the thalassemias, and the structural globin chain variants such as Hb C, E, S, Lepore and Constant Spring (Table 41-3).

Hemoglobin is a tetrameric protein bound to four organometallic heme units (Fig. 41-16).[56] The protein portion consists of two pairs of related polypeptide globin chains, α,β,δ,γ,ε, and ζ, held together by relatively weak van der Waal's forces. Each of the four polypeptide chains forms a "pocket" in which the ferroporphyrin unit, heme, resides.[57] The heme portion of the complex is composed of a ferrous ion chelated to a non-peptide, organic protoporphyrin 9 ring.

The main function of hemoglobin is oxygen transport; the efficiency of this is reflected in the hemoglobin oxygen affinity curve. This unusual sigmoidal curve is a function of intrinsic and extrinsic factors (Fig. 41-17).[58] Intrinsic factors include the overall heterotetrameric structure of hemoglobin, the composition of the globin units surrounding the heme ring, and the amino acid residues in contact with the porphoryin ring. Extrinsic factors include pH and 2,3-diphosphoglycerate (2,3-DPG) concentration of the red blood cell. Under physiologic conditions, the oxygen affinity of embryonic and fetal (Hb F) hemoglobins is greater than that of adult hemoglobin, Hb A, an effect largely due to the increased sensitivity of Hb A to 2,3-DPG.[59]

Table 41-3 Inherited disorders of hemoglobin synthesis

Quantitative
β-Thalassemia
α-Thalassemia
δβ-Thalassemia
Hereditary persistence of fetal hemoglobin
Structural
Hemoglobin S
Hemoglobin C
Quantitative/Structural
Hemoglobin E
Hemoglobin Lepore
Hemoglobin Constant Spring

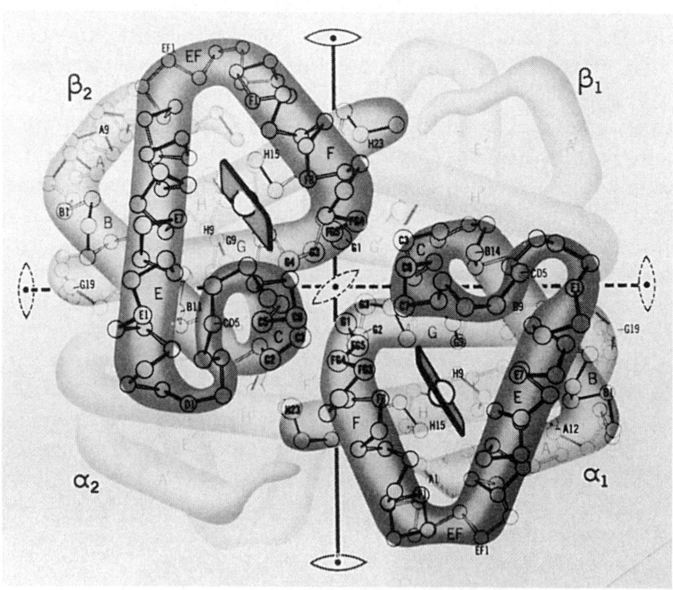

Fig. 41-16 Diagram of tetrameric structure of adult hemoglobin (Hb A; α2β2). One α and one β chain each with a heme subunit (rectangles) are highlighted. (From Dickerson RE, Geis I: *Hemoglobin: structure, function, evolution, and pathology,* Menlo Park, Calif., 1983, Benjamin/Cummings.)

Globin chain gene expression changes sequentially through gestation. The changes follow the linear sequence of the globin chain genes on the respective chromosomes (Fig. 41-18).[57] The genes encoding α and ζ chains are located on chromosome 16 and the genes for the ε, γ, δ and β chains on chromosome 11. The ζ and ε genes are the 5′ most globin genes of their respective chromosomes and are the first globin genes to be expressed in the developing embryo. This is suceeded by α and γ gene expression. The last developmental switch occurs on chromosome 11 with the change in production from γ to β and δ chains. This corresponds to the switch in production of Hb F to Hb A and HbA_2, respectively. The exact mechanism controlling these switching events is unknown.

The type of hemoglobin synthesized depends on the relative proportions of the six different globin chains produced (Fig. 41-18). The first hemoglobins synthesized are at 5 weeks of gestation and are Gower 1 (ζ2ε2), Gower 2 (α2ε2) and Hemoglobin Portland (ζ2γ2). Concentrations of these hemoglobins decrease as globin chain synthesis switches from ζ and ε to α and γ, resulting in increasing fetal hemoglobin levels (Hb F: α2γ2). This globin chain switch coincides with the onset of hepatic hematopoiesis. By the second trimester, Hb F accounts for more than 90% of hemoglobin. The remainder is adult hemoglobin (Hb A, α2β2) which is the product of a small population of β chain- producing erythroid precursors. Between the 30th week of gestation and the 12th postnatal week, β chain producing normoblasts expressing Hb A become the predominant population. This conversion coincides with a shift to medullary hematopoiesis. Hb F production declines to about 1 to 2% of total hemoglobin by the first year of post-natal life. Delta chain synthesis begins in the third

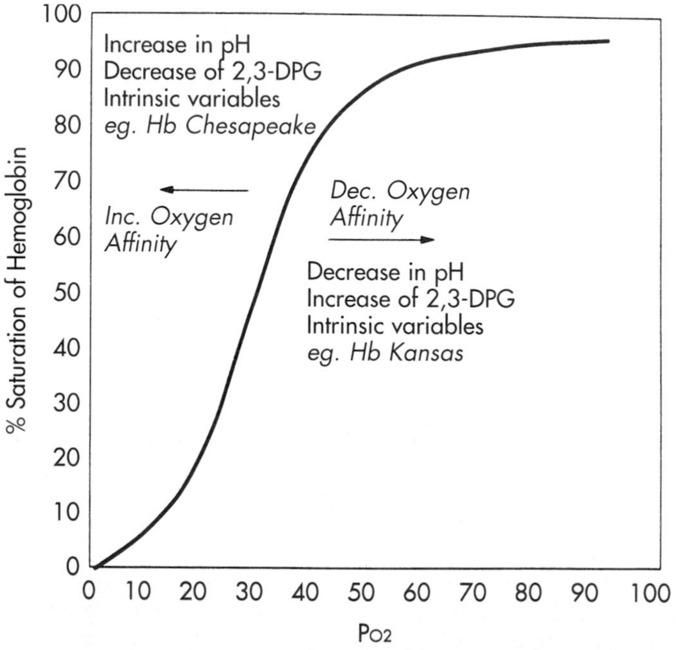

Fig. 41-17 Oxygen affinity curve for adult hemoglobin. Parameters affecting the curve and hemoglobin oxygen affinity are illustrated. Examples are given. (Modified from Steinberg MH, Benz EJ: Hemoglobin synthesis, structure, and function. In Hoffman R, Benz EJ, Shattil SJ, Furie B, Cohen HJ, editors: *Hematology: basic principles and practice,* New York, 1991, Churchill-Livingstone.)

trimester and gradually increases during the first year of life combining with α chains to produce Hb A_2 (α2δ2). After this time it accounts for 1.5% to 3.5% of the total hemoglobin. The composition of hemoglobin after the first year of life remains stable and consists of Hb A (>95%), Hb A_2 (<3.5%) and Hb F (<1%).

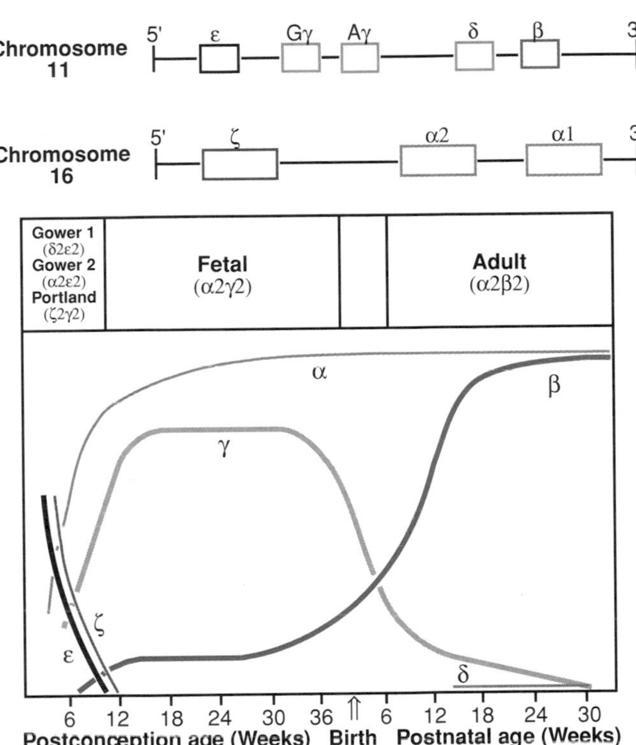

Fig. 41-18 Genomic orientation and temporal expression patterns of globin chain genes. Globin genes are shown as boxes on the respective chromosomes in the upper panel. Temporal patterns of globin gene expression and hemoglobin production are shown in lower panel. (Modified from Weatherall DJ, Clegg JB, Higgs DR, Wood WG: The hemoglobinopathies. In Scriver CR, Beaudet AL, Sly WS, Valle D, editors: *The metabolic basis of inherited disorders,* ed 6, New York, 1989, McGraw-Hill.)

Thalassemias

The thalassemias are inherited disorders of reduced globin chain synthesis that result in unbalanced erythrocytic concentrations of the globin components of hemoglobin. These defects result from perturbations in globin chain mRNA production.[57,60] The clinical manifestations vary from asymptomatic to lethal, depending on the defective globin chain type and the degree of reduction in globin chain production. Common to all thalassemias is a decreased mean corpuscular hemoglobin (MCH) and mean corpuscular volume (MCV) due to the primary defect in hemoglobin synthesis. Shortened red blood cell survival results from the deposition of unpaired globin chain precipitates on the red cell membrane. Thalassemias are classified by the deficient globin chain: α thalassemia represents a deficiency of α globin production and β thalassemia, deficient β globin production. Subclassification of the thalassemias has historically been based on clinical severity (Table 41-4 and 41-5). The three types of β thalassemia are major, intermedia, and minor. The four clinical types of α thalassemia are Hb Bart's hydrops fetalis syndrome, Hb H disease, α thalassemia trait, and the silent carrier state.

β-Thalassemia. The most common molecular genetic basis for β thalassemia is point mutation on chromosome 11 involving a regulatory region of the β globin gene affecting transcriptional promoter regions, RNA splice sites, and the polyadenylation signal site. Deletions of portions of the β globin gene have been described but are less common.[61] These genetic defects result in deficient transcription, processing, or intracellular transport of β globin mRNA, ultimately leading to deficient β globin chain polypeptide production. The severity of the deficiency depends on the specific mutation. The clinical manifestations of β thalassemia occur after birth, coinciding with the switch from unimpaired γ to impaired β chain production. The low cytoplasmic concentration of γ and β globin chains results in unpaired α chains. The tendency of these intracytoplasmic free α chains to polymerize into insoluble precipitates on the red blood cell membranes produces most of the clinical symptomatology. Once formed, these precipitates cause unusual cellular rigidity leading to increased intramedullary destruction of red cell precursors, ineffective erythropoiesis. These precipitates also lead to premature splenic destruction of the circulating red blood cells. The ineffective erythropoiesis, splenic-based hemolysis, and primary deficiency in hemoglobin production all contribute to the anemia,

Table 41-4 Genotypes, hemoglobin composition, and ethnic origin of major subtypes of β thalassemias

Subtype	Major ethnic origin*	Hemoglobin g/dL	Common genotypes	Significant hemoglobin electrophoresis findings†
Major	A,M	<5	β°/β° β°/β^+ β^+/β^+	Hb A 0-50% Hb F 50-98%
Intermedia	A,M,AF	5-10	Diverse	Variable
Minor	A,M,AF	10-12	β°/β β^+/β	Hb A2 4-9% Hb F 1-5%

*A, Equatorial Asia; *M,* Mediterranean basin; *AF,* Equatorial Africa

†Adult values derived from Weatherall DJ, Clegg JB, Higgs DR, Wood WG: The hemoglobinopathies. In Scriver CR, Beaudet AL, Sly WS, Valle D, editors: *The metabolic basis of inherited disease,* ed 6, New York, 1989, McGraw-Hill; Fairbanks VF: *Hemoglobinopathies and thalassemias: laboratory methods and case studies,* New York, 1980, Thieme.

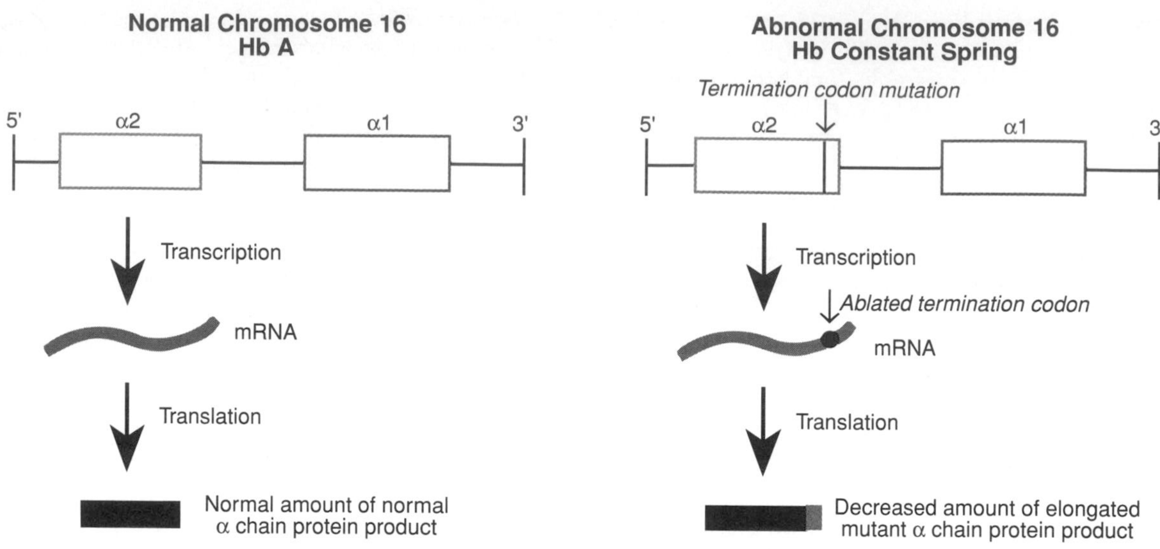

Fig. 41-19 Schematic representation of the molecular pathogenesis of Hemoglobin Constant Spring.

the degree of which depends on the severity of the globin chain imbalance.[57] Morbidity and mortality in severely affected individuals relate to hemosiderosis resulting from repeated transfusions. The major laboratory findings are listed in Table 41-4. Hemoglobin electrophoresis is necessary for diagnosis of this disease.

In β thalassemia major, the red blood cells show marked anisopoikilocytosis and are microcytic and hypochromic. Target cells, basophilic stippling, and Pappenheimer bodies (siderotic granules) are present. The marrow shows marked erythroid hyperplasia. The changes in β thalassemia minor may be subtle and are characterized by microcytosis, minimal hypochromasia, and basophilic stippling. Iron stores are normal to increased.

α-Thalassemia. In contrast to the DNA point mutations responsible for β thalassemia, deficient α chain mRNA production results in most cases from the deletion of one or both α globin genes on chromosome 16 producing the α^+ (- α) or α^o (- -) haplotypes, respectively (Table 41-5). There are, however, notable exceptions to this "deletion rule" such as the thalassemic hemoglobinopathy, Hb Constant Spring, which is due to point mutation (Fig. 41-19).[60]

Alpha thalassemia begins in the fetus with the switch from unimpaired ζ to impaired α globin chain synthesis. As the total concentration of α and ζ globin chains decreases, the excess unbound γ and β chains form the semi-soluble tetramers, Hb Bart's (γ4) and Hb H (β4), that precipitate in and damage only senescent red blood cells. Anemia results from impaired hemoglobin synthesis and increased splenic-based hemolysis.

Hemoglobin Bart's hydrops fetalis syndrome is the most severe form of α thalassemia. This syndrome initially manifests *in utero* and is associated with the absence of α chain production. It is nearly always due to the inheritance of two α^o (- -) genes, resulting in the complete deletion of the α chain genes. As ζ chain synthesis subsides, Hb Portland (ζ2γ2) is replaced by the high oxygen affinity hemoglobins, Bart's (γ4) and H (β4), which produce severe fetal hypoxia with resulting cardiac failure and anasarca. Hepatosplenomegaly, pronounced extramedullary hematopoiesis and placental enlargement are virtually always present. Death usually occurs either

Table 41-5 Genotypes, hemoglobin composition, and ethnic origin of major subtypes of α thalassemias

Subtype	Major ethnic origin	Hemoglobin g/dL	Common genotypes	Significant hemoglobin electrophoresis findings†
Hb Bart's Hydrops Fetalis	A,M	3 to 10	—/—	Hb Bart's 100%‡
Hb H	A,M	2.6 to 12.4	—/—α	Hb F 10%‡ Hb H 10-15%
Trait or Silent Carrier	A,M,AF	10 to 14	—/αα -α/αα -α/-α	Normal‡

A, Equatorial Asia; *M*, Mediterranean basin; *AF*, equatorial Africa

†Adult values derived from Weatherall DJ, Clegg JB, Higgs DR, Wood WG: The hemoglobinopathies. In Scriber CR, Beaudet AL, Sly WS, Valle D, editors: *The metabolic basis of inherited disease*, ed 6, New York, 1989, McGraw-Hill; Fairbanks VF: *Hemoglobinopathies and thalassemias: laboratory methods and case studies*, New York, 1980, Thieme.

‡Hb Bart's in varying amounts may be seen in all α thalassemias in newborn period (see text).

in utero between 30 to 40 weeks gestation or shortly after birth. This disease is prevalent in populations of Southeast Asian and Mediterranean origin and is a common cause of stillbirth in the former group (Table 41-5).

Structural hemoglobin variants

Structural hemoglobin variants result from globin gene mutation and have electrophoretic mobilities distinct from HbA. These hemoglobins may be associated with hematologic findings of thalassemia or hemolytic anemia.

Structural hemoglobin variants resembling thalassemia The structural hemoglobin variants associated with thalassemia are characterized by a mutation in one of the globin chain genes of Hb A. An electrophoretically distinct globin chain is synthesized in decreased amounts resulting in a globin chain imbalance with clinical and hematologic findings of thalassemia. Examples of this are Hb E, Hb Constant Spring, and Hb Lepore (Table 41-6).

Hb E is a variant where a point mutation in the β chain gene leads to the substitution of lysine for glutamine at amino acid 26 of the β globin molecule.[62] The mutation leads to decreased β chain synthesis and a hemoglobin that has a different electrophoretic mobility from Hb A on cellulose acetate gel.[63] Homozygotes for Hb E generally manifest a mild microcytic anemia with numerous target cells and show 99% Hb E; the balance is Hb F. Heterozygotes are asymptomatic with normal hemoglobin levels. The red cells are microcytic. Hemoglobin electrophoresis shows approximately 30% Hb E.

Hb Lepore results from a hybrid globin gene consisting of the 5′ portion of the δ globin gene and the 3′ portion of the β globin gene (Fig. 41-20).[59] The hybrid globin gene produces small amounts of a δ/β fusion protein. Hb Lepore (α2δβLepore2) has an electrophoretic mobility distinct from Hb A (α2β2). Homozygotes for Hb Lepore generally have a severe anemia resembling β thalassemia major or intermedia. Heterozygotes for Hb Lepore have a mild microcytic anemia; electrophoresis shows 10% to 15% Hb Lepore and 2% to 10% Hb F.[63]

Hemoglobin Constant Spring results from a mutation in the termination codon of one α chain gene producing a polypeptide chain that is 31 amino acids longer than the normal α chain (Fig. 41-19).[64] The aberrant α chain is synthesized in low amount. Heterozygotes have no or a mild microcytic anemia. Electrophoresis shows approximately 1% Hb Constant Spring. Double heterozygotes for Hb Constant Spring gene and α thalessemia gene manifest symptomatology of Hb H disease. Electrophoresis is identical to Hb H disease except for the presence of 1% to 5% Hb Constant Spring.

Structural hemoglobin variants associated with hemolysis The structural hemoglobin variants associated with hemolytic anemia are characterized by the presence of a mutant hemoglobin which results from an amino acid substitution. HbS and HbC are the most common disorders of this type.

Hemoglobin S ($\alpha 2\beta^s 2$) results from a mutation in the sixth codon of the β chain gene on chromosome 11 leading to the substitution of a valine for a glutamic acid.[65,66] It is the most common hemoglobin variant in the United States; 8% of African-Americans are heterozygotes and 0.2%, homozygotes.[67] The gene is rare in individuals of other ethnic backgrounds (Table 41-6).

When high concentrations of Hb S deoxygenate in the microvasculature, an insoluble Hb gel forms leading to the characteristic red cell sickling (Fig. 41-21).[57] This shape change hinders passage through the microvasculature and may result in vasoocclusion with tissue ischemia. Red cell sickling depends on several variables. In general, decreased pH, low pO_2, and high ionic strength promote sickling. Such conditions exist in the spleen and renal medulla and these sites frequently undergo infarction in patients homozygous for Hb S leading to autosplenectomy and renal papillary necrosis. Hb F inhibits Hb S gel formation and sickling. Individuals who coinherit hereditary persistence of fetal hemoglobin and HbS generally exhibit mild or no symptoms of sickle cell anemia.

Homozygotes for Hb S have hemoglobin levels between 7 and 11 g/dL. Repeated vasoocclusive events in these patients result in myocardial, hepatic and skeletal damage. Infection is the major cause of death. Aplastic crisis may result from viral infections, such as parvovirus B19, leading to marrow erythroid hypoplasia and severe anemia.[68] Heterozygotes are hematologically normal.

Hemoglobin C ($\alpha 2\beta^c 2$) results from a mutation in the sixth codon of the β globin gene leading to a substitution of lysine

Table 41-6 Mutations, genotype, and ethnic origin of common structural hemoglobin variants

Disease	Mutation (chain)	Mutation (protein)*	Genotype	Ethnic Origin	Prevalence†
Hb S	β	6 Glu→Val	S/S	African	0.14% of African-Americans
Hb C	β	6 Glu→Lys	C/C	West African	0.02% of African-Americans
Hb SC	β	6 Glu→Val/6 Glu→Lys	S/C	West African	0.13% of African-Americans
Hb E	β	26 Glu→Lys	E/E	Southeast Asian	15-30% in Southeast Asian populations
Hb Lepore	β	δβ Deletion/fusion	See text	Italian and Greek	Infrequent
Hb Constant Spring	α	α Termination codon ablation	See text	Southeast Asian	3% in some Southeast Asian populations

*Number indicates the amino acid residue of globin chain; left hand abbreviations indicate normally present amino acid and right hand abbreviations show amino acid present in disease state.

†From Fairbanks VF: *Hemoglobinopathies and thalassemias: laboratory methods and case studies:* New York, 1980, Brian C. Decker, Inc; Schwartz E, Benz EJ: The thalassemia syndromes. In Hoffman R, Benz EJ, Shattil SJ, Furie B, Cohen HJ, editors: *Hematology: basic principles and practice,* New York, 1991, Churchill-Livingstone; Schneider RG et al: Abnormal hemoglobins in a quarter million people, *Blood* 48: 629, 1976.

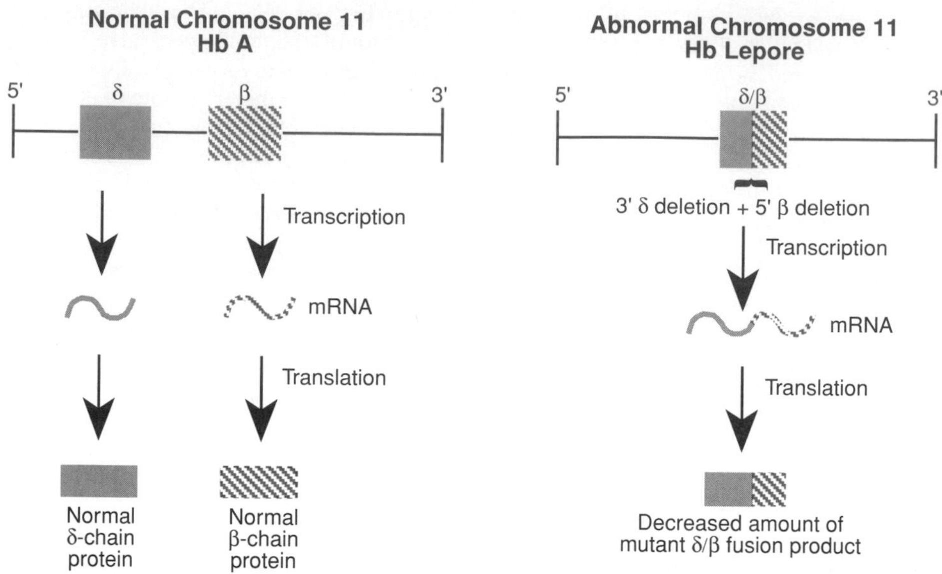

Fig. 41-20 Schematic representation of the molecular pathogenesis of Hemoglobin Lepore.

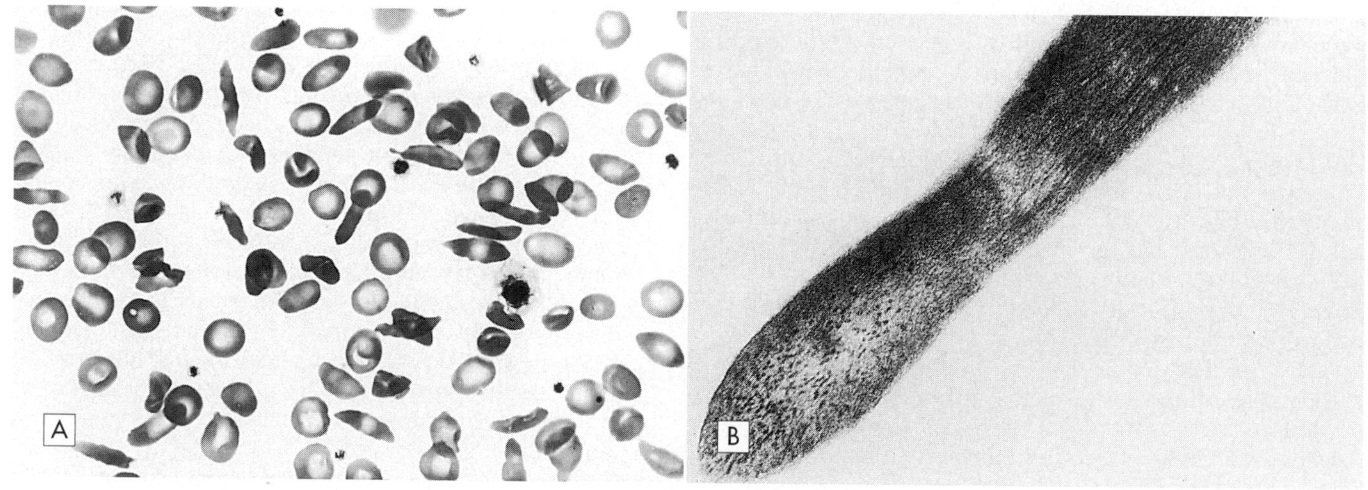

Fig. 41-21 Hemoglobin S light microscopic and ultrastructural findings **A,** Sickle shaped red cells characteristic of Hemoglobin S (Wright-Giemsa.) **B,** Transmission electron micrograph of deoxygenated, polymerized Hemoglobin S (X50,000). (Courtesy Dr. C. Rozman. From Rozman C et al: *Cell ultrastructure for hematologists,* Barcelona, 1993, Ediciones Doyma, S.A.)

for a glutamic acid. Overall, 2.4% of African-Americans are heterozygous and 0.02% are homozygous for Hb C. Double heterozygotes for HbS (b^s) and Hb C (b^c) genes are found in 0.13% of African-Americans (Table 41-6).[69]

Hb C has a tendency to form rhomboid intraerythrocytic crystals that increase hemolysis (Fig. 41-22).[57] Hb F inhibits Hb C crystal formation. Homozygotes have a hemoglobin level of 8 to 12 g/dL. Target cells predominate. Heterozygotes have no anemia, but 10% to 30% of red blood cells are target cells.

Double heterozygotes for Hb S and Hb C have a mild hemolytic anemia with hemoglobin levels of 11 to 13 g/dL and a mild reticulocytosis. Pseudo-sickled cells and elongated red cells with rhomboid crystals may be present in blood smears.

Hemolytic anemias

The hemolytic anemias are due to an increased rate of erythrocyte destruction. These anemias are generally normocytic, normochromic; there is an increased number of polychromatic erythrocytes in the blood reflecting increased input of young red blood cells into the blood in response to the increased rate of destruction. In the bone marrow, there is hyperplasia of the erythroid precursors. Blood tests reveal elevated lactic acid dehydrogenase, increased unconjugated bilirubin and carboxyhemoglobin, and decreased serum haptoglobin concentration, a hemoglobin-binding protein.

The site of destruction of the red blood cells in the hemolytic anemias may be intravascular or extravascular. The latter occurs via macrophages, primarily in the spleen and liver. The site of destruction in the hemolytic anemias due to

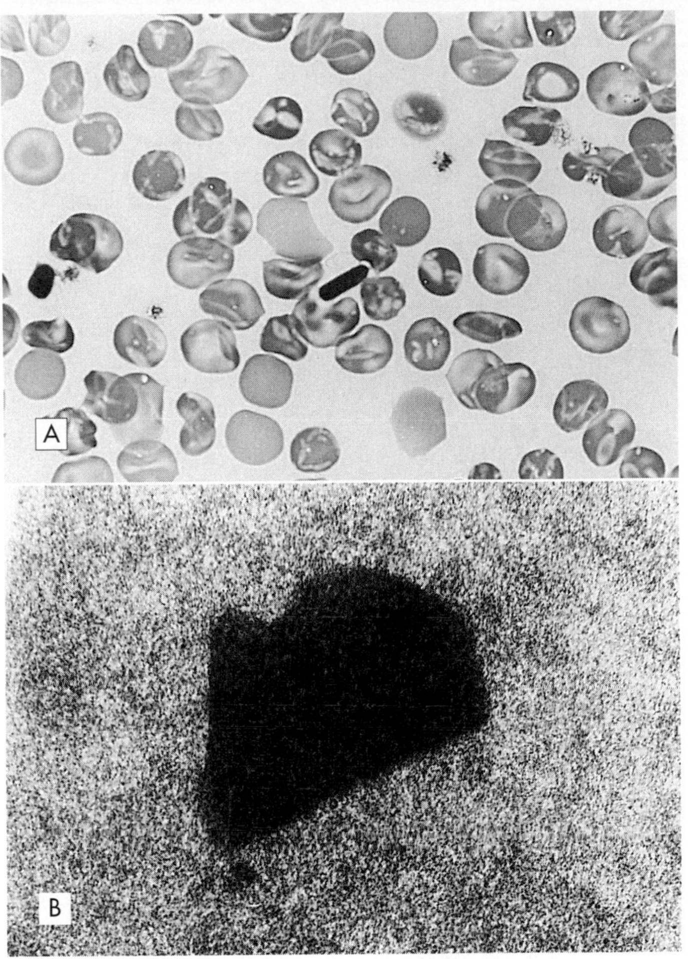

Fig. 41-22 Hemoglobin C: Light microscopic and ultrastructural findings. **A,** Red cells showing intraerythrocytic rhomboid crystals of Hemoglobin C (Wright-Giemsa). (Courtesy of Virginia L. Kubic, M.D., Hennepin County Medical Center, Minneapolis, Minn). **B,** Transmission electron micrograph of Hemoglobin C crystals. (Courtesy of Dr. C. Rozman. From Rozman C, Woessner S, Feliu E, Lafuente R, Berga LI: *Cell ultrastructure for hematologists,* Barcelona, 1993, Ediciones Doyma, S.A.)

the major cytoskeletal defects is primarily the fixed macrophage system of the spleen. As a result, splenectomy is beneficial in these patients. Hemolysis due to red blood cell enzyme defects and microangiopathic type are primarily intravascular. Severe intravascular hemolytic anemias are accompanied by hemoglobinemia, hemoglobinuria, and hemosiderinuria. The major categories of anemias due to an increased rate of destruction are listed in Table 41-7.

Table 41-7 Anemias caused by increased erythrocyte destruction*

Cytoskeletal defects
Enzymatic defects
Immune mediated
Microangiopathic
Paroxysmal nocturnal hemoglobinuria

*Hemolytic anemias caused by structural hemoglobin variants are excluded.

Anemias associated with erythrocyte cytoskeletal defects

The major forms of inherited cytoskeletal abnormalities are clinically classified by the predominant red cell shape: hereditary spherocytosis (HS), hereditary elliptocytosis (HE), and hereditary pyropoikilocytosis (HPP) (Table 41-8).[70-75]

The components of the erythrocyte membrane cytoskeleton are illustrated in Fig. 41-23. The major proteins, α and β spectrin, constitute a flexible scaffold, which is held together and anchored to the membrane via attachment to ankyrin, actin, band 3 protein, protein 4.1, adducin and glycophorin C.[70,71] Both quantitative and qualitative abnormalities, especially those affecting contact sites between these proteins, may lead to an unstable cytoskeleton and shortened erythrocyte survival.

Common hereditary spherocytosis (HS) is usually an autosomal dominant disorder characterized by slight to moderately severe hemolytic anemia usually associated with splenomegaly. The rare cases due to recessive inheritance are generally associated with more severe disease. The spherical shape of the erythrocytes is acquired in the circulation following dissociation of membrane lipids from the unstable cytoskeleton leading to a decreased surface area to volume ratio.[70,71] Spherocytes are rigid, slowing passage through the splenic red pulp, leading to premature destruction.

The anemia is usually mild with hemoglobin levels in the range of 12 to 13g/dL. The mean corpuscular hemoglobin concentration (MCHC) is elevated in approximately half of the patients.[72] Spherocytes may be difficult to identify in the blood smear. The osmotic fragility test is a sensitive assay for detection of spherocytes. The osmotic lysis of spherocytes is a reflection of the decreased surface area to volume ratio and not the primary cytoskeletal instability. In HS, there is commonly a population of hypersensitive erythrocytes that have been conditioned by the spleen.[73] The sensitivity of the test is increased by preincubation of affected red blood cells at 37° C for 24 hours. The increased sensitivity of the "incubated osmotic fragility" results from the accelerated metabolic depletion of HS erythrocytes and may be necessary to detect the abnormal red blood cells in up to 25% of cases of HS.[72] *Aplastic crisis* in patients with hereditary spherocytosis is usually due to normoblast hypoplasia resulting in severely uncompensated hemolysis; parvovirus B19 infection may be a causative agent.[29]

Common hereditary elliptocytosis (HE) is an autosomal dominant disorder. Elliptocytes generally constitute more than 25% of the erythrocytes.[70,71] Affected patients are usually asymptomatic and have a normal hemoglobin; there may be mild, compensated chronic hemolysis. The elliptical shape is acquired after release from the marrow. Mutations have been identified in multiple genes, including the spectrin genes, impairing the formation of spectrin dimers and tetramers, and in the protein 4.1 gene, affecting spectrin or actin binding.[71,74]

Hereditary pyropoikilocytosis (HPP) is usually inherited as an autosomal recessive disorder and is regarded as a severe form of hereditary elliptocytosis.[74] In HPP, lysis of erythrocytes occurs rapidly at 44-46° C in contrast to normal erythrocytes which lyse at 49° C.[70,73] Red blood cell changes similar to those

Table 41-8 Differential diagnosis of common poikilocytes

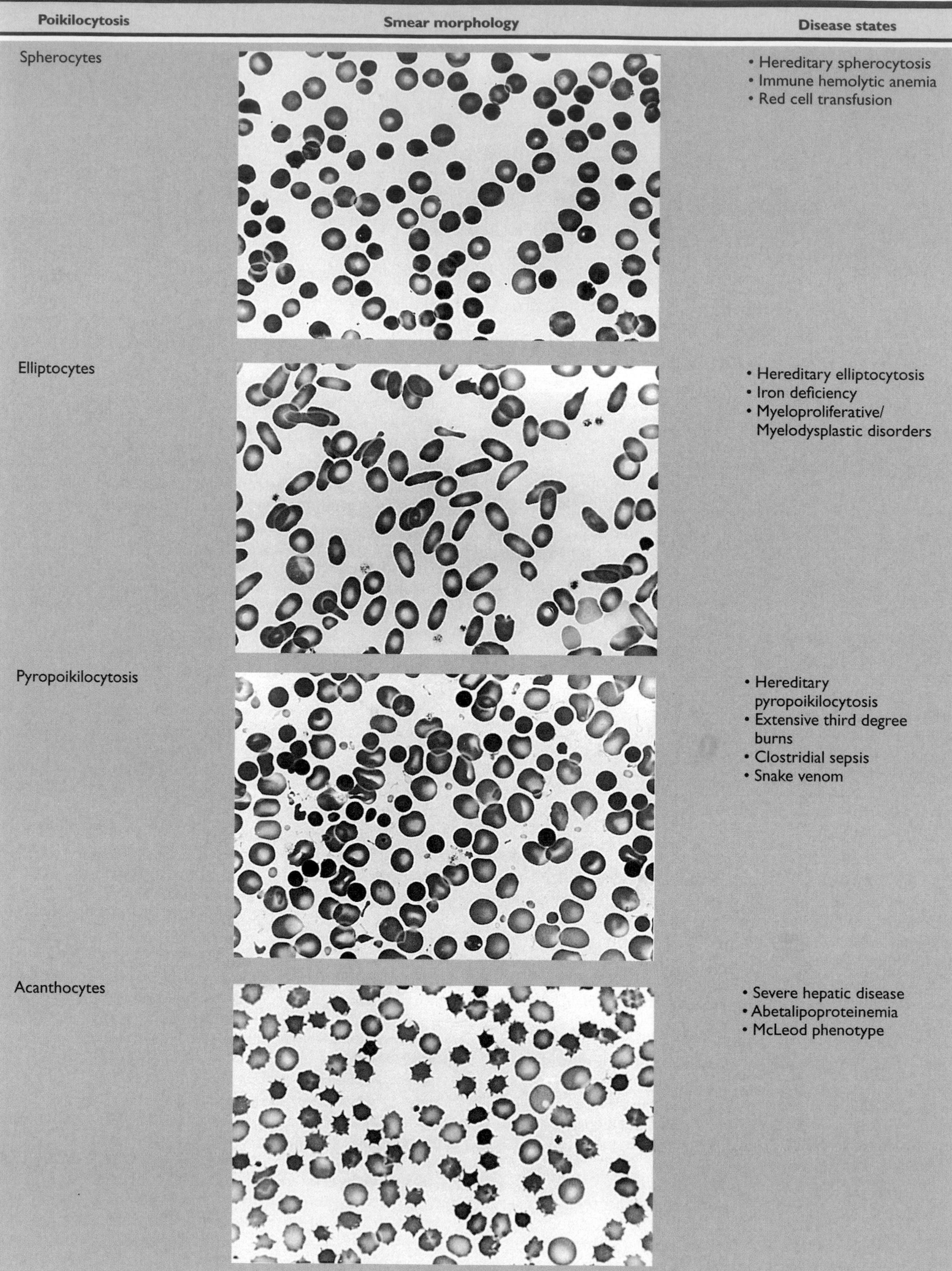

Poikilocytosis	Smear morphology	Disease states
Spherocytes		• Hereditary spherocytosis • Immune hemolytic anemia • Red cell transfusion
Elliptocytes		• Hereditary elliptocytosis • Iron deficiency • Myeloproliferative/ Myelodysplastic disorders
Pyropoikilocytosis		• Hereditary pyropoikilocytosis • Extensive third degree burns • Clostridial sepsis • Snake venom
Acanthocytes		• Severe hepatic disease • Abetalipoproteinemia • McLeod phenotype

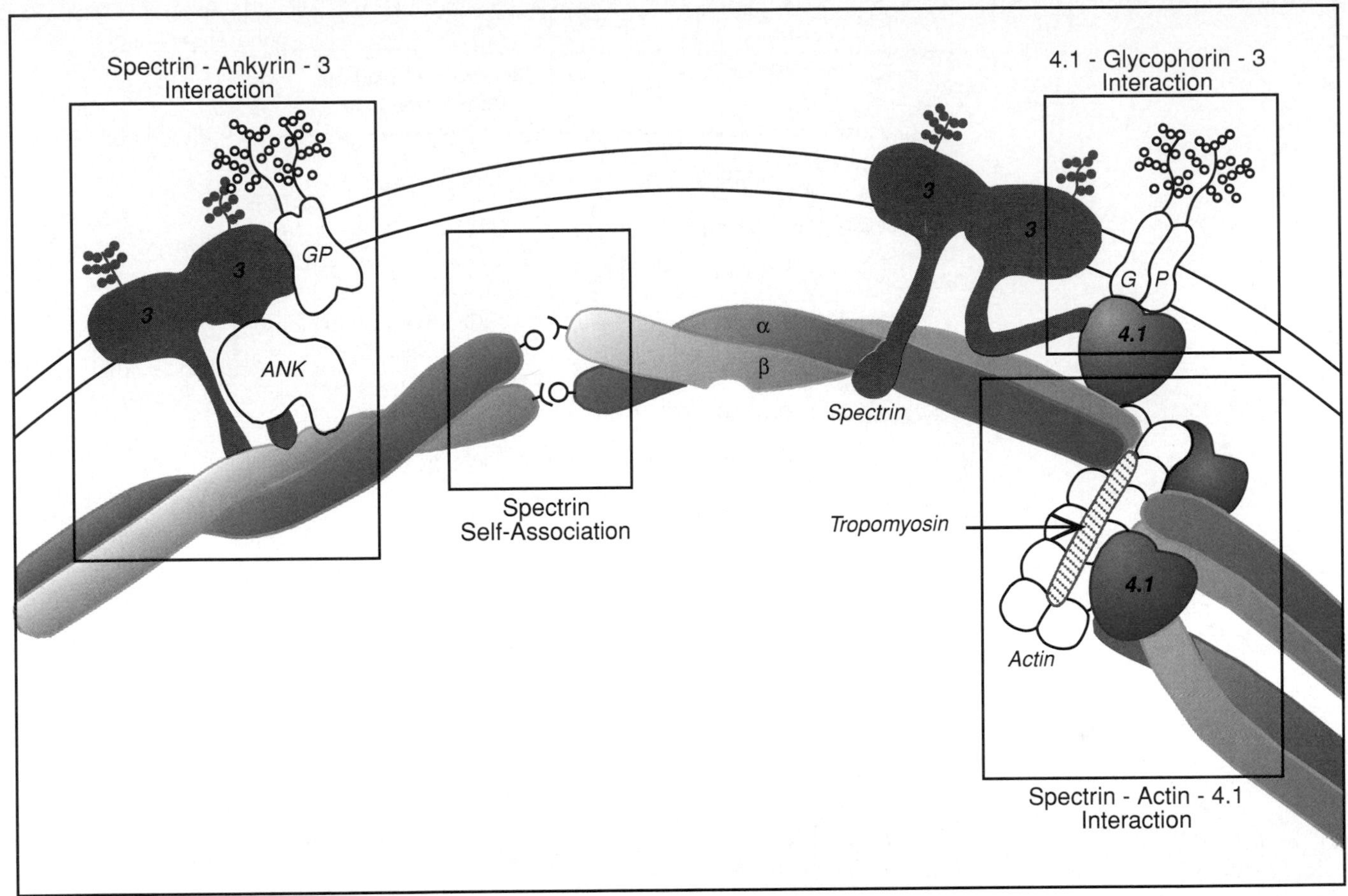

Fig. 41-23 Components of the erythrocyte cytoskeleton. *Ank*, Ankyrin; *GP*, glycophorin. (From Lux SE, Becker PS: Disorders of the red cell membrane skeleton: hereditary spherocytosis and hereditary elliptocytosis. In Scriver CR, Beaudet AL, Sly WS, Valle D, editors: *The metabolic basis of inherited disease*, ed 6, New York, 1989, McGraw-Hill.)

in pyropoikilocytosis may be observed in the blood of patients with extensive third degree burns and clostridial sepsis.

Acanthocytosis arises from diverse causes including both hereditary and acquired abnormalities (see Table 41-8). In abetalipoproteinemia, there is a deficiency of apolipoprotein B and a resultant decrease in plasma cholesterol, phospholipid and triglycerides; the mechanism of the erythrocyte destruction is unclear. In contrast, a minority of patients with severe liver disease develop a markedly elevated cholesterol to phospholipid ratio in the erythrocyte membrane. These lipid abnormalities lead to rigid, spiculated membranes that are predisposed to early destruction.

Although the identification of spherocytosis, elliptocytosis, acanthocytosis, or pyropoikilocytosis may suggest an inherited membrane abnormality, none of these morphologic patterns are specific (Table 41-8). The presence of spherocytes represents the most common diagnostic problem and suggests a differential diagnosis of hereditary spherocytosis and immune hemolytic anemia. This distinction is usually made by a combination of the direct antiglobulin test and clinical and family histories. The etiology of elliptocytosis, acanthocytosis and pyropoikilocytosis will usually be apparent from the red cell indices and the clinical history. Splenectomy is beneficial in most patients with hemolytic anemia due to cytoskeletal defects. Although the erythrocyte cytoskeletal defect remains, erythrocyte survival generally approaches normal.

Anemias associated with enzyme deficiencies

The hemolytic anemias due to enzymatic defects are a result of disruption of either anaerobic glycolysis or the hexose monophosphate shunt. Anaerobic glycolysis, the Embden-Meyerhoff pathway, is necessary for the generation of ATP; the hexose-monophosphate shunt (HMS) is necessary for the generation of the reducing compound, NADPH (Fig. 41-24). The most common HMS defect is glucose-6-phosphate dehydrogenase (G6PD) deficiency and the most common glycolytic defect is pyruvate kinase deficiency. Defects in G6PD and phosphoglycerate kinase are X-linked; the remaining defects are autosomal recessive.[76]

Glucose-6-phosphate dehydrogenase deficiency is the most commonly described enzymatic defect in humans and affects 400 million people worldwide.[76] It is most prevalent in African, Middle Eastern, Asian, and Mediterranean populations. The geographic distribution overlaps with *P. falciparum* malaria and in a mild state the deficiency appears to confer some degree of resistance to infection. The inability of the erythrocyte to generate NADPH exhausts the supply of reduced glutathione, which is necessary to protect hemoglobin from oxidant stress (Fig. 41-24). Accumulation of hydrogen peroxide, superoxide, and free radicals causes membrane damage and denaturation of hemoglobin. The denatured hemoglobin adheres to the membrane as a Heinz body, which is detected by supravital staining (Fig. 41-25).[77] The severity of hemoly-

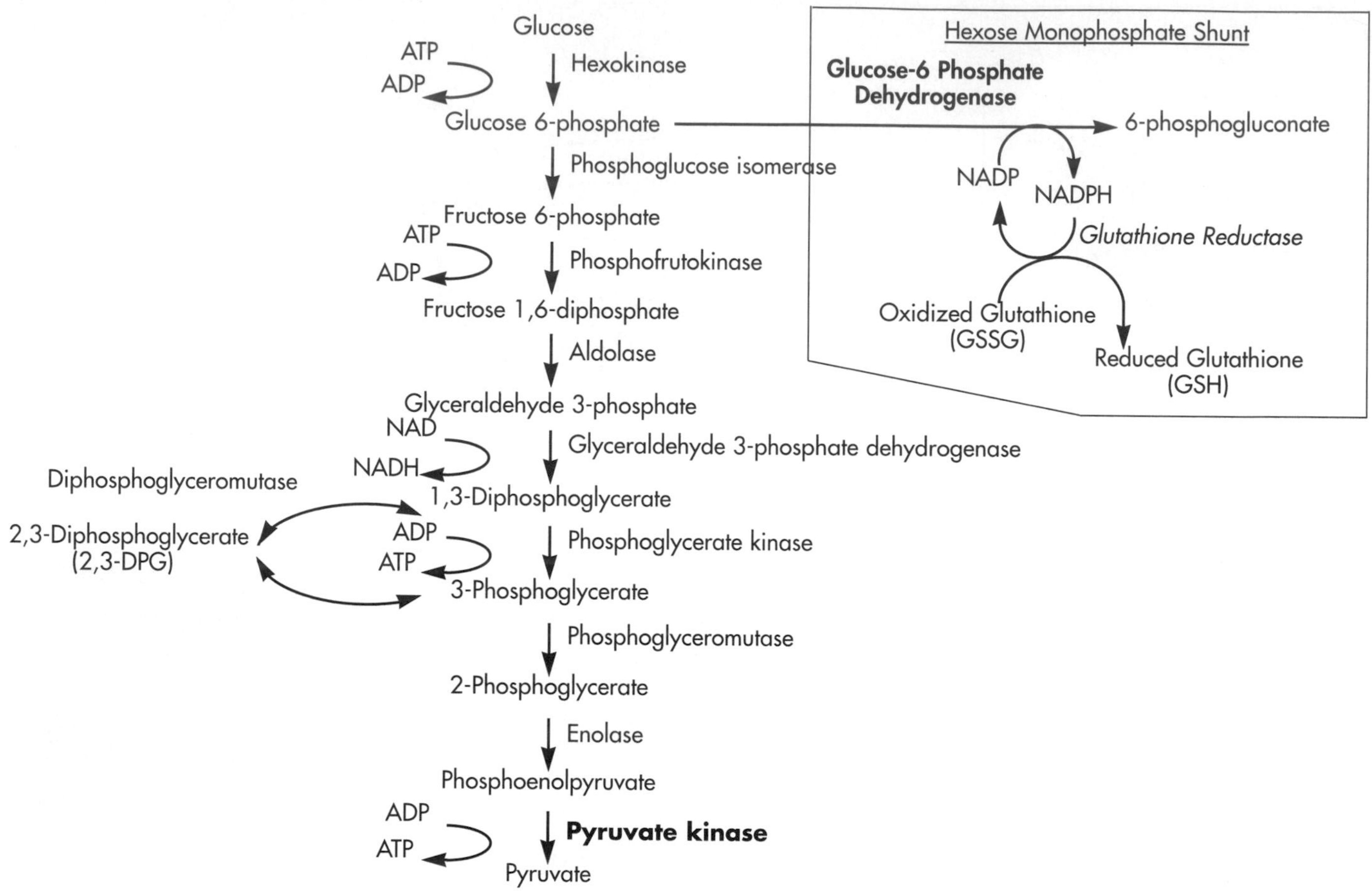

Fig. 41-24 Erythrocyte enzymes. Glycolysis and the first step of the hexose monophosphate shunt. The enzymatic defects discussed are shown in bold type.

sis depends, in part, on the level of enzyme activity. In many G6PD variants, enzyme activity is normal in reticulocytes but decays rapidly in mature red blood cells. Most G6PD-deficient patients are asymptomatic unless exposed to agents that induce oxidant stress, such as those listed in Table 41-9. The blood smear after a hemolytic episode may not have distinctive morphologic features. There may be red blood cells with a portion missing, so-called bite cells. In some instances, the red blood cell changes resemble a microangiopathic hemolytic anemia.

Pyruvate kinase deficiency is the most common anemia due to an inherited defect in anaerobic glycolysis.[78,79] The defect results in decreased production of pyruvate and ATP, and leads to an accumulation of 2,3-DPG (Fig. 41-24). The ATP deficiency impairs red blood cell membrane ion pumps, causing cell shrinkage and echinocyte formation. The anemia is usually moderate to severe; the clinical symptoms of anemia are partially ameliorated by increased levels of 2,3-DPG.[78] The morphologic changes are nonspecific; the most common poikilocyte is the spiculated erythrocyte. The disease generally manifests in childhood, shows some exacerbation during viral infections and pregnancy, and may be ameliorated by splenectomy.[79]

Immune related hemolytic anemias

Increased destruction of erythrocytes by immune mechanisms occurs in diverse settings; examples include an idiosyncratic reaction to a drug, an autoimmune disorder such as systemic lupus erythematosus, or in patients with malignant lymphoproliferative disorders. Common features of immune hemolytic anemias are reticulocytosis, spherocytosis, and marrow erythroid hyperplasia. The direct antiglobulin test (DAT) identifies immunoglobulin molecules or complement components bound to the erythrocyte membrane. The immune hemolytic anemias are subclassified by the temperature dependence of the antibody binding to antigen: warm autoimmune hemolytic anemia, cold agglutinins, and paroxysmal cold hemoglobinuria.[80]

The autoantibodies associated with warm autoimmune hemolytic anemia are usually IgG, bind at 35 to 40°C and frequently recognize antigens that appear to be related to the Rh system.[81,82] These antibodies do not usually fix complement, but antibody-coated erythrocytes are bound via Fc receptors to splenic and hepatic macrophages.

Cold agglutinins are IgM antibodies that bind to the erythrocyte at temperatures less than 30°C and are usually directed against the I or i antigen.[82] Antibody binds to erythrocytes, causing agglutination and a characteristic peripheral blood smear (Fig. 41-26). Complement is fixed and activated, usually coating the erythrocytes with C3b without activation of the membrane attack complex of the cascade. The C3b is preferentially bound by hepatic macrophages, leading to extravascular hemolysis.[83] Polyclonal cold agglutinin antibodies are associated with *Mycoplasma pneumoniae* and infectious mononucleosis.[82] Chronic cold agglutinin disease is most

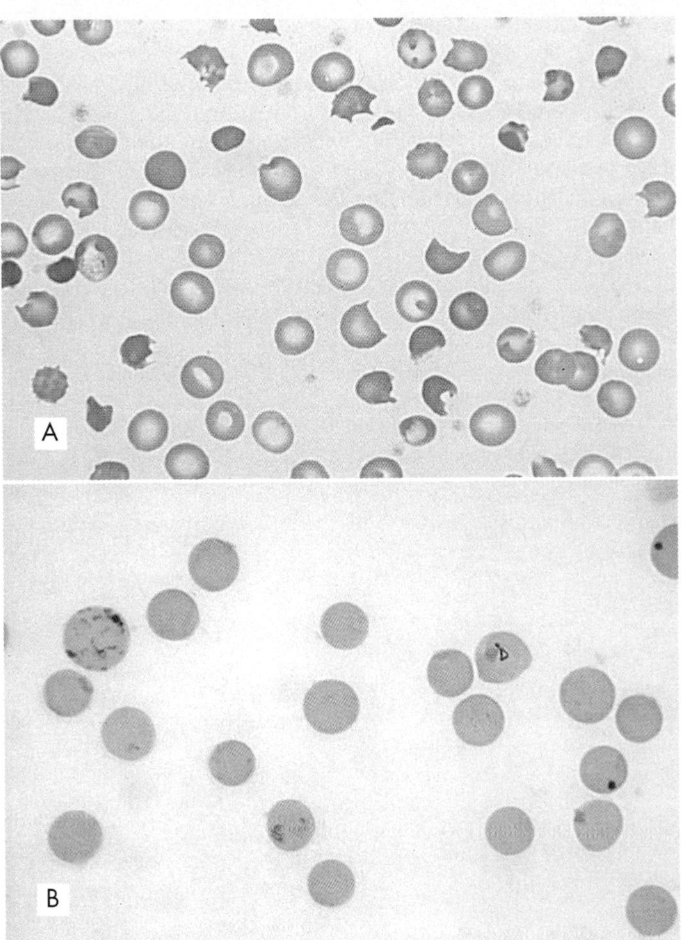

Fig. 41-25 Heinz body hemolytic anemia. **A,** Numerous "bite cells", in a blood smear from a patient with low glucose 6-phosphate dehydrogenase activity who was treated with dapsone (Wright-Giemsa). **B,** Heinz bodies, denatured hemoglobin, are bright green. Reticulocytes contain delicate red granular deposits of RNA (Neutral Red-Brilliant Green).

commonly due to a monoclonal IgM antibody; there is frequently an underlying lymphoproliferative disorder.[80]

Paroxysmal cold hemoglobinuria is due to IgG antibodies, so-called Donath-Landsteiner antibodies, that bind to the erythrocyte at cold temperatures and activate the complete complement cascade. Intravascular hemolysis occurs only following warming. Historically, Donath-Landsteiner antibodies were associated with tertiary syphilis; most of the present cases arise in the context of a viral infection and are self-limited.[80]

Several mechanisms have been described for drug-induced hemolytic anemia. Antibodies may be produced during penicillin therapy that recognize metabolites of penicillin bound to the erythrocyte membrane. These IgG antibodies usually lead to extravascular hemolysis.[80] Alpha methyldopa-induced autoimmune hemolytic anemia appears to arise from alteration in immune regulation allowing autoantibody production very similar to other forms of warm autoimmune hemolytic anemia. The incidence of DAT positivity is significantly higher than the incidence of hemolysis in patients treated with α-methyldopa.

Table 41-9 Representative agents implicated in hemolytic crises in glucose 6-phosphate dehydrogenase deficient patients

Drugs
Antimalarials (e.g., Primaquine)
Sulfonamides (e.g., Sulfamethoxazole)
Sulfones (e.g. Dapsone)
Nitrofurans
Nalidixic acid
Infections
Bacterial infection: *S. typhi, E. coli*
Rickettsiae
Viral hepatitis
Influenza A (in vitro)
Miscellaneous
Fava beans
Diabetic ketoacidosis

Modified from Lukens JN: Glucose-6-phosphate dehydrogenase deficiency and related deficiencies involving the pentose phosphate pathway and glutathione metabolism. In Lee GR et al, editors: *Wintrobe's clinical hematology,* ed 9, Philadelphia, 1993, Lea and Febiger.

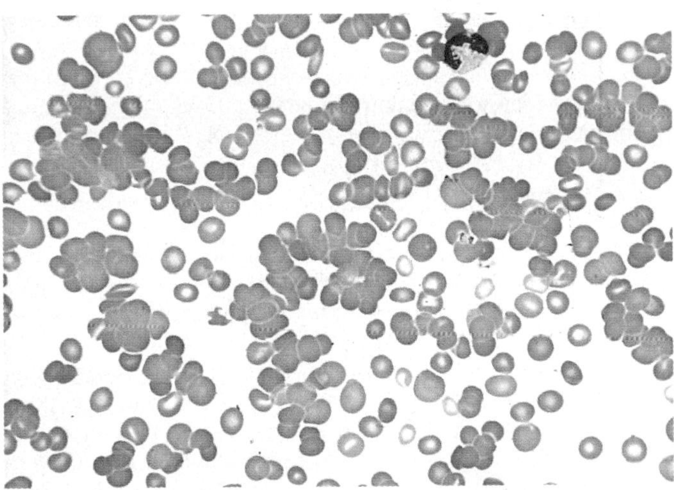

Fig. 41-26 Peripheral blood smear from a patient with chronic cold agglutinin disease showing prominent aggregation of erythrocytes (Wright-Giemsa).

Microangiopathic hemolytic anemia

The microangiopathic hemolytic anemias result from erythrocyte fragmentation due to mechanical trauma during passage through the microvasculature. Often, this is the result of erythrocyte passage through the fibrin/platelet strands in a low pressure, low flow circuit, such as the microvasculature in disseminated intravascular coagulation (DIC). Similar forces may be present in mechanical heart valve prostheses. Other etiologies are listed in Table 41-10.

Blood smears have characteristic red cell fragments or schistocytes and microspherocytes (Fig. 41-27). Laboratory evidence of intravascular hemolysis includes hyperbilirubinemia, elevated lactic acid dehydrogenase, and decreased haptoglobin. Coagulation abnormalities and thrombocytopenia may be present.

The two most well-defined pathologic syndromes with primary vascular pathology and a microangiopathic hemolytic anemia are thrombotic thrombocytopenic purpura (TTP) and hemolytic uremic syndrome (HUS).

Thrombotic thrombocytopenic purpura is a systemic disease of uncertain etiology in which a microangiopathic hemolytic anemia and thrombocytopenia are the principal hematologic manifestations.[84] The disease has a peak incidence in the fourth decade and is more common in females than males. The major pathology is the presence of widespread hyalin thrombi composed of fibrin and platelets in the arterioles and capillaries.[85] All organs are affected. Thrombotic thrombocytopenic purpura may have an insidious or abrupt onset. Because of the widespread organ involvement, it is a disease of protean manifestations. A diagnostic triad of microangiopathic hemolytic anemia, thrombocytopenia, and neurologic manifestations has been used to characterize the disease; the addition of renal abnormalities and fever constitute a diagnostic pentad.[84] In addition to fragmented red blood cells and thrombocytopenia, the blood smear usually contains nucleated red blood cells, microspherocytes, and an increased number of polychromatic red blood cells. There is usually a neutrophilic leukocytosis. In the bone marrow there are increased numbers of erythroid precursors and normal to increased numbers of megakaryocytes. Untreated TTP has a very high fatality rate, approximately 90%. Treatment with plasma exchange reduces the mortality to 20% to 30%.[86]

Hemolytic uremic syndrome of childhood (HUS) is a multisystem disorder with principal manifestations of microangiopathic hemolytic anemia, thrombocytopenia, and acute renal injury. Usually, HUS has an abrupt onset following an episode of gastroenteritis.[87] HUS may be typical (epidemic) or atypical (sporadic).

Typical HUS most commonly occurs in infants and young children; it may also present in adults. The clinical findings include anuria, vomiting, prostration, and neurologic abnormalities. Several mechanisms have been proposed for the pathogenesis of HUS. The common pathology is damage to the endothelium of the microvasculature followed by deposition of fibrin and platelets resulting in microthrombi and vascular occlusion. This sequence of events results in shearing of the red blood cells as shown in Fig. 41-27, *B*. Several microorganisms have been implicated as causes of the vascular injury in HUS. The most frequent association is with veratoxin-producing *Escherichia coli; Shigella spp.* and *Streptococcus pneumoniae* are less frequently implicated. The blood findings in HUS include a microangiopathic hemolytic anemia, thrombocytopenia, normoblastemia, reticulocytosis, and neutrophilic leukocytosis. The marrow shows erythroid hyperplasia and normal to increased number of megakaryocytes. Associated laboratory findings reflect renal failure and include elevated urea nitrogen and creatinine. The prognosis in the HUS depends on the causative agent and the severity of the process. More than 90% of patients recover from the acute event.[87] A significant number of patients develop end stage chronic renal failure.

Table 41-10 Causes of microangiopathic hemolytic anemia

Thrombotic thrombocytopenic purpura (TTP)
Hemolytic uremic syndrome (HUS)
Disseminated intravascular coagulation (DIC) (*e.g., adenocarcinoma, sepsis*)
Mechanical heart valve*
Vasculitis (*e.g., collagen vascular disease, polyarteritis nodosa, Wegner's granulomatosis, R. rickettsii*)
Malignant hypertension
Drugs (*e.g., Mitomycin, Cyclosporin A*)
Congenital vascular malformation (Kasabach-Merritt syndrome)

*Although not related to changes in microvasculature, this etiology is included due to the similar pathogenesis and morphologic appearance.

Acute blood loss

The anemia of acute blood loss is normocytic, normochromic unless complicated by other factors. Because acute hemorrhage results in the loss of both red blood cells and plasma, the effects of acute hemorrhage are not immediately reflected in the hematocrit or hemoglobin, which relate to unit volume. The reduced hemoglobin is only apparent after the blood vol-

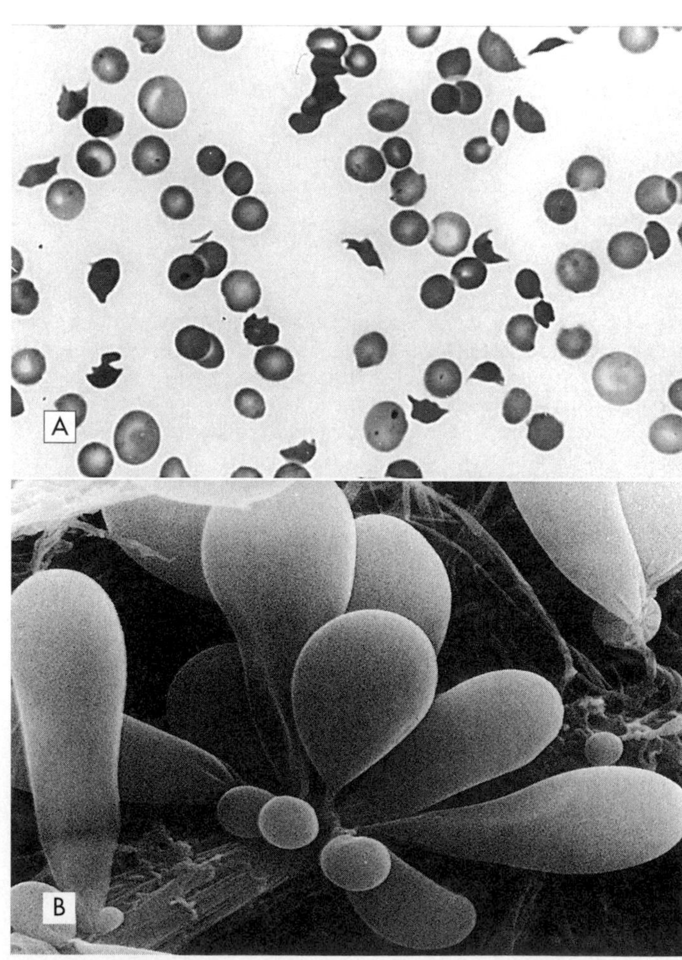

Fig. 41-27 Microangiopathic hemolytic anemia. **A,** Light micrograph of a blood smear from a patient with metastatic adenocarcinoma with disseminated intravascular coagulation. There are numerous fragmented red blood cells (schistocytes) (Wright-Giemsa). **B,** Scanning electron micrograph of red blood cells being sheared by fibrin strands. (Electron micrograph courtesy Brian S. Bull, M.D., Loma Linda University School of Medicine, Loma Linda, Calif)

ume has been reconstituted by fluid from the extravascular space; this normally occurs over a period of 48 to 72 hours or sooner if intravenous fluids are administered. The reticulocyte response is delayed for approximately 5 days because of maturation of erythroid precursors. The maximum reticulocytosis is seen at 8 to 10 days, but continuing blood loss or replacement therapy may alter this time frame. Acute hemorrhage can also be accompanied by a thrombocytosis and neutrophilic leukocytosis.

Paroxysmal nocturnal hemoglobinuria

Paroxysmal nocturnal hemoglobinuria (PNH) is an acquired, clonal disorder of a hematopoietic progenitor cell that is characterized by intravascular hemolysis due to abnormal susceptibility of erythrocytes to complement. The defect affects all myeloid cell lines in the majority of patients, and lymphoid cell lines in a subset of patients, suggesting origin in a stem cell or early progenitor cell.[88]

The disease is due to defective synthesis of a glycosylphosphatidylinositol (GPI) molecule, which anchors several membrane-associated proteins that protect the red blood cell from complement-mediated lysis, such as decay accelerating factor (DAF,CD55), membrane inhibitor of reactive lysis (MIRL, CD59) and C8-binding protein (C8bp). Deficiency of these molecules, especially of MIRL, due to the defective anchoring, leads to increased susceptibility to intravascular lysis by the complement system.[89]

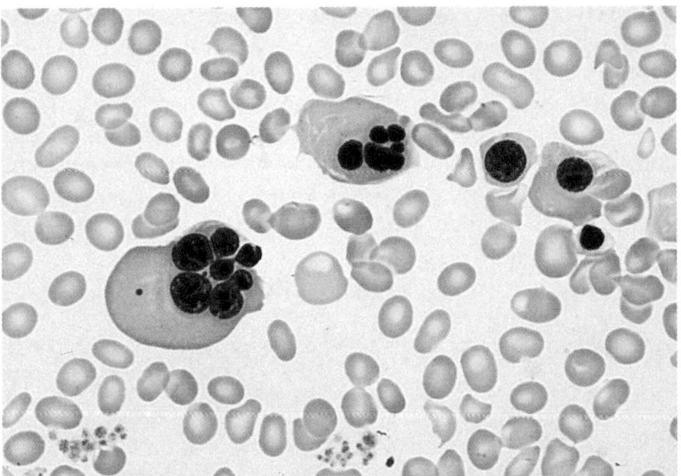

Fig. 41-28 Marrow aspirate from a patient with Type III congenital dyserythropoietic anemia. Giant multinucleated erythroid precursors with nuclear/cytoplasmic asynchrony are prominent (Wright-Giemsa).

PNH most commonly presents in adult life with anemia and frequently pancytopenia. Overt hemoglobinuria occurs in less than 25% of patients; nocturnal hemoglobinuria is less frequent.[90] The classic diagnostic tests for PNH are the Ham and sucrose water hemolysis tests in which there is hemolysis of erythrocytes when complement is activated by either low pH or low ionic strength, respectively.[91,92] Deficiencies of CD55 and CD59 can be identified immunologically.[93] The neutrophil alkaline phosphatase score and erythrocyte acetylcholinesterase activity are also usually decreased. Bone marrow iron stores are commonly decreased because of intravascular hemolysis and hemosiderinuria.[91]

Thrombotic complications, especially in the mesenteric, hepatic, and cerebral veins, are important causes of morbidity and mortality. Approximately 20% of patients with PNH develop myeloproliferative or myelodysplastic disorders; a lesser number develop acute myeloid leukemia.[94,95]

Congenital dyserythropoietic anemias

The congenital dyserythropoietic anemias are a rare group of inherited disorders characterized by anemia, ineffective erythropoiesis, and dyserythropoiesis (Fig. 41-28). There are three generally recognized types of CDA, I, II, and III, based on mode of inheritance and morphologic and serologic findings (Table 41-11).[96-98] Because some cases of CDA do not fit into any of these categories, additional types have been proposed.[99]

In type II CDA, also known as hereditary erythroblastic multinuclearity associated with a positive acidified serum test (HEMPAS), the red blood cells lyse in the presence of acidified donor serum resembling paroxysmal nocturnal hemoglobinuria (PNH).[96] In contrast to PNH, type II CDA red blood cells are not lysed by their own acidified serum or in the sucrose hemolysis test. The lysis in type II CDA is mediated by a complement-fixing IgM antibody that is present in 30% of normal control sera but absent in patients with this type of CDA.

NEUTROPENIA AND AGRANULOCYTOSIS

Neutropenia is a decrease in the absolute number of blood neutrophils; in adults, less than 1.5×10^9/L in white individuals and 1.3×10^9/L in black individuals. Neutropenia may be a component of generalized bone marrow failure, pancytopenia, or an isolated finding. Isolated neutropenias may be either congenital or acquired.

Congenital neutropenia

The congenital neutropenias encompass a clinical spectrum of diseases from the severe form, infantile genetic agranulocytosis or Kostman syndrome, which is a lethal, autosomal reces-

Table 41-11 Mode of inheritance and morphologic and laboratory findings of the major types of congenital dyserythropoietic anemias (CDA)

CDA	Inheritance	Hb	Marrow erythroid precursors	Lysis in acidified serum
Type I	Autosomal recessive	8-13g/dL	Erythroblast nuclei connected by chromatin strand	−
Type II	Autosomal recessive	5-15g/dL	Up to 20% multinucleated erythroblasts	+
Type III	Autosomal dominant	9-15g/dL	Multinucleated giant erythroblasts	−

sive form of neutropenia with neutrophil counts less than 0.2×10^9/L, to the milder forms such as cyclic neutropenia, chronic benign neutropenia of childhood, Chediak-Higashi syndrome, and the autosomal recessive neutropenia associated with exocrine pancreatic insufficiency known as Schwachman syndrome.[40] Neutropenia also occurs with some congenital immune deficiency syndromes, such as reticular dysgenesis and X-linked agammaglobulinemia.

The blood and marrow findings vary in the different disorders. In Schwachman syndrome in which the neutrophils are morphologically unremarkable, there is thrombocytopenia in 70% and an anemia in 50% of cases.[40] In Chediak-Higashi syndrome, the granulocytes contain large clumps of primary and secondary cytoplasmic granules (Fig. 41-29). Lymphocytes contain large azurophilic granules. Monocytes do not appear affected. Congenital neutropenia is usually accompanied by a monocytosis except in patients with Schwachman syndrome. Eosinophilia may be present. A concomitant lymphocytopenia is present in reticular dysgenesis; platelet counts and hemoglobin values are usually normal.

Marrow aspirates from patients with neutropenia can be categorized into one of three primary patterns: (1) virtual aplasia of the neutrophilic precursors as occurs in reticular dysgenesis, (2) a predominance of promyelocytes, and early myelocytes with no or few mature neutrophils, the so-called maturation arrest as found in infantile genetic agranulocytosis, Schwachman syndrome, chronic benign neutropenia of childhood and some cases of cyclic neutropenia, and (3) granulocytic hyperplasia with all stages of maturation as in Chediak-Higashi syndrome.

An unusual form of congenital neutropenia is cyclical.[100] It presents primarily in childhood, shows no sex predilection, and is familial in 25% of cases. Characteristically, each cycle consists of recurrent 8- to 10-day episodes of profound neutropenia followed by 12 to 14-day transitional periods with normal or near normal neutrophil numbers. Cycles are approximately 21 days in length. During neutropenic periods patients are generally symptomatic with ulcers, adenopathy, and fevers. The marrow shows granulocytic hyperplasia during neutropenic periods and right-shifted neutrophil maturation later in the cycle.

Acquired neutropenia

The most common etiologies of acquired, isolated neutropenia are idiosyncratic drug reaction, autoimmune disease, infection, and malignancy.

Drugs causing neutropenia may destroy neutrophils by a dose-dependent, direct cytotoxic effect, an idiosyncratic toxic effect, or by eliciting an abnormal immune response. The morphologic appearance of the marrow is similar to congenital neutropenia; a "maturation arrest" is a common finding (Fig. 41-30). Prototypical drugs with toxic effects are cancer chemotherapeutic drugs, chloramphenicol, and the phenothiazines; drugs that produce neutropenia by the immune mechanisms include procainamide, aminopyrine, penicillin, and propylthiouracil.

Autoimmune diseases associated with neutropenia are systemic lupus erythematosus and Sjögren syndrome. Neutropenia may also occur in patients with rheumatoid arthritis and splenomegaly, a triad of findings referred to as Felty's syndrome. Individuals infected with viruses, including Epstein Barr virus, hepatitis A and B, respiratory syncytial virus, influenza A and B, measles, rubella, and varicella, frequently develop transient neutropenia; this may be one component of pancytopenia. Typhoid fever, tuberculosis, rickettsial, and malarial infection may also be associated with significant neutropenia. Parvovirus B19 is a cause of chronic neutropenia.[101] Sepsis is a common cause of neutropenia, especially in individuals with limited marrow reserve, such as neonates and the aged. An isolated neutropenia may be observed in myelodysplastic syndromes. The advent of monocytosis in acquired neutropenia frequently heralds recovery phase.

Neutropenia places the patient at risk for bacterial infection. In general, the risk of infection is inversely proportional to the neutrophil count, and increases with the duration of neutropenia. The susceptibility to infection first becomes apparent at absolute neutrophil counts less than 1×10^9/L; absolute neutrophil counts less than 0.5×10^9/L are associated with a high risk of infection.

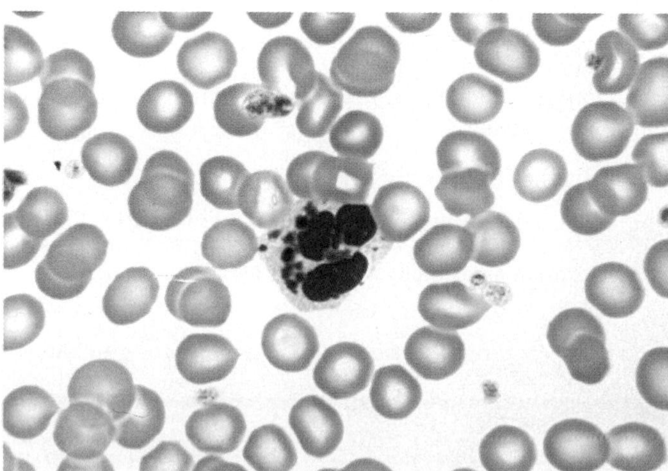

Fig. 41-29 Blood smear from a patient with Chediak-Higashi syndrome showing a neutrophil with large purple-blue cytoplasmic granules. These represent abnormal aggregates of azurophilic and specific granules (Wright-Giemsa).

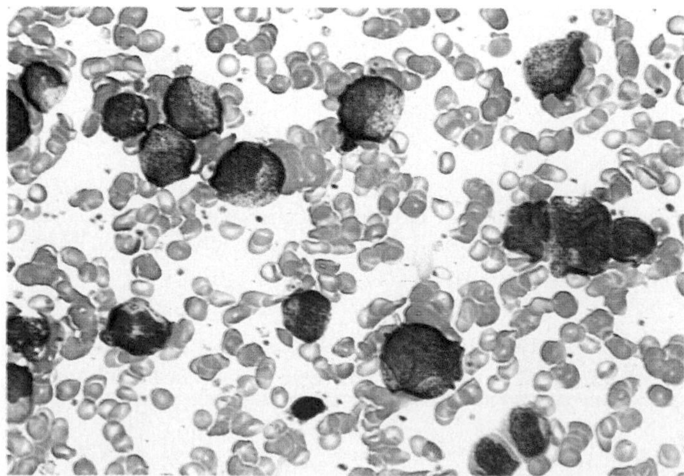

Fig. 41-30 Promyelocyte "maturation arrest" in immune-mediated neutropenia. Numerous granulocytic precursors are present with little evidence of maturation beyond the promyelocyte and myelocyte stages (Wright-Giemsa).

THROMBOCYTOPENIA

Thrombocytopenia similar to decreases in other constituents of the blood may result from decreased platelet production or decreased platelet survival. Decreased production is usually due to generalized marrow failure, as occurs in aplastic anemia or the replacement of marrow by leukemic cells. Thrombocytopenia due to decreased production may also result from abnormal myelopoiesis, as occurs in some myeloid leukemias, myelodysplastic syndromes, and megaloblastic anemias. Selective megakaryocyte hypoplasia or aplasia is rare. One example, megakaryocytic hypoplasia and thrombocytopenia associated with bilateral absence of the radii (TAR syndrome), occurs as an uncommon, autosomal recessive disorder.[102] It usually manifests in the first 4 months of life. Associated findings include short stature and cardiac and/or renal abnormalities. The megakaryocytes are small and dysplastic. The thrombocytopenia improves with increasing age with near normal platelet counts by adult age.

Thrombocytopenia due to decreased platelet survival reflects increased platelet consumption, immune-related destruction, or hypersplenism. Consumptive thrombocytopenia occurs in thrombotic thrombocytopenic purpura (TTP), hemolytic uremic syndrome (HUS), and disseminated intravascular coagulation (DIC).

The immunologic destruction of platelets occurs in a diverse group of diseases (Table 41-12). Idiopathic immune-related thrombocytopenia usually occurs as an acute form in children and a chronic form in adults. Acute idiopathic thrombocytopenic purpura (ITP) often follows a viral infection. There is no or slight splenomegaly.[103,104] Serious hemorrhage, such as intracranial hemorrhage, is rare. More than 90% of cases of ITP remit spontaneously. Chronic idiopathic thrombocytopenic purpura usually presents insidiously in adults; women are affected more frequently than men. In contrast to the acute type, there are few spontaneous remissions.

In ITP there is increased destruction of IgG antibody-coated platelets by splenic macrophages.[103,105] Antibodies directed against platelet glycoproteins IIb or IbX have been reported.[105-107] The destruction of platelets by splenic macrophages is inhibited by glucocorticoids and androgens and accentuated by estrogens. Destruction of platelets by splenic macrophages can be inhibited by infusion of hyperimmune globulin that saturates macrophage Fc receptors.[108]

Table 41-12 Classification of immune thrombocytopenia

Idiopathic thrombocytopenic purpura (ITP)
Acute ITP
Chronic ITP
Secondary immune thrombocytopenia
Drug Induced
Systemic autoimmune disease
Acquired immunodeficiency syndrome (AIDS)
Malignancy
Neonatal
Congenital ITP
Neonatal alloimmune thrombocytopenia

The pathogenesis of secondary immune thrombocytopenia is heterogeneous (Table 41-12). In systemic lupus erythematosus, thrombocytopenia may occur before other symptoms or at any time in the disease and is usually associated with antiplatelet antibodies. The thrombocytopenia may be associated with immune hemolytic anemia.[103] In patients with AIDS, thrombocytopenia due to autoantibodies and immune complex deposition have been implicated.[109] The antiplatelet antibodies in congenital isoimmune thrombocytopenia are formed by PI^{A1}-negative mothers in response to foreign fetal PI^{A1} in 85% to 90% of cases.[110] The pathophysiology is analogous to alloimmune hemolytic anemia of the newborn; however, first-born infants are commonly affected.

Several drugs are implicated in immune thrombocytopenia. The precise mechanisms are, for the most part, not well understood. Quinidine therapy can induce antibodies that appear to bind specifically to a complex of the drug and platelet glycoprotein IX.[111]

Idiosyncratic heparin-induced thrombocytopenia appears to be related to binding of heparin-IgG immune complexes to the platelet surface. The immune complexes may interact with platelet membrane Fc receptors and lead to platelet activation.[112] Heparin-induced thrombocytopenia is distinct from other immune-mediated thrombocytopenias in that thrombotic events are more common than hemorrhagic complications. Arterial thromboses in the peripheral vascular system, coronary arteries, and cerebrovascular system, the *white clot syndrome,* may be associated with significant morbidity. Thrombocytopenia remits within several days of discontinuance of heparin therapy.

The pathologic findings in the autoimmune and secondary thrombocytopenias are nonspecific. The platelets are generally larger than normal platelets and normally granulated. The bone marrow in both types contains normal to increased number of normally maturing megakaryocytes.

Splenomegaly can cause splenic sequestration of platelets and thrombocytopenia; the major mechanism is considered to be passive platelet pooling rather than destruction.

LEUKEMIAS AND RELATED DISORDERS

The leukemias are neoplastic proliferations of hematopoietic cells that manifest primarily in the blood and bone marrow. They are classified into two major cytologic types, myeloid or lymphocytic, based on the primary cell of origin. Within each cytologic type, the leukemias are further classified as acute or chronic, based on the degree of maturation of the major cell population. In the acute leukemias, there is a marked increase in the percentage of blast cells in the marrow and usually in the blood. Evidence of marrow failure is frequently a presenting finding. In the chronic leukemias, the predominant cells are mature or maturing cells with only a slight or no increase in blasts. The chronic leukemias are generally characterized by a marked leukocytosis; manifestations of marrow failure are not usually present at the onset.

The annual incidence of leukemia of all types, in all races, in the United States in 1987-88 was 9.5 per 100,000 population.[113] The incidence of the major types per 100,000 population was: acute lymphoblastic leukemia 1.5, acute myeloid leukemia 2.2, chronic lymphocytic leukemia 2.6, and chronic myeloid leukemia 1.3. The incidence in males for all types was 12.5 and for females 7.3. The annual incidence of leukemia of all types in the black population, both sexes, in the same period was 8.7 per 100,000 population. The rate of acute lymphoblastic leukemia was 1.0, acute myeloid leukemia 1.9, chronic lymphocytic leukemia 2.6, and chronic myeloid leukemia 1.5. The incidence in black males was 11.3 and in black females 6.8. The annual incidence of leukemias of all types in the white population, both sexes, in 1987-88 was 9.6 per 100,000: acute lymphoblastic leukemia 1.5, chronic lymphocytic leukemia 2.6, acute myeloid leukemia 2.2 and chronic myeloid leukemia 1.3. The incidence in white males was 12.7 and in white females 7.3.

Acute myeloid leukemias

The acute myeloid leukemias are primarily bone marrow derived neoplasias that originate in the myeloid stem cell or a more differentiated precursor cell. Eight major types of acute myeloid leukemia (AML) are recognized (Table 41-13).[114-116] The classification of the acute myeloid leukemias, as presented, is based primarily on cytologic characterisitics of the proliferating cells augmented by cytochemical, immunologic, and ultrastructural data in some types.

The clinical findings of patients with AML are a consequence of the displacement of the normal hematopoietic cells in the marrow by the leukemic cells and the dysfunctional nature of neoplastic hematopoietic cells. The major manifestations are bleeding disorders related to thrombocytopenia, infections resulting from decreased normal neutrophils, and fatigue from anemia. Leukemic cells may infiltrate organs, but this feature is less marked than in the chronic leukemias.

As illustrated in Fig. 41-2, the normal myeloid system is composed of several different cell types that vary in morphologic and functional characteristics. This rich diversity is recapitulated in the acute leukemias. In general, AML is principally expressed as a proliferation of the precursors or immature cells of one of the major myeloid lineages. In some leukemias, most notably acute myelomonocytic leukemia and erythroleukemia, there is involvement of two or more cell lineages. Occasionally, several major myeloid lineages are involved in the neoplastic process (e.g., myeloblasts, erythroblasts, and megakaryoblasts), and these leukemias are termed panmyeloses.

Thirty percent blasts in marrow or blood is required for a diagnosis of AML.[114-116] The leukemic cell population may consist principally of blasts, as occurs in AML-MO and AML-M1, or there may be substantial evidence of cell maturation as in cases of AML with maturation (AML M2). The maturing cells frequently show abnormalities of nuclear and cytoplasmic development, dysplastic changes. These abnormalities may be present in one or all of the myeloid cell types. The major blast populations in the acute myeloid leukemias include the myeloblast, monoblast, erythroblast, and megakaryoblast. Two types of myeloblasts are generally recognized: type I and type II (Fig. 41-31). The type I myeloblast has no cytoplasmic granules; the type II myeloblast has a few to 20 scattered, azurophilic granules. The monoblasts and promonocytes are the major immature cells in the *acute monocytic leukemias,* and the megakaryoblast is the major blast in acute megakaryoblastic leukemia (Fig. 41-32). The promyelocyte is the predominant abnormal cell in acute *promyelocytic leukemia* (Fig. 41-33). *Erythroleukemia* involves both the

Table 41-13 Classification of acute myeloid leukemias

Acute myeloblastic leukemia, minimally differentiated (AML-M0)
Acute myeloblastic leukemia without maturation (AML-M1)
Acute myeloblastic leukemia with maturation (AML-M2)
Acute promyelocytic leukemia (AML-M3)
Hypergranular type
Microgranular variant
Acute myelomonocytic leukemia (AML-M4)
Increased marrow eosinophils (AML M4-E0)
Acute monocytic leukemia (AML)
Acute monoblastic leukemia (AML-M5A)
Acute monocytic leukemia, differentiated (AML-M5B)
Erythroleukemia (AML-M6)
Acute megakaryoblastic leukemia (AML-M7)

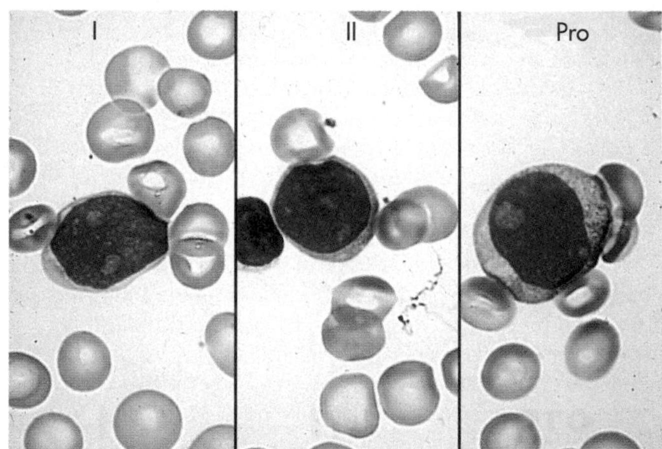

Fig. 41-31 Type I and II myeloblasts, promyelocytes. The type I myeloblast *(I)* is agranular. The type II myeloblast *(II)* has a few azurophilic granules in the cytoplasm at the lower right. The promyelocyte *(Pro)* has numerous azurophilic granules in the cytoplasm (Wright-Giemsa).

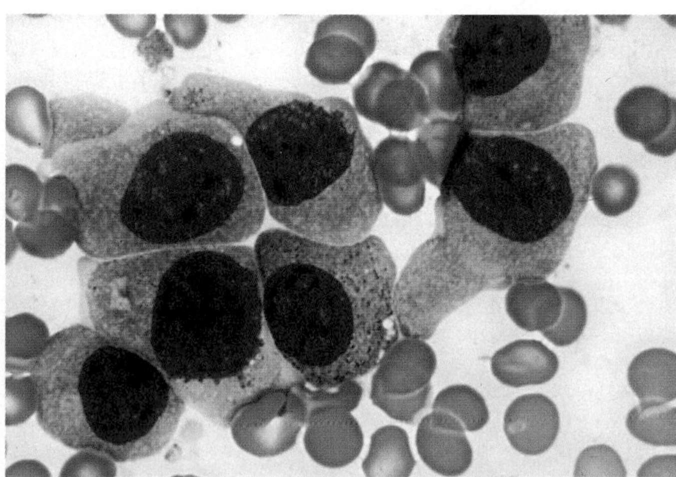

Fig. 41-32 Monoblasts in a marrow smear from a patient with acute monoblastic leukemia (M5A). The monoblasts are larger than myeloblasts and usually have abundant cytoplasm, frequently with delicate scattered azurophilic granules (Wright-Giemsa).

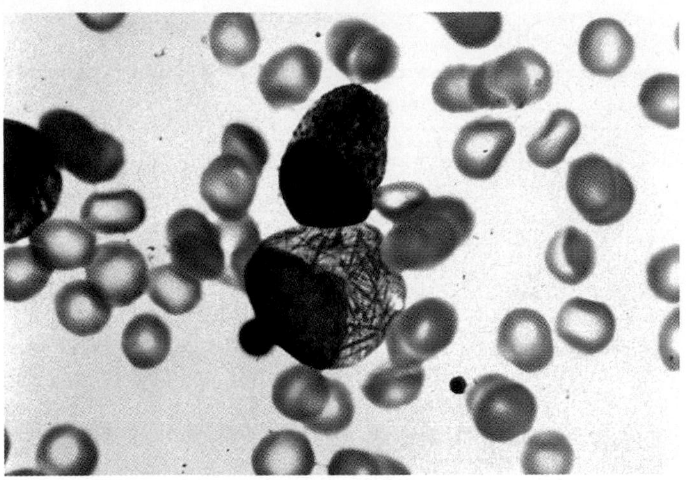

Fig. 41-33 Bone marrow smear from a patient with hypergranular acute promyelocytic leukemia; the cell with multiple intertwining Auer rods is referred to as a "faggot" cell and is a characteristic finding in this type of leukemia (Wright-Giemsa).

myeloblasts and erythroid precursors, but the diagnosis is based only on the percent of myeloblasts in the non-erythroid cell population.

In approximately 60% of cases of AML, Auer rods are identified in myeloblasts; the Auer rod is a linear, azurophilic structure composed of coalesced azurophilic granules (Fig. 41-34). The Auer rod is found only in the AMLs or high-grade myelodysplastic syndromes.

The principal laboratory features of the AMLs are listed in Table 41-14. The leukocyte count varies and patients may present with either marked leukocytosis, marked leukopenia, or normal count; in patients with a marked leukocytosis blast cells usually predominate (Table 41-15).

The marrow sections are markedly hypercellular in the majority of cases and the cellular composition reflects the degree of maturation (Fig. 41-35). Normal myeloid cells are usually markedly reduced; this leads to bone marrow failure. In 10% to 15% of cases of AML, primarily in older individuals, the marrow is hypocellular and, in some instances, may resemble the marrow in hypoplastic or aplastic anemia; this is referred to as hypocellular acute leukemia (Fig. 41-36). Myelofibrosis may be present; it appears to be more frequent in acute megakaryoblastic leukemia than other types. Acute myelofibrosis is a form of AML in which there is proliferation of all major myeloid cells and associated fibrosis. Megakaryocyte proliferation in this entity may be particularly prominent. The myelofibrosis is an epiphenomenon; the fibroblasts are not malignant.

There are several cytogenetic abnormalities in AML, some of which are associated with specific morphologic types. A notable example of this association is the t(15;17) (q11; q11-12), which occurs in 90% to 100% of cases of acute promyelocytic leukemia and is considered specific for this morphologic type of leukemia.[117] Other abnormalities, such as inv 16 (p13q22) and t(16:16) (p13; q22), that usually occur in acute myelomonocytic leukemia with increased marrow eosinophils, appear to be associated with a more prolonged survival. The t(8;21) (q22; q22) abnormality is identified in approximately 20% of cases of acute myeloblastic leukemia with maturation (M2). The translocation involves the AML-1 gene on chromosome 21 and the ETO gene on chromosome 8.[118]

The AMLs are generally aggressive diseases. Without therapy, most patients die within a few months. Multiagent chemotherapy results in remission in 50% to 75% of patients. The median survival for all types is 8.7 to 12.7 months with multiagent regimens.[119] Bone marrow transplantation is being increasingly used in the therapeutic approach to this disease.

Myelodysplastic syndromes

The myelodysplastic syndromes (MDS) are bone marrow disorders with the unifying feature of dysplasia in one or more of the myeloid cell lines, with or without a concurrent increase in myeloblasts.[120-124] In those myelodysplastic syndromes with increased blasts, the number in the blood or marrow is less than the 30% requisite for a diagnosis of AML. The clinical symptoms usually relate to bone marrow failure. The laboratory findings vary, but most patients are anemic. A substantial number of patients has bicytopenia or pancytopenia. A classification of the myelodysplastic syndromes and the major features of each are summarized in Table 41-16.

The dysplastic changes that characterize MDS may be present in one or more myeloid cell lines. Megaloblastoid erythropoiesis with macrocytosis is frequent (Fig. 41-37). Ringed sideroblasts may be present in all types and is the major finding in refractory anemia with ringed sideroblasts (Fig. 41-38). Neutrophils may show nuclear hypolobulation and diminished or abnormal granule production. Small dysplastic megakaryocytes with hypolobulated nuclei are frequent. The marrow in most cases of primary MDS is hypercellular; occasional cases may be hypocellular.

Cytogenetic abnormalities in the myeloid cells are evidence of the clonal nature of the disease. Relatively frequent chromosomal abnormalities are -5, 5q-, -7, 7q-, +8 and 20q-.[117,121-124] Complex abnormalities have been associated with a poor prognosis. Certain chromosomal abnormalities appear to define clinical pathologic syndromes. A de novo, isolated 5q-abnor-

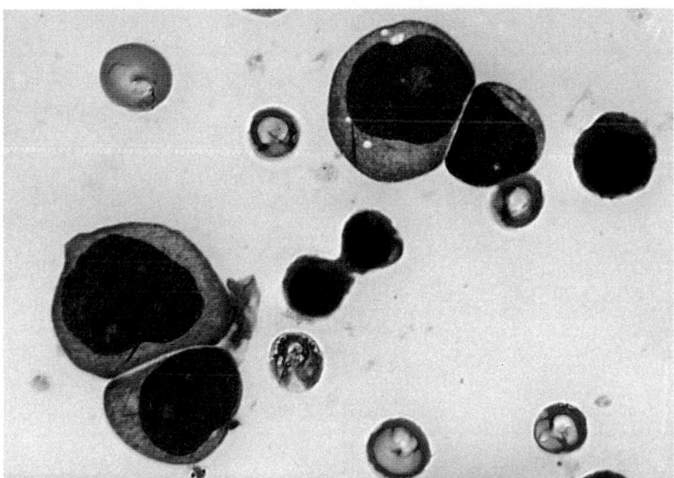

Fig. 41-34 Four myeloblasts in a bone marrow smear from a patient with acute myeloblastic leukemia with maturation (M2). These blasts vary in size and amount of cytoplasm. The blast at the upper right is small with sparse cytoplasm and more coarse nuclear chromatin and inconspicuous nucleoli. All of the blasts contain Auer rods (Wright-Giemsa).

Table 41-14 Summary of diagnostic features of acute myeloid leukemias

FAB type	Bone marrow findings	Immunophenotype
AML-M0	≥30% blasts; <3% blasts reactive for MPO, SBB, or NSE	≥20% blasts express one or more myeloid antigens: CD13, CD14, CD33; may be TdT positive; blasts negative for lymphocytic antigens
AML-M1	≥30% blasts; ≥3% blasts reactive for MPO or SBB; <10% of marrow nucleated cells are promyelocytes or more mature neutrophils	Blasts express myeloid antigens: CD13, CD14, CD33
AML-M2	≥30% of blasts; ≥3% blasts reactive for MPO or SBB; ≥ 10% of marrow nucleated cells are promyelocytes or more mature neutrophils	Blasts myeloid antigen positive; blasts in 40% to 80% of t(8;21) associated cases are CD19 positive; blasts in approximately 20% of t(8; 21) associated cases are TdT positive
AML-M3	≥ 30% blasts and abnormal promyelocytes; intense MPO and SBB reactivity; promyelocytes and blasts with multiple Auer rods (faggot cells); t(15;17) cytogenetic abnormality	Blasts and promyelocytes express myeloid antigens; promyelocytes are HLA-DR negative in most cases
AML-M4	≥30% myeloblasts, monoblasts, and promonocytes; ≥20% monocytic cells in marrow; ≥ 5 × 10^9/L monocytic cells in blood; ≥20% neutrophils and precursors in marrow; monocytic cells reactive for NSE; abnormal eosinophils in M4 with associated inv (16) chromosome abnormality	Varying proportions of blasts and monocytic cells express CD13, CD14, CD15, CD33; monocyte cells express CD36.
AML-M5A	≥80% monocytic cells; monoblasts ≥80% of monocytic cells; monoblasts and promonocytes NSE positive (approximately 10 to 20% of cases are negative or equivocally positive); monoblasts usually MPO and SBB negative (may be positive in a minority of cases)	Varying proportions of CD13, CD14, CD15, and CD33-positive cells; monoblasts express CD36 and may express CD4.
AML-M5B	≥80% of monocytic cells; monoblasts < 80% of monocytic cells; promonocytes predominate; monoblasts and promonocytes NSE positive; promonocytes may have scattered MPO-and SBB-positive granules.	Varying proportions of monoblasts and promonocytes express CD13, CD14, CD15, CD33; monoblasts and promonocytes express CD36.
AML-M6	≥50% erythroid precursors; ≥30% of nonerythroid precursors are myeloblasts; Auer rods may be present in myeloblasts; dyserythropoiesis; erythroid precursors frequently PAS positive.	Myeloblasts express myeloid antigens; erythroid precursors express glycophorin A, react with antibody to hemoglobin A, and express CD36.
AML-M7	≥30% blasts; ≥50% megakaryocytic cells by morphology, immunophenotype studies, or electron microscopy	Megakaryocytic cells express panmyeloid antigen CD33, and platelet glycoproteins (CD41 and CD61) and CD36.

MPO, Myeloperoxidase; *SBB,* Sudan black B; *NSE,* nonspecific esterase; *PAS,* periodic acid-Schiff; *TdT,* terminal deoxynucleotidyltransferase.

Table 41-15 Leukocyte count in patients with acute lymphoblastic and acute myeloid leukemias

Blood leukocyte count (X10^9/L)	ALL (%)	AML (%)
<5	25	29
5-10	15	15
10-49	34	28
50-99	15	13
>100	11	15

Modified from Wintrobe MM: *Clinical hematology,* ed 7, Lea and Febiger, 1974.

mality is associated with a MDS that occurs primarily in older women who present with a severe macrocytic anemia, normal or increased platelets, and hypolobated megakaryocytes; these patients usually have a prolonged survival (Fig. 41-39).[125] An isolated monosomy 7 in children is associated with an aggressive form of MDS.[126]

The evolution and survival for the major types of MDS are summarized in Table 41-17. Most patients who do not progress to acute myeloid leukemia generally develop marrow failure and succumb to complications of neutropenia and/or thrombocytopenia. However, as evident in Table 41-17, there is considerable variability in median survival between the various types of MDS, and a wide range of survival within some types. Refractory anemia with ringed sideroblasts has a low incidence of evolution to AML and a long median survival; it is probable that in a high percentage of these patients the hematologic findings are due to a metabolic abnormality and not neoplasia.

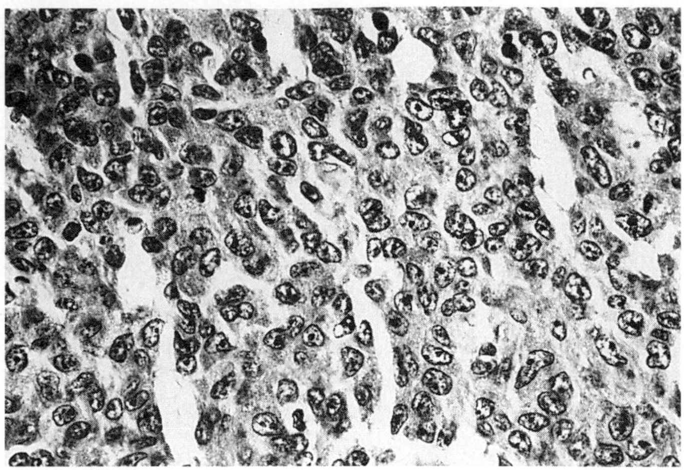

Fig. 41-35 Bone marrow biopsy from a patient with acute monoblastic leukemia. The marrow is markedly hypercellular due to replacement of normal hematopoietic cells by leukemic cells.

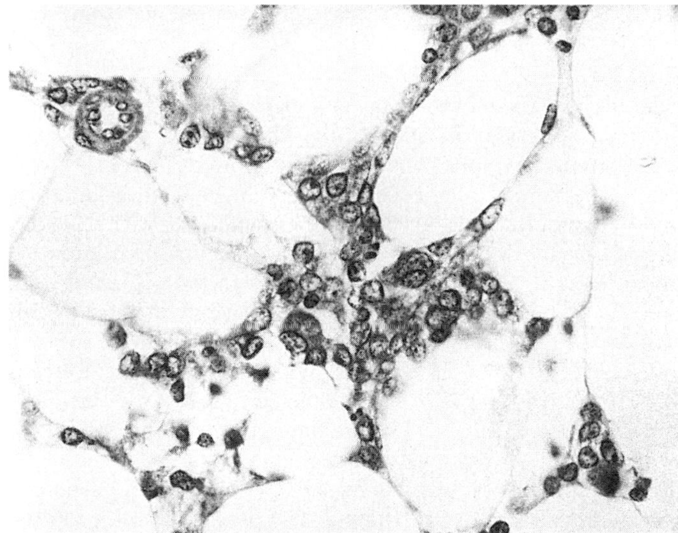

Fig. 41-36 Hypocellular bone marrow biopsy from a patient with acute myeloblastic leukemia without maturation (MI). The marrow interstitium contains a high percent of blasts in contrast to aplastic anemia in which the interstitium contains well-differentiated lymphocytes and plasma cells.

The therapy-related myelodysplastic syndromes occur in patients previously treated with chemotherapy and radiation.[123,127-129] The peak period of occurrence is 5 to 6 years after the initiation of therapy. These types of MDS frequently involve all the major myeloid cell lines and are basically stem cell disorders that manifest as a panmyelosis (Fig. 41-40). Clonal cytogenetic abnormalities involving chromosomes 5 and/or 7 are frequent. The clinical course is generally more aggressive than in the primary type. A form of therapy-related myelodysplastic syndrome occurring in patients treated with etoposide has a high association with abnormalities of 11q23 and frequently evidence of monocytic differentiation.

Chronic myeloproliferative disorders

Chronic myeloproliferative disorders (CMPDs) are stem cell disorders that manifest primarily as clonal expansions of predominantly mature myeloid cells in the bone marrow and blood. These disorders have a relatively long chronic phase, and usually evolve into an accelerated phase or an acute phase resembling acute leukemia with survival measured in months. In other instances the evolution is characterized by bone marrow failure without blastic transformation. Myelofibrosis is a common feature in the progression of these disorders.

Table 41-16 Classification of primary myelodysplastic syndromes

Refractory anemia (RA)	Anemia refractory to hematinic therapy; dyserythropoiesis +/–; granulocytes and megakaryocytes usually normal; marrow blasts less than 5%; no blasts in blood
Refractory anemia with ringed sideroblasts (RARS)	More than 15% of red cell precursors in marrow "ringed" sideroblasts; less than 5% blasts in marrow Dyserythropoiesis +/–; granulocytes and megakaryocytes usually normal
Refractory anemia with excess blasts (RAEB)	5% to 20% blasts in marrow; less than 5% blasts in blood
Refractory anemia with excess blasts in transformation (RAEB-T)	1. 20% to 29% blasts in marrow 2. 5% to 29% blasts in blood 3. Auer rods (any one criterion suffices)
Chronic myelomonocytic leukemia (CMML)	>1 × 10^9/L monocytes in blood; <20% blasts in marrow; dysgranulopoiesis +/–
Chronic myelomonocytic leukemia in transformation (CMML-T)	>1 × 10^9/L monocytes in blood and one of the criteria listed for RAEB-T
Myelodysplastic syndrome, unclassified	Less than 5% blasts in marrow; significant dysplasia in two or more myeloid cell lines

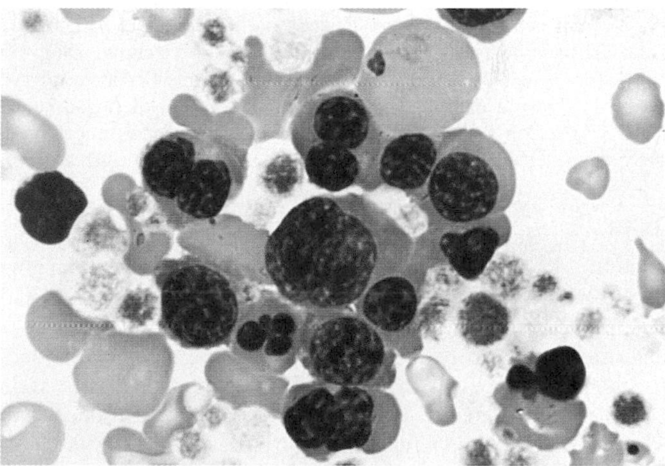

Fig. 41-37 Bone marrow smear from a patient with a therapy related myelodysplastic syndrome. There is marked dyserythropoiesis with megaloblastoid and lobulated nuclei (Wright-Giemsa).

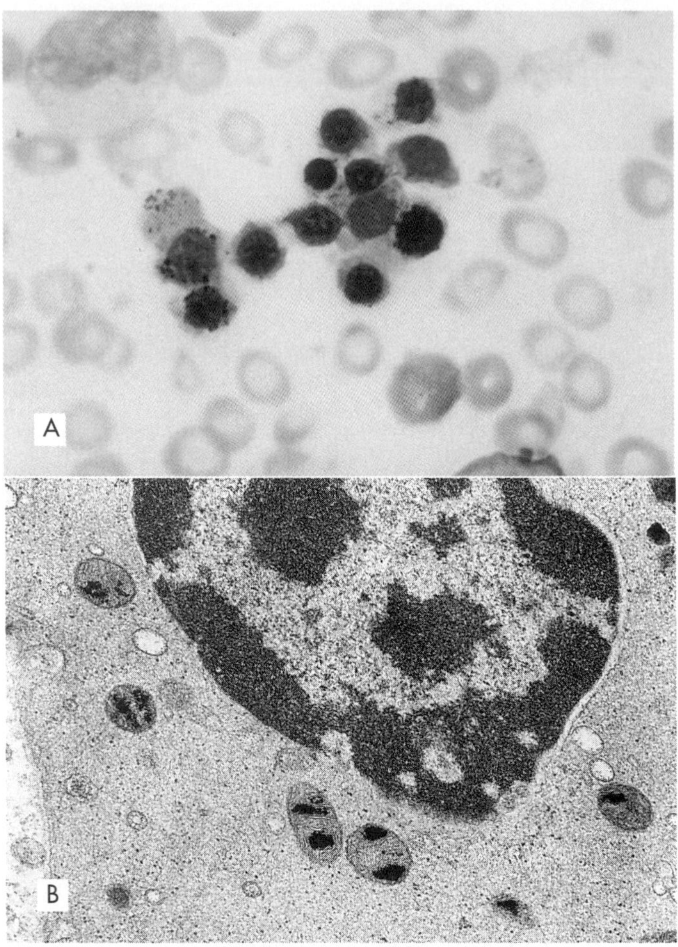

Fig. 41-38 Ringed Sideroblast: light microscopy and ultrastructure. **A,** Marrow smear showing a cluster of erythroblasts. The ringed sideroblasts have many blue-green iron granules circumscribing the nuclei (Prussian blue/Saffron). **B,** Electron micrograph of an erythroid precursor from a patient with refractory anemia with ringed sideroblasts. The iron appears as black deposits (ferruginous micelles) in the cristae of the mitochondria (Uranyl acetate, lead citrate).

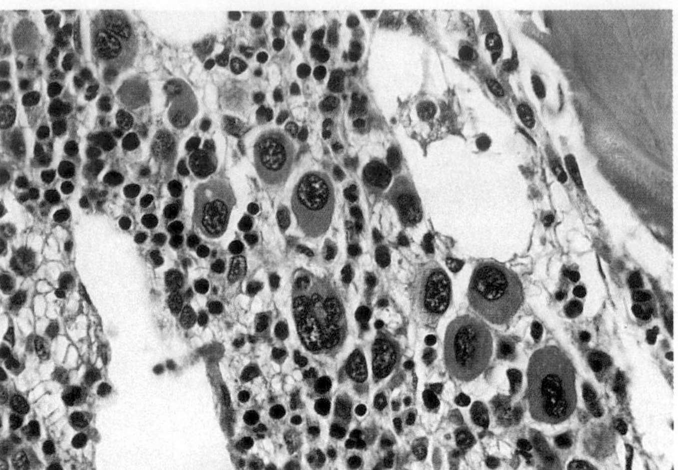

Fig. 41-39 Refractory anemia with excess of blasts associated with a de novo isolated $5q^-$ chromosome abnormality. Bone marrow biopsy from a 57-year-old woman with macrocytic anemia, 6% myeloblasts in the marrow smear and a de novo isolated $5q^-$ cytogenetic abnormality. Megakaryocytes are numerous, and some have hypolobulated nuclei.

The four generally recognized CMPDs are: chronic myeloid leukemia (CML), polycythemia vera (PV), chronic idiopathic myelofibrosis (CIM or agnogenic myeloid metaplasia), and essential thrombocythemia (ET). The historical basis for subclassification has been the predominating cell type in the blood. It is generally accepted that the CMPDs are hematopoietic stem cell disorders, capable of multi-lineage differentiation in any given patient. Recent advances in the understanding of the biology of these lesions has led to a multidisciplinary approach to the diagnosis and classification of these malignancies which includes hematologic and physical findings, cytogenetic and molecular analysis, and blood chemistry profiles.

Juvenile chronic myeloid leukemia (JCML) and chronic myelomonocytic leukemia-myeloproliferative are in the differential diagnosis of CMPD.

Chronic myeloid leukemia

The diagnostic features of CML are splenomegaly, a marked leukocytosis, basophilia, and the Philadelphia chromosome by cytogenetic analysis.[130] Although the vast majority of patients present with white blood cell counts above 50 x 10^9/L, the disease may be diagnosed with leukocyte counts less than 10 x 10^9/L with the identification of the Philadelphia chromosome, t (9;22), or its molecular equivalent, the BCR-ABL hybrid gene. The annual incidence of CML in the United States is approximately 1 to 2 per 100,000 individuals.[131] The median age of onset is 53 years.[132] The disease occurs in children but is uncommon. Splenomegaly is present in more than 70% of patients at presentation, and symptomatology related to this finding is frequently the presenting chief complaint.[133]

In 70% to 90% of patients the leukocyte count exceeds 100x10^9/L (Fig. 41-41). Marked leukocytosis is particularly common in children.[134] The predominant leukocytes are neutrophils at the myelocyte and segmented stages; myeloblasts do not generally exceed 2% to 3%.[133] An absolute basophilia is present in virtually all patients. The platelet count is normal to increased with a mean of 484x10^9/L; some patients present with a marked thrombocythemia as the initial manisfestation.[135] The hemoglobin is generally slightly to moderately decreased. The neutrophil alkaline phosphatase (NAP) score is decreased in 90% to 95% of cases.[136]

The bone marrow is markedly hypercellular with a neutrophilic hyperplasia. Megakaryocytes are increased in number with a spectrum of maturation from small nonlobulated forms to larger polylobulated forms. Reticulin fibers may be increased. Sea blue histiocytes and pseudo-Gaucher cells may be present.

The Philadelphia (Ph) chromosome [t(9;22) (q34;q11)] is present in 95% of cases and is the earliest recognized manifestation of this disease. This acquired abnormality results from the reciprocal translocation between the c-*abl* oncogene (ABL) on chromosome 9 and the major breakpoint cluster region (M-bcr) of the breakpoint cluster region gene (BCR) on chromosome 22 (Fig. 41-42).[130] In those cases of CML that are negative for the Ph by cytogenetics, BCR/ABL rearrangement is identified by molecular studies.

The usual biologic course of CML is a chronic phase of 3 to 4 years followed by a more aggressive phase of relatively short duration.[137] The aggressive phase manifests as an overt transformation to an acute leukemia, *blast crisis,* or a more

Table 41-17 Myelodysplastic syndromes: median survival and incidence of leukemic evolution

Type	Percent developing acute leukemia	Median survival in months (range)
Refractory anemia (RA)	12	50 (18-64)
Refractory anemia with ringed sideroblasts (RARS)	8	51(14-76+)
Refractory anemia with excess of blasts (RAEB)	44	11 (7-16)
Refractory anemia with excess of blasts in transformation (RAEB-T)	60	8 (2.5-11)
Chronic myelomonocytic leukemia (CMML)	40	11 (9-60+)

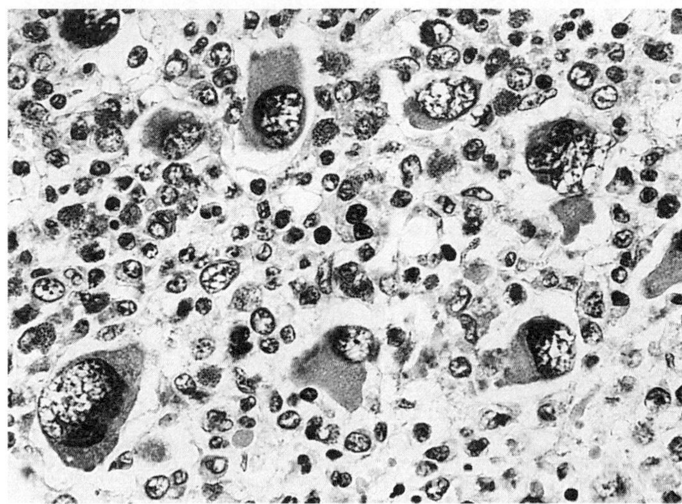

Fig. 41-40 Bone marrow section from a patient with a therapy related acute panmyelosis. All major myeloid cell lines are increased. The megakaryocytes appear dysplastic with dispersed nuclear chromatin and hypolobulated nuclei.

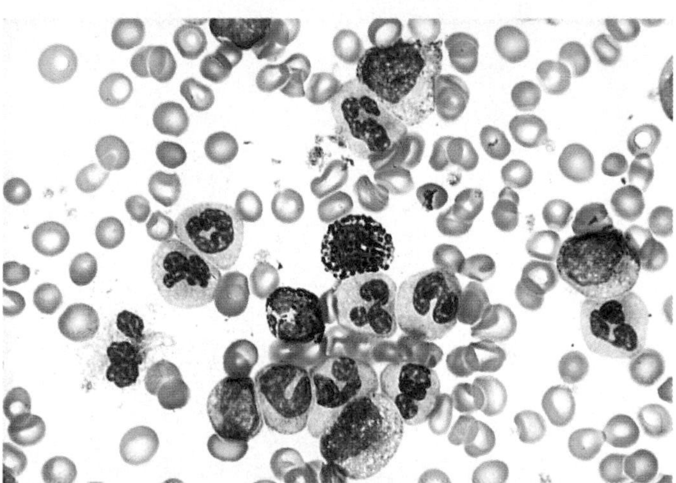

Fig. 41-41 Blood smear from a child with chronic myeloid leukemia showing marked leukocytosis and basophilia. Karyotype analysis identified a Philadelphia chromosome (Wright-Giemsa).

insidious change, *accelerated phase,* that heralds marrow failure.[132,138-140] The blast crisis is defined as 30% or more blasts in the blood or marrow or a focus of blasts in a marrow biopsy or extramedullary site. In 70% of cases the blasts are cytochemically and/or immunophenotypically myeloid.[139] Maturation into any one or all of the three myeloid cell lines may be apparent. Dysgranulocytopoiesis is frequently present. The blasts in 30% of blast crises are morphologically and immunophenotypically lymphoblastic.[141,142]

The accelerated phase is characterized by one or more of the following findings: increase of marrow or blood blasts but less than 30%, karyotypic evolution, significant and progressive myelofibrosis, or greater than 20% basophils in the blood.[139,140] The accelerated phase may evolve to blast crisis. Blast crisis and accelerated phase are often accompanied by cytogenetic evolution. The most common additional cytogenetic abnormalities are a second Ph, trisomy 8, trisomy 19, and isochromosome 17q.[143]

Polycythemia vera

Polycythemia vera is characterized by an increased red cell mass and splenomegaly (Table 41-18). There is no evidence of the Philadelphia chromosome by cytogenetic or molecular analysis. The annual incidence is 0.5 to 1.0 cases per 100,000 individuals, and the median age of onset is 60 years.[144,145] There is a slight male predominance. Symptoms are related primarily to the increased blood viscosity due to increased red blood cell mass and include headache, dizziness, and weakness; postbathing pruritus occurs in some patients. Splenomegaly is present in 90% of cases.

Hematocrits are markedly elevated in most cases. The leukocyte count is usually 10 to 20 $\times$ 10^9/L with left-shifted neutrophilic leukocytosis. Absolute basophilia is present in two thirds of the patients. Platelet counts are normal or elevated. The bone marrow is markedly hypercellular with increased numbers of all three myeloid cell types (Fig. 41-43). Megakaryocytes are frequently disproportionately increased and may occur in clusters. Iron stores are usually absent or decreased. The neutrophil alkaline phosphatase (NAP) score is elevated or high normal.[146]

Secondary causes of elevated hematocrit must be excluded before a diagnosis of PV is established (Table 41-19). The diagnosis of PV should be made with caution in patients with decreased arterial oxygen saturation.

Polycythemia vera is characterized by a long stable phase of 5 to 20 years' duration. In 10% to 20% of patients the stable phase is followed by a "spent phase" (myeloid metaplasia) marked by decreasing red cell mass, myelofibrosis, increasing splenomegaly and extramedullary hematopoiesis. Ten percent of patients eventually develop acute myeloid leukemia; risk factors include therapeutic administration of chlorambucil or ^{32}P and the presence of the spent phase.[147]

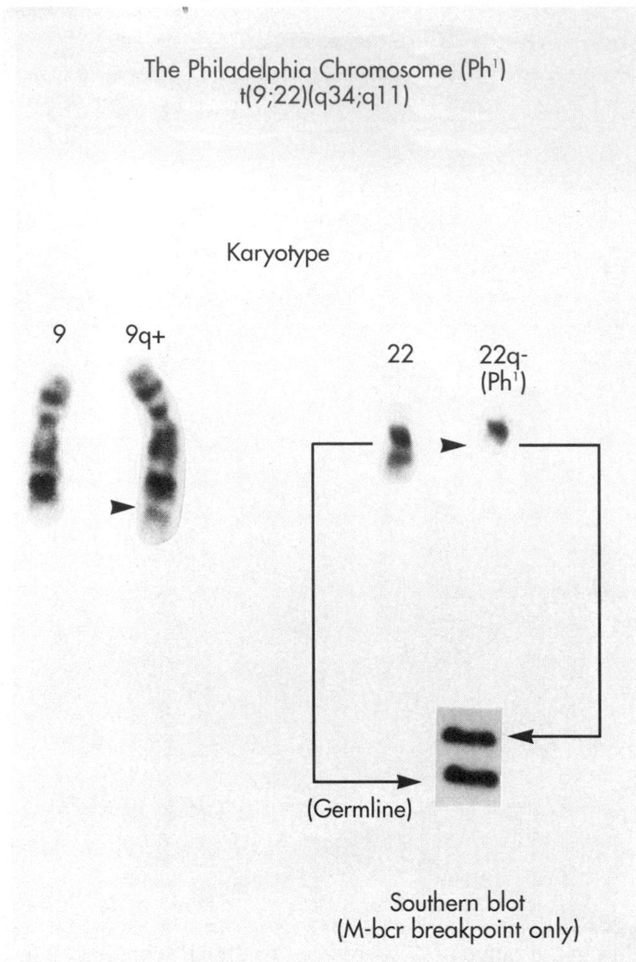

Fig. 41-42 Chronic myeloid leukemia: Philadelphia chromosome. Karyotype of a cell and southern blot of the DNA from a marrow specimen of a patient with CML. The two arrows denote chromosomes 9 and 22 breakpoints in the t(9;22). In the lower right is an autoradiogram of a Southern blot of BglII digested DNA hybridized to a probe recognizing sequences in the major breakpoint cluster region (M-bcr) on chromosome 22. The upper and lower bands are from the rearranged and unrearranged chromosomes 22, respectively.

Table 41-18 Polycythemia Vera Study Group criteria for the diagnosis of polycythemia vera*

A Criteria
1. Increased red blood cell mass
males: ≥36 ml/kg
females: ≥32 ml/kg
2. Normal arterial oxygen saturation
3. Splenomegaly
B Criteria
1. Thrombocytosis: ≥400 $\times 10^9$/L
2. Leukocytes: ≥12 $\times 10^9$/L†
3. Increased neutrophil alkaline phosphatase†
4. Increased serum vitamin B_{12} or unsaturated B_{12} binding protein

*To diagnose PV the patient must have all A criteria or A1, A2, and two B criteria.
†In the absence of fever or infection.
Modified from Hoffman R, Wasserman LR: *Adv Intern Med* 24:255, 1974.

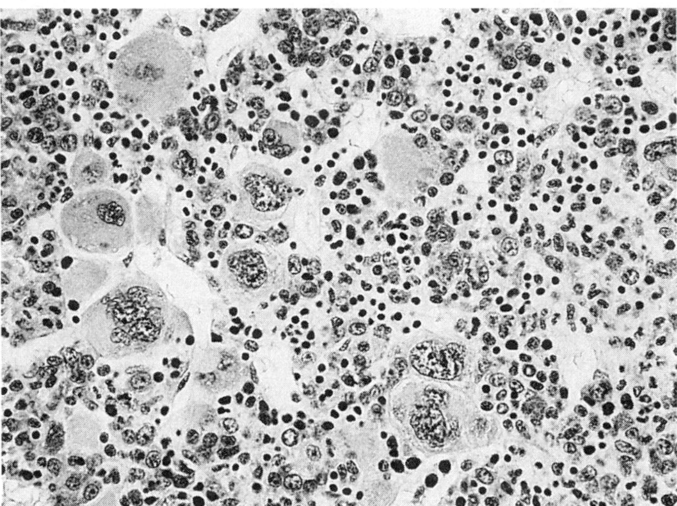

Fig. 41-43 Hypercellular marrow biopsy from a patient with polycythemia vera showing pan myeloid hyperplasia.

Essential thrombocythemia

Essential thrombocythemia is characterized by marked thrombocytosis; the presence of a Philadelphia chromosome or molecular evidence of the BCR/ABL hybrid gene is exclusionary for the diagnosis (Table 41-20).[148] The median age of onset is 61 years. There is no sex predominance; a younger subset of predominantly female patients is affected in the fourth and fifth decades.[149]

Patients frequently present with abnormal bleeding or microvasculature vaso-occlusive events. Splenomegaly is present in one third of patients. The majority of patients have platelet counts in excess of 1000 × 10^9/L; the median leukocyte count is 11.5 × 10^9/L. The bone marrow is usually hypercellular but may be normal or hypocellular; hypocellular marrows are more common in older individuals. The principal findings are in the megakaryocytes, which may show changes similar to those in PV; the latter is usually characterized by a panhyperplasia with an increase in erythroid precursors and granulocytes. In some patients the distinction between PV and ET is not possible on the basis of marrow morphology. The major distinguishing laboratory and clinical features are listed in Tables 40-18 and 40-20

Patients with ET have a prolonged course with 80% survival at 5 to 8 years. Patients under 40 years of age generally have a more indolent disease than older patients.[149] Morbidity and mortality are related to thromboembolic and hemorrhagic events; these are controlled by agents such as hydroxyurea and anagrelide, which reduce the platelet number.[150]

Chronic idiopathic myelofibrosis (agnogenic myeloid metaplasia)

Chronic idiopathic myelofibrosis is a panmyelosis with varying degrees of myelofibrosis, splenomegaly, and extramedullary hematopoiesis. There is no Philadelphia chromosome or BCR/ABL hybrid gene. The median age of onset is 60 to 67 years, with a male predominance.[151] Presenting complaints are

Table 41-19 Causes of elevated hematocrit

Normal red cell mass (relative polycythemia)
- Dehydration
- Smoking
- Idiopathic

Increased red cell mass
- Primary
  - Polycythemia vera
- Secondary (due to increased erythropoietin secretion)
  - Low O_2 saturation
    - Cardiopulmonary disease
    - High altitude
  - Normal or elevated O_2 saturation
    - Inappropriate erythropoietin secretion
      - Renal vascular impairment
      - Hydronephrosis
      - Neoplasia
        - Hepatoma
        - Renal cell carcinomas and cysts
        - Cerebellar hemangiomas
        - Uterine leiyomyomas
    - High O_2 affinity hemoglobins
      - Fetal hemoglobin
      - Hemoglobin chesapeake
      - Hemoglobin malmo

Modified from Berlin NI, *Semin Hematol* 12:340, 1975.

Table 41-20 Polycythemia Vera Study Group criteria for the diagnosis of essential thrombocythemia

Platelet count >600 $\times 10^9$/L
Hemoglobin ≤13 gm/dL or normal red cell mass
No stainable marrow iron or no response to iron therapy
No cytogenetic or molecular evidence of the Ph chromosome
Collagen fibrosis
- Absent
- Involving less than 1/3 of biopsy specimen in patients lacking both splenomegaly and a leukoerythroblastic reaction

No demonstrable cause for a thrombocytosis

Modified from Murphy et al, *Semin Hematol* 23:178, 1986.

fatigue, weight loss, and fever. Hepatosplenomegaly is virtually always present.

Most patients are anemic.[152] The leukocyte count ranges from 1 to 62 $\times 10^9$/L (mean: 15 $\times 10^9$/L). Rarely, patients may present with leukocyte counts in excess of 100 $\times 10^9$/L. Leukoerythroblastosis and increased red blood cell poikilocytosis with dacryocytes are characteristic of CIM. Atypical, large, hypogranular platelets and micromegakaryocytes are generally noted. The marrow is hypercellular in most cases with varying proportions of hematopoietic cells and fibrosis. Dense fibrosis with coarse bundles of collagen and osteosclerosis may be present (Fig. 41-44). The sinusoids may be markedly dilated with prominent hematopoiesis. Megakaryocytes are increased and show dysplastic changes, which include condensed chromatin and distorted nuclei. Although fibrosis is prominent, the fibroblastic proliferation is an epiphenomenon; the fibrocytes are not derived from the malignant stem cell.

There are variable degrees of extramedullary hematopoiesis in the spleen, liver, and lymph nodes involving all three myeloid cell lines; megakaryocytes are generally most conspicuous (Fig. 41-45).[153] It has generally been viewed that the degree of marrow fibrosis and splenomegaly parallels the duration of disease. Ward and Block described three temporally-related morphologic stages in the marrow.[154] The initial stage was characterized by a panmyeloid hyperplasia; the second by myeloid cell atrophy with increasing fibrous tissue, and the third by marked fibrosis and possibly osteosclerosis. Other investigators have not found this close temporal relationship.[155]

Patients with CIM have a median survival of 5 years.[156,157] Occasionally, transformation to acute myeloid leukemia occurs.

Juvenile chronic myeloid leukemia

Juvenile chronic myeloid leukemia is a myeloid disorder occurring in children, usually less than 2 years of age.[158] The hematologic features are more those of a myelodysplastic syndrome than of a chronic myeloproliferative disorder. There is no cytogenetic or molecular evidence of the Philadelphia chromosome or monosomy 7. The male to female ratio is 2:1. Hepatosplenomegaly, lymphadenopathy, and a skin rash, frequently facial, are common presenting findings. There is moderate anemia and leukocytosis ranging from 27 to 77 $\times 10^9$/L. The leukocyte differential generally shows a higher percentage of myeloblasts, monocytes, lymphocytes and nucleated red blood cells than Ph-positive CML. Thrombocytopenia is generally present. Basophilia may be present. The marrow is hypercellular; megakaryocytes are generally decreased. An important diagnostic feature of JCML is elevated fetal hemoglobin in the range of 40% to 55%. The NAP score in JCML is usually decreased.

Juvenile chronic myeloid leukemia is characterized by progressive bone marrow failure without overt blast crisis. The median survival is 10 to 12 months.[159,160]

Hypereosinophilic syndrome

The hypereosinophilic syndrome is a rare disorder of unexplained persistent eosinophilia; the eosinophils usually exceed 1.5 $\times 10^9$/L.[161,162]

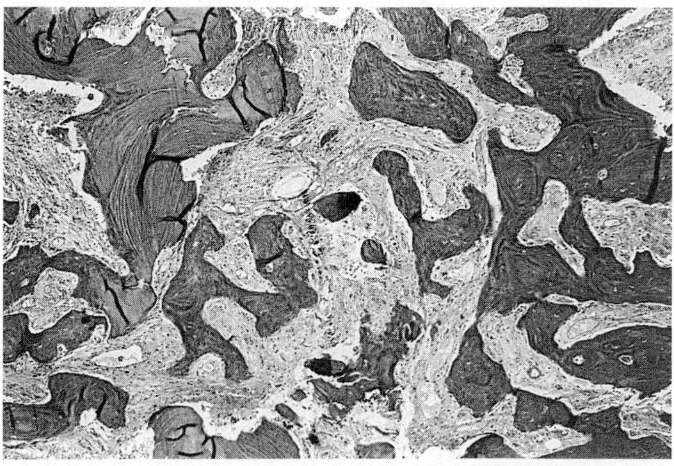

Fig. 41-44 Marrow biopsy with marked myelofibrosis and osteosclerosis from a patient with chronic idiopathic myelofibrosis.

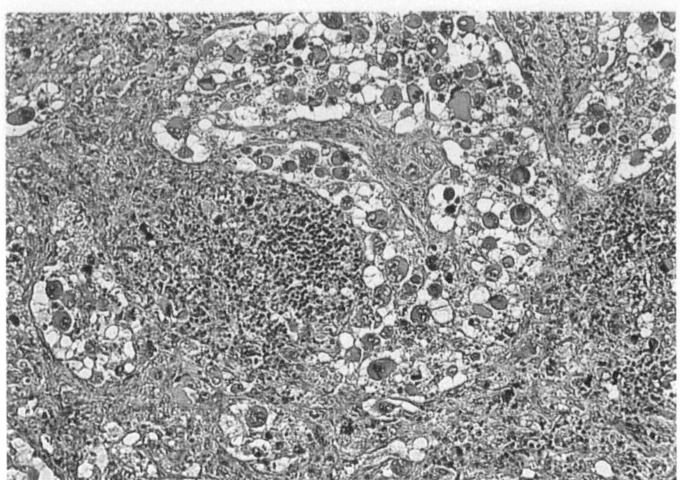

Fig. 41-45 Lymph node from a patient with chronic idiopathic myelofibrosis, showing intrasinusoid extramedullary hematopoiesis; megakaryocytes are prominent.

The symptomatology relates to organ dysfunction as a result of tissue damage by injurious products released by the eosinophil granules in the form of major basic protein and eosinophil cationic protein.[162,163] The organs most frequently involved are the heart, lungs, and central nervous system. Hematologic findings may include anemia, thrombocytopenia, marrow fibrosis, and possible evolution to acute leukemia.

Systemic mastocytosis

Systemic mastocytosis is an uncommon disorder marked by mast cell proliferation in several organs, including bone marrow and spleen. It usually presents in the context of urticaria pigmentosa but may occur in the absence of cutaneous manifestations. The median age of onset for patients with urticaria pigmentosa is 45 years; the median age of onset for patients without urticaria pigmentosa is 75 years.[164] The clinical findings include weakness, fractures, weight loss, arthralgias, episodic flushing, bronchospasm, and diarrhea. Radiologic changes include osteoblastic, osteolytic, or concurrent osteoblastic/osteolytic lesions of bone.

The bone marrow is the most common noncutaneous site of involvement.[164-166] The lesions may be focal or diffuse and consist predominantly of mast cells, or may be polycellular, consisting of mast cells, lymphocytes, histiocytes, and eosinophils (Fig. 41-46). The noninvolved marrow frequently shows a granulocytic hyperplasia. There appears to be an increased incidence of myeloproliferative disorders in patients with systemic mastocytosis.[167]

Granulocytic sarcoma

Granulocytic sarcoma is a tumor of myeloid cells occurring in an extramedullary site.[168,169] The tumors are more common in children than adults. The term *chloroma* has been used for these lesions because of the green color of the cut surface due to the myeloperoxidase content. Granulocytic sarcomas may occur as isolated lesions, or in conjunction with an acute or chronic myeloproliferative disorder. An association with AML-M2 with the t(8;21) chromosome abnormality has been reported.[170] The most common sites are the subperiostium of the bones of the skull, paranasal sinuses, sternum, ribs, vertebrae, and pelvis; skin and lymph nodes are additional, relatively frequent sites of occurrence. The cytology of the tumors varies from a uniform population of poorly differentiated blasts to lesions in which there is maturation to more mature cells, including promyelocytes and myelocytes. Immature eosinophils are frequently present in lesions showing maturation. In most instances where granulocytic sarcoma occurs as an isolated lesion, the process evolves to acute myeloid leukemia after months to years. In other instances, recurrence of the disease is characterized by granulocytic sarcomas at additional sites.[168] Local radiation therapy is curative in some patients.

Acute lymphoblastic leukemia

Acute lymphoblastic leukemia (ALL) is a form of acute leukemia in which the proliferating cells are lymphoblasts.[171] There are three morphologic types, based on the predominant blast morphology: L1, L2, and L3. The L1 lymphoblast is a small cell, approximately twice the size of a normal lymphocyte, with a high nuclear/cytoplasmic ratio, a homogenous, smooth nuclear chromatin, and no identified or inconspicuous nucleoli (Fig. 41-47). The L2 lymphoblasts are larger than the L1 lymphoblast, with moderate amounts of lightly basophilic cytoplasm and fine nuclear chromatin with distinct and sometimes prominent multiple nucleoli (Fig. 41-47).

L3 lymphoblasts have a moderate amount of intensely basophilic cytoplasm that contains sharply defined, clear vacuoles, which are usually oil red O positive and periodic acid Schiff negative. The nucleus is round to oval and contains two to four distinct nucleoli; the chromatin is slightly coarse (Fig. 41-48). Mitotic figures are numerous. Approximately 95% of ALLs are L1 or L2; L1 is the predominant type in childhood, and L2 is the predominant type in adults; 2% to 5% of both adult and childhood ALL has L3 morphology.[171]

The intertrabecular space of the bone marrow is usually replaced by lymphoblasts. Mitotic figures are sparse in ALL-L1; in a minority of cases, particularly those with T-cell phenotype or those associated with the Philadelphia chromosome, mitotic figures may be abundant. In ALL-L2 mitotic activity is

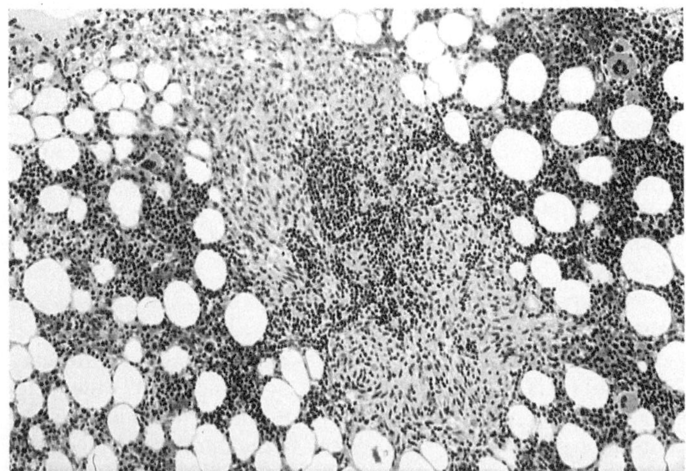

Fig. 41-46 Focal mast cell lesion in a marrow biopsy from a patient with systemic mastocytosis. There is a central focal infiltrate of well-differentiated lymphocytes. The mast cells are slightly elongated and have lightly staining cytoplasm.

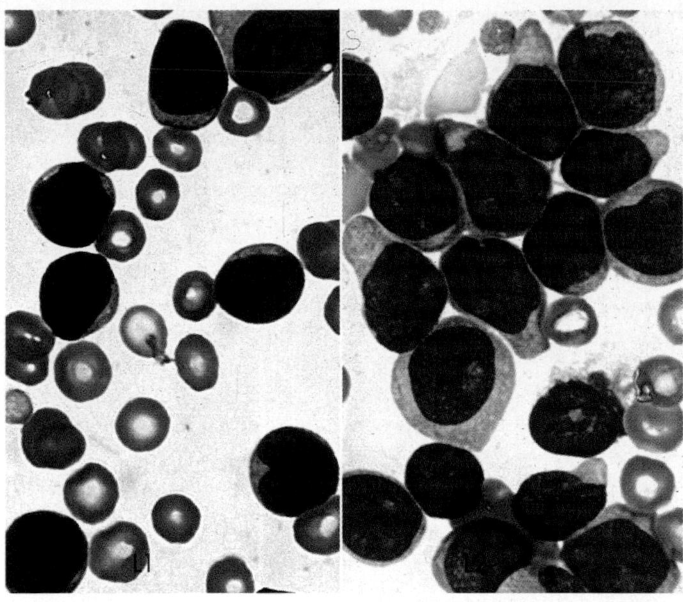

Fig. 41-47 Acute lymphoblastic leukemia. Characteristic morphology of L1 and L2 lymphoblasts in marrow aspirates (Wright-Giemsa).

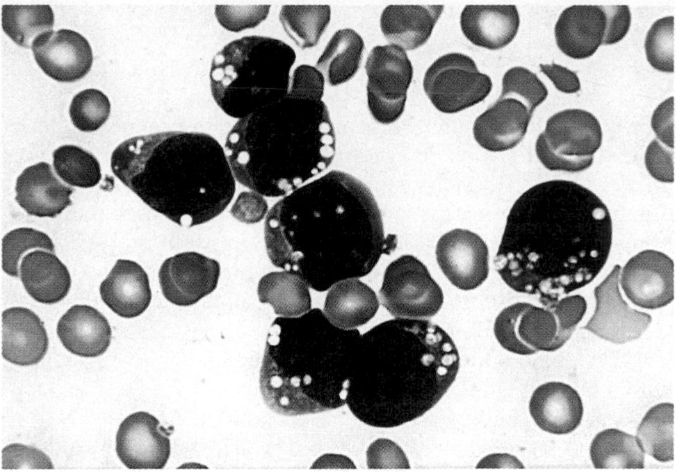

Fig. 41-48 Acute lymphoblastic leukemia. L3 lymphoblasts in a marrow aspirate. The cytoplasm contains sharply outlined cytoplasmic vacuoles (Wright-Giemsa).

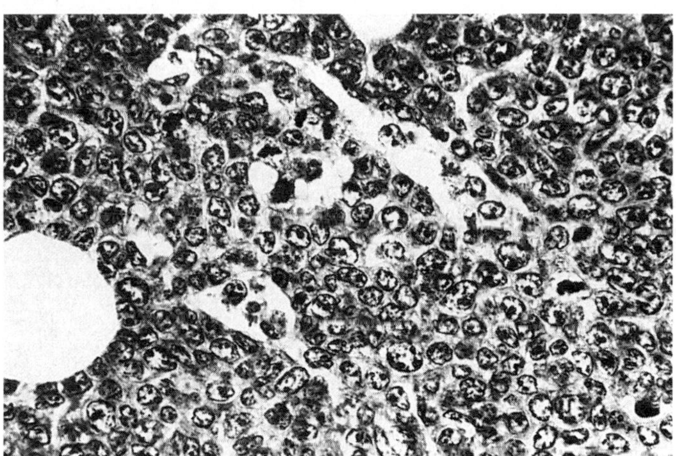

Fig. 41-49 Acute lymphoblastic leukemia. L3 lymphoblasts in trephine biopsy section. Several mitotic figures are present.

variable. The marrow histology in ALL-L3 is that of a small noncleaved cell lymphoma, Burkitt's or non-Burkitt's type. Mitotic figures are numerous. The starry sky appearance encountered in lymph nodes is usually not recapitulated in the marrow (Fig. 41-49).

There are three major immunophenotypic groups of ALL: B-cell precursor, T-cell, and B-cell.[172-176] The lymphoblasts in B-cell precursor ALL express pan B-cell antigens but lack cell surface immunoglobulin; these cells express the nuclear enzyme, terminal deoxynucleotidyltransferase (TdT). B-cell precursor ALL has either L1 or L2 morphology. This group accounts for 85% of ALLs and is clinically diverse. B-cell precursor ALL may be further divided into three immunophenotypic groups: null cell, common, and pre-B (Table 41-21).[173,174,176] The lymphoblasts of "common" B-cell precursor ALL are positive for CD10 (CALLA) and do not express cytoplasmic μ heavy chains. Lymphoblasts in "pre-B" B-cell precursor ALL are distinguished by the expression of cytoplasmic μ heavy chains and, usually CD10 positivity.[176] "Null cell" lymphoblasts lack both CD10 and cytoplasmic μ chain. Acute lymphoblastic leukemia arising in infants is frequently of the "null cell" type.

The lymphoblasts of T-cell ALL variably express pan T-cell surface antigens; cytoplasmic CD3 and nuclear TdT are expressed in a majority of cases. T-cell ALL accounts for 15% of all ALLs and has either L1 or L2 morphology. Patients with T-cell ALL are predominantly male, adolescent, and present with a marked leukocytosis.[175] Approximately half of the cases present with a mediastinal mass, and central nervous system involvement is frequent.

The lymphoblasts of B-cell ALL express pan–B-cell antigens, cell surface immunoglobulin, and have L3 morphology; however, they lack nuclear TdT. There is a male predilection in B-cell ALL with a male to female ratio of 5: 1.[175] Virtually all cases of B-cell ALL are associated with the t(8;14) or the variant translocations, t(2;8) or t(8;22). Each of these translocations represents the juxtaposition of an immunoglobulin heavy chain locus (chromosome 14) or kappa (chromosome 2) or lambda (chromosome 22) light chain locus to the c-*myc* oncogene on chromosome 8. This results in increased c-*myc* transcription and is fundamental in the pathogenesis of this malignancy, as discussed in Chapter 24.[177] There is a strong association of ileocecal lymphoma of small, non-cleaved cell type (SNCL) in patients with ALL-L3. Acute lymphoblastic leukemia-L3 and SNCL are cytologically, immunologically, and cytogenetically identical; these two disorders are either closely related or represent different manifestations of the same process.

Lymphoblastic lymphomas of the T-cell and B-cell precursor types frequently involve the marrow and/or blood. The distinction between marrow involvement by lymphoblastic lymphoma and ALL-L1 or ALL-L2 may not be completely clear in some patients. Evidence of marrow sparing, as reflected by normal or near normal hematologic parameters, and partial involvement of the marrow on trephine biopsy suggest an extramedullary origin of the tumor.

Symptoms of ALL are related to bone marrow failure due to marrow replacement by lymphoblasts. Organomegaly and lymphadenopathy are present in approximately 75% of patients.

Fifty to seventy percent of children with B-cell precursor ALL achieve long-term disease-free survival with contemporary chemotherapeutic protocols.[178] Adverse prognostic determinants in ALL include age at diagnosis of less than 1 year or greater than 10 years, marked leukocytosis at diagnosis, organomegaly, and the presence of chromosomal translocations. Cytogenetic abnormalities are frequent in ALL, and some are of independent prognostic significance. Hyperdiploid karyotypes with more than 50 chromosomes are usually associated with a good prognosis; those with translocations such as t(9;22), t(8;14), t(4;11), and t(1;19) are generally associated with a poor prognosis.[179]

Approximately 5% of cases of childhood ALL and 20% to 30% of cases of adult ALL are associated with the Philadelphia chromosome.[180] The blasts are morphologically L1 or L2, TdT^+, $CD10^+$, B-cell precursors that may express cytoplasmic immunoglobulin. Marked leukocytosis is common. Rarely the neoplasia arises in an extramedullary site. The breakpoints of the t(9;22) associated with ALL may be located in one of two major regions in the BCR gene on chromosome 22 (Fig. 41-50). Fifty to ninety percent of cases have a breakpoint location in the BCR gene in the first intron; younger patients have a higher incidence of the breakpoint in this location.[181] The BCR breakpoints in most of the remaining cases are located in introns 13 or 14 of the BCR gene, the same introns most commonly involved in the t(9;22) of CML.[130] Breakpoints in either location juxtapose the BCR gene on chromosome 22 with the c-*abl* oncogene on chromosome 9 and result in a BCR-ABL fusion protein product considered essential to the pathogenesis of the leukemia.

The t(4;11) occurs in approximately 2% of childhood ALL, usually in infants less than 1 year of age.[182] There is frequently a marked leukocytosis. The lymphoid blasts are B-cell precursors, generally of the null cell type. In contrast to other B-cell precursor ALLs, the lymphoblasts in a high percentage of cases do not express CD10 or CD24. CD15 and, occasionally, other myeloid antigens may be expressed. The TdT is positive in this type of ALL, but the percentage of reactive blasts varies. The t(4:11) acute leukemia may involve a common, hematopoietic progenitor cell and manifest as a biphenotypic leukemia (Fig. 41-51).[183]

Table 41-21 Subtypes of B-cell precursor ALL

Type	CD10 (CALLA)	Cytoplasmic µ	Surface Ig	TdT
Null cell	–	–	–	+
Common	+	–	–	+
Pre B	+/–	+	–	+

µ, Immunoglobulin IgM heavy chains; TdT, Terminal deoxynucleotidyltransferase

Mixed phenotype acute leukemia

Mixed phenotype acute leukemia is a form of leukemia in which the blasts have characteristics of lymphoid and myeloid lineages.[184] The leukemia may be classified as either mixed lineage or bilineal, depending on the expression patterns in the individual blasts. In mixed lineage acute leukemias the blasts coexpress the myeloid and lymphoid characteristics; in bilineal acute leukemia two populations of blasts are noted, those that express lymphoid characteristics and those that express myeloid characteristics.

Myeloid antigen positive ALL is a specific type of mixed phenotype acute leukemia with blasts having the morphologic and immunophenotypic features of lymphoblasts, but that coexpress one or more myeloid antigens. This may occur in both B-cell precursor and T-lineage ALL. In the B-cell precursor leukemias it is a more frequent occurrence in adult patients

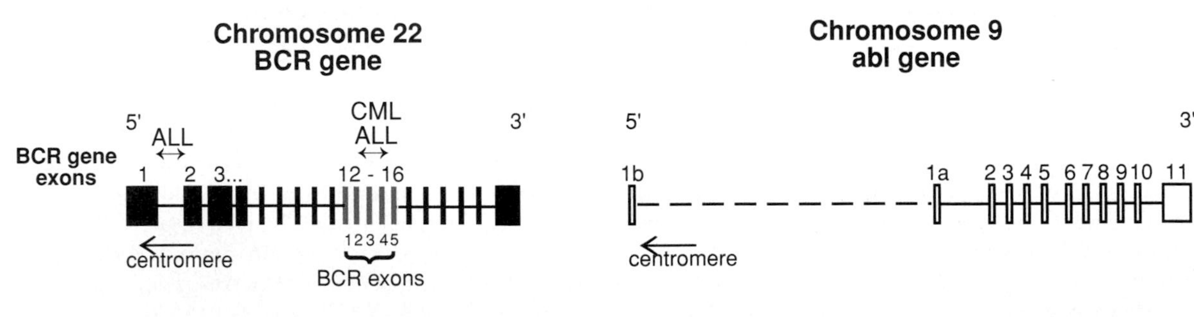

CML BCR-abl gene (Ph chromosome)

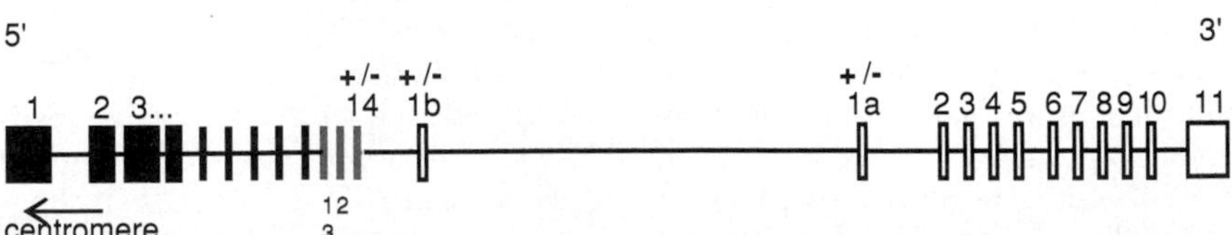

Fig. 41-50 Schematic diagram of the Philadelphia chromosome. The upper portion shows the unrearranged BCR gene and *c-abl* oncogene on chromosomes 22 and 9, respectively. The lower portion shows the relationship of the two genes on the Philadelphia chromosome. The boxes represent the exons. The locations of the ALL and CML breakpoints in the BCR gene are indicated. (Modified from Kurzrock et al: *N Engl J Med* 319:990, 1988.)

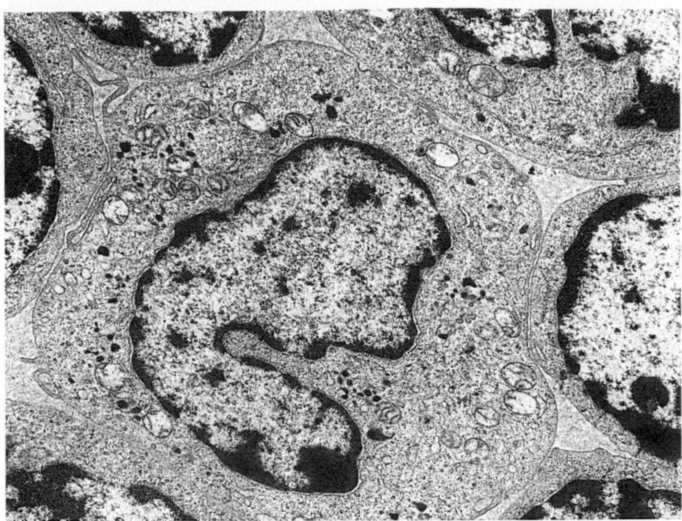

Fig. 41-51 Transmission electron micrograph of monocytoid cells in a bone marrow specimen from a case of acute lymphoblastic leukemia associated with the t(4;11) chromosome abnormality. The leukemia associated with this translocation has the potential of concurrent lymphoid and myeloid differentiation (Uranyl Acetate/Lead Citrate).

and ALLs associated with the t(9;22) and t(4;11).[185,186] This aberrant phenotype may reflect a malignant transformation of a pluripotential hematopoietic stem cell.

Chronic lymphoproliferative disorders

The chronic lymphoproliferative disorders include a very heterogeneous group of diseases that are generally characterized as proliferations of small well-differentiated lymphocytes. In some of these diseases, most notably prolymphocytic leukemia, the proliferative process involves larger lymphocytes. Immunologically, this group of leukemias includes B-cell and T-cell types that are clinically and morphologically heterogeneous.

B-cell chronic lymphoproliferative disorders

Table 41-22 is a classification of the major small B-lymphocyte proliferations.

B-cell chronic lymphocytic leukemia is a sustained lymphocytosis of light chain-restricted lymphocytes.[187,188] The annual incidence in the United States is 2.6 cases per 100,000 individuals.[113] The disease is more common in older individuals; the male to female ratio is 3:1. The clinical findings include lymphadenopathy, splenomegaly, and hepatomegaly. Clinical staging systems for CLL based on hematologic parameters and degree of organ involvement reflect the extent of disease and correlate with prognosis.[187]

The degree of lymphocytosis varies and ranges from 4×10^9/L to counts in excess of 400×10^9/L. In the majority of cases the lymphocytes are relatively uniform in appearance; the cells are small with condensed nuclear chromatin and sparse cytoplasm (Fig. 41-52). Damaged cells are usually present. Nucleoli are inconspicuous or not visible. In the mixed cell type, the cells are more heteromorphous, with both small and large lymphocytes. The marrow involvement may be diffuse, focal, interstitial, or a combination of these findings. A diffuse pattern of involvement is associated with more aggressive disease.[189,190]

The lymphocytes of B-cell CLL express pan–B-cell antigens and sparse amounts of light chain-restricted cell surface immunoglobulin.[191,192] In addition, the lymphocytes in most cases express CD5, a pan–T-cell antigen, and form spontaneous rosettes with mouse erythrocytes.[188] Approximately 50% to 75% of patients with B-cell CLL are hypogammaglobulinemic.[193] Fifteen to thirty percent of patients develop autoimmune hemolytic anemia, neutropenia, or thrombocytopenia. In some cases of B-cell CLL there is evolution to a more aggressive phase referred to as Richter transformation which is marked by pyrexia, increasing fatigue, weight loss, and a large cell, frequently polymorphous lymphoma. This is usually a terminal event.

Hairy cell leukemia is an uncommon, B-cell lymphoproliferative disorder with a peak incidence in the fifth and sixth decades.[194] The male to female ratio is 4 to 1. Patients usually present with splenomegaly and pancytopenia.

The characteristic cell of hairy cell leukemia is of medium size with an oval to lobated nucleus.[194,195] (Fig. 41-53). The cytoplasm is characterized as shaggy; on phase contrast microscopy the cytoplasm appears as hairy projections. Histochemical studies show leukemic cells to contain tartrate-resistant acid phosphatase. The marrow shows a loosely structured infiltrate that may be diffuse or focal. There is generally an increase in reticulin fibers.[196,197] The spleen shows predominant infiltration of the red pulp with infringement on the white pulp; pseudo-sinuses are a characteristic feature as discussed in Chapter 43.[196]

Table 41-22 B-cell chronic lymphoproliferative disorders

Chronic lymphocytic leukemia
Typical
Mixed cell type
Prolymphocytic leukemia
Chronic lymphocytic leukemia/prolymphocytic leukemia
Hairy cell leukemia
Splenic lymphoma with villous lymphocytes

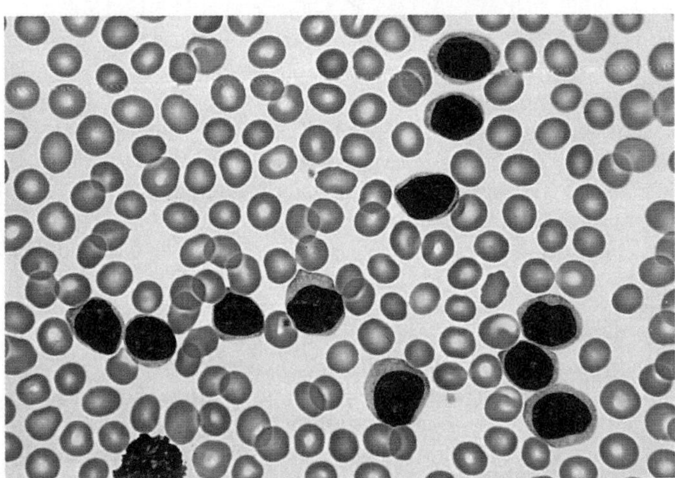

Fig. 41-52 Blood smear from a patient with B-cell chronic lymphocytic leukemia and autoimmune hemolytic anemia. There are numerous well-differentiated lymphocytes with a high nuclear cytoplasmic ratio and condensed nuclear chromatin (Wright-Giemsa).

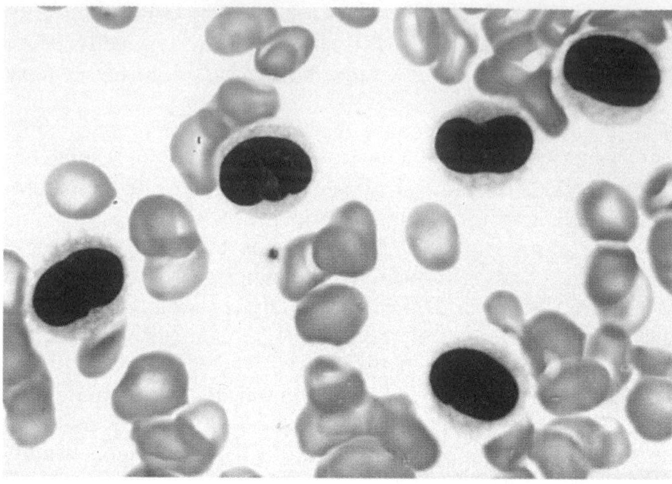

Fig. 41-53 Blood smear from a patient with hairy cell leukemia. The hairy cells have shaggy cytoplasm (Wright-Giemsa).

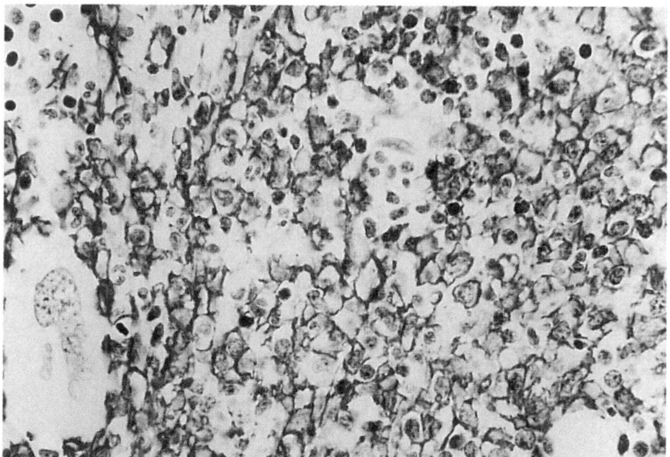

Fig. 41-54 Bone marrow biopsy from a patient with hairy cell leukemia reacted with antibody to CD20 (L26). The membrane of the hairy cells is intensely positive. Several negative myeloid cells are scattered throughout the leukemic infiltrate.

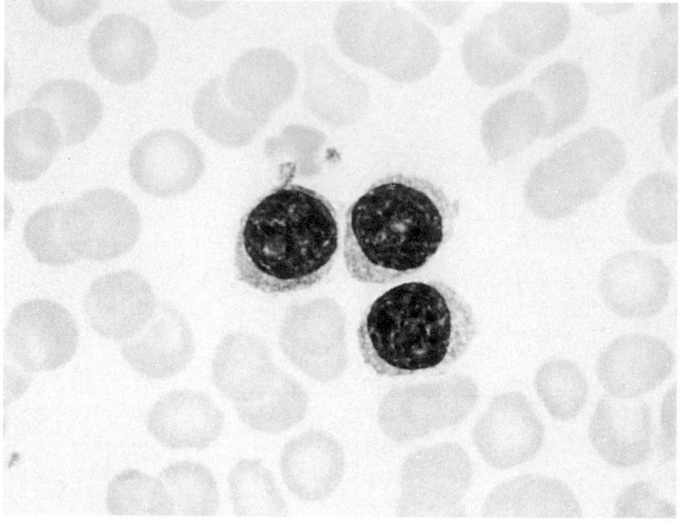

Fig. 41-55 Three abnormal lymphocytes in a blood smear from a patient with marked splenomegaly. The lymphocytes have a distinct nucleolus and cytoplasmic projections (Wright-Giemsa).

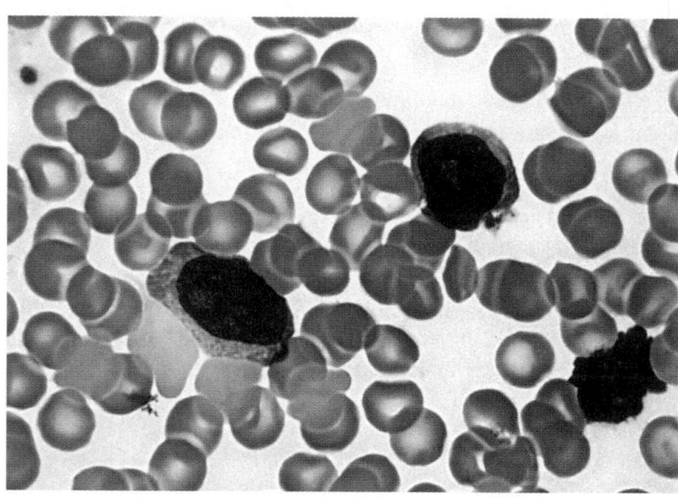

Fig. 41-56 Blood smear from an adult male with B-cell prolymphocytic leukemia. The prolymphocytes are large with abundant basophilic cytoplasm, coarse nuclear chromatin and an unusually prominent single nucleolus (Wright-Giemsa).

The immunophenotype of the hairy cells is that of a mature B-cell with intense cell surface and cytoplasmic immunoglobulin and intense expression of pan–B-cell antigens (Fig. 41-54). Unlike the lymphocytes of CLL, hairy cells do not express CD5 but react with antibodies to CD11c, CD25, and B ly-7.[188,194,198]

Splenic lymphoma with villous lymphocytes is a disorder of older individuals. There are abnormal lymphocytes in the blood and marrow, and pronounced splenomegaly with minimal or no lymphadenopathy.[188,199,200] Approximately 60% of patients have a modest IgM monoclonal gammopathy.

The lymphocytes in the blood are small to medium size with a moderate amount of slightly to moderately basophilic cytoplasm (Fig. 41-55). Some of the lymphocytes have villous cytoplasmic projections. The nuclear chromatin is coarse and there may be a distinct nucleolus.

The lymphoma cells express moderate to intense light chain restricted surface immunoglobulin and pan–B-cell antigens; unlike the lymphocytes in chronic lymphocytic leukemia, the lymphocytes in only a minority of cases of splenic lymphoma express CD5. The spleen may show both red and white pulp involvement. The bone marrow shows varying degrees of lymphocytic infiltration. In approximately 20% to 25% of cases, there is a t(11;14) chromosome abnormality.

B-cell prolymphocytic leukemia is a very rare disorder; the predominant lymphocyte is the prolymphocyte, a medium-sized cell with moderate to abundant basophilic cytoplasm, slightly coarse nuclear chromatin, and a prominent nucleolus.[188,200,201] (Fig. 41-56) The lymphocyte count is usually markedly elevated; the leukocyte count in 67% of patients is in excess of 100 $\times 10^9$/L and in excess of 200 $\times 10^9$/L in 40%.[202] There is marked splenomegaly and minimal or no peripheral lymphadenopathy. Prolymphocytes, in contrast to the lymphocytes of typical B-cell CLL, express intense surface immunoglobin and do not form spontaneous rosettes with mouse red blood cells. The pattern of bone marrow involvement is usually focal, or focal and interstitial. The clinical course is usually aggressive.

T-cell chronic lymphoproliferative disorders

The T-cell leukemias are generally categorized into two major groups based on the origin of the lymphocyte: thymic and post-thymic. The leukemias that arise from the thymic-based lymphocytes manifest as acute lymphoblastic leukemia or lymphoblastic lymphoma and are terminal deoxynucleotidyltransferase (TdT) positive. The post-thymic leukemias are clinically and morphologically heterogeneous diseases; the lymphocytes are terminal deoxynucleotidyltransferase negative (Table 41-23).[188,200] Except for adult T-cell leukemia/lymphoma, which is endemic in some areas of the world, the post-thymic T-cell leukemias are rare. Post-thymic lymphocytes express pan-T-cell antigens, and generally segregate into helper, $CD4^+$ or cytotoxic, $CD8^+$ entities.

T-cell prolymphocytic leukemia (T-PLL) is a disease of older individuals.[203] The median age of onset is 69 years; there is a slight male predominance. Individuals with ataxia telangiectasia appear to have an increased incidence of T-PLL.[203] The major clinical findings include splenomegaly, hepatomegaly, lymphadenopathy, serous effusions, and skin lesions. The disease usually follows an aggressive clinical course.

There is usually, but not invariably, a marked lymphocytosis; the leukocyte count ranges from 16 to 1000×10^9/L, with a median of 200×10^9/L. The predominant lymphocyte in most cases has slightly condensed nuclear chromatin, a prominent single nucleolus, and a moderate amount of basophilic cytoplasm. A small cell variant with more condensed nuclear chromatin and a less conspicuous nucleolus is recognized. The bone marrow shows varying degrees of infiltration and may be only minimally involved.

Usually the T-prolymphocyte expresses pan–T-lymphocyte surface antigens and helper cell phenotype, CD4. The prolymphocytes in a minority of cases express CD8 or the aberrant phenotype, $CD4^+$, $CD8^+$. The prolymphocytes in approximately 75% of cases have an abnormality of chromosome 14 involving bands q11 and q32. Trisomy for isochromosome 8q is present in 50% of patients.[203]

Granulated T-cell lymphocyte leukemia is a disorder primarily of adults.[204-206] There is usually an associated neutropenia, which may be marked; recurrent bacterial infections are frequent. The disease may have an indolent clinical course.

The predominant lymphocytes are medium to large; their distinctive feature is abundant cytoplasm which contains coarse azurophilic granules (Fig. 41-57). The granulated T-lymphocytes express pan–T surface antigens and CD8. The neoplastic nature of the disorder is confirmed by molecular studies that show T-cell receptor rearrangement. There may be only minimal leukemic infiltration of the marrow.[207]

A variant of granulated lymphocyte leukemia is of natural killer (NK) cell origin.[204] The lymphocytes in this disorder are CD2 positive and CD3, CD4, and CD8 negative and express NK cell antigens such as CD56. The cells lack T-cell receptor rearrangement.

Sézary syndrome is an uncommon disorder in which atypical T-lymphocytes infiltrate the skin, causing a generalized, pruiritic exfoliative erythroderma described fully in Chapter 71.[188,208] The average age of onset is approximately 60 years, and the disease is more common in males. In most patients

Table 41-23 T-cell chronic lymphoproliferative disorders

T prolymphocytic leukemia
Granulated T-lymphocyte leukemia
Sézary syndrome
Adult T-cell leukemia

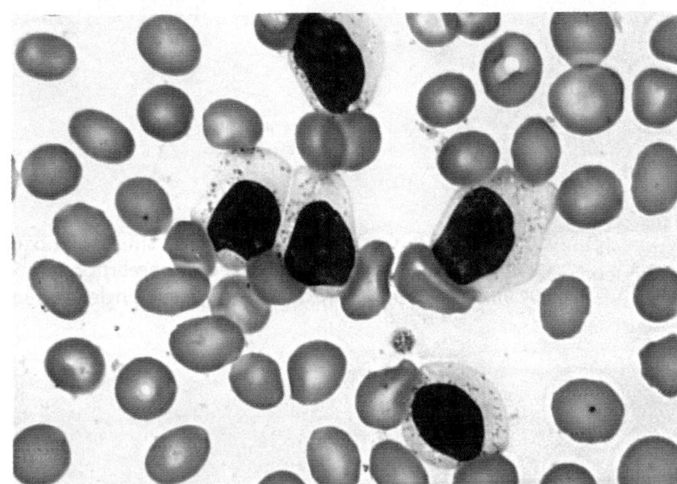

Fig. 41-57 Five granulated lymphocytes in a blood smear from a patient with $CD8^+$ granulated lymphocyte leukemia. The cytoplasm is abundant and contains coarse azurophilic granules (Wright-Giemsa).

the disorder is relatively indolent. The Sezary cell, as it occurs in blood smears, is a large cell with a high nuclear to cytoplasmic ratio. The nucleus is described as cerebriform because of complex convolutions (Fig. 41-58, *A* and *B*).[209] Small cell variants occur. The number of cells in the blood varies, and counts up to 70×10^9/L have been reported.[208] The marrow is usually minimally, almost imperceptibly, involved. The Sezary cells express pan–T-cell antigens and are of helper cell phenotype.

Adult T-cell leukemia/lymphoma is a post-thymic T-cell proliferation that occurs principally in adults. The disease is associated with infection with the human T-cell leukemia/lymphoma virus, HTLV-1, in most cases.[210-212] Adult T-cell leukemia/lymphoma may present as a leukemia or lymphoma; some patients present with overlapping features. The disease generally follows an acute course; smoldering and chronic forms have been described. Approximately 30% of patients present with hypercalcemia due to increased osteoclastic activity.[211]

The disease is most common in southwestern Japan but is also reported from the Caribbean basin, the southeastern United States, and parts of West Africa. The mean age at diagnosis is 57 years; there is a slight female predominance. Lymphadenopathy is the major clinical finding. Skin lesions and splenomegaly are present in approximately half of the patients.

The leukocyte count varies, with levels up to 500×10^9/L in some patients.[211] The morphology of the abnormal lymphocytes is one of the most unusual in hematologic neoplasia. The cells vary in size, and the nuclei may be markedly convoluted. The term *flower shaped* has been applied to the unusual

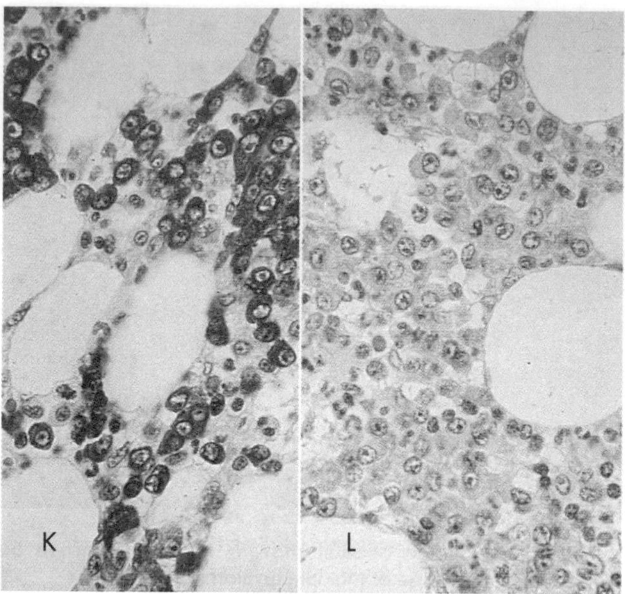

Fig. 41-63 Bone marrow biopsy from a patient with multiple myeloma reacted with antibodies to κ (k) and λ (l) light chains. The plasma cells are κ light chain restricted.

paraffin-embedded tissues with anti-κ and anti-λ antibodies show a light chain–restricted population of plasma cells (Fig. 41-63). The plasma cells in the majority of cases of myeloma do not express pan–B-cell antigens or CD45 (leukocyte common antigen). Epithelial membrane antigen is detected in approximately 60% of cases; cytokeratin is present in 25% of cases. This immunohistochemical profile may lead to ambiguity in anaplastic myeloma where the morphologic differential may include carcinoma; kappa and lambda staining are definitive.[222] PCA-1, CD38, and CD56 are expressed in the majority of cases. Membrane CD10 and myelomonocytic antigens may be expressed in occasional cases.

The serum beta-2 (β-2) microglobulin level at the time of presentation and the plasma cell–labeling index have been proposed as prognostic factors.[223,224] The β-2 microglobulin (β-2) is usually elevated in multiple myeloma and has been found to correlate with prognosis; levels greater than 4 mg/ml have been associated with short survival. The elevated B-2 microglobulin may be a direct effect of the myeloma or due to decreased renal filtration. The plasma cell-labeling index reflects the fraction of plasma cells undergoing DNA replication, the S phase. Cases of myeloma in which the labeling index is equal to or greater than 4.0 have a median survival of 18 months compared with a median survival of 38 months for those cases in which the labeling index is less than 4.0.[224] The labeling index has been utilized to distinguish multiple myeloma from monoclonal gammopathy of undetermined significance; values of greater than 0.4% are usually associated with a diagnosis of multiple myeloma. A labeling index of more than 1.0% is predictive of shorter survival.[223]

The term *smoldering myeloma* has been proposed for patients with the diagnostic laboratory features of myeloma, but in whom there is no evidence of lytic lesions or bone marrow failure.[223]

Plasma cell leukemia

Plasma cell leukemia is a form of plasma cell dyscrasia in which there is more than 20% or $2.0X10^9$/L plasma cells in the blood at presentation.[225] There is an increased incidence of organomegaly when compared with myeloma without plasma cell leukemia. The bone marrow is generally diffusely involved with evidence of bone marrow failure.[226] This type of plasma cell dyscrasia has an unfavorable prognosis.[225,226]

Monoclonal gammopathy of undetermined significance

Monoclonal gammopathy of undetermined significance (MGUS) encompasses a spectrum of patients with a monoclonal gammopathy who lack the morphologic and radiologic evidence of myeloma.[227] Diagnostic criteria for MGUS are listed in Table 41-25. Approximately 3% of individuals over the age of 70 have a detectable monoclonal immunoglobulin in the absence of recognizeable disease. Approximately 20% of patients with MGUS have a stable clinical course. Twenty years after onset, about one third of patients have overt multiple myeloma, amyloidosis, or a lymphoproliferative disorder.[227]

Solitary plasmacytoma

Plasmacytoma is a localized proliferation of light chain–restricted plasma cells. The plasmacytomas are generally classified according to location, solitary plasmacytoma of bone, or extramedullary plasmacytoma.[228-230] The majority of patients have no detectable monoclonal protein in the serum or urine at presentation; if a monoclonal protein is present it is usually less than 2g/dL.[228,229] Solitary plasmacytoma of bone occurs most frequently in the vertebrae, ribs, pelvis, and pectoral girdle; extramedullary plasmacytoma occurs most frequently in mucosal sites in the nasal sinuses, oropharynx, and larynx.[229,231] The diagnosis requires exclusion of marrow disease (Table 41-24). Approximately 75% of patients with solitary plasmacytoma of bone develop multiple myeloma within 10 years.[230] A minority of extramedullary plasmacytomas evolve to multiple myeloma.[231]

Heavy-chain disease

The heavy-chain diseases are a group of B-cell immunoproliferative disorders in which the monoclonal protein is the

Table 41-25 Diagnostic criteria for monoclonal gammopathy of undetermined significance (MGUS)

Criteria
Monoclonal immunoglobulin present but < 3.5 g/dl
Marrow plasma cells < 10% without discrete aggregates
Normal Hb, Ca^{2+}, renal function
No lytic bone lesions
No or minimal monoclonal immunoglobulin in the urine
Normal β-2-microglobulin
No evidence of amyloidosis
No plasmacytoma

Modified from Grogan TM, Spier CM: The B-cell immunoproliferative disorders, including multiple myeloma and amyloidosis. In Knowles DM, editor: *Neoplastic hematopathology*, Baltimore, 1992, Williams and Wilkins; Greipp PR: Advances in the diagnosis and management of myeloma, *Semin Hematol* 29: 24, 1992; Kyle RA: Diagnostic criteria of multiple myeloma, *Hematol Oncol Clin North Am* 6: 347, 1992.

heavy-chain component of the immunoglobulin molecule. The different heavy chain classes are correlated with different disease manifestations. Alpha heavy chain disease is particularly distinctive in its predilection for younger individuals and its association with a small intestinal lymphoplasmacytoid lymphoma, so-called Mediterranean lymphoma or immunoproliferative small intestinal disease.[232] Remissions following antibiotic therapy have been reported.[233] The other heavy chain diseases are less well-characterized.

Waldenström macroglobulinemia

Waldenström macroglobulinemia refers to a monoclonal gammopathy of the IgM class usually associated with a plasmacytoid lymphoma.[234] The median age at diagnosis is 60 years, and there is a male predominance. Clinical findings include signs and symptoms related to hyperviscosity or coagulopathies, cold sensitivity due to cryoglobulinemia, and peripheral neuropathies.[234,235] Lymphadenopathy and organomegaly are common. The lymphoma cells, typically small lymphocytes or plasmacytoid lymphocytes, are present in the blood in 30% of cases. The marrow is involved in 85% of cases; the infiltrates may be focal or diffuse. The lymphocytes are well differentiated or plasmacytoid; Dutcher bodies may be present in these cells.

The disease is usually slowly progressive, with median survival of approximately 5 years.

Amyloidosis

Primary amyloidosis is the accumulation of amyloid in the absence of a coexisting disease.[236] The amyloid is generally composed of the complete or partial immunoglobulin light chain molecules, AL amyloid. AL amyloid also occurs in patients with multiple myeloma.[236] Lambda light chains are more frequently associated with the formation of amyloid than kappa light chains.[217] The AL amyloid is deposited throughout many tissues; the major sites are the myocardium, kidney, tongue, GI tract, peripheral nervous system, and blood vessels.[237]

Patients present with a variety of findings: fatigue, weight loss, congestive heart failure, macroglossia, purpura, peripheral neuropathies, renal insufficiency, and proteinuria. The median survival is approximately one year; significantly shorter survivals occur when amyloidosis is associated with multiple myeloma or congestive heart failure.[237]

A serum monoclonal protein is detectable in less than half of the patients by routine electrophoresis; immunoelectrophoresis or immunofixation reveal an M-protein in approximately two thirds of patients.[237] Patients without overt multiple myeloma usually have a modest, less than 10%, bone marrow plasmacytosis. Aspiration of abdominal fat reveals amyloid in over 70% of patients, and bone marrow biopsy reveals amyloid in slightly less than 50% of patients. Rectal biopsy is diagnostic in 80% of cases.[236,237]

DISORDERS OF THE MONOCYTE/MACROPHAGE SYSTEM

Lipid storage diseases

The disorders collectively referred to as *lipid storage disease* are inborn errors of metabolism in which enzyme defects lead to the accumulation of abnormal amounts of metabolic products in various cells of the body, including cells of the monocyte/macrophage system, resulting in large lipid-laden histiocytes. The major disorders with manifestations in the bone marrow and other hematopoietic tissues include Gaucher disease, Niemann-Pick disease, and sea blue histiocytes.

Gaucher disease is an autosomal recessive disorder characterized by an accumulation of glucosylceramide in various body cells as a result of a deficiency in lysosomal glucocerebrosidase.[238] There are three clinical forms: type I, chronic nonneuropathic (adult type); type II, acute neuropathic (infantile type); and type III, subacute neuropathic (juvenile type). The features of each are discussed in Chapter 14, but hepatosplenomegaly and bone marrow involvement are common to all three types.

Gaucher cells are present in all organs and are abundant in the bone marrow, spleen, lymph nodes, and liver. The characteristic Gaucher cell results from the accumulation of glucocerebroside in the lysosomes of cells of the monocyte/macrophage system. The typical Gaucher cell is large, 30 to 50 um, with one or more eccentrically located nuclei and expanded cytoplasm that has a fibrillary or striated pattern (Fig. 41-64).[239] Gaucher cells are periodic acid-Schiff (PAS)-positive and usually contain abundant iron. The cells are positive for tartrate-resistant acid phophastase similar to the leukemic cells in hairy cell leukemia. The bone marrow usually shows extensive replacement by Gaucher cells; the infiltration is associated with varying degrees of fibrosis.

Type I Gaucher disease may be associated with a normal life span. Patients with type II disease usually die in the first 2 years of life of neurologic deterioration; patients with type III disease have a variable clinical course.

Niemann-Pick disease is composed of an autosomal recessive group of sphingomyelin cholesterol lipidoses caused by a deficiency of lysosomal sphingomyelinase, as discussed in Chapter 14.[240] The major features are hepatosplenomegaly and accumulation of storage cells in the bone marrow and other organs.

The Niemann-Pick cell, as it occurs in the bone marrow from patients with the spingomyelin cholesterol lipidoses, is derived from the monocyte/macrophage system and measures 20 to 50 μm in diameter; the cytoplasm is expanded by the accumulation of varying sized clear vacuoles (Fig. 41-65, *A*).[239] The usually single nucleus is randomly located. In biopsy sections, the cells are diffusely distributed in the interstitium and have the appearance of foam cells (Fig. 41-65, *B*); the cytoplasm stains for neutral lipid and is non-reactive with PAS. The foam cell as identified in Niemann-Pick disease is not unique to that disorder; similar cells may be observed in other diseases of lipid metabolism, including hypercholesterolemia and Tangier disease.

The *sea blue histiocyte* is a macrophage that contains a substance or substances that stain blue in Romanowsky-stained preparations and tan to lightly eosinophilic in hematoxylin and eosin–stained sections.[239] The substance has not been well characterized but appears to result from cell breakdown products, primarily nuclear. The term ceroid storage disease has been applied to some of these findings. This type of macrophage may be observed in several unrelated disorders, and the finding lacks diagnostic specificity. This type of cell has been identified in some cases of Niemann-Pick disease.[239]

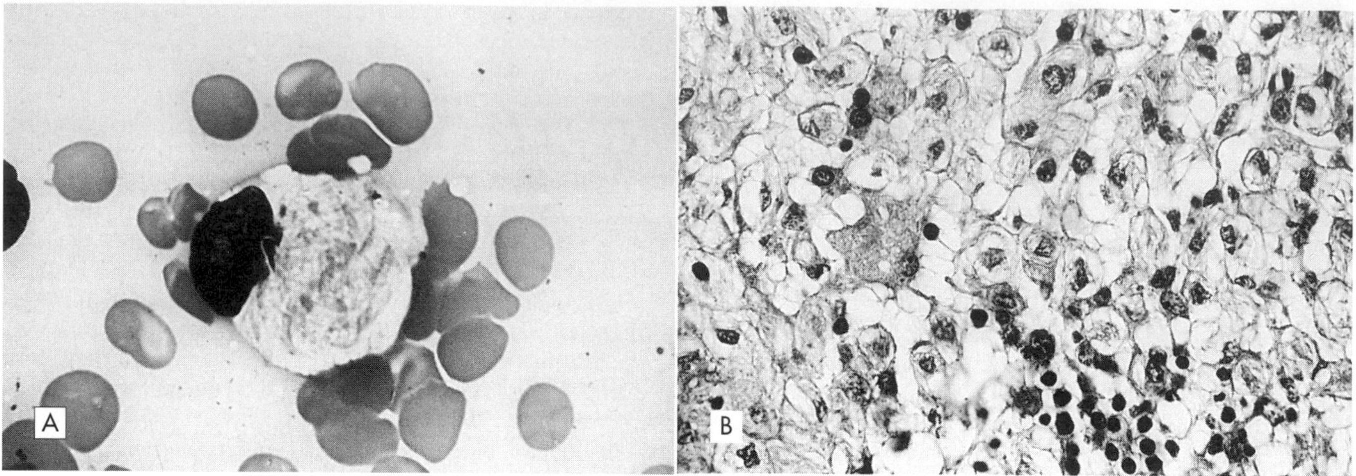

Fig. 41-64 **A,** Gaucher cell in a bone marrow smear from an adult with type I nonneuropathic Gaucher disease (Wright-Giemsa). **B,** Bone marrow biopsy from the same patient showing extensive marrow infiltration by Gaucher cells. The cytoplasmic contents are marked by a fibrillar pattern.

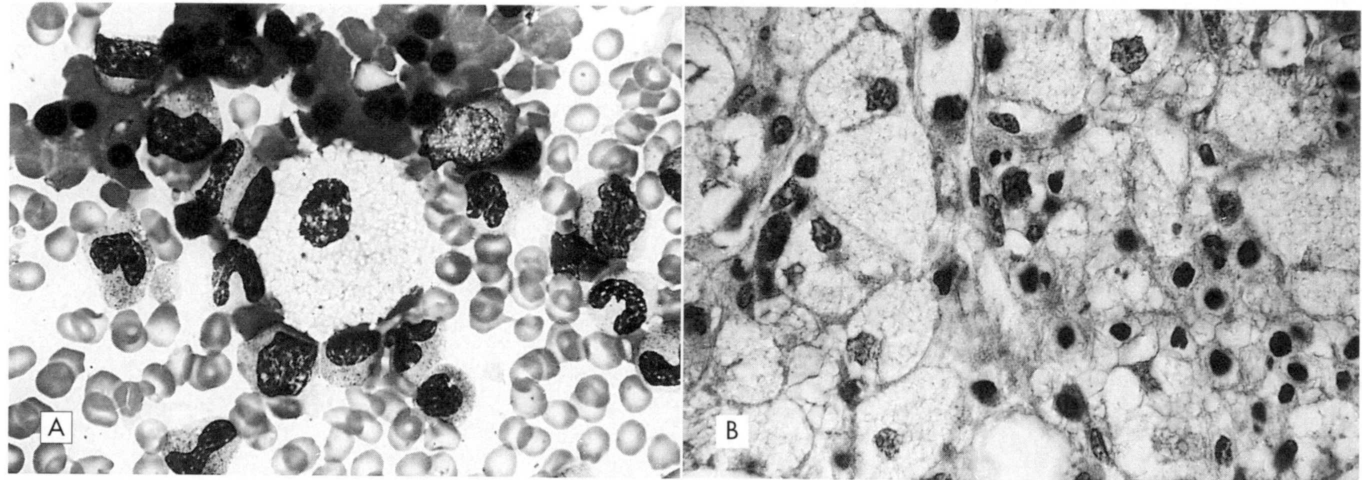

Fig. 41-65 Niemann-Pick disease. **A,** Foam cells in a marrow aspirate smear from a child with Niemann-Pick disease. The cytoplasm is filled with clear vacuoles (Wright-Giemsa). **B,** Bone marrow section from the same patient showing numerous closely packed foam cells and intermingled hematopoietic cells.

HEMOPHAGOCYTIC DISORDERS

The hemophagocytic disorders have, as a unifying feature, a marked increase in hemophagocytic histiocytes in the hematopoietic organs, including the bone marrow, spleen, and lymph nodes (Table 41-26).[241,242] The histiocytes in these disorders show varying degrees of phagocytosis of hematopoietic cells. In some cases, the phagocytic activity is marked. There are usually associated cytopenias and frequently pancytopenia, which may be severe. Coagulation abnormalities, hypofibrinogenemia, and hypertriglyceridemia are associated laboratory findings. Splenomegaly and hepatomegaly are frequent clinical manifestations.

The underlying mechanisms of the hemophagocytic processes are not well understood, but the histiocytic hyperplasia and hemophagocytosis are probably epiphenomena resulting from the elaboration of cytokines that lead to stimulation of the monocyte/macrophage system. The findings may occur in the context of immunosuppression, viral, bacterial and protozoan infections and lymphoproliferative disorders.[242] An association with T-cell lymphoma and leukemia has been reported (Fig. 41-66).[243] This relationship probably involves the elaboration of cytokines by the T-cells, which leads to heightened activation of the monocyte/macrophage system.

A familial form of the disease, familial lymphohistiocytosis, which may be related to a congenital immune deficit is recognized.[244] The cause of the hemophagocytosis in this disorder may be similar to that in the secondary types in that a congenital or acquired immune defect may lead to an increased susceptibility to some type of infectious process and activation either directly or indirectly of the monocyte/macrophage system.

The bone marrow in the hemophagocytic disorders usually, but not invariably, shows histocytic hyperplasia with numerous phagocytic histiocytes. Lymph nodes show histiocytic

Table 41-26 Hemophagocytic disorders

Hemophagocytic lymphohistiocytosis
familial
sporadic
Secondary
infections
viral
bacterial
protozoan
T-cell lymphoproliferative disorders

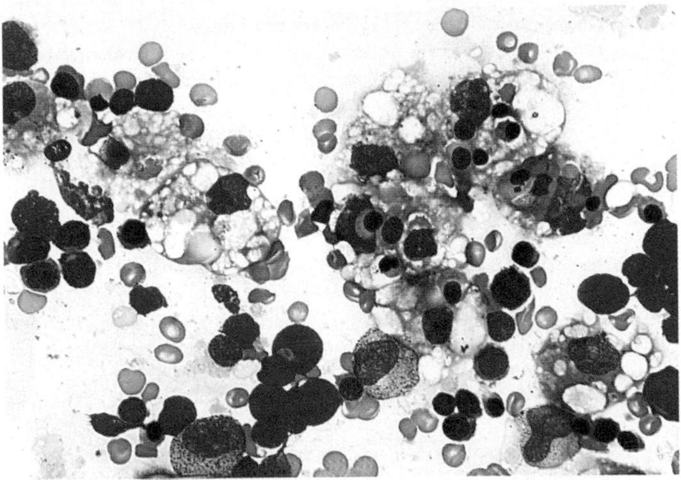

Fig. 41-66 Bone marrow aspirate from a child with a Ki-1 positive T-cell lymphoma in a lymph node biopsy. There is marked histiocytic hyperplasia. Two of the histiocytes contain phagocytosed red cells. The histiocytic hyperplasia regressed with disease remission and recurred with relapse of the lymphoma (Wright-Giemsa).

hyperplasia in the sinuses and T-cell areas. Lymphocyte depletion may be present. The spleen shows diffuse involvement by the histiocytic proliferation.

The clinical course in the hemophagocytic syndromes is variable. There is a high mortality in those cases associated with infections and immunosuppression.[245]

METASTATIC TUMOR

In adults the most common metastatic tumors to the marrow originate in the breast, prostate, lung, thyroid, kidney, and gastrointestinal tract.[246] In children, neuroblastoma, rhabdomyosarcoma, and retinoblastoma are the most common; Wilm's tumor does not metastasize to the marrow with any frequency.[247] Sarcomas, other than rhabdomyosarcoma, are infrequently detected in marrow biopsies.

A leukoerythroblastosis is frequently present; fifteen percent of patients with this finding have a metastatic tumor.[32] Marrow failure due to marrow replacement by tumor and circulating tumor cells occurs very rarely and usually reflects massive tumor burden.

In smear preparations, the tumor cells usually occur in clusters (Fig. 41-67). In the marrow biopsy, metastatic tumor may show focal or diffuse involvement. The tumor may show fewer differentiating features than the primary site. A desmoplastic reaction is frequently present.

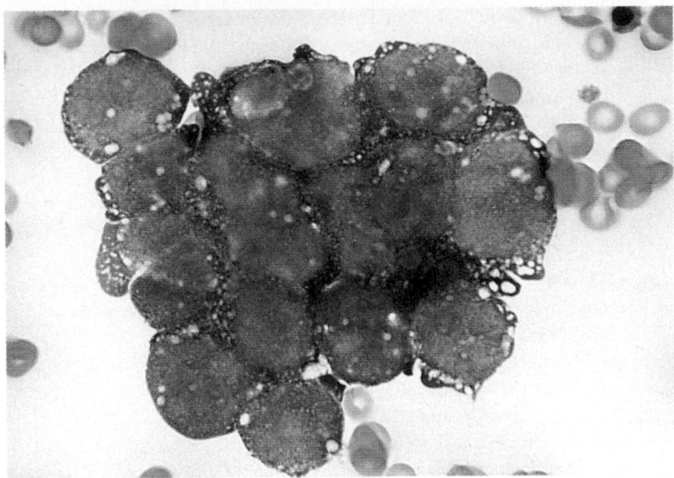

Fig. 41-67 Marrow aspirate from a child showing a cluster of metastatic rhabdomyosarcoma cells (Wright-Giemsa).

REFERENCES

Normal hematopoiesis

1. Bloom W, Fawcett D: *A textbook of histology,* ed 10, Philadelphia, 1975, W.B. Saunders.
2. Wintrobe MM, Lee RG, Boggs DR, Bithell TC, et al: *Clinical hematology,* ed 8, Philadelphia, 1981, Lea & Febiger.
3. Campbell AD, Wicha MS: Extracellular matrix and the haematopoietic microenvironment, *J Lab Clin Med* 112:140, 1988.
4. Lambertson RH, Weiss L: A model of intramedullary hematopoietic microenvironments based on stereologic study of the distribution of endoclonal marrow colonies, *Blood* 63:287, 1984.
5. Weiss LP: Functional organization of the hematopoietic system. In Hoffman R, Benz EJ, Shattil SJ et al, editors: *Hematology: basic principles and practice,* New York, 1991, Churchill Livingstone.
6. Johnston RB: Current concepts: immunology, monocytes and macrophages, *New Engl J Med* 318:747, 1988.
7. Groopman JE, Molina JM, Scadden DT: Hematopoietic growth factors: biology and clinical applications, *N Engl J Med* 321:1449, 1989.
8. Metcalf D, Morstyn G: Colony stimulating factors: general biology. In DeVita VT, Hellman S, Rosenberg SA, editors: *Biologic therapy of cancer,* Philadelphia, 1991, J.B. Lippincott.
9. McDonald TP: Thrombopoietin: its biology, clinical aspects, and possibilities, *Am J Pediat Hematol Oncol* 14:8, 1992.
10. Finch CA: Erythropoiesis, erythropoietin, and iron, *Blood* 60:1241, 1982.
11. Ishiashi T, Koziol JA, Burstein SA: Human recombinant erythropoietin promotes differentiation of murine megakaryoctyes in vitro, *J Clin Invest* 79:286, 1987.
12. Radtke HW, Erbes PM, Schippers E, Koch KM: Serum erythropoietin concentration in anephric patients, *Nephron* 22:361, 1978.
13. Lieschke GJ, Burgess AW: Granulocyte colony stimulating factor and granulocyte-macrophage colony-stimulating factor, *N Engl J Med* 327:28, 1992.
14. Knapp W, Dorken B, Gills WR et al: Leucocyte typing IV: *white cell differentiation antigens,* New York, 1989, Oxford University Press.
15. Loken MR, Shah VO Dattilio KL, Civin CI: Flow cytometric analysis of human bone marrow. II. Normal B-lymphocyte development, *Blood* 70:1316, 1987.
16. Felix CA, Poplack DG: Characterization of acute lymphoblastic leukemia of childhood by immunoglobulin and T-cell receptor gene patterns, *Leukemia* 5:1015, 1991.

17. Loken MR, Civin CI, Fackler MJ et al: Characterization of erythroid, lymphoid and monomyeloid lineages in normal human bone marrow. In Laerum OD, Bjerknes R, editors: *Flow cytometry in hematology,* Boston, 1992, Academic Press.
18. LeBien TW, Villablanca JG: Ontogeny of normal human B-cell and T-cell precursors and its relation to leukemogenesis, *Hematol Oncol Clinics N A* 4:835, 1990.
19. Anderson KC, Bates MP, Slaughenhoupt BB et al: Expression of human B-cell-associated antigens on leukemias and lymphomas: a model of human B-cell differentiation, *Blood* 63:1424, 1984.
20. Lassoued K, Nunez CA, Billips L et al: Expression of surrogate light chain receptors is restricted to a late stage in pre-B-cell differentiation, *Cell* 73:73, 1993.
21. van Noesel CJM, van Lier RAW: Architecture of the human B-cell antigen receptors, *Blood* 82: 363, 1993.
22. Terstappen LWMM, Johnsen S, Segers-Nolten IMJ, Loken MR: Indentification and characterization of plasma cells in normal human bone marrow by high-resolution flow cytometry, *Blood* 76: 1739, 1990.
23. Bertho JM, Mossalayi MD, Dalloul AH, Mouterde G, Debre P: Isolation of an early T-cell precursor (CFU-TL) from human bone marrow, *Blood* 75:1064, 1990.
24. Chabannon C, Wood P, Torok-Storb B: Expression of CD7 on normal human myeloid progenitors, *Immunol* 149:2110, 1992.
25. Knowles DM, Chadburn A, Inghirami G: Immunophenotypic markers useful in the diagnosis and classification of hematopoietic neoplasms. In Knowles DM, editor: *Neoplastic hematopathology,* Baltimore, 1992, Williams and Wilkins.
26. Labeta M, Landmann R, Obrecht JP, Obrist R: Human B-cells express membrane-bound and soluble forms of the CD14 myeloid antigen, *Molecular Immunol* 28:115, 1991.
27. Terstappen LWMM, Safford M, Loken MR: Flow cytometric analysis of human bone marrow. III. Neutrophil maturation, *Leukemia* 4:657, 1990.
28. Hartsock RJ, Smith EB, Petty CS: Normal variations with aging of the amount of hematopoietic tissue in bone marrow from the anterior iliac crest, *Am J Clin Pathol* 43:326, 1965.
29. Young N: Hematologic and hematopoietic consequences of B 19 parvovirus infection, *Semin Hematol* 25:159, 1988.
30. Dessypris EN: The biology of pure red cell aplasia, *Semin Hematol* 28:275, 1991.
31. Seaman JP, Kjeldsberg CR, Linker A: Gelantinous transformation of the marrow, *Human Pathol* 6:685, 1978.
32. Weick JK, Hagedorn AB, Linman JW: Leukoerythroblastosis: diagnostic and prognostic significance, *Mayo Clin Proc* 49:110, 1974.
33. Lofsness KG, Houlihan PM, Brunning RD: Hematologic parameters and leukocyte histogram patterns in infectious mononucleosis, *Am J Clin Pathol* 87:485, 1987.

Processing of bone marrow specimens

34. Brunning RD, McKenna RW: *Atlas of tumor pathology: tumors of the bone marrow,* Armed Forces Institute of Pathology, Washington, D.C., 1994, 475.

Inflammation

35. Sverdlow SH, Collins RD: Marrow granulomas. In Ioachim HL, editor: *Pathology of granulomas*, New York, 1983, Raven Press.
36. Okun DB, Sun NC, Tanaka KR: Bone marrow granulomas in Q Fever, *Am J Clin Path* 71: 117, 1979.

Anemias

37. International Agranulocytosis and Aplastic Anemia Study: Risks of agranulocytosis and aplastic anemia: a first report of their relation to drug use with special reference to analgesics, *J Am Med Assoc* 256:1749, 1986.
38. Gordon-Smith EC, Rutherford TR: Fanconi anaemia-constitutional, familial aplastic anaemia, *Bailliere's Clin Haematol* 2:139, 1989.
39. Nissen C: The pathophysiology of aplastic anemia, *Semin Hematol* 28:313, 1991.
40. Evans DIK: Congenital defects of the marrow stem cell, *Bailliere's Clin Haematol* 2:163, 1989.
41. Szklo M, Sensenbrenner C, Markowitz J et al: Incidence of aplastic anemia in metropolitan Baltimore: a population-based study, *Blood* 66:115, 1985.
42. Kurtzman G, Young N: Viruses and bone marrow failure, *Bailliere's Clin Haematol* 2:51, 1989.
43. Storb R: Bone marrow transplanatation for aplastic anemia. In Forman SJ, Blume KG, Donnell Thomas DE: *Bone marrow transplantation*, Blackwell Scientific, Boston, 1994.
44. Freedman MH: Pure red cell aplasia in childhood and adolescence: pathogenesis and approaches to diagnosis, *Br J Haematol* 85:246, 1993.
45. Lee GR: Megaloblastic and nonmegaloblastic macrocytic anemias. In Lee GR, Bithell TC, Foerster J et al, editors: *Wintrobe's clinical hematology,* ed 9, Philadelphia, 1993, Lea and Febiger.
46. Lee GR: Nutritional factors in the production and function of erythrocytes. In Lee GR, Bithell TC, Foerster J et al, editors: *Wintrobe's clinical hematology,* ed 9, Philadelphia, 1993, Lea and Febiger.
47. Antony AC: Megaloblastic anemias. In Hoffman R, Benz EJ, Shattil SJ et al, editors: *Hematology: basic principles and practice,* New York, 1991, Churchill Livingstone.
48. Fenton WA, Rosenberg LE: Inherited disorders of cobolamin transport and metabolism. In Scriver CR, Beaudet AL, Sly WS, Valle D, editors: *The metabolic basis of inherited disease,* ed 6, New York, 1991, McGraw-Hill.
49. Rosenblatt DS: Inherited disorders of folate transport and metabolism. In Scriver CR, Beaudet AL, Sly WS, Valle D, editors: *The metabolic basis of inherited disease*, ed 6, New York, 1989 McGraw Hill.
50. Brittenham GM: Disorders of iron metabolism: iron deficiency and overload. In Hoffman R, Benz EJ, Shattil SJ et al, editors: Hematology: basic principles and practice, New York, 1991, Churchill Livingstone.
51. Cartwright GE, Lee GR: The anaemia of chronic disorders, *Br J Haematol* 21:147, 1971.
52. Lee GR: The anemia of chronic disease, *Semin Hematol* 20:61, 1983.
53. Lee GR: The anemia of chronic disorders. In Lee GR, Bithell TC, Foerster J et al, editors: *Wintrobe's clinical hematology,* ed 9, Philadelphia, 1993, Lea and Febiger.
54. Sears DA: Anemia of chronic disease, *Med Clin N A* 76:567, 1992.
55. Cash JM, Sears DA: The anemia of chronic disease: spectrum of associated diseases in a series of unselected hospitalized patients, *Am J Med* 87:638, 1989.
56. Dickerson R, Geis I: Hemoglobin: structure, function, evolution, pathology, Menlo Park, Calif, 1983, Benjamin-Cummings.
57. Weatherall DJ, Clegg JB, Higgs DR, Wood WG: The hemoglobinopathies. In Scriver CR, Beaudet AL, Sly WS, Valle D, editors: *The metabolic basis of inherited disease*, ed 6, New York, 1989, McGraw-Hill.
58. Steinberg M, Benz E: Hemoglobin synthesis, structure, and function. In Hoffman R, Benz E, Shattil SJ et al, editors: *Hematology: basic principles and practice,* New York, 1991, Churchill Livingstone.
59. Bunn HF, Forget BG: *Hemoglobin: molecular, genetic, and clinical aspects*, Philadelphia, 1986, W. B. Saunders.
60. Schwartz E, Benz EJ: The thalassemia syndromes. In Hoffman R, Benz EJ, Shattil SJ et al, editors: *Hematology: basic principles and practice*, New York, 1991, Churchill Livingstone.
61. Kazazian HH, Boehm CD: Molecular basis and prenatal diagnosis of β-thalassemia, *Blood* 72: 1107, 1988.
62. Orkin SH, Kazazian HH, Antonarakis SE et al: Abnormal RNA processing due to the exon mutations of b^e globin gene, *Nature* 300: 768, 1982.
63. Fairbanks VF: Thalassemias and hereditary persistence of fetal hemoglobin (HPHF). In Fairbanks VF editor: Hemoglobinopathies and thalassemias: laboratory methods and case studies, New York, 1980, Thieme.
64. Weatherall DJ, Clegg JB: The α-chain termination mutants and their relationship to the α-thalassemias, *Philos Trans R Soc Lond.* (B) 271:440, 1975.
65. Pauling L, Itano HA, Singer SJ, Wells IG: Sickle cell anemia, a molecular disease, *Science* 110:543, 1949.
66. Ingram VM: Specific chemical difference between the globins of normal human and sickle-cell anaemia haemoglobin, *Nature* 178: 792, 1956.
67. Beutler E: The sickle diseases and related disorders. In Williams WJ, Beutler E, Erslev AJ, Lichtman MA editors: *Hematology,* ed 4, New York, 1990, McGraw-Hill.

68. Saarinen UM, Chorba TL, Tattersall P et al: Human parvovirus B-19 induced epidemic acute red cell aplasia in patients with hereditary hemolytic anemia, *Blood* 67: 1411, 1986.
69. Schneider RG, Hightower B, Hosty TS et al: Abnormal hemoglobins in a quarter million people, *Blood* 48: 629, 1976.
70. Palek J, Lambert S: Genetics of the red cell membrane skeleton, *Semin Hematol* 27: 290, 1990.
71. Palek J, Sahr KE: Mutations of the red blood cell membrane proteins: from clinical evaluation to detection of the underlying genetic defect, *Blood* 80: 308, 1992.
72. Lux SE, Becker PS: Disorders of the red cell membrane skeleton: hereditary spherocytosis and hereditary elliptocytosis. In Scriver CR, Beaudet AL, Sly WS, Valle D editors: *The metabolic basis of inherited disease,* ed 6, New York, 1989, McGraw-Hill.
73. Palek J: Red cell membrane disorders. In Hoffman R, Benz EJ, Shattil SJ et al, editors: *Hematology: Basic principles and practice,* New York, 1991, Churchill Livingstone.
74. Mohandas N, Chasis JA: Red blood cell deformity, membrane material properties and shape: regulation by transmembrane skeletal and cytosolic proteins and lipids, *Semin Hematol* 30: 171, 1993.
75. Lukens JN: Hereditary spherocytosis and other hemolytic anemias associated with abnormalities of the red cell membrane and cytoskeleton. In Lee GR, Bithell TC, Foerster J et al, editors: *Wintrobe's clinical hematology,* ed 9, Philadelphia, 1993, Lea and Febiger.
76. Luzzatto L, Mehta A: Glucose-6-phosphate dehydrogenase deficiency. In Scriver CR, Beaudet AL, Sly WS, Valle D, editors: *The metabolic basis of inherited disease,* ed 6, 1989, New York.
77. Saltman P: Oxidative stress: a radical view, *Semin Hematol* 26:249, 1989.
78. Lukens JN: Hereditary hemolytic anemias associated with abnormalities of erythrocyte anaerobic glycolysis and nucleotide metabolism. In Lee GR, Bithell TC, Foerster J et al, editors: *Wintrobe's clinical hematology,* ed 9, Philadelphia, 1993, Lea and Febiger.
79. Valentine WN, Tanaka KR, Paglia DE: Pyruvate kinase and other enzyme deficiency disorders of the erythrocyte. In Scriver CR, Beaudet AL, Sly WS, Valle D, editors: *The metabolic basis of inherited disease,* ed 6, New York, 1989, McGraw-Hill.
80. Schwartz RS, Berkman EM, Silberstein LE: The autoimmune hemolytic anemias. In Hoffman R, Benz EJ, Shattil SJ, Furie B, Cohen HJ, editors: *Hematology: Basic principles and practice,* New York, 1991, Churchill Livingstone.
81. Engelfriet CP, Overbeeke MAM, von dem Borne AEGK: Autoimmune hemolytic anemia, *Semin Hematol* 29: 3, 1992.
82. Garratty G: Target antigens for red-cell-bound autoantibodies. In Nance SJ editor: *Clinical and basic science aspects of immunohematology,* Arlington, 1991, American Association of Blood Banks.
83. Rosse WF, Adams JP: The variability of hemolysis in the cold agglutinin syndrome, *Blood* 56:409, 1980.
84. Kwaan HC: Clinicopathologic features of thrombotic thrombocytopenia purpura, *Semin Hematol* 24:71, 1987.
85. Lian E C-Y: Pathogenesis of thrombotic thrombocytopenia purpura, *Semin Hematol* 24: 82, 1987.
86. Rock GA, Shumak KH, Buskard NA et al: Comparison of plasma exchange with plasma infusion in the treatment of thrombotic thrombocytopenic purpura, *N Eng J Med* 325: 393, 1991.
87. Kaplan BS, Proesmans W: The hemolytic uremic syndrome of childhood and its variants, *Semin Hematol* 24: 148, 1987.
88. Rosse WF: The glycolipid anchor of membrane surface proteins, *Semin Hematol* 30: 219, 1993.
89. Wilcox LA, Ezzell JL, Bernshaw NJ, Parker CJ: Molecular basis of the enhanced susceptibility of the erythrocytes of paroxysmal nocturnal hemoglobinuria to hemolysis in acidified serum, *Blood* 78: 820, 1991.
90. Lee GR: Paroxysmal nocturnal hemoglobuinuria, In Lee GR, Bithell TC, Foerster J, Athens JW et al, editors: *Wintrobe's clinical hematology,* ed 9, Philadelphia, 1993, Lea and Febiger.
91. Beutler E: Paroxysmal nocturnal hemoglobinuria, In Williams WJ, Beutler E, Erslev AJ, Lichtman MA, editors: *Hematology,* ed 4, New York, 1990, McGraw-Hill.
92. Hartman RC, Jenkins DE, Arnold AB: Diagnostic specificity of sucrose hemolysis test for paroxysmal nocturnal hemoglobinuria, *Blood* 35: 462, 1970.
93. Schubert J, Alvarado M, Uciechowski P et al: Diagnosis of paroxysmal nocturnal haemoglobinuria using immunophenotyping of peripheral blood cells, *Brit J Haematol* 79:487, 1991.
94. Graham DL, Gastineau DA: Paroxysmal nocturnal hemoglobinuria as a marker for clonal myelopathy, *Am J Med* 93: 671, 1991.
95. Rosse WF: Paroxysmal nocturnal hemoglobinuria: the biochemical defects and the clinical syndrome, *Blood Reviews* 3:192, 1989.
96. Crookston JH, Crookston MC, Burnie KL et al: Hereditary erythroblastic multinuclearity associated with a positive acidified serum test: a type of congenital dyserythropoietic anaemia, *Brit J Haematol* 17:11, 1969.
97. Wolff JA, von Hofe FH: Familial erythroid multinuclearity, *Blood* 6:1274, 1951.
98. Heimpel H, Forteza-Vila J, Queisser W, Spiertz E: Electron and light microscopic study of the erythroblasts of patients with congenital dyserythropoietic anemia, *Blood* 37: 299, 1971.
99. Bird AR, Karabus CD, Hartley PS: Type IV congenital dyserythropoietic anemia with an unusual response to splenectomy, *Am J Ped Hematol Oncol* 7:196, 1985.

Neutropenia and agranulocytosis

100. Dale DC, Hammond WP IV: Cyclic neutropenia: a clinical review, *Blood Rev* 2:178, 1988.
101. McClain K, Estrov Z, Chen H, Mahoney D: Chronic neutropenia of childhood: frequent association with parvovirus infection and correlations with bone marrow culture studies, *Br J Haematol* 85: 57, 1993.

Thrombocytopenia

102. Hall JG: Thrombocytopenia and absent radius (TAR) syndrome, *J Med Genet* 24: 79, 1987.
103. Bithell TC: Thrombocytopenia caused by immunologic platelet destruction: Idiopathic thrombocytopenic purpura (ITP), drug-induced thrombocytopenia, and miscellaneous forms. In Lee GR, Bithell TC, Foerster J et al, editors: *Wintrobe's clinical hematology,* ed 9, Philadelphia, 1993, Lea and Febiger.
104. Waters AH: Autoimmune thrombocytopenia: clinical aspects, *Semin Hematol* 29:18, 1992.
105. Kiefel V, Santoso S, Mueller-Eckhardt C: Serological, biochemical and molecular aspects of platelet autoantigens, *Semin Hematol* 29: 26, 1992.
106. George JN: Platelet IgG: measurement, interpretation, and clinical significance, *Prog Hemostasis Thrombosis* 10:97, 1991.
107. Bussel JB: Autoimmune thrombocytopenic purpura, *Hematol Oncol Clinics N A* 4:179, 1990.
108. Blanchette VS, Kirby MA, Turner C: Role of intravenous immunoglobulin G in autoimmune hematologic disorders, *Semin Hematol* 29(3supp2): 72, 1992.
109. Kaplan C, Morinet F, Carton J: Virus-induced autoimmune thrombocytopenia and neutropenia, *Semin Hematol* 29(3supp2): 34, 1992.
110. von dem Borne AEGK, Kuijpers RWAM, Goldschmeding R: Platelet antigens in alloimmune thrombocytopenia. In Nance SJ editor: Clinical and Basic Science Aspects of Immunohematology, Arlington, Vir, 1991, American Association of Blood Banks.
111. Murphy WG, Kelton JG: Idiosyncratic drug-induced thrombocytopenia, *Current Studies in Hematology and Blood Transfusion* 54:71, 1988.
112. Warkentin TE, Kelton JG: Heparin-induced thrombocytopenia, *Prog Hemostasis and Thrombosis* 10:1, 1991.

Leukemias and related disorders

113. Ries LAG, Hankey BF, Miller BA et al: *Cancer Statistics Review* 1973-88, National Cancer Institute, NIH Pub. No. 91-2789, 1991.
114. Bennett JM, Catovsky D, Daniet MT et al: Proposals for the classification of the acute leukemias, French-American-British (FAB) co-operative group, *Br J Haematol* 33: 451, 1976.
115. Litz CE, Brunning RD: Acute myeloid leukemias. In DM Knowles, editor: *Neoplastic hematopathology,* Baltimore, 1992, Williams & Wilkins.

116. Cheson BD, Cassilith PA, Head D et al: Report of the National Cancer Institute sponsored workshop on definitions of diagnosis and response in acute myeloid leukemia, *J Clin Oncol* 8:813, 1990.
117. Yunis JJ, Brunning RD: Prognostic significance of chromosomal abnormalities in acute leukaemias and myelodysplastic syndromes, *Clinics Haematol* 15:597, 1986.
118. Nucifora G, Birn DJ, Erickson P et al: Detection of DNA rearrangements in the AML1 and ETO loci and of an AML/ETO fusion mRNA in patients with t(8;21) acute myeloid leukemia, *Blood* 81:883, 1993.
119. Wiernik PH, Banks PLC, Case DC: Cytrabine plus idarubicin or daurorubican as induction and consolidation therapy for previously untreated adult patients with acute myeloid leukemia, *Blood* 79:313, 1992.
120. Bennett JM, Catovsky D, Daniel MT et al: Proposals for the classification of the myelodysplastic syndromes, *Brit J Haematol* 51:189, 1982.
121. List AF, Garewal HS, Sandberg AA: The myelodysplastic syndromes: biology and implications for management, *J Clin Oncol* 8:1424, 1990.
122. Noel P: Management of patients with myelodysplastic syndromes, *Mayo Clinic Proc* 66:485, 1991.
123. Third MIC Cooperative Study Group: Recommendations for a morphologic, immunologic, and cytogenetic (MIC) working classification of the primary and therapy related myelodysplastic disorders, *Canc Genet and Cytogenet* 32:1, 1988.
124. Brunning RD: Myelodysplastic Sydromes. In DM Knowles, editor: *Neoplastic hematopathology,* Baltimore, 1992, Williams & Wilkins.
125. Mathew P, Tefferi A, Dewald GW et al: The 5-q Syndrome: a single institution study of 43 consecutive cases, *Blood* 81:1040, 1993.
126. Evans JP, Czepulkowski B, Gibbons B et al: Childhood monosomy 7 revisited, *Br J Haematol* 69:41, 1988.
127. Foucar K, McKenna RW, Bloomfield CD et al: Therapy related leukemia, a panmyelosis, *Cancer* 43:1285, 1979.
128. Kantarijan HM, Keating MJ: Therapy-related leukemia and myelodysplastic syndrome, *Semin Oncol* 14:435, 1987.
129. Michels SD, McKenna RW, Arthur DC et al: Therapy related acute myeloid leukemia and myelodysplastic syndrome: a clinical and morphologic study of 65 cases, *Blood* 65:1364, 1985.
130. Kurzrock R, Gutterman JR, Talpaz M: The molecular genetics of Philadelphia chromosome-positive leukemias, *N Engl J Med* 319:990, 1988.
131. Cutler SJ, Young JL: *Third national cancer survey: incidence data,* Washington, D.C., 1975, U.S. Government Printing Office.
132. Moloney WC: Natural history of chronic granulocytic leukaemia, *Clin Haematol* 6:41, 1977.
133. Medical Research Council's Working Party for Therapeutic Trials in Leukaemia: Chronic granulocytic leukaemia: comparison of radiotherapy and busulfan therapy, *Br Med J* 1:201, 1968.
134. Rowe JM, Lichtman MA: Hyperleukocytoisis and leukostasis: common features of childhood chronic myelogenous leukemia, *Blood* 63: 1230, 1984.
135. Spiers ASD, Bain BJ, Turner JE: The peripheral blood in chronic granulocytic leukaemia: study of 50 untreated Philadelphia positive cases, *Scand J Haematol* 18:25, 1977.
136. Wachstein M: Alkaline phosphatase activity in normal and abnormal human blood and bone marrow, *J Lab Clin Med* 31:1, 1946.
137. Kantarjian HM, Deisseroth A, Kurzrock R et al: Chronic myelogenous leukemia: a concise update, *Blood* 3:691, 1993.
138. Canellos GP: Clinical characteristics of the blast phase of chronic granulocytic leukemia, *Hematol Oncol Clin North Am* 4:359, 1990.
139. Muehleck SD, McKenna RW, Arthur DC et al: Transformation of chronic myelogenous leukemia: clinical, morphologic, and cytogenetic features, *Am J Clin Pathol* 82: 1, 1984.
140. Kantarjian HM, Dixon D, Keating MJ: Characteristics of accelerated disease in chronic myelogeous leukemia, *Cancer* 61:1441, 1988.
141. Bakhshi A, Minowada J, Arnold A: Lymphoid blast crises of chronic myelogenous leukemia represent stages in the development of B-cell precursor, *N Engl J Med* 309: 826, 1983.
142. Janossy G, Greaves MF, Revesz T: Blast crisis of chronic myeloid leukaemia. II. Cell surface marker analysis of lymphoid and myeloid cases, *Br J Haematol* 34:179, 1976.
143. Rowley JD: Chromosomes in leukemia and lymphoma, *Semin Hematol* 15:301, 1984.
144. Najean Y, Mugnier P, Dresch C, Rain JD: Polycythaemia vera in young people: an analysis of 58 cases diagnosed before 40 years, *Br J Haematol* 67:285, 1987.
145. Anger B, Haug U, Seidler R, Heimpel H: Polycythemia vera, a clinical study of 141 patients, *Blut* 59: 493, 1989.
146. Ellis JT, Peterson P, Geller SA, Rappaport H: Studies of the bone marrow in polycythemia vera and the evolution of myelofibrosis and secondary hematologic malignancies, *Semin Hematol* 23:144, 1986.
147. Landaw SA: Acute leukemia in polycythemia vera, *Semin Hematol* 23:156, 1986.
148. Murphy S, Iland H, Rosenthal D, Laszlo J: Essential thrombocythemia: an interim report from the Polycythemia Vera Study Group, *Semin Hematol* 23: 177, 1986.
149. McIntyre KJ, Hoagland HC, Silverstein MN, Petitt RM: Essential thrombocythemia in young adults, *Mayo Clin Proc* 66:149, 1991.
150. Silverstein MN, Petitt RM, Solberg LA et al: Anagrelide: a new drug for treating thrombocytosis, *N Engl J Med* 318:1292, 1988.
151. Weinstein IM: Idiopathic myelofibrosis: historical review, diagnosis, and management, *Blood* Rev 5:98, 1991.
152. Thiele J, Zankovich R, Steinberg T et al: Agnogenic myeloid metaplasia (AMM) - correlation of bone marrow lesions with laboratory data: a longitudinal clinicopathological study on 114 patients, *Hematol Oncol* 7: 327, 1989.
153. Rappaport H: Tumors of the hematopoietic system. In *Atlas of tumor pathology,* Washington, D.C. 1966, Armed Forces Institute of Pathology.
154. Ward HP, Block MH: The natural history of agnogenic myeloid metaplasia (AMM) and a critical evaluation of its relationship with the myeloproliferative syndrome, *Medicine* (Baltimore) 50:357, 1971.
155. Wolf BC, Neiman RS: Myelofibrosis with myeloid metaplasia: pathophysiologic implications of the correlation between bone marrow changes and progression of splenomegaly, *Blood* 1985: 803, 1985.
156. Varki A, Lottenberg R, Griffith R, Reinhard E: The syndrome of idiopathic myelofibrosis: a clinicopathologic review with emphasis on the prognostic variables predicting survival, *Medicine* (Baltimore) 62: 353, 1983.
157. Visani G, Fineli C, Castelli U: Myelofibrosis with myeloid metaplasia: clinical and haematological parameters predicting survival in a series of 133 patients, *Br J Haematol* 75: 4, 1990.
158. Hardisty RM, Speed DE, Till M: Granulocytic leukaemia in childhood, *Br J Haematol* 10: 551, 1964.
159. Freedman MH, Estrov Z, Chan HS: Juvenile chronic myelogenous leukemia, *Am J Pediatr Hematol Oncol* 10:261, 1988.
160. Sanders JE, Buckner CD, Thomas ED: Allogeneic marrow transplantation for children with juvenile chronic myelogenous leukemia, *Blood* 71:1144, 1988.
161. Fauci AS, Harley JB, Roberts WC et al: The idiopathic hypereosinophilic syndrome: clinical, pathologic, and therapeutic considerations, *Ann Int Med* 97: 78, 1982.
162. Schwartz LB: Hypereosiniophilic syndrome, *Virginia Medicine* 111:350, 1984.
163. Weller PF: The immunobiology of eosinophils, *N Eng J Med* 324:1110, 1991.
164. Brunning RD, McKenna RW, Rosai J et al: Systemic mastocytosis, extracutaneous manifestations, *Am J Surg Pathol* 7:425, 1983.
165. Lawrence JB, Friedman BS, Travis WD et al: Hematologic manifestations of systemic mast cell disease: a prospective study of laboratory and morphologic features and their relation to prognosis, *Am J Med* 91: 612, 1991.
166. Travis WD, Li CY, Bergstralh EY et al: Systemic mast cell disease: analysis of 58 cases and literature review, *Medicine(Baltimore)* 67: 345, 1988.
167. Horny HP, Rick M, Wehrmann M, Kaiserling E: Blood findings in generalized mastocytosis: evidence of frequent simultaneous occurrence of myeloproliferative disorders, *Brit J Haematol* 76:186, 1990.
168. Meis JM, Butler JJ, Osborne BM et al: Granulocytic sarcoma in non leukemic patients, *Cancer* 44:2697, 1979.
169. Nieman RS, Barcos M, Berard C et al: Granulocytic sarcoma, *Cancer* 48: 1426, 1981.

170. Tallman MS, Hakamian D, Shaw JM et al: Granulocytic sarcoma is associated with the t(8;21) translocation in acute myeloid leukemia, *J Clin Oncol* 11:690, 1993.
171. Bennett JM, Catovsky D, Daniel MT et al: The morphologic classification of acute lymphoblastic leukaemia: concordance among observers and clinical correlations, *Br J Haematol* 47:553, 1981.
172. Foon KA, Todd RF: Immunologic classification of leukemia and lymphoma, *Blood* 68:1, 1986.
173. Greaves M, Janossy G, Peto J, Kay H: Immunologically defined subclass of acute lymphoblastic leukaemia in children: their relationship to presentation features and prognosis, *Brit J Haematol* 48:179, 1981.
174. Vogler L, Crist WM, Bockman DE et al: Pre-B leukemia: a new phenotype of childhood lymphoblastic leukemia, *N Engl J Med* 298:872, 1978.
175. Pui CH, Behm FG, Crist WM: Clinical and biologic relevance of immunologic marker studies in childhood acute lymphoblastic leukemia, *Blood* 82:343, 1993.
176. Vogler LB, Crist WM, Sarrif AM et al: An analysis of clinical and laboratory features of acute lymphocytic leukemias with emphasis on 35 children with pre-B leukemia, *Blood* 58:135, 1981.
177. Magrath I: The pathogenesis of Burkitt's lymphoma, *Adv Cancer Res* 55:133, 1990.
178. Gaynon PS: Primary treatment of childhood acute lymphoblastic leukemia of non-T-cell lineage (including infants) *Hematol Oncol Clin N A* 1990, 4:915.
179. Le Beau MM: The role of cytogenetics in the diagnosis and classification of hematopoietic neoplasms, In Knowles DM, editor: *Neoplastic hematopathology*, Baltimore, 1993, Williams and Wilkins.
180. Ribeiro RC, Abromowitch M, Raimondi SC et al: Clinical and biological hallmarks of the Philadelphia chromosome in childhood acute lymphoblastic leukemia, *Blood* 70:948, 1987.
181. Westbrook CA, Hooberman AL, Spino C et al: Clinical significance of the BCR-ABL fusion gene in adult acute lymphoblastic leukemia: a cancer and leukemia group B study (8762), *Blood* 80:2983, 1992.
182. Pui CH, Frankel LS, Carroll AJ et al: Clinical characteristics and treatment outcome of childhood acute lymphoblastic leukemia with the t(4;11) (q21;q23): a collaborative study of 40 cases, Rosai J, editor: *Blood* 77:440, 1991.
183. Parkin JL, Arthur DC, Abramson CS et al: Acute leukemia associated with the t(4;11) chromosome rearrangement: ultrastructural and immunologic characteristics, *Blood* 60:1321, 1982.
184. Brunning RD, McKenna RW: Acute Leukemia. In Rosai J, editor: Atlas of tumor pathology: tumors of the bone marrow, 1994, American Registry of Pathology.
185. Sobol RE, Mick R, Royston I et al: Clinical importance of myeloid antigen expression in adult acute lymphoblastic leukemia, *N Engl J Med* 316:1111, 1987.
186. Drexler HG, Thiel E, Ludwig WD: Review of the incidence and clinical relevance of myeloid antigen positive acute lymphoblastic leukemia, *Leukemia* 8:637, 1991.
187. International Workshop on Chronic Lymphocytic Leukemia: Chronic lymphocytic leukemia: recommendations for diagnosis, staging, and response criteria, *Ann Int Med* 110:236, 1989.
188. Bennett JM, Catovsky D, Daniel MT et al: Proposals for the classification of chronic (mature) B and T lymphoid leukaemias, *J Clin Pathol* 42:567, 1989.
189. Lipshutz MD, Mir R, Rai KR, Sawitsky A: Bone marrow biopsy and clinical staging in chronic lymphocytic leukemia, *Cancer* 46:1422, 1980.
190. Rozman C, Montserrat E, Rodriguez-Fernandez J et al: Bone marrow histologic pattern-the best single prognostic parmeter in chronic lymphocytic leukemia: a multivariate survival analysis of 329 cases, *Blood* 64:642, 1984.
191. Batata A, Shen B: Immunophenotyping of subtypes of B-chronic (mature) lymphoid leukemia, *Cancer* 70:2436, 1992.
192. Geisler CH, Larsen JK, Hansen NE et al: Prognostic importance of flow cytometric immunophenotyping of 540 consecutive patients with B-cell chronic lymphocytic leukemia, *Blood* 78:1795, 1991.
193. Dighiero G, Travade P, Cheveret S et al: B-cell chronic lymphocytic leukemia: present status and future directions (French Cooperative Group on CLL), *Blood* 78:1901, 1991.
194. Paoletti M, Bitter MA, Vardiman JW: Hairy cell leukemia-morphologic cytochemical, and immunologic features, *Clin in Lab Med* 8:179, 1988.
195. Bouroncle BA: Leukemic reticuloendotheliosis (hairy cell leukemia), *Blood* 53:412, 1979.
196. Burke JS, Rappaport H: The diagnosis and differential diagnosis of hairy cell leukemia in bone marrow and spleen, *Semin Oncol* 11:334, 1984.
197. Burke JS: The value of the bone marrow biopsy in the diagnosis of hairy cell leukemia, *Am J Clin Pathol* 70:876, 1978.
198. Robbins BA, Ellison DJ, Spinosa JC et al: Diagnostic application of two-color flow cytometry in 161 cases of hairy cell leukemia, *Blood* 82:1277, 1993.
199. Mulligan SP, Catovsky D: Splenic lymphoma with villous lymphocytes, *Leukemia and Lymphoma* 6:97, 1992.
200. Litz CE, Brunning RD: Chronic lymphoproliferative disorders: classification and diagnosis, *Bail Clin Haematol* 6:767, 1993.
201. Galton DAG, Goldman JM, Wiltshaw E et al: Prolymphocytic leukaemia, *Brit J Haematol* 27:7, 1974.
202. Catovsky D: Prolymphocytic leukemia, *Nouv Rev Fr Hematol* 24:343, 1982.
203. Matutes E, Brito-Babapulle V, Swansbury J et al: Clinical and laboratory features of 78 cases of T-prolymphocytic leukemia, *Blood* 78:3269, 1991.
204. Chan WC, Link S, Mawle A, Check J, Brynes RK, Winton EF: Heterogeneity of large granular lymphocyte proliferations: delineation of two major subtypes, *Blood* 68:1142, 1986.
205. Loughran TPJ: Clonal disease of large granular lymphocytes, *Blood* 82: 1, 1993.
206. McKenna RW, Arthur DC, Gajl-Peczalska KJ, Flynn P, Brunning RD: Granulated T-cell lymphocytosis with neutropenia: malignant or benign chronic lymphoproliferative disorder? *Blood* 66:259, 1985.
207. Agnarsson BA, Loughran TP, Starkebaum G, Kadin ME: The pathology of large granular lymphocyte leukemia, *Human Pathol* 20:643, 1989.
208. Flandrin G, Brouet JC: The Sezary cell; cytologic, cytochemical and immunologic studies, *Mayo Clin Proc* 49:575, 1974.
209. Lutzner MA, Jordan HW: The ultrastructure of an abnormal cell in Sezary syndrome, *Blood* 31:719, 1968.
210. Uchiyama T, Yodoi J, Sagawa K et al: Adult T-cell leukemia: clinical and hematologic features of 16 cases, *Blood* 50:481, 1977.
211. Kinoshita K, Kamihira S, Ikeda S et al: Clincal, hematologic and pathologic features of leukemic T-cell lymphoma, *Cancer* 50:1554, 1982.
212. Shimamoto Y, Ono K, Sano M et al : Comparison of CHOP versus VEPA therapy in patients with lymphoma type of adult of T-cell leukemia, *Leukemia and Lymphoma* 2:335, 1990.

Plasma cell dyscrasias

213. Durie BG: Staging and kinetics of multiple myeloma, *Semin Oncol* 13: 300, 1986.
214. Riedel DA, Pottern LM: The epidemiology of multiple myeloma, *Hematol Oncol Clin N A* 6: 225, 1992.
215. Foerster J: Multiple Myeloma. In Lee GR, Bithell TC, Foerster J et al, editors: *Wintrobe's clinical hematology*, ed 9, Philadelphia, 1993, Lea and Febiger.
216. Kyle RA: Diagnostic criteria of multiple myeloma, *Hematol Oncol Clin N A* 6: 347, 1992.
217. Feiner HD: Pathology of dysproteinemia: light chain amyloidosis, non-amyloid immunoglobulin deposition disease, cryoglobulinemia syndromes, and macroglobulinemia of Waldenstrom, *Human Pathol* 19:1255, 1988.
218. Jancelewicz Z, Takatsuki K, Sugai S, Pruzanski W: IgD multiple myeloma, *Arch Int Med* 135: 87, 1975.
219. Kyle RA, Lust JA: Monoclonal gammopathies of undetermined significance, *Semin Hematol* 26:176, 1989.
220. Greipp PR, Raymond NM, Kyle RA, O'Fallon WM: Multiple myeloma: significance of plasmablastic subtype in morphologic classification, *Blood* 65: 305, 1985.
221. Sukpanichnant S, Cousar JB, Leelasiri A et al: Diagnostic criteria and histologic grading in multiple myeloma: histologic and immunohistologic analysis of 176 cases with clinical correlation, *Hum Pathol* 25:308, 1994
222. Pileri S, Poggi S, Baglioni P et al: Histology and immunohistology of bone marrow biopsy in multiple myeloma, *Europ J Haematol* 51: 52, 1989.

223. Greipp PR: Advances in the diagnosis and management of myeloma, *Semin Hematol* 29(suppl 2): 24, 1992.
224. Greipp PR, Katzmann JA, O'Fallon WM, Kyle RA: Value of $\beta 2$ microglobulin level and plasma cell labeling indices as prognostic factors in patients with newly diagnosed myleoma, *Blood* 72:219, 1988
225. Kosmo MA, Gale RP: Plasma cell leukemia, *Semin Hematol* 24:202, 1987.
226. Woodruff RK, Malpas JS, Paxton AM, Lister TA: Plasma cell leukemia (PCL): a report on 15 patients, *Blood* 52:839, 1978.
227. Kyle RA: "Benign" monoclonal gammopathy-after 20-35 years of follow-up, *Mayo Clin Proc* 68:26, 1993.
228. Grogan TM, Spier CM: The B-cell immunoproliferative disorders, including multiple myeloma and amyloidosis. In Knowles DM, editor: *Neoplastic hematopathology,* Baltimore, 1992, Williams and Wilkins.
229. Meis JM, Butler JJ, Osborne BM, Ordoniz G: Solitary plasmacytomas of bone and extramedullary plasmacytomas, a clinicopathologic and immunohistochemical study, *Cancer* 59:1475, 1987.
230. Dimopoulos MA, Moulopoulos A, Delasalle K, Alexanian R: Solitary plasmacytoma of bone and asymptomatic multiple myeloma, *Hematol Oncol Clin N A* 6: 359, 1992.
231. Woodruff RK, Whittle JM, Malpas JS: Solitary plasmacytoma I: extramedullary soft tissue plasmacytoma, *Cancer* 43:2340, 1979.
232. Galian A, Lecestre M-J, Scotto J et al: Pathological study of alpha-chain disease with special emphasis on evolution, *Cancer* 39:2081, 1977.
233. Ben-Ayed F, Halphen M, Najjar T et al: Treatment of alpha heavy chain disease: results of a prospective study in 21 Tunisian patients by the Tunisian-French intestinal lymphoma study group, *Cancer* 63:1251, 1989.
234. Waldenstrom JG: Macroglobulinemia: a review, *Haematologica* 71: 437, 1986.
235. MacKenzie MR, Fudenberg HH: Macroglobulinemia: an analysis for forty patients, *Blood* 39:874, 1972.
236. Buxbaum J: Mechanisms of disease: monoclonal immunoglobulin deposition, amyloidosis, light chain deposition disease, and light and heavy chain deposition disease, *Hematol Oncol Clin N A* 6:323, 1992.
237. Kyle RA, Gertz MA: Systemic amyloidosis, *Critical Reviews in Oncol/Hematol* 10:49, 1990.

Disorders of the monocyte/macrophage system

238. Barranger JA, Ginns BI: Glucosylceramide lipidoses: Gaucher disease. In Scriver CR, Beaudet AL, Sly WS, Valle D, editors: *The metabolic basis of inherited disease,* ed 6, New York, 1989, McGraw-Hill.
239. Hansen HG, Graucob E: Hematologic cytology of storage disease, New York, 1985, Springer Verlag.
240. Spence MW, Calahan JW: Spingomyelin-cholesterol lipidoses: the Niemann-Pick group of diseases. In Scriver CR, Beaudet AL, Sly WS, Valle D, editors: The metabolic basis of inherited disease, ed 6, New York, 1989, McGraw-Hill.

Hemophagocytic disorders

241. Reiner AP, Spivak JL: Hematophagocytic histiocytosis: a report of 23 new patients and a review of the literature, *Medicine(Baltimore)* 67:345, 1988.
242. Woda BA, Sullivan JL: Reactive histiocytic disorders, *Am J Clin Pathol* 99: 459, 1993.
243. Jaffee ES, Costa J, Fauci AS et al: Malignant lymphoma and erythrophagocytosis simulating malignant histiocytosis, *Am J Med* 75:741, 1983.
244. Henter JI, Elinder G, Ost A: Diagnostic guidelines for hemophagocytic lymphohistocytosis, *Semin Oncol* 18:29, 1991.
245. Risdall RJ, McKenna RW, Nesbit ME et al: A benign histiocyte proliferation distinct from malignant histiocytosis, *Cancer* 44:993, 1979.

Metastatic tumor

246. Anner RM, Drewinko B: Frequency and significance of bone marrow involvement by metastatic solid tumors, *Cancer* 39: 1337, 1976.
247. Finklestein JZ, Ekert H, Isaacs H, Higgins G: Bone marrow metastases in children with solid tumor, *Amer J Dis Child* 119: 49, 1970.

42 Lymph Nodes

Lawrence M. Weiss
Wing (John) C. Chan
Bertram Schnitzer

PATHOLOGIC EVALUATION OF A LYMPH NODE

In most cases, an abnormal lymph node will be surgically excised intact. In general, the surgeon should obtain the most enlarged lymph node that is accessible to removal. The specimen should be sent fresh, and not initially placed in fixative, so appropriate tissue can be taken for special studies. This usually includes fresh tissue for possible frozen section immunophenotypic studies, flow cytometry, or molecular studies, and may also include sterile tissue for cytogenetic or microbiologic cultures. Frozen sections may be helpful to determine whether adequate diagnostic tissue have been obtained, and may often, but not always, distinguish a nonhematolymphoid from a hematolymphoid process. In conjunction with touch preparations (to better demonstrates cytologic features), one may be able to establish a diagnosis of Hodgkin's disease (HD) or non-Hodgkin's lymphoma (NHL), assign a rough estimate of grade in NHL, and recognize some specific lymphoma types at the time of frozen section. Nonetheless, we recommend deferring specific diagnosis in most cases, unless there is an immediate clinical need, since optimal morphology and ancillary studies are often necessary for a precise and completely accurate diagnosis.

Since optimal evaluation of lymphoid lesions depends upon attention to fine nuclear detail, prompt and proper fixation is important. Some hematopathologists prefer metal-based fixatives such as B5 for fixation of lymph nodes in addition to neutral-buffered formalin. Tissues should be promptly fixed to preserve cytologic detail, and should also not be overfixed, as this tends to hinder immunohistochemistry. Thin sections are helpful in evaluating nuclear features.

Occasionally, fine needle aspiration biopsy (FNAB) is used to sample abnormal lymph nodes. These studies can be useful in determining whether an enlarged mass is actually a lymph node, and can often be used to determine benign vs. malignant and hematolymphoid vs. nonhematolymphoid. We do not recommend FNAB when there is a high suspicion of lymphoma, unless the patient is a poor candidate for surgical biopsy or the abnormal lymph node is in an inaccessible location. Nonetheless, one can often establish a diagnosis of HD, separate low-grade from high-grade NHL, and may recognize a variety of subtypes of NHL.[1] However, accurate specific subtyping may be difficult, and both false positive and false negative results can occur. FNAB can be used to obtain tissue for special studies such as immunophenotypic and molecular studies, and may be particularly useful in the staging and follow-up of patients with known malignant lymphoma.

The availability of monoclonal antibodies that detect leukocyte antigens in routinely fixed, paraffin-embedded tissue sections and modern antigen retrieval techniques such as heating in citrate buffer have dramatically changed the practice of hematopathology.[2-9] Table 42-1 lists selected antigens that may be detected in paraffin-embedded tissues. Use of these antibodies allows identification of a lesion as hematolymphoid, assessment of immunoarchitecture, and phenotypic analysis of neoplastic hematolymphoid populations (Fig. 42-1). In some circumstances, these studies may be useful in distinguishing a neoplastic from a reactive population. Examples include the demonstration of light chain restriction in B-cell lymphomas expressing cytoplasmic immunogloblin, the reactivity of follicular B-cells with *bcl*-2 in follicular lymphoma, or the aberrant co-expression of the T-cell/myeloid marker CD43 with B lineage markers on the neoplastic cells in diffuse B-cell lymphomas (Fig. 42-2).[2-9] Usually, the neoplastic cells can be assigned to the B or T lineage using paraffin section antibodies. Antibodies such as Ki-67 can also be used to provide indirect measures of cellular proliferation.[10]

Despite the advances in paraffin section immunohistochemistry, a much greater array of antibodies reacting against a much wider variety of leukocyte antigens is available when acetone-fixed cell frozen sections or cell suspensions are used.[11-13] Table 42-2 summarizes some of the more important antigens useful in hematopathology. In addition to being able to distinguish neoplastic proliferations from reactive infiltrates by the same methods as used in paraffin section immunophenotyping, one may determine light chain restriction in B-cell lymphomas expressing surface immunoglobulin and may identify both B- and T-cell lymphomas with aberrant expression or loss of antigens, such as the loss of one or more pan–T-cell antigens in peripheral T-cell lymphomas. In addition, one may use the pattern of antigen reactivity as an aid in the subclassification of NHLs, such as in distinguishing the low-grade lymphomas from one another by evaluating reactivity for CD5, CD10, and CD23.

Advantages to performing these studies in frozen sections include the ability to evaluate immunoarchitecture and a greater ability to identify focal lesions. Advantages to performing these studies by flow cytometry on cell suspensions include the ability to easily quantitate results, important for example in assessing the kappa to lambda ratio; the ability to easily perform double-labeling studies; and the ability to gate on specific cell populations by cell size. One disadvantage to flow cytometry is the potential to preferentially lose certain cell populations that may be more susceptible to destruction during the preparation of the cell suspensions. Additional studies that can be performed by flow cytometry include measures of DNA content and S-phase fraction. Up to one-third of NHLs have an aneuploid line, with the incidence of aneuploidy increasing with increasing histologic grade.[14] In general, the proliferative rate of lymphomas is also related to its histologic grade.[14,15] Moreover, within certain categories of lymphoma, the S-phase fraction has been related to prognosis.

Molecular studies have become increasingly important in the evaluation of lymphoid lesions in the last ten years, including the assessment of the B- and T-lymphocyte antigen receptor genes and the detection of specific chromosomal aberrations.[16-20] The immunoglobulin heavy chain gene on chromosome 14 and the kappa and lambda light chain genes on chromosomes 2 and 22, respectively, comprise the B-cell

Table 42-1 Major leukocyte antigens detectable in paraffin sections

Antigen	Predominant expression
TdT	Lymphoblastic neoplasms
Myeloperoxidase	Myeloid cells and myeloid leukemia
Lysozyme	Histiocytes and myeloid cells, histiocytic neoplasms, and myeloid leukemia
Immunoglobulin light and heavy chain	Plasma cells, plasma cells and plasmacytoid neoplasms, some follicular lymphomas
bcl-2	Non-germinal center B-cells, most T-cells, most follicular lymphomas, many low-grade and some higher grade B-cell lymphomas
Epithelial membrane antigen	Plasma cells and plasma cell neoplasms, many nodular L&H lymphocyte predominance, anaplastic large cell lymphoma, and T-cell rich B-cell lymphoma
EBV latent membrane protein	Some EBV-infected cells (most notably EBV$^+$ Hodgkin's cells)
CD3	T-cells and many T-cell lymphomas
CD15	Myeloid cells, Hodgkin's disease, some non-Hodgkin's lymphomas
CD20	B-cells and B-cell lymphomas, nodular L&H lymphocyte predominance
CD21	Follicular dendritic cells, mantle and marginal zone B-cells and neoplasms
CD30	Activated lymphoid cells, Hodgkin's disease, anaplastic large cell lymphoma
CD34	Progenitor cells, some myeloid leukemias, some lymphoblastic neoplasms
CD40	B-cells and Hodgkin's disease
CD43	T-cells, myeloid cells, mast cells, T-cell lymphomas, some B-cell lymphomas, myeloid leukemia, mast cell neoplasms
CD45/CD45RB	Hematolymphoid cells
CD45RA	B-cells and subset of T-cells, B-cell lymphomas, nodular L&H lymphocyte predominance
CD45R0	Most T-cells, histiocytes, myeloid cells, T-cell lymphomas
CD57	Subset of T-cells and natural killer cells, subset of T-cell lymphomas
CD68	Histiocytes, myeloid cells, mast cells and neoplasms, some non-Hodgkin's lymphomas

TDT, Terminal deoxynbonucleotidal transferase

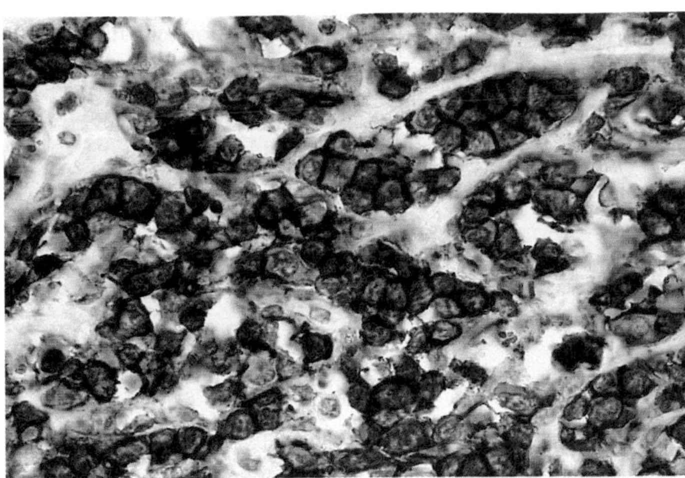

Fig. 42-1 B-cell lymphoma. This lymphoma was initially mistaken for a carcinoma, because of the pattern of fibrosis. Immunohistochemical stains such as this CD20 stain for B-cells helped to established the correct diagnosis.

antigen receptor genes. The T-cell receptor genes include the alpha/delta complex on chromosome 14q11, and the beta and gamma genes present on chromosomes 7q35 and 7p13, respectively. Somatic DNA rearrangement of the antigen receptor genes is one of the earliest known processes to occur during lymphocyte differentiation. Each antigen receptor gene is composed of families of two or more gene segments, termed variable (V), diversity (D), joining (J), and constant (C) regions. These gene segments are separated by long stretches of DNA which are deleted during the process of gene rearrangement (Fig. 42-3). Once these rearrangements have occurred, they are relatively stable markers of the individual lymphocyte and all its progeny.

Antigen receptor gene rearrangements are detected by two main molecular techniques: Southern blotting and polymerase chain reaction (PCR). With Southern blotting, gene rearrangement is detected by a change in the pattern of bands detected using a hybridization probe to a portion of the antigen receptor gene after application of DNA-restriction enzymes. Since the sensitivity of Southern blotting is 1% to 5%, the detection of an abnormal band indicates the presence of a monoclonal population of at least 1% to 5%, which in almost all cases indicates a neoplastic process. Since reactive populations are composed of mixed clones of cells each comprising less than 1% of the infiltrate, their rearranged antigen receptor genes cannot be detected. Southern blotting generally requires fresh tissue to obtain high-quality DNA and takes about 2-3 weeks for the procedure.

With PCR, primers are used that are homologous to sequences flanking the sites where the various gene segments are joined to each other. In the nonrearranged states the primers are too far apart for amplification to occur, but after somatic gene rearrangement has occurred, amplification can take place. PCR is somewhat more sensitive than Southern blotting, but its sensitivity may be limited by the background of non-clonally rearranged genes that also may be amplified. PCR is faster to perform than Southern blotting, with results obtainable in 1-5 days, and it may be performed in paraffin-embedded tissues in many cases. However, PCR also has one disadvantage in that not all gene segments may be recognized by a single set of

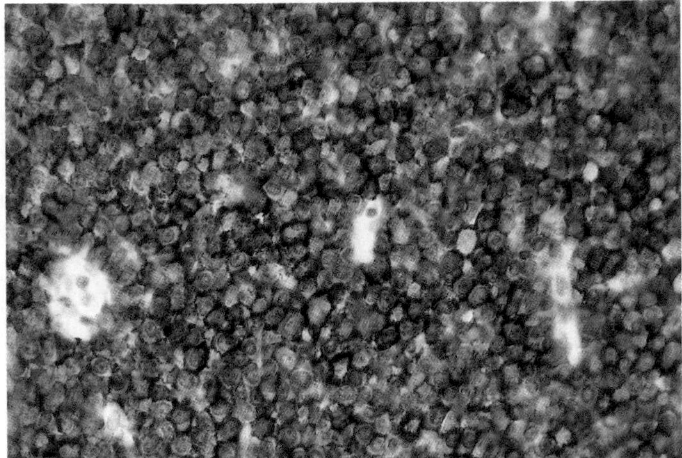

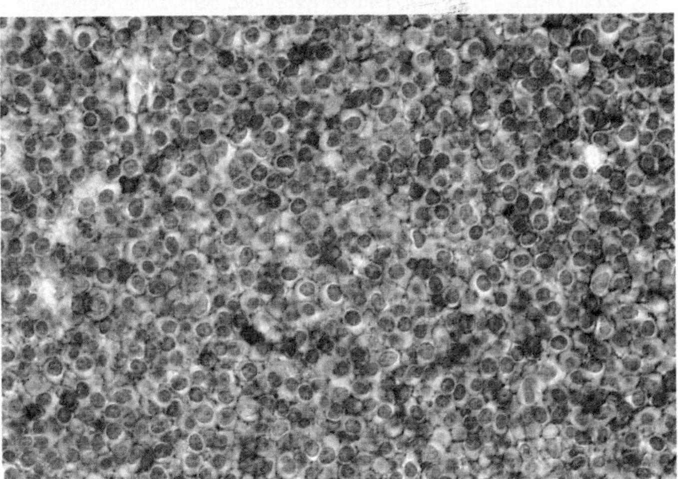

Fig. 42-2 Small lymphocytic lymphoma. **A,** Diffuse membrane staining for the B-cell antigen CD20 is seen. **B,** Aberrant coexpression of the T-cell/myeloid marker CD43 is seen.

primers. This may lead to false negative results that may be minimized if a cocktail of several primers is used. With PCR, one may also design specific primers to individual tumors. This may enhance sensitivity, and may be particularly useful in assessing the presence of residual disease.

Antigen receptor gene rearrangement may be used for the diagnosis of malignancy as well as the determination of cell lineage. Although the detection of rearranged bands usually implies a malignant process, it is not completely specific. Monoclonal bands may be detected in some clinically benign diseases, such as lymphomatoid papulosis.[21] Thus, the results of gene rearrangement studies must be interpreted in the context of all clinical, histologic, and immunologic data available.

Assessment of the presence of specific chromosomal translocations may also be done by Southern blotting or PCR, using probes or primers, respectively, homologous to genes flanking the sites of translocation. These studies may be easier to perform than classical cytogenetics and do not require fresh sterile tissue. The molecular approach to the identification of specific translocations also has the advantage of great potential sensitivity and specificity. However, the DNA adjacent to the translocations must be well characterized (to obtain the appropriate probes and primers). Another potential problem is that

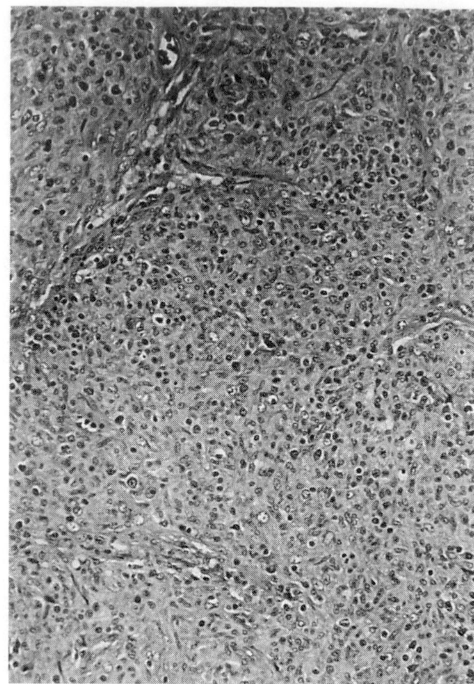

Fig. 42-10 Mycobacterial spindle cell pseudotumor. The pattern of fibrosis and the presence of numerous chronic inflammatory cells is very reminiscent of inflammatory pseudotumor. A high level of suspicion and the performance of appropriate special stains are necessary to establish the diagnosis.

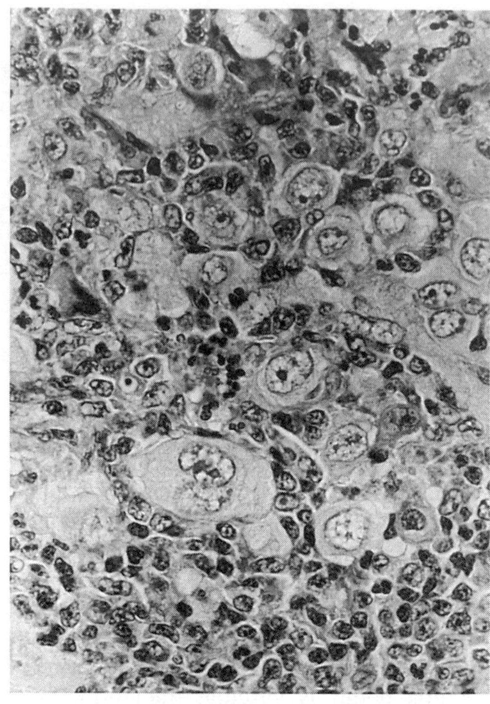

Fig. 42-11 Metastatic nasopharyngeal carcinoma. This tumor was initially mistaken for nodular sclerosing Hodgkin's disease. Keratin immunostaining confirmed the diagnosis of carcinoma.

The lesion is benign, but rarely may recur. It probably represents the end-stage of a variety of inflammatory lesions that may affect the lymph node. A histologically similar lesion is mycobacterial spindle cell pseudotumor (Fig. 42-10).[60] This lesion occurs in HIV-infected patients and represents an infection by atypical mycobacteria; appropriate special stains demonstrate the presence of numerous bacilli with the proliferating histiocytes.

Metastatic tumors

Metastatic tumors are by far the most common nonhematopoietic elements to involve lymph nodes. Carcinoma is the most common tumor type to metastasize to lymph nodes, but lymph node metastases are also a common occurrence in malignant melanoma, germ cell tumors, and certain types of sarcomas. In general, the presence of lymph node metastases will significantly adversely affect the prognosis; therefore, removal of local lymph nodes, often by formal lymph node dissection, is common practice in many standard surgical cancer resections. Lymph nodes involved by metastatic tumor usually show total or subtotal replacement, often with extension to adjacent perinodal lymphatics and soft tissues. Early involvement of lymph nodes usually manifests in the subcapsular sinuses. In general, the prognosis decreases with the number of involved nodes, and the presence of extracapsular soft tissue extension may indicate a need for subsequent radiation therapy.[61] Some investigators have shown that more metastases to lymph nodes can be detected by the performance of immunohistochemistry to identify occult foci of tumor, but it has not yet been convincingly demonstrated that their detection improves prognostication.[62]

Often an enlarged lymph node is removed from a patient, and unexpectedly, an undifferentiated malignant neoplasm is found. Even if some differentiating features are present, the differential diagnosis can still be quite large. For example, signet ring cells can be found in carcinomas, lymphomas, and malignant melanomas. Undifferentiated neoplasms are often large cell lymphomas, but a significant number will represent poorly differentiated carcinoma, malignant melanoma, germ cell tumor, or even sarcoma (Fig. 42-11). Although electron microscopy (EM) may be helpful in selected cases, the great majority of cases can be resolved by histochemical stains such as mucin and particularly immunohistochemical studies performed in paraffin-embedded tissues. Leukocyte common antigen (CD45) will identify over 90% of malignant lymphomas;[7] and CD30 (a marker of Hodgkin's disease, anaplastic large cell lymphoma, and some other lymphomas), the B lineage marker CD20, and the T-cell/myeloid marker CD43 will identify most $CD45^-$ hematolymphoid tumors.[3-5] Keratin will identify almost all cases of carcinoma, while S-100 is a sensitive (but not completely specific) marker for malignant melanoma. Use of a battery of immunostains is important in differential diagnosis, since so many tumors can have overlapping reactivities and for cross-validation of staining reactions. For example, many breast carcinomas are S-100-positive; a strongly keratin-positive, S-100-positive tumor is likely to be breast carcinoma and not malignant melanoma. However, a keratin-negative, S-100 positive tumor that is also found to be positive for the melanoma marker HMB45 is very likely to be a malignant melanoma and not breast carcinoma. Placental alkaline phosphatase is a relatively sensitive (although not completely specific) marker for germ cell tumors.

Metastatic carcinoma of unknown primary is not uncommon. The possible primary site may be suggested by the site of the involved lymph node. Location in the neck should raise consideration of a primary within the upper aerodigestive tract. Location in the axilla in a woman should raise strong consideration for breast carcinoma. Involvement of the supraclavicular region should raise consideration for an abdominal primary. Paraffin section immunohistochemistry can also be very helpful in determining the possible primary site.

REACTIVE LYMPHADENOPATHIES

The main function of lymph nodes is to process antigen and present the altered antigen to B- or T-lymphocytes.[26] The altered antigen may cause proliferation of B- or T-lymphocytes in one or more of the nodal compartments, leading to expansion of these compartments, and subsequently resulting in nodal enlargement or lymphadenopathy. The response to many different antigens leads to proliferations of different subsets or combinations of subsets of B- and T-cells, sinus histiocytes, or occasionally the specialized accessory cells (dermatopathic lymphadenitis). Proliferations in lymph nodes of different individuals vary according to the person's age, immunologic make-up, and past experience with the offending antigen and the duration of the proliferation. Histologically, this series of events leads to the development of one of the benign lymphoid proliferations or hyperplasias (see below).

Acute and chronic lymphadenitis

The term *lymphadenitis* is generally used to indicate infection in a lymph node with the infectious agent being present. The infectious agent can cause acute or chronic lymphadenitis. Acute lymphadenitis, which is rarely, if ever, diagnosed by the surgical pathologist, is most commonly caused by local septic infections that spread to lymph nodes, for example: tonsillitis, skin and oral cavity infections and abscesses, and the usual etiologic agents are pyogenic bacteria, particularly streptococci and staphylococci. The primary site of infection is usually known and draining lymph nodes are not examined through biopsy. Chronic lymphadenitis is a general term and includes numerous disorders instigated by a variety of infectious agents that result in a broad spectrum of nonacute reactions. Granulomatous disorders and lymphadenopathy caused by viruses, rickettsiae, mycoses, and other agents can all be called chronic lymphadenitis but are usually designated by the name of the etiologic agent if it is known (e.g., tuberculous lymphadenitis, toxoplasmosis lymphadenitis).

In contrast to lymphadenitis, the term *lymphoid hyperplasia* is applied to lymphoid proliferations in response to antigenic stimulation without evidence of infectious involvement of the node.

Enlarged peripheral lymph nodes are among the most frequently excised structures in both children and adults, because they are readily accessible and may yield diagnoses of disorders that are distant from them, thereby obviating the need for biopsy of less amenable sites. Such lymph node biopsies may yield evidence of benign reactive lymphadenopathies, metastatic tumors, infectious processes, or metabolic disorders, or else these nodes may be the sites of primary lymph node neoplasms, namely, malignant lymphomas.

Although lymphomas have elicited much literature, most lymph nodes biopsy specimens, in fact, reveal of one the many types of reactive hyperplasias.[63] In the vast majority of cases, the etiology of the reactive lymphadenopathy is unknown, and, thus, a diagnosis of nonspecific reactive hyperplasia is made. In some cases, however, the pathologist is able to offer an etiology or render a differential diagnosis as to etiology and suggest additional laboratory tests or stains for microorganisms to confirm or dismiss the suspicion. Disorders showing characteristic but not entirely etiologically diagnostic proliferations include the hyperplasias associated with rheumatoid arthritis,[64] HIV infection,[65] toxoplasmosis,[66] syphilis,[67] infectious mononucleosis,[68] nonnecrotizing and necrotizing or suppurative granulomas,[63] and the characteristic histologic changes that may be associated with systemic lupus erythematosus,[69] Kikuchi's disease,[70] and Whipple's disease.[71] The histologic findings and results of laboratory tests correlated with the clinical findings may then result in a definitive and specific diagnosis.

In general, features of a benign lymphoid proliferation include retention of the lymph node architecture, a polymorphous cell population, and lack of atypicality of the lymphocytes, whereas Hodgkin's disease and non-Hodgkin's lymphomas are most often recognized by effacement of the nodal architecture and the presence of atypical cells. However, there are many exceptions. Reactive hyperplasias may efface the nodal architecture, and atypical cells may be present, while the converse may be seen in lymphomatous lymph nodes. When it is not possible to differentiate benign lymphoproliferative processes from lymphomas on morphological grounds alone, ancillary techniques such as immunophenotyping and, occasionally, genotypic analysis are required to distinguish between a monoclonal (presumably, but not invariably, malignant) from a polyclonal (benign) lymphoproliferation.

Reactive lymphadenopathies are divided on the basis of the normal lymph nodal compartments into five patterns: 1) follicular; 2) interfollicular; 3) mixed follicular and interfollicular; 4) diffuse; and 5) sinus pattern (Table 42-3).

Follicular hyperplasia

Microscopic examination of all lymph node biopsy specimens should start under low magnification. Thus, the pathologist can assess the nodal architecture and detect alterations in the various compartments, which can then be examined more closely. Follicular hyperplasia is the most common type of reactive lymphoid proliferation. Particularly common in children and adolescents, its etiology is largely unknown. It is defined as an increase in the number and size of follicles (Fig. 42-12). The follicles frequently also vary in shape. Fusion of adjacent germinal centers may take place, resulting in large, bizarre geographic structures (Fig. 42-13). The hyperplastic follicles consist of expanded germinal centers, usually at the expense of the mantle zone, which may be thin and attenuated. The hyperplastic germinal center usually contains mixtures of small and large cleaved and noncleaved cells (Figs. 42-4 and 42-5). In some cases the reactive germinal centers consist almost exclusively of large transformed cells. Mitotic figures are often numerous and a "starry sky" appearance, which also indicates a high proliferative rate, is characteristic of a hyperplastic germinal center. Polarity of the germinal centers, which is a good indicator of a benign follicle, is visualized in some but not all of the follicles. This polarity is formed by a predominance of

Table 42-3 Patterns of reactive lymphadenopathies

Follicular pattern
Nonspecific follicular hyperplasia
Rheumatoid arthritis/Sjögren's syndrome
Syphilis
Angiofollicular hyperplasia (Castleman's disease)
HIV-related
Progressive transformation of germinal centers
Interfollicular pattern
Nonspecific interfollicular hyperplasia
Dermatopathic lymphadenitis
Histiocytic necrotizing lymphadenitis (Kikuchi's disease)
Granulomatous lymphadenitis
Mixed follicular and interfollicular pattern
Toxoplasmosis lymphadenitis
Cat-scratch disease
Lymphogranuloma venereum
Mesenteric lymphadenitis
Kimura's disease
Diffuse pattern
Infectious mononucleosis and other viral lymphadenitis
Abnormal immune response/angioimmunoblastic lymphadenopathy
Drug-induced hypersensitivity reactions
Systemic lupus erythematosus
Mucocutaneous lymph node syndrome (Kawasaki's disease)
Sinus pattern
Sinus histiocytosis
Hemophagocytic syndrome
Sinus histiocytosis with massive lymphadenopathy
Lymphangiography effect
Whipple's disease

large transformed germinal center cells that have a high mitotic rate and are interspersed with tingible body macrophages at one pole, while the remainder of the germinal center consists primarily of small cleaved cells and dendritic reticulum cells (Figs. 42-4, 42-5, and 42-14). The portion of the germinal center composed of the large cells is also referred to as the "dark zone," because the lymphoid cells have deeply staining cytoplasm and they are closely apposed to one another. The "light zone" or "pale zone" that makes up the remainder of the germinal center consists primarily of small cleaved and dendritic reticulum cells, both of which have pale-staining cytoplasm and a low mitotic rate.[25] Few if any tingible body macrophages are present among these cells. Plasma cells may be found within the germinal center and they are easily identified by staining for kappa and lambda light chains (Fig. 42-14). Varying numbers of small T-lymphocytes are identified among the germinal center cells by immunostaining (Fig. 42-15). The germinal centers are sharply demarcated from the surrounding rim of mantle zone cells, except in some cases of florid follicular hyperplasia, as, for example, in lymph nodes of HIV-infected individuals.[65] In such cases, small lymphocytes infiltrate and disrupt germinal centers, a phenomenon known as *follicle lysis*. The mantle zone may be decreased in width or attenuated when the germinal centers become larger, and in florid follicular hyperplasia, the mantle zone may be totally absent. The interfollicular areas contain varying mixtures of small lymphocytes, plasma cells, and immunoblasts (large transformed lymphocytes), and high endothelial vessels may be prominent.

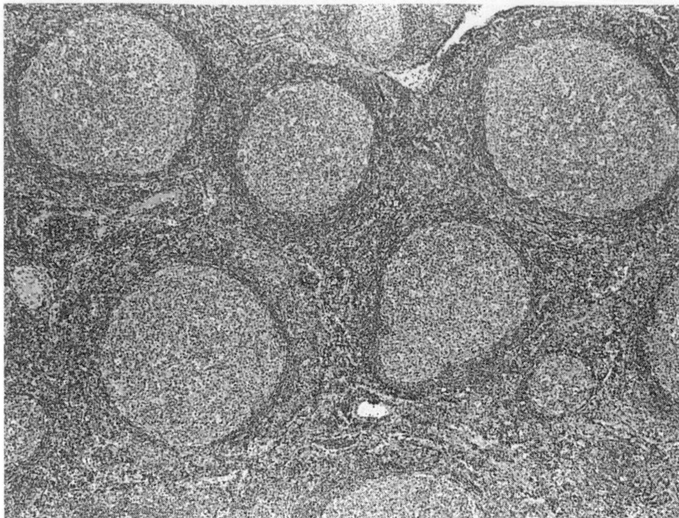

Fig. 42-12 Follicular hyperplasia. The number of follicles is increased; the germinal centers are enlarged, have a starry-sky appearance and are surrounded by an attenuated mantle zone.

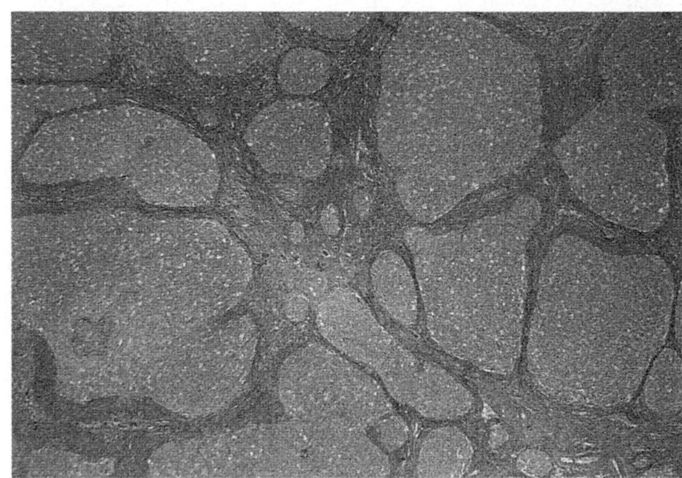

Fig. 42-13 Follicular hyperplasia. Fusion of adjacent germinal centers resulting in large bizarre structures in a lymph node from a

Differential diagnosis of follicular hyperplasia

The major diagnostic difficulty is in distinguishing follicular hyperplasia from follicular lymphoma. Some of the criteria that are useful, but far from foolproof, originally established by Rappaport,[72] are listed in Table 42-4. It must be emphasized that no single criterion can be used to distinguish between follicular hyperplasia and follicular lymphoma in an individual case. All of the listed morphological features must be considered in order for the pathologist to make the correct diagnosis. The difficulties encountered in the differential diagnosis are compounded by suboptimal sections.

The most reliable single morphological criterion in differentiating follicular hyperplasia from follicular lymphoma is the distribution and density of follicles per unit area, a factor readily determined by scanning the slide under very low magnification.[73] The neoplastic follicles tend to be closely apposed

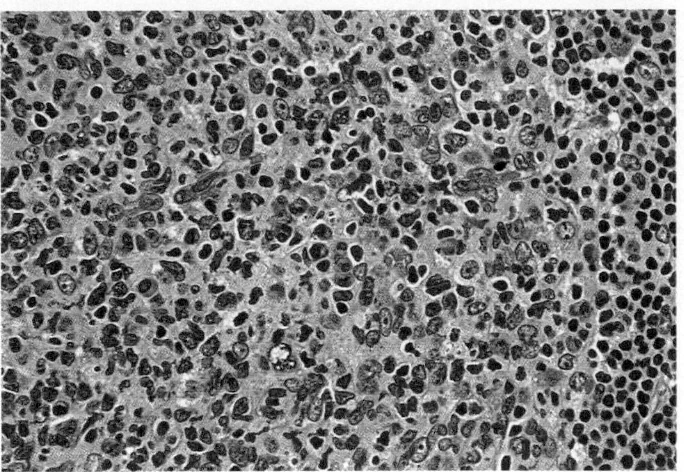

Fig. 42-14 Large and small cleaved and noncleaved germinal center cells, tingible body macrophages, and scattered plasma cells within a hyperplastic germinal center.

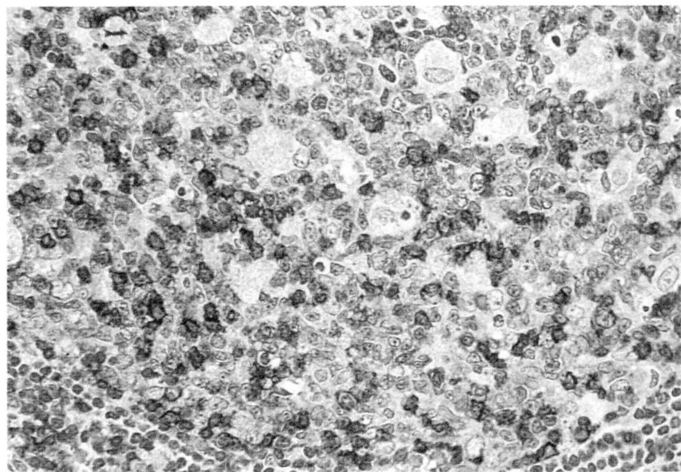

Fig. 42-15 Small T-lymphocytes are readily detected in the germinal center by immunostaining with antibody to CD45R0.

to one another, lending a "back to back" appearance. An equally useful and reliable feature that helps distinguish follicular hyperplasia from follicular lymphoma is the demonstration of polarity.[74] Polarity denotes organization of the follicle into an antigen-presenting zone that is rich in dendritic reticulum cells and a zone in which lymphocytes proliferate; this zonation is absent in neoplastic follicles. In addition, the neoplastic follicles tend to be more uniform than the benign follicles, which often vary considerably in size and shape. The amount of interfollicular tissue is smaller in follicular lymphomas, and neoplastic cells may infiltrate these areas, which is a feature diagnostic of lymphoma. Plasma cells tend to be present in interfollicular areas as well as within follicles more frequently in hyperplasias than in follicular lymphomas. Other features favoring lymphoma include absence of tingible body macrophages, a lower mitotic rate, and attenuation or complete absence of mantle zones. Follicular large cell lymphomas may have a high mitotic rate and a starry sky appearance, thereby resembling hyperplastic germinal centers, but diffuse areas of lymphoma are often present, which help in distinguishing this least common type of follicular lymphomas from

Table 42-4 Architectural and cytologic features of follicular hyperplasia and follicular lymphoma

Follicular hyperplasia	Follicular lymphoma
Nodal architecture preserved	Nodal architecture effaced
Germinal centers vary in size and shape	Follicles uniform
Low density of follicles	High density of follicles
Polarization of large transformed cells in germinal centers	Absence of polarization in follicles
Mitotic rate moderate to high in germinal centers	Mitotic rate low in follicles
Tingible body macrophages in germinal centers	Absence of tingible body macrophages
Sharp demarcation of germinal centers from mantle zone lymphocytes	Borders of follicles not well defined; mantle zones incomplete, breached or absent
Ample interfollicular areas containing inflammatory cells	Sparse interfollicular areas that may contain neoplastic cells

follicular hyperplasia. Also, mantle zones are usually lacking in this type of lymphoma. There are always exceptions to the characteristic features distinguishing benign from neoplastic follicular proliferations, and it is sometimes not possible to differentiate with certainty between them. In such instances, determination of light chain restriction or, if this is not possible, genotyping may be necessary.[20,35] Staining for *bcl-2* protein may also be helpful. Neoplastic follicular center cells usually stain for *bcl-2* protein, while benign follicle center cells do not.[75] In addition, about 85% to 90% of follicular lymphomas have the structural cytogenetic t(14;18), which is absent in follicular hyperplasia.[75] If frozen tissue is unavailable to indicate clonality, bone marrow biopsy to determine whether involvement by lymphoma is present, or repeat lymph node biopsy may be required.

Other disorders that are occasionally considered in the differential diagnosis include mantle cell lymphoma, especially mantle zone lymphoma, and, rarely, small lymphocytic lymphoma/chronic lymphocytic leukemia (CLL) with proliferation centers. In mantle cell lymphoma, which is a B-cell neoplasm, small lymphocytes, some with irregular nuclear contours (mantle zone derived), form nodules of expanded mantles around benign germinal centers, or "naked" germinal centers are isolated in a diffuse proliferation of mantle-zone cells.[76] Such expanded mantle zones or "naked" germinal centers without interfollicular areas are not seen in follicular hyperplasia. The proliferation centers in small lymphocytic lymphoma/CLL are composed of loosely arranged mixtures of small and large transformed monoclonal B-cells, but cleaved cells and tingible body macrophages, which are present in reactive follicles, are absent in this low-grade lymphoma.[74] Also, there are no mantle zones surrounding proliferation centers, whereas these are usually present in follicular hyperplasia. Histologically, the plasma cell variant of Castleman's disease may be indistinguishable from the changes associated with rheumatoid arthritis. A clinical history is helpful to enable the pathologist to differentiate between the two disorders. Patients with the plasma cell variant of Castleman's disease may have a variety of symptoms and abnormal laboratory tests, which are usually absent in patients with rheumatoid arthritis.[63]

It is always prudent to carefully scan under low magnification interfollicular areas for interfollicular HD, which may be masked by the prominent follicular hyperplasia.[77] Slight expansion of those areas may reveal the polymorphous infiltrate of HD that can be easily missed, especially when one is not aware of this entity. Immunostaining with CD15 may assist one in identifying Reed-Sternberg cells.

Rheumatoid arthritis and Sjögren's syndrome

Lymphadenopathy, which may be generalized, is common during the course of these diseases.[63,78] Sometimes there is waxing and waning of the enlarged nodes. There is an increased risk of development of B-cell lymphoma, particularly in patients with Sjögren's syndrome.[79] Because the nodes can reach a considerable size and the possibility of lymphoma cannot be excluded clinically, a lymph node biopsy may be carried out. The histologic features of lymph nodes in rheumatoid arthritis and Sjögren's syndrome are: 1) follicular hyperplasia; and 2) interfollicular plasmacytosis. Follicular hyperplasia is often present throughout the entire node.[64,78,80] The prominent germinal centers contain tingible body macrophages and a mitotic high rate is present. Mantle zones may be attenuated. Some polarized germinal centers are usually present. The interfollicular plasmacytosis is striking (Fig. 42-16). Sometimes, solid sheets of plasma cells in the interfollicular areas together with the follicular hyperplasia resemble, or are indistinguishable from, the histologic picture seen in the plasma cell variant of Castleman's disease.[81] Immunostaining shows that the plasma cells are polyclonal. The sinuses may be compressed by the enlarged germinal centers, and they usually contain some polymorphonuclear leukocytes (PMLs). Immunoblasts and vascular proliferation in the interfollicular areas are present but usually not prominent. In secondary syphilis, follicular hyperplasia and interfollicular plasmacytosis are usually seen in addition to the thickening of the capsule and the fibrous trabeculae, which are absent in lymph nodes of rheumatoid arthritis.[67,52]

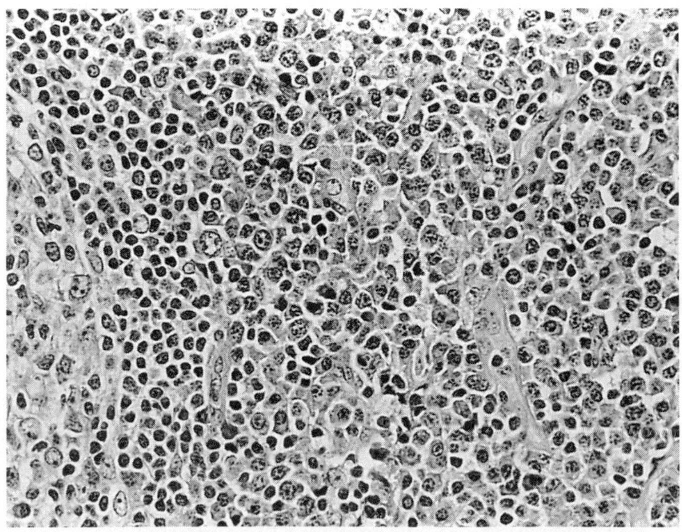

Fig. 42-16 Portion of germinal center, attenuated mantle zone, and adjacent interfollicular area composed of a dense plasma cell infiltrate in a lymph node from a patient with rheumatoid arthritis.

Although the histologic changes in rheumatoid arthritis and Sjögren's syndrome may be identical, a sinusoidal and/or paracortical monocytoid B-cell proliferation that can cause distortion of the nodal architecture may be present in nodes of patients with Sjögren's syndrome.[82] It is sometimes difficult to distinguish on morphologic grounds benign (polyclonal) monocytoid B-cell proliferations from malignant (monoclonal) low grade monocytoid B-cell lymphomas that are associated with Sjögren's syndrome. Immunophenotypic or genotypic studies may be helpful in such cases.

Syphilis

Although primary or secondary syphilis is rarely diagnosed from a lymph node biopsy, this diagnosis is undoubtedly occasionally missed. The pathologist should be aware of the characteristic, although not specific, histologic findings in syphilitic or luetic lymphadenitis, whose incidence is on the rise. In most of the reported cases, biopsies of the inguinal lymph nodes have been done, although in secondary syphilis, lymphadenopathy is often generalized. Histologically, luetic lymphadenitis is characterized by follicular hyperplasia and interfollicular plasmacytosis resembling that seen in rheumatoid arthritis.[52,67] It differs from the latter disorder in that the capsule and trabeculae are thickened and infiltrated by plasma cells, and perivenular plasmacytosis, and clusters of epithelioid histiocytes and epithelioid granulomas with multinucleated giant cells may be present. Endarteritis, phlebitis, and, occasionally, abscesses are noted. The histologic impression of syphilitic lymphadenitis is confirmed by demonstrating the causative spirochetes by the Warthin-Starry silver stain, by immunohistologic methods, and by serologic studies. In lymph nodes, the spirochetes are often found within the walls and around postcapillary venules and sometimes within germinal centers.[67]

Castleman's disease

Castleman's disease, named after the pathologist who first described the entity,[83] is also known by the descriptive terms *angiofollicular lymph node hyperplasia* or *giant lymph node hyperplasia*.[81,84,85] In Castleman's initial report, the lesions were solitary and confined to the mediastinum, still the most frequent site of involvement. Since then, the disease has been reported in many other locations including the abdominal cavity, which is the second most common site, the pulmonary parenchyma, axillary and cervical regions, and skeletal muscle.[81] We have also seen involvement of the kidney in a case with abdominal cavity lesions that necessitated nephrectomy. Two forms of the disease exist: the localized type, which is by far the more common, and the more recently described multicentric or generalized form.[84-87]

Histologically, there are two major types of localized Castleman's disease: the much more common hyaline vascular type and the plasma cell type.[81] There is also a third, the least common mixed type, showing features of both hyaline vascular and plasma cell types.[88] The two major forms of the disease vary not only in their histologic appearances but also in their clinical presentations. Patients with the plasma cell type may present with a wide variety of unexplainable symptoms and/or abnormal laboratory findings. After excision of their solitary lesion, the patient's symptoms disappear and their abnormal laboratory test results return to normal.[81]

Hyaline vascular type. More than 90% of cases are of the hyaline vascular histologic type.[81] There is no sex predilection and this type has been reported in patients ranging in age from 8 to 69 years (median 33 years). Grossly, the lesion consists of a single rounded mass ranging in size from 1.5 to 16 cm. Patients with the hyaline vascular type of disease are generally asymptomatic unless the large mass abuts or partially obstructs a structure such as a bronchus. Microscopically, the lesions are distinctive, consisting of 1) regressively transformed, involuted, or atrophic germinal centers surrounded by variably-sized mantle zones, often arranged in concentric rings referred to as "onion skin layers"; and 2) a prominent interfollicular vascularity that accounts for the reported profuse bleeding when the mass is incised during the surgical procedure, and sinuses are absent (Fig. 42-17). The germinal centers are depleted of lymphocytes and consist predominantly of dendritic reticulum cells and some endothelial cells (Fig. 42-18). Vessels, which often become hyalinized, can be seen entering the germinal center from the interfollicular zone. These abnormal germinal centers may have a squamous cell-like appearance and may superficially resemble Hassall's corpuscles and, with their penetrating hyalinized vessel entering at right angles to the follicle, have been likened to a lollipop[81] (Fig. 42-17). In some cases, the palisading, small mantle-zone lymphocytes almost completely obscure the small residual germinal centers. When this histologic feature predominates, the lesion is referred to as the *lymphoid variant of the hyaline vascular type* (Fig. 42-19).[81] Another characteristic finding is the presence of more than one small germinal center within a single follicle (Fig. 42-20). The interfollicular areas contain small lymphocytes, occasional eosinophils, some plasma cells, and few immunoblasts. Clusters of plasmacytoid monocytes (plasmacytoid T-cells) are not infrequently seen.[89] Large, dense fibrotic masses, usually around larger vessels, are often but not always scattered in interfollicular areas. Sinuses are usually obliterated but may be seen at the periphery of the lesion.

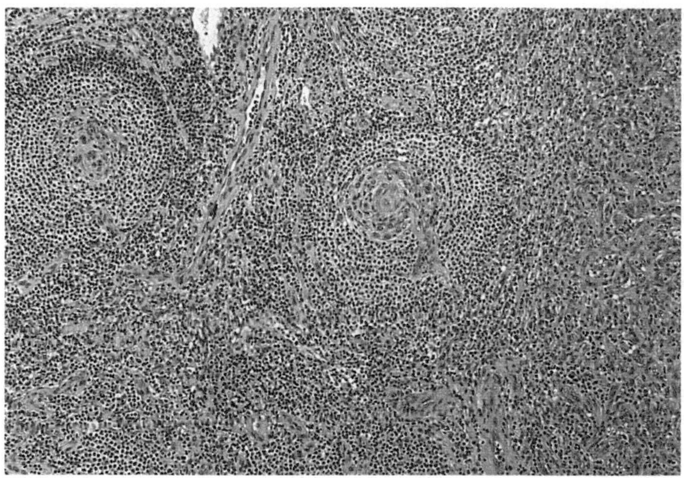

Fig. 42-17 Hyaline vascular Castleman's disease showing two follicles with regressively transformed germinal centers surrounded by concentrically arranged mantle zone lymphocytes. "Lollipop" appearance of a follicle is evident (right). Interfollicular vascularity is prominent.

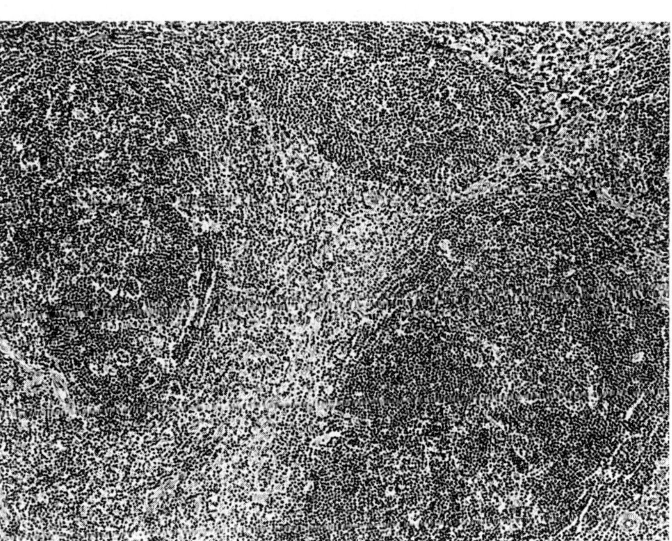

Fig. 42-19 Lymphoid variant of Castleman's disease. The follicles are composed entirely of concentrically arranged small mantle cell lymphocytes. Interfollicular vascularity is present.

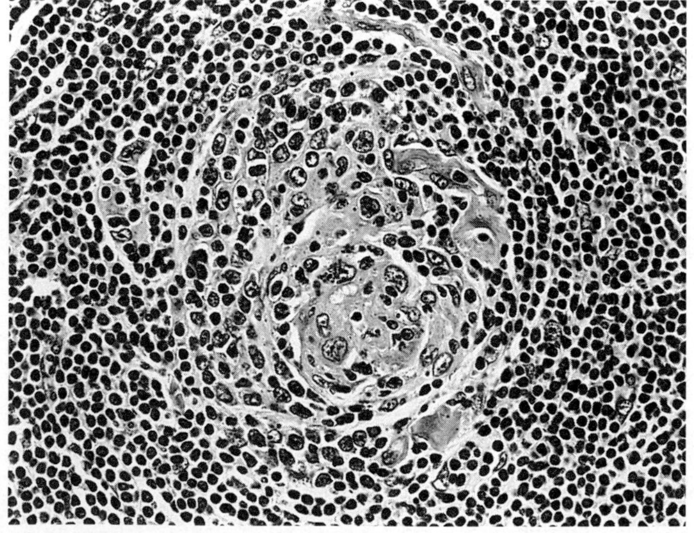

Fig. 42-18 Atrophic germinal center is devoid of lymphocytes and consists primarily of dendritic cells. A hyalinized vessel is present at the periphery of the germinal center.

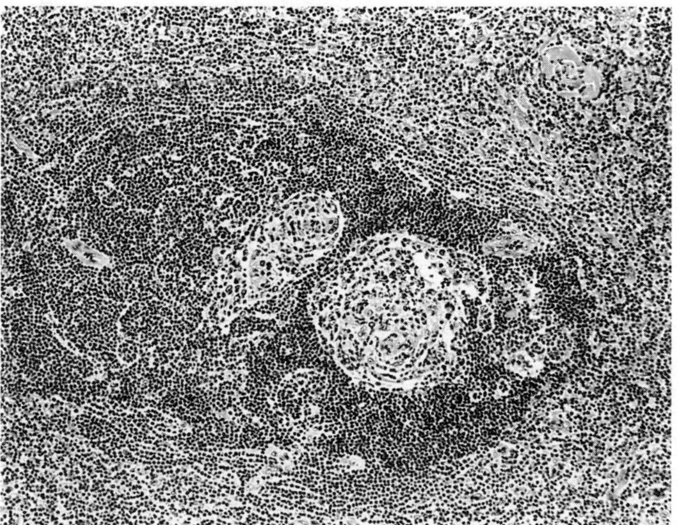

Fig. 42-20 Two atrophic germinal centers depleted of lymphocytes within a single follicle. Vascularity with sclerosis around a vessel is present in the interfollicular area.

The differential diagnosis of the hyaline vascular type of Castleman's disease includes the Castleman's-like lesions seen in HIV-related, persistent generalized lymphadenopathy.[85] In both diseases, the small germinal centers may be identical, but the interfollicular vascularity is greater, and the cellular polymorphism and plasmacytosis in the interfollicular areas are less pronounced in Castleman's disease. Also, the mantle zones are more prominent in Castleman's disease, while they tend to be small or even absent in HIV-related adenopathy.

Plasma cell type. The ages of patients with this type of Castleman's disease reported in the literature ranged from 8 to 62 (median 22 years) and no predilection for either sex was noted.[81] There are a number of significant differences between the two types of Castleman's disease. In contrast to patients with the hyaline vascular type, those with the plasma cell type frequently have a variety of unexplainable symptoms and abnormal laboratory tests. These include anemia, often microcytic, polyclonal hypergammaglobulinemia, thrombocytosis, and a number of other abnormalities which somewhat mysteriously all return to normal following excision of the solitary lesion.[81,85] Although the anterior mediastinum may be involved, an abdominal location, particularly the mesentery of the small bowel, is a favorite site of the plasma cell lesion, especially in symptomatic individuals. Also, the plasma cell variant often consists of a group of enlarged nodes rather than a single, rounded mass characteristic of the hyaline vascular type. Approximately 10% of cases are of the plasma cell type.

Histologically, the nodal architecture is partly intact because occasional sinuses are preserved. Follicular hyperplasia is prominent, displaying all the features of a reactive follicle, although occasional atrophic germinal centers may be present. Mantle zones may be intact and are invariably surrounded by sheets of plasma cells (Fig. 42-21). The plasma cells are polyclonal in most cases, although monoclonal plasma cells have occasionally been reported.[90] The vascular proliferation characteristic of the hyaline vascular variant is inconspicuous or absent.

The differential diagnosis of the plasma cell variant includes other follicular hyperplasias with prominent interfollicular plasmacytosis, such as those associated with rheumatoid arthritis and other autoimmune disorders, and syphilis. In Castleman's disease, there is a greater degree of obliteration of sinuses than in other disorders and the thick, fibrosed capsule and trabeculae seen in syphilis are lacking. The diagnosis of the plasma cell variant of Castleman's disease should not be conclusively made until other disorders are excluded by means of clinical findings and laboratory tests.[85]

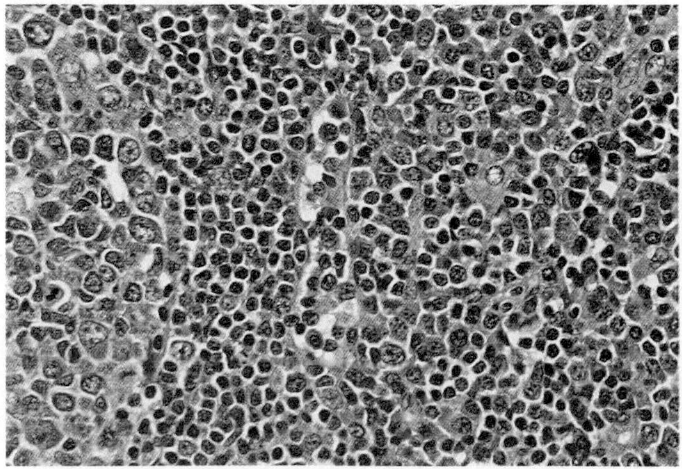

Fig. 42-21 Plasma cell variant of Castleman's disease showing part of a follicle adjacent to a dense interfollicular plasma cell infiltrate.

Transitional type. The transitional or mixed variant is an uncommon localized lesion.[88] Patients are usually asymptomatic, and, histologically, the lesion resembles the hyaline vascular type except that there are foci of plasmacytosis and possibly some hyperplastic germinal centers. Marked interfollicular plasmacytosis with hyaline vascular germinal centers is even less common.

Systemic (multicentric) Castleman's disease

There are a number of synonyms for the disease including the descriptive and more apt term *systemic lymphoproliferative disorder with morphologic features of Castleman's disease.*[84] The diagnosis of this disease is one of exclusion, and other disorders that cause similar histologic changes must be ruled out.[85] The patients are older (57 years, median age) than those with the localized disease, most are male, peripheral lymph nodes are always involved, and the development of malignancies is common. The clinical course of this disorder varies. It may behave like a chronic disease with a persistent or relapsing pattern or else like an unremitting aggressive lymphoproliferative disorder that may be fatal.[87] The disorder may be associated with Kaposi's sarcoma or with POEMS or Crow-Fukase syndrome.[91,92] Lymph nodes with similar histologic changes have also been reported in patients with AIDS.[93]

The histologic changes of multicentric Castleman's disease are nonspecific and resemble those of the plasma cell variant of the localized lesion, except that follicles with hyaline-vascular germinal centers may be present. Other organs frequently involved by the systemic disorder include bone marrow, liver, kidney, skin, and central and peripheral nervous system. Frizzera defines this disorder by a combination of four clinicopathologic criteria: 1) the characteristic histologic features of the plasma cell type of the disease; 2) a predominantly lymphadenopathic disease, involving multiple lymph node sites, mostly peripheral nodes; 3) various manifestations of multisystem involvement; and 4) an idiopathic nature.[85] In contrast to the plasma cell variant of the localized disease, there is greater architectural preservation of the node and sinuses are often dilated and filled with deeply-staining lymph. The germinal centers vary from regressively transformed to hyperplastic. The interfollicular areas show plasmacytosis, but the plasma cells may be admixed with immunoblasts, and some areas may show vascular proliferation. The plasma cells in most cases are polyclonal, although cases with monoclonal plasma cell have also been reported.[84,90]

The differential diagnoses, as listed above, include those disorders that cause similar histologic changes, particularly autoimmune disorders, HIV-related lymphadenopathy, lymph nodal or disseminated Kaposi's sarcoma, and reactive clinical processes secondary to other malignancies.[84-86,92] Clinical history and laboratory findings are essential in the differential diagnosis.

HIV-related lymphadenopathy

Enlarged lymph nodes, often widespread, are a frequent finding in HIV-infected patients, a condition known as *persistent generalized lymphadenopathy*. Associated splenomegaly and hepatomegaly may also be present. Persistent generalized lymphadenopathy is defined as: 1) lymph node enlargement of at least 3 months' duration; 2) the absence of any illness or drug use known to cause lymph node enlargement; and 3) histologic evidence of follicular hyperplasia in the node obtained at biopsy.[93] Biopsies should be done on enlarged lymph nodes in HIV-patients to determine whether the adenopathy is due to lymphoid hyperplasia, infection, lymphoma, or Kaposi's sarcoma.

Three major histologic patterns that correspond to the temporal progression of the disease and that appear to correlate with the immune status and the prognosis of HIV-positive patients have been described.[65,94-97,99] Follicular hyperplasia or a combination of follicular hyperplasia and follicular involution are the early lesions, while follicular involution is a more advanced pattern followed by the last stage lymphocyte depletion. Most lymph nodes show severe follicular hyperplasia or a combination of follicular hyperplasia and follicular involution.[65,96] Follicular involution without follicular hyperplasia is less common, and the least common histologic finding in lymph nodes is lymphocyte depletion. Follicular involution and lymphocyte depletion may follow lymph node biopsy showing follicular hyperplasia and may provide pertinent prognostic information. Patients with lymph nodes showing follicular involution and lymphocyte depletion tend to develop some of the stigmata of AIDS, while those whose lymph nodes demonstrate follicular hyperplasia appear to have a less symptomatic course.[65,95,96]

The hyperplastic follicles, which often become extremely large, are present throughout both cortex and medulla and may even extend outside of the lymph node capsule. In fact, most of the lymph node consists of hyperplastic germinal centers with little intervening interfollicular tissue.[96,97] These large germinal centers are composed mostly of transformed large noncleaved and small noncleaved follicle center cells and have a high mitotic rate and a prominent starry sky appearance (Fig. 42-22). This type of follicular hyperplasia is referred to as *florid* or *explosive*.[96,98] The mantle zones around the large germinal centers are attenuated, disrupted or entirely absent, and the "naked" germinal centers are surrounded by cells of the interfollicular areas (Fig. 42-23). Coalescence of neighboring follicles may result in the formation of giant-sized germinal centers, which may have bizarre outlines referred to as *geographic* follicles.[96,98] A characteristic, although not specific, finding seen in some follicles is the invagination of small mantle zone lymphocytes into the germinal centers, which is termed *follicular lysis*.[65,94] This follicular lysis or follicular fragmentation disrupts the germinal center, leaving irregular collections of germinal center cells among swaths of small mantle-zone lymphocytes (Fig. 42-24). The absence of mantle zones and the irregular clusters of large cells may be misinterpreted as representing large cell lymphoma.[97] Extravasation of red blood cells from germinal center vessels is also encountered.[96] Multinucleated giant cells, some of the Warthin-Finkeldey type, may be seen in follicles or interfollicular areas.[94] Another characteris-

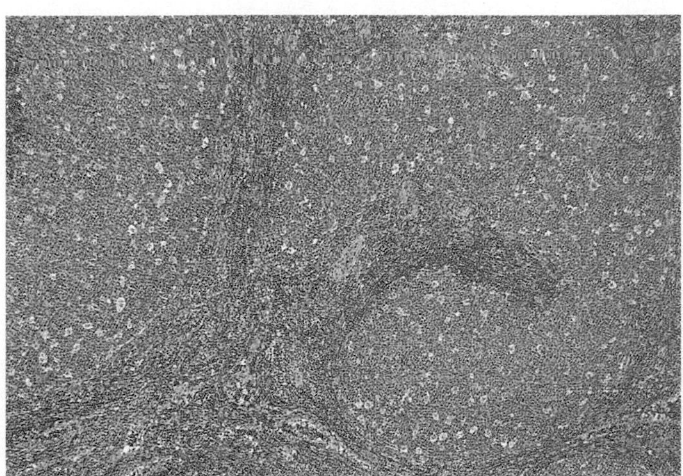

Fig. 42-22 Florid follicular hyperplasia in HIV-related lymphoadenopathy. Most of the node is replaced by large germinal centers in which there is a prominent starry sky appearance.

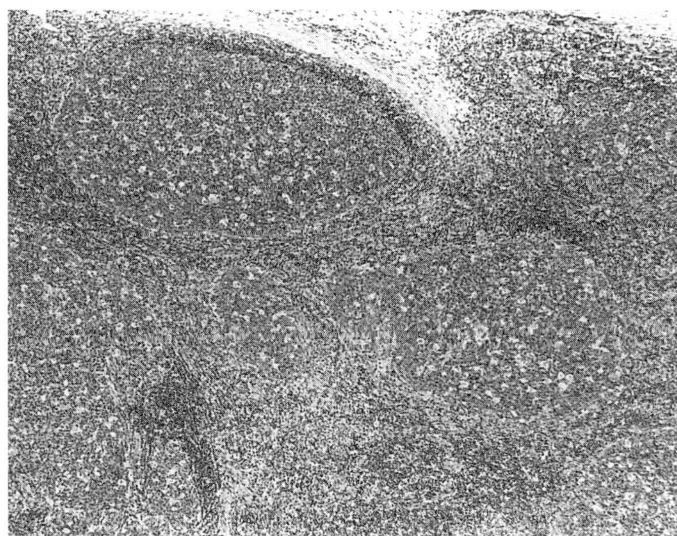

Fig. 42-23 Follicular hyperplasia in HIV-related lymphadenopathy. The mantle zone around some of the large germinal centers is absent and the "naked" germinal centers are surrounded by cells of the interfollicular area.

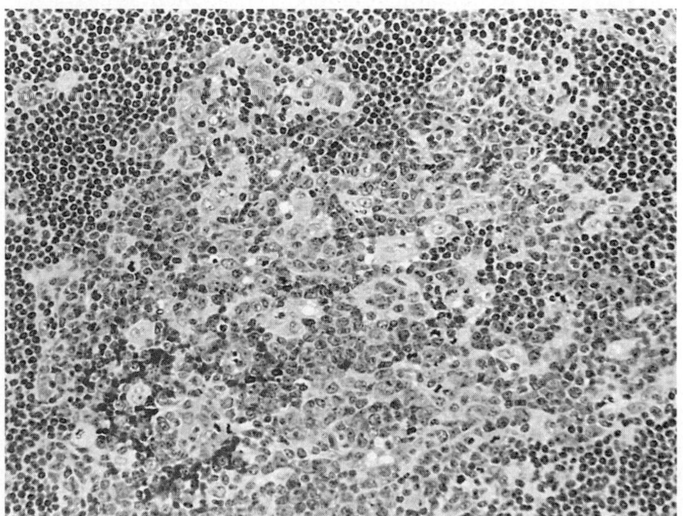

Fig. 42-24 Fragmentation of the germinal center (follicular lysis) leaves irregular collections of large germinal center cells among small mantle zone lymphocytes.

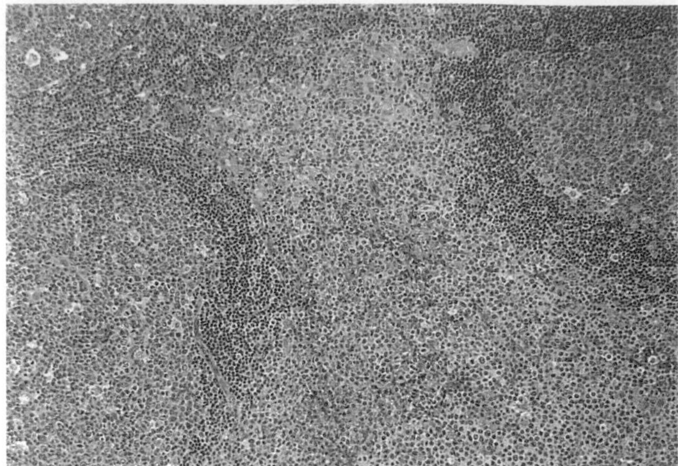

Fig. 42-25 Monocytoid B-cells in the paracortex between two large germinal centers in a lymph node from an individual with HIV infection.

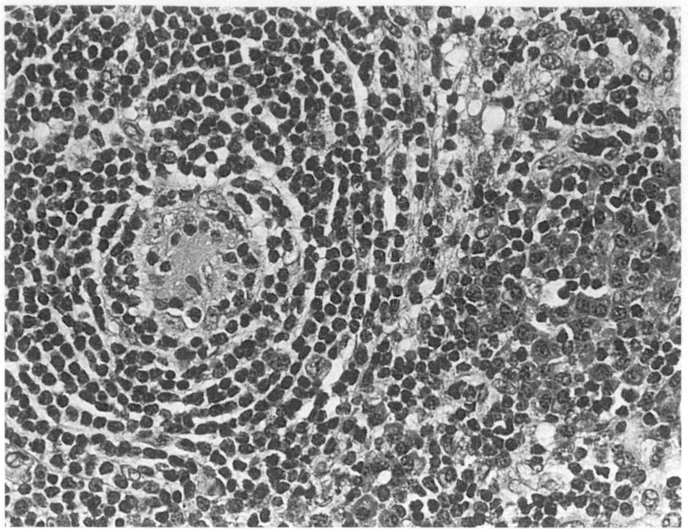

Fig. 42-26 Follicular involution in a lymph node from an HIV-positive patient showing a regressively transformed germinal center indistinguishable from that seen in Castleman's disease, and a focus of interfollicular plasmacytosis.

tic, but again not specific, find-ing is the distention of sinuses filled with polyclonal monocytoid B-cells, usually accompanied by scattered neutrophils (Fig. 42-25).[94,96,98-100] The monocytoid B-cell proliferation may also be seen in paracortical areas, sometimes partially encircling germinal centers.[100] The monocytoid B-cells have ample clear cytoplasm and a bland oval, slightly indented nucleus with inconspicuous nucleoli. The interfollicular areas usually contain a polymorphous inflammatory cell infiltrate consisting of varying numbers of lymphocytes, plasma cells, eosinophils, immunoblasts, and histiocytes, as well as a vascular proliferation with prominent endothelial cells.[96,98] Also occasionally seen are focal dermatopathic changes, often without demonstrable melanin, although the patient may have no skin lesions. As already mentioned, the constellation of histologic changes described is not specific but should alert the pathologist to the possibility that the patient may have an HIV infection.

Less frequently seen and sometimes noted following a lymph node biopsy with florid follicular hyperplasia, are the changes of follicular involution.[65] This pattern is characterized by small germinal centers which are also referred to as *regressively transformed* or *burnt-out* germinal centers.[93-95,98] They may closely resemble the small compact follicles seen in the hyaline vascular type of Castleman's disease, and they consist primarily of concentrically arranged dendritic reticulum cells and a few residual lymphocytes. As in Castleman's disease, hyalinized vessels may be seen entering the small germinal centers at right angles, giving rise to the characteristic "lollipop" appearance.[95] Some follicles may have a surrounding rim of mantle zone lymphocytes, while others completely lack mantle zones and consist of "naked" germinal centers. The interfollicular areas are prominent and expanded and lymphocytes, although present, are decreased in number. Focal or diffuse plasmacytosis (Fig. 42-26) and increased histiocytes are usually present in interfollicular areas, as are immunoblasts and a vascular proliferation with prominent endothelial cells.[65,94,95] Sinus histiocytosis may be present or absent. Fibrosis of the capsule with obliteration of the subcapsular sinus is common, and there may be fibrosis of the medullary areas.[95]

The lymph nodes in mixed follicular hyperplasia and follicular involution are usually enlarged and histologically show

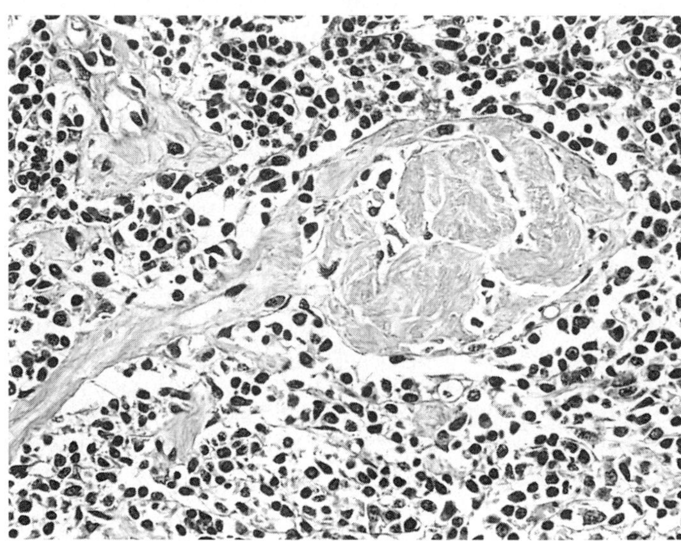

Fig. 42-27 HIV-related lymphadenopathy, lymphocyte depletion displaying paucity of lymphocytes and increased numbers of plasma cells. A hyalinized remnant of a germinal center with a vessel leading into it is present.

features of both follicular hyperplasia and involution.[65,97] The percentage of involuted follicles is usually less than 50%.[96] The interfollicular areas are larger than those in nodes with florid follicular hyperplasia. Monocytoid B-cells in sinuses and paracortex are usually also present. The interfollicular areas contain a mixture of lymphocytes, plasma cells, immunoblasts, and histiocytes.[97]

Biopsies are not usually done on lymph nodes characteristic of lymphocyte depletion because they are small, but they are often obtained at autopsy. Histologically, the capsule is fibrosed, and fibrous tissue extends into the node. Follicles and germinal centers are no longer seen, and there is severe lymphocyte depletion (Fig. 42-27).[65,98] Most of the cells that remain are histiocytes and plasma cells. Most of the remaining small node consists of medulla and sinuses that contain histiocytes, often with phagocytosed blood cells, predominantly erythrocytes. When many histiocytes with granular cytoplasm are present within the node, acid-fast stains usually show them to be packed with *Mycobacterium avium–intracellulare*.

Progressive transformation of germinal centers

Progressive transformation of germinal centers is an uncommon nonspecific reactive process that is usually associated with follicular hyperplasia in the same lymph node. It is important for the pathologist to be aware of and recognize this process because it may closely resemble nodular lymphocyte predominance (LP) HD. In fact, a relationship between progressively transformed germinal centers and HD has been proposed, and it is likely that nodular LPHD arises from these altered germinal centers.[101-104]

Histologically, the progressively transformed germinal center consists of very large oval structures or nodules that are three to four times the size of the hyperplastic follicles with which these transformed germinal centers are associated (Fig. 42-28). Because of their size, progressively transformed germinal centers are readily identified under very low magnification examination of the node. The fully developed transformed germinal center consists predominantly of small lymphocytes among which scattered, residual germinal center cells and dendritic cells remain[101,103,104] (Fig. 42-29). The small lymphocytes appear to be mostly polyclonal mantle zone-B-cells, which express IgM and IgD, and usually small numbers of helper T-cells, both of which have infiltrated and gradually replaced germinal center cells.[101] Various stages or transitions in this transformation may be seen. The earlier lesion consists of germinal centers fragmented by the infiltrating small lymphocytes, and, as the name implies, the germinal center cells are progressively replaced until only few of them remain.

As mentioned, the most important disorder that must be differentiated from progressive transformation of germinal centers is nodular LPHD.[101-104] Both disorders have a similar appearance under low magnification and both consist predominantly of small B-lymphocytes. Although HD more often has varying numbers of epithelioid histiocytes within or surrounding the nodules, occasional cases of transformed germinal centers also have epithelioid histiocytes, especially around the periphery of the nodules. Another confounding feature of the two disorders is that progressive transformation may precede, be present simultaneously with, or develop after a diagnosis of LP HD has been established. Both disorders tend to recur, and subsequent biopsies may show either one or the other process. The presence of L & H Reed-Sternberg variants is diagnostic of this type of HD. However, residual large germinal center cells within the transformed germinal center may closely resemble the L & H Reed-Sternberg variants in this type of HD, and since both of these cell types stain with the B-cell antibody CD20 and are negative for CD15, they cannot be differentiated immunologically.[101] The most useful clue that the large cells are the Reed-Sternberg variants is that these cells are usually surrounded by T-cells ($CD4^+$, $CD57^+$), while residual large germinal center cells are not.[105] Also, in many cases, Reed-Sternberg variants in nodular LPHD stain positive with anti-epithelial membrane antigen, while residual germinal center cells are negative. In addition, progressive transformation of germinal centers is almost invariably associated with follicular hyperplasia, while HD is not. When follicles remain in this type of HD, they are compressed as a rim around the periphery of the node.

Less common problems in the differential diagnosis of this benign process are follicular lymphoma of small cleaved cells and mantle cell lymphoma. The former lymphoma is a monoclonal B-cell (SIg^+, $CD5^-$, $CD10^+$) proliferation, and the neoplastic follicles are never as large as the nodules of transformed germinal centers. Also, they are composed predominantly of small cleaved cells, which are absent in the benign process. The follicular hyperplasia that is associated with progressive transformation of germinal centers is absent in follicular lymphomas. Mantle cell lymphoma may also have a vaguely nodular appearance, but it too is a monoclonal B-cell (SIg^+, $CD5^+$, $CD10^-$) process.[76] In addition, the nuclear contours of many of the lymphocytes in mantle cell lymphoma are irregular, in contrast to those in progressively transformed follicle centers.

Interfollicular pattern

The monotonous interfollicular or paracortical region of an unstimulated lymph node is much less conspicuous than the

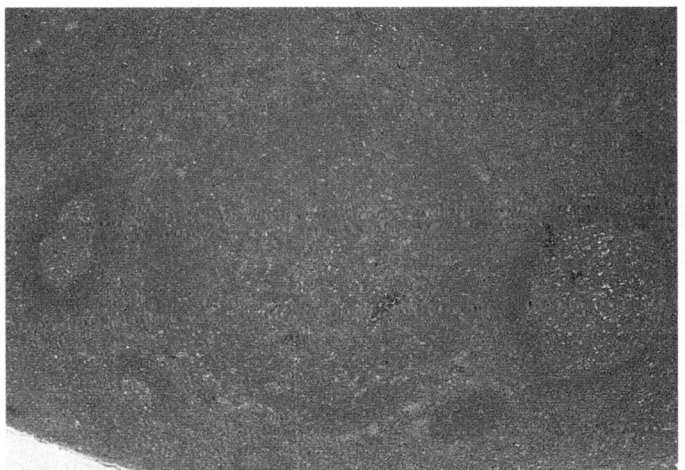

Fig. 42-28 Lymph node with progressive transformation of a germinal center. The hyperplastic follicles are dwarfed by a progressively transformed germinal center composed predominantly of small lymphocytes.

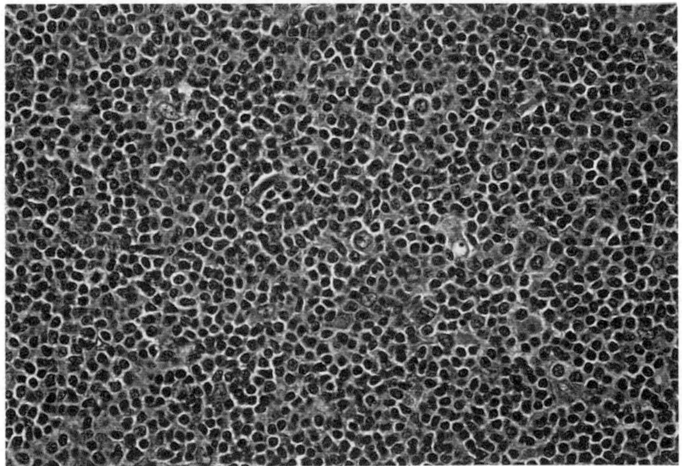

Fig. 42-29 Higher magnification of Figure 42-28 showing residual large germinal center cells and a tingible body macrophage among the small lymphocytes.

circumscribed follicles with their polymorphous cellular germinal centers. The paracortex is populated primarily by small T-cells, postcapillary venules that bring circulating T-cells to that region, and interdigitating reticulum cells that are not easily seen without immunostains.

Although interfollicular hyperplasia is not always readily distinguishable from the diffuse pattern of hyperplasia, germinal centers and sinuses tend to be preserved, while these structures are less likely to be as prominent or they may be completely obliterated in the diffuse pattern. Interfollicular hyperplasia may be barely perceptible when there is only a mild proliferation of small paracortical T-cells, or else it may be easily identified under the scanning lens, particularly when larger cells make up part of the proliferation. The paracortex is expanded, separating or displacing follicles, and its cellular composition varies according to the nature of the stimulus and its duration. Viral infections, especially early in the course of the illness, may be associated with both follicular and paracortical hyperplasia, while later in the course of a viral process, a diffuse pattern of proliferation may dominate (viral infections are discussed under diffuse pattern). Disorders described as interfollicular include dermatopathic lymphadenitis,[106] in which the proliferation of Langerhans' cells and histiocytes displaces follicles; histiocytic necrotizing lymphadenitis,[107-110] in which the distinctive patches of necrosis are localized to interfollicular areas; and the granulomatous inflammations,[111] which are characteristically between follicles.

Dermatopathic lymphadenitis

Dermatopathic lymphadenitis is associated with a variety of benign skin disorders and also with mycosis fungoides/Sezary syndrome.[106,112] Histologic findings identical to those in patients with skin lesions are occasionally noted in individuals without apparent skin disorders. Dermatopathic change in patients with mycosis fungoides is an ominous prognostic sign whether or not the node is involved by the neoplastic T-cells.

Histologically, the fully developed lesion can be easily recognized under low magnification. The paracortex is expanded by cells with ample pale-staining cytoplasm (Fig. 42-30). The large pale-staining cells consist of histiocytes, a minority of which contain melanin and Langerhans cells.[113] Langerhans cells are identified under high magnification by their nuclei, which have complex and delicately folded membranes, and by their positive staining with S-100 protein, HLA/DR and CD2 (frozen section).[114] Small lymphocytes among the histiocytes and Langerhans' cells have irregular nuclear contours and cannot always be reliably distinguished from early involvement of lymph nodes by the neoplastic cells of mycosis fungoides. Early involvement by this cutaneous T-cell lymphoma can be ascertained morphologically with confidence only when at least partial effacement of the lymph node is present.[112] The follicles are often displaced to the outer cortex by the paracortical expansion. They may be atrophic or hyperplastic. Large transformed lymphoid cells (immunoblasts) and plasma cells may also be present in the paracortex. Sinus histiocytosis is often present in medullary sinuses. These sinus histiocytes are readily distinguished from Langerhans' cells by their abundant cytoplasm, their round or oval nuclei, and their absence of immunostaining with S-100 and CD1.

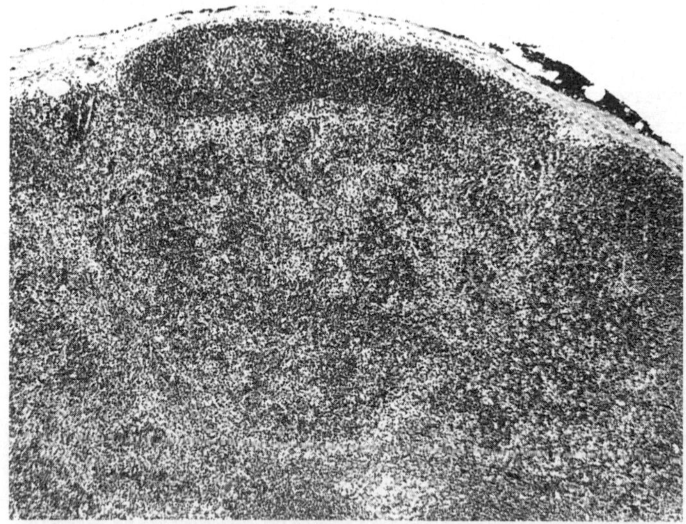

Fig. 42-30 Dermatopathic lymphadenitis showing nodular expansion of the paracortex by pale-staining cells that include histiocytes and Langerhans' cells. The follicle is displaced beneath the capsule of the node.

Histiocytic necrotizing lymphadenitis

Histiocytic necrotizing lymphadenitis, also known as histiocytic necrotizing lymphadenitis without granulocytic infiltration and Kikuchi-Fujimoto or Kikuchi's disease, was first described in Japan and is now recognized throughout the world as a distinct clinicopathologic entity.[70,107-110,115] It is a benign self-limiting disease primarily affecting young women. Isolated cervical lymphadenopathy is common and may be associated with fever, or the presenting symptom may be fever of unknown origin. The disorder may be a *forme fruste* of systemic lupus erythematosus (SLE), since a small number of patients later develop lupus and, histologically, the lesions are similar.[70]

Microscopically, the disease is characterized by patchy areas of necrosis confined to the paracortical and cortical areas with prominent karyorrhectic and karyolytic debris and a virtual absence of PMLs[70,107-110,115] (Fig. 42-31). These necrotic areas are surrounded by atypical-appearing mononuclear cells. These consist of a mixture of cells including histiocytes with "twisted" or "curved" nuclei, phagocytic macrophages (histiocytes), immunoblasts, plasmacytoid monocytes (plasmacytoid T-cells), and foamy histiocytes (Fig. 42-32). Because of the atypical appearance of the large cells, some cases have been misdiagnosed as large cell lymphomas. Binucleate immunoblasts resembling Reed-Sternberg cells may result in an erroneous diagnosis of HD. A stage in the development of the typical necrotic lesion referred to as the "proliferative phase" is characterized by a focal lesion consisting of a mixture of immunoblasts, histiocytes, and plasmacytoid monocytes. It is in this stage that the differential diagnosis from lymphoma may be particularly difficult to make. Plasma cells are usually sparse or absent. The remainder of the lymph node usually contains immunoblasts scattered among small paracortical lymphocytes, imparting a mottled appearance not unlike that seen in viral infections. Follicles are usually not prominent. Close follow-up of patients with Kikuchi's disease is indicated because of the possibility of their developing SLE.

As mentioned, the differential diagnosis includes large cell lymphoma, HD and SLE.[69] NHLs can usually be excluded because of the heterogeneity of the large cells, the focal patchy nature of the lesion, and the presence of plasmacytoid monocytes. Although necrosis is often associated with HD, it usu-

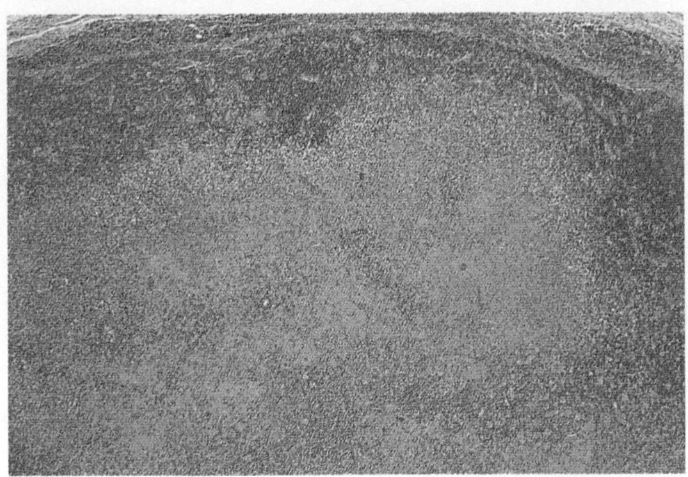

Fig. 42-31 Kikuchi's disease. An irregular patchy focus of paracortical necrosis devoid of neutrophils is characteristic of this disorder.

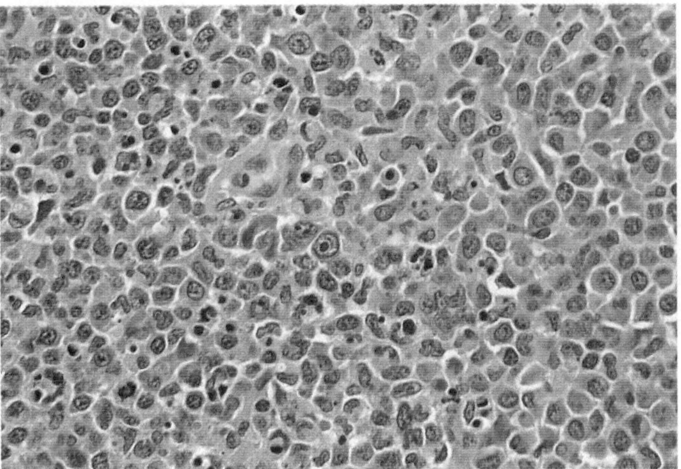

Fig. 42-32 Higher magnification of Fig. 42-31 adjacent to the necrotic focus showing a mixture of large cells including histiocytes, some with curved nuclei, immunoblasts, and plasmacytoid monocytes.

ally contains neutrophils, and a polymorphous inflammatory infiltrate is characteristic. Many Reed-Sternberg cells may surround the necrotic foci in HD, and these can be distinguished from the atypical large cells seen in Kikuchi's disease morphologically by their positive staining with CD15. Also, the presence of hyperplastic follicles and the mottled appearance in the uninvolved part of the node suggest that the process is benign. The necrosis with karyorrhectic debris seen in SLE may be identical to that in Kikuchi's disease, while hematoxylin bodies, when present, are characteristic of lupus. Larger areas of lymph node necrosis and the presence of plasma cells also favor the latter disease. Other necrotizing lesions, including cat scratch disease, lymphogranuloma venereum (LGV), and yersinia infections, all contain numerous segmented neutrophils in areas of necrosis.

Granulomatous lymphadenitis

There are numerous causes of infective and noninfective granulomatous lymphadenitis. Histologically, the granulomas are identical to those seen in other tissues. They may have areas of necrosis, caseation or suppuration, or the granulomas may be nonnecrotizing. The nonnecrotizing or epithelioid granulomas are characteristic of, but not specific for, sarcoidosis.[111] Necrotizing or caseating granulomas are seen in mycobacterial or fungal infections, and suppurative granulomas are characteristic of disorders such as cat scratch disease,[63,116] LGV,[63,117] tularemia,[63,74] yersinia[63,74,118] and certain fungal infections.[74] Special stains for acid-fast organisms and fungi or silver stains are necessary to determine the etiology of granulomatous lymphadenitis. Culture of lymph node biopsy specimens is also important in establishing a specific etiologic diagnosis. Despite staining for organisms and taking cultures of node biopsy specimens, one cannot always be sure of the etiology of granulomatous lymphadenitis.

Sarcoidosis is a multisystem granulomatous disease in which the causative agent and the pathogenic mechanisms are unknown.[111] In contrast, the clinical presentation, course of the disease, and laboratory and histologic features are well recognized. Histologically, the lesion of sarcoidosis is characterized by discrete, nonnecrotizing epithelioid granulomas, although occasional small foci of central fibrinoid necrosis are seen. The granulomas may be surrounded by sclerosis and older granulomas may become progressively hyalinized. Langhans giant cells may or may not be present. Asteroid bodies, Schaumann's bodies, and crystals of calcium oxalate are rarely seen within giant cells and are not specific of sarcoidosis. Small, needle-like or oval periodic acid-Schiff (PAS)-positive, acid-fast structures may be found in the cytoplasm of giant cells and are known as Hamazaki-Wesenberg bodies.[63] Sarcoid-like granulomas are not specific, and the diagnosis of sarcoidosis is one of exclusion. The etiology of these granulomas is often unknown. They may be seen in lymph nodes of patients with HD, where, because of their number, they may mask Reed-Sternberg cells present in the small amount of intervening lymphoid tissue. These granulomas may also be a prominent feature of some NHLs. They may be found in mesenteric lymph nodes of patients with Crohn's disease and in nodes draining carcinomas, and they are also associated with beryl-liosis. Staining for acid-fast bacilli and fungi should always be carried out to exclude an infectious etiology of any granulomatous lymphadenitis. The granulomas in tuberculosis usually, but not always, have areas of necrosis surrounded by epithelioid histiocytes and Langhans giant cells, while granulomas of fungal infections show similar necrosis or sometimes suppurative granulomas and, rarely, nonnecrotizing epithelioid granulomas.

Mixed follicular and interfollicular pattern

The disorders with a mixed pattern involve more than one lymph nodal compartment, and the most common type of mixed pattern hyperplasia involves the follicles and interfollicular areas. Many of these mixed patterns are associated with reactions to infectious agents. The most common are toxoplasmosis lymphadenitis,[66] cat scratch disease,[116] LGV,[117] mesenteric lymphadenitis[74,118] and the involvement of lymph nodes by Kimura's disease,[119,120] uncommon in the United States, however. Another common mixed proliferation includes follicular hyperplasia and sinus histiocytosis.

Toxoplasmosis lymphadenitis

Approximately 50% of adults in the United States are infected with *Toxoplasma gondii,* which has a worldwide distribution. Individuals with acute acquired toxoplasmosis may be totally asymptomatic, experience flu-like symptoms, or present with an infectious mononucleosis-like picture including atypical lymphocytes in the peripheral blood. In humans, the disease is transmitted through exposure to cat feces that contain the oocyst or through handling or ingestion of uncooked meat.[121] Enlargement of a single lymph node, especially of the posterior cervical region, may occur or, less commonly, multiple nodes may become enlarged.

Histologically, the features of toxoplasmosis lymphadenitis are distinctive. They consist of 1) follicular hyperplasia; 2) collections of single or small clusters of epithelioid histiocytes in the interfollicular areas, encroaching upon and also within germinal centers; and 3) focal dilatation of sinuses which are filled with monocytoid B-cells[66] (Fig. 42-33). These histologic findings are consistent with a diagnosis of toxoplasmosis lymphadenitis, which must then be confirmed by serologic studies.

The follicular hyperplasia is pronounced and the enlarged follicles contain mostly large, transformed lymphoid cells, a high mitotic rate, and numerous tingible body macrophages. Characteristically, the germinal centers have ragged, indistinct margins. The clusters of histiocytes in the paracortex do not form granulomas, and multinucleate giant cells and necrosis are not present. Parasitic cysts have only rarely been reported in lymph nodes. The medullary cords contain many plasma cells. Scattered neutrophils are usually seen among the monocytoid B-cells.

The differential diagnosis of toxoplasmosis lymphadenitis includes the florid or explosive follicular hyperplasia and the sinusoidal and parafollicular monocytoid B-cell proliferation seen in HIV-associated lymphadenopathy.[65,100] Clusters of epithelioid histiocytes are usually absent in HIV-associated lymphadenopathy, and follicular lysis and hemorrhage, which are absent in toxoplasmosis, are usually present. The hyperplastic germinal centers are usually much larger in HIV-associated lymphadenopathy. Also considered in the differential diagnosis is interfollicular HD. The prominent follicular hyperplasia may mask HD, in which single or small clusters of epithelioid histiocytes are common. Eosinophils are not seen in toxoplasmosis lymphadenitis but are often present in HD, so their presence should alert the pathologist to the possibility of interfollicular HD. Coexistence of the two disorders has been reported.[122] Rarely, monocytoid B-cell proliferations have been described in Hodgkin's disease but not in the interfollicular type. Clusters of histiocytes, especially involving germinal centers similar to those in toxoplasmosis, have been described in patients with leishmaniasis.

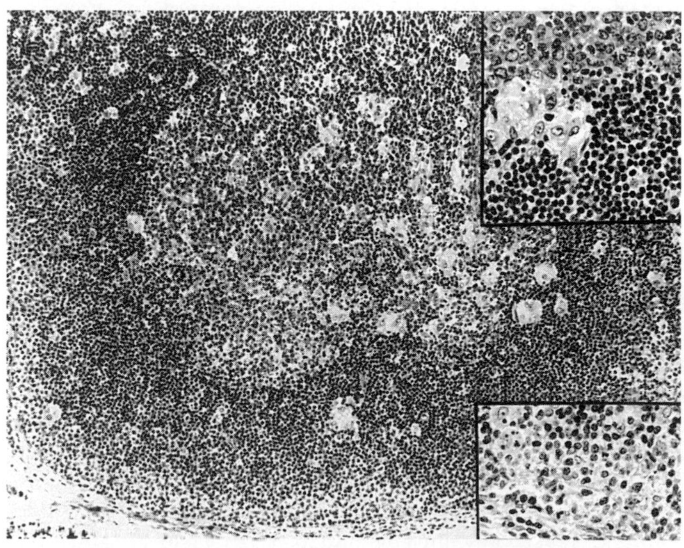

Fig. 42-33 Toxoplasmosis lymphadenitis. The subcapsular and intermediate sinuses are distended by monocytoid B-cells. Small clusters of epithelioid histiocytes in the paracortex encroach upon a germinal center which has irregular borders. Insets. Higher magnification showing a cluster of histiocytes at the edge of a germinal center *(top)* and monocytoid B-cells *(bottom)*.

Cat-scratch disease and lymphogranuloma venereum

Cat-scratch disease was first recognized more than 60 years ago. Clinically, it is a self-limited disorder characterized by development of regional lymphadenopathy, usually but not always occurring after a cat scratch or bite distal to the affected lymph node. Lymph nodes in the axilla, groin, and neck are most commonly affected. It is estimated that 22,000 cases are diagnosed each year in the United States, and more than 2000 victims are hospitalized. Although most cases of cat scratch disease resolve spontaneously within several months, there are occasional severe complications including encephalitis, neuroretinitis, and follicular conjunctivitis. The long-sought etiologic agent of cat scratch disease is *Rochalimaea henselae*. An indirect fluorescent-antibody test that may be useful diagnostically has recently been developed.[123] It has a high sensitivity (88%) and specificity (94%) for cat scratch disease. Cat scratch disease can now be differentiated in tissue sections from similar histologic lesions (particularly LGV) caused by other etiologic agents by demonstrating the causative organisms which are gram-negative but positive upon Warthin-Starry silver impregnation.[116,124]

LGV is a sexually transmitted disease caused by *Chlamydia* and may be histologically indistinguishable from cat scratch disease.[117] This disorder is diagnosed most frequently in inguinal lymph nodes. Histologically, the fully developed suppurative granuloma of cat scratch disease and LGV is distinctive. It consists of a central area of suppurative necrosis surrounded by palisading histiocytes and fibroblasts (Fig. 42-34).

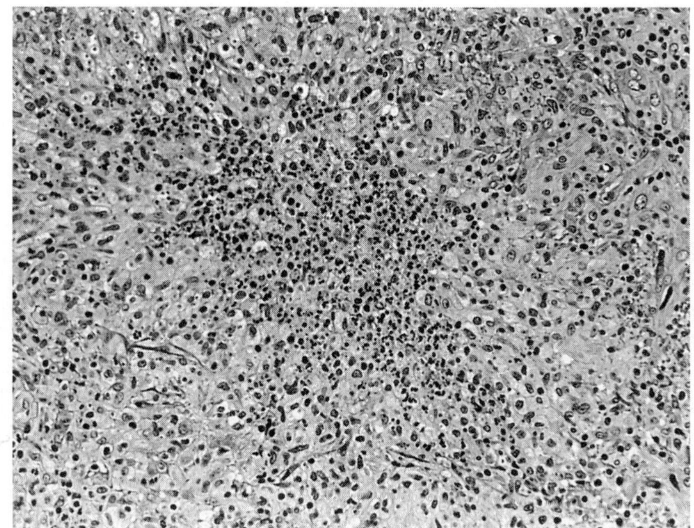

Fig. 42-34 Lymph node in a patient with a history of multiple cat scratches. Central suppurative necrosis surrounded by palisading histiocytes and fibroblasts.

Less characteristic are the earlier lesions in cat scratch disease, which may show only small foci of necrosis and small clusters of neutrophils surrounded by histiocytes. Those early lesions usually start near the subcapsular sinuses and the small developing abscesses may also involve germinal centers, which often show a pronounced degree of follicular hyperplasia. It is in the early lesions that the causative organisms are most likely to be detected, especially within walls of capillaries, histiocytes and areas of necrosis. They are rarely seen in the fully developed suppurative granulomas. The suppurative granulomas usually increase in size and may extend into the medullary region. In the later stages of the disease, the neutrophils gradually disappear and the necrotic areas are no longer suppurative. Frequently, all stages of development of the suppurative granuloma are seen within the same lymph node. The sinuses may be distended and contain monocytoid B-cells.

Rochalimaea species[123] has also been implicated as the cause of bacillary angiomatosis, a disorder that is characterized by proliferation of small blood vessels and endothelial cells in skin, visceral organs, and occasionally lymph nodes and that occurs almost exclusively in individuals with AIDS.[110]

Differential diagnosis of cat scratch disease on routine sections includes LGV, tularemia, brucellosis, yersinia infections and certain fungal or, less commonly, mycobacterial infections. Clinical findings, staining for the organism causing cat scratch disease, and culture of organisms are all important in differentiating among these disorders. Necrotic foci in HD, especially in the syncytial variant, may mimic the suppurative granulomas of cat scratch disease. The cells surrounding the necrotic foci often consist of a mixture of epithelioid histiocytes, Hodgkin's cells and Reed-Sternberg cells.

Yersinia *(mesenteric)* lymphadenitis

This disorder is seen predominantly in children and occasionally in young adults who present with symptoms of acute appendicitis. The appendix itself shows no evidence of acute infection. Mesenteric lymph nodes are enlarged and show either nonspecific follicular hyperplasia or there may be associated epithelioid cell clusters, small necrotizing epithelioid cell clusters, or small necrotizing epithelioid granulomas. When the latter changes are present, it is believed that the disorder is caused by the gram-negative organisms *Yersinia enterocolitica* or, less frequently, the related organism *Y. pseudotuberculosis*.[74,118] Additional histologic changes include a thickened capsule, follicular hyperplasia, dilated sinuses filled with lymphocytes, and an immunoblastic proliferation in the paracortex. The diagnosis should be confirmed by appropriate cultures.

Kimura's disease

Kimura's disease is a benign chronic inflammatory disorder of unknown etiology.[119,120] It is endemic in Asians and is seen predominantly in young to middle-aged men, occurring only sporadically in Caucasians. The patients present with deep-seated masses involving the subcutis of the head and neck region, and sometimes submandibular or parotid glands are infiltrated. Regional lymph nodes may be involved and occasionally lymph node enlargement may be the sole initial presentation.[119] Peripheral blood eosinophilia is characteristic, as are elevated levels of serum IgE. The pathologic features of Kimura's disease are different from those of angiolymphoid hyperplasia with eosinophilia (epithelioid hemangioma) with which it is often confused. The prognosis of Kimura's disease is excellent even with conservative therapy, although recurrences are common.[119,120] Therefore, it is important for pathologists to recognize the lymph node changes in Kimura's disease to differentiate it from disorders requiring more aggressive therapy.

The individual histologic features are not pathognomonic for the disease, but the total histologic picture should alert the pathologist to consider this disorder in the differential diagnosis. Follicular hyperplasia that may be florid is a constant finding, as is eosinophilic infiltration of paracortex and sinuses. Increased numbers of post-capillary venules are also seen in these cases. These venules together with eosinophils may form circumscribed nodules in the paracortex. Features that are frequently present include: sclerosis that obliterates sinuses and paracortex; polykaryocytes of the Warthin-Finkeldey type, which may be present in germinal centers and paracortex; vascularization of germinal centers; proteinaceous material in germinal centers; and eosinophilic abscesses, particularly in the paracortex. "Folliculolysis" associated with eosinophilic infiltrates has been described and partial necrosis of germinal centers may be seen. Another characteristic feature is the presence of IgE in the germinal centers and IgE on the surface of non-degranulated mast cells in the paracortex.

Included in the differentiated diagnosis of Kimura's disease is Hodgkin's disease. Although sclerosis and eosinophilia are present in both disorders, Reed-Sternberg cells are not seen in Kimura's disease. In addition, the architecture is preserved in Kimura's disease, whereas, with the exception of interfollicular HD, the nodal architecture or part of the architecture is effaced in HD. Massive eosinophilia in lymph nodes may also be seen in allergic or drug reactions.[74] Also, in parasitic infestation of lymph nodes there is often severe eosinophilia including eosinophilic abscesses. The florid follicular hyperplasia and Warthin-Finkeldey giant cells seen in Kimura's disease are usually absent in the other disorders.

Diffuse pattern

The architecture of the lymph node in diffuse hyperplasias is often partly or occasionally totally effaced, and the composition of the proliferating cell population varies according to the type of stimulus and its duration. There is generally a polymorphous population of cells that include lymphocytes, immunoblasts, plasma cells, eosinophils, and histiocytes in varying proportions. Proliferation of immunoblasts is characteristically associated with viral infections and is also seen in idiosyncratic reactions to drugs. The presence of immunoblasts among the small paracortical T-cells lends a mottled appearance to the expanded area, which is usually accompanied by a proliferation of postcapillary venules lined by prominent endothelial cells. The large transformed cells may be of T- or B-cell type, the latter having migrated from hyperplastic follicles that may have been present at an earlier stage of the process. The severe types of diffuse hyperplasias with their polymorphous or occasionally monomorphous (immunoblastic) proliferations can cause pathologists problems in differentiating a benign process from both HD and NHLs.

The most common causes of diffuse hyperplasias include infectious mononucleosis and other viral disorders,[68] immunoblastic/angioimmunoblastic lymphadenopathy[125,126] and related abnormal immune reactions, drug-induced hypersensitivity reactions,[127,128] and uncommon disorders diagnosed by lymph node biopsy, namely, SLE[69] and the rare disorder, mucocutaneous lymph node syndrome (Kawasaki's disease).[129]

Infectious mononucleosis

Infectious mononucleosis is usually diagnosed on the basis of clinical findings, the presence of atypical lymphocytes in the peripheral blood, and a positive mono-spot test or other Epstein-Barr virus (EBV) serologic studies. Rarely, the surgical pathologist is confronted with a lymph node biopsy, a tonsil, or a ruptured spleen from a patient who has not been diagnosed by the usual means, often because the presentation of the disease was atypical or the adenopathy persisted. It is of utmost importance to remember that infectious mononucleosis is a great imitator. Histologically, it may show nonspecific follicular and/or paracortical hyperplasia, or it may mimic and may be difficult to distinguish from both HD and NHL.[68,130-132] The histologic changes may be similar to those described in such other viral disorders as herpes lymphadenitis and postvaccinial lymphadenitis.[133] The microscopic picture also varies according to the time of biopsy during the course of the disease. Although the basic architecture may be severely distorted, it is usually intact. If the lymph node is fragmented, partial architectural preservation may be difficult to appreciate. The most remarkable and characteristic finding of infectious mononucleosis and of many other viral disorders, best identified under low magnification, is an expansion of the paracortex, partly due to a proliferation of large transformed cells (immunoblasts) among the small, predominantly T-lymphocytes (Fig. 42-35). In addition, plasma cells, plasmacytoid cells, and a brisk vascular (post-capillary venules) proliferation with prominent, hyperplastic endothelial cells are apparent in the paracortex. Foci of necrosis are not unusual. In some cases, follicles are readily identified, while in others they are ill-defined and small. The sinuses may be dilated and contain the same cells that populate the paracortex (immunoblasts, plasma cells and plasmacytoid cells) or the dilated sinuses may contain monocytoid B-cells or mixtures of these cells and immunoblasts (Fig. 42-36). In some nodes the sinuses may be compressed. Binucleate immunoblasts that may be indistinguishable from Reed-Sternberg cells are often seen in the paracortex, thus suggesting the possibility of HD, and the occasional presence of eosinophils, again, points to that diagnosis. In some cases, the immunoblasts form clusters or even sheets (Fig. 42-35), suggesting the possibility of large cell immunoblastic lymphoma.[134] In situ hybridization studies for EBV may be of use, but positive results do not rule out other EBV-associated diseases such as HD.[135]

As already mentioned, the differential diagnosis of infectious mononucleosis includes both HD and NHL in addition to other viral infections.[68,132,134] Although the Reed-Sternberg-like immunoblasts in infectious mononucleosis may be indistinguishable from true Reed-Sternberg cells in HD, the cellular environment in which they are found (predominantly lymphocytes, plasmacytoid cells, plasma cells and immunoblasts) is different from that characteristic of one of the subtypes of HD. Both Reed-Sternberg cells and the proper inflammatory cell infiltrate are required for the pathologist to establish a diagnosis of HD. It should be stressed that examination under low magnification of the entire lymph node often reveals the tell-tale mottled appearance of the paracortex, absent in HD but characteristic of viral disorders. Immunostaining of the Reed-Sternberg cells may be of additional help. Unlike Reed-Sternberg cells in HD ($CD15^+$, $CD30^+$), the imposter Reed-Sternberg cells in infectious mononucleosis are $CD15^-$, although they are often $CD30^+$.[68,130,131] They may also stain with T- or B-cell antibodies, or occasionally they stain with neither.

Large cell immunoblastic lymphoma can usually be distinguished from clusters and sheets of immunoblasts in infectious mononucleosis when an intact node is obtained by biopsy, but identification may be more troublesome when the node is fragmented. Examination under low magnification will clearly show that portions of the node reveal benign reactive changes. Although large cell lymphomas may occasionally partially

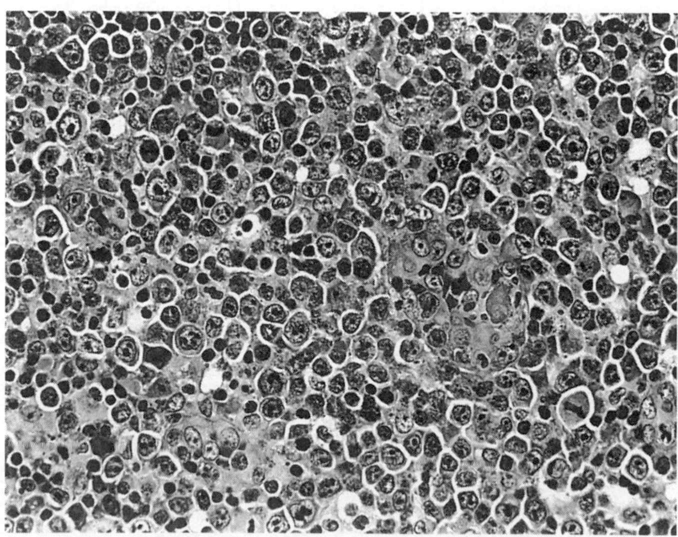

Fig. 42-35 Mottled appearance (left) and solid area of immunoblasts surrounding a high endothelial venule in a lymph node from a patient with infectious mononucleosis.

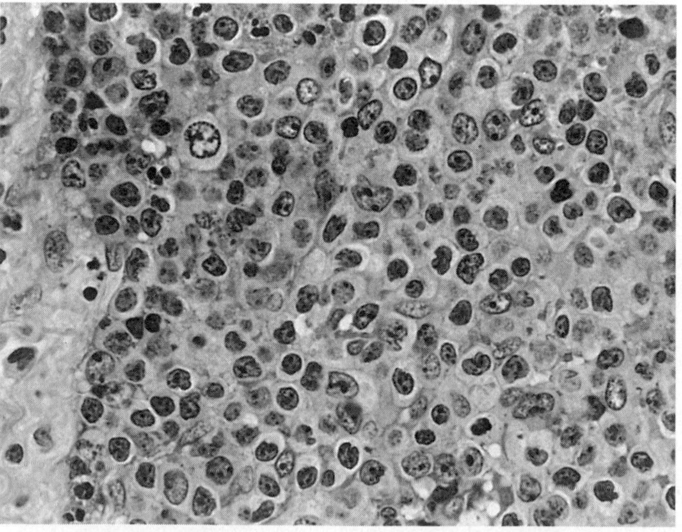

Fig. 42-36 Subcapsular sinus (capsule left) in a lymph node from a patient with infectious mononucleosis showing a mixture of monocytoid B-cells and immunoblasts.

involve a lymph node, the presence of a mottled paracortex with a polymorphous infiltrate in areas not involved by lymphoma would be unusual. Demonstration of clonality may again be helpful, although oligoclonal proliferation of T-cells has been demonstrated in infectious mononucleosis.

Cytomegalovirus (CMV) infections in nonimmunosuppressed individuals may resemble changes seen in infectious mononucleosis, or they may show a histologic picture including a pronounced follicular hyperplasia with a monocytoid B-cell proliferation with or without an interfollicular hyperplasia.[74,136] The characteristic CMV inclusions in both nucleus and cytoplasm, together with serologic, immunohistochemical and in-situ hybridization techniques, will establish a specific diagnosis of CMV infection.[137]

Herpes simplex or herpes zoster infections may cause enlargement of regional lymph nodes.[138,139] These nodes are rarely taken for biopsy because herpes infections are readily diagnosed from the characteristic skin lesion almost always present. Histologically, changes are similar to those described in other viral disorders showing a paracortical polymorphous infiltrate in which immunoblasts may predominate. Reed-Sternberg-like cells may also be present. Necrosis, multinucleated giant cells, and viral inclusions may be found. The diagnosis can be confirmed by immunohistochemical stains and in situ hybridization.

Postvaccinial lymphadenitis is rarely seen today because vaccination against smallpox is no longer routinely required for international travel. Most of the patients reported by Hartsock complained of painful lymph node enlargement, especially of left supraclavicular nodes, which drained the site of vaccination.[133] Biopsies were done on the lymph nodes 7 to 15 days after the patients had been inoculated, and, for unknown reasons, a history of vaccination was not elicited. Histologically, the general nodal architecture remains intact, although it is distorted to varying degrees. The findings, which resemble those in other viral infections, include: 1) a mottled appearance of the expanded paracortex; 2) follicular and/or diffuse hyperplasia; 3) vascular and sinusoidal changes; and 4) a polymorphous cellular infiltrate consisting of lymphocytes, eosinophils, plasma cells, and mast cells.

A histologic picture similar to that seen in postvaccinial lymphadenitis may be seen in regional lymph nodes after intramuscular or subcutaneous inoculation of attenuated measles virus.[140] Warthin-Finkeldey giant cells characteristic of measles may be present.

Abnormal immune reactions

Angioimmunoblastic lymphadenopathy (AILD) and immunoblastic lymphadenopathy (IBL) are closely related disorders, which, together with similar atypical immunoblastic proliferations, are included in the category of abnormal immune response of lymph nodes.[125,126] These entities were initially described as benign lymphoproliferative disorders occurring most often in middle-aged to older males. AILD/IBL is often associated with fever, weight loss, skin rash, lymphadenopathy that is usually generalized, and abnormal laboratory findings including Coombs-positive hemolytic anemia and polyclonal hypergammaglobulinemia. The disorder may follow intake of antibiotics and other medications or exposure to viral infections. The clinical course varies from case to case. Some patients fully recover, but in other instances, the disorder has an aggressive and sometimes fatal course. Some investigators have postulated that AILD/IBL is a premalignant disorder of altered immunoregulation characterized by clonal expansions of B- and T-cells.[126] Evolution to malignant lymphomas has been described.[141,126] In recent years, it has become increasingly difficult to diagnose the disease and it is likely that many cases previously diagnosed as AILD/IBL were actually lymphomas from the onset rather than abnormal immune reactions.[141] This point is further discussed in the section on AILD-like peripheral T-cell lymphoma, in this chapter.

The histologic features of AILD/IBL include effacement of the nodal architecture, except that "burnt-out" germinal centers may be present and some sinuses can be identified.[125,126] There is a polymorphous cellular proliferation consisting of immunoblasts, plasma cells, single or small clusters of histiocytes, and sometimes eosinophils, accompanied by a prominent proliferation of arborized postcapillary venules with prominent endothelial cells that are readily identified with PAS staining (Figs. 42-37 and 42-38). Amorphous interstitial PAS positive material is noted in some cases. Lymphocytes are pres-

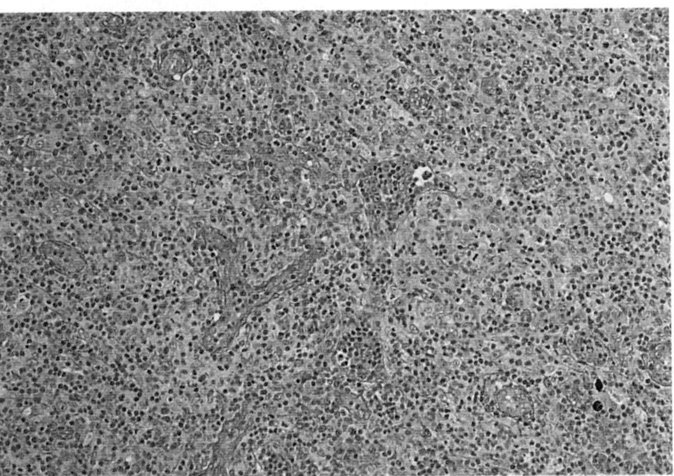

Fig. 42-37 Lymph node from a patient diagnosed as having AILD. The nodal architecture is effaced by a diffuse polymorphous cellular infiltrate containing many branching vessels. (PAS.)

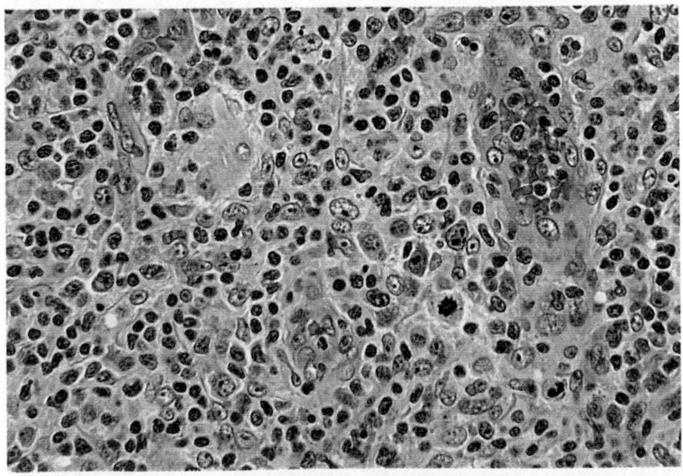

Fig. 42-38 Higher magnification of Fig. 42-37 showing high endothelial vessels within a polymorphous infiltrate of lymphocytes, plasma cells, immunoblasts, histiocytes and a Reed-Sternberg-like cell.

ent but depleted, giving the node an overall hypocellular appearance. Occasionally, clusters, islands or sheets of immunoblasts are present, and this finding may indicate a more aggressive course. Most immunophenotypic studies in AILD/IBL have shown a T-cell proliferation. With few exceptions the lymphocytes have a helper cell phenotype.[142-144] Occasional B-cell lymphomas arising in AILD/IBL have been reported.[145,146]

Atypical immunoblastic proliferations resembling lymphomas but differing from AILD/IBL in clinical presentation and histologic features have been referred to by a variety of different names including *abnormal immune responses of lymph nodes*.[141] They differ histologically from typical AILD/IBL in that there may be a greater degree of architectural preservation and less vascular proliferation; residual germinal centers may be more prominent; and there may be fewer immunoblasts and more plasma and plasmacytoid cells.

The histologic features of AILD/IBL are not specific. Japanese investigators described a peripheral T-cell lymphoma which is now known as AILD-like, peripheral T-cell lymphoma whose histologic characteristics closely resemble or are indistinguishable from those of AILD-IBL.[147] This T-cell lymphoproliferative process showed a spectrum of histologic changes ranging from not obviously malignant T-cell dysplasia to peripheral T-cell lymphoma.[142] The absence of reliable histologic features that distinguish AILD/IBL from AILD-like peripheral T-cell lymphoma has made interpretation of subsequent immunologic, molecular and cytogenetic studies difficult.[141,148,149] Gene rearrangement studies to assess clonality of AILD/IBL and associated lymphomas have most often shown T-cell receptor gene rearrangements, although rearrangements of immunoglobulin genes have also been reported.[141,144,148-150]

Frizzera has proposed a pragmatic approach to the definition of lymphoproliferative disorders with histologic features of AILD/IBL.[141] By correlating clonality data obtained from these different techniques, namely, immunophenotyping, molecular (genotypic) and cytogenetic studies, these abnormal immunoblastic proliferations can be divided into three groups: 1) polyclonal, benign proliferations that may be called AILD/IBL; 2) AILD-like lymphomas of T-cell type and much less frequently, B-cell type; and 3) AILD-like dysplasias. Proliferations lacking clonality by all three techniques (immunophenotyping, genotyping and cytogenetic analysis) belong to the first, benign group, those showing clonality by all three methods are AILD-like T-cell lymphomas or occasionally B-cell lymphomas, while the third group shows discordance among the three parameters used. In the latter, indeterminate group of disorders, clones of cells may proliferate and regress, or the lesion may develop into a true lymphoma.

The differential diagnosis of the abnormal immune proliferations includes, as stated above, NHLs as well as HD. Lymph nodes in AILD-like peripheral T-cell lymphoma tend to be more cellular (less lymphocyte depleted) than those in AILD/IBL and often have clusters of atypical cells with clear cytoplasm, which are absent in AILD/IBL. Because of the polymorphous cellular proliferation, AILD/IBL may mimic mixed cellularity Hodgkin's disease. However, Reed-Sternberg-like immunoblasts in AILD/IBL and AILD-like T-cell lymphomas do not stain with anti-CD15, while true Reed-Sternberg cells do, and the prominent vascularity characteristic of AILD/IBL and AILD-like T-cell lymphoma is not found in HD. Also, the number of immunoblasts seen in the other disorders are absent in HD. Multicentric Castleman's disease may resemble AILD/IBL and other hyperimmune reactions, but the follicular hyperplasia and the degree of plasmacytosis found in Castleman's disease are greater than those usually present in AILD/IBL.[84]

Drug-induced hypersensitivity reactions

A number of drugs are associated with enlargement of lymph nodes in susceptible individuals, but the most widely known substance causing lymphadenopathy is Dilantin (diphenylhydantoin).[74,127,128] More recently the anticonvulsant carbamazepine has also been implicated in this type of hypersensitivity reaction.[151] The lymph node enlargement may be associated with fever, skin rash, and sometimes joint pains, or else symptoms may be completely lacking, especially in individuals taking Dilantin. The cervical lymph nodes are most often affected, but axillary and inguinal nodes may also become enlarged. With Dilantin, lymphadenopathy usually develops two to three weeks after the start of therapy, but occasionally it may not be detected for several months. Lymphadenopathy usually subsides within two weeks of stopping the medication.

Histologically, the major change in the lymph nodes is an expansion of the paracortex due to a diffuse polymorphous proliferation of a variety of cells including lymphocytes, immunoblasts, plasma cells, eosinophils, and histiocytes (Fig. 42-39). These histologic features may resemble those seen in infectious mononucleosis. In some cases, when numerous immunoblasts are present, the proliferation may resemble or be indistinguishable from that seen in AILD/IBL or even in NHL or HD.[52] A number of patients have developed lymphoma of both types after long-term hydantoin therapy.[152] Follicular hyperplasia may accompany paracortical expansion in the early stages, while later in the course of the disease the paracortical expansion may partly or completely overrun the

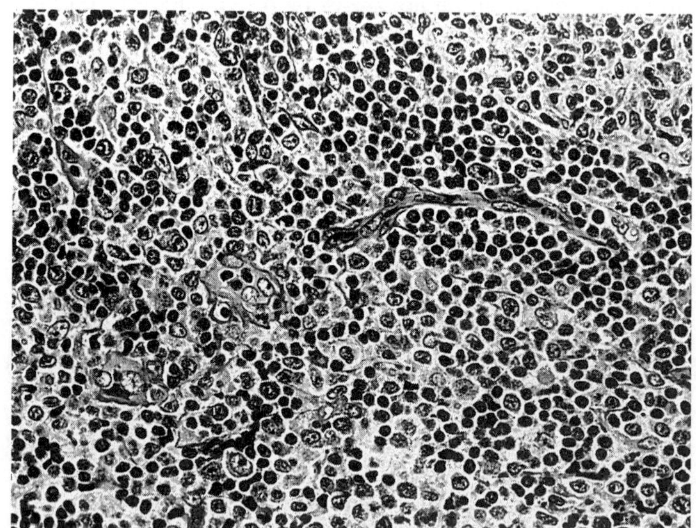

Fig. 42-39 Hypersensitivity reaction in a 40-year-old man taking Dilantin. High endothelial vessels are present within a diffuse polymorphous infiltrate consisting of lymphocytes, plasma cells, eosinophils, and immunoblasts, and a part of a follicle is present (upper right).

follicles. A proliferation of high endothelial vessels is common, and, when combined with many immunoblasts, the proliferation may resemble AILD/IBL, except that reactive germinal centers are often still present. Such proliferations may be interpreted as representing abnormal immune reactions. When sheets of immunoblasts are present, the proliferation may resemble large cell lymphoma. Binucleate immunoblasts may be indistinguishable from Reed-Sternberg cells, thus calling to mind HD. However, in most instances, examination by low magnification reveals partial retention of the nodal architecture, which is much less commonly seen in lymphomas than in benign proliferations.

Systemic lupus erythematosus

Enlarged lymph nodes, especially cervical nodes, occur in 30 to 60% of patients with SLE. Because patients with autoimmune disorders are at risk for development of lymphoma, biopsies are often done on the enlarged lymph nodes in these patients. Histologically, the nodes most often show nonspecific hyperplasias, particularly follicular hyperplasia with plasmacytosis.[63,69,74,153] Findings characteristic of SLE include areas of necrosis containing karyorrhectic debris and usually absence of neutrophils, but plasmacytosis is present. The necrosis may, therefore, be identical to that in Kikuchi's disease. In many instances, necrosis is more extensive and may be of the coagulative type. Blood vessels may be necrotic and thrombosed. In addition to the absence of plasmacytosis, hematoxylin bodies, which are found in lupus, especially at the edge of the necrotic areas, within sinuses, and around or within walls of blood vessels (Fig. 42-40), are absent in Kikuchi's disease.[69,70] Hematoxylin bodies consist of amorphous hematoxophilic structures of altered DNA, 5 to 12 mm in diameter and stainable with Feulgen and PAS.[74] The histologic interpretation of SLE should always be confirmed by clinical history and serologic studies.

Mucocutaneous lymph node syndrome (Kawasaki's disease)

Kawasaki's disease or mucocutaneous lymph node syndrome was first described in Japan but is now recognized in other parts of the world.[63,74,129,154,155] It is an acute, febrile exanthematous disease of undetermined etiology seen in children mostly under the age of four. It is characterized clinically by fever, erythematous rash, lesions of the conjunctiva and oral mucosa, cervical adenopathy, and coronary arteritis. One to three percent of children die of coronary arteritis during the acute phase of the disease, and some die several years after apparent recovery. The dominant histologic feature in lymph nodes includes multiple foci of necrosis associated with vascular lesions. Small blood vessels contain thrombi, fibrinoid necrosis, and infiltration of their walls by lymphocytes and histiocytes. The vascular lesions are associated with focal or widespread necrosis of the node that may include follicles. The necrosis of the nodes may be indistinguishable from that seen in lymph nodes of patients with SLE, which can be excluded from the differential diagnosis on clinical grounds.

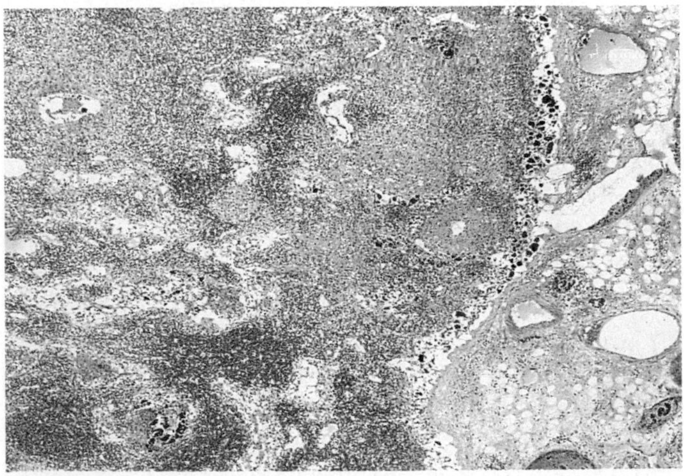

Fig. 42-40 Lymph node from a patient with systemic lupus erythematosus showing extensive necrosis without neutrophils and hematoxylin bodies within sinuses and vessels.

Sinus pattern

Benign disorders in which sinuses are primarily involved include: the common and completely nonspecific sinus histiocytosis; avidly phagocytic histiocytes in lymph node sinuses that are seen in the hemophagocytic syndromes caused most often by viruses but less often by a variety of infectious agents; the rare but morphologically distinctive and mysterious sinus histiocytosis with massive lymphadenopathy, or Rosai-Dorfman disease; the effects of lymphangiography; the proliferation of Langerhans' cells known as *Langerhans' cell histiocytosis (histiocytosis-X)*; and Whipple's disease with its characteristic PAS-positive sickle-like particles in the cytoplasm of histiocytes.[34,63,71,74,156-159] Since Langerhans' cell histiocytosis has been found to be a monoclonal process and therefore probably truly neoplastic, it is considered in detail later in this chapter.

Sinus histiocytosis

Sinus histiocytosis is a common nonspecific finding in lymph node biopsies.[74] It may be combined with follicular or interfollicular hyperplasia. It may be seen in lymph nodes draining sites of inflammation or tumors, especially breast and gastrointestinal carcinomas. It is also frequently seen in lymph nodes from the abdomen. Histologically, the sinuses are dilated and filled with histiocytes, which are large cells with ample cytoplasm and bland-appearing nuclei (Fig. 42-41). Phagocytes of red cells and hemosiderin deposition may be seen in the cytoplasm after transfusions or in cases of hemolytic anemia, and lymph nodes from the mediastinum usually contain sinus histiocytes with anthracotic pigment.

Hemophagocytic syndromes

In 1939, Robb-Smith reported a disease which he called *histiocytic medullary reticulosis* that is probably the same as or similar to what was later described as *virus-associated hemophagocytic syndrome*.[158,160] The term was changed to *infection-associated hemophagocytic syndrome* when it became clear that the syndrome was associated with bacterial, fungal and parasitic infections as well.[157] It is a benign but often fatal disorder that occurs in immunocompromised hosts but may also be seen in patients without a history of immunodeficiency. The immunodeficiency associated with this disorder may be secondary to immunosuppression in transplant patients, or it may occur in individuals with congenital immunodeficiency or in patients with acute lymphoblastic

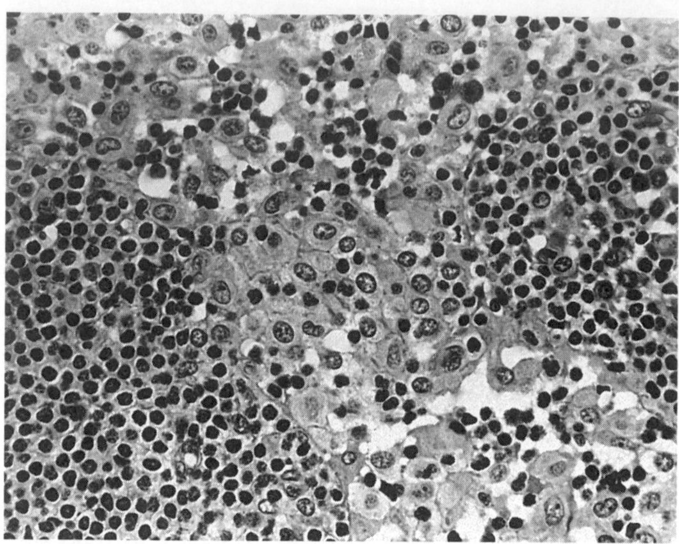

Fig. 42-41 Sinus histiocytosis. Histiocytes with ample cytoplasm, bland-appearing nuclei, and inconspicuous nucleoli fill dilated sinuses.

leukemia and T-cell lymphomas.[161-163] The clinical findings include high fever, constitutional symptoms, anemia, hepatosplenomegaly, abnormal liver function tests, and coagulopathy.

The diagnosis of this disorder is most often made from a bone marrow aspirate in which histiocytes containing phagocytosed blood cells are readily seen. In lymph node biopsy specimens, the sinuses are often dilated and filled with bland-appearing benign sinus histiocytes containing phagocytosed red blood cells (Fig. 42-42). Neutrophils, lymphocytes, and platelets are also within the cytoplasm of the histiocytes but are not as prominent nor as easily detected. The remainder of the node may show depletion of lymphocytes and vascular proliferation. The red pulp of the spleen is usually greatly expanded by phagocytic histiocytes that are also present in the hepatic sinuses.

The major entities that should be differentiated from infection-associated hemophagocytic syndrome include: 1) malignant histiocytosis, 2) large cell lymphomas with a sinusoidal pattern, including Ki-1 anaplastic large cell lymphoma; 3) metastatic nonhematolymphoid neoplasms; and, by virtue of their sinusoidal and/or parafollicular pattern of involvement, 4) monocytoid B-cell proliferations; and 5) hairy cell leukemia.[161,164-168] Another entity that can often be differentiated on clinical grounds is familial hemophagocytic lymphohistiocytosis.[74]

Malignant histiocytosis is rarely diagnosed in the 1990s. Most of the cases previously reported were probably examples of the viral-associated hemophagocytic syndrome. Those cases in which the cells had obvious malignant features cytologically were most likely examples of large cell lymphomas, including $CD30^+$ anaplastic large cell lymphomas, which have a sinusoidal localization in lymph nodes.[167-169] In these lymphomas, erythrophagocytosis, which is usually not pronounced, is present almost exclusively in benign histiocytes and is rarely noted in obviously neoplastic cells. Monocytoid B-cell lymphomas, reactive monocytoid B-cell proliferations, and hairy cell leukemia are not associated with hemophagocytosis and resemble the syndrome only in their sinusoidal and parafollicular pattern of nodal involvement. Metastatic carcinomas and melanomas in sinuses can be differentiated from the avidly phagocytic, benign-appearing histiocytes by their malignant cytologic features.

Sinus histiocytosis with massive lymphadenopathy

Sinus histiocytosis with massive lymphadenopathy, or Rosai-Dorfman disease, is a rare disorder.[153,159] It affects males slightly more often than females and is seen in all age groups, but most cases occur in the first two decades of life, and its distribution is worldwide. Massive bilateral cervical adenopathy is the most common presentation, while other sites of involvement include inguinal, axillary, and mediastinal nodes. Extranodal involvement, especially skin, upper respiratory tract, ocular adnexa, and bone, has been described. Polyclonal hypergammaglobulinemia, elevated erythrocyte sedimentation rate, and anemia are included among the abnormal laboratory tests that may be seen. The etiology of the disorder is unknown, but recent findings suggest that it is a disorder of altered immunity.

Grossly, the excised tissue typically consists of a multinodular mass of nodes separated by bands of fibrosis.[159] Histologically, the capsule is markedly thickened, and the fibrosis extends into the pericapsular tissue. The sinuses are markedly dilated and contain many histiocytes with abundant clear or foamy cytoplasm along with a vesicular nucleus that has a distinct nucleolus. Some histocytes may contain atypical hyperchromatic nuclei with a prominent nucleolus. The characteristic finding of this entity is the presence of numerous lymphocytes within the histiocyte cytoplasm, and, less frequently, plasma cells, neutrophils, and even red cells (Fig. 42-43). These cells are apparently not phagocytosed and appear to be viable within the cytoplasm of the histiocytes (emperipolesis). Also characteristic is a heavy plasma cell infiltrate of the medullary cords. In many cases, only remnants of intersinusoidal lymph node tissue remain. Follicles are not prominent. The sinusoidal histiocytes are S-100 and $CD1^+$ like the cells of Langerhans' cell histiocytosis, which are positive with both these antibodies.[153,170,171]

Whipple's disease

Whipple's disease is a bacterial infection involving the small intestine and is most commonly seen in middle-aged males. Clinically the patients have variable symptoms including

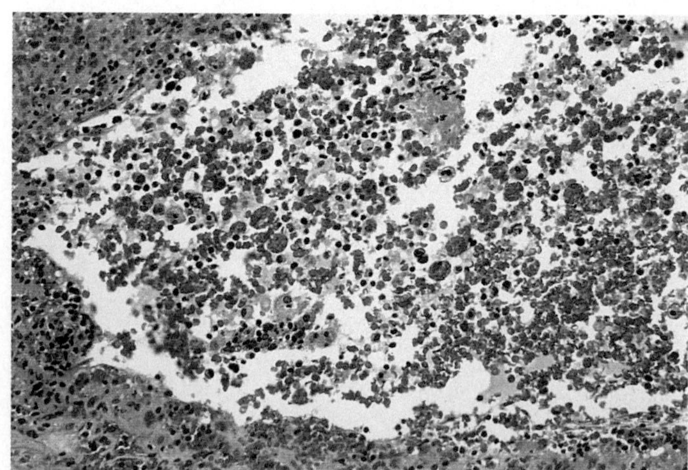

Fig. 42-42 Infection associated hemophagocytic syndrome showing histiocytes containing many phagocytosed red cells within a distended sinus.

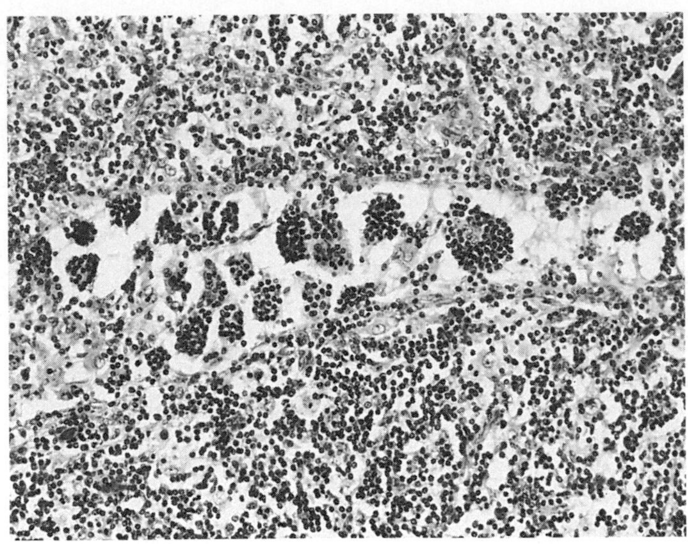

Fig. 42-43 Sinus histiocytosis with massive lymphadenopathy. The cytoplasm of the histiocytes within the dilated sinuses is filled with small lymphocytes.

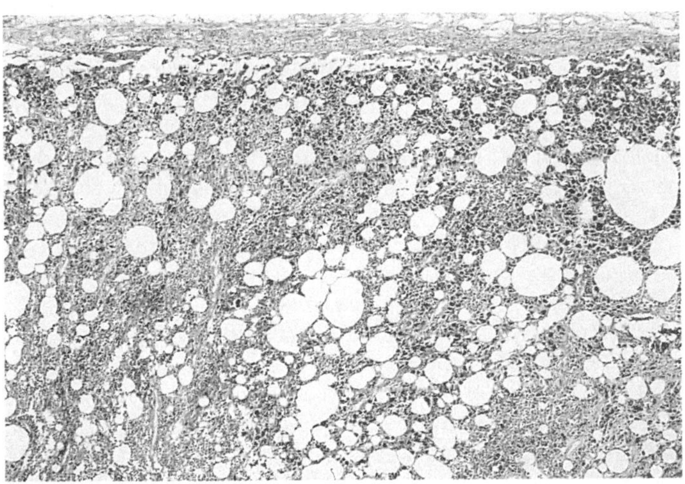

Fig. 42-44 Whipple's disease showing distention of sinuses by vacuoles and histiocytes containing PAS-positive particles.

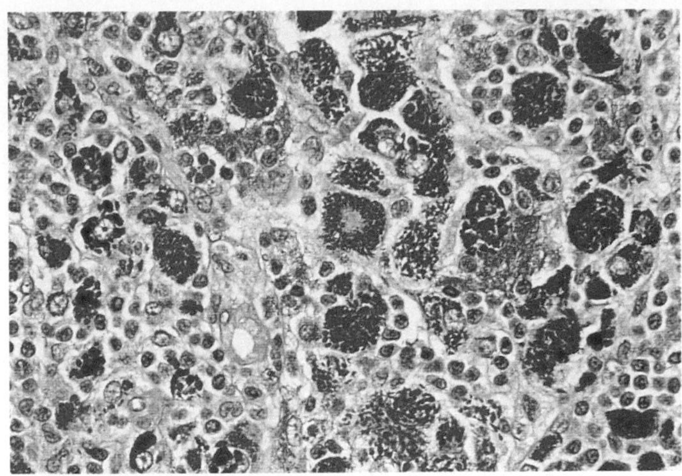

Fig. 42-45 Higher magnification of PAS-positive sickle-form particles within histiocyte cytoplasm.

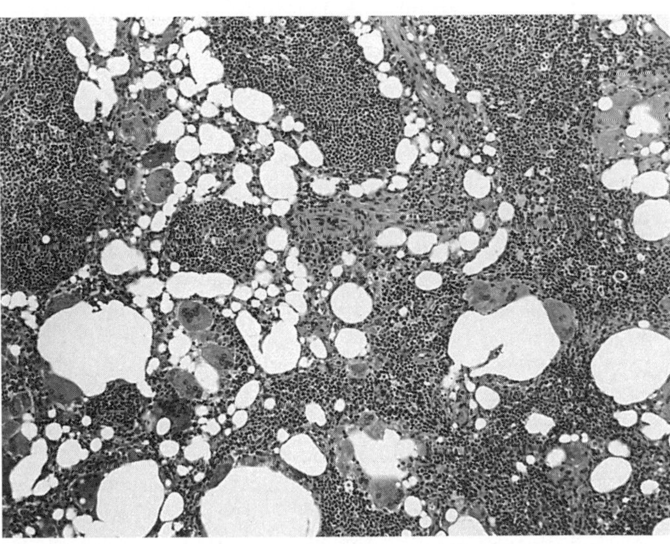

Fig. 42-46 Large vacuoles, histiocytes, and multinucleate giant cells within the diluted sinuses of a patient who had undergone lymphangiography.

weight loss, diarrhea, and arthralgias, or they may have no specific complaints.[172] In addition, the patients often have steatorrhea, hypoalbuminemia, and low serum carotene levels. Abdominal lymph nodes are frequently involved and peripheral lymphadenopathy may be seen in about 50% of patients. Histologically, the lymph node sinuses are dilated and contain large vacuoles formed by loss of lipid materials during tissue processing. The sinuses also contain large histiocytes with abundant vacuolated cytoplasm (Fig. 42-44) and nonnecrotizing granulomas. These features may resemble the changes seen after lymphangiography. Characteristic of Whipple's disease is the presence of diastase-resistant PAS-positive sickle-form particles in the cytoplasm of the histiocytes (Fig. 42-45).[63,71,172] These PAS-positive particles correspond to the causative bacillary organisms that can be easily demonstrated by EM.[173] The uncultured bacillus of Whipple's disease has recently been identified.[174]

The differential diagnosis of Whipple's disease includes infection by *Mycobacterium avium–intracellulare,* which is seen in patients with AIDS. The histiocytes in this infection also contain PAS-positive material. An acid-fast stain must always be carried out to distinguish between these two infections. The histiocytes are packed with acid-fast bacilli in the mycobacterial infection.

Lymphangiography effect

Lymphangiography, which was once routinely carried out for staging of Hodgkin's disease, is now much less commonly utilized, and node biopsy specimens showing the changes caused by injection of the radiopaque lipid-based material are rarely seen. The injected medium is dissolved during tissue processing, leaving behind large vacuoles within sinuses.[175] Many large multinuclear foreign-body type giant cells, some stretched around vacuoles, are characteristic (Fig. 42-46). Eosinophils may be seen within the sinuses and in medullary cords.

Lymph nodes in the porta hepatis and celiac axis often contain lipophagic vacuolization of sinus histiocytes and multinucleate giant cells. The vacuoles are much smaller than those associated with lymphangiography. Lipid granulomas are also seen in these nodes. Lymph node sinuses in cases of pneumatosis intestinalis contain large gas vacuoles surrounded by a granulomatous reaction.[74]

HODGKIN'S DISEASE (HD)

Historical background and definition

In 1832, Thomas Hodgkin first described the clinical and gross autopsy findings of a series of patients with enormous enlargement of the lymph nodes and involvement of the spleen.[176] Wilkes subsequently published a series of 15 similar cases and coined the term *Hodgkin's disease* for this entity.[177] The nature of HD had been controversial until fairly recently. While many believed that it was a malignant neoplasm, others favored an infectious, perhaps tuberculous, or an inflammatory disease. Cytogenetic studies have shown the presence of aneuploid cells, often in the tetraploid range, in tissues involved by HD. Furthermore, cases with clonal chromosomal abnormalities have been well documented. These observations lend support to the neoplastic nature of HD.[178,179]

It is difficult to give a short and precise definition of HD. Current evidence, in fact, suggests that HD may be a syndrome consisting of several entities. However, there are a number of clinical and pathologic features that unite the various forms of HD and set them apart from non-Hodgkin's lymphomas. HD presents in lymph nodes and tends to spread to contiguous lymph nodes in a rather predictable pattern as the disease progresses. Histologically, the tumor tissue contains a large admixture of reactive elements such as small lymphocytes, histocytes, eosinophils, neutrophils, and plasma cells. The neoplastic cell that characterize this disease, the diagnostic Reed-Sternberg (RS) cell, should always be present. This cell is a large cell and by light microscopy contain two or more nuclei or nuclear lobes with large inclusion body-like eosinophilic nucleoli surrounded by a halo of clear nucleoplasm. There is a moderate amount of eosinophilic to amphophilic cytoplasm (Fig. 42-47, *A*). In addition, varying numbers of large pleomorphic neoplastic cells with distinctive features in each subtype of HD (the RS cell variants) are scattered in this milieu (Figs. 42-47, *B* through 42-47, *E*).[180,181]

Epidemiology and etiology

There are about 7900 new cases of HD per year in the United States, with an overall incidence rate of about 3/100,000 person-year.[182] The disease has a bimodal age distribution with a young age peak between 15 and 35 years and then a subsequent gradual increase with age after 45.[183] However, there are geographical variations in the age distribution with an increase in childhood cases and a decrease in incidence of the young adult group in less developed countries and in lower socioeconomic groups of developed nations (Fig. 42-48).[184-186] The incidence of HD is low in all age groups studied in several Asian countries.[185,186]

In the United States, HD shows a male predominance (1.3:1) with the exception of the nodular sclerosis subtype in young adults. Young adults tend to have a predominance of nodular sclerosis (NS) and lymphocytic predominance (LP) subtypes while the mixed cellularity (MC) and lymphocytic depletion (LD) subtypes are more prevalent in the older age group. In less developed countries, MC and LD subtypes predominate in both children and adults. There is probably an increase in incidence of HD, MC subtype, in patients with AIDS, especially in the group with a history of intravenous drug use.[187-189]

The etiology of HD is still unknown. The epidemiological data show that HD in young patients shares certain characteristics with the disease epidemiology of certain viral infections such as poliomyelitis and infectious mononucleosis, suggesting the involvement of a viral agent.[190,191] This putative agent, similar to the EBV, causes a low incidence of disease in early childhood but a much greater chance of clinical disease when encountered later in life. Under poor socioeconomic conditions, childhood infection is prevalent, while with improved sanitation, more individuals will encounter the organism later, with the disease peak in late adolescence and early adult life. There have also been some reports of time-space clustering of cases but no clear conclusion can be drawn from the data.[192]

Other evidence that favors a common source exposure or genetic factors in the pathogenesis of HD include the occurrence of familial cases.[193-197] In one of the reports, there is a seven-fold excess risk of HD in siblings, with a greater concordance of sex than expected, suggesting interpersonal transmission or common source exposure.[194] There are some slight increases in the frequency of HD in HLA types A1, B5, B8 and B18.[198] The significance of the weak association is unclear and it is hoped that further studies on familial cases will shed some light on the possible role of HLA in HD.[195,197]

Of the possible infectious agents, three have received special attention. Retroviruses are prime candidates for consideration since many animal leukemias and lymphomas are caused by retroviruses and recently two T-lymphotropic viruses (HTLV-I and HTLV-II) have been associated with human lymphoproliferative disorders. There was, in fact, an early report on the presence of reverse transcriptase (a retrovirus encoded enzyme) in HD tissue,[199] but so far, no retrovirus has been linked to HD.[200] The role of HIV in the increased incidence of HD in AIDS is probably indirect, as a consequence of the damage to the immune system. Since the disease seems to be more prevalent among intravenous drug users, an agent transmitted through the parenteral route, in addition to HIV, may be involved in its pathogenesis.[187,188]

There was some recent interest in the possible involvement of human herpes virus 6 (HHV-6).[201,202] HHV-6 sequences were detectable in a small proportion of HD but its role in the pathogenesis of HD is unclear.[203-205] Evidence for the involvement of EBV is much stronger. Persons with prior infectious mononucleosis are at increased risk of HD and those who are seropositive for EBV infection have a three- to four-fold increase in incidence of HD.[206,207] The antibody titer to viral capsid antigen is higher in patients with HD,[191] and the EBV antibody pattern in sera of patients before diagnosis suggests enchanced viral activation.[208] Recently, HD tissue has been studied for the presence of EBV genome. Using Southern blot hybridization technique, 17 to 29% of cases studied are positive for EBV and in many cases, the tumor appears to contain a clonal viral population, suggesting that the infection occurs before the neoplastic transformation of the cell.[209 213] EBV is detectable in about 60% of the cases when examined by assays utilizing PCR.[213-216] In many cases where EBV was detected by the above methods, it has been shown unequivocally that the RS cell and its variants contain EBV genome by in situ hybridization (Fig. 42-49).[210,217-220] Using specific monoclonal antibodies, the viral latent membrane protein-1 has also been demonstrated in RS cells and vari-

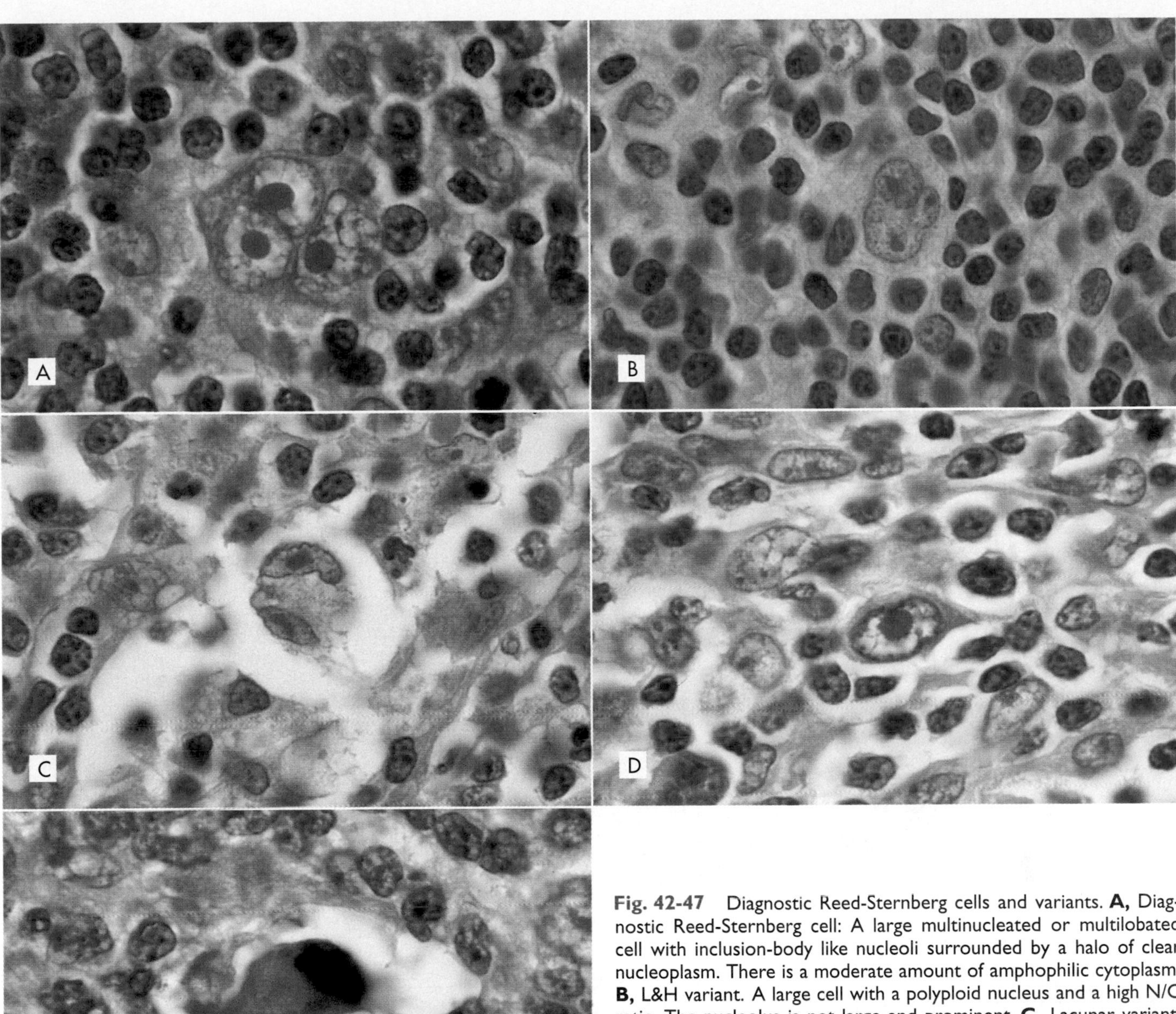

Fig. 42-47 Diagnostic Reed-Sternberg cells and variants. **A,** Diagnostic Reed-Sternberg cell: A large multinucleated or multilobated cell with inclusion-body like nucleoli surrounded by a halo of clear nucleoplasm. There is a moderate amount of amphophilic cytoplasm. **B,** L&H variant. A large cell with a polyploid nucleus and a high N/C ratio. The nucleolus is not large and prominent. **C,** Lacunar variant: the cell has a lobated nucleus with small to moderately prominent nucleoli in a clear lacuna produced by the retraction of cytoplasm from the plasm membrane. A small amount of cytoplasm is often observed around the nucleus. **D,** Mononuclear variant. This cell has the characteristic of a diagnostic Reed-Sternberg cell but with a single round or oval nucleus. **E,** Mummified (necrobiotic) cells frequently seen in NSHD with pyknotic nucleus and darkly eosinophilic cytoplasm.

ants.[219,221,222] The type of HD most frequently associated with EBV is the MC type, while the LP type is usually negative. In the LP type, EBV is probably of little pathogenetic significance. In the other types where EBV is present in a higher proportion of cases, the role of the virus is still far from clear. Many cases are not EBV positive, suggesting that the virus is not essential for the pathogenesis of the disease. In HD developing in patients with HIV infection, the incidence of EBV positivity is very high (80-90%).[223] There is also a high incidence of EBV positivity in HD occurring in some developing countries, particularly in children.[224,225] However, there is a higher proportion of the MC type in these populations, which may partially account for the high incidence of EBV detection.

Histopathologic classification

The pathologic classification used continues to be the one proposed by Lukes and Butler in 1966.[180,181] The relationship of this classification with the older one by Jackson and Parker[226] and the simplified version adopted at the Rye Conference is shown in Table 42-5.[227] The relative frequencies of the various types of HD in the United States reported from Stanford University are also included.[228] These figures vary to some extent depending on the age range, socioeconomic status and the existence of any predisposing factors in the population under consideration as mentioned in the epidemiology section.

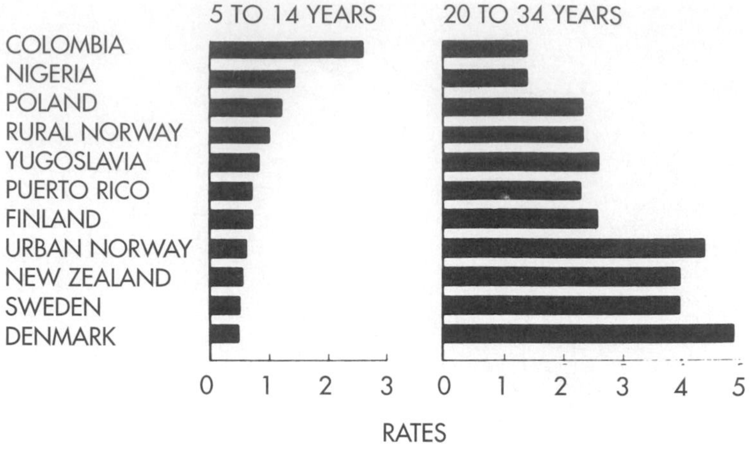

Fig. 42-48 Average annual incidence rates/100,000 population for children (5-14 years) and young adults (20-34 years). Calculated for males in selected countries. (From Correa P, O'Conor GT: *Int J Cancer* 8:192, 1971.)

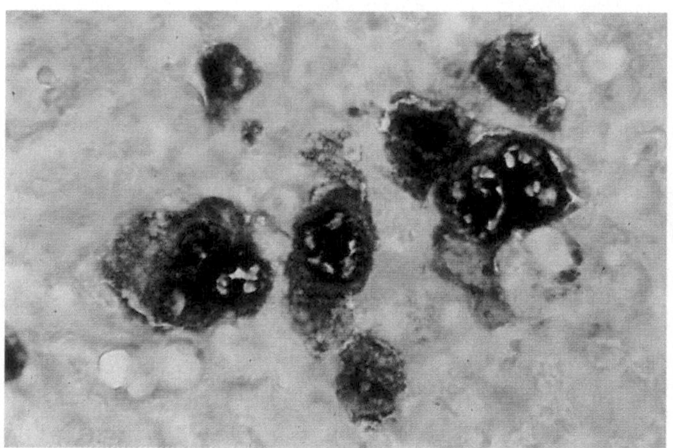

Fig. 42-49 Hodgkin's disease. In situ hybridization for Epstein-Barr–encoded RNA (EBER) immuohistochemistry for CD15. The nuclei of Reed-Sternberg cells are black, indicating the presence of Epstein-Barr–encoded RNA while the cytoplasm is brown, indicating reactivity of the cells for CD15. Other cells in the field are unstained.

Lymphocytic predominance type

As its name implies, the cellular background consists of numerous small lymphocytes and admixed histiocytes, which may be quite abundant (Fig. 42-50). A type of RS cell variant, the L&H variants are seen scattered among this lymphohistiocytic infiltrate. The L&H cells are large cells with a large, often lobulated (popcorn-like) nucleus and a high N/C ratio. Nuclear chromatin is very fine and the nucleoli are not prominent (Fig. 42-47, *B*). Cells frequently seen in other types of HD, such as eosinophils, plasma cells, and neutrophils, are rarely observed. Diagnostic RS cells are very difficult to find and in fact some authorities believe that they are no longer necessary for diagnosis when other typical features are present.[229] L&H cells, however, can be very prominent, even forming focal aggregates in some cases. In the nodular form, the lymph node architecture is replaced by numerous large neoplastic nodules, which bear a close resemblance to the large altered germinal centers called progressively transformed germinal centers (PTGCs) occasionally seen interspersed with hyperplastic germinal centers in reactive lymph nodes (Fig. 42-51). PTGCs have been observed in lymph nodes biopsy

Table 42-5 The pathologic classification of Hodgkin's disease

Jackson & Parker	Lukes & Butler	Rye Conference	Frequency (%)*
Paragranuloma	1. Lymphocytic and histiocytic a. Nodular b. Diffuse	Lymphocytic predominance	5
Granuloma	2. Nodular sclerosis	Nodular sclerosis	70
	3. Mixed cellularity	Mixed cellularity	22
Sarcoma	4. Diffuse fibrosis 5. Reticular	Lymphocytic depletion	1

From Colby TV, Hoppe RT, Warnke RA: *Cancer* 49:1848, 1981.
*2% of the cases were considered unclassifiable.

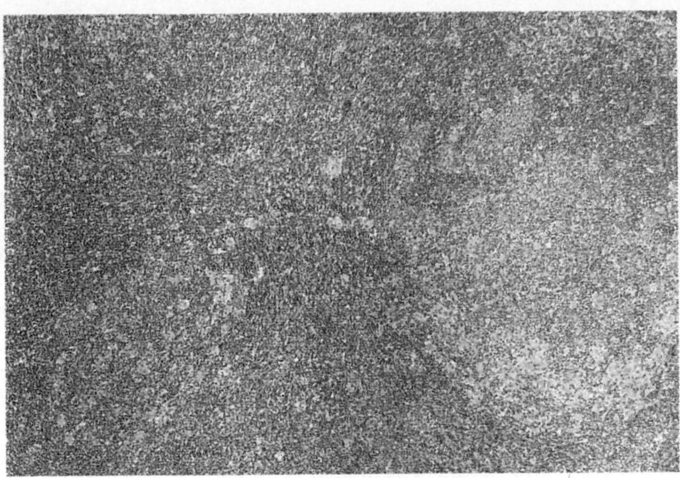

Fig. 42-50 L&H HD, nodular type. Large nodules with small round lymphocytes, histiocytes, and scattered L&H cells.

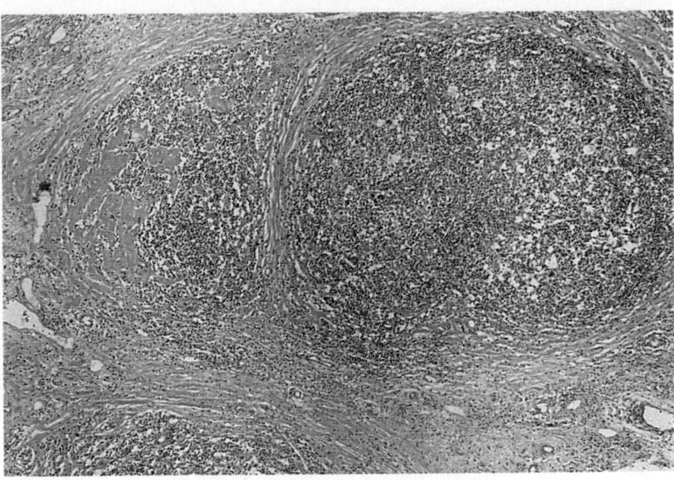

Fig. 42-52 NSHD. Bands of thick collagen fibers extending from a thickened capsule to divide the lymph node into multiple cellular nodules.

Fig. 42-51 Progressively transformed germinal centers. Note the large nodule among normal germinal centers. Many small round lymphocytes from the mantle zone intermix with follicular center cells.

specimens obtained before, after or concurrent with the diagnosis of HD,[101,104,230] and may be confused with focal involvement of the lymph node by nodular L&H HD.

In the diffuse subtype, nodules are not discernable in H&E sections. The node is replaced by a diffuse proliferation with a cellular composition similar to the neoplastic nodules in the nodular subtype. Sometimes, an involved lymph node may show both nodular and diffuse areas. The L&H cells have a unique immunophenotype distinct from that seen in RS cell variants in other forms of HD and this difference is useful in the differential diagnosis in difficult cases.

Nodular sclerosis (NS) type

This type of HD is the only subtype with a slight female predominance. It is characterized by the presence of a thickened lymph node capsule with well-formed bands of collagen extending inwards separating the tumor tissue into cellular nodules that contain variable proportions of lymphocytes, histiocytes, eosinophils, plasma cells, and neutrophils in addition to RS variants called lacunar cells (Fig. 42-52). The lacunar cells consist of a multilobated nucleus with moderately prominent nucleoli surrounded by a clear space caused by the artifactual retraction of the cytoplasm from the nuclear membrane (Fig. 42-47, *C*). This lacunar artifact is much less prominent in Zenker or B5 fixed tissue than in formalin-fixed material. Necrosis and microabscess formation can be quite prominent in this form of HD (Fig. 42-53). Necrobiotic (mummified) neoplastic cells are also frequently observed. These cells show a pyknotic nucleus surrounded by dense dark eosinophilic cytoplasm (Fig. 42-47, *E*). Sclerosis may be so prominent that much of the cellular nodule or much of the tumor consists of dense collagen. In other cases, fibrosis can be minimal but the presence of at least one single well-formed birefringent collagen band extending from the capsule should be observed to classify the case as NSHD. The term *cellular phase* has been applied to such cases. The classification of cases with features of NSHD (even with vague nodularity) but no birefringent collagen bands as described is difficult,[231] but would be put into the mixed cellularity category according to the original criteria.[181]

There have been attempts to classify NSHD into subtypes. Several studies suggest that cases with >25% of cellular nodules showing lymphocyte depletion due to large numbers of RS variants or contain numerous highly pleomorphic cells or >80% of the nodules composed largely of fibrohistiocytic cells (NS-grade II) have a poorer prognosis than cases not showing these features (NS-grade I).[232-234] The clinical value and the reproducibility of this subclassification among pathologists require some additional studies.

Mixed cellularity (MC) type. This type of HD shows a mixed cellular background of lymphocytes, histiocytes, eosinophils and plasma cells (Fig. 42-54). There are interspersed RS variants called the mononuclear variants (Fig. 42-47, *D*), which resemble diagnostic RS cells but having a single round or oval nucleus. Diagnostic RS cells are also readily identified. Areas of disorderly fibrosis and necrosis may be seen but not prominent. This type of HD is the one most likely confused with peripheral T-cell lymphomas and when there is a prominent component of epithelioid histiocytes, the distinc-

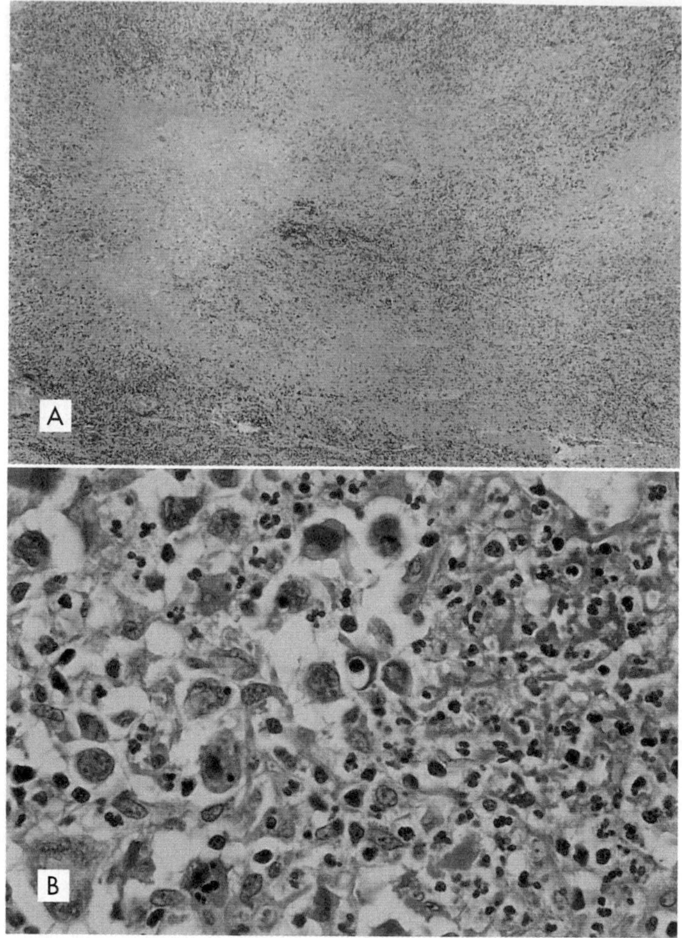

Fig. 42-53 NSHD. **A,** Necrosis and **B,** Microabscess formation can be prominent features. These foci may be surrounded by a rim of RS variants.

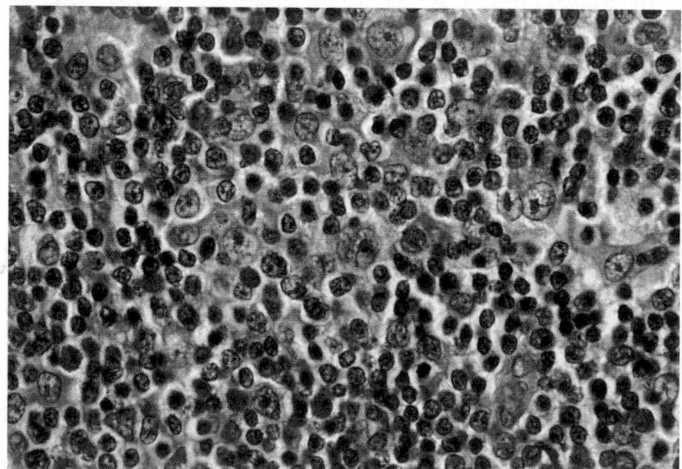

Fig. 42-54 MCHD. The tumor shows a mixed cellular background with scattered mononuclear RS variants.

tion between Lennert's lymphoma may be difficult (Fig. 42-55). It is also noteworthy that this is the predominant type of HD seen in patients with AIDS.[189,235,236]

Lymphocytic depletion (LD) type. This is an uncommon type of HD accounting for 5% or less of cases and often present at an older age with systemic symptoms, advanced disease and prominent subdiaphragmatic involvement.[237,238] Other authors felt that patients with LDHD are in many ways similar to patients with MC and the constellation of clinical features just mentioned are not that prevalent.[239,240] The diffuse fibrosis type is rare and is characterized by replacement of the node by a disorderly nonbirefringent fibrosis with a consequent decrease in lymphocytes (Fig. 42-56). RS cells are not necessarily numerous. In contrast, the reticular subtype shows a prominent proliferation of RS cells (Fig. 42-57). In some cases, there are abundant extremely pleomorphic, bizarre RS cells and these cases have been referred to as the sarcomatous subtype. The reticular type of LDHD may be confused with NSHD with lymphocyte depletion and also with non-Hodgkin's lymphomas with many large anaplastic tumor cells and cells simulating RS cells.[240] In some patients, a lymph node may show features of both diffuse fibrosis and reticular

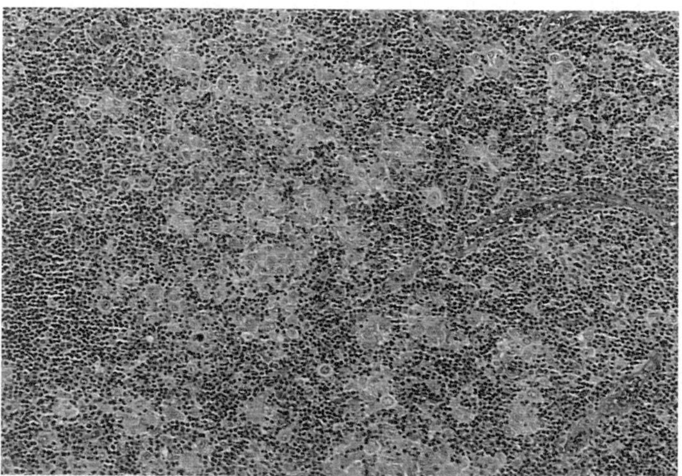

Fig. 42-55 MCHD with a high content of epithelioid histiocytes. Note the loose aggregates of epithelioid histiocytes scattering throughout the section resembling the background of a lymphoepitheloid cell lymphoma ("Lennert's lymphoma").

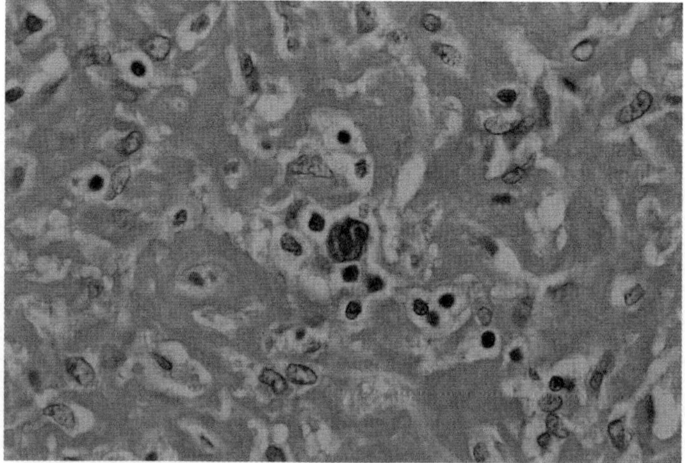

Fig. 42-56 LDHD, diffuse fibrosis type. Much of the lymph node has been replaced by a pink, eosinophilic amorphous material with depletion of lymphocytes. Scattered RS cell variants are seen.

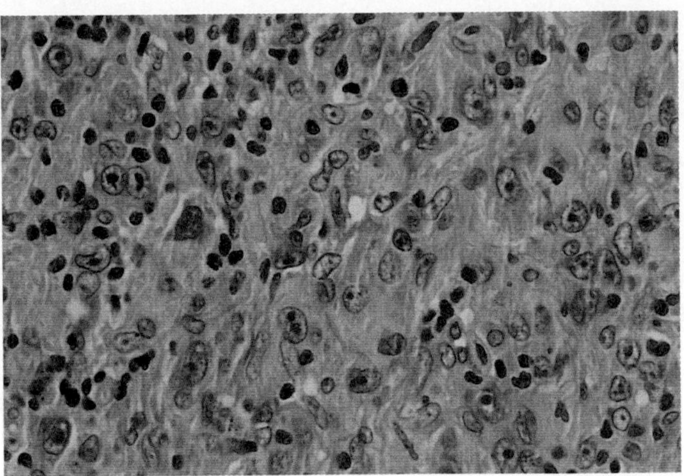

Fig. 42-57 LDHD, reticular type. The lymph node is largely replaced by a proliferation of Reed-Sternberg cells and variants.

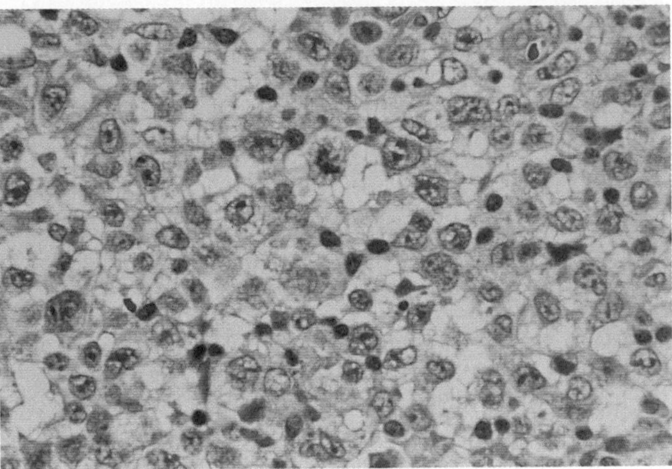

Fig. 42-58 NSHD, Syncytial variant. Cohesive sheets of RS variants occupy much of this lymph node. These cells may surround a necrotic focus. While some of the cells have the appearance of lacunar cells, others might just show pale cytoplasm around a nucleus which may or may not show multilobation.

type or the two histologic types may be seen in lymph nodes from different regions.[181]

Histopathologic variants

HD with unusual histopathologic features has been described. The name interfollicular HD has been applied to lymph nodes with follicular hyperplasia and foci of HD in the interfollicular area.[77] The diagnostic criteria are the same as other forms of HD but such foci may be missed on casual examination, resulting in an erroneous diagnosis. The foci may be quite small, and the subtyping of HD may be difficult or impossible. In some cases of NSHD variant, RS variants may occur in cohesive aggregates which often surround a necrotic focus; this has been termed the *syncytial variant* of NSHD (Fig. 42-58).[241] Many of the cells in these aggregates may not have the classic appearance of lacunar cells and if the biopsy does not include areas morphologically typical of NSHD, it may easily be confused with other neoplasms such as metastatic carcinoma or even germ cell tumors. The diagnosis of the syncytial variant of NSHD is especially difficult in B5-fixed material or in small biopsies. Immunohistochemical studies can be very useful in correctly identifying this form of HD under such circumstances.

Association of HD with other lymphoproliferative diseases

HD may precede, follow, or exist concurrently with another lymphoproliferative disorder, including NHL and CLL (Fig. 42-59).[242-251] As cells resembling RS cells may be seen in a variety of neoplastic and reactive condition, it is important that the diagnosis of HD be well substantiated. Immunohistochemical studies may be useful in confirming the diagnosis but it should be noted that none of the markers available is specific for HD. In cases where cells resembling RS cells are seen scattered in an otherwise typical NHL or CLL without a proper HD milieu, the diagnosis of HD is difficult to establish.[252] In situ hybridization studies have demonstrated that the RS cells are almost always EBV-postiive when they arise in a setting of CLL/small lymphocytic lymphoma.[251]

There have been a number of reports describing patients with CLL developing a clinicopathologic picture suggestive of

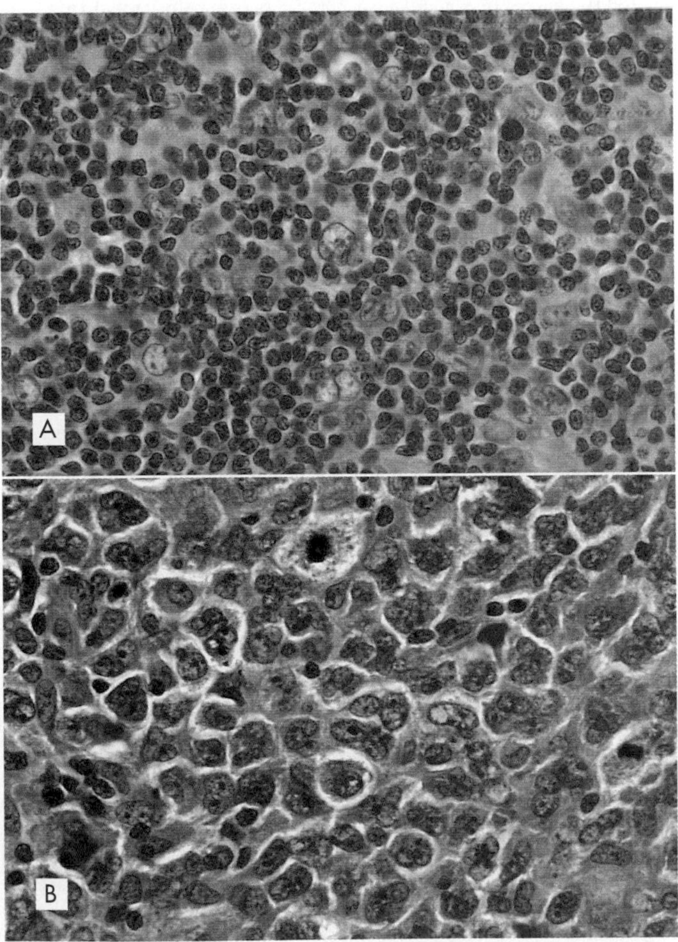

Fig. 42-59 A case of HD, **A,** followed by the development of a large cell lymphoma **B.**

Richter's transformation but a biopsy of the lymph node shows features consistent with HD disease (Fig. 42-60). Some of these cases have also been shown to be immunophenotypically characteristic of HD. Patients with this "Hodgkin type of Richter's syndrome" appeared to have a better prognosis than the typical Richter's syndrome with large cell lymphoma emerging in CLL.[253]

In addition to the above lymphoproliferative disorders, Langerhans' cell histiocytosis have also been associated with HD.[254,255]

Pathology of staging laparotomy[181,256]

Abdominal lymph nodes may be distorted by large amounts of lipoid material with an accompanying foreign body reaction due to the injection of contrast for lymphangiogram. Lymph node involvement by HD may be extensive and easily identified or it may be focal with involvement of only a small area in the paracortex. Criteria for diagnosis is similar to what has been described above except that diagnostic RS cells are not an absolute requirement when RS variants are seen in the proper cellular milieu. In doubtful cases, deeper sections may reveal more diagnostic areas and immunohistochemical studies may occasionally be helpful by demonstrating the classical pattern of markers in the large pleomorphic cells.

Splenic involvement is focal and sometimes the foci are very small. Therefore, it is important that the spleen should be thinly sliced at 0.2-0.3 cm intervals and the slice examined carefully for any enlarged white-tan foci which should be submitted for histologic examination. The small foci of involvement appear to start in the white pulp (Fig. 42-61). Diagnostic criteria are similar to those outlined for lymph nodes.

In the liver, involvement is also focal with the initial involvement starting in the portal triad (Fig. 42-62). Foci of marrow involvement show accompanying stromal fibrosis in addition to the cellular infiltrate (Fig. 42-63). Diagnosis is again based on finding typical RS variants in the proper cellular background. Any area of fibrosis in the bone marrow should be scrutinized carefully for involvement and deeper sections obtained to find more diagnostic areas.

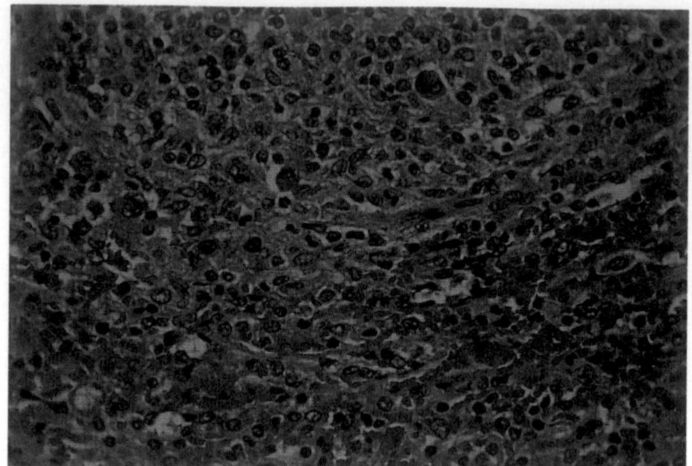

Fig. 42-61 HD, splenic involvement. An early focus involving the malpighian corpuscle of the spleen.

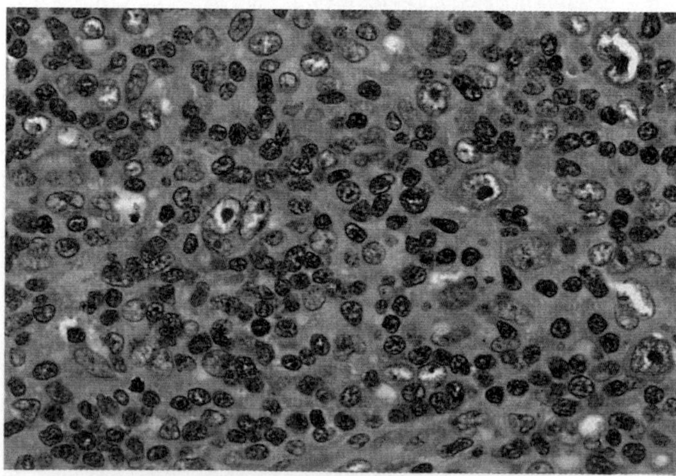

Fig. 42-60 A case of "HD transformation" in a B-chronic lymphocytic leukemia. The large pleomorphic cells resemble RS cells and variants and in this case, have the usual immunophenotype of RS cells ($CD15^+$, $CD30^+$, $CD20^-$).

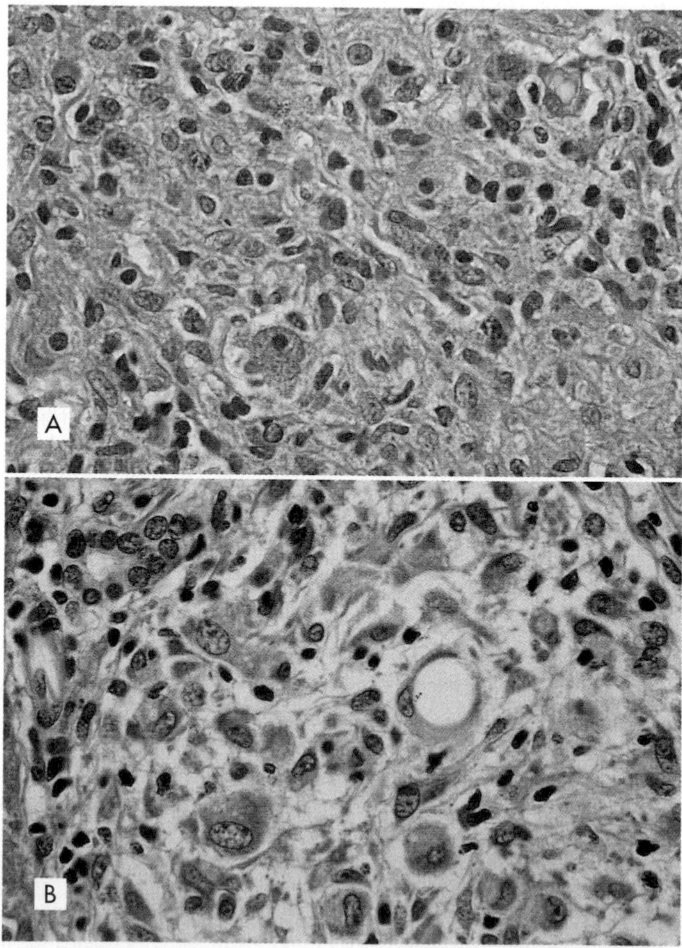

Fig. 42-62 HD, liver involvement. **A,** Involvement of the portal triad in contrast to **B,** Another case with portal epithelioid granulomas without HD.

Epithelioid granulomas may be found in any of the above organs.[257] Their presence per se is not indicative of involvement (Fig. 42-62). On the other hand, HD may be accompanied by a granulomatous reaction, and evidence of involvement should be sought in areas with granulomas (Fig. 42-64).

Pathology of relapse

When Hodgkin's lymphoma relapses in sites that have not been irradiated, the histology in general is similar to that of the original biopsy. This is especially well documented in the nodular sclerosis type.[258,259] Interconversion between NS type and NS, cellular phase, is frequently observed, supporting the concept that the two belong to the same subgroup of HD. Occasional relapses showing a different histologic type have been described. However, even when the histologic type is preserved, there is usually a decrease in lymphocytes with an increase in RS cells, eosinophils, and histiocytes in the relapsed lymphoma.[259]

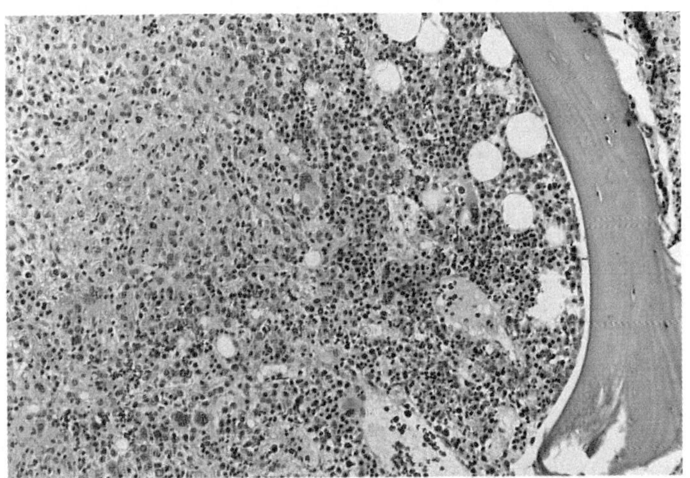

Fig. 42-63 HD, bone marrow involvement. Patchy marrow involvement, note the fibrosis and polymorphic cellular background as well as presence of RS variants.

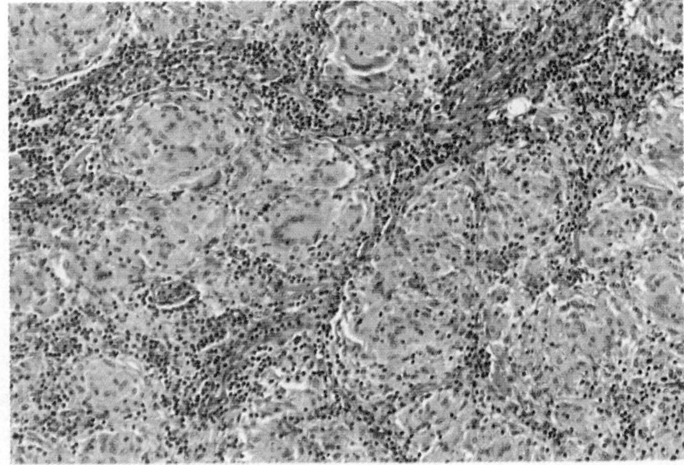

Fig. 42-64 HD with sarcoid-like granulomas. Typical mixed cellularity HD is observed in between the granulomas.

When the lymphoma relapses in a previously treated area, the morphology often differs significantly from the original biopsy.[260,261] Lymphocytes and other inflammatory elements are usually decreased with a corresponding increase in RS cells and RS cell variants. Necrosis is often more prominent and the lymphoma is often difficult to subclassify. However, the morphology of the relapsed lymphoma does not predict patient survival after relapse.[260] It should be pointed out that after treatment, involved lymph nodes may be converted to fibrous tissue which may persist as a mass, raising the concern of residual disease. A stable residual mass post-therapy often does not contain any tumor and a biopsy may need to be performed to determine its nature.[262]

In the era of curative therapy for HD, the extent of disease at autopsy is much reduced compared with earlier times. The extent of involvement is still related to the original histologic subgroup, with lymphocytic predominance type showing the least and lymphocytic depletion type showing the most extensive involvement.[261] Oropharyngeal and meningeal involvement is more frequently found with patients with short survival, while spinal, peripheral nerve, female genital tract, and breast involvement is more frequently found in autopsies of longer-term survivors. Vascular invasion at the time of diagnosis is correlated with increased extranodal involvement at autopsy. The histologic appearance of the tumor is often altered in treated patients, with a decrease in lymphocytes and inflammatory cells giving rise to a more monomorphic proliferation of RS cells and variants at autopsy. Focal sclerosis is often observed.

Differential diagnosis

A variety of reactive and neoplastic proliferation may simulate HD. Since HD possesses such a wide variety of morphologic appearances, it would be helpful to consider the differential diagnosis for each subtype of HD.

The nodular variety of L&H HD may be confused with follicular hyperplasia or a follicular center cell lymphoma.[101] The nodules in HD are large and contain small round lymphocytes, variable numbers of histocytes and L&H variants. Most reactive follicles are smaller and contain numerous follicular center cells without a histiocytic component aside from tingible body macrophages. Typical L&H cells are not observed. PTGC may resemble the nodules in L&H HD, and they sometimes coexist in the same lymph node. Focal aggregates of follicular center cells can still be found in PTGC while typical L&H cells are absent. Furthermore, only scattered PTGC are observed among typical reactive follicles, whereas the nodules in L&H HD usually predominate in the involved region of the lymph node and L&H cells are detectable in the internodular areas. The neoplastic follicles of a follicular center cell lymphoma contain mostly follicular center cells rather than small lymphocytes and typical L&H cells are not present.

The diffuse variety of L&H HD may be confused with a small lymphocytic, a diffuse mantle cell or a T-cell rich B-cell lymphoma. A small lymphocytic lymphoma generally has well-defined pseudofollicular centers and the large cell in the lymphoma is quite distinctive from L&H cells. They are smaller, with a regular, round-to-oval nucleus containing a prominent central nucleolus and a small to moderate amount of basophilic cytoplasm. The small lymphocytes in a mantle cell lymphoma are considerably more irregular than those seen in L&H HD. Large cells are very infrequent or absent. In both of these NHLs, histocytes are generally not a significant component. Immunohistochemically, the small lymphocytes are mostly B-cells, sometimes with paradoxical CD43 expression. If frozen tissue is available, CD5 expression and monoclonality can be readily demonstrated. T-cell rich B-cell lymphoma may present a diagnostic dilemma. In some cases, the large B-cells do not resemble L&H cells, making a diagnosis of L&H HD unlikely, whereas in other cases, the large cells bear some resemblance to L&H cells (Fig. 42-65). In the latter situation, several morphologic features are useful in the differential diagnosis. The small lymphocytes in T-cell rich B-cell lymphoma show a considerable degree of pleomorphism in some cases and are often almost exclusively T-cells. Vasculature can also be very prominent in T-cell rich B-cell lymphoma. Immunohistochemistry may be helpful when the morphology is equivocal. If a significant proportion of T-cells in the lesion are $CD57^+$, it favors the diagnosis of L & H HD, while monoclonality of the B-cell population demonstrated immunohistochemically or by Southern blot analysis, confirms the diagnosis of T-cell rich B-cell lymphoma.

HD, NS type frequently presents as a mediastinal mass in a young female. Mediastinal large-cell lymphoma is also prevalent in this population. The morphologic distinction between the two can be very difficult, especially in small biopsy specimens, which are quite often crushed and distorted due to the accompanying fibrosis. An adequate rebiopsy of the largest mass should be performed if the initial specimen is inadequate. Almost all mediastinal large-cell lymphomas are of B-cell lineage, whereas most NSHD would have an immunohistochemical pattern characteristic of HD ($CD20^-$, $CD15^+$, $CD30^+$). A strong clonally-rearranged IgH band in Southern analysis supports the diagnosis of a B-cell lymphoma.

The syncytial variant of NSHD may be mistakenly diagnosed as a large-cell lymphoma, a metastatic carcinoma, melanoma, or even a seminoma or vice versa. The diagnosis of HD is suggested when some areas with the typical morphology of NSHD is present. If the entire biopsy specimen is composed of syncytial aggregates of large pleomorphic cells, the suspicion of HD is raised when at least some of the cells show typical features of lacunar cells such as hyperlobation of the nucleus, a low N/C ratio, and a clear or pale staining cytoplasm.

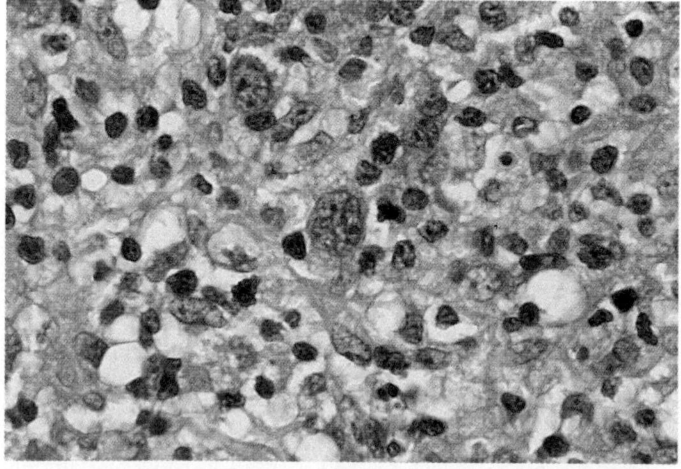

Fig. 42-65 T-cell rich B-cell lymphoma. In this case, the large neoplastic B-cells bear some resemblance to L&H Reed-Sternberg variants.

Diagnosis is especially difficult in B5-fixed tissue. A panel of monoclonal antibodies may be helpful in the differential diagnosis (Table 42-6).

Peripheral T-cell lymphoma may be confused with HD, especially the MC type, as it can have a polymorphic background with large cells resembling RS cells. In general, vascular proliferation is more prominent in T-cell lymphomas and there are many pleomorphic small and medium-sized lymphoid cells in addition to large cells. Immunohistochemical studies performed on paraffin tissue may be helpful. The authors have not seen definite staining of RS cells with anti-CD43 or anti-CD45R0, whereas, CD15, 30 and 74 are frequently positive. In most reported series, clonal T-beta gene rearrangement cannot be detected in HD. The demonstration of clonal T-beta gene rearrangement, especially with a strong signal would very much favor the diagnosis of a peripheral T-cell lymphoma.

Some reactive conditions may have immunoblasts with prominent nucleoli resembling RS cells (Fig. 42-66). HD is an unlikely diagnosis without the proper milieu. Difficulties may arise when cells resembling RS cells occur in a polymorphic infiltrate. Reactive conditions, but not MCHD, are often accompanied by many typical immunoblasts. RS cells often react with both anti CD15 and CD30, but not with anti CD20 or CD3, an unlikely pattern for immunoblasts. Furthermore, the clinical history may also suggest a reactive condition such as a drug reaction or a viral infection.

It has been pointed out that a significant proportion of LDHD may, in fact, represent NHL. Aside from peripheral T-cell lymphomas as discussed earlier, anaplastic large-cell lymphoma[166] and occasionally immunoblastic lymphoma of the plasmacytoid (IBL-PC) type may cause confusion with HD. IBL-PC may have many large cells with very prominent nucleoli that resemble RS cells but it is generally more monomorphic with few background small lymphocytes and other reactive elements. Phenotypically, the cells are B-cells with clonal Ig gene rearrangement and/or expression. Anaplastic large-cell lymphomas may be related to HD, but there are a number of clinical, morphologic, and immunophenotypic differences that allow the differentiation between the two in most cases (Table 42-7).

Immunophenotyping

HD, L&H type with a nodular growth pattern is immunophenotypically distinctive. The nodules contain a dense network of follicular dendritic cells and many small IgM^+, IgD^+ B-lymphocytes.[263,264] Interestingly, the T-cells in the nodules are mostly $CD4^+$, $CD57^+$ cells, resembling T-cells seen in normal germinal centers.[264] The L&H cells react with antibodies against CD45, CD20, CD74 and CDW75 in paraffin-embedded tissues[7,264-267] and CD22 in tissue specially processed to preserve more labile antigens (Fig. 42-67). Furthermore, the J-chain of multimeric immunoglobulins have been demonstrated in the L&H cells of many cases[264,268] and individual cells contain either kappa or lambda light chain, but not both.[264] These findings suggest that the L&H cells are derived from the B-cell lineage and the immunoarchitecture of the lesion is very similar to that of progressively transformed germinal centers.

The relationship of the nodular and the diffuse type is still somewhat controversial. Cases with nodular areas coexisting

Table 42-6 Immunohistochemical profile useful in the diagnosis of an anterior mediastinal tumor

	Hodgkin's disease*	Mediastinal LCL	Seminoma	Thymoma	Metastatic carcinoma	Metastatic melanoma
Tumor cells						
Paraffin section						
CD45	–	+	–	–	–	–
CD20 L26	–	+	ID	–	–	–
LN1	+/–	+/–	ID	ID	+/–	ID
LN2	+	+	ID	ID	+/–	ID
CD15	+	ID	ID	ID	+/–	ID
CD30	+	–	–	–	–	–
Cytokeratin	–	–	–	+	+	–
S-100	–	–	–	–	–	+
Frozen section						
B-cell markers:						
(CD19, 20, 22)	–	+	–	–	–	–
Monotypic Ig	–	+/–	–	–	–	–
T-cell markers:						
(CD2, CD3, TCAR)	–	–	–	–	–	–
Small lymphocytes†						
CD1	–	–	–	+	–	–
TdT	–	–	–	+	–	–

*Lymphocyte predominant type of Hodgkin's disease has a different immunophenotypic profile.
†This should be assessed in areas away from thymic tissue.
+/–, Some cases positive; +, all or majority positive; –, all or majority negative; *TCAR,* T-cell antigen receptor; *ID,* insufficient data

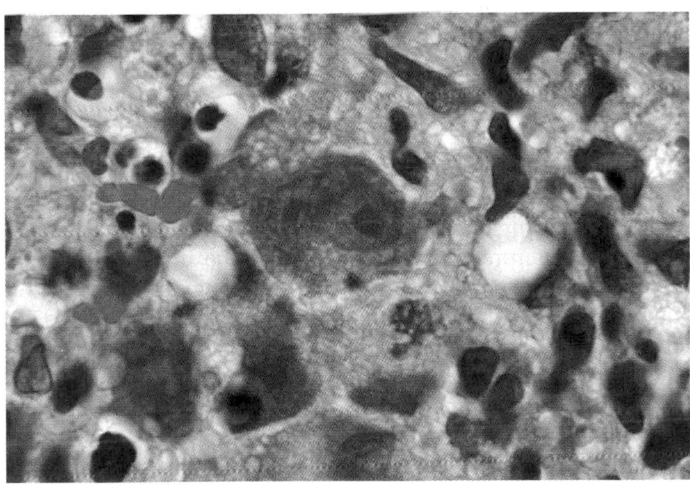

Fig. 42-66 A case of infectious mononucleosis with large pleomorphic cells resembling RS cells and RS variants.

Table 42-7 Features useful in differentiating Hodgkin's disease and anaplastic large cell lymphoma

Feature	HD	ALCL
Morphology		
Sinusoidal infiltration	–	+
Cohesive clusters	–	+
Immunohistochemistry		
CD45	–	+/–
CD43	–	+/–
CD30	+	+
CD15	+	+/–
EMA	–	+
Clinical		
Extranodal presentation	–	+/–
Molecular		
t(2;5)	–	+/–
Tβ rearrangement	–	+/–

+, Frequently observed; +/–, observed in some; –, infrequent

with diffuse areas can be seen, suggesting that some diffuse cases may be derived from an initially nodular growth. Primary diffuse variants may also exist,[269] but it is not clear whether a primary diffuse growth represents just a different growth pattern from the nodular type or a basically different entity. It is also possible that the diffuse subtype is heterogeneous, with some cases being the diffuse counterpart of the nodular type and other cases representing distinct entities. Immunohistochemically, the follicular dendritic cell networks are small and ill defined in the diffuse variant.[263] The number of small B-lymphocytes is much diminished but there are still many small $CD4^+$ and $CD57^+$ T-cells present.[269] The L&H cells are less consistently $CD20^+$.[263,270]

In formalin-fixed, paraffin-embedded sections, the RS cells and variants of the other histologic types of HD are frequently CD15 and CD30 positive (Fig. 42-68), but the usually employed T- and B-cell markers such as CD45RO (UCHLI), CD43 (L60, Leu 22, MT1), polyclonal anti-CD3, CD20 (L26), and CDw75 (LN-1) are generally negative.[2,3,5,7,265,266,271,272] The small lymphocytes are predominantly T-cells except in

Table 42-10 Recommended guidelines for investigation of patient with Hodgkin's disease

Recommended
- History and examination
  - B symptoms: weight loss >10% during previous 6 mo, documented fever, night sweats
- Radiology
  - Plain chest radiograph
  - CT thorax
  - CT abdomen and pelvis
  - Bipedal lymphogram
- Hematology
  - Full blood count*
  - Lymphocyte count*
  - Erythrocyte sedimentation rate*
  - Bone marrow biopsy†
- Biochemistry
  - Tests of liver function*
  - Albumin, LDH, calcium*
- Under special circumstances
  - Ultrasound scanning
  - Magnetic resonance imaging
- Other imaging techniques
  - Isotope scanning
  - Gallium
  - Technetium

Both CT abdomen and pelvis and bipedal lymphogram not usually required.
*Do not determine stage: may not influence management.
†Not for stage IA or IIA with "favourable features."
(From Lister TA et al: *Semin Oncol* 17:696, 1990)

of a parenchymal organ by a lymph node is not considered dissemination and the disease stage is not altered but a suffix "E" should be added to indicate extranodal involvement. Hematogenous spread to distant organs are more commonly observed in MC and LD forms of HD.[178,323] Liver involvement is always accompanied by disease in the spleen and it is postulated that splenic involvement allows ready access to the hematogenous route and facilitates widespread dissemination. However, infiltration of the spleen is not a necessary prelude to hematogenous dissemination. Vascular invasion in lymph nodes has been observed in tissue sections, and it has been suggested that this finding is associated with a higher incidence of distant dissemination probably via the hematogenous route.[324]

While advanced disease is more common in MC and LD HD, splenic and abdominal lymph node involvement are not uncommon in patients with the NS and LP subtypes.[325] Abdominal disease tends to involve paraaortic and splenic hilar lymph nodes. Mesenteric lymph node involvement is uncommon. Patients with NSHD have a high frequency of mediastinal involvement and neighboring pulmonary tissue may be infiltrated.[325,326] It is rare to find HD presenting in an extranodal organ and disseminated involvement of parenchymal organs liver: (5% to 10%) and bone marrow (5% to 15%) is also infrequent at presentation.[327]

There is no general agreement on the use of staging laparotomy.[327,328] Detection of splenic and upper abdominal lymph node involvement by various radiological methods is still quite inaccurate and staging laparotomy has been shown to change the clinical stage in 35% to 40% of patients.[327] However, for an individual patient, staging laparotomy is useful only when the information obtained from the more accurate staging would alter the treatment plan. Otherwise, the added morbidity, possible long-term complications and cost do not justify the procedure. For example, a patient with LP or NSHD and clinical stage IA disease affecting high cervical lymph nodes has little chance of subdiaphragmatic disease and a staging laparotomy is of little value. Most patients with clinical stage IVB & IIIB disease would require chemotherapy and a staging laparotomy seldom downstage the disease sufficiently to warrant treatment with radiotherapy alone.[329] There is some evidence that stage IIIA disease limited to the upper abdomen (Stage III_1A) has a better disease-free and overall survival than

Table 42-11 Clinical and pathologic findings of Hodgkin's disease by subclassification

					Symptoms		Pathologic stage (Ann Arbor)			
Histology	No.	M	F	Mean age (range)	A	B	I	II	III	IV
LP	34	26	8	30.9 (9-64)	31	3	11	13	8	2
NS	397	203	194	27.9 (2-73)	255	142	29	196	120	52
NSCP	63	43	20	34.4 (8-69)	41	22	5	34	21	3
MC	146	106	40	32.1 (4-71)	97	49	21	43	56	26
LD	9	7	2	33.9 (13-61)	5	4	0	5	1	3
Uncl.	10	8	2	31.6 (13-51)	6	4	2	4	3	1
TOTAL	659	393	266	29.7 (2-73)	435	224	68	295	209	87

From Colby TV et al: *Cancer* 49:1848, 1981.

disease with involvement of the lower abdomen (Stage III_2A) when treated with radiotherapy. This difference is not apparent with more aggressive treatment. In this situation, it is important to determine the stage if radiotherapy alone is considered.

Treatment and prognosis

Radiotherapy has been employed to treat patients with HD since the 1920s. The earlier machines could only deliver kilovolt energy beams and damage to superficial tissues limited the dosages and the field that could be irradiated. Despite these limitations, Peters and co-workers reported a 51% 5-year survival and a 35% 10-year survival for all patients but those with advanced disease were all dead by 10 years.[330] With the availability of megavoltage machines, increased experience of treating these patients and knowledge of adverse factors that would require modification of therapy, curative radiotherapy can be delivered with less complications and greater efficacy.[178] Adequate radiotherapy incorporates the concept of extended field irradiation to treat not only involved nodal groups but also lymph node groups likely to be involved from our knowledge of the pattern of spread of HD from the initial site of involvement. In general, patients with pathologic stage I, II and some with stage IIIA, can be adequately treated with radiotherapy. Exceptions include patients with a large mediastinal mass (defined as greater than one-third of the maximum intrathoracic diameter of a regular PA film) which has a high incidence of relapse after standard radiotherapy. Patients with clinical stage IIB disease, spleen showing greater than four separate sites of involvement, stage III_2A disease, pathologic stage IIB subdiaphragmatic disease and patients with systemic symptoms including both weight loss and fever may not be adequately treated with radiotherapy alone. Based on the knowledge gained from previous studies with laparotomy staged patients, it is possible to design radiotherapy on patients with good prognostic factors based on clinical stage alone.[331,332] Such predictions are, of course, not always accurate but relapse after radiotherapy can usually be effectively salvaged by multiagent chemotherapy with no adverse effect on overall survival.[333]

Disseminated disease cannot be adequately treated with radiotherapy. Early trials using nitrogen mustard, or another alkylating agent,[334,335] often gave a good initial response but the disease invariably relapsed. Other single agents similarly failed to achieve lasting remissions. The success of the National Cancer Institute trial using a four-drug combination regimen: mechlorethamine, vincristine, procarbazine and prednisone (MOPP) drastically changed the prognosis of advanced stage HD with about half of the patients achieved a failure-free-survival at 5 years.[336] A number of different MOPP variants have been introduced but the most widely employed alternative regimen is the one introduced by Bonadonna and colleagues containing doxorubicin, bleomycin, vinblastine, and dacarbazine (ABVD).[337] ABVD is as effective, if not more so, than MOPP,[338] but it has also been argued that the apparent superior results from ABVD may be due to the more frequent acute toxicity of MOPP leading to dosage reduction and consequent reduced therapeutic efficacy.[339] ABVD contains non-crossreacting drugs and may be used for therapy in cases of failure of response to MOPP. It has also been suggested that the use of alternate cycles of non-crossreacting regimens may reduce the likelihood of developing tumor resistance. This has led to trials of regimens alternating MOPP with ABVD. A recent trial has shown that MOPP-ABVD combination is no more effective than ABVD alone.[338] More studies need to be performed to determine the place of such alternating regimen in the treatment of HD.

Combined modality therapy (the combination of radiotherapy and chemotherapy) is the treatment of choice in some situations such as in patients with bulky mediastinal disease and in many pediatric patients, to decrease the complications of full-dose radiotherapy and to avoid staging laparotomy.[340]

In a survey of hospitals in the USA with cancer programs approved by the Cancer Commission of the American College of Surgeons,[341] the overall 10-year survival rate for HD patients was 51.5% (65.4% if deaths unrelated to HD were excluded). It is apparent that the stage of the disease and the age at diagnosis have major impacts on survival (Fig. 42-71).

Currently, about 20%-30% of patients will fail to achieve a complete remission or will relapse after treatment.[333] Of these, only about half will achieve a durable second remission on treatment.

As mentioned earlier, HD relapsing after radiotherapy can generally be salvaged by one of the standard chemotherapy regimens such as MOPP, with 5-year freedom from second relapse of 60% to 80%.[333] Those who relapsed after chemotherapy with a complete remission (CR) of 1 year or longer before relapse have a much better prognosis than those with shorter remissions. However, salvage chemotherapy often fails to achieve a lasting CR even in the former group of patients.[333,339] This has led to the use of high-dose chemotherapy combined with autologous bone marrow or peripheral blood stem cell transplantation (ABMT/PSCT) in patients who relapsed after chemotherapy.[342] For patients with poor prognostic features such as a first remission interval of less than one year, B symptoms at first relapse, relapse after stage IV disease and, the third or later relapses and patients who fail to achieve a complete remission with standard chemotherapy, high-dose chemotherapy with ABMT/PSCT may give the best chance of a long-term survival. However, the result achievable is still very dependent on patient selection and those with drug sensitive disease and good performance status at the time of transplantation are more likely to have a lasting CR.[342]

For the group of patients with AIDS and HD, the lymphoma tends to be at an advanced stage with systemic symptoms at presentation. The disease is more prone to involve extranodal sites and the course is much more aggressive. The patient generally requires treatment with chemotherapy due to advanced disease but the compromised immune system makes infectious complications more likely. Survival is short with a median of around 14 months.[343]

It is not clear whether cases of LPHD behave similarly to other types of HD. Some studies have found that patients with lymphocyte predominance generally have a very slow course of disease, with single or multiple relapses, independent of stage or treatment and equally distributed up to 10 years after initial therapy, unusual behavior for classical HD.[344-346] However, other investigations have not found a unique behavior for this subtype.[347]

Complications of treatment

Modern radiochemotherapy for HD is associated with significant acute and late complications.[348-352] The acute toxicity of multiagent chemotherapy is much more pronounced compared with radiotherapy and is dependent on the dose and drug com-

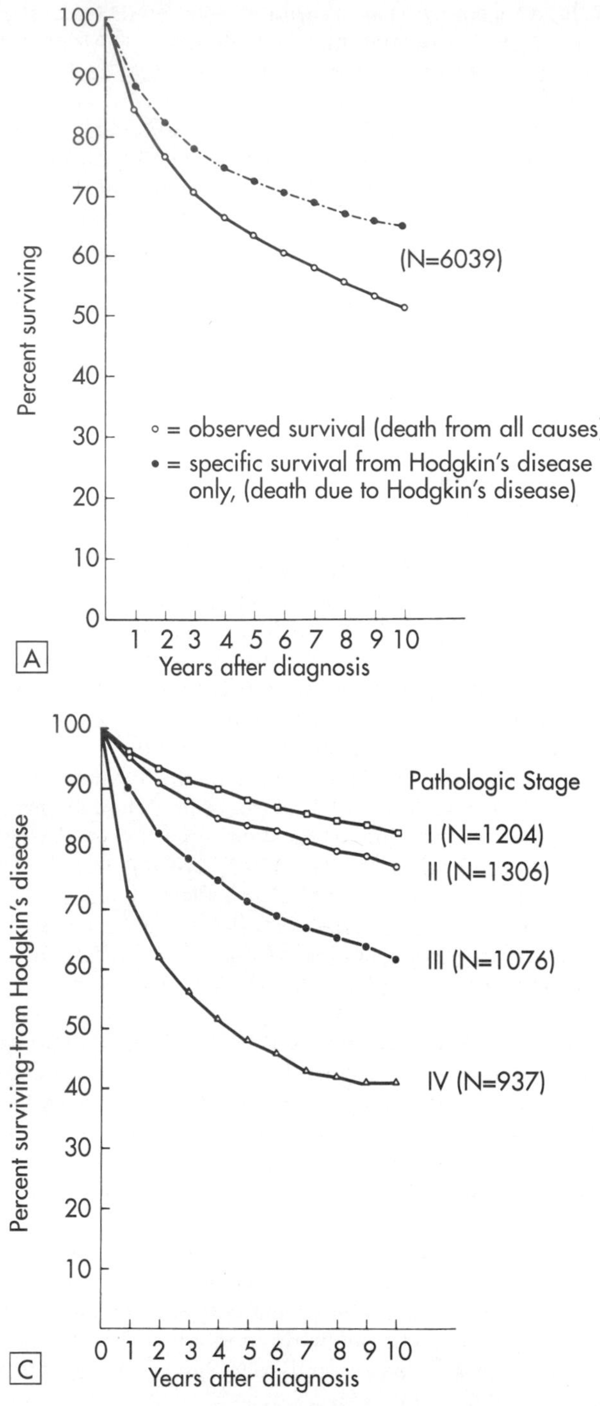

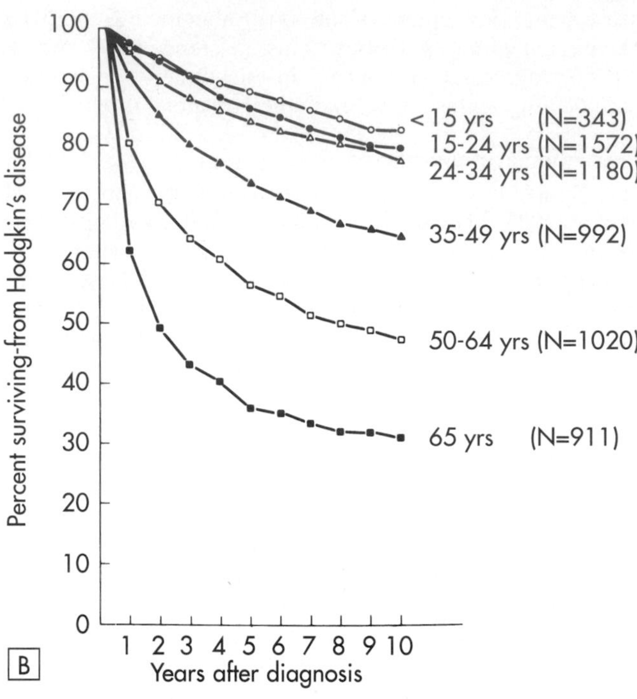

Fig. 42-71 **A,** Ten-year survival of patients with Hodgkin's disease. **B,** Ten-year survival by age at diagnosis, specific to Hodgkin's disease only. **C,** Ten-year survival by pathologic stage, specific to Hodgkin's disease only (Kennedy BJ et al: *Cancer* 56:2547, 1985.)

bination used. Chemotherapy is associated with nausea, vomiting, and temporary alopecia. Bone marrow suppression is dose dependent but the duration of cytopenia may be reduced with the administration of cytokines. Neurotoxicity could be troublesome but reversible in Vinca alkaloid-containing regimens.

One of the most serious complications of therapy for HD is the development of a second malignancy. Acute nonlymphocytic leukemia (ANLL) shows a peak incidence between 3-9 years (mean 76 months) after the diagnosis of HD. It is uncertain whether there is still an excess of cases after 10 years. Radiotherapy alone gives rise to little or no increase in the incidence of ANLL. Chemotherapy regimens containing alkylating agents and nitrosourea are leukemogenic and the risk increases with the length of administration but it is still unclear whether the combination of radiotherapy and chemotherapy is worse than chemotherapy alone. It has been suggested that patients with age >40, prior splenectomy or extensive (total or subtotal) nodal irradiation when combined with chemotherapy, have an increased risk of developing ANLL,[350] but these risk factors need further substantiation.[351,352]

The incidence of NHL is increased in patients with HD, especially the LP subtype.[351-354] There is no clear association with specific types of therapy. It is possible that the development of NHL is part of the natural course of HD or the underlying immunocompromised state predisposes to the development of the second lymphoma. B-cell lymphomas predominate,[351,352,354] but T-cell lymphomas have been reported.[355]

Carcinomas and sarcoma are also increased in HD, usually with a long latency and showing an increase in incidence with time.[350,351] Tumors with the most striking increase are those from the salivary gland, thyroid gland, and soft tissue, but the most common tumors are carcinomas from the lung, gastrointestinal tract, skin, and soft tissue sarcomas. Radiation probably plays an important role in the pathogenesis in these tumors and many of them arise in radiation fields. Smoking may be a cofactor in the development of lung cancer. Patients who subsequently develop thyroid carcinomas and soft tissue or bone sarcomas are significantly younger at the time of diagnosis of HD.

Permanent sterility is an important complication in male patients treated with MOPP. Although female patients may suffer from transient amenorrhea and premature menopause, fertility is much less affected and children from treated patients appear to have no increase in incidence of congenital anomalies or abnormalities in postnatal development.[350]

Other complications include the development of subclinical (with increased level of thyroid stimulating hormone) and clinical hypothyroidism in patients with the thyroid included in the irradiation field. The incidence of pulmonary and cardiovascular complications postirradiation is dependent on the radiation dose, dose rate, and the volume of tissue irradiated. Symptomatic complications are nowadays infrequent. Acute radiation pneumonitis usually develops in 2 to 3 months and usually subsides without specific treatment or with a tapering course of steroid therapy. Chronic restrictive pulmonary fibrosis may manifest 9 to 12 months after treatment and most cases are mild. Bleomycin is the drug most commonly associated with pulmonary toxicity which is dose related. Nitrosourea may also cause pulmonary fibrosis. Acute pericarditis occurs most commonly between 5 to 9 months after radiotherapy. It may be asymptomatic but severe cases require reduction of the effusion, steroid treatment or even pericardiectomy. Chronic constrictive pericarditis may develop 53 to 124 months after radiotherapy. Although cardiac failure post radiotherapy is rare, laboratory evidence for functional impairment is common. Doxorubicin is cardiotoxic but seldom causes clinical symptoms if the cumulative dose is below 400 mg/m^2. Radiation damage to the heart and some other drugs, such as cyclophosphamide potentiate the cardiac toxicity of doxorubicin. Accelerated coronary atherosclerosis, thrombosis of the internal carotid artery, and aortic regurgitation due to endocardial fibrosis have also been attributed to irradiation damage.

Laparotomy with splenectomy predisposes the patient to overwhelming sepsis when infected with encapsulated bacteria such as *S. pneumonia* and *H. influenzae*. Intensive therapy, by depressing the titers of protective antibodies, potentiate the risk. This complication is especially likely to occur in young children, and splenectomy should be avoided in this age group if possible.[356] Multivalent pneumococcal vaccine may be useful in prophylaxis against strept pneumonia infection in splenectomized patients. Failure may be due to an inadequate antibody response or infection with organisms of serotypes not included in the vaccine.[348]

Treatment administered to children may have additional effects on growth and development. Radiotherapy affects bone growth and if a significant portion of the spine is included in the radiation field, the child would have stunted growth. Growth of other bones may be affected depending on the radiotherapy applied. Avascular necrosis of bone, most commonly affecting the femoral head, is an uncommon complication of chemotherapy containing steroids. This complication is not limited to any age group but the potential impact would be greatest in children.

NON-HODGKIN'S LYMPHOMA

Non-Hodgkin's lymphomas are defined as all malignant lymphomas other than Hodgkin's disease. The vast majority of NHLs represent B-, and less commonly, T-lineage neoplasms. Rare cases do not express B- or T- lineage makers and are termed null-cell, and extremely rare neoplasms may be of true histiocytic lineage.

Approximately 40,000 new cases of NHLs will be diagnosed in the United States during 1995, accounting for approximately 3% of all cancers and cancer deaths.[182] The overall male: female ratio is about 1.3:1, and the median age at presentation is about 55 years. However, NHL is a relatively common cancer in children, and is the third most common cause of cancer death in this age group. Whites are more commonly affected than nonwhites. The incidence of NHL is somewhat higher in North America than in Europe and South America, and much higher than in Asia (with the notable exception of Israel, which has an incidence rate similar to North America.)[357] Europe has a much lower incidence of follicular lymphoma than in the United States, and Asia has a lower incidence of B-cell lymphomas in general. NHLs are relatively more common in patients with immunodeficiencies, both inherited and acquired (such as HIV-associated and after transplantation).

Since 1970, there has been a documented increase in the incidence of NHLs, at the rate of 3% to 4% per year, occurring in both sexes, in all racial groups, both within and outside of the United States, and in all age groups except the youngest.[357] Some of the increase within the United States may be due to the increase in the HIV-associated population. Data have been presented linking exposure to hair dyes, herbicides, and organic chemicals.[358-360] In general, low doses of radiation do not predispose to the development of NHLs. HTLV-1 virus has been found to be the etiologic agent of a distinct subset of NHL called adult T-cell leukemia/lymphoma.[361] EBV is associated with some types of NHL, including many lymphoma arising in patients with immunodeficiency, endemic Burkitt's lymphoma, and some types of T-cell lymphoma, especially angiocentric T-cell lymphomas arising in the upper respiratory tract.[362,363]

Henry Rappaport devised the first modern classification system for NHLs, recognizing that lymphomas with a nodular pattern behave differently than those with a diffuse pattern and that cell type also affects prognosis.[364] Lukes and Collins and the original Kiel classification pioneered by Lennert and colleagues introduced the first biologically relevant classification systems.[365,366] Other classification systems soon followed. In 1982, a large National Cancer Institute sponsored study of the classifications of NHLs devised a Working Formulation for Clinical Usage as a means of translation among the various systems (Table 42-12).[367] However, it was found to be practi-

Table 42-12 Working formulation of non-Hodgkin's lymphomas for clinical usage

Low grade
A. Small lymphocytic
Consistent with CLL, plasmacytoid
B. Follicular predominantly small cleaved cell
Diffuse areas, sclerosis
C. Follicular mixed small cleaved and large cell
Diffuse areas, sclerosis
Intermediate grade
D. Follicular predominantly large cell
Diffuse areas, sclerosis
E. Diffuse small cleaved cell
Sclerosis
F. Diffuse mixed, small and large cell
Sclerosis, epithelioid cell component
G. Diffuse large cell
Cleaved cell, noncleaved cell, sclerosis
High grade
H. Large cell, immunoblastic
Plasmacytoid, clear cell, polymorphous, epithelioid cell component
I. Lymphoblastic
Convoluted, nonconvoluted
J. Small noncleaved cell
Burkitt's, follicular areas
Miscellaneous
Composite, mycosis fungoides, histiocytic, extramedullary plasmacytoma, unclassifiable, other

From *Cancer* 49:2112, 1982.

Table 42-13 Updated Kiel classification of non-Hodgkin's lymphomas

B-cell	T-cell
Low grade	
Lymphocytic—chronic lymphocytic and prolymphocytic leukemia; hairy cell leukemia	Lymphocytic—chronic lymphocytic and prolymphocytic leukemia
Lymphoplasmacytic/cytoid	Lymphoepithelioid
Plasmacytic	Angioimmunoblastic
Centroblastic/centrocytic	T zone
Centrocytic	Pleomorphic, small cell
High grade	
Centroblastic	Pleomorphic, medium and large cell
Immunoblastic	Immunoblastic
Large cell anaplastic	Large cell anaplastic
Burkitt lymphoma	
Lymphoblastic	Lymphoblastic
Rare types	Rare types

From Stansfield AG, Diebold J, Kapanci Y et al: *Lancet* 1:292, 1988.

cal and clinically relevant as a classification system in its own right and is the classification system for NHLs most used in the United States today. It listed major categories of lymphomas based upon purely morphologic criteria, grouped into three histologic grades: low, intermediate, and high. It must be kept in mind that the grading system was based on the treatment of patients by protocols carried out in the 1970s. Treatments have dramatically improved, blurring the differences in the current overall survival between the three groups. The revised Kiel classification has also utilized a grading system, separating B- and T-cell lymphomas into lymphomas of low and high grade (Table 42-13).[368] Recently, another classification based upon discrete clinicopathologic entities organized within a biologic framework has been proposed (Table 42-14).[369] However, it does not attempt to grade lymphomas, and its clinical relevance is at this time still untested.

Patients with NHL are staged by the Ann Arbor staging system similar to HD.[319] However, it is not as useful in NHLs as it is for HD, since NHLs spread in a much more unpredictable way than in HD.[370] Age, bulk of disease, performance status, number of extranodal sites of disease, and the involvement of certain sites such as the central nervous system are all important determinants of prognosis in addition to grade and stage.[371] Most NHLs present in lymph nodes, but there is a much higher incidence of extranodal involvement than in HD. In certain lymphomas such as small, noncleaved cell lymphoma and lymphoblastic lymphoma, extranodal presentation such as the gastrointestinal tract and the thymus, respectively, are more common than nodal presentations. In addition, involvement of Waldeyer's ring lymphoid tissue is much more common in NHLs than in HD.[372]

Virtually all malignant lymphomas are monoclonal populations of B- or, less commonly, T-lymphocytes. Therefore, they usually show monoclonal rearrangements of the immunoglobulin heavy and light chain genes or T-cell receptor genes, respectively (Table 42-15) (Figs. 42-72 and 42-73). A common theme in the pathogenesis of many types of NHL is the presence of characteristic translocations. Typically, a cellular oncogene is translocated to adjacent to one of the antigen receptor genes, leading to deregulation of the oncogene (Table 42-16). Overexpression of the protein coded by the oncogene generally leads to a proliferative advantage for the affected cells. Other genetic events such as mutations in additional oncogenes or tumor suppressor genes give the cell the full neoplastic phenotype and determine the ultimate aggressiveness of the lymphoma.

In the following sections, major subtypes of NHL are discussed. Rather than following the Working Formulation, the discussion is organized by clinicopathologic entities, with references to the corresponding category or categories in the Working Formulation. A single lymphoma subtype is usually present in a given patient. Rarely, two distinctly different and well demarcated types of lymphoma are present in a single specimen; this situation has been termed *composite lymphoma*. A more common occurrence is the appearance of two different subtypes of lymphoma in separate sites, termed discordant lymphoma. This usually manifests as the occurrence of an intermediate grade lymphoma in a lymph node biopsy, with a low grade lymphoma present in the bone marrow. In these cases, the same clone of tumor can usually be demonstrated by immunologic or molecular studies, despite the differences in morphology.

Small lymphocytic lymphoma

Small lymphocytic lymphoma is defined as a diffuse B-cell lymphoma with the morphologic features of small, mature lymphocytes. It is a low grade malignant lymphoma in the Working Formulation.[367] There is an arbitrary distinction between small lymphocytic lymphoma and chronic lymphocytic leukemia,

Table 42-14 Lymphoid neoplasms recognized by the International Lymphoma Study Group

B-cell neoplasms
I. Precursor B-cell neoplasm: B-precursor lymphoblastic leukemia/lymphoma
II. Peripheral B-cell neoplasms
  1. B-cell chronic lymphocytic leukemia/prolymphocytic leukemia/small lymphocytic lymphoma
  2. Lymphoplasmacytoid lymphoma/immunocytoma
  3. Mantle cell lymphoma
  4. Follicle center lymphoma, follicular
     Provisional cytologic grades: small cell, mixed small and large cell, large cell
     Provisional subtype: diffuse, predominantly small cell type
  5. Marginal zone B-cell lymphoma
     Extranodal (MALT type +/– monocytoid B-cells)
     Provisional category: Nodal (+/– monocytoid B-cells)
     Provisional category: Splenic (+/– villous lymphocytes)
  6. Hairy cell leukemia
  7. Plasmacytoma/myeloma
  8. Diffuse large cell B-cell lymphoma
     Subtype: primary mediastinal (thymic) B-cell lymphoma
  9. Burkitt lymphoma
  10. Provisional category: High-grade B-cell lymphoma, Burkitt-like

T-cell and putative NK-cell neoplasms
I. Precursor T-cell neoplasm: T-precursor lymphoblastic lymphoma/leukemia
II. Peripheral T-cell and NK-cell neoplasms
  1. T-cell chronic lymphocytic leukemia/prolymphocytic leukemia
  2. Large granular lymphocyte leukemia (LGL)
  3. Mycosis fungoides/Sézary syndrome
  4. Peripheral T-cell lymphoma
     Provisional subtypes: medium-sized cell, mixed medium and large cell, large cell, lymphoeithelioid cell
  5. Angioimmunoblastic T-cell lymphoma (AILD)
  6. Angiocentric lymphoma
  7. Intestinal T-cell lymphoma (+/– enteropathy associated)
  8. Adult T-cell lymphoma/leukemia (ATL/L)
  9. Anaplastic large cell lymphoma (ALCL), $CD30^+$, T- and null-cell types
  10. Provisional subtype: Anaplastic large-cell lymphoma, Hodgkin's-like

Unclassifiable
1. B-cell lymphoma, unclassifiable (low grade/high grade)
2. T-cell lymphoma, unclassifiable (low grade/high grade)
3. Malignant lymphoma, unclassifiable

From Harris NL, Jaffe ES, Stein H et al: *Blood* 84:1361, 1994.

Table 42-15 Non-Hodgkin's lymphomas and typical pattern of gene rearrangements

	Ig heavy	Ig light	T beta
Most B-cell lymphomas	100%	100%	5-10%
B-lymphoblastic	100%	40%	20-30%
Peripheral T-cell lymphoma	5-10%	<1%	90%
T-lymphoblastic	20-30%	1%	90%

which appear to represent two clinical syndromes, but one biologic disease. One working group has recommended designating cases as chronic lymphocytic leukemia if patients have greater than 5,000/mm^3 circulating lymphocytes and greater than 30% lymphocytes in the bone marrow,[373] but the specific criteria used for differentiation can vary.

Small lymphocytic lymphoma constitutes approximately 5% of all NHLs.[367] This lymphoma has the highest median age at presentation of any of the major categories of NHL, at about 60 years, and is rare in childhood. Patients usually present with generalized lymphadenopathy.[374,375] B symptoms are infrequent, and serum gammopathy is usually not present. Patients are found to have stage IV disease in over 80% of cases. This is usually the result of marrow involvement, present in about 70% of cases at presentation, but involvement of the liver and spleen is also common, and usually evident on physical examination. The disease generally follows an indolent course, even in untreated patients. Involvement of the peripheral blood in patients without such involvement at presentation occurs in about 10% to 20% of patients. In about 10% of cases, there is transformation to a large cell lymphoma (Richter's syndrome).[376] Rarely, there is transformation to HD.[251,253]

Involved lymph nodes usually show diffuse effacement of architecture (Fig. 42-74).[377] In many cases, extensive infiltration of perinodal adipose tissue is present. A minority of cases show subtotal involvement of the lymphoid, with sparing of follicles or sinuses. About one-third to one-half of cases show vague pale areas, termed proliferation centers (pseudofollicles, growth centers), although a distinct follicular pattern is not seen. Proliferation centers are even more common in cases associated with a peripheral lymphocytosis, found in about three-quarters of these cases.[378,379]

autoantigens and not *H. pylori,* it is has been found that non-neoplastic T-cell are activated by the bacteria. This may lead to the production of cytokines by the T-cells, stimulating a B-cell proliferation.[400]

In general, extranodal marginal zone lymphoma has an excellent prognosis, when localized. Patients with marginal zone lymphoma of gastric origin have been successfully treated by antibiotic therapy to eradicate *H. pylori,* with regression of the lymphoma.[401] Patients with nodal marginal zone lymphoma as well as patients with extranodal disease that eventually disseminates to systemic sites have indolent, but incurable disease, similar to other low-grade lymphomas. Involvement of the bone marrow or peripheral blood, and particularly the development of large cell lymphoma, are adverse prognostic signs.[396]

Mantle cell lymphoma

Mantle cell lymphoma (centrocytic lymphoma, intermediately differentiated lymphocytic lymphoma, mantle zone lymphoma, germinocytoma) is a low to intermediate grade lymphoma composed of small- to medium-sized lymphocyte with a mature chromatin pattern and slightly irregular nuclear membranes.[402] Before their proper recognition, most cases were probably classified as intermediate grade, diffuse small cleaved cell type in the Working Formulation.

The epidemiology of mantle cell lymphoma is not well delineated since it has only been fully clarified as a discrete entity relatively recently. It constitutes approximately 5 to 10% of NHLs in the United States, and may be more common in Europe.[367,376] It appears to be most frequent in the older population, and is rare in children. There is a male:female ratio of about 2:1. Patients usually present with generalized lymphadenopathy, and most patients are found to be in stage IV. Bone marrow involvement at presentation is found in about one-third of patients. Other sites of frequent involvement include spleen, Waldeyer's ring, and peripheral blood. Gastrointestinal tract involvement may manifest as multiple polypoid masses (lymphomatous polyposis). A small proportion of cases may transform to a high-grade lymphoma, termed the blastic variant of mantle cell lymphoma, although patients may also present de novo with this variant.[403] Transformation to large cell lymphoma does not commonly occur.

Architecturally, several patterns may be seen. Usually, there is diffuse effacement or, at most, a vaguely nodular appearance. Another common pattern of involvement is as a broad and expansile mantle around reactive germinal centers (mantle zone pattern); this pattern may be seen focally or exclusively (Fig. 42-80). Finally, there may be complete replacement of follicles including both the follicular center and mantle, yielding a pseudofollicular appearance. Generally, fibrosis and necrosis is not found in this lymphoma.

Cytologically, the lymphoma is composed of a homogeneous population of lymphoid cells that are the same size or slightly larger than normal small lymphocytes (Fig. 42-81). The nuclear membranes are usually slightly irregular and indented, but not usually as irregular as the small cleaved cells of follicular lymphoma; however, some cases have been reported in which predominantly round nuclei are found. The chromatin is generally mature, but slightly more dispersed than usually found in normal small lymphocytes. Nucleoli are generally inconspicuous, and when present, are not large. Cytoplasm is scant. Cases of the blastic variant contain cells with nuclei that are slightly larger that have a very fine chromatin pattern, more closely resembling the lymphoblasts of lymphoblastic lymphoma. The mitotic rate is high in the blastic variant, but is usually less than 20 per 10 high-power fields in the majority of cases. Large lymphoid cells and immunoblasts are not generally a part of this tumor. The tumor cells are present admixed with small, round lymphocytes which represent a host infiltrate. In addition, scattered epithelioid histiocytes may be found.

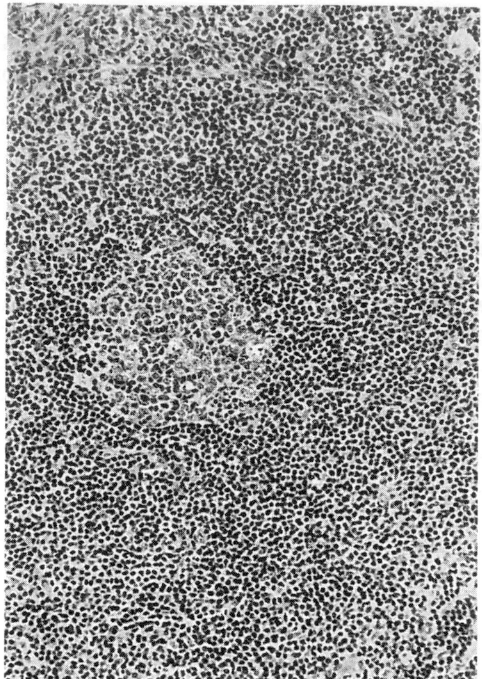

Fig. 42-80 Mantle cell lymphoma. A mantle zone pattern is demonstrated.

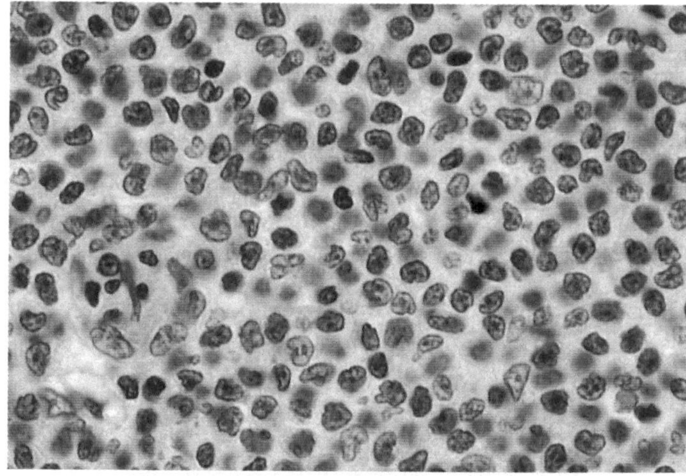

Fig. 42-81 Mantle cell lymphoma. There is a monotonous population of small lymphocytes with a mature chromatin pattern and slightly irregular nuclear outlines.

The neoplastic cells of mantle cell lymphoma are invariably of B-lineage, expressing the B-cell marker CD20 in addition to leukocyte common antigen (CD45) in paraffin sections.[383] There is usually coexpression of the T-cell/myeloid marker

CD43. In frozen sections, the cells express monoclonal surface immunoglobulin, usually IgM and also often IgD. Unique among B-cell lymphomas, there is a slight predilection for lambda light chain. Residual germinal centers are polyclonal. There is expression of the pan-B-cell markers CD19, CD20, and CD22, and in contrast to small lymphocytic lymphoma, CD23 is negative. CALLA (CD10) may be positive or negative. Similar to small lymphocytic lymphoma, there is usually aberrant coexpression of the T-lineage marker CD5. Stains for follicular dendritic cells demonstrate a prominent but disrupted pattern.

Classical cytogenetics can detect a t(11;14)(q13;q32) in approximately 50% of cases of mantle cell lymphoma.[404] This translocation can also be detected by Southern blotting. Molecular studies have demonstrated that the t(11;14) involves juxtaposition of the *bcl*-1 locus on the long arm of chromosome with the an immunoglobulin heavy chain gene enhancer sequence.[405] Although the chromosome breakpoints are found in a wide variety of sites along chromosome 11q13, more than 80% are clustered in a specific region known as the major translocation cluster. Almost all of the translocations in the major translocation cluster occur within a 300 bp segment amenable to detection by the polymerase chain reaction.[406]

The *bcl*-1 translocation results in deregulation and overexpression of the PRAD1/cyclinD1 (CCND1) gene, which codes for a cell-cycle protein that is not normally expressed in lymphoid cells.[407] This overexpression is thought to perturb the G_1-S transition of the cell cycle, leading to uncontrolled mitotic cycling of t(11;14)-carrying cells at a point in differentiation when B-cells need to exit from the cell cycle to become resting lymphocytes or differentiate into IgM-secreting plasma cells.[402,407] Additional genetic events may occur subsequent to this defect, leading to full tumor development.

Tentatively, mantle cell lymphoma is regarded by most hematopathologists to be an intermediate grade lymphoma.[402,403] The median survival is about 4 to 5 years, but unlike most other intermediate grade lymphomas, patients are usually not cured by chemotherapy, and show a continual drop-off in the survival curve over time, without a plateau. Patients whose tumors show a predominantly mantle zone architecture may have a better prognosis, while the presence of a high mitotic rate predicts a worse prognosis.[408] The blastic variant of mantle cell lymphoma has a poor prognosis more similar to high grade lymphomas, whether it occurs de novo, or as a transformation of preceding mantle cell lymphoma of usual type.

Follicular lymphoma

Follicular lymphoma is a low to intermediate grade lymphoma that shows a follicular architecture and represents the neoplastic counterpart of germinal center B-lymphocytes.[367] There are three major variants recognized, the predominantly small cleaved cell variant, the mixed small cleaved and large cell variant, and the predominantly large cell variant, defined by the cytologic characteristics of the proliferating cells. The predominantly small cleaved cell variant and the mixed small cleaved and large cell variant are recognized as low-grade lymphomas in the Working Formulation, while the predominantly large cell variant is regarded as an intermediate grade lymphoma.[367]

Follicular lymphoma is a relatively common lymphoma in the United States, representing approximately 40% of cases of NHL. The small cleaved cell variant accounts for about two-thirds of cases of follicular lymphoma, while the mixed small cleaved cell and large cell and predominantly large cell variants constitute approximately 25% and 10% of cases, respectively. Follicular lymphoma is less common in Europe and Asia, constituting approximately 20% and 10% of all NHLs, respectively.[367,409] In the Working Formulation study, the mean age of patients with follicular lymphoma was approximately 55 years. Follicular lymphoma is very uncommon under the age of 40 and extremely rare in childhood.[410] Similar to most NHLs, the male-to-female ratio is about 1.3:1.

Patients most often present with one or several enlarged lymph nodes, but are found to have stage IV disease in about two-thirds of cases, usually due to bone marrow involvement. Splenic and hepatic involvement are also common at presentation. Despite the widespread disease, patients usually have an indolent course with slow progression.[411] Occasional cases of spontaneous regression occur, although the disease usually returns. Over time, there is a tendency to transform to a higher-grade lymphoma, usually diffuse large cell lymphoma; this eventually occurs in about 30% to 40% of cases.[412]

On histologic examination, a follicular architecture is seen which may be present through the involved tissue or may be focal (follicular and diffuse) (Fig. 42-82). The neoplastic follicles are usually densely packed, with little intervening interfollicular area, and typically of relatively uniform size. Mantle zones are usually absent, but may be retained, usually as a thin rim.

Cytologically, several different types of follicular lymphoma are recognized. In the most common variant, the small cleaved cell type, a relatively homogeneous population of small lymphoid cells with irregular, often elongated, nuclei with coarse chromatin and indistinct nucleoli (termed small cleaved cells or centrocytes) is present, without the usual mixture of larger germinal center B-cells, tingible-body macrophages, and follicular dendritic cells (Fig. 42-83). Occasional larger cells are almost always present, but constitute a clear minority. Mitotic figures are usually not numerous in this subtype.

In the mixed, small cleaved cell and large cell variant, there is a second population of large cells (two to three times the diameter of normal lymphocytes) with vesicular nuclei (Fig. 42-84). These large cells have been separated into cleaved cells and noncleaved cells. Cleaved cells (also termed *centro-*

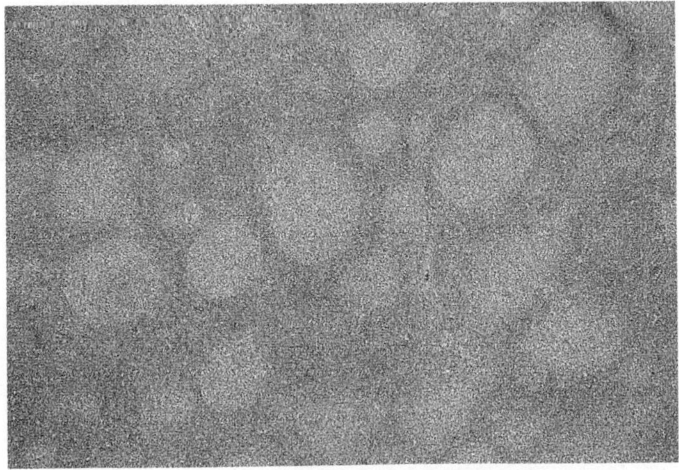

Fig. 42-82 Follicular lymphoma. Many crowded nodules of relatively even size and lacking well-defined mantle zones are present.

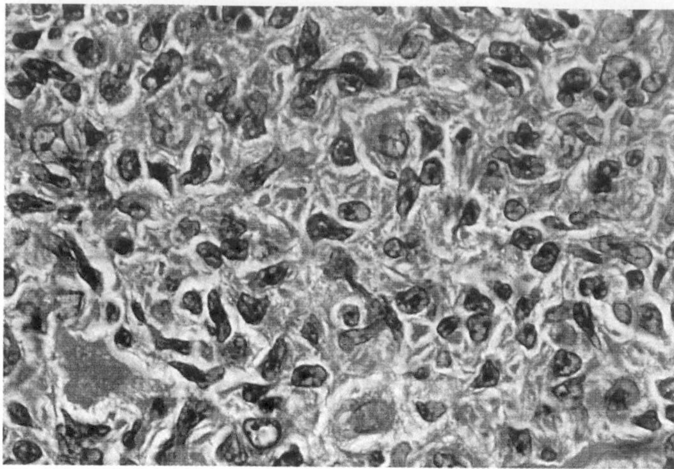

Fig. 42-83 Follicular, predominantly small cleaved cell lymphoma. There is a monotonous population of small cells with contorted nuclear outlines (cleaved cells).

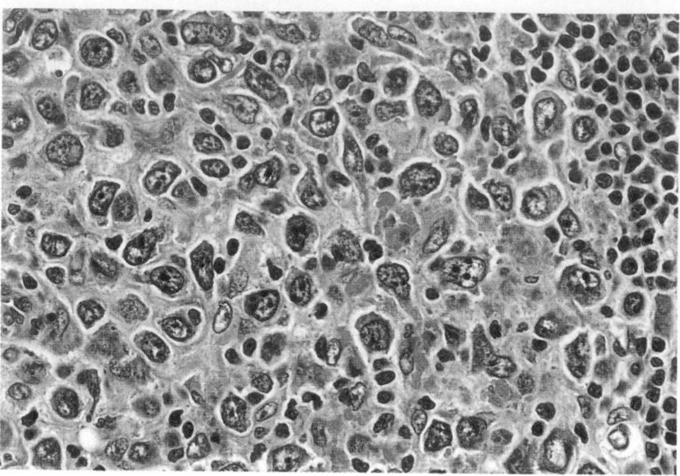

Fig. 42-85 Follicular, predominantly large cell lymphoma. Large noncleaved cells predominate.

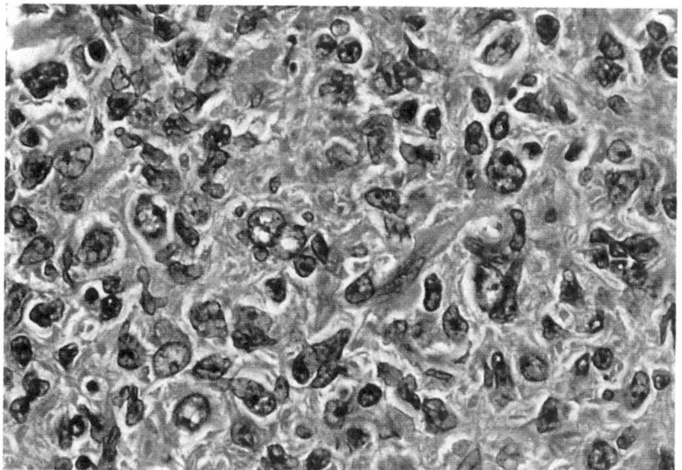

Fig. 42-84 Follicular, mixed small cleaved and large cell lymphoma.

cytes) have irregular nuclear membranes, lack discernable nucleoli, and usually have minimal cytoplasm. Noncleaved cells (also termed centroblasts) usually have rounded nuclear outlines, possess round to oval nuclei that contain one to three nucleoli, often apposed to the nuclear membrane, usually situated at the short axis of the oval nucleus. A rim of amphophilic or basophilic cytoplasm is usually present. In the mixed variant of follicular lymphoma, there is no clear preponderance of small or large cells over the other.

In the predominantly large cell category, the majority of neoplastic cells within the follicles are large cells, although large noncleaved cells usually predominate (Fig. 42-85). Mitotic figures may be numerous in this subtype. Although not present in all follicular lymphomas, many contain areas with diffuse effacement of architecture. These areas are more common in cases with a higher percentage of large cells, and tend to show sclerosis.

There is no uniform method used to separate the three cytologic types of follicular lymphoma. Most hematopathologists make the distinctions arbitrarily, with the predominantly small cleaved cell type diagnosed when there are greater than 75% small, cleaved cells, the mixed type diagnosed when there are between 25% and 75% large cells, and the predominantly large cell type diagnosed when there are greater than 75% large cells.[413] Mann and Berard proposed counting large noncleaved cells per high-power field (×10 eyepiece and ×40 objective), with predominantly small cleaved cell type diagnosed when there are 0 to 5 large cells, the mixed type diagnosed when there are between 6 and 15 large cells, and the predominantly large cell type diagnosed when there are greater than 15 large cells per high-power field.[414] In general, there is poor reproducibility in the cytologic divisions among different observers.

At times, the neoplastic cells in follicular lymphomas can take on unusual appearances. Rarely, neoplastic cells may contain clear or eosinophilic cytoplasmic inclusions, imparting a signet-ring-like appearance (Fig. 42-86).[415] In other rare cases, cells with cerebriform nuclei (more typical of mycosis fungicides) may be found instead of the usual cleaved cells.[416] The neoplastic cells may rarely have a fine, chromatin appearance, suggestive of a more blastic lymphoma.[417] Another unusual manifestation is the presence of plasmacytoid differentiation in the neoplastic population.[418] Finally, another rare appearance is the presence within the neoplastic follicles of a uniform population of small, round lymphocytes similar that seen in small lymphocytic lymphoma, without a population of cleaved cells.[419]

All follicular lymphomas are B-lineage neoplasms; moreover, over 90% express surface or cytoplasmic immunoglobulins with light chain restriction.[420] IgM with or without IgD is the most common heavy chain isotype, but IgG and, most rarely, IgA may be expressed. In addition, the neoplastic cells are usually $CD10^+$, and virtually always $CD5^-$ and $CD43^-$. *Bcl*-2 protein, a protein demonstrable in paraffin sections, is positive in approximately 80% to 90% of cases (Fig. 42-87).[75,421] Monoclonal antibodies against CD35 and CD21 demonstrate a rich and organized network of follicular dendritic cells in the neoplastic follicles, analogous of that observed in reactive follicles. In addition, scattered T-lymphocytes, mostly T-helper cells, are present in the follicles. Numerous T-cells are present in the interfollicular areas.

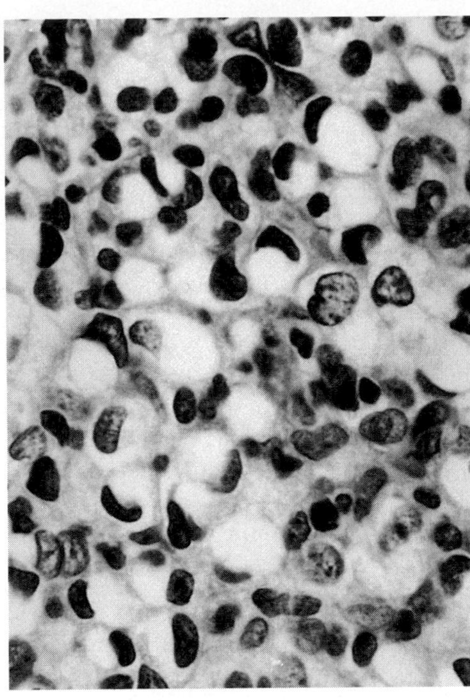

Fig. 42-86 Follicular lymphoma, signet ring cell type. There are numerous clear cytoplasmic vacuoles, many of which are indenting the nucleus.

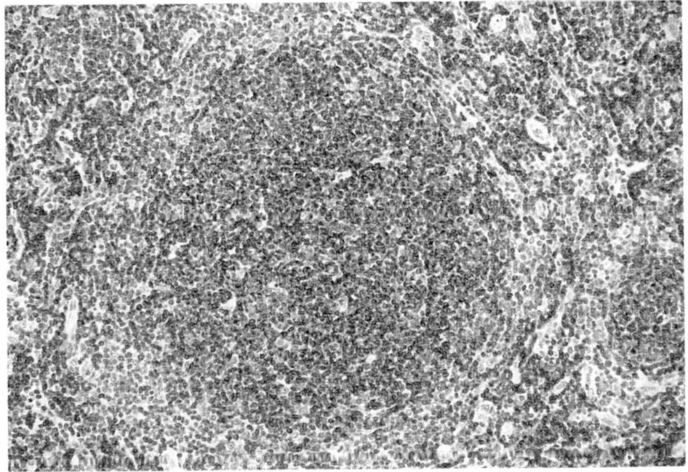

Fig. 42-87 Follicular lymphoma, *bcl-2* stain. Cytoplasmic *bcl-2* staining is present in the neoplastic follicles.

Classical cytogenetics has demonstrated that a t(14;18)(q32;q21) occurs in 80% to 90% of cases of follicular lymphoma (Fig. 42-88).[422] Molecular studies have demonstrated that the *bcl*-2 gene on chromosome 18 is translocated to the joining region of the immunoglobulin heavy chain gene, suggesting an error at the time of somatic recombination, early in B-cell differentiation.[423] At the molecular level, the exact breakpoints on chromosome 18 are clustered at several loci. Approximately 50% to 60% of translocations occur at the major breakpoint region (mbr), and about 10% to 20% of translocations occur at the minor cluster region (MCR).[424] Thus a limited number of primers and probes can be used to perform polymerase chain reaction assays or Southern blot

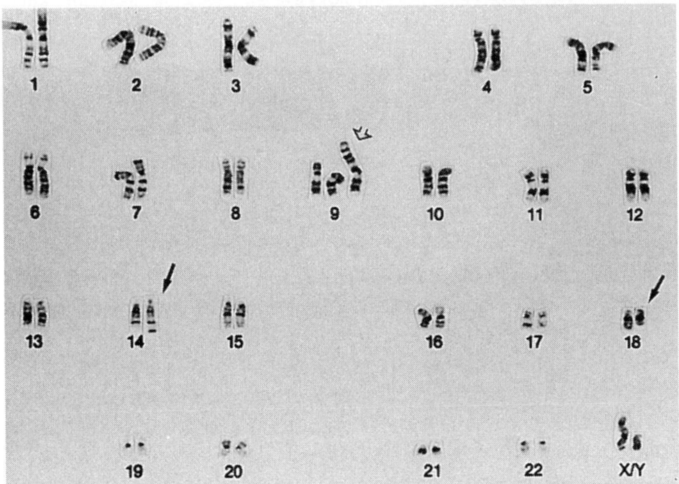

Fig. 42-88 Follicular lymphoma. This karotype shows a t(14;18)(q32;q21). In addition, there is a der(9)t(1;19)(q21;p22).

hybridization that will detect a majority of the translocations. These assays, particularly polymerase chain reaction studies, can be used for initial diagnosis, staging, assessment of residual disease following therapy, and the assessment of occult disease during clinical remission.

The *bcl*-2 gene is an integral membrane protein that inhibits apoptosis (programmed cell death).[9,425] Present in a wide variety of cell types of fetal and adult tissues, *bcl*-2 protein is thought to be of physiologic importance in morphogenesis and in preventing long-lived postmitotic and stem cells from undergoing programmed cell death. As a result of the t(14;18), the *bcl*-2 gene becomes deregulated and expressed in abnormally high levels. In follicular lymphoma, *bcl*-2 may act by providing an abnormal pool of long-lived cells at risk for secondary genetic abnormalities. Transgenic mice with the fusion *bcl*-2/immunoglobulin heavy-chain gene overexpress *bcl*-2 in lymphoid tissues, leading to polyclonal follicular lymphoproliferations of non-cycling B-cells.[426] Genomic events additional to the t(14;18), including abnormalities of chromosome regions 1p21-22, 6q23-26, and the short arm of chromosome 17 determine the biological aggressiveness of a given follicular lymphoma.[427] Mutation of the tumor suppressor gene p53 has been demonstrated in 25% to 30% of the intermediate-to high-grade lymphomas that arise as a transformation of follicular lymphoma, suggesting that p53 mutation is associated with progression in follicular lymphomas.[428,429] In these cases, immunohistochemical studies carried out on the antecedent follicular lymphomas have demonstrated a rare population of p53 positive cells, suggesting that it is these cells that give rise to the transformed lymphoma.[428] A smaller subset of cases of progressed follicular lymphomas have acquired abnormalities of the *myc* gene.[430]

The low-grade follicular lymphomas are rarely cured by conventional therapies.[412] Therefore, mild chemotherapeutic regimens are generally used. There is also a role for radiation therapy in follicular lymphoma. In relatively asymptomatic patients, a trial of no therapy may be undertaken, with the understanding that treatment will probably be required as the disease progresses. Once conversion to diffuse large cell lymphoma occurs, the prognosis is poor. Experimental therapies such as monoclonal antibodies and particularly bone marrow transplantation represent promising areas for possible disease eradication. The intermediate-grade follicular lymphoma, follicular predominantly large cell lymphoma, is generally treated more aggressively, with more intensive chemotherapeutic regimens that include anthracycline, since these patients may enjoy sustained remissions.[431]

Besides the cytologic characteristics of the follicular lymphoma, the degree of follicular architecture may also be a prognostic factor. One study found that the low-grade follicular lymphomas with a predominantly follicular pattern had a significantly longer survival than patterns with greater than 25% diffuse areas.[432] A significantly worse prognosis has been found in follicular, mixed small cleaved cell and large cell lymphomas with a diffuse component greater than 75% as compared to cases with a greater degree of follicularity.[433] Similarly, increasing areas of diffuse histology predicts a worse survival in follicular large cell lymphoma.[431] Although the presence of absence of a t(14;18) has no correlation with clinical outcome, the presence of a higher percentage of cells with abnormal metaphases, and a number of chromosomal breaks higher than 6 are associated with a poor survival.[427] Chromosomal breaks at either 6q23-26 or 17p are independent poor prognostic factors; the presence either abnormality is also significantly associated with transformation into a diffuse large cell lymphoma.

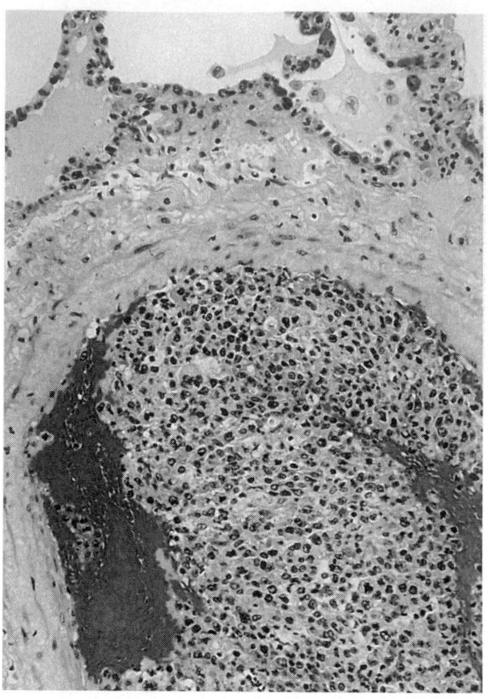

Fig. 42-89 Lung with intravascular large cell lymphoma. The lymphoma is entirely intraluminal, with no extension into the wall or adjoining pulmonary parenchyma.

Diffuse mixed, diffuse large cell, and large cell immunoblastic lymphomas of B lineage

Diffuse mixed small cleaved and large cell lymphoma, diffuse large cell lymphoma, and large cell immunoblastic lymphoma of B lineage are all B-lineage lymphomas with a significant component of large lymphoid cells. Large cells are larger than the nuclei of histiocytes and generally have a vesicular chromatin pattern. Diffuse mixed lymphoma and diffuse large cell lymphoma are intermediate-grade lymphomas in the Working Formulation whereas large cell immunoblastic lymphoma is of high-grade.[367] Rare cases of anaplastic large cell lymphoma of B lineage are discussed in a subsequent section.

These three lymphoma types constitute approximately 35% of NHLs.[367] They are most common in adulthood, with the median age at presentation about 55 years. However, they occur in all age groups, including the pediatric population in which they constitute one-quarter to one-third of NHLs. There is a slight male predominance. Most patients present without a significant prior history. Some patients have a history of a prior lymphoma, usually follicular lymphoma or small lymphocytic lymphoma, but including a wide variety of types. Some patients have a history of an immune disorder such as a collagen vascular disease or an overt immunodeficiency. Many of these latter lymphomas are associated with EBV (see later section on immunodeficiency-related lymphomas).

Patients generally present with a single, fast-growing mass, usually nodal or extranodal, the latter occurring in about 40% of cases. Neck, axillary, and mediastinal lymph node presentations are relatively common. Common sites of extranodal disease include the gastrointestinal tract, particularly the stomach and small intestine, skin, and Waldeyer's ring, although any organ can be affected. About one-quarter of patients have B symptoms.[434] Approximately 50% of patients have stage III or stage IV disease at presentation. This often manifests as involvement of the liver or spleen. Bone marrow involvement is relatively uncommon, occurring in about 10% to 15% of cases. Similarly, involvement of the peripheral blood is rare.

Partial or complete diffuse effacement of lymph node architecture is almost always seen. Occasionally, areas of follicular involvement may be found, indicating an origin from a follicular lymphoma. Other architectural patterns include a prominent paracortical or sinusoidal distribution (the latter termed *sinusoidal large cell lymphoma*). Rarely, the lymphoma may be present exclusively within vascular spaces in extranodal sites, usually in the skin, lung, adrenal, or central nervous system) designated intravascular lymphoma (also termed *angiotropic lymphoma* or formerly *malignant angioendotheliomatosis*) (Fig. 42-89).[435]

The hallmark of these lymphomas is the presence of a significant component of large lymphoid cells or immunoblasts. Large lymphoid cells have nuclei as least as large as the size of histiocyte nuclei, and usually two to three times larger than a small lymphocyte (Fig. 42-90). The nuclei may be round, oval, or elongated; and may have a round, slightly irregular, or highly irregular nuclear contour (multilobated). The chromatin pattern is usually vesicular, with condensation of chromatin beneath the nuclear membrane. Cytoplasm may be inconspicuous or may be moderate in amount, occasionally with plasmacytoid features. Often, the large lymphoid cells have a close resemblance to the large cleaved and noncleaved cells of follicular lymphoma. The atypical large lymphoid cells are usually pleomorphic within a given case, but may be monomorphic. Immunoblasts generally have large nuclei which have uniformly round to oval nuclear membranes and possess a vesicular chromatin pattern. Characteristically, there is a centrally placed prominent nucleolus, which may be basophilic or eosinophilic (Fig. 42-91). Cytoplasm is generally abundant and may be plasmacytoid, or pale to clear. There is generally a

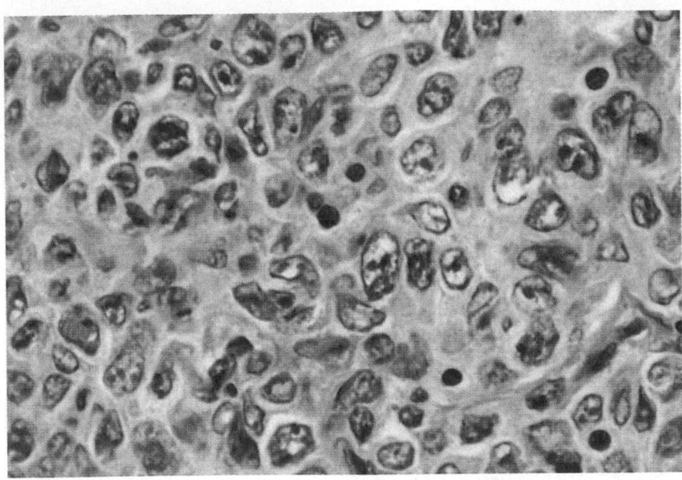

Fig. 42-90 Diffuse large cell lymphoma. Scattered small lymphocytes are present for comparison of nuclear size.

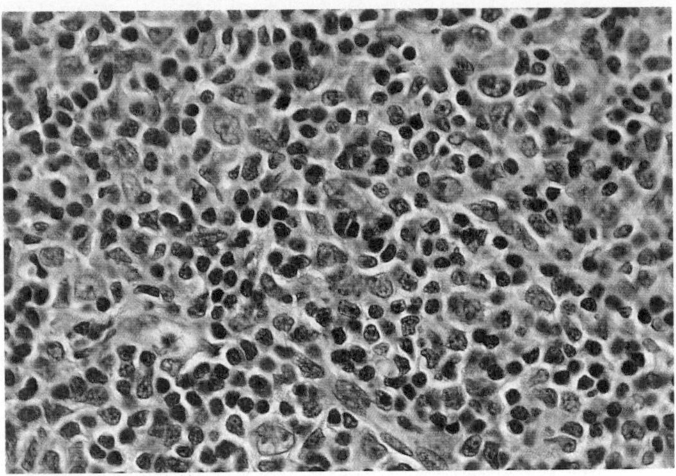

Fig. 42-92 Diffuse mixed small and large cell lymphoma. A relatively even admixture of small and large atypical lymphoid cells is seen.

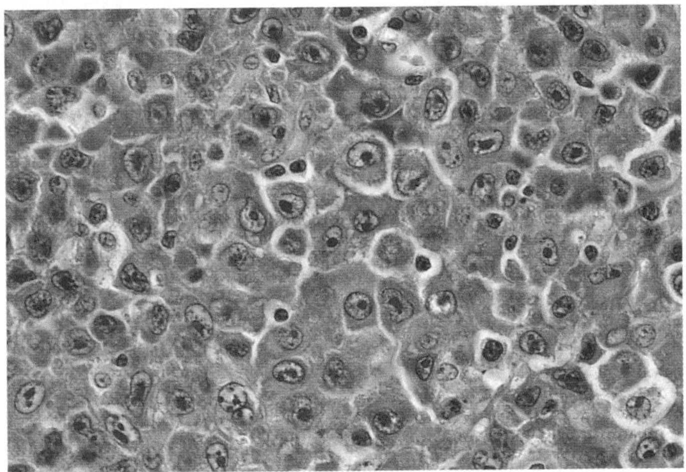

Fig. 42-91 Large cell immunoblastic lymphoma. The cells are large with vesicular nuclei containing a single centrally located prominent nucleolus. The cytoplasm is abundant and shows plasmacytoid features.

greater degree of monomorphism in immunoblastic lymphoma as opposed to large cell lymphoma. In the Working Formulation, a subtype of polymorphous was also included in the category of large cell immunoblastic, but this was intended to encompass cases of peripheral T-cell lymphoma, considered in a separate section of this chapter.

In diffuse mixed lymphoma, there is a significant admixture of small lymphoid cells, such that neither element dominates (Fig. 42-92). The small cells may be truly cleaved and part of the neoplastic process, usually indicating a relationship to follicular lymphoma. In other cases, the small cells may be round and regular. In some of these latter cases, the small, round lymphoid cells are part of the neoplastic process, often a clue to an underlying small lymphocytic lymphoma that is undergoing conversion to a large cell lymphoma (Richter's syndrome). In other cases, the small, round cells can be demonstrated to represent reactive T-lymphocytes, and not part of the neoplastic process. These cases are usually designated T-cell rich B-cell lymphoma;[436] many hematopathologists consider these cases more properly designated as large cell lymphoma with a reactive component, despite the histologic appearance of a mixture of small and large cells (Fig. 42-93). In other cases, histiocytes may predominate, prompting the designation histiocyte-rich B-cell lymphoma.[437] Even in histologically evident diffuse large cell lymphomas, there is usually an admixture of cell types, including small lymphocytes, polyclonal plasma cells, histiocytes, and occasionally eosinophils. Immunoblastic lymphoma tends to have a lesser number of admixed reactive cells, usually histiocytes.

Necrosis may be a focal or prominent feature in large cell lymphomas, usually in the subtype. Sclerosis is also common, either broad fibrous bands, compartmentalizing fibrosis, separating the lymphoid cells into small aggregates which may simulate other neoplasms, or a diffuse sclerosis enveloping individual cells (Fig. 42-94). Sclerosis tends to be less common in the immunoblastic subtype.

Expression of leukocyte common antigen (CD45) is found in over 95% of cases, with most of the negative cases found within the category of plasmacytoid immunoblastic lymphoma.[7] By definition, all of these lymphomas are B-lineage neoplasms, exhibiting expression of the B-cell markers and in paraffin sections, and CD20 in frozen sections.[438] Approximately two-thirds of cases express surface immunoglobulin demonstrable in frozen sections, usually of IgM isotype, although other isotypes may be found. Cases with plasmacytoid features, usually of the immunoblastic subtype, often express cytoplasmic immunoglobulin which may be demonstrated in paraffin sections. Coexpression of the T-cell marker CD5 is found in about 10% of cases, and a similar percentage may show coexpression of the T-cell/myeloid marker CD43, the latter usually found in plasmacytoid immunoblastic lymphoma.[11]

Virtually all cases, including immunoglobulin-negative cases, have detectable clonal immunoglobulin heavy and light chain gene rearrangements. Concurrent rearrangement of the Tβ-cell receptor gene can be found in about 5% to 10% of cases. About 10% to 25% of cases have a rearrangement involving the *bcl*-6 (*laz*-3, *bcl*-5) locus on chromosome 3q27.[439] These cases may be demonstrated by Southern blotting, but

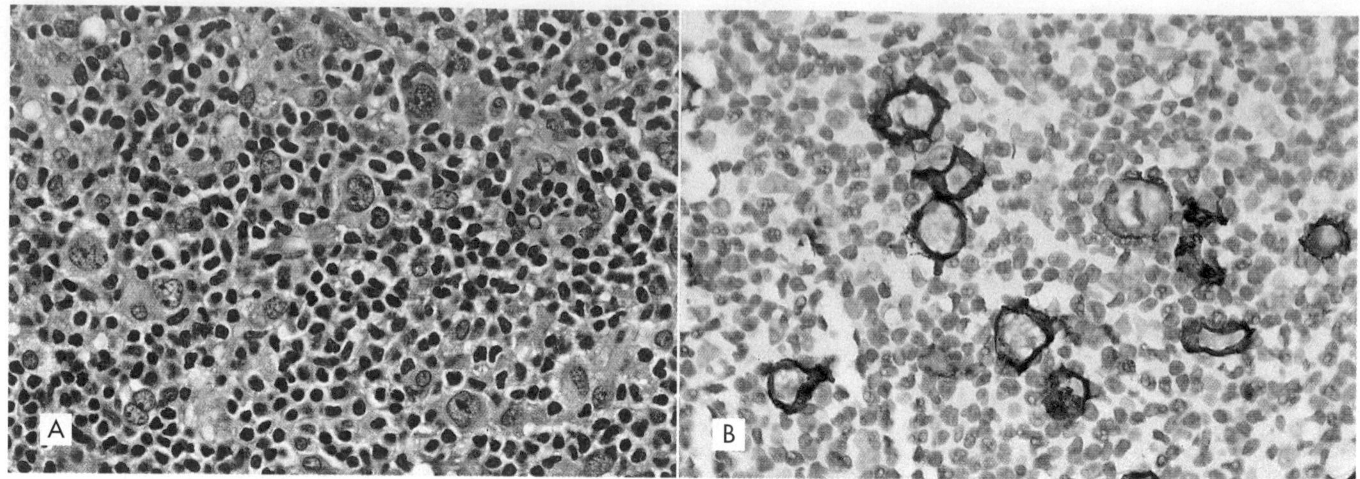

Fig. 42-93 T-cell rich B-cell lymphoma. **A,** A predominantly small cell population is present, with scattered larger cells. **B,** The large cells express the B-lineage marker CD20.

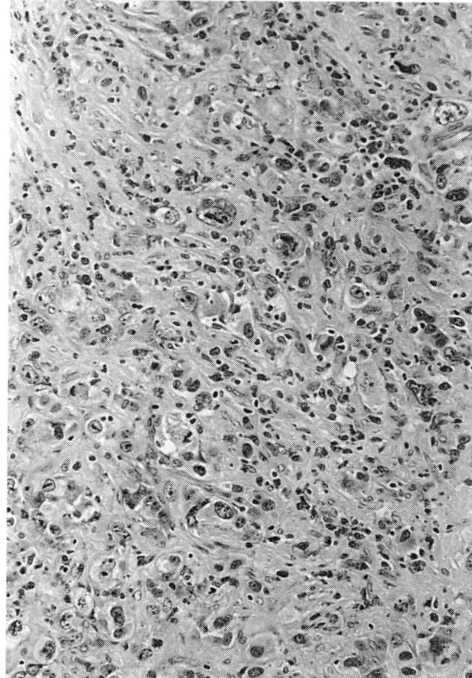

Fig. 42-94 Diffuse large cell lymphoma with sclerosis. Single tumor cells and small nests of tumor cells are embedded in a fibrous stroma containing host cells.

are difficult to detect by classical cytogenetics because of the localization at the tip of the long arm of chromosome.[440] The translocation involves the immunoglobulin heavy chain gene, either light chain gene, or other uncharacterized loci on other chromosomes. The presence of *bcl*-6 rearrangements correlates with clinical presentation at extranodal sites. All lymphomas with *bcl*-6 breakpoints express *bcl*-6 protein in large amounts. The functional of *bcl*-6 protein is not well characterized, but it is a member of the zinc-finger family proteins that regulate differentiation and development.[440A]

Approximately 30% of cases of diffuse large cell lymphoma have evidence for a t(14;18); many of these cases have a previous history of follicular lymphoma.[424] Although p53 mutation is not a common characteristic of de novo diffuse large cell lymphoma, it is seen in about 25% to 30% of cases of diffuse large cell lymphomas that have arisen as a transformation of previous follicular lymphoma, as discussed above in the section on follicular lymphoma.[428,429] Approximately 10 to 20% of cases of diffuse large cell lymphoma have evidence of c-myc rearrangements, including a small subset of cases arising as a transformation of follicular lymphoma.[430]

The large cell lymphomas generally respond well to aggressive chemotherapeutic regimens including multiple drugs, with a remission rate of about 80%, and an overall survival rate of 60%.[441] Those patients who do not achieve complete remission generally die within the first few years, yielding a survival curve with an initially steep decline. However, most of those patients who do achieve successful remission are cured, leading to an eventual plateau in the survival curve over time. In some patients treated for large cell lymphoma, the large cell component may disappear, leaving a low-grade component that may or may not have been initially not evident. There is a role for radiation therapy or surgery in patients with localized disease. There may be a role for high-dose chemotherapy and bone marrow transplantation for patients with relapsed disease.

Although large cell immunoblastic lymphoma was separated from the intermediate-grade large cell lymphomas as a high-grade lymphoma,[367] several subsequent studies have not found significant differences in survival between the two groups.[442] Factors that have been shown to have prognostic significance include stage, age, performance status, number of extranodal sites of disease, and bulk of disease as identified by serum lactate dehydrogenase levels. These factors have been combined into an International Prognostic Index for Aggressive Lymphomas (IPI), an index that is now being widely used to stratify large-cell lymphoma patients before treatment in prospective randomized trials.[371] In some studies, an aberrant immunophenotype, a high proliferative fraction, and a low percentage of $CD8^+$ cells in the reactive component has been correlated with poorer survival.[443-445] In one study, the presence of a *bcl-6* rearrangement is associated better overall survival and survival without disease progression.[439] In addition, the presence of a t(14;18) has been correlated with a shorter survival without disease progression in some but not all studies.

Peripheral T-cell lymphoma (PTCL)

Peripheral T-cell lymphoma (PTCL) (also called *post-thymic T-cell lymphomas*) is defined as a malignant lymphoma derived from T-lymphocytes whose morphologic appearance and immunophenotype are consistent with mature T-cells. Although an immunologic approach is not employed in the Working Formulation, virtually all cases of PTCL would be classified as intermediate to high grade.[446] The term PTCL encompasses several clinicopathologic entities, including mycosis fungoides/Sézary syndrome, adult T-cell leukemia/lymphoma, angioimmunoblastic lymphadenopathy with dysproteinemia (AILD)-like T-cell lymphoma, lymphoepithelioid T-cell lymphoma, angiocentric T-cell lymphoma, intestinal T-cell lymphoma, T-cell lymphoma associated with erythrophagocytosis, hepatosplenic T-cell lymphoma, erythrophagocytic T-gamma lymphoma, and many cases of anaplastic $CD30^+$ lymphoma (covered in a later section).

PTCL is a relatively uncommon lymphoma, accounting for approximately 10% to 15% of all diffuse lymphomas in the United States. It occurs in all age groups, but is most common in the elderly. The male:female ratio is about 3:2.[447-449] It is more common among Asian populations, and is particularly common in areas where HTLV-1 infection is endemic.[450] In these areas, which include the southernmost islands of Japan, the Caribbean, the southeastern United States, equatorial Africa, and possibly Southern Italy, HTLV-1 is the etiologic agent of adult T-cell leukemia/lymphoma. HTLV-1 is a retrovirus which travels by blood transfusion, intravenous drug abuse, from mother to child (probably during breast-feeding), and from male to female via sexual transmission. The virus remains latent for many years, but about 1 in 1000 adult male carriers and 1 in 2000 adult female carriers develop adult T-cell leukemia/lymphoma each year.[451] A minority of PTLD may be associated with Epstein-Barr infection, particularly those developing in the upper respiratory tract, especially the nasal region.[363] These latter cases also appear to be more frequent among Asian populations.

Patients with PTCL may have a history of a prior immune disorder.[447-449] They usually present with generalized lymphadenopathy, and often have skin involvement. Approximately two-thirds of patients present with stage III or IV disease, due to involvement of visceral organs such as bone marrow, spleen, liver and lung. Patients often present with anemia and not uncommonly have systemic "B-type" symptoms. The clinical course is variable, with some having rapidly progressive disease and others following an indolent course.

PTCL are difficult to recognize morphologically, because they can assume a wide variety of histologic appearances.[446,452] They never show a follicular architecture, but may show diffuse effacement, preferential paracortical infiltration, or preferential sinusoidal involvement. The neoplastic population varies widely from case to case. Usually, a mixture of atypical intermediate to large lymphoid cells is seen (Fig. 42-95). The atypical cells often have irregular nuclear contours, which vary from one cell to another, and may include highly pleomorphic forms, including cells with multilobated nuclei (Fig. 42-96). Cells with pale or clear cytoplasm may be a feature of PTCL, but similar cells may found as the neoplastic element of B-cell lymphomas. Typically, there is an admixture of reactive cells, particularly epithelioid and nonepithelioid histiocytes, nonneoplastic small lymphocytes, eosinophils, and polyclonal plasma cells. Often, there is increased vascularity and an unusual prominence of the high-endothelial venules. If categorized according to the Working Formulation, many PTCL would be classified as intermediate grade, diffuse mixed small and large cell or predominantly large cell type, with most others classified as high-grade, large cell immunoblastic type (clear cell or polymorphous subtypes); a small minority might be classified as intermediate-grade, diffuse, small "cleaved" type.

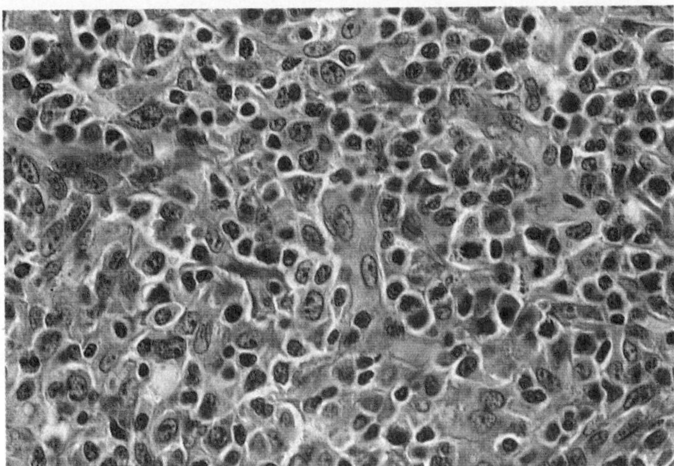

Fig. 42-95 Peripheral T-cell lymphoma. A mixed population is present, including intermediate- to large-sized atypical lymphoid cells. Note the prominent vascularity and presence of eosinophils.

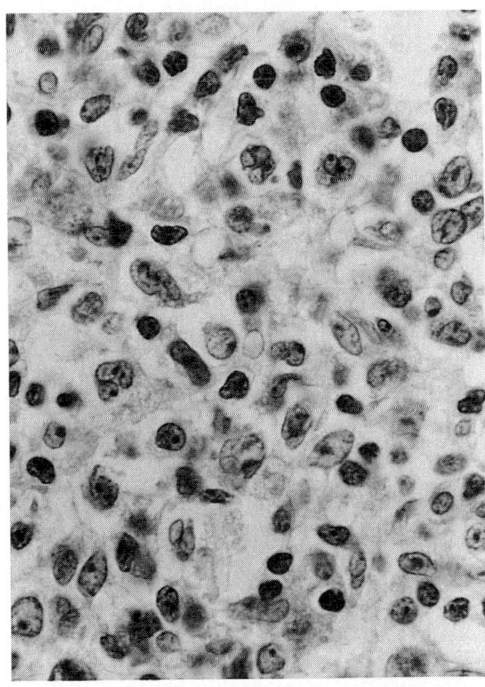

Fig. 42-96 Peripheral T-cell lymphoma. This lymphoma contains a mixed population of small, intermediate, and large atypical lymphoid cells. Many of the large lymphoid cells have hyperlobated nuclear outlines.

In paraffin sections, leukocyte common antigen (CD45) is expressed in about 90 percent of cases.[7] The T-lineage associated antigens CD45R0, CD3, and CD43 (the latter not highly specific) are expressed in 80% to 85% of cases.[3,7] Expression of B-lineage markers in not seen, and, in contrast to T-lymphoblastic neoplasms, terminal deoxynucleotidyl transferase (TdT), is negative. In frozen sections, PTCL usually express the pan–T-antigens CD2, CD3, and CD5, and the majority-cell antigen CD7, although aberrant loss of one or more these antigens is common in individual PTCL.[11,446,453] This aberrant loss of pan–T-antigens is found in about 75% of cases, and may be exploited to distinguish neoplastic from reactive T-cell infiltrates. CD7 is the antigen most frequently absent, followed by CD5, CD3, and CD2. PTCL usually express helper/inducer antigens ($CD4^+$, $CD8^-$), but may be have a cytotoxic/suppressor phenotype ($CD4^-$, $CD8^+$, or more rarely, $CD4^+$, $CD8^+$ or $CD4^-$, $CD8^-$. A subset of T-cell lymphomas expresses the neural cell adhesion molecule N-CAM (CD56).[454] These cases have a predilection for unusual anatomic sites of involvement, particularly the central nervous system.

The large majority of PTCL possess clonal Tβ cell receptor gene rearrangements.[455] Approximately 10% of cases also show clonal rearrangements of the immunoglobulin heavy chain gene. The karyotypes of these neoplasms tend to be complex, with many nonrecurring structural abnormalities.[456] The sites of the T-cell receptor genes show a predilection for involvement, being found in about 5% of cases. Abnormalities of 6q, 1p, and 1q are also more commonly associated with PTCL.

Patients with PTCL are generally treated with the same agents used for diffuse large cell lymphoma. It is a matter of great controversy wither PTCL have a worse clinical outcome than B-lineage neoplasms of similar histologic grade. Multiple studies have been performed, with many studies showing PTCL having a worse clinical outcome than B-lineage neoplasms,[457] and just as many studies showing no significant differences in survival.[458] The latter studies often employ the most aggressive chemotherapeutic regimens, suggesting that these regimens minimize any differences in survival that may naturally exist between the two groups of neoplasms. Some studies suggest that histologic grading of PTCL may have prognostic significance, but stage is a much stronger predictor of outcome.[452]

Adult T-cell leukemia/lymphoma (ATL)

This variant of PTCL is invariably associated with HTLV-1 infection (see above). Patients are usually adults, but tend to be younger than patients with PTLD as a whole.[459] They virtually always present with widespread disease, usually with generalized lymphadenopathy and skin, liver, spleen, and bone involvement. Patients are often hypercalcemic, and characteristic hyperlobated cells are found in the peripheral blood. Histologically, there are no specific features to distinguish ATL from other PTCL, although a high degree of pleomorphism is often seen.[460] Characteristically, cases of ATL are $CD7^-$, and usually $CD25^+$ (IL-2 receptor).[461] By molecular analysis, all cases can be demonstrated to have clonal integration of HTLV-1. Patients with ATL generally have a poor prognosis, with a median survival of less than 1 year.

AILD-like T-cell lymphoma

AILD was described as an atypical lymphoproliferative disorder characterized by a cell-poor diffuse effacement of architecture, numerous arborizing vessels, absence or regression of germinal centers, and often containing intercellular deposits of a PAS-positive amorphous substance.[125,126] Because clonal T-cell populations can often be identified by either Southern blotting or classical cytogenetics in tissues histologically consistent with AILD,[144,148-150] some hematopathologists believe that all cases of AILD actually represent PTCL at inception.[452] Other hematopathologists prefer to retain the concept of AILD and diagnose AILD-like T-cell lymphoma only when clear morphologic evidence of lymphoma is present or when dominant clonal T-cell populations are identified.[141] When the cellularity is increased, and a greater number of atypical cells and immunoblasts are present, particularly cells containing clear cytoplasm and often forming clusters around vessels, the diagnosis of AILD-like lymphoma can generally be made (Fig. 42-97).[462] A proportion of cases of both AILD and AILD-like lymphoma terminate in diffuse large cell lymphoma, of either B- or T-cell phenotype.[145,146] At least some of the B-cell lymphomas have been associated with EBV.[146] In situ hybridization studies of AILD and AILD-like lymphoma have revealed increased numbers of EBV-infected B- and T-cells, probably a result of the decreased cellular immunity present.[463] These cells may eventually give rise to clones which escape immunologic control.

Lymphoepithelioid T-cell lymphoma

This neoplasm, also termed *T-cell lymphoma* with high content of epithelioid histiocytes or Lennert lymphoma, is defined by its characteristic histologic appearance.[464] The lymph node architecture is effaced by a diffuse proliferation in which epithelioid histiocytes, in single cells and in small clusters, dominate (Fig. 42-98). Well-formed granulomas and multinucleated Langhans-type giants cells are usually not present. In the background, there is always a population of small, medium, and large-sized atypical lymphoid cells, representing the neoplastic population, and plasma cells and eosinophils are also usually present (Fig. 42-99). In the Working Formulation, most cases are characterized as intermediate grade, diffused mixed small "cleaved" and large cell.

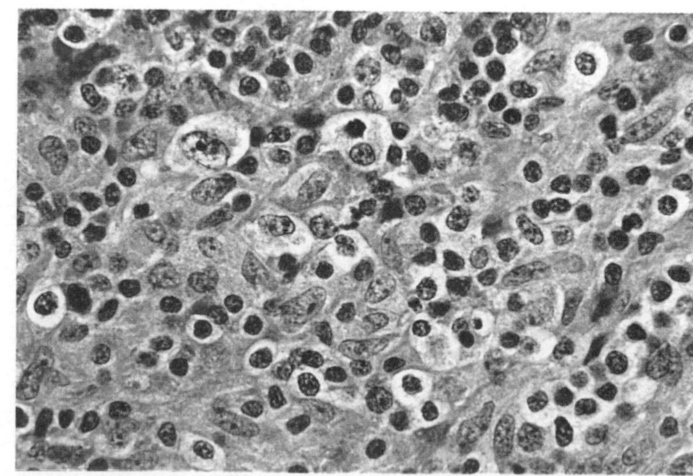

Figure 42-97 AILD-like T-cell lymphoma. Intermediate-sized atypical lymphoid cells with pale cytoplasm are present singly and in small clusters.

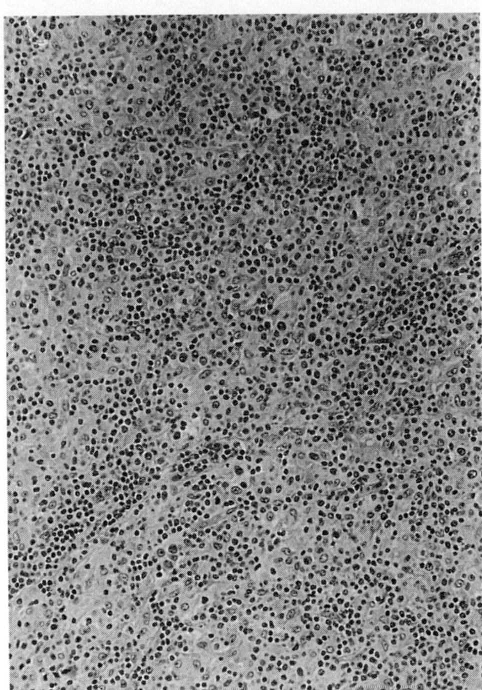

Fig. 42-98 Lymphoepithelioid T-cell (Lennert's) lymphoma. There is a diffuse proliferation of epithelioid histiocytes, leading to a pale appearance at low magnification.

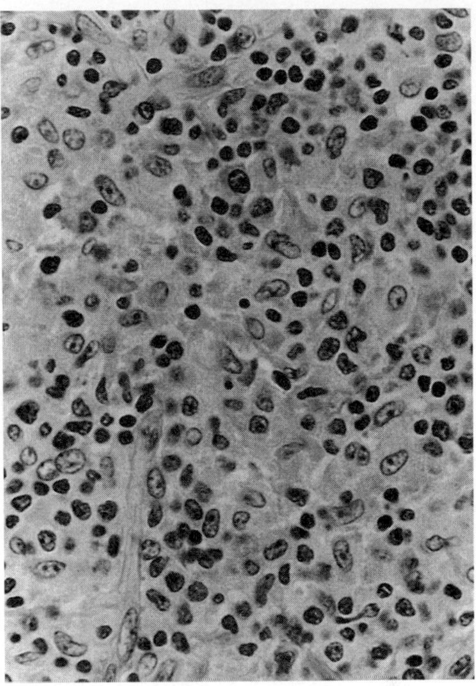

Fig. 42-99 Lymphoepithelioid T-cell (Lennert's) lymphoma. In between the numerous epithelioid histiocytes are scattered atypical lymphoid cells.

Angiocentric T-cell lymphoma

Angiocentric T-cell lymphoma is a term that encompasses a group of previously poorly characterized entities, such as lymphomatoid granulomatosis and polymorphic reticulosis.[465,466] This lymphoma occurs in extranodal sites, and is particularly common in the upper and lower respiratory tract and the skin. It appears to be more common in Asian than Western populations. There is a significant association with EBV in the lymphomas involving the upper respiratory tract, particularly the nasal passages.[363,466,467] Occasional cases are associated with hemophagocytic syndrome. There is a strong tendency for the disease to recur at extranodal sites.

The unifying feature for this lymphoma is infiltration of the walls of small arteries and veins (Fig. 42-100). The cellular infiltrate consists of a mixture of atypical lymphoid cells along with small lymphocytes, plasma cells, histiocytes, and often eosinophils. Necrosis is often present, usually paralleling the amount of vascular infiltration and destruction. A grading system has been developed for these lesions, with Grade I lesions showing infrequent or absent large lymphoid cells (benign lymphocytic angiitis and granulomatosis), Grade II lesions showing evidence of clear cytologic atypia, and Grade III lesions showing a more monomorphic appearance with greater numbers of large lymphoid cells.[465]

A significant number of angiocentric lymphomas involving the upper respiratory tract, particularly those involving the nose and associated with EBV, lack detectable clonal T-cell receptor gene rearrangements, even in those cases in which clonality can be demonstrated by other means.[363,468] Many of these cases lack the most pan–T-cell antigens, with the exception of CD2, and express the natural killer-associated antigen CD56.[363] These findings raise the possibility that these cases actually represent lymphomas derived from NK cells rather than T-cells. However, they usually lack other NK markers such as CD16 and CD57; thus, the true lineage is still unclear.

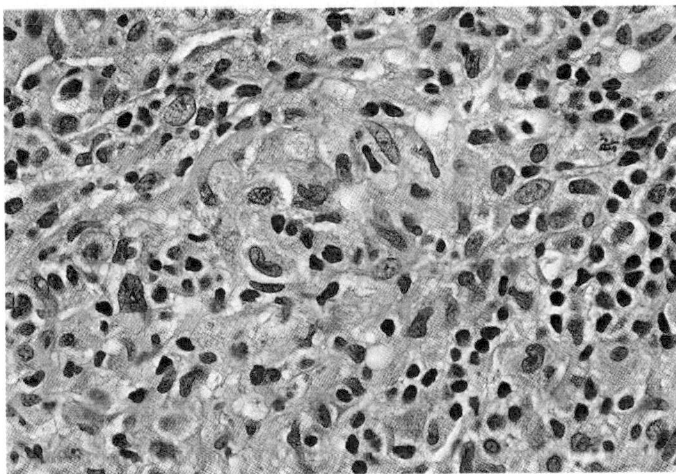

Fig. 42-100 Angiocentric T-cell lymphoma. This small artery is infiltrated by atypical lymphoid cells, with occlusion of the lumen.

Recent reappraisal of pulmonary lymphomatoid granulomatosis has provided evidence that many cases represent a monoclonal proliferation of EBV-infected B-cells with a prominent T-cell reaction and vasculitis and thus may be distinct from other angiocentric T-cell lymphomas arising in other sites.[468a]

Intestinal T-cell lymphoma (ulcerative jejunitis, malignant "histiocytosis" of the intestine)[469,470]

This is a rare variant of PTLD that usually occurs in patients with a long history of malabsorption. It affects the jejunum most commonly, but also may occur in the colon; multifocal involvement is common. Grossly, ulceration, with or without a mass, is generally present. Microscopically, the neoplastic cells are similar to those of other PTCL. However, the cells typically infiltrate the overlying epithelium and tend to spread along the adjacent mucosa. The proliferating cells often express HML-1 (CD103), a marker of normal mucosal associated T-lymphocytes.[471]

PTCL with erythrophagocytosis, hepatosplenic T-cell lymphoma, and erythrophagocytic T-γ lymphoma

These are rare variants of PTCL, all of which have been confused with malignant histiocytosis in the past. PTCL with erythrophagocytosis generally occurs as either of two clinical presentations. In the first, patients with a history of lymphoma develop symptom of a hemophagocytic syndrome, i.e., hepatosplenomegaly, fever, and pancytopenia.[162] Bland phagocytizing histiocytes are found in the bone marrow, lymph nodes, spleen, and liver, without lymphoma present at these sites. In the second presentation, patients without a prior history of lymphoma develop hemophagocytic syndrome.[161] In this case, a PTCL, often angiocentric, is found in apposition with benign lymphophagocytizing histiocytes. In both cases, cytokine production by either tumor or other cells has been postulated to be responsible for the hemophagocytic syndrome.[472]

Hepatosplenic T-cell lymphoma is a rare PTCL with preferential involvement of the sinusoids of the liver, the red pulp of the spleen, and the sinusoids of the bone marrow.[473] Tumor cells usually lack CD5 and CD7 antigens and display clonal rearrangement of the δ and γ rather than α or β T-cell receptor genes.

In erythrophagocytic T-γ lymphoma, infiltration is seen in the red pulp of the spleen, the sinusoids of the liver, diffusely throughout the bone marrow, and in the paracortical regions of lymph nodes.[474] Although said to derive from normal T-γ cells, the tumor cells lack the prominent azurophilic granules usually present in those cells. It is possible that this entity actually represents hepatosplenic T-cell lymphoma.

Anaplastic large cell lymphoma

Anaplastic large cell lymphoma is a neoplastic proliferation of lymphoid cells with highly pleomorphic cytologic features, often present in a sinusoidal distribution and almost always expressing the lymphocyte activation marker CD30.[166,475] In the past, many cases had been diagnosed as malignant histiocytosis.[169] In the Working Formation, these tumors are best classified as high grade, large cell immunoblastic type.

Primary anaplastic large cell lymphoma is a rare lymphoma, representing about 2% to 5% of NHLs.[476,477] There is a bimodal age distribution, with one peak in childhood and another in adulthood. There is a 2:1 male:female ratio. Some cases have been reported in patients with immunodeficiencies but this constitutes a clear minority of cases. Although initial reports suggested a strong association with EBV,[478] later studies have not confirmed that relationship outside of the setting of immunodeficiency.[479] Occasional cases of anaplastic large cell lymphoma occur as a complication of another lymphoma, including HD and a variety of types of NHL.[480]

Patients generally present with an enlarged lymph node (systemic form), although extranodal presentations are common. Patients with the systemic form usually present with stage I or II disease, with a low incidence of bone marrow involvement.[477] Some cases may present with systemic symptoms and generalized involvement, producing the clinical syndrome previously associated with malignant histiocytosis. Primary presentation limited to skin (primary cutaneous form) is another common presentation of anaplastic large cell lymphoma.[475,481] Usually, patients present with one or several papules or nodules, occasionally with a history of spontaneous regression, similar to the clinical presentation of lymphomatoid papulosis.

Architecturally, a prominent sinusoidal pattern of involvement of lymph nodes is characteristic, but preferential paracortical infiltration and complete diffuse effacement are also commonly seen.[476] The neoplasm is defined by its cytologic characteristics. The proliferating cells are large, with large, highly pleomorphic nuclei. The nuclei may be round, but are more often irregular and may include multilobated forms (Fig. 42-101). Multinucleated cells, particularly with nuclei forming a wreath-like appearance ("doughnut" cells), may be found. The chromatin pattern is highly irregular, with coarse clumped areas interspersed with vesicular areas. Nucleoli may be single or multiple and are usually very prominent. The cytoplasm is usually abundant, and may be basophilic, amphophilic, eosinophilic, or pale. The cytoplasm of one cell may abut closely with that of an adjacent cell, giving a cohesive appearance reminiscent of carcinoma or melanoma.

Fibrosis may be prominent, and focal necrosis is often present. Occasionally, the stroma may be spindled or myxoid, mimicking a sarcoma.[482] Characteristically, there are admixed reactive cells, including numerous plasma cells, scattered neutrophils, histiocytes, and occasionally, eosinophils.

Anaplastic large cell lymphoma expresses leukocyte common antigen (CD45) in about two-thirds of cases, the lowest percentage of any major category of lymphoma.[7] The most

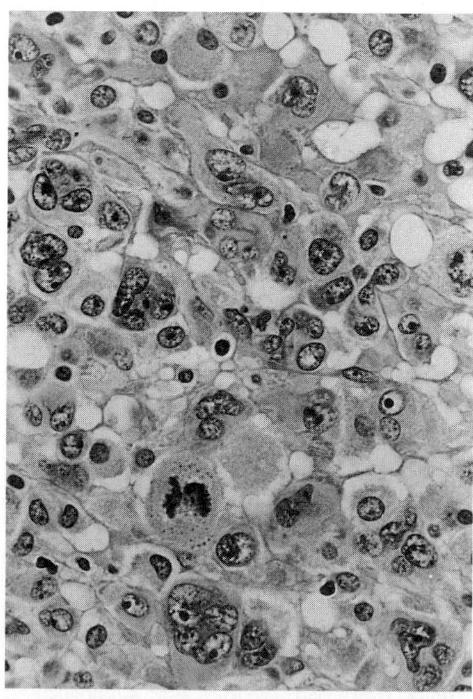

Fig. 42-101 Anaplastic large cell lymphoma. Highly anaplastic features are seen which could raise confusion with poorly differentiated carcinoma or malignant melanoma. Note the presence of mutlilobated cells which could mimic the Reed-Sternberg cells of Hodgkin's disease.

consistent finding is the demonstration of the CD30 antigen, a marker of lymphocyte activation, in almost all cases, and generally easily demonstrated in paraffin sections.[5,166] CD30 is a member of the tumor necrosis factor/nerve growth factor receptor superfamily whose ligand is a protein in a family of cytokines that includes TNF-∝ and TNF-β.[5] Usually, there is also expression of other markers of lymphocyte activation, including HLA-DR, the transferrin receptor (CD71), and the interleukin-2 receptor (CD25). A high percentage of cases also show expression of epithelial membrane antigen, although this antigen is usually absent on primary cutaneous cases.[483,484] In contrast, primary cutaneous cases express the cutaneous lymphocyte antigen HECA-452.[484] Immunologic studies demonstrate a T lineage (usually with loss of multiple pan-T antigens) in about two-thirds of cases, a B lineage in about 15% of cases, and no clear demonstration of T- or B-cell lineage in about 15% of cases.[166,477]

Gene rearrangement studies demonstrate approximately 60% of cases to have rearrangements of the Tβ receptor gene, 20% of cases to have rearrangements of the immunoglobulin heavy chain gene, and about 20% to have a germline configuration.[167,485,486] Occasionally, there are discrepancies between the results of immunophenotyping and immunogenotyping studies. A characteristic translocation involving the long arm of chromosome 5 is found in anaplastic large cell lymphoma; this is most often a t(2;5)(p23;q35), but may also be a t(5;6) or t(3;5).[487] It has been recently shown that, in the t(2;5), the nucleophosmin (NPM) gene on chromosome 5q35 becomes fused to the catalytic domain of the anaplastic lymphoma kinase (ALK) gene on chromosome 2p23.[488] Deregulation of the truncated ALK may contribute to malignant transformation. The incidence of these translocations in anaplastic large cell lymphoma is still not clear. Preliminary work on selected cases suggested the association was high, but a recent Southern blot hybridization study on unselected cases found an incidence of 13%.[489]

Preliminary data suggests that patients with anaplastic large cell lymphoma have a better overall survival than patients with other diffuse large cell lymphomas, both in children and adults.[490,491] The better overall survival appears to be related to the success of salvage therapy.[491,492]

Lymphoblastic lymphoma

Lymphoblastic lymphoma is a high grade malignant lymphoma that the tissue equivalent of acute lymphoblastic leukemia.[367] The neoplastic cells have a close resemblance to immature thymocytes. Lymphoblastic lymphoma is relatively uncommon, constituting about 4% of all NHLs in the Working Formulation study. Although it occurs in all age groups, it is particularly common in children and young adolescents, and constitutes approximately one-third of all pediatric NHLs.[493] There is a 2:1 male:female ratio.

The typical presentation is that of a mediastinal mass, often associated with pleural or pericardial effusions.[494,495] The mass is usually large, and may be responsible for respiratory compromise. Other less common sites of initial presentation include supradiaphragmatic lymph nodes, Waldeyer's ring, and the gonads. Lymphoblastic lymphoma and acute lymphoblastic leukemia represent biologic ends of one spectrum. When greater than 10% circulating blasts are found in the peripheral blood or greater than 25% bone marrow involvement is seen, the disease is best characterized as acute lymphoblastic leukemia.[493,496] Untreated, the diseases shows rapid progression, with frequent involvement of the bone marrow, central nervous system, and gonads.

Lymphoblastic lymphoma shows diffuse effacement of lymph node architecture, often with extensive spread into the pericapsular soft tissues. When lymphoblastic lymphoma infiltrates soft tissues, it often evokes a fibrous response that tends to trap the tumor cells forming a single file pattern of infiltration (Fig. 42-102). The mitotic rate is high, and extensive single cell necrosis may be present. At high magnification, there is a very monotonous population of small to medium-sized cells containing a nucleus with a very fine chromatin pattern, and generally without discernible nucleoli (Fig. 42-103). In many cases, the nuclear outlines are highly irregular (the convoluted subtype), while in other cases, the nuclear outlines are rounded (the nonconvoluted subtype). Occasionally, the nucleoli may be slightly larger, and may possess small, but discernible nucleoli (atypical or large cell variant). Cytoplasm is uniformly scant, and usually not visualized at all in routine sections. With the exception of tingible-body macrophages, there is usually no accompanying host infiltrate.

Almost all lymphoblastic neoplasms are terminal deoxynucleotidyl transferase positive (a marker now demonstrable in paraffin sections), whether of B or T lineage (Fig. 42-104).[497-499] Approximately 85% of lymphoblastic lymphomas are of T lineage, particularly those presenting with a mediastinal mass.[499-500] In paraffin sections these neoplasms are positive for leukocyte common antigen (CD45) in about 80% of cases and positive for CD43 and cytoplasmic CD3 in about 90% of cases.[3,7] In contrast, T-lymphoblastic lymphomas lacks expression of B lineage antigens. In frozen sections, an immature thymic phenotype is usually found (Fig. 42 105).[499,500] The most immature T-lymphoblastic neoplasms may express only CD7 (prethymic phenotype). Slightly more mature neoplasms express other pan–T-cell antigens such as CD2, CD3 (cytoplasmic) and CD5 (stage I

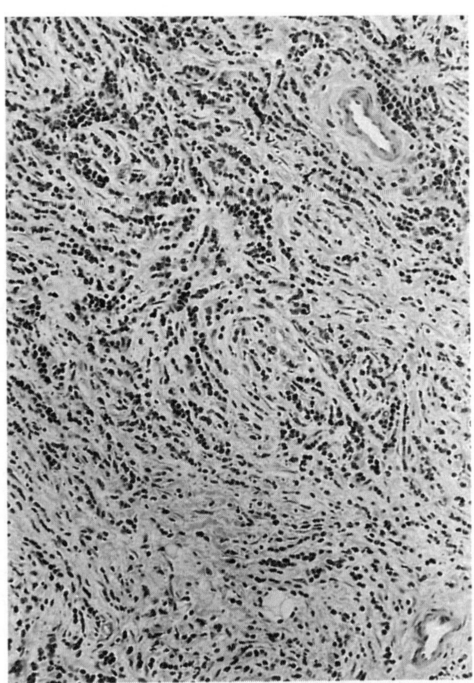

Fig. 42-102 Lymphoblastic lymphoma. A single cell file pattern of infiltration is seen in the perinodal tissues of this case.

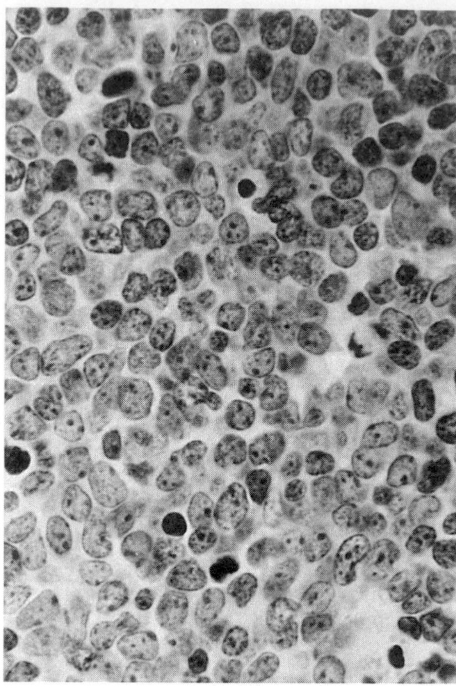

Fig. 42-103 Lymphoblastic lymphoma. There is a uniform population of medium-sized lymphoid cells with a fine chromatin pattern and indistinct nucleoli. Note the presence of scattered mitotic figures.

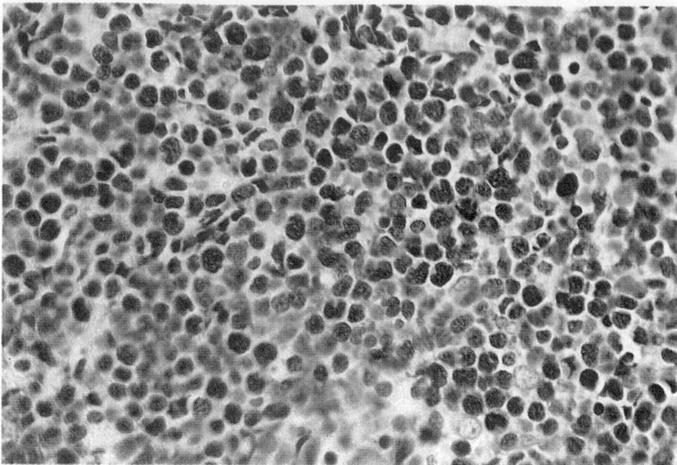

Fig. 42-104 Lymphoblastic lymphoma, TdT stain. A nuclear pattern of staining is seen in this paraffin section study.

thymic phenotype). A larger subset of T-lymphoblastic lymphomas express a stage II thymic phenotype, characterized by CD1 expression, either with absence of both the T-cell subset markers CD4 and CD8 or with coexpression of both. Another major subset of T-lymphoblastic lymphomas express a more mature T-cell phenotype, with either a helper ($CD4^+$, $CD8^-$) phenotype or a cytotoxic/suppressor ($CD4^-$, $CD8^+$) phenotype, with absent CD1 (stage III thymic phenotype). T-lymphoblastic lymphoma tends to occur in male patients and be associated with a mediastinal mass. Approximately 20 of the T lineage cases may show strong positivity for CD16 and CD57, markers of natural killer cells; these cases tend to occur in females and may be more aggressive clinically.[501]

Approximately 15% of lymphoblastic lymphomas are of B lineage, expressing the B lineage markers CD19, CD20, CD21, and CD10 (CALLA).[498,499,501] Their immature phenotype is reflected in their patterns of immunoglobulin expression, either lacking cytoplasmic immunoglobulin (pre-pre-B-cell), or only expressing cytoplasmic immunoglobulin (pre-B-cell). Rare cases may express surface immunoglobulin;[502] many of these cases, which may lack TdT expression, may be indistinguishable from the blastic variant of mantle cell lymphoma. Cases of B lineage lymphoblastic lymphoma tend to present in skin and bone, and are not found as a mediastinal mass.[503]

The most immature T-lymphoblastic lymphomas, expressing only CD7, generally show a germline configuration for the T-cell receptor β chain gene.[504] However, other T-lymphoblastic lymphomas do have detectable Tβ receptor gene rearrangements; a subset may also clonally rearrange the immunoglobulin heavy chain gene.[505] Most T-lymphoblastic lymphomas contain cytogenetic abnormalities, mostly chromosomal translocations.[506] Multiple recurrent translocations have been described, often involving the sites of the T-cell receptor genes. The most common type described, occurring in up to one-third of cases, involves the TAL/SCL gene on chromosome 1p32.[507] The TAL gene probably codes for a transcription factor that may activate a wide variety of other genes.

B-lineage lymphoblastic lymphomas generally show clonal rearrangements of the immunoglobulin heavy chain gene.[505] Up to 25% of cases may also show clonal rearrangements of the β T-cell receptor gene. Recurring translocations have also been reported, identical to that seen in B-acute lymphoblastic leukemia (see chapter on bone marrow).

Although a high-grade lymphoma, lymphoblastic lymphoma responds very well to multidrug chemotherapeutic regimens effective in acute lymphoblastic leukemia, with modern therapies giving survival rates over 50%.[496] Intrathecal chemotherapy or intracranial radiotherapy is often used, since the central nervous system is a frequent site of relapse. Prognostic factors include high stage with bone marrow or central nervous system involvement and a high serum lactate dehydrogenase. Bone marrow transplantation may be an option in high risk or other patients.

Small noncleaved cell lymphoma

Small noncleaved cell lymphoma (SNCL) is a high grade malignant lymphoma that consists of two closely related morphologic subtypes: Burkitt's type and non-Burkitt's type.[367] Burkitt's lymphoma is endemic in Africa, and occurs primarily in children, representing the most common childhood malignancy in the malarial belt of equatorial Africa. In the United States, SNCL lymphomas are relatively uncommon, comprising approximately 2% of NHLs. The Burkitt subtype has a peak incidence in children, while the non-Burkitt subtype has a peak later in adulthood.[508-510] In South America, an intermediate incidence of SNCL is seen. In all areas, the male-to-female ratio is about 2.5:1. African Burkitt's lymphoma has a high association with EBV, with a distribution correlating with the malarial belt being present in up to 95% of cases in these areas.[511] In contrast, in the United States, only about 5% to 15% of cases are associated with EBV.[512]

Endemic Burkitt's lymphoma usually presents in extranodal sites, particularly the bones of the jaw.[513] In the United States,

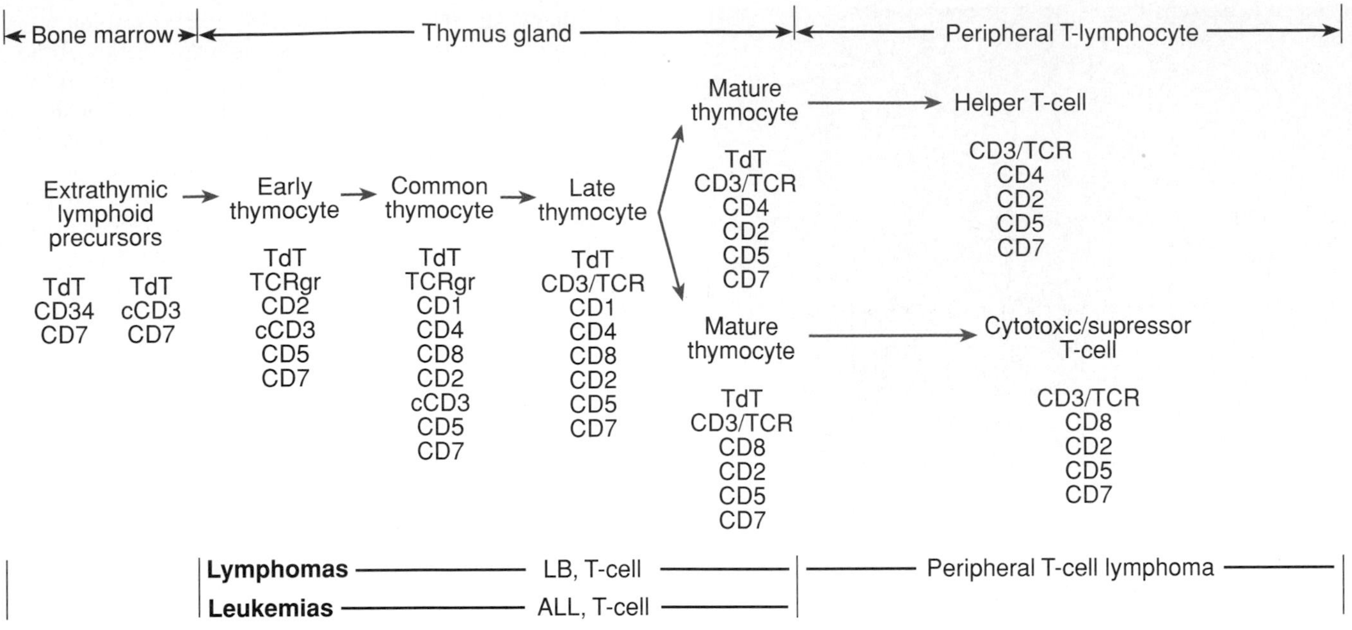

Fig. 42-105 Expression of antigens by normal developing and neoplastic T-lymphocytes in a hypothetical model of differentiation. *C*, Cytoplasmic; *gr*, gene rearrangement; *TCR*, T-cell receptor.

an abdominal presentation is most frequent, although the non-Burkitt subtype may have a relatively higher incidence of peripheral lymphadenopathy.[509,510,514] Bone marrow involvement occurs in 10% to 30% of cases, with a relatively higher incidence of bone marrow involvement in the non-Burkitt subtype. The mediastinum, liver, and spleen are almost always uninvolved in SNCL.[514] There may be overlap between SNCL with extensive involvement of the bone marrow and the L3 subtype of acute lymphoblastic leukemia; they may represent different manifestations of one biologic disease.

At low magnification, there is almost always diffuse effacement of architecture by a relatively monotonous population of cells (Fig. 42-106); rarely selective involvement of germinal centers is seen. The mitotic rate is extremely high; SNCL has the shortest doubling times of all studied tumors. Consistent with the high cell turnover, numerous tingible-body macrophages are evenly dispersed among the neoplastic cells, usually imparting a "starry-sky" appearance. At high magnification, the cells of Burkitt's lymphoma have intermediately-sized nuclei with coarsely reticulated chromatin, relatively clear parachromatin, and two to five basophilic nuclei (Fig. 42-107). There is a moderate rim of amphophilic cytoplasm which often squares off with the cytoplasm of adjacent cells. Touch preparations may demonstrate cytoplasmic vacuoles, representing lipid. The neoplastic cells of the non-Burkitt subtype are similar to those of the Burkitt type, except that there is greater pleomorphism from cell to cell and fewer, but often more prominent, nucleoli (Fig. 42-108). The histologic distinction between the Burkitt's and non-Burkitt's subtype may be quite subtle, particularly in suboptimal preparations.

Virtually all SNCL are B-lineage neoplasms, expressing surface immunoglobulins. They usually carry the IgM and/or IgD heavy chain and are usually CD10 (CALLA) positive, consistent with neoplasm of relatively immature B-cells.[515] In contrast to lymphoblastic neoplasms, however, SNCL is negative for TdT.

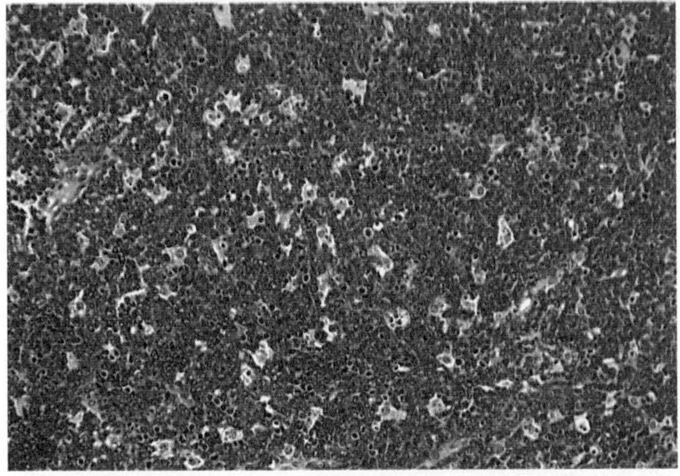

Fig. 42-106 Burkitt's lymphoma. A starry sky pattern is seen at low magnification.

Almost all cases of the endemic Burkitt's lymphoma carry a translocation involving chromosome 8: a t(8;14)(q23;q21) is present in about 80% of cases, a t(8;22) is present in about 15% of cases (all with lambda light chain expression), and a t(2;8) is present in about 5% of cases (all with kappa light chain expression).[516] The breakpoint on chromosome 8 is at the site of the *myc* gene, while the breakpoints on chromosomes 14, 22, and 8 are the sites of the immunoglobulin heavy chain gene, the lambda light chain gene, and kappa light chain gene, respectively. Molecular analyses have demonstrated that, in most cases, the breakpoint on chromosome 14 involves the D_H or J_H region of the immunoglobulin heavy chain gene, suggesting that translocation occurs as a result of a recombinase error.

A somewhat lower incidence of translocation involving chromosome 8 is seen in sporadic Burkitt lymphoma.[512] More-

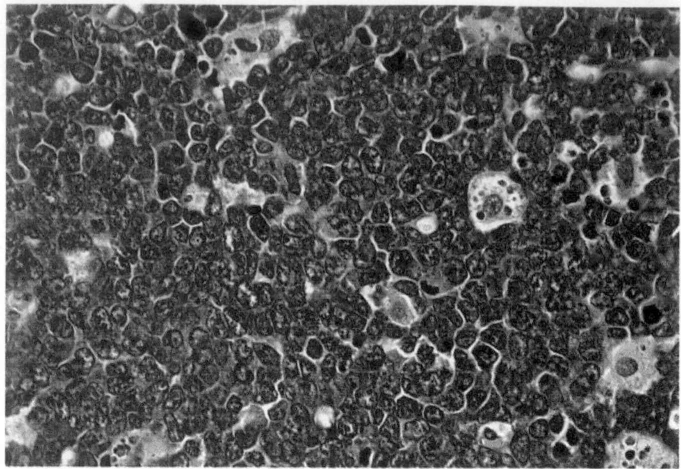

Fig. 42-107 Burkitt's lymphoma. There is a homogenous population of medium-sized lymphoid cells. The nuclei have a chromatin pattern that is not as fine as seen in lymphoblastic lymphoma, and several nucleoli are event in each nucleus.

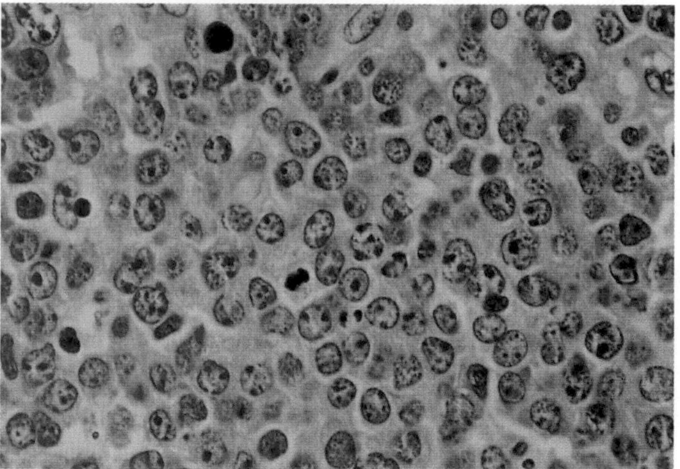

Fig. 42-108 Small noncleaved cell lymphoma, non-Burkitt's type. A population of intermediate-sized lymphoid cells with a high mitotic rate is present. The cells are somewhat more pleomorphic than typically seen in Burkitt's lymphoma.

over, the breakpoint on chromosome 14 usually involves the switch region of the immunoglobulin heavy chain gene, suggesting that translocation occurs at a later stage of B-cell development than in endemic Burkitt's lymphoma.[517] *C-myc* translocations have not been found in the non-Burkitt's subtype of SNCL.[512]

At the molecular level, the breakpoints at the *myc* gene are heterogeneous; they may occur far 5′ of the *myc* gene, immediately upstream of the first exon, or within the first exon of the gene.[516] Despite this molecular heterogeneity, the result of all of the translocations is to deregulate the *myc* gene, possibly by the influence of enhancer elements from the immunoglobulin heavy chain gene.[518] In addition, there are often mutations in the *c-myc* gene that cluster within regions of *c-myc* associated with phosphorylation and transactivation.[519] The *myc* gene codes for a nuclear protein that acts as a transcription factor, with an important role in B-lymphocyte proliferation and differentiation.

For diagnostic purposes, the t(8;14) and the variant translocations are usually detected by classical cytogenetics. Although Southern blot hybridization may detect many of the translocations, the great molecular heterogeneity of the breakpoints make negative results by Southern blotting of limited utility.

Although it is clear that *myc* deregulation is of crucial importance in the pathogenesis of SNCL, additional genetic events must also be important. The frequent presence of EBV in endemic Burkitt's lymphoma suggests a role for this virus, perhaps acting as a B-cell proliferation factor increasing the pool of cells at risk for *myc* rearrangements. In addition, mutations in the p53 gene are found in a significant percentage of cases of SNCL, perhaps accounting for the aggressive behavior exhibited by this neoplasm.[385]

SNCL is generally treated with combination chemotherapy, although there is also a role for surgical debulking with this lymphoma.[520] Modern regimens have led to cure rates up to 70% to 90%. Adverse prognostic factors include large unresected bulk, a high serum lactate dehydrogenase, or involvement of the central nervous system or bone marrow. The prognostic significance of Burkitt's vs. non-Burkitt's subtypes is unclear, with most studies reporting no significant differences in survival.[509,510] Relapse, if it occurs, usually manifests within the first year. Although Burkitt's lymphoma is usually cured if relapse does not occur within 2 years, late relapses may occur in the non-Burkitt's subtype.[510]

Lymphoproliferations in immunodeficient hosts

There is a greatly increased risk of development of a lymphoproliferative disorder in patients with immunodeficiencies, whether primary or acquired. These lymphomas have many common features. First, they are usually NHLs, most often diffuse large cell lymphomas or small noncleaved lymphomas of B lineage. There is a very high association of these neoplasms with EBV infection; the level of the association varies with the particular immunodeficiency. There is a marked tendency for involvement of extranodal sites, including the gastrointestinal tract, central nervous system, and soft tissue.

The primary immunodeficiencies most associated with the development of malignant lymphoma include X-linked lymphoproliferative syndrome, Wiskott-Aldrich syndrome, ataxia telangiectasia, common variable immunodeficiency, and severe combined immunodeficiency syndrome.[521,522] In X-linked lymphoproliferative syndrome, there is a marked susceptibility to EBV infection. Most patients develop severe or fatal infectious mononucleosis on their initial exposure to EBV, and about 30% develop acquired hypo- or agammaglobulinemia.[523] B-lineage malignant lymphoma arises in about 25% of patients, and is invariably associated with EBV, often of low stage, and with a prediction for the ileocecal region. A somewhat wider variety of lymphomas arises in the other syndromes, with a risk of lymphoma of 10% to 20% in Wiskott-Aldrich syndrome, 10% in ataxia-telangiectasia, 1% to 7% in common variable immunodeficiency syndrome, and 1% to 4% in severe combined immunodeficiency.[522] In severe combined immunodeficiency, patients with NHL usually present in infancy, and often have involvement of multiple sites, including extranodal sites.

AIDS-associated NHL has become a major problem in patients with HIV infection.[524] Already, HIV-related lymphomas represent over 10% of NHLs diagnosed in the United

States.[525] In one study of asymptomatic HIV-infected patients on anti-viral therapy, there was a 3.2% probability of developing lymphoma at two years, with an additional 0.8% rise for each subsequent 6-month period.[526] Thus, as more HIV-infected patients live longer, the incidence of this lymphoma will likely continue to rise. The risk for lymphomas is highest in HIV-infected hemophiliacs and lowest in those HIV-infected patients who acquired the disease by heterosexual contact.[527]

Virtually all the NHLs arising in HIV-infected patients represent diffuse, intermediate, or high-grade lymphomas.[343,528,529] Most patients present with widespread disease, often involving extranodal sites. Common sites of extranodal disease include the central nervous system, the gastrointestinal tract (particularly the rectum and anus), liver, and bone marrow, but virtually any organ may be affected.

Histologically, most of the lymphomas can be classified as small noncleaved cell type or large cell lymphoma, particularly immunoblastic type. Small noncleaved cell lymphomas tend to be seen at a younger age and occur with higher mean CD4 counts than the large cell lymphomas.[527,530] In addition, they tend to occur in lymph node, bone marrow, and muscle, while the large cell lymphomas are more common in extranodal sites such as the gastrointestinal tract, brain, and oral cavity.

Immunologically, almost all AIDS-associated NHLs are B-cell neoplasms, with clonal rearrangements of the immunoglobulin heavy and light chain genes,[343] although some unusual polyclonal lymphomas have been reported.[531] Since an oligoclonal pattern has been demonstrated in HIV-associated benign lymphadenopathy, and a multiclonal pattern has been demonstrated when multiple sites of lymphoma have been studied from a single patient, it has been postulated that an unrestrained polyclonal B-cell proliferation progresses to oligoclonal proliferations, and multiclonal lymphomas result when additional genetic changes occur.[532]

Approximately 50% of AIDS-associated NHLs are associated with EBV, including about 80% of cases of large cell immunoblastic lymphoma, 30% of small noncleaved cell lymphoma, and 20% of intermediate grade large cell lymphoma.[533-535] Site of involvement is of some significance; for example, virtually all central nervous system lymphomas are EBV positive.[536] Both EBV type 1 and 2 are found, and the pattern of EBV gene expression has similarities and differences with both Burkitt lymphoma and post-transplantation lymphoproliferative disease.

Recently, it has been shown that rearrangements of the bcl-6 gene can be detected in about 20% of AIDS-related large cell lymphomas, but not in small noncleaved cell lymphoma.[537] In contrast, structural lesions, mostly t(8;14) translocations, indicative of *c-myc* oncogene are uniformly present in small noncleaved cell lymphoma, but found in less than half of cases of large cell lymphoma.[538] The location of the *c-myc* breakpoints on chromosome 8 and the preferential involvement of the immunoglobulin gene switch region is similar to sporadic Burkitt's lymphoma. Mutations of the *c-myc* gene in its coding region are found in many cases, particularly those associated with a t(8;14); mutations in the first intron are also found in some cases.[539] In addition p53 loss or mutation and ras mutation are found in about 40% and 15% of cases of AIDS-associated small noncleaved cell lymphoma, but not in the large cell lymphomas. These results suggest that there may be two separate pathogenetic mechanisms, one primarily involving EBV and/or *bcl*-6 and another involving mutations in oncogenes or tumor suppressor genes.

The median survival of patients with AIDS-associated NHL is less than one year. Treatment is difficult to deliver effectively, as significant toxicity to multiagent chemotherapy is seen.[524] Many patients are treated with low-dose chemotherapy or standard-dose chemotherapy with hematopoietic growth factors, with intrathecal chemotherapy for central nervous system prophylaxis. Poor prognostic factors include history of AIDS prior to the development of lymphoma, very low CD4 counts, poor Karnofsky performance status, the presence of bone marrow involvement, and the presence of extranodal disease.[528,540]

There is also an increase in NHLs in patients who have received immunosuppressive therapy for a variety of reasons including treatment of malignant neoplasms and connective tissue disorders (such as rheumatoid arthritis),[541,542] but the most important group of patients are those who have been placed on intensive immunosuppressive regimens after organ transplantation. The risk for development of lymphoma varies with the organ transplanted as well as the immunosuppressive regimen employed, but ranges from about 1% to 12%. Additional risk factors in the development of lymphoma include the pretransplant history, the number of rejection episodes, younger age at transplantation, and evidence of abnormally high numbers of EBV-infected cells in prelymphoma biopsy specimens.[543-547]

Typically, the lymphoproliferative disorders occur within 1 year of transplantation, usually presenting as a systemic infectious mononucleosis-like syndrome, often centered upon the head and neck, or as localized tumor masses. Extranodal sites are more frequent than nodal presentations, and may involve any site, including the allograft organ. The central nervous system, liver, lung, gastrointestinal tract, and soft tissue are all common sites of involvement.

A wide variety of histologic features can be encountered.[548] Involved sites show diffuse effacement by a population of lymphoid cells with varying degrees of atypia and monomorphism. In some cases, termed the polymorphic variant, there is a complete spectrum of B-lymphocytes and plasma cells, ranging from small lymphocytes, small lymphoplasmacytoid cells, mature plasma cells, plasmacytoid immunoblasts, and germinal center cells. In the monomorphic variant, the lesions are more typical of diffuse NHLs of B-cell type, either large cell, especially the plasmacytoid immunoblastic variant, or, less commonly, small noncleaved cell type (Fig. 42-109). Necrosis is common, particularly in the monomorphic type, and may manifest as extensive and geographic coagulative necrosis or as single-cell apoptosis. Rare cases may have histologic features of low-grade B-cell lymphoma or plasmacytoma.

Although occasional peripheral T-cell lymphomas have been reported, almost all post-transplantation lymphoproliferations are B-lineage processes. The polymorphic lesions may have a monoclonal or polyclonal pattern of immunoglobulin expression.[549,550] The monomorphic lesions usually express monoclonal immunoglobulin or are immunoglobulin-negative.[550,551] By Southern blot studies, polymorphic lesions may show no demonstrable immunoglobulin gene rearrangements consistent with a polyclonal proliferation, multiple faint rearrangement bands consistent with an oligoclonal proliferation, or patterns consistent with a monoclonal prolifera-

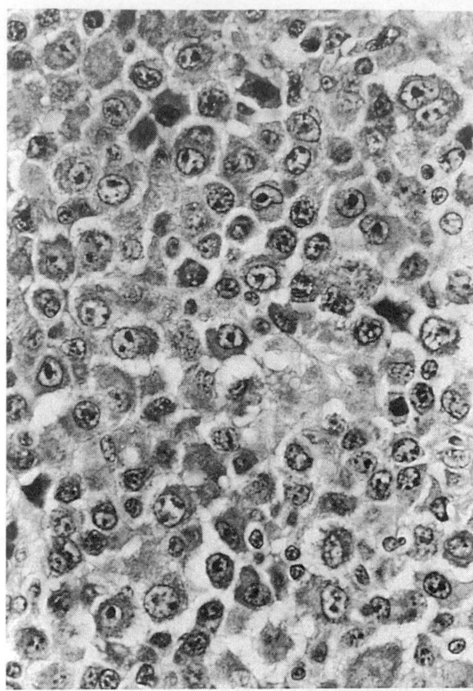

Fig. 42-109 Immunoblastic lymphoma, arising in a patient on immunosuppressive therapy, after cardiac transplantation.

tion.[549,550] The monomorphic lesions generally show a monoclonal pattern of immunoglobulin gene rearrangement.[550,551] However, different but monoclonal patterns of immunoglobulin gene rearrangement may be seen at different sites of disease in the same patients, implying a multiclonal process.[552]

In contrast to AIDS-associated lymphoma in which only about 50% of cases are associated with EBV, virtually all cases of post-transplantation lymphoproliferations are EBV-positive.[543,544,553] Another difference is that *c-myc* gene rearrangements are not common in post-transplantation lymphoproliferations; when present, they occur in monoclonal proliferations.[550] In sum, the data support a progression from a polyclonal to an oligoclonal to a monoclonal B-cell proliferation, probably driven by EBV, in a host who cannot mount a sufficient T-cell response to keep the proliferation in check.

Patients who develop post-transplantation lymphoproliferations are often initially treated by withdrawal of the immunosuppressive therapy. This alone may lead to regression of the lesions. There also may be a response to acyclovir, a drug effective in blocking EBV lytic infection. Some cases, however, progress, particularly those lesions with a monomorphic histology, sparse numbers of host T-cells, significant monoclonal populations as detected by molecular studies, and evidence of *c-myc* rearrangement.[550,554]

OTHER HEMATOPOIETIC PROLIFERATIONS IN LYMPH NODES

True histiocytic lymphoma

True histiocytic lymphoma (malignant histiocytosis) is defined as a malignant lymphoma derived from monocytes/histiocytes, without evidence of marrow involvement (either concurrent or subsequent. Although previously thought to be not uncommon, true histiocytic lymphomas are now thought to be rare, on the order of 0.5% of all large cell lymphomas.[555] Modern immunophenotyping studies have demonstrated that most cases previously thought to represent true histiocytic lymphoma or malignant histiocytosis actually are B-, T-, or null large cell lymphomas, and often anaplastic large cell lymphoma.[169]

There are few well-documented cases; therefore the clinical and histologic features are not well delineated. Most patients are adults, with a male predominance. Patients usually present with multiple sites of disease, with lymph node and skin involvement most common. However, a variety of organs have been reported to be involved, including small intestine, spleen, and liver.[555-557] The bone marrow is commonly involved. Patients generally have a poor response to multidrug chemotherapy, and death usually occurrs within 1 year.

Histologically, cases of true histiocytic lymphoma generally show effacement of lymph node architecture, sometimes with preferential sinusoidal involvement. The cytologic features are usually those of a diffuse large cell lymphoma, usually with pleomorphic nuclei with prominent nucleoli. The cytoplasm is often abundant, but only occasionally is hemophagocytosis or other phagocytosis seen. All cases of suspected true histiocytic lymphoma need confirmation by a large battery of immunohistochemical studies for confirmation. The neoplastic cells often show staining for CD45 and should show positivity for at least two relatively specific markers of histiocytic differentiation, such as CD68, CD4, CD11c, and lysozyme.[55] In addition, the neoplastic cells should lack expression of any truly specific markers of T- or B-cell differentiation. Preferably, the cases should have a germline configuration for the immunoglobulin and T-cell receptor genes, although some investigators accept their presence.

Langerhans' cell histiocytosis

Langerhans' cell histiocytosis, formerly known as histiocytosis X, may be confined to lymph nodes, but it often signals involvement of other organs, particularly skin, lung, and bones.[34,558] Most patients who present with lymph node enlargement are children or young adults. Isolated lymphadenopathy is most common, although some patients present with widespread adenopathy, and they are often febrile.[34] Spontaneous resolution may be seen in patients with involvement of single nodes, but recurrences either in lymph nodes or other sites may occasionally be seen. Coexistence of Langerhans' cell histiocytosis with HD and NHL has been reported.[254,255]

In lymph nodes, the infiltrate is within sinuses (Fig. 42-110). The cells have distinctive morphologic, immunophenotypic, and ultrastructural features that may help one in making a definitive diagnosis. The mononuclear cells have characteristic grooved nuclei with complex, folded delicate nuclear membranes, which have been likened to coffee beans. Nucleoli are inconspicuous, and mitoses are essentially absent. Rare multinucleate giant cells may be seen and varying numbers of eosinophils, which may be numerous, are found among the Langerhans' cells. Eosinophilic abscesses, occasionally with central necrosis, may be present. The cells are S-100 protein and CD74 positive in a diffuse nuclear and cytoplasmic pattern, and they also stain with CD1 (frozen section) and in many cases with HLA/DR and vimentin.[170] Ultrastructurally, Langerhans' cells contain the characteristic Langerhans' or Birbeck gran-

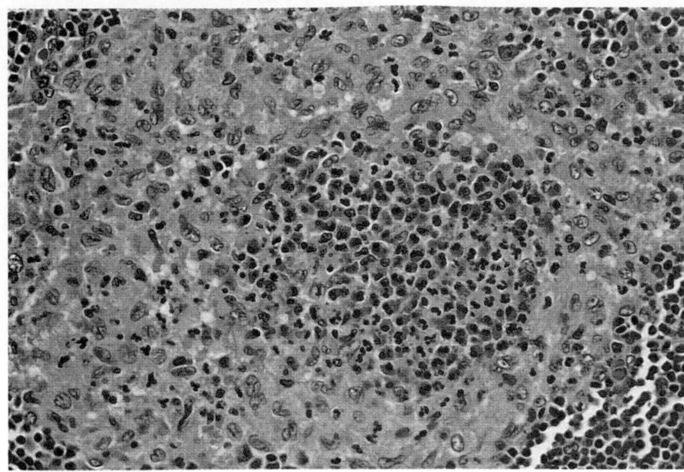

Fig. 42-110 Lymph node involved by Langerhans' cell histiocytosis. A sinus is distended by Langerhans' cells and eosinophils that form an abscess. The nuclei of the Langerhans' cells have delicate folds.

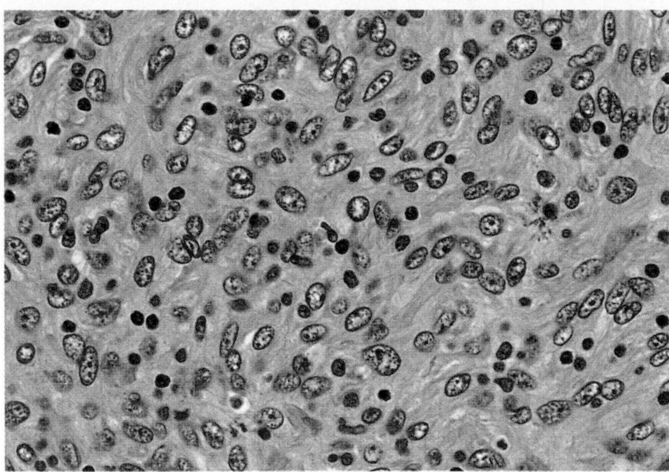

Fig. 42-111 Follicular dendritic cell sarcoma. There is a spindle cell proliferation, with scattered small lymphocytes.

ules. Recently, it has been shown that Langerhans' cell histiocytosis represents a monoclonal disorder, even in monostotic lesions.[559] Thus it probably represents a true neoplasm.

Langerhans' cell histiocytosis is usually readily differentiated from other disorders associated with a proliferation of cells in sinuses, such as: sinus histiocytosis, sinus histiocytosis with massive lymphadenopathy (also S-100 positive), and cytologically malignant cells in sinuses including Ki-1 anaplastic large cell lymphoma and metastatic tumors.[29]

Dendritic cell sarcoma

The dendritic cell sarcomas include follicular dendritic cell sarcoma and interdigitating cell sarcoma. Follicular dendritic cell sarcoma is a rare neoplasm that shows differentiation similar to nonneoplastic dendritic reticulum cells, the antigen-processing cells of normal germinal centers.[560,561] The neoplasm is very rare, with less than 20 reported cases. It usually presents in adults as enlargement of a single lymph node, although involvement of extranodal sites has been reported.[562] Histologically, a spindle cell tumor is seen, often with fascicles and storiforming (Fig. 42-111). The individual cells possess relatively bland nuclei with a low mitotic rate. Cytoplasm is pale to slightly eosinophilic. A characteristic feature is the presence of numerous scattered small lymphocytes. The tumor is defined by its immunophenotype.[560-562] The tumor cells show the staining pattern of normal dendritic reticulum cells, including reactivity for the complement markers CD21 and CD35 as well as the lysosomal marker CD68 (Fig. 42-112). The tumors may or may not be positive for CD45 and S-100. Electron microscopy will demonstrate numerous cell processes attached to one another by desmosomes. The tumor behaves as a low-grade sarcoma, usually with local recurrence, although metastatic disease has also been reported.

Interdigitating dendritic cell sarcoma is a related neoplasm that shows differentiation toward interdigitating dendritic cells, the antigen-processing cells of the paracortical region of the lymph node. It is also a rare tumor, with fewer than 30 reported cases.[561,563] It occurs in adults, and involves lymph nodes as well as extranodal sites. Histologically, the neoplasm is usually a spindle cell tumor similar to follicular dendritic cell sarcoma, although some cases have shown cells with a more rounded appearance. Immunohistochemical studies demonstrate CD45, S-100, and CD68 positivity, similar to normal interdigitating dendritic cells.[561] Although the known experience is small, cases of interdigitating dendritic cell sarcoma may have a more aggressive course than follicular dendritic cell sarcoma, with a higher incidence of involvement of multiple sites, including visceral organs, with death due to disease occurring in approximately one-half of patients, generally within 1 year of diagnosis.

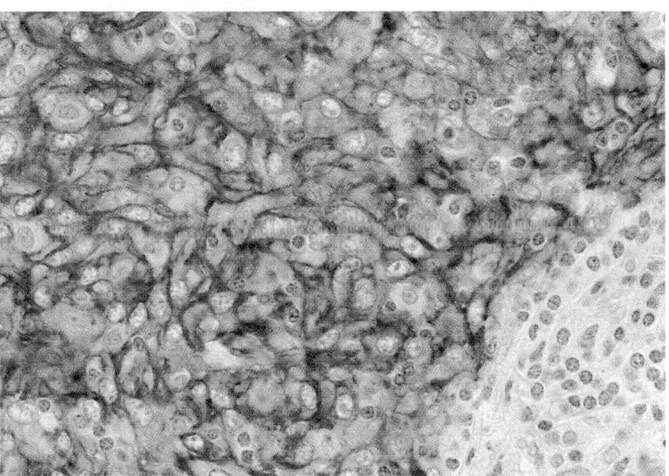

Fig. 42-112 Follicular dendritic cell sarcoma, CD21 stain. The neoplastic cells show strong membrane staining for C3d (CD21).

Myeloid leukemia

Myeloid leukemias may involve the lymph nodes. Often termed extramedullary myeloid tumor, granulocytic sarcoma, or chloroma, lymph node involvement may occur in patients with known myeloid leukemia, both acute and chronic, as well as in patients without a known history of leukemia. It may be the first presentation of disease or may be the first sign of relapse (including the first sign of blastic transformation), but usually occurs in patients with known active disease. Involved lymph nodes may show partial involvement, either sinusoidal

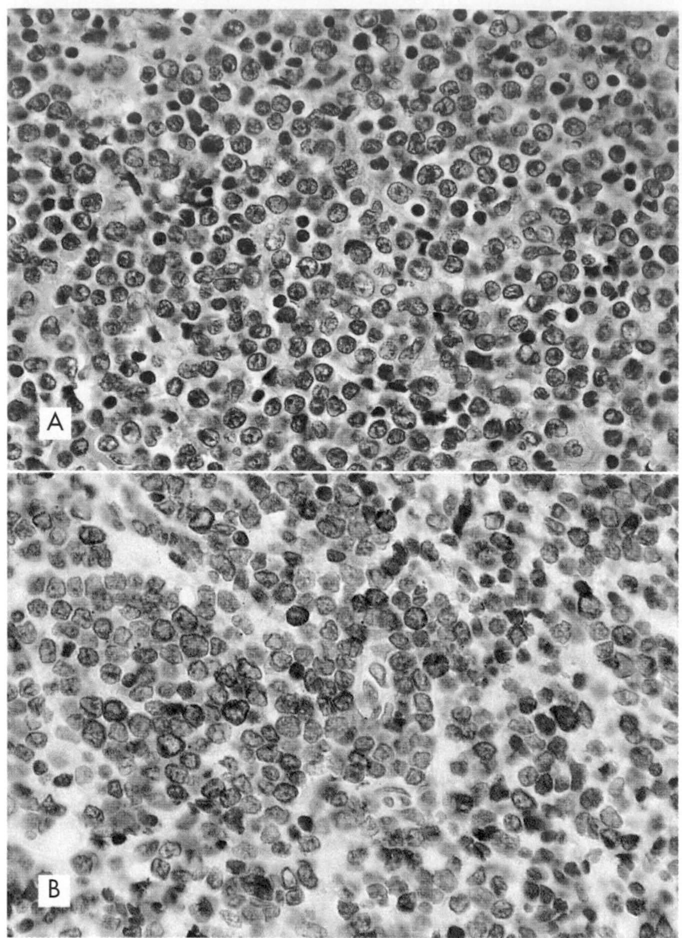

Fig. 42-113 Acute myeloid leukemia, involving a lymph node. **A,** A diagnosis of "atypical" lymphoblastic lymphoma was favored histologically, as this patient did not have a history of leukemia. **B,** This myeloperoxidase stain shows cytoplasmic positivity in a majority of the tumor cells.

or interfollicular, or diffuse effacement of architecture. A uniform population of cells is present, usually with a high mitotic rate, and occasionally with a starry-sky appearance. The nuclei are generally intermediate in size, may have fine or vesicular chromatin, and generally have moderately sized nucleoli (Fig. 42-113). Cytoplasm may be scanty or moderate in amount, and may contain granules. Occasionally, admixed myelocytes will be identified. The Leder stain will be positive in about two-thirds of cases. Immunohistochemistry is very helpful, with myeloperoxidase, CD43, and CD68 each positive in a high percentage of cases (Fig. 42-114).[564]

Myeloid leukemias can easily be histologically confused with NHL, particularly lymphoblastic or large cell types. Myeloid cells are often slightly larger than the cells of lymphoblastic lymphoma and usually contain more prominent nucleoli; and their chromatin pattern is usually finer than the cells of typical large cell lymphoma. The identification of myelocytes or cytoplasmic granules or the recognition that the proliferating cells do not have classical features of a specific type of NHL should prompt the application of a battery of histochemical and immunohistochemical studies, which includes specific myeloid markers such as myeloperoxidase.

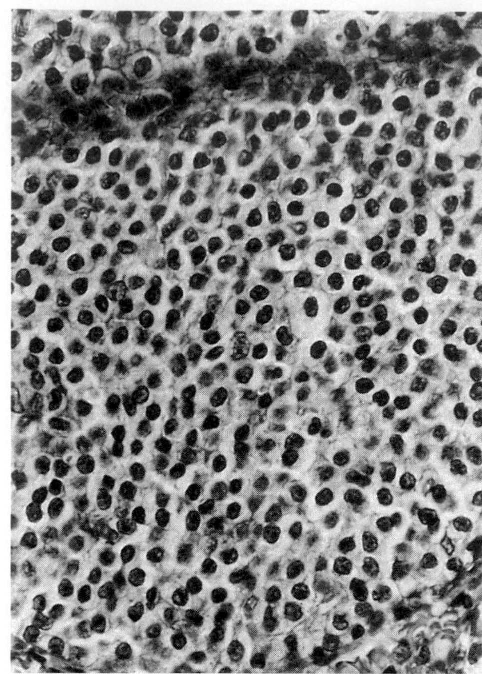

Fig. 42-114 Hairy cell leukemia. There is a monotonous population of small lymphoid cells with abundant clear cytoplasm. This patient had a longstanding history of hairy cell leukemia.

Plasmacytoid monocytic lymphoma (plasmacytoid T-cell lymphoma) may represent a lesion related to myeloid leukemia.[565] The patients are usually elderly, and present with generalized lymphadenopathy and hepatosplenomegaly. The patients almost always have myelomonocytic leukemia, either at the time of diagnosis or shortly after, and therefore plasmacytoid monocytic lymphoma probably represents an unusual manifestation of myeloid leukemia. Involved nodes show focal or diffuse infiltration by a mormorphous proliferation of medium-sized cells with round to oval eccentric nuclei and a moderate amount of cytoplasm. Immunohistochemical studies demonstrate the characteristic phenotype of plasmacytoid monocytic cells, with reactivity for histiocytic markers, often combined with the aberrant expression of CD5.

Other proliferations

Hairy cell leukemia may also involve the lymph nodes, but the involvement is usually insignificant in comparison to involvement of the bone marrow and spleen.[566] The outer cortex is usually preferentially involved, and the cytologic features are identical to that found in other sites (Fig. 42-114). The histologic appearance may be easily confused with monocytoid B-cell lymphoma, but the clinical circumstances should be able to resolve the diagnostic dilemma. Plasmacytoma of lymph node can occur rarely as an isolated finding, as part of multiple myeloma, or as regional involvement of a solitary plasmacytoma.[567] Occasional cases are associated with amyloidosis of the lymph node.[568] Lymph nodes may also be involved in systemic mastocytosis.[569] The infiltrate preferentially involves the medullary cords and perivascular sites. The cells are usually bland, with small, oval or indented nuclei, fine chromatin, and a moderate amount of pale cytoplasm (Fig. 42-115). The infiltrate is often accompanied by eosinophils and sclerosis, clues that should prompt additional studies. Giemsa, chloroacetate

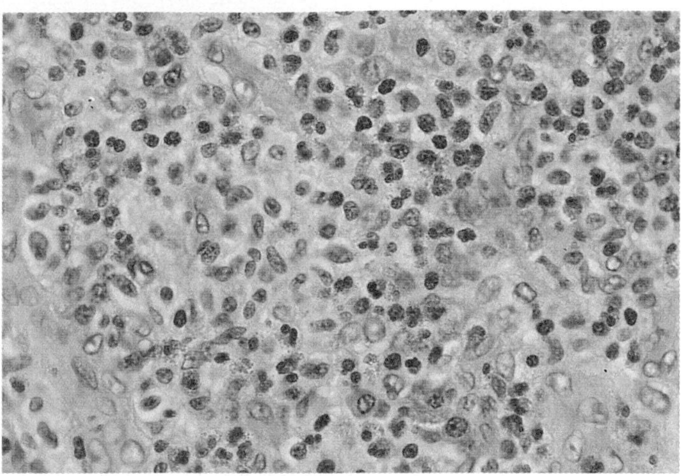

Fig. 42-115 Mast cell disease. There is a proliferation of cells with small to intermediate-sized nuclei with bland cytologic features and a moderate rim of pale cytoplasm. Note the numerous eosinophils, which are often a helpful clue to the diagnosis.

esterase, and toluidine blue stains are helpful to identify mast cell granules.

REFERENCES

Pathologic evaluation of a lymph node

1. Russell J, Skinner J, Orell S, Seshadri R: Fine needle aspiration cytology in the management of lymphoma, *Aust NZ J Med* 13:365, 1983.
2. Arber DA, Weiss LM: CD15: A review, *Appl Immunohistochem* 1:17, 1993.
3. Arber DA, Weiss LM: CD43: A review, *Appl Immunohistochem* 1:88, 1993.
4. Cartun RW, Coles FB, Pastuszak WT: Utilization of monoclonal antibody L26 in the identification and confirmation of B-cell lymphomas: a sensitive and specific marker applicable to formalin-and B-5-fixed, paraffin-embedded tissues, *Am J Pathol* 129:415, 1987.
5. Chang KL, Arber DA, Weiss LM: CD30: A review, *Appl Immunohistochem* 1:244, 1993.
6. Davy FR, Gatter KC, Ralfkiaer E et al: Immunophenotyping of non-Hodgkin's lymphomas using a panel of antibodies on paraffin-embedded tissues, *Am J Pathol* 129:43, 1987.
7. Weiss LM, Arber DA, Chang KL: CD45: A review, *Appl Immunohistochem* 1:166, 1993.
8. Weiss LM, Arber DA, Chang KL: CD68: A review, *Appl Immunohistochem* 2:2, 1994.
9. Weiss LM, Chang KL: The *bcl-2* proto-oncogene, *Appl Immunohistochem* 1:163, 1993.
10. Weiss LM, Medeiros LJ, Strickler JG et al: Non-Hodgkin's lymphomas: proliferative rate as assessed by Ki-67 antibody, *Hum Pathol* 18:1155, 1987.
11. Picker LJ, Weiss LM, Medeiros LJ et al: Immunophenotypic criteria for the diagnosis of non-Hodgkin's lymphoma, *Am J Pathol* 128:181, 1987.
12. Knapp W, Dorken B, Gilks WR et al: *Leukocyte Typing IV: white Cell Differentiation Antigens*, Oxford, 1989, Oxford Press.
13. Stein H, Lennert K, Feller A, Mason D: Immunohistological analysis of human lymphoma: correlation of histological and immunological categories, *Adv Cancer Res* 42:67, 1984.
14. Juneja SK, Cooper IA, Hodson GS et al: DNA ploidy patterns and cytokinetics of non-Hodgkin's lymphoma, *J Clin Pathol* 39:987, 1986.
15. Braylan RC, Benson NA, Nourse VA: Cellular DNA of human neoplastic B-cells measured by flow cytometry, *Cancer* Res 44:5010, 1984.
16. Cossman J, Uppenkamp M, Sundeen J et al: Molecular genetics and the diagnosis of lymphoma, *Arch Pathol Lab Med* 112:117, 1988.
17. Griesser H, Feller A, Lennert K et al: Rearrangement of the beta chain of the T-cell antigen receptor and immunoglobulin genes in lymphoproliferative disorders, *J Clin Invest* 78:1179, 1986.
18. Sklar J and Weiss LM: Applications of antigen receptor gene rearrangements to the diagnosis and characterization of lymphoid neoplasms, *Ann Rev Med* 39:315, 1988.
19. Weiss LM, Spagnolo DV: Assessment of clonality in lymphoid proliferations, *Am J Pathol* 142:1579, 1993.
20. Davis RE, Warnke RA, Dorfman RF, Cleary ML: Utility of molecular genetic analysis for the diagnosis of neoplasia in morphologically an immunophenotypically equivocal hematolymphoid lesions, *Cancer* 67:2890, 1991.
21. Weiss LM, Wood GS, Trela MJ et al: Clonal T-cell populations in lymphomatoid papulosis. Evidence for a lymphoproliferative etiology in a clinically benign disease, *N Engl J Med* 315:475, 1986.
22. Aster J, Kobayashi Y, Shiota M et al: Detection of the t(14;18) at similar frequencies in hyperplastic lymphoid tissues from American and Japanese Patients, *Am J Pathol* 141:291, 1992.
23. Segal GH, Scott M, Jorgensen T, Braylan RC: Standard polymerase chain reaction analysis does not detect a t(14;18) in reactive lymphoid hyperplasia, *Arch Pathol Lab Med* 118:791, 1994.

Normal lymph nodes

24. Roitt I: Essential Immunology, ed 7, London, 1991, Blackwell Scientific Publications, 1991.
25. Liu Y-J, Johnson GD, Gordon J, MacLennan JCM: Germinal centers in T-cell-dependent antibody responses, *Immunol Today* 13:17, 1992.
26. Hall JG: The functional anatomy of lymph nodes. In Stansfeld AG, editors: *Lymph node biopsy interpretation*, Edinburgh, 1985, Churchill Livingstone.
27. Van der Valk P, Meijer CJLM: The histology of reactive lymph nodes, *Am J Surg Pathol* 11:866, 1987.
28. Nieuwenhuis P, Keuning FJ: Germinal centers and the origin of the B-cell system. II. Germinal centers in the rabbit spleen and popliteal lymph nodes, *Immunology* 26:509, 1974.
29. van den Oord JJ, de Wolf-Peeters C, Desmet VJ: The marginal zone in the human reactive lymph node, *Am J Clin Pathol* 86:475, 1986.
30. Van Krieken JHJM, von Schilling C, Kluin M, Lennert K: Splenic marginal zone lymphocytes and related cells in the lymph node: a morphologic and immunohistochemical study, *Hum Pathol* 20:320, 1989.
31. van der Valk P, van der Loo EM, Jansen J et al: Analysis of lymphoid and dendritic cells in human lymph node, tonsil and spleen: a study using monoclonal and heterologous antibodies, *Virchows Arch B (Cell Pathol)* 45:169, 1984.
32. Stein H, Bank A, Tolksdorf G et al: Immunohistologic analysis of the organization of normal lymphoid tissue and non-Hodgkin's lymphomas, *J Histochem Cytochem* 28:746, 1980.
33. Nossal GJV, Abbot A, Mitchell J, Lummos Z: Antigens in immunity-XV: ultrastructural features of antigen capture in primary and secondary lymphoid follicles, *J Exp Med* 127:277, 1968.
34. Motoi M, Helbron D, Kaiserling E, Lennert K: Eosinophilic granuloma of lymph nodes: a variant of histiocytosis X, *Histopathology* 4:585, 1980.
35. Stein H: The immunologic and immunochemical basis for the Kiel classification. In Lennert K, editor: *Malignant lymphomas other than Hodgkin's disease*, Berlin, Springer-Verlag, 1978.
36. Gowans JL, Knight EJ: The route of recirculation of lymphocytes in the rat, *Proc R Soc Biol* 159:257, 1964.
37. Pals ST, Horst E, Scheper RJ, Meijer CJLM: Mechanisms of human lymphocyte migration and their role in the pathogenesis of disease, *Immunol Rev* 108:111, 1989.
38. Facchetti F, De Wolf-Peeters C, Mason DY et al: Plasmacytoid T-cells: immunohistochemical evidence for their monocyte macrophage origin, *Am J Pathol* 133:15, 1988.

Nonhematopoietic lesions in lymph nodes

39. Karp LA, Czernobilsky B: Glandular inclusions in pelvic and abdominal paraaortic lymph nodes: a study of autopsy and surgical material in males and females, *Am J Clin Pathol* 52:212, 1969.
40. Clement PB: Pathology of endometriosis, *Pathol Annu* 25(1):245, 1990.
41. Mills SE: Decidual and squamous metaplasia in abdomino-pelvic lymph nodes, *Int J Gynecol Pathol* 2:209, 1983.

42. Holdsworth PJ, Hopkinson JM, Leveson SH: Benign axillary epithelial lymph node inclusions—a histological pitfall, *Histopathology* 13:226, 1988.
43. Rosai J, Carcangiu ML, DeLellis RA: Tumors of the thyroid gland. In *Atlas of tumor pathology*, ed 3, Washington, D.C., 1992, Armed Forces Institute of Pathology.
44. Bautista NC, Cohen S, Anders KH: Benign melanocytic nevus cells in axillary lymph nodes: a prospective incidence and immunohistochemical study with literature review, *Am J Clin Pathol* 102:102, 1994.
45. Epstein JI, Erlandson RA, Rosen PP: Nodal blue nevi: a study of three cases, *Am J Surg Pathol* 8:907, 1984.
46. McCarthy SW, Palmer AA, Bale PM, Hirst E: Naevus cells in lymph nodes, *Pathology* 6:351, 1971.
47. Rodriguez HA, Ackerman LV: Cellular blue nevus: clinicopathologic study of forty-five cases, *Cancer* 21:393, 1968.
48. Finkbeiner WE, Egbert BM, Groundwater JR, Sagebiel RW: Kaposi's sarcoma in young homosexual men: a histopathologic study with particular reference to lymph node involvement, *Arch Pathol Lab Med* 106:261, 1982.
49. Chen KTK: Multicentric Castleman's disease and Kaposi's sarcoma, *Am J Surg Pathol* 8:287, 1984.
50. Chan JKC, Frizzera G, Fletcher CDM, Rosai J: Primary vascular tumors of lymph nodes other than Kaposi's sarcoma: analysis of 39 cases and delineation of two new entities, *Am J Surg Pathol* 16:335, 1992.
51. Chan JKC, Warnke RA, Dorfman RF: Vascular transformation of sinuses in lymph nodes, a study of its morphologic spectrum and distinction from Kaposi's sarcoma, *Am J Surg Pathol* 14:732, 1991.
52. Dorfman RF, and Warnke R: Lymphadenopathy simulating the malignant lymphomas, *Hum Pathol* 5:519, 1974.
53. Haferkamp O, Rosenau W, Lennert K: Vascular transformation of lymph node sinuses due to venous obstruction, *Arch Pathol* 92:81, 1971.
54. Chan JKC, Lewin KJ, Lombard CD et al: The histopathology of bacillary angiomatosis of lymph nodes, *Am J Surg Pathol* 14:430, 1991.
55. Warnke RA, Weiss LM, Chan JKC et al: Tumors of the lymphoid system. In *Atlas of tumor pathology*, Washington, D.C., 1995, Armed Forces Institute of Pathology.
56. Suster S, Rosai J: Intranodal hemorrhagic spindle cell tumor with "amianthoid" fibers: report of six cases of a distinctive mesenchymal neoplasm of the inguinal region that simulates Kaposi's sarcoma, *Am J Surg Pathol* 13:347, 1989.
57. Weiss SW, Gnepp DR, Bratthauer GL: Palisaded myofibroblastoma: a benign mesenchymal tumor of lymph node, *Am J Surg Pathol* 13:341, 1989.
58. Perrone T, de Wolf-Peeters C, Frizzera G: Inflammatory pseudotumors of lymph nodes: a distinctive pattern of nodal reaction, *Am J Surg Pathol* 12:351, 1988.
59. Davis RE, Warnke RA, Dorfman RF: Inflammatory pseudotumor of lymph nodes: additional observations and evidence for an inflammatory etiology, *Am J Surg Pathol* 14:744, 1991.
60. Chen KTK: Mycobacterial spindle cell pseudotumor of lymph nodes, *Am J Surg Pathol* 16:276, 1992.
61. Fisher ER, Gregorio RM, Redmond C et al: Pathologic findings from the National Surgical Adjuvant Breast Project (Protocol No. 4). III. The significance of extrandoal extension of axillary micrometastases, *Am J Clin Pathol* 65:439, 1976.
62. Wells CA, Heryet A, Brochier J et al: The immunocytochemical detection of axillary micrometastases in breast cancer, *Br J Cancer* 50:193, 1984.

Reactive lymphadenopathies

63. Schnitzer B: Reactive lymphoid hyperplasia. In Jaffe ES, editor: *Surgical pathology of the lymph nodes and related organs*, Philadelphia, 1985, Saunders.
64. Nosanchuk JS, Schnitzer B: Follicular hyperplasia in lymph nodes from patients with rheumatoid arthritis, *Cancer* 24:343, 1969.
65. Chadburn A, Metroka C, Mouradian J: Progressive lymph node histology and its prognostic value in patients with acquired immunodeficiency syndrome and AIDS-related complex, *Hum Pathol* 20:579, 1989.
66. Stansfeld AG: The histologic diagnosis of toxoplasmic lymphadenitis, *J Clin Pathol* 14:565, 1961.
67. Hartsock RJ, Halling LW, King FM: Luetic lymphadenitis: a clinical and histologic study of 20 cases, *Am J Clin Pathol* 53:304, 1970.
68. Childs CC, Parham DM, Berard CW: Infectious mononucleosis: the spectrum of morphologic changes simulating lymphoma in lymph nodes and tonsils, *Am J Surg Pathol* 11:122, 1987.
69. Medeiros LJ, Kaynor B, Harris NL: Lupus lymphadenitis: report of a case with immunohistologic studies on frozen sections, *Hum Pathol* 20:295, 1989.
70. Dorfman RF, Berry GJ: Kikuchi's histiocytic necrotizing lymphadenitis: an analysis of 108 cases with emphasis on differential diagnosis, *Semin Diagn Pathol* 5:329, 1988.
71. Sieracki JC, Fine G: Whipple's disease—observations on systemic involvement. II. Gross and histologic observations, *Arch Pathol* 67:81, 1959.
72. Rappaport H, Winter WJ, Hicks EB: Follicular lymphoma: a re-evaluation of its position in the scheme of malignant lymphoma, based on a survey of 253 cases, *Cancer* 9:792, 1956.
73. Nathwani BN, Winberg CD, Diamond LW, Bearman RM, Kim H: Morphologic criteria for the differentiation of follicular lymphoma from florid reactive follicular hyperplasia: a study of 80 cases, *Cancer* 48:1794, 1981.
74. Symmers W St C: The lymphoreticular system. In Henry K, Symmers W St C, editors: *Systemic pathology*, Edinburgh, 1992, Churchill Livingstone.
75. Ngan B-Y, Chen-Levy Z, Weiss LM et al: Expression in non-Hodgkin lymphoma of the *bcl-2* protein associated with the t(14;18) translocation, *N Engl J Med* 318:1638, 1988.
76. Weisenburger, DD: Mantle-zone lymphoma: an immunohistologic study, *Cancer* 53:1073, 1984.
77. Doggett RS, Colby TV, Dorfman RF: Interfollicular Hodgkin's disease, *Am J Surg Pathol* 7:145, 1983.
78. Schnitzer B: Pathology of lymphoid tissue in rheumatoid arthritis and allied diseases. In Glynn LE, Schlumberger HD, editor: *Bayer Symposium VI. Experimental models of chronic inflammatory diseases*, New York, 1977 Springer-Verlag.
79. Symmons, DPM: Neoplasms of the immune system in rheumatoid arthritis, *Am J Med* 78:22, 1985.
80. Kondratowicz GM, Symmons DP, Bacon PA et al: Rheumatoid lymphadenopathy: a morphological and immunohistochemical study, *J Clin Pathol* 43:106, 1990.
81. Keller AR, Hochholzer L, Castleman B: Hyaline-vascular and plasma-cell types of giant lymph node hyperplasia of mediastinum and other locations, *Cancer* 29:670, 1972.
82. McCurley TJ, Collins RD, Ball E, Collins RD: Nodal and extranodal lymphoproliferative disorders in Sjögren's syndrome: a clinical and immunopathologic study, *Hum Pathol* 21:482, 1990.
83. Castleman B, Iverson I, Menendez VP: Localized mediastinal lymph node hyperplasia resembling thymoma, *Cancer* 9:822, 1956.
84. Frizzera G, Peterson BA, Bayrd ED, Goldman A: A systemic lymphoproliferative disorder with morphologic features of Castleman's disease: clinical findings and clinicopathologic correlations in 15 patients, *J Clin Oncol* 3:1202, 1985.
85. Frizzera G: Castleman's disease and related disorders, *Semin Diagn Pathol* 5:346, 1988.
86. Frizzera G: Castleman's disease: more questions than answers, *Hum Pathol* 16:202, 1985.
87. Weisenburger DD, Nathwani BN, Winberg CD, Rappaport H: Multicentric angiofollicular lymph node hyperplasia: a clinicopathologic study of 16 cases, *Hum Pathol* 16:162, 1985.
88. Flendrig JA: Benign giant lymphoma: clinicopathologic correlation study. In Clark RL, Cumley RW, editor: The year book of cancer, Chicago, 1970, Mosby.
89. Harris NL, Bahn AK: "Plasmacytoid T-cells" in Castleman's disease, *Am J Surg Pathol* 11:109, 1987.
90. Radaszkiewicz T, Hansmann ML, Lennert K: Monoclonality and polyclonality of plasma cells in Castleman's disease of the plasma cell variant, *Histopathology* 14:11, 1989.
91. Bitter MA, Komaiko W, Franklin WA: Giant lymph node hyperplasia with osteoblastic bone lesions and the POEMS (Takatsuki's) syndrome, *Cancer* 56:188, 1985.

92. Dickson D, Ben-Ezra JM, Reed J et al: Multicentric giant lymph-node hyperplasia, Kaposi's sarcoma, and lymphoma, *Arch Pathol Lab Med* 109:1013, 1985.
93. Centers for Disease Control and Prevention: Persistent, generalized lymphadenopathy among homosexual males, *MMWR* 31:249, 1982.
94. Brynes RK, Chan WC, Spira TJ, Ewing E, Chandler FW: Value of lymph node biopsy in unexplained lymphadenopathy in homosexual men, *JAMA* 250:1313, 1983.
95. Ioachim HL, Cronin W, Roy M, Maya M: Persistent lymphadenopathies in people at high risk for HIV infection: clinicopathologic correlations and long-term follow-up in 79 cases, *Am J Clin Pathol* 93:208, 1990.
96. Knowles DM, Chadburn A: Lymphadenopathy and the lymphoid neoplasms associated with the acquired immune deficiency syndrome (AIDS). In Knowles DM, editor: *Neoplastic hematopath,* Baltimore, 1992, Williams and Wilkins.
97. Pileri S, Rivano MT, Raise E et al, editors: The value of lymph node biopsy in patients with acquired immunodeficiency syndrome (AIDS) and the AIDS-related complex (ARC): a morphological and immunohistochemical study of 90 cases, *Histopathology* 10:1107, 1986.
98. Ewing EP, Chandler FW, Spira TJ et al: Primary lymph node pathology in AIDS and AIDS-related lymphadenopathy, *Arch Pathol Lab Med* 109:977, 1985.
99. Said JW: AIDS related lymphadenopathies, *Semin Diagn Pathol* 5:365, 1988.
100. Sohn CC, Sheibani K, Winberg CD, Rappaport H: Monocytoid B-lymphocytes: their relation to the patterns of the acquired immunodeficiency syndrome (AIDS) and AIDS-related lymphadenopathy, *Hum Pathol* 16:979, 1985.
101. Burns BF, Colby TV, Dorfman RF: Differential diagnostic features of nodular L&H Hodgkin's disease, including progressive transformation of germinal centers, *Am J Surg Pathol* 8:253, 1984.
102. Hansmann M-L, Fellbaum C, Hui PK, Moubayed P: Progressive transformation of germinal centers with and without association to Hodgkin's disease, *Am J Clin Pathol* 93:219, 1990.
103. Osborne BM, Butler JJ: Clinical implications of progressive transformation of germinal centers, *Am J Surg Pathol* 8:725, 1984.
104. Poppema S, Kaiserling E, Lennert K: Hodgkin's disease with lymphocytic predominance nodular type (nodular paragranuloma) and progressively transformed germinal centers: a cytohistological study, *Histopathology* 3:295, 1979.
105. Poppema S, Visser L, De Leij L: Reactivity of presumed anti-natural killer cell antibody Leu 7 with intrafollicular T-lymphocytes, *Clin Exp Immunol* 54:834, 1983.
106. Gould E, Porto R, Albores-Saavedra J, Ibe MJ: Dermatopathic lymphadenitis: the spectrum and significance of its morphologic features, *Arch Pathol Lab Med* 112:1145, 1988.
107. Chamulak GA, Brynes RK, Nathwani BN: Kikuchi-Fujimoto disease mimicking malignant lymphoma, *Am J Surg Pathol* 14:514, 1990.
108. Fujimoto Y, Kozima Y, Yamaguchi K: Cervical subacute necrotizing lymphadenitis: a new clinicopathologic entity, *Naika* 20:920, 1972.
109. Kikuchi M: Lymphadenitis showing focal reticulum cell hyperplasia with nuclear debris and phagocytes: a clinico-pathological study (in Japanese), *Nippon Ketsueki Gakkai Zasshi* 35:379, 1972.
110. Koehler JE, Quinn FD, Berger GT, LeBoit PE, Tappero JW: Isolation of Rochalimaea species from cutaneous and osseous lesions of bacillary angiomatosis, *N Engl J Med* 327:1625, 1992.
111. Bascom R, Johns CJ: The natural history and management of sarcoidosis, *Adv Intern Med* 31:213, 1986.
112. Burke JS, Colby TV: Dermatopathic lymphadenopathy: comparison of cases associated and unassociated with mycosis fungoides, *Am J Surg Pathol* 5:343.
113. Rausch E, Kaiserling E, Goos M: Langerhans cells and interdigitating reticulum cells in the thymus-dependent region in human dermatopathic lymphadenitis, *Virchows Arch B (Cell Pathol)* 25:327, 1977.
114. Weiss LM, Beckstead JH, Warnke RA, Wood GS: Leu 6 expressing lymph node cells are dendritic cells and closely related to interdigitating cells, *Hum Pathol* 17:179, 1986.
115. Pileri S, Kikuchi M, Helbron D, Lennert K: Histiocytic necrotizing lymphadenitis without granulocytic infiltration, *Virchows Arch A (Pathol Anat Histol)* 395:257, 1982.
116. Wear DJ, Margileth AM, Hadfield TL, Fischer GW, Schlagel CJ, King FM: Cat scratch disease: a bacterial infection, *Science* 221:1403, 1983.
117. Walzer PD, Armstrong D: Lymphogranuloma venereum presenting as supraclavicular and inguinal lymphadenopathy, *Sex Transm Dis* 4:12, 1977.
118. Schapers RFM, Reif R, Lennert K, Knapp W: Mesenteric lymphadenitis due to Yersinia enterocolitica, *Virchows Arch A (Pathol Anat Histol)* 390:127, 1981.
119. Hui PK, Chan JKC, Ng CS, Kung ITM, Gwi E: Lymphadenopathy in Kimura's disease, *Am J Surg Pathol* 13:177, 1989.
120. Kuo T-T, Shih L-Y, Chan H-L: Kimura's disease: involvement of regional lymph nodes and distinction from angiolymphoid hyperplasia with eosinophilia, *Am J Surg Pathol* 12:843, 1988.
121. Hutchinson WM, Dunachie JF, Work K: The faecal transmission of Toxoplasma gondii, *Acta Pathol Microbiol Scand* 74:462, 1968.
122. McCabe RE, Brooks RG, Dorfman RF, Remington JS: Clinical spectrum in 107 cases of toxoplasmic lymphadenopathy, *Rev Infect Dis* 9:754, 1987.
123. Zangwill KM, Hamilton DH, Perkins BA et al: Cat scratch disease in Connecticut: epidemiology, risk factors, and evaluation of a new diagnostic test, *N Engl J Med* 329:8, 1993.
124. Miller-Catchpole R, Variakojis D, Vardiman JW et al: Cat-scratch disease: identification of bacteria in seven cases of lymphadenitis, *Am J Surg Pathol* 10:276, 1986.
125. Frizzera G, Moran EM, Rappaport H: Angio-immunoblastic lymphadenopathy. Diagnosis and clinical course, *Am J Med* 59:803, 1975.
126. Lukes RJ, Tindle BH: Immunoblastic lymphadenopathy: a hyperimmune entity resembling Hodgkin's disease, *N Engl J Med* 292:1, 1975.
127. Gams RA, Neal JA, Conrad FG: Hydantoin-induced pseudo-pseudolymphoma, *Ann Intern Med* 69:557, 1968.
128. Saltzstein SL, Ackerman LV: Lymphadenopathy induced by anticonvulsant drugs clinically and pathologically mimicking malignant lymphomas, *Cancer* 12:164, 1959.
129. Kawasaki T: Acute febrile mucocutaneous syndrome with lymphoid involvement with specific desquamation of fingers and toes in children, *Jpn J Allerg* 16:178, 1967.
130. Abbondanzo SL, Sato N, Straus SE, Jaffe ES: Acute infectious mononucleosis. (CD30) (KI-1) antigen expression and histologic correlations, *Am J Clin Pathol* 93:698, 1990.
131. Fellbaum C, Hansmann ML, Parwaresch MR, Lennert K: Monoclonal antibodies Ki-B3 and Leu M1 discriminate giant cells of infectious mononucleosis and of Hodgkin's disease, *Hum Pathol* 19:1168, 1988.
132. Tindle BH, Parke JW, Lukes RJ: "Reed-Sternberg cells" in infectious mononucleosis, *Am J Clin Pathol* 58:607, 1972.
133. Hartsock RJ: Postvaccinial lymphadenitis: hyperplasia of lymphoid tissue that simulates malignant lymphomas, *Cancer* 21:632, 1968.
134. Otteman LA, Greipp PR, Ruiz-Argüelles GJ et al: Infectious mononucleosis mimicking a B-cell immunoblastic lymphoma associated with an abnormality in regulatory T-cells, *Am J Med* 78:885, 1985.
135. Shin SS, Berry GJ, Weiss LM: Infectious mononucleosis: diagnosis by in situ hybridization in two cases with atypical features, *Am J Surg Pathol* 7:625, 1991.
136. Vago JF, Titman WE, Swerdlow SH: CMV-associated lymphadenopathy in the "normal" host: a histopathologic and immunophenotypic description (abstract), *Lab Invest* 60:100A, 1989.
137. Younes M, Podesta A, Helie M, Buckley P: Infection of T but not B lymphocytes by cytomegalovirus in lymph nodes: an immunophenotypic study, *Am J Surg Pathol* 15:75, 1991.
138. Tamaru J, Atsuo M, Horie H et al: Herpes simplex lymphadenitis: report of two cases with review of the literature, *Am J Surg Pathol* 14:571, 1990.
139. Gaffey MJ, Ben-Ezra J, Weiss LM: Herpes simplex lymphadenitis, *Am J Clin Pathol* 95:709, 1991.
140. Dorfman RF, Herweg J: Live, attenuated measles virus vaccine: inguinal lymphadenopathy complicating administration, *JAMA* 198:320, 1966.

241. Strickler JG, Michie SA, Warnke RA, Dorfman RF: The "syncytial variant" of nodular sclerosing Hodgkin's disease, *Am J Surg Pathol* 10:470, 1986.
242. Travis LB, Gonazalez CL, Hankey BF, Jaffe ES: Hodgkin's disease following non-Hodgkin's lymphoma, *Cancer* 69:2337, 1992.
243. Kim H, Hendrickson MR, Dorfman RF: Composite lymphoma, *Cancer* 40:959, 1977.
244. Casey TT, Cousar JB, Mangum M et al: Monomorphic lymphomas arising in patients with Hodgkin's disease: correlation of morphologic, immunophenotypic, and molecular genetic findings in 12 cases, *Am J Pathol* 136:81, 1990.
245. Chan WC, Griem ML, Grozea PN et al: Mycosis fungoides and Hodgkin's disease occurring in the same patient: report of three cases, *Cancer* 44:1408, 1979.
246. Simrell CR, Boccia RV, Longo DL, Jaffe ES: Coexisting Hodgkin's disease and mycosis fungoides. Immunohistochemical proof of its existence, *Arch Pathol Lab Med* 110:1029, 1986.
247. Han T: Chronic lymphocytic leukemia in Hodgkin's disease: report of a case and review of the literature, *Cancer* 28:300, 1971.
248. Choi H, Keller RH: Coexistence of chronic lympyhocytic leukemia and Hodgkin's disease, *Cancer* 48:48, 1981.
249. Grossman DM, Hanson CA, Schnitzer B: Simultaneous lymphocyte predominant Hodgkin's disease and large-cell lymphoma, *Am J Surg Pathol* 15:668, 1991.
250. Sundeen JT, Cossman J, Jaffe ES: Lymphocyte predominant Hodgkin's disease nodular subtype with coexistent "large cell lymphoma": histological progression or composite malignancy? *Am J Surg Pathol* 12:599, 1988.
251. Momose H, Jaffe ES, Shin SS, Chen YY, Weiss LM: Chronic lymphocytic leukemia/small lymphocytic lymphoma with Reed-Sternberg-like cells and possible transformation to Hodgkin's disease: mediation by Epstein-Barr virus, *Am J Surg Pathol* 16:859, 1992.
252. Tsang WYW, Chan JKC, Ng CS: The nature of Reed-Sternberg-like cells in chronic lymphocytic leukemia, *Am J Clin Pathol* 99:317, 1993.
253. Brecher M, Banks PM: Hodgkin's disease variant of Richter's syndrome: report of eight cases, *Am J Clin Pathol* 93:333, 1990.
254. Burns BF, Colby TV, Dorfman RF: Langerhans' cell granulomatosis (histiocytosis X) associated with malignant lymphomas, *Am J Surg Pathol* 7:529, 1983.
255. Neuman MP, Frizzera G: The coexistence of Langerhans' cell granulomatosis and malignant lymphoma may take different forms: report of seven cases with a review of the literature, *Hum Pathol* 17:1060, 1986.
256. Rappaport H, Berard CW, Butler JJ et al: Report of the committee on histopathological criteria contributing to staging of Hodgkin's disease, *Cancer Res* 31:1864, 1971.
257. Sacks EL, Donaldson SS, Gordon J, Dorfman RF: Epithelioid granulomas associated with Hodgkin's disease: clinical correlations in 55 previously untreated patients, *Cancer* 41:562, 1978.
258. Strum SB, Rappaport H: Interrelations of the histologic types of Hodgkin's disease, *Arch Pathol* 91:127, 1971.
259. Colby TV, Warnke RA: The histology of the initial relapse of Hodgkin's disease, *Cancer* 45:289, 1980.
260. Dolginow D, Colby TV: Recurrent Hodgkin's disease in treated sites, *Cancer* 48:1124, 1981.
261. Grogan TM, Berard CW, Steinhorn SC et al: Changing patterns of Hodgkin's disease at autopsy: a 25-year experience at the National Cancer Institute, 1953-1978. *Cancer Treat Rep* 66:653, 1982.
262. Chen JL, Osborne BM, Butler JJ: Residual fibrous masses in treated Hodgkin's disease, *Cancer* 60:407, 1987.
263. Hansmann ML, Stein H, Dallenbach F, Fellbaum C: Diffuse lymphocyte-predominant Hodgkin's disease (diffuse paragranuloma): a variant of the B-cell-derived nodular type, *Am J Pathol* 138:29, 1991.
264. Timens W, Visser L, Poppema S: Nodular lymphocyte predominance type of Hodgkin's disease is a germinal center lymphoma, *Lab Invest* 54:457, 1986.
265. Chittal SM, Caveriviere P, Schwarting R et al: Monoclonal antibodies in the diagnosis of Hodgkin's disease: the search for a rational panel, *Am J Surg Pathol* 12:9, 1988.
266. Ree HJ, Neiman RS, Martin AW et al: Paraffin section markers for Reed-Sternberg cells: a comparative study of peanut agglutinin, Leu-M1, LN-2, and Ber H2, *Cancer* 63:2030, 1989.
267. Coles FB, Cartun RW, Pastuszak WT: Hodgkin's disease, lymphocyte-predominant type: immunoreactivity with B-cell antibodies, *Mod Pathol* 1:274, 1988.
268. Stein H, Hansmann ML, Lennert K et al: Reed-Sternberg and Hodgkin cells in lymphocyte-predominant Hodgkin's disease of nodular subtype contain J chain, *Am J Clin Pathol* 86:292, 1986.
269. Poppema S: Lymphocyte-predominance Hodgkin's disease, *Int Rev Exp Pathol* 33:53, 1992.
270. Tefferi A, Zellers RA, Banks PM et al: Clinical correlates of distinct immunophenotypic and histologic subcategories of lymphocyte-predominance Hodgkin's disease, *J Clin Oncol* 8:1959, 1990.
271. Hsu SM, Jaffe ES: Leu-M1 and peanut agglutinin stain the neoplastic cells of Hodgkin's disease, *Am J Clin Pathol* 82:29, 1984.
272. Stein H, Gerdes J, Schwab U et al: Identification of Hodgkin and Sternberg-Reed cells as a unique cell type derived from a newly-detected small-cell population, *Int J Cancer* 30:445, 1982.
273. Poppema S, Elema JD, Halie MR: The localization of Hodgkin's disease in lymph nodes: a study with immunohistological, enzyme histochemical and rosetting techniques on frozen sections, *Int J Cancer* 24:532, 1979.
274. Mir R, Kahn LB: Immunohistochemistry of Hodgkin's disease: a study of 20 cases, *Cancer* 52:2064, 1983.
275. Casey TT, Olson SJ, Cousar JB, Collins RD: Immunophenotypes of Reed-Sternberg cells: a study of 19 cases of Hodgkin's disease in plastic-embedded sections, *Blood* 74:2624, 1989.
276. Agnarsson BA, Kadin ME: The immunophenotype of Reed-Sternberg cells: a study of 50 cases of Hodgkin's disease using fixed frozen tissues, *Cancer* 63:2083, 1989.
277. Weiss LM: Gene analysis and Epstein-Barr viral genome studies of Hodgkin's disease, *Int Rev Exp Pathol* 33:165, 1992.
278. Sundeen J, Lipford E, Uppenkamp M et al: Rearranged antigen receptor genes in Hodgkin's disease, *Blood* 70:96, 1987.
279. Feller AC, Griesser H: DNA gene rearrangement studies in Hodgkin's disease and related lymphomas: a contribution to their cellular origin, *Recent Results Cancer Res* 117:27, 1989.
280. Jacobson JO, Wilkes BM, Harris NL: Polyclonal rearrangement of the T-cell antigen receptor genes in Hodgkin's disease: implications for diagnosis, *Mod Pathol* 4:172, 1991.
281. Thangavelu M, LeBeau MM: Chromosomal abnormalities in Hodgkin's disease, *Hematol Oncol Clin N Am* 3:221, 1989.
282. Tilly H, Bastard C, Delastre T et al: Cytogenetic studies in untreated Hodgkin's disease, *Blood* 77:1298, 1991.
283. Ladanyi M, Parsa NZ, Offit L et al: Clonal cytogenetic abnormalities in Hodgkin's disease, *Genes Chromsomes & Cancer* 3:294, 1991.
284. Poppema S, Kaleta J, Hepperle B: Chromosomal abnormalities in patients with Hodgkin's disease: evidence for frequent invovlement of the 14q chromosomal region but infrequent *bcl-2* gene rearrangement in Reed-Sternberg cells, *JNCI* 84:1789, 1992.
285. Cabanillas F, Pathak S, Trujillo J et al: Cytogenetic features of Hodgkin's disease suggest possible origin from a lymphocyte, *Blood* 71:1615, 1988.
286. Stetler-Stevenson M, Crush-Stanton S, Cossman J: Involvement of the *bcl-2* gene in Hodgkin's disease, *J Natl Cancer Inst* 82:855, 1990.
287. Gupta RK, Whelan JS, Lister TA et al: Direct sequence analysis of the t(14;18) chromosomal translocation in Hodgkin's disease, *Blood* 79:2084, 1992.
288. Said JW, Sassoon AF, Shintaku IP et al: Absence of *bcl-2* major breakpoint region and J_H gene rearrangement in lymphocyte predominance Hodgkin's disease: results of Southern blot analysis and polymerase chain reaction, *Am J Pathol* 138:261, 1991.
289. Athan E, Chadburn A, Knowles DM: The *bcl-2* gene translocation is undetectable in Hodgkin's disease by Southern blot hybridization and polymerase chain reaction, *Am J Pathol* 141:193, 1992.
290. Algara P, Martinez P, Sanchez L et al: Lymphocyte predominance Hodgkin's disease (nodular paragranuloma)—a *bcl-2* negative germinal centre lymphoma, *Histopathology* 19:69, 1991.

291. Hsu, SM, Xie SS, Hsu PL, Waldron JA Jr: Interleukin-6, but not interleukin-4, is expressed by Reed-Sternberg cells in Hodgkin's disease with or without histologic features of Castleman's disease, *Am J Pathol* 141:129, 1992.
292. Jücker M, Abts H, Li W et al: Expression of interleukin-6 and interleukin-6 receptor in Hodgkin's disease, *Blood* 77:2413, 1991.
293. Merz H, Houssiau FA, Orscheschek K et al: Interleukin-9 expression in human malignant lymphomas: unique association with Hodgkin's disease and large cell anaplastic lymphoma, *Blood* 78:1311, 1991.
294. Samoszuk M, Nansen L: Detection of interleukin-5 messenger RNA in Reed-Sternberg cells of Hodgkin's disease with eosinophilia, *Blood* 75:13, 1990.
295. Kadin ME, Agnarsson BA, Ellingsworth LR, Newcom SR: Immunohistochemical evidence of a role for transforming growth factor beta in the pathogenesis of nodular sclerosing Hodgkin's disease, *Am J Pathol* 136:1209, 1990.
295a. Delabie J, Tierens A, Wu G et al: Lymphocyte predominance Hodgkin's disease: lineage and clonality determination using a single cell assay, Blood 84:3291, 1994.
296. Diehl V, von Kalle C, Fonatsch C et al: The cell of origin in Hodgkin's disease, *Sem Oncol* 17:660, 1990.
297. Gregory CD, Kirchgens C, Edwards CF et al: Epstein-Barr virus-transformed human precursor B-cell lines: altered growth phenotype of lines with germ-line or rearranged but nonexpressed heavy chain genes, *Eur J Immunol* 17:1199, 1987.
298. Klein G: Epstein-Barr virus-carrying cells in Hodgkin's disease, *Blood* 80:299, 1992.
299. Harris NL: Epstein-Barr virus in lymphoma protagonist or passenger? *Am J Clin Path* 98:278, 1992.
300. Hsu SM, Hsu PL: Aberrant expression of T-cell and B-cell markers in myelocyte/monocyte/histiocyte-derived lymphoma and leukemia cells: is the infrequent espression of T/B-cell markers sufficient to establish a lymphoid origin for Hodgkin's Reed-Sternburg cells? *Am J Pathol* 134:203, 1989.
301. Hsu SM: The never-ending controversies in Hodgkin's disease, *Blood* 75:1742, 1990.
302. Drexler HG: More on the origin of the Reed-Sternberg cell, *Blood* 76:1665, 1990.
303. Slivnick DJ, Ellis TM, Nawrocki JF, Fisher RI: The impact of Hodgkin's disease on the immune system, *Sem Oncol* 17:673, 1990.
304. Fuks Z, Strober S, Kaplan HS: Interaction between serum factors and T-lymphocytes in Hodgkin's disease, *N Engl J Med* 295:1273, 1976.
305. Tullgren O, Grimfors G, Holm G et al: Lymphocyte abnormalities predicting a poor prognosis in Hodgkin's disease: a long-term follow-up, *Cancer* 68:768, 1991.
306. Posner MR, Reinherz EL, Breard J et al: Lymphoid subpopulations of peripheral blood and spleen in untreated Hodgkin's disease, *Cancer* 48:1170, 1981.
307. Goodwin JS, Messner RP, Bankhurst AD et al: Prostaglandin-producing suppressor cells in Hodgkin's disease, *N Engl J Med* 297:963, 1977.
308. Vanhaelen CPJ, Fisher RI: Increased sensitivity of lymphocytes from patients with Hodgkin's disease to concanavalin A-induced suppressor cells, *J Immunol* 127:1216, 1981.
309. Roux M, Schraven B, Roux A et al: Natural inhibitors of T-cell activation in Hodgkin's disease, *Blood* 78:2365, 1991.
310. Ford RJ, Tsao J, Kouttab NM et al: Association of an interleukin abnormality with the T-cell defect in Hodgkin's disease, *Blood* 64:386, 1984.
311. Pizzolo G, Chilosi M, Vinante F et al: Soluble interleukin-2 receptors in the serum of patients with Hodgkin's disease, *Br J Cancer* 55:427, 1987.
312. Wahl SM, McCartney-Frances N, Mergenhagen SE: Inflammatory and immunomodulatory roles of TGF-β, *Immunol Today* 10:258, 1989.
313. van Rijswijk REN, Sybesma JPHB, Kater L: A prospective study of the changes in immune status following radiotherapy for Hodgkin's disease, *Cancer* 53:62, 1984.
314. Liberati AM, Ballatori E, Fizzoti M et al: Immunologic profile in patients with Hodgkin's disease in complete remission, *Cancer* 59:1906, 1987.
315. Weitzman SA, Aisenberg AC, Siber GR, Smith DH: Impaired humoral immunity in treated Hodgkin's disease, *N Engl J Med* 297:245, 1977.
316. Minor DR, Schiffman G, McIntosh LS: Response of patients with Hodgkin's disease to pneumococcal vaccine, *Ann Int Med* 90:887, 1979.
317. Levy S, Tempe JL, Aleksijevic A et al: Depressed NK cell activity of peripheral blood mononuclear cells in untreated Hodgkin's disease: enhancing effect of interferon in vitro, *Scand J Haematol* 33:386, 1984.
318. Macklis RM, Mauch PM, Burakoff SJ, Smith BR: Lymphoid irradiation results in long-term increases in natural killer cells in patients treated for Hodgkin's disease, *Cancer* 69:778, 1992.
319. Carbone PP, Kaplan HS, Musshoff K et al: Report of the committee on Hodgkin's disease staging classification, *Cancer Res* 31:1860, 1971.
320. Lister TA, Crowther D, Sutcliffe SB et al: Report of a committee convened to discuss the evaluation and staging of patients with Hodgkin's disease: cotswolds meeting, *J Clin Oncol* 7:1630, 1989.
321. Lister TA, Crowther D: Staging for Hodgkin's disease, *Sem Oncol* 17:696, 1990.
322. Kaplan HS, Dorfman RF, Nelsen TS, Rosenberg SA: Staging laparotomy and splenectomy in Hodgkin's disease: analysis of indications and patterns of involvement in 285 consecutive, unselected patients, *Natl Cancer Inst Monogr* 36:291, 1973.
323. Kaplan HS: *Hodgkin's disease*, ed 2, Cambridge, Mass, 1980, Harvard University Press.
324. Rappaport H, Strum SB, Hutchison G, Allen LW: Clinical and biological significance of vascular invasion in Hodgkin's disease, *Cancer Res* 31:1794, 1971.
325. Dorfman RF: Relationship of histology to site in Hodgkin's disease, *Cancer Res* 31:1786, 1971.
326. Berard CW, Thomas LB, Axtell LM et al: The relationship of histopathological subtype to clinical stage of Hodgkin's disease at diagnosis, *Cancer Res* 31:1776, 1971.
327. Moormeier JA, Williams SF, Golomb HM: The staging of Hodgkin's disease, *Hematol Oncol Clin N Am* 3:237, 1989.
328. Rosenberg SA: Exploratory laparotomy and splenectomy for Hodgkin's disease: a commentary, *J Clin Oncol* 6:574, 1988.
329. Mauch P, Larson D, Osteen R et al: Prognostic factors for positive surgical staging in patients with Hodgkin's disease, *J Clin Oncol* 18:257, 990.
330. Peters MV: A study of survivals in Hodgkin's disease treated radiologically, *Am J Roentgenol Rad Therapy* 63:299, 1950.
331. Hoppe RT: Early-stage Hodgkin's disease: a choice of treatments or a treatment of choice? *J Clin Oncol* 9:897, 1991.
332. Farah R, Weichselbaum RR: Management of stage I and II Hodgkin's disease, *Hematol Oncol Clin N Am* 3:253, 1989.
333. Hoppe RT: Development of effective salvage treatment programs for Hodgkin's disease: an ongoing clinical challenge, *Blood* 77:2093, 1991.
334. Jacobson LO, Spurr CL, Barron ESG, Smith T, Lushbaugh C, Dick GF: Nitrogen mustard therapy: studies on the effect of methylbis-(b-chloroethyl) amine hydrochloride on neoplastic diseases and allied disorders of the hemopoietic system, *JAMA* 132:263, 1946.
335. Goodman LS, Wintrobe MM, Dameshek W, Goodman MJ, Gilman A, McLennan MT: Nitrogen mustard therapy: use of methyl-bis-(b-chloroethyl) amine hydrochloride and tris-(b-chloroethyl) amine hydrochloride for Hodgkin's disease, lymphosarcoma, leukemia and certain allied and miscellaneous disorders, *JAMA* 132:126, 1946.
336. DeVita VT Jr, Serpick AA, Carbone PP: Combination chemotherapy in the treatment of advanced Hodgkin's disease, *Ann Int Med* 73:881, 1970.
337. Bonadonna G, Zucali R, Monfardini S, De Lena M, Uslenghi C: Combination chemotherapy of Hodgkin's disease with adriamycin, bleomycin, vinblastine, and imidazole carboxamide versus MOPP, *Cancer* 36:252, 1975.
338. Canellos GP, Anderson JR, Propert KJ et al: Chemotherapy of advanced Hodgkin's disease with MOPP, ABVD, or MOPP alternating with ABVD, *N Engl J Med* 327:1478, 1992.
339. DeVita VT, Jr, Hubbard SM: Hodgkin's disease, *N Engl J Med* 328:560, 1993.

340. Pao WJ, Kun LE: Hodgkin's disease in children, *Hematol Oncol Clin N Am* 3:345, 1989.
341. Kennedy, BJ, Loeb V Jr, Peterson VM et al: National survey of patterns of care for Hodgkin's disease, *Cancer* 56:2547, 1985.
342. Kessinger A, Nademanee A, Forman SJ, Armitage JO: Autologous bone marrow transplantation for Hodgkins and non-Hodgkin's lymphomas, *Hematol Oncol Clin N Am* 4:577, 1990.
343. Knowles DM, Chamulak GA, Subar M et al: Lymphoid neoplasia associated with the acquired immunodeficiency syndrome (AIDS): the New York University Medical Center experience with 105 patients (1981-1986), *Ann Intern Med* 108:744, 1988.
344. Hansmann M-L, Zwingers T, Böske A et al: Clinical features of nodular paragranuloma (Hodgkin's disease, lymphocyte predominance type, nodular), *J Cancer Res Clin Oncol* 108:321, 1984.
345. Regula DP, Hoppe RT, Weiss LM: Nodular and diffuse types of lymphocyte predominance Hodgkin's disease, *N Engl J Med* 318:214, 1988.
346. Regula DP, Weiss LM, Warnke RA, Dorfman RF: Lymphocyte predominance Hodgkin's disease: a reappraisal based upon histological and immunophenotypical findings in relapsing cases, *Histopathology* 11:1107, 1987.
347. Borg-Grech A, Radford JA, Crowther D et al: A comparative study of the nodular and diffuse variants of lymphocyte-predominant Hodgkin's disease, *J Clin Oncol* 7:1303, 1989.
348. Bookman MA, Longo DL: Concomitant illness in patients treated for Hodgkin's disease, *Cancer Treatment Rev* 13:77, 1986.
349. van Rijswijk REN, Verbeek J, Haanen C et al: Major complications and causes of death in patients treated for Hodgkin's disease, *J Clin Oncol* 5:1624, 1987.
350. Urba WJ, Longo, DL: Hodgkin's disease, *N Engl J Med* 326:678, 1992.
351. Zarrabi MH, Rosner F: Second neoplasms in Hodgkin's disease: current controversies, *Hematol Oncol Clin N Am* 3:303, 1989.
352. Swerdlow AJ, Douglas AJ, Vaughan Hudson G et al: Risk of second primary cancers after Hodgkin's disease by type of treatment: analysis of 2846 patients in the British National Lymphoma Investigation, *BMJ* 304:1137, 1992.
353. Miettinen M, Franssila KO, Saxen E: Hodgkin's disease, lymphocytic predominance nodular: increased risk for subsequent non-Hodgkin's lymphomas, *Cancer* 51:2293, 1983.
354. Zarate-Osorno A, Medeiros LJ, Longo DL, Jaffe ES: Non-Hodgkin's lymphomas arising in patients successfully treated for Hodgkin's disease: a clinical, histologic, and immunophenotypic study of 14 cases, *Am J Surg Pathol* 16:885, 1992.
355. Gowitt GT, Chan WC, Brynes RK, Heffner LT: T-cell lymphoma following Hodgkin's disease, *Cancer* 56:1191, 1985.
356. Chilcote RR, Baehner RL, Hammond D, The Investigators and Special Studies Committee of the Children's Cancer Study Group: septicemia and meningitis in children splenectomized for Hodgkin's disease, *N Engl J Med* 295:798, 1976.

Non-Hodgkin's lymphoma

357. Devesa SS, Fears T: Non-Hodgkin's lymphoma time trends: United States and international data, *Cancer Res* 52 (suppl):5432s, 1992.
358. Scherr PA, Hutchison GB, Neiman RS: Non-Hodgkin's lymphoma an occupational exposure, *Cancer Res* 52 (suppl):5503s, 1992.
359. Hoar SK, Blair A, Holmes FF et al: Agricultural herbicide and risk of lymphoma and soft tissue sarcoma, *JAMA* 256:1141, 1986.
360. Cantor KP, Blair A, Everett G et al: Hair dye use and risk of leukemia and lymphoma, *Am J Public Health* 78:570, 1988.
361. Blayney DW, Jaffe ES, Fisher RI et al: The human T-cell leukemia/lymphoma virus (HTLV), lymphoma, lytic bone lesions, and hypercalcemia, *Ann Intern Med* 98:144, 1983.
362. Gaffey MJ, Weiss LM: Association of Epstein-Barr virus with human neoplasia, *Pathol Annual* 27:55, 1992.
363. Weiss LM, Arber DA, Strickler JG: Nasal T-cell lymphoma, *Ann Oncol* 5 (suppl 1):S39, 1994.
364. Rappaport H: Tumors of the hematopoietic system. In Atlas of tumor pathology, 1st series, fascicle 8, Washington, D.C., 1966, Armed Forces Institute of Pathology.
365. Lukes RJ, Collins RD: Immunological characterization of human malignant lymphomas, *Cancer* 34:1488, 1974.
366. Gerard-Marchant R, Hamlin I, Lennert K et al: Classification of non-Hodgkin's lymphomas, *Lancet* ii:406, 1974.
367. The Non-Hodgkin's Lymphoma Pathologic Classification Project: National Cancer Institute sponsored study of classifications of non-Hodgkin's lymphomas: summary and description of a working formulation for clinical usage, *Cancer* 49:2112, 1982.
368. Stansfield AG, Diebold J, Kapanci Y et al: Updated Kiel classification (letter), *Lancet* i:292, 1988.
369. Harris NL, Jaffe ES, Stein H et al: A revised European-American classification of lymphoid neoplasms: a proposal from the International Lymphoma Study Group, *Blood* 84:1361, 1994.
370. Rosenberg SA: Validity of the Ann Arbor Staging Classification for the non-Hodgkin's lymphomas, *Cancer Treat Rep* 61:1023, 1977.
371. The International Non-Hodgkin's Lymphoma Prognostic Factors Project: A predictive model for aggressive non-Hodgkin's lymphoma, *N Engl J Med* 329:987, 1993.
372. Kim H, Dorfman RF: Morphological studies of 84 untreated patients subjected to laparotomy for the staging of non-Hodgkin's lymphomas: 33:657, 1974.
373. Cheson BD, Bennett JM, Rai KR et al: Guidelines for clinical protocols for chronic lymphocytic leukemia: recommendations of the National Cancer Institute-sponsored working group, *Am J Hematol* 29:152, 1988.
374. Pangalis GA, Boussiotis VA, Kittas C: Malignant disorders of small lymphocytes. Small lymphocytic lymphoma, lymphoplasmacytic lymphoma, and chronic lymphocytic leukemia: their clinical and laboratory relationship, *Am J Clin Pathol* 99:402, 1993.
375. Morrison WH, Hoppe RT, Weiss LM et al: Small lymphocytic lymphoma, *J Clin Oncol* 7:598, 1989.
376. Berger F, Felman P, Sonet A et al: Nonfollicular small B-cell lymphomas: a heterogeneous group of patients with distinct clinical features and outcome, *Blood* 83:2829, 1994.
377. Ben-Ezra J, Burke JS, Swartz WG et al: Small lymphocytic lymphoma: a clinicopathologic anlaysis of 268 cases, *Blood* 73:579, 1989.
378. Lennert K, Feller AC: Histopathology of non-Hodgkin's lymphomas (based on the updated Kiel classification), ed 2, Berlin, 1992, Springer-Verlag.
379. Dick F, Maca RD: The lymph node in chronic lymphocytic leukemia, *Cancer* 41:283, 1978.
380. Pugh WC, Manning JT, Butler JJ: Paraimmunoblastic variant of small lymphocytic lymphoma/leukemia, *Am J Surg Pathol* 12:970, 1988.
381. Contos M, Kornstein M, Innes D, Ben-Ezra J: The utility of CD20 and CD43 in subclassification of low-grade B-cell lymphoma on paraffin sections, *Mod Pathol* 5:631, 1992.
382. Ngan BY, Picker LJ, Medeiros LJ, Warnke RA: Immunophenotypic diagnosis of non-Hodgkin's lymphoma in paraffin sections: co-expression of L60 (leu-22) and L26 antigens correlated with malignant histologic findings, *Am J Clin Pathol* 91:579, 1989.
383. Zukerberg L, Medeiros L, Ferry J, Harris N: Diffuse low-grade B-cell lymphomas: four clinically distinct subtypes defined by a combination of morphologic and immunophenotypic features, *Am J Clin Pathol* 100:373, 1993.
384. Juliusson G, Gahrton G, Oscier D et al: Cytogenetic findings and survival in B-cell chronic lymphocytic leukemia: second IWCLL compilation of data on 662 patients, *Leukemia Lymphoma* 5 (suppl):21, 1991.
385. Gaidano G, Ballerini P, Gong JZ et al: p53 mutations in human lymphoid malignancies: association with Burkitt lymphoma and chronic lymphocytic leukemia, *Proc Natl Acad Sci USA* 88:5413, 1991.
386. Medeiros LJ, Picker LJ, Gelb AB et al: Numbers of host "helper" T-cells and proliferating cells predict survival in diffuse small-cell lymphomas, *J Clin Oncol* 7:1009, 1989.
387. Pangalis GA, Nathwani BN, Rappaport H: Malignant lymphoma, well differentiated lymphocytic type: its relationship with chronic lymphocytic leukemia and macroglobulinemia of Waldenström, *Cancer* 39: 999, 1977.

388. Harris NL, Bhan AK: B-cell neoplasms of the lymphocytic, lymphoplasmacytoid, and plasma cell types: immunohistologic analysis and clinical correlation, *Hum Pathol* 16:829, 1985.
389. Offit K, Parsa NZ, Filippa D et al: t(9;14)(p13;q32) denotes a subset of low-grade non-Hodgkin's lymphoma with plasmacytoid differentiation, *Blood* 80:2594, 1992.
390. Isaacson PG: Lymphomas of mucosa-associated lymphoid tissue (MALT), *Histopathology* 16:627, 1990.
391. Shin SS, Sheibani K: Monocytoid B-cell lymphoma, *Am J Clin Pathol* 99:421, 1993.
392. Isaacson PG, Wright DH: Malignant lymphoma of mucosa associated lymphoid tissue, *Cancer* 52:1410, 1983.
393. Pelstring RJ, Essell JH, Kurtin PJ et al: Diversity of organ site involvement among malignant lymphomas of mucosa-associated tissues, *Am J Clin Pathol* 96:748, 1991.
394. Parsonnet J, Hansen S, Rodriguez L et al: Helicobacter pylori infection and gastric lymphoma, *N Engl J Med* 330:1267, 1994.
395. Shin SS, Sheibani K, Fishleder A et al: Monocytoid B-cell lymphoma in patients with Sjogren's syndrome: a clinicopathologic study of 13 patients, *Hum Pathol* 22:422, 1991.
396. Ngan BY, Warnke RA, Wilson M et al: Monocytoid B-cell lymphoma: a study of 36 cases, *Hum Pathol* 22:409, 1991.
397. Nathwani BN, Mohrmann RL, Brynes RK et al: Monocytoid B-cell lymphomas: an assessment of diagnostic criteria and a perspective on histogenesis, *Hum Pathol* 23:1061, 1992.
398. Chan JKC: Antibiotic-responsive gastric lymphoma? *Adv Anat Pathol* 1:33, 1994.
399. Wotherspoon AC, Finn TM, Isaacson PG: Trisomy 3 in low-grade B-cell lymphomas of mucosa-associated lymphoid tissue, *Blood* 85:2000, 1995.
400. Hussell T, Isaacson PG, Crabtree JE, Spencer J: The response of cells from low-grade B-cell gastric lymphomas of mucosa-associated lymphoid tissue to Helicobacter pylori, *Lancet* 342:571, 1993.
401. Wotherspoon A, Doglioni C, Diss T et al: Regression of primary low-grade B-cell gastric lymphoma of mucosa-associated lymphoid tissue type after eradication of Helicobacter pylori, *Lancet* 342:575, 1993.
402. Banks PM, Chan J, Cleary ML et al: Mantle cell lymphoma: a proposal for unification of morphologic, immunologic, and molecular data, *Am J Surg Pathol* 16:637, 1992.
403. Lardelli P, Bookman MA, Sundeen J et al: Lymphocytic lymphoma of intermediate differentiation: morphologic and immunophenotypic spectrum and clinical correlations, *Am J Surg Pathol* 14:752, 1990.
404. Raffeld M, Jaffe ES: Bcl-2, t(11;14), and mantle cell-derived lymphomas, *Blood* 78:259, 1991.
405. Williams ME, Swerdlow Sh, Rosenber CL, Arnold A: Chromosome 11 translocation breakpoints at the PRAD1/Cyclin D1 gene locus in centrocytic lymphoma, *Leukemia* 7:241, 1993.
406. Rimokh R, Berger F, Delsol G et al: Detection of the chromosomal translocation t(11;14) by polymerase chain reaction in mantle cell lymphomas, *Blood* 83:1871, 1994.
407. Rimokh R, Berger F, Delsol G et al: Rearrangement and overexpression of the BCL-2/PRAD-1 gene in intermediate lymphocytic lymphomas and in t(11q13)-bearing leukemias, *Blood* 81:3063, 1993.
408. Duggan MJ, Weisenburger DD, Ye YL et al: Mantle zone lymphoma: a clinicopathologic study of 22 cases, *Cancer* 66:522, 1990.
409. Liang R, Like SL, Ho FCS et al: Histologic subtypes and survival of Chinese patients with non-Hodgkin's lymphomas, *Cancer* 66:1850, 1990.
410. Pinto A, Hutchison RE, Grant LH et al: Follicular lymphomas in pediatric patients, *Mod Pathol* 3:308, 1990.
411. Horning SJ, Rosenberg SA: The natural history of initially untreated low grade non-Hodgkin's lymphomas, *N Engl J Med* 311:1471, 1984.
412. Rosenberg SA: The low-grade non-Hodgkin's lymphomas: challenges and opportunities, *J Clin Oncol* 3:299, 1985.
413. Harris NL, Ferry JA: Follicular lymphoma and related disorders (Germinal center lymphomas). In Knowles DM, editor *Neoplastic hematopathology,* Baltimore, 1992.
414. Mann RB, Berard CW: Criteria for the cytologic subclassification of follicular lymphomas: a proposed alternative method, *Hematol Oncol* 1:187, 1982.
415. Kim H, Dorfman RF, Rappaport H: Signet-ring lymphoma: a rare morphologic and functional expression of nodular (follicular) lymphoma, *Am J Surg Pathol* 2:119, 1978.
416. Nathwani BN, Sheibani K, Winberg CD, Burke JS, Rappaport H: Neoplastic B-cells with cerebriform nuclei in follicular lymphomas, *Hum Pathol* 16:173, 1985.
417. Come SE, Jaffe ES, Andersen JC et al: Non-Hodgkin's lymphomas in leukemic phase: clinicopathologic correlations, *Am J Med* 69:667, 1980.
418. Vago JF, Hurtubise PE, Redden-Borowski MN, Martelo OJ, Swerdlow SH: Follicular center-cell lymphoma with plasmacytic differentiation, monoclonal paraprotein, and peripheral blood involvement. Recapitulation of normal B-cell development, *Am J Surg Pathol* 9:764, 1985.
419. Chang KL, Arber DA, Shibata D, Rappaport H, Weiss LM: Follicular small lymphocytic lymphoma: a rare but distinct clinicopathologic entity, *Am J Surg Pathol* 18:99, 1994.
420. Warnke R, Levy R: Immunopathology of follicular lymphomas: a model of B-lymphocyte homing, *N Engl J Med* 298:481, 1978.
421. Pezzella F, Tse AGD, Cordell JL et al: Expression of the BCL-2 oncogene protein is not specific for the 14;18 chromosomal translocation, *Am J Pathol* 137; 225, 1990.
422. Yunis JJ, Oken MM, Kaplan ME et al: Distinctive chromosomal abnormalities in histologic subtypes of non-Hodgkin's lymphoma, *N Engl J Med* 307:1231, 1982.
423. Tsujimoto Y, Cossman J, Jaffe E, Croce CM: Involvement of the BCL-2 gene in human follicular lymphoma, *Science* 228:1440, 1985.
424. Weiss LM, Warnke RA, Sklar J, Cleary ML: Molecular analysis of the t(14;18) chromosomal translocation in malignant lymphomas, *N Engl J Med* 317:1185, 1987.
425. Hockenbery D, Nunez G, Milliman C et al: Bcl-2 is an inner mitochondrial protein that blocks programmed cell death, *Nature* 348:334, 1990.
426. McDonnell TJ, Deane N, Platt FM et al: Bcl-2-immunoglobulin transgenic mice demonstrate extended B-cell survival and follicular lymphoproliferation, *Cell* 57:79, 1989.
427. Tilly H, Rossi A, Stamatoullas A et al: Prognostic value of chromosomal abnormalities in follicular lymphoma, *Blood* 84:1043, 1994.
428. Sander CA, Yano T, Clark HM et al: p53 mutation is associated with progression in follicular lymphomas, *Blood* 82:1994, 1993.
429. Lo Coco F, Gaidano G, Louie DC et al: p53 mutations are associated with histologic transformation of follicular lymphoma, *Blood* 92:2289, 1994.
430. Yano T, Jaffe ES, Longo DL, Raffeld M: MYC rearrangements in histologically progressed follicular lymphomas, *Blood* 80:758, 1992.
431. Bartlett, Rizeq M, Dorfman RF et al: Follicular large-cell lymphoma: intermediate or low grade? *J Clin Oncol* 12:1349, 1994.
432. Ezdinli EZ, Costello WG, Kucuk O, Berard CW: Effect of the degree of nodularity on the survival of patients with nodular lymphomas, *J Clin Oncol* 5:413, 1987.
433. Hu E, Weiss LM, Hoppe RT, Horning SJ: Follicular and diffuse mixed small cleaved and large cell lymphoma—a clinicopathologic study, *J Clin Oncol* 3:1183, 1985.
434. Simon R, Durrelman S, Hoppe RG et al: The non-Hodgkin lymphoma pathologic classification project, long-term follow-up of 1153 patients with non-Hodgkin lymphomas, *Ann Intern Med* 104:757, 1986.
435. Sheibani K, Battifora H, Winberg CD et al: Further evidence that "malignant angioendotheliomatosis" is an angiotropic large cell lymphoma, *N Engl J Med* 314:943, 1986.
436. Macon WR, Williams ME, Greer JP et al: T-cell-rich B-cell lymphomas: a clinicopathologic study of 19 cases, *Am J Surg Pathol* 16:351, 1992.
437. Delabie J, Vandenberghe E, Kennes C et al: Histiocyte-rich B-cell lymphoma: a distinct clinicopathologic entity possibly related to lymphocyte predominant Hodgkin's disease, paragranuloma subtype, *Am J Surg Pathol* 16:37, 1992.
438. Doggett RS, Wood GS, Horning S et al: The immunologic characterization of 95 nodal and extranodal diffuse large cell lymphomas in 89 patients, *Am J Pathol* 115:245, 1984.
439. Offit K, Lo Coco F, Louie DC et al: Rearrangement of the *bcl-6* gene as a prognostic marker in diffuse large-cell lymphoma, *N Engl J Med* 331:74, 1994.

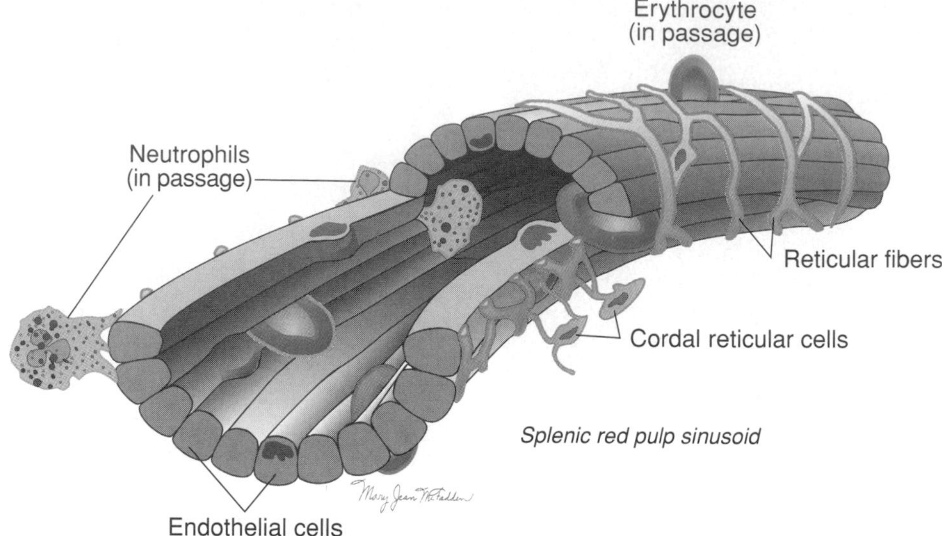

Fig. 43-5 Sinus wall of the human spleen. The sinus-lining cells are arranged in parallel and are held together loosely by a discontinuous meshwork of ring fibers, which provides stability for the sinus wall and anchors the sinuses to the dendritic macrophages of the cords of Billroth. Notice the leukocytes and red blood cells passing through the sinus wall. The ability of these cells to deform is crucial for them to traverse the sinus. (Modified from a drawing by Dr. Richard Rosales.)

Table 43-1 Functions of the spleen

Filtration
Culling (cell destruction)
Physiologic (senescent red blood cells)
Pathologic
- Destruction of structurally abnormal red blood cells
- Destruction of antibody-coated cells
- Destruction of normal blood cells by pathologically altered spleen

Pitting ("face-lifting" of red blood cells)
Physiologic
- Removal of red blood cell inclusions (such as Howell-Jolly bodies, siderotic granules, Heinz bodies)
- Temporary sequestration of reticulocytes

Pathologic
- Removal of intracellular parasites (e.g., *Plasmodium, Babesia*)
- Erythroclasis (fragmentation of abnormal red blood cells with release of fragments into the blood)
- Removal of extracellular particulate material (such as bacteria, antigen-antibody complexes)

Immunologic function
Physiologic
Antigen trapping and processing
Activation of complement system
Lymphocyte transformation and activation
Immunoglobin and lymphokine production
Pathologic: production of autoantibodies
Reservoir
Sequestration and storage of hematologic cells (except for platelets minor function in human beings)
Iron storage and recycling
Hematopoietic function
Lymphocyte and macrophage production (erythropoiesis, granulopoiesis, and megakaryopoiesis probably do not occur in humans)

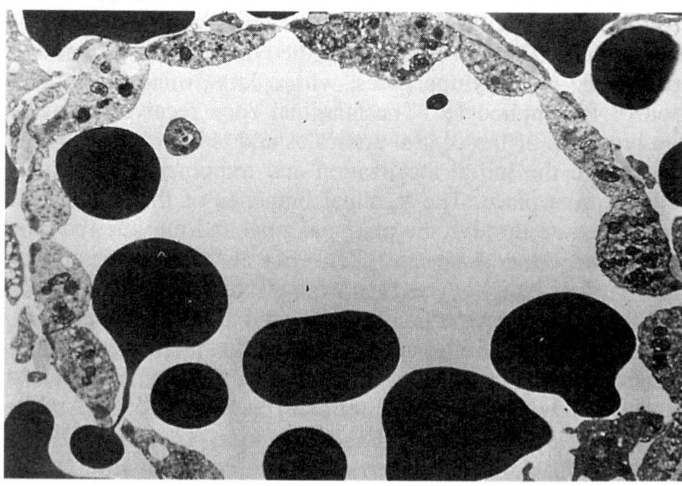

Fig. 43-6 Transmission electron micrograph of a normal red blood cell traversing the sinus wall in a human spleen. Notice how it must deform to reenter the sinus.

Billroth, which are rich in lysosomal acid hydrolase, these cells become more susceptible to destruction.

Besides the low oxygen tension in the cords of Billroth, a naturally occurring phenomenon of red blood cell aging further contributes to the selective destruction of older red blood cells. As red blood cells age, they lose their surface membrane and become spherocytes, which are less deformable and less capable of traversing the spaces between the sinus-lining cells in the red pulp of the spleen (Fig. 43-6). When preferentially sequestered in the cords of Billroth, they are subject to destruction. Other factors may affect the plasticity of red cells. Cytoplasmic inclusions render cells less deformable, as does antibody coating. This explains the cellular destruction that takes place in such disorders as autoimmune hemolytic anemias and immune thrombocytopenic purpura (ITP).

The spleen also performs a function called *erythroclasis*,[17] which is the destruction of red blood cells by fragmentation. The cellular fragments are then returned to the peripheral blood and removed on subsequent passage through the spleen. This phenomenon occurs in a variety of autoimmune hemolytic anemias and beta-thalassemia, and in many hemoglobinopathies.

The immunologic functions of the spleen are similar to those of other lymphoid organs—trapping and processing of antigens, the production of antibodies and lymphokines, and activation of the complement system. However, unlike other lymphoid tissues, which respond to localized immunologic stimulation, the spleen functions in reaction to disseminated blood-borne immunologic processes.

REACTIVE LESIONS

Hypersplenism

Hypersplenism refers to the (excessive) destruction of blood cells by the spleen, resulting in cytopenias of one or more blood cell lines.[18,19] Most cases of hypersplenism associated with pathologic enlargement of the spleen are attributable to disorders involving the red pulp, which result in an increased portion of the total blood flow passing through the spleen and undergoing filtration. Hypersplenism may result from abnormalities inherent in the blood cells themselves (intracorpuscular defects) such as hereditary spherocytosis or ITP, or may be attributable to the increased sequestration of blood cells. Hypersplenism is of clinical importance because it is the only major functional abnormality of the spleen, and it is the most frequent indication for splenectomy. Dameshek initially postulated that hypersplenism could result from a humoral factor produced by the spleen, but there has been no persuasive evidence to prove his theory.

Hyposplenism

Hyposplenism is defined as the decreased or absent function of the spleen (Table 43-2),[20,21] either its filtration function or its immunologic function. It may be congenital or acquired. Congenital hyposplenism is rare and usually is the result of absence of the spleen (asplenia). This is typically found with several other congenital malformations. Polysplenia may produce the same results. Acquired hyposplenism is much more common and is usually the result of splenectomy. Another example of acquired hyposplenism is sickle-cell disease, in which the spleen becomes progressively fibrotic and nonfunctional because of autoinfarction. Vasculitides such as polyarteritis nodosa are associated with autoinfarction. The spleen may atrophy without infarction, as is reported to occur in ulcerative colitis and celiac disease.[22] There are other conditions in which the spleen may be functionally deficient without decreasing in weight. These conditions include amyloidosis, extensive granulomatous infiltration, and some neoplastic vascular diseases of the spleen. Functional hyposplenism may also result when the spleen is massively infiltrated by malignant cells, as occurs in the settings of leukemia and lymphoma. However, this was more frequent before the advent of multiagent chemotherapy.

The absence of the spleen, whether congenital or acquired, increases the risk of overwhelming sepsis, a condition referred to as the "syndrome of overwhelming postsplenectomy infection (OPSI)."[23] The incidence of this syndrome is greatest in young patients and in patients with underlying immunologic abnormalities such as ITP or Hodgkin's disease. It occurs most frequently within 2 years of splenectomy but can also occur many years after removal of the organ. The organisms usually responsible for the syndrome are strains of *Streptococcus pneumoniae* and *Haemophilus influenzae*. However, non–polysaccharide-encapsulated bacteria such as *Staphylococcus* and *Meningococcus* are occasionally responsible, and the syndrome has also been described with *Babesia* as the offending organism.[24] The pathophysiologic mechanism underlying this condition relates to the absence of bacteria-specific, opsonizing antibodies, particularly IgM, that are not synthesized effectively in organs other than the spleen, and by the absence of a specific filtration mechanism to eliminate such antibody-coated bacteria from the circulation. Because the splenic synthesis of an opsonizing antibody is specific only for each antigenically distinct bacterial subtype, patients who undergo splenectomy at a young age are usually treated thereafter with a polyvalent antipneumococcal vaccine, and this has led to a reduced incidence of this complication of the asplenic state. Typically, splenectomy for the treatment of physically induced rupture and splenectomy in older adults do not carry the same increased risk of infection that affects children and patients with an underlying immunodeficiency. The probable reason for this is that, as persons age, specific antibodies to a larger number of organisms are more likely to be synthesized.

Hyposplenism also includes the depressed immunologic function of the spleen.[25] This occurs in many clinical congenital and acquired conditions in which the lymphoid system of the spleen is defective. The spleen's ability to respond to antigenic stimuli is affected by a variety of intrinsic and extrinsic factors. Children with congenital immunodeficiency disorders usually have hypoplasia of the white pulp. Spleens from

Table 43-2 Conditions associated with hyposplenism

Congenital
Prematurity (transient)
Asplenia
Immunodeficiency disorders
Acquired
Splenectomy
Associated with atrophy or infarction, or both
Irradiation
Cytotoxic and immunosuppressive drugs
Sickle-cell disease
Systemic vasculitides
Essential thrombocythemia
Malabsorption syndromes
Autoimmune disorders
Acquired autoimmune disease
Endocrine disorders
Associated with normal or increased splenic size
Chronic alcoholism
Infiltration by leukemia or lymphoma
Amyloidosis
Granulomatous infiltration
Vascular tumors

characteristic macrophages. Such patients have decreased red blood cell survival times.

Perhaps the most common example of disorders associated with an increased number of cordal macrophages is *fibrocongestive splenomegaly,* a condition usually associated with portal hypertension and liver cirrhosis. Increased numbers of the macrophages are seen early in this disease, but they are usually not present later when progressive fibrosis of the cords of Billroth occurs.

Cordal macrophages containing ceroid accumulate in the spleen in both congenital and acquired conditions.[43] The sea-blue histiocyte syndrome, so named because of the intensely blue macrophages in Romanovsky-stained smears,[44-47] has been described as a familial disorder involving phospholipid metabolism (the Hermansky-Pudlak syndrome).[48] However, this pigment may also be found in the spleen in unrelated disorders that have as a common basis an increased destruction and turnover of cells, resulting in an increased lipid burden presented to the spleen. Such conditions include hyperlipidemias,[49] chronic myelogenous leukemia, chronic granulomatous disease, infection-associated hemophagocytic syndrome, and ITP. They may also occur as an incidental finding.

Ceroid is a product of lipid oxidation and polymerization. As it ages, it stains with PAS, acid-fast, and Prussian blue stains. Ceroid-containing macrophages frequently appear somewhat dirty brown in hematoxylin and eosin–stained sections. Regardless of the underlying disease responsible for ceroid macrophages in the spleen, the morphologic picture appears the same. However, in some conditions such as the infection-associated hemophagocytic syndrome,[50,51] the clinical presentation and associated erythrophagocytosis may make the diagnosis apparent. In this disorder, which occurs primarily in children and in immunocompromised adults, there is a proliferation of benign-appearing macrophages, some of which contain ceroid pigment, as well as phagocytised red cells (Fig. 43-15), platelets, and granulocytes. Most cases of the infection-associated hemophagocytic syndrome are associated with herpesvirus, Epstein-Barr virus, or adenovirus infection. Cases associated with bacterial, fungal, or even parasitic infections have also been reported.[50,51]

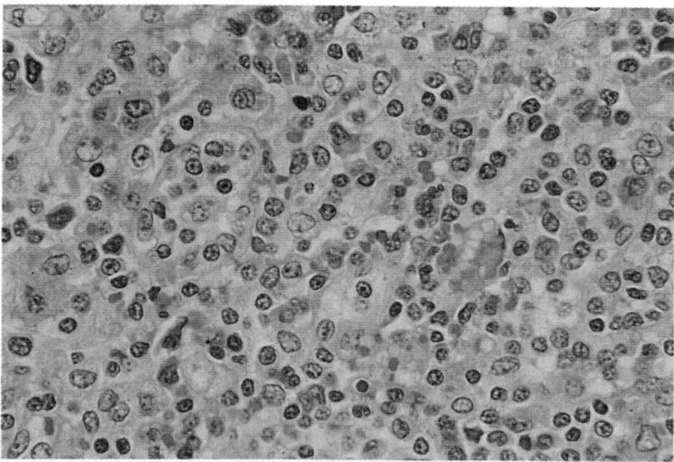

Fig. 43-15 Infection-associated hemophagocytic syndrome. The red pulp contains numerous macrophages with ingested red blood cells. Notice the associated infiltration of plasma cells and transformed lymphocytes. These cells are frequently present, particularly in cases associated with viral disease.

A disorder historically known as *malignant histiocytosis* is also characterized by the significant proliferation of macrophages, frequently with erythrophagocytosis, in association with the formation of more primitive hematopoietic cells, which for many years were believed to be primitive neoplastic macrophages (Fig. 43-16). Recent studies indicate, however, that most cases previously deemed "malignant histiocytosis" were actually either the infection-associated hemophagocytic syndrome or an unusual form of malignant lymphoma, usually of T-cell type,[52,53] accompanied by the formation of reactive macrophages. "True" malignant histiocytosis has, however, been reported, albeit rarely.[53] A localized process, called *histiocytoma,* has also been described.[54]

Circulatory disturbances

The most common circulatory disturbance affecting the spleen is splenic infarction (Fig. 43-17). Infarctions may occur as the result of either of two mechanisms. The first involves occlusion of the splenic artery or one of its tributaries as the result of embolization, usually originating from valvular lesions in the left side of the heart. Septic infarctions may also occur as a result of infective endocarditis. Nonembolic infarctions, secondary to focal stasis and thrombosis in the spleen, are probably more

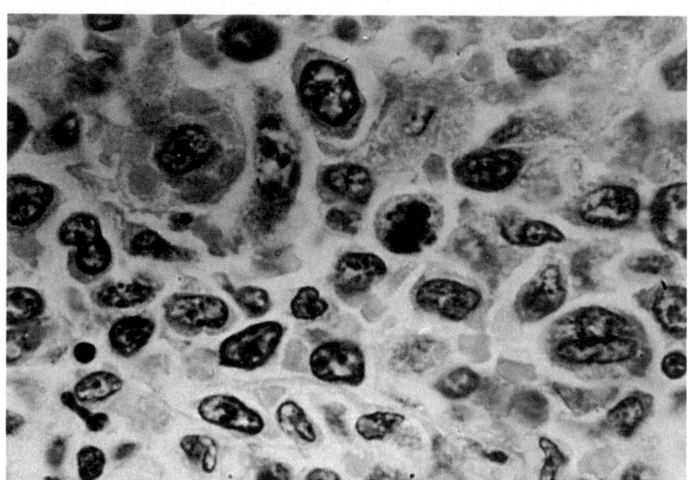

Fig. 43-16 T-cell lymphoma mimicking malignant histiocytosis. Erythrophagocytosis *(upper left)* may be a prominent feature in this disorder, prompting an erroneous diagnosis of hemophagocytic syndrome. The other infiltrating cells, however, appear neoplastic, and display the immunophenotype of T lymphocytes.

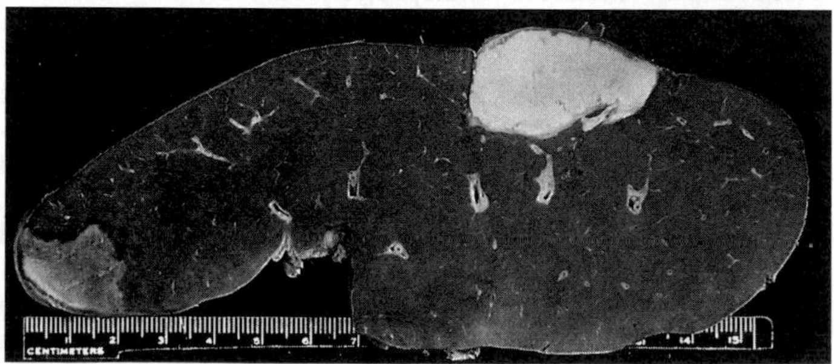

Fig. 43-17 Cross section of a spleen showing two infarcts. The one *on the right* is older and is well demarcated. The other, *on the left,* is more recent and shows a peripheral area of hyperemia.

common. They may be caused by local vascular occlusion, by the infiltration of tumor cells, as in hemangiosarcoma or metastatic carcinoma, or by the stasis of sequestered and abnormal blood cells, as in sickle-cell disease. Infarctions are also common in massively enlarged spleens, regardless of the cause.

Vasculitis in the spleen is similar to that seen in other organs of the body and occurs in similar conditions such as polyarteritis nodosa, systemic lupus erythematosus, and hypersensitivity (leukocytoclastic) angiitis.[55] In addition, there may be fibrin thrombi in small arterioles in the spleen in the setting of thrombotic thrombocytopenic purpura.[56] However, such thrombi may also occur as an isolated phenomenon in the absence of an associated underlying disease.

NEOPLASMS

Malignant lymphoma

True primary malignant lymphomas of the spleen are uncommon.[57,58] Most cases of lymphomatous involvement of the spleen are part of a disseminated disorder.[15,59-61] Among the cases of disseminated lymphoma that involve the spleen are those in which the spleen is predominantly involved and in which the patients manifest significant splenomegaly in the absence of clinically detectable disease in the lymph nodes or bone marrow.[62-64] Regardless of the clinical presentation, malignant lymphomas of the spleen usually involve the white pulp, though rarely there are malignant lymphomas of either the B- or T-cell type that involve the red pulp predominantly or exclusively. There are two general patterns of white pulp involvement. The first is the miliary pattern in which all the white pulp is involved to some degree[15,61] (Fig. 43-18). This produces an enlarged spleen with expansion of all the white pulp nodules, such that these are multiple nodules with a diameter ranging from 1 mm to 10 cm seen on cut sections. The malignant lymphomas responsible for this pattern of involvement are usually of the low-grade B-cell type, including malignant lymphomas of the small lymphocytic (with or without plasmacytoid differentiation), mantle cell, marginal zone cell, small cleaved cell, and mixed cell types. Large cell lymphomas, on the other hand, usually produce one or more tumorlike masses that may or may not involve the white pulp and that spare many of the malpighian corpuscles. This gross feature more closely resembles that of a metastatic tumor. Red pulp involvement by malignant lymphoma most commonly occurs in the low-grade lesions and is accompanied by blood and bone marrow involvement (Fig. 43-19).

Although the finding of splenomegaly in patients with malignant lymphoma usually implies splenic involvement by tumor, the converse is not true. There are numerous examples of lymphomatous involvement of the spleen without splenomegaly. In addition, malignant lymphomas cannot be classified as follicular or diffuse on the basis of splenic involvement. Most lymphomas, regardless of their origin from follicular center cells, involve the spleen in a nodular (miliary) pattern, reflecting the anatomic structure of the white pulp. The cytomorphology of malignant lymphomas involving the spleen, however, is essentially identical to that of other organs.

Several recent studies have pointed up the existence of a clinical syndrome of malignant lymphoma that presents with massive splenomegaly in the absence of clinically apparent

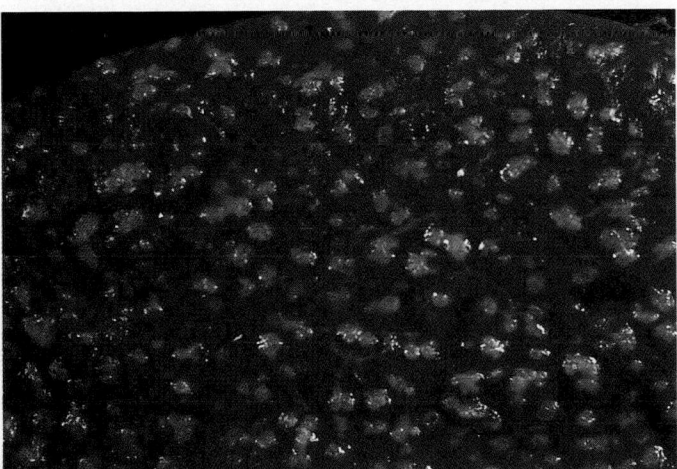

Fig. 43-18 Splenic cross section in a case of malignant lymphoma of the mantle cell type. Notice that much of the white pulp is involved, creating a miliary pattern (that is, small nodules). This is characteristic of splenic involvement in the low-grade malignant lymphomas.

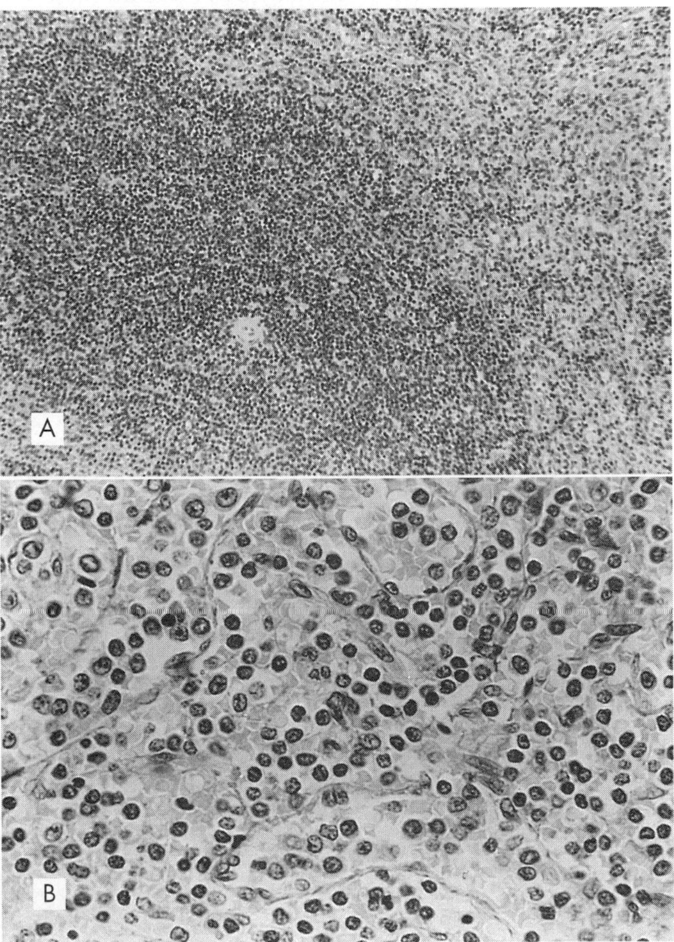

Fig. 43-19 **A,** Malignant lymphoma of the small lymphocytic type. Notice the replacement of the white pulp by a homogeneous infiltrate of small lymphocytes. The red pulp is also involved. **B,** Notice the involvement of both cords and sinuses of the red pulp in this example of malignant lymphoma of the small lymphocytic type. All low-grade malignant lymphomas exhibit some degree of red pulp involvement. It is greatest in the setting of chronic lymphocytic leukemia or of a significant peripheral blood involvement.

lymphadenopathy.[61,62,64] These cases have been referred to as *malignant lymphoma presenting with prominent splenomegaly,*[62] *splenic lymphoma with villous lymphocytes,*[65] *malignant lymphoma mimicking hairy cell disease,*[64] *splenic marginal zone cell lymphoma,*[66] and *splenic monocytoid B-cell lymphoma.*[67] This clinical syndrome is caused by a variety of low-grade B-cell malignancies, including malignant lymphoma of small lymphocytic (with or without plasmacytoid features), mantle cell, and marginal zone types. These lesions can be differentiated from one another by their cytomorphologic features, the pattern of splenic involvement, and their immunophenotypes. Occasionally some of these cases are limited to the spleen, but in the vast majority of cases careful staging reveals disease in the splenic hilar lymph nodes, bone marrow, or peripheral blood. Some cases may be associated with the presence of a paraprotein.[64,68]

Most malignant lymphomas of the spleen are of B-cell type, and there are relatively few studies of immunologically confirmed T-cell lymphomas in this organ. Malignant lymphomas of T-cell type may involve the red pulp (Fig. 43-20), and occasionally these may be accompanied by a rich macrophage component that may erroneously indicate a possible diagnosis of malignant histiocytosis. This is a rare disease involving malignant histiocytes that has occasionally been found to affect the spleen.[54,69] Other forms of malignant lymphoma of T-cell type do appear to exhibit characteristic patterns of involvement in the spleen. Mycosis fungoides may affect both the red and white pulp,[70] and lymphoblastic lymphoma tends to involve the areas of the white pulp next to the periarteriolar lymphoid sheath.

The therapeutic value of splenectomy in malignant lymphoma is unclear. If the disease is limited to the spleen, particularly in cases of large cell lymphoma, splenectomy appears appropriate. Splenectomy may also be appropriate in a patient with malignant lymphoma who has hypersplenism. With these exceptions, there appears to be no great benefit from splenectomy.

Hodgkin's disease

Hodgkin's disease involves the spleen in approximately one third of all cases; the spleen is the most common site of extranodal organ involvement and this is typical of stage III or IV disease.[15,71] Although all histologic subtypes of Hodgkin's disease may involve the spleen, the frequency of this differs. Nodular sclerosis and mixed-cellularity Hodgkin's disease most often affect the spleen, whereas the least common types are lymphocyte predominance and lymphocyte depletion. Hodgkin's disease that involves the spleen always occurs in the white pulp and is usually grossly visible in the form of small nodules of tumor larger than the normal malpighian corpuscles. In the spleen Hodgkin's disease may cause miliary nodules or a few large tumor masses, thereby mimicking non-Hodgkin's lymphoma (Fig. 43-21).[72] Splenic involvement by Hodgkin's disease may not cause marked splenomegaly. As a result splenectomy specimens must be carefully examined so that small foci are not missed (Fig. 43-22). If the spleen is involved, other organs such as the liver and bone marrow may also be involved. It is crucial to document splenic involvement in patients with Hodgkin's disease because, if found, this has a

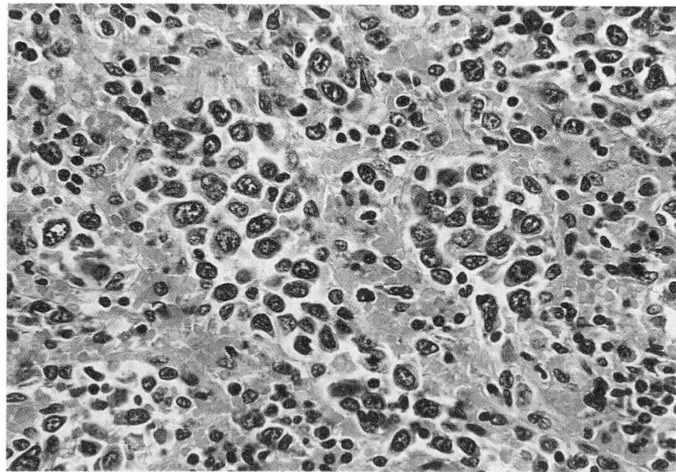

Fig. 43-20 High-grade malignant lymphoma simulating malignant histiocytosis. In this case, as in many others, the neoplastic cells are T lymphocytes. True malignant histiocytosis is rare in the spleen.

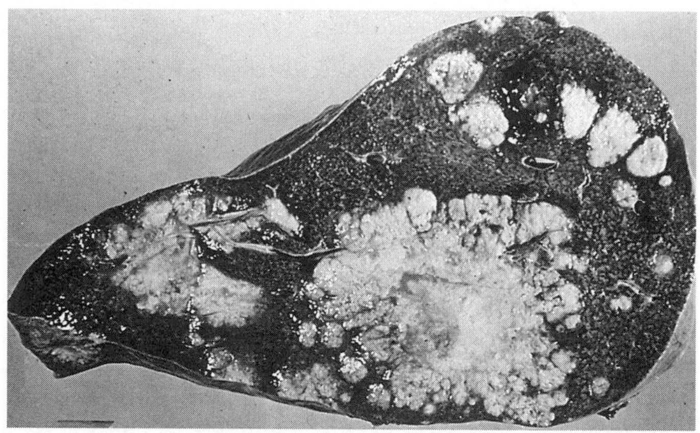

Fig. 43-21 Cross section of a spleen showing the multiple nodules characteristic of Hodgkin's disease. Such massive involvement has negative prognostic implications.

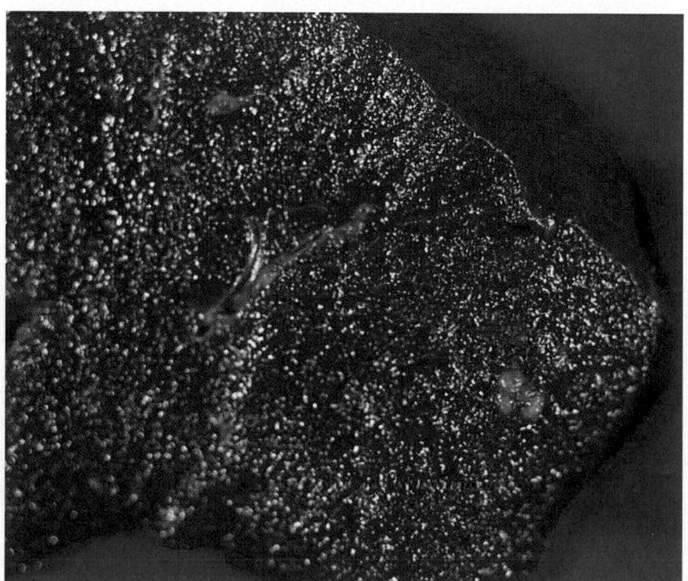

Fig. 43-22 Involvement of the spleen by Hodgkin's disease can be quite subtle, as in this case showing a single tiny focus in an otherwise normal organ. Examination of the spleen must be meticulous to find such foci.

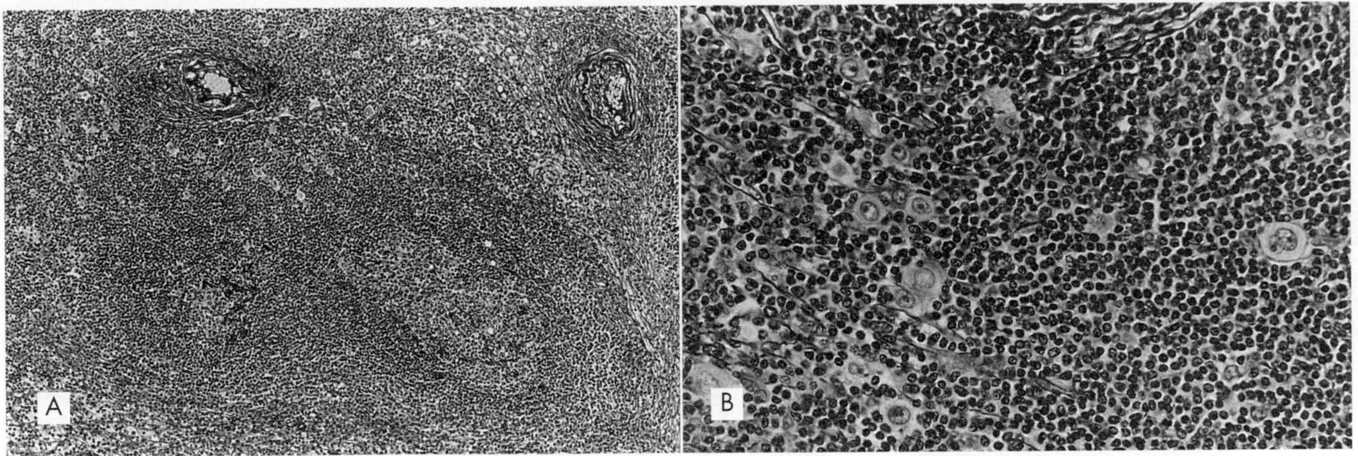

Fig. 43-23 Splenic involvement in Hodgkin's disease always occurs in the white pulp. **A,** In this case an expanded perifollicular zone of lymphoid cells is noted, which appears only slightly larger than the normal malpighian corpuscle. **B,** Examination of this area under higher magnification reveals characteristic lacunar cells.

considerable effect on the method of treatment and on the risk of involvement of other organs.

The histologic criteria for determining splenic involvement in Hodgkin's disease depend on whether a prior histologic diagnosis has been established based on lymph node findings.[72-74] If the diagnosis is established, the finding of Reed-Sternberg variants, such as lacunar cells, in an appropriate cellular background is sufficient to establish the diagnosis of splenic Hodgkin's disease. (Fig. 43-23) However, without a prior diagnosis based on lymph node biopsy findings, the finding of Reed-Sternberg cells is required to make the diagnosis. Infiltration of the red pulp by single Reed-Sternberg cells or other inflammatory cells does not occur in Hodgkin's disease.[72] Noncaseating sarcoid granulomas form fairly frequently in the spleens of patients with Hodgkin's disease, but their presence does not signify involvement.[30]

Dysproteinemias

Dysproteinemias are a heterogeneous group of lymphoid proliferations that includes morphologically benign lesions that develop in association with polyclonal or monoclonal immunoglobulin production; and morphologically atypical proliferations that occur in association with paraproteinemia that do not appear to involve the spleen in a manner similar to that typical of most malignant lymphomas.[15] The morphologically benign lesions include a poorly defined group of immunologic reactions referred to as *immunoblastic proliferations,* and these frequently occur in association with autoimmune diseases. These lesions may also occur in primary amyloidosis and angiofollicular lymph node hyperplasia (Castleman's disease),[75] though in some cases of the latter disorder careful examination often reveals the presence of atypical plasma cells. A common feature in these disorders is hyperplasia of the white pulp, together with the presence of a variety of immunologically active cells. These infiltrations may also involve the red pulp. Similar lesions associated with monoclonal immunoglobulin production include most cases of primary amyloidosis.[76,77] Amyloidosis may either involve the white or red pulp (see Chapter 20). In both instances careful examination frequently reveals plasma cells and plasmacytoid lymphocytes in either the red or white pulp. In many of these cases immunohistologic studies show that the plasma cells and plasmacytoid lymphocytes display cytoplasmic monoclonal light chains.[76]

Other conditions associated with morphologically benign appearing infiltrations in the spleen include gamma heavy-chain disease and cold agglutinin disease.[78] However, in both primary and secondary cold agglutinin disease careful immunohistologic staining may reveal a clone of lymphoid cells displaying light chain restriction. In addition, a B-cell lymphoma may be manifested as the disease progresses.

The morphologically atypical proliferations associated with paraproteinemia include multiple myeloma and Waldenström's macroglobulinemia.[79,80] In these disorders the red pulp is usually affected more severely than the white pulp. Despite being defined as atypical, most cells appear morphologically benign in most cases. In Waldenström's disease, lymphocytes, plasma cells, immunoblasts, and plasmacytoid lymphocytes infiltrate both the cords of Billroth and the trabecular arteries.

Leukemia

The most common malignancy involving the splenic red pulp is leukemia[15] (Fig. 43-24). The degree of involvement in a given patient depends on the duration of the leukemia and the degree of peripheral blood involvement because leukemic infiltration probably occurs mainly by way of the sequestration of leukemic cells as they circulate through the spleen. Therefore the red pulp is involved in all instances. Initially, individual leukemic cells accumulate in both the cords of Billroth and in the sinuses, but eventually the pattern of infiltration becomes diffuse (Fig. 43-25). Although the spleen is usually involved in untreated cases of acute leukemia, splenomegaly is uncommon because therapy is instituted before considerable involvement occurs. In the chronic leukemias, on the other hand, substantial splenic involvement usually occurs before therapy is instituted.[81] In chronic myeloid leukemia (CML) the red pulp is infiltrated by myeloid cells in varying stages of maturation, with a preponderance of myelocytes and promyelocytes.[82] In addition, one may find occasional clusters of normoblasts and megakaryocytes, particularly when there is significant reticulin fibrosis in the bone marrow. Clusters of blast cells are a not characteristic finding in CML, except during blastic transformation. The spleen is the most common site of extramedullary blastic transformation. Rapid enlargement

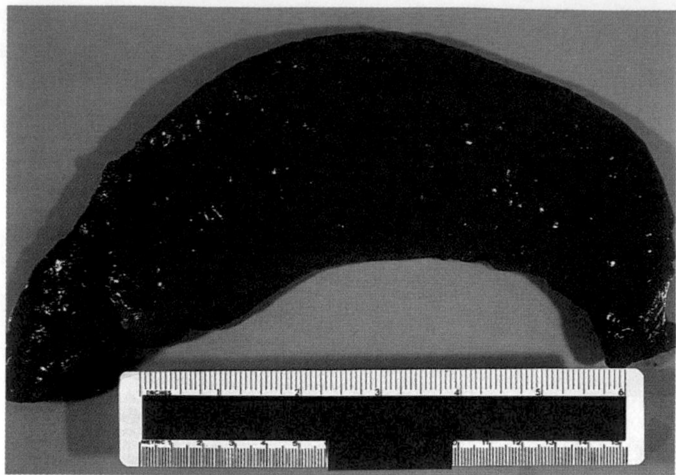

Fig. 43-24 Cross section of a spleen in an untreated case of acute myeloid leukemia. Notice the absence of normal white pulp. It is unusual to see cases of acute leukemia with this degree of splenic enlargement.

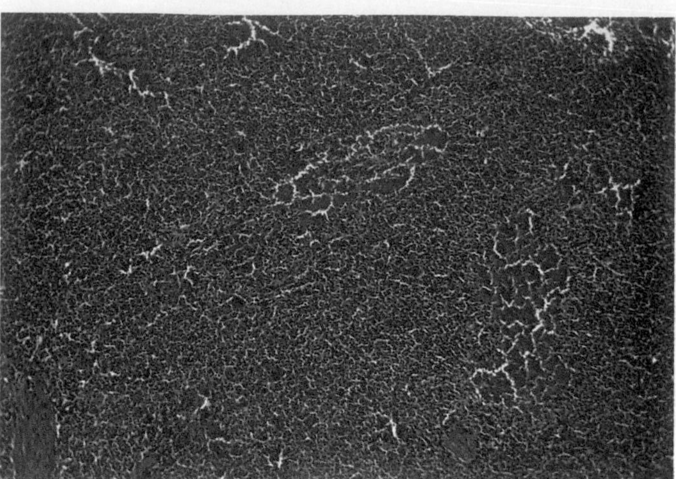

Fig. 43-26 Hairy cell leukemia. Notice the "blood lakes," which are characteristic but not diagnostic of hairy cell leukemia.

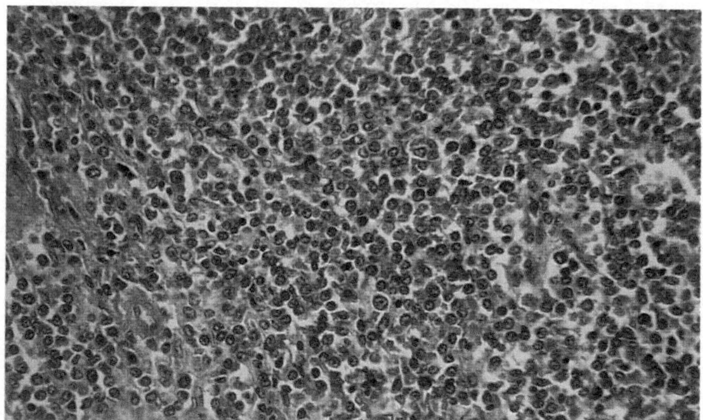

Fig. 43-25 Acute myeloid leukemia. The cords and sinuses are filled with blast cells.

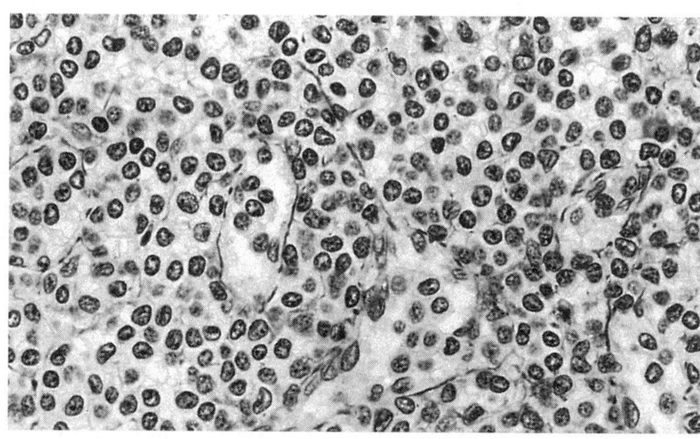

Fig. 43-27 Hairy cell leukemia. The cords and sinuses of the red pulp are infiltrated by a population of bland-appearing mononuclear cells with a fairly copious amount of cytoplasm and little if any mitotic activity.

of the spleen stemming from a proliferation of myeloblasts and promyelocytes may be the first evidence of such transformation.[15] In monocytic leukemias there is also significant involvement of the spleen. The splenic infiltrate in most types of acute leukemia involves both the red pulp cords and sinuses. In acute erythroleukemia, on the other hand, the leukemic cells preferentially cluster in the red pulp sinuses.[15]

The most characteristic leukemic disorder involving the spleen is *hairy cell leukemia*.[83] The usual presenting signs of this malignancy of B-lymphocytes are massive splenomegaly, inconspicuous lymphadenopathy, invariable bone marrow involvement, and cytopenias of one or more peripheral blood cell lines. Paradoxically, leukemic cells may be difficult to find in the peripheral blood. The diagnosis is frequently made on the basis of the findings yielded by splenectomy specimens recovered for therapeutic reasons to ameliorate the cytopenias. The hairy cells infiltrate into the red pulp and surround the trabecular vessels in the white pulp. The proliferation is associated with considerable blood pooling because of the formation of venous lakes, which are attributable to the substitution of hairy cells for normal sinus-lining cells. The resultant structures have been referred to as *pseudosinuses* (Fig. 43-26). The neoplastic cells possess a rather bland morphology, with round to oval or bean-shaped nuclei, somewhat compact chromatin, and abundant pale cytoplasm. Mitotic activity is virtually absent (Fig. 43-27).

Chronic lymphocytic leukemia (CLL) is most often of B-cell type (B-CLL), and it involves the white pulp of the spleen. In common with other leukemic disorders, there is also extensive red pulp involvement in CLL.[61,81] A somewhat unusual characteristic of the T-cell type of CLL is that it may involve the red pulp exclusively, with no apparent evidence of expansion of the white pulp.

Prolymphocytic leukemia, a rare variant of CLL, usually of B-cell type, causes massive splenomegaly and high blood cell counts.[84,85] The circulating cells and those infiltrating the spleen have the features typical of prolymphocytes, such as abundant cytoplasm and nuclei, with the peripheral condensation of chromatin and a single, large nucleoli. A recently recognized variant of CLL, referred to as *large granular lymphocytosis,* may present with massive splenomegaly and may be morphologically mistaken for prolymphocytic leukemia.[86] The two may be distinguished on both clinical and immunologic grounds because large granular lymphocytosis is usually not associated with a significant lymphocytosis and is frequently also accompanied by neutropenia. In addition, immunologic studies usually reveal a T-cell or natural killer cell origin of the tumor cells in the setting of large granular lymphocytosis.

Systemic mastocytosis may involve the spleen. This may happen with or without mast cell leukemia, which is present with the splenomegaly.[87,88] The mast cells infiltrate into the periphery of the white pulp in the marginal zone, with extension into the red pulp, or they may diffusely infiltrate into the red pulp alone. A characteristic accompanying feature is diffuse fibrosis similar to that observed in the setting of mast cell disease in the bone marrow.

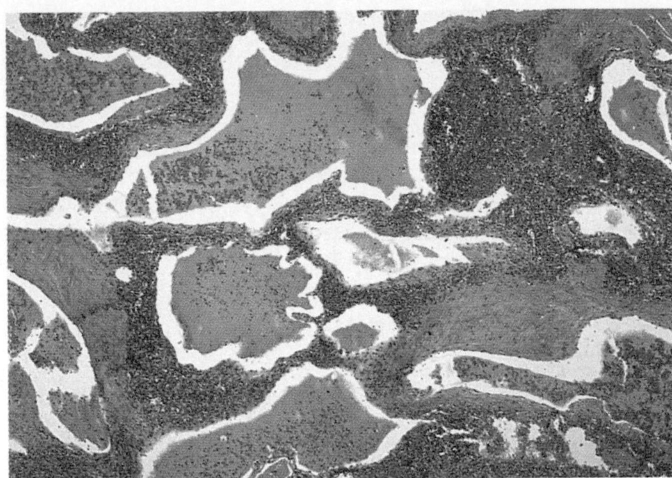

Fig. 43-28 Hemangioma. This is the most common tumor of the spleen and is usually of little significance.

Myeloproliferative disorders

The myeloproliferative disorders (polycythemia vera, agnogenic myeloid metaplasia, essential thrombocythemia, and CML) cause splenomegaly.[81,82] However, the mechanism responsible for causing splenomegaly is significantly different in each of these disorders. Essential thrombocythemia and CML have been discussed previously. In polycythemia vera approximately three fourths of the cases are associated with splenomegaly. In uncomplicated polycythemia vera splenomegaly is caused by plethora alone.[89] The splenic red pulp shows significant engorgement with blood, with little, if any, evidence of myeloid metaplasia. In the spent phase of polycythemia vera, also called *post–polycythemic myeloid metaplasia,* one sees extramedullary hematopoiesis.[89]

The most dramatic example of splenomegaly in the myeloproliferative diseases occurs in agnogenic myeloid metaplasia, also called *myelofibrosis with myeloid metaplasia.* This disorder is characterized by fibrosis of the bone marrow, the presence of nucleated erythrocytes and immature granulocytes in the peripheral blood, and progressive splenomegaly with extramedullary hematopoiesis in the spleen. The spleen may become massive, and weights of 7 kg or more have been reported.[81] As already commented on, the red pulp proliferation consists of cordal macrophages and a varying number of nucleated red cells, megakaryocytes, and granulocytic precursors in the cords of Billroth and the sinuses.[81,82] It has been postulated that the hematopoietic precursor cells in the spleen originate in the bone marrow and enter the peripheral blood because of the alterations in the bone marrow stroma that occur in this disorder.[90,91] The hematopoietic precursors in the spleen in agnogenic myeloid metaplasia therefore appear to be colonized from the bone marrow, and their formation is not caused by the reactivation of endogenous fetal hematopoiesis.

Although the leukemic and myeloproliferative disorders display characteristic abnormalities in the spleen, this is not so of the preleukemic or myelodysplastic disorders. In these conditions there are no specific abnormalities in the spleen.

Vascular tumors

Hemangiomas are the most common tumors of the spleen (Fig. 43-28).[92] They occur as small incidental lesions in as many as 10% of all persons. They are usually cavernous and, if large enough, may cause thrombocytopenia or other cytopenias. An apparently benign vascular lesion of the spleen that has recently been described has been termed *littoral cell angioma.*[93] Hemangiosarcomas and malignant hemangioendotheliomas[94] are uncommon neoplasms that present clinically with thrombocytopenia and splenic enlargement, with or without pain in the left upper quadrant. Microscopically they may exhibit diverse morphologic patterns, ranging from low-grade lesions with little mitotic activity, well-defined vascular channels, and foci of extramedullary hematopoiesis; to highly anaplastic, solid and spindle cell sarcomas. There is little correlation between the histologic grade of an angiosarcoma in the spleen and its clinical behavior. Bad prognostic features include thrombocytopenia, splenic infarcts, and metastases. In addition, splenic rupture is an ominous complication.

Tumorlike conditions

Other conditions mimicking vascular tumors are occasionally encountered in the spleen. They include peliosis, which is usually associated with peliosis of the liver and with the ingestion of androgenic-anabolic steroids.[95] This lesion consists of venous lakes that result from the cystic dilatation of the sinuses of the red pulp. In a given case one may see lesions in varying stages of development, ranging from early cystic dilatation to the early organization of blood clots within the lesion, and finally to organization with fibrous scar formation.[95]

Inflammatory pseudotumors are rare tumorlike conditions of the spleen that are usually composed of fibroblasts, lymphocytes, plasma cells, and macrophages.[96,97] They resemble inflammatory pseudotumors (or plasma cell granulomas) in other organs. *Hamartomas* are lesions that are composed of mature red pulp elements and only scattered lymphoid cells.[98,99] Most are small and incidental. However, on rare occasions they may produce splenomegaly and thrombocytopenia secondary to the sequestration of platelets.

Several types of cysts have been noted in the spleen.[100-102] These include epidermoid, mesothelial (or epithelials), false or traumatic, and echinococcal cysts, all of which are rare.

Metastatic tumors

Metastatic tumors rarely involve the spleen. If they do, they are usually a sign of disseminated malignancy, most often melanoma or carcinomas of the lung and breast.[103] Splenic involvement typically involves the formation of one or more tumor masses, but on rare occasions a diffuse or miliary infiltration may simulate leukemia or lymphoma. In our experience this is most commonly seen in the setting of small cell carcinoma of the lung.

REFERENCES

Normal spleen

1. Harrington WJ Jr, Harrington TJ, Harrington WJ Sr: Is splenectomy an outmoded procedure?, *Adv Intern Med* 35:415, 1990.
2. McCormick WF, Kashgarian M: The weight of the adult human spleen, *Am J Clin Pathol* 43:332, 1965.
3. Myers J, Segal RJ: Weight of the spleen. I. Range of normal in a nonhospital population, *Arch Pathol* 98:33, 1974.
4. Weiss L: The structure of the normal spleen, *Semin Hematol* 2:205, 1965.
5. Millikin PD: The nodular white pulp of the human spleen, *Arch Pathol* 87:247, 1969.
6. Grogan TM, Jolley CS, Rangel CS: Immunoarchitecture of the human spleen, *Lymphology* 16:72, 1983.
7. Grogan TM et al: Further delineation of the immunoarchitecture of the human spleen, *Lymphology* 17:61, 1984.
8. Weiss L: A scanning electron microscopic study of the spleen, *Blood* 43:665, 1974.
9. Chen L-T, Weiss L: Electron microscopy of the red pulp of the human spleen, *Am J Anat* 134:425, 1972.
10. Hirasawa Y, Tokuhiro H: Electron microscopic studies on the normal human spleen: especially on the red pulp and reticulo-endothelial cells, *Blood* 35:201, 1970.
11. Burke JS, Simon GT: Electron microscopy of the spleen. I, Anatomy and microcirculation, *Am J Pathol* 58:127, 1970.
12. King JT, Puchtler H, Sweat F: Ring fibers in human spleens, *Arch Pathol* 85:237, 1968.
13. Chen L-T: Microcirculation of the spleen: an open or closed circulation?, *Science* 20:157, 1978.
14. Weiss L, Tavassoli M: Anatomical hazards to the passage of erythrocytes through the spleen, *Semin Hematol* 7:372, 1970.
15. Wolf BC, Neiman RS: Disorders of the spleen. In Bennington J, editor: *Major problems in pathology,* vol 23, Philadelphia, 1989, Saunders.
16. Wolf BC, Luevano E, Neiman RS: Evidence to suggest that the human fetal spleen is not a hematopoietic organ, *Am J Clin Pathol* 80:140, 1983.
17. Crosby WH: Normal functions of the spleen relative to red blood cells: a review, *Blood* 14:399, 1959.

Reactive lesions

18. Jacobs HS: Hypersplenism: mechanisms and management, *Br J Haematol* 27:1, 1974.
19. Jandl JH, Aster RH: Increased splenic pooling and the pathogenesis of hypersplenism, *Am J Med Sci* 253:383, 1967.
20. Crosby WH: Hyposplenism: an inquiry into normal functions of the spleen, *Annu Rev Med* 14:349, 1963.
21. Corrigan JJ, Van Wyck DB, Crosby WH: Clinical disorders of the splenic function: the spectrum from asplenism to hypersplenism, *Lymphology* 16:101, 1983.
22. Martin JB, Bew HE: The association of splenic atrophy and intestinal malabsorption: report of a case and review of the literature, *Can Med Assoc J* 92:875, 1965.
23. Holdsworth RJ, Irving AD, Cuschieri A: Postsplenectomy sepsis and its mortality rate: actual versus perceived risks, *Br J Surg* 78:1031, 1991.
24. Rosner F et al: Babesiosis in splenectomized adults. *Am J Med* 76:696, 1984.
25. Wardrop CAJ et al: Immunologic abnormalities in splenic atrophy, *Lancet* 2:4, 1975.
26. Mobley K et al: Autopsy findings in the acquired immunodeficiency syndrome, *Pathol Annu* 1:197, 1985.
27. Urmacher C, Nielsen S: The histopathology of the acquired immunodeficiency syndrome, *Pathol Annu* 1:45, 1985.
28. Lipson RL, Bayrd FD, Watkins CH: The postsplenectomy blood picture, *Am J Clin Pathol* 35:526, 1959.
29. Neiman RS: Incidence and importance of splenic sarcoid-like granulomas, *Arch Pathol Lab Med* 101:518, 1977.
30. Collins RD, Neiman RS: Granulomatous diseases of the spleen. In Ioachim HL, editor: *Pathology of granulomas,* New York, 1983, Raven Press.
31. Rappaport H, Crosby WH: Auto-immune hemolytic anemia. II. Morphologic observations and clinicopathologic correlations, *Am J Pathol* 33:429, 1957.
32. Molnar Z, Rappaport H: Fine structure of the spleen in hereditary spherocytosis, *Blood* 1:81, 1972.
33. MacPherson AIS et al: The role of the spleen in congenital spherocytosis, *Am J Med* 50:35, 1971.
34. Hathorn M: Patterns of red cell destruction in sickle-cell anaemia, *Br J Haematol* 13:746, 1967.
35. Schwartz AD: The splenic platelet reservoir in sickle cell anemia, *Blood* 40:678, 1972.
36. Schnitzer B et al: An ultrastructural study of the red pulp of the spleen in malaria, *Blood* 41:205, 1973.
37. Wyler DJ: Splenic functions in malaria, *Lymphology* 16:121, 1983.
38. Hassan NMR, Neiman RS: Pathology of the spleen in steroid treated immune thrombocytopenic purpura, *Am J Clin Pathol* 84:433, 1985.
39. Chang C-S, Li C-Y, Cha SS: Chronic idiopathic thrombocytopenic purpura, splenic pathologic features and their clinical correlation, *Arch Pathol Lab Med* 117:981, 1993.
40. Evans RS et al: Primary thrombocytopenic purpura and acquired hemolytic anemia: evidence for a common etiology, *Arch Intern Med* 87:48, 1951.
41. Lee RE, Peters SP, Glew RH: Gaucher's disease: clinical, morphologic, and pathogenetic considerations, *Pathol Annu* 2:309, 1977.
42. Peters SP, Lee RE, Glew RH: Gaucher's disease: a review, *Medicine* 56:425, 1977.
43. Rywlin AM et al: Ceroid histiocytosis of the spleen and bone marrow in idiopathic thrombocytopenic purpura (ITP): a contribution to the understanding of the sea-blue histiocyte, *Blood* 37:587, 1971.
44. Sawitsky A, Rosner F, Chodsky S: The sea-blue histiocyte syndrome, a review—genetic and biochemical studies, *Semin Hematol* 9:285, 1972.
45. Silverstein MN, Ellefson RD: The syndrome of the sea-blue histiocyte, *Semin Hematol* 9:299, 1972.
46. Silverstein MN, Ellefson RD, Ahern FJ: The syndrome of the sea-blue histiocyte, *N Engl J Med* 282:1, 1970.
47. Rywlin AM et al: Ceroid histiocytosis of the spleen in hyperlipidemia: relationship to the syndrome of the sea-blue histiocyte, *Am J Clin Pathol* 56:572, 1971.
48. Schinella RA et al: Hermansky-Pudlak syndrome: a clinicopathologic study, *Hum Pathol* 16:366, 1985.
49. Parker AC et al: Sea-blue histiocytosis associated with hyperlipidaemia, *J Clin Pathol* 29:634, 1976.
50. Risdall RJ et al: Virus-associated hemophagocytic syndrome: a benign histiocytic proliferation distinct from malignant histiocytosis, *Cancer* 44:993, 1979.
51. Risdall RJ et al: Bacteria-associated hemophagocytic syndrome, *Cancer* 54:2968, 1984.
52. Neiman RS: Immunoblastic sarcoma, *Am J Surg Pathol* 6:755, 1982.
53. Warnke RA, Kim H, Dorfman RF: Malignant histiocytosis (histiocytic medullary reticulosis). I. Clinicopathologic study of 29 cases, *Cancer* 35:215, 1975.
54. Franchino C et al: A clinicopathologically distinctive primary splenic histiocytic neoplasm: demonstration of its histiocytic derivation by immunophenotypic and molecular genetic analysis, *Am J Surg Pathol* 12:398, 1988.
55. Alarcón-Segovia D: The necrotizing vasculitides: a new pathogenetic classification, *Med Clin North Am* 61:241, 1977.
56. Saracco SM, Farhi DC: Splenic pathology in thrombotic thrombocytopenic purpura, *Am J Surg Pathol* 14:223, 1990.

Neoplasms

57. Falk S, Stutte HJ: Primary malignant lymphomas of the spleen: a morphologic and immunohistochemical analysis of 17 cases, *Cancer* 66:2612, 1990.
58. Harris NL et al: Diffuse large cell (histiocytic) lymphoma of the spleen: clinical and pathological characteristics of 10 Cases, *Cancer* 54:2460, 1984.
59. Burke JS: Surgical pathology of the spleen: an approach to the differential diagnosis of splenic lymphomas and leukemias. I. Diseases of the white pulp, *Am J Surg Pathol* 5:551, 1981.
60. Kim H, Dorfman RF: Morphologic studies of 84 untreated patients subjected to laparotomy for the staging of non-Hodgkin's lymphomas, *Cancer* 33:657, 1974.
61. Kraemer BB, Osborne BM, Butler JJ: Primary splenic presentation of malignant lymphoma and related disorders: a study of 49 cases. *Cancer* 54:1606, 1984.
62. Narang S, Wolf BC, Neiman RS: Malignant lymphoma presenting with prominent splenomegaly: a clinicopathologic study with reference to intermediate cell lymphoma, *Cancer* 55:1948, 1985.
63. Ahmann DL et al: Malignant lymphoma of the spleen: a review of 49 cases in which the diagnosis was made at splenectomy, *Cancer* 19:461, 1966.
64. Neiman RS, Sullivan AL, Jaffe R: Malignant lymphoma simulating leukemic reticuloendotheliosis, *Cancer* 43:329, 1979.
65. Melo JV et al: Splenic B-cell lymphoma with circulating villous lymphocytes: differential diagnosis of B-cell leukaemias with large spleens, *J Clin Pathol* 40:642, 1987.
66. Schmid C et al: Splenic marginal zone cell lymphoma, *Am J Surg Pathol* 16:455, 1992.
67. Sheibani K: Monocytoid B-cell lymphoma. In Knowles DM, editor: *Neoplastic hematopathology,* Baltimore, 1992, Williams & Wilkins.
68. Spriano P et al: Splenomegalic immunocytoma with circulating hairy cells: report of eight cases and revision of the literature, *Haematologica* 71:25, 1986.
69. Wilson MS et al: Malignant histiocytosis: a reassessment of cases previously reported in 1975 based on paraffin section immunophenotyping studies, *Cancer* 66:530, 1990.
70. Rappaport H, Thomas LB: Mycosis fungoides: the pathology of extracutaneous involvement, *Cancer* 34:1198, 1974.
71. Kehoe JE et al: Value of splenectomy in non-Hodgkin's lymphoma, *Cancer* 55:1256, 1985.
72. Neiman RS: Current problems in the histopathologic diagnosis and classification of Hodgkin's disease, *Pathol Annu* 2:289, 1978.
73. Farrer-Brown G et al: The diagnosis of Hodgkin's disease in surgically excised spleens, *J Clin Pathol* 25:294, 1972.
74. Kadin ME, Glatstein E, Dorfman RF: Clinicopathologic studies of 117 untreated patients subjected to laparotomy for the staging of Hodgkin's disease, *Cancer* 27:1277, 1971.
75. Gaba AR et al: Multicentric giant lymph node hyperplasia, *Am J Clin Pathol* 69:86, 1978.
76. Wolf BC et al: Bone marrow morphology and immunology in systemic amyloidosis, *Am J Clin Pathol* 86:84, 1986.
77. Wu BD et al: The predictive value of bone marrow morphology and immunostaining in primary (AL) amyloidosis, *Am J Clin Pathol* 96:95, 1991.
78. Frangione B, Franklin FC: Heavy chain disease: clinical features and molecular significance of the disordered immunoglobulin structure, *Semin Hematol* 10:53, 1973.
79. Dutcher TF, Fahey JL: The histopathology of the macroglobulinemia of waldenström, *J Natl Cancer Inst* 22:887, 1959.
80. MacKenzie MR, Fudenberg HH: Macroglobulinemia: an analysis for forty patients, *Blood* 39:874, 1972.
81. Wolf BC, Neiman RS: The histopathologic manifestations of the lymphoproliferative and myeloproliferative disorders involving the spleen. In Knowles, Daniel M, editors: *Neoplastic hematopathology,* Baltimore, 1992, Williams & Wilkins.
82. Wolf BC, Neiman RS: The myeloproliferative disorders. In Bick RL, editor: *Principles of hematology: clinical and laboratory practice,* St. Louis, 1993, Mosby.
83. Bitter MA: Hairy cell leukemia, In Knowles DM, editor: *Neoplastic hematopathology,* Baltimore, 1992, Williams & Wilkins.
84. Bearman RM, Pangalis GA, Rappaport H: Prolymphocytic leukemia: clinical, histopathological, and cytochemical observations, *Cancer* 42:2360, 1978.
85. Galton DAG et al: Prolymphocytic leukemia, *Br J Haematol* 24:7, 1974.
86. Pandolfi F et al: Clinical course and prognosis of the lymphoproliferative disease of granular lymphocytes: a multicenter study, *Cancer* 65:341, 1990.
87. Webb TA, Li C-Y, Yam LT: Systemic mast cell disease: a clinical and hematopathologic study of 26 cases, *Cancer* 49:927, 1982.
88. Travis WD, Li C-Y: Pathology of the lymph node and spleen in systemic mast cell disease, *Mod Pathol* 1:4, 1988.
89. Wolf BC et al: Splenic hematopoiesis in polycythemia vera: a morphologic and immunohistologic study, *Am J Clin Pathol* 89:69, 1988.
90. Wolf BC, Neiman RS: Myelofibrosis with myeloid metaplasia: pathophysiologic implication between bone marrow changes and progression of splenomegaly, *Blood* 65:803, 1985.
91. Wolf BC, Neiman RS: Hypothesis—splenic filtration and the pathogenesis of extramedullary hematopoiesis in agnogenic myeloid metaplasia, *Hematol Pathol* 1:77, 1987.
92. Pines B, Rabinovitch J: Hemangioma of the spleen, *Arch Pathol* 33:487, 1942.
93. Falk S, Stutte HJ, Frizzera G: Littoral cell angioma. A novel splenic vascular lesion demonstrating histiocytic differentiation, *Am J Surg Pathol* 15:1023, 1991.
94. Wick MR et al: Primary nonlymphoreticular malignant neoplasms of the spleen, *Am J Surg Pathol* 6:229, 1982.
95. Lacson A, Berman LD, Neiman RS: Peliosis of the spleen, *Am J Clin Pathol* 71:586, 1979.
96. Cotelingham JD, Jaffe ES: Inflammatory pseudotumor of the spleen, *Am J Surg Pathol* 8:375, 1984.
97. Sheahan DK, Wolf BC, Neiman RS: Inflammatory pseudotumor of the spleen: a clinicopathologic study of 3 cases, *Hum Pathol* 19:1024, 1988.
98. Silverman ML, LiVolsi VA: Splenic hamartoma, *Am J Clin Pathol* 70:224, 1978.
99. Ross CF, Schiller KFR: Hamartoma of spleen associated with thrombocytopenia, *J Pathol* 105:62, 1971.
100. Shousha S: Splenic cysts: a report of 6 cases and a brief review, *Postgrad Med J* 54:265, 1978.
101. Robbins FG et al: Splenic epidermoid cysts, *Ann Surg* 187:231, 1978.
102. Tsakraklides V, Hadley TW: Epidermoid cysts of the spleen: a report of five cases, *Arch Pathol* 96:251, 1973.
103. Marymont JH Jr, Gross S: Patterns of metastatic cancer in the spleen, *Am J Clin Pathol* 40:58, 1963.

44 Thymus and Mediastinum

A. THYMUS

Hans Konrad Müller-Hermelink
Alexander Marx
Thomas Kirchner

Abbreviations

ALL	Acute lymphoblastic lymphoma
AChR	Acetylcholine receptor
BMT	Bone marrow transplantation
CD	Cluster-of-differentiation antigen
EBV	Epstein-Barr virus
EBERs	Epstein-Barr virus early RNAs
EMA	Epithelial membrane antigen
GC	Germinal center
GVHD	Graft-versus-host disease
GVH	Graft-versus-host reaction
HLA	Human leukocyte antigen
IDC	Interdigitating reticulum cells
LMP	Latent membrane protein (of EBV)
MALT	Mucosa-associated lymphoid tissue
MG	Myasthenia gravis
MHC	Major histocompatibility complex
SCID	Severe combined immunodeficiency
TCR	T-cell receptor
TdT	Terminal deoxynucleotidyl transferase
TET	Thymic epithelial tumor
WDTC	Well-differentiated thymic carcinoma

The thymus is a lymphoepithelial organ that has the central role in T-lymphocyte development. Originally believed to be the seat of the soul[1] and more recently to be the "clock for immunologic aging,"[2] the thymus remained with an unknown function until the 1960s when it was discovered after neonatal thymectomy in rodents that the thymus is an important component of the immune system.[3-6] The pathology of the thymus has been reviewed recently in several reviews and monographs.[7-12]

NORMAL THYMUS

Embryology

The epithelial component of the thymus anlage is derived from ectoderm endoderm of the cervical sinus and the third pharyngeal pouch, respectively.[13-17] During embryonal development at stage Carnegie 22 (23 mm SCL), ectoderm-derived tissue from the cervical vesicle fuses with and surrounds the descending proliferation of the third pharyngeal pouch–derived entoderm, giving rise to a solid paired epithelial primordium of the thymus.[18,19] This tubelike structure is obliterated by epithelial proliferation and loses its open connections to the pharynx by the end of the second embryonal month.[20] Two thymic lobes derived from each side of the neck fuse into a single organ behind the sternum and ventral to the brachiocephalic vein, neighboring the aortic arch at its posterior surface and its large vessels. Both lobes are tightly fixed to each other by their connective tissue capsule in the thoracic portion, forming a plump body that overrides the pericardium and gives rise to two cervical "horns" that are neighboring the trachea at their medial faces and the two pleural cavities laterally. There are many variations in the cervical portion that remains in contact with the lateral or posterior face of the thyroid gland even at birth. Also the caudal extension of the thoracic part of the thymus may vary significantly, reaching usually the height of the fourth intercostal space but sometimes extending even to the diaphragm.[21,22]

The epithelial cells of the thymic anlage at the eighth gestational week form nests enclosed by a basal lamina that separates them from the surrounding mesenchyme. Both cell types are interconnected by desmosomes. Myoid cells, derived from the prechordal mesenchyme,[23,24] are already present at this stage of development. This epithelial anlage is then colonized by blood-borne lymphohemopoietic precursors, which first become visible at the ninth gestational week.[18,25,26] The influx of precursor cells into the thymus appears to occur in several waves during embryonal life and may persist, albeit at a much lower level, throughout the whole postnatal life.[27-29] The precursors reaching the thymus through blood vessels are derived from sites of hemopoiesis, that is, the yolk sac, the fetal liver, and finally the bone marrow.[27] It is not known how many lymphoid cells colonize the epithelial thymic anlage, but it appears that almost all cortical thymocytes are formed locally. Rapidly dividing lymphoid precursors and their descendants fill up the epithelial meshwork, forming cortical pseudolobules separated from each other by interlobular septa. The demarcation of the cortex from the medulla becomes apparent by the twelfth gestational week.[20] Hassall's corpuscles first appear as whorled epithelial structures in the presumptive medulla at the tenth to twelfth gestational week. The morphogenesis of cortex and medulla is completed by the sixteenth gestational week. The thymus will continue to grow until the first month of neonatal life. Lymphoid and epithelial cell maturation and differentiation occur simultaneously and are definitely interdependent.

The initial colonization of the thymus by lymphoid cells involves precursors of T-lymphocytes and also B-lymphocytes, which home in on mainly the vicinity of Hassall's corpuscles.[30-34] Thymic B-lymphocytes are found by the sixteenth gestational week, when other B-cell compartments in the periphery are just emerging (such as lymph node, tonsil) or still absent (spleen). Thymic macrophages and precursors of dendritic cells and Langerhans' cells are also blood-borne.[18,35,36] Invasion of the medulla by dendritic cells is seen at the end of the third month of gestation.

Significant cellular export of naïve T-cells out of the thymus starts at about the thirteenth gestational week,[20] reflected by the invasion of high endothelial venules by lymphoid cells in the paracortical areas of lymph nodes with the formation of nodular T-zones.[37,38]

Structure

The two lobes of the thymus are subdivided by connective tissue septa into numerous small lobules (Fig. 44-1). Each lobule consists of a cortex and medulla. The narrow perivascular space[39] defined by the basement membrane of thymic epithelial cells on the one hand and the vascular basement membrane on the other is the third thymic component. The perivascular space is filled by migratory lymphoid cells. It is highly interconnected with the medullary area and cannot be distinguished from it in routinely stained slides. These three compartments can be distinguished by silver impregnation; the epithelial space of the cortex is devoid of stainable material, whereas perivascular spaces contain a dense fibrillar network. Short basement membranes surround medullary epithelial cells. The perivascular space (Fig. 44-1, *C*) merges with the perilobular adipose tissue, which increases in volume and finally surrounds the entire lobules when the epithelial part shrinks because of age-related involution.

The thymus consists of many cell types, the most notable of which are epithelial cells, lymphocytes, macrophages, dendritic cells, myoid cells, blood vessels, and connective tissue stromal cells. There are also scattered neutrophils, eosinophils, and occasional neuroendocrine cells and erythroid precursors. Postpubertal thymus consists mostly of fat cells.

The thymus contains four morphologically distinct types of epithelial cells. Each of these cell types has an unique localization, light microscopic and ultrastructural morphology, and immunologic phenotype.[40-45]

1. The *subcapsular epithelium* surrounds the cortical portion of the lobules abutting on the fibrous capsule. At the base of the mesenchymal and fibrous septa at the cortical medullary boundary, these epithelial cells merge with the perivascular epithelium and give rise to medullary epithelial cells.

2. The *cortical epithelium* forms a three-dimensional network in contact with developing immature thymocytes. In the outer cortex epithelial cells are very large. These cells have round to oval nuclei with distinct nucleoli surrounded only by a small rim of cytoplasm. The small cytoplasmic extensions and invaginations enclose lymphoid precursors, thus forming large lymphoepithelial complexes. These epithelial cells are called *thymic nurse cells*.[46,47] In the deeper cortex, epithelial cells become smaller, often oriented perpendicularly to the thymic surface. Their nuclei are smaller and their nucleoli are less prominent than those in thymic nurse cells.

3. *Medullary epithelial cells* are spindle shaped. The nuclei are fusiform with a much denser chromatin structure than that of cortical epithelial cells. Nucleoli are inconspicuous. Cytoplasmic processes are often densely stained and contain numerous cytoplasmic filaments, composed of smooth muscle actin and myosin as well as high molecular weight keratins. Medullary epithelial cells are attached to basement membranes and are continuous to the medullary perivascular epithelial cells.

4. Keratinizing squamous epithelial cells form *Hassall's corpuscles*. These concentrically layered cells form nests with central keratinization though occasionally there is evidence of a glandular differentiation.

In addition, rare endocrine cells may be identified in the medulla by electron microscopy and immunohistochemistry.[8,9,48,49] These cells are argyrophilic and can be demonstrated by silver staining.

Findings in thymic tumors indicate that at least two separate epithelial cell lineages exist in the thymus: (1) the *cortical*

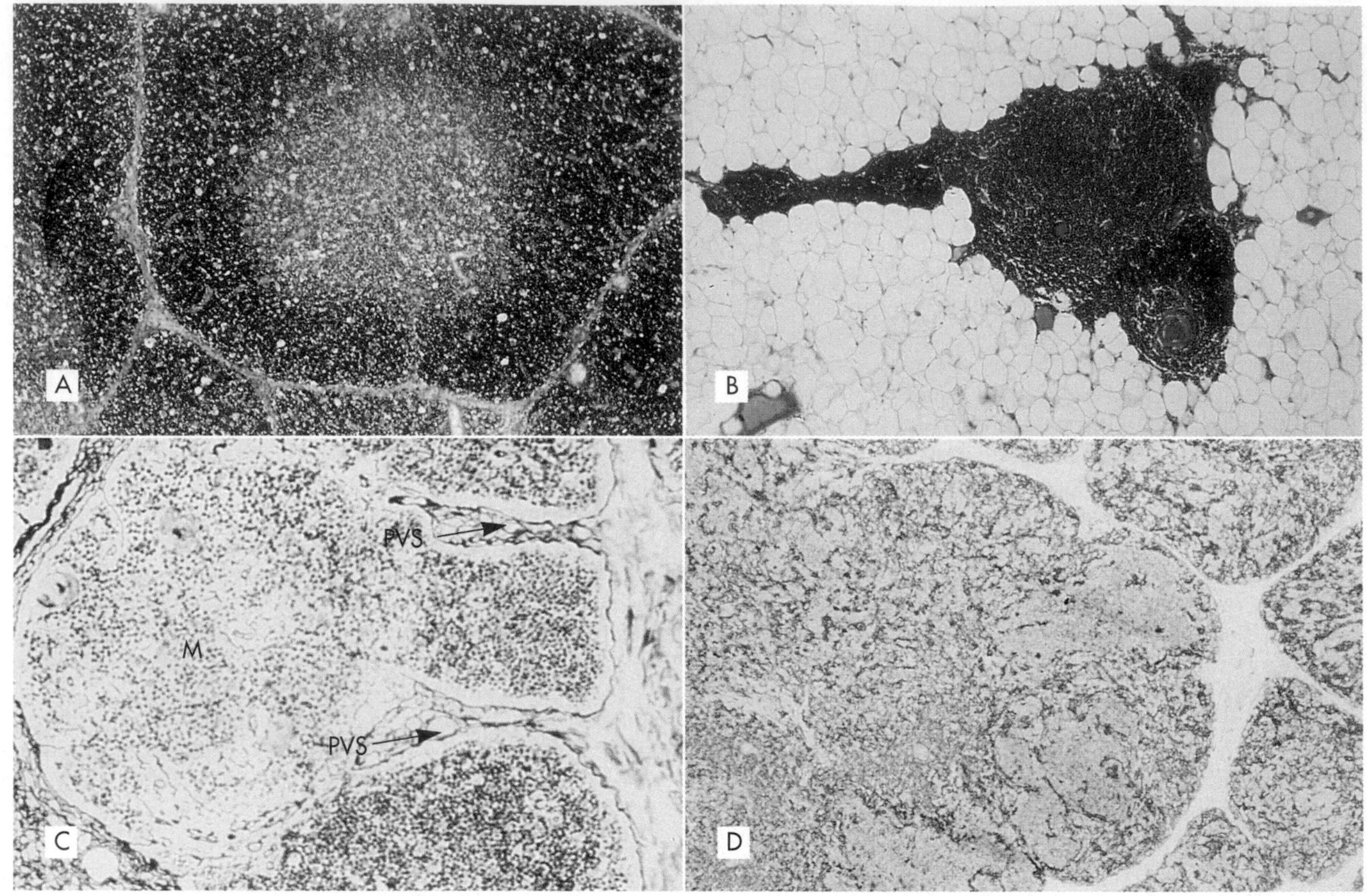

Fig. 44-1 Normal structure of the thymus. **A,** Histology of the normal human thymus in the newborn. **B,** Thymus in an 80-year-old person. **C,** Perivascular space in the normal thymus characterized by a dense reticulin network and a continuous basement membrane separating the perivascular space, *PVS,* from the thymic medulla, *M.* **D,** Focal epithelium-free areas in the thymic cortex are a regular finding in the noramal human thymus (anti–HLA-DR, immunoperoxidase).

program, starting with subcapsular and periseptal epithelium giving rise to large cortical epithelial cells (including thymic nurse cells), finally differentiating to squamous epithelium of Hassall's corpuscles, and (2) the *medullary program,* starting from perivascular epithelium, differentiating to spindle-shaped medullary epithelial cells.[49,50] Subpopulations of thymic epithelial cells can be recognized with specific monoclonal antibodies.[51]

Most of the thymic lymphocytes belong to the T-cell lineage. However, there are also B-cells and NK-cells. Although a small number of T-cells seems to differentiate by an extrathymic pathway, the maturation of most T-lymphocyte precursors takes place within the meshwork of thymic epithelial cells. Different steps of this process can be defined by immunologic phenotyping.[52-56] The prothymocytes are positive for the terminal deoxynucleotidyl transferase (TdT) and give rise to cortical thymocytes, which express CD1, CD2, CD3, CD5, and both CD4 and CD8.[57-61] These CD4 and CD8 double-positive cortical thymocytes differentiate into two lineages: $CD4^+$ or $CD8^+$ lymphocytes of the thymic medulla. The T-cell receptor (TCR) that is linked to CD3 appears first in cortical thymocytes. The genes encoding the TCR subunits are rearranged within the population of CD4/CD8 double-positive thymocytes, which results in the formation of functional TCR molecules composed of an alpha and a beta polypeptide chain. An alternative cell lineage with the gamma/delta TCR phenotype evolves in parallel.[62-66]

Only a small proportion of cells derived from cortical thymocytes will reach the periphery as mature T-lymphocytes. Most probably, more than 95% of the thymocytes will die by still incompletely understood mechanisms[67-69] that by their functional result are termed *positive* and *negative selection.*[70-73] Positive selection takes place in the cortex by interaction of immature thymocytes expressing the TCR at low levels with cortical epithelial cells expressing MHC determinants.[74-77] As a result of TCR recognition of self MHC determinants, selected precursor cells will survive (positive selection) whereas those not recognizing a self MHC determinant are prone to apoptotic cell death.

Negative selection takes place through the interaction of positively selected precursors that mature into TCR-positive cells with bone marrow–derived mesenchymal cells at the corticomedullary junction.[78-82] The essential mesenchymal cells mediating negative selection are believed to be the dendritic cells or B-lymphocytes.[70,83-89] These cells are "professional" antigen-presenting cells that, through surface MHC class I and class II antigens, present all varieties of self peptides.[90] Maturing T-lymphocytes that are activated by self peptides will die (negative selection), whereas nonreacting T-lymphocytes may be liberated from the thymus and go to the periphery building up the repertoire of TCRs recognizing self MHC determinants as well as nonself peptides, or sequestered tissue-specific antigens. The process of T-cell maturation and selection is highly regulated by cytokines and other hormones as well as specific thymic hormones produced by epithelial cells.[91-94]

B-lymphocytes of particular phenotype ($CD19^+$, $CD20^+$, $CD37^+$, $CD40^+$, $CD21^-$, $CD10^-$, $CD70^-$) and morphology are distributed mainly around Hassall's corpuscles in the thymic medulla, whereas plasma cells and other B-cells are seen in the perivascular space sometimes forming lymphoid follicles and germinal centers.[30,95-98] Medullary B-lymphocytes may show significant proliferative activity.

The epithelial structure of the cortical lobules varies: in some lobules the epithelial cells are abundant and in contact with individual lymphoid cells, whereas others are almost devoid of epithelial cells[98] (Fig. 44-1, *D*). These two structural patterns of epithelial cells may merge one into another. Epithelial cells are best demonstrated immunohistochemically with antibodies to keratins or MHC class II antigens.

Lymphoid cells are similar in both the cortex and medulla. Within the meshes of the spindle-shaped medullary epithelial cells there are dendritic (interdigitating) cells and mature lymphocytes of T and B phenotype resulting in a cellular composition that is similar to that of peripheral lymphoid tissue.[98,99] Other nonlymphoid cells are also distributed in distinct localizations. Macrophages are present in cortex and medulla, whereas dendritic cells and Langerhans' cells are particularly common at the corticomedullary junction and throughout the medullary area but not in the cortex.[100,101] Myoid cells are found only in the medulla.[102-109] Tissue mast cells may be present in the perivascular and epithelial space of the medulla.[110] Melanocytes can also be present.[111,112]

INVOLUTION OF THE THYMUS

Age-related involution

In contrast to those of some other species the size of the thymus in humans does not change significantly after the age of 1 year. However, the amount of lymphoid tissue decreases and is replaced by adipose tissue[113] (Fig. 44-1, *B*). Remnants of thymic lymphoid tissue or epithelial strands are found in this fat tissue even in very old persons. These remnants show the characteristic structure of cortex and medulla (Fig. 44-1) and contain proliferating lymphocytes that have TdT and CD1.[114]

The gradual loss of lymphoid thymic tissue starts soon after birth and is not influenced by any specific functional event. The atrophy of thymus occurs at the same rate in both sexes.[115] The so-called pubertal atrophy reported in the older literature has not been scientifically documented. Exceptionally large thymuses were considered as a pathologic condition (the so-called status thymolymphaticus) and were therefore excluded from the "normal material," especially in children between 1 and 6 years.[116] Subsequently it was shown that even these "enlarged" thymuses were within the normal ranges. Sudden death reported in some cases could not be causally linked to thymic enlargement.[117]

Various tissue compartments of the thymus change at a different rate during age-related involution. The epithelial space and in particular the thymus cortex shows a steady and almost linear decline at a rate of about 5% per year until 40 years of age (Fig. 44-2). By the fortieth year less than 10% of the total volume is composed of lymphoid cortical tissue. The amount of lymphoid cells in the perivascular space increases over the first two decades and then declines exponentially.

The reasons for this steady decrease of thymic cortical volume are unclear.[118] The mitotic activity of lymphoid precursors remains constant throughout life, and the ratio of lymphoid cells to thymic epithelial cells declines only very late in life. There is, however, a progressive loss of thymic cortical epithelial cells. Since these cells are responsible for the specific intrathymic homing and proliferation of lymphoid precursors, loss of the epithelial cells probably affects lymphopoiesis and contributes to overall atrophy of the thymus.

The age-related involution of cortical lymphoid tissue is also independent from some nonneoplastic processes involving the thymic medulla. For example, the formation of large germinal centers in lymphofollicular thymitis of myasthenia gravis has no effect on the volume of cortical lymphoid tissue[98] (Fig. 44-2). On the other hand, infiltration of the thymic medulla by malignant lymphoma leads to a rapid loss of cortical lymphoid tissue.

Accidental involution

Accidental involution can be acute or chronic. Acute involution of the thymus may occur in response to any form of acute stress. It may be associated with acute respiratory distress syndrome, trauma or sepsis, chemotherapy, or irradiation.[119-122] In contrast to primary immunodeficiency it is reversible, at least in its early stages. Acute accidental involution appears to be mediated by endogenous corticosteroids, which are released in stress. Corticosteroids promote apoptotic cell death of cortical thymocytes, which express steroid receptors.[123]

Early accidental thymic involution is histologically characterized by diffuse apoptotic cell death of cortical thymocytes and phagocytosis of altered pyknotic cell remnants by macrophages.[119-121] These macrophages account for the starry-sky appearance of the cortex. The cortical volume shrinks, but the thymic medulla remains unaltered, since mature T- and B-lymphocytes are corticosteroid resistant.

At later stages of involution, the thymic epithelial cells become more visible, unmasked by a loss of lymphocytes (Fig. 44-3). The cortex may be almost devoid of any lymphoid cells and contain only lipid-rich foamy macrophages between the cords of epithelial cells. Since the cortex is shrunken to a small rim surrounding the unaltered thymic medulla, the normal ratio of cortex to medulla is reversed. Within the thymic medulla cystic Hassall's corpuscles become prominent, and the fibrous capsule of the thymus is usually broader than usual.

In chronic wasting conditions and in malnutrition the thymus is severely atrophic.[119,124-126] In such cases the cortex may disappear completely, and no remnants of cortical epithelium are found beneath the thickened capsule. Foamy macrophages may still be present; however, even they are less prominent than in subacute involution. The medulla contains cystic Hassall's corpuscles and spindle-shaped medullary epithelial cells. The lymphoid content of the medulla is also diminished, and the medulla may be reduced to solid strands of epithelial cells. This end-stage thymic atrophy has the same morphology irrespective of its cause.

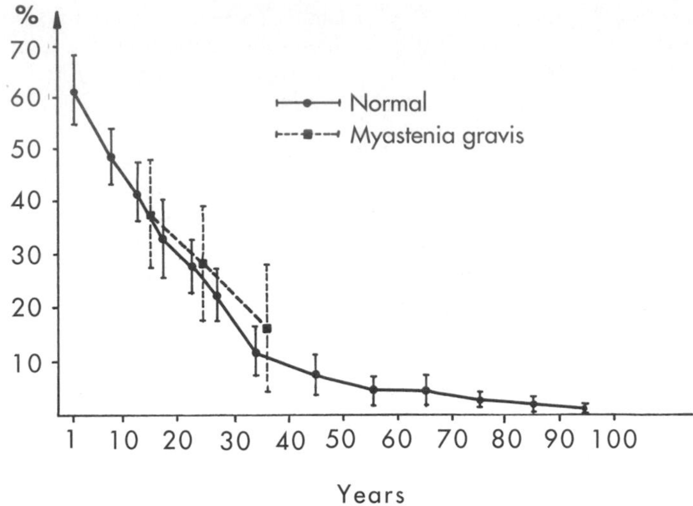

Fig. 44-2 Age-related involution of the thymus in the normal population *(solid line)* and patients suffering from myasthenia gravis with a lymphofollicular thymitis *(dashed line)*. Bars indicate standard deviation from the mean.

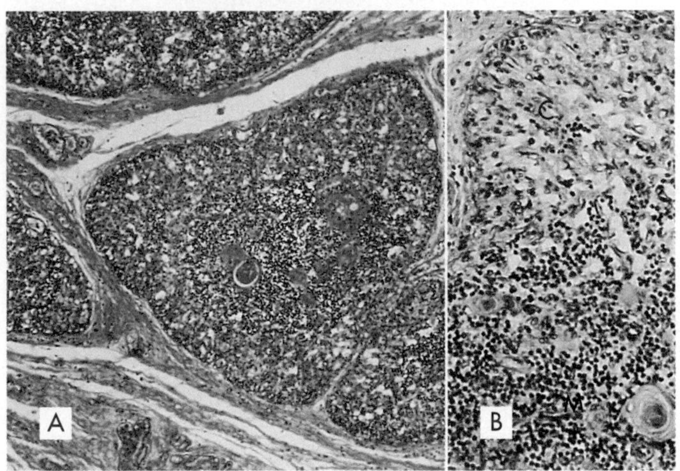

Fig. 44-3 Accidental thymic involution after prolonged stress, **A,** Almost complete lack of lymphoid cells in the atrophic thymic cortex surrounding the unaltered thymic medulla. **B,** Higher magnification of atrophic thymic cortex and unaltered medulla.

PRIMARY IMMUNODEFICIENCY DISEASES

Severe combined immunodeficiency

Severe combined immunodeficiency (SCID) results from different genetic defects affecting enzymes involved in the nuclear metabolism, the formation of effective TCR rearrangements, and T-cell differentiation and function. In many cases of typical SCID the cause remains unclear.[127-129]

In SCID the thymus is in its normal position but usually very small (0.5 to 4 g)[130] (Fig. 44-4, *A*). Histologically it appears lobular but shows no distinct cortical and medullary parts. Hassall's corpuscles are absent. The arrangement of epithelial cells may be nodular or reminiscent of glandular acini. Sometimes a rim of cortical epithelial cells surrounds the centrally located spindle-shaped medullary epithelium. The last pattern showing the highest resemblance to the normal thymic structure is often found in adenosine deaminase or nucleosid phosphorylase deficiency.

Lymphocyte populations are invariably severely depleted, and often there are no lymphoid cells at all. Thymic changes in SCID have been classified into either five[131] or four[132] different categories. These observations have led to the following terminology:[110]

1. *Simple dysplasia* (Fig. 44-5, *A*). Simple dysplasia is the most common pattern where epithelial lobules are small and separated by fibroadipose tissue. The lobules are composed of nodules of polyhedral epithelial cells with eosinophilic cytoplasm and ovoid nucleoli. There are no Hassall's corpuscles and no corticomedullary demarcation. Lymphoid cells are scarce and scanty and resemble mature lymphocytes. This pattern corresponds to the "pinealoid form"[133] and the "partial dysplasia with phagocytosis."[131]

2. *Dysplasia with stromal corticomedullary differentiation* (Fig. 44-5, *B*). Here, lobules are larger. The outlines of the gland are more regular than those in simple dysplasia. Some corticomedullary differentiation is seen. No Hassall's corpuscle are found. Sometimes large foamy cells are found in the central part of each lobule. This aspect corresponds to the "late fetal pattern"[131] and is more frequently found with the above-mentioned enzyme defects.

3. *Dysplasia with pseudoglandular appearance.* This pattern is very distinctive and probably represents the most primitive aspect of thymic dysplasias. The arrangement of epithelial cells resembles an acinar or glandular structure. No Hassall's corpuscles or lymphoid cells are found. Sometimes, peripheral lymph nodes are lacking.

4. *Pattern similar to severe atrophy.* In these cases the thymic structure is normal, and Hassall's corpuscles are present.

The different histologic patterns can not be correlated to the various causes of SCID. *Thymus dysplasia* in itself is not the cause of immunodeficiency, since allogeneic bone marrow transplantation (BMT) can restore full immunoreactivity in up to 70% of treated cases within a few months.[134] This is well illustrated by a typical SCID case of a patient dying 3 months

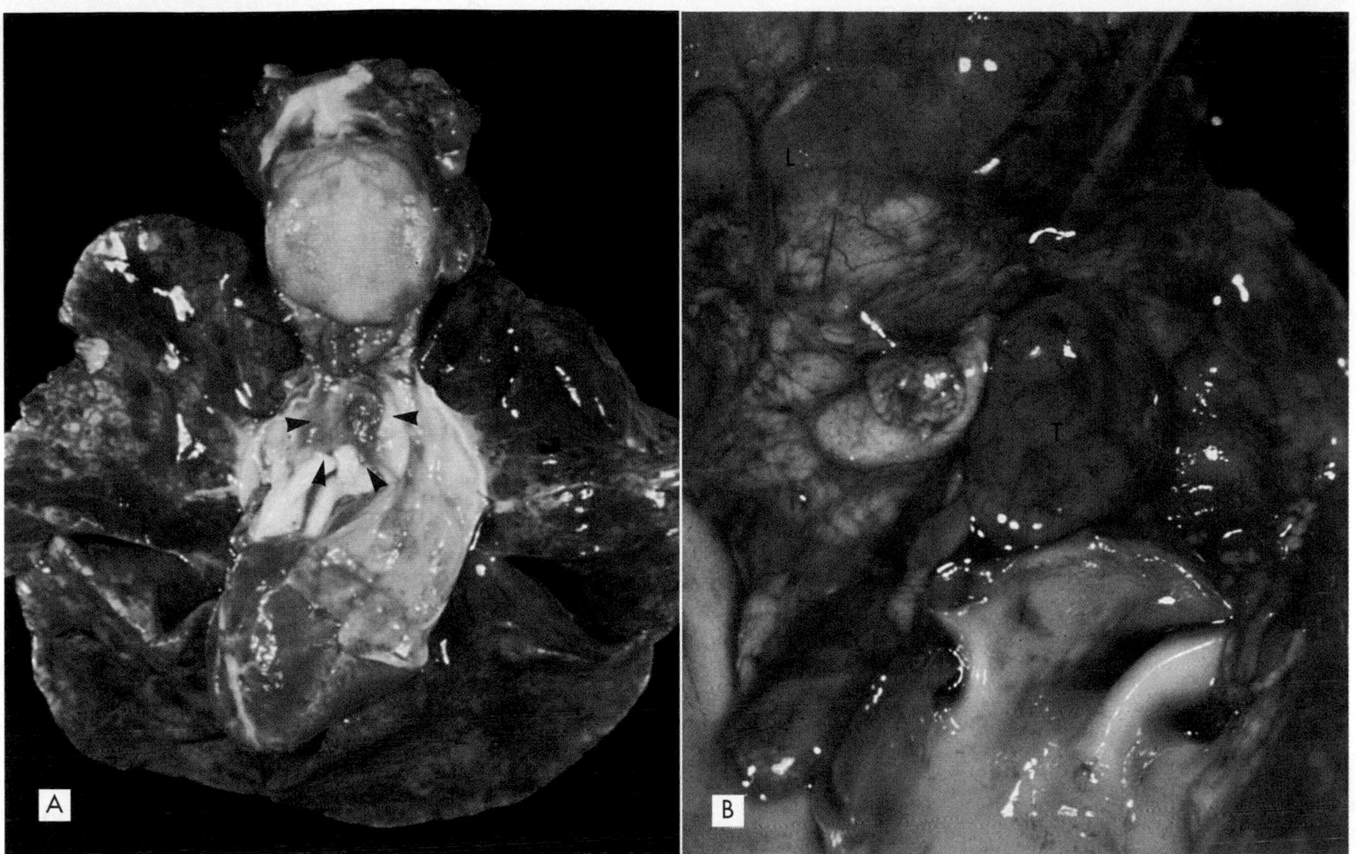

Fig. 44-4 Thymus in primary immunodeficiency diseases. **A,** Severe combined immunodeficiency (SCID) in a 6-month-old boy dying of severe sepsis. Extremely hypoplastic thymus in an orthotopic position, *arrowheads,* in the mediastinal midline close to the aortic arch. **B,** Incomplete DiGeorge's syndrome: extremely hypoplastic and incompletely descended thymus, *T,* in the left cervical region posterior to the (here removed) thyroid gland and below the larynx, *L.*

after BMT who showed fully restored cortical and medullary portions of the thymus, though at that time Hassall's corpuscles were still missing.[110] It is thus safe to conclude that the thymus in most cases of SCID is immature, frozen at the state of the embryonal epithelial thymic rudiment, which is capable of acquiring full function within months after appropriate colonization by healthy bone marrow precursor cells.

This rudimentary epithelial thymus of SCID may be damaged further by intrauterine infections and by allogeneic maternal lymphocytes crossing into the fetal circulation. In extreme cases, massive maternofetal transfusion may lead to acute graft-versus-host disease (GVHD) apparent at birth.[135-138] Since 40% of children with SCID harbor maternal lymphocytes in their circulation, sometimes in high quantities,[139,140] the epithelial rudiment of the thymus may be further altered by resultant GVHD in its acute or chronic form.[141] In these cases the thymus rudiment is infiltrated by macrophages, some of which are laden with hemosiderin (Fig. 44-6). The whole structure becomes obscured by infiltrating lymphocytes and capsular neovascularization. Similar changes may also happen after BMT (see below). Intrauterine GVH-reaction may lead to thymus alterations that are very similar if not identical to the findings in SCID patients.[141] Moreover, it was proposed that given the appropriate genetic setting (maternal:parental) the transplacental passage of maternal lymphocytes could cause SCID.

DiGeorge's syndrome

The hallmarks of the DiGeorge's syndrome are agenesis of thymus and parathyroid glands accompanied by facial and cardiovascular malformations. These malformations reflect a defect in the development of the third and fourth pharyngeal pouches,[142] hence the acronym "Catch 22" for cardiac defects, abnormal facies, thymic hypoplasia, cleft palate, and hypocalcemia.[143,144] In most cases the thymus is not absent, since a detailed search in the cervical tissues will reveal small ectopic remnants of the thymus (Fig. 44-4, *B*). These remnants consist of histologically normal thymic tissue showing, at most, some degree of atrophy. Almost all cases show deletion of chromosome segment 22g-KIW 11.

Maldescent and ectopia of the thymus

The anomaly of maldescent and ectopia of the thymus may be seen very rarely in the absence of the DiGeorge's syndrome. Among 3236 pediatric necropsies over 23 years Bale and colleagues[145] recorded an abnormal position of thymic tissue in 34 cases. Twenty-four children showed typical anomalies of the DiGeorge's syndrome, 3 had noncardiac anomalies, and the remaining 7 cases had isolated thymic anomalies. The maldescended and ectopic tissue was localized near the thyroid gland or lower in the neck, but also at more cranial locations, including seven cases found medial to the submandibular sali-

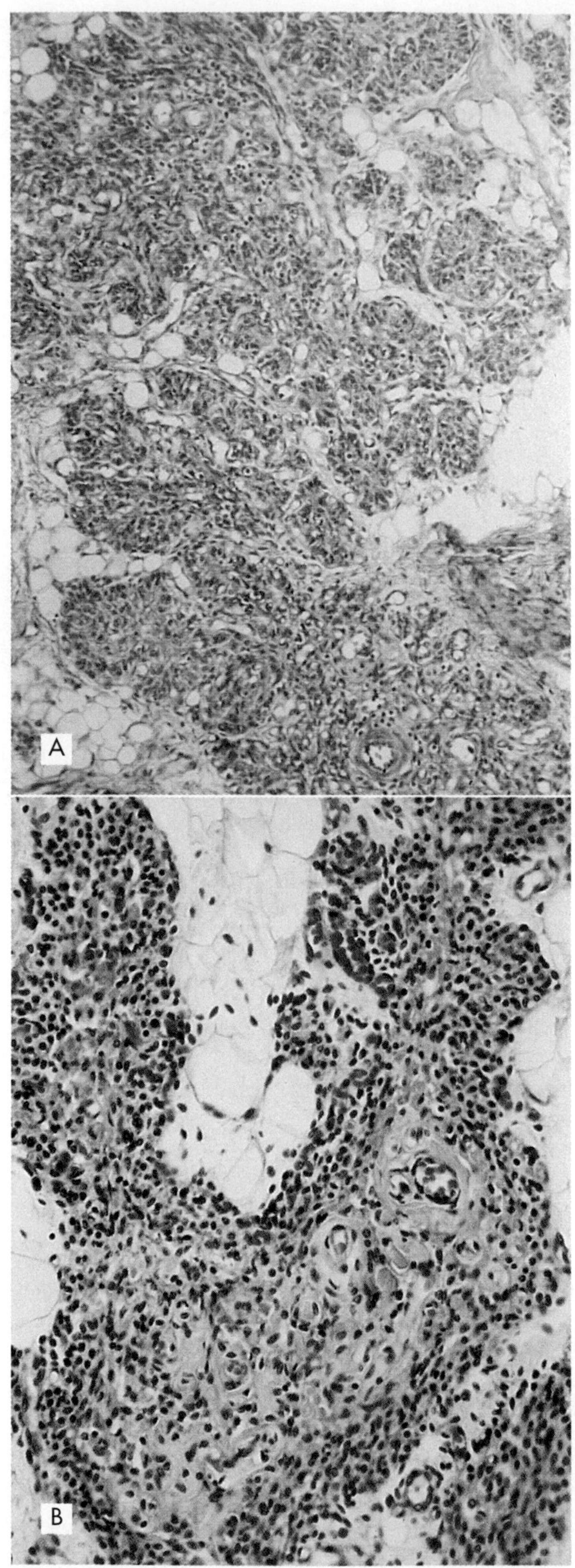

Fig. 44-5 Thymus in primary immundeficiency disease. **A,** Simple thymic dyplasia. Epithelial thymic lobules almost devoid of lymphoid cells, without corticomedullary demarcation and with a lack of Hassall's corpuscles. **B,** Dysplasia with stromal corticomedullary differentiation. Rudimentary cortical medullary demarcation is evident, but no Hassall's corpuscles are seen. Patient had SCID caused by purine nucleoside phosphorylase (PNP) deficiency.

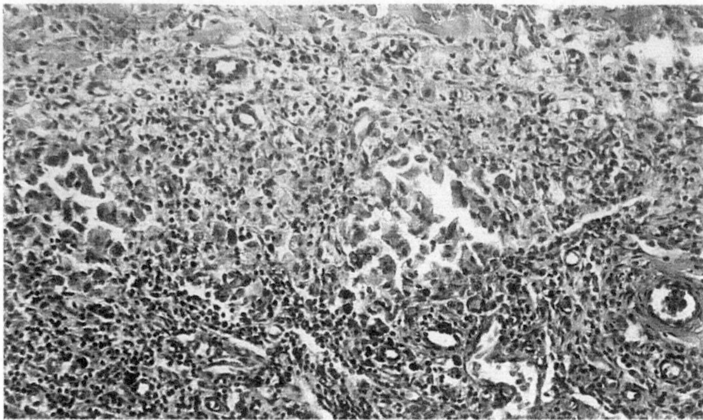

Fig. 44-6 Thymus in graft-versus-host disease (GVHD). Spontaneous thymic GVHD in an SCID patient. Infiltration of the dysplastic thymus by lymphoid cells, monocytes, and siderin-laden macrophages.

vary gland and one at the base of the skull. Some ectopic thymuses were cystic and classified as thymopharyngeal cysts or pouches. The size of an ectopic thymus varies and may even mimic a tumor, prompting surgical intervention.

Other primary immunodeficiencies

Primary immunodeficiency combined with typical thymus dysplasia may be found in concert with other diseases or malformative syndromes, such as short limb dwarfism[146] and Omenn's syndrome (familial eosinophilic reticulosis).[147,148] The changes in the thymus are variable. *Ataxia telangiectasia*[149] includes T-cell defects of late onset and thymic atrophy. The thymus appears very small and lipomatous. The remaining thymic lobes are small and do not show distinct separation of cortex from the medulla. Hassall's corpuscles are missing.[110,130] *Wiscott-Aldrich syndrome* which recently was shown to result from a defect of CD43 receptor[150] also affects the thymus. The histologic findings are variable and range from normal to slight atrophy to an almost complete depletion of lymphocytes. Such epithelial thymic remnants often contain calcified Hassall's corpuscles.[130]

Bruton's agammaglobulinemia[151] and other B-cell–related immunodeficiencies do not affect thymic development directly. However, the thymus may exhibit changes of stress involution secondary to repeated infections.

ACQUIRED IMMUNODEFICIENCY DISEASES

Bone marrow transplantation

Most bone marrow allograft recipients show atrophy and a hyperinvolution of the thymus.[152-155] The outcome and fate of the thymic restitution depends on the type of conditioning pretreatment, age of the recipient, and posttransplantation complications, such as viral infection (as by CMV) or GVHD.[153,155] The early normalization of peripheral blood lymphocyte counts is attributable to donor T-cells in the bone marrow graft. At that time the thymus of the host is still depleted of lymphocytes. Late restitution, evidenced by normalization of $CD4^+$ cell counts and full immunoreactivity, is thymus dependent and involves an interaction between donor's lymphocytes and host thymic epithelial cells. Donor-derived dendritic cells and macrophages of thymic medulla also participate in this process, leading to an immunologic chimerism.

In the *early posttransplantation phase* the changes in the thymus depend on the pretransplantation treatment. In patients transplanted for aplastic anemia who were conditioned only with drugs, the epithelial structure of the thymus appears to be largely preserved. The thymus consists only of epithelial cells and large, sometimes cystic Hassall's corpuscles in the center of the thymic medulla. In leukemic patients receiving total body irradiation the epithelial component of the thymus is much more atrophic and Hassall's bodies are inconspicuous. Up to 3 months after BMT no thymic lymphopoiesis is found. However, the medulla, especially around Hassall's corpuscles, is infiltrated by mature T-lymphocytes probably of donor origin. Individual epithelial cell necrosis and apoptosis of epithelial cells at the rim of Hassall's corpuscles may be seen in patients who develop a GVH reaction. These alterations are especially prominent 30 days after transplantation and usually correlate with generalized GVHD, which by 2 months after BMT causes pronounced atrophy of the thymus and a considerable destruction of thymic epithelial cells.

Signs of thymic restitution such as reappearance of lymphoid cells are seen in some specimens 3 to 4 months after BMT. Lymphoid cells appear immature and are intermixed with epithelial cells, forming cortical lymphoid nodules. Many patients dying of GVHD at that time, however, still show severe and extreme thymic atrophy. The complete restitution of thymic structures has been documented in a patient 4½ years after BMT who died in a car accident. MHC class II–positive cortical epithelial cells cannot be detected in the atrophic thymic remnants later than 1 week after transplantation. Although such conclusions could be based on inappropriately sampled tissue and negative selection of material, it is, however, obvious that lymphoid reconstitution requires intact cortical epithelium. Whether this epithelium can differentiate from still unknown precursor cells before or simultaneously with lymphoid cells remains to be shown. The speed of peripheral restitution of immune function and the repopulation of lymph nodes and spleen is also dependent on the age and functional stage of the thymus.[156]

HIV infection and AIDS

Autopsy studies of patients dying of AIDS invariably show a severely involuted thymus, consisting only of solid strands of epithelial cells devoid of lymphocytes and lacking Hassall's corpuscles.[157-159] This end-stage thymic atrophy is not different from chronic accidental involution from other causes.[160,161] Thymic biopsy specimens in children with AIDS show precocious involution and involution mimicking dysplasia. Thymitis with infiltration of the thymus by plasma cells and giant cells may also be present. In the final stages of AIDS very few epithelial cells contain the viral genome.

Experimental studies indicate that the thymus is an important target for HIV. Progressive thymus atrophy has been observed in rhesus monkeys infected with the simian immunodeficiency virus (SIV).[162,163] The atrophy of thymus precedes lymphocyte depletion in peripheral lymphoid tissues and the onset of clinical symptoms of AIDS.[162,163] Histologically there is a progressive apoptosis of cortical epithelial cells and dendritic cells at the corticomedullary junction.[163] Since the viral genome is present only in very few cells, the progressive loss of thymic function may be induced by an indirect mechanism.[163,164] A similar effect is shown also in another experimental model of human HIV infection, that is, the SCID-hu mouse, in which SCID mice are repopulated by human lymphohemopoietic cells. HIV infections in these animals cause a suppressed human thymopoiesis precluding the regeneration of the peripheral T-cell compartment.[165-167] Therefore the mechanism and role of the thymus in the pathogenesis of HIV-induced immune system dysfunction needs to be further evaluated.

INFECTIONS OF THE THYMUS

Viral infections

Involvement of the thymus in inflammatory and infectious diseases is extremely rare.[168-172] Nevertheless histologic signs of thymic infection may be found at autopsy, especially in generalized viral infection.

Cytomegalovirus inclusion bodies and giant cells may be found in generalized CMV infection after bone marrow transplantation. In lethal *varicella-zoster* infection the thymus may show features of accidental involution as well as a spongiolytic lesion leading to the formation of small vesicular spaces in the thymic epithelium. The viable cells may contain intranuclear herpesvirus inclusions, which can be detected by electron microscopy. In a case of *measles giant cell pneumonia* the thymus was severely atrophic, showing thickened PAS-positive basement membranes in the perivascular spaces and individual giant cells. In fetal *infectious mononucleosis* thymus may show pronounced lymphohistiocytic infiltration with loss of corticomedullary demarcation. In some cases multinucleated giant cells were found in the medullary areas. If there are no infiltrates of atypical lymphoid cells, the thymus is usually atrophic, showing signs of acute or chronic accidental involution. These pathologic changes are not accompanied by significant functional defects. If infection were to take place during the crucial phases of thymic development, as in intrauterine *rubella* infection, long-lasting defects of thymic function could follow.

Bacterial infections

Bacterial infections of the thymus are extremely rare. Thymus may be affected in bacterial mediastinitis. The older literature contained descriptions of so-called *Dubois's abscesses* in neonatal syphilis.[12] These lesions are, however, more typical of acute accidental involution, that is, apoptosis of thymocytes and infiltration of Hassall's corpuscles by lymphoid cells. However, in *neonatal syphilis* the thymus may become infected with spirochetes and show spongiolytic alterations, which can be demonstrated by special stains (Dieterle stain or Warthin-Starry stain).

AUTOIMMUNE DISEASES

Myasthenia gravis

Myasthenia gravis (MG) is an autoimmune disease characterized by autoantibodies against the acetylcholine receptor (AChR), which may impair the function of the neuromuscular junction causing progressive muscle weakness.[173,174] Since 75% to 85% of MG patients exhibit pathologic changes of the thymus[8] (Table 44-1), it is thought that thymic abnormalities are linked pathogenetically to MG.[175-178] Furthermore, each of the three main thymic alterations—thymitis, thymic epithelial tumors, and thymic atrophy—is associated with such distinct age, sex, and immunogenetic findings that different mechanisms of tolerance breakdown have been predicted.[179,180] Thymic pathology has become one of the main criteria for classifying myasthenic syndromes[181] (Table 44-2).

The most frequent thymic alteration—lymphofollicular thymitis—is assumed to be pathogenetically related to MG. The same changes have been encountered in several other autoimmune diseases. However, the etiologic or pathogenetic link between thymic disease and these autoimmune diseases has not yet been elucidated (Table 44-3). The association between thymoma and MG is also enigmatic but statistically significant. Other autoimmune diseases such as polymyositis, rheumatoid arthritis, systemic lupus erythematosus, Sjögren's disease, Hashimoto's thyroiditis, and ulcerative colitis or disturbances of immune functions such as mucocutaneous candidiasis[184-188] are occasionally associated with thymic epithelial tumors. However, these occur at such a low frequency that a more than fortuitous association is difficult to prove.

Lymphofollicular thymitis

Lymphofollicular thymitis is defined as an increased number of lymphoid follicles with germinal centers (GCs) within the thymus. Since this thymic alteration is often associated with a slight thymic hyperplasia, it has also been called *lymphoid follicular hyperplasia of the thymus.*[189] However, to stress the inflammatory nature of the process and to clearly distinguish it from *true thymic hyperplasia*[190] we prefer the generic term *thymitis,* which was originally suggested by Goldstein.[191]

Clinical findings. Lymphofollicular thymitis, though not specific for MG, is the most common thymic alteration in MG and is encountered in 50% to 70% of MG cases.[8,174,192] It is typically found in young females 40 years of age and is associated with the HLA A1, B8, DR3 haplotypes[179,193] (Table 44-2).

Pathology. Macroscopically the thymus is in most cases not different from the thymus in age-matched controls. Only occasionally the thymus is slightly enlarged and shows a gray, lymph node–like cut surface. Microscopically, lymphofollicular thymitis is characterized by the formation of intrathymic GCs, which are clearly evident in routinely stained slides (Fig. 44-7). GCs may be present only in parts of the thymus,[194] but usually GCs are numerous and evenly distributed.[195] GC formation in thymitis begins in the perivascular spaces that become extended, resulting in a club-shaped widening at the corticomedullary junction. In the normal thymus the perivascular spaces can easily be delineated by reticulin stains or immunohistochemically with antibodies to keratin. This continuous border between the perivascular spaces and the medulla is disrupted because of the enlargement of GCs in the course of lymphofollicular thymitis and an increased number of small vessels entering the medulla. The number of reticulin fibers appears increased both in the perivascular spaces and in the medulla, and so these two compartments become indistinguishable one from another. Finally, GCs extend into the medulla close to Hassall's corpuscles. However, the width and thymocyte content of the cortex remain unaltered.

Immunohistochemistry. The intrathymic GCs have the same immunohistochemical features as the GCs in lymph nodes or tonsils.[196,197] GCs contain $CD19^+$, $CD20^+$, and $CD22^+$ B-cells intermingled with some $CD4^+$ and a few $CD8^+$ mature T-cells in a network of $KiM4^+$ follicular dendritic cells. In addition, the thymus contains infiltrates of B-cells in the perivascular spaces and in the medulla, leaving

Table 44-1 Pathologic thymic alterations and their frequencies in patients with myasthenia gravis

Thymic disorder	Frequency %
Thymitis	
Lymphofollicular thymitis	50-60
Thymitis with diffuse B-cell infiltration	10
Thymic epithelial tumors	10-25
Normal thymus or mild thymic atrophy	10-20
Thymolipoma	<1
True thymic hyperplasia	<1

Table 44-2 Age and sex distribution and immunogenetic findings in the three most frequent thymic abnormalities encountered in myasthenia gravis patients

Thymic pathology	Typical age (years)	Sex ratio (M:F)	HLA haplotype
Thymitis	10-40	1:3	A1, B8, DR3
Thymoma	30-80	1:1	DR2
Normal thymus or mild thymic atrophy	40-80	2:1	B7, DR2

Data from DeBaets MH, Vincent A: Myasthenia gravis In Bona CA, Siminovitch KA, Zanetti M, Theofilopoulos AB, editors: *The molecular pathology of autoimmune diseases,* Chur, Switzerland, 1993, Harwood Academic Publishers.
Degli-Esposti MA, Andreas A, Christiansen FT et al: An approach to the localization of the susceptibility genes for generalized myasthenia gravis by mapping recombinant ancestral haplotypes, *Immunogenetics* 35:355, 1992.
Demaine A. Willcox N, Janer M et al: Immunglobulin heavy chain gene associations in myasthenia gravis: new evidence for disease heterogeneity, *J Neurol* 239:53, 1992.

Table 44-3 Autoimmune diseases for which a pathogenetic role of thymic pathology is assumed

Thymic disorder	Associated autoimmune disease
Cortical type of thymic epithelial tumor (TET)	Myasthenia gravis (frequent)
Mixed/composite thymoma	Myasthenia gravis (frequent)
Medullary thymoma	Myasthenia gravis (rare)
	Pure red blood cell aplasia
	Pancytopenia
	Neutropenia
	Hypogammaglobulinemia

Data from Souadijian JV, Enriques P, Silverstein MN, Pepin JM: The spectrum of diseases associated with thymoma. *Arch Intern Med* 134:374, 1974.
Mathieson PW, O'Neill JH, Durrant ST et al: Antibody-mediated pure neutrophil aplasia, recurrent myasthenia gravis and previous thymoma: case report and literature review, *QJ Med* 74:57, 1990.
Ackland SP, Bur ME, Adler SS, Bur ME, Adler SS et al: White blood cell aplasia associated with thymoma, *Am J Clin Pathol* 89:260, 1988.

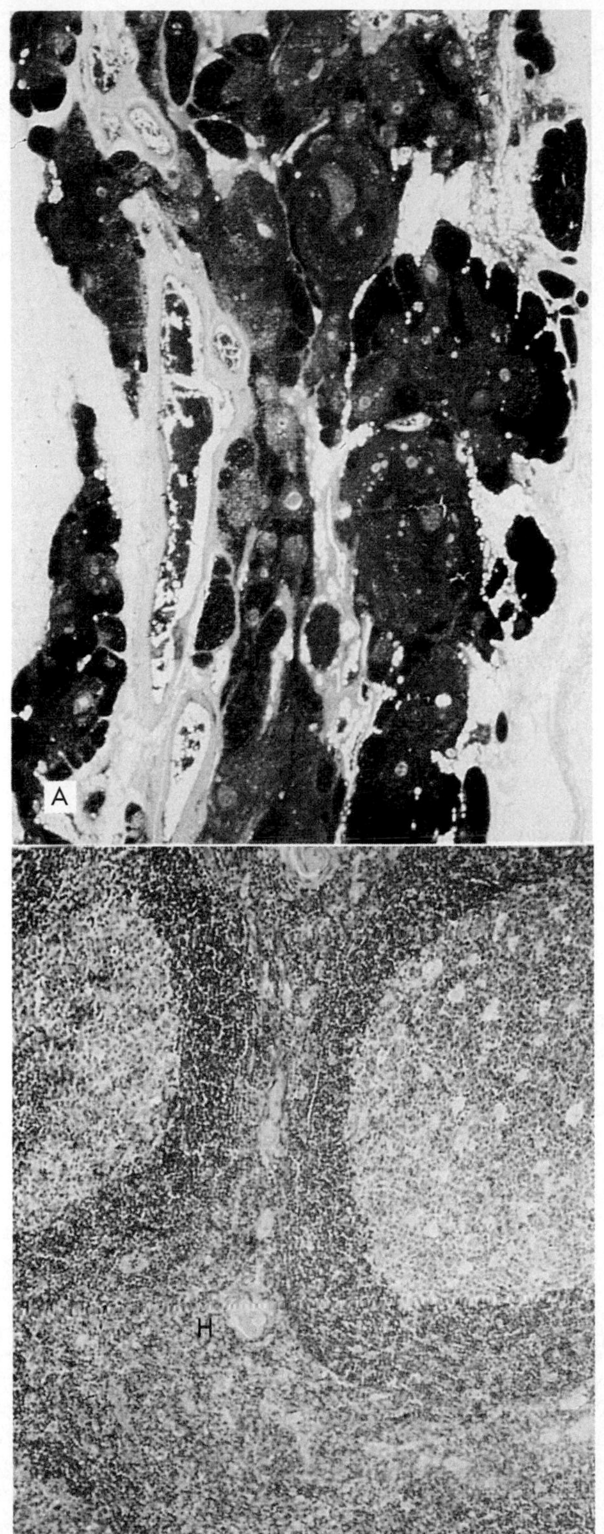

Fig. 44-7 Lymphofollicular thymitis in myastenia gravis. **A,** Low-power view of lymphofollicular thymitis with numerous lymphoid follicles in the perivascular spaces and medulla. **B,** Prominent lymphoid follicles with germinal center formation in perivascular spaces and the medulla close to a Hassall's corpuscle, *H*.

only the cortex free of B-cells.[195] The indistinct borders between the perivascular spaces and the medulla can be highlighted by antibodies to keratins and laminin that demonstrate a disruption of the normally continuous epithelial lining on the outer side of the perivascular spaces and the laminin-positive basal lamina of the vessels.[8,195,198] Medullary epithelium sometimes may surround lymphoid follicles completely, but keratin-positive cells are never found within GCs. As in the normal thymus the subcortical epithelium in thymitis exhibits CD56-positivity. In close association with GCs and diffuse B-cell infiltrates, mature $CD3^+$ T-cells with a predominance of the $CD4^+$ subset can be identified.[99] $CD11c^+$, $S\text{-}100^-$ interdigitating reticulum cells (IDCs) are found in increased numbers admixed with T-cells. In contrast to the normal thymus, these $CD11c^+$ IDCs become $CD1^+$ in lymphofollicular thymitis, an indication of a state of activation as in peripheral lymphoid organs.[199] In addition, $CD1^+$ and $S\text{-}100^+$ Langerhans' cells are centered around Hassall's corpuscles.[195] IDCs, Langerhans' cells, and the thymic epithelium of cortex and medulla are MHC class II (HLA-DR) positive as many lymphoid cells are. In contrast, thymic myoid cells are MHC class II negative. As in the normal thymus, myoid cells in lymphofollicular thymitis are confined to the medulla where they occur just outside GCs but never within them.[200,201] Myoid cells, which become less frequent with age and are barely detectable after 50 years of age tend to be less numerous in lymphofollicular thymitis than in age-matched control thymuses. These cells can be demonstrated by antibodies against desmin,[201] the AChR[200,202,203] or titin.[204] In lymphofollicular thymitis myoid cells exhibit an abnormally close association with MHC class II^+, $CD11c^+$ dendritic cells as can be shown by double labeling.[201] Finally, multinucleated $CD11c^+$ and $CD68^+$ histiocytic giant cells occur in the medulla in lymphofollicular thymitis in one half of the cases.[195] Such cells are not seen in normal thymuses or MG-associated thymic atrophy.

Lymphofollicular thymitis and the pathogenesis of myasthenia gravis. Thymectomy is of doubtful benefit to MG patients who have a normal thymus, thymic atrophy, thymoma, or seronegative MG.[174,205] In seropositive MG patients with lymphofollicular thymitis thymectomy has a beneficial effect both clinically and serologically.[174,206-209] These clinical data have suggested a pathogenetic role for the thymus.[210] This hypothesis has been supported by the identification of the autoantigen, that is, AChR on thymic myoid cells,[175,200,211-213] by the detection of AChR-specific T-cells[214,215] that are enriched in MG thymuses,[216,217] and by the finding that the thymus itself showing lymphofollicular thymitis is the main source of autoantibodies.[218,219] Considering the abnormal association between activated interdigitating reticulum cells and myoid cells in lymphofollicular thymitis,[202] the detection of the fetal type of AChR exclusively on thymic myoid cells but not on innervated skeletal muscle,[213,220] and the preferential reactivity of anti-AChR autoantibodies with fetal-type AChR,[221] it has been concluded that AChR peptides and AChR may be presented by IDCs and follicular dendritic cells to T-cells and B-cells respectively and that activated AChR-specific T-cells may provide help to anti-AChR autoantibody-producing B-cells.[175,201,213] However, these findings do not resolve the enigma, whether the autoimmune process starts inside the thymus because of immunoregulatory disturbances[175,212,222] or the thymus is involved secondarily by a systemic immune process.[174,217,223-225] However, since AChR-specific T-cells are constituents of the T-cell repertoire of healthy persons,[226,227] disturbances of immune tolerance probably play a major role in the pathogenesis of MG.[227] Thymic GC formation also has been described in Graves' disease, Hashimoto's thyroiditis, Addison's disease, autoimmune hemolytic anemia, systemic lupus erythematosus, progressive systemic sclerosis, ulcerative colitis, Behçet's disease, rheumatoid arthritis,[212] and Wegener's granulomatosis.[201] Lymphofollicular thymitis in these diseases is morphologically similar to the MG-associated thymitis.

Differential diagnosis. GC formation may be found in nonmyasthenic and apparently *healthy individuals* at a frequency ranging from 1% to 50%.[228-230] GCs were present in 13% of our patients who underwent heart surgery.[213] In contrast to MG-associated lymphofollicular thymitis, GCs in nonmyasthenic healthy persons are not preferentially located in the vicinity of myoid cells and contacts between IDCs and myoid cells are quite rare.[201] Finally, the number of GCs is usually much lower than that in MG.

Thymuses in the vicinity of MG-associated thymomas exhibit GC formation in up to 60% of cases, that is, up to 10 times more frequently than thymuses from nonmyasthenic controls.[9,231,232] Furthermore, lymphofollicular thymitis is usually more pronounced in peritumorous thymic remnants than in normal thymuses, a finding indicating that the immune process in these cases is similar to thymitis in nonparaneoplastic MG.[9] In support of this idea, B-cells producing anti-AChR autoantibodies could be isolated from peritumorous thymic tissue.[233,234]

True thymic hyperplasia is distinguished from lymphofollicular thymitis by a lack of GCs, a normal number of medullary B-cells, and a considerable increase of weight of the thymus as compared to age-matched controls.

Thymitis with diffuse B-cell infiltration

Thymitis with diffuse B-cell infiltration of the medulla is encountered in about 10% of MG patients. The majority of these patients are between 10 and 20 years of age, that is, on average 10 years younger than MG patients with lymphofollicular thymitis.[195] Compared with age-matched controls this condition is characterized by an increased number of B-cells in the thymic medulla and perivascular spaces but a lack of GCs in routine stains. By immunohistochemistry, a few small aggregates of KiM4$^+$ follicular dendritic cells may be detectable.[195] Since B-cells are normal constituents of the thymic medulla and become more numerous with age,[195,235,236] such an increased number of B-cells is not easily documented without appropriate studies.

This condition shares with lymphofollicular thymitis certain features that may be useful in diagnosis: the distention of perivascular spaces, the interruption of the epithelial lining and reticulin fibers at the border between perivascular spaces and the medulla, the increase of medullary reticulin fibers and of KiM1$^+$ (CD11c$^+$) IDCs, and an increased number of contacts between myoid cells and IDCs. As in lymphofollicular thymitis the cortex is unaltered in thymitis with diffuse B cell infiltration. This form of thymitis is typically observed after long-term corticosteroid and azathioprin treatment,[237] and therefore it is assumed that it can either be a precursor or a residual form of lymphofollicular thymitis.[201,237] MG patients with this type of thymitis profit most by thymectomy,[231] which is usually accompanied by disappearances of autoimmune phenomena.

Thymic atrophy

Thymic atrophy is the third most common thymic finding in MG patients. However, such atrophy is generally mild and evident only on histologic examination. The weight of the thymus may not be different from that in age-matched controls. Except for a slight widening of the perivascular spaces, no abnormalities may be encountered by routine light microscopy. By immunohistochemistry a slightly increased number of B-cells in the perivascular spaces and medulla and a higher number of KiM1$^+$ IDCs may be present in some cases.[195] GCs and myoid cells are generally absent. The pathogenetic link between thymic atrophy and MG is unclear.

Thymolipoma and thymic hyperplasia

Thymolipoma is a rare thymic abnormality in MG patients[238-240] as is *true thymic hyperplasia* (personal observation). Both are described in detail below.

TUMOR-LIKE LESIONS OF THE THYMUS

Thymic cysts

Microscopic thymic cysts measuring up to 3 mm in diameter are a frequent finding in atrophic thymuses, in thymic epithelial tumors,[50] and in thymuses of patients exposed to chemotherapy or long-term immunosuppression.[8]

Clinically relevant thymic cysts may either be congenital or acquired.[241] Such cysts measure up to 18 cm in diameter and are usually found unrelated to MG. Most patients are 20 to 50 years of age and have symptoms pertaining to the local mass lesion and its obstructive complications.[242]

Acquired thymic cysts result from reactive proliferation of thymic epithelium and are not considered benign cystic tumors. Cyst development after surgery, irradiation, or chemotherapy or as a complication of Hodgkin's disease has been observed.[243-246] Cysts may be located either within the body of the thymus or are connected to it by a thin stalk.

Pathology. *Congenital* thymic cysts are usually unilocular and thin walled, are filled with serous fluid, and lack concomitant fibrous adhesions. The *acquired* thymic cysts are usually multilocular and thick walled, are filled with hemorrhagic fluid or semisolid necrotic material, and are sometimes calcified and adherent to other mediastinal structures by a pericystic fibrosis.[241,247] Microscopically, congenital cysts are lined by a few layers of nonkeratinized squamous epithelium and have an acellular delicate fibrous wall. By contrast, multilocular (acquired) cysts have a squamous, cuboidal, columnar, or mixed epithelial lining that may be unilayered or multilayered and may exhibit papillary projections. Remnants of Hassall's corpuscles or thymic tissue in the cyst walls are not a regular finding, whereas chronic inflammatory infiltrates and hemosiderin deposits are consistently present. Rarely pseudoepithelial hyperplasia of the epithelial lining with rare mitoses may occur, with epithelial strands extending into the fibrous cyst wall.[247,248] The absence of numerous and atypical mitoses and the lack of atypia distinguish these cysts from well-differentiated squamous carcinoma of the thymus. True malignant transformation of a thymic cyst is an extremely rare event.[249]

Differential Diagnosis. Thymic cysts must be distinguished from other cystic processes such as intrathymic parathyroid cysts or cystic germ cell tumors. Parathyroid cysts contain parathyroid cells in their wall.[250] Cystic germ cell tumors may contain malignant cells or components of teratomas.[242,243] Extrathymic cysts of the mediastinum such as pericardial cysts or bronchogenic cysts should also be considered in the differential diagnosis.[251]

True thymic hyperplasia

In true thymic hyperplasia the thymus is enlarged beyond the upper normal limit of age-matched controls[252] but has retained its normal histologic features. The *idiopathic form* has mainly been reported in otherwise healthy children.[190,253] We have observed two adult cases, one a 28-year-old myasthenic male, the other a 56-year-old healthy female. Since there was no significant alteration of thymic histology in the former case, it is unclear whether this kind of thymic disorder is causally related to MG.

In the *rebound type* of true thymic hyperplasia an enlargement of the thymus is observed in the recovery phase after irradiation or chemotherapy for Hodgkin's disease or non-Hodgkin's lymphoma.[254-256] Obviously, it may be very difficult to distinguish this benign condition from relapse of the respective neoplasm, and biopsy may be necessary in some cases.

Thymolipoma

Thymolipomas are tumors composed of mature adipose tissue and tubular remnants of epithelial tissue. The epithelial strands may contain Hassall's corpuscles but usually no germinal centers. They are often extremely large tumors that have an ill-defined lobulated appearance and a thin fibrous capsule.[239] Some tumors are associated with autoimmune diseases such as Graves' disease, aplastic anemia, and surprisingly also MG.[239] Thymolipomas exhibit no sex predilection, and although they occur at all ages, most are diagnosed in adolescence and young adults. Malignant change has been documented very rarely so far.[239a]

THYMIC EPITHELIAL TUMORS

The term *thymoma,* "as a tumor, benign or malignant, derived from the thymic epithelium," was introduced by Bell in 1917.[257] Several classifications were proposed since then[258-260] until Rosai and Levine divided thymus tumors into different categories on the basis of invasiveness and metastatic potential.[9] Completely encapsulated tumors and spindle cell tumors with no cytologic atypia have been considered to be probably benign, whereas invasive tumors were divided into two categories of malignancy: category I tumors with no or minimal cytologic atypia were usually only locally invasive and rarely showed lymphatic or hematogenous spread. Category II thymomas were cytologically malignant and also were called "thymic carcinomas." Within the latter category different histologic types of thymic carcinomas have been established, most of which showed a highly aggressive behavior and a bad prognosis.[261-263] Grade I squamous cell carcinoma and mucoepidermoid carcinoma may show a better prognosis.[245,261] The unequivocal value of invasivity as a major clinical and pathologic criterion of outcome[264,265] was also appreciated in the most widely accepted staging system for thymic tumors according to Masaoka and associates.[266] However, definite histologic and cytologic criteria relevant to prediction of the invasiveness or metastatic behavior especially in category I tumors of the thymus were not established.[9]

We consider cortical epithelial differentiation as an indicator of invasiveness[242,267-270] and use this criterion for classifying thymic epithelial tumors.

In this chapter the epithelial tumors of the thymus are histologically classified into several types based on the histologic relationships between distinct tumor entities and their normal thymic counterparts: medullary thymoma, mixed (composite) thymoma, predominantly cortical thymoma (organoid thymoma), cortical thymoma, and well-differentiated thymic carcinoma. In addition to these "organotypic" tumors,[270] the thymus may give rise to adenocarcinomas, squamous carcinomas, and neuroendocrine carcinomas, which are indistinguishable from extrathymic tumors of the same name. Using the criteria provided below, one can assign most if not all thymic epithelial tumors to distinct tumor entities and can include them in the preexisting classes of benign or category I and category II malignant thymoma (Table 44-4).

Benign thymoma

Medullary thymoma

Medullary thymomas are composed of spindle-shaped epithelial cells and contain only a low-to-moderate number of mainly mature lymphocytes (Fig. 44-8). The epithelial cells have uniform nuclei with small nucleoli and a rather dense chromatin pattern. Often these flat or cylindroid cells are arranged in a storiform pattern or form rosette-like or glandular structures. In slides treated with PAS or reticulin stains a distinct fibrillar extracellular material is noted. In glandular areas condensed PAS-positive secretory material may be found. In the center of these tumors only a small amount of fibrous tissue is found even though they have a thick capsule. At the inner margin of this capsule sheets of epithelial cells may show a pseudoinvasive pattern. Only in a minority of cases an extension of lobular or fingerlike projections of epithelial cells into the capsule will reach the mediastinal fat. In a given case of medullary thymoma different growth patterns may be present, including a storiform, hemangiopericytoma-like, rosette-forming, and glandular pat-

Table 44-4 Clinicopathologic and histologic classification of thymic epithelial tumors

Clinicopathologic category	Histologic type
Benign thymoma	Medullary thymoma Mixed/composite thymoma
Malignant thymoma (category I)	Predominantly cortical thymoma Cortical thymoma Well-differentiated thymic carcinoma (WDTC)
Malignant thymoma (category II)	*Low grade:* Squamous cell carcinoma (I to III) Basaloid carcinoma Mucoepidermoid carcinoma *High grade:* Lymphoepithelioma-like carcinoma Clear cell carcinoma Sarcomatoid carcinoma Small cell/neuroendocrine carcinoma Anaplastic carcinoma

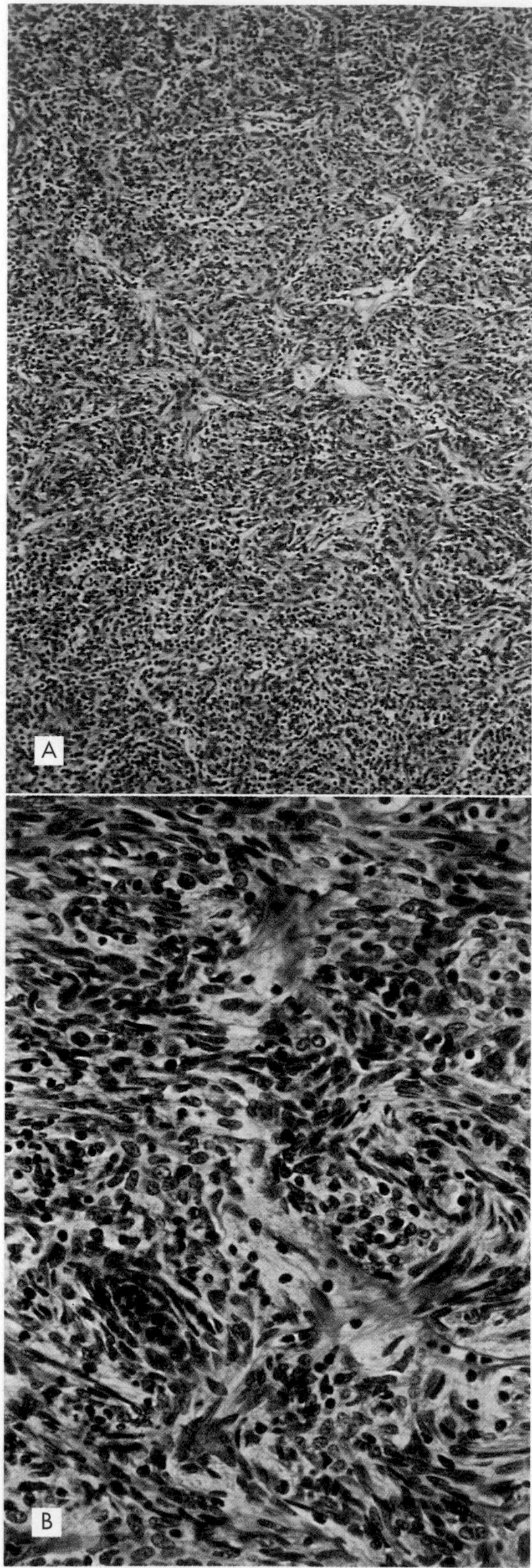

Fig. 44-8 Medullary thymoma. Spindle cell area in a medullary thymoma. Lymphoid cells among spindle-shaped neoplastic epithelial cells are mainly mature T-cells, but some immature, $CD1^+$ thymocytes are usually present.

tern. The different growth patterns have no prognostic significance.

The lymphoid component consists of small mature T-cells. The CD4:CD8 ratio is about 2 to 1, that is, similar to the ratio of helper to suppressor T-lymphocytes in the normal thymic medulla. Some focal clusters of asteroid or small B-lymphocytes expressing CD20 may be present. In addition, also epithelial cells may express the CD20 antigen.[271,272] IDCs are also demonstrable immunohistochemically in rather high numbers with antibodies to S-100, CD11c, and CD1. Hassall's corpuscles or foci of squamous differentiation are not seen. The proliferative activity of epithelial cells is very low, and mitoses are almost never found.

Mixed (composite) thymoma

Mixed thymoma is composed of epithelium-rich, spindle-cell areas and lymphocyte-rich areas. On gross examination mixed thymoma is very similar to medullary thymoma, but it may be surrounded by a fibrous capsule. The inner capsular lining is usually also indistinct because of local extensions of epithelial sheets into the capsule. Histologically, mixed thymomas are composed of two distinct components: spindle-shaped epithelial cells identical to those in medullary thymoma, and lymphocyte-rich lobules containing large stellate epithelial cells, some of which may show open nuclei and distinct nucleoli as in cortical thymoma (Fig. 44-9, *A*). These areas may be highlighted by reticulin stain (Fig. 44-9, *B*). The amount of each of these components may vary significantly.[232] Furthermore, the two components may be found in separate lobules of the tumor, or there may be a predominance of lymphocyte-rich areas with only small nests of oval or spindle-shaped medullary cells, or the two components may be intermixed one with another. As in medullary thymoma microcystic or glandular areas may be present. Mixed (composite) thymoma may exhibit cystic or dilated perivascular space that can be packed with lymphocytes. As in medullary thymoma no Hassall's corpuscles or epidermoid foci are found.

The ultrastructural features of epithelial cells in the medullary type and lymphocyte-rich areas of mixed thymoma show similarities to the features of normal thymic epithelial cells of the inner cortex and medulla surrounding the perivascular spaces at the corticomedullary junction.

Malignant thymoma (category I)

Predominantly cortical (organoid) thymoma

The predominantly cortical thymoma recapitulates histologically the full range of differentiation of the thymic cortex including medullary islands. Therefore this type of thymoma has been called "thymus-like"[9] or "organoid."[232] The tumors are composed of well-formed lobules that are separated by delicate thin fibrous septa. There is a predominance of the lymphocyte-rich inner cortical type of differentiation with epithelial cells with round to oval nuclei and small nucleoli. The cellular extensions are usually hidden by densely packed lymphoid cells of small to medium size. The epithelial cells are less numerous and less prominent and usually smaller than those of cortical thymoma.

In medullary islands the lymphoid cells are less densely packed. These areas thus appear lighter, yet they contain Hassall's corpuscles. Although medullary islands appear roughly similar to the normal thymic medulla, a more detailed analysis shows distinct differences. Ultrastructurally[273] the epithelial cells of medullary islands differ from the typical medullary

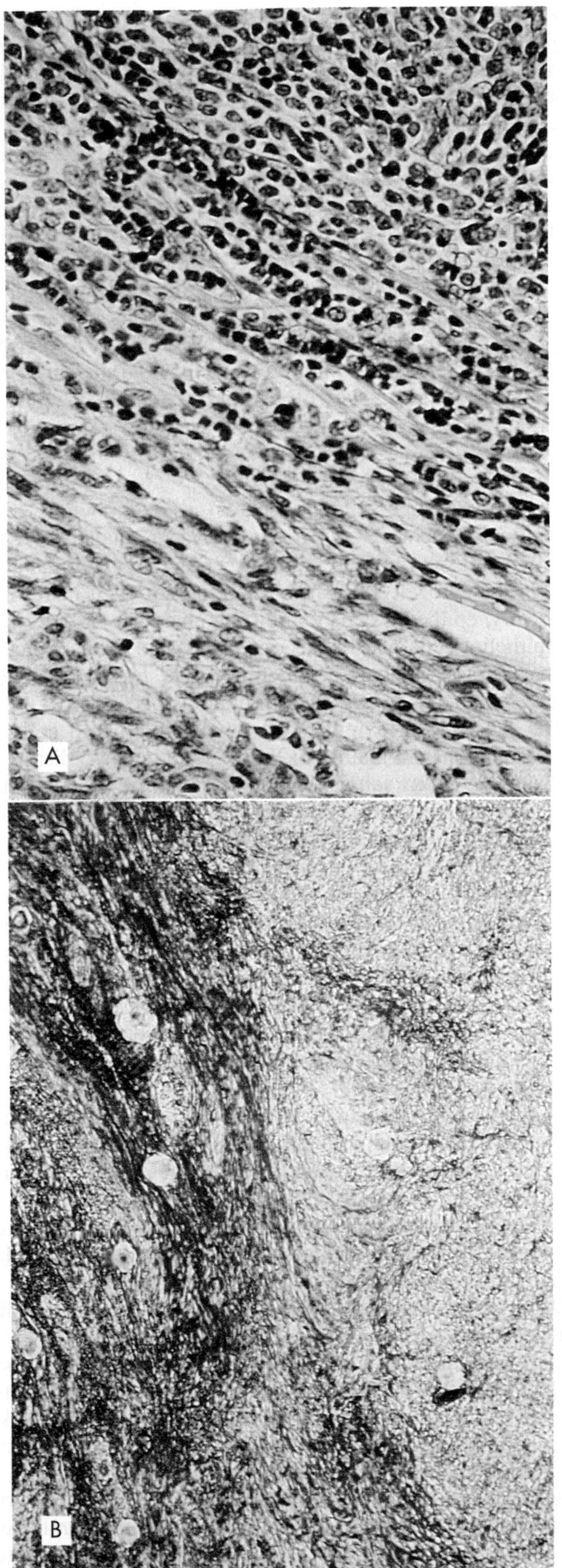

Fig. 44-9 Mixed (composite) thymoma. **A,** Sharp juxtaposition of spindle cell areas and lymphocyte-rich areas are the histologic hallmark of mixed thymoma. **B,** Silver impregnation highlights spindle cell areas and lymphocyte-rich tumor regions.

spindle-shaped epithelial cell, since they lack the high intermediate filament content in cytoplasmic extensions and are not associated with basement membrane as in the normal medulla. Tumor cells actually have features of smaller and more elongated cortical epithelial cells, which are found at the corticomedullary junctions in the normal thymus. In addition, thymic myoid cells are never found in thymoma in contrast to the normal thymic medulla. On the other hand, interdigitating cells and scattered solitary mature $CD4^+$ and $CD8^+$ T-cells, which are normally found in the thymic medulla, are also present in the tumors. Perivascular spaces are usually present and may be dilated and cystic or packed with lymphoid cells.

Predominantly cortical thymomas are usually large tumors (average diameter 10 cm). A continuous fibrous capsule is usually not present, and the tumors invade adjacent structures.

Cortical thymoma

Cortical thymomas are composed of large sheets of epithelial cells. These cells have round to oval nuclei, vesicular chromatin, and prominent central nucleoli (Fig. 44-10, *A*). These features are similar to those of epithelial cells in the outer cortex of the normal thymus. However, the cells are much larger, and the cytoplasmic rim is broader. The cytoplasm of these epithelial cells is usually faintly eosinophilic or clear and sometimes vacuolated. Within the cytoplasm of these cells often single or multiple and sometimes densely packed immature lymphoid cells are found. Similar lymphoid cells are also seen between the epithelial cell processes. The number of lymphocytes is approximately equal to the number of neoplastic thymic epithelial cells (Fig. 44-10, *B*) but always less than in predominantly cortical thymoma. Epithelial cells and lymphoid cells may be clearly distinguished. Areas of medullary differentiation (medullary islands) may be present but are much less distinct and less frequent than in predominantly cortical thymoma. If present, they are distributed irregularly throughout the tumor tissue. Epithelial cell clusters simulating Hassall's corpuscles may be seen in the periphery of the tumor, sometimes beneath the fibrous capsule at the junction with normal thymic tissue or within areas of medullary differentiation. Perivascular spaces are often narrow and filled with lymphoid cells. Around perivascular spaces epithelial cells show palisading along a thin basement membrane separating the epithelial space from the perivascular space. The formation of small cystic spaces may be lined by EMA-positive cylindroid cells, whereas cortical epithelial cells are EMA negative.

Lymphoid follicles with typical GCs are not uncommon, especially in cases associated with MG. Starry-sky macrophages are rather frequent but sometimes difficult to distinguish from epithelial cells with clear cytoplasm without histochemistry. Focal accumulations of foam cells may occur. Cortical thymoma have a lobular architecture with conspicuous fibrous septa. Invasion of adjacent structures is typical.

Corticosteroids, irradiation, or cytostatic treatment before surgery may cause microcystic degeneration of thymoma. Numerous apoptotic cells are then seen with their fragments included within cytoplasmic vacuoles. Such cases may be difficult to distinguish from well-differentiated thymic carcinoma.

On the ultrastructural level, epithelial cells in cortical thymomas resemble those in the outer thymic cortex. Some tumor cells also show differentiation toward thymic nurse cells.

Lymphoepithelioma-like carcinoma

Lymphoepithelioma-like carcinoma is a high-grade carcinoma of the thymus and the second most frequent of this subgroup. Morphologically this tumor is identical to lymphoepithelial carcinoma of the nasopharynx. A network of large, spindle-shaped, and keratin-positive tumor cells with large and sharply delineated nuclei and prominent, large, and round acidophilic nucleoli are typical. Reactive dense lymphoid infiltrates are made up of mature T-cells that are either $CD4^+$ or $CD8^+$. Double-positive $CD4^+/CD8^+$ immature thymocytes are not present among the tumor cells.[276] Keratinization and intercellular bridges are not encountered. Lymphoepithelioma-like carcinomas contain Epstein-Barr virus, which is detectable by in situ hybridization or immunohistochemistry.[277-280]

Clear cell carcinoma

Clear cell carcinoma, a rare high-grade tumor of the thymus, is characterized by large polygonal tumor cells with a clear, glycogen-rich cytoplasm and a moderate nuclear atypia. These histologic features are reminiscent of renal cell carcinoma.[262,281,282]

Sarcomatoid carcinoma and carcinosarcoma

Sarcomatoid carcinoma is a high-grade tumor composed of spindle-shaped and anaplastic tumor cells. Foci of epithelial cells with a solid growth pattern may give a hint to the diagnosis.[262] True carcinosarcomas contain epithelial cells and cells showing cartilaginous and rhabdomyomatous differentiation.[283] The epithelial nature of these tumors is best recognized by immunohistochemistry with antibodies to keratin. The differential diagnosis should include spindle cell–rich medullary thymomas, which, however, lack solid epithelial foci, show no mitoses, and are cytologically bland. Teratomas of the thymus and malignant schwannomas with a striated muscle cell component (triton tumor) enter also the differential diagnosis, especially in small biopsy samples, but are easily excluded by their typical features recognized upon examination of the entire tumor.

Thymic carcinoid and small cell carcinoma

Thymic carcinoids are tumors of neuroendocrine cells that are invasive and have a tendency for distant metastasis.[284] These tumors may be associated with the multiple endocrine neoplasia (MEN) syndrome type 1 or 2a.[285-287] Approximately 30% of cases are associated with paraneoplastic endocrine symptoms, most often in the form of Cushing's syndrome.[284,286,288] Hormonally active tumors have a worse prognosis than tumors without endocrine function.

Histologically, thymic carcinoids are composed of small cells with round or oval nuclei. The cytoplasm is scant or well developed, and granular cells grow in ribbons or form islands. Rosettes may be seen.[289] Focal necrosis and calcification are sometimes encountered. Tumor cells invade blood and lymphatic vessels and grow into adjacent organs. Some carcinoids may contain melanin.[290] Generic endocrine markers like neuron-specific enolase, chromogranin, and synaptophysin are detectable immunohistochemically in almost all cases. Specific secretory products like ACTH, metenkephalin, somatostatin, cholecystokinin, calcitonin, and serotonin are found less frequently.[285,288,291]

Small cell carcinomas (oat cell carcinomas) are indistinguishable from similar carcinomas of the lung.[292] Therefore the diagnosis of a thymic small cell carcinoma requires the clinical exclusion of an extrathymic primary.

Anaplastic carcinoma

Anaplastic carcinoma is a high-grade tumor with pronounced cellular and nuclear atypia and usually neoplastic giant cells. The tumors in this group exhibit no recognizable differentiation and thus cannot be classified otherwise.

Clinicopathologic correlations

Prognosis and histologic type. Subtyping of thymic epithelial tumors according to their lymphocyte content into predominantly lymphocytic, mixed, and predominantly epithelial thymomas has no prognostic significance.[293,294] In contrast, histologic subtyping according to the histologic classification given in Table 44-5 was shown to be an independent prognostic factor despite its high correlation with stage.[232] In this study WDTC recurred more often and earlier than predominantly cortical and cortical thymoma.[232] Five of 7 relapses and 6 of 7 deaths from thymic epithelial tumors were in patients with WDTC. The actuarial survival rate of patients with WDTC was 80% at 5 years and 54% at 10 years, whereas survival of patients with medullary, mixed, predominantly cortical, and cortical thymoma was 100% after 5 and 10 years. In our own cases there was no death in medullary and mixed thymomas, and the one relapse in a mixed thymoma 9 years after surgery was probably attributable to incomplete resection with subcutaneous implantation of tumor cells by a drainage tube during the operation.[270] Thus, mixed thymoma may behave similar to pleomorphic adenoma of salivary glands, which may recur after incision of the tumor capsule and local implantation of tumor cells.

The 5-year survival for category II thymomas, when all tumor types were considered and some WDTC were included was 33%.[245] Subdivision into low-grade carcinomas (squamous cell carcinoma, basaloid carcinoma, mucoepidermoid carcinoma) and high-grade tumors demonstrated no deaths in the former and a death rate of 84.6% for the latter subgroup,[245] which is in accordance with previous results.[261,292,295,296] The median survival for lymphoepithelioma-like thymic carcinoma, small cell, and clear cell carcinoma was reported to be 15 to 19.5 months.[245,295]

Paraneoplastic syndromes in thymic epithelial tumors. Thymic epithelial tumors are often associated with paraneoplastic syndromes and especially with immunologic disorders. Myasthenia gravis is most often observed, usually with cortical thymoma and WDTC. Myasthenia gravis is uncommonly associated with mixed and medullary thymoma. Category II malignant thymomas are not associated with autoimmunity. In our series 82% of cases with paraneoplastic MG were associated with predominantly cortical thymoma, cortical thymoma, or WDTC, whereas only 18% of the cases were related to mixed or medullary thymomas.[270] In another series 85% of all cases with paraneoplastic MG were detected in patients with predominantly cortical thymoma, cortical thymoma, and WDTC, but only 15% were found in patients with mixed or medullary thymomas.[232] Follicular lymphoid hyperplasia, either within the tumor, in the residual tumor-free thymus, or both, is significantly associated with MG.[232,269] Recent findings indicate that an abnormal expression of a 153 kD protein, which shares a very immunogenic epitope with the alpha-subunit of the muscle AChR and is mainly expressed in cortical thymomas and WDTC, is significantly associated with the occurrence of MG.[202,203,297,298] It is possible that this protein can cause paraneoplastic MG by a false-positive selection of intratumorous AChR-specific T-cells, which are activated and thus initiate the disease in extrathymic lymphoid tissues.[176,178,298,299,300] Still undefined pathogenetic mechanisms are probably relevant for the development of pure red cell anemia and hypogammaglobulinemia, which are mostly found in mixed and medullary thymomas.

LYMPHOMAS OF THE THYMUS

Malignant lymphomas are the most frequent malignant tumors of the upper anterior mediastinum. They can involve the thymus or the lymph nodes. Lymphomas originating in the thymus are classified as (1) lymphoblastic lymphoma of T-cell type, (2) primary mediastinal B-cell lymphoma of high-grade malignancy, (3) low grade malignant B-cell lymphoma of MALT type, and (4) Hodgkin's disease. The most common of these is Hodgkin's disease. Other thymic lymphomas are relatively rare.

Lymphoblastic lymphoma of T-cell type

Lymphoblastic lymphoma of T-cell origin makes up to 20% of lymphoblastic lymphoma. It is found predominantly in older children, most of whom are male. Lymphoblastic lymphoma often evolves into acute lymphoblastic leukemia (ALL). ALL infiltrating the thymus is indistinguishable by light microscopy or ultrastructurally from primary lymphoblastic lymphoma.

Histopathology. The thymus is densely infiltrated with medium-sized lymphoid cells. Infiltrates are first found in the cortex and comprise medium-sized cells, which are larger than lymphocytes in small lymphocytic lymphoma or mature lymphocytes in the thymic medulla. Tumor cells exhibit a lose chromatin pattern and irregular, sometimes lobulated nuclear contours, called the "convoluted type"[301] (Fig. 44-12). Ki-67 immunostaining shows that 80% to 90% of neoplastic lymphoid cells are in the S-phase of the mitotic cycle. Reactive macrophages may be present, accounting for the starry-sky pattern. Subsequently, lymphoma cells infiltrate the thymic medulla around Hassall's corpuscles, the thymic capsule, perivascular spaces, and the surrounding mediastinal fat. The lobular structure of thymic tissue may thus disappear. Usually the infiltrated connective tissue shows moderate-to-significant sclerosis.

Cytologic smears reveal medium-sized blast cells with irregular to round nuclei and a small clear cytoplasmic rim. Nucleoli are not prominent. A very typical feature is the focal acid phosphatase activity, and no evidence of nonspecific esterase.

Immunophenotypic characteristics. Mediastinal lymphoblastic lymphoma is composed of precursor T-cells, which have a phenotype similar to fetal thymocytes of the 12th to 16th gestational weeks. The neoplastic cells express $CD1^+$, TdT^+ and both $CD4^+$ and $CD8^+$, together with a rearranged T-cell receptor and common T-cell antigens, such as CD2, CD3, and CD5.

Differential diagnosis. The most important differential diagnosis is cortical thymoma, since the rare cases of thymoma found in childhood are of cortical thymoma type. At the light microscopic level it is important to look at the infiltrating

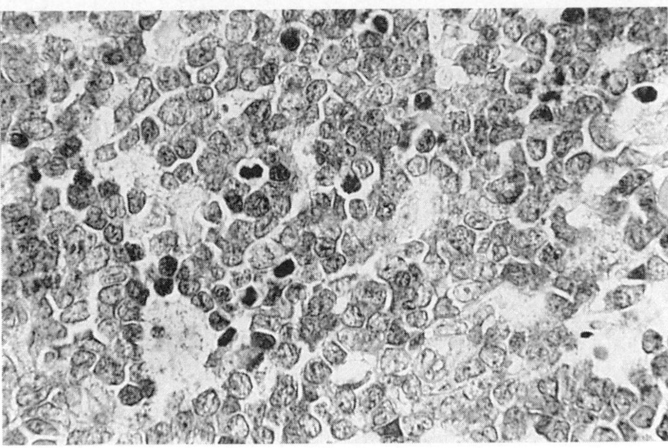

Fig. 44-12 Lymphoblastic lymphoma of the thymus. Characteristic cytologic appearance of T-lymphoblasts of a lymphoblastic lymphoma. Tumor cells with characteristic convoluted nuclei, a finely dispersed chromatin, and inconspicuous nucleoli.

edge, which in cortical thymoma, and even in invasive parts, show the primary epithelial character of thymoma proliferation, whereas lymphoblastic lymphoma shows invasion of perivascular spaces and mediastinal fat. In lymphoblastic lymphoma, thymic cortical epithelium is largely destroyed. Usually keratin stains are negative and reveal only the remnants of Hassall's corpuscles. In contrast the network of epithelial cells is clearly evident in cortical thymoma.

Very difficult diagnostic problems are thymectomy specimens obtained after chemotherapy. Such thymectomy is usually performed if there is a residual tumor after completed chemotherapy. In many of these cases a central necrotic tumor mass without viable cells is found surrounded by broad fibrosclerotic tissue if there is rebound hyperplasia. In these cases it is sometimes impossible to rule out minimally residual disease or early recurring tumor infiltration by histologic means. The almost synchronized repopulation of the thymic remnant by precursor cells and the fibrotic and sclerotic change of surrounding tissue caused by earlier tumor infiltration make the diagnostic decision very complex. It is important to note whether immature thymocytes are confined to the epithelial space, whether epithelial cells of cortical type are present, and whether perivascular spaces are infiltrated by lymphoblasts. Some help can be gained if one compares the exact phenotype with that of previous lymphoblastic lymphoma and by molecular biologic analysis of T-cell receptor rearrangement.

Primary mediastinal B-cell lymphoma of high-grade malignancy

The diffuse large cell lymphoma called *primary mediastinal B-cell lymphoma of high-grade malignancy* has some unique clinicopathologic features that are suggestive that it is a distinct entity. Most patients are 20- to 40-year-old women, who, as a group, are distinct from other patients with large cell lymphoma. The hypothesis of a thymic origin for this lymphoma was formulated by Addis and Isaacson[302] and confirmed by later studies.[303,304] Primary mediastinal B-cell lymphoma accounts for about 1% of all non-Hodgkin's lymphomas and 2% to 4% of large cell lymphomas. At clinical presention the tumors are usually large and locally invasive. An interesting feature of this lymphoma is its early infiltration of large mediastinal veins and its tendency to metastasis by a hematogenous route, leading to secondary tumors in many organs. The lymph nodes and bone marrow are usually spared.

Histopathology. The tumor is composed of medium to large lymphoid cells that infiltrate the thymus diffusely. The infiltrating edge of the tumor may not contain thymic tissue but may show a lymphoid tumor arranged in cohesive sheets with interstitial fibrosclerosis resulting in a pseudoalveolar pattern. Necrosis is present occasionally, and mitoses are frequent. Residual thymic tissue in the form of cysts lined by cuboidal or respiratory epithelium may be found (Fig. 44-13, *A*). Lymphoepithelial lesions may be found in such areas. In other instances the epithelial reticulum may be covered by infiltrating lymphoma cells and can be recognized only by immunohistochemistry (Fig. 44-13, *B*). The demonstration of an epithelial meshwork should not lead to the erroneous diagnosis of thymoma, since lymphoid cells are of B-cell phenotype and also infiltrate the surrounding mediastinal tissue.

Cytologically tumor cells are medium to large showing some pleomorphism (Fig. 44-13, *C*). The cytoplasm is often clear, in other cases slightly basophilic. Nucleoli are inconspicuous and, if present, small and sometimes localized to the nuclear membrane, giving a resemblance to centroblasts. The typical alveolar sclerosis of primary tumors in the mediastinum usually is absent in the metastases.

Immunophenotyping. In paraffin-sections the B-cell phenotype can be demonstrated by anti-CD20 (L26). On frozen sections $CD19^+$, $CD20^+$, $CD22^+$, and $CD37^+$ can usually be demonstrated (Fig. 44-13, *D*), whereas MHC class II antigens are often lacking, and CD21, CD10, surface immunoglobulins, CD30, CD25, und CD70 are almost always negative.[303-307] CD21-negativity has been interpreted as an indication for the thymic origin of this lymphoma because also thymic B-cells lack this antigen. Negativity for CD10 and CD70 almost certainly excludes a germinal center origin.

Immunoglobulin heavy-chain and light-chain genes have shown a clonal rearrangement by Southern blot[308] or PCR analysis.

Unusual structural changes of the c-*myc* gene were found in three of six primary mediastinal B-cell lymphomas.[309] No rearrangements were found involving the *bcl*-2 gene and the major or minor break points involved in the 14;18 translocation.

Differential diagnosis. *Hodgkin's lymphoma* may be a difficult differential diagnosis, since some of primary mediastinal B-cell lymphomas contain individual Reed-Sternberg–like cells, which usually also are of B-cell phenotype. We have seen one case of combined lymphoma (simultaneous occurrence of primary mediastinal B-cell lymphoma and Hodgkin's disease). Hodgkin's disease often shows cystic alterations of the thymic structure, which may persist after successful treatment.

Anaplastic large cell lymphoma may be distinguished from primary B-cell lymphoma, which lacks CD30 but expresses B-cell markers.[310] *Carcinoma of the thymus,* an important differential diagnostic point, is usually excluded by immunostaining for keratins. *Seminoma* must be considered in the differential diagnosis because its cells, like those of primary mediastinal B-cell lymphoma, have clear and abundant cytoplasm. Immunohistologically seminomas express placental alkaline phosphatase and lack all lymphoma markers.

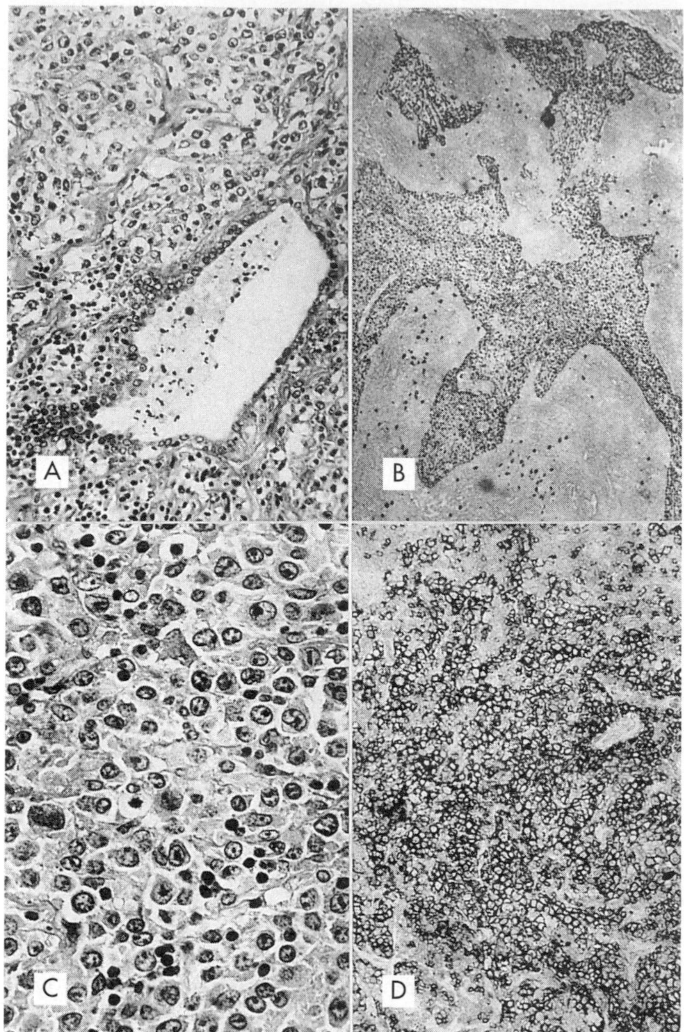

Fig. 44-13 Sclerosing mediastinal B-cell lymphoma of thymic origin. **A,** Characteristic secondary cyst formation inside the tumor infiltration. **B,** Thymic remnant within the lymphoma highlighted by antikeratin immunohistochemistry (immunoperoxidase). **C,** Anaplastic tumor cells with pleomorphic nuclei, prominent irregular nucleoli and a faintly basophilic or clear cytoplasm. **D,** Confluent infiltrates of B-cells expressing CD22 (alkaline phosphatase, immunohistochemistry).

Hodgkin's disease

Hodgkin's disease often involves the thymus, which is infiltrated in about 30% of cases with mediastinal disease. Hodgkin's disease infiltrates contain calcified Hassall's corpuscles or involve mostly the thymic medulla, causing cystic enlargement of Hassall's corpuscles. This may give rise to large cystic tumor masses.[311-314] The peculiar interaction of a pleomorphic infiltrate simulating an inflammatory disease and the proliferation of epithelium has previously been erroneously designated as "granulomatous thymoma" and was a topic of significant controversy. Today this discussion has been settled by immunohistochemistry.

Hodgkin's disease of the thymus is more frequent in young female patients. It is notable that patients with Hodgkin's disease of the thymus seldom have splenomegaly or peripheral lymphadenopathy.

Histopathology. Hodgkin's disease of the thymus is usually of the nodular sclerosing variant. The syncytial subset of this variant is not uncommon. The tumors may reach large size and show partial necrosis. At the time of diagnosis infiltrates of the pleura or lung, mediastinal fat, local lymph nodes, and the pericardium are not uncommon.

Infiltration of the thymus by Hodgkin's disease may be found in close vicinity to cysts, which are lined by simple or squamous epithelium and sometimes by respiratory epithelium that has keratin. These cysts may persist also after successful chemotherapy. Interestingly even early infiltration of the thymic medulla by Hodgkin's disease leads to rapid disappearance of all cortical thymocytes in the infiltrated lobules.

Immunophenotyping. Hodgkin's disease cells express typically CD15, CD30, and sometimes the CD20 (L26) antigen. The EMA is not expressed in almost all cases but may be found in some cases of the syncytial variant. In these cases differential diagnosis of large cell anaplastic lymphoma (Hodgkin-related type) has to be considered.[315,316] The p53 protein can be demonstrated by immunohistology in paraffin sections in all cases of Hodgkin's disease, indicating a mutated p53 gene.[317-320] About 40% of cases will express the "latent membrane protein" (LMP) of the EBV, and "Epstein-Barr virus early RNAs" (EBERs) can be demonstrated in some cases similar to nodular sclerosing Hodgkin's disease elsewhere.[321-325] No consistent rearrangements of immunoglobulin or T-cell receptor genes are found.

Small-cell B-cell lymphoma of MALT type

Very rare cases of a primary low-grade B-cell lymphoma of MALT type have been described in the thymus.[326,327] The tumor shows a lymphoid infiltration present around residual Hassall's corpuscles, some of which are cystic and may show typical lymphoepithelial lesions as in salivary gland lymphomas or stomach lymphoma. Cytologically the tumor cells are small to medium-sized cleaved (centrocyte-like) lymphoid cells. Infiltration pattern and immunophenotype indicate a relationship to the unique B-cell population of the thymic medulla.

Histiocytosis X

Histiocytosis X of the thymus is a rare disease.[328-330] It may accompany histiocytosis X in other tissues such as lung. Rarely, histiocytosis X also occurs as a solitary mediastinal mass. The latter form is found in the pediatric age group. In that case the thymus is infiltrated by large masses of atypical Langerhans' cells, which by immunophenotyping show the presence of S-100$^+$, CD1$^+$, and CD11c$^+$ phenotype and may be associated with a variable number of eosinophilic granulocytes. The prognosis for children with unifocal mediastinal histiocytosis X is excellent, whereas the prognosis of disseminated histiocytosis X is guarded. The most relevant differential diagnosis is the exclusion of a combined Hodgkin's disease, which has been documented in some cases of mediastinal histiocytosis X. Tumoral forms of histiocytosis X in the thymus or mediastinum has to be distinguished from a reactive increase of Langerhans' cells, which may be found in thymoma and lymphofollicular thymitis of myasthenia gravis.

REFERENCES

General

1. Hyrtl J: *Onomatologia Anatomica: Geschichte und Kritik der anatomischen Sprache der Gegenwart,* Vienna, 1880, Wilhelm Braumüller; Photographic reprint, Hildesheim and New York, 1970, Georg Oms.
2. Kay MMB: The thymus: clock for immunologic aging? *J Invest Dermatol* 73:29, 1979.
3. Miller JFAP: Immunological function of the thymus, *Lancet* 2:748, 1961.
4. Miller JFAP: Experimental thymology has come to age: review article, *Thymus* 1:3, 1979.
5. Miller JFAP, Osoba D: Current concepts of the immunological function of the thymus, *Physiol Rev* 47:437, 1967.
6. Michalke WD, Hess MW, Riedwyl H et al: Thymic lymphopoiesis and cell loss in newborn mice, *Blood* 33:541, 1969.
7. van Ewijk W, Shores EW, Singer A: Crosstalk in the mouse thymus, *Immunol Today* 15:214, 1994.
8. Müller-Hermelink HK: The human thymus. In *Curr Top Pathol,* fasc 75, Berlin, 1986, Springer-Verlag.
9. Rosai J, Levine GD: Tumors of the thymus. In *Atlas of tumor pathology,* series 2, fasc 13, Washington, D.C., 1975, Armed Forces Institute of Pathology.
10. Ritter MA, Crispe IN: *The thymus,* IRL in focus series, Oxford, 1991, Oxford University Press.
11. Henry K, Farrer-Brown G: *A colour atlas of thymus and lymph node histopathology with ultrastructure,* London, 1981, Wolf Medical Publications.
12. Otto HF: *Pathologie des Thymus,* Berlin, 1984, Springer-Verlag.

Normal thymus

13. Norris EH: The morphogenesis and histogenesis of the thymus gland in man in which the origin of the Hassall's corpuscles of the human thymus is discovered, *Contrib Embryol* 27:191, 1938.
14. Moore MWS, Owen JJT: Experimental studies on the development of the thymus, *J Exp Med* 126:715, 1967.
15. Owen JJT, Ritter MA: Tissue interaction in the development of thymus lymphocytes, *J Exp Med* 129:431, 1969.
16. Le Douarin NM, Jotereau FV: Tracing of cells of the avian thymus through embryonic life in interspecific chimeras, *J Exp Med* 142:17, 1975.
17. Cordier AC, Haumont SA: Development of thymus, parathyroids and ultimo-branchial bodies in NMRI and nude mice, *Am J Anat* 157:227, 1980.
18. von Gaudecker B, Müller-Hermelink HK: Ontogeny and organization of the stationary non-lymphoid cells in the human thymus, *Cell Tissue Res* 207:287, 1980.
19. Müller-Hermelink HK, von Gaudecker B: Ontogenese des lymphatischen Systems beim Menschen, *Verh Anat Ges* 74:235, 1980.
20. von Gaudecker B, Müller-Hermelink HK: Ontogeny and organization of the stationary non lymphoid cells in the human thymus, *Cell Tissue Res* 207:287, 1986.
21. Gruber GB: Über Variationen der Thymusform und -lage, *Z Angew Anat* 6:320, 1920.
22. Gruber GB: Die Entwicklungsstörungen der Thymusdrüse. In Schwalbe E, Gruber GB, editors: *Die Morphologie der Missbildungen des Menschen und der Tiere.* III. Die Einzelmissbildungen: Jena, 1932, Fischer.
23. van de Velde RL, Friedman NB: Thymic myoid cells and myasthenia gravis, *Am J Pathol* 59:347, 1970.
24. Seifert R, Christ B: On the differentiation and origin of myoid cells in the avian thymus, *Anat Embryol* 181:287, 1990.
25. von Gaudecker B, Müller-Hermelink HK: Ontogenetic differentiation of epithelial and non-epithelial cells in the human thymus, *Adv Exp Med Biol* 114:19, 1979.
26. Haynes BF, Martin ME, Kay HH, Kurtzberg J: Early events in human T cell ontogeny, phenotypic charcterization and immunohistologic localization of T cell precursors in early human fetal tissues, *J Exp Med* 168:1061, 1988.
27. Dunon D, Imhof A: Mechanisms of thymus homing, *J Am Soc Hematol* 81:1, 1993.
28. Scollay R, Smith J, Stauffer V: Dynamics of early T cells: prothymocyte migration and proliferation in the adult mouse thymus, *Immunol Rev* 91:129, 1986.

29. Jotereau F, Heuze F, Salomon-Vie V, Gascan H: Cell kinetics in the fetal mouse thymus: precursor cell input, proliferation and emigration, *J Immunol* 138:1026, 1987.
30. Isaacson PG, Norton AJ, Addis BI: The human thymus contains a novel population of B lymphocytes, *Lancet* 2:1488, 1987.
31. Hofmann WJ, Momburg F, Möller P: Thymic medullary cells expressing B lymphocyte antigens, *Hum Pathol* 19:1280, 1988.
32. Shortman K, Scollay R, Andrews P, Boyd R: Development of T lymphocytes within the thymus and within thymic nurse cells, *Curr Top Microbiol Immunol* 126: 5, 1986.
33. Agus DB, Surh CHD, Sprent J: Reentry of T cells to the adult thymus is restricted to activated T cells, *J Exp Med* 173: 1039, 1991.
34. Surh CHD, Sprent J, Webb SR: Exclusion of circulating T cells from the thymus does not apply in the neonatal period, *J Exp Med* 177: 379, 1993.
35. Kaiserling E, Stein H, Müller-Hermelink HK: Interdigitating reticulum cells in the human thymus, *Cell Tissue Res* 155:47, 1974.
36. Ardavin C, Wu L, Li CHL, Shortman K: Thymic dendritic cells and T cells develop simultaneously in the thymus from a common precursor population, *Nature* 362:761, 1993.
37. Markgraf R, von Gaudecker B, Müller-Hermelink HK: The development of the human lymph node, *Cell Tissue Res* 225:387, 1982.
38. Campana D, Janoosy G, Coustan-Smith E: The expression of T cell receptor-associated proteins during T cell ontogeny in man, *J Immunol* 142:57, 1989.
39. Clark SL: The intrathymic environment, *Contemp Top Immunobiol* 4:77, 1976.
40. Ritter MA, Sauvage CA, Cotmore SF: The human thymus microenvironment: in vivo identification of thymic nurse cells and other antigenically-distinct subpopulations of epithelial cells, *Immunology* 44:439, 1981.
41. Ritter MA, Haynes BF: Summary of thymic epithelium workshop. In McMichael M et al, editors: *Leukocyte typing III,* Oxford, 1987, Oxford University Press.
42. Singh J: The ultrastructure of epithelial reticular cells. In Kendall MD, editor: *The thymus gland,* London, 1981, Academic Press.
43. Haynes BF, Shimizu K, Eisenbarth GS: Identification of human and rodent thymic epithelium using tetanus toxin and monoclonal antibody A2B5, *J Clin Invest* 71:9, 1983.
44. McFarland EJ, Scearce RM, Haynes BF: The human thymic microenvironment: cortical thymic epithelium is an antigenically distinct region of thymic microenvironment, *J Immunol* 133:1241, 1984.
45. Wijngaert FP van den, Kendall D, Schuurman HJ et al: Heterogeneity of epithelial cells in the human thymus, *Cell Tissue Res* 237:227, 1984.
46. Wekerle H, Ketelsen UP: Thymic nurse cells: Ia-bearing epithelium involved in T-lymphocyte differentiation, *Nature* 283:402, 1980.
47. Wekerle H, Ketelsen UP, Ernst M: Thymic nurse cells: lymphoepithelial cell complexes in murine thymuses: morphological and serological characterization, *J Exp Med* 151: 925, 1980.
48. Rosai J, Higa E, Davie J: Mediastinal endocrine neoplasm in patients with multiple endocrine adenomatosis: a previously unrecognized association, *Cancer* 29:1075, 1972.
49. Müller-Hermelink HK, Marino M, Palestro G: Pathology of thymus epithelial tumors. In Müller-Hermelink HK, editor: The human thymus, *Curr Top Pathol,* 75:208, Berlin, 1986, Springer-Verlag.
50. Müller-Hermelink HK, Marx A, Kirchner T: Advances in the diagnosis and classification of thymic epithelial tumors. In Anthony PP, McSween RNM, editors: *Recent Advances in Histopathology,* fasc 16:49, Edinburgh, 1994, Churchill Livingstone.
51. Haynes BF: Human thymic epithelium and T cell development: current issues and future directions, *Thymus* 16:143, 1990.
52. Haynes BF, Denning SM, Singer KH, Kurtzberg J: Ontogeny of T-cell precursors: a model for the initial stages of human T-cell development, *Immunol Today* 10:87, 1989.
53. Terstappen WMM, Huang S, Picker LJ: Flow cytometric assessment of human T-cell differentiation in thymus and bone marrow, *Blood* 79:666, 1992.
54. Godfrey DI, Zlotnik A: Control points in early T-cell development, *Immunol Today* 14:547, 1993.
55. Chervenak R, Dempsey D, Soloff R et al: The expression of CD4 by T cell precursors resident in both the thymus and the bone marrow, *J Immunol* 151:4486, 1993.
56. Ezine S, Ceredig R: Haemopoieses and early T-cell differentiation, *Immunol Today* 15:151, 1994.
57. Haynes BF, Martin ME, Kay HH, Kurtzberg J: Early events in human T cell ontogeny: phenotypic characterization and immunohistologic localization of T cell precursor in early human fetal tissues, *J Exp Med* 168:1061, 1988.
58. Sotzik F, Boyd A, Shortman K: Surface antigens of human thymocyte populations defined by CD3, CD4 and CD8 expression: CD1a is expressed by mature thymocytes but not peripheral T cells, *Immunol Lett* 36:101, 1993.
59. Haynes BF, Denning SM, Le PT, Singer KH: Human intrathymic T cell differentiation, *Semin Immunol* 2:67, 1990.
60. Patel D, Haynes BF: Cell adhesion molecules involved in intrathymic T cell development, *Immunology* 5:283, 1993.
61. Marx A, Schömig D, Schultz A et al: Distribution of molecules mediating thymocyte-stroma interactions in human thymus, thymitis and thymic epithelial tumors, *Thymus* 24:321, 1994.
62. Purdoll DM, Fowlkes BJ, Lew AM et al: Thymus-dependent and thymus-independent developmental pathways for peripheral T cell receptor gamma/delta-bearing lymphocytes, *J Immunol* 140:4091, 1988.
63. Raulet DH: The structure, function, and molecular genetics of the gamma/delta T cell receptor, *Annu Rev Immunol* 7:175, 1989.
64. Mackall CL, Granger L, Sheard MA et al: T-cell regeneration after bone marrow transplantation: differential CD45 isoform expression on thymic-derived versus thymic-independent progeny, *Blood* 82:2585, 1993.
65. Rocha B, Vassalli P, Guy-Brand D: The extrathymic T-cell development pathway, *Immunol Today* 13: 449, 1992.
66. Poussier P, Teh HS, Julius M: Thymus-independent positive and negtive selection of T cells expressing a major histocompatibility complex class I restricted transgenic T cell receptor alpha/beta in the intestinal epithelium, *J Exp Med* 178:1947, 1993.
67. Murphy KM, Heimberger AB, Loh DY: Induction by antigen of intrathymic apoptosis of CD4+CD8+ TCRlo thymocytes in vivo, *Science* 250:1720, 1990.
68. Boyd RL, Hugo P: Towards an integrated view of thymopoiesis, *Immunol Today* 12:71, 1991.
69. Zhou T, Bluethmann H, Eldridge J et al: Origin of CD4-CD8-B220+ T cells in MRL-lpr/lpr mice: clues from a T cell receptor beta transgenic mouse, *J Immunol* 150:3651, 1993.
70. von Boehmer H: Developmental biology of T cells in T cell receptor transgenic mice, *Annu Rev Immunol* 8:531, 1990.
71. Ohasi PS, Pircher H, Burki K et al: Distinct sequence of negative or positive selection implied by thymocyte T-cell receptor densities, *Nature* 346:861, 1990.
72. Marrack P, Parker DC: A little of what you fancy, *Nature* 368:397, 1994.
73. Bevan MJ, Hogquist KA, Jameson SC: Selecting the T cell receptor repertoire, *Science* 264: 796, 1994.
74. Teh HS, Kisielow P, Scott B et al: Thymic major histocompatibility complex antigens and the α/β T-cell receptor determine the CD4/CD8 phenotype of T cells, *Nature* 335: 229, 1988.
75. Nikolic-Zugic J, Bevan M: Role of self-peptides in positively selecting the T cell repertoire, *Nature* 344:65, 1990.
76. Benoist C, Mathis D: Positive selection of the T cell repertoire: where and when does it occur? *Cell* 58:1027, 1989.
77. Hogquist KA, Jameson WR, Heath WR et al: T cell receptor antagonist peptides induce positive selection, *Cell* 76:17, 1994.
78. Speiser DE, Lees RK, Hengartner H et al: Positive and negative selection of T cell receptor V beta domains controlled by distinct cell populations in the thymus, *J Exp Med* 170:2165, 1989.
79. Fairchild P, Austyn JM: Thymic dendritic cells: phenotype and function, *Immunology* 6.187, 1990.
80. Carlow DA, van Oers NSC, Teh SJ, Teh HS: Deletion of antigen-specific immature thymocytes by dendritic cells requires LFA-1/ICAM interactions, *J Immunol* 148: 1595, 1992.
81. Pircher H, Brduscha K, Steinhoff U et al: Tolerance induction by clonal deletion of CD4+8+ thymocytes in vitro does not require dedicated antigen-presenting cells, *Eur J Immunol* 23:669, 1993.

82. Page DM, Kane LP, Allison JP, Hedrick STM: Two signals are required for negative selection of CD4+/CD8+ thymocytes, *J Immunol* 151:1868, 1993.
83. Owen JJ, Jenkinson FT: Apoptosis and T-cell repertoire selection in the thymus, *Ann N Y Acad Sci* 663:305, 1992.
84. Ferrick DA, Ohashi PS, Wallace V et al: Thymic ontogeny and selection of α/β and γ/δ T cells, *Immunol Today* 10:403, 1989.
85. Palacios R, Sidera P, von Boehmer H: Recombinant interleukin 4/BSF-1 promotes growth and differentiation of intrathymic T cell precursors from fetal mice in vitro, *EMBO J* 6:91, 1987.
86. Le PT, Kurtzberg J, Brandt SJ et al: Human thymic epithelial cells produce granulocyte and macrophage colony-stimulating factors, *J Immunol* 141:1211, 1988.
87. Haynes BF, Singer KH, Denning SM, Martin ME: Analysis of expression of CD2, CD3, and T cell antigen receptor molecules during early fetal thymic development, *Exp Med* 141:3776, 1988.
88. Hadden JW, Malec PH, Coto J, Hadden EM: Thymic involution in aging: prospects for correction, *Ann N Y Acad Sci* 673:231, 1992.
89. Quik M, Philie J, Goldstein G: Thymopoietin, a thymic polypeptide, prevents nicotinic agonist–induced morphological changes in neonatal muscle cells in culture, *Brain Res* 599:117, 1992.
90. Kyewski BA, Fathmann CG, Rous RV: Intrathymic presentation of circulating non-MHC antigens by medullary dendritic cells: an antigen-dependent microenvironment for T cell differentiation, *J Exp Med* 163:231, 1986.
91. Mizutani S, Watt SM, Robertson D et al: Cloning of human thymic subcapsular cortex epithelial cells with T-lymphocyte binding sites and hemopoietic growth factor activity, *Proc Natl Acad Sci USA* 84:4999, 1987.
92. Quik M, Philie J, Goldstein G: Thymopoietin, a thymic polypeptide, prevents nicotinic agonist–induced morphological changes in neonatal muscle cells in culture (retraction of Quik M, Philie J, Goldstein G), *Brain Res* 599:117, 1992.
93. Kurtzberg J, Denning S, Nycum LM et al: Immature human thymocytes can be driven to differentiate into nonlymphoid lineages by cytokines from thymic epithelial cells, *Proc Natl Acad Sci USA* 86:7575, 1989.
94. Murphy WJ, Durum SK, Anver M et al: Recombinant human growth hormone promotes human lymphocytes engraftment in immunodeficient mice and results in an increased incidence of human Epstein-Barr virus–induced B-cell lymphoma, *Brain Behav Immun* 6:355, 1992.
95. Möller P, Moldenhauer G, Momburg F et al: Mediastinal lymphoma of clear cell type is a tumor corresponding to terminal steps of B cell differentiation, *Blood* 69:1087, 1987.
96. Kirchner TH, Hoppe F, Schalke B, Müller-Hermelink HK: Microenvironment of thymic myoid cells myasthenia gravis, *Virchows Arch [B] (Cell Pathol)* 54:295, 1988.
97. Fend F, Kirchner TH, Marx A, Müller-Hermelink HK: B-cells in thymic epithelial tumours, *Virchows Archiv [B] (Cell Pathol)* 63:241, 1993.
98. Kirchner TH, Schalke B, Melms A et al: Immunohistological patterns of non-neoplastic changes in the thymus in Myasthenia gravis, *Virchows Arch [B] (Cell Pathol)* 52:237, 1986.
99. Janossy G, Bofill M, Trejdosiewicz LK et al, editors: Cellular differentiation of lymphoid subpopulations and their microenvironments: the human thymus, *Curr Top Pathol* 75:89, Berlin, 1986, Springer-Verlag.
100. Janossy G, Thomas JA, Bollum FJ et al: The human thymic microenvironment: an immunohistological study, *J Immunol* 125:202, 1980.
101. Janossy G, Tidman N, Papageorgiou ES, Goldstein G: Distribution of T lymphocyte subsets in the human bone marrow and thymus—an analysis with monoclonal antibodies, *J Immunol* 126:1608, 1981.
102. van der Geld HWR, Strauss AJL: Myasthenia gravis: immunological relationship between striated muscle and thymus, *Lancet* 1:57, 1966.
103. Kamo I, Kunishita T, Kikuchi A et al: Characterization of a macrophage lineage cell colony-stimulating factor produced by thymic myoid cells, *Immunology* 79:103, 1993.
104. Iseki M, Tsuda N, Kishikawa M et al: Thymolipoma with striated myoid cells: histological, immunohistochemical and ultrastructural study, *Am J Surg Pathol* 14:395, 1990.
105. Kao I, Drachman DB: Thymus muscle cells bear acetylcholine receptors: possible relation to myasthenia gravis, *Science* 195:74, 1977.
106. Schluep M, Willcox N, Vincent A et al: Acetylcholine receptors in human thymic myoid cells in situ: an immunohistological study, *Ann Neurol* 22:212, 1987.
107. Kirchner TH, Hoppe F, Schalke B, Müller-Hermelink HK: Microenvironment of thymic myoid cells in myasthenia gravis, *Virchows Arch [B] (Cell Pathol)* 54:295, 1988.
108. Mayer S: Zur Lehre von der Schilddrüse und Thymus bei den Amphibien, *Anat Anz* 3:97, 1888.
109. Müller-Hermelink HK, Kirchner TH, Hoppe F, Demel S: Thymic myoid cells—stimulants and/or targets of autoimmune myasthenia gravis, *Monogr Allergy* 25:68, 1988.
110. Nezelof CH: Pathology of the thymus in immunodeficiency states. In Müller-Hermelink, editor: The human thymus, *Curr Top Pathol* 75:151, Berlin, 1986, Springer-Verlag.
111. Lagrange W, Dahm HH, Karstens J et al: Melanocytic neuroendocrine carcinoma of the thymus, *Cancer* 59:484, 1987.
112. Markert CL, Silvers WK: The effect of genotype and cell environment on melanoblast differentiation in the house mouse, *Genetics* 41:429, 1956.
113. Steinmann GG: Changes in the human thymus during aging. In Müller-Hermelink HK, editor: The human thymus, *Curr Top Pathol* 75:43, Berlin, 1986, Springer-Verlag.

Involution of the thymus

114. Steinmann GG, Müller-Hermelink HK: Lymphocyte differentiation and its microenvironment in the human thymus during aging, *Monogr Dev Biol* 17:142, 1984.
115. Steinmann GG, Klaus B, Müller-Hermelink HK: The involution of the aging human thymic epithelium is independent of puberty, *Scand J Immunol* 22:563, 1985.
116. Young M, Turnbull HM: An analysis of the data collected by the status lymphaticus investigation committee, *J Pathol Bacteriol* 34:213, 1931.
117. Goldstein G, Mackay IR: *The human thymus,* London, 1970, William Heinemann Medical Books.
118. Fabris N: Biomarkers of aging in the neuroendocrine-immune domain. Time for a new theory of aging? *Ann N Y Acad Sci* 663: 335, 1992.
119. Dourov B: Thymic atrophy and immune deficiency in malnutrition. In Müller-Hermelink, editor: The human thymus, *Curr Top Pathol* 75:127, Berlin, 1986, Springer-Verlag.
120. Veis DJ, Sorenson CM, Shutter JR, Korsemeyer SJ: *Bcl*-2–deficient mice demonstrate fulminant lymphoid apoptosis, polycystic kidneys, and hypopigmented hair, *Cell* 75:229, 1993.
121. Concordet JP, Ferry A: Physiological programmed cell death in thymocytes is induced by physical stress (exercise), *Am J Physiol* 265:626, 1993.
122. Henry L: "Accidental" involution of the human thymus, *J Pathol Bacteriol* 96:337, 1968.
123. Cowan WK, Sorenson GD: Electron microscopic observations of acute thymic involution produced by hydrocortisone, *Lab Invest* 13:353, 1964.
124. Mugerwa JW: The lymphoreticular system in kwashiorkor, *J Pathol* 105:105, 1971.
125. Smythe PM, Schonland M, Brereton-Stiles GG et al: Thymolymphatic deficiency and depression of cell-mediated immunity in protein calorie malnutrition, *Lancet* 2:939, 1971.
126. Schonland M: Depression of immunity in protein-calorie malnutrition: a post-mortem study, *Environ Child Health* 18:217, 1972.

Primary immunodeficiency

127. Huber J, Zegers BJM, Schuurman HJ: Pathology of congenital immunodeficiencies, *Semin Diagn Pathol* 9:31, 1992.
128. Buckley RH: Immunodeficiency diseases, *JAMA* 268:2797, 1932.
129. Stiehm FR: New and old immundeficiencies, *Pediatr Res* 33:87, 1993.
130. Nezelof C: Thymic pathology in primary immunodeficiences, *Histopathology* 21:499, 1992.
131. Borzy MS, Schulte-Wissermann H, Gilbert E et al: Thymic morphology in immunodeficiency diseases: results in thymic biopsies, *Clin Immunol Immunopathol* 12:31, 1979.

229. Middleton G: The incidence of follicular structures in the human thymus at autopsy, *Aust J Exp Biol Med Sci* 45:189, 1967.
230. Vetters JM, Barclay RS: The incidence of germinal centres in thymus glands in patients with congenital heart disease, *J Clin Pathol* 26:583, 1976.
231. Alpert LI, Papatestas A, Kark A et al: A histologic reappraisal of the thymus in myasthenia gravis, *Arch Pathol* 91:55, 1971.
232. Quintanilla-Martínez L, Wilkins EW, Ferry JA, Harris NL: Thymoma: morphologic subclassification correlates with invasiveness and immunohistologic features in a study of 122 cases, *Hum Pathol* 24:958, 1993.
233. Fujii Y, Mondon Y, Nakahara K et al: Antibody to acetylcholine receptor in myasthenia gravis: production by lymphocytes from thymus and thymoma, *Neurology* 34:1182, 1984.
234. Newsom-Davis J, Willcox N, Schluep M et al: Immunological heterogeneity and cellular mechanisms in myasthenia gravis, *Ann NY Acad Sci* 505:12, 1987.
235. Isaacson PG, Norton AJ, Addis BJ: The human thymus contains a novel population of B lymphocytes, *Lancet* 2:1488, 1987.
236. Fend F, Kirchner T, Marx A, Müller-Hermelink HK: B-cells in thymic epithelial tumors: phenotype, distribution and relation to the intramedullary B-cell population of the normal thymus, *Verh Dtsch Ges Pathol* 76:253, 1993.
237. Schalke B, Mertens HG, Kircher T et al: Long-term treatment with azathioprine abolishes thymic lymphoid follicular hyperplasia in myasthenia gravis, *Lancet* 2:682, 1987.
238. Reintgen D, Fetter BF, Roses A, McCarty KS: Thymolipoma in association with myasthenia gravis, *Arch Pathol Lab Med* 102:463, 1978.
239. Otto HF, Löning T, Lachenmayer L et al: Thymolipoma in association with myasthenia gravis, *Cancer* 50:1623, 1982.
239a. Havlicek F, Rosai J: A sarcoma of thymic stroma with features of liposarcoma, *Am J Clin Pathol* 82:217, 1984.
240. Le Marc'hadour F, Pinel N, Pasquier B et al: Thymolipoma in association with myasthenia gravis, *Am J Surg Pathol* 15:802, 1991.

Tumor-like lesions of the thymus

241. Suster S, Rosai J: Multilocular thymic cyst: an acquired reactive process: study of 18 cases, *Am J Surg Pathol* 15:388, 1991.
242. Leong ASY: Thymic cysts. In Givel JC, editor: *Surgery of the thymus,* Berlin, 1990, Springer-Verlag.
243. Wick MR: Mediastinal cysts and intrathoracic thyroid tumors, *Semin Diagn Pathol* 7:285, 1990.
244. Baron RL, Sagel SS, Baglan RJ: Thymic cysts following radiation therapy for Hodgkin's disease, *Radiology* 41:593, 1981.
245. Lewis CR, Manoharan A: Benign thymic cysts in Hodgkin's disease: report of a case and review of published cases, *Thorax* 42:633, 1987.
246. Jaramillo P, Pérez-Atayde A, Griscom NT: Apparent association between thymic cysts and prior thoracotomy, *Radiology* 172:207, 1989.
247. Suster S, Barbuto D, Carlson G, Rosai J: Multilocular thymic cysts with pseudoepitheliomatous hyperplasia, *Hum Pathol* 22:455, 1991.
248. Michal M, Havlicek F: Pseudo-epitheliomatous hyperplasia in thymic cysts, *Histopathology* 19:281, 1991.
249. Suster S, Rosai J: Thymic carcinoma: a clinicopathologic study of 60 cases, *Cancer* 67:1025, 1991.
250. Clark OH: Mediastinal parathyroid tumors, *Arch Surg* 123:1096, 1988.
251. Salyer DC, Salyer WR, Eggleston JC: Benign developmental cysts of the mediastinum, *Arch Pathol Lab Med* 101:136, 1977.
252. Hammar JA: Die Menschenthymus in Gesundheit und Krankheit: Ergebnisse der numerischen Analyse von mehr als tausend menschlichen Thymusdrüsen. Teil I: Das normale Organ. Zugleich eine kritische Beleuchtung der Lehre des "Status Thymicus," *Z Mikr Anat Forsch* 6(suppl):1, 1926.
253. Balcom RJ, Hakanson DO, Werner A, Gordon LP: Massive thymic hyperplasia in an infant with Beckwith-Wiedemann syndrome, *Arch Pathol Lab Med* 109:153, 1985.
254. Carmosino L, DiBenedetto A, Feffer S: Thymic hyperplasia following successful chemotherapy: a report of two cases and review of the literature, *Cancer* 56:1526, 1985.
255. Simmonds P, Silberstein P, McKendrick J: Thymic hyperplasia in adults following chemotherapy for malignancy, *Aust NZ J Med* 23:264, 1993.
256. Small EJ, Venock AP, Damond LE: Gallium-avid thymic hyperplasia in an adult after chemotherapy for Hodgkin disease, *Cancer* 72:905, 1993.

Thymic epithelial tumors

257. Bell ET: Tumors of the thymus in myasthenia gravis, *J Nerv Ment Dis* 45:130, 1917.
258. Castleman B: Tumors of the thymus gland. In *Atlas of tumor pathology,* sec. V, fasc 19, Washington, D.C., 1955, Armed Forces Institute of Pathology.
259. Lattes R: Thymoma and other tumors of the thymus: an analysis of 107 cases, *Cancer* 15:1224, 1962.
260. Bernatz PE, Harrison EG, Clagett OT: Thymoma: a clinicopathologic study, *J Thorac Cardiovasc Surg* 42:424, 1961.
261. Shimosato Y, Kameya T, Nagai K, Suemasu K: Squamous cell carcinoma of the thymus: an analysis of eight cases, *Am J Surg Pathol* 1:109, 1977.
262. Snover DC, Levine GD, Rosai J: Thymic carcinoma: five distinctive histological variants, *Am J Surg Pathol* 6:451, 1982.
263. Wick MR: Assessing the prognosis of thymomas [editorial comment], *Ann Thorac Surg* 50:521, 1990.
264. Wick MR, Weiland LH, Scheithauer BW, Bernatz PE: Primary thymic carcinomas, *Am J Surg Pathol* 6:613, 1982.
265. Lewis JE, Wick MR, Scheithauer BW et al: Thymoma: a clinicopathologic review, *Cancer* 60:2727, 1987.
266. Masaoka A, Yasumasa M, Nakahara K, Tanioka T: Follow-up study of thymomas with special reference to their clinical stages, *Cancer* 48:2485, 1981.
267. Marino M, Müller-Hermelink HK: Thymoma and thymic carcinoma: relation of thymoma epithelial cells to the cortical and medullary differentiation of thymus, *Virchows Arch [A] (Pathol Arch)* 407:119, 1985.
268. Müller-Hermelink HK, Kirchner T: The diagnosis of thymic epithelial tumors. In Sarrazin R, Vrousos C, Vincent F, editors: *Thymic tumors,* Basel, 1989, Karger.
269. Kirchner T, Müller-Hermelink HK: New approaches to the diagnosis of thymic epithelial tumors. In Fenoglio Preiser CM, Wolff M, Rilke F, editors: *Progress in surgical pathology* 10:167, Philadelphia, 1989, Field & Wood.
270. Kirchner T, Schalke B, Buchwald J et al: Well-differentiated thymic carcinoma: an organotypical low-grade carcinoma with relationship to cortical thymoma, *Am J Surg Pathol* 16:1153, 1992.
271. Chilosi M, Castelli P, Martignoni G et al: Neoplastic epithelial cells in a subset of human thymomas express the B cell–associated CD20 antigen, *Am J Surg Pathol* 16:988, 1992.
272. Masunaga A, Sugawara I, Nakamura H et al: Strong expression of L26 antigen in epithelial cells of human neonatal thymus: an immunohistochemical study using light and electron microscopy, *Thymus* 21:65, 1993.
273. Arnold B, Marx A, Kirchner Th, Müller-Hermelink HK: Ultrastrukturelle Differenzierung von Thymomen und hochdifferenzierten Thymuskarzinomen, *Verh Dtsch Ges Pathol* 75:260, 1991 25:21, 1994.
274. Ho FCS, Fu KH, Lam SY et al: Evaluation of a histogenetic classification of thymic epithelial tumours, *Histopathology* 25:21, 1994.
275. Tanaka M, Shimokawa R, Matsubara O et al: Mucoepidermoid carcinoma of the thymic region, *Acta Pathol Jpn* 32:703, 1982.
276. Sato Y, Watanabe S, Mukai K et al: An immunohistochemical study of thymic epithelial tumors, *Am J Surg Pathol* 10:862, 1986.
277. Leyvraz S, Henle W, Chahinian AP et al: Association of Epstein-Barr virus with thymic carcinoma, *N Engl J Med* 312:1296, 1985.
278. Weiss LM, Movahed LA, Butler EA et al: Analysis of lymphoepithelioma and lymphoepithelioma-like carcinomas for Epstein-Barr viral genomes by in situ hybridization, *Am J Surg Pathol* 13:625, 1989.
279. Inghirami G, Chilosi M, Knowles DM: Western thymomas lack Epstein-Barr virus by Southern blotting analysis and by polymerase chain reaction, *Am J Pathol* 136:1429, 1990.
280. Borisch B, Kirchner T, Marx A, Müller-Hermelink HK: Absence of the Epstein-Barr virus genome in the normal thymus, thymic epithelial tumors, thymic lymphoid hyperplasia in a European population, *Virchows Arch [B] (Cell Pathol)* 59:359, 1990.
281. Stephens M, Khalil J, Gibbs AR: Primary clear cell carcinoma of the thymus gland, *Histopathology* 11:763, 1987.
282. Wolfe JT III, Wick MR, Banks PM, Scheithauer BW: Clear cell carcinoma of the thymus, *Mayo Clin Proc* 58:365, 1983.

283. Rosai J: *Ackerman's surgical pathology*, ed 8, St. Louis, 1996, Mosby.
284. Wick MR, Carney JA, Bernatz PE, Brown LR: Primary mediastinal carcinoid tumors, *Am J Surg Pathol* 6:195, 1982.
285. Rosai J, Higa E, Davie JM: Mediastinal endocrine neoplasm in patients with multiple endocrine adenomatosis: a previously unrecognized association, *Cancer* 29: 1075, 1972.
286. Rosai J, Levine G, Weber WR, Higa E: Carcinoid tumors and oat cell carcinomas of the thymus, *Pathol Annu* 11:201, 1976.
287. Rosai J, Higa E: Mediastinal endocrine neoplasm, of probable thymic origin, related to carcinoid tumor: clinicopathologic study of 8 cases, *Cancer* 29:1061, 1972.
288. Wick MR, Scheithauer BW: Thymic carcinoid: a histologic, immunohistochemical and ultrastructural study of 12 cases, *Cancer* 53:475, 1984.
289. Levine GD, Rosai J: A spindle cell variant of thymic carcinoid tumor: a clinical histologic and fine structural study with emphasis on its distinction from spindle cell thymoma, *Arch Pathol* 100:293, 1976.
290. Lagrange W, Dahm HK, Karstens J et al: Melanocytic neuroendocrine carcinoma of the thymus, *Cancer* 59:484, 1987.
291. Herbst WM, Kummer W, Hofmann W et al: Carcinoid tumors of the thymus: an immunohistochemical study, *Cancer* 60:2465, 1987.
292. Wick MR, Scheithauer BW: Oat-cell carcinoma of the thymus, *Cancer* 49:1652, 1982.
293. Pescarmona E, Rendina EA, Venuta F et al: The prognostic implication of thymoma histologic subtyping: a study of 80 consecutive cases, *Am J Clin Pathol* 93:190, 1990.
294. Pescarmona E, Rendina EA, Venuta F et al: Analysis of prognostic factors and clinico-pathological staging of thymoma, *Ann Thorac Surg* 50:534, 1990.
295. Kuo TT, Chang JP, Lin FJ et al: Thymic carcinomas: histopathologic varieties and immunohistochemical study, *Am J Surg Pathol* 34:14, 1990.
296. Truong LD, Mody DR, Cagle PT et al: Thymic carcinoma: a clinicopathologic study of 13 cases, *Am J Surg Pathol* 14:151, 1990.
297. Marx A, Kirchner Th, Hoppe F et al: Proteins with epitopes of the acetylcholine receptor in epithelial cell cultures of thymomas in myasthenia gravis, *Am J Pathol* 134:865, 1989.
298. Marx A, O'Connor R, Geuder K et al: Characterization of a protein with an acetylcholine receptor epitope from myasthenia gravis-associated thymomas, *Lab Invest* 62:279, 1990.
299. Marx A, Geuder K, Schoepfer R et al: Analysis of the acetylcholine receptor epitope bearing protein p153 in thymomas favors false-positive T-cell selection as a mechanism of paraneoplastic myasthenia gravis. In Imhof BA, Berrih-Aknin S, Ezine S, editors: *Lymphatic tissues and in vivo immune responses*, New York, 1991, Marcel Decker.
300. Marx A, Kirchner Th, Greiner A et al: Neurofilament epitopes in thymoma and antiaxonal autoantibodies in myasthenia gravis, *Lancet* 339:707, 1992.

Lymphomas of the thymus

301. Barcos MP, Lukes RJ: Malignant lymphoma of convoluted lymphocytes: a new entitiy of possible T cell type. In Sinks LF, Godden JO, editors: *Conflicts in childhood cancer: an evaluation of current management*, New York, 1975, Alan R Liss.
302. Addis BJ, Isaacson PG: Large cell lymphoma of the mediastinum: a B cell tumour of probable thymic origin, *Histopathology* 10:379, 1986.
303. Isaacson PG, Norton AJ, Addis B: The human thymus contains a novel population of B lymphocytes, *Lancet* 2:1488, 1987.
304. Davis RE, Dorfman RF, Warnke RA: Primary large-cell lymphoma of the thymus, *Hum Pathol* 21:1262, 1990.
305. Menestrina F, Chilos M, Bonetti F et al: Mediastinal large-cell lymphoma of B-type, with sclerosis: histopathological and immunohistochemical study of eight cases, *Histopathology* 10:589, 1986.
306. Möller P, Lämmler B, Erberlein-Gonska M et al: Primary mediastinal clear cell lymphome of B-cell type, *Virchows Arch [A] (Anat Pathol)* 409:79, 1986.
307. Möller P, Moldenhauer G, Momburg F et al: Mediastinal lymphoma of clear cell type is a tumor corresponding to terminal steps of B cell differentiation, *Blood* 69:1087, 1987.
308. Scarpa A, Bonetti F, Menestrina F et al: Mediastinal large cell lymphoma with sclerosis, genotypic analysis establishes its B nature, *Virchows Arch* 412:17, 1987.
309. Scarpa A, Borgato L, Chilosi M et al: Evidence of c-*myc* gene anormalities in mediastinal large B cell lymphoma of young adult age, *Blood* 78:780, 1991.
310. Frizzera G: Pathology and clinical correlations of the non-Hodgkin's lymphomas. In Benz EJ et al, editors: *Hematology: basic principles and practice*, New York, 1990, Churchill Livingstone.
311. Kim HC, Nosher J, Haas A et al: Cystic degeneration of thymic Hodgkin's disease following radiation therapy, *Cancer* 55:354, 1985.
312. Fechner RE: Hodgkin's disease of the thymus, *Cancer* 23:16, 1969.
313. Katz A, Lattes R: Granulomatous (24 cases) thymoma or Hodgkin's disease of thymus? A clinical and histologic study and re-evaluation, *Cancer* 23:1, 1969.
314. Keller AR, Castleman B: Hodgkin's disease of the thymus gland, *Cancer* 33:1615, 1974.
315. Delsol G, Saati TA, Gatter KC et al: Coexpression of epithelial membrane antigen (EMA), Ki-1, and interleukin-2 receptor by anaplastic large cell lymphomas: diagnostic value in so-called malignant histiocytosis, *Am J Pathol* 130:59, 1988.
316. Rosso R, Paulli M, Magrini U et al: Anaplastic large cell lymphoma, CD30/Ki-1 positive, expressing the CD15/Leu-M1 antigen: immunohistochemical and morphological relationships to Hodgkin's disease, *Virchows Arch [A] (Anat Pathol)* 416:229, 1990.
317. Gupta RK, Patel K, Bodmer WF, Bodmer JG: Mutatin of p53 in primary biopsy material and cell lines from Hodgkin disease, *Proc Natl Acad Sci USA* 90:2817, 1993.
318. Trumper LH, Brady G, Gagg A et al: Single-cell analysis of Hodgkin and Reed-Sternberg cells: molecular heterogeneity of gene expression and p53 mutations, *Blood* 81:3097, 1993.
319. Doussis IA, Pezzella F, Lane DP et al: An immunocytochemical study of p53 and *bcl*-2 protein expression in Hodgkin's disease, *Am J Clin Pathol* 99:663, 1993.
320. Niedobitek G, Rowlands DC, Young LS et al: Overexpression of p53 in Hodgkin's disease: lack of correlation with Epstein-Barr virus infection, *J Pathol* 169:207, 1993.
321. Weiss LM, Mohaved LA, Warnke RA, Sklar J: Detection of Epstein-Barr viral genomes in Reed-Sternberg cells of Hodgkin's disease, *N Engl J Med* 302:502, 1989.
322. Jiwa NM, Kanavaros P, van der Valk P et al: Expression of c-*myc* and *bcl*-2 oncogene products in Reed-Sternberg cells independent of presence of Epstein-Barr virus, *J Clin Pathol* 46:211, 1993.
323. Herndier BG, Sánchez HC, Chang KL et al: High prevalence of Epstein-Barr virus in the Reed-Sternberg cells of HIV-associated Hodgkin's disease, *Am J Pathol* 142:1073, 1993.
324. Lin JC, Lin SC, De BK et al: Precision of genotyping of Epstein-Barr virus by polymerase chain reaction using three gene loci (EBNA-3C, and EBER): predominance of type A virus associated with Hodgkin's disease, *Blood* 81:3372, 1993.
325. Brousset P, Rochaix P, Chittal S et al: High incidence of Epstein-Barr virus detection in Hodgkin's disease and absence of detection in anaplastic large-cell lymphome in children, *Histopathology* 23:189, 1993.
326. Isaacson PG, Chan JK, Tang C, Addis BJ: Low grade B-cell lymphoma of mucosa-associated lymphoid tissue arising in the thymus: a thymic lymphoma mimicking myoepithelial sialadenitis, *Am J Surg Pathol* 15:342, 1990.
327. Nakagawa A, Nakamura S, Koshikawa T et al: Clinicopathologic study of primary mediastinal non-lymphoblastic non-Hodgkin's lymphomas among the Japanese, *Acta Pathol Jpn* 43:44, 1993.
328. Pescarmona E, Rendina EA, Ricci C, Baroni CD: Histiocytosis X and lymphoid follicular hyperplasia of the thymus in myasthenia gravis, *Histopathology* 14:465, 1989.
329. Drut R: Multivisceral dysplastic lesions in a patient with tuberous sclerosis and Langerhans cell histiocytosis, *Pediatr Pathol* 10:633, 1990.
330. Ben Ezra J, Bailey A, Azumi N et al: Malignant histiocytosis X: a distinct clinicopathologic entity, *Cancer* 68:1050, 1991.

B. MEDIASTINUM

Alberto Marchevsky
Neal S. Goldstein

NORMAL MEDIASTINUM

The mediastinum is the part of the thorax located between the two pleural cavities. It is bounded anteriorly by the sternum, posteriorly by the thoracic vertebra, inferiorly by the diaphragm, and superiorly by the first thoracic ribs, first thoracic vertebra, and manubrium.[1,2]

The mediastinum has been traditionally subdivided into four compartments that can be identified on chest roent-genogram: superior, anterior, middle, and posterior.[1] This classification is useful for diagnostic purposes in that certain pathologic conditions are more frequent in particular locations. The *superior mediastinum* extends from the manubrium of the sternum through the lower edge of the fourth thoracic vertebral body. The *anterior mediastinum* lies immediately below the superior mediastinum compartment, anteriorly to the pericardium, and posteriorly to the chest wall. The *posterior mediastinum* is located behind the pericardium and diaphragm. The *middle mediastinum* is the space found between the anterior and the posterior divisions of the mediastinum. Most consider it to contain only the pericardium and contents.[1-3]

The anterior and middle mediastinum contain the superior vena cava, pulmonary arteries, phrenic nerves, right recurrent laryngeal and buccal nerves, left and right main bronchi, esophagus, tracheal bifurcation, and other tissues anterior to the trachea. The superior mediastinum contains the thymus glands, internal mammary vessels and lymph nodes, and fibroadipose connective tissue. Rarely it can contain thyroid and parathyroid tissue. The posterior mediastinum encompasses the descending portion of the thoracic aorta, lower end of the esophagus, thoracic duct, sympathetic ganglia, and numerous lymph nodes.

More recent anatomic classifications of the mediastinum are based on computerized tomographic (CT) scans and divide the area into the thoracic inlet, anterior mediastinum, supra-aortic, infra-aortic, supra-azygous, infra-azygous, and hilar areas (Fig. 44-14). Many lesions occur primarily in one compartment (Table 44-5).

NONNEOPLASTIC DISEASES

Acute mediastinitis

Acute mediastinitis is a bacterial infection involving one of the mediastinal compartments, most often the middle mediastinum. It is frequently a lethal complication of esophageal perforation secondary to postoperative dehiscence of a recent esophageal anastomosis but may follow other thoracic surgical procedures as well. Because the normal esophagus contains bacteria, its perforation usually results in a highly virulent necrotizing acute inflammation with frequent abscess formation.[4,5] Less frequently, acute mediastinitis is secondary to sternal osteomyelitis, dental abscess, and pulmonary or pleural infections.[5-8]

Patients with acute mediastinitis present clinically with severe chest pain associated with fever, leukocytosis, and other signs of acute infection. A widening of the mediastinum is seen on chest x-ray films (Fig. 44-15). Histologically, acute mediastinitis is characterized by severe acute inflammation with numerous polymorphonuclear leukocytes that permeate diffusely the connective tissues of the mediastinum. Pockets of pus may accumulate, with secondary abscess formation. The mediastinum is usually surgically drained or debrided. Cultures frequently yield a mixed bacterial flora with beta-hemolytic and anaerobic streptococci, *Staphylococcus aureus*, or various aerobic and anaerobic gram-negative bacilli.[9]

Chronic fibrosing mediastinitis

Chronic fibrosing mediastinitis (also known as *sclerosing mediastinitis* and *granulomatous mediastinitis*) is an unusual condition characterized by the formation of a firm, ill-

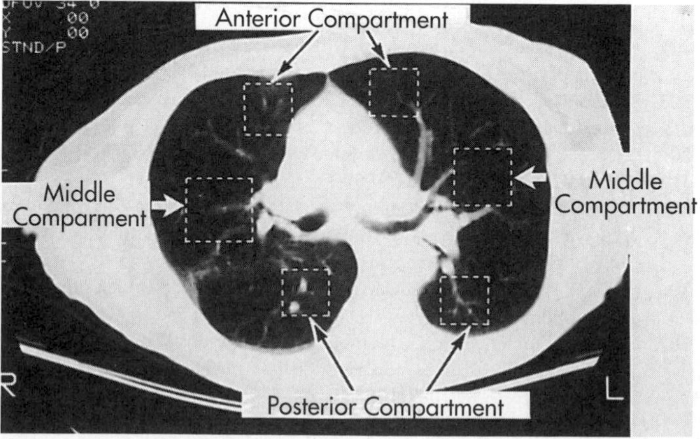

Fig. 44-14 Location of mediastinal lesions.

Table 44-5 Location of lesions by mediastinal compartment

Superior compartment
Metastatic tumors
Thyroid lesions
Parathyroid lesions
Anterior compartment
Metastatic tumors
Thymic lesions
Thyroid lesions
Parathyroid lesions
Cysts
Lymphoproliferative disorders
Middle mediastinum
Cysts
Mesothelial and pericardial lesions
Chronic fibrosing mediastinitis
Posterior mediastinum
Cysts
Neurogenic tumors
Spinal lesions

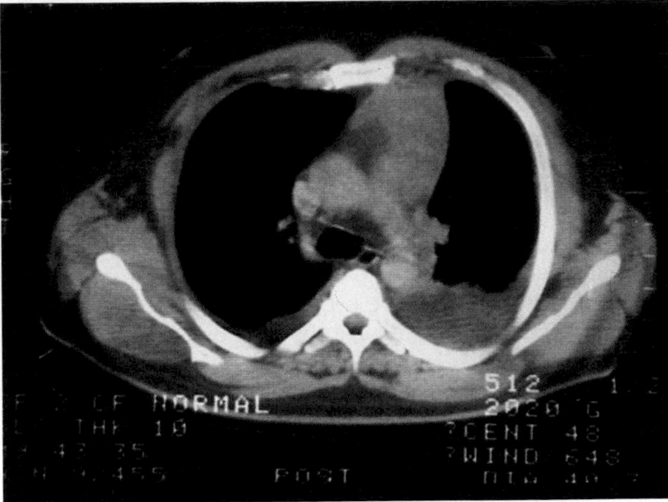

Fig. 44-16 CT scan of the chest showing a large, ill-defined anterior mediastinal mass and left pleural effusion. A biopsy was performed on the mass, which was diagnosed as sclerosing mediastinitis.

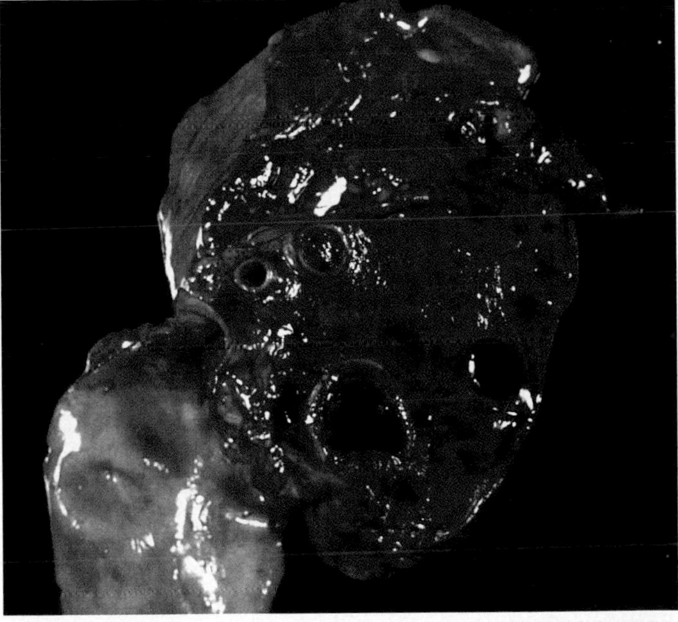

Fig. 44-15 Acute mediastinitis caused by mucormycosis. The patient was a diabetic who developed a rapidly expanding anterior mediastinal mass that caused death. The lesion has ill-defined borders and a hemorrhagic appearance.

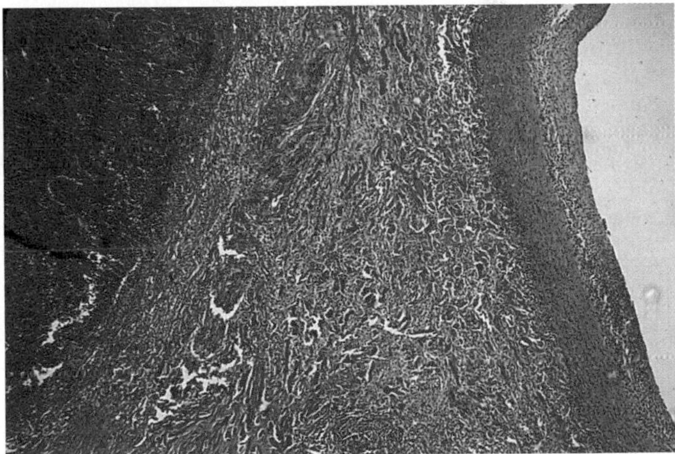

Fig. 44-17 Sclerosing mediastinitis characterized histologically by dense fibrous tissue infiltrating mediastinal structures.

defined mediastinal mass (Fig. 44-16). Histologically it presents as dense fibrosis with focal granulomatous inflammation (Fig. 44-17).[10]

Chronic sclerosing mediastinitis may be an idiopathic condition or is associated with fungal *(Histoplasma capsulatum, Cryptococcus neoformans)*, mycobacterial *(Mycobacterium tuberculosis, Mycobacterium avium–intracellulare)*, and bacterial infections *(Nocardia asteroides, Actinomyces israelii)*. It has also been reported in patients with autoimmune diseases, sarcoidosis, rheumatic fever, distal neoplasms, traumatic hemorrhage, and drugs such as methysergide.[10-13] In the United States, histoplasmosis is the most common pathogen identified. Some patients with sclerosing mediastinitis can also develop fibrosis in extrathoracic locations including the retroperitoneum, orbit, thyroid (Riedel's thyroiditis), and liver (sclerosing cholangitis).[14]

The pathogenesis of noninfectious sclerosing mediastinitis is unknown, but a delayed-hypersensitivity autoimmune reaction mechanism has been postulated. In patients with histoplasmosis, it has been postulated that some unidentified antigen of *Histoplasma* sp. diffuses from infected lymph nodes with granulomatous lymphadenitis into the adjacent tissues, inciting an immunologic reaction and subsequent fibrosis at the periphery of the granulomas.

Chronic fibrosing mediastinitis affects patients of both sexes and all ages, but it is most prevalent among young (19 to 25 years), white women. Approximately 40% of patients are asymptomatic at the time of initial diagnosis and are identified by abnormal findings on a chest x-ray film. Other patients present with nonspecific complaints such as cough, dyspnea, chest pain, fever, wheezing, hemoptysis, or other symptoms secondary to the extension of fibrosis into adjacent structures. For example, chronic fibrosing mediastinitis is the most common cause of the superior vena cava syndrome.

Invasion of the pulmonary veins at the left atrium results in a clinical syndrome that closely mimics mitral valve stenosis with pulmonary hypertension.[15] Secondary thrombosis of the pulmonary veins may be associated with pulmonary infarcts.[16] Thrombosis of the pulmonary artery encased or involved by the fibrosis results in pulmonary infarcts.[17,18] Bronchial and tracheal obstruction are rare because the airway cartilage usually acts as a barrier against fibrous tissue invasion. The esophagus, which is relatively movable, is usually not infiltrated by fibrous tissue but rather displaced by it.

Chronic fibrosing (sclerosing) mediastinitis presents grossly as an ill-defined, firm, gray mass that surrounds and infiltrates mediastinal structures (Fig. 44-16). It usually involves the middle mediastinum. Histologically it consists of dense fibrous tissue with variable infiltrates of lymphocytes, macrophages, and plasma cells (Fig. 44-17). Caseating or noncaseating granulomas can be focally present, particularly in mediastinal lymph nodes enclosed by the fibrotic process. Impregnation with methenamine-silver and Ziehl-Neelsen's acid-fast stains should be routinely done to establish or exclude an infectious cause.

Chronic fibrosing mediastinitis is usually a self-limited process that tends to regress with time. However, it may also progress and cause complications, in which case surgical resection is indicated.

Endocrine masses

The mediastinum may contain aberrant thyroid or parathyroid tissue. Paragangliomas are also occasionally found. All these lesions are most often present in the anterior and superior mediastinal compartments.

Mediastinal thyroid lesions

True ectopic or aberrant intrathoracic thyroid lesions not contiguous with the thyroid itself are uncommon. Most represent mediastinal extension of the pathologic processes involving the thyroid in the neck. Thyroid nodular hyperplasia (nodular goiter) often has an intrathoracic component, accounting for approximately 10% of mediastinal masses. It is usually found in the anterior mediastinum but may involve the posterior mediastinum in 25% of patients.[19] The thyroid gland is enclosed in the neck superiorly by the hyoid bone and posteriorly by the larynx and is surrounded by rigid structures that normally prevent its downward expansion into the mediastinum. However, an enlarged thyroid gland with nodular hyperplasia can grow into the right side of the superior mediastinum. Extension into the left side of the thorax is less likely because the aortic arch and other great vessels serve as a mechanical barrier and prevent extension into the mediastinum.[20]

Mediastinal thyroid nodular hyperplasia is most frequent in women. Symptoms of compression of thoracic structures by the enlarged thyroid tissue, include cough, retrosternal pain, and sensation of weight in the chest.[20] The patients are usually euthyroid but may rarely develop thyrotoxicosis. On physical examination, a palpable cervical goiter or mass is usually detected.

Grossly, multinodular or adenomatous goiter is characterized by an enlarged thyroid gland that is greatly distorted by multiple nodules surrounded by a fibrous capsule.[20] The nodules are composed of thyroid follicles of various sizes lined by amphophilic or oxyphilic follicular cells. They frequently exhibit areas of hemorrhage, calcification, or cystic degeneration.

Diffuse hyperplasia of the thyroid gland (Graves' disease) is less frequent in the mediastinum.[21-23] Other thyroid lesions, such as follicular adenomas, thyroiditis, and malignancies infrequently extend into the thorax.[20]

Mediastinal parathyroid

There are normally four parathyroid glands, located on the posterior aspects of the thyroid lobes. The parathyroid glands develop from the third and fourth branchial clefts and extend caudally during embryogenesis. The final location of parathyroids may vary individually.[24] In approximately 10% of persons the parathyroid glands are located not only in the typical retrothyroid position, but also in the submaxillary areas, within the thyroid gland, or in the thymus, mediastinum, and pericardium.[25-28]

In the thorax, ectopic parathyroids are usually found in the anterior mediastinum, adjacent to the thymus or enclosed within its capsule. This information is important clinically because approximately 38% of patients requiring reoperation for persistent or recurrent hyperparathyroidism are found to have ectopic parathyroid glands in the mediastinum.[27]

Adenoma is the most common lesion of mediastinal parathyroids. Histologically it is indistinguishable from parathyroid adenomas in the usual neck location.[24] Most parathyroid adenomas are solitary nodules that weigh over 75 mg and measure over 1 cm in diameter. Histologically they are well encapsulated and composed of chief cells, oncocytic cells, or clear cells arranged into trabeculas, solid nests, and microacini. A rim of normal parathyroid tissue is frequently found in the capsule. Parathyroid adenomas, similar to those in the neck, cannot be distinguished histologically from parathyroid hyperplasia by histologic examination of a single parathyroid. Although parathyroid hyperplasia is rare in the mediastinum, the differential diagnosis of adenoma requires that other normal parathyroids be identified in addition to the adenomatous gland. Parathyroid carcinoma is extremely rare in the mediastinum.[25]

TUMORS AND MASS LESIONS

Paraganglioma

Mediastinal paragangliomas usually originate from the supra-aortic and aorticopulmonary bodies and are found in the superior mediastinum.[29-33] They can also develop in the posterior mediastinum, arising from the periaortic sympathetic paraganglia.[29-36] These tumors occur in all age groups (mean age, 47 years) and are slightly more frequent in women (1.8:1).[36] Approximately half of patients with mediastinal paragangliomas are asymptomatic at the time of the initial diagnosis and are found to have a superior mediastinal tumor on routine chest roentgenograph. The other half of these patients present with hoarseness, dysphagia, chest pain or discomfort, cough, or hemoptysis. Mediastinal paragangliomas can be multiple and are occasionally associated with gastric stromal tumors and pulmonary chondromas (Carney's triad).[37,38]

Paragangliomas are well encapsulated, gray-pink, highly vascular tumors composed histologically of nests of polygonal to cuboidal cells *(Zellballen),* surrounded by vascularized septa. The tumor cells have round nuclei and clear or eosinophilic, granular cytoplasm. The tumor cells contain intracytoplasmic neurosecretory granules that stain with immunocytochemical methods using antibodies to chromogranin, somatostatin, Leu-7, or neuron-specific enolase.[33] The neurosecretory granules can also be demonstrated by electron microscopy; they measure 100 to 300 nm in diameter and exhibit characteristic ultrastructural features with an electron-dense core and a single membrane. The fibrous stroma separating the nests of polygonal cells has spindle sustentacular cells that stain with antibodies to S-100 protein.

Most paragangliomas are benign neoplasms. Malignant transformation occurs in approximately 10% of lesions. The diagnosis of malignancy cannot be established reliably by histologic characteristics alone. Cellular pleomorphism with occasional bizarre giant tumor cells, rare mitotic figures, and focal vascular invasion can be seen in benign lesions and are not diagnostic of malignancy. The final diagnosis of malignant paraganglioma is based on demonstrating extensive local neoplastic invasion of adjacent tissues or distant metastases.[33,39]

Lymphoproliferative and hematopoietic disorders

Mediastinal lymph nodes and the thymus can be involved by a variety of lymphoproliferative disorders ranging from reactive lymphoid hyperplasia to malignant lymphomas. Indeed, lymphoid proliferations are among the most common causes of mediastinal masses, and malignant lymphomas are the most frequent malignant tumors of the mediastinum.[40,41]

Malignant lymphomas

The range of benign and malignant lymphadenopathies involving the mediastinum is listed in Table 44-6. The mediastinum is involved in approximately 15% to 20% of patients with malignant lymphoma.[42-44]

Hodgkin's disease of the nodular sclerosis or mixed cellularity type is the most common form of malignant lymphoma involving the mediastinum in adult patients, whereas lymphoblastic lymphoma is the most common in children. The disease presents as a mediastinal mass (Fig. 44-18, *A*). Histologically it has the features typical of Hodgkin's disease in other anatomic sites (Fig. 44-18, *B*).

Hodgkin's disease involving the mediastinum generally has a favorable prognosis. Patients with stage I and stage II disease and mediastinal involvement at the time of initial diagnosis have an 88% 5-year survival rate compared with 98% survival rates for individuals with similar tumor stage but lacking mediastinal masses.[45] However, presence of a large mediastinal mass in a patient with Hodgkin's disease is an unfavorable prognostic factor that requires aggressive multimodal therapy.[46]

Mediastinal non-Hodgkin's lymphomas are unusual, except for lymphoblastic lymphoma in children. Only 6% of patients with non-Hodgkin's lymphomas present initially with mediastinal disease.[47] Mediastinal non-Hodgkin's lymphomas occur in all age groups, with the highest incidence in the fourth decade of life. They are somewhat more frequent in

Table 44-6 Mediastinal lymphadenopathies

Granulomatous lymphadenitis
Tuberculosis
Fungal infections
Histoplasmosis
Coccidioidomycosis
Sarcoidosis
Silicosis
Wegener's granulomatosis
Neoplasms
Non-Hodgkin's lymphomas
Hodgkin's lymphoma
Metastatic tumors
Granulocytic sarcoma
Others
Reactive
Nonspecific follicular or parafollicular lymphoid hyperplasia
Systemic lupus erythematosus
Rheumatoid arthritis
Viral infections (especially infectious mononucleosis)
Angiofollicular hyperplasia (Castleman's disease)

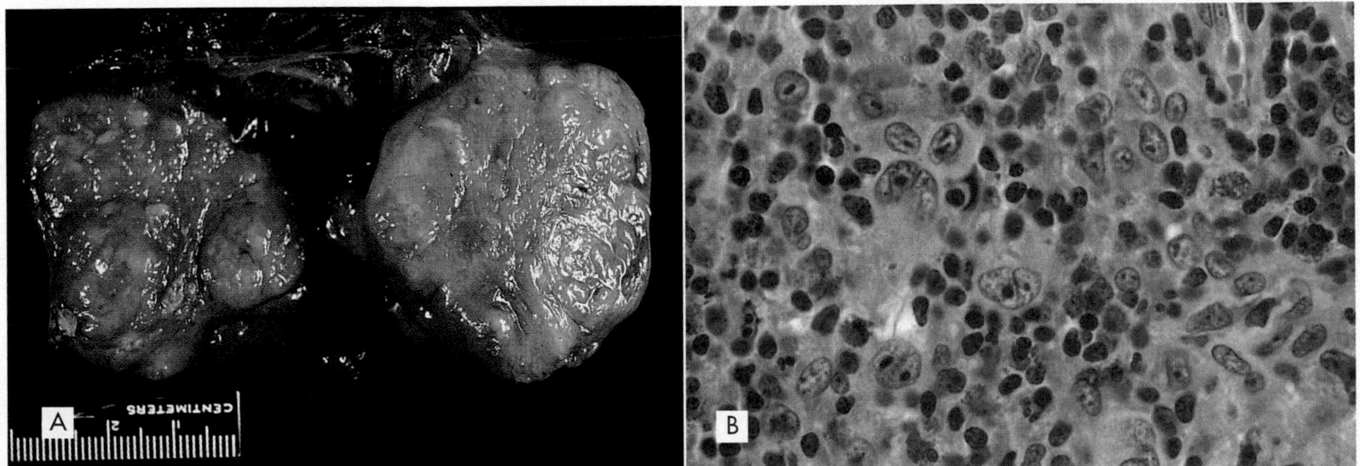

Fig. 44-18 Hodgkin's disease of the mediastinum. **A,** The lymph nodes are enlarged and matted together by soft, yellow necrotic tissues. **B,** Histologically, the lesion is characterized by a mixed infiltrate composed of small lymphoid cells, eosinophils, and large Reed-Sternberg cells. The latter have double nuclei with prominent nucleoli.

women, with the female-to-male ratio being 1:5. Most of these lymphomas are B-cell–lineage neoplasms that presumably originate from mediastinal lymph nodes or from B-lymphocytes that are normally present in the medulla and septa of the thymus. Histologically, the majority of non-Hodgkin's lymphomas of the mediastinum are classified as diffuse, large cell type and are often associated with sclerosis.[48]

Mediastinal lymphoma in children

Lymphoblastic lymphoma is the most common childhood neoplasm of the thorax.[49] Mediastinal involvement is found in approximately 50% of all cases. This lymphoma is biologically closely related to acute lymphoblastic leukemia (ALL),[49] as discussed in greater detail in Chapter 41.

Granulocytic sarcoma (chloroma)

Granulocytic sarcomas develop in patients with acute monoblastic and myelogenous leukemia.[50] Such mediastinal masses are composed of malignant myeloid cells. In the past, granulocytic sarcomas have posed difficult diagnostic problems for the surgical pathologist because the neoplastic hematopoietic cells resemble normal lymphoid cells in routine histologic slides. However, the distinction between lymphoid cells and granulocytes can now be readily established with the aid of immunohistochemical stains for lymphocyte antigens, such as leukocyte common antigen (CD45) and L26 (CD20). Myeloperoxidase can be demonstrated with enzyme histochemistry methods in malignant myeloblastic cells, when one uses a reaction to naphthol ASD chloroacetate esterase (Leder's stain). Myeloid and monocytic cells contain intracytoplasmic lysozyme, which is also detectable with immunohistochemical methods.[51,52]

Lymphadenitis

Enlarged mediastinal lymph nodes attributable to granulomatous lymphadenitis and other inflammatory lymphadenopathies are common.[53,54] Infectious granulomas are most often caused by bacteria such as *Mycobacterium tuberculosis* or fungal infections such as histoplasmosis and coccidioidomycosis. Noninfectious granulomas are features of many diseases, most notably sarcoidosis, silicosis, and Wegener's granulomatosis (Table 44-6).[55]

Tuberculous mediastinal and hilar lymphadenitis is common in children with primary tuberculosis but is unusual in adults.[56,57] Lymph nodes appear enlarged, soft, and matted and contain white areas of friable, caseating, necrotic material. These lymph nodes are frequently adherent to blood vessels and other mediastinal structures. Acid-fast bacilli can be demonstrated in smears of caseous material with Ziehl-Neelsen stain or Fite stain.

In chronic tuberculous lymphadenitis the lesions are firm, gray-white, and calcified. Histologically the lymph nodes contain multiple, confluent epithelioid granulomas at different stages of development. Small granulomas are composed of giant cells, epithelioid cells, and lymphocytes. Large granulomas have central caseous, acellular, eosinophilic necrosis, whereas older lesions have areas of fibrosis with calcification.

Fungal lymphadenitis caused by *Histoplasma capsulatum, Coccidioides immitis, Cryptococcus neoformans* and other fungi also present as granulomatous lymphadenitis. Fungal caseating granulomatous reactions are indistinguishable morphologically from tuberculosis. The etiologic diagnosis is established by fungal cultures or morphologic identification of the organisms in tissue sections using the periodic acid–Schiff reaction (PAS stain) or Gomori's methenamine silver stains (GMS stain).

Sarcoidosis of the mediastinum is usually part of the systemic granulomatous disease that often involves other lymph nodes and lungs and less often bones, soft tissue, eyes, and salivary glands.[58] It is more frequent in black women in the third through fifth decades of life. The disease is approximately 10 times more frequent in black patients than in white patients and the women-to-men ratio is 2:1. Patients with sarcoidosis have elevated levels of serum lysozyme and angiotensin-converting enzyme, believed to be derived from epithelioid macrophages.[59] The mediastinal lymph nodes, particularly the hilar and paratracheal nodes, are involved in 60% to 90% of patients with sarcoidosis. These lymph nodes are uniformly enlarged and soft and exhibit grossly small nodules on cut section. Histologically the lymph nodes are partially or completely replaced by multiple, usually discrete, round, and relatively uniform in size noncaseating granulomas composed of epithelioid cells. The epithelioid and multinucleated giant cells of sarcoid granulomas can exhibit various intracellular and extracellular inclusion bodies such as asteroid, Schaumann, or Hamazaki-Weisenberg bodies. These inclusion bodies are not pathognomonic of sarcoidosis and can be seen in other granulomatous conditions as well. Asteroid bodies are eosinophilic, spiderlike intracytoplasmic inclusions composed of lipoproteins. Schaumann bodies are intracellular, round, calcified, concentrically laminated structures. Hamazaki-Weisenberg bodies are giant lysosomes that appear as extracellular clusters of yellow-brown, spindle-shaped structures. They can resemble fungal yeasts on histologic slides stained with GMS stain.

Sarcoid granulomas can have focal central areas of necrosis, but extensive caseous necrosis or calcifications are unusual.[58]

Other granulomatous lymphadenopathies

Silicosis is a form of pneumoconiosis caused by inhalation of silica particles. The pulmonary disease is frequently associated with granulomatous mediastinal lymphadenopathy. The enlarged lymph nodes contain silicotic nodules composed of epithelioid cell granulomas. Within these granulomas there are birefringent particles of silicon dioxide that can be demonstrated with polarized light microscopy.[60] The nodules become hyalinized in concentric layers, giving the lesion a characteristic "onionskin" appearance. These lymph nodes are also frequently calcified and are readily recognized on chest x-ray films.

Wegener's granulomatosis is a disease of unknown cause characterized by granulomatous lesions and necrotizing angiitis in the upper respiratory tracts, lungs, and kidneys. Mediastinal lymph node enlargement is common.[60] Carcinomas can be associated with sarcoid epithelioid cell granulomas in lymph nodes.[61] The pathogenesis of these granulomas is unknown.

Angiofollicular hyperplasia (Castleman's disease)

Angiofollicular hyperplasia was described in 1954 as a form of benign lymph node hyperplasia simulating thymoma.[62] It usually presents as a solitary mediastinal mass, or, less frequently, in extrathoracic form. No age or sex predominance has been described.[63] Patients with localized angiofollicular hyperplasia are often asymptomatic and are found to have a large mediastinal mass on routine chest roentgenogram. Localized symptoms in patients with large mediastinal masses secondary to compression of mediastinal structures are less frequent (Fig. 44-19, *A*). Two histopathologic variants are distinguished: the hyaline vascular and the plasma cell variants (Fig. 44-19, *B*). Both histopathologic variants are characterized by the presence of increased nodal vascularity and development of venous channels in lymph node follicles (so-called lollipop follicles). More details about Castleman's disease are found in Chapter 42.

Mediastinal cysts

Mediastinal cysts are infrequent benign intrathoracic lesions that constitute 10% to 27% of all mediastinal masses (Table 44-7). They can be congenital or acquired in origin; most mediastinal cysts result from developmental anomalies of the foregut or related embryologic structures.[64-69] A small number of intrathoracic lesions secondary to cystic degeneration of mediastinal neoplasms or intrathoracic extensions of pancreatic pseudocyst have also been described.[64]

Table 44-7 Mediastinal cystic lesions

True cysts
Bronchogenic
Esophageal
Gastroenteric
Pericardial
Mesothelial
Thymic
Neoplasms with cystic change
Thymomas
Teratoma
Germ cell tumors
Hodgkin's lymphoma
Other
Lymphangiomas (cystic hygromas)
Pancreatic pseudocyst
Hydatid (echinococcal) cyst

Bronchogenic cysts

Bronchogenic cysts are the most frequent congenital cystic lesions of the mediastinum and account for approximately half of all congenital cysts of the area.[64,70-76] They occur in all age groups but are most frequent in adult patients in their third and fourth decades of life; they are 1.5 times more frequent in men than in women.[70,71,74-79] Patients are usually asymptomatic at the time of initial diagnosis and are found to have a mediastinal mass on chest x-ray film.[67] Rarely, bronchogenic cysts located in the carina cause death in early life as a result of compression of the trachea or a major bronchus.[67]

Bronchogenic cysts result from abnormal branching of the bronchopulmonary tree during intrauterine development.[67] The primitive tracheal tube develops from a medial ventral outgrowth of the foregut during the third and fourth weeks of intrauterine life. It bifurcates during the sixth intrauterine week of life, giving rise to the primitive lung buds. These lung buds continue to bifurcate dichotomously, resulting in the formation of the bronchi and smaller airways.[67] It has been postulated that bronchogenic cysts develop after the fourth intrauterine week of life, from supernumerary lung buds that arise from the primitive airways after separation of the trachea from the esophagus by the esophagotracheal septum.[65,67] They can be intrapulmonary or extrapulmonary.[67] Intrapulmonary cysts result from abnormal branches of the bronchial tree that remain attached to the bronchial wall during embryogenesis and become enveloped by the developing lung parenchyma. Extrapulmonary cysts result from abnormal buds that lose contact with the airways during embryogenesis. They remain in the mediastinum and gradually increase in size as a result of the secretions of the cyst epithelium into a closed cavity.

Bronchogenic cysts are spherical, cystic, and usually unilocular.[65,67] They can be loculated or multiple and usually measure only a few centimeters in diameter. Some cysts may expand and reach a diameter of 15 to 20 cm. Grossly, bronchogenic cysts characteristically have thin walls with trabeculated inner surfaces (Fig. 44-20). Histologically they are lined

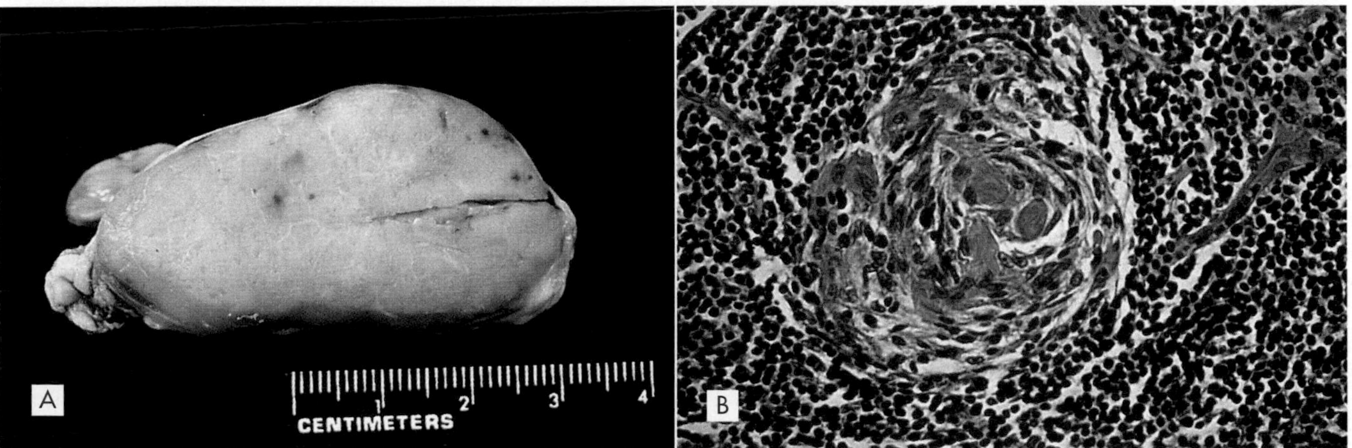

Fig. 44-19 A, Castleman's disease of the mediastinum (angiofollicular hyperplasia) presenting as a nodular mass. **B,** Castleman's disease of the mediastinum. The photomicrograph shows a lymphoid follicle with multiple proliferating capillaries, characteristic of the lesion. A small vessel is seen entering the lymphoid follicle *(right)*.

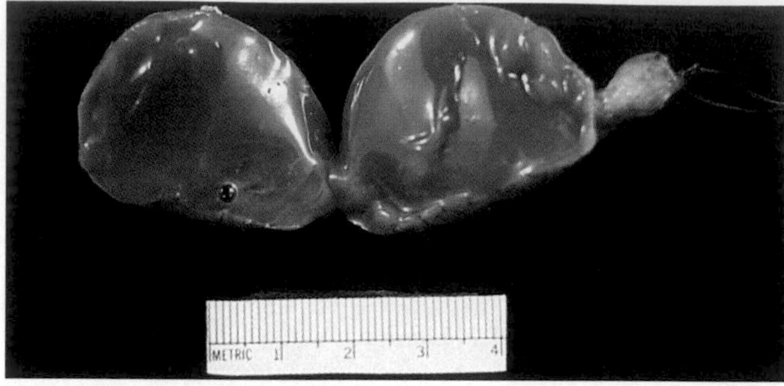

Fig. 44-20 Bronchogenic cyst of the mediastinum.

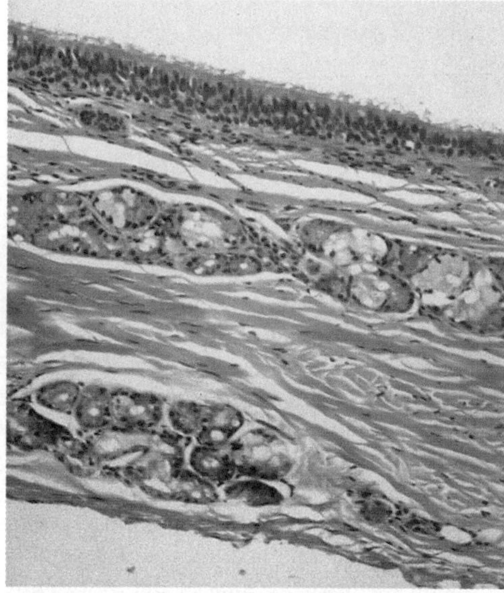

Fig. 44-21 Bronchogenic cyst of the mediastinum lined by respiratory type of epithelium with bronchial type glands.

by pseudostratified, ciliated respiratory epithelium with bronchial glands, smooth muscle, connective tissue, and cartilage in the lamina propria[76] (Fig. 44-21, *A*). In focal areas the epithelium can undergo squamous metaplasia, or it can become attenuated into a simple flattened epithelial layer. Bronchogenic cysts are benign lesions amenable to surgical resection. Malignant transformation is very unusual.[64]

Thymic cysts

Cysts of the thymus are usually congenital lesions that result from cystic degeneration of Hassall's corpuscles. They are found in patients of all ages and represent approximately 1% of mediastinal masses. Pathologically they present as multiloculated cysts lined by a thin fibrous wall with focal calcification. They contain clear or bloody material in the lumen. Histologically they are lined by flattened, columnar, cuboidal, ciliated, or stratified epithelium and are characterized by the presence of thymic tissue in the cyst wall.[76] These benign lesions are readily cured by surgery.

Esophageal cysts

Esophageal cysts derived from primitive foregut are less frequent than bronchogenic cysts, even though these cysts are embryologically closely related to each other. Esophageal cysts are usually found in patients under 20 years of age and are more common in males. In newborns they can be associated with other congenital anomalies such as tracheoesophageal fistulas.[65,67]

Esophageal cysts are unilocular and round and have mucus material in their lumens.[65,67] They are located in the esophageal wall or in the mediastinum immediately adjacent to the esophagus. Histologically the cyst wall is lined predominantly by nonkeratinizing, stratified squamous epithelium; it can also exhibit areas of pseudostratified ciliated epithelium. The cyst wall has a lamina propria with a muscularis propria, esophageal type of glands, and a muscularis propria composed of two well-defined layers of smooth muscle.[67,76]

The pathologic distinction between bronchogenic and esophageal cysts can be difficult because of similarities in location and morphology. Bronchogenic cysts can be attached to the esophageal wall during development and are occasionally found within the esophageal wall.[65,76] The presence of cartilage in a cyst wall in the absence of a well-defined muscularis propria composed of two layers of smooth muscle strongly supports the diagnosis of bronchogenic cyst. Clinical symptoms caused by esophageal cysts are similar to those caused by bronchogenic cysts.

Tracheoesophageal cysts

Tracheoesophageal cysts are rare mediastinal lesions that exhibit mixed features of bronchogenic and esophageal cysts.[67,76] They are lined by squamous epithelium and ciliated columnar epithelium and can have esophageal glands, cartilage, or two layers of smooth muscle in the cyst wall. These cysts probably result from partially obliterated tracheoesophageal fistulas that continue growing slowly after birth.[67,76]

Occasionally, developmental mediastinal cysts cannot be categorized with certainty. Some lesions lack a clear relationship to either the airways or the esophagus and are lined by a simple, ciliated, columnar epithelium without cartilage or a muscularis propria in the cyst wall. These cysts probably develop during early embryogenesis before the generation of the esophagus or the airways.

Gastroenteric cysts

Gastroenteric cysts are unusual lesions of the posterior mediastinum typically associated with vertebral abnormalities.[76,80] They have been reported under various names such as "gastric cysts," "foregut duplications" and "esophageal duplications."[76,81,82] They are more frequent in males and are usually diagnosed in infancy. Approximately 60% of patients are infants younger than 1 year of age. Gastroenteric cysts usually present as large, spherical, unilocular lesions that are frequently attached to the vertebral column by fibrous strands. The cyst wall is pink-grey and thin. The lumen contains clear, bloody, or yellow-green fluid. Histologically the cyst is lined by a gastric, ciliated-columnar, respiratory, squamous, small intestinal, large intestinal, or duodenal epithelium. Gastric mucosa with fundic (body) gland epithelium is the most common component. The cyst wall also has a lamina propria and a submucosa, separated by a muscularis mucosa. The muscularis propria is composed of two to three distinct layers of smooth muscle; sympathetic ganglion cells and nerves are frequently found in this muscularis propria.

Gastroenteric cysts are benign lesions that usually present with pain and signs of compression of mediastinal and thoracic structures. Occasionally they cause acute mediastinitis. They are usually cured by surgical excision. To our knowledge, no malignant transformation has been reported.

Pericardial and mesothelial cysts

Pericardial and mesothelial cysts are relatively common congenital lesions of the mediastinum that have been described under various names, such as "spring water cysts," "hydrocele of the mediastinum," "mesothelial cysts," "cardiophrenic angle cysts," and "pleural cysts of the mediastinum."[76,83,84] They are best classified as pericardial cysts when they are attached to the pericardium and as mesothelial cysts when they are encountered in other mediastinal locations. Pericardial cysts probably develop from persistent segments of the pericardial ventral-parietal recess that fail to establish contact with the pericardial cavity during embryogenesis.[85] Pericardial cysts also can be acquired after pericarditis.[86] Mesothelial cysts develop as a result of a developmental abnormality of the pleuroperitoneal coelom or the dorsal recesses of the pericardial coelom.

Pericardial and mediastinal mesothelial cysts are most often diagnosed in adults, with a peak incidence in the fourth to fifth decades. No sex predilection has been described.[64] Approximately half of the patients are asymptomatic at the time of initial diagnosis. The others present with cough, dyspnea, and other signs of compression of mediastinal structures.[67] Pericardial and mesothelial cysts are spherical, unilocular, seldom multilocular, lesions that can measure up to 30 cm in diameter. Their thin walls are semitranslucent; their lumens contain clear, watery fluid (Fig. 44-22, *A*). Histologically, these cysts are lined by a single layer of cuboidal or flattened epithelial cells with an underlying connective tissue stroma, which can contain rare, smooth muscle fibers (Fig. 44-22, *B*).

Pericardial and mesothelial cysts are benign lesions that are cured by surgical drainage or excision. They are not known to undergo malignant transformation.

Thoracic duct cysts

Thoracic duct cysts are unusual mediastinal lesions; most are found at autopsy.[76,87] They are classified as degenerative or lymphangiomatous thoracic duct cysts. The more common degenerative variety is usually encountered incidentally at autopsy of elderly women. The cyst wall and the remainder of the thoracic duct appear thickened, fibrotic, and calcified.[88] Lymphangiomatous cysts occur in younger individuals in their fourth to fifth decades of life. They present as single or multiple spaces filled with chyle.[76,89] They can have a distinct connection with the thoracic duct and are probably caused by congenital weakness of the thoracic duct wall, with progressive dilatation of its lumen and aneurysmal formation resulting in cyst formation.

Other mediastinal cysts

Hydatid cysts caused by the larval stage of the dog tapeworm *(Echinococcus granulosus),* and a few patients with pancreatic pseudocyst extending into the mediastinum have been described.[90-95] Patients with pancreatic pseudocyst usually have a history of previous pancreatitis and are found to have pleural effusion, a pancreatic mass, and a posterior mediastinum cyst.

Mesenchymal tumors

Mesenchymal tumors are unusual in the thorax, accounting for fewer than 10% of all mediastinal masses (Table 44-8). Unusual examples of practically all histopathologic variants of

Table 44-8 Mesenchymal tumors of the mediastinum

Benign	Malignant
Lymphangioma	Malignant hemangioendothelioma
Hemangioma	Malignant fibrous histiocytoma
Epithelioid hemangioendothelioma	Liposarcoma
	Leiomyosarcoma
Hemangiopericytoma	Synovial sarcoma
Lipoma	Osteogenic sarcoma
Lipomatosis	Chondrosarcoma
Leiomyoma	Granulocytic sarcoma
Rhabdomyoma	Others
Chondroma	
Solitary fibrous tumors	
Myxoma	
Meningioma	
Others	

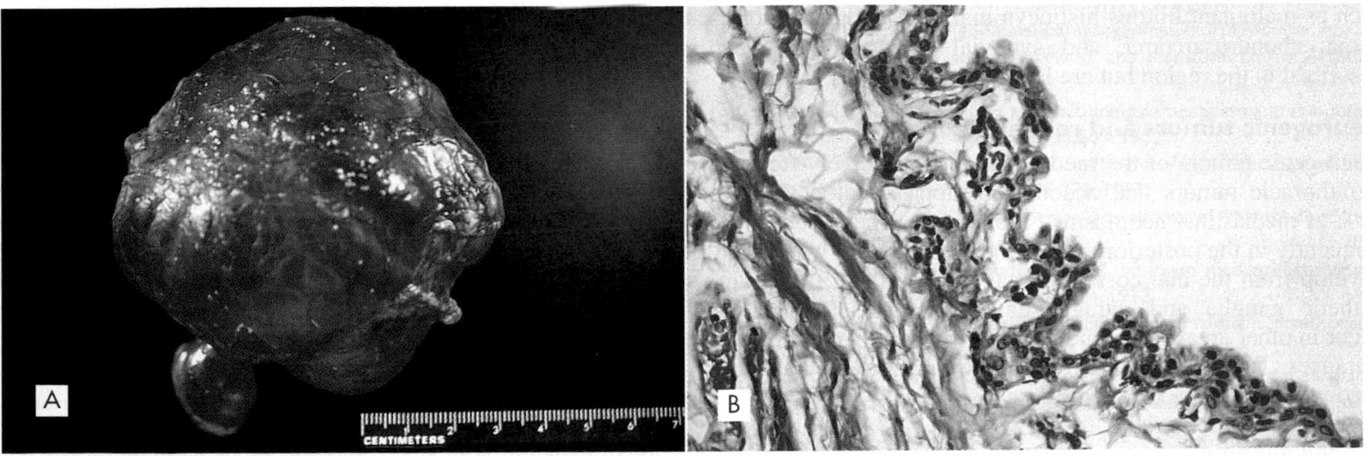

Fig. 44-22 A, Pericardial cyst. The large lesion is uniloculated and filled with clear, watery fluid. **B,** Pericardial cyst lined by mesothelial cells with small round nuclei and amphophilic cytoplasm.

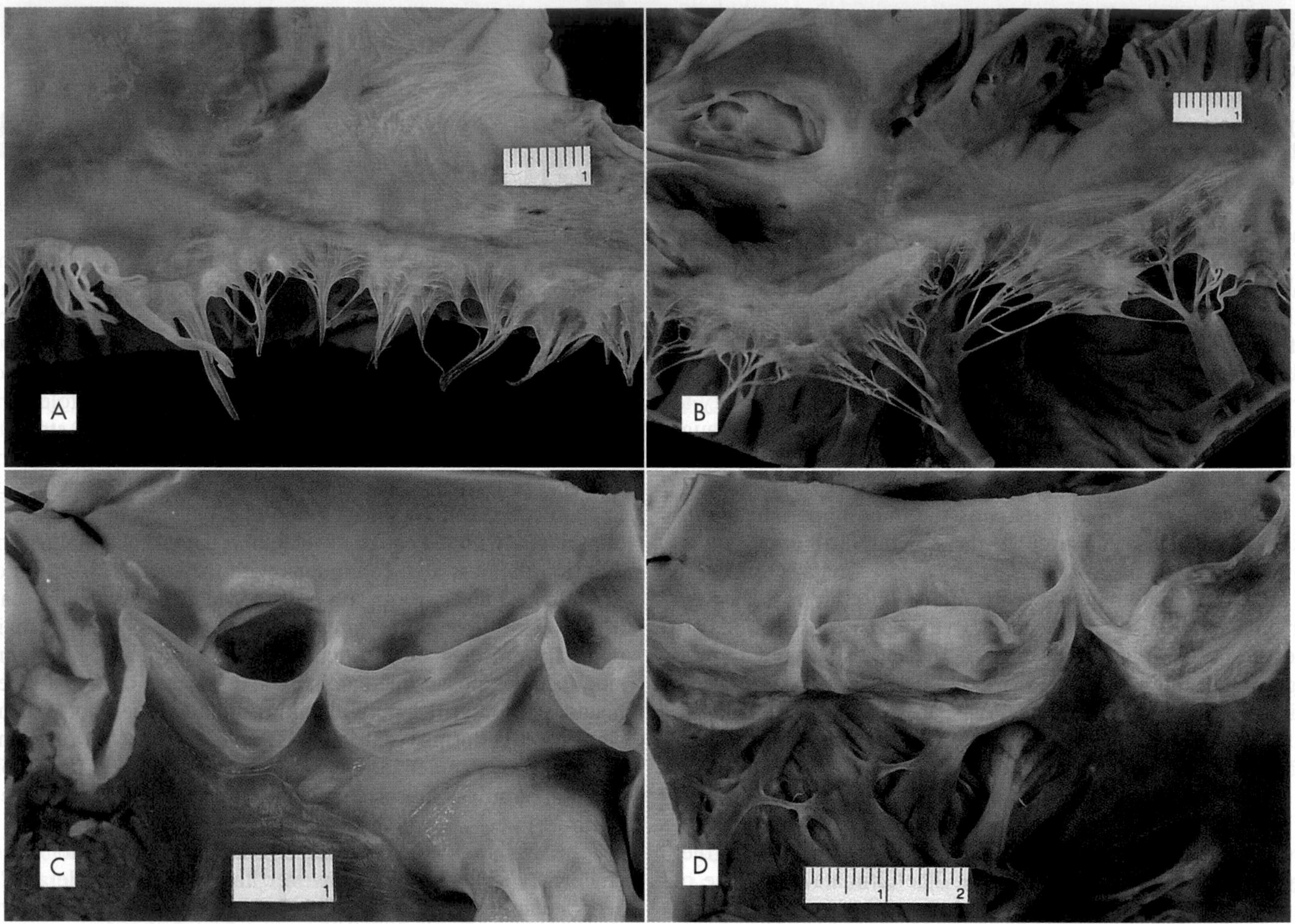

Fig. 45-1 Representative examples of structurally normal adult cardiac valves. **A,** Mitral valve. The opened mitral valve is not so delicate as the tricuspid valve, either in leaflet or chordal constituency. However, there is no hooding or redundancy and an appearance of uniformity of coloration and texture. As often noted, one or two of the chordae tendineae attached to the anterior leaflet *(leftward)* are thicker than the remaining chordae. The open left atrium is seen superiorly. **B,** Tricuspid valve. The delicate, virtually transparent nature of the normal tricuspid valve leaflet is depicted, as well as the fine, thin chordae tendineae. The prominent chordal attachment to multiple (anterior, posterior, and septal) papillary muscles is also depicted. Superior and to the left, the fossa ovalis and underlying coronary sinus orifice are seen. **C,** Aortic valve. The three-cusped aortic valve has somewhat more prominent and distinct nodules of Arantius than the pulmonic valve. As well, the leaflets are translucent but somewhat thicker and the definition of the sinotubular junction is more discrete. Indeed, in this photograph there is a small fibrofatty plaque at the superior border of the sinotubular junction overlying the right sinus of Valsalva. The fibrous continuity of the anterior leaflet of the mitral valve with the aortic valve is depicted in the lower right of the image. **D,** Pulmonic valve. The three-cusped pulmonic valve has characteristic delicacy and thinness of the tissues with a slight appearance of cuspal redundancy.

by the ventricular septum, whereas the left cusp is continuous with the base of the anterior mitral leaflet. The sinuses of Valsalva are expanded reservoirs behind the cusps caudal to the sinotubular junction designed to provide a catchment for diastolic filling of the coronary arteries. Pulmonary valve characteristics are similar to those of the aortic valve except for the significant delicacy of the pulmonary structures.

Histologically the base of mitral leaflet attachment is invested in bundles of cardiac myocytes. The atrialis begins basally with a prominent, discontinuous layer of smooth muscle cells arranged in tight aggregates. Within this region there are prominent elastic fibrils that decrease in number toward the midportion of the leaflet and are even less dense and organized toward the free margin. A membrane-like band of connective tissue underlies the surface endothelium of the atrialis and is thicker than a typical basement membrane. In the region of thickening related to leaflet apposition, variable swirls of dense collagenized tissue and loose cellular zones are present. The spongiosa is narrow relative to the thickness of the atrialis or ventricularis and has less dense connective tissue elements with slightly more mesenchymal cells, most of which are immunohistochemically and ultrastructurally consistent with myofibroblasts. They are elongate, neuroid to polygonal, and are termed *valvular interstitial cells* (VICs). These large, branching mesenchymal cells with large oval nuclei, morphologically consistent with VICs, are found in normal leaflets.

The ventricularis is a well-organized, sheath-like layer of laminar collagen, and over the basal half of the leaflets there is a discrete subendothelial elastin membrane. Rare small vessels are found at the base of attachment; some are muscular arteries, whereas others are venous or lymphatic structures. Chordae have a dense collagenized, tendinous structural core with a thin, overlying loose connective tissue and covering endothelium. The superficial connective tissue layer contains a small but distinct amount of elastin.

Normal aortic valve cusps have similar microscopic architectural features as mitral valve leaflets. The elastotic layer is more prominent on the ventricular aspect of the cusps, and small aggregates of macrophage-like mononuclear cells are present in the base of attachment to the aortic wall or myocardium. Tricuspid valve leaflets are a delicate rendition of mitral valve leaflets, and they are approximately one third to one half as thick. Otherwise, the approximate trilaminar structure is comparable.

Acute rheumatic fever and rheumatic heart disease

Definition, etiology, and clinical presentation. Acute rheumatic fever is a systemic, nonsuppurative, inflammatory disease that affects the tendons, joints, fasciae, muscles, arteries, subcutaneous tissue, connective tissues, serous membranes, lungs, brain, and heart. Primary sequelae of rheumatic fever include arthritis, chorea, and carditis, either in combination or isolation. Cardiac complications, grouped under the nomenclature of *rheumatic heart disease* (RHD), constitute the most enduring and potentially devastating lesions associated with acute rheumatic fever.

Migratory polyarthritis, subcutaneous nodules, erythema marginatum, and Sydenham's chorea are the chief extracardiac symptoms and signs. Additional criteria (according to Jones[3]) such as joint pain (arthralgia), fever, or a previous history of rheumatic fever or rheumatic heart disease, may help to confirm a diagnosis of rheumatic fever when only one of the major manifestations of the disease is present in a given patient. In isolation, these minor criteria may not necessarily point to rheumatic disease. Extracardiac features of acute rheumatic fever may be present to varying degrees of severity over the course of the illness; they do not result in lasting deformity or damage and normally disappear with or without treatment. Cardiac injury, by contrast, can be highly destructive; RHD disease, often impinging on the heart over several decades, remains the primary cause of acquired valvular heart disease in the world.[4]

The myocardium, pericardium, and endocardium are involved in approximately half of all cases of acute rheumatic fever.[4] Myocarditis is the most common affliction; however, diseases of the endocardium, either parietal or valvular, are the most serious. Valvulitis, associated with rheumatic endocarditis, is the most devastating cardiac lesion resulting from acute rheumatic fever, since it is rarely confined to the endocardium but instead affects the entire valve including chordae tendineae. Unlike myocarditis and pericarditis, endocarditis typically results in chronic heart disease.[5]

The majority of valvular diseases attributed to RHD involve the mitral valve. Almost all mitral valve stenoses and a significant proportion of insufficient mitral valves have their origin in rheumatic disease. Aortic valves, too, are commonly affected. RHD rarely attacks pulmonary or tricuspid valves in isolation, though multivalvular disease involving these valves is not uncommon.

Only in the past few years have scientists managed to approach a consensus on the etiology of acute rheumatic fever. The involvement of group A streptococci in acute rheumatic fever has been definitively confirmed. Although the primary etiologic factor[6] has been identified, the precise mechanisms by which it initiates rheumatic fever remain elusive. Over the past century, additional causes, such as viral infections[7,8] trauma, fatigue, cold[6] and genetic and environmental factors, acting either in isolation or in combination with Streptoccocus pyogenes, are proposed as possible instigators of disease. Few, if any, of the hypotheses regarding complicating factors in the development of rheumatic fever have been discarded entirely. Recent advances in research, however, have resulted in the positive identification of particular M-protein serotypes, which are believed to be primary markers of rheumatogenic potential in virulent strains of streptococci. Future exploration of the M-protein serotypes may enable clarification as to which of the apparently rheumatogenic strains are best able to elicit rheumatic fever.

Difficulties inherent in resolving the enigmatic etiology of rheumatic fever have preoccupied investigators since the early seventeenth century[9]; in recent years, an additional problem has arisen over difficulty in consistently recognizing symptoms and signs. As progress in understanding and proper application of public health measures accelerated, particularly over the last few decades, the incidence of rheumatic fever in developed countries declined dramatically. As a result, many physicians trained in the 1970s and 1980s and practicing in the Western world are not fully acquainted with the essential signs and symptoms of acute rheumatic fever and RHD.[9-13]

The Jones criteria for the clinical identification of rheumatic fever and RHD, first published in 1944, have been revised several times, with the most recent revision in 1992 being sponsored by the American Heart Association[3] (Table 45-1). Serial revisions have received varying degrees of criti-

Table 45-1 Guidelines for the diagnosis of initial attack of rheumatic fever; Jones criteria* (1992 update[3])

Major manifestations
Carditis
Polyarthritis
Chorea (Sydenham's chorea)
Erythema marginatum
Subcutaneous nodules
Minor manifestations
Clinical findings
Arthralgia
Fever
Laboratory findings
Elevated acute phase reactions
Erythrocyte sedimentation rate
C-reactive protein
Prolonged PR interval
Supporting evidence of antecedent group A streptococcal infections
Positive throat culture or rapid streptococcal antigen test
Elevated or rising streptococcal antibody titer

*If supported by evidence of preceding group A streptococcal infection, the presence of two major manifestations or of one major and two minor manifestations indicates a high probability of acute rheumatic fever.

cism over the years[6,9,14,15]; however, the changes made in the original document stand in themselves as testimony to advances toward understanding the disease process. At the same time, vigilant revisions of identification criteria cannot fully accommodate the diversity of symptoms with which the disease may present in any particular patient. As Bisno has pointed out,[6] acquaintance with the "clinical personality" of the disease must accompany an understanding of the Jones criteria, which enable users only to rule out rheumatic fever. They don't exclude another disorder mimicking the disease.

Finally, presentations of the disease vary according to the severity of the attack, whether they are manifest in the patient as isolated or combined arthritis, carditis, or chorea. Arthritis is the most frequent manifestation, but again carditis, in both the acute and chronic phases of the disease, is the most serious.[10] Presentation of these sequelae are varied and differ greatly according to the additional lesions with which they are associated. Moreover, as several observers have noted, the dramatic decline in incidence of rheumatic fever in the West has been accompanied by a change in presentation of the disease.[6,16] As a result, the apparent infrequency with which acute rheumatic fever is found in the United States, Canada, and Western Europe may be attributable in part to the problem of recognizing new or altered representations of the disease, but, at the same time, its decreased incidence exaggerates the difficulty of routine identification.

Scope and epidemiology. The geographical occurrence and historical incidence of acute rheumatic fever remains one of the most important aspects of the disease. Although the number of patients diagnosed with rheumatic fever has declined dramatically in North America and developed nations worldwide in the second half of the twentieth century, economically depressed regions, particularly in Asia, Central and South America, and Africa, have continued to suffer a greater burden from the disease. Efforts by international agencies like the World Health Organization in those regions with poor public health have initiated a perceptible decline of the disease.[17] Nevertheless, rheumatic fever and rheumatic heart disease continue to be the most common causes of acquired cardiac dysfunction and death in underdeveloped countries.

It is generally agreed that the higher incidence of acute rheumatic fever in specific geographical regions is linked to socioeconomic factors and is not associated with climate.[18,21] Greater population density, poverty, inadequate living conditions, undernourishment and malnutrition, close person-to-person contact, and restricted access to medical aid are believed to contribute to the prevalence of the acute rheumatic fever in areas where these conditions are commonplace.

Other issues, such as age, sex, race, and heredity, appear to differ in their individual importance as potential predisposing factors. However, children 6 to 15 years of age are the most frequently afflicted with acute rheumatic fever.[22] The disease is uncommon in children younger than 5 years old. Initial onset of rheumatic fever in adulthood is a rare but well-documented event.[14,23-26] At one time, rheumatic fever was believed to occur more frequently in women than in men, though current views reject this claim.[27] It is important, however, to note that specific valvular diseases resulting from RHD may demonstrate sex predilection. Studies of race-related differences in the incidence of rheumatic fever have pointed to a higher frequency of disease in nonwhites.[28] These discrepancies are believed to be the product of socioeconomic and environmental factors and not an indication of true racial predisposition.[9,29] The issues of heredity and genetics and their relative roles in the epidemiology of rheumatic fever have not been resolved, though several reports note an increased susceptibility to rheumatic fever within families.[6,9,30-33]

Although continued improvements in public health may be important, a variety of theories have been proposed to explain the dramatic decrease in incidence of rheumatic fever and RHD over the past 40 years in Western nations. For certain, the phenomenon is attributed in part to the amelioration of living standards and health care, most notably in the United States, Canada, Britain, and Japan. Advances in medicine, commencing with the introduction of sulfonamide prophylaxis (for secondary rheumatic attacks) in the 1930s and ultimately the discovery and application of penicillin therapy in the 1940s and, more specifically, benzathine penicillin G in the 1950s[34] are believed to have greatly accelerated the decline of disease. Current data indicate that natural mutations occurring within streptococcal bacteria may also have assisted in restricting the disease. Several authors report that strains of group A streptococci prevalent in the United States in recent decades have not demonstrated high rheumatogenicity.[35-37]

Given the virtual eradication of acute rheumatic fever over the last half century, its "resurgence" in the United States in the past 10 years[10,11,31,38,39] was totally unexpected (Fig. 45-2). Although the number of cases reported is nowhere near the figures recorded before and during the Second World War, the sudden return of the disease has drawn considerable attention within the health professions. Particularly significant is that a large proportion of the patients described are from relatively affluent backgrounds in suburban and rural areas. For a disease long associated with impoverished living conditions and the overcrowding of inner cities, its appearance among a population with better access to healthcare and a lower risk of hygiene-associated infection was utterly unforeseen.

One explanation is that, as the incidence of rheumatic fever dropped to insignificant levels throughout the Western world, hospitals and practitioners became less rigorous in their man-

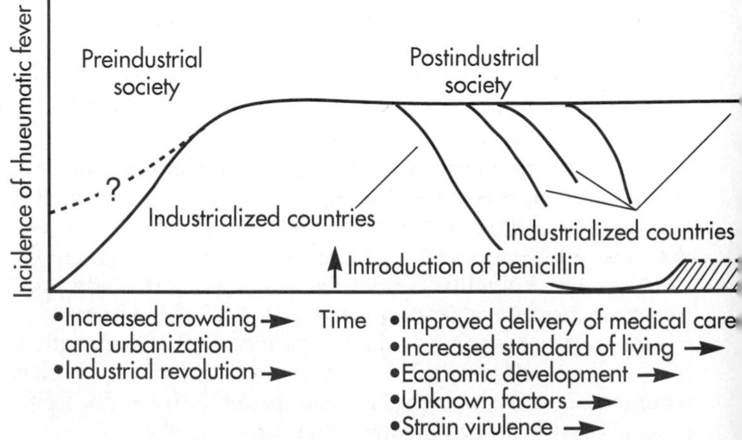

Fig. 45-2 Chronology of changes in the incidence of rheumatic fever in industrializing and industrialized countries as influenced by changes in standard of living and delivery of primary health care, and by the introduction of antibiotics into clinical medicine. The hatched area under the curve *(right)* reflects the recent recrudescence of rheumatic fever in industrial and postindustrial societies. (From Kaplan EL: *Circulation* 88:1964, 1993.)

agement and prophylaxis of streptococcal pharyngitis. Bisno notes that present-day postinfection therapy, typically consisting of 10 days of oral penicillin V, is not nearly as comprehensive or effective as the stringent methods used in the past.[31] Therapy used to include intramuscular benzathine penicillin G, in addition to the procurement of throat cultures, both from the patient after treatment (to verify that the bacteria had been eliminated) and from family contacts (to rule out further infection).[31] Moreover, because many physicians are unfamiliar with the primary symptoms of rheumatic fever, patients potentially at high risk of developing rheumatic fever after streptococcal infection are not treated accordingly. Thus resumption of more meticulous practices with regard to diagnosis and treatment of acute streptococcal infections may help to limit the further reemergence of the disease.

Several researchers have pointed out, however, that relaxation on prophylaxis and lack of proper diagnosis cannot fully account for all the new patients with rheumatic fever reported since 1984. Of all patients ultimately diagnosed with acute rheumatic fever, only one third to one half[9] do not have a history of streptococcal infection. Others can recall experiencing sore throats for which they never sought medical attention. In either scenario, the subsequent onset of rheumatic fever is not associated with a deficiency in medical acumen.

A second theory, currently dominating the study of rheumatic disease, is based on the premise of strain mutation, previously used to explain the decline of acute rheumatic fever. Recent data indicate that the resurgence of acute rheumatic fever may have been matched by the simultaneous emergence of new, highly virulent serotypes of group A streptococcal bacteria.[38] Other studies report a concomitant resurgence of particular rheumatogenic strains of group A streptococci; the highly mucoid M types[1,3,5,6,18] are among the strains described.[9,40] The precise manner in which these particular strains are able to elicit rheumatic fever remains unclear. It is likely that specific changes in the rheumatogenic potential of particular strains, occurring at a time when the medical profession has somewhat relaxed its vigilance over the symptoms of rheumatic fever, have produced the current revival of disease.

Pathology. Pathologic effects of acute rheumatic fever are concentrated in the connective tissues, primarily those of the heart, skin, and joints, though additional organs may also be affected. Proliferative inflammation is usually conspicuous in these sites. Although the course of illness in acute rheumatic fever is relatively short, rarely lasting 4 months, recurrent attacks are common. Extracardiac features of acute rheumatic fever have been well documented elsewhere[9,41]

Rheumatic heart disease, rheumatic valvular disease in particular, results from chronic damage to the heart. When death follows an initial attack of rheumatic fever, the cardiac valves may appear largely unaffected at autopsy. By contrast, heart valves in chronic RHD are radically disfigured and scarred.[42] As a pancarditis, acute rheumatic fever affects the "layers" of the heart in different ways and to varying degrees.

PERICARDIUM. Pericarditis is normally the least serious lesion associated with acute rheumatic fever, typically reflecting the effects of an acute, nonspecific inflammatory infiltrate on the serous membranes including ample fibrin. Unlike the endocardium and myocardium, the pericardium is much more likely to repair itself fully after injury without lasting sequelae.[43]

In rheumatic pericarditis, the surface of the heart may appear slightly reddened or, in more severe cases, display a dense, shaggy exudate with adhesions, the so-called cor villosum, or 'shaggy heart.' The latter state is typical of patients suffering from repeated rheumatic attacks. Development of chronic pericarditis depends largely on the degree of thickening and adhesion—resulting from abundant fibrin and edema—within the pericardial layers, or between the pericardium and neighboring extracardiac structures.

Microscopic examination of rheumatic pericarditis reveals accumulation of fibrin, plasma cells, lymphocytes, histiocytes, and, in rare cases, the presence of neutrophils. Arrays of fibroblasts and Aschoff cells are evident adjacent to areas with fibrinoid.

MYOCARDIUM. The gross pathologic features of severe rheumatic myocarditis include a globular heart and ventricular cavity enlargement. Small, grossly visible fibrous scars, identifiable in late-stage chronic RHD, are suggestive that areas of active inflammation including Aschoff bodies evolve to scar as the inflammatory process subsides.

Aschoff bodies are the most telling histologic lesions of rheumatic myocarditis (Fig. 45-3). They are most dramatic in their granulomatous state, normally reached 3 to 4 weeks after the onset of acute rheumatic fever. Aschoff nodules are found in the interstitial tissue of the myocardium and may also be prominent in the subendocardial connective tissue. They rarely occur in the valves. Aschoff cells, multinucleated giant cells, may be as large as 1 mm in diameter. They are typically found in the ventricular septum, LV free wall, and left atrial free wall.[44] Aschoff bodies may be arrayed in a roughly linear fashion and are typically perivascular.

In the later stages of RHD mononuclear cells or multinucleated Aschoff cells are conspicuous throughout the interstitial tissue. Associated infiltrates include plasma cells, lymphocytes, histiocytes, and occasionally neutrophils. Additional muscle lesions, easily confused with Aschoff bodies, may develop as a result of parenchymal damage. Thus, degenerative or necrotic muscle tissue is normally surrounded by a variety of cells including cardiac histiocytes and multinucleated giant cells.[45]

ENDOCARDIUM. The most serious form of rheumatic endocarditis is *rheumatic valvulitis.* Endocarditis affecting the parietal (mural) endocardium is less common and rarely as devastating as the valvular lesions characteristic of chronic RHD. Parietal endocarditis is evident primarily in the free wall of the left atrium superior to the posterior mitral valve leaflet. The surface of the endocardium becomes discolored and furrowed as fibrosis heals, evolving over time to a thick, ridged gray-white plaque. Endocardial thickening, extensive formation of Aschoff bodies, and overlying thrombosis are common.

Valvular lesions resulting from RHD are discussed in detail in the section on mitral stenosis; however, several nonspecific pathologic features may be observed.

Verrucous endocarditis, constituted by tiny, translucent nodules, is the characteristic vegetation of RHD. Over time, nodules typically become more opaque, turning a tan-gray color. In comparison with the extensive and proliferative lesions typical of bacterial endocarditis, verrucous vegetations are minimal and normally confined to the lines of cuspal apposition. They rarely result in gross abnormality.[43] Vegetations may appear on the atrial surfaces of the atrioventricular (AV) valves or on the ventricular surfaces of the semilunar valves. Vegetations may also extend onto the left atrial parietal endo-

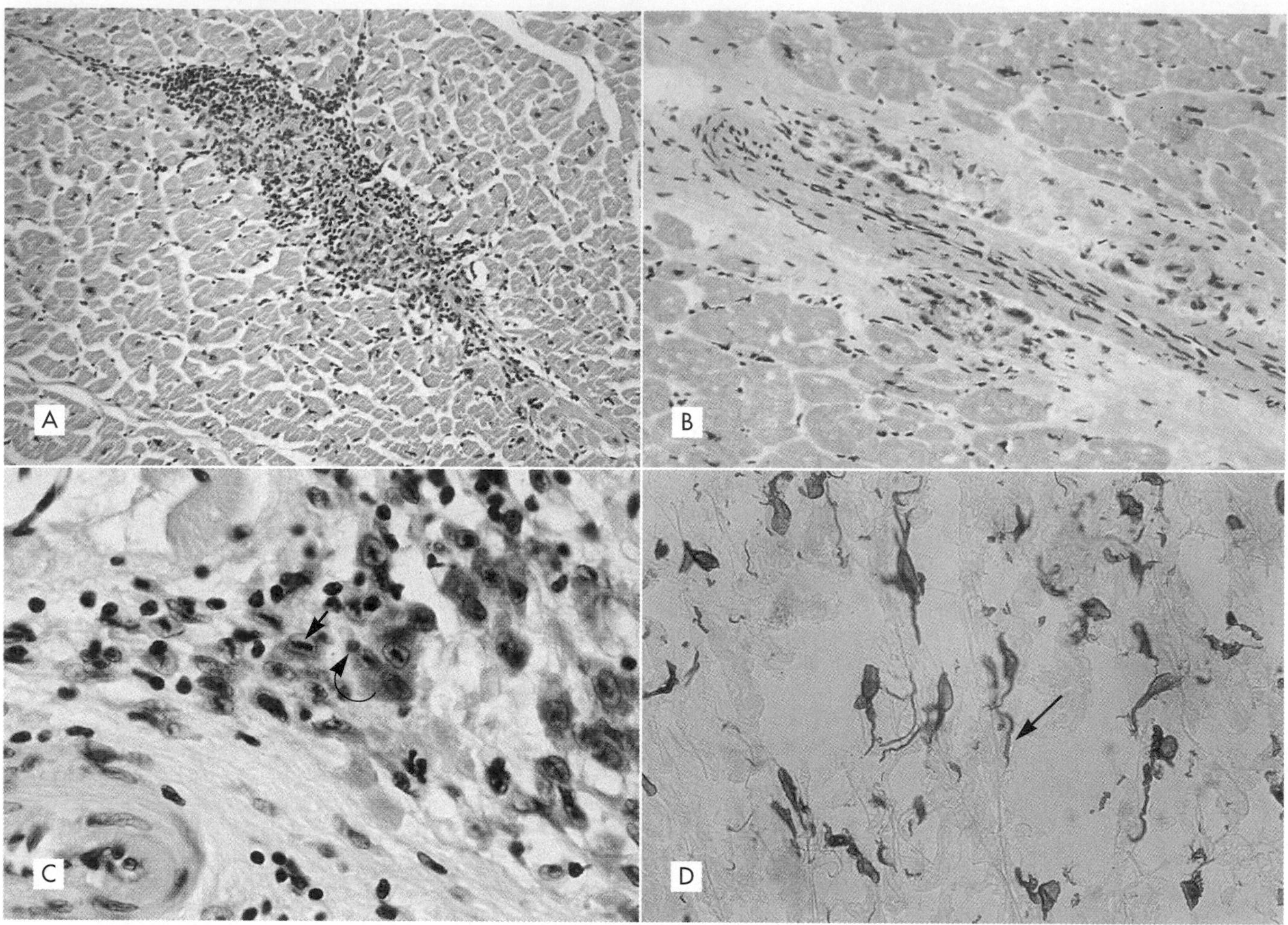

Fig. 45-3 **A,** Ventricular myocardium in active rheumatic carditis. Here, an active Aschoff lesion includes numerous histiocytes surrounded by lymphocytes. This collection of cells is in an interstitial plane and in a perivascular distribution. Rheumatic carditis tends to be interstitial. **B,** The Aschoff bodies or lesions are adjacent to a small longitudinally cut intramural artery of the myocardium. A variety of large cells are noted in the perivascular lesions, including those with characteristics of Anichkov's cells. Small amounts of fibrinous material are present in these perivascular aggregates, an indication that these lesions are subacute. No vasculitis is evident. **C,** An Aschoff lesion with caterpillar cells *(arrow),* owl's eye cells *(curved arrow),* and associated lymphocytes. This edematous, active lesion was found in an explanted heart with active rheumatic carditis. **D,** Valvular interstitial cells *(VICs)* are from mitral valve stained by immunoperoxidase technique for reactivity of antistreptococcal antibodies. These cells are vividly positive and have numerous long and unusual cytoplasmic projections *(arrow).* They are probably the matrix-producing cells in proliferative processes of heart valves.

cardium and, in rare instances, onto the chordae tendineae or papillary muscles. Verrucous vegetations usually form in rows and clusters, though they may occur as isolated lesions. Resolution of vegetations typically results in thickening of the cusp and partial or total obliteration of valve commissures. The mitral valve is the most common site for verrucous endocarditis, though the aortic valve, either in combination with the mitral valve or in isolation, is also frequently affected. Rheumatic vegetations involving the tricuspid and pulmonary valves are rare.

Microscopic investigation of rheumatic endocarditis reveals lymphocyte infiltration throughout the endocardium. The primary microscopic features of RHD within the endocardium are edema and swelling of the valve cusps. Cusp vascularization appears within days of the initial illness, and, within 6 to 8 weeks, thick-walled muscular arteries and arterioles develop. These arterioles are most prominent in the region of attachment of the root of a cusp. Evidence of inflammation or necrosis of connective tissue is often found underlying verrucous clusters. Neutrophils, plasma cells, and fibroblasts may be present. Severe rheumatic endocarditis is punctuated by the appearance of Aschoff bodies within the valves or by necrosis of valvular collagen or rupture of the chordae tendineae.

Pathobiology. Acute rheumatic fever typically has its onset within 6 weeks after untreated β-hemolytic group A streptococcal infection and may present as early as 10 days after infection.[27] Only 1% to 3%[46,47] of all streptococcal infections lead to rheumatic fever.

Researchers postulate that the link between streptococcal infection and rheumatic fever is an immune response, after a period in which the streptococcal organism colonizes and proliferates in the oropharyngeal mucosa of a susceptible host.

Significant immunologic abnormalities develop during the time separating the initial sore throat and streptococcal infection from the development of acute rheumatic fever.

The precise mechanisms by which acute rheumatic fever develops in a susceptible host consequent to streptococcal infection have not been identified. The prevailing theory postulates that virulent streptococcal organisms, absorbed by the hypersensitive patient, bind with the connective tissues, provoking an immunologic reaction in the host. Several investigators have identified specific human tissue components that demonstrate immunologic cross-reactivity to group A streptococci, several of which are located within the heart or are closely associated with it.[48-51]

Early responses to streptococcal infection occur principally in the connective tissues, normally in the form of edema and increased acid mucopolysaccharides. Collagen fibers are parted and become progressively swollen, fragmented, and frayed. As the disease progresses, pathologic changes are dominated by infiltration of lymphocytes, plasma cells, histiocytes, and fibroblasts and proliferation of the Aschoff bodies as a hallmark of the granulomatous phase.

Mitral stenosis

Definition and clinical presentation. Rheumatic fever is by far the most common cause of mitral valve stenosis. Other causes are extremely rare; these include rheumatoid arthritis,[52] malignant metastatic carcinoid, systemic lupus erythematosus (SLE)[53] infective endocarditis,[54,55] calcification of the mitral annulus, atrial septal defect (as a component of Lutembacher syndrome,[56] Whipple's disease,[57] and amyloid deposits.[58] Bana and associates[59] and Misch[60] describe instances of mitral valve stenosis developing as a result of fibrous tissue deposition consequent to methysergide therapy. Mitral stenosis induced by deposition of ceramide trihexoside in Fabry's disease[61] or of mucopolysaccharides associated with the Hunter-Hurler[62] Hurler-Scheie,[27] and Maroteaux-Lamy[63,64] syndromes has also been reported. Left atrial tumors, myxomas in particular, impinging on left atrial outflow can simulate a stenotic mitral valve. Commissurotomy sites may heal with residual stenosis or even exaggerated stenosis.

Rheumatic disease is responsible for well over 90% of all mitral valve stenoses; however, only one half of patients diagnosed with such valve lesions provide a history of acute rheumatic fever.[54] Moreover, most individuals who develop stenotic mitral valves remain asymptomatic for long periods after an initial episode of rheumatic carditis.[54] The findings of Wood's study,[65] published in 1954, indicated an average latency period of 19 years between the onset of RHD and the manifestation of mitral stenosis. Rheumatic mitral stenosis, as with mitral valve diseases in general,[66] is preponderant in women.

Patients with stenotic mitral valves display progressive dyspnea on exertion as a result of diminished pulmonary compliance. Additional presentations may include acute pulmonary edema precipitated by pregnancy, febrile illness, sudden onset of atrial fibrillation,[67] emotional stress, sexual intercourse, or respiratory infection.[68] In advanced disease, right-sided heart failure may result. Mitral stenosis can be identified by a loud first heart sound, opening snap, or a diastolic rumble. The latter is often accompanied by apical presystolic accentuation. Complications typically accompanying mitral stenosis include hemoptysis, thromboembolism, and infective endocarditis. Infective endocarditis has also been reported to exacerbate preexisting mitral stenosis.[69]

Pathology. Mitral valve leaflets are directly affected by the initial episode of rheumatic carditis. At this time, tiny, translucent nodules form on the closure margin of the leaflets (Fig. 45-4). Entering its symptomatic phase, rheumatic mitral stenosis is characterized by diffuse thickening of the valve cusps, potentially accompanied by calcific deposits, which may in turn extend to and thereby rigidify the valve ring. As the disease progresses, the valve may assume a funnel-like shape and foster valve commissure fusion and chordae tendineae fusion, thickening, and retraction. Chordal fusion with or without shortening contributes to the "fishmouth" or "buttonhole" configuration of the valve orifice. Excessive adherence and rigidity in the valve leaflets can lead to reduction or, in exceptional instances, negation of normal leaflet excursion, producing combined mitral regurgitation and stenosis.

Microscopically, dense, nonuniformly layered collagenized connective tissue is diffusely present in all three layers of the thickened valve leaflets. Numbers of VICs in the leaflets are increased in the spongiosa.

Immunohistochemically, VICs, smooth muscle cells and endothelial cells in a rheumatic valve cross-react with anti-streptococcal monoclonal antibodies, 36.2.2, 49.8.9, and 54.2.8.[4] Such reactivity may reflect sites at which immune stimulation of cell growth or matrix synthesis can occur. Immune dysregulation of matrix production or turnover remains as one central hypothesis underlying valvular distortion and fibrosis after acute rheumatic fever.

Therapy. Given the often lengthy asymptomatic period typical of rheumatic mitral valve stenosis, controversy exists regarding the timing and necessity of intervention.[70] Normally, patients are viewed as requiring intervention when their symptoms have developed to a moderate level, that is, displaying paroxysmal nocturnal dyspnea, dyspnea and orthopnea, with or without pulmonary edema.[54] Both open mitral valve commissurotomy and percutaneous balloon valvuloplasty are used with comparable success[70] in the alleviation of pliable, noncalcific, nonregurgitative stenotic valves. When regurgitation is a factor, valve replacement is normally required. Despite the acclaim that has supported the use of balloon valvuloplasty since its advent in 1984 as an alternative to surgical methods, valve replacement is at times necessitated by the onset of mitral regurgitation occurring after valvular balloon dilatation.[71] A comparative study conducted by Röthlisberger and associates[72] in 1993 suggests that the incidence of regurgitation resulting from balloon valvuloplasty for mitral stenosis may be lower with the *Inoue* single-balloon method than with the double-balloon *Mansfield* technique.

Mitral insufficiency

Definition and clinical presentation. Although mitral valve regurgitation, like mitral valve stenosis, is most commonly linked to RHD, a significant percentage of regurgitative mitral valves can be attributed to nonrheumatic causes.[73] Of these, the most common include rupture of the chordae tendineae, ischemic papillary muscle dysfunction, mitral valve prolapse, and infective endocarditis.[73] Iatrogenic mitral regurgitation, subsequent to percutaneous balloon valvuloplasty for mitral stenosis, has been reported. Some researchers estimate that severe mitral regurgitation occurs in up to 15% of all patients

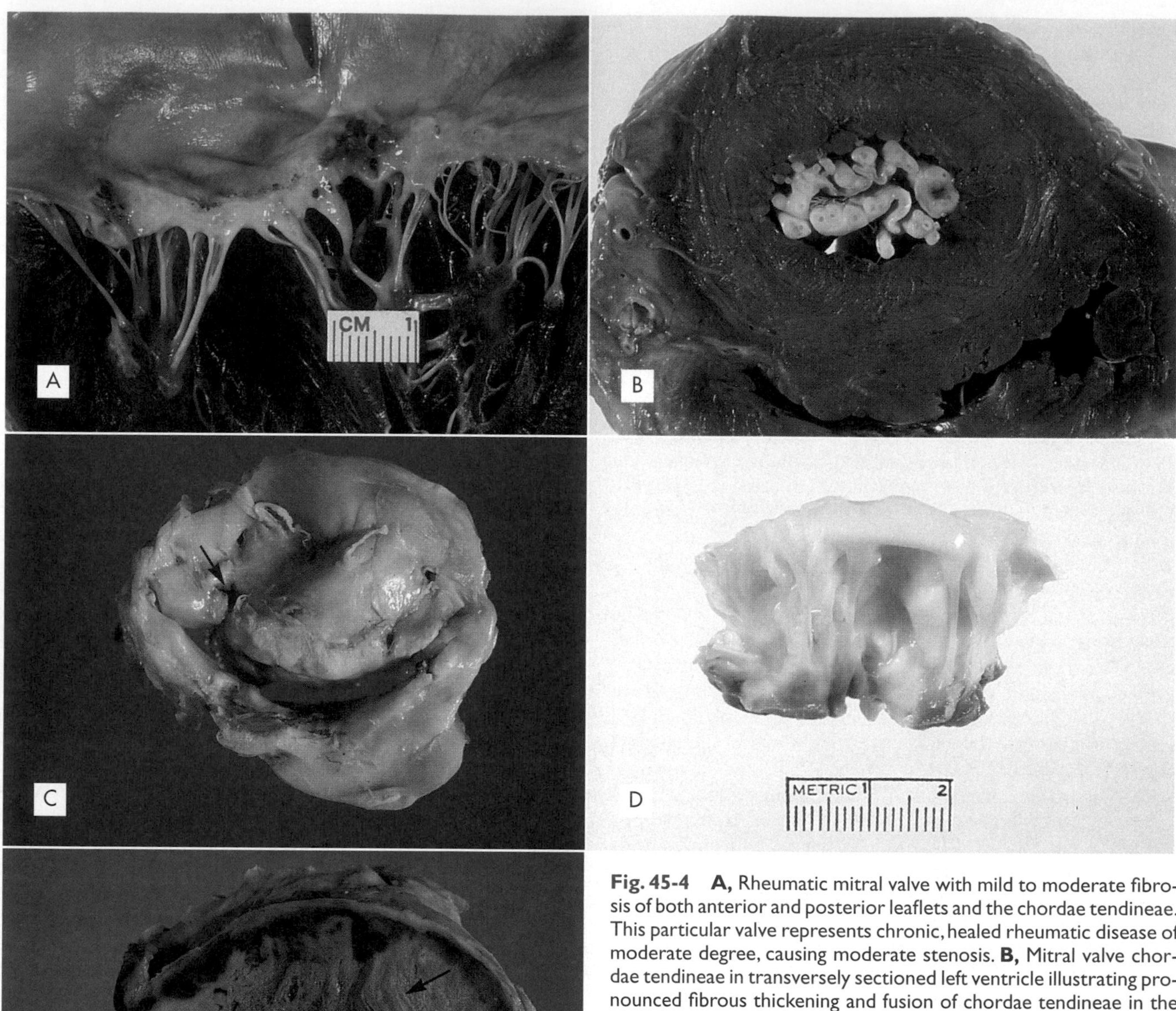

Fig. 45-4 **A,** Rheumatic mitral valve with mild to moderate fibrosis of both anterior and posterior leaflets and the chordae tendineae. This particular valve represents chronic, healed rheumatic disease of moderate degree, causing moderate stenosis. **B,** Mitral valve chordae tendineae in transversely sectioned left ventricle illustrating pronounced fibrous thickening and fusion of chordae tendineae in the setting of healed rheumatic mitral disease. There is circumferential left ventricular hypertrophy. The right ventricular cavity is to the lower right. **C,** Atrial view of an excised, severely fibrotic rheumatic mitral valve with previous commissurotomy site *(arrow)*. The valve is both stenotic and regurgitant. **D,** Transverse view of a rheumatic mitral valve with severe chordal fusion and thickening associated with diffuse leaflet fibrosis and projection of fibrous tissue onto the tips of the papillary muscles. **E,** Laminated, unorganized "ball" thrombus from left atrium is found in association with rheumatic mitral stenosis. Gross representation of lines of Zahn is quite obvious *(arrows)*. The site of atrial attachment is along the upper border.

who undergo balloon valvuloplasty for acquired mitral valve obstruction.[74-77]

The nature and severity of mitral regurgitation varies according to the nature of the disease impinging on the valve and the particular feature or region of the valve it affects. Rheumatic mitral regurgitation typically affects the mitral valve leaflets, chordae tendineae, and papillary muscles. Rheumatic fever may result in rupture of the chordae tendineae, though this may also occur spontaneously[78] or subsequent to floppy valve syndrome, connective tissue disorders (that is, the Marfan syndrome), chest trauma or surgery,[73] myocardial infarction, infective endocarditis, myxomatous proliferation, osteogenesis imperfecta, or nonspecific mechanical strain.[68]

Coronary artery disease (CAD) is the most common cause of ischemic papillary muscle dysfunction leading to mitral regurgitation, though papillary muscle "failure" may also result from severe anemia or shock[68] In the context of myocardial infarcts, necrosis of the papillary muscles and their subjacent free wall is common, often initiating a legacy of chronic mitral regurgitation. Dysfunction of the papillary muscles attributable to an inconstant blood supply may be transient, for example, during attacks of angina pectoris, producing temporary mitral regurgitation. Altered contractile capacity of the papillary muscles or rupture of all or part of a papillary muscle can also result in acute mitral regurgitation. Altered angulation of papillary muscles to nonparallel alignments as a result of ventricular dilatation is also important as a factor in mitral regurgitation.

Infective endocarditis, primarily associated with the valve leaflets, can lead to mitral regurgitation when the infection progresses to the point of destroying the leaflets or when vegetations prevent the leaflets from closing normally.[69]

Calcification of the mitral valve ring occurs idiopathically or secondary to aortic stenosis, systemic hypertension, diabetes mellitus, and Marfan or Hurler syndromes[68] Such deposits can lead to mitral regurgitation, normally only of significance in elderly patients.[68,79]

Presentation of symptomatic mitral regurgitation differs depending on whether the condition is acute or chronic. In acute cases, LV overload is sudden, resulting from abrupt disruption or failure of the valve. Patients typically present with pulmonary edema and pulmonary hypertension. It is important to note, however, that the symptoms displayed will differ greatly based on the cause of the sudden onset. In chronic mitral regurgitation, patients usually remain asymptomatic until LV failure occurs, a period potentially in excess of several decades.[80] Low cardiac input resulting in persistent weakness and fatigue are the chief symptoms of chronic mitral regurgitation.

Pathology. In chronic rheumatic mitral regurgitation, mitral valve cusps typically become thickened, retracted, fibrotic, and calcific. In combined mitral valve stenosis and regurgitation, chordae tendineae and papillary muscles may fuse and retract, preventing the leaflets from achieving normal closure during ventricular systole. In pure mitral regurgitation, by contrast, chordae tendineae may be characterized by elongation resulting in prolapse of the anterior or posterior mitral leaflets.[81] When mitral regurgitation results primarily from valve prolapse, the disease is characterized by thinning and elongation of chordae and valve leaflets, in accompaniment of their myxomatous degeneration. In infective endocarditis, vegetations proliferate primarily on the valve leaflets, thereby restricting leaflet closure. Isolated rupture of chordae tendineae is an obvious manifestation of endocarditic destruction and a cause of severe mitral regurgitation; sudden chordal rupture may also be associated with mitral valve prolapse. Incomplete or partial rupture of the chordae is normally reflected as chronic mitral regurgitation, though partial chordal destruction by endocarditic vegetations may also produce chronic mitral regurgitation. Pathologic processes producing mitral regurgitation as a result of papillary muscle dysfunction manifest chiefly as ischemic papillary muscle damage or necrosis. Partial or total rupture of the papillary muscle apical heads can produce severe mitral regurgitation. Total rupture of a papillary muscle normally results in sudden death.[80]

Therapy. Regurgitant mitral valves that are not excessively damaged, rigid, or fibrotic and are free from calcification are normally repaired or reconstructed through valvuloplasty. When mitral regurgitation has resulted from RHD (without calcification), floppy mitral valve syndrome, or ruptured chordae tendineae, valve repair is now a common therapeutic choice. When this is not possible, valve replacement is considered.[73]

At present, patients are considered for surgery when their symptoms are classified as NYHA (New York Heart Association) class III or IV.[73] However, debate surrounding the question of timing of intervention in progressively regurgitant valvular disease persists, comparable to controversy over the same issue pertinent to mitral stenosis. In mitral regurgitation, the asymptomatic phase is normally longer than that with mitral stenosis.[68] Indeed, patients with mild mitral regurgitation may remain asymptomatic their whole lives.[82]

Mitral valve prolapse

Definition and clinical presentation. Valve prolapse occurs primarily in the mitral valve, though associated tricuspid and aortic valve prolapses have been observed.[83,84] The syndrome has been described by various nomenclature, the more common being floppy valve syndrome, mitral valve prolapse, billowing or ballooning mitral valve syndrome, midsystolic click-murmur condition, and Reid's or Barlow's syndrome. Mild valve prolapse in humans is extremely common; 5% to 10% of the population are afflicted.[85,86] It is important to distinguish valve prolapse in general from the floppy valve syndrome, however. Most persons with prolapse are asymptomatic, never develop complications, and, indeed, never seek diagnosis. Cardiomyopathic processes, ischemic heart disease leading to papillary muscle dysfunction, and rupture of chordae tendineae may produce clinically significant mitral valve prolapse[87] without inherent connective tissue abnormalities in the valve.

Clinically significant mitral valve prolapse is, however, usually associated with myxomatous transformation (mucoid degeneration) of the valve tissue. This is "true" floppy valve syndrome. In many instances, the primary cause is never known. Diseases and syndromes known to be associated with myxomatous transformation are summarized in Table 45-2. Mitral valve prolapse has also been reported to develop consequent to mitral commissurotomy for rheumatic mitral stenosis.[88]

Patients with mitral valve prolapse secondary to myxomatous transformation (mucoid degeneration) are more likely to develop complications than those in whom the condition is not

Table 45-2 **Conditions associated with mitral valve prolapse including those factors associated with frank floppy valve syndrome**

Connective tissue abnormalities
Marfan syndrome
Ehlers-Danlos syndrome
Osteogenesis imperfecta
Pseudoxanthoma elasticum
Ebstein's anomaly
Asthenic habitus
Rheologic and physiological factors
Polyarteritis nodosa
Myotonic dystrophy
Duchenne's muscular dystrophy
Cardiomyopathy
von Willebrand's disease
Keratoconus
Hyperthyroidism
Atrial septal defect (ostium secundum)
Holt-Oram syndrome

associated with a clear syndrome.[87] Progressive mitral regurgitation is the most common complication, though associated or isolated rupture of the chordae tendineae, infective endocarditis, and arrhythmias may also result. Sudden death, as an extremely rare complication of mitral valve prolapse, has been reported.[89,90]

Thus, with exceptions, patients with mitral valve prolapse are usually asymptomatic and rarely experience serious complications. When symptomatic, patients may experience lightheadedness, fatigue, dizziness, chest pain, or dyspnea, or all these. The most common physical findings are asthenic habitus, skeletal anomalies, or a combination of hyperextensible joints, arachnodactyly, and a high-arched palate, the latter potentially pointing to Marfan's syndrome. In that syndrome most patients develop mucoid degeneration of the mitral valve. The auscultatory trademark of floppy valve syndrome is the distinct midsystolic click, often accompanied by a late systolic murmur. As prolapse increases, permitting greater mitral regurgitation, the murmur may become pansystolic. Very rarely, a floppy valve may be identified by a so-called honk during systole, believed to be caused by vibration of the chordae tendineae and valve leaflets.[91,92]

Pathology. In floppy valve syndrome, the valve cusps expand, chordae lengthen and possibly rupture, and one or both cusps, as a result, "billow" or prolapse into the atrium during ventricular systole (Fig. 45-5). Medial, lateral, or middle scallops of the posterior leaflet or the anterior leaflet, either singly or in combination, may be involved. Over time, if the mechanical strain produced by an expanded cusp becomes extreme, chordae may rupture; dissolution of collagen in the chordae may also contribute to this potential complication. Mitral valve regurgitation typically results, often with a regurgitant volume warranting clinical attention. Mitral valve ring may become dilated and eventually calcific as a result of

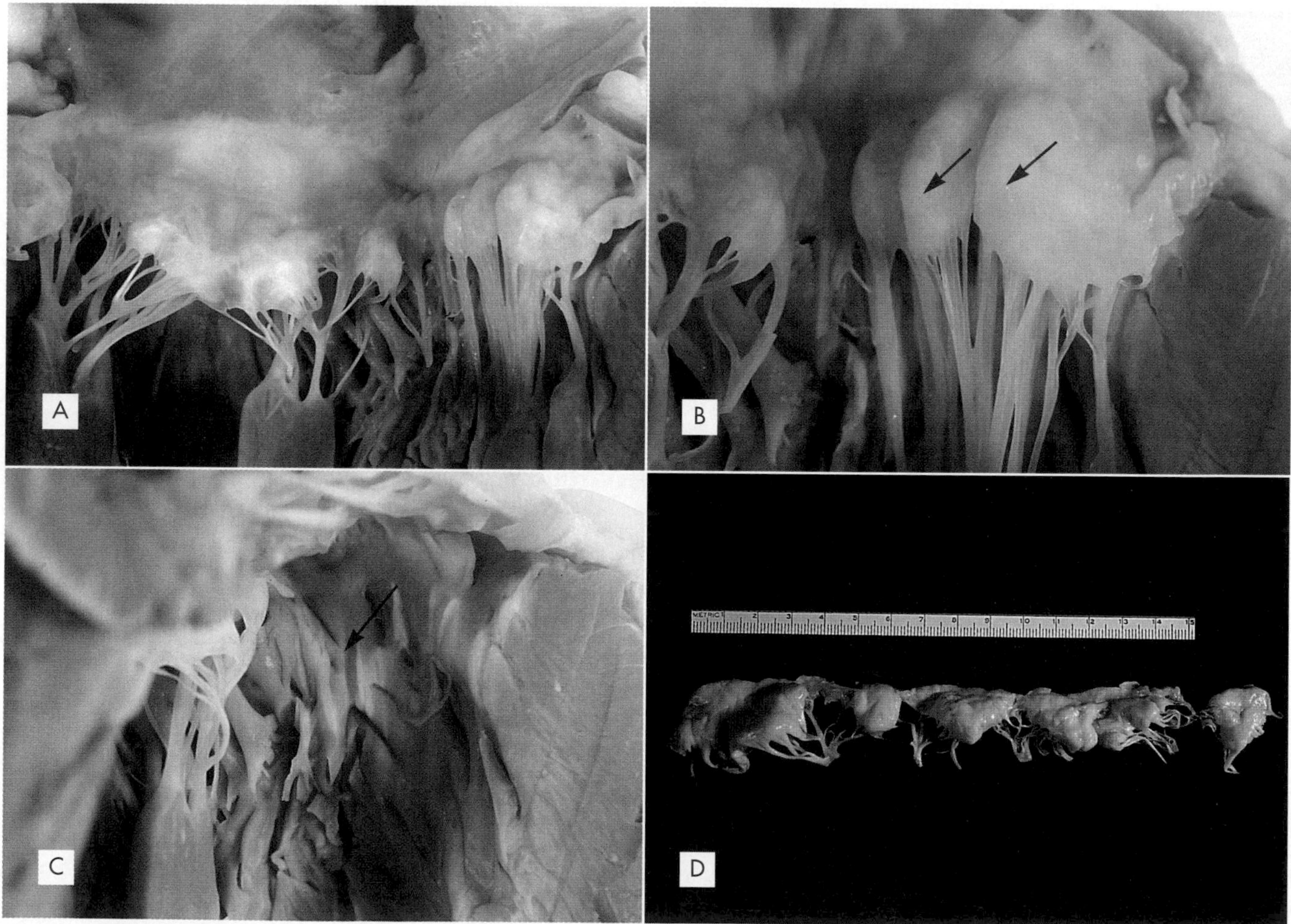

Fig. 45-5 **A,** Floppy mitral valve. The greatest redundancy and gelatinous change are noted in the posterior leaflet (to the right), but there is also localized thickening along the free margin of the anterior mitral leaflet. Chordae are variably thickened. **B,** Closer view of posterior leaflet of mitral valve with noticeable gelatinous thickening, redundancy, and hooding *(arrows)* typical of floppy mitral valves. Again, the chordae are variably thickened. There is focal brown discoloration over one of the smaller redundancies. **C,** Left ventricular endocardium underlying (behind) the posterior mitral leaflet in the same heart with a floppy mitral valve. Notice the classical appearance of fibrous contact (friction) sites *(arrow)* where chordae tendineae rub against the endocardial surface adjacent to the prolapsing floppy valve. This heart was cut in a four-chamber echocardiographic plane. **D,** An operatively excised mitral valve with severe floppiness. There are numerous hoods, redundancies, and thickenings throughout the leaflet tissue and variable chordal thickening. The thickenings are gelatinous. Annular length is also greatly increased.

mucoid changes affecting the annulus. Excessive mobility of the "floppy" leaflets and chordae may lead to friction lesions on the posterior wall of the LV endocardium. These linear fibrous reactions are virtually pathognomonic of prolapse. In some instances, endocardial fibrosis, produced by an expanded anterior cusp may in turn cause adjacent chordae tendineae to thicken and fuse.[43] Increased superficial leaflet fibrosis resulting from friction between ballooning cusps is a common feature in mitral valve prolapse. Accumulation of platelets at the coaptation line of the valve cusps is also expected.

Microscopic observations reveal prominent changes in leaflet structure and characteristic mucoid degeneration of the fibrosa and spongiosa. Cystic "spaces" containing acid mucopolysaccharides are prominent in the expanded spongiosa of leaflets and in the sheath of the chordae tendineae. Collagenous laminae appear disrupted and fragmented,[43] and valve leaflets, the annulus, and chordae tendineae all show evidence of myxomatous thickening.

Therapy. Mitral valve prolapse rarely requires intervention. Patients who develop mitral valve regurgitation, experience rupture of chordae tendineae, or have arrhythmias should be treated accordingly. Patients who develop arrhythmias secondary to a myxomatous mitral valve may require antiarrhythmic drug therapy, though arrhythmias linked to mitral valve prolapse usually require no more than routine observation. The minimal risk of prolapse-associated infective endocarditis can be further reduced through the prescription of antibiotic prophylaxis. Rupture of chordae tendineae is rare though the immediate consequence, namely, acute mitral regurgitation, is much more severe. If rupture has occurred, patients usually require immediate surgical intervention; valvuloplasty is used effectively in most cases. Progressive mitral regurgitation should be monitored closely. The condition may become acutely severe, mandating the use of vasodilatory drugs, intra–aortic balloon–pump therapy, and ultimately valve repair or replacement. Cohn and associates[93] have reviewed the relative success of various surgical methods of therapy for myxoma–related mitral regurgitation.

Aortic valve stenosis

Definition and clinical presentation. Aortic valve stenosis is the chief cause of LV outflow obstruction. RHD is the most common cause of acquired aortic stenosis when rheumatic complications also involve the mitral valve. However, when acquired aortic stenosis presents as an isolated, "pure" lesion, unassociated with additional valvular lesions (though accompanying aortic regurgitation may or may not be manifest), RHD is involved in a much smaller proportion of cases. Instead, degenerative aortic valve disease, producing progressive calcification along the flexion lines of the valves and potentially spreading into the valve cusps, is the major cause of acquired, nonrheumatic aortic stenosis. This is particularly so in the elderly. Calcification in degenerative aortic stenosis may copresent with calcific deposits in the mitral valve ring and coronary arteries. Aortic regurgitation, on the other hand, rarely accompanies aortic stenosis of degenerative origin. Such valvular incompetence much more frequently accompanies rheumatic aortic stenosis. Other rare causes of acquired aortic stenosis include severe atherosclerosis, ochronosis,[94] rheumatoid syndrome,[68] SLE,[95-97] Fabry's disease,[98] type II hyperlipoproteinemia,[99,100] infective endocarditis,[101,102] and injury resulting from radiation.[103-105] Yost and colleagues[106] suggest that calcific aortic stenosis may at times be associated with Paget's disease of bone. Rare instances of calcific aortic stenosis related to immunologic disorders have also been reported.[107]

In most patients, the symptoms of aortic stenosis do not appear until the sixth decade or later.[108] This is particularly true for degenerative valve disease in which sclerosis and calcification build up over a lifetime with superimposed normal "wear and tear" of the valve. Eventually, increasing obstruction of the valve orifice and mounting intracavitary pressure and strain on the myocardium produce symptoms that initially manifest on exertion. Dizziness and syncope, resulting from decreased cardiac output during effort, are often the earliest symptoms. Angina pectoris, precipitated by exertion, occurs in approximately two thirds of patients with severe aortic stenosis and is frequently accompanied by CAD.[109,110] When the disease has progressed to a critical stage, patients often display debilitation and peripheral cyanosis, typical of reduced cardiac output, in addition to symptoms characteristic of LV failure: coughing, fatigue, progressive dyspnea on exertion, orthopnea, and paroxysmal nocturnal dyspnea. Gastrointestinal bleeding associated with calcific aortic stenosis, first reported by Heyde[111] and Schwartz[112] in 1958, is now recognized as a common accompaniment of aortic stenosis. Physical manifestations of aortic valve stenosis include systolic murmur, thrill, delayed carotid upstroke, delayed second heart sound, occasionally conspicuous jugular venous A waves, and a prominent left atrial "kick," discernible through palpation or auscultation.

Pathology. In aortic stenosis of rheumatic origin, valve cusps retract and stiffen as valve leaflets and annulus undergo neovascularization, commissures fuse, and cusps thicken and become fibrous. Calcific nodules may form on the valve cusps. Calcification of the aortic valve may occur secondary to inflammation and commissural fusion in aortic stenosis of rheumatic origin, though it is associated primarily with degenerative aortic stenosis. In degenerative aortic stenosis, stenosis does not involve commissural fusion but is instead the result of large calcium deposits within the aortic cusps, which extend into the sinuses of Valsalva (Fig. 45-6). The sinotubular junction usually has associated fibrocalcific changes in patients with degenerative aortic valve stenosis. Although certain bicuspid valves develop calcific changes more quickly than normal aortic valves, the likelihood of such degeneration is unpredictable. As in aortic stenosis of rheumatic origin, degenerative valve cusps become fibrous and thickened, thereby contributing to a narrowed orifice.

Therapy. Surgical treatment is required when a patient with aortic stenosis is diagnosed as experiencing moderately severe to severe obstruction.[98] LV failure, syncope, dizziness, and angina pectoris are the chief clinical indications that the stenosis has reached a stage of operability. Noninvasive methods of study, such as Doppler ultrasound and echocardiography, are used to confirm the clinical presentation, though the efficacy of the latter in detecting abnormalities in the asymptomatic patient has been questioned.[80,113] Regular follow-up examination is advised in asymptomatic patients to monitor the advance of the disease and ensure the prevention of associated infections, particularly infective endocarditis. The rate of disease progression is higher in calcific aortic stenosis than in stenotic aortic valves of rheumatic origin.[80,113-115] Given the rapidity of disease progression, particularly in the degenerative and calcific types, patients with mild aortic stenosis undergoing surgery for coexistent coronary or mitral valve

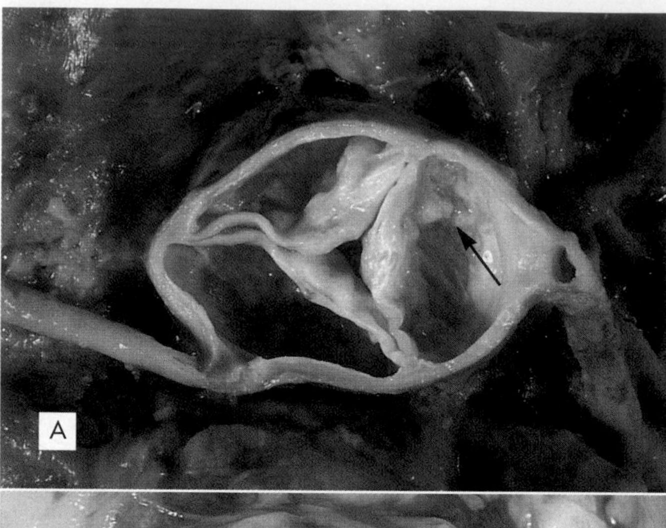

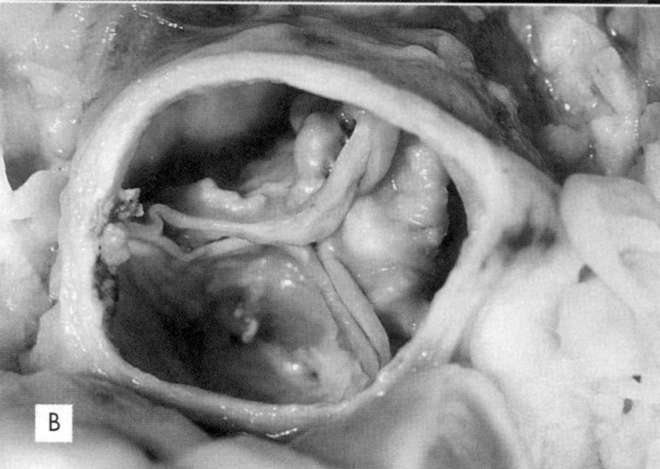

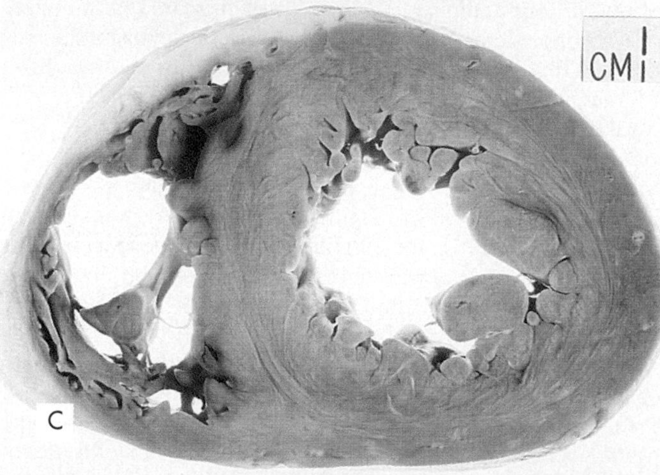

Fig. 45-6 **A,** Superior view of tricuspid, fibrocalcific, mild to moderately stenotic aortic valve. As noted, there are numerous calcific deposits *(arrow)* accompanying fibrous thickening of the cusps. The commissures are focally fused, with the posterior left cuspal commissure being most severely so. This is an example of degenerative aortic valve stenosis. The left main and right coronary arteries arise to the right and left respectively. **B,** Superior view of tricuspid, fibrocalcific, severely stenotic aortic valve. The calcific deposits are larger, more numerous, and more fibrotic. **C,** Transverse section of the ventricular myocardium from a heart with severe aortic stenosis. Both left hypertrophy and dilatation are evident, and right ventricular dilatation caused by chronic parenchymal lung disease is also prominent.

lesions should be considered for aortic valve replacement.[114] Open commissurotomy or balloon valvuloplasty are possible only in adult patients with noncalcific stenosis.[98]

Aortic valve insufficiency

Definition and clinical presentation. Aortic valve regurgitation may be acute or chronic. As with other diseases affecting the valves of the heart, the point at which chronic aortic regurgitation requires surgical intervention depends on the rate of disease progression. Individual patients differ greatly in this regard.

Rheumatic fever is one of the more common causes of aortic regurgitation. As fibrous matrix expands the valve cusps, they retract, allowing regurgitation into the left ventricle. Rheumatic aortic regurgitation is often combined with aortic stenosis and with diseases of the mitral valve. Syphilitic (luetic) heart disease produces aortic insufficiency through inflammation in the region of the aortic commissures. The inflammatory process is associated with adventitial and medial damage, with weakening and expansion of the aortic wall. This dilatation along with retraction of the valve cusps produces valvular incompetence.[116] Infective endocarditis, affecting the valve cusps, both body and base, is another major cause of chronic aortic regurgitation and is by far the most common cause of acute aortic regurgitation. Other inflammatory diseases that lead, on rare occasions, to aortic regurgitation include SLE,[117] ankylosing spondylitis,[118,119] rheumatoid arthritis,[120] Reiter's syndrome,[121,122] Behçet's syndrome,[123] Takayasu's arteritis,[124,125] methysergide therapy,[60] Whipple's disease,[126] relapsing polychondritis,[127] and giant cell arteritis.[128] Aortic dissection or aortic trauma can cause an aortic laceration precipitating aortic cusp prolapse and aortic regurgitation; both events are of primary importance in acute aortic regurgitation. Myxomatous transformation of the aortic valve has been reported as an increasingly important cause of aortic regurgitation.[129,130] Other rare causes are connective tissue disorders including Marfan's syndrome,[131] Ehlers-Danlos IV syndrome,[132] osteogenesis imperfecta,[133] pseudoxanthoma elasticum,[134] annuloaortic ectasia,[135] and "cystic medionecrosis" of the aorta. All these disorders may be associated with cuspal myxomatous degeneration. Hypertension and renal failure may also produce aortic incompetence,[136] the result of both root dilatation and cuspal prolapse. Acute aortic regurgitation can occur subsequent to aortic valve replacement (for a stenotic aortic valve) for a variety of reasons.[134]

Patients with chronic aortic valve regurgitation may remain asymptomatic for decades.[137] Acute aortic regurgitation, on the other hand, normally presents with highly conspicuous symptoms of left–sided heart failure, namely, exhaustion, fatigue, dyspnea, orthopnea, and paroxysmal nocturnal dyspnea. The onset of these signs and symptoms can usually be pinpointed precisely. Similar symptoms are evident in patients with chronic aortic regurgitation in whom the disease has progressed to an advanced stage, though it is rarely possible to specify the duration since onset. During the asymptomatic period, patients with aortic regurgitation may notice audible heart sounds, forceful pulsations in the neck vessels, or slight orthostatic dizziness.[134] Symptomatic aortic regurgitation typically presents in the form of angina pectoris or congestive heart failure in which LV failure precedes RV failure.[134] Dyspnea and fatigue are often the first symptoms.

Physical signs of aortic regurgitation include LV enlargement and hyperactivity, low diastolic blood pressure, displaced apical impulse (typically found below and to the left of its normal location), and ejection clicks, normally heard in early systole. Aortic regurgitation usually produces a soft, high-pitched, blowing murmur, though the so-called seagull or cooing dove murmur, much louder in tone, can also indicate aortic regurgitation.

Pathologic features. The gross pathologic features of an insufficient aortic valve vary according to the primary disease involved (Fig. 45-7). In all instances, however, chronic aortic regurgitation results in dilatation and hypertrophy of the left ventricle and eventual dilatation of the mitral valve annulus. Hypertrophy and dilatation of the left atrium, in addition to the development of LV endocardial "pockets," may also occur.

In rheumatic aortic regurgitation, valve cusps become fibrotic and contracted. Contracture may not be equally distributed among the three cusps, further resulting in malalignment.[138] Calcification associated with aortic regurgitation is rare.[118] Commissural fusion may occur producing combined aortic regurgitation and aortic stenosis. When aortic insufficiency results from infective endocarditis, the lesion is characterized by perforation of valve cusps or destruction of cuspal tissue. Vegetative growth along the lines of cuspal closure may also cause aortic regurgitation. Syphilitic heart disease, as with most of inflammatory diseases, causes commissural widening, cusp contracture, and aortic valve annulus dilatation. Features of myxomatous change in the aortic valve leading to regurgitation have been emphasized by Tonnemacher and associates,[130] who describe discontinuity of the fibrosa and widening of the zona spongiosa by excess acid mucopolysaccharides. This deformation of cuspal tissue often involves more than 50% of the valve cuspal volume.

Microscopically, an excess of ground substance consistent with glycosaminoglycan accumulation is observed in valves from connective tissue syndromes. Microscopic lesions of healing or healed infective or noninfective endocarditis are localized to regions of valvular damage and are characterized by typical tissue destruction and repair, with variable foci of granulation tissue, neovascularity, and surface thrombosis.

Therapy. Patients with asymptomatic mild-to-moderate aortic regurgitation are normally not considered for operative intervention. Instead, regular echocardiographic surveillance of disease progression is recommended, coupled with antibiotic prophylaxis for endocarditis. In patients with severe aortic regurgitation, sinus rhythm may be disrupted, and LV dilatation may progress. Antiarrhythmic and inotropic agents may be required. Where syphilitic heart disease is the primary cause of regurgitation, a full course of penicillin therapy may be prescribed.[68] However, active infection is long past by the time that the aortic sequelae are apparent.

Operative intervention is generally undertaken in severe, symptomatic, chronic aortic regurgitation and in acute aortic regurgitation. Clinical consensus as to the appropriate timing of intervention in patients with progressively worsening regurgitation has not been definitively reached. Operative correction must be particularly appropriate in the latter instance, since the risk of sudden death is much higher.[139]

Tricuspid stenosis

Definition and clinical presentation. Acquired tricuspid valve stenosis seldom occurs as an isolated lesion but is found pre-

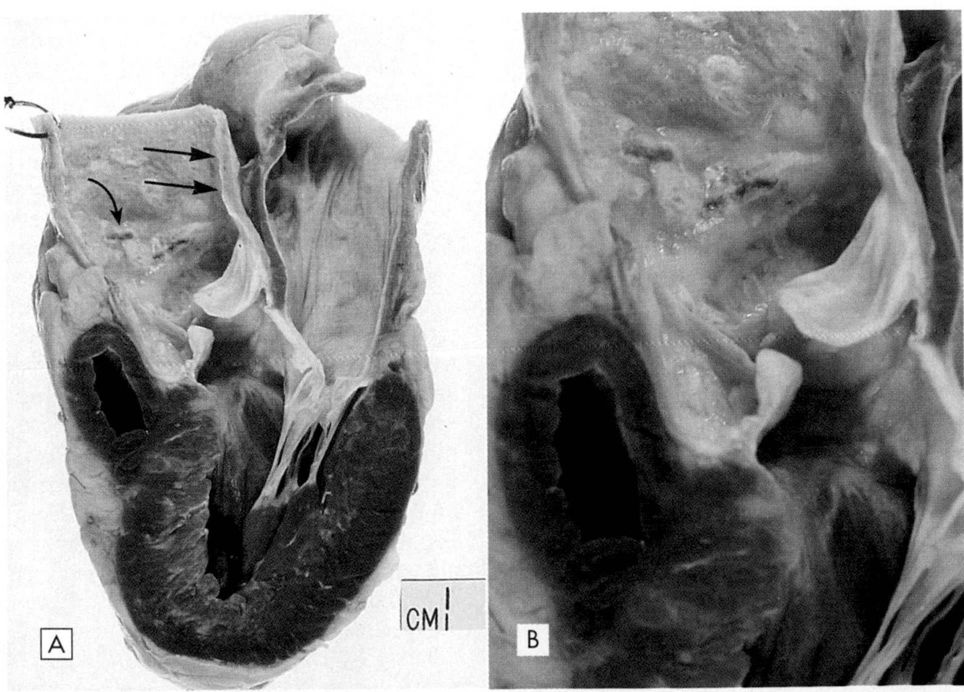

Fig. 45-7 **A,** Parasternal long-axis view of a heart from an elderly person with considerable dilatation and wall thickening of the aortic root *(arrows)*. These latter changes are associated with multiple fibrous plaques and focal sinotubular ulcerative calcific changes *(curved arrow)* most consistent with healed aortitis. There is also mild left ventricular outflow tract endocardial thickening and interstitial fibrosis in the ventricular septum. **B,** Evidence of aortic valve insufficiency is seen better in a closer view, including focal endocardial thickening below the aortic valve. The infundibulum of the right ventricle is seen to the left.

dominantly in association with mitral stenosis.[140,141] Rheumatic fever is responsible for approximately one third of all stenotic tricuspid valves.[140] Other valvular diseases may also be present. As with mitral valve stenosis, tricuspid stenosis occurs more frequently in women than in men. Isolated tricuspid stenosis is highly exceptional, and most cases are rheumatic in origin.[140] Rare causes of tricuspid stenosis include right atrial tumors, pericardial tumors, tricuspid atresia, carcinoid syndrome,[68] and metabolic or enzymatic abnormalities.[27] Endocarditis as a factor in tricuspid stenosis is extremely uncommon though stenosis can occur in association with right-sided endocarditis in intravenous (IV) drug users, and Weyman and colleagues[142] recount one patient with Loeffler's endocarditis presenting with combined mitral and tricuspid stenosis. Enia and colleagues[143] describe endocarditis-related tricuspid stenosis, arising 5 years after pacemaker insertion. Two additional patients with pacemaker-induced tricuspid stenosis have been reported.[144,145] Ridker and associates[146] described tricuspid stenosis associated with massive carcinoid plaque deposition after the surgical implantation of a porcine bioprosthetic valve.

Patients with tricuspid stenosis typically display accentuated jugular venous A waves unrelated to pulmonary hypertension. Edema, hepatomegaly, ascites, abdominal swelling, or anasarca may be present. Fatigue resulting from low cardiac outflow is often reported. Significantly, when tricuspid stenosis is accompanied by mitral stenosis, symptoms characteristic of mitral stenosis such as hemoptysis, paroxysmal nocturnal dyspnea, and acute pulmonary edema are rarely present, and their absence may point to multivalvular rheumatic disease.

Pathology. Rheumatic tricuspid valve stenosis is characterized by leaflet fibrosis, architectural disruption of connective tissue laminae and neovascular changes. As well, there is chordal fusion, thickening, and retraction. Commissural fusion is typically most conspicuous at the anteroseptal commissure. When all three commissures are affected, flow is impeded by the rigidity of both cusps and chordae, and accentuated by reduction in orifice size because of commissural fusion. The appearance of the valve is usually distinctive, with diffuse thickening of leaflet and cusps, without intrinsic or "onlay" gelatinous changes characteristic of floppiness or carcinoid valve disease.

Therapy. Surgery is usually required in significant tricuspid valve stenosis. Valvulotomy and annuloplasty (in the setting of combined tricuspid stenosis and tricuspid regurgitation) are performed. Several recent studies have explored the efficacy of balloon valvuloplasty in the treatment of stenotic tricuspid valves.[147-150]

Tricuspid insufficiency

Definition and clinical presentation. Insufficiency of the native tricuspid valve may occur for many reasons. Among conditions presenting early in life, dysplasia of the tricuspid valve is the most common. Dysplasia in the absence of downward displacement (apical displacement) is more likely to present in early childhood. When displacement of the tricuspid valve occurs in association with various degrees of dysplasia (Ebstein's malformation), the presentation may be in childhood or early or late adulthood. Other lesions of the tricuspid valve that may lead to insufficiency or regurgitation include the "unguarded" tricuspid orifice and a straddling tricuspid valve. These lesions are typically noted in association with complex congenital heart disease and present early in life.

The presence of tricuspid valve atresia without downward displacement may lead to giant right atrium and regurgitant reflux into the hepatic veins. A congested pulsatile liver is likely to result. The patient will be viewed as having RV failure. Ebstein's malformation is much more protean in its presentation, depending on the degree of displacement, the degree of dysplasia, and associated malformation of the right ventricle. Such a valvular lesion may also be associated with functional stenosis of the inflow as well as the outflow of the right ventricle. Arrhythmias, at times life threatening, are a concomitant of Ebstein's anomaly.

Acquired causes of regurgitation through the tricuspid valve will present according to the situation at hand. Thus the possibility of tricuspid regurgitation after chest trauma[151] may be reflected in a near-term accident or other traumatic event. It is also noted that such trauma may lead to delayed tricuspid valve regurgitation or recognition at a distant time. Elevated jugular-venous pressure with a V wave may be the most common physical sign in such patients. A tricuspid valve murmur will be noted in the majority as well. Hepatomegaly and liver pulsation are also frequently observed. Patients typically present with dyspnea and fatigue with a lesser frequency of palpitations and other complaints. Other circumstances in which acquired tricuspid valve regurgitation may occur are less common. Acute rheumatic fever and subsequent development of rheumatic valvular disease may be manifest as tricuspid insufficiency. Even less common is prominent tricuspid regurgitation subsequent to operative pericardiectomy for constrictive pericarditis.[152] Similarly, tricuspid regurgitation may occur after balloon valvuloplasty for rheumatic tricuspid valve stenosis; however, the frequency of this potential complication is not yet well studied.[147] The decision to replace or not replace the tricuspid valve when operative removal of rheumatic mitral valves is undertaken remains uncertain. However, many patients (86%) undergoing removal of stenotic mitral valves have purely regurgitant tricuspid valves. These valves may be anatomically normal or abnormal.[153] Rarely, in complication of an inferior wall acute myocardial infarct, tricuspid insufficiency may necessitate valve replacement.[154] Such an occurrence is typically in association with an acquired ventricular septal defect.

Pathology. The congenitally regurgitant tricuspid valve typically lacks normal chordal structures and connections. The free margins are variably rolled and thickened, are gelatinous and opaque in appearance, and have irregularities of the margin (Fig. 45-8). These thickenings can be accompanied by other diaphanous regions of the leaflets. The chordae may be rudimentary or partially normal. When the valve is regurgitant on the basis of displacement in the Ebstein's malformation, it is typically large and sail-like with numerous aberrant chordal attachments causing insufficiency and narrowing of the orifice in certain parts. When affected by trauma, the chordae, the valve itself, or both, may be disrupted. When the valve is affected by rheumatic disease, a combination of stenosis and regurgitation is expected. Functional regurgitation of the tricuspid valve is not infrequent when there is increased pressure and volume of the right ventricle. There is also the possibility of functional regurgitation when operative procedures affect the geometry of both ventricles, as with valve replacements on the left side. Thus a Carpentier ring may be necessary to fortify and restrain the dilated tricuspid valve annulus.

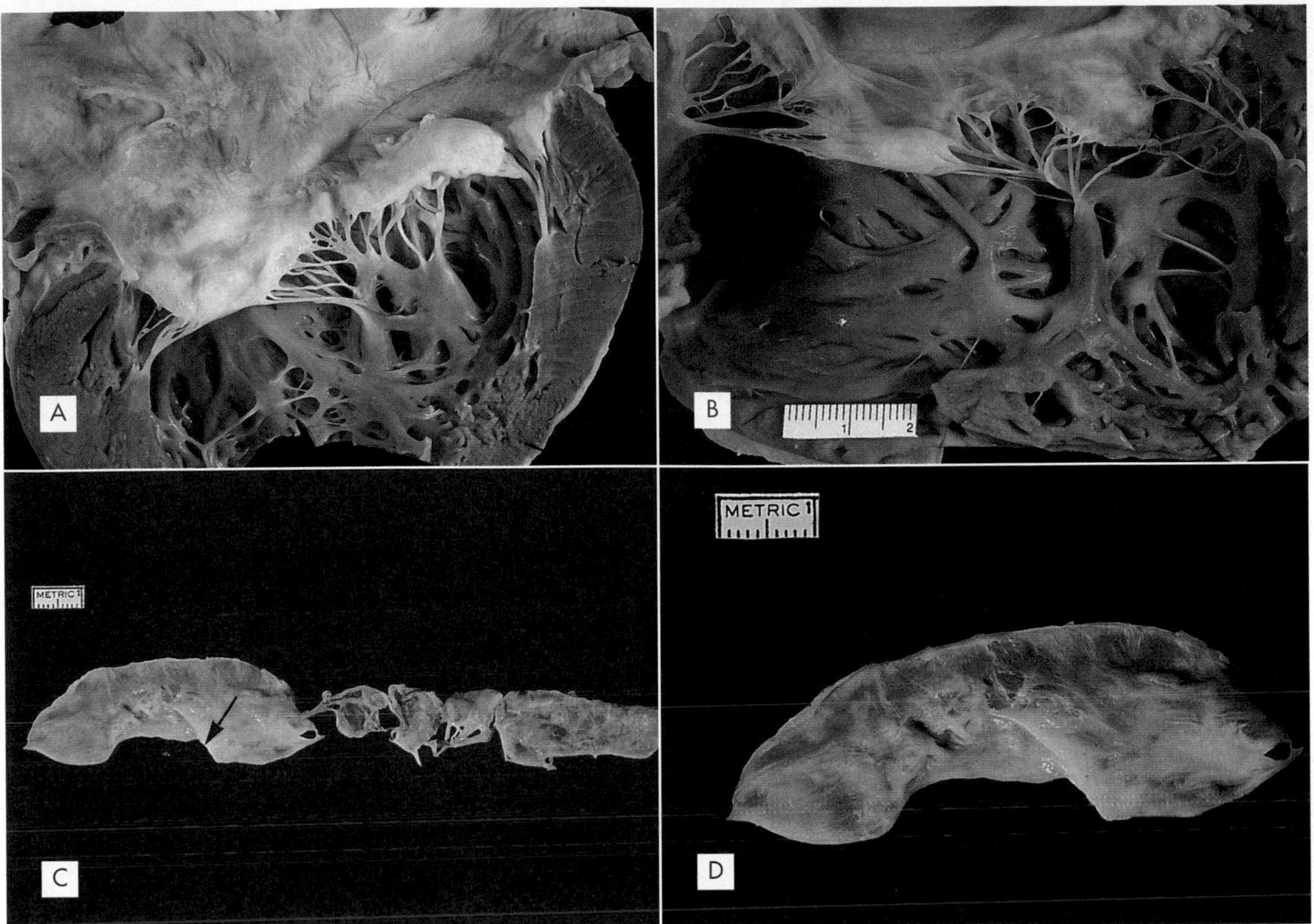

Fig. 45-8 In situ view of mitral, **A,** and tricuspid, **B,** valves, both affected by floppiness, including gelatinous thickening, hooding, and redundancy. Both ventricular cavities are dilated. The posterior leaflet of the mitral valve is by far the most severely affected. **C,** Operatively removed congenitally regurgitant tricuspid valve. The valve has virtually no normal chordae tendineae with a scalloped and thickened free margin of the anterior leaflet *(arrow)*. The remainder of the leaflet tissue was also variably thickened and translucent without normal chordal structures. **D,** In a closer view, the anterior leaflet of the tricuspid valve is seen to be greatly abnormal without chordal projections and with a scalloped free margin, variable thickening, and accentuated translucency.

Histologically the congenitally regurgitant tricuspid valve has variably increased matrix with a preponderance of glycosaminoglycan and proteoglycan–rich material. An increased number of valvular interstitial cells may be seen as well. There is typically no inflammation. The histologic changes associated with Ebstein's anomaly may be similar. The effect of rheumatic valvulitis is typically one in which more collagen is synthesized, and the matrix is less myxoid. When carcinoid heart disease occurs and combined stenosis and regurgitation of the tricuspid valve may accompany alterations in function of the pulmonary valve, an onlay of elastin-lacking, glycosoaminoglycan-rich ground substance is expected, with rare inflammatory cells and an otherwise intact underlying valve leaflet. Only in active or healing infective endocarditis may there be a combination of microthrombi, microorganisms, and active and chronic inflammatory responses. These are similar to those seen on any valve surface affected by infective endocarditis.

Pulmonary stenosis

Definition and clinical presentation. Pulmonary valve stenosis in the adult is normally the result of a congenital lesion. Less frequently, RHD affecting the pulmonary valve can lead to stenosis; however, it is typically associated with rheumatic disease involving other cardiac valves and rarely results in severe deformity.[155] In some instances, malignant carcinoid tumors arising in the lower gut and metastatic to the liver lead to endocardial carcinoid plaques in the outflow tract of the right ventricle and can result in a combination of pulmonary stenosis and pulmonary regurgitation. Constriction of the pulmonary valve ring and retraction and fusion of valve cusps may occur.[68] Aneurysm of the sinus of Valsalva or cardiac tumors may also lead to pulmonary obstruction.[155]

In pulmonary stenosis, RV hypertrophy, secondary to impediment of the RV outlet, results in decreased ventricular distensibility and compliance, and in turn may eventually impair right atrial emptying during systole. Indications of this valvular malfunction include a giant A wave in the jugular venous system.[156]

Balloon valvuloplasty remains the most effective surgical means of palliating a congenitally stenotic pulmonary valve. Recent data[157] contradict those of several earlier studies[158,159] and indicate that for *carcinoid* pulmonary stenosis, balloon dilatation is not as effective as pulmonary valvotomy, valvectomy, or valve replacement.

Pathology. The stenotic pulmonary valve affected by RHD is very rare. When present, it has all the features of other heart valves affected by this slowly progressive diffusely fibrosing process. Neovascularity may be observed, and rare monocyte macrophages may be present within the thickened cusps. Congenital pulmonary valve stenosis may be of two distinct types. In the first the valve is a three-cuspid one with fusion along the commissures creating a domelike configuration and a central orifice ranging from atretic to pinpoint to moderately narrowed. The valve may also be of a severely dysplastic nature. When this occurs, the cusps are considerably thickened and have redundant, somewhat gelatinous appearing tissue within the sinuses of Valsalva. The excessive tissue mass of such a valve and the tissue within the sinuses prevent proper opening or closure of the valve cusps. The findings with respect to carcinoid disease are similar to those seen on the tricuspid valve.

Microscopically the features in the rheumatic, dysplastic, or carcinoid valve are comparable to those seen in other valves affected by the same disorders.

Pulmonary insufficiency

Definition and clinical presentation. Adult acquired pulmonary valvular regurgitation (PVR) is rare, primarily resulting from dilatation of the pulmonary valve trunk and annulus. The latter results either from various forms of pulmonary arterial systolic hypertension or from primary dilatation of the pulmonary artery. Pulmonary arterial dilatation may in turn occur idiopathically[160] or as a result of connective tissue disorders such as the Marfan syndrome[161] or Ehlers-Danlos syndrome.[162] Additional causes of PVR include infective endocarditis,[163-165] carcinoid syndrome,[68] chest trauma,[165] syphilis,[160] long–standing pulmonary hypertension,[166] and rheumatic disease.[167] Involvement by rheumatic disease is now highly unusual.[168] Iatrogenically induced PVR can occur after surgical treatment of pulmonary valve stenosis or tetralogy of Fallot, or as a result of trauma by balloon–tipped catheters. Patients with PVR are normally asymptomatic, though auscultation may detect a low-frequency rumbling diastolic murmur along the left sternal border.[169]

Pathology. Primary disease affecting the pulmonary valve is unusual, with regurgitation occurring in some bicuspid valves. The pathologic substrate leading to pulmonary regurgitation is the same in most cases, that is, hereditary or degenerative dilatation of the pulmonary artery or of the valve annulus. Dilatation is typically fusiform in absence of trauma or infection. The symmetrical dilatation seen in the aortic root in Marfan syndrome may be mimicked in the pulmonary trunk. Associated intimal tears (stretch marks) may be visible.

Therapy. Syndromic causes of pulmonary trunk dilatation bear follow-up study to ensure intervention before dissection. Unless complications arise, that is, indications of RV failure, PVR may not require intervention apart from routine follow-up examination and infective endocarditis prophylaxis.

Endocarditis

Endocarditis, or inflammation of the endocardial lining of the heart, may involve any surface within the cardiac chambers. Indeed, endocarditic lesions have been observed on all valvular, chordal, trabecular, and papillary muscle structures. Most lesions occur on the heart valves. This is particularly true for noninfective forms of endocarditis. In such bland conditions the vegetations tend to be arranged along the appositional margin of leaflets or cusps. These are sites of repetitive contact and continuous locuses of minor endothelial disruption and endocardial injury. Vegetations arising as an infective process are typically larger, more friable, and extensive. They involve extravalvular sites and may be a significant cause of tissue destruction, obstruction, or embolism.

In general, endocarditic lesions are viewed as noninfective or infective. The infective vegetations may be caused by any number of organisms or precipitated by a prior bacterial infection (*Streptococcus pyogenes* in the case of acute rheumatic fever) or may emerge from initially bland vegetations that become seeded secondarily. The processes of inflammation may involve entire leaflets or cusp, this being true for noninfective endocarditides like rheumatic fever and for infective endocarditis.

Rheumatic valvulitis (endocarditis)

The acute valvulitis of rheumatic fever is discussed under the section on rheumatic heart disease. During the acute inflammatory phase of the disease there is a pancarditis, which includes a diffusely edematous valvulitis with generally small wartlike (verrucous) vegetations along the coadaptational margin leaflets or cusps. These vegetations are sterile. They may remain seeded on the valves or in rare circumstances mobilize. The vegetations may undergo healing and resorption, as is typical, leaving nearly no trace of the acute disease.

When rheumatic endocarditis heals, a valve is not typically injured further unless acute rheumatic fever recurs. However, a small percentage of patients with acute rheumatic valvulitis will progress over several decades to structurally and clinically important valvular defects causing stenosis or regurgitation. Some observers have said that RHD is mitral valve stenosis! However, rheumatic valvular disease may involve all heart valves. Detailed discussion of the lesions that follow from rheumatic valvulitis is presented elsewhere in this chapter.

Libman-Sacks endocarditis

Disseminated lupus erythematosus has many morbid consequences. One is the endocarditic involvement of AV valves by bland, medium-sized, somewhat flat, granular vegetations distributed not only along the lines of valve closure, but also over both inflow and outflow surfaces and with extension onto the atrial and ventricular endocardium.[170] These lesions occur in less than half of patients with SLE. Verrucae in the recesses behind the mitral or tricuspid valves are significant diagnostic features of these endocarditic lesions. The vegetations typically involve more than one valve concurrently, with particular predilection for the AV valves. Generally, the tricuspid valve is the most important singular site of involvement followed by mitral and pulmonic and a lesser frequency of aortic involvement. These vegetations are not so prone to emboli as others.

From a microscopic point of view, the lesions can vary from planar areas of edema, to fibrinoid change, and a mixed inflammatory infiltrate including *hematoxylin bodies*.[170] The latter constitutes a specific feature of this disorder with focuses of chromatin material. When more grossly visible, the vegetations include rather amorphous fibrinoid material as well as sites of superficial valvular necrosis and microthrombi. Again, hematoxylin bodies may be embedded within the thrombic material. The inflammatory valvulitis characteristic of Libman-Sacks endocarditis includes plethoric small blood vessels.

The condition is similar to acute RHD in that a pancarditis often is present. Thus the myocardium may have focal mixed infiltrates with localized necrosis, edema, and fibrinoid alteration. A distinction is that this condition does not have Aschoff bodies. The pericardium has similar fibrinoid changes and a variable fibrinous or serofibrinous pericarditis. The amount of pericardial fluid is typically small but may range to a very large effusion (500 to 1000 g).[171] When the acute episode subsides, the fibrinous material may organize and produce obliteration of the pericardial cavity and a form of chronic adhesive pericarditis.

Nonbacterial thrombotic endocarditis (NBTE)

The bland form of noninfective endocarditis, nonbacterial thrombotic endocarditis, occurs in association with inanition, cachexia, and chronic debilitating disease.[172,173] The vegetations range from small isolated spherical lesions of a few millimeters to those that are large, friable, and tan in coloration. Although the smaller vegetations may resemble those of rheumatic valvulitis, the larger ones may mimic infective endocarditis. In either situation the vegetations are located along the line of coaptation of leaflets or cusps and may involve commissures. When healed, these verrucae may be partially resorbed and remain as an irregular nodular or planar lesion with focal thickening of the valve margin. Lambl's excrescences may represent healed, small NBTE lesions. Certainly they represent microthrombic materials that have healed, whether they are specifically NBTE or not.[172]

In general, like rheumatic valvular disease, NBTE has a predilection for the mitral valve (Fig. 45-9). There is a similar

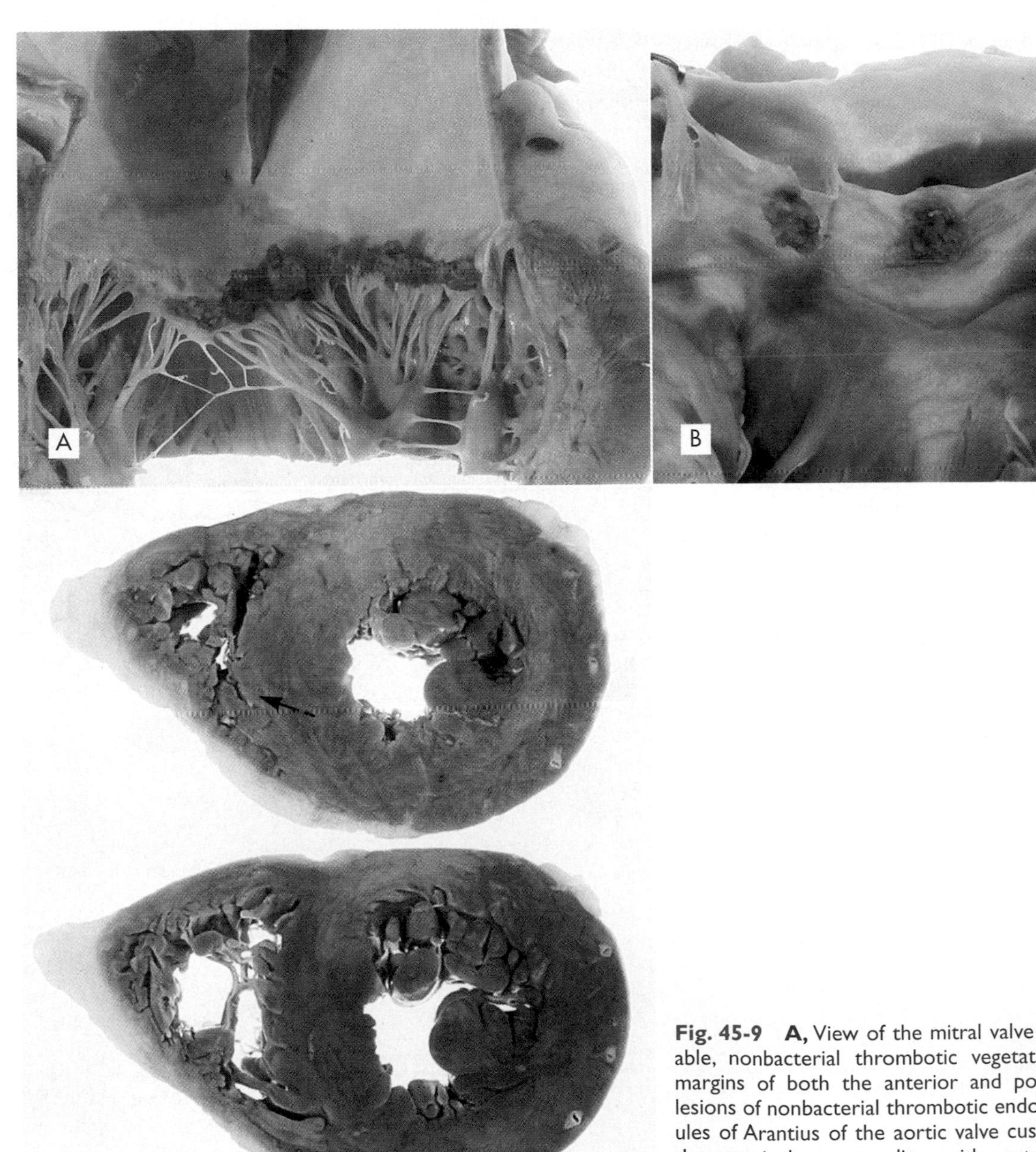

Fig. 45-9 **A,** View of the mitral valve with an extensive line of friable, nonbacterial thrombotic vegetations along the coaptational margins of both the anterior and posterior leaflets. **B,** "Kissing" lesions of nonbacterial thrombotic endocarditis on the zones of nodules of Arantius of the aortic valve cusps. **C,** Transverse sections of the ventricular myocardium with acute infarcts, particularly prominent in the posterior septal region, and highlighted *(nonstaining areas)* by the triphenyltetrazolium chloride stain *(upper section)*.

decreasing frequency from the aortic through tricuspid and pulmonic valves, though all four valves may be involved. The lesions are virtually limited to the valvular tissue, and the mural endocardium is spared. Of note, the presence of chronic rheumatic valvular disease increases the likelihood that NBTE lesions will form in a given patient.

Extracellular edema with expanded interstitial space, fibrinoid change, and capillary prominence may disrupt normal collagenous and matrix architecture. Inflammatory cells are sparse. The bland lesions arise as microthrombi on focally injured or degenerative valvular surfaces. The precise pathogenesis of these lesions is unknown; however, allergic, nutritional, hemodynamic, and structural factors have been impuned.[172] The possibility that coagulation is altered in patients with inanition and cachexia leading to increased likelihood of microthrombus formation has been proposed.[174] Such is well argued in patients with malignancy in whom hypercoagulability may be present. The association of NBTE with chronic debilitating disease[173] has been borne out in many observations. Certain patients who do not fall into this category also have NBTE lesions. The most important clinical relationship lies in their propensity to embolize and cause infarcts throughout the body. In addition, they are indistinguishable by echocardiography from the vegetations of infective endocarditis. Further, these lesions may become infected secondarily. Certain investigators have observed a concordant decrease in the frequency of infective and noninfective endocarditis in recent decades, held as evidence in support of the idea that infective endocarditis is often a sequela of NBTE.[175]

Infective endocarditis

The term *bacterial endocarditis* was used for years to describe infective vegetations that localized on any endocardial structure within the heart. Because bacteria were the most important pathogens, fungi and other nonbacterial organisms were placed in a subsidiary category. With the evolution of medical care and the significant number of patients with various forms of immunodeficiency, the frequency of fungal endocarditis has increased significantly (Table 45-3).

Involvement of the endocardium by microorganisms reflects one nidus of localization in otherwise systemic infections that have multiple possible portals of entry. As well, infected lesions may embolize readily to distant sites, further disseminating the infection and complicating interpretation of clinical status as well as the process of eradication of the organism.

Changing concepts of infective endocarditis have reduced the emphasis on acute versus subacute disease. As implied in the terminology, the acute forms are more fulminant, invariably fatal without treatment, associated with virulent organisms, and run a course of 2 to 8 weeks; subacute and chronic disease runs from weeks to months.[176] At times the delayed and persistent nature of the latter forms are associated with a milder course and less morbid outcome. It is possible that certain of the latter endocarditic lesions heal themselves in vivo, even without particular therapy.[177] The distinction between acute and subacute forms of infective endocarditis has diminished, partly because of modulation by therapy. Ultimately, the effect of an organism on host structures and the extent of tis-

Table 45-3 Many and changing faces of infective endocarditis

Era	Preantibiotic	Postantibiotic	Intravenous drug abuse	Prosthetic valves*	Modern
Site	Community at large		Community	Hospital and community	Hospital (nosocomial)
Main Organisms		*Streptococcus viridans* > others (65%) *Staphylococcus aureus* (25%) Culture negative (10%)†	*Staphylococcus aureus* (60%) *Streptococcus* species (20%) *Pseudomonas aeruginosa* (10%)	Coagulase negative, methacillin resistant *Staphylococcus* (60%) *Staphylococcus aureus* Gram-negative bacilli Diphtheroids Fungi Streptococcus	*Pseudomonas aeruginosa* *Enterococcus* *Staphylococcus aureus epidermidis warneri* Fungi *Candida* *Aspergillus* *Mucor*
Treatment	None	Antimicrobials	Antimicrobials	Surgery or antimicrobials, or both‡	Surgery, antibiotics, and antifungals
Mortality	~100%	~30%	~40%	20%–30%	~65%
Risk groups	Young adult, RHD, CHD, alcoholics, malnourished	Old adult, adults and children with CHD	Addicts in "shooting galleries"; previous IE infective endocarditis	Hospitalized, operative patients	Patients with inherent or iatrogenic immunodeficiency with or without antibosis
Location of lesions	MV>AV>MV+AV	MV>AV>MV+AV	TV>AV>MV>AV+MV	Site of prosthesis	Multivalvular, mural, pancarditis

AV, Aortic valve; *CHD*, congestive heart disease; *MV*, mitral valve; *RHD*, rheumatic heart disease; *TV*, tricuspid valve. Intravenous drug abuse includes mainly heroin, cocaine†

*Two peaks: early—nosocomial; late—community.

†Includes infection by fastidious organisms, *Coxiella burnetii*, *Chlamydia* species, and uremia and noninfective processes.

‡Fungal infective endocarditis (IE) demands surgery, but intravenous drug abuse IE-related on the tricuspid valve may receive antimicrobials alone.

sue destruction will determine the significance of a given bout of endocarditis. The tendency for staphylococci rapidly to destroy heart valves, erode valve annuli, and spread widely emphasizes the critical necessity of early recognition and treatment. Less virulent organisms may produce a more tolerable and indolent form of disease but, then again, in a given host may be highly destructive. It is important to note the changing patterns of endocarditis since the introduction of antibiotic therapy and as the last few decades have unfolded. A broader diversity of unusual organisms have been recognized as a significant cause of infective endocarditis. The frequency of IV drug abuse and various forms of systemic immunodeficiency have contributed to the emergence of entirely new pathogenetic agents.

The distribution of endocarditic processes by age and sex have changed over the twentieth century. Infective endocarditis caused by bacteria in the first half of the century was predominantly seen in patients over 50 years of age. This preponderance actually increased in the 1950s, 1960s and 1970s. The frequency of endocarditis[178-180] in older patients has been matched recently by that in IV drug users at risk and in immunocompromised patients in various programs requiring transplantation and cancer chemotherapy. Each of these two latter groups have their own unique susceptibility to infections and now represent a significant cohort of patients with infective endocarditis. The frequency of infection in men and women and boys and girls is era specific and cohort specific.

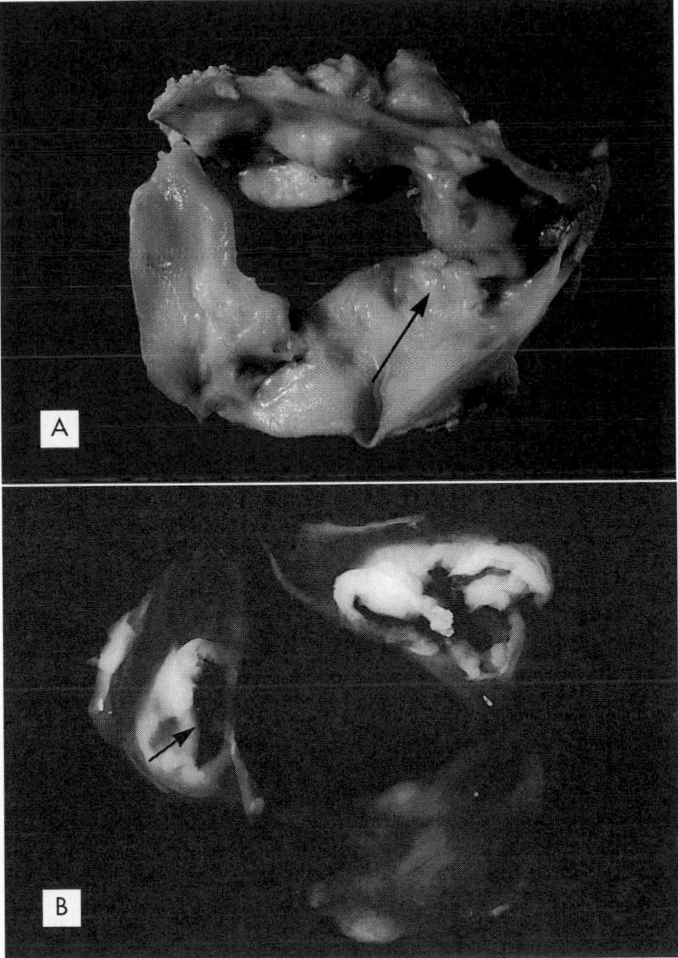

Fig. 45-10 **A,** Caudad (ventricular) view of aortic valve cusps with noticeable deformity, nodularity, and fibrocalcific deposits *(arrow)* consistent with healed infective endocarditis. The irregularity of fibrocalcific changes is the most telling gross characteristic of endocarditis. The valve was regurgitant. **B,** Ex vivo radiograph of operatively excised pulmonic valve from a patient with gonococcal pulmonic valve endocarditis. Variable areas of thickening are related to distortion and edema of valvular tissue with superimposed vegetative lesions, whereas the radiolucent areas *(arrow)* reflect cuspal loss caused by the infection.

The importance of *Streptococcus* organisms *(S. viridans,* enterococci, and microaerophilic strains) and staphylococci[179,181] is still evident in the overall proportion of patients with infective endocarditis. However, the recent emergence of fungal endocarditis has changed the demography of the disease. Until a few years ago, perhaps as many as 90% of bacterial endocarditides[21,176,182,183] were attributable to *Streptococcus viridans.* Thus the trend has been for other forms of the disease to become more prominent. *Staphylococcus aureus* is among the most vicious of bacterial organisms causing endocarditis, precipitating fulminant syndromes of sepsis, valvular destruction and regurgitation, extension into the valve ring, pericardial effusion, ventricular excavation, and embolization.[180,182] Pneumococcal and gonococcal endocarditis are relatively rare though in certain groups at risk such events still occur. Gonococcal endocarditis can be a very destructive form of the disease (Fig. 45-10). Additional causes of endocarditis are listed in Table 45-4.[184-188]

The increased invasiveness of procedures including major operative intervention on the heart and vascular system, the placement of conduits, valves, and other devices within the

Table 45-4 **Organisms causing infective endocarditis in humans**

Staphylococcus
S. aureus
S. epidermidis
Streptococcus
Enterococci
E. faecalis
E. faecium
E. durans
S. viridans
S. bovis
HACEK groups: *Haemophilus* species (usually not *Haemophilus influenzae)*
Actinobacillus actinomycetemcomitans
Cardiobacterium hominis
Eikenella corrodens
Klingella sp
Escherichia coli
Klebsiella sp
Salmonella sp
Serratia marcescens
Listeria monocytogenes
Other gram-negative bacteria
Fungi or yeasts
Candida sp
Aspergillus sp
Zygomycetes *(Mucor, Absidia, Rhizopus)*
Polymicrobial infections
Culture negative

Table 45-5 Location of active infective endocarditic (IE) lesions: experience in 137 patients in the 1970s

Location	Patients Number (%)
Right-sided valves	23 (17)
1. Isolated = 13	
2. Combined with left-sided IE = 10	
Left-sided valves	74 (54)
1. Aortic valve (AV) = 34	
2. Mitral valve (MV) = 22	
3. AV + MV = 18	
Prosthetic valves	22 (16)
1. Aortic valve = 15	
2. Mitral valve = 7	
Valvulotomy or valvuloplasty	4 (3)
1. Aortic valve = 1	
2. Mitral Valve = 3	
Complicating congenital cardiac shunt	6 (4)
Limited to mural endocardium	8 (6)
TOTAL	137 (100)

Modified from Arnett EN, Roberts WC: *Thorac Cardiovasc Surg* 30:327, 1982.

Table 45-6 Factors predisposing to endocarditis

Transient bacteremia related to tooth brushing, dental procedures, manipulation of the genitourinary or gastrointestinal tracts, delivery of a child[184]
Upper respiratory tract infections.[183]
Localized infection elsewhere in the body—pneumonia, skin infections, renal infections
Intravenous drug use without asepsis
Invasive operative or interventional procedures including resections for cancer and various kinds of catheterizations.[180]
Cardiovascular surgery for valvular or congenital disease.[185]
Implantation of prosthetic valves[186,187]
Underlying heart disease—rheumatic valvular disease,[187] bicuspid aortic valves, intracardiac shunts, atrial septal defects < ventricular septal defects < aortopulmonary windows or patent ductus arteriosus)[188]
Unknown source

milieu of the blood-surface interface (Table 45-5), the lack of sterile needle programs for drug addicts, and, as noted, the immunosuppression involved in modern therapies for malignancy and other hematologic disorders has created opportunities for endocarditis previously not seen in such numbers or in type. The predisposing factors of greatest significance are listed in Table 45-6.

The mechanism by which endocarditis is initiated, becomes fully established, and progresses relates to the presence of an abnormal endothelial surface, an unusual titer or type of microorganism in the blood, and the presence of agglutinating antibodies. Certainly hemodynamic factors contribute to the disruption of normal surface integrity, and the development of endocarditis is directly related to jetting and turbulence of blood flow in many types of preexistent heart diseases and in normal hearts. Whether NBTE is a progenitor of infective endocarditis remains unknown.[189]

Endocarditic lesions range from small to large multilobulated, friable, shaggy, giant aggregates (Fig. 45-11). The mitral valve is most commonly affected in community-acquired, non–IV drug related endocarditis. The aortic valve is also involved with high frequency. Right-sided heart valves are affected particularly when there is evidence of IV drug use.

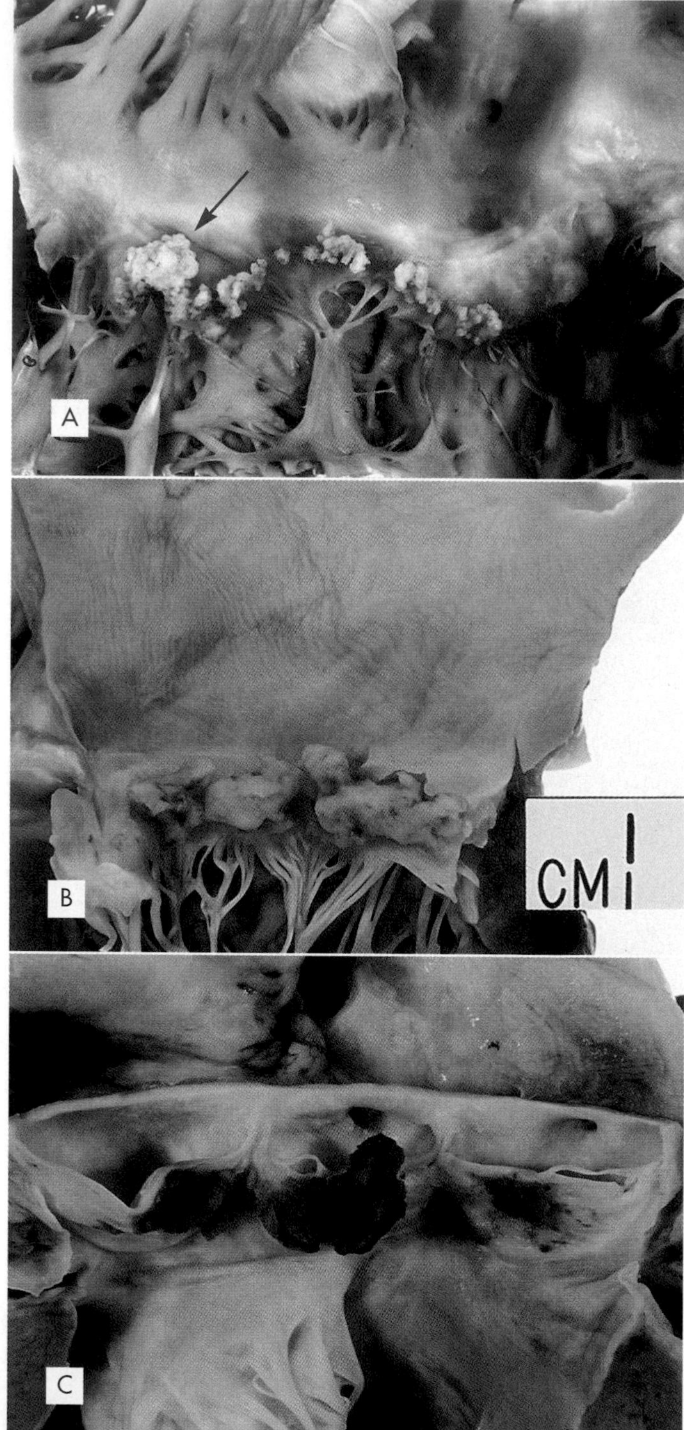

Fig. 45-11 **A,** Tricuspid valve with variable and, at times, exceedingly large *(arrow)* pale, friable vegetations along the coaptational margins of the leaflets. **B,** Huge, friable, infective endocarditic lesions involving the mitral valve posterior leaflet. These vegetations would be an excellent source for thromboemboli. **C,** Opened aortic valve with multiple shaggy and friable vegetations. The back side of the anterior mitral leaflet is seen at the lower left, whereas the upper ventricular septum is seen at the right. These vegetations are infective.

The widely variable location, appearance, size, and shape of endocarditic lesions relates to the diversity of organisms involved and the range of immune competencies encountered by these organisms (Fig. 45-11). Thus patients may have a virtual smattering of endocarditic lesions on heart valves, chordae, and mural endocardial surfaces concurrently. This is particularly so with fungal endocarditis (Fig. 45-12). Bacterial forms tend to localize more discretely on a valve where the process began and progress more by extension than by multifocal cardiac involvement. The disruption of valvular cuspal, leaflet, and chordal structures leading to regurgitant jets further exacerbates the infection by secondarily infecting a site of jet contact (Fig. 45-13). On occasion, endocarditis may lead to stenosis of a valve or exaggeration of a preexistent stenotic orifice.[69]

The histologic appearance of active infective endocarditis is one of fibrin, platelets, and entrapped red blood cells and leukocytes with bacteria or fungi or other organisms in clusters and clumps, often superficial with erosion and with invasion of the underlying valvular or mural surface by the necrotizing inflammatory process (Fig. 45-12). Frank microabscess formation is characteristic, and this necrotizing process can lead to any number of unusual anatomic defects, including frank valve ring abscesses, erosion into the conduction system with heart block, aneurysm formation, and fistulas. Foreign-body giant cell reaction in an endocarditic vegetation[190] may reflect the fulminance of the process or the involvement of granulomatous organisms. The aging of an infective endocarditic vegetation involves the development of a granulation tissue at the base, ultimately rendering a fibrotic or calcific nodule with deformation of the corresponding valve leaflet or cusp. The risk of complications does not diminish immediately after an active endocarditic episode. Healing of a vegetation depends on the virulence of the organism, the timing of therapy, and the extent of the endocarditic process at the time therapy is begun. A certain frequency of endocarditic lesions occurring in the community will be culture negative. It may

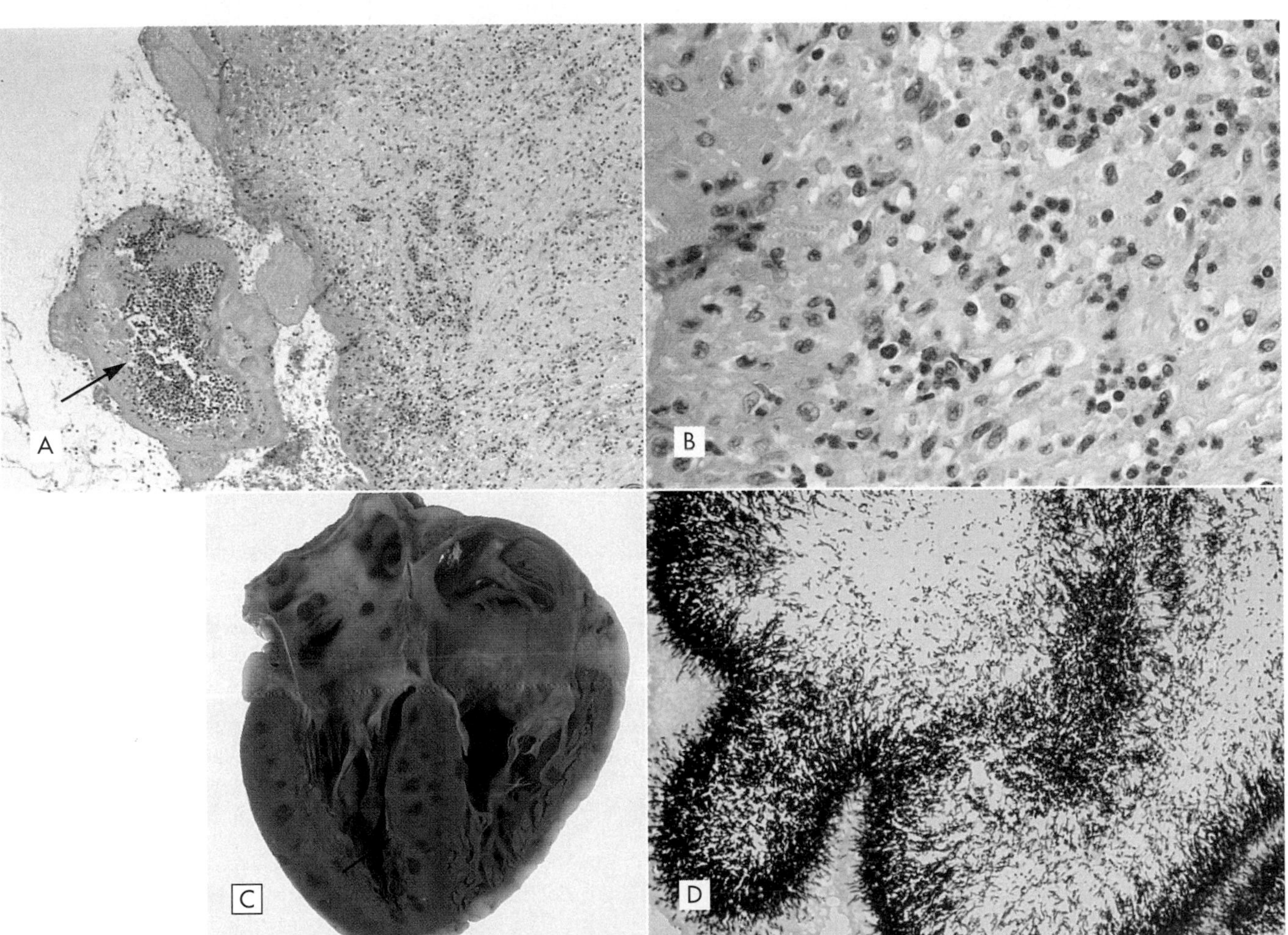

Fig. 45-12 **A,** Photomicrograph of active infective endocarditis with almost polypoid microvegetation on top of a broad-based healing vegetation. The portion of the vegetation to the lower left constitutes a microabscess *(arrow)* surrounded by fibrin and platelets. The portion to the right includes more mononuclear cells than polymorphonuclear leukocytes and neovascular channels and early fibroplasia as a component of healing. **B,** Photomicrograph of vegetation involved by active infective endocarditis. The field includes components of fibrin and polymorphonuclear leukocytes, as well as mononuclear cells and a few small blood vessels indicative of early healing within components of this lesion. **C,** Four-chamber echocardiographic view of anterior half of an autopsy heart with characteristic and widely disseminated cardiac fungal infection. Multifocal myocardial *(arrow)* as well as epicardial and endocardial infective lesions are evident. Four-chamber dilatation is also apparent. **D,** Fungi involving a vegetation on a heart valve. (Gomori methenamine silver stain.)

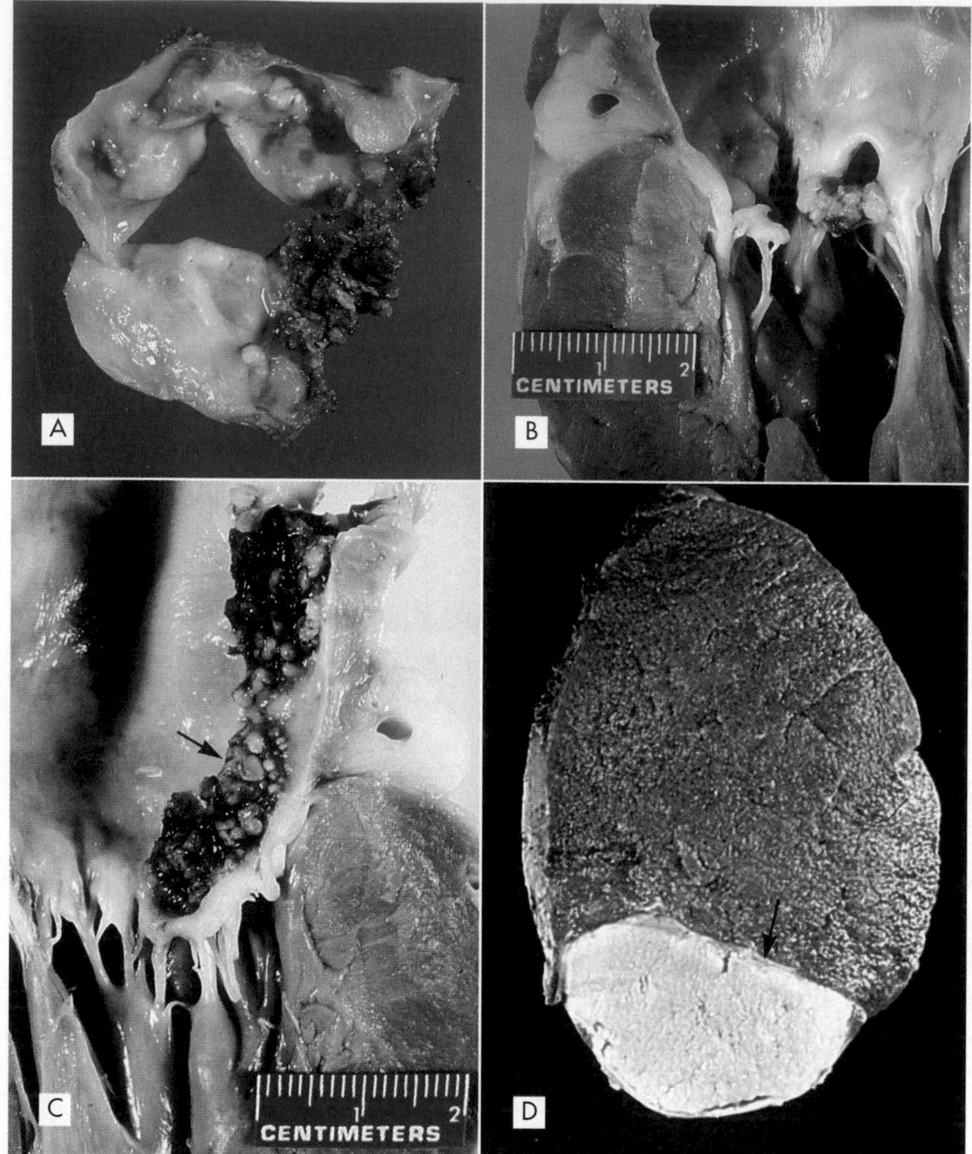

Fig. 45-13 **A,** Infective vegetative material involving a previously malformed and fibrocalcific, probably bicuspid, aortic valve. There has been significant destruction. **B,** Mitral valve area depicting region of tissue loss in the anterior mitral leaflet caused by a previous endocarditic episode and a superimposed vegetation of active infective endocarditis. The left ventricular free wall *(LVFW)* is to the left. **C,** Posterior lateral left atrial wall of patient with active infective endocarditis on a previously injured mitral valve and striking jet lesion *(arrow)*. The remarkable vegetative material has spewed retrogradely through an opening in the damaged anterior mitral leaflet. The vegetation here starts at the free margin of the posterior mitral leaflet. The *LVFW* is denoted. **D,** Cut section of spleen from a patient with septic embolic infarct *(arrow)* consequent to infective endocarditis. The infarcted area is pale and soft as represented particularly on the photograph at higher power.

include as many as 17% of bacterial endocarditides.[183] The more acute the syndrome, the less frequent sterile cultures will be found.[180] The lack of positive blood cultures, even as obtained in appropriate laboratory conditions [191] does not exclude the possibility of finding organisms by stain or culture at autopsy[21] or explant. Administration of antibiotics before obtainment of a blood culture will contribute to culture-negative results, whereas postimmunization factors may prevent bacteremia from being detected by routine culture. The balance between organisms entering the bloodstream and immune responses will determine the likelihood of culture negativity in the face of an active infective endocarditis.[190]

Occult endocarditis may also be found on the pulmonic valve. The uncommonness of singular involvement of the pulmonic valve by endocarditis may lead to a delay in recognition of the infection. The use of echocardiography and other imaging modalities and a high level of suspicion for patients with somewhat atypical presentations will reduce the chances that such patients are missed.[163]

The complications and sequelae of infective endocarditis are protean (Table 45-7). The heart itself may be involved, as noted earlier, by "metastatic" infection involving multiple sites along the mural and valvular endocardium, as well as in the myocardium and pericardium. The extent of spread may

Table 45-7 Potential complications of infective endocarditis

Direct damage to heart
Perforation of valve cusps/leaflets causing insufficiency
Valve ring or myocardial abscess and fistula formation
Suppurative and obliterative pericarditis
Dehiscence of prosthetic valves, conduits, and patch components
Late valve fibrosis causing stenosis (accompanied by insufficiency)
Septic embolization
Cerebral abscess
Mycotic aneurysm
Lung abscess
Systemic sepsis with metastatic infections
Osteomyelitis
Disseminated abscesses
Infectious arteritis with thrombotic occlusion
Infarcts—brain, myocardium, spleen, kidneys, other viscera
Ischemia in distribution of ileofemoral or other major arteries
Circulating immune complexes
Focal or diffuse glomerulonephritis

depend on the development of ring abscesses,[193] the overwhelming nature of a given infection, or embolization to coronary arteries leading to secondary seeding of the myocardium. Development of significant valvular regurgitation in the setting of high fever and other circulating cytokines and endotoxin will precipitate a syndrome of progressive heart failure and central and peripheral shock. When perforations occur in relationship to necrotizing vegetations, not only are valve cusps or leaflets involved, but also infection of the membranous septum, proximal great arteries, chordae tendineae, and other structures may produce unusual ruptures or aneurysms.[194,195] The chances of continued progression in cardiac or valvular dysfunction after healing of infective endocarditis may lead to significant noninfective clinical problems months to years after the acute episode.

Beyond causing systemic shock, the seeding of the bloodstream periphery by emboli will lead to new focuses of continued infection with infarction of vital organs including the brain, spleen, kidneys, and bowel. Also, the possibility of arterial infection and the development of mycotic aneurysms must be remembered. When lesions are predominantly on the right side of the heart, involving primarily the tricuspid and pulmonic valves, the possibility of pneumonia and pulmonary abscesses is increased.

Classical clinical signs of systemic sepsis related to endocarditis include various petechiae in the hands and feet and fingertips, subungually, and in conjunctivae and eye grounds. Tender, red, raised punctate lesions on hands and feet (Osler's nodes) may also be accompanied by painless hemorrhagic raised areas on the palms and soles (Janeway lesions). These lesions likely are endotoxic in origin or related to immune complexes. Similarly, focal necrotizing glomerulonephritis in association with infective endocarditis is most likely immunologically mediated and not a consequence of embolization.[196]

The outcome of infective endocarditis depends on the organism, the setting, and the patient. Since the introduction of antibiotics and other antimicrobials, expectation of survival has ranged as high as 90% to 100%. The acuteness of the infection and the promptness of recognition determine the prognosis. The decision to combine antimicrobial therapy with operative intervention also is crucial. The judgment as to how delayed operative intervention should be relative to the inception of antibiotic therapy has evolved over the years and the decision-making process remains difficult considering the number of divergent organisms and settings in which endocardial infection may occur. Certainly the more acute the disease, the less the likelihood of full recovery.[180,197] whereas in those with more slowly evolving disease[198] the results can be decidedly better. As mentioned, despite the eradication of infection, numerous delayed complications may occur.[182] In fact, now that infective endocarditis is treated quite effectively from the microbiologic point of view, congestive heart failure related to valvular incompetence, associated pancarditis, or coronary embolization has become more important. The systemic sequelae of the disease also play a major role in determining the viability of the patient with such an acute episode. Infection remains a significant cause of death.[199] Opportunistic organisms including various mycobacteria, typical and atypical, may involve the endocardium,[191] and these may be reflected in histologic appearance of acute necrotizing vegetations or granulomatous lesions. The frequency of such organisms as syphilis and gonorrhea involving the valves or the heart has significantly diminished. However, with the reprise of all sorts of venereally transmitted diseases, the likelihood that *Treponema pallidum* and the gonococcus will be responsible for their share of endocarditis seems likely. As noted, various yeasts and fungi are well known to cause large multifocal friable and hemorrhagic, vegetative lesions.[200-203] Although viruses have been suspected of causing endocarditis in humans, with part of the suspicion being based on evidence in experimental animals,[204,205] such lesions have not been documented. The possibility that adenovirus or other viruses are involved in initiating endocardial fibroblastosis was pursued for years. Certainly rickettsial organisms have been known to cause infective endocarditis.[206] They should not be forgotten.

MYOCARDIAL DISEASES

Hypertrophy and dilatation

The normal heart undergoes a process of myocardial cell hypertrophy and hyperplasia before birth. At birth significant cell division of ventricular myocytes ceases, and henceforth atrial myocytes divide infrequently. Thus postnatal growth of the human heart is a reflection of myocyte hypertrophy and increasing amounts of interstitial cellularity, matrix, and vascularity. There is also a general increase in the amount of fibroelastotic endocardial lining tissue with age. The overall increase in heart size reaches a plateau under normal circumstances in the late postpubertal period or early adulthood. In general, the normal human adult heart weighs less than 350 g, though certain men have normal hearts that weigh somewhat more. Throughout the remainder of life, in the absence of aberrant stimuli, the heart may undergo modest hypertrophy (increased mass), especially in response to exercise training. In old age the heart may actually atrophy with concomitant atrophy and loss of cardiac myocytes.

Physiologic hypertrophy associated with exercise training is associated with mild thickening of the RV and LV free walls and ventricular septum. The cardiac chambers may be dilated, particularly as a consequence of dynamic rhythmic exercise training. These changes may be detected by imaging techniques. Hypertrophy may be substantial in athletes who pursue intensive training regimens and perform a considerable amount of high-resistance, low-repetition work. Such hypertrophy may be confused with hypertrophy seen in pathologic conditions such as hypertrophic cardiomyopathy. However, absence of other features of cardiomyopathy, including localization of hypertrophy and family or environmental histories that imply disease, assist in clarifying normal from abnormal.

Pathologic hypertrophy of the heart is a fascinating and unresolved issue. The nature of hypertrophy may be such that there is considerable wall thickening with little or no chamber dilatation (hypertensive heart disease, hypertrophic cardiomyopathy, aortic valve stenosis, subaortic and supra-aortic valve stenoses), or such hypertrophy may occur in the face of pronounced chamber dilatation (after myocardial infarction or in idiopathic dilated cardiomyopathy, toxic cardiomyopathy, myocarditis, valvular insufficiency, and intracardiac shunts). Of interest, those hearts with pressure overload undergo, on average, the least increase in total cardiac mass, whereas hearts that experience volume overload will undergo the greatest increase in mass. Distinction between hypertrophy as a cellular process and hypertrophy as an organ-based process is clearly important pathologically. The regulatory mechanisms involved in cardiac hypertrophy under different circumstances remain to be confirmed. Certainly, alterations in modulation of receptor expression and signal transduction, isoform expression of cardiac contractile proteins, induction of the "fetal" gene program in cardiac myocytes, alterations in metabolism, and changes in nucleic acid and protein synthesis are all involved. The interstitium is also "plastic" in composition and quantity during hypertrophy, and in injury and repair processes. The factors that regulate the response of the myocardium to either hypertrophy alone or hypertrophy dilated have not been fully clarified.

Cardiomyopathy

Cardiomyopathies are diseases characterized by cardiac dysfunction in which the main abnormality lies in the working myocardium. Cardiomyopathies can be divided into two groups: primary (idiopathic, unknown causes) and secondary (known causes). In defining the cardiomyopathies clinically, it is useful to recognize the varied types of pathophysiology that are expressed. Both the primary and secondary categories have three possible functional states: (1) hypertrophic, hyperdynamic; (2) dilated, congestive; and (3) restrictive, constrictive (Fig. 45-14). To designate a cardiomyopathy as primary, one must exclude acquired valvular, coronary, pericardial, and aortic diseases and congenital cardiac defects. Myocardial storage diseases and secondary endocardial diseases also must be sought and excluded as major causes of cardiac dysfunction. Although therapy at times may be similar for primary and secondary myocardial diseases, it is often distinctly different, and the prognosis may depend on the specific diagnosis.

Known causes

Cor pulmonale

Definition and clinical presentation. Cor pulmonale is hypertrophy or dilatation of the right side of the heart caused by pulmonary disease involving the lung parenchyma or the pulmonary circulation. Cor pulmonale can occur as an acute or chronic disease. In the acute stages, a rapid dilatation of the pulmonary trunk, conus, and right ventricle occurs, whereas in the chronic stage, hypertrophy of the right ventricle predominates. The structural and functional characteristics present according to the nature of ventricular overload and the length of time involved. Chronic cor pulmonale is more common as it relates to diseases causing chronic pulmonary hypertension. Multiple diseases can cause cor pulmonale, and these can be divided into three major groups[207,208] (Table 45-8). Chronic obstructive pulmonary disease is the major cause of cor pulmonale.

Pathologic features. The thickened RV free wall of the heart with cor pulmonale typically is constituted by myocytes with hypertrophy and accompanying nuclear changes. If hypertrophy occurs in the setting of coronary atherosclerotic disease, scarring or other evidence of infarction may be observed as accompaniments (Fig. 45-15). The possibility of mural thrombi is also enhanced as the ventricle becomes more dysfunctional and dilated. Diseases causing pulmonary hypertension and cor pulmonale may also directly involve the heart. Sarcoidosis is a good example of a condition with such multifocality.

Systemic hypertension

Definition and clinical presentation. A hypertrophic state of the left ventricle is commonly associated with long-standing systemic hypertension or valvular aortic stenosis, less often with supra-aortic stenosis and aortic coarctation, and infrequently with hypertrophic cardiomyopathy. Discerning the distinctive nature of the hypertrophic process associated with systemic hypertension as distinct from other causes of hypertrophy remains a challenge. As already discussed, hypertensive heart disease is a form of secondary myocardial disease. Patients with this type of cardiomyopathy may present with arrhythmias resulting in sudden death,[209] and this liability may be compounded by concurrent ischemic heart disease.[210]

Pathologic features. The major pathologic feature of hypertensive hypertrophy is the striking involvement of the left ventricle. The distribution of this hypertrophy is characteristically "concentric" with all portions of the LV walls being about the same thickness,[211] in contrast to primary forms of hypertrophy, which may be characterized by asymmetry. This general distinction does not always hold true, and older patients may have a combined hypertensive and obstructive type of hypertrophy. In hypertensive hypertrophy, the cardiac chamber is typically very small; however, once cardiac failure develops, the chamber may dilate (Fig. 45-16).

The histopathologic features of the hypertensive left ventricle include moderate to pronounced myocyte hypertrophy and nuclear enlargement, irregularity, hyperchromasia, and vesicular changes. In addition, the hypertensive ventricle typically has increased interstitial (perimyocytic) connective tissue, as well as increased perivascular connective tissue. The increased connective tissue is most prominent in the inner half of the ventricular wall toward the LV cavity. When hypertrophy is accompanied by coronary atherosclerotic disease, replacement fibrosis related to ischemic injury may be observed. Similarly, the hypertensive heart is more susceptible to acute injury in the process of an acute myocardial infarction.

Toxic injury

Definition and clinical presentation. Although recognized only for a little over two decades,[212-214] the causal relationship

TYPE OF CARDIOMYOPATHY	SPECIFIC CAUSE (SECONDARY)	INDIRECT CAUSE OF MYOCARDIAL DYSFUNCTION
Dilated (systolic disorder)	Infective myocarditis; hemochromatosis; chronic anemia; alcohol; adriamycin; sarcoidosis	Ischemic heart disease; valvular heart disease; hypertensive heart disease; congenital heart disease
Hypertrophic (diastolic disorder)	Friedreich's ataxia; glycogen storage disease; infants of diabetic mothers	Hypertensive heart disease, especially in older patients; aortic stenosis
Restrictive (diastolic and systolic disorder)	Amyloidosis; pancardiac radiation-induced fibrosis	Pericardial fibrosis, effusion (constriction)

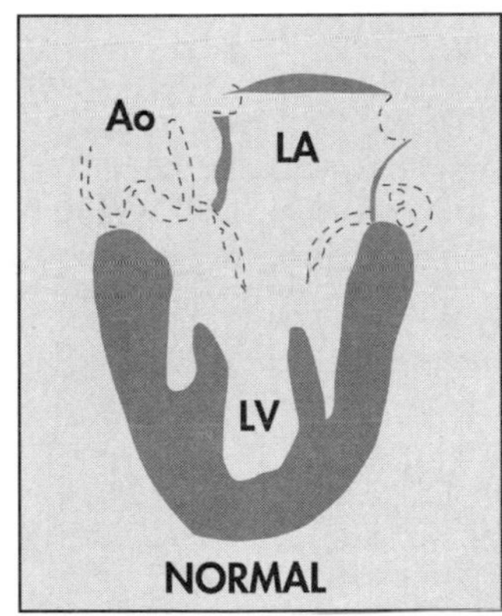

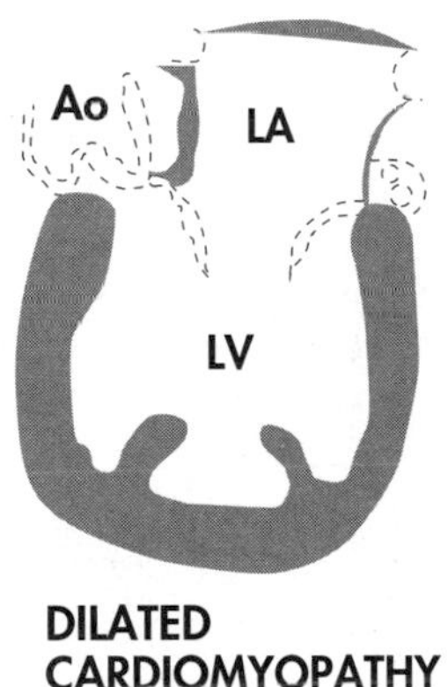

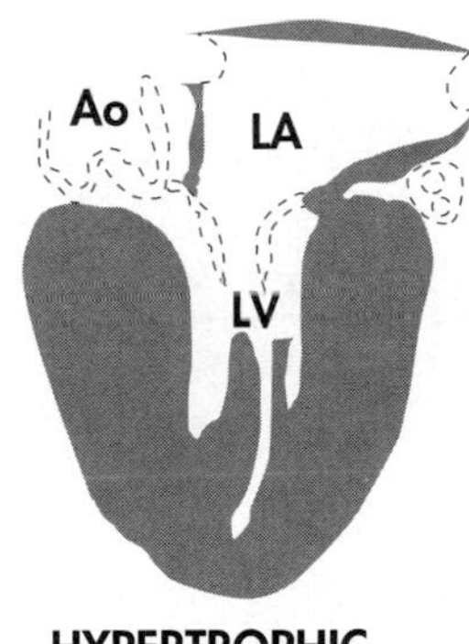

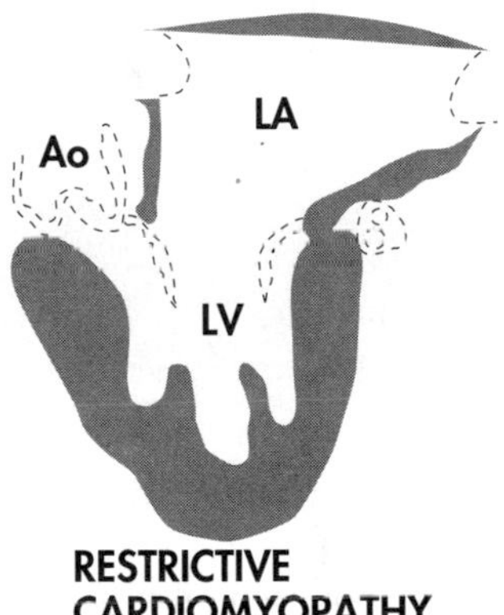

Fig. 45-14 Enumerative and diagrammatic illustrations of the types and specific and less-specific causes of dilated, hypertrophic, and restrictive cardiomyopathy. The nature of these cardiopathies is discussed further in the text.

between anthracycline administration and cardiomyopathy is firmly established and well studied. Cardiotoxicity is the major harmful side effect of doxorubicin and the anthracycline family of compounds. The toxicity may be asymptomatic and manifest only by nonspecific T-wave changes, or it may evolve into florid cardiomyopathy with rapidly progressive biventricular heart failure. Cardiotoxicity is almost always related to the total dose of drug administered, and if the dosage is kept below a 450 to 550 mg/m^2 body surface area, cardiomyopathy is unlikely to occur.[215]

Numerous otherwise highly effective therapeutic agents have drug-related cardiac side-effects.[216] A number of these are summarized in Table 45-9. As noted, agents that are used to treat neoplasms, particularly anthracyclines, have a well-known and well-defined cardiotoxicity. Certain drugs impair sinoatrial and AV nodal function including digoxin and tricyclic antidepressants. Other drugs may produce myocardial ischemia, whereas others are more particularly arrhythmogenic. In the latter category, numerous antiarrhythmics are indeed proarrhythmic in certain settings and doses. Some drugs inflame the myocardium or pericardium on the basis of hypersensitivity responses or an autoimmune-like phenomenon. Yet other agents may injure heart valves directly. Methysergide is a historical example, producing fibrotic reactions, which lead to valvular dysfunction. Other agents, notably including alcohol, have cardiomyopathic and cardiodepressive effects.

The mechanism or mechanisms of anthracycline toxicity with respect to the heart remain under study.[213,214] Adriamycin (doxorubicin) may cause cellular damage by way of lipid peroxidation, intercalation into nuclear or mitochondrial DNA, alteration of cellular calcium regulation, or initiation of bioreductive changes leading to the formation of oxygen free radicals and alkyating species with secondary mitochondrial dysfunction. The role of cardiolipin-doxorubicin interaction in altering the function of mitochondrial oxidative substrate translocators remains of interest.[214] The potential for development of less cardiotoxic anthracyclines has recently been revisited by Mross.[213] He emphasized the evidence that supports a

Table 45-8 Causes of cor pulmonale

Pathobiologic condition	Diseases
Chronic hypoxemia	Chronic obstructive pulmonary disease Idiopathic pulmonary fibrosis Sarcoidosis Bronchiectasis Sleep apnea After a cerebrovascular accident Kyphoscoliosis Extreme obesity Guillain–Barré syndrome
Vascular obliteration	Primary pulmonary hypertension Chronic pulmonary thromboemolism Pulmonary arteritis including collagen vascular diseases Pulmonary veno-occlusive diseases
Hypoxemia and obliteration	Diffuse pulmonary emphysema Tuberculosis Pneumoconiosis Scleroderma Multiple, organized, small pulmonary emboli

different mechanism for the cardiotoxic versus anticancer activity of anthracyclines. Thus, free radical formation appears to be involved in cardiotoxicity but not in anticancer activity.

Cocaine is an alkaloid compound derived from the leaves of the coca plant. Multiple pathways of potential toxicity have postulated as a basis for the observation of acute myocardial infarction, cardiomyopathic and myocarditic presentations, and arrhythmias and conduction disturbances.[212] The most frequently observed histopathologic finding in the setting of cocaine abuse is multifocal contraction band necrosis and microscars within the myocardium. It is common also to observe thrombotic occlusion in coincidence with atherosclerotic plaques in cocaine users who experience myocardial infarction. The likelihood that cocaine may produce significant coronary spasm is supported by various experimental models including aortic strips, atrial wall, and vascular preparations.[212] Potential mechanisms of cocaine-induced cardiac disease are synopsized in Table 45-10.

Pathologic features. Unlike many cardiomyopathies, doxorubicin cardiomyopathy is associated with distinctive morphologic abnormalities, including focal myocardial cell necrosis, vacuolar degeneration, and myofibrillar dropout. Moreover, these structural abnormalities, as detected by RV biopsies, have been shown to correlate roughly with the functional abnormalities of myocardium.

Details of the light and electron microscopic features of anthracycline toxicity in the myocardium have been rendered by different observers[217,218] (Fig. 45-17). The limitation of light microscopy in the grading of anthracycline toxicity has been emphasized, and the need for both thick sections and electron micrographs is reflected in the ultrastructural basis of

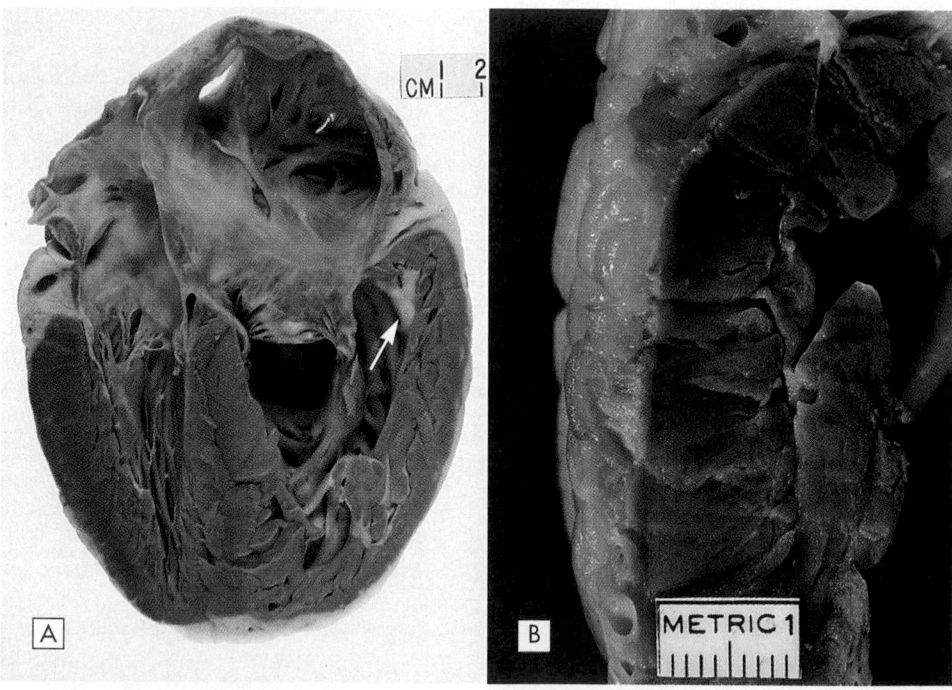

Fig. 45-15 **A,** Four-chamber echocardiographic view of an autopsy heart with right ventricular hypertrophy and dilatation. This is related to primary pulmonary hypertension. There is also considerable right atrial dilatation, and the right-sided heart chambers dwarf the left. There is focal endocardial thickening in several areas in the right ventricle *(arrow)* consistent with healed mural thrombi. **B,** Right ventricular free wall of an autopsy heart with patent ductus arteriosus persistently open into midadulthood. The patient had irreversible pulmonary vascular obstructive disease. The obvious hypertrophy of this wall is a reflection of the pressure overload.

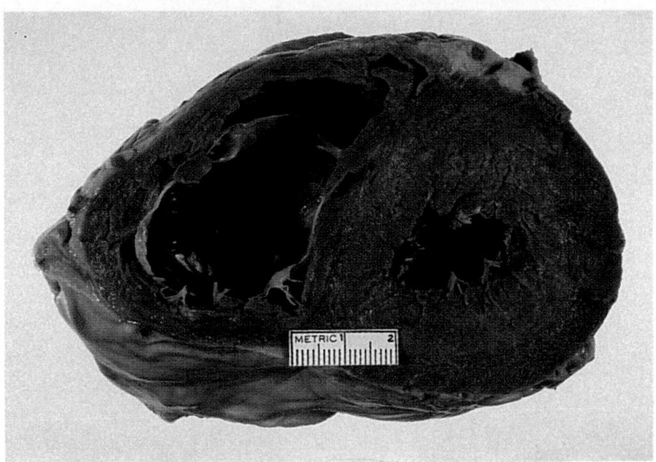

Fig. 45-16 Transverse ventricular section, viewed toward the base of the heart, illustrating left ventricular hypertrophy. There is also moderate right ventricular hypertrophy and moderate to pronounced right ventricular dilatation. Thus in this heart there is evidence of concentric left ventricular hypertrophy related to systemic hypertension and right ventricular changes consistent with cor pulmonale.

Table 45-9 Therapeutic agents associated with cardiomyopathy

Anthracyclines
Adriamycin (doxorubicin)
Daunomycin
Amphetamines
Arsenicals
Catecholamines (endogenous or exogenous)
Chloroquine
Ephedrine
Lithium carbonate
Mitomycin C
Rubidazone
Tricyclic antidepressants
Emetine
Chlorpromazine
Procainamide
Quinidine

Table 45-10 Potential mechanisms of cocaine-induced cardiac arrest

Peripheral and coronary vasoconstriction → coronary spasm
Sympathomimetic activity
Hypersensitivity responses
Direct toxicity
Increased myocardial oxygen demand

a classification of anthracycline-related injury.[217] The combination of myofibrillar loss and sarcoplasmic reticular dilatation (vacuolar degeneration) serves as a basis for the classification system (Table 45-11).

Radiation injury

Definition and clinical presentation. Radiation injury to the heart may be the dose-limiting factor for thoracic irradiation.[219] The main incidence of radiation heart disease has been seen in Hodgkin's patients, followed by those with metastatic seminoma, breast cancer, and lung cancer.[220] All anatomic parts of the heart can be affected by radiation heart disease including the pericardium, myocardium, endocardium, valves, conduction system, and coronary arteries (Fig. 45-18). Microcirculatory injury has been deemed a common pathogenetic factor in the pathologic state of the irradiated heart;[221-224] such injury may include membrane abnormalities and cytoplasmic swelling in endothelial cells with subsequent platelet and fibrin deposition, thrombus formation, and capillary rupture as observed in rabbit models.[221] Indeed, the fundamental work of Stewart and Fajardo[221-224] has demonstrated by light microscopy and ultrastructural analysis that the endothelial cells of small blood vessels are frequently injured by cardiac irradiation.

The frequency of heart involvement in radiation depends on several factors, including the dosage, time and type of delivery of the radiation doses (expressed in rad), and time and intensity of follow-up study of the patient.[220] Multiple studies have been reported on the prevalence of radiation heart disease.[225–229]

Accidental radiation exposure with acute radiation poisoning can result in circulatory collapse and shock unresponsive to fluids and pressor agents.[230-232] Hypotension and hemoconcentration develop in hours, followed by diffuse vascular injury and capillary leak, with pulmonary edema and effusions.

Carlson and colleagues[105] discussed the increasing prevalence of radiation-associated cardiac disease in long survivors after mediastinal irradiation. They summarized information on 35 patients with radiation-associated valvular disease from five published reports and observations in their own patients. Only one patient had undergone valve replacement in the follow-up period. The difficulty in dealing operatively with radiation-induced cardiac fibrosis was emphasized in a patient who required aortic valve replacement. Patients received between 3500 and 5000 centiGrays of irradiation, three had Hodgkin's disease, one lymphoma, and one seminoma. All patients had either aortic or mitral valve disease or both, including both stenotic and regurgitant lesions secondary to radiation injury.

Lesions in human radiation-induced heart disease simulate those in the rabbit experience. After initial polymorphonuclear leukocytic infiltration, the injured tissues undergo healing responses, which include fibrotic proliferation with unusual fibroblasts, fibrin deposition in pericardial effusions, and an ultimate increase in cardiac mass. Mural thrombi are common. Fibrosis of valvular endocardium with thickening and contracture are observed. The accelerated radiation-induced coronary disease is somewhat different from typical atherosclerosis in that it has less lipid in plaques. There is a predominance of plasma cells, as well as fibrosis of the media and dropout of corresponding smooth muscle cells.

Pericardial involvement. The most clinically significant form of radiation heart disease is, in general, pericarditis with a high frequency of pericardial effusion [220,233,234] (Fig. 45-19). Bloody pericardial effusions are common, and a fibrinous exudate is present from damaged leaky capillaries and impaired fibrinolysis.[219,235] Grossly the pericardium is thickened, and such thickening may be associated with fibrosis of the underlying epicardium.[236] The parietal pericardium is most frequently and severely involved. Microscopically, collagenous

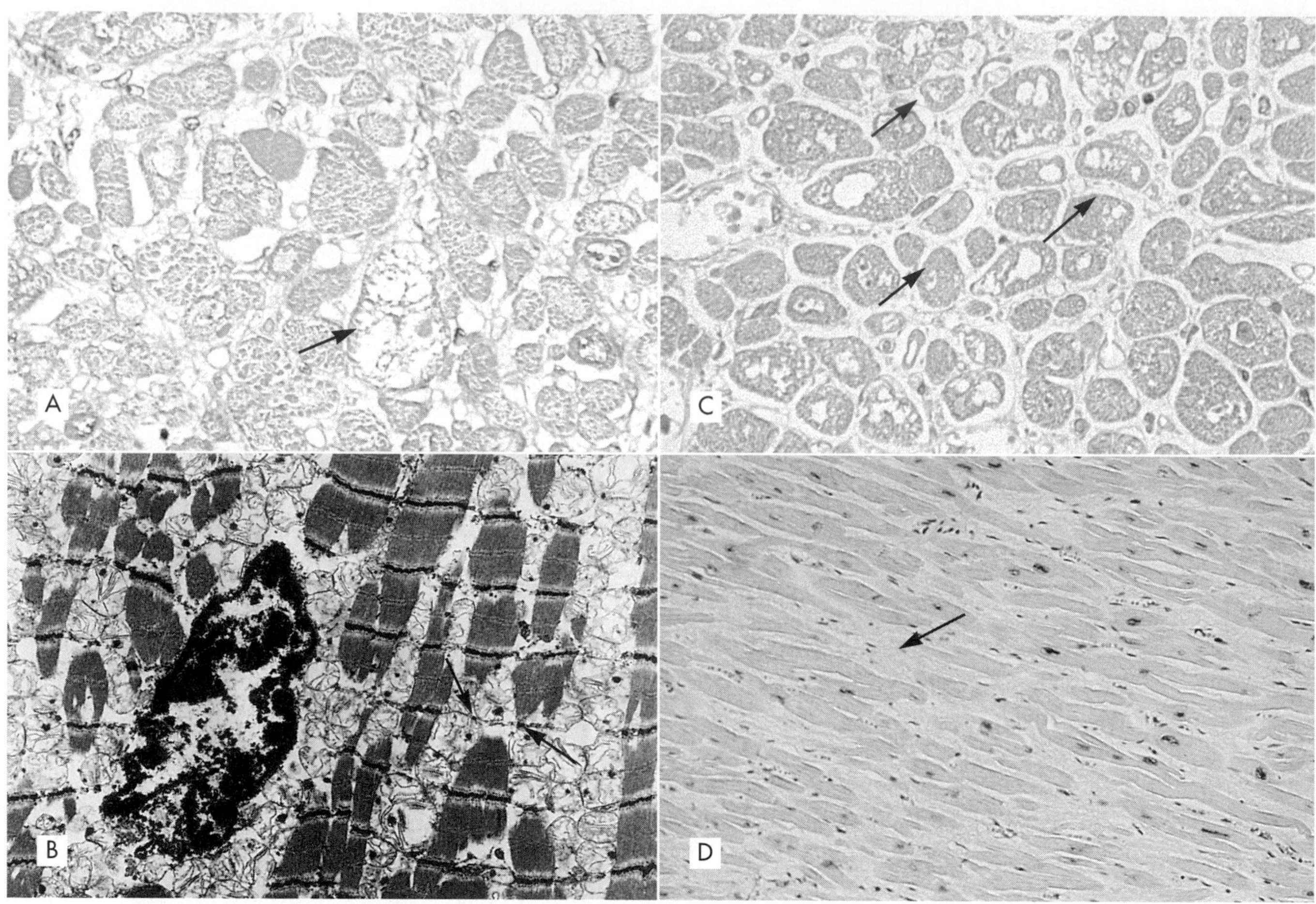

Fig. 45-17 A, Photomicrograph of ventricular myocardium with enlarged cardiac myocyte and coalescent vacuoles *(arrow)* consistent with anthracycline toxicity. Variable myocyte size is noted, and variable myofilament density reflects, in part, artifactual contraction bands and perhaps, in part, myofilament loss. **B,** Photomicrograph of ventricular myocardium from a patient with anthracycline toxicity. There are numerous cardiac myocytes with coalescent cytoplasmic vacuoles *(arrows)*. These vacuoles are most readily seen on Epon-embedded sections and on electron micrographs. At times, they may be seen readily on standard paraffin sections as shown here. The vacuoles reflect sarcoplasmic reticular dilatation. **C,** Electron micrograph of a ventricular myocyte with loss of sarcomeres in the setting of anthracycline cardiotoxicity. The Z band persists where sarcomeres have been lost in this field *(arrows)*. Loss of myofilament proteins is well described in anthracycline toxicity and is reflected here. **D,** Photomicrograph of ventricular myocardium with extensive interstitial fibrosis *(arrow)* in association with myocyte hypertrophy and nuclear hyperchromatism. This appearance is consistent with chronic effects of anthracycline toxicity with injury and repair.

replacement of normal pericardium is seen with large bizarre fibroblasts, mixed inflammation, and neovascular channels.[237]

Myocardial involvement. The myocardial tissue may be characterized by increased interstitial and perivascular fibrous tissue. In a similar fashion to the pericardia, there may be actual inflammation and a degree of vessel hyperemia. The visible extent of the involvement of the myocardium is usually minimal, unless an unusually large dose of radiation has been delivered. However, the myocardium would certainly be more stiff after significant anterior mediastinal radiation than before. The degree of inflammation is directly related to the intensity of the radiation and the duration of time from irradiation until examination. Thus, engorged neovessels and the inflammatory responses will tend to subside in the weeks after irradiation.

Endocardial involvement. The endocardium of the irradiated heart is often thickened by fibrous tissue (Fig. 45-20). This fibroblastic response to irradiation is rather universal. Thickening of the endocardium is not usually associated with frank thrombus formation. Similar changes occur in the valves of the irradiated heart. Irregular fibrosis of leaflets and cusps may be accompanied by dystrophic calcification in areas of most severe injury. Again, a degree of inflammation and neovascular response may be observed.

Conduction system involvement. In a fashion similar to the remainder of the heart, the conducting components of the myocardium may be affected by irradiation. Most commonly, the left bundle branches may be involved by fibrosis. Deeper components of the conduction network may be spared, given the usual location of the heart and its spatial orientation, as well as the field and direction of radiation.

Coronary artery involvement. The epicardial coronary arteries have been found to develop accelerated atherosclerotic disease in the face of irradiation. This change is typically fibrocalcific and may have an eggshell quality. Similar changes are noted in the thoracic aorta. Thus the intima, media, and adventitia of irradiated blood vessels are very responsive to the injury, and occlusive disease may be significantly enhanced.

Table 45-11 Histopathologic and ultrastructural evidence of major toxic effects of anthracyclines on cardiac myocytes

Atrophy
Nuclear chromatin condensation
Shrinkage or disappearance of nuclei
Accumulation of myelin figures
"Ghost" cells—myocytolysis, vacuolization
Myofibrillar changes
Frank loss
Irregularity, expansion of Z bands
Separation of myofilaments
Endoplasmic reticular changes
Dilatation (vacuolization)
Increased sarcoplasmic reticulum
Free ribosomes
Basophilic degeneration
Increased lipofuscin
Loss of cytoplasmic glycogen
Eventual interstitial and replacement fibrosis

Metabolic abnormalities

Protein metabolism

BROWN ATROPHY. As the human heart ages, accumulation of lipofuscin pigments may accompany general cell atrophy. The excess accumulation of lipofuscin (from Latin *fuscus* 'brown' pigment as a function of apparent lipid peroxidation of those lipids in subcellular membranes results in a characteristic enhancement of brown coloration in older heart muscle. The basis of accelerated accumulation of indigestible oxidative by-products in the aging heart is uncertain. The rate of accumulation may be considerably accelerated beyond the usual accumulation of such by-products as a person's heart reaches senescence. Although the lipofuscin pigments are not in themselves known to be cardiotoxic, they signal the progressive loss of structural and functional integrity of the heart muscle and are typically associated with mild degrees of myocardial compromise in the elderly patient.

PARENCHYMATOUS AND HYDROPIC DEGENERATION. Extraordinary conditions including infectious diseases, high fevers, intoxications from chemical and metallic substances, extensive burns, and anoxia may result in parenchymatous or hydropic degeneration. In this condition the myocardium is soft, and there is dilatation of the ventricles. The muscle of the ventricles may appear gray-brown and have a swollen, opaque appearance (that is, cloudy swelling). The microscopic appearance is that of swollen indistinct muscle cells with granularity of the cytoplasm. When severe, the cytoplasm is vacuolated in relation to intracellular edema.

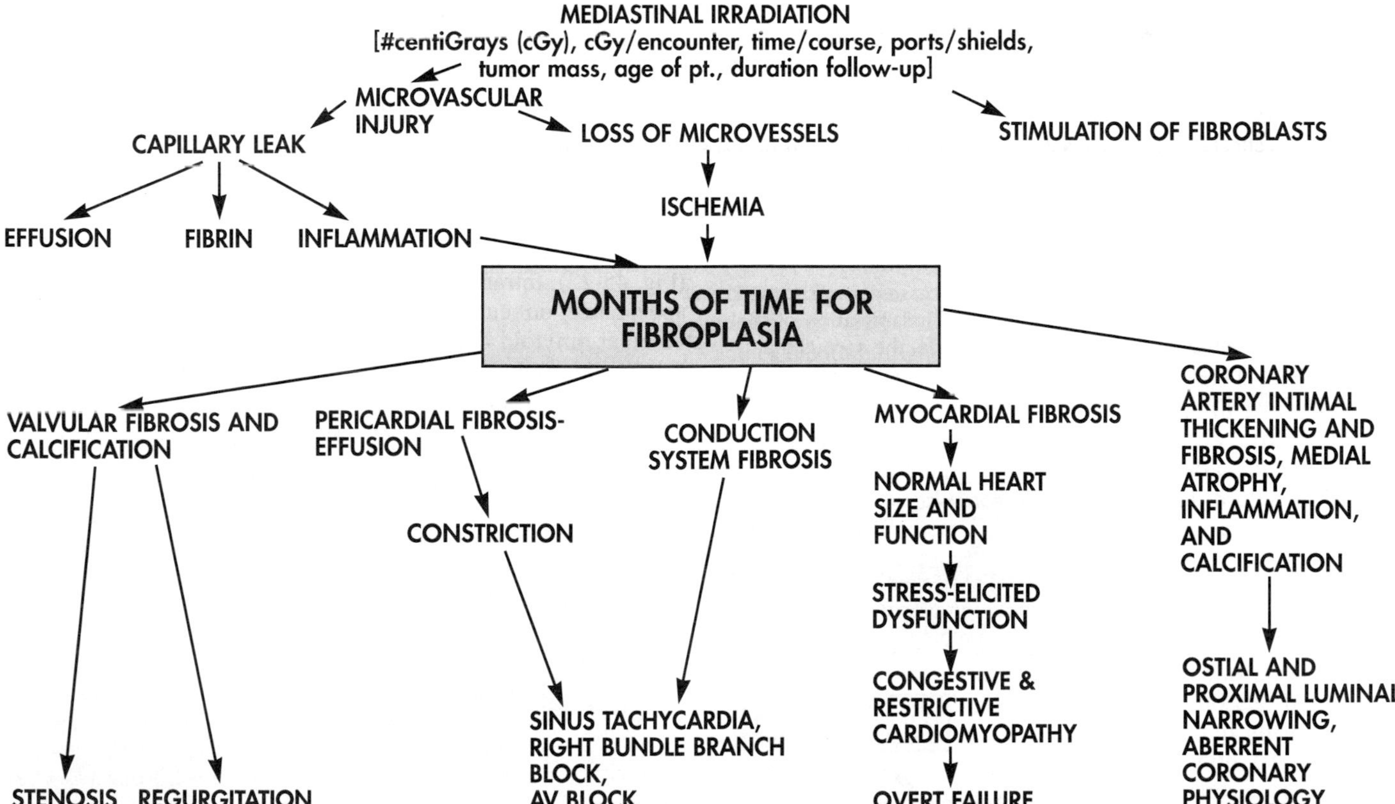

Fig. 45-18 Mediastinal irradiation for primary or secondary tumors results in macrovascular injury and alteration in fibroblast behavior. Over a period of months, a wide variety of pathobiologic consequences may ensue with a similarly diverse number of clinical consequences involving valvular, pericardial, conductive, myocardial, and vascular structures.

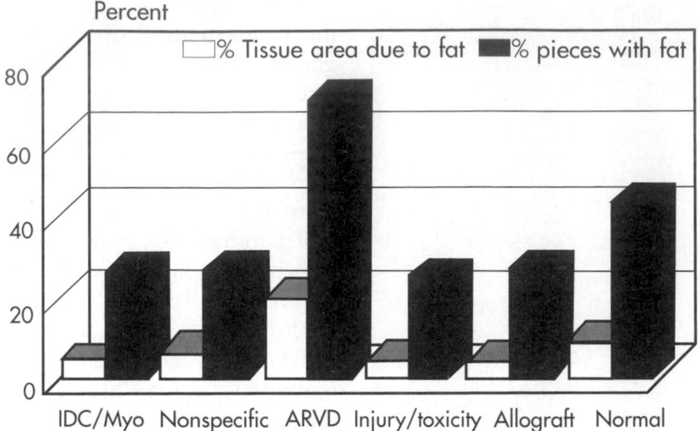

Fig. 45-24 Percentage of tissue area with fat and percentage of pieces with fat present in endomyocardial biopsy samples from patients in different clinicopathologic groups. A significantly greater amount of fat is present in arrhythmogenic right ventricular dysplasia than in any other group. (From Dembinski AS, Dobson JR, Wilson JE, et al: *Cardiovasc Pathol* 3:33, 1994.)

Table 45-13 The mucopolysaccharidoses and their cardiovascular effects

Type	Syndromes	Defect	Major cardiovascular consequences
I	Hurler-Scheie	α-L-Iduronidase deficiency	Thickened, dysfunctional valves and chordae; Severe coronary artery narrowing
II	Hunter	Iduronate sulphatase	Thickened, dysfunctional valves; altered cardiac interstitium, ventricular function
III	Sanfilippo A	Heparan sulphatase	Thickened valves
	B	*N*-Acetyl-α-D-glucosaminidase	
IV	Morquio	Hexosamine-6-sulphatase	Thickened valves
VI	Maroteaux-Lamy	Arylsulphatase B	Thickened valves
VII	—	β-Glucuronidase	Thickened valves; narrowed blood vessels

mechanically alter cardiac function and lead to obstructions or arrhythmias.

Calcification and ossification. When myocardial cells die, it is usually in the setting of ischemia. Also, in valvular structures wherein injury and repair phenomenon have been at play, there is cell death. Inflammatory diseases of pericardia will also lead to cell death. The extent of injury and repair and the rapidity of cell death contribute to the possibility of dystrophic calcification. Such calcification can be seen in areas of myocardial infarction, particularly when patients have been hypercalcemic during the before-death period. Calcification in rheumatic valves and in valves with degenerative stenoses is eventually the rule rather than the exception. There is also an indication that flexure points in heart valves are susceptible to dystrophic calcification. This may explain the phenomenon of mitral annular calcification. The evolution of calcific deposits within atherosclerotic plaques in epicardial coronary arteries reflects the same fundamental processes as seen in other cardiac locations (Fig. 45-26). Irradiation injury accelerates this process. As well, tuberous calcifications of the pericardia reflect the intense inflammatory and injurious processes that evolve to hyalinized fibrosis and calcification. Although uncommon, bone formation may be found in any cardiac locations where calcification occurs. Similarly, trabecular bone formation may be found in cardiac myxomas.

Metastatic calcification in the setting of metabolic abnormalities including hyperparathyroidism, malignant destruction of bone, hypervitaminosis D, or renal disorders, may lead to multiorgan calcification. The elastica of blood vessels and of endocardium is calciphilic and is among the first sites to reflect metastatic calcific processes.

Hemochromatosis and hemosiderosis. Iron-overload heart disease is another infiltrative disorder that may be seen as a cardiomyopathy of the restrictive or congestive form. Hemochromatosis (and iron-overload hemosiderosis), like amyloidosis, may be diagnosed by endomyocardial biopsy. Hereditary abnormalities in iron handling and environmentally induced (transfusion-related) iron overload may result in excessive iron deposits within the cardiac myocytes, as well as in their neighboring interstitial fibroblasts. The ventricular myocardium is most dramatically affected, with a gradient from epicardium to endocardium (most to least). The positiv-

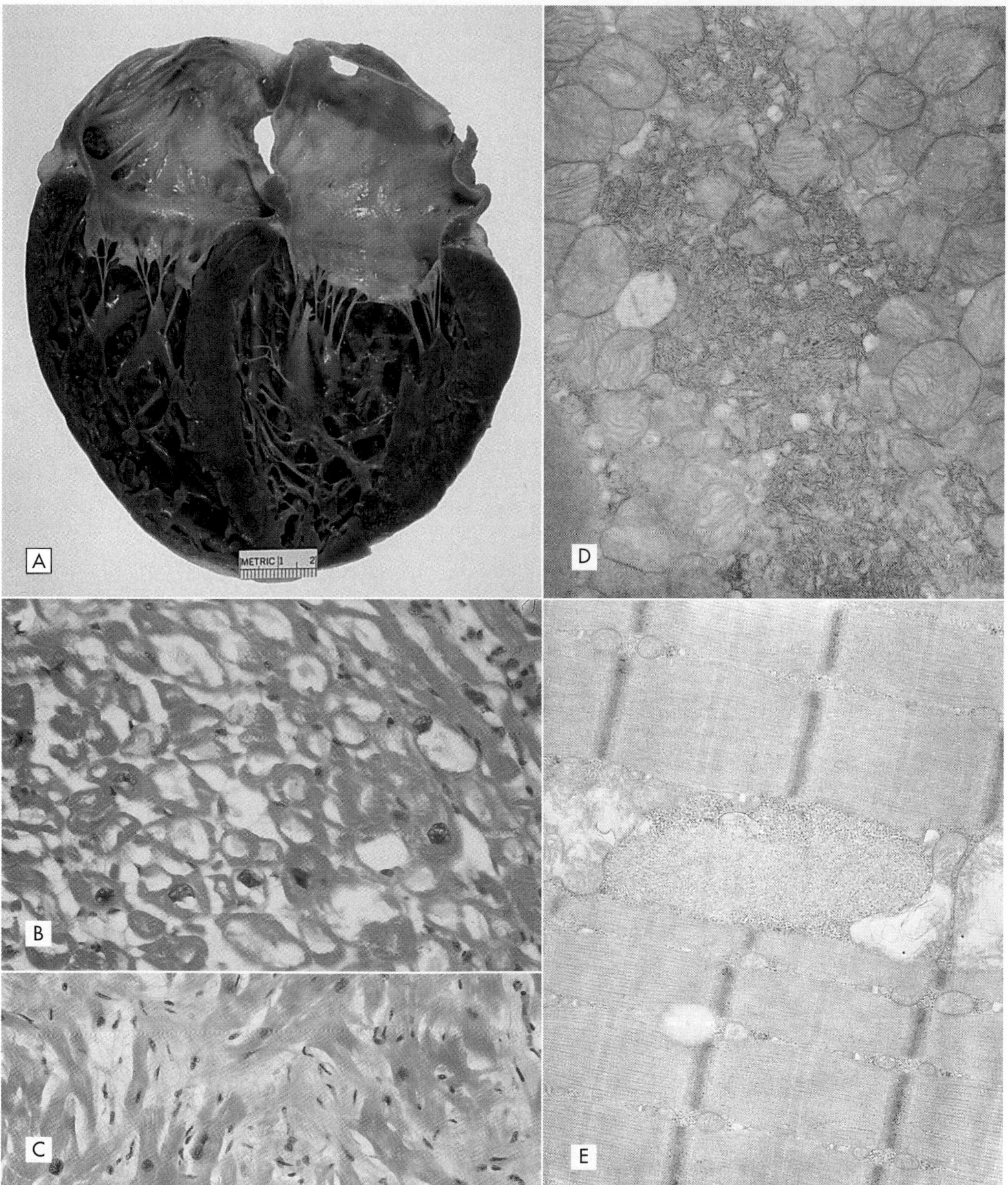

Fig. 45-25 The heart in type IV glycogenosis. **A,** Four-chamber echocardiographic view of an autopsy heart from a 12-year-old boy with pronounced four-chamber dilatation and bowing of the ventricular septum from left to right. **B,** Ventricular myocardium illustrating numerous cytoplasmic vacuoles with glycogen material present. In certain cells, the storage material has been removed by processing whereas others are completely loaded. Myocyte nuclear enlargement and hyperchromatism is noted in a few cells. **C,** Ventricular myocardium from the same patient stained with PAS to highlight the glycogen-rich storage material. **D,** Electron micrograph of a cardiac myocyte with accumulated fibrillar glycogen material surrounded by mitochondria. The fibrillar glycogen is typical of type IV glycogenosis **E,** Electron micrograph of skeletal muscle from the same patient depicting normal sarcomeres and glycogen material. The glycogen is mixed with alpha granules as well as fibrillar components.

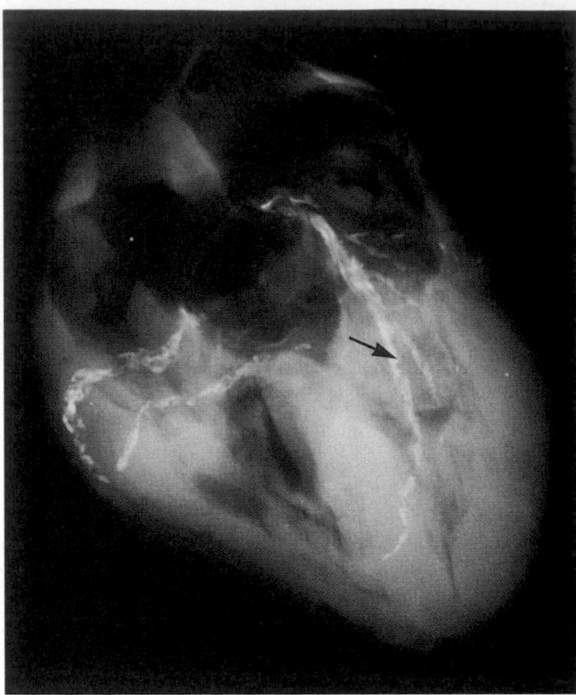

Fig. 45-26 Postmortem radiograph of heart with severe atherosclerotic disease and accompanying calcific changes. This impressive example of dystrophic calcification in atherosclerotic plaques provides a silhouette of the coronary artery distribution. The left anterior descending is depicted *(arrow),* whereas the right coronary artery loops to the lower left in the atrioventricular groove.

ity of Prussian blue stains may confirm an impression of gross "brownness," seen in the fresh state of organs affected by iron overload. Ultrastructural evidence indicates probable lysosomal localization. When hemolysis is induced by such processes as rigid or abnormal prosthetic heart valves, the same picture may be seen.[258] The myocardial function of the hemochromatotic heart may be significantly depressed.[259] Arrhythmias may also be observed.[260] It is possible with chelating agents to reverse the extent of myocardial iron deposition and improve structure and function. Detection of iron may be achieved by x-ray microanalysis and more recently by magnetic resonance injury. The role of iron in altering gene expression of myocyte structural and enzymatic proteins is a contemporary focus of interest.

ANEMIA. Iron-deficiency anemia or macrocytic anemia may lead to high-output heart failure. When anemia is long standing and untreated, the heart will work harder to maintain proper oxygenation and in the process will ultimately fail. The marginal oxygenation of the heart muscle itself will be reflected in fibrosis of the end artery-supplied papillary muscles. Thus it is common to find fibrous tips of papillary muscles in both right and left ventricles in the heart of the anemic patient.

When sickle cell trait (SA) is present, the extent of injury to the myocardium is often not profound. Thrombotic events may involve the coronary arteries or extracardiac vessels. The same is true for sickle cell disease (SS), only to a greater extent. The ventricles may become myopathic, dilated, and iron overloaded, the last from transfusional support. The same vascular events that lead to infarcts and ischemia will be manifest in the heart and other organs including the brain, spleen, kidneys, and eyes. Thus patients with sickle cell disease often develop a dilated cardiomyopathy, at least partly attributable to multiple infarcts and partly attributable to generalized myocardial ischemia.[261]

Nutritional disturbances

MALNUTRITION. In severe nutritional deprivation the heart may undergo brown atrophy. The heart becomes smaller, the cardiac myocytes become smaller, and the amount of lipofuscin pigment increases. Serous fat atrophy may be seen on the epicardial surface. The latter change may also be seen in patients with chronic diseases such as leukemias and lymphomas; it is also seen in acquired immunodeficiency syndrome. Heart failure in protein-deficient, carbohydrate-sufficient disease, kwashiorkor, is associated with a dilated cardiomyopathy with endomyocardial fibrosis and mural thrombus formation. Generalized myocytolytic changes and interstitial fibrosis are seen histologically. Similar findings may be observed in protein-calorie deficiency (marasmus).

Patients undergoing open heart surgery in whom *cardiac cachexia* has ensued because of underlying valvular disease are known to be at risk for poor outcome.[262] However, in efforts to improve nutritional status of such patients by repletion postoperatively the investigators were unable to alter outcomes.

VITAMIN DEFICIENCIES. In deficiency of vitamin B_1 (thiamine), also called *beriberi* (meaning in sinhalese 'I cannot, I cannot,' for the severe constipation such patients have), the possibility of congestive heart failure is certainly present. Hypoproteinemia as well as the failing heart may contribute to peripheral edema in such patients. Decreased afterload caused by peripheral vasodilatation accentuates cardiac output and cardiac work, ultimately leading to cardiac failure. This consequence is not unlike that seen with anemia. Thus the heart of the beriberi patient is grossly indistinguishable from idiopathic dilated cardiomyopathy. The interstitial edema of the heart with beriberi[263,264] is accompanied by slight endomyocardial fibrosis. It is not a surprise that some investigators have had difficulty separating the appearance of beriberi heart disease from that attributable to chronic alcoholism. The cardiomyopathy of alcohol abuse is also indistinguishable from idiopathic dilated cardiomyopathy.

Vitamin C deficiency (scurvy) may lead to multiple skeletal changes that contribute to pulmonary hypertension.[265] Thus, deaths in these patients are particularly related to RV hypertrophy, a form of cor pulmonale.

Selenium–vitamin E deficiency is now recognized as an important form of systemic disease that also involves the heart.[266] In this condition, originally termed *Keshan disease* for the city in Manchuria, China, where it was most endemic, relates to the deficiency of selenium in the soil and the essential interaction between vitamin E and selenium in normal cell physiology. Thus, in patients who die with Keshan's disease, there is impressive multigenerational evidence of injury with a unique and most profound form of contraction band formation that leads the remainder of each myocyte appearing virtually transparent on light microscopy. These acute lesions are associated with areas of healing. The role of vitamin E as an antioxidant has been revived, and the possibility that aberrant redox states that lead to myofiber necrosis are linked to a deficiency of vitamin E or other antioxidants is certainly tenable.

POTASSIUM. Regulation of myocardial potassium, as well as that level in the bloodstream, is crucial for normal physiologic processes. Severe hypokalemia leads to profound alterations in cardiac cell depolarization and action potential formation. Bradycardias and standstill may ensue. Myocyte necrosis and fibrosis may be observed. On the other hand, hyperkalemia may exacerbate ventricular arrhythmias and lead to fibrillation. Potassium homeostasis thus is delicate, reflected in the fact that potassium as an ion is the most implicated in otherwise unexplained hospital-related deaths.[267]

Endocrine disturbances

Hypothyroidism

DEFINITION AND CLINICAL PRESENTATION. Hypothyroidism occurs generally as a result of reduced secretion of thyroxine (T_4) and triiodothyronine (T_3) by the thyroid gland. Cardiac manifestations of thyroid deficiency are normally referred to as myxedema heart disease. Almost all hypothyroidism results from damage to the thyroid gland, usually mediated by inflammatory processes. Less commonly, hypothyroidism is linked to either hypothalamic or pituitary disease in which a reduction in thyrotropin secretion can produce the hypothyroid state.

The clinical signs of hypothyroidism often evolve gradually over a period of several years before the disorder is recognized. Patients experience weakness, fatigue, dry skin, cold intolerance, memory impairment, shortness of breath, constipation, personality inconsistency, and menorrhagia or other menstrual abnormalities. In severe hypothyroidism, patients demonstrate speech impairment, decreased hearing, puffy facial features, myxedema of the lower extremities, and yellow skin resulting from reduced conversion of carotene into vitamin A.

Cardiovascular manifestations of hypothyroidism are common. The chief findings are cardiac enlargement and dilatation, increased systemic vascular resistance, decreased stroke volume, weak arterial pulse, hypotension, increased systolic and presystolic ejection period, distant heart sound, and sinus bradycardia. Paroxysmal atrial tachycardias, atrial fibrillation, and pericardial effusions have also been reported.[268-270] The precise relationship between atherosclerosis and thyroid deficiency is not fully understood though a significantly higher incidence of atherosclerosis in hyperthyroid patients has been observed.[271,272]

As with thyroid disorders in general, hypothyroidism is more common in women than in men, occurring at least twice as often in female patients.[68] Hypothyroidism is less common in children and adolescents, though congenital thyroid deficiency is found in infants, and is normally detected within the first 3 months of life. In adults, the incidence of hypothyroidism is highest between the third and sixth decades.

PATHOLOGY. Overt cardiac enlargement and dilatation of the individual chambers are the primary gross pathologic features of myxedema heart disease. Enlargement is attributable to myocardial damage, and the enlarged heart may be accompanied by pericardial effusion.[273] A flabby, pale myocardium is also typical. Ventricular wall hypertrophy (thickening) is rare, usually evident only in patients with coexistent hypertension.

Microscopic evidence of myxedema heart disease is reflected primarily in the cardiac myocytes. Histologic changes include myofiber vacuolization, swelling, degeneration, and loss of cross-striations. Interstitial edema and fatty infiltration may also be apparent. Interstitial connective tissue may be somewhat gelatinous. Basophilic (mucoid) degeneration occurs in myxedema, and, as discussed earlier, is characterized by fine granular accumulations in the cytoplasm of individual myocytes. Basophilic degeneration in hypothyroid heart disease is found primarily in the LV free wall myocardium and ventricular septum. Ultrastructural features of the granular material that constitutes basophilic degeneration reveals fibrillar elements digestible by amylase.

THERAPY. For younger patients with minor cardiovascular complications, administration of daily oral doses of L–thyroxine usually restores normal function and returns serum hormone levels to stable euthyroidism within a few months. In elderly or severely ill patients, or patients with underlying cardiac disorders, care must be taken in augmenting hormone replacement to avoid potentially devastating effects on the cardiovascular system. Thus, more gradual T_4 replacement is recommended in patients with CAD or congestive heart failure. In these patients, surgical revascularization of the diseased arteries may be performed successfully before full thyroid hormone replacement. Propranolol management of angina in the setting of serious myxedema can induce severe bradycardia.

Hyperthyroidism

DEFINITION AND CLINICAL PRESENTATION. Hyperthyroidism denotes an overabundance of the thyroid hormones T_4 and T_3. Although multiple human organs are typically affected by hyperthyroidism, the heart is the most sensitive human organ to thyroid imbalance. As such, cardiac manifestations are, in most instances, the primary clinical indicators of hyperthyroidism. Cardiac involvement in thyroid imbalance varies significantly depending on the extent of thyroid excess; the most serious cardiac sequelae of hyperthyroidism are acute angina pectoris and congestive heart failure, both of which must be promptly addressed.

Graves' disease (diffuse toxic goiter) and Plummer's disease (nodular toxic goiter) are the most common causes of hyperthyroidism. In rare instances, hyperthyroidism may occur secondarily to a thyroid hormone–producing carcinoma. Other infrequent causes include subacute thyroiditis (namely, Hashimoto's thyroiditis, or painless lymphocyte thyroiditis), a single, toxic adenoma, excessive thyroid hormone ingestion, excessive iodine or iodide ingestion, or McCune-Albright syndrome[68,274]

Patients with hyperthyroidism normally demonstrate a range of general symptoms, including fatigue, hyperactivity, insomnia, heat and exercise intolerance, dyspnea, increased appetite with weight loss, nocturia, diarrhea, oligomenorrhea, muscle weakness, tremor, hyperthermia, emotional lability, and eyelid retraction. Cardiac manifestations of hyperthyroidism (Table 45-14) provide the most definitive evidence of thyroid hormone excess.

In certain patients, particularly older adults, clinical signs of hyperthyroidism may not be apparent. In these instances especially, cardiac manifestations are essential features for accurate diagnosis. Elevated T_3 and, in most cases, T_4 levels in the blood also provide telltale evidence of thyroid excess.

Auscultatory findings in hyperthyroidism include a midsystolic murmur along the left sternal border and a hyperactive precordium accompanied by a loud first heart sound. The so-called Means-Lerman systolic scratch heard in the second left intercostal space during expiration may also be present.[68]

Hyperthyroidism occurs in varying degrees of severity, depending on the amount of excess thyroid hormones present in the patient. It is a relatively common disorder, particularly in adults between ages 30 and 50; women are four to eight times more likely to develop hyperthyroidism than men.[68] Hyperthyroidism is less common in children, normally developing during puberty or early adolescence.

Table 45-14 Cardiac manifestations of hyperthyroidism

Increased heart rate; tachycardia
Atrial fibrillation, palpitations
Increased cardiac output and cardiac work
Increased coronary blood flow
Enhanced left ventricular contractility
Abbreviated systolic ejection period and preejection period
Decreased systemic vascular resistance
Widened pulse pressure
Systolic and diastolic (less common) hypertension
Cardiac hypertrophy
Serum enzyme abnormalities

PATHOLOGY. Moderate cardiac hypertrophy is the main gross pathologic characteristic of hyperthyroidism. Heart size in hyperthyroid patients is typically 30% to 50% greater than a normal heart.[275] Early on, the heart is primarily hypertrophied without chamber dilatation. Once hypermetabolism has been prolonged, the heart will begin to fail and dilate.

Microscopically, myofiber hypertrophy, foci of eosinophilic and lymphocytic inflammation, mild interstitial fibrosis, and fatty infiltration may be apparent. Necrosis or fibrosis of papillary muscle tips may be observed as well. Investigation of cardiac involvement in hyperthyroidism reveals specific mitochondrial changes within the heart. Mitochondria are often increased in number and size and are often vacuolated with disorientation of cristae.[276]

THERAPY. Cardiac complications of hyperthyroidism normally recede or are erased when the source of the thyroid imbalance is swiftly identified and treated. However, given the pathogenesis of the various sequelae, precise diagnosis is essential for effective reduction of the influence on the heart. The specific cardiovascular manifestations and the severity of the hyperthyroid state are additional determinants of appropriate therapy. It is also important to eliminate the possibility of additional factors, acting independently or in association with thyroid hormones, which mimic hyperthyroidism. Catecholamine excess, induced endogenously or exogenously, produces clinical and cardiac symptoms almost identical to those associated with hyperthyroidism, as does enhanced sympathoadrenal activity in general.[274,277,278] The relationship between sympathoadrenal processes and hyperthyroidism and their influence on the cardiovascular system are discussed comprehensively elsewhere.[277,278]

Surgical removal of the thyroid gland is the definitive therapy for uncomplicated hyperthyroidism, normally used in younger patients (less than 25 years). Radioactive iodine(^{131}I) therapy is used in older patients. Neither method, however, is applicable in critically ill patients, nor in patients with Hashimoto's thyroiditis. In the latter instance, the thyrotoxic phase is quickly terminated on administration of antithyroid drugs or beta-blockade therapy.[275] Beta-adrenoreceptor blocking agents are also effective in reducing thyroid production and influence in severely ill patients and are particularly important in reversing atrial fibrillation, tachycardia, palpitations, heat intolerance, fatigue, and weakness. In patients with congestive heart failure unassociated with tachycardia, Beta-blockade may not be appropriate, since interference with sympathetic stimulation of the heart may worsen cardiac congestion. Simultaneous administration of cardiac glycosides or other inotropes with appropriate doses of beta-blocking agents may reduce the risk of heart failure.

Beta-adrenergic blockade is the most effective pharmaceutical method for diminishing the cardiac complications of hyperthyroidism; it does not, however, reverse the elevated rate of oxidation associated with the accelerated metabolic rate. Treatment of the fundamental thyroid imbalance can be achieved only through the concomitant administration of agents that limit overall thyroid hormone production.

Pituitary disease

ACROMEGALY. Excessive secretion of growth hormone (GH) somatotropin results in acromegaly, the only disease of the pituitary gland capable of producing significant cardiovascular malfunction. GH deficiency, by contrast, has no known particular cardiac sequelae.

In most patients, acromegaly is the result of GH production by an eosinophilic or chromophobe pituitary adenoma. Clinical evidence of acromegaly evolves gradually; symptoms often go unrecognized for more than a decade. The clinical manifestations are produced by the effect of excessive GH levels on muscle, bone, and connective tissues. Broadening and coarsening of hands, feet, and facial features are the most pronounced external features of the disease. Organomegaly, in which the heart often exceeds other organs in proportional enlargement, is a common finding. Metabolic alterations, including glucose intolerance (sometimes in the form of full-blown diabetes mellitus), and osteoporosis may also present as coindications of GH excess. Coexisting hyperthyroidism occurs in up to 10% of acromegalic patients.[279]

Cardiac complications occur in approximately one third of all acromegalic patients[279] and are a primary cause of mortality in acromegaly.[208,280,281] Gross hypertrophy and dilatation of the heart are seen in most cases. Moreover, the incidence of a coexisting cardiac dysfunction in various forms is significantly higher in acromegalic patients than in control populations. Hypertension is one of the chief cardiovascular disorders associated with GH excess; 25% to 35% of patients with acromegaly present with systemic hypertension, a rate almost four times higher than in the general population.[279] Additional cardiovascular manifestations of acromegaly include congestive heart failure, ischemic heart disease, and CAD, namely, angina, infarction, and atherosclerosis, though this last, in most cases, is relatively mild. Arrhythmias, particularly premature ventricular contractions and AV conduction defects, are also found.

Acromegaly, by definition, is an adult disease. Excessive GH secretion in children is normally referred to as *gigantism* (or *giantism*) and produces different effects.[108] In adults, GH excess may occur at any age, though the slow progression of the disease and the almost imperceptible development of its clinical manifestations ensures that most cases are not recognized until the third to fifth decade of life. Cardiomegaly as the primary cardiac sequela of acromegaly normally presents after the fifth decade.[282] Acromegaly occurs in both sexes; however, pituitary adenomas, which may result in acromegaly, are slightly more common in men than in women.

PATHOLOGIC FEATURES. The most striking gross pathologic characteristic of the cardiovascular system in acromegaly is the noticeable enlargement of the heart. Heart weights in excess of 1000 g are not uncommon in acromegaly.[283] Hypertrophy and dilatation occurs in all cardiac chambers, and the myocardium of both ventricles is often greatly thickened. Thus, concentric LV hypertrophy is a common finding.

Increased interstitial fibrous tissue ranges from moderate to extensive. The somewhat myxoid connective tissue is a distinctive microscopic feature of acromegalic heart disease. Other frequent changes include myocyte hypertrophy and myofibrillar degeneration. Less commonly, intimal and medial fibromuscular hyperplasia may be present in intramural coronary arteries.

PATHOBIOLOGY CONSIDERATIONS. The specific mechanisms by which GH excess (acromegaly) produces various cardiac disorders are not fully understood. The etiology and pathogenesis of cardiomegaly in particular has been a major debate among investigators of acromegaly over the last decade, and, despite the number of hypotheses proposed, no consensus has been reached.[283] Cardiomegaly may be related in part to the generalized effect of GH on protein synthesis; however, the lack of a direct correlation between the extent of heart enlargement and the level of circulating somatotropin indicates that other factors must be involved. Thus it is possible that additional pituitary products trigger heart enlargement. The ambiguity surrounding these ideas has led several researchers to propose the existence of an distinct "acromegalic cardiomyopathy." This concept accounts for the cardiomegaly and depressed cardiac function present in absence of hypertension, valvular disease, and CAD.[283-286]

The precise interaction of hypertension and GH excess is equally uncertain. There is no consistent relationship linking the level of circulating GH to blood pressure in the acromegalic patient.[279] The process by which hypertension develops remains unknown; however, sodium retention, resulting from the direct effect of somatotropin on the kidney, is at least partly responsible.

THERAPY. Surgery and proton-beam irradiation are the two methods of treatment most often used on acromegalic patients. The choice of therapy depends largely on the specific condition in the individual patient, the severity of illness, and the severity and combination of accompanying cardiac disorders. Surgical procedures entail greater risk; however, they are much more expedient in halting and in reversing, at least in part, the progression of the disease. GH secretion levels decrease within hours or days after surgical removal of a pituitary tumor, whereas the results of radiation therapy may take months to years. Isotope implantation, used independently or in conjunction with other methods, has been used with variable success in acromegalic patients. Medical therapy, normally in the form of dopamine agonists, bromocriptine, or somatostatin, can assist in the suppression of GH secretion.

Treatment of associated cardiovascular disease normally involves the same measures used in nonacromegalic patients. Significantly, patients with acromegaly-associated hypertension are particularly responsive to volume-depleting approaches involving diuretics and sodium restriction.[282] The efficacy of these methods is likely attributable to their ability to counteract the effect of somatotropin in the kidney. By contrast, patients in whom so-called acromegalic cardiomyopathy appears to be the underlying cause of congestive heart disease are highly resistant to conventional cardiac therapy.[282]

Catecholamines effects

DEFINITION AND CLINICAL PRESENTATION. Catecholamines, produced endogenously at normal levels, play an important role in regulating myocardial function and metabolism. Catecholamine toxicity results from catecholamine secretion by the adrenal medullary tumor, pheochromocytoma, or from therapeutic administration of catecholamines (normally for the treatment of pump failure) at levels exceeding the body's physiologic milieu.

Because physicians today are aware of the toxic effects of excessive doses of catecholamines, most catecholamine-induced cardiomyopathies result from pheochromocytomas. These tumors are sympathoadrenal masses derived from chromaffin cells. Although rare, they have received considerable attention primarily because of their poor prognosis without early diagnosis.

Most pheochromocytomas occur sporadically, though a small proportion (approximately 10%) are familial, inherited as an autosomal trait, typically associated with a pluriglandular neoplastic syndrome.[287] The most commonly secreted catecholamines associated with pheochromocytomas are norepinephrine and epinephrine, normally elaborated in combination, though hypersecretion of both, and especially norepinephrine, may occur in isolation. Pheochromocytoma production of dopamine alone has been reported,[288] though this particular form of catecholamine excess may not have significant cardiac implications.

The primary clinical manifestation of catecholamine toxicity is hypertension. Hypertension associated with catecholamine excess is sustained in most patients and is often distinguished by paroxysmal "attacks." Patients with catecholamine toxicity may also present with intermittent or sustained hypertension without paroxysms.[108] The sudden elevation in blood pressure may also be associated with additional symptoms during paroxysmal attacks. These include sweating, headaches, anxiety, tremor, fatigue, nausea, vomiting, abdominal pain, and visual field disturbances.[108] Additional clinical symptoms include increased basal metabolism, decreased skeletal muscle function and calcium turnover, emotional lability, and eyelid retraction.[277] The most severe, noncardiac complications of catecholamine-related hypertension are pulmonary edema, cerebral hemorrhage, and death.

Cardiovascular sequelae of hypertension secondary to catecholamine toxicity are various, including congestive heart failure, myocardial infarction, ventricular fibrillation, contraction band necrosis, acute myocarditis, and cardiac arrest. Any of the clinical features associated with these particular cardiac disorders may be linked to underlying catecholamine excess.

Pheochromocytomas can occur in both sexes at any age, though, in both men and women, pheochromocytomas occur most frequently in the fourth and fifth decades.

PATHOLOGY. The chief gross pathologic characteristic of the heart in protracted catecholamine excess is LV hypertrophy. The degree of hypertrophy depends on the severity of associated hypertension. Subendocardial hemorrhages, found along the LV papillary muscles, and intramyocardial hemorrhages are common as early lesions.

Microscopic features include myocyte hypertrophy and nuclear polyploidy (Fig. 45-27). In acute hypercatecholaminemia, areas of eosinophilic traverse banding begin to appear, with alternating granular zones within the cytoplasm and with loss of definition of the linear myofibrillar arrangement and normal cross–striations. Approximately half the patients with advanced pheochromocytomas also have myocardial necrosis with contraction bands. As the lesion progresses, microscopic examination reveals infiltration by polymorphonuclear leukocytes, lymphocytes, and histiocytes and phagocytosis of necrotic cell debris accompanied by small hemorrhages and edema.[289] In certain settings, a basophilic, finely granular

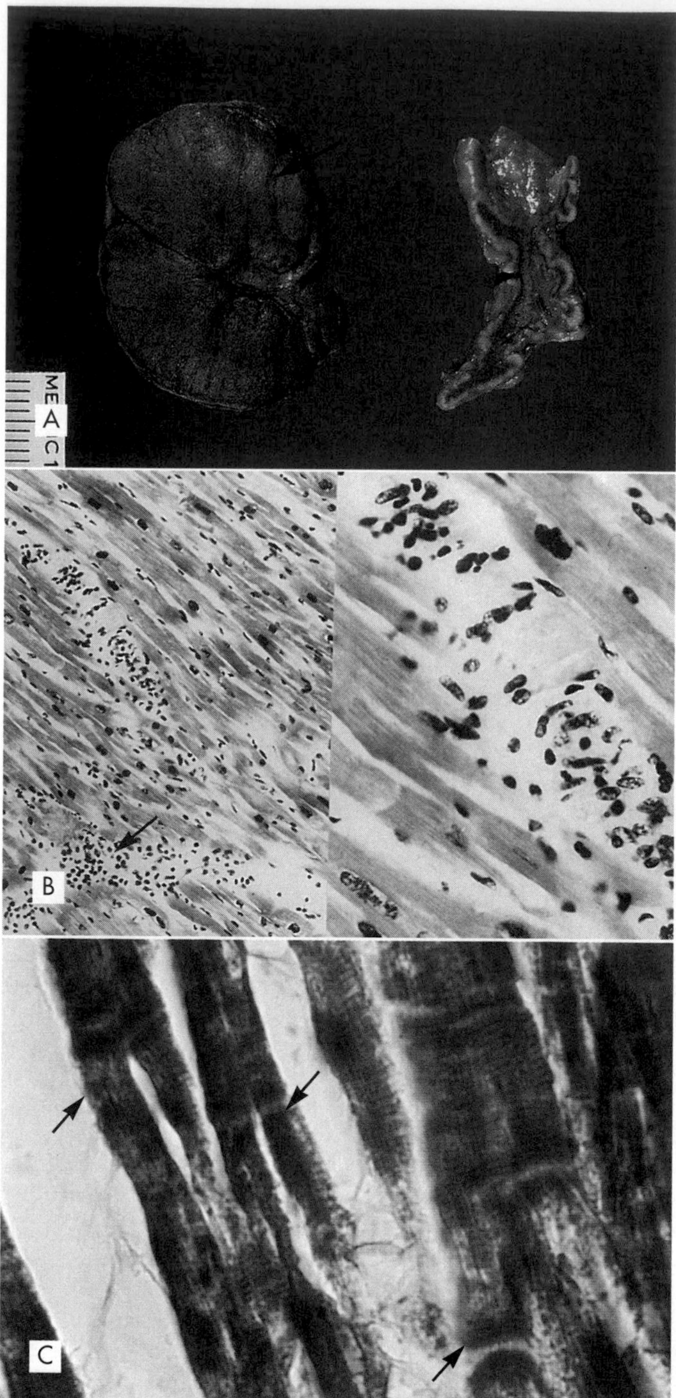

Fig. 45-27 **A,** Left and right adrenal glands from a young woman with sudden cardiac death and extensive catecholamine toxic lesions in the myocardium. Here the left adrenal gland has a greatly expanded medulla *(arrow)* capable of producing excess catecholamines. Such causes of elevated serum catecholamine levels and catecholamine cardiotoxicity are rare but must be considered. **B,** Photomicrographs of ventricular myocardium from a patient with pheochromocytoma and sudden cardiac death. An early but rather extensive interstitial infiltrate, predominated by polymorphonuclear leukocytes *(arrow),* is associated with numerous contraction band lesions in myocytes. The tissue also has an edematous appearance. **C,** Photomicrograph of ventricular myocardium with extensive myocyte contraction bands *(arrows).* This type of change may be reversible or irreversible but is associated with catecholamine toxicity, either exogenously or endogenously derived. (Phosphotungstic acid–hematoxylin stain.)

material representing dislocated mitochondria is found between the eosinophilic myocyte contraction bands.

Ultrastructurally, hypercontracted sarcomeres with swollen mitochondria and endoplasmic reticulum are evident. Amorphous calcium phosphate deposits are found in mitochondria, with these latter lesions typically containing calcium hydroxyapatite. Calcium deposits are regarded as indications of irreversible myocardial damage.

PATHOBIOLOGY. Disease progression in catecholamine toxicity is related, in part, to the particular type and quantity of catecholamine present in overabundance. As reviewed, endogenous norepinephrine and epinephrine and synthetic isoproterenol, each differ considerably in the manner and intensity with which they influence on the heart.[290] In addition, a range of coexisting physiologic factors may contribute to or accelerate myocardial injury.[290]

The primary process by which catecholamine toxicity elicits its cardiovascular malfunction involves excessive adrenergic stimulation of both alpha- and beta-adrenoreceptors in the coronary bed. In normal myocardial activity, alpha-receptors are generally responsible for mediating vasoconstriction, whereas beta-receptors instigate vasodilatation and cardiac myocyte contractility. Catecholamine overabundance and associated adrenoreceptor overstimulation depletes muscle cell energy reserves causing biochemical and ultimately structural alteration of cardiac cells, the most important being myocardial hypercontraction. Hypertension is a consequence of central and peripheral adrenergic stimulation.

THERAPY. Swift intervention is required in catecholamine toxicity in order to halt the progression of what is otherwise a deadly disease. Prompt recognition and management greatly improve the prognosis. Before therapy can begin, however, a definitive diagnosis is imperative, normally made on the basis of excess levels of catecholamines in urine or plasma samples. Imaging may help. Clinical presentations are confusing because of the remarkable similarities in the clinical picture of both hyperthyroidism and catecholamine excess.

After catecholamine toxicity has been confirmed, administration of pharmacologic adrenergic-receptor blockers help to reduce the effect of circulating catecholamines. The varying efficacy of some of the more common antagonists is discussed elsewhere.[289] When a pheochromocytoma is the underlying cause of catecholamine excess, surgical removal of the tumor is normally performed after the adrenergic blockade therapy has stabilized the patient thereby increasing the chances of intraoperative and postoperative survival. Dramatic improvement in cardiovascular state is normally reached after removal of the pheochromocytoma.

Carcinoid heart disease

DEFINITION AND CLINICAL PRESENTATION. Cardiac abnormalities associated with the carcinoid syndrome are caused by circulating hormonal substances secreted by a carcinoid tumor. Carcinoid tumors arise from enterochromaffin cells and are usually found in the gastrointestinal or respiratory tracts, though other locations have been described.[291,292] Cardiac manifestations are seen in approximately half of all patients with carcinoid tumors.[293] The right side of the heart is the most commonly affected, whereas left–sided cardiac involvement is seen in only one third of all patients with fatal carcinoid syndrome and rarely induces hemodynamic complications like those found in right-sided involvement.[293] Carcinoid syndrome is found equally in both sexes, with the highest incidence of disease occurring in the sixth decade.[294]

The presentation of patients with metastatic midgut carcinoid tumors includes diarrhea, episodic flushing, mottling and cyanosis, telangiectasias, and bronchospasm. Serum levels of serotonin are elevated and 5-hydroxyindoleacetic acid is in excess in the urine. Diarrhea, bronchoconstriction, cutaneous flushing, and endocardial plaques are the primary characteristics of carcinoid syndrome. Less commonly, patients may present with respiratory problems including episodic asthma or hyperventilation, normally during flushing attacks.[294] Cardiac manifestations normally develop much more gradually than other symptoms and often go unrecognized for several years. Clinical markers of carcinoid heart disease include increased venous pressure, RV hypertrophy and right-sided cardiac murmurs, indications of tricuspid insufficiency or stenosis, and pulmonary stenosis. Over time, right-sided cardiac failure develops and peripheral edema becomes increasingly conspicuous.

When cardiac structures are involved, typically the tricuspid and pulmonary valves have focal and diffuse plaques of glycosaminoglycan-rich, elastin-free connective tissue onlayed over the valve leaflets and cusps and over the neighboring mural endocardium. Similar deposits may be seen anywhere in the right-sided chambers of the heart. The underlying structure of the heart valves is generally intact, including the elastic lamina on which the plaques lay. Occasional neovessels with rare mononuclear cells may be evident in association with the plaques. The plaques are present on both sides of the cusps or leaflets, more often upstream on the tricuspid valve and downstream on the pulmonic valve. Combined tricuspid valve regurgitation and pulmonary valve stenosis are the most common complications. Fusion and thickening of chordae tendineae by the same process may contribute to valvular dysfunction. Rarely, the left-sided valve structures will be involved. The pulmonary circulation apparently metabolizes the circulating substance responsible for the development of the succulent plaques. Left-sided cardiac lesions have been observed in patients without a left-to-right cardiovascular shunt, an indication that the probable causative substance is not totally inactivated in the lungs. It remains to be clarified as to what other circulating peptides beyond serotonin might be involved in a metabolic alteration of the leaflets leading to plaques.

PATHOLOGY. The gross pathologic characteristics of the heart in carcinoid syndrome include right atrial enlargement, right-axis deviation, and RV hypertrophy. Focal or diffuse plaque-like thickening is seen in the valvular and mural endocardium and occasionally in the intima of the great veins, coronary sinus, pulmonary trunk, and main pulmonary arteries. Fibrous tissue is located primarily on the ventricular aspect of the posterior and septal leaflets of the tricuspid valve (Fig. 45-28). When the atrial aspect is involved, fibrous tissue may be evident to comparable degrees on both the ventricular and atrial aspects of the anterior leaflet.

Unknown causes

Congestive (dilated) cardiomyopathy

Definition and clinical presentation. Congestive cardiomyopathy is clinically noted by the presence of cardiomegaly, progressive and recurrent heart failure, and signs of systemic or pulmonary embolism. It occurs most frequently in adult men.

Pathology. Grossly, the most prominent feature is dilatation of both ventricles (Fig. 45-29). The weight of the heart, however, can be heavier than normal, or in the normal range. A common finding is that of mural thrombi, either in one or both of the ventricles. Microscopically the most common finding is an increase in the size of myocardial fibers.

Hypertrophic cardiomyopathy

Definition and clinical presentation. Hypertrophic cardiomyopathy (HCM) has received much attention since it was first described as an unequivocal pathologic entity over 30

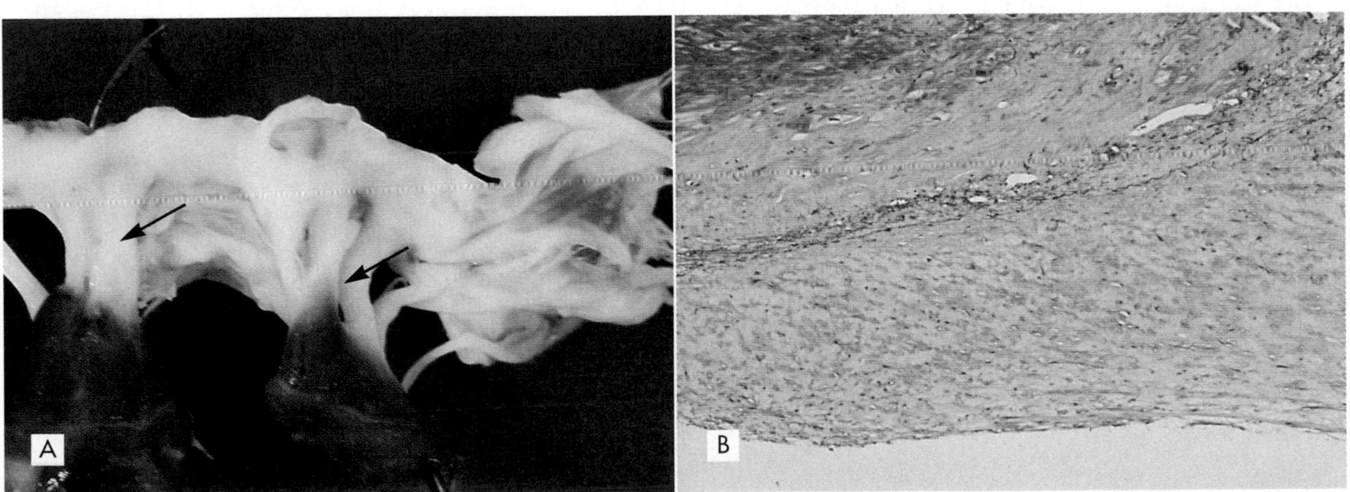

Fig. 45-28 A, Greatly and variably thickened valvular and chordal tissue of a tricuspid valve removed from a patient with carcinoid heart disease. The very white connective tissue *(arrow)* overlying the chordae tendineae is typical of the involvement seen on tricuspid and pulmonic valves in patients with midgut carcinoids metastatic to the liver. The tissue is an "onlay" of glycosaminoglycan-rich material. The papillary *(PAP)* muscle is designated. It is also apparent that portions of the valve leaflet are relatively spared (notice translucent region to the upper right). **B,** Photomicrograph of the junction of the elastica *(E)* of tricuspid valve papillary muscle with glycosaminoglycan *(GAG)*–rich connective tissue onlay *(sea green)* in the setting of carcinoid heart disease. The papillary muscle is partially fibrotic and collagen-rich as reflected in the yellow coloration. (Movat's stain.)

years ago. In this disorder the heart is hypertrophied and hyperdynamic. Systolic ejection generally is in the range of 70% to 80% of LV end-diastolic volume, and "heart failure" results partly from difficulty in diastolic filling of the hypertrophied, poorly compliant, small-cavity ventricle. Impaired relaxation and increased wall stress contribute to diminished rate and degree of diastolic filling. The left atrium is typically dilated. Because a midsystolic subaortic gradient frequently is present, HCMs are usually subdivided into those with and those without obstruction. It has never been clarified whether the gradient reflects a real obstruction to blood flow or the finding is incidental in a hyperdynamic heart that obliterates the left ventricle in systole. Since patients with gradients do no worse and possibly even better than patients without gradients and since gradients tend to vary in the same patient, the subclassification by "obstruction" has become less meaningful in management.

The pathogenesis of HCM is unresolved, and the morphologic and clinical forms are varied. In about 50% to 60% of patients, HCM is a familial. Regardless, the disorder is typically associated with asymmetrical hypertrophy of the ventricular septum. The extent and location of hypertrophic involvement can, however, be quite variable.

Pathologic features. Thickening of the anterior (and posterior) mitral valve leaflets because of septal contact induced by anterior systolic motion is complemented by mirror-image fibrous plaque formation in the LV outflow tract. The anterior mitral valve area is increased. As well, variable scarring may be present in the ventricular septum, suggestive of ischemic episodes. The myocardial histologic appearance is abnormal, highlighted by disarray (disorganization) of myocardial fibers and abnormally thick-walled intramural coronary arteries (Fig. 45-29).

Pathobiology. HCM was described categorically by Donald Teare in 1958,[295] who observed it at autopsy as the cause of sudden death in young adults. Earlier observers had suggested a distinct disease entity with asymmetrical LV hypertrophy, but interest was not piqued until Teare's description.[296] Familial studies support the idea that HCM may reflect an underlying genetic defect, ultimately manifest in abnormal cardiac structure and function. Nearly 40 point mutations have been found in the beta-myosin heavy-chain gene[297] and in the troponin T gene[298] (Fig. 45-30). The muscle fiber disarray may reflect abnormal wall stress and tension created by the abnormality of cardiac shape or genetically determined functional abnormalities of LV contraction. If present early enough in embryonic life, functional abnormalities could result in the congenital abnormality of heart structure. The precise interaction of structure and function in this condition remains unknown. However, this interplay may determine why the disease is manifest in some people very early in life and in others much later.

Arrhythmogenic right ventricular dysplasia

Definition and clinical presentation. Arrhythmogenic right ventricular dysplasia (ARVD), first described in 1977, affects children beginning in infancy and adults into old age.[300,301] The average age of patients with a clinical diagnosis of ARVD is 36 years. Although arrhythmias, syncope, and sudden death are

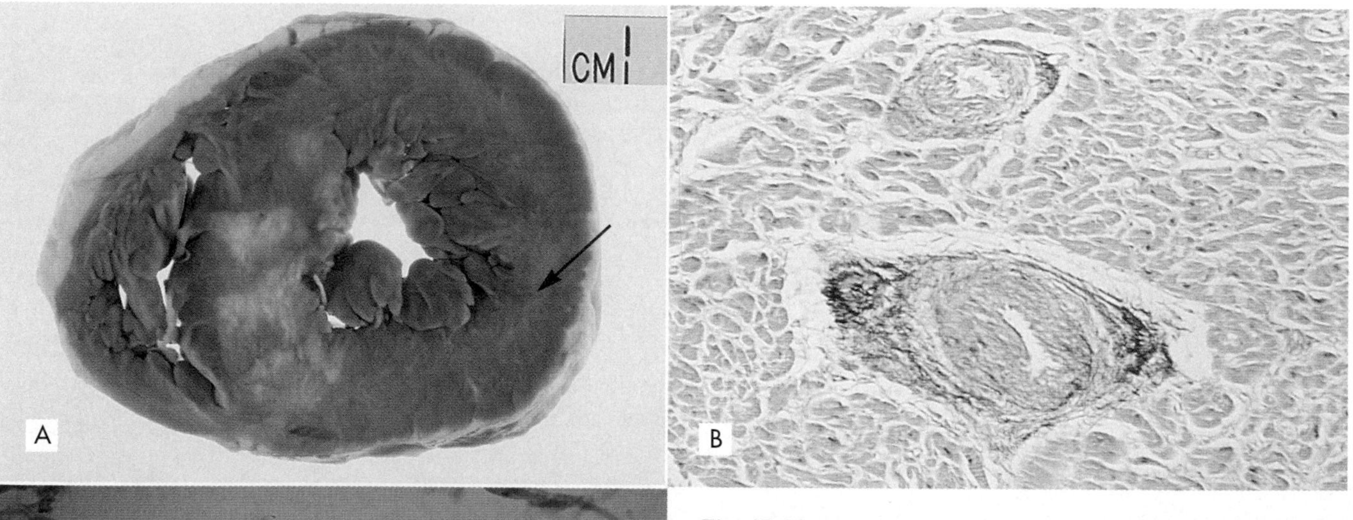

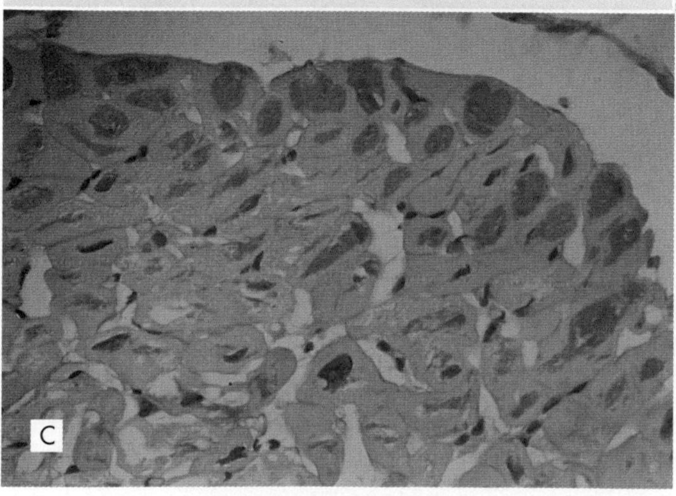

Fig. 45-29 **A,** Transverse ventricular myocardial section from an autopsy heart with hypertrophic cardiomyopathy here illustrating patchy collagenized scarring of the ventricular septum and extensive hypertrophic process in the ventricular septum and anterior left ventricular free wall *(top).* A less hypertrophic and somewhat thinner left ventricular free wall region in the lateral and posterolateral free wall is denoted *(arrow).* **B,** Photomicrograph of an intramural coronary artery in the region of the atrioventricular node from an autopsy heart of a young person with sudden death during exercise. There is considerable thickening of the arterial walls, primarily intimal and medial, but with a slightly increased adventitial fibrous cuff. The relationship of this type of arterial change to the actual sudden death event remains speculative. (Elastic von Gieson stain.) **C,** Ventricular septal myocardium illustrating hypertrophied and disorganized (interlacing) cardiac myocytes typical of those found in large numbers in hearts with hypertrophic cardiomyopathy. There is nuclear enlargement and associated interstitial fibrosis.

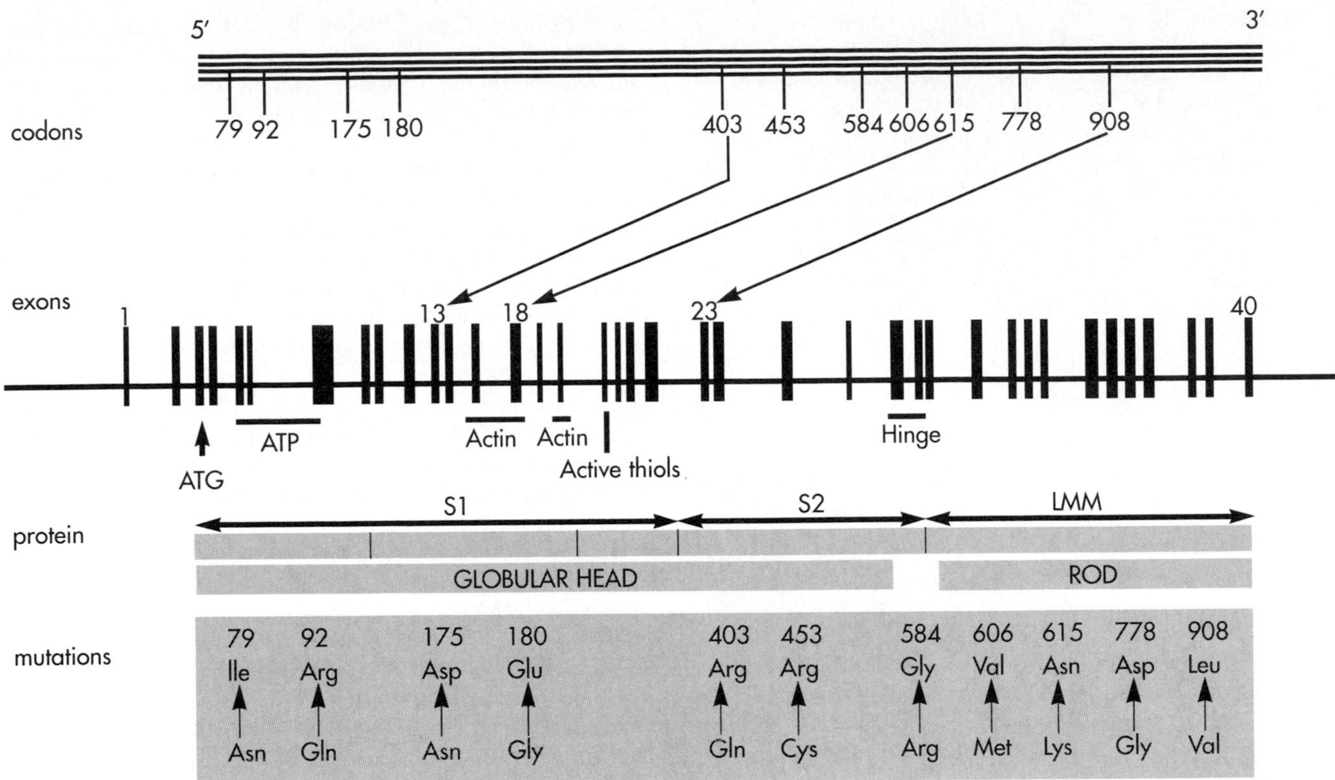

Fig. 45-30 Highly diagrammatic illustration of the general location of exemplary point mutations in the beta-myosin heavy-chain associated with hypertrophic cardiomyopathy in reported kindreds. (From Seidman CE, Seidman JG: *Mol Biol Med* 8:159.1991; Marian AJ, Robert R: *Texas Heart J* 21:6,1994.)

hallmarks of this condition, RV failure may also be a prominent feature. The massive dilatation of the right ventricle that may attend the arrhythmias is frequently reflected in cardiomegaly on chest x-ray film and in RV dilatation on echocardiographic examination. The condition was initially believed to involve only the right ventricle, however, Manyari and associates[302] have established the presence of latent LV dysfunction in patients with other features of ARVD. Thus the more widespread involvement, reflected in an abnormal LV ejection fraction, may be uncovered by exercise in a large number of ARVD patients[302] or may be present at rest. Not surprisingly, the right ventricle has segmental and global dysfunction during exercise.

Webb and colleagues[303] lend additional support for more widespread cardiomyopathy in ARVD patients in their observations on four patients with a clinical diagnosis of ARVD. Beyond RV functional abnormalities, the patients had evidence of LV dilatation or wall-motion abnormalities on radionuclide angiography or catheterization. LV dysfunction has been explained in one of three ways. It may be secondary to the same dysplastic process as that affecting the right ventricle, or to an enlarged and poorly functioning right ventricle. In addition, recurrent arrhythmias may cause systemic hypotension leading to endocardial hypoxia and myocardial damage.

In the experience of Marcus and colleagues[304] who reported an extensive study of 24 patients with ARVD, the most common sites of RV involvement are the anterior RV infundibulum, the RV apex, and the posterior RV free wall. This triad of sites has been coined the *triangle of dysplasia*. The arrhythmogenic sites involved are important clinically since surgery may be aimed at electrical isolation or ablation of one or multiple sites involved.[304,305] Diffuse involvement of the left or right ventricles may lead to recurrent ventricular tachycardia and progression of disease despite medical or surgical intervention.[305]

Pathologic features. Perhaps because ARVD was described only recently, its morphologic features are less widely known than other forms of arrhythmogenic heart disease. Indeed, a few autopsy, surgical, or biopsy reports have detailed the precise distribution of lesions in hearts affected by ARVD or the comparative nature of lesions within a heart or between hearts, or the occurrence of related structural cardiac abnormalities. In ARVD, the RV myocardium is partially or totally absent, being replaced by fibrous or fatty tissue in areas of myocardial absence (Fig. 45-31). When the condition is severe, the endocardium and epicardium are opposed.

Little information is available about the histologic features of ARVD. Some reports have briefly described areas of fibrosis and fatty infiltration with sparse myocytes.[306] Atypical myocytes with enlarged hyperchromatic nuclei and prominent aggregates of mast cells along borders between fatty and muscular tissue have been found in our experience (Fig. 45-31). These changes have been similar to the right and left ventricles as well as in atrial sections. They are also similar to features described in Uhl's anomaly (congenital RV hypoplasia and as seen in lipomatous hypertrophy of the atrial septum). The possibility that these myopathies are an expression of common denominators of myocardial hypoplasia with fibrofatty replacement has been raised.[307]

Pathobiology. The wide range of ages at which ARVD may surface clinically behooves the pathologist to be on guard for

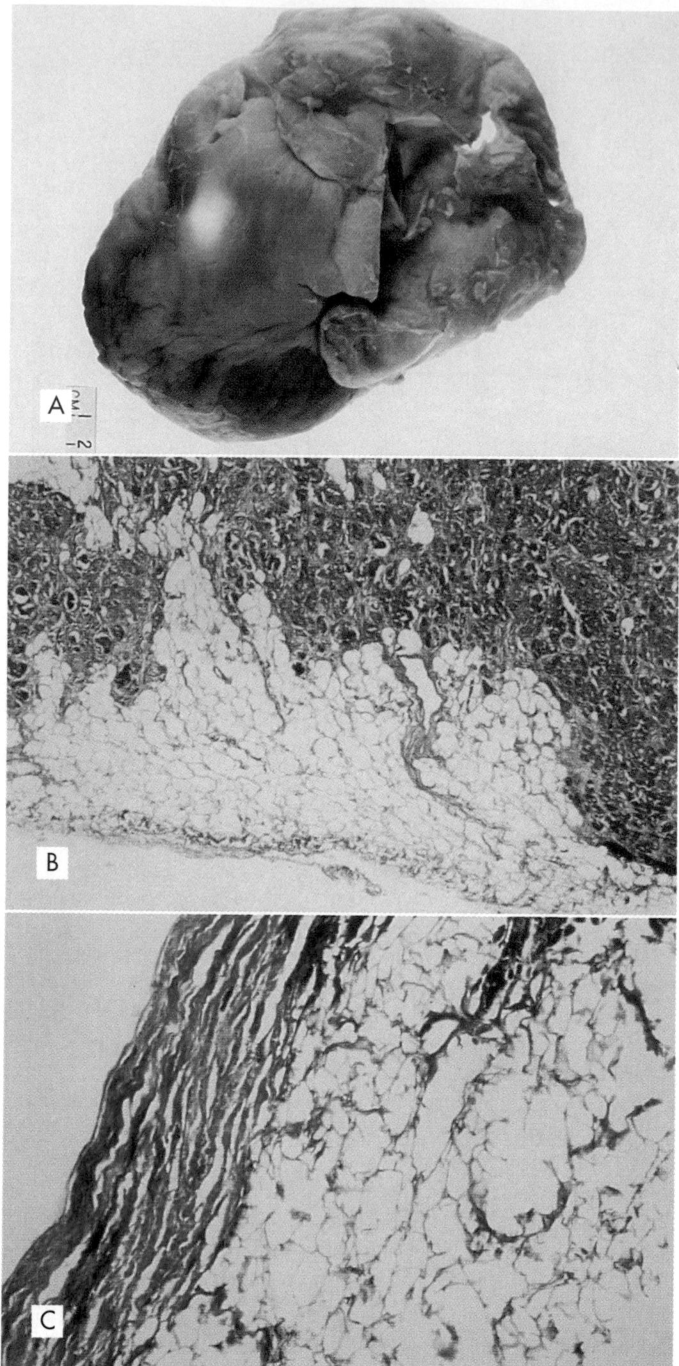

Fig. 45-31 Arrhythmogenic right ventricular dysplasia (ARVD). **A,** Anterior view of autopsy heart with ARVD depicting extensive fat with transillumination of an area in the anterior right ventricular free wall where no muscle is present. **B,** Epicardial and subepicardial region of the left ventricular free wall illustrating the partial absence of the outer portion of the muscular wall and "infiltration" by fat. Thus the left ventricular free wall, though not as involved as the right ventricular free wall, is abnormal insofar as the amount of fat and the associated interstitial fibrosis and cardiac myopathic changes are concerned. **C,** Anterior right ventricular free wall with adipose tissue *(rightward)* and collagenous fibrous tissue *(blue)* and absence of myocardium. (Masson's trichrome stain).

subtle forms of the disease. ARVD in children may be reflected clinically in bundle branch patterns of ventricular tachycardia similar to those seen in adults[308]; however, the diagnosis may be missed clinically or morphologically because of its rarity.

The possibility of familial occurrence emphasizes the need for family follow-up study when ARVD is diagnosed at autopsy and was not suspected clinically. Since 1974[309] several observers have documented familial occurrence of the diseases.[310,311] Most recently, Laurent and associates[312] found 4 of 21 members of a family to have definite ARVD, with 2 others to have abnormal RV morphology on echocardiography but no arrhythmias, and 5 with arrhythmias but no apparent morphologic abnormality. As well, Nava and colleagues[313] studied 32 of 40 family members and found 14 to have ARVD. Two of those affected had an autopsy. Twelve were diagnosed by two-dimensional echocardiography or hemodynamics and angiography.

Imaging modalities similar to those used in other forms of heart disease have been applied in efforts to confirm the clinical impression of ARVD.[314] Up to now, two-dimensional echocardiography, contrast ventriculography, gated equilibrium radioventriculography with Fourier analysis, digital subtraction angiography, ciné computed tomography, tomodensitometry, and technetium-99m and thallium-201 scanning have been used in studies of ARVD. However, the variability in involvement of the heart and the meager amount of published morphologic information on patients who die of ARVD offered a fertile area for additional studies including biopsy-autopsy correlation and comparative assessment of hearts of patients deemed clinically to have ARVD and Uhl's disease.

Endocardial fibroelastosis

Definition and clinical presentation. Endocardial fibroelastosis occurs most often in infancy and childhood. The cause of the disease is unknown; however, many factors including mechanical, inflammatory, and hereditary have been noted.[315] Clinical diagnosis is often made by exclusion of other conditions, including myocarditis, idiopathic dilated cardiomyopathy, carnitine deficiency or other metabolic disorders, and anomalous origin of the left coronary artery.[296,315] Several studies of the survival of patients diagnosed with endocardial fibroelastosis have been done.[316-318,320] Survival rates range from 65% to 70% over 10 years of follow-up. Ino and colleagues[315] also found that more than 50% of their patients had persistent congestive heart failure.

Pathologic features. Gross examination of hearts reveals a rapid increase in size that is predominantly left-sided and has a globular cardiac shape. The LV endocardium has a typical opaque, porcelain-like surface with diffuse thickening in the outflow tract (Fig. 45-32). This thickening can range from less than a millimeter to several millimeters in thickness. The ventricular architecture is significantly altered resulting in flat trabeculae carneae cordis, thickened and shortened chordae tendineae, and fibrotic papillary muscles. Histologically the endocardium demonstrates hyperplasia with prominent collagenous and elastic fibers.[319,320]

Endomyocardial fibrosis. Endomyocardial fibrosis (EMF) is a relatively rare condition in the Western world. It is characterized by the development of a variably inflamed, fibrous reaction along the endomyocardium of the ventricles. Since Löffler's description of "endocarditis parietalis fibroplastica" in 1936,[321] the association of the fibrotic process with

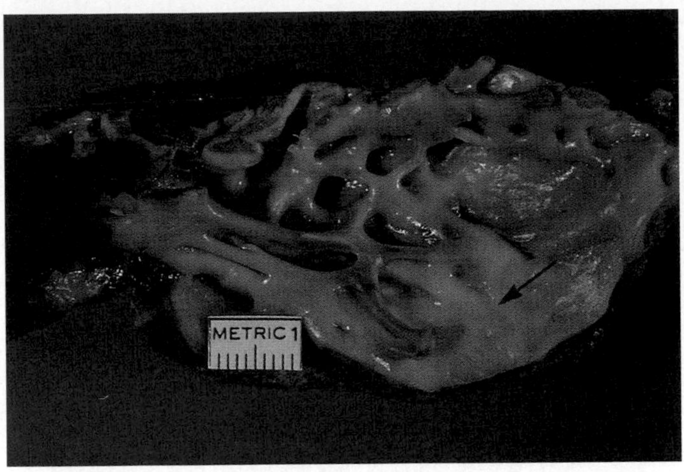

Fig. 45-32 View of endocardial surface of operatively resected left ventricular aneurysm. The endocardial surface is rather diffusely thickened by fibroelastic endocardial tissue *(arrow)*. This type of secondary fibroelastotic change is related to turbulence and reaction to the previous acute injury.

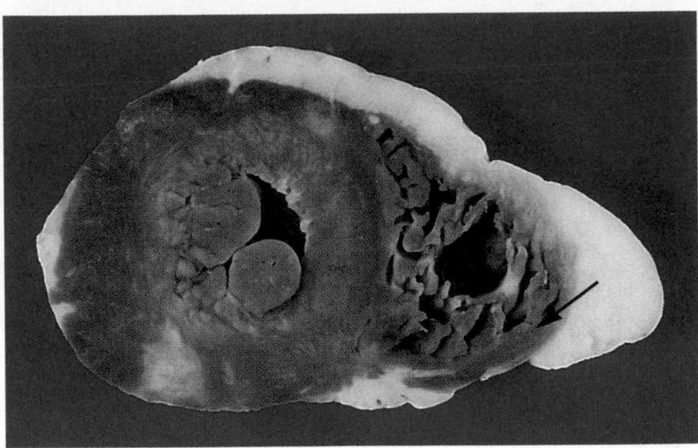

Fig. 45-33 Transverse ventricular section of an autopsy heart with areas of granulomatous infiltration by sarcoidosis. The lesions are most prominent in the posterior left ventricular free wall *(cream colored)* and less so in a patchy distribution in the anterior left ventricular free wall. The anterior surface of the heart is toward the top.

eosinophilia in the heart and systemically was identified. This eosinophilic form of EMF was recognized to be the same as "Davies's endomyocardial fibrosis (tropical type)." The hypereosinophilia of EMF occurring in temperate climes, as well as that associated with tropical EMF, has become recognized as the pathogenetic link between diverse conditions in which EMF occurs. Thus, certain hematologic malignancies, lymphomas, carcinomas, parasitic diseases, hypersensitivity disorders, or granulomatous and vasculitic diseases may have associated EMF. When frank hypereosinophilia syndrome (HES) (blood eosinophilic count $>1.5 \times 10^9$ per liter) occurs, the development of restrictive cardiomyopathic physiologic processes, hypercoagulability, and gammaglobulinemia is the rule. Large intracavitary thrombi, particularly in the left ventricle, may give rise to systemic emboli. Thus, anticoagulation is necessary. Later in the disease process, the fibrotic tissues may interfere not only with ventricular relaxation, filling, and contraction, but also with the function of the mitral or tricuspid valves. Eosinophils secrete highly toxic cationic proteins and also are capable of producing important peroxidases. The eosinophil-derived major basic protein, eosinophil-derived cationic protein, eosinophil-derived neurotoxin, and eosinophil peroxidase all may play a role in the injury process of EMF. Eosinophils also lead to the release of leukotriene C_4. Vascular tone will secondarily be altered. Interleukin (IL)-3, GM-CSF, and IL-5 all stimulate eosinophil production by bone marrow. Their consequences insofar as the heart is concerned are uncertain. The major granule products of eosinophils have been identified immunohistochemically in the acute thrombic stage and later necrotic stage of EMF disease, with small amounts remaining in the fibrotic phase. It remains to be determined why the endomyocardium is particularly susceptible to eosinophilic injury and to establish the role of inhibitors of eosinophil-derived proteins in protecting the heart.

Sarcoidosis

Definition and clinical presentation. Sarcoidosis may involve the heart by direct infiltration of the myocardium with granulomas. These infiltrative lesions may be extensive enough to replace large portions of the myocardium and lead to cardiac dilatation, dysrhythmias, heart failure, and sudden death. As such, the entity may mimic congestive cardiomyopathy.

Pathology. Grossly, ventricular myocardium is replaced by patchy gray-white infiltrates, and associated thinning of ventricular free walls or of the ventricular septum corresponds to sites of intense fibroinflammatory changes. The diagnosis of sarcoidosis is most often made by histologic findings of fibrosis and noncaseating granulomatous inflammation. Lesions consist of numerous multinucleated giant cells containing intracytoplasmic inclusions like asteroid bodies (Fig. 45-33). The histopathologic features of sarcoidosis includes "hard" granulomas with central giant cells and a halo of leukocytes. The white cells are presumably $CD4^+$ lymphocytes.

Carditis

Myocarditis

Definition and clinical presentation. Myocarditis is an inflammatory disease of the myocardium constituted by various subsets of inflammatory cells and at times having known causes but at others having unknown causes. The actual frequency of myocarditis as a clinical entity is difficult to establish, particularly because of the range of presentations from subclinical, virtually innocuous, to fulminant failure or arrhythmia-generating inflammation and injury. It is also known that patients may present with symptoms of heart failure or arrhythmia only to have these disappear in a few hours to days. Thus the range of clinical syndromes makes establishment of cardiac involvement a big challenge. Propensity to perform a biopsy on the endomyocardium varies from institution to institution and depends on the point of view of the local cardiologist. If exclusionary information on the biopsy as well as positive information[322] is considered valuable in management, it is likely that patients presenting in idiopathic heart failure of short duration will undergo biopsy.

Pathology. The definition of myocarditis has rested primarily in histopathologic criteria established and published in 1987.[323] These criteria are briefly summarized in Table 45-15. Recognition of the normal constituency of the endomy-

Table 45-15 Histopathologic criteria of myocarditis

First biopsy
Myocarditis
Borderline myocarditis (?Rebiopsy)
No myocarditis
Subsequent biopsy
Ongoing myocarditis
Resolving myocarditis
Resolved myocarditis

ocardium is obviously crucial to making an appropriate interpretation of endomyocardial biopsy specimens. Myocarditis may be constituted by an infiltrate that is monomorphic (such as lymphocytic, eosinophilic, monocyte-macrophage) or, more typically, is mixed with a predominance of one cell type or another (Fig. 45-34). The convention of calling idiopathic myocarditis "lymphocytic" is probably not a good one when one considers that the infiltrates in myocarditis are most commonly a prominent mixture of T-lymphocytes and macrophages.[324] When infiltrates are present, injury of the cardiac myocytes or other tissue constituents may be readily visible or difficult to ascertain. This difficulty is one of the bases of the category of borderline myocarditis in the original Dallas criteria. The possibility of interstitial edema and accompanying vasculitis and tissue hemorrhage must be considered. The possibility of innocuous sentinel lymphocytes[325] must be recognized. Subsets of myocarditis from the histopathologic standpoint are defined, once again, on the basis of the infiltrative cells. The patterns and distribution of the infiltrates and the injury can be protean and may or may not be clearly associated with the degree or localization of ventricular dysfunction. Several considerations must be accommodated at the time of biopsy (Table 45-16).

Pathobiology. The role of viruses in the causation of myocarditis that otherwise is considered idiopathic has attracted a great deal of attention during the last decade. Certainly enteroviruses are known as significant causes of human myocarditis, and as indicated by the experience at the Glasgow Infirmary,[326] the enteroviruses are among viruses most likely to cause cardiac disease. Detection of enteroviruses within human endomyocardial biopsy specimens, in explanted end-stage hearts, or at autopsy has been achieved by use of a wide range of molecular strategies and has generally indicated that about 25% of those people with active myocarditis beyond the pediatric age group will have enterovirus genome present.[327] The role of the virus in direct injury of the myocardium has been established,[328] whereas the possibility that immune mechanisms are at play in the dysfunction of the myocardium or in the actual injury of myocardial elements remains a contestable and important issue. Other causes of myocarditis, particularly other infectious agents and toxic agents, must be considered.

Therapy. The treatment of idiopathic myocarditis remains somewhat unresolved. Most patients with mild symptoms improve spontaneously, though the course and likelihood of such improvement in a given patient is obviously not known. The myocarditis treatment trial recently completed in North America revealed no significant difference in outcomes of patients treated or not treated with immunosuppressives, prednisone, and cyclosporin A. Thus, conventional cardiovascular support therapy is still the rule. Experimental evidence in popular murine models of enteroviral myocarditis indicates that if coxsackievirus variants are the cause of myocarditis, immunoenhancement may be the best strategy.[327]

Cardiac rejection

Acute rejection

Definition and clinical presentation. Allointolerance of transplanted tissues or organs is the result of immunogenetic mismatches between donor and recipient at various "major" and "minor" histocompatibility loci. Over the years, immunosuppressive regimens have steadily evolved and have reduced the likelihood of biopsy-detected rejection and the severity of rejection when present. However, acute rejection still represents a significant risk after transplantation, and in the first few months this risk is highest.

The clinical presentation of a patient with rejection may be one of occult, nonhemodynamically important rejection or one in which there is prominent acute heart failure. In consideration of this variability, and in consideration of the standardized criteria for histopathologic evaluation of heart muscle rejection,[329] the management of patients has been guided to a significant degree by the endomyocardial biopsy. No other measure of immunologic, hemodynamical, physiologic, or biochemical derangement has been more useful than the biopsy in this regard.

Pathology. The Billingham classification of heart allograft rejection has been adapted and modified by various centers and ultimately by the working group for the International Society for Heart and Lung Transplantation (ISHLT)[329,330] and has undergone a very recent revision. The working classification is synopsized in Table 45-17. Most recently, grades 1a, 1b, and 2 have been collapsed into one grade. This is based on the observation that these three grades have similar prognostic implications. The basis of the classification system as it evolves is related to the number of infiltrating inflammatory cells and the number of inflammatory foci associated with parenchymal or vascular damage (Fig. 45-35). The possibility of frank vasculitis and considerable interstitial edema with hemorrhage exists in the higher grades of acute rejection (3a, 3b, 4). Thus, allograft rejection is progressively more severe as the number and size of infiltrates increases and the amount of associated damage is amplified. Determination of myocyte damage may be made by use of routine hematoxylin and eosin stains but is usually made more clear with Masson's trichrome stain.

In the diagnosis of acute rejection, the possibility of a previous site of alloinjury that is in the process of healing must be considered. Numerous other artifacts, mimickers, and lesions also must be accounted for in arriving at a histopathologic diagnosis of acute rejection. Recognition of biopsy sites, appreciation that opportunistic infections can produce an inflammatory picture that mimics rejection, and understanding that endocardial infiltrates (Quilty effects) may appear very similar to rejection need to be gained. Indeed, Quilty lesions, which are usually endocardially based, may be cut in such a plane as to appear deep within the tissue and more significantly mimic allograft rejection.[331] Recently recognition of posttransplantation lymphoproliferative disorder (PTLD) has focused attention on posttransplantation potential for malignancy. Although the exact trigger for PTLD is not known, the

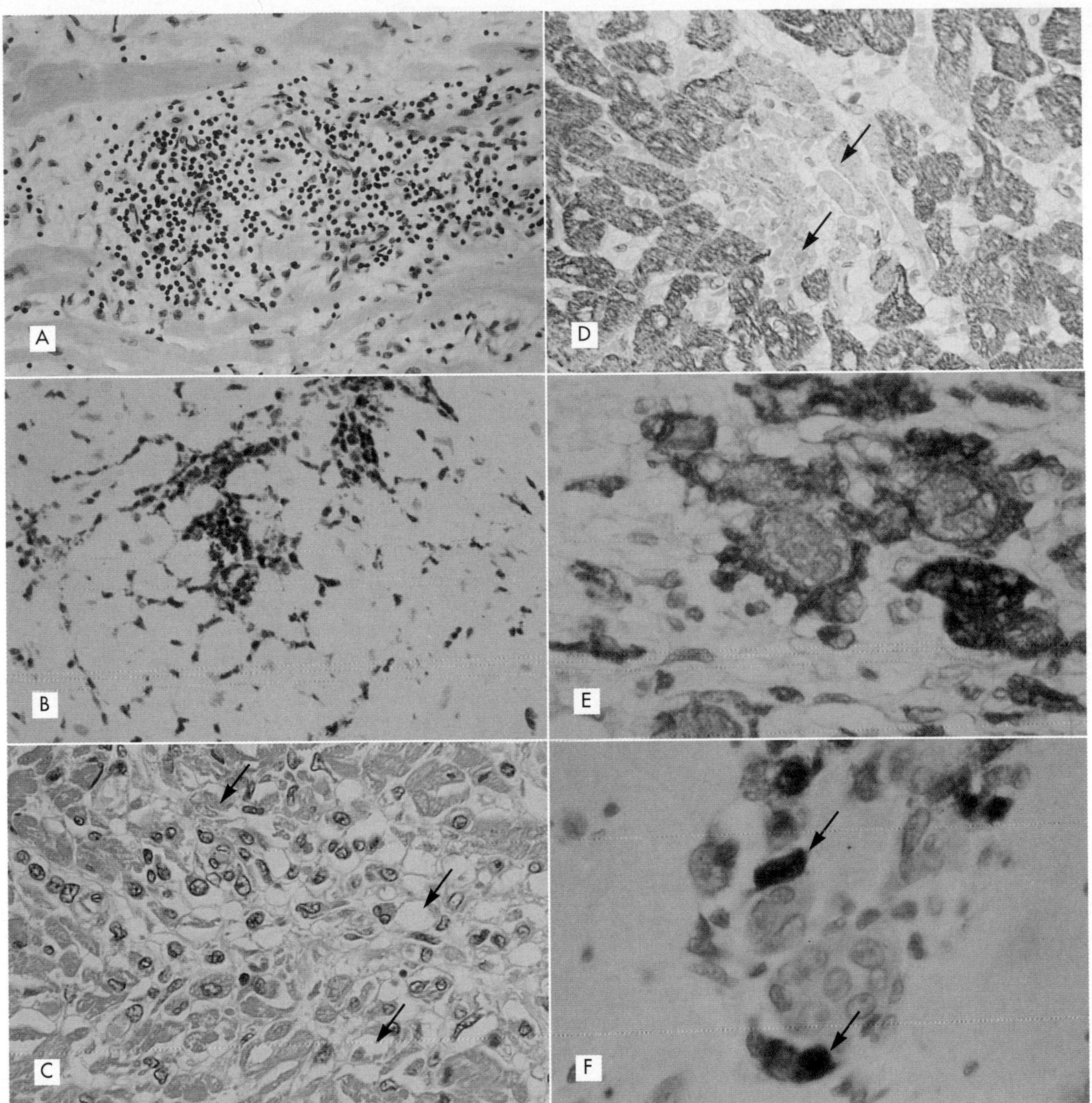

Fig. 45-34 Microscopic appearances of myocarditis. **A,** Active myocarditis of the predominantly lymphocytic type. Isolated myocytes are surrounded by the infiltrate in a background of what appears to be edema. **B,** Ventricular myocardium with myocarditis and clusters of cells immunoreactively positive as monocyte macrophages. **C,** Ventricular myocardium with active myocarditis and myocytolysis *(arrows)*. The cytolysis is associated with an infiltrate of activated immune cells in a child with suspected viral myocarditis. **D,** Ventricular myocardium with influenza A–related myocarditis in a young child. The "punched-out" lesions of myocyte necrosis are best defined by lack of positive staining *(arrows)* with monoclonal antibody to muscle-specific alpha-actin. Focal hyperemia and red blood cell extravasation is appreciated. **E,** Giant cell myocarditis with multinucleated giant cells positive for muscle-specific alpha-actin monoclonal antibody staining. Some of the giant cells in the same heart were derived from muscle cells, whereas others were of monocyte-macrophage lineage. **F,** Giant cell myocarditis with multinucleated giant cell and neighboring immunoreactively positive monocyte macrophages *(MAC) (arrows)*. Although this multinucleated cell is immunonegative, others in this case were immunopositive with the same antibody. (**B** and **F,** Immunoperoxidase stain MAC387; **D** and **E,** alpha-actin.)

Table 45-16 Considerations in endomyocardial biopsy

Essential matters
Obtain adequate tissue with rapid/consistent triage
Prepare representative sections with appropriate use of stains, antibodies, probes, primers
Archive of frozen tissue, cells, and serum
Biopsy early in an illness
Record information on
- History of drug use
- Atherosclerotic risk

Consider systemic diseases
- Malignant
- Metabolic
- Infiltrative
- Inflammatory

Tissue artifacts
Contraction bands
Compression (squeeze)
Hemorrhage
Telescoped blood vessels
Appearance of interstitial edema
Sites of previous biopsy
Sites of contact by indwelling catheters
Vasopressive lesions including cocaine-induced changes
Acute or healed ischemic lesions
Micro-thrombi
MICE
Appearance of endomyocardial fibrosis due to tangential sectioning
Portions of chordae
Valve leaflets
Noncardiac tissue

Other caveats
Amount of fibrous tissue or adipose tissue will vary from biopsy encounter to encounter
The sensitivity of detection of certain diseases is disease-specific and is related to:
- Patterns of lesion distribution
- Size of lesions
- Criteria for diagnosis
- Evaluative techniques applied
- Stage of disease when biopsy is performed

intensity of anti–T-cell antibody therapy during the induction period may be important.[332] Ischemic injury related to advancing graft vascular disease may also be confusing and must be remembered when one is reviewing biopsy material. The acute injury (coagulation necrosis) and healing or healed lesions tend to have a distribution typical for ischemic processes.

Pathobiology. Infiltrating cells in acute rejection are predominated by T-lymphocytes and monocyte macrophages. A surprisingly low percentage of these T-lymphocytes are antigen specific. Thus there is large amplification of the immune response, and a considerable amount of the immune response to the allograft is a secondary phenomenon. Increased expression of class I histocompatibility antigens on cardiac myocytes and class II histocompatibility antigens on interstitial and endothelial cells play a role in the localization of antigen–specific alloreactive T-cells. The grade of rejection histopathologically is related to the ability to grow lymphocytes from cultured biopsy specimens.[333] The role of antibody in mediating injury in acute rejection remains unsettled except in the xenography.

Table 45-17 ISHLT* working classification of allograft rejection on endomyocardial biopsy

Grade	Classification
0	No rejection
1a	Focal mild
1b	Diffuse mild
2	Focal moderate
3a	Multifocal moderate
3b	Diffuse moderate to severe
4	Severe

*International Society for Heart and Lung Transplantation, Dallas Tex.

Therapy. Several immunosuppressive regimens are available to treat acute rejection. Typically grades 1a, 1b, and 2 are reversible with or without augmentation of immunosuppressive therapy. Rebiopsy may be indicated for moderate rejection (grade 2). Severe rejection (grade 3 and above) is reversible but with greater difficulty and definitely requires augmentation of immunosuppressive therapy.

Chronic rejection

Definition and clinical presentation. Chronic rejection is a term typically used to designate the transplant vascular disease that accompanies allointolerance and the targeting of blood vessels by immune responses. This form of rejection begins within hours of implant of an allograft, and the histopathologic evidence of "chronic rejection" is available in allografts removed within the first few days or weeks after transplantation. The disease is now known to be a variant of atherosclerosis with a large lipid and lipoprotein overload involving both intima and media. The intimal thickening is of uniform severity both proximally and distally in the coronary arterial tree, and it reflects prominent matrix deposition along with lipid insudation, as well as a more modest mesenchymal cell migration and proliferation. "Chronic rejection" is a process present early after transplantation but is often thought of as an end point reflected in the disease reaching a clinical horizon of symptoms and signs. When a patient develops significant chronic rejection, the result is typically either small-scale or large-scale vessel narrowing to the point of causing myocardial ischemia. This ischemia may result in heart failure, sudden death, or acute myocardial infarction. When ischemia occurs in the transplanted heart, significant chest pain often is absent and the presentation may be somewhat elusive. Differentiating between an ischemic cause of acute failure without chest pain and severe acute rejection depends on endomyocardial biopsy results and a keen clinical acumen.

Pathology. Chronic rejection defined as a pathobiologic process is illustrated by an early mononuclear cell infiltrate in the superficial intima, subendothelial bandlike infiltrates, and a "looseness" of the intima that is in part attributable to lipid insudation and also possibly attributable to cytotoxic phenomena (Fig. 45-36). As the chronic rejection process unfolds, there is a rapid increase in intimal thickness with elevated lipid content, rapid increase in extracellular matrix, continued superficial inflammatory infiltrates predominated by T-lymphocytes and monocyte-macrophages, and, as well, deep focally localized infiltrates, frank atheromas with extracellular cholesterol deposits, and ultimate partial disruption of the

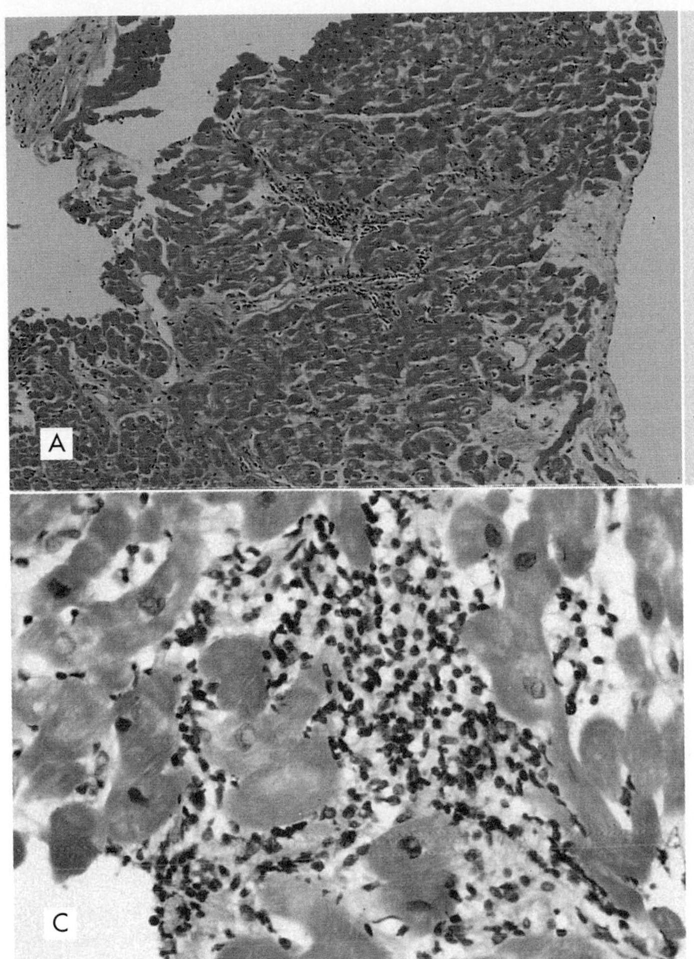

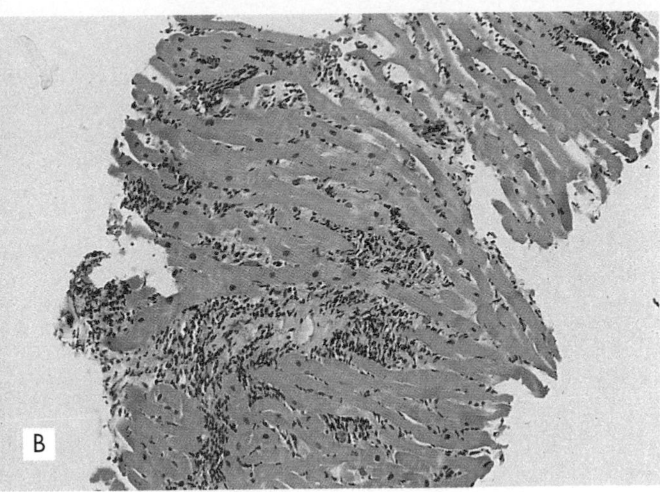

Fig. 45-35 Cellular rejection. **A,** Photomicrograph of right ventricular endomyocardial biopsy specimen with focal moderate (grade II) rejection. There is a single, quite well-defined focus of inflammation that, at higher power, is associated with myocyte degeneration. There is no other significant infiltrate in the field. **B,** Multifocal, invasive mononuclear cell infiltrates in a right ventricular endomyocardial biopsy specimen from a human heart allograft. This pattern is typical of moderate rejection (grade 3A). **C,** Higher power view of a cellular infiltrate in a right ventricular endomyocardial biopsy specimen illustrating the percolation of infiltrating cells in and around ventricular myocytes.

internal elastic lamina. Although the internal elastic lamina often is intact as compared to native atherosclerotic processes with the same degree of luminal narrowing, this is only a relative truism. The arteriopathic process proceeds rapidly, and the intimal proliferative component is more dominant than both the proliferative and destructive components that characterize a more long-standing, indolent course of native atherosclerosis. The tunica media is involved by lipid transformation of medial smooth muscle cells into foam cells and by variable incursion of mononuclear cells from the adventitial connective tissue inward into the outer media. Thus, the media is not spared in this disease and its physiologic and anatomic aberrancy must play different roles in consequences to the heart muscle itself. The involvement of small blood vessels within the myocardium is generally less visible than the larger epicardial coronary arteries are; however, when involvement is present, it is usually severe and results in profound local ischemia. Detection of such arteriopathic "chronic rejection" changes on endomyocardial biopsy (Fig. 45-36, *C*) has been demonstrated as a poor prognostic sign.[334-336] Pathologic changes in intramural vessels have been associated with more prominent lesions on angiographic evaluation of epicardial vessels.[337,338] The possibility that thrombus may be superimposed on the arteriopathic process has been recognized and observed in certain fatalities. Generally, the pathologic features do not include calcification, though in more long-standing grafts the lesions begin to take on characteristics more typical of native atherosclerosis.

Pathobiology. It is widely recognized that transplant vascular disease occurs in all solid organ grafts and has a similar set of features in all organs in the setting of suppression of immune intolerance by immunosuppressive regimens. These features have been noted above. The important concepts about the disease include its exceedingly rapid development more rapid than the most severe, naturally occurring, genetically based atheromatous disease as in type II homozygote hypercholesterolemia–LDL receptor defects. The process is initiated by alloimmunity to the foreign organ and is related in part to demonstrable histocompatibility mismatches such that the disease spares no particular vascular field within the transplanted organ. The devastating consequences of the disease relate primarily to the impressive proliferative thickening of the intima. This intimal thickening is dominated by matrix and includes areas of increased cellularity.

Therapy. The use of therapeutic modalities applied to hearts with native atherosclerotic disease have found less efficacy in the transplanted heart. Thus, coronary artery bypass grafting, atherectomy, balloon angioplasty, stenting, and other mechanical interventions are thwarted by the diffuseness of the disease process and the generally concentric nature of lesions. The aggressive use of newer antirejection therapeutic agents has suggested the possibility of reduced chronic rejection in the human heart. However, most observations up to now are experimental in animal models or are anecdotal. The ultimate goal of inducing tolerance to the grafted organ will most likely be the avenue to prevention of graft vascular dis-

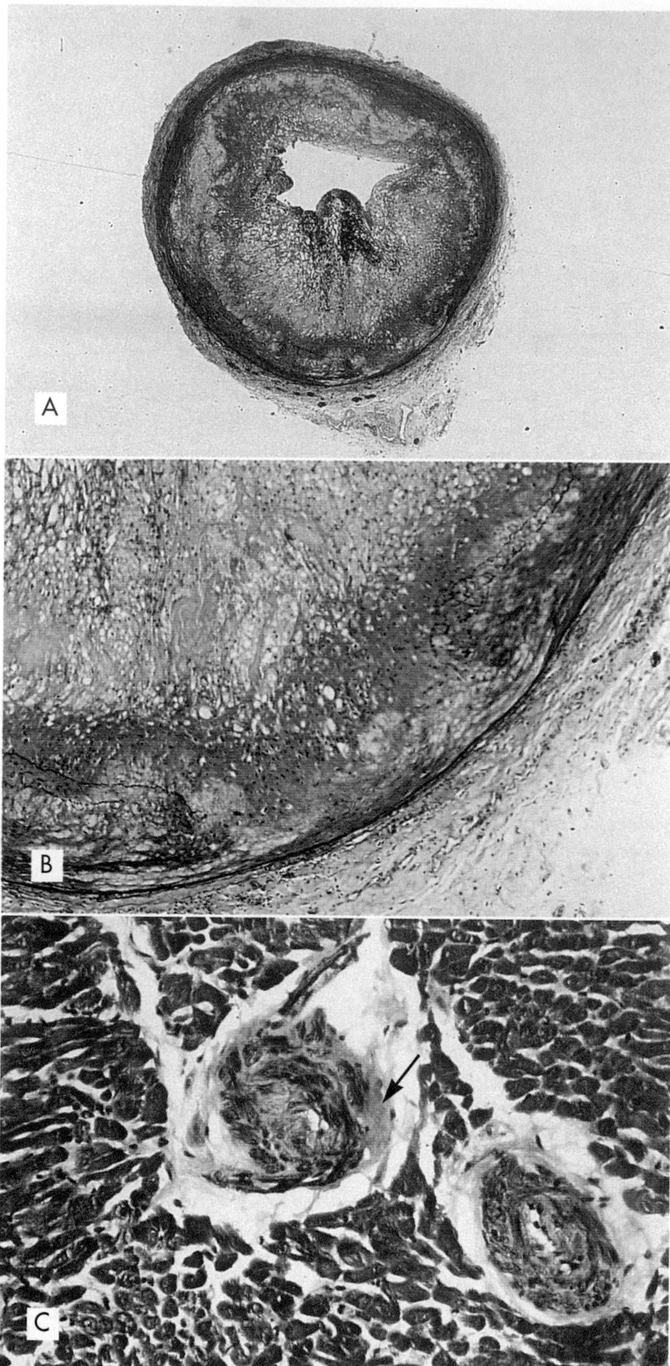

Fig. 45-36 Microscopic appearances of transplant vascular disease (chronic rejection). **A,** Transverse section of epicardial coronary artery from a human heart allograft illustrating rather concentric advanced intimal thickening. On the elastin stain, glycosaminoglycan material remains pale cream–colored, and the intima is apparently rich in such matrix. There is also evidence of vacuoles in the intima *(white,* more superficial*)* indicative of lipid deposits. **B,** Lipid richness of evolving atheromas in transplant vascular disease including foam cells and cholesterol clefting that extends into the media. **C,** Intramural coronary artery from human heart allograft with pronounced fibromuscular thickening leading to near occlusion of the small vessel. There is increased collagen in the adventitia *(arrow),* as well as disruption and fibrosis of the proliferative intima and media. (**A** and **B,** Elastic van Gieson stain; Masson's trichrome stain.)

ease. Reducing proliferative tendencies in response to immune triggers and particular attention to "conventional" coronary risk factors after transplantation will also aid in slowing the process.

Conduction system disturbances

Key features of normal anatomy

The sinoatrial node (SAN) lies in the sulcus terminalis subepicardially and approaches the junction of right atrial appendage and superior vena cava.[339-341] It is the shape of an upside-down, pyramidal, teardrop, 1 to 1.5 cm in length by 0.5 by 0.3 cm transversely. Whorled, interlacing, small, pale myofibers with interspersed collagenous matrix are present that are typically circumscribed, with transitional areas. The node is supplied by the sinus nodal artery from the right coronary (about 50%), left circumflex (40%), or dually (10%). It is innervated by postganglionic parasympathetic nerve fibers. Aging leads to increased collagen and decreased nodal bulk.

At the anterior leftward apex of *Koch's triangle,* along the vector of *Todaro's tendon,* anterior to the coronary sinus, and superior to the membranous septum, both subendocardially and subepicardially lies the atrioventricular node.[339-343] More spherical than the SAN, it projects into the penetrating *His bundle.* Whorled, interlacing, small, pale myofibers lay in a collagenous matrix. Transitional, superficial (loose) and deep (compact) zones are evident with an atrial myofiber overlay. Connections may occur between atrial transitional cells ("last" cells) and the proximal node. Variable archipelagos extending into the central fibrous body may be observed, the exact significance of which remains unclear. The node is supplied by an AV nodal artery from the crux of the heart. Neural projections are found in the lower atrial septum. Collagen weave like the SAN increases with age.

The main bundle of His projects through the central fibrous body.[339-344] Fasciculoventricular connections may occur. Bundle fibers run parallelly, and on exit from the central fibrous body, multifascicular (trifascicular) branching of the left bundle occurs. The right bundle continues as a geometric extension of the main bundle (and may run deep to the endocardium initially). Proximally, as extensions of the bundle branches, the *Purkinje fibers* are only slightly larger than working myofibers. Distally, Purkinje fibers are even larger, with cleared cytoplasm, numerous mitochondria, and prominent positive PAS staining. Purkinje fibers are generally in the immediate subendocardium and may run in fine trabeculas.

As aging progresses, the SAN becomes more fibrotic and has thicker elastic fibers around nodal myocytes.[345,346] The specialized nodal myocytes are lost, and fatty replacement occurs. The AV node has an increase in nodal collagen and elastic tissue, slight infiltration by mononuclear cells, and focal degeneration of nodal myocytes. The bundle of *His* and the bundle branches have an increase in elastic tissue. In addition, the bundle branches may undergo fatty infiltration or fibrous replacement. Replacement by fibrous tissue with linear formation of fibroelastic tissue may also occur.

Clinical presentation

Associated with cardiac arrhythmias. *Sinus bradycardia* has no pathologic correlate, and so there may be aberrant innervation. Sick sinus syndrome may be accompanied by SAN atrophy and fibrosis and rarely amyloidosis with variable abnormalities in the AV nodal system and a normal SAN artery.

Sinoatrial block may occur from an intrathoracic tumor, with invasion of the vagus nerve. First- and second-degree AV block is without visible anatomic defects. Third-degree block may also reflect acute injury (myocardial infarct, trauma, surgery, infection, autoimmunity, tumor), chronic progressive incursion (calcification, fibrosis), or bilateral bundle-branch fibrosis (in the elderly, Lev's disease and Lenègre's disease). Right bundle branch block may be familial and may be induced by right ventriculotomy.[347] Left bundle branch block is a concomitant of hypertrophy and occurs in association with bilateral bundle branch fibrosis[348]

Supraventricular arrhythmias may occur with atrial fibrillation and is often in association with mitral valve stenosis.[349] It also occurs with diverse factors—hyperthyroidism, ischemia, pericardial constriction, or systemic hypertension—and may occur in the absence of structural heart disease. There is a possible replacement of the SAN by fibrofatty tissue, and embolic events may ensue or occur on cardioversion.

Paroxysmal atrial tachycardia is consequent to ischemia, hypertensive hypertrophy, aortic valvular stenosis, infections, or drugs. The therapy is uncertain, and the morphology is undefined.

Ventricular tachycardia may be paroxysmal, recurrent, and intractable.[350,351] *Torsade de pointes* has variable morphology. Preexcitation may be from Wolff-Parkinson-White (accessory atrial to ventricular pathway, ?Kent bundles), Lown-Ganong-Levine (atrial septum to ventricular septum AVN or His bundle (?James tract), or the PR interval may be normal and the QRS wide (with delta wave) in nodo-His-ventricular connections, Mahaim fibers[352] (Fig. 45-37).

Ventricular fibrillation may be related to neurogenic factors (?left stellate ganglion stimulation), which may cause tachyarrhythmias without structural heart disease. The morphology of the heart is related directly to the circumstances of fibrillation.[353]

Sudden cardiac death in specific patient populations

Young adults including athletes. Physiologic responses to exercise training include enhanced oxidation capacity, central and peripheral, adaptive myocardial hypertrophy and ventricular function, resting sinus bradycardia, intermittently enhanced fibrinolysis, improved lipid profile, weight control, body composition, self-image, and reduced blood pressure.

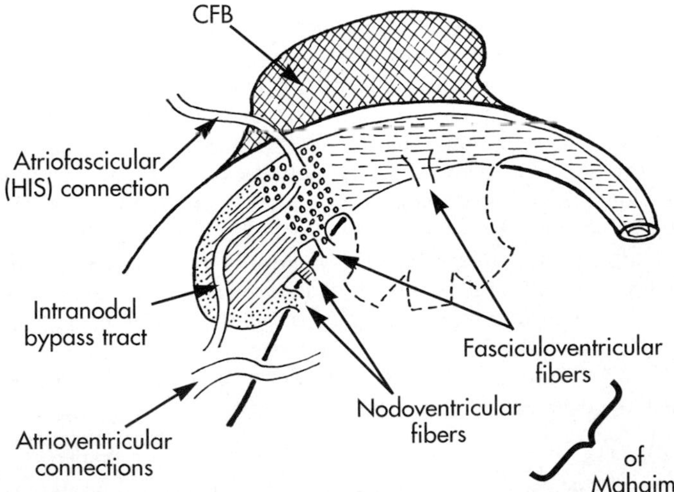

Fig. 45-37 Depiction of the atrioventricular node and the numerous possibilities for "bypass" tracts. As seen, accessory connections may occur from atria to ventricles, from atria to node, from node to ventricles, or from His to ventricles. Any of these avenues could be the substrate for preexcitation.

Athlete's heart syndrome has revolved around a popular misconception.[354,355] The following facts are important: (1) a truly normal heart in an otherwise healthy person does not develop pathologic lesions with exercise unless severe metabolic or electrolytic alterations have occurred as in heat disorders, and (2) aberrant cardiovascular function or structure in an athlete may relate to ecogenetic factors. The collision of inherent susceptibilities and environmental triggers is undoubtedly central to exercise-related deaths.

Sudden death and exercise are linked. Suddenness of death ranges from instantaneous to as long as 24 hours after the event. It is important to document association of the strenuous event with the onset of symptoms or signs. The expected incidence of sudden cardiac arrest in exercising adults and children is low (6 to 13 per 100,000 population); however, the hourly rate of sudden death associated with exercise surpasses that for rest. Neither static nor dynamic forms of exercise seem to be excluded as possible contributors to death in athletes with abnormal hearts. Sudden death during exercise or an athletic event is more common than at rest; however the period after acute exercise is potentially life threatening as well. In general, the younger the person exercising, the greater the likelihood that the cause of associated cardiac death is congenital or hereditary. Those who undertake very vigorous activity but only for a short time per week appear to have the greatest increase in relative risk. Extensive discussions have been held regarding whether to, how to, and what to evaluate or screen in people undertaking athletic competition.

Cardiomyopathies. Hypertrophic cardiomyopathy has a prominent association with sudden death in young adults.[356,357] The risk of sudden death is related to severity of ventricular arrhythmias.[358] As noted earlier, HCM is heritable and linked with genetic point mutations in myosin heavy-chain genes and troponin T. Scarring in the thickened ventricular septum is typical in those with sudden death. The prototypic pathological phenotype includes hypertrophy, prominent ventricular septum, mitral valve leaflet thickening, and endocardial plaque in the LV outflow tract, as well as excess myofiber disorganization and thick-walled intramural coronary arteries.

Idiopathic dilated cardiomyopathy presents 25% of the time with arrhythmias or sudden death. Bundle branch fibrosis is common, as is interstitial fibrosis, but precise correspondence between rhythm and dilatation, fibrosis, and mass is often lacking.

ARVD presents with heart failure or arrhythmia.[358,359] The heart weight is increased. Myopathic myocytes, transmural areas of myocardial absence with adipose accumulation and associated fibrous tissue, with or without extensive inflammation in the fat and fibrous tissue are the key features. The inflammatory type may be mistaken for myocarditis. Many loci for possible reentry exist.

Coronary artery diseases. Atherosclerotic diseases have a higher frequency of superimposed thrombus on a plaque fissure in association with transmural myocardial infarcts; however, this phenomenon is least associated with "instantaneous" sudden death[360] In both settings, infarcts and sudden death, severe three-vessel disease is the rule.

Anomalous origin of the right coronary artery from the left sinus of Valsalva, or vice versa, can cause electrical disturbances. Flaplike ostia and constraint of the proximal portion of the aberrant coronary artery by adventitia are the two most likely factors promoting sudden death. Anomalous origin of left coronary artery from pulmonary trunk may present in adulthood.

Vascular dissections. Spontaneous coronary artery dissections, particularly in reproductive-aged women, may be accompanied by accumulation of medial glycosaminoglycans or medioadventitial eosinophilia as the main feature. Aortic dissections may lead to angina pectoris, acute myocardial infarction, or sudden death, with accompanying arrhythmias.[358,361]

Valvular heart disease. LV pressure overload, as seen with aortic valve stenosis, results in myocardial hypertrophy, increased collagen in the heart muscle, and prominent transmural gradients. All these factors may contribute to arrhythmogenesis.[346,358]

The mechanism of sudden death in mitral valve prolapse remains unresolved. Undue tension on papillary muscles by prolapsing leaflets may contribute, and irritation or ischemia in the papillary muscles is suggested by loci of arrhythmogenesis or fibrosis in the sites. Contact of chordae against endomyocardium is another candidate arrhythmogenic irritant.

Pathologic features

Infection. All forms of infection that include a tropism for the heart tissues may result in conductive or arrhythmogenic alterations.[362,363] At times these alterations are particularly related to the actual conduction tissues. The consequences of involvement of the conductive tissues are obvious; however the protean presentation of infections of working myocardium including a variety of viruses, bacteria, and parasites that can lead to automaticity problems, conductive problems, or both. The role of the infectious agents versus the associated immune response in the actual injury of myocardium and conductive tissue depends on the inciting agent and the stage of disease. For the most part, all infective conditions can produce a variable myocarditis, the extent and distribution of which is dictated by the extent and distribution of the offending antigens. Viral infections (enteroviruses, mumps), borreliosis (Lyme disease),[364] trypanosomiasis (Chagas' disease), mycobacterioses, and diphtheria have all been implicated in conduction system disorders.

Inflammation. Other inflammatory conditions of unknown, autoimmune, or postinfectious causes may result in automaticity and conductive problems.[365-367] Of particular significance and as alluded to earlier in this chapter, cardiac sarcoidosis can produce a broad range of clinical syndromes including heart failure, valvular regurgitation, variable degrees of heart block, arrhythmias, and sudden death. The distribution of sarcoid nodules and granulomas tends to be multiple and may lead to weakening and distortion of the wall, imposition on the conductive pathways, or provocation of local reentry focuses. Other granulomatous conditions that are systemic and involve other organs as well as the heart may have arrhythmic consequences. Wegener's granulomatosis is a case in point. Polymyositis and dermatomyositis may be associated with a myocarditic process and consequent disruption of structure and function including rhythm disturbances. Enteroviruses have been associated with the latter disorders.

Infarction. The consequences of ischemic heart disease with reversible and irreversible myocardial injury and acute, subacute, and chronic processes of myocardial injury and repair may manifest as subtle reflections of ischemia (ST-segment depression), variable degrees of heart block, ventricular premature contractions, ventricular tachycardia, and ventricular fibrillation, or ventricular standstill.[368-371] The risk of infarction to AV conduction differs for posterior and anterior wall infarcts. The possibility of heart block is greater with the former, whereas a much larger infarct is necessary to cause heart block when the anterior coronary circulation is involved.

Infiltration. Deposits of eosinophilic, amorphous amyloid protein (characteristic relationship to cardiac myocytes) (squeezing, surrounding, hugging) is seen with all forms of amyloid involving the heart muscle. Association of amyloid deposits with multiple myeloma or chronic inflammatory conditions (infectious or noninfectious) and neoplasms results in atrial fibrillation, heart block, and, less often, ventricular rhythm disturbances. Arrhythmias may be related to direct infiltration of the myocardium and the conduction system, occlusion of intramural coronary arteries (with secondary ischemia), or infiltration of cardiac nerves.

Iron deposits in hemochromatosis occur in all working and conductive myocardial tissues, producing a continuum of atrial and ventricular arrhythmias including automaticity and conductive problems. Associated scarring may also contribute to inhomogeneity in the myocardium.

Common tumors involving the conduction system include rhabdomyomas with the clinical results reflecting the location of the tumor nodules and, most emphatically, mesotheliomas of the AV node (endotheliomas), which interrupt the AV conductive axis. Secondary tumor involvement may lead to protean exhibition of arrhythmias and block.

Fibrous tissue occurring in response to clear-cut injury, unexplained fibrous proliferations, and the aging process certainly participate in the attenuation of nodal as well as His bundle and Purkinje tissues. The coarse or delicate encasement or isolation of conductive components or of individual islands of myocardial tissue may be sufficient substrate for arrhythmogenesis.

Anatomic-electrophysiologic correlation

Opportunities to relate clinical arrhythmias, sudden death, and pathologic findings are still crucial.[372-376] It is worth emphasizing that arrhythmogenesis *most often* has only a speculative anatomic basis, *less frequently* a definitive anatomic lesion. As well, arrhythmogenesis is more frequently attributable to lesions outside of the conduction system proper than within. Correlation of successful or unsuccessful radiofrequency ablation with autopsy findings should be pursued when possible. Correlative studies in animal models are also of great importance. Finally, conductive block postoperatively or postprocedurally will depend on the complexity of the operation or procedure and the susceptibility of certain pathways to injury.

Tumors

Tumors that arise in the heart are relatively rare; even myxomas, the most common primary tumors, have been estimated to occur in less than 0.02% to 0.03% of the population. The incidence is higher for secondary tumors, where approximately 10% of extracardiac primary tumors may have metastases to the heart. Both primary and secondary tumors have a wide variety of presentations, not necessarily reflective of their pathologic nature or histogenetic origin. Cardiac tumors present primarily as rhythm disturbances, contractility abnormalities, obstructions, valvular regurgitation, embolic events, or pericardial effusion with tamponade.[377] Additionally, tumors may present as conventional ischemia, cardiomyopathy, systemic or local infections, or intrinsic valvular disease, or less often, as mimicry of noninfectious and inflammatory diseases, pulmonary vascular diseases, endocrinopathies, and intrinsic shunts. Current availability of numerous imaging modalities, including two-dimensional and M-mode echocardiography, computerized tomography, radionuclide imaging, angiography, or cardiac catheterization, has enhanced the likelihood that the presence and nature of a given tumor may be established during life[377] and may lead to endomyocardial biopsy or resection at operation. These modalities may all increase the chances for definitive or adjunctive therapy, and advisement of patients and their families is made possible.

Primary tumors

Definition and clinical presentation. Morbid or mortal consequences are frequent with primary cardiac tumors, dependent on the involvement of important cardiac structures. Undesirable effects are dependent on location, size, mobility, friability, or invasiveness of a tumor. Primary tumors of the heart and pericardia are more important for local effects than for the potential of metastatic behavior. The frequency of malignant primary tumors is extremely low. Clinical presentation is directly related to the site of primary cardiac tumor involvement. The general correspondence of symptoms and clinical signs to tumor site is illustrated in Table 45-18, emphasizing the effects of tumors dependent on their location.

The frequency of benign and malignant primary tumors of the heart and pericardium is distinct for particular age groups, and the outcome is age dependent. Extended courses are more likely when tumors of similar histologic appearance arise in the hearts of adults. The data in Fig. 45-38 represent cumulative experience of the Armed Forces Institute of Pathology (AFIP)[378] and three other investigators[379-381] covering nearly 75 years and over 41,000 autopsies. A total of 265, 82, and 49 benign cardiac tumors and 117, 9, and 3 malignant tumors were found in adults, children, and infants respectively.

The most common tumor found in adults (predominantly middle-aged females) is the primary, benign myxoma, of which most occur sporadically.[380] Myxomas may be familial, in which case they occur in younger patients, and this subset of tumors is often multiple at the time of presentation. Systemic symptoms may include fever, weight loss, fatigue, anemia (may be hemolytic), increased immunoglobulin levels, leukocytosis, thrombocytopenia, erythrocytosis, Raynaud's phenomenon, clubbing, and breast fibroadenomas.[380]

Myxoma. Grossly, myxomas are pedunculated and typically polypoid with an irregular and glistening surface and may also have a gelatinous appearance accompanied by substantial hemorrhage. There is a short stalk that forms the attachment to the endocardium of the heart (Fig. 45-39).

Histologically, abundant, eosinophilic myxoid matrix contains polygonal to stellate myxoma cells distributed singly, in small groups, and around thin-walled vascular channels (Fig. 45-39). The myxoma cells embedded within the matrix are often termed *lipedic cells.* Mononuclear cells (macrophages, lymphocytes, plasma cells) are seen as focal collections. Myxomas may also have areas of recent and old hemorrhage, calcification, and metaplastic bone formation. Large quantities of acid mucopolysaccharide are present in the myxoma matrix, primarily in the vicinity of vascular channels. Cells forming the vascular channels show endothelial differentiation with positivity for factor VIII–related antigen. Myxomas contain a diverse population of cells with positivity for different differentiation markers such as S-100, a protein present in Schwann cells and melanocytes, and neuron-specific enolase, a cytoplasmic protein in axons.[384] Ultrastructurally, myxoma cells resemble multipotential mesenchymal cells.

Pathobiology. In patients with cardiac myxomas, a high serum concentration of the circulating cytokine 6 IL-6 produces systemic symptoms[382] including headache, syncope, dysarthria, and hemiparesis, and fever, weight loss, elevation of erythrocyte sedimentation rate, serum C-reactive protein, and serum gammaglobulin levels have also been demonstrated.[382] These symptoms as well as high levels of IL-6 have been demonstrated. Once the myxoma is resected, elevated serum IL-6 levels revert to normal, and systemic symptoms are relieved. Thus, evidence up to now indicates the key role IL-6 may play in the immunologic alterations associated with cardiac myxomas.

Rhabdomyomas. Rhabdomyomas may vary in size (from millimeters to several centimeters in diameter) and number (are multiple in over 90% of patients).[378] The small rhabdomyomas are usually found intramurally, whereas larger tumors may extend into the ventricular cavity.[386]

Microscopically, large, vacuolated "spider" cells are the predominant cell in which the vacuolated appearance is an artifactual consequence of glycogen removal during routine histologic processing. The spider cell typically has a central nucleus and spherical, glycogen-rich cytoplasmic mass. Postfixation cytoplasmic strands extend to the cell periphery. This cell is the hallmark of rhabdomyoma and is present in all tumors. Bundles of myofilaments and a cytoplasm rich in mitochondria and glycogen have been demonstrated by electron microscopy.[384]

Fibromas. On gross examination, fibromas are solid and fibrous and without necrosis or hemorrhage. Fibromas are nonencapsulated and extend into the surrounding myocardium.[378] They typically range in size from 3 to 10 cm in diameter when discovered. The tumors may be cellular. However, they are typically composed of firm fibrous tissue. In the central portion, dystrophic calcification and cystic degeneration occur, probably because of poor blood supply.

On histologic examination, fascicles of spindle cells (fibroblasts) with abundant extracellular collagen are present with variable cellularity and rare mitotic figures. Fibrous tissue at the tumor periphery contains prominent elastin admixed with the collagenous tissue. A fibroma typically contains rare myocytes and limited vascularity.

Secondary (metastatic) tumors

Definition and clinical presentation. Metastases or tumor extension to the heart may occur on the epicardial surface, within the cardiac chambers, or as an infiltrative process in the myocardial wall. The frequency of involvement of the heart by metastatic tumor is strikingly higher than the occurrence of primary cardiac tumors.[378] Nearly all malignant tumors from every organ or tissue can metastasize to the heart with one exception, tumors primary to the central nervous system.[378,385-397] This diverse origin of metastases reflects geo-

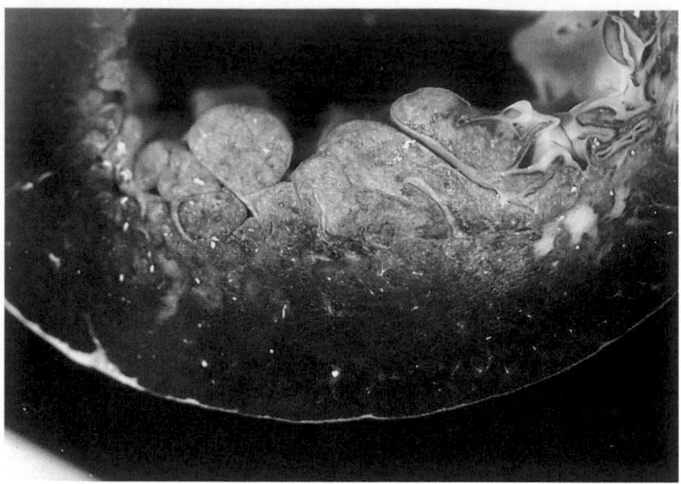

Fig. 45-49 Human myocardial infarction. The tissue has been stained for succinic dehydrogenase activity. The area of enzyme loss is subendocardial but confined to one region. The infarct appears to be made up of coalescence of smaller areas of necrosis of differing age.

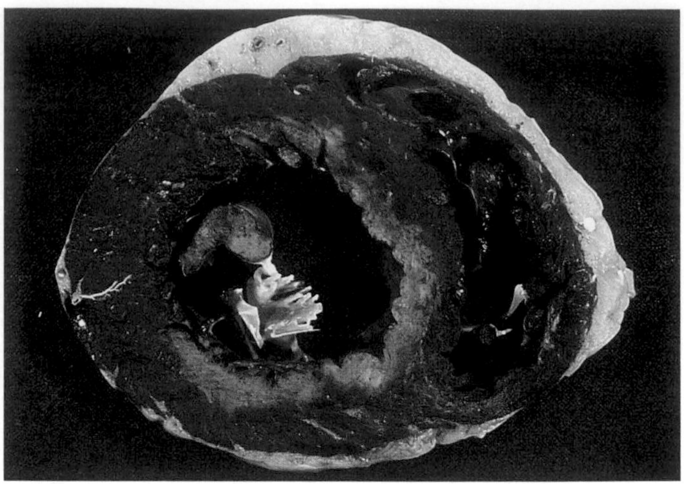

Fig. 45-50 Human myocardial infarction. The tissue has been stained for succinic dehydrogenase activity. Enzyme loss is subendocardial and extends across the areas supplied by at least three coronary arteries. This form of diffuse subendocardial necrosis is not related necessarily to coronary thrombosis.

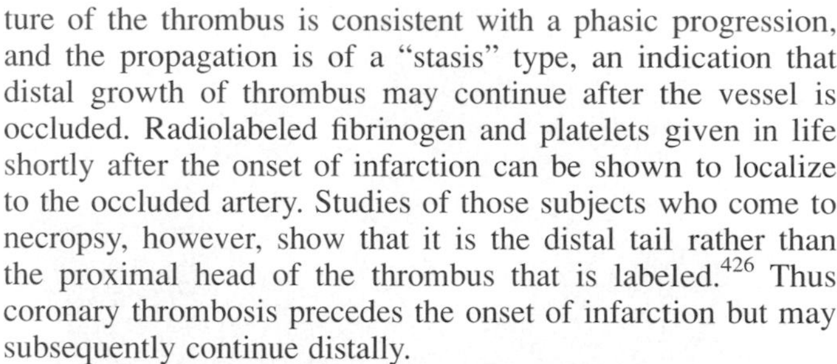

ture of the thrombus is consistent with a phasic progression, and the propagation is of a "stasis" type, an indication that distal growth of thrombus may continue after the vessel is occluded. Radiolabeled fibrinogen and platelets given in life shortly after the onset of infarction can be shown to localize to the occluded artery. Studies of those subjects who come to necropsy, however, show that it is the distal tail rather than the proximal head of the thrombus that is labeled.[426] Thus coronary thrombosis precedes the onset of infarction but may subsequently continue distally.

Autopsy studies show that regional subendocardial (nontransmural) infarction in man is not uncommon, particularly in association with unstable angina or in sudden ischemic death. Pathologic studies of regional subendocardial infarction show there is recent plaque disruption in the supplying artery. In contrast to transmural infarction there is a lower incidence of total arterial occlusion and a higher incidence of the distal segment of the artery being patent and filling either by antegrade flow over mural thrombus or by well-developed collateral flow.[427] Distal propagation of thrombus is virtually never found in nontransmural infarction.

Diffuse (nonregional) subendocardial necrosis is attributable to an overall fall in myocardial perfusion and can occur in the absence of any structural coronary artery disease. The subendocardial zone is particularly vulnerable to ischemic damage and, when compared with subpericardial muscle, has a 20% higher oxygen utilization per gram of tissue. Significant decreases in aortic diastolic pressure, reduction in diastolic duration and any increase in LV diastolic pressure decrease the proportion of blood flow entering the subendocardial muscle. Subendocardial necrosis may also occur in carbon monoxide poisoning and prolonged hypoglycemia. Diffuse subendocardial necrosis is common in end-stage triple-vessel coronary disease. Diffuse subendocardial necrosis may develop when regional infarction is complicated by cardiogenic shock. The central zones of the papillary muscle are the most vulnerable component of the subendocardial tissues.

Multifocal microscopic foci of necrosis have many causes. In the subendocardial zone, they represent an early stage of more confluent necrosis and also occur at the margins of larger areas of infarction. In the subpericardial zone microscopic foci of necrosis are related to intramyocardial platelet emboli. Any patient dying after prolonged hypoxia or hypotension will have microscopic foci of necrosis as a preliminary stage of diffuse ischemic damage. In severe LV hypertrophy microscopic foci of necrosis are common without obvious impairment of coronary blood flow or hypoxia. High catecholamine levels, both iatrogenic or natural, and raised intracranial pressure are also causes of these small foci of myocardial necrosis. Therapy with very high doses of inotropic agents to sustain cardiac output leads to such foci of necrosis.

Pathologic features of atherosclerosis

Morphologic types of plaque

In arteries opened longitudinally, fatty streaks or dots (Fig. 45-51) are yellow and barely raised above the intimal surface. Fatty streaks have a predilection for the flow dividing downstream areas at branching points. *Fatty streaks* consist histologically of cells containing abundant intracellular lipid (foam cells), which can be shown by immunohistochemistry to be of macrophage origin.

Fibrolipid plaques are oval and raised above the intimal surface (Fig. 45-52). They range in color from white to yellow. Raised (advanced) fibrolipid plaques consist of collagen and other connective tissue matrix proteins produced by smooth muscle cells, extracellular lipid (predominantly cholesterol and esters), and lipid-containing macrophage foam cells. There is considerable heterogeneity in the composition of raised plaques even in one artery. Plaques may be white and solid with a very high proportion of collagen or, at the other extreme, soft and yellow plaques with over 75% of their volume made up of extracellular lipid. The yellow color of the lipid is caused by carotenoid pigment.

In fibrolipid plaques the extracellular lipid is aggregated into the center as a lipid core (Fig. 45-53). This core is surrounded and encapsulated by collagen. The portion of the plaque that separates the core from the lumen of the artery is the cap. The collagenous tissue and particularly the cap con-

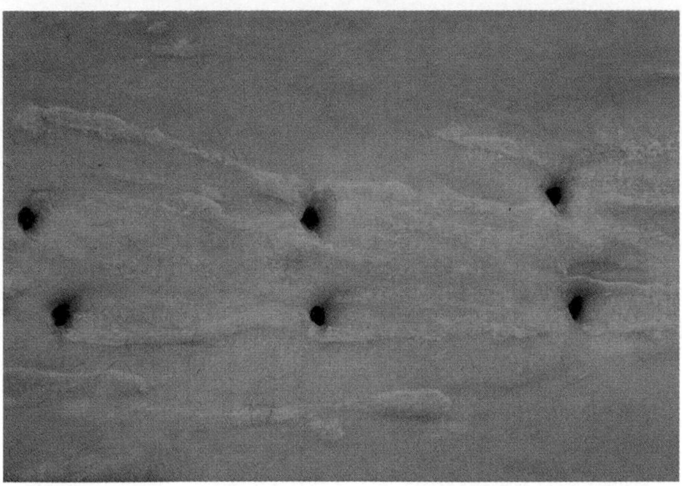

Fig. 45-51 Fatty streaks in a human aorta. The lesions are flat and yellow.

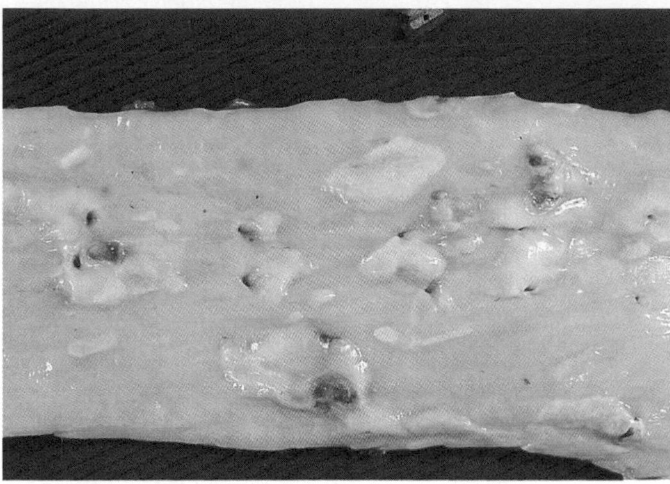

Fig. 45-52 Fibrolipid plaques in a human aorta. In addition to fatty streaks, this aorta contains raised lesions. Some are yellow, others are white. The long axis of each lesion is in the direction of flow. One plaque is complicated by red thrombus deposition.

tain smooth muscle cells lying in lacunas (Fig. 45-54). The lipid core contains extracellular lipid and debris with cholesterol clefts and is usually acellular. At the margins of the core there is a zone of lipid-filled macrophages, and many plaques also contain T-lymphocytes. Many fibrolipid plaques undergo calcification. Plates of calcification develop in collagenous tissue close to the intimal-medial junction at the base of the plaque. In another form nodules of calcification develop within the lipid core itself. Although atherosclerosis is an intimal disease, secondary changes develop in the media. Plaque formation induces new capillary vessels to enter the media and the base of the plaque from the adventitia. The medial smooth muscle cells atrophy and vanish immediately behind the plaque leading to medial thinning. An adventitial infiltrate of B- and T-lymphocytes is common behind plaques.

Complicated plaques are those that are undergoing thrombosis and at necropsy thrombus can be seen within or on the surface of the plaque (Fig. 45-53).

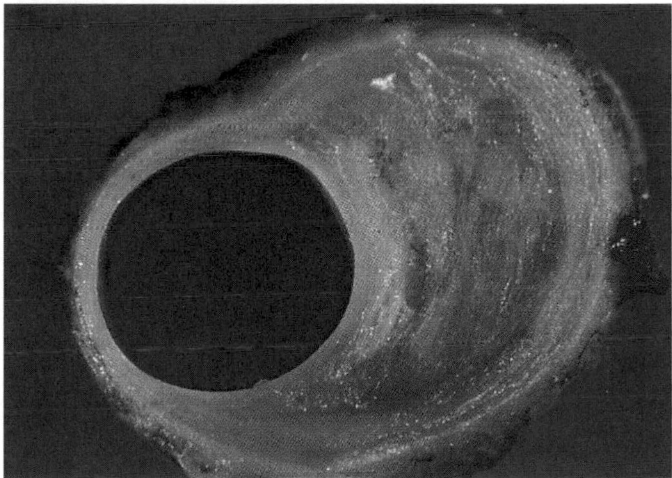

Fig. 45-53 A cross section of a human coronary artery with a fibrolipid plaque stained by Sudan Red. The plaque contains a core of lipid, which is separated from the lumen by a white fibrous cap. The plaque projects outward rather than inward. The artery was angiographically normal. There is a segment of normal vessel wall opposite the plaque.

Evolution of human atherosclerotic plaques

Necropsy studies are limited by being observations at one point in time. The plethora of plaque types found in adult aortas led to the view that new lesions continued to be generated throughout life, and several schemes of plaque evolution were proposed. Stary,[428] who examined age cohorts of individuals who died early in life and could therefore devise an evolutionary pattern based on the age at which lesions of a particular type first appeared, has clarified the matter. Fibromuscular thickening and smooth muscle cells in the intima of the coronary arteries, often accentuated at branching points, is universal in humans. This is an adaptive response and not atherosclerosis. Human coronary arteries differ from those of many animals in whom the coronary intima does not contain smooth muscle cells. The first atherosclerotic lesions to appear are composed entirely of lipid-filled foam cells predominantly of macrophage origin. Some lipids, however, can be shown within smooth muscle cells. The next stage is associated with the appearance of extracellular lipid including cholesterol crystals. This is followed by the accumulation of more smooth muscle cells, leading to the formation of a lipid core enclosed by fibromuscular tissue. The first observable event in human atherogenesis is the accumulation of lipid-filled macrophages in the intima.

Animal models of atherogenesis

Atherosclerotic lesions with extracellular lipid and fibromuscular proliferation can be produced in many animal species when plasma lipid levels are raised.[429,430] This may be achieved by high fat diets or by genetic defects such as that found in the Watanabe rabbit. Such models show that the first observable event is monocyte migration through the intact endothelium followed by the appearance of lipid-filled foam cells in the intima. Endothelial denudation with exposure of the intimal matrix and platelet adhesion is not present in the early phase of atherogenesis in animal models or human disease. A very important facet of animal models is that lesions containing lipid can be produced only when plasma lipids are raised. Lesions produced by denuding of the endothelium after balloon injury are followed by smooth muscle proliferation alone. They are thus a good model of vascular injury but not of atherogenesis.

Processes in atherogenesis

Atherosclerosis is now regarded as a response of the intima to damage and injury caused by lipid deposition.[431] A wide range of processes such as smoking or viral infection may enhance the process.

Although epidemiologic evidence linked an increased risk of human atherosclerosis to elevated plasma lipids, there was a paradox. The monocyte does not have a receptor enabling it to take up normal plasma low density lipid (LDL). Thus, although it was known that LDL entered the intima from the plasma, it was uncertain how lipid appeared inside foam cells.

Native LDL within the intima undergoes modification in a process requiring metal ions and possibly binding to proteoglycan or to the surface of endothelial cells.[432,433] Minimally modified LDL acts as an inflammatory mediator invoking the expression of molecules such as ICAM, VCAM, and ELAM on the endothelial cells and the production of MCP–I. These invoke monocyte migration. Minimally modified LDL undergoes further oxidation and is now readily taken up by the scavenger receptor of macrophages.[434] This receptor does not downregulate, and the cells become stuffed with lipid to form foam cells (Fig. 45-55). Macrophages are also induced to divide and become immobilized and activated leading to the production of a wide range of cytokines and growth factors including TNF-α and platelet-derived growth factor (PDGF).[431,435] Macrophage death by apoptosis allows release of lipid and particularly cholesterol into the tissues to form the lipid core (Fig. 45-56). The whole process invokes proliferation and collagen production by smooth muscle cells involving a host of cytokines and growth factors. Immune responses to oxidized lipid are responsible for the T- and B-cell adventitial inflammation. Fibrinogen enters the intima; production of thrombin and conversion to fibrin occurs because of the high concentration of tissue factor in macrophages. Fibrin and thrombin complexes are a further stimulus to smooth muscle proliferation within the plaque.[436]

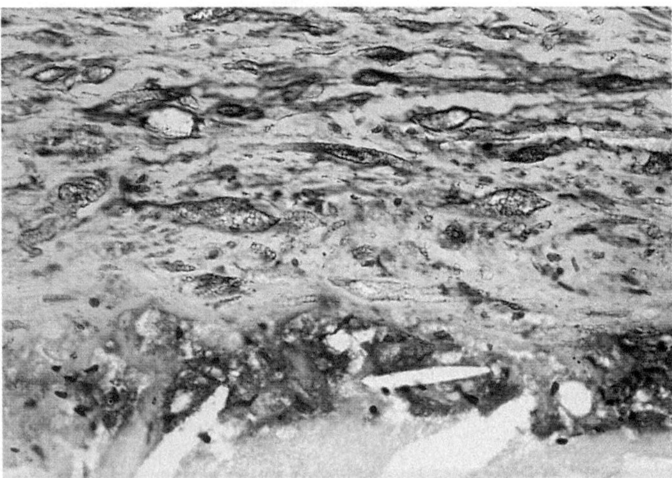

Fig. 45-54 Cell types in a fibrolipid plaque. The section was stained for smooth muscle actin *(brown)* by immunohistochemistry. An antibody to a macrophage antigen, CD68, has been stained red. The plaque cap contains numerous elongated smooth muscle cells, some of which contain lipid. The macrophages are clustered at the edge of the core in relation to cholesterol clefts.

Role of platelets in plaque evolution

Both human studies and animal models agree that the endothelium over fatty streaks is intact.[431,437] Platelet reactions thus play no part in plaque initiation. Once advanced plaques have formed, endothelial denudation with the deposition of platelets on the exposed intimal matrix does occur. PDGF may thus have an important role in plaque growth. Endothelial denudation is associated with the clustering of lipid-filled macrophages (Fig. 45-57) just below the surface, and many appear to be reentering the circulation through a damaged endothelial surface.

Causes of thrombosis in atherosclerosis

Two mechanisms cause thrombosis on atherosclerotic plaques.[438] In superficial injury there is endothelial denudation over a plaque with thrombus formation superimposed on an otherwise intact plaque. At an ultramicroscopic degree this process is almost ubiquitous over fibrolipid plaques. Larger thrombi are associated with more extensive denudation. Superficial thrombi that significantly narrow the lumen occur at points of previous high-grade stenosis and in smaller coronary arteries. There is an association with foam cell infiltration immediately beneath the endothelial surface (Fig. 45-58). Approximately one in four occlusive coronary thrombi are related to superficial injury.

In deep injury there is major disruption of a plaque with tearing of the cap. The disruption allows blood to enter the lipid core itself where thrombus forms, distorting and expanding the plaque from within (Fig. 45-45). The lipid core is highly thrombogenic because of tissue factor released by macrophages and exposed fragments of collagen. Although thrombosis is initially within the plaque, it may subsequently extend into the lumen and 3 out of 4 occlusive thrombi are caused by disruption.

The magnitude of an episode of disruption varies widely. At one extreme the tear is a fissure into the edge of a plaque allowing only a small intraplaque thrombus to form. At the other extreme the whole cap of a plaque may be lost extruding cholesterol into the lumen and invoking occluding thrombosis.

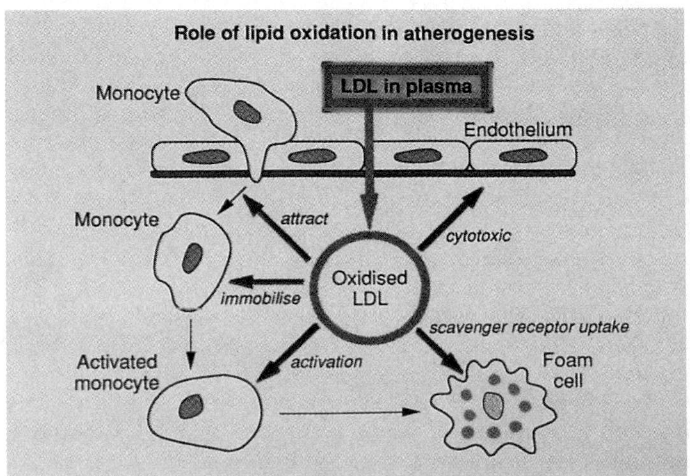

Fig. 45-55 Diagram of foam cell formation.

Outcome of plaque disruption and thrombosis

Plaque disruption invokes a repair response of fibrinolysis and smooth muscle proliferation (Fig. 45-59). The potential outcome is very variable ranging from resolution without an increase in stenosis to chronic total occlusion. Many variables determine this outcome. In some patients relatively minor disruption is associated with major ultraluminal thrombus formation (Fig. 45-60). These patients may have a high thrombotic potential or low lytic activity. In such cases fibrinolytic therapy often restores a good lumen. Other disruptions are a major stimulus to thrombosis, and where the lumen is occluded by a mass of thrombus containing fragments of plaque cap and cholesterol, lytic therapy may not reopen the vessel (Fig. 45-61). The whole process of thrombosis is very dynamic, and angiography in life clearly shows that thrombi wax and wane in size over minutes. Pathologists cannot be dogmatic about vessel patency based on a necropsy examination, which simply reflects the state of the vessel at the moment of death.

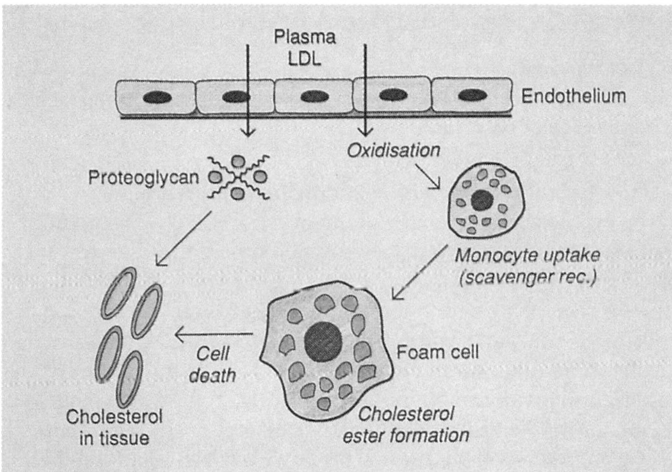

Fig. 45-56 Diagram of lipid core formation. Much of the cholesterol in the lipid core is derived from macrophage death. A small portion may be derived from metabolism of low density lipoprotein bound to proteoglycan.

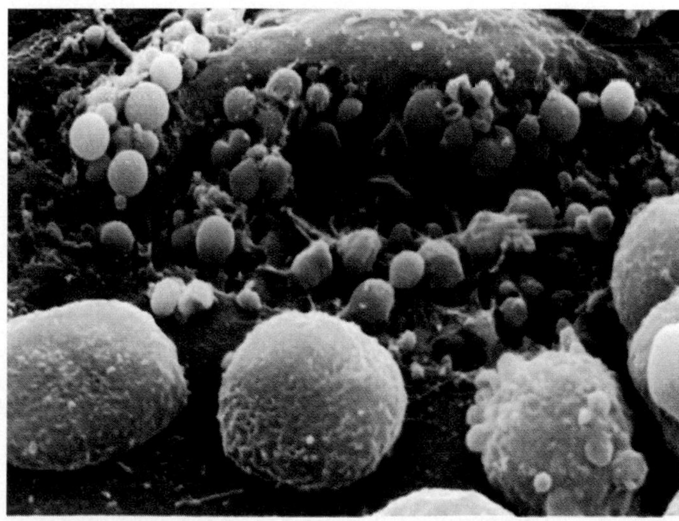

Fig. 45-57 Endothelial denudation demonstrated in a scanning electron micrograph of a human coronary artery. An endothelial cell has been lost, and the exposed matrix is covered by platelets. Numerous monocytes are adherent to the endothelium.

Causes of plaque disruption

There is a subgroup of plaques that are particularly vulnerable to disruption. Such plaques are characterized by a lipid core that occupies more than 50% of overall plaque volume, a cap in which there are focal areas of thinning with macrophage infiltration and plaques in which the numbers of macrophages exceed that of smooth muscle cells. Active dissolution of the collagen of the cap by macrophages releasing proteolytic enzymes such as stromelysin and gelatinase under the influence of cytokines such as TNF-α are a postulated mechanism for cap tears.

Intramyocardial vasculature

The epicardial arteries throughout their courses send penetrating branches into the myocardium. The distribution of these vessels can be studied only by microinjection techniques.

The intramyocardial arteries that supply the arteriolar bed fall into two distinct groups. One has straight nontapering ves-

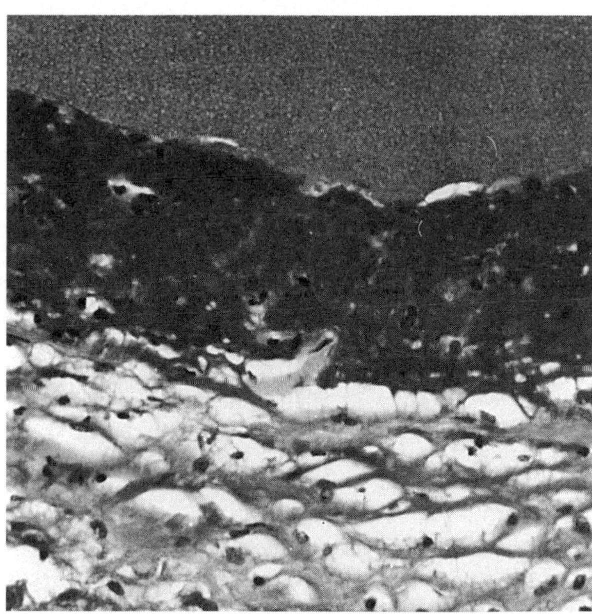

Fig. 45-58 Superficial thrombus formation. A mass of dark-staining thrombus is adherent to the surface of a plaque. The underlying intima is infiltrated with foam cells.

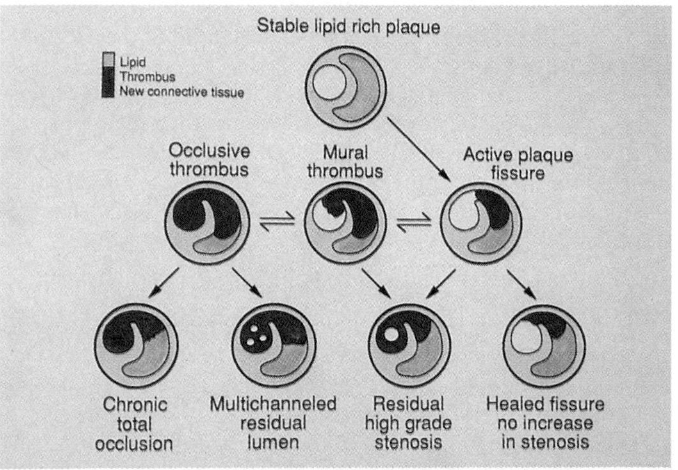

Fig. 45-59 Diagram of the potential outcomes of an episode of plaque disruption.

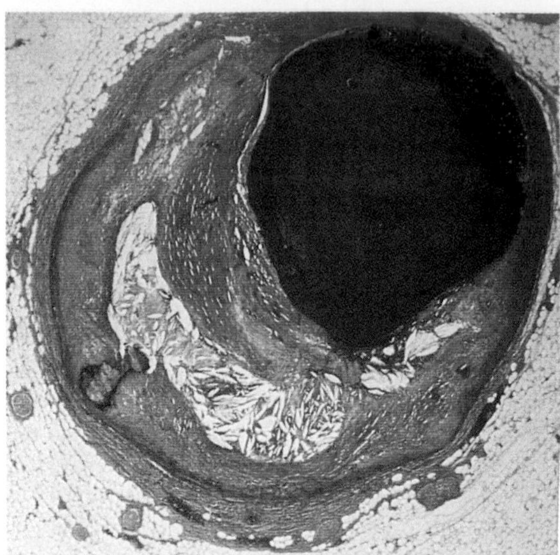

Fig. 45-60 Coronary thrombus stained by the picro–Mallory trichrome method. Thrombus is red and collagen blue. There is a small fissure in a plaque to which there has been a major thrombotic response in the lumen.

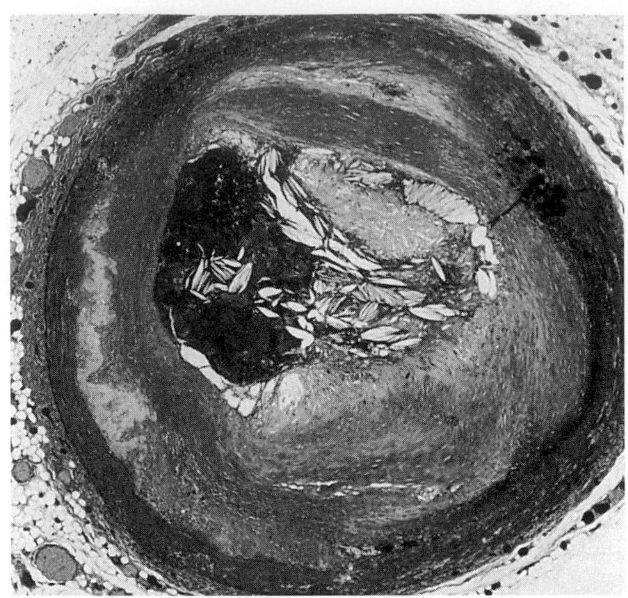

Fig. 45-61 Coronary thrombosis. There has been plaque disruption with extrusion of cholesterol into the lumen. This has invoked a massive thrombotic response.

sels of an approximately 400 to 800 μm external diameter with a well-developed media. These extend to the endocardial surface before breaking up into a plexus of smaller arteries. This system also supplies an artery to the center of each papillary muscle. The second system branches throughout the full thickness of the ventricular wall; tapering down rapidly to arteries with an external diameter of approximately 50 μm. Accompanying these vessels are veins, which also have well-developed medial muscle though a thinner wall and a larger external diameter than those of the arteries.

Collateral flow

The epicardial coronary arteries are functionally end vessels, meaning that sudden occlusion leads to ischemic myocardial damage. In a normal heart, if a low-viscosity fluid is injected into one coronary artery orifice, it however emerges from the other; thus anatomically connections exist between adjacent coronary beds.

Stenosis or occlusion of a coronary artery creates a pressure differential between the distal vessel and adjacent normal coronary arteries. Such pressure differences invoke collateral flow. It is not possible to demonstrate collaterals at autopsy other than by injection techniques.

There are three levels of collateral development. Short segments of complete occlusion of a major epicardial artery may be bridged by the enlargement of vessels in the adventitia at the site. Connections between adjacent, separate arteries may involve the enlargement of smaller epicardial arteries, including those in the atria. Finally anastomatic corrections develop within the myocardium itself, between subendocardial arteries and veins.

Metabolic and structural consequences of experimental coronary artery occlusion

The model used most frequently is ligation of the left circumflex coronary artery in the anesthetized dog.[439] Within 1 or 2 minutes of ligation, a portion of the lateral wall of the left ventricle ceases to contract. In those that survive a minimum of 8 to 12 hours, autopsy reveals an area of infarcted muscle in the lateral wall of the left ventricle.

Functional changes in myocardial infarction

Myocardial ischemia can be defined as a level of ATP consumption above that which can be provided by a particular coronary blood flow.[440] Within myocytes such ischemia is translated into structural damage within a relatively short time. Within 20 seconds after complete coronary occlusion systolic regional contraction diminishes and ceases by 1 to 2 minutes. The electrocardiogram changes by 30 seconds. If flow is reestablished within 20 to 40 minutes, necrosis can be totally prevented; if flow is not reestablished, some myocyte necrosis is inevitable.

Biochemical changes

Seconds after coronary arterial occlusion myocardial tissue oxygen levels fall and mitochondrial aerobic glycolysis ceases. Anaerobic glycolysis becomes the only source of new high-energy phosphates using glycogen as a substrate. Creatinine phosphate levels fall to virtually zero within 2 to 3 minutes. ATP levels within the cell begin to fall significantly only after 2 to 3 minutes. Intracellular acidosis develops in part, because of lactate production from glycogen stores; the depletion of stainable glycogen granules is the first morphologic evidence of ischemia. Phosphate also accumulates rapidly after the breakdown of creatinine phosphate.

Within seconds of ischemia, there is also evidence of a membrane-functional abnormality with loss of intracellular potassium ions. The intracellular sodium levels do not change initially. Brief periods of ischemia can be reversed without leading to tissue necrosis. The best indication of irreversible cell damage is disruption of the cell membrane; such changes can be detected by electron microscopy after 40 minutes of ischemia.

Structural changes after experimental infarction

Ultrastructural changes can be observed within the reversible phase of ischemia, including mitochondrial swelling and glycogen depletion. Within 40 minutes of total occlusion the changes are more severe, including disruption of cristae within swollen mitochondria, sarcoplasmic swelling, clumping of chromatin within the nuclei, and total loss of glycogen; irreversible change has occurred once granular electron-dense deposits of calcium appear within mitochondria and there are breaks in the cell membrane.[441]

Although ultrastructural changes occur within 40 minutes of occlusion, changes visible on light microscopy cannot be recognized before at least 4 to 8 hours have elapsed. The first recognizable histologic feature is an accumulation of polymorphonuclear leukocytes within the interstitial tissues, which may start as early as 4 hours and last for up to 3 days. Beyond this time, macrophages are the dominant cells. Individual muscle cells become hypereosinophilic (coagulative necrosis) with nuclear pyknosis followed by loss of cross-striations, and by 4 to 5 days they have disintegrated to be phagocytosed by macrophages. Perfusion within the central zone of an infarct is absent because of persistent occlusion of the major artery and destruction of the capillary bed by the necrotic process. Thus, within this central zone, the changes described above are retarded or absent. Repair of infarcts is dependent on a rim of granulation tissue at the junction with viable tissue, which contains intact perfused capillaries. Fibroblasts extend inward into the infarct from about 7 to 10 days; the whole process takes up to 8 weeks to produce a solid mass of fibrous tissue.

Animal models allow an occluded coronary artery to be reopened and flow reestablished at varying intervals. A comparison of infarcted areas that have been reperfused with those in which flow was not reestablished shows significant differences. Within minutes of reperfusion, the myocardial cells undergo explosive swelling because of water entering the cell. Calcium ions also pour into the cell invoking focal hypercontraction and shunting together of sarcomeres forming "contraction bands" within the cell, recognizable on light microscopy. Contraction band necrosis is recognizable histologically within 20 minutes of the onset of infarction in contrast to the traditional form of "coagulative" necrosis, which requires survival for at least 4 to 6 hours before it is recognizable.

Morphologic changes in human myocardial infarction

The microscopic appearances of human myocardial infarcts are similar in principal to those in animal models. Some regional infarcts are a single area of necrosis, which is apparently homogeneous in structure, though there is always an irregular lateral border with focal areas of viable myocardium mixed with necrotic areas. A surviving subendocardial band of muscle up to 10 cells in thickness is almost universal. The central zone of some infarcts comprises totally necrotic myocytes with no vascular perfusion. In contrast, other infarcts appear to represent the confluence of multifocal areas of necrosis of different ages. Such appearances are suggestive that in some cases arterial obstruction is complete and sudden, whereas in others it is staccato in origin with repeated episodes of occlusion and reperfusion. Although there are complicated descriptions of the microscopic changes designed to date exactly the onset of infarct, they can provide a rough approximation only. This inexactitude is the result of the intermittent occlusion that precedes many human infarcts and produces a more complex picture than the simple animal-ligation model.

Coagulation necrosis (Fig. 45-62) is the typical appearance of myocardial muscle cells seen in well-established regional transmural infarction after complete cessation of blood flow to the area. The muscle cells become hypereosinophilic but otherwise appear little affected until 24 hours, after which the cross-striations vanish and the myofibrils begin to coalesce. The earliest histologically recognizable changes at 12 to 24 hours is the accumulation of polymorphs within the interstitial tissue.

In contraction band necrosis (Fig. 45-63), dense eosinophilic transverse bands are present within the muscle cell. These represent telescoped sarcomeres, and the cell is often greatly shortened. This form of necrosis is more common when flow has been restored.

In any area of necrosis, a distinction has to be made between those instances in which the whole tissue is dead, including the stroma and vascular component and those in which only the muscle cells have died. The former is found in the center of regional transmural infarcts. The reparative process takes place only at the margins where the infarct abuts onto tissue with viable stroma and vessels. Amorphous hyaline muscle fibers, which have undergone little change other than total loss of striations, and nuclei may persist for many weeks or months incarcerated in the center of such infarcts. From 3 to 5 days, macrophages, fibroblasts, and capillaries begin to extend into the infarct from the periphery. Collagen deposition begins by 7 to 10 days and may take many weeks to transform the infarct into a fibrous scar. The ingrowth of capillaries into the area of infarction is mediated by release, within the infarct, of a myocardial angiogenesis factor closely related in structure to angiogenesis factors elaborated by tumor cells.

In areas of infarction in which the stroma has not undergone necrosis, the reparative process is far more rapid. In part, this may stem from the smaller size of the foci of necrosis, but it is also attributable to the presence of viable stromal cells within the area. In such areas, the myofibrillary structure of the muscle is lost, leading to the formation of hyaline masses after which macrophages appear within the sheath of the original muscle cells. The stroma collapses and coalesces to allow some proliferation of collagen to leave ultimately a small focal scar often containing some residual lipofuscin.

In myocytolysis (Fig. 45-64) the cells become large and vacuolated with loss of myofibrils, but the nuclei persist and mitochondrial enzyme activity remains. The appearance is often seen immediately beneath the endocardium or around blood vessels within areas that otherwise show conventional coagulative necrosis. The change is believed to indicate sublethal ischemic damage.

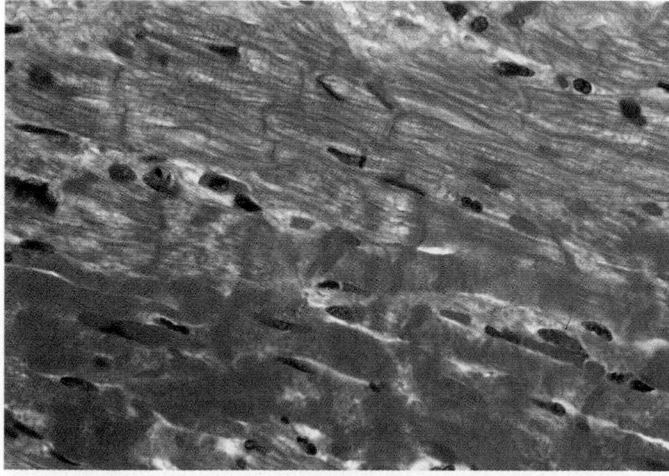

Fig. 45-62 Human myocardial infarction. The histologic section shows the edge of an area of regional necrosis. The necrotic myocytes show amorphous deeply eosinophilic appearance. Adjacent surviving cells appear pale and vacuolated.

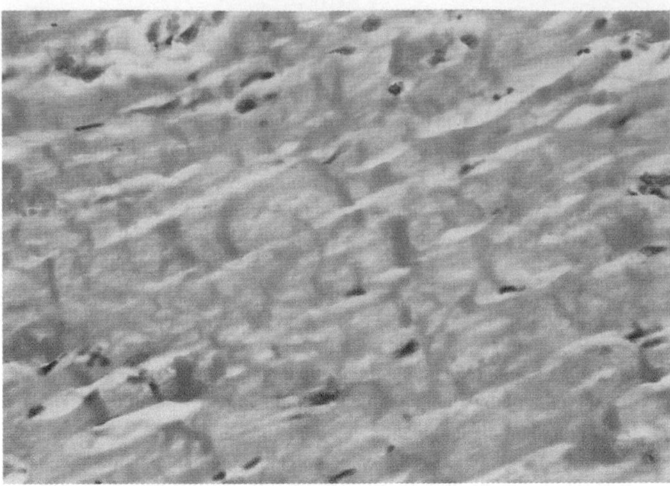

Fig. 45-63 Human myocardial infarction. In contraction band necrosis each myocyte has deeply eosinophilic cross banding.

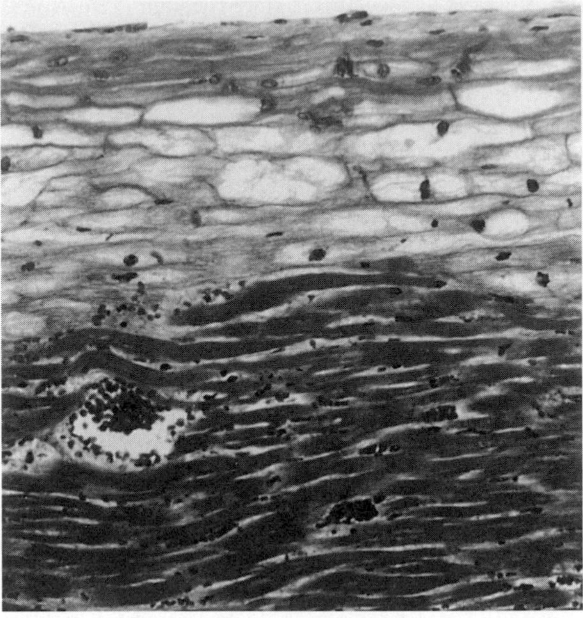

Fig. 45-64 Human myocardial infarction. The subendocardial area of a transmural regional infarct is shown. The immediately subendocardial surviving layer of myocytes shows loss of myofibrils, but the nuclei are preserved (myocytolysis). The deeper area of necrosis shows deeply eosinophilic myocytes that have lost their nuclei.

Complications and prognosis after regional transmural infarction

In the first 48 hours of acute myocardial infarction ventricular fibrillation causes sudden death. Even small infarcts can cause such sudden ventricular fibrillation. By 48 hours, the risk of ventricular arrhythmias is virtually over. Infarct size, that is, the proportion of the total LV muscle mass that has been lost, is directly related to the subsequent mortality. Cardiogenic shock occurs in patients whose infarcts involve more than 40% of the total LV muscle mass.[442] It is these patients who develop progressive subendocardial infarction.

Infarct extension and expansion

Stretching and thinning (expansion) of the infarcted tissue (Figs. 45-65 and 45-66) is associated with a high mortality and may progress to cardiac rupture. Such expansion is a feature of anterior transmural infarcts that involve more than 30% of the total left ventricular mass. The stretching of the infarct is attributable to combinations of tearing or sliding of muscle bundles relative to each other. Repair by fibrosis of an infarct that has expanded leads to a permanent globular dilatation of the ventricle.[443,444] Expansion must be separated from extension; in the latter further necrosis occurs; in expansion the volume of dead myocardium does not increase.

External cardiac rupture

Pericardial tamponade caused by external cardiac rupture is responsible up to 20% of the acute mortality and is the most common cause of death after ventricular arrhythmias and cardiogenic shock. Rupture is a complication only of transmural infarction.

There are two forms of rupture.[445] In one there is a slitlike tear between viable and nonviable muscle in an infarct that has not undergone expansion. Such ruptures occur within the first 2 days. In infarcts that have undergone expansion the endocardium may tear with extravasation of blood between the muscle bundles. This form of rupture occurs typically from the fifth to the tenth day. One report links accumulation of eosinophils within the infarct with an increased risk of rupture.[446] Rupture is more common in elderly women.[447]

Ventricular septal defects

Anterior or posterior septal transmural infarcts of the interventricular septum may rupture (Fig. 45-66) leading to the sudden acquisition of a left-to-right shunt.[448] Left anterior descending coronary occlusion is above the first septal branch, and in a patient in whom collateral flow is minimal, it is the most common cause. The resulting infarct is large and, in association with the hemodynamic burden of a shunt, causes a high mortality. The shunt takes place initially through a ragged hole ranging from 1 to 3 cm^2 in size. It is rare for patients to survive. It is usually those with smaller defects who will develop a smooth-edged hole as the infarct heals. In posterior septal infarction, the septal defects occur behind the posterior medial papillary muscle on the left side and open into the right ventricle close to the septal cusp of the tricuspid valve. These defects are associated with aneurysms of the posterior wall of the left ventricle and with RV infarction.

Papillary muscle infarction

Necrosis of the papillary muscles is common during acute infarction, being present to some degree in 15% to 30% of anterior and up to 50% of posterior infarctions. The greater frequency of posterior medial papillary muscle infarction reflects the blood supply from the right coronary artery, whereas the anterolateral group of papillary muscles is predominantly supplied by the left circumflex artery, a less common site of thrombosis. In less than 1% of fatal infarcts a portion of a papillary muscle avulses.[449,450] In the most severe form, the whole papillary muscle ruptures and the stump attached to the chordae passes in a flail-like motion across the mitral valve orifice associated with torrential mitral regurgitation. Rupture of a subhead of a papillary muscle, to which only one or two chordae are attached, is less catastrophic and leads to prolapse of a portion of the cusp only. Partial tears

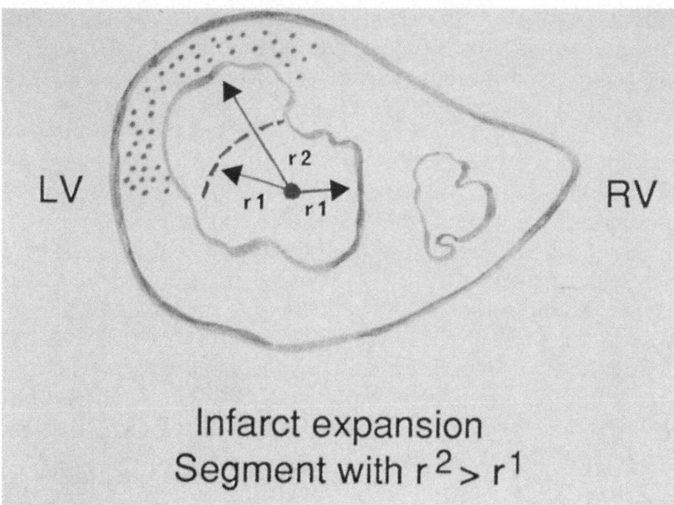

Fig. 45-65 Diagram of the concept of infarct expansion in the acute phase.

may heal to leave an elongated papillary muscle with a central fibrous isthmus and chronic regurgitation. Rupture of the posterior papillary muscle is 4 to 7 times more frequent than rupture of the anterolateral papillary muscle, but in neither case is the infarct necessarily large or transmural.

Right ventricular infarction

Between 20% and 50% of patients with posteroinferior infarcts of the left ventricle have some concomitant RV necrosis.[451] The incidence of RV infarction in association with anterior infarction is far lower. The RV myocardium is supplied by the right coronary artery, and the more proximal and the more complete the occlusion caused by thrombosis the more likely it is for infarction to occur in the right ventricle. Concomitant RV infarction leads to severe heart failure and an enlarged liver without evidence of left-sided failure and pulmonary edema.

Ventricular aneurysms

An aneurysm is a convex protrusion of the ventricular wall composed of collagen (Fig. 45-67). Such ischemic aneurysms result only from transmural infarction. There is a range of aneurysms from those with very diffuse bulges and a wide base to very localized saccular bulges with a narrow neck. Aneurysms present clinically with persistent ventricular arrhythmias, cardiac failure, and systemic emboli from mural thrombosis within the aneurysm. Late cardiac rupture is rare. The presence of mural thrombus is not a constant feature; aneurysms apparently identical in shape and size may be full of thrombus, contain some mural thrombus, or have no thrombus. The wall of ventricular aneurysms is composed predominantly of collagen, but calcification may occur,[452] particularly where the sac is lined by a thin coat of old thrombus. The pathogenesis of aneurysm formation can be either expansion of the infarct in the acute phase with subsequent replacement fibrosis stabilizing the new expanded shape, or the later expansion of an infarct that had already undergone fibrous replacement. A clinical study[453] using serial two-dimensional echocardiography found that aneurysms developed in 35 of 158 patients (22%) with infarction. Early aneurysms developed within the period in intensive care in 15 patients, and all were anterior and apical.

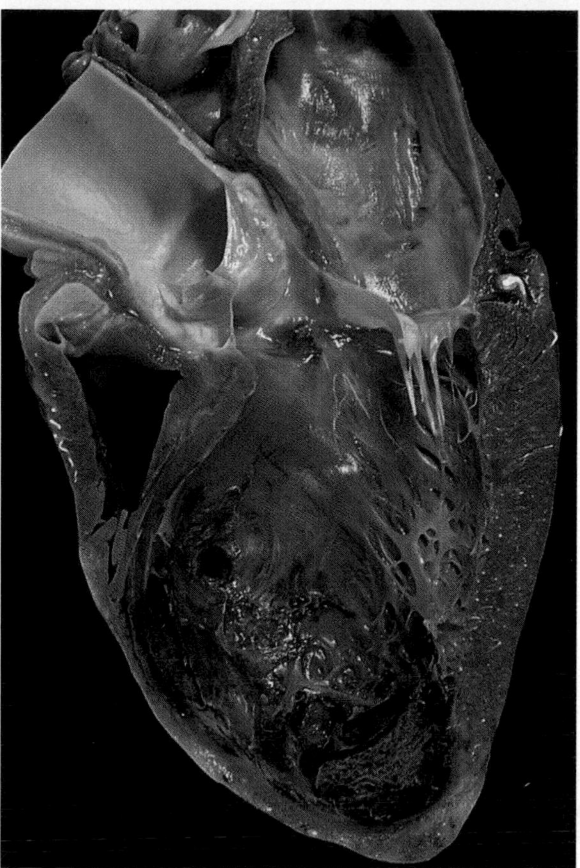

Fig. 45-66 Acute infarction with expansion. In a long-axis transection of the left ventricle an acute anterior infarct has thinned and is bowed outward. Mural thrombus has formed. In addition, there is a ventricular septal rupture.

Aneurysms developed within 3 months in a further 14 patients including some on the posterior wall.

A different pathogenesis has been proposed for aneurysms that have a very narrow neck opening into a large fibrous sac.[454] This form of aneurysm results from a ventricular tear that has led to a subpericardial hematoma, stopping just short of rupture into the pericardium. Organization of the hematoma results in an aneurysmal sac to which the name *pseudoventricular aneurysm* has been applied because the wall did not wholly derive from ventricular myocardium. Ventricular aneurysms with a narrow neck and large external sac are also found in patients without CAD and must be presumed to be congenital. Penetrating trauma such as knife wounds also leads to similar aneurysms.

Myocardial infarction with normal coronary arteries

The prevalence of myocardial infarction in which subsequent angiography is normal is between 1% and 3%.[455] The number of pathologic studies is small, and it is possible to list only potential causes. In some cases, the development of thrombosis is out of proportion with the degree of underlying atheroma, and so lysis restores a vessel outline that, at worse, is slightly irregular. In others thrombosis appears to have occurred in arteries that have no morphologic evidence of prior atherosclerosis. Other possible precipitating mechanisms are coronary emboli and spontaneous coronary artery dissection. Most cases, however, probably are attributable to spasm

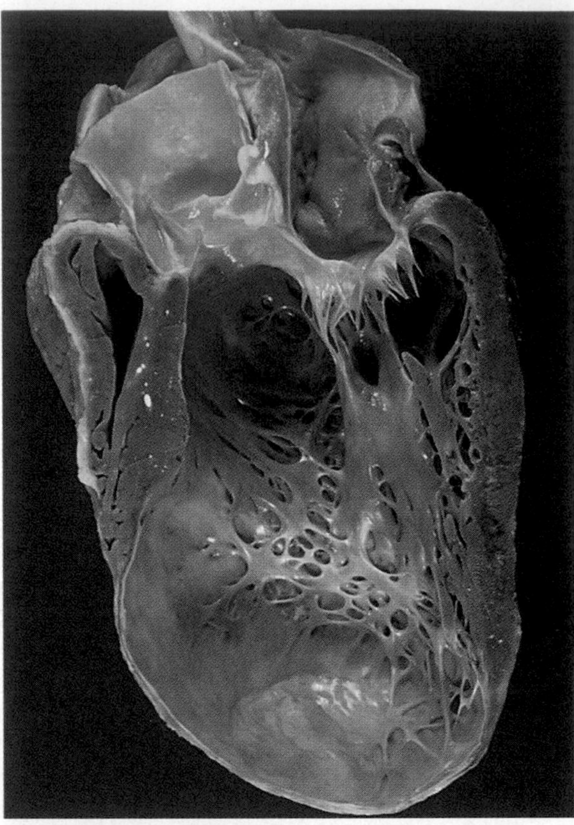

Fig. 45-67 Ischemic ventricular aneurysm. In a long-axis view of the left ventricle there is a large thin-walled apical aneurysm that does not contain thrombus.

and are forms of variant angina. Spasm is not a phenomenon that can be recognized at autopsy and is a presumptive diagnosis when there is a regional infarct supplied by a morphologically normal artery. Cocaine is a potent coronary vasoconstrictor and should always be excluded.

Coronary ostial stenosis

Angiographic studies in vivo[456,457] emphasizes the rarity of ostial stenosis and that the majority of cases are found in association with coronary stenosis elsewhere. In 6105 angiograms carried out for chest pain only 62 cases were found. In only 10 of these was the ostial stenosis isolated; all were relatively young women who had a low incidence of atheroma-related risk factors. Such findings lead to speculation that isolated ostial stenosis might be caused by aortic root dysplasia, intimal hyperplasia, or a sphincter-like ring of smooth muscle. The results of the few pathologic studies available,[458] however, are suggestive of an unusual distribution of atheroma rather than a separate pathogenesis for ostial stenosis. Ostial stenosis in association with aortic regurgitation is a complication of syphilitic aortitis.

Nonatheromatous coronary artery disease

Congenital anomalies

A vast number of variations in the origins of the coronary arteries exist. Some cause no physiologic abnormality; others are dangerous.[459,460]

The origin of both arteries from one aortic sinus or a single coronary orifice has no functional significance unless a coronary artery crossing from right to left or vice versa passes between the aorta and the pulmonary trunk. In this case, progressive intimal proliferation may occur leading to occlusion. One coronary orifice situated in the pulmonary trunk has serious sequelae because in patients who survive infancy a significant left-to-right shunt develops and the artery opening into the pulmonary trunk becomes aneurysmally dilated. Subendocardial fibrosis and calcification develop in infancy, making heart failure a common presentation. Late sudden death as the presenting symptom in adult life is also common.

Aneurysmal dilatation of a coronary artery that opens as a congenital fistula into atria, ventricles, or coronary sinus also occurs. Mural thrombosis may develop at the shunt sites leading to a risk of bacterial endocarditis.

In infants, sudden death may be associated with atresia of a segment of coronary artery but the ostia are normal. The commonest pattern is for the first portion of the left anterior descending coronary artery to be a threadlike structure with a tiny lumen and a disorganized thick intima and media. The distal part of the vessel is often fed by large collateral vessels crossing the outflow tract of the right ventricle from the right coronary. The condition is usually associated with considerable papillary muscle fibrosis and calcification.

Spontaneous dissection of coronary arteries

Dissection confined to the coronary artery may develop as a complication of surgery or be spontaneous.[461] In isolated coronary dissection it is uncommon to find an intimal tear, and the process is initially a hematoma between the media and adventitia rather than within the media (Fig. 45-68). A review of the cases of spontaneous coronary dissection in the literature indicates characteristic features. There is a preponderance of women; 40% of cases occur in the puerperium. Presentation is with acute infarction, sudden death, or unstable angina, with the left anterior descending artery being affected more commonly than the right, by a ratio of 4 to 1. Postmortem studies, however, show that multiple dissections are common, an indication that the basis may lie in a generalized abnormality of the coronary arteries. Pathologic studies also indicate that the process may begin as a subadventitial hematoma caused by bleeding from vessels crossing into the most superficial layer of the media. Such hematomas may compress the arterial lumen leading to ischemic myocardial damage or may invoke local arterial spasm. Resolution and organization of the hematoma at this stage can lead to a return to normal angiographic appearances. In other cases, the hematoma leads to the development of an intimal tear and more major arterial disruption. Intimal tears can be invoked easily by apparently uneventful angiography in patients who have subadventitial hematomas.

Medial cystic change analogous to the changes seen in the aortic media with dissection are inconsistent; in a different morphologic manifestation an infiltrate of the adventitia with inflammatory cells including eosinophils is frequently described.

Arterial bridging

At some sites the epicardial arteries are covered by a layer of subepicardial myocardium. The phenomenon occurs in varying degrees in up to 50% of normal hearts. External compression of the artery during systole can be detected angiographically and can be responsible for myocardial infarction, or sudden death,[462,463] or may induce angina in hypertrophied ventricles. It must be emphasized, however, that bridging is common in normal hearts from subjects without any history of

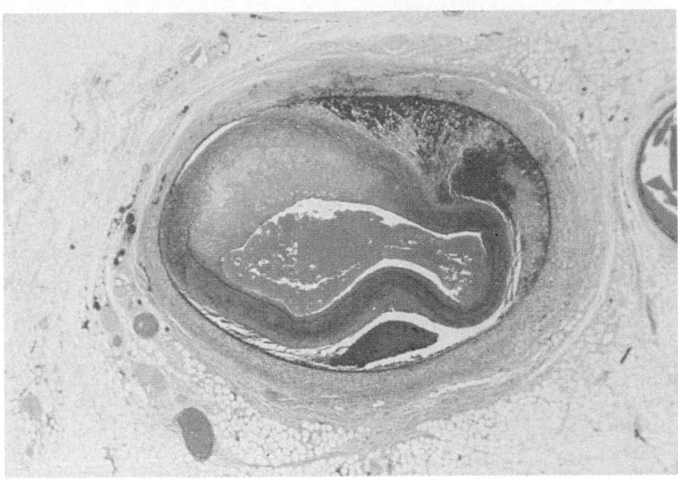

Fig. 45-68 Spontaneous coronary artery dissection. A dissection plane containing red blood cells and thrombus is present between the adventitia and the media. The lumen of the artery contains gray angiographic material. Since no angiographic material enters the dissection track, it indicates that there was no intimal tear. Sudden death in a young woman.

cardiac symptoms. Bridged arterial segments appear to be protected from atheromatous disease.

Coronary aneurysms

The terms *aneurysm,*[464] *aneurysmal dilatation*, and *coronary ectasia* describe different parts of a continuum running from localized bulges in an angiographically normal artery through localized areas of dilatation in an artery with areas of stenosis to diffuse dilatation of the whole artery. There is considerable overlap and inconsistency in the use of these terms. About 1.5% of coronary arteriograms in adults show appearances falling within this range. In all cases, the basic pathologic process is one of medial loss. The commonest form is dilated ectatic segments of artery alternating with stenotic segments. Diffuse dilatation does cause pronounced medial atrophy, but the reason why stenosis should occur in some areas and dilatation in others is not known. Diffuse ectasia in old age without stenosis is associated with diffuse loss of medial muscle often with some intimal calcification and minor lipid deposition. Diffuse dilatation of one artery in young individuals usually is caused by a high-flow fistula into the pulmonary artery, atria, or ventricles.

Localized saccular coronary aneurysms represent destruction or loss of the media in part of the circumference of the artery. A minority are attributable to congenital defects in the media, but most represent the end stage of an inflammatory process. Classic polyarteritis nodosa affects the coronary arteries as part of a systemic involvement of muscular arteries, but in Kawasaki's disease[465-467] the coronary arteries are extensively involved (Fig. 45-69). Kawasaki's disease, endemic in Japan but occurring as sporadic cases worldwide, presents as an acute febrile illness in children, associated with a skin rash, oral ulceration, and cervical lymphadenopathy easily mistaken for rubella. Cardiac involvement may develop after a short latent period and is characterized by coronary aneurysms leading to thrombosis and myocardial infarction as a cause of sudden death. Coronary arterial involvement may be less severe, leaving a residual aneurysm, which may be detected by angiography or thrombose and lead to infarction in later adult life. The cause is assumed to be viral though the exact agent is unknown.

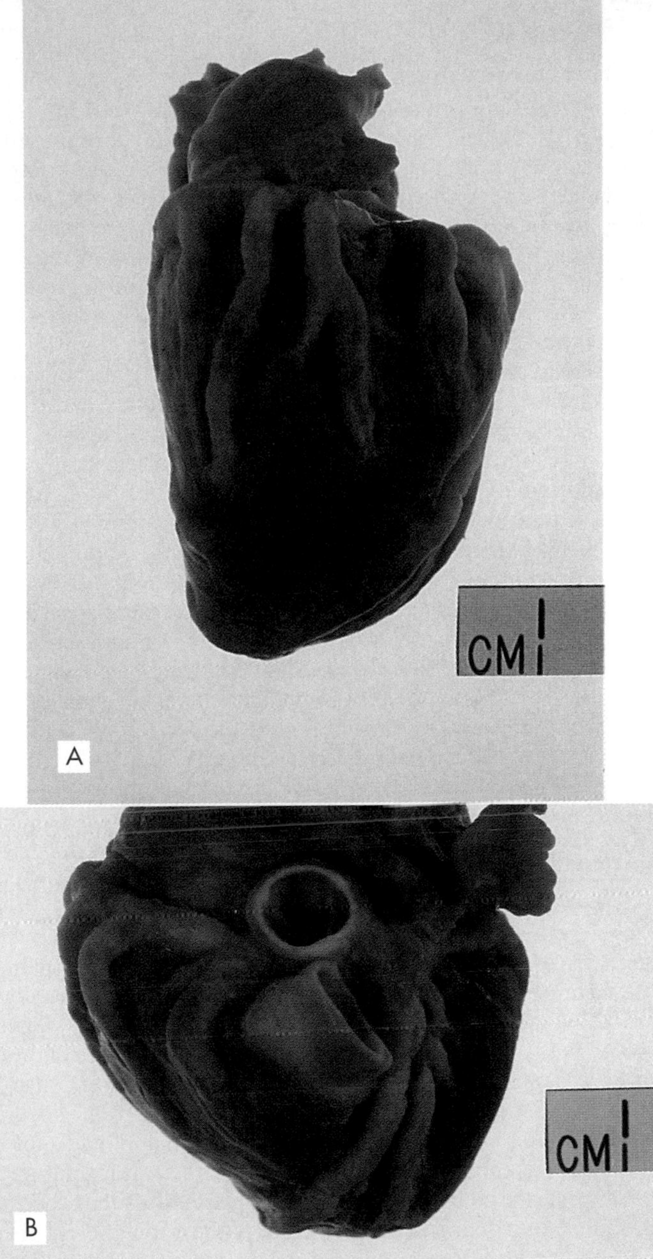

Fig. 45-69 Kawasaki disease. **A,** Anterosuperior view of the epicardial surface of an infant autopsy heart from a patient with fatal Kawasaki coronary arteriopathy. The arteritis processes led to pronounced thickening and immense prominence of virtually all the epicardial coronary arteries shown. The dramatic appearance is attributable to a combination of ectasia with accompanying intimal thickening. The adventitia is fibrotic, casting a whiter than normal hue to the vessels. **B,** Right lateral view of the same heart as depicted in **A,** illustrating further the prominence of the various acute marginal coronary branches descending over the right ventricular surface. The greatly narrowed lumen of the coronary arteries in this heart was further compromised acutely by superimposed thrombosis of the distal, dominant right coronary artery.

PERICARDIAL DISEASES

Normal pericardium

The pericardium is a fibrous sac that surrounds the heart. It has two layers; the *epicardium,* which is a single layer of mesothelial cells covering the heart, is continuous with the lining of the inner surface of the second pericardial layer, the *fibrosa.* Only in rare instances are there partial or complete congenital absences of the parietal pericardium.[468] Histologically, the pericardial lining consists of a single layer of mesothelial cells, which have microvilli. The fibrosa consists of collagen tissue arranged in thick wavy bands.

An increase in volume of the pericardial fluid does not immediately lead to a rise in pressure within the pericardial cavity. This lag is the result of the straightening of the collagen bundles that constitute the fibrosa layer. Distending the pericardial cavity post mortem requires around 150 ml of fluid; in a living human subject, however, acute increases of smaller amounts of fluid may result in hemodynamic changes. However, larger amounts of fluid accumulating slowly can be accommodated without symptoms. The normal amount of fluid in the pericardial sac is around 20 ml. The pericardial fluid has a similar composition to plasma, with a slightly lower protein concentration and a relatively higher albumen level. Tamponade is an acute phenomenon and occurs when the volume of fluid in the pericardial sac exerts sufficient pressure on the heart to impede ventricular filling. Constriction is the result of chronic pericardial fibrosis preventing atrial and later ventricular filling.

Pericarditis

Acute and chronic pericarditis

Acute pericarditis is inflammatory in origin with a significant fibrinous component. Tamponade rarely occurs. Chest pain is the dominant symptom. The causes are viral infection, tuberculosis, uremia, postinfarction state and postcardiac surgery. Acute pericarditis may be a self-limiting short-term condition or persist as chronic forms that develop fibrosis with constriction over some years.

The term *chronic pericarditis* can also be applied to infections such as tuberculosis or to the later effects of resolution of acute pericarditis by fibrosis. Chronic pericarditis that does not produce constriction is an incidental autopsy diagnosis. There are many causes of chronic constrictive pericarditis.[469] Some are relatively common; others very rare (Table 45-19).

Tuberculous pericarditis

Pericardial involvement in tuberculosis[470] is attributable to either hematogenous spread or to direct extension from the lung or mediastinal lymph nodes. During the first 2 weeks, there is fibrin deposition as well as a mild degree of pericardial effusion. The pericardial fluid is hemorrhagic and has a high concentration of proteins and neutrophils. After the first 2 weeks, the inflammatory cell population consists mostly of mononuclear cells. Later, typical tuberculous granulomas are seen, with formation of epithelioid cells, Langhans' giant cells, and caseous necrosis. Tubercle bacilli are present in the lesions. In the more advanced stage, there is a striking increase in the thickness of the pericardium, with fusion of both layers and the development of dense fibrosis and calcification resulting in constrictive pericarditis.

Tuberculous pericarditis is now reported in AIDS patients.[471] In general, tuberculosis appears as part of a disseminated disease in AIDS patients, but there are a few reports in which pericarditis was the presenting symptom.

Viral pericarditis

The most common viruses causing acute pericarditis are coxsackieviruses A and B, echoviruses, and polioviruses. Diagnosis is made by a significant rise in viral antibodies titers in blood. Acute viral pericarditis is generally accompanied by pericardial effusions, which range from straw colored to hemorrhagic. The episode tends to be short lived (1 to 2 weeks) in most cases.

Recurrent attacks may occur, and it is this group that may progress to chronic constrictive pericarditis.[472] Recurrent episodes have been particularly linked to coxsackievirus infection.

Nonviral infectious pericarditis

Neisseria gonorrhoeae can cause pericarditis.[473] Histoplasmosis may also cause a pericarditis that can progress to restriction.[474] Surgical procedures in the chest particularly when a sternal wound is infected can lead to acute pericarditis. Penetrating chest injury caused by knives or bullets can also become infected.

Pericarditis in connective tissue diseases

An acute fibrinous pericarditis is always present in acute rheumatic fever but resolves rapidly and does not progress to restriction.

Pericarditis is a relatively common finding in patients with rheumatoid arthritis. Autopsy data show that approximately 30% to 50% of the patients have mild chronic pericarditis. In life, however, patients with rheumatoid arthritis only rarely manifest symptoms of pericarditis. Chronic constriction[475] can occur in older patients who have long and extraarticular disease.

SLE, pericarditis is the most common manifestation of cardiac involvement.[476] Up to a third of patients with SLE have symptoms of pericardial involvement, and this figure increases to 80% when one includes autopsy cases. In general, cardiac tamponade is rare, and the clinical signs of pericarditis disappear after treatment.

Other causes

Any patient with uremia can develop a fibrinous pericarditis. Acute pericarditis is a common complication of renal trans-

Table 45-19 Causes of chronic pericarditis and constriction

- Infective
  - Postinfection nonresolution and persistent viral infection (coxsackievirus)
  - Tuberculosis
  - Histoplasmosis
- Connective tissue disorders
  - Scleroderma
  - Systemic lupus
  - Rheumatoid
- Postradiotherapy state
- Post–cardiac surgery
- Uremia
- Asbestosis
- Sarcoidosis

plantation.[477] Recent reviews of nearly 1500 patients covering a 27-year period have shown an incidence of pericarditis of 2.4%. The cause of the pericarditis was uremia in 40%, both uremia and cytomegalovirus in 12%, cytomegalovirus in 9%, and bacterial infections in 9%. Some cases remained without an etiologic diagnosis.

Pericarditis after cardiac surgery is common. During the first few days, there is a minor degree of hemorrhage together with fibrin deposition and an acute inflammatory cell infiltrate. With time, however, the fibrin becomes organized, and the pericardium thickens and may result in constrictive pericarditis.[478] Exposure to asbestos is associated with pericardial as well as pleural fibrosis, and constriction is reported.[479] After mediastinal radiotherapy dense fibrosis and calcification of either the visceral or parietal pericardium can lead to restriction.

Surgical excision in chronic constrictive pericarditis

In the relief of pericardial constriction the simplest procedure is the removal of a window of the anterior wall of the parietal pericardium. Fibrosis in the visceral pericardium requires stripping from the fibrous tissue of the myocardium itself and is more difficult.

The material the pathologist receives from surgical excision of the pericardium should be examined when a tissue diagnosis is being attempted. It is advisable to examine a large proportion of the material to look for granulomas indicating tuberculosis or the palisaded granulomas of rheumatoid disease. Most cases, however, will prove negative, and the cause remains unknown. In the developed world most are probably viral.

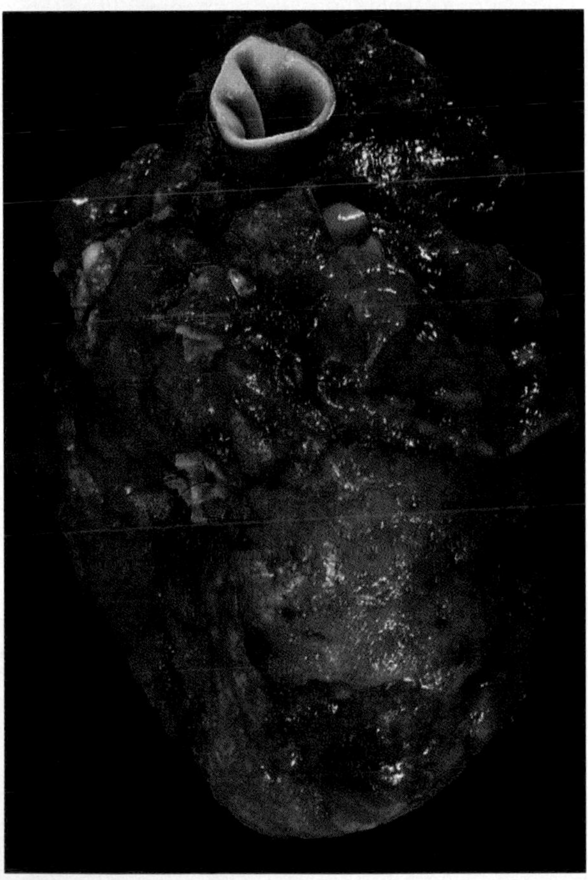

Fig. 45-70 Pericardial hemangiosarcoma. The patient was a young woman who presented with sudden tamponade as a result of a hemorrhagic pericardial effusion. A needle biopsy specimen showed hemangiosarcoma. Death occurred in 4 months with widespread metastasis and right atrial invasion. The clinical history is typical. At necropsy the visceral pericardium was completely covered by a sheet of hemorrhagic tumor.

Pericardial tumors

Approximately 10% of patients with terminal malignancy will have cardiac involvement, of these 85% will have pericardial involvement. The presence of tumor cells in the pericardium leads to a hemorrhagic pericarditis and cardiac tamponade.[480]

Secondary carcinoma is the most common cause of acute cardiac tamponade in patients who do not have myocardial infarction. Cytologic examination of the pericardial fluid is usually diagnostic. The frequency of positive results is around 80%, with a false positive rate of around 3%. The most common tumors to metastasize to the pericardium are lung, breast melanomas, and lymphomas.

Primary pericardial tumors are very rare. Benign mesothelial and pericardial cysts are the most common and are diagnosed by being seen on chest radiographs as an incidental finding. They consist of a fibrous capsule lined by mesothelial cells and are more usually unilocular than multiple. Hemangiosarcomas (Fig. 45-70) characteristically present as sudden tamponade caused by hemorrhagic effusions. Fibrosarcomas and liposarcomas are very rare. Primary mesotheliomas of the pericardium are recorded but are too rare to be certain if there is a link to asbestosis.

CARDIOGENIC SHOCK

Definition and clinical presentation. Cardiogenic shock is produced when myocardial function fails to maintain systemic blood flow at a level capable of fulfilling metabolic requirements. Because of the severity of many of the causative factors and resulting complications, cardiogenic shock is indisputably one of the most serious cardiac conditions. Even in patients met with swift diagnosis and therapy, the mortality is extremely high.

Acute myocardial infarction is by far the most common cause of cardiogenic shock, though numerous other cardiac and extracardiac entities associated with myocardial dysfunction may lead to cardiac pump failure. When infarction is the cause, the timing of onset and the severity of shock are directly related to the degree of myocardial damage.[68,481,482] Three-vessel coronary artery disease and acute infarction of the left ventricular myocardium are normally present in patients with cardiogenic shock secondary to this form of myocardial injury.[483] Concomitants of myocardial infarction that contribute to cardiogenic shock include extensive LV damage, ventricular septal rupture, acute mitral valve regurgitation (as a result of papillary muscle or chordal rupture), and RV infarction. The latter problem occurs in one fourth of all patients who suffer inferior wall myocardial infarction; isolated RV infarction is uncommon.[484]

As suggested, cardiogenic shock may result from cardiac disorders linked to insufficient ventricular performance other than ischemic infarction. These include severe myocarditis or dilated cardiomyopathy, severe valvular lesions (namely, stenosis or regurgitation of either the aortic or mitral valves), AV block, bradyarrhythmias, or tachyarrhythmias. Inadequate ventricular function secondary to coronary bypass surgery may be implicated in cardiogenic shock.[485]

Cardiac compression or constriction can also produce cardiogenic shock. Intracardiac obstruction is normally produced by valvular stenoses, though ball valve thrombus and atrial myxoma or other tumors must be considered. Pericardial tamponade, pulmonary embolism, severe pulmonary hypertension, aortic coarctation, hypertrophic cardiomyopathy, and tension pneumothorax are additional obstructive or compressive causes.[485]

Chief presentations of cardiogenic shock are hypotension, hypoperfusion, and extensive organ and cellular dysfunction.[485] In cardiogenic shock, hypotension may be defined as a mean blood pressure 30 mm Hg below previous basal values.[486] Cool, clammy skin; restlessness, agitation or obtundation, and decreased urine output are the chief clinical indicators of hypoperfusion.[487] Sinus tachycardia, weak peripheral pulse, tachypnea, and hypothermia or hyperthermia may also present.[487] In most settings, the symptoms of cardiogenic shock are accompanied by the primary manifestations of the etiologic condition.

One of the few epidemiologic studies of cardiogenic shock was conducted by Goldberg and colleagues in 1991.[488] Their research focused solely on the incidence and mortality of cardiogenic shock associated with acute myocardial infarction within a specific community and revealed no improvement in prognosis or incidence over time. Additional epidemiologic studies of cardiogenic shock are rare.[489]

The mortality for cardiogenic shock depends in part on the primary conditions that led to myocardial failure; on average, it is 80% or greater.[490] As with other forms of circulatory shock, this rate increases dramatically with age.[490]

Pathology. In cardiogenic shock, as with circulatory collapse of any nature, the pathologic features are dominated by extensive hypoperfusion of tissues and cells (Fig. 45-71). Increased production of lactate and, potentially, lacticacidosis result from cellular hypoxia.

Pathobiology. Cardiogenic shock is a syndrome of progressive deterioration (Fig. 45-71). Emergence of symptoms, however, may take anywhere from a few hours to several days after

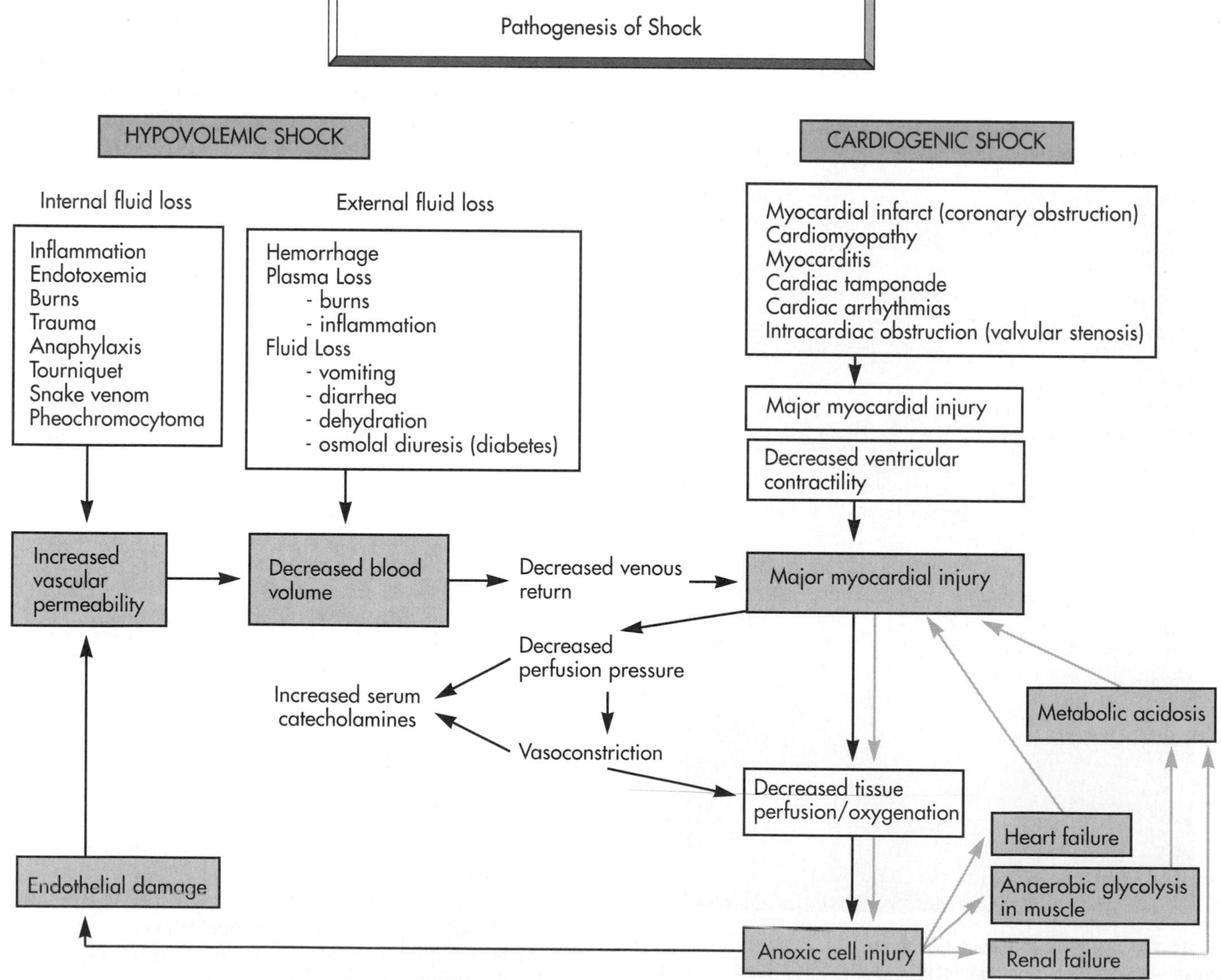

Fig. 45-71 Pathogenetic interrelationships in circulatory shock. The diagram emphasizes the multitude of internal and external processes that may lead to fluid loss and hypovolemic shock as well as the numerous common causes of cardiogenic (heart pump) shock. The vicious cycle of decreased cardiac function and escalating malperfusion with acidosis and multiorgan injury is also emphasized.

the onset of severe myocardial insufficiency before gradual hemodynamic deterioration results in cardiogenic shock. In the initial phase, cellular injury as a result of hemodynamic and metabolic disturbances can be halted and, if treated in time, reversed. If the condition is allowed to persist, irreversible cell damage and death are the inevitable result (Table 45-20).

After the onset of cardiogenic shock, tissue hypoperfusion develops, ultimately leading to organ dysfunction, which in turn exacerbates the initial symptoms of shock. Lungs, liver, kidneys, stomach, intestine, pancreas, and brain may all be affected secondarily to ineffective circulation. Tissue perfusion is further impaired as elevated circulating catecholamine produces systemic arteriolar vasoconstriction. Multiple lipid and carbohydrate metabolic abnormalities may develop, and various vasoactive substances are released.[487] With every passing minute, the extent of cell necrosis and tissue damage escalates and the likelihood of full recovery disappears.

Therapy. Therapy for cardiogenic shock cannot commence until a precise diagnosis has been made regarding its primary cause or causes. Diagnosis, however, may not take place until the patient has been stabilized. Cardiogenic shock, regardless of its cause, involves considerable pain for the patient, which must be alleviated as much as possible before additional measures are undertaken. Reestablishment of circulatory homeostasis and aggressive treatment of hypotension are necessary stabilizing procedures. Hypotension may be relieved in part through volume expansion on its own, or in addition to the administration of pressor agents.

In pinpointing the specific cause of cardiac shock in a single patient, one must distinguish acute myocardial infarction from other cardiac conditions that may mimic its presentation, such as massive pulmonary embolism, tension, pneumothorax, or pericardial tamponade.[490] Likewise, it is equally important to isolate specific disorders complicating myocardial infarction that may lead to sudden heart failure.[491] Rupture of the ventricular septum, injury or rupture of a papillary muscle, or damage to the valve apparatus, all of which produce acute mitral insufficiency, are prime examples of the many serious complications associated with myocardial infarction that require prompt recognition and correction. In most settings, the primary cause of cardiogenic shock can be elicited after obtainment of a brief patient history, physical examination, electrocardiogram, echocardiogram, portable chest radiograph, and arterial blood gases.[487]

As mentioned, various vasodilatory agents are used in cardiogenic shock characterized by severe, persistent systemic hypotension. Patients presenting with poor peripheral perfusion and an elevated pulmonary capillary wedge pressure, in addition to hypotension, are normally recommended for pharmacologic therapy. Where inotropic agents are insufficient, various interventional methods may be applicable. Intra-aortic balloon counterpulsation has been used increasingly to provide mechanical support for a failing pump. Intra-aortic intervention is particularly successful where cardiogenic shock has resulted from mechanical defects such as papillary muscle or ventricular septal rupture, or from extensive myocardial ischemia or infarction.[487] Surgical procedures, involving correction or replacement of isolated heart mechanisms, are normally undertaken for valvular lesions responsible for cardiogenic shock. The diverse mechanical, percutaneous, and surgical procedures used in the amelioration and restoration of normal circulatory function have been reviewed by Goldenberg.[492] Cardiac transplant for treatment of cardiogenic shock is less common than other methods described. Transplantation may involve the implantation of temporary or permanent ventricular assist devices or the substitution of a total artificial heart, until a donor heart is obtained. Unfortunately the survival rate of patients provided with mechanical devices is tempered by the scarcity of donor hearts.

Table 45-20 Complications of circulatory shock

- Fever, ultimate hypoxemic brain death
- Adult respiratory distress syndrome (ARDS)
- Necrosis
  - Myocardial, multifocal, particularly subendocardial
  - Liver, centrilobular, hemorrhagic
  - Intestine, superficial, hemorrhagic
  - Kidney, acute tubular
- Congestion and hyperfunction of spleen
- Stress (corticosteroid) ulcers of stomach
- Vasodilatation and splanchnic pooling

ACKNOWLEDGMENT

The authors wish to acknowledge the excellent journalistic assistance of Shelley Wood, Janet Wilson, and Shelina Babul in the completion of this chapter. Their diligence and expertise are deeply appreciated.

REFERENCES

1. US Bureau of the Census, Department of Commerce: *Mortality statistics—1920,* Washington, D.C., 1922, US Government Printing Office.
2. Hogg RS, Schechter MT, Montaner JS: Impact of HIV infection and AIDS on death rates in British Columbia and Canada, *Can Med Assoc J* 150:711, 1994.

Valvular lesions

3. Special Writing Group of the Committee on Rheumatic Fever E and Kawasaki Disease of the Council on Cardiovascular Disease in the Young of the American Heart Association: Guidelines for the diagnosis of rheumatic fever: Jones criteria, 1992 update, *JAMA* 268:2069, 1992.
4. Gulizia JM: *Cellular and molecular mechanisms of inflammatory heart disease,* doctoral thesis, Department of Pathology and Microbiology, University of Nebraska Medical Center, Omaha, Neb, 1991.
5. Feinstein AR, DiMassa R: Prognostic significance of valvular involvement in acute rheumatic fever, *N Engl J Med* 260:1001, 1959.
6. Waksman BH: The etiology of rheumatic fever: a review of theories and evidence, 1949, *Medicine* 72:262, 1993.
7. Pomerance A: *The pathology of the heart,* London, 1975, Blackwell.
8. Burch GE, Giles TD, Colcolough HL: Pathogenesis of "rheumatic" heart disease: critique and theory, *Am Heart J* 80:556, 1970.
9. Homer C, Shulman ST: Clinical aspects of acute rheumatic fever, *J Rheumatol* 29:2, 1991.
10. Ayoub EM: Resurgence of rheumatic fever in the United States: the changing picture of a preventable illness, *Postgrad Med* 92:133, 1992.
11. Alto WA, Gibson R: Acute rheumatic fever: an update, *Am Fam Physician* 45:613, 1992.
12. Griffiths SP, Gersony WM: Acute rheumatic fever in New York City (1969 to 1988): a comparative study of two decades, *J Pediatr* 116:882, 1990.
13. Kaplan EL, Hill HR: Return of rheumatic fever: consequences, implications, and needs, *J Pediatr* 111:244, 1987.
14. Whitelaw DA, Rayner BL, Willcox PA: Community-acquired bacteremia in the elderly: a prospective study of 121 cases, *J Am Geriatr* Soc 40:996, 1992.
15. Sergent JS: Acute rheumatic fever, *Trans Am Clin Climatol Assoc* 104:15, 1992.
16. Vyse T: Rheumatic fever: changes in its incidence and presentation, *Br Med J* 302:518, 1991.

17. WHO Cardiovascular Diseases Unit and Principal Investigators: WHO programme for the prevention of rheumatic fever/rheumatic heart disease in 16 developing countries: Report from Phase I (1986–90), *Bull World Health Organ* 70:213, 1992.
18. Garcia-Palmiere MR: Rheumatic fever and rheumatic heart disease as seen in the tropics, *Am Heart J* 64:577, 1962.
19. Shaper AG: Cardiovascular disease in the tropics. I. Rheumatic heart, *Br Med J* 3:683, 1972.
20. Shefferman MM, Goodman JS, Ultan LB et al: Acute rheumatic fever in Puerto Rico, *Am J Dis Child* 110:239, 1965.
21. Cates JE, Christie RV: Subacute bacterial endocarditis: review of 442 patients treated in 14 centres appointed by Penicillin Trials Committee of Medical Research Council, *Q J Med* 20:93, 1951.
22. Bland EF, Jones TD: Rheumatic fever and rheumatic heart disease: a twenty year report on 1000 patients followed since childhood, *Circulation* 4:837, 1951.
23. Friedberg CK: Rheumatic fever in the adult: criteria and implications, *Circulation* 19:161, 1959.
24. Stollerman GH: Factors determining the attack rate of rheumatic fever, *JAMA* 177:823, 1961.
25. Ben Dov I, Berry E: Acute rheumatic fever in adults over 45 years, *Semin Arthritis Rheum* 10:100, 1980.
26. McDanald EC, Weisman MH: Articular manifestations of rheumatic fever in adults, *Ann Intern Med* 89:917, 1978.
27. Silver MD: Blood flow obstruction related to tricuspid, pulmonary, and mitral valves. In *Cardiovascular pathology*, New York, 1991, Churchill Livingstone.
28. Stollerman GH: Rheumatic and hereditable connective tissue diseases of the cardiovascular system. In Braunwald E, editor: *Heart disease: a textbook of cardiovascular medicine*, Philadelphia, 1988, Saunders.
29. Stamler J: Cardiovascular diseases in the United States, *Am J Cardiol* 10:319, 1962.
30. Wilson MG: *Advances in rheumatic fever*, New York, 1962, Harper & Row.
31. Bisno AL: The resurgence of acute rheumatic fever in the United States, *Annu Rev Med* 41:319, 1990.
32. Spagnuolo M, Taranta A: Rheumatic fever in siblings: similarity of its clinical manifestations, *N Engl J Med* 278:183, 1968.
33. Wilson MG, Schweitzer MD, Lubschez R: Familial epidemiology of rheumatic fever: genetic and epidemiological studies, *J Pediatr* 22:468, 1943.
34. Stollerman GH: Variation in group A streptococci and the prevalence of rheumatic fever: a half-century vigil, *Ann Intern Med* 118:467, 1993.
35. Stollerman GH: Nephritogenic and rheumatogenic group A streptococci, *J Infect Dis* 120:259, 1969.
36. Bisno AL, Pearce IA, Wall HP et al: Contrasting epidemiology of acute rheumatic fever and acute glomerulonephritis, *N Engl J Med* 283:561, 1970.
37. Bisno AL, Pearce IA, Stollerman GH: Streptococcal infections which fail to cause recurrences of rheumatic fever, *J Infect Dis* 136:276, 1977.
38. Kaplan EL: T. Duckett Jones Memorial Lecture: Global assessment of rheumatic fever and rheumatic heart disease at the close of the century: influences and dynamics of populations and pathogens: a failure to realize prevention? *Circulation* 88:1964, 1993.
39. Congeni BL: The resurgence of acute rheumatic fever in the United States, *Pediatr Ann* 21:816, 1992.
40. Bisno AL: Group A streptococcal infections and acute rheumatic fever, *N Engl J Med* 325:783, 1991.
41. Amigo MC, Martínez-Lavín M, Reyes PA: Acute rheumatic fever, *Rheum Dis Clin North Am* 19:333, 1993.
42. Pape LA: Pathogenesis and etiology of valvular heart disease. In Dalen JE, Alpert JS, editors: *Valvular heart disease*, Boston, 1987, Little, Brown & Co.
43. Davies MJ: *Pathology of cardiac valves*, London, 1980, Butterworth.
44. Virmani R, Roberts WC: Aschoff bodies in operatively excised atrial appendages and in papillary muscles: frequency and clinical significance, *Circulation* 55:559, 1977.
45. Gulizia JM, Cunningham MW, McManus BM: Immunoreactivity of anti-streptococcal monoclonal antibodies to human heart valves: evidence for multiple cross-reactive epitopes, *Am J Pathol* 138:285, 1991.
46. Siegel AC, Johnson EE, Stollerman GH: Controlled studies of streptococcal pharyngitis in a pediatric population. I. Factors related to the attack rate of rheumatic fever, *N Engl J Med* 265:559, 1961.
47. Rammelkamp CH Jr, Wannamaker LW, Denny FW: Epidemiology and prevention of rheumatic fever, *Bull NY Acad Med* 28:321, 1952.
48. Kaplan MH: The cross-reaction of group A streptococci with heart tissue and its relations to autoimmunity in rheumatic fever, *Bull Rheum Dis* 19:560, 1969.
49. Van de Rijn I, Zabriskie JB, McCarthy M: Group A streptococcal antigens cross-reactive with myocardium: purification of heart-reactive antibody and isolation and characterization of the streptococcal antigen, *J Exp Med* 146:579, 1977.
50. Goldstein I, Halpern B, Robert L: Immunologic relationship between streptococcus A polysaccharide and the structural glycoproteins of heart valves, *Nature* 213:44, 1967.
51. Gulizia JM, Cunningham MW, McManus BM: Evolving issues regarding the immunopathogenesis of rheumatic heart disease. *Cor Notes, Soc Cardiovasc Pathol* 5:9, 1990.
52. Bortolotti U, Valente M, Agozzino L et al: Rheumatoid mitral stenosis requiring valve replacement, *Am Heart J* 107:1049, 1984.
53. Evans DTP, Sloman JG: Mitral stenosis and mitral incompetence due to Libman-Sacks endocarditis and mitral valve replacement, *Aust NZ J Med* 11:526, 1981.
54. Dalen JE: Mitral stenosis. In Dalen JE, Alpert JS, editors: *Valvular heart disease*, Boston, 1987, Little, Brown & Co.
55. Charney R, Keltz TN, Attai L et al: Acute valvular obstruction from streptococcal endocarditis, *Am Heart J* 125:544, 1993.
56. Steinbrunn W, Cohn DE, Selzer A: Atrial septal defect associated with mitral stenosis: the Lutembacher syndrome revisited, *Am J Med* 48:295, 1970.
57. McAllister HA Jr, Fenoglio JJ Jr: Cardiac involvement in Whipple's disease, *Circulation* 52:152, 1975.
58. Ladefoged C, Rohr N: Amyloid deposits in aortic and mitral valves, *Virchows Arch [A] (Pathol Anat Histopathol)* 404:301, 1984.
59. Bana DS, MacNeal PS, LeCompte PM: Cardiac murmurs and endocardial fibrosis associated with methysergide therapy, *Am Heart J* 88:640, 1974.
60. Misch KA: Development of heart valve lesions during methysergide therapy, *Br Med J* 2:345, 1974.
61. Leder AA, Bosworth WC: Angiokeratoma corporis diffusum universale (Fabry's disease) with mitral stenosis, *Am J Med* 38:814, 1965.
62. Johnson GL, Vine DL, Cottrill CM et al: Echocardiographic mitral valve deformity in the mucopolysaccharidoses, *Pediatrics* 67:401, 1981.
63. Marwick TH, Bastian B, Hughes CF et al: Mitral stenosis in the Maroteaux-Lamy syndrome: a treatable cause of dyspnea, *Postgrad Med J* 68:287, 1992.
64. Tan CT, Schaff HV, Miller FA Jr et al: Valvular heart disease in four patients with Maroteaux-Lamy syndrome, *Circulation* 85:188, 1992.
65. Wood P: An appreciation of mitral stenosis. Part I. Clinical features, *Br Med J* 1(1051):1954, 1954.
66. White PD: *Heart disease*, New York, 1951, MacMillan.
67. McKay CR: Catheter balloon valvuloplasty treatment of adult patients with mitral stenosis, *Chest* 95:410, 1989.
68. Braunwald E: Valvular heart disease. In Braunwald E, editor, *Heart Disease: A Textbook of Cardiovascular Medicine*, Philadelphia, 1988, WB Saunders.
69. Waller BF, McManus BM, Roberts WC: Mitral valve stenosis produced by or worsened by active infective endocarditis, *Chest* 83:498, 1982.
70. Essop MR: Relief of rheumatic mitral stenosis—when and how?, *Am J Cardiol* 73:85, 1994.
71. Essop MR, Turner E, Wisenbaugh T et al: Surgery for significant mitral regurgitation following mitral balloon valvotomy, *J Am Coll Cardiol* 19:113, 1992.
72. Röthlisberger C, Essop MR, Skudicky D et al: Results of percutaneous balloon mitral valvotomy in young adults, *Am J Cardiol* 72:73, 1993.
73. Rippe JM, Howe JP III: Acute mitral regurgitation. In Dalen JE, Alpert JS, editors: *Valvular heart disease*, Boston, 1987, Little, Brown & Co.
74. Sancho M, Medina A, Suárez de Lezo J et al: Factors influencing progression of mitral regurgitation after transarterial balloon valvuloplasty for mitral stenosis, *Am J Cardiol* 66:737, 1990.

75. Herrmann HC, Kleaveland JP, Hill JA et al: The M-Heart percutaneous balloon mitral Valvuloplasty Registry: initial results and early follow-up: the M-Heart Group, *J Am Coll Cardiol* 15:1221, 1990.
76. Roth RB, Block PC, Palacios IF: Predictors of increased mitral regurgitation after percutaneous mitral balloon valvotomy, *Cathet Cardiovasc Diagn* 20:17, 1990.
77. Essop MR, Wisenbaugh T, Skoularigis J et al: Mitral regurgitation following mitral balloon valvotomy: differing mechanisms for severe versus mild-to-moderate lesions, *Circulation* 84:1669, 1991.
78. Scott-Jupp W, Barnett NL, Gallagher PJ et al: Ultrastructural changes in spontaneous rupture of mitral chordae tendineae, *J Pathol* 133:185, 1981.
79. Korn D, DeSanctis RW, Sell S: Massive calcification of the mitral annulus, *N Engl J Med* 267:900, 1962.
80. Braunwald E, Goldblatt A, Ayen MM et al: Congenital aortic stenosis: clinical and hemodynamic findings in 100 patients, *Circulation* 27:420, 1963.
81. Marcus RH, Sareli P, Pocock WA et al: The spectrum of severe rheumatic mitral valve disease in a developing country: correlations among clinical presentation, surgical pathologic findings, and hemodynamic sequelae, *Ann Intern Med* 120:177, 1994.
82. Stapleton JF: Natural history of chronic valvular disease. In Likoff W, editor: *Valvular heart disease: comprehensive evaluation and managment,* Philadelphia, 1986, FA Davis.
83. Gooch AS, Maranhao V, Scampardonis G et al: Prolapse of both mitral and tricuspid leaflets in systolic murmur-click syndrome, *N Engl J Med* 287:1218, 1972.
84. Rippe JM, Angoff G, Sloss LJ et al: Multiple floppy valves: an echocardiographic syndrome, *Am J Med* 66:817, 1979.
85. Savage DD, Garrison RJ, Devereux RB et al: Mitral valve prolapse in the general population. I. Epidemiologic features: the Framingham Study, *Am Heart J* 106:577, 1983.
86. Procacci PM, Savran SV, Schreiter SL et al: Prevalence of clinical mitral valve prolapse in 1,169 young women, *N Engl J Med* 294:1086, 1976.
87. Weiner BH, Alpert JS: Mitral regurgitation: Mitral valve prolapse. In Dalen JE, Alpert JS, editors: *Valvular heart disease,* Boston, 1987, Little, Brown & Co.
88. Gottdiener JS, Sherber HS, Harvey WP: Midsystolic click and mitral valve prolapse following commissurotomy, *Am J Med* 64:295, 1978.
89. Chesler E, Gornick CC: Maladies attributed to myxomatous mitral valve, *Circulation* 83:328, 1991.
90. Jeresaty RM: *Mitral valve prolapse,* New York, 1979, Raven Press.
91. Felner JM, Harwood S, Mond H et al: Systolic honks in young children, *Am J Cardiol* 40:206, 1977.
92. DeSa'Neto A, Tye KH, Desser KB et al: Precordial "honk" during atrial tachyarrhythmia, *Chest* 75:1, 1979.
93. Cohn LH, Couper GS, Aranki SF et al: Long-term results of mitral valve reconstruction for regurgitation of the myxomatous mitral valve, *J Thorac Cardiovasc Surg* 107:143, 1994.
94. Ptacin M, Sebastian J, Bamrah VS: Ochronotic cardiovascular disease, *Clin Cardiol* 8:441, 1985.
95. Bulkley BH, Roberts WC: The heart in systemic erythematosis and the changes induced in it by corticosteroid therapy: a study of 36 necropsy patients, *Am J Med* 48:243, 1975.
96. Pritzker MR, Ernst JD, Caudill C et al: Acquired aortic stenosis in systemic lupus erythematosus, *Ann Intern Med* 93:434, 1980.
97. Lerman BB, Thomas LC, Abrams GD et al: Aortic stenosis associated with systemic lupus erythematosus, *Am J Med* 72:707, 1982.
98. Levinson GE: Aortic stenosis. In Dalen JE, Alpert JS, editors: *Valvular heart disease,* Boston, 1987, Little, Brown & Co.
99. Roberts WC, Ferrans VJ, Levy RI et al: Cardiovascular pathology in hyperlipoproteinemia: anatomic observations in 42 necropsy patients with normal or abnormal serum lipoprotein patterns, *Am J Cardiol* 31:557, 1973.
100. Dinsmore RE, Lees RS: Vascular calcification in types II and IV hyperlipoproteinemia: radiographic appearance and clinical significance, *Am J Roentgenol* 144:895, 1985.
101. Roberts WC, Ewy GA, Glancy DL et al: Valvular stenosis produced by active infective endocarditis, *Circulation* 36:449, 1967.
102. Arnett EN, Roberts WC: Pathology of active infective endocarditis: a necropsy analysis of 192 patients, *Thorac Cardiovasc Surg* 30:327, 1982.
103. Detrano RC, Yiannikas J, Salcedo EE: Two-dimensional echocardiographic assessment of radiation-induced valvular heart disease, *Am Heart J* 107:584, 1984.
104. Warda M, Khan A, Massumi A et al: Radiation-induced valvular dysfunction, *J Am Coll Cardiol* 2:180, 1983.
105. Carlson RG, Mayfield WR, Normann S et al: Radiation-associated valvular disease, *Chest* 99:538, 1991.
106. Yost JH, Spencer-Green G, Krant JD: Vascular steal mimicking compression myelopathy in Paget's disease of bone: rapid reversal with calcitonin and systemic steroids, *J Rheumatol* 20:1064, 1993.
107. Tentolouris C, Kontozoglou T, Toutouzas P: Familial calcification of aorta and calcific aortic valve disease associated with immunologic abnormalities, *Am Heart J* 126:904, 1993.
108. Cotran RS, Kumar V, Robbins SL: *Pathologic basis of disease,* Philadelphia, 1989, Saunders.
109. Hakki AH, Kimbiris D, Iskandrian AS et al: Angina pectoris and coronary artery disease in patients with severe aortic valvular disease, *Am Heart J* 100:441, 1980.
110. Green SJ, Pizzarello RA, Padmanabhan VT et al: Relation of angina pectoris to coronary artery disease in aortic valve stenosis, *Am J Cardiol* 55:1063, 1985.
111. Heyde EC: Gastrointestinal bleeding in aortic stenosis, *N Engl J Med* 259:196, 1958.
112. Schwartz BM: Additional note on bleeding in aortic stenosis, *N Engl J Med* 259:456, 1958.
113. Gamboa R, Hugenholz PG, Nadas AS: Accuracy of the phonocardiogram in assessing severity of aortic and pulmonary stenosis, *Circulation* 30:35, 1964.
114. Davies SW, Gershlick AH, Balcon R: Progression of valvar aortic stenosis: a long-term retrospective study, *Eur Heart J* 12:10, 1991.
115. Wagner S, Selzer A: Patterns of progression of aortic stenosis: a longitudinal hemodynamic study, *Circulation* 65:709, 1982.
116. Prewitt TA: Syphilitic aortic insufficiency: its increased incidence in the elderly, *JAMA* 211:637, 1970.
117. Oh WMC, Taylor RT, Olsen EGJ: Aortic regurgitation in systemic lupus erythematosus requiring aortic valve replacement, *Br Heart J* 36:413, 1974.
118. Olson LJ, Subramanian R, Edwards WD: Surgical pathology of pure aortic insufficiency: a study of 225 cases, *Mayo Clin Proc* 59:835, 1984.
119. Reid GD, Patterson MWH, Patterson AC et al: Aortic insufficiency in association with juvenile ankylosing spondylitis, *J Pediatr* 95:78, 1979.
120. Roberts WC, Kehoe JA, Carpenter DF: Cardiac valvular lesions in rheumatoid arthritis, *Arch Intern Med* 122:141, 1968.
121. Rodnan GP, Benedek TG, Shaver JA et al: Reiter's syndrome and aortic insufficiency, *JAMA* 189:889, 1964.
122. Paulus HE, Pearson CM, Pitts W: Aortic Insufficiency in five patients with Reiter's syndrome: a detailed clinical and pathological study, *Am J Med* 53:464, 1972.
123. Rae SA, Vandenburg M, Scholtz CL: Aortic regurgitation and false aneurysm in Behçet's disease, *Postgrad Med J* 56:438, 1980.
124. Roberts WC, MacGregor RR, DeBlanc HJ Jr et al: The pre-pulseless phase of pulseless disease, or pulseless disease with pulses: a newly recognized cause of cardiac disease, monoclonal gammopathy and "fever of unknown origin," *Am J Med* 46:313, 1969.
125. Shelhamer JH, Volkman DJ, Parrillo JE et al: Takayasu's arteritis and its therapy, *Ann Intern Med* 103:121, 1985.
126. Bostwick DG, Bensch KG, Burke JS et al: Whipple's disease presenting as aortic insufficiency, *N Engl J Med* 305:995, 1981.
127. Esdah J, Hawkins D, Gold P et al: Vascular involvement in relapsing polychondritis, *Can Med Assoc J* 116:1019, 1977.
128. Vered Z, Pras M, Horowitz A et al: Severe aortic regurgitation: a rare clinical presentation of giant cell arteritis, *Clin Cardiol* 9:509, 1986.
129. Allen WM, Matloss JM, Fishbein MC: Myxoid degeneration of the aortic valve and isolated severe aortic regurgitation, *Am J Cardiol* 55:439, 1985.
130. Tonnemacher D, Reid C, Kawanishi D et al: Frequency of myxomatous degeneration of the aortic valve as a cause of isolated aortic regurgitation severe enough to warrant aortic valve replacement, *Am J Cardiol* 60:1194, 1987.

131. Wagenvoort C, Neufeld HN, Edwards JE: Cardiovascular system in Marfan's syndrome and in idiopathic dilatation of the ascending aorta, *Am J Cardiol* 9:496, 1962.
132. Edmindson O, Nellen M, Ross DN: Case reports—aortic valve replacement in a case of Ehlers-Danlos syndrome, *Br Heart J* 42:103, 1979.
133. Weisinger B, Glassman E, Spencer FC et al: Successful aortic valve replacement with osteogenesis imperfecta, *Br Heart J* 37:475, 1975.
134. Alpert JS: Chronic aortic regurgitation. In Dalen JE, Alpert JS, editors: *Valvular heart disease,* Boston, 1987, Little, Brown & Co.
135. Lemon DK, White CW: Anuloaortic ectasia: angiographic, hemodynamic and clinical comparison with aortic valve insufficiency, *Am J Cardiol* 41:482, 1978.
136. Waller BF, Kishel JC, Roberts WC: Severe aortic regurgitation from systemic hypertension (without aortic dissection) requiring aortic valve replacement: analysis of four patients, *Am J Cardiol* 49:473, 1982.
137. Goldschlager N, Pfeifer J, Cohn K et al: The natural history of aortic regurgitation: a clinical and hemodynamic study, *Am J Med* 54:577, 1973.
138. Edwards JE: Pathology of aortic incompetence. In Silver MD, editor: *Cardiovascular pathology,* New York, 1991, Churchill Livingstone.
139. Benotti JR: Acute aortic insufficiency. In Dalen JE, Alpert JS, editors: *Valvular heart disease,* Boston, 1987, Little, Brown & Co.
140. Ockene IS: Tricuspid valve disease. In Dalen JE, Alpert JS, editors: *Valvular heart disease,* Boston, 1987, Little, Brown & Co.
141. Wooley CF, Fontana ME, Kilman JW et al: Tricuspid stenosis: atrial systolic murmur, tricuspid opening snap and right atrial pressure pulse, *Am J Med* 78:375, 1985.
142. Weyman AE, Rankin R, King H: Loeffler's endocarditis presenting as mitral and tricuspid stenosis, *Am J Cardiol* 40:438, 1977.
143. Enia F, Lo Mauro R, Meschisi F et al: Right-sided infective endocarditis with acquired tricuspid valve stenosis associated with transvenous pacemaker: a case report, *PACE (Pacing Clin Electrophysiol)* 14:1093, 1991.
144. Old WP, Paulsen W, Lewis SA et al: Pacemaker lead-induced tricuspid stenosis: diagnosis by Doppler echocardiography, *Am Heart J* 117:1165, 1989.
145. Lee M, Chaux A: Unusual complications of endocardial pacing, *J Thorac Cardiovasc Surg* 80:934, 1980.
146. Ridker PM, Chertow GM, Karlson EW et al: Bioprosthetic tricuspid valve stenosis associated with extensive plaque deposition in carcinoid heart disease, *Am Heart J* 121:1835, 1991.
147. Orbe LC, Sobrino N, Arcas R et al: Initial outcome of percutaneous balloon valvuloplasty in rheumatic tricuspid valve stenosis, *Am J Cardiol* 71:353, 1993.
148. Al Zaibag M, Ribeiro P, Al Kasab S: Percutaneous balloon valvotomy in tricuspid stenosis, *Br Heart J* 57:51, 1987.
149. Ribeiro PA, Al Zaibag M, Al Kasab S et al: Percutaneous double balloon valvotomy for rheumatic tricuspid stenosis, *Am J Cardiol* 61:660, 1988.
150. Shrivastava S, Radhakrishnan S, Vishva D: Concurrent balloon dilatation of tricuspid and calcific valve in a patient of rheumatic heart disease, *Int J Cardiol* 20:133, 1988.
151. Hirata K, Kyushima M, Asato H et al: Tricuspid regurgitation due to blunt chest trauma: report of a case and review of the literature, *Jpn Heart J* 34:361, 1993.
152. Johnson TL, Bauman WB, Josephson RA: Worsening tricuspid regurgitation following pericardiectomy for constrictive pericarditis, *Chest* 104:79, 1993.
153. Eways EA, Roberts WC: Clinical and anatomic observations in patients having mitral valve replacement for mitral stenosis and simultaneous tricuspid valve replacement, *Am J Cardiol* 68:1367, 1991.
154. Feng WC, Singh AK, Moran JM: Tricuspid regurgitation with postinfarction ventricular septal defect, *Ann Thorac Surg* 49:659, 1990.
155. Seymour J, Emanuel R, Pattinson N: Acquired pulmonary stenosis, *Br Heart J* 30:776, 1968.
156. Kaplan S, Adolf RJ, Murphy DJ: Pulmonary valve stenosis. In Roberts WC, editor: *Adult congenital heart disease,* Philadelphia, 1987, FA Davis.
157. Grant SC, Scarffe JH, Levy RD et al: Failure of balloon dilatation of the pulmonary valve in carcinoid pulmonary stenosis, *Br Heart J* 67:450, 1992.
158. Mullins PA, Hall JA, Shapiro LM: Balloon dilatation of tricuspid stenosis caused by carcinoid heart disease, *Br Heart J* 63:249, 1990.
159. Cheng TO: Nonsurgical treatment of carcinoid heart disease, *Ann Thorac Surg* 51:1046, 1991.
160. Runco V, Levin HS: The spectrum of pulmonic regurgitation, *Am Heart Assoc Monogr* 46:175, 1975.
161. Childers RS, McCrea PC: Absence of the pulmonary valve: a case occurring in Marfan's syndrome, *Circulation* 29:598, 1964.
162. Chandraratna PA, Wilson D, Imaizumi T et al: Invasive and noninvasive assessment of pulmonic regurgitation: clinical, angiographic, phonocardiographic, echocardiographic, and Doppler ultrasound correlations, *Clin Cardiol* 5:360, 1982.
163. Cassling RS, Rogler WC, McManus BM: Isolated pulmonic valve infective endocarditis: a diagnostically elusive entity, *Am Heart J* 109:558, 1985.
164. Cremieux AC, Witchitz S, Malergue MC et al: Clinical and echocardiographic observations in pulmonary valve endocarditis, *Am J Cardiol* 56:610, 1985.
165. DePace NL, Nestico PF, Iskandrian AS et al: Acute severe pulmonic valve regurgitation: pathophysiology, diagnosis, and treatment, *Am Heart J* 108:567, 1984.
166. Kirshenbaum HD: Pulmonic valve disease. In Dalen JE, Alpert JS, editors: *Valvular heart disease,* Boston, 1987, Little, Brown & Co.
167. Jacoby WJ, Tucker DH, Sumner RG: The second heart sound in congenital pulmonary valvular insufficiency, *Am Heart J* 69:603, 1965.
168. Ansari A: Isolated pulmonary valvular regurgitation: current perspectives, *Prog Cardiovasc Dis* 33:329, 1991.
169. Harvey WP: Auscultatory features. In Roberts WC, editor: *Adult congenital heart disease,* Philadelphia, 1987, FA Davis.
170. Gross L: Cardiac lesions in Libman-Sacks disease, with consideration of its relationship to acute diffuse erythematosus, *Am J Pathol* 16:375, 1940.
171. Humphreys EM: Cardiac lesions of the acute disseminated lupus erythematosus, *Ann Intern Med* 28:12, 1948.
172. Allen AC, Sirota JH: Morphogenesis and significance of degenerative verrucal endocardiosis (terminal endocarditis, endocarditis simplex, nonbacterial thrombotic endocarditis), *Am J Pathol* 20:1025, 1944.
173. Gross L, Griedberg CR: Nonbacterial thrombotic endocarditis: classification and general description, *Arch Intern Med* 58:620, 1936.
174. McKay DG: *Disseminated intravascular coagulation,* New York, 1965, Harper & Row.
175. Angrist AA, Marquiss J: Changing morphologic picture of endocarditis since advent of chemotherapy and antibiotic agents, *Am J Pathol* 30:39, 1954.
176. Kerr A Jr: *Subacute bacterial endocarditis,* Springfield, Ill, 1955, Charles C Thomas.
177. McManus BM, Rogler WC, Rogers JG et al: Spontaneously healing infective endocarditis: an unrecognized phenomena? *Eur Heart J* 8(supp J): 327, 1987.
178. Hayward GW: Infective endocarditis: A changing disease, *Br Med J* 2:706, 1973.
179. Lerner PI, Weinstein L: Infective endocarditis in the antiobiotic era, *N Engl J Med* 274:199, 1966.
180. Pankey GA: Acute bacterial endocarditis at the University of Minnesota Hospitals, *Am Heart J* 64:583, 1962.
181. Chase RM Jr: Infective endocarditis today, *Med Clin North Am* 57:1383, 1973.
182. Morgan WL, Bland EF: Bacterial endocarditis in the antibiotic era: with special reference to the later complications, *Circulation* 19:753, 1959.
183. Pankey GA: Subacute bacterial endocarditis at the University of Minnesota Hospital, 1939 through 1959, *Ann Intern Med* 55:550, 1961.
184. Glaser RJ, Rifkind D: The diagnosis and treatment of bacterial endocarditis, *Med Clin North Am* 47:1285, 1963.
185. Braimbridge MV: Cardiac surgery and bacterial endocarditis, *Lancet* 1:1307, 1969.
186. Madison J, Wang K, Gobel FL et al: Prosthetic aortic valvular endocarditis, *Circulation* 51:940, 1975.
187. Weinstein L: "Modern" infective endocarditis, *JAMA* 233:260, 1975.
188. McManus BM: Patent ductus arteriosus in adults. In: Roberts WC, editor: Adult *congenital heart disease,* Philadelphia, 1987, FA Davis.

189. Roberts WC, Arnett E: Active infective endocarditis: a clinicopathologic analysis of 137 necropsy patients, *Curr Probl Cardiol* 1:2, 1976.
190. Angrist AA, Oka M: Pathogenesis of bacterial endocarditis, *JAMA* 183:249, 1963.
191. Saphir O: Nonrheumatic inflammatory diseases of the heart. In *Pathology of the heart*, Springfield, Ill, 1960, Charles C Thomas.
192. Keefer CS: Subacute bacterial endocarditis: Active cases without bacteremia, *Ann Intern Med* 11:714, 1937.
193. Sheldon WH, Golden A: Abscesses of valve rings of heart, frequent but not well recognized complication of acute bacterial endocarditis, *Circulation* 4:1, 1951.
194. McManus BM, Katz MF, Blackbourne BD et al: Acquired cor triatriatum (left ventricular false aneurysm): A complication of active infective endocarditis of the aortic valve with ring abscess treated by valve replacement, *Am Heart J* 104:312, 1982.
195. Sobczyk WL, Johes JW, McManus BM: Clinically occult "false-on-true" left ventricular aneurysm: Association with late sudden death following mitral valve replacement, *Am Heart J* 112:1090, 1986.
196. Allen AC: *The Kidney*, New York, 1962, Grune and Stratton.
197. Friedberg CK, Goldman HM, Field LE: Study of bacterial endocarditis, *Arch Intern Med* 107:6, 1961.
198. Uwaydah MM, Weinberg AN: Bacterial endocarditis - a changing pattern, *N Engl J Med* 273:1231, 1965.
199. Robinson MJ, Greenberg JJ, Korn M et al: Infective endocarditis at autopsy, *Am J Med* 52:492, 1972.
200. Cornell A, Shookhoff HB: Actinomyocosis of heart simulating rheumatic fever: Report of 3 cases of cardiac actinomycosis with review of literature, *Arch Intern Med* 74:11, 1944.
201. Soler-Bechara J, Soscia JL, Kennedy RJ et al: *Candida* endocarditis, *Am J Cardiol* 13:820, 1964.
202. Merchant RK et al: Fungal endocarditis: review of the literature and report of three cases, *Ann Intern Med* 48:242, 1958.
203. Bainbridge MV: Cardiac surgery and bacterial endocarditis, *Lancet* 1:1307, 1969.
204. Pearce JM: Heart disease and filterable viruses, *Circulation* 21:448, 1960.
205. Burch GE, De Pasquale NP: Viral endocarditis, *Am Heart J* 67:721, 1964.
206. Grist NR: Rickettsial endocarditis, *Br Med J* 53:8, 1963.

Myocardial diseases

207. Vandiviere HM: Pulmonary hypertension and cor pulmonale, *South Med J* 86(10):2S7, 1993.
208. Sherman S: Cor pulmonale: treatment implications of right versus left ventricular impairment, *Postgrad Med* 91:227, 1992.
209. Pringle SD, Dunn FG, Macfarlane PW et al: Significance of ventricular arrhythmias in systemic hypertension with left ventricular hypertrophy, *Am J Cardiol* 69:913, 1992.
210. Houghton JL, Carr AA, Prisant LM et al: Morphologic, hemodynamic and coronary perfusion characteristics in severe left ventricular hypertrophy secondary to systemic hypertension and evidence for nonatherosclerotic myocardial ischemia, *Am J Cardiol* 69:219, 1992.
211. Lewis JF, Maron BJ: Diversity of patterns of hypertrophy in patients with systemic hypertension and marked left ventricular wall thickening, *Am J Cardiol* 65:874, 1990.
212. Isner JM, Chokshi SK: Cardiovascular complications of cocaine, *Curr Probl Cardiol* 16:89, 1991.
213. Mross K: New anthracycline derivatives: What for? *Eur J Cancer* 27:1542, 1991.
214. Fu LX, Waagstein F, Hjalmarson A: A new insight into adriamycin-induced cardiotoxicity, *Int J Cardiol* 29:15, 1990.
215. Rosenthal DS, Braunwald E: Hematological oncological disorders and heart disease. In Braunwald E, editor: *Heart disease: a textbook of cardiovascular medicine*, Philadelphia, 1988, Saunders.
216. Horowitz JD: Drugs that induce heart problems. Which agents? What effects? *J Cardiovasc Med* 8:308, 1983.
217. Rowan RA, Masek MA, Billingham ME: Ultrastructural morphometric analysis of endomyocardial biopsies: idiopathic dilated cardiomyopathy, anthracycline cardiotoxicity, and normal myocardium, *Am J Cardiovasc Pathol* 2:137, 1988.
218. Buja LM, Ferrans VJ, Mayer RJ et al: Cardiac ultrastructural changes induced by daunorubicin therapy, *Cancer* 32:771, 1973.
219. Stewart JR, Fajardo LF: Radiation-induced heart disease: an update, *Prog Cardiovasc Dis* 27:173, 1984.
220. Arsenian MA: Cardiovascular sequelae of therapeutic thoracic radiation, *Prog Cardiovasc Dis* 33:299, 1991.
221. Fajardo LF, Stewart JR: Pathogenesis of radiation-induced myocardial fibrosis, *Lab Invest* 29:244, 1973.
222. Fajardo LF, Stewart JR: Experimental radiation-induced heart disease. I. Light microscopic studies, *Am J Pathol* 59:299, 1970.
223. Stewart JR, Fajardo LF, Cohn KE: Experimental radiation-induced heart disease in rabbits, *Radiology* 91:814, 1968.
224. Fajardo LF: Radiation-induced coronary artery disease, *Chest* 71:563, 1977.
225. Applefield MM, Wiernik PH: Cardiac disease after radiation therapy for Hodgkin's disease: analysis of 48 patients, *Am J Cardiol* 51:1679, 1983.
226. Stewart JR, Fajardo LF: Dose response in human and experimental radiation-induced heart disease, *Radiology* 99:403, 1971.
227. Byhardt R, Brace K, Ruckdeschel J et al: Dose and treatment factors in radiation related pericardial effusion associated with the mantle technique for Hodgkin's disease, *Cancer* 75:795, 1975.
228. Martin RG, Ruckdeschel JC, Chang P et al: Radiation-related pericarditis, *Am J Cardiol* 35:216, 1975.
229. Ruckdeschel JC, Chang P, Martin RG et al: Radiation-related pericardial effusions in patients with Hodgkin's disease, *Medicine* 54:245, 1975.
230. Karas JS, Stanbury JB: Fatal radiation syndrome from an accidental nuclear excursion, *N Engl J Med* 272:755, 1965.
231. Fanger H, Lushbaugh CC: Radiation death from cardiovascular shock following a criticality accident, *Arch Pathol* 83:446, 1987.
232. Lushbaugh CC: Gross and microscopic pathology and neuropathology in acute radiation death resulting from an accidental nuclear critical excursion, *J Occup Med* 3:160, 1961.
233. Cohn KE, Stewart JR, Fajardo LF et al: Heart disease following radiation, *Medicine* 46:281, 1967.
234. Bradley EW, Zook BC, Casarett GW et al: Coronary arteriosclerosis and atherosclerosis in fast neutron or photon irradiated dogs, *Int J Radiat Oncol Biol Phys* 7:1103, 1981.
235. Fleming WH, Szakacs TE, King ER: The effects of gamma radiation on the fibrinolytic system of the dog lung and its modification by certain drugs: relationship to radiation pneumonitis and hyaline membrane formation in the lung, *J Nucl Med* 3:34, 1962.
236. Fajardo LF, Stewart JR, Cohn KE: Morphology of radiation-induced heart disease, *Arch Pathol* 86:512, 1968.
237. Hurst DW: Radiation fibrosis of pericardium with cardiac tamponade, *Can Med Assoc J* 81:377, 1959.
238. Haust MD, Rowlands DT Jr, Garancis JC et al: Histochemical studies on cardiac "colloid," *Am J Pathol* 40:185, 1962.
239. Roy PE: Basophilic degeneration of myocardium, *Lab Invest* 32:729, 1975.
240. Koske JC, Angell W: Fine structure of basophilic myocardial degeneration, *Arch Pathol* 89:491, 1970.
241. Rosai J, Lascano EF: Basophilic (mucoid) degeneration of myocardium, *Am J Pathol* 61:99, 1970.
242. Manion WC: Basophilic mucoid degeneration of the heart, *Med Ann DC* 34:60, 1965.
243. Glenner GG: Amyloid deposits and amyloidosis: I. The fibrilloses, *N Engl J Med* 302:1283, 1980.
244. Glenner GG: Amyloid deposits and amyloidosis: II. The fibrilloses, *N Engl J Med* 302:1333, 1980.
245. Ganeval D, Noel LH, Homme JLP: Light-chain deposition disease: its relation with AL-type amyloidosis, *Kidney Int* 26:1, 1984.
246. Gertz MA, Kyle RA, Edwards WD: Recognition of congestive heart failure due to senile cardiac amyloidosis, *Biomed Pharmacother* 43:101, 1989.
247. Cohen AS: Amyloidosis, *N Engl J Med* 277:522, 1967.
248. Dembinski AS, Dobson JR, Wilson JE et al: Frequency, extent, and distribution of endomyocardial adipose tissue: morphometric analysis of

endomyocardial biopsy specimens from 241 patients, *Cardiovasc Pathol* 3:33, 1994.

249. Meckel CR, Wilson JE, Sears TD et al: Myocardial fibrosis in endomyocardial biospy specimens: Do different bioptomes affect estimation? *Am J Cardiol* 2:309, 1989.
250. Scott JM: Fatty change in the myocardium of newborn infants, *Am Heart J* 64:283, 1962.
251. Dible JH: Is fatty degeneration of heart muscle a phanerosis? *J Pathol Bacteriol* 39:197, 1934.
252. Batsakis JG: Degenerative lesions of the heart. In Gould SE, editor: *Pathology of the heart and blood vessels,* ed 3, Springfield, Ill., 1968, Charles C Thomas.
253. Ross CF, Belton EM: A case of isolated cardiac lipidosis, *Br Heart J* 30:726, 1968.
254. Dawson IMP: Histology and histochemistry of gargoylism, *J Pathol Bacteriol* 67:587, 1954.
255. Strauss L: The pathology of gargoylism: report of case and review of the literature, *Am J Pathol* 24:855, 1948.
256. di Sant'Agnese PA: Diseases of glycogen storage with special reference to the cardiac type of generalized glycogenosis, *Ann N Y Acad Sci* 72:439, 1959.
257. Greene GM, Weldon DC, Cheatham FP et al: Juvenile polysaccharidosis with cardioskeletal myopathy, *Arch Pathol Lab Med* 111:977, 1987.
258. Radio SJ, Suvalsky SD, Hofschire PJ et al: Rapid calcification of the bovine pericardial valve in adolescence: critical aortic stenosis, hemolytic anemia, and quantitative renal hemosiderosis, *Arch Pathol Lab Med* 109:1118, 1985.
259. Levin EB, Golum A: Heart in hemochromatosis, *Am Heart J* 45:277, 1953.
260. Vigorito VJ, Hutchins GM: Cardiac conduction system in hemochromatosis, *Am J Cardiol* 44:418, 1979.
261. Bertrand E: Les cardiomyopathies en région tropicale, *Ann Cardiol Angeiol* 35:305, 1986 (with English abstract).
262. Abel RM, Fischer JE, Buckley MJ et al: Malnutrition in cardiac patients: results of a prospective, randomized evaluation of early postoperative total parenteral nutrition (TPN), *Acta Chir Scand* 466:77, 1976.
263. Benchimol AB, Schlesinger P: Beriberi heart disease, *Am Heart J* 46:245, 1953.
264. Blankenhorn MA, Vilter CF, Scheinker IM, Austin RS: Occidental beriberi heart disease, *JAMA* 131:717, 1946.
265. Follis RH Jr: Sudden death in infants with scurvy, *J Pediatr* 20:347, 1942.
266. Diplock AT: Metabolic and functional defects in selenium deficiency, *Philos Trans R Soc Lond* 294:105, 1981.
267. Brown RS: Potassium homeostasis and clinical implications, *Am J Med* 77:3, 1984.
268. Sander GE, Thomas MG, Giles TD: Endocrine diseases associated with cardiomyopathy. In Giles TD, Sander GE, editors: *Cardiomyopathy,* Littleton, Mass., 1988, PSG Publishing.
269. Kurtzman RS, Otto D, Chepey JJ: Myxedema heart disease, *Radiology* 84:624, 1965.
270. Hardisty CA, Naik DR, Munro DS: Pericardial infusions in hypothyroidism, *Clin Endocrinol* 13:349, 1980.
271. Steinberg AD: Myxedema and coronary artery disease—a comparative autopsy study, *Ann Intern Med* 68:338, 1968.
272. Vanhaelst L, Neve P, Chailly P et al: Coronary-artery disease in hypothyroidism: observations in clinical myxoedema, *Lancet* 2:800, 1967.
273. Aber CP, Thompson GS: Factors associated with cardiac enlargement in myxoedema, *Br Heart J* 25:421, 1963.
274. Zimmerman D, Gan-Gaisano M: Hyperthyroidism in children and adolescents, *Pediatr Clin North Am* 37:1273, 1990.
275. Christy JH, Clements SD Jr: The heart and endocrine disease. In Hurst JW, editor: *The heart,* New York, 1982, McGraw-Hill.
276. Callas G, Hayes Jr: Alterations in the fine structure of cardiac muscle mitochondria induced by hyperthyroidism, *Anat Rec* 178:539, 1974.
277. Levey GS, Klein I: Catecholamine-thyroid hormone interactions and the cardiovascular manifestations of hyperthyroidism, *Am J Med* 88:642, 1990.
278. Skelton CL: The heart and hyperthyroidism, *N Engl J Med* 307:1206, 1982.
279. Molitch ME: Clinical manifestations of acromegaly, *Endocrinol Metab Clin North Am* 21:597, 1992.
280. Wright AD, Hill DM, Lowy C et al: Mortality in acromegaly, *Q J Med* 39:1, 1970.
281. deGroot WJ: Acromegaly associated with endocrine disorders, *Cardiovasc Clin* 4:319, 1972.
282. Williams GH, Braunwald E: Endocrine and nutritional disorders and heart disease. In Braunwald E, editor: *Heart disease: a textbook of cardiovascular medicine,* Philadelphia, 1988, Saunders.
283. Lie JT: Pathology of the heart in acromegaly: anatomic findings in 27 autopsied patients, *Am Heart J* 100:41, 1980.
284. Hradec J, Marek J, Kral J et al: Heart in pituitary diseases, *Cor Vasa* 34:101, 1992.
285. Jonas EA, Aloia JF, Lane FJ: Evidence of subclinical heart muscle dysfunction in acromegaly, *Chest* 67:190, 1975.
286. Pepine CJ, Alcia J: Heart muscle disease in acromegaly, *Am J Med* 48:530, 1970.
287. Goldsmith RE: Polyendocrine syndromes and the heart, *Primary Cardiol* 7:153, 1981.
288. Manger WM, Gifford RWJ: *Pheochromocytoma,* New York, 1977, Springer-Verlag.
289. Imperato-McGinley J, Gautier T, Ehlers K et al: Reversibility of catecholamine-induced dilated cardiomyopathy in a child with a pheochromocytoma, *N Engl J Med* 316:793, 1987.
290. Rona G: Catecholamine cardiotoxicity, *J Mol Cell Cardiol* 17:291, 1985.
291. Grahame-Smith DG: *The carcinoid syndrome,* London, 1972, William Heineman Medical Books.
292. Oei SG, Kloosterman MD, Verhoeven AT: Primary ovarian carcinoid tumor in combination with carcinoid heart disease: a case report, *Eur J Obstet Gynecol Reprod Biol* 31:185, 1989.
293. Wynne J, Braunwald E: The cardiomyopathies and myocarditides. In Braunwald E, editor: *Heart disease: a textbook of cardiovascular medicine,* Philadelphia, 1988, Saunders.
294. Clarke B, Hodgson HJ: Carcinoid syndrome: medical management, *Br J Hosp Med* 35:146, 1986.
295. Teare D: Hypertrophy of the heart in young adults, *Br Heart J* 20:1, 1958.
296. Maron BJ: Hypertrophic cardiomyopathy, *Curr Probl Cardiol* 18:639, 1993.
297. Seidman CE, Seidman JG: Mutations in cardiac myosin heavy chain genes cause familial hypertrophic cardiomyopathy, *Mol Biol Med* 8:159, 1991.
298. Marian AJ, Roberts R: Molecular basis of hypertrophic and dilated cardiomyopathy, *Texas Heart Inst J* 21:6, 1994.
299. Thierfelder L, Watkins H, MacRae C et al: Alpha-tropomyosin and cardiac troponin T mutations cause familial hypertrophic cardiomyopathy: a disease of the sarcomere, *Cell* 77:701, 1994.
300. Fontaine G et al: Stimulation studies and epicardial mapping in ventricular tachycardia: study of mechanisms and selection for surgery. In Kulbertus HE, editor: *Re-entrant arrhythmias,* Lancaster, Engl., 1977, MTP Press.
301. Fontaine G, Frank R, Tonet JL et al: Arrhythmogenic right ventricular dysplasia: a clinical model for the study of chronic ventricular tachycardia, *Jpn Circ J* (Eng) 48:515, 1984.
302. Manyari DE, Klein GJ, Gulamhusein S et al: Arrhythmogenic right ventricular dysplasia: a generalized cardiomyopathy, *Circulation* 68:251, 1983.
303. Webb JG, Kerr CR, Huckell VF et al: Left ventricular abnormalities in arrhythmogenic right ventricular dysplasia, *Am J Cardiol* 58:568, 1986.
304. Marcus FI, Fontaine GH, Guiraudon G et al: Right ventricular dysplasia: a report of 24 adult cases, *Circulation* 65:384, 1982.
305. Guiraudon GM, Klein GJ, Gulamhusein SS et al: Total disconnection of the right ventricular free wall: surgical treatment of right ventricular tachycardia associated with right ventricular dysplasia, *Circulation* 67:463, 1983.
306. Grigg LE, Vohra JK, Chan W et al: Arrhythmogenic right ventricular dysplasia: clinical, electrophysiological, and pathological features, *Aust NZ J Med* 15:634, 1985.
307. Gaffney FA, Nicod P, Lin JC et al: Noninvasive recognition of the parchment right ventricle (Uhl's anomaly arrhythmogenic right ventricular dysplasia) syndrome, *Clin Cardiol* 6:235, 1983.

308. Dungan WT, Garson A Jr, Gillette PC: Arrhythmogenic right ventricular dysplasia: a cause of ventricular tachycardia in children with apparently normal hearts, *Am Heart J* 102:745, 1981.
309. Waynberger M, Coutadon M, Peltier JM et al: Tachycardies ventriculaires familiales. A propos de 7 observations, *Nouv Presse Med* 3:1857, 1974.
310. Ruder MA, Winston SA, Davis JC et al: Arrhythmogenic right ventricular dysplasia in a family, *Am J Cardiol* 56:799, 1985.
311. Lundquist CB, Eneström S, Edvardsson N et al: Arrhythmogenic right ventricular dysplasia presenting with ventricular tachycardia in a father and son, *Clin Cardiol* 10:277, 1987.
312. Laurent M, Descaves C, Biron Y et al: Familial form of arrhythmogenic right ventricular dysplasia, *Am Heart J* 113:827, 1987.
313. Nava A, Scognamiglio R, Thiene G et al: A polymorphic form of familial arrhythmogenic right ventricular dysplasia, *Am J Cardiol* 59:1405, 1987.
314. Rossi P, Massumi A, Gillette P et al: Arrhythmogenic right ventricular dysplasia: clinical features, diagnostic techniques, and current management, *Am Heart J* 103:415, 1982.
315. Ino T, Benson LN, Freedom RM et al: Natural history and prognostic risk factors in endocardial fibroelastosis, *Am J Cardiol* 62:431, 1988.
316. Keith JD, Rose V, Manning JA: Endocardial fibroelastosis. In Keith JD et al, editors: ed 3, *Heart disease in infancy and childhood,* New York, 1978, MacMillan.
317. Rowe RD, Benson LN, Wilson G et al: Clinical diagnosis of left ventricular endocardial fibroelastosis of the dilated type: the Keith criteria and tissue confirmation, *Pediatr Cardiol* 8:231, 1987.
318. Griffin ML, Hernandez A, Martin TC et al: Dilated cardiomyopathy in infants and children, *J Am Coll Cardiol* 11:139, 1988.
319. Fishbein MC, Ferrans VJ, Roberts WC: Histologic and ultrastructural features of primary and secondary endocardial fibroelastosis, *Arch Pathol Lab Med* 101:49, 1977.
320. Lewis AB, Neustein HB, Takahashi M et al: Findings on endomyocardial biopsy in infants and children, *Am J Cardiol* 55:143, 1985.
321. Loeffler W: Endocarditis parietalis fibroplastica mit Bluteosinophilie, ein eigenartiges Krankheitsbild, *Schweiz Med Wochenschr* 17:817, 1936.
322. Kasper EK, Agema WRP, Hutchins GM et al: The causes of dilated cardiomyopathy: a clinicopathological review of 673 consecutive patients, *J Am Coll Cardiol* 23:586, 1994.
323. Aretz HT, Billingham ME, Edwards WD et al: Myocarditis: a histopathological definition and classification, *Am J Cardiovasc Pathol* 1:3, 1987.
324. Chow LH, Ye YL, Linder J et al: Phenotypic analysis of infiltrating cells in human myocarditis, *Arch Pathol Lab Med* 13:1357, 1989.
325. Tazelaar HD, Billingham MB: Leukocytic infiltrates in idiopathic dilated cardiomyopathy: a source of confusion with active myocarditis, *Am J Surg Pathol* 10:405, 1986.
326. Grist NR, Reid D: Epidemiology of viral infections of the heart. In Banatrala JE, editor: *Viral infections of the heart,* Boston, 1993, Little, Brown & Co.
327. McManus BM, Kandolf R: Myocarditis: evolving concepts of cause, consequence, and control, *Curr Opin Cardiol* 6:418, 1991.
328. McManus BM, Chow LH, Wilson JE et al: Direct myocardial injury by enterovirus: a central role in the evolution of murine myocarditis, *Clin Immunol Immunopathol* 68:159, 1993.
329. Billingham ME, Cary NR, Hammond ME et al: A working formulation for the standardization of nomenclature in the diagnosis of heart and lung rejection: Heart Rejection Study Group, The International Society for Heart Transplantation, *J Heart Lung Transplant* 9:587, 1990.
330. Billingham ME: Diagnosis of cardiac rejection by endomyocardial biopsy, *J Heart Transplant* 1:25, 1982.
331. Bell G, Lones M, Czer LSC et al: Grade 2 cellular cardiac rejection: Does it exist? [Abstract], *Lab Invest* 70:26A, 1994.
332. Swinnen LJ, Costanzo-Nordin MR, Fisher SG et al: Increased incidence of lymphoproliferative disorder after immunosuppression with the monoclonal antibody OKT3 in cardiac transplant recipients, *N Engl J Med* 323:1723, 1990.
333. Weber T, Kaufman C, Zeevi A et al: Lymphocyte growth from cardiac allograft biopsy specimens with no or minimal cellular infiltrates: association with subsequent rejection episode, *J Heart Transplant* 8:233, 1989.
334. Herskowitz A, Soule LM, Ueda K et al: Arteriolar vasculitis on endomyocardial biopsy: a histologic predictor of poor outcome in cyclosporine-treated heart transplant recipients, *J Heart Transplant* 6:127, 1987.
335. Koskinen PK, Nieminen MS, Krogerus LA et al: Cytomegalovirus infection and accelerated cardiac allograft vasculopathy in human cardiac allografts, *J Heart Lung Transplant* 12:724, 1993.
336. Koskinen PK, Krogerus LA, Nieminen MS et al: Quantitation of cytomegalovirus infection-associated histologic findings in endomyocardial biopsies of heart allografts, *J Heart Lung Transplant* 12:343, 1993.
337. Keogh AM, Valantine HA, Hunt SA et al: Impact of proximal or midvessel discrete coronary artery stenoses on survival after heart transplantation, *J Heart Lung Transplant* 11:892, 1992.
338. Alderman EL, Wexler L: Angiographic implications of cardiac transplantation, *Am J Cardiol* 64:16E, 1989.
339. Waller BF, Gering LE, Branyas NA et al: Anatomy, histology, and pathology of the cardiac conduction system: Part II, *Clin Cardiol* 16:347, 1993.
340. Waller BF, Gering LE, Branyas NA et al: Anatomy, histology, and pathology of the cardiac conduction system: Part VI, *Clin Cardiol* 16:623, 1993.
341. Waller BF, Gering LE, Branyas NA et al: Anatomy, histology, and pathology of the cardiac conduction system: Part IV, *Clin Cardiol* 16:507, 1993.
342. Thaemert JC: Fine structure of the artrioventricular node as viewed in serial sections, *Am J Anat* 136:43, 1973.
343. Thaemert JC: Atrioventricular node innervation in ultrastructural three dimensions, *Am J Anat* 128:239, 1970.
344. Mahaim I: Kent's fibers and the AV paraspecific conduction through the upper connections of the bundle of His—Tawara, *Am Heart J* 33:651, 1947.
345. Bharati S, Lev M: The pathologic changes in the conduction system beyond the age of ninety, *Am Heart J* 124:486, 1992.
346. Pomerance A: Age-related cardiovascular changes and mechanically induced endocardial pathology. In Silver MD, editor: *Cardiovascular pathology,* New York, 1991, Churchill Livingstone.
347. Alpman A, Guldal M, Erol C et al: The role of arrhythmia and left ventricular dysfunction in patients with acute myocardial infarction and bundle branch block, *Jpn Heart J* 34:145, 1993.
348. Schneider JF, Thomas E, Kreger BE et al: Newly acquired left bundle-branch block: the Framingham study, *Ann Intern Med* 90:303, 1979.
349. Marinchak RA, Friehling TD, Kowey PR: A clinician's approach to diagnosing supraventricular tachycardia, *J Crit Illness* 3:39, 1988.
350. Myerburg RJ, Conde C, Ships DS et al: Antiarrhythmic drug therapy in survivors of prehospital cardiac arrest: comparison of effects of chronic ventricular arrhythmias and recurrent cardiac arrest, *Circulation* 59:855, 1979.
351. Lo KS, Gantz KB, Stetson PL et al: Disopyramide-induced ventricular tachycardia, *Arch Intern Med* 140:413, 1980.
352. Silver MA: Morphologic substrates of ventricular arrhythmias, *Clin Prog Electrophys Pacing* 4:1, 1986.
353. Sugrue DD, Holmes DR, Gersh BJ et al: Cardiac histologic findings in patients with life-threatening ventricular arrhythmias of unknown origin, *J Am Coll Cardiol* 4:952, 1984.
354. Zehender M, Meinertz T, Keul J et al: ECG variants and cardiac arrhythmias in athletes: clinical relevance and prognostic importance, *Am Heart J* 119:1378, 1990.
355. Aoki T, Motoyasu M, Simizu Y et al: A case of dilated cardiomyopathy manifested by exercise-induced left bundle branch block, *Jpn Circ J* 57:573, 1993.
356. Maron BJ, Fananapazir L: Sudden cardiac death in hypertrophic cardiomyopathy, *Circulation* 85(suppl I):157, 1992.
357. Silver MM, Silver MD: Cardiomyopathies. In Silver MD, editor: *Cardiovascular pathology,* New York, 1991, Churchill Livingstone.
358. Lie JT: Sudden death from diseases of the cardiovascular system. In Silver MD, editor: *Cardiovascular pathology,* New York, 1991, Churchill Livingstone.
359. Sabel KG, Blomström-Lundqvist C, Olsson B et al: Arrhythmogenic right ventricular dysplasia in brother and sister: Is it related to myocarditis? *Pediatr Cardiol* 11:113, 1990.
360. Hurwitz J, Josephson ME: Sudden cardiac death in patients with chronic coronary heart disease, *Circulation* 85(suppl I):143, 1992.

361. Matoba R, Shikata I, Iwai K et al: An epidemiologic and histopathological study of sudden cardiac death in Osaka medical examiner's office, *Jpn Circ J* 53:1581, 1989.
362. Woo KS: Bradytachyarrhythmia as the first manifestation of acute rheumatic carditis in an adult, *West J Med* 156:413, 1992.
363. Inoue S, Shinohara F, Sakai T et al: Myocarditis and arrhythmia: a clinicopathological study of conduction system based on serial section in 65 cases, *Jpn Circ J* 53:49, 1989.
364. De Koning J, Hoogkamp-Korstanje JAA, van der Linde MR et al: Demonstration of spirochetes in cardiac biopsies of patients with lyme disease, *J Infect Dis* 160:150, 1989.
365. Foerster A: The conduction system in human cardiac allografts: a histological and immunopathological study, *Pathol Res Pract* 188:783, 1992.
366. Bharati S, Billingham M, Lev M: The conduction system in transplanted hearts, *Chest* 102:1182, 1992.
367. Bharati S, Engle MA, Fatica NS et al: The heart and conduction system in acute Kawasaki disease: report of fraternal cases—one lethal, one relapsing, *Am Heart J* 120:359, 1990.
368. Moss J: Clinical significance of ventricular arrhythmias in patients with and without coronary artery disease, *Prog Cardiovasc Dis* 23:33, 1980.
369. Okabe M, Fukuda K, Nakashima Y et al: Pathological extent of interventricular septal infarction in patients with acute anteroseptal myocardial infarction with and without right bundle branch block, *Jpn Heart J* 34:121, 1993.
370. Kyriakidis M, Barbetseas J, Antonopoulos A et al: Early atrial arrhythmias in acute myocardial infarction, *Chest* 101:944, 1992.
371. James TN, Riddick L: Sudden death due to isolated acute infarction of the his bundle, *J Am Coll Cardiol* 15:1183, 1990.
372. Kasanuki H, Ohnishi S, Tanaka E et al: Mechanism and prediction of sudden cardiac death in arrhythmia patients using electrophysiological studies, *Jpn Circ J* 53:1565, 1989.
373. Archie Lo YS, Billingham M, Rowan RA et al: Histopathologic and electrophysiologic correlation in idiopathic dilated cardiomyopathy and sustained ventricular tachyarrhythmia, *Am J Cardiol* 64:1063, 1989.
374. Fragola PV, Autore C, Magni G et al: Limitations of the electrocardiographic diagnosis of left ventricular hypertrophy: the influence of left anterior hemiblock and right bundle branch block, *Int J Cardiol* 34:41, 1992.
375. Brugada P, Brugada J: Right bundle branch block, persistent ST segment elevation and sudden cardiac death: a distinct clinical and electrocardiographic syndrome, *J Am Coll Cardiol* 20:1391, 1992.
376. Wilson GJ: The pathology of cardiac pacing. In Silver MD, editor: *Cardiovascular pathology,* New York, 1991, Churchill Livingstone.
377. Colucci WS, Braunwald E: Primary tumors of the heart. In Braunwald E, editor: *Heart disease: a textbook of cardiovascular medicine,* Philadelphia, 1980, Saunders.
378. McAllister HA, Fenoglio JJ: *Tumors of the cardiovascular system,* Washington, DC, 1977, Armed Forces Institute of Pathology.
379. Nada AS, Ellison RC: Cardiac tumors in infancy, *Am J Cardiol* 21:363, 1968.
380. Fine G: *Neoplasms of the pericardium and heart,* Springfield Ill., 1968, Gould, SE.
381. Lam KYL, Dickens P, Chan ACL: Tumors of the heart, *Arch Pathol Lab Med* 117:1027, 1993.
382. Peters MN, Hall RJ, Cooley DA et al: The clinical syndrome of atrial myxoma, *JAMA* 230:694, 1974.
383. Allard MF, Taylor GP, Wilson JE et al: Primary tumors. In Braunwald E, Goldhaber SZ, editors: *Atlas of heart diseases,* Philadelphia, 1995, Current Medicine.
384. Krikler DM, Rode J, Davies MJ et al: Atrial myxoma: a tumor in search of its origins, *Br Heart J* 67:89, 1992.
385. Wada A, Kanda T, Hayashi R et al: Cardiac myxoma metastasized to the brain: potential role of endogenous interleukin-6, *Cardiology* 83:208, 1993.
386. Heath D: Pathology of cardiac tumors, *Am J Cardiol* 21:315, 1968.
387. Colucci WS, Braunwald E: Primary tumors of the heart. In Braunwald E, editor: *Heart disease: a textbook of cardiovascular medicine,* Philadelphia, 1992, Saunders.
388. Fine G: Neoplasms of the pericardium and heart. In Gould SE, editor: *Pathology of the heart and blood vessels,* Springfield, Ill., 1968, Charles C Thomas.
389. Chan HSL, Sonley MJ, Moës CAF et al: Primary and secondary tumors of childhood involving the heart, pericardium, and great vessels: a review of 75 cases and review of the literature, *Cancer* 56:825, 1985.
390. Goudie RB: Secondary tumors of the heart and pericardium, *Br Heart J* 17:183, 1955.
391. Malaret GE, Aliaga P: Metastatic diseases to the heart, *Cancer* 22:457, 1968.
392. Roberts WC, Glancy DL, DeVita VT: Heart in malignant lymphoma (Hodgkin's disease, lymphosarcoma, reticulum cell sarcoma and mycosis fugoides): a study of 196 autopsy cases, *Am J Cardiol* 22:85, 1968.
393. MacGee W: Metastatic and invasive tumors involving the heart in a geriatric population: a necropsy study, *Virchows Arch [A] (Pathol Anat Histopathol)* 419:183, 1991.
394. Lam KY, Dickens P, Chan ACL: Tumors of the heart: a 20 year experience with a review of 12485 consecutive autopsies, *Arch Pathol Lab Med* 117:1027, 1993.
395. Abraham K, Reddy V, Gattuso P: Neoplasms metastatic to the heart: a review of 3314 consecutive autopsies, *Am J Cardiovasc Pathol* 3:195, 1990.
396. Young JM, Goldman IR: Tumor metastasis to the heart, *Circulation* 9:220, 1954.
397. Prichard RW: Tumors of the heart: a review of the subjects and report of one hundred and fifty cases, *Arch Pathol* 51:98, 1951.
398. Scott RW, Garvin CF: Tumors of the heart and pericardium, *Am Heart J* 17:431, 1939.
399. Deloach JF, Haynes JW: Secondary tumors of the heart and pericardium: a review of the subject and report of 137 cases, *Arch Intern Med* 91:224, 1953.
400. Harrer WMV, Lewis PL: Metastatic tumors involving the heart and pericardium, *Penn Med* 74:57, 1971.
401. Couetil JP, McGoldrick JP, Wallwork J et al: Malignant tumors after heart transplantation, *J Heart Transplant* 9:622, 1990.
402. Penn I: Tumors after renal and cardiac transplantation, *Hematol Oncol Clin North Am* 7:431, 1993.
403. Nalesnik MA, Jaffe R, Starzl TE et al: The pathology of posttransplant lymphoproliferative disorders occurring in the setting of cyclosporine A–prednisone immunosuppression, *Am J Pathol* 133:173, 1988.
404. Armitage JM, Kormos RL, Stuart RS et al: Posttransplant lymphoproliferative disease in thoracic organ transplant patients: ten years of cyclosporine-based immunosuppression, *J Heart Lung Transplant* 10:877, 1991.
405. Flipse TR, Tazelaar HD, Holmes DR: Diagnosis of malignant cardiac disease by endomyocardial biopsy, *Mayo Clin Proc* 65:1415, 1990.
406. Franciosa JA, Lawrinson J: Coronary artery occlusion due to neoplasm: a rare cause of myocardial infarction, *Arch Intern Med* 128:797, 1971.
407. Ackerman DM, Hyma BA, Edwards WD: Malignant neoplastic emboli to the coronary arteries: a report of two cases and review of the literature, *Hum Pathol* 18:955, 1987.
408. Aylwin JA: Avoidable vascular spread in resection for bronchial carcinoma, *Thorax* 6:250, 1951.
409. Karlsberg RP, Sagel SS, Ferguson TB: Myocardial infarction due to tumor embolization following pulmonary resection, *Chest* 74:582, 1978.

Coronary artery diseases

410. Tejada C, Strong J, Montenegro M et al: Distribution of aortic and coronary atherosclerosis by geographic location, race and sex, *Lab Invest* 18:509, 1968.
411. PDAY Research Group: Relationship of atherosclerosis in young men to serum lipoprotein, cholesterol concentrations and smoking: a preliminary report from the Pathological Determinants of Atherosclerosis in Youth Study, *JAMA* 264:3018, 1990.
412. Glagov S, Weisenberd E, Zarins C et al: Compensatory enlargement of human atherosclerotic coronary arteries, *N Engl J Med* 316:1371, 1987.
413. Hangartner J, Charleston A, Davies M et al: Morphological characteristics of clinically significant coronary artery stenosis in stable angina, *Br Heart J* 56:501, 1986.

414. Roberts W: The coronary arteries and left ventricle in clinically isolated angina pectoris: a necropsy analysis, *Am J Med* 67:792, 1979.
415. Saner H, Gobel F, Salomonowitz E et al: The disease free wall in coronary atherosclerosis: its relation to degree of obstruction, *J Am Coll Cardiol* 6:1096, 1985.
416. Roberts W, Virmani R: Formation of new coronary arteries within a previously obstructed epicardial coronary artery (intra-arterial arteries): a mechanism for occurrence of angiographically normal coronary arteries after healing of acute myocardial infarction, *Am J Cardiol* 54:1361, 1984.
417. Levin D, Fallon J: Significance of the angiographic morphology of localized coronary stenosis: histopathologic correlations, *Circulation* 66:316, 1982.
418. Falk E: Unstable angina with fatal outcome: dynamic coronary thrombosis leading to infarction and/or sudden death, *Circulation* 66:316, 1985.
419. Davies M, Thomas A, Knapman P et al: Intramyocardial platelet aggregation in patients with unstable angina suffering sudden ischaemic cardiac death, *Circulation* 73:418, 1986.
420. Roberts W, Curry R, Isner J: Sudden death in Prinzmetal's angina with coronary spasm documented by arteriography: analysis of three necropsy cases, *Am J Cardiol* 50:203, 1982.
421. Kohchi K, Takebayashi S, Hiroki T et al: Significance of adventitial inflammation of the coronary artery in patients with unstable angina: results at autopsy, *Circulation* 71:709, 1985.
422. Forman M, Oates J, Robertson D: Increased adventitial mast cells in a patient with coronary spasm, *N Engl J Med* 313:1138, 1985.
423. Davies M, Thomas A: Plaque fissuring—the cause of acute myocardial infarction, sudden ischaemic death and crescendo angina, *Br Heart J* 53:363, 1985.
424. Falk E: Plaque rupture with severe pre-existing stenosis precipitating coronary thrombosis: characteristics of coronary atherosclerotic plaque underlying fatal occlusive thrombi, *Br Heart J* 50:127, 1983.
425. Horie T, Sekiguchi M, Hirosawa K: Coronary thrombosis in pathogenesis of acute myocardial infarction: histopathological study of coronary arteries in 108 necropsied cases using serial section, *Br Heart J* 40:153, 1978.
426. Fulton W: Pathological concepts in acute coronary thrombosis: relevance to treatment, *Br Heart J* 70:403, 1993.
427. Piek JJ, Becker AE: Collateral blood supply to the myocardium at risk in human myocardial infarction: a quantitative post mortem assessment, *J Am Coll Cardiol* 11:1290, 1988.
428. Stary H: Composition and classification of human atherosclerotic lesions, *Virchows Arch [A] (Pathol Anat Histopathol)* 421:277, 1992.
429. Faggiotto A, Ross R, Harker L: Studies of hypercholesterolaemia in the non-human primate. I. Changes that lead to fatty streak formation, *Arteriosclerosis* 4:323, 1984.
430. Faggiotto A, Ross R: Studies of hypercholesterolaemia in non-human primates. II. Fatty streak conversion to fibrous plaque, *Arteriosclerosis* 4:341, 1984.
431. Ross R: The pathogenesis of atherosclerosis—a perspective for the 1990's, *Nature* 362:801, 1993.
432. Witztum J: Role of oxidised low density lipoprotein in atherogenesis, *Br Heart J* 69:S12, 1993.
433. Ylä-Herttuala S, Palinski W, Rosenfeld M et al: Evidence for the presence of oxidatively modified low density lipoprotein in atherosclerotic lesions of rabbit and man, *J Clin Invest* 84:1086, 1989.
434. Naito M, Suzuki H, Mori T et al: Coexpression of type I and type II human macrophage scavenger receptors in macrophages of various organs and foam cells in atherosclerotic lesions, *Am J Pathol* 141:591, 1992.
435. Liao F, Berliner J, Mehrabian M: Minimally modified low density lipoprotein is biologically active in vivo, *J Clin Invest* 87:2253, 1991.
436. Bini A, Fenoglio J, Mesa-Tejada R et al: Identification and distribution of fibrinogen, fibrin and fibrin(ogen) degradation products in atherosclerosis: use of monoclonal antibodies, *Arteriosclerosis* 9:109, 1989.
437. Davies M, Woolf N, Rowles P et al: Morphology of the endothelium over atherosclerotic plaques in human coronary arteries, *Br Heart J* 60:459, 1988.
438. Davies M: A macroscopic and microscopic view of coronary thrombi, *Circulation* 82:1138, 1990.
439. Reimer K, Jennings R, Cobb F: Animal models for protecting myocardium: results of the NHLBI cooperative study, *Circ Res* 56:651, 1985.
440. Poole-Wilson P: Haemodynamic and metabolic consequences of angina and myocardial infarction. In Fox KM, editor: *Ischaemic heart disease*, Lancaster, Engl., 1987, MTP Press.
441. Jennings R, Reimer K: Lethal myocardial ischaemic injury, *Am J Pathol* 102:241, 1981.
442. Alonso D, Scheidr S, Post M et al: Pathophysiology of cardiogenic shock, quantifications of myocardial necrosis, clinical pathologic and electrocardiographic correlation, *Circulation* 48:588, 1973.
443. Pirolo S, Hutchins GM, Moore W: Infarct expansion: pathologic analysis of 204 patients with a single myocardial infarct, *J Am Coll Cardiol* 7:349, 1986.
444. Gaudron P, Eilles C, Kugler I et al: Progressive left ventricular dysfunction and remodelling after myocardial infarction, *Circulation* 87:755, 1993.
445. Becker AE, van Mantgem JP: Cardiac tamponade: a study of 50 hearts, *Eur J Cardiol* 3:349, 1975.
446. Atkinson J, Robinowitz M, McCallister H et al: Association of eosinophils with cardiac rupture, *Hum Pathol* 16:562, 1985.
447. Dellborg M, Held P, Swedberg K et al: Rupture of the myocardium: occurrence and risk factors, *Br Heart J* 54:11, 1985.
448. Mann JM, Roberts WC: Acquired ventricular septal defect during acute myocardial infarction: analysis of 38 unoperated necropsy patients and comparison with 50 unoperated necropsy patients without rupture, *Am J Cardiol* 62:8, 1988.
449. Nishimura RA, Schaff H, Shub C et al: Papillary muscle rupture complicating acute myocardial infarction: analysis of 17 patients, *Am J Cardiol* 51:373, 1983.
450. Barbour D, Roberts W: Rupture of a left ventricular papillary muscle during acute myocardial infarction, *J Am Coll Cardiol* 8:548, 1986.
451. Isner J, Roberts W: Right ventricular infarction complicating left ventricular infarction secondary to coronary artery disease: frequency, location, associated findings and significance from analysis of 236 necropsy patients with acute or healed myocardial infarction, *Am J Cardiol* 42:885, 1978.
452. Roberts W, Kaufman R: Calcification of healed myocardial infarcts, *Am J Cardiol* 60:28, 1987.
453. Visser C, Kan G Meltzer G, et al: Incidence, timing and prognostic value of left ventricular aneurysm formation after infarction, *Am J Cardiol* 57:729, 1986.
454. Van Tassel R, Edwards J: Rupture of the heart complicating myocardial infarction: analysis of 40 cases including nine examples of left ventricular false aneurysm, *Chest* 61:104, 1972.
455. Legrand V, Deliege M, Henrard L et al: Patients with myocardial infarction and normal coronary arteriogram, *Chest* 82:678, 1982.
456. Thompson R: Isolated coronary ostial stenosis in women, *J Am Coll Cardiol* 7:997, 1986.
457. Miller A, Honey M, El Sayed H: Isolated coronary stenosis, *Cathet Cardiovasc Diagn* 12:30, 1986.
458. Stewart J, Ward D, Davies M et al: Isolated coronary ostial stenosis: observations on the pathology, *Eur Heart J* 8:917, 1987.
459. Lipsett J, Byard RW, Carpenter BF et al: Anomalous coronary arteries arising from the aorta associated with sudden death in infancy and early childhood: an autopsy series, *Arch Pathol Lab Med* 115:770, 1991.
460. Taylor AJ, Rogan KM, Virmani R: Sudden cardiac death associated with isolated congenital coronary artery anomalies, *J Am Coll Cardiol* 20:640, 1992.
461. Mathieu D, Lardé D, Vasile N: Primary dissecting aneurysms of the coronary arteries: case report and literature review, *Cardiovasc Intervent Radiol* 7:71, 1984.
462. Corrado D, Thiene G, Cocco P et al: Non–atherosclerotic coronary artery disease and sudden death in the young, *Br Heart J* 68:601, 1992.
463. Ishall T, Hosoda Y, Osaka T, et al: The significance of myocardial bridge upon atherosclerosis in the left anterior descending coronary artery, *J Pathol* 148:279, 1986.
464. Daoud A, Pankin D, Tulgan H et al: Aneurysms of the coronary artery: report of 10 cases and review of the literature, *Am J Cardiol* 11:228, 1963.

465. Yanagawa H, Nakamura Y, Kawasaki T et al: Nationwide epidemic of Kawasaki disease in Japan during the winter of 1985-1986, *Lancet* 2:1138, 1986.
466. Kato H, Ichinose E, Yoshioka F et al: Fate of coronary aneurysms in Kawasaki disease, serial coronary angiography and long-term follow-up study, *Am J Cardiol* 49:1758, 1982.
467. Fujiwara H, Hamashima Y: Pathology of the heart in Kawasaki disease, *Pediatrics* 61:100, 1978.

Pericardial diseases

468. Van Son JA, Danielson GK, Schaff HV et al: Congenital partial and complete absence of the pericardium, *Mayo Clin Proc* 68:743, 1993.
469. Scully RE, Mark EJ, NcNelly WF et al: Case records of the Massachusetts General Hospital: weekly clinicopathological exercises, *N Engl J Med* 330:126, 1994.
470. Fowler NO: Tuberculous pericarditis, *JAMA* 266:99, 1991.
471. Horn DL, Hewlett D, Alfalla C et al: Fatal hospital-acquired multi-drug resistant tuberculous pericarditis in two patients with AIDS, *N Engl J Med* 327:1816, 1992.
472. Muir P, Nicholson F, Tilzey AJ et al: Chronic relapsing pericarditis and dilated cardiomyopathy: serological evidence of persistent entero–virus infection, *Lancet* 1:804, 1989.
473. Wilson J, Zaman AG, Simmons AV: Gonococcal arthritis complicated by acute pericarditis and pericardial effusion, *Br Heart J* 63:134, 1990.
474. Picardi J, Kauffman C, Schwarz J et al: Pericarditis caused by *Histoplasma capsulatum, Am J Cardiol* 37:82, 1976.
475. Hara KS, Ballard DJ, Ilstrup DM et al: Rheumatoid pericarditis: clinical features and survival, *Medicine* 69:81, 1990.
476. Kahl LE: The spectrum of pericardial tamponade in systemic lupus erythematosus, *Arthritis Rheum* 35:1343, 1992 (comment: *Arthritis Rheum* 36:1029, 1993).
477. Sever MS, Steinmuller DR, Hayes JM et al: Pericarditis following renal transplantation, *Transplantation* 51:1229, 1991.
478. Cimino J, Kogan A: Constrictive pericarditis after cardiac surgery: report of three cases and review of the literature, *Am Heart J* 118:1292, 1989.
479. Davies D, Andrews M, Jones J: Asbestos induced pericardial effusion and constrictive pericarditis, *Thorax* 46:429, 1991.
480. Wilding G, Green HL, Longo DL et al: Tumors of the heart and pericardium, *Cancer Treat Rev* 15:165, 1988.

Cardiogenic shock

481. Page DL, Caulfield JB, Kastor JA et al: Myocardial changes associated with cardiogenic shock, *N Engl J Med* 285:133, 1971.
482. Caulfield JB, Dunkman WB, Leinbach RC: Cardiogenic shock: myocardial changes associated with and without artificial left ventricular counterpulsation, *Arch Pathol* 93:532, 1972.
483. Weil MH, Von Plata M, Rackow EC: Acute circulatory failure (shock). In Braunwald E, editor: *Heart disease: a textbook of cardiovascular medicine,* Philadelphia, 1987, Saunders.
484. Roberts N, Harrison DG, Reimer KA et al: Right ventricular infarction with shock but without significant left ventricular infarction: a new clinical syndrome, *Am Heart J* 110:1047, 1985.
485. Alpert JS, Becker RC: Cardiogenic shock: elements of etiology, diagnosis, and therapy, *Clin Cardiol* 16:182, 1993.
486. McCall D, O'Rourke RA: Hypotension and cardiogenic shock. In Stein JH, editor: *Internal medicine,* Boston, 1990, Little, Brown & Co.
487. Alpert JS, Becker RC: Mechanisms and management of cardiogenic shock, *Crit Care Clin* 9:205, 1993.
488. Goldberg RJ, Gore JM, Alpert JS et al: Cardiogenic shock after acute myocardial infarction: incidence and mortality from a community-wide perspective, 1975 to 1988, *N Engl J Med* 325:1117, 1991.
489. Moosvi AR, Gheorghiade M, Goldstein S et al: Management of cardiogenic shock complicating acute myocardial infarction: the Henry Ford Hospital experience and review of the literature, *Henry Ford Hosp Med J* 39:240, 1991.
490. Teba L, Banks DE, Balaan MR: Understanding circulatory shock. Is it hypovolemic, cardiogenic, or vasogenic? *Postgrad Med* 91:121, 1992.
491. McGhie AI, Golstein RA: Pathogenesis and management of acute heart failure and cardiogenic shock: role of inotropic therapy, *Chest* 102:626S, 1992.
492. Goldenberg IF: Nonpharmacologic management of cardiac arrest and cardiogenic shock, *Chest* 102:596S, 1992.

46 Congenital Heart Disease

William D. Edwards

Abbreviations used in figures

Ao	Aorta	*PDA*	Patent ductal artery
ARV	Atrialized right ventricle	*PT*	Pulmonary trunk
CAVV	Common atrioventricular valve	*PVC*	Pulmonary venous confluence
ICV	Inferior caval vein	*RA*	Right atrium
IL	Inferior limb (of septal band)	*RCA*	Right coronary artery
LA	Left atrium	*RPA*	Right pulmonary artery
LBV	Left brachiocephalic vein	*RPV*	Right pulmonary vein
LPA	Left pulmonary artery	*RV*	Right ventricle
LPV	Left pulmonary vein	*RVOT*	Right ventricular outflow tract
LV	Left ventricle	*SB*	Septal band
LVOT	Left ventricular outflow tract	*SCV*	Superior caval vein
OF	Oval fossa (fossa ovalis)	*SL*	Superior limb (of septal band)
OS	Outlet (infundibular) septum	*TA*	Truncal artery
PB	Parietal band	*V*	Ventricle

BACKGROUND

Definition and demographics

Congenital heart disease encompasses disorders of the cardiovascular system that result from faulty embryogenesis and that are present at birth. Cardiomyopathies and storage diseases are not included. This chapter is necessarily limited in scope, and only the most commonly encountered anomalies are discussed. For additional information see the recent textbooks of pediatric cardiology and cardiac surgery.[1-5]

The incidence of congenital heart disease per 1000 live births is approximately 7.0 overall and 3.5 for anomalies requiring intervention in infancy. It is higher in premature babies than in full-term infants and is tenfold higher in stillbirths than live births. These figures do not include floppy mitral valves or congenitally bicuspid aortic valves, which occur in 5% to 10% and 1% to 2% of the population, respectively, but which usually are not clinically significant until adult life.

Excluding these two disorders, ventricular septal defects represent the most prevalent form of congenital heart disease and account for about one third of the cases among live births.[6] Atrial septal defect, pulmonary stenosis, tetralogy of Fallot, and patent ductal artery (ductus arteriosus) together constitute an additional one third of the cases (Table 46-1). Because these anomalies are generally associated with prolonged survival, whereas other disorders are often associated with a high mortality, their relative frequencies noted in autopsy series are appreciably different.[7]

Most anomalies show no sex predilection. However, atrial septal defect and patent ductal artery occur more often in girls, and complete transposition, aortic coarctation, and aortic stenosis or atresia more commonly affect boys. In fact virtually all congenital forms of left-sided obstructions occur predominantly in male offspring.

Syndromes that include combinations of cardiac and extracardiac malformations are often associated with either gross chromosomal anomalies (such as trisomy 21) or with single mutant genes.[8] They can occur sporadically or may be transmitted as autosomal or X-linked traits with a mendelian pattern of inheritance. Cardiac malformations that are not part of a syndrome are rarely associated with gross chromosomal abnormalities.

In addition to hereditary factors, exposure of the embryo to drugs, infections, or maternal conditions may also result in cardiac malformations. Drugs that presumptively can act as cardiovascular teratogens include alcohol, amphetamines, anticonvulsants, chemotherapeutic agents, lithium, sex hormones, thalidomide, and retinoic acid. The postrubella syndrome is associated with peripheral pulmonary artery stenosis, a patent ductal artery, and septal defects. The risk of cardiac anomalies among the offspring of women with diabetes mellitus, systemic lupus erythematosus, or phenylketonuria is also higher than that in the general population.

Approximately 90% of congenital cardiac anomalies in human beings are believed to be associated with a multifactorial mode of transmission, particularly if there are no extracardiac malformations. In such cases the occurrence of the anomaly is determined by interactions between either a single-gene or polygenic predisposition and various environmental factors. The disorder usually shows familial aggregation without a mendelian pattern of inheritance. In general the likelihood of unaffected parents having a second child with congenital heart disease ranges from 2% to 6%.[6,9] The risk is tripled if there are two affected first-degree relatives. Interestingly the likelihood of having affected offspring is about 6% if the mother has a cardiac anomaly but only 3% if the father does.

Historical background

The twentieth century has witnessed remarkable advances in the diagnosis and treatment of congenital heart disease. Surgical closure of a patent ductal artery was first accomplished in the late 1930s, and the creation of a subclavian-to-pulmonary artery shunt to increase pulmonary blood flow was first performed during the 1940s. The development of a pump-oxygenator (heart-lung machine) in the early 1950s represented one of the great medical achievements of the twentieth century, and transformed the vision of open-heart surgery into reality. By the late 1950s creative teams had devised techniques for the patch closure of septal defects and for the repair of Fallot's tetralogy.

Table 46-1 **Relative frequency and distribution of selected cardiac malformations**

Cardiac malformation	Approximate frequency %	Male-to-female ratio
Ventricular septal defect	32	1:1
Atrial septal defect	8	1:2
Pulmonary stenosis	8	1:1
Tetralogy of Fallot (including pulmonary atresia)	8	1:1
Patent ductal artery (ductus arteriosus)	8	1:2
Aortic stenosis	6	3:1
Coarctation of the aorta	6	2:1
Complete transposition of the great arteries	5	2:1
Atrioventricular septal defect	4	1:1
Tricuspid atresia	2	1:1
Aortic atresia (hypoplastic left heart syndrome)	2	3:1
Total anomalous pulmonary venous connection	2	1:1
Persistent truncal artery (truncus arteriosus)	1	1:1
Pulmonary atresia with intact ventricular septum	1	1:1
Double inlet left ventricle	1	1:1
Double outlet right ventricle	<1	1:1
Corrected transposition of the great arteries	<1	1:1
Ebstein's anomaly of the tricuspid valve	<1	1:1
Other malformations	<5	—

From Emmanouilides GC, Riemenschneider TA, Allen HD, Gutgesell HP, editors: *Moss and Adams' heart disease in infants, children, and adolescents, including the fetus and young adult*, ed 5, Baltimore, 1995, Williams & Wilkins; Freedom RM, Benson LN, Smallhorn JF, editors: *Neonatal heart disease*, London, 1992, Springer-Verlag; Moller JH, Neal WA, editors: *Fetal, neonatal, and infant cardiac disease*, Norwalk, Conn, 1990, Appleton & Lange; Anderson RH, Macartney FJ, Shinebourne EA, Tynan M, editors: *Paediatric cardiology*, Edinburgh, 1987, Churchill Livingstone; Kirklin JW, Barratt-Boyes BG, editors: *Cardiac surgery: morphology, diagnostic criteria, natural history, techniques, results, and indications*, ed 2, New York, 1993, Churchill Livingstone.

With the introduction of cadaveric and synthetic conduits during the 1960s, a means for the reconstruction of the right ventricular outflow tract was provided, and this revolutionized the surgical treatment of complex conotruncal anomalies. Similarly, with the creation and modification of atriopulmonary shunts, accomplished in the 1970s, the repair of hearts with only one functional ventricle became possible. The 1980s were highlighted by the refinement of reparative procedures for use during early infancy, by the development of numerous catheter-based nonsurgical interventional procedures, and by the advent of neonatal cardiac transplantation. As the 1990s usher in the twenty-first century, ingenious and creative minds are at work modifying and refining current techniques and are devising new technologies for the intrauterine repair of malformed fetal hearts.

Role of pathologist

The role of pathologists in the evaluation of patients with congenital heart disease has changed dramatically over the past 50 years. During the first half of this century, Maude Abbott[10] categorized hundreds of malformed hearts obtained from autopsy, and thereby established the foundation for those who would later devise the operative interventions just described.[11] During the second half of this century, pathologists such as Lev[12] and Edwards[13,14] described the anatomic details of malformed hearts that were of particular interest to surgeons, including various subgroups of specific anomalies, the location of the coronary arteries and specialized conduction tissues, and the secondary effects of cardiac malformations on the pulmonary circulation. More recently Van Praagh and Takao[15] have emphasized embryology and morphology; Anderson and Becker[16] have stressed nomenclature and morphology; and Edwards[17] has reviewed the pathologic consequences of interventional procedures.

Pathologists now rarely encounter unoperated forms of congenital heart disease in persons from industrialized countries. Consequently an evaluation of cardiopulmonary specimens at autopsy entails not only a detailed inspection of the underlying malformation and its secondary effects on the heart and lungs, but also an identification of the specific procedures that were performed and an evaluation of the postprocedural effects or complications.[18] Moreover, chronic lesions such as aortic root dilatation or floppy valves, which have developed only as patients have survived into adulthood, may also be encountered.

Perspective on nomenclature

Numerous classification systems have been proposed to categorize the great diversity of malformed hearts. Moreover, systems of nomenclature have been adopted for groups of anomalies, such as hearts with a single functional ventricle, and for individual anomalies, such as ventricular septal defects. Investigators have emphasized various features of these defects in their terminology, including embryogenesis, spatial relationships (between atriums, ventricles, and great arteries), clinical aspects (cyanosis or altered pulmonary blood flow), and surgical anatomy.[19]

However, as newer terms have been added, older ones have rarely been abandoned. As a result, the field of congenital heart disease has become a sea of synonyms, adding further confusion to an already complex subject. In this chapter the system of nomenclature suggested by Anderson and colleagues[20] is employed, with some modification. Also favored are anglicized terms (see Appendix 46-1), which are used here with their Latin counterparts in parentheses—for example, *ductal artery (ductus arteriosus).*

UNIFYING CONCEPTS OF CONGENITAL HEART DISEASE

Segmental analysis

For the evaluation of cardiac malformations, the heart is best considered as having three segments (atriums [atria], ventricles, and great arteries), each of which is normally partitioned into two components (usually right-sided and left-sided). Atrioventricular valves connect atriums to ventricles, and semilunar valves connect ventricles to great arteries. Thus there are only a limited number of possible connections between the three major segments, regardless of their spatial orientations.

Right-sided and left-sided structures at each level are evaluated, in a systematic manner, from the standpoint of their morphology, relative positions, connections to proximal and distal segments, and the presence and locations of shunts, obstructions, and valvular regurgitation. The sequential segmental method for investigating congenital cardiac malformations represents a diagnostic cornerstone for both clinicians and pathologists.[15,20] In general the cardiac position and visceral sidedness are determined before this method is applied.

Cardiac position

Within the chest the heart can be described positionally as left-sided (normal), right-sided, or midline. Independently the direction of the ventricular apex can be designated as leftward (levocardia), rightward (dextrocardia), or inferiorly directed (mesocardia). In contrast, displacement of the heart by adjacent structures is designated as levoposition, dextroposition, or mesoposition. Very rarely sternal or diaphragmatic defects are associated with an extrathoracic, or ectopic, heart (ectopia cordis).[21]

Visceral sidedness

Because the cardiovascular, respiratory, and digestive systems are asymmetric, they are characterized by sidedness or handedness, which appears to be determined genetically. Sidedness may be normal (situs solitus), mirror image (situs inversus), isomeric (situs ambiguus), or indeterminate (situs ambiguus). Right isomerism denotes bilateral right-sided symmetry, whereas left isomerism indicates bilateral left-sidedness. Abnormalities can affect the entire body, as in total mirror-image sidedness (situs inversus totalis), or may involve the asymmetric organ systems individually. Accordingly the sidedness of the cardiovascular, respiratory, and digestive systems should be evaluated separately.

The relationship between isomerism and splenic anomalies is intriguing and is possibly related to the left-sided nature of the splenic anlage embryologically. Thus, when right isomerism pertains, the spleen is usually absent, indicative of the asplenia syndrome.[22] In contrast, left isomerism is generally associated with the presence of multiple spleens, restricted to one side of the vertebral column, as part of the polysplenia syndrome.[23]

Cardiac sidedness is determined by the position of the morphologic right atrium. It is *not* determined by the direction of the cardiac apex, the positions of the ventricles or great arteries, or the sidedness of noncardiac viscera. Likewise, pulmonary sidedness is defined by the positions of the morphologic right and left lungs.[19] Abdominal sidedness is determined by the position of the liver and inferior caval vein (vena cava), which is usually opposite that of the stomach, pancreas, spleen, and abdominal aorta.

Morphology of cardiac segments

The most reliable anatomic criteria for distinguishing between morphologic right and left atriums are the connections of the inferior caval vein, the presence of a large pyramidal appendage, and identification of the limb of the oval fossa (fossa ovalis), all of which are indicative of a morphologic right atrium[19,24] (Table 46-2). A common atrium is the result of absence, or near absence, of the atrial septum and is almost always associated with an atrioventricular septal defect, with or without asplenia (right isomerism).

Atrioventricular valves connect atriums to ventricles. Because the valves travel with their respective ventricles, a morphologic tricuspid valve is almost invariably joined to a morphologic right ventricle, whereas the mitral valve is connected to the left ventricle. Thus, if both atrioventricular valves join the left ventricle, they both tend to exhibit mitral morphology. A common atrioventricular valve exists when the mitral and tricuspid valves are not separated from one another and produce a single valvular orifice.

A ventricle consists of an endocardium-lined chamber within the ventricular myocardium. Although normal ventricles are characterized by inlet, trabecular, and outlet regions, hypoplastic ventricles frequently consist of only one or two components. Because virtually all human hearts contain two ventricles, the terms *single ventricle* and *univentricular heart* are inaccurate. The most reliable features that allow distinction between morphologic right and left ventricles are the nature of the apical trabeculations, the morphology of the adjacent atrioventricular valve, and the state of the continuity between the atrioventricular and semilunar valves (Table 46-2). Normal differences in ventricular wall thickness and chamber shape do not necessarily pertain in malformed hearts. A true common ventricle with an absent septum is exceedingly rare.

A semilunar valve serves to connect a ventricle to a great artery. It is named after the artery into which it empties and *not* the ventricle from which it arises. The truncal valve represents a common semilunar valve that results when the truncal artery (truncus arteriosus) fails to divide into the ascending aorta and pulmonary trunk.

Position of cardiac segments

Once the cardiac segments (atriums, ventricles, and great arteries) are identified morphologically, their spatial orientations are determined next. The positions of the valves are addressed later when segmental connections are discussed. The position of the morphologic right atrium, which determines cardiac sidedness, can be right-sided, left-sided, bilateral (right isomerism), or absent (left isomerism).

The location of the ventricles is determined by the position of the cardiac apex (levocardia, dextrocardia, or mesocardia) and the plane of the ventricular septum. Normally the septum is roughly vertical. However, it can be angled, horizontal, or twisted in the settings of double inlet left ventricles, superoinferior ventricles, or crisscross hearts, respectively. The positions of the ventricles may also be designated as normal or as mirror image (L-loop, inverted ventricles).

Table 46-2 Comparison of anatomic features for right-sided and left-sided structures at each cardiac segmental level

Right side of heart	Left side of heart
Right atrium	**Left atrium**
Limb of oval fossa (limbus fossae ovalis)	Second ostium (ostium secundum)
Large pyramidal appendage	Small fingerlike appendage
Terminal crest (crista terminalis)	No terminal crest
Pectinate muscles	No pectinate muscles
Receives caval veins and coronary sinus*	Receives pulmonary veins*
Tricuspid valve	**Mitral valve**
Low septal annular attachment	High septal annular attachment
Septal cordal attachments	No septal cordal attachments
Triangular orifice (midleaflet level)	Elliptical orifice (midleaflet level)
Three leaflets and commissures	Two leaflets and commissures
Three papillary muscles	Two large papillary muscles
Empties into right ventricle	Empties into left ventricle
Right ventricle	**Left ventricle**
Receives tricuspid valve	Receives mitral valve
Tricuspid–pulmonary valve discontinuity	Mitral-aortic valve continuity
Muscular outflow tract	Muscular-valvular outflow tract
Septal and parietal bands	No septal or parietal band
Large apical trabeculations	Small apical trabeculations
Coarse septal surface	Smooth upper septal surface
Crescentic in cross section*	Circular in cross section*
Thin free wall (3-5 mm)*	Thick free wall (12-15 mm)*
Pulmonary valve	**Aortic valve**
Empties into pulmonary trunk	Empties into ascending aorta

*Variable features.

The position of the ascending aorta is generally described in terms of its relationship to the pulmonary trunk and is normally posterior and rightward. Dextroposition of the aorta indicates a slightly anterior shift, between right-posterior and right-lateral, and is commonly a feature of tetralogy of Fallot, a double outlet right ventricle, and atrioventricular septal defects. In contrast, a right-anterior aorta occurs most frequently in association with complete transposition of the great arteries. A left-anterior aorta is encountered less often and is usually associated with congenitally corrected transposition of the great arteries or with a double inlet left ventricle.

The position of the aortic arch is defined by the bronchus over which it travels. Thus, in the normal state a left aortic arch courses over the left main bronchus. Conversely, a right aortic arch travels over the right main bronchus and exhibits mirror image branching of the arch vessels. It is most commonly associated with pulmonary atresia with a ventricular septal defect, a persistent truncal artery, or tetralogy of Fallot. The rare double aortic arch travels over both bronchuses (bronchi) and forms a vascular ring around the trachea and esophagus.

Connections of cardiac segments

After the cardiac segments have been evaluated from the standpoint of their morphology and position, the venoatrial, atrioventricular, and ventriculoarterial connections can be determined. The cardiac valves form the mortar that joins atriums to ventricles and ventricles to great arteries. However, the presence of connections does not necessarily imply patency. In the setting of aortic atresia, for example, the identification of an imperforate valve between the left ventricle and ascending aorta indicates a concordant connection, despite the absence of blood flow between the two.

Venoatrial connections

Abnormal venoatrial connections stem from malformations of the embryologic sinus vein (sinus venosus), common pulmonary vein, or their derivatives. Thus, anomalies can involve the systemic veins, pulmonary veins, or both, and they can involve all or only some of the veins. Consequently the connection of each vein should be evaluated separately.

Atrioventricular connections

The atriums can connect to the ventricles in four possible ways—concordant, discordant, univentricular, or ambiguous (Fig. 46-1). Concordance represents the normal state, whereas discordance represents ventricular inversion. A univentricular connection exists when both atriums connect to only one ventricle, and it can be of the double, single, or common inlet type. When valvular atresia exists, it is important to distinguish between complete absence of an atrioventricular connection on that side (that is, a single inlet heart) and the presence of an imperforate fibrous membrane (*not* representing a single inlet connection).

Ventriculoarterial connections

The possible modes of connection between the ventricles and two great arteries can be concordant, discordant, or double outlet, and their connection to only one great artery can consist of a single or common outlet (Fig. 46-2). Concordance represents the normal state, whereas discordance connotes transposed great arteries. Because the term *great vessels* can refer to either arteries or veins, the term *great arteries* is favored for the nomenclature pertaining to transposition complexes. Occasionally in the setting of pulmonary or aortic atresia, the ventricle from which the corresponding great artery once arose cannot be established with certainty, and the connection is considered indeterminate.

Shunt connections

A congenital shunt is defined as an abnormal communication between two cardiac chambers, between a chamber and a great artery, or between two great arteries. As such it represents another form of connection to be assessed segmentally. For example, in an atrial septal defect the left atrium connects not only to the left ventricle but also to the right atrium.

Overriding valves (septal malalignments)

Overriding is defined as the biventricular emptying of an atrioventricular valve or the biventricular origin of a semilunar valve. It is a property of the valve annulus and is always associated with a malalignment type of ventricular septal defect.[19] Moreover, annular overriding may interfere with an accurate determination of cardiac connections. In general a cardiac valve is assigned to the ventricle into which it drains or from which it empties by more than 50% (the so-called 50% rule). Similarly, if a common atrioventricular valve overrides one ventricle by more than 75%, the connection is considered a common inlet.

Straddling valves (contralateral insertions)

Straddling is defined as the anomalous insertion of tendinous cords (chordae tendineae) or papillary muscles into the contralateral ventricle, and its severity depends on the extent of the insertions, along either the septum or the free wall[25] (Fig. 45-3). Consequently, straddling affects only the atrioventricular valves and also requires the presence of a ventricular septal defect. Cordal straddling may occur alone or in conjunction with annular overriding.

Effects of congenital lesions on the heart

The altered hemodynamic states associated with most forms of congenital heart disease characteristically produce secondary changes in the muscle mass and volume of the cardiac chambers. With time, myocardial injury and cardiac failure may ensue.

Hypertrophy and dilatation

Cardiac hypertrophy represents an adaptive response to an increased work load, and it affects atriums as well as ventricles. It may be physiologic, as in conditioned athletes, or pathologic, as in the setting of congenital heart disease. Conditions such as aortic or pulmonary stenosis, which impose a ventricular pressure overload, induce *pressure* hypertrophy without causing appreciable dilatation. In contrast, disorders that cause a volume overload, such as an atrial septal defect or tricuspid regurgitation, are attended by *volume* hypertrophy with chamber dilatation.[26] Volume hypertrophy is considered a form of ventricular remodeling.

In the context of volume hypertrophy, dilatation masks the degree of hypertrophy, and wall thickness is often normal.[27] Consequently, when a chamber is dilated, its wall thickness cannot be used as an indicator of hypertrophy. Rather the myocardial mass (or weight) must be determined and com-

bly less than the systemic vascular resistance. In contrast, if severe pulmonary hypertension develops, shunt reversal will eventually occur and produce a right-to-left shunt with peripheral cyanosis.

Atrial septal defect

A congenital atrial septal defect represents an interatrial communication that allows blood to flow potentially in either direction. Although its size and the extent of its shunt are important clinically, an atrial septal defect is classified according to its location relative to the oval fossa (fossa ovalis). First, however, a patent oval foramen warrants a separate discussion.

Patent oval foramen

After the first year of life the oval foramen remains potentially patent, or valvular competent, in about one third of normal hearts.[43] Postnatally, however, this flap valve is closed functionally because the pressure in the left atrium exceeds that in the right atrium. Consequently a patent oval foramen does not represent a congenital atrial septal defect, though it *does* represent a potential site for paradoxical embolization. An atrial septal aneurysm most commonly forms in patients with a patent oval foramen and may also be associated with mitral valve prolapse.

General features

A defect at the oval fossa is known as a *fossa* or *secundum atrial septal defect* (see Appendix 46-2). This form accounts for about 85% of the atrial septal defects and results from a deficient or fenestrated valve of the oval fossa (Fig. 46-7). Most fossa defects occur as isolated anomalies, some of which produce heart failure in infancy, but most of which remain asymptomatic until adulthood. Most cases are sporadic, but some are familial or occur with syndromes such as the Holt-Oram syndrome.[44] If the defect coexists with another cardiac anomaly, the latter is generally the more severe lesion; examples include ventricular septal defect, patent ductal artery, valvular atresia, and conotruncal anomalies. Mitral valve prolapse may also be observed clinically, though floppy features are uncommon pathologically.

An outlet or primum atrial septal defect is located anterior to the oval fossa (see Appendix 46-2). It is associated with a cleft anterior mitral leaflet and represents a partial form of atrioventricular septal defect, to be discussed in the next section in this chapter.

Inlet atrial septal defects involve the region of the embryologic sinus vein (sinus venosus) posterior to the oval fossa and are also called *sinus venosus defects*. They are associated with an anomalous connection of the right pulmonary veins and are discussed in another section (Anomalous pulmonary venous connection).

The rarest form of atrial septal defect occurs at the coronary sinus ostium and results when the coronary sinus is unroofed and merges with the left atrium. Coronary sinus atrial septal defects are often associated with the left atrial connection of a persistent left superior caval vein.

Some hearts exhibit multiple atrial septal defects. The most frequent combination is that of fossa (secundum) and outlet (primum) defects. In patients with right isomerism or asplenia, the only remnant of atrial septum is a muscular cord that separates a combined fossa-inlet defect, above, from a combined outlet–coronary sinus defect, below. This represents a common atrium.

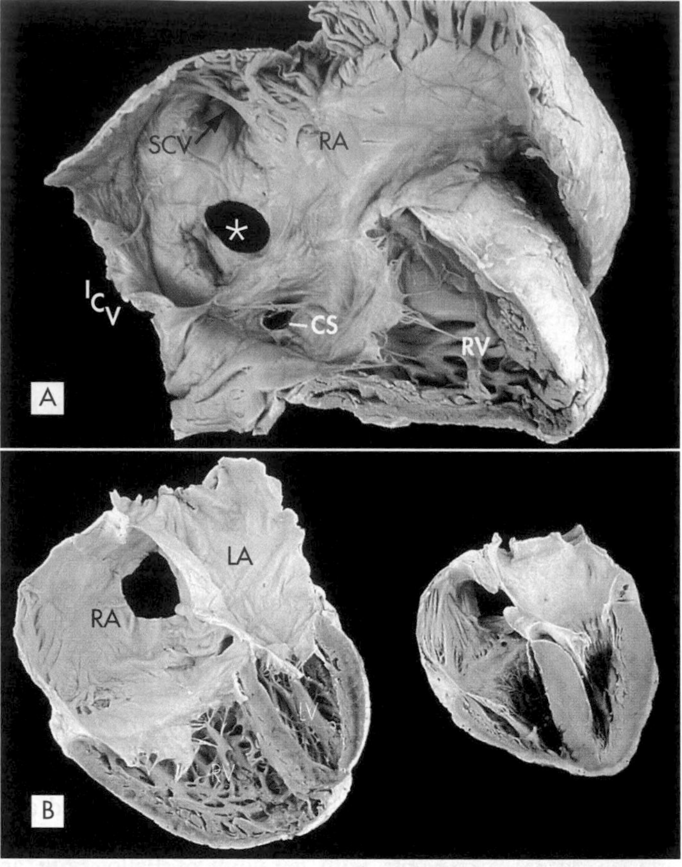

Fig. 46-7 Atrial septal defect, fossa (secundum) type, as seen in adults. **A,** Large defect (*) (opened right atrium). **B,** Volume hypertrophy of right atrium and right ventricle, with normal heart at right for comparison (four-chamber view).

Secondary cardiopulmonary effects

A left-to-right shunt occurs during ventricular diastole because the right ventricle is more compliant and thereby fills more readily than does the left ventricle. This in turn occurs because pulmonary vascular resistance is substantially less than systemic vascular resistance. As a result of the left-to-right shunt, a right-sided volume overload develops and is associated with prominent dilatation of the right atrium, right ventricle, and entire pulmonary circulation. Moreover, right atrial dilatation causes further enlargement of the septal defect. Eventually, volume hypertrophy involves the right ventricle, and the resulting chamber enlargement produces annular dilatation and tricuspid and pulmonary regurgitation. However, despite appreciable dilatation, the formation of a right-sided mural thrombus is rare. Microscopically the right ventricle is characterized by myocyte hypertrophy and focal interstitial fibrosis.

Hemodynamically, atrial septal defects are characterized by increased pulmonary blood flow, which is usually well tolerated because of the great capacity for the pulmonary vasculature to dilate and open additional capillary beds. With time mild medial hypertrophy and eccentric intimal fibrosis develop in pulmonary arteries and veins.[45] Organized arterial thrombus may also be observed in adults with the defect. Among patients with isolated atrial septal defects, the likelihood of *irreversible* plexogenic pulmonary hypertension developing is less than 10%.[46] The most common causes of death among the other 90% of adults with unoperated atrial septal defects are congestive heart failure, occurring in 20% (often resulting from atrial arrhythmias), and ischemic heart disease or other causes unrelated to the defect, affecting 70%.

Pathology of interventions

Because atrial septal defects rarely close spontaneously, symptomatic lesions are closed either surgically with the placement of sutures or a patch or interventionally with the placement of a clamshell occluder, delivered by a transvenous catheter.[47-49] Serious postoperative complications are uncommon but include persistent right ventricular dilatation, atrial arrhythmias, embolization of mural thrombus along the surgical patch, and persistent or progressive pulmonary hypertension. Residual interatrial shunts are rare, and patients are not at risk for infective endocarditis.

The surgical mortality for isolated defects is less than 1% for all age groups.[5] Though rare, early postoperative deaths are generally related to pulmonary hypertension or, in the elderly, to coexistent disorders such as mitral regurgitation, ischemic heart disease, or heart failure. Late deaths generally result from cerebral infarction, heart failure, or arrhythmias.

In some newborns the presence of an unobstructed interatrial communication is necessary for survival. Examples of disorders in which this is critical include complete transposition with an intact ventricular septum and a closing ductal artery, as well as tricuspid atresia, mitral atresia, or total anomalous pulmonary venous connection. Balloon atrial septostomy generally affords excellent palliation. The most common cause of procedural failure is stretching, rather than tearing, of the valve of the oval fossa.[17] Complications are rare and are usually related to damage to adjacent structures. If the balloon method fails, either a transcatheter blade septostomy or a surgical Blalock-Hanlon atrial septectomy can be performed (Table 46-5).

Atrioventricular septal defect

Because the level of the septal insertion of the mitral annulus is normally higher than that of the tricuspid valve, an atrioventricular septum exists that separates the right atrium from the left ventricle. The right side of this septum corresponds roughly to the anatomic triangle of Koch, within whose boundaries lies the atrioventricular node.[27]

Congenital shunts in this region are referred to as *atrioventricular septal defects,* and two major forms are recognized—partial and complete. Both are associated not only with a septal defect but also with abnormalities of the atrioventricular valves and with posteroinferior displacement of the atrioventricular conduction tissues. Synonyms for them

Table 46-5 **Eponymous surgical procedures for malformed hearts**

Eponym	Description of procedure	Cardiovascular anomalies
Blalock-Hanlon shunt	Partial atrial septectomy (posterosuperior region)	Complete TGA with intact ventricular septum
Blalock-Taussig shunt	Subclavian-to–pulmonary artery (classic: end-to-side anastomosis; modified: interposed synthetic graft)	Conditions with decreased pulmonary blood flow (tetralogy, PA-VSD, and DORV or DILV with PS)
Damus-Kaye-Stansel procedure	Proximal PT to ascending aorta (end-to-side anastomosis); conduit from RV to distal PT; VSD closure	Complete TGA without PS and with or without VSD
Glenn anastomosis	SCV to RPA (end-to-side); ligation of SCV at RA; ligation of proximal RPA (bidirectional Glenn: no ligation of RPA)	Tricuspid atresia, or DILV with PS
Fontan procedure (modified)	Anastomosis of SCV, RA, or RV to RPA or LPA; may include intraatrial conduit from ICV to SCV	Hearts with single functional ventricle (for example, tricuspid atresia, and DILV)
Jatene procedure	Transection and switching of great arteries and coronary arteries	Complete TGA, and DORV with subpulmonary VSD
Konno procedure	Outlet (infundibular) septostomy, with patch enlargement of LV and RV outflow tracts, and aortic valve replacement	Tunnel subaortic stenosis, and severe hypertrophic cardiomyopathy
Mustard procedure	Resection of atrial septum; intraatrial baffle directing caval blood to LV, and pulmonary venous blood to RV	Complete TGA
Norwood procedure	Stage 1 (atrial septectomy; PDA ligation; PT transection; aortic incision; reconstruction of aorta with allograft; aorta-PT shunt) Stage 2 (modified Fontan operation)	Aortic atresia (hypoplastic left heart syndrome)
Potts shunt	Descending thoracic aorta to LPA (side-to-side anastomosis)	Same as for Blalock-Taussig shunt
Rastelli procedure	VSD closure directing LV blood to aorta; conduit from RV to distal PT; ligation of proximal PT	PA-VSD, PTA, complete TGA with VSD and PS, and DORVwith PS
Senning procedure	Use of atrial septum to fashion intraatrial baffle, similar to Mustard procedure	Complete TGA
Waterston shunt	Ascending aorta to RPA (side-to-side anastomosis)	Same as for Blalock-Taussig shunt

DILV, Double inlet left ventricle; *DORV,* double outlet right ventricle; *ICV,* inferior caval vein; *LPA,* left pulmonary artery; *LV,* left ventricle; *PA-VSD,* pulmonary *atresia* with a ventricular septal defect; *PDA,* patent ductal artery; *PS,* pulmonary stenosis; *PT,* pulmonary trunk; *PTA,* persistent truncal artery; *RA,* right atrium; *RPA,* right pulmonary artery; *RV,* right ventricle; *SCV,* superior caval vein; *TGA,* transposition of the great arteries; *VSD,* ventricular septal defect.

include *atrioventricular canal defects, endocardial cushion defects,* and others (see Appendix 46-2).

General features

The most commonly observed form of partial atrioventricular septal defect manifests as an outlet (primum) atrial septal defect and a cleft in the anterior mitral lealfet. Deficiency of the atrioventricular septum is accompanied by downward displacement of the mitral valve to the level of the tricuspid annulus, such that the shunt is interatrial in location rather than atrioventricular. The valvular cleft, which differs from a commissure by having no subjacent papillary muscle, prevents adequate closure and is associated with mitral regurgitation. Partial defects often remain asymptomatic until adulthood.

In contrast, complete forms of atrioventricular septal defect are more common than the partial forms and almost always become symptomatic during the first year of life. They are characterized by a large septal defect and a common atrioventricular valve that usually contains five leaflets (see Fig. 46-6). The effect of the septal defect on left ventricular morphology is a foreshortened inflow tract and a lengthened outflow tract[50] (Fig. 46-8). The valve, which lies in a plane perpendicular to the defect, is usually regurgitant, and with time a focal hooding deformity and microscopic features of a floppy valve may develop.[51] About 35% of the cases occur in patients with Down syndrome, and 15% to 20% of the patients with Down syndrome have complete atrioventricular septal defects. This cardiac malformation has also been associated with the asplenia (right isomerism) and polysplenia (left isomerism) syndromes.

In the setting of a complete atrioventricular septal defect, the most common coexistent anomalies are a fossa (secundum) atrial septal defect, a persistent left superior caval vein, and pulmonary stenosis. Conotruncal anomalies occurring in conjunction with the complete form include tetralogy of Fallot, often in patients with Down syndrome, and a double outlet right ventricle, usually in patients with the polysplenia syndrome.[52] Other associated malformations include coarctation of the aorta, patent ductal artery, discrete subaortic stenosis, a common atrium (usually with right isomerism), and an abnormal mitral component of the common atrioventricular valve. Common inlet ventricles are usually associated with hypoplasia of the contralateral ventricle.

Secondary cardiopulmonary effects

The major hemodynamic effects of partial atrioventricular septal defects are mitral regurgitation and an interatrial left-to-right shunt. These impose a volume overload on the left ven-

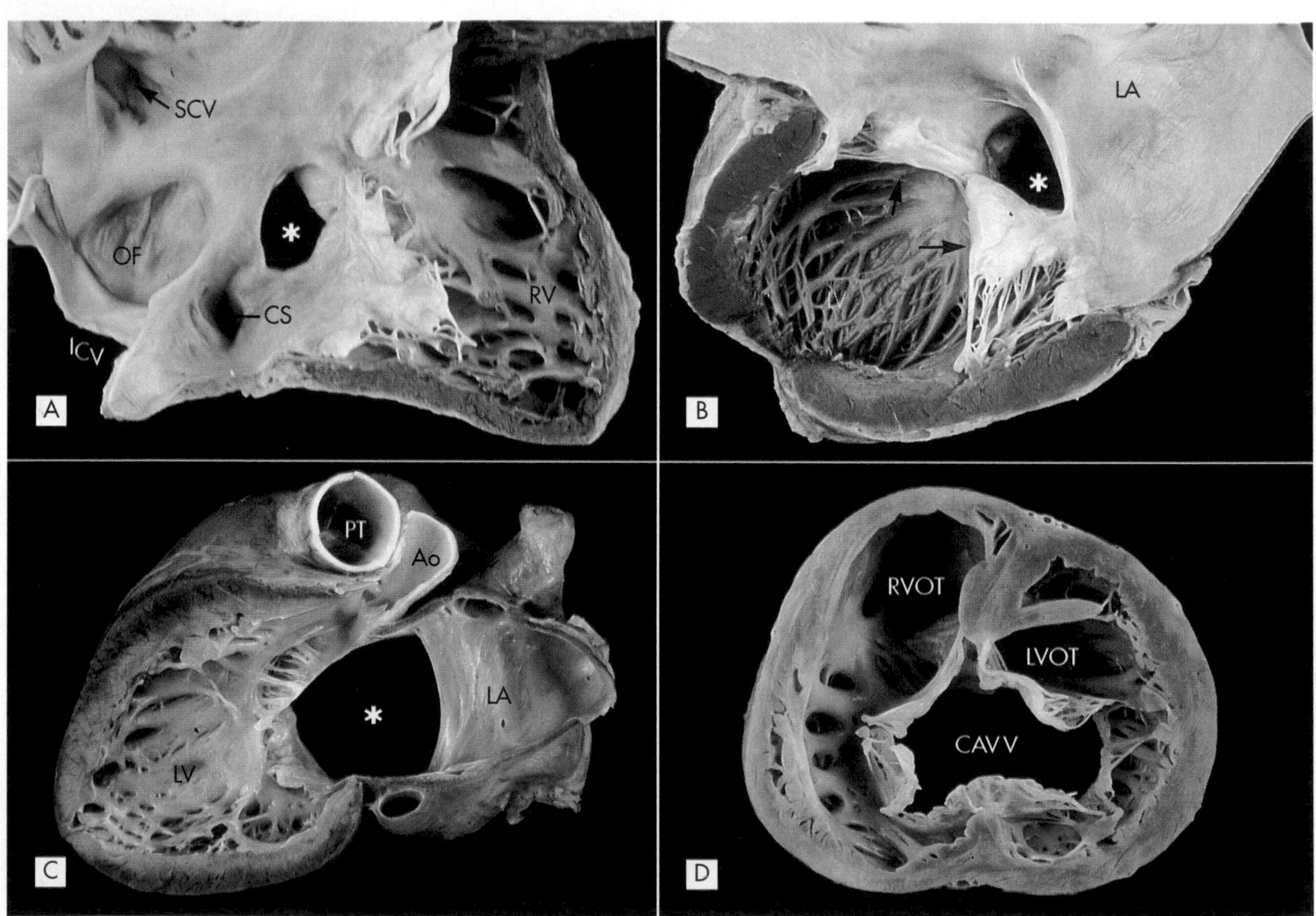

Fig. 46-8 Atrioventricular septal defects. **A,** and **B,** Partial form in an adult showing an outlet (primum) atrial septal defect (*) and a cleft *(arrow)* in the anterior mitral leaflet (right-sided and left-sided views). **C,** and **D,** Complete form in children, showing a large septal defect (*) and the common atrioventricular valve (long-axis and short-axis views).

tricle and the right-sided cardiac chambers and produce an element of pulmonary venous hypertension. Consequently the secondary cardiac effects are similar to those resulting from a fossa (secundum) atrial septal defect. In contrast, the complete form is associated not only with the hemodynamic features already described but also with an interventricular left-to-right shunt. As a result, there is equalization of ventricular pressures and considerable right ventricular hypertrophy.

In patients with the partial form, pulmonary hypertension occurs because of the increase in pulmonary blood flow that is produced by the atrial septal defect, and pulmonary venous hypertension arises because of the mitral regurgitation. In the complete form of the defect, the increased pulmonary arterial pressure is related to the ventricular septal defect, and this increase in pressure accelerates the development of plexogenic pulmonary hypertension.

Moreover, hypertensive pulmonary vascular disease develops at a younger age in patients with Down syndrome than in those who do not have this syndrome.[53] In these patients, the ability of their muscular pulmonary arteries to develop medial hypertrophy is impaired, such that obstructive intimal hyperplasia becomes the primary early response to elevated pressure.[54] Rarely, irreversible disease can occur within the first year. Chronic hypoxia is also commonly associated with Down syndrome and contributes to the severity of the pulmonary hypertension.[40]

Pulmonary hypertension and valvular regurgitation lead to heart failure, recurrent pneumonia, and growth retardation. Among patients with unoperated complete atrioventricular septal defects, 80% die of heart failure or pneumonia by 2 years of age, and irreversible pulmonary hypertension usually develops in the remainder by 5 years of age.[5,17]

Pathology of interventions

The surgical procedure used to repair both the partial and complete forms is remarkably similar and entails patch closure of the septal defect and reconstruction of the mitral component. The latter may be fashioned into either a bileaflet or trileaflet valve in order to establish a competent valve and to prevent left ventricular outflow tract obstruction.[5,55,56] Mitral valve replacement is necessary in some patients with the complete defect and a severely malformed valve.

Postoperative complications in patients with partial defects include arrhythmias, the need for pacemaker insertion, residual mitral regurgitation, a residual atrial septal defect, and fixed subaortic stenosis.[17] Operative deaths occur in fewer than 1% of the patients with only mild mitral incompetence, and the mortality rate is less than 4% overall.

Among patients with the complete form of atrioventricular septal defect, the early postoperative mortality rate is less than 5%.[5] The primary cause of postoperative morbidity and mortality is mitral valve dysfunction, with either regurgitation or stenosis.[17,18] Other complications include fixed subaortic stenosis, supraventricular arrhythmias, complete heart block, mitral prosthetic valve dysfunction, and progressive pulmonary hypertension.[57] Early postoperative death usually results from acute heart failure, and the mortality rate is higher for patients with conotruncal anomalies than for those without. Additional surgical risks include severe symptoms preoperatively, severe regurgitation of the common atrioventricular valve, substantial deformity of the mitral component, a hypoplastic ventricle, and the coexistence of Down syndrome and tetralogy of Fallot.

Ventricular septal defect

A congenital ventricular septal defect is characterized by an anomalous communication between the two ventricles (see Fig. 46-6). It results from inadequate growth and focally absent fusion of the embryologic septal components. Although most cases occur sporadically, some are associated with trisomy or with maternal exposure to teratogens or infections. Extracardiac malformations coexist in about 25% and usually affect the musculoskeletal and central nervous systems, and less frequently the respiratory, genitourinary, and digestive systems.

Ventricular septal defects represent the most common form of congenital heart disease. They may occur as an isolated lesion or with other cardiac malformations, such as an atrial septal defect, patent ductal artery, conotruncal anomaly, or single functional ventricle. Ventricular septal defects may be categorized according to their location, size, or association with valvular overriding, and several classification systems have been devised.[58-60]

General features

Among the ventricular septal defects observed at operation or autopsy, 75% to 80% involve the membranous septum and are called *membranous defects* (see Appendix 46-2). Defects in this location are generally large and can extend in an outlet, inlet, or apical direction. They are bordered superiorly by the right and posterior aortic cusps and posteriorly by the continuity between the mitral and tricuspid valves (that is, by the central fibrous body, or right fibrous trigone) (Fig. 46-9). Their anterior and inferior borders are muscular, and the atrioventricular (His) bundle travels along the inferior border as it forms the left and right bundle branches.

Outlet defects are located beneath the right and left cusps of both semilunar valves and account for 5% to 10% of all ventricular septal defects. Synonyms for the anomaly include *infundibular defect* and others (see Appendix 46-2). Most occur with conotruncal anomalies such as tetralogy of Fallot, double outlet right ventricle, and persistent truncal artery (truncus arteriosus). Inadequate support for the overlying semilunar valves can lead to prolapse, particularly of the right aortic cusp, with secondary regurgitation.[61]

Inlet ventricular septal defects involve the inlet septum, beneath the septal tricuspid leaflet, and represent about 5% of all defects. They generally occur with other cardiac malformations.

In contrast to membranous, outlet, and inlet defects, the borders of muscular ventricular septal defects are entirely myocardial and do not include a cardiac valve. Single defects tend to occur along lines of junction between septal regions, whereas multiple muscular defects usually involve the anteroapical trabecular septum and produce a so-called Swiss-cheese septum. Although muscular defects account for only 10% to 20% of the cases observed at operation or autopsy, they actually represent the most common form of ventricular septal defect. However, because most are small and close spontaneously, they are not often encountered by surgeons or pathologists.

A ventricular septal defect is considered small if its area is substantially less than that of the aortic valve orifice or if it is associated with an interventricular pressure gradient. With time restrictive defects may become even smaller as the result of progressive endocardial fibrotic thickening and can eventu-

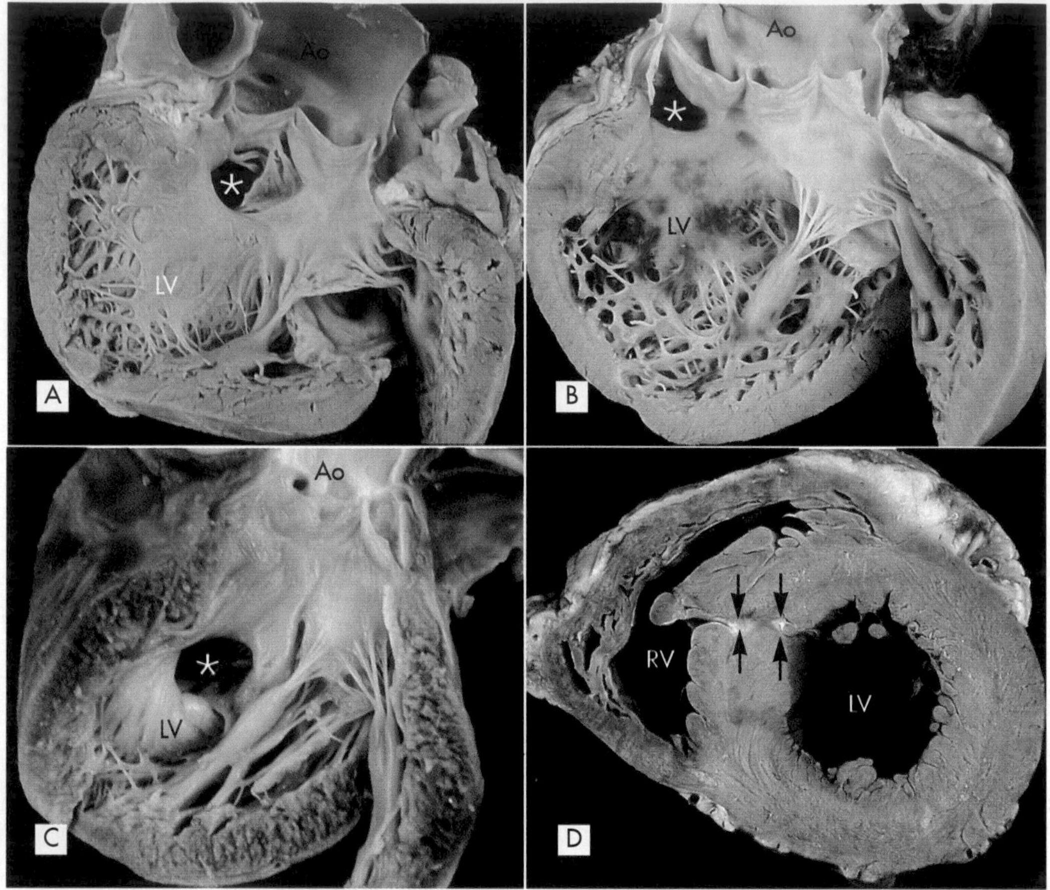

Fig. 46-9 Ventricular septal defects. **A** to **C**, Defects (*) of membranous **(A)**, outlet **(B)**, and muscular **(C)** types (opened left ventricles). **D**, Spontaneously closed muscular defect *(arrows)* (short-axis view).

ally close completely. Some restrictive defects, such as those associated with tricuspid atresia or a double inlet left ventricle, are necessary for survival.

Occasionally hearts exhibit two large ventricular septal defects. The most commonly encountered combination is a membranous defect and an inlet muscular defect. In this situation the His bundle and both bundle branches travel along the bar of myocardium between the two defects. A true common ventricle, with an absent septum and with morphologically right and left ventricular free walls, is extraordinarily rare.

Ventricular septal defects are dynamic lesions that can change appreciably over time. Approximately 50% close spontaneously within the first 2 years of life. As expected, the frequency of closure is higher for small defects (>60%) than for large ones (<10%). A small muscular defect closes when the opposite sides of its muscular walls adhere, with the attendant formation of a dense fibrous plug. In contrast, the spontaneous closure of a membranous defect occurs when the septal tricuspid leaflet adheres to the rim of the defect, forming a scalloped structure that is sometimes misinterpreted to be an aneurysm of the membranous septum.

As discussed previously, annular overriding is always associated with a malalignment ventricular septal defect. Malalignment of the atrial and ventricular septums can affect inlet or membranous defects in conjunction with overriding of an atrioventricular valve. Similarly, malalignment of the ventricular and outlet septums may be a feature of membranous or outlet defects in conjunction with overriding of a semilunar valve. A rightward shift of the outlet septum most commonly occurs with the conotruncal anomalies, whereas a leftward shift generally produces subaortic stenosis and is usually associated with hypoplasia, coarctation, or interruption of the aortic arch.

Secondary cardiopulmonary effects

Nonrestrictive defects are attended by the equalization of pressures within the two ventricles in conjunction with prominent right ventricular hypertrophy. The direction of the shunt is determined not by the ventricular compliance but by the levels of pulmonary and systemic vascular resistance. Thus, in the presence of relatively low pulmonary vascular resistance, the shunt is from left to right; if obstructive pulmonary vascular disease develops, shunt reversal, and hence peripheral cyanosis, will occur. The secondary cardiac effects consist of pressure and volume hypertrophy of the right ventricle, dilatation of the pulmonary valve and pulmonary arteries, volume hypertrophy of the left atrium and left ventricle, mild dilatation of the mitral valve, and pressure hypertrophy of the right atrium.

In the setting of a large and unoperated ventricular septal defect, the pulmonary vascular bed is exposed to an increase in both flow and pressure. A persistent elevation in pulmonary artery pressure is not well tolerated and is associated with the development of plexogenic disease, with the appearance of grade 1 and 2 lesions during the first 2 years of life.[62,63] In contrast to patients with atrial septal defects, those with large ventricular septal defects are at a high risk for the development of irreversible pulmonary hypertension during childhood. Virtually all such patients who do not die of heart failure or infective endocarditis will eventually succumb to the ravages of plexogenic pulmonary hypertension, usually during the third or fourth decade of life.

The natural history of a ventricular septal defect is influenced by the size and location of the defect and by the presence of other cardiac anomalies. For those subjects with large defects that do not close spontaneously and are not closed surgically, death occurring during infancy generally results from congestive heart failure or recurrent pneumonias, whereas death in young adults is most commonly the result of irreversible pulmonary hypertension. Infective endocarditis, usually resulting from *Streptococcus viridans* or *Staphylococcus aureus,* is most frequently associated with small defects and tends to affect men older than 20 years.[64]

Pathology of interventions

Surgical closure is recommended for the treatment of ventricular septal defects that neither decrease in size nor close spontaneously. Most are membranous defects, and most are repaired with a synthetic patch. With time the patch acquires a neoendocardium that may contain mural thrombus or calcium. The most frequent complication is a residual shunt, although fewer than 5% of these require reoperation.[5,17] Other complications include conduction disturbances, ventricular arrhythmias, and aortic or tricuspid regurgitation.[65] For children undergoing surgical closure between 6 and 12 months of age, the likelihood of progressive and irreversible plexogenic pulmonary hypertension developing is essentially nil.

The surgical mortality is less than 1% for infants with isolated defects and about 10% overall.[5] Early postoperative deaths usually result from acute heart failure, whereas late deaths are often sudden and associated with residual pulmonary hypertension or ventricular arrhythmias. Recently, ventricular septal defects have been closed by nonsurgical means using a clamshell device.[66]

For patients with a restrictive defect and other cardiac malformations, the surgical repair may entail enlarging rather than closing the defect. Examples include the Rastelli type of repair for patients with complete transposition or a double outlet right ventricle and the Fontan operation for patients with tricuspid atresia or a double inlet left ventricle and origin of the aorta from a hypoplastic right ventricle. Potential surgical complications include damage to the atrioventricular conduction tissues and injury to the ventricular free wall or overlying epicardial coronary arteries.[17]

Ventriculoarterial septal defect

In a sense ventriculoarterial (conotruncal) septal defects are analogous to atrioventricular septal defects (see Fig. 46-6). They are characterized by a large defect and by a common truncal valve. The valve in turn empties into a persistent truncal artery (truncus arteriosus), which is also the name for the entire malformation. This entity is discussed in detail in the section dealing with conotruncal anomalies.

Aortopulmonary septal defect

An aortopulmonary septal defect consists of an anomalous communication between the ascending aorta and the pulmonary trunk (see Fig. 46-6). Synonyms for it include *aortopulmonary window* and others (see Appendix 46-2).

General features

The defect is large in about 90% of the cases, and it may occur proximally (near the semilunar valves) or distally (near the origin of the right pulmonary artery). It is an isolated lesion in about 50% of the patients. In the remainder it is most commonly associated with aortic obstruction stemming from coarctation, hypoplasia, or an interrupted arch that is unrelated to the DiGeorge's syndrome.[67] In some patients the right pulmonary artery originates from the ascending aorta; in others a coronary artery arises from the pulmonary trunk. Other anomalies that may accompany the defect include tetralogy of Fallot, pulmonary atresia, a bicuspid aortic valve, a ventricular septal defect, subaortic stenosis, a right aortic arch, a patent ductal artery, and an atrial septal defect.

Secondary cardiopulmonary effects

As with ventricular septal defects, the shunt is initially directed from left to right. This results in volume hypertrophy of the left ventricle and dilatation of the pulmonary circulation and left atrium. Aortopulmonary septal defects generally produce severe heart failure during infancy and, if surgical treatment is not instituted, lead to intractable heart failure or irreversible pulmonary hypertension.

Pathology of interventions

Because such defects rarely close spontaneously, most are repaired during the first year of life using a transaortic approach. Large defects are repaired with a patch of Dacron or pericardium. Care is taken to not injure the semilunar valves and the coronary ostiums. In general the surgical mortality is less than 5%, although it is increased for infants with obstructive aortic lesions and for patients with appreciable pulmonary hypertension.[68]

Patent ductal artery

During fetal life the ductal artery provides an avenue for blood to flow between the right ventricle and the systemic circulation. Because this communication is unnecessary postnatally, it functionally closes within 24 hours of a full-term birth. This is a result of the higher oxygen tension in the ductal blood than was present prenatally. Anatomic ductal closure is generally accomplished within 2 to 8 weeks after birth and is accompanied by proliferation and fibroelastic thickening of intimal pads, luminal thrombosis, and eventually, calcification.[69,70]

Persistent postnatal patency of the ductal artery is observed more frequently in babies born at high altitude than at sea level and in premature infants than in full-term infants. With the exception of premature infants, if the ductal artery has not closed by 3 months of age, it is unlikely to close thereafter. A patent ductal artery may be an isolated anomaly or associated with other cardiac malformations. Though usually sporadic, it can also be familial or related to the postrubella syndrome.

In the presence of a left aortic arch, the term *ductal artery* implies the left ductal artery (that is, the vessel connecting the undersurface of the aortic arch to the proximal left pulmonary artery) (see Fig. 46-6). The right ductal artery, which normally involutes during embryologic development, connects the proximal right subclavian artery to the right pulmonary artery. In the setting of a mirror-image right aortic arch, a persistent patent

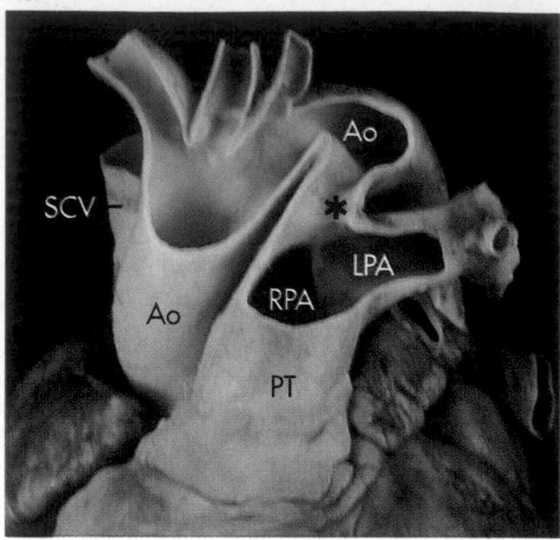

Fig. 46-10 Patent ductal artery (*) in an adult with plexogenic pulmonary hypertension.

ductal artery is as likely to be right-sided as left-sided. Finally, congenital absence of the ductal artery occurs among some patients with tetralogy of Fallot or persistent truncal artery.

General features

A patent ductal artery is an isolated anomaly in about 75% of infants and almost all adults (Fig. 46-10). Coexistent lesions, when present, include atrial or ventricular septal defects, conotruncal anomalies, and valvular or vascular obstructions. Persistent ductal arteries vary considerably in size and shape; they can be short or long, conical or tubular, or involved by single or multiple constrictions.[71] In contrast to an aortopulmonary septal defect, the ductal artery does not involve the ascending aorta. Furthermore, as a nonbranching structure it also differs from the collateral arteries that form in association with pulmonary atresia and a ventricular septal defect.

Secondary cardiopulmonary effects

Because pulmonary vascular resistance is less than the systemic resistance, blood flow through a patent ductal artery is initially from left to right. This produces volume hypertrophy of the left ventricle and dilatation of the pulmonary arteries and left atrium. The development of plexogenic pulmonary hypertension occurs somewhat later in patients with a patent ductal artery than in those with isolated ventricular septal defects.[36]

Patients with a large unoperated ductal artery usually die in infancy of heart failure or pneumonia. In those with a ductal artery of moderate size, death generally occurs during young adult life most commonly from heart failure or pulmonary hypertension, although sudden death and fatal pulmonary embolism have also been reported in such patients.[17] Finally, patients with a small ductal artery are particularly prone to develop infective endarteritis during the second or third decade.

Pathology of interventions

Because the ductal artery is an extrapericardial structure, its closure does not require a pericardial incision. Ductal closure in premature infants is associated with a decreased frequency of necrotizing enterocolitis and is generally performed with a vascular clip.[72] In full-term infants and children, the artery is usually either ligated or transected and oversewn, whereas special procedures have been developed for adults with calcified ductal arteries.[5,17] In virtually all patients undergoing surgical closure before 2 years of age, the pulmonary vascular resistance and left ventricular size return to normal and the risk for infective endarteritis or endocarditis becomes no greater than that for the general population.

Postoperative complications are uncommon and are usually related to the existence of cardiomegaly or pulmonary hypertension preoperatively. Although pulmonary hypertension may persist after ductal closure in adults, it does not necessarily preclude a long survival. Other reported surgical complications include injury to the phrenic or left recurrent laryngeal nerve, paraplegia, aortobronchial fistula, and others.[17]

In premature infants the mortality associated with ductal closure is less than 1%, though about 20% will later die of disorders related to their prematurity. Excluding these deaths, the surgical death rate approaches zero for patients younger than 2 years and is less than 2% for adults.[5]

Among premature infants, closure of the ductal artery may be induced nonsurgically with indomethacin. Ductal closure can be accomplished in older patients by nonsurgical embolotherapy; however, the occlusion device is currently investigational in the United States and operation may be a less expensive option.[73] Complications are uncommon and include residual shunts, infective endocarditis, and hemolysis.

Patency of the ductal artery is necessary for the survival of patients with certain cardiac malformations. Examples of such defects include aortic atresia, an interrupted aortic arch, pulmonary atresia without collateral arteries, and complete transpositon of the great arteries with an intact ventricular septum. Nonetheless, ductal closure generally progresses in such patients, despite the likelihood of a fatal outcome. For these patients, treatment with prostaglandin E_1 is commonly employed to maintain ductal patency. However, after prolonged therapy degenerative lesions can develop that weaken the ductal wall.[69] If ductal closure is performed later, ductal hemorrhages or pseudoaneurysms may form and complicate the postoperative course.

CONOTRUNCAL ANOMALIES

Conotruncal anomalies share in common the abnormal development of their ventricular outflow tracts (Fig. 46-11). Most are associated with an overriding great artery, and one or both arteries arise from the contralateral ventricle in some cases. Many patients harbor a ventricular septal defect of the membranous or outlet type as well as valvular or subvalvular pulmonary stenosis. In contrast to the septal defects discussed in the previous section, conotruncal anomalies are frequently associated with right-to-left shunts and peripheral cyanosis. Detailed discussions of the various conotruncal malformations are available in recent textbooks.[1-5]

Tetralogy of Fallot

Tetralogy of Fallot is characterized by subpulmonary stenosis, a ventricular septal defect, an overriding aorta, and right ventricular hypertrophy. The hypertrophy is a secondary lesion, however, and not a congenital malformation. As a rule the ventricular septal defect is large and is associated with equal-

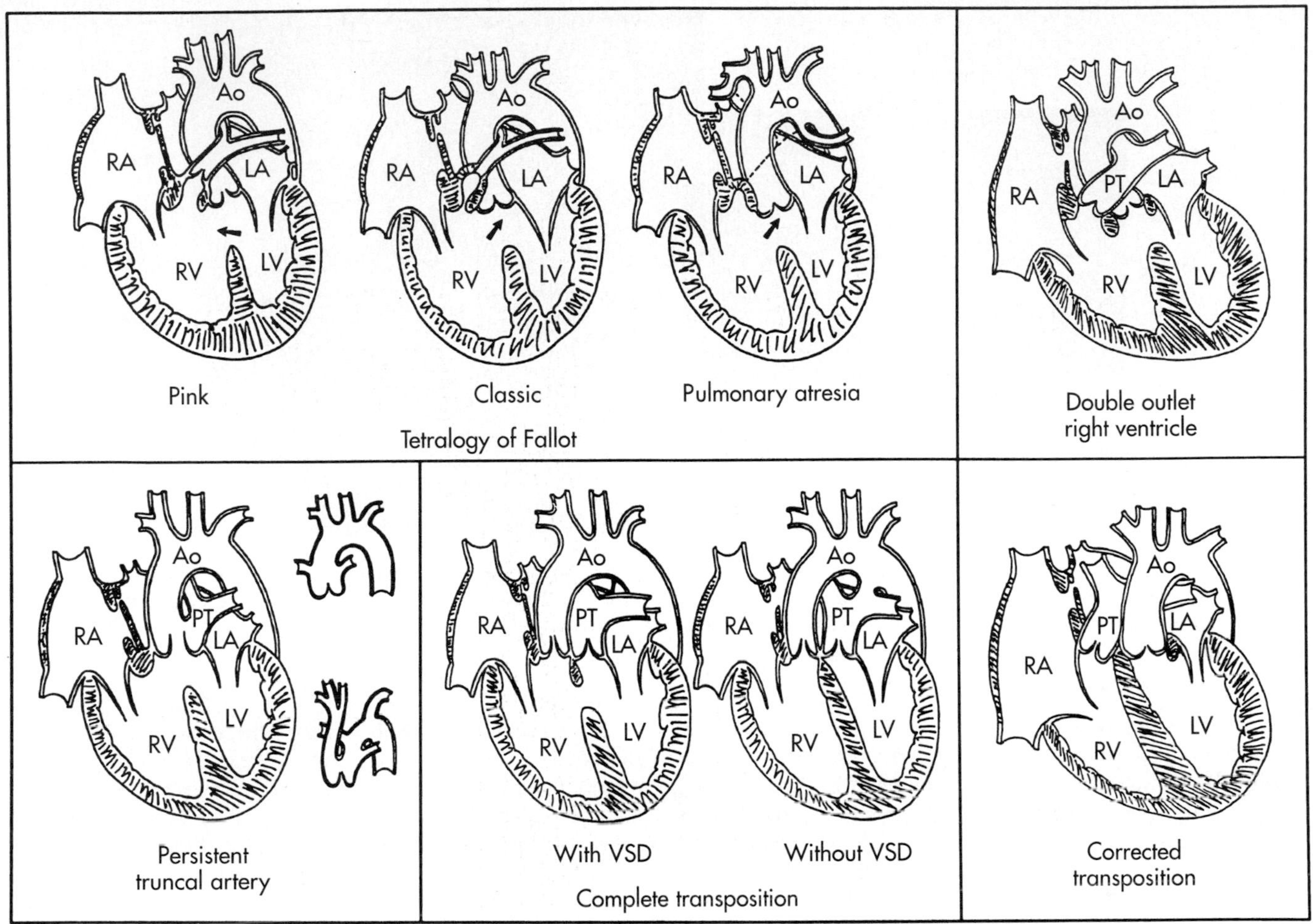

Fig. 46-11 Conotruncal anomalies.

ization of left and right ventricular pressures. Although the degree of aortic overriding is quite variable, it has little effect on the underlying hemodynamic state. Thus it is the extent of the subpulmonary stenosis that largely determines the clinical hemodynamic presentation of patients with tetralogy of Fallot. In fact any malformation that includes subpulmonary stenosis and a ventricular septal defect can produce clinical features that mimic those of classic tetralogy.

Tetralogy with mild stenosis behaves like an isolated large ventricular septal defect with a left-to-right shunt (so-called pink tetralogy). Much more frequently, however, the subpulmonary stenosis is moderate or severe and is associated with a right-to-left shunt and peripheral cyanosis (classic tetralogy). In fact Fallot's tetralogy is the most common form of cyanotic congenital heart disease (see Table 46-1). Its most severe variant, which includes pulmonary atresia, often exhibits a complex pulmonary blood supply, and this defect is discussed as a separate entity in the next section.

Embryologically, anterosuperior and leftward displacement of the infundibular septum results not only in the development of subpulmonary stenosis, but also in the production of a malalignment ventricular septal defect and an overriding aorta. Thus each of the characteristic abnormalities that occur in tetralogy can be attributed to a single malformation.[74]

General features

Insertion of the outlet septum anterior to the superior limb of the septal band represents the morphologic hallmark of tetralogy of Fallot and serves to distinguish it from the entity known as a *double outlet right ventricle.* Pulmonary blood flow can be obstructed at one or more levels along the right ventricular outflow tract, from its orifice (ostium infundibuli) to the pulmonary valve (Fig. 46-12). The outflow tract often forms an infundibular chamber that varies from ellipsoid to tubular, is longer than it is in normal hearts, and is generally lined by thickened endocardium.[75] Microscopically, myocytes appear hypertrophied and exhibit myofiber disarray, a feature that should not be misinterpreted as hypertrophic cardiomyopathy in surgical or autopsy specimens. Hypertrophied myocytes, as well as autonomic factors, constitute the morphologic abnormality responsible for the dynamic outflow tract obstruction.[76]

The pulmonary valve characteristically exhibits annular hypoplasia, dysplastic cuspid thickening, and in about half of the cases, bicuspid morphology.[77] Consequently the valve also represents a site of stenosis, which can worsen over time as the patient grows. In some patients stenosis is transformed into atresia as the result of fibrosis, thrombosis, or endocarditis. There is a direct relationship between the severity of pul-

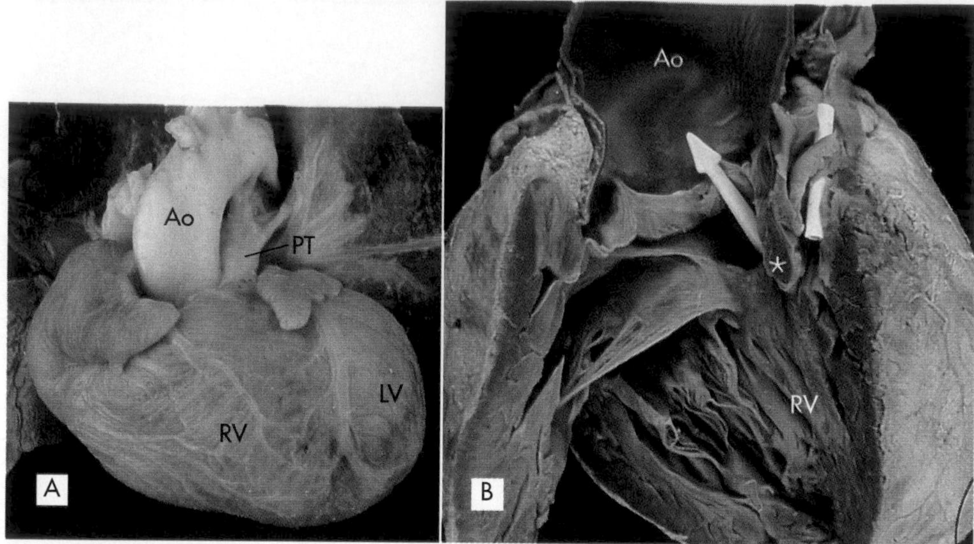

Fig. 46-12 Tetralogy of Fallot. **A,** Hypoplastic pulmonary trunk and enlarged ascending aorta (anterior view). **B,** Displaced outlet septum (*) with subpulmonary stenosis *(probe),* a ventricular septal defect *(arrow probe),* and an overriding aorta (opened, hypertrophied right ventricle).

monary stenosis, particularly at the valvular level, and the degree of hypoplasia affecting the pulmonary arteries.

Rarely the pulmonary cusps are congenitally absent and associated with severe regurgitation rather than stenosis. This syndrome, known as *tetralogy with an absent pulmonary valve,* is generally associated with massive dilatation of the pulmonary arteries and with secondary bronchial compression.[42]

The ventricular septal defect is of the membranous type in about 75% of the cases and of the outlet (infundibular) type in the remainder. As a malalignment defect, roofed by an overriding aortic valve, it extends more superiorly and is generally larger than defects without malalignment. The aorta usually arises either predominantly from the right ventricle or approximately 50% of it arises from each ventricle (so-called biventricular origin). Thus the ventriculoarterial *connection* may be a double outlet right ventricle even though the *malformation* is tetralogy of Fallot.

Dextroposition of the aorta is a characteristic feature of tetralogy. There tends to be an inverse relationship between the diameter of the ascending aorta and that of the pulmonary trunk, and in patients with hypoplastic pulmonary arteries, dilatation of the aortic root may result in aortic regurgitation. In about 25% of hearts with tetralogy, the aortic arch is right-sided and exhibits mirror-image brachiocephalic branching. The ductal artery is congenitally absent in another 25%.

The oval fossa is the site of a patent foramen in 50% of the cases and an atrial septal defect in 20%, a condition known as *pentalogy of Fallot.* Coronary anomalies affect about 5% of the patients, and most commonly the left anterior descending or right coronary artery originates from the contralateral aortic sinus or coronary artery. Other associated anomalies include vascular rings, origin of the left pulmonary artery from the ascending aorta, a persistent left superior caval vein, and a complete atrioventricular septal defect (often in patients with Down syndrome).[52]

Secondary cardiopulmonary effects

In patients with the classic form of tetralogy of Fallot, pressure hypertrophy of the right atrium and right ventricle produces an enlarged heart with an upturned apex. The tricuspid and mitral valves are generally somewhat smaller than normal, and the aortic valve is often dilated. Although the left atrium and left ventricle are initially normal in size, if the cardiac anomaly is not treated surgically, substantial hypertrophy and dilatation will develop in both ventricles. In contrast, hearts from patients with the acyanotic form of tetralogy resemble those from patients with large ventricular septal defects.

Pulmonary perfusion is inadequate in patients with classic tetralogy of Fallot. The elastic pulmonary arteries (that is, from the level of the pulmonary valve to intrapulmonary arteries about 1 mm in diameter) are generally hypoplastic and thin walled, and the muscular pulmonary arteries distally are also thin walled. With time, especially in patients with polycythemia, in situ thrombus may develop and undergo partial lysis and recanalization to form delicate luminal fibrous webs. If adequate blood flow is established surgically, the elastic arteries will usually dilate, thicken, and approach normal size.[78]

Among patients with unoperated tetralogy of Fallot, the mortality rates are 25% at 1 year, 40% at 3 years, 70% at 10 years, and 95% at 40 years.[5] Natural history studies have documented that most deaths result from chronic heart failure, sudden fatal arrhythmia, infective endocarditis, or cerebral thrombosis or abscess.[17] Maternal death may also occur during pregnancy.

Pathology of interventions

Between 1945 and 1965 the natural history statistics just cited were altered dramatically with the advent of palliative shunts and reparative procedures. The purpose of creating a systemic-to-pulmonary artery shunt is to increase pulmonary blood flow and enlarge the pulmonary arteries in preparation for a reparative operation. Of the Blalock-Taussig, Waterston, and Potts anastomoses (see Table 46-5), the modified Blalock-Taussig is preferred because it is associated with the least serious complications and is technically the easiest to create and take down.

Currently the most commonly encountered complication is shunt failure resulting from thrombosis, kinking, or anastomotic stricture as the child grows.[17] Shunt failure is inversely related to patient age and the diameter of the shunt. Other complications are rare. The surgical mortality for modified Blalock-Taussig shunts is less than 5% overall and is significantly lower for patients with classic tetralogy of Fallot.[5]

Surgical repair of tetralogy is usually performed at 6 to 18 months of age and consists of closure of the ventricular septal defect and relief of the subpulmonary stenosis. This entails the performance of several procedures, including the take-down of previous shunts, patch closure of the septal defect, a right ventriculotomy, resection of infundibular myocardium, a pulmonary valvotomy, and reconstruction of the right ventricular outflow tract with an infundibular or transannular patch of pericardium or Dacron. The three most common causes of postoperative disability are ventricular tachycardia, occurring in 10% of the patients, residual subpulmonary stenosis, occurring in 10%; and residual ventricular septal defect affecting about 5%.[17] Right ventricular dysfunction and aortic regurgitation are late occurrences.[79] Other postopertative complications are rare.

The early postoperative mortality is less than 5%, and late deaths claim an additional 5% of the patients by 20 years after operation.[5,17] Recent results of repairs performed during the first few months of life indicate an even lower mortality. Risk factors for early death include severe annular hypoplasia, use of a transannular patch, multiple previous shunt procedures, major associated anomalies, and age younger than 2 months or older than 4 years. Early postoperative deaths are associated with acute heart failure in 50% of the patients and with diffuse alveolar damage in 25%, as well as with injury to the cardiac conduction system, a residual ventricular septal defect, residual subpulmonary stenosis, and other technical factors.[18,80] Overall, late postoperative sudden death occurs in about 2% of the cases and correlates with postoperative arrhythmias and persistent cardiomegaly. However, among those who survive to adulthood, sudden death becomes rare.[81]

Pulmonary atresia with ventricular septal defect

The combination of pulmonary atresia with a ventricular septal defect is considered the most severe form of tetralogy of Fallot (see Appendix 46-2), and occasionally it occurs as part of the velocardiofacial syndrome.[82] It is characterized by a malalignment ventricular septal defect, an overriding aorta, and the absence of a direct connection between the right ventricle and pulmonary arteries (see Fig. 46-11). The pulmonary blood supply, arising as it does from the ductal or systemic collateral arteries, is the most variable and distinguishing feature of this entity, and its embryologic derivation is complex.[83]

To clarify the discussion that follows, it is important to emphasize several general concepts and definitions. First, ductal and collateral sources may coexist in the same patient but rarely coexist in the same lung. Second, a single arterial source of blood supply to a lung is considered unifocal, whereas numerous channels constitute a multifocal blood supply. And third, central pulmonary arteries include those within the mediastinum but outside the lungs.

General features

The right ventricular outflow tract terminates as a short blind pouch in about 70% of the patients with pulmonary atresia and a ventricular septal defect, and is absent altogether in 30%.[84] Rarely only the pulmonary valve is imperforate. More commonly the atretic segment affects both the valve and a variable length of the pulmonary trunk (Fig. 46-13). In this setting, free communication exists between the right and left pulmonary arteries and the vessels are considered confluent. In contrast, if atresia extends beyond the bifurcation, this communication is lost and the central pulmonary arteries are nonconfluent. The distinction between confluence and nonconfluence is important surgically.

In most cases a cordlike structure can be identified grossly as the remnant of an atretic pulmonary trunk. In other cases, perhaps related to previous surgical dissection, no such structure can be found. Even so, microscopic examination of the tissues taken from the expected site of the pulmonary trunk may reveal a minute vascular remnant that differs from small muscular nutrient arteries by its distinctly elastic media.

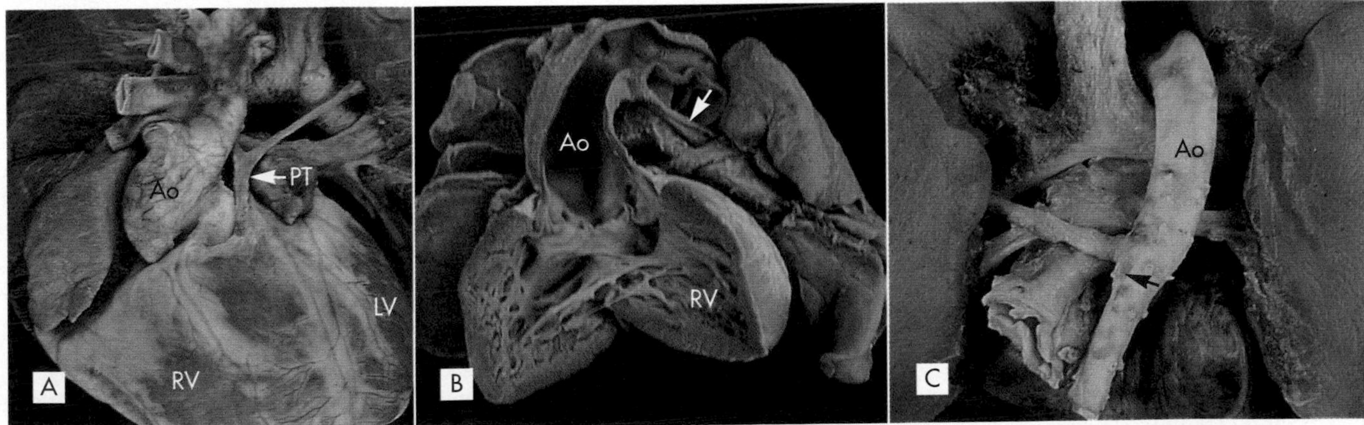

Fig. 46-13 Pulmonary atresia with a ventricular septal defect. **A,** Atretic cordlike pulmonary trunk *(arrow)* and dilated ascending aorta (anterior view). **B,** Ventricular septal defect (*), overriding aorta, and ductal origin *(arrow)* of the left pulmonary artery (opened right ventricle). **C,** Systemic collateral artery *(arrow)* arising from descending thoracic aorta (posterior view).

The caliber of the central pulmonary arteries is quite variable but tends to be nearly normal if unobstructed ductal or collateral arteries anastomose centrally or with the lobar branches. However, if multiple collateral arteries anastomose more distally within the lungs, the central pulmonary arteries will generally show moderate to severe hypoplasia. In addition, hypoplastic central arteries can result if the collateral artery that supplies them is focally stenotic.

When a ductal artery is present, it is unilateral and associated with confluent pulmonary arteries in more than 80% of the cases.[85] In this situation the arterial distribution to both lungs is normal and the central pulmonary arteries is of normal size because of the wide patency of the ductal artery during fetal life. However, the ductal artery is not a stable sole source of pulmonary blood supply and closes postnatally in 50% to 65% of the patients, necessitating the surgical creation of a shunt. In the remaining 35% to 50% it becomes stenotic and the pulmonary arteries progressively atrophy as the child grows.

When the central arteries are nonconfluent, the ductal supply to the ipsilateral lung is unifocal and its intrapulmonary distribution is normal. Only rarely are nonconfluent pulmonary arteries associated with bilateral ductal arteries. More commonly the ipsilateral lung is supplied by the ductal artery and the contralateral lung is supplied by multiple collateral arteries.

When the ductal arteries are absent bilaterally, the intrapulmonary patterns of blood supply are often quite complex. Each lung then usually exhibits a multifocal blood supply, coming from several collateral arteries, with a fragmented intrapulmonary arterial distribution (a so-called arborization abnormality). In such cases each collateral vessel supplies one or more bronchopulmonary segments. Collateral arteries anastomose with central pulmonary arteries in 40% of the cases and with intrapulmonary vessels in 60%. Within the lungs, loop anastomoses can form between collateral arteries, and these are not always detectable angiographically because of the competitive blood flow that obscures them. Accordingly, such cases require careful dissection at autopsy to document and clarify the morphologic patterns of blood supply to the lungs.

Collateral arteries arise most commonly from the descending thoracic aorta, less frequently from the subclavian arteries, and rarely from the abdominal aorta or its branches or from the coronary arteries. Their number varies from one to six, their diameters range from 1 to 20 mm, and focal stenoses occur in nearly 60%.[84,85] Although the central pulmonary arteries are confluent in about 65% of patients, they usually only supply a portion of each lung because multiple collateral arteries usually supply the larger remaining portions of the lungs.

Generally the aorta emanates predominantly from the right ventricle, although the degree of dextroposition is less than that occurring in classic tetralogy of Fallot. The ascending aorta is also dilated, a feature that contributes to the development of aortic regurgitation in adulthood.[79] A right aortic arch, observed in about 40% of the cases, occurs more frequently in the setting of pulmonary atresia with a ventricular septal defect than in any other form of congenital heart disease.

A fossa (secundum) atrial septal defect is present in 50% of the cases. Coronary anomalies are rare and include origin of the right coronary artery from the left aortic sinus. Other associated malformations include persistent left superior caval vein, an anomalous pulmonary venous connection, tricuspid stenosis or atresia, a complete atrioventricular septal defect, complete or corrected transposition of the great arteries, a double inlet left ventricle, and isomerism (asplenia and polysplenia syndromes).

Secondary cardiopulmonary effects

Grossly the cardiac chambers and valves resemble those seen in patients with classic tetralogy of Fallot. With time both ventricles exhibit prominent hypertrophy and dilatation. Among patients treated surgically during childhood or adulthood, the hypertrophy generally does not regress to a significant degree and persistent cardiomegaly is the rule. Microscopically, myocyte hypertrophy and subendocardial fibrosis are the morphologic abnormalities responsible for the decreased ventricular compliance.

In most cases stenotic lesions within the ductal or collateral arteries tend to protect the pulmonary circulation from constant exposure to systemic pressure. In some patients, however, hypertensive pulmonary vascular disease can develop in a region of the lung that is supplied by a nonstenotic collateral artery. Similarly, a ductal artery may occasionally remain widely patent and expose one or both lungs to systemic pressure.

The natural history studies conducted in patients who have pulmonary atresia with a ventricular septal defect have revealed that the mortality at 1 year is 50%, at 3 years is 75%, and at 10 years is 90%.[17] These statistics are significantly worse than those for classic tetralogy of Fallot. Death most often results from congestive heart failure, sudden fatal arrhythmia, infective endocarditis, or in adults, hemoptysis.

Pathology of interventions

The Rastelli-type repair has revolutionized the surgical approach used for patients with cyanotic congenital heart disease (see Table 46-5). In this procedure the ventricular septal defect is closed with an intraventricular patch that directs left ventricular blood into the ascending aorta, and an extracardiac conduit is then interposed between the right ventricle and the pulmonary arteries. Shunt procedures may first be necessary not only to relieve the peripheral cyanosis but also to enlarge the hypoplastic or atrophic pulmonary arteries to a size sufficient for a reparative procedure to be carried out, as discussed in a previous section (Tetralogy of Fallot).[82] For patients with multiple collateral arteries, staged procedures are often necessary to "unifocalize" the pulmonary blood supply to each lung.

Extracardiac conduits include cadaveric aortic or pulmonary homografts and Dacron tube grafts that contain bioprosthetic valves. Over time the calcification of homografts causes them to have an eggshell fragility, such that fracture and rupture may occur during the median sternotomy at subsequent operations. Cryopreserved pulmonary allografts appear less prone to calcification than do aortic homografts.[86,87]

Among the various potential complications of the Rastelli procedure, conduit stenosis is the most common and necessitates reoperation within 5 years in 5% to 10% of the patients. Calcification of the bioprosthetic valve, associated with the high calcium turnover in growing children, is the leading cause of conduit stenosis. Neointimal hyperplasia within the tube graft represents another source of obstruction. Taken together, valvular and neointimal stenoses account for about

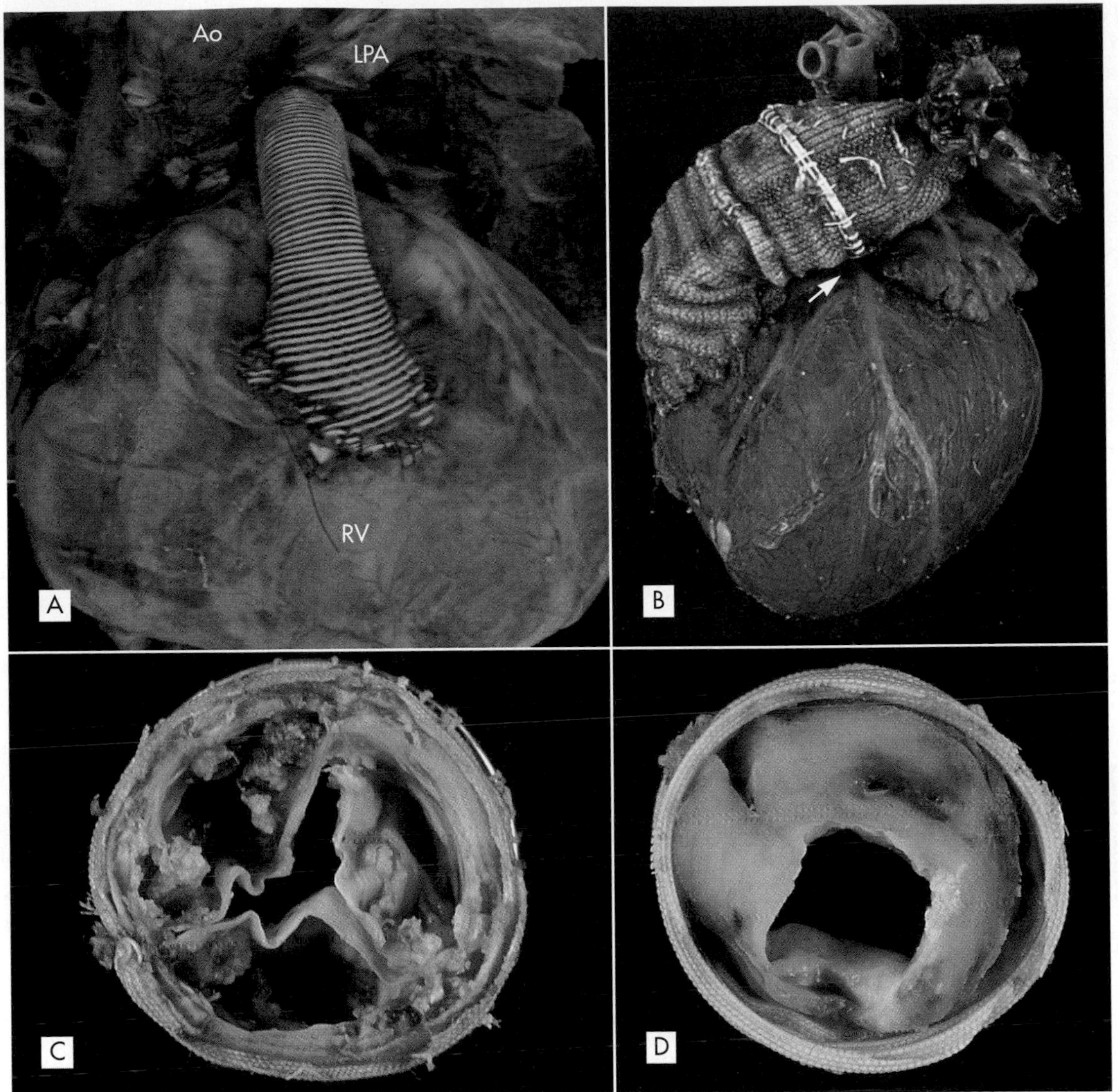

Fig. 46-14 Conduit repair of conotruncal anomalies. **A,** Rastelli procedure for tetralogy with pulmonary atresia (anterior view). **B,** Coronary compression *(arrow)* by metallic valve ring (left lateral view). **C,** and **D,** Conduit stenosis as a result of valvular calcification **(C)** and severe neointimal fibroplasia **(D)**.

90% of the obstructed conduits[88] (Fig. 46-14). Other causes include extrinsic sternal compression, the patient's outgrowing the conduit, and anastomotic stenosis, either proximally at the right ventricle or distally at the pulmonary arteries.

Conduit valves may also become regurgitant as a result of degeneration, and the causes include torn or flail cusps, thrombosis with retracted cusps, and infective endocarditis with perforated cusps. Finally the bioprosthetic annulus may compress an underlying coronary artery and produce myocardial ischemia or sudden death.

Postoperative complications related to the intraventricular patch can also occur.[17] Partial dehiscence may arise, necessitating reoperation to close the residual ventricular septal defect. In patients with restrictive defects that are not enlarged adequately at the time of operation, subaortic stenosis can develop and become progressively more severe as the patient grows.

Other potential complications include complete heart block, coronary artery injury, mediastinal infection, and progressive pulmonary hypertension. It is encouraging that the latter does not occur among patients undergoing operation before 6 months of age.[5] However, in most patients who undergo a Rastelli type of repair, some degree of residual left ventricular hypertrophy and dilatation, as well as diminished biventricular function remains.

The early mortality in patients with pulmonary atresia and a ventricular septal defect who undergo a Rastelli repair is about 10%, versus an overall rate of 20%.[5] Moreover, the early death rate appears to be lower in patients with homografts than in those with valved conduits. The most important surgical risk factors are the patient's preoperative functional class, the presence of small central pulmonary arteries, and the existence of multiple collateral arteries. Early postoperative deaths are usually attributable to acute heart failure, conduit compression, or sepsis.

Late postoperative deaths claim less than 10% of the patients and are usually attributable to chronic heart failure or sudden fatal arrhythmia.[5] Among patients undergoing reoperation for the relief of conduit stenosis, the mortality is less than 5% overall and less than 1% for those with no other complicating factors.

Double outlet right ventricle

The term *double outlet right ventricle* may be used to describe either a general type of ventriculoarterial connection (see Fig. 46-2) or a specific type of congenital heart disease (see Fig 46-11), but the two conditions are not synonymous. Unnecessary confusion can be prevented if the intended usage is clearly stated.

A double outlet connection exists when both great arteries arise by more than 50% from only one ventricle. Thus most cases of tetralogy also exhibit this type of ventriculoarterial connection. The feature that distinguishes tetralogy from the entity known as *double outlet right ventricle* is the site where the outlet (infundibular) septum inserts relative to the superior limb of the septal band. In tetralogy of Fallot the insertion is anterior and leftward, whereas in a double outlet right ventricle it is posterior and rightward (Fig. 46-15). The two disorders also differ in their embryogenesis.[74,89]

For the remainder of this section, the specific entity and not the ventriculoarterial connection is discussed. Even so, a double outlet right ventricle represents a widely diverse group of malformations that can be categorized further on the basis of the type and position of the ventricular septal defect, the position of the great arteries relative to each other and to the septal defect, the presence or absence of subarterial stenosis, and the presence or absence of other significant malformations.

General features

In most cases the ventricular septal defect is large and is cradled by the two limbs of the septal band (Fig. 46-16). The defect is also of malalignment type, and the position of the displaced outlet septum determines whether the defect is subaortic, subpulmonary, or doubly committed.[90] Most commonly the malalignment defect is subaortic and either membranous or outlet (infundibular) in type. Rarely it is small and restrictive, is absent, or is remote from the great arteries, as in the setting of a double outlet right ventricle with a complete atrioventricular septal defect.[52]

An overriding semilunar valve, with biventricular origin of its great artery, may also occur. The position of the ascending aorta relative to the pulmonary trunk is usually normal, dextroposed, or right lateral (the so-called side-by-side arrangement). Less commonly it is a right anterior or left anterior

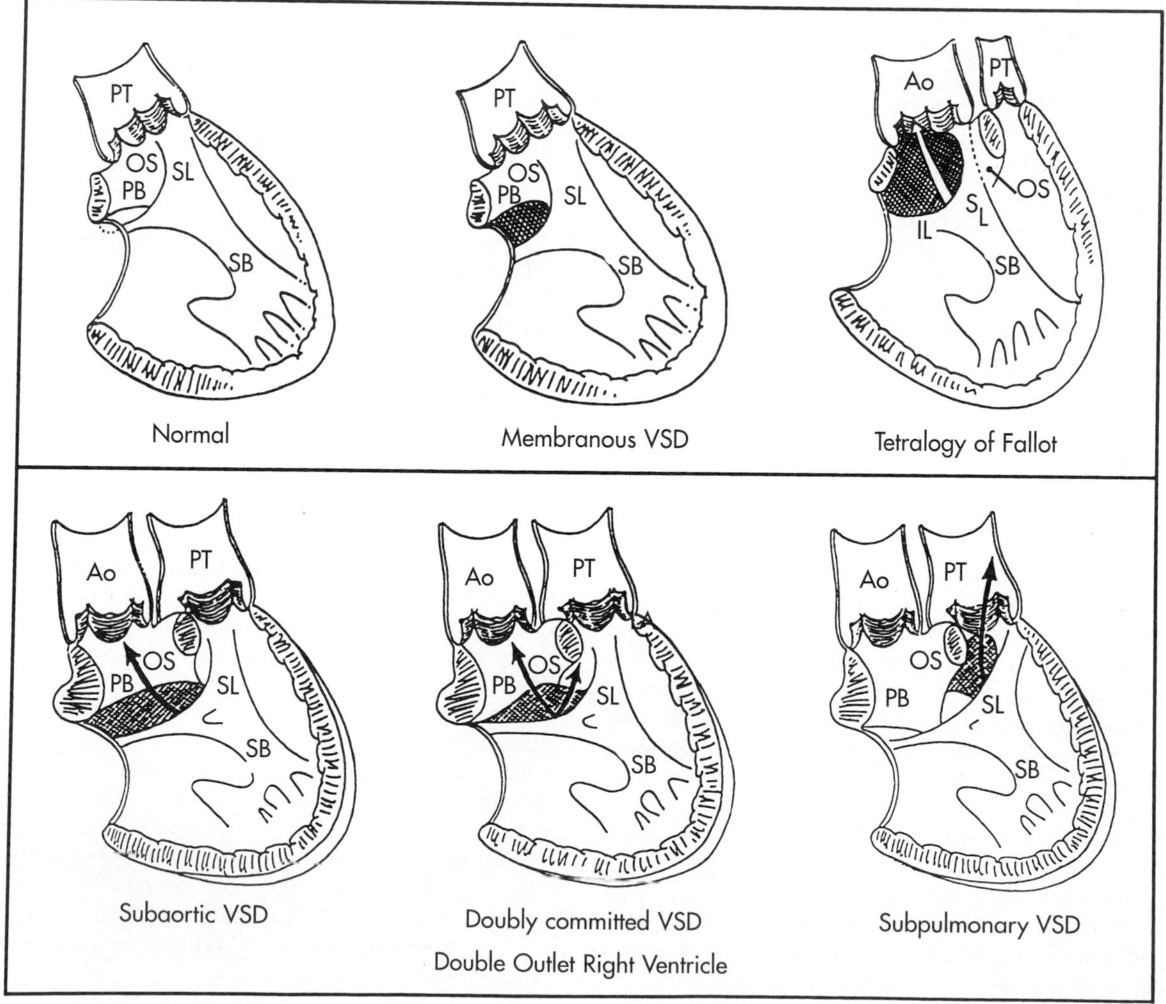

Fig. 46-15 Comparison of tetralogy of Fallot *(upper panel)* and double outlet right ventricle *(lower panel)*.

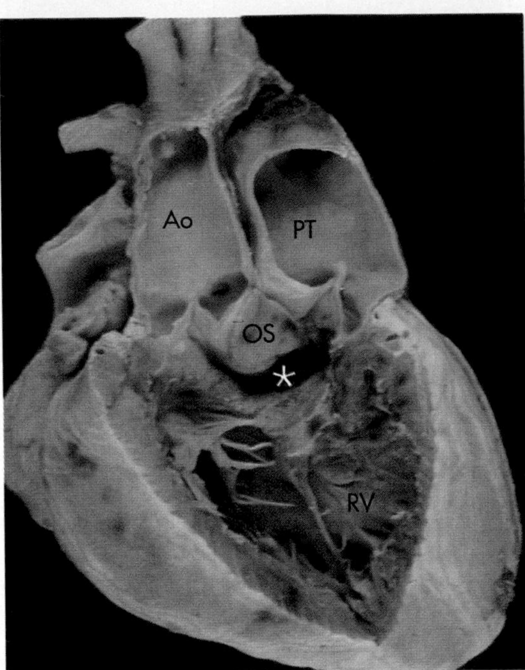

Fig. 46-16 Double outlet right ventricle with a doubly committed ventricular septal defect (*), with a portion of the right ventricular free wall removed (anterior view).

structure. However, regardless of the ascending aortic position, the aortic arch tends to be left-sided (that is, it travels over the left main bronchus).

Subarterial obstruction generally results from narrowing produced by the displaced outlet septum and is more often subpulmonary than subaortic in location.[91] Appreciable hypertrophy of this muscular bar may be associated with an element of dynamic outflow tract obstruction that can persist, or even first develop, postoperatively once the ventricular septal defect is closed and the right ventricular pressure decreases.

In many cases a ridge of myocardium separates the mitral and semilunar valves, in contrast to the direct fibrous continuity that exists between the mitral and aortic valves in normal hearts. However, this is not a constant feature and therefore is not pathognomic for hearts with double outlet right ventricle.

Anomalous origin of the coronary arteries represents a commonly observed additional malformation, particularly if the spatial relationship of the great arteries is also abnormal. Patients that have both a double outlet right ventricle and a complete atrioventricular septal defect often have other cardiac anomalies as part of the polysplenia syndrome. The combination of a double outlet right ventricle with atrioventricular discordance and dextrocardia constitutes the Mayo syndrome. Other associated anomalies, such as straddling mitral valves, are rare.

Secondary cardiopulmonary effects

The hearts of patients with a double outlet right ventricle exhibit right ventricular hypertrophy and right atrial dilatation. With time both ventricles may become hypertrophied and dilated. The risk of plexogenic pulmonary hypertension developing is low in patients with subpulmonary stenosis and high in those without.

The most frequently encountered form of double outlet right ventricle is characterized by a subaortic ventricular septal defect and subpulmonary stenosis. It resembles tetralogy of Fallot in terms of its morphologic and hemodynamic characteristics and its natural history. In contrast, in those patients with no obstruction to pulmonary blood flow, the chance of survival without surgery is similar to that in patients with an isolated ventricular septal defect. Finally, the natural history of a subpulmonary defect and an overriding pulmonary valve (Taussig-Bing anomaly) resembles that of complete transposition of the great arteries.[92] Other forms of double outlet right ventricle are rare.

Pathology of interventions

In patients with a double outlet right ventricle and a subaortic ventricular septal defect, a patch is sewn along the inferior rim of the defect to form an intraventricular tunnel that serves to direct left ventricular blood into the ascending aorta. Because the ventricular septal defect forms the opening into this tunnel, restrictive defects must be enlarged. Infundibular resection is performed when subpulmonary stenosis is present. In some cases reconstruction of the right ventricular outflow tract entails placement of a transannular patch or insertion of an extracardiac conduit.

Postoperative complications occur in 1% of the patients and most commonly stem from patch dehiscence or tunnel obstruction. The early mortality rate is less than 5% overall and about 10% for procedures employing an extracardiac conduit.[5,17] The actuarial postoperative survival is approximately 85% at 15 years. However, sudden death occurs relatively frequently in the late postoperative period and is associated with ventricular tachyarrhythmias or complete heart block.[93]

Persistent truncal artery

By definition a persistent truncal artery consists of a single great artery that emanates from the base of the heart and gives rise to the pulmonary, systemic, and coronary circulations (see Fig 46-11). A ventricular septal defect is almost always present. Synonyms for it include *persistent arterial trunk*, *truncus arteriosus*, and others (see Appendix 46-2). This anomaly may be familial or associated with the DiGeorge's syndrome.[94]

The morphologic features of pulmonary atresia with a ventricular septal defect can resemble those of a persistent truncal artery, particularly if the pulmonary trunk is atretic and cannot be identified. The distinguishing feature, however, is the derivation of its pulmonary blood supply from the ductal artery or collateral arteries, rather than from a truncal artery. These two entities also appear to have a different embryogenesis.[74]

Similarly, at autopsy, hearts affected by aortic atresia may bear a superficial resemblance to those with a persistent truncal artery. However, careful dissection will reveal a hypoplastic ascending aorta traveling beside a dilated pulmonary trunk and sharing a common adventitia.

General features

The manner in which the pulmonary arteries arise from the truncal artery varies considerably (Fig. 46-17). In about 55% of the patients a short pulmonary trunk arises and then bifurcates. In the others the right and left pulmonary arteries arise independently from the truncal root, and are close to one another in 35% and separated by some distance in the remaining 10%. These correspond to types I, II, and III, respec-

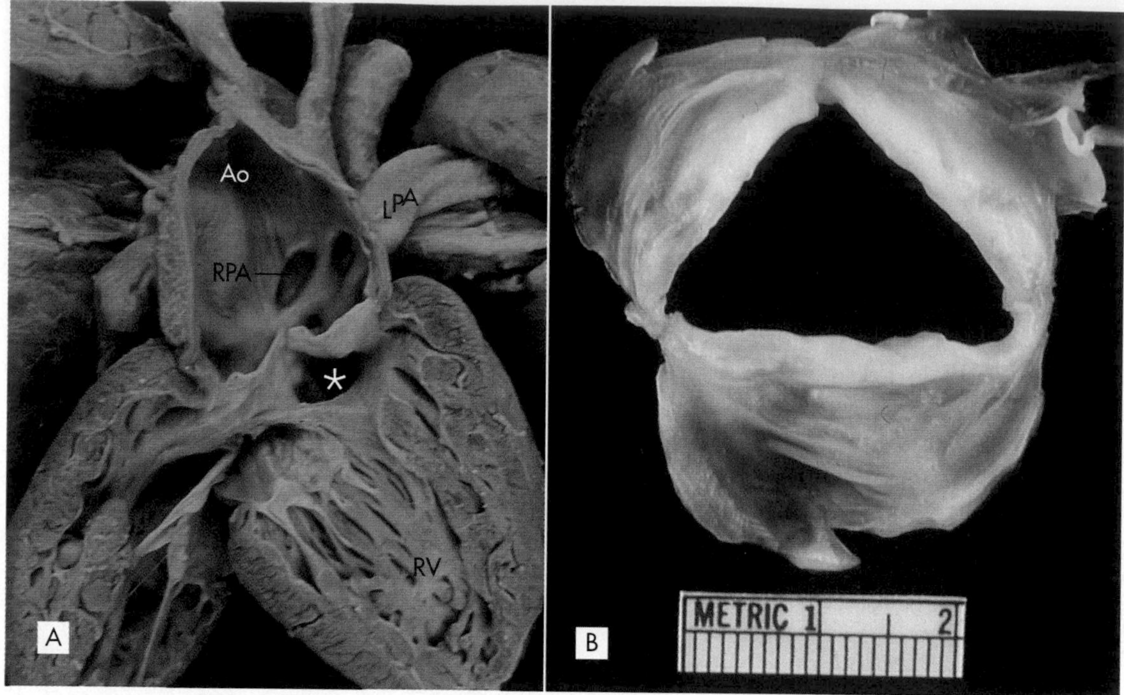

Fig. 46-17 Persistent truncal artery. **A,** Above the ventricular septal defect (*) the overriding truncal artery gives rise to the ascending aorta and both pulmonary arteries (opened right ventricle). **B,** Surgically resected regurgitant truncal valve, resulting from progressive postoperative "aortic" root dilatation.

tively.[95] Other classification systems have been proposed.[96,97] Unilateral absence (atresia) of one pulmonary artery occurs in 15%.

A right aortic arch with mirror image brachiocephalic branching occurs in about 30% of the patients with a persistent truncal artery. Interruption of the aortic arch is observed in 15%, is accompanied by ductal continuity of the descending thoracic aorta, and is frequently associated with the DiGeorge's syndrome. Otherwise the ductal artery is absent in approximately 50% of the patients. Infrequently the aortic arch is hypoplastic or associated with coarctation, and very rarely there is a double aortic arch.

Coronary artery anomalies are common and affect the ostial origin more often than the epicardial distribution.[98] Ostial abnormalities are observed in 40% and are important surgically. Coronary arteries may arise from the same truncal sinus, or above the sinotubular junction, or just above a commissure in association with a slitlike and functionally stenotic ostium. Rarely one coronary artery arises from a pulmonary artery. Abnormalities in the epicardial distribution most commonly involve a prominent conus branch from the right coronary artery or origin of the posterior descending branch from the circumflex artery (so-called left coronary dominance).

The truncal valve is tricuspid in about 70%, quadricuspid in 20%, and bicuspid in 10%.[99] Only very rarely is it pentacuspid or unicommissural. The truncal valve is in direct fibrous continuity with the mitral valve in all cases but with the tricuspid valve only infrequently. It overrides the venticular septum in approximately 60% of the cases, has a predominantly right ventricular origin in 30%, and arises primarily from the left ventricle in only 10%. Regurgitation can result from cuspid deformity, prolapse, and inequality in size; from commissural abnormalities; or from annular dilatation. The annular dilatation may also contribute to the development of "aortic" regurgitation as a late postoperative complication.[79] Truncal valve stenosis is rare and is usually attributable to nodular dysplasia of the cusps.

In the setting of a persistent truncal artery, the ventricular septal defect is usually large and of a malalignment outlet (infundibular) type. Thus it is cradled between the two limbs of the septal band and is roofed by the overriding truncal valve cusps. Infrequently it represents a membranous defect with an outlet extension. Only rarely is the defect restrictive or absent. Atrioventricular conduction tissues travel along the inferior aspect of the defect.[100]

Associated anomalies include a fossa (secundum) atrial septal defect, occurring in 15% of the patients; an aberrant retroesophageal subclavian artery, in 7%; a persistent left superior caval vein, in 7%, and mild tricuspid stenosis, in 6%. Other associated malformations, such as tricuspid atresia or anomalous pulmonary venous connection, are rare. However, extracardiac anomalies are found in 25% of the autopsy cases and include skeletal deformities, malrotation of the bowel, and hydroureter.

Secondary cardiopulmonary effects

A persistent truncal artery with a large ventricular septal defect imposes a pressure overload on the right ventricle and, with time, a volume overload on both ventricles and the left atrium, particularly if the truncal valve is regurgitant. Moreover, ventricular perfusion with desaturated blood flowing at a low diastolic pressure, resulting from runoff through the pulmonary arteries, leads to subendocardial ischemia within the first year of life. As a result, biventricular hypertrophy and subendocardial fibrosis can become prominent. Eventually poor ventricular compliance leads to biatrial dilatation. In adults, medial degeneration (so-called cystic medial necrosis) represents the microscopic counterpart of the truncal root dilatation that is observed grossly.

Long-term exposure of the pulmonary circulation to systemic arterial pressure results in the development of plexogenic pulmonary hypertension. High-grade irreversible lesions form more rapidly and to a greater extent in patients with a persistant truncal artery than in those with an isolated ventricular septal defect.[101] This is especially true for patients who are lacking one pulmonary artery because of atresia. Moreover, in the event of chronic truncal valve regurgitation, pulmonary venous hypertension may coexist with plexogenic disease.

The prognosis for patients with an unoperated persistent truncal artery is dismal. The mortality rates are 20% at 1 week of age, 40% at 1 month, 80% at 6 months, and 90% at 1 year.[5] Death usually results from heart failure or pneumonia. Among those who survive to adulthood, irreversible pulmonary hypertension is usually fatal in the third decade.

Pathology of interventions

Repair of a persistent truncal artery is generally performed during the first few months of life. Most commonly the repair entails a Rastelli type of procedure with insertion of either a synthetic conduit or a cadaveric homograft, though repairs without conduits have been described.[5] The potential complications of conduits are described in detail in a previous section (Pulmonary atresia with ventricular septal defect).

Early postoperative death rates are higher in patients with a persistent truncal artery than in those with pulmonary atresia with a ventricular septal defect, those with a double outlet right ventricle, or those with complete transposition of the great arteries. The rates are 15% overall, 40% for those who have undergone a pulmonary artery banding procedure, and about 65% for those with unilateral absence of a pulmonary artery.[5,17] However, early and late death rates of 10% are being reported for neonates without extracardiac anomalies who undergo operative repair within the first month of life. Causes of early and late postoperative deaths are the same as those noted for the Rastelli procedure.

Complete transposition of the great arteries

Complete transposition of the great arteries is characterized by ventriculoarterial discordance in the presence of atrioventricular concordance (see Fig. 46-2). Thus systemic venous blood travels from the right atrium to the right ventricle and into the aorta, and pulmonary venous blood travels from the left atrium to the left ventricle and into the pulmonary trunk. Synonyms for this anomaly include “d-transposition” and others (see Appendix 46-2). Several different hypotheses have been proposed to explain the embryogenesis of transposition.[15,89,102]

Because the systemic and pulmonary circulations are completely separated, a shunt must exist for the infant to survive after birth. The most commonly observed interatrial communication is a patent oval foramen, which tends to close after birth, as does a patent ductal artery. Thus the only stable shunts are large ventricular septal defects and less frequently atrial septal defects. For practical purposes, patients with complete transposition are divided into two categories—those with a ventricular septal defect and those with an intact ventricular septum (see Fig. 46-11). Those with an intact septum generally require the creation of a shunt within the first few days of life, as the ductal artery closes.

Left ventricular outflow tract obstruction is also observed relatively frequently. Thus there are four major categories of complete transposition of the great arteries, based on the presence or absence of a ventricular septal defect and subpulmonary stenosis:

1. Transposition with an intact ventricular septum (65%)
2. Transposition with a ventricular septal defect (20%)
3. Transposition with a ventricular septal defect and subpulmonary stenosis (10%)
4. Transposition with an intact ventricular septum and subpulmonary stenosis (5%)

Hearts with an intact ventricular septum and no left-sided obstruction have a thin-walled left ventricle, whereas those in the other three categories each exhibit left ventricular hypertrophy.

General features

In most cases of complete transposition there is a right anterior aorta with parallel great arteries, in contrast to their normally intertwined state (Fig. 46-18). Furthermore, the orifices of the two semilunar valves lie in the same plane, rather than positioned perpendicular to one another. Other arrangements of the great arteries are possible, including a right lateral aorta or a posterior aorta, but these are rare.

As a result of faulty development of the infundibulum, the ventricular outflow tracts are abnormal, and the outlet (infundibular) septum is skewed relative to the subjacent ventricular septum and the overlying great arteries. In about 90% of the cases a subaortic infundibulum (conus) exists, such that the right ventricular outflow tract represents a complete encirclement of myocardium, and the subpulmonary infundibulum is absent, such that the pulmonary and mitral valves are in direct continuity.[102]

Among patients with complete transposition, ventricular septal defects occur in 30% and, when present, are membranous in about 60%, muscular in 25%, outlet (infundibular) in 5%, and a combination of two or more defects in 10%. Restrictive features are observed in 40% of the cases of muscular defects but in only 15% of the membranous cases. At least half of the nonrestrictive defects are associated with appreciable malalignment of septal structures.

Malalignment in turn influences whether the ventricular outflow tracts become obstructed.[103,104] Anterior and rightward displacement of the outlet septum is associated with an overriding pulmonary valve and dynamic subaortic stenosis. Moreover, because of the decreased blood flow in the ascending aorta during fetal life, coarctation or interruption of the aorta occurs in most of these cases. Posterior and leftward malalignment of the outlet septum produces subpulmonary stenosis that may become dynamic and progressive with increasing age. The pulmonary arteries, however, are not hypoplastic because of ductal patency during fetal life.

Left ventricular outflow tract obstruction affects a third of the patients with a ventricular septal defect but only 5% of those with an intact ventricular septum, for an overall frequency of about 15%. Obstruction can result not only from malalignment of the outlet septum but also from the discrete or tunnel forms of subpulmonary stenosis, from a cleft anterior

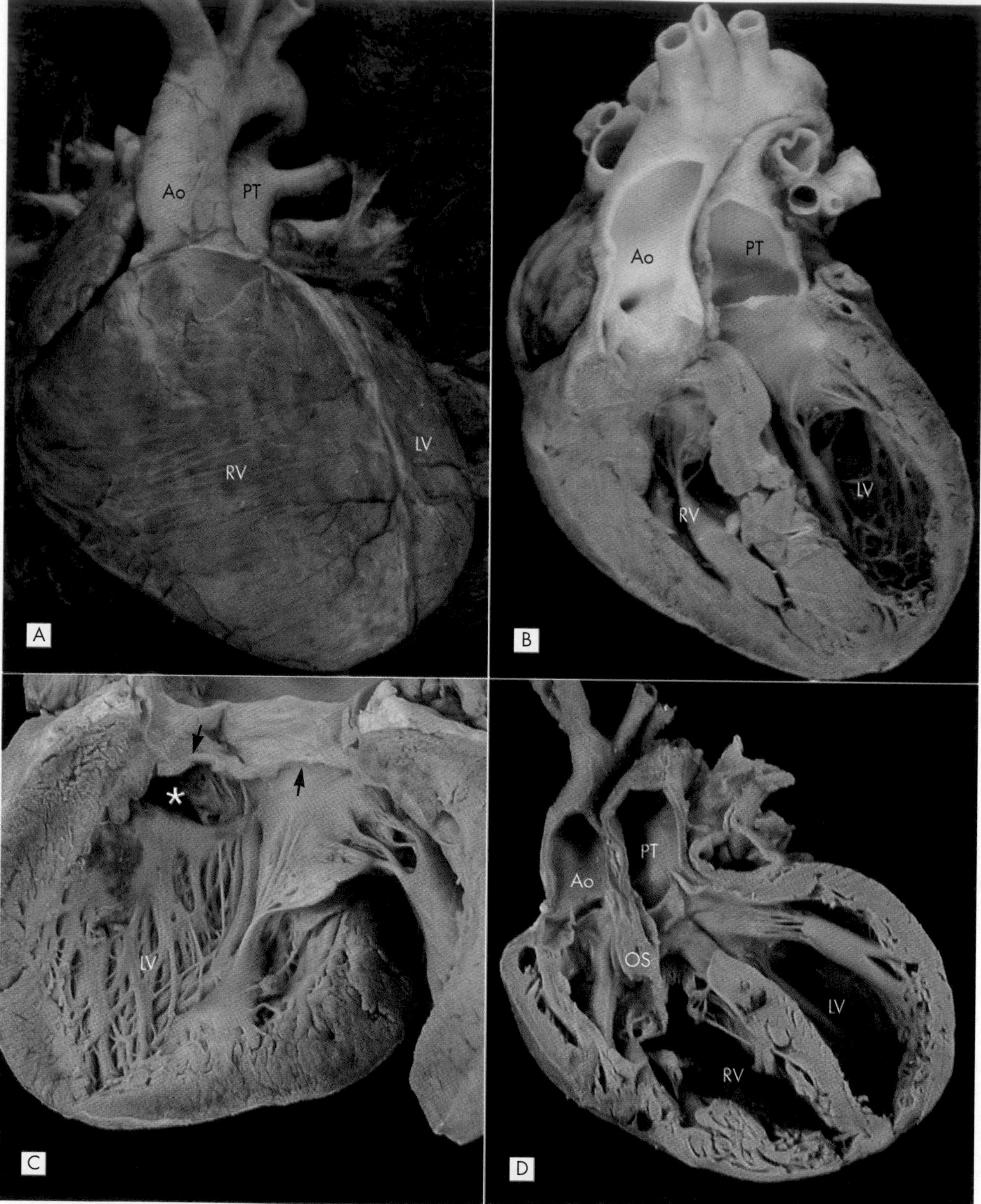

Fig. 46-18 Complete transposition of the great arteries. **A,** Right anterior aorta (anterior view). **B,** Ventriculoarterial discordance (long-axis view). **C,** Left ventricular outflow tract obstruction due to discrete subpulmonary stenosis *(arrows)* (opened left ventricle). **D,** Malalignment ventricular septal defect with an overriding pulmonary valve, considered clinically to represent a Taussig-Bing double outlet right ventricle (long-axis view).

mitral leaflet, from redundant mitral leaflet tissue, or from a straddling tricuspid valve.[105,106] Rarely, stenosis can occur at the level of the pulmonary valve, usually in conjunction with subpulmonary stenosis, and may be associated with a hypoplastic and dysplastic bicuspid valve.

Although right ventricular outflow tract obstruction is usually the result of a malaligned and hypertrophied outlet septum, abnormalities of the tricuspid valve can also contribute to its formation and may be important surgically.[107] In some cases, cordal straddling or anomalous cordal insertions into the outlet septum prevent a Rastelli type of repair from being performed because they interfere with positioning of the intraventricular patch that directs left ventricular blood into the ascending aorta.

The coronary arteries almost always arise from the two aortic sinuses closest to, or facing, the pulmonary trunk, with the right artery originating from the right-sided aortic sinus and the left artery from the left-sided sinus. This pattern, with the circumflex artery originating from either the left or right coronary artery, accounts for 90% of the cases of complete transposition.[108] Variations in this pattern are more common in patients with an aortic position other than right anterior. Even so, only 1% of the patients exhibit coronary origins that might preclude performance of an arterial switch operation, and in most of these the artery proximally travels within the aortic wall.

With regard to associated anomalies, a ventricular septal defect and subpulmonary stenosis occur with such frequency that they are used to subclassify patients with complete transposition of the great arteries. Disorders of the pulmonary, mitral, and tricuspid valves have already been described, as have subaortic stenosis and coarctation or interruption of the aorta. Other associated conditions include a fossa (secundum) atrial septal defect, which occurs in 5% of the patients, and juxtaposed atrial appendages, which affect 4%. These comprise the so-called *simple* cases of complete transposition. In contrast, *complex* cases include the existence of other major malformations such as complete atrioventricular septal defect, tricuspid atresia, mitral atresia, or a double inlet left ventricle.[52] The preceding discussion applies to simple rather than complex cases.

Secondary cardiopulmonary effects

In patients with an intact ventricular septum but without subpulmonary stenosis, the left ventricular wall becomes progressively atrophic as it assumes its postnatal function as a low-pressure pulmonary ventricle.[109] Although the left ventricular wall thickness is normal at birth, it will generally decline below the lower limits of normal by 3 months of age and will resemble the normal right ventricular wall thickness by the age of 6 months. Consequently, surgical repairs that recruit the left ventricle as the systemic pumping chamber are performed before the infant is 3 months old.

In the setting of transposition of the great arteries and a ventricular septal defect, there is volume hypertrophy of the right ventricle and pressure hypertrophy of the left ventricle. In the event of coexistent subpulmonary stenosis, both ventricles are hypertrophied and dilated. Disproportionate septal thickening may develop in patients with severe biventricular hypertrophy and resemble hypertrophic cardiomyopathy.

Regardless of the presence of a ventricular septal defect, the pulmonary blood flow is generally excessive, such that the pulmonary trunk is dilated and substantially larger than the ascending aorta. This mismatch in diameters may pose technical difficulties during the arterial switch operation. In many patients the bronchopulmonary collateral circulation is prominent; in some it may remain enlarged after an operative repair.

The pulmonary vascular bed in patients with complete transposition of the great arteries behaves like that described for patients with Down's syndrome and an atrioventricular septal defect. Plexogenic disease tends to progress more rapidly in these two settings than it does patients with isolated ventricular septal defects, and it occasionally becomes irreversible within the first year of life.[110] Severe pulmonary hypertension can even develop at an early age in patients with an intact ventricular septum and a closed ductal artery. In patients with complete transposition the ability of muscular pulmonary arteries to produce medial hypertrophy is impaired, such that obstructive intimal hyperplasia is the primary early response to elevated pressure.[111]

Natural history studies conducted in patients with transposition of the great arteries show overall mortalities of 50% at 1 month of age, 85% at 6 months, 90% at 1 year, and 95% at 5 years.[5] Thus, if left untreated, this condition is as devastating as a persistent truncal artery. However, the mortality rate varies depending on the associated conditions, and at 1 year of age is 95% in patients with an intact ventricular septum, 70% in those with a ventricular septal defect, and 30% in those with a ventricular septal defect and subpulmonary stenosis.

Pathology of interventions

The creation of a palliative atrial septal defect is usually necessary during the first few days of postnatal life in patients with transposed great arteries and an intact ventricular septum. The procedures for accomplishing this include transcatheter atrial septostomy or surgical septectomy, as discussed in a previous section (Atrial Septal Defects). Even with a septostomy, however, about 15% of the patients die before 3 months of age unless a reparative procedure is performed.

The reparative operations available for patients with complete transposition of the great arteries are both numerous and ingenious and include the Mustard, Senning, Rastelli, Damus-Kaye-Stansel, and Jatene operations[5,17] (see Table 46-5). The Mustard and Senning atrial switch operations entail the creation of an intraatrial baffle that produces atrioventricular discordance (Fig. 46-19). In contrast, the Rastelli and Damus-Kaye-Stansel procedures require a rerouting of left ventricular blood into the aorta and the insertion of a valved conduit between the right ventricle and pulmonary arteries. However, the best way of restoring near-normal anatomy is the modified Jatene arterial switch procedure. If these various repairs are performed before the patient is 6 months old, severe progressive pulmonary hypertension does not occur postoperatively.

Overall, the incidence of complications associated with the Senning operation is less than that with the Mustard procedure, and the early postoperative death rate is 10%. After the Mustard operation normal sinus rhythm is progressively lost in approximately half of the patients as a result of damage to the sinus node or its artery, and either supraventricular arrhythmias or atrioventricular conduction disturbances develop. Obstruction to systemic or pulmonary venous blood flow represents another potential complication, but its frequency has been reduced to less than 10% with the introduction of modifi-

dilated. The right-sided left ventricle shows volume hypertrophy in patients with a ventricular septal defect but exhibits generalized atrophy in those without a defect or subpulmonary stenosis.

Plexogenic pulmonary hypertension develops in the setting of a ventricular septal defect without coexistent subpulmonary stenosis. In patients with tricuspid regurgitation, the microscopic features of chronic pulmonary venous hypertension are also commonly observed.

Natural history studies have shown that survival into adulthood is common and that death is usually related to right ventricular failure.[115] Anything that increases right ventricular work load, such as tricuspid regurgitation or a ventricular septal defect, has an adverse effect on survival. The presence of a ventricular septal defect also adds the complication of pulmonary hypertension.

Pathology of interventions

The objectives of surgical procedures in patients with congenitally corrected transposition are primarily to close the ventricular septal defect, relieve the tricuspid regurgitation, and relieve the ventricular outflow tract obstruction. Risk factors for early postoperative death include preoperative heart failure, right ventricular dysfunction, heart block, and young age at the time of surgery.[116] Overall postoperative mortalities are 10% at 1 month, 20% at 1 year, and 25% at 10 years.[5] In contrast to the state of the right ventricle in complete transposition, the right ventricle in corrected transposition may function well as a systemic ventricle for many years, once the valvular regurgitation and congenital obstructions are relieved.[117]

SINGLE FUNCTIONAL VENTRICLES

Among the patients with congenitally malformed hearts there exists a group with only one functional ventricle. Within this group are two categories of hearts: (1) those with a univentricular atrioventricular connection, which can be of a double, single, or common inlet type, and (2) those with atresia or severe stenosis of a semilunar valve but with an intact ventricular septum (Figs. 46-1, 46-21). Although there is only one *functional* ventricle in such patients, the other ventricle is still present but hypoplastic. This is in keeping with the observation that virtually all human hearts contain two ventricles, regard-

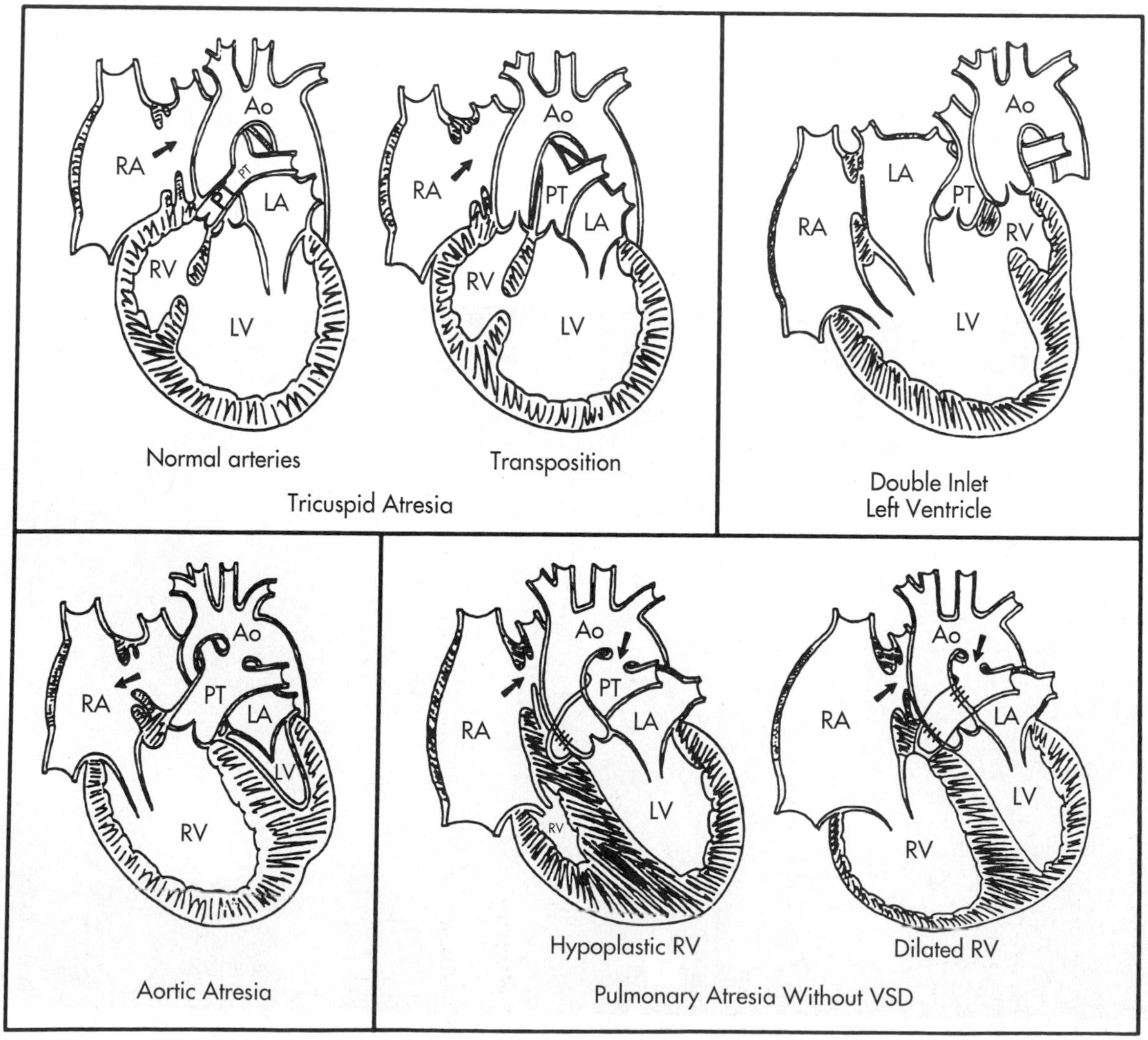

Fig. 46-21 Single functional ventricles. *Upper panel,* Univentricular atrioventricular connections. *Lower panel,* Atresia of semilunar valves with an intact ventricular septum.

less of the complexity of the underlying malformations. Thus the terms *univentricular heart* and *single ventricle* are anatomically inaccurate. A detailed discussion of this topic can be found in various textbooks.[1-5]

Because the functional ventricle must serve as the systemic pumping chamber and because the other ventricle is either too small or technically unusable as a pulmonary pumping chamber, most surgical repairs involve the creation of atriopulmonary or cavopulmonary anastomoses to deliver systemic venous blood to the lungs. Postoperatively, sufficient forward blood flow depends more on an adequate thoracic bellows action and low pulmonary vascular resistance than on atrial contractility. Thus a patient with appreciable coexistent scoliosis or pulmonary hypertension would not be a proper candidate for this type of surgical repair.

Tricuspid atresia

By definition tricuspid atresia is the absence of a direct communication between either atrium and the right ventricle (Fig. 46-21). Hearts may be further categorized according to their ventriculoarterial connection, which is usually either concordant or discordant, and according to the presence or absence of subpulmonary stenosis. An interatrial communication, a hypoplastic right ventricle, and in most cases a ventricular septal defect are part of the disorder. Anomalies of the musculoskeletal or digestive systems are present in about 20% of the cases. Tricuspid atresia may also be associated with Down, asplenia, or other syndromes. Embryologically the disorder is believed to result from obstruction of the tricuspid orifice by rightward malalignment of the ventricular septum.[15]

General features

Externally the heart is characterized by a hypoplastic right ventricle, as indicated by a rightward shift in the position of the left anterior descending coronary artery. In about 85% of the cases the right atrium can be dissected free from the underlying right ventricle, thus demonstrating that there is a true absence of the right atrioventricular connection[118] (Fig. 46-22). In only about 15% of the cases is there an imperforate valve between the two chambers in the form of a visible fibrous plug. The ascending aorta may be normally positioned or may constitute a right anterior structure. Only rarely are other aortic positions encountered.

Internally a dimplelike depression is present at the base of the right atrium but represents a remnant of the membranous septum rather than an atretic tricuspid valve.[119] The nearby eustachian valve is prominent in 40% of the cases. An interatrial communication, which is necessary to allow the egress of systemic venous blood from the right atrium, takes the form of a patent oval foramen in 80% of the patients, a fossa (secundum) atrial septal defect in about 20%, and rarely an outlet (primum) defect. The patent oval foramen becomes obstructive in 15% of the children as they grow.

A ventricular septal defect is present in 90% of the cases and is of muscular type in almost all. It typically occurs along the junction between the outlet (infundibular) and trabecular septums and frequently is elliptical rather than circular. As such the defect is restrictive in about 85% of the cases and often becomes even smaller over time. At birth there is a direct relationship between the size of the defect and that of the right ventricular chamber.

The ventriculoarterial connection is concordant in nearly 75% of the cases, discordant in nearly 25%, and double outlet or other in less than 5%. In those with a concordant connection, pulmonary blood flow is obstructed in 85% (stenosis in 75%; atresia in 10%) and a restrictive ventricular septal defect is the most common cause of subvalvular stenosis.[120] In contrast, in those with a discordant connection, pulmonary obstruction is present in only 35% (stenosis in 25%; atresia in 10%) and is usually caused either by a narrowed outflow tract or by accessory mitral valvular tissue.

Although the left ventricle is generally normal, the membranous septum is inapparent and the mitral valve is mal-

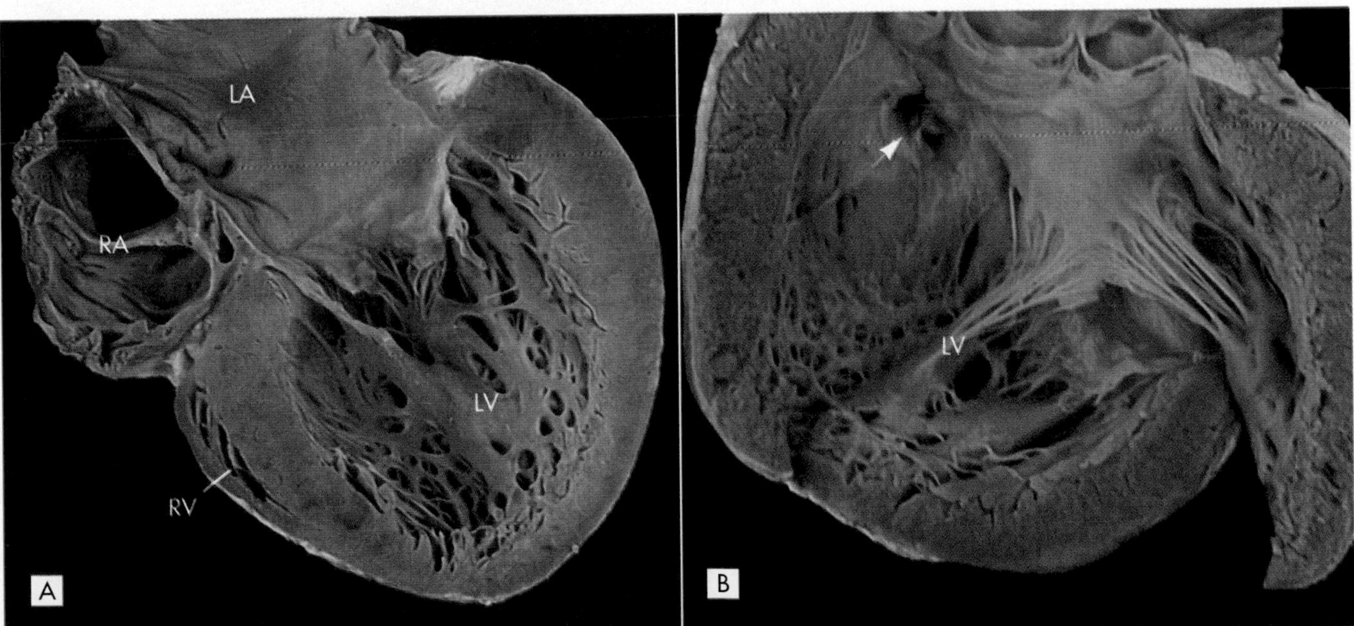

Fig. 46-22 Tricuspid atresia. **A,** Absent right atrioventricular connection with a hypoplastic right ventricle (four-chamber view). **B,** Restrictive ventricular septal defect *(arrow)* (opened left ventricle).

formed in half of the cases. Most commonly the valve has a cleft in the anterior leaflet, the cordal insertions within the left ventricle are abnormal, or there is cordal straddling into the hypoplastic right ventricle.[121]

In 35% of the patients with transposed great arteries and a restrictive ventricular septal defect, diminished aortic blood flow during intrauterine life leads to the combination of a patent ductal artery, tubular hypoplasia of the aortic arch, and coarctation of the aorta. The right ventricle is extremely hypoplastic in patients with coexistent tricuspid and pulmonary atresia, and patent ductal or systemic collateral arteries supply the lungs. Other associated malformations include a left superior caval vein, juxtaposed atrial appendages, a persistent truncal artery, and an absent pulmonary valve.

Secondary cardiopulmonary effects

The right atrium in patients with tricuspid atresia is both hypertrophied and dilated, and volume hypertrophy characterizes the left atrium and left ventricle. Annular dilatation is a feature of the mitral valve and may also affect the pulmonary valve if it arises unobstructed from the left ventricle. Although the right ventricular chamber is hypoplastic, its free wall is hypertrophied if the ventricular septal defect is nonrestrictive.

The likelihood of the plexogenic form of pulmonary hypertension developing in patients depends on whether pulmonary blood flow is unobstructed. If the relationship of the great arteries is normal, this condition exists in fewer than 15% of the patients. However, unobstructed pulmonary blood flow occurs in about 65% of those with transposed great arteries. Chronic heart failure and mitral valve anomalies generally lead to the development of pulmonary venous hypertension.

Among patients with tricuspid atresia and normally related great arteries who have not undergone surgery, the mortality at 1 year of age is 90% for those with obstructed pulmonary blood flow and 25% for those with unobstructed flow.[5] In contrast, among patients with transposed great arteries, the rate is 95% for those without subpulmonary stenosis and 50% for those with obstruction. Death in infancy is usually the result of severe systemic hypoxia, and later death is most often the result of left ventricular failure. Thus a shunt procedure or pulmonary artery banding is often necessary in infancy to ensure both adequate blood pulmonary flow and patient survival until a Fontan operation can be performed at an older age.[122]

Pathology of interventions

The Glenn cavopulmonary anastomosis (see Table 46-5) is recommended for older children with complex cyanotic congenital heart disease in whom a Fontan repair is not feasible and for younger children who will later undergo a second-stage Fontan operation. Complications are usually related to the nonpulsatile nature of pulmonary blood flow into the right lung and include preferential flow to the lower lobe and the development of pulmonary arteriovenous fistulas. Numerous other complications have also been reported.[17] The operative mortality is 3%.

Refinement of the Fontan procedure, with its many variations and modifications, has revolutionized the surgical treatment of patients with only a single functional ventricle (Fig. 46-23).[123] In general a modified Fontan atriopulmonary anastomosis is performed when patients are about 2 years old. Complications are related primarily to the to-and-fro blood flow in a system lacking a pumping chamber or valves. Ascites

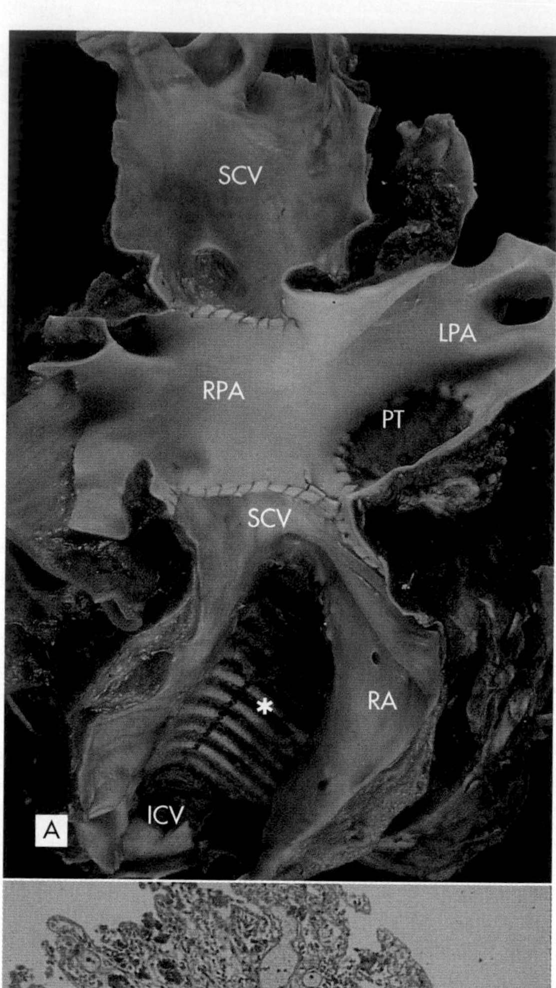

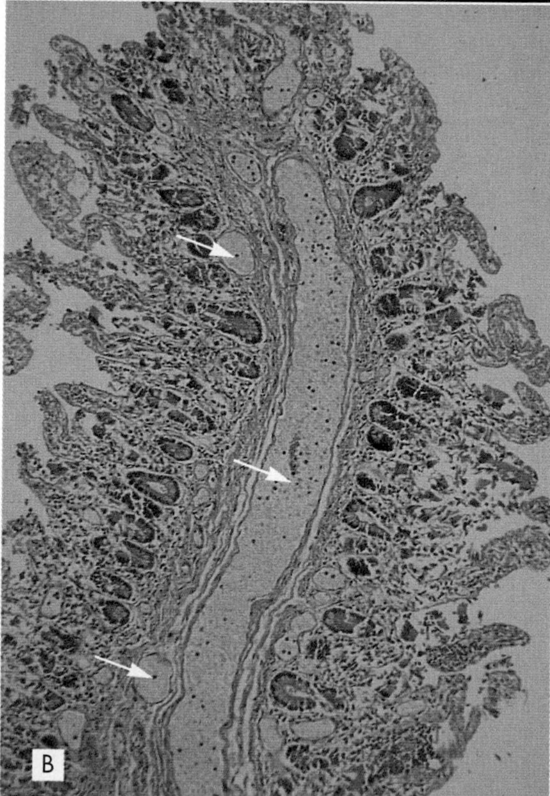

Fig. 46-23 Modified Fontan operation for single functional ventricle. **A,** Intra-atrial conduit (*) and a bidirectional cavopulmonary anastomosis. **B,** Dilated lymphatics *(arrows)* in the small bowel, associated with a postoperative protein-losing enteropathy.

and edema occur in 15% of the patients and may be accompanied by a chylothorax. In addition, caval and hepatic venous reflux can cause impaired liver function, dilated enteric lymphatics, and a protein-losing enteropathy. Right atrial stasis may result in obstructive mural thrombus, and patch dehiscence is usually associated with the development of an interatrial shunt. Recurrent ventricular tachycardia can also occur.

The hospital mortality is less than 10% among patients with tricuspid atresia, in contrast to the 25% rate in patients with the asplenia syndrome (right isomerism), and the late mortality is an additional 15%.[5] In general the surgical risk factors for a modified Fontan operation include anomalies other than tricuspid atresia, atrioventricular valve dysfunction, ventricular dysfunction or pronounced hypertrophy, asplenia or polysplenia syndromes, a previous pulmonary artery banding procedure, and pulmonary hypertension.[124,125] Postoperative death usually results from chronic heart failure, persistent fluid accumulation, reoperation, infection, arrhythmias, or a protein-losing enteropathy.[17] Arrhythmic deaths may be sudden.

Double inlet left ventricle

Hearts with a single inlet connection include tricuspid atresia, which is discussed in the previous section, and mitral atresia, which is beyond the scope of this chapter. Hearts with a common inlet connection often have a dominant right ventricle, from which both great arteries arise, and a markedly hypoplastic left ventricle along the posteroinferior aspect of the heart. Common inlet ventricles are rare and are often a part of the asplenia or polysplenia syndrome.

At least 75% of the hearts with a double inlet connection have a prominent left ventricle and a hypoplastic right ventricle, which is located along the anterosuperior aspect of the heart and gives rise to at least one great artery.[126,127] The remainder of this section is limited to a discussion of double inlet left ventricles (see Fig. 46-21). Embryologically it results from malalignment of the ventricular septum, such that the tricuspid component of the atrioventricular canal and its ventricular inlet remain directed into the developing left ventricle.

General features

Externally, hearts with a double inlet left ventricle may resemble those with tricuspid atresia. Both anomalies have a distinctive hypoplastic right ventricle that provides an origin for a great artery and is bordered by the anterior descending and conus coronary arteries. Internally the hypoplastic chamber, like that in tricuspid atresia, consists primarily of an outlet (infundibular) component and an apical trabecular component of variable size, with virtual absence of the inlet portion in most hearts.

The ventriculoarterial connection is discordant in 90% of the cases, and the transposed aorta is a left anterior structure in 65% and a right anterior one in 35%.[127,128] In the setting of a right anterior aorta the pulmonary trunk arises from a normal (noninverted) left ventricle, whereas in the setting of a left anterior aorta the left ventricle assumes an inverted mirror image appearance, similar to that encountered in congenitally corrected transposition. In the remaining 10% the ventriculoarterial connection is double outlet, common outlet (persistent truncal artery), or single outlet (pulmonary atresia), or is concordant (Holmes heart).

The feature that distinguishes a double inlet left ventricle from either tricuspid atresia or corrected transposition is the presence of two atrioventricular valves that connect primarily to the morphologic left ventricle (Fig. 46-24). In most cases both valves possess a mitral morphology, one being the mirror image of the other, and both are associated with two sets of papillary muscles. Less commonly one valve exhibits a tricuspid morphology, with cordal attachments to the ventricular septum or straddling into the right ventricle. In about a third of the hearts one valve has a hybrid structure that is neither mitral nor tricuspid.[129] A cleft in the anterior mitral leaflet may produce appreciable regurgitation.

Direct continuity between the atrioventricular and semilunar valves establishes the identity of the main chamber as a morphologic left ventricle. Even so, the apical region may have a heavily trabeculated appearance, due to the presence of four sets of papillary muscles. The ventricular septum assumes an angled position, rather than its normal vertical orientation, and is grossly malaligned with respect to the atrial septum. The ventricular septal defect is usually muscular and elliptical, similar to that encountered in tricuspid atresia.[130]

There tends to be an inverse relationship between the size of the ventricular septal defect and that of the left ventricular outflow tract. Thus, subpulmonary stenosis occurs frequently in patients with transposed great arteries and a large defect, and this most often results from malalignment of the outlet septum, as well as from the presence of endocardial tissue tags. The pulmonary valve may also be stenotic. In contrast, subaortic stenosis is likely in patients with transposed great arteries and a restrictive defect, and may be associated with hypoplasia, coarctation, or interruption of the thoracic aorta.

As both the patient and the heart grow, changes in the sizes of various structures may bring about dramatic changes in the observed hemodynamic state. The ventricular septal defect frequently becomes restrictive over time as the result of progressive endocardial fibrosis along its rim, and ventricular outflow tract obstructions can also become more severe. Moreover, with ongoing annular dilatation and floppy changes, an atrioventricular valve may become regurgitant. Finally, heart block often develops in patients with inverted ventricles, as it does in those with corrected transposition.

Secondary cardiopulmonary effects

Volume hypertrophy affects the left ventricle and may become severe over time, particularly in the presence of a regurgitant atrioventricular valve. Microscopically, myocyte hypertrophy and interstitial fibrosis constitute the morphologic abnormalities responsible for reduced ventricular compliance. In such hearts intraoperative protection from ischemic injury can be difficult. Biatrial dilatation may develop with time as well.

As with tricuspid atresia, the likelihood of irreversible plexogenic pulmonary hypertension developing is increased in patients with unobstructed pulmonary blood flow who are older than 2 years at the time of operative intervention.[131] Regurgitation of the left-sided atrioventricular valve and poor ventricular compliance often result in pulmonary venous hypertension.

Natural history studies have revealed an overall mortality of 25% at 1 month of age, 45% at 1 year, and 55% at 5 years.[5] Early death is particularly likely in patients with subaortic stenosis, heart failure, or severe acidosis. In contrast, the mortality is only 10% at 10 years of age in patients with transposed great arteries, a left anterior aorta, and mild subpulmonary stenosis.

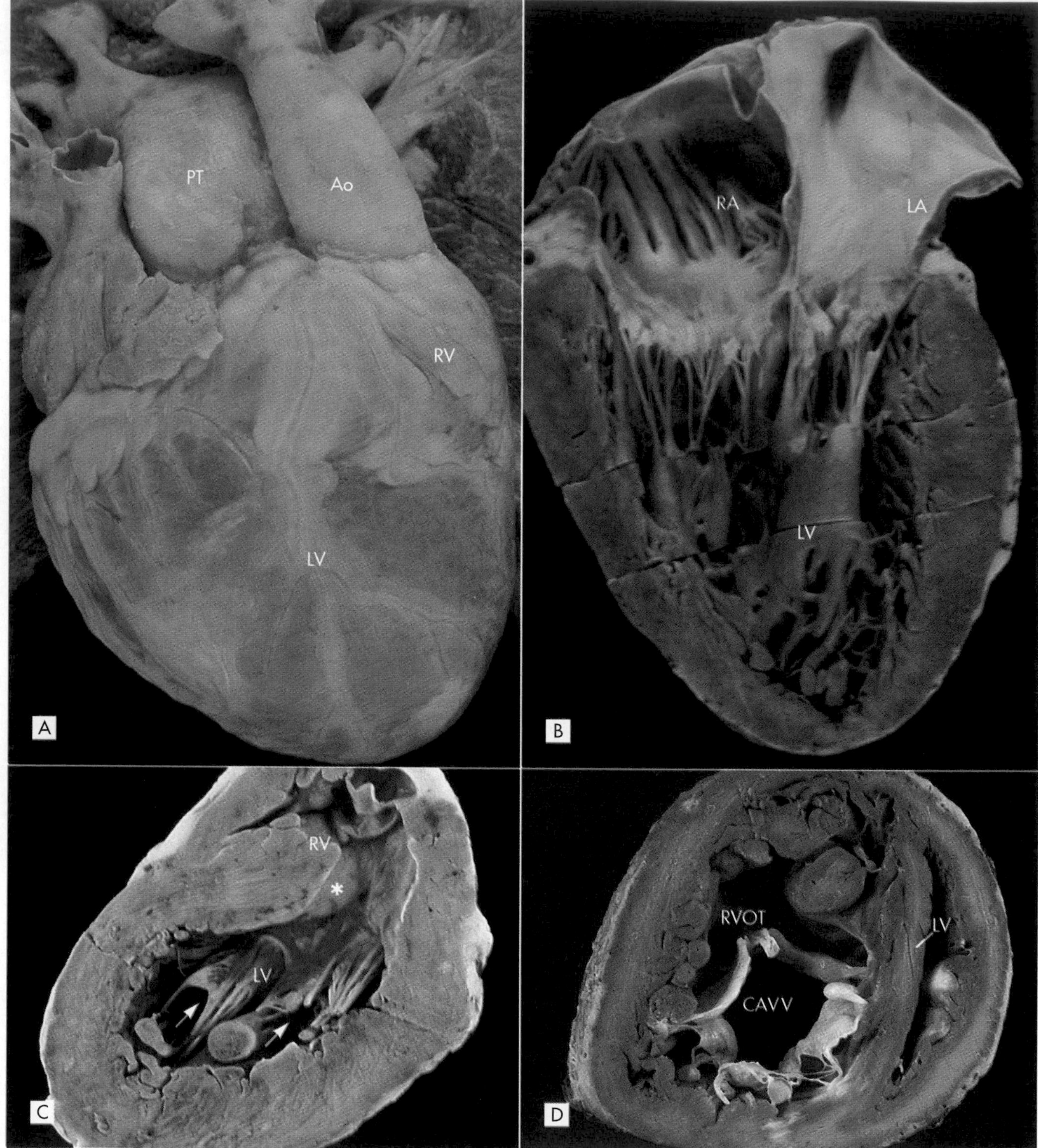

Fig. 46-24 Double inlet left ventricle. **A,** Left anterior aorta with a hypoplastic subaortic right ventricle (anterior view). **B,** Double inlet atrioventricular connection (three-chamber view). **C,** Hypoplastic right ventricle, large ventricular septal defect (*), and two atrioventricular valves *(arrows)* in the left ventricle (short-axis view). **D,** Common inlet right ventricle, shown for comparison (short-axis view).

Pathology of interventions

Among selected patients with favorable morphologic features, a synthetic patch may be used to divide the left ventricle into systemic and pulmonary pumping chambers. Complications from ventricular septation include patch dehiscence, the formation of a ventricular pseudoaneurysm, incompetence of an atrioventricular valve, and damage to the conduction system.[17] The postoperative mortality at 1 month is 35% overall but less than 10% for uncomplicated cases.[5] Hospital deaths are usually the result of acute heart failure, and late deaths are either sudden or occur at reoperation.

Palliative banding of the pulmonary trunk may be necessary to alleviate pulmonary hypertension in patients with transposed great arteries, so that a Fontan operation can be performed at about 2 years of age. However, when there is aortic coarctation, pulmonary artery banding is contraindicated because of the high risk of rapid obstruction of the ventricular septal defect and pronounced left ventricular hypertrophy.[132]

Most patients with a double inlet left ventricle benefit from a modified Fontan operation, the details of which are discussed in another section (Tricuspid Atresia). Among those undergoing such a procedure during early childhood, their left ventricular hypertrophy and dilatation tend to regress, and ventricular contractility improves.[133]

Aortic atresia (hypoplastic left heart syndrome)

Among patients with aortic valve atresia and an intact ventricular septum, the diminished left-sided blood flow that occurs during cardiac embryogenesis, perhaps related to premature narrowing of the oval foramen, results in hypoplasia of all left-sided structures from the level of the left atrium to the aortic arch at the level of the ductal artery[134] (see Fig. 46-21). Thus aortic atresia is virtually synonymous with the hypoplastic left heart syndrome. Postnatal survival depends on whether there are shunts at the atrial septum and ductal artery, and coronary perfusion depends on whether there is adequate retrograde blood flow in the ascending aorta. As expected, ductal narrowing heralds the patient's demise.

General features

Externally the hypoplastic left ventricle forms a distinct bulge along the left posterobasal aspect of the heart.[134] Because the ascending aorta and pulmonary trunk are enveloped by a common adventitia, the hypoplastic aorta may not be readily visible and the pulmonary trunk can be misinterpreted as a persistent truncal artery. Careful dissection, with identification of the origins of the coronary arteries, allows the two entities to be readily distinguished from one another. A ridgelike coarctation at the junction of the hypoplastic aortic arch with the dilated descending thoracic aorta, just opposite the patent ductal artery, is apparent in nearly 75% of the cases.[135] As the ductal artery begins to close, prominent longitudinal ridges develop along its luminal surface. The oval foramen is usually patent but restrictive.

If the mitral valve is hypoplastic but competent, high pressure is generated in the left ventricular cavity, and the only route of escape for the blood is through intramural coronary veins and arteries. Consequently the left ventricle has hypertrophied walls, a hypoplastic chamber, and secondary endocardial fibroelastosis of variable severity (Fig. 46-25), and the overlying epicardial coronary vessels may be enlarged and tortuous.[136,137] Mitral atresia occurs in about 35% of the cases and is associated with an extremely hypoplastic left ventricle. In contrast, a regurgitant mitral valve is associated with a somewhat larger left ventricular chamber and normal endocardium.

Secondary cardiopulmonary effects

The right ventricle and right atrium in patients with a double inlet left ventricle exhibit volume hypertrophy, and the tricuspid and pulmonary valves are dilated. Microscopically, right ventricular myocytes are hypertrophied, and the myocardial interstitium may be involved by edema or mild fibrosis. The pulmonary vasculature exhibits the characteristic features of pulmonary venous hypertension. Hepatic congestion may be associated with centrilobular (zone 3) necrosis terminally.

Death most commonly occurs within the first 2 weeks of life and is related to ductal closure. In those patients whose ductal artery remains patent, death resulting from right ventricular failure generally occurs within the first 6 weeks of life.

Pathology of interventions

The surgical options for patients with aortic atresia and the hypoplastic left heart syndrome are limited and include com-

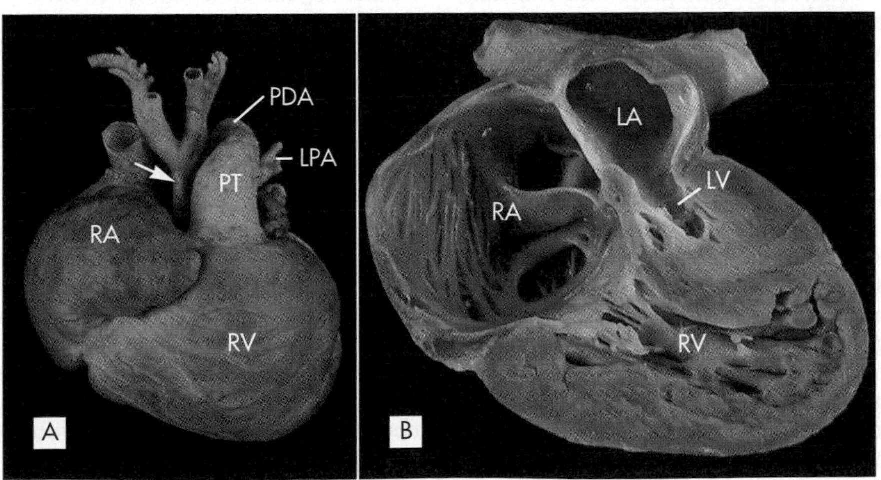

Fig. 46-25 Aortic atresia (hypoplastic left heart syndrome). **A,** Hypoplastic ascending aorta *(arrow)* (anterior view). **B,** Hypoplastic left ventricle and mitral valve (four-chamber view).

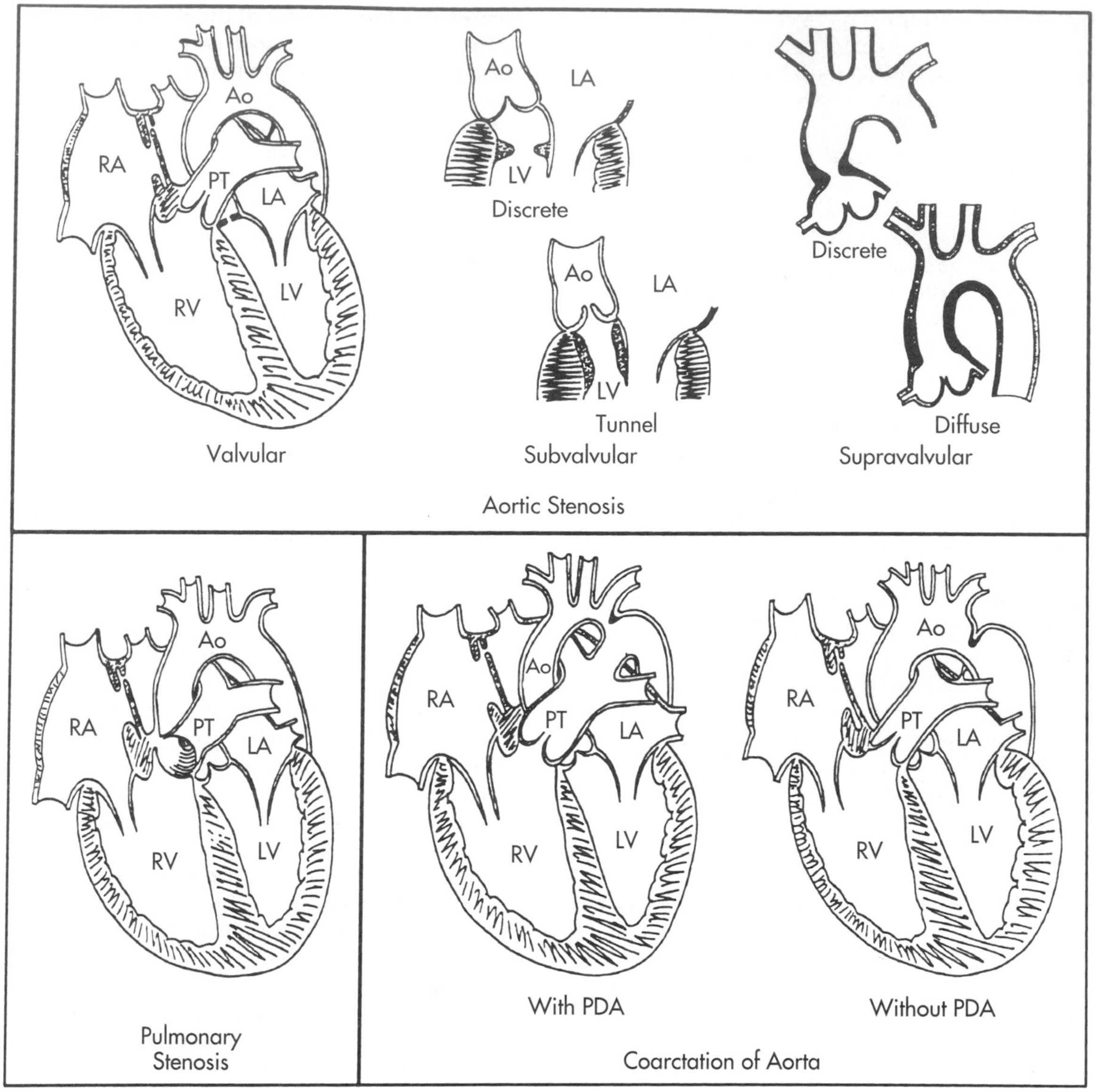

Fig. 46-27 Valvular and arterial stenosis. *Upper,* Aortic stenosis. *Lower,* Pulmonary stenosis and aortic coarctation.

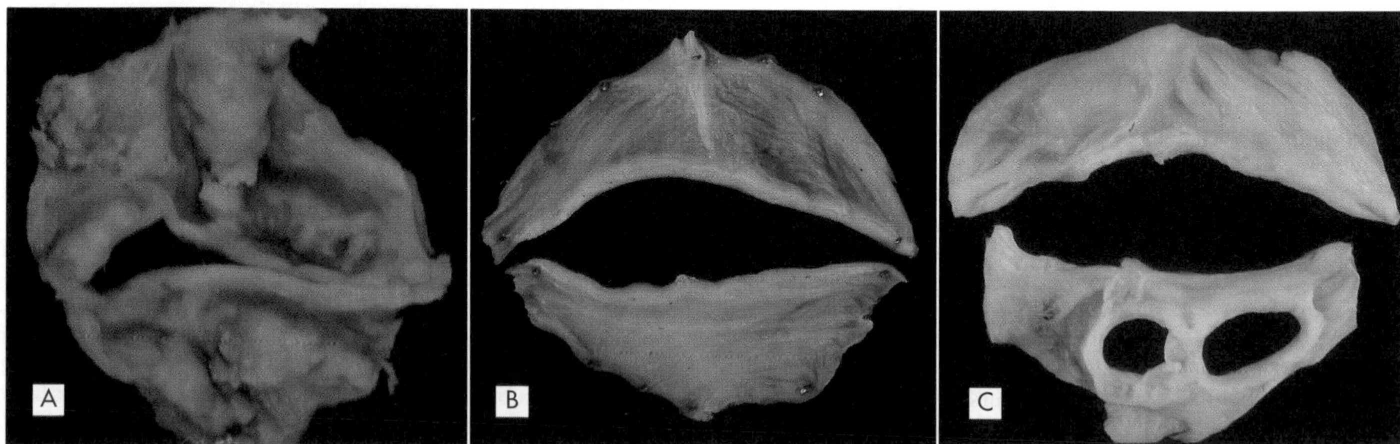

Fig. 46-28 Congenitally bicuspid aortic valve (surgical specimens). **A,** Stenosis resulting from calcification. **B,** Regurgitation resulting from cuspid prolapse and annular dilatation. **C,** Regurgitation resulting from healed infective endocarditis with cuspid perforations.

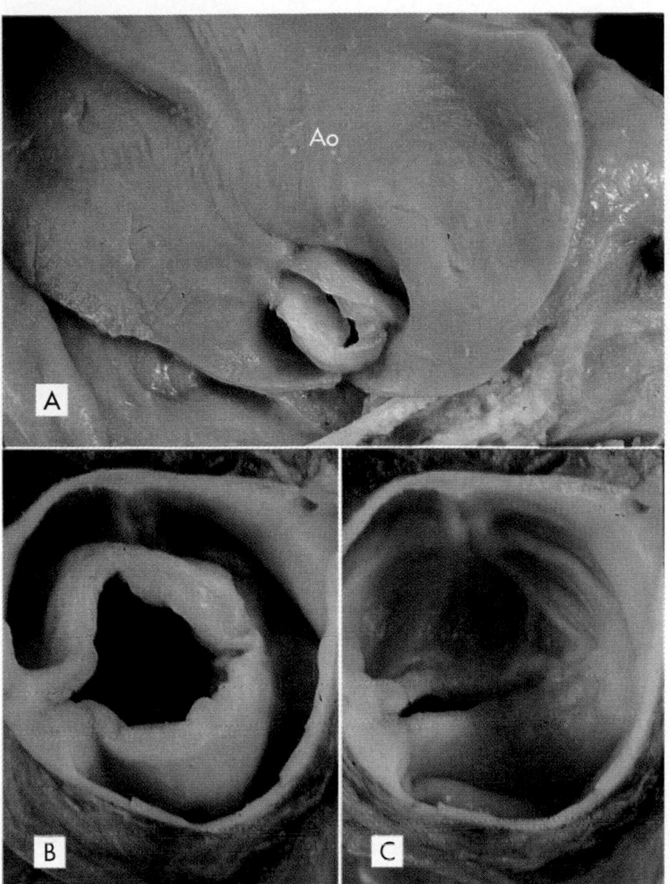

Fig. 46-29 Aortic stenosis. **A,** Critical stenosis of a unicommissural valve in an infant. **B,** and **C,** Mild stenosis of a unicommissural valve in a young adult (opened and closed positions).

branous septum, and septal hypertrophy, occurring in infants of diabetic mothers.

Supravalvular aortic stenosis may result from discrete narrowing at the aortic sinotubular junction or diffuse narrowing of the entire ascending aorta and aortic arch. The aortic valve is thickened, and the coronary ostiums can become stenotic. Involvement of the coronary arteries may be associated with focal or diffuse luminal obstruction and secondary myocardial ischemia. Discrete or diffuse stenosis also affects the mediastinal pulmonary arteries in some patients. Microscopically, thickened arterial walls are affected by fibromuscular dysplasia, with merging of the medial and intimal layers and with a whirled and haphazard, rather than parallel, arrangement of smooth muscle cells and elastic fibers.[155] Many cases are associated with the Williams-Beuren syndrome, which includes hypercalcemia and elfinlike facies.[156]

Secondary cardiopulmonary effects

In critical aortic stenosis, decreased blood flow during fetal life often results in hypoplasia of the left ventricle, ascending aorta, and aortic arch, as well as aortic coarctation. Moderate aortic stenosis, whether valvular, subvalvular, or supravalvular in location, causes pressure hypertrophy of the left ventricle, together with subendocardial fibrosis. Decreased ventricular compliance in turn causes left atrial dilatation and pulmonary venous hypertension.

Critical aortic stenosis in neonates is almost always associated with intractable heart failure and death within the first few days to weeks after birth. In contrast, noncritical stenosis has a much more protracted course. Within 10 years of diagnosis severe stenosis will develop in 20% of the patients with initially mild disease and in 60% of those with initially moderate stenosis.[5] Sudden death occurs in about 10% of the patients whose aortic stenosis has become severe. Infective endocarditis affects fewer than 1%. In general, subaortic stenosis behaves like mild valvular disease, and patients with supravalvular obstruction have a natural history similar to that in patients with moderate valvular stenosis.

Pathology of interventions

Balloon valvuloplasty is successful in 90% of the patients with valvular aortic stenosis. The early postprocedural mortality is about 15%, and death usually results from cusp tears with acute aortic regurgitation.[157] Surgical valvuloplasty also carries a 15% early mortality, with most deaths attributable to acute heart failure, especially in those patients with a hypoplastic left ventricle.[5,18] Aortic valve replacement in neonates carries a particularly poor prognosis.

In patients with discrete subaortic stenosis, resection of the obstructive ridge requires the avoidance of atrioventricular conduction tissues. The early mortality rate is 3%, and 90% of the patients are alive after 15 years.[5] Death stems from residual or recurrent stenosis or from infective endocarditis. Tunnel subaortic stenosis is a complex lesion that requires complex and creative repairs. Left ventricular apicoaortic conduits have not been particularly successful, because of the complications related to inadequate retrograde aortic perfusion of the cerebral and coronary arteries. Better results have been achieved with the Konno aortoventriculoplasty procedure (see Table 46-5), which is associated with a mortality rate of 20% in young children and 10% in adults. Other forms of subaortic stenosis are alleviated by resection of the obstructing tissues.

The repair of supravalvular aortic stenosis entails patch enlargement of the involved arteries. Early postoperative mortalities are 1% for the discrete form and 15% for the diffuse form.[158] Excluding operative deaths, the 10-year survival rate is about 95% and the 20-year rate is 90%.

Pulmonary stenosis

Like its left-sided counterpart, pulmonary stenosis can be valvular, subvalvular, or supravalvular in location. Valvular stenosis can occur as an isolated lesion or as part of a more complex malformation, including conotruncal anomalies and atrioventricular septal defects. Isolated forms may be sporadic, familial, or part of a syndrome, such as Noonan's syndrome.[159] In contrast, subpulmonary stenosis almost always coexists with conotruncal anomalies or hearts with a univentricular atrioventricular connection, and supravalvular pulmonary stenosis is generally a feature of the Williams-Beuren syndrome.[156] Only valvular stenosis is discussed in this section (Fig. 46-27).

General features

In autopsy series isolated pulmonary stenosis has been noted to be associated with a dome-shaped acommissural valve in about 45% of the cases, a dysplastic tricuspid pulmonary valve in 25%, a unicommissural valve in 15%, a bicuspid valve in 10%, and a hypoplastic annulus in 5%[160] (Fig. 46-30). These

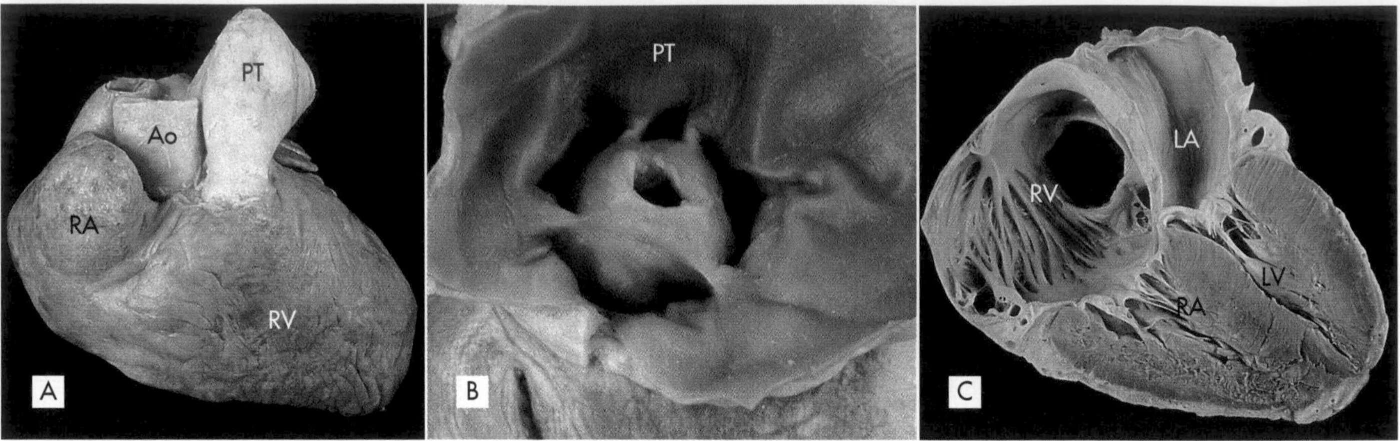

Fig. 46-30 Pulmonary stenosis. **A,** Poststenotic dilatation of the pulmonary trunk (anterior view). **B,** Dome-shaped acommissural valve. **C,** Pronounced right ventricular hypertrophy (four-chamber view).

percentages vary somewhat in surgical series.[77] Fibrous ridges, or raphes, of variable height are characteristically present along the arterial aspect of the malformed valves and indicate the sites of congenitally fused commissures. Focal valvular calcification may occur in adults, especially after an episode of infective endocarditis.

Secondary cardiopulmonary effects

Only in neonates with critical pulmonary stenosis are the right ventricle and tricuspid valve hypoplastic. Otherwise, pressure hypertrophy of a normal-sized right ventricle constitutes the primary cardiac effect of pulmonary stenosis. The wall thicknesses of the two ventricles may become similar, and the ventricular septum can straighten, such that both ventricles exhibit a D shape in cross section. In some cases leftward bowing of the septum adversely affects left ventricular function.[161] Decreased ventricular compliance (caused by myocyte hypertrophy and interstitial fibrosis) and tricuspid regurgitation (caused by annular dilatation) both contribute to the development of a dilated right atrium. Patency of the oval foramen is attended by a right-to-left shunt. Poststenotic dilatation of the pulmonary trunk is a characteristic feature in about 70% of the cases, though the pulmonary vasculature within the lungs is essentially normal.

Without treatment, neonates with critical pulmonary stenosis die of hypoxemia or heart failure within the first few weeks or months after birth.[5] In contrast, those with mild or moderate stenosis who become symptomatic during infancy or early childhood generally die of congestive heart failure during late childhood or adolescence. Finally, if symptoms do not occur until adulthood, the likelihood of progression is low and the long-term prognosis is excellent.

Pathology of interventions

Currently, transcatheter balloon valvuloplasty is the treatment of choice for isolated pulmonary stenosis, though successful relief of the obstruction may be difficult if the valves are severely dysplastic.[162] Complications are rare. The early mortality approaches zero, and the 5-year postprocedural results are excellent.[163]

Similarly, for patients with noncritical pulmonary stenosis the operative mortality is nearly zero. and survival after 25 years is about 95%. Reoperation for the relief of residual stenosis is necessary in fewer than 5% of the patients. Postoperative pulmonary insufficiency may occur but is usually well tolerated.

In contrast, the operative repair of critical pulmonary stenosis in neonates is associated with an early mortality of about 10% and an additional late mortality of 10%, such that 80% of the patients are alive 4 years after operation.[5] Death is usually the result of hypoxemia or acute heart failure.

Coarctation of the aorta

Embryologically, obstruction of the aortic arch opposite the ductal artery is believed to result from decreased blood flow into the ascending aorta, increased pulmonary and ductal arterial blood flow, the extension of contractile ductal tissue into the aorta, or a combination of these factors.[164-166] So-called coarctation of the distal thoracic or abdominal aorta usually represents the aftermath of Takayasu's aortitis rather than a true congenital malformation.

If coarctation is considered analogous to valvular stenosis, then interruption of the aortic arch corresponds to valvular atresia; there are three types, as determined by the site of the interruption: type A, between the ductal and left subclavian arteries; type B, between the left subclavian and left common carotid arteries; and type C, between the left common carotid and brachiocephalic arteries. Type A interruption is considered the most severe form of coarctation, whereas type B is probably related to an abnormality of neural crest tissue and is often associated with the DiGeorge syndrome.[94,164] A type C interruption is extremely rare.

Coarctation becomes symptomatic soon after birth in about 70% of the cases. This infantile or preductal form is associated with tubular hypoplasia of the aortic arch (or aortic isthmus) in 45%, a patent ductal artery in 70%, and other cardiac anomalies in 90%.[167] In the remaining 30% of the cases the coarctation is an isolated lesion that is usually diagnosed in older children or adults as the adult or postductal form (see Fig. 46-27). Coarctation may also be associated with Turner's or Shone's syndrome.

General features

Externally, coarctation produces a V-shaped invagination along the aortic wall just opposite the ductal artery (or liga-

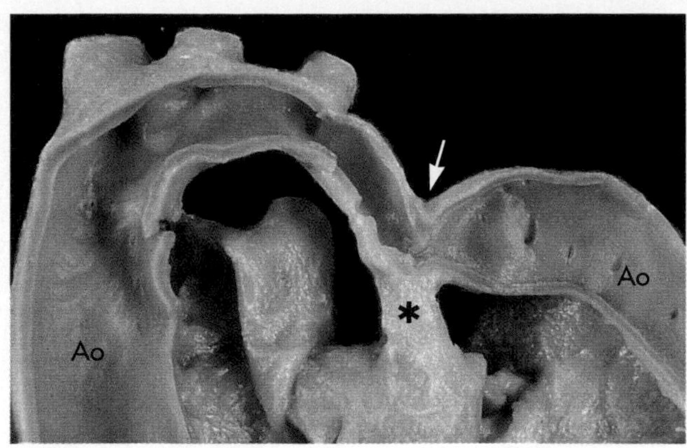

Fig. 46-31 Coarctation of the aorta with a typical indentation of the aortic wall *(arrow)* opposite the ductal arterial ligament (*).

ment); internally it represents an arterial infolding that initially consists primarily of medial tissue but later also includes proliferative fibrointimal thickening[168] (Fig. 46-31). Because luminal obstruction may become more severe with time, even to the point of an acquired occlusion (a type A interruption), its severity cannot always be predicted accurately by the depth of the external notch alone.

Among neonates with coarctation of the aorta, including those with a type A interruption, a congenitally bicuspid aortic valve occurs in about 50%, a ventricular septal defect (usually of the malalignment membranous type) in 30%, subaortic stenosis in 25%, and mitral valve anomalies in 25%. Other malformations include complete transposition of the great arteries, occurring in about 10%; aortic valve stenosis or atresia, afflicting 5%; complete atrioventricular septal defect, affecting 5%; and congenital cerebral artery aneurysms. Coarctation is *not* a feature of right-sided obstructions such as tetralogy of Fallot or pulmonary atresia with an intact ventricular septum. Type B interruption of the aorta is associated with the DiGeorge's syndrome in 50% of the cases and with an aberrant retroesophageal right subclavian artery in about 50%.

Shone's syndrome is characterized by multiple congenital left-sided obstructions, one of which is coarctation of the aorta. Stenosis at the level of the mitral valve may be related to an annular ridge (the so-called supravalvular mitral ring) or a parachute mitral valve (with only one well-formed papillary muscle).[169] Subaortic stenosis results from hypertrophy and malalignment of the ventricular septum, rather than from the discrete or tunnel forms or coexistent hypertrophic cardiomyopathy. Not all patients with Shone's syndrome exhibit all levels of obstruction. Other commonly observed anomalies include a bicuspid aortic valve and a ventricular septal defect.

Secondary cardiopulmonary effects

In patients with moderate to severe coarctation or with interruption of the aorta, blood pressure in the descending thoracic aorta and abdominal aorta is low, and inadequate renal perfusion leads to the development of hypertension in the preductal portion of the aorta. Intercostal arteries provide an avenue for ascending aortic blood to bypass the obstructed region and enter the descending thoracic aorta. Over time these pulsating and tortuous vessels produce rib notching that can be detected radiographically.

Because of hypertension within the ascending aorta, concentric pressure hypertrophy of the left ventricle is the rule. Right ventricular hypertrophy is also observed in patients with a patent ductal artery. Grossly the ascending aorta is often dilated, and microscopically it may be affected by appreciable medial degeneration (so-called cystic medial necrosis). Plexogenic pulmonary hypertension may develop in patients with a patent ductal artery, whereas those without it often show features of pulmonary venous hypertension.

Although infants with critical coarctation may die of congestive heart failure, most patients survive to adulthood. The mortality for patients who go untreated is 25% at 20 years of age, 50% at 30 years, 75% at 45 years, and 90% at 60 years. Death is most commonly the result of aortic rupture, aortic dissection, rupture of a congenital cerebral artery aneurysm, infective endocarditis or endarteritis, or chronic heart failure stemming from hypertension, bicuspid aortic stenosis, or premature coronary atherosclerosis.[5,17] Among patients with an interrupted aortic arch, the mortality rate is 75% at 1 month of age and 90% at 1 year.

Pathology of interventions

The surgical repair of aortic coarctation entails either a subclavian flap aortoplasty or a segmental resection and end-to-end anastomosis, or a combination of these two techniques. Postoperative paradoxical hypertension is the rule, and ischemic abdominal pain and recurrent chylothorax occur relatively frequently. Persistent or recurrent coarctation is observed in about 25% of infants after an end-to-end anastomosis but in fewer than 5% after a subclavian flap repair.[170] The frequency of this complication is also less than 5% in older children and adults. The best results are achieved when the subclavian flap repair is performed in infants between 6 and 12 months of age and when the end-to-end anastomosis is carried out in children between 2 to 9 years of age. Infective endocarditis or endarteritis, paraplegia, aortic aneurysms, dissection, and rupture represent other reported postoperative complications.

The early mortalities are about 5% for infants and 1% for other age groups, and the cumulative late mortalities are 3% at 1 year, 10% at 10 years, and 20% at 25 years.[5] Early deaths are generally attributable to acute heart failure, and late deaths result from essentially the same disorders as those noted in the natural history studies. The early postoperative mortality is about 35% in patients with an interrupted aortic arch.

In the setting of persistent or recurrent coarctation, percutaneous balloon aortoplasty is usually the treatment of choice and good to excellent results are achieved in 75% of the patients.[171] Recently this nonsurgical method has been applied to neonates as well as older adults with coarctation, and the results have been encouraging.[172,173] Although the likelihood of balloon or surgical interventions relieving the coarctation is the same for both, the morbidity and complication rates are lower in those who undergo balloon valvuloplasty than in those who have surgical repairs.

OTHER CARDIOVASCULAR ANOMALIES

Among the various venous malformations, only anomalous pulmonary venous connection is discussed in this chapter. Defects not discussed include atresia of the common pulmonary vein, isolated pulmonary vein stenosis, triatrial heart (cor triatriatum), and systemic venous anomalies. Similarly, the only form of congenital valvular regurgitation discussed in detail is Ebstein's malformation. The reader is directed to the recent textbooks for a review of other disorders.[1-5]

Anomalous pulmonary venous connection

Anomalous pulmonary venous connection involves a lack of direct continuity between the pulmonary veins and the left atrium. The entity is partial if only some veins connect anomalously and complete if they all do (Fig. 46-32). Embryologically the total form is believed to result from atresia of the common pulmonary vein, with retention of venous channels between the lungs and the sinus vein (sinus venosus), common cardinal veins, or umbilicovitelline veins.[174]

Distinction is made between *connection* and *drainage* because the two terms are not synonymous when it comes to the partial forms of the disorder. *Connection* is an anatomic term that implies the existence of a direct link between two structures. In contrast, *drainage* is a hemodynamic term that refers to the direction of blood flow.

General features

In most cases of partial anomalous pulmonary venous connection, the left pulmonary veins connect normally to the left atrium, and the right pulmonary veins join in an anomalous fashion to either the right atrium or the superior caval vein (Fig. 46-33). This is almost invariably associated with an inlet (sinus venosus) atrial septal defect. Thus blood flow from the right-sided pulmonary veins is directed into the left atrium across the septal defect, such that the connection is anomalous but the drainage generally is not. Usually there are no other malformations.

The scimitar syndrome represents a rare form of partial anomalous pulmonary venous connection that is characterized

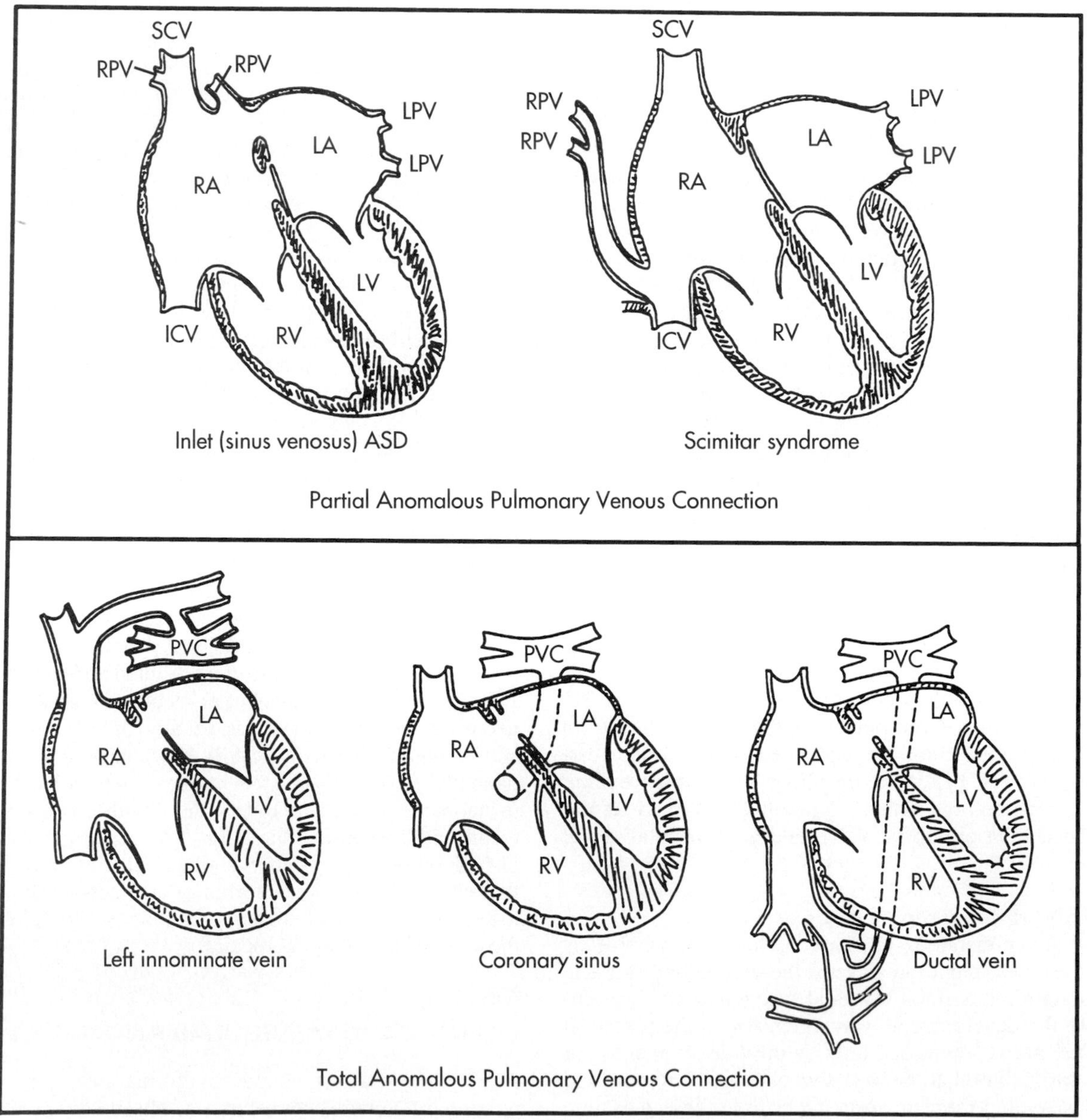

Fig. 46-32 Anomalous pulmonary venous connection. *Upper,* Partial forms. *Lower,* Total forms.

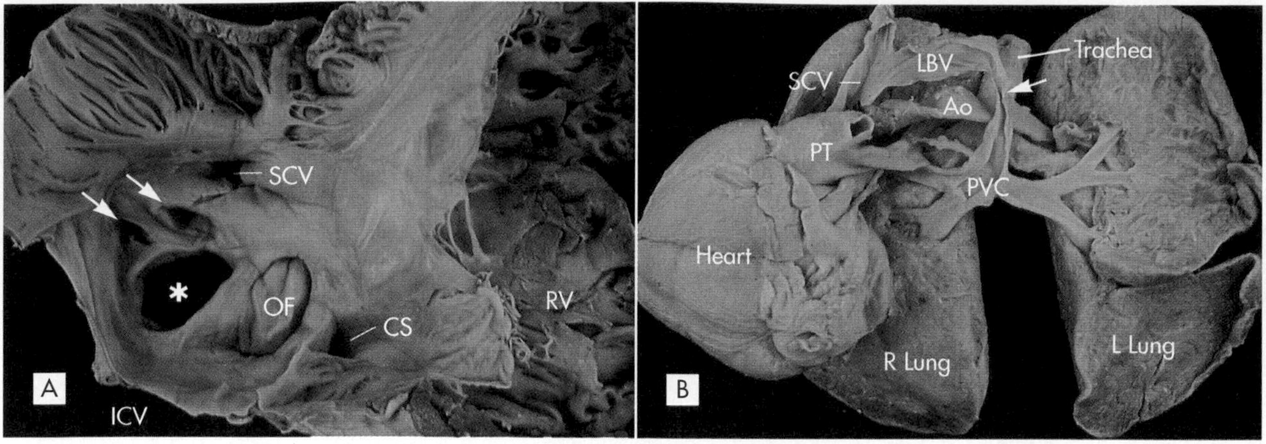

Fig. 46-33 Anomalous pulmonary venous connection. **A,** Partial form with an inlet (sinus venosus) atrial septal defect (*) and an anomalous connection of the right pulmonary veins *(arrows)* (opened right atrium). **B,** Total form showing an anomalous connection *(arrow)* of the pulmonary venous confluence to the left brachiocephalic vein. (The left pulmonary artery has been severed and the heart has been rotated to the rightward to demonstrate the malformation.)

by connection of the right-sided veins to the suprahepatic portion of the inferior caval vein, just above the diaphragm. It is generally associated with a hypoplastic right lung and secondary dextroposition of the heart *(not* dextrocardia). The syndrome is isolated in 75% of the cases and occurs with other cardiac anomalies in 25%.[175]

In the complete form all pulmonary veins join together behind the left atrium to form a venous confluence that then connects with systemic veins either above or below the diaphragm.[176] Anomalous connections include the left brachiocephalic, superior caval, or azygos vein, above the heart, or the coronary sinus or right atrium, at the level of the heart. When the connection is subdiaphragmatic, it generally involves the inferior caval, hepatic, portal, or left gastric vein or the ductal vein (ductus venosus). Connections to more than one systemic vein may also be observed. In more than half of the cases, however, the pulmonary veins are joined either to the left brachiocephalic vein or to the coronary sinus (Fig. 46-33). Obstruction to pulmonary venous blood flow, resulting from either intrinsic or extrinsic factors, affects all patients with connection below the diaphragm and 50% of those with connection above the diaphragm.[177]

Either a patent oval foramen or a fossa (secundum) atrial septal defect is always present to allow blood flow into the left atrium. The anomaly is otherwise isolated in about 65% of the cases. Its coexistence with other major malformations, such as the conotruncal anomalies or a single functional ventricle, often occurs as a part of the asplenia or polysplenia syndrome.

Secondary cardiopulmonary effects

The right atrium and right ventricle are characterized by volume hypertrophy, and the valve rings and pulmonary arteries on the right side are also dilated. Although the left ventricular size is normal, the left atrium is usually hypoplastic, with its volume about half the normal one because of the lack of incorporation of the pulmonary veins into its wall.

Microscopically the pulmonary circulation exhibits the features typical of chronic pulmonary venous hypertension.[178] These changes are particularly pronounced in patients with a subdiaphragmatic connection and obstructed pulmonary venous blood flow. Although medial hypertrophy of the muscular pulmonary arteries and veins is potentially reversible, it can still be the source of acute vasospastic pulmonary hypertension in the early postoperative period.

The partial form of anomalous pulmonary venous connection behaves much like a large atrial septal defect and often does not become symptomatic until adulthood. In contrast, patients with the total form have a poor prognosis, with mortalities of 20% at 1 month of life, 50% at 3 months, and 80% at 1 year.[5,179] The risk of early death is greatest for those with obstructed pulmonary venous blood flow. Sudden death may be the first manifestation of this anomaly and therefore may be discovered at the time of a forensic autopsy.[180]

Pathology of interventions

For patients with an inlet (sinus venosus) atrial septal defect and anomalous right-sided pulmonary veins, the early postoperative mortality is less than 1%, similar to that for patients who undergo repair of an isolated fossa (secundum) atrial septal defect.[5] Patients undergoing repair in the first few years of life enjoy survival rates as adults that are similar to those in the general population. In contrast, the surgical risk for patients with the scimitar syndrome is higher and is related more to the hypoplastic right lung than to the anomalous pulmonary venous connection.

The surgical repair of a total anomalous pulmonary venous connection entails anastomosis of the pulmonary venous confluence to the left atrium. The early hospital mortality is about 15% and is related to the critically ill state of the neonate at the time of operation and to episodes of severe vasospastic pulmonary hypertension that occur in the immediate postoperative period.[5] Late deaths are rare and are usually related to pulmonary vein stenosis.

Ebstein's anomaly

Ebstein's malformation represents a congenital disorder of the tricuspid valve that is associated with valvular regurgitation and conduction abnormalities, particularly the Wolff-Parkin-

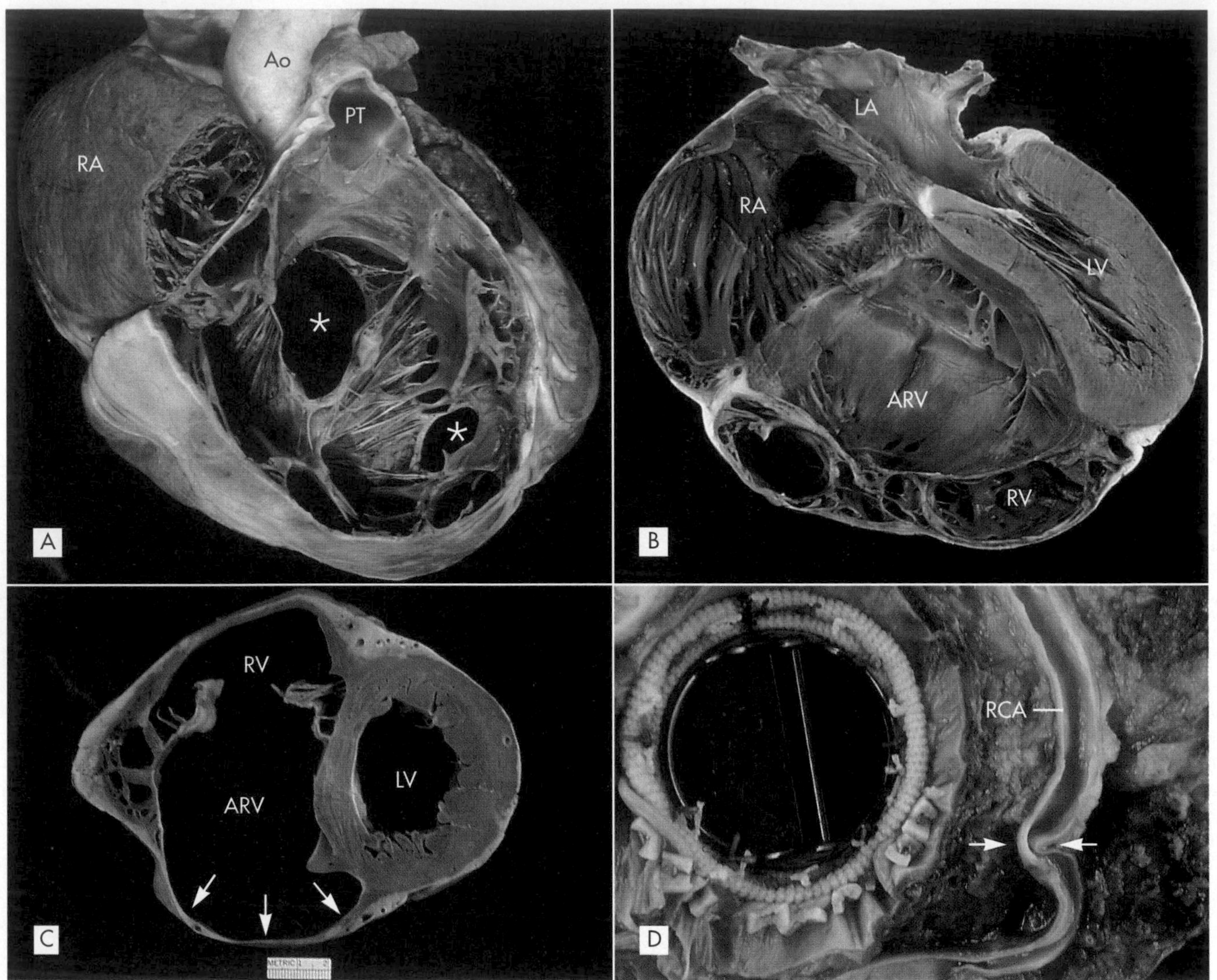

Fig. 46-34 Ebstein's malformation. **A,** Fenestrations (*) of the anterior tricuspid leaflet (anterior view, with a portion of the right ventricular wall removed). **B,** Downward displacement of the tricuspid annulus, atrialization of the right ventricular inlet, and right ventricular and right atrial dilatation (four-chamber view). **C,** Marked right ventricular dilatation and aneurysm formation *(arrows)* (short-axis view). **D,** Surgical plication annuloplasty and tricuspid valve replacement, with kinking *(arrows)* of right coronary artery (base-of-heart view).

son-White syndrome. Grossly the valve is characterized by downward displacement of its septal and posterior leaflets, a sail-like redundancy of the anterior leaflet, and dilatation of its annulus.[181,182] Because each of these features can be expressed to variable degrees, the morphologic appearance of the valve is highly variable, as is the severity of regurgitation.

Although most cases are sporadic, familial cases have been reported. However, an association with syndromes other than Wolff-Parkinson-White is rare. Its relationship to maternal exposure to lithium is currently unsettled.[183,184] Embryologically, Ebstein's anomaly is thought to result from incomplete undermining of the right ventricular myocardium.

General features

In hearts with Ebstein's anomaly, the septal and posterior tricuspid leaflets are adherent to the underlying right ventricular myocardium. In moderate to severe cases the leaflets are thickened, dysplastic, and focally attached to the ventricular wall by numerous short muscular stumps (Fig. 46-34). Tendinous cords are generally short and malformed, or absent altogether. As a result the two leaflets and the functional annulus are displaced downward.

In contrast, the anterior tricuspid leaflet forms a redundant intracavitary curtain that separates the right ventricular inflow and outflow tracts. It not only contributes to the formation of the true valvular orifice but also contains several fenestrations of variable size that serve as accessory orifices. Tendinous cords that are attached to the anterior leaflet are characteristically short and malformed, such that valvular excursion at the midleaflet level is wide, whereas that at the true orifice is quite limited. As a result, valve closure is hindered and tricuspid regurgitation is often moderate to severe, especially if the accessory orifices are also relatively large.

The annulus at the atrioventricular junction is poorly formed and tends to be appreciably dilated. This contributes to the development of valvular regurgitation. Furthermore, the incomplete nature of the annulus promotes the formation of direct muscular connections between the right atrium and right ventricle, thereby providing the morphologic substrate for ventricular preexcitation.

In some cases the anterior tricuspid leaflet is obstructive and causes subpulmonary stenosis. Occasionally the mitral valve is also abnormal and exhibits a cleft anterior leaflet, a parachute deformity with only one papillary muscle, or prolapse and other features of a floppy valve.[185] Although the atrial septum is usually the site of a patent oval foramen, it is involved by a fossa (secundum) atrial septal defect in some patients. Other associated anomalies are rare, and include pulmonary stenosis or atresia, congenitally corrected transposition, ventricular septal defect, atrioventricular septal defect, tetralogy of Fallot, and coarctation of the aorta.

Included in the differential diagnosis for Ebstein's malformation are Uhl's anomaly, right ventricular dysplasia, tricuspid valve dysplasia, an unguarded tricuspid orifice, and hypoplasia of the right ventricular apex.[181] Occasionally Ebstein's anomaly may exist on the left side of the heart. Examples of this include mirror-image cardiac sidedness (cardiac situs inversus), atrioventricular discordance with a left-sided morphologic right ventricle and tricuspid valve, and the very rare condition in which Ebstein's anomaly involves a morphologic mitral valve.

Secondary cardiopulmonary effects

Cardiomegaly can be massive, especially in infants with severe tricuspid regurgitation. Cardiac enlargement is primarily a result of right atrial and right ventricular dilatation related to a chronic volume overload. Moreover, downward displacement of the septal and posterior tricuspid leaflets leads to aneurysmal thinning and dilatation of the right ventricular inflow tract. This region, which commonly exhibits right atrial pressure, is referred to as the *atrialized portion* of the right ventricle. In some cases leftward bowing of the ventricular septum occurs and causes the cross-sectional shapes of the two ventricles to be reversed, such that the right ventricle is circular and the left ventricle is crescentic. Interestingly, in hearts with Ebstein's anomaly, mural thrombus does not tend to develop within the right-sided chambers, regardless of their size.

In the setting of chronic and severe tricuspid regurgitation, the liver and portal circulations become the most extensively affected extracardiac tissues. Congestive hepatomegaly is commonly encountered and may be characterized microscopically not only by centrilobular (zone 3) congestion but also by patchy and bandlike areas of fibrosis, without regenerative nodules. Thus chronic congestion produces hepatic fibrosis but not true cirrhosis. Congestive splenomegaly may also be prominent, and a few cases of hypersplenism have been reported.

Patients whose defect is diagnosed during infancy tend to have a more severely deformed tricuspid valve and a higher mortality than do patients whose defect is diagnosed later in life. Among neonates with symptomatic disease, the risk factors for death before 3 months of age include tethered attachments of the anterior tricuspid leaflet, dysplastic features of the right ventricle, and left ventricular compression by the dilated right ventricle. Death is most commonly the result of right heart failure or a fatal arrhythmia. It is of interest that infective endocarditis rarely affects the malformed tricuspid valve.

Pathology of interventions

Surgical interventions for Ebstein's malformation include either valve repair or valve replacement, accompanied by a reduction right atrioplasty, plication of the atrialized portion of the right ventricle, and closure of the interatrial communication.[186] Ebstein's anomaly is the most common reason for tricuspid valve replacement among patients younger than 40 years.[187] In severe cases, which include massive right ventricular dilatation and failure, a Fontan procedure may be performed, though palliative operations overall have not been particularly successful.

When the intent is to repair the valve, annular plication is performed to reduce the size of the orifice. Kinking of the right coronary artery, though rare, represents one of the most serious potential complications of this procedure and generally results in acute infarction of the inferoseptal wall of the left ventricle and the inferior wall of the right ventricle. Prosthetic dysfunction and infection are recognized complications of valve replacement procedures. Persistent right ventricular dysfunction can occur after either operation and is related to the presence of appreciable dilatation and fibrosis preoperatively.[188] Other complications include damage to the atrioventricular node or His bundle and a residual interatrial communication. The most common causes of postoperative death are heart failure and fatal arrhythmias, the same as those for unoperated cases.

Coronary and conduction anomalies

Anomalies of the coronary arteries and the conduction system may occur alone or in conjunction with other cardiac malformations. However, a detailed presentation of these two topics is beyond the scope of this chapter. For additional information on them, the reader is referred to books or review articles.[1-5,189-192]

EVALUATION OF CONGENITAL HEART DISEASE AT AUTOPSY

Pathologists who evaluate autopsy specimens from patients with congenital heart disease treated surgically must often function as a "medical archeologist," identifying alterations associated not only with the underlying malformations but also resulting from previous interventional procedures. To provide useful information for one's surgical and clinical colleagues, the following should be evaluated in detail:

1. Underlying congenital cardiac malformations
2. Secondary hypertensive pulmonary vascular disease
3. Extracardiac anomalies suggestive of a syndrome
4. The effects of all interventional procedures, including takedowns
5. Postinterventional enlargement of hypoplastic structures
6. Postinterventional regression of pulmonary vascular disease
7. Postinterventional regression of hypertrophy or dilatation
8. Postinterventional complications, including ischemia
9. Late development of valvular regurgitation,
10. Evidence of acute or chronic heart failure
11. Evidence of cardiac or extracardiac infections

12. Correlation of the findings with clinical imaging findings.

Practical considerations

At the time of autopsy, before organ removal, the location and number of spleens should be determined, as well as whether there are malrotations of the bowel. By knowing these features and the location and morphology of the liver, the sidedness of the abdominal viscera can be established, as described in an earlier section (Visceral Sidedness). In the thorax the number of lung lobes should be determined and recorded, although this does not always allow correct identification of pulmonary sidedness. Similarly, the external appearance of the atrial appendages usually, but not always, corresponds to cardiac sidedness. The apical direction should also be recorded.

A standard form is used at the Mayo Clinic for recording this information and the other morphologic data obtained during a detailed sequential segmental analysis of the heart (see Appendix 46-3). Descriptions of interventional procedures are recorded on the back of the form. Such information can then be entered easily into a computer data base.

Before organ removal the thoracic organs should be inspected for evidence of an anomalous origin of the pulmonary arteries or anomalous connections of the pulmonary veins. If such anomalies are present, or if visceral isomerism exists, the thoracic and abdominal organs should be removed as one tissue block and the relative positions of the aorta and the inferior caval, azygos, and hemiazygos veins should be identified along the posterior surface.[193] Otherwise the two sets of organs can be removed separately from the body. Once this is accomplished, the relationship of the pulmonary arteries to the bronchial tree can be used to establish pulmonary sidedness unequivocally. Similarly, after the heart has been opened, cardiac sidedness can be established based on the internal morphology of the atriums.

Initially the heart and lungs are kept together as one tissue specimen, along with the entire thoracic aorta and appreciable lengths of the arch vessels. Some investigators advocate the dissection of fresh tissues; others recommend dissection only after fixation.[193,194] For the latter purpose, the lungs should be distended to their total capacity by transtracheal gravity perfusion and the heart should be distended by syringe perfusion of the chambers or by a continuous perfusion system. For continuous perfusion, cannulas are inserted into one of the caval veins and into the descending thoracic aorta and pins are used to hold corks in the other vessels.

If the pulmonary arterial and venous connections are normal, the lungs can be removed, but not discarded, from the cardiac specimen. For the microscopic evaluation of pulmonary vascular and parenchymal disease, the upper and lower lobes of each lung should be sampled, with arteries and airways cut in crosssection. Sections of myocardium from each ventricle should also be submitted for the evaluation of ischemia, inflammation, and fibrosis.

Specimens from fetuses and from patients older than 50 years present special challenges. Use of a dissecting microscope is strongly recommended for the evaluation of a malformed fetal heart and detailed correlation with premortem fetal echocardiographic findings, if available, is important. For older adults, the coronary arteries should be cut in cross-section to identify not only anomalies of origin and distribution but also the location and extent of atherosclerosis.

Methods of dissection

Although various methods of cardiac dissection have been proposed, those that have withstood the test of time include the inflow-outflow, window, base-of-heart, and tomographic methods, as illustrated throughout this chapter. Moreover, the tomographic planes of section (short-axis, long-axis, and four-chamber) correspond to the views most commonly obtained by two-dimensional echocardiography.

Nontomographic methods

Among the various methods that have been described for the dissection of hearts with congenital malformations, the inflow-outflow technique is perhaps the easiest to learn and the quickest to perform. In this method the heart is opened according to the direction of blood flow. Some investigators recommend this approach for the investigation of virtually all forms of congenital heart disease.[193]

In selected cases congenital malformations are best visualized by removing windows of tissue from the cardiac chambers or great vessels. Results are most satisfactory when specimens prepared by perfusion-fixation, paraffin-infiltration, or plastination are used.[195]

Tomographic methods

The bread-slice method is recommended not only for the evaluation of ischemic heart disease, but also for that of congenitally malformed hearts with appreciable hypertrophy, dilatation, or susceptibility to ischemic injury.[194] Ventricular slices, viewed from an apical perspective, correspond to the echocardiographic short-axis plane. The valves are demonstrated by removing the atriums and great arteries from the basal slice.

Other tomographic methods of dissection entail bisection of the heart using a single plane of section. The left ventricular long-axis method nicely demonstrates septal defects and valvular interrelationships, whereas four-chamber dissections are particularly useful for comparing changes in the relative sizes of the cardiac chambers.

From a practical standpoint, the best tomographic cross sections are achieved in perfusion-fixed specimens that are bisected by one continuous slice with a very sharp knife. Sawing motions produce a serrated surface and should not be used. After a section has been made and photographed, both halves of the specimen can be glued back together and resectioned along another plane.[196] Any of the commercially available cyanoacrylate glues (such as Krazy Glue or Superglue) will suffice. The best results are obtained with smooth and dry surfaces.

Specimen photography

In the field of congenital heart disease, formal lectures, case presentations, and informal workshops all rely heavily on visual images, and diagrams are indispensible for giving an overview of a topic and for categorizing various groups of disorders. However, gross specimens are necessary for an appreciation of the three-dimensional morphology. Because a review of actual specimens is not always feasible, photographs of gross specimens often serve to demonstrate the structural details. In this regard, the success of one's teaching efforts is based in large part on the quality of one's photographs. Careful planning and attention to detail are generally more important for achieving good results than is having access to the most expensive photographic equipment.

Camera and film

For medical photography, a 35 mm single-lens-reflex (SLR) camera with through-the-lens light-metering is recommended.[197,198] One may use a standard 50 mm lens, a macrolens, or a lens with a longer focal length that is attached to a barrel mount or a bellows. The aperture should be small (generally an *f*-stop of 16 or greater) to achieve an adequate depth of field of focus. Finally, the importance of attention to sharp focusing cannot be overemphasized.

To achieve high-resolution (nongrainy) photographs, film with an ISO (formerly ASA) rating of 100 or less is recommended. The choice of daylight or tungsten film depends on the type of lighting being used. Kodachrome, Ektachrome, and Fujichrome films are all currently archival in quality (stable for at least 25 years) if properly stored in a cool, dry, and dark area. Ektachrome and Fujichrome have the advantage of rapid E-6 processing, whereas Kodachrome requires a more complex and time-consuming process.

With these suggestions in mind, it is also important to recognize that the methods for storing visual information are changing dramatically. With improvements in the processing speed of computers and the development of high-resolution monitors, cameras and film may become obsolete for the acquisition and storage of visual images in the not-too-distant future. Even now, at some institutions gross and microscopic images are being stored in a digitized format, and selected lectures are being presented using CD-ROM rather than a carousel projector.

Copy stand and specimen layout

Regardless of these changes, however, a copy stand will remain a necessary item. Any of the commercially available copy stands that are equipped with stationary or movable floodlamps or flash units should be adequate for use with 35-mm cameras. If the color temperature of the lights does not match that of the film, one or the other may be changed or inexpensive corrective filters can be purchased. To reduce reflective glare (specular reflections), diffusion screens can be constructed of milky-white translucent Mylar plastic or other similar material and placed between the light source and the specimen.[197] Rotatable polarizing filters can also be employed to eliminate glare, but they are generally somewhat cumbersome and time-consuming to use. Axial light can be used to illuminate specimens with deep cavities, and ultraviolet light may be added to enhance the surface details.[199,200]

To retain realistic colors, hearts can be placed in nonformalin fixatives such as Kaiserling or Jores or kept in formalin for less than 15 minutes. For specimens fixed in formalin less than 1 week, colors can be restored by soaking them in 80% ethanol for 15 to 30 minutes. The use of diffusion screens

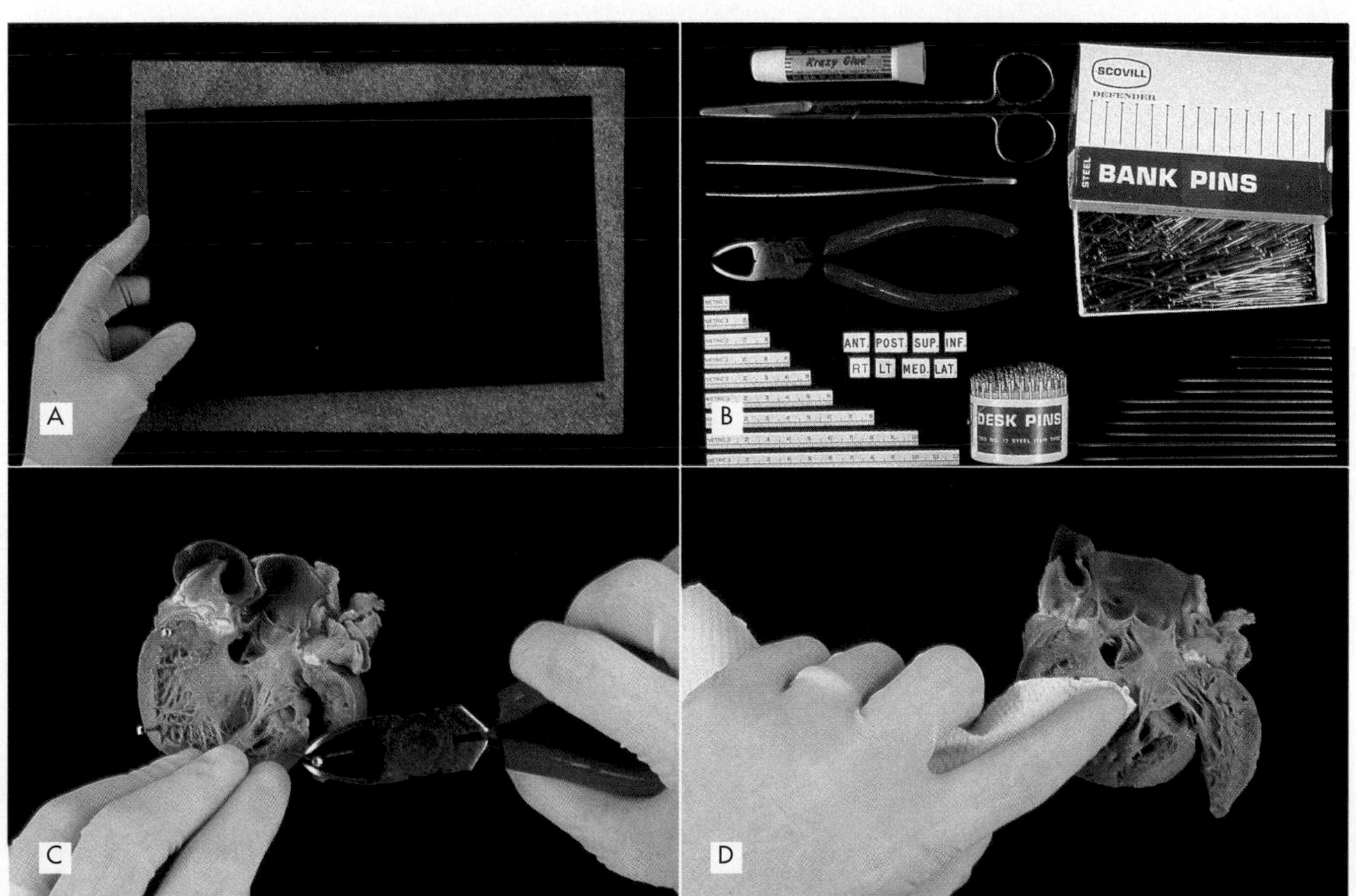

Fig. 46-35 Preparation of specimens for photography. **A,** Black cardboard is placed on a corkboard. **B,** Tools are assembled for pinning the specimen. **C,** Pins of various sizes are used to hold the specimen in position. **D,** After cutting off the exposed portions of the pins, the specimen is carefully dried and then photographed (see Fig. 46-9, *A,* for the result). (From Edwards WD: *Mayo Clin Proc* 63:42, 1988.)

with fixed and dried specimens virtually eliminates any reflective glare. In general the most pleasing results are obtained when hearts are photographed against a black background, rather than on backlit translucent sheets of colored plastic. At the Mayo Clinic, specimens are pinned to black cardboard (made with water-insoluble ink) that is placed over a sheet of corkboard (Fig. 46-35). The heads of the pins are then removed with cutting pliers so that they will not be visible in the photograph, as described in detail in a recent publication.[197]

Appendix 46-1 Latin terms and their anglicized equivalents

Latin term (plural)	Anglicized equivalent (plural)
Annulus (annuli); anulus (anuli)	Annulus (annuluses), or anulus, or ring
Aorta (aortae)	Aorta (aortas)
Atrium (atria)	Atrium (atriums)
Chorda tendinea (chordae tendineae)	Tendinous cord (cords)
Conus arteriosus	Right ventricular outflow tract, or infundibulum
Cor triatriatum	Triatrial heart, or double chamber left atrium
Cor triatriatum dexter	Double chamber right atrium
Crista supraventricularis	Supraventricular crest or ridge
Crista terminalis	Terminal crest or ridge
Ductus arteriosus (ductus, *not* ducti)	Ductal artery, or arterial duct
Ductus venosus	Ductal vein, or venous duct
Ectopia cordis	Ectopic heart, or extrathoracic heart
Foramen ovale	Oval foramen
Fossa ovalis	Oval fossa
Inferior vena cava	Inferior caval vein
Infundibulum (infundibuli)	Infundibulum (infundibulums)
Ligamentum arteriosum	Arterial ligament
Ligamentum venosum	Venous ligament
Limbus fossae ovalis, or anulus ovalis	Limb or rim of the oval fossa
Ostium (ostia)	Ostium (ostiums), or orifice
Ostium primum	First ostium or orifice
Ostium secundum	Second ostium or orifice
Patent ductus arteriosus	Patent ductal artery, or patent arterial duct
Patent foramen ovale	Patent oval foramen
Septum (septa, *not* septae or septi)	Septum (septums)
Septum primum	First septum
Septum secundum	Second septum
Sinus venosus	Venous sinus, or sinus vein
Situs ambiguus	Isomerism, or indeterminate sidedness
Situs inversus	Mirror image sidedness
Situs solitus	Normal sidedness
Superior vena cava	Superior caval vein
Trabecula septomarginalis	Septal band, or moderator band
Trabecula carnea (trabeculae carneae)	Trabeculation(s)
Truncus arteriosus	Truncal artery, or arterial trunk

Appendix 46-2 Synonyms for commonly used diagnostic terms

Preferred term	Synonyms
Anomalous pulmonary venous connection	Anomalous pulmonary venous drainage or return (not always anatomically accurate)
Aortopulmonary septal defect	Aortopulmonary window or fenestration; aorticopulmonary window or septal defect
Asplenia syndrome	Right isomerism; visceral heterotaxy; Ivemark's syndrome (eponyms should be avoided)
Atrioventricular discordance	Ventricular inversion; l-loop ventricles
Atrioventricular septal defect	AV canal defect; endocardial cushion defect; AV commune; common AV orifice
Common inlet right ventricle	Cor biloculare (no longer an acceptable term)
Complete transposition of the great arteries	d-Transposition; d-loop transposition; simple regular transposition; complete transposition of the great vessels
Congenitally corrected transposition of the great arteries	l-Transposition; corrected transposition of the great arteries; physiologically corrected transposition
Double outlet right ventricle with subpulmonary VSD	Taussig-Bing heart (eponyms should be avoided)
Double chamber left atrium	Subdivided left atrium; triatrial heart; cor triatriatum (a term to avoid)
Double inlet left ventricle	Single left ventricle; univentricular heart; common ventricle (exceedingly rare); cor triloculare biatriatum (no longer an acceptable term)
Double inlet left ventricle with normally related great arteries	Holmes heart (eponyms should be avoided)
Extrathoracic heart	Ectopic heart; ectopia cordis
Fossa or secundum ASD	Ostium secundum or fossa ovalis ASD
Inlet or sinus venosus ASD	Juxtacaval ASD; sinoseptal defect
Inlet VSD	Subtricuspid, AV canal, or AV commune VSD
Membranous VSD	Paramembranous, perimembranous, or infracristal VSD
Muscular VSD	Persistent bulboventricular foramen
Outlet or primum ASD	Ostium primum ASD; partial AV septal defect
Outlet or infundibular VSD	Subarterial, subaortic, subpulmonary, supracristal, conal, or doubly committed juxta-arterial VSD
Patent ductal artery	Patent arterial duct; patent ductus arteriosus; persistent ductal artery
Persistent truncal artery	Persistent arterial trunk; truncus arteriosus; truncus arteriosus communis
Polysplenia syndrome	Left isomerism; visceral heterotaxy
Pulmonary atresia with VSD	Tetralogy with pulmonary atresia (pseudotruncus and type IV truncus are no longer acceptable)
Right or left pulmonary artery from ascending aorta	Hemitruncus (no longer acceptable)
Superoinferior ventricles	Over-and-under heart; upstairs-downstairs heart
Tricuspid atresia	Single inlet left ventricle; absent right atrioventricular connection
Twisted atrioventricular connection	Crisscross heart

ASD, Atrial septal defect; *AV*, atrioventricular; *d*, dextro; *l*, levo; *VSD*, ventricular septal defect.

Appendix 46-3 Standardized form for the autopsy evaluation of congenital heart disease

GENERAL INFORMATION

Patient Name: ______ CASE NO.: ______

Patient I.D. No.: ______ Age, Gender: ______

Date of Death: ______

CARDIAC ARRANGEMENT

Thoracic Position: □ Left-Sided □ Right-Sided □ Midline □ Unknown □ Ectopic ______

Apical Direction: □ Levocardia □ Dextrocardia □ Mesocardia □ Other: ______

Displacement: □ None □ Levoposition □ Dextroposition □ Mesoposition □ Unknown

Morphologic RA: □ Right-sided □ Left-Sided □ Bilateral □ Absent □ Indeterminate

PULMONARY ARRANGEMENT

Morphology of Right-Sided Lung: □ Right □ Left □ Indeterminate Lobes (No.): ______

Morphology of Left-Sided Lung: □ Left □ Right □ Indeterminate Lobes (No.): ______

ABDOMINAL ARRANGEMENT

Spleen: □ Single □ Accessory □ Polysplenia □ Asplenia □ Unknown

Liver: □ Right-Sided □ Left-Sided □ Midline □ Unknown □ Other: ______

Bowel: □ Normal □ Malrotation: ______

VISCERAL SIDEDNESS

Cardiac: □ Normal □ Mirror-Image □ R. Isomerism □ L. Isomerism □ Indeterminate □ Unknown

Pulmonary: □ Normal □ Mirror-Image □ R. Isomerism □ L. Isomerism □ Indeterminate □ Unknown

Abdominal: □ Normal □ Mirror-Image □ R. Isomerism □ L. Isomerism □ Indeterminate □ Unknown

ATRIUMS

Right-Sided: □ RA □ LA ______

Left-Sided: □ LA □ RA ______

Septum: □ Intact □ Patent □ ASD: ______

Coronary Sinus: □ Present □ Absent ______

ATRIOVENTRICULAR VALVES

Right-Sided: _____ % to RV _____ % to LV Morphology: ______

Left-Sided: _____ % to RV _____ % to LV Morphology: ______

Common: _____ % to RV _____ % to LV ______

VENTRICLES

Morphologic RV: Orientation: □ Normal □ Mirror-Image □ Position: ______

Morphologic LV: Orientation: □ Normal □ Mirror-Image □ Position: ______

Hypoplastic Chamber: □ RV □ LV ______

Septal Position: □ Vertical □ Angled □ Horizontal □ Twisted □ Other: ______

Septum: □ Intact □ VSD: ______

SEMILUNAR VALVES

Pulmonary: _____ % from RV _____ % from LV Morphology: ______

Aortic: _____ % from RV _____ % from LV Morphology: ______

Truncal: _____ % from RV _____ % from LV Morphology: ______

AORTIC VALVE POSITION RELATIVE TO PULMONARY VALVE

□ R. Post. □ Dextroposed □ R. Lat. □ R. Ant □ Ant. □ L. Ant. □ L. Lat. □ L. Post. □ Post.

GREAT ARTERIES

Pulmonary Artery: □ Present □ Hypoplastic □ Atretic □ Absent □ Other: ______

□ Systemic Collaterals ______

Thoracic Aorta: □ L. Arch □ R. Arch □ Coarctation □ Other: ______

Ductal Artery: □ Ligament □ Patent □ Absent □ Other: ______

CORONARY ARTERIES

Ostiums: □ Normal □ Other: ______

Distribution: □ Normal □ Mirror-Image □ Other: ______

Appendix 46-3 **Standardized form for the autopsy evaluation of congenital heart disease—cont'd**

CONNECTIONS

Venoatrial: Systemic Veins: □ Normal □ Other: ____

Pulmonary Veins: □ Normal □ Other: ____

Atrioventricular: Biventricular: □ Concordance □ Discordance □ Ambiguous: ____

Univentricular: □ Double Inlet ____ □ Single Inlet ____ □ Common Inlet ____

Ventriculoarterial: Two Arteries: □ Concordance □ Discordance □ Double Outlet ____

One Artery: □ Single Outlet (Atretic PT) □ Common Outlet (Persistent Truncal Artery)

CARDIAC MEASUREMENTS

Body Size: Height (cm) ____ Weight (kg) ____ BSA (m^2) ____

Weights (g): Heart & Lungs ____ R. Lung ____ L. Lung ____

Heart ____ (Normal Mean ____ and Range ____)

Wall Thickness (cm): LV ____ RV ____ VS ____

Valves (cm): Aortic ____ Pulmonary ____ Truncal ____

Mitral ____ Tricuspid ____ Common ____

Shunts (cm): POF ____ ASD ____ AVSD ____ VSD ____ PDA ____

SECONDARY CARDIAC EFFECTS

	Hypertrophy	Dilatation	Atrophy	Fibrosis	Mural Thrombus
LV:	____	____	____	____	____
RV:	____	____	____	____	____
LA:	____	____	____	____	____
RA:	____	____	____	____	____

SECONDARY PULMONARY EFFECTS

Plexogenic Pulmonary Hypertension: ____

Pulmonary Venous Hypertension: ____

Other Pulmonary Hypertension: ____

Pulmonary Infection: ____

Other Microscopic Features: ____

INTERVENTIONAL PROCEDURES

Procedure (Date): ____

Appearance at Autopsy: ____

Procedure (Date): ____

Appearance at Autopsy: ____

Procedure (Date): ____

Appearance at Autopsy: ____

Procedure (Date): ____

Appearance at Autopsy: ____

Procedure (Date): ____

Appearance at Autopsy: ____

DIAGRAMS

REFERENCES

General references

1. Emmanouilides GC, Riemenschneider TA, Allen HD, Gutgesell HP, editors: *Moss and Adams' heart disease in infants, children, and adolescents, including the fetus and young adult,* ed 5, Baltimore, 1995, Williams & Wilkins.
2. Freedom RM, Benson LN, Smallhorn JF, editors: *Neonatal heart disease,* London, 1992, Springer-Verlag.
3. Moller JH, Neal WA, editors: *Fetal, neonatal, and infant cardiac disease,* Norwalk, Conn, 1990, Appleton & Lange.
4. Anderson RH, Macartney FJ, Shinebourne EA, Tynan M, editors: *Paediatric cardiology,* Edinburgh, 1987, Churchill Livingstone.
5. Kirklin JW, Barratt-Boyes BG, editors: *Cardiac surgery: morphology, diagnostic criteria, natural history, techniques, results, and indications,* ed 2, New York, 1993, Churchill Livingstone.
6. Hoffman JI: Congenital heart disease: incidence and inheritance, *Pediatr Clin North Am* 37:25, 1990.
7. Samánek M: Children with congenital heart disease: probability of natural survival, *Pediatr Cardiol* 13:152, 1992.
8. Lin AE: Congenital heart defects in malformation syndromes, *Clin Perinatol* 17:641, 1990.
9. Driscoll DJ, Michels VV, Gersony WM et al: Occurrence risk for congenital heart defects in relatives of patients with aortic stenosis, pulmonary stenosis, or ventricular septal defect, *Circulation* 87(suppl):I, 1993.
10. Abbott ME: *Atlas of congenital cardiac disease,* New York, 1936, American Heart Association.
11. Waugh D: Maudie: the life and times of McGill's Maude Abbott, *Mod Pathol* 5:597, 1992.
12. Lev M: Congenital heart disease. In Saphir O, editor: *A text on systemic pathology,* New York, 1958, Grune & Stratton.
13. Wagenvoort CA, Heath D, Edwards JE: *The pathology of the pulmonary vasculature,* Springfield, Ill, 1964, Charles C Thomas.
14. Edwards JE: Congenital malformations of the heart and great vessels. In Gould SE, editor: *Pathology of the heart,* ed 3, Springfield, Ill, 1968, Charles C Thomas.
15. Van Praagh R, Takao A: *Etiology and morphogenesis of congenital heart disease,* Mount Kisco, NY, 1980, Futura.
16. Becker AE, Anderson RH: *Pathology of congenital heart disease,* London, 1981, Butterworths.
17. Edwards WD: Congenital heart disease. In Schoen FJ, editor: *Interventional and surgical cardiovascular pathology: clinical correlations and basic principles,* Philadelphia, 1989, Saunders.
18. Becker AE, Essed CE: The heart after surgery for congenital heart disease, *Am J Cardiovasc Pathol* 1:301, 1988.
19. Edwards WD: Classification and terminology of cardiovascular anomalies. In Emmanouilides GC, Riemenschneider TA, Allen HD, Gutgesell HP, editors: *Moss & Adams' heart disease in infants, children, and adolescents, including the fetus and young adult,* ed 5, Baltimore, 1995, Williams & Wilkins.

Unifying concepts of congenital heart disease

20. Anderson RH, Becker AE, Freedom RM et al: Sequential segmental analysis of congenital heart disease, *Pediatr Cardiol* 5:281, 1984.
21. Leca F, Thibert M, Khoury, W et al: Extrathoracic heart (ectopia cordis): report of two cases and review of the literature, *Int J Cardiol* 22:221, 1989.
22. Anderson C, Devine WA, Anderson RH, Zuberbuhler JR: Abnormalities of the spleen in relation to congenital malformations of the heart: a survey of necropsy findings in children, *Br Heart J* 63:122, 1990.
23. Peoples WM, Moller JH, Edwards JE: Polysplenia: a review of 146 cases, *Pediatr Cardiol* 4:129, 1983.
24. Sharma S, Devine W, Anderson RH, Zuberbuhler JR: The determination of atrial arrangement by examination of appendage morphology in 1842 autopsied specimens, *Br Heart J* 60:227, 1988.
25. Rice MJ, Seward JB, Edwards WD et al: Straddling atrioventricular valve: two-dimensional echocardiographic diagnosis, classification and surgical implications, *Am J Cardiol* 55:505, 1985.

Secondary cardiac and pulmonary lesions

26. Schoen FJ, Lawrie GM, Titus JL: Left ventricular cellular hypertrophy in pressure- and volume-overload valvular heart disease, *Hum Pathol* 15:860, 1984.
27. Edwards WD: Cardiac anatomy and examination of cardiac specimens. In Emmanouilides GC, Riemenschneider TA, Allen HD, Gutgesell HP, editors: *Moss and Adams' heart disease in infants, children, and adolescents, including the fetus and young adult,* ed 5, Baltimore, 1995, Williams & Wilkins.
28. Scholz DG, Kitzman DW, Hagen PT et al: Age-related changes in normal human hearts during the first 10 decades of life. Part I (growth): a quantitative anatomic study of 200 specimens from subjects from birth to 19 years old, *Mayo Clin Proc* 63:126, 1988.
29. Kitzman DW, Scholz DG, Hagen PT et al: Age-related changes in normal human hearts during the first 10 decades of life. Part II (maturity). A quantitative anatomic study of 765 specimens from subjects 20 to 99 years old, *Mayo Clin Proc* 63:137, 1988.
30. Goodman LC, Epling S, Kelly S et al: DNA flow cytometry of myocardial cell nuclei in paraffin-embedded, human autopsy, cardiac tissue, *Am J Cardiovasc Pathol* 3:55, 1990.
31. Eghbali M: Molecular and cellular mechanisms of induction and regression of cardiac fibrosis in various models of myocardial hypertrophy, *Cardiovasc Pathol* 2:199, 1993.
32. Donnelly WH: Ischemic myocardial necrosis and papillary muscle dysfunction in infants and children, *Am J Cardiovasc Pathol* 1:173, 1987.
33. Heath D, Edwards JE: The pathology of hypertensive pulmonary vascular disease: a description of six grades of structural changes in the pulmonary arteries with special reference to congenital cardiac septal defects, *Circulation* 18:533, 1958.
34. Wagenvoort CA: Hypertensive pulmonary vascular disease complicating congenital heart disease: a review, *Cardiovasc Clin* 5(1):43, 1973.
35. Rabinovitch M, Haworth SG, Vance Z et al: Early pulmonary vascular changes in congenital heart disease studied in biopsy tissue, *Hum Pathol* 11:499, 1980.
36. Yamaki S, Mohri H, Haneda K et al: Indications for surgery based on lung biopsy in cases of ventricular septal defect and/or patent ductus arteriosus with severe pulmonary hypertension, *Chest* 96:31, 1989.
37. Braunlin EA, Moller JH, Patton C et al: Predictive value of lung biopsy in ventricular septal defect: long-term follow-up, *J Am Coll Cardiol* 8:1113, 1986.
38. Wagenvoort CA: Open lung biopsies in congenital heart disease for evaluation of pulmonary vascular disease: predictive value with regard to corrective operability, *Histopathology* 9:417, 1985.
39. Bush A, Busst CM, Haworth SG et al: Correlations of lung morphology, pulmonary vascular resistance, and outcome in children with congenital heart disease, *Br Heart J* 59:480, 1988.
40. Spicer RL: Cardiovascular disease in Down syndrome, *Pediatr Clin North Am* 31:1331, 1984.
41. Edwards WD: Pathology of pulmonary hypertension, *Cardiovasc Clin* 18:321, 1988.
42. Fischer DR, Neches WH, Beerman LB et al: Tetralogy of Fallot with absent pulmonic valve: analysis of 17 patients, *Am J Cardiol* 53:1433, 1984.

Cardiovascular shunts

Atrial septal defect

43. Hagen PT, Scholz DG, Edwards WD: Incidence and size of patent foramen ovale during the first 10 decades of life: an autopsy study of 965 normal hearts, *Mayo Clin Proc* 59:17, 1984.
44. Lin AE, Perloff JK: Upper limb malformations associated with congenital heart disease, *Am J Cardiol* 55:1576, 1985.
45. Haworth SG: Pulmonary vascular disease in secundum atrial septal defect in childhood, *Am J Cardiol* 51:265, 1983.
46. Steele PM, Fuster V, Cohen M et al: Isolated atrial septal defect with pulmonary vascular obstructive disease: long-term follow-up and prediction of outcome after surgical correction, *Circulation* 76:1037, 1987.
47. Horvath KA, Burke RP, Collins JJ, Cohn LH: Surgical treatment of adult atrial septal defect: early and long-term results, *J Am Coll Cardiol* 20:1156, 1992.

48. Chan KC, Godman MJ: Morphological variations of fossa ovalis atrial septal defects (secundum): feasibility for transcutaneous closure with the clam-shell device, *Br Heart J* 69:52, 1993.
49. Ferriera SM, Ho SY, Anderson RH: Morphological study of defects of the atrial septum within the oval fossa: implications for transcatheter closure of left-to-right shunt, *Br Heart J* 67:316, 1992.

Atrioventricular septal defect

50. Ebels T, Anderson RH, Devine W et al: Anomalies of the left atrioventricular valve and related ventricular septal morphology in atrioventricular septal defects, *J Thorac Cardiovasc Surg* 99:299, 1990.
51. Fugelstad SJ, Danielson GK, Puga FJ, Edwards WD: Surgical pathology of the common atrioventricular valve: a study of 11 cases, *Am J Cardiovasc Pathol* 2:49, 1988.
52. Bharati S, Kirklin JW, McAllister HA Jr, Lev M: The surgical anatomy of common atrioventricular orifice associated with tetralogy of Fallot, double outlet right ventricle and complete regular transposition, *Circulation* 61:1142, 1980.
53. Clapp S, Perry BL, Farooki ZQ et al: Down's syndrome, complete atrioventricular canal, and pulmonary vascular obstructive disease, *J Thorac Cardiovasc Surg* 100:115, 1990.
54. Yamaki S, Horiuchi T, Sekino Y: Quantitative analysis of pulmonary vascular disease in simple cardiac anomalies with the Down syndrome, *Am J Cardiol* 51:1502, 1983.
55. Chang CI, Becker AE: Surgical anatomy of left ventricular outflow tract obstruction in complete atrioventricular septal defect: a concept for operative repair, *J Thorac Cardiovasc Surg* 94:897, 1987.
56. Ebels T, Ho SY, Anderson RH et al: The surgical anatomy of the left ventricular outflow tract in atrioventricular septal defect, *Ann Thorac Surg* 41:483, 1986.
57. Thiene G, Mazzucco A, Grisolia EF et al: Postoperative pathology of complete atrioventricular defects, *J Thorac Cardiovasc Surg* 83:891, 1982.

Ventricular septal defect

58. Anderson RH, Wilcox BR: The surgical anatomy of ventricular septal defects associated with overriding valvar orifices, *J Cardiac Surg* 8:130, 1993.
59. Soto B, Ceballos R, Kirklin J: Ventricular septal defects: a surgical viewpoint, *J Am Coll Cardiol* 14:1291, 1989.
60. Hagler DJ, Edwards WD, Seward JB, Tajik AJ: Standardized nomenclature of the ventricular septum and ventricular septal defects, with applications for two-dimensional echocardiography, *Mayo Clin Proc* 60:741, 1985.
61. Ando M, Takao A: Pathological anatomy of ventricular septal defect associated with aortic valve prolapse and regurgitation, *Heart Vessels* 2:117, 1986.
62. Hall SM, Haworth SG: Onset and evolution of pulmonary vascular disease in young children: abnormal postnatal remodelling studied in lung biopsies, *J Pathol* 166:183, 1992.
63. Haworth SG: Pulmonary vascular disease in ventricular septal defect: structural and functional correlations in lung biopsies from 85 patients, with outcome of intracardiac repair, *J Pathol* 152:57, 1987.
64. Saiman L, Prince A, Gersony WM: Pediatric infective endocarditis in the modern era, *J Pediatr* 122:847, 1993.
65. Moller JH, Patton C, Varco RL, Lillehei CW: Late results (30 to 35 years) after operative closure of isolated ventricular septal defect from 1954 to 1960, *Am J Cardiol* 68:1491, 1991.
66. Bridges ND, Lock JE: Transcatheter closure of ventricular septal defects, *Prog Pediatr Cardiol* 1(2):72, 1992.

Aortopulmonary septal defect

67. Kutsche LM, Van Mierop LHS: Anatomy and pathogenesis of aorticopulmonary septal defect, *Am J Cardiol* 59:443, 1987.
68. Prasad T, Valiathan M, Shyamakrishnan K, Venkitachalam C: Surgical management of aortopulmonary septal defect, *Ann Thorac Surg* 47:877, 1989.

Patent ductal artery

69. Gittenberger-de Groot AC, Strengers JL: Histopathology of the arterial duct (ductus arteriosus) with and without treatment with prostaglandin E_1. *Int J Cardiol* 19:153, 1988.
70. Tada T, Wakabayashi T, Nakao Y et al: Human ductus arteriosus: a histological study on the relation between ductal maturation and gestational age, *Acta Pathol Jpn* 35:23, 1985.
71. Krichenko A, Benson LN, Burrows P et al: Angiographic classification of the isolated, persistently patent ductus arteriosus and implications for percutaneous catheter occlusion, *Am J Cardiol* 63:877, 1989.
72. Cassady G, Crouse DT, Kirklin JW et al: A randomized, controlled trial of very early prophylactic ligation of the ductus arteriosus in babies who weighed 1000 g or less at birth, *N Engl J Med* 320:1511, 1989.
73. Gray DT, Fyler DC, Walker AM et al: Clinical outcomes and costs of transcatheter as compared with surgical closure of patent ductus arteriosus, *N Engl J Med* 329:1517, 1993.

Conotruncal anomalies

Tetralogy of Fallot

74. Bartelings MM, Gittenberger-de Groot AC: Morphogenetic considerations on congenital malformations of the outflow tract. Part 1. Common arterial trunk and tetralogy of Fallot, *Int J Cardiol* 32:213, 1991.
75. Howell CE, Ho SY, Anderson RH, Elliott MJ: Variations within the fibrous skeleton and ventricular outflow tracts in tetralogy of Fallot, *Ann Thorac Surg* 50:450, 1990.
76. McGrath LB, Chen C, Gu J et al: Determination of infundibular innervation and amine receptor content in cyanotic and acyanotic myocardium: relation to clinical events in tetralogy of Fallot, *Pediatr Cardiol* 12:155, 1991.
77. Altrichter PM, Olson LJ, Edwards WD et al: Surgical pathology of the pulmonary valve: a study of 116 cases spanning 15 years, *Mayo Clin Proc* 64:1352, 1989.
78. Rosenberg HG, Williams WG, Trusler GA et al: Structural composition of central pulmonary arteries: growth potential after surgical shunts, *J Thorac Cardiovasc Surg* 94:498, 1987.
79. Dare AJ, Veinot JP, Edwards WD et al: New observations on the etiology of aortic valve disease: a surgical pathologic study of 236 cases from 1990, *Hum Pathol* 24:1330, 1993.
80. Thiene G, Mazzucco A, Anderson RH et al: Tetralogy of Fallot after surgery: autopsy review of 14 cases, *Hum Pathol* 15:1018, 1984.
81. Murphy JG, Gersh BJ, Mair DD et al: Long-term outcome in patients undergoing surgical repair of tetralogy of Fallot, *N Engl J Med* 329:593, 1993.

Pulmonary atresia with ventricular septal defect

82. Jedele KB, Michels VV, Puga FJ, Feldt RH: Velo-cardio-facial syndrome associated with ventricular septal defect, pulmonary atresia, and hypoplastic pulmonary arteries, *Pediatrics* 89:915, 1992.
83. Rabinovitch M: Pathology and anatomy of pulmonary atresia and ventricular septal defect, *Prog Pediatr Cardiol* 1(1):9, 1992.
84. Anderson RH, Devine WA, del Nido P: The surgical anatomy of tetralogy of Fallot with pulmonary atresia rather than pulmonary stenosis, *J Cardiac Surg* 6:41, 1991.
85. Liao PK, Edwards WD, Julsrud PR et al: Pulmonary blood supply in patients with pulmonary atresia and ventricular septal defect, *J Am Coll Cardiol* 6:1343, 1985.
86. Pearl JM, Laks H, Drinkwater DC Jr et al: Repair of conotruncal abnormalities with the use of the valved conduit: improved early and midterm results with the cryopreserved homograft, *J Am Coll Cardiol* 20:191, 1992.
87. Albert JD, Bishop DA, Fullerton DA et al: Conduit reconstruction of the right ventricular outflow tract: lessons learned in a twelve-year experience, *J Thorac Cardiovasc Surg* 106:228, 1993.
88. Edwards WD, Agarwal KC, Feldt RH et al: Surgical pathology of obstructed, right-sided, porcine-valved extracardiac conduits, *Arch Pathol Lab Med* 107:400, 1983.

Double outlet right ventricle

89. Bartelings MM, Gittenberger-de Groot AC: Morphogenetic considerations on congenital malformations of the outflow tract. Part 2. complete transposition of the great arteries and double outlet right ventricle, *Int J Cardiol* 33:5, 1991.
90. de la Cruz MV, Cayre R, Martínez OAS et al: The infundibular interrelationships and the ventriculoarterial connection in double outlet right ventricle: clinical and surgical implications, *Int J Cardiol* 35:153, 1992.
91. Howell CE, Ho SY, Anderson RH, Elliott MJ: Fibrous skeleton and ventricular outflow tracts in double-outlet right ventricle, *Ann Thorac Surg* 51:394, 1991.

92. Stellin G, Zuberbuhler JR, Anderson RH, Siewers RD: The surgical anatomy of the Taussig-Bing malformation, *J Thorac Cardiovasc Surg* 93:560, 1987.
93. Shen WK, Holmes DR Jr, Porter CJ et al: Sudden death after repair of double-outlet right ventricle, *Circulation* 81:128, 1990.

Persistent truncal artery

94. Radford DJ, Perkins L, Lachman R, Thong YH: Spectrum of DiGeorge syndrome in patients with truncus arteriosus: expanded DiGeorge syndrome, *Pediatr Cardiol* 9:95, 1988.
95. Butto F, Lucas RV Jr, Edwards JE: Persistent truncus arteriosus: pathologic anatomy in 54 cases, *Pediatr Cardiol* 7:95, 1986.
96. Van Praagh R: Truncus arteriosus: what is it really and how should it be classified?, *Eur J Cardiothorac Surg* 1:65, 1987.
97. Anderson RH, Thiene G: Categorization and description of hearts with a common arterial trunk, *Eur J Cardiothorac Surg* 3:481, 1989.
98. de la Cruz MV, Cayre R, Angelini P et al: Coronary arteries in truncus arteriosus, *Am J Cardiol* 66:1482, 1990.
99. Fuglestad SJ, Puga FJ, Danielson GK, Edwards WD: Surgical pathology of the truncal valve: a study of 12 cases, *Am J Cardiovasc Pathol* 2:39, 1988.
100. Bharati S, Karp R, Lev M: The conduction system in truncus arteriosus and its surgical significance: a study of five cases, *J Thorac Cardiovasc Surg* 104:954, 1992.
101. Juaneda E, Haworth SG: Pulmonary vascular disease in children with truncus arteriosus, *Am J Cardiol* 54:1314, 1984.

Complete transposition of the great arteries

102. Pasquini L, Sanders SP, Parness IA et al: Conal anatomy in 119 patients with d-loop transposition of the great arteries and ventricular septal defect: an echocardiographic and pathologic study, *J Am Coll Cardiol* 21:1712, 1993.
103. Hoyer MH, Zuberbuhler JR, Anderson RH, del Nido P: Morphology of ventricular septal defects in complete transposition: surgical implications, *J Thorac Cardiovasc Surg* 104:1203, 1992.
104. Milanesi O, Ho SY, Thiene G et al: The ventricular septal defect in complete transposition of the great arteries: pathologic anatomy in 57 cases with emphasis on subaortic, subpulmonary, and aortic arch obstruction, *Hum Pathol* 18:392, 1987.
105. Silberbach M, Castro WL, Goldstein MA et al: Comparison of types of pulmonary stenosis and the state of the ventricular septum in complete transposition of the great arteries, *Pediatr Cardiol* 10:11, 1989.
106. Moene RJ, Oppenheimer-Dekker A: Congenital mitral valve anomalies in transposition of the great arteries, *Am J Cardiol* 49:1972, 1982.
107. Huhta JC, Edwards WD, Danielson GK et al: Abnormalities of the tricuspid valve in complete transposition of the great arteries with ventricular septal defect, *J Thorac Cardiovasc Surg* 83:569, 1982.
108. Sim EKW, van Son JAM, Edwards WD et al: Coronary artery anatomy in complete transposition of the great arteries, *Ann Thorac Surg* 57:890, 1994.
109. DiDonato RM, Fujii AM, Jonas RA, Castaneda AR: Age-dependent ventricular response to pressure overload: considerations for the arterial switch operation, *J Thorac Cardiovasc Surg* 104:713, 1992.
110. Haworth SG, Radley-Smith R, Yacoub M: Lung biopsy findings in transposition of the great arteries with ventricular septal defect: potentially reversible pulmonary vascular disease is not always synonymous with operablility, *J Am Coll Cardiol* 9:327, 1987.
111. Yamaki S, Wagenvoort CA: Plexogenic pulmonary arteriopathy: significance of medial thickness with respect to advanced pulmonary vascular lesions, *Am J Pathol* 105:70, 1981.
112. Akiba T, Neirotti R, Becker AE: Is there an anatomic basis for subvalvular right ventricular outflow tract obstruction after an arterial switch repair for complete transposition? A morphometric study and review, *J Thorac Cardiovasc Surg* 105:142, 1993.

Congenitally corrected transposition of the great arteries

113. Allwork SP, Bentall HH, Becker AE et al: Congenitally corrected transposition of the great arteries: morphologic study of 32 cases, *Am J Cardiol* 38:910, 1976.
114. Anderson KR, Danielson GK, McGoon DC, Lie JT: Ebstein's anomaly of the left-sided tricuspid valve: pathologic anatomy of the valvular malformation, *Circulation* 58(suppl I):87, 1978.
115. Huhta JC, Danielson GK, Ritter DG, Ilstrup DM: Survival in atrioventricular discordance, *Pediatr Cardiol* 6:57, 1985.
116. Lundstrom U, Bull C, Wyse RK, Somerville J: The natural and "unnatural" history of congenitally corrected transposition, *Am J Cardiol* 65:1222, 1990.
117. Dimas AP, Moodie DS, Sterba R, Gill CC: Long-term function of the morphologic right ventricle in adult patients with corrected transposition of the great arteries, *Am Heart J* 118:526, 1989.

Single functional ventricles

Tricuspid atresia

118. Anderson RH, Rigby ML: The morphologic heterogeneity of "tricuspid atresia," *Int J Cardiol* 16:67, 1987.
119. Thoele DG, Ursell PC, Ho SY et al: Atrial morphologic features in tricuspid atresia, *J Thorac Cardiovasc Surg* 102:606, 1991.
120. Ottenkamp J, Wenink ACG, Quaegebeur JM et al: Tricuspid atresia: morphology of the outlet chamber with special emphasis on surgical implications, *J Thorac Cardiovasc Surg* 89:597, 1985.
121. Ottenkamp J, Wenink ACG: Anomalies of the mitral valve and of the left ventricular architecture in tricuspid valve atresia, *Am J Cardiol* 63:880, 1989.
122. Franklin RCG, Spiegelhalter DJ Sullivan ID et al: Tricuspid atresia presenting in infancy: survival and suitability for the Fontan operation, *Circulation* 87:427, 1993.
123. Castaneda AR: From Glenn to Fontan: a continuing evolution, *Circulation* 86(suppl II):80, 1992.
124. Driscoll DJ, Offord KP, Feldt RH et al: Five- to fifteen-year follow-up after Fontan operation, *Circulation* 85:469, 1992.
125. Caspi J, Coles JG, Rabinovitch M et al: Morphological findings contributing to a failed Fontan procedure, *Circulation* 82(suppl IV):177, 1990.

Double inlet left ventricle

126. Ho SY, Zuberbuhler JR, Anderson RH: Pathology of hearts with a univentricular atrioventricular connection, *Perspect Pediatr Pathol* 12:69, 1988.
127. Van Praagh R, Plett JA, Van Praagh S: Single ventricle: pathology, embryology, terminology and classification, *Herz* 4:113, 1979.
128. Bevilacqua M, Sanders SP, Van Praagh S et al: Double-inlet left ventricle: echocardiographic anatomy with emphasis on the morphology of the atrioventricular valves and ventricular septal defect, *J Am Coll Cardiol* 18:559, 1991.
129. Doherty A, Ho SY, Anderson RH, Rigby ML: Morphological nature of the atrioventricular valves in hearts with double inlet left ventricle, *Pediatr Pathol* 9:521, 1989.
130. Anderson RH, Penkoske PA, Zuberbuhler JR: Variable morphology of ventricular septal defect in double inlet left ventricle, *Am J Cardiol* 55:1560, 1985.
131. Juaneda E, Haworth SG: Double inlet ventricle: lung biopsy findings and implications for management, *Br Heart J* 53:515, 1985.
132. Franklin RCG, Sullivan ID, Anderson RH et al: Is banding of the pulmonary trunk obsolete for infants with tricuspid atresia and double inlet ventricle with a discordant ventriculoarterial connection? Role of aortic arch obstruction and subaortic stenosis, *J Am Coll Cardiol* 16:1455, 1990.
133. Sluysmans T, Sanders SP, van der Velde M et al: Natural history and patterns of recovery of contractile function in single left ventricle after Fontan operation, *Circulation* 86:1753, 1992.

Aortic atresia (hypoplastic left heart syndrome)

134. Bharati S, Lev M: The surgical anatomy of hypoplasia of the aortic tract complex, *J Thorac Cardiovasc Surg* 88:97, 1984.
135. Aiello VD, Ho SY, Anderson RH, Thiene G: Morphologic features of the hypoplastic left heart syndrome: a reappraisal, *Pediatr Pathol* 10:931, 1990.
136. Baffa JM, Chen SL, Guttenberg ME et al: Coronary artery abnormalities and right ventricular histology in hypoplastic left heart syndrome, *J Am Coll Cardiol* 20:350, 1992.
137. Sauer U, Gittenberger-de Groot AC, Gieshauser M et al: Coronary arteries in hypoplastic left heart syndrome: histopathologic and histo-

metrical studies and implications for surgery, *Circulation* 80(suppl I):168, 1989.

138. Pigott JD, Murphy JD, Barber G, Norwood WI: Palliative reconstructive surgery for hypoplastic left heart syndrome, *Ann Thorac Surg* 45:122, 1988.
139. Chiavarelli M, Gundry SR, Razzouk AJ, Bailey LL: Cardiac transplantation for infants with hypoplastic left heart syndrome, *JAMA* 270:2944, 1993.
140. Backer CL, Zales VR, Idriss FS et al: Heart transplantation in neonates and in children, *J Heart Lung Transplant* 11:311, 1992.
141. Baum D, Bernstein D: Pediatric heart transplantation: complications, *Progr Pediatr Cardiol* 2(4):29, 1993.

Pulmonary atresia with intact ventricular septum

142. Kutsche LM, Van Mierop LHS: Pulmonary atresia with and without ventricular septal defect: a different etiology and pathogenesis for the atresia in the 2 types?, *Am J Cardiol* 65:261, 1983.
143. Stellin G, Santini F, Thiene G et al: Pulmonary atresia, intact ventricular septum, and Ebstein anomaly of the tricuspid valve: anatomic and surgical considerations, *J Thorac Cardiovasc Surg* 106:255, 1993.
144. Anderson RH, Silverman NH, Zuberbuhler JR: Congenitally unguarded tricuspid orifice: its differentiation from Ebstein's malformation in association with pulmonary atresia and intact ventricular septum, *Pediatr Cardiol* 11:86, 1990.
145. Bulkley BH, D'Amico B, Taylor AL: Extensive myocardial fiber disarray in aortic and pulmonary atresia: relevance to hypertrophic cardiomyopathy, *Circulation* 67:191, 1983.
146. O'Connor WN, Stahr BJ, Cottrill CM et al: Ventriculocoronary connections in hypoplastic right heart syndrome: autopsy serial section study of six cases, *J Am Coll Cardiol* 11:1061, 1988.
147. Kasznica J, Ursell PC, Blanc WA, Gersony WM: Abnormalities of the coronary circulation in pulmonary atresia and intact ventricular septum, *Am Heart J* 114:1415, 1987.
148. Parsons JM, Rees MR, Gibbs JL: Percutaneous laser valvotomy with balloon dilatation of the pulmonary valve as primary treatment for pulmonary atresia, *Br Heart J* 66:36, 1991.
149. Hanley FL, Sade RM, Blackstone EH et al: Outcomes in neonatal pulmonary atresia with intact ventricular septum: a multi-institutional study, *J Thorac Cardiovasc Surg* 105:406, 1993.
150. Pawade A, Capuani A, Penny DJ et al: Pulmonary atresia with intact ventricular septum: surgical management based on right ventricular infundibulum, *J Cardiac Surg 8:371, 1993.*

Cardiovascular obstructions

Aortic stenosis

151. Roberts CS, Roberts WC: Dissection of the aorta associated with congenital malformation of the aortic valve, *J Am Coll Cardiol* 17:712, 1991.
152. Larson EW, Edwards WD: Risk factors for aortic dissection: a necropsy study of 161 cases, *Am J Cardiol* 53:849, 1984.
153. Anderson RH, Devine WA, Ho SY et al: The myth of the aortic annulus: the anatomy of the subaortic outflow tract, *Ann Thorac Surg* 52:640, 1991.
154. Maizza AF, Ho SY, Anderson RH: Obstruction of the left ventricular outflow tract: anatomical observations and surgical implications, *J Heart Valve Dis* 2:66, 1993.
155. van Son JAM, Edwards WD, Danielson GK: Pathology of coronary arteries, myocardium, and great arteries in supravalvular aortic stenosis: report of five cases with implications for surgical treatment, *J Thorac Cardiovasc Surg* 108:21, 1994.
156. Zalstein E, Moes CA, Musewe NN, Freedom RM: The spectrum of cardiovascular anomalies in Williams-Beuren syndrome, *Pediatr Cardiol* 12:219, 1991.
157. Roth SJ, Keane JF: Balloon aortic valvuloplasty, *Prog Pediatr* Cardiol 1(2):3, 1992.
158. van Son JAM, Danielson GK, Puga FJ et al: Supravalvular aortic stenosis: long-term results of surgical treatment, *J Thorac Cardiovasc Surg* 107:103, 1994.

Pulmonary stenosis

159. Burch M, Sharland M, Shinebourne E et al: Cardiologic abnormalities in Noonan syndrome: phenotypic diagnosis and echocardiographic assessment of 118 patients, *J Am Coll Cardiol* 22:1189, 1993.
160. Gikonyo BM, Lucas RV Jr, Edwards JE: Anatomic features of congenital pulmonary valvar stenosis, *Pediatr Cardiol* 8:109, 1987.
161. Sholler GF, Colan SD, Sanders SP: Effect of isolated right ventricular outflow obstruction on left ventricular function in infants, *Am J Cardiol* 62:778, 1988.
162. Musewe N, Robertson MA, Benson LN et al: The dysplastic pulmonary valve: echocardiographic features and results of balloon dilation, *Br Heart J* 57:364, 1987.
163. Masura J, Burch M, Deanfield JE, Sullivan ID: Five-year follow-up after balloon pulmonary valvuloplasty, *J Am Coll Cardiol* 21:132, 1993.

Coarctation of the aorta

164. Van Mierop LHS, Kutsche LM: Aortic obstructions in infants and children: pathogenesis of aortic arch obstructions, *Prog Pediatr Cardiol* 3(1):28, 1994.
165. Russell GA, Berry PJ, Watterson K et al: Patterns of ductal tissue in coarctation of the aorta in the first three months of life, *J Thorac Cardiovasc Surg* 102:596, 1991.
166. Rosenberg HS: Coarctation as a deformation, *Pediatr Pathol* 10:103, 1990.
167. Bharati S, Lev M: The surgical anatomy of the heart in tubular hypoplasia of the transverse aorta (preductal coarctation), *J Thorac Cardiovasc Surg* 91:79, 1986.
168. Glancy D, Morrow A, Simon A, Roberts WC: Juxtaductal aortic coarctation: analysis of 84 patients studied hemodynamically, angiographically, and morphologically after age 1 year, *Am J Cardiol* 51:537, 1983.
169. Tandon R, Moller JH, Edwards JE: Anomalies associated with the parachute mitral valve: a pathologic analysis of 52 cases, *Can J Cardiol* 2:278, 1986.
170. Kappetein AP, Zwinderman AH, Bogers AJ et al: More than thirty-five years of coarctation repair: an unexpected high relapse rate, *J Thorac Cardiovasc Surg* 107:87, 1994.
171. Rocchini AP: Balloon angioplasty of postoperative aortic recoarctation, *Prog Pediatr Cardiol* 1(2):28, 1992.
172. Rao PS, Chopra PS, Koscik R et al: Surgical versus balloon therapy for aortic coarctation in infants, *J Am Coll Cardiol* 23:1479, 1994.
173. Phadke K, Dyet JF, Aber CP, Hartley W: Balloon angioplasty of adult aortic coarctation, *Br Heart J* 69:36, 1993.

Other cardiovascular anomalies

Anomalous pulmonary venous connection

174. Rammos S, Gittenberger de Groot AC, Oppenheimer-Dekker A: The abnormal pulmonary venous connexion: a developmental approach. *Int J Cardiol* 29:285, 1990.
175. Gikonyo DK, Tandon R, Lucas RV Jr, Edwards JE: Scimitar syndrome in neonates: report of four cases and review of the literature, *Pediatr Cardiol* 6:193, 1986.
176. Delisle G, Ando M, Calder AL et al: Total anomalous pulmonary venous connection: report of 93 autopsied cases with emphasis on diagnostic and surgical considerations, *Am Heart J* 91:99, 1976.
177. Lucas RV Jr, Lock JE, Tandon R, Edwards JE: Gross and histological anatomy of total anomalous pulmonary venous connection, *Am J Cardiol* 62:292, 1988.
178. Yamaki S, Tsunemoto M, Shimada M et al: Quantitative analysis of pulmonary vascular disease in total anomalous pulmonary venous connection in sixty infants, *J Thorac Cardiovasc Surg* 104:728, 1992.
179. Raisher BD, Grant JW, Martin TC et al: Complete repair of total anomalous pulmonary venous connection in infancy, *J Thorac Cardiovasc Surg* 104:443, 1992.
180. Byard RW, Moore L: Total anomalous pulmonary venous drainage and sudden death in infancy, *Forensic Sci Int* 51:197, 1991.

Ebstein's anomaly

181. Edwards WD: Embryology and pathologic features of Ebstein's anomaly, *Prog Pediatr Cardiol* 2(1):5, 1993.
182. Zuberbuhler JR, Becker AE, Anderson RH, Lenox CC: Ebstein's malformation and the embryological development of the tricuspid valve: with a note on the nature of "clefts" in the atrioventricular valves, *Pediatr Cardiol* 5:289, 1984.
183. Zalstein E, Koren G, Einarson T, Freedom RM: A case-control study on the association between first trimester exposure to lithium and Ebstein's anomaly, *Am J Cardiol* 65:817, 1990.

184. Sipek A: Lithium and Ebstein's anomaly, *Cor Vasa* 31:149, 1989.
185. Castaneda-Zuniga W, Nath HP, Moller JH, Edwards JE: Left-sided anomalies in Ebstein's malformation of the tricuspid valve, *Pediatr Cardiol* 3:181, 1982.
186. Danielson GK: Surgical management of Ebstein's anomaly, *Prog Pediatr Cardiol* 2(1):51, 1993.
187. Hauck AJ, Freeman DP, Ackermann DM et al: Surgical pathology of the tricuspid valve: a study of 363 cases spanning 25 years, *Mayo Clin Proc* 63:851, 1988.
188. Celermajer DS, Dodd SM, Greenwald SE et al: Morbid anatomy in neonates with Ebstein's anomaly of the tricuspid valve: pathophysiologic and clinical implications, *J Am Coll Cardiol* 19:1049, 1992.

Coronary and conduction anomalies

189. Neufeld HN, Schneeweiss A: *Coronary artery disease in infants and children,* Philadelphia, 1983, Lea & Febiger.
190. Vlodaver Z, Neufeld HN, Edwards JE: *Coronary arterial variations in the normal heart and in congenital heart disease,* New York, 1975, Academic Press.
191. Anderson RH, Ho SY: The disposition of the conduction tissues in congenitally malformed hearts with reference to their embryologic development, *J Perinat Med* 19(Suppl 1):201, 1991.
192. Davies MJ, Anderson RH, Becker AE: *The conduction system of the heart.*, London, 1983, Butterworth.

Evaluation of congenital heart disease at autopsy

Methods of dissection

193. Devine WA, Debich DE, Anderson RH: Dissection of congenitally malformed hearts, with comments on the value of sequential segmental analysis, *Pediatr Pathol* 11:235, 1991.
194. Ackermann DM, Edwards WD: Anatomic basis for tomographic analysis of the pediatric heart at autopsy, *Perspect Pediatr Pathol* 12:44, 1988.
195. Russell GA, Berry PJ: Approaches to the demonstration of congenital heart disease, *J Clin Pathol* 39:503, 1986.
196. Edwards WD, Tajik AJ, Seward JB: Standardized nomenclature and anatomic basis for regional tomographic analysis of the heart, *Mayo Clin Proc* 56:479, 1981.

Specimen photography

197. Edwards WD: Photography of medical specimens: experiences from teaching cardiovascular pathology, *Mayo Clin Proc* 63:42, 1988.
198. Vetter JP: Gross specimen photography. In Vetter JP, editor: *Biomedical photography*, Boston, 1992, Butterworth-Heineman.
199. Fredrickson RM: A method of using axial light in gross specimen photography, *J Biol Photogr* 57:69, 1989.
200. Cutignola L, Bullough PG: Photographic reproduction of anatomic specimens using ultraviolet illumination, *Am J Surg Pathol* 15:1096, 1991.

47 Vascular System

A. BLOOD VESSELS AND LYMPHATICS

Sean Moore

ARTERIES

Normal arteries and age-related changes

Arteries conventionally are divided into three types depending on their size and certain histologic features: (1) large, elastic arteries; (2) medium-sized, distributing, muscular arteries; and (3) arterioles, which connect to capillaries. The three types are not sharply divided; elastic arteries gradually merge with muscular arteries and muscular arteries with arterioles. Histologically all arteries have three layers: the tunica intima on the luminal side of the vessel, the tunica media as a middle layer, and the tunica adventitia as the outermost layer. These three layers become less definite as the arteries diminish in size and usually are not clearly identifiable in arterioles. Arteries and veins of all sizes and types are lined by an endothelium, which is a single layer of cells. The endothelial cells, basement membranes, and different amounts of connective tissues in different vessels form the tunica intima. Endothelial cells are not well demonstrated in routine histologic preparations. Endothelial cells react with antibodies to factor VIII antigen and can be also demonstrated with *Ulex europaeus* pectin. On electron microscopy preparations endothelial cells appear as flattened cells containing specialized junctions, intracellular organelles for the transport of substances, and typical Weibel-Palade bodies.

The elastic arteries include the aorta and its major branches and the major pulmonary arteries. In the first decade of life the tunica intima of these vessels is composed of endothelial cells with their basement membranes, a scanty amount of ground substance, collagen and elastic fibers, and the internal elastic lamina (lamella). The intima is bounded by the internal elastic lamina, a fenestrated sheet of elastic fibers that may be regarded both as part of the intima and as the beginning of the tunica media. The tunica media of elastic arteries constitutes the bulk of the arterial wall and consists chiefly of concentrically arranged, fenestrated laminae of elastic tissue with intervening smooth muscle cells and a histologically amorphous ground substance, which biochemically is a proteoglycan. An elastic lamella and the adjacent interlamellar zone is called a *lamellar unit*.[1] The elastic laminas become thicker and more numerous in adulthood than they are in childhood. The outermost elastic lamina of the media is the external elastic lamina. The tunica adventitia consists of irregularly arranged collagen and elastic fibers. Small nutrient vessels of the arteries themselves, the vasa vasorum, are present in the adventitia, together with lymphatics and nerves. In human beings the outer portion of the media of the thoracic aorta also has vasa vasorum.

Muscular arteries are generally branches of elastic arteries, with internal diameters ranging from 0.3 to 3 mm. The definition of a muscular artery is mainly a histologic one and is related to the near absence of well-defined elastic laminas in the media. The intima of a muscular artery is similar to that of an elastic artery, but thinner. The internal elastic lamina in muscular arteries in usual light microscopic preparations appears to be a single, continuous, wavy line; it is not continuous, however, but fenestrated, and is not wavy in life, the waviness being a postmortem artifact. The tunica media of the muscular arteries is thick compared with the other two layers and consists primarily of circularly disposed, spindle-shaped smooth muscle cells, fine collagen and elastic fibers, and ground substance organized in an orderly fashion. The external elastic lamina is less prominent than that of elastic arteries and is not present in cerebral arteries. The tunica adventitia is thinner than the tunica media and consists of collagen fibers, coarse and irregular elastic fibers, vasa vasorum, lymphatics, and nerves.

The intima and the inner parts of the media in both elastic and large muscular arteries derive nutrition from the vascular lumen by perfusion, whereas the nourishment of the outer media is derived from the vasa vasorum. There is therefore a nutritional boundary zone (watershed area) within the media that is especially susceptible to damage resulting from changes such as increased thickness of the intima, mural thrombosis within the arterial lumen, impaired oxygenation of or oxygen release by the circulating blood, and obstruction of the vasa vasorum.

Arterioles are the smallest arteries, with an internal diameter of 0.3 mm or less. The larger arterioles have the usual three tissue layers, including a poorly defined internal elastic lamina. The media in the smaller arterioles is one or two smooth muscle cells thick. The adventitia, consisting chiefly of collagen and elastic fibers, is relatively thick in larger arterioles and less prominent in smaller ones.

Changes that are roughly proportional to age occur in arteries as a result of the constant hemodynamic stresses produced by intraluminal blood pressure and flow. With time the walls of all arteries become more rigid, thus the term *senile arteriosclerosis.* These age-related changes are reflected in the dilatation (ectasia) of some large elastic arteries and in the tortuosity of some large muscular arteries. The structural basis of arterial aging, which may be regarded as an inevitable physiologic process, is most conspicuous in the intima but also involves the media.

In the fetus and neonate the intima is composed almost exclusively of endothelial cells with basement membranes. In older infants some splitting of the internal elastic lamina and accumulation of fine elastic fibrils between the internal elastic lamina and the basement membrane of the endothelium are found. These changes represent the beginning of intimal thickening that is a part of the normal growth and remodeling processes. By 6 to 12 months of age, smooth muscle cells are found in the intima adjacent to the internal elastic lamina, creating a musculoelastic intimal layer. These smooth muscle cells synthesize basement membrane material, collagen, elastin, and the proteoglycan (ground substance) of extracellular material.[2] However, considerable intimal thickening can be found in some infants and neonates, and this has been related to a family history of coronary artery disease, indicating that intimal thickening is a morphologic manifestation of a predisposition to coronary artery disease.[3] Intimal thickening progresses throughout life with the addition of more elastic and collagen fibers and the eventual loss of cellular elements. These changes are seen most commonly in coronary arteries, the abdominal aorta (more on the dorsal than the ventral aspect), and the larger arteries of the lower extremities, all of which tend to manifest severe atherosclerotic lesions.

Arteriosclerosis

Arteriosclerosis is a generic inclusive term that describes thickening and hardening of the arterial wall. Included in this term are four pathologic entities: arteriolosclerosis, hypertensive arteriosclerosis, Mönckeberg's medial calcific sclerosis, and atherosclerosis. Some confusion results from use of the term *arteriosclerosis* to refer to the more specific disease *atherosclerosis,* and the use of the unqualified term in reference to the arterial changes associated with aging (senile arteriosclerosis), hypertension (hypertensive arteriosclerosis), and the reparative response of the artery to injuries (reparative arteriosclerosis). The term *hyaline arteriosclerosis* usually means 'hyaline arteriolosclerosis.'

Arteriolosclerosis

Two morphologic abnormalities of arterioles, hyaline arteriosclerosis (arteriolar hyalinosis) and hyperplastic (proliferative) arteriolosclerosis, constitute arteriolosclerosis.

Hyaline arteriolosclerosis. Hyaline arteriolar thickening (sclerosis) is a common pathologic lesion. Arteriolar hyalinosis pathologically is manifested by a subendothelial, homogeneous, glassy pink material in hematoxylin-eosin–stained sections (Fig. 47-1). It may accompany hypertensive disease, be a physiologic phenomenon of aging, or occur in patients with diabetes mellitus. The usual hyalinosis of visceral arterioles begins as a focal, segmental process that spreads to involve the entire circumference of the vessel. Some of the hyaline material, which is not homogeneous chemically, appears to be derived from precipitated plasma proteins, the major component being the inactive form of complement C3b.[4] Moderate reduplication and thickening of the endothelial basement membranes are usually present. The hyaline arteriolosclerosis of aging cerebral arterioles differs from that of visceral arterioles in that it appears to result from progressive fibrotic thickening of the adventitia and from fibrosis of the media leading to the hyalinized vessel.

Hyperplastic (proliferative) arteriolosclerosis. The intimal thickening with consequent luminal reduction that takes place in the setting of hyperplastic arteriolosclerosis is a characteristic lesion of malignant hypertension, but identical changes may be found in patients with the hemolytic-uremic syndrome, progressive systemic sclerosis (scleroderma), homocystine-

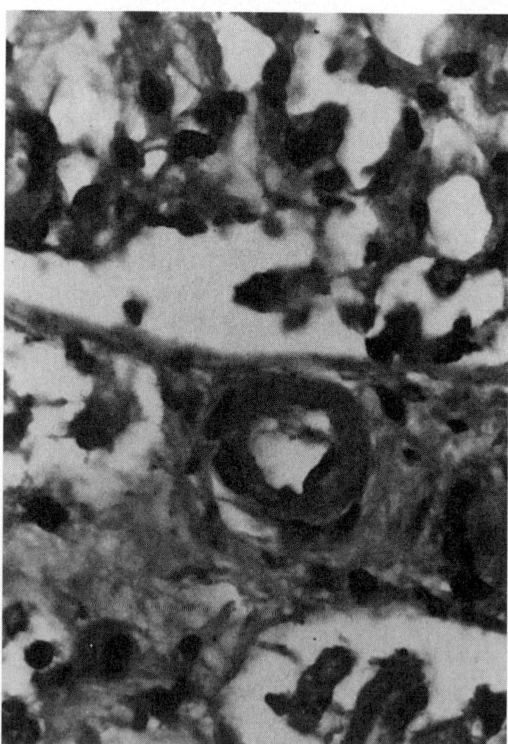

Fig. 47-1 Hyaline arteriolosclerosis.

mia, congenital rubella, chronic rejection, and malignant atrophic papulosis (Degos's disease), as well as in those exposed to radiation.[5] The process has been studied most extensively in the setting of accelerated hypertension, especially in renal interlobular arterioles and small arteries. Three main intimal morphologic patterns that can be distinguished are the "onionskin lesion," mucinous intimal thickening, and the fibrous intimal thickening.[6] The onionskin intimal lesion consists of loosely disposed layers of modified smooth muscle cells (Fig. 47-2). The mucinous intimal thickening consists mainly of lucent amorphous material, probably proteoglycans, with few cells. Fibrous intimal thickening, which is less common, has hyaline deposits, reduplicated elastic fibers, and coarse bundles of collagen. The fine structural features of the cells of the thickened intima are those of modified smooth muscle cells, including a basement membrane, pinocytotic vesicles, cytoplasmic myofilaments, and most characteristically and constantly, spindle-shaped dense bodies or attachment devices associated with myofilaments. The pathogenesis of these intimal changes is unclear, but the plasma proteins probably gain entry into the intima after endothelial injury such as that caused by increased pressure (hypertension), hypoxia, or immunologic damage. Similar morphologic lesions can be induced experimentally by emboli of platelet aggregates derived from a thrombogenic source in the thoracic aorta of rabbits.[7] The common pathway responsible for these changes is endothelial injury with increased permeability followed by a healing reaction of the vessel wall that involves the migration of smooth muscle cells from the media and the proliferation of these cells with fibrosis.

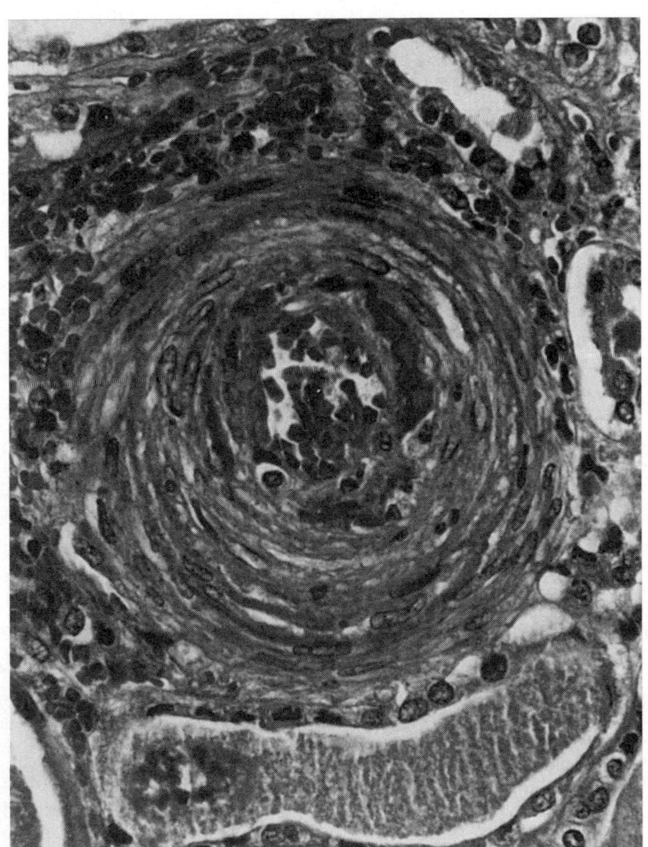

Fig. 47-2 Hyperplastic arteriolosclerosis.

Hypertensive arteriosclerosis

Regardless of its cause, hypertension may be divided clinically and to some degree pathologically into chronic (benign) and accelerated (malignant) types. Accelerated hypertension may occur de novo, or it may supervene in patients who are chronically hypertensive. A sustained elevation of the arterial blood pressure is associated with apparently adaptive structural changes in arteries of all sizes. The changes in the larger arteries are similar in all types of hypertension, but different processes come into play in the smaller arteries and arterioles in the settings of chronic and accelerated hypertension.

The classic hypertensive arterial change of large and medium-sized arteries found in young persons is medial hypertrophy resulting from increased numbers and enlargement of the smooth muscle cells and elastic fibers. The intima of these vessels may have more numerous longitudinally oriented smooth muscle fibers. With time these hyperplastic and hypertrophic changes are replaced by collagen, with the thickened arterial wall becoming less resilient and the lumen becoming dilated and tortuous.

In patients with benign hypertension smaller arteries may show medial thickening like that seen in the larger arteries, but the intimal thickening is more pronounced and results in luminal narrowing. The major change is hyaline arteriolosclerosis. Reduplication of basement membranes, elastosis, fibrosis, and hyaline deposits commonly are present in both the benign and malignant forms of hypertension.

In malignant hypertension the intima of smaller arteries and arterioles is thickened by hyperplastic (proliferative) lesions, which have been described previously. In addition to the hyperplastic and hyaline changes, arterioles, especially in the kidney, may undergo fibrinoid necrosis, and this is manifested by the presence of pyknotic nuclei, an accumulation of polymorphonuclear leukocytes, and the intramural extravasation of red blood cells (see Fig. 47-2). Fibrin thrombi within the narrowed lumens may be present and may be an additional cause of ischemia.

Mönckeberg's medial calcific sclerosis

Mönckeberg's medial calcification is an age-related degenerative process in which the media of large and medium-sized muscular arteries calcify, and it is a fundamentally different process from occlusive atherosclerosis and has little or no clinical significance.[8] The vessels most commonly affected are the femoral, tibial, radial, ulnar, and uterine arteries. This calcific arteriosclerotic lesion may coexist with atherosclerosis in the same vessels. Affected vessels, which are hard when palpated and are demonstrable on roentgenograms, generally are dilated and show transverse ridges of medial calcification under the intima. Sometimes medial calcification exhibits osseous metaplasia containing marrow elements (Fig. 47-3). The cause is unknown, but it is probably a misconception to consider Mönckeberg's medial calcification a disease process. Similar medial calcific lesions have been produced in experimental animals by the repeated infusion of vasoactive pharmacologic agents such as epinephrine or nicotine.

Medial calcification also occurs in the setting of *arterial calcification of infancy.* In pseudoxanthoma elasticum, a recessively inherited disease, changes occur in the elastic fibers of the skin, eyes, and vessels. The earliest detectable histologic vascular lesion is an accumulation of calcium in elastic fibers, followed by fragmentation of the fibers. Calcification is often found in the internal elastic lamina of the gastric arteries and

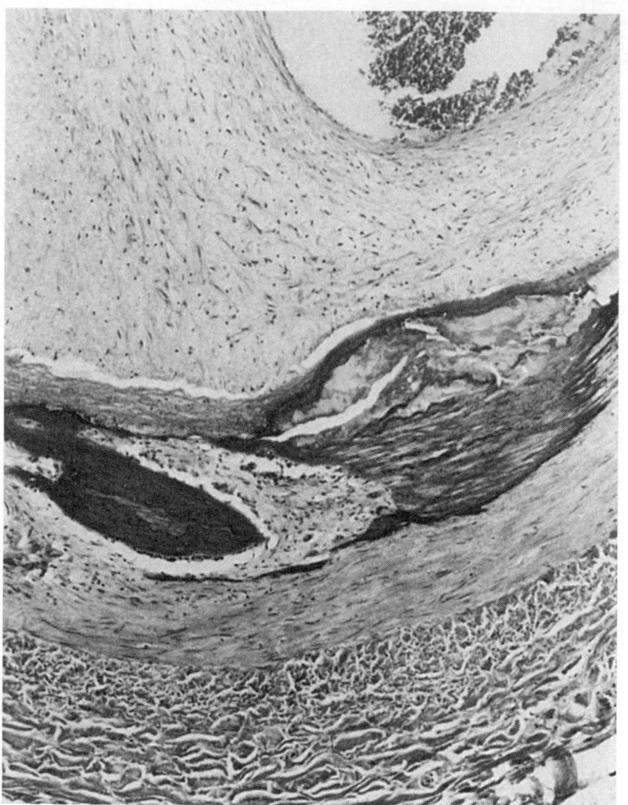

Fig. 47-3 Medial calcification (Mönckeberg's medial calcific sclerosis). Calcification of inner media is associated with osseous metaplasia.

in all medial elastic tissue of the coronary and large peripheral arteries. Coronary arterial occlusion may occur. Idiopathic arterial calcification of infancy is a rare but serious disease often involving coronary and systemic arteries[9] in babies less than 6 months old. The calcification is found in the internal elastic lamina and in the media, often associated with fibrous intimal thickening. When the coronary arteries are involved, the heart becomes enlarged and myocardial infarction may cause death. No pathogenic mechanism is known; the results of studies of calcium and other mineral metabolism, lipid metabolism, and endocrine functions have all been normal.

Atherosclerosis

Atherosclerosis is a distinctive form of arteriosclerosis. The disease begins in and primarily involves the intima of the aorta and its musculoelastic branches. There is variability in the vessels involved and in the distribution from one person to another. However, some generally valid observations are possible. When the disease becomes more severe and extensive, the focal nature of the process may be somewhat overshadowed by a more generalized destruction of the arterial wall, associated with extension of the lesions from the intima into the media. This leads to a generalized increase in vessel diameter, and in advanced atherosclerosis it is usual for the aorta and its branches to show a diffuse ectasia. In areas where the disease is even more advanced, aneurysms may form, and again the abdominal aorta is the primary site for this.

The abdominal aorta is involved earlier and more extensively than the thoracic aorta, the dorsal surface of the aorta is more affected than the ventral surface, and the inflow tract of flow dividers is more involved than the areas just distal to branch orifices. Some straight running vessels, such as the internal mammary and renal arteries, are spared even in the most advanced cases of the disease. Although arising as the result of diffuse intimal thickening, atherosclerosis is a focal disease. The major components of plaques are smooth muscle cells that are set in a connective tissue matrix, with variable amounts of lipid in both intracellular and intercellular locations. Most of the intracellular lipid occurs in smooth muscle cells. A lesser proportion of intracellular lipid is present in macrophages, usually most abundantly surrounding a central pool of lipid at the base of the plaque or in relation to surface endothelial disruption and thrombus formation.

Rupture or disruption of the localized plaque causes the clinical manifestations of the disease.[10] Rupture exposes collagen in the plaque to the bloodstream, initiating platelet aggregation and thrombosis with resultant thromboembolic sequelae or occlusion.[11] Alternatively blood dissecting into the plaque from the lumen may enlarge the lesion sufficiently to block the lumen.[12] It is the soft, lipid core of the plaque that is responsible for the disease being named "atherosclerosis," *athērē* being the Greek word for 'porridge' or 'gruel' and *sclerosis* connoting 'scar formation.' The latter aspect is responsible for the colloquial designation of the disease as "hardening of the arteries."

Morphology of atherosclerotic lesions

Many lesions have been described as being early lesions or precursors to the fully developed lesions. It seems clear that all lesions arise in a setting of intimal thickening. Although this is an almost universal condition of the musculoelastic arteries of human beings, at least in late childhood, adolescence, and adult life, there is debate about whether this diffuse intimal thickening represents a normal process of aging or is in fact the first stage of the development of atherosclerosis. The Committee on Vascular Lesions of the Council on Arteriosclerosis of the American Heart Association considers it to be a normal development, presumably related to aging.[13] However, the view of Wilens[14] that "in general arteries that are commonly the seat of atherosclerotic change are those that at an early age show relatively pronounced, diffuse, fibrous intimal thickening" seems valid. Wilens further observed that such intimal thickening was never encountered in animals that do not show spontaneous atherosclerosis.

In areas near branch vessel orifices, the intimal thickening is focally pronounced, giving rise to eccentric intimal thickenings or cushions.[15] These are similar to the eccentric intimal thickenings or cushions observed near branch vessel orifices in swine. "Spontaneous" atherosclerosis also develops in swine, and these cushions are the site of smooth muscle cell proliferation and lipid deposition when the animals are fed a lipid-rich diet.[16] Other species such as the rabbits have virtually no intimal tissue and only an occasional smooth muscle cell between the endothelium and the internal elastic lamina.

The occurrence of localized intimal thickening at sites near branch vessel orifices, an event associated with low shear stress, has led to the concept that these are areas of "adaptation" thickening. These areas have been described as having a superficial compartment (the luminal aspect) that is rich in proteoglycans. The thickenings are composed predominantly of smooth muscle cells. Macrophages are seen as isolated cells that are few in number but are three times more numerous in these areas of eccentric thickening than they are in diffuse intimal thickening. It is in these areas that lipid deposition becomes noticeable and in which progression to raised fibro-fatty plaques occurs.

Fatty dots and streaks. Most consideration has been given to fatty streaks or dots as initial lesions. They occur in the aortas of young children of all races and geographic locations, irrespective of the propensity for advanced lesions to develop in some groups and not in others (Fig. 47-4). To the naked eye they are apparent on the luminal surface as slightly raised areas that are yellower than the surrounding intima. Microscopically they are composed almost exclusively of lipid-containing smooth muscle cells (Fig. 47-5). This observation has been repeatedly made on morphologic grounds and has recently been confirmed by immunohistochemical staining.[18] Lipid is also present in the interstitium of the lesions,[19] and small amounts of lipid have also been observed in areas of intimal thickening.[20]

In contrast, the lesions induced in experimental animals by feeding them lipid or cholesterol are composed exclusively of macrophage foam cells only later acquiring a component of smooth muscle cells below the macrophage-rich superficial zone.[21] This has caused some confusion, because many authors writing on experimental atherosclerosis equate these diet-induced lesions in animals with those seen in human beings and use the presumed similarity of the lesions to support hyperlipidemia or dyslipidemia as the prime cause.

Fatty streaks and fibrous plaques. The evolution of fatty streaks into fibrous plaques has been much discussed.[22] This progression is suggested by the declining extent of fatty streak involvement, which, after reaching a peak between 24 and 34 years of age, is apparently gradually replaced by more advanced lesions. Findings from the recent PDAY (Pathological Determinants of Atherosclerosis in Youth) study[23] indicate that raised lesions occur in areas where there is a high probability of sudanophilia, although not all sudanophilia is associated with such areas. This suggests that the course of the evolution of fatty streaks to fibrous plaques may be different in different anatomic locations. A close relationship between raised lesions and areas of previous sudanophilic lesions has been observed.[23]

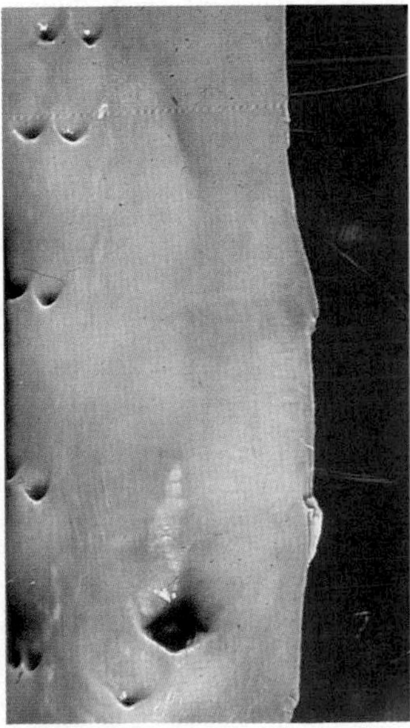

Fig. 47-4 Aorta of an adolescent boy showing intimal fatty streaks.

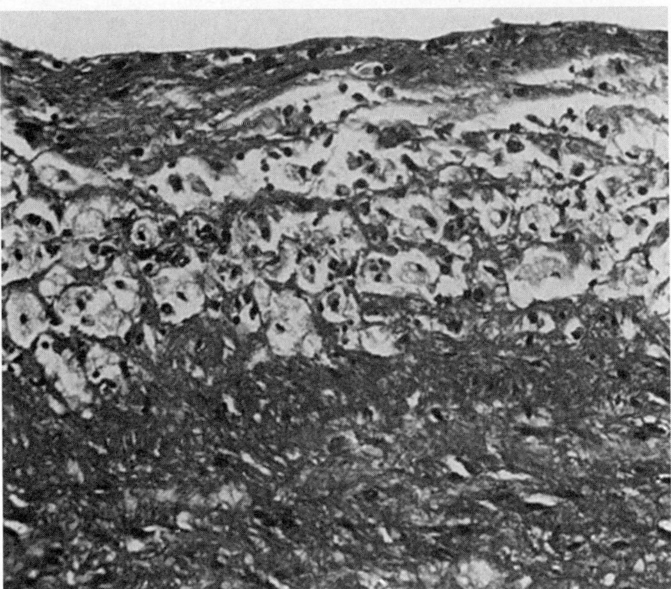

Fig. 47-5 Foam cells in intima of aorta. Lumen and endothelium are above.

Microthrombus. Another early type of lesion is the microthrombus, which is composed chiefly of platelets with some admixed white blood cells. Such lesions are difficult to find and tend to be seen only infrequently on microscopic sections. The organization of such thrombi is likely to give rise to foam cell–rich lesions. Microthrombi have been found on the surfaces of human and animal arteries.[24,25]

Gelatinous lesion. Another early lesion is the gelatinous lesion, which mainly shows a fluid expansion of the intima. This disruptive, serous, inflammatory lesion was first described by German pathologists.[26] Edematous lesions of the intima have been observed to be associated with an increased deposition of leukocytes and platelets in both human subjects and experimental animals.[27]

It is of interest that all these early lesions (namely, fatty streaks, mural thrombi, and gelatinous lesions) can be induced by injury to the vessel wall, caused either by the effects of an indwelling catheter or by repeated immunologic injury, without any dietary manipulation of lipid intake, and that the main and frequently the only cellular component in fatty streaks and gelatinous lesions is the smooth muscle cell.[27]

Fibrous plaques. Fibrous plaques are presumed to be intermediate in terms of both time and severity between early lesions and advanced, raised lesions, and consist of slightly raised, gray lesions located on the intimal surface. Microscopically a fibrous cap, composed of smooth muscle cells and related connective tissue fibers, covers and surrounds a central lipid core or pool. The intimal surface is covered by an intact layer of endothelium. There is great variability in the thickness of the lesions, but the thickness tends to increase with age. In addition, the thicker the intima, the more likely it is that it will have a lipid core.[28]

Vascular territories involved

Atherosclerosis, as already described, is a disease of the aorta and its musculoelastic branches. Although in advanced disease the entire intimal surface may be involved, the disease has a characteristic and stereotypical distribution in the initial stages. The abdominal aorta is more involved than the thoracic aorta, the dorsal surface is more affected than the ventral, and the inflow tract of the flow dividers of branch vessels is involved, in contrast to the area just distal to the branch vessel orifice. This distribution must be in part determined by flow characteristics, and it is widely believed that the areas of initial and eventually heaviest involvement are those where low flow, flow separation, and reattachment occur,[29] whereas rapid flow or high shear areas, such as those just distal to branch vessels, are relatively spared. There is increased endothelial cell turnover in areas of low shear or disturbed flow.[30] Normally the longitudinally placed endothelial nuclei, like the keel of a ship, are oriented in the long axis of the vessel. They lose this orientation in areas of disturbed flow, the cells also changing shape to become more polygonal and perhaps exhibiting subtle features of injury.[31]

In some forms of atherosclerosis, such as that associated with diabetes, there is evidence that the distribution in the vascular tree may differ from the usual, with coronary arteries and peripheral limb vessels being more involved than the aorta. In the atherosclerosis associated with immunologic injury, such as transplant atherosclerosis, the thickening of the intima is concentric rather than eccentric. This may mean that, if the damage to the endothelium, which may initiate the process, is sufficiently severe, the flow characteristics are of little importance in lesion development and progression.

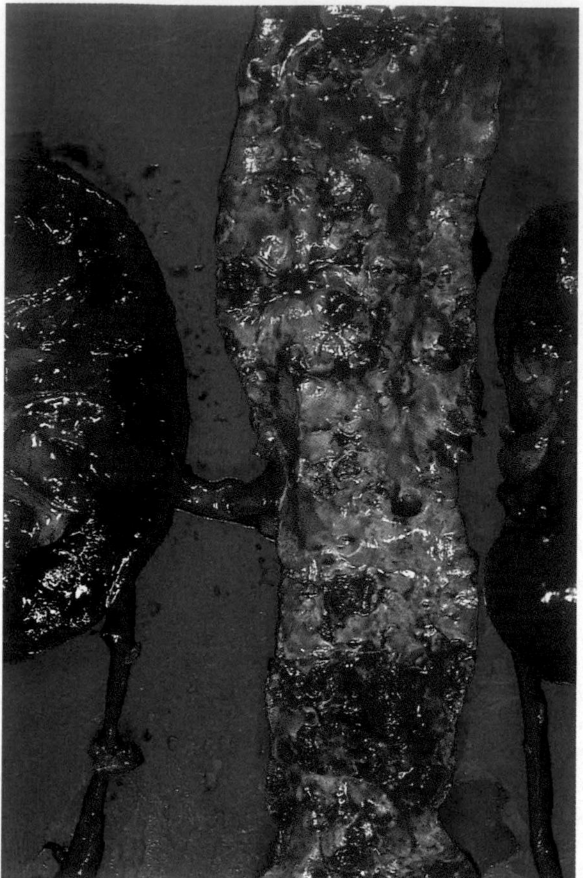

Fig. 47-6 Severe atherosclerosis of abdominal aorta.

Progression of atherosclerosis

The process by which these lesions progress to become complicated lesions is not fully understood. One recognized feature of progression is the deposition of thrombus, often on a "shoulder" of the lesions. This is facilitated by a flow disturbance in the form of a vortex, and this flow disturbance is possibly precipitated by endothelial disruption. In artificial flow systems, an object placed on the wall of a straight tube has been observed to cause eddy currents to form distal to the partial obstruction; in this current, formed elements such as platelets repeatedly collide with each other and the vessel wall.[32] This may account for the occurrence of layers of thrombus of differing ages often seen microscopically on fibrous plaques.

Expansion may also occur through the further deposition of lipid in the core of the lesions. Growth factors released by either of these processes may further stimulate the proliferation of smooth muscle cells. Atheroma formation, calcification of the arterial wall, ulceration of the intima, and mural thrombosis then ensue (Fig. 47-6).

Regression of atherosclerosis

Much of the experimental data on atherosclerosis regression have come from studies of animals fed diets with a high lipid or cholesterol content or both. In many such studies it has been convincingly shown that lesions regress when lipid is mobilized from lesions and the numbers of lipid-filled macrophages decrease.[33,34] What relevance these findings have to human atherosclerosis is not clear. The development in recent years of more sophisticated techniques to monitor lesion size or vessel lumen size has led to the performance of a number of studies attempting to demonstrate regression. It should be recognized, however, that in all such studies there are important technical limitations that may compromise or invalidate results.[35] Lipid-lowering drugs as well as dietary lipid restriction have been employed in most studies. Very few trials of diet alone have shown that it has an effect on progression. The Leiden Intervention Trial has yielded possibly the most convincing data. It showed progression in 21 of 30 subjects and no growth in lesion size in 18. Progression is associated with a total cholesterol–to–high-density lipoprotein (HDL) ratio of more than 6:9. There was no enlargement of the lesion when the ratio was lower than this.[36]

A review of the radiographic studies documenting the response of coronary artery disease to diet and drugs in general showed a reduction in the incidence of clinical events, but the evidence for reduced disease progression and increased regression was at best marginal.[37] For example, in the Familial Atherosclerosis Treatment Study, which involved the use of intensive drug regimens in men with coronary artery disease, who had elevated levels of apolipoprotein B, the mean reduction in proximal stenosis severity was 1% and only 12% of all lesions showed convincing regression.[38] However, the incidence of coronary events was reduced by 75%, an outcome estimated to be attributable to a 93% reduction in the likelihood that a mildly or moderately diseased arterial segment would undergo substantial progression to a severe lesion causing a clinical event.

Clinical events and their pathologic counterparts

Atherosclerosis of the arteries serving the myocardium, brain, and lower limbs gives rise to various manifestations of the disease that result from stenosis of the vessels or the effects of thromboembolism, or both. Vessel stenosis is attributable to severe encroachment on the lumen and causes various anginal syndromes. Stenosis of the vessels to the lower limbs is associated with intermittent claudication. Fixed stenosis of the coronary arteries causes angina of effect, and a similar process, affecting the mesenteric arteries, causes intestinal angina. Peripheral vascular disease of the lower limbs is particularly frequent in diabetics and cigarette smokers. Diabetes also equalizes the sex-related difference in the incidence of coronary heart disease that is normally seen between premenopausal women and men of comparable age.[39] Enlargement of the plaque, causing it to encroach on the lumen, is probably related, in part, to repeated episodes of thrombus formation and incorporation. The formation of a thrombus may relate more to the presence of fissures on the plaque surface than to disruption of the plaque, which is more likely to occur when severely stenotic lesions are present.[40] As the plaque becomes larger, the tendency for thrombosis to occur is increased by the disturbed flow and by the fact that more platelets tend to adhere to a surface in fast-flowing systems with a high shear stress than they do when the shear stress is less.[41]

Plaque fissure and rupture. The reason or reasons for a plaque fissuring or rupturing are unknown. It is widely believed that plaques with a large lipid core and a correspondingly thin fibrous cap are more likely to rupture. They are estimated to represent 10% to 20% of the overall lesion population but account for 80% to 90% of the acute clinical events. It has been shown that such plaques rupture at the shoulder, where the thin fibrous cap overlying the lipid pool joins the thickened intima at the edge of the raised lesion.[40] What causes the connective tissue, which usually at this stage of lesion development is rich in collagen, to disintegrate is unknown. However, the macrophages that proliferate, representing the characteristic response to platelet-fibrin thrombus formation,[41] are known to contain proteolytic enzymes, such as metalloproteinases, that are capable of degrading many of the connective tissue proteins. This indicates that plaque rupture might follow one or many episodes of mural thrombus formation related to plaque fissure.[42] However, why plaque fissure with accompanying mural thrombosis occurs is not readily explained.

Thrombosis on plaques. The thrombus that forms in relation to fissured or ruptured atherosclerotic plaques has a prominent fibrin component that probably results from the activation of thrombin. This contrasts with the almost exclusively platelet containing thrombus, which is deposited as a monolayer or carpet of platelets when endothelium is removed from a normal vessel.[43] "Normal" in this context means a vessel in which the endothelium lies directly on the internal elastic lamina. When a neointima has formed after such platelet deposition, induced by balloon catheter removal of the endothelium, subsequent removal of the endothelium results in the formation of a platelet-fibrin thrombus, presumably related to the large amount of collagen present and the generation of abundant thrombin.[44] Because atheromatous plaques also have an abundant collagen content, their rupture is also associated with the formation of a thrombus in which fibrin is a conspicuous component. Plaques express more tissue factor and plasminogen activator inhibitor than normal intima does.[45,46]

Sequelae of mural thrombus. As a thrombus forms on an arterial wall, pieces of its superficial aspect are discharged continuously into the bloodstream. We have known of emboli formed of aggregated platelets for many years, especially in relation to the rupture of plaques of the internal carotid artery in the settings of amaurosis fugax and transient ischemic attacks.[47]

Coronary thromboembolism

Only in the past few years has the same mechanism been recognized to be at work in the coronary circulation. The sudden discharge of emboli into the myocardial microcirculation results in ventricular tachycardia or ventricular fibrillation and "sudden cardiac death," or both events. Autopsy studies have shown the existence of platelet aggregate emboli in the myocardial microcirculation of people who have died suddenly, often preceded by the clinical syndrome of unstable angina.[48] Of practical importance, awareness of this mechanism led to the use of aspirin, a drug which inhibits platelet aggregation, to prevent death in patients with unstable angina. This treatment is responsible for saving the lives of a significant number of people. The experimental induction of coronary artery thrombosis in dogs, accomplished by placing a thrombogenic wire in the left anterior descending coronary artery, was observed to cause the development of occlusive thrombosis or mural thrombosis, associated with emboli in the microcirculation, or areas of focal ischemic damage to the myocardium similar to the lesions described in people suffering sudden cardiac death. Both mural thrombosis with embolism and complete thrombotic occlusion were associated with arrhythmic cardiac death.[49]

Crescendo angina leading to myocardial infarction is also likely associated with a mural thrombus. Completion of the arterial occlusion is probably brought about by growth of the thrombus and by spasm of the artery caused by the release of thromboxane A_2, serotonin, and other cytokines from the thrombus. Whether the occlusion persists for sufficient time to cause a myocardial infarction may depend on the extent of the endothelial disruption at the thrombotic site. The endothelium has been shown to become damaged when thrombus is induced by the injection of thrombin into a segment of rabbit aorta.[50] Accordingly, the release of thrombin may cause further damage to the endothelium on the side of the lumen opposite the site of thrombus formation. This is probably important because the release of prostacyclin from intact endothelium may be a critical factor in opposing thrombus extension and facilitating vessel dilatation.

Thrombus and infarct extension. When an occlusive thrombus has formed, factors facilitating reopening of the lumen may then come into play. If they do not, or are not effective, thrombus extension may occur, resulting in enlargement of the infarct territory. The factors tending to open the lumen are release of the vessel spasm and fibrinolysis, which results from the release of tissue plasminogen activator (tPA). Again, preservation of some viable endothelium is probably important in securing this outcome.

Effects of thrombotic occlusion

Treatment of an impending or actual acute myocardial infarction with thrombolytic agents such as tPA or streptokinase has proved able to salvage myocardium, even when administered up to 6 hours after the clinical onset of chest pain or other symptoms of heart attack. This contrasts with the results from experimental studies of myocardial infarction, in which irreversible damage was found to occur between 20 and 40 minutes after ligation of a coronary artery in dogs. It is not clear why there should be this great disparity in the time required for irreversible myocardial damage to take place in the human form of the disease, compared with the time observed in the setting of experimental coronary occlusion. One possible explanation may be that symptoms develop before the mural thrombus becomes a completely occlusive lesion. The presence of a rich collateral circulation, induced by vessel stenosis, may also afford some protection to the human heart. It is of interest that an infarct does not develop in all dogs subjected to experimental coronary ligation, whereas an experimentally induced occlusive thrombus always results in a full-thickness myocardial infarct. The difference may relate to the release of vasospastic agents from the forming coronary thrombus.[49]

Intermittent coronary artery occlusion. It has been shown experimentally that the creation of a significant (<70%) stenosis of the lumen of a coronary artery in dogs by a ligature, which also causes some endothelial damage, is associated with the formation of a platelet mass that is readily disrupted, either spontaneously or by the effect of drugs that inhibit platelet aggregation in response to agonists. The platelet plug tends to build up to the point of occlusion and then is disrupted by distal embolization of the mass. This cycle is repeated a number of times. It is likely that such a process occurs in humans and may account for some cases of unstable angina, or crescendo angina, or sudden arrhythmic death.

Cerebral ischemia

The same ischemic mechanisms described for the coronary arteries presumably are also at work in other vascular territories. The atherosclerotic lesion responsible for ocular and cerebrovascular events usually forms at the bifurcation of the carotid artery and preferentially involves the internal carotid artery origin.[51] Emboli arising mainly from this site cause the majority of cerebral ischemic lesions. However, similar lesions in the vertebral arteries, the ascending aorta, or the aortic arch are also sources of emboli. It is now well established that amaurosis fugax and transient ischemic attacks result from emboli, usually composed mainly of platelets, but sometimes also of cholesterol crystal–laden debris from excavated plaques. These clinical syndromes often precede the development of a completed stroke, caused when a thrombus containing a large proportion of fibrin lodges firmly in a cerebral vessel, most commonly the middle cerebral artery. Such thrombi, unlike those largely composed of aggregated platelets, are less likely to be disrupted after lodgment and are probably larger than the small platelet aggregates that are shed by a forming mural thrombus. The latter are more likely to temporarily block smaller vessels such as the retinal arteries (as in amaurosis fugax) or smaller vessels in the microcirculation.

Atherosclerosis in other vascular territories

Disease manifestations related to vessel stenosis and thromboembolism are especially prominent in tissues served by the abdominal aorta and its branches. Embolism in the leg vessels may cause the blue toe syndrome or gangrene of the toes and feet. Stenosis of the leg vessels, if severe, may cause leg cramps and intermittent claudication.

Similar processes affecting the gut may cause intestinal angina or segmental necrosis. Because of the rich collateral blood supply to the intestine, severe disease of several of the supplying vessels is usually present before ischemic manifestations become apparent.

Stenosis of renal artery orifices may lead to a Goldblatt type of hypertension and is typically associated with the hypersecretion of renin.

Cholesterol embolism

With severe, complicated atherosclerosis of the aorta, particularly in the elderly, emboli composed of atheromatous debris frequently lodge in the vessels supplying skeletal muscles in the lower limbs and are often found at autopsy in the kidneys, spleen, and pancreas[52] (Fig. 47-7). When the process is extensive and severe, an arteritis may occur in the embolized vessels, sometimes mimicking polyarteritis nodosa clinically.[53]

Atherosclerotic aneurysms

Aneurysm formation caused by extensive replacement of the medial coat, as the result of extension of the atheromatous disease, most frequently involves the abdominal aorta between the take-off of the renal arteries and the iliac bifurcation, but may arise in any vessel where atherosclerosis occurs, such as in the basilar artery or coronary arteries. The aneurysms are saccular and their cavities are filled with old, largely structureless unorganized thrombus material (Fig. 47-8).

Abdominal aortic aneurysms are likely to rupture when they reach a certain size, generally agreed to be 5 to 6 cm in diameter. There is, however, some debate about the likelihood of rupture, and it may be that this has been overestimated in studies consisting of patients referred to centers having surgical expertise, versus the incidence observed in community practices.[54] In recent reports of a relatively high familial incidence of aortic aneurysms, a genetic basis, apart from atherosclerosis, has been suggested, specifically mutations in the gene for type III collagen.[55] If this is confirmed by the results of more extensive studies, it would not exclude atherosclerosis

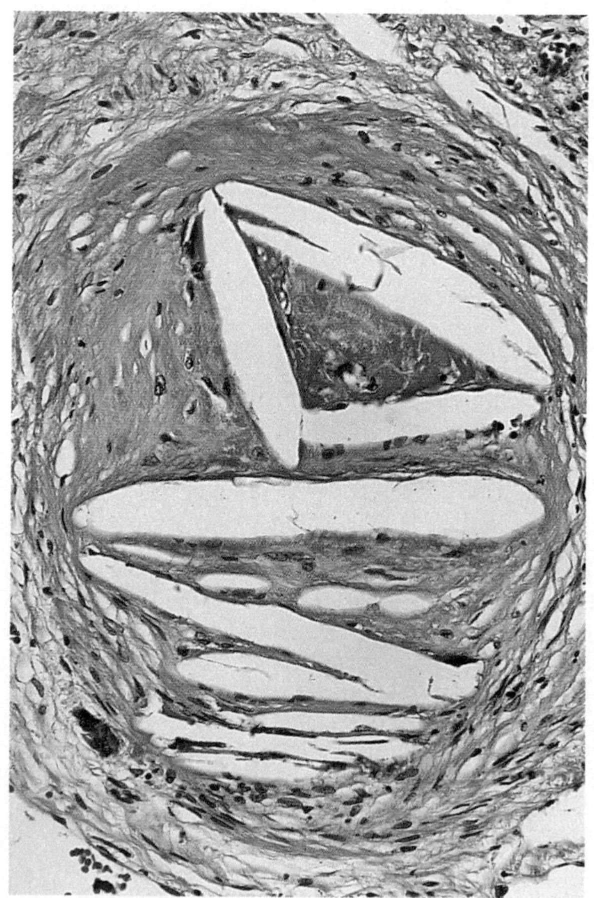

Fig. 47-7 Cholesterol embolism.

as the main cause but would implicate a significant accessory risk factor. Often a relatively slow leakage of blood, attended by symptoms related to the site of rupture, precedes a massive, fatal hemorrhage. The hemorrhage may be peritoneal or retroperitoneal in location, usually the latter. The interval between the onset of hemorrhage and fatal, full-scale rupture may last from 2 to 6 days. It is in this interval that diagnosis and surgical repair may be accomplished, if the diagnosis is suspected. Many cases, however, go unrecognized, with the diagnosis made only at autopsy. There may be other manifestations of atherosclerotic disease, such as peripheral vascular disease or myocardial ischemia, as the aneurysm is an indication of severe, usually generalized involvement.

Atherosclerotic aneurysms occasionally rupture into the gastrointestinal tract, most commonly the duodenum. This is usually accompanied by fever.

Abdominal aortic aneurysms may be coextensive with iliac artery aneurysms. Those aneurysms that form elsewhere in the aorta as a result of the atheroscleroic process only occur when an abdominal aneurysm is present. Aneurysms of the thoracic aorta that form in the absence of abdominal aortic involvement are characteristic of syphilitic aortitis and most commonly involve the ascending aorta and arch of the aorta.

Other forms of atherosclerosis related to known vascular injury

Lesions closely resembling atherosclerosis arise in a number of situations in which physical injury, surgical interventions, or inflammation produce arterial wall damage. Radiation-induced damage to arteries and "transplant" atherosclerosis are examples. The placement of catheters in the aortas of neonates, for the monitoring of blood gas levels gives rise to thromboatherosclerotic lesions similar to those induced experimentally by indwelling catheters in rabbit aortas.[56]

Scribner shunts connecting a radial artery to an arm vein, placed for dialysis access, cause extensive thrombosis in the vein. A marked intimal thickening containing lipid develops beneath this thrombus. In some instances a lipid pool with cholesterol crystal clefts has been observed.[57] These lesions are similar to ones induced experimentally in sheep by the creation of arteriovenous anastomoses.[58]

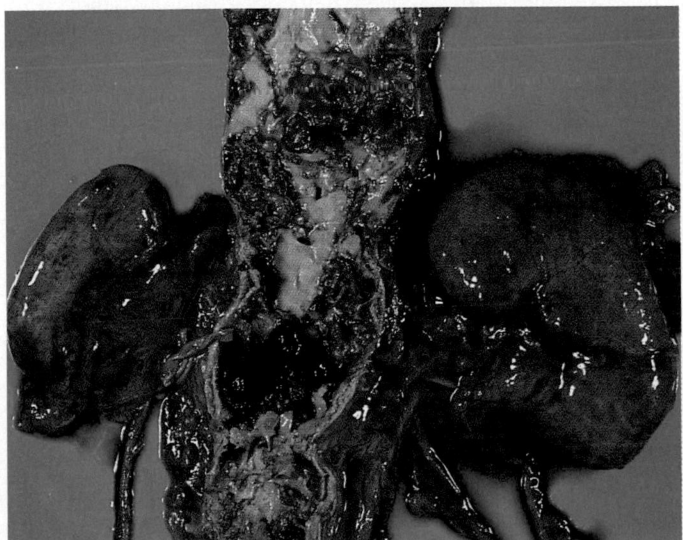

Fig. 47-8 Abdominal atherosclerotic aneurysm.

Pulmonary hypertension provides an instructive "experiment of nature." In such cases it is common to find fatty streaks in the intima, especially of the main pulmonary arteries. Occasionally, fully developed atheromatous lesions are encountered. In one such case, a complex congenital heart disease, characterized by atrial and ventricular septal defects, and tetralogy of Fallot was found at autopsy in a 44-year old woman who clinically was thought to have Eisenmenger's syndrome. The left main pulmonary artery was atretic. The arteries of the right lung, which were supplied by the right pulmonary artery, showed large fibrous plaques with a basal lipid pool. The aorta showed only some slight intimal thickening. This case illustrates that presumably hemodynamically mediated damage to the wall of an artery in the lesser circulation can cause atherosclerosis when the systemic arteries are "normal."

Epidemiology

In terms of morbidity and mortality, atherosclerosis is the most important disease affecting the populations of industrialized countries. However, there has been a sharp decline in coronary heart disease mortality in the United States in recent years.[59] This was accompanied by the finding of less extensive coronary atherosclerosis postmortem in person 25 to 44 years old in 1968 to 1972 compared with the findings from 1960 to 1964 in a study conducted in New Orleans.[60] Populations moving from a place where the incidence is low to one where the incidence is high become subject to the higher rates of the country of adoption. This has been interpreted to mean that environmental influences are more important than genetic factors.

Age. The incidence of the disease increases as people age. Although in general the clinical manifestations are age related, the disease, especially in the form of sudden cardiac death, may afflict middle-aged or young adults. Precocious onset is associated with other known risk factors, such as familial hyperlipidemia, diabetes mellitus, homocystinuria, and progeria. As people age, the intima of the musculoelastic arteries becomes progressively thicker, and this correlates with lipid deposition.[61]

Sex. There is a striking difference between the incidence of atherosclerosis in male and female patients. Up until the time of menopause in women, there is a strong predominance in men of comparable age. The incidence in postmenopausal women increases, and elderly of both sexes are more equally affected.[62] There is a tendency to underdiagnose and perhaps to undertreat coronary heart disease in women. The role of estrogen in providing protection is suggested by some decrease in the incidence of the disease in women treated with estrogen to delay or prevent the onset of the menopause, though the mechanism responsible for this is unclear.[63] Women on hormone replacement therapy have shown a lower concentration of fibrinogen and high levels of plasminogen.[64] Premenopausal women in general have higher levels of HDL and an increase in the HDL–to–low-density lipoprotein (LDL) ratio compared with that in men.

Fibrinogen and other coagulation factors. Increased levels of fibrinogen and factor VII in white men between 40 and 64 years of age, as observed over a 5 year period, have been noted to be more strongly predictive of ischemic heart disease than blood cholesterol levels.[65] High fibrinogen levels were more predictive of coronary heart disease in younger men.

In middle-aged men there are associations among high platelet count, an increased tendency of platelets to aggregate, and coronary heart disease.[66]

Hyperlipidemia. There is considerable epidemiologic research showing that an increased serum level of cholesterol (specifically LDL cholesterol) is an etiologic risk factor for the development of coronary heart disease and that the pharmacologic reduction in the LDL cholesterol level in men with pronounced hypercholesterolemia reduces the incidence. What is less clear is whether such intervention in persons with marginally elevated LDL levels is effective. Many patients who suffer coronary heart disease have normal plasma lipid and lipoprotein cholesterol levels, though many of these have an elevated beta-lipoprotein level.[67] The association of coronary heart disease with the total cholesterol–to–HDL cholesterol ratio is much stronger than its association with the LDL level alone.[68] A high HDL level appears to afford some protection, and this is consistent with the relative benefit seen in premenopausal women who exercise consistently[69] and consume a moderate amount of alcohol,[70] especially wine.[71]

Cigarette smoking. Cigarette smoking is associated with at least twice the risk of cardiovascular events, including myocardial infarction, sudden death, and stroke,[72] and increases the mortality resulting from coronary disease by 70%. Smoking has deleterious effects on lipid metabolism, especially lowering the HDL level. In addition, elevated levels of fibrinogen and plasminogen activator inhibitor might promote thrombotic events.

Diabetes mellitus. Diabetes mellitus is associated with an increased incidence of the clinical manifestation of atherosclerosis. Peripheral vascular disease and coronary heart disease are especially common. Diabetes tends to equalize the sex-related difference in the incidence of coronary heart disease, with diabetic women affected as frequently as nondiabetic men. There is no shortage of the metabolic and coagulation factors that are adversely affected by diabetes. Triglyceride and very low density lipoprotein levels are elevated, and the HDL level is lowered. The production of von Willebrand factor from endothelial cells and thromboxane A_2 from platelets is increased. Prostacyclin production by the vessel wall has been observed to be diminished in experimentally induced diabetes. Insulin stimulates the proliferation of smooth muscle cells, which in turn fosters the growth of plaques. Serum is more stimulatory to smooth muscle cell proliferation in patients with type I diabetes than it is in nondiabetics, probably stemming from stimulation by growth hormone.[73] Alterations in glycosaminoglycan metabolism may promote the binding of lipoprotein to proteoglycan in the vessel wall. Finally, the formation of immune complexes to glycosylated LDL and the formation of advanced glycoslyation end-products may influence the process. Nonenzymatic glycosylation of collagen may provide a more potent stimulus to platelet aggregation in the diabetic.[73]

Physical inactivity. There is increasing evidence of the benefits from habitual physical activity in the primary prevention of coronary heart disease.[74] It is recognized that such activity is associated with an elevation in the HDL level, a known protective factor.[74] Modifications in the thrombotic process, specifically increases in tPA activity and the levels of tPA in the active form and decreases in plasminogen activator inhibitor-I activity and the fibrinogen level, have also been observed. These effects were restricted to older men, however.[75] Although exercise is part of the regimen followed by patients in numerous intervention studies, no study has assessed the role of physical training alone in secondary prevention.

Genetic influences. A familial predisposition to atherosclerosis, which is well recognized, probably depends on a large number of known, or as yet unknown, risk factors. As noted previously, there appear to be differences among different racial groups in terms of the susceptibility to and localization of the disease. However, these tend to be modified or overshadowed by environmental influences.

Hypertension. Many patients with the clinical manifestations of atherosclerosis are also hypertensive. Hypertension usually commences several decades before atherosclerotic disease becomes apparent clinically. Hypertension has been noted to enhance the experimental atherosclerosis induced by a lipid diet. The relationship between the two conditions is complicated, and there is the possibility that atherosclerosis may be responsible for causing some cases of hypertension of renal ischemic origin. Splinting of the carotid baroreceptors resulting from calcification when the atherosclerosis is advanced may contribute to causing systolic hypertension in the elderly. Persons who were previously hypertensive may be unable to sustain the elevated pressure if coronary heart disease supervenes. Treatment of mild to moderate hypertension (diastolic pressure 90 to 114 mm Hg) can bring about a reduction in the incidence of stroke, but has little if any effect on the incidence of coronary heart disease.

Obesity is an important but minor risk factor. Its association with other risk factors such as physical inactivity may explain its influence.

Social class. There are large differences in the risk of ischemic heart disease among the members of different social classes,[76] those in the lowest class being at highest risk. Whether this is mediated by another presumptive risk factor—stress—is debatable. In one report the authors conclude that the self-reported inability to relax after work was associated with an increased risk of coronary heart disease.[77]

Etiology and pathogenesis

The development of a coherent theory explaining the origin and progression of atherosclerosis is compromised by lack of agreement about what constitutes the early stage or stages, and to some extent by a lack of consensus about the true nature of the lesions. Built on this insecure foundation, attempts to explain or rationalize the meaning of various known disease associations possess varying degrees of credibility. Some see lipid in the lesions as the key to the initiation, progression, and complications of the disease. Others are more impressed by the proliferative aspects, especially the proliferation of smooth muscle cells, and the inflammatory nature of lesions appears central to the thinking of some investigators. Still others attempt to meld all these aspects together, maintaining that the diversity of the disease results from its multifactorial nature.

Current concepts. Currently the most widely accepted theory explaining the initiation and development of the disease is the so-called modified response-to-injury hypothesis[78] (Fig. 47-9). The response is "modified" by incorporating lipid entry into arterial walls as the initial injury stimulus, which then gives rise to the migration and proliferation of smooth muscle cells from the medial coat into the intimal lesion already

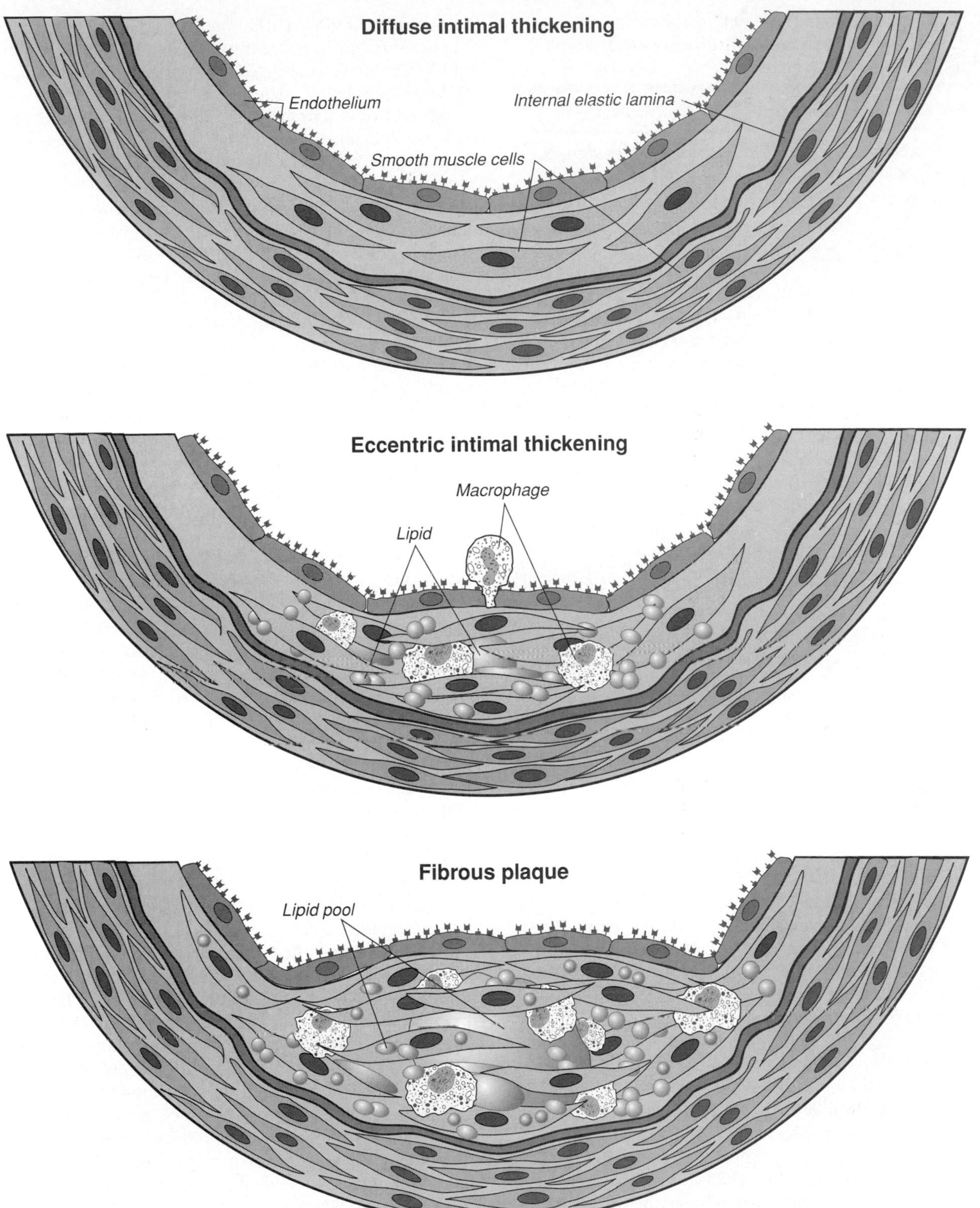

Fig. 47-9 Pathogenesis of atherosclerosis.

formed by the accumulation of lipid-filled macrophages. In the original, unmodified response-to-injury hypothesis,[79] endothelial injury or dysfunction was considered the primary event, which was then followed by the migration and proliferation of medial smooth muscle cells that formed an intimal plaque, which subsequently accumulated lipid.

It can be seen that a principal difference between these two theories is that, in the modified response-to-injury hypothesis, the cell making up the bulk of the early lesions is the macrophage, whereas in the unmodified hypothesis the cell most involved is the smooth muscle cell (Table 47-1). The modified response-to-injury hypothesis postulated that lipo-

Table 47-1 Comparison of response to injury hypothesis and modified response to injury hypothesis

Modified response to injury	Response to injury
Monocytes adhere to endothelium and enter the intima	Endothelial injury or stimulus causes release of PDGF or EDGF
↓	↓
Lipid accumulates in macrophages in the intima	Smooth muscle cells migrate from media and proliferate in intima
↓	↓
Fatty streak disrupts endothelium	Lipoproteins form complexes with structural proteins, e.g., proteoglycans
↓	↓
Platelets adhere and release PDGF	Lipoprotein-proteoglycan complexes taken up by smooth muscle cells and macrophages
↓	↓
Smooth muscle cells migrate from media and proliferate in intima	Plaque composed mainly of lipid-laden smooth muscle cells
↓	
Plaque composed mainly of macrophage foam cells with smooth muscle cells at base	—

EDGF, Endothelial cell-derived growth factor; *PDGF,* platelet-derived growth factor.

protein entry into the intima was the initial event and that this was followed by the uptake of lipoprotein by monocytes attracted to the areas of lipid deposition, resulting in a macrophage-rich fatty streak lesion. There are several problems with this explanation. First, not all those who have clinically significant atherosclerosis have elevated blood lipid levels or dyslipidemia. Those who favor hyperlipidemia as the initiating injury mechanism admit to a paradox—that monocytes do not have receptors for and do not take up unmodified LDL.[80] The rationalization they propose to explain this paradox is that the oxidation of lipoprotein causes the migration of monocytes that are able to take up the oxidized lipid mainly by way of the "scavenger" receptor, which is not downregulated by intracellular lipid; the cell then becomes laden with lipid to form a foam cell. Although it is likely that some oxidation of lipoprotein occurs after it is deposited,[81] this does not explain why the lipid accumulated in the intima in the first place.

Possibly the most compelling argument against this concept of pathogenesis is that early human lesions, including fatty streaks, have a cellular content that is overwhelmingly composed of smooth muscle cells.[82-84] If hyperlipidemia is the underlying pathogenetic mechanism responsible for the development of fatty streaks, it is indeed curious that infants in geographic areas where the populace does not suffer advanced atherosclerosis, and whose blood cholesterol levels are much lower than those of the residents of most industrialized countries, are found at necropsy to have large numbers of fatty streaks.[85]

Experimental evidence supporting the modified response-to-injury hypothesis rests on the results of experiments involving the consumption of dietary lipid supplements. In these experiments the blood cholesterol levels are usually very high, of the order of 900 to 1000 mg/dl or more. These are the kind of levels found in the setting of homozygous familial hyperlipidemia, in Watanabe rabbits,[86] or in the St. Thomas' Hospital strain of rabbits.[87] The lesions in these instances are mainly composed of macrophage type foam cells. Macrophage foam cells also accumulate in organs and structures such as the liver, spleen, bone marrow, and renal glomeruli.

Synergy of injury and hyperlipidemia. There is good evidence for the synergy of injury and hyperlipidemia in inducing atherosclerotic changes in vessels.[88] Most of the experiments that have shown this combine immunologically induced damage with dietary lipid excess. The lesions so caused differ in an important respect from naturally occurring human atherosclerosis, in that the lipid-laden intimal thickening is distributed equally around the vessel lumen, rather than eccentrically.[89] A probable human example of this type of immunologically induced atherosclerosis is transplant atherosclerosis.[90] Immunologically induced damage to vessels, brought about by instilling human serum into a carotid artery of normally fed rabbits every week for several weeks, has been found to lead to the formation of lipid-rich lesions, which subsequently regress to become fibrous intimal thickenings without a lipid content.[91]

Atherosclerosis induced by injury. All the lesions seen in the human form of atherosclerosis can be induced in animals by injury involving either the mechanical or immunologic disruption of the endothelial layer.[92] Thus fatty streaks (composed of lipid-laden smooth muscle cells), fibrous intimal thickenings without lipid, fibrous plaques (with lipid), and raised lesions with a basally placed lipid pool can all be seen after endothelial injury in normolipemic, normally fed animals. The development and progression of the lesions differ somewhat among the animals, depending on the method used to produce endothelial injury. These lesions have abundant cholesteryl ester and lesser amounts of free cholesterol, similar to the lesions seen in human beings.

When the injury in rabbits is caused by an indwelling catheter in the aorta or by repeated immunologic damage to the carotid artery, the lesions become smaller and the lipid content diminishes after removal of the injury stimulus. Those lesions caused by removal of the endothelium with a balloon catheter not only persist but continue to become thicker for as long as they have been observed—2 years.[93] The reason for the difference in the outcome of these two lesions is not apparent but may relate to tissue remodeling caused by the release of proteolytic enzymes from macrophages in the thrombus-rich lesions induced by mechanical or immunologic injury.[94]

There are numerous macrophages in the superficial part of raised lesions induced by an indwelling aortic catheter, and very little proteoglycan, collagen, or elastica is detectable in the interstitial tissue around them. Thrombin may also play a part in degrading the other matrix elements.[94] The formation of lesions induced both by an indwelling catheter[95] and by balloon catheter deendothelialization[96] can be greatly inhibited or prevented by the administration of antiplatelet serum to severely depress the number of circulating platelets before the injury is inflicted. Given as little as 1 hour after the injury, or if the platelet count is allowed to rise at any time, the lesion develops as if no thrombocytopenia had been induced. Platelet-derived growth factor is chemotactic for smooth muscle cells,[97,98] and some have claimed that this is its main activity, the smooth muscle cell proliferation being attributable to the action of other cytokines such as basic-fibroblast growth factor.[99] However, the sustained release of this growth factor has not been shown, and it is likely that its release early in the course of balloon injury results from its discharge from necrotic muscle cells in the media of the ballooned rat carotid artery.[100]

Intimal thickening and restenosis after angioplasty. The occurrence of intimal proliferation caused by endothelial injury has taken on added interest because of the problem of restenosis in patients who undergo coronary angioplasty.

Little or no intimal thickening is found in the rabbit aorta injured by a balloon catheter that is distended to the point where the pressure on the wall causes necrosis of smooth muscle cells in the media.[101] Presumably this is because of damage to the medial cells that provide the cells that migrate into the intima and proliferate there.

Encroachment on the newly distended lumen, to the point where the narrowing is clinically significant, arises in 20% to 40% of the patients who undergo angioplasty.[102] Presumably some degree of stenosis develops in all patients. This is analogous to the progressive intimal thickening that occurs in the rabbit aorta after balloon catheter removal of the endothelium,[101] with a continuing, increased proliferative capacity observed in tissue cultures of smooth muscle cells from the neointima 3 months after the injury.[103]

Accumulation of lipid in the neointima after endothelial injury. Because lipid-rich, typical atheromatous lesions can be induced in normolipemic animals by simply removing the endothelium,[101] it is of interest to know why this occurs. The lipid accumulates in those parts of the intima that have been covered by regenerated endothelium. Paradoxically, in disagreement with conventional views about lipid deposition being related to increased permeability, the areas not covered by regenerated endothelium[104] show little or no lipid, except to a slight extent in the deepest part of the neointima.

Kinetic studies of lipoprotein entry and retention, though showing some acceleration in the entry rate into the neointima covered by regenerated endothelium, show a sharp increase in the initial uptake of lipoprotein by the areas not covered by endothelium. However, this rate rapidly slows, with the lipoprotein level appearing to equilibrate with that in the medium; this was observed in an organ culture experiment and presumably also occurs in the bloodstream in vivo.[105] However, the lipoprotein content of the endothelium-covered areas rapidly increases and is maintained at a high level. These kinetics parallel the content of glycosaminoglycans in the neointima, in that their concentration increases in the endothelium-covered areas and decreases in the uncovered areas.[106] There are also qualitative changes in the proteoglycans produced, making them more capable of binding lipoproteins.[107]

Mechanism of lipid accumulation in injury-induced lesions. These foregoing observations indicate the probable existence of a mechanism by which lipoprotein normally entering the intima is trapped in the neointima covered by regenerated endothelium. Proteoglycans rich in chondroitin sulfate, found predominantly in the neointima covered by regenerated endothelium, have a stronger affinity for lipoproteins than do the proteoglycans present in uninjured aorta.[107] Lipoproteins from the sera of animals rendered hypercholesterolemic by cholesterol feeding bind more avidly with proteoglycans than lipoproteins from normally fed animals do.[108] It is of interest that HDL does not bind at all to proteoglycan.[106] Complexes formed of LDL and chondroitin sulfate are more actively taken up by smooth muscle cells[109] and macrophages[110] than are native lipoproteins, and the complexes extracted from neointima are more avidly taken up than are those extracted from normal aortic tissue. The uptake is mainly accomplished by means of the apoliproprotein B and E receptor pathway, with phagocytosis as the second important route of uptake and a minor part occurring by way of the scavenger receptor.[111]

The co-localization of chondroitin sulfate and endogenous apo-lipoprotein B in the endothelium-covered neointima occurring after balloon deendothelialization has been demonstrated in normally fed rabbits (i.e., without a dietary lipid supplement.)[112] The formation of complexes between lipoproteins and other proteins has been described. Complexes with fibrinogen[113] and elastin[114] may be especially important.

Relevance of injury-induced atherosclerosis to human disease. What relevance do these observations on atherosclerosis induced by injury have to the human form of the disease? It is unlikely that large areas of endothelial cover are lost, and it is known that very small areas of denudation are quickly recovered through endothelial spreading or replication.[115] However, the presence of small areas of injury, as evidenced by the observation of intimal microthrombi[116] and formed elements of the blood accumulating in areas of intimal edema[117] may indicate that such injuries do occur and that possibly their repetition precipitates the development of smooth muscle cell migration and proliferation in the intima. This would then form the substrate for lipid deposition and the development of more advanced lesions.

Lesions in relation to flow patterns. Raised atherosclerotic lesions form first at sites of blood flow separation and turbulence.[118] The endothelium in these areas lacks the characteristic regular orientation in which the cells are oriented in the long axis of flow. In contrast, the cells are organized haphazardly and tend to be polygonal.[119] It may be that the endothelial cells in these regions are more prone to injury or to be affected by stimuli that might result in their producing cytokines such as endothelial cell–derived growth factor (EDGF),[120] which might be instrumental in causing lesion growth.

Injury mechanisms and risk factors. The concept of lipid accumulation in relation to the changes in the neointima that take place in response to injury provides a rationale for the influence of life-style or risk factors. Proliferating smooth muscle cells synthesize extracellular proteins such as proteoglycans at a more rapid rate than do the nonproliferating cells of the contractile phenotype.[121] This increased matrix synthesis could then cause entering lipoprotein to be readily trapped, accounting for the appearance and accumulation of lipid in the lesions. In conditions of hyperlipemia or dyslipidemia, (such as increased blood levels of apolipoprotein B[122] or of Lp(a)[123]), the tendency for lipid to accumulate would be greater. Metabolic disorders such as diabetes mellitus[124] and homocystinemia,[125] both of which are associated with abnormal proteoglycan production, would in this situation render the vessel more prone to lipid accumulation. Homocystinemia might also act by causing endothelial damage,[126] and "spontaneous" thromboses are a clinically important feature of those with the homozygous defect.[127] Radiation-induced damage, especially that involving the coronary arteries, in patients treated for malignant tumors with high-dose irradiation to the anterior chest is another clinical example of injury-induced atherosclerosis.[128]

Infections and immune injury

Viruses and infectious agents. The concept of the disease representing a response to injury also fits well with the behavior of other potentially damaging agents such as antibodies and viruses. Marek's disease virus in chickens causes the formation of lipid-rich lesions that closely resemble atherosclerosis, especially in coronary and mesenteric arteries.[129] There is seroepidemiologic evidence indicating an association between *Chlamydia pneumoniae* and coronary heart disease,[130] and this organism has been identified in coronary artery atheromas by electron microscopy.[131] Various herpes II viruses, including cytomegalovirus, have been identified in human lesions.[132]

Immunologic injury. The prominence of T-cells in some early lesions of human atherosclerosis has led to speculation about the immunologic reactions occurring in the disease process.[133]

Thrombosis and injury. The injury theory also fits well with the frequently reported alterations in coagulation observed in patients with atherosclerotic disease.[134] The Northwick Park study, which showed a stronger epidemiologic association of elevated fibrinogen levels than of elevated blood cholesterol levels to coronary heart disease,[135] has led the way to exploration of the possible role of other factors such as factor VII and tissue plasminogen activator inhibitor-I[136] in atherogenesis or atherosclerosis progression.

Apart from overt structural or morphologically detectable endothelial injury, the possibility of functional damage or stimulation of the endothelium does exist. Damage induced metabolically could cause the release of EDGF, leading to smooth muscle cell migration and proliferation in the intima, thus setting the stage for lipid accumulation. That lesions develop first and progress more rapidly in certain parts of the arterial tree indicates that the endothelium in these areas may be more vulnerable to such damage or stimulation. These susceptible areas are those where blood flow has been observed to separate in model flow systems,[137] and where morphologic alterations of the endothelium are observed. These alterations consist of a loss in the orientation of the long axis of the cells in the direction of blood flow and other features suggestive of alterations, such as an increased turnover of the cells.

Diabetes mellitus provides an example of a metabolic disturbance causing alterations in endothelial function[138] and thrombosis. These alterations include increased production of the von Willebrand factor and decreased production of prostacyclin, plasminogen activator, and EDGF. Alloxan diabetes is associated with an increased uptake of ^{3}H-thymidine, indicating increased cell turnover.[139] Diabetes also alters the proportion of various glycosaminoglycans in proteoglycans, which might facilitate the binding of lipoproteins.[124]

Thrombotic aspects of atherogenesis. Continuing injury to the inner lining of the vessel wall, associated with the continuing deposition of platelet-fibrin thrombus, has been found to lead to the development of lipid-rich atheromatous lesions in rabbits fed a normal diet, unsupplemented with lipid or cholesterol.[140] These lesions regress to non–lipid containing intimal thickenings when the injury stimulus is removed. Paradoxically the lesions induced by the removal of the endothelium with a balloon catheter do not regress but continue to accumulate lipid.[101]

Human atheromatous lesions have an increased neointimal content of fibrin at all stages of development, and coincidentally plasminogen activator-inhibitor-1 tissue factor expression and thrombin receptor activity within the plaque are also increased. It has also become apparent recently that high plasma PA1-1 levels are associated with coronary heart disease, especially in those who have had a myocardial infarction or present with unstable angina.[141]

The presence of fibrinogen in early lesions has been noted,[142] and the ability of fibrinogen to bind lipoproteins may be important in sequestering lipid in lesions. It is possible that the role played by proteoglycans in lipid binding may become more prominent later in lesion development. In older lesions, in which the content of proteoglycans decreases relative to that of other matrix elements,[143] collagen and elastic tissue could serve as agents to bind lipoproteins. In this regard it is of interest that a heritable disorder of connective tissue, pseudoxanthoma elasticum, is associated with the premature onset of clinically overt manifestations of atherosclerosis.

Aneurysms

Diffuse dilatation of an artery is referred to as *ectasia* and is usually seen in the setting of advanced atherosclerosis of the aorta and its main branches. As a consequence, it is a frequent concomitant of old age in populations that suffer significant atherosclerotic disease.

Localized dilatation of an artery is referred to as an *aneurysm.*[144] Classified as to their shape and morphology, such lesions may be saccular, fusiform, or dissecting. Abnormal communications between arteries and veins composed of distorted, thin-walled vessels are referred to as *cirsoid aneurysms* and are of particular clinical importance when they arise in the brain.

Most aneurysms occur in the aorta and are mostly atherosclerotic; these are discussed under the complications of atherosclerosis. Other major forms of aneurysms include infectious aneurysms and those caused by hereditary metabolic disorders of connective tissue.

Syphilitic aneurysm

Syphilitic aneurysms have declined greatly in incidence and are now a pathologic curiosity. Most are saccular, occur in the thoracic aorta, and mainly involve the arch. Symptoms are related to the compression of structures in the vicinity of the aneurysm, and these include hoarseness resulting from recurrent laryngeal nerve compression and pupillary changes resulting from sympathetic nerve involvement. Exsanguinating hemorrhage resulting from rupture is the cause of death.

Apart from the localized saccular aneurysm, the ascending aorta may be greatly ectatic (Fig. 47-10). The intimal surface characteristically shows an irregular wrinkled appearance, described as resembling a tree bark (Fig. 47-11). A usual accompaniment is incompetence of the aortic valve stemming from retraction of the cusps, characterized by a rolled appearance of their free margins and widening of the commissures.

The wall of the aorta involved by syphilis exhibits a characteristic infiltration of lymphocytes and plasma cells around the vasa vasorum, with related lenticular areas where the muscle and elastic tissue of the media have been replaced by collagen-producing cells of a more fibroblastic than myogenic character. Although this leads to a weakening of the wall and eventual aneurysm formation, dissecting aneurysm does not occur as it does in Erdheim's disease.

Dissecting aneurysms

Although dissecting aneurysms can form in any artery, the aorta is the most common location (Fig. 47-12). There is bleeding into the wall in a planar fashion, usually between the outer and middle two thirds of the media, and this is associ-

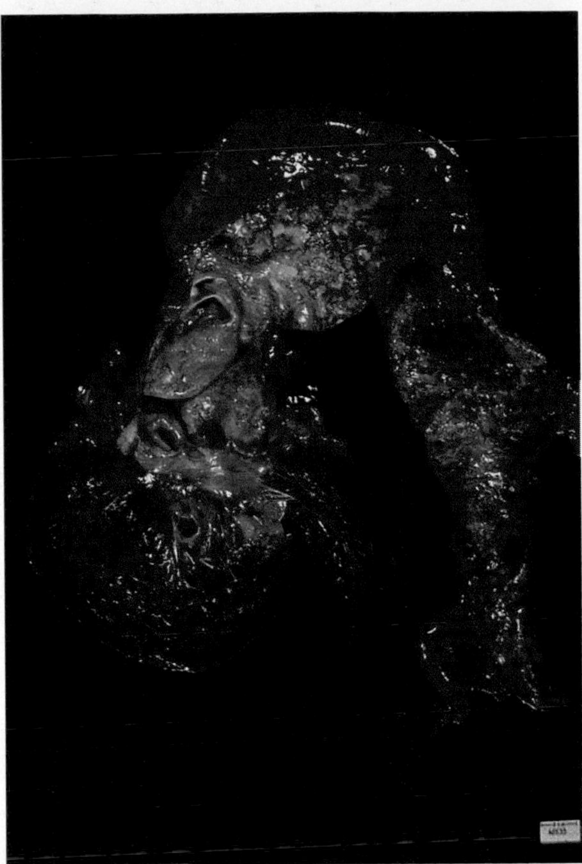

Fig. 47-10 Syphilitic aneurysm. (Courtesy Dr. Antonio Martínez-Hernández, Memphis, Tenn.)

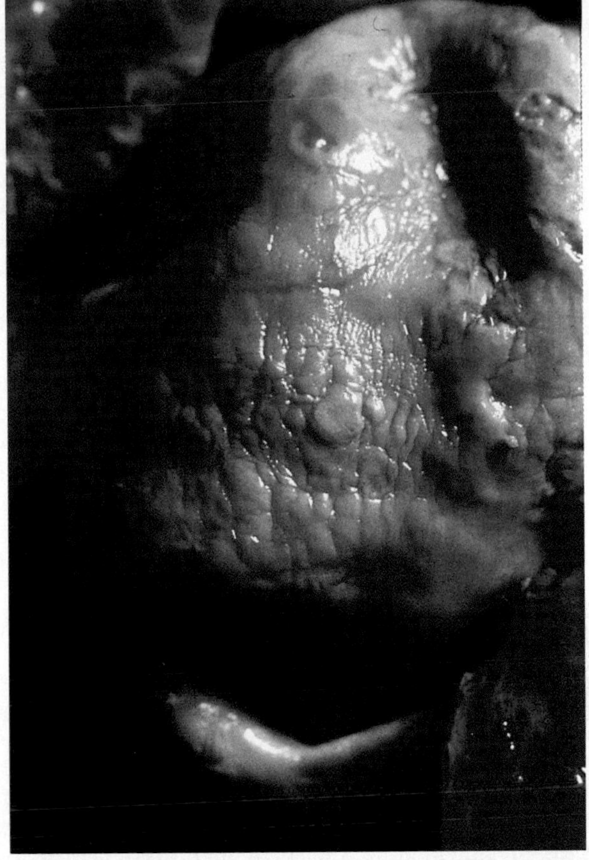

Fig. 47-11 Intima of a syphilitic aneurysm showing "tree-bark" appearance.

ated with an intimal tear in 95% of the cases. The dissection extends proximally and distally from the tear and usually ruptures externally, causing a fatal outcome. Most tears occur in the ascending aorta, and the external rupture most often extends into the pericardium, resulting in pericardial tamponade. The next most common site of external hemorrhage is the pleural cavity, followed by the mediastinum and lung. Instead of rupturing externally, the dissecting column of blood can reenter through a distal tear in the aorta or one of its large branches, such as an iliac artery. Reentry sites occur in 10% to 20% of the cases. The presence of a reentry site does not preclude the existence of an external rupture.

Most intimal tears occur in the ascending aorta less than 4 cm from the aortic valve.[145] It is common to refer to dissections involving or beginning in the ascending aorta and arch as type A dissections. Type B dissections commence in the descending aorta, beyond the orifice of the left subclavian artery.

Clinical manifestations may be the result of a dissection extending to major branches of the aorta, thereby compromising blood flow to such areas as the brain, myocardium, and intestine.

The pathologic substrate considered responsible for causing dissecting aneurysms is believed to be an alteration in the connective tissue of the medial coat, first described by Erdheim as idiopathic cystic medionecrosis,[146] although Erdheim noted these changes in patients with rupture of an ascending aortic aneurysm. The name is something of a misnomer, because

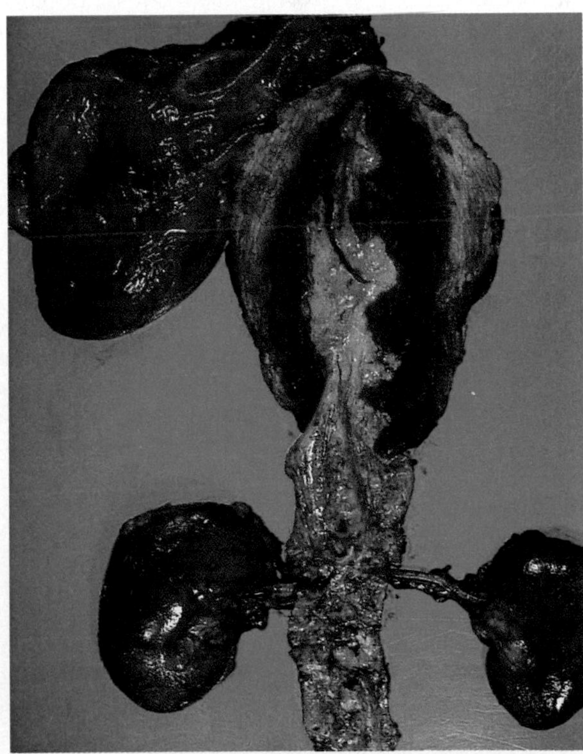

Fig. 47-12 Dissecting aneurysm of thoracic aorta.

frank necrosis of tissue is not a feature. Smooth muscle cells and elastica may be lost and replaced by material described as mucoid or myxoid, and consisting of proteoglycans. It has not been determined whether the structure or chemical characteristics of the proteoglycans are altered or whether molecules with a normal content and distribution of glycosaminoglycans are simply produced in excess. Because proteoglycans are often considered the "glue" that binds normal tissue elements, it may well be that the proteoglycan production is dysregulated.

No intimal tear can be found in up to 10% of the cases of dissecting aneurysm. This has been used as an argument to support the belief that the dissection commences as bleeding into the media, the seat of altered or abnormal structure. This structural alteration varies considerably as noted in different series and cases.[147] In some patients the defect principally consists of a loss of muscle tissue; in others there is a deficiency in elastica and in some a loss of both. It has been reported that degeneration of elastic tissue is the more prominent feature in younger patients. These degenerative changes in the media associated with dissection are more pronounced in the ascending portion of the aorta than elsewhere.

Although there is some statistical relationship of dissecting aneurysms to hypertension, the pressure elevation needed to cause artificial dissection is much higher than occurs in hypertension. Hypertension has been cited as a predisposing factor, because of its high incidence among patients who suffer aortic dissection and because of the frequent autopsy finding of left ventricular hypertrophy. However, its role in the pathogenesis of the disorder is questionable, as dissection can occur in the absence of either clinical or pathologic evidence of hypertension.

Marfan's syndrome. Marfan's syndrome is a heritable disorder of connective tissue that is characterized by a typical body habitus, arachnodactyly, and dislocation of the lens of the eye, and is frequently associated with disease of the aorta, especially affecting the proximal part.[148] The weakening of vessels has been related to a defect in the synthesis of fibrillin.[149] The medial defect, which is often more distinct in patients with the syndrome than in those who suffer a dissecting aneurysm but do not have Marfan's syndrome, may cause aneurysmal dilatation of the proximal aorta with rupture of the dissecting aneurysm as a terminal event. The proximal aortic dilatation may also cause aortic insufficiency. Histologically, areas in the media may show a prominent loss of elastica, with pools of metachromatic material or actual cystic degeneration.

The importance of degenerative changes in the media in the pathogenesis of a dissecting aneurysm has been questioned on the basis that "no one of the features can be termed [a] basic pathological process." Similar features may be observed in the settings of atherosclerosis, senile aortas, and Marfan's syndrome, as well as in cases of incomplete or complete dissection.[150]

The role of dissection as the primary event has been promoted on the basis of the absence of an intimal tear in some cases. However, in one series of 161 cases an intimal tear was found in every patient.[150] It may be that some separation occurs in the media as a first event, followed by lifting or breaking of the detached inner part of the wall, possibly then culminating in a tear (Fig. 47-13).

Most intimal tears occur in the ascending aorta or the arch. Some more distal tears, especially those in the lower abdominal aorta or iliac arteries, arise in disrupted atherosclerotic plaques. Iatrogenic causes, such as procedures in which catheters are passed into these vessels, are likely to increase in frequency as these procedures become more popular.

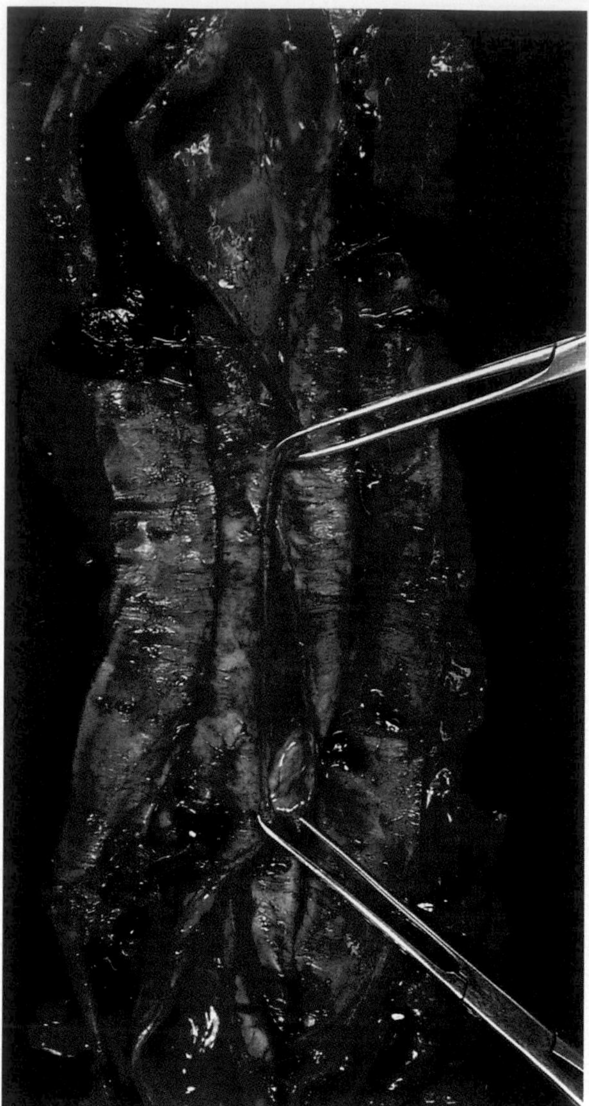

Fig. 47-13 Dissecting aneurysm. The space formed by the separation of layers of the aortic wall contains clotted blood.

Another condition associated with dissecting aneurysms is pregnancy, though the incidence of dissecting aneurysms in pregnant women varies widely. Rupture is most likely to occur in the third trimester.[150]

A dissecting aneurysm may complicate giant cell aortitis[151] and also occurs in patients with congenital aortic stenosis, especially when associated with aortic valve malformations. The risk is increased nine times in patients with a congenitally bicuspid valve and 18 times in those with a unicommisural valve.[150]

Dissecting aneurysm has also been reported to occur in association with fibromuscular dysplasia that involves many vessels, including the aorta.[152] The association is of interest, as this is another condition in which morphologic damage occurs in the arterial wall elastica.

Traumatic aneurysm

Traumatic aneurysms may occur after penetration or rupture of an artery. Compression injuries may cause the aorta to rupture, more often just distal to the obliterated ductus arteriosus; less commonly the ascending aorta is affected. Most patients die of hemorrhage, with 239 of the 275 patients in the series reported on by Parmley succumbing within the first hour. Only 5 (2%) survived long enough for a chronic traumatic aneurysm to develop.[153] For the hemorrhage to be contained long enough to permit a "false" aneurysm to develop, the adventitia or the surrounding tissues must provide a boundary or capsule that contains the pulsating hematoma.

Once a false aneurysm has formed, it may remain for a long time without causing symptoms, and may be observed radiologically as a dense, possibly calcified mass. Enlargement and rupture may occur at any time. Some aneurysms of arteries caused by blunt trauma are not false but have components of the arterial wall in their structure.[154]

Arteriovenous aneurysm

The term *arteriovenous aneurysm* is somewhat arbitrarily applied to any communication existing between systemic arteries and veins, whether as a result of congenital malformation, a spontaneous process, or surgery or trauma. Congenital arteriovenous aneurysms consist of a congeries of abnormal vessels with multiple arteriovenous fistulas. There may be hypertrophy of the affected part, such as a limb. Lesions of the brain, often referred to as *cirsoid aneurysms,* may give rise to life-threatening hemorrhages.

Acquired arteriovenous fistulas occur as a result of trauma or more rarely as a result of infection of an arterial wall caused by infected embolic material from bacterial endocarditis.

Surgically created communications between arteries and veins are made to provide access for dialysis. Clinically significant arteriovenous fistulas resulting from trauma arise in areas where large arteries and veins are close to each other. Cardiac decompensation may ensue if the opening is large.

Surgically created arteriovenous fistulas between the iliac or femoral vessels of dogs were found to lead to the development of bacterial endocarditis in 75%.[155] It was concluded that the increased load on the heart rendered the valves susceptible to colonization by any circulating organisms.

Mycotic aneurysm

When an artery wall becomes the seat of an acute inflammatory reaction that is caused by bacteria, the resulting destruction of muscle and elastic tissue may weaken the wall, causing an aneurysm to form. The source in small arteries may be infected emboli from infective endocarditis or any other source of infection.[156] In large vessels such as the aorta, which is the most common location, the bacteria may gain access through the vasa vasorum either in association with septicemia or as microemboli from bacterial endocarditis. The term, hallowed by usage, is clearly a misnomer, as the lesion is usually not caused by fungal infection. It is worth noting in this connection, however, that certain fungi, especially *Mucor* and *Aspergillus,* are capable of invading blood vessels. This often causes thrombosis. The lungs are the usual sites for the fungal involvement of vessels, and the "target" lesions, produced by a central area of necrosis surrounded by inflammation, are a characteristic finding.

Other aneurysms that result from an inflammatory process in the arterial wall are those that complicate various kinds of vasculitis. Examples are periarteritis nodosa, in which mesenteric vessel involvement is common, or Kawasaki disease, in which it is common for aneurysms of the coronary arteries to occur.

Berry aneurysm refers to a small round aneurysm that occurs on a bifurcation of the circle of Willis. The aneurysm develops in association with a defect in the medial muscular layer. Rupture, which is more likely to occur when the aneurysm's diameter exceeds 10 mm, results in subarachnoid hemorrhage. (For more details on these aneurysms see Chapter 77.)

Fibromuscular dysplasia

Fibromuscular dysplasia is considered to be a nonatherosclerotic and noninflammatory disease of arterial walls. It most commonly involves the renal arteries and less often other musculoelastic arteries. The process involves a fibromuscular proliferation that may affect the intima, media, or adventitia; of these, the medial type is the most common.[157] The process is usually segmental, involving portions of the arterial wall, with intervening areas, which are not stenotic. A characteristic pattern seen on x-ray studies of the contrast-filled, affected vessel is referred to as a "rosary" or "string of beads" sign.

The etiology of the condition is speculative. An interesting possibility is that it might be a sequel to a process known as *segmental mediolytic arteritis.* This is characterized by necrosis in the arterial wall and affects the same range of vessels involved in fibromuscular dysplasia. This condition was first reported in 1976,[158] and in a recent review the author proposes that it is a variant of fibromuscular dysplasia.[159] A similar lesion of the coronary arteries has been observed in stillborn and liveborn infants.

Fibromuscular dysplasia preferentially involves the renal arteries. Five subtypes are recognized[157] (Table 47-2). The most common is medial fibroplasia, which accounts for 60% to 90% of the cases. Perimedial fibroplasia accounts for 20% to 25% of the cases, whereas other forms are very rare.

One conspicuous feature is the apparent rupture and retraction of the internal elastic lamina. Another is the formation of prominent masses or cushions composed of smooth muscle cells and related connective tissue elements, which project into the lumen. The arterial wall may be thinned out between the stenosis or appear to be aneurysmal.

The symptoms and signs of fibromuscular dysplasia are related to the vascular territories involved. Renal artery involvement affecting either the main renal artery or some of its segmental branches is an important cause of renovascular hypertension, especially in young women. The involvement is

Table 47-2 Pathologic classification of fibromuscular dysplasia

Subtype	Pathologic appearance
Intimal fibroplasia	Proliferation of intimal cells
Medial fibroplasia	Fibromuscular protrusions alternate with aneurysmal areas of thinned media ("string of beads" sign on angiogram)
Perimedial fibroplasia	Proliferation of fibroblasts in outer portion of media
Medial hyperplasia	Hyperplasia of smooth muscle in the media
Periaterial fibroplasia	Proliferation of fibroblasts in adventitia with scattered lymphocytes

bilateral in half the cases, and when it is unilateral, the right renal artery is involved three times more often than the left. The affected kidney or portion of the kidney is atrophic and consists of small atrophic tubules. The glomeruli appear to be crowded together.

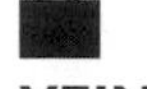

VEINS

Normal structure and age-related changes

Normal veins differ from arteries of the same size in that the wall of a vein is thinner, the three tunicae are less well demarcated, elastic tissue is scanty and not clearly organized into distinct internal and external elastic laminas, and medial smooth muscle cells are relatively fewer in number, widely separated by collagen fibers, and arranged in both circular and longitudinal fashion. All veins, except the venae cavae and common iliac veins, have valves. The valves, which are best developed in the leg veins, are paired folds of intimal tissue with collagen and elastin but little smooth muscle. Valves occur every 1 to 6 cm, often just distal to the point of entry of a tributary vein, and prevent retrograde venous blood flow. The venous system is a reservoir or capacitance unit for the cardiovascular system, containing 60% to 75% of the blood volume.

The principle age change in veins is the development of a definite fibromuscular intimal layer, which often is eccentric in thickness at a given site. This intimal fibromuscular layer hyalinizes with age and may calcify focally. Although this change rarely produces luminal narrowing, the advanced forms create phlebosclerosis.

Varicosities

Varicose veins

Varicose veins are abnormally dilated and tortuous veins. Although this pathologic condition of veins may occur in any part of the body, including the lower esophagus, anal region, and spermatic cord, the most common sites are the superficial veins of the lower extremities, particularly the long saphenous vein and its tributaries. More than 20 million people in the United States are affected by varicose veins of the legs, with the peak occurrence being in the fourth and fifth decades. Women are affected three to six times more often than men. The condition appears to be more prevalent in Western countries. The etiology and pathogenesis of varicosities are multifactorial. Major considerations include hereditary (familial) weakness of the venous wall and valves, increased intraluminal pressure in leg veins from the upright posture with incompetence of the valves resulting from dilatation of the vessel, pregnancy because of compression of iliac veins and increased blood volume, and hormonal effects on smooth muscle. Less common etiologic and pathogenic factors are obesity and aging with atrophy of perivenous soft tissues. Scarring changes and thrombotic or neoplastic obstructions may be associated with varicosities distal to the involved venous segment.

Varicose veins of the legs are dilated, tortuous, elongated, and nodular. Histologic changes are similar to those of age but more pronounced. Calcific foci related to degeneration of medial elastic fibers may be present. Thrombosis is common, and organization of the thrombi may lead to intimal fibrous and hyaline plaques. All these changes are considered to be secondary, not causal. Prolonged venous stasis leads to skin changes of edema, stasis dermatitis, cellulitis, erosion, and ulceration and is a major factor in the development of thrombophlebitis in varicose veins. Pulmonary thromboembolism from varicose veins is uncommon.

Esophageal varices

Esophageal varices are tortuous and distended coronary veins of the distal esophagus and cardia of the stomach. They are almost always the result of obstruction of portal venous flow, most often caused by cirrhosis, since the coronary veins serve as collateral channels. In addition to hepatic cirrhosis, esophageal varices result from superior vena cava obstruction, portal vein thrombosis, hepatic vein thrombosis (Budd-Chiari syndrome), pylephlebitis, and tumor compression of the major portal trunk. Rupture and bleeding are the problems related to esophageal varices. Treatment includes sclerotherapy or shunt surgery.[160]

Hemorrhoids

Hemorrhoids are varicosities of the hemorrhoidal venous plexuses. External hemorrhoids are varicosities of the inferior hemorrhoidal plexus, which is located below the dentate line of the anal canal, is covered by squamous epithelium, and drains to the internal iliac veins of the systemic venous system. Internal hemorrhoids are varicose veins of the submucosal internal hemorrhoidal plexus, which is located above the dentate line, is covered by transitional and columnar epithelium, and drains to the portal venous system. Factors implicated in hemorrhoidal disease are hereditary, erect posture, obstruction of venous return caused by increased intraabdominal pressure as with pregnancy, straining during bowel movement and diarrhea, and portal hypertension by virtue of the hemorrhoidal plexus serving as a collateral channel. Thrombosis, ulceration, hemorrhage, and perianal infection are frequent complications of hemorrhoids.

Varicocele

A varicocele is a mass of varicose veins of the pampiniform plexus of the spermatic cord. This plexus is formed by the veins draining the testes and epididymis and drains by a single channel into the renal vein on the left and into the inferior vena cava on the right side of the body. Primary (idiopathic) varicocele is common on the left side but rare on the right. Secondary (symptomatic) varicocele may occur on either side and results from increased pressure on or in the spermatic veins as with hepatosplenomegaly, pronounced hydronephrosis, and abdominal tumors.

Phlebothrombosis and thrombophlebitis

In the past, two types of venous thrombosis were recognized: thrombophlebitis resulting from inflammation of the vein caused by injury or by neighboring inflammation, and phlebothrombosis as a primary condition related to hemodynamic and coagulation alterations. Today this distinction is recognized to be more theoretical than practical, since in most cases the initial problem is phlebothrombosis and the thrombus itself causes inflammatory reaction in the wall of the affected vein, manifested by local and systemic signs and symptoms of an inflammatory state. The terms commonly are used synonymously.

The pathogenesis of venous thrombosis is summarized in Virchow's triad, which emphasizes the importance of changes in the vessel, particularly endothelial damage; changes in the composition of the blood; and disturbance of blood flow, especially stasis. Thrombosis is augmented if the fibrinolytic mechanism is defective or inhibited. One or more of these pathogenic factors are likely to be present in certain clinical situations, including use of estrogen-containing compounds, malignancy, cardiac disease with congestive heart failure or arrhythmia, postoperative states, and inactivity or immobilization for any reason.

Phlebographic, pathologic, and radioactive tracer studies in the legs have shown that venous thrombosis develops initially in calf veins, mainly in the valvular sinuses and the related valves. Most of these spontaneously lyse or organize. Only some enlarge to form a thrombus of sufficient size to cause luminal obstruction or embolize. Thrombosis of larger veins, such as those of the iliofemoral system, which may be an extension of thrombi originating in calf veins, has a higher risk of pulmonary thromboembolism. Pulmonary thromboemboli originate from veins of the legs in approximately 95% of cases. Approximately half of patients with acute venous thrombosis will have pulmonary thromboembolic episodes, but the majority of these are clinically inapparent.[161]

The affected vein may appear normal or may be distended and firm to palpation. Internally a mural or an occlusive thrombus is present. The attachment of the thrombus to the wall may be delicate and easily separated. If the initial site of attachment of the thrombus can be determined, most often it is in the sinus of a valve. At the point of attachment an inflammatory-reparative process is present in thrombi that have been present for more than several hours. This reaction initially consists of an ingrowth of fibroblasts into the thrombus from the venous intima, along with the deposition of scattered lymphocytes, macrophages, and a few polymorphonuclear leukocytes. Later, granulation tissue organizes the thrombus; the complete resolution may lead to a focus of fibrous intimal thickening or to an organized, recanalized thrombus.

Special types of venous thrombosis

Superficial thrombophlebitis. Superficial venous thrombosis of the legs usually results from varicose veins, whereas that of the arms usually is caused by the administration of intravenous fluids. The local inflammatory response generally is aseptic. Pulmonary thromboembolism is rare, and when it occurs, it is most often the result of extension of the thrombotic process into the common femoral vein or of the coexistence of deep vein thrombosis.

Thrombophlebitis migrans. Thrombophlebitis migrans is a clinical, but not morpholigic, condition characterized by recurrent episodes of venous thrombosis of the extremities and viscera. It is most commonly associated with malignant tumors, Buerger's disease, connective tissue disorders, and blood disorders such as polycythemia rubra vera and sickle cell disease, with the use of intravenous catheters.[162] Malignant neoplasms particularly associated with migratory thrombophlebitis are carcinomas of the lung, female reproductive tract, pancreas, gastrointestinal tract, prostate, and breast. Frequently this syndrome is accompanied by nonbacterial thrombotic endocarditis of the cardiac valves.

Phlegmasia alba dolens. The clinical finding of "white, painful leg" refers to massive swelling of the leg that is associated with some, but not all, cases of iliofemoral venous thrombosis.[163] The massive swelling is postulated to result from blockage of veins and perivenous lymphatics by an inflammatory process. The condition is much more common in the left than in the right leg, probably because the left iliac vein is compressed by the right common iliac artery or by the aortic bifurcation. It occurs most often in women in the third trimester of pregnancy or after childbirth, or in patients who have had extensive pelvic surgery. The frequent absence of valves within the iliac veins and the proximity of the iliofemoral system to the inferior vena cava may account for the development of pulmonary embolism in this condition.

Phlegmasia cerulea dolens. In some patients with massive iliofemoral venous thrombosis, the extremity is greatly swollen, the skin is blue, and bullae or superficial gangrene develop. The basis for this complication of venous thrombosis is thrombosis of collateral channels and decreased arterial blood flow. It is a serious condition with a mortality that ranges from 27% to 42%, depending on the presence or absence of venous gangrene.

Superior vena cava syndrome. Obstruction of the superior vena cava (SVC) most often results from external compression. Thrombosis is present in less than half of the patients and most often results from the process that compresses or invades the wall of the SVC. Although in the past the SVC syndrome was caused by syphilitic aortic aneurysm or tuberculous mediastinitis in 40% of patients, today most instances result from malignant disease. Bronchogenic carcinoma accounts for 75% of patients with the SVC syndrome, and about half of these have small-cell carcinoma, 15% have lymphoma, and 7% have metastatic neoplasms from various sites. Rare causes of the SVC syndrome include primary SVC thrombosis, pericardial constriction, idiopathic sclerosing mediastinitis, and goiter. The clinical syndrome of obstruction of the SVC consists of dilatation of veins of the upper part of the thorax and neck; edema and plethora of the face, neck, and upper part of the torso including the breasts; edema of the conjunctiva; and central nervous system symptoms of headache, visual distortion, and disturbed state of consciousness.

Inferior vena cava syndrome. The most common cause of obstruction of the inferior vena cava (IVC) is thrombosis, usually by extension from thrombosed iliac and femoral veins. Neoplastic involvement by external compression, invasion, or direct intraluminal extension is the other major cause of IVC obstruction. Renal cell carcinoma is the tumor that most commonly causes IVC obstruction. Less frequent causes are external pressure from abdominal aortic aneurysm, ascites, pregnancy, retroperitoneal fibrosis, paravertebral lymphadenopathy, pelvic lipomatosis, pelvic inflammatory disease, and extension of hepatic and renal vein thrombi into the IVC. In childhood, IVC obstruction may result from right-sided Wilms' tumor, neuroblastoma, or multicystic kidneys. Symptoms and signs of IVC obstruction are swelling and edema of the lower extremities, distention of the superficial veins of the lower limbs, and the appearance of collateral venous channels in the lower abdomen.

Thrombosis of hepatic veins (Budd-Chiari syndrome). The Budd-Chiari syndrome is thrombotic obstruction of the major hepatic veins resulting in hepatic congestion and portal hypertension. The IVC may be involved by direct extension. Secondary slowing of blood flow in the portal vein may lead to thrombosis of the portal system. The cause can be identified in about two thirds of cases. The most frequent underlying conditions are hematologic disorders (polycythemia rubra vera, paroxysmal nocturnal hemoglobinuria, and myeloproliferative diseases) and use of oral contraceptives. Various drugs, pregnancy and the postpartum state, primary and secondary tumors of the liver, and trauma are other causes.[164] Worldwide, the most common cause of hepatic outflow obstruction is a membranous web of the inferior vena cava.[165] Intense hepatic congestion with a "nutmeg" appearance, centrilobular or panlobular necrosis and hemorrhage, and replacement fibrosis are the major pathologic features in the liver. Acute forms, characterized by abdominal pain, ascites, and acute hepatic failure, are associated with complete sudden obstruction. Subacute to chronic forms, characterized by abdominal pain, ascites, and hepatosplenomegaly, are associated with incomplete occlusion of the veins.

Portal vein obstruction. Extrahepatic obstruction of the portal vein may be caused by thrombosis (pylethrombosis), compression by intra-abdominal tumors or cysts, congenital venous atresia with cavernous malformation in childhood, and inflammation (pylephlebitis) that usually results from an intra-abdominal infection. Thrombosis of the portal vein may be a complication of cirrhosis, visceral carcinoma, or polycythemia rubra vera. The thrombus may undergo organization and become a fibrous cord or undergo cavernous transformation to form a spongy, trabeculated venous lake involving the area of the portal vein and extending into the gastroduodenal ligament. Acute complete thrombosis of the portal vein in the absence of formed collaterals is catastrophic, leading to hemorrhagic infarction of the small bowel. Chronic forms have signs of portal hypertension with abdominal pain, ascites, splenomegaly, hematemesis, and melena.

Aortocoronary vein bypass grafts

Segments of veins, usually autologous saphenous veins, are used to bypass obstructed coronary arteries, as well as peripheral arteries, with generally good results for long periods. Changes in these venous grafts influence their long-term function. The major morphologic alteration is fibromuscular intimal proliferation that begins a few days after operation but is not necessarily steadily progressive with time, although it may cause severe luminal narrowing or total occlusion of the bypass graft.[166] Occlusion of these grafts in the early postoperative period is thrombotic and is mainly related to arterial disease distal to the coronary anastomosis or to technical surgical factors. The proliferating intimal cells are longitudinally oriented smooth muscle cells similar to those found in atherosclerotic lesions. They are capable of synthesizing collagen, elastin, and glycosaminoglycans. With time, the intimal lesion becomes less cellular and has more collagen fibers and ground substance. Factors implicated in the ubiquitous intimal proliferation in coronary artery bypass vein grafts are arterial intravascular pressure and flow, angle of anastomosis, tension on the graft, ischemic insult caused by severance of vasa vasorum of the graft, and mural deposits of fibrin that accumulate as a result of endothelial demage. True atherosclerotic changes in saphenous vein bypass grafts are uncommon until years after operation, though they are more common and appear earlier in patients with hyperlipidemic states.[166]

LYMPHATICS

Normal structure

The lymphatic system consists of lymphatic capillaries, lymphatic vessels (collecting vessels), and lymph nodes. Lymphatic capillaries are similar but not identical to blood capillaries. They consist of a single layer of endothelium with an interrupted basal lamina and scattered single smooth muscle cells. Lymphatic vessels resemble veins, and those larger than 200 to 500 μm in external diameter have poorly defined intimal, medial, and adventitial layers whose structure quantitatively shows great variations. Virtually all lymphatic vessels have valves, which may be either bicuspid or tricuspid. The vessels often are dilated in the segments between valves. Lymphatic capillaries and vessels unite to form superficial and deep plexuses in and about many tissues and organs. The larger lymphatic vessels, such as the thoracic duct, have nerves and small blood vessels in their adventitia.

Lymphangitis

Acute lymphangitis results from the introduction of microorganisms, especially pyogenic bacteria, into the subcutaneous tissue. The superficial lymphatics are affected. Common organisms are β-hemolytic streptococci and staphylococci. The affected lymphatics are visible as cutaneous erythematous streaks that spread up the arm or leg to the axillary or inguinal lymph nodes. Microscopically the lymphatics are dilated and contain leukocytes, cell debris, and coagulated lymph. The perilymphatic tissues are hyperemic and edematous with an inflammatory exudate. Recovery from acute lymphangitis with or without treatment usually is complete and without sequelae, but recurrent acute lymphangitis or incomplete resolution may lead to chronic lymphangitis. Chronic lymphangitis may cause permanent lymphatic obstruction by fibrosis resulting in chronic lymphedema.

Lymphedema

Lymphedema is swelling of soft tissue, especially the limbs, caused by a localized increase in the quantity of lymph.

Congenital lymphedema. Abnormal development of the lymphatic system has been noted in several congenital disorders, such as Turner's syndrome.[167] A familial-hereditary form *(Milroy's disease)* and a nonfamilial (simple) form of congenital lymphedema are recognized. In both forms, from birth, part or all of one extremity is diffusely swollen but is not painful or ulcerated. Milroy's disease, which also may be associated with other congenital anomalies, appears to be transmitted as an autosomal dominant trait with high penetrance, variable expression, and a predilection for males. Histologic study of the involved region in either form shows dilatation of the subcutaneous lymphatics, increased interstitial fluid, and some fibrosis in long-standing cases.

Lymphedema praecox. In lymphedema praecox, which primarily affects females in the second or third decade of life, lymphedema begins in the foot or ankle and progresses slowly up the leg to involve the entire extremity in months or years. The skin of the extremity becomes roughened, and the edema becomes nonpitting. Other abnormalities have been observed in patients with lymphedema praecox, including yellow nails, pleural effusion, primary pulmonary hypertension, bronchiectasis, cerebrovascular malformations, small pelvis, hypospadias, abnormal bone length, osteosclerosis, pes cavus, fused lumbar vertebrae, fixed flexion of the finger, distichiasis, hemangiomas of the feet and hands, and micrognathism. The cause is unknown, but a relationship to the reproductive system in suspected because of age of onset, female preponderance, and increased swelling during menses.

Secondary (obstructive) lymphedema

The most common cause of obstructive lymphedema is a malignant tumor that occludes the lymphatic vessels or the lymph nodes. Surgical removal of lymphatics or lymph nodes and destruction of lymphatics by irradiation also are frequent causes.

Less common causes include sclerosing retroperitoneal fibrosis, granulomatous processes such as sarcoidosis and tuberculosis of retroperitoneal or inguinal lymph nodes, nematodal parasitic infestation (filariasis) of lymphatics producing elephantiasis, and rheumatoid arthritis. Because of the numerous anastomotic connections among lymphatic vessels, obstruction must be widespread or involve a critical site for draining lymph nodes, such as the axilla or the groin, for secondary lymphedema to develop. Lymphatics distal to the point of obstruction are greatly dilated, and the interstitial vessels are edematous and become fibrotic with time. Rupture of distended large lymphatics may occur, permitting the escape of milky lymphatic fluid, which may create, depending on site of drainage, chylous ascites (chyloperitoneum), chylothorax, chylopericardium, or chyluria.

Lymphangioma

Lymphangiomas are benign overgrowths of lymphatic vessels; whether these are congenital malformations, hamartomas, or true neoplasms is not certain. Lymphangiomas are classified as capillary, cavernous, or cystic (hygroma) types, and combinations are frequent.

Capillary lymphangioma *(lymphangioma simplex)* is an apparently congenital lesion of the skin or mucous membranes of the head and neck that grows slowly if at all. The small, circumscribed, pale white to pink tumors are composed of a network of endothelium-lined, thin-walled lymphatic spaces often separated by lymphoid aggregates.

Lymphangiomyoma, which can be regarded as a variant of capillary lymphangioma, has proliferating smooth muscle cells and branching, slitlike lymphatic channels. It is a rare, acquired or congenital lesion most commonly involving abdominal and thoracic lymphatics of females[169] that may be associated with chylothorax.

Cavernous lymphangioma is more common than the capillary variety. It also is an apparently congenital lesion that grows slowly and is composed of numerous dilated lymphatic spaces filled with lymph (chylangioma), which may be coagulated and hyalinized or calcified. The distinction from capillary lymphangioma on the basis of size of channels is somewhat arbitrary. Mixed lesions of cavernous lymphangioma and hemangioma are more common.

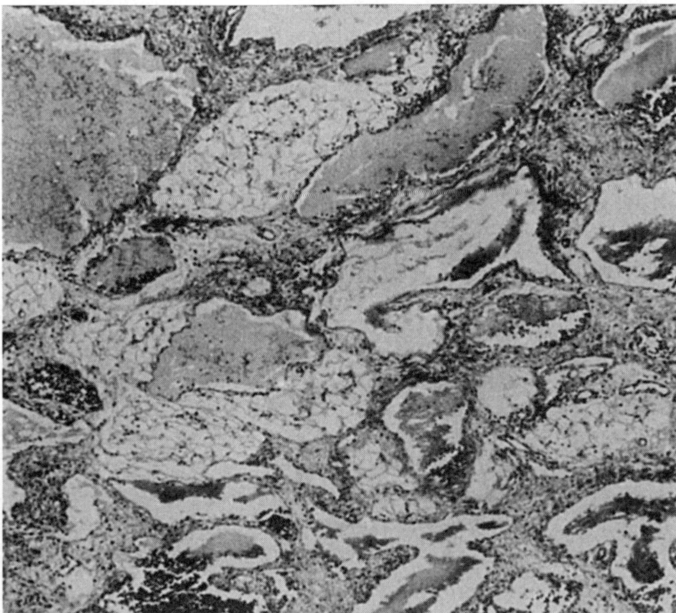

Fig. 47-14 Cystic hygroma from the neck of a child is composed of dilated lymphatic spaces surrounded by connective tissue that contains lymphocytes.

Cystic lymphangioma (hygroma) occurs principally in the neck *(hygroma colli cysticum)* as a disfiguring congenital lesion. The cystic mass usually is multilocular and contains serous fluid or lymph. The histologic structure is similar to that of cavernous lymphangioma except for the large size of the spaces (Fig. 47-14). Large collections of lymphocytes may be present in the stroma. Total excision of large lesions may be difficult, and incomplete excision leads to recurrence. Infection of cystic hygroma is a serious problem.

REFERENCES

Arteries

1. Clark JM, Glagov S: Transmural organization of the aortic media; the Lamellar Unit revised, *Arteriosclerosis* 5:19, 1985
2. Majack RA, Bornstein P: Biosynthesis and modulation of extracellular components by cultured vascular smooth muscle cells. In Campbell JH, Campbell GR, editors: *Vascular smooth muscle in culture,* Boca Raton, Fla, 1986, CRC Press.
3. Kaprio J, Norio R, Pesonen E, Sarna S: Intimal thickening of coronary arteries in infants in relation to family history of coronary artery disease, *Circulation* 87:1960, 1993.

Arteriosclerosis

4. Gamble CN: The pathogenesis of hyaline arteriosclerosis, *Am J Pathol* 122:140, 1986.
5. Rao RN, Hilliard K, Wray CH: Widespread intimal hyperplasia of small arteries and arterioles, *Arch Pathol Lab Med* 107:254, 1993.
6. Sinclair RA, Antonovych TT, Mostofi FK: Renal proliferative arteriopathies and associated glomerular changes: a light and electron microscopic study, *Hum Pathol* 7:565, 1976.
7. Lough J, Moore S: Platelet embolic injury: the healing process, *Exp Mol Pathol* 17:133, 1972.
8. Mönkeberg JG: Über die reine Mediaverkalkung der Extremitätenarterien und ihr Verhalten zur arteriosclerose, *Virchows Arch A Pathol Anat* 171:141, 1903.
9. Moran JJ: Idiopathic arterial calcification of infancy: a clinico-pathologic study, *Pathol Annu* 10:393, 1975.

Atherosclerosis

10. Davies MJ, Thomas AC: Plaque fissuring: the cause of acute myocardial infarction, sudden ischaemic death and crescendo angina, *Br Heart J* 53:363, 1985.
11. Falk E: Plaque rupture with severe pre-existing stenosis precipitating coronary thrombosis: characteristics of coronary atherosclerotic plaques underlying fatal occlusive thrombi, *Br Heart J* 50:127, 1983.
12. Chapman I: Morphogenesis of occluding coronary artery thrombosis, *Arch Pathol Lab Med* 80:256, 1965.
13. Stary HC, Blankenhorn DH, Chandler AB et al: A definition of the intima of human arteries and of its atherosclerosis-prone regions: a report from the Committee on Vascular Lesions of the Council on Arteriosclerosis, American Heart Association, *Circulation* 85:391, 1992.
14. Wilens SL: The nature of diffuse intimal thickening of coronary arteries, *Am J Pathol* 27:825, 1951.
15. Ku DN, Giddens DP, Zarins CK, Glagov S: Pulsatile flow and atherosclerosis in the human carotid bifurcation: positive correlation between plaque location and low and oscillating shear stress, *Arterioscler Thromb* 5:293, 1985.
16. Scott RF, Reidy MA, Kim DN et al: Intima cell mass–derived atherosclerotic lesions in the abdominal aorta of hyperlipemic swine. Part 2: Investigation of endothelial cell changes and leukocyte adherence associated with early smooth muscle cell proliferative activity, *Atherosclerosis* 62:27, 1986.
17. Stary H: Evolution and progression of atherosclerotic lesions in coronary arteries of children and young adults, *Arteriosclerosis* 9:1, 1989.

18. Katsuda S, Boyd HC, Fligner C et al: Human atherosclerosis III: Immunohistochemical analysis of the cell composition of lesions of young adults, *Am J Pathol* 140:907, 1992.
19. Smith E, Keene GA, Grant A et al: Fate of fibrinogen in human arterial intima, *Arterioscler Thromb* 10:263, 1990.
20. Hoff MF, Heideman CI, Gaubatz JW et al: Quantification of apo B in grossly normal human aorta, *Circ Res* 40:56, 1977.
21. Faggiotto A, Ross R, Harker L: Studies of hypercholesterolemia in the non-human primate. I. Changes that lead to fatty streak formation, *Arteriosclerosis* 4:323, 1984.
22. McGill HC Jr: Persistent problems in the pathogenesis of atherosclerosis, *Arteriosclerosis* 4:443, 1984.
23. The PDAY Research Group. Natural history of aortic and coronary atherosclerotic lesions in youth. Findings from the PDAY Study, *Arterioscler Thromb* 13:1291, 1993.
24. Haerem JW: Mural platelet microthrombi and major acute lesions of main epicardial arteries in sudden cardiac death, *Atherosclerosis* 19:539, 1974.
25. Geissinger M, Mustard JF, Rowsell HC: The occurrence of microthrombi on the aortic endothelium of swine, *Can Med Assoc J* 87:405, 1962.
26. Doerr W: Perfusion Theorie der Arteriosklerose. In Bagmann W, Doerr W, editors: *Zwanglose Abhandlungen aus dem Gebiet der normalen und pathologischen Anatomie,* Heft 13, Stuttgart, 1963, George Thieme Verlag.
27. Moore S: Responses of the arterial wall to injury, *Diabetes* 20(suppl 2): 1, 1981.
28. Tracy R, Kissling GE: Age and fibroplasia as preconditions for atheronecrosis in human coronary arteries, *Arch Pathol Lab Med* 111:957, 1987.
29. Herem RM, Levesque MJ: Fluid dynamics as a factor in localization of atherogenesis, *Ann NY Acad Sci* 416:709, 1983.
30. Davies PF, Remuzzi A, Gordon EI, Gimbrone MA: Turbulent fluid shear stress induces vascular endothelial cell turnover in vitro, *Proc Natl Acad Sci USA* 83:2114, 1986.
31. Wright HP: Mitosis pattern in aortic endothelium, *Atherosclerosis* 15:93, 1972.
32. Goldsmith HL: Blood flow and thrombosis, *Thromb Diath Haemorrh* 32:35, 1974.
33. Hoff H, Yamauchi Y, Bond MG: Regulation in tissue LDL accumulation during coronary artery regression in cynomolgus monkeys, *Atherosclerosis,* 56:51, 1985.
34. St. Clair RW: Atherosclerosis regression in animal models, *Prog Cardiovasc Dis* 26:109, 1983.
35. DeFeyter PJ, Serruys PW, Davies MJ et al: Qualitative coronary angiography to measure progression and regression of coronary atherosclerosis: value, limitations and implications for clinical trials, *Circulation* 84:412, 1991.
36. Arntzenius AC, Kromhout D, Barth JD: Diet, lipoproteins and the progression of coronary atherosclerosis: the Leiden Intervention Trial, *N Engl J Med* 312:805, 1985.
37. Brown BG, Zhao XG, Sacco DE, Albers JJ: Lipid lowering and plaque regression: new insights into prevention of plaque disruption and clinical events in coronary disease, *Circulation* 87:1781, 1993.
38. Brown BG, Albert JJ, Fisher LD et al: Regression of coronary artery disease as a result of intensive lipid-lowering therapy in men with high levels of apolipoprotein B, *N Engl J Med* 323: 1289, 1990.
39. Keen M, Jarrett RJ, Fuller SH, McCartney P: Hyperglycemia and arterial disease, *Diabetes* 30(suppl 2) 49, 1981.
40. Richardson PD, Davies MJ, Born GVR: Influence of plaque configuration and stress distribution on fissuring of coronary atherosclerotic plaques, *Lancet* 2:947, 1989.
41. Baumgartner HB, Turitto VT, Weiss JH: Effect of shear rate on platelet interaction with subendothelium in citrated and native blood. II. Relationships among platelet adhesion, thrombus dimension and fibrin formation, *J Lab Clin Med* 95:208, 1980.
42. Hand RA, Chandler AS: Atherosclerotic metamorphosis of analogous pulmonary thromboemboli in the rabbit, *Am J Pathol* 49:469, 1962.
43. Groves HL, Kinlough-Rathbone RL, Richard M et al: Platelet interaction with damaged rabbit aorta, *Lab Invest* 40:194, 1979.
44. Groves HL, Kinlough-Rathbone RL, Richardson M et al: Thrombin generation and fibrin formation following injury to rabbit neo-intima: studies of vessel wall reactivity and platelet survival, *Lab Invest* 46:605, 1982.
45. Wilcox JM, Smith KM, Schwartz SM, Gordon D: Localization of tissue factor in the normal vessel wall and in the atherosclerotic plaque, *Proc Natl Acad Sci USA* 86:2839, 1989.
46. Juhan-Vague I, Alessi MC: Plasminogen activator inhibitor and atherothrombosis, *Thromb Haemost* 70:138, 1993.
47. Gunning AJ, Pickering GW, Robb-Smith AM, Ross-Russel RW: Mural thrombosis of the internal carotid artery and subsequent embolism, *Q J Med* 33:155, 1964.
48. Davies MJ, Thomas AC, Knapman PA, Hangartner JR: Intramyocardial platelet aggregation in patients with unstable angina suffering ischemic cardiac death, *Circulation* 73:418, 1986.
49. Moore S, Belbeck LW, Evans G, Pineau S: Effects of complete or partial occlusion of a coronary artery, *Lab Invest* 44:151, 1981.
50. Lough J, Moore S: Endothelial injury induced by thrombin or thrombi, *Lab Invest* 33:130, 1976.
51. Harrison MJG, Marshall J: Angiographic appearance of carotid bifurcation in patients with completed stroke, transient ischemic attacks and cerebral tumors, *Br Med J* 205, 1976.
52. Maurizi CP, Barker AE, Truehart RE: Atheromatous emboli, a postmortem study with special reference to the lower extremities, *Arch Pathol Lab Med* 86:528, 1968.
53. Anderson WR: Necrotizing angitis associated with embolization of cholesterol, *Am J Clin Pathol* 43:65, 1965.
54. Nevitt MP, Ballard DJ, Hallett JW: Prognosis of abdominal aortic aneurysms: a population based study, *N Engl J Med* 321:1009, 1989.
55. Kuivaniemi H, Tromp G, Prockop DJ: Genetic causes of aortic aneurysms. Unlearning at least part of what the textbooks say, *J Clin Invest* 88:1441, 1991.
56. Tyson JE, DeSa DJ, Moore S: Thrombo-atheromatous complications of umbilical arterial catheterization in the newborn period; clinico-pathological study, *Arch Dis Child* 51:744, 1976.
57. Moore S: Clinical correlations, *Thromb Diath Haemorrh* 33:417, 1975.
58. Stehbens WE, Karmody AM: Venous atherosclerosis associated with arteriovenous fistulas for hemodialysis, *Arch Surg* 110:176, 1975.
59. Stamler J: The marked decline in coronary heart disease mortality rates in the United States 1968-1981. Summary of findings and possible explanations, *Cardiology* 72:11, 1985.
60. Strong JP, Guzman MA: Decrease in coronary atherosclerosis in New Orleans, *Lab Invest* 43:297, 1980.
61. Tracy R, Kissling GE: Age and fibroplasia as preconditions for atherosclerosis in human coronary arteries, *Arch Pathol Lab Med* 111:957, 1987.
62. Gordon T, Kannell WB, Hjortland MC, McNamara PN: Menopause and coronary heart disease: the Framingham Study, *Ann Nutr Metab* 89:158, 1987.
63. Bush TL, Barrett-Connor E, Cowan LD et al: Cardiovascular mortality and non-contraceptive use of estrogen in women: results from the Lipid Research Clinics Program Follow-up Study, *Circulation* 75:1102, 1987.
64. Meilahn EN, Kuller LH, Matthews KA, Kiss JE: Hemostatic factors according to menopausal states and use of hormone replacement therapy, *Epidemiology* 2:445, 1992.
65. Meade TW, Brozovic M, Chakrabarti RR et al: Haemostatic function and ischemic heart disease: principal results of the Northwick Park Heart Study, *Lancet* 2:533, 1986.
66. Thauzow E, Erikssen J, Sandvik L et al: Blood platelet count and function are related to total and cardiovascular death in apparently healthy men, *Circulation* 84:936, 1991.
67. Sniderman A, Shapiro AS, Marpole D, Skinner B et al: Association of coronary atherosclerosis with hyperapobetalipoproteinemia (increased protein but normal cholesterol levels in human plasma low density [β] lipoproteins), *Proc Natl Acad Sci USA* 72:604, 1980.
68. Grundy SM: Cholesterol and coronary heart disease: a new era, *JAMA* 256:2844, 1986.
69. Powell KE, Thompson PD, Caspersen CJ, Kendrick JS: Physical activity and the incidence of coronary heart disease, *Annu Rev Public Health* 8:253, 1987.

70. Thomson J, Symes C, Heaton K: Moderate alcohol intake reduces bile cholesterol saturation and raises HDL cholesterol, *Lancet* 2:819, 1983.
71. Renaud S, de Logeril M: Wine, alcohol, platelets and the French paradox for coronary heart disease, *Lancet* 2:819, 1983.
72. Department of Health and Human Services: *Reducing the heart consequences of smoking: 25 years of progress: a report of the Surgeon General,* Washington, DC, 1989, Government Printing Office (DHHS publication no [CDC] 89-8411).
73. Moore S: The pathogenesis of atherosclerosis, *Metabolism* 34(suppl 1):13, 1985.
74. Berlin JA, Colditz GA: A meta-analysis of physical activity in the prevention of coronary heart disease, *Am J Epidemiol* 136:612, 1990.
75. Stratton JR, Chandler WL, Schwartz RS et al: Effects of physical conditioning on fibrinolytic variables, *Circulation* 83:1692, 1991.
76. Marmot M: Psychosocial factors and cardiovascular disease, *Eur Heart J* 9:690, 1988.
77. Saudicani P, Hein HO, Gyntelberg F: Are social inequalities as associated with the risk of ischemic heart disease a result of psychosocial working conditions? *Atherosclerosis* 106:165, 1993.
78. Ross R: The pathogenesis of atherosclerosis: a perspective for the 1990's, *Nature* 362:801, 1993.
79. Ross R, Glomset JA: The pathogenesis of atherosclerosis, *N Engl J Med* 295:369, 420, 1976.
80. Steinberg D: Lipoproteins and the pathogenesis of atherosclerosis, *Circulation* 76:508, 1987.
81. Parthasarathy S, Quinn MC, Schwenke DC, Carew T et al: Oxidative modification of beta–very low density lipoprotein. Potential role in monocyte recruitment and foam cell formation, *Arteriosclerosis* 9:398, 1988.
82. Geer JC: Fine structure of human aorta intimal thickening and fatty streaks, *Lab Invest* 14:1764, 1965.
83. Gown AM, Toyohiro T, Ross R: Human atherosclerosis II: immunocytochemical analysis of the cellular composition of human atherosclerotic lesions, *Am J Pathol* 125:191, 1968.
84. Katsuda S, Boyd HC, Fligner C et al: Human atherosclerosis III: immunohistochemical analysis of the cell composition of lesions of young adults, *Am J Pathol* 140:907, 1992.
85. Restropo C, Tracy R: Variations in human aortic fatty streaks among geographic locations, *Atherlosclerosis* 21:179, 1975.
86. Watanabe Y: Serial inbreeding of rabbits with hereditary hyperlipidemia (WHHL-rabbit): incidence and development of atherosclerosis and xanthoma, *Atherosclerosis* 36:261, 1980.
87. LaVille A, Turner PR, Pittilo M et al: Hereditary hyperlipidemia in the rabbit due to over-production of lipoproteins. I. Biochemical studies, *Arteriosclerosis* 7:105, 1987.
88. Minick CR, Murphy GE, Campbell WG Jr: Experimental induction of atheroarteriosclerosis by the synergy of allergic injury to arteries and lipid rich diet, *J Exp Med* 124:635, 1966.
89. Wissler R: Theories and new horizons in the pathogenesis of atherosclerosis and the mechanisms of clinical effects, *Arch Pathol Lab Med* 116:1281, 1992.
90. Hruban RH, Beschorner WE, Baumgartner WA et al: Accelerated arteriosclerosis in heart transplant recipients is associated with a T-lymphocyte–mediated endothelialitis, *Am J Pathol* 137:871, 1990.
91. Friedman RJ, Moore S, Singal DP: Repeated endothelial injury and induction of atherosclerosis in normolipemic rabbits by human serum, *Lab Invest* 32:404, 1974.
92. Moore S: Responses of the arterial wall to injury, *Diabetes* 30(suppl): 8-13, 1981.
93. Moore S: Injury mechanisms in atherosclerosis. In Moore S, editor: *Vascular injury and atherosclerosis,* New York, 1981, Marcel Dekker.
94. Richardson M, Hatton MWC, Moore S: The plasma proteases thrombin and plasmin degrade the proteoglycan of rabbit aorta segments in vitro: an integrated ultrastructural and biochemical study, *Clin Exp Med* 11:139, 1988.
95. Moore S, Friedman RJ, Singal DP et al: Inhibition of injury-induced thromboatherosclerotic lesions by antiplatelet serum in rabbits, *Thromb Haemost* 35:70, 1976.
96. Friedman RJ, Stemerman MB, Wenz B et al: The effect of thrombocytopenia on experimental arteriosclerotic lesion formation in rabbits. I. Smooth muscle cell proliferation and re-endothelialization, *J Clin Invest* 61:722, 1977.
97. Ihnatowycz, IO, Winocour PD, Moore S: A platelet-derived factor chemotactic for rabbit arterial smooth muscle cells, *Artery* 9:316, 1982.
98. Grotendorst GR, Seppa HE, Kleinman MK, Martin GD: Attachment of smooth muscle cells to collagen and their migration toward platelet-derived growth factor, *Proc Natl Acad Sci USA* 78:3669, 1981.
99. Lindner V, Majack RA, Reidy MA: Basic fibroblast growth factor stimulates endothelial regrowth and proliferation in denuded arteries, *J Clin Invest* 85:2004, 1990.
100. Olson HE, Chao S, Lindner V, Reidy MA: Intimal smooth muscle cell proliferation after balloon catheter injury; the role of basic fibroblast growth factor, *Am J Pathol* 140:1023, 1992.
101. Moore S, Belbeck LW, Richardson M, Taylor W: Lipid accumulation in the neointima in normal fed rabbits in response to 1 or 6 removals of the aortic endothelium, *Lab Invest* 47:37, 1982.
102. Forrester JS, Fishbein MC, Helfant R, Fagin T: A paradigm for restenosis based on cell biology: clues for development of new preventive therapies, *J Am Coll Cardiol* 17:758, 1991.
103. Li Z, Alavi MZ, Moore S: The proliferation of neointimal smooth muscle cells cultured from rabbit aortic explants 15 weeks after de-endothelialization by a balloon catheter, *Int J Exp Pathol* 75:169 1994.
104. Day AJ, Alavi MZ, Moore S: Influx of $^{3}H/^{14}C$-cholesterol labelled lipoprotein in re-endothelialized and de-endothelialized areas of ballooned aortas of normal-fed and cholesterol-fed rabbits, *Atherosclerosis* 55:339, 1985.
105. Alavi, MZ, Moore S: Kinetics of low density lipoprotein interactions with rabbit aortic wall following balloon catheter de-endothelialization, *Arteriosclerosis* 4:395, 1984.
106. Alavi MZ, Moore S: Glycosaminoglycan composition and biosynthesis in the endothelium-covered neointima of de-endothelialized rabbit aorta, *Exp Mol Pathol* 42:389, 1985.
107. Alavi MZ, Richard M, Moore S: The in-vitro interactions between serum lipoproteins and proteoglycans of the neointima of rabbit aorta, following a single balloon catheter injury, *Am J Pathol* 134:287, 1989.
108. Alavi MZ, Galis Z, Li Z, Moore S: Dietary alterations of plasma lipoproteins influence their interaction with proteoglycan enriched extracts from neointima of rabbit aorta, *Clin Invest Med* 14:419, 1991.
109. Ismail NA, Alavi MZ, Moore S: Lipoprotein: proteoglycan complexes from injured aortas accelerate lipoprotein uptake by arterial smooth muscle cells, *Atherosclerosis*, 105:79, 1994.
110. Ismail NA, Alavi MZ, Moore S: Isolation of lipoprotein-proteoglycan complexes from balloon catheter deendothelialized aortas and uptake of these complexes by blood monocyte–derived macrophages, *Pathology*, 26:145, 1994.
111. Ismail NAE, Alavi MZ, Moore S: Lipoprotein-proteoglycan complexes from injured rabbit aortas accelerate lipoprotein uptake by arterial smooth muscle cells, *Atherosclerosis* 105:79, 1994.
112. Galis Z, Alavi MZ, Moore S: Co-localization of aortic apolipoprotein B and chondroitin sulfate in an injury model of atherosclerosis, *Am J Pathol* 142:1432, 1993.
113. Smith EB, Staples EM, Dietz HS, Smith RH: Role of endothelium in sequestration of lipoprotein and fibrinogen in aortic lesions, thrombi and graft pseudo-intimas, *Lancet* 2:812, 1979.
114. Podet EJ, Shaffer DR, Gianturco SH et al: Interaction of low density lipoproteins with human aortic elastin, *Arterioscler Thromb* 11:116, 1991.
115. Wong MK, Gotlieb AI: In vitro re-endothelialization of a single cell wound: role of microfilament bundles in rapid filopodia-mediated wound closure, *Lab Invest* 51:75, 1984.
116. Spurlock BO, Chandler AB: Adherent platelets and surface microthrombi of the human aorta and left coronary artery: a scanning electron microscopy study, *Scanning Microsc* 1:1359, 1987.
117. Jorgensen L, Packham MA, Rowsell HC, Mustard JF: Deposition of formed elements on the blood of the intima and signs of intimal injury in the aorta of rabbit, pig and man, *Lab Invest* 27:341, 1972.
118. Ku DN, Giddems DP, Zarins K, Glagov S: Pulsatile flow and atherosclerosis in the human carotid bifurcation: positive correlation between plaque

location and low and oscillating shear stress, *Arterioscler Thromb* 5:293, 1985.
119. Levesque MJ, Liepsch D, Moravec S, Nerem RM: Correlation of endothelial cell shape and wall shear stress in a stenosed dog aorta, *Arteriosclerosis* 5:220, 1985.
120. Dicorleto PE, Bowen-Pope DF: Cultured endothelial cells produce a platelet-derived growth factor-like protein, *Proc Natl Acad Sci USA* 80:1919, 1983.
121. Chamley-Campbell JH, Campbell Gr, Ross R: Phenotype dependent response of cultured aortic smooth muscle to serum mitogens, *J Cell Biol*, 89:379, 1981.
122. Wasty F, Alavi MZ, Li Z et al: In vitro interaction between low density lipoprotein from hyper betalipoproteinemic plasma and arterial wall proteoglycans, *Can J Cardiol* 8:605, 1992.
123. Kostner GM, Bihari-Varga M: Is the atherogenicity of Lp(a) caused by its reactivity with proteoglycans? *Eur Heart J* 11(suppl E):184, 1990.
124. Wasty F, Alavi MZ, Moore S: Distribution of glycosaminoglycans in the intima of human aortas: changes in atherosclerosis and diabetes, *Diabetologia* 36:316, 1993.
125. McCully KS: Importance of homocysteine-induced abnormalities in proteoglycan structure in arteriosclerosis, *Am J Pathol* 59:181, 1970.
126. Harker LA, Ross R, Slichter J, Scott CR: Homocysteine induced arteriosclerosis: the role of endothelial cell injury and platelet response in its genesis, *J Clin Invest* 58:763, 1976.
127. Bienvenu T, Ankri A, Chadefaux B et al: Elevated total plasma homocysteine, a risk factor for thrombosis: relation to coagulation and fibrinolytic parameters, *Thromb Res* 70:123, 1993.
128. Orzan F, Brusca A, Conte M et al: Severe coronary artery disease after radiation therapy of the chest and mediastinum: clinical presentation and treatment, *Br Heart J* 69:496, 1993.
129. Fabricant CG, Fabricant J, Litrenta MM et al: Virus induced atherosclerosis, *J Exp Med* 148:336, 1978.
130. Saikku P, Mattila K, Nieminen MS et al: Serological evidence of an assocation of a novel *Chlamydia* TWAR, with chronic coronary heart disease and acute myocardial infarction, *Lancet* 2:983, 1988.
131. Kuo CC, Gown AM, Benditt EP, Grayston JT: Detection of *Chlamydia pneumoniae* in aortic lesions of atherosclerosis by immunocytochemical stains, *Arterioscler Thromb* 13:1501, 1993.
132. Benditt EP, Barret T, McDougall JK: Viruses in the etiology of atherosclerosis, *Proc Natl Acad Sci USA* 80:6396, 1983.
133. Hansson GK, Jonasson L, Seifert PS, Stemme S: Immune mechanisms in atherosclerosis, *Arterosclerosis* 9:567, 1989.
134. Loscalzo J: The relation between atherosclerosis and thrombosis, *Circulation* 86 (suppl II): 93, 1992.
135. Meade TW, Mellows S, Brozovic M et al: Haemostatic function and ischemic heart disease, *Lancet* 2:533, 1986.
136. Mehta Z, Mehta P, Lawson D, Saldeen T: Plasma tissue plasminogen activator inhibitor levels in coronary artery disease: correlation with age and serum triglyceride concentrations, *J Am Coll Cardiol* 9:263, 1989.
137. Goldsmith HL, Turitto VT: Rheological aspects of thrombosis and haemostasis: basic principles and applications, *Thromb Haemost* 55:415, 1986.
138. Moore S: Pathogenesis of atherosclerosis. *Metabolism* 34(suppl 1):13, 1985.
139. Hadcock S, Richardson M, Winocour PD, Hatton MWC: Intimal alterations in rabbit aortas during six months of alloxan-induced diabetes, *Arterioscler Thromb* 11:517, 1991.
140. Moore S: Thrombo-atherosclerosis in normolipemic rabbits; a result of continued endothelial damage, *Lab Invest* 29:478, 1973.
141. Cortellaro M, Cofrancesco E, Boschetti C et al: Increased fibrin turnover and high PA1-1 activity as predictors of ischemic events in atherosclerotic patients: a case-control study, *Arterioscler Thromb* 13:1412, 1993.
142. Greco C, DiLoreto M, Ciavolella M, Banci M et al: Immunodetection of human atherosclerotic plaque with ^{125}I-labelled monoclonal antifibrin antibodies, *Atherosclerosis* 100:133, 1993.
143. Stevens RL, Colombo M, Gonzales JJ et al: The glycosaminoglycans of the human artery and their changes in atherosclerosis, *J Clin Invest* 58:470, 1976.

Aneurysms

144. Ernst CB: Abdominal aortic aneurysm, *N Engl J Med* 328:1167, 1993.
145. Roberts WC: Aortic dissection: anatomy of aneurysms: consequences and causes, *Am Heart J* 101:195, 1981.
146. Erdheim J: Medionecrosis aortae idiopathica cystica, *Virchows Arch Pathol Anat* 275:187, 1930.
147. Schlatman MD, Becker AE: Pathogenesis of dissecting aneurysm of aorta: comparative histopathological study of significance of medial changes, *Am J Cardiol* 39:21, 1977.
148. Sinclair RJG, Kitchen AH, Turner RWD: The Marfan syndrome, *J Med* 29:19, 1960.
149. Francke U, Furthmayr H: Marfan's syndrome and other disorders of fibrillin, *N Engl J Med* 330:1383, 1994.
150. Larson, EW, Edwards WD: Risk factors for aortic dissection: necropsy study of 161 cases, *Am J Cardiol* 58:849, 1984.
151. Harris M: Dissecting aneurysm of the aorta due to giant cell arteritis, *Br Heart J* 30:840, 1968.
152. Gatalica Z, Gibas Z, Martínez-Hernández A: Dissecting aortic aneurysm as a complication of generalized fibromuscular disease, *Hum Pathol* 23:586, 1992.
153. Parmley LF, Mattingly TW, Manion WC, Jahnke EJ Jr: Non-penetrating traumatic injury of the aorta, *Circulation* 17:1086, 1968.
154. Heggtveit HA, Campbell JS, Hooper GD: Innominate arterial aneurysms occurring after blunt trauma, *Am J Clin Pathol* 42:69, 1964.
155. Lillehei CW, Bobb JRR, Fisscher MB: The occurrence of endocarditis with vascular deformities in dogs with arterio-venous fistulas, *Ann Surg* 132:577, 1950.
156. Adlaka A, Yale Sh, Patel R et al: *Haemophilus influenzae* serotype F: an unusual cause of a mycotic aneurysm in an adult, *Mayo Clin Proc* 69:467, 1994.

Fibromuscular dysplasia

157. Luscher TF, Lie JT, Stanson AW et al: Arterial fibromuscular dysplasia, *Mayo Clin Proc* 62:931, 1987.
158. Slavin RE, González-Vitale JC: Segmental mediolytic arteritis: a clinicopathological study, *Lab Invest* 35:23, 1976.
159. Lie JT: Segmental mediolytic arteritis: not an arteritis but a variant of arterial fibromuscular disease, *J Vasc Surg* 16:66, 1992.

Veins

160. Rikkers LF, Jin G, Burnett DA et al: Shunt surgery versus endoscopic sclerotherapy for variceal hemorrhage: late results of a randomized trial, *Am J Surg* 165:27, 1993.
161. Saeger W, Genzkow M: Venous thromboses and pulmonary embolism in postmorten series: probable causes by correlations of clinical data and basic diseases, *Pathol Res Pract* 190:394, 1994.
162. Raad II, Luna M, Khalil SM et al: The relationship between the thrombotic and infectious complications of central venous catheters, *JAMA* 271:1014, 1994.
163. Wong WT: Surgical management of the post-phlebitic leg syndrome, *Am J Surg* 165:163, 1993.
164. Mitchell MC, Boitnott JK, Kaufman S et al: Budd-Chiari syndrome: etiology, diagnosis and management, *Medicine* 61:199, 1982.
165. Rector WG, Xu YH, Goldstein L, Peters RL et al: Membranous obstruction of the inferior vena in the United States, *Medicine* 64:134, 1985.
166. Titus JL: The heart after surgery for ischemic heart disease, *Am J Cardiovasc Pathol* 1:339, 1988.

Lymphatics

167. Greenlee R, Hoyme H, Witte M et al: Developmental disorders of the lymphatic system, *Lymphology* 26:156, 1993.
168. Joos E, Bourgeois P, Famaey JP: Lymphatic disorders in rheumatoid arthritis, *Semin Arthritis Rheum* 22:392, 1993.
169. McCarty KS, Mossler JA, McLelland R et al: Pulmonary lymphangiomyomatosis repressive to progesterone, *N Engl J Med* 303:1461, 1980.

B. VASCULITIS

J. Charles Jennette
Seymour Rosen

Vasculitis is inflammation of blood vessels. It can be confined to a single organ, such as the skin, or can affect multiple organ systems. Systemic vasculitides can affect any organ and can mimic many diseases clinically. Therefore vasculitis is often considered in the differential diagnosis of various multisystem diseases.

As is true of other tissues, the gross and histologic expressions of inflammatory injury in blood vessels are limited in number. Because of the nonspecificity of gross and histologic features of vasculitides, many of which have similar or overlapping clinical manifestations, the definitive diagnosis is based on correlation of the gross and histologic features with clinical, serologic, microbiologic, and immunopathologic data.

ETIOLOGY AND PATHOGENESIS

Vasculitides can be categorized on the basis of known or putative pathogenic mechanisms (Table 47-3). Although the initiating causes vary, most vasculitides share common pathogenic pathways that lead to the activation of leukocytes in vessel walls, with resultant injury. Inflammatory mediators act on both circulating leukocytes and endothelial cells to induce the adhesion of leukocytes to endothelial cells, with subsequent diapedesis. In contrast to the margination and diapedesis of leukocytes that occur at sites of nonvasculitic inflammation, which do not cause significant vessel wall injury, vasculitis is characterized by actual inflammatory injury to vessel walls that results from the activation of leukocytes and other inflammatory mediators within and adjacent to vessel walls. This is caused by the presence of pathogenic factors that can drive leukocytes to complete activation as they are adhering to and penetrating vessel walls. Such pathogenic factors include infectious pathogens, immune complexes, and autoantibodies with specificity for autoantigens on vessel walls or leukocytes.

Infection-induced vasculitis

As in other tissues, invasion of vessel walls by infectious pathogens causes inflammation. Infectious organisms reach vessel walls by (1) direct extension from adjacent extravascular sites of infection, such as the extension of a pulmonary fungal infection into the walls of pulmonary vessels; (2) septic embolization of thrombotic material containing pathogens, such as emboli released from valvular vegetations in a patient with bacterial endocarditis; and (3) hematogenous dissemination of pathogens, such as that occurring in neisserial septicemia and spotted fever rickettsial diseases. Vascular inflammation results not only from the activation of inflammatory mediators by microorganisms or their degradation products, such as bacterial formyl tripeptides and glycolipids, but also from the host's immune response to the invading microorganisms.

Vascular inflammation caused by pyogenic bacteria is characterized by the presence of numerous neutrophils during the acute phase, resulting in focal vascular necrosis, hemorrhage, and sometimes thrombosis. The bacteria, such as *Neisseria*, may be detected in tissue sections at the site of inflammation. Systemic vasculitis caused by direct invasion of the vessels by pyogenic bacteria is the result of bacteremia.

Products of bacteria attract and activate leukocytes, especially neutrophils, and also activate humoral inflammatory mediator systems, such as the complement system. Although in acute septicemic vasculitis most of the inflammation is induced by nonimmune inflammatory events, immune responses to the bacteria can cause the generation of antibodies that bind to bacterial antigens and amplify the acute inflammatory response. As is discussed later, antibody responses to microbial antigens also cause vasculitis by causing immune complex deposits to be produced in vessels that are not invaded by viable pathogens.

Rickettsial, spirochetal, mycobacterial, and fungal invasion of vessels induces inflammation that has a predominance of

Table 47-3 Types of vasculitis categorized on the basis of proposed pathogenic mechanisms

Direct infection of vessels
Bacterial vasculitis (such as neisserial)
Mycobacterial vasculitis (such as tuberculous)
Spirochetal vasculitis (such as syphilitic)
Rickettsial vasculitis (such as Rocky Mountain spotted fever)
Fungal vasculitis (such as aspergillosis)
Viral vasculitis (such as herpes zoster)
Immunologic injury
Immune complex–mediated vasculitis
- Henoch-Schönlein purpura
- Cryoglobulinemic vasculitis
- Lupus vasculitis
- Rheumatoid vasculitis
- Serum sickness vasculitis
  - Induced by whole serum
  - Induced by heterologous proteins
- Infection-induced immune complex vasculitis
  - Viral (such as hepatitis B and C)
  - Bacterial (such as group A *Streptococcus*)
- Paraneoplastic vasculitis
- Behçet's disease
- Some drug-induced vasculitides (such as sulfonamide-induced vasculitis)

Direct antibody attack–mediated vasculitis
- Goodpasture's syndrome (mediated by anti–basement membrane antibodies)
- Kawasaki disease (possibly mediated by antiendothelial antibodies)

Antineutrophil cytoplasmic autoantibody–mediated vasculitis
- Wegener's granulomatosis
- Microscopic polyangiitis (microscopic polyarteritis)
- Churg-Strauss syndrome
- Some drug-induced vasculitides (such as thiouracil-induced vasculitis)

Cell-mediated vasculitis
- Allograft cellular vascular rejection

Unknown
Giant cell (temporal) arteritis
Takayasu arteritis
Polyarteritis nodosa
Behçet's disease

mononuclear leukocytes rather than neutrophils. This parallels the pattern of inflammation caused by these pathogens in other tissues.

Immune-mediated vasculitis

Antibody-mediated and cell-mediated immune mechanisms are involved in the pathogenesis of vasculitis (see Table 47-3). Immune responses may be initiated by heterologous antigens, such as injected proteins in serum sickness and viral antigens in hepatitis C–associated vasculitis, and by autoantigens, such as immunoglobulins in cryoglobulinemic vasculitis and proteinase-3 (PR 3) in Wegener's granulomatosis.

More than fifty years ago Arnold Rich[1] suspected that hypersensitivity (immune) responses cause vasculitis after he observed vasculitis in patients who had been injected with horse serum or sulfonamide antibiotics. He confirmed this by inducing vasculitis in rabbits with intravenous injections of horse serum.[2] In the 1950s and 1960s, Frank Dixon and his associates[3] elucidated the immune pathogenesis of serum sickness in rabbits by demonstrating that the development of vasculitis was temporally related to the generation of circulating immune complexes and the deposition of these complexes in vessel walls. The localization of immune complexes in vessel walls causes the activation of both inflammatory effector cells (such as neutrophils, monocytes, mast cells, platelets and endothelial cells) and humoral inflammatory mediator systems (such as complement, kinin, plasmin, and coagulation systems).[4-6] The activation of neutrophils and monocytes results in the release of lytic enzymes and toxic oxygen metabolites that cause injury to the vessel walls. In severe disease this results in vascular necrosis, hemorrhage, and thrombosis.

Pathogenic immune complexes may contain heterologous antigens or autoantigens. Heterologous antigens can come from injected therapeutic agents or infectious pathogens. Therapeutic agents that have been associated with the development of vasculitis include drugs (such as sulfonamides) and heterologous proteins (such as antitoxin horse serum, mouse monoclonal antibodies, and cloned streptokinase). Localized infections such as hepatitis B, hepatitis C, and streptococcal infections can cause systemic vasculitis by releasing antigens that participate in the formation of pathogenic immune complexes. Occasionally, vasculitis occurring in patients may result from the immune response to tumor antigens, but the pathogenesis of such paraneoplastic vasculitis is obscure. A variety of autoantibodies are believed to cause immune complex–mediated vasculitis, such as antinuclear antibodies in lupus vasculitis and antiimmunoglobulins (rheumatoid factors) in cryoglobulinemic and rheumatoid vasculitis.

Vascular immune complexes are either derived from preformed immune complexes deposited from the circulation or formed in situ as a result of the binding of uncomplexed antibodies from the circulation to antigens within vessel walls. Antigens eliciting in situ immune complex formation are constitutive components of the vessel wall (that is, an autoantigen) or are secondarily planted in the vessel wall. The former in essence constitutes a direct autoimmune attack on vessels. The first-described and best-documented example of this autoimmune mechanism of vascular injury is Goodpasture's syndrome. In patients with this syndrome autoantibodies with specificity for the type IV collagen in renal glomerular and pulmonary alveolar capillaries bind to vessel walls and induce acute necrotizing inflammation.[7] This causes a pulmonary-renal vasculitic syndrome that includes pulmonary hemorrhage and glomerulonephritis. A less well documented example of direct autoantibody attack on vessels has been proposed in Kawasaki disease, which may be caused by circulating autoantibodies specific for endothelial antigens that are expressed only after endothelial stimulation by cytokines.[8] These anti–endothelial cell autoantibodies are capable of binding to and killing endothelial cells in vitro and thus may be involved in the pathogenesis of the vasculitis in vivo.

Recently it has been proposed that autoantibodies with specificity for antigens in the granules of neutrophils and the lysosomes of monocytes, called *antineutrophil cytoplasmic autoantibodies (ANCAs)*, are able to activate these leukocytes and cause vasculitis.[9] ANCAs occur in patients with Wegener's granulomatosis, microscopic polyangiitis (microscopic polyarteritis), and Churg-Strauss syndrome. In these aggressive forms of systemic necrotizing vasculitis, there is no evidence of immunoglobulin deposition in the vessel walls.

There is experimental evidence that ANCAs can interact with circulating neutrophils and monocytes after these leukocytes have been primed by cytokines, such as interleukin-1 or tumor necrosis factor, or by microbial products, such as formyl tripeptides. The primed neutrophils and monocytes express ANCA target antigens at their surfaces, making them accessible to the autoantibodies. This results in neutrophil and monocyte activation, with the degranulation and release of toxic oxygen metabolites. In vitro these events cause the adherence to and destruction of cultured endothelial cells.[9]

Immune complex localization in vessel walls, direct binding of autoantibodies to antigens in vessel walls, and the ANCA-induced activation of leukocytes would all lead to a final common pathway of vascular inflammation, characterized by the adhesion of leukocytes to endothelial cells, the invasion of vessel walls by inflammatory cells, and necrotizing injury that could lead to hemorrhage and thrombosis. The histologic appearance and clinical manifestation of these antibody-mediated mechanisms would be similar. An accurate diagnosis can be made only by performing studies in addition to routine histologic studies; for example, the immunohistologic identification of immune complex deposits in vessel walls would indicate an immune complex pathogenesis, the immunohistologic or serologic detection of anti–basement membrane antibodies would indicate anti–basement membrane antibody–mediated vascular injury, and serologic detection of ANCA would indicate ANCA-associated vasculitis.

A primary pathogenic role for T-cell–mediated immunity has been suggested for some types of vasculitis, but the evidence supporting this is inconclusive. The presence of predominantly T-lymphocytes in the inflammatory infiltrates of some vasculitides and the presence of granulomatous inflammation with multinucleated giant cells in others has been the major basis for incriminating cell-mediated immunity. The only form of vasculitis that is clearly directly mediated by T-lymphocytes is acute cellular vascular rejection of allografts. In this process activated T-lymphocytes attach to endothelial cells and penetrate the intima of arteries (Fig. 47-15) and in severe rejection the muscularis. This pattern of vasculitis is not observed in any setting other than allograft rejection. Lymphomatoid granulomatosis, which is characterized by angiocentric and angiodestructive infiltrates of atypical lymphocytes, was once believed to be a type of vasculitis caused by a cell-mediated immune response, but it is now known to be an angiotropic lymphoma.

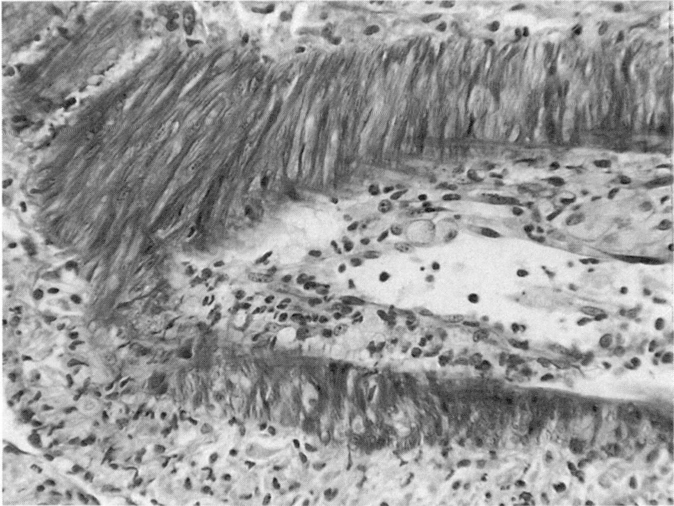

Fig. 47-15 Rejection vasculitis in a renal allograft arcuate artery. Notice the intimal edema and infiltration by mononuclear leukocytes.

NOMENCLATURE OF VASCULITIDES

Historical overview

Pathologic descriptions of noninfectious vasculitis began to appear in the medical literature during the nineteenth century. The first convincing gross pathologic description of a systemic arteritis was published by Rokitansky in 1852, who described the case of a 23-year-old patient with multiple aneurysms in small arteries throughout the body, except for the brain.[10] Thirty-five years later, Eppinger[11] reported the histologic findings in Rokitansky's patient, which confirmed the presence of necrotizing arteritis at sites of aneurysm formation.

The first definitive report of noninfectious systemic necrotizing arteritis, however, was published in 1866 by Kussmaul and Maier,[12] who named the disease *periarteritis nodosa.* Subsequently it was realized that the inflammation was transmural rather than perivascular, and the term was modified to *polyarteritis nodosa.*[13,14]

The early reports of polyarteritis nodosa emphasized the grossly discernible arterial nodules, but soon the importance of the microscopic variant of polyarteritis became obvious.[15,16] In fact, Davson and others[16] concluded that the "form of the disease in which the diagnosis can be made only after histologic examination is the commoner." Microscopic polyarteritis was initially considered a variant of polyarteritis nodosa, but over the past decade it has become apparent that microscopic polyarteritis (microscopic polyangiitis) and polyarteritis nodosa are sufficiently different from one another clinically, pathologically and pathogenetically to be considered different diseases.[17,18]

Additional patterns of arteritis with features that distinguished them from the initial descriptions of polyarteritis nodosa also emerged; these include (1) granulomatous arteritis with prominent temporal artery involvement (giant cell [temporal] arteritis)[19,20]; (2) granulomatous arteritis with extensive involvement of the aorta (Takayasu arteritis)[21,22]; (3) necrotizing arteritis associated with mucosal and cutaneous inflammation and lymphadenopathy (Kawasaki disease)[23]; (4) necrotizing arteritis with respiratory tract necrotizing granulomatous inflammation (Wegener's granulomatosis)[24-26]; and (5) necrotizing arteritis with granulomatous inflammation, eosinophilia, and asthma (Churg-Strauss syndrome).[27-29] The latter two diseases also include vasculitis affecting vessels smaller than arteries.

Small-vessel vasculitis affecting arterioles, venules, and capillaries was found to be the basis for the manifestations of a type of vasculitis described by Johann Schönlein[30] and more completely by his student Eduard Henoch.[31] This syndrome, Henoch-Schönlein purpura, is characterized by purpura, arthralgias, abdominal pain, and nephritis. Small-vessel vasculitis was also recognized to be a manifestation of hypersensitivity responses, such as serum sickness and drug allergy,[1] and to be an occasional accompaniment to systemic rheumatic and autoimmune diseases, neoplasms, and infections.[32,33]

Table 47-4 Names and definitions of vasculitis adopted by the Chapel Hill Consensus Conference on the Nomenclature of Systemic Vasculitis

Name	Definition
Large-vessel vasculitis*	
Giant cell (temporal) arteritis	Granulomatous arteritis of the aorta and its major branches, with a predilection for the extracranial branches of the carotid artery. *Often involves the temporal artery. Usually occurs in patients older than 50 and often is associated with polymyalgia rheumatica.*
Takayasu arteritis	Granulomatous inflammation of the aorta and its major branches. *Usually occurs in patients younger than 50.*
Medium-sized–vessel vasculitis*	
Polyarteritis nodosa (classic polyarteritis nodosa)	Necrotizing inflammation of medium-sized or small arteries without glomerulonephritis or vasculitis in arterioles, capillaries, or venules.
Kawasaki disease	Arteritis involving large, medium-sized, and small arteries and associated with mucocutaneous lymph node syndrome. *Coronary arteries are often involved. Aorta and veins may be involved. Usually occurs in children.*
Small-vessel vasculitis*	
Wegener's granulomatosis†‡	Granulomatous inflammation involving the respiratory tract and necrotizing vasculitis affecting small to medium-sized vessels (e.g., capillaries, venules, arterioles, and arteries). *Necrotizing glomerulonephritis is common.*
Churg-Strauss syndrome†‡	Eosinophil-rich and granulomatous inflammation involving the respiratory tract and necrotizing vasculitis affecting small to medium-sized vessels, associated with asthma and blood eosinophilia.
Microscopic polyangiitis (microscopic polyarteritis)†‡	Necrotizing vasculitis with few or no immune deposits affecting small vessels (i.e., capillaries, venules, or arterioles). *Necrotizing arteritis involving small and medium-sized arteries may be present. Necrotizing glomerulonephritis is very common. Pulmonary capillaritis often occurs.*
Henoch-Schönlein purpura‡	Vasculitis with IgA-dominant immune deposits affecting small vessels (i.e., capillaries, venules, or arterioles). *Typically involves skin, gut, and glomeruli and is associated with arthralgias or arthritis.*
Essential cryoglobulinemic vasculitis‡	Vasculitis with cryoglobulin immune deposits affecting small vessels (i.e., capillaries, venules, or arterioles) and associated with cryoglobulins in serum. *Skin and glomeruli are often involved.*
Cutaneous leukocytoclastic angiitis	Isolated cutaneous leukocytoclastic angiitis without systemic vasculitis or glomerulonephritis.

Modified from Jennette JC et al: *Arthrit Rheum* 37:187, 1994.

**Large artery* refers to the aorta and the largest branches directed toward major body regions (e.g., to the extremities and the head and neck); *medium-sized artery* refers to the main visceral arteries (e.g., renal, hepatic, coronary, and mesenteric arteries); and *small artery* refers to the distal arterial radicals that connect with arterioles (e.g., renal arcuate and interlobular arteries).

†Strongly associated with antineutrophil cytoplasmic autoantibodies.

‡May be accompanied by glomerulonephritis and can manifest as nephritis or pulmonary-renal vasculitic syndrome.

In 1952, based on a careful review of the world's literature and experience with over 50 patients and 100 experimental animals with vasculitis, Pearl Zeek[32] categorized the noninfectious vasculitides into five groups: (1) periarteritis nodosa, (2) allergic granulomatous angiitis, (3) hypersensitivity angiitis, (4) rheumatic arteritis, and (5) temporal arteritis. Zeek preferred the term *hypersensitivity angiitis* for small-vessel arteritis because of the relationship to hypersensitivity in some patients, such as those in whom vasculitis developed after they were injected with horse serum or sulfonamides and because of its similarities to serum sickness vasculitis in experimental animals. Although this landmark attempt at classifying systemic vasculitis demonstrated that vasculitides could be divided into clinically and pathologically distinctive categories, Zeek failed to include some important categories of vasculitis that had been described before her publication, most notably Wegener's granulomatosis and Henoch-Schönlein purpura. Over the ensuing 50 years, important observations have been made that have further elucidated the categories of vasculitis described by Zeek and that have revealed additional distinctive types of vasculitis.

Chapel Hill Consensus Conference on the Nomenclature of Systemic Vasculitis

Subsequent to the seminal classification attempt by Zeek, there have been numerous publications dealing with the nomenclature of the noninfectious systemic vasculitides.[18,32-39] Although most of these proposed approaches have been workable, a major problem has been the lack of international adoption of a standardized nomenclature approach, which further complicates the difficult task of diagnosing vasculitides. A recent international consensus conference addressed this problem and proposed the nomenclature system that is used in the discussions that follow in this chapter.[18]

Table 47-4 gives the names and definitions of some of the most common noninfectious vasculitides in accord with Chapel Hill Consensus Conference on the Nomenclature of Systemic Vasculitis, and Fig. 47-15 depicts the predominant types of vessels involved by these vasculitides. Note that there is substantial overlap among the vasculitides, not only with respect to vessel involvement but also with respect to the clinical and histologic features. Nevertheless, there are distinguishing features that allow identification of the various categories of vasculitis. Resolving this differential diagnosis is important for predicting the natural history and response to treatment of the vasculitis in an individual patient.

LARGE-VESSEL VASCULITIDES

The large-vessel vasculitides affect the aorta and its major branches (Table 47-4, Fig. 47-16). The two major vasculitides that involve these vessels are Takayasu arteritis and giant cell (temporal) arteritis. Both of these vasculitides are characterized histologically by chronic granulomatous inflammation. Understanding the relationship of these two diseases to each other has been difficult because little is known of their etiology or pathogenesis. Other observations, however, indicate that they are different diseases; for example, Takayasu arteritis begins in the first three decades of life, whereas the onset of giant cell (temporal) arteritis is extremely rare before age 50. In addition, giant cell (temporal) arteritis is more common in whites, whereas Takayasu arteritis is more common in persons of Oriental or Indian ancestry and in mestizos in Mexico. The distinction between Takayasu arteritis and giant cell (temporal) arteritis is based on multiple factors, including the patient's age, the vessels involved, and the gross and microscopic appearance of the lesions.

Takayasu arteritis

Takayasu arteritis is a granulomatous inflammation of the aorta and its major branches that almost always occurs in patients younger than 50 years old.[18,40-42] The pulmonary trunk may also be involved. The earliest complete description of the disease was that published by Savory in 1856,[21] but it has been named after the Japanese ophthalmologist, Mikito Takayasu, who in 1908 reported on a patient with the ocular manifestations of the disease.[22] Because of the frequent involvement of the aortic arch and the large arteries to the extremities, this disease has also been called *aortic arch syndrome* and *pulseless disease*.

Etiology and pathogenesis. The cause of Takayasu arteritis is unknown. It has been hypothetically linked to tuberculosis, syphilis, streptococcal infection, parasitic infections, rheumatic fever, rheumatoid arthritis, collagen vascular disease, ankylosing spondylitis, genetic factors, hypersensitivity, and

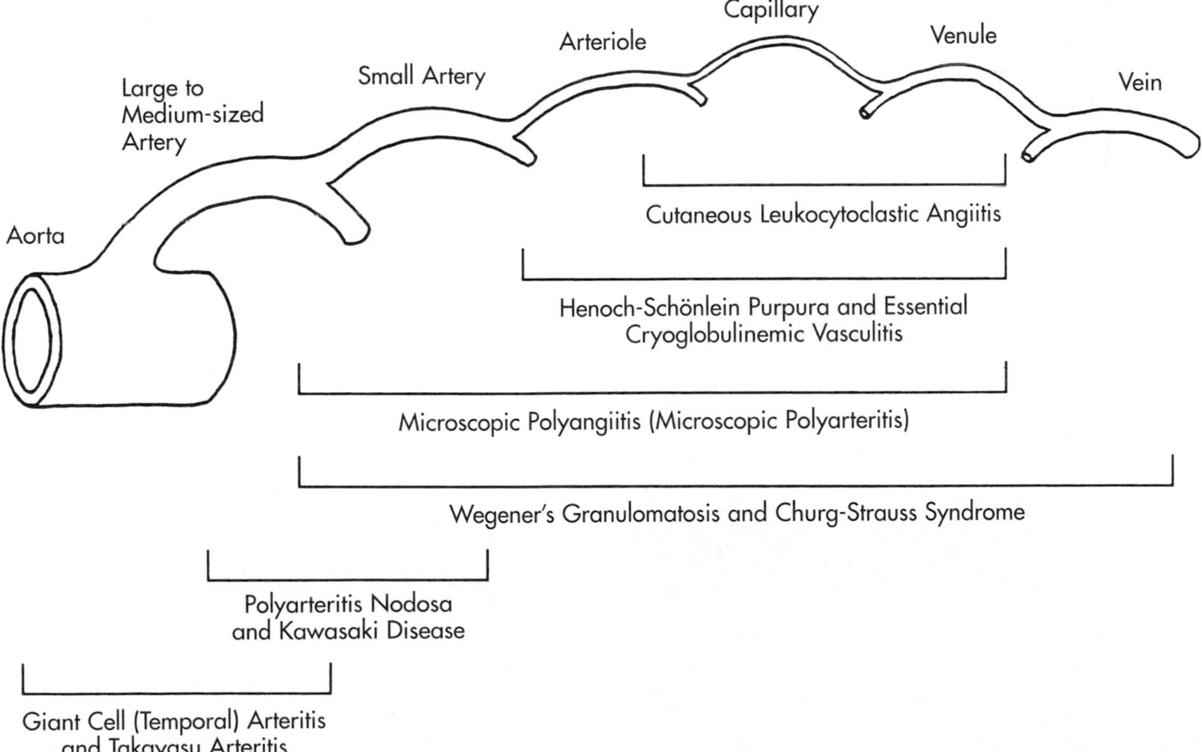

Fig. 47-16 Predominant distribution of vascular involvement by selected vasculitides (see Table 47-4 for definitions). *Large artery* refers to the aorta and the largest branches directed toward major body regions (such as those to the extremities and the head and neck); *medium-sized artery* refers to the main visceral arteries (such as renal, hepatic, coronary, and mesenteric arteries); and *small artery* refers to the distal arterial radicals (such as intraparenchymal arteries). Notice that some small- and large-vessel vasculitides may involve medium-sized arteries but large- and medium-sized–vessel vasculitides typically do not involve vessels smaller than arteries. (Modified from Jennette JC, Falk RJ, Andrassy K et al: *Arthritis Rheum* 37:187, 1994.)

autoimmunity, but none of these proposed causes has been documented. Current opinion favors an immune mechanism, but there is no compelling evidence to support this either.

Pathology. Takayasu arteritis primarily involves the aorta and large elastic arteries. Histologically the earliest vascular changes are focal inflammation and necrosis of the media of involved arteries, with later extension of the inflammation into the adventitia and intima (Fig. 47-17). The inflammatory cell infiltrates are composed predominantly of lymphocytes and mononuclear phagocytes, with admixed eosinophils, neutrophils, and plasma cells. Multinucleated giant cells are often but not always present. The inflammation causes the irregular focal destruction of medial elastic lamellas and muscle cells, which results in medial fibrosis. Inflammation in the adventitia and intima also induces fibrosis. Contraction of the fibrotic media and fibroblastic expansion of the intima lead to progressive luminal narrowing. Thrombosis of injured arterial segments precipitates acute obstruction. In advanced stages of the disease the mural injury is characterized by dense fibrosis without inflammatory cells.

The most common gross changes exhibited by patients with Takayasu arteritis are mural thickening and luminal narrowing, but aneurysms may form in these patients as well. When involved segments of vessels are opened longitudinally, the irregular intimal thickening often has the appearance of raised plaques. Takayasu arteritis is categorized into four types on the basis of the gross distribution of disease, as follows: type I, involvement localized to the aortic arch and its branches; type II, thoracic, descending, and abdominal aorta involvement; type III, combined features of types I and II; and type IV, pulmonary artery involvement (Fig. 47-18). Type III is most common. The subclavian artery is involved in approximately 85% of the patients, the renal artery in 60%, the carotid artery in 45%, the vertebral artery in 20%, the iliac artery in 15%, the innominate artery in 15%, and the pulmonary artery in 15%.

Clinical Features. Most cases of Takayasu arteritis have been reported from Asia (especially Japan) and Africa, but the disease occurs worldwide. A rough estimate of the incidence in the United States is 3 cases per million population. There is a strong female predominance, with a female-to-male ratio of approximately 9:1. The age of onset is usually between 10 and 20 years.

Takayasu arteritis typically has two clinical phases: (1) an initial phase manifesting as systemic symptoms of inflammation (such as fever, weakness, anorexia, malaise, weight loss, night sweats, and arthralgias) followed by an asymptomatic interval lasting from several months to many years; and (2) a vasoocclusive phase during which the signs and symptoms of the obstructive vasculopathy become evident. These include claudication and diminished pulses in extremities, a systolic blood pressure difference of more than 10 mm Hg between the arms, bruits over involved arteries or the aorta, irregular narrowing and poststenotic dilatation of the aorta and its major branches, shown by arteriography, visual disturbances, renovascular hypertension, and congestive heart failure. When the pulmonary arteries are affected, pulmonary hypertension and pulmonary infarction may develop. Laboratory-detected abnormalities are nonspecific and include an elevated erythrocyte sedimentation rate, anemia, and hypergammaglobulinemia.

Symptoms may be ameliorated with corticosteroid treatment, but cyclophosphamide may be required for patients with progressive disease that is unresponsive to this. Surgical intervention is sometimes needed to eliminate vascular narrowing or occlusion. Aneurysms, aortic regurgitation, and retinopathy are predictors of a poor prognosis. In the absence of these indicators, the10-year survival is greater than 90%.

Differential diagnosis. Diseases that must be considered in the pathologic differential diagnosis of Takayasu arteritis include atherosclerosis, arteriosclerosis, fibromuscular dysplasia, thromboangiitis obliterans, syphilitic aortitis, and giant cell (temporal) arteritis. The fibrotic vascular lesions that occur in the chronic "burned-out" form of Takayasu arteritis pose the greatest diagnostic difficulty and the disease cannot be then diagnosed on the basis of the morphology alone.

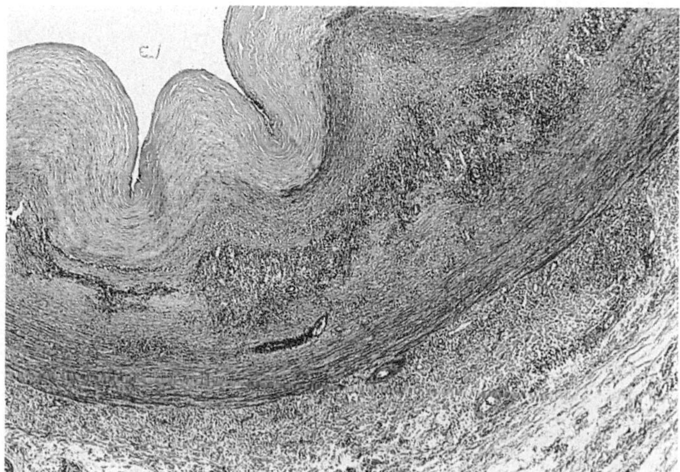

Fig. 47-17 Takayasu arteritis involving the aorta. Notice the transmural inflammation, the disruption of the muscularis, and the fibrosis in the intima and adventitia. (Masson trichrome stain.)

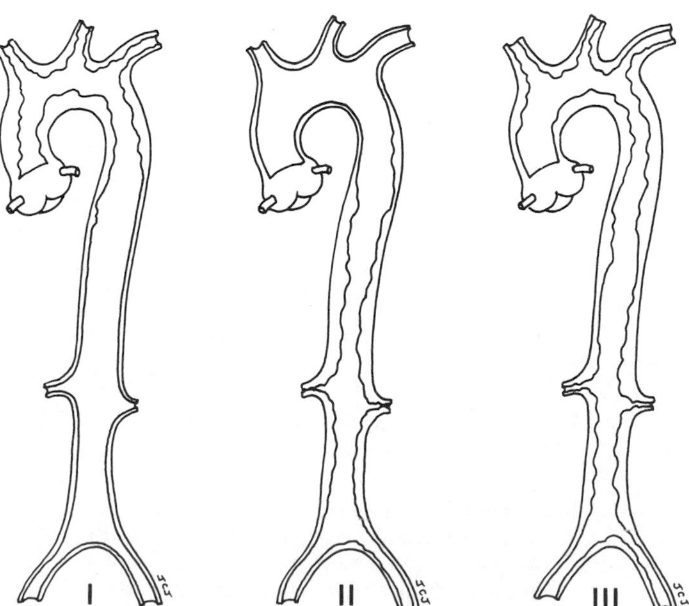

Fig. 47-18 Distribution of aortic involvement in types I, II, and III Takayasu arteritis.

Giant cell (temporal) arteritis

Giant cell (temporal) arteritis is a granulomatous arteritis of the aorta and its major branches, with a predilection for the extracranial branches of the carotid artery. It usually occurs in patients older than 50 and often is associated with polymyalgia rheumatica. Giant cell (temporal) arteritis is the most common form of vasculitis in older patients. At the Chapel Hill conference it was proposed to place "temporal" in parentheses because the temporal artery is frequently but not always involved.[18] In addition, some other forms of systemic vasculitis, such as Wegener's granulomatosis or microscopic polyarteritis, occasionally involve the temporal arteries.

Temporal arteritis was first reported in 1890 by Hutchinson,[19] who described an elderly man with painful red streaks over his temporal arteries. The disease was more completely described in 1932 by Horton, Magath, and Brown,[20] who not only described the clinical manifestations but also identified histologically that granulomatous arteritis was the basis of the symptoms. In 1941 Gilmour[43] described the pathologic findings in four patients, reviewed the descriptions of others in the literature, and concluded that the disease affected the aorta and its branches as well as the temporal artery. In the 1950s and 1960s, the strong association between giant cell (temporal) arteritis and polymyalgia rheumatica was recognized.[44-46]

Etiology and pathogenesis. The etiology and pathogenesis of giant cell (temporal) arteritis are unknown. The presence of activated CD4 T-lymphocytes is suggestive of an immune mechanism, but the inciting event has not been determined. Support for an immunologic pathogenesis is provided by the increased prevalence of certain major histocompatibility complex HLA-DR antigens, especially HLA-DR4, in patient populations.[47,48] The higher frequency of involvement of vessels with a high elastin content and the prominence of inflammation around disrupted elastica and phagocytosed fragments of elastica in macrophages have raised the possibility that giant cell (temporal) arteritis results from an immune-mediated inflammatory response to elastin. For example, Wilkinson and Russell[49] observed that giant cell (temporal) arteritis involvement of the vertebral and internal carotid arteries terminates at the site where the vessels penetrate the dura mater, at which point they also lose their elastica.[49] However, experimental studies have not demonstrated a cell- or antibody-mediated autoimmune response to elastin or other arterial wall constituents in patients with giant cell (temporal) arteritis.[50]

Pathology. The granulomatous arteritis with giant cells has a predilection for the aorta and its major branches, especially the extracranial branches of the carotid artery.[42,49,51-53] Small arteries are less commonly affected. The lesions are typically segmental, in that vessels may have focally injured segments adjacent to uninjured segments. Histologically the lesions are characterized by a panarteritis, which begins in the media but extends to involve the intima and adventitia (Fig. 47-19). The typical inflammatory infiltrate consists primarily of mononuclear leukocytes, with lymphocytes and macrophages predominating. Multinucleated giant cells are frequently but not always present. Eosinophils and neutrophils usually are not numerous. Although focal fibrinoid necrosis may occur, if extensive, this should raise the possibility of the presence of another type of systemic arteritis, such as Wegener's granulomatosis or polyarteritis with temporal artery involvement. Granulomatous inflammation with giant cells may be centered on the internal and less often external elastic lamina, which typically shows fragmentation. Fragments of elastica sometimes can be seen within the cytoplasm of giant cells and other macrophages. Intimal expansion can cause luminal narrowing, but thrombosis is uncommon. Whereas the arterial branches of the aorta are characteristically narrowed, involvement of the aorta may lead to aneurysmal dilatation, resulting in aortic valve insufficiency or dissection or rupture of the aneurysm.

Giant cell arteritis has been observed, either as a localized disease or as a component of disseminated disease, in many organs that are not frequently affected by the disease, including the female genital tract,[54] breast,[55] heart,[56] thyroid,[57] liver,[58] small bowel,[59] gallbladder,[60] kidney,[61] pancreas,[56] esophagus,[61] bone marrow,[62] spinal cord,[63] nerve,[64] and prostate.[61] Either temporal arteritis or polymyalgia rheumatica, or both, have been found in many of these patients, indicating that the vasculitic involvement of these organs is an unusual expression of giant cell (temporal) arteritis.

A temporal artery biopsy specimen often is obtained as part of the investigation in patients with giant cell arteritis. In patients with signs and symptoms of giant cell (temporal) arteritis, the biopsy findings are often diagnostic, even when there is no clinical evidence of temporal artery involvement. In addition, histologically typical giant cell (temporal) arteritis is often identifiable histologically in the temporal arteries of patients with polymyalgia rheumatica who do not have signs or symptoms of arteritis.[45,46] Because of the segmental nature of vascular involvement, to ensure adequate sensitivity a 3 cm or more segment of artery should be obtained for examination. If no abnormality is identified at the levels of the section initially examined, the tissue should be step-sectioned for maximum diagnostic yield. After 1 week of corticosteroid treatment, the diagnostic yield of temporal artery biopsy specimens declines.[65]

Based on pathologic observations, the term *polymyalgia rheumatica* is a misnomer. The inflammation that causes the aching and stiffness in the neck, shoulders, and hips is in fact a synovitis rather than a myositis.[66] Involved synovium exhibits a mild to moderate focal infiltration of mononuclear leuko-

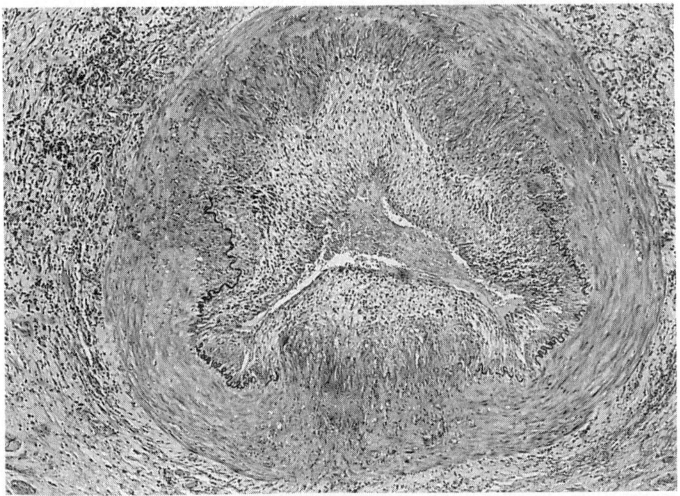

Fig. 47-19 Giant cell (temporal) arteritis involving a temporal artery. Notice the disruption of the internal elastica, the transmural inflammation, and the considerable intimal expansion with luminal narrowing. (Elastic stain.)

cytes and neutrophils and slight synovial proliferation, but no destructive pannus formation.

Clinical features. Giant cell (temporal) arteritis has a strong predilection for whites, especially those of northern European extraction, including persons of this ethnic background who live in the northern United States. The incidence rate in the population of Sweden aged 50 and older is 25/100,000 for women and 9.4/100,000 for men.[67] This is similar to the incidence in the residents of Minnesota, where many are of northern European origin, but the incidence is ten times greater than that in the residents of southern United States. Over 95% of the patients with giant cell (temporal) arteritis are 50 years old or older.

The clinical manifestations of giant cell (temporal) arteritis include nonspecific constitutional signs and symptoms of inflammatory disease, such as fever, malaise, anorexia, weight loss, night sweats, and fatigue, as well as signs and symptoms caused by arterial injury. The most common symptom is headache. Temporal artery inflammation (50% of patients) causes temporal artery tenderness, induration, nodularity, and decreased pulsation. Narrowing of extracranial arteries in the head may result in jaw claudication (50% of patients), tongue dysfunction, earache, deafness, and blindness. Disease in arteries to the extremities causes intermittent claudication of both upper and lower extremities, Raynaud's phenomenon, and decreased or absent pulses of the upper or lower extremities, or both. Involvement of the aortic arch and thoracic aorta can cause dilatation of the aortic root with regurgitation, as well as aneurysm formation with dissection or rupture.

More than 50% of patients with giant cell (temporal) arteritis have polymyalgia rheumatica. This is characterized by aching and stiffness in the neck and proximal muscles of the shoulders and hips. Polymyalgia rheumatica can occur at the same time, before or after the onset of other signs and symptoms of giant cell (temporal) arteritis.

Giant cell (temporal) arteritis usually responds well to corticosteroid therapy. Because most patients require at least a year of treatment before the disease resolves, adverse results of steroid treatment are common. Rupture of an aortic aneurysm, the most life-threatening direct effect of giant cell (temporal) arteritis, is uncommon.

Differential diagnosis. The histologic features of Takayasu arteritis and giant cell (temporal) arteritis are indistinguishable, though giant cells and elastica lamina disruption are more pronounced in the latter. The vascular distribution of the two diseases overlaps too much for this to be a useful differential feature. The only relatively reliable gross difference is the absence of aortic narrowing in patients with giant cell (temporal) arteritis and its frequency in those with Takayasu arteritis. The best discriminator between Takayasu arteritis and giant cell (temporal) arteritis, however, is patient age, because the former rarely develops after 40 years of age and the latter rarely occurs before 50 years of age.

The histologic alterations of chronic giant cell (temporal) arteritis may be difficult to distinguish from aging changes. Lie and others[67] have noted that progressive thickening of the intima of arteries occurs with age, along with fragmentation, fraying, stretching, and calcification of the internal elastic lamina. All of these changes occur in the chronic phase of giant cell (temporal) arteritis. In chronically injured vessels, careful histologic examination of multiple levels of section may be required to identify the presence of inflammation or giant cells that supports a diagnosis of giant cell (temporal) arteritis.

MEDIUM-VESSEL VASCULITIDES

Medium-vessel vasculitides are characterized by the predominant involvement of main visceral arteries, such as the coronary, hepatic, renal, and mesenteric arteries and their branches. These same vessels, however, also can be involved with large-vessel and small-vessel vasculitides (see Fig. 47-16). Therefore the differential diagnosis in a patient with inflammatory injury in a medium-sized artery is quite lengthy. Pathologic changes in vessels are useful in resolving this differential diagnosis, but as with other vasculitides, correlation of the pathologic changes with other data often is required for an accurate diagnosis to be made.

Thromboangiitis obliterans, also known as *Buerger's disease,* is an uncommon form of vascular inflammation that affects small and medium-sized arteries and veins almost exclusively in the extremities. Whether this disease is more closely related to arteriosclerotic and thrombotic diseases than to vasculitic diseases is unsettled.

Kawasaki disease

Kawasaki disease is an acute febrile illness of childhood associated with the mucocutaneous lymph node syndrome that includes arteritis involving large, medium-sized, and small arteries. Coronary arteries are often affected, and the aorta and veins may be involved. It usually occurs in children less than 5 years of age. Although Kawasaki disease was first described in the Japanese,[23] it occurs worldwide.[68]

Etiology and pathogenesis. The etiology and pathogenesis of Kawasaki disease are unknown. Infectious causes of the disease have been explored because of its tendency to sometimes occur in epidemics and to develop after upper respiratory tract infections. Two epidemic outbreaks in the United States were carefully investigated by Bell and others,[69] but no evidence of person-to-person transmission, common-source exposure, or a common etiologic agent was identified. Most cases are sporadic, however.

Because of several immunologic abnormalities reported in patients with Kawasaki disease, immune mechanisms have been implicated in its pathogenesis. These abnormalities include a decrease in the number of circulating CD8 T-lymphocytes, an increase in the number of circulating activated CD4 T-lymphocytes, an increased level of circulating cytokines, and hyperactivity of B-lymphocytes with increased immunoglobulin secretion. Leung and others[8] identified the existence of cytotoxic antibodies reactive with cultured endothelial cells that have been activated with cytokines. This led to the hypothesis that these autoantibodies cause the vascular injury of Kawasaki disease. An immune pathogenesis, however, has not been proved.

Pathology. The vasculitic lesions of Kawasaki disease predominantly involve small and medium-sized arteries, especially the coronary arteries. As a result, Kawasaki disease is the most common cause of myocardial infarction in children. Veins are involved occasionally. The histologic lesions of Kawasaki disease are characterized by segmental mural necrosis with the infiltration of neutrophils or mononuclear leukocytes (Fig. 47-20), with the latter predominating in older lesions.[68,70,71] All layers of the arteries are involved, including the intima, which may become considerably thickened, resulting in luminal narrowing. Areas of necrosis occur but typically

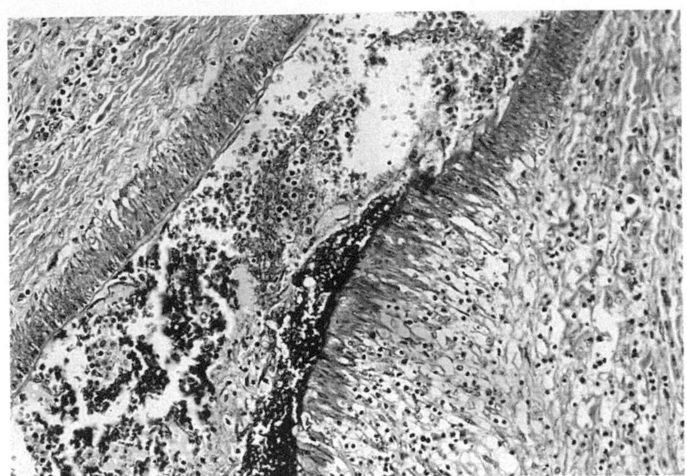

Fig. 47-20 Kawasaki disease affecting a small coronary artery. Notice the focal intimal destruction with thrombosis and fibrinoid necrosis and the subjacent medial and adventitial inflammation. (Specimen courtesy Drs. S.J. Qualman and D.D. Sedmak, Columbus, Ohio.) (Masson trichrome stain.)

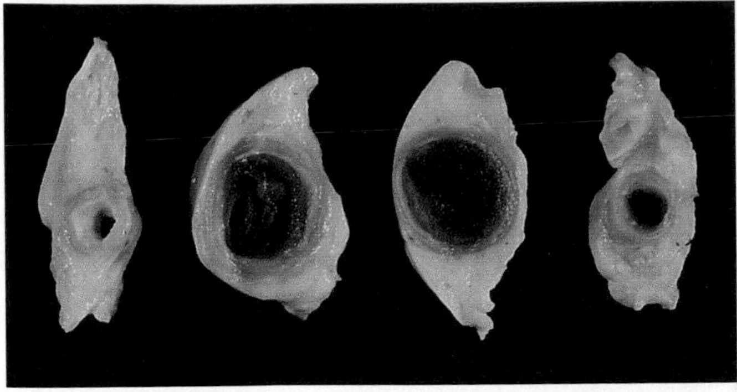

Fig. 47-21 Coronary artery aneurysm with thrombosis from a patient with Kawasaki disease who died of acute myocardial infarction.

contain more leukocytes and more leukocyte debris than do the areas of fibrinoid necrosis seen in the settings of polyarteritis nodosa and the ANCA-associated vasculitides. Aneurysms and thrombosis may develop (Fig. 47-21). Aneurysms are most common in the coronary arteries, but they also form in other arteries. For example, in patients with coronary aneurysms secondary to Kawasaki disease, Inoue and others identified aneurysms in the axillary arteries of 82%, the iliac arteries of 73%, the renal arteries of 27%, the internal mammary arteries of 14%, and the mesenteric arteries of 9%. Healing often leads to fibrotic narrowing of arteries.

In addition to arteritis, some patients with Kawasaki disease have inflammatory visceral lesions, including mononuclear leukocyte–rich infiltrates in the myocardium, endocardium, cardiac valves, and hepatic portal tracts.[68] The lymph node lesions of Kawasaki disease are variable and nonspecific and include hyperplasia of the follicles and paracortex, vascular thrombosis, focal necrosis, and focal fibrosis.

Clinical features. Most cases of Kawasaki disease are sporadic, but epidemics also occur. In the United States there is a peak incidence in the spring. The disease is more common in Asians and Polynesians than in whites and blacks. The disease is most frequent in children less than 5 years old.

The clinical manifestations of Kawasaki disease include fever, a polymorphous erythematous rash, a diffuse mucosal inflammation, nonsuppurative lymphadenopathy, indurative edema of the extremities, erythema of the palms and soles, and desquamation of the tips of the digits. This grouping of features is called the *mucocutaneous lymph node syndrome,* which is sometimes used as a synonym for Kawasaki disease. Evidence of arteritis in patients with Kawasaki disease includes the radiographic demonstration of visceral artery aneurysms or the signs and symptoms of myocardial infarction. Kawasaki disease should always be at the top of the differential diagnosis in a child with myocardial infarction.

The most life-threatening feature, especially in untreated patients, is coronary arteritis, which may result in myocardial infarction. Corticosteroid treatment is contraindicated because it may increase the risk of coronary artery aneurysm formation. Aspirin combined with intravenous gamma globulin is the preferred treatment.[73] The mortality associated with treated cases is less than 5%, and recurrence is very rare.

Differential diagnosis. Kawasaki disease must be differentiated from polyarteritis nodosa and microscopic polyangiitis (microscopic polyarteritis), both of which are rare in children. Histologically the arteritis of Kawasaki disease consists of less fibrinoid necrosis than do polyarteritis nodosa and microscopic polyangiitis. Microscopic polyangiitis often includes small-vessel disease that is not found in Kawasaki disease, such as glomerulonephritis, pulmonary alveolar capillaritis, and cutaneous leukocytoclastic angiitis. None of these diseases except Kawasaki disease presents as a mucocutaneous lymph node syndrome.

Polyarteritis nodosa

Polyarteritis nodosa manifests as necrotizing inflammation of medium-sized or small arteries. As discussed earlier, however, the term *polyarteritis nodosa* has been used quite variably over the years, with some definitions including the involvement of vessels smaller than arteries. According to the Chapel Hill nomenclature system, the name "polyarteritis nodosa" is used to refer to necrotizing vasculitis that affects arteries but not vessels smaller than arteries[18] (see Table 47-4, Fig. 47-16). The name *microscopic polyangiitis* (or alternatively *microscopic polyarteritis*) is used to refer to necrotizing vasculitis that involves vessels smaller than arteries (i.e., arterioles, venules, and capillaries), with or without small-artery and medium sized–artery involvement. According to these definitions either type of vasculitis can affect small and medium-sized arteries, but polyarteritis nodosa does not affect vessels smaller than arteries and microscopic polyangiitis always includes the involvement of vessels smaller than arteries. When defined in this way, polyarteritis nodosa is much less common than microscopic polyangiitis.

Etiology and pathogenesis. Arterial immune complex deposition has been incriminated in the pathogenesis of polyarteritis nodosa, but the evidence supporting this is limited. In addition, immune complex–mediated vasculitis predominantly involves small arteries, as well as vessels smaller than arteries, especially glomerular capillaries. Patients with extensive involvement of medium-sized arteries, that is, those with classic polyarteritis nodosa, typically do not exhibit evidence of immune complex deposition.

Infections have been proposed as the sources of the antigens in immune complexes in patients with "polyarteritis nodosa," especially hepatitis B infection in adults[74,75] and group A streptococcal infection in children.[76] However, hepatitis B–associated vasculitis often involves small vessels. This led Gocke and his collaborators, who in 1970 were the first to report the association between hepatitis B and vasculitis, to change their designation for the vasculitis in patients with hepatitis B from *polyarteritis nodosa*[74] to the more generic term *necrotizing vasculitis*.[75]

Even if infection-induced immune complex–mediated injury can cause polyarteritis nodosa in some patients, in most there is no evidence of infection or immune complexes. Therefore most cases of polyarteritis nodosa remain idiopathic.

Pathology. Polyarteritis nodosa primarily involves the main visceral arteries, such as the coronary, hepatic, renal, and mesenteric arteries, and their major branches, including intraparenchymal radicals. The segmental inflammation and necrosis in an artery wall often causes an aneurysm (actually a pseudoaneurysm) to form, and this is responsible for causing the grossly visible arterial nodules that prompted the term *nodosa* as initially proposed by Kussmaul and Maier[12] (Figs. 47-22, 47-23). Grossly identifiable tender erythematous nodules in the skin are caused by arteritis in the dermis or subcutaneous tissue. Rupture of arteritic aneurysms may result in massive hemorrhage. Thrombosis may develop at the site of arteritis, and occlusion of the artery can produce infarction, most often in the kidneys and spleen. Inflammatory narrowing or thrombotic occlusion of arteries in the gut and skin causes superficial necrosis and ulceration, which is analogous to the infarction occurring within the viscera. Gut perforation is caused by transmural intestinal infarction. Inflammation, necrosis, and thrombosis of arteries in the digits may cause distal gangrene.

The histologic lesions of polyarteritis nodosa are characterized by mural fibrinoid necrosis and accompanying inflammation. The fibrinoid character of the necrosis results from the insudation of plasma proteins into zones of mural and perivascular necrosis, leading to activation of the coagulation cascade and the deposition of fibrin. Immunohistochemical staining with antifibrin antibodies demonstrates intense staining for fibrin in acute lesions (see Fig. 47-23). Early in the course of inflammation, neutrophils and sometimes eosinophils are conspicuous, often with substantial leukocytoclasia. Mononuclear leukocytes predominate in older lesions. Ultimately the injured vascular segments undergo fibrosis.

In addition to grossly visible lesions, there may also be small-artery involvement. For example, polyarteritis nodosa can involve small arteries in the hepatic portal tracts, dermis, subcutaneous tissue, skeletal muscle, perineural connective tissues, myocardium, pancreas, spleen, and kidney (such as interlobar, arcuate, and interlobular arteries) (Fig. 47-24). The fibrinoid necrosis and inflammation in these small arteries is histologically indistinguishable from that caused by small-vessel vasculitides such as microscopic polyangiitis, Wegener's granulomatosis, and Churg-Strauss syndrome; therefore additional clinical or pathologic data are required for a definitive diagnosis to be made if small-artery necrotizing inflammation is observed in a biopsy specimen.

Clinical features. The epidemiologic and clinical features of polyarteritis nodosa are difficult to determine accurately from the literature because so many different criteria have been used to define this disease. Polyarteritis nodosa is most common in adults, but it does occur in childhood,[77] in which case it must be distinguished from Kawasaki disease. As with most systemic vasculitides, polyarteritis nodosa causes both nonspecific constitutional signs and symptoms of inflammatory disease, as well as signs and symptoms of the tissue injury resulting directly from the arteritis. Constitutional symptoms include fever, malaise, arthralgias, myalgias, and anorexia. Signs and symptoms of the tissue injury caused by the arteritis include localized muscle pain or weakness, peripheral neuropathy, bowel pain or bleeding, hypertension, tender cutaneous nodules, skin ulceration, and peripheral gangrene. Imaging studies may disclose aneurysms or occlusions of the main visceral arteries. The most life-threatening complications

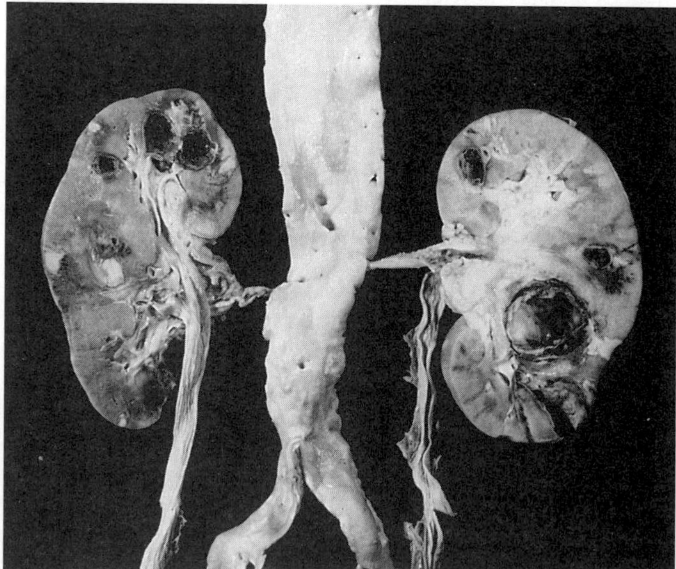

Fig. 47-22 Polyarteritis nodosa causing aneurysms of the renal lobar and arcuate arteries. Notice the cortical infarcts and the dissection tract that resulted in fatal retroperitoneal hemorrhage.

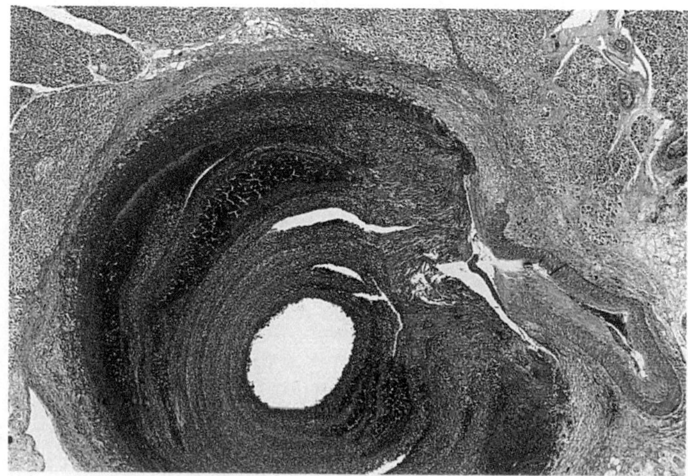

Fig. 47-23 Polyarteritis nodosa causing an aneurysm in the pancreas. Notice the uninvolved segment of artery leading up to the necrotizing lesion and the thrombosis within the aneurysm.

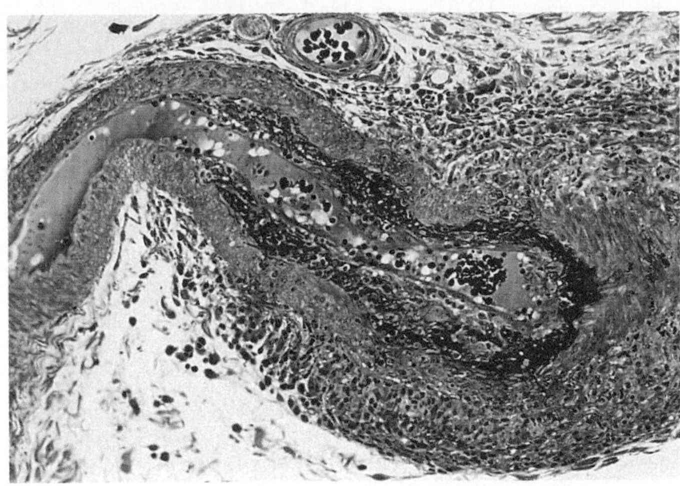

Fig. 47-24 Polyarteritis nodosa affecting a small subcutaneous artery. There is segmental injury, fibrinoid necrosis in the intima, and transmural inflammation extending into the perivascular tissue.

of polyarteritis nodosa are myocardial infarction and massive hemorrhage secondary to rupture of an aneurysm.[78]

Because different vessels can be involved in different patients, the clinical presentations of polyarteritis nodosa are extremely varied. Fever, abdominal pain, and muscle pain are the most common initial symptoms. Although most patients have multisystem disease, isolated organ polyarteritis nodosa does occur. This has been documented best in patients with so-called cutaneous polyarteritis nodosa in whom the arteritis is confined to the skin and subjacent tissue.[79] Some patients who initially appear to have disease limited to one organ may eventually manifest systemic disease, however.[77]

Treatment with high-dose corticosteroids, usually in combination with cytotoxic drugs, usually yields good results. Surgery is sometimes carried out to repair a ruptured aneurysm, remove an aneurysm before rupture, or eliminate occlusions.

Differential diagnosis. As illustrated in Fig. 47-16, the vascular distribution of polyarteritis nodosa overlaps with that seen in several vasculitides. The differential diagnosis includes other diseases that affect medium-sized and small arteries, such as Kawasaki disease, microscopic polyangiitis (microscopic polyarteritis), Wegener's granulomatosis, Churg-Strauss syndrome, Takayasu arteritis, giant cell (temporal) arteritis, Buerger's disease, fibromuscular dysplasia, and arteriosclerosis. The chronic arterial lesions found in patients with Takayasu arteritis, giant cell (temporal) arteritis, Buerger's disease, fibromuscular dysplasia, and arteriosclerosis can be difficult to distinguish from the chronic fibrotic lesions seen in patients with polyarteritis nodosa, but the distribution of involved vessels and the clinical features of the disease usually allow accurate differentiation among these diseases.

Because many vasculitides affect medium-sized arteries, angiographic demonstration of aneurysms in main visceral arteries is not very useful for making a specific diagnosis. Such aneurysms can be caused not only by polyarteritis nodosa, but also by microscopic polyangiitis, Wegener's granulomatosis, Churg-Strauss syndrome, Kawasaki disease, giant cell (temporal) arteritis, and Takayasu arteritis.

Kawasaki disease is distinguished from childhood polyarteritis nodosa by the presence of the mucocutaneous lymph node syndrome. In addition, histologically the arteritis of Kawasaki disease usually exhibits less fibrinoid necrosis.

The most problematic differential diagnosis is that between polyarteritis nodosa and microscopic polyangiitis (microscopic polyarteritis). As noted earlier, in some classifications of vasculitides these diseases are grouped together under the term "polyarteritis nodosa" and thus they are not differentiated. However, necrotizing arteritis not accompanied by vasculitis in vessels smaller than arteries appears to be pathologically, pathogenetically, and clinically different from the necrotizing arteritis that is accompanied by vasculitis affecting vessels smaller than arteries. Features of vasculitic lesions that can be used to distinguish polyarteritis nodosa from microscopic polyangiitis include the presence, only in the latter, of glomerulonephritis, pulmonary alveolar capillaritis, and post-capillary venular leukocytoclastic angiitis. In line with this approach, Heptinstall[80] has pointed out the utility of identifying arteritis in the kidney based on the presence or absence of glomerulonephritis.

ANCAs are a sensitive serologic marker for microscopic polyangiitis but are not associated with necrotizing arteritis that does not include small-vessel disease (that is, polyarteritis nodosa). Therefore necrotizing arteritis in ANCA-positive patients is usually accompanied by vasculitis in vessels smaller than arteries, whereas necrotizing arteritis in ANCA-negative patients typically is not.

Necrotizing arteritis that is histologically indistinguishable from polyarteritis nodosa occurs not only in microscopic polyangiitis, but also in the other ANCA-associated vasculitides, Wegener's granulomatosis, and Churg-Strauss syndrome. As with microscopic polyangiitis, these diseases are distinguished from polyarteritis nodosa by the finding of vasculitis in vessels smaller than arteries and ANCA in the serum. In addition, patients with Wegener's granulomatosis have necrotizing granulomatous inflammation and patients with Churg-Strauss syndrome have asthma and eosinophilia.

Thromboangiitis obliterans (Buerger's disease)

Buerger's disease, which also is called "thromboangiitis obliterans," causes inflammation and thrombosis of small and medium-sized arteries and veins in the extremities.[81,82] Although described earlier by Felix von Winiwater,[83] the disease has been named after the pathologist Leo Buerger,[84] who in 1908 described the pathologic features of the disease in detail. Whether Buerger's disease is more closely related to atherosclerosis and arteriosclerosis than to the vasculitides is not clear; however, because it causes inflammation of the small and medium-sized arteries, it is considered here.

Etiology and pathogenesis. The cause of Buerger's disease is unknown. A genetic predisposition, toxic exposure to cigarette smoke, hypercoagulability, and autoimmunity have all been proposed as participants in the pathogenesis. There is a very strong association between this disease and cigarette smoking, but this may be a synergistic factor rather than a cause. The most intriguing evidence of an autoimmune pathogenesis is the detection of cellular and humoral immune reactivity to collagen in some patients with Buerger's disease.[85] However, this may be secondary to the vascular injury rather than the primary cause of disease, and a similar reactivity may occur in patients with other types of vascular inflammation.

Pathology. The arteries in the lower extremities, such as the tibial, femoral, peroneal, and popliteal arteries, are most often involved, but arteries in the upper extremities, such as the radial and ulnar arteries, may also be affected. Veins may be involved as well. The injury is typically segmental. The characteristic histologic lesion is thrombotic occlusion, initially accompanied by prominent neutrophilic infiltration of both the thrombus and vessel wall. The thrombus may contain focal dense accumulations of neutrophils (microabscesses). As the lesions age, the infiltrates in the thrombus and vessel wall become predominantly mononuclear, occasionally containing a few multinucleated giant cells. The giant cells sometimes appear to be located at sites of earlier microabscess formation. The media then returns to normal, the intima expands, and the thrombus organizes. The fibroblastic proliferation in the intima and the thrombus may result in a continuous zone of young fibrous tissue containing proliferating blood vessels completely filling the area demarcated by the internal elastic lamina (Fig. 47-25). In a fashion analogous to the recanalization that takes place in any thrombus, this evolves through the deposition of more collagen and enlargement of the vascular channels.

Clinical features. Buerger's disease occurs predominantly in men under 40 years of age who smoke cigarettes. Approximately 80% of the patients with Buerger's disease are men, but the incidence in women is rising. The disease is most common in the residents of Asia and the Middle East, while its frequency in the United States population is decreasing.

The most common clinical manifestations are claudication, Raynaud's phenomenon, migratory superficial thrombophlebitis, and distal gangrene. In one series 54% of the patients had disease confined to the lower extremities, 38% had disease confined to the upper extremities, and 8% had disease in both upper and lower extremities.[81] In contrast to other vasculitides, which have constitutional symptoms, fever and malaise are not features of Buerger's disease. It becomes difficult clinically to distinguish Buerger's disease from the complications of atherosclerosis in patients older than 45.

Buerger's disease is not life threatening except in patients with superimposed infection and sepsis stemming from gangrenous tissue. Nevertheless, major amputation may be required in some cases. The cessation of tobacco abuse correlates with disease abatement.

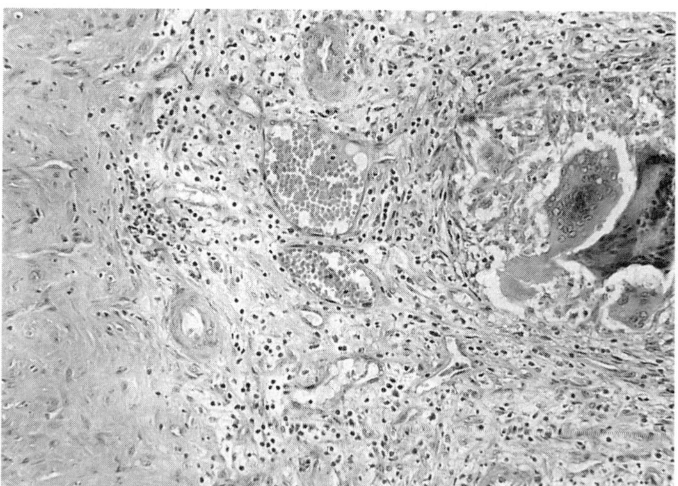

Fig. 47-25 Thromboangiitis obliterans in a medium-sized artery from the leg. The muscularis is on the left and the lumen is completely occluded by an organizing thrombus. Notice the cluster of multinucleated giant cells on the right.

Differential diagnosis. Buerger's disease must be differentiated pathologically from arteriosclerosis, atherosclerosis, and a form of arteritis that can affect medium-sized arteries. All of these diseases can cause segmental thrombosis of arteries. Histologically the most useful distinguishing features of Buerger's disease are the numerous neutrophils in the thrombi of the acute lesions and the preservation of the elastic lamina and media in the mature lesions. Unlike atherosclerosis, no calcification or lipid accumulation occurs in patients with Buerger's disease. Although there may be transmural inflammation in early lesions of Buerger's disease, this inflammation does not cause medial necrosis and fibrosis, whereas the arteritides typically cause fragmentation of the elastic lamina and focal destruction of the media. This confinement of the major injury internal to the elastic lamina is shown very nicely in the drawings that were published with von Winiwater's case report in 1879.[83]

SMALL-VESSEL VASCULITIDES

Small-vessel vasculitis can be documented by light microscopy, but for a more specific diagnosis, immunohistologic studies and serologic testing for autoimmune or infectious diseases must also be performed. It is also useful to know whether the patient has been exposed to drugs or other exogenous causes of vasculitis. The distribution of vasculitis in the organ system and the presence or absence of the components of various vasculitic syndromes also are important for establishing the final diagnosis.

Henoch-Schönlein purpura

Henoch-Schönlein purpura is a vasculitis characterized by IgA-dominant immune deposits in small vessels (that is, capillaries, venules, or arterioles). It typically involves the skin, gut, and glomeruli and is associated with arthralgias or arthritis.[86-89] "Schönlein-Henoch purpura" and "anaphylactoid purpura" are synonyms for this disease.

Henoch-Schönlein purpura was one of the first small-vessel vasculitides recognized clinically. Schönlein[30] described part of the syndrome in 1837 and Henoch[31] described the complete syndrome in 1874. The disease was first defined on the basis of the clinical manifestations alone. Because numerous pathogenetically different small-vessel vasculitides produce similar signs and symptoms, Henoch-Schönlein purpura has been redefined and limited to vascular lesions that have IgA-dominant immune deposits.[18] In patients with purpura, nephritis, arthralgias, and abdominal pain who fulfill the clinical criteria for Henoch-Schönlein purpura, immunopathologic analysis can identify numerous distinctive vasculitides, such as vasculitis with IgA-dominant immune complex deposits (that is, Henoch-Schönlein purpura), vasculitis with IgG and IgM immune complex deposits (such as cryoglobulinemic vasculitis), and vasculitis with no deposits but with ANCA in the serum (such as microscopic polyangiitis).

Etiology and pathogenesis. Henoch-Schönlein purpura is often preceded by an infectious disease, especially an upper respiratory tract infection. The infection, however, appears to be more of a synergistic factor than a precipitant of the expression of underlying immunopathogenic events, possibly by upregulating mucosal IgA antibody production and leukocyte reactivity. The presence of vascular deposits of immune complexes composed predominantly of IgA and C3, along with varying amounts of IgG and IgM, indicates that the inflammation is induced by these immune complexes. Because IgA does not activate complement by the classic pathway, the alternative activation pathway may be most important in recruiting inflammatory cells. IgA in the immune complexes appears to be derived predominantly from the lymphoid tissue in the respiratory tract and gut mucosa in response to some antigen. Hypothetical antigens include microbes and ingested materials, including food.

Pathology. The typical acute histologic lesion of Henoch-Schönlein purpura is a leukocytoclastic angiitis affecting postcapillary venules, capillaries, and arterioles. This is characterized by a focal necrosis of the vessel walls as well as necrosis of infiltrating neutrophils, which results in the accumulation of conspicuous leukocytoclastic debris at the sites of injury (Fig. 47-26). Perivascular hemorrhage, fibrinoid material, and luminal thrombosis may be present. This histologic lesion is observed most often in the dermis and intestinal wall. IgA-dominant immune complexes can be demonstrated by immunohistologic studies performed on both injured as well as uninjured vessels (Fig. 47-27).

The lesion in the kidney is a proliferative glomerulonephritis that is identical to IgA nephropathy. Immunohistologically there is a mesangial accumulation of IgA-dominant immune complex deposits. In the most severe lesions, immune complex deposits also involve the glomerular capillary loops. The immune complex deposits appear as electron-dense deposits on electron microscopy studies.

Focal proliferative glomerulonephritis is the most common glomerular lesion. Some patients with hematuria have well-defined IgA-dominant mesangial immune deposits revealed by immunohistologic studies but no glomerular abnormalities are shown by light microscopy. Severe diffuse proliferative glomerulonephritis and crescentic glomerulonephritis occur in a few patients, and their presence indicates an unfavorable prognosis.

Clinical features. The incidence of Henoch-Schönlein purpura peaks around 5 years of age and is the most common type of vasculitis in children. It occurs in adults but much less often. Onset is most common in the winter and spring and often follows an upper respiratory tract infection. There is a slight male predominance.

Clinical signs and symptoms include fever, arthralgias, nonthrombocytopenic purpura, colicky abdominal pain, blood in the stool, hematuria, and proteinuria. The purpura has a predilection for the extensor surfaces of the lower legs, buttocks, and forearms.

Because of the good prognosis for spontaneous recovery, supportive management is usually adequate. A persistent or recurrent course or the development of progressive renal failure is an indication for the need for treatment with corticosteroids or cytotoxic drugs.

Differential diagnosis. The differential diagnosis of Henoch-Schönlein purpura includes microscopic polyangiitis (microscopic polyarteritis), cryoglobulinemic vasculitis, Wegener's granulomatosis, drug-induced vasculitis, paraneoplastic vasculitis, rheumatoid vasculitis, and infectious vasculitis, especially *Neisseria*-induced vasculitis.

On the basis of light microscopy findings alone, the leukocytoclastic angiitis of Henoch-Schönlein purpura cannot be differentiated from that of cryoglobulinemic vasculitis, microscopic polyangiitis, Wegener's granulomatosis, Churg-Strauss syndrome, and the cutaneous leukocytoclastic angiitis associated with drug hypersensitivity, neoplasms, and collagen-vascular diseases. Therefore, when dermal leukocytoclastic angiitis is identified on the basis of skin biopsy specimen findings, additional clinical, serologic, or immunohistologic data should be obtained to determine what type of vasculitis is most likely present.

If a clinical definition of Henoch-Schönlein purpura is used to establish the diagnosis, which does not require the demonstration of IgA-dominant vascular deposits, some patients, including children, who in fact have ANCA-associated microscopic polyangiitis or Wegener's granulomatosis may be missed.[90,91] It is very important to make this distinction because of the greatly different treatments for the two disorders. If tissue is not available for immunohistologic analysis, the results of serologic analysis for ANCA can help resolve this differential problem.[92]

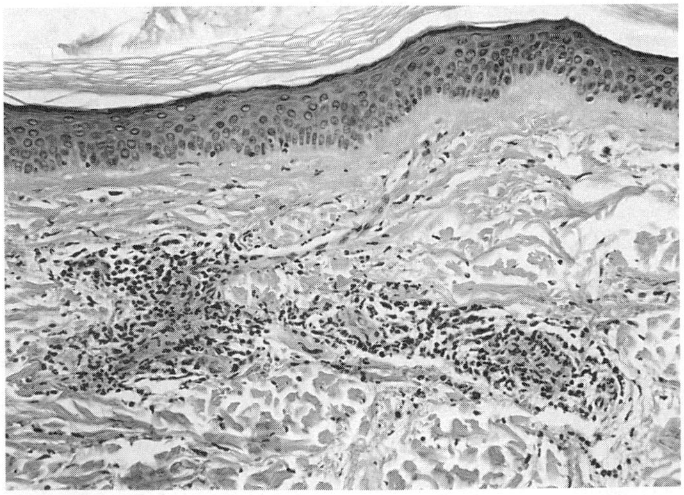

Fig. 47-26 Henoch-Schönlein purpura causing dermal leukocytoclastic angiitis.

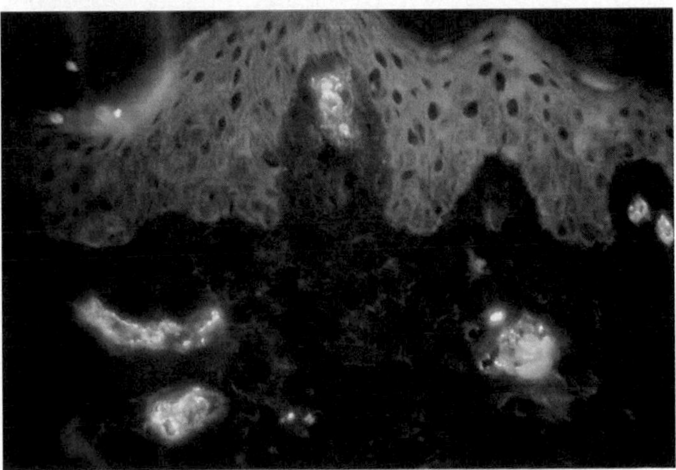

Fig. 47-27 IgA-dominant immune deposits in dermal vessels from a patient with Henoch-Schönlein purpura. (Fluorescein isothiocyanate–anti-IgA.)

The characteristics of Henoch-Schönlein purpura cannot be differentiated from those of IgA nephropathy in renal biopsy specimens, except in the extremely rare instance when extraglomerular vasculitis is observed in a specimen from a patient with Henoch-Schönlein purpura. Therefore, when glomerulonephritis with IgA-dominant immune complexes is identified in a renal biopsy specimen, additional data about the nature of small-vessel vasculitis in other tissues are required to determine whether the patient has Henoch-Schönlein purpura.

Cryoglobulinemic vasculitis

Cryoglobulinemic vasculitis is characterized by cryoglobulinemia and deposits of cryoglobulins in small vessels (that is, capillaries, venules, or arterioles).[93-95] Skin and glomeruli are often involved.

Cryoglobulins are serum immunoglobulins that precipitate at 4° C and redissolve at 37° C. There are three major types of cryoglobulins: type I is monoclonal, type II is mixed monoclonal-polyclonal, and type III is polyclonal. Monoclonal cryoglobulins usually occur in patients with plasma cell dyscrasias or B-cell lymphomas and cause morbidity primarily by precipitating within vessels and producing occlusion. Type I monoclonal cryoglobulins are not effective activators of inflammatory mediator systems and therefore rarely cause overt vasculitis. Type II cryoglobulins usually contain monoclonal IgM kappa antibodies with an antiimmunoglobulin specificity (that is, rheumatoid factor activity) that are bound to polyclonal IgG. Occasionally the monoclonal antiimmunoglobulin component is IgG or IgA. Type III cryoglobulins contain only polyclonal immunoglobulins. Types II and III cryoglobulins, also called *mixed cryoglobulins*, are immune complexes that are capable of activating inflammatory mediators, including the complement system, and thus characteristically cause systemic small-vessel vasculitis. Approximately half of the patients with cryoglobulins have type III, a fourth have type II, and a fourth have type I cryoglobulins.

Etiology and pathogenesis. The precise basis for the immune dysregulation and clonal B-cell proliferation that results in the production of autoantibodies with antiimmunoglobulin specificity is not known, but many conditions have been identified that appear to incite this process. Pathologic levels of cryoglobulins can be detected in blood of patients with lymphoproliferative diseases (such as Waldenström's macroglobulinemia, multiple myeloma, chronic lymphocytic leukemia, and lymphocytic lymphomas), infections (such as hepatitis C, hepatitis B, and infectious mononucleosis), and collagen-vascular diseases (such as systemic lupus erythematosus, rheumatoid arthritis, and Sjögren's syndrome). Hepatitis C infection may be a particularly important cause of mixed cryoglobulinemia.[96,97] Mixed cryoglobulinemia occurring in the absence of any identifiable inciting disease is called "essential cryoglobulinemia."

Cryoglobulin immune complexes deposited in vessel walls cause the activation of complement and other inflammatory mediator systems. This results in an influx of neutrophils and vessel wall necrosis in postcapillary venules and arterioles.

Pathology. Mixed cryoglobulinemic vasculitis affects arterioles, postcapillary venules, and capillaries. The postcapillary venules in the dermis are the most often involved. Glomerular lesions arise less often. Alveolar capillaritis is uncommon, and small arteries are rarely affected.

Involved vessels exhibit segmental necrosis and neutrophilic infiltration with leukocytoclasia. This leukocytoclastic angiitis is histologically similar to that seen in other small-vessel vasculitides, such as Henoch-Schönlein purpura, microscopic polyangiitis and Wegener's granulomatosis. The most specific histologic finding is the presence of "hyaline thrombi," which are aggregates of cryoglobulins within vessel lumens.

Direct immunofluorescence microscopy can demonstrate the existence of granular deposits of immunoglobulins and complement in vessel walls and sometimes luminal aggregates of cryoglobulins and complement. In contrast to true thrombi, these hyaline thrombi do not contain fibrin.

The glomerular lesions usually possess the features of type I membranoproliferative glomerulonephritis and are caused by the deposition of immune complexes (that is, cryoglobulins) in glomerular capillary walls and mesangium. Hyaline thrombi may be found in capillary lumens. Other patterns of glomerulonephritis may occur, such as focal or diffuse proliferative glomerulonephritis. On electron microscopy preparations, the immune complex dense deposits are often seen to contain arrays of microtubular (immunotactoid) structures. Similar ultrastructural dense deposits appear in other vessels involved by cryoglobulinemic vasculitis, such as dermal postcapillary venules.

Clinical features. The incidence of cryoglobulinemic vasculitis peaks in the fifth and sixth decades of life and is more common in women than in men. Clinical manifestations include purpura, Raynaud's phenomenon, arthralgias, hematuria and proteinuria, muscle pain and weakness, and peripheral neuropathy. The most typical finding is purpura affecting the lower extremities, which may evolve into skin ulcers.

Cryoglobulinemias are usually associated with a high titer of rheumatoid factor and low serum levels of CH50, C1q, and C4 levels. The C3 level is less often and less severely depressed, and the terminal complement components are normal or elevated in quantity. Serologic testing should be performed to identify the causes of secondary cryoglobulinemia, such as hepatitis C, hepatitis B, and systemic lupus erythematosus.

The prognosis is best if vasculitis is confined to the skin. Ominous findings are severe glomerulonephritis and pulmonary hemorrhage, though the latter is rare. High-dose corticosteroids, cytotoxic drugs, plasmapheresis and alpha-interferon have been used for treatment, with variable results. Some patients recover spontaneously.

Differential diagnosis. The differential diagnosis of cryoglobulinemic vasculitis includes Henoch-Schönlein purpura, hypocomplementemic urticarial vasculitis, microscopic polyangiitis, Wegener's granulomatosis, drug-induced vasculitis, paraneoplastic vasculitis, rheumatoid vasculitis, and infectious vasculitis. As with the other small-vessel vasculitides, the final diagnosis cannot be made on the basis of light microscopy findings alone but requires serologic studies to confirm the existence of cryoglobulins. Immunohistologic data are useful but not diagnostic because other forms of small-vessel vasculitis may have immunoglobulin and complement deposits in vessel walls.

Many persons have detectable low levels of circulating cryoglobulins that are not causing disease. Therefore the detection of very small amounts of cryoglobulins (<100 mg/L; cryocrit, <5%) in a patient with small-vessel vasculitis does not prove that they are the cause of the vasculitis. In addition, cryoglobulins must be distinguished from other cryoproteins, such as cryofibrinogen and C-reactive protein-albumin complexes.

Microscopic polyangiitis (microscopic polyarteritis)

Microscopic polyangiitis (microscopic polyarteritis) is a necrotizing vasculitis in which few or no immune deposits affect small vessels (that is, capillaries, venules, or arterioles). Necrotizing glomerulonephritis and pulmonary capillaritis are common. Necrotizing arteritis involving small and medium-sized arteries is present in some but not all patients. Because not all patients with this disease have arteritis, the term *microscopic polyangiitis* is more appropriate than *microscopic polyarteritis*.[18] Microscopic polyangiitis shares many clinical, pathologic, serologic, and probably pathogenetic features with Wegener's granulomatosis and Churg-Strauss syndrome.[98]

As discussed earlier, some classification systems categorize microscopic polyangiitis with polyarteritis nodosa, but there is substantial evidence indicating that necrotizing vasculitis confined to small and medium-sized arteries (that is, polyarteritis nodosa as defined by the Chapel Hill nomenclature system) is a clinically and pathogenetically different disease from necrotizing vasculitis that has a predilection for vessels smaller than arteries and only occasionally affects medium-sized arteries (that is, microscopic polyangiitis as defined by the Chapel Hill nomenclature system).[18,17,80,98]

Etiology and pathogenesis. The definition of microscopic polyangiitis adopted by the Chapel Hill conference requires that there be few or no immune deposits in vessel walls. This criterion is necessary for distinguishing microscopic polyangiitis from histologically similar immune complex–mediated small-vessel vasculitides, such as Henoch-Schönlein purpura, cryoglobulinemic vasculitis, and serum sickness vasculitis. Most patients with microscopic polyangiitis have ANCAs.[98]

ANCAs are autoantibodies that are specific for constituents of neutrophil granules and monocyte lysosomes. The two most common specificities in patients with vasculitis are those for PR3 and myeloperoxidase (MPO). ANCAs are usually detected by either indirect immunofluorescence microscopy or enzyme-linked immunosorbent assay. When detected using alcohol-fixed normal human neutrophils as the substrate for indirect immunofluorescence microscopy, ANCAs exhibit two staining patterns: cytoplasmic staining and perinuclear staining (Fig. 47-28). Autoantibodies that cause cytoplasmic staining (C-ANCA) are usually specific for PR3, and those that cause perinuclear staining (P-ANCA) are usually specific for MPO. The perinuclear ANCA staining of alcohol-fixed neutrophils results from the diffusion and binding of a cytoplasmic antigen, such as MPO, to the nucleus during substrate preparation. More than 80% of the patients with microscopic polyangiitis have either P-ANCA (MPO-ANCA) or C-ANCA (PR3-ANCA).

There is mounting evidence that ANCAs are able to activate neutrophils and monocytes in the circulation.[9] The target antigens of ANCA, such as PR3 and MPO, are in the cytoplasm of quiescent neutrophils and monocytes. To be accessible for interaction with ANCAs, the antigens must be expressed at the surface of the cells. This happens when neutrophils and monocytes are exposed to certain cytokines, such as interleukin-1 and tumor necrosis factor-alpha, and to microbial products, such as lipopolysaccharide and formyl tripeptides. In one hypothesis proposed to explain ANCA-mediated vasculitis, a synergistic event, such as a respiratory tract infection, is thought to prime the neutrophils and monocytes to express ANCA target antigens at the cell surface. Circulating ANCAs then interact with the antigens and activate the leukocytes, causing them to adhere to and penetrate vessel walls. The activated leukocytes also release toxic oxygen metabolites and lytic granule enzymes, which cause vascular necrosis. These pathogenetic events have been documented in vitro but not in vivo.[9] Circumstantial support for this hypothesis comes from the epidemiologic observation that the signs and symptoms of microscopic polyangiitis, as well as of the other ANCA-associated vasculitides, often begin shortly after a flu-like illness, which could be the event that precipitates increased cytokine release and leukocyte priming.

Pathology. Microscopic polyangiitis affects predominantly arterioles, capillaries, and venules (see Fig. 47-16).[26,98] Small arteries are occasionally affected and medium-sized arteries

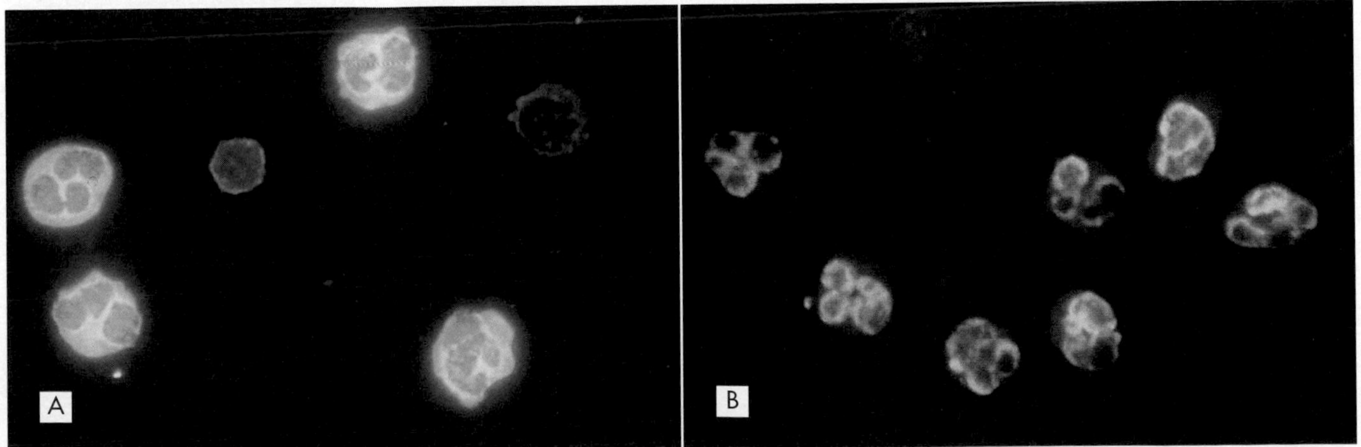

Fig. 47-28 Indirect immunofluorescence microscopy detection of antineutrophil cytoplasmic autoantibodies (ANCAs) using alcohol-fixed normal human neutrophils as the substrate. **A,** Cytoplasmic staining pattern caused by ANCA specific for proteinase-3 (C-ANCA). **B,** Perinuclear staining caused by ANCA specific for myeloperoxidase (P-ANCA).

are affected least often. Many patients, however, suffer no arterial involvement, which is the reason the name *microscopic polyangiitis* is preferable to *microscopic polyarteritis* for this disease.

Histologically the acute vascular lesions, no matter where they are, are characterized by segmental fibrinoid necrosis[98] (Fig. 47-29). Mural and perivascular neutrophilic infiltration with leukocytoclasia is prominent in acute lesions (Fig. 47-30). Eosinophils may be conspicuous, and when they are, Churg-Strauss syndrome should be ruled out clinically. Thrombosis may occur. Older lesions contain mononuclear leukocytes and undergo fibrosis.

Necrotizing glomerulonephritis and necrotizing alveolar capillaritis are common in patients with microscopic polyangiitis. The glomerulonephritis is characterized by focal, segmental, glomerular fibrinoid necrosis associated with crescent formation. Arterioles and arteries in the cortex and vasa recta in the medulla may be affected by segmental necrotizing inflammation. The acute alveolar capillaritis is characterized by septal neutrophilic infiltration and leukocytoclasia (Fig. 47-31), by focal necrosis with the dissolution of septal basement membranes (seen well with silver staining), and by hemorrhage into air spaces, which is manifested clinically as hemoptysis. In the chronic phase of capillaritis there is septal fibrosis with the appearance of hemosiderin-laden macrophages.

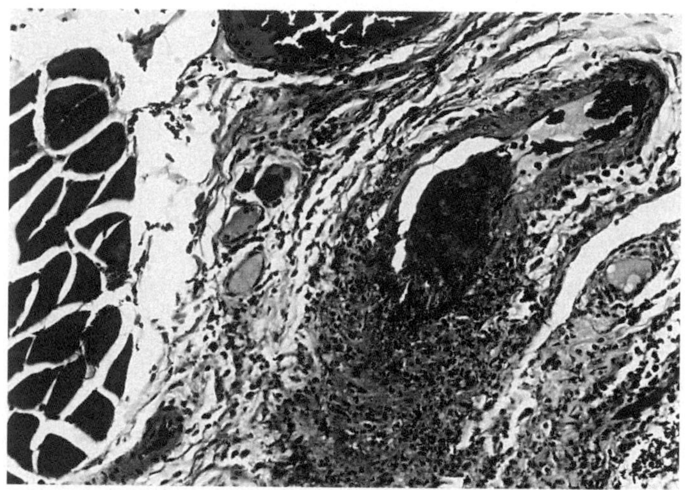

Fig. 47-29 Microscopic polyangiitis affecting a small artery in a skeletal muscle biopsy specimen. Notice the segmental fibrinoid necrosis, the mural and perivascular inflammation with leukocytoclasia, and the thrombosis.

By definition immunohistologic studies demonstrate an absence or paucity of immunoglobulin deposition. This distinguishes the vascular inflammation of microscopic polyangiitis from immune complex and anti–glomerular basement membrane antibody–mediated disease. There is a nonspecific entrapment of immunoglobulins and complement at the sites of necrosis and sclerosis, which should not be confused with immune complex deposition. Immunohistologic analysis shows the foci of fibrinoid necrosis to contain fibrin.

Electron microscopic examination of vessels does not reveal typical immune complex–type electron-dense deposits. The earliest ultrastructural changes are endothelial injury and the subendothelial accumulation of fibrin.[99]

Clinical features. Although microscopic polyangiitis can occur at any age, it has a predilection for older patients, with the mean age at onset in the 6th decade of life.[17,100] There is no sex-related predisposition. The disease is more common in whites than blacks, and initial onset of the disease is most common in the winter and spring.[100]

In approximately 90% of patients, signs and symptoms of vascular inflammation begin after what is usually described as a flu-like illness. Common clinical manifestations include fever, arthralgias, myalgias, weakness, peripheral neuropathy, purpura, hematuria and proteinuria, pulmonary infiltrates, hemoptysis, sinusitis, abdominal pain, and gastrointestinal hemorrhage. The clinical presentations are extremely varied because of differences in the organ systems involved among different patients. Some patients present with vascular inflammation apparently confined to one organ, but eventually manifestations of multisystem disease develop.

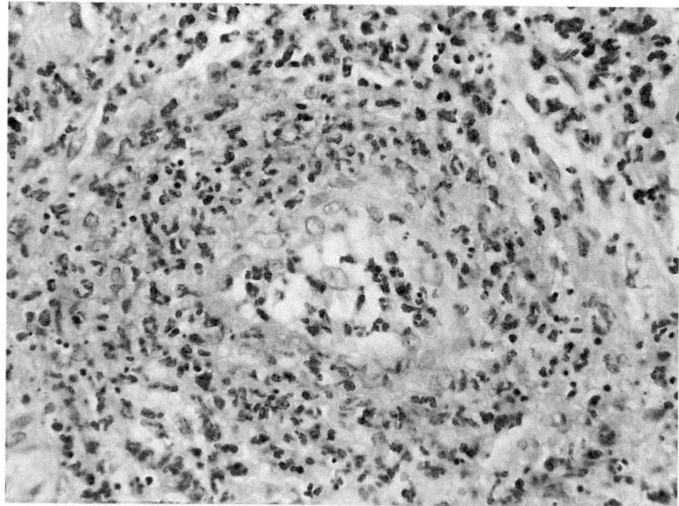

Fig. 47-30 Microscopic polyangiitis affecting a postcapillary venule in the dermis. There is intense neutrophilic infiltration and leukocytoclasia. (From Jennette JC: *Am J Kidney Dis* 18:164, 1991.)

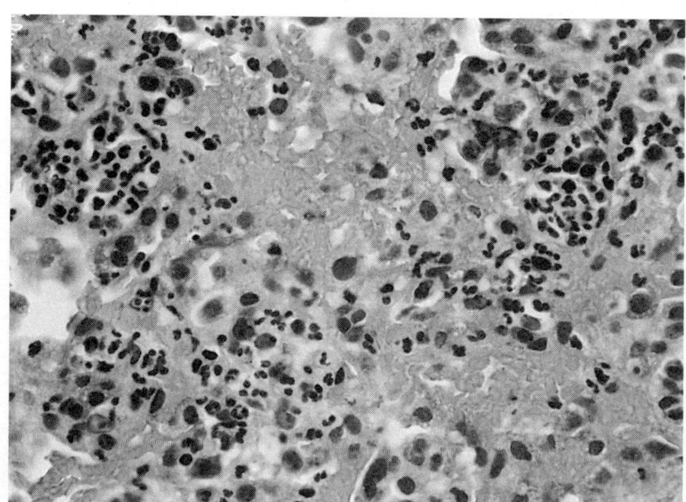

Fig. 47-31 Microscopic polyangiitis causing a pulmonary alveolar capillaritis. Notice the intense neutrophilic infiltration, the leukocytoclasia, and the massive hemorrhage.

Unless appropriately treated, microscopic polyangiitis can cause irreversible injury to critical organs, such as the lungs or kidneys. Treatment is with high-dose corticosteroids such as intravenous methylprednisolone and cytotoxic drugs such as cyclophosphamide.[100]

Differential diagnosis. The differential diagnosis of microscopic polyangiitis includes Henoch-Schönlein purpura, cryoglobulinemic vasculitis, Wegener's granulomatosis, Churg-Strauss syndrome, polyarteritis nodosa, systemic lupus erythematosus, Goodpasture's syndrome, drug-induced vasculitis, paraneoplastic vasculitis, rheumatoid vasculitis, and infectious vasculitis.

The histologic and clinical features of microscopic polyangiitis are similar to those of many other types of small-vessel vasculitis. In certain respects, therefore, microscopic polyangiitis must be diagnosed not only by recognizing its characteristic pathologic features, but also by ruling out the other diseases in the differential diagnosis. For example, a patient with systemic disease whose biopsy results indicate leukocytoclastic angiitis in the skin, liver, and kidney should be diagnosed as having microscopic polyangiitis only after other types of small-vessel vasculitis are excluded, such as Wegener's granulomatosis, Churg-Strauss syndrome, Henoch-Schönlein purpura, cryoglobulinemic vasculitis, lupus vasculitis, rheumatoid vasculitis, and serum sickness vasculitis.

Patients with microscopic polyangiitis may present with the pulmonary-renal vasculitic syndrome. There are other causes of the pulmonary-renal vasculitic syndrome, however, such as Goodpasture's syndrome, Wegener's granulomatosis, and Henoch Schönlein purpura. Serologic and immunohistologic studies can be useful in differentiating between these diseases (Fig. 47-32).

As discussed earlier, most patients with microscopic polyangiitis have ANCA: either P-ANCA (MPO-ANCA) or C-ANCA (PR3-ANCA). This is a useful serologic marker for distinguishing microscopic polyangiitis from the small-vessel vasculitides that are not associated with ANCA (see Table 47-3), but does not differentiate it from Wegener's granulomatosis or Churg-Strauss syndrome. Those patients who have P-ANCA, however, are unlikely to have Wegener's granulomatosis because more than 90% of those with Wegener's granulomatosis have C-ANCA and less than 5% have P-ANCA (see Fig. 47-32).

Wegener's granulomatosis

Wegener's granulomatosis is characterized by granulomatous inflammation, often involving the upper or lower respiratory tract, and frequently accompanied by necrotizing vasculitis affecting small to medium-sized vessels, such as capillaries, venules, arterioles, and arteries. Necrotizing glomerulonephritis is common. Limited variants that do not exhibit all of these features occur as well, including granulomatous inflammation with no vasculitis.

Although early reports of this disease were published by Klinger[24] and Wegener,[25] the definitive description of Wegener's granulomatosis was published by Godman and Churg in 1954.[26] They recognized the classic triad of features: (1) systemic necrotizing vasculitis, (2) necrotizing granulomatous inflammation of the upper or lower respiratory tract, or both, and (3) necrotizing glomerulonephritis. Subsequently it was realized that some patients manifest the characteristic necrotizing granulomatous inflammation of Wegener's granulomatosis without the full triad.[101,102] Such patients are often said to have "limited" Wegener's granulomatosis.

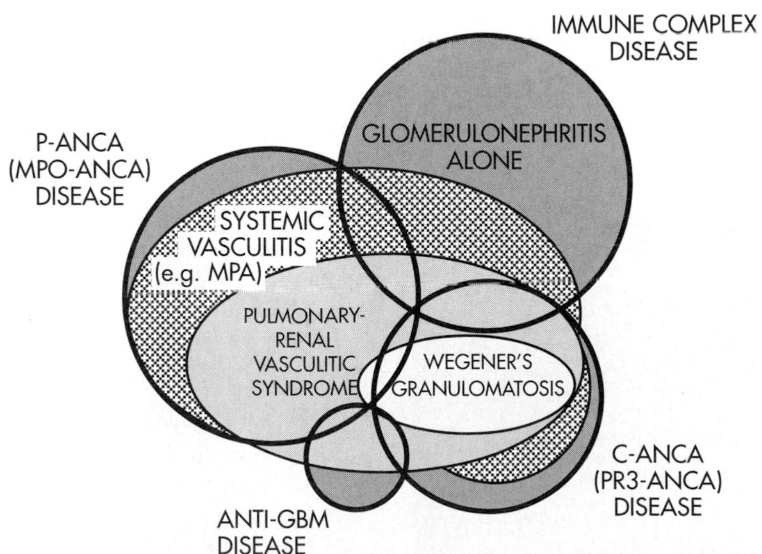

Fig. 47-32 The immunopathologic categories of small-vessel vasculitis are depicted as *circles,* with the relative size of each circle representing the frequency of each category among patients with severe (crescentic) glomerulonephritis. The *ovals* represent different clinicopathologic manifestations of vasculitis. Some clinicopathologic manifestations can be caused by more than one immunopathologic category of injury; for example, pulmonary-renal vasculitic syndrome can be caused by anti-glomerular basement membrane antibodies, antineutrophil cytoplasmic autoantibodies (ANCA) specific for proteinase-3 (such as Wegener's granulomatosis), ANCA specific for myeloperoxidase (such as microscopic polyangiitis), or immune complexes (such as cryoglobulinemia). Also notice that a minority of patients have overlapping immunopathologic findings, such as ANCA and anti–glomerular basement membrane antibodies. (From Jennette JC: *Am J Kidney Dis* 18:164, 1991.)

Etiology and pathogenesis. Theories about the etiology and pathogenesis of Wegener's granulomatosis have centered on immunologic mechanisms.[103] An immune complex pathogenesis received considerable support, until it was shown that there is very little immunohistologic evidence of vascular immune deposits in patients with the disease.[104] Because of the conspicuous numbers of activated lymphocytes and mononuclear phagocytes in the fully developed lesions of Wegener's granulomatosis, a T-lymphocyte–mediated immune injury also has been considered. There is no strong evidence, however, that lymphocytes and macrophages have a primary pathogenetic role, and it is believed that ANCAs are much more likely to be the pathogenic culprits. This is based on the very high frequency of ANCAs in patients with Wegener's granulomatosis, the correlation of ANCA titers with disease activity, and the evidence that ANCAs can activate leukocytes in vitro.[9]

Pathology. Necrotizing granulomatous inflammation is the constant feature of Wegener's granulomatosis and is observed most often in the upper and lower respiratory tracts, but occasionally in other tissues, such as the orbit, skin, and kidneys. A few patients have the typical granulomatous inflammation without evidence of vasculitis. The lesions are not as compact as the granulomas of sarcoidosis, but rather consist of loosely arranged mononuclear and polymorphonuclear leukocytes with scattered multinucleated giant cells (Fig. 47-33). In small lesions there is often an irregular central zone of necrosis and neutrophils surrounded by the mixed inflammatory infiltrate. Large lesions contain extensive areas of liquefactive necrosis, which typically exhibit an irregular geographic pattern at low magnification and contain large amounts of nuclear dust and basophilic debris from disrupted nuclei of parenchymal cells and leukocytes. In the lungs the tissue debris from large necrotic zones may be expectorated through the airways, resulting in cavity formation. The granulomatous inflammation may be vasocentric or bronchocentric. When small airways are involved, the injury evolves into a bronchiolitis fibrosa obliterans pattern. In the lungs, besides granulomatous vasculitis, nongranulomatous necrotizing vasculitis and alveolar capillaritis that are identical to those seen in the setting of microscopic polyangiitis may occur.

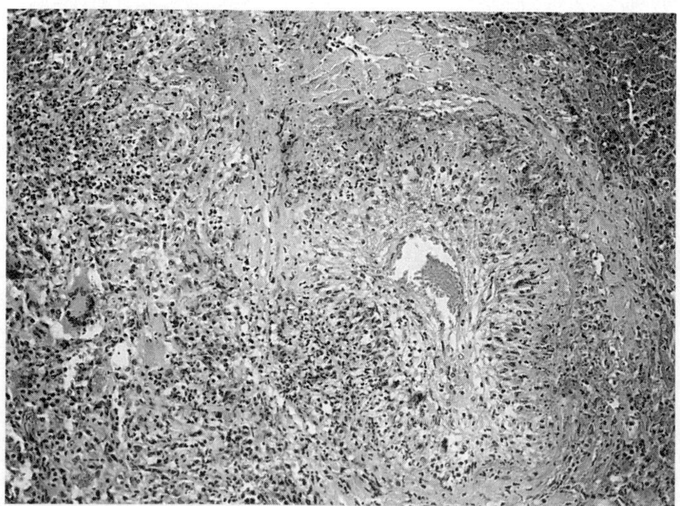

Fig. 47-33 Wegener's granulomatosis in lung tissue. Necrotizing granulomatous inflammation with scattered multinucleated giant cells affect the parenchyma, *left,* and a small pulmonary artery, *right.*

The vasculitis in the lungs and elsewhere can involve arteries, arterioles, veins, venules, and capillaries (see Fig. 47-16) and can be granulomatous or nongranulomatous. The latter is histologically identical to other types of necrotizing vasculitis, such as microscopic polyangiitis (microscopic polyarteritis). The glomerulonephritis of Wegener's granulomatosis is a pauciimmune necrotizing and crescentic glomerulonephritis that is pathologically indistinguishable from the glomerulonephritis of microscopic polyangiitis. Even the multinucleated giant cells involved in the glomerular and periglomerular inflammation are not a totally specific feature of Wegener's granulomatosis.

The chronic phases are characterized by nonspecific chronic inflammation and fibrosis. Acute and chronic lesions can occur simultaneously.

Clinical features. Wegener's granulomatosis occurs most often in the fifth decade of life[102,103,105] but can occur at any age, including childhood.[90,91] As is true of many systemic vasculitides, patients with Wegener's granulomatosis often exhibit the constitutional manifestation of inflammatory disease, such as fever, malaise, anorexia, weight loss, arthralgias, and myalgias. More direct manifestations of the inflammatory tissue injury include rhinitis, sinusitis, and epistaxis; shortness of breath; hemoptysis and nodules, infiltrates, or cavities (shown by chest radiographs); hematuria, proteinuria, and renal insufficiency; purpura and skin nodules; mononeuritis multiplex; otitis; keratoconjunctivitis and orbital pseudotumor; and subglottic stenosis. Because of the varied expression of Wegener's granulomatosis, the ELK (upper respiratory tract, lungs, kidneys) staging system, or some variation of it, is often used to stage disease.[102]

More than 90% of the patients with active, untreated, systemic Wegener's granulomatosis who have histologically documented granulomatous inflammation have C-ANCA (PR3-ANCA); less than 5% have P-ANCA; and less than 5% have no ANCA. Of the patients whose Wegener's granulomatosis is diagnosed on clinical grounds alone, as on the basis of the presence of sinusitis, pulmonary infiltrates, purpura, and a rapidly progressive glomerulonephritis, without histological documentation of the granulomatous inflammation, a higher proportion will prove to have P-ANCA (MPO-ANCA). Most of these patients in fact have microscopic polyangiitis rather than Wegener's granulomatosis. The frequency of ANCAs in patients with limited disease and treated disease is lower, and the ANCA titer is also lower.

Although some patients, especially those with disease limited to the upper respiratory tract, have indolent disease, the mortality is high in many patients with the classic triad of Wegener's granulomatosis who are not treated aggressively with immunosuppressive agents. The usual treatment is with high-dose corticosteroids in combination with cytotoxic drugs. Recurrences are common after initial control of the disease and require additional treatment.

Differential diagnosis. Wegener's granulomatosis must be distinguished from Churg-Strauss syndrome, microscopic polyangiitis, lymphomatoid granulomatosis, necrotizing sarcoid granulomatosis, and infection.

Infections, especially fungal and mycobacterial ones, can cause a granulomatous inflammation similar to that caused by Wegener's granulomatosis. Infections can also occur secondarily in patients with Wegener's granulomatosis, especially those treated with immunosuppressive drugs. Special staining and cultures for pathogens are prudent measures if there is any suspicion of infection.

Wegener's granulomatosis has many pathologic features in common with microscopic polyangiitis and Churg-Strauss syndrome. It is distinguished from the former by the presence of granulomatous inflammation and from the latter by the absence of eosinophilia and of asthma.

The diagnosis in patients with Wegener's granulomatosis affecting sites other than the lungs or sinuses, for example, those presenting with orbital pseudotumor or subglottic stenosis, may not be as apparent clinically, and histologic and serologic data are then very important for reaching the correct diagnosis.

Churg-Strauss syndrome

Churg-Strauss syndrome is characterized by an eosinophil-rich and granulomatous inflammation involving the respiratory tract and a necrotizing vasculitis affecting small to medium-sized vessels that is associated with asthma and blood eosinophilia.[106-108]

The disease was initially considered a distinctive form of polyarteritis nodosa that affected patients with asthma.[27,28] The clinical and pathologic features were definitively described by Churg and Strass in 1951.[29] The most widely used synonym for Churg-Strauss syndrome is "allergic granulomatosis and angiitis."

Etiology and pathogenesis. The etiology of Churg-Strauss syndrome is unknown. ANCAs are found in the blood and are believed to play a role in the pathogenesis. Asthma and other forms of atopy may influence the phenotype of ANCA-induced injury, thus giving Churg-Strauss syndrome pathologic features not observed in Wegener's granulomatosis or microscopic polyangiitis.

Pathology. The vasculitis of Churg-Strauss syndrome is histologically very similar to that of Wegener's granulomatosis and microscopic polyangiitis; however, there is a tendency for there to be more eosinophils among the infiltrating leukocytes (Fig. 47-34). The vasculitis of Churg-Strauss syndrome can affect many organ systems, with the lungs, heart, peripheral nervous system, skin, gut, and kidneys the most frequent targets. A pauciimmune focal necrotizing glomerulonephritis may occur, but this is usually less severe than the glomerulonephritis occurring in Wegener's granulomatosis or microscopic polyangiitis. The necrotizing granulomatous inflammation of Churg-Strauss syndrome resembles that of Wegener's granulomatosis, but once again there tend to be more eosinophils (Fig. 47-35). In early lesions the central focus of necrosis sometimes contains degenerating eosinophils or cellular debris containing eosinophil granules and Charcot-Leyden crystals.

The asthma and blood eosinophilia predate the signs and symptoms of vasculitis and tissue inflammation. Eosinophil-rich pulmonary inflammation (such as eosinophilic pneumonia) and gastrointestinal inflammation (such as eosinophilic enteritis) may appear before evidence of actual vasculitis. A diagnosis of Churg-Strauss syndrome cannot be made at this time.

Clinical features. The clinical features of Churg-Strauss syndrome include asthma, eosinophilia (>10% of cases), peripheral neuropathy, pulmonary infiltrates, sinusitis, rhinitis, hematuria and proteinuria, and bowel pain and bleeding. Allergic rhinitis and asthma are the first features to appear. These may precede the vasculitis by decades and may resolve when the vasculitis develops. An eosinophilic inflammation of tissues, especially of the lungs and gut, can also precede the vasculitis. The vasculitic phase of Churg-Strauss syndrome usually begins in the fourth or fifth decade of life and produces signs and symptoms similar to those caused be microscopic polyangiitis and Wegener's granulomatosis. Cutaneous involvement is common during the vasculitic phase, with approximately half of the patients having purpura caused by dermal leukocytoclastic angiitis, and a third having nodules caused by granulomatous inflammation and arteritis.

ANCAs, usually P-ANCAs, are present in patients in the vasculitic phase of Churg-Strauss syndrome, but these disappear with treatment. Peripheral blood eosinophilia is an important diagnostic feature. Most patients also have elevated serum IgE levels.

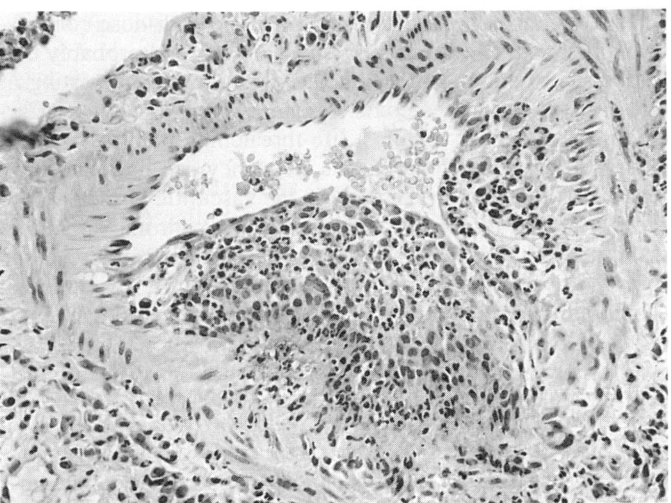

Fig. 47-34 Churg-Strauss syndrome causing necrotizing inflammation in a pulmonary artery. There are numerous eosinophils in the vascular and perivascular inflammation.

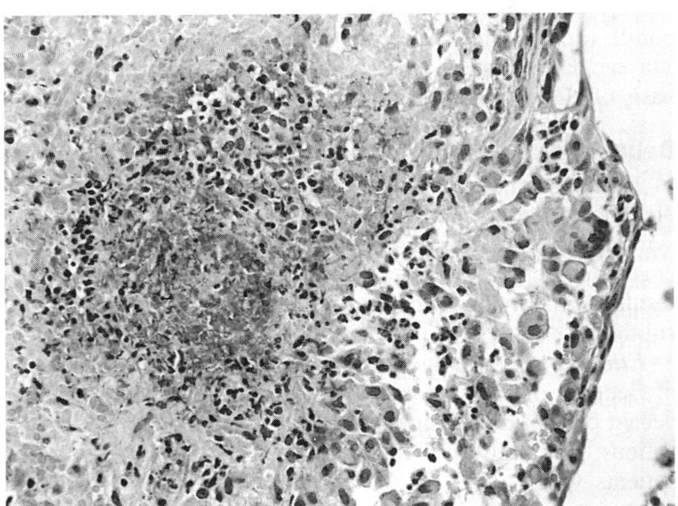

Fig. 47-35 Churg-Strauss syndrome causing necrotizing granulomatous pulmonary inflammation. Notice the central focus of necrotic debris.

The *vasa vasorum* become severely stenotic secondary to an endarteritic inflammatory and fibrotic process. Small mural gummas occasionally form and spirochetes are rarely identified in patients with syphilitic aortitis.

Bacterial vasculitis

Bacterial infection causes vasculitis by means of several processes: the invasion of vessels adjacent to and within localized sites of infection, the hematogenous spread of infected emboli, and the systemic infection of small vessels secondary to bacteremia.

The bacteremia caused by *Neisseria meningitidis* and *Neisseria gonorrhoeae* causes small-vessel vasculitis that is manifested as purpura.[129,130] The acute dermal lesion is a leukocytoclastic angiitis. *Neisseria* organisms can be seen in the endothelial cells and neutrophils and in Gram-stained smears of blood from the acute lesions.[129]

Patients with functional or anatomic asplenia can suffer bacteremic small-vessel vasculitis with purpura. This is usually secondary to *Streptococcus pneumoniae* infection.[129] Staphylococcal bacteremia, such as that caused by endocarditis and infected shunts, can also cause leukocytoclastic angiitis with purpura.[131]

Direct invasion of vessels occasionally occurs at sites of necrotizing inflammation, especially in *Pseudomonas* or *Klebsiella pneumoniae* infection.

Embolization of infected thrombotic material can result in the formation of "mycotic aneurysms" in any type of vessel. The aorta and medium-sized and small arteries, including the cerebral arteries, are the vessels most commonly affected.

Rickettsial vasculitis

The skin rash of typhus and Rocky Mountain spotted fever results from vascular invasion by the *Rickettsia* organisms. *Rickettsia* organisms have a predilection for the endothelial cells of capillaries, postcapillary venules, arterioles, and to a lesser extent small arteries. Smooth muscle cells may also be invaded. Some vascular injury results from direct vascular cytotoxicity and some from the mononuclear leukocyte inflammatory response to the infection.

The earliest vascular lesion is endothelial swelling, followed by endothelial necrosis, infiltration by mononuclear leukocytes, hemorrhage, and sometimes thrombosis (Fig. 47-38). In patients with Rocky Mountain spotted fever, *Rickettsia* organisms can be demonstrated in vessel walls by direct immunofluorescence microscopy[132] (Fig. 47-39).

Mycobacterial vasculitis

Although tuberculous aortitis and arteritis have been recognized for centuries, they are uncommon in the United States today. Tuberculous phlebitis is somewhat more common. It is not clear whether vascular involvement arises as the result of direct extension from adjacent tuberculomas or by means of hematogenous or lymphatic spread.

Histologically, involved vessels are affected by a granulomatous inflammation that resembles the appearance of tuberculous lesions elsewhere, although the amount of caseous

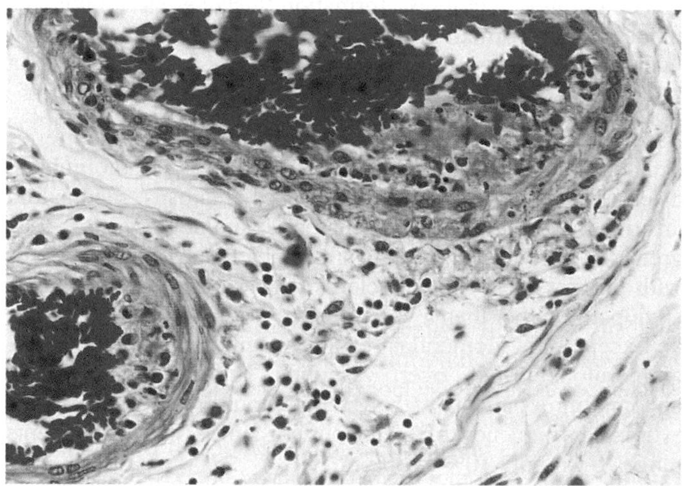

Fig. 47-38 Small artery in the peritesticular tissue of a patient with Rocky Mountain spotted fever. Notice the segmental inflammation, necrosis, and thrombosis.

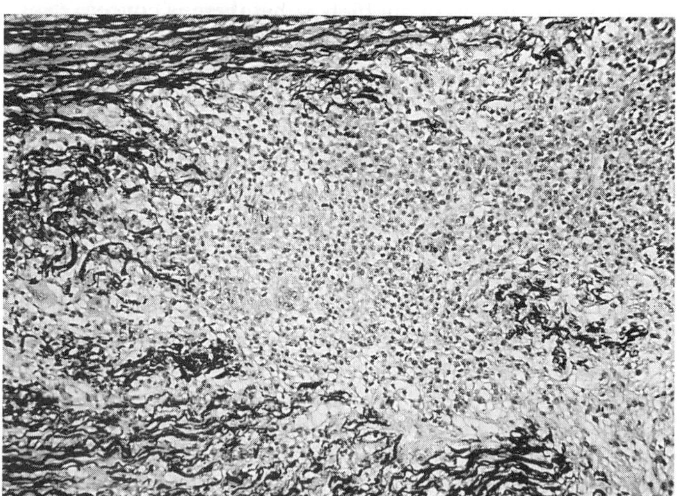

Fig. 47-37 Syphilitic aortitis with focal disruption of the medial elastic tissue by inflammation with a predominance of mononuclear leukocytes. (Elastic tissue stain.)

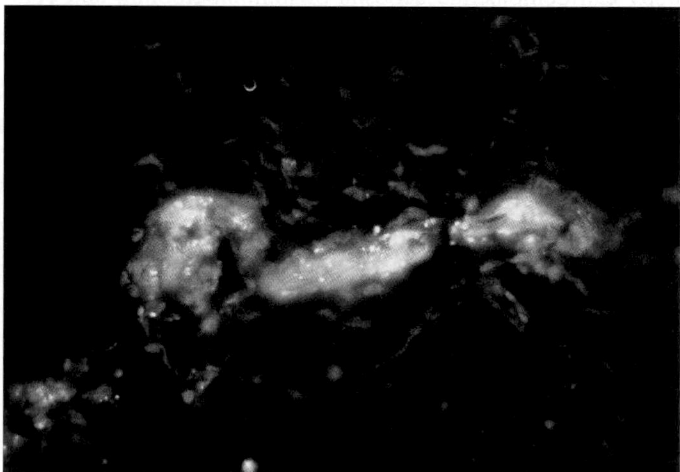

Fig. 47-39 Direct immunofluorescence microscopy study of a skin biopsy specimen from a patient with Rocky Mountain spotted fever demonstrating *Rickettsia* organisms in a small dermal vessel. (Fluorescein isothiocyanate–conjugated anti–*Rickettsia rickettsii*.)

necrosis generally is less. Mycobacteria can usually be detected within the inflamed vessel walls.

Mycobacterium tuberculosis can also cause acute and chronic vasculitis of central nervous system vessels by direct invasion associated with tuberculous meningitis.[133,134] Arteries at the base of the brain are the most susceptible vessels.

Fungal vasculitis

Fungal vasculitis can be caused by a variety of fungi, including *Aspergillus, Mucor, Candida, Cryptococcus, Nocardia, Actinomyces,* and *Coccidioides.*[134] It usually occurs in immunocompromized hosts. Fungal vasculitis is caused by direct extension of infection from the surrounding tissue.

Rhinocerebral mucormycosis, which usually occurs in poorly controlled diabetics, is a distinctive syndrome that is characterized clinically by ptosis, exophthalmos, ophthalmoplegia, headaches, and a black nasal discharge. A major pathologic feature of the disease is direct invasion of blood vessels by hyphae.[134]

Viral vasculitis

Vascular inflammation resulting from direct vessel wall invasion by viruses is uncommon. As discussed earlier, viral infections, especially hepatitis B and C infection, can cause vasculitis by participating in immune complex formation.[74,75,96,97] In addition, viral diseases can predispose a patient to the development of vasculitis that apparently does not involve viral proliferation in vessel walls. This is best documented in the setting of human immunodeficiency virus infection, which is associated with the development of polyarteritis nodosa, microscopic polyangiitis, and central nervous system angiitis.[135]

The best-known example of a vasculitis caused by direct invasion of the vessel walls by a virus is the arteritis that occurs with *herpes zoster ophthalmicus.*[134,136] In this disease, herpes zoster infection of the trigeminal nerve, including the ophthalmic branch, is followed in a few weeks by arteritis in the ipsilateral internal carotid and middle cerebral arteries, which results in cerebral ischemia and contralateral hemiplegia. There is evidence that the arteritis is caused by direct invasion of the artery walls by the virus, followed by a cell-mediated immune response. In support of this, virus particles have been demonstrated in smooth muscle cells from involved arteries in patients with herpes zoster ophthalmicus.[136] Viral infection may also cause granulomatous angiitis of the central nervous system, even when there is no clinically recognized viral infection.[137]

Granulomatous small-vessel vasculitis has been found in the involved dermatome after a cutaneous *herpes zoster* infection. Although the virus could not be identified in the tissue by polymerase chain reaction, the inflammatory response could be secondary to an immune response to the presence of residual viral proteins.[138]

REFERENCES

Etiology and pathogenesis

1. Rich AR: The role of hypersensitivity in periarteritis nodosa. As indicated by seven cases developing during serum sickness and sulfonamide therapy, *Bull Johns Hopkins Hosp* 71:123, 1942.
2. Rich AR, Gregory JE: The experimental demonstration that periarteritis nodosa is a manifestation of hypersensitivity. *Bull Johns Hopkins Hosp* 72:65, 1943.
3. Dixon FJ, Vázquez JJ, Weigle WO et al: Pathogenesis of serum sickness, *Arch Pathol* 65:18, 1958.
4. Cochrane CG, Koffler D: Immune complex disease in experimental animals and man, *Adv Immunol* 16:185, 1973.
5. Jennette JC, Charles LA, Falk RJ: The neutrophil and its role in systemic vasculitis. In LeRoy EC, editor: *The biologic basis of systemic vasculitis,* New York, 1992, Marcel Dekker.
6. Cotran RS, Pober JS: Cytokine-endothelial interactions in inflammation, immunity, and vascular injury, *J Am Soc Nephrol* 1:225, 1990.
7. Lerner RA, Glassock RJ, Dixon FJ: The role of anti-glomerular basement membrane antibody in the pathogenesis of human glomerulonephritis, *J Exp Med* 126:989, 1967.
8. Leung DYM, Collins T, Lapierre LA et al: Immunoglobulin M antibodies present in the acute phase of Kawasaki syndrome lyse cultured vascular endothelial cells stimulated by gamma interferon, *J Clin Invest* 77:1428, 1986.
9. Jennette JC, Falk RJ: Pathogenic potential of anti-neutrophil cytoplasmic autoantibodies, *Lab Invest* 70:135, 1994.

Nomenclature

10. Rokitansky K: Üeber einige der wichtigsten Krankheiten der Arterien, *Denkschrift Kais Akad der Wissensch* 4:49, 1852.
11. Eppinger H: Pathogenesis (Histogenesis und Aetiologie) der Aneurysmen einschliesslich des Aneurysma equi verminosum: pathologisch-anatomische Studien, *Arch Klin Chir* 35(suppl):1:563, 1887.
12. Kussmaul A, Maier R: Über eine bisher nicht beschreibene eigenthümliche Arterienerkrankung (Periarteriitis nodosa), die mit Morbus Brightii und rapid fortschreitender allgemeiner Muskellähmung einhergeht, *Dtsch Arch Klin Med* 1:484, 1866.
13. Ferrari E: Über Polyarteriitis acuta nodosa (sogenannte Periarteriitis nodosa) und ihre Beziehungen zur Polymyositis und Polyneuritis acuta, *Beitr Pathol Anat* 34:350, 1903.
14. Dickson WEC: Polyarteritis acuta nodosa and periarteritis nodosa. *J Pathol Bact* 12:31, 1908.
15. Arkin A: A clinical and pathological study of periarteritis nodosa: a report of five cases, one histologically healed, *Am J Pathol* 6:401, 1930.
16. Davson J, Ball J, Platt R: The kidney in periarteritis nodosa, *Q J Med* 17:175, 1948.
17. Savage COS, Winearls CG, Evans DJ et al: Microscopic polyarteritis: presentation, pathology and prognosis, *Q J Med* 56:467, 1985.
18. Jennette JC, Falk RJ, Andrassy K et al: Nomenclature of systemic vasculitides: the proposal of an international consensus conference, *Arthritis Rheum* 37:187, 1994.
19. Hutchinson J: Diseases of the arteries: on a peculiar form of thrombotic arteries of the aged which is sometimes productive of gangrene, *Arch Surg* [Lond] 1:323, 1890.
20. Horton BT, Magath TB, Brown GE: An undescribed form of arteritis of the temporal vessels, *Mayo Clin Proc* 7:700, 1932.
21. Savory WS: Case of a young woman in whom the main arteries of both upper extremities and of the left side of the neck were throughout completely obliterated, *Med Chir Trans Lond* 39:205, 1856.
22. Takayasu M: Case with unusual changes of the central vessels in the retina, *Acta Soc Ophthalmol Jpn* 12:554, 1908.
23. Kawasaki T, Kosaki F, Okawa S et al: A new infantile febrile mucocutaneous lymph node syndrome (MLNS) prevailing in Japan, *Pediatrics* 54:271, 1974.
24. Klinger H: Grenzformen der Periarteriitis nodosa, *Frankf Z Pathol* 42:455, 1931.
25. Wegener F: Über eine eigenartige rhinogene Granulomatose mit besonderer Beteiligung des Arteriensystems unter der Nieren, *Beitr Pathol Anat* 102:36, 1939.
26. Godman GC, Churg J: Wegener's granulomatosis: pathology and review of the literature, *Arch Pathol* 58:533, 1954.
27. Rackemann FM, Greene CC: Periarteritis nodosa and asthma, *Trans Assoc Am Physicians* 54:112, 1939.
28. Wilson KS, Alexander HL: The relation of periarteritis nodosa to bronchial asthma and other forms of human hypersensitiveness, *J Lab Clin Med* 30:195, 1945.
29. Churg J, Strauss L: Allergic granulomatosis, allergic angiitis, and periarteritis nodosa, *Am J Pathol* 27:277, 1951.

30. Schönlein JL: *Allegemeine und specielle Pathologie und Therapie*, ed 3, vol 2, Herisau, Germany, 1837, Literatur-Comptoir.
31. Henoch EH: Über eine eigenthümliche Form von Purpura, *Berl Klin Wochenschr* 11:641, 1874.
32. Zeek PM: Periarteritis nodosa: a critical review, *Am J Clin Pathol* 22:777, 1952.
33. Fauci AS, Haynes BF, Katz P: The spectrum of vasculitis. Clinical, pathologic, immunologic, and therapeutic considerations, *Ann Intern Med* 89:660, 1978.
34. McCluskey RT, Fienber R: Vasculitis in primary vasculitides, granulomatoses, and connective tissue diseases, *Hum Pathol* 14:305, 1983.
35. Lie JT: Systemic and isolated vasculitis: a rational approach to classification and pathologic diagnosis, *Pathol Annu* 24(Part 1):25, 1989.
36. Churg J, Churg A: Idiopathic and secondary vasculitis: a review, *Mod Pathol* 2:144, 1989.
37. Waldherr R, Eberlein-Gonska M, Noronha IL: Histopathological differentiation of systemic necrotizing vasculitides, *APMIS* 19(suppl):17, 1990.
38. Hunder GG, Arend WP, Bloch DA et al: The American College of Rheumatology 1990 criteria for the classification of vasculitis, *Arthritis Rheum* 33:1065, 1990.
39. Lie JT: Vasculitis, 1815 to 1991: classification and diagnostic specificity, *J Rheumatol* 24:25, 1992.

Large-vessel vasculitides

40. Arend WP, Michel BA, Bloch DA et al: The American College of Rheumatology 1990 criteria for the classification of Takayasu arteritis, *Arthritis Rheum* 33:1134, 1990.
41. Lie JT: Takayasu arteritis. In Churg A, Churg J, editors: *Systemic vasculitides,* New York and Tokyo, 1991, Igaku-Shoin.
42. Churg J: Large vessel vasculitis, *Clin Exp Immunol* 93(suppl 1):11, 1993.
43. Gilmour JR: Giant-cell chronic arteritis, *J Pathol* 53:263, 1941.
44. Paulley JW: Anarthritic rheumatoid diseases, *Lancet* 2:946, 1956.
45. Alestig K, Barr J: Giant-cell arteritis: a biopsy study of polymyalgia rheumatica including one case of Takayasu's disease, *Lancet* 1:1228, 1963.
46. Hamrin B, Jonsson N, Landberg T: Arteritis in polymyalgia rheumatica, *Lancet* 1:397, 1964.
47. Richardson JE, Gladman DD, Fam A et al: HLA-DR4 in giant cell arteritis: an association with polymyalgia rheumatica syndrome, *Arthritis Rheum* 30:1293, 1987.
48. Andersson R: Immunological studies in giant cell arteritis, *Baillière's Clin Rheumatol* 5:405, 1991.
49. Wilkinson IM, Russell RW: Arteries of the head and neck in giant cell arteritis—a pathological study to show the pattern of involvement, *Arch Neurol* 27:378, 1972.
50. Papaionnou CC, Hunder GG, McDuffie FC: Cellular immunity in polymyalgia rheumatica and giant cell arteritis: lack of response to muscle or artery homogenates, *Arthritis Rheum* 22:740, 1979.
51. Hamilton CR, Shelley WM, Tumulty PA: Giant cell arteritis: including temporal arteritis and polymyalgia rheumatica, *Medicine* 50:1, 1971.
52. Jacobs MR, Allen NB: Giant cell arteritis. In Churg A, Churg J, editors: *Systemic vasculitides,* New York and Tokyo, 1991, Igaku-Shoin.
53. Hunder GG, Bloch DA, Michel BA et al: The American College of Rheumatology 1990 criteria for the classification of giant cell arteritis, *Arthritis Rheum* 33:1122, 1990.
54. Lhote F, Mainguene C, Griselle-Wiseler V et al: Giant cell arteritis of the female genital tract with temporal arteritis, *Ann Rheum Dis* 51:900, 1992.
55. McKendry RJR, Guindi M, Hill DP: Giant cell arteritis (temporal arteritis) affecting the breast: report of two cases and review of published reports, *Ann Rheum Dis* 49:1001, 1990.
56. Hamrin B: Polymyalgia rheumatica, *Acta Med Scand Suppl* 533:1, 1972.
57. How J, Bewsher PD, Walker W: Giant-cell arteritis and hypothyroidism, *Br Med J* 2:99, 1977.
58. Dickson ER, Maldonado JE, Sheps SG et al: Systemic giant-cell arteritis with polymyalgia rheumatica: reversible abnormalities of liver function, *JAMA* 224:1496, 1973.
59. Srigley JR, Gardiner GW: Giant cell arteritis with small bowel infarction: a case report and review of the literature, *Am J Gastroenterol* 73:157, 1980.
60. Papaionnou CC, Hunder GG, Lie JT: Vasculitis of the gallbladder in a 70-year-old with giant cell (temporal) arteritis, *J Rheumatol* 6:71, 1979.
61. Elling H, Kirstensen IB: Fatal renal failure in polymyalgia rheumatica caused by disseminated giant cell arteritis, *Scand J Rheumatol* 9:206, 1980.
62. Enos WF, Pierre RV, Rosenblatt JE: Giant cell arteritis detected by bone marrow biopsy, *Mayo Clin Proc* 56:381, 1981.
63. Engelke WD, Dorstmann D: Highly located transverse lesion of the cord with quadriplegia caused by giant cell arteritis, *Fortschr Neurol Psychiatr* 47:91, 1979.
64. Merianos P, Smyrnis P, Tsomy K: Giant cell arteritis of the median nerve simulating carpal tunnel syndrome, *J Hand Surg* [Br] 15:249, 1983.
65. Allison MC, Gallagher PJ: Temporal artery biopsy and corticosteroid treatment, *Ann Rheum Dis* 43:416, 1984.
66. Chou CT, Schumacher HR: Clinical and pathologic studies of synovitis in polymyalgia rheumatica, *Arthritis Rheum* 27:1107, 1984.
67. Lie JT, Brown AL, Carter ET: Spectrum of aging changes in temporal arteries. Its significance in interpretation of biopsy of temporal artery, *Arch Pathol* 90:278, 1970.

Medium-sized–vessel vasculitides

68. Gribetz D, Landing BH, Larson EJ: Kawasaki disease: mucocutaneous lymph node syndrome (MCLNS). In Churg A, Churg J, editors: *Systemic vasculitides,* New York and Tokyo, 1991, Igaku-Shoin.
69. Bell DM, Brink EW, Nitzkin JL et al: Kawasaki syndrome: description of two outbreaks in the United States, *N Engl J Med* 304:1568, 1981.
70. Hirose S, Hamashima Y: Morphological observations on the vasculitis in the mucocutaneous lymph node syndrome, *Eur J Pediatr* 129:17, 1978.
71. Fujiwara H, Hamashima Y: Pathology of the heart in Kawasaki disease, *Pediatrics* 61:100, 1978.
72. Inoue O, Akagi T, Ichinose E et al: Systemic artery involvement in Kawasaki disease. In *Proc 3rd Int Kawasaki Disease Symp,* Tokyo, 1988.
73. Newburger JW, Takahashi M, Burns JC et al: The treatment of Kawasaki syndrome with intravenous gamma globulin, *N Engl J Med* 315:789, 1987.
74. Gocke DJ, Hsu K, Morgan C et al: Association between polyarteritis and Australia antigen, *Lancet* 2:1149, 1970.
75. Sergent JS, Lockshin MD, Christian CL et al: Vasculitis with hepatitis B antigenemia: long-term observations in nine patients, *Medicine* 55:1, 1976.
76. Fink CW: The role of *Streptococcus* in poststreptococcal reactive arthritis and childhood polyarteritis nodosa, *J Rheum* 18(suppl 29):14, 1991.
77. Magilvay DB, Petty RE, Cassidy JT et al: A syndrome of childhood polyarteritis, *J Pediatr* 91:25, 1977.
78. Smith DL: Spontaneous rupture of a renal artery aneurysm in polyarteritis nodosa: critical review of the literature and report of a case, *Am J Med* 87:464, 1989.
79. Moreland LW, Ball CV: Cutaneous polyarteritis nodosa, *Am J Med* 88:426, 1990.
80. Heptinstall RH: Polyarteritis (periarteritis) nodosa, Wegener's syndrome, and other forms of vasculitis. In Heptinstall RH, editor: *Pathology of the kidney,* vol 2, Boston, 1992, Little, Brown & Co.
81. Mills JL, Taylor LM, Porter JM et al: Buerger's disease in the modern era, *Am J Surg* 154:123, 1987.
82. Joyce JW: Buerger's disease (thromboangiitis obliterans), *Rheum Dis Clin North Am* 16:463, 1990.
83. von Winiwater F: Ueber eine eigenthümliche Form von Endarteritis und Endophlebitis mit Gangrän des Fusses, *Arch Klin Chir* 23:202, 1879.
84. Buerger L: Thromboangiitis obliterans: a study of the vascular lesions leading to presenile spontaneous gangrene, *Am J Med Sci* 136:567, 1908.
85. Adar R, Papa MZ, Halpern Z et al: Cellular sensitivity to collagen in thromboangiitis obliterans, *N Engl J Med* 308:1113, 1983.

Small-vessel vasculitides

86. Cream JJ, Gumpel JM, Peachey RDG: Schönlein-Henoch purpura in adults: a study of 77 adults with anaphylactoid or Schönlein-Henoch purpura, *Q J Med* 39:461, 1970.

87. Hurley RM, Drummond KN: Anaphylactoid purpura nephritis: clinicopathologic correlations, *J Pediatr* 81:904, 1972.
88. Heng MC: Henoch-Schönlein purpura, *Br J Dermatol* 112:235, 1985.
89. Roth DA, Wilz DR, Theil GB: Schönlein-Henoch syndrome in adults, *Q J Med* 55:145, 1985.
90. Hall SL, Miller LC, Duggan E et al: Wegener's granulomatosis in pediatric patients, *J Pediatr* 106:739, 1985.
91. Katsanis E, McLaine PN, Hellerstein S: Wegener's granulomatosis, *J Pediatr* 108:792, 1986.
92. Jennette JC, Tuttle R, Falk RJ: The clinical, serologic and immunohistologic heterogeneity of cutaneous leukocytoclastic angiitis, *Adv Exp Med Biol* 536:323, 1993.
93. Brouet JC, Clauvel JP, Danon T et al: Biological and clinical significance of cryoglobulins: a report of 86 cases, *Am J Med* 57:775, 1974.
94. Gorevic PD, Kassab HJ, Levo Y et al: Mixed cryoglobulinemia: clinical aspects and long-term follow-up of 40 patients, *Am J Med* 69:287, 1980.
95. Churg J: Cryoglobulinemic vasculitis. In Churg A, Churg J, editors: *Systemic vasculitides,* New York and Tokyo, 1991, Igaku-Shoin.
96. Agnello V, Chung RT, Kaplan LM: A role for hepatitis C virus infection in type II cryoglobulinemia, *N Engl J Med* 327:1490, 1992.
97. Marcellin P, Descamps V, Martinot-Peignoux M et al: Cryoglobulinemia with vasculitis associated with hepatitis C virus infection, *Gastroenterology* 104:272, 1993.
98. Jennette JC: Anti-neutrophil cytoplasmic autoantibody–associated disease: a pathologist's perspective, *Am J Kidney Dis* 18:164, 1991.
99. D'Agati V, Chander P, Nash M et al: Idiopathic microscopic polyarteritis nodosa: ultrastructural observations on the renal vascular and glomerular lesions, *Am J Kidney Dis* 7:95, 1986.
100. Falk RJ, Hogan S, Carey TS et al: The clinical course of patients with antineutrophil cytoplasmic autoantibody associated glomerulonephritis and systemic vasculitis, *Ann Intern Med* 1990, 113:656.
101. Carrington CB, Liebow AA: Limited forms of angiitis and granulomatosis of Wegener's type, *Am J Med* 41:497, 1966.
102. Deremee RA, McDonald TJ, Harrison EG et al: Wegener's granulomatosis: anatomic correlates, a proposed classification, *Mayo Clin Proc* 51:777, 1976.
103. Lieberman K, Churg A: Wegener's granulomatosis. In Churg A, Churg J, editors: *Systemic vasculitides,* New York and Tokyo, 1991, Igaku-Shoin.
104. Ronco P, Verroust P, Mifnon F et al: Immunopathological studies of polyarteritis nodosa and Wegener's granulomatosis: a report of 43 patients with 51 renal biopsies, *Q J Med* 52:212, 1983.
105. Leavitt RY, Fauci AS, Bloch DA et al: The American College of Rheumatology 1990 criteria for the clarification of Wegener's granulomatosis, *Arthritis Rheum* 33:1101, 1990.
106. Lanham JG, Elkon KB, Pusey CD et al: Systemic vasculitis with asthma and eosinophilia: a clinical approach to the Churg-Strauss syndrome, *Medicine* 63:65, 1984.
107. Lanham JG, Churg J: Churg-Strauss syndrome. In Churg A, Churg J, editors: *Systemic vasculitides,* New York and Tokyo, 1991, Igaku-Shoin.
108. Masi AT, Hunder GG, Lie JT et al: The American College of Rheumatology 1990 criteria for the classification of Churg-Strauss syndrome, *Arthritis Rheum* 33:1094, 1990.
109. Behçet H: Über rezidivierende Aphthöse, durch ein Virus verursachte Geschwüre am Mund, am Auge und an den Genitalien, *Dermatol Wochenschr* 105:1152, 1937.
110. O'Duffy JD: Vasculitis in Behçet's disease, *Rheum Dis Clin North Am* 16:423, 1990.
111. Arbesfeld SJ, Kurban AK: Behçet's disease, New perspectives on an enigmatic syndrome, *J Am Dermatol* 19:767, 1988.
112. Jorizzo JL, Solomon AR, Cavallo T: Behçet's syndrome: immunopathologic and histopathologic assessment of pathergy lesions is useful in diagnosis and follow-up, *Arch Pathol Lab Med* 109:747, 1985.
113. James DG, Thomson A: Recognition of the diverse cardiovascular manifestations of Behçet's disease, *Arch Intern Med* 145:1047, 1985.
114. Zax RH, Hodge SJ, Callen JP: Cutaneous leukocytoclastic vasculitis: serial histopathologic evaluation demonstrates the dynamic nature of the infiltrate, *Arch Dermatol* 126:69, 1990.
115. Davies KA, Mathieson P, Winearls CG et al: Serum sickness and acute renal failure after streptokinase therapy for myocardial infarction, *Clin Exp Immunol* 80:83, 1990.
116. Patel A, Prussick R, Buchanan WW et al: Serum sickness–like illness and leukocytoclastic vasculitis after intravenous streptokinase, *J Am Acad Dermatol* 24:652, 1991.
117. Giger U, Werner LL, Millichamp NJ et al: Sulfadiazine-induced allergy in six Doberman pinschers, *J Am Vet Med Assoc* 86:479, 1985.
118. Dolman KM, Gans ROB, Vervaat TJ et al: Vasculitis and anti-neutrophil cytoplasmic autoantibodies associated with propylthiouracil therapy, *Lancet* 2:651, 1993.
119. Grishman E, Spiera H: Vasculitis in connective tissue diseases, including hypocomplementemic vasculitis. In Churg A, Churg J, editors: *Systemic vasculitides,* New York and Tokyo, 1991, Igaku-Shoin.
120. Watson R: Cutaneous lesions in systemic lupus erythematosus, *Med Clin North Am* 73:1091, 1989.
121. Korbet SM, Schwartz M, Lewis EJ: Immune complex deposition and coronary vasculitis in systemic lupus erythematosus: report of two cases, *Am J Med* 77:141, 1984.
122. Myers JL, Katzenstein AA: Microangiitis in lupus-induced pulmonary hemorrhage, *Am J Clin Pathol* 85:552, 1986.
123. Mehregan DR, Hall MJ, Gibson LE: Urticarial vasculitis: a histopathologic and clinical review of 72 cases, *J Am Acad Dermatol* 26:441, 1992.
124. Jorizzo JL, Apisarnthanarax P, Subrt P et al: Bowel-bypass syndrome without bowel bypass: bowel-associated dermatosis-arthritis syndrome, *Arch Intern Med* 143:457, 1983.
125. Sánchez-Guerrero J, Gutiérrez-Ureña S, Vidaller A et al: Vasculitis as a paraneoplastic syndrome: report of 11 cases and review of the literature, *J Rheumatol* 17:1458, 1990.
126. Lacour JP, Castanet J, Perrin C et al: Cutaneous leukocytoclastic vasculitis and renal cancer: two cases, *Am J Med* 4:104, 1993.

Infectious vasculitides

127. Berkmen YM: Historical background of aortitis. In Lande A, Berkmen YM, McAllister HA Jr, editors: *Aortitis: clinical, pathologic, and radiographic aspects,* New York, 1986, Raven Press.
128. Jackman JD, Randolf JD: Cardiovascular syphilis, *Am J Med* 87:425, 1989.
129. Kingston ME, Mackey D: Skin clues in the diagnosis of life-threatening infections, *Rev Infect Dis* 8:1, 1986.
130. Sotto MN, Langer B, Hoshino-Shimizu S et al: Pathogenesis of cutaneous lesions in acute meningococcemia in humans: light, immunofluorescent, and electron microscopic studies of skin biopsy specimens, *J Infect Dis* 133:506, 1976.
131. Dodd HJ, Goldsmith HJ, Verbov JL: Necrotizing cutaneous vasculitis occurring as an early feature of 'shunt nephritis'. *Clin Exp Dermatol* 10:284, 1985.
132. Walker DH, Cain BG, Olmstead PM: Laboratory diagnosis of Rocky Mountain spotted fever by immunofluorescent demonstration of *Rickettsia rickettsii* in cutaneous lesions, *Am J Clin Pathol* 69:619, 1978.
133. Dastur CK, Wadia NH: Spinal meningitides with radiculopathy: part 2 (pathology and pathogenesis), *J Neuro Sci* 8:261, 1969.
134. Kurent JE, Moore PM: Vasculitis of the nervous system. In LeRoy EC, editor: *The biologic basis of systemic vasculitis,* New York, 1992, Marcel Dekker.
135. Calabrese LH: Vasculitis and infection with the human immunodeficiency virus, *Rheum Dis Clin North Am* 17:131, 1991.
136. Doyle PW, Gibson G, Dolman CL: Herpes zoster ophthalmicus with contralateral hemiplegia; identification of cause, *Ann Neurol* 14:85, 1983.
137. Reyes MG, Fresco R, Chokroverty S et al: Virus-like particles in granulomatous angiitis of the central nervous system, *Neurology* 26:797, 1976.
138. Langenberg A, Yen TSB, LeBoit PE: Granulomatous vasculitis occurring after cutaneous herpes zoster despite absence of viral genome, *J Am Acad Dermatol* 24:429, 1991.

48 Upper Respiratory Tract

Jerome B. Taxy

NOSE AND PARANASAL SINUSES

Development and normal anatomy

The embryonic nose appears during the fourth week of gestation as a frontonasal elevation, just above the invaginating stomodaeum. By the end of the fourth week, the nasal placodes appear as symmetric ectodermal thickenings on either side of the central mound. During the fifth week, the placodes are surrounded by ectomesenchymal nasal elevations and become the nasal pits, which progressively invaginate as nasal sacs and become the definitive nasal cavities by the end of the sixth embryonic week. The nasal cavities connect, by means of the patent nasal choanae, with the pharynx, after rupture of the oronasal membrane.[1] A merging of the medial nasal elevations during this process yields the philtrum, part of the anterior palate and middle maxilla. The alae nasi result from the lateral nasal elevations and define the lateral nasal folds.

The paranasal sinuses form as diverticula from the lateral wall of the nasal cavity around the third fetal month (Fig. 48-1). The three pairs of cavities and series of ethmoid air cells occupy paramedian positions within the maxillary, frontal, ethmoid, and sphenoid bones but drain into the main nasal cavity. The definitive enlargement and pneumatization of these structures occurs around puberty.[2,3]

The nasal lining epithelium is of two types. Anteriorly, in the nares, it is keratinized stratified squamous epithelium with prominent pilosebaceous units. This gives way abruptly in the nasal cavities to a pseudostratified columnar epithelium with numerous goblet cells, beneath which are scattered minor salivary gland acini and ducts.

The mucosa of the nasal cavities and paranasal sinuses is often referred to as *Schneiderian mucosa* to emphasize its ectodermal origin as opposed to the endodermal origin of the morphologically identical mucosa lining the rest of the respiratory tract. A local specialization of this mucosa is in the region of the cribriform plate, high in the nasal cavity, where there are ciliated, bipolar olfactory neural cells that connect to the central olfactory apparatus.

The nasal stroma is a well-vascularized fibromuscular tissue, histologically similar to the erectile tissue of the external genitalia (Fig. 48-2). This is occasionally misinterpreted as a vascular malformation or vascular tumor. In the paranasal sinuses, a layer of thin cancellous bone supports this mucosal and stromal arrangement.

Malformations

Minor malformations and deformities of the nasal septum are common. Major malformations are rare but important because a dysmorphic nose, as a prominent feature of the facial midline, may indicate a recognizable syndrome.

Teratogens may cause facial anomalies involving the nose. The *fetal alcohol syndrome* results in a short, upturned nose, broad, low nasal bridge, thin upper lip, and hypoplastic philtrum.[4] In syndromes of holoprosencephaly, the small nose may be in its normal position but with a single nostril and nasal cavity (Fig. 48-3). In the cyclops anomaly there may be complete nasal aplasia or a nasal rudiment that occurs above the eye (Fig. 48-4). The failure of the medial nasal and the medial maxillary prominences to merge to form the upper lip may result in clefting. This clefting may also involve the developing palatal ridges and result in various combinations of clefting of the lip and palate, which will then also involve the integrity of the nasal cavity. Such abnormalities occur as frequently as 1:1000 births.[4] Hypoplasia of the maxillary sinus, usually as a unilateral occurrence, is the most common anomaly of the paranasal sinuses.[5] The significance of this or any other malformation is the dysfunction of drainage or mucociliary clearance as contributory factors in the development of sinusitis.

Choanal atresia, an anomaly occurring in about 1:60,000 births,[6] is attributable to a persistent oronasal membrane. If unilateral, it may escape clinical attention. However, because of the obligate nasal respirations of newborns, bilateral

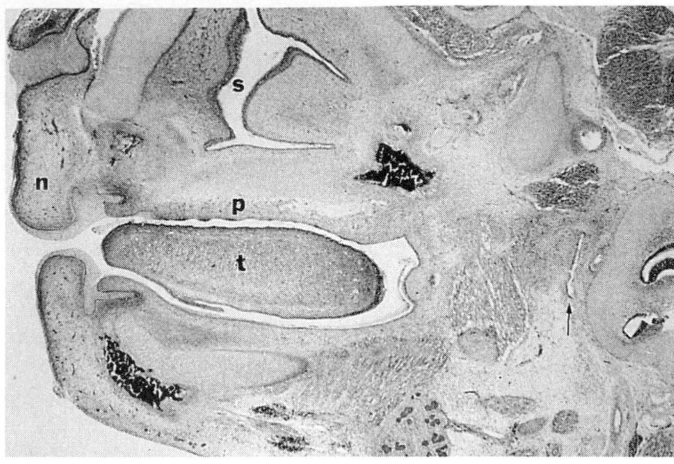

Fig. 48-1 Sagittal section of the fetal head at approximately 7 weeks gestation. *S*, Area of developing paranasal sinuses; *N*, nose; *P*, palate; *T*, tongue. Slit-like space behind the tongue is the pharynx, *arrow*.

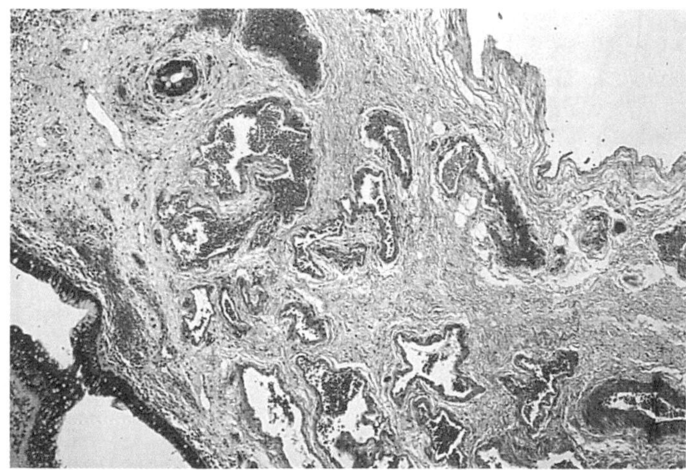

Fig. 48-2 Normal nasal mucosa and stroma. The thin-walled vessels are of variable size and shape and are invested by ample fibromuscular tissue, similar to erectile tissue of the genitalia.

choanal atresia can be fatal. The integrity of the posterior choanae should be ascertained at autopsy in each fetal or newborn death.

Nasal glioma is a rare congenital anomaly related to the abnormal development of the frontal lobe of the brain. This lesion is encountered almost exclusively in young children. In approximately 60% of cases the lesions occur anterior to the nasal bone and present clinically as masses over the nasal bridge; in 30% they are posterior to the nasal bone and are appreciated as intranasal or intraoral tumors producing respiratory distress, cerebrospinal fluid (CSF) rhinorrhea, and epistaxis. About 10% of cases have combined anatomic locations (Fig. 48-5). A connection to the central nervous system remains in about one fourth of cases.[7,8]

Histologically, nasal glioma consists of mixtures of glia, neurons, and occasionally ependyma and may be considered the anterior counterpart to the encephalocele (Fig. 48-6). Microcalcifications may also be present. Excessive scar tissue

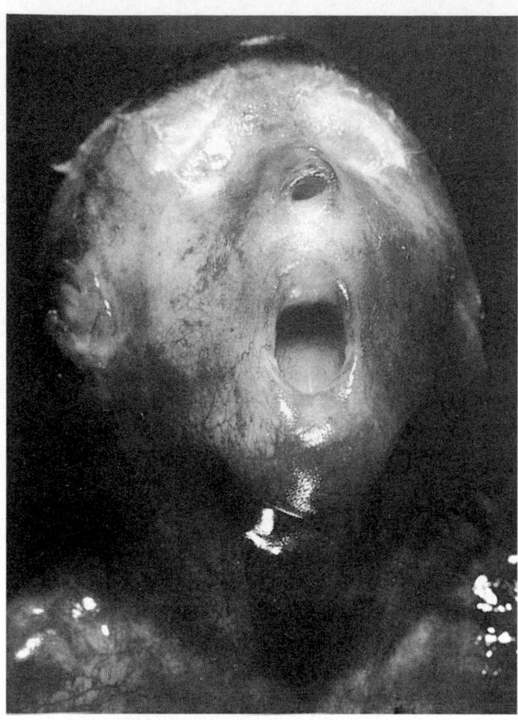

Fig. 48-3 Fetus, about 20 weeks of gestation, with single nostril. An encephalocele (not shown) and polydactyly of all extremities are also present.

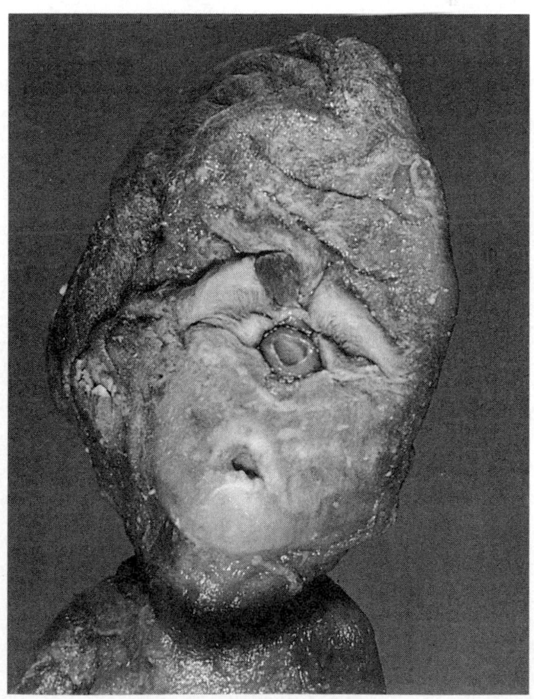

Fig. 48-4 Macerated cyclops fetus about 16 weeks of gestation with nasal rudiment above the eye.

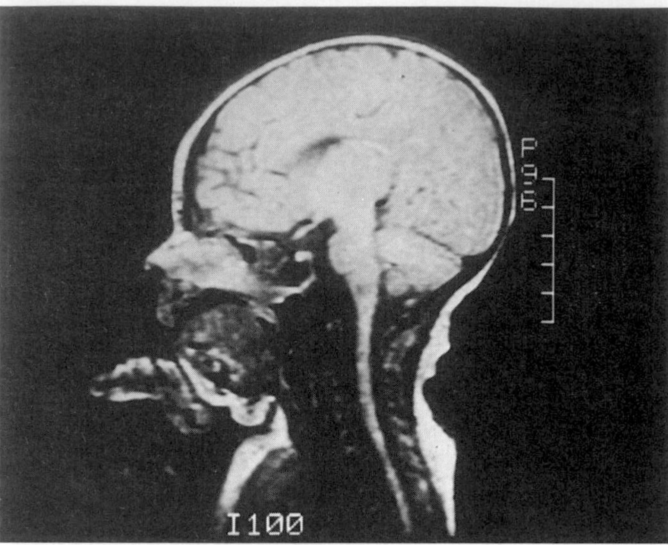

Fig. 48-5 Magnetic resonance image of a nasal glioma in a newborn with respiratory distress. Mass fills the nasal cavity and produces a bulge at the nasal bridge. No central nervous system connection is demonstrated.

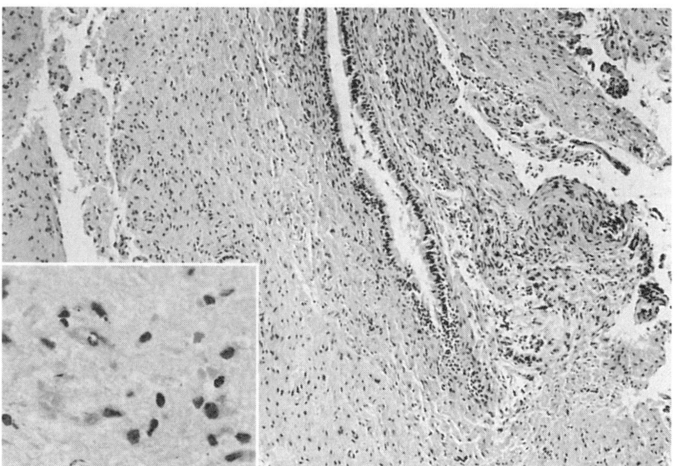

Fig. 48-6 Nasal glioma. Nasal mucosa infiltrated by cytologically bland glial cells. *Inset*, Glia with small dark nuclei set in a fibrillary background.

may obscure the glial component, which can be effectively detected by immunohistochemical staining for glial fibrillary acidic protein. Extranasal lesions can be treated by simple excision; intranasal lesions usually require a lateral rhinotomy. Excision is usually curative, though a 10% to 15% recurrence has been reported for intranasal lesions. Rarely, a neoplasm may present with the clinical features of a nasal glioma.[9]

Inflammatory disease

Sinusitis

Most upper respiratory infections, typified by the common cold, affect the nose and the paranasal sinuses but do not result in clinical sinusitis. These diseases are usually self-limited. The transition into chronic sinusitis may occur depending on the nature of the organism and host immune status. Drainage problems of the sinuses, allergies, ciliary dysfunction, and tumefactions of inflammatory tissue are among the more common contributory factors.

Sinusitis causes symptoms when excessive mucus production and edema obstruct the ostia and impede drainage from the sinuses into the nasal cavity. With the common cold this occurs in approximately 0.5% of cases[10] but may be more frequent in primary bacterial infections. The fluid stasis and inflammation within the sinuses result in headache, facial pain and pressure, and tooth tenderness. The stenosis or closure of the ostia further interferes with gas exchange, lowers the oxygen tension, and should favor anaerobic bacterial growth, though these organisms are isolated in less than 10% of cases.[10,11]

The most common bacteria recovered in an acute infection are *Haemophilus influenzae* and *Streptococcus pneumoniae*.[10] In chronic sinusitis, the cultures are frequently polymicrobial and often represent contaminant organisms, an indication that the underlying pathogen has not been successfully detected.[11] Previous antibiotic therapy may interfere with the successful identification of organisms.

Mucocele

Mucocele is a complication of chronic sinusitis. Bone erosion, sclerosis, intrasinus fluid, and debris accumulation contribute to an expansile process, which may or may not be epithelialized. These are most common in the frontal sinus, producing headache, proptosis, and diplopia. The maxillary sinus is affected in 10% of cases, where the process may be asymptomatic.[10] In the rare circumstance of sphenoid and ethmoid involvement, the process is typically contiguous with other sinuses.[12] Similar lesions can be produced by obstructed minor salivary gland ducts. Intracranial involvement is not common but may occur either by direct extension or by hematogenous spread.

Ciliary dysfunction

A normal cilium consists of nine peripheral pairs of microtubules surrounding a central doublet (Fig. 48-7). The peripheral tubules are each connected to the central pair by a radial spoke; the doublets are connected to each other by dynein arms. Dynein allows the sliding of microtubules over each other. Each cilium is anchored below the plasma membrane to a basal body and a rootlet, which are interconnected by transverse bundles of filaments. These complex interconnections allow for the synchronous beating of the cilia, which moves mucus, debris, and other particulate matter over the mucosal surface en route to disposal. Abnormalities of ciliary structure, including compound cilia and focal absences of dynein arms or microtubules, occur focally in about 1% to 3% of cilia in normal individuals.[13,14] Abnormal ciliary morphology may be induced by viruses or environmental pollutants[13,15] but is probably reversible. Impaired ciliary function is seen in 60% to 70% of patients with chronic sinusitis.[16]

The widespread absence of ciliary dynein arms is encountered in *Kartagener's syndrome*. This inherited condition includes in its typical form situs inversus, chronic sinusitis, bronchiectasis, and male infertility. It has an incidence of 1:20,000. These patients have ciliary dysfunction, variously termed "ciliary dyskinesia" or "immotile cilia." Ciliary abnormality can be diagnosed by electron microscopy of nasal biopsy material.[15]

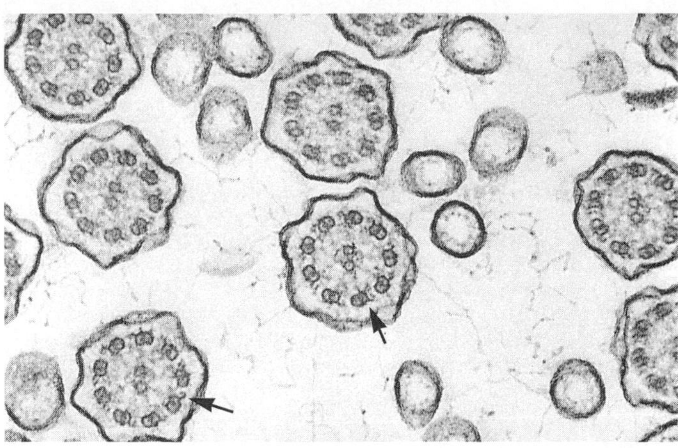

Fig. 48-7 Normal cilia and interspersed (smaller) microvilli, all in cross section. Cilia show circular arrangement of nine pairs of tubules and a central doublet from which radial spokes emanate. External dynein arms, *arrows,* are absent in ciliary dyskinesia.

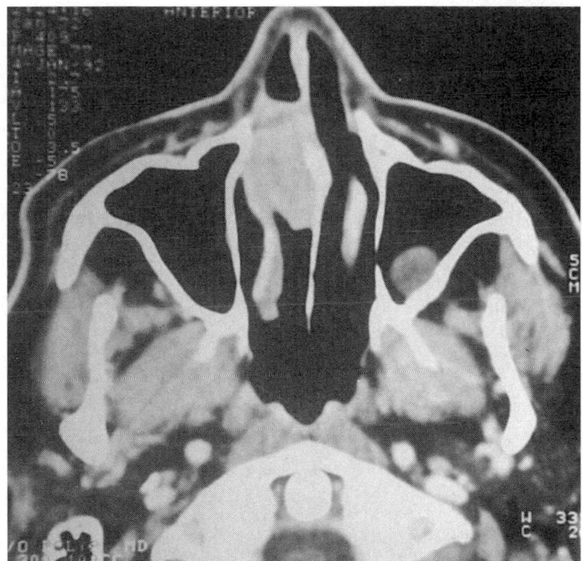

Fig. 48-8 CT scan of paranasal sinus in 43-year-old man with rhinoscleroma. Right nasal cavity and posterior wall of left maxillary sinus are involved.

The ultrastructural assessment of ciliary function is problematic. The sample should be obtained from noninflamed respiratory mucosa, since a chronically inflamed surface may have been replaced by metaplastic squamous epithelium. The ultrastructural examination is technically difficult, requiring high magnifications, sharp visual acuity, and an almost perfect cross section of the cilia. Also, an optimal number of cilia to be examined has yet to be defined. Cilia of normal structure and beat frequency may still be ineffective if the beating is not synchronous. Whether defects in dynein arms in patients without Kartagener's syndrome are congenital or acquired because of infection is not clear.[14,15]

Infections of uncommon cause

Granulomas of the nose have been traditionally considered evidence of mycobacterial or fungal infection, or sarcoidosis.

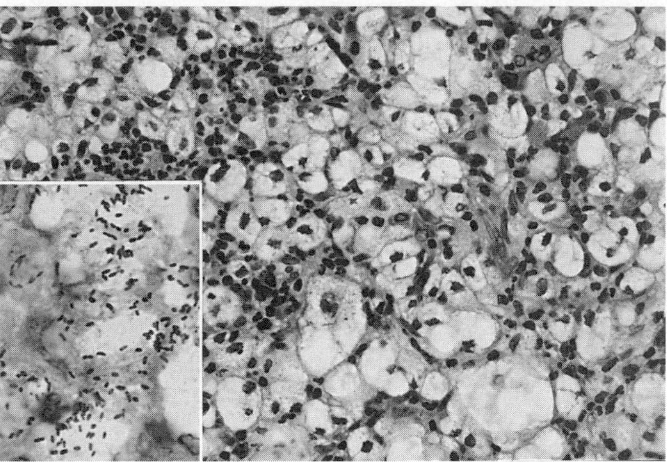

Fig. 48-9 Nasal biopsy sample of patient in Fig. 48-8, showing numerous foamy histiocytes (Mikulicz cells) and lymphocytes. Inset, Numerous bacteria are seen within Mikulicz cells (Warthin-Starry stain).

Tuberculosis or leprosy of the nose and paranasal sinuses is extremely rare in the United States, and fungal infection may not elicit granuloma formation at all. *Sarcoidosis* produces granulomas, though its occurrence in this location is unusual. In 2319 patients with sarcoid studied over a 31-year period, 17 had histologically proved nasal involvement.[17] The clinical manifestations included nasal crusting, sinus opacification, or a mass. Nasal involvement does not herald the diagnosis but occurs as part of well-established clinical disease.

Rhinoscleroma

Rhinoscleroma is an uncommon chronic, destructive infection inexplicably restricted to the respiratory mucosa, usually of the nasal cavity and paranasal sinuses. It is caused by a gram-negative coccobacillus, *Klebsiella rhinoscleromatis,* which grows aerobically on MacConkey's or blood agar. Endemic areas for this disease include Latin America, Egypt, Indonesia, and central and eastern Europe. The paucity of cases in the West may be changing because of immigration from these areas.[18]

There are three stages of clinical disease, which correlate with the ease in identifying organisms. The early (exudative) and late (sclerotic) stages are histologically nonspecific, and although organisms are demonstrable, they may be obscured by the response itself.

In the proliferative (granulomatous) stage, which is when most patients come to clinical attention, the disease almost always affects the nose, producing obstructing masses or destroying the nasal bones. Radiographic studies show a high incidence of multifocal involvement of the paranasal sinuses, nasal cavity, and nasopharynx (Fig. 48-8).[19] Laryngeal involvement is rare.[18,19] It is in this second stage that a plethora of organisms is found within the sheets of foamy non–lipid containing histiocytes, the Mikulicz cells (Fig. 48-9). An accompanying lymphoplasmacytic infiltrate, can be intense. By routine light microscopy, tuberculous leprosy may be considered, but the diagnosis can be resolved by simple special stains, since the rhinoscleroma organisms appear positive with the Giemsa and Warthin-Starry stains and negative with Fite's method. There is no cure for this infection, which can, however, be controlled by antibiotics and surgery.

Rhinosporidiosis

Rhinosporidiosis is a chronic infection caused by *Rhinosporidium seeberi,* probably a spore-producing fungus that has never been cultured.[20] The appearance of the spores within a large sporangium is similar to that seen in *Coccidiodes imitis*. The disease is endemic in India and Sri Lanka where the patients are predominantly male (male/female ratio of 2:1 to 6:1) and appears as a nasal obstruction, a watery nasal discharge, and epistaxis. A review of 23 cases from Europe revealed only 6 native Europeans.[21] Approximately 80% of cases involve a solitary, friable, polypoid lesion of the nose; orbital involvement is seen in 15% of patients.[22] Although this infection does not undergo dissemination, it has been reported to occur in, for example, skin, bone, and urethra, the latter possibly by self-inoculation.

Histologic examination of the polypoid masses demonstrates thick-walled sacs or sporangia, about 250 μm in diameter. The sporangium contains numerous spores (each about the size of an erythrocyte), which, when released by rupture of the sac, escape into the nasal secretions or into surrounding tissue to germinate into a trophocyte. A granulomatous response may be seen. Spores and sporangia can be seen on conventional sections and are effectively highlighted by periodic acid–Schuff (PAS) stain or methenamine silver stain (Fig. 48-10). This disease does not respond to antibiotics and usually requires surgical intervention.

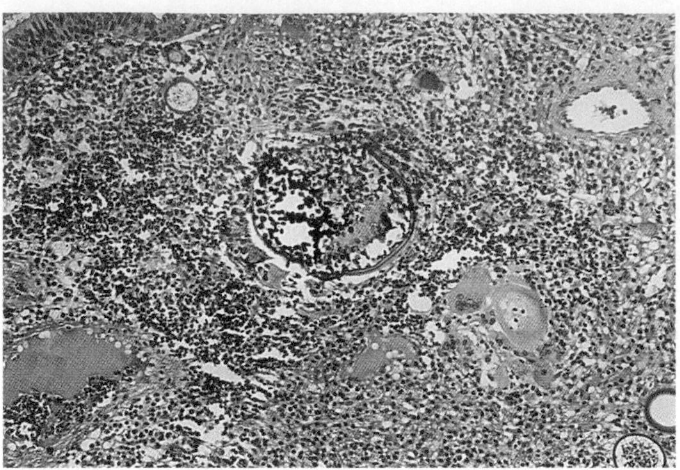

Fig. 48-10 Rhinosporidiosis. Nasal mucosa contains a sporangium, filled with spores and surrounded by multinucleated giant cells.

Mucormycosis

Mucormycosis, or *zygomycosis*, is a term applied to infection with a fungus from any of three pathogenic genera of the Mucoracea family: *Mucor, Rhizopus,* and *Absidia*. These saprophytic fungi are found in soil, dust particles, fruits, starchy foods, and manure. They can be cultured from the nose, nasopharynx, and stool of healthy people.[23] Symptoms usually occur under conditions that favor opportunistic infection, such as chronic disease or cancer. Diabetes mellitus is the predisposing cause in 70% of cases.[23] Healthy individuals are not commonly infected. In experimental studies, rats made diabetic by alloxan and then infected with *Rhizopus* by direct inoculation of the ethmoid sinus died within 2 weeks. Infected, non–alloxan treated animals did not become ill.[24] Diabetes probably promotes the infection in humans as well.

The initial stages of infection are similar to those for an acute sinusitis with a bloody discharge. A crusted, black necrotic layer forms over the turbinate mucosa. Orbital involvement and facial necrosis may ensue. Histologic examination of debrided tissues demonstrates angioinvasive, broad, nonseptate, branching hyphae. Although hematogenous dissemination may occur, the most common complication is direct intracranial invasion, which has a mortality of almost 70%.[24] Overall survival has improved in recent years because of early diagnosis and treatment. Although the optimal management is controversial, surgical débridement is essential.

Allergic fungal sinusitis

In 1983, Katzenstein and colleagues[25] reported seven patients with a fungal sinusitis characterized by copious amounts of "allergic" mucin and the presence of branching septate hyphae. These were noninvasive infections in immunocompetent young adults typically with an atopic history, nasal polyps, and sinus opacification. Although no cultures were available, the morphology was consistent with *Aspergillus,* and the disease was considered analogous to allergic bronchopulmonary aspergillosis.

Table 48-1 Allergic fungal sinusitis: pathologic features

Allergic mucin
Viscous
Inflammatory debris
Sloughed epithelium
Charcot-Leyden crystals
Branching septate hyphae
Organisms recovered
Alternaria
Aspergillus
Bipolaris
Curvularia
Drechslera
Exserohilum
Helminthosporium

The current designation applied to these patients is *allergic fungal sinusitis* (Table 48-1), since subsequent reports with culture data have demonstrated that in immunologically competent hosts with refractory chronic sinusitis the fungus recovered may be *Aspergillus* or a dematiaceous fungus such as *Alternaria* or *Curvularia*.[26,27] In a review of 70 cases, only 42 were caused by *Aspergillus*.[28] This condition affects both children and adults with no gender preference. The causal relationship between atopy and fungal infection is unclear; antibiotic usage and environmental pollution may be factors as well.[27] Skin tests may be reactive for the fungus recovered from the sinus, but peripheral eosinophil counts and serum IgE levels may not correlate with active infection.[28]

Multiple sinus involvement is typical (Fig. 48-11). The "allergic" mucinous debris is thick, almost gluelike, with numerous Charcot-Leyden crystals. Organisms are sparsely distributed within the mucin and are identified often with great difficulty, special stains notwithstanding. Regardless of the eventual microbiologic identification, the hyphae are branching and septate. The treatment for these patients is adequate nasal drainage, which usually requires surgical intervention.

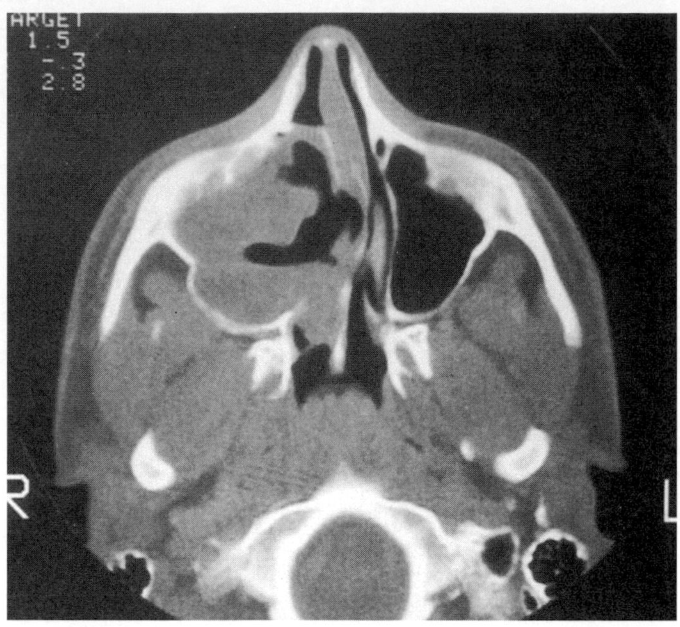

Fig. 48-11 Allergic fungal sinusitis. CT scan of a 17-year-old man showing pronounced polypoid edema involving the right nasal cavity and maxillary sinus with bone erosion.

Fungal sinusitis in immunologically compromised patients is more likely to disseminate. In this setting, *Aspergillus* is a commonly recovered organism with extensive sinus involvement and angioinvasiveness.[29]

Inflammation of noninfectious origin

Myospherulosis

Myospherulosis occurs in the upper respiratory tract in patients whose nasal cavities have been packed with gauze containing petroleum jelly. The granulomatous tissue response includes numerous large (20 to 100 μm) sacs containing a variable number of spherules between 4 and 7 μm in diameter (Fig. 48-12). Despite the striking resemblance of these pale to brown spherules to sporulating fungi, histochemical and electron microscopic analysis has shown these bodies to be degenerated erythrocytes.[30,31] The changes are probably induced by the reaction of blood and lipid material in the petroleum jelly.

Wegener's granulomatosis

Wegener's granulomatosis is a systemic vasculitis principally affecting the upper and lower respiratory tracts and kidneys. Approximately 15% of patients will present with respiratory tract symptoms only; however, about 90% of patients will have nasal or nasal sinus involvement, which makes a biopsy of this easily accessible site a frequent procedure in the workup of such patients. However, because the biopsy specimens often lack specificity and because the disease has protean clinical manifestations, a thorough clinicopathologic approach to this diagnosis is required.

The diagnostic evaluation of nasal biopsy specimens is often a frustrating issue. It has been recommended that a biopsy specimen of at least 5 mm be submitted,[32] though an appropriate amount of tissue from a representative area is a matter of surgical judgment. The patient's nasal symptoms include rhinorrhea, bloody or purulent nasal discharge,

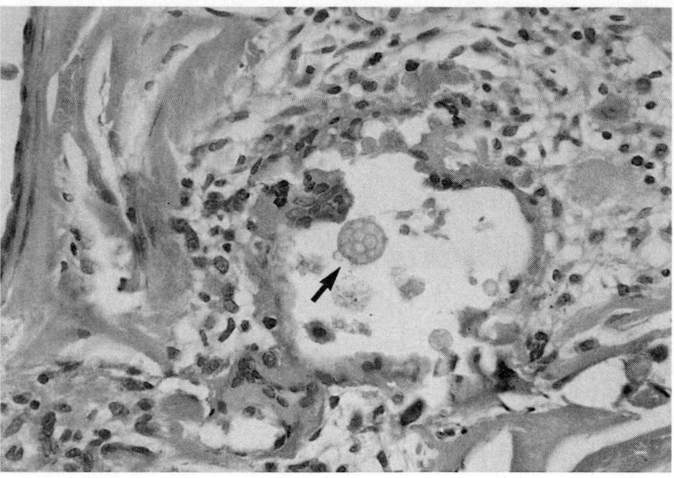

Fig. 48-12 Myospherulosis. This focus of inflammation with a multinucleated giant cell contains a central sac containing a cluster of sporelike bodies that represent altered erythrocytes. Smaller, single bodies are also in the vicinity. (Courtesy Dr. S.E. Mills, Charlottesville, Virg.)

mucosal ulcers, and sinus pain. The crusting, inflammation, and ulceration of the nasal mucosa compromise the acquisition of tissue for diagnosis, and so biopsy samples under these circumstances tend to be small and artifactually crushed. Only about a half of the samples may be adequate for diagnosis.[32]

The classic pathologic triad of necrosis, granulomas and vasculitis are seen together infrequently[33,34] (Fig. 48-13). In one large study, all three were present in 16% of the biopsy specimens, but any two were seen in only about 20%[33] (Table 48-2). The necrosis of Wegener's granulomatosis typically has a geographic pattern, but this may not be commonly observed; the granulomas are not usually well formed, as in sarcoid, and the vasculitis varies in its histologic components.[33] The tissue changes observed in the biopsy are therefore often nonspecific.

The differential diagnosis includes granuloma-producing infections, for which stains and cultures should be performed for identification of the organism. Clinical entities such as midfacial destruction produced by cocaine snorting or by allergic angiitis and granulomatosis (Churg-Straus syndrome) may yield biopsy findings similar to those of Wegener's granulomatosis and should be excluded on clinical grounds. Angiocentric T-cell lymphoma (previously called *polymorphic reticulosis* or *malignant midline reticulosis*) involves the presence of malignant lymphocytes.

Antineutrophil cytoplasmic antibodies (ANCA) are useful in the diagnosis of Wegener's granulomatosis and for estimating the activity of the disease. The antibody in the majority of patients is an IgG autoantibody directed against proteinase 3, a neutrophilic serine protease, which can be seen on indirect immunofluorescence as granular deposits in the cytoplasm of ethanol-fixed, cytocentrifuged neutrophils. A few patients will have antibody directed against myeloperoxidase, which gives a perinuclear staining reaction.[35] ANCA is positive in 96% of patients with generalized disease and 67% of patients with active limited disease.[32,35] This test may be helpful in confirming a diagnosis of Wegener's granulomatosis that has typical or suggestive clinical features but nonspecific histologic findings.

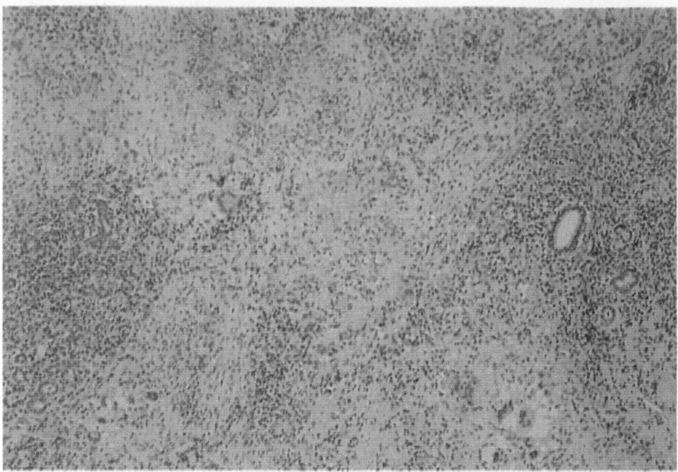

Fig. 48-13 Wegener's granulomatosis. Nasal biopsy with some preserved nasal glands distorted by intense inflammation. Central vessel is obliterated and surrounded by poorly formed granulomatous infiltrate. (Courtesy Dr. R. Zarbo, Detroit.)

Table 48-2 Inflammatory features in Wegener's granulomatosis*

Feature	Occurrence (% of specimens)
Necrosis	33
Geographic	28
Granuloma	42
Poorly formed	16
Scattered giant cells	42
Vasculitis	26
Granulomatous	6
Fibrinoid necrosis	8
Acute	17
Chronic	22

Modified from Devany KO, Travis WD, Hoffman G et al: *Am J Surg Pathol* 14:555, 1990.

*All three major features were present in 16%, vasculitis and granulomas were present in 21%, and vasculitis and necrosis were present in 23% of the biopsy specimens respectively.

Benign tumors

Nasal polyps

Nasal polyps are nonneoplastic tumefactions usually associated with chronic inflammation. Intense tissue eosinophilia correlates with a history of allergic or atopic disease, which are frequent in these patients.[36] In one series of 224 patients with nasal polyps, 32% had a history of allergy and 26% were asthmatic; aspirin sensitivity has also been etiologically implicated.[37] In cystic fibrosis and Kartagener's syndrome polyps are related to chronic infection. Finding nasal polyps in children under 10 years of age is suggestive of cystic fibrosis. Some patients with cystic fibrosis may even have concurrent allergies.[38]

Histologically, nasal polyps are represented by an edematous submucosa infiltrated by inflammatory cells, especially eosinophils and plasma cells. The overlying respiratory mucosa is usually intact. Although most nasal polyps are not a diagnostic problem, an occasional lesion will contain cytologically atypical stromal cells with dysplastic and bizarre features (Fig. 48-14). This may be especially true if the polyp surface has ulcerated and produced a granulation tissue reaction, as may be seen in the more mobile antrochoanal polyps. The proximity of these cells to blood vessel lumina indicates that some may be endothelial. Nasal polyps with atypical stromal cells are benign lesions as noted in a recent series of patients with a prolonged follow-up study.[39] This histologic observation is therefore just a morphologic curiosity and should not be mistaken for malignancy.

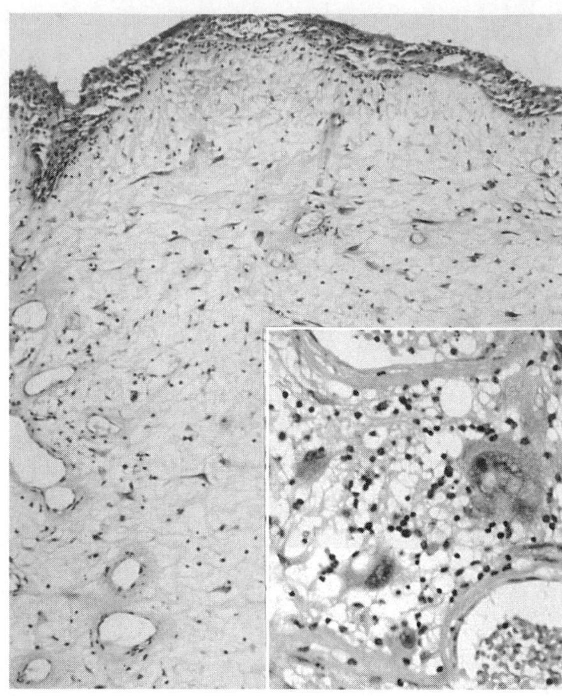

Fig. 48-14 Nasal polyp. Overlying intact mucosa is inflamed. Edematous stroma contains many scattered atypical stromal cells. Stromal cells can exhibit pronounced atypia, especially in association with an ulcerated surface, *inset*.

Papillomas

Papillomas of the schneiderian mucosa are of three histologic varieties: exophytic (fungiform), endophytic (inverted), and oncocytic (cylindrical cell). The terminology is somewhat confusing because the diagnostic subclassification uses macroscopic features and epithelial growth patterns for the first two and a specific cell type for the third. In addition, the designation *inverted papilloma* is often used generically for all three.[40] Human papillomavirus (HPV), particularly HPV 6 and 11, has recently been documented, either by in situ hybridization or polymerase chain reaction, in 20% to 76% of fungiform or inverted lesions.[41-43] The presence of viral genome raises additional questions regarding the cause and biologic behavior.

Fungiform and inverted papillomas, whether pure lesions or histologically mixed, account for about 95% of all schneiderian papillomas. These tumors predominate in males in an age range from adolescence to the elderly, an average being around 50 years. The usual symptoms of nasal stuffiness, epistaxis, and nasal discharge may be accompanied by pain and facial distortion. Symptoms may be present for a few weeks or even years.[41,44] Rapid growth may reflect bone destruction.[45]

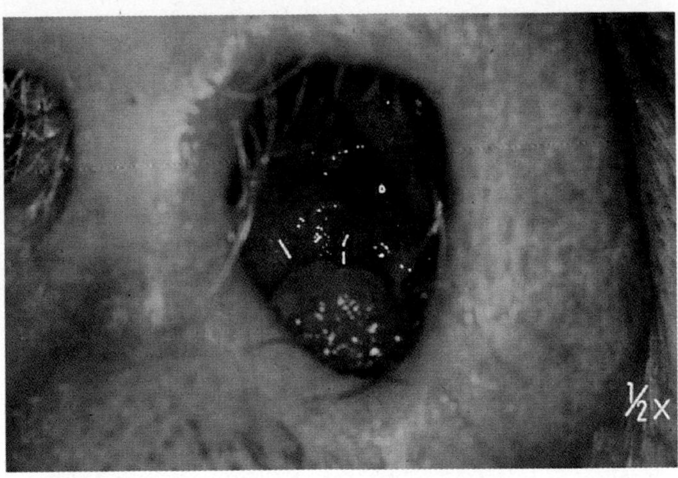

Fig. 48-15 Schneiderian papilloma involving the nasal cavity extending onto the septum and lateral wall. (Courtesy Dr. R. Sirota, Oak Park, Ill.)

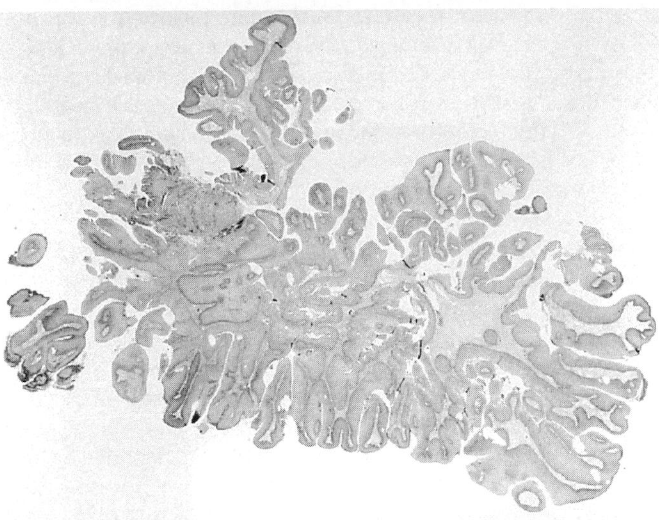

Fig. 48-16 Schneiderian papilloma with exophytic and inverted features.

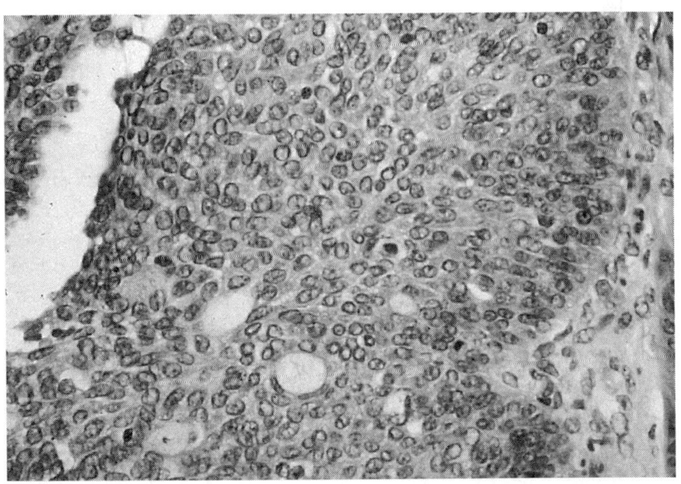

Fig. 48-17 Proliferation of monotonous, bland, basaloid cells with clear spaces representing mucinous residua or "microcysts."

Exophytic lesions are typically located on the nasal septum, and are grossly wartlike. Inverted lesions, which invaginate into an edematous stroma and involve the lateral nasal wall and sinuses, are broadly based, resilient masses (Fig. 48-15 and 48-16). The growth patterns are often mixed regardless of the anatomic location of the lesion. The histology of fungiform and inverted lesions includes intramucosal proliferation of basaloid cells with occasional squamous differentiation, which may spare isolated mucin-containing respiratory cells as "microcysts" (Fig. 48-17).

Cytologic atypia of varying degrees and mitotic figures are common; recurrent lesions may show more cytologic atypia and mitoses when compared with previous lesions from the same patient.[46] There are no reliable indicators of recurrence, a phenomenon observed in 28% to 67% of cases over a period ranging from 1 to 23 years.[44,46,47] The high rate of recurrence and the multifocality of these lesions often require lateral rhinotomy, medial maxillectomy, and mucosal stripping for optimal results.

In situ or invasive squamous cell carcinoma may develop either in the original lesion or in association with progressive recurrences. There are no reliable histologic features in a given papilloma to allow prediction of this development, and its frequency is uncertain. The criteria of malignancy, as applied in historical retrospective, are not uniform. In one literature review, 18 malignant cases were found between 1897 and 1972.[44] However, more recent surveys suggest an incidence of malignancy of about 10% of cases.[40,46] Although carcinoma is a recognized complication of sinonasal papillomas, it is also clear that death caused by tumor is uncommon.[44,46,47]

Cylindrical cell or oncocytic papillomas constitute about 5% of all schneiderian papillomas.[48] They are similar demographically and clinically to the other types and exhibit both exophytic and inverted growth patterns but present a distinctive cytologic pattern, since the constituent cells are oncocytes. Carcinoma has also been documented to arise from oncocytic papillomas.[49]

Miscellaneous benign tumors

Benign *salivary gland tumors* are uncommon in the nasal cavity. These tumors show occasional secondary sinus extension.[50] Among 81 primary, benign minor salivary gland tumors collected over a 44 year period, only 4 were in a paranasal sinus.[51] One report summarized 40 cases of intranasal *mixed tumor* collected over a 25 year period.[52] The patients were mostly female and the mean age was 42 years. All patients had the usual obstructive symptoms, and all tumors involved the nasal cavity. Most were based on the nasal septum. Three secondarily involved the maxillary sinus. Histologically, the tumors were more cellular than mixed tumors in the major salivary glands, but an adequate surgical excision appeared curative. Of 34 patients followed for an average of 7.5 years, 31 experienced no recurrence.

Most nonepithelial tumors are reported as case reports. In one comprehensive collection, there were 156 benign tumors, most of which were vascular or fibro-osseous.[53] *Meningiomas* are slowly growing and locally invasive and histologically demonstrate intranuclear pseudoinclusions similar to intracranial meningiomas.[54] Some sinonasal *hemangiopericytomas* have been reported recently.[55,56] Hemangiopericytoma in this location appears in all aspects of its morphology, as well as in its biologic behavior, to be similar to hemangiopericytoma in conventional soft-tissue locations.[55] The sinonasal lesions tend to be smaller (possibly because of the anatomic location), often low grade, and with diploid DNA content.[56] The relationship of this tumor to the recently described, morphologically similar *solitary fibrous tumor*[57] is unresolved.

Benign *fibro-osseous lesions* of the facial bones are also known as *fibrous dysplasia, ossifying fibroma,* and *cementifying fibroma.* Histopathologic examination of these lesions demonstrates a cellular, bland, swirling fibrous stroma with considerable degrees of overlap in the appearances of woven bone, bony trabeculae surrounded by osteoblasts, and calcospherules suggestive of cementicles. A clinically reliable radiographic diagnosis is based on a sharply delineated image, regardless of the histologic composition. These lesions, especially those of large size, may produce facial distortion, pain, visual changes, and contribute to infection. They are locally extensive but slowly growing, averaging about 2 years of preclinical growth, and affect a young age group (average 21 years).[58] Fibro-osseous lesions should not be confused with *osteomas,* benign bony tumors consisting of thick trabeculae of mature bone typically occurring in the frontal sinus.[59]

Malignant tumors

Epithelial tumors: general considerations

The statistics cited for epithelial malignancy of the head and neck often group the nasal vestibule, nasal cavity, and nasal sinuses together. Even acknowledging this dilutional factor, tumors in these locations are uncommon, representing 3% of the approximately 43,000 head and neck cancers diagnosed annually in the United States.[60-62] There may be some geographic variation, since by comparison the incidence in Japan, Nigeria, and Jamaica is two times higher than that in the general world population.[61]

The environmental factors influencing the development of nasal cancer are well known (Table 48-3), though the exact mechanisms of the individual agents may not be fully understood. Although the strong carcinogenic effect of tobacco and alcohol has been established for squamous carcinoma of the oral cavity, pharynx, and larynx, the role of these agents in nasal cancer is less well understood.[61,63] Nasal cancer also manifests a lower rate of multiple primary tumors. In a study of 1297 patients with a primary nasal carcinoma, a second, usually metachronous, head and neck lesion occurred in 3.4% of patients.[64] This contrasts with a 14% occurrence in one large study of nonnasal upper aerodigestive tract tumors, a figure that itself may be conservative.[65]

Radium-dial painting and mustard gas production were linked with nasal cancer in industrial workers but are of historic interest only. By contrast, nickel smelting and refining remain the main contemporary industrial risks.[61,66] The involvement of human papillomavirus is suggested by the histologic observation of koilocytotic change within the squamous mucosa associated with nasal squamous carcinomas and by studies using the techniques of modern molecular biology.[67] The exact role of the virus and any of its gene products remains putative.[68]

The association of primary (nonsalivary) adenocarcinoma of the nasal sinuses with wood dust is well known.[66] It is unclear whether this association is caused solely by natural softwood or hardwood resins or the chemicals involved in wood finishing, such as benzene, formaldehyde, and isopropanol. Chronic exposure to leather tanning agents may also contribute to adenocarcinoma.[61]

Regardless of the histologic type, malignant tumors in the nose and paranasal sinuses most often present with symptoms of chronic sinusitis, are refractory to conservative management, and are diagnosed at an advanced stage.[60,69-71] Table 48-4 lists the tumors most likely to be encountered in this region. Squamous cell carcinoma, the most common tumor, accounts for as many as 67% of all cases; other tumors occur significantly less frequently.

Squamous cell carcinoma of the nasal vestibule

The nasal vestibule is that space anatomically defined by the lower border of the upper nasal cartilage, the nasal septum, the ala nasi, and the anterior naris. Few studies deal specifically with carcinoma in this location.[60] Although the lining of the nasal vestibule is cutaneous, almost all the malignant tumors are squamous cell carcinomas, and they are rare. Patel and colleagues[72] reported 31 nasal vestibule cancers (30 squamous, 1 basal cell) out of 4747 head and neck tumors accessioned between 1975 and 1990.

This is a tumor predominantly of elderly men, appearing as a mass lesion or a nonbleeding ulcer, which may require a complete nasal amputation (Fig. 48-18). Radiotherapy has been employed advantageously, though the primary or combined roles of these two modalities are debated. Histologically, the tumor is typically keratinizing (Fig. 48-19). There is no

Table 48-3 Environmental agents implicated in nasal cancer

Squamous cell carcinoma
Radium-dial painting
Mustard gas
Nickel
Human papillomavirus
Adenocarcinoma
Wood dust
Leather tanning agents
Chromium
Isopropanol

Table 48-4 Malignant tumors of the nose and paranasal sinuses*

Tumor type	Incidence (% range)
Squamous cell carcinoma	24-67
Anaplastic, undifferentiated, or unspecified tumor	8-11
Adenocarcinoma	8-14
Salivary gland (mostly adenoid cystic carcinoma)	2-16
Melanoma	1-5
Olfactory neuroblastoma (small cell carcinoma)	0.2-9
Lymphoma/plasmacytoma	2-9
Sarcoma	8-10

*Modified from references 61, 69, 70, 73, and 75.

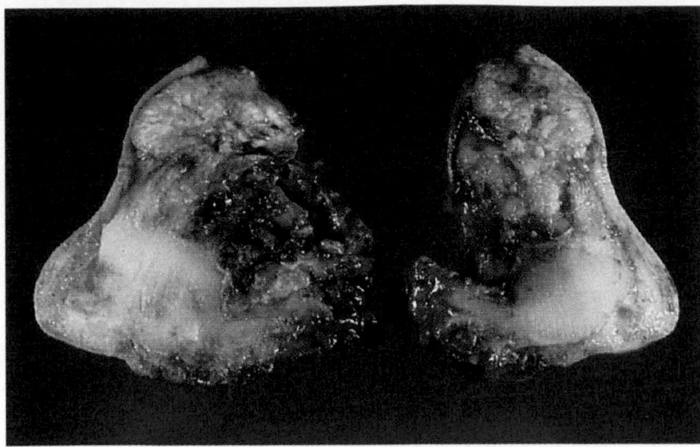

Fig. 48-18 Nasal amputation for squamous cell carcinoma of the nasal vestibule. The friable exophytic tumor has extended high into the anterior nasal cavity on both sides of the septum, S.

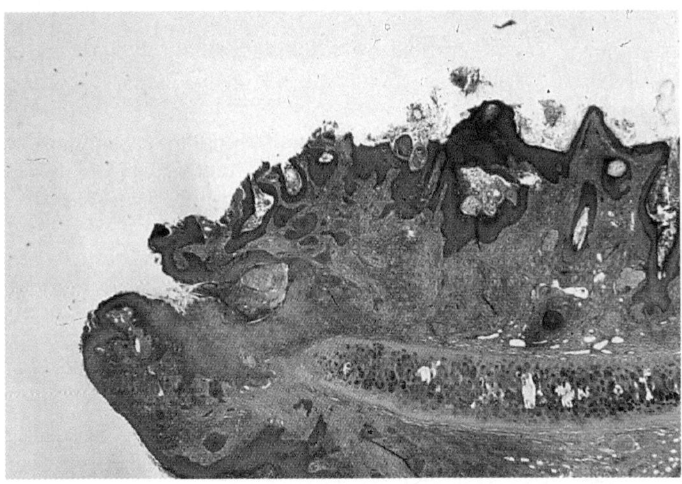

Fig. 48-19 Invasive squamous cell carcinoma of the nasal vestibule encroaching on the hyaline cartilage of the septum, *arrow*.

currently accepted uniform staging system for this anatomic location; it is therefore difficult to assess the significance of extent of disease with respect to recurrence, metastasis, or survival. Almost 80% of tumors recur, but reported 5-year survival rates are in the range of 75% to 100%. Positive cervical nodes occur in about 10% of patients and may diminish the 5-year survival rate to as low as 38%.[72]

Squamous carcinoma of the nasal cavity and paranasal sinus

The nasal cavity and paranasal sinuses have a common mucosal lining, and are interconnected. Carcinomas of this region are often multifocal and are discussed together.

Men of an average age of 60 account for one half to two thirds of invasive tumors; 40% to 75% of cases affect the nasal cavity or the maxillary sinus. In one study, fewer than 2% of all in situ carcinomas of the head and neck were found in this location.[73] The difficulty in visualizing the mucosal surfaces of this region may explain the infrequent clinical observation of leukoerythroplakia, which in other parts of the upper aerodigestive tract is indicative of dysplastic mucosal change.

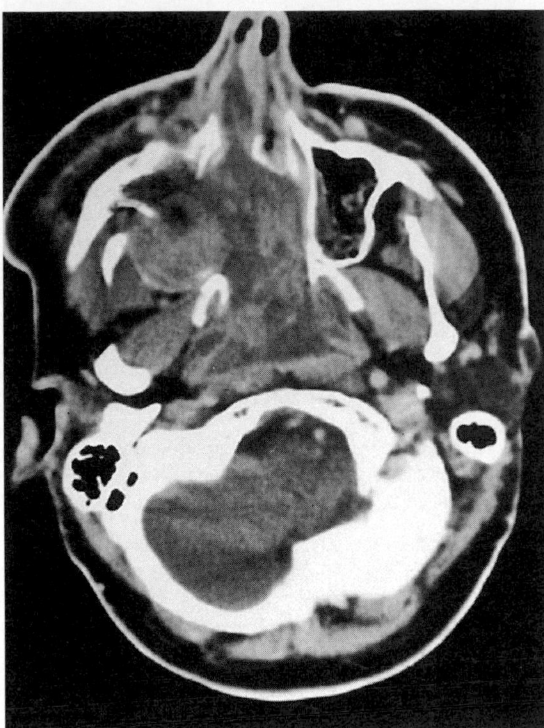

Fig. 48-20 Squamous cell carcinoma of the right maxillary sinus. CT scan showing the tumor extending anteriorly into the nasal cavity, eroding the anterior sinus wall into the facial soft tissue and posteriorly to the skull base.

Most patients with tumors of the maxillary sinus are at the T3 or T4 stage at diagnosis.[74-76] Nodal metastases are more frequent in tumors at the T3 or T4 stage. The advanced clinical stage is also evidenced by facial asymmetry, with a facial, oral, or orbital mass or a tumor being visible in the nasal cavity (Fig. 48-20). Radiographic evidence of extension into these areas is present in 20% to 60% of cases.[71,77] Surgical treatment entails radical maxillectomy (Fig. 48-21).

Histologically the tumors are typical squamous cell carcinomas. Although metastases to cervical nodes occur in 10% to 15% of cases, distant metastases are uncommon, and principally affect the lung and liver. Most deaths are attributable to local recurrences, about 70% of which become apparent within the first 2 years.[74] It is alleged that the best survivals are achieved for patients with low-stage disease; however, the reported 5-year survival rate after surgery, radiation, and inconsistently administered chemotherapy has a broad range. In a literature summary of 766 patients, the survival rate ranged from 8% to 42%;[60] other series report 32% to 43% 5-year survival rates.[69,71,74-77]

Adenocarcinoma

Adenocarcinomas in the paranasal sinuses originate from salivary glands or from mucoid cells. Histologically, most salivary gland tumors are adenoid cystic carcinomas or adenocarcinomas of no specific histologic type.[78-81] Adenoid cystic carcinoma is morphologically identical to its major salivary gland counterpart. The tumor exhibits no sex preference, occurs in the sixth decade of life, and is located most often in the maxillary sinus and nasal cavity.[51,80] The expected infiltrative growth may account for its often incomplete surgical

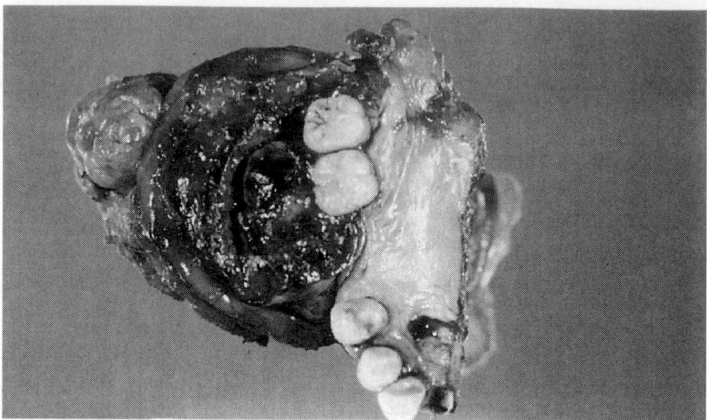

Fig. 48-21 Lateral view of a radical maxillectomy for squamous cell carcinoma. The maxilla and palate are everted and partially overlie a poorly circumscribed dark, friable mass that has destroyed the lateral maxillary wall.

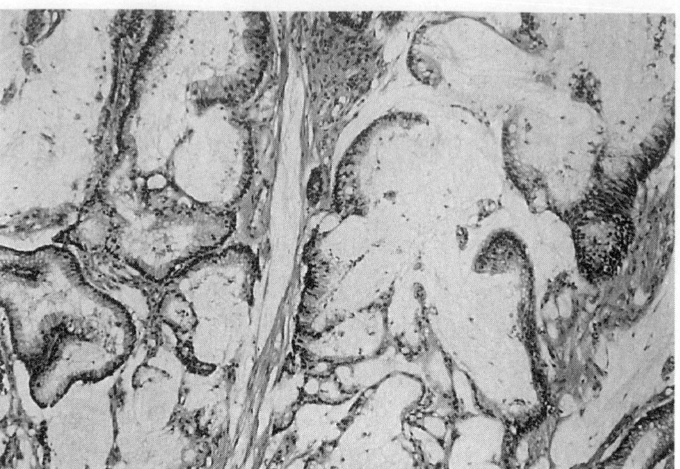

Fig. 48-22 Colonic type, mucinous adenocarcinoma of paranasal sinus (Courtesy Dr. S.E. Mills, Charlottesville, Virg.)

extirpation and contributes to morbidity by extending to the nearby sensory organs and brain. It has been regarded as a high-grade tumor[51] but may exhibit indolent growth characterized by recurrences with a 10-year survival rate of approximately 50%.[51,80]

Nonsalivary adenocarcinomas are rare tumors that may show occupational association or occur sporadically.[82] Histologically they are divided into low- and high-grade lesions.[78,83] Wood dust exposure is strongly associated with these tumors, especially with so-called adenocarcinoma of the intestinal or colonic type.[78,82-84] A historical survey of 213 cases found that 19% of the tumors occurred in woodworkers,[82] though the incidence in smaller series ranges from 33% to 71%.[83,84] Some reports do not implicate an occupational exposure.[85] For those tumors associated with such an exposure, there is a predominance of males around 60 years of age, with the ethmoid sinus being the favored location.[82-84] The tumors are unilateral, friable masses producing nonspecific symptoms.

Histologically, some studies have attempted to subclassify or grade tumors on architectural or cytologic grounds.[78,82,83] Colonic and papillary types appear to be the most common (Fig. 48-22). Most tumors are mucin positive, and there are some with argentaffin granules, ultrastructural neuroendocrine granules, and exocrine (Paneth cell type) granules.[82,86] Cervical node metastases have been noted in 8% to 12% of cases,[82] an observation that would appear not to justify routine neck dissection. Distant metastases have been reported in 30% of high-grade tumors.[78] The 5-year survival for occupationally related cases is about 50%[82] and is similar to those reports not employing histologic grading.[84,85] In one study, 78% of patients with high-grade tumors died of tumor, most within 3 years,[78] but survivals of up to 20 years have been reported.[85]

Other malignant tumors

Olfactory neuroblastoma (ONB) is the best recognized entity in an unusual group of nasal and sinus tumors that includes small cell carcinoma[87] and sinonasal undifferentiated carcinoma (SNUC).[88] ONB occurs in both children and adults, with an average age of onset of about 40 years. Males and females are equally affected. Predominant symptoms are nasal stuffiness and epistaxis but may include proptosis and facial asymmetry. It is typified by a unilateral nasal mass with involvement of a sinus cavity and the cribriform plate (Fig. 48-23).

Historically, there has been a histologic range recognized for ONB as represented by the former terminology: "esthesioneuroblastoma," "esthesioneuroepithelioma," and "esthesioneurocytoma." The morphologic range is, however, best represented by two groups. The well-differentiated tumors are those that most closely resemble the typical pediatric visceral neuroblastomas and manifest as confluent nests of small, monotonous nuclei set in an abundant pink, fibrillary stroma (Fig. 48-24). Pseudorosettes may be common. The poorly differentiated variety exhibits a scant or absent fibrillary background. In such tumors broad sheets of epithelial-like cells contain occasional true rosettes. Areas of hemorrhage and necrosis are prominent. The fibrillary background corresponds ultrastructurally to axonal processes containing dense and lucent vesicles, microtubules, and filaments. Ultrastructural granules and cell processes may be seen in the poorly differentiated variant but are less common.

Both variants exhibit positive staining for cytokeratin, neurofilament, and S-100 protein.[89] The cytokeratin reactivity in well-differentiated ONB has no ultrastructural correlate and is unexplained. In both types, the S-100–positive cells exhibit a sustentacular distribution and correlate with the identification of Schwann cells by electron microscopy.[89] Although Schwann cells are seen in both pediatric neuroblastoma and ONB, the former often exhibits ganglion cell differentiation and has not been found reactive to cytokeratin.

The morphologic distinction of poorly differentiated ONB and small cell carcinomas in this region can be subtle so that clinical relevance is questionable. The most important clinical issue remains the resectability of the tumors.[90] Staging systems[91,92] help to assess prognosis, though no staging system has received uniform clinical acceptance. The 5-year survival rate for low-stage neuroblastomas ranges from 77% to 100%; for advanced tumors, the survival rate drops to 50% or less.[91,92] Patients treated with combinations of surgery and radiation seem to do best.[92]

In the nose and paranasal sinuses, *melanoma* is rare. These tumors account for about 1% of all melanomas.[93] Two thirds

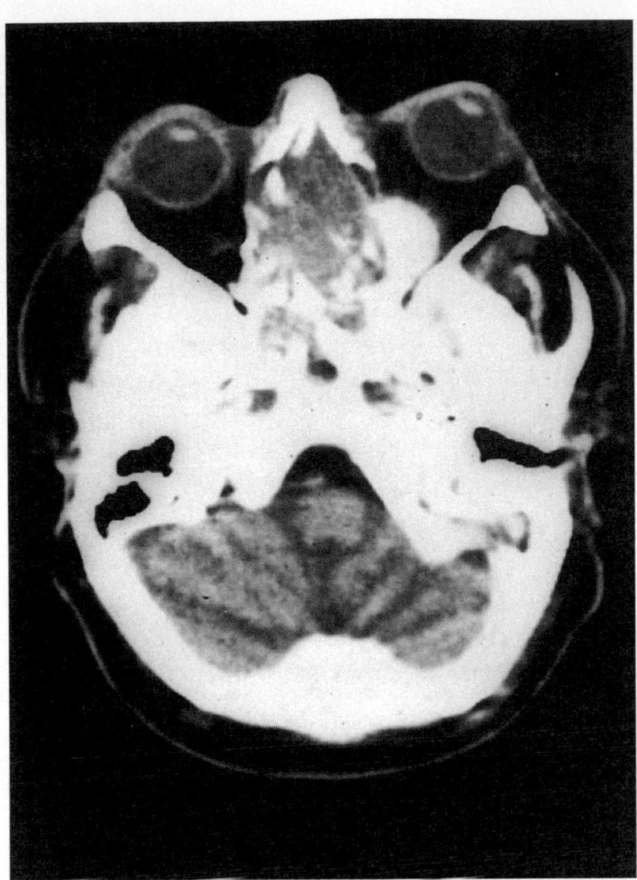

Fig. 48-23 Olfactory neuroblastoma. CT scan showing a destructive nasal mass involving the cribriform plate.

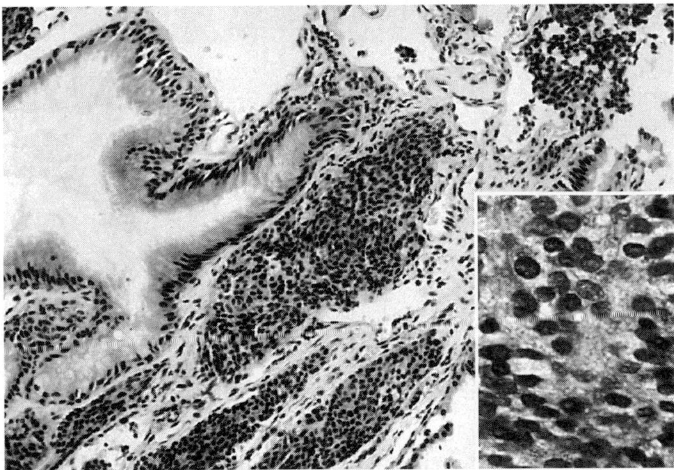

Fig. 48-24 Well-differentiated olfactory neuroblastoma. Nasal mucosa with nests of small tumor cells and scant intercellular fibrillary material. *Inset,* small tumor cells with more abundant fibrillary material.

of these melanomas are on the lateral nasal wall or septum.[94] The maxillary antrum is most frequently affected. Even in this location, whites are disproportionately affected, though in Japanese and blacks the rates are higher than would be anticipated from the respective cutaneous incidence in these populations.[94]

In contrast to their cutaneous counterparts, nasal melanomas show no association with sun exposure and a rarity of histologic precursor lesions. Junctional activity was seen in 5 of 14 cases in one report.[95] Historically, pigmentation of the tumor was an important diagnostic criterion, and therefore the number of reported cases may not be accurate. Nasal melanoma occurs equally in elderly males and females, though the older literature indicates a male predominance, with a median age of about 70 years.[95,96] Light microscopic morphology is not prognostically significant. Small-cell, spindle-cell, epithelioid, and pleomorphic variants of melanoma can be misinterpreted for carcinoma with similar morphology.[95] Immunohistochemistry for S-100 protein and melanoma antigen HMB-45 can be useful to identify melanocytic differentiation. In recent literature, the tumor demonstrates a high rate of local recurrence and disseminated metastases. Five-year survival rates range from 0% to 33%.[95-97]

Primary sinonasal *lymphoma* differs from other extranodal lymphomas by the higher incidence of T-cell phenotypes. T-cell lymphoma in Asian populations is a relatively common tumor and includes its occurrence in the nose. However, even in the West, where nasal lymphoma is uncommon, there are more T-cell lymphomas than would be expected based on their occurrence in peripheral lymph nodes.[98] In both populations, there is an unexplained association of Epstein-Barr virus (EBV) antigens in these lymphomas, detected by in situ hybridization in 13 out of 14 cases in one study.[99] The pathogenetic role of EBV in this context is not yet defined. About 40% of sinonasal lymphomas are of the large cell type.[98,99] This high-grade morphology may signify an aggressive tumor.[100]

Extramedullary *plasmacytoma* of the sinonasal region is histologically similar to plasmacytomas of bone or multiple myeloma. Clinically, extramedullary plasmacytoma appears as a locally aggressive tumor without serum abnormalities. There may be a slight male predominance, and the patients are elderly. Grossly the tumors are raised, submucosal lesions with fleshy, dark red-gray surfaces, primarily involving the nasal cavity.[101,102] The monoclonal plasma cell proliferation can be detected immunohistochemically by staining for kappa and lambda light chains, thus helping to differentiate extramedullary plasmacytoma from other inflammatory lesions containing nonneoplastic plasma cells. These lesions may recur locally and occasionally evolve into systemic myeloma, but this usually occurs over a period of years.

NASOPHARYNX

Development and normal anatomy

The nasopharynx (NP) is an endodermally derived, pouchlike cranial extension of the developing foregut (Fig. 48-1). It is the most superiorly located portion of the pharynx just above the level of the soft palate. Anteriorly, the NP is defined by the nasal choanae, communicating directly with the nasal cavities. Posteriorly is the skull base; laterally located are the eustachian tubes. Just posterior and lateral to the eustachian tubes is the pharyngeal recess, or fossa of Rosenmüller, lined by respiratory mucosa with partial cartilaginous support.

The NP is lined by a pseudostratified ciliated epithelium with occasional patches of squamous cells. On the posterior wall beneath the respiratory mucosa is the lymphoid tissue of the pharyngeal tonsils, which when enlarged are recognized pathologically as adenoids. Lymphatic drainage is via the retropharyngeal and high internal jugular nodes, which are of clinical importance in evaluating primary malignancies in this area. Remnants of Rathke's pouch and notochord are common in the roof of the NP,[3,103] though their pathologic significance as sources of tumors is minor.

Benign tumors

Benign neoplasms of the NP are rare. Possibly the most common is the *juvenile nasopharyngeal angiofibroma*, which is peculiarly restricted to adolescent and young adult men. Because of these demographics and a few reports of tumor shrinkage in response to exogenous estrogens, it has been alleged that these tumors are related to the fluctuating androgenic stimulation and hormonal imbalance of puberty. The patients do not manifest clinical evidence of endocrine dysfunction. Serum measurements of estrogen are normal, and assays of tumors for estrogen and progesterone receptors are negative.[104] Androgen receptors have been demonstrated in the tumor.[104] Tumors were successfully transplanted to both male and female nude mice but did not continue to grow spontaneously and failed to grow in response to androgen administration.[105] In vitro, the tumor was likewise not successfully stimulated by androgens.[105] The effect of androgens on the occurrence and growth of this tumor is therefore still unclear.

Juvenile nasopharyngeal angiofibroma originates in the region of the sphenopalatine foramen and affects individuals ranging in age from about 5 years to the early 30s (mean age of about 15 years). The major symptoms are obstruction and epistaxis, which can be brisk and occasionally life threatening. The tumor easily fills the NP and extends along natural planes and foramina to involve contiguous nasal and sinus cavities, producing bone erosion and occasionally intracranial extension. Historically, anterior bowing of the posterior wall of the maxillary sinus on plain films or tomography was considered a diagnostic radiographic finding. Most modern imaging is done by computerized tomography or magnetic resonance imaging, which are more sensitive indicators of the distribution of the lesion. Nevertheless, many patients are diagnosed with advanced disease; in one series, 50% of patients had intracranial involvement at the time of diagnosis.[106]

The tumors appear as firm, smoothly contoured, pink-tan masses with clinically apparent prominent surface vascularity (Fig. 48-25). Histologically, the lesions are composed of staghorn and irregularly shaped thin-walled vascular spaces together with a fibrous stroma of variable cellularity (Fig. 48-26). The nuclei of the stromal cells exhibit dense inclusions (probably composed of nucleic acid), clearly visible by electron microscopy. These inclusions are especially prominent in virgin tumors and can also be visualized by light microscopy[107] (Fig. 48-27).

Surgery is the usual treatment, with blood loss a common complication.[108,109] Recurrences are usually apparent within 18 months of the initial surgery. The recurrence rates vary and can be as high as 36%.[109] Radiotherapy is usually reserved for tumors (or recurrences) with intracranial extension.

Pituitary adenomas may appear in the NP or sphenoid sinus. The most common mechanism is by direct extension of an intrasellar lesion; this occurs in about 2% of pituitary adenomas.[110] Tumors typically occur in elderly patients who have the usual nasal symptoms of obstruction and epistaxis but also

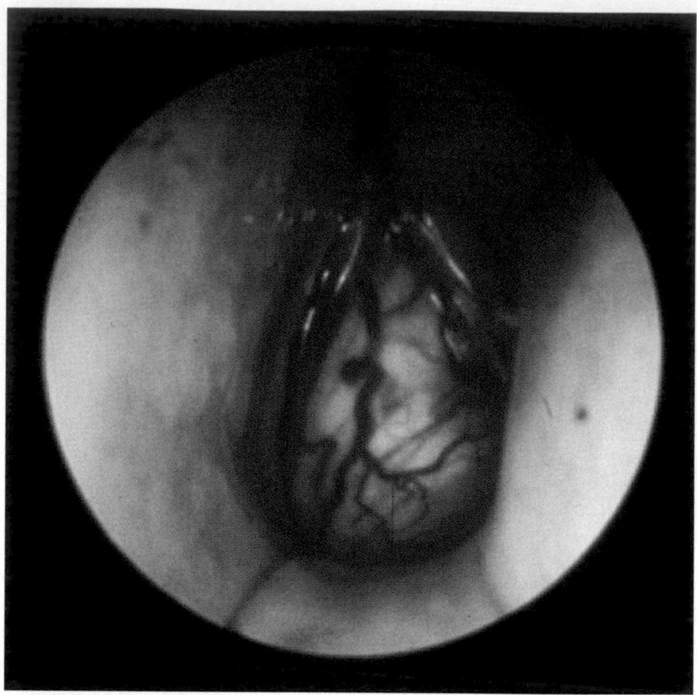

Fig. 48-25 Juvenile nasopharyngeal angiofibroma as viewed through a nasal speculum. Mass with obvious prominent surface vascularity fills the nasal cavity.

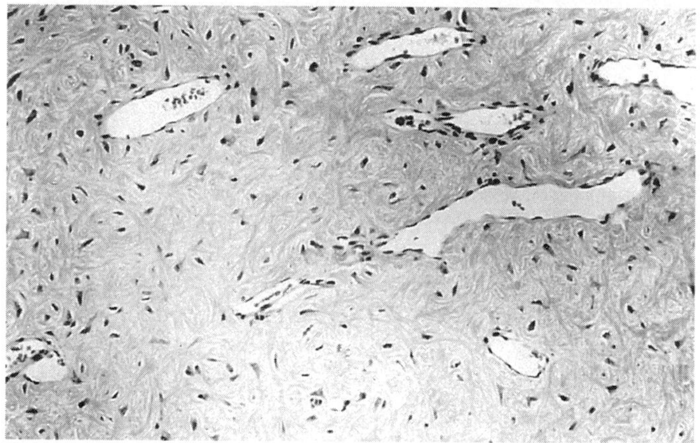

Fig. 48-26 Juvenile nasopharyngeal angiofibroma with numerous gaping, irregular vessels and dense fibrous stroma.

exhibit clinical features of a pituitary adenoma: various hormonal dysfunctions, impotence, and visual-field abnormalities. A more unusual finding is a nasopharyngeal or sphenoid sinus pituitary adenoma with a normal anterior pituitary.[111] The explanation for this phenomenon centers on embryologic residua from the migration of Rathke's pouch. These patients are approached by standard transsphenoidal surgery. The normal array of major pituitary hormones has been found, though the clinical significance of the pattern of hormone expression is speculative.[112]

Nasopharyngeal carcinoma

Nasopharyngeal carcinoma (NPC) accounts for 85% of malignant tumors in this anatomic site. Historically, this biologically

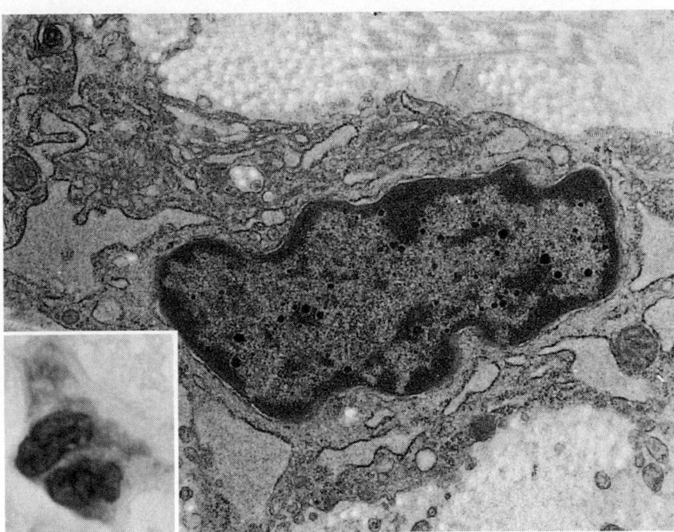

Fig. 48-27 Juvenile nasopharyngeal angiofibroma. Electron micrograph of stromal cell with numerous intranuclear inclusions, characteristic of this tumor. *Inset,* JNA binucleate stromal cell with intranuclear inclusions photographed under oil immersion.

Table 48-5 WHO histologic classification of nasopharyngeal carcinoma

Squamous cell carcinoma
Keratinization or intercellular bridges, or both
Nonkeratinizing carcinoma
Defined cell borders, pavement-like pattern
Undifferentiated carcinoma
Syncytial growth, large polygonal cells (with occasional spindle-shaped cells), prominent nucleoli, lymphoid stroma

distinct form of head and neck cancer has been described under many terms. The present preferred World Health Organization (WHO) terminology regards NPC as a continuum in the differentiation of squamous cell carcinoma (Table 48-5).[113] In this classification, undifferentiated carcinoma (UC) corresponds to what has been historically recognized by pathologists as *lymphoepithelioma,* the most generic but best-understood term among physicians treating this neoplasm. Of the three categories of NPC, UC is the most common, regardless of the patient's age or race, and accounts for 60% to 80% of cases.[114-117]

Few human tumors have been studied epidemiologically as much as NPC has. Males predominate (male/female ratio of 2:1 to 3:1), with the average age of onset being about 50; The tumor is unusual in children.[115,118,119] It is a relatively common malignancy in the provinces of southeast China, where it constitutes about 30% of all cancers and 63% of all malignant head and neck tumors.[119] An increased familial risk for NPC has been suggested to be attributable to HLA-B17 and HLA-Bw46 phenotypes. The nitrosamine-laden brine used by southern Chinese in salting fish may have a carcinogenic influence. Among other Asians, Filipinos have an incidence less than that of the Chinese but greater than that of other Asians or of whites.[118,120] The use of herbal medicines containing phorbol esters has been linked to the relatively high incidence of NPC in the Philippines.[120] Cigarette smoking and alcohol consumption, though not commonly implicated in the genesis of this tumor, may in fact predispose the individual to the development of NPC.[121] NPC is much less common in whites, and in the Western world it accounts for less than 1% of all cancers.

Table 48-6 Epstein-Barr virus expression in nasopharyngeal carcinoma

Epstein-Barr nuclear antigen (EBNA)*
Latent protein
Types 1, 2, 3a-3c, and leader protein
Latent cycle membrane proteins*
Latent membrane protein (LMP)
Terminal protein 1
Terminal protein 2
EB early RNA†

*Genome is 10 to 40 kilo–base pairs in length.
†Short RNA segment (<170 nucleotides).

The most investigated factor in the development of NPC is EBV. Once acquired, this ubiquitous virus remains latent in B-lymphocytes and epithelial cells of the oral, pharyngeal, cervical, and salivary gland epithelia for the life of the host. In NPC, the virus is reactivated, and its products can be detected serologically in the form of greatly elevated levels of IgA antibodies to viral capsid antigen and IgG antibodies to early antigen.[116,122] Virus may be demonstrated within the tumor itself, either immunohistochemically or by application of molecular biology techniques to detect gene products or nucleotide sequences (Table 48-6). Of the several antigens expressed by reactivated latent cells, the EB nuclear antigens (EBNAs) and latent membrane proteins (LMPs) have been the most studied.[123-125] EBV DNA sequences have been identified within tumor cells.[126] In situ hybridization has detected an EBV-associated RNA nucleotide segment (EBER) within tumor cells.[127] One or more of these virus-related macromolecules will be expressed by virtually all NPC, primary or metastatic. Although their function or functions are unknown, they may be regarded as diagnostic markers for NPC in cases for which the histopathologic features are difficult or the clinical setting is unusual.

NPC is usually clinically advanced by the time of diagnosis, regardless of age or race and despite symptoms of only a few months in duration.[116,117,122,128] The presumed origin in the fossa of Rosenmüller produces local bulk within the nasopharynx and results in ear symptoms (fullness, tinnitus, or deafness) in 40% to 70% of cases. Nasal bleeding occurs in 30% to 80% of cases. A neck mass, indicating nodal metastasis, is present in 60% to 80% of patients.[114-117] Similar to squamous cancer of the paranasal sinus, in situ carcinoma is detected infrequently. In one series of 187 patients, only 18 had NPC in situ.[129]

The primary lesion, even in patients with nodal metastasis, may be small or clinically difficult to visualize. The diagnosis is usually made by examination of an excised cervical lymph node, or possibly by a nodal aspiration. This may be followed by endoscopic examination of the NP together with a biopsy. Histologically the typical undifferentiated carcinoma appears as broad sheets of large cells with vesicular nuclei, large

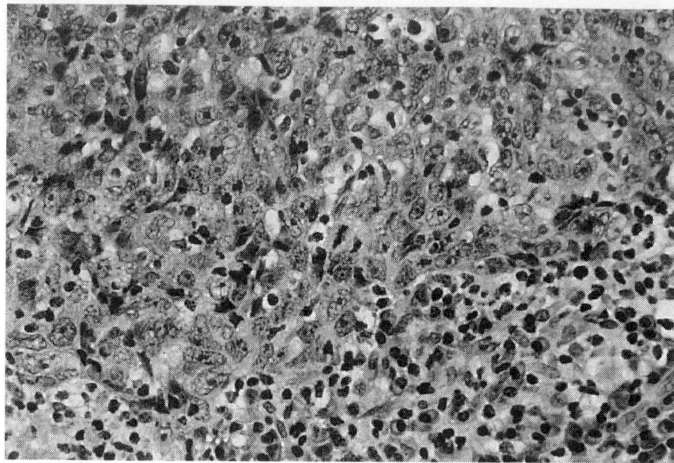

Fig. 48-28 Nasopharyngeal carcinoma, undifferentiated type. Broad sheet of large, polygonal cells with vesicular nuclei and prominent nucleoli. There is no evidence of cytoplasmic differentiation. Tumor cells are surrounded by a prominent mature lymphoid infiltrate.

prominent nucleoli, and indistinct cell borders (Fig. 48-28). Fusiform tumor cells are not unusual. Despite this high-grade appearance, immunohistochemistry for keratin is strongly positive; electron microscopy uniformly demonstrates well-formed desmosomes and tonofilaments.[130] These features support the squamous epithelial nature of this light-microscopically undifferentiated tumor. The density of the lymphoid stroma is variable but typically intense. The lymphocytes are small, mature cells, forming the local milieu, and are not part of the neoplasm.

The advanced clinical stage at diagnosis notwithstanding, most patients will respond initially to radiation. However, the 5-year survival rate is about 50%, with bone being a frequent site of distant metastases.[115,116,126]

LARYNX

Development and normal anatomy

The larynx first appears around the third embryonic week as the developing endoderm is being divided by a groove, separating the digestive (dorsal) from the respiratory (ventral) tracts. The cranial portion of the ventral division becomes the epiglottis and larynx with mesenchymal contributions (hyoid bone, external cartilage plates, skeletal muscle) from branchial arches 3, 4 (epiglottis), and 6 (larynx). Between the seventh and tenth weeks the larynx is closed but becomes recanalized, during which process the true and false cords are formed.[1] Laryngeal atresia and the webs or bands encountered in newborns with stridor may be attributed to abnormalities in this recanalization.[2]

The fully developed larynx extends from the tip of the epiglottis to the inferior margin of the cricoid cartilage. Functionally, there are three parts: (1) the supraglottis, consisting of the epiglottis, false cord, ventricle, and saccule; (2) the glottis, consisting of the true cord and anterior commissure; and (3) the subglottis, consisting of the lower border of the true cord to the end of the cricoid cartilage. This classification is useful when one is considering the lymphatic drainage pattern, which determines the route of tumor spread—cranial from the supraglottis and caudal from the subglottis. True glottic lymphatics are scant.[3]

Histologically, nonkeratinizing squamous epithelium lines the lingual aspect of the epiglottis and its upper laryngeal aspect. This gradually merges with a pseudostratified ciliated columnar epithelium, which continues along the false cord and lines the ventricle. Squamous epithelium also occupies the superior and glottic aspects of the true cord and then blends with respiratory epithelium on the inferior surface. Seromucinous glands are diffusely present, except on the true cord, and connect to the surface.

Nonneoplastic disease

Acute laryngitis

Acute laryngitis, part of the syndrome of clinical croup, is a common pediatric condition of seasonal cold weather occurrence and of viral origin. The principal agents, parainfluenza virus or respiratory syncytial virus, can be detected by direct immunofluorescence on respiratory epithelium[131] (Fig. 48-29).

Acute epiglottitis

Acute epiglottitis is a more serious and primarily pediatric condition, though adults may also be severely affected. An indurated, hyperemic epiglottis causes airway obstruction in patients with fever and stridor. Blood cultures most often recover *H. influenzae* type b, which may also cause sepsis and prostration.[132,133] This disease can be fatal though it responds to antibiotic treatment. Fungi may afflict the laryngeal structures, but such affliction is exceptionally rare.[134]

Laryngeal inflammation also occurs in the setting of systemic disease. *Relapsing polychondritis,* possibly an autoimmune disease, is an intermittently active chronic inflammatory process that is progressively invasive and destroys cartilaginous tissue, especially in the head and neck. It is probably related to and may be clinically concurrent with other autoimmune diseases, especially vasculitis.[135,136]

Laryngeal ulcers

Laryngeal ulcers may be related to prior intubation, radiation, or gastroesophageal reflux.[137-139] In most instances, the clinical history will obviate the need for biopsy. Reflux may be responsible for so-called contact ulcers, typically occurring on

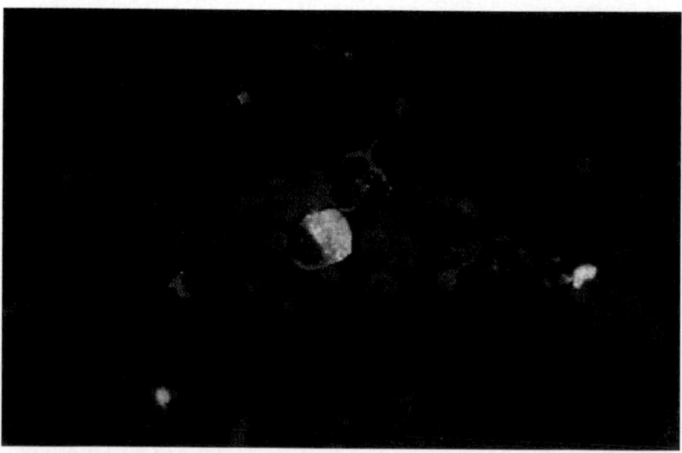

Fig. 48-29 Croup. Respiratory epithelial cells with positive direct immunofluorescence for respiratory syncytial virus.

the posterior third of the true cord. Vocal abuse or chronic throat clearing also play an etiologic role.[138] Radiation-related lesions may exhibit atypical stromal cells within florid granulation tissue.[137]

Vocal nodules and polyps

Vocal nodules and polyps are common nonneoplastic tumefactions related to vocal abuse. Although nodules occur on the anterior true cord or anterior commissure and polyps may, in addition, originate from the ventricle, they are covered by an intact or slightly hyperplastic squamous epithelium (Fig. 48-30). The lesion is composed of edematous, loose connective tissue with occasional atypical cells, and deposits of fibrinoid material, not to be confused with amyloid (Fig. 48-31). These pathologic features are similar to the findings in *polypoid degeneration,* a chronic condition involving the entire length of one or both vocal folds, and probably related to cigarette smoking.[140]

Amyloid

Amyloid deposits in the larynx may present as slowly growing mass lesions. Although an underlying cause is rarely found, occasional rare cases of primary systemic amyloidosis and multiple myeloma have been recorded.[141] Histologically, submucosal confluent nodules of pink, hyaline material are surrounded by a foreign body giant cells chronic inflammatory cells. These lesions may recur, and repeated surgical excisions may result in periglottic scarring with vocal cord dysfunction.[141,142]

Cysts

Cysts in the larynx occur over a broad age range, mainly affecting people in their 60s without any sex preference. Most cysts are encountered in the region of the true cord, vallecula-epiglottis, or ventricle and are solitary. Hoarseness, pain, and foreign-body sensation are prominent symptoms.

The classification of these lesions has traditionally been clinically based on location, size, and relationship to the surface mucosa.[143] In this system, *ductal cysts* are the most common and occur typically in adults. These small (<0.5 cm) lesions occur close to the surface at any location and are assumed to arise as retention cysts from minor salivary gland ducts (Fig. 48-32). *Saccular cysts* are supraglottic and range in diameter from 1 to 7 cm. They are assumed to arise congeni-

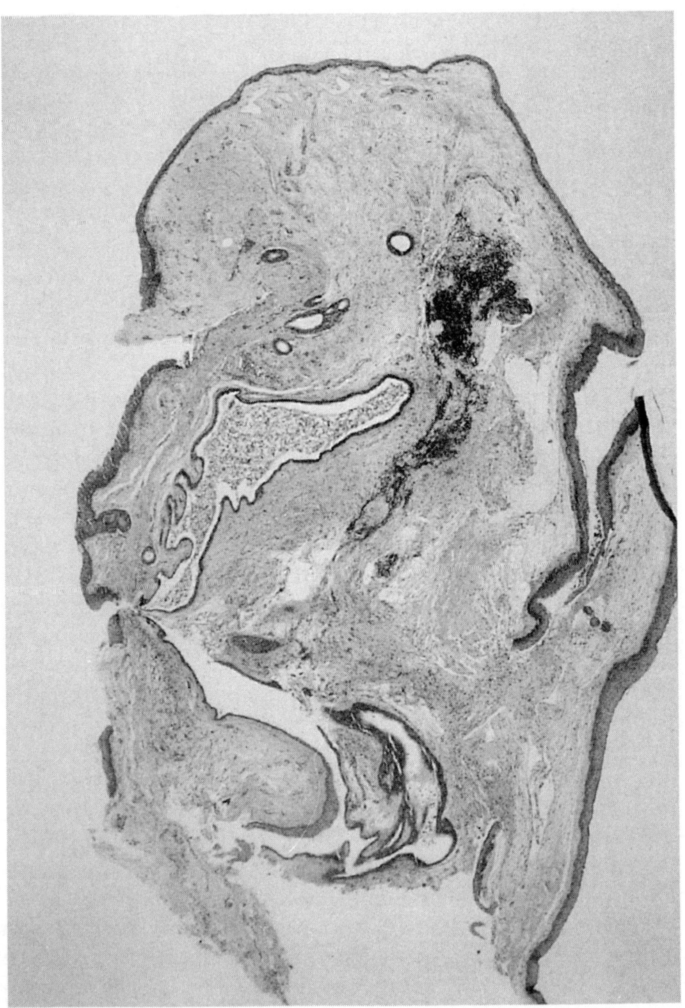

Fig. 48-30 Vocal nodule (singer's node). Polypoid mass with intact epithelium and edematous stroma.

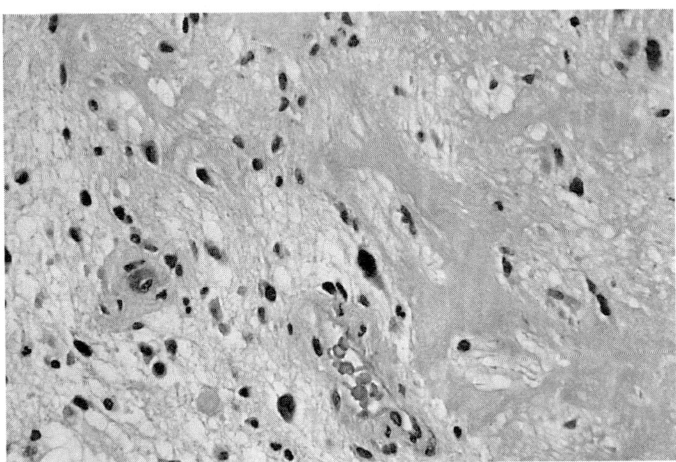

Fig. 48-31 Vocal nodule. Hyaline deposits within the stroma appear similar to amyloid. An occasional stromal cell with reactive atypia is common.

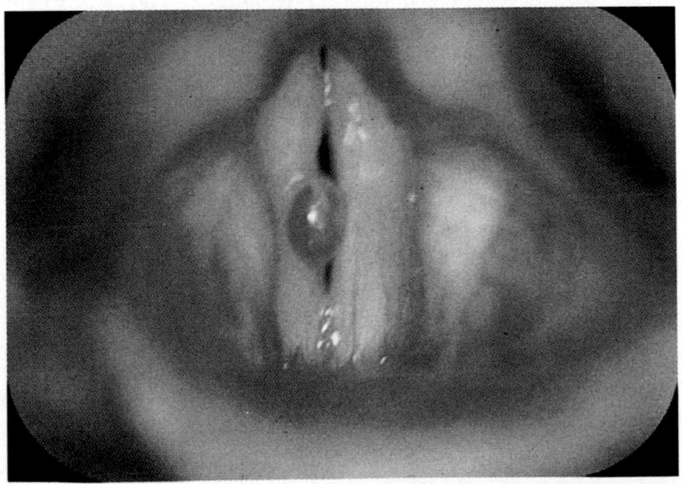

Fig. 48-32 Endoscopic view of a cyst of the left true cord.

Table 48-7 Respiratory papillomatosis: locations

Site	Frequency of involvement (%)
Lung	2.5
Nasal vestibule	2.6
Nasopharynx	3.0
Bronchi	5.2
Palate	10.3
Trachea	10.9
Epiglottis	11.6
Larynx	97.9

Modified from Kashima H, Mounts P, Leventhal B et al: *Ann Otol Rhinol Laryngol* 102:580, 1993.

tally from the laryngeal saccule, which may account for their tendency to overhang the glottis. Cysts in this location are more common in children and may require numerous endoscopies with drainage of air or inspissated contents that may be occasionally infected. The course may be complicated by subglottic stenosis.[144]

The histologic features of the cysts have not generally been emphasized but may have clinical significance. In one study of adult cases, almost one half of the cysts were lined by squamous epithelium and associated with patches of lymphoid tissue, similar to tonsillar crypts. Other "tonsillar cysts" were lined by cuboidal or respiratory epithelium overlying lymphoid aggregates of variable sizes.[145] No recurrences were noted. Cysts lined by oncocytic epithelium probably represent part of a diffuse metaplastic change, the stimulus for which is not known but may be related to age. Oncocytic cysts predominate in the ventricle and the false cord and have a small rate of recurrence.[145,146]

Benign tumors and tumorlike conditions

Respiratory papillomatosis

Respiratory papillomatosis, a benign, multifocal distribution of *squamous papillomas,* involves the larynx in nearly 98% of cases[147] (Table 48-7). This is a chronically remitting and relapsing condition affecting both children and adults with an equal sex distribution. The long-standing suspicion that this disease is virally mediated has been supported by the ultrastructural finding of viral particles.[148] More recently, HPV types 6 and 11 have been identified either by Southern blotting, polymerase chain reaction, or in situ hybridization in almost every lesion studied[149-152] (Fig. 48-33). HPV DNA as well as HPV types 6 and 11 have also been detected in laryngeal mucosa that is uninvolved by tumor.[149,150] However, the etiologic significance of HPV is controversial.

In children, the assumption has been that the virus is acquired by fetal aspiration during vaginal delivery from mothers who carry HPV. Retrospective analyses indicate that 30% to 50% of affected children had an HPV-carrying mother.[150,153] However, as recently summarized, the incidence of laryngeal papillomatosis in prospective population studies is zero.[153] Furthermore, the female genital tract harbors other viral types in addition to types 6 and 11, none of which have been identified in the laryngeal lesions. Adult lesions would have to be explained by a prolonged latency of the virus,

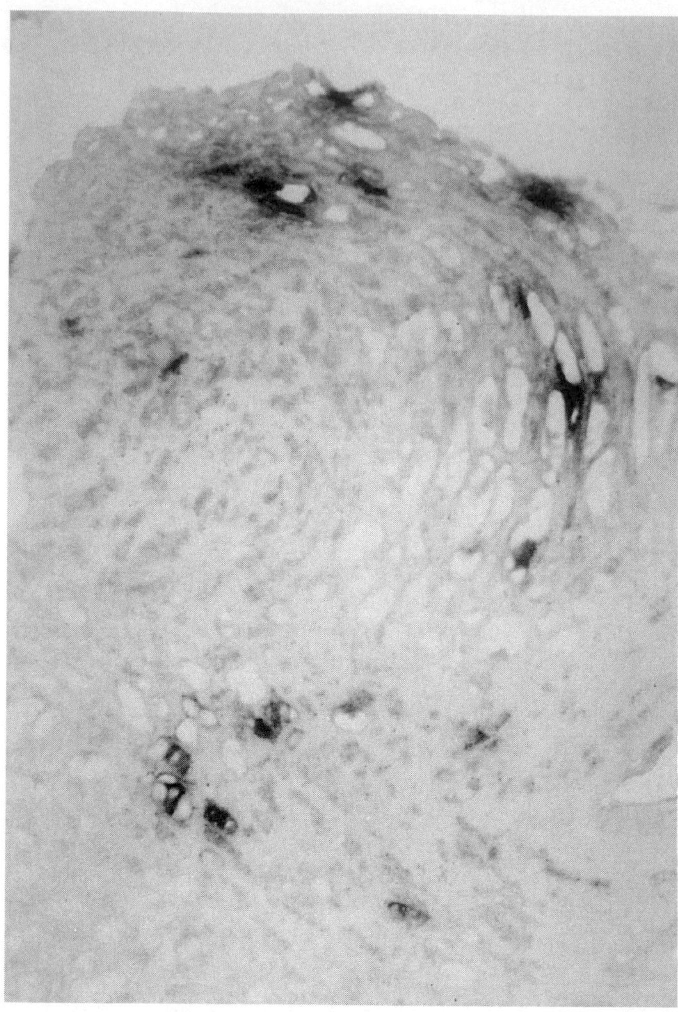

Fig. 48-33 Laryngeal papilloma. Positive immunostain using a biotinylated probe for HPV 6/11. (Alkaline phosphatase chromogen.)

which was indeed acquired at birth. It is possible that HPV is a relevant but not the only factor in the genesis and recurrent behavior of laryngeal papillomatosis. There appears to be no correlation between the type of HPV and the nature of the subsequent clinical course.

In children, the incidence of laryngeal papillomatosis peaks at 2 to 3 years of age and is characterized by multiple small lesions on and about the true cords and supraglottis. Adult cases, most common at 20 to 45 years of age, are usually solitary and less extensive if multifocal. Recurrences are less prominent in adults but remain a potential, serious clinical issue. In children regrowth may occasionally occur in periods as short as 1 or 2 months. There is a suggestion that recurrences appear at junctions of squamous and respiratory mucosa.[147] Unproved in this context is the contribution of the continued trauma of surgery, including tracheostomy, to the induction of recurrences as it promotes development of metaplastic squamous epithelium. Nevertheless, the management strategy is the resection of lesions as symptoms warrant with minimizing of long-term scarring. Radiation should be avoided, since it has been linked to the development of laryngeal squamous carcinoma.[154]

Histologically, most papillomas are exophytic, consisting of a delicate fibrovascular core covered by maturing, nonkeratinizing squamous epithelium with occasional dyskeratosis (Fig. 48-34). Koilocytosis, reflecting the presence of virus, is easily identified in such lesions. A nagging issue for pathologists has been the biologic significance of intramucosal dysplasia often seen in these lesions, represented by increasing cellularity, cytologic atypia, and mitotic activity (Fig. 48-35). The appearance of dysplasia can be confusing, but despite the alarming histopathology, invasive squamous carcinoma develops only rarely.[150,151,155] Dysplastic features may in fact correlate with rapid papilloma regrowth, not with impending malignancy, and probably do not require more than conservative removal and continued clinical surveillance.[155]

The disease may run a lifetime course. The remission rates for both children and adults are at about 35%.[150] Rarely, there is extensive local disease together with involvement of the lower respiratory tract, namely, the trachea, bronchi, and lungs. The reason for such extensive distribution is not clear, but it can result in pneumonia, abscess, destruction of pulmonary parenchyma, and death. It is in this aggressive clinical context that cytologically benign papillomatous growths invade vascular channels, lymph nodes, and soft tissue. Some of these nonirradiated cases also manifest the spontaneous development of invasive squamous carcinoma.[156,157] HPV type 11 has been identified in such malignancy and in the coexistent papillomas.[157,158]

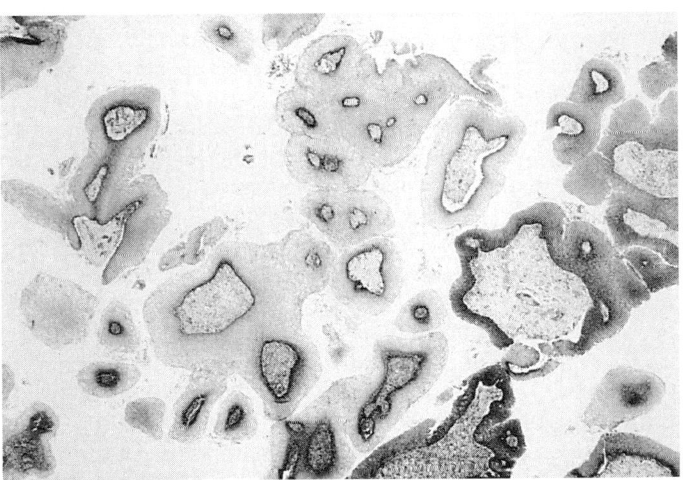

Fig. 48-34 Laryngeal papillomatosis. Numerous squamous papillomas from a 1-year-old girl. Notice differences in cell densities: less cellular papillomas on left have more obvious koilocytosis; more densely cellular on right exhibit dysplasia.

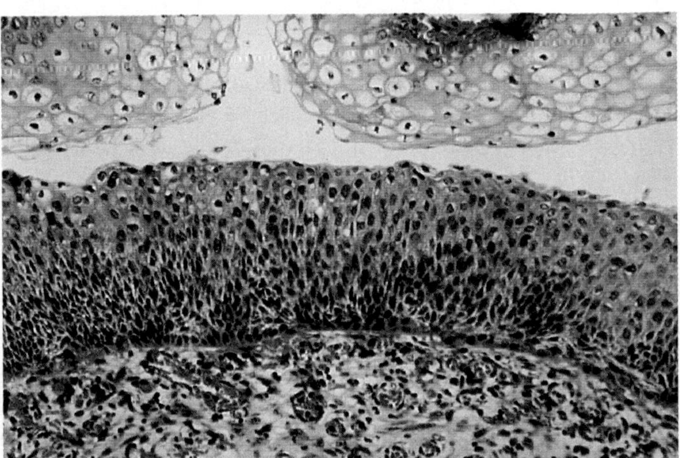

Fig. 48-35 Close apposition of a dysplastic papilloma with residual superficial viral changes, *bottom,* and two top fragments with only viral changes.

Verruca vulgaris

Verruca vulgaris is an unusual, recently described entity that is histologically similar to its cutaneous counterpart. HPV types 6 and 11 have been localized to this lesion.[159] Its distinction from verrucous carcinoma is problematic and controversial. The range of soft-tissue tumors and salivary gland tumors is seen, but rarely.[160] *Benign vascular tumors,* including pyogenic granuloma, are perhaps the most common soft-tissue lesions.

Malignant tumors

Squamous cell carcinomas

Squamous carcinomas account for 95% of laryngeal cancers.[63] Although it is the most common malignancy of the upper airway in adults, it accounts for only about 1.5% of all cancers.[161] Most patients are in their 60s and 70s with 80% to 90% being men.[162-164] In fact, many studies deal exclusively with men.[165-169] Cigarette smoking is the strongest environmental influence, both as an initiator and as a promoter of carcinomatous changes. Nonsmokers with laryngeal carcinoma are an exception. The incidence of second primary tumors in these patients varies but further emphasizes the role of smoking. In one study, 41 of 218 patients with laryngeal carcinoma developed a second primary tumor, 20 of which were lung cancers and 5 of which were separate head and neck lesions.[163]

Heavy alcohol consumption has a significant additive effect with smoking, especially for supraglottic tumors.[167] Other occupational exposures, for example, to asbestos, wood dust, heavy metals, and coal, are associated with a slightly higher risk when adjusted for smoking and alcohol.[164,167] Although several HPV types have been demonstrated in laryngeal carcinoma using a variety of methods, the infrequency of this observation indicates that the carcinogenic influence of HPV in this tumor system is not a strong one.[170] The consumption of carotene containing fruits and vegetables may have a moderating effect on the development of this tumor.[63,164,168]

For the diagnostic pathologist, intraepithelial laryngeal dysplasia presents some controversy. The full-thickness loss of polarity and the absence of maturation and mitoses in the upper strata, which are expected for carcinoma in situ, are not uniformly encountered in the larynx, since disordered growth is often accompanied by surface keratinization[171-173] (Fig. 48-36). Nevertheless, such lesions are often aneuploid, especially those cases manifesting the most severe degrees of cytologic atypia.[171,172] The biologic potential of dysplastic keratinized lesions, both as precursors to histologically typical in situ squamous carcinoma and to invasive cancer, is uncertain.

The frequency of progression of in situ disease is debated. A literature review indicates that untreated carcinoma in situ progresses in 33% to 90% of cases; even treated cases progress to invasive cancer in up to 36% of cases.[174] Progression to invasive disease seems to be a slow process. In an autopsy study of 942 high-risk individuals, the 16% incidence

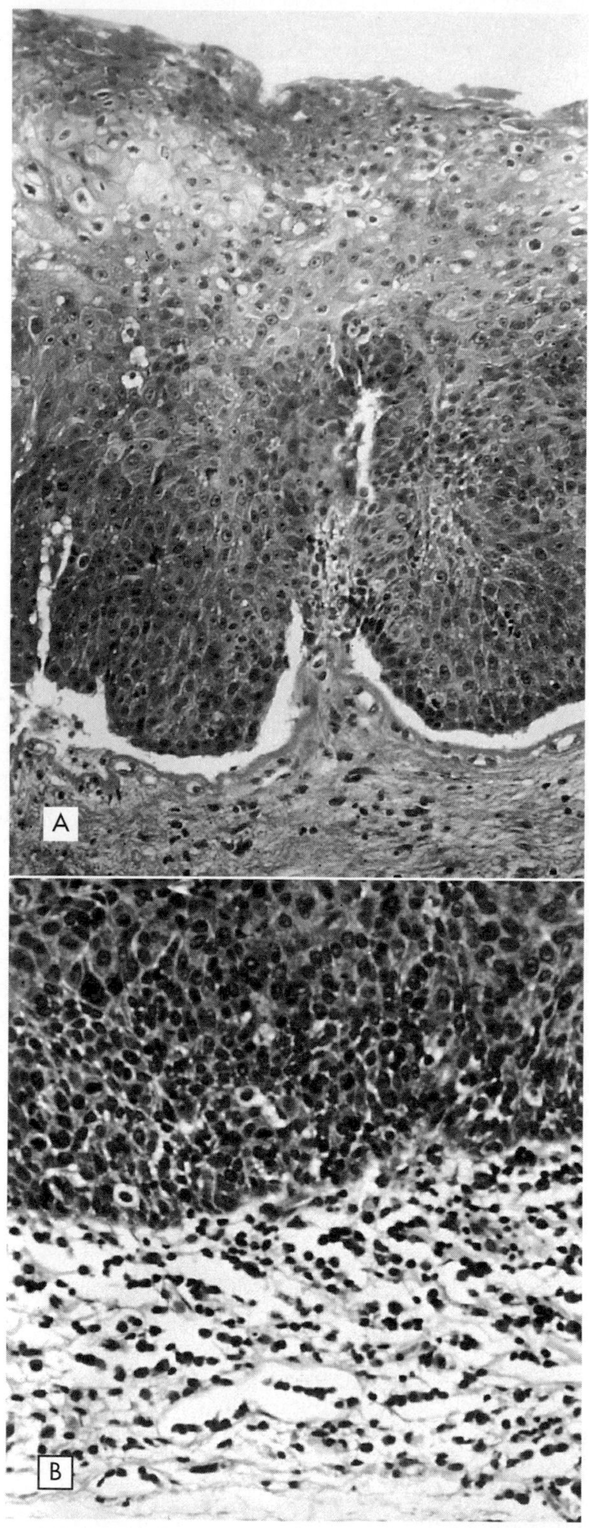

Fig. 48-36 A, Keratinizing intraepithelial dysplasia of larynx. Such lesions are often aneuploid. **B,** Typical in situ squamous carcinoma of larynx. Full-thickness proliferation of primitive cells without maturation.

of in situ carcinoma was accompanied by only 8 cases of invasive squamous carcinoma.[175] In another study, invasive disease supervened over a mean period of more than 50 months and there was only one tumor-related death.[173]

Approximately 75% of invasive laryngeal carcinomas are associated with a recognizable in situ component. Dysphonia, sore throat, foreign-body sensation, and dysphagia frequently bring the patient to clinical attention, though the type and severity of the symptoms depend on the anatomic location. For these typically exophytic or ulcerative lesions, voice quality may be distorted even by small glottic tumors (Fig. 48-37). Supraglottic tumors may grow silently and become apparent when there is grossly bulky disease (Fig. 48-38). Older literature indicated that 60% to 65% of tumors were glottic, 30% to 35% were supraglottic, and the remainder subglottic. Recent literature suggests a distributional change, with nearly half the cases being supraglottic and a more substantial number being transglottic tumors (Table 48-8). Subglottic tumors remain the least frequent.

The TNM staging system is widely utilized to classify laryngeal carcinomas and is the most clinically relevant (Chapter 3). Stage I or stage II lesions are candidates for primary irradiation with or without conservative surgery such as a supraglottic laryngectomy. Stages III or IV may require laryngectomy and node dissections. The direct invasion of the various laryngeal cartilages is uncommon. Factors such as the paucity of glottic or a plethora of supraglottic lymphatics, age, or tumor ulceration are not independently significant.[166,176] Histologic grading has been infrequently and inconsistently employed. Cervical metastatic disease at presentation ranges from 24% to 52%[165,166,169]; distant metastases are uncommon, even in the late stages of disease.

There are two important variants of squamous carcinoma in the larynx. *Verrucous carcinoma* is a broadly based warty growth usually of the glottis, constituting 1% to 4% of all laryngeal carcinomas.[177,178] Despite impressive tumor bulk, cytologic malignancy is absent, and there is no vascular or neural invasion. There is an impressive inflammatory infiltrate at the stromal interface with foreign-body granulomas as a result of extravasated keratin. Earlier fears of inducing anaplastic transformation because of radiation therapy appear unfounded. Metastases are unusual; death is secondary to uncontrolled local disease.

Spindle cell carcinoma

Spindle cell carcinoma is a grossly polypoid or infiltrative lesion composed of malignant spindle cells with a conventional in situ or invasive squamous carcinoma. The spindle cell component gives a positive immunostaining reaction for keratin[179,180] and shows ultrastructural evidence of epithelial differentiation.[179,181] Monophasic spindle cell tumors occasionally demonstrate mesenchymal differentiation and are indistinguishable from true sarcomas.[182]

Miscellaneous malignant tumors

Fewer than 1% of all laryngeal cancers are of nonsquamous epithelial origin.[183] The most common are *neuroendocrine carcinomas,* which range histologically from carcinoids to small cell carcinoma.[184] In addition to histologic features shared with similar tumors in more typical locations, laryngeal tumors are immunohistochemically positive for neuropeptides and serotonin, are associated with paraneoplastic syndromes,

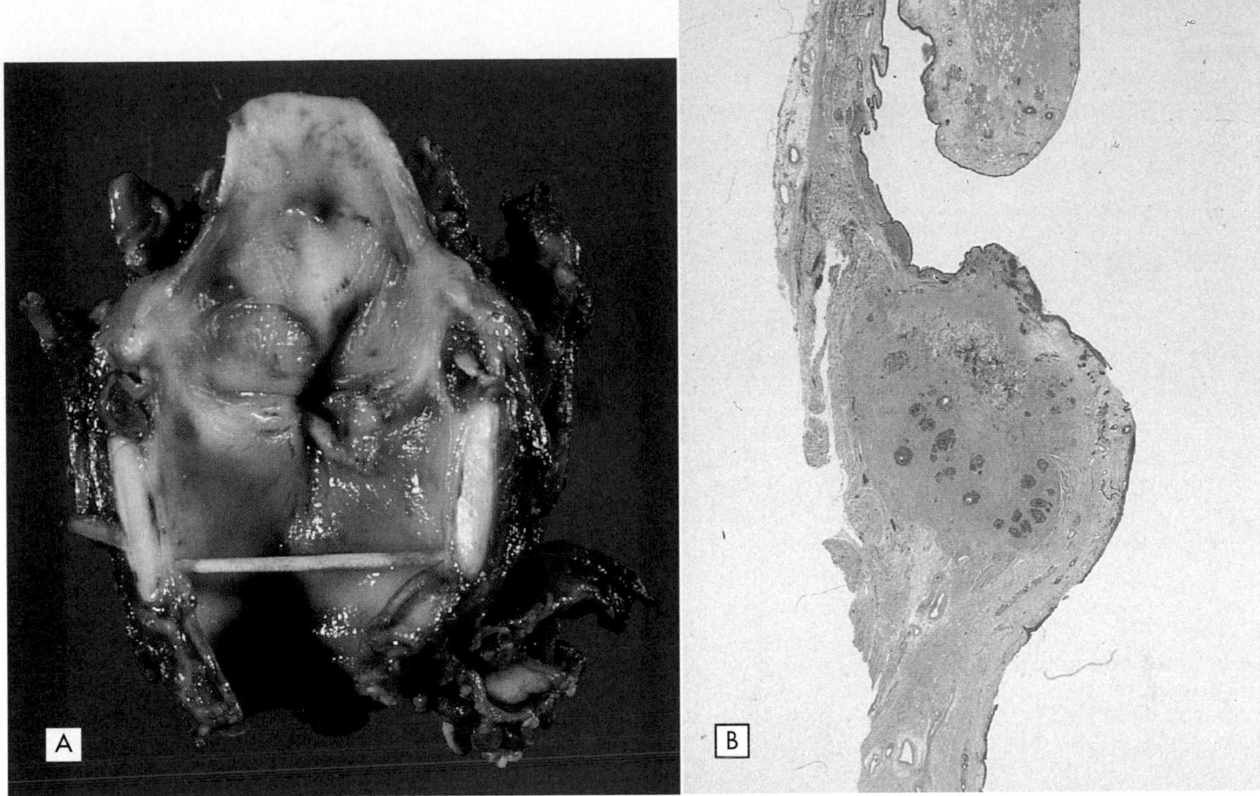

Fig. 48-37 **A,** Laryngectomy for an invasive squamous cell carcinoma of the right true cord, recurrent after initial radiation therapy. Notice small caudal extension but absence of midline crossover. **B,** Vertical section through a squamous carcinoma localized to the true cord. Invasive, keratinized foci can be seen. False cord and ventricle are free of tumor.

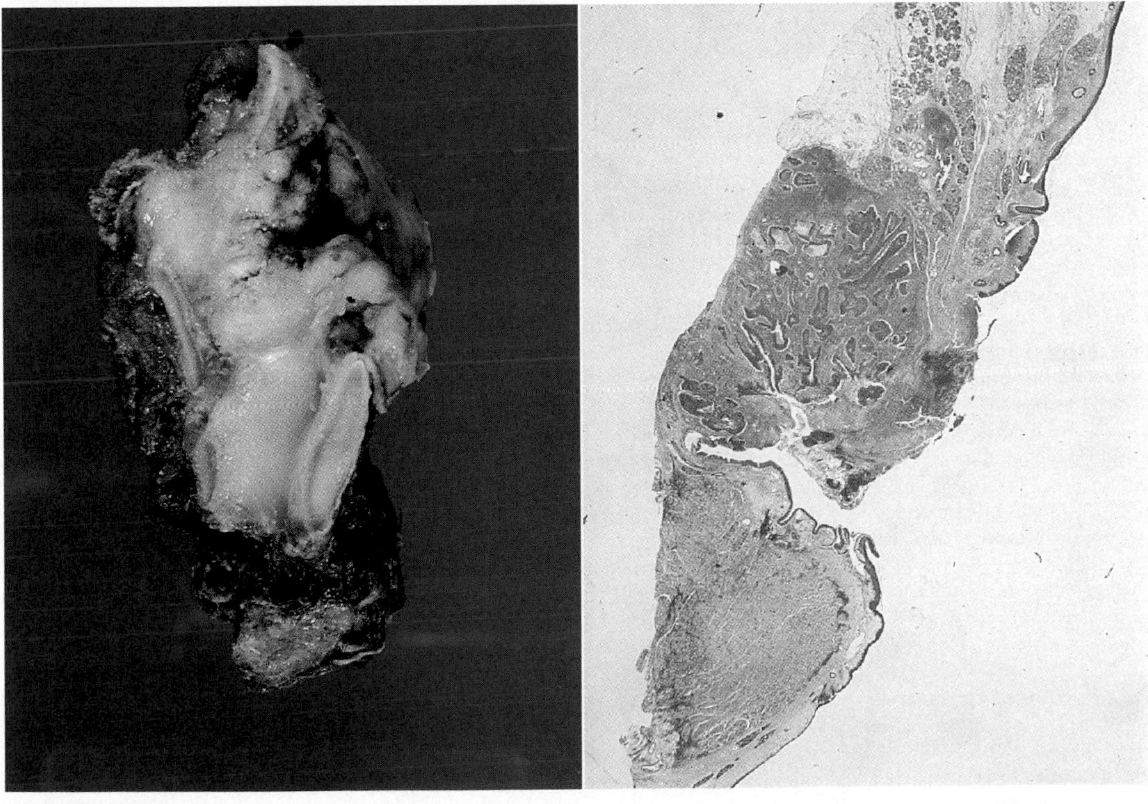

Fig. 48-38 **A,** Sagittal section of a laryngectomy for invasive supraglottic carcinoma involving the epiglottis extending to the region of the false cord. **B,** Vertical section through a supraglottic squamous carcinoma. Mucosal focus of hemorrhage and ulceration is adjacent to a large invasive tumor focus, extending into the ventricle. The true cord is not involved.

Table 48-8 Carcinoma of the larynx: anatomic location

Ref. #	Number of tumors	Location of tumors: Supraglottic	Glottic	Subglottic	Transglottic
165	416	195	137	43	41
166	378	180	83	5	110
168	194	92	94	8	0
169	296	163	127	0	0
TOTAL	1284	630 (49%)	441 (34%)	56 (4%)	151 (11%)

and may even exhibit stromal amyloid.[184,185] Clinical behavior of these tumors is determined by their histology. *Adenoid cystic carcinomas,* 67% of which are subglottic, are morphologically identical to their major salivary gland counterparts.

REFERENCES

Nose and paranasal sinuses

Development and normal anatomy

1. Moore KL, Persaud TVN: *The developing human: clinically oriented embryology,* ed 5, Philadelphia, 1993, Saunders.
2. O'Rahilly R, Muller F: *Human embryology and teratology,* New York, 1992, Wiley-Liss.
3. Fechner RE, Mills SE: Larynx and pharynx. In Sternberg SS, editor: *Histology for pathologists,* New York, 1992, Raven Press.

Malformations

4. Gorlin RJ, Cohen MM Jr, Levin LS: *Syndromes of the head and neck,* ed 2, New York, 1990, Oxford University Press.
5. Milczuk HA, Dalley RW, Wessbacher FW et al: Nasal and paranasal sinus anomalies in children with chronic sinusitis, *Laryngoscope* 103:247, 1993.
6. Stocker JT: The respiratory tract. In Stocker JT, Dehner LP, editors: *Pediatric pathology,* Philadelphia, 1992, Lippincott.
7. Patterson K, Kapur S, Chandra, RS: Nasal gliomas and related brain heterotopias: a pathologist's perspective, *Pediatr Pathol* 5:353, 1986.
8. Gorenstein A, Kern EB, Facer GW et al: Nasal gliomas, *Arch Otolaryngol* 106:536, 1980.
9. Bossen EH, Hudson WR: Oligodendroglioma arising in heterotopic brain tissue of the soft palate and nasopharynx, *Am J Surg Pathol* 11:571, 1987.
10. Friedman RA, Harris JP: Sinusitis, *Annu Rev Med* 42:471, 1991.

Inflammatory disease

11. Orobello PW, Park RI, Belcher LS et al: Microbiology of chronic sinusitis in children, *Arch Otolaryngol Head Neck Surg* 117:980, 1991.
12. Holt GR, Standefer JA, Brown WE Jr et al: Infectious diseases of the sphenoid sinus, *Laryngoscope* 94:330, 1984.
13. Carson JL, Collier AM, Hu SS: Acquired ciliary defects in nasal epithelium of children with acute viral upper respiratory infections, *N Engl J Med* 312:463, 1985.
14. Smallman LA, Finils JG: Ultrastructural abnormalities of cilia in the human respiratory tract, *Hum Pathol* 17:848-855, 1986.
15. Boat TF, Carson JL: Ciliary dysmorphology and dysfunction: primary or acquired, *N Engl J Med* 323:1700, 1990.
16. Sakakura Y, Majima Y, Harada T et al: Nasal mucociliary transport of chronic sinusitis in children, *Arch Otolaryngol Head Neck Surg* 118:1234, 1992.

Infections of uncommon cause

17. McCaffrey TV, McDonald TJ: Sarcoidosis of the nose and paranasal sinuses, *Laryngoscope* 93:1281, 1983.
18. Batsakis JG, el-Naggar AK: Rhinoscleroma and rhinosporidiosis, *Ann Otol Rhinol Laryngol* 101:879, 1992.
19. Abou-Seif SG, El-Ebrashy F, Gaafar HA: Scleroma of the upper respiratory passages: a CT study, *J Laryngol Otol* 105:198, 1991.
20. Thianprasit M, Thagerugpol K: Rhinosporidiosis, *Curr Top Med Mycol* 3:64, 1989.
21. van der Coer JMGI, Marres HAM, Wielinga EWJ et al: Rhinosporidiosis in Europe, *J Laryngol Otol* 106:440, 1992.
22. Ratnaker C, Madhavan M, Sankaran V et al: Rhinosporidiosis in Pondicherry, *J Trop Med Hyg* 95:280, 1992.
23. Tyson JC, Gittelman PD, Jacobs JJ et al: Recurrent mucormycosis of the paranasal sinuses in an immunologically competent host, *Otolaryngol Head Neck Surg* 107:115, 1992.
24. Anand VK, Alemar G, Griswold JA Jr: Intracranial complications of mucormycosis: an experimental model and clinical review, *Laryngoscope* 102:656, 1992.
25. Katzenstein ALA, Sale SR, Greenberger PA: Pathologic findings in allergic aspergillus sinusitis: a newly recognized form of sinusitis, *Am J Surg Pathol* 7:439, 1983.
26. Friedman GC, Hartwick RWJ, Ro JY et al: Allergic fungal sinusitis: report of 3 cases associated with dematiaceous fungi, *Am J Clin Pathol* 96:368, 1991.
27. Manning SC, Schaefer SD, Close LG et al: Culture positive allergic fungal sinusitis, *Arch Otolaryngol Head Neck Surg* 117:174, 1991.
28. Goldstein MF, Dvorin DJ, Dunsky EH: Allergic *Rhizomucor* sinusitis, *J Allergy Clin Immunol* 90:394, 1992.
29. Viollier AF, Peterson DE, DeJongh CA et al: *Aspergillus* sinusitis in cancer patients, *Cancer* 58:366, 1986.

Inflammation of noninfectious origin

30. Rosai J: The nature of myospherulosis of the upper respiratory tract, *Am J Clin Pathol* 69:475, 1978.
31. Kakizaki H, Shimada K: Experimental study of the cause of myospherulosis, *Am J Clin Pathol* 99:249, 1993.
32. Colby TV, Tazelaar HD, Specks U et al: Nasal biopsy in Wegener's granulomatosis, *Hum Pathol* 22:101, 1991.
33. Devaney KO, Travis WD, Hoffman G et al: Interpretation of head and neck biopsies in Wegener's granulomatosis: a pathologic study of 126 biopsies in 70 patients, *Am J Surg Pathol* 14:555, 1990.
34. DelBuono EA, Flint A: Diagnostic usefulness of nasal biopsy in Wegener's granulomatosis, *Hum Pathol* 22:107, 1991.
35. Fienberg R, Mark EJ, Goodman M et al: Correlation of antineutrophil cytoplasmic antibodies with the extrarenal histopathology of Wegener's (pathergic) granulomatosis and related forms of vasculitis, *Hum Pathol* 24:160, 1993.

Benign tumors

NASAL POLYPS

36. Perkins JA, Blakeslee D, Pierre A: Nasal polyps: a manifestation of allergy? *Otolaryngol Head Neck Surg* 101:641, 1989.
37. Granström G, Jacobsson E, Jeppsson PH: Influence of allergy, asthma and hypertension on nasal polyposis, *Acta Otolaryngol* 492(suppl):21, 1992.
38. Drake-Lee AB, Morgan DW: Nasal polyps and sinusitis in children with cystic fibrosis, *J Laryngol Otol* 103.753, 1989.
39. Compagno J, Hyams VJ, Lepore ML: Nasal polyposis with stromal atypia: review and follow-up of 14 cases, *Arch Pathol Lab Med* 100:224, 1976.

PAPILLOMAS

40. Phillips PP, Gustafson RO, Facer GW: The clinical behavior of inverting papilloma of the nose and paranasal sinuses: report of 112 cases and review of the literature, *Laryngoscope* 100:463, 1990.

41. Weber RS, Shillitoe EJ, Robbins KT et al: Prevalence of human papillomavirus in inverted nasal papillomas, *Arch Otolaryngol Head Neck Surg* 114:23, 1988.
42. Judd R, Zaki SR, Coffield LM et al: Sinonasal papillomas and human papillomavirus: human papillomavirus 11 detected in fungiform Schneiderian papillomas by in-situ hybridization and the polymerase chain reaction, *Hum Pathol* 22:550, 1991.
43. McLachlin CM, Kandel RA, Colgan TJ et al: Prevalence of human papillomavirus in sinonasal papillomas: a study using polymerase chain reaction and in-situ hybridization, *Mod Pathol* 5:406, 1992.
44. Lasser A, Rothfeld PR, Shapiro RS, Epithelial papilloma and squamous cell carcinoma of the nasal cavity and paranasal sinuses: a clinicopathological study, *Cancer* 38:2503, 1976.
45. Youssem DM, Fellows DW, Kennedy DW et al: Inverted papilloma: evaluation with MR imaging, *Radiology* 185:501, 1992.
46. Christensen WN, Smith RRL: Schneiderian papillomas: a clinicopathologic study of 67 cases, *Hum Pathol* 17:393, 1986.
47. Ridolfi RL, Lieberman PH, Erlandson RA et al: Schneiderian papillomas: a clinicopathologic study of 30 cases, *Am J Surg Pathol* 1:43, 1977.
48. Barnes L, Bedetti C: Oncocytic Schneiderian papilloma: A reappraisal of cylindrical cell papilloma of the sinonasal tract, *Hum Pathol* 15:344, 1984.
49. Ward BE, Fechner RE, Mills SE: Carcinoma arising in oncocytic Schneiderian papilloma, *Am J Surg Pathol* 14:364, 1990.

MISCELLANEOUS BENIGN TUMORS

50. Manning JT, Batsakis JG: Salivary-type neoplasms of the sinonasal tract, *Ann Otol Rhinol Laryngol* 100:691, 1991.
51. Spiro RH, Thaler HT, Hicks WF et al: The importance of clinical staging of minor salivary gland carcinoma, *Am J Surg* 162:330, 1991.
52. Compagno J, Wong RT: Intranasal mixed tumors (pleomorphic adenomas): a clinicopathologic study of 40 cases, *Am J Clin Pathol* 68:213, 1977.
53. Fu YS, Perzin KH: Non-epithelial tumors of the nasal cavity, paranasal sinuses and nasopharynx: a clinicopathologic study. I. General features and vascular tumors, *Cancer* 33:1275, 1974.
54. Taxy JB: Meningioma of the paranasal sinuses: a report of two cases, *Am J Surg Pathol* 14:82, 1990.
55. Eichhorn JH, Dickersin GR, Bhan AK et al: Sinonasal hemangiopericytoma: a reassessment with electron microscopy, immunohistochemistry and long-term follow-up, *Am J Surg Pathol* 14:856, 1990.
56. El-Naggar AK, Batsakis JG, García GM et al: Sinonasal herangiopericytomas: a clinocopathologic and DNA content study, *Arch Otolaryngol Head Neck Surg* 118:134, 1992.
57. Witkin GB, Rosai J: Solitary fibrous tumor of the upper respiratory tract: a report of six cases, *Am J Surg Pathol* 15:842, 1991.
58. Johnson LC, Yousefi M, Vinh TN et al: Juvenile ossifying fibroma: its nature, dynamics and origin, *Acta Otolaryngol,* suppl pp 1-40, 1991.
59. Dragoslav LJS, Dragoslava RD: Indications for the surgical treatment of osteoma of the frontal and ethmoid sinuses, *Clin Otolaryngol* 15:397, 1990.

Malignant tumors

GENERAL

60. Barnes L, Verbin RS, Gnepp DR: Diseases of the nose, paranasal sinuses and nasopharynx. In Barnes L, editor: *Surgical pathology of the head and neck,* New York, 1985, Marcel Dekker.
61. Lund VJ: Malignancy of the nose and sinuses: epidemiological and aetiological considerations, *Rhinology* 29:57, 1991.
62. Vokes EE, Weichselbaum RR, Lippman SM et al: Head and neck cancer, *N Engl J Med* 328:184, 1993.
63. Cann CI, Fried MP, Rothman KJ: Epidemiology of squamous cell cancer of the head and neck, *Otolaryngol Clin North Am* 18:367, 1985.
64. Miyaguchi M, Sakai S, Mori N et al: Multiple primary malignancies in patients with malignant tumours of the nasal cavities and paranasal sinuses, *J Laryngol Otol* 104:696, 1990.
65. Gluckman JL, Crissman JD: Survival rates in 548 patients with multiple neoplasms of the upper aerodigestive tract, *Laryngoscope* 93:71, 1983.
66. Reith A, Boysen M, Voss R: Environmental pathology of the upper respiratory tract. In Gnepp DR, editor: *Pathology of the head and neck,* New York, 1988, Churchill Livingstone.
67. Furuta Y, Takasu T, Asai T et al: Detection of human papillomavirus DNA in carcinomas of the nasal cavities and paranasal sinuses by polymerase chain reaction, *Cancer* 69:353, 1992.
68. Furuta Y, Takasu T, Asai T et al: Clinical significance of the epidermal growth factor receptor gene in squamous cell carcinomas of the nasal cavities and paranasal sinuses, *Cancer* 69:358, 1992.
69. Bush SE, Bagshaw MA: Carcinoma of the paranasal sinuses, *Cancer* 50:154, 1982.
70. Kenady DE: Cancer of the paranasal sinuses, *Surg Clin North Am* 66:119, 1986.
71. Chow JM, Leonetti JP, Mafee MF: Epithelial tumors of the paranasal sinuses and nasal cavity, *Radiol Clin North Am* 31:61, 1993.

SQUAMOUS CARCINOMA OF THE NASAL CAVITY AND PARANASAL SINUS

72. Patel P, Tiwari R, Karim ABMF et al: Squamous cell carcinoma of the nasal vestibule, *J Laryngol Otol* 106:332, 1992.
73. Bouquot JE, Kurland LT, Weiland LH: Carcinoma in-situ of the upper aerodigestive tract: incidence, time trends and follow-up in Rochester, Minnesota, 1935-1984, *Cancer* 61:1691, 1988.
74. Kondo M, Inuyama Y, Ando Y et al: Patterns of relapse of squamous cell carcinoma of the maxillary sinus, *Cancer* 53:2206, 1984.
75. Sisson GA, Toriumi DM, Atiyah RA: Paranasal sinus malignancy: a comprehensive update, *Laryngoscope* 99:143, 1989.
76. Spiro JD, Soo KC, Spiro RH: Squamous carcinoma of the nasal cavity and paranasal sinuses, *Am J Surg* 158:328, 1989.
77. Weber AL, Stanton AC: Malignant tumors of the paranasal sinuses: radiologic, clinical and histopathologic evaluation of 200 cases, *Head Neck Surg* 6:761, 1984.

ADENOCARCINOMA

78. Heffner DK, Hyams VJ, Hanck KW et al: Low grade adenocarcinoma of the nasal cavity and paranasal sinuses, *Cancer* 50:312, 1982.
79. Gnepp DR, Heffner DK: Mucosal origin of sinonasal tract adenomatous neoplasms, *Mod Pathol* 2:365, 1989.
80. Tran L, Sidrys J, Horton D et al: Malignant salivary gland tumors of the paranasal sinuses and nasal cavity: the UCLA experience, *Am J Clin Oncol* 12:387, 1989.
81. Andersen LJ, Therkildsen MH, Ockelmann HH et al: Malignant epithelial tumors in the minor salivary glands, the submandibular gland and the sublingual gland: prognostic factors and treatment results, *Cancer* 68:2431, 1991.
82. Barnes L: Intestinal-type adenocarcinoma of the nasal cavity and paranasal sinuses, *Am J Surg Pathol* 10:192, 1986.
83. Franquemont DW, Fechner RE, Mills SE: Histological classification of sinonasal intestinal-type adenocarcinoma, *Am J Surg Pathol* 15:368, 1991.
84. Klintenberg C, Olofsson J, Hellquist H et al: Adenocarcinoma of the ethmoid sinuses: a review of 28 cases with special reference to wood dust exposure, *Cancer* 54:482, 1984.
85. Alessi DM, Trapp TK, Fu YS et al: Nonsalivary sinonasal adenocarcinoma, *Arch Otolaryngol Head Neck Surg* 114:996, 1988.
86. Batsakis JG, Mackay B, Ordóñez NG: Enteric-type adenocarcinoma of the nasal cavity: an electron microscopic and immunocytochemical study, *Cancer* 54:855, 1984.

OTHER MALIGNANT TUMORS

87. Weiss MD, deFries HO, Taxy JB et al: Primary small cell carcinoma of the paranasal sinuses, *Arch Otolaryngol* 109:341, 1983.
88. Frierson HF Jr, Mills SE, Fechner RE et al: Sinonasal undifferentiated carcinoma: an aggressive neoplasm derived from Schneiderian epithelium and distinct from olfactory neuroblastoma, *Am J Surg Pathol* 10:771, 1986.
89. Taxy JB, Bharani NK, Mills SE et al: The spectrum of olfactory neural tumors: a light microscopic, immunohistochemical and ultrastructural analysis, *Am J Surg Pathol* 10:687, 1986.
90. Mills SE, Frierson HF Jr: Olfactory neuroblastoma: a clinicopathologic study of 21 cases, *Am J Surg Pathol* 9:317, 1985.
91. Kadish S, Goodman M, Wang CC: Olfactory neuroblastoma: a clinical analysis of 17 cases, *Cancer* 67:1571, 1976.
92. Dulguerov P, Calcaterra T: Esthesioneuroblastoma: the UCLA experience, 1970-1990, *Laryngoscope* 102:843, 1992.

93. Lund V: Malignant melanoma of the nasal cavity and paranasal sinuses, *J Laryngol Otol* 96:347, 1982.
94. Batsakis JG, Regezi JA, Solomon AR et al: The pathology of head and neck tumors. 13. Mucosal melanomas, *Head Neck Surg* 4:404, 1982.
95. Franquemont DW, Mills SE: Sinonasal malignant melanoma: a clinical and immunohistochemical study of 14 cases, *Am J Clin Pathol* 96:698, 1991.
96. Panje WR, Moran WJ: Melanoma of the upper aerodigestive tract: a review of 21 cases, *Head Neck Surg* 8:309, 1986.
97. Lund VJ: Malignant melanoma of the nasal cavity and paranasal sinuses, *Ear Nose Throat* 72:285, 1993.
98. Campo E, Cardesa A, Alos L et al: Non-Hodgkin's lymphoma of the nasal cavity and paranasal sinuses: an immunohistochemical study, *Am J Clin Pathol* 96:184, 1991.
99. Arber DA, Weiss LM, Albujar PF et al: Nasal lymphomas in Peru: high incidence of T-cell immunophenotype and Epstein-Barr virus infection, *Am J Surg Pathol* 17:392, 1993.
100. Shibuya H, Kamiyama R, Watanabe I et al: Waldeyer's ring and oral sinonasal non-Hodgkin's lymphoma, *Cancer* 59:940, 1987.
101. Fu YS, Perzin KH: Non-epithelial tumors of the nasal cavity, paranasal sinuses and nasopharynx: a clinicopathologic study. IX. Plasmacytoma, *Cancer* 42:2399, 1978.
102. Meis JM, Butler JJ, Osborn BM, Ordóñez NG: Solitary plasmacytomas of bone and extramedullary plasmacytomas: a clinicopathologic and immunohistochemical study, *Cancer* 59:1475, 1987.

Nasopharynx

Development and normal anatomy

103. Hyams VJ, Batsakis JG, Michaels L: Tumors of the upper respiratory tract and ear, *Atlas of tumor pathology*, ser 2, Fasc 25, Washington DC, 1988, AFIP.

Benign tumors

JUVENILE NASOPHARYNGEAL ANGIOFIBROMA

104. Lee DA, Rao BR, Meyer JS et al: Hormonal receptor determination in juvenile nasopharyngeal angiofibromas, *Cancer* 46:547, 1980.
105. Shikami AH, Richtsmeier WJ: Juvenile nasopharyngeal angiofibroma tumor models: failure of androgens to stimulate growth in nude mice and in vitro, *Arch Otolaryngol Head Neck Surg* 118:256, 1992.
106. Sessions RB, Bryan RN, Naclerio RM et al: Radiographic staging of juvenile angiofibroma, *Head Neck Surg* 3:279, 1981.
107. Taxy, JB: Juvenile nasopharyngeal angiofibroma: an ultrastructural study, *Cancer* 39:1044, 1977.
108. Waldman SR, Levine HL, Astor F et al: Surgical experience with nasopharyngeal angiofibroma, *Arch Otolaryngol* 107:677, 1981.
109. Gullane PJ, Davidson J, O'Dwyer T et al: Juvenile angiofibroma: a review of the literature and a case series report, *Laryngoscope* 102:928, 1992.

PITUITARY ADENOMA

110. Van der Mey AGL, van Krieken JHJM, van Dulken H et al: Large pituitary adenomas with extension into the nasopharynx: report of 3 cases with a review of the literature, *Ann Otol Rhinol Laryngol* 98:618, 1989.
111. Lloyd RV, Chandler WF, Kovacs K et al: Ectopic pituitary adenomas with normal anterior pituitary glands, *Am J Surg Pathol* 10:546, 1986.
112. Scheithauer BW, Kovacs KT, Laws ER Jr et al: Pathology of invasive pituitary tumors with special reference to functional classification, *J Neurosurg* 65:733, 1986.

Nasopharyngeal carcinoma

113. Shanmugaratham K, Sobin LH, *Histologic typing of upper respiratory tract tumors,* No 19, *International histological classification of tumors,* Geneva, 1978, WHO, pp 32-33.
114. Easton JM, Levine PH, Hyams VJ: Nasopharyngeal carcinoma in the United States: a pathologic study of 177 US and 30 foreign cases, *Arch Otolaryngol* 106:88, 1980.
115. Jenki RDT, Anderson JR, Jereb B et al: Nasopharyngeal carcinoma: a retrospective review of patients less than 30 years of age: a report from Children's Cancer Study Group, *Cancer* 27:360, 1981.
116. Neel HB III: Nasopharyngeal carcinoma: clinical presentation, diagnosis, treatment and prognosis, *Otolaryngol Clin North Am* 18:479, 1985.
117. Shan JST, Poon YF, Wei WI et al: Nasopharyngeal carcinoma in young patients, *Cancer* 65:2606, 1990.
118. Burt RD, Vaughan TL, McKnight B: Descriptive epidemiology and survival analysis of nasopharyngeal carcinoma in the United States, *Int J Cancer* 52:549, 1992.
119. Wang AY: Analysis of 26,826 patients with tumors in the head and neck, *Chung-Hua Chung Liu Tsa Chih* 14:308, 1992 (in Chinese).
120. Hildesheim A, West S, DeVeyra E et al: Herbal medicine use, Epstein-Barr virus and risk of nasopharyngeal carcinoma, *Cancer Res* 52:3048, 1992.
121. Nam J, McLaughlin JK, Blot WJ: Cigarette smoking, alcohol and nasopharyngeal carcinoma: a case-control study among U.S. whites, *J Natl Cancer Inst* 84:619, 1992.
122. Neel HB III, Nasopharyngeal carcinoma: diagnosis, staging and management, *Oncology* 6:87, 1992.
123. Feinmesser R, Miyazaki I, Cheung R et al: Diagnosis of nasopharyngeal carcinoma by DNA amplifications of tissue obtained by fine needle aspiration, *N Engl J Med* 326:17, 1992.
124. Brousset P, Butet V, Chittal S et al: Comparison of in-situ hybridization using different non-isotopic probes for detection of Epstein-Barr virus in nasopharyngeal carcinoma and immunohistochemical correlation with anti-latent membrane protein antibody, *Lab Invest* 67:457, 1992.
125. Stewart JP, Arrand JR: Expression of the Epstein-Barr virus latent membrane protein in nasopharyngeal carcinoma biopsy specimens, *Hum Pathol* 24:239, 1993.
126. Hawkins EP, Krischer JP, Smith BE et al: Nasopharyngeal carcinoma in children: a retrospective review and demonstration of Epstein-Barr viral genomes in tumor cell cytoplasm: a report of the Pediatric Oncology Group, *Hum Pathol* 21:805, 1990.
127. Wu TC, Mann RB, Epstein JI et al: Abundant expression of EBER-1 small nuclear RNA in nasopharyngeal carcinoma: a morphologically distinctive target for detection of Epstein-Barr virus in formalin fixed paraffin embedded carcinoma specimens, *Am J Pathol* 138:1461, 1991.
128. Cvitkovic E, Bachouchi M, Armand JP: Nasopharyngeal carcinoma: biology, natural history and therapeutic implications, *Hematol Oncol Clin North Am* 5:821, 1991.
129. Chan CW, Nicholls JM, Sham JST et al: Nasopharyngeal carcinoma in situ in nasopharyngeal carcinoma, *J Clin Pathol* 45:898, 1992.
130. Taxy JB, Hidvegi DF, Battifora H: Nasopharyngeal carcinoma: antikeratin immunohistochemistry and electron microscopy, *Am J Clin Pathol* 83:320, 1985.

Larynx

Nonneoplastic disease

131. Costello MJ, Swernoff NT, Yungbluth M: Laboratory diagnosis of viral respiratory tract infections, *Lab Med* 24:150, 1993.
132. Trollfors B, Nylen O, Strangert K: Acute epiglottitis in children and adults in Sweden, 1981-1983, *Arch Dis Child* 65:491, 1990.
133. Kass EG, McFadden EA, Jacobson S et al: Acute epiglottitis in the adult: experience with a seasonal presentation, *Laryngoscope* 103:841, 1993.
134. Reder PA, Neel HB III: Blastomycosis in otolaryngology: review of a large series, *Laryngoscope* 103:53, 1993.
135. Batsakis JG, Manning JT: Relapsing polychondritis, *Ann Otol Rhinol Laryngol* 98:83, 1989.
136. Michet CJ: Vasculitis and relapsing polychondritis, *Rheum Dis Clin North Am* 16:441, 1990.
137. Weidner N, Askin FB, Berthrong M et al: Bizarre (pseudomalignant) granulation tissue reactions following ionizing radiation exposure: a microscopic, immunohistochemical and flow cytometric study, *Cancer* 59:1509, 1987.
138. Wenig BM, Heffner DK: Contact ulcers of the larynx: a reacquaintance with the pathology of an often underdiagnosed entity, *Arch Pathol Lab Med* 114:825, 1990.
139. Gould SJ, Young M: Subglottic ulceration and healing following endotracheal intubation in the neonate: a morphometric study, *Ann Otol Rhinol Laryngol* 101:815, 1992.
140. Lumpkin SMM, Bennett S, Bishop SG: Post-surgical follow-up study of patients with severe polypoid degeneration, *Laryngoscope* 100:399, 1990.
141. Talbot AR: Laryngeal amyloidosis, *J Laryngol Otol* 104:147, 1990.

142. Godbersen GS, Leh JF, Hansmann ML et al: Organ-linked laryngeal amyloid deposits: clinical, morphological and immunohistochemical results of five cases, *Ann Otol Rhinol Laryngol* 101:770, 1992.
143. DeSanto LW, Devine KD, Weiland LH: Cysts of the larynx: classification, *Laryngoscope* 80:145, 1970.
144. Civantos FJ, Holinger LD: Laryngoceles and saccular cysts in infants and children, *Arch Otolaryngol Head Neck Surg* 118:296, 1992.
145. Newman BH, Taxy JB, Laker HI: Laryngeal cysts in adults: a clinicopathologic study of 20 cases, *Am J Clin Pathol* 81:715, 1984.
146. Ophir D, Lifschitz-Mercer B: Oncocytic cystic lesions of the upper respiratory tract, *Ear Nose Throat J* 68:237, 1989.

Benign tumors

147. Kashima H, Mounts P, Leventhal B et al: Sites of predilection in recurrent respiratory papillomatosis, *Ann Otol Rhinol Laryngol* 102:580, 1993.
148. Incze JS, Lui PS, Strong MS, Vaughan CW et al: The morphology of human papillomas of the upper respiratory tract, *Cancer* 39, 1634, 1977.
149. Steinberg BM, Topp WC, Schneider PS et al: Laryngeal papillomavirus infection during clinical remission, *N Engl J Med* 308:1261, 1983.
150. Abramson AL, Steinberg BM, Winkler B: Laryngeal papillomatosis: clinical, histopathologic and molecular studies, *Laryngoscope* 97:678, 1987.
151. Crissman JD, Kessis T, Shah KV et al: Squamous papillary neoplasia of the adult upper respiratory tract, *Hum Pathol* 19:1387, 1988.
152. Kashima HK, Kessis T, Mounts P et al: Polymerase chain reaction identification of human papillomavirus DNA in CO_2 laser plume from recurrent respiratory papillomatosis, *Otolaryngol Head Neck Surg* 104:191, 1991.
153. Gutman LT, Herman-Giddons ME, Phelps WC: Transmission of human genital papillomavirus disease: comparison of data from adults and children, *Pediatrics* 91:31, 1993.
154. Gindhart TD, Johnston WH, Chism SE et al: Carcinoma of the larynx in childhood, *Cancer* 46:1683, 1980.
155. Quick CA, Foucar E, Dehner LP: Frequency and significance of epithelial atypia in laryngeal papillomatosis, *Laryngoscope* 89:550, 1979.
156. Schnadig VJ, Clar WD, Clegg TJ et al: Invasive papillomatosis and squamous carcinoma complicating juvenile laryngeal papillomatosis, *Arch Otolaryngol Head Neck Surg* 112:966, 1986.
157. Guillou L, Sahli R, Chaubert P et al: Squamous cell carcinoma of the lung in a nonsmoking, nonirradiated patient with juvenile laryngotracheal papillomatosis: evidence of human papillomavirus-11 DNA in both carcinoma and papillomas, *Am J Surg Pathol* 15:891, 1991.
158. Byrne JC, Tsao MS, Fraser RS et al: Human papillomavirus-11 DNA in a patient with chronic laryngotracheobronchial papillomatosis and metastatic squamous cell carcinoma of the lung, *N Engl J Med* 317:873, 1987.
159. Barnes L, Yunis EJ, Krebs FJ III et al: Verruca vulgaris of the larynx: demonstration of human papillomavirus types 6/11 by in situ hybridization, *Arch Pathol Lab Med* 115:895, 1991.
160. Mills SE, Fechner RE: Pathology of the larynx. In *Atlas of head and neck pathology*, Chicago, 1985, American Society of Clinical Pathologists Press.

Malignant tumors

SQUAMOUS CELL CARCINOMA

161. Steele GD Jr, Winchester DP, Menck HR et al: *National cancer data base: annual review of patient care 1993*, Atlanta, 1993, American Cancer Society, p 107.
162. *Cancer in Illinois-1989: an incidence report by 107 hospitals*, Chicago, 1991, American Cancer Society, Illinois Division.
163. Roberts TJ, Epstein B, Lee DJ: Second neoplasms in patients with carcinoma of the vocal cord: incidence and implications for survival, *Int J Radiat Oncol Biol Phys* 21:583, 1991.
164. Zheng W, Blot WJ, Shu XO et al: Diet and other risk factors for laryngeal cancer in Shanghai, China, *Am J Epidemiol* 136:178, 1992.
165. Pera E, Morena A, Galindo L: Prognostic factors in laryngeal carcinoma: a multifactorial study of 416 cases, *Cancer* 58:928, 1986.
166. Barra S, Talamini R, Proto E et al: Survival analysis of 378 surgically treated cases of laryngeal carcinoma in south Sardinia, *Cancer* 65:3521, 1990.
167. Maier H, Gewelke V, Dietz A et al: Risk factors of cancer of the larynx: results of the Heidelberg case-control study, *Otolaryngol Head Neck Surg* 107:577, 1992.
168. Muscat JE, Wynder EL: Tobacco, alcohol, asbestos and occupational risk factors for laryngeal cancer, *Cancer* 69:2244, 1992.
169. Pradier R, González A, Matos E et al: Prognostic factors in laryngeal carcinoma: experience in 296 male patients, *Cancer* 71:2472, 1993.
170. Brandwein MS, Nuovo GJ, Biller H: Analysis of prevalence of human papillomavirus in laryngeal carcinoma: study of 40 cases using polymerase chain reaction and consensus primers, *Ann Otol Rhinol Laryngol* 102:309, 1993.
171. Crissman JD, Fu YS: Intraepithelial neoplasia of the larynx: a clinicopathologic study of 6 cases with DNA analysis, *Arch Otolaryngol Head Neck Surg* 112:522, 1986.
172. Crissman JD, Zarbo RJ: Quantitation of DNA ploidy in squamous intraepithelial neoplasia of the laryngeal glottis, *Arch Otolaryngol Head Neck Surg* 117:182, 1991.
173. Stenersen TC, Hoel PS, Boysen M: Carcinoma in-situ of the larynx: an evaluation of its natural clinical course, *Clin Otolaryngol* 16:358, 1991.
174. Bouquot JE, Kurland LT, Weiland LH: Carcinoma in situ of the upper aerodigestive tract: incidence, time trends and follow-up in Rochester, MN, 1935-1984, *Cancer* 61:1691, 1988.
175. Auerbach O, Hammon EC, Garfinkel L: Histologic changes in the larynx in relation to smoking habits, *Cancer* 25:92, 1970.
176. Shvero J, Hadar T, Segal K et al: Laryngeal carcinoma in patients 40 years of age and younger, *Cancer* 60:3092, 1987.

VERRUCOUS CARCINOMA

177. Ferlito A, Recher G: Ackerman's tumor (verrucous carcinoma) of the larynx: a clinicopathologic study of 77 cases, *Cancer* 46:1617, 1980.
178. Luna MA, Tortoledo ME: Verrucous carcinoma. In Gnepp DR, editor: *Pathology of the head and neck*, New York, 1988, Churchill-Livingstone.

SPINDLE CELL CARCINOMA

179. Zarbo RJ, Crissman JD, Venkat H et al: Spindle cell carcinoma of the upper aerodigestive tract mucosa: an immunohistologic and ultrastructural study of 18 biphasic tumors and comparison with 7 monophasic spindle cell tumors, *Am J Surg Pathol* 10:741, 1986.
180. Ellis GL, Langloss JM, Heffner DK et al: Spindle cell carcinoma of the aerodigestive tract: an immunohistochemical analysis of 21 cases, *Am J Surg Pathol* 11:335, 1987.
181. Nappi O, Wick MR: Sarcomatoid neoplasms of the respiratory tract, *Semin Diag Pathol* 10:137, 1993.
182. Gorenstein A, Neel HB III, Weiland LH et al: Sarcomas of the larynx, *Arch Otolaryngol* 106:8, 1980.

NEUROENDOCRINE CARCINOMA

183. Batsakis JG, Luna MA, El-Naggar AK: Nonsquamous carcinomas of the larynx, *Ann Otol Rhinol Laryngol* 101:1024, 1992.
184. Wenig BM, Gnepp DR: The spectrum of neuroendocrine carcinomas of the larynx, *Semin Diag Pathol* 6:329, 1989.
185. Ferlito A, Friedmann I: Review of neuroendocrine carcinomas of the larynx, *Ann Otol Rhinol Laryngol* 98:780, 1989.

49 Lungs

Charles Kuhn III
William W. West
John E. Craighead
Allen R. Gibbs

NORMAL LUNG

Anatomy and histology

The lung consists of airways, blood vessels, the connective tissue framework, and the external delimiting envelope, the pleura.[1] The airways include the trachea, bronchi, bronchioli, and acini. The lungs have dual blood supply, and the vessels belong to either the pulmonary or the bronchial circulatory system. The pleura overlying the lungs, called *visceral pleura,* is continuous with the parietal pleura lining the inside of the chest cavity.

Airways. The pulmonary airways begin as the left and right major bronchus, which are anatomic extensions of the trachea. The main bronchi branch dichotomously give rise to gradually smaller and smaller bronchi (Fig. 49-1). On average, there are 16 generations of bronchi and bronchioles before the first respiratory bronchioles are reached, but the number of generations varies from approximately 8 to 23 in different regions of the lung.

The walls of the trachea and main bronchi are reinforced by C-shaped rings of cartilage anteriorly and laterally with a sheet of transversely arranged smooth muscle filling the gap posteriorly. Within the lung, as successive generations of bronchi become smaller, they are reinforced by progressively smaller and fewer islands of cartilage. The smooth muscle continues as bundles that wind in a spiral down the intrapulmonary bronchi, which extend into gradually narrower and narrower airways.

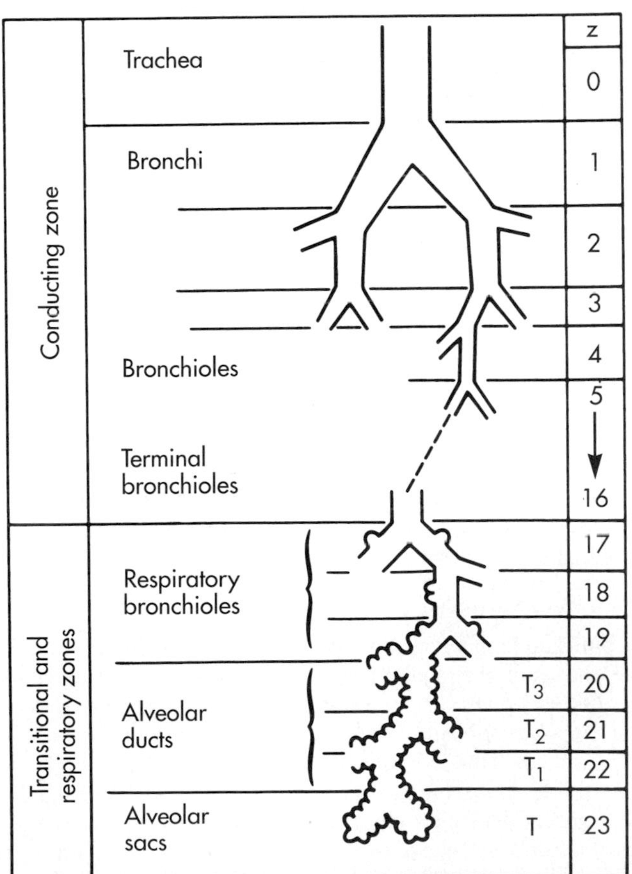

Fig. 49-1 Diagram of the lower respiratory tract. Gas exchange occurs in the transitional and respiratory zones where velocity of air flow is nil. It is at these sites where direct damage to the airways occurs as a result of environmental pollutants. (From Craighead JE, editor: *Pathology of environmental and occupational disease,* St. Louis, 1995, Mosby.)

The mucosa of the *trachea* and *bronchi* is lined by a pseudostratified ciliated columnar epithelium. Although all the epithelial cells rest on the basal lamina, at least two layers of nuclei are evident by light microscopy. By electron microscopy four cell types can be recognized in the bronchial epithelium: ciliated cells, mucous cells, neuroendocrine (Kulchitsky) cells, and basal cells (Fig. 49-2). Ciliated cells account for more than 90% of all bronchial cells. Mucous cells are filled with mucin-rich granules. Their cytoplasm extends to the luminal surface. Neuroendocrine cells contain round neuroendocrine cytoplasmic granules. The basal cells are small, triangular cells with relatively few organelles, which are attached to the basal lamina with hemidesmosomes and to neighboring columnar cells by desmosomes. These latter two cell types are located along the basal lamina, and their cytoplasm does not extend to the lumen of the airways.

The *bronchial glands* are located in the lamina propria of the bronchi. Most glands occupy the space between the cartilage and surface epithelium, but some extend between cartilages deep into the bronchial wall. These glands are compound tubuloacinar structures composed of three cell types: (1) mucous cells, the cytoplasm of which is filled with weakly basophilic secretory vacuoles; (2) serous cells, the apical cytoplasm of which contains eosinophilic granules 1 to 2 μm in diameter, and such granules contain biologically active substances such as proteases inhibitors, lysozyme, and lactoferrin; (3) myoepithelial cells, which form a contractile network enclosing the glands. The myoepithelial cells resemble smooth muscle ultrastructurally and contain smooth muscle actin isoforms but are joined to the secretory epithelial cells by desmosomes. The gland acini empty into ducts lined by mucus-secreting cells except near the bronchial lumen, where they become ciliated.

Bronchi, which contain cartilage in their wall, extend into *bronchioli,* airways that measure 2 down to 0.5 mm in width. The walls of bronchioli are devoid of both cartilage and glands and consist only of smooth muscle cells and connective tissue. The simple columnar epithelium lining the bronchioli is composed mainly of ciliated epithelial cells interspersed with nonciliated secretory cells called *Clara cells.* Clara cells contain secretory granules visible by electron microscopy, but their function remains controversial. The bronchioli give rise to respiratory bronchioles, cuboidal, and nonciliated cells. The epithelium of respiratory bronchioli is continuous with the epithelium lining the alveoli.

The alveoli are air spaces lined by thin walls composed of capillaries covered by epithelium and supported by a delicate mesh of connective tissue. The alveolar lining consists predominantly of type I epithelial cells, which cover 98% of the alveolar surface. Interspersed between these cells are small cuboidal epithelial cells, type II cells. The type II cells are characterized by a microvillous surface and cytoplasmic lamellar bodies, which contain the alveolar surfactant. Pulmonary surfactant consists of nearly 85% lipid, predominantly saturated phosphatidylcholine, and 15% protein with four unique proteins designated surfactant proteins (SP) A, B, C, and D.

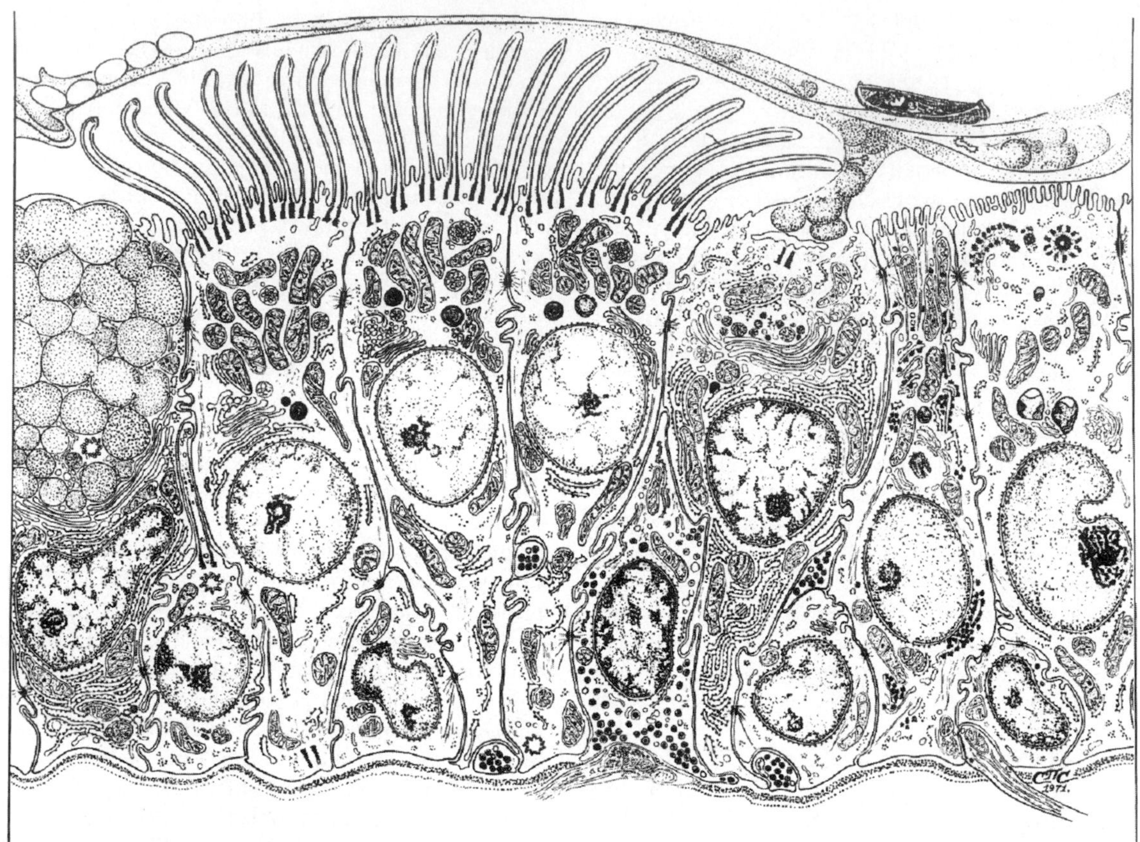

Fig. 49-2 Diagram of bronchial epithelium. Four cell types can be recognized: ciliated cells, mucous cells, neuroendocrine cells, and basal cells. (From Weiss L, Greep RO: *Histology,* ed 4, New York, 1977, McGraw-Hill.)

Pulmonary vasculature. The lungs have a dual blood supply: the functional circulatory system comprising the pulmonary artery and its branches and the nutritional system originating from bronchial arteries. The venous blood is brought from the right ventricle to the lung by the pulmonary arteries, which originate from the pulmonary trunk. The pulmonary artery extends into branches that enter the lung accompanying the bronchi and run with them in the lung enclosed by a common sheath of adventitial connective tissue. The smallest branches of the pulmonary artery enter the acinus with the respiratory bronchioles, giving rise to precapillary arterioles, which accompany the alveolar ducts. The pulmonary veins lie at the periphery of the acini, often within connective tissue septa that divide the parenchyma into lobules. One vein drains two or more acini.

The bronchial arteries originate from the thoracic aorta. One or two bronchial arteries supply arterial blood to each lung. The branches of the bronchial arteries run along the bronchial tree down to the level of respiratory bronchioli, whereupon they form capillaries that anastomose with the branches of the pulmonary artery.

Bronchus–associated lymphoid tissue (BALT). The immune system in the lung is represented by lymphoid nodules associated with the bronchioles, lymph nodes at the bifurcations of the bronchi, and by lymphocytes, plasma cells, and mast cells diffusely scattered through the mucosa of the bronchi. The lymphoid nodules of BALT consist predominantly of B-cells. T-cells are also present in considerable numbers. Macrophages, the principal resident phagocytes, are found in small numbers in the interstitium as well as within alveolar spaces and on the surface of the airway mucosa. Macrophages represent more than 90% of all cells obtained by bronchioloalveolar lavage, whereas lymphocytes account for 1% to 5% of all cells.[2]

Pleura. The pleural investment of the lung is composed of alternating layers of collagen and elastic fibers covered by a single layer of epithelium called *mesothelium* because of its mesodermal origin. Flat nearly to the point of invisibility in normal lungs, mesothelial cells become cuboidal and easily visible in response to injury. Long, slender microvilli are their principal ultrastructural specialization.

Lung development

Intrauterine lung development can be conveniently divided into five phases: embryonal phase, pseudoglandular phase, canalicular (acinar) phase, saccular phase, and alveolar phase.[3-10]

Embryonal phase (weeks 4 to 6 of gestation) begins with formation of a bud of the primitive foregut. The single lung bud divides into two primary bronchial buds, and each of those subsequently divide. *Pseudoglandular phase (weeks 7 to 16 of gestation)* is so called because during this phase the lungs have a glandular appearance. The asymmetric dichotomous airway branching initiated in the embryonal phase continues throughout the pseudoglandular period. By the end of this phase, all the conducting (nonrespiratory) airways have formed down to the level of the terminal bronchioles. *Canalicular (acinar) phase (weeks 17 to 27 of gestation)* is characterized by the formation of the basic framework of the acinus (the portion of the lung that is distal to the terminal bronchiole). Although the first two stages of intrauterine development revolve around the conducting airways, the canalicular phase and subsequent phases (saccular and alveolar) focus on the development of the gas-exchange portion of the lung, the acinus. During the canalicular phase, the airways continue to branch beyond the terminal bronchioles. Small blood vessels canalize the acinar mesenchyma, and this interstitial tissue begins to mature and thin. The glycogen-rich cuboidal epithelium of the distal air spaces begins to differentiate. At approximately 20 weeks, some of these distal air-space epithelial cells begin to show cytoplasmic features of type II pneumocytes with evidence of surfactant production and storage (lamellar and multivesicular bodies) as their cytoplasmic glycogen diminishes. The vascular meshwork begins in the interstitium, and the capillaries then approach the epithelial surfaces of the nearby air space. As a capillary approaches the overlying epithelium, the epithelial cells differentiate into flattened type I pneumocytes with the characteristically thinned cytoplasm.

During this exponential increase in the number of pulmonary capillaries and in potential air-exchange surface area, the interstitial mesenchyma also forms the outlines of the pulmonary lobule, and the type II cells begin to produce surfactant. Although surfactant is detectable in the type II cell cytoplasm by 20 to 22 weeks, there is insufficient airspace surfactant to stabilize the lung until at least 24 to 26 weeks. By the end of the canalicular period (27 weeks) the maturing gas-exchange sites and surfactant system result in the first potential for life-sustaining extrauterine respiration.

Saccular phase (weeks 28 to 35 of gestation) is characterized by an expansion of the pulmonary gas-exchange surface area. The thinning of the interstitium is accompanied by the appearance of numerous secondary crests that arise from the air space walls and subdivide the primitive distal air spaces (saccules) into smaller units (subsaccules), at the same time increasing the potential gas-exchange area. Elastic fibers form the netlike framework of the acinus.[6]

Alveolar phase (week 36 to term) is characterized by the formation of alveoli, which become apparent by 36 weeks of gestation. Some alveoli may appear as early as 32 weeks. In contrast to many laboratory animals, which develop alveoli only postnatally, in humans there is significant prenatal alveolar development during this phase of intrauterine development. Alveoli continue to develop throughout late gestation and early childhood. At term the gas-exchange surface area of the lungs approximates 4 square meters.[7]

At birth the number of alveoli, though highly variable, averages 50 million, whereas adult numbers range from 300 million to 600 million. This dramatic increase in the number of alveoli predominantly occurs during the first 2 years of life.[8] Although alveolar acquisition ceases at 2 to 3 years of age, the gas-exchange surface area of the lung continues to increase as the child grows. After 2 years of age, the number of alveoli remains relatively constant while lung volume and alveolar size increase as the individual grows. Lung volume and the number of alveoli appear to be related to body height in the adult.

Reid[9] has succinctly summarized the most important features of lung development as follows: (1) the conducting airways (tracheobronchial tree through the terminal bronchioles) are developed by the sixteenth week of gestation, (2) alveoli develop mainly after birth, particularly in the first 2 years of life, and (3) preacinar arteries follow the development of the airways, whereas intra-acinar vessels follow that of alveoli.

DEVELOPMENTAL ANOMALIES

The larynx, lungs (including trachea), and esophagus develop as derivatives of the primitive foregut. It is not surprising to find that congenital abnormalities involving one often are accompanied by abnormalities in one or more of the others as well as defects in other organ systems, since the respiratory system develops close to the branchial arches and pouches.[11-13]

Tracheal anomalies

Tracheoesophageal fistula is frequently (95% of cases) associated with esophageal atresia resulting in the clinical picture of maternal polyhydramnios and excessive oropharyngeal secretions with paroxysms of choking and coughing with feeding attempts in the often premature neonate.[10] There are five types of tracheoesophageal fistula and esophageal atresia; however, one type, esophageal atresia with a fistula from the trachea or carina to the lower esophageal segment, accounts for 85% of the cases. Over 50% of patients with tracheoesophageal fistula have associated congenital anomalies, often involving multiple systems.[14]

Tracheal agenesis is a rare, fatal anomaly which may be associated with a tracheoesophageal or bronchoesophageal fistula, and congenital anomalies of the larynx, heart, genitourinary tract, gastrointestinal tract, or central nervous system.[15-16] *Tracheal stenosis* is rarely congenital in origin because most cases are related to prior intubation.[17] Congenital tracheal stenosis may be related to abnormalities in the trachea itself, such as complete tracheal cartilaginous rings (absence of the *pars mebranacea*), or extrinsic compression of the trachea, most frequently attributable to anomalous blood vessels.[18-20] *Tracheobronchomegaly* refers to considerable dilatation of the trachea and major bronchi, possibly because of a congenital defect in connective tissue.[21,22]

Bronchial anomalies

There is a wide range of congenital bronchial anomalies, often with variations within each type.[13,23] The minor anomalies are often asymptomatic incidental findings; however, the association with congenital anomalies in other organ systems continues when one looks at many of the congenital defects of the major bronchi.[24,25] Bronchial anomalies include abnormal bronchial branching patterns, abnormalities in size, abnormal connections with other structures, and cartilage plate abnormalities.[26]

Bronchial isomerism refers to bilaterally symmetric lobar bronchial patterns described as bilateral right lung or bilateral left lung; remember, the bronchial branching pattern is generally characterized by asymmetric dichotomous branching, and so the right lung is not normally a mirror image of the left or vice versa. Bronchial isomerism is associated with at least five variants of polysplenia-asplenia syndromes with significant cardiac and gastrointestinal anomalies.[27] Although true supernumerary bronchi are rare, abnormally placed bronchi, such as the tracheal bronchus, are more common. The tracheal bronchus is a displaced bronchus that originates from the trachea.[28] The most common tracheal bronchus is the right upper lobe apical segment bronchus (pre-eparterial bronchus), which is usually an asymptomatic incidental finding; a minority may be associated with recurrent infections. The bridging bronchus involves a bronchial connection between the left main bronchus and the right lower lobe, which traverses ("bridges") the mediastinum.[29] This pattern may also be seen with a sling left pulmonary artery.

Bronchial atresia most often involves the left upper lobe and may be associated with distal hyperinflation (congenital pulmonary overinflation) in infants or is more commonly asymptomatic in adults.[30] Radiologic studies may demonstrate mucus plugs in the bronchial lumen distal to the atretic site, though the distal parenchyma is aerated by collateral pathways.[31]

Bronchial stenosis may be intrinsic or extrinsic.[10] Intrinsic congenital stenosis of a mainstem bronchus is rare compared to extrinsic compression by abnormal blood vessels, cysts, or tumors.

Congenital bronchobiliary fistula likely represents a duplication of a portion of the foregut resulting in an abnormal communication between a bronchus (usually the right mainstem) and the biliary system.[10] Within days of birth, focal areas of pneumonia, atelectasis, or even hyperinflation may be associated with production of a yellow-green bilious sputum. *Congenital bronchoesophageal fistula* usually involves the right main bronchus and is frequently associated with esophageal atresia and tracheoesophageal fistula.[32,33]

Bronchogenic cyst

Bronchogenic cyst is usually an extrapulmonary cyst formed as the result of an accessory lung bud from the foregut that becomes isolated from the rest of the tracheobronchial tree producing a usually solitary cyst whose lining imitates the lining of a bronchus.[12] Most bronchogenic cysts are located near the midline of the thorax, some paratracheal or parabronchial, others paraesophageal or even in the subcutaneous tissue over the sternum.[34,35] Unusual cases can range from the hypopharynx to below the diaphragm. The cysts range from a few centimeters in infants up to 10 cm in adults (Fig. 49-3). The cyst is discrete, smooth walled, generally unilocular, and lined by ciliated cuboidal to pseudostratified columnar epithelium overlying a fibromuscular wall that may contain islands of cartilage and seromucinous glands. A watery fluid or mucus fills the cyst though secondary infection may produce a purulent nature to the cyst contents. Bronchogenic cyst should be differentiated from an enteric cyst, esophageal cyst, or pericardial cyst. Although secondary infection can distort the histologic features of any of these cysts, the intact esophageal cyst generally has a stratified squamous epithelial lining over a muscular cyst wall, and the enteric cyst lining usually consists of columnar epithelium with areas of gastric glandular differentiation. An intraparenchymal pulmonary cyst believed to be bronchogenic must be differentiated from the large cyst variety of congenital cystic adenomatoid malformation as well as a lung abscess.

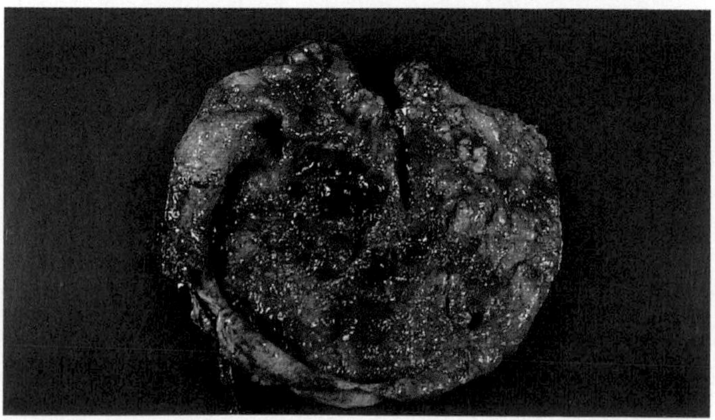

Fig. 49-3 Large bronchogenic cyst from an adult. The inside lining appears rugged.

Many bronchogenic cysts are noted as an incidental finding in a child or young adult; however, some may produce congenital pulmonary overinflation or respiratory distress in an infant because of airway obstruction. Secondary infection may also produce symptoms. In addition to congenital pulmonary hyperinflation, bronchogenic cyst may be associated with bronchial atresia or extralobar sequestration.

Pulmonary parenchymal anomalies

Congenital anomalies of the pulmonary parenchyma range from clinically insignificant aberrations in the lobar configuration of the lungs to the obviously fatal bilateral pulmonary agenesis. Upwards of 25% of individuals have variations in the anatomy of the fissures, including absent fissures, incomplete fissures, or supernumerary fissures.[13] The variations result in curiosities such as bilobed right lung or trilobed left lung; however, the associated bronchial branching patterns are most often normal. Recognition of most of these variants is important for the radiologist, but most do not result in clinical disease unless they are associated with other anomalies. The pattern and density of the interlobular septa also varies between individuals; the septa are most numerous and readily recognized in the subpleural regions of the lung, especially along the edges or angles of a lobe or along the diaphragmatic surface. Septa are less common along the lateral costal subpleural margins. The septal variations are not clinically significant.

Herniation of lung tissue is uncommon but may be the cause of apparent "ectopic" lung tissue, which must be differentiated from extralobar sequestration. Herniation into the neck is associated with some congenital syndromes affecting the cervical skeletomuscular system (iniencephaly, Klippel-Feil syndrome) and the 5p– (cri du chat) syndrome.[36] Lung tissue may also herniate through the diaphragm or into the intercostal space.[13]

Horseshoe lung refers to congenitally fused lungs. The right and left lung bases are joined at the midline by a fused portion of parenchyma located posterior to the pericardium but anterior to the aorta and esophagus. Significant pulmonary vascular anomalies, including scimitar syndrome, are associated with horseshoe lung.[37] A *crossover lung segment* also crosses the midline behind the heart, but in this disorder, the right lung extends into the left lower area of the thorax by an expansion of the right pleura behind the heart. Radiographically, crossover lung segment may mimic horseshoe lung; however, in crossover lung segment the right lung is not fused with the left lung. Like horseshoe lung, crossover lung segment is associated with scimitar syndrome.

Agenesis refers to the absence of both the distal pulmonary parenchyma and the associated bronchial branch. *Aplasia* is characterized by the presence of a rudimentary bronchial branch but the absence of the distal pulmonary tissue.[13,38]

Congenital absence of a lobe, lung, or both lungs should raise the suspicion of associated congenital anomalies including cardiovascular anomalies, skeletal defects, tracheal atresia, tracheoesophageal fistula, genitourinary defects, and gastrointestinal maldevelopment.[39] Bilateral congenital absence of the lungs is rare and fatal.[40] Unilateral absence of a lung is also associated with a variety of anomalies in other systems in up to 75% of cases.[41] The associated anomalies generally dictate the prognosis because isolated unilateral absence of a lung may not affect long-term survival. Uncomplicated unilateral absence may present with recurrent pulmonary infections during childhood or may be discovered incidentally in an asymptomatic adult. Although either the right or left lung may fail to develop, absence of the right lung generates a higher mortality because of a higher incidence of accompanying serious cardiovascular abnormalities.[12]

Congenital alveolar capillary dysplasia presents as progressive hypoxemia in the newborn with a clinical picture suggestive of persistent pulmonary hypertension.[42,43] Pathologically this rare entity is characterized by thickened alveolar septa, decreased acinar complexity, poor vascularization of the interstitial tissue and apparent failure of capillarization of the alveolar air-blood barrier. Alveolar capillary dysplasia may accompany misalignment of the pulmonary vessels where some of the pulmonary veins run centrally in the lobule instead of the normal location at the periphery of the lobule in the interlobular septa. *Congenital acinar dysplasia* may also present with neonatal hypoxemia.[44] In this disorder the morphology is suggestive of abortive development of the pulmonary acinus because the lungs are composed of numerous bronchus-like structures embedded in a cellular mesenchyma; no true pulmonary acinar tissue develops, with the obvious implications of minimal extrauterine survival. Some authors suggest that congenital acinar dysplasia may represent a rare variant of congenital adenomatoid malformation.[12]

Heterotopic tissues that may be found in the lung include ectopic adrenocortical tissue, thyroid, neuroglial tissue, and striated muscle. Infants with anencephaly account for cases of neuroglial heterotopia. *Rhabdomyomatous heterotopia* (rhabdomyomatous dysplasia) may accompany horseshoe lung, pulmonary sequestrations, or congenital adenomatoid malformation, or it may be seen as a diffuse infiltration of the pulmonary interstitium.[10,12]

Pulmonary hypoplasia

Pulmonary hypoplasia is defined as the incomplete or defective development that results in an overall decrease in relative volume or weight of the lung because of a reduction in the number or size of the acini.[10] The decrease in lung size or volume may result from any one or more of the following: a decrease in the number of alveoli, a decrease in the size of alveoli, or a decrease in the number of airway branches. Hypoplasia may be unilateral or bilateral. Etiologic factors include a limitation of space in the thoracic cavity, metabolic defects, abnormal or absent fetal breathing movements, diminished pulmonary blood flow, loss of intrauterine lung fluid, or primary mesodermal defects.[12] Many cases represent combinations of these etiologic factors. A minority of cases of hypoplasia are idiopathic, some sporadic, and a few familial. More than half of the cases of pulmonary hypoplasia are ascribed to a variety of intrauterine insults that result in diminished thoracic space for the developing lung. Diaphragmatic hernia, usually left sided, accounts for many of these cases. In Bochdalek's hernia, which is the most common form of congenital diaphragmatic hernia, portions of the abdominal viscera herniate into the thoracic cavity through a relatively central defect in the affected hemidiaphragm (usually the left). The ipsilateral lung is hypoplastic, and the contralateral lung may also be affected.[45,46] Pleural effusions, ascites, intrathoracic or abdominal masses (tumors, cysts, malformations), oligohydramnios, and chest wall deformities may result in insufficient intrathoracic space for appropriate lung development.[47] Normal intrauterine lung fluid volumes and fetal breathing movements are necessary for normal lung development. Oligohydramnios resulting from renal agenesis, renal dysplasia, polycystic renal disease, congenital urinary tract obstruction, or prolonged amniotic fluid leaks can produce pulmonary hypoplasia. Renal disorders may also work by a metabolic pathway to cause pulmonary hypoplasia because there is evidence that these disorders may affect fetal collagen metabolism. Chromosomal anomalies such as trisomy 8, trisomy 21, or trisomy 13 produce pulmonary hypoplasia; the mechanism has not been identified, though some researchers have hypothesized a generalized mesodermal defect. The defect associated with trisomy 21 (Down syndrome) results in pulmonary hypoplasia that develops during the first few months of life, since the lung development at birth is reportedly within normal limits.[48] CNS defects or skeletomuscular disorders that preclude normal intrauterine respiratory movements are associated with hypoplastic lungs.

Hypoplastic lungs are smaller than normal, as evidenced by a decrease in lung volume or lung weights. Comparison with expected values for lung weight and lung weight–body weight ratios are useful in substantiating the diagnosis. Although routinely available, lung weights can be distorted by variations in the amount of fluid and inflammatory processes such that care must be used in basing the lung assessment on the weight alone. Lung volume compared to crown-rump length, alveolar counts, radial alveolar counting, airway counts, and analysis of lung DNA content have all been used in the diagnosis of pulmonary hypoplasia.[49] Hypoplasia may range from a mild decrease in lung weight or volume to life-threatening deficits in gas-exchange tissue. In cases where hypoplasia has been identified as the cause of death, lung weights less than 30% to 40% of normal are not uncommon.

Pulmonary hypoplasia has been identified in 10% to 15% of neonatal autopsies where the lungs are systematically examined and in approximately 50% of cases with other significant congenital anomalies. On the other hand, in over 85% of cases pulmonary hypoplasia is associated with other congenital anomalies, most commonly diaphragmatic hernia or renal disorders.[10] The diagnosis of pulmonary hypoplasia should raise the suspicion of associated congenital anomalies. Pulmonary hypoplasia clinically presents as respiratory distress within minutes of delivery. The clinical picture may be overshadowed by the associated congenital anomalies. In severe cases the infants are difficult to ventilate, and death is often caused by progressive hypoxemia.

Bronchopulmonary sequestration

Bronchopulmonary sequestration is defined as a mass of pulmonary parenchyma that does not communicate with the tracheobronchial tree through a normally located bronchus and the isolated parenchyma usually has an anomalous arterial supply, usually from a systemic vessel. In essence, the mass of pulmonary tissues is "sequestered" from the normal airways of the lung. Sequestrations may be intralobar or extralobar. There are significant clinical and pathologic differences between the two. Extralobar sequestration is defined as a sequestration that is completely separate from the normal pleural investment of the lung, whereas intralobar sequestration is located within the pleural investment of the lung.[13]

Historically, both forms of sequestrations were theorized to have originated from abnormal fetal lung development involving the acquisition of an accessory lung bud from the foregut distal to the normal tracheobronchial bud. The proposals suggested that earlier origin of the accessory bud, which was closer to the normal tracheobronchial bud, would lead to an intralobar sequestration, whereas later development of the accessory bud, farther from the normal tracheobronchial bud, would result in an extralobar sequestration. The accessory lung bud theory could account for extralobar sequestration and its frequent association with other congenital anomalies but does not explain adequately intralobar sequestration. Apparently, most intralobar sequestrations are acquired lesions that develop in neonatal lungs damaged by recurrent pneumonias. The affected lung segment is revascularized by systemic arteries from the pulmonary ligament, or less often the diaphragm. As the systemic arterial supply takes over, the usual bronchial connections are obliterated, resulting in the picture of an isolated segment of pulmonary tissue with a systemic vascular supply.[50]

Extralobar sequestration (accessory lobe) is located within the thorax in approximately 85% of cases, usually the left lower thorax between the left lower lobe and the diaphragm and occasionally within the mediastinum.[51] Extrathoracic sites include locations within or below the diaphragm.[52,53] Both the arterial supply and the venous drainage are usually through systemic vessels.[12] By definition extralobar sequestration is a discrete mass of pulmonary parenchyma that lies outside the pleural investment of the lung. Extralobar sequestrations vary considerably in size ranging from 0.5 to 15 cm in greatest dimension. The anomalous tissue usually consists of a round to ovoid discrete mass of pink-tan spongy tissue that closely resembles immature lung. The extralobar sequestration is covered by thin translucent wrinkled pleura, and there may be a pseudohilum with a localized collection of irregular bronchi and vessels at one pole. Microscopically the lesion consists of pulmonary parenchyma that resembles immature lung with dilated bronchioles and occasional small cystic spaces formed by abortive bronchi. Areas histologically resembling congenital adenomatoid malformation are not uncommon. In contrast to the acquired intralobar sequestration, extralobar sequestration usually does not demonstrate significant inflammatory and fibrotic changes related to recurrent infection.

Extralobar sequestrations predominantly appear in infants and children and only rarely in adults.[54,55] Symptoms usually appear during the first few days to months of life. The clinical picture can vary from neonatal respiratory distress to the childhood presentation of an upper abdominal mass.[56,57] Some perinatal cases present with varying degrees of edema and associated maternal polyhydramnios, whereas others portray a picture resembling lobar emphysema with associated unaerated lung. There is a 3:1 male-to-female predominance. There is a frequent association (65% of cases) with coexisting congenital anomalies such as diaphragmatic defects and eventrations, *pectus excavatum*, anomalous connections with the gastrointestinal system (bronchopulmonary foregut malformations), and cardiovascular defects (such as scimitar syndrome).

Intralobar sequestration usually can be traced to recurrent inflammation and scarring. Almost always (98% of cases) it involves a lower lobe of the lung, most frequently the posterobasal segment of the left lower lobe.[10,58] One or more systemic arteries feed the inflamed focus most often by means of the hypertrophied pulmonary ligament arterial system, whereas the venous side drains via the pulmonary system. The overriding pathologic findings, both gross and microscopic, are those of a chronic recurring pneumonia with varying degrees of fibrosis and bronchiectasis (Fig. 49-4). The lesions range from solid fibrotic to partially cystic areas that irregularly blend with the surrounding intact pulmonary parenchyma. The normal communications between the sequestration and the tracheobronchial tree are obliterated, though the frequent identification of air-fluid levels is radiologically suggestive that the lesion somehow communicates with the airways, possibly by means of collateral channels. The overlying visceral pleura reflects the inflammatory nature of the lesion with variable pleural thickening and fibrovascular adhesions to adjacent structures.[59]

The clinical picture of an intralobar sequestration is that of a recurrent localized pneumonia or a lung abscess with intermittent fevers, cough, and an irregular lower lobe mass on chest roentgenogram.[60] In contrast to the extralobar sequestration, the intralobar sequestration rarely presents before 5 years of age and is infrequently associated with other congenital anomalies.[61]

Congenital cystic adenomatoid malformation

Congenital cystic adenomatoid malformation (CCAM) encompasses a continuum of hamartomatous cystic lung lesions characterized by the presence of abnormal bronchiolar structures of varying sizes or distribution. These relatively common congenital masses of abnormal lung tissue are classified on the basis of the sizes of the cysts and the microscopic features of the cyst walls. The cause of CCAM is unknown, though some investigators have suggested that the range of cases represents a malformation that mimics the differentiation of the airways, ranging from bronchial structures to distal acinar structures, possibly related to an underlying defect in bronchial development as evidenced by reports of associated bronchial atresia.[62]

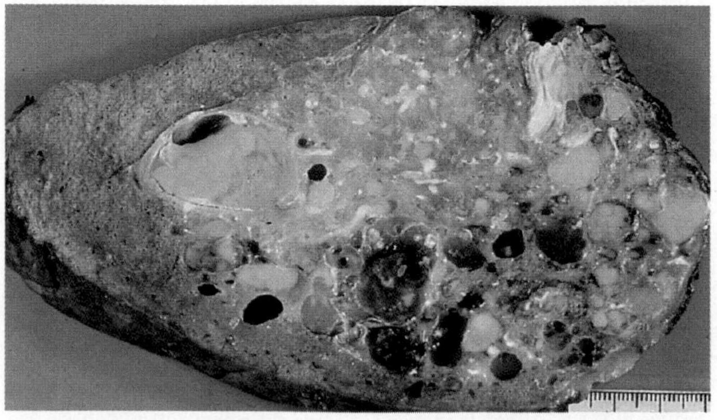

Fig. 49-4 Intralobar sequestration. The lung shows fibrosis and bronchiectasis.

CCAM is generally a unilateral lesion that is most commonly (90% of cases) confined to a single lobe, though occasionally it may involve most of one lung. Bilateral or multiple lesions are rare.[63] The right and left lungs are almost equally affected. There is a slightly higher incidence of lower lobe lesions than that of other lobes. CCAM is usually cuffed by at least a partial rim of intact lung parenchyma, though the margins of the lesion may not be distinct. Although CCAM encompasses a range of lesions, most cases conform to one of three categories.[12,64]

Type 1 is the large cyst category and accounts for approximately 50% of cases. The lesion consists of an irregular cystic mass in which the larger cysts (3 to 10 cm in greatest diameter) dominate, though smaller cysts are frequently noted in the background (Fig. 49-5). The cysts are lined by pseudostratified columnar ciliated epithelium overlying a relatively prominent fibromuscular layer that mimics the walls of proximal bronchiolar structures or small bronchi (Fig. 49-6). Cartilage and foci of mucous cells are noted in some cases.[65] The morphology is suggestive of a lesion that imitates the differentiation at the distal bronchial–proximal bronchiolar level of the lung.

Type 2 consists of numerous smaller cysts (0.5 to 2 cm) throughout the lesion without a predominant large cyst component. Approximately 40% of the cases of CCAM fit into this category. It is often difficult to distinguish grossly where the type 2 CCAM ends and the normal lung parenchyma begins. Cuboidal to columnar epithelial cells may line a relatively thin fibromuscular layer in the larger cysts; however, most of the lesion is composed of thin-walled bronchiole-like structures. The lining of the cysts is histologically reminiscent of the bronchiolar level of the airways. Unusual variants have skeletal muscle fibers (rhabdomyomatous differentiation) scattered through the interstitium; reportedly these variants have a higher incidence of associated congenital anomalies.

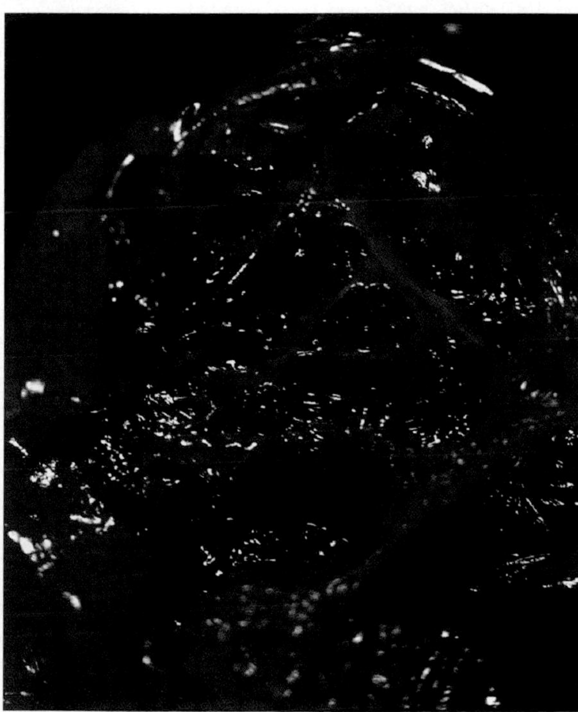

Fig. 49-5 Congenital cystic adenomatoid malformation.

Type 3 grossly appears as the most solid variant of the three because it consists of innumerable evenly distributed small cysts that measure less than 0.2 cm in greatest dimension. Type 3 accounts for approximately 10% of CCAM cases. The type 3 lesion tends to be larger and not uncommonly occupies an entire lobe or most of one lung. The microscopic appearance is suggestive of immature lung with a predominant background of alveoli-like structures lined by cuboidal cells that appear to be type II pneumocytes by electron microscopy. Occasional randomly scattered irregular thin-walled bronchiole-like structures are interspersed between the alveoli-like zones. The histologic appearance mimics that of the proximal acinus with terminal bronchiole-like structures and structures resembling alveoli. Cartilage and skeletal muscle are absent.

Unusual cystic lung lesions that do not fit well into any of the three categories have been reported. An expanded classification based on the hamartomatous components of the CCAM has been proposed. Rare lesions composed of bronchus-like structures with few bronchioles have been reported, as well as lesions that more closely mimic the distal acinus.[63]

CCAM is a disorder of infancy because over 85% of cases are identified before 2 years of age. Many cases present between 1 day and 1 month of age, though rare adult cases have been reported.[66] In utero diagnosis by ultrasound is not unusual.[67] Respiratory distress in an infant is the most common presenting clinical picture, often with an expanding cystic lung mass. Cough, fever, and repeated respiratory infection are less common presentations. Almost half of the infants with CCAM are premature.[13] Nonimmune fetal hydrops (anasarca) and stillbirth are common, and maternal polyhydramnios frequently accompanies CCAM, especially the generally bulky type 3 lesions. The severity of symptoms generally correlates with the size of the lesion, since the larger the lesion the more symptomatic the patient is. Although CCAM lacks intact bronchi, the frequent air-trapping after birth produces an expanding cystic mass and serves as evidence that the lesions communicate with the tracheobronchial tree.[68] The expansion with concomitant compression of adjacent lung tissue and frequent mediastinal shift produces the often observed respiratory distress that may lead to the death of the infant. CCAM, especially type 2, may be associated with a variety of

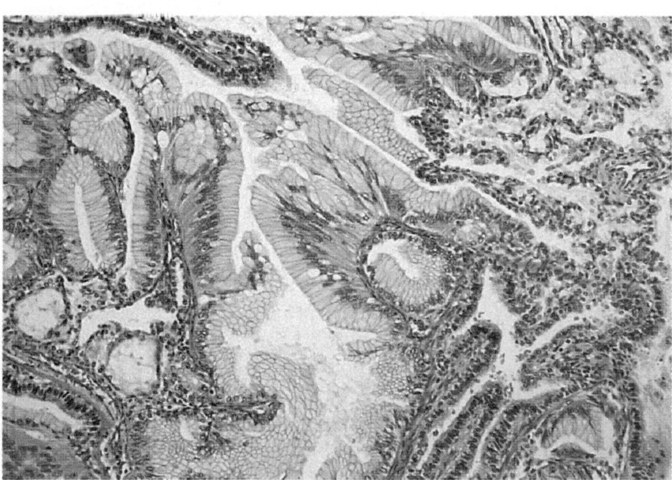

Fig. 49-6 Histologic appearance of congenital cystic adenomatoid malformation. Cleft-like spaces are lined by columnar epithelium.

other congenital anomalies including bilateral renal agenesis/dysgenesis, extralobar sequestration, diaphragmatic hernia, cardiovascular malformations, and pulmonary hypoplasia in the uninvolved lung. Surgical resection of the involved lobe is the recommended treatment. The associated congenital anomalies may adversely affect the prognosis.

Congenital pulmonary lymphangiectasis

Congenital pulmonary lymphangiectasis (CPL) is a rare, often fatal congenital disorder characterized by the diffuse distention of the pulmonary lymphatics.[69,70] Primary and secondary categories have been described. Most cases are considered to be secondary forms of CPL and are predominantly associated with serious cardiovascular anomalies, especially forms with significant pulmonary venous obstruction such as total anomalous pulmonary venous return. Uncommon cases reflect the pulmonary lymphatic involvement as part of a generalized disorder of lymphangiectasia with chylous effusions, lymphangiomas in various organs, and bone destruction. Although primary forms with only lung involvement have been described, the diagnosis of CPL should be seriously questioned in the absence of associated congenital anomalies such as significant cardiovascular defects.

Diffuse pronounced distention of the entire pulmonary lymphatic system characterizes the pathologic appearance in CPL. Grossly the lungs are enlarged, heavy, and noncompliant with prominent dilatation of the pleural, interlobular, and bronchovascular lymphatic networks. Microscopically the process is an ectasia of lymphatics because the dilated spaces are lined by endothelium and correspond to the distribution of the normal pulmonary lymphatic system. CPL must be distinguished from interstitial pulmonary "emphysema" where there is interstitial infiltration of air but the air-filled dilated spaces are often irregular and are not lined by endothelium. Dilated lymphatics are also noted in the setting of hyaline membrane disease. The diagnosis of CPL should be made cautiously in the setting of interstitial emphysema or pneumothorax.

CPL is usually a neonatal disorder with respiratory symptoms often developing within hours of birth. Some newborns present with pleural effusions, chylothorax, or a history of maternal polyhydramnios. Most cases are fatal within days to weeks because of progressive respiratory failure. Stillborns account for 10% of cases. Over 80% of the cases are assocated with multiple congenital anomalies, especially cardiovascular lesions. There is a 2:1 male-to-female predominance. The pathologically dilated pulmonary lymphatics correlate with the prominent Kerley B lines seen on chest roentgenograms and the linear and reticular densities that appear to radiate from the hilum.[69]

Congenital pulmonary overinflation ("emphysema")

Congenital pulmonary overinflation is a relatively common congenital pulmonary disorder characterized by hyperinflation of the pulmonary parenchyma of a lobe or segment secondary to bronchial obstruction, either intrinsic or extrinsic.[10,12] Although historically termed *congenital emphysema,* that term implies a destructive process of the acinus. In most cases of congenital pulmonary overinflation, the affected paren-chyma is significantly hyperinflated but lacks a component of acinar destruction such that it is best titled *overinflation*. The bronchial obstruction may be attributable to intrinsic defects such as bronchial stenosis, bronchial atresia, abnormal origin of a bronchus, or abnormal amount or distribution of bronchial cartilage, or the obstruction may be related to extrinsic compression of the airway by aberrant vessels (such as pulmonary artery sling) or masses (such as bronchogenic cyst). Similar finding of overinflation may rarely be secondary to acquired bronchial obstruction as in bronchial mucus plugs, intrabronchial granulation tissue secondary to the trauma of repeated airway suctioning, or aspirated meconium. There is a 2:1 male predominance.

Congenital pulmonary overinflation most often involves a lobe or a segment of a lobe.[71] Multilobe involvement is rare. Over 90% of cases involve one of the upper lobes or the middle lobe. The involved lobe is significantly enlarged because of the hyperinflation of the parenchyma. Even after surgical excision, the affected parenchyma often remains overinflated as evidence of the underlying airway obstruction. The hyperinflated parenchyma can be traced to the point of bronchial obstruction in many cases. Microscopically the overinflation is substantiated by alveolar ducts and alveoli that are several times larger than normal. Significant fibrosis or destruction of the alveolar parenchyma is generally not part of this disorder. Examination of the involved bronchus may reveal focal or diffuse abnormalities in the cartilage, stenotic areas or extrinsic lesions that compress the bronchus. Congenital pulmonary overinflation caused by obstruction must be differentiated from rare cases of apparent overinflation caused by polyalveolar lobe (pulmonary hyperplasia) where the abnormality lies in the alveolar parenchyma instead of the bronchus. In polyalveolar lobe, lobar expansion is secondary to a significant increase in the number of alveoli. Congenital pulmonary overinflation is associated with other congenital anomalies in approximately 40% of the cases, especially cardiovascular anomalies.[70] Most cases require lobar resection.[72]

Anomalies of pulmonary vasculature

A wide range of congenital anomalies may involve the pulmonary arterial system or the venous system.[73] The anomalous pulmonary arteries may arise from the ductus arteriosus, the aorta, or its branches to provide systemic blood flow and accompanying systemic pressures to the lungs. The *left pulmonary artery "sling"* refers to the aberrant origin of the left pulmonary artery from the right.[13] The anomalous vessel runs anterior to the esophagus but posterior to the trachea and may be associated with tracheal stenosis as a result of the compression by the vessel combined with abnormal ring-shaped tracheal cartilages. This anomaly is also associated with a bridging bronchus that connects the right middle and lower lobes to the left main bronchus. There are other vascular anomalies that may compromise airflow by compression of the trachea or major bronchi. The proximal portion of the pulmonary arterial system may be absent even in the face of an intact intrapulmonary arterial system.[74] Peripheral stenotic lesions may also be seen in Down syndrome, Ehlers-Danlos syndrome, and cutis laxa. Focal stenotic arterial lesions can be part of a wide range of disorders including associated congenital cardiac defects. Arteriohepatic dysplasia (Alagille's syndrome) manifests as peripheral stenotic lesions of the pulmonary arteries associated with cholestasis, and a paucity of intrahepatic bile ducts in children with peculiar facies.[75]Congenital rubella may result in similar peripheral stenotic lesions in the pulmonary system.

Anomalous pulmonary venous return may be partial or total. The anomalous venous system may drain into the innominate vein, the coronary veins, the right atrium, or the inferior vena cava anywhere between the hepatic vein and the right atrium, often below the diaphragm. Total anomalous venous return involves the anomalous drainage of all four main pulmonary veins into the aberrant site.[76] In partial anomalous venous return only a portion of the pulmonary venous return is aberrant. The *scimitar syndrome* is one example of partial anomalous venous return.[77,78] This syndrome manifests as a hypoplastic right lung, at least a partial systemic arterial supply to the right lung, dextroposition (mediastinal shift to the right) of the heart, and an anomalous pulmonary vein that drains the right lung to the inferior vena cava, usually below the diaphragm.[13] The anomalous vein usually runs inferiorly parallel to the right border of the heart. The scimitar anomaly is named for the similarity of the bandlike chest roentgenographic outline of the large anomalous pulmonary vein along the right heart border to a curved Turkish saber known as a scimitar. Associated anomalies include congenital cardiac defects, abnormal lung lobation, and accessory diaphragm. This complicated syndrome may overlap with horseshoe lung and pulmonary sequestration.

The pulmonary venous system may be focally stenotic, or segments of the system may be missing. Unilateral pulmonary venous stenosis has been noted in association with ventricular septal defects. With significant compromise of the venous system, associated areas of hemorrhage, hemosiderin pigmentation, and lymphangiectasis may develop as markers of the compromised venous outflow.

Arteriovenous fistulas represent an abnormal communication between the pulmonary arteries and veins, though occasionally systemic arteries are involved. The fistulas may be single or multiple. In most cases the fistulas are the pulmonary manifestation of familial hemorrhagic telangiectasias (Osler-Weber-Rendu syndrome) and are usually multiple. Occasionally isolated arteriovenous fistulas are noted without evidence of familial hemorrhagic telangiectasia, and other fistulas may be traumatically acquired. Many fistulas are asymptomatic; some produce symptoms related to the arteriovenous shunting of blood (exertional dyspnea, cyanosis, digital clubbing, polycythemia).[13]

ADAPTATION TO EXTRAUTERINE LIFE

Dramatic pulmonary physiologic changes characterize the abrupt transition from the relatively protected environment of the fetus to the extrauterine existence of the neonate. In utero, the lungs are fluid filled, receive only a fraction of the cardiac output, and do not serve as a gas-exchange organ.[79] After separation of the placenta, the neonate is dependent on adequate pulmonary oxygen and carbon dioxide exchange for survival. Birth serves as the final test of fetal lung maturation because survival of the newborn depends on the coordinated maturation of the pulmonary anatomic, physiologic, and biochemical systems.[80] Fetal lungs are distended by fluid in utero. Adaptation to extrauterine life requires the removal of lung liquid from the potential air spaces, the inflation of these spaces with air, and the stabilization of air-space surface tension in order to maintain an acceptable gas-filled functional residual capacity.[81]

During the last half of gestation fetal lung epithelium actively secretes into the potential air-space a chloride-rich, protein-poor fluid that is biochemically distinct from amniotic fluid.[82] Fetal lung fluid contributes to the composition of amniotic fluid, because the secreted lung fluid mixes with amniotic fluid during intrauterine respiratory movements. This mixing accounts for the not infrequent finding of fetal squames from the amniotic fluid in the small air spaces of otherwise normal neonates.[83] The balance between fetal lung fluid production and drainage is important, because obstruction to fluid drainage may lead to increased lung size and complexity, and excessive removal of lung fluid can lead to pulmonary hypoplasia.[81,84] At birth, this air-space fluid must be rapidly cleared in order to sustain oxygenation and ventilation. Although a small amount of lung fluid may be extruded from the lungs and upper respiratory tract as the infant squeezes through the birth canal, evidence indicates that a significant decrease in pulmonary fluid secretion actually precedes labor. This decrease in lung fluid production, and possibly even fluid reabsorption, progresses through labor and delivery so that only 30% to 40% of the air-space fluid remains to be resolved after delivery of the neonate. Preterm delivery or cesarean section without prior labor results in an increase in residual lung fluid that must be resolved to establish normal respiration. During the first few hours of air breathing, residual lung fluid is rapidly cleared from the distal air space into the pulmonary interstitium. From there the fluid is cleared from the lungs predominantly by reabsorption into the now expanded pulmonary vasculature while a smaller fraction drains by means of the pulmonary lymphatic system. This dramatic movement of fluid is aided by the significant protein concentration gradient from the protein-poor air-space fluid into the relatively protein-rich pulmonary interstitium, by the active sodium reabsorption on the part of the pulmonary epithelium and by the increase in pulmonary blood flow and drop in pulmonary vascular pressure. Air-space fluid clearance is maximal during the first 30 to 60 minutes of neonatal life, as the air-space fluid is moved from the gas side of the alveolar epithelium into the pulmonary interstitium. Elimination of the excess pulmonary interstitial fluid load is normally complete by approximately 6 hours after delivery.[81,82]

The first breath of the newborn may be one of the most important, yet most difficult, respiratory events of life, as the fluid-filled lungs are transformed into air-breathing organs of respiration after the maternally derived oxygen source is abruptly ended by the separation of the placenta. With the first breath comes a sharp increase in pulmonary blood flow, a progressive drop in pulmonary artery pressure, and the establishment of a functional residual capacity of lung gas that replaces the fetal air-space fluid volume.[85] There is a rapid change from a low-flow, high-resistance pulmonary vascular system to a low-resistance, high-flow system with the closure of the *ductus arteriosus*.

The biochemical maturation of the surfactant system is crucial to neonatal respiratory function as the newborn functional residual capacity approaches the closing volume. Maturation of the surfactant system stabilizes the residual volume of gas in the lung after the first few breaths and prevents expiratory collapse of the newly opened small airways and alveoli.[83] Surfactant is a unique surface-active lipoprotein that is produced by pulmonary type 2 cells and secreted into the distal air spaces where it forms a monolayer at the air-water interface.

Surfactant serves to dramatically diminish surface tension, thus preventing distal air-space collapse on expiration. The surface tension–lowering properties of surfactant are important because surface tension accounts for almost two thirds of the total retractile force in an air-inflated lung.[81] Without the surface tension–lowering capability of surfactant, the small air spaces of the neonatal lung are unstable at low lung gas volumes and tend to collapse, seriously impairing the newborn's ability to breath. In essence, surfactant serves as an antiatelectasis factor.

By weight, surfactant is composed of 80% phospholipid, 10% protein, and 10% neutral lipids. The phospholipid component consists largely of a lecithin, dipalmitoylphosphatidylcholine (DPPC), which serves as the major surface-active component. At least 4 surfactant proteins have been identified.[86-89] Like the phospholipids, these proteins are produced by type 2 pneumocytes. The proteins appear at different stages of fetal lung development and parallel the maturation of the phospholipid fraction of surfactant. The proteins significantly interact with the phospholipid components of surfactant to reduce alveolar surface tension, aid in the recycling of secreted surfactant, and assist in the activation of alveolar macrophages.[87,89]

Surfactant is generally not detectable in amniotic fluid during the first two trimesters of gestation.[90] During the third trimester, type 2 pneumocytes produce progressively increasing amounts of surfactant.[89] Early in the third trimester DPPC (lecithin) approximately equals the amount of sphingomyelin present in amniotic fluid. At approximately 34 weeks of gestation there is a substantial increase in the amount of DPPC (lecithin) produced and a concomitant stabilization or slow fall in the sphingomyelin level. This increase in the ratio of amniotic fluid lecithin (L) to sphingomyelin (S) continues to term and marks the maturation of the surfactant system. At approximately 35 or 36 weeks of gestation another phospholipid, phosphatidylglycerol (PG), appears in amniotic fluid in clinically significant amounts.[90] In addition to the amniotic fluid L:S ratio, several other tests on amniotic fluid are designed to detect the maturation of the fetal pulmonary surfactant system including tests to detect the presence of PG, biophysical tests of the surface-lowering properties such as foam stability tests, optical absorbance tests, "microviscosity" tests, and lamellar body counts. Some of these tests promise to replace the time-consuming classical L:S ratio in the preterm assessment of fetal lung maturity.[90,91] Maturation of the surfactant system may be affected by several hormones, and some pharmacologic methods are aimed at hastening the maturation of the surfactant-producing system.[89]

Failure of the neonate to adapt physiologically to the new environment or failure in the maturation of the lung anatomy or the surfactant system may result in a variety of neonatal respiratory disorders including hyaline membrane disease, bronchopulmonary dysplasia, persistent pulmonary hypertension (persistent fetal circulation), massive pulmonary hemorrhage, and meconium aspiration. Prematurity accounts for most acquired pulmonary disorders in the neonate, since many of these infants suffer from a failure in the maturation of the pulmonary surfactant-producing system. Although full-term newborns may infrequently develop respiratory disease, the pulmonary findings in this mature group are often a manifestation of an underlying problem such as infection, stress, or other external insult.[83]

PERINATAL LUNG DISEASE

Transient tachypnea of the newborn ("neonatal wet lung")

Normally the mature newborn rapidly clears the residual air-space lung fluid into the pulmonary interstitium within minutes to an hour of birth. The fluid is normally cleared from the pulmonary interstitium within 6 hours of birth. Transient tachypnea of the newborn (TTN), also called *neonatal wet lung disease* or *type II respiratory distress syndrome,* is a relatively common cause of often mild, self-limited respiratory distress in the newborn that is believed to be attributable to the delayed clearance of air space and interstitial fluid from the lungs after birth. This delayed removal of lung fluid is reflected in the chest x-ray film of alveolar filling and prominent interstitial pulmonary markings. Uncomplicated cases of TTN appear with the early onset of respiratory distress almost from the time of birth with tachypnea, retractions, and grunting. Some infants will require ventilatory support or other supportive measures including supplemental oxygen; however, the clinical picture is one of gradual improvement over 12 to 24 hours as the excess lung fluid is cleared. The prognosis is excellent with only supportive therapy. The incidence of TTN is increased with prematurity, cesarean section (especially without antecedent labor), and maternal diabetes. Most affected newborns are term infants or the larger premature infants with birth weights usually greater than 1500 g.[83,92]

Hyaline membrane disease

Hyaline membrane disease (HMD) is a clinical and pathologic perinatal disorder related to the deficiency of pulmonary surfactant. The pathologic pattern morphologically resembles diffuse alveolar damage, whereas the clinical picture is that of the respiratory distress syndrome of the newborn associated with a deficiency of pulmonary surfactant.[92-94] Most infants with HMD are premature, with inadequate production of functional surfactant leading to perinatal respiratory distress and the formation of hyaline membranes in the parenchymal lung tissue. The incidence of HMD increases dramatically as the gestational age falls. At 28 weeks of gestation, frequently with birth weights of less than 1000 g, the incidence of HMD is as high as 60% to 80%, whereas it is less than 1% at 38 weeks of gestation.[90,91] Because neonatal weight varies with gestational age, the incidence of HMD also varies inversely with the birth weight. Although gestational prematurity is the most common cause of HMD, other forms of morphologic prematurity such as pulmonary hypoplasia may present a similar pathologic picture. Uncommonly, HMD may be seen in term or postterm infants, where it is associated with a variety of disorders that secondarily affect the lungs, such as meconium aspiration, intrauterine or perinatal asphyxia, septicemia, and pulmonary hypoplasia.[95,96]

Several risk factors are associated with HMD, including prematurity (especially if the mother has a history of prior premature infants that were affected), white race, male sex, absence of intrauterine growth retardation, maternal diabetes, multiple gestation, and delivery by cesarean section. The risk of HMD is actually reduced in infants who withstand a variety of prenatal stresses such as those with intrauterine growth retardation or amniotic fluid infection, in those who pass meconium before delivery, in uncomplicated prolonged rupture of membranes, in subacute placental abruption, and in maternal chronic hypertension.[83,92,97] The intrauterine stress appears to produce a premature maturation of the surfactant system.

HMD is largely associated with prematurity: insufficient development of the surfactant system in combination with varying degrees of anatomic immaturity of the lungs. In HMD the premature newborn suffers from a relative lack of surfactant, which leads to high internal surface forces within the lung and subsequent collapse of alveoli and small airways.[83] The atelectasis leads to inefficient ventilation in the newborn with ventilation to perfusion mismatch, distention and damage of the compliant distal bronchioles, and leak of a protein-rich edema fluid from the damaged surfaces into the air spaces. The high surface tension in the distal air spaces substantially increases the work of breathing.

Many of the pathologic features described in HMD were noted before the modern era of neonatal ventilators, intensive oxygen therapy, and neonatal intensive care units. In uncomplicated, untreated HMD, the pathologic state correlates with the age of the process. During the first 6 to 8 hours after birth, grossly detectable patchy atelectasis (Fig. 49-7) and edema are associated with the microscopic findings of distal bronchiolar epithelial necrosis and basophilic necrotic debris in the distal airways accompanied by an abnormal expansion pattern.[59,98] The poorly inflated lungs are heavy and usually sink in water. Very immature infants with anatomically immature lungs who die in the first few hours after birth may be difficult to identify as HMD, since the characteristic hyaline membranes are not formed for several hours and the immature lung histologic features complicate recognition of the usual pattern of HMD. Hyaline membranes, which are microscopic eosinophilic membranes that line the air-space surfaces of respiratory bronchioles and alveolar ducts, begin to appear in significant numbers after 6 to 8 hours, and peak at approximately 24 to 36 hours (Fig. 49-8). Hyaline membranes result from the mechanical forces of ventilation on the exuded air-space fluid, necrotic cellular debris, and remnants of amniotic fluid that remain in the distal lung parenchyma.[83,97]

By 24 to 36 hours the lungs are firm, poorly expanded, and liverlike because of the widespread zones of atelectasis, widespread congestion, and the proteinaceous fluid in the distal air spaces. Microscopic foci of hemorrhage are common. Bronchioles more proximal to the atelectatic parenchyma are dilated, as are many of the pulmonary lymphatics. From 24 to 48 hours a cellular response becomes progressively more prominent as macrophages migrate into the distal air spaces and begin to clean up the hyaline membranes and cellular debris, and much of the edema is reabsorbed.[97,98] Resolution of HMD, which generally begins at 48 to 72 hours after birth, is characterized by the continued cleanup by macrophages with an associated proliferation of hyperplastic epithelial cells that attempt to resurface the damaged distal bronchiolar epithelium.[59] At the same time, an increasing quantity of surfactant is produced and released into the distal air spaces by the type 2 pneumocytes, substantially improving ventilation.[99]

The above pathologic findings of untreated, uncomplicated HMD were described before the establishment of modern neonatal intensive care units. The pathologist rarely sees untreated HMD in the United States today. Oxygen therapy and mechanical ventilation can produce a series of overlying changes in the neonatal lungs already damaged by HMD. The pathologic changes attributable to the medical intervention are often difficult to separate from those of the underlying disease.[83]

Variations in the appearance of hyaline membranes also exist. Yellow hyaline membranes may be seen in some infants if unconjugated bilirubin leaks into the distal air spaces from the foci of mucosal damage and binds to the pro-

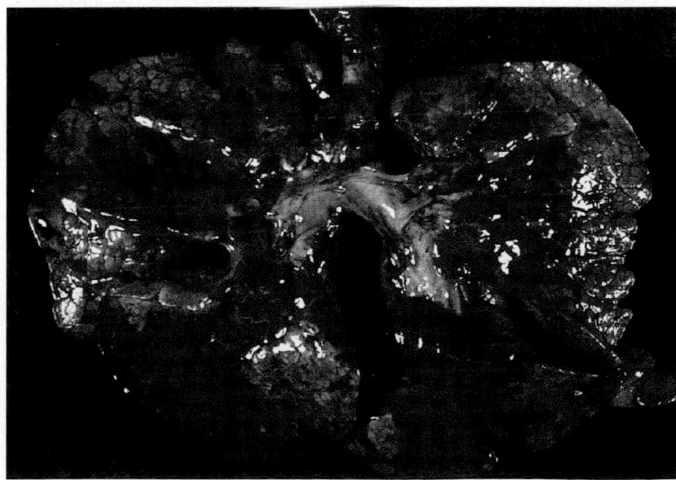

Fig. 49-7 Patchy atelectasis of neonatal lungs.

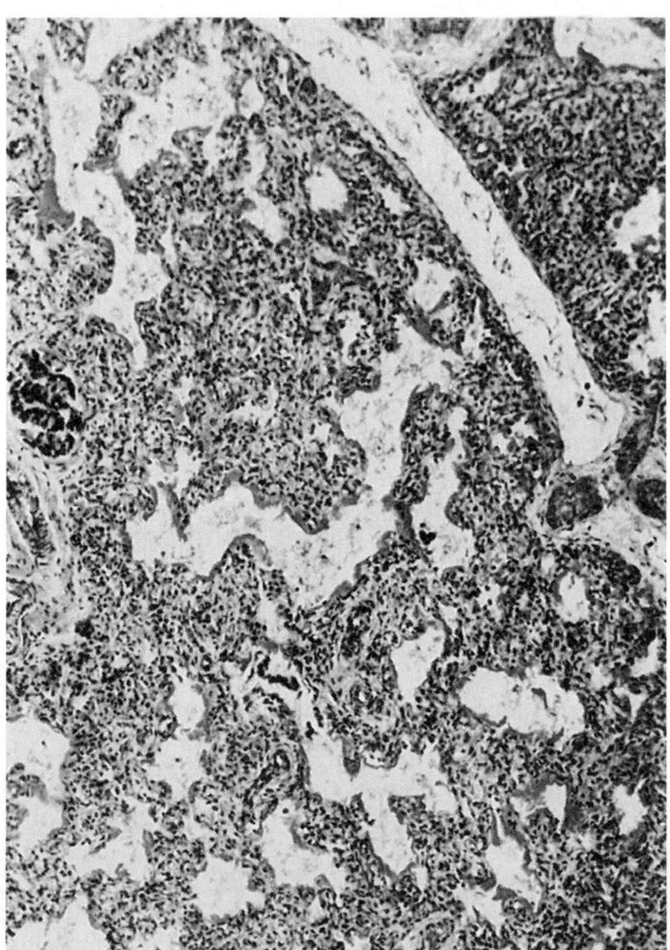

Fig. 49-8 Hyaline membranes line the alveolar ducts. The alveoli are atelectatic, and the lymphatics are dilated.

tein and cellular debris of the hyaline membrane. Yellow hyaline membranes have been associated with kernicterus, intraventricular cerebral hemorrhage, intrahepatic bile stasis, pulmonary hemorrhage, and disseminated intravascular coagulation.[97,100,101] Although hyaline membranes are characteristic of HMD, they are not specific for HMD, because perinatal infection can also produce hyaline membranes. Granular, fragmented, or faintly basophilic hyaline membranes are sometimes associated with significant neonatal bacterial lung infections caused by organisms such as *Streptococcus* or *Escherichia coli*.[59] Although acute inflammatory cells may not be prominent, gram stain of the hyaline membranes in these cases reveals numerous bacterial organisms embedded in the proteinaceous background of the membrane.

After transient tachypnea of the newborn, HMD is the most common cause of neonatal respiratory distress, affecting an estimated 1% of all newborns.[92,102] The typical neonate with respiratory distress syndrome and HMD is a premature infant who develops tachypnea, intercostal and subcostal retractions, grunting and cyanosis shortly after birth. In contrast to transient tachypnea of the newborn, in HMD oxygen requirements progressively increase and the infant's respiratory status progressively worsens over the interval between birth and 48 hours. The pathologic changes correlate with the radiologic and functional abnormalities. Hypoxia with poor pulmonary compliance reflects the ventilation-perfusion mismatch and the deficiency of surfactant.[83,103] A chest roentgenogram displays bilateral, diffuse "ground-glass" opacification of the fields of both lungs and air bronchograms. Clinical improvement, corresponding to the resolution phase of HMD, often begins at 48 to 72 hours in uncomplicated HMD with progressive improvement over the ensuing 3 to 5 days. Before the availability of mechanical ventilation, most infants recovered or died within the first 3 days after birth.[92]

The prognosis is good for infants who weigh more than 2500 g at birth. During the early 1990s, the widespread clinical use of surfactant replacement therapy and newer modes of mechanical ventilation in the neonatal intensive care units substantially improved the survival of even more immature newborns.[102,104] With the recent advances in therapy, HMD is uncommonly seen at autopsy in a neonate except for extremely premature infants or neonates with other complicating disorders such as congenital anomalies, infections, or gastrointestinal or CNS complications.[83] HMD, largely associated with immaturity, appears to be the initial insult to the lungs, whereas the occurrence of bronchopulmonary dysplasia appears to be the result of aggressive supportive respiratory therapy for infants who would otherwise have died of HMD. Complications of HMD include bronchopulmonary dysplasia, intraventricular cerebral hemorrhage, necrotizing enterocolitis, patent ductus arteriosus, and dissection of air into the interstitium of the lung (interstitial air, pneumothorax, mediastinal emphysema, air embolism).[59,93]

Bronchopulmonary dysplasia

Bronchopulmonary dysplasia (BPD) is the chronic pulmonary disease of infancy that follows ventilator and oxygen therapy for HMD.[83,105] BPD entails a combination of clinical, radiographic, and pathologic changes that generally follow the more severe cases of hyaline membrane disease. It results from the therapeutic rescue of a group of newborns that would otherwise have died. The clinical, radiographic, and pathologic definitions of BPD in the literature vary considerably, producing significant variability in the incidence and survival data.[59,93]

Recent advances in surfactant-replacement therapy and high-frequency ventilation have significantly decreased morbidity and mortality in newborns with HMD; however, these same advances have salvaged smaller, even more immature neonates who are at risk for BPD. In the mid-1960s the average infant with BPD was born at 34 weeks of gestational age with a birth weight just over 2200 g. By the mid-1990s, most infants who develop BPD weigh less than 1000 g at birth.[105] The highest incidence and the most severe forms of BPD occur in the most immature lungs.[106,107]

The cause of BPD is multifactorial.[108] BPD appears to be the result of an extended acute injury in a structurally and biochemically immature lung. The pathologic and functional pulmonary changes result from a complex interaction between the exposure to high oxygen levels, the barotrauma associated with the respiratory support, and the pulmonary reparative process, all during an important phase of lung growth and development.[106,108] The biochemical state of the neonate is not sufficiently equipped with antioxidant defenses to withstand exposure to prolonged or high oxygen levels. The relatively noncompliant, surfactant-deficient, distal lung parenchyma, with its patchy atelectasis, is exposed to the same mechanical ventilatory pressures and frequencies as the more proximal but relatively compliant tracheobronchial tree. The bronchiolar damage of HMD leaves some bronchioles obstructed with debris, some partially obstructed, and others relatively intact. The net result is varying degrees of parenchymal collapse alternating with patchy areas of hyperinflation.[107]

There is significant heterogeneity in the severity of pathologic changes and clinical findings in infants with BPD. The pathologic findings in the lung in BPD resemble the variety and chronology of changes seen in diffuse alveolar damage. BPD can be sequentially divided into three overlapping phases: (1) an early reparative phase, (2) a subacute fibroproliferative phase, and (3) a chronic fibroproliferative phase.

The continuum of pathologic changes of BPD begins during the latter half of the first week of life, where it merges almost imperceptibly with the picture of organizing hyaline membrane disease. At this point the lungs are firm, heavy, and irregularly atelectatic. The microscopic picture includes irregularly distributed zones of atelectasis interspersed with hyperexpanded acini. Bronchiolar and bronchial epithelial necrosis, luminal debris, scattered organizing hyaline membranes in the distal parenchyma, airspace macrophages, and activated interstitial fibroblasts are evident at this time.[59,83]

With progression to the subacute fibroproliferative stage from about the second week to the fourth week of life, attempts to organize and repair the bronchiolar damage are evident. Some bronchioles remain, whereas others appear to drop out secondary to the ongoing peribronchiolar fibrosis and luminal organization *(bronchiolitis obliterans)*. Interstitial fibrosis becomes prominent and hyaline membranes scarce by the end of this phase (Fig. 49-9).

As the process further organizes and enters the chronic fibroproliferative phase, the areas of atelectasis become less prominent while the hyperexpanded acini remodel around the obliterated parenchymal zones. This remodeling, over the ensuing few months, leads to the appearance of deep "pseudofissures" along the pleural surfaces, a hallmark of chronic BPD. Infants with BPD have significantly fewer alveoli than

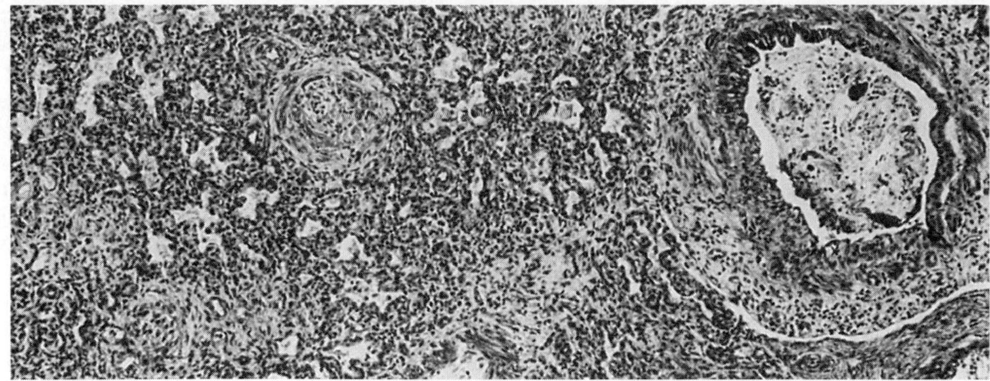

Fig. 49-9 Bronchopulmonary dysplasia in acute phase. Some bronchioles show epithelial necrosis and squamous metaplasia. Lighter nodules represent bronchioles obliterated by fibrous tissue.

normal with evidence that they do not "catch up" with their peers with respect to postnatal lung development. Fatal BPD is characterized by considerable impairment of lung development with alveolar hypoplasia and a significant reduction in the gas-exchange internal surface area of the lung.[109,110] The usual postnatal alveolar development is substantially interrupted and altered in the infant with BPD.

Infants dying with complications of BPD at this point demonstrate somatic growth retardation. The lung volumes are small, even corrected for the body weight, with abnormal development of individual lung lobe volumes. (Abnormally enlarged lobes may alternate with unusually small lobes). The central airway changes include submucosal gland hypertrophy, smooth muscle hyperplasia, and varying degrees of squamous metaplasia. Bronchiolar smooth muscle hyperplasia and irregular areas of interstitial fibrosis are common.[111,112]

The spectrum of clinical presentations of BPD is wide, reflecting the continuum of pathologic changes seen in the lung repair process. BPD affects from 5% to 20% of newborns treated by artificial ventilation.[59,105] However, differing clinical and pathologic definitions along with varying neonatal management protocols and referral patterns result in a wide variation in the reported incidence. The risk of BPD varies inversely with the neonate's gestational age and weight. With current therapies, BPD develops in over 80% of neonates that weigh less than 700 g at birth, whereas less than 5% of neonates over 1500 g are affected.[105] Although predominantly a disorder of prematurity, BPD may uncommonly be seen in term infants who require ventilatory support for a variety of underlying disorders such as meconium aspiration, congenital heart disease, pneumonia, and persistent pulmonary hypertension of the newborn.[59,105]

Most premature infants with respiratory distress and uncomplicated HMD rapidly improve after the second or third day of life such that minimal or no supplemental respiratory support is required by the end of the first week. Those that do not significantly improve by the end of the first week often evolve into the clinical picture of BPD.[108] By clinical definition, infants with BPD have signs of respiratory distress, hypoxia, and chest roentgenographic abnormalities that persist beyond 1 month of age. Affected infants suffer from varying degrees of hypoxia, CO_2 retention, airflow obstruction, and reduced pulmonary compliance. The radiologic features of BPD vary with the course and the pathologic changes. During the first week such features resemble HMD, but that picture gradually gives way to the picture of hyperexpanded acini and lobules alternating with irregularly collapsed parenchymal foci. Pulmonary interstitial air, or one of its complications, may further complicate the chest roentgenographic features in BPD.[105,113]

Many infants with BPD survive, and the pulmonary abnormalities substantially diminish as the infant reaches childhood.[106] However, up to 40% of infants with severe BPD die, with most of these deaths occurring during a prolonged initial hospitalization as a result of progressive respiratory failure, sepsis, or cardiovascular complications.[113] In the majority that survive into childhood and adolescence, there is evidence that most have some residual pulmonary functional abnormalities (airway obstruction, airway hyperreactivity, and hyperinflation) despite the significant overall clinical improvement.[106,113] Some of the subtle persistent functional abnormalities may be related to prematurity, with its effect on lung growth and development, and not necessarily to the therapy for HMD. Long-standing BPD patients suffer from recurrent, often severe, lower respiratory infections.[114]

Complications of BPD include pulmonary interstitial air, pneumothorax, pneumomediastinum, pulmonary hypertension, cor pulmonale, systemic hypertension, and right- or left-sided or biventricular cardiac hypertrophy.[112] Oral structures, the trachea, or the larynx may be damaged in BPD.[59] Pulmonary vascular changes in BPD-associated pulmonary hypertension include a reduction in the total cross-sectional perfusion area and an abnormal muscularization of the more peripheral pulmonary arteries.[115] Intravenous lipid infusion, as part of the nutritional support of these infants, has uncommonly been reported to result in a distinctive pulmonary arterial lipid lesion.

Pulmonary interstitial air

Pulmonary interstitial air (PIA), also called *pulmonary interstitial emphysema* (PIE), is the presence of air in the connective tissue planes of the lung. Although PIA may occur spontaneously during the perinatal period, it is most often seen in premature infants receiving ventilatory support for HMD or BPD. Entry of air into the connective tissue of the lung may result in a variety of clinical signs, symptoms, and radiographic appearances, called the *pulmonary air-leak syndromes*. Once in the pulmonary interstitium, the air may resorb uneventfully over a few days or persist for multiple days to weeks.[59,116,117]

The uneven lung-expansion patterns seen in HMD and BPD serve as evidence of the significant variations in ventilatory pressures and regional compliances in the lung parenchyma. The delicate premature acinar lung tissue may focally rupture at the base of an alveolus or air may break through the thin walls of the more proximal and compliant small airways to gain access to the interstitium.[117] Once air gains entry to the connective tissue planes of the lung, it may dissect along the bronchovascular bundles or along the interlobular septa. If the air dissects to the hilum, it may extend into the mediastinum, the pericardium, the thoracic soft tissues or even into the subcutaneous tissues. In the other direction, the interstitial pulmonary air may dissect to the pleural surface and rupture through the pleura to produce a pneumothorax.[116]

PIA produces multiple, variably sized, round to oval cysts distributed along the connective tissue planes of the lung (such as the interlobular septa or the bronchovascular bundles). Microscopically, the cysts of PIA lack a recognizable endothelial or epithelial lining. Based upon the pathologic findings and the age of the infant, two categories of PIA are recognized[59,116]: acute PIA, seen in infants less than 7 days old, and chronic (persistent) PIA, seen in infants more than 7 days old.

Acute PIA most often diffusely involves the lungs with relatively regular, small (< 0.5 cm) rounded cysts, somewhat linearly arranged along bronchovascular bundles and interlobular septa. Chronic PIA may be diffuse (involving all lobes), or it may be localized, often involving only one or two lobes (Fig. 49-10). The cysts in chronic diffuse PIA tend to consist of a combination of cysts and intercommunicating channels, most less than 1.0 cm in diameter. In the chronic localized form of PIA, the cysts tend to vary significantly in size, and some interstitial collections of air may reach 3 to 4 cm.

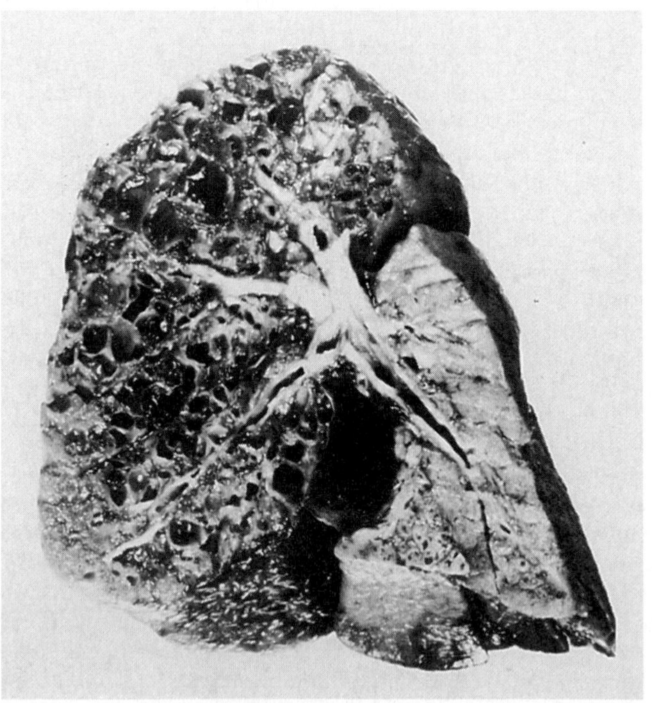

Fig. 49-10 Chronic pulmonary interstitial air. The lung contains large cystic spaces surrounded by fibrosis.

Microscopically, cysts in the chronic (persistent) forms of PIA, especially the localized form, often demonstrate a histologic reaction to the presence of air in the lung interstitium. In chronic PIA the cysts are at least partially lined by activated fibroblasts, occasional multinucleated giant cells, and scattered macrophages, analogous to the findings in pneumatosis cystoides intestinalis. The mural reaction to the interstitial air imparts a more irregular and ragged microscopic appearance to the cystic spaces.[59,116]

Diffuse forms of PIA must be distinguished from lymphangiectasis where the cystic spaces are lined by endothelium. Chronic, localized PIA may grossly and radiographically resemble congenital cystic adenomatoid malformation, congenital lobar emphysema, and postinfectious pneumatocele.[116]

Clinically, PIA is most commonly found in preterm infants receiving artificial ventilation for HMD or BPD. PIA may result from meconium aspiration, or pulmonary hypoplasia, or uncommonly interstitial air may occur spontaneously in a newborn without a recognizable underlying cause.[118] The incidence of PIA rises as the birth weight and gestational age fall, reaching approximately 40% with birth weights of less than 1000 g. PIA and its complications are associated with significant morbidity and mortality.[59,116] The clinical presentation of PIA varies considerably with the pattern and rapidity of air dissection. Findings may vary from the incidental radiographic discovery of PIA in an otherwise stable infant to a critical, clinical decompensation in an infant whose respiratory system is already taxed. Pneumothorax, pneumomediastinum and pneumopericardium are important and not infrequent complications of PIA.[118,119] Rarely pneumoperitoneum may be seen as part of the continuum of PIA; however, abdominal sources of the peritoneal air should be excluded first because they are more likely. Entry of PIA into the lymphatics of the lung can produce an air embolus. In "air block" PIA accumulates around the hilar blood vessels in sufficient quantity to interrupt pulmonary blood flow, resulting in circulatory collapse.[116]

Radiographically, PIA consists of linearly arranged, translucent cysts that seem to radiate from the hilum. Localized forms of PIA may form larger subpleural cystic structures ("pseudocysts"), which may be mistaken for a pneumothorax.[118] Chronic localized PIA may progressively enlarge and displace adjacent lung and mediastinal structures sometimes requiring surgical intervention, though they may respond to more conservative management.[120] Chronic diffuse PIA is closely associated with BPD and appears to carry a poor prognosis.[59]

Massive pulmonary hemorrhage in the newborn

Patchy zone of parenchymal hemorrhage are common in neonates dying of a wide variety of disorders. HMD and BPD frequently exhibit microscopic foci of hemorrhage; however, the small foci of hemorrhage are usually overshadowed by the pathologic changes of the underlying disease process. Massive pulmonary hemorrhage (MPH) of the newborn refers to a clinical syndrome of respiratory distress and acute collapse associated with large confluent zones of pulmonary hemorrhage that involves at least two lobes of the lung and often more.[121] In this uncommon disorder, the hemorrhage dominates the clinical picture and is often the principal cause of death. The usual setting is one of dramatic deterioration in an infant mechanically ventilated for a variety of reasons such as perinatal asphyxia, HMD, or BPD. Sudden deterioration in the clinical status is accompanied by the appearance of coarse pulmonary infiltrates on chest roentgenogram, reflecting the massive nature of the bleeding. Frothy blood is suctioned from the endotracheal tube and blood-stained fluid pours from the nose and mouth.[122]

MPH most likely represents a catastrophic but nonspecific terminal event with a wide variety of underlying causes.[59] MPH can affect infants of all sizes, but preterm, small for gestational age male infants are the most often affected.[121] Significant perinatal anoxia, often with cerebral edema or hemorrhage, cardiac disorders, or twin gestations are also significant predisposing factors.[121] MPH is also seen in stillborn infants. Neonatal pneumonia may produce MPH. Although the underlying mechanism has not been defined, the wide variety of clinical associations indicates that MPH may be a nonspecific result of a wide variety of insults to the capillary integrity of the lung. In some cases, the low hematocrit of the tracheal blood reported in MPH is suggestive that the hemorrhage represents a hemorrhagic form of pulmonary edema.[122] High microvascular pressure and damage to the pulmonary epithelium are also factors etiologically related to MPH.

Pathologically the lungs are consolidated by widespread zones of hemorrhage. The cut surface exudes a hemorrhagic, often frothy fluid. The lungs may also demonstrate changes of the underlying disorder, if one is associated with the MPH. Microscopically the alveolar spaces and small airways are filled with red blood cells and associated with variable foci of interstitial hemorrhage and pulmonary edema. The widespread bleeding may obscure the underlying disease process.[83] Histologic evidence of pneumonia should be sought as well as any evidence of disseminated intravascular coagulation.[59] MPH secondary to serious neonatal infections may be associated with evidence of coagulopathy, though most infants with MPH do not demonstrate coagulation defects. Cardiac defects and cerebral edema or hemorrhage are also common associations in MPH.

Based upon the 1958 British Perinatal Mortality Survey, the estimated frequency of MPH is 1 per 1000 live births, once hemorrhagic pneumonia is excluded. The onset of bleeding is most often between birth and 14 days, most frequently in the first week of life. Fortunately, MPH is uncommon because the mortality is high and survivors uncommon. Most infants die within hours to a few days of the onset of bleeding.[122]

Meconium aspiration syndrome

Meconium aspiration is defined as the presence of meconium in the respiratory tract of the neonate below the level of the vocal cords. Aspiration of large amounts of thick, tenacious meconium may be associated with hypoxia, significant respiratory distress, and even death in the neonate.[123] Meconium-stained amniotic fluid is not uncommon; from 10% to 20% of all live births are associated with the passage of meconium from the fetal gastrointestinal tract into the amniotic fluid. Meconium-stained amniotic fluid is usually noted in the mature or postmature neonate. Meconium passage may represent physiologic defecation in a mature or postmature infant, or it may be a sign of significant fetal distress.[124,125] It is rare before 38 weeks of gestation, but meconium staining is noted in over 30% of infants more than 42 weeks of gestational age.[123,125] Despite the relatively frequent occurrence of meconium-stained amniotic fluid, only one out of 20 (5%) of infants with meconium-stained amniotic fluid will develop the respiratory disorder of meconium aspiration syndrome (MAS).[92]

Once meconium is passed into the amniotic fluid, perinatal aspiration may occur with the first few breathes of life or in utero with the gasping efforts of a compromised fetus.[92,125] Meconium produces the deleterious respiratory effects largely through mechanical obstruction of the airways of the lungs by viscid meconium. Large airway obstruction with abundant, tenacious meconium may cause the rapid demise of the infant. With complete obstruction of smaller airways of the lung, distal atelectasis results; with partial obstruction there may be expiratory air trapping resulting in focal parenchymal hyperinflation. Meconium also acts to inhibit and displace surfactant in the distal airways and alveoli. The inflammatory picture of a chemical pneumonitis may follow meconium aspiration in some cases within 24 to 48 hours of birth, though the inflammatory pattern is variable because in some cases large amounts of meconium may be noted with minimal to no inflammatory response.[123]

Infants dying with MAS may grossly display variable amounts of thick, green-gray meconium within the large and small airways. Patchy, bilateral atelectasis alternates with focal areas of parenchymal overinflation. Microscopically the air ways at various levels are filled with fetal squames, mucus, and pigmented acellular debris. Small aggregates of fetal squames alone are not sufficient for a diagnosis of meconium aspiration because they are often observed in the distal air spaces of stillborn infants and neonates without meconium aspiration. Postmortem inflation of the neonatal lung may compromise the microscopic search for evidence of meconium aspiration.[124] After 12 to 24 hours, there may be an associated inflammatory response manifesting as acute inflammatory cells and macrophages as well as scattered hyaline membranes. In the postmature infant with hyaline membranes, MAS is a common finding.[123] Excessive muscularization of the acinar pulmonary arteries has been reported in severe cases of MAS, though some reports question this finding.[124] PIA, pneumomediastinum, or pneumothorax are found in many of the infants dying of MAS.

MAS is a disorder of mature or postmature infants, and in this group it is a common cause of respiratory distress during the first few days of life. Meconium aspiration spans a wide variety of respiratory disease from clinically asymptomatic radiographic findings to the severely depressed, hypoxic neonate in respiratory failure with associated persistent pulmonary hypertension who requires mechanical ventilation and high levels of supplemental oxygen.[92] Most infants who develop respiratory disease caused by MAS exhibit fetal heart rate pattern abnormalities or other evidence of intrauterine stress during labor and delivery. The thicker the consistency of the meconium-stained amniotic fluid, the higher is the probability of subsequent clinical respiratory disease caused by meconium aspiration. Oropharyngeal and nasopharyngeal suctioning at the time of birth and suctioning of the trachea in selected cases have decreased the incidence and mortality caused by MAS.[125] Respiratory compromise as the result of MAS generally appears within the first few hours of birth and in severe cases may even present at the time of delivery. The radiographic picture mirrors the pathologic condition: patchy bilateral areas of atelectasis and consolidation are interspersed between zones of hyperinflation. Pulmonary interstitial air, pneumomediastinum, and pneumothorax are common complications.[123] Supplemental oxygen and mechanical ventilation suffice for most cases, whereas extracorporeal membrane oxygenation (ECMO) may be necessary in the most severe cases. Rapid clinical and radiographic improvement characterize the first 24 to 48 hours of life in most survivors, whereas more severe cases may require a week or more to show clinical improvement.[92,125]

Fatalities may occur within a few minutes of birth to a few days. Meconium aspiration syndrome is fatal in 5% to 10% of cases with current therapy.[123] Children who survive MAS as a neonate may have clinical evidence of obstructive airway disease, wheezing, and bronchospasm on subsequent pulmonary function testing.[125]

Persistent pulmonary hypertension of the newborn

Persistent pulmonary hypertension of the newborn (PPHN), also known as *persistent fetal circulation,* is a clinical syndrome characterized by cyanosis and respiratory distress in the first few days of life associated with a postnatal persistence of a high pulmonary vascular resistance resulting in pulmonary hypertension. PPHN was initially called "persistent fetal circulation" because the postnatal circulatory pattern resembled the fetal pattern of right to left shunting in association with a high-resistance pulmonary vascular system. Under normal circumstances the pulmonary vascular resistance falls in the immediate postnatal period with the oxygenation of the pulmonary parenchyma and the initiation of extrauterine existence. This fall in resistance is accompanied by a substantial increase in pulmonary blood flow and a functional end to the fetal right to left shunting through the foramen ovale and ductus arteriosus. In PPHN, the normal drop in pulmonary vascular resistance either does not occur or occurs only to be followed by a subsequent rise in resistance. The resultant inadequate pulmonary blood flow is associated with significant right to left shunting of blood at the atrial level through the foramen ovale and, in some cases, at the level of the ductus arteriosus.[126,127]

PPHN is a clinical syndrome that results from a complex group of disorders of diverse causes that result in the clinical picture of persistent pulmonary hypertension in the newborn. There is an idiopathic, primary form of PPHN that must be differentiated from a variety of secondary forms of PPHN, because some of the underlying disorders in the secondary forms are amenable to therapy. Secondary PPHN is associated with a variety of clinical conditions including meconium aspiration, severe perinatal asphyxia, diaphragmatic hernia, nonbacterial endocardial thrombosis, neonatal sepsis, and pulmonary hypoplasia.[92] Alveolar capillary dysplasia (misalignment of pulmonary veins), an unusual developmental anomaly of the pulmonary vascular system and the pulmonary lobule, may also present as a secondary form of PPHN.

The problem in PPHN may be a functional vasoconstriction of the pulmonary arteries resulting in pulmonary hypertension, but in many cases the structure of the pulmonary arterial system is also abnormal with excessive muscularization of the small, distal pulmonary arterial branches. PPHN may be functionally classified into three categories[83]: (1) acute pulmonary vasoconstriction or hyperviscosity without structural pulmonary arterial changes, (2) excessive muscularization of the distal pulmonary arterial system, and (3) structurally deficient total cross-sectional area of the pulmonary vascular bed.

The *pulmonary vasoconstrictive-hyperviscosity type of hypertension* may be the result of a wide variety of pulmonary disorders such as acute perinatal asphyxia, pulmonary immaturity with HMD, polycythemia, or neonatal infections. The "idiopathic" forms of PPHN and occasional secondary forms, such as some cases of meconium aspiration, generally exhibit the *excessive muscularization* of the smaller pulmonary arteries of the neonatal acinus. These intra-acinar pulmonary arteries are generally nonmuscularized in the newborn. The excessive muscularization in infants with the "idiopathic" forms of PPHN and in some cases of meconium aspiration indicates that these infants may suffer from a form of intrauterine insult that results in the in utero proliferation of medial smooth muscle into the distal pulmonary arterial tree.[128] This form may also be seen in infants of mothers who chronically ingested prostaglandin inhibitors (such as aspirin, indomethacin) during the pregnancy.[129] PPHN in association with a deficient total cross-sectional area of the pulmonary vascular bed may be seen in pulmonary hypoplasia, congenital diaphragmatic hernia, chronic oligohydramnios, and congenital alveolar capillary dysplasia.

Congenital alveolar capillary dysplasia results in a deficit in the total number of alveolar capillaries and small pulmonary arterioles as well as an associated misplacement of the pulmonary venous system alongside the pulmonary arteries at the center of the pulmonary lobules instead of the usual location away from the arteries in the interlobular septa. This disorder reportedly is also associated with varying degrees of underdevelopment of the alveolar parenchyma. PPHN secondary to congenital alveolar capillary dysplasia portends a dismal prognosis. These infants usually die within days to a few weeks of birth.[130]

PPHN usually occurs in full-term or postmature infants, often with perinatal asphyxia.[127] The initial clinical picture of a cyanotic neonate with respiratory distress must be differentiated from the various forms of cyanotic congenital heart disease as well as significant pulmonary parenchymal disease that may secondarily result in pulmonary hypertension. The pulmonary hypertension of PPHN is accompanied by significant right to left shunting through the *foramen ovale* and often through the ductus arteriosus as well as clinical evidence of right ventricular overload in the absence of an identifiable cardiovascular malformation.[92] The primary form of PPHN radiologically presents with lung fields that appear hyperinflated and undervascularized. The early onset of significant pulmonary hypertension, which appears out of proportion to the parenchymal lung changes, as assessed by chest roentgenographic observation, and the lack of an underlying cardiovascular malformation are clinically helpful in differentiating PPHN from other forms of neonatal respiratory distress.[92,127]

Artificial ventilation, supplemental oxygen, drugs, and even ECMO have been used in the treatment of infants with PPHN. In cases that recover, the pulmonary artery pressures gradually diminish over the first 5 days of life, and the associated right to left shunting disappears as the clinical condition improves.[92] PPHN associated with alveolar capillary dysplasia, pulmonary hypoplasia, and the forms associated with excessive muscularization of the pulmonary acinar arteries generally do poorly with high mortality rates within the first few days to weeks of life, whereas infants with normal pulmonary vessels generally have a better prognosis.[127]

Infectious disorders of the newborn lung

Pulmonary infections produce significant morbidity and mortality in the neonatal period. More than 10% of infants in modern neonatal intensive care units develop pneumonia during the neonatal period, and the mortality approaches 20%.[83] Pneumonia is a common finding in neonatal autopsies.[59] The causative organism and the clinical picture of neonatal lung infections vary with the mechanism by which the neonate acquires the infection. Infectious organisms that cause neonatal pulmonary disease may be acquired by several routes,[131] including (1) transplacental spread of a maternal infection, (2) intrauterine ascending amniotic fluid infection, (3) intrapartum exposure to organisms as the infant passes through the birth canal, or (4) postnatal exposure to organisms from the environment.

Transplacental initiation of neonatal pneumonia is uncommon and is usually part of a generalized congenital infection with hematogenous spread of the organism from the mother across the placenta to systemically infect the fetus in utero. In these cases the neonatal pneumonia is just one aspect of a generalized infectious process often involving multiple organ systems of the fetus. Rubella (*Rubivirus*), herpes zoster (varicella-zoster virus), cytomegalic inclusion disease, and herpes simplex are examples of diseases by viruses that may transplacentally infect the fetus during maternal viremia.[132,133] Bacterial organisms are less common, but *Listeria monocytogenes, Mycobacterium tuberculosis,*[134] and *Treponema pallidum* may be associated with transplacentally acquired neonatal pulmonary infection. *Toxoplasma gondii*, a parasite, also crosses the placenta during pregnancy to infect the fetus. The presentation of the transplacentally acquired pulmonary infection may vary from respiratory failure at birth to a more chronic picture of pneumonia that persists for multiple weeks, depending on the causative organism and the timing of the infection during gestation.

Most neonatal pneumonias are acquired in the perinatal period, during the labor and delivery process, and result from maternally derived organisms. Amniotic fluid infection with aspiration of the infected fluid by the fetus accounts for 20% to 40% of cases of early onset neonatal sepsis and pneumonia.[135] Organisms from the lower genital tract of the mother may ascend into the amniotic cavity after rupture of the placental membranes, or the organisms may pass through intact membranes. The organisms in the infected amniotic fluid gain access to the neonatal lungs with the respiratory movements of the fetus. Acute inflammatory cells from the infected amniotic fluid may be aspirated into the perinatal lungs and appear in the airways and alveoli of the infant (Fig. 49-11). Amnionitis with associated neonatal pneumonia is more frequent with prematurity, prolonged labor, frequent digital exams during labor and in cases where there is a history of maternal urinary tract infection within a few weeks of delivery.[92] The neonatal pneumonias that result from these intrauterine ascending amniotic fluid infections are frequently severe and may be associated with stillborns, abortions, and early postnatal death in full-term infants. Blood culture results are often positive. The mortality in these early-onset pneumonias is substantially higher than that in the neonatal pneumonias that begin several days after birth. Group B *Streptococcus* and *E. coli* are two of the more common bacterial causes of amnionitis with postamnionitis neonatal pneumonia.[92]

Pneumonias acquired in the perinatal period include ascending infections that produce the amniotic fluid infection syndrome, as well as infections that begin as the infant passes through the birth canal and is exposed to the variety of organisms that are found in the cervical canal and vagina. As these organisms are acquired during the intrapartum period, the onset of clinical respiratory disease may be later than in the amniotic fluid infection syndrome. Organisms acquired during the intrapartum period may take a few days to a few weeks to cause clinical respiratory disease. The intrapartum infections may be viral or bacterial. Group B *Streptococcus, E. coli, Chlamydia,* and viruses such as herpes simplex virus may be acquired as the infant passes through the birth canal. A wide variety of clinical illness may be seen in the viral infections, and the severity of the subsequent neonatal infection may be related to the presence or absence of protective maternally derived antibodies in the neonatal circulation.[131,136]

Postnatally, infants may acquire pulmonary infections from the environment, including other humans. Offending organisms associated with pneumonias acquired in the postnatal period vary with the source of the infection. Gram-negative bacterial organisms such as *Pseudomonas, Klebsiella, Serratia,* and *Flavobacterium* may be associated with contaminated respiratory equipment, whereas *Staphylococcus aureus* and other gram-negative enteric organisims may be acquired from contaminated caregivers or family members. A variety of viral agents may spread in the nursery environment such as respiratory syncytial virus, influenza virus, parainfluenza viruses, and adenovirus.[136] Nosocomially acquired fungal infections may produce neonatal pulmonary disease, most often as part of a systemic neonatal fungal infection. Most neonatal fungal infections are caused by opportunistic fungi (such as *Candida, Malassezia*) rather than true pathogenic fungi.[137,138] Very low birth weight infants, prolonged administration of antibiotics, prolonged intubation, and vascular access devices, such as indwelling catheters, are risk factors for fungal infections.[139] Invasive procedures, intubation with mechanical ventilation, hyperoxic damage, and barotrauma all predispose the neonate to pneumonia. The infant may acquire a nosocomial pneumonia from contaminated equipment, caregivers, or the hospital nursery environment.[131,140] Late-onset pneumonias are commonest in preterm infants who require prolonged artificial ventilation. These late-onset pneumonias are generally less fulminant than the perinatally acquired pneumonias.

Although there may be overlap, the histopathologic pattern of neonatal pneumonia generally fits into one of three cate-

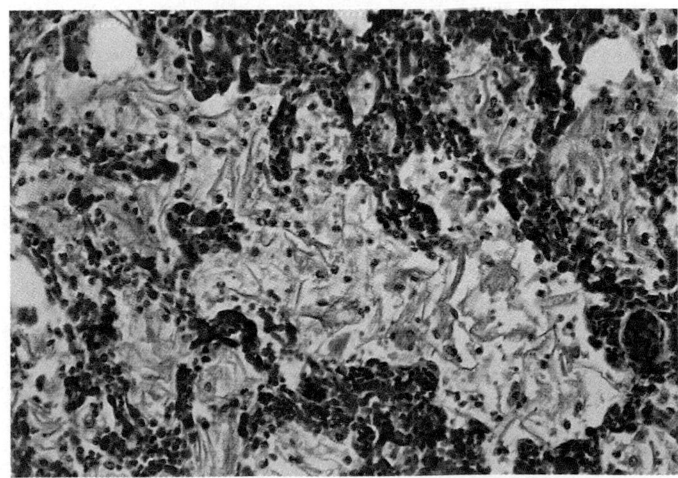

Fig. 49-11 Aspiration of infected amniotic fluid. Alveoli contain squamous and inflammatory cells.

gories: (1) hyaline membrane formation, (2) a suppurative inflammatory pattern, or (3) an interstitial pneumonitis. The causative organism and the time of onset of the pneumonia determine the pattern. Perinatally acquired group B streptococcal infections as well as some gram-negative enterics and some viruses may produce a pathologic pattern of hyaline membrane formation that must be distinguished from HMD caused by immaturity. Although these pneumonias resemble HMD, the pulmonary parenchymal expansion pattern differs from HMD, and more acute inflammatory cells are generally noted in the pneumonias. The chest roentgenographic findings of neonatal pneumonia and neonatal respiratory distress syndrome may be identical, though small pleural effusions are more common in pneumonia. In the cases of early-onset pneumonia, the hyaline membranes may be associated with a minimal acute inflammatory exudate, especially pneumonias in preterm infants that present at birth or within a day or two of birth. In these cases, large numbers of infecting bacteria can often be identified within the hyaline membranes with appropriate stains. Neonatal bacterial pneumonias that begin more than a few days after birth tend to produce a more classical picture of an acute inflammatory exudate filling distal bronchioles and alveoli, similar to suppurative bacterial pneumonias in the adult.[59] Interstitial neonatal pneumonias are typically the consequence of viral infection or *Chlamydia*.[131] Appropriate cultures of lung and blood should be submitted when pneumonia is a pathologic consideration.

Group B streptococcus is the most frequently identified bacterial organism causing neonatal pneumonia in the United States and accounts for more than half of all pneumonias that present during the first 48 hours of life.[59,132,141] Found in the genital tract and lower gastrointestinal tract of 10% to 30% of pregnant females, approximately 50% of the infants of these culture-positive mothers are colonized with group B streptococci. Only 1% of these colonized infants will develop invasive infections, and almost all of these will have neonatal pneumonia. Prolonged rupture of the membranes and chorioamnionitis are predisposing factors. Group B streptococci most often produce a fulminant, often fatal, pneumonia within the first 24 hours of life; however, this organism may also be acquired postnatally with the onset of infectious symptoms 1 to 6 weeks after birth.

Chlamydia trachomatis may cause neonatal pneumonia as well as neonatal inclusion conjunctivitis.[142] Sexually transmitted chlamydial genital tract infections of the adult are prevalent, affecting 5% to 10% of reproductive-age females. The infant acquires the organisms during the birth process through the infected lower genital tract of the mother. Respiratory symptoms begin at 2 to 8 weeks of age and include tachypnea, nasal congestion, and a staccato cough. An antecedent chlamydial conjunctivitis is observed in 50% of these infants.[83,131] Although the course may extend over weeks, recovery is the rule. Chlamydial pneumonias in infants are histologically characterized by a bronchiolitis accompanied by interstitial lymphoplasmacytic inflammatory infiltrates.

Ureaplasma urealyticum and *Mycoplasma hominis* are common isolates from the lower genital tract of reproductive-age females and have been isolated from cases of chorioamnionitis. It has been argued that these fastidious organisms may cause neonatal pneumonia and even chronic lung disease in infants,[132,143] but the evidence is inconclusive.

INFECTIONS OF THE LUNG

Influenza and pneumonia together are the sixth leading cause of death in the United States. They account for 2.8% of hospitalizations or more than 500,000 admissions per year. Nosocomial pneumonia develops in 0.5% to 1% of all patients hospitalized but in as many as 13% of critically ill patients admitted to intensive care units.

Routes of infection. Organisms reach the lung through the airways, by means of the bloodstream, by traumatic implantation, or by direct spread across the diaphragm from a subphrenic source. Inhalation of infected aerosols spreads exogenous organisms either from environmental sources or person-to-person by droplets that are generated by coughing or speaking. Pneumonia can also develop when the endogenous organisms of the upper respiratory flora are aspirated into the lower respiratory tract of a susceptible subject. Nosocomial pneumonia is often endogenous because of several factors in the hospital that promote colonization of upper airways by potential pathogens.[144] Antibiotics eliminate interference by the normal flora, promoting colonization by resistant strains. The use of nasogastric tubes and antacid regimens common in intensive care units permit enteric gram-negative rods access to the upper respiratory tract.[145] In critically ill patients, proteolytic alterations in cell surface molecules of nasopharyngeal epithelium promote the binding of gram-negative bacilli, an essential step in colonization.[146]

Pulmonary defenses. Several mechanisms protect the respiratory tract from infection. The mucus coating the airway mucosa provides a mechanical barrier that is propelled toward the oropharynx by ciliary action at a rate of 1 to 2 cm per minute in the central airways, rapidly removing organisms and other insoluble matter. The mechanical cleansing is bolstered by specific soluble antibacterial molecules, secretory immunoglobulin A, fibronectin, lysozyme, and lactoferrin produced in the bronchial mucosa. At the alveolar level, the primary defense is the alveolar macrophage. Most organisms reaching the alveoli are engulfed and killed long before they are physically cleared from the lung. Clinically important factors that depress macrophage function include starvation, ethanol ingestion, hypoxia, uremia, air pollutants, cigarette smoke, and antecedant viral infection. The alveolar lining fluid contains some immunoglobulin and complement components. Surfactant itself influences the phagocytosis and killing of some organisms, and one of the so-called surfactant proteins, SPD, is homologous to conglutinin and probably serves an antibacterial function rather than enchancing surface activity. Alveolar macrophages, when stimulated, can produce a variety of cytokines to recruit and activate other inflammatory cells. The lymphoid nodules located at the bifurcations of bronchioles and along the perilobular septa are part of the mucosa-associated lymphoid system and participate in specific immune reactions.

Viral infections

The biology of viral infections is discussed in Chapter 36. The major viruses that infect the lower respiratory tract and their pathologic manifestations are listed in Table 49-1.

In viral bronchitis, notably that caused by the influenza and parainfluenza viruses, the columnar epithelial cells show the most severe damage and are often sloughed, leaving behind a

Table 49-1 Viral infections of the lower respiratory tract

Virus	Nucleic acid	Family	Tracheo-bronchitis	Bronchiolitis	Interstitial pneumonia	Focal necrosis	Intranuclear inclusion	Cytoplasmic inclusion
Influenza	RNA	Orthomyxoviridae	+	+	+	−	−	−
Parainfluenza	RNA	Paramyxoviridae	+	+	+	−	−	+
Measles	RNA	Paramyxoviridae	+	+	+	−	+	+
Respiratory syncitial virus	RNA	Paramyxoviridae	+	+	+	−	−	+
Adenovirus	DNA	Adenoviridae	+	+	+	−	+	−
Herpes simplex	DNA	Herpetoviridae	+	+	+	+	+	−
Varicella-zoster virus	DNA	Herpetoviridae	+	+	+	+	+	−
Cytomegalovirus	DNA	Herpetoviridae	−	+	+	+	+	+

layer of basal cells. Regeneration from the basal cells can lead transiently to squamous metaplasia. The bronchioles are involved pathologically in many viral infections. Infection of the bronchioles is especially common in the first 2 years of life, when it produces a characteristic clinical picture with the acute onset of tachypnea, dyspnea, coughing, and wheezing, often with sternal retraction. Patients are usually afebrile. Most cases are caused by respiratory syncytial virus (RSV), but parainfluenza type III, adenovirus, and mycoplasma can produce a similar syndrome.[147] Epidemics of RSV bronchiolitis occur in the winter months and are especially common in day-care centers where susceptible infants assemble. The disease is ordinarily mild and only 1% to 2% of children require hospitalization.

When the rare lethal cases of RSV bronchiolitis come to autopsy, the lungs may be considered to be normal on gross examination, but close inspection reveals thickening of the small airways, which appear on the cut surface of the lung as 2 to 4 mm gray nodules with a barely visible pinpoint lumen. Microscopically, the walls of the bronchioles are densely infiltrated with mononuclear inflammatory cells (Fig. 49-12). Early, there is necrosis of the epithelial cells with the formation of plugs of necrotic material and leukocytes in the bronchiolar lumen. Regeneration of the epithelium begins after 3 to 4 days and is complete by 15 days with the regeneration of the cilia. The parenchyma shows alternating areas of air trapping and atelectasis, but parenchymal inflammation is limited to extension of the inflammatory infiltrate from the bronchioles into the walls of abutting alveoli.

Bronchiolitis caused by adenovirus tends to be more severe than that caused by RSV. Necrosis of the bronchiolar epithelium is extensive and may extend into the bronchiolar wall.[148] This probably explains the higher mortality of adenoviral bronchiolitis (5% to 7%) and the high frequency of sequelae.

Viral pneumonias occur at any age. Most viruses that produce pneumonia infect epithelial cells either exclusively or in addition to infecting other types of cells. The predominant tissue response is an acute interstitial pneumonia (Fig. 49-13). The walls of the air spaces are thickened by edema, congestion, and an infiltrate predominantly of mononuclear cells. The air spaces contain edema, fibrin, and a scanty cellular exudate of monocytes, macrophages, occasional neutrophils, and sloughed epithelial cells. In fatal cases, hyaline membranes are usually present along alveolar ducts, and the histologic pattern resembles diffuse alveolar damage (DAD) from other causes. Alveolar epithelial cells are enlarged and hyperplastic. Patients who have been ill for more than a few days show evidence of tissue repair and organization. Exudate in alveolar spaces is invaded by fibroblasts and converted to buds of fibrous tissue similar to organizing bacterial pneumonia or the reparative phase of DAD. Foci of epithelial hyperplasia and metaplasia to a squamous or bronchiolar type are found even in alveoli. Discrete foci of necrosis are often seen in pneumonia caused by herpes simplex viruses or varicella-zoster virus but are unusual with other viruses.

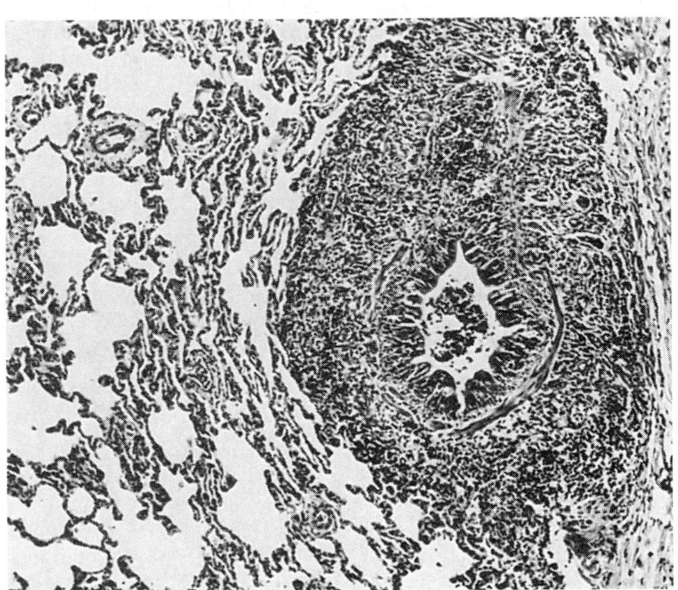

Fig. 49-12 Viral bronchiolitis. The wall of bronchiole is infiltrated with mononuclear cells. The alveoli are collapsed partially but not inflamed.

The specific infecting virus determines the cytologic features of the infected cells including the presence and morphology of inclusions and the tendency to form syncytia and giant cells. A specific etiologic diagnosis is often possible with routine histologic examination in the giant cell pneumonia of measles (Fig. 49-14), or the use of inclusions and cytologic

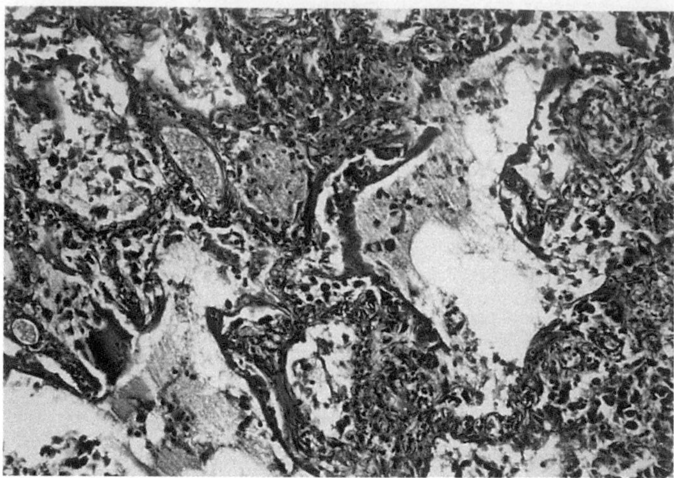

Fig. 49-13 Viral pneumonia. The alveolar septa are widened. The alveoli contain edema fluid, hyaline membranes, and mononuclear cells.

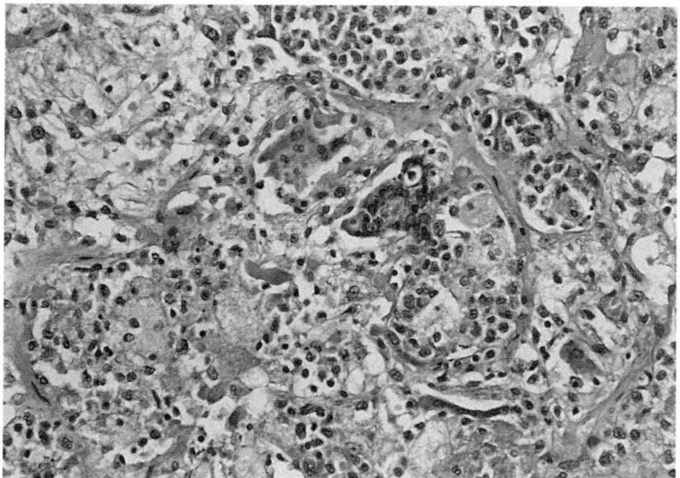

Fig. 49-14 Measles pneumonia. The exudate contains multinucleated giant cells.

features of cytomegalovirus- or adenovirus-infected epithelium. At the other extreme, influenza pneumonia has no distinguishing morphologic features and requires demonstration of the virus by culture, serology, immunohistochemistry, or nucleic acid hybridization.[149]

Viral respiratory infections can cause both acute and chronic sequelae. Acutely they predispose to infection by other viruses and to bacterial superinfection. Measles or adenoviral infection in childhood can lead to bronchiectasis, and some epidemiologic data link early respiratory infection to the subsequent development of chronic airflow obstruction.

Mycoplasmal, chlamydial, and rickettsial infections

Mycoplasmal pneumonia

Mycoplasma pneumoniae is a common cause of both sporadic and epidemic upper respiratory infections in otherwise healthy populations. The disease it causes lacks any striking seasonal incidence and predominantly affects older children and young adults. It appears that pneumonia develops in less than 10% of infected subjects. Clinically, mycoplasmal pneumonia is a benign, self-limited disease with few complications. Usually only one lung is involved, and the radiographic infiltrate is patchy or segmental in distribution.

The causative agents are small free-living organisms measuring 20 by 200 nm that can be cultured on simple media in vitro. They are enclosed by a membrane but lack a cell wall and therefore cannot be stained in histologic sections except by immunohistochemical methods. During infection, the flask-shaped organisms attach to respiratory epithelial cells by a specialized electron-dense structure at the tip of which there is contained the major adhesin P1. The bound organisms inhibit the catalase of the host cells causing a toxic buildup of intracellular peroxide, which results in lysis of the cells.[150]

Because of the benign course of mycoplasmal pneumonia, pathologic features of only a few cases have been described.[151] Grossly the lungs show a fibrinous pleurisy and patchy consolidations. Microscopic findings are bronchiolitis and interstitial pneumonia. The walls of bronchioles are congested, edematous, and infiltrated with mononuclear cells. Epithelial cells degenerate and slough. In some cases, inflammatory infiltrates occur mainly in the pleura and perilobular septa, whereas in others the alveolar walls are infiltrated with mononuclear cells. In fatal cases, edema and hyaline membranes may be seen. The histologic changes are indistinguishable from those of viral pneumonia and culture or immunohistochemical demonstration of the organisms is required for diagnosis.

A variety of immunologic phenomena accompany mycoplasmal infection, including the appearance of circulating immune complexes, rheumatoid factor, and biologic false-positive serological test results for syphilis. Cold agglutinins appear in approximately 50% of patients. These are IgM antibodies with anti-I specificity that agglutinate the patient's erythrocytes at 4° C but not at 37° C. Occasionally they may cause Raynaud's pnenomenon or hemolytic anemia. Nonrespiratory manifestations of *Mycoplasma pneumoniae* have been described in the skin, gastrointestinal tract, musculoskeletal system, heart, and nervous system. It is unclear whether they are caused by immunologic mechanisms or spread of infection.

Chlamydial pneumonia

All pathogenic *Chlamydia* organisms can cause pneumonia. *Chlamydia trachomatis* infection acquired at birth is a well-documented cause of pneumonia in infants. *Chlamydia pneumoniae* infection of adults is accompanied by upper respiratory tract symptoms and less often by atypical pneumonia. It has been estimated that 10% of all pneumonias in adults are caused by *C. pneumoniae*.[152] *Chlamydia psittaci* infection is a zoonosis acquired by close contact with pet birds or in the poultry industry.[153]

Chlamydial pneumonias of adults are mild and respond well to treatment. Hence, the pathology remains poorly understood. Histopathologic changes in rare cases of lethal chlamydial pneumonias were nonspecific. Focal bronchiolitis, interstitial and intra-alveolar pneumonia have been reported, but some of these changes could be attributed to secondary bacterial infection, which may complicate severe disease.

Rickettsial pneumonia

The most important pulmonary pathogens are *Coxiella burnetii* and *Rickettsia rickettsii*. *C. burnetii,* the cause of Q fever, may cause pneumonia, which is characterized by multiple foci of consolidation that appear round on x-ray examination.[154] The disease usually responds well to treatment, and therefore the pathologic features of typical Q fever pneumonia remain incompletely documented. A few cases that were examined at autopsy had severe necrotizing bronchiolitis and hemorrhagic pneumonia.[155]

The infection with *R. rickettsii,* the cause of Rocky Mountain spotted fever, is associated with respiratory symptoms in 30% to 40% cases. Histologically the infection is characterized by mononuclear cell infiltration of alveolar septa and the walls of small blood vessels. The intra-alveolar accumulation of edema fluid, macrophages, and fibrin is believed to be secondary to increased permeability of damaged blood vessels.[156]

Bacterial infections

Acute tracheobronchitis

Acute bacterial infections of the large airways are a frequent complication of viral infections. In young children with small-caliber airways, bacterial infection can cause severe obstruction. In children below 6 years of age, acute bacterial tracheitis produces a characteristic syndrome resembling croup but with stridor, high fever, and toxicity.[157] Epiglottitis is absent. Most cases are caused by *Staphylococcus aureus,* but other bacteria may also be responsible. Tracheal obstruction by subglottic edema and mucopurulent exudate can be lethal unless treated. Although bacterial tracheitis seldom occurs in adults, it has been reported in patients infected with human immunodeficiency virus (HIV).[158]

Pneumococcal pneumonia

Streptococcus pneumoniae, commonly called the "pneumococcus," is a gram-positive facultative anaerobe that produces alpha-hemolysis when cultured on blood agar. In smears and tissue sections, it appears as lancet-shaped diplococci and in short chains and clumps. Although more than 80 strains can be distinguished based on the antigens of their capsular polysaccharides, only eight strains account for two thirds of pneumonias. Currently, 4% to 5% of isolates are penicillin resistant.

The pneumococcus continues to be the commonest cause of community-acquired pneumonia requiring hospitalization, accounting for 30% to 80% of cases.[159,160] Groups at high risk include the very old and the very young, alcoholics, poorly controlled diabetics, splenectomized subjects, and patients with multiple myeloma or sickle cell disease. In HIV-infected patients, pneumococcal pneumonia is 5 to 18 times more common than that in the general population. In HIV-infected subjects, the first episode of pneumococcal pneumonia usually occurs before all the criteria for AIDS have been met.[161]

Pathology. The pneumococcus can cause either lobar or bronchopneumonia (Fig. 49-15). In the preantibiotic era, two thirds of cases were lobar pneumonia, but currently fewer cases present this classical picture. In lobar pneumonia, one or occasionally several lobes of the lung are involved. Individual lobes are uniform in appearance because the process spreads rapidly through the whole lobe until contained by the lobar fissure. Traditionally the process is separated into four stages: edema, red hepatization, gray hepatization, and resolution or organization.

Pneumococci colonize the upper respiratory tract and reach the lower respiratory tract by aspiration. Commonly this occurs several days after a viral respiratory infection that paves the way by damaging the ciliated epithelium and stimulating copious secretions. The initial response is an outpouring of edema fluid, which provides a rich broth in which the organisms proliferate and then spreads them throughout the lobe through pores of Kohn and bronchioles. At this stage, the involved lobe appears distended, moist, and deep red-purple. The pleura is shiny, and fluid exudes from the cut surface. With the passage of time, progressively more fibrin is deposited. Neutrophils enter the alveoli recruited by chemoattractants, some derived from complement and some from macrophages by the arachidonic acid cascade.[162] Phagocytosis of bacteria begins, and within 24 hours most of the bacteria are found within neutrophils. At first engorged capillaries and diapedesis of erythrocytes into the alveoli give the lobe a red color, and the filling of the air spaces with fibrin and leukocytes gives the tissue a firm, liverlike consistency. This phase is classically described by the term *red hepatization.* With time, increasing amounts of fibrin and leukocytes enter the air spaces, the alveolar capillaries appear compressed, and the lobe becomes progressively grayer in its gross appearance, evolving into the stage of gray hepatization (Fig. 49-16). In untreated individuals, organisms decrease in number progressively after approximately 5 days.

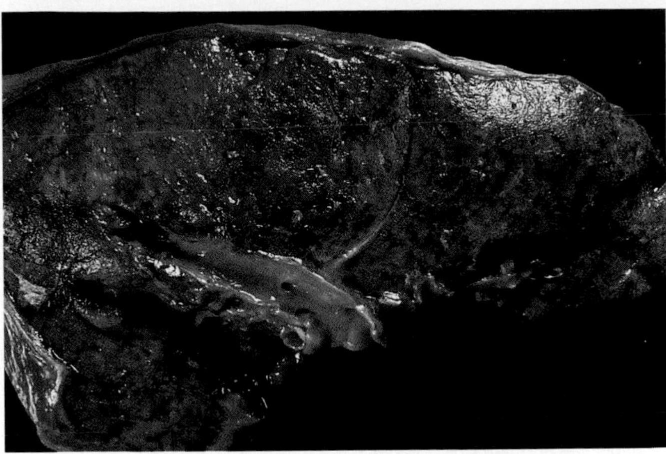

Fig. 49-15 Lobar pneumonia. The lungs are consolidated, and the parenchyma appears bulging on the cross section.

In the usual course, the final stage is resolution. As a rule, necrosis of alveolar walls is not a feature of pneumococcal pneumonia except with serotype 3. Since the exudation is intra-alveolar, it can be cleared through the bronchial tree, restoring the lung to normal. Macrophages are the predominant cell during this process. Beginning as early as 48 hours after onset, monocytes can be found in the alveolar exudate, and by 5 to 10 days, monocytes and macrophages become the predominant type of inflammatory cell. The neutrophils undergo apoptosis and are taken up by the macrophages while the fibrin network breaks down under the influence of proteases released from the neutrophils and newly arrived macrophages. The exudate is gradually removed by phagocytosis or expectorated, and the alveolar architecture ultimately returns to normal.

In a small proportion of cases, resolution is incomplete, and unresolved areas undergo organization. Fibroblasts invade the air spaces and lay down a provisional matrix rich in proteogly-

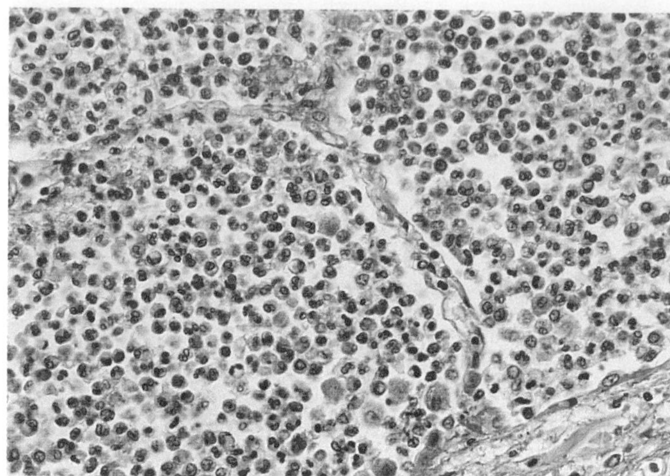

Fig. 49-16 Lobar pneumonia in stage of gray hepatization. The alveoli are filled with neutrophils. Alveolar walls are relatively normal.

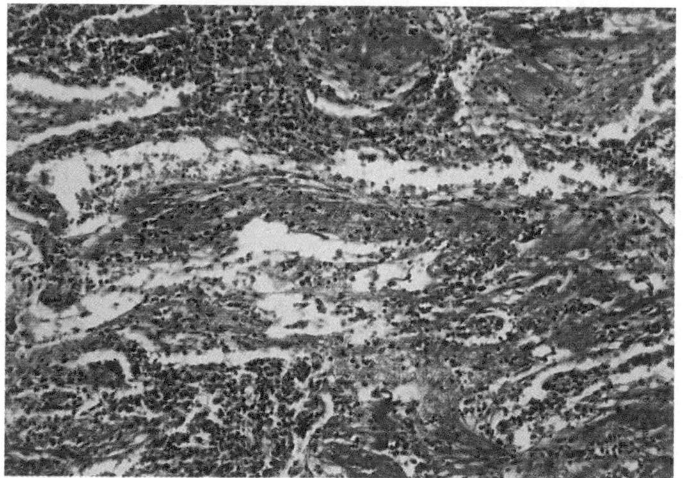

Fig. 49-17 Organizing pneumonia. The fibroblasts invade the intraalveolar fibrin.

cans and glycoproteins, which is gradually converted to collagenous tissue (Fig. 49-17). In some areas, alveolar epithelium migrates over the organizing exudate within air spaces incorporating it into alveolar walls, giving rise to an appearance indistinguishable from interstitial fibrosis. In other areas, the air spaces remain filled, and the lung is converted to fleshy gray glistening solid tissue whose meaty consistency accounts for the old term for the process, carnification. Factors that promote organization rather than resolution include bronchial obstruction and necrosis of alveolar walls.

The pneumococcus is more likely to produce bronchopneumonia rather than lobar pneumonia when patients are very young or are older than 50 and if they have underlying disease, such as chronic airflow obstruction or serious extrathoracic disease. The pneumonia is commonly bilateral and has an appearance similar to that of other bronchopneumonias, notably multiple foci of consolidation centered on terminal airways.

Complications. In most patients with lobar pneumonia, there is a fibrinous pleuritis and effusion without infection of

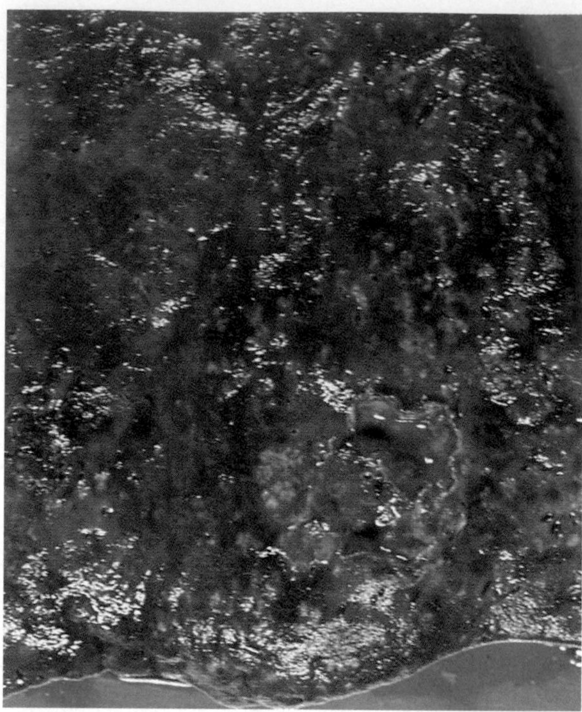

Fig. 49-18 Lung abscesses. The large abscess cavity contains viscous pus. The surrounding parenchyma appears consolidated and contains scattered smaller abscesses, which are whitish yellow.

the pleural fluid (*parapneumonic effusion*). In 15% to 25% of patients, infection of the pleural space develops (*empyema*). The pleural fluid becomes turbid and then frankly purulent with loculated collections of pus. Exudate in the pleural cavity cannot be cleared readily, and empyemas heal by organization rather than resolving. The lung becomes encased by a fibrous peel, which can be sufficiently thick to restrict expansion of the lung.

Bacteremia occurs in 15% to 30% of patients with pneumococcal pneumonia, more often with lobar than with bronchopneumonia. It occurs in those with serious underlying disease, especially infection by HIV. Bacteremic spread can lead to meningitis or, less commonly, to bacterial endocarditis, arthritis, or pericarditis. The mortality remains high despite antibiotics: 15% in those without meningitis and 33% with meningitis.[163]

Lung abscess results from the breakdown of alveolar walls (Fig. 49-18). The frequency of this complication is twice greater with type 3 pneumococcus than with other strains, evidently because type 3 pneumococcus is protected from phagocytosis by its abundant production of capsular polysaccharide.

Clinical correlations. The onset of pneumococcal pneumonia is usually abrupt with a shaking chill followed by high fever, systemic symptoms, and pleuritic chest pain. Most patients cough up rusty or purulent sputum. Leukocytosis up to 20×10^9/L (20,000/mm^3) is common, and leukopenia is a grave prognostic sign. Most patients respond rapidly to antibiotics, and improvement is evident within 24 hours.

Other gram-positive pneumonias

Beta-hemolytic streptococci are an uncommon cause of pneumonia at present. Lancefield group A streptococci were formerly the most prominent strains, but recently group B stains have assumed greater importance. Infections caused by group B streptococci in the newborn have been discussed earlier. In adults, pulmonary infection caused by beta-hemolytic streptococci is usually seen in severely debilitated patients, often as part of a polymicrobial pneumonia. Beta-hemolytic streptococci cause bronchopneumonia with a greater degree of interstitial involvement than in other bacterial pneumonias.

Staphylococcus aureus commonly colonizes the nose and skin. Pneumonia usually occurs either in the presence of an extrapulmonary source of bacteremia or after a viral infection. Hematogenous pneumonia is seen in those with soft-tissue infections, intravenous lines, and hemodialysis shunts and in parenteral narcotic users, especially those with right-sided bacterial endocarditis.[164] Hematogenous dissemination to the lung produces multiple peripheral lung lesions, most numerous in the lower lobes where the blood flow is greatest.[165] The lesions may be septic infarcts that appear yellow and purulent but retain to some extent the wedge-shaped configuration of infarcts and are associated with thrombosed vessels, or they may be rounded patches of necrotizing pneumonia that break down, giving rise to abscesses.

Aerogenous staphylococcal pneumonia follows the spread of organisms from the colonized nasopharynx after viral infections or, in hospitalized patients, after endotracheal intubation. The lesions are those of a bronchopneumonia accompanied by a severe hemorrhagic and necrotizing bronchitis. Purulent exudate fills the bronchioles and spreads into the adjacent acini. Early necrosis and breakdown of alveolar walls may result in hemorrhage in the surrounding lung (Fig. 49-19).

Staphylococcal pneumonia in small children is often complicated by the development of pneumatoceles, air containing spaces that are seen roentgenographically within areas of consolidation and enlarge very rapidly, often over hours. They are thin walled and can disappear over several weeks without residua. Most radiologists assume that they arise from the trapping of air distal to partial obstruction of a bronchus, which acts as a check valve. Other local complications of staphylococcal pneumonia include parapneumonic pleural effusion, empyema, and bronchopleural fistula.

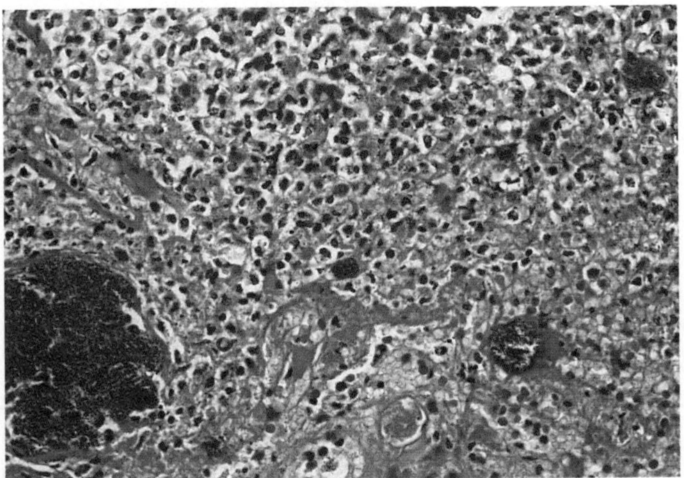

Fig. 49-19 Necrotizing pneumonia. There is necrosis of alveolar septa. Large bacterial colonies *(blue)* are also present.

Pneumonia caused by gram-negative bacteria

In the preantibiotic era, gram-negative bacteria accounted for 0.5% to 5% of pneumonias, and most were caused by *Klebsiella* and *Enterobacter* organisms. The incidence of gram-negative pneumonias has increased, and currently they account for 5% to 30% of community-acquired bacterial pneumonia requiring hospitalization and for the majority of nosocomial pneumonias. Even when community acquired, they are virtually limited to persons with underlying illnesses.[166,167]

The pathologic pattern of gram-negative pneumonias is influenced by the route of infection as well as by the causative organism and underlying disease (Table 49-2). Microaspiration commonly occurs during sleep, and infection favors dependent regions of the lung, the right lung over the left one because of the straighter course of the right bronchus, and the posterior segments, which are dependent when a patient is supine. Hematogenous dissemination most often produces a bilateral lower lobe distribution. The amount of hemorrhage and necrosis varies with the organism, with abscesses being common with *Klebsiella, E. coli,* and *Pseudomonas* and rare with *Haemophilus influenzae* or *Branhamella* organisms. The intra-alveolar exudate contains polymorphonuclear neutrophils, monocytes, and macrophages in varying proportions, but monocytes and macrophages frequently predominate.

Pseudomonas aeruginosa causes two distinct forms of pneumonia. One pattern common in critically ill, ventilator-dependent patients is confluent bronchopneumonia resulting from aspiration. The other, usually seen in burn patients and in those who are leukopenic from chemotherapy of leukemia or solid tumors, is a consequence of hematogenous spread from a nonrespiratory source.[168] Grossly the hematogenous lesions begin as small peripheral hemorrhages enlarging into rounded foci of necrosis still surrounded by a rim of hemorrhage.[169] Microscopically, established lesions consist of eosinophilic coagulative necrosis in which the outlines of the underlying tissue structure remain and inflammatory cells are few. The walls of arteries, and veins are faintly basophilic and hazy, and Gram stain that shows that they are teeming with bacilli. The necrosis and hemorrhage are not the result of ischemia but rather are caused by toxins including exotoxin A, elastase, and alkaline protease released by the bacteria.

The mortality of gram-negative pneumonia is around 30% overall but is widely variable depending on the causative organism and underlying disease.

Pneumonia caused by Legionella

Since their discovery during the investigation of an epidemic of pneumonia at an American Legion convention in 1976, the *Legionella* species have emerged as a leading cause of sporadic and epidemic community-acquired pneumonia as well as an occasional cause of nosocomial pneumonia.[170] At present, there are more than 20 known species of *Legionella*, some with multiple serotypes. At least 10 species cause pneumonia in man. The legionellae are slow-growing, motile bacteria 2 to 4 μm in length that resemble gram-negative bacilli ultrastructurally. Their slow growth, fastidious nutritional requirements, and failure to stain by Gram's method explain how they escaped discovery until recently.

The normal habitat for the bacteria is warm water, and epidemics usually occur during the summer months. The route of transmission is controversial. Epidemics have usually been

Table 49-2 Some features of gram-negative pneumonias in adults

Organism	Predisposing condition	Pathogenesis	Mortality* (%)
Klebsiella pneumoniae	Alcoholism, CAO, DM, cirrhosis, therapeutic immunosuppression	Aspiration	35-50
Proteus spp.	Alcoholism, CAO, DM	Aspiration	18
Escherichia coli	Urinary tract, gastrointestinal, or biliary infection	Hematogenous	30
Haemophilus influenzae	CAO, viral infection, HIV	Aspiration	10-20
Pseudomonas aeruginosa	Intensive care, CAO	Aspiration	50
	Malignancy, leukopenia, burns	Hematogenous	80-100
	Cystic fibrosis	Endobronchial colonization	
Branhamella catarrhalis	CAO, malnutrition	Aspiration	<5%
Acinetobacter spp.	Alcoholism, ventilators	Aspiration	45

CAO, Chronic airflow obstruction; *DM,* diabetes mellitus; *HIV,* human immunodeficiency virus.
* Mortality is approximate and strongly influenced by the severity of the predisposing condition.

attributed to inhalation of infected aerosols, but recent outbreaks traced to potable water are suggestive of a sequence of colonization of the oropharynx and aspiration.[171] As with other infections, impaired host defenses play a role. In the original epidemic, most of those affected were cigarette smokers over 50 years of age. Hospital epidemics have mainly affected those with chronic illness, especially subjects receiving corticosteroids.

L. pneumophila, the species responsible for the original epidemic, causes two clinical syndromes: Pontiac fever, which is an acute influenza-like febrile illness with a short incubation period, high attack rate, and negligible mortality and pneumonia with a low attack rate, a serious and prolonged course, and 25% mortality.[170] Although pathologic changes of patients with pneumonia are usually limited to the lungs, the onset of the disease is often dominated by systemic symptoms, fever, diarrhea, leukopenia, and hyponatremia. Cough, dyspnea, sputum production, and signs of pneumonia may not appear until the fifth to seventh day.

The gross findings in the lungs of fatal cases are a confluent bronchopneumonia usually involving multiple lobes. Entire lobes may be consolidated, but areas of early involvement usually show a lobular involvement. Small pleural effusions and a fibrinous pleuritis are commonly present. The histologic findings are not distinctive. The alveoli are filled with an exudate of fibrin, neutrophils, and mononuclear phagocytes in varying proportions. Most alveolar septa show only minor changes manifesting as foci of hyperplasia of the alveolar epithelium. Thrombosis of vessels and necrosis of alveolar walls are present in some cases. In cases of long duration, organization of the intra-alveolar exudate occurs. The diagnosis can be suspected when the Gram stain shows negative results, but methods that stain all bacteria, such as Dieterle's silver stain, show numerous organisms. The diagnosis should be confirmed by culture or by immunohistochemical analysis, which can be satisfactorily applied to formalin-fixed paraffin sections. *L. micdadei,* a species that causes nosocomial pneumonia in the immunosuppressed, is weakly acid fast and can be stained with a modified Kinyoun's stain.

The relentless progression and resistance to therapy of *Legionella* pneumonia is probably the result of the organism's ability to survive and proliferate within phagocytes. The organisms produce several factors that impair signal transduction during phagocyte activation.[172,173] As a result, phagocytes may show impairment of oxidative burst and superoxide production, and some strains produce impaired lysosome-phagosome fusion.

Lung lesions caused by anaerobic bacteria

Anaerobic bacteria are plentiful in the oral cavity, where they colonize beneath the gum margins and in the tonsillar crypts. They gain access to the lung by aspiration. Consequently the usual clinical context for anaerobic pulmonary infections is a combination of severe gingival disease (pyorrhea) and an altered state of consciousness, as occurs with alcohol intoxication, drug overdose, anesthesia, or a seizure disorder.

Aspiration introduces a mixed flora into the lung, and many infections are polymicrobial—some with several species of anaerobes, others with a mixture of aerobic and anaerobic organisms. The most frequent organisms are anaerobic and microaerophilic streptococci, *Fusobacterium nucleatum,* and various species of *Bacteroides.*

Anaerobes cause four types of lung lesions, abscesses, necrotizing pneumonia, pneumonitis, and empyema.[174] Aspirational lung abscesses are often called "primary lung abscesses" to distinguish them from abscesses complicating another disease such as an obstructing lesion of a bronchus or pneumonia caused by one of the more usual pathogens. They occur in the dependent regions of the lung, the posterior segments of the upper lobes, which are dependent if the subject is supine or a basal segment if the patient is erect, and more often on the right than on the left. The lesions are usually solitary with a cavity up to several centimeters in diameter with a shaggy, irregular lining. Often they have a dirty brown appearance and fetid odor. The cavity may contain sloughed necrotic tissue. Microscopically the cavity is lined by a pyogenic membrane and enclosed by granulation tissue or in cases of long standing, a fibrous capsule. Partial reepithelialization of the cavity, usually by metaplastic squamous epithelium, may occur. Large arteries and veins in the wall show fibrous intimal thickening and even complete obliteration of their lumen. Occasionally they may be thrombosed or necrotic.

Sequential roentgenographic observations indicate that abscesses begin as areas of pneumonia that undergo necrosis and cavitate over a period of several weeks. Patients often show signs of chronic disease such as weight loss or anemia. The prognosis for primary lung abscess is excellent, and more than 95% of patients are cured. Deaths occur rarely and result from either massive hemoptysis or occasionally from extrathoracic spread of infection. The course of secondary lung abscess is strongly influenced by the underlying disease and is generally poorer than that of primary lung abscess.

Chronic destructive pneumonia is another possible result of aspiration. It too is usually seen in those with oral sepsis and a predisposition to aspiration. Typically more than one lobe is involved, and the process produces areas of different ages and degrees of activity. The lung parenchyma is consolidated with multiple cavities containing pus or sloughed necrotic tissue. Histologic examination shows a mixture of exudative and organizing pneumonia with areas of necrosis. The bronchi show changes from acute bronchitis with ulceration to bronchiectasis. The organisms responsible are the same as those causing primary lung abscess. The clinical picture is highly variable from asymptomatic to chronic disease with fever, anemia, and weight loss to acute fulminant pneumonia. The mortality is 5% to 10%.

Acute pneumonitis produced by anaerobes is difficult to distinguish from other causes of bacterial pneumonia because the fetid sputum typical of anaerobic infection is usually absent. The disease is usually of short duration and responds well to antibiotics. Untreated, it would probably evolve into abscesses.

Empyema is usually associated with underlying lung abscess or pneumonia and can cause bronchopleural fistula. Less commonly, empyema results from spread of anaerobes from a subphrenic source.

Pneumocystis carinii pneumonia

The classification of *Pneumocystis carinii* has been controversial, but the sequence of its ribosomal RNA places it among the fungi.[175] The ecology of the organism is not well understood. It is probably widespread in the environment, since nearly all adults and even small children have antibodies to the organism. *Pneumocystis* organisms can probably colonize the lung without causing disease. Treatment of rabbits or rats with corticosteroids induces an interstitial pneumonia containing organisms, and such an effect indicates that latent infection may be widespread in these species.

Pneumonia caused by *Pneumocystis* was first recognized in severely malnourished infants in Europe at the end of World War II. Currently, *Pneumocystis* pneumonia is seen in severely immunodeficient patients with impaired cell-mediated immunity whether hereditary or caused by disease or therapy. In subjects infected with HIV, it is one of the defining manifestations of AIDS and is usually not seen until the $CD4^+$ lymphocyte count falls below 200 cells/mm^3. Before prophylaxis became widespread, at least 80% of patients with AIDS in Western countries developed *Pneumocystis* pneumonia. In East Africa it is uncommon in the AIDS population.

The development of *Pneumocystis* pneumonia is manifested clinically by the rapid onset of dyspnea, tachypnea, and cyanosis, sometimes accompanied by a mild nonproductive cough. There are few physical signs, but the chest roentgenogram usually shows diffuse alveolar and interstitial infiltrates. Atypical manifestations are most frequent in AIDS patients, including localized lesions, the formation of cysts, and pneumothorax.[176] "Breakthrough" pneumonia in patients receiving aerosolized pentamidine for prophylaxis is often restricted to the upper lobes.

At autopsy, the lungs, in typical cases, are firm and heavy. The pleura is blue-gray without exudate. The interlobular septa are edematous. The cut surface of the lung is dry, dusky, and uniform. The typical histologic appearance is an interstitial pneumonia with thickening and mononuclear infiltration of the alveolar walls and hyperplasia of the epithelium. The alveolar spaces are filled with a characteristic frothy exudate that is eosinophilic or amphophilic with round holes up to 6 to 8 μm in diameter (Fig. 49-20). Some of the holes contain one or a few weakly basophilic dots no more than 1 μm in diameter. Organisms can most easily be seen in sections stained with Gomori's methenamine silver or sulfonated toluidine blue, which stain only the cysts, or by immunochemical analysis. Giemsa's stain or Gram stain demonstrates intracystic bodies in imprints or clinical fluids but are difficult to interpret on sections. In sections, the cysts are 4 to 6 μm in diameter and often appear collapsed or cup shaped.

Histologic findings may be atypical in up to 50% of cases. Histologic variants including diffuse alveolar damage, nonspecific interstitial pneumonia, bronchiolitis obliterans–organizing

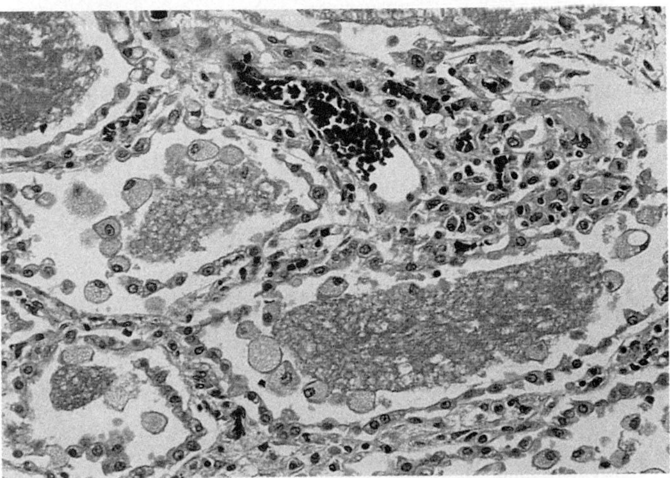

Fig. 49-20 *Pneumocystis carinii* pneumonia. The alveoli contain floccular material.

pneumonia, and granulomas were recognized before the AIDS epidemic.[177,178] Cyst formation and vascular invasion are almost limited to AIDS patients. Infection is restricted to the lungs in most cases, but instances of systemic dissemination are documented and have become more frequent since AIDS appeared.

The clinical diagnosis can sometimes be made by examination of induced sputum and efficiently by bronchoalveolar lavage. Some investigators find that immunohistochemical methods that stain both cysts and trophozoites are more sensitive than silver stains, which blacken cysts selectively, but others find little difference. Where available, PCR with Southern blotting is orders of magnitude more sensitive than staining.

Bronchiectasis

Bronchiectasis is irreversible dilatation of the bronchi. It is usually accompanied by infection of the bronchial wall and obliteration of the distal airways. It occurs in several clinical settings: (1) after damage to the bronchi by acute infection early in life; (2) distal to an obstruction of a major bronchus; (3) in a heterogeneous group of conditions in which the bronchial antibacterial defenses are defective such as agammaglobulinemia, cystic fibrosis, and the immotile cilia syndrome; (4) as a manifestation of allergy to certain molds; (5) after the inhalation of certain toxic gases.[179]

The onset of bronchiectasis is usually early in life. Formerly, in most cases it manifested after an acute childhood respiratory illness such as whooping cough or scarlet fever. Currently, 60% of cases are of insidious onset ("idiopathic") and adenovirus is the major cause of those with a clear postinfectious manifestation. The disease characteristically affects the first three generations distal to the segmental bronchi. The more distal airways are obliterated. The involved bronchi are dilated nearly to the pleura, are irregular in contour, and are filled with mucus or mucopus (Fig. 49-21). The bronchial walls may be thickened, or, in dilated saccules, abnormally thinned. The normal longitudinal mucosa ridges are replaced with transverse folds.

Microscopically the bronchial epithelium may be normal, or ulcerated, or show mucous cell hyperplasia or squamous metaplasia. In the wall are varying degrees of fibrosis, chronic inflammation, and destruction of normal elements. The smooth muscle elastic tissue and even the cartilage may be destroyed and replaced by fibrous tissue. The inflammatory infiltrate is mononuclear, composed of lymphocytes, macrophages, and dendritic cells. The lymphocytes diffusely infiltrating the bronchus are T-lymphocytes, mainly of the CD8 type. In some cases, germinal centers composed of B-lymphocytes are numerous. Whitwell has termed this variant *follicular bronchiectasis*.[180] The lung parenchyma adjacent to the diseased bronchus usually shows fibrosis.

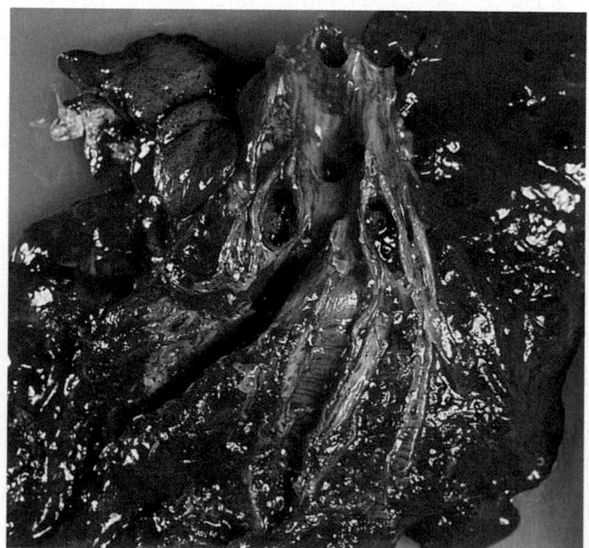

Fig. 49-21 Bronchiectasis. The dilated bronchi and bronchioli can be dissected almost to the pleural surface.

The distribution of bronchiectasis varies with its cause. That associated with hereditary defects in lung defenses can be diffuse. Postinfectious bronchiectasis has an unexplained predilection for the left lower lobe and lingula. Bronchiectasis distal to obstruction depends on the cause of the obstruction. Bronchiectasis caused by compression of the bronchus by granulomatous lymph nodes is most common in the right middle lobe because the right middle lobe bronchus is relatively long and its origin is surrounded by nodes that are wedged against it by the lower lobe bronchi. The nodes at this location receive drainage from both the lower lobe and the middle lobe, contributing to the frequency with which they are involved as part of a primary tuberculous complex.

Formerly the clinical picture of bronchiectasis was dramatic. Patients were young, debilitated, and cyanotic with clubbed fingers and produced large volumes of fetid sputum. Death before 40 years of age was common. Currently the disease is of insidious onset, often beginning as wheezy bronchitis followed by repeated chest infections, chronic rhinosinusitis, and tiredness. Hemoptysis may occur. Currently, most patients with bronchiectasis die of unrelated processes. Respiratory failure and cor pulmonale, rather than suppurative infection, are the major causes of death from bronchiectasis. However, 80% of patients with bronchiectasis have no greater annual loss of pulmonary function than normals.

Ciliary dyskinesia

In the syndrome of ciliary dyskinesia (immotile cilia syndrome), airway clearance mechanisms are defective because of diminished and ineffective ciliary beating. The syndrome is caused by several hereditary defects in the axoneme, the internal machinery of the cilia (Fig. 49-22). The axoneme is formed of nine peripheral doublet microtubules enclosing two central singlet microtubules. Arrayed in two rows along each doublet microtubule are paired adenosine triphosphatase-rich dynein arms. The power of ciliary beating is provided by the hydrolysis of ATP, which produces changes in the configuration of the dynein arms, which in turn produces sliding between doublets. The sliding shear is converted to bending waves by radial spokes that project inward from the doublet tubules intermittently linking them to short projecting structures along the central pair.

At least 20 structural abnormalities of the axoneme have been described, including absence of the whole axoneme. The commonest abnormalities in ciliary dyskinesia are absence of either the outer or the inner dynein arm, or both arms, followed by defects of the radial spokes. The defect within an affected family is consistent.

Symptoms begin soon after birth. Patients have repeated bouts of otitis, sinusitis, and recurrent chest infections. Clearance of radiolabeled aerosols from the airways is absent, except

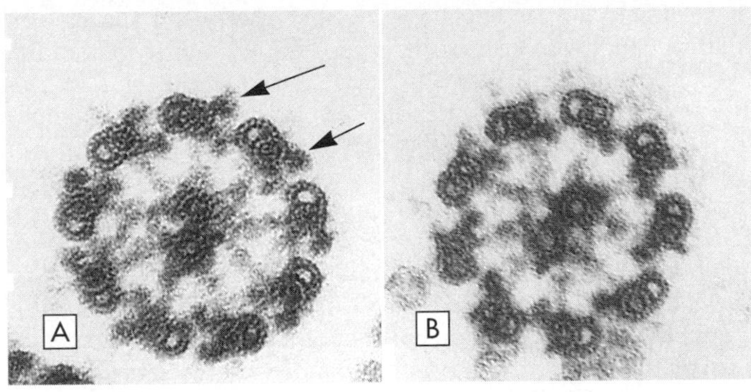

Fig. 49-22 Electron micrographs of cross-sectioned cilia. **A,** Normal cilium shows dynein arms *(arrows).* ***B,*** Immotile cilia syndrome. Dynein arms are missing.

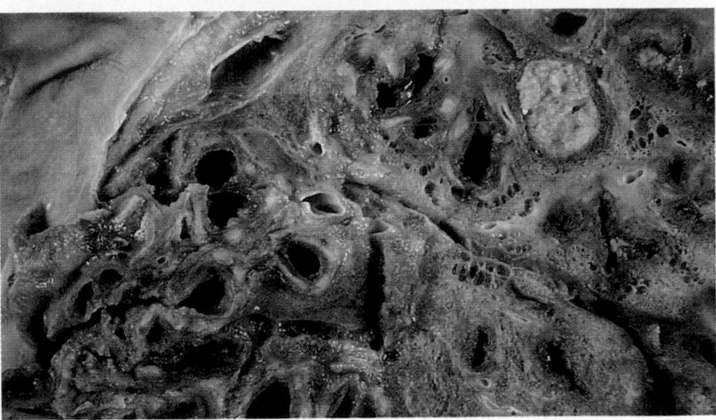

Fig. 49-23 Cystic fibrosis. This lung from a 20-year-old man shows diffuse bronchiectasis.

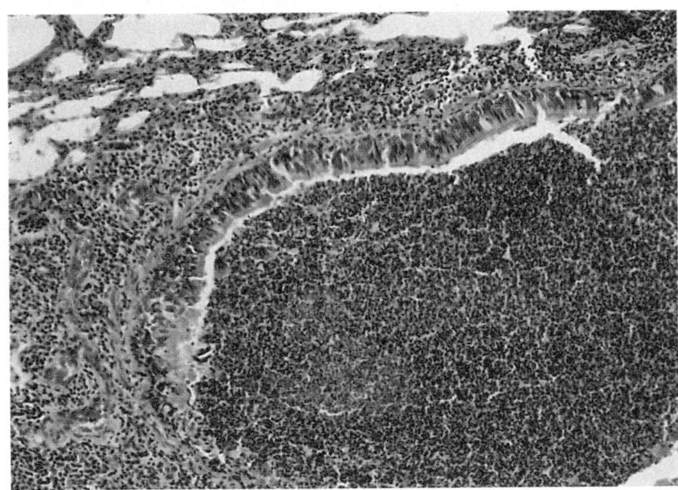

Fig. 49-24 Cystic fibrosis. The bronchiole is filled with an exudate composed of neutrophils.

during coughing. Bronchiectasis and nasal polyps develop gradually. In 50% of patients, there is situs inversus. Kartagener's triad of sinusitis, bronchiectasis, and situs inversus is thus found only in a subset of patients with ciliary dyskinesia.

Because sperm flagellae are powered by the same mechanism as cilia, men are usually infertile. Curiously, women are able to conceive despite the fact that the fallopian tube is lined by ciliated epithelium.

The diagnosis of ciliary dyskinesia syndrome can be made by phase microscopy of living ciliated cells obtained from the nasal cavity by curetting or brushing, followed by electron microscopy. A variety of abnormalities of the axoneme can be acquired as a result of injury, and so a diagnosis of primary ciliary dyskinesia should not be made unless a consistent defect is present in virtually every cilium and the clinical findings are supportive.[181,182]

Cystic fibrosis

Cystic fibrosis (CF) is an autosomal, recessive, hereditary, systemic disease. Despite widespread organ involvement, pulmonary disease dominates the clinical picture in those who survive the neonatal period. Therapy has improved the median survival from 5 years in 1960 to the late twenties currently. In older patients, pulmonary involvement is present in nearly all and is the cause of death in over 95%.

The pathology of the pulmonary disease in fatal cases is well documented.[183,184] The lungs are overtly normal at birth. In patients dying after the first month of life, progressively severe changes develop with metaplasia of bronchiolar epithelium to a mucus-secreting type followed by mucous plugging, bronchitis, and bronchopneumonia. Past 4 months of age, mucopurulent plugging of the large and small airways is universal at autopsy, and bronchiectasis is the rule (Fig. 49-23). Histologically the bronchi and bronchioli contain neutrophils (Fig. 49-24). The peripheral lung shows pneumonia and focal fibrosis. Emphysema is common when lungs of older children and adults are examined by adequate morphologic methods but is mild.

The propensity of patients with CF to develop infections and bronchiectasis can be attributed to impaired mucociliary clearance. Nevertheless, the propensity of specific infectious agents to be involved, notably staphylococci, mucoid variants of *Pseudomonas aeruginosa,* and *Pseudomonas cepacia* remains poorly understood.[185] Colonization of airways is difficult to eradicate; the consequences are repeated bouts of pneumonia, repeated purulent exudation into alveoli, and ultimately parenchymal fibrosis, acinar dilatation and simplication and, not infrequently, formation of bullae. Considerable variation in the expression of CF has been noted. Although some patients survive for only a few months, others reach 18 years of age with normal chest roentgenographic findings and pulmonary function test results. Although some mutations in the responsible gene are typically associated with severe disease and others with mild disease, patients with the same genotype can show variable severity, indicating that factors other than genotype also influence expression of the disease.[186,187]

Cystic fibrosis is caused by mutations in the gene *cftr* (for *c*ystic *f*ibrosis *t*ransmembrane conductance *r*egulator), which is located on the long arm of chromosome 7. It codes for an anion channel CFTR, which is expressed in many tissues, including the apical plasma membrane of the bronchial epithelium Clara cells and bronchial glands.[188] Efficient mucociliary clearance requires optimal amounts of periciliary fluid and a correct degree of hydration of the mucus. These properties are governed by ion transport by the bronchial epithelium, which absorbs sodium from the airway lumen and secretes chloride into it.[189] The chloride secretion in normal airways is stimulated by factors such as beta-adrenergic agonists and prostaglandins that raise intracellular cyclic adenosine 3′, 5′–monophosphate (cAMP). In CF, cAMP fails to activate normal chloride secretion.

The molecular basis for many cases of CF is now understood. The anion channel CFTR belongs to a family of transport proteins that bind and hydrolyze ATP in order to function. The mutation that is present in 70% of the abnormal genes causing CF in whites is the deletion of the entire codon for the phenylalanine residue at position 508 in the first ATP binding domain (delta F508). This deletion has several effects: Intracellular processing of the mutant CFTR is impaired, and so little protein is inserted into the membrane and most is degraded intracellularly.[190,191] That portion that undergoes membrane insertion is unstable and is rapidly turned over.[192,193] And finally, because the mutation affects a domain required for functioning of the channel, even a channel that is correctly inserted into the membrane fails to remain open normally.[194] This mutation causes severe disease with early appearance of pancreatic insufficiency. Some mutations associated with milder CF phenotypes affect charged amino acids in the transmembrane domains of CFTR that form the ion channel proper. These lead to diminished rates of chloride flux through the channel.[195]

Diminished chloride and water secretion coupled with a poorly understood excessive sodium transport away from the lung impair mucociliary clearance in CF patients, and such impairment permits colonization by bacteria, particularly by mucoid pseudomonas. Bacterial products, such as elastase and pyocyanin, stimulate hypersecretion of mucus and damage the cilia. Local cytokines recruit neutrophils whose products also have damaging effects and further impair the efficiency of clearance leading to chronic, relentless infection of the airways with hyperreactivity of the airways, recurrent bronchopneumonia, and diffuse bronchiectasis.

Pulmonary hypertension with cor pulmonale is a late complication of the lung disease in CF. Its main cause is hypoxia, but shunts between the bronchial and pulmonary arteries in the walls of ectatic bronchi may also contribute.

PULMONARY CIRCULATORY DISEASES

Pulmonary thromboembolism

It is estimated that approximately 600,000 patients have pulmonary emboli in the United States each year but that only one third this number are diagnosed clinically. More than 90% of clinically significant emboli form in the deep veins of the legs, especially the iliac, femoral, and popliteal arteries. Emboli have been detected in 50% to 60% of hospital deaths at autopsy, but most were small and probably not of major clinical significance.

The clinical effects of thromboembolism vary depending on the volume of emboli and on the condition of the pulmonary and systemic circulations. Emboli may cause no symptoms, acute transient dyspnea with a normal chest radiograph, pulmonary infarcts, acute cor pulmonale, or even sudden death. Many of the physiologic consequences of thromboembolism are attributable to mechanical obstruction of the vascular bed. These can be exacerbated by smooth muscle contraction caused by platelet aggregation on the clot surface with release of vasoactive mediators. The immediate effects on gas exchange are increased dead space, ventilation, pneumoconstriction, hypoxemia, and hyperventilation. The hypoxemia is attributed to decreased cardiac output leading to widening of the systemic arteriovenous difference in oxygen tension coupled with the production of the regions of low ventilation/perfusion ratio by diversion of blood flow to unobstructed portions of the parenchyma. Later, surfactant synthesis may be impaired as a result of depletion of metabolic substrates. This produces edema and atelectasis, which lead to reversible roentgenographic infiltrates in areas of embolism. The hemodynamic effects of emboli are slight unless 40% or more of the vascular bed is occluded. They include a rise in pulmonary artery pressure and, in severe cases, congestive heart failure and shock.[196,197]

Massive pulmonary embolism is a well-recognized cause of sudden death, which may be virtually instantaneous or extend over several minutes. The pulmonary arteries are distended by clots that are often coiled and twisted and bear the imprints of venous valves. The parenchyma shows little change except for congestion, which presumably comes by way of the bronchial circulation. Sublethal thromboemboli are usually recurrent. Consequently it is usual to find emboli of various ages at autopsy. Fresh emboli are poorly adherent but can be distinguished from postmortem clots because they distend the artery and have a drier, more granular surface. Lines of Zahn and imprints of valves are diagnostic. Older thrombi are adherent and retracted to various degrees (Fig. 49-25).

The fate of nonfatal emboli is variable. Retraction of the clot followed by activation of thrombolytic mechanisms will restore the circulation and remove most clots over a period of several days. Organization and recanalization of the thrombus occur more slowly. The thrombus is invaded by smooth muscle from the arterial wall, and the fibrin is removed and replaced with connective tissue while endothelial cells migrate over the surface of the clot and invade the thrombotic material to form new vascular channels. The clot is gradually transformed into fibrous ridges or webs with multiple points of attachment to the vessel wall[198] (Fig. 49-26).

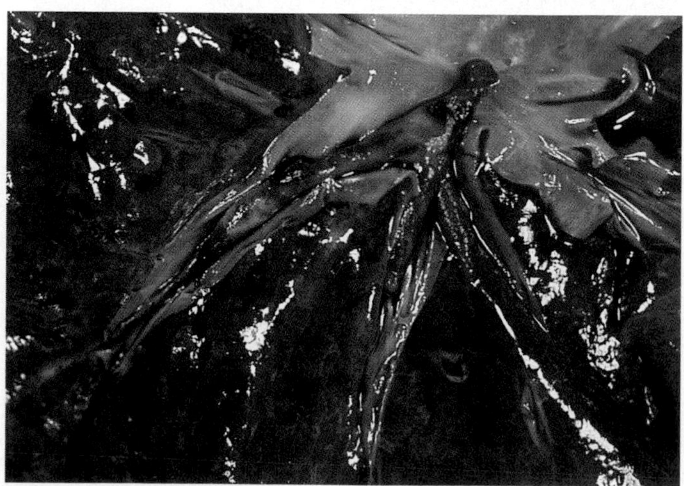

Fig. 49-25 Pulmonary embolus. The embolus extends into major branches of the pulmonary artery.

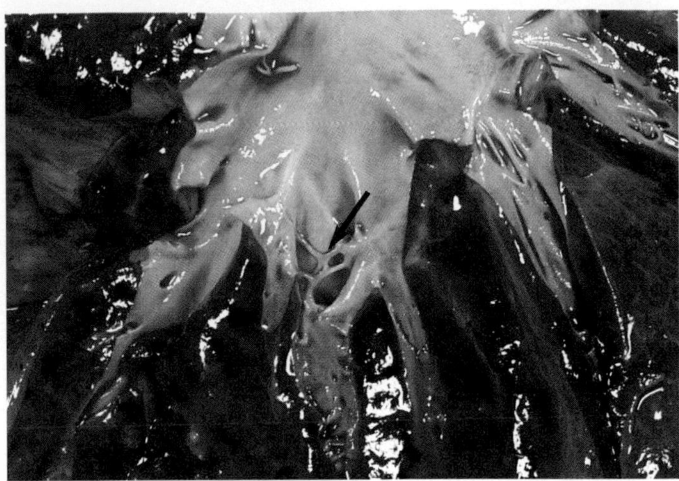

Fig. 49-26 Webs in pulmonary artery *(arrow)*. Such webs result from organization of pulmonary thromboemboli.

Pulmonary infarcts

A pulmonary artery can become obstructed without necrosis of the tissue it supplies. The tissue can obtain its oxygen from the alveolar gas and its metabolic substrates through the bronchial circulation. Infarcts develop in only 10% to 15% of episodes of emboli. Curiously, the emboli are usually relatively small, affecting vessels of 3 mm in diameter or less. The major risk factors associated with infarcts are general debility, heart failure, and multiplicity of emboli.[199,200]

Pulmonary infarcts are typically wedge-shaped, pleura-based, hemorrhagic foci, usually in the lower lung zones where blood flow is greatest. Fibrinous exudate is present on the overlying pleura after several hours. With time, the center of the infarct becomes brown and then pale as the hemorrhage is broken down and removed. Alveolar walls undergo necrosis and neutrophils may be present. Over the next few weeks, granulation tissue surrounds and invades the necrotic tissue, gradually replacing it and converting the infarct into a linear scar.

Other types of emboli

Fat emboli occur, almost invariably, after severe trauma accompanied by multiple fractures of long bones. Abrupt pressure changes during fracture of the bones rupture the thin-walled venous sinuses in the marrow and force marrow fat into them, whence it embolizes to the lung. In addition, levels of plasma triglycerides, free fatty acids, and lipase rise as part of the stress response. Other causes of fat embolism include orthopedic procedures, such as joint replacement, that involve insertion of an intramedullary rod or stem, liposuction, acute pancreatitis, and diabetes mellitus. The emboli travel to the lung at the time of trauma, but the onset of symptoms is delayed 12 to 24 hours. Probably the elapsed time is required for hydrolysis of the embolized fat to release fatty acids, which damage the endothelium and activate blood coagulation. This results in a high-permeability pulmonary edema and clinical manifestations of the adult respiratory distress syndrome.[201]

Fat emboli can be suspected in ordinary histologic sections as distended empty-appearing capillary loops and arterioles, but frozen sections stained for fat are required for confirmation.

Trauma to bones with hematopoietically active marrow produces bone marrow emboli. They are common at autopsy in patients who have received vigorous cardiopulmonary resuscitation. Like thrombotic emboli, they become adherent, endothelialized, and eventually organized.

Amniotic fluid embolism is a rare but catastrophic complication of pregnancy. Risk factors include multiparity, premature separation of the placenta, and rupture of the cervix.[202] Tetanic uterine contractions occurring when the infant's head is in the birth canal force the amniotic fluid through a rupture in the chorion into the maternal venous sinuses, precipitating immediate dyspnea, tachypnea, and hypotension, often followed by disseminated intravascular coagulation.[203] At autopsy, the lungs are hemorrhagic. Clumps of squamous cells are lodged in the arterioles, and mucus and lipid, which are also components of amniotic fluid, can be identified with appropriate stains.[204]

Foreign-body embolism may result from many materials introduced into the body that can embolize to the lung. Intravenous drug abusers inject themselves with impure preparations of narcotics to which substances have been added as "fillers." The insoluble additives lodge in arterioles and small muscular arteries where they cause thrombosis and proliferation of intimal cells. They often migrate into the perivascular space where they elicit a foreign-body response with macrophages, multinucleated giant cells, and occasionally a few lymphocytes. Although these lesions are usually asymptomatic, widespread thrombi can result in pulmonary hypertension, and widespread perivascular granulomas can cause roentgenographic nodularity and restriction of ventilation. In cases where lesions are not numerous, their detection is aided by the use of polarizing filters, since cornstarch and talc, two of the materials commonly used as fillers, are strongly birefringent.[205]

Air embolism is produced when negative intrathoracic pressure draws air into an open vein, an event most likely to occur during neurosurgical or otolaryngologic procedures in which the patient sits upright and the operative wound is above the level of the heart. Air bubbles that lodge in the pulmonary arteries and right ventricle mechanically obstruct blood flow, trigger blood clotting, and activate neutrophils. In turn, these changes produce pulmonary edema, hypoxemia, systemic hypotension, and myocardial ischemia. Embolism of more than 100 ml of air can be fatal.[206]

Pulmonary hypertension

The normal pressure in the pulmonary artery is 16/7 mm Hg (mean 12 mm Hg) at rest and rises with exercise. A mean pressure of greater than 25 mm Hg at rest or 30 with exercise is considered to be clinical pulmonary hypertension. The pulmonary artery pressure is determined by the left atrial pressure and the pressure drop across the pulmonary vascular bed, which equals the product of the pulmonary vascular resistance and the pulmonary blood flow:

$$P_{pa} = QR + P_{LA}$$

where P_{pa} is the mean pressure in the pulmonary artery, Q and R are the pulmonary blood flow and resistance respectively, and *PLA* is left atrial pressure measured in clinical practice as the pulmonary wedge pressure. Hence pulmonary hypertension can be caused by increased flow as occurs with left-to-right intracardiac shunts, by lesions that elevate vascular resistance, or by elevations in wedge pressure such as those occurring with mitral stenosis and left ventricular failure, or by lesions that obstruct pulmonary veins. Many disease processes change more than one variable.[207]

Pulmonary circulation in congenital heart disease

Pulmonary hypertension caused by increased flow develops at variable rates in patients with left-to-right shunts. In atrial septal defects, large increases in flow can occur with only small increases in pulmonary artery pressure because of recruitment of the vascular bed. Hypertension develops only over decades as a consequence of gradual arterial damage with an attendant rise in vascular resistance. In contrast, with ventricular septal defect or patent ductus arteriosus, hypertension develops rapidly because increased flow is accompanied by the direct transmission of systemic pressure through the anatomic defect. Hence in patients with ventricular septal defects or patent ductus, the combined elevation of pressure and flow can produce vascular damage leading to fixed pulmonary hypertension by the time a patient is several years old.[207]

The structural changes in the muscular pulmonary arteries in congenital heart disease are important in determining whether surgical correction of the cardiac defects alleviate the pulmonary hypertension. In 1958 Heath and Edwards described the vascular changes in the muscular pulmonary arteries in congenital heart disease, dividing them into the six grades listed in Table 49-3. Grades I through III are reversible, but grades IV through VI generally are not.[208]

The early changes in this scheme are hypertrophy of the media of the muscular pulmonary arteries and extension of the smooth muscle of the arterioles down the alveolar ducts. Without systematic quantitative studies on uniformally expanded lungs, grade I changes are difficult to recognize. Grade II changes include the preceding, but in addition some arteries show reduplication of the elastic lamina and proliferation of smooth muscle in the intima. The intimal thickening of grade III is much more severe, with narrowing and even obliteration of the lumen (Fig 49-27). The media may be thin, suggestive of atrophy, in a few vessels with considerably thickened intimas. The arterioles may show extreme concentric intimal proliferation in a pattern called "onionskin thickening."

Grade IV hypertensive changes are characterized by complex structures called "plexiform lesions." These usually occur just distal to the branch point of a muscular artery. The proximal segment of the lesion consists of an artery with a distinct muscular tunica media and severe concentric intimal thickening and fibrosis. The segment of artery downstream is dilated, thin walled, and tortuous with little tunica media. At the junction between these segments, there is pronounced cellular proliferation superficially resembling a renal glomerulus, with complex interweaving of vascular channels between groups of endothelial cells. Often there are deposits of fibrin between the endothelial cells or within the vascular channels. The elastic lamina is often destroyed in the proliferative zone. Small numbers of B- and T-lymphocytes are present in the adventitia of the vessel.[209] Grade V lesions include not only plexiform lesions, but also thin-walled, tortuous vessels that serial sections show to be arteries but in which the reorganization of the wall of the vessel with severe atrophy of the media leads to a pattern of elastic tissue resembling that in veins. The hallmark of grade VI is fibrinoid necrosis of arteries, which may be accompanied by acute inflammation resembling acute vasculitis (Fig. 49-28).

Table 49-3 The Heath-Edwards grades of pulmonary hypertension

Grade I:	Muscular extension into arterioles Medial hypertrophy of muscular arteries
Grade II:	Medial hypertrophy with intimal cellular proliferation
Grade III:	Progressive intimal fibrosis and occlusion
Grade IV:	Plexiform lesions and dilation of arteries
Grade V:	Chronic dilatation lesions with veinlike arteries
Grade VI:	Arterial necrosis and arteritis

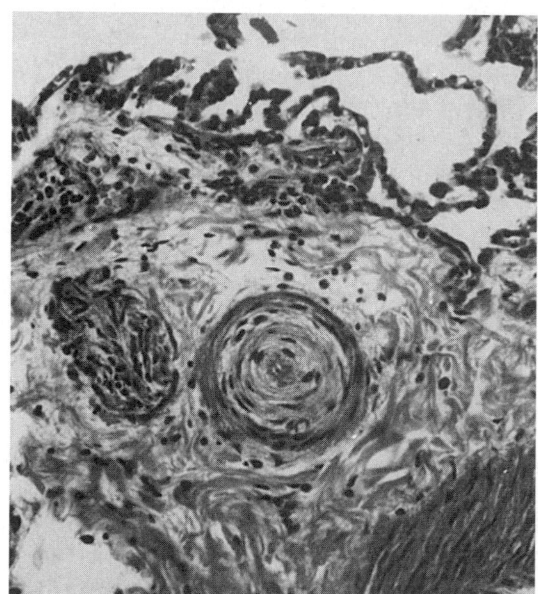

Fig. 49-27 Grade III pulmonary hypertensive changes. Onionskin hyperplasia of intima of small pulmonary artery.

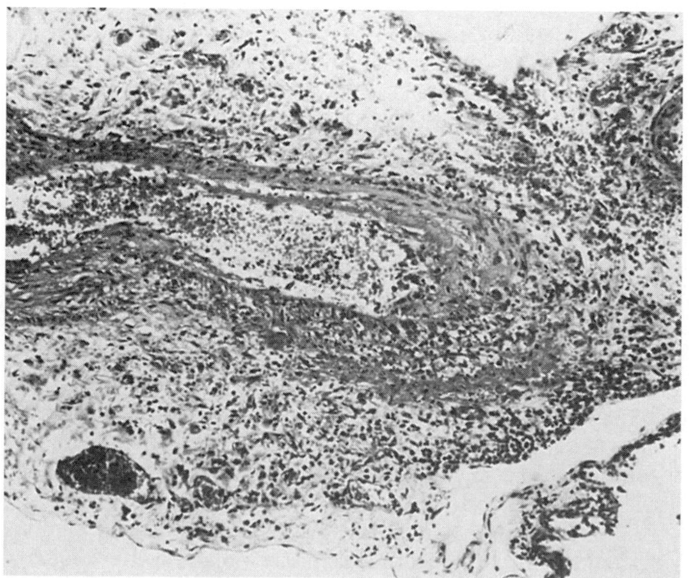

Fig. 49-28 Grade VI pulmonary hypertension. The muscular artery shows fibrinoid necrosis.

The Heath-Edwards scheme has been criticized on three grounds.[210] First, grade is assigned based on qualitative features of the most severe lesions and no account is taken of the extent of vascular damage. Second, numbering the grades IV through VI implies a progression through stages that may be the opposite of the actual morphogenetic sequence. There is experimental evidence that plexiform lesions form as a consequence of necrosis of the artery, and such formation triggers endothelial proliferation in response.[211] The dilated thin-walled downstream vessels arise in part from poststenotic dilatation of a pulmonary artery with damaged media and in part from bronchial vessels enlarging in response to the obstruction. Furthermore, a loss of arteries or failure of their development can be detected only by quantitative study. Despite these limitations, the Heath-Edwards classification has proved to be a simple first estimate of prognosis.

Hypoxic vascular remodeling

A major difference between the systemic and pulmonary circulation is that hypoxia dilates systemic resistance vessels but constricts the small pulmonary arteries.[212] Because this reflex shunts flow away from poorly ventilated lung, it aids matching of perfusion to ventilation. The beneficial effects of this reflex are subverted when hypoxia is widespread and chronic. In chronic hypoxia, the initial vasoconstriction is followed by remodeling of the pulmonary arteries, which results in pulmonary hypertension. Many muscular arteries develop a layer of longitudinal muscle in the intima and smooth muscle, which normally is restricted to arterioles in the proximal alveolar duct, extending distally along the arterioles. Electron microscopy of experimental animals indicates that muscle in the distal arterioles arises in part by the differentiation of pericytes, which are inconspicuous when viewed by light microscopy and in part by the recruitment and differentiation of perivascular fibroblasts into the arteriolar wall. Autocrine or paracrine signals responsible for these changes are under active investigation. Because hypoxia simulates release of endothelin and platelet-derived growth factor by endothelium, these two mediators are attractive candidates. More proximal vessels also become thickened. The thickening is accompanied by increased synthesis of extracellular matrix, induction of matrix-degrading proteases, and smooth-muscle proliferation. Clinical conditions associated with hypoxic vascular remodeling include residence at high altitude, chronic lung disease, and impaired ventilation as a result of neuromuscular disease, severe kyphoscoliosis, morbid obesity (Pickwickian syndrome), or sleep apnea syndrome.

Primary pulmonary hypertension

In some individuals, pulmonary hypertension develops in the absence of underlying disease. Such patients complain of dyspnea and syncopal episodes associated with exertion. Hypoxemia and reduced cardiac output eventually appear. The hypertension is usually severe and poorly responsive to therapy, and the median survival without transplantation is only 3 years from the time of diagnosis. Most patients die of right-sided cardiac failure or die suddenly presumably of an arrhythmia.[213] The pathologic changes are variable, but in 85% of cases one of three patterns is seen.[214] Some patients have only muscular hypertrophy, concentric or eccentric intimal thickening, and distal extension of arteriolar smooth muscle. More often, patients show the range of changes seen in patients with congenital heart disease including severe concentric laminar onionskin intimal proliferation and plexiform lesions. In the third pattern, the intimal thickening is most often eccentric and is accompanied by organizing thrombi including so-called colander lesions in which an occluded vessel is recanalized by multiple new vascular channels. Some patients may have both plexiform lesions and organizing thrombi.

The full range of pathologic changes seen in primary pulmonary hypertension can be seen in patients with chronic emboli to their central pulmonary arteries, even including plexiform lesions in some instances.[215] Nevertheless, most patients with unexplained pulmonary hypertension have no evidence of emboli to large vessels, and careful autopsies show no source for emboli. As a result, authorities now believe that thrombi found in the muscular pulmonary arteries of patients with primary pulmonary hypertension form in situ as a consequence of endothelial injury.[214] In support of this view, biochemical studies have shown elevated plasma levels of fibrinopeptide A in patients with primary pulmonary hypertension that fall with heparin administration.[216] Such patients also show increased excretion of thromboxane metabolites, suggestive of activation of platelets with decreased excretion of prostacyclin metabolites and increased endothelial production of endothelin, implicating dysfunction of the endothelium.[217,218]

No clear clinical separation between the three pathologic patterns is evident. Primary pulmonary hypertension occurs at any age from childhood to the elderly, though the majority of patients are in the third or fourth decades and women outnumber men by a substantial margin. Patients with plexiform arteriopathy tend to be younger than those with thrombotic lesions, have a stronger female predominance, and have a more rapidly progressive course, but there is a substantial overlap between groups. Response to vasodilators is similar.

Pulmonary veno-occlusive disease (PVOD) is a rare anatomic lesion that also presents the clinical picture of primary pulmonary hypertension. In PVOD, the sex incidence is equal or in some series male patients predominate. The chest roentgenogram features may be suggestive of the diagnosis. There are signs of interstitial edema with Kerley's lines, but the pulmonary veins are not visible, and there is no left atrial enlargement. The pressure measured with a wedged catheter may be normal or increased.

In PVOD, fibrous obliteration of small veins is believed to be the cause of pulmonary hypertension, and changes in the arteries and lung parenchyma are secondary. There is widespread obliteration of the veins and venules by eccentric or concentric intimal fibrosis. Often fibrous septa divide the lumens of veins into two or several vascular channels. In some cases, recent and organizing thrombi are present in veins, and it is likely that organization of thrombi is responsible for the intimal fibrosis in many patients. In a few reports, granulomatous or other inflammatory processes were responsible for the obliteration of veins. The arteries show intimal thickening and medial hypertrophy. Thrombi have been reported in the arteries in a few cases and may represent emboli or in situ thrombosis. The perilobular septa are widened and lymphatics dilated. The parenchyma is congested and may show nodular areas of hemosiderosis and fibrosis or occasionally venous infarcts, which typically are centered on perilobular septa.[214]

The cause of PVOD is unknown. Familial cases have been reported. A few features indicate that it may be triggered by infection. In many patients, onset has followed an episode of influenza-like illness. Some patients have had serologic evidence of recent viral infection, and one had immunofluorescent and electron microscopic evidence of immune complex deposition in the veins. Rarely, similar pathologic changes complicate chemotherapy. Obstruction of large pulmonary veins in the hilum of the lung or mediastinum by sclerosing mediastinitis produces morphologic change in the lung parenchyma similar to PVOD.[219]

The clinical syndrome of primary pulmonary hypertension can also be caused by a rare vascular proliferative process, known as *pulmonary capillary hemangiomatosis,* in which there is an overgrowth of thin-walled capillary-sized or small cavernous blood vessels in the pleura, perilobular septa, peribronchial and periarterial connective tissue sheaths, and lung parenchyma. The disease affects children and young adults. Symptoms and signs may also be caused by pulmonary bleeding or interstitial involvement. The abnormal vascular channels compress or invade and obliterate small veins in the periloblar septa producing a secondary pulmonary veno-occlusive disease that is responsible for pulmonary hypertension. Pulmonary arteries uninvolved by the angiomatosis show hypertensive intimal and medial thickening. Hemosiderin-laden macrophages and a few spindle cells and vascular slits may be suggestive of a diagnosis of Kaposi's sarcoma, but the preponderance of well-formed capillary spaces and the clinical setting should enable a correct diagnosis tc be made.[220,221]

Pulmonary hypertension with a severe course and histopathologic changes of plexiform pulmonary arteriopathy occurs in several settings. One association is with collagen vascular diseases, notably scleroderma and systemic lupus erythematosus, indicating that primary pulmonary hypertension may sometimes be immunologically mediated. The anorexigenic drug aminorex and toxic chemicals associated with rapeseed oil ingestion were associated with epidemics of pulmonary hypertension in Europe. Pulmonary hypertension with plexiform lesions occurs in patients with cirrhosis and portal hypertension and in subjects infected with HIV.[222,223]

Consequences of pulmonary hypertension. In the pulmonary trunk, pulmonary hypertension present from the time of birth prevents the fragmentation of elastic laminae and thinning of the wall, which normally take place postnatally, and the trunk retains its aorta-like structure. When pulmonary hypertension appears later in life after the trunk has regressed, the trunk hypertrophies and can approach the thickness of the aorta if the hypertension is severe but the fragmented pattern of elastic fibers persists. The elastic arteries hypertrophy and develop atherosclerosis.

The right ventricle of the heart hypertrophies in response to increased afterload. One can most reliably evaluate right ventricular hypertrophy at autopsy by dissecting away the atria and epicardial fat and separating the free wall of the right ventricle from the left ventricle and septum. In adult men, the weight of the free wall of the right ventricle in excess of 70 g indicates hypertrophy. In children or adults in whom a cause of left ventricular hypertrophy can be excluded, the ratio of the weight of the left ventricle and septum to the right ventricle can be used. A ratio less than 2 indicates right ventricular hypertrophy. Measurement of the thickness of the right ventricle is lcss reliable than weighing it because dilation of a hypertrophied ventricle will thin its wall.

Pulmonary edema and congestion

There are few organs in which the development of edema causes greater functional impairment than in the lung. Flooding of the air spaces by edema produces severe abnormalities of gas exchange. Fortunately, the lung can accommodate a substantial increase in fluid filtration across the alveolar capillaries before the alveolar space becomes involved.

Pathophysiology. The epithelial cells that form the barrier between the air spaces and the interstitium are joined by tight junctions (zonulae occludentes), which form a nearly impermeable barrier to the passage of proteins and small solutes. The endothelium of the pulmonary capillaries is nonfenestrated, but the zonulae occludentes between endothelial cells are less tight than those of the epithelium. In consequence, the capillary endothelium is more permeable than the epithelium, and so fluid filtered across the endothelium tends to be retained in the interstitium.

The forces governing fluid filtration are related by the Starling equation:

$$Q_f = K_f\,(P_{mv} - P_i) - \sigma(\pi_{mv} - \pi_i)$$

where Q_f is the fluid filtration rate, K_f is the filtration coefficient of the microvessels, P_{mv} is the hydrostatic pressure in the microvessels, P_i is the hydrostatic pressure in the interstitial tissue, σ is a coefficient measuring the resistance of the microvascular endothelium to the flow of protein, π_{mv} is the colloid osmotic pressure of the plasma, and π_i is the colloid osmotic pressure of the interstitial fluid surrounding the microvessels. Thus the main force driving fluid out of the vascular bed is the hydrostatic pressure across the vessel wall and that retaining it is the gradient in osmotic pressure between the vessel lumen and the perivascular space.

Filtered interstitial fluid is cleared by the lymphatics located in the loose connective tissue spaces surrounding the bronchioles, muscular arteries, and veins. There are no lymphatics in the alveolar walls themselves, but the interstitial pressures are lower in the junctions between alveoli, and such reduction helps to drain the interstitial fluid first to the junctions and thence to the perivascular and peribronchial connective tissue spaces.

The development of edema is a dynamic process.[224] At first, as the filtration of fluid across the pulmonary vascular bed increases, the fluid is efficiently conducted to the lymphatics and removed. Once the capacity of the lymphatics is exceeded, excess fluid first accumulates in the loose connective tissue spaces surrounding the bronchioles, arteries, and the perilobular connective tissue septa. The thickened septa can be seen in roentgenograms as Kerly's lines. At this stage, clinical manifestations are mild, but early closure of the small airways, because of the peribronchiolar edema, can be detected by sensitive physiologic tests.

Thickening of the alveolar walls by edema produces little impairment of *gas* exchange because the excess fluid in the interstitial connective tissue of the alveolar wall does not materially widen the barrier for gaseous diffusion. In a section through a normal alveolar wall, the capillaries lie to one side of the connective tissue space containing collagen and elastic fibers, sharing a basement membrane with the alveolar epithelium (Fig. 49-29). When excess fluid builds up in the alveolar walls, it accumulates in the connective tissue space while the capillary remains attached to the alveolar epithelium through their common basement membrane.

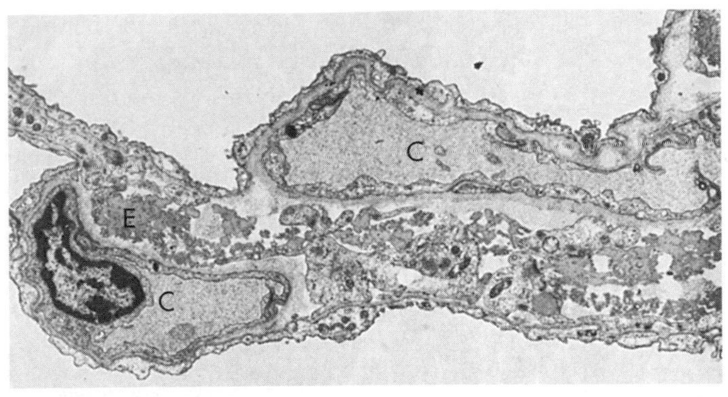

Fig. 49-29 Electron micrograph of alveolar septum of human lung. *C*, Capillary; *E*, elastic fibers.

Severe hemodynamic stress directly damages the alveolar epithelial cells and separates intercellular junctions, permitting fluid and protein to flood the alveolar space.[224-226] Thus, the traditional distinction between hemodynamic and permeability edema, though useful clinically, is not absolute.

Removal of alveolar edema fluid is brought about in part by clearance up the airways and in part by transport back to the interstitium for removal by the lymphatics and circulating blood. Type II alveolar epithelial cells and airway epithelial cells actively transport ions from the lumen to the interstitium providing the driving force for fluid absorption.[227]

The lung in left-sided heart failure

Acute elevation of the pulmonary venous pressure is transmitted to the capillaries, where it can provoke pulmonary edema. Its causes include left ventricular failure, disease of the mitral valve, or obstructing lesions of the veins. The lungs are heavy and moist, and frothy fluid exudes from the cut surface. Microscopically the alveolar capillaries are congested, the perivascular spaces and interlobular septa are dilated, and the lymphatics are distended. The alveolar spaces contain an eosinophilic coagulum of protein, often with a few extravasated erythrocytes.

Chronically elevated venous pressure produces the condition known as *chronic passive congestion,* or *brown induration of the lung*. The lungs are heavy and firm, and the sectioned surface has a brown hue. The alveolar septa are thickened and often lined by cuboidal epithelium. Clusters of hemosiderin-laden macrophages are present in the alveolar spaces.

Particularly severe chronic passive congestion occurs with rheumatic mitral stenosis. The very gradual rise in the pressure in the left atrium and pulmonary veins allows time for the lymphatics to hypertrophy, providing a measure of compensation for the increased fluid filtration and permitting high venous pressures to develop without severe alveolar edema. Chronic interstitial edema leads to fibrosis of the alveolar and interlobular septa. Fibrous intimal thickening occurs in the veins, and the smooth muscle sometimes becomes organized into a distinct circumferential band separating elastic lamellae resembling the tunica media of the muscular arteries. Venous distention also produces reflex constriction of the pulmonary arteries. Although the resultant increase in precapillary resistance gives a measure of protection to the capillary bed, it also produces pulmonary hypertension with concomitant changes in the pulmonary arteries. The muscular pulmonary arteries develop medial hypertrophy and intimal fibrosis while smooth muscle extends into the distal precapillary arterioles.[228]

In the lungs of patients with mitral stenosis or other causes of severe chronic pulmonary congestion, repeat diapedesis of erythrocytes produces iron encrustation of the elastic fibers of the small veins and arteries, which can then act as foreign bodies leading to the formation of giant cells. Small trabeculas of bone can form in alveolar spaces by an unknown mechanism.

Other causes of edema with a hemodynamic component

High-altitude pulmonary edema develops in some individuals who ascend rapidly to altitudes above 10,000 feet, usually appearing within 48 hours of arrival. The hypoxia of high altitude produces pulmonary arteriolar constriction and hypertension in normal subjects, but in those with high-altitude pulmonary edema, this response is greatly exaggerated. Despite the high pulmonary arterial pressure, the pulmonary wedge pressures reflecting left atrial pressures are normal. Electron microscopic studies of animals exposed to simulated high altitude have shown damage to the alveolar capillaries.[229] Edema fluid suctioned from the lungs of humans with high-altitude edema contains inflammatory mediators and has a higher protein concentration than the edema fluid from patients in cardiac failure, indicating increased permeability.[230] The few autopsy cases reported had not only edema of the perivascular connective tissue septa and alveolar spaces, but also hyaline membranes, confirming that the alveolar walls were damaged.[231]

Massive pulmonary edema is seen after head injury, seizures, and subarachnoid hemorrhage. This neurogenic pulmonary edema can develop within seconds, or more gradually. In the early phase of the edema, there is intense systemic vasoconstriction, increased venous return to the heart, and constriction of pulmonary veins, which together shift blood volume from the systemic circulation to the pulmonary capillaries. In some subjects there is evidence of cardiac damage, but in most the cause of the edema is damage to pulmonary capillaries.[232,233]

Patients with renal failure may develop edema with a characteristic perihilar distribution seen roentgenographically. Histologic features are hemorrhagic and fibrin-rich edema of the air spaces with focal hyaline membranes. Although this disorder is commonly called "uremic pneumonia," its occurrence is not closely correlated with the degree of azotemia. Hemodynamic factors that may contribute include hypertension with left ventricular failure, fluid overload, and decreased colloid osmotic pressure in those with the nephrotic syndrome and hypoproteinuria.

Drugs of abuse including heroin and freebase cocaine give rise to pulmonary edema with a high protein content indicative of increased permeability.

Diffuse alveolar damage and the adult respiratory distress syndrome

Acute injury to the alveolar capillary endothelium and epithelium leads to edema rich in proteins. The edema tends to be more prolonged than hemodynamic edema, in part because leakage of protein decreases the osmotic forces favoring reabsorption of fluid and in part because of the deposition of fibrin within the air spaces. Because the morphology and pathophysiology are simi-

Idiopathic organizing pneumonia

Idiopathic organizing pneumonia, also called *bronchiolitis obliterans with patchy organizing pneumonia (BOOP),* or *cryptogenic organizing pneumonitis,* is a less fulminant form of fibrosing lung disease.[252,253] The illness often begins with symptoms suggestive of a viral pneumonitis followed by cough, dyspnea, and frequently fever and weight loss that fail to resolve after several weeks. The chest roentgenograph shows patchy alveolar infiltrates, often peripherally or subpleurally distributed and sometimes migratory. Pulmonary function tests show a restrictive pattern.

Pathology. Pulmonary changes are patchy but temporally uniform (Fig. 49-32). Typically, there are numerous polypoid protrusions *(Masson bodies)* composed of fibroblasts in a pale-staining proteoglycan-rich extracellular matrix within the lumens of respiratory bronchioles, alveolar ducts, and even alveoli (Fig. 49-33). Clusters of lymphocytes, macrophages, and plasma cells may form a nidus in the center of Masson bodies. Membranous bronchioles often are inflamed but generally are not filled with connective tissue. The alveolar septa vary from nearly normal in some biopsy specimens to variably thickened in others. Alveoli between Masson bodies are often atelectatic and may contain lipid-laden macrophages, a consequence of obstruction by Masson bodies in the more proximal part of the acinus. The alveolar epithelium is hyperplastic and enlarged atypical epithelial cells migrate onto the surface of the Masson bodies.[254-256]

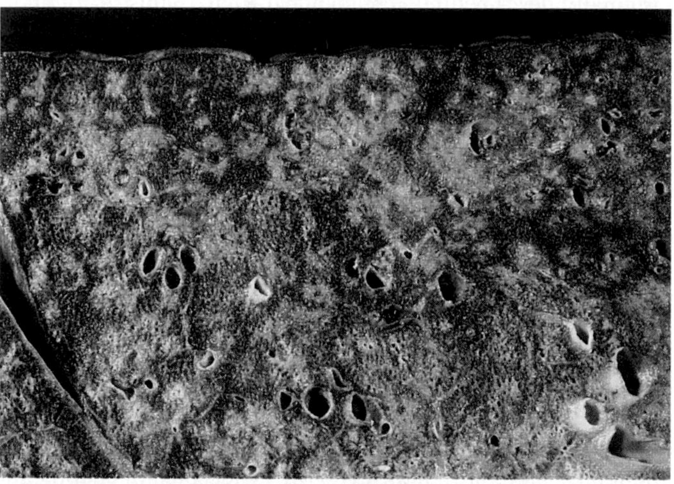

Fig. 49-32 Bronchiolitis obliterans. The obliterated bronchioli surrounded with consolidated pulmonary parenchyma impart to the cross section of lung parenchyma a micronodular pattern.

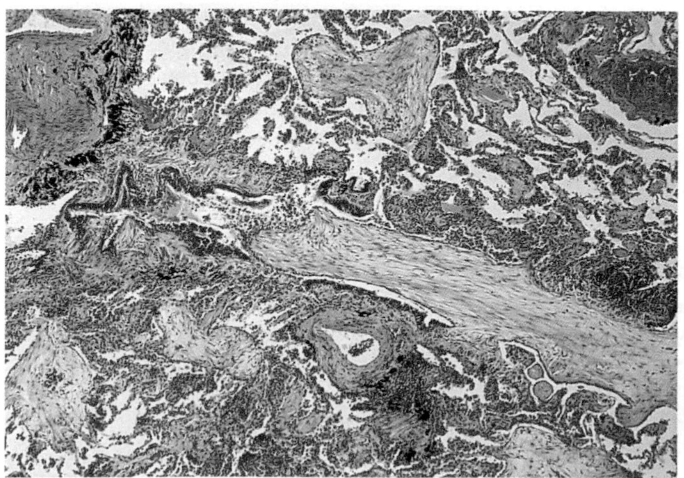

Fig. 49-33 Bronchiolitis obliterans. Masson bodies obliterate the lumen of bronchioli.

These histologic findings are nonspecific, and similar abnormalities occur in organizing infections or chemical pneumonias. Patients usually have failed a trial of antibiotics before biopsy, and many respond promptly to corticosteroids. Steroid responsiveness indicates that the process may not be infectious. Although most patients do respond favorably to steroids, some relapse when the therapy is tapered, and others follow a progressive course despite treatment.[257]

Chronic idiopathic pulmonary fibrosis

Clinical features. The majority of patients who ultimately are found to have pulmonary fibrosis have a disease of insidious onset. Persons of any age can be affected, but most are middle aged or older. Symptoms develop gradually with cough and increasing dyspnea, which initially is noticeable only with vigorous exercise but later appears on mild exertion or at rest. Clubbing of the fingers is observed in many patients, and a few basilar crackles can be heard on auscultation of the chest. Chest roentgenogram usually shows bilateral infiltrates but may be normal early in the course. Computerized tomography shows a mixture of linear and ground-glass opacity, often with a symmetrical subpleural predominance. The rate of progression is highly variable. The median survival is 5 years, and improvement is rare.

Pathology. At autopsy, the lungs are heavier than normal but reduced in volume, and the pleural surface often has a hobnail appearance. The tissue is abnormally firm and holds its shape during slicing. The process is variable in character even within a given lung. Normal areas are interspersed with foci of scarring in which air spaces are obliterated and other areas where air spaces are abnormally large and thick walled (Fig. 49-34).

The microscopic changes are varied, and although some regions are normal, others show thickened and inflamed alveolar walls, and still others show greatly abnormal air spaces with thick collagenous walls, infiltration in inflammatory cells and focally lymphoid follicles (Fig. 49-35). Typically there are widely scattered subepithelial foci of hypertrophied fibroblasts aligned parallel to the epithelial surface and embedded in a proteoglycan and fibronectin–rich stroma. Immunohistochemical and ultrastructural studies have shown these to be sites of organization of intra-alveolar exudate which become incorporated into the air-space wall, contributing to the thickening.[258] As the air-space walls become increasingly fibrous, alveolar capillaries disappear and are replaced by scar. The number of inflammatory cells is variable but tends to decrease in the more scarred areas. The epithelial changes are also varied.[259] The lining of relatively acutely inflamed alveoli shows predominantly hyperplastic alveolar epithelial cells whereas the more fibrotic air spaces become lined by a bronchiolar type of epithelium either by extension of epithelium from the bronchioles or by metaplasia of the alveolar epithelium. Foci of squamous metaplasia can also be found. Arteries are thickened by a combination of medial hypertrophy and the development of a longitudinal intimal layer of smooth muscle. Smooth muscle hyperplasia can also be striking in the interstitium where it probably arises mainly from hyperplasia of the smooth muscle of the alveolar ducts and respiratory bronchioles but possibly also from differentiation of septal connective tissue cells.

Two approaches have been used in an effort to aid clinicians in predicting prognosis and response to therapy. One is to define morphologic patterns with particular natural histories; the other is to grade specific morphologic features.

In the 1960s, Liebow devised a morphologic classification of interstitial pneumonias that appeared to have clinical utility.[260] His category *usual interstitial pneumonia* (UIP) corresponds to the heterogeneous grouping of abnormalities described above as the histologic appearance of most cases of *chronic idiopathic pulmonary fibrosis* (IPF). Accumulated experience and newer technology have distinguished others of his categories from chronic idiopathic pulmonary fibrosis, but one remains, *desquamative interstitial pneumonia* (DIP).

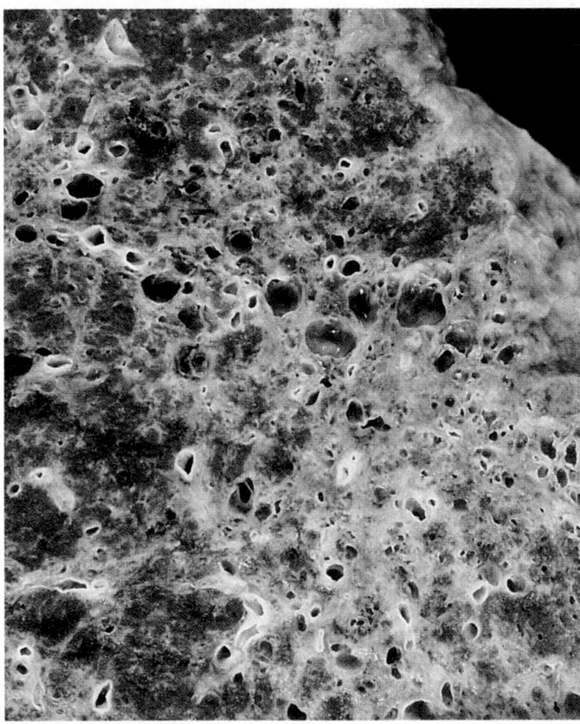

Fig. 49-34 Idiopathic pulmonary fibrosis. Cross section of the lung shows fibrosis with microcystic dilatation of air spaces.

DIP describes a histologic pattern characterized by modest interstitial fibrosis accompanied by hyperplasia of type II alveolar epithelial cells and the filling of the alveolar spaces with large numbers of alveolar macrophages (Fig. 49-36). The uniformity of the histologic appearance contrasts with the variegated appearance of UIP. Uniformity is also evident radiographically. The existence of DIP as a distinct subset of IPF is controversial, and some consider it one end of a morphological continuum.[261] A few patients with biopsy diagnoses of DIP may have pneumoconioses and some have respiratory bronchiolitis with interstitial lung disease (see later section). Nevertheless, a follow-up study of patients with biopsy specimens showing DIP demonstrated a greatly more favorable prognosis than UIP (which is virtually always progressive).[262] Because of this prognostic difference, DIP remains a clinically useful category.

Another pattern that does not fit the well-known categories described above has been termed *nonspecific interstitial pneumonia,* or *cellular interstitial pneumonia* (CIP). Biopsy specimens of CIP differ from those of UIP in that the appearance is uniform, with all areas appearing approximately the same age, and the acinar pattern of lung architecture is retained without the severe remodeling seen in the honeycombed regions of UIP. The walls of air spaces are thickened by an infiltrate of mononuclear cells, alveolar epithelial cells are enlarged, and hyperplastic and fibrosis is variable but usually not severe. Patients usually complained of dyspnea for several months and had bilateral infiltrates in their chest roentgenogram. These patients rarely follow the progressive course typical of UIP. This same histologic pattern can be produced by a varity of causes such as hypersensitivity pneumonitis, drug reactions, or collagen vascular disease.[263]

Several observers have graded various histologic changes in an effort to predict prognosis and response to therapy.

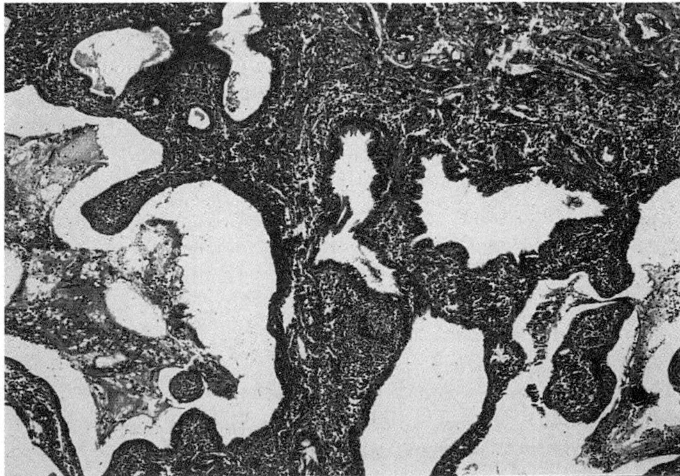

Fig. 49-35 Idiopathic pulmonary fibrosis. The lung parenchyma has a simplified structure because of a loss of alveoli, which have been replaced by fibrous tissue.

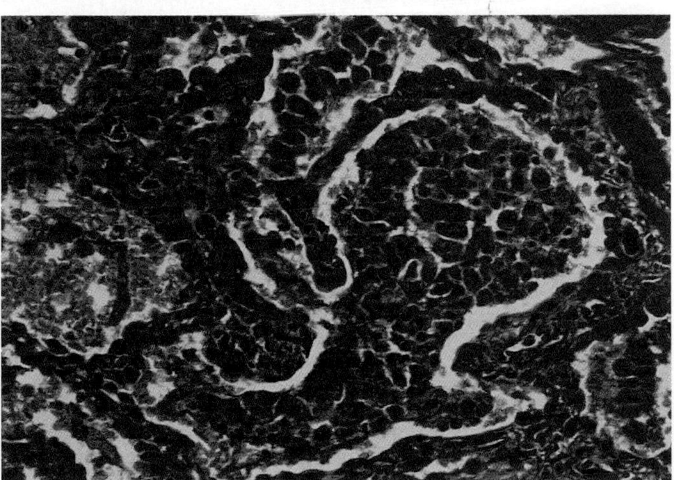

Fig. 49-36 Desquamative interstitial pneumonia. The septa are thickened, and the alveoli contain numerous macrophages.

Fibrosis, honeycombing, and arterial intimal thickening commonly occur together and correlate with poor response to therapy.[264,265] Some investigators have found that the intensity of inflammatory cell exudation (termed "cellularity") correlate with a favorable response to therapy.[266] Many studies failed to define "cellularity" adequately, and when inflammatory cell infiltration was examined in detail, its prognostic utility was not confirmed.[261]

Pathophysiology. The major physiologic abnormalities of lungs with IPF are decreased lung volumes, decreased compliance, and impaired gas exchange. In advanced disease, reduced lung volumes and compliance are readily explained by the obliteration of air spaces by fibrous tissue and decreased distensibility of the tissue because of its excess collagen content and replacement of the more pliable type III collagen by type I. Edema and fibrin deposition may also alter the surface-tension properties of the lung. The irregular deposition of connective tissue produces uneven tissue compliance that, combined with inflammation around small airways, produces abnormal distribution of the inhaled air. Destruction of capillary bed in scarred areas leads to decreased perfusion and loss of diffusion surface. The result of these changes is poor matching of ventilation to perfusion, which is measured in the pulmonary function laboratory as widening of the gradient of oxygen tension between alveolus and arterial blood and a decreased diffusion capacity; these ultimately result in hypoxemia.

Pathogenesis. The course and morphology of IPF are suggestive of slowly progressive injury. Even in patients in whom biopsies are performed long after the onset of symptoms, electron microscopy and immunohistochemistry show widely scattered tiny foci of epithelial necrosis and sloughing, fibrin exudation, and ongoing organization of intra-alveolar exudates. Inflammatory cells probably contribute to the smoldering injury by the release of oxidants and proteases. Several observations implicate immunologic mechanisms of injury: (1) Similar patterns of clinical and morphologic lung disease occur as manifestations of collagen vascular diseases that are immunologically mediated; (2) autoantibodies such as antinuclear factors and rheumatoid factor are common; (3) patients with IPF often have elevated circulating levels of immune complexes; (4) the involved tissue is infiltrated with immunologically competent cells, including antibody-producing B-cells arranged in lymphoid follicles, helper and suppressor T-lymphocytes forming dense infiltrate, and HLA-DR–positive dendritic cells that are more numerous than in normal lungs;[267] (5) the alveolar epithelium often expresses the class II major histocompatibility antigens HLA-DR and DQ.[268] Specific immunologic mechanisms of tissue injury have not been defined.

The local exudation that follows upon the injury may inactivate surfactant resulting in local collapse of alveoli. Fibrin exudates persist and provide a scaffold for fibrous organization because fibrinolytic mechanisms that remove fibrin from normal lungs are impaired in IPF.[269] Organization of the fibrin occurs by recruitment, proliferation, and stimulation of fibroblasts, which may be brought about by a variety of signals. The deposition of the fibrin itself results in the generation of thrombin, release of fibrinopeptides, and deposition of plasma fibronectin, which all influence fibroblast activity. Alveolar and interstitial macrophages and alveolar epithelial cells in IPF lesions produce tumor necrosis factor–alpha, platelet-derived growth factor (PDGF), transforming growth factor–beta (TGF-β), and other cytokines, which are potent signals for proliferation of fibroblasts and formation of extracellular matrix.[270-272] Connective tissue deposition within collapsed alveolar spaces can lead to permanent closure and loss of alveoli.

IMMUNOLOGIC LUNG DISEASE

Immunologic mechanisms participate in a variety of lung diseases. Many of the entities discussed in this section are induced by immune reactions to identifiable antigens that are not themselves directly pathogenic. Asthma is included though immunologic reactions are only one among several groups of inciting agents.

Asthma

Asthma is a disorder characterized by increased responsiveness of the airways to various stimuli as manifested by episodes of wheezing and increased resistance to expiratory air flow. The stimuli vary and include antigens, infection, air pollutants, respiratory irritants, exercise, and emotional factors. Asthma is a common condition affecting approximately 4% of the population. Since 1980 the rates of hospitalization and mortality have been rising.

Clinical features. Asthma has been traditionally divided into two subsets, intrinsic and extrinsic, though the distinction is not always sharp and cases with mixed features are common. In extrinsic asthma, attacks are often triggered by specific identifiable allergens. Patients are usually children or young adults with an atopic history. Many patients have high levels of IgE in their serum and peripheral blood eosinophilia. Asthmatic attacks typically become less frequent with time, often disappearing in adulthood. In contrast, many asthmatics whose symptoms develop in middle age or older do not have a history of atopy, and their asthmatic episodes are not triggered by identifiable allergens. Eosinophilia of the blood is less common and serum IgE is not so severely elevated as in the early asthmatics. This intrinsic asthma often becomes worse with time.

Deaths occur in approximately 0.1% of asthmatics per year. Death may be sudden, allowing insufficient time for hospitalization, or may occur during status asthmaticus, a severe, unremitting asthmatic episode that fails to give the usual prompt response to therapy.[273] The lungs at autopsy are distended with air and do not collapse when the chest is opened. On the sectioned surface of the lung, the bronchi of segmental size and smaller are plugged with mucus, which may appear clear and gelatinous or yellow and opaque. The parenchyma appears normal, and emphysema is ordinarily absent. In histologic sections, the bronchi are filled with mucus, which may appear eosinophilic or faintly basophilic (Fig. 49-37). Typically the mucus contains clumps of sloughed bronchial epithelial cells, degenerating eosinophils, and crystals derived from the eosinophil lysophospholipase (Charcot-Leyden crystals) and so-called Curshman spirals (Fig. 49-38). The bronchial epithelium shows an increase in goblet cells at the expense of ciliated cells. Often there is extensive sloughing of the columnar epithelium, leaving regions of basal lamina covered only by a discontinuous layer of basal cells. The epithelium rests on a compact eosinophilic hyaline structure 5 to 20 μm thick

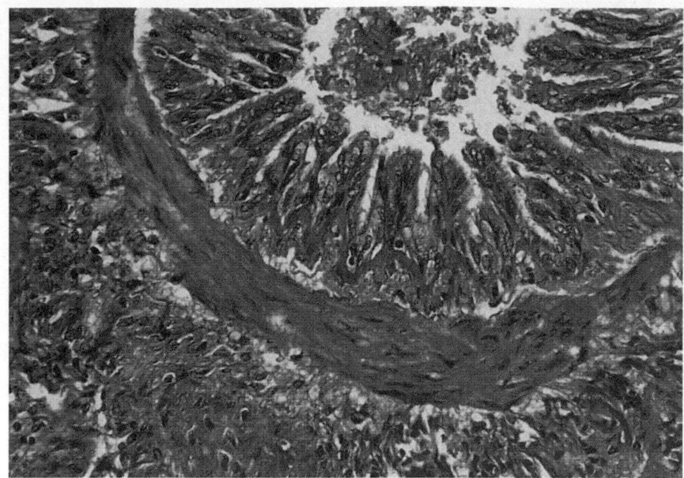

Fig. 49-37 Asthma. The bronchiole has a hyperplastic epithelium and a thickened basement membrane and shows prominent smooth muscle cells in its wall. The lumen contains mucus.

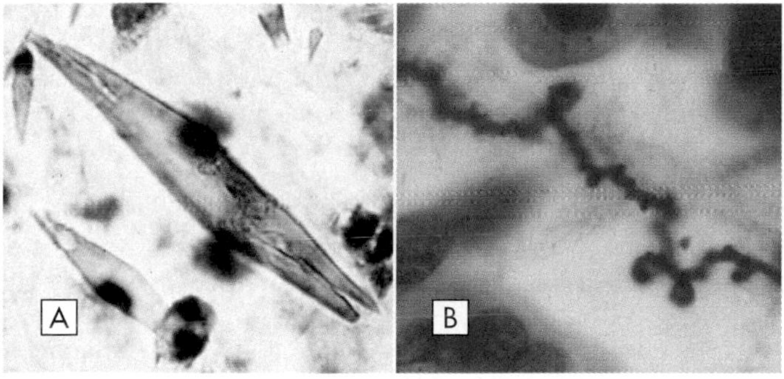

Fig. 49-38 Asthma. **A,** Charcot-Leyden crystal. **B,** Curshman spiral.

compared with 1 to 2 µm in normals. By electron microscopy, this structure consists of a basal lamina of normal thickness overlying a zone of closely packed cross-banded collagen fibers responsible for the abnormal thickening.[274] The mucous glands show hypertrophy, dilated ducts, and an increased proportion of mucous cells. The submucosa is thickened by edema and infiltration of inflammatory cells, and inflammation also extends into the smooth muscle layer. In most patients, the inflammatory infiltrate consists mainly of eosinophils and lymphocytes, but in those with very acute asthma who die before they can be hospitalized, neutrophils and plasma cells may be also numerous. Some studies indicate that mast cells may be increased, whereas others have found normal or even decreased numbers. Those present appear to be degranulating. Smooth muscle hypertrophy has been documented in quantitative studies of patients dying of asthma[275] but was not found in asthmatics dying of other causes.[276]

Recent biopsy studies of airways of living asthmatics indicate that, even between attacks, asthmatic airways show epithelial damage, mucosal edema, and infiltration of activated lymphocytes and eosinophils. The changes are similar but less severe than those observed at autopsy.[274]

In atopic asthma, the pathogenesis is initiated by the exposure of a genetically predisposed subject to specific antigens. In the nonatopic subjects, environmental stimuli such as viral infection, air pollutants, tobacco smoke, or occupational exposure to irritant chemicals damage the airway epithelium and initiate inflammation. In both types of patients, the process involves reciprocal interplay between inflammation, epithelial injury, and abnormal regulation of airway functions such as mucus secretion and bronchoconstriction.[277]

A role for mast cells is well established in atopic asthma. Atopic subjects synthesize cytophilic antibodies, mainly IgE, which sensitize mast cells and other inflammatory cells by binding to specific FcE receptors. Binding of antigen to the IgE cross-links the receptors that activates the mast cells to release preformed granule-associated mediators such as histamine, chymase, tryptase, and peptides chemotactic for neutrophils and eosinophils and to synthesize new mediators, platelet activating factor, prostaglandin D_2, thromboxane, and leukotriene C_4 and D_4. These mediators are potent bronchoconstrictors and mucus secretogogues as well as having proinflammatory activity.[277,278]

The predominant lymphocytes in asthmatic airways are $CD4^+$ helper T-cells of the TH2 subtype, active in the synthesis of interleukins (IL-2, IL-3, IL-4, and IL-5) and GM-CSF.[279,280] These cytokines promote the growth and influx of mast cells and eosinophils. Eosinophil granules, in turn, contain products such as major basic protein, eosinophil cationic protein, peroxidase, and eosinophil neurotoxin, which damage airway epithelial cells in vitro and have been localized in proximity to epithelial cells in biopsy material. Activated eosinophils produce oxidants, which augment tissue injury, and leukotrienes, which contribute to mucus hypersection and bronchoconstriction.[281] Epithelial injury when mild opens intercellular junctions[282] and when more severe causes sloughing of columnar cells.[283] Both effects increase permeability, permitting greater exposure of mast cells and lymphocytes to specific antigens, as well as having other effects detailed below.

The airflow obstruction of asthma results from mucus plugging, abnormal regulation of bronchial tone, and inflammatory thickening of the airway mucosa. Mucus plugging is caused by hypersecretion exacerbated by loss of ciliated cells and ultrastructural damage to remaining cilia. Mucus secretion and bronchial tone are regulated by both neural and extraneural elements. In human airways, the main autonomic innervation of the mucus glands and smooth muscle is cholinergic by means of the vagus nerve. Acetylcholine is both a bronchoconstrictor and a stimulant of mucus section by its effect on muscarinic receptors. The cholinergic effects are modulated by nonadrenergic noncholinergic (NANC) nerves that produce inhibitory transmitters such as vasoactive intestinal peptide (VIP) and nitrogen oxide.[284] The sensory innervation of the bronchi is provided by small nonmyelinated afferent C-fibers that terminate between the columnar epithelial cells. The C-fibers are irritant receptors that contain the physiologically active peptides substance P, neurokinin A, and calcitonin gene-related peptide. The neuropeptides are released locally by axon reflexes when the irritant receptors are stimulated, triggering cough, bronchoconstriction, and local edema.[284] Bronchial tone is also influenced by the products of bronchial epithelium, endothelin 1, which has a bronchoconstrictor, and an as-yet incompletely characterized relaxing activity. The increased responsiveness of asthmatic airways to acetylcholine and other bronchoconstrictors may result from loss of inhibitory VIP-containing NANC nerves,[285] increased production of endothelin by epithelial cells,[286] and epithelial damage that exposes the irritant receptors, thereby facilititating the axon reflexes that release the tachykinins substance P and neurokinin A. Sloughing of epithelial cells may also lead to loss of relaxing activity and to loss of enzymes associated with the epithelium that inactivate substance P and neurokinin A. Furthermore, because the inflammatory edema thickens the airway mucosa, shortening of the bronchial smooth muscle produces a great increase in air flow resistance in asthmatics when compared with normals.[287,288]

Peribronchial edema and inflammation may facilitate airway narrowing by diminishing the traction of the surrounding lung parenchyma on the airways.

Other pathophysiologic mechanisms are important in particular asthmatic subjects. In asthmatics whose attacks are triggered by exercise or cold, cooling of the airway may provoke mediator release and reflex dilatation of bronchial arteries.[289] In aspirin-induced asthma, leukotriene C4 and D4 play a prominent role, probably because aspirin inhibits the cyclooxygenase pathway of arachidonic acid metabolism increasing its metabolism by the competing lipoxygenase pathway.[290]

Allergic bronchopulmonary mycosis

Colonization of the airways by certain fungi can lead to asthma complicated by proximal bronchiectasis and parenchymal infiltrates. The colonizing fungus is usually *Aspergillus fumigatus* or one of the other *Aspergillus* species, but rarely *Candida, Helminthosporium,* or *Curvularia* have been isolated. Allergic aspergillosis is distinct from other lesions caused by *Aspergillus*—invasive aspergillosis, chronic necrotizing aspergillosis, hypersensitivity pneumonitis, or *Aspergillus* fungus ball.

Allergic bronchopulmonary aspergillosis usually develops in atopic individuals. Asthmatic episodes are accompanied by eosinophilia, high serum IgE levels, and the appearance of parenchymal infiltrates on the chest roentgenogram. Some patients expectorate characteristic bronchial casts containing organisms, mucus, and fibrin. Early in the course of the illness, roentgenograms show plugging of the bronchi and bronchiectasis involving segmental and subsegmental bronchi and sparing those more peripheral. In the late stages with fibrosis, the peripheral airways are obliterated.[291]

Resected tissue shows severe bronchiectasis with bronchi plugged by brown to yellow casts. The plugs consist of mucus and fibrin containing large numbers of degenerating eosinophils, Charcot-Leyden crystals, and sloughed epithelium. Organisms can be found in the mucus in the majority of cases and do not invade the bronchial wall. The bronchi show mucus hypersecretion and infiltration with chronic inflammatory cells. The lung may show obstructive pneumonia with fibrosis and lipid-laden macrophages or infiltration with eosinophils and macrophages. Small granulomas are common and consist of nodular collections of foreign-body giant cells surrounding degenerated material, which includes products of cell breakdown and often degenerated eosinophils.[292]

The immunologic mechanisms are believed to involve immediate hypersensitivity and either an immune complex or cell-mediated reaction. Patients typically have high levels of IgE and IgA antibodies to *Aspergillus* extracts, and their basophils degranulate in response to *Aspergillus* antigens. They respond to skin tests with an immediate wheal and flare followed in many cases by a second reaction 4 to 6 hours later, proper timing for an Arthus reaction. Similarly, patients challenged with *Aspergillus* antigen by inhalation show an immediate fall in forced vital capacity, from which they recover followed by a second fall several hours later. The histologic features offer little support for an Arthus type of reaction, however, and the presence of activated T-lymphocytes is suggestive of participation of cell-mediated mechanisms.[293]

Bronchocentric granulomatosis

Bronchocentric granulomatosis is a response of the lung in which small airways are the site of necrotizing granulomatous inflammation. One third to one half of patients with this lesion have asthmatic episodes, eosinophilia, and evidence of sensitization to *Aspergillus* organisms.[294] In the rest, the cause is unknown and eosinophilia is absent. Initially the mucosal lining of the bronchioles and bronchi is replaced by palisading epithelioid cells. Later, the bronchioles themselves are destroyed, completely replaced by granulomas,[294,295] the nature of which can be recognized only by their location adjacent to a pulmonary artery that is either normal or involved only by contiguity with the bronchial granuloma. The center of the granuloma may contain necrotic neutrophils, eosinophils, or simply amorphous debris surrounded by palisading histiocytes. Rarely fungal hyphae can be identified in the necrotic center. Central airways are relatively spared. In addition to a nonspecific chronic inflammatory infiltrate, they may have small granulomas in the mucous glands and destruction of cartilage by a mononuclear infiltrate.

Hypersensitivity pneumonia (extrinsic allergic alveolitis)

The clinical picture of hypersensitivity pneumonia varies depending on the nature of the inciting antigen and the intensity of exposure. An abrupt exposure to a high dose of antigen produces an acute onset, whereas repetitive low-dose exposure results in the insidious development of an illness that is more difficult for the clinician to associate with exposure. Acute hypersensitivity pneumonia typically begins 4 to 8 hours after exposure with the abrupt onset of malaise, fever, myalgia, dyspnea, and cough. The chest roentgenogram shows patchy or miliary parenchymal infiltrates bilaterally. Manifestations gradually subside if further exposure is avoided. In other patients, however, the onset is more insidious, and a physician may not be consulted until the patient has had several attacks or chronic dyspnea has already developed.

Early in the disease, lesions tend to be localized around terminal and respiratory bronchioles. Alveolar walls are infiltrated with lymphocytes, plasma cells, and macrophages. In at least two thirds of cases, there are granulomas composed of loose aggregates of histiocytes and giant cells of either the foreign-body or the Langhans type. The granulomas are less well formed than those of sarcoidosis; necrosis is not seen (Fig. 49-39). Buds of organizing fibrous tissue (Masson bodies) often fill respiratory bronchioles and alveolar ducts[296-298] (Fig. 49-40). Alveoli may contain macrophages engorged with lipid, a nonspecific change associated with obstruction of air passages. Eosinophils and neutrophils are few, and vasculitis is rarely seen.

In chronic cases, the lungs show fibrosis with or without honeycombing. Involvement is most severe in the upper lobes. The histologic changes may be entirely nonspecific with interstitial and intra-alveolar fibrosis and some inflammatory infiltrate, though frequently a few granulomas may be found.

The physiologic abnormalities are those common to interstitial lung disease: reduction in total lung capacity and its subdivisions, a low diffusing capacity, hypoxemia, and low compliance. A minority of patients have airflow obstruction because of inflammation, organizing exudate in small airways, or, more rarely, granulomas in their walls.

A variety of antigens can give rise to hypersensitivity pneumonia (Table 49-6). In farmer's lung, the antigens are the spores of thermophilic actinomycetes, *Thermoactinomyces vulgaris* and *Micropolyspora faeni* (or *Faenia rectivigula*), which thrive in wet hay. Thermophilic actinomycetes also grow in the fibrous residues of processing sugar cane (bagasse) and in mushroom compost giving rise to clinical syndromes of bagassosis and mushroom worker's lung respectively. Hypersensitivity pneumonia caused by thermophilic actinomycetes contaminating furnace filters or domestic humidifiers can be of insidious onset leading to fibrosis by the time of clinical examination. Bird fancier's lung is caused by antigens from avian serum or bird droppings, and in the plastics industry simple chemicals such as isocyanates and phthalic anhydride are responsible. Despite the variety of antigens and types of environmental exposure involved, the clinical syndromes and histopathology vary more with the intensity and duration of exposure than with the inciting antigen.

The immunologic mechanisms responsible for hypersensitivity pneumonia are incompletely understood. Generally, only 5% to 15% of exposed subjects become ill. The lag of 4 to 8 hours between exposure and onset of symptoms is appropriate

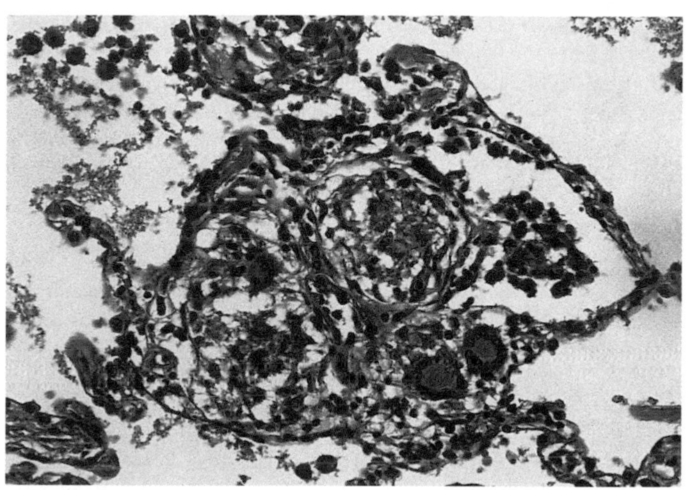

Fig. 49-39 Hypersensitivity pneumonia. Loosely structured granulomas with giant cells.

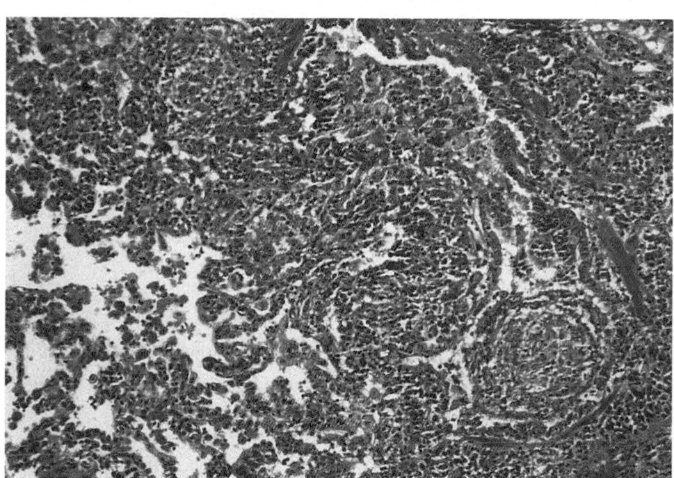

Fig. 49-40 Hypersensitivity pneumonia in later stages shows obliterative changes.

Table 49-6 Common etiologic (or suspected) agents of hypersensitivity pneumonitis

Agent	Disease	Exposure
Thermophilic actinomycetes		
Micropolyspora faeni	Farmer's lung	Moldy hay
Thermoactinomyces viridis	Farmer's lung	Moldy hay
Thermoactinomyces vulgaris	Mushroom worker's lung	Moldy compost
Thermoactinomyces sacchari	Bagassosis	Moldy sugar cane
Thermoactinomyces candidus	Ventilator pneumonitis	Contaminated forced-air system
Fungi		
Cryptostroma corticale	Maple bark stripper's disease	Moldy maple bark
Aspergillus clavatus	Malt worker's lung	Moldy malt
Penicillium frequentans	Suberosis	Moldy cork dust
Penicillium casei	Cheese worker's lung	Cheese mold
Alternaria spp. (*Cryptostroma corticale*)	Woodworker's lung	Moldy wood chips
Pullularia spp. (*Aureobasidium* spp.)	Sequoiosis	Moldy redwood dust
Mucor spp.	Paprika splitter's lung	Paprika dust
Lycoperdon spp.	Mushroom picker's lung	Puffballs
Arthropods		
Sitophilus granarius	Wheat weevil disease	Infested wheat
Animal proteins		
Avian proteins	Bird breeder's lung	Avian droppings
Animal fur	Furrier's lung	Animal furs

Modified from Fink J: Hypersensitivity pneumonitis. In Merchant J, editor: *Occupational respiratory disease,* publ no. 86-102, Washington, D.C., 1981, US Public Health Service, Department of Health and Human Services.

for an Arthus reaction. Since biopsies are not performed on patients who have been ill for only a few hours, it is not known whether the vasculitis and neutrophilic exudate typical of an Arthus reaction are present early. Stronger evidence favors the involvement of cell-mediated immunity.[299] The presence of precipitating antibodies to causative antigens are widespread in exposed populations but are markers of exposure and correlate poorly with the presence of disease. Tests of cellular immune reactivity such as lymphocyte transformation and cytokine production by mononuclear cells exposed to antigen in vitro correlate more closely with respiratory symptoms. The microscopic characteristics of hypersensitivity pneumonia, that is, the presence of granulomas and mononuclear cells, the elevation in T-lymphocytes observed in bronchoalveolar lavage specimens,[300] and the results of experiments inducing hypersensitivity pneumonia in animals all support the involvement of cell-mediated immunity. A defect in suppressor T-cell function in symptomatic persons offers a plausible explanation for their abnormal immune response.[301]

Pulmonary infiltration and eosinophilia

The combination of elevated counts of eosinophils in the peripheral blood and infiltration of the lungs seen in the chest roentgenogram constitutes the syndrome of pulmonary infiltration and eosinophilia (PIE syndrome). The syndrome has numerous causes (Table 49-7).

When PIE syndrome is attributable to infestation with worms such as *Ascaris lumbricoides, Toxocara canis,* or *Strongyloides* spp. the infiltrates are seen radiographically during larval migration through the lung en route to the intestine. At that time, stool examination may not show ova. To make a diagnosis, one may need to reexamine stool several weeks later when the larvae have matured to adults that shed ova.

Tropical eosinophilia is a hypersensitivity reaction to infestation with the filarial worms *Wuchereria bancrofti or Brugia malayi.* The filaria reside in lymphatics, and circulating microfilaria are seldom identified. The extreme eosinophilia, presence of antifilarial antibodies, and prompt response to treatment with diethylcarbamazine are diagnostic. The histopathologic features, in the acute phase, are similar to those of eosinophilic pneumonia, becoming granulomatous later.[302]

Among the more common lesions causing infiltration of the lung in the PIE syndrome is eosinophilic pneumonia. The predominant morphologic feature of eosinophilic pneumonia is an exudate of monocytes, macrophages, and eosinophils within the air spaces. Infiltration of alveolar walls takes place to a variable extent, but the predominant exudation is intra-alveolar (Fig. 49-41). Organizing fibrous exudate infiltrated with eosinophils may be present within respiratory bronchioles. When extensive, this feature may be suggestive of a diagnosis of bronchiolitis obliterans–organizing pneumonia. Collections of degenerating eosinophils known as eosinophilic abscesses are a useful diagnostic feature of eosinophilic pneumonia.[303]

Table 49-7 Causes of pulmonary infiltration and eosinophilia (PIE) syndrome

Diseases with PIE as a major component
Allergic bronchopulmonary aspergillosis
Chronic eosinophilic pneumonia
Drug reactions
Helminth infestations
Tropical eosinophilia
Vasculitis (Churg-Strauss syndrome)
Illnesses infrequently associated with PIE
Bacterial and fungal infections
Sarcoidosis
Tumors
Other

Known causes of eosinophilic pneumonia include drug reaction, inhalation of crack cocaine, and ingestion of L-tryptophan, but most cases are idiopathic. Clinical presentation may be severe and acute[304] or more commonly subacute and relapsing.[305]

Some patients have a history of asthma or atopy. Symptoms include cough, fever, sweats, dyspnea, and weight loss. Occasionally, blood eosinophilia is absent. Radiographic infiltrates are patchy and typically subpleural in distribution. Bronchoalveolar lavage readily allows detection of eosinophils in air spaces. The response to treatment with corticosteroids is so prompt and dramatic that a trial of therapy is accepted as a diagnostic maneuver.

Lung transplantation

Improvements in immunosuppression, surgical technique, and lung preservation have made lung transplantation or combined heart-lung transplantation acceptable treatment for end-stage disease of the lung or pulmonary circulation. The immunosuppression required to prevent immunologic rejection of the graft place the transplanted lung and (host lung in single-lung transplants) at risk for infection and drug-induced lesions. In addition, the graft is subject to specific pathologic processes.[306]

The implantation response is a form of high-permeability edema affecting the graft in the first few days after transplantation, as a result of surgical trauma, denervation of the graft, disruption of its lymphatic drainage, ischemia, and reperfusion injury. The pathologic characteristics resemble those of diffuse alveolar damage from other causes. Allograft rejection should be suspected when a patient with a previously functioning lung graft develops respiratory symptoms and deterioration of

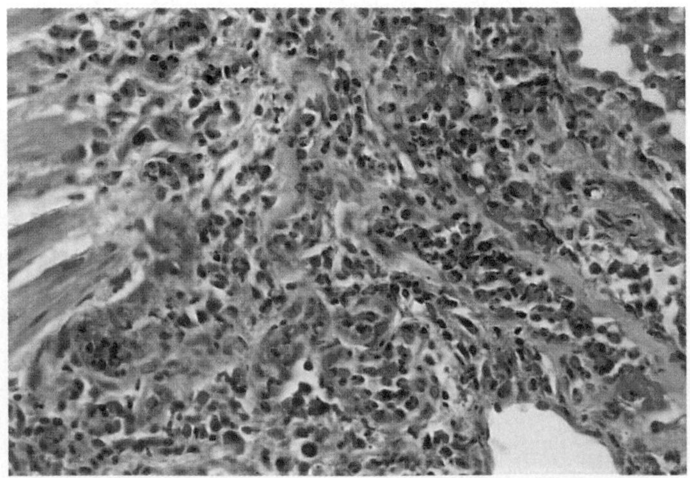

Fig. 49-41 Eosinophilic pneumonia. Alveoli contain eosinophils. The septa appear thickened.

pulmonary function, once infection is ruled out. The histologic hallmark of acute rejection is the finding of perivascular infiltrates of mature lymphocytes, immunoblasts, and occasionally a few eosinophils in veins and arteries. Lymphocytes may invade the subendothelial space, causing the endothelium to separate from the vessel wall, a feature known as *endothelialitis*.[307] Lymphocytic infiltration of the mucosa of the bronchioles sometimes accompanied by neutrophils ("acute on chronic inflammation") is also common.[308] Severe examples of acute rejection may also show vasculitis, lymphocytic infiltration of alveolar walls, and alveolar epithelial damage with fibrinous exudate.

Chronic allograft rejection is manifested by obliterative bronchiolitis and accelerated arteriosclerosis. Obliterative bronchiolitis usually begins several months after a sucessful transplant with symptoms of cough and dyspnea and rapidly progresses to severe irreversible airflow obstruction. The bronchioles are the seat of an acute bronchiolitis that begins with sloughing of the bronchiolar epithelium and infiltration of inflammatory cells and proceeds to concentric fibrosis of the lamina propria often leading to complete filling of the lumen of the bronchiole with granulation tissue. Although it is difficult to exclude infection, drug-induced injury, or aspiration as causes of the bronchiolitis, it is widely believed to be a consequence of chronic rejection. This possibility is reinforced by the occurrence of an identical lesion in patients who have undergone bone marrow transplantation for hematologic disease and in whom graft-versus-host disease has occurred.[309] Indeed in both types of patients, infection may trigger immunologic rejection by increasing the expression of class 2 histocompatibility antigens on the airway epithelium.[306]

Arteriosclerosis in the allografted lung resembles that in chronic rejection of other allografts. It begins as a mucinous thickening of the intima accompanied by an influx of smooth muscle cells from the media. Over time, the intimal thickening becomes fibrotic, and lipid and cholesterol are deposited. The lesions may be concentric or eccentric, and arteries of all sizes may be affected.

Cartilage in central airways of lung allografts are irregular and show calcification, ossification, and focal resorption by vascular ingrowth. These abnormalities occur in all grafts irrespective of the presence or absence of rejection and are attributed to the impaired bronchial blood supply.[310]

Epstein-Barr virus induces polyclonal and monoclonal B-cell lymphoproliferative disorders in heart-lung transplant recipients. The disorder can arise in the grafted lung or elsewhere in the recipient. Monoclonal disorders usually resemble immunoblastic lymphomas with cells resembling Reed-Sternberg cells. Often the lesions disappear when immunosuppression is decreased, though some behave as progressive lymphomas.[311]

Sarcoidosis

Sarcoidosis is a systemic disease of unknown cause characterized by the presence of noncaseating granulomas in affected organs.[312] The thoracic organs are involved in more than 90% of patients. The disease is most common in young adults between 20 and 40 years of age and is rare below 10 years. It occurs worldwide. In the United States, the prevalence is 10 times higher in blacks than in whites and greater in women than in men. In South Africa, the prevalence is also higher in blacks. In Europe, the prevalence is highest in Scandinavians, and there is no distinct sex predilection.[313]

Pathology. The diagnostic feature of sarcoidosis is the noncaseating granuloma, a compact nodule of epithelioid cells with a few lymphocytes, monocytes, and macrophages (Figure 49-42). Necrosis is nearly always absent, but a small amount of granular eosinophilic necrosis may be present in the center of an occasional granuloma in an otherwise typical case. The epithelioid cells are generally similar to those of tuberculosis when viewed by light and electron microscopy. By electron microscopy, two types of epithelioid cells have been described, one with extensively developed endoplasmic reticulum and few granules or vacuoles, the other with many vacuoles containing finely granular material. The epithelioid cells are derived from monocytes and macrophages in response to cytokines. Because of their extensive endoplasmic reticulum and paucity of phagosomes, they have been interpreted as poorly phagocytic secretory variants.

Giant cells of either foreign-body or Langhans type are common. Their ultrastructure and thymidine labeling studies show that they form by fusion of epithelioid cells. They may contain inclusions such as asteroid bodies (Fig. 49-43), cal-

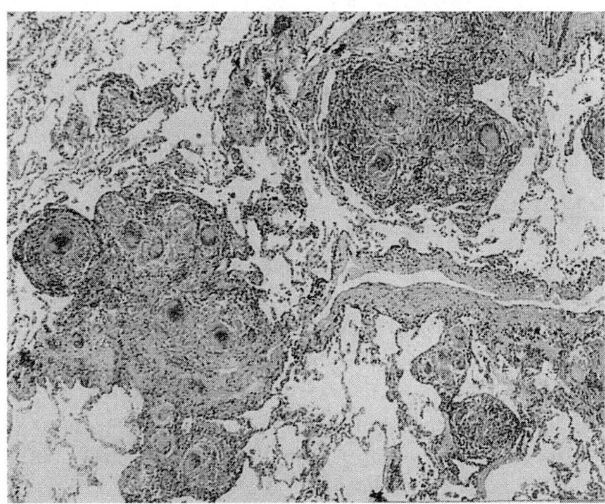

Fig. 49-42 Sarcoidosis. Multiple noncaseating granulomas in the lung parenchyma.

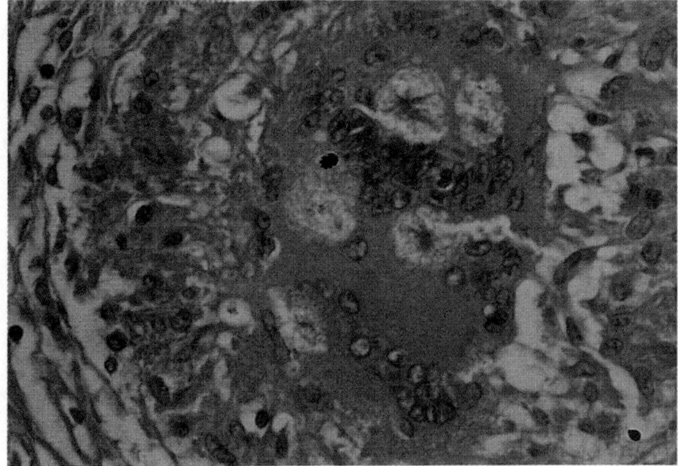

Fig. 49-43 Sarcoidosis. Giant cells are multinucleated and contain asteroid bodies.

cium oxalate crystals, or concentric lamellae of calcium and iron-containing material (conchoid bodies, or Schaumann bodies), but these inclusions are not pathognomonic.[314]

The earliest stages of pulmonary sarcoidosis are not well known. Rosen and associates have observed a nonspecific interstitial infiltrate of mononuclear cells accompanying nonfibrotic granulomas of early sarcoidosis.[315] They propose that the granulomas evolve from a nonspecific alveolitis.

The healing of the granulomas begins with the appearance of an encircling fibrous capsule that gradually becomes thicker and more hyaline, replacing the granuloma until only a few macrophages and giant cells persist in the center. Eventually these, too, are replaced by fibrous tissue.

Sarcoid granulomas involve any of the structures of the lung. Often they are most numerous near lymphatic vessel-containing structures, large or small airways, blood vessels, or the perilobular septa and pleura. Conglomeration of granulomas matted together by fibrosis can give rise to large nodules. Healing and scarring can produce honeycombing, bullae, or upper lobe cavities that lack the caseous or liquified contents of tuberculous cavities.

Natural history. The clinical course of thoracic sarcoidosis can be followed sequentially from study of the chest radiographs.[316] The stages are as follows:

Stage 1: Bilateral hilar adenopathy
Stage 2a: Hilar adenopathy with pulmonary infiltrates
Stage 2b: Parenchymal infiltrates without adenopathy
Stage 3: Interstitial fibrosis

The earliest manifestation of sarcoidosis is bilateral hilar lymph node enlargement without roentgenographic changes in the parenchyma. Most patients at this stage are asymptomatic. Some have cutaneous lesions of erythema nodosum. Despite the normal appearance of the parenchyma roentgenographically, patients may have mild abnormalities of pulmonary function or show the presence of granulomas in transbronchial biopsy specimens. Sixty percent to 80% of patients who present with stage 1 disease show regression without therapy in 6 months to 2 years. In only 10% does parenchymal disease of sufficient severity to be roentgenographically detectable develop. Patients with both parenchymal infiltrates and hilar adenopathy usually have pulmonary dysfunction, and in only half will the chest roentgenogram return to normal. Patients with parenchymal disease without hilar adenopathy rarely improve and usually have dysfunction. Reduced diffusing capacity and restriction of ventilation are the rule, but concomitant airflow obstruction is also common because of involvement of bronchi and bronchioles by granulomas.

Diagnosis. The diagnosis of sarcoidosis is based on the clinical findings and the demonstration of noncaseating granulomas in any involved tissue. Transbronchial biopsy discloses granulomas in 90% of patients with roentgenographic lung involvement, and 50% of those with stage 1 disease. The histologic findings are not distinguishable from infectious granulomas. Stains and cultures for mycobacteria and fungi must always be done. The most a pathologist can say is, "consistent with sarcoidosis."

There are abnormalities in the serum of sarcoidosis patients, but none is specific. Hyperglobulinemia is common, hypercalcemia less so. Hypercalcemia is the result of 1-hydroxylation of circulating 25-hydroxyvitamin D_3 to the biologically active 1,25-dihydroxy vitamin D_3 by activated macrophages in the granulomas. Elevation of serum angiotensin-converting enzyme (ACE) occurs in 40% to 80% of patients with sarcoidosis, usually those with active disease. Because ACE is also elevated in a small proportion of patients with infectious granulomas or noninfectious interstitial lung disease, it is more useful as a measure of disease activity than as a specific diagnostic test. The Kveim-Siltzbach reaction is a skin test using an antigen prepared from involved lymph node and spleen. With correctly prepared antigen, the test is specific, but the antigen is not approved by the U.S. Food and Drug Administration and is not generally available.

Etiology and pathogenesis. The cause of sarcoidosis is unknown. The presence of granulomas is suggestive of a cell-mediated immune response. Cells lavaged from the lung include increased numbers of helper T-lymphocytes that express HLA-DR and interleukin-2 receptors, secrete interleukin-2, interferon-gamma, and monocyte chemoattractants, and use a restricted T-cell antigen receptor repertoire. The mononuclear phagocytes in the bronchoalveolar lavage display an immature phenotype, present antigen efficiently, secrete interleukin-1 and tumor necrosis factor, and often form rosettes with the lymphocytes. This evidence of lymphocyte-macrophage interaction also supports the hypothesis of a cell-mediated immune reaction in the lung.[317] The antigen, if any, is unknown. By definition, the results of stains and cultures for mycobacteria are negative. Sensitive molecular techniques have demonstrated the presence of mycobacterial nucleic acid in some patients,[318,319] but some investigators have failed to confirm this, and the topic is one of active current investigation.

Necrotizing sarcoid granulomatosis

The term *necrotizing sarcoid granulomatosis* describes nodular pulmonary lesions consisting of a collection of epithelioid granulomas united in a background of fibrous tissue and inflammatory cells in which irregular, sometimes extensive areas of fibrinoid or coagulative necrosis occur. The necrosis is quite different from the central necrosis surrounded by epithelioid cells that is common in infectious granulomas. Vasculitis involving both arteries and veins is usually present. Vessels can be invaded or obliterated by granulomas, involved by an inflammatory process resembling giant cell arteritis, or the vasculitis can be a nonspecific mononuclear inflammatory infiltration of the vessel wall.[320] The lesions are multiple and bilateral, but extrapulmonary manifestations are rare. Hilar adenopathy has been reported infrequently. A few patients have had hepatic granulomas or uveitis. Patients usually complain of chest discomfort, and 50% have systemic symptoms such as fever, malaise, or weight loss. The course of the disease has generally been favorable. Most patients have either remained stable or had regression of lesions on steroid or cytotoxic therapy.

It is uncertain whether necrotizing sarcoid granulomatosis is an atypical manifestation of sarcoidosis or a separate disease entity.[321] Although necrosis is not a feature of the granulomas of classical sarcoidosis, the necrosis of necrotizing sarcoid granulomatosis is explicable as infarction secondary to the vasculitis rather than a property of the individual granulomas. Kveim testing has not been reported.

Acquired immunodeficiency syndrome

The lung is a major target organ in AIDS. The most common form of clinical involvement is infection, directly traceable to the impaired cell-mediated immunity. Formerly 85% of lung infections in developed nations were caused by *Pneumocystis carinii.* Because of widespread prophylaxis against *Pneumocystis,* bacterial pneumonia caused by common community-acquired bacteria have become the most common. Cytomegalovirus and mycobacterial infections are also common. A wide variety of exotic organisms also infect the lungs of AIDS patients.[322]

AIDS also predisposes to neoplastic involvement of the lung, most often by Kaposi's sarcoma, malignant lymphoma, or smooth muscle tumors.[323]

Lymphoid interstitial pneumonia (LIP) occurs in children or adults infected with HIV manifesting either AIDS-related complex or full-fledged AIDS. Both the peribronchial and perivascular spaces and the interalveolar septa are infiltrated with small lymphocytes with a variable proportion of plasma cells and often germinal centers. LIP is sometimes associated with generalized lymphadenopathy, sicca syndrome, and lymphoid infiltrates in other organs.

Many HIV-infected patients with neither pulmonary symptoms nor abnormal roentgenogram features nevertheless have reduced diffusing capacity, abnormal permeability to inhaled radionuclides, or histologic evidence of nonspecific interstitial pneumonitis. This HIV-related pneumonitis is manifest by lymphocytic infiltrates around bronchioles and blood vessels. Germinal centers may be present, but infiltration of alveolar septa is minimal or absent. Focal type II cell hyperplasia and intra-alveolar organization may be present.[324]

In both LIP and nonspecific interstitial pneumonia, most of the lymphocytes are $CD8^+$ T-lymphocytes. The few B-cells are polyclonal. Scattered mononuclear cells contain HIV virus, and both LIP and the milder nonspecific interstitial pneumonitis may represent immunologic host responses to the virus.[325]

Rare manifestations of HIV infection include severe pulmonary hypertension[223] and the premature development of emphysema.[326]

COLLAGEN-VASCULAR DISEASES

Acute rheumatic fever

Pulmonary involvement in acute rheumatic fever is not uncommon, occurring in 12% to 50% of autopsies with that disease. Patients show tachypnea, hypoxemia, and patchy migratory infiltrates in the chest roentgenogram.[327] Pathologic changes are nonspecific, resembling organizing diffuse alveolar damage. The alveolar walls are thickened by edema and a mixed mononuclear infiltrate. Alveolar ducts are lined by hyaline membranes. Fibrin in various stages of organization is present in alveoli. Thrombosis of small arteries, alveolar septal necrosis, vasculitis, and patchy areas of infarct-like necrosis are found in occasional cases.[328]

Rheumatoid lung disease

Pulmonary involvement in rheumatoid disease takes several forms including pleural effusion, infiltrative lung disease, bronchiolitis, necrobiotic nodules, vasculitis, and rheumatoid pneumoconiosis.[329] Pleural effusions commonly occur in men with high titers of rheumatoid factor. Characteristically the pleural fluid glucose is reduced below 30 mg/dl, and the pH is low. RA cells, neutrophils with cytoplasmic inclusions containing phagocytized rheumatoid factor, may be present in fluid.[330] Thoracoscopy shows a characteristic granular appearance to the pleural surface, and a biopsy specimen may show palisading histiocytes and giant cells like those of a rheumatoid nodule lining the pleural surface.[331]

The frequency of infiltrative lung disease in rheumatoid arthritis (RA) is difficult to gauge. Roentgenographic changes are infrequent, whereas 30% to 40% of patients have been reported to have abnormalities of diffusion often without symptoms. The pathologic features of parenchymal infiltrates are diverse and include lymphoid hyperplasia, organizing pneumonia, CIP, UIP, and rarely even diffuse alveolar damage.[332] Several of the drugs used to treat rheumatoid arthritis also cause infiltrative lung disease, and sometimes it may be impossible to be certain whether pathologic changes are caused by the primary disease or by a drug.

Severe progressive obstructive lung disease caused by obliterative bronchiolitis is a recognized complication of RA.[333] Although a relationship to penicillamine therapy has been suggested, not all patients with bronchiolitis obliterans have received this drug. Lesser degrees of bronchitis and bronchiolitis probably are not unusual in rheumatoid arthritis, since many patients with RA have small airways dysfunction detectable by sensitive physiologic tests. Full-blown bronchiectasis, while not common in RA, seems to occur more often than would be expected by chance.[334]

Necrobiotic nodules are the most specific pathologic manifestation of rheumatoid disease. They closely resemble the more common subcutaneous nodules. They occur in patients with active disease and high titers of rheumatoid factor, may be single or multiple, and may occur as an isolated form of lung disease or against a background of pulmonary fibrosis. The center of the nodules may consist of fibrinoid necrosis or degenerating neutrophils. A band of palisading histiocytes surrounds the necrotic center. External to the palisading cells is a zone of fibrous tissue, lymphocytes, and plasma cells (Fig. 49-44).

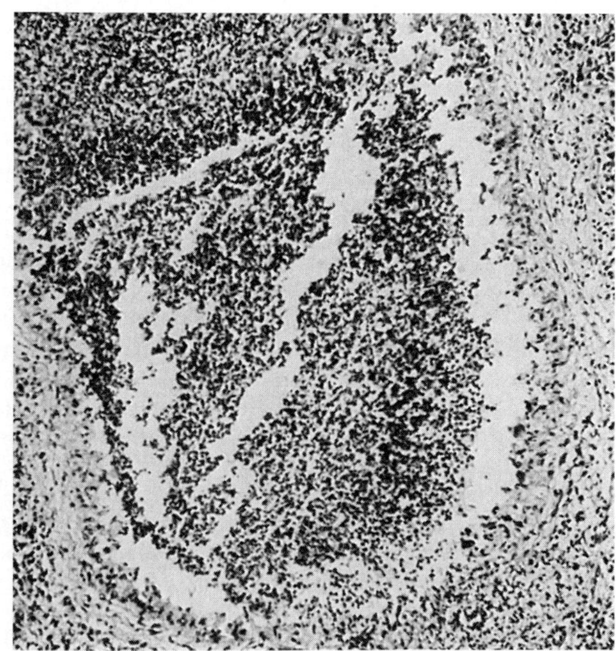

Fig. 49-44 Rheumatoid lung disease. Necrobiotic subpleural nodule.

Miners exposed to various mineral dusts develop a modified form of nodule known as rheumatoid pneumoconiosis, or Caplan's syndrome. Over a few months, round opacities from 0.3 cm to several centimeters in diameter appear in the chest roentgenogram mainly in the peripheral lung fields. The lesions may be solitary, or several may fuse to form a large conglomerate mass. Macroscopically they are pale gray with concentric darker layers of pigment. The pale areas tend to liquify, leaving clefts. Histologically the center is necrotic and often contains foci of calcification. Concentric bands of dust are seen in the necrotic center. A zone of palisading histiocytes encloses the necrotic center, and the whole is encapsulated by a layer of circumferential collagen bundles with lymphocytes and plasma cells. Rheumatoid pneumoconiosis occasionally occurs in miners without articular disease, but circulating rheumatoid factor is invariably present, and some will subsequently develop arthritis.

Necrotizing vasculitis is rare in rheumatoid disease. Pulmonary involvement usually accompanies systemic vasculitis, but isolated pulmonary vasculitis has been reported.

Systemic lupus erythematosus

Lung disease occurs in many patients with systemic lupus erythematosus (SLE). Often the lung disease is attributable to infection that was a recognized complication of SLE even before modern intensive immunosuppressive therapy. Leukopenia, hypocomplementemia, and general debility are predisposing factors. Patients with lupus anticoagulant or antiphospholipid antibodies are paradoxically prone to thrombosis, which may give rise to pulmonary emboli. The most common manifestation of SLE in the chest is pleurisy, which occurs in 30% of patients. It may be painful and is accompanied by small effusions. The fluid has the properties of an exudate and may contain LE cells and immune complexes.[330] The histologic findings are a nonspecific organizing fibrinous exudate. Although pulmonary hemorrhage in SLE can result from coagulation abnormalities, uremia, or infection, it can also be a direct manifestation of the primary disease. Histologically the lungs show extensive intra-alveolar hemorrhage, usually with siderophages. Abnormalities of the alveolar walls, small arteries, and veins may be minimal, but often there is a mild thickening of the alveolar septa by edema accompanied by infiltration of neutrophils and focal hyperplasia of type II cells (Fig. 49-45). Electron microscopy shows subendothelial dense deposits in the alveolar capillaries, and immunohistochemical analysis shows granular staining for immunoglobulin and complement, both indicative of deposition of immune complexes.[335]

Interstitial pneumonia occurs in less than 10% of patients with SLE and may be acute or chronic. Biopsy examination in a few cases of acute lupus pneumonitis has shown organizing diffuse alveolar damage.[336] Immunohistochemical studies have shown the presence of DNA and immune complexes in the alveolar walls. Eluted antibody had anti-DNA activity.[337] Less commonly, the pneumonia is chronic, with morphologic features of UIP. Chronic interstitial pneumonia is especially common in a subset of SLE patients with serologic features overlapping those of scleroderma.

Pulmonary hypertension can develop in patients with SLE in the absence of significant parenchymal lung disease. Its morphologic basis may be active or healed vasculitis, or plexiform arteriopathy indistinguishable from primary pulmonary hypertension.[338] Immune complexes deposited in the intima and media of arteries probably are responsible for the vascular damage. Raynaud's phenomenon is often present in patients with SLE and pulmonary hypertension, suggestive of a component of altered vascular reactivity in the pathogenesis.

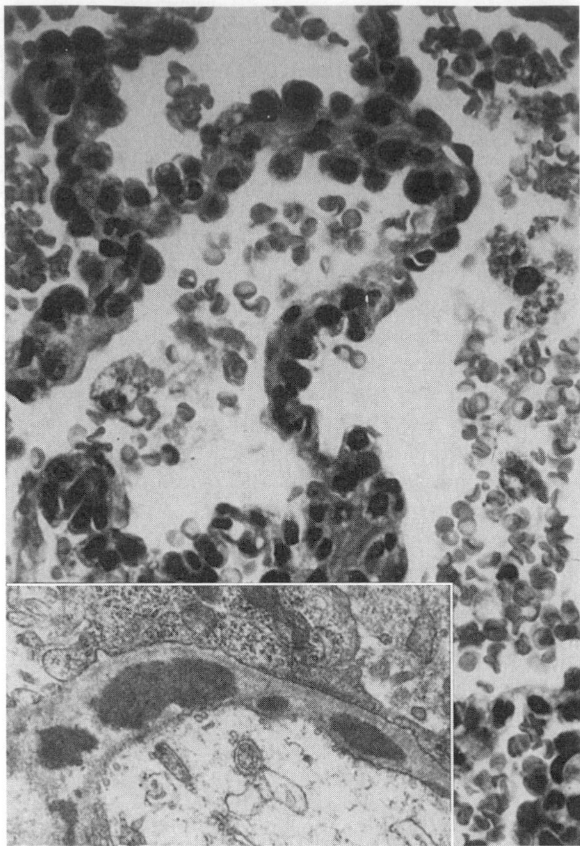

Fig. 49-45 Systemic lupus erythematosus. Alveoli are lined with hyperplastic epithelial cells. *Inset,* Electron microscopic details of the basal lamina with dense deposits.

Sjögren's syndrome

Sjögren's syndrome combines lymphoid infiltration of the salivary and lacrimal glands with other manifestations of collagen vascular disease, most commonly, arthritis and hyperglobulinemia. Involvement of the bronchial mucous glands by a process similar to that in the salivary glands can lead to failure of bronchial clearance and repeated infections.[339] Chronic airflow obstruction associated with bronchiolitis is common and can be disabling (Fig, 49-31). In the lung parenchyma, a nonspecific interstitial pneumonia is present in approximately 3% to 45% of patients. A variety of lymphoproliferative lesions occur in lungs and elsewhere in Sjögren's syndrome. In the lungs these range from lymphoid interstitial pneumonia in which the interstitium of the lung is heavily infiltrated by lymphocytes and plasma cells to pseudolymphomas with nodules and masses of benign lymphoid tissue with germinal centers and a well-differentiated polyclonal mature lymphoplasmacytic infiltration to frankly malignant lymphoma, usually of the large cell type.[340] Most lymphomas developing in Sjögren's syndrome are of the B-cell type.

Scleroderma

In scleroderma, the respiratory tract is the fourth most commonly involved organ system, after the skin, kidney, and gastrointestinal tract. As clinical management of the renal complications has improved, pulmonary involvement has emerged as the leading cause of death.[341]

Lung changes include primarily pulmonary fibrosis and vascular disease (Fig. 49-46). In addition, esophageal involvement by scleroderma leads to aspiration. Pulmonary fibrosis is the commoner type of involvement by scleroderma. The clinical manifestations are similar to idiopathic pulmonary fibrosis (IPF), but the course is more protracted. Roentgenographs of the chest show bibasilar reticulonodular infiltrates. Pulmonary function tests show a restrictive ventilatory defect in 60% of patients, but as many as one third may have obstruction, and 10% are normal. The histopathologic characteristics resemble those of UIP and are not distinctive unless there are characteristic vascular changes.[341]

Vascular lesions are the most characteristic pathologic features of pulmonary scleroderma and can occur with or without an associated pulmonary fibrosis. In typical cases there is concentric myxoid or fibrous intimal thickening of small muscular arteries. When the intimal changes are relatively mild, the tunica media is hypertrophied, but as the intimal change becomes severe, the media atrophies. Some arteries also show mononuclear cell infiltration of the intima. The milder degrees of pulmonary vascular disease are associated with isolated reduction in the diffusing capacity for carbon monoxide, whereas more severe degrees cause pulmonary hypertension.[342] Studies disagree as to whether pulmonary hypertension is more or less common in the CREST variant of scleroderma than in progressive systemic sclerosis.[343]

Other collagen vascular diseases

Pulmonary dysfunction in polymyositis and dermatomyositis results from the involvement of the respiratory muscles or from infiltrative lung disease. Infiltrative lung disease develops in only 5% to 10% of all patients but in more than 50% of those patients with antibodies to aminoacyl t-RNA (anti-Jo-1). Several histologic patterns can occur with important prognostic differences. As is the case with idiopathic lung disease, patients with organizing pneumonia or cellular interstitial pneumonia have a better prognosis than those with UIP, whereas the few with diffuse alveolar damage have a rapidly progressive downhill course.[344]

Pulmonary symptoms in ankylosing spondylitis usually result from ventilatory restriction caused by chest wall disease, but apical bullous lesions also occur. Pulmonary involvement in primary biliary cirrhosis is rare and varied. Lesions include infiltrative lung disease, obliterative bronchiolitis, and primary pulmonary hypertension. Noncaseating granulomas, when present, are diagnostically useful.[345] Infiltration of the lung parenchyma and small blood vessels by eosinophils and mononuclear cells occurs in the eosinophilia-myalgia syndrome caused by L-tryptophane ingestion.[346]

PULMONARY VASCULITIDES

Wegener's granulomatosis

The four components of Wegener's granulomatosis are granulomas of the upper respiratory tract, granulomas of the lung, systemic vasculitis, and a focal usually necrotizing glomerulonephritis.[347] Granulomas may be present in other organs as well. Not all components need be present in a given patient. DeRemee classified the disease according to the sites involved—*E* for upper respiratory, *L* for lung, *K* for kidney. Thus a patient with only lung granulomas and glomerulonephritis had the LK variant.[348] Wegener's granulomatosus is one of several causes of the clinical syndrome of lethal midline granulomatosus.

Grossly, the pulmonary lesions may have the appearance of pale infarcts or vary from small to bulky necrotic nodules (Fig 49-47). The histologic features manifest as of necrotizing granulomas with an associated vasculitis (Fig. 49-48). The granulomas often form against a background of nonspecific inflammation. Palisading histiocytes enclose microabscess or larger zones of geographic necrosis, which may be bland and infarctlike with partial preservation of the underlying tissue architecture or may be softer and contain abundant cellular debris.[349] Giant cells may be scanty or numerous and are usually of the foreign-body type. Bronchi and bronchioles are

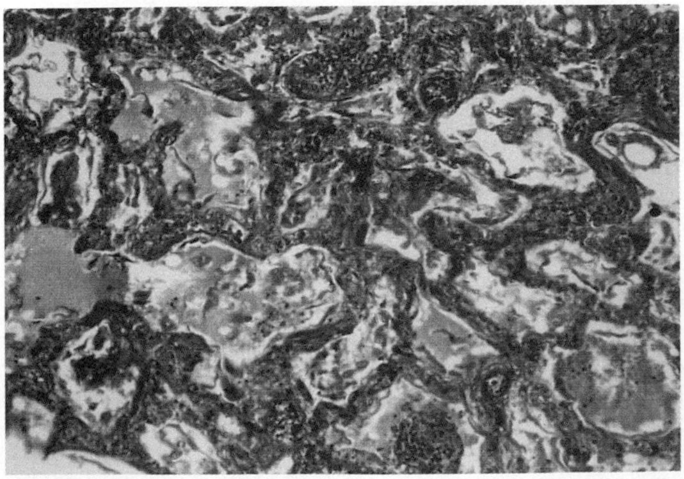

Fig. 49-46 Scleroderma. Lung shows interstitial fibrosis. Alveoli contain protein-rich edema.

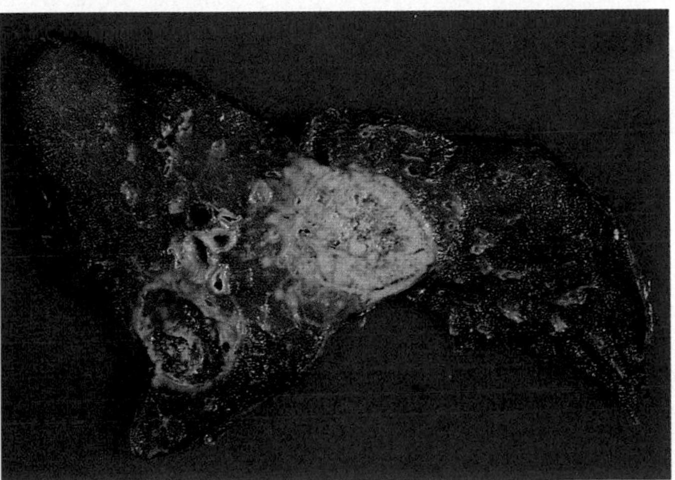

Fig. 49-47 Wegener's granulomatosis. The lung parenchyma contains two nodules that show central necrosis.

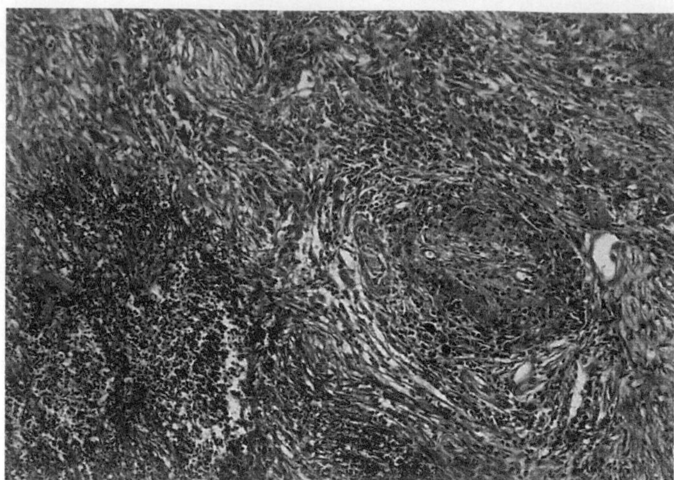

Fig. 49-48 Wegener's granulomatosis. The section shows areas of necrosis, inflammation, and vasculitis.

often involved. Compact epithelioid granulomas, like those of sarcoidosis or tuberculosis, are distinctly unusual.

Vasculitis involves both veins and arteries and vessels from millimeter to tens of micrometers in size. Usually the vasculitis is manifested by mononuclear cell invasion of all coats of the vessel wall. In larger vessels, the granulomatous quality of the inflammation may be obvious with palisading histiocytes and giant cells. Fibrinoid necrosis of vessels is uncommon but may be seen in active cases. Pulmonary capillaritis may present as diffuse pulmonary hemorrhage.[350]

Wegener's granulomatosis can affect patients of any age. Men outnumber women by a small margin. The clinical manifestations vary according to the sites involved. Pulmonary symptoms are nonspecific and include cough, dyspnea, and pleurisy. Systemic manifestations such as fever, weight loss, anemia, and leukocytosis are common in multifocal disease but are infrequent when disease is limited to one or a few sites. A chest roentgenogram shows one or more large rounded densities that may cavitate. These lesions occur predominantly in the lower lobes.

The diagnosis depends on the integration of clinical and pathologic information. The histologic diagnosis in the lung requires the presence of both vasculitis and necrotizing granulomatous inflammation. The combination is not specific, however, and special stains and cultures are needed to rule out infection, since vasculitis is not rare in contiguity with infectious granulomas. Vasculitis in vessels remote from actual granulomas is helpful in making the diagnosis but is not always found, especially in small biopsy specimens. The discovery that most patients with Wegener's granulomatosis have antineutrophil cytoplasmic antibodies (ANCA) directed against a lysosomal serine proteinase, proteinase 3, has provided a clinical test with greater than 90% specificity.[351]

The pathogenesis of Wegener's granulomatosis is uncertain. Immunofluorescent studies of the kidney and lung have given variable results, some supporting immune complex deposition, others not. Cell-mediated immunity may play a role because the predominant inflammatory cells are T-lymphocytes, with a predominance of the helper T-cell subset.[352] In vitro, the ANCA stimulates primed neutrophils to secrete oxidants and lysosomal enzymes. They may play a role in the production of tissue necrosis.[353]

Allergic granulomatosis and angiitis

Allergic granulomatosis and angiitis, or the Churg-Strauss syndrome, is a distinctive vasculitic syndrome that resembles polyarteritis nodosa with asthma and granulomatous and nongranulomatous pulmonary involvement.[354-356] In the prodromal phase of the illness, patients often have nonspecific allergic upper respiratory manifestations such as rhinitis, sinusitis, or nasal polyps. Asthma is present, usually for several years, before the appearance of a systemic illness with blood eosinophilia and pulmonary infiltrates. In the third phase, a systemic, necrotizing vasculitis with extravascular granulomas develops.[354] Antineutrophil cytoplasmic antibodies may be present and usually take on a stain with a perinuclear distribution (p-ANCA). Serum IgE concentration may be elevated to above 1000 mg/dl. Many tissues can be involved, including the heart, gastrointestinal tract, kidney, skin, muscles, joints, and central and peripheral nervous systems. Rarely only a single tissue is involved. Unlike Wegener's granulomatosis and many vasculitides, renal failure is not prominent, and 50% of deaths are attributable to cardiac involvement.

Radiographic pulmonary infiltrates are caused by lesions of two types: (1) eosinophilic pneumonia with patchy eosinophilic infiltrates and foci of degenerating eosinophils and Charcot-Leyden crystals, or (2) granulomas. The granulomas consist of foci of necrosis or eosinophilic abscesses surrounded by palisading histiocytes and giant cells. The associated vasculitis involves arteries more than veins. In typical lesions, the tunica media of muscular arteries are replaced by giant cells and all coats of the artery are infiltrated by eosinophils.[356]

Goodpasture's syndrome

The development of antibodies to antigens in the basal lamina can produce either glomerulonephritis alone or pulmonary hemorrhage and glomerulonephritis, a combination known as Goodpasture's syndrome. Goodpasture's syndrome usually occurs in men between 16 and 30 years of age. The majority of cases have been reported to have the HLA-DRw2 haplotype. Hemoptysis is the initial symptom, often accompanied by exertional dyspnea, fatigue, and weakness. Iron-deficiency anemia, hematuria, and proteinuria follow. Without therapy the disease is usually lethal within a year, but spontaneous remissions can occur.

The lung shows acute hemorrhage usually accompanied by hemosiderin-laden macrophages. Alveolar septa are widened by interstitial edema accompanied by a capillaritis manifest as infiltration of neutrophils either within the septal interstitium or within the air spaces but clinging to the septa. The alveolar epithelium is hyperplastic. Focally there may be hyaline membranes or organizing fibrous tissue within air spaces.[357] In cases of longer duration, elastic fibers in arteries and veins become encrusted by iron salts accompanied by foreign-body giant cells (so-called endogenous pneumoconiosis). The histologic pattern is not specific, and the diagnosis requires the demonstration of anti-basement membrane antibodies either in the serum or deposited in the tissue where immunofluorescent staining of either lung or renal glomeruli shows linear staining for immunoglobulin and often complement.

The pathogenesis of the disease is clearly related to the production of the antibodies that are directed against a noncollagenous epitope near the carboxyl terminus of the $\alpha 3$ chain of type IV collagen. Neither the stimulus for antibody formation nor the reason for the restricted organ distribution of its reactivity are understood. Most patients with Goodpasture's syndrome are smokers, and sometimes the onset of disease has followed influenzal infection or inhalation exposure to hydrocarbon solvents. These environmental insults may damage the nonfenestrated endothelium, allowing the antibodies access to the pulmonary basal lamina.[358]

Diffuse pulmonary hemorrhage

The syndrome of diffuse pulmonary hemorrhage has several causes and associations in addition to Wegener's granulomatosis and Goodpasture's syndrome, among them small vessel polyarteritis nodosa, Henoch-Schönlein purpura, and various other immune complex-mediated diseases, including SLE and the glomerulonephritides. The pathologic basis in nearly all such cases is capillaritis, identified by the clustering of neutrophils in the alveolar septa. They may be within the interstitium or within the adjacent air space, but even when free in the air space, they do not fill the space but remain near the alveolar septa as though attracted there. Fibrin thrombi in capillaries or even necrosis of alveolar walls may be present in acute cases. The pulmonary hemorrhage is often accompanied by nonspecific changes, that is, hemosiderosis, "endogenous pneumoconiosis," hyaline membranes, or air space organization. Immunofluorescent studies of lung or other tissues may or may not show immune complex deposition.[359]

There remains a small group of patients who have repeated pulmonary hemorrhage in the absence of a systemic disease. To this group the term *idiopathic pulmonary hemorrhage* (or hemosiderosis) applies. More than 80% of patients with idiopathic pulmonary hemorrhage are children, and most of the remainder are young adults. Usually the disease begins with mild episodes of intrapulmonary bleeding associated with cough, dyspnea, and rapidly changing pulmonary infiltrates. Occasionally the first episode is one of brisk hemoptysis. Iron-deficiency anemia is common because of sequestration of blood in the lung. In a few cases of idiopathic pulmonary hemorrhage in adults, the underlying pathologic state has been reported to be capillaritis.[359] More commonly, no abnormalities of the alveolar septa or vessels are seen by light microscopy. Ultrastructural abnormalities of the alveolar or capillary basal laminae have been reported, but none has been consistent, and many cases appear ultrastructurally normal. The course of idiopathic pulmonary hemorrhage is variable. Patients can die during an initial episode or survive for many years with recurring episodes of hemorrhage leading to fibrosis and respiratory insufficiency. Remissions of many years in duration may occur either spontaneously or after therapy.

MISCELLANEOUS LUNG DISEASES

Langerhans' cell histiocytosis (histiocytosis X)

The Langerhans' cells are bone-marrow-derived members of the mononuclear phagocyte system closely allied to the dendritic cells. Like the dendritic cells, they are specialized for antigen presentation and accessory cell function but particularly within epithelium. In normal lung they are found within bronchiolar epithelium but not in the alveoli.[360] The Langerhans' cell histiocytoses (also called *histocytosis X*) are clonal proliferations of Langerhans' cells that vary greatly in extent.[361] Disseminated histiocytosis mainly affects children, whereas localized forms are usually indolent and predominantly affect young adults. Lung involvement is typically widespread or diffuse in acute disseminated Langerhans' cell histiocytosis (Letterer-Siwe type) and can produce striking honeycomblike change (Fig. 49-49).

Langerhans' cell histiocytosis limited to the lung (pulmonary eosinophilic granuloma) is a disease of young adults, and nearly all are cigarette smokers. Symptoms are variable. Some patients are asymptomatic, and the process is discovered accidentally by chest roentgenography. Others are first seen because of pneumothorax, whereas still others have gradually worsening cough and dyspnea as a result of interstitial involvement. The chest roentgenogram early shows nodular infiltrates, which may resolve or become reticular with subsequent appearance of bullae or honeycombing. Sparing of the costophrenic angles is characteristic but not specific.[362]

The pathologic features were well described by Auld[363] and confirmed by subsequent observers.[364] At low power, a striking feature is the nodular pattern with normal intervening tissue. Many lesions are centered on terminal bronchioles. Early lesions are interstitial nodules composed of a mixed cell population consisting of typical Langerhans' histiocytes along with varying proportions of eosinophils, neutrophils, plasma cells lymphocytes, and ordinary pigmented macrophages. Langerhans' cells have an indistinct pale pink or amphophilic cytoplasm and a nucleus that is reniform, notched, or highly folded with open chromatin (Fig. 49-50). By electron microscopy,

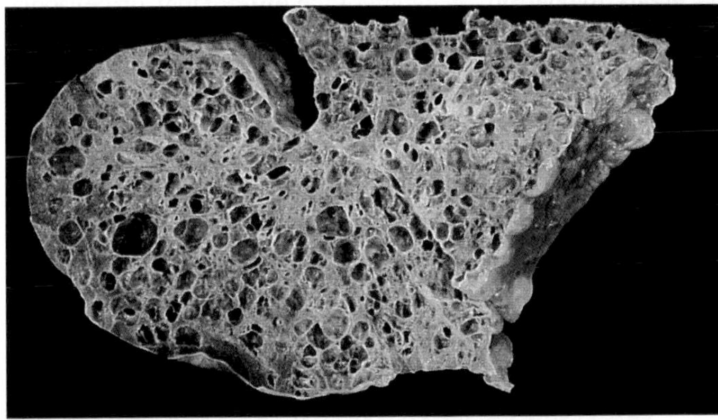

Fig. 49-49 Disseminated Langerhans' histiocytosis, Letterer-Siwe type, shows honeycomb-like changes in the lung.

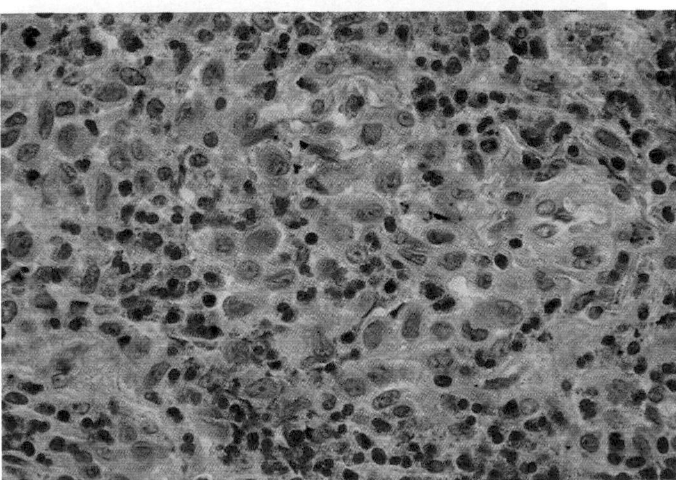

Fig. 49-50 Langerhans' histiocytosis. The infiltrate consists of histiocytes that have reniform nuclei and eosinophils.

drome or Ehlers-Danlos syndrome, in most the cause is unknown. The pleura responds to the presence of pneumothorax by exudation of fibrin accompanied by a proliferation and infiltration of macrophages, eosinophils, multinucleated giant cells, and mesothelial cells known as *reactive eosinophilic pleuritis.*[400] This response is nonspecific and does not indicate underlying disease.

Behind a totally occluded bronchus, the lung collapses as the intra-alveolar gas is absorbed. This can happen rapidly when mucus plugs a bronchus in someone breathing 100% oxygen. In persons breathing room air, obstruction of a bronchus causes only minor volume loss because absorption of the nitrogen in the air is gradual and the gas is replaced by edema fluid. Gradual occlusion of a bronchus leads to bronchiectasis, organizing pneumonia, and endogenous lipid pneumonia, rather than simple collapse.

Shallow respiration leads to alveolar collapse as a result of rising surface tension in the alveolar lining. The process is poorly understood, but deep ventilation is a stimulus for surfactant secretion by type II cells and is required for the formation of a stable surface film. Collapse because of shallow ventilation is common in postoperative patients whose respiration is depressed by anesthesia and incisional pain.[401]

CHRONIC AIRFLOW OBSTRUCTION

Chronic airflow obstruction (CAO) is a term used to describe abnormal slowing of expiratory airflow as measured by physiologic tests. Ordinarily, it refers to slowing that is not completely reversed by bronchodilators and hence is not usually applied to asthma. In practice, some patients have obstruction that is partially reversible, and in them distinction from asthma is difficult.

Chronic airflow obstruction is associated with abnormalities in the bronchi, bronchioles, or acini and with numerous different structural abnormalities at each level.[402] Commonly, abnormalities at several levels are present in the same patient, reflecting the tissue response to inhaled irritants at each level. An international committee in 1959 defined chronic bronchitis as excessive sputum production and spelled out operational criteria for use in epidemiologic studies. These criteria were sputum production on most days for at least 3 months a year for at least 2 successive years, if not caused by another specific disease such as tuberculosis, bronchiectasis, or cancer. Emphysema was defined in terms of its pathologic anatomy, as abnormal dilatation of air spaces distal to the terminal nonrespiratory bronchiole with destruction of air space walls. Later the qualification was added that there not be significant fibrosis to exclude honeycomb lungs, which behave very differently from emphysematous lungs.[403] In fact, minor degrees of fibrosis are the rule in some types of emphysema. Advances in pulmonary physiology led to the recognition that increased resistance to airflow through bronchioles less than 2 mm was present in patients with CAO and could often be detected before the forced expiratory volume in 1 second (FEV_1) was abnormal. The term "small airways disease" is often used to encompass various intrinsic anatomic abnormalities of the bronchioles that may contribute to this dysfunction.

Incidence. The disease processes associated with CAO are often merged under the term *chronic obstructive pulmonary disease,* COPD. COPD is the fifth leading cause of death in the United States and accounts for 3.5% of deaths annually. The mortality is roughly 2½ times greater for men than women and has trebled since 1950. Because COPD progresses slowly over many years, it causes enormous disability. Two million hospitalizations and 17 million visits to physician offices are caused by COPD annually in the United States. Overwhelmingly the major cause of COPD is cigarette smoking, though industrial causes and community air pollution have also been implicated.

Chronic bronchitis

Pathologic changes observed in the large airways of subjects with cough and excess mucous production include enlargement of the mucous glands, an increase in the proportion of mucous cells relative to serous cells, an increase in the amount of sulfated and acidic mucous by histochemical staining, and dilatation of the ducts of the mucus glands with mucous plugs. Assessment of mucous gland volume for research purposes is rigorously accomplished by stereologic testing, but a simple assessment in diagnostic practice can be made by the gland to wall ratio, or Reid index, the thickness of the lobules of mucous glands divided by the distance between the basement membrane of the bronchial epithelium and perichondrium (Fig. 49-54). Originally, Reid obtained values of the ratio between 0.14 to 0.36 in normals whereas subjects clinically diagnosed as bronchitic averaged 0.59. Subsequent studies have established that the Reid index and other measures of gland volume are unimodally distributed on a bell-shaped curve with no clear separation between normal and diseased. As Thurlbeck has pointed out, the situation is similar in regard to blood pressure measurements where the distinction between normotensive and hypertensive is also arbitrary.[402] Inflammatory infiltration of the bronchial mucosa is common in persons with excess sputum production but is not closely correlated with gland volume.

Although mucous gland enlargement correlates well with cigarette smoking and sputum production, most studies have found only a weak correlation with physiologic measures of

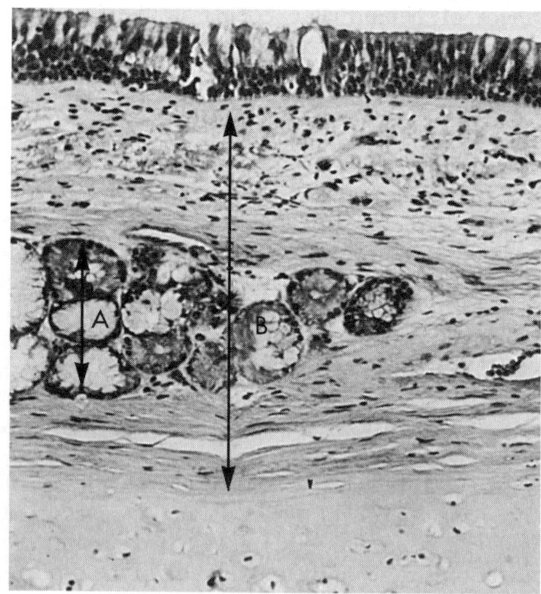

Fig. 49-54 Normal bronchus. Gland-to-wall ratio (A/B) is quick measure of mucous gland volume. It increases in chronic bronchitis.

airflow obstruction. Clinical studies that show that excess mucus production is not related to mortality from COPD also support the conclusion that excess sputum production and its anatomic counterpart gland enlargement are not a major cause of CAO.[404]

Some patients with chronic hypersecretion of mucus have repeated episodes of chest infection with increased cough and sputum production, sputum purulence, and dyspnea. Episodes are characterized by the appearance of bacteria in the sputum or, in subjects whose airways are permanently colonized, an increase in the number of organisms. The commonest species associated with these exacerbations are unencapsulated strains of *Haemophilus influenzae,* followed by *Streptococcus pneumoniae* and *Branhamella catarrhalis*. The trigger in one third of such episodes is an identifiable viral or mycoplasmal infection. During the acute episode there is often deterioration of pulmonary function, but it is reversible and in most studies the long-term development of chronic airflow obstruction is little influenced by intercurrent infections.[405]

Small airway lesions

In normal lungs, the aggregate area of the peripheral airways is large, the flow is correspondingly low. Only 20% of the normal airflow resistance resides in the small airways less than 2 mm in diameter. In CAO, there is a pronounced increase in the resistance in small airways, which may contribute more than 80% of the total.[406]

The function of small airways is influenced both by the structure and reactivity of the airways themselves and by their interaction with the surrounding lung parenchyma. Severe CAO can result from either intrinsic bronchiolar abnormalities or parenchymal changes, specifically, changes in elastic recoil and emphysema. Thurlbeck has pointed out that many studies of the pathologic basis of CAO have used lungs resected for localized peripheral tumors that have only mild CAO permitting major surgery, whereas others used lungs obtained at autopsy from patients dying of COPD who had severe disease. In the former group, changes in small airways correlate most closely with functional abnormalities, whereas in the latter emphysema usually predominates.[402]

Anatomic abnormalities identified in small airways of smokers include bronchiolar narrowing, goblet cell metaplasia, mucus plugging, inflammation, fibrosis, and increased muscle and tortuosity of the airways.[407] These changes are often subtle and difficult to appreciate during the diagnostic inspection of histologic slides. Their importance has been shown by quantitative analysis of large series of cases.

Correlations between various physiologic tests and summed pathologic scores document the importance of these small airway lesions in causing CAO. Uncertainties remain regarding the relative importance of particular morphologic abnormalities in causing abnormalities in particular pulmonary function tests. The relatively low order of correlation between fixed structural changes and tests of expiratory function point to the importance of superimposed functional effects. Epithelial injury and inflammation may cause hyperreactivity of small airways. Inflammatory exudate interferes with surfactant function, and loss of alveolar attachments facilitates airway closure.[408]

Specific forms of small airways disease

Several types of bronchiolitis are specific in terms of cause, clinical associations, or pathologic characteristics (Table 49-9).

Table 49-9 Specific types of bronchiolitis

Postinfectious
Toxic chemicals
Mineral dust
Transplant bronchiolitis
Collagen-vascular disease
Rheumatoid arthritis
Sjögren's syndrome
Other
Idiopathic obliterative or constrictive bronchiolitis
Follicular bronchitis and bronchiolitis
Diffuse panbronchiolitis
Respiratory bronchiolitis

Bronchiolitis associated with mineral dust, transplantation, and collagen vascular disease are discussed elsewhere. There is evidence that bronchial infections early in life may predispose to later COPD. In addition, severe viral bronchitis and bronchiolitis associated with relatively destructive organisms such as influenza, measles, adenovirus, or mycoplasma can lead to rapidly progressive narrowing or even total obliteration of small airways.[409] When widespread, this obliterative bronchiolitis causes generalized airflow obstruction. Postinfectious bronchiolitis obliterans can also be localized. Unilateral lung transradiancy (Swyer-James or McLeod's syndrome) results from obliterative bronchiolitis mostly limited to one side or one lobe causing air trapping and diminished blood flow on the affected side.[410] Obliteration in more proximal airways precludes collateral ventilation and produces absorption atelectasis.[411]

Bronchiolitis obliterans after the inhalation of toxic fumes can either appear as a sequela of ARDS or develop several weeks after the episode of inhalation without earlier overt clinical lung disease. Various toxic chemicals, including inhalation of smoke, NO_2 in silo filler's disease, and sundry industrial chemicals, cause similar patterns of injury.[412] The disease is manifest as cough, progressive dyspnea, and airflow obstruction. The histopathologic examination may show either constrictive bronchiolitis or endobronchiolar polyps of fibrous tissue similar to the Masson bodies of organizing pneumonia.[413]

Some nonsmokers without a clear history of viral infection, toxic exposure, or collagen vascular disease develop cough, dyspnea and progressive CAO.[414] In the few cases reported, women outnumber men. Chest roentgenograms are relatively normal except for slight bronchial thickening and overexpansion of the lungs. The pathologic changes manifest as either complete obliteration of small airways or a pattern described as constrictive bronchiolitis in which there is inflammation with submucosal and peribronchial fibrosis.[415] Epithelial changes are variable but usually appear as ulceration and squamous or cuboidal metaplasia. The sharp increase in fibrous tissue betwween the smooth muscle and epithelium is a useful histologic feature. The lung parenchyma is spared. Pulmonary function tests show irreversible obstruction with air trapping. Diffusing capacity overall is reduced, but the diffusion coefficient that corrects for the volume of lung inaccessible to the test gas (carbon monoxide) is normal.[414] The course of the disease is variable: a few patients have improved on therapy, most have remained relatively stable, and a few have had progressive fatal illnesses.

Follicular bronchitis/bronchiolitis refers to chronic airway inflammation with the occurrence of lymphoid follicles in the walls of the bronchi and bronchioles. In some cases, there is neutrophilic exudate in the airway lumens. Follicular bronchitis and bronchiolitis occurs in three clinical settings: with collagen vascular disease, with immune deficiency, and with eosinophilia suggestive of an allergic basis. The lymphoid hyperplasia often produces lymphoid nodules along the perilobular septa as well as in the peribronchial tissue. The chest roentgenogram usually shows a reticulinodular infiltrate, and the ventilatory dysfunction may be obstructive, restrictive, or mixed.[416]

Diffuse panbronchiolitis is common in Japan, where it was first described, whereas few cases have been reported in the West.[417] The disease predominantly involves the transitional zone between conductive airways and acini. Mononuclear interstitial inflammatory exudate infiltrates the respiratory bronchioles in cases with minimal involvement and extends proximally into the terminal and membranous bronchioles in those with more extensive disease. Later bronchiectasis may develop. Foamy macrophages often accompany the mononuclear inflammatory infiltrate.[418] There may be neutrophils in the bronchiolar lumens. Patients experience a gradual dyspnea accompanied with cough and sputum production. The chest roentgenogram shows miliary nodularity, and spirometry shows an obstructive or mixed obstructive and restrictive defect in ventilation. Two thirds of patients have an associated sinusitis. Colonization of airways with bacteria including *Pseudomonas* organisms is common. The course is progressive and can eventuate in respiratory failure.[419]

Another lesion that predominantly affects the respiratory bronchioles, and which is nearly universal in regular cigarette smokers, has been termed *respiratory bronchiolitis.* The lumens of the respiratory bronchioles contain aggregates of alveolar macrophages containing a brown autofluorescent pigment. The walls of the respiratory bronchioles are mildly thickened by a combination of chronic inflammation and fibrosis. Wisps of intraluminal mucus are often seen in terminal bronchioles proximal to the aggregates of macrophages. Respiratory bronchiolitis is usually clinically silent and is associated with a normal FEV_1, but mild abnormalities can be shown with more sensitive tests of pulmonary function. In a few very heavy cigarette smokers, it causes an infiltrative pattern on the chest roentgenogram and mild ventilatory restriction, which can lead to the need for performance of a lung biopsy.[420] Its course is not progressive, and cessation of smoking reverses the clinical manifestations. Respiratory bronchiolitis with infiltrative lung disease overlaps with mild DIP, and the distinction may be arbitrary in some cases.[421]

Emphysema

With the passage of years, the lung gradually loses elastic recoil, alveolar ducts dilate, and the fraction of lung that is composed of alveolar duct increases at the expense of alveoli. These changes are part of the normal process of aging and are not emphysema, which is by definition an abnormal enlargement of air spaces.

Mild degrees of emphysema are difficult to recognize in fresh lung. Distending the lung by instillation of a fixative through the bronchi improves recognition of emphysema and is adequate for routine purposes. Slices of the fixed lung can be impregnated with barium sulfate, and such a procedure takes only minutes and provides optimum detection and photography. Paper-mounted whole-lung sections, which are permanent and easily stored, are also useful. In the inflation-fixed lung, the alveolar ducts are at the limit of resolution of the unaided eye, though in the aged they form holes of tenths of a millimeter in size. Spaces in the parenchyma over 1 mm in size are abnormal.

Emphysema is common at autopsy, with a prevalence of 20% to 100%, depending on the population studied and the technique and criteria used. The prevalence and severity increases with age and are greater in men than women. Minor degrees of emphysema are clinically inapparent, and as a rule subjects with less than 20% of the lung involved have no symptoms.

Classification

On the sectioned surface of the lung, connective tissue septa extend inward from the pleura and outline units of parenchyma, termed *secondary lobules,* that are 1 to 2 cm in diameter and contain 2 to 5 acini. The acini are the functional gas-exchanging units of lung and consist of three to five generations of respiratory bronchioles and a variable number of alveolar ducts and alveolar sacs. Emphysema is classified according to the portion of the acinus it involves.[422]

Centriacinar emphysema. Emphysema that initially involves the respiratory bronchioles is termed *centriacinar,* or *centrilobular emphysema" (CLE)* The lesions of CLE appear grossly as roughly spherical holes 1 to 5 mm in diameter near the center of the lobules and separated from the perilobular septa by a rim of normal tissue (Fig. 49-55). Usually dark pigment is associated with lesions, and in advanced lesions the emphysematous spaces are crossed by strands of tissue containing vessels that remain after destruction of alveolar walls. Usually the upper lobes are involved more severely than the lower and the superior segments more than the basilar ones. The bronchioles supplying centriacinar emphysema often are inflamed, distorted, and stenotic. CLE is usually the type of emphysema found when chronic bronchitis and emphysema coexist. Patients with CLE are almost invariably smokers.

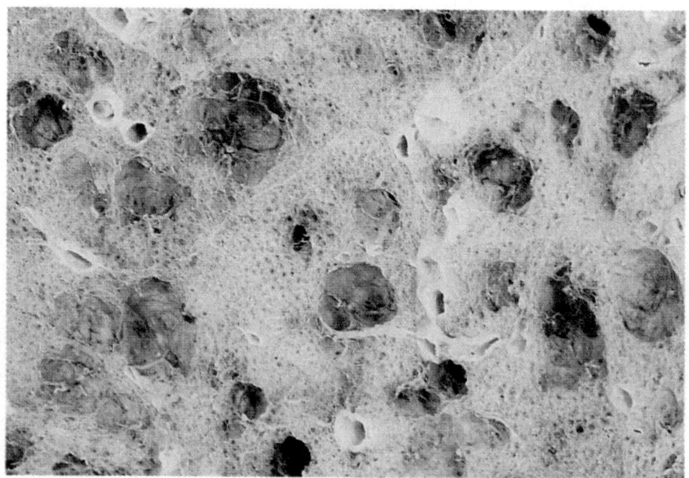

Fig. 49-55 Centriacinar emphysema.

Panacinar emphysema. In panacinar emphysema, all portions of the acinus are affected, but usually the alveolar ducts are involved more severely than the respiratory bronchioles. Individual lobules are variably involved, but even in minimally involved lobules abnormally enlarged air spaces reach the perilobular septa (Fig. 49-56). Both upper and lower lobes are usually involved to a comparable degree, but the lower lobes may have the more severe lesions. Panacinar emphysema occurs most often in middle-aged cigarette smokers, but it is also the characteristic type of emphysema in rare familial cases occurring in young adults whose serum antitrypsin levels may be normal or reduced. Small airway lesions are less severe than in centriacinar emphysema.

Distal acinar (paraseptal) emphysema. In distal acinar emphysema, the lesions are localized along the pleura and perilobular septa (Fig. 49-57). As an isolated finding, it is not associated with CAO but does predispose to pneumothorax. It can be associated with CLE.

Mixed and unclassified emphysema. It is not unusual to find emphysema of more than one type in a given lung, for example, centriacinar emphysema in the upper lobes and panacinar in the lower lobes. Many cases of emphysema do not fit unambiguously into one of the above types, either because the lesions are atypical or because they are so severe that it is impossible to recognize the portion of the acinus that was involved initially. In one study, only 27 of 122 emphysematous lungs examined by three expert pathologists unequivocally showed centriacinar or panacinar emphysema, with the remainder being mixed or unclassifiable. There is agreement that centriacinar emphysema is most severe in the upper lobes, whereas panacinar is more uniformly distributed, but there are no other clinical differences that consistently distinguish them, and whether they have a similar pathogenesis has not been established.[423]

Bullae. Bullae are subpleural air-filled cystic regions of severe emphysema greater than 1 cm in diameter. They are found most frequently along the sharp margins of the lungs anteriorly and near the apices. In pathologic specimens, they protrude like bubbles from the surface of the lung, but during life they are confined by the chest wall and indent and compress the lung. They are found in association with each of the forms of emphysema and sometimes, especially in young people, in otherwise normal lungs. Some bullae appear essentially empty, but most contain strands or remnants of tissue, indicating that they represent severely damaged lung that has lost its elastic recoil. Microscopically the walls of bullae show fibrosis and chronic inflammation. The most common cause of spontaneous pneumothorax in young people is rupture of apical bullae, but rupture is fortunately rare in generalized emphysema. Large bullae that occupy more than 30% of a hemithorax cause pulmonary dysfunction by compression of the remaining lung.

Morphogenesis of emphysema

There seem to be at least two ways that destruction of alveolar walls takes place. One, first described by Waters in 1862, is through the departition of air spaces by the enlargement and coalescence of holes. In both humans and animals, there are small holes (pores of Kohn) in normal alveolar septa that generally lie in the spaces between capillaries. Some enlargement of pores takes place with aging even in nonemphysematous lungs, but the process is exaggerated in emphysema. The pores encroach on and obliterate capillaries and coalesce, and gradually alveolar walls disappear, leaving behind strands of tissue that often contain the more resistant arteries. The abnormally large holes called "fenestrae" can be easily observed in barium sulfate-inpregnated lungs by use of a stereomicroscope, and in histologic sections they can be recognized because segments of airspace wall between fenestrae appear to be detached from the rest of the lung when the plane of section passes through the fenestrae.

Another type of emphysematous destruction is recognized as "loss of the orderly appearance of the acinus and its components."[423] In early panacinar emphysema, Heppleston and Leopold described dilatation of alveolar ducts with shortening

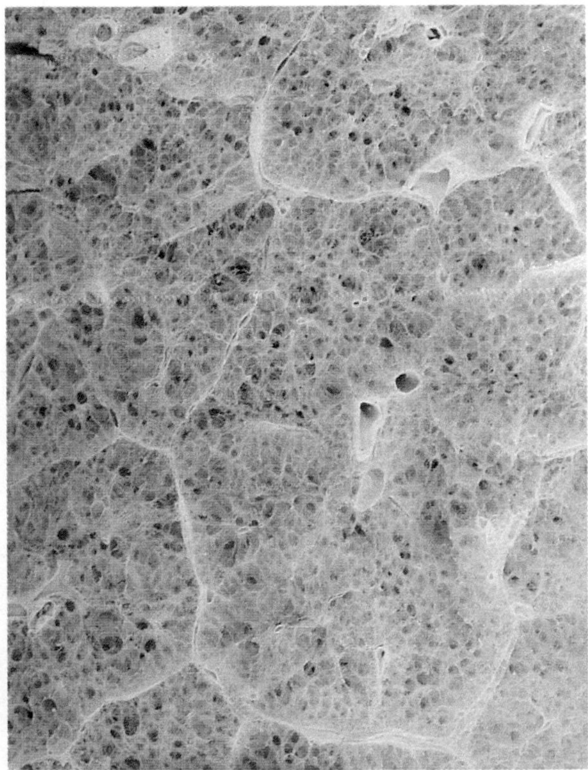

Fig. 49-56 Panacinar emphysema.

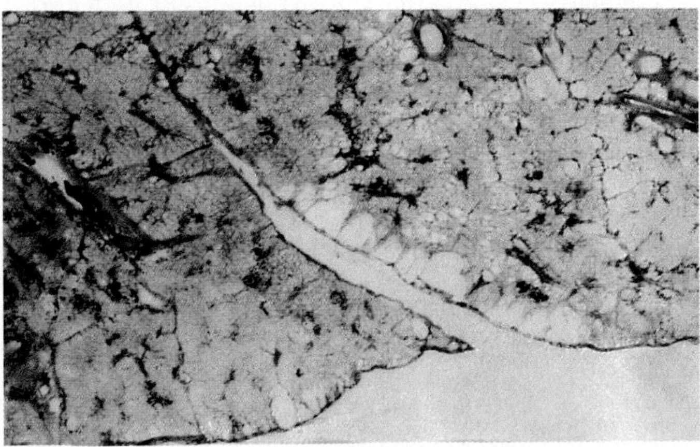

Fig. 49-57 Paraseptal emphysema.

and effacement of interalveolar septa,[424] and similar morphologic changes occur in experimental models of emphysema. The surface area of the lung is diminished, and such reduction indicates tissue loss, but fenestration is not prominent.

Pathophysiology

The most specific physiologic abnormality of the emphysematous lung is loss of elastic recoil. Lung recoil derives in part from surface forces and in part from the connective tissue. One might expect that the lost surface in emphysematous tissue and disrupted connective tissue account for the reduced recoil. In fact, some evidence indicates that gross emphysematous lesions are noncompliant, and it may be subtle alterations in the more normal lung that are more important.[425,426] Loss of gas-exchanging surface and the accompanying vascular bed caused by destruction of air space walls in emphysema explains the loss of diffusing capacity. Of the many abnormal pulmonary function tests in chronic obstructive pulmonary disease (COPD), loss of diffusing capacity correlates best with the extent of emphysema.

The basis for airflow obstruction in emphysema has been studied intensively. Hogg and coworkers showed that the major site of obstruction is in the small airways.[406] The decreased elastic recoil of the lung is one factor causing expiratory narrowing of the bronchioles. The thin-walled bronchioles are held open during expiration by the outward recoil of the surrounding lung, which is greater the more the lung is expanded. Physiologic studies of carefully selected emphysematous patients have shown that the conductance of their airways (the reciprocal of resistance) is normal for the elastic recoil of their lungs, but to generate a given recoil, the lungs must be at a higher volume than normal. In contrast, patients with intrinsic airways narrowing (asthma) had reduced conductance for any given degree of elastic recoil. Morphologic studies of emphysematous lungs show that there are fewer alveolar walls attached to the bronchioles than normal and such a reduction provides an anatomic basis for the diminished support, tortuosity, and premature closure of small airways in emphysema.

Emphysematous patients also have associated epithelial changes, inflammation, and fibrosis in the small airways, which contribute to airflow obstruction.[408] The resultant airway narrowing has been well documented in centriacinar emphysema using casts.

Etiology

The evidence that cigarette smoking is the major cause of emphysema is overwhelming.[428] A variety of autopsy populations from hospitals and coroners' offices has been studied, and a rough dose-response relationship holds true. Emphysema is seldom seen in the lungs of nonsmokers and when present is generally of low grade. In smokers over 40 years of age, normal lungs are unusual, and heavy smokers have more extensive and severe emphysema than light smokers have. Between 20% and 40% of those who smoke more than a pack per day have emphysema of relatively high grade. In all studies, however, some heavy smokers escape emphysema. This indicates that there are other factors that determine individual susceptibility or that cigarette smoke acts additively with other factors in the environment.

Air pollution is often considered as a cause of emphysema. One study controlled for smoking showed that patients autopsied in a relatively industrialized city, St. Louis, Missouri, had more severe emphysema than patients in Winnepeg, Manitoba, where pollution was less.[429] Comparable studies are few.

There are poorly understood familial influences in COPD. In addition, emphysema is a complication of several rare inherited diseases. One group of diseases directly affects the connective tissues and includes cutis laxa, Marfan's syndrome, and Menke's syndrome. Emphysema is also closely linked to deficiency of the serum protein alpha-1-antitrypsin or alpha-1-protease inhibitor (α_1-PI).[430] Although deficiency of α_1-PI is responsible for only about 1% of cases of emphysema, the recognition of the association has had a pivotal role in shaping the modern theory of the pathogenesis of emphysema.

Alpha-1-protease (α_1-PI) inhibitor deficiency

α_1-PI, or alpha-1-antitrypsin, is a 52-kilodalton plasma glycoprotein that is synthesized mainly in the liver but also by macrophages and a few other cells. In vitro it inhibits a group of proteases with serine at their active site, which includes trypsin, thrombin, plasmin, elastase, and others. The inhibitor is encoded by a gene on chromosome 14 with at least 75 known alleles. The normal allele, designated *M,* is found in 90% of the population. Severe deficiency is rare and is usually associated with homozygosity for an allele designated *Z.* Such individuals have less than 15% of the normal serum concentration of α_1-PI and a high incidence of emphysema and liver disease. The emphysema is panacinar in type with a lower lobe predominance. Respiratory symptoms appear at an earlier age than for most COPD, often by the fifth decade, and they develop 15 years earlier for smokers than for nonsmokers. COPD may develop in as much as 85% of deficient subjects.[430]

The basis for emphysema in α_1-PI deficiency is now well understood. The common (Z type) deficiency is caused by a point mutation that substitutes a lysine for a glutamic acid at position 342 in the α_1-PI molecule.[431] As a result, the mutant protein cannot fold normally. The mutant α_1-PI forms large polymers by a process called loop-sheet polymerization in the endoplasmic reticulum of the hepatocyte.[432] As a result, little inhibitor is processed to the Golgi apparatus or secreted. Some protein accumulates in the endoplasmic reticulum of hepatocytes as periodic acid Schiff-positive globules and some is degraded intracellularly.

The principal target of α_1-PI in vivo is an elastase from the azurophil granules of neutrophils that is capable of producing emphysema in experimental animals. Much evidence indicates that degradation of elastic tissue and other connective tissue proteins by unopposed activity of neutrophil elastase occurs in the lung, either because of chronic low-level release of the enzyme from phagocytes or episodic release during pulmonary inflammation. The degradation of connective tissue triggers the remodeling of lung architecture ultimately producing emphysema.

Emphysema in smokers

Whether an imbalance of proteases and protease inhibitors is involved in the pathogenesis of emphysema in ordinary smokers is less certain. Neither cigarette smoke dosage nor levels of α_1-PI in plasma or of elastase in leukocytes account for the variation in pulmonary function among smokers. It is possible that the mechanism of centrilobular emphysema differs fundamentally from that of the panlobular emphysema of α_1-PI deficiency. Nevertheless, cigarette smoke influences several biochemical and cellular responses that affect the integrity of the elastic fiber network.[433]

Cigarette smoke increases the phagocyte burden in the lung by altering the kinetics of neutrophils margining in the pulmonary capillaries, increasing the number of macrophages in the lung and causing release of chemoattractants from macrophages. Both neutrophils and alveolar macrophages are sources of enzymes capable of degrading extracellular matrix. At least two enzymes from neutrophils and five from macrophages degrade elastin, the connective tissue protein most strongly implicated in emphysema. There are several different protease inhibitors in lung, and at least two of them, both active against neutrophil elastases, are inactivated as inhibitors when oxidized by cigarette smoke.[434]

In animals, destruction of elastic tissue is followed by resynthesis. Cigarette smoke inhibits this repair and increases the severity of the emphysema that results. In humans, there is evidence for the binding of elastase in emphysematous tissue and evidence supporting increased turnover of elastin in some smokers and a greater and more consistent increase in smokers with CAO. Such data support a mechanism wherein tobacco smoke produces emphysema by promoting the release of proteases from inflammatory cells and modifying the defenses that protect the lung from proteolytic damage.

Natural history of chronic airflow obstruction. In normal persons, pulmonary function gradually declines starting around 20 years of age. For the majority of the smokers, including many with cough, phlegm, and even recurrent chest infections, the annual rate of decline is little greater than normal. In a small number of more sensitive smokers, the rate of decline is accelerated, and the accelerated decline can be detected by spirometry by 30 or 40 years of age, well before overt COPD develops. If the smoker stops smoking, the cough may disappear, and the rate of decline in pulmonary function returns to normal, but the lost function is not regained and the ex-smoker functions at a lower level than that predicted for his or her age. With the normal rate of decline, the decrease in ventilatory function does not reach clinical significance even in advanced age. COPD develops only in that sensitive minority of subjects.

By the time symptoms develop, the pathologic process and abnormal decline in pulmonary function have been going on for many years. Survival once symptoms appear is variable but is often for many years. Respiratory failure heralds the terminal phase of the disease, and although many patients survive their first episode of respiratory failure, two thirds will be dead within 2 years.

Hypertrophy and eventual failure of the right ventricle are terminal events in some COPD patients. The major factor that raises pulmonary vascular resistance in CAO and contributes to cor pulmonale is hypoxic vasoconstriction. Hypoxia causes endothelial abnormalities, including impaired synthesis of the vasodilator NO and increased release of the vasoconstricor endothelin. Other contributing factors are restriction of capillary recruitment because of emphysema, increased viscosity of the blood as a result of secondary polycythemia, elevated alveolar pressures that compress the alveolar capillaries during expiration against high airway resistance, and in some patients left ventricular dysfunction.[435]

INORGANIC AND ORGANIC DUST-ASSOCIATED RESPIRATORY DISEASES

The term *pneumoconiosis* was coined by the pathologist Zenker in 1866 to refer to diseases of the lung parenchyma attributable to the inhalation of inorganic mineral dust. Humans are exposed to these minerals in the form of dust particulates during (1) mining and milling (primary exposure); (2) their utilization in construction and manufacturing (secondary exposure); and (3) the renovation and restoration of buildings and the repair or destruction of manufactured products (tertiary exposure)[436] (Table 49-10).

Mineral dusts of health importance are found in several physical forms (Table 49-11) over a range of particle sizes. Although the larger particles usually compose the bulk of a product by weight, the smaller inhalable particles are substantially more numerous and of greater health importance. Aerosolized, relatively large particles are readily cleared and expelled from the nasal cavities and oral pharynx. On the other hand, the fine particles of dust (less than 5 mm in diameter) are those that are inhaled deep into the lungs and reach the

Table 49-10 Common sources of exposure to pathogenic mineral dusts in industrialized countries

Nature of exposure	Asbestos	Silica	Coal	Talc
Primary	Miners and millers of primary product	Miners of other minerals, quarriers of granite	Miners and millers	Miners and millers
Secondary	Shipbuilding, insulation, friction products and textile manufacturers	Sandblasters, stone masons, polishers, potters, Abrasive manufacturers	Firemen, steam plant operators	Pharmaceutical and cosmetic manufacturers
Tertiary	Insulators, construction workers, firefighters	NA	NA	Users of cosmetics

NA, not applicable

Table 49-11 Characteristics of common potentially pathogenic mineral particles

Granular
Silica
Feldspar
Nonfibrous zeolite
Nonfibrous tremolite
Platy
Mica
Talc
Kaolinite
Vermiculite
Mixtures
Slate and shale
China clay
Volcanic ash
Fibrous
Asbestos
Fiberglass
Erionite

acini where disease occurs. Inorganic dust particles differ substantially in toxicity and pathogenicity. Most of the dust particulates to which humans are exposed are believed to be nonpathogenic and are classified as nuisance dusts by governmental agencies. They are primarily irritants in the respiratory tract when inhaled in large amounts. Other dusts are mildly fibrogenic and cause disease only when the exposure is heavy and the clearance mechanisms for the dust in the lungs are overwhelmed (see below). The fine particles of silica and asbestos are the major fibrogenic particles to which humans are exposed (Table 49-12).

Table 49-12 Disease-producing capacity of common pathogenic mineral particulates

Highly fibrogenic
Asbestos (amphibole > chrysotile)
Silicon dioxide (cristobalite > alpha quartz)
Mildly fibrogenic
Talc
Kaolinite and related platy aluminum silicates
Mica
Graphite
Nonfibrogenic particles ("nuisance" dusts)
Titanium dioxide (rutile)
Feldspar and related granular aluminum silicates
Aluminum silicate combustion product (mullite)
Metal particles
Carbon particles

Silicosis

Silicosis (a term derived from the Latin *silex* meaning 'flint') is an inflammatory and fibrotic lung disease caused by the inhalation of crystalline silica.[437,438] The term was first used in 1870 by Visconti, but people have probably suffered from silicosis since prehistoric times. An outbreak of acute silicosis among the Gauley Bridge (West Virginia) tunnelers exposed to high concentrations of aerosolized pure quartz in the 1930s led to the establishment of occupational dust standards in the United States for the first time. Over subsequent decades, the risk of silicosis and its severity in the developed countries of the world has decreased because of governmental regulations, increased general awareness of the hazard by industry, and better dust-control measures in the workplace. The exact prevalence of silicosis worldwide is not known.

Pathogenesis. Silica (silicon dioxide) is most frequently found geologically in the crystalline form known as alpha quartz. There are other much less common crystalline forms (tridymite and cristobalite) that occur naturally in volcanic rocks or form when alpha quartz is heated in industrial processes. These forms are more fibrogenic than alpha quartz. In addition, there are amorphous forms (diatomite and vitreous silica) that are not fibrogenic, though the fibrogenic crystalline forms are created if amorphous silicon dioxide is heated to greater than 1000° C.

The toxicity of silica is not so intense in vivo as might be expected from in vitro tests, probably because the particles in vivo become coated with surfactant lipids and lung fluids.[438] Particle toxicity also is attenuated by extraneous minerals such as feldspar, kaolin, and mica that frequently accompany silica in naturally occurring minerals. Thus exposure to pure silica rarely occurs. Weathered silica particles prove to be less pathogenic than those with freshly fractured surfaces. Particle size is also important. Small particles have greater surface area than larger particles relative to their mass. This enhances the ability of the particle to bind to cell membranes, an event believed to be important in the genesis of the biologic effects that result in lung fibrosis. Silicosis develops in response to inhaled silica particles. The factors that determine whether disease will develop and how severe it will be are not understood completely. Cumulative dose and the duration of exposure play a major role. The admixture of other minerals and coexistence of tuberculosis are important. Genetic factors that determine the individual response must be considered as well.

Workers in many occupations risk exposure to silica. These include mining, quarrying, tunneling, stonemasonry, sandblasting, foundry work, and the manufacture of ceramics, refractories, abrasives, and fillers. The disease silicosis can be categorized in three forms (Table 49-13).

Acute silicosis

Acute silicosis (silicotic alveolar proteinosis, silicoproteinosis) is rare and results from inadvertent, heavy exposure to dust composed of fine particulates of silica. It has been described in sandblasters and workers exposed to the fine dust particles used in abrasive products.[439,440] The pulmonary parenchymal lesions are similar to idiopathic alveolar proteinosis.[441] Post mortem, the lungs are heavy and firm and exude fluid from the cut surface. Nodules are either absent or poorly developed. Microscopically the alveolar spaces are filled by a granular, eosinophilic material that is periodic acid-Schiff reactive and rich in lipid. There are variable amounts of alveolar cell hyperplasia, interstitial inflammation, and fibrosis. Poorly developed silicotic nodules occasionally are present. Accumulation of large quantities of silica dust is demonstrated in the lung parenchyma in analytical studies of lung tissue.

Accelerated silicosis

The term *accelerated silicosis* refers to pulmonary disease developing after periods of heavy exposure to particulate silica

Table 49-13 Clinical forms of silicosis

	Acute	Accelerated	Chronic
Exposure	Heavy	Heavy	Low
Clinical onset	<3 years	5 to 10 years	>20 years
Radiology	Alveolar filling with exudates	Indistinct nodularity	Well-defined nodules
Pathology	Proteinosis	Immature nodules	Classical nodules

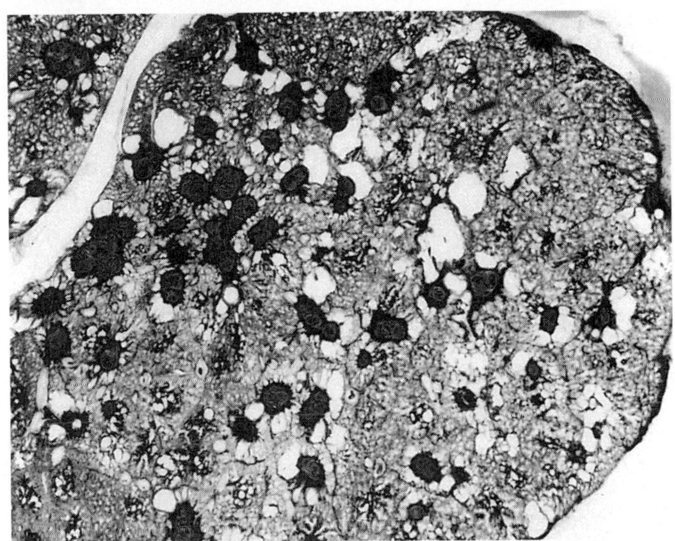

Fig. 49-58 Simple silicosis in a coal worker. The black color of the nodules represents carbon particles that have accumulated at these sites. Notice the absence of a pleural reaction and the upper lobe predominance of the nodules. The nodules are associated with a localized emphysematous process which is termed *scar emphysema.* (From Craighead JE, editor: *Pathology of environmental and occupational disease,* St. Louis, 1995, Mosby)

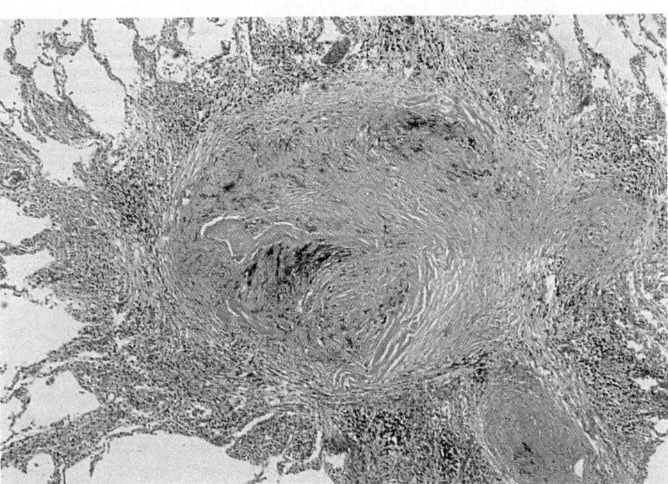

Fig. 49-59 Typical silicotic nodule from a slate worker. Notice the central whorled collagen deposits interspersed with dust. The accumulations of macrophages and small amounts of collagen at the periphery of the nodule represent lesions caused by nonquartz silicate particles and carbon dust.

for roughly 5 to 10 years. The lesions are not well characterized pathologically, but one finds nodules throughout the lung in various stages of development. As a result, the radiograph of the lungs exhibits a diffuse nodular, fibrotic pattern with a predominance of changes in the upper lung lobes.

Chronic silicosis

Chronic (or simple) silicosis is characterized radiographically by multiple rounded nodules that are less than 1 cm in diameter and predominantly located in the upper lobes of the lung (Fig. 49-58). They may be calcifed and heavily pigmented with carbon. Irregular opacities are often present because substantial amounts of silicate mineral particulates often accompany the silica in the inhaled dust. Lesions caused by these silicates develop around the silicotic nodule, resulting in this radiologic picture. "Eggshell" calcification of hilar nodes is a radiologic feature that is highly suggestive of silicosis. Complicated silicosis, by definition, exhibits nodules greater than 1 cm in diameter. They often represent coalescent nodules.

Grossly the lung tissue usually reveals foci of pleural fibrosis to a variable extent and the so-called candle-wax lesions that represent silicotic nodules developing adjacent to lymphatics in the pleura. The hilar lymph nodes are hard, grayish black, whorled, and often calcified. This accounts for the "eggshell" appearance of the nodes in roentgenograms. On cut sections, the lungs show well-demarcated, firm, oval, whorled nodules, particularly in the upper zones. Microscopic examination reveals the classical silicotic nodules with a central whorled, fibrous layered area, an intermediate zone of concentrically arranged collagen fibers, and a peripheral zone composed of dust-laden macrophages and randomly arranged collagen (Fig. 49-59). The central area is variably calcified and hyalinized. Polarization microscopy of the nodule reveals fine, weakly birefringent silica particles in the central zone that can best be seen after the eye is dark adapted by reducing ambient lighting. Typically the brightly birefringent particles in the peripheral zone represent accumulations of silicates of various types. Hilar lymph nodes also contain silicotic nodules, but such nodules can be found even in patients who have no evidence of pulmonary silicosis. Extrapulmonary silicosis has been described also in extrathoracic lymph nodes, liver, spleen, and bone marrow.

Progressive massive fibrosis

Progressive massive fibrosis is manifest as a conglomeration of nodules having a diameter of greater than 1 cm. It develops in a background of silicotic nodules or coal workers' pneumoconiosis (see later section). They usually occur in the upper lung lobes and frequently exhibit areas of avascular necrosis (Fig. 49-60). In the past, *Mycobacterium tuberculosis* infection often was found in these lesions. Although occasionally seen in the elderly, this is primarily of historical interest, for the lesion does not develop when airborne dust exposure is regulated.

Parasilicosis syndromes

There are three clinical entities claimed to be associated with silica exposure: (1) scleroderma,[442,443] (2) rheumatoid arthritis,[444] and (3) glomerulonephritis.[445] The strongest evidence for the link between silica exposure and scleroderma comes from case-control studies[443] where a pattern of consistent, heavy exposure (but not an increased prevalence of radiologic silicosis) was associated with scleroderma among South African gold and coal miners. In another South African case-control study, the rate of progression of silicosis in subjects with active rheumatoid arthritis was greater than in those without arthritis. In addition, the nodules tended to be larger. Occasional case reports have linked silica exposure with the occurrence of glomerulonephritis and renal tubular lesions.

Silica and lung cancer

Epidemiologic and experimental studies of the role of crystalline silica in the development of lung cancer have yielded conflicting evidence.[446,447] A recent review of the literature by a committee of experts resulted in the following conclusions: (1) the published data from in vitro experiments are insufficient to conclude that silica is either genotoxic or carcinogenic; (2) there is evidence of a carcinogenic effect of crystalline silica in rats (but not mice and guinea pigs); and (3) the epidemiologic studies are difficult to interpret because they have not properly accounted for confounding factors such as smoking and exposure to occupational carcinogens.[448] Therefore the evidence still is insufficient to permit conclusions regarding the effect of silica exposure on the development of lung cancer.

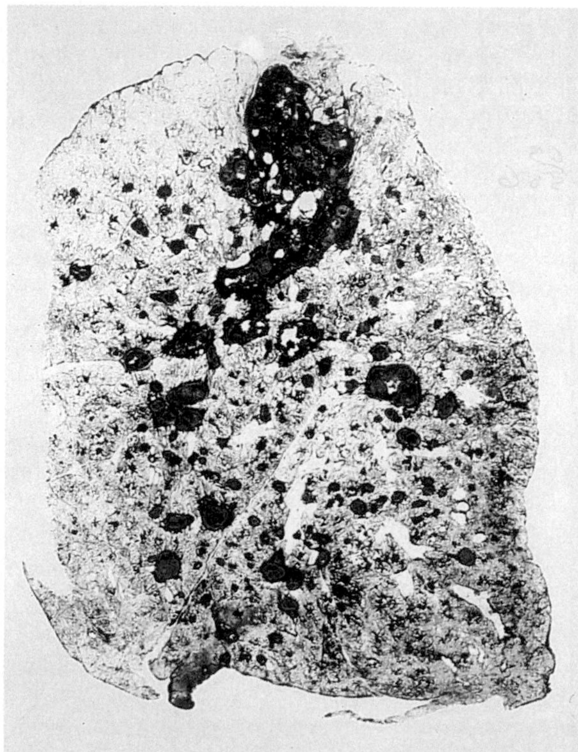

Fig. 49-60 Progressive massive fibrosis in the upper lobes of a coal worker with silicosis. Again, notice the predominance of the lesions in the upper lobes and the absence of pleural thickening. The lung was examined after autopsy by the Gough-Wentworth technique.

Silicatosis

The term *silicatosis* refers to pulmonary disease consequent to the inhalation of dust containing particulates of nonfibrous silicate minerals occurring in the absence of silica dust. Silicate minerals constitute approximately one third of the known mineral species and are ubiquitous. They have widespread commercial importance and a vast range of industrial uses. They also make up a substantial proportion of the ambient dust encountered in the air of urban and rural environments. Included in this group are the platy magnesium silicate talc[449] and the aluminum silicates-mica,[450] kaolin,[450] fuller's earth,[451] feldspars, sepiolite, attapulgite, and woolastonite.[452,453] The major commercial minerals are granular or platy, though some proportion of the particles in some commercial preparations of talc and mica may have a fibrous composition. A few, such as woolastonite, attapulgite, and sepiolite, are fibrous. There have been relatively few systematic studies of the pathologic effects of these minerals per se because exposure is commonly confounded by concomitant exposure to silica or asbestos (or both). Some of the published studies are flawed by inadequate analysis of the mineral in lung tissue. Thus, care must be taken in interpreting the results of epidemiologic studies.

The lesions caused by the various silicates are similar and are described together here.[453] Macroscopically, multiple gray-white stellate lesions are observed at the centers of the lobules, usually in the upper lung lobes. Dust also is present in lesions that develop in the subpleural tissue, the interlobular septa, and in hilar lymph nodes. Palpable nodules ranging in size from a few millimeters to 1 cm in diameter are found less frequently and in an irregular distribution. Progressive massive fibrosis, described rarely, has been associated with heavy, prolonged exposures occurring before the advent of satisfactory dust control. In some cases, there may be diffuse interstitial fibrosis with honeycombing.

Microscopically the earliest lesions are seen adjacent to the bronchi and blood vessels and consist of accumulations of macrophages heavily laden with dust and associated with focal fibrosis (Fig. 49-61). Polarization microscopy reveals highly birefringent particulate material that appears granular, platy, or lancet shaped (Fig. 49-62). As the dust burden of the lungs

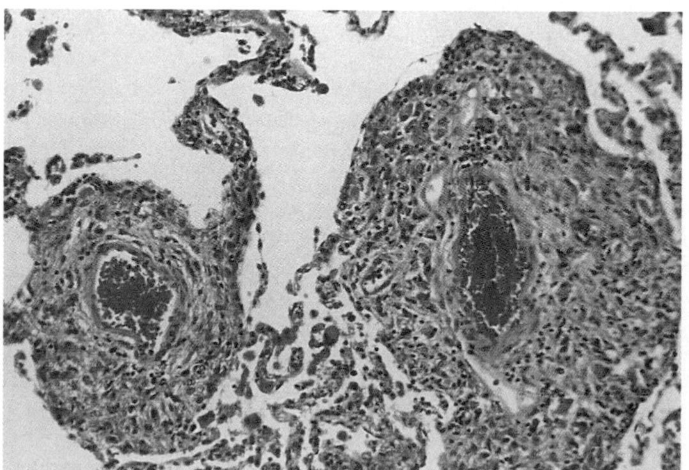

Fig. 49-61 Perivascular fibrosis and chronic inflammation in the lung of a slate worker. Typically the lesions of silicatosis develop adjacent to lymphatics that accompany small blood vessels and bronchi in the lungs. Polarization microscopy usually demonstrates prominent lancet-shaped or granular particulates.

increases, adjacent lesions link, yielding a more diffuse interstitial pattern. In some cases, prominent collections of foreign-body giant cells containing the dust particles are found. These are particularly conspicuous in lesions because of talc or mica. Rarely, sarcoid-like granulomatous lesions have been described. It is unclear what causes this reaction. Pleural thickening has been reported in association with several of the silicate minerals.

Asbestos-associated diseases

Asbestos became important as a commercial mineral in the late 1800s when its value as a fire retardant and insulant was recognized. Asbestosis was first demonstrated at autopsy in 1900. In the mid-1920s, the asbestos body was described. Although the health risks associated with exposure were recognized before World War II, it was generally concluded that asbestos was dangerous only when exposure was exceedingly heavy. During World War II, large amounts of asbestos were used in the construction of naval and merchant marine vessels and a wide variety of war vehicles. After the war, the usefulness of asbestos was recognized industrially, and it was incorporated into consumer products and in insulation of all types. In the 1970s, the health risks of asbestos resulting from occupational exposure during and after the war became evident. Since that time, asbestos utilization has plummeted as governments have promulgated increasingly restrictive regulations, and litigation by those alleging injury has grown.

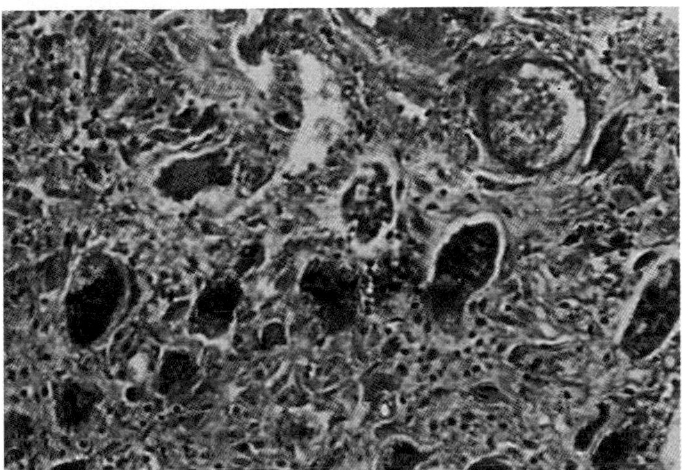

Fig. 49-62 Talcosis. Notice the accumulation of the irregular, plate-like and lancet-shaped particles of talc demonstrated by polarization microscopy in the illustration at right. Many of the particulates are found within the multinucleate giant cells, which are characteristic of talcosis. Despite the dense accumulations of particulates, the amount of collagen deposition is relatively modest in comparison to silicosis or asbestosis. This tissue section was prepared from the lung of a talc miner, accounting for the crudeness of the particles. Individuals who are exposed to talc of a cosmetic or pharmaceutical grade by inhalation or intravenous use exhibit smaller granular particulates of this platy mineral.

The term *asbestos* refers to a family of minerals comprising two subfamilies, the amphiboles and serpentines (Fig. 49-63). The commercial amphibole asbestos types are extracted from the earth in South Africa and, to a more limited extent, in Bolivia and Australia. These fibers are rigid, long, and straight. They differ dramatically from the serpentine fibers as represented by the mineral chrysotile. These latter fibers are variable in length and breadth, and are pliable. They exhibit a curly or wavy configuration. Over 95% of the asbestos used throughout the world today is of the chrysotile type. Noncommercial amphiboles in low concentrations contaminate certain seams of chrysotile.

Chrysotile is mined in localized deposits in many parts of the world, with the Russian Federation and Canada being the major producers. The ore undergoes a rigorous process of purification to eliminate contaminants before marketing. The biologic effects of the amphibole and serpentine types of asbestos differ. The latter material is generally believed to be less pathogenic than the former, most probably because it breaks down over time and is not retained in the lung tissue. In contrast, amphiboles persist in the lungs indefinitely.

Pleural disease

Four forms of disease of the pleural cavity develop in asbestos-exposed individuals. They differ in clinical impor-

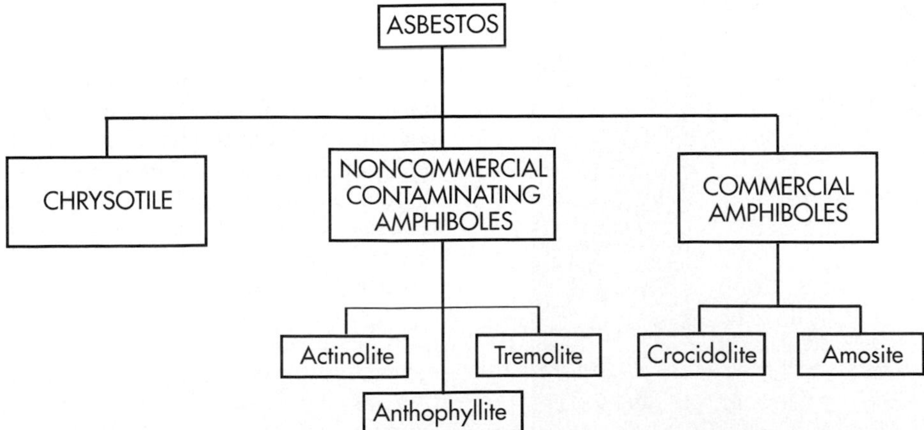

Fig. 49-63 Diagram of the different types of commercial and noncommercial asbestos. Chrysotile is the most commonly used mineral, whereas the amphiboles, crocidolite and amosite, are of historical importance, since they are no longer imported for commerce into the United States, and Western Europe. Yet the amphiboles are responsible for a substantial proportion of mesotheliomas that have occurred in the United States and Western Europe during the last several decades. Noncommercial amphiboles contaminate some seams of chrysotile asbestos. Anthophyllite was formerly mined in Finland, but it is no longer of commercial importance.

tance and often occur in the absence of pulmonary parenchymal lesions (asbestosis).

Pleural plaques

Circumscribed plaques composed of dense fibrous tissue commonly develop on the parietal pleural surface and diaphragms of individuals exposed to asbestos of all types (Fig. 49-64). In certain geographic areas (Finland and Central Europe), plaques are common in the general population in the absence of an association with commercial asbestos exposure. The plaque appears to be the most sensitive clinical marker of asbestos exposure and is found in 1% to 2% of males in routine autopsy series in the United States and in a substantially larger proportion of the population in heavily industrialized regions of Europe and in Canada. Plaques develop over the lifetime of the asbestos-exposed individuals. Their temporal evolution is difficult to define inasmuch as they are detected by radiologic means during life, a measure that is imprecise. At autopsy, the plaques are located in the intercostal spaces, particularly in the lateral aspects of the chest cavity and on the dome of the diaphragm. On gross examination, they exhibit the appearance of ivory and the consistency of leather and have well-delineated margins with irregular bosselations on the surface. Microscopically they are composed of dense, avascular, collagenous tissue, but at the margin of plaques, small blood vessels, and variable numbers of mature lymphocytes accumulate. The plaques are situated on a base of loose connective tissue and adipose on the parietal pleural surface.

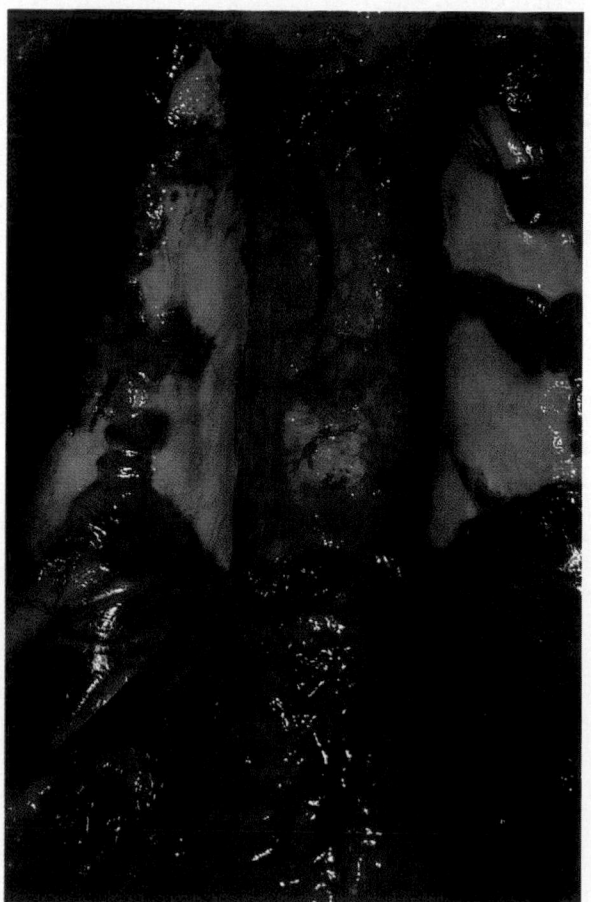

Fig. 49-64 Pleural plaques covering the parietal pleura.

Attempts to isolate asbestos fibers and asbestos bodies from plaques are not always successful, but in the hands of some investigators, small numbers of particulates have been recovered.

Visceral pleural thickening

Diffuse thickening of the visceral pleural surface is observed in some individuals exposed occupationally to asbestos. Frequently, this pleural lesion develops in association with asbestosis, but it can be observed in individuals who exhibit no fibrotic pulmonary lung disease. Pleural fibrosis can contribute to the development of restrictive pulmonary functional disease.

In comparison to parietal pleural plaques, visceral pleural thickening is an inconsistent finding among those exposed to asbestos. The pathogenesis is obscure, but we envision the response to be consequent to the accumulation of asbestos fibers in or subjacent to the pleura. At this location, asbestos might be expected to provoke an inflammatory reaction associated with the generation of growth factors and cytokines by macrophages, which stimulate fibroblastic activity.

Pleural effusions

To a variable extent, individuals heavily exposed to asbestos occasionally develop benign effusions in the pleural cavity 5 to 20 years after their initial exposure. The effusions persist for variable periods of time and often fail to reoccur if the fluid is removed by thoracentesis. The pathogenesis of the asbestos-associated pleural effusions is uncertain, but it would be reasonable to assume that they develop as a consequence of asbestos injury to pleural tissue, since they often occur in those with visceral pleural fibrosis.

Malignant mesothelioma

One of the most serious outcomes of asbestos exposure is mesothelioma, an invariably fatal tumor that usually develops in the pleural cavity, though not unknown in the peritoneum or pericardium of asbestos-exposed individuals.[454] Roughly 20% to 40% of mesotheliomas are not associated with asbestos exposure and are of unknown cause.[455-457] The remaining tumors almost invariably develop in individuals exposed to the commercial amphibole asbestos types, crocidolite and amosite, but an occasional lesion may be caused by a fibrous form of amphibole known as tremolite.[458] This last asbestos type occurs as a contaminant of chrysotile,[459] talc,[460] and vermiculite.[461] Experimental studies strongly indicate that the long, thin fibers of amphibole asbestos that lodge in the pleural lining of the chest are responsible for the development of the disease, but the exact pathogenesis of malignant mesothelioma remains obscure. The latency period of malignant mesothelioma is almost invariably longer than 20 years and, on the average, somewhat over 30 years in duration.[462]

Massive effusions are the principal clinical sign of malignant mesotheliomas. These effusions that harbor malignant cells are recurrent and appear to be caused by the elaboration of a vascular leakage factor by the tumor cells. At the time of surgical exploration, the neoplastic process is widespread in the body cavities (Fig. 49-65). The tumor invests and surrounds the major organs, but customarily it only superficially invades their external surfaces. This indicates that the lesion develops over an extended period of time before it becomes clinically evident. After diagnosis, the majority of patients

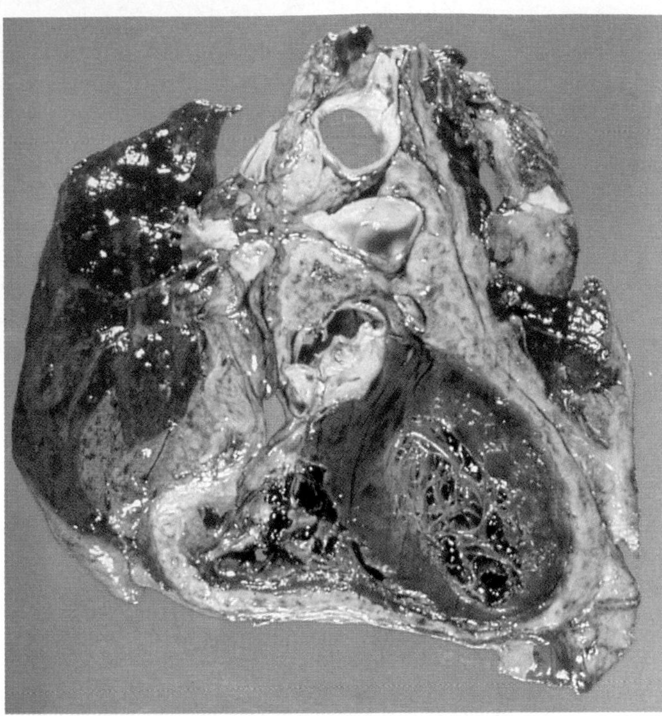

Fig. 49-65 Mesothelioma involving the mediastinum and pericardium. This lesion originated in one of the pleural cavities but manifests many of its pathologic effects by its involvement and encroachment upon the heart.

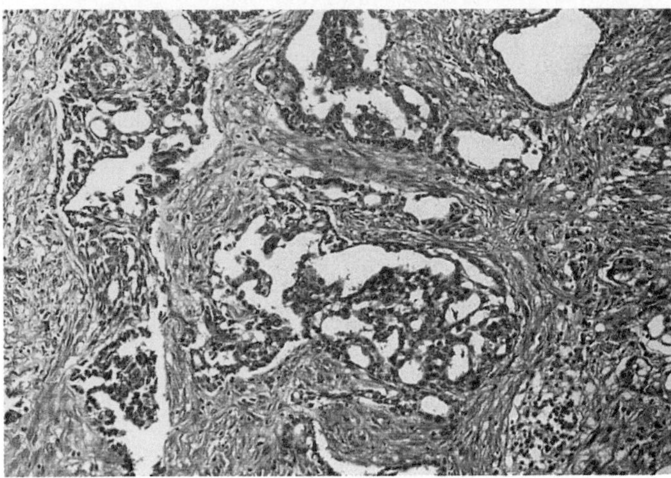

Fig. 49-66 Glandulopapillary epithelial malignant mesothelioma. Notice the dense collagenous tissue, some of which is formed by the tumor cells.

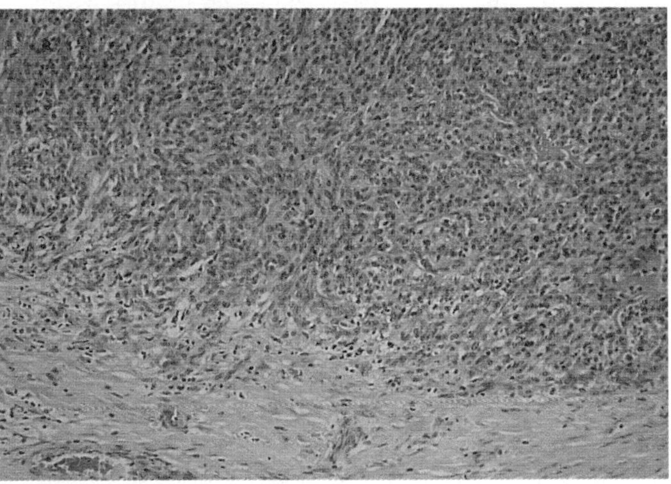

Fig. 49-67 Fibrosarcomatous mesothelioma extending into an area of dense collagenous tissue deposition. Notice the spindle cells which are characteristic of these lesions. The demonstration of cytokeratins within the cytoplasm of these fibroblastoid-like tumor cells is helpful in the diagnosis of malignant mesothelioma. The dense band of connective tissue adjacent to the accumulations of tumor cells is typical of these tumors.

succumb within a 12-month period, and over 85% are dead before the end of the second year.[456,457] The disease is invariably fatal; at autopsy, metastases are commonly found in the mediastinum, the opposite chest, and abdominal cavity and in the liver, adrenals, and vertebral bodies. Aggressive chemotherapy and radiation therapy, as well as surgery, have failed to influence dramatically the outcome of the disease.

Malignant mesotheliomas exhibit a wide variety of morphologic patterns[463] (Figs. 49-66 and 46-67). A substantial proportion of the tumors are epithelial in nature; these lesions range in appearance from sheets of malignant mesothelial cells exhibiting a monotonous pattern to complex glandulopapillary cancers that resemble adenocarcinomas.[464] It is the latter pattern that often puts the pathologist into a diagnostic quandary. A minority of malignant mesotheliomas exhibit a sarcomatous pattern, and in this regard, simulate fibrosarcoma.[457] Rarely the tumors exhibit myxomatous morphology or osteoid formation in patterns that simulate sarcomas of these differentiated types. The most common histologic pattern of malignant mesothelioma is the so-called biphasic lesion, comprising a mixture of morphologic types, the proportions of which vary among microscopic fields. These lesions can be confused with carcinosarcomas, synovial cell sarcoma, spindle-cell variants of melanoma, and renal cell carcinoma. Accumulations of stromal elements often are prominent in mesotheliomas; in some the stroma is dense collagen, but in others it exhibits a hyaline or cartilaginous appearance. The factors influencing the variable morphologic expressions of this tumor are not known, but it does not appear to represent clonal expansion of different morphologic entities.

Because mesotheliomas simulate adenocarcinomas on the one hand and sarcomas on the other, pathologists may require histochemical or immunohistochemical stains to assist the diagnosis. In tumor tissue fixed in the absence of water, hyaluronic acid can be demonstrated in the cytoplasm of cells and in the lumen of glands using either an Alcian blue stain at low pH or the colloidal iron stain. This approach, however, usually is not useful, since most tumors are fixed in formalin. Immunohistochemistry may be useful, since both epithelial and sarcomatous mesotheliomas contain keratin, which is often demonstrable in form of perinuclear cytoplasmic dots or aggregates. No mesothelioma-specific immunoreagents are available, but a battery of staining could be informative and could sway one to decide whether a tumor is a mesothelioma or an adenocarcinoma.[465-467] For example, mesotheliomas usually but not invariably lack carcinoembryonic antigen and neutral mucin. Electron microscopy is also useful, especially in tumors composed of cells that exhibit on their surface (Fig. 49-68) and prominent aggregates of cytoplasmic tonofilaments.[468] The cells of malignant mesotheliomas often exhibit only modest degrees of pleomorphism, a feature that makes the cytologic diagnosis of the tumor difficult. However, some tumors demonstrate considerable pleomorphism and the presence of tumor giant cells.

Asbestosis

Asbestosis in its classical form is a diffuse fibrotic disease process of the lung consequent to exposure to asbestos of all types over extended periods of time.[469,470] The disease is rare today because of the almost universal introduction of regulations in developed countries that limit the concentrations of asbestos in the air of the workplace.

Typically the fibrotic changes of asbestosis are focal and are most prominent in the lower lung lobes. Variable degrees of visceral pleural fibrosis is also usually present. Although severe asbestosis does not pose diagnostic problems for the pathologist when the disease is localized and of minimal severity, considerable difficulty may be experienced in differentiating it from other forms of pulmonary fibrosis. The presence of asbestos bodies in or adjacent to the walls of fibrotic respiratory bronchioles is the hallmark of the disease (Fig. 49-69). Their presence in the lung tissue in small numbers is not sufficient for the diagnosis of asbestosis but is only a marker of exposure.

Asbestos bodies exhibit a variety of morphologic forms but have, as their common characteristic, a core of asbestos, which is coated by ferroprotein (Fig. 49-70). Almost invariably, this core is an amphibole fiber; only rarely does chrysotile form asbestos bodies. The mechanism whereby asbestos bodies develop is obscure, but they seem to be formed by macrophages that attempt to phagocytize long fibers of asbestos in the lungs. Asbestos bodies are mimicked when ferruginous accumulations develop on other types of foreign material in the lung. These structures, commonly known as "ferruginous bodies," are formed on particles of talc, graphite, mica, fiberglass, and other less common material in the lung. In contrast to true asbestos bodies, which are clear, the core of these particles is dark. Asbestos bodies represent only a portion of the asbestos fiber burden of the lung. The remainder of the fibers in the lung tissue are uncoated and are demonstrable only by ultrastructural means after digestion of the lung parenchyma. Attempts have been made to relate quantitatively the number of asbestos fibers and bodies in digests of lung tissue with the presence of fibrotic disease. Because some forms of asbestos break down and are eliminated from the lungs after inhalation and because there appear to be differences in host reactivity, a wide range of asbestos fiber concentrations have been found in association with fibrotic disease attributable to asbestos. Thus the pathologist cannot rely solely on asbestos fiber or body counts to establish the diagnosis.

The pathogenesis of asbestosis has been illuminated by numerous experimental studies during the past decade. The disease develops initially in the region of the respiratory bronchioles where inhaled asbestos fibers typically deposit. These foreign particles initiate an inflammatory response composed of macrophages and polymorphonuclear leukocytes. The

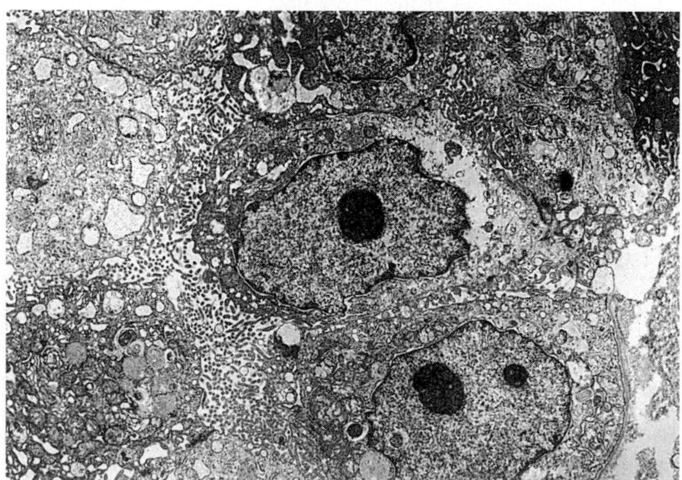

Fig. 49-68 Electron micrograph of an epithelial mesothelioma, demonstrating the complex, thin surface microvilli that characterize these tumors. Electron microscopy is a sensitive means for establishing the diagnosis of mesothelioma, since microvilli of this type are not seen in adenocarcinomas and sarcomas.

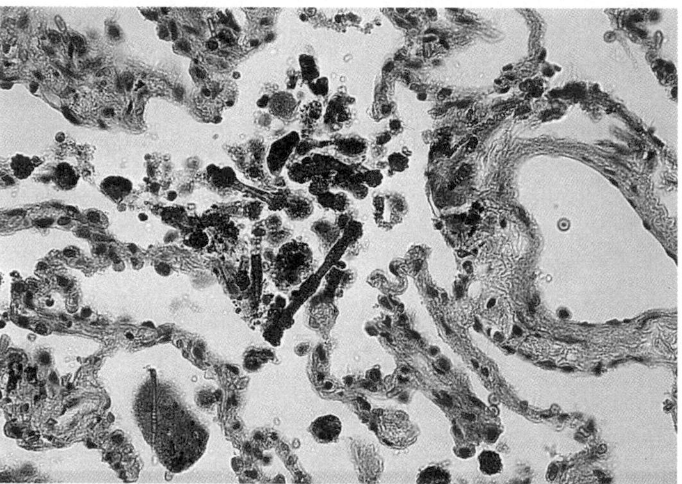

Fig. 49-69 Asbestosis. Asbestos bodies are found in the air spaces.

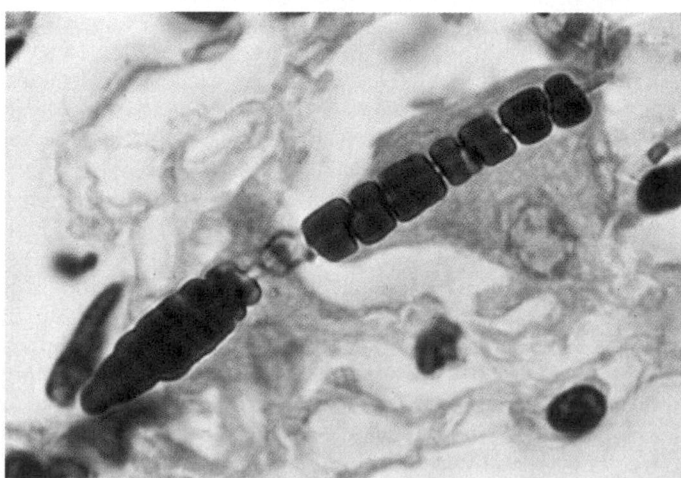

Fig. 49-70 Asbestos body.

inflammatory cells then generate oxygen free radicals and proteases, which have the potential to damage the lung parenchyma. When exposure to asbestos is light, these elements are neutralized by naturally occurring antioxidants such as superoxide dismutase and catalase, as well as other antioxidants and antiproteases in the tissue. Heavy asbestos exposure, however, overwhelms these lung defense mechanisms and scarring develops. Growth factors elaborated by the macrophages appear to contribute to the development of fibrosis. These events, occurring in multiple respiratory units, ultimately evolve to the point of diffuse fibrosis accompanied by respiratory insufficiency and are associated with linear and irregular densities when the lung tissue is examined radiologically. Concomitantly a proportion of the asbestos fibers develop into asbestos bodies where they mark the fibrous tissue by their presence. It is the microscopical finding of scarring in the acinus intimately associated with asbestos bodies that serves as the key diagnostic criterion of asbestosis. With continued exposure, confluent areas of fibrosis develop, ultimately resulting in the "honeycombing" that is so characteristic of advanced fibrotic pulmonary disease.

Asbestos-related lung cancer

Epidemiologic studies demonstrate an increased prevalence of bronchogenic carcinoma occurring among individuals exposed to asbestos who smoke.[471] Although this observation doubtlessly is correct, the effect of asbestos most probably is only manifest when and if the exposure is of sufficient duration and intensity to result in asbestosis. The latency period for asbestos-related lung cancer is said to be shorter than the latency of tumors related to tobacco smoke. In the absence of asbestosis, the prevalence of bronchogenic carcinoma is no higher than that in the general population of cigarette smokers. An epidemiologic association of bronchogenic carcinoma with the presence of pleural plaques has not been documented.

Several decades ago, the literature suggested that adenocarcinomas were found with increased prevalence in the asbestos-exposed individual. Although this may in fact be the case among those with severe asbestosis, recent studies have failed to demonstrate an association of a specific morphologic type of cancer with asbestos exposure. Unfortunately, these investigations have not critically analyzed the degrees of fibrosis in relation to tumor histologic type.

Epidemiologic evidence indicating that asbestos is an initiator of cancer (that is, a complete carcinogen) in the airways is limited. Rather, in the smoker it appears to act as a promoter substance, enhancing the carcinogenic effects of cigarette smoke. In doing so, it shortens the latency period for the development of the tumor or increases the likelihood that cancer will occur.[472-475]

Coal workers' pneumoconiosis

Coal workers' pneumoconiosis (CWP) is defined as "fibrosis of the lungs due to exposure to coal dust.[476] Pneumoconiosis has been associated with coal mining since the 1880s. In the early part of this century, it was believed to be caused by exposure to quartz, but studies of Welsh coal trimmers, whose job was to load ships with coal and who had no exposure to quartz, demonstrated that inhalation of coal dust alone can result in a pneumoconiosis. A similar disease occurs in those exposed to other carbonaceous dusts such as carbon black and graphite. The term *simple CWP* refers to lung disease in which the lesions are less than 1 cm in diameter, whereas *complicated CWP,* or *progressive massive fibrosis,* applies to lesions that are larger.[436] As a result of improved dust control measures in the coal mines of Western Europe and the United States, there has been a dramatic decrease in the prevalence of CWP in these areas. It is now rare to find CWP in miners under 50 years if age.

Pathogenesis. Coal is a general term referring to a complex group of minerals that are rich in carbon. Coal contains many organic materials (benzenes, phenols, naphthalenes, and polycyclic aromatic hydrocarbons) in addition to carbon. The major inorganic mineral components of coal are clays (such as kaolinite, muscovite and illite), sulfides, and chlorides. Common trace elements include arsenic, lead, manganese, and titanium. Because coal seams often are thin or variable in depth, miners often are exposed to silica and silicate dusts from the adjacent rock deposits.

The formation of coal occurs through a continuous transformation of plant material that results in an increase in hardness and the content of carbon with time. The oldest coal (anthracite) has the highest content of carbon, the greatest calorific value, and the lowest percentage of quartz, ash, and volatile matter. The youngest coal (lignite) has the lowest carbon content, the least calorific value, the highest percentage of quartz and ash, and greater than 30% volatile matter. Bituminous coal is intermediate in age between anthracite and lignite. In the industry, coals are classified by "rank." Anthracite coal is accorded a high rank and lignite a low rank.

The profusion of small radiologic opacities in simple CWP correlates with the cumulative lifetime exposure to respirable coal dust.[436] The density of opacities, in turn, correlates with the concentration of dust retained within the lung tissues. However, the risk of developing simple CWP varies from mine to mine despite similar degrees of dust exposure.[477] The risk of developing CWP is greatest in collieries mining high-rank coals. In this regard, it is interesting to note that the in vitro cytotoxicity of dusts has been shown to increase with the geologic age and rank of the coal.

The role of quartz in coal mine dusts and the development of CWP has been extensively researched with inconsistent findings. As stated above, the risk of CWP increases with coal rank, whereas the quartz content tends to decrease. However, coal workers who are exposed to dusts with high quartz content develop radiologic changes with unusual rapidity, and there is an increased risk of progressive massive fibrosis.[478-480]

Pathology. In CWP the external surfaces of the lungs show increased black pigmentation, but pleural thickening usually is not conspicuous (Fig. 49-71). The hilar lymph nodes often are enlarged and appear homogeneously black, though sometimes they are grayish black, with whorled nodules resembling silicotic nodules, even when there is no evidence of silicosis in the lung parenchyma. Simple CWP is characterized by the presence of numerous small, focal, impalpable, stellate, black lesions termed *macules,* or *primary dust foci* (Fig. 49-72). They are distributed throughout the lung, though there is a preponderance in the upper lobes of the lung. The lesions range in diameter from about 1 to 5 mm. They are often associated with dilated air spaces measuring 1 to 3 mm across, the so-called focal emphysema.[481,482] Nodules (secondary dust foci), which are most commonly observed on a background of macules, are less consistently present and usually few in number (Fig. 49-73). They are firm, palpable, stellate, or round. The smaller

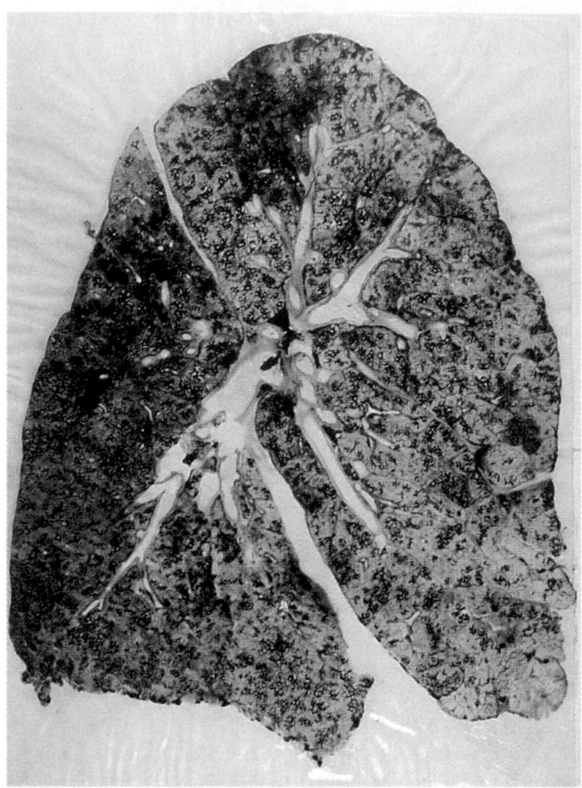

Fig. 49-71 Coal workers' pneumoconiosis. The lungs show increased black pigmentation.

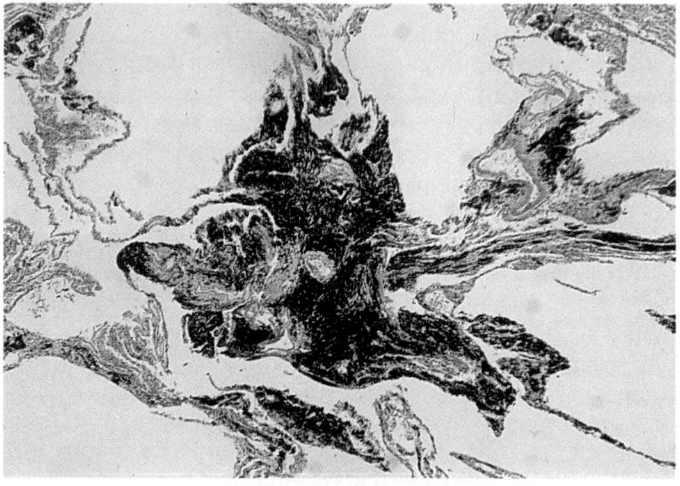

Fig. 49-72 A macule associated with scar emphysema. The lesions are nondescript but represent the accumulation of carbon particles associated with modest deposits of collagen.

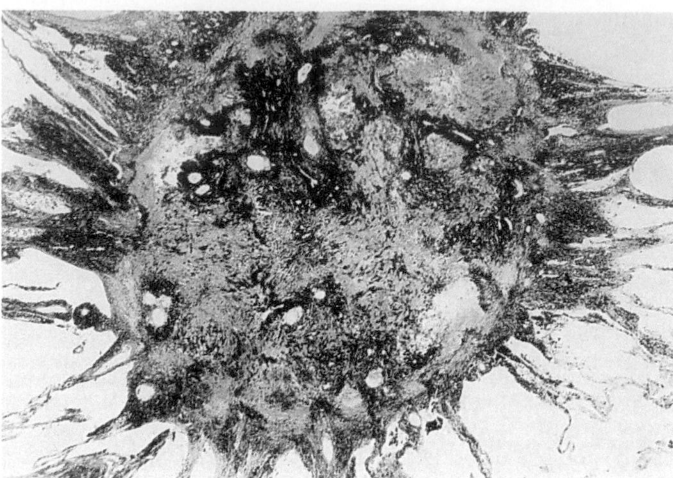

Fig. 49-73 A nodule in the lung of a coal miner. The nodules are a prominent and advanced feature of coal workers' pneumoconiosis and may on occasion represent the consolidation of several macules.

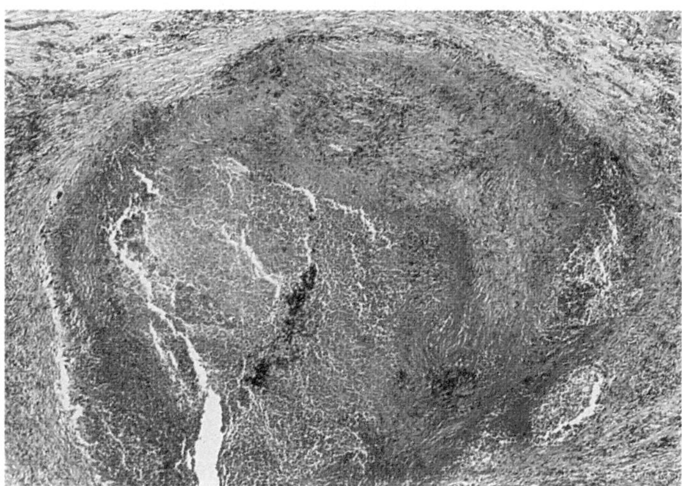

Fig. 49-74 Caplan's lesion in the lung of a coal miner. These lesions exhibit certain features of the rheumatoid nodule, specifically the palisading of fibroblasts at the margin and the central necrosis associated with dust deposits.

nodules frequently are uniformly pigmented, but those greater than 3 mm in diameter usually possess central fibrotic areas that contain relatively little dust.

In 1953, Caplan observed that the prevalence of complicated CWP was greater in Welsh coal miners with rheumatoid arthritis than in those without. In about one fourth of these cases, there were unusual rounded opacities on chest roentgenograms.[483] In 1955, Gough and colleagues[484] described the pathology of these lesions. They usually are large, circumscribed nodules that may be discrete or confluent and occur on a background of simple CWP (Fig. 49-74). When fully developed, they show concentric, alternating gray and black bands. Microscopically the center of the lesions is necrotic, with a variable amount of cellular debris, cavitation, and calcification. At the margin of this zone, there is a narrow rim of neutrophils and nuclear debris, which, in turn, is usually surrounded by a palisaded layer of histiocytes. A zone of collagen, lymphocytes, and plasma cells (which, in areas, cuff small blood vessels) surrounds this layer. The lesions have been reported much less frequently in the United States than in Europe.

Interstitial fibrosis occurring in coal workers has received little attention, yet there is evidence that it is more common in this group than one would expect.[485] Autopsy studies of coal workers from Wales and West Virginia demonstrate a prevalence of about 16% to 18%. Additional studies are required to establish why and under what conditions coal dust exposures result in interstitial fibrosis.

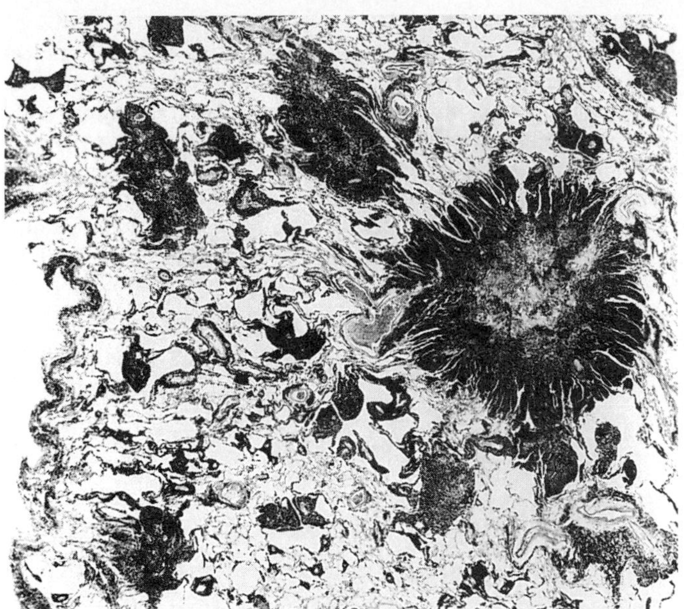

Fig. 49-75 A mixed-dust lesion illustrating the "Medusa head" appearance of the typical scar. The central portion of the lesion represents dense collagenous tissue encompassing silica particles. These lesions develop as a result of exposure to a mixture of environmental dusts. (From Craighead JE, editor: *Pathology of environmental and occupational disease*, St. Louis, 1995, Mosby.)

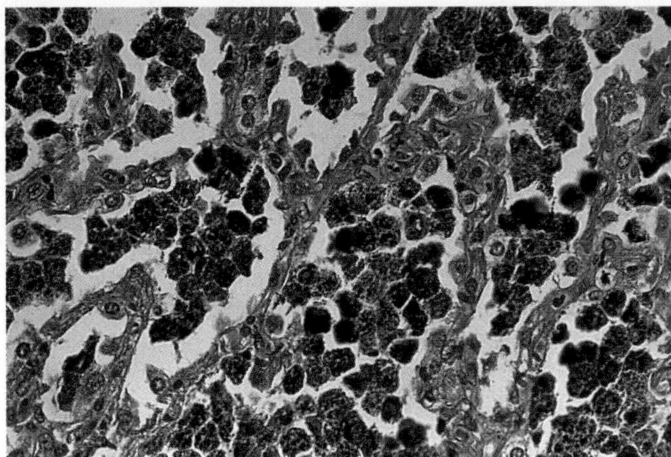

Fig. 49-76 Siderosis. There are dense accumulations of iron-containing macrophages in the lung of this iron ore miner.

Mixed-dust fibrosis

The term *mixed-dust fibrosis* usually is applied to pneumoconiotic lesions occurring in workers exposed to silica concomitantly with significant amounts of less fibrogenic dusts such as iron, silicates, and carbon.[486] Examples include (1) foundry workers, welders, and hematite workers in whom there is exposure to silica and iron, (2) slate workers exposed to silica and mica, (3) shale miners and china stone and ceramic workers exposed to silica and kaolinite, and (4) coal workers who may be exposed to silica in addition to coal dust (Fig. 49-75).

The lesions are characterized microscopically by a stellate shape with the collagen and reticulin fibers arranged linearly rather than concentrically. This yields an irregular configuration to the lesions in radiography. The centers of the lesions show a variable amount of fibrosis and hyalinization. Large numbers of dust-laden macrophages are present. The distinction from silicosis is somewhat arbitrary, since it is not unusual to see typical silicotic nodules in other areas of the same lung. Polarization microscopy often reveals a mixture of particle types.

Siderosis

Siderosis applies to the deposition of iron oxides in the lung without significant exposure to other minerals.[487] It is seen in arc welders, silver polishers, iron and steel workers, and miners of iron-containing ores such as ochre.[486] Since iron oxide is either not or only very weakly fibrogenic, loss of lung function does not occur. However, multiple small densities may be observed in the chest roentgenogram.

Grossly the lungs exhibit macules that are red, reddish brown, or grayish black, depending on the amounts of iron and carbon present. Microscopically, centrilobular collections of dust-laden macrophages predominate with little fibrosis being evident (Fig. 49-76). Numerous nonfibrous ferruginous bodies having round or irregularly shaped black cores are present.

Welding

Welders are exposed to a wide variety of substances including oxides of iron, zinc, cadmium, beryllium, chromium, and nickel and gases such as oxides of nitrogen, ozone, and isocyanates. The exposure depends on the composition of the electrodes used for welding, the flux, and the composition of the base metal and its coating. Welders also can be exposed to silica influx and asbestos as bystanders.

A diversity of pathologic lesions have been described in the lungs of welders, including siderosis, mixed-dust fibrotic lesions, bronchiolitis, lung cancer, and mesothelioma.[487] However, it remains a matter of debate as to whether welding fumes per se cause pulmonary disease. The term *welders' lung* therefore is inappropriate, since structural pulmonary changes in the welder, if they occur at all, are not specific. On the other hand, the lungs of arc welders frequently exhibit accumulations of tiny, dense, spherical bodies, the so-called welders' bodies.

Metal-induced lung diseases

The effects of metals on the human lung have been poorly studied. There have been numerous case reports associating certain metals with various types of pathologic reactions, but the exposures and pathologic reactions are poorly documented. A selected few are briefly discussed below.

Hard metal disease

Hard metal disease develops sporadically in workers employed in industries in which synthetic hard metal bits are manufactured or used in the cutting and fabrication of metal parts and equipment.[488,489] It also has been reported in diamond polishers.[490] Since only a small proportion of those potentially exposed are affected and because symptoms often are variable and ill defined, the prevalence of the condition is unknown. Hard metal disease is believed to develop as a result of the inhalation of cobalt salts that are employed in fusing fine particles of tungsten, tantalum, and titanium into the hard metal bits and diamond-polishing disks used in a wide variety of industries. The disease often but not invariably first becomes evident within days or weeks of the time of initial exposure.[491] In some, it is expressed as a dermatitis and, in others, as chronic bronchitis. However, its most profound manifestation is diffuse interstitial pulmonary fibrosis associated with restrictive pulmonary functional abnormalities. Microscopically the pulmonary lesions exhibit variable degrees of interstitial fibrosis and mononuclear inflammation accompanied by the accumulation of variable numbers of multinucleate cells in air spaces.[492] These cells appear to form from those lining air spaces and pulmonary alveolar macrophages, which are found in large numbers (Fig. 49-77). Fine opaque granules that are believed to be hard metal particles are scattered within the cytoplasm of these cells.[493] Many, if not all the cases of giant cell pneumonia (GCP) originally described by Liebow may represent examples of this disease.

The mechanism whereby the disease develops is unknown, but it would appear to be based on hypersensitivity that is reflected in only a few of the many exposed workers. With the general recognition of the hazards posed by hard metal dust, industrial controls have substantially reduced the number of cases that occur.

Berylliosis

The inhalation of a variety of beryllium-containing materials in particulate aerosolized form results in pulmonary granulomatous disease in a small proportion of those exposed.[494] Beryllium metal is widely used in industrial products and has found recent application in the atomic energy and space programs. Because the toxicity of beryllium is now widely appreciated, the disease occurs only rarely. Yet, because a diversity of industries use products containing beryllium oxides or salts, effective control by regulation is difficult.

The lesions of berylliosis are histologically indistinguishable from those of sarcoidosis (Fig. 49-78). In contrast to sarcoidosis, which is a systemic disease, berylliosis is limited to lung and the skin at sites of local inoculation. Since morphologic and analytical techniques for differentiating the two disease conditions are not available, the patient's employment history is critical to establishing the diagnosis.

Chromium

Excessive rates of lung and nasal cancer have been found in workers exposed to hexavalent but not trivalent chromium compounds, such as chromate production workers and chromium platers.[495,496] The risk increased with the severity and duration of exposure. No specific histologic type of lung cancer has been associated with exposure to chromium compounds. The carcinogenicity of chromium and nickel compounds is of interest because they may be present in the polluted air of urban areas.

Nickel

An increased rate of lung and nasal cancer has been found in workers in the refining, smelting, and mining industries.[497,498] The pathogenesis is not understood, and there is still debate as to which nickel compounds are carcinogenic to humans.

Organic dust disease

Pulmonary diseases caused by exposure to organic dust can result entirely from allergic or toxic mechanisms or both. The diseases attributable to hypersensitivty to organic dusts are described elsewhere.

Humidifier fever

Humidifiers and air conditioners contaminated by microorganisms have been associated with both hypersensitivity pneumonitis and a syndrome called "humidifier fever."[499] It is characterized by fever and sweat, headache, malaise, cough, and dyspnea that commences in the worker 4 to 8 hours after exposure. Unlike hypersensitivity pneumonitis, resolution of the symptoms usually occurs within 24 to 48 hours even in the presence of continuing exposure. The pathogenesis and pathology of the disease are unknown.

Acute organic dust toxic syndrome

Originally called *mycotoxicosis,* this term now describes a complex of acute symptoms (including chills, malaise, myalgia, dry cough, breathlessness, headache, and nausea) occurring a few hours after a heavy exposure to organic dust. For example, it has been described after exposure to moldy hay, grain, straw, and silage. It differs from hypersensitivity pneu-

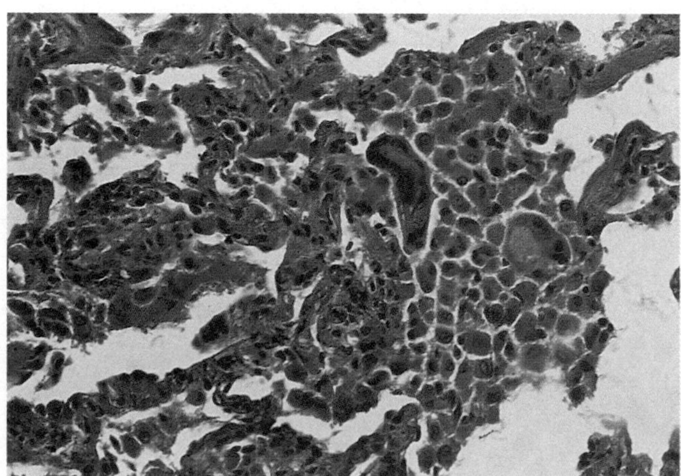

Fig. 49-77 Hard metal disease. Notice the accumulations of macrophages and multinucleate cells. Lesions of this type exhibit variable degrees of interstitial fibrosis.

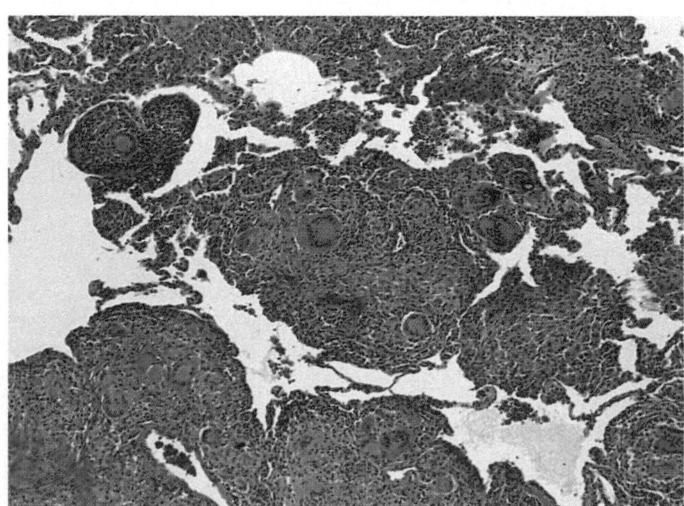

Fig. 49-78 Berylliosis. The lung contains numerous noncaseating granulomas.

monitis in that prior sensitization is not required and the chest roentgenagram fails to exhibit infiltrates. Complete recovery usually occurs in 2 to 3 days.[500]

PULMONARY NEOPLASMS

Tumors of the lungs can be classified clinically, histogenetically, or pathologically into several categories.[501-505] *Clinically* the tumors may be symptomatic or asymptomatic, benign or malignant. Most of those diagnosed clinically are malignant. *Histogenetically* the tumors may be classified according to their provenience, as originating from the bronchi, bronchioli, pulmonary connective tissue and blood vessels, or pleura. *Pathologic* classification may be based on microscopic or microscopic features. On the basis of location the tumors may be classified as central or peripheral, localized or diffuse, solitary or multiple. Most current histologic classifications are based on the second edition of the World Health Organization Histologic Typing of Lung Tumors (Table 49-14).[506-507]

Epidemiology. Lung cancer is at the present time the most common fatal malignancy in men and women in the United States. The age-adjusted death rate attributable to lung cancer in men increased 121%, from 33.4 per 100,000 in 1956 to 1958 to 73.7 per 100,000 in 1986 to 1988, and in 1990 increased to 75.6 per 100,000. Lung cancer death rates in women increased by 425%, from 5.4 per 100,000 in 1956 to 1958 to 28.2 per 100,000 in 1986, and in 1990 continued to increase to 31.7 per 100,000. Current estimates predict over 150,000 new cases per year and over 140,000 deaths from lung cancer per year during this decade.[508] The incidence of lung cancer in younger men has leveled off in the last decade, and a slight decrease has been noted in younger men, which probably related to the antismoking campaign.[509] However, the incidence of lung cancer seems to be on the increase in Asia and many other parts of the world, and currently death caused by lung cancer is the leading cause of neoplasia-related mortality worldwide.[503]

Lung cancer has a peak incidence in the group 50 to 70 years of age, and only 3% to 8% of all patients are younger than 40 years.[507,508]

Etiology. Irrespective of the age, more than 90% of all patients registered worldwide are smokers. This implies that smoking is the major cause of lung cancer.[510] The genetic predisposition[511] could play a significant modifying role, but the hereditary determinants of pulmonary carcinogenesis are not fully understood. Other environmental factors could adversely influence the carcinogenicity of tobacco smoke. Among those, the best known are asbestos[471] and radon,[512] which have a multiplicative effect. Other environmental and industrial carcinogens are less important. Cancer among uranium miners[513] has been well documented. Several other heavy metals such as nickel, copper, beryllium, chromium, and arsenic have also been implicated as possible pulmonary carcinogens.[436,503]

The role of viruses in the pathogenesis of lung cancer has not been studied adequately. Yousem and colleagues[514] found human papillomavirus DNA in 30% of squamous cell carcinomas but also in the adjacent metaplastic bronchial epithelium, an indication that this virus could have a pathogenetic role. The role of oncogenes and tumor-suppressor genes is currently under investigation.[515-519] The most promising leads point to p53, K-*ras*, *bcl*-2 and *N-myc*, but the current evidence is far from conclusive. The relationship between the action of oncogenes and chromosomal changes that commonly occur in lung cancer[520] is also under study.

Clinical features. The clinical assessment of patients with lung cancer must take into consideration the size and location of the tumor, the extent of spread, the histologic characteristics of the tumor, and the presence or absence of other diseases, infections, and systemic symptoms attributable to the tumor. The age of the patient is also important, since lung cancer is rare under 40 years of age. Pulmonary tumors in children are biologically and clinically distinct from those in adults.[521]

The clinical and radiologic findings at the time of diagnosis are used for staging of lung tumors, which provide the most important prognostic information and is essential for the planning of treatment. The staging is best done using the interna-

Table 49-14 Abbreviated WHO histologic classification of primary lung tumors

I. Epithelial tumors
  A. Benign tumors
    1. Papillomas
    2. Adenomas
      a. Pleomorphic adenoma
      b. Monomorphic adenoma
  B. Dysplasia/carcinoma in situ
  C. Malignant tumors
    1. Squamous cell carcinoma (epidermoid carcinoma)
    2. Small cell carcinoma
      a. Oat cell carcinoma
      b. Intermediate cell type
      c. Combined oat cell carcinoma
    3. Adenocarcinomas
      a. Acinar adenocarcinoma
      b. Papillary adenocarcinoma
      c. Bronchioloalveolar carcinoma
      d. Solid carcinoma with mucus formation
    4. Large cell carcinoma
      variants:
      a. Giant cell carcinoma
      b. Clear cell carcinoma
    5. Adenosquamous carcinoma
    6. Carcinoid tumor
    7. Bronchial gland carcinomas
      a. Adenoid cystic carcinoma
      b. Mucoepidermoid carcinoma
    8. Others
II. Soft tissue tumors primary in the lung
III. Pleural tumors
  A. Benign mesothelioma
  B. Malignant mesothelioma
IV. Miscellaneous tumors
  A. Benign tumors
  B. Malignant tumors
    1. Carcinosarcoma
    2. Pulmonary blastoma
    3. Malignant melanoma
    4. Malignant lymphoma
    5. Others
V. Unclassified tumors
VI. Tumorlike lesions

Modified from Colby TV, Koss MN, Travis WD: Tumors of the lower respiratory tract. *Atlas of tumor pathology,* series 3, fasc. 13, Washington, D.C., 1995, Armed Forces Institute of Pathology; and The World Health Organization Histological Typing of Lung Tumors, *Am J Clin Pathol* 77:123-126, 1982.

tional TNM system, as outlined by Mountain.[522] Histologic data are also important, but in most instances it suffices to know whether the tumor is a cell carcinoma or some other malignancy. Small cell carcinomas require chemotherapy and are not treated surgically in contrast to non-small cell lung carcinomas (NSCLC), which are treated according to other protocols.[523]

Local and systemic symptoms of most lung cancers are related to the mass effect of the tumor. Local symptoms include coughing, hemoptysis, dyspnea, and chest pain. Systemic symptoms include weight loss, cachexia, and pain attributable to metastases. Lung cancer is often associated with paraneoplastic syndromes caused by ectopic production of polypeptide hormones.[524] Small cell carcinomas secrete most often antidiuretic hormone and ACTH, whereas squamous cell carcinomas produce most often parathyroid hormone-related peptide.

Lung cancer has a poor prognosis. The survival depends on the clinical stage and the histologic type of tumor, and although some tumors have a better prognosis than others, the overall 5-year survival is 5% to 10%.

Benign epithelial tumors

Benign tumors are rare. Such tumors can originate from several pulmonary cells and are thus localized either in the central or peripheral part of the lungs. *Squamous papillomas* typically arise in the larger bronchi and are most often found in children.[505] Papillomas may be multiple, and in such cases they are often associated with laryngeal papillomatosis. *Alveolar adenomas* are peripheral cystic tumors composed of epithelial cells resembling normal alveolar cells lying on delicate fibrous septa.[525] *Mucinous cystadenomas*[526,527] may be located centrally or peripherally. Some mucinous cystic tumors may be of borderline malignancy.[528]

Bronchial glands can give rise to benign and malignant tumors, which resemble those arising from salivary glands.[529] Pulmonary *myoepitheliomas* are probably of the same origin.[530] Some pleomorphic adenomas of the salivary gland type are located in the peripheral parts of the lungs.[531]

Carcinoma of the lung

Most of the malignant tumors of the lower respiratory tract are called *bronchogenic carcinomas* because they originate from the epithelium of bronchi (Fig. 49-79). They result from the malignant transformation of bronchial stem cells or their immediate descendants and are therefore composed of cells that are normally found in the bronchial epithelium. Tumors composed of ciliated or mucous cells are classified as adenocarcinomas; those composed of neuroendocrine cells, as small cell carcinomas; whereas those that are not committed or do not show such differentiation are classified as large cell carcinomas. Squamous cell carcinomas do not have a corresponding cell type in the bronchial epithelium. These tumors originate from foci of squamous metaplasia that are common in smokers. Malignant tumors evolve through a preinvasive stage *(carcinoma in situ)* resembling the incipient carcinoma of the vulva, cervix, or the oral mucosa.

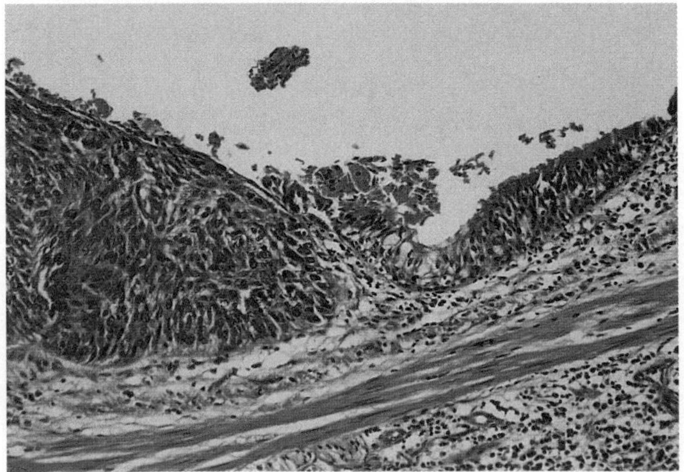

Fig. 49-79 Carcinoma of the bronchus. Histologic focus of early carcinoma.

The diagnosis of lung tumors may be made on tissue specimens obtained by bronchial or open surgical and transthoracic biopsy. Diagnosis may be established cytologically by examination of the sputum, bronchial brushings, bronchialoalveolar lavage specimens, or fine-needle aspirates. Experienced pathologists will usually agree whether a tumor is a small cell carcinoma or a NSCLC, but there is less agreement on the subclassification of tumors belonging to the latter group.[507] Approximately 20% to 30% of lung cancers are small cell carcinomas.[502,503] In the NSCLC group squamous cell carcinomas and adenocarcinomas predominate and are represented in approximately equal ratios, which vary from one study to another in the range from 20% to 35%.

Squamous cell carcinoma

Approximately 20% to 35% of all lung tumors are squamous cell carcinomas. Two thirds of squamous carcinomas are central tumors, involving the main or lobar bronchi (Fig. 49-80), whereas one third arise in the lung periphery, either in small bronchi or in association with scars.[532] However, in some patients with large bronchi involved at the time of diagnosis, serial roentgenographic observations indicate that the tumor actually arose in a more peripheral location and grew to involve the central bronchi late in its course. Bronchial involvement may take the form of a warty endobronchial protrusion, or the tumor may ulcerate the bronchus and grow outward. If the tumor obstructs a large bronchus, the lung distal to the tumor will often be the site of obstructive pneumonia and bronchiectasis.

The gross appearance of most squamous carcinomas is not distinctive, but large, well-differentiated tumors may have

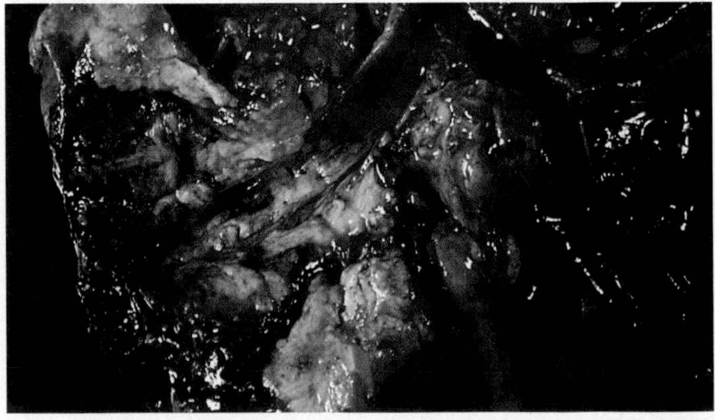

Fig. 49-80 Squamous cell carcinoma. This hilar tumor originates from the main bronchus.

shiny caseous yellow foci that correspond to heavily keratinized tumor tissue. The expectoration of keratinous or necrotic material may produce cavities within the tumor. Indeed, the majority of cavitary lung carcinomas are of the squamous cell type.

The microscopic diagnosis of squamous carcinoma depends on the identification of either intercellular bridges or keratinization. Keratinized cells can be recognized in sections by their brightly eosinophilic cytoplasm and pyknotic nuclei. Squamous carcinomas of the lung tend to be poorly differentiated and often vary from one area to another. Typically they are composed of nests of cells that palisade at the periphery of the lobules and become enlarged and flattened centrally. Whorls or eddies of cells may be keratinized (epidermoid pearls); the whole center of the lobule may be filled with keratin, or at the other extreme only a few single cells may be keratinized.

Although most squamous cell carcinomas have at least some areas of large cells with plentiful cytoplasm, some tumors are composed of spindle cells or consist only of relatively small basophilic cells resembling those of basal cell carcinoma in the skin.[533] The distinction from small cell carcinoma is difficult in such cases. Electron microscopy may be helpful since the cells of squamous carcinoma contain tonofilaments and are joined with adjacent cells by desmosomes on short projections of cytoplasm. These tumor cells contain neither neuroendocrine granules nor mucin.

Adenocarcinoma

Adenocarcinomas account for approximately one third of all lung tumors. Previously, adenocarcinoma was the most common form of lung tumors in women. Although adenocarcinoma is the most common type of bronchogenic carcinoma in nonsmokers, most patients with adenocarcinoma are smokers.

Most of adenocarcinomas arise in the periphery of the lung[534,535] (Fig. 49-81). Some tumors arise in scars, though recent investigations indicate that the fibrosis associated with some adenocarcinomas is stroma laid down in the tumor rather than preexisting scar. Adjacent alveoli often contain hyperplastic or atypical alveolar cells indicative of a "field effect" of carcinogenesis. Some of these atypical cells could represent precursor lesions that have not progressed to cancer.[536] Many tumors, especially of the bronchioloalveolar type, are multiclonal.[537] Such tumors typically infiltrate the lungs diffusely and on cross section of lung parenchyma may appear as pneumonia with abscesses (Fig. 49-82) or miliary tuberculosis.

Adenocarcinoma appears as discrete masses, usually at the lung periphery, where they often cause retraction of the overlying pleura. The borders of the tumor may be smooth, or stellate protrusions may extend into the surrounding lung. Irregular pigmentation of the tumor is not unusual, since inhaled dust and soot are not easily cleared from areas of tumor and the lymphatics are often obstructed.

Microscopically, adenocarcinomas are highly variable in appearance. According to the WHO classification, four histologic subtypes are recognized: (1) acinic or glandular, (2) papillary, (3) bronchioloalveolar, and (4) solid adenocarcinoma.

Other subtypes of adenocarcinoma have also been described, some of which could represent variants of these subtypes, whereas others are probably of bronchial gland origin.[538]

Among the subtypes of pulmonary adenocarcinoma, bronchioloalveolar carcinomas have been studied most extensively.[537] This cancer has a tendency to spread through the lungs along the existing air-space walls, which serve as the stroma for the tumor (Fig. 49-83). The walls of alveoli, alveolar ducts, and to a variable extent bronchioles are lined by malignant epithelial cells that vary in shape from cuboidal to columnar. The alveolar walls over which the tumor cells spread may be normal or may be thickened by fibrosis. When they are thickened, an abrupt transition to normal thickness usually occurs precisely where the neoplastic epithelium ends, an indication that the thickening is a reaction to the tumor rather than preexisting fibrosis. The malignant epithelium may be highly atypical or closely resemble normal bronchiolar or alveolar lining cells. Some bronchioloalveolar carcinomas are

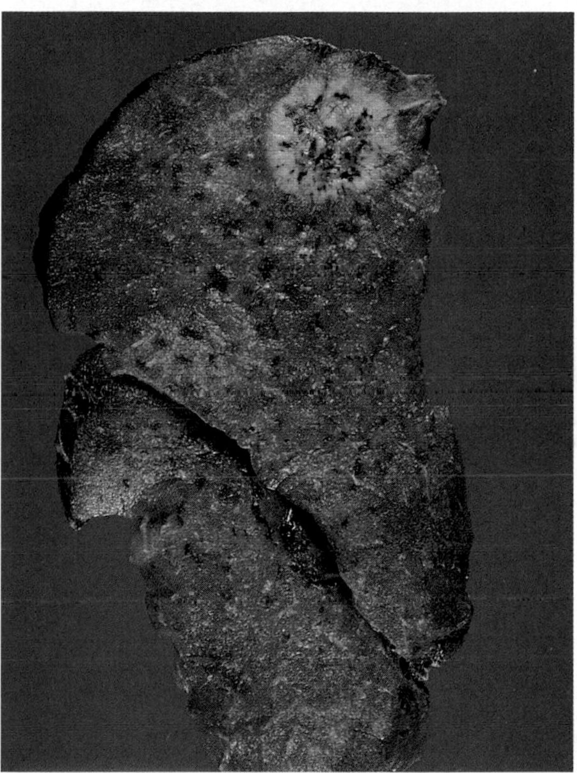

Fig. 49-81 Peripheral adenocarcinoma. The tumor shows prominent black pigmentation, suggestive of its having evolved in anthracotic scar.

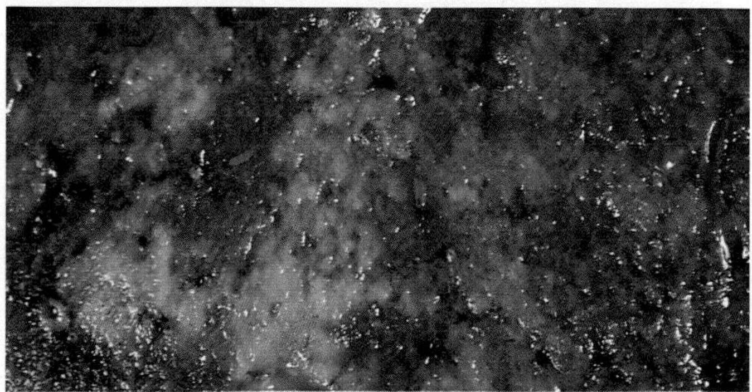

Fig. 49-82 Bronchioloalveolar carcinoma. The tumor infiltrates diffusely the lung parenchyma. There is no grossly visible dominant tumor mass, and the lesion may be confused with pneumonia.

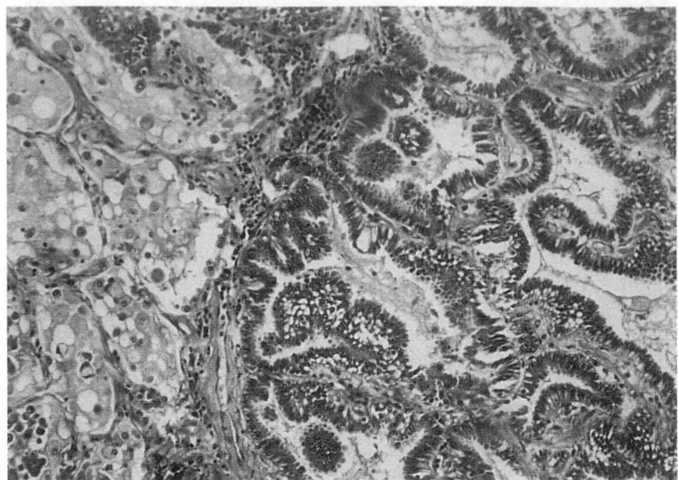

Fig. 49-83 Bronchioloalveolar tumor. The tumor cells grow along the existing alveolar septa. The alveolar spaces are filled with mucin.

composed of tall mucin-producing cells that fill the involved air spaces with mucus.

Electron microscopic studies of bronchioloalveolar carcinomas have shown differentiation along several lines. Tumors with ultrastructural features of type II alveolar epithelial cells have been described, and the cells of some tumors have been shown to contain the antigens of the protein portion (apoprotein) of alveolar surfactant. Other tumors are composed mainly of cells with granules like those of Clara cells or cells filled with mucin.

Metastatic adenocarcinomas found in the lungs may mimic primary lung adenocarcinoma and often it is not possible to determine whether a tumor is a primary tumor or a metastasis. Epithelial mesotheliomas have also many features in common with adenocarcinomas of the lung. Concurrent adenocarcinoma and mesothelioma has been reported, but such coincidence is rare.[539]

The prognosis of adenocarcinomas is unfavorable. Attempts to predict the outcome by grading the tumors have not been successful. Newer studies indicate that the invasiveness of the tumor, as assessed by immunohistochemical analysis, could provide valuable predictive information.[540,541]

Large cell undifferentiated carcinoma

Large cell undifferentiated carcinoma is a diagnosis by default.[542,543] Approximately 7% and 15% of carcinomas of the lung are composed of relatively large cells (greater than 12 μm in diameter) that lack specific features by which they could be assigned to either the squamous or the adenocarcinoma group. The tumors vary in microscopic appearance from lobules of well-formed epithelium lacking evidence of gland formation, secretion, or keratin to anaplastic tumors formed of poorly cohesive cells scarcely recognizable as epithelium. These tumors are considered undifferentiated, but if electron microscopy or other special techniques are used, the majority of such tumors show some evidence of differentiation, indicating that they are really poorly differentiated variants of adenocarcinoma, squamous cell carcinoma, combined adenosquamous carcinoma, or neuroendocrine carcinoma.

Large cell undifferentiated carcinomas arise either at the lung periphery or centrally. They grow rapidly and are usually large tumors by the time of diagnosis.

The WHO classification[506] recognizes two variants of large cell carcinoma. *Giant cell carcinoma* is a highly malignant form of undifferentiated carcinoma composed of huge, poorly cohesive cells with eosinophilic cytoplasm and one or several large convoluted nuclei. The tumors are often infiltrated with polymorphonuclear leukocytes, and collections of neutrophils appear within the cytoplasm of the tumor cells as if phagocytosed. *Clear cell carcinomas* are composed of cells with clear cytoplasm that is rich in glycogen.

Adenosquamous carcinoma

By light microscopy 1% to 3% of lung carcinomas have clear evidence of both keratinization and glandular or secretory differentiation. Most are peripheral tumors associated with scars. Adenosquamous carcinomas should be distinguished from mucoepidermoid carcinoma of the mucous glands located in the large bronchi.

Small cell carcinoma

Small cell carcinomas account for 15% to 20% of lung carcinomas.[544-549] On gross examination they appear as fleshy encephaloid tumors (Fig. 49-84) forming nodules or infiltrating and destroying the wall of a major bronchus. Hilar and mediastinal lymph node involvement is usually extensive in untreated patients and is often more conspicuous than the primary tumor. Microscopically several patterns are recognized.[544,545] The oat cell type consists of round or elongated poorly cohesive cells 10 to 12 μm in length or slightly larger than lymphocytes. The tumor cells have dark clumped chromatin and little recognizable cytoplasm. Nucleoli are absent or inconspicuous. Necrosis is usually present and is widespread in larger tumors (Fig. 49-85). Blood vessels in necrotic areas become encrusted with DNA, staining blue with hematoxylin in routine sections. The pattern of tumor growth is diffuse but with some division into lobules by vessels and stroma, which helps to distinguish oat cell carcinoma from lymphoma. The intermediate cell type of small cell carcinoma is composed of cells slightly larger than those of the oat cell type and with somewhat better intercellular cohesion and organization into lobules. Some tumors are composed of large or spindle-shaped cells.[547] Most tumors contain ribbons of cells or pseudorosettes closely associated with vessels, making their endocrine origin easy to recognize.[546,547]

By electron microscopy, 70% to 80% of small cell carcinomas contain small secretory granules of neuroendocrine

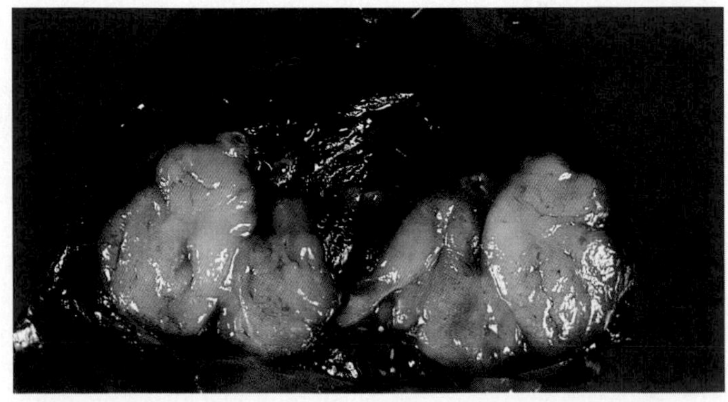

Fig. 49-84 Small cell carcinoma. The tumor forms confluent nodules. On cross sectioning the nodules have an encephaloid appearance.

type.[548,549] The characteristic granules are membrane bound, with an electron-lucent "halo" between the membrane and the dense granule matrix (Fig. 49-86). The granules are not present in every cell, and sometimes extensive search is required to find them. Immunohistochemical analysis is helpful for diagnosis, since many small cell carcinomas contain peptides such as bombesin, ACTH, or synaptophysin. Cytokeratin is usually present as well.

Spread of bronchogenic carcinoma

Carcinoma of the lung can invade contiguous structures directly and metastasize by the lymphatics and bloodstream. Lymphatic metastasis usually takes place in the hilar lymph nodes initially with spread to contiguous groups leading to mediastinal, cervical, and para-aortic involvement. When pleural adhesions are present, spread to the lymphatic plexus of the parietal pleura can lead to the appearance of tumor in axillary or supraclavicular nodes.

The brain, liver, bone, and adrenal glands are the most common sites of hematogenous dissemination. Adrenal involvement may also develop by lymphatic connections across the diaphragm. With small cell carcinoma, bone marrow involvement is common even in the absence of overt bone destruction; therefore, bone scanning and marrow aspiration are useful as staging procedures.

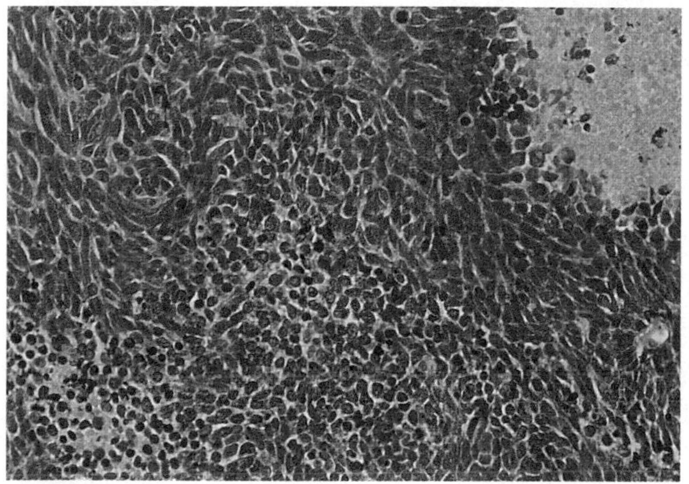

Fig. 49-85 Small cell carcinoma. The small blue cells appear elongated or round depending on the plane of sectioning. The tumor shows prominent necrosis.

Carcinoids

Bronchial carcinoids are tumors of low-grade malignancy with neuroendocrine differentiation.[550] They tend to occur at a younger age than bronchogenic carcinomas, often appearing below 40 years of age and sometimes in childhood. Bronchial carcinoids are not related to cigarette smoking and have an equal sex incidence. The majority of carcinoids arise in central bronchi (Fig. 49-87) where they form a smooth-surfaced endobronchial polypoid growth. However, the major portion of the tumor lies outside the bronchial wall, the so-called iceberg pattern of growth. The tumor tissue often has a yellow-tan color, especially after fixation with formaldehyde. Microscopically carcinoids are formed of uniform cells with a fairly abundant, finely granular cytoplasm and oval, centrally located nuclei with clumped chromatin (Fig. 49-88). These cells form ribbons, trabeculae, or nests and are usually grouped around capillaries. The stroma is usually scant but may be plentiful and may contain hyalinized connective tissue or more rarely amyloid or bone. Mitoses are rare, and necrosis is usually absent.

Twenty percent of carcinoids arise in small bronchi or bronchioles and occur as peripheral lung nodules. Often the peripheral carcinoids are composed of spindle-shaped cells

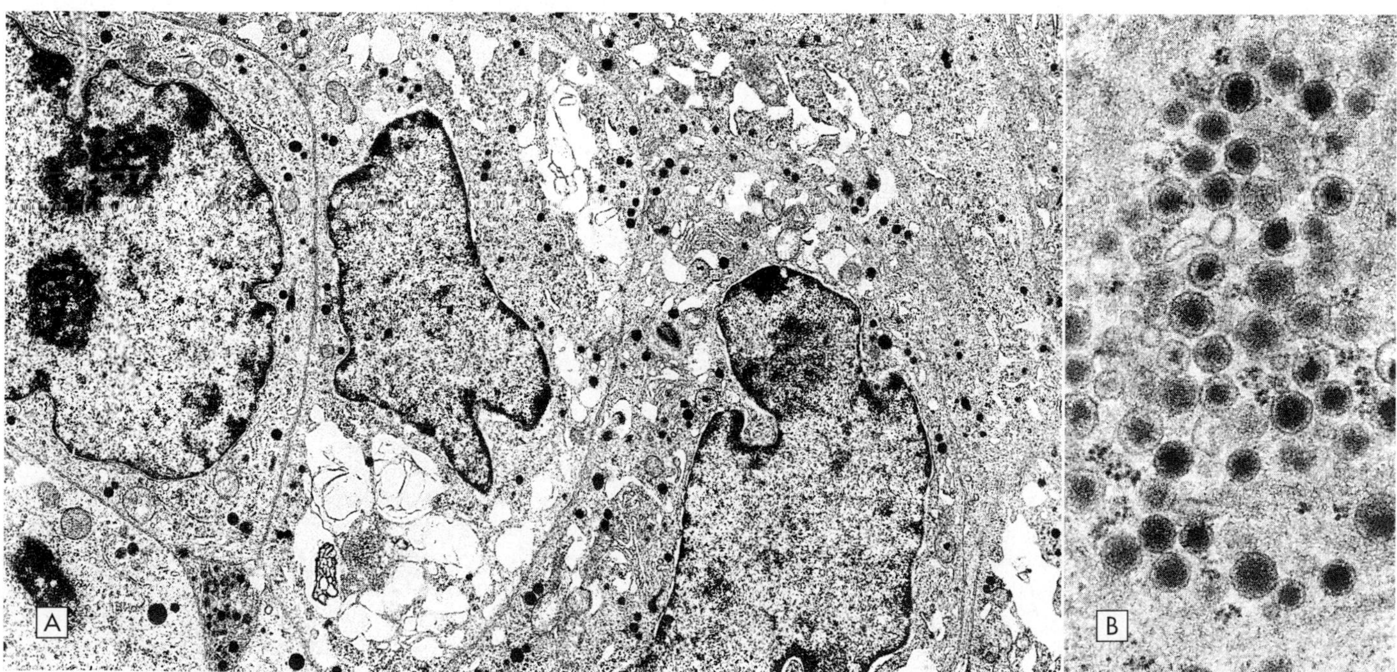

Fig. 49-86 Electron microscopy of a small cell carcinoma. **A,** The tumor cells have elongated nuclei and contain dense granules in their cytoplasm. **B,** Detail at higher magnification shows neuroendocrine granules. The granules have a central dense core separated from the limiting membrane by a clear halo.

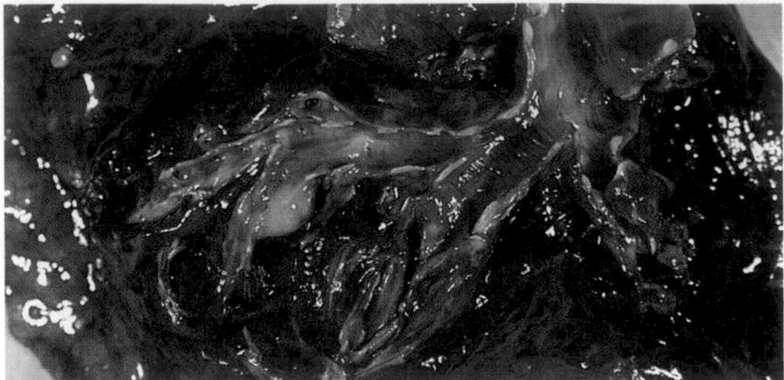

Fig. 49-87 Carcinoid. The tumor presented as a small nodule attached to the bronchus.

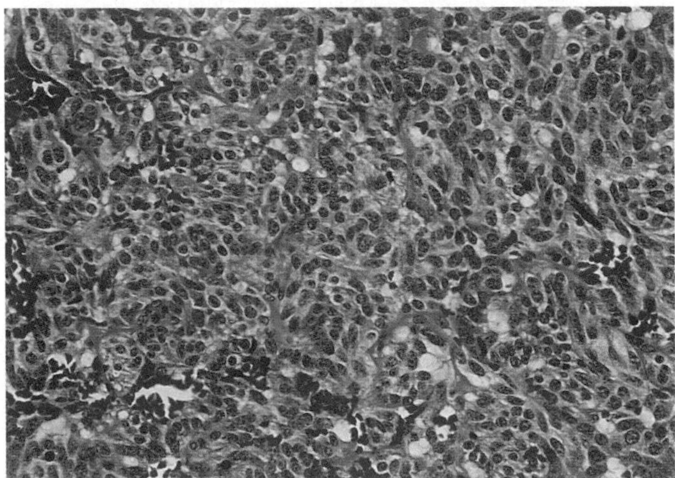

Fig. 49-88 Carcinoid tumor. The tumor is composed of uniform cells that have round nuclei.

with little cytoplasm. Such tumors can be mistaken for small cell carcinoma but are distinguishable by the uniformity of the cells and the absence of necrosis or mitosis.

The secretory granules of bronchial carcinoids resemble those of other foregut carcinoids. They do not reduce silver in the argentaffin reaction and stain only erratically with argyrophil stains in which the reducing agent is added. Electron microscopy, however, consistently shows abundant, electron-dense, spherical granules with an average diameter of 200 nm. The carcinoids contain neuropeptide hormones (Table 49-15). The prognosis for bronchial carcinoids is in stark contrast to that of small cell carcinoma: 90% of treated patients survive 10 years after operation.

A small number of tumors combine an architectural pattern similar to the usual carcinoid with greater cytologic atypism and more mitotic activity or necrosis. Such tumors are known as atypical carcinoids or well-differentiated neuroendocrine carcinomas. They express the same immunohistochemical markers as ordinary carcinoids but more often contain ectopic peptide hormones. Their behavior is more aggressive than that of ordinary carcinoids but less than that of small cell carcinoma.

Mesenchymal tumors

Mesenchymal tumors of the lungs are rare. These tumors have the same histologic features as their counterparts in the soft tissues. Such tumors may be benign[551-553] or malignant.[554,555]

Table 49-15 Expression of neuroendocrine markers in lung carcinoids

Marker	Percentage of cases positive
Neuron-specific enolase	88
Chromogranin A	86
Bombesin	67
Serotonin	65
Leu-enkephalin	32
Somatostatin	25
Calcitonin	9
Vasoactive intestinal polypeptide	24
Beta–human chorionic gonadotropin (β-hCG)	36
Met-enkephalin	18
Adrenocorticotropic hormone (ACTH)	13
Pancreatic polypeptide	20
Substance P	20
Gastrin	13

Modified from Mackay B, Lukeman JM, Ordóñez NG: *Tumors of the lung,* Philadelphia, 1991, Saunders

Sarcomas grow as bulky masses (Fig. 49-89) and invade into the surrounding organs. Such tumors have poor prognosis. Malignant tumors must be differentiated from metastatic sarcomas, which tend to metastasize to lungs. The diagnosis of primary pulmonary sarcoma should be made only if there is no evidence that the lung lesion is a metastasis.

Mixed epithelial-mesenchymal tumors

According to the WHO classification, *carcinosarcoma* is defined as a malignant tumor with an admixture of carcinoma and sarcoma, growing as a polypoid structure in a large bronchus.[506] The same term and several closely related names, such as *carcinoma with sarcomatoid elements,* or *sarcomatoid carcinoma,* have been used for other histologically mixed neoplasms, adding to the confusion of the terminology.[556-561] It is obvious that some of those carcinosarcomas are actually epithelial tumors, and the proposal has been made that the terms *biphasic sarcomatoid carcinoma* and *monophasic sarcomatoid carcinoma* be used for them.[560]

Lymphoma

Pulmonary lymphoma may present as a primary lung disease or more often as an extension of the disease from the lymph nodes and the bone marrow into the lungs. Secondary involvement is much more common than primary pulmonary lymphoma: it occurs in 30% to 40% of cases of chronic lymphocytic leukemia and in 45% of cases of high-grade lymphoma.[504] Primary pulmonary lymphoma accounts for less than 0.5% of all lymphomas.

Most primary lymphomas of the lung originate from the mucosa-associated lymphoid tissue (MALT) and present as slow-growing solitary lesions.[562,563] Less commonly, the disease presents as a multifocal or diffuse process.[564] Primary high-grade lymphomas of the lungs are rare. Such lesions usually represent secondary involvement and are associated with lymph node disease. Lymphomatoid granulomatosis, an angiocentric lymphoproliferative disorder described by Liebow in the 1970s, has proven to be an Epstein-Barr virus related, pulmonary, B-cell lesion rich in T-cells.[565]

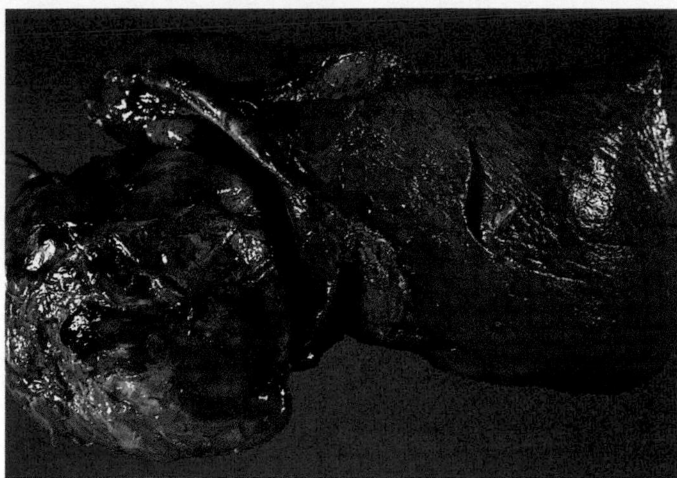

Fig. 49-89 Sarcoma of the lung. The tumor presented as a large mass.

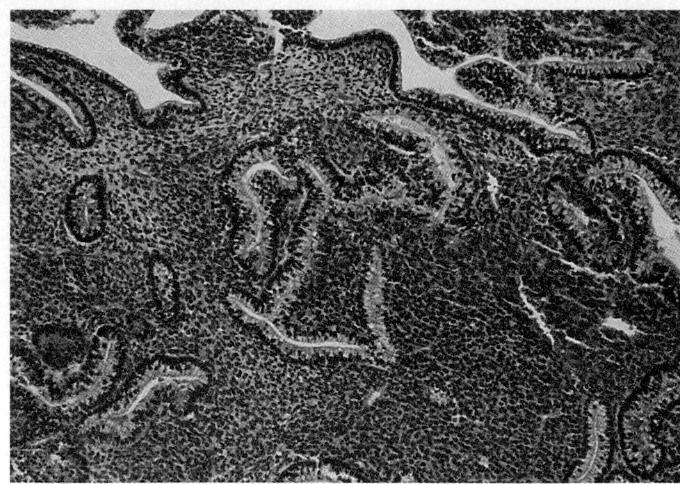

Fig. 49-90 Pulmonary blastoma. The tumor is composed of branching ducts surrounded by stroma composed of densely arranged small blue cells reminiscent of developing fetal lung.

Mesothelioma

Mesotheliomas are tumors of the pleura. These tumors have been epidemiologically linked to asbestos exposure and have been discussed earlier in this chapter. Histologically mesotheliomas can be subdivided into three groups: epithelial, sarcomatoid, and biphasic tumors. The epithelial mesotheliomas may show several histologic patterns but most often grow as tubulopapillary tumors. Solid, microcystic, pseudoglandular patterns are less common. Such tumors may be indistinguishable from adenocarcinoma. Sarcomatous tumors have usually the features of fibrosarcoma, or malignant fibrous histiocytoma. Biphasic tumors resemble synovial sarcoma.

Miscellaneous rare tumors and tumorlike lesions

A variety of benign and malignant tumors and tumorlike lesions may be encountered in the lungs. These include pulmonary blastoma[566] (Fig. 49-90), pulmonary endodermal tumor resembling fetal lung,[567] primary malignant melanoma,[568] malignant ependymoma,[569] meningioma,[570] malignant melanotic schwannoma of the bronchus,[571] and many others.

Hamartomas are the most common benign tumors of the lung.[572] Despite their name, which implies a developmental defect, they appear to be acquired lesions, since they are not found in infancy and their maximum incidence is not reached until 60 years of age. They produce no symptoms but are often discovered incidentally on chest roentgenograms. Hamartomas present as well-circumscribed nodules, 1 to 4 cm in diameter (Fig. 49-91), that shell out readily and are easily recognized grossly by their translucent cartilage-like appearance, cauliflower-like clefts, and rubbery consistency. They consist of lobules of connective tissue, usually containing cartilage, often with fat or fibrous tissue. The lobules are separated by clefts or tubules lined with columnar or cuboidal epithelium growing in from the surface of the tumor. The epithelium is probably entrapped respiratory epithelium, and the connective tissue may be the neoplastic component. Hamartomas may occasionally give rise to malignant tumors.[573]

Mesenchymal cystic hamartomas are rare lesions that begin in infancy and childhood but usually become symptomatic in adulthood. Only exceptionally are they diagnosed in children.[574] Histologically, these hamartomas consist of cysts lined by epithelia and immature vascular stroma.

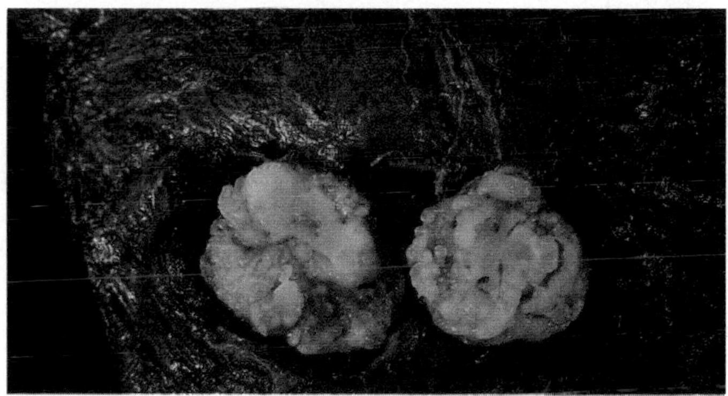

Fig. 49-91 Hamartoma. The nodule has a prominently clefted appearance on cross section.

The so-called *sclerosing hemangioma* also causes few symptoms and is usually discovered accidentally on the chest roentgenogram as a rounded nodule which are occasionally multiple.[574] These lesions are of controversial histogenesis. They consist of a circumscribed unencapsulated nodule formed by the proliferation in the interstitium of epithelium-like cells with an oval central nucleus and a clear or pale eosinophilic cytoplasm with distinct cytoplasmic margins. Individual cells may be surrounded by fibrous tissue that in some areas compresses and replaces the tumor cells, resulting in foci of sclerosis. Where cellular or sclerotic tumor abuts air spaces, it is covered with hyperplastic alveolar epithelium composed mainly of type II pneumocytes.[575] In some areas, involved alveolar walls protruding into alveolar ducts give the tumor a papillary appearance; hemorrhage into alveolar spaces remaining in the tumor may mimic vascular spaces; hence, the original name *hemangioma*.

Benign clear cell tumor is known informally as the "sugar tumor" because of its high glycogen content.[576] These lesions are circumscribed masses in the lung parenchyma formed of cords or nests of large cells with a cytoplasm sometimes

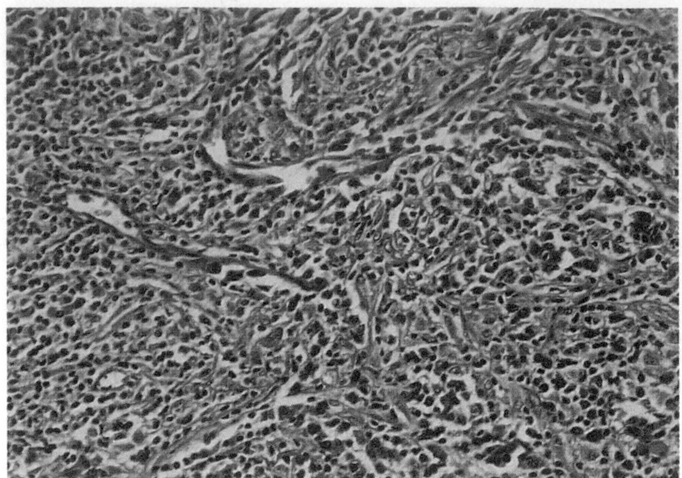

Fig. 49-92 Inflammatory pseudotumor. The lesion is composed of a variety of cell types. Plasma cells and fibrosis predominate.

entirely clear and sometimes empty but with wispy eosinophilic strands radiating from the nucleus (spider cells). The cords and nests are separated by delicate capillaries that lead into characteristic dilated sinusoids. At first glance the lesions resemble metastic renal cell carcinoma, but extended follow-up observation has proven their benign nature. The cytoplasm of renal cell carcinoma is clear, mainly because of fat, whereas that of benign clear cell tumor is filled with glycogen. Electron microscopy characteristically shows glycogen-filled lysosomes as well as free cytoplasmic glycogen. These features do not provide clues about the histogenesis of the tumors.

Inflammatory pseudotumors (plasma cell granulomas, fibrous xanthomas) are tumorlike lesions that are usually entirely intraparenchymal but may be attached to the pleura or are even endobronchial.[577] They occur at any age but are most common in adolescents and children. They are morphologically heterogeneous, usually consisting of a background of edematous or hyalinized fibrous tissue infiltrated with varying numbers of plasma cells, Russell bodies, and lymphocytes (Fig. 49-92). Although the plasma cells are mature and well differentiated, they are often greatly distorted by fibrous tissue. Histiocytes with or without fat may be part of the solid lesions or fill adjacent obstructed air spaces.

Additional new entities are being described every so often. Most recent additions are the so-called placentoid bullous lesions[578,579] and bronchial blue nevus.[580] It is important to know such lesions in order to avoid confusion with true neoplasms.

Metastatic tumors

Lungs are commonly involved by metastatic tumors, which could originate from any site. Both carcinomas and sarcomas metastasize to the lungs. The metastases may reach the lungs hematogenously, through the lymphatics, or by direct extension from adjacent structures. Histologically, many of these tumors cannot be distinguished from primary pulmonary neoplasms.

REFERENCES

Normal lung

1. Kuhn C: Normal anatomy and histology. In Thurlbeck WM, Churg AM, editors: *Pathology of the lung,* ed 2, New York, 1995, Thieme Medical Publishers.
2. Crapo JD, Barry BE, Gehr P et al: Cell number and cell characteristics of the normal human lung, *Am Rev Respir Dis* 126:332, 1982.
3. Thurlbeck WM: Lung growth. In Thurlbeck WM, Churg AM, editors: *Pathology of the lung,* ed 2, New York, 1995, Thieme Medical Publishers.
4. Thurlbeck WM: Prematurity and the developing lung, *Clin Perinatol* 19:497, 1992.
5. DiMaio M, Gil J, Ciurea D, Kattan M: Structural maturation of the human fetal lung: a morphometric study of the development of air-blood barriers, *Pediatr Res* 26:88, 1989.
6. Nakamura Y, Fukuda S, Hashimoto T: Pulmonary elastic fibers in normal human development and in pathological conditions, *Pediatr Pathol* 10:689, 1990.
7. Hislop A, Wigglesworth JS, Desai R: Alveolar development in the human fetus and infant, *Early Hum Dev* 13:1, 1986.
8. Thurlbeck WM: Postnatal human lung growth, *Thorax* 37:564, 1982.
9. Reid LM: Lung growth in health and disease, *Br J Dis* Chest 78:113, 1984.
10. Stocker JT: The respiratory tract. In Stocker JT, Dehner LP, editors: *Pediatric pathology,* Philadelphia, 1992, Lippincott.

Developmental anomalies

11. Landing BH: Congenital malformations of the larynx and trachea. In Saldana, MJ, editor: *Pathology of pulmonary disease,* Philadelphia, Lippincott.
12. Stocker JT: Congenital and developmental diseases. In Dail DM, Hammar SP, editors: *Pulmonary pathology,* 1994, Springer-Verlag.
13. Landing BH, Dixon LG: Congenital malformations and genetic disorders of the respiratory tract, *Am Rev Respir Dis* 120:151, 1979.
14. Berkhoff WBC, Scholtmeyer RJ, Tibboel D, Molenaar JC: Urogenital tract abnormalities associated with esophageal atresia and tracheoesophageal fistula, *J Urol* 141:362, 1989.
15. Evans JA, Reggin J, Greenberg C: Tracheal agenesis and associated malformations: a comparison with tracheoesophageal fistula and the VACTERL association, *Am J Med Genet* 21:21, 1985.
16. Diaz EM Jr, Adams JM, Hawkins HK, Smith RJH: Tracheal agenesis: a case report and literature review, *Arch Otolaryngol Head Neck Surg* 115:741, 1989.
17. Streitz JM Jr, Shapshay SM: Airway injury after tracheotomy and endotracheal intubation, *Surg Clin North Am* 71:1211, 1991.
18. Loeff DS, Filler RM, Vinograd I et al: Congenital tracheal stenosis: a review of 22 patients from 1965 to 1987, *J Pediatr* Surg 23:744, 1988.
19. deLorimier AA, Harrison MR, Hardy K et al: Tracheobronchial obstructions in infants and children: experience with 45 cases, *Ann Surg* 212:277, 1990.
20. Laing MR, Albert DM, Quinney RE, Bailey CM: Tracheal stenosis in infants and young children, *J Laryngol Otol* 104:229, 1990.
21. Shin MS, Jackson RM, Ho K-J: Tracheobronchomegaly (Mournier-Kuhn syndrome): CT diagnosis, *AJR* 150:777, 1988.
22. Van Schoor J, Joos G, Pauwels R: Tracheobronchomegaly: the Mounier-Kuhn syndrome: report of two cases and review of the literature, *Eur Respir J* 4:1303, 1991.
23. Bailey PV, Tracy T Jr, Connors RH, DeMello D et al: Congenital bronchopulmonary malformations, *J Thorac Cardiovasc Surg* 99:597, 1990.
24. Landing BH: Syndromes of congenital heart disease with tracheobronchial anomalies, *Am J Roentgenol Radium Ther Nucl Med* 123:679, 1975.
25. Evans JA: Aberrant bronchi and cardiovascular anomalies, *Am J Med Genet* 35:46, 1990.
26. Landing BH, Wells TR: Tracheobronchial anomalies in children. In Rosenberg HS, Bolande RP, editors: *Perspectives in pediatric pathology,* St. Louis, 1973, Mosby.
27. Landing BH: Five syndromes (malformation complexes) of pulmonary symmetry, congenital heart disease and multiple spleens, *Pediatr Pathol* 2:125, 1984.
28. Cope R, Campbell JR, Wall M: Bilateral tracheal bronchi, *J Pediatr* Surg 21:443, 1986.
29. Gonzalez-Crussi F, Padilla L-M, Miller JK, Grosfield JL: "Bridging bronchus": a previously undescribed airway anomaly, *Am J Dis Child* 130:1015, 1976.

30. Montague NT, Shaw RR: Bronchial atresia, *Ann Thorac Surg* 18:337, 1974.
31. Jederlinic PJ, Sicilian LS, Baigelman W, Gaensler EA: Congenital bronchial atresia: a report of 4 cases and a review of the literature, *Medicine* 65:73, 1986.
32. Leithiser RE Jr, Capitanio MA, Macpherson RI, Wood BP: "Communicating" bronchopulmonary foregut malformations, *AJR* 146:227, 1986.
33. Srikanth MS, Ford EG, Stanley P, Mahour GH: Communicating bronchopulmonary foregut malformations: classification and embryogenesis, *J Pediatr* Surg 27:732, 1992.
34. Alshabkhoun S, Starkey GWB, Asnes RA: Bronchogenic cysts of the mediastinum in infancy: a cause of acute respiratory distress, *Ann Thorac Surg* 4:532, 1967.
35. Fraga S, Helwig EB, Rosen SH: Bronchogenic cysts in the skin and subcutaneous tissue. *Am J Clin Pathol* 56:230, 1971.
36. Cunningham MD, Peters ER: Cervical hernia of the lung associated with the cri du chat syndrome, *Am J Dis Child* 118:769, 1969.
37. Frank JL, Poole CA, Rosas G: Horseshoe lung: clinical, pathologic, and radiologic features and a new plain film finding, *AJR* 146:217, 1986.
38. Campanella C, Odell JA: Unilateral pulmonary agenesis: a report of 4 cases, *S Afr Med J* 71:785, 1987.
39. Knowles S, Thomas RM, Lindenbaum RH et al: Pulmonary agenesis as part of the VACTERL sequence, *Arch Dis Child* 63:723, 1988.
40. Engellenner W, Kaplan C, Van de Vegte GL: Pulmonary agenesis association with nonimmune hydrops, *Pediatr Pathol* 9:725, 1989.
41. Booth JB, Berry CL: Unilateral pulmonary agenesis, *Arch Dis Child* 42:361, 1967.
42. Janney CG, Askin FB, Kuhn C III: Congenital alveolar capillary dysplasia: an unusual cause of respiratory distress in the newborn, *Am J Clin Pathol* 76:722, 1981.
43. Cater G, Thibeault DW, Beatty EC et al: Misalignment of lung vessels and alveolar capillary dysplasia: a cause of persistent pulmonary hypertension, *J Pediatr* 114:293, 1989.
44. Rutledge JC, Jensen P: Acinar dysplasia: a new form of pulmonary maldevelopment, *Hum Pathol* 17(12):1290, 1986.
45. George DK, Cooney TP, Chiu BK, Thurlbeck WM: Hypoplasia and immaturity of the terminal lung unit (acinus) in congenital diaphragmatic hernia, *Am Rev Respir Dis* 136:947, 1987.
46. Nakamura Y, Yamamoto I, Fukuda S, Hashimoto T: Pulmonary acinar development in diaphragmatic hernia, *Arch Pathol Lab Med* 115:372, 1991.
47. Nakamura Y, Harada K, Yamamoto I et al: Human pulmonary hypoplasia: statistical, morphological, morphometric, and biochemical study, *Arch Pathol Lab Med* 116:635, 1992.
48. Cooney TP, Wentworth PJ, Thurlbeck WM: Diminished radial count is found only postnatally in Down's syndrome, *Pediatr Pulmonol* 5:204, 1988.
49. Wigglesworth JS, Desai R, Aber V: Quantitative aspects of perinatal lung growth, *Early Hum Dev* 15:203, 1987.
50. Stocker JT, Malczak HT: A study of pulmonary ligament arteries: relationship to intralobar pulmonary sequestration, *Chest* 86:611, 1984.
51. Piccione W Jr, Burt ME: Pulmonary sequestration in the neonate, *Chest* 97:244, 1990.
52. Savic B, Birtel FJ, Tholen W et al: Lung sequestration: report of seven cases and review of 540 published cases, *Thorax* 34:96, 1979.
53. Ke F-J, Chang S-C, Su W-J, Perng R-P: Extralobar pulmonary sequestration presenting as an anterior mediastinal tumor in an adult, *Chest* 104:303, 1993.
54. Stocker JT, Kagan-Hallet K: Extralobar pulmonary sequestration: analysis of 15 cases, *Am J Clin Pathol* 72:917, 1979.
55. Hruban RH, Shumway SJ, Orel SB et al: Congenital bronchopulmonary foregut malformations: intralobar and extralobar pulmonary sequestrations communicating with the foregut, *Am J Clin Pathol* 91:403, 1989.
56. Lager DJ, Kuper KA, Haake GK: Subdiaphragmatic extralobar pulmonary sequestration, *Arch Pathol Lab Med* 115:536, 1991.
57. Dolkart LA, Reimers FT, Helmuth WV et al: Antenatal diagnosis of pulmonary sequestration: a review, *Obstet Gynecol Surv* 47:515, 1992.
58. Ikezoe J, Murayama S, Godwin JD et al: Bronchopulmonary sequestration: CT assessment, *Radiology* 176:375, 1990.
59. Stocker JT, Dehner LP: Acquired neonatal and pediatric diseases. In Dail DH, Hammar Sp, editors: *Pulmonary pathology,* New York, 1994, Springer-Verlag.
60. Landing BH: Emphysematous and cystic lesions. In Saldana MJ, editor: *Pathology of pulmonary disease,* Philadelphia, Lippincott.
61. Louie HW, Martin SM, Mulder DG: Pulmonary sequestration: 17-year experience at UCLA, *Am Surg* 59:801, 1993.
62. Moerman P, Fryns JP, Vandenberghe K et al: Pathogenesis of congenital cystic adenomatoid malformation of the lung, *Histopathology* 21:315, 1992.
63. Cloutier MM, Schaeffer DA, Hight D: Congenital cystic adenomatoid malformation, *Chest* 103:761, 1993.
64. Stocker JT, Madewell JE, Drake RM: Congenital cystic adenomatoid malformation of the lung: classification and morphologic spectrum, *Hum Pathol* 8:155, 1977.
65. Benning TL, Godwin JD, Roggli VL, Askin FB: Cartilaginous variant of congenital adenomatoid malformation of the lung, *Chest* 92:514, 1987.
66. Miller RK, Sieber WK, Yunis EJ: Congenital adenomatoid malformation of the lung: a report of 17 cases and review of the literature, *Pathol Annu* 15 (pt. 1): 387, 1980.
67. Revillon Y, Jan D, Plattner V et al: Congenital cystic adenomatoid malformation of the lung: prenatal management and prognosis, *J Pediatr Surg* 28:1009, 1993.
68. Bainbridge TC, Solimano A, Rotschild A et al: Waxing and waning hyperinflation in congenital cystic adenomatoid malformation of the lung, *J Perinatol* 12:237, 1992.
69. Gardner TW, Domm AC, Brock CE, Pruitt AW: Congenital pulmonary lymphangiectasis, *Clin Pediatr* 22:75, 1983.
70. Gilbert EF, Opitz JM: Malformations and genetic disorders of the respiratory tract. In Stocker JT editor: *Pediatric pulmonary disease,* New York, 1989, Hemisphere Publishing Corp.
71. Man DWK, Hamdy MH, Hendry GMA et al: Congenital lobar emphysema: problems in diagnosis and management, *Arch Dis Child* 58:709, 1983.
72. Schneider JR, St Cyr JA, Thompson TR et al: The changing spectrum of cystic pulmonary lesions requiring surgical resection in infants, *J Thorac Cardiovasc Surg* 89:332, 1985.
73. Patterson K, Donnelly WH, Dehner LP: The cardiovascular system. In Stocker JT, Dehner, LP editors: *Pediatric pathology,* Philadelphia, 1992, Lippincott.
74. Presbitero P, Bull C, Haworth SG, DeLaval M: Absent or occult pulmonary artery, *Br Heart J* 52:178, 1984.
75. Landing BH: Vascular lesions of the respiratory tract and disorders of the chest wall and diaphragm. In Saldana MJ, editor: *Pathology of pulmonary disease,* Philadelphia, 1994, Lippincott.
76. Haworth SG, Reid L: Structural study of pulmonary circulation and of the heart in total anomalous pulmonary venous return in early infancy, *Br Heart J* 39:80, 1977.
77. Canter CE, Martin TC, Spray TL et al: Scimitar syndrome in childhood, *Am J Cardiol* 58:652, 1986.
78. Dupuis C, Charaf LA, Breviere GM et al: The "adult" form of the scimitar syndrome, *Am J Cardiol* 70:502, 1992.

Perinatal lung disease

79. Godfrey S: Growth and development of the respiratory system: functional development. In Dobbing J, Davis JA, editors: *Scientific foundations of paediatrics,* ed 2, Baltimore, 1981, University Park Press.
80. Perelman RH, Engle MJ, Farrell PM: Perspectives on fetal lung development, *Lung* 159:53, 1981.
81. Bland RD: Lung liquid clearance before and after birth, *Semin Perinatol* 12:124, 1988.
82. Walther FJ, Taeusch HW: Pathophysiology of neonatal surfactant insufficiency: clinical aspects. In Robertson B, van Golde LMG, Batenburg JJ, editors: *Pulmonary surfactant: from molecular biology to clinical practice,* Amsterdam, 1992 Elsevier Science Publishers.
83. Langston C, Askin FB: Pulmonary disorders in the neonate, infant, and child. In Thurlbeck WM, Churg AM, editors: *Pathology of the lung,* New York, 1995, Thieme Medical.

84. Wigglesworth JS, Desai R, Hislop AA: Fetal lung growth in congenital laryngeal atresia, *Pediatr Pathol* 7:515, 1987.
85. Truog WE III: Pulmonary gas exchange. In Chernick V, Mellins RB, editors: *Basic mechanisms of pediatric respiratory disease: cellular and integrative,* St. Louis, 1991, Mosby.
86. Williams MC: Morphologic aspects of the surfactant system. In Robertson B, van Golde LMG, Batenburg JJ, editors: *Pulmonary surfactant: from molecular biology to clinical practice,* Amsterdam, 1992, Elsevier Science Publishers.
87. Lacaze-Masmonteil T: Pulmonary surfactant proteins, *Crit Care Med* 21(suppl):S376, 1993.
88. Cochrane CG, Revak SD: Protein-phospholipid interactions in pulmonary surfactant, *Chest* 105(suppl):57S, 1994.
89. Mendelson CR, Alcorn JL, Gao E: The pulmonary surfactant protein genes and their regulation in fetal lung, *Semin Perinatol* 17:223,235, 1993.
90. Dubin SB: Assessment of fetal lung maturity by laboratory methods, *Clin Lab Med* 12:603, 1992.
91. Tanasijevic MJ, Wybenga DR, Richardson D et al: A predictive model for fetal lung maturity employing gestational age and test results, *Am J Clin Pathol* 102:788, 1994.
92. Corbet A: Respiratory disorders in the newborn. In Chernick V, Kendig EL, editors: *Disorders of the respiratory tract in children,* ed 5, Philadelphia, 1990, Saunders.
93. Fagan DG, Emery JL: A review and restatement of some problems in histological interpretation of the infant lung, *Semin Diagn Pathol* 9:13, 1992.
94. Obladen M: History of surfactant research. In Robertson B, van Golde LMG, Batenburg JJ, editors: *Pulmonary surfactant: from molecular biology to clinical practice,* Amsterdam, 1992, Elsevier Science Publishers.
95. Seo IS, Gillim SE, Mirkin LD: Hyaline membranes in postmature infants, *Pediatr Pathol* 10:539, 1990.
96. Pfenninger J, Tschaeppeler H, Wagner BP et al: The paradox of adult respiratory distress syndrome in neonates, *Pediatr Pulmonol* 10:18, 1991.
97. Reyes-Mugica M, Gonzalez-Crussi F: Pulmonary disease in the pediatric age group. In Saldana MJ, editor: *Pathology of pulmonary disease,* Philadelphia, 1994, Lippincott.
98. Lauweryns JM: "Hyaline membrane disease" in newborn infants: macroscopic, radiographic, and light and electron microscopic studies, *Hum Pathol* 1:175, 1970.
99. Nakamura Y, Saitoh Y, Yamamoto I et al: Regenerative process of hyaline membrane disease, *Arch Pathol Lab Med* 112:821, 1988.
100. Doshi N, Klionsky B, Fujikura T, MacDonald H: Pulmonary yellow hyaline membranes in neonates, *Hum Pathol* 11(suppl):520, 1980.
101. Morgenstern B, Klionsky B, Doshi N: Yellow hyaline membrane disease: identification of the pigment and bilirubin binding, *Lab Invest* 44:514, 1981.
102. Jobe A, Ikegami M: Surfactant for the treatment of respiratory distress syndrome, *Am Rev Respir Dis* 136:1256, 1987.
103. Cotton RB: A model of the effect of surfactant treatment on gas exchange in hyaline membrane disease, *Semin Perinatol* 18:19, 1994.
104. Jobe AH: Pulmonary surfactant therapy, *N Engl J Med* 328:861, 1993.
105. Abman SH, Groothius JR: Pathophysiology and treatment of bronchopulmonary dysplasia: current issues, *Pediatr Clin North Am* 41:277, 1994.
106. Nickerson BG: Bronchopulmonary dysplasia: chronic pulmonary disease following neonatal respiratory failure, *Chest* 87:528, 1985.
107. Truog WE, Jackson JC: Alternative modes of ventilation in the prevention and treatment of bronchopulmonary dysplasia, *Clin Perinatol* 19:621, 1992.
108. O'Brodovich HM, Mellins RB: Bronchopulmonary dysplasia: unresolved neonatal acute lung injury, *Am Rev Respir Dis* 132:694, 1985.
109. Margraf LR, Tomashefski JF Jr, Bruce MC, Dahms BB: Morphometric analysis of the lung in bronchopulmonary dysplasia, *Am Rev Respir Dis* 143:391, 1991.
110. Bonikos DS, Bensch KG, Northway WH Jr, Edwards DK: Bronchopulmonary dysplasia: the pulmonary pathologic sequel of necrotizing bronchiolitis and pulmonary fibrosis, *Hum Pathol* 7:643, 1976.
111. Anderson WR, Engel RR: Cardiopulmonary sequelae of reparative stages of bronchopulmonary dysplasia, *Arch Pathol Lab Med* 107:603, 1983.
112. Stocker JT: Pathologic features of long-standing "healed" bronchopulmonary dysplasia: a study of 28 3- to 40-month-old infants, *Hum Pathol* 17:943, 1986.
113. Northway WH Jr, Moss RB, Carlisle KB et al: Late pulmonary sequelae of bronchopulmonary dysplasia, *N Engl J Med* 323:1793, 1990.
114. Myers MG, McGuinness GA, Lachenbruch PA et al: Respiratory illnesses in survivors of infant respiratory distress syndrome, *Am Rev Respir Dis* 133:1011, 1986.
115. Gorenflo M, Vogel M, Obladen M: Pulmonary vascular changes in bronchopulmonary dysplasia: a clinicopathologic correlation in short- and long-term survivors, *Pediatr Pathol* 11:851, 1991.
116. Askin FB: Pulmonary interstitial air and pneumothorax in the neonate. In Stocker JT, editor: *Pediatric pulmonary disease,* New York, 1989, Hemisphere Publishing Corp.
117. Caldwell EJ, Powell RD Jr, Mullooly JP: Interstitial emphysema: a study of physiologic factors involved in experimental induction of the lesion, *Am Rev Respir Dis* 102:516, 1970.
118. Brewer LL, Moskowitz PS, Carrington CB, Bensch KG: *Pneumatosis pulmonalis:* a complication of the idiopathic respiratory distress syndrome, *Am J Pathol* 95:171, 1979.
119. Greenough A, Dixon AK, Roberton NRC: Pulmonary interstitial emphysema, *Arch Dis Child* 59:1046, 1984.
120. Swingle HM, Eggert LD, Bucciarelli RL: New approach to management of unilateral tension pulmonary interstitial emphysema in premature infants, *Pediatrics* 74:354, 1984.
121. Esterly JR, Oppenheimer EH: Massive pulmonary hemorrhage in the newborn. I. Pathologic considerations, *J Pediatr* 69:3, 1966.
122. Trompeter R, Yu VYH, Aynsley-Green A, Roberton NRC: Massive pulmonary haemorrhage in the newborn infant, *Arch Dis Child* 50:123, 1975.
123. Katz VL, Bowes WA: Meconium aspiration syndrome: reflections on a murky subject, *Am J Obstet Gynecol* 166:171, 1992.
124. Perlman EJ, Moore GW, Hutchins GM: The pulmonary vasculature in meconium aspiration, *Hum Pathol* 20:701, 1989.
125. Wiswell TE, Bent RC: Meconium staining and the meconium aspiration syndrome: unresolved issues, *Pediatr Clin North Am* 40:955, 1993.
126. Gersony WM: Neonatal pulmonary hypertension: pathophysiology, classification, and etiology, *Clin Perinatol* 11:517, 1984.
127. Walsh-Sukys MC: Persistent pulmonary hypertension of the newborn: the black box revisited, *Clin Perinatol* 20:127, 1993.
128. Murphy JD, Rabinovitch M, Goldstein JD, Reid LM: The structural basis of persistent pulmonary hypertension of the newborn infant, *J Pediatr* 98:962, 1981.
129. Haworth SG: Primary and secondary pulmonary hypertension in childhood: a clinicopathological reappraisal, *Curr Top Pathol* 73:91, 1983.
130. Cullinane C, Cox PN, Silver MM: Persistent pulmonary hypertension of the newborn due to alveolar capillary dysplasia, *Pediatr Pathol* 12:499, 1992.
131. Whitsett JA, Pryhuber GS, Rice WR et al: Acute respiratory disorders. In Avery GB, Fletcher MA, MacDonald MG, editors: *Neonatology: pathophysiology and management of the newborn,* Philadelphia, 1994, Lippincott.
132. Zeichner SL, Plotkin SA: Mechanisms and pathways of congenital infections, *Clin Perinatol* 15:163, 1988.
133. Toltzis P: Current issues in neonatal herpes simplex virus infection, *Clin Perinatol* 18:193, 1991.
134. Jacobs RF, Abernathy RS: Management of tuberculosis in pregnancy and the newborn, *Clin Perinatol* 15:305, 1988.
135. Newton ER: Chorioamnionitis and intra-amniotic infection, *Clin Obstet Gynecol* 36:795, 1993.
136. Pinto A, Beck R, Jadavji T: Fatal neonatal pneumonia caused by adenovirus type 35: report of one case and review of the literature, *Arch Pathol Lab Med* 116:95, 1992.
137. Shek YH, Tucker MC, Viciana AL et al: *Malassezia furfur:* disseminated infection in premature infants, *Am J Clin Pathol* 92:595, 1989.
138. Nicholls JM, Yuen KY, Tam AYC: Systemic fungal infections in neonates, *Br J Hosp Med* 49:420, 1993.
139. Nicholls JM, Yuen KY, Saing H: *Malassezia* furfur infection in a neonate, *Br J Hosp Med* 49:425, 1993.

140. St. Geme JW III, Harris MC: Coagulase-negative staphylococcal infection in the neonate, *Clin Perinatol* 18:281, 1991.
141. Katz VL: Management of group B streptococcal disease in pregnancy, *Clin Obstet Gynecol* 36:832, 1993.
142. Rettig PJ: Perinatal infections with *Chlamydia trachomatis*, *Clin Perinatol* 15:321, 1988.
143. Waites KB, Crouse DT, Cassell GH: Therapeutic considerations for *Ureaplasma urealyticum* infections in neonates, *Clin Infect Dis* 17(suppl):S208, 1993.

Infections of the lung

144. A'Court C, Garrard SC: Nosocomial pneumonia in the intensive care unit: mechanisms and significance, *Thorax* 47:465, 1992.
145. Tryba M: The gastropulmonary route of infection—fact or fiction? *Am J Med* 91(suppl 2A):135S, 1991.
146. Woods DE, Straus DC, Johanson WG, Bass JA: Role of salivary protease activity in adherence of gram-negative bacilli to mammalian buccal epithelial cells in vivo, *J Clin Invest* 68:1435, 1981.
147. Wohl MED, Chernick V: Bronchiolitis, *Am Rev Respir Dis* 118:759, 1978.
148. Becroft DMO: Histopathology of fatal adenovirus infection of the respiratory tract in young children, *J Clin Pathol* 20:561, 1967.
149. Yeldandi AV, Colby TV: Pathologic features of lung biopsy specimens from influenza pneumonia cases, *Hum Pathol* 25:47, 1995.
150. Kahane I: In vitro studies on the mechanism of adherence and pathogenicity of mycoplasmas, *Isr J Med Sci* 20:874, 1984.
151. Rollins S, Colby T, Clayton F: Open lung biopsy in *Mycoplasma pneumoniae* pneumonia, *Arch Pathol Lab Med* 110:34, 1986.
152. Grayston JT, Thom DH: The chlamidial pneumonias, *Curr Clin Top Infect Dis* 11:1, 1991.
153. Yung AP, Grayson ML: Psittacosis: a review of 105 cases, *Med J Aust* 148:228, 1988.
154. Sawyer LA, Fishbein DB, McDade JE: Q-fever: current concepts, *Rev Infect Dis* 9:935, 1987.
155. Urso FP: The pathologic findings in rickettsial pneumonia, *Am J Clin Pathol* 64:335, 1975.
156. Walker DH, Crawford CG, Cain BG: Rickettsial infection of pulmonary microcirculation: the basis for interstitial pneumonitis in Rocky Mountain spotted fever, *Hum Pathol* 11:263, 1980.
157. Donnelly BW, McMillan JA, Weiner LB: Bacterial tracheitis: report of eight new cases and review, *Rev Infect Dis* 12:729, 1990.
158. Valor PR, Polnitsky CA, Tanis DJ, Sherter CB: Bacterial tracheitis with upper airway obstruction in a patient with the acquired immunodeficiency syndrome, *Am Rev Respir Dis* 146:1598, 1992.
159. Pachon J, Prados MD, Capote F et al: Severe community-acquired pneumonia: etiology, prognosis and treatment, *Am Rev Respir Dis* 142:369, 1990.
160. Fang GD, Fine M, Orloff J et al: New and emerging etiologies for community-acquired pneumonia with implications for therapy: a prospective multicenter study of 359 cases, *Medicine* 69:307, 1990.
161. Janoff EN, Breiman RF, Daley CL, Hopewell PC: Pneumococcal disease during HIV infection: epidemiologic, clinical and immunologic perspectives, *Ann Intern Med* 117:314, 1992.
162. Tuomanen E, Rich, R, Zak O: Induction of pulmonary inflammation by components of the pneumococcal cell surface, *Am Rev Respir Dis* 135:869, 1987.
163. Burman LA, Norrby R, Trollfors B: Invasive pneumococcal infections: incidence, predisposing factors and prognosis, *Rev Infect Dis* 7:133, 1985.
164. Musher DM, Lamm N, Darouiche RO et al: The current spectrum of *Staphylococcus aureus* infection in a tertiary care hospital, *Medicine* 73:186, 1994.
165. Tsai TC, Tsai YH, Lan RS et al: Pulmonary manifestations of *Staphyloccus aureus* septicemia, *Chest* 101:574, 1992.
166. Rouby JJ, Martin de Lassale E, Poete P et al: Nosocomial pneumonia in the critically ill: histologic and bacteriologic aspects, *Am Rev Respir Dis* 146:1059, 1992.
167. Fagon J, Chastre J, Hance AJ et al: Nosocomial pneumonia in ventilated patients: a cohort study evaluating attributable mortality and hospital stay, *Am J Med* 94:281, 1993.
168. Bodey GP, Ladeja L, Elting L: *Pseudomonas* bacteremia: retrospective analysis of 410 episodes, *Arch Intern Med* 145:1621, 1985.
169. Fetzer AE, Werner AS, Hagstrom JWC: Pathology features of pseudomonal pneumonia, *Am Rev Respir Dis* 96:1121, 1967.
170. Winn WC Jr: Legionnaires disease: historical perspective, *Clin Microbiol Rev* 1:60, 1988.
171. Blatt SP, Parkinson MD, Pace E et al: Nosocomial Legionnaire's disease: aspiration as a primary mode of disease acquisition, *Am J Med* 95:16-22, 1993; comment in 95:13, 1993.
172. Dowling JN, Saha AK, Glew RH: Virulence factors of the family Legionellaceae, *Microbiol Rev* 56:32, 1992.
173. Belyi YF: Intracellular parasitism of *Legionella* and signaling in eukaryotic cells, *FASEB J* 7:1011, 1993.
174. Bartlett SG, Finegold SM: Anaerobic infections of the lung and pleural space, *Am Rev Respir Dis* 110:56, 1974.
175. Edman JC, Kovacs JA, Masur H et al: Ribosomal RNA sequence shows *Pneumocystis carinii* to be a member of the fungi, *Nature* 334:519, 1988.
176. Travis WD, Pittaluga S, Lipschik GY et al: Atypical pathologic manifestations of *Pneumocystis carinii* pneumonia in the acquired immunodeficiency syndrome: review of 123 lung biopsies from 76 patients with emphasis on cysts, vascular invasion, vasculitis and granulomas, *Am J Surg Pathol* 14:615, 1990.
177. Luna MA, Cleary KR: Spectrum of pathologic manifestations of *Pneumocystis carinii* pneumonia in patients with neoplastic diseases, *Semin Diagn Pathol* 6:262, 1989.
178. Foley NM, Griffiths MH, Miller RF: Histologically atypical *Pneumocystis carinii* pneumonia, *Thorax* 48:996, 1993.
179. Barker AF, Bardana EJ: Bronchiectasis: update of an orphan disease, *Am Rev Respir Dis* 137:969, 1988.
180. Whitwell F: A study of the pathology and pathogenesis of bronchiectasis, *Thorax* 7:213, 1952.
181. Mierau GW, Agostini R, Beals TF et al: The role of electron microscopy in evaluating ciliary dysfunction: report of a workshop, *Ultrastruct Pathol* 16:245, 1992.
182. Lurie M, Rennert G, Goldenberg S, Rivlin J et al: Ciliary ultrastructure in primary ciliary dyskinesia and other chronic respiratory conditions: the relevance of microtubular abnormalities, *Ultrastruct Pathol* 16:547, 1992.
183. Bedrossian CWM, Greenberg SD, Singer DB et al: the lung in cystic fibrosis: a quantitative study including the prevalance of pathologic findings among different age groups, *Hum Pathol* 7:195, 1976.
184. Vawter GF, Schwachman H: Cystic fibrosis in adults: an autopsy study, *Pathol Annu* 14(pt 2):357, 1979.
185. Buret A, Cripps AW: The immunoevasive activities of *Pseudomonas aeruginosa:* relevance for cystic fibrosis. *Am Rev Respir Dis* 148:793, 1993.
186. Burke W, Aitken ML, Chen SH, Scott CR: Variable severity of pulmonary disease in adults with identical cystic fibrosis mutations, *Chest* 102:506, 1992.
187. The cystic fibrosis genotype-phenotype consortium: correlation between genotype and phenotype in patients with cystic fibrosis, *N Engl J Med* 329:1308, 1993.
188. Riordan JR: The cystic fibrosis transmembrane conductance regulator, *Annu Rev Physiol* 55:609, 1993.
189. Boucher RC: Human airway ion transport, *Am J Respir Crit Care Med* 150:271, 581, 1994.
190. Cheng SH, Gregory RJ, Marshall J et al: Defective intracellular transport and processing of CFTR is the molecular basis of most cystic fibrosis, *Cell* 63:827, 1990.
191. Puchelle E, Gaillard D, Ploton D et al: Differential localization of the cystic fibrosis transmembrane conductance regulator in normal and cystic fibrosis airway epithelium, *Am J Respir Cell Molec Biol* 7:485, 1992.
192. Lukacs GL, Change XB, Bear C et al: The delta F508 mutation decreases the stability of cystic fibrosis transmembrane conductance regulator in the plasma membrane—determination of functional half-lives on transfected cells, *J Biol Chem* 268:21592, 1993.
193. Yang YP, Janich S, Cohn JA, Wilson JM: The common variant of cystic fibrosis transmembrane conductance regulator is recognized by HSP70 and degraded in a pre-Golgi nonlysosomal compartment, *Proc Natl Acad Sci USA* 90:9480, 1993.

194. Dalemans W, Barbry P, Champigny G et al: Altered ion channel kinetics associated with the delta F508 cystic fibrosis mutation, *Nature* 354:526, 1991.
195. Sheppard DN, Rich DP, Ostegaard LS et al: Mutations in CFTR associated with mild disease form chloride channels with altered pore properties, *Nature* 362:160, 1993.

Pulmonary circulatory diseases

196. Moser KM: Venous thromboembolism, *Am Rev Respir Dis* 141:235, 1990.
197. Rosenow EC, Osmundson PJ, Brown ML: Pulmonary embolism, *Mayo Clin Proc* 56:161, 1981.
198. Korn D, Gore I, Blenke A, Collins DP: Pulmonary arterial bands and webs: a previously unrecognized manifestation of organized pulmonary emboli, *Am J Pathol* 40:129, 1962.
199. Tsao M-S, Schraufnagel D, Wang NS: Pathogenesis of pulmonary infarction, *Am J Med* 72:599, 1982.
200. Schraufnagel DE, Tsao M-S, Yao TT, Wang NS: Factors associated with pulmonary infarction: a discriminant analysis study, *Am J Clin Pathol* 84:15, 1985.
201. Fabian TC: Unraveling the fat embolism syndrome, *N Engl J Med* 329:961, 1993.
202. Sperry K: Amniotic fluid embolism: to understand an enigma, *JAMA* 255:2183, 1986.
203. Clark SL: New concepts of amniotic fluid embolism: a review, *Obstet Gynecol Surv* 45:360, 1990.
204. Attwood HD: The histological diagnosis of amniotic-fluid embolism, *J Pathol Bacteriol* 76:211, 1958.
205. Tomashefski JF, Hirsch CS: The pulmonary vascular lesions of intravenous drug abuse, *Hum Pathol* 11:133, 1980.
206. O'Quinn RJ, Kakshminarayan S: Venous air embolism, *Arch Intern Med* 142:2173, 1982.
207. Edwards JE: Pathology of chronic pulmonary hypertension, *Pathol Annu* 1, 1974.
208. Heath D, Edward JE: The pathology of hypertensive pulmonary vascular disease, *Circulation* 18:533, 1958.
209. Tuder RM, Groves B, Badesch DB, Voelkel NF: Exuberant endothelial cell growth and elements of inflammation are present in plexiform lesions of pulmonary hypertension, *Am J Pathol* 144:275, 1994.
210. Wagenvoort CA: Grading of pulmonary vascular lesions—a reappraisal, *Histopathology* 5:595, 1981.
211. Saldana ME, Harley RA, Liebow AA, Carrington CB: Experimental extreme pulmonary hypertension and vascular disease in relation to polycythemia, *Am J Pathol* 52:935, 1968.
212. Cutaia M, Rounds S: Hypoxic pulmonary vasoconstriction: physiologic significance, mechanism and clinical relevance, *Chest* 97:706, 1990.
213. Rubin LJ: ACCP consensus statement: primary pulmonary hypertension, *Chest* 104:236, 1993.
214. Pietra GG, Edwards WD, Kay JM et al: Histopathology of primary pulmonary hypertension: a qualitative and quantitative study of pulmonary blood vessels from 58 patients in the National Heart, Lung and Blood Institute primary pulmonary hypertension registry, *Circulation* 80:1198, 1989.
215. Moser KM, Bloor CM: Pulmonary vascular lesions occurring in patients with chronic major vessel thromboembolic pulmonary hypertension, *Chest* 103:685, 1993.
216. Eisenberg PR, Lucore C, Kaufman L et al: Fibrinopeptide A levels indicative of pulmonary vascular thrombosis in patients with primary pulmonary hypertension, *Circulation* 82:841, 1990.
217. Christman BW, McPherson CD, Newman JH et al: An imbalance between the excretion of thromboxane and prostacyclin metabolites in pulmonary hypertension, *N Engl J Med* 327:70, 1992.
218. Giaid A, Yanagisawa M., Langleben D et al: Expression of endothelin-1 in the lungs of patients with pulmonary hypertension, *N Engl J Med* 328:1732, 1993.
219. Espinosa RE, Edwards WD, Rosenow EC, Schaff HV: Idiopathic pulmonary hilar fibrosis: an unusual cause of pulmonary hypertension, *Mayo Clin Proc* 68:778, 1993.
220. Tron V, Magee F, Wright JL et al: Pulmonary capillary hemangiomatosis, *Hum Pathol* 17:1144, 1986.
221. Canny GS, Cutz E, MacLusky IB, Levison H: Diffuse pulmonary angiomatosis, *Thorax* 46:851, 1991.
222. McDonnell PJ, Toye PA, Hutchins GM: Primary pulmonary hypertension and cirrhosis: are they related? *Am Rev Respir Dis* 127:437, 1983.
223. Petitpretz P, Brenot F, Azarian R et al: Pulmonary hypertension in patients with human immunodeficiency virus infection: comparison with primary pulmonary hypertension, *Circulation* 89:2722, 1994.
224. Crapo JD: New concepts in the formation of pulmonary edema, *Am Rev Respir Dis* 147:790, 1993.
225. Bachofen H, Schurch S, Weibel ER: Experimental hydrostatic pulmonary edema in rabbit lungs: barrier lesions, *Am Rev Respir Dis* 147:997, 1993.
226. West JB, Mathieu-Costello O: Stress failure of pulmonary capillaries: role in lung and heart disease, *Lancet* 340:762, 1992.
227. Barker PM: Transalveolar Na^+ absorption: a strategy to counter alveolar flooding? *Am J Respir Crit Care Med* 150:302, 1994.
228. Heath D, Edwards JE: Histological changes in the lung in diseases associated with pulmonary venous hypertension, *Br J Dis Chest* 53:8, 1959.
229. Heath D, Moosavi H, Smith P: Ultrastructure of high altitude pulmonary edema, *Thorax* 28:694, 1973.
230. Schoene RB, Hakett PH, Henderson WR et al: High-altitude pulmonary edema: characteristics of lung lavage fluid, *JAMA* 256:63, 1986.
231. Arias-Stella J, Kruger H: Pathology of high altitude pulmonary edema, *Arch Pathol* 76:147, 1963.
232. Bekemeyer WP, Pinstein M: Neurogenic pulmonary edema: new concepts, *South Med J* 82:380, 1989.
233. Colice GL, Matthay MA, Bass E, Matthay RA: Neurogenic pulmonary edema, *Am Rev Respir Dis* 130:941, 1984.
234. Tomashefski JF: Pulmonary pathology of the adult respiratory distress syndrome, *Clin Chest Med* 11:593, 1990.
235. Fukuda Y, Ishizaki M, Masuda Y et al: The role of intra-alveolar fibrosis in the process of pulmonary structural remodeling in patients with diffuse alveolar damage, *Am J Pathol* 126:171, 1987.
236. Snow RL, Davies P, Pontoppidan H et al: Pulmonary vascular remodeling in adult respiratory distress syndrome, *Am Rev Respir Dis* 126:887, 1982.
237. Suchyta MR, Clemmer TP, Elliott CG, Orme JF et al: The adult respiratory distress syndrome: a report of survival and modifying factors, *Chest* 101:1074, 1992.
238. Bone RC: The pathogenesis of sepsis, *Ann Intern Med* 115:457, 1991.
239. Heffner JE, Sahn SA, Repine JE: The role of platelets in the adult respiratory distress syndrome: culprits or bystanders? *Am Rev Respir Dis* 135:482, 1987.
240. Swank DW, Moore SB: Roles of the neutrophil and other mediators in adult respiratory distress syndrome, *Mayo Clin Proc* 64:1118, 1989.
241. Lewis JF, Jobe AH: Surfactant and the adult respiratory distress syndrome, *Am Rev Respir Dis* 147:218, 1993.
242. Wispe JR, Clark JC, Warner BB, Fajardo D et al: Tumor necrosis factor—alpha inhibits expression of pulmonary surfactant protein, *J Clin Invest* 86:1954, 1990.
243. Bertozzi P, Astedt B, Zenius L et al: Depressed bronchoalveolar urokinase activity in patients with adult respiratory distress syndrome, *N Engl J Med* 322:890, 1990.
244. Idell S, James KK, Levin EG et al: Local abnormalities in coagulation and fibrinolytic pathways predispose to alveolar fibrin deposition in the adult respiratory distress syndrome, *J Clin Invest* 84:695, 1989.

Interstitial pneumonia and pulmonary fibrosis

245. Crouch EC: Pathobiology of pulmonary fibrosis, *Am J Physiol* 259(Lung Cell Mol Physiol):L159, 1990.
246. Katzenstein A-LA: Idiopathic interstitial pneumonia: classification and diagnosis. In Churg A, Katzenstein A-LA, editors: *The lung: current concepts,* Baltimore, 1993, Williams & Wilkins.
247. Hamman L, Rich AR: Acute diffuse interstitial fibrosis of the lungs, *Bull Johns Hopkins Hosp* 74:177, 1994.
248. Askin FB: Back to the future: the Hamman-Rich syndrome and acute interstitial pneumonia, *Mayo Clin Proc* 65:1624, 1990.
249. Olson J, Colby TV, Elliott CG: Hamman-Rich syndrome revisited, *Mayo Clin Proc* 65:1538, 1990.

250. Katzenstein A-LA, Myers JL, Mazur MT: Acute interstitial pneumonia: a clinicopathologic ultrastructural and cell kinetic study, *Am J Surg Pathol* 10:256, 1986.
251. Pratt DS, Schwartz MI, May JJ, Dreisen RB: Rapidly progressive pulmonary fibrosis: the accelerated variant of interstitial pneumonitis, *Thorax* 34:587, 1979.
252. Epler GR, Colby TV, McLoud TC et al: Bronchiolitis obliterans organizing pneumonia, *N Engl J Med* 312:152, 1985.
253. Davidson AG, Heard BE, McAllister, WAC, Turner-Warwick MEH: Cryptogenic organizing pneumonitis, *Q J Med* 52:383, 1983.
254. Katzenstein A-LA, Myers JL, Prophet WD, Corley LS et al: Bronchiolitis obliterans and usual interstitial pneumonia: a comparative clinicopathologic study, *Am J Surg Pathol* 10:371, 1986.
255. Colby TV: Pathologic aspects of bronchiolitis obliterans organizing pneumonia, *Chest* 102(S):385, 1992.
256. Kitaichi M: Differential diagnosis of bronchiolitis obliterans organizing pneumonia, *Chest* 102(S): 445, 1992.
257. Belloma R, Finlay M, McLaughlin P, Tai E: Clinical spectrum of cryptogenic organizing pneumonitis, *Thorax* 46:554, 1991.
258. Basset F, Ferrans UJ, Soler P et al: Intraluminal fibrosis in interstitial lung disorders, *Am J Pathol* 122:443, 1986.
259. Hammar SP, Bockus D, Pemington F, Friedman S: Idiopathic fibrosing alveolitis: a review with emphasis on ultrastructural and immunohistochemical features, *Ultrastruct Pathol* 9:345, 1985.
260. Liebow AA: New concepts and entities in pulmonary disease. In Liebow AA, Smith DE, editors: *The lung*, Baltimore, 1968, Williams & Wilkins.
261. Winterbauer RH, Hammar SP, Hallman KO et al: Diffuse interstitial pneumonitis: clinicopathologic correlations in 20 patients treated with prednisone/azathioprine, *Am J Med* 65:661, 1978.
262. Carrington CB, Gaensler EA, Coutu RE et al: Natural history and treated course of usual and desquamative interstitial pneumonia, *N Engl J Med* 298:801, 1978.
263. Katzenstein A-LA, Fiorelli RF: Nonspecific interstitial pneumonia/fibrosis: histologic features and clinical significance, *Am J Surg Pathol* 18:136, 1994.
264. Cherniack RM, Colby TV, Flint A et al: Quantitative assessment of lung pathology in idiopathic pulmonary fibrosis, *Am Rev Respir Dis* 144:892, 1991.
265. Hyde DM, King TE, McDermott T et al: Idiopathic pulmonary fibrosis: quantitative assessment of lung pathology; comparison of a semiquantitative and morphometric histopathologic scoring system, *Am Rev Respir Dis* 146:1042, 1992.
266. Wright PH, Heard BE, Steel SJ, Turner-Warwick M: Cryptogenic fibrosing alveolitis: assessment by graded trephine lung biopsy histology compared with clinical, radiographic and physiological features, *Br J Dis Chest* 75:61, 1981.
267. duBois RM: Recent advances in immunology of interstitial lung disease, *Clin Exp Allergy* 21:9, 1991.
268. Kallenberg CGM, Schilizzi BM, Beaumont F, DeLey L et al: The expression of class II major histocompatibility complex antigens on alveolar epithelium in interstitial lung disease: relevance to pathogenesis of idiopathic pulmonary fibrosis, *J Clin Pathol* 40:725, 1987.
269. Chapman HA, Bertozzi P, Reilly JJ: Role of enzymes mediating thrombosis and thrombolysis in lung disease, *Chest* 93:1256, 1988.
270. Piguet PF, Ribaux C, Karpuz V et al: Expression and localization of tumor necrosis factor–alpha and its mRNA in idiopathic pulmonary fibrosis, *Am J Pathol* 143:651, 1993.
271. Elias JA, Freundlich B, Kern JA, Rosenbloom J: Cytokine networks in the regulation of inflammation and fibrosis in the lung, *Chest* 97:1439, 1990.
272. Gauldie J: Cytokines and pulmonary fibrosis, *Thorax* 48:931, 1993.

Immunologic lung diseases

273. Benatar SR: Fatal asthma, *N Engl J Med* 314:423, 1986.
274. Jeffery P: Morphology of the airway wall in asthma and in chronic obstructive pulmonary disease, *Am Rev Respir Dis* 143:1152, 1991.
275. Takizawa T, Thurlbeck WM: Muscle and mucous gland size in the major bronchi of patients with chronic bronchitis, asthma and asthmatic bronchitis, *Am Rev Respir Dis* 104:331, 1971.
276. Sobonya RE: Quantitative structural alterations in long-standing allergic asthma, *Am Rev Respir Dis* 130:289, 1984.
277. Djukanovic R, Roche WR, Wilson JW et al: Mucosal inflammation in asthma, *Am Rev Respir Dis* 142:434, 1990.
278. Holgate S: Mediator and cytokine mechanisms in asthma, *Thorax* 48:103, 1993.
279. Azzawi M, Johnston PW, Majumdar S, Kay AB et al: T-lymphocytes and activated eosinophils in airway mucosa in fatal asthma and cystic fibrosis, *Am Rev Respir Dis* 145:1477, 1992.
280. Robinson DS, Hamid Q, Ying S et al: Predominant T_{H2}-like bronchoalveolar T-lymphocyte population in atopic asthma, *N Engl J Med* 326:298, 1992.
281. Gleich GJ, Adolphson CR, Leiferman KM: The biology of the eosinophilic leukocyte, *Annu Rev Med* 44:85, 1993.
282. Ohashi Y, Motogima S, Fukuda T, Makimo S: Airway hyperresponsiveness, increased intercellular spaces of bronchial epithelium and increased infiltration of eosinophils and lymphocytes in bronchial mucosa in asthma, *Am Rev Respir Dis* 145:1469, 1992.
283. Laitinen LA, Heino M, Laitinen A et al: Damage of the airway epithelium and bronchial reactivity in patients with asthma, *Am Rev Respir Dis* 131:599, 1985.
284. Barnes PJ, Baraniuk J, Belvisi MG: Neuropeptides in the respiratory tract, *Am Rev Respir Dis* 144:1187, 1991.
285. Ollerenshaw S, Jarvis D, Woolcock A et al: Absence of immunoreactive vasoactive intestinal polypeptide in tissue from the lungs of patients with asthma, *N Engl J Med* 320:1244, 1989.
286. Springall DR, Wowarth PH, Counihan H et al: Endothelin immunoreactivity of airway epithelium in asthmatic patients, *Lancet* 337:697, 1991.
287. Kuwano K, Bosken CH, Pare PD et al: Small airway dimensions in asthma and in chronic obstructive pulmonary disease, *Am Rev Respir Dis* 148: 1220, 1993.
288. Wiggs BR, Bosken C, Pare PD et al: A model of airway narrowing in asthma and in chronic obstructive pulmonary disease, *Am Rev Respir Dis* 145:1251, 1992.
289. Hendrickson CD, Lynch JM, Gleeson K: Exercise-induced asthma: a clinical perspective, *Lung* 172:1, 1994.
290. Israel E, Fischer AR, Rosenberg MA et al: The pivotal role of 5-lipoxygenase products in the reaction of aspirin-sensitive asthmatics to aspirin, *Am Rev Respir Dis* 148:1447, 1993.
291. Greenberger PA, Patterson R: Allergic bronchopulmonary aspergillosis: model of bronchopulmonary disease with defined serologic, radiologic, pathologic and clinical findings from asthma to fatal destructive lung disease, *Chest* 91:165S, 1987.
292. Bosken CH, Myers JL, Greenberger PA, Katzenstein A-L: Pathologic features of allergic bronchopulmonary aspergillosis, *Am J Surg Pathol* 12:216, 1988.
293. Slavin RG, Bedrossian CW, Hutchison PS et al: A pathologic study of allergic bronchopulmonary aspergillosis, *J Allergy Clin Immunol* 81:718, 1988.
294. Katzenstein A-L, Liebow AA, Friedman PJ: Bronchocentric granulomatosis, mucoid impaction and hypersensitivity reactions to fungi, *Am Rev Respir Dis* 111:497, 1975.
295. Koss MN, Robinson RG, Hochholzer L: Bronchocentric granulomatosis, *Hum Pathol* 12:632, 1981.
296. Seal RME, Hapke EJ, Thomas GO et al: The pathology of the acute and chronic stages of farmer's lung, *Thorax* 23:469, 1968.
297. Hammar S: Hypersensitivity pneumonitis, *Pathol Annu* 23(pt 1):193, 1988.
298. Coleman A, Colby TV: Histologic diagnosis of extrinsic allergic alveolitis, *Am J Surg Pathol* 12:514, 1988.
299. Rose C, King TE: Controversies in hypersensitivity pneumonitis, *Am Rev Respir Dis* 145:1, 1992.
300. Costabel U, Bross JK, Marxen J, Matthys H: T-lymphocytosis in bronchoalveolar lavage fluid of hypersensitivity pneumonitis: changes in profile of T-cell subsets during the course of disease, *Chest* 85:514, 1984.
301. Keller RH, Calvanico NJ, Stevens JO: Hypersensitivity pneumonitis in nonhuman primates: (1) studies on the relationship of immunoregulation and disease activity, *J Immunol* 128:116, 1982.

302. Otteson EA, Nutman TB: Tropical pulmonary eosinophilia, *Annu Rev Med* 43:417, 1992.
303. Carrington CB, Addington WW, Geoff AM et al: Chronic eosinophilic pneumonia, *N Engl J Med* 280:787, 1969.
304. Bodesch DB, King TE, Schartz MI: Acute eosinophilic pneumonia: a hypersensitivity phenomenon? *Am Rev Respir Dis* 139:249, 1989.
305. Jederlinic PJ, Sicilian L, Gaensler EA: Chronic eosinophilic pneumonia: a report of 19 cases and a review of the literature, *Medicine* 67:154, 1988.
306. Randhawa P, Youssem SA: The pathology of lung transplantation, *Pathol Annu* 27(pt 2):247, 1992.
307. Marchevsky A, Hartman G, Walts A et al: Lung transplantation: the pathologic diagnosis of pulmonary complications, *Mod Pathol* 4:133, 1991.
308. Higgenbottam T, Stewart S, Penketh A, Wallork J: Transbronchial lung biopsy for the diagnosis of rejection in heart-lung transplant patients, *Transplantation* 46:532, 1988.
309. Urbanski SJ, Kossakowska AE, Curtis J et al: Idiopathic small airways pathology in patients with graft-versus-host disease following allogeneic bone marrow transplantation, *Am J Surg Pathol* 11:965, 1987.
310. Yousem SA, Dauber JH, Griffith BP: Bronchial cartilage alterations in lung transplantation, *Chest* 98:1121, 1990.
311. Yousem SA, Randhawa P, Locker J et al: Post-transplant lymphoproliferative disorders in heart-lung transplant recipients: primary presentation in the allograft, *Hum Pathol* 20:361, 1989.
312. James GD, Neville E: Pathology of sarcoidosis, *Pathobiol Annu* 7:31, 1977.
313. Rosen Y, Vuletin JC, Pertschuk LP, Silverstein E: Sarcoidosis from the pathologist's vantage point, *Pathol Annu* 14:405, 1979.
314. Rosen Y, Athanassiades TJ, Moon S, Lyons HA: Nongranulomatous interstitial pneumonitis in sarcoidosis, *Chest* 74:122, 1978.
315. Perry A, Vuitch F: Causes of death in patients with sarcoidosis: a morphologic study of 38 autopsies with clinicopathologic correlations, *Arch Pathol Lab Med* 119:167, 1995.
316. DeRemee RA: The roentgen staging of sarcoidosis: historic and contemporary perspectives, *Chest* 83:128, 1981.
317. Thomas PD, Hunninghake GW: Current concepts of the pathogenesis of sarcoidosis, *Am Rev Respir Dis* 135:747, 1987.
318. Mitchell IC, Turk JL, Mitchell DN: Detection of mycobacterial DNA in sarcoidosis with liquid phase hybridization, *Lancet* 339:1015, 1992.
319. Saboor SA, Johnson NM, McFadden J: Detection of mycobacterial DNA in sarcoidosis and tuberculosis with polymerase chain reaction, *Lancet* 339:1012, 1992.
320. Koss MN, Hochholzer L, Feigin DS et al: Necrotizing sarcoid-like granulomatosis: clinical, pathologic and immunopathologic findings, *Hum Pathol* 11Suppl:510, 1980.
321. Churg A, Carrington CB, Gupta R: Necrotizing sarcoid granulomatosis, *Chest* 76:406, 1979.
322. Murray JF, Mills J: Pulmonary infectious complications of human immunodeficiency virus infection, *Am Rev Respir Dis* 141:1356, 1582, 1990.
323. White DA, Matthay RA: Non-infectious pulmonary complication of infection with human immunodeficiency virus, *Am Rev Respir Dis* 140:1763, 1989.
324. Travis WD, Fox CH, Devaney KO et al: Lymphoid pneumonitis in 50 adult patients infected with the human immunodeficiency virus: lymphocytic interstitial pneumonitis versus nonspecific interstitial pneumonitis, *Hum Pathol* 23:529, 1992.
325. Itescu S, Brancato LJ, Buxbaum J et al: A diffuse infiltrative CD8 lymphocytosis syndrome in human immunodeficiency virus (HIV) infection: a host immune response associated with HLA DR 5, *Ann Intern Med* 112:3, 1990.
326. Diaz PT, Clanton TL, Pacht ER: Emphysema-like pulmonary disease associated with human immunodeficiency virus infection, *Ann Intern Med* 116:124, 1992.

Collagen vascular diseases

327. Brown G, Goldring D, Behrer R: Rheumatic pneumonia, *J Pediatr* 52:598, 1958.
328. Scott RF, Thomas WA, Kissane JM: Rheumatic pneumonitis: pathologic features, *J Pediatr* 54:60, 1959.
329. Wiedeman HP, Matthay RA: Pulmonary manifestations of the collagen vascular diseases, *Clin Chest Med* 10:677, 1989.
330. Sahn S: The pleura, *Am Rev Respir Dis* 138:184, 1988.
331. Faurschou P, Francis D, Fuarup P: Thoracoscopic, histological and clinical findings in nine cases of rheumatoid pleural effusion, *Thorax* 40:371, 1985.
332. Yousem SA, Colby TV, Carrington CB: Lung biopsy in rheumatoid arthritis, *Am Rev Respir Dis* 131:770, 1985.
333. Geddes DM, Corrin B, Brewerton DA et al: Progressive airway obliteration in adults and its association with rheumatoid disease, *Q J Med* 46:427, 1977.
334. Shadick NA, Fanta CH, Weinblatt ME et al: Bronchiectasis: a late feature of severe rheumatoid arthritis, *Medicine* 73:161, 1994.
335. Eagan J, Memoli VA, Roberts SL et al: Pulmonary hemorrhage and systemic lupus erythematosus, *Medicine* 57:545, 1978.
336. Matthay RA, Schwartz MI, Petty TL et al: Pulmonary manifestations of systemic lupus erythematosus: review of twelve cases of acute lupus pneumonitis, *Medicine* 54:397, 1974.
337. Inoue T, Kanayama Y, Ohe A et al: Immunopathologic studies of pneumonitis in systemic lupus erythematosus, *Ann Intern Med* 91:30, 1979.
338. Nair SS, Askari AD, Popelka CG, Kleinerman JF: Pulmonary hypertension and systemic lupus erythematosus, *Arch Intern Med* 140:109, 1980.
339. Strimlan CV, Rosenow EC III, Divertie MB et al: Pulmonary manifestations of Sjögren's syndrome, *Chest* 70:354, 1976.
340. McCurley TL, Collins RD, Ball E, Collins RD: Nodal and extranodal lymphoproliferative disorders in Sjögren's syndrome: a clinical and immunopathologic study, *Hum Pathol* 21:482, 1990.
341. McCarthy DS, Baragar FD, Dhingra S et al: The lungs in systemic sclerosis (scleroderma): a review and new information, *Semin Arthritis Rheum* 17:271, 1988.
342. Ungerer RG, Tashkin DP, Fust D et al: Prevalence and clinical correlates of pulmonary arterial hypertension in progressive systemic sclerosis, *Am J Med* 75:65, 1983.
343. Yousem SA: The pulmonary pathologic manifestations of the CREST syndrome, *Hum Pathol* 21:467, 1990.
344. Tazalaar H, Viggiano RW, Pickersgill J, Colby TV: Interstitial lung disease in polymyositis and dermatomyositis: clinical features and prognosis as correlated with histologic findings, *Am Rev Respir Dis* 141:727, 1990.
345. Wallace JG, Tong MJ, Ueki BH, Quismorio FP: Pulmonary involvement in primary biliary cirrhosis, *J Clin Gastroenterol* 9:431, 1987.
346. Martin RW, Duffy J, Engel AG et al: The clinical spectrum of the eosinophilia myalgia syndrome associated with L-tryptophane ingestion, *Ann Intern Med* 113:124, 1990.

Pulmonary vasculitides

347. Colby TV, Specks U: Wegener's granulomatosis in the 1990's: a pulmonary pathologist's perspective. In Churg A, Katzenstein A-LA, editors: *The lung: current concepts,* Baltimore, 1993, Williams & Wilkins.
348. Sneller MC: Wegener's granulomatosis, *JAMA* 273:1288, 1995.
349. Travis WD, Hoffman GS, Leavitt RY et al: Surgical pathology of the lung in Wegener's granulomatosis: review of 87 open lung biopsies from 67 patients, *Am J Surg Pathol* 15:315, 1991.
350. Mark EJ, Ramirez JF: Pulmonary capillaritis and hemorrhage with systemic vasculitis, *Arch Pathol Lab Med* 109:413, 1985.
351. Jennette JC: Antineutrophil cytoplasmic antibody-associated diseases: a pathologist's perspective, *Am J Kidney Dis* 18:164, 1991.
352. Gephardt GN, Shah LF, Tubbs RR, Ahmad M: Wegener's granulomatosis: immunomicroscopic and ultrastructural study of four cases, *Arch Pathol Lab Med* 114:961, 1990.
353. Ewert BH, Jennette JC, Falk RJ: The pathogenic role of antineutrophil cytoplasmic autoantibodies, *Am J Kidney Dis* 18:188, 1991.
354. Lanham JG, Elkon KB, Pusey CD, Hughes GR: Systemic vasculitis with asthma and eosinophilia: a clinical approach to the Churg-Strauss syndrome, *Medicine* 63:65, 1984.
355. Lie JT: Limited forms of Churg-Strauss syndrome, *Pathol Annu* 28(pt 2): 199, 1993.
356. Koss MN, Antonovych T, Hochholzer L: Allergic granulomatosis (Churg-Strauss syndrome): pulmonary and renal morphologic findings, *Am J Surg Pathol* 5:21, 1981.

357. Lombard CM, Colby TV, Elliott CG: Surgical pathology of the lung in antibasement membrane antibody–associated Goodpasture's syndrome, *Hum Pathol* 20:445, 1989.
358. Kelly PT, Haponik EF: Goodpasture's syndrome: molecular and clinical advances, *Medicine* 73:171, 1994.
359. Travis WD, Colby TV, Lombard C, Carpenter HA: A clinicopathologic study of 34 cases of diffuse pulmonary hemorrhage with lung biopsy confirmation, *Am J Surg Pathol* 14:1112, 1990.

Miscellaneous lung diseases

360. Soler P, Moreau A, Basset F, Hance AJ: Cigarette smoking induced changes in number and differentiated state of pulmonary dendritic cells/Langerhans cells, *Am Rev Respir Dis* 139:1112, 1989.
361. Willman CL, Busque L, Griffith BB et al: Langerhans-cell histiocytosis (histiocytosis-X): a clonal proliferative disease, *N Engl J Med* 331:154, 1994.
362. Basset F, Corrin B, Spencer H et al: Pulmonary histiocytosis-X, *Am Rev Respir Dis* 118:811, 1978.
363. Auld D: Pathology of eosinophilic granuloma of the lung, *Arch Pathol* 63:113, 1957.
364. Travis WD, Borok Z, Roum JH et al: Pulmonary Langerhans cell granulomatosis (histiocytosis X): a clinicopathologic study of 48 cases, *Am J Surg Pathol* 17:971, 1993.
365. Webber D, Tron V, Askin F, Churg A: S-100 staining in the diagnosis of eosinophilic granuloma of lung, *Am J Clin Pathol* 84:447, 1985.
366. Colasante A, Poletti V, Rosini S et al: Langerhans cells in Langerhans cell histiocytosis and peripheral adenocarcinoma of the lung, *Am Rev Respir Dis* 148:752, 1993.
367. Soler P, Kambouchner M, Valeyre D, Hance AJ: Pulmonary Langerhans cell granulomatosis (histiocytosis X), *Annu Rev Med* 43:105, 1992.
368. Corrin B, Liebow AA, Friedman PJ: Pulmonary lymphangiomyomatosis: a review, *Am J Pathol* 79:347, 1975.
369. Bonetti F, Chiordera PL, Pea M et al: Transbronchial biopsy in lymphangiomyomatosis of the lung: HMB 45 for diagnosis, *Am J Surg Pathol* 17:1092, 1995.
370. Carrington CB, Cugell DW, Gaensler EA et al: Lymphangioleiomyomatosis: physiologic-pathologic-radiologic correlations, *Am Rev Respir Dis* 116:977, 1977.
371. Taylor JR, Ryu J, Colby TV, Raffin TA: Lymphangiomyomatosis: clinical course in 32 patients, *N Engl J Med* 323:1254, 1990.
372. Colley MH, Geppert E, Franklin WA: Immunohistochemical detection of steroid receptors in a case of pulmonary lymphangioleiomyomatosis, *Am J Surg Pathol* 13:803, 1989.
373. Rosen SH, Castleman B, Liebow AA: Pulmonary alveolar proteinosis, *N Engl J Med* 258:1123, 1958.
374. Kuhn C, Gyorkey F, Levine BE, Ramírez-Rivera J: Pulmonary alveolar proteinosis, *Lab Invest* 15:492, 1966.
375. Bell DY, Hook GER: Pulmonary alveolar proteinosis: analysis of airway and alveolar proteins, *Am Rev Respir Dis* 199:979, 1979.
376. Singh G, Katyal SL, Bedrossian CWM, Rogers RM: Pulmonary alveolar proteinosis: staining for surfactant apoprotein in alveolar proteinosis and in conditions simulating it, *Chest* 83:82, 1983.
377. Nogee LM, Garnier G, Dietz HC et al: A mutation in the surfactant protein B gene responsible for fatal neonatal respiratory disease in multiple kindreds, *J Clin Invest* 93:1860, 1994.
378. Bedrossian CMW, Luna MA, Couklin RH, Miller WC: Alveolar proteinosis as a consequence of immunosuppression: a hypothesis based on clinical and pathologic observations, *Hum Pathol* 11:527, 1980.
379. Ruben FL, Talamo TS: Secondary pulmonary alveolar proteinosis occurring in two patients with acquired immune deficiency syndrome, *Am J Med* 80:1187, 1986.
380. Witty LA, Tapson VF, Piantadosi CA: Isolation of mycobacteria in patients with pulmonary alveolar proteinosis, *Medicine* 73:103, 1994.
381. Ramirez RJ, Savard EV, Hawkins JE: Biological effect of pulmonary washings from cases of alveolar proteinosis, *Am Rev Respir Dis* 94:244, 1966.
382. Golde DW, Territo M, Finley TN, Cline MJ: Defective lung macrophages in pulmonary alveolar proteinosis, *Ann Intern Med* 85:304, 1976.
383. Chen KT: Amyloidosis presenting in the respiratory tract, *Pathol Annu* 24(1):253, 1989.
384. Knapp MJ, Roggli VL, Kim J et al: Pleural amyloidosis, *Arch Pathol Lab Med* 112:57, 1988.
385. Minra K, Shirasawa H: Lambda III subgroup immunoglobulin light chains are precursor proteins of nodular pulmonary amyloidosis, *Am J Clin Pathol* 100:561, 1993.
386. Kijner CH, Yousem SA: Systemic light chain deposition disease presenting as multiple pulmonary nodules, *Am J Surg Pathol* 12:405, 1988.
387. Conger JD, Hammond WS, Alfrey AC et al: Pulmonary calcifications in chronic dialysis patients: clinical and pathologic studies, *Ann Intern Med* 83:330, 1975.
388. Popelka CG, Kleinerman J: Diffuse pulmonary ossification, *Arch Intern Med* 137:523, 1977.
389. Joines RW, Roggli VL: Dendriform pulmonary ossification: report of two cases with unique features, *Am J Clin Pathol* 91:398, 1989.
390. Prakash UBS, Barham SS, Rosenow EC III et al: Pulmonary alveolar microlithiasis: a review including ultrastructural and pulmonary function studies, *Mayo Clin Proc* 58:290, 1983.
391. Sears MR, Chang AR, Taylor AJ: Pulmonary alveolar microlithiasis, *Thorax* 26:704, 1971.
392. Rosenow E, Myers J, Swenson S, Pisani R: Drug-induced pulmonary disease: an update, *Chest* 102:239, 1992.
393. Myers JL: Diagnosis of drug reactions in the lung. In Churg A, Katzenstein A, editors: *The lung: current concepts,* Baltimore, 1993, Williams & Wilkins.
394. Jennings FL, Arden A: Development of radiation pneumonitis: time and dose, factors, *Arch Pathol* 74:351, 1962.
395. Roberts CM, Foulcher E, Zaunders JJ et al: Radiation pneumonitis: a possible lymphocyte-mediated hypersensitivity reaction, *Ann Intern Med* 118:696, 1993.
396. Morgan GW, Breit SY: Radiation and the lung: a re-evaluation of the mechanisms mediating pulmonary injury, *Int J Radiat Oncol Biol Physics* 31:361, 1995.
397. Wynne JW, Modell JH: Respiratory aspiration of stomach contents, *Ann Intern Med* 87:466, 1977.
398. Borrie J, Gwynne JF: Paraffinoma of lung: lipoid pneumonia, *Thorax* 28:214, 1973.
399. Licter I, Gwynne JF: Spontaneous pneumothorax in young subjects: a clinical and pathological study, *Thorax* 26:409, 1971.
400. Askin FB, McCann BF, Kuhn C: Reactive eosinophilic pleuritis: a lesson to be distinguished from pulmonary eosinophilic granuloma, *Arch Pathol Lab Med* 101:187, 1977.
401. Rigg SRA: Pulmonary atelectasis after anesthesia: pathophysiology and management, *Can Anaesth Soc J* 28:305, 1981.

Chronic airflow obstruction

402. Thurlbeck WM: Pathology chronic airflow obstruction. In Cherniack NS, editor: *Chronic obstructive pulmonary disease,* Philadelphia, 1991, Saunders.
403. Snider GL, Kleinerman J, Thurlbeck WM, Bengali ZK: The definition of emphysema: a report of a National Heart Lung and Blood Institute Division of lung disease workshop, *Am Rev Respir Dis* 132:182, 1985.
404. Peto R, Speizer FE, Cochrane AL et al: The relevance in adults of airflow obstruction but not of mucus hypersecretion, to mortality from chronic lung disease: results from 20 years of prospective observation, *Am Rev Respir Dis* 128:491, 1983.
405. Murphy TF, Sethi S: Bacterial infection in chronic obstructive pulmonary disease, *Am Rev Respir Dis* 146:1067, 1992.
406. Hogg JC, Macklem PT, Thurlbeck WM: Site and nature of airway obstruction in chronic obstructive lung disease, *N Engl J Med* 278:1355, 1968.
407. Wright JL, Cagle P, Churg A et al: Diseases of the small airways, *Am Rev Respir Dis* 146:240, 1992.
408. Saetta M, Finkelstein M, Cosio MG: Morphologic and cellular basis for airflow limitation in smokers, *Eur Respir J* 7:1505, 1994.
409. Hardy KA, Schidlow DV, Zaeri N: Obliterative bronchiolitis in children, *Chest* 93:460, 1988.
410. Reid L, Simon G: Unilateral lung translucency, *Thorax* 9:147, 1954.

411. Kargi A, Kuhn C: Bronchiolitis obliterans: unilateral fibrous obliteration of the lumen of bronchi with atelectasis, *Chest* 93:1107, 1988.
412. King TE: Bronchiolitis obliterans, *Lung* 167:69, 1989.
413. Wright JL: Inhalational lung injury causing bronchiolitis, *Clin Chest Med* 14:635, 1993.
414. Turton CW, Williams G, Green M: Cryptogenic obliterative bronchiolitis in adults, *Thorax* 36:805, 1981.
415. Kraft M, Mortenson RL, Colby TV et al: Cryptogenic constrictive bronchiolitis: a clinicopathologic study, *Am Rev Respir Dis* 148:1093, 1993.
416. Yousem SA, Colby TV, Carrington CB: Follicular bronchitis/bronchiolitis, *Hum Pathol* 16:700, 1985.
417. Homma H, Yamanaka A, Tanimoto S et al: Diffuse *panbronchiolitis:* a disease of the transitional zone of the lung, *Chest* 83:63, 1983.
418. Iwata M, Colby TV, Kitaichi M: Diffuse panbronchiolitis: diagnosis and distinction from various pulmonary diseases with centrilobular interstitial foam cell accumulations, *Hum Pathol* 25:357, 1994.
419. Sugiyama Y: Diffuse panbronchiolitis, *Clin Chest Med* 14:765, 1993.
420. Myers J, Veal C, Shin M, Katzenstein A-LA: Respiratory bronchiolitis causing interstitial lung disease: a clinicopathologic study of six cases, *Am Rev Respir Dis* 135:880, 1987.
421. Yousem S, Colby T, Gaensler E: Respiratory bronchiolitis-associated interstitial lung disease and its relationship to desquamative interstitial pneumonia, *Mayo Clin Proc* 64:1373, 1989.
422. Snider GL: Emphysema: The first two centuries and beyond: a historical overview with suggestions for future research, *Am Rev Respir Dis* 146:1334, 1615, 1992.
423. Mitchell RS, Silvers GW, Goodman N et al: Are centrilobular and panlobular emphysema two different diseases? *Hum Pathol* 1:433, 1970.
424. Heppleston AG, Leopold JG: Chronic pulmonary emphysema: anatomy and pathogenesis, *Am J Med* 31:279, 1961.
425. Thurlbeck WM: Emphysema then and now, *Can Respir J* 1:21, 1994.
426. Hogg JC, Wright SL, Wiggs BR et al: Lung structure and function in cigarette smokers, *Thorax* 49:473, 1994.
427. Depierre A, Bignon J, Lebeau A et al: Quantitative study of parenchyma and small conductive airways in chronic nonspecific lung disease, *Chest* 62:699, 1972.
428. Surgeon General: *The health consequences of smoking: chronic obstructive lung disease,* Rockville, Md., 1984, US Department of Health and Human Services.
429. Ishikawa S, Bowden D, Fisher V, Wyatt J: The "emphysema profile" in two midwestern cities in North America, *Arch Environ Health* 18:660, 1969.
430. Ericksson S: Alpha-1-antitrypsin deficiency: lessons learned from the bedside to the gene and back again, *Chest* 95:181, 1989.
431. Crystal RG: Alpha-1-antitrypsin deficiency, emphysema and liver disease: genetic basis and strategies for therapy, *J Clin Invest* 85:1343, 1990.
432. Lomas DA, Carrell RW: A protein structural approach to the solution of biological problems: alpha-1-antitrypsin as a recent example, *Am J Physiol* 265(Lung Cell Mol Physiol):L211, 1993.
433. Janoff A: Elastases and emphysema: current assessment of the protease-antiprotease hypothesis, *Am Rev Respir Dis* 132:417, 1985.
434. Evans MD, Pryor WA: Cigarette smoking, emphysema, and damage to alpha-1-proteinase inhibitor, *Am J Physiol* 226:L593, 1994.
435. Macnee W: Pathophysiology of cor pulmonale in chronic obstructive pulmonary disease, *Am J Respir Crit Care Med* 150:833, 1994.

Pneumoconioses and dust-associated respiratory diseases

436. Craighead JE, editor: *Pathology of environmental and occupational disease,* St. Louis, 1995, Mosby.
437. Craighead JE, Kleinerman J, Abraham JL et al: Diseases associated with exposure to silica and nonfibrous silicate minerals, *Arch Pathol Lab Med* 112:673, 1988.
438. Begin R, Cantin A, Masse S: Recent advances in the pathogenesis and clinical assessment of mineral dust pneumoconioses: asbestosis, silicosis and coal pneumoconiosis, *Eur Respir J* 2:988, 1989.
439. Suratt PM, Winn WC, Brody AR et al: Acute silicosis in tombstone sandblasters, *Am Rev Respir Dis* 115:521, 1977.
440. Banks DE, Morring KL, Boehlecke BA et al: Silicosis in silica flour workers, *Am Rev Respir Dis* 124:445, 1981.
441. Buechner HA, Ansari A: Acute silicoproteinosis: pathologic variant of acute silicosis in sandblasters, characterized by histologic features resembling alveolar proteinosis, *Chest* 55:274, 1969.
442. Cowie RL: Silica-dust–exposed mine workers with scleroderma (systemic sclerosis), *Chest* 92:260, 1987.
443. Sluis-Kremer GK: Silica, silicosis and progressive systemic sclerosis, *Br J Ind Med* 41:838, 1987.
444. Sluis-Kremer GK, Hessel PA, Hnizdo E et al: Relationship between silicosis and rheumatoid arthritis, *Thorax* 41:596, 1986.
445. Banks DE, Milutinovic J, Desnick RJ et al: Silicon nephropathy mimicking Fabry's disease, *Am J Nephrol* 3:279, 1983.
446. Pairon JC, Brochard P, Jaurand MC, Bignon J: Silica and lung cancer: a controversial issue, *Eur Respir J* 4:730, 1991.
447. Craighead JE: Do silica and asbestos cause lung cancer? *Arch Pathol Lab Med* 116:16, 1992.
448. McDonald JC: Silica, silicosis and lung cancer, *Br J Ind Med* 46:289, 1989.
449. Gibbs AR, Pooley FD, Griffiths DM et al: Talc pneumoconiosis: a pathologic and mineralogic study, *Hum Pathol* 23:1344, 1992.
450. Vallyathan NV, Craighead JE: Pulmonary pathology in workers exposed to nonasbestiform talc, *Hum Pathol* 12:28, 1981.
451. Sakula A: Pneumoconiosis due to fuller's earth, *Thorax* 16:176, 1961.
452. Huuskonen MS, Tossavainen A, Koskinen H et al: Wollastonite exposure and lung fibrosis, *Environ Res* 30:291, 1983.
453. Bignon J, editor: *Health related effects of phyllosilicates,* NATO ASI series, v G 21, Berlin, 1990, Springer-Verlag.
454. Craighead JE: Current pathogenetic concepts of diffuse malignant mesothelioma, *Hum Pathol* 18:544, 1987.
455. Pisani RJ, Colby TV, Williams DE: Malignant mesothelioma of the pleura, *Mayo Clin Proc* 63:1234, 1988.
456. Ruffie P, Feld R, Minkin S et al: Diffuse malignant mesothelioma of the pleura in Ontario and Quebec: a retrospective study of 332 patients, *J Clin Oncol* 7:1157, 1989.
457. Hillerdal G: Malignant mesothelioma 1982: review of 4710 published cases, *Br J Dis Chest* 77:321, 1983.
458. Weill H, Abraham JL, Balmes JR et al: Health effects of tremolite, *Am Rev Respir Dis* 142:1453, 1990.
459. Churg A: Chrysotile, tremolite, and malignant mesothelioma in man, *Chest* 93:621, 1988.
460. Reger R, Morgan WKC: On talc, tremolite, and tergiversation, *Br J Ind Med* 47:505, 1990.
461. Amandus HE, Wheeler R, Armstrong BG et al: Mortality of vermiculite miners exposed to tremolite, *Ann Occup Hyg* 32:459, 1988.
462. Peto J, Seldman H, Selikoff IJ: Mesothelioma mortality in asbestos workers: implications for models of carcinogenesis and risk assessment, *Br J Cancer* 45:124, 1982.
463. McCaughey WTE, Kannerstein M, Churg J: Tumors and pseudotumors of the serous membranes, *Atlas of tumor pathology,* fasc 20, Washington, D.C., 1985, Armed Forces Institute of Pathology.
464. Koss M, Travis W, Moran C, Hochholzer L: Pseudomesotheliomatous adenocarcinoma: a reappraisal, *Semin Diagn Pathol* 9:117, 1992.
465. Miettinen M, Kovatic AJ: HBME-1: a monoclonal antibody useful in the differential diagnosis of mesothelima, adenocarcinoma, and soft tissue and bone tumors, *Appl Immunohistochem,* 1995. (In press.)
466. Bedrossian CWM, Bonsib S, Moran C: Differential diagnosis between mesothelioma and adenocarcinoma: a multimodal approach based on ultrastructure and immunocytochemistry, *Semin Diagn Pathol* 9:124, 1992.
467. Sheibani K, Esteban JM, Bailey A et al: Immunopathologic and molecular studies as an aid to the diagnosis of malignant mesothelioma, *Hum Pathol* 23:107, 1992.
468. Warhol MJ, Hickey WF, Corson JM: Malignant mesothelioma: ultrastructural distinction from adenocarcinoma, *Am J Surg Pathol* 6:307, 1982.
469. Craighead JE, Abraham JL, Churg A et al: The pathology of asbestos-associated diseases of the lungs and pleural cavities: diagnostic criteria and proposed grading schema, *Arch Pathol Lab Med* 106:544, 1982.
470. Roggli VL, Greenberg SD, Pratt PC, editors: *Pathology of asbestos-associated diseases,* Boston, 1992, Little, Brown.

471. Churg A: Asbestos, asbestosis, and lung cancer [editorial], *Mod Pathol* 6:509, 1993.
472. Kipen HM, Lilis R, Suzuki Y et al: Pulmonary fibrosis in asbestos insulation workers with lung cancer: a radiological and histopathological evaluation, *Br J Ind Med* 44:96, 1987.
473. Sluis-Cremer GK, Bezuidenhout BN: Relationship between asbestosis and bronchial cancer in amphibole asbestos miners, *Br J Ind Med* 46:537, 1989.
474. Edelman DA: Does asbestosis increase the risk of lung cancer? *Int Arch Occup Environ Health* 62:345, 1990.
475. Hughes JM, Weill H: Asbestosis as a precursor of asbestos related lung cancer: results of a prospective mortality study, *Br J Ind Med* 48:229, 1991.
476. Kleinerman J, Green F, Laquer W et al: Pathology standards for coal workers' pneumoconiosis, *Arch Pathol Lab Med* 103:373, 1979.
477. Hurley JF, Burns J, Copland L et al: Coalworkers' simple pneumoconiosis and exposure to dust at ten British coalmines, *Br J Ind Med* 39:120-127, 1982.
478. Davis JMG, Addison J, Brown GM et al: *Further studies on the importance of quartz in the development of coalworkers' pneumoconiosis,* Edinburgh, 1991, Institute of Occupational Medicine.
479. Seaton A, Lapp NL, Morgan WKC: The relationship of pulmonary impairment in simple coal workers' pneumoconiosis to type of radiological opacity, *Br J Ind Med* 29:50, 1972.
480. Ruckley VA, Fernie JM, Champman JS et al: Comparison of radiographic appearances with associated pathology and lung dust content in a group of coal workers, *Br J Ind Med* 41:459, 1984.
481. Seaton A: Coal-mining, emphysema, and compensation, *Br J Ind Med* 47:433, 1990.
482. Cockcroft A, Seal RME, Wagner JC et al: Postmortem study of emphysema in coal workers and noncoal workers, *Lancet* 2:600, 1982.
483. Caplan A, Payne RB, Withley JL: A broader concept of Caplan's syndrome related to rheumatoid factors, *Thorax* 17:205, 1962.
484. Gough J, Rivers D, Seal RME: Pathological studies of modified pneumoconiosis in coal miners with rheumatoid arthritis (Caplan's syndrome), *Thorax* 10:9, 1955.
485. McConnachie K, Green FHY, Vallyathan V et al: Interstitial fibrosis in coal miners: experience in Wales and West Virginia, *Ann Occup Hyg* 32:553, 1988.
486. McLaughlin AIG, Harding HE: Pneumoconiosis and other causes of death in iron and steel foundry workers, *Arch Ind Health* 14:350, 1956.
487. Morgan WKC, Kerr HD: Pathologic and physiologic studies of welders' siderosis, *Ann Intern Med* 58:293, 1963.
488. Coates EO, Watson JHL: Diffuse interstitial lung disease in tungsten carbide workers, *Ann Intern Med* 75:709, 1971.
489. Coates EO, Watson JHL: Pathology of the lung in tungsten carbide workers using light and electron microscopy, *J Occup Med* 15:280, 1973.
490. Nemery B, Nagels J, Verbeken E et al: Rapidly fatal progression of cobalt lung in a diamond polisher, *Am Rev Respir Dis* 141.1373, 1990.
491. Fischbein A, Luo J-C L, Solomon SJ et al: Clinical findings among hard metal workers, *Br J Ind Med* 49:17, 1992.
492. Davison AG, Haslam PL, Corrin B et al: Interstitial lung disease and asthma in hard-metal workers: bronchoalveolar lavage, ultrastructural, and analytical findings and results of bronchial provocation tests, *Thorax* 38:119, 1983.
493. Demedts M, Gheysens B, Nagels J et al: Cobalt lung in diamond polishers, *Am Rev Respir Dis* 130:130, 1984.
494. Freiman DG, Hardy HL: Beryllium disease: the relation of pulmonary pathology to clinical course and prognosis based on a study of 130 cases from the U.S. Beryllium Case Registry, *Hum Pathol* 1:25, 1970.
495. Hayes RB: Review of occupational epidemiology of chromium chemicals and respiratory cancer, *Sci Total Environ* 71:331, 1988.
496. Norseth T: The carcinogenicity of chromium and its salts, *Br J Ind Med* 43:649, 1986.
497. Doll R, Mathews JD, Morgan LG: Cancers of the lung and nasal sinuses in nickel workers, *Br J Ind Med* 34:102, 1977.
498. Sunderman FW Jr: Recent advances in metal carcinogenesis, *Ann Clin Lab Sci* 14:93, 1984.
499. Sherwood Burge P: Humidifier fever. In Brewis RAL, Gibson GJ, Geddes DM, editors: *Respiratory medicine,* London, 1990, Balliere Tindall.
500. Von Essen S, Robbins RA, Thompson AB, Rennard SI: Organic dust toxic syndrome: an acute febrile reaction to organic dust exposure distinct from hypersensitivity pneumonitis, *J Toxicol Clin Toxicol* 28:389, 1990.

Neoplasms

501. Mackay B, Lukeman JM, Ordóñez NG: *Tumors of the lung,* Philadelphia, 1991, Saunders.
502. Saldana MJ, editor: *Pathology of pulmonary disease,* Philadelphia, 1994, Lippincott.
503. Dail DH, Hammar SP, editors: *Pulmonary pathology,* ed 2, New York, 1994, Springer-Verlag.
504. Shimosato Y, Miller RR: *Biopsy interpretation of the lung,* New York 1995, Raven Press.
505. Colby TV, Koss MN, Travis WD: *Tumors of the lower respiratory tract, Atlas of tumor pathology,* series 3, fasc 13, Washington D.C., 1995, Armed Forces Institute of Pathology.
506. The World Health Organization Histological Typing of Lung Tumours, *Am J Clin Pathol* 77:123, 1982.
507. Burnett RA, Swanson Beck J, Howatson SR et al: Observer variability in histopathologic reporting of malignant bronchial biopsy specimens, *J Clin Pathol* 47:711, 1994.
508. Wingo PA, Tong T, Bolden S: Cancer statistics 1995, *CA Cancer J Clin* 45:8, 1995.
509. Samet JM: Epidemiology of lung cancer, *Chest* 103:20, 1993.
510. Davila DG, Williams DE: The etiology of lung cancer, *Mayo Clin Proc* 68:170, 1993.
511. Law MR: Genetic predisposition to lung cancer, *Br J Cancer* 61:195, 1990.
512. Pershagen G, Akerblom G, Axelson O et al: Residential radon exposure and lung cancer in Sweden, *N Engl J Med* 330:159, 1994.
513. Auerbach O, Saccomanno G, Kuschner M et al: Histologic findings in the tracheobronchial tree of uranium miners and non-miners with lung cancer, *Cancer* 42:483, 1978.
514. Yousem SA, Ohori P, Sonmez-Alpan E: Occurrence of human papillomavirus DNA in primary lung neoplasms, *Cancer* 69:693, 1992.
515. Richardson GE, Johnson BE: The biology of lung cancer, *Semin Oncol* 20:105, 1993.
516. Brambilla E, Gazzeri S, Moro D et al: Immunohistochemical study of p53 in human lung carcinomas, *Am J Pathol* 143:199, 1993.
517. Tenaud C, Negoescu A, Labat-Moleur F et al: p53 immunolabeling in archival paraffin-embedded tissues: optimal protocol based on microwave heating for eight antibodies on lung carcinomas, *Mod Pathol* 7:853, 1994.
518. Rosenhuis S, Slebos RJC, Boot AJM et al: Incidence and possible significance of K-*ras* oncogene activation in adenocarcinoma of the human lung, *Cancer Res* 48:5738, 1988.
519. Pezzella F, Turley H, Kuzu I et al: *bcl*-2 protein in non–small cell lung carcinoma, *N Engl J Med* 369:690, 1993.
520. Merlo A, Gabrielson E, Mabry M et al: Homozygous deletion on chromosome 9p and loss of heterozygosity on 9γ, 6p and 6γ in primary human small cell lung cancer, *Cancer Res* 54:2322, 1994.
521. Cohen MC, Kaschula RO: Primary pulmonary tumors in childhood: review of 31 years' experience and the literature, *Pediatr Pulmonol* 14:222, 1992.
522. Mountain CF: The new international staging system for lung cancer, *Surg Clin North Am* 67:925, 1987.
523. Feigal EG, Christian M, Cheson B et al: New chemotherapeutic agents in non-small-cell lung cancer, *Semin Oncol* 20:185, 1993.
524. Patel A: Paraneoplastic syndromes associated with lung cancer, *Mayo Clin Proc* 68:278, 1993.
525. Yousem SA, Hochholzer L: Alveolar adenoma, *Hum Pathol* 17:1066, 1986.
526. Kragel PJ, Devaney KO, Meth BM et al: Mucinous cystadenoma of the lung: a report of two cases with immunohistochemical and ultrastructural analysis, *Arch Pathol Lab Med* 114:1053, 1990.
527. Dixon AY, Moran JF, Wesselius LJ, McGregor DH: Pulmonary mucinous cystic tumor: case report with review of the literature, *Am J Surg Pathol* 17:722, 1993.

528. Graeme-Cook F, Mark EJ: Pulmonary mucinous cystic tumors of borderline malignancy, *Hum Pathol* 22:185, 1991.
529. Moran CA, Suster S, Askin FB, Koss MN: Benign and malignant salivary gland-type mixed tumors of the lung: clinicopathologic and immunohistochemical study of eight cases, *Cancer* 73:2481, 1994.
530. Strickler JG, Hegstrom J, Thomas MJ, Yousem SA: Myoepithelioma of the lung, *Arch Pathol Lab Med* 111:1082, 1987.
531. Sakamoto H, Uda H, Tanaka T et al: Pleomorphic adenoma in the periphery of the lung: report of a case and review of the literature, *Arch Pathol Lab Med* 115:393, 1991.
532. Carter D: Squamous cell carcinoma of the lung: an update, *Semin Diagn Pathol* 2:226, 1985.
533. Suster S, Huszar M, Herczeg E: Spindle cell squamous carcinoma of the lung: immunocytochemical and ultrastructural study of a case, *Histopathology* 11:871, 1987.
534. Shimosato Y, Noguchi M, Matsuno Y: Adenocarcinoma of the lung: its development and malignant progression, *Lung Cancer* 9:99, 1993.
535. Cagle PT, Cohle SD, Greenberg SD: Natural history of pulmonary scar cancers, clinical and pathologic implications, *Cancer* 56:2031, 1985.
536. Rao SK, Fraire AE: Alveolar cell hyperplasia in association with adenocarcinoma of lung, *Mod Pathol* 8:165, 1995.
537. Barsky SH, Grossman DA, Ho J, Holmes EC: The multifocality of bronchioloalveolar lung carcinoma: evidence and implications of a multiclonal origin, *Mod Pathol* 7:633, 1994.
538. Moran CA, Suster S, Loss MN: Acinic cell carcinoma of the lung ("Fechner tumor"): a clinicopathologic, immunohistochemical and ultrastructural study of five cases, *Am J Surg Pathol* 16:1039, 1992.
539. Cagle PT, Wessels R, Greenberg SD: Concurrent mesothelioma and adenocarcinoma of the lung in a patient with asbestosis, *Mod Pathol* 6:438, 1993.
540. Yamashiro K, Yasuda S, Nagase A et al: Prognostic significance of an interface pattern of central fibrosis and tumor cells in peripheral adenocarcinoma of the lung, *Hum Pathol* 26:67, 1995.
541. Matsui K, Kitagawa M, Sugiyama S, Yamamoto K: Distribution pattern of the basement membrane components is one of the significant prognostic correlates in peripheral lung adenocarcinomas, *Hum Pathol* 26:186, 1995.
542. Fishback NF, Travis WD, Moran CA et al: Pleomorphic (spindle and giant cell) carcinomas of the lung: a clinicopathologic study of 78 cases, *Cancer* 73:2936, 1994.
543. Ishida T, Kaneko S, Tateishi M et al: Large cell carcinoma of the lung: prognostic implications of his pathologic and immunohistochemical subtyping, *Am J Clin Pathol* 93:176, 1990.
544. Hirsch FR, Matthews MJ, Aisner S et al: Histopathologic classification of small lung cell lung cancer: changing concepts and terminology, *Cancer* 62:973, 1988.
545. McCue PA, Finkel GC: Small-cell lung carcinoma: an evolving histopathological spectrum, *Semin Oncol* 20:153, 1993.
546. Travis WD, Linnoila RI, Tsokos MG et al: Neuroendocrine tumors of the lung with proposed criteria for large-cell neuroendocrine carcinoma: an ultrastructural, immunohistochemical, and flow cytometric study of 35 cases, *Am J Surg Pathol* 15:529, 1991.
547. Wick MR, Berg LC, Hertz MT: Large cell carcinoma of the lung with neuroendocrine differentiation: a comparison with large cell "undifferentiated" pulmonary tumors, *Am J Clin Pathol* 94:796, 1992.
548. Warren WH, Faber LP, Gould VE: Neuroendocrine neoplasms of the lung: a clinicopathologic update, *J Thorac Cardiovasc Surg* 98:321, 1989.
549. Warren WH, Memoli VA, Gould VE: Well differentiated and small cell neuroendocrine carcinomas of the lung: two related but distinct clinicopathologic entities, *Virchows [B] Arch (Cell Pathol)* 55:299, 1988.
550. Yousem SA, Taylor SR: Typical and atypical carcinoid tumors of the lung: a clinicopathologic and DNA analysis of 20 tumors, *Mod Pathol* 3:502, 1990.
551. Matsuba K, Saito T, Ando K, Shirakusa T: Atypical lipoma of the lung, *Thorax* 46:685, 1991.
552. Moran CA, Suster S, Koss MN: Endobronchial lipomas: a clinicopathologic study of four cases, *Mod Pathol* 7:212, 1994.
553. Guinee DG Jr, Thornberry DS, Azumi N et al: Unique pulmonary presentation of an angiomyolipoma, analysis of clinical radiographic and histopathologic features, *Am J Surg Pathol* 19:476, 1995.
554. Guccion JG, Rosen SH: Bronchopulmonary leiomyosarcomas and fibrosarcomas: a study of 32 cases and review of the literature, *Cancer* 30:835, 1972.
555. Nappi O, Wick MR. Sarcomatoid neoplasms of the respiratory tract, *Semin Diagn Pathol* 10:137, 1993.
556. Ishida T, Tateishi M, Kaneko S et al: Carcinosarcoma and spindle cell carcinoma of the lung: clinicopathologic and immunohistochemical studies, *J Thorac Cardiovasc Surg* 100:844, 1990.
557. Humphrey PA, Scroggs MW, Roggli VL, Shelburne JD: Pulmonary carcinomas with a sarcomatoid element: an immunocytochemical and ultrastructural analysis, *Hum Pathol* 19:155, 1980.
558. Ro JY, Chen JL, Lee JS et al: Sarcomatoid carcinoma of the lung: immunohistochemical and ultrastructural studies of 14 cases, *Cancer* 69:376, 1992.
559. Rainosek DE, Ro JY, Ordóñez NG et al: Sarcomatoid carcinoma of the lung: a case with atypical carcinoid and rhabdomyosarcomatous components, *Am J Clin Pathol* 102:360, 1994.
560. Nappi O, Glasner SD, Swanson PE, Wick MR: Biphasic and monophasic sarcomatoid carcinomas of the lung: a reappraisal of "carcinosarcomas" and "spindle cell carcinomas," *Am J Clin Pathol* 102:331, 1994.
561. Ro JY, Chen JL, Lee JS et al: Sarcomatoid carcinoma of the lung: immunohistochemical and ultrastructural studies of 14 cases, *Cancer* 69:376, 1992.
562. Addis BJ, Hyjek E, Isaacson PG: Primary pulmonary lymphoma: a reappraisal of its histogenesis and its relationship to pseudolymphoma and lymphoid interstitial pneumonia, *Histopathology* 13:1, 1988.
563. Nicholson AG, Wotherspoon AC, Diss T et al: Pulmonary B-cell non-Hodgkin's lymphomas: the value of immunohistochemistry and gene analysis in diagnosis, *Histopathology* 26:395, 1995.
564. Elenitoba-Johnson K, Medeiros LJ, Khorsand J, King TC: Lymphoma of the mucosa-associated lymphoid tissue of the lung, *Am J Clin Pathol* 103:341, 1995.
565. Guinee D Jr, Jaffe E, Kingma D et al: Pulmonary lymphomatoid granulomatosis: evidence for a proliferation of Epstein-Barr virus infected B-lymphocytes with a prominent T-cell component and vasculitis, *Am J Surg Pathol* 18:753, 1994.
566. Cohen RE, Weaver MG, Montenegro HD, Abdul-Karim FW: Pulmonary blastoma with malignant melanoma component, *Arch Pathol Lab Med* 114:1076, 1990.
567. Nakatani Y, Dickersin GR, Mark EJ: Pulmonary endodermal tumor resembling fetal lung: a clinicopathologic study of five cases with immunohistochemical and ultrastructural characterization, *Hum Pathol* 21:1097, 1990.
568. Jennings TA, Axiotis CA, Kress Y, Carter D: Primary malignant melanoma of the lower respiratory tract: report of a case and literature review, *Am J Clin Pathol* 94:649, 1990.
569. Crotty TB, Hooker RP, Swensen SJ et al: Primary malignant ependymoma of the lung, *Mayo Clin Proc* 67:373, 1992.
570. Drlicek M, Grisold W, Lorber J et al: Pulmonary meningioma immunohistochemical and ultrastructural features, *Am J Surg Pathol* 15:455, 1991.
571. Rowlands D, Edwards C, Collins F: Malignant melanotic schwannoma of the bronchus, *J Clin Pathol* 40:1449, 1987.
572. Salminen US: Pulmonary hamartoma: a clinical study of 77 cases in a 21-year period and review of literature, *Eur J Cardiothorac Surg* 4:15, 1990.
573. Basile A, Gregoris A, Antoci B, Romanelli M: Malignant change in benign pulmonary hamartoma, *Thorax* 33:232, 1989.
574. van Klaveren RJ, Hassing HHM, Wiersma-van Tilburg JM et al: Mesenchymal cystic hamartoma of the lung: a rare case of relapsing pneumothorax, *Thorax* 49:1175, 1994.
575. Yousem SA, Wick MR, Singh G et al: So-called sclerosing hemangiomas of lung: an immunohistochemical study supporting a respiratory epithelial origin, *Am J Surg Pathol* 12:582, 1988.

576. Gaffey MJ, Mills SE, Askin FB et al: Clear cell tumor of the lung: a clinicopathologic, immunohistochemical, and ultrastructural study of eight cases, *Am J Surg Pathol* 14:248, 1990.
577. Matsubara O, Tan-Liu NS, Kenney RM, Mark E: Inflammatory pseudotumors of the lung: progression from organizing pneumonia to fibrous histocytoma or to plasma cell granuloma in 32 cases, *Hum Pathol* 19:807, 1988.
578. Mark EJ, Muller KM, McChesney T et al: Placentoid bullous lesions of the lung, *Hum Pathol* 26:74, 1995.
579. Fidler ME, Koomen M, Sebek B et al: Placental transmogrification of the lung, a histologic variant of giant bullous emphysema: clinicopathogical study of three further cases, *Am J Surg Pathol,* 19:563, 1995.
580. Ferrara G, Boscaino A, de Rosa G: Bronchial blue naevus: a previously unreported entity, *Histopathology* 26:581, 1995.

Index

Page numbers in *italics* indicate illustrations. Page numbers followed by a t indicate tables.

D

F

G

J

K

L

N

P

Q

R

S

T

U

V

W

X